a LANGE medical book

2027 CURRENT Medical Diagnosis & Treatment

SIXTY-SIXTH EDITION

Edited by

Kenneth R. McQuaid, MD
Professor of Medicine, Emeritus
Department of Medicine
University of California, San Francisco

Maxine A. Papadakis, MD
Professor of Medicine, Emeritus
Department of Medicine
University of California, San Francisco

Michael W. Rabow, MD
Professor of Medicine and Urology
Division of Palliative Medicine
Department of Medicine
University of California, San Francisco

Associate Editor

Paul L. Nadler, MD
Clinical Professor of Medicine
Division of General Internal Medicine
Department of Medicine
University of California, San Francisco

With Contributing Authors

Mc Graw Hill

Current Medical Diagnosis & Treatment 2027, Sixty-Sixth Edition

1 2 3 4 5 LBC 30 29 28 27 26

ISBN 978-1-264-82471-7
MHID 1-264-82471-8
IE ISBN 978-1-264-82450-2
IE MHID 1-264-82450-5
ISSN 0092-8682

Notice

Medicine is an ever-changing science. As new research and clinical experience broaden our knowledge, changes in treatment and drug therapy are required. The authors and the publisher of this work have checked with sources believed to be reliable in their efforts to provide information that is complete and generally in accord with the standards accepted at the time of publication. However, in view of the possibility of human error or changes in medical sciences, neither the authors nor the publisher nor any other party who has been involved in the preparation or publication of this work warrants that the information contained herein is in every respect accurate or complete, and they disclaim all responsibility for any errors or omissions or for the results obtained from use of the information contained in this work. Readers are encouraged to confirm the information contained herein with other sources. For example and in particular, readers are advised to check the product information sheet included in the package of each medication they plan to administer to be certain that the information contained in this work is accurate and that changes have not been made in the recommended dose or in the contraindications for administration. This recommendation is of particular importance in connection with new or infrequently used medications.

This book was set in Minion Pro by KnowledgeWorks Global Ltd.
The editors were Kay Conerly, Jennifer Bernstein, and Sylvia Choi.
The production supervisor was Jeffrey Herzich.
The digital production manager was Priscilla Beer.
Project management was provided by Radhika Jolly at KnowledgeWorks Global Ltd.
The copyeditors were Greg Feldman, Kathryn Whitley, Allison Scerbo, and Kerri Fitzgerald.
The index was prepared by Susan Hunter.

This book is printed on acid-free paper.

Contents

Authors

Rime Abbas, MD
Clinical Assistant Professor, Division of Pulmonary, Allergy, Critical Care, and Sleep Medicine, Department of Medicine, University of Pittsburgh School of Medicine, Pittsburgh, Pennsylvania
Pulmonary Disorders

James H. Acuff, MD
Infectious Diseases Fellow, Baylor College of Medicine, Houston, Texas
Viral & Rickettsial Infections

Michael J. Aminoff, MD, DSc, FRCP
Distinguished Professor Emeritus, Department of Neurology, University of California, San Francisco
Nervous System Disorders

Charalambos Babis Andreadis, MD, MSCE
Professor of Clinical Medicine, Division of Hematology/Oncology, Department of Medicine, University of California, San Francisco
Blood Disorders

Kevin L. Ard, MD, MPH
Faculty, Division of Infectious Diseases, Massachusetts General Hospital; Medical Director, National LGBTQIA+ Health Education Center, Fenway Institute; Assistant Professor of Medicine, Harvard Medical School, Boston, Massachusetts
Sexual & Gender Minority Health

John Benjamin Jess Arevalo, MD, MBA
Assistant Clinical Professor, Department of Anesthesia and Perioperative Care, University of California, San Francisco
Palliative Care & Pain Management

Nayan Arora, MD, FASN
Associate Professor of Medicine, Division of Nephrology, Oregon Health & Science University, Portland, Oregon
Electrolyte & Acid-Base Disorders

Soraya Azari, MD
Physician Specialist, San Francisco Department of Public Health; Professor of Medicine, Zuckerberg San Francisco General and Trauma Center, University of California, San Francisco,
Substance Use Disorders

Emma D. Bainbridge, MD, MPH
Assistant Clinical Professor, Division of Infectious Diseases, Department of Medicine, University of California, San Francisco
Bacterial & Chlamydial Infections

Kara E. Bischoff, MD
Professor and Associate Division Chief for Outpatient Palliative Care, University of California, San Francisco
Palliative Care & Pain Management

Michael J. Blaha, MD, MPH
Professor of Medicine, Division of Cardiology, Department of Medicine; Director of Clinical Research, Ciccarone Center for the Prevention of Cardiovascular Disease, Johns Hopkins University School of Medicine, Baltimore, Maryland
Lipid Disorders

Jill Brown, MD, MPH, MHS, FACOG
Associate Professor, Department of Gynecologic Surgery and Obstetrics, Uniformed Services University of the Health Sciences, Bethesda, Maryland
Gynecologic Disorders

Mandy Brown, PharmD
Associate Clinical Professor, School of Pharmacy, University of California, San Francisco
Drug References

James Buxbaum, MD
Professor of Medicine (Clinical Scholar), Executive Director, Digestive Health Institute, Keck School of Medicine, University of Southern California, Los Angeles, California
Liver, Biliary Tract, & Pancreas Disorders

Hugo Q. Cheng, MD
Clinical Professor of Medicine, Division of Hospital Medicine, Department of Medicine, University of California, San Francisco
Preoperative Evaluation & Perioperative Management

Peter V. Chin-Hong, MD
Associate Dean for Regional Campuses, Professor of Medicine, Division of Infectious Diseases, Department of Medicine, University of California, San Francisco
Common Problems in Infectious Diseases & Antimicrobial Therapy

Russ Cucina, MD, MS
Professor of Hospital Medicine, Department of Medicine; Vice President, Genetic and Genomic Services, and Chief Health Information Officer, UCSF Health System, University of California, San Francisco
CMDT on AccessMedicine—Information Technology in Patient Care

Marc A. Dall'Era, MD
Professor of Urology, Department of Urologic Surgery, UC Davis Health, University of California, Davis
Cancer

Lloyd E. Damon, MD
Professor Emeritus of Hematology, Division of Hematology/Oncology, Department of Medicine, University of California, San Francisco
Blood Disorders

Tiffany O. Dea, PharmD, BCOP
Oncology Pharmacist, Veterans Affairs Health Care System, San Francisco, California; Adjunct Professor, Thomas J. Long School of Pharmacy and Health Sciences, Stockton, California
Cancer

Charles DeBattista, DMH, MD
Professor of Psychiatry and Behavioral Sciences, Department of Psychiatry and Behavioral Sciences; Director, Depression Clinic and Research Program; Director of Medical Student Education in Psychiatry, Stanford University School of Medicine, Stanford, California
Psychiatric Disorders

Monara Dini, DPM
Associate Clinical Professor of Orthopedics, Department of Orthopedic Surgery, University of California, San Francisco
CMDT on AccessMedicine —Podiatric Disorders

Tonja C. Dirkx, MD
Chief, Nephrology Section, Veterans Affairs Portland Health Care System; Associate Professor of Medicine, Division of Nephrology, Department of Medicine, Oregon Health & Science University, Portland, Oregon
Kidney Disease

Vanja C. Douglas, MD
Sara & Evan Williams Foundation Endowed Neurohospitalist Chair, Professor of Clinical Neurology, Department of Neurology, University of California, San Francisco
Nervous System Disorders

Jacque L. Duncan, MD
Chair and Distinguished Professor, Department of Ophthalmology, University of California, San Francisco
Disorders of the Eyes & Lids

Amy Eby, MD
Clinical Assistant Professor, Division of Internal Medicine, University of Washington, Seattle, Washington
Diabetes Mellitus & Hypoglycemia

Sarah Adler Fink, RD, CDN, CNSC
Dietetic Internship Program Coordinator, Department of Food and Nutrition, New York-Presbyterian Hospital, New York, New York
Nutrition, Nutritional Disorders, & Obesity

Paul A. Fitzgerald, MD
Clinical Professor of Medicine, Division of Endocrinology, Department of Medicine, University of California, San Francisco
Disorders of the Pituitary, Thyroid, & Adrenal Glands

Meghan E. Fitzpatrick, MD
Associate Professor of Medicine, Division of Pulmonary and Critical Care Medicine, Department of Medicine, University of Pittsburgh School of Medicine, Pittsburgh, Pennsylvania
Pulmonary Disorders

Monica Fung, MD, MPH
Associate Professor, Division of Infectious Diseases, Department of Medicine, University of California, San Francisco
Common Problems in Infectious Diseases & Antimicrobial Therapy

Monica Gandhi, MD, MPH
Professor, Division of HIV, Infectious Diseases, and Global Medicine, Zuckerberg San Francisco General Hospital, University of California, San Francisco
HIV Infection & AIDS

Warren J. Gasper, MD
Associate Professor of Clinical Surgery, Division of Vascular and Endovascular Surgery, Department of Surgery, University of California, San Francisco
Blood Vessel & Lymphatic Disorders

Armando E. Giuliano, MD, FACS, FRCSEd
Professor of Surgery, Linda and Jim Lippman Chair in Surgical Oncology; Director, Surgical Oncology; Associate Director, Cedars-Sinai Cancer Center, Los Angeles, California
Breast Disorders

Ralph Gonzales, MD, MSPH
Professor of Medicine, Division of General Internal Medicine, Department of Medicine; Associate Dean, Clinical Innovation and Chief Innovation Officer, UCSF Health; University of California, San Francisco
Common Symptoms

Christopher B. Granger, MD
Fred Cobb, MD Distinguished Professor of Medicine, Professor of Nursing, Division of Cardiology, Duke University Medical Center Duke Clinical Research Institute, Durham, North Carolina
Heart Failure & Cardiomyopathy

Katherine Gruenberg, PharmD, MAEd
Associate Professor of Clinical Pharmacy, School of Pharmacy, University of California, San Francisco
Common Problems in Infectious Diseases & Antimicrobial Therapy; CMDT on AccessMedicine—Anti-Infective Treatment: Antibiotic, Antifungal, & Antiviral Agents

Ashley Gutierrez, MD
Department of Dermatology, Keck School of Medicine, University of Southern California, Los Angeles, California,
References

Richard J. Hamill, MD, FIDSA
Professor, Departments of Medicine and Molecular Virology and Microbiology, Vice-Chair for Education, Department of Medicine, Baylor College of Medicine; Staff Physician, Infectious Disease Section, Michael E. DeBakey VA Medical Center, Houston, Texas
Mycotic Infections

G. Michael Harper, MD
Professor, Division of Geriatrics, Department of Medicine, University of California, San Francisco School of Medicine; San Francisco Veterans Affairs Health Care System, San Francisco, California
Geriatric Disorders

Mitzi Hawkins, MD
Assistant Professor, Obstetrics, Gynecology & Reproductive Sciences, University of California, San Francisco
Sexual & Gender Minority Health

Marah C. Hehemann, MD
Associate Professor, Department of Urology, University of Washington, Seattle, Washington
Urologic Disorders

J. Janet Ho, MD, MPH, FASAM, FAAHPM
Associate Professor, University of California, San Francisco
Substance Use Disorders

Elaine Hsiang, MD
Clinical Instructor, Department of Emergency Medicine, Stanford University School of Medicine, Stanford, California
Sexual & Gender Minority Health

Sara A. Hurvitz, MD
Professor of Medicine, Smith Family Endowed Chair in Women's Health; Head, Division of Hematology and Oncology, University of Washington Department of Medicine; Senior Vice President, Clinical Research Division, Fred Hutchinson Cancer Center, Seattle, Washington
Breast Disorders

James C. Iannuzzi, MD, MPH
Associate Professor of Surgery, Division of Vascular and Endovascular Surgery, Department of Surgery, University of California, San Francisco
Blood Vessel & Lymphatic Disorders

Leon I. Igel, MD, FACP, FTOS, DABOM
Clinical Assistant Professor of Medicine, Division of Endocrinology, Diabetes and Metabolism, Department of Medicine, Weill Cornell Medical College, New York, New York; Chief Medical Officer, FlyteHealth, New Canaan, Connecticut
Nutrition, Nutritional Disorders, & Obesity

Kevin P. Jackson, MD
Associate Professor of Medicine, Division of Cardiology, Department of Medicine; Director of Electrophysiology Lab, Duke University Hospital, Duke University Medical Center, Durham, North Carolina
Disorders of Cardiac Rhythm

J. Ashley Jefferson, MD, FRCP
Professor of Medicine, Division of Nephrology, Department of Medicine; Section Head, Nephrology, University of Washington Medical Center, Seattle, Washington
Electrolyte & Acid-Base Disorders

Kelly A. Johnson, MD, MPH
Assistant Professor of Medicine, Division of Infectious Diseases; Medical Director, California Prevention Training Center, University of California, San Francisco
Bacterial & Chlamydial Infections

Meshell D. Johnson, MD
Professor of Medicine, University of California, San Francisco; Chief, Division of Pulmonary, Critical Care, Sleep, and Allergy Medicine, San Francisco Veterans Affairs Health Care System
Blood Vessel & Lymphatic Disorders

Marianne A. Juarez, MD
Associate Clinical Professor, Department of Emergency Medicine, University of California, San Francisco
Disorders Related to Environmental Emergencies

Emily Kaip, PharmD
Pharmacist Specialist, Infectious Diseases, University of California, San Francisco Medical Center; Assistant Clinical Professor, University of California, San Francisco School of Pharmacy
CMDT on AccessMedicine—Anti-infective Treatment: Antibiotic, Antifungal, & Antiviral Agents

Andrew Ko, MD
Professor and Associate Chief, Division of Hematology/Oncology, University of California, San Francisco
Cancer

Elliott D. Kozin, MD
Assistant Professor of Otolaryngology—Head and Neck Surgery, Harvard Medical School; Physician and Surgeon, Massachusetts Eye and Ear, Boston, Massachusetts
Otolaryngology Disorders

Mildred Kwan, MD, PhD
Associate Professor of Medicine, Division of Rheumatology, Allergy & Immunology, Department of Medicine, University of North Carolina School of Medicine, Chapel Hill, North Carolina
Rheumatologic, Immunologic, & Allergic Disorders

Rossana Lau-Ng, MD
Assistant Professor, Section of Geriatrics, Department of Medicine, Boston University Chobanian & Avedisian School of Medicine, Boston, Massachusetts
Geriatric Disorders

Andrew D. Leavitt, MD
Professor, Departments of Medicine (Hematology) and Laboratory Medicine; Medical Director, Adult Hemophilia Treatment Center, University of California, San Francisco
Disorders of Hemostasis, Thrombosis, & Antithrombotic Therapy

Chuanyi Mark Lu, MD
Professor and Vice Chair, Department of Laboratory Medicine, University of California, San Francisco; Chief, Lab Medicine Service, Veterans Affairs Health Care System, San Francisco, California
CMDT on AccessMedicine—Diagnostic Testing & Medical Decision-Making; CMDT on AccessMedicine—Appendix: Therapeutic Drug Monitoring, Pharmacogenetic Tests, Laboratory Reference Intervals, & Commonly Used Blood Specimen Collection Tubes

Anthony Luke, MD, MPH
Benioff Distinguished Professor in Sports Medicine, Department of Orthopaedics; Director, UCSF Primary Care Sports Medicine; Director, Human Performance Center at the Orthopaedic Institute, University of California, San Francisco
Orthopedic Disorders & Sports Medicine

Lawrence R. Lustig, MD
Howard W. Smith Professor and Chair, Department of Otolaryngology—Head & Neck Surgery, Columbia Vagelos College of Physicians and Surgeons, Columbia University Irving Medical Center & New York Presbyterian Hospital, New York, New York
Otolaryngology Disorders

C. Benjamin Ma, MD
Professor and Chair, Department of Orthopaedic Surgery, Dr. Peter and Sophie Pappas Endowed Chair, V-nee Yeh Endowed Professor of Orthopaedic Surgery, University of California, San Francisco
Orthopedic Disorders & Sports Medicine

Rebecca L. Manno, MD, MHS
Adjunct Assistant Professor, Division of Rheumatology, Johns Hopkins University School of Medicine, Baltimore, Maryland
Rheumatologic, Immunologic, & Allergic Disorders

Mohamad Matout, MD, CM, MSc, DABPN
Clinical Assistant Professor, Stanford University, Palo Alto, California
Psychiatric Disorders

Kenneth H. Mayer, MD
Professor of Medicine, Harvard Medical School; Co-Chair and Medical Research Director, The Fenway Institute; Attending Physician, Beth Israel Deaconess Medical Center, Boston, Massachusetts
Sexual & Gender Minority Health

Molly McCallum, MD
Endocrinology Fellow, University of California, San Francisco
References

Kenneth R. McQuaid, MD
Professor Emeritus of Medicine, Department of Medicine, University of California, San Francisco
Gastrointestinal Disorders

Paul L. Nadler, MD
Clinical Professor of Medicine, Division of General Internal Medicine, Department of Medicine; Director, UCSF Health Urgent Care at Parnassus; University of California, San Francisco
Common Symptoms

Jacqueline A. Nemer, MD, FACEP
Professor of Emergency Medicine, Department of Emergency Medicine; Medical Director, Clinical Documentation Integrity, Department of Quality and Safety, University of California, San Francisco
Disorders Related to Environmental Emergencies

Sarah Nouri, MD, MPH
Assistant Professor, University of California, San Francisco
Palliative Care & Pain Management

Neeti B. Parikh, MD
Associate Professor of Ophthalmology, Department of Ophthalmology, University of California, San Francisco
Disorders of the Eyes & Lids

Ina Park, MD, MS
Professor, Department of Family and Community Medicine and Department of Obstetrics, Gynecology, and Reproductive Sciences, University of California, San Francisco
Spirochetal Infections

Charles B. Parks, DPM
Associate Clinical Professor, Chief of Podiatric Surgery Division, Department of Orthopedic Surgery, University of California, San Francisco
CMDT on AccessMedicine—Podiatric Disorders

Chloe E. Peters, MD
Assistant Professor, Department of Veterans Affairs, University of Washington, Seattle, Washington
Urologic Disorders

Logan Peterson, MD, FACOG
Assistant Professor, Uniformed Services University of the Health Sciences, Bethesda, Maryland
Gynecologic Disorders

Michael Pignone, MD, MPH
Professor of Medicine, Vice Chair for Quality and Innovation, Department of Medicine, Duke University School of Medicine, Durham, North Carolina
Disease Prevention & Health Promotion

Erika Leemann Price, MD, MPH
Clinical Professor, Department of Medicine, University of California, San Francisco; Hospitalist, San Francisco Veterans Affairs Health Care System
Disorders of Hemostasis, Thrombosis, & Antithrombotic Therapy

Reed E. Pyeritz, MD, PhD
William Smilow Professor of Medicine and Genetics, Emeritus, Raymond and Ruth Perelman School of Medicine of the University of Pennsylvania, Philadelphia
Genetic & Genomic Disorders

Kristin S. Raj, MD
Clinical Professor of Psychiatry, Department of Psychiatry and Behavioral Sciences, Stanford University School of Medicine, Stanford, California
Psychiatric Disorders

Jessica Ristau, MD
Assistant Professor, University of California, San Francisco
Substance Use Disorders

Belinda Rivera-Lebron, MD, MS, FCCP
Professor of Medicine, Division of Pulmonary, Allergy and Critical Care Medicine, Department of Medicine, University of Pittsburgh School of Medicine, Pittsburgh, Pennsylvania
Pulmonary Disorders

Scott W. Roberts, MD
Professor of Obstetrics and Gynecology, Department of Obstetrics and Gynecology, University of Texas Southwestern Medical Center, Dallas, Texas
Obstetrics & Obstetric Disorders

Patricia A. Robertson, MD
Professor of Obstetrics and Gynecology, Department of Obstetrics, Gynecology, and Reproductive Sciences, University of California, San Francisco
Sexual & Gender Minority Health

Vanessa L. Rogers, MD
Professor of Obstetrics and Gynecology, Department of Obstetrics and Gynecology; Vice Chair of Education and Faculty Development, University of Texas Southwestern Medical Center, Dallas, Texas
Obstetrics & Obstetric Disorders

Nathan W. Rojek, MD
Associate Professor of Dermatology, Department of Dermatology, University of California, Irvine
Dermatologic Disorders

Stacey R. Rose, MD, FACP, FIDSA
Associate Professor, Department of Medicine, Division of Infectious Diseases and the Huffington Department of Education, Innovation and Technology; Director, Center for Professionalism, Baylor College of Medicine, Houston, Texas
Mycotic Infections

Philip J. Rosenthal, MD
Professor of Medicine, Department of Medicine, University of California, San Francisco; Associate Chief, Division of HIV, Infectious Diseases, and Global Medicine, Zuckerberg San Francisco General Hospital
Protozoal & Helminthic Infections

Tina R. Sadarangani, PhD, RN, ANP-C, GNP-BC, FAAN
Assistant Professor, New York University Grossman School of Medicine & Rory Meyers College of Nursing, New York, New York
Geriatric Disorders

Katherine H. Saunders, MD, FTOS, DABOM
Clinical Assistant Professor of Medicine, Division of Endocrinology, Diabetes and Metabolism, Department of Medicine, Weill Cornell Medicine, New York, New York; Co-Founder, FlyteHealth, New Canaan, Connecticut
Nutrition, Nutritional Disorders, & Obesity

Anne Schafer, MD
Professor of Medicine, University of California, San Francisco
Disorders of Parathyroid Glands & Bone Metabolism

Gerami D. Seitzman, MD
Professor of Ophthalmology, Department of Ophthalmology, Francis I. Proctor Foundation, University of California, San Francisco
Disorders of the Eyes & Lids

Ann Cai Shah, MD
Associate Clinical Professor of Anesthesia and Pain Medicine, Director, Cancer Pain Service, Department of Anesthesia and Perioperative Care, University of California, San Francisco
Palliative Care & Pain Management

Wayne X. Shandera, MD
Associate Professor of Medicine, Department of Medicine, Baylor College of Medicine, Houston, Texas
Viral & Rickettsial Infections

Robert T. Short III, MD
Cardiovascular Disease Fellow, Beth Israel Deaconess Medical Center, Harvard Medical School, Boston, Massachusetts
Heart Failure & Cardiomyopathy

Katerina Shvartsman, MD, FACOG
Associate Professor of Obstetrics and Gynecology, Department of Gynecologic Surgery and Obstetrics, Uniformed Services University of the Health Sciences, Bethesda, Maryland
Gynecologic Disorders

Karin Sinavsky, MD, MS
Assistant Clinical Professor, Department of Anesthesia and Perioperative Care, University of California, San Francisco
Palliative Care & Pain Management

Craig Smollin, MD
Professor of Emergency Medicine, Department of Emergency Medicine, University of California, San Francisco; Medical Director, California Poison Control System—San Francisco Division
Poisoning

Mathew Sorensen, MD, MS, FACS
Professor of Urology, Vice Chair of Education, Department of Urology, University of Washington, Seattle; Director, Comprehensive Metabolic Stone Clinic, Puget Sound Veterans Affairs Health Care System, Seattle, Washington
Urologic Disorders

Matthew A. Spinelli, MD, MAS
Associate Professor, Division of HIV, Infectious Diseases, and Global Medicine, Zuckerberg San Francisco General Hospital, University of California, San Francisco
HIV Infection & AIDS

Savitha Subramanian, MD
Professor of Medicine, Division of Metabolism, Endocrinology and Nutrition, University of Washington, Seattle, Washington
Diabetes Mellitus & Hypoglycemia

Michael Sutters, MD, MRCP (UK)
Attending Nephrologist, Virginia Mason Medical Center, Seattle, Washington
Systemic Hypertension

John Szumowski, MD, MPH
Associate Clinical Professor, Division of Infectious Diseases, Department of Medicine, San Francisco VA Medical Center and University of California, San Francisco
Viral & Rickettsial Infections

Elliot B. Tapper MD, FAASLD
Associate Professor and Chief, Hepatology Division of Gastroenterology and Hepatology, University of Michigan, Ann Arbor, Michigan
Liver, Biliary Tract, & Pancreas Disorders

Teresa K. Tarrant, MD
Associate Professor, Division of Rheumatology and Immunology, Department of Medicine,, Duke University Health System, Durham, North Carolina
Rheumatologic, Immunologic, & Allergic Disorders

Judith Walsh, MD, MPH
Professor of Clinical Medicine, Division of General Internal Medicine, Women's Health Center of Excellence, University of California, San Francisco
Women's Health Issues

Sunny Wang, MD
Professor of Clinical Medicine, Division of Hematology/Oncology, University of California, San Francisco; Chief of Hematology/Oncology, San Francisco Veterans Affairs Health Care System
Cancer

Zachary K. Wegermann, MD
Assistant Professor of Medicine—Cardiology, Duke University School of Medicine, Durham, North Carolina
Coronary Artery Disease, Valvular Disease, & Other Key Topics in Cardiology

Nolan R. Williams, MD
Associate Professor of Psychiatry and Behavioral Sciences (Major Labs & Translational Neuroscience Incubator) and, by courtesy, of Radiology (Neuroimaging and Neurointervention); Director, Brain Stimulation Laboratory; Director, Interventional Psychiatry Clinical Research, Department of Psychiatry and Behavioral Sciences, Stanford University, Stanford, California
Psychiatric Disorders

Leah J. Witt, MD
Associate Professor, Division of Geriatrics and Division of Pulmonary, Critical Care, Allergy and Sleep Medicine, Department of Medicine, University of California, San Francisco
Geriatric Disorders

Rachel Wojcik, MD, MS
Assistant Professor, University of Pittsburgh School of Medicine, Pittsburgh, Pennsylvania
Pulmonary Disorders

Tyler B. Woodell, MD, MCR
Associate Professor of Medicine, Division of Nephrology-Hypertension, Department of Medicine, University of California, San Diego
Kidney Disease

Scott Worswick, MD
Clinical Associate Professor of Dermatology, Department of Dermatology, Keck School of Medicine, University of Southern California, Los Angeles, California
Dermatologic Disorders

Jinoos Yazdany, MD, MPH
Alice Betts Endowed Professor, Department of Medicine, University of California, San Francisco; Chief, Division of Rheumatology, Zuckerberg San Francisco General Hospital
Rheumatologic, Immunologic, & Allergic Disorders

Emmanuelle Yecies, MD, MS
Clinical Assistant Professor, Stanford University, Stanford, California
Women's Health Issues

Preface

CURRENT Medical Diagnosis & Treatment 2027 (CMDT 2027) is the 66th edition of this single-source reference for practitioners of adult medicine in both hospital and ambulatory settings. The book emphasizes the practical features of clinical diagnosis and patient management in all fields of internal medicine and in specialties of interest to primary care practitioners and to subspecialists who provide general care.

The editors of *CMDT* have committed to a thorough examination of our content to remove biased language, research, and recommendations. Annually since 2020, we have been pursuing an ongoing, formal process of review and revision in an effort to recognize and correct biases and to promote equity in our book and thus in the practice of medicine. While we, the editors, take this on as our responsibility, we also invite readers to share with us any *CMDT* content that they find problematic or biased. Please email comments to CMDT@mheducation.com.

We have tried to describe populations used in the studies that form the basis of the information in *CMDT* and use appropriate language where we can (eg, persons of sub-Sahara African descent, rather than African Americans). We continue, however, to use terms from original sources when study populations are broad.

INTENDED AUDIENCE FOR *CMDT*

House officers, medical students, and all other health professions learners will find the descriptions of diagnostic and therapeutic modalities, with citations to the current literature, of everyday usefulness in patient care.

Internists, family physicians, hospitalists, nurse practitioners, physician associates, and all primary care providers of adult medicine will appreciate *CMDT* as a ready reference and refresher text. Physicians in other specialties, pharmacists, and dentists will find the book a useful basic medical reference text. Nurses, nurse practitioners, and physician associates will welcome the format and scope of the book as a means of quickly referencing medical diagnosis and treatment modalities.

Patients and their family members who seek information about the nature of specific diseases and their diagnosis and treatment may also find this book to be a valuable resource.

NEW IN THIS EDITION OF *CMDT*

The **"Year in Review: Key Clinical Updates in *CMDT 2027*"** highlights what the editors consider to be the most significant clinical changes over the last year, providing page numbers and reference citations for easy access. This tool is meant to get users "current" quickly but does not reflect all the changes since the last edition.

OUTSTANDING FEATURES OF *CMDT*

- National and international authorities distilling current evidence and deep experience into reliable recommendations
- Medical advances up to time of annual publication
- Detailed presentation of internal medicine disciplines, plus key primary care topics
- At-a-glance format, facilitating efficient use in any practice setting
- Coverage of more than 1000 diseases and disorders
- Specific disease prevention information
- Easy access to medication dosages, with trade names indexed and updated in each annual edition
- Recent references, with unique identifiers (PubMed, PMID numbers) for rapid downloading of article abstracts and, in some instances, full-text reference articles

BONUS E-CHAPTERS, *CMDT* ON ACCESSMEDICINE

Five ***e-chapters*** listed in the Table of Contents can be accessed at **www.AccessMedicine.com/CMDT.** These online-only chapters (available without the need for subscription) include

- Anti-infective Treatment: Antibiotic, Antifungal, & Antiviral Agents
- Diagnostic Testing & Medical Decision-Making
- Information Technology in Patient Care
- Podiatric Disorders
- Appendix: Therapeutic Drug Monitoring, Pharmacogenetic Tests, Laboratory Reference Intervals, & Commonly Used Blood Specimen Collection Tubes

ACKNOWLEDGMENTS

We wish to thank our authors for participating once again in the annual updating of this important book. We are especially grateful to:

Tyler Brehm, MD

Brigid M. Dolan, MD, MEd

Mazen El Ali, MD

Lawrence S. Friedman, MD

Brian Jordan, MD

Todd Kiefer, MD

Umesh Masharani, MBBS

Julian A. Mitton, MD, MPH

Lawrence Poree, MD, MPH, PhD

Nicole Rosendale, MD

Jishna Shrestha, MBBS

Carling Ursem, MD

who are passing the baton this year. We have all benefited from their clinical wisdom and commitment.

Many students and physicians have contributed useful suggestions to this and previous editions, and we are grateful. We continue to welcome comments and recommendations for future editions via email at CMDT@mheducation.com.

Kenneth R. McQuaid, MD
Maxine A. Papadakis, MD
Michael W. Rabow, MD
Paul L. Nadler, MD
San Francisco, California

YEAR IN REVIEW: KEY CLINICAL UPDATES IN *CMDT* 2027

Entries presented in the Year in Review are curated by the editors as being extremely impactful to daily clinical practice. These highlighted entries are only a fraction of all the updates included across this edition of *CMDT*.

Topic	Page Number	Key New Advances Affecting Clinical Practice*
CHAPTER 1: DISEASE PREVENTION & HEALTH PROMOTION		
Prevention of Cardiovascular Disease	5	• The recent PREVENT™ equations appear to more accurately predict 10-year atherosclerotic cardiovascular disease (ASCVD) risk than older risk equations. *Zhou H et al. J Am Heart Assoc. [PMID: 39921505]*
Prevention of Physical Inactivity	10	• For patients taking GLP-1 medications, aerobic physical activity (at recommended levels) combined with resistance training at 60–90 minutes per week may help preserve lean muscle mass and enhance weight loss and metabolic outcomes. *Mehrtash F et al. JAMA Intern Med. [PMID: 40658434]*
CHAPTER 2: COMMON SYMPTOMS		
Chest Pain	24	• The 0/1-hour accelerated protocol using high-sensitivity cardiac troponin 1 for evaluation of MI compared to a 0/3-hour standard care protocol and application of a modified HEART score did not lead to safer ED discharges. *Miller J et al. Ann Emerg Med. [PMID: 38888531]*
Hemoptysis	22	• Bronchial artery embolization has a technical success rate of 97% and is more effective than conservative treatment in controlling hemoptysis, but there is no difference in all-cause mortality. *Fan S et al. BMC Pulm Med. [PMID: 39215233]*
Palpitations	27	• Symptom-rhythm correlation in long-term continuous ambulatory monitoring is 18% overall (highest for atrial fibrillation and isolated ectopic beats). Median time to actionable arrhythmia was > 48 hours, limiting the utility of the Holter monitor even with daily symptoms. *Battisti AJ et al. Heart Rhythm. [PMID: 41205886]*
CHAPTER 3: PREOPERATIVE EVALUATION & PERIOPERATIVE MANAGEMENT		
Management of Endocrine Diseases	50	• GLP-1 agonists delay gastric emptying and may increase the risk of aspiration during sedation and anesthesia. A multi-specialty consensus statement recommends an individualized approach to determining how long to hold these agents before surgery. *American Diabetes Association Professional Practice Committee. Diabetes Care. [PMID: 39651972]*
Pulmonary Evaluation in Non-Lung Resection Surgery	47	• Formal polysomnography to diagnose obstructive sleep apnea (OSA) before surgery is recommended for patients with evidence of impaired gas exchange or end-organ damage. Patients using positive airway pressure devices should continue to do so after surgery. Patients with OSA should be closely monitored for respiratory decompensation after surgery. *Ceban F et al. J Clin Anesth. [PMID: 38718686]*

*See chapter for further details and references.

(continued on following page)

Topic	Page Number	Key New Advances Affecting Clinical Practice*
CHAPTER 4: GERIATRIC DISORDERS		
Dementia	56	• The emergence of FDA-cleared and commercially available CSF and blood-based biomarker tests are most useful to confirm a diagnosis of Alzheimer disease for patients with mild cognitive impairment (MCI) or early dementia who may be candidates for immunotherapy targeting amyloid-β. *Kim BH et al. Transl Neurodegener. [PMID: 39865265]*
	56	• For patients whose initial neuroimaging does not find a structural cause of cognitive impairment and who may be candidates for anti-amyloid therapy because of symptoms suggestive of MCI or early dementia due to Alzheimer disease, PET scans that detect amyloid-β in the brain can confirm a diagnosis of Alzheimer disease with a high degree of accuracy. *Expert Panel on Neurological Imaging. J Am Coll Radiol. [PMID: 40409878]*
	58	• In small short-term clinical trials of sleep disturbances in patients with Alzheimer disease and related dementias, the dual orexin receptor antagonists, suvorexant and lemborexant, modestly improved total sleep time, wakefulness after sleep onset, and sleep efficiency. *Alshiban A et al. Am J Geriatr Psychiatry. [PMID: 39462720]*
CHAPTER 5: PALLIATIVE CARE & PAIN MANAGEMENT		
Novel Nonopioid Analgesics	83	• In 2025, the new nonopioid analgesic suzetrigine was approved for the short-term treatment of moderate-to-severe *acute* pain only and can reduce the need for opioid analgesics in the setting of recent surgery or injury. *McCoun J et al. J Pain Res. [PMID: 40165940]*
CHAPTER 6: DERMATOLOGIC DISORDERS		
Bullous Pemphigoid	146	• In 2025, dupilumab became the first targeted biologic to be FDA-approved to treat bullous pemphigoid and should be considered for first-line therapy. *Olbrich H, Sadik CD. Expert Opin Emerg Drugs. [PMID: 40878514]*
Malignant and Premalignant Lesions	112	• In patients with nodular basal cell carcinoma, combination treatment with superficial curettage followed by imiquimod yielded a 22% 5-year recurrence rate compared with 2% following surgical excision. *Verkouteren BJA et al. JAMA Dermatol. [PMID: 39878970]*
Pompholyx	143	• In 2025, delgocitinib cream 2%, a topical JAK-inhibitor, became the first FDA-approved treatment for adults with moderate-to-severe chronic hand eczema (CHE). *Abdelhalim A et al. J Dermatolog Treat. [PMID: 40096745]*
CHAPTER 7: DISORDERS OF THE EYES & LIDS		
Retinal Disorders Associated with Systemic Diseases	190	• The first US Food and Drug Administration–approved treatment for macular telangiectasia (MacTel) type 2 is revakinagene taroretcel. *Chew EY et al. NEJM Evid. [PMID: 40693847]*
CHAPTER 9: PULMONARY DISORDERS		
Asthma	244	• ICS-formoterol combinations are gaining preference as both reliever medications and controller medications because formoterol is a LABA that has rapid onset (within 1–3 minutes), is longer-acting than SABAs, and provides increased therapeutic benefit in conjunction with an ICS. *Beasley R et al. J Allergy Clin Immunol Pract. [PMID: 36639054]; Dubin S et al. Mo Med. [PMID: 39421468]; Rayner DG et al. JAMA. [PMID: 39465893]*
Bronchiectasis	260	• For those with recurrent exacerbations (≥ 3 annually), a preventive macrolide (eg, azithromycin) or long-term inhaled antibiotics (colistin, gentamycin) have been found to decrease the frequency of exacerbations. *Barker AF et al. JAMA. [PMID: 40293759]; Chalmers JD et al. Eur Respir J. [PMID: 41016738]*

*See chapter for further details and references.

Topic	Page Number	Key New Advances Affecting Clinical Practice*
Chronic Obstructive Pulmonary Disease	258	• Ensifentrine, a first-in-class inhaled dual PDE3/4 inhibitor, has demonstrated significant improvements in lung function, symptoms, and exacerbation reduction in COPD, offering a novel anti-inflammatory and bronchodilatory option for patients with persistent symptoms despite standard therapy. *GOLD Committee. 2025 Report.* https://goldcopd.org/2025-gold-report/; *Patel N. Nurse Pract. [PMID: 38941078]; Singh D et al. Drugs. [PMID: 40392521]*
Idiopathic Interstitial Pneumonia	286	• Nerandomilast, a phosphodiesterase 4B with antifibrotic and immunomodulatory properties, has recently been shown to slow the progression of idiopathic pulmonary fibrosis (IPF) and has been approved by the FDA. *Richeldi L et al. N Engl J Med. [PMID: 40387033]*
Pneumonia	267	• New data in outpatients suggest equal effectiveness of shorter duration of antibiotics (but not < 3 days) in immunocompetent adult patients without comorbidities if patients have reached clinical stability at day 3.
	268	• Approach to pneumococcal vaccination depends on prior history of pneumococcal vaccination. *Kobayashi M et al. MMWR. [PMID: 39773952]*
Pulmonary Tuberculosis	279	• Some guidelines now recommend a shorter (6-month) treatment regimen as equivalent to a 15-month regimen in patients with drug-resistant tuberculosis. *Saukkonen JJ et al. Am J Respir Crit Care Med. [PMID: 40693952]*
	279	• For the treatment of latent tuberculosis infection, the CDC recommends the rifamycin-containing regimens (3 or 4 months) over WHO-favored isoniazid monotherapy (6 or 9 months), due to higher rates of completion of the shorter courses.
Sarcoidosis	289	• A 2025 open-label trial comparing corticosteroids with methotrexate for 24 weeks in moderate-to-severe pulmonary sarcoidosis showed similar lung function improvement. Therefore, methotrexate now is preferred to avoid the long-term effects of steroid use. *Kahlmann V et al. N Engl J Med. [PMID: 40387020]*
Solitary Pulmonary Nodule	283	• Robotic-assisted bronchoscopy has significantly improved access to peripheral lung lesions, with pooled diagnostic yields of ~77–88%, low complication rates, and enhanced success in assessment of nodules < 2 cm. *Zhang C et al. Thorac Cancer. [PMID: 38286133]*
CHAPTER 10: CORONARY ARTERY DISEASE, VALVULAR DISEASE, & OTHER KEY TOPICS IN CARDIOLOGY		
Acute Coronary Syndromes without ST-Segment Elevation	326	• While treatment guidelines recommend at least 1 year of treatment with dual antiplatelet therapy (DAPT) after acute coronary syndrome (ACS), more recent data suggests a 3-month duration may be safer (less bleeding) with improved survival. With current generation drug-eluting stents, there is data that DAPT can be discontinued after 1 month in high-bleeding-risk patients without an appreciable increase in mortality. *Newby D et al. Dual-ACS Trial, presented at ESC Congress 2025*
Acute MI with ST-Segment Elevation	332	• The more recent REDUCE-AMI trial found no long-term benefit from β-blockers in uncomplicated acute myocardial infarction (AMI) patients with a normal left ventricular (LV) ejection fraction. *Yndigegn T et al. N Engl J Med. [PMID: 38587241]*
	334	• Recent data from the DanGer Shock study suggests patients with cardiogenic shock in acute myocardial infarction (AMI-CS) benefit from use of an Impella (percutaneous ventricular assist device) compared to intra-aortic balloon pump (IABP) and pressors/inotropes alone. Prior studies of IABPs have found no benefit in the setting of AMI-CS. *Møller JE et al. N Engl J Med. [PMID: 40888722]*

*See chapter for further details and references.

(continued on following page)

Topic	Page Number	Key New Advances Affecting Clinical Practice*
Aortic Stenosis	341	• A recent clinical trial showed benefit for transcatheter aortic valve replacement (TAVR) in asymptomatic severe aortic stenosis, mainly by reduction in heart failure hospitalizations when an Edwards SAPIEN valve was used. *Généreux P et al. Am Heart J. [PMID: 38056546]*
Tricuspid Regurgitation	353	• Transcatheter edge-to-edge repair of the tricuspid valve (T-TEER) was recently shown to be safe and effective at reducing the degree of tricuspid regurgitation and improving quality of life in patients with severe tricuspid regurgitation. Transcatheter tricuspid valve replacement with the EVOQUE valve also demonstrated similar results. *Hajj J et al. Future Cardiol. [PMID: 40779241]*
CHAPTER 11: HEART FAILURE & CARDIOMYOPATHY		
Heart Failure	384	• While all of the following classes of medications may be useful in managing patients with HF, a 2025 meta-analysis showed that "quadruple therapy" (ARNI, β-blocker, MRA, and SGLT-2 inhibitor) provides the greatest mortality reduction in HFrEF. *Van Essen BJ, J Am Coll Cardiol. [PMID: 40892608]*
	385	• The 2024 FINEARTS-HF trial showed that finerenone significantly reduces the risk of HF hospitalizations and death among patients with heart failure with mildly reduced ejection fraction (HFmrEF) and heart failure with preserved ejection fraction (HFpEF). This was also the first study to show definitive benefit of an MRA in HFpEF. *Solomon SD et al. N Engl J Med. [PMID: 39225278]*
	387	• The VICTOR trial comprised stable outpatients and did not show reduction in HF hospitalizations or cardiovascular death with vericiguat but did show reduction in all-cause mortality. *Chen SH et al. Diabetes Obes Metab. [PMID: 41588709]*
Hypertrophic Cardiomyopathy	397	• In 2024, an ACC/AHA joint committee issued updated clinical practice guidelines for the diagnosis and treatment of hypertrophic cardiomyopathy (HCM). *Ommen SR et al. J Am Coll Cardiol. [PMID: 38727647]*
	398	• In 2025 the FDA approved a novel agent for the treatment of symptomatic obstructive HCM: aficamten. It has been shown to improve exercise capacity and symptoms. *Maron MS et al. N Engl J Med. [PMID: 38739079]*
CHAPTER 12: DISORDERS OF CARDIAC RHYTHM		
Paroxysmal Supraventricular Tachycardia	407	• Etripamil is a novel self-administered intranasal calcium channel blocker approved for termination of paroxysmal supraventricular tachycardia (PSVT). The medication has rapid pharmacokinetics with peak plasma concentration by 8 minutes and 60% of patients converting to sinus rhythm by 30 minutes. *Pokorney SD et al. JAMA Cardiol. [PMID: 40202738]*
CHAPTER 13: SYSTEMIC HYPERTENSION		
Resistant Hypertension	446	• Aprocitentan, an FDA-approved dual endothelin receptor antagonist for treatment of resistant hypertension, is an option in patients uncontrolled on three drugs, including a diuretic. • Renal sympathetic nerve ablation is a consideration for patients who have failed or are intolerant to maximal medical therapy. *Zeng W et al. Expert Rev Cardiovasc Ther. [PMID: 39258872]*

*See chapter for further details and references.

Topic	Page Number	Key New Advances Affecting Clinical Practice*
Uncontrolled Hypertension and Hypertensive Emergency	447	• In the inpatient setting escalation of oral antihypertensive therapy or the addition of intravenous medications for treatment of asymptomatic uncontrolled hypertension increases the risk of mortality, stroke, troponin release, and transfer to the ICU. As-needed antihypertensives prescribed during hospital admission carry a high risk of hypotensive organ injury and are best avoided. *Bress AP et al. Hypertension. [PMID: 38804130]; Miller JB et al. BMJ. [PMID: 39059997]*
CHAPTER 14: BLOOD VESSEL & LYMPHATIC DISORDERS		
Chronic Occlusive Disease: Femoral & Popliteal Arteries	453	• The SWEDEPAD 2 clinical trial and meta-analyses of device-approval clinical trials found significantly increased mortality at 5 years in patients with intermittent claudication treated with paclitaxel-coated devices. *Nordanstig J et al. Lancet. [PMID: 40902614]*
Occlusive Cerebrovascular Disease	457	• In the CREST-2 trial a durable reduction in the rate of stroke was seen at 4 years in patients treated with medical therapy plus carotid stent (2.8%) vs medical therapy (6.0%) and in patients treated with medical therapy plus carotid endarterectomy (3.7%) vs medical therapy (5.3%). *Brott TG et al. N Engl J Med. [PMID: 41269206]*
Shock	476	• A recent study demonstrated no difference in incidence of death or hospital readmission within 90 days for patients receiving balanced (lactated Ringer solution or Plasma-Lyte) or unbalanced (0.9% saline) crystalloid solutions. *McIntyre L et al. N Engl J Med. [PMID: 40503714]*
	478	• A systematic review and meta-analysis analysed 43 RCTs with > 10,000 patients with severe community-acquired pneumonia or acute respiratory distress syndrome and found that early initiation (within 72 hours of ICU admission) of low-dose corticosteroids (< 400 mg/day hydrocortisone equivalent) for a prolonged period (≥ 7 days) reduced short-term mortality by nearly 15% without increasing the incidence of secondary infections or GI bleeding. *Cao L et al. BMC Anesthesiol. [PMID: 40597594]*
CHAPTER 15: BLOOD DISORDERS		
Acute Leukemia	508	• Newer agents—venetoclax (bcl2 inhibitor), ivosidenib (targeting IDH1 mutations), enasidenib (targeting IDH2 mutations), gilteritinib (targeting FLT3 mutations), and revumenib or ziftomenib (menin inhibitors)—are being incorporated in the care of patients in the relapsed/refractory setting but also increasingly being studied in front-line combinations. *Chen EC et al. Am J Hematol. [PMID: 39901865]; Sabakhtarishvili G et al. Am J Clin Oncol. [PMID: 39238120]; Shimon S et al. Am J Hematol. [PMID: 39936576]*
Essential Thrombocytosis	501	• An antibody targeting the mutant calreticulin molecule on the cell surface in patients with Type 1 CALR mutations, INCA033989, showed promise in early trials with rapid, durable hematological responses and a favorable safety profile and received breakthrough designation by the FDA.
Hodgkin Lymphoma	514	• The response-adapted combination regimen BrECADD (Brentuximab Vedotin, Etoposide, Cyclophosphamide, Doxorubicin, Dacarbazine, Dexamethasone) has shown promise as a shorter regimen for high-risk patients. *Borchmann P et al. Lancet. [PMID: 38971175]*
Myelodysplastic Neoplasms	505	• Mutations in the *UBA1* gene can cause the recently identified VEXAS syndrome (Vacuoles, E1 enzyme, X-linked, Autoinflammatory, Somatic), a severe inflammatory condition primarily affecting older men, and leading to fevers, rashes, chondritis, and, importantly, myelodysplasia and other hematologic abnormalities. *Nakajima H, Kumimoto H. Int J Hematol. [PMID: 38819628]*

*See chapter for further details and references.

(continued on following page)

Topic	Page Number	Key New Advances Affecting Clinical Practice*
CHAPTER 16: DISORDERS OF HEMOSTASIS, THROMBOSIS, & ANTITHROMBOTIC THERAPY		
Antithrombotic Therapy	550	• Apixaban carries the lowest bleeding risk of the direct-acting oral anticoagulants (DOACs). *Mahé I et al. N Engl J Med. [PMID: 40162636]; Piazza G et al. N Engl J Med. [PMID: 40888734]*
Congenital Disorders of Coagulation	536	• Non-factor products (rebalancing agents) for treatment of hemophilia A and B with and without inhibitors include fitusiran, an siRNA therapeutic that reduces antithrombin expression, and two tissue factor pathway inhibitors, marstacimab and concizumab. *Mahlangu J et al. Blood Adv. [PMID: 41499759]; Matino D et al. Blood. [PMID: 41351884]; Young G et al. Blood. [PMID: 40053895]*
Increased Platelet Destruction	527	• Rilzabrutinib, a Bruton tyrosine kinase inhibitor, is a treatment option for refractory immune thrombocytopenia (ITP). *Kuter DJ et al. Blood. [PMID: 40090011]*
CHAPTER 17: GASTROINTESTINAL DISORDERS		
Atrophic Gastritis with Intestinal Metaplasia	601	• A recent AGA guideline recommends that screening for gastric cancer be considered in high-risk groups, including non-White racial and ethnic groups, first-generation immigrants from high-incidence regions, and those with a family history of gastric cancer in first-degree relatives. *Morgan DR et al. Am J Gastroenterol. [PMID: 40072510]; Shah S et al. Gastroenterology. [PMID: 39718517]*
Complications of Peptic Ulcer Disease	607	• A recent meta-analysis of 8 RCTs reported similar rates of initial hemostasis and recurrent bleeding between topical hemostatic powder and conventional endoscopic therapies for nonmalignancy-related GI bleeding. *Liu K et al. Gastrointest Endosc. [PMID: 39265743]*
Crohn Disease	633	• The anti-IL23p19 antibodies risankizumab and guselkumab are preferred to ustekinumab in patients with moderate-to-severe Crohn disease who have failed or lost response to prior biologic agents. *Panaccione R et al. Lancet. [PMID: 40684778]; Peyrin-Biroulet L et al. N Engl J Med. [PMID: 39018531]*
	633	• In a 52-week trial, mirikizumab vs ustekinumab demonstrated non significant but numerically higher clinical remission (51% vs 42%) and endoscopic response (45% vs 40%). *Ferrante M et al. Lancet. [PMID: 39581202]*
Diarrhea	573	• Measurement in a single stool specimen of total bile acid concentration > 1.88 μmol/g with > 4.6% primary bile acids is strongly suggestive of bile acid diarrhea. *Camilleri M. Am J Gastroenterol. [PMID: 39480027]; Dilmaghani S et al. Clin Gastroenterol Hepatol. [PMID: 40378992]*
Intestinal Tuberculosis	619	• When there is diagnostic uncertainty, an empiric trial of anti-TB therapy should be administered for 4–8 weeks (followed by clinical and endoscopic reassessment) before considering immunosuppressive therapy for possible Crohn disease. *Mouli V et al. Gastroenterology. [PMID: 40840713]*
Stress Gastritis	598	• In a trial of 4821 critically ill patients undergoing mechanical ventilation, clinically significant bleeding occurred in 1% of patients who received an intravenous PPI (pantoprazole 40 mg daily) versus 3.5% who received placebo. *Cook D et al. N Engl J Med. [PMID: 38875111]*

*See chapter for further details and references.

Topic	Page Number	Key New Advances Affecting Clinical Practice*
Whipple Disease	612	• A treatment regimen for Whipple disease, alternative to intravenous ceftriaxone followed by oral trimethoprim-sulfamethoxazole, is doxycycline 100 mg orally twice daily and hydroxychloroquine 200 mg orally twice daily for 12 months. *Moos V et al. Lancet Infect Dis. [PMID: 39978372]*
CHAPTER 18: LIVER, BILIARY TRACT, & PANCREAS DISORDERS		
Acute Pancreatitis	705	• Oral intake of fluid and solid foods can be resumed early in the disease course when the patient expresses an appetite, is largely free of pain, and has bowel sounds (even if the serum amylase is still elevated), and has been demonstrated to shorten length of hospitalization. • A "step-up" approach to treatment of walled-off pancreatic necrosis increasingly is used in which nonsurgical catheter drainage by either endoscopic transluminal (transgastric or transduodenal) or percutaneous placement under radiologic guidance (possibly performed < 4 weeks after development) reduces major complications and mortality relative to traditional open surgical approaches. *IAP/APA/EPC/IPC/JPS Working Group. Pancreatology. [PMID: 40651900]*
	705	• Placement of a stent across the pancreatic duct or orifice has been shown to reduce the risk of post-endoscopic retrograde cholangiopancreatography (ERCP) pancreatitis in high-risk patients; a combination of a pancreatic stent and NSAIDs provides more protection than NSAIDs alone and is recommended. *Elmunzer BJ et al. Lancet. [PMID: 38219767]*
Alcohol-Associated Liver Disease	671	• For patients with alcohol-associated hepatitis who respond to prednisone (up to 40 mg daily or the equivalent for up to 1 month), prednisone should be tapered by 10 mg per week without reductions in effectiveness. *Kulkarni AV et al. Am J Gastroenterol. [PMID: 40079479]*
Asymptomatic Pancreatic Cysts	710	• Recent studies indicate that most cases of neoplastic progression of intraductal papillary mucinous neoplasms (IPMNs) and mucinous cystic neoplasms (MCNs) occur within the first year following detection. It is therefore recommended, for suspected branch duct IPMNs and MCNs, that repeat cross-sectional CT or MRI be performed at 6 months. *Han Y et al. JAMA Surg. [PMID: 38231494]*
Chronic Viral Hepatitis	665–666	• Patients who wish to discontinue antiviral therapy for hepatitis B should meet all of the following criteria: no cirrhosis, HBeAg-negative and anti-HBe positive for > 1 year (if HBeAg-positive at start of treatment), HBV DNA undetectable > 2 years, no HIV or HDV co-infection, and agreement to participate in frequent laboratory monitoring. (The AASLD 2025 guideline also recommends that the HBsAg level be < 100 IU/mL but this test may not be widely available.) • Alanine aminotransferase (ALT) with HBV DNA levels should be monitored monthly for 6 months, every 3 months for a year and then every 3–6 months thereafter with treatment reinitiated if an increase of the ALT or DNA > 10,000 IU/mL. *Ghany MG et al. Hepatology. [PMID: 41186418]*
Cirrhosis	679	• The results of the 2025 UK ASEPTIC trial demonstrated no benefit from primary prophylaxis using trimethoprim-sulfamethoxazole in patients with ascites who have not had bacterial peritonitis.
	682	• For cirrhotic patients with cirrhosis admitted with acute decompensations, the MELD score and presence of extrahepatic organ failures known as "acute-on-chronic liver failure" (ACLF) predict mortality. *Karvellas CJ et al. Hepatology. [PMID: 37939273]*

*See chapter for further details and references.

(continued on following page)

Topic	Page Number	Key New Advances Affecting Clinical Practice*
Chronic Pancreatitis	708	• Strong opioids are sometimes necessary for those with more severe or frequent pain patterns. *Phillips AE et al. Clin Transl Gastroenterol. [PMID: 39907252]*
	709	• Targeted immunotherapy with monoclonal antibodies to immunoglobulin G components shows promise for systemic IgG_4-associated disease. *Stone JH. N Engl J Med. [PMID: 39541094]*
	709	• Patients who step up from endoscopic to surgical therapy may be less likely to exhibit long-term complete pain relief than those who start with operative therapy, and should be counseled about both options at the outset of treatment. *Sheth S et al. Gastrointest Endosc. [PMID: 39115496]; van Veldhuisen CL et al. JAMA Surg. [PMID: 39565607]*
Metabolic Dysfunction-Associated Steatotic Liver Disease	675	• In 2025 semaglutide, a GLP-1 analog, was approved for metabolic dysfunction-associated steatohepatitis (MASH) based on its ability to improve the resolution of MASH and fibrosis. *Sanyal AJ et al. N Engl J Med. [PMID: 40305708]*
CHAPTER 19: BREAST DISORDERS		
Carcinoma of the Female Breast: Curative Treatment	724	• ASCO guidelines state clinicians should not recommend routine sentinel lymph node biopsy in postmenopausal patients > age 50 who have grade 1–2, small (< 2 cm), hormone-receptor-positive, HER2-negative breast cancer, and negative findings on preoperative axillary ultrasonography who undergo breast-conserving therapy. *Park KU et al. J Clin Oncol. [PMID: 40209128]; Reimer T et al. N Engl J Med. [PMID: 39665649]*
	725	• Radiation alone may be preferable to the combination of radiation and hormone therapy in older women with low-risk breast cancer. • Radiation may be avoided in women who have complete disappearance of their cancer after neoadjuvant systemic therapy. *Ghannam Y et al. Cancer Radiother. [PMID: 41270649]; Hibon J et al. Cancer Radiother. [PMID: 40774101]; Mamounas EP et al. N Engl J Med. [PMID: 40466065]; Meattini I et al. Lancet Oncol. [PMID: 39675376]*
	725	• The SUPREMO trial showed that post-mastectomy radiotherapy is unnecessary for women with 1–3 involved axillary nodes who receive adjuvant systemic therapy. *Kunkler IH et al. N Engl J Med. [PMID: 41191939]*
	726	• The 2025 DESTINY-Breast05 study demonstrated a significant improvement in invasive disease-free survival with adjuvant trastuzumab deruxtecan (T-DXd) compared to trastuzumab emtansine (T-DM1) in high-risk patients who have residual disease after standard neoadjuvant therapy. This treatment may soon become standard of care for select patients. *Loibl S et al. N Engl J Med. [PMID: 41370739]*
Carcinoma of the Female Breast: Lobular Carcinoma In Situ & Noninvasive Cancer	722	• The COMET trial examined the nonoperative management of selected patients with low-risk ductal carcinoma in situ (DCIS) (grade 1 or 2, hormone-receptor-positive). Two-year follow-up demonstrated no difference in the risk of ipsilateral invasive breast cancer recurrence between patients randomized to active monitoring or surgery (with or without radiation). *Hwang S et al. JAMA. [PMID: 39665585]*

*See chapter for further details and references.

Topic	Page Number	Key New Advances Affecting Clinical Practice*
Carcinoma of the Female Breast: Palliative Treatment	731	• In selected patients it may be appropriate to start with single-agent endocrine therapy and defer use of the CDK4/6 inhibitor to the second-line setting. *Sonke GS et al. Nature. [PMID: 39604725]*
	731	• An oral SERD, imlunestrant, showed an improved progression-free survival compared to standard endocrine therapy and received regulatory approval. *Jhaveri KL et al. N Engl J Med. [PMID: 39660834]*
	731	• The VIKTORIA-1 trial evaluated the combination of gedatolisib plus fulvestrant, with or without palbociclib, compared to single-agent fulvestrant in patients who had received a prior CDK4/6i and who did not have a mutation in the gene encoding PI3K, PIK3CA. The progression-free survival was improved with both the triplet and doublet compared to fulvestrant alone. *Hurvitz SA et al. J Clin Oncol. [PMID: 41802242]*
	732	• T-DXd, in combination with pertuzumab (T-DXd/P), is FDA-approved as a first-line HER2-directed therapy based on the DESTINY-Breast09 trial. *Tolaney SM et al. N Engl J Med. [PMID: 41160818]*
	732	• The ASCENT 03 study showed that sacituzumab govitecan is of benefit as first-line treatment. *Cortés J et al. N Engl J Med. [PMID: 41124233]*
	733	• The TROP-2-directed antibody drug conjugate, datopotamab deruxtecan, demonstrated significant benefits compared to chemotherapy in two phase 3 clinical trials for hormone-receptor-positive breast cancer (TROPION-Breast01) and triple-negative breast cancer (TROPION-Breast02). Datopotamab deruxtecan is FDA-approved for hormone-receptor–positive metastatic breast cancer. *Bardia A et al. Clin Oncol. [PMID: 39265124]*
CHAPTER 21: GYNECOLOGIC DISORDERS		
Cervical Intraepithelial Neoplasia (CIN)	774	• Self-collected vaginal specimens for primary HPV testing were added as a screening option in 2025. The ACS recommends screening with self-collection be repeated every 3 years. *Perkins RB et al. CA Cancer J Clin. [PMID: 41342729]*
Postmenopausal Uterine Bleeding	751	• Transvaginal sonography may be a less reliable modality for initial screening in Black individuals. *Dell KM et al. JAMA Oncol. [PMID: 38935372]; Doll KM et al. JAMA Oncol. [PMID: 34264304]; Slaager FC et al. Eur J Obstet Gynecol Reprod Biol. [PMID: 40294513]*
Vaginitis	771–772	• The ACOG updated its clinical recommendations to advise concurrent partner therapy with a combined oral and topical antimicrobial for male sexual partners of adult patients with recurrent, symptomatic bacterial vaginosis. *No authors listed. Obstet Gynecol. [PMID: 41100865]; Powell AM et al. Obstet Gyncecol Clin North Am. [PMID: 37149312]; Vodstrcil LA et al. N Engl J Med. [PMID: 40043236]*
CHAPTER 23: RHEUMATOLOGIC, IMMUNOLOGIC, & ALLERGIC DISORDERS		
Antiphospholipid Syndrome	826	• Those with all three antiphospholipid antibodies ("triple positivity") have the highest risk of thrombosis and pregnancy loss, higher recurrence rates, and usually require lifelong anticoagulation. *Devreese KMJ et al. J Thromb Haemost. [PMID: 39510414]*
Microscopic Polyangiitis	844	• Patients with severe disease, typically involving pulmonary hemorrhage and glomerulonephritis, require urgent induction treatment with corticosteroids, avacopan, and either rituximab or cyclophosphamide. *Merkel PA et al. ACR Open Rheumatol. [PMID: 40192160]*

*See chapter for further details and references.

(continued on following page)

Topic	Page Number	Key New Advances Affecting Clinical Practice*
Polymyalgia Rheumatica & Giant Cell Arteritis	839	• Methotrexate (15–25 mg orally weekly) may have a steroid-sparing role in refractory polymyalgia rheumatica. *Bolhuis TE et al. Ann Rheum Dis. [PMID: 41423373]*
	839–840	• Upadacitinib 15 mg orally daily with a 26-week corticosteroid taper showed superior efficacy (sustained remission of giant cell arteritis) compared with placebo and a 52-week corticosteroid taper. • Giant cell arteritis treatment guidelines are to initiate a steroid-sparing therapy along with corticosteroids for all patients with new or relapsing giant cell arteritis. *Blockmans D et al. N Engl J Med. [PMID: 40174237]*
Rheumatoid Arthritis	820	• Tocilizumab can be used alone or in combination with methotrexate in patients with disease refractory to TNF inhibitor therapy. *Liu T et al. JAMA Netw Open. [PMID: 40388166]*
Systemic Lupus Erythematosus	824	• Obinutuzumab, a B-cell depleting agent, is approved to treat active lupus nephritis when used in combination with mycophenolate mofetil. *Fanouriakis A et al. Ann Rheum Dis. [PMID: 41107121]; Sammaritano LR et al. Arthritis Rheumatol. [PMID: 40331662]*
CHAPTER 24: ELECTROLYTE & ACID-BASE DISORDERS		
Hyponatremia	868	• Interpretation of a urine sodium level post-saline administration has been shown to improve diagnostic yield, differentiating between hypovolemic hyponatremia and the syndrome of inappropriate antidiuresis. *Chienwichai K et al. Sci Rep. [PMID: 40775013]*
CHAPTER 25: KIDNEY DISORDERS		
Diabetic Kidney Disease	924	• The combination of MRAs and SGLT-2 inhibitors leads to greater reduction in proteinuria than either treatment alone; non steroidal MRAs (eg, finerenone) are less likely to cause hyperkalemia. *Agarwal R et al. N Engl J Med. [PMID: 40470996]*
Interstitial Nephritis	901	• Immune checkpoint inhibitor (ICI)-associated acute kidney injury (AKI) is becoming increasingly common. General recommendations include holding therapy and treating with a course of corticosteroids. Based on consideration of treatment benefit, re-introduction of ICI therapy after AKI resolution may be considered with careful monitoring. Avoidance of concomitant potentially allergenic medications (eg, proton pump inhibitors [PPIs], sulfonamides, and ciprofloxacin) may help prevent acute interstitial nephritis (AIN) due to ICIs. *Herrmann SM et al. Kidney Int. [PMID: 39455026]*
Nephritic Spectrum Glomerular Diseases	916	• Iptacopan, which inhibits factor B in the complement alternative pathway, leads to a clinically meaningful reduction in proteinuria in C3 glomerulopathies. *Kavanagh D et al. Lancet. [PMID: 41016405]*
Renal Artery Stenosis	911	• Angioplasty with stenting is no better than optimal medical management in most patients. Stenting may not be the hoped-for "panacea" due to its inability to address underlying small vessel disease and renal scarring, which are often present at the time of diagnosis. *Shao C et al. Kidney Blood Press Res. [PMID: 40064159]*

*See chapter for further details and references.

Topic	Page Number	Key New Advances Affecting Clinical Practice*
CHAPTER 26: UROLOGIC DISORDERS		
Acute Cystitis	934	• Gepotidacin is a novel antibiotic that received FDA approval in 2025 for use in uncomplicated UTIs. *Wagenlehner F et al. Lancet. [PMID: 38342126]*
Acute Pyelonephritis	937	• Shorter antibiotic courses are now recommended; duration should be 5–7 days for a fluoroquinolone and 7 days for a non-fluoroquinolone. Patients with bacteremia who are improving clinically should be treated for 7 days. *Geyer AC et al. Antimicrob Steward Healthc Epidemiol. [PMID: 37771747]; Veillette JJ et al. Open Forum Infect Dis. [PMID: 38665174]*
Urinary Stone Disease: Renal Calculi	947	• New vacuum aspiration sheaths and scopes have expanded the limits of ureteroscopic treatment of stones. *Bargagli M et al. Nat Rev Nephrol. [PMID: 40790363]; Pearle MS et al. J Urol. [PMID: 41263323]*
CHAPTER 27: NERVOUS SYSTEM DISORDERS		
Essential (Familial) Tremor	994	• Transcutaneous electrical stimulation of the median and radial nerves modestly improves function and is an option for tremors that are not controlled by medications or suitable for surgical treatment. *Shih LC. Continuum (Minneap Minn). [PMID: 40748121]*
Multiple Sclerosis	1012–1013	• Teriflunomide and dimethyl fumarate delay time to first clinical attack in patients with radiologically isolated syndrome. *Gonzalez-Lorenzo M et al. Cochrane Database Syst Rev. [PMID: 38174776]*
Myasthenia Gravis	1031	• Nipocalimab and rozanolixizumab are approved by the FDA for acetylcholine antibody–positive myasthenia and MuSK-positive myasthenia.
Neurofibromatosis	993–994	• In patients with neurofibromatosis type 1, two mitogen-activated protein kinase inhibitors are approved by the FDA for treatment of inoperable plexiform neurofibromas: selumetinib in children 1 year of age and older and mirdametinib in adults and children. *Sato AA et al. Am J Med Genet C Semin Med Genet. [PMID: 40968507]*
CHAPTER 28: PSYCHIATRIC DISORDERS		
Neurocognitive Disorders	1075	• In 2025, the first blood test (Lumipulse) to assist in the diagnosis of Alzheimer disease was approved by the FDA. The test measures the ratio of Tau p217 to β-amyloid 1-42.
Schizophrenia Spectrum Disorders	1055	• For patients with schizophrenia who are taking clozapine, updated 2025 guidelines recommend weekly absolute neutrophil count (ANC) monitoring for the first 18 weeks, biweekly through 1 year, and monthly thereafter, if stable.
Sleep-Wake Disorders	1070	• Contemporary guidelines reinforce cognitive behavioral therapy for insomnia (CBT-I) as the first-line intervention for chronic insomnia, with pharmacotherapy reserved for adjunctive use or when CBT-I is inaccessible or insufficient. *Hwang JW et al. NPJ Digit Med. [PMID: 40075149]*
	1070	• Dual orexin receptor antagonists and melatonin receptor agonists play a growing role in the management of chronic insomnia due to their more physiologic modulation of sleep-wake pathways and reduced risk for dependence. *Kishi T et al. Transl Psychiatry. [PMID: 40555730]*

*See chapter for further details and references.

(continued on following page)

Topic	Page Number	Key New Advances Affecting Clinical Practice*
Trauma & Stressor-Related Disorders	1038	• While the α-blocking agent prazosin (2–10 mg orally at bedtime) has been widely used to decrease nightmares and improving quality of sleep in PTSD, recent large-scale trials have not consistently demonstrated superiority over placebo for this indication. *Zhao YF et al. BMC Psychiatry. [PMID: 40665297]*
CHAPTER 29: DISORDERS OF THE PITUITARY, THYROID, & ADRENAL GLANDS		
Acromegaly & Gigantism	1087	• In a placebo-controlled trial, 83% of patients taking paltusotine, a somatostatin receptor ligand, achieved a normal serum IGF I level, compared to 4% of the placebo group. *Biller BMK et al. J Clin Endocrinol Metab. [PMID: 41128642]*
Cushing Syndrome	1122	• Osilodrostat 2 mg orally twice daily can normalize urine free cortisol and improve the manifestations of hypercortisolism. *Fleseriu M et al. J Endocr Soc. [PMID: 40226519]*
Primary Aldosteronism	1124	• Updated endocrine society guidelines suggest that all hypertensive patients be screened for primary aldosteronism (PA). *Adler GK et al. J Clin Endocrinol Metab. [PMID: 40658480]*
	1124	• Imaging with ^{11}C-MTO PET-CT is an alternative to adrenal vein sampling to detect a small unilateral adenoma. *Teo AED et al. J Clin Endocrinol Metab. [PMID: 40690719]*
	1125	• Finerenone, a nonsteroidal mineralocorticoid antagonist with no anti-androgenic effects, has been used successfully for patients with primary aldosteronism. *Hu J et al. Circulation. [PMID: 39804908]*
	1125	• Treatment with baxdrostat, a highly selective aldosterone synthase inhibitor, is started at 2 mg per day orally for the first 4 weeks, then increased to 4 mg or 6 mg daily. *Flack JM et al. N Engl J Med. [PMID: 40888730]*
Thyroiditis	1093	• Dietary supplementation with selenium 200 mcg/day reduces serum levels of TPO Ab and may be associated with improvements in mood. The favored formulation is selenomethionine. *Zhang H et al. Medicine (Baltimore). [PMID: 40898469]*
CHAPTER 30: DISORDERS OF PARATHYROID GLANDS & BONE METABOLISM		
Multiple Endocrine Neoplasia (MEN)	1154	• MEN-4 may mimic MEN-1, so screening should be considered in patients with an MEN-1–like phenotype who do not have an MEN-1 gene mutation. *Chevalier B et al. J Clin Endocrinol Metab. [PMID: 38288531]*
Primary Hyperparathyroidism	1144	• Definitive treatment with parathyroidectomy is recommended for patients with primary hyperparathyroidism who are symptomatic or who have nephrolithiasis, osteoporotic fracture, or other symptoms of parathyroid bone disease, unless there is a contraindication to surgery. *Kongsaree N et al. J Clin Endocrinol Metab. [PMID: 38739762]; Liu Y et al. J Clin Endocrinol Metab. [PMID: 39319404]; Silva BC et al. Best Pract Res Clin Endocrinol Metab. [PMID: 30477754]*

*See chapter for further details and references.

Topic	Page Number	Key New Advances Affecting Clinical Practice*
CHAPTER 31: DIABETES MELLITUS & HYPOGLYCEMIA		
Diabetes Mellitus	1165	• In a recent pooled analysis of patients from four RCTs, compared to medical management, bariatric surgery was associated with better long-term improvement of glycemic control, use of fewer medications, and greater weight loss at 7 to 12 years of follow-up. *Courcoulas AP et al. JAMA. [PMID: 38411644]*
	1168	• Both subcutaneous and oral semaglutide significantly reduce the risk of major adverse cardiovascular events in patients with type 2 diabetes at high cardiovascular risk. • Studies on metabolic-associated steatotic liver disease (MASLD) have demonstrated improvement of liver enzymes, decrease in liver fat content, and improved systemic and hepatic inflammation without effect on fibrosis.
	1169	• Links between GLP-1 receptor agonist use and pancreatitis, pancreatic cancer, and metabolic bone disease have not been supported by several large-scale trials, meta-analyses, or real-world data. *Nauck MA et al. Lancet. [PMID: 41547366]*
	1169	• In patients with type 2 diabetes and major atherosclerotic cardiovascular events, tirzepatide was noninferior to dulaglutide for the composite endpoint of death from cardiovascular causes, myocardial infarction, and stroke. *Nicholls SJ et al. N Engl J Med. [PMID: 41406444]*
	1170	• Landmark clinical trials have demonstrated that several SGLT-2 inhibitors have cardiovascular benefits that extend beyond their glucose lowering effects, including reduced cardiovascular mortality and hospitalization for heart failure. *O'Hara DV et al. Nat Rev Nephrol. [PMID: 38671190]*
	1183	• Some GLP-1 receptor agonists are linked to an increased risk of non-arteritic anterior ischemic optic neuropathy and age-related macular degeneration, but further studies are needed. *Amini A et al. Acta Ophthalmol. [PMID: 40055951]*
Diabetic Ketoacidosis	1193	• The anion gap is no longer used as a criterion to assess DKA resolution. *Umpierrez GE et al. Diabetes Care. [PMID: 39052901]*
CHAPTER 32: LIPID DISORDERS		
High Blood Triglycerides	1211	• Olezarsen and plozasiran (which was approved in 2025 for familial chylomicronemia syndrome) may soon be approved for severe hypertriglyceridemia. *Watts GF et al. N Engl J Med. [PMID: 39225259]*
Treatment of High LDL Cholesterol	1209	• The VESALIUS trial extended the benefits of PCSK9 inhibitors to patients without prior MI or stroke; in VESALIUS, among 12,257 patients with no prior ASCVD but established advanced atherosclerosis, evolocumab decreased the primary cardiovascular endpoint by 25%. *Bohula EA et al. N Engl J Med. [PMID: 41211925]*
	1209	• The 2025 ESC cholesterol guidelines recommend consideration of targeting to an LDL < 40 mg/dL for patients experiencing a second CVD event while already on maximally tolerated statin therapy ("extreme risk"). *Mach F et al. Eur Heart J. [PMID: 40878289] [Erratum: PMID: 41417047]*
	1209	• The newest PCSK9 inhibitor lerodalcibep-liga is a recombinant fusion protein that blocks the PCSK9 protein and can be given as a monthly subcutaneous injection.

*See chapter for further details and references.

(continued on following page)

Topic	Page Number	Key New Advances Affecting Clinical Practice*
CHAPTER 33: NUTRITION, NUTRITIONAL DISORDERS, & OBESITY		
Complications of Parenteral Nutritional Support	1230	• The use of peripheral parenteral nutrition over central parenteral nutrition when appropriate is another useful strategy to prevent catheter-related bloodstream infections. *Bidgood E et al. Nutr Clin Pract. [PMID: 39467781]*
Obesity	1219	• In 2025, semaglutide 2.4 mg was approved for the treatment of noncirrhotic MASH in adults with moderate to advanced liver fibrosis. • In 2025, oral semaglutide was the first oral GLP-1 receptor agonist to receive FDA approval to reduce excess body weight and maintain long-term weight reduction long term in adults with obesity or overweight with at least one weight-related comorbid condition; it was also approved to reduce the risk of major adverse cardiovascular events (MACE) in adults with obesity or overweight who have established cardiovascular disease. • In the OASIS 4 trial, oral semaglutide was associated with 13.6% total body weight loss at 64 weeks compared to 2.2% with placebo in adults without diabetes who had obesity or overweight with one or more weight-related comorbidities. *Jordan G et al. Gastrointest Endosc Clin N Am. [PMID: 39277293]; McGowan B et al. Nat Med. [PMID: 41039115]; Thomsen RW et al. Diabetes Obese Metab. [PMID: 40196933]*
CHAPTER 35: HIV INFECTION & AIDS		
Complications: Skin Manifestations	1293	• Tecovirimat is safe but not effective in reducing the severity and duration of mpox lesions. There is now no effective antiviral for mpox, and prevention relies on vaccination. *Zucker J et al. N Engl J Med. [PMID: 41740032]*
Prevention	1297	• An isolated positive HIV RNA at cabotegravir PrEP follow-up, particularly if it is at the limit of detection (ie, < 20, but detected), should be repeated and the patient should be counseled that there is a higher probability of false positives than a true positive. *Landovitz RJ et al. HPTN 083 Abstract, Conference on Retroviruses and Opportunistic Infections.*
	1297	• Approval of a new long-acting PrEP agent, biyearly subdermal lenacapavir (LEN), occurred in June 2025. *Bekker LG et al. N Engl J Med. [PMID: 39046157]; Kelley CF et al. N Engl J Med. [PMID: 39602624]*
Treatment	1314	• The International Antiviral Society-USA and DHHS recommend cabotegravir/rilpivirine among those at high risk of HIV progression who cannot take oral ART, with virus susceptible to both agents. For individuals with HIV resistant to rilpivirine, some clinicians are using cabotegravir and lenacapvir together off-label. *Gandhi M et al. Open Forum Infect Dis. [PMID: 38628952]; Hickey MD et al. Clin Infect Dis. [PMID: 39367871]*
CHAPTER 36: VIRAL & RICKETTSIAL INFECTIONS		
Epstein-Barr Virus & Infectious Mononucleosis	1328	• Rituximab is shown to be a useful supplement to chemotherapy for patients in Africa with Burkitt lymphoma. *Mawalla WF et al. Blood Adv. [PMID: 39983056]*

*See chapter for further details and references.

Topic	Page Number	Key New Advances Affecting Clinical Practice*
Herpes Zoster (Shingles)	1326	• In studies from 2 San Francisco Bay area medical schools, those vaccinated with the recombinant vaccine (now replaced with Shingrix) show a decrease over several years in the onset of Alzheimer disease. *Eyting M et al. Nature. [PMID: 40175543]*
Respiratory Syncytial Virus (RSV) & Other Paramyxoviruses	1370	• The prophylactic monoclonal antibody palivizumab was the first monoclonal released for RSV and shows an excellent record as a highly effective preventive agent for RSV in high-risk infants. *Carbonell-Estrany X et al. Expert Rev Anti Infect Ther. [PMID: 40111069]*
	1370	• Clesrovimab-cfor (Enflonsia) received FDA approval for use in infants during their first season at risk for RSV.
Seasonal Influenza	1372	• A meta-analysis among those 65 or greater shows improved efficacy with high-dose, adjuvanted, or recombinant influenza vaccines compared with standard-dose unadjuvanted influenza vaccines. *Ferdinands JM et al. J Am Geriatr Soc. [PMID: 39230284]*
Severe Acute Respiratory Syndrome—Coronavirus 2019 (SARS-CoV-2)	1367	• Vaccines against COVID all show good efficacy against variants other than the original target, although nucleic acid vaccines offer the most protection. *Hoang TNA et al. Trans R Soc Trop Med Hyg. [PMID: 39495246]; Janes H et al. J infect Dis. [PMID: 39225478]*
CHAPTER 37: BACTERIAL & CHLAMYDIAL INFECTIONS		
Gonococcal Infections	1427	• As of late 2025, two new oral medications, gepotidacin and zoliflodacin, have been demonstrated in RCTs to be non inferior to the combination of ceftriaxone and azithromycin for the treatment of uncomplicated urogenital gonorrhea. These newer oral medications may be incorporated into treatment guidelines in the future. *Luckey A et al. Lancet. [PMID: 41391465]*
CHAPTER 39: PROTOZOAL & HELMINTHIC INFECTIONS		
Lymphatic Filariasis	1489	• Moxidectin (approved for onchocerciasis) plus albendazole improved clearance of microfilariae compared to ivermectin plus albendazole. *Koudou GB et al. Lancet Infect Dis. [PMID: 40345209]*
Schistosomiasis	1479	• A divided dose of 80 mg/kg of praziquantel yielded improved cure rates for *S mansoni* infections. *Bustinduy AL et al. Lancet. [PMID: 40412398]*
CHAPTER 40: MYCOTIC INFECTIONS		
Candidiasis	1495	• The 2025 global guidelines for the diagnosis and management of candidiasis recommend an intravenous echinocandin as first-line therapy (ie, caspofungin [70 mg once, then 50 mg daily], micafungin [100 mg daily], or anidulafungin [200 mg once, then 100 mg daily]). *Cornely OA et al. Lancet Infect Dis. [PMID: 39956121]*
Histoplasmosis	1496	• Specific therapy can be withheld in immunocompetent individuals with asymptomatic noncalcified pulmonary nodules and mild acute pulmonary disease. *Pappas P et al. Clin Infect Dis. [PMID: 40637160]*

*See chapter for further details and references.

(continued on following page)

Topic	Page Number	Key New Advances Affecting Clinical Practice*
CHAPTER 43: CANCER		
Bladder Cancer	1593	• TAR-200, a novel intravesical gemcitabine-releasing system, has been approved for use in Bacillus Calmette-Guérin–unresponsive high-risk non–muscle-invasive bladder cancer. *Daneshmand S et al. J Clin Oncol. [PMID: 40737582]*
Carcinoma of the Anus	1581	• Retifanlimab (an ICI) was approved by the FDA in 2025 for advanced squamous cell carcinoma of the anal canal. *Rao S et al. Lancet. [PMID: 40517007]*
Colorectal Cancer	1576	• Patients with MSI-H/dMMR tumors benefit from the addition of the ICI atezolizumab to standard adjuvant chemotherapy, with an improvement in 3-year disease-free survival from 76.6% to 86.4%. *Sinicrope FA et al. N Engl J Med. [PMID: 41880612]*
	1576	• Compelling evidence suggests that even an abbreviated course of preoperative immunotherapy alone (nivolumab plus ipilimumab), without chemotherapy, may be an appropriate strategy for patients with MSI-H/dMMR tumors. *Chalabi M et al. N Engl J Med. [PMID: 38838311]*
	1577	• A recent phase 3 study showed that in this group of patients, the addition of cetuximab plus encorafenib (an oral RAF inhibitor) to standard chemotherapy (FOLFOX) led to improvements in objective response rate, progression-free survival, and overall survival compared to standard treatment (FOLFOX with or without bevacizumab). *Elez E et al. N Engl J Med. [PMID: 40444708]*
	1577	• For the 3–5% of patients with metastatic MSI or dMMR colorectal cancer, immunotherapy alone with either a single (anti-PD1 monoclonal antibody) or doublet ICI combination (anti-PD1 plus anti-CTLA4 mAbs) represents the preferred front-line therapy, as it has demonstrated improved progression-free survival, more durable responses, and fewer severe adverse events compared to standard chemotherapy. *Andre T et al. N Engl J Med. [PMID: 39602630]*
	1578	• Select patients who achieve a complete clinical response to total neoadjuvant therapy may be candidates for non operative management, with close surveillance by endoscopy and cross-sectional imaging to ensure no local regrowth (or metastatic dissemination). *Amatu A et al. Lancet Oncol. [PMID: 41308677]*
Gastric Adenocarcinoma	1570	• Recent evidence from the phase 3 MATTERHORN trial in patients with resectable (stage II–IVA) gastric and gastroesophageal junction cancer indicated that the addition of an ICI (durvalumab) to fluorouracil, leucovorin, oxaliplatin, and docetaxel (FLOT) chemotherapy further improves clinical outcomes, including a 2-year event-free survival of 67.4% compared to 58.5% with chemotherapy alone. *Janjigian YY et al. N Engl J Med. [PMID: 40454643]*
Hepatocellular Carcinoma	1560	• A dual immune-checkpoint inhibitor combination, nivolumab plus ipilimumab, was approved in 2025 as a front-line treatment option for patients in whom large or bleeding esophageal varices are present. *Yau T et al. Future Oncol. [PMID: 41981891]*

*See chapter for further details and references.

Topic	Page Number	Key New Advances Affecting Clinical Practice*
	1561	• A large phase 3 trial evaluating transarterial chemoembolization (TACE) in combination with lenvatinib plus pembrolizumab has demonstrated a significant improvement in median progression-free survival when compared to TACE plus placebo. *Kudo M et al. Lancet. [PMID: 39798578]*
Prostate Cancer	1589	• The 2024 AUA/ASTRO/SUO Salvage Therapy for Prostate Cancer Guideline recommends PSA monitoring after treatment with early salvage therapy (PSA < 0.5) for recurrence. • PSMA PET scans before salvage therapy are shown to change treatment in up to 34% of men and may lead to improved outcomes. *Morgan TM et al. J Urol. [PMID: 38421253]*
	1591	• Based on data from the Amplitude trial, the FDA recently approved niraparib with abiraterone acetate as first-line therapy for men with BRCA 1/2-mutated metastatic castrate-sensitive prostate cancer, which supports upfront genomics testing for all men presenting with metastatic disease. *Attard G et al. Nat Med. [PMID: 41057655]*
	1591	• Lutetium-177-PSMA-617, the first theranostic radioligand agent for metastatic castration-resistant prostate cancer approved for use in men with PSMA-producing tumors who have progressed on other lines of therapy, is now approved for earlier use before chemotherapy.
CHAPTER 45: ORTHOPEDIC DISORDERS & SPORTS MEDICINE		
Adhesive Capsulitis	1627	• Hydrodissection by intraarticular injection of large volumes of saline or anesthetic may improve symptoms. *Vita F et al. Musculoskelet Surg. [PMID: 41444457]*
Ankle Injuries	1653	• Icing acutely after an ankle sprain can help with early pain and swelling; however, it does not appear to help with recovery from injury, so ice can be used with caution if it is more than 12 hours after injury. *Wu V et al. Am Fam Physician. [PMID: 41533404]*
Anterior Cruciate Ligament Injury	1646	• There is strong support for using neuromuscular training programs to significantly reduce (by almost half) the risk of anterior cruciate ligament rupture among athletes. *Watson SL et al. Am J Sports Med. [PMID: 41486737]*
Lateral & Medial Epicondylosis	1634	• Compared to prolotherapy, extracorporeal shock wave and physiotherapy, PRP had better clinical and functional outcomes for chronic lateral epicondylosis over a 2-year follow-up. *Lhee SH et al. Am J Sports Med. [PMID: 40815854]*
Low Back Pain	1629	• Self-management strategies including pain education, exercises (postural strength, core stabilization, mobility, stretches), cognitive-behavioral strategies (relaxed breathing, progressive muscle relaxations, guided imagery, cognitive restructuring), and social strategies (pleasant activity scheduling, communication for navigating social roles) were better than medical care or spinal manipulation. *Bronfort G et al. JAMA. [PMID: 41460638]*
Lumbar Disc Herniation	1632	• Platelet-rich plasma (PRP), bone marrow aspirate concentrate, and chemonucleolysis have demonstrated potential in delaying disc degeneration and enhancing tissue repair when injected alone or an adjunct to surgical procedures. *Tong Y et al. Front Neurol. [PMID: 41487424]*

*See chapter for further details and references.

(continued on following page)

Topic	Page Number	Key New Advances Affecting Clinical Practice*
Meniscus Injuries	1649	• Neuromuscular exercises including lower extremity strengthening, balance, hip and core strengthening, and patient education are first-line non operative treatments. An RCT showed that physical therapy and home exercises were both helpful in cases of degenerative meniscus tears. *Katz JN et al. N Engl J Med. [PMID: 41160820]*
Neck Pain	1633	• A recent meta-analysis of 25 RCTs showed that cervical disc arthroplasty was superior to anterior discectomy and fusion for the treatment of symptomatic cervical disc disease, with better success, fewer secondary surgeries, and fewer adverse events. *Yakdan S et al. J Neurosurg Spine. [PMID: 40882232]*
Spinal Stenosis	1631	• Lumbar epidural spinal injections are effective for immediate improvement in pain and function and provide short-term benefits in lumbar radiculopathy and some spinal stenosis cases. *Soin A et al. Cureus. [PMID: 41487815]*
CHAPTER 47: SUBSTANCE USE DISORDERS		
Other Drugs & Substances	1703	• Benzodiazepines (eg, diazepam) are first-line treatment for GHB withdrawal, given in scheduled tapers and symptom-triggered doses. Other adjuncts include baclofen (GABA-B agonist), barbiturates (pentobarbital, phenobarbital), propofol, or dexmedetomidine for severe cases, and antipsychotics for severe psychosis. Severe withdrawal may require ICU care with mechanical ventilation, sedative infusions (midazolam), and multi-modal pharmacotherapy. *Borelli CM et al. Am J Addict. [PMID: 39953704]*

*See chapter for further details and references.

Disease Prevention & Health Promotion

1

Michael Pignone, MD, MPH[1]

GENERAL APPROACH TO THE PATIENT

The medical interview serves several functions. It is used to collect information to assist in diagnosis (the "history" of the present illness), to understand patient values and goals, to assess and communicate prognosis, to establish a therapeutic relationship, and to reach agreement with the patient about further diagnostic procedures and therapeutic options. It also serves as an opportunity to influence patient behavior, such as in motivational discussions about smoking cessation or medication adherence. Interviewing techniques that promote shared decision making increase patient involvement and satisfaction. Effective clinician-patient communication and increased patient involvement can improve health outcomes.

Patient Adherence

For many illnesses, successful prevention and treatment depend on difficult fundamental behavioral changes, including altering diet, taking up exercise, giving up smoking, cutting down drinking, wearing masks to prevent infection, and adhering to complex medication regimens. Adherence is a common problem; up to 50% of patients fail to achieve full adherence, and one-third never take their medicines. Many patients with medical problems, even those with access to care, do not seek appropriate care or may drop out of care prematurely. Adherence rates for short-term, self-administered therapies are higher than for long-term therapies and are inversely correlated with the number of interventions, their complexity and cost, and the patient's perception of overmedication.

As an example, in persons with HIV, adherence to antiretroviral therapy is a crucial determinant of treatment success. Studies have unequivocally demonstrated a close relationship between patient adherence and plasma HIV RNA levels, CD4 cell counts, and mortality. High adherence levels are needed to maintain virologic suppression. However, studies show that adherence varies over time, and inconsistent adherence is associated with incomplete viral suppression.

Patient reasons for suboptimal adherence include simple forgetfulness, being away from home, being busy, and changing daily routine. Other reasons include psychiatric disorders (depression or substance misuse), uncertainty about the effectiveness of treatment, lack of knowledge about the consequences of poor adherence, regimen complexity, and treatment side effects. The rising costs of medications, including generic medications, and the increase in patient cost-sharing burden have made adherence even more difficult, particularly for patients with lower incomes.

Patients seem better able to take prescribed medications than to adhere to recommendations to change their diet, exercise habits, or alcohol intake or to perform various self-care activities (such as monitoring blood glucose levels at home). For short-term regimens, adherence to medications can be improved by giving clear instructions. Writing out advice to patients, including changes in medication, may be helpful. Because low functional health literacy is common (*almost half of English-speaking US patients are unable to read and understand standard health education materials*), other forms of communication—such as illustrated simple text, videotapes, or oral instructions—may be more effective. Clinicians and health care delivery systems must provide culturally and linguistically appropriate health services.

To help improve adherence to long-term regimens, clinicians can work with patients to reach agreement on the goals for therapy, provide clear, concise information about the regimen, ensure understanding by using the "teach-back" method, counsel about the importance of adherence and how to organize medication-taking, reinforce self-monitoring, provide more convenient care, prescribe a simple dosage regimen for all medications (preferably no more than one or two doses daily), suggest ways to help in remembering to take doses (time of day, mealtime, alarms) and to keep appointments, prescribe lower-cost generic medications when available, and provide ways to simplify dosing (medication boxes). Single-unit doses supplied in foil wrappers can increase adherence but should be avoided for patients who have difficulty opening them. Medication boxes with compartments (eg, Medisets) that are filled

[1]Dr. Pignone is a former member of the US Preventive Services Task Force (USPSTF). The views expressed in this chapter are his and not necessarily those of the USPSTF.

weekly by the patient, caregiver, or pharmacy are useful. Devices can provide feedback to show patients whether they have taken doses as scheduled or to notify patients (or others) within a day if doses are skipped. Reminders, including cell phone text messages and mobile apps, are another effective means of encouraging adherence. The clinician can also enlist social support from family and friends, recruit an adherence monitor, provide a more convenient care environment with fewer barriers, and provide rewards and recognition for the patient's efforts to follow the regimen. Collaborative programs in which pharmacists help ensure adherence are also effective. Motivational interviewing techniques can be helpful when patients are ambivalent about their therapy.

Adherence is also improved when a trusting clinician-patient relationship has been established and when patients actively participate in their care. Clinicians can improve patient adherence by inquiring about specific behaviors and barriers in a nonjudgmental manner. When asked, many patients admit to incomplete adherence with medication regimens, plans for giving up cigarette smoking, or engaging only in "safer sex" practices, offering an opportunity for joint problem-solving. Although difficult, sufficient time must be made available for communication.

Medication adherence can be assessed generally with a single question: "In the past month, how often did you take your medications as your clinician prescribed?" Other ways of assessing medication adherence include pill counts and refill records; monitoring serum, urine, or saliva levels of medications or metabolites; watching for appointment nonattendance and treatment nonresponse; and assessing predictable medication effects, such as weight changes with diuretics or bradycardia from beta-blockers. In some conditions, even partial adherence, as with medication treatment of hypertension and diabetes mellitus, improves outcomes compared with nonadherence; in other cases, such as HIV antiretroviral therapy or tuberculosis treatment, partial adherence may be *worse* than complete nonadherence.

Guiding Principles of Care

Ethical practices are called for in medical care at both the "micro" level of the individual patient-clinician relationship and the "macro" level of allocation of resources or the adoption of infection-reducing public health interventions. *Ethical principles that guide the successful approach to diagnosis and treatment are honesty, beneficence, justice, avoidance of conflict of interest, and the pledge to do no harm.* Increasingly, Western medicine involves partnership with patients in important decisions about medical care, eg, which colorectal screening test to obtain or which modality of therapy for breast cancer or how far to proceed with treatment attempts for patients who have end-stage illnesses (see Chapter 5).

The clinician's role does not end with diagnosis and treatment. The importance of the empathic clinician in helping patients and their families face serious illness and death cannot be overemphasized. *"To cure sometimes, to relieve often, and to comfort always"* is a French saying as apt today as it was five centuries ago—as is Francis Peabody's admonition: *"The secret of the care of the patient is in caring for the patient."* Training to improve mindfulness and enhance patient-centered communication increases patient satisfaction and may also improve clinician satisfaction.

Cabezas MF et al. The effect of health literacy interventions on self-management in chronic diseases: a systematic review. Ann Behav Med. 2025;59:kaaf073. [PMID: 41176327]

Chan AHY et al. Effect of electronic adherence monitoring on adherence and outcomes in chronic conditions: a systematic review and meta-analysis. PLoS One. 2022;17:e0265715. [PMID: 35312704]

Lanke V et al. Evaluating the effectiveness of mobile apps on medication adherence for chronic conditions: systematic review and meta-analysis. J Med Internet Res. 2025;27:e60822. [PMID: 40743450]

HEALTH MAINTENANCE & DISEASE PREVENTION

Preventive medicine can be categorized as primary, secondary, or tertiary. *Primary prevention* aims to remove or reduce disease risk factors (eg, immunization, giving up or not starting smoking). *Secondary prevention* techniques promote early detection of disease or precursor states (eg, routine cervical Papanicolaou screening to detect carcinoma or dysplasia). *Tertiary prevention* measures are aimed at limiting the impact of established disease (eg, partial mastectomy combined with radiation therapy to remove and control localized breast cancer).

Table 1–1 shows leading causes of death in the United States for 2024 and Figure 1–1 compares leading causes of death in 1990, 2010, and 2021. The 2024 mortality data are notable for the continued reduction in COVID-19-related deaths relative to other leading causes

Table 1–1. Leading causes of death in the United States, 2024.

Category	Estimate
All causes	**3,072,039**
1. Heart disease	683,037
2. Cancer	619,812
3. Unintentional injuries	196,488
4. Stroke	166,783
5. Chronic lower respiratory diseases	145,612
6. Alzheimer disease	116,016
7. Diabetes mellitus	94,382
8. Kidney disease	55,070
9. Chronic liver disease and cirrhosis	52,259
10. Suicide	48,683

Data from Ahmad FB et al. Mortality in the United States: provisional data, 2024. Vital Statistics Rapid Release. 2025;39:1. https://dx.doi.org/10.15620/cdc/174621

Leading risks, 1990	Age-standardised rate of death per 100 000 (95% UI)	Leading risks, 2010	Age-standardised rate of death per 100 000 (95% UI)	Leading risks, 2021	Age-standardised rate of death per 100 000 (95% UI)
1 High systolic blood pressure	140.0 (113.9 to 161.3)	1 Tobacco	77.1 (63.6 to 91.0)	1 High systolic blood pressure	73.1 (58.2 to 86.8)
2 Tobacco	123.9 (104.2 to 144.3)	2 High systolic blood pressure	76.4 (60.5 to 90.3)	2 High fasting plasma glucose	61.3 (48.9 to 75.1)
3 Dietary risks	103.0 (29.0 to 156.7)	3 Dietary risks	68.0 (27.0 to 98.2)	3 Tobacco	60.6 (49.1 to 72.8)
4 High LDL cholesterol	74.2 (47.5 to 101.7)	4 High fasting plasma glucose	59.2 (46.9 to 72.2)	4 Dietary risks	59.0 (26.0 to 83.7)
5 High fasting plasma glucose	56.1 (47.2 to 65.2)	5 High body-mass index	52.4 (23.6 to 80.8)	5 High body-mass index	55.5 (26.9 to 83.7)
6 High body-mass index	52.7 (22.1 to 85.4)	6 Kidney dysfunction	37.1 (30.8 to 42.6)	6 Kidney dysfunction	40.5 (34.0 to 45.9)
7 Kidney dysfunction	45.1 (35.3 to 54.4)	7 High LDL cholesterol	31.6 (19.4 to 44.9)	7 Drug use	27.7 (25.1 to 30.5)
8 Air pollution	44.3 (20.4 to 72.0)	8 High alcohol use	19.9 (17.6 to 22.7)	8 High LDL cholesterol	26.9 (16.4 to 38.2)
9 Non-optimal temperature	24.6 (21.1 to 29.4)	9 Non-optimal temperature	19.2 (15.9 to 22.7)	9 High alcohol use	22.3 (19.6 to 25.3)
10 High alcohol use	20.8 (18.5 to 24.4)	10 Air pollution	18.7 (12.7 to 24.9)	10 Non-optimal temperature	15.7 (13.2 to 18.3)
11 Occupational risks	16.4 (13.6 to 19.1)	11 Drug use	16.6 (15.5 to 17.7)	11 Occupational risks	10.6 (8.9 to 12.0)
12 Other environmental risks	12.1 (1.0 to 23.2)	12 Occupational risks	13.3 (11.0 to 15.1)	12 Air pollution	10.3 (6.0 to 15.3)
13 Unsafe sex	10.1 (9.7 to 10.4)	13 Other environmental risks	8.1 (0.9 to 15.8)	13 Other environmental risks	6.9 (0.6 to 13.6)
14 Child and maternal malnutrition	9.2 (9.0 to 9.5)	14 Child and maternal malnutrition	6.8 (6.6 to 6.9)	14 Child and maternal malnutrition	6.8 (6.2 to 7.4)
15 Drug use	8.0 (7.2 to 9.0)	15 Low physical activity	5.0 (2.2 to 8.2)	15 Low physical activity	5.0 (2.0 to 8.1)

▲ **Figure 1–1.** Leading causes of death in 1990, 2010, and 2021 in the United States for all ages and sexes combined (causes are ranked by number of deaths in each year). (Reproduced from GBD 2021 US Burden of Disease Collaborators. The burden of diseases, injuries, and risk factors by state in the USA, 1990-2021: a systematic analysis for the Global Burden of Disease Study 2021. *Lancet.* 2024;404:2314.)

of death, as well as a reduction in unintentional injuries (due to continued progress in reducing opiate-related overdose deaths). Recent increases in mortality and decreased life expectancy have been larger in the United States than in Western European countries; this discrepancy has been driven partially by differences in COVID-19 mortality as well as ongoing trends in other midlife preventable mortality, particularly deaths from heart disease, unintentional injuries (including overdoses), and liver disease.

Many effective preventive services are underutilized, and few adults receive all of the most strongly recommended services. Several methods, including the use of provider or patient reminder systems (including interactive patient health records), reorganization of care environments to reduce barriers, and possibly provision of financial incentives to clinicians (though this remains controversial), can increase utilization of preventive services, but such methods have not been widely adopted.

Ahmad FB et al. Leading causes of death in the US, 2019–2023. JAMA. 2024;332:957. [PMID: 39116093]

Ahmad FB et al. Mortality in the United States: provisional data, 2024. Vital Statistics Rapid Release. 2025;39:1. https://dx.doi.org/10.15620/cdc/174621

GBD 2021 US Burden of Disease Collaborators. The burden of diseases, injuries, and risk factors by state in the USA, 1990–2021: a systematic analysis for the Global Burden of Disease Study 2021. Lancet. 2024;404:2314. [PMID: 39645376]

Woolf SH. Increasing mortality rates in the US, but not from COVID-19. JAMA. 2024;332:959. [PMID: 39207745]

PREVENTION OF INFECTIOUS DISEASES

Much of the historic decline in the incidence and fatality rates of infectious diseases is attributable to public health measures—especially immunization, improved sanitation, nonpharmacologic interventions (eg, mask-wearing to prevent respiratory-transmissible conditions, improvements in indoor air quality), and better nutrition. This observation has been reinforced by the experience during the global COVID-19 pandemic.

Immunization remains the best means of preventing many infectious diseases. Recommended immunization schedules for children and adolescents can be found online at https://www.cdc.gov/vaccines/schedules/hcp/child-adolescent.html, and the schedule for adults is available at https://www.cdc.gov/vaccines/hcp/imz-schedules/adult-age.html (see also Chapters 34 and 36). In addition to the severe toll in morbidity and mortality from COVID-19, substantial morbidity and mortality continue to occur from vaccine-preventable diseases, such as hepatitis A, hepatitis B, influenza, and pneumococcal infections. *The high incidence and mortality rates from COVID-19 and other recent outbreaks of vaccine-preventable diseases in the United States highlight the need to better understand vaccine hesitancy or refusal and methods for mitigating it.*

The Advisory Committee on Immunization Practices recommendations for the following vaccines appear in Table 1–2: influenza; MMR; 23-valent pneumococcal; tetanus, diphtheria, and acellular pertussis; hepatitis B; HPV; RSV; meningococcal; mpox; and Zoster (shingles). Updated guidance for COVID-19 vaccination also is provided.

Persons traveling to countries where infections are endemic should take the precautions described in Chapter 34 and at https://wwwnc.cdc.gov/travel/destinations/list. Immunization registries—confidential, population-based, computerized information systems that collect vaccination data about all residents of a geographic area—can be used to increase and sustain high vaccination coverage.

Globally, COVID-19 has resulted in > 7.1 million deaths through November 2025, including > 1.2 million in the United States, according to World Health Organization (WHO) data. Estimates of total excess deaths from COVID-19 may be twice as high. In addition to its tremendous overall health impact, the COVID-19 pandemic has revealed and exacerbated profound inequities in health and health care. In the United States, the COVID-19 mortality rates are higher in Black, Latina/Latino, and American Indian patients compared with White patients. Currently, the CDC recommends that persons aged 6 months and older consider COVID-19 vaccination (through receiving a

Table 1–2. Advisory Committee on Adult Immunization Practices selected vaccine recommendations, 2025 (listed in alphabetical order by vaccine).

Vaccine	Recommendation	Comment
COVID-19	Routine vaccination for all persons 19 and older. For previously unvaccinated persons: • 1 dose of updated (2025–2026 Formula) Moderna or Pfizer-BioNTech vaccine • 2-dose series of updated (2024–2025 Formula) Novavax at 0, 3–8 weeks For previously vaccinated with one or more doses of any COVID-19 vaccine: one dose of any updated (2025–2026 Formula) COVID-19 vaccine administered at least 8 weeks after the most recent COVID-19 vaccine dose. A second dose of 2024–2025 COVID-19 is recommended for adults aged 65 years and older and for ages 6 months to 64 years who are moderately or severely immunocompromised.	New addition of recommended second dosing for older adults and immunocompromised; option for third dose for immunocompromised as well
Hepatitis B	Two-, three-, or four-dose primary series recommended for all adults aged 19–59 years who have not been previously vaccinated or infected. Recommended for patients aged 60 years and older who are at increased risk or who wish to be vaccinated.	Prevents chronic hepatitis B and cirrhosis and their predispositions to HCC
HPV VLP	Routine HPV vaccination for children and adults aged 9–26 years. Shared decision making is recommended for unvaccinated individuals aged 27–45 years (vaccine is not licensed for adults older than 45 years).	Prevents persistent HPV infections effectively and thus may impact rate of CIN II–III
Influenza	Routine vaccination for all persons aged 6 months and older, including all adults. An alternative high-dose inactivated vaccine is available for adults aged 65 years and older.	When vaccine supply is limited, certain groups should be given priority, such as adults aged 50 years and older, individuals with chronic illness or immunosuppression, and pregnant women
Meningococcal	MenB-4C (Bexsero) administered as a 2-dose series (0 and 6 months) for young adults aged 16–23 years based on shared clinical decision-making for the prevention of serogroup B meningococcal disease and as a 3-dose series at 0, 1–2, and 6 months when given to persons aged ≥ 10 years at increased risk for serogroup B meningococcal disease.	New recommendation
MMR	Two doses for adults at high risk for exposure and transmission (eg, college students, health care workers); otherwise, one dose for adults aged 18 years and older.	Physician documentation of disease is not acceptable evidence of MMR immunity
Mpox	Any person at risk for mpox infection: complete 2-dose series, 28 days apart. Risk factors for mpox infection include: • Persons who are gay or bisexual and other MSM, transgender, or nonbinary people who in the past 6 months have had a new diagnosis of at least 1 sexually transmitted disease; > 1 sexual partner; sex at a commercial sex venue; or sex in association with a large public event in a geographic area where mpox transmission is occurring • Persons who are sexual partners of persons described above • Persons who anticipate experiencing any of the situations described above	
Pneumococcal	One dose of PCV15 followed by PPSV23 *or* One dose of PCV20 or PCV21 For all adults aged 50 years and older plus those aged 19–64 years who are at increased risk.	New recommendation to start at age 50 years
RSV	Routine RSV vaccination (one dose) for pregnant persons at 32 weeks 0 days through 36 weeks 6 days gestation from September through January in most of the continental United States. Shared decision making for adults aged 60 and older. Those who are immunocompromised or who have chronic conditions are most likely to benefit.	
Tdap	Routine use of a single dose of Tdap for adults aged 19–64 years.	Replaces next booster dose of Td vaccine
Zoster (shingles)	Two doses (2–6 months apart) of recombinant zoster vaccine to prevent shingles and related complications in adults aged ≥ 50 years and for adults aged ≥ 19 years who are or will be immunodeficient or immunosuppressed.	

CIN, cervical intraepithelial neoplasia; VLP, virus-like particle; MSM, men who have sex with men; PCV15, 15-valent pneumococcal conjugate; PCV20, 20-valent pneumococcal conjugate; PCV21, 21-valent pneumococcal conjugate; PPSV23, 23-valent pneumococcal polysaccharide; Td, tetanus and diphtheria toxoids; Tdap, tetanus, diphtheria, and five-component acellular pertussis.

primary series and appropriate boosters) to help protect against COVID-19 (see Chapter 36 and Table 1–2) using one of the CDC-approved vaccines. The CDC notes that vaccination "is especially important if you are ages 65 and older, are at high risk for severe COVID-19, or have never received a COVID-19 vaccine."

The USPSTF recommends **behavioral counseling** for adolescents and adults who are sexually active and at increased risk for STIs. Sexually active women aged 24 years or younger and older women who are at increased risk for infection should be **screened for chlamydia and gonorrhea**. Screening HIV-positive men or men who have sex with men for syphilis every 3 months is associated with improved syphilis detection.

The CDC recommends universal **HIV screening** of all patients aged 13–64, and the USPSTF recommends that clinicians screen adolescents and adults aged 15–65 years. Clinicians should integrate biomedical and behavioral approaches for HIV prevention. In addition to reducing sexual transmission of HIV, initiation of antiretroviral therapy reduces the risk for AIDS-defining events and death among patients with less immunologically advanced disease.

Daily **preexposure prophylaxis (PrEP)** with the fixed-dose combination of tenofovir disoproxil 300 mg and emtricitabine 200 mg (Truvada) should be considered for persons who are HIV-negative but at substantial risk for HIV infection. Studies of men who have sex with men suggest that PrEP is very effective in reducing the risk of contracting HIV. Patients taking PrEP should be encouraged to use other prevention strategies, such as consistent condom use, to maximally reduce their risk. **Postexposure prophylaxis (PEP)** with combinations of antiretroviral medications is widely used after occupational and nonoccupational contact and may reduce the risk of transmission by about 80%. PEP should be initiated within 72 hours of exposure.

Herpes zoster, caused by reactivation from previous varicella zoster virus infection, affects many older adults and persons with immune system dysfunction. The Advisory Committee on Immunization Practices recommends that the **herpes zoster subunit vaccine** (HZ/su; Shingrix) be used for the prevention of herpes zoster and related complications in immunocompetent adults aged 50 and older and in individuals who previously received Zostavax.

Centers for Disease Control and Prevention (CDC). https://covid.cdc.gov/covid-data-tracker/#datatracker-home

Centers for Disease Control and Prevention (CDC). Preventing HIV with PrEP, 2024. https://www.cdc.gov/hiv/prevention/prep.html?CDC_AAref_Val=https://www.cdc.gov/hiv/basics/prep.html

Centers for Disease Control and Prevention (CDC). Recommended adult immunization schedule for ages 19 years or older, United States, 2025. https://www.cdc.gov/vaccines/hcp/imz-schedules/downloads/adult/adult-combined-schedule.pdf

Melgar M et al. Use of respiratory syncytial virus vaccines in older adults: recommendations of the Advisory Committee on Immunization Practices—United States, 2023. MMWR Morb Mortal Wkly Rep 2023;72:793. [PMID: 37471262]

Msemburi W et al. The WHO estimates of excess mortality associated with the COVID-19 pandemic. Nature. 2023;613:130. [PMID: 36517599]

Qaseem A et al; Population Health and Medical Science Committee of the American College of Physicians; Haeme R et al. Influenza vaccines for 2025-2026 in adults who are not pregnant or immunocompromised: rapid practice points from the American College of Physicians. Ann Intern Med. 2026;179:110. [PMID: 41248504]

PREVENTION OF CARDIOVASCULAR DISEASE

Cardiovascular disease, including CHD and stroke, is the leading cause of death globally, with over 20 million deaths in 2021, nearly one-third of all deaths. Over three-quarters of all cardiovascular deaths occur in low- and middle-income countries; however, CHD and stroke remain top causes of death in the United States as well. Several risk factors increase the risk for coronary disease and stroke. These risk factors can be divided into those that are modifiable (eg, lipid disorders, hypertension, cigarette smoking) and those that are not (eg, age, sex, family history of early coronary disease). Impressive declines in age-specific mortality rates from heart disease and stroke were achieved in all age groups in North America from 1980 to 2015, in large part through improvement of modifiable risk factors: reductions in cigarette smoking, improvements in lipid levels, and more aggressive detection and treatment of hypertension. However, the past several years have seen a disturbing increase in cardiovascular deaths in the United States and a plateau in the reduction in cardiovascular mortality rates. This section considers the role of screening for cardiovascular risk and the use of effective therapies to reduce such risk. Key USPSTF recommendations for cardiovascular prevention are shown in Table 1–3. Guidelines encourage regular assessment of global cardiovascular risk in adults 40–79 years of age without known CVD using standard cardiovascular risk factors and in younger adults at increased risk. The role of nontraditional risk factors for improving risk estimation and therapeutic decision making remains uncertain. However, current guidance recommends considering cardiovascular risk prevention within the context of cardiovascular-kidney-metabolic health. The recent PREVENT equations appear to perform more accurately than older risk equations.

Di Cesare M et al. The heart of the world. Glob Heart. 2024;19:11. [PMID: 38273998]

Khan SS et al; American Heart Association. Novel prediction equations for absolute risk assessment of total cardiovascular disease incorporating cardiovascular-kidney-metabolic health: a scientific statement from the American Heart Association. Circulation. 2023;148:1982. [PMID: 37947094]

Zhou H et al. Evaluation and comparison of the PREVENT and pooled cohort equations for 10-year atherosclerotic cardiovascular risk prediction. J Am Heart Assoc. 2025;14:e039454. [PMID: 39921505]

Abdominal Aortic Aneurysm

One-time screening for AAA by ultrasonography is recommended by the USPSTF (B recommendation) in men aged 65–75 years who have ever smoked. One-time screening for AAA is associated with a relative reduction in odds of

Table 1–3. Expert recommendations for cardiovascular risk prevention methods: USPSTF.[1]

Prevention Method	Recommendation [Year Issued]
Screening for AAA	Recommends one-time screening for AAA by ultrasonography in men aged 65–75 years who have ever smoked. (B) Selectively offer screening for AAA in men aged 65–75 years who have never smoked. (C) Current evidence is insufficient to assess the balance of benefits and harms of screening for AAA in women aged 65–75 years who have ever smoked or have a family history of AAA. (I) Recommends against routine screening for AAA in women who have never smoked and have no family history of AAA. (D) [2019]
Aspirin use	The decision to initiate low-dose aspirin use for the primary prevention of CVD in adults aged 40–59 years who have a 10% or greater 10-year CVD risk should be an individual one. Evidence indicates that the net benefit of aspirin use in this group is small. Persons who are not at increased risk for bleeding and are willing to take low-dose aspirin daily are more likely to benefit. [C] Recommends against initiating low-dose aspirin use for primary prevention of CVD in adults aged 60 years or older. [D] [2022]
Blood pressure screening	Recommends screening for hypertension in adults aged 18 years or older with office blood pressure measurement. Recommends obtaining blood pressure measurements outside of the clinical setting for diagnostic confirmation before starting treatment. (A) [2021]
Serum lipid screening and use of statins for prevention	Recommends that clinicians prescribe a statin for primary prevention of CVD for adults aged 40–75 years who have one or more CVD risk factors (ie, dyslipidemia, diabetes, hypertension, or smoking) and an estimated 10-year risk of a cardiovascular event of 10% or greater. [B] Recommends that clinicians selectively offer a statin for primary prevention of CVD for adults aged 40–75 years who have one or more CVD risk factors (ie, dyslipidemia, diabetes, hypertension, or smoking) and an estimated 10-year risk of a cardiovascular event of 7.5% to <10%. The likelihood of benefit is smaller in this group than in persons with a 10-year risk of 10% or greater. [C] Current evidence is insufficient to assess the balance of benefits and harms of initiating a statin for the primary prevention of CVD events and mortality in adults aged 76 years or older. [I] [2022]
Counseling about healthful diet and physical activity for CVD prevention	Recommends offering or referring adults with CVD risk factors to behavioral counseling interventions to promote a healthy diet and physical activity. (B) [2020] Recommends that primary care professionals individualize the decision to offer or refer adults without CVD risk factors to behavioral counseling interventions to promote a healthy diet and physical activity. (C) [2022]
Screening for diabetes mellitus	Recommends screening for prediabetes and type 2 diabetes in adults aged 35–70 years who have overweight or obesity. Clinicians should offer or refer patients with prediabetes to effective preventive interventions. (B) [2021]
Screening for smoking and counseling to promote cessation	Recommends that clinicians ask all adults about tobacco use, advise them to stop using tobacco, provide those who use tobacco behavioral interventions, and prescribe US FDA–approved pharmacotherapy to nonpregnant adults. (A) [2021]

[1]USPSTF recommendations available at http://www.uspreventiveservicestaskforce.org/BrowseRec/Index/browse-recommendations.
Recommendation A: The USPSTF strongly recommends that clinicians routinely provide the service to eligible patients. (The USPSTF found good evidence that the service improves important health outcomes and concludes that benefits substantially outweigh harms.)
Recommendation B: The USPSTF recommends that clinicians routinely provide the service to eligible patients. (The USPSTF found at least fair evidence that the service improves important health outcomes and concludes that benefits substantially outweigh harms.)
Recommendation C: The USPSTF makes no recommendation for or against routine provision of the service.
Recommendation D: The USPSTF recommends against routinely providing the service to asymptomatic patients. (The USPSTF found at least fair evidence that the service is ineffective or that harms outweigh benefits.)
Recommendation I: The USPSTF concludes that the evidence is insufficient to recommend for or against routinely providing the service.

AAA-related mortality over 12–15 years and a similar reduction in AAA-related ruptures. For men aged 65–75 years who have never smoked, individualized and shared decision making is warranted. Women who have never smoked and who have no family history of AAA do not appear to benefit from such screening (D recommendation); the current evidence for women who have ever smoked or who have a family history of AAA is insufficient to assess the balance of risks versus benefits (I recommendation) (Table 1–3).

Premji S et al. Population health and health inequality impacts of the National Abdominal Aortic Aneurysm Screening Programme (NAAASP) in England. Med Decis Making. 2026;46:202. [PMID: 41230943]

Cigarette Smoking

Cigarette smoking remains the most important cause of preventable morbidity and early mortality. In 2023, tobacco use accounted for an estimated 7.36 million deaths worldwide. Cigarettes are responsible for one in every five deaths in the United States, or over 480,000 deaths annually. The most frequent causes of smoking-related deaths are cancer, CVD, and respiratory disease (COPD). The annual cost of smoking-related health care is about $240 billion in the United States, with another $372 billion in productivity losses. In 2024, survey data showed that 11% of adults were cigarette smokers, with lower rates among young adults.

Although tobacco use constitutes one of the most serious common medical problems, it is undertreated. Of the estimated 28.8 million adult smokers (11.6% of the population) in 2022, 67% wanted to quit and 77% saw a health care provider in the past year. Of these, only 50% received advice or assistance. Several effective clinical interventions are available to promote smoking cessation, including counseling, pharmacotherapy, and a combination of the two.

Persons whose clinicians advise them to quit are 1.6 times as likely to attempt quitting. Use of evidence-based interventions is low: only one-third of persons used medication assistance and <10% received evidence-based counseling, while only 5.3% used both.

More than half of smokers attempt to quit each year, but only 5–10% are successful. Factors associated with successful cessation include having a rule against smoking in the home, younger age, having a higher income, being insured, and having a higher education. Mental health counseling in the past year was also associated with successful smoking cessation.

Helpful counseling strategies are shown in Table 1–4. Additionally, a system should be implemented to identify smokers, and advice to quit should be tailored to the patient's level of readiness to change. *All patients trying to quit should be offered pharmacotherapy* (Table 1–5) *except those with medical contraindications, women who are pregnant or breastfeeding, and adolescents.* Weight gain occurs in most patients (80%) following smoking cessation. Average weight gain is 2 kg, but for some (10–15%), major weight gain—over 13 kg—may occur. Planning for the possibility of weight gain, and means of mitigating it, may help with maintenance of cessation.

Several pharmacologic therapies shown to be effective in promoting cessation are summarized in Table 1–5. Nicotine replacement therapy doubles the chance of successful quitting. The nicotine patch, gum, and lozenges are available over the counter, and nicotine nasal spray and inhalers are available by prescription. The sustained-release antidepressant drug bupropion (150–300 mg/day orally) is an effective smoking cessation agent and is associated with minimal weight gain, although seizures are a contraindication. It acts by boosting brain levels of dopamine and norepinephrine, mimicking the effect of nicotine. Varenicline, a partial nicotinic acetylcholine-receptor agonist, also has been shown to improve cessation rates; however, its adverse effects, particularly its effects on mood, are not completely understood and warrant careful consideration, although recent safety data have provided reassurance. A head-to-head trial found varenicline to be more effective than other pharmacologic therapies and all pharmacologic therapies to be more effective than placebo. Combination therapy is more effective than a single pharmacologic modality. The efficacy of e-cigarettes in

Table 1–4. Inquiries to help in support of smoking cessation.

Component	Helpful Clinician Statements and Inquiries
Communicate your caring and concern	"I am concerned about the effects of smoking on your health… • and want you to know that I am willing to help you quit." • and so how do you feel about quitting?" • do you have any fears or ambivalent feelings about quitting?"
Encourage the patient to talk about the quitting process	"Tell me… • why do you want to quit smoking?" • when you tried quitting smoking in the past, what sort of difficulties did you encounter?" • were you able to succeed at all, even for a while?" • what concerns or worries do you have about quitting now?"
Provide basic information about smoking (eg, its addictive nature) and successful quitting (eg, nature and time course of withdrawal)	"Did you know that… • the nicotine in cigarette smoke is highly addictive?" • within a day of stopping, you will notice nicotine withdrawal symptoms, such as irritability and craving?" • after you quit, any smoking (even a single puff) makes it likely that you will fully relapse into smoking again?"
Encourage the patient to make a quit attempt	"I want to reassure you that… • as your clinician, I believe you are going to be able to quit." • many effective smoking cessation treatments are now available." • more than half the people who have *ever* smoked have now successfully quit."

Table 1–5. Medications for tobacco dependence and smoking cessation (categories listed in order of frequency of use).

Medication	Some Formulations	Usual Adult Dosage[1,2]
Nicotine Replacement Therapies (NRTs)		
Nicotine transdermal patch[3] – generic (NicoDerm CQ)	7, 14, 21 mg/24-h patches	1 patch/day
Nicotine polacrilex gum[3] – generic (Nicorette gum)	2, 4 mg/pieces	8–24 pieces/day[4,5]
Nicotine polacrilex lozenge[3,6] – generic (Nicorette lozenge)	2, 4 mg/lozenges	8–20 lozenges/day[4,7]
Nicotine oral inhaler – Nicotrol[8]	10 mg cartridges	4–16 cartridges/day
Nicotine nasal spray – Nicotrol NS	200 sprays/10 mL bottles (0.5 mg/spray)	2 sprays 8–40×/day (max 10 sprays/h)
Dopaminergic-Noradrenergic Reuptake Inhibitor		
Bupropion SR – generic	100, 150, 200 mg SR tablets[9]	150 mg orally once daily × 3 days, then 150 mg orally twice daily
Nicotinic Receptor Partial Agonist		
Varenicline tartrate – Chantix	0.5, 1 mg tablets	0.5 mg orally once daily × 3 days, then 0.5 mg twice daily on days 4–7, then 1 mg twice daily

SR, sustained-release.
[1]Dosage reductions may be needed for liver or kidney impairment.
[2]Patients should receive a minimum of 3–6 months of effective therapy. In general, the dosage of NRTs can be tapered at the end of treatment; bupropion SR and varenicline can usually be stopped without a gradual dosage reduction, but some clinicians recommend a taper.
[3]Available over the counter for persons ≥ 18 years old.
[4]Avoid eating or drinking within 15 minutes of using a gum or lozenge.
[5]A second piece of gum can be used within 1 hour. Continuously chewing one piece after another is not recommended.
[6]Also available in a mini-lozenge.
[7]Maximum of 5 lozenges in 6 hours or 20 lozenges/day. Use of > 1 lozenge at a time or continuously using one after another is not recommended.
[8]Not currently available from the manufacturer.
[9]Only the generic 150-mg SR tablets are FDA-approved as a smoking cessation aid.

smoking cessation has not been well evaluated, and some users may find them addictive. "E-cigarette or vaping use–associated lung injury" (EVALI) should prompt additional caution in the use of unregulated nicotine delivery devices for smoking cessation (see Chapter 9).

Clinicians should not show disapproval of patients who fail to stop smoking or who are not ready to make a quit attempt. Thoughtful advice that emphasizes the benefits of cessation and recognizes common barriers to success can increase motivation to quit and quit rates. An upcoming medical procedure or intercurrent illness or hospitalization may motivate even the most addicted smoker to quit.

Individualized or group counseling is very cost-effective, even more so than treating hypertension. Smoking cessation counseling by telephone ("quitlines") and text messaging have both proved effective. An additional strategy is to recommend that any smoking take place outdoors to limit the effects of passive smoke on housemates and coworkers. This can lead to smoking reduction and quitting.

Public policies, including higher cigarette taxes and more restrictive public smoking laws, have also been shown to encourage cessation, as have financial incentives directed to patients.

GBD 2021 Tobacco Forecasting Collaborators. Forecasting the effects of smoking prevalence scenarios on years of life lost and life expectancy from 2022 to 2050: a systematic analysis for the Global Burden of Disease Study 2021. Lancet Public Health. 2024;9:e729. [PMID: 39366729]
GBD 2023 Disease and Injury and Risk Factor Collaborators. Burden of 375 diseases and injuries, risk-attributable burden of 88 risk factors, and healthy life expectancy in 204 countries and territories, including 660 subnational locations, 1990-2023: a systematic analysis for the Global Burden of Disease Study 2023. Lancet. 2025;406:1873. [PMID: 41092926]

Lipid Disorders

Higher LDL cholesterol concentrations and lower HDL levels are associated with an increased risk of CHD (see Chapter 32). Measurement of total and HDL cholesterol levels can help assess the degree of CHD risk. The best age to start screening is controversial, as is its frequency. Cholesterol-lowering therapy reduces the relative risk of CHD events, with the degree of reduction proportional to the reduction in LDL cholesterol achieved, at least at initial LDL levels > 100 mg/dL. The absolute benefits of screening for—and treating—abnormal lipid levels depend on the presence and level of other cardiovascular risk factors, including hypertension, diabetes mellitus, smoking, age, and sex (see Chapter 32). If other risk factors are present, atherosclerotic CVD risk is higher and the potential benefits of therapy are greater. Patients with known CVD are at higher risk and have larger benefits from reduction in LDL cholesterol. The optimal risk threshold for initiating statins for primary prevention remains somewhat controversial, although most guidelines now suggest statin therapy when 10-year atherosclerotic cardiovascular risk is > 10%. Use of a cardiovascular risk calculator can help inform decision making for primary prevention.

Evidence for the effectiveness of statin-type medications is better than for the other classes of lipid-lowering agents or dietary changes specifically for improving lipid levels. Multiple large, randomized, placebo-controlled trials have demonstrated important reductions in total mortality, major coronary events, and strokes with lowering levels of LDL cholesterol by statin therapy for patients with known CVD. Statins also reduce cardiovascular events for patients with diabetes mellitus. For patients with no previous history of cardiovascular events, meta-analyses have shown important reductions of cardiovascular events and all-cause mortality.

Antilipidemic monoclonal antibody agents (eg, evolocumab and alirocumab) lower LDL cholesterol by 50–60% by binding proprotein convertase subtilisin kexin type 9 (PCSK9), which decreases the degradation of LDL receptors. PCSK9 inhibitors also decrease Lp(a) levels. These medications are expensive and so are often used mainly in high-risk patients when statin therapy does not reduce LDL cholesterol sufficiently at maximally tolerated doses or when patients are intolerant of statins. Few side effects have been reported with PCSK9 inhibitor use.

Guidelines for statin and PCSK9 therapy are discussed in Chapter 32.

Writing Committee Members; Blumenthal RS et al. 2026 ACC/AHA/AACVPR/ABC/ACPM/ADA/AGS/APhA/ASPC/NLA/PCNA Guideline on the management of dyslipidemia: A report of the American College of Cardiology/American Heart Association Joint Committee on Clinical Practice Guidelines. Circulation. 2026 Mar 13. [Epub ahead of print][PMID: 41824552]

Khan SS et al; American Heart Association. Novel prediction equations for absolute risk assessment of total cardiovascular disease incorporating cardiovascular-kidney-metabolic health: a scientific statement from the American Heart Association. Circulation. 2023;148:1982. [PMID: 37947094]

US Preventive Services Task Force; Mangione CM et al. Statin use for the primary prevention of cardiovascular disease in adults: US Preventive Services Task Force Recommendation Statement. JAMA. 2022;328:746. [PMID: 35997723]

Hypertension

The most recent data from the National Health and Nutrition Examination Survey estimated the adult prevalence of hypertension at 47.7%, using a 130/80 mm Hg threshold or current medication use. Less than 60% of persons were aware of their hypertension and about half were being treated, with only 20% being controlled at the 130/80 mm Hg threshold. These patterns have been stable over the past 10 years.

In every adult age group, higher values of systolic and diastolic blood pressure carry greater risks of stroke and HF. Systolic blood pressure is a better predictor of morbid events than diastolic blood pressure. Home monitoring is better correlated with target organ damage than clinic-based values. Clinicians can apply specific blood pressure criteria, such as those of the Joint National Committee or American Heart Association guidelines, along with consideration of the patient's cardiovascular risk and personal values, to decide at what levels treatment should be considered in individual cases.

Primary prevention of hypertension can be accomplished by strategies aimed at both the general population and special high-risk populations. The latter include persons with high-normal blood pressure or a family history of hypertension; Black persons; and individuals with various behavioral risk factors, such as physical inactivity; excessive consumption of salt, alcohol, or calories; and deficient intake of potassium. Effective interventions for primary prevention of hypertension include reduced sodium and alcohol consumption, weight loss, and regular exercise. Diets high in fresh fruits and vegetables and low in saturated fat and sugar-containing beverages are associated with lower blood pressure.

Improved identification and treatment of hypertension has been a major cause of the decline in stroke deaths as well as the reduction in incidence of HF-related hospitalizations; more recently, stalled progress in control of hypertension has led to slowing of improvements in cardiovascular outcomes. *Because hypertension is usually asymptomatic, screening is strongly recommended to identify patients for treatment.* Elevated office readings should be confirmed with repeated measurements, ideally from ambulatory monitoring or home measurements. Despite strong recommendations in favor of screening and treatment, hypertension control remains suboptimal. Several types of interventions, including telehealth applications, have been shown to be effective in increasing adherence and blood pressure control. An intervention that included both patient and provider education was more effective than provider education alone in achieving control of hypertension, suggesting the benefits of patient participation; another trial found that home monitoring combined with telephone-based nurse support was more effective than home monitoring alone for blood pressure control. Pharmacologic management of hypertension is discussed in Chapter 13.

Fryar CD et al. Hypertension prevalence, awareness, treatment, and control among adults age 18 and older: United States, August 2021–August 2023. NCHS Data Brief, no 511. Hyattsville, MD: National Center for Health Statistics. 2024.

Hardy ST et al. Prevention of cardiovascular disease events and deaths among black adults via systolic blood pressure equity. JAMA Netw Open. 2025;8:e2541336. [PMID: 41186946]

Mikulski BS et al. Mobile health applications and medication adherence of patients with hypertension: a systematic review and meta-analysis. Am J Prev Med. 2022;62:626. [PMID: 34963562]

Writing Committee Members; Jones DW et al. 2025 AHA/ACC/AANP/AAPA/ABC/ACCP/ACPM/AGS/AMA/ASPC/NMA/PCNA/SGIM guideline for the prevention, detection, evaluation and management of high blood pressure in adults: a report of the American College of Cardiology/American Heart Association Joint Committee on Clinical Practice Guidelines. Circulation. 2025;152:e114. [PMID: 40811497] Erratum in: Circulation. 2025;152:e403. [PMID: 41212942]

Chemoprevention

Regular use of low-dose aspirin (81–325 mg) can reduce cardiovascular events but increases GI bleeding and hemorrhagic stroke. The potential benefits of aspirin may exceed the possible adverse effects among middle-aged adults who are at increased cardiovascular risk, which can be defined as a 10-year risk of > 10%, and who do not have an increased risk of bleeding. However, a large trial in older healthy adults did not find clear benefit from aspirin for reduction of cardiovascular events and saw an increase in all-cause mortality with aspirin. Therefore, aspirin should *not* be routinely initiated in healthy adults over age 70.

NSAIDs may reduce the incidence of colorectal adenomas and polyps but may also increase heart disease and GI bleeding and thus are *not* recommended for colon cancer prevention in average-risk patients.

Antioxidant vitamin (vitamin E, vitamin C, and β-carotene) supplementation produced no significant reductions in the 5-year incidence of—or mortality from—vascular disease, cancer, or other major outcomes in high-risk individuals with CAD, other occlusive arterial disease, or diabetes mellitus.

US Preventive Services Task Force; Davidson KW et al. Aspirin use to prevent cardiovascular disease: US Preventive Services Task Force Recommendation Statement. JAMA. 2022;327:1577. [PMID: 35471505]

PREVENTION OF OSTEOPOROSIS

See Chapter 30.

Osteoporosis, characterized by low bone mineral density, is common and associated with an increased risk of fracture. The lifetime risk of an osteoporotic fracture is about 50% for women and 30% for men. Osteoporotic fractures can cause significant pain and disability. As such, research has focused on means of preventing osteoporosis and related fractures. Primary prevention strategies include calcium supplementation, vitamin D supplementation, and exercise programs. The effectiveness of calcium and vitamin D for fracture prevention remains controversial, particularly in noninstitutionalized individuals.

Screening for osteoporosis on the basis of low bone mineral density is recommended for women over age 65, based on indirect evidence that screening can identify women with low bone mineral density and that treatment of women with low bone density with bisphosphonates is effective in reducing fractures. However, real-world adherence to pharmacologic therapy for osteoporosis is low: one-third to one-half of patients do not take their medication as directed. Screening for osteoporosis is also recommended in younger women who are at increased risk. The effectiveness of screening in men has not been established. Bisphosphonates reduce fracture risk but may increase the risk of certain uncommon, atypical types of femoral fractures and rare osteonecrosis of the jaw and are associated with some nonserious GI symptoms. As such, consideration of the benefits and risks of therapy, as well as the importance of consistent adherence, is important when deciding about screening.

Calikyan A et al. Osteoporosis screening disparities among ethnic and racial minorities: a systematic review. J Osteoporos. 2023;2023:1277319. [PMID: 37138642]
Kahwati LC et al. Screening for osteoporosis to prevent fractures: a systematic evidence review for the US Preventive Services Task Force. JAMA. 2025;333:509. [PMID: 39808441]
US Preventive Services Task Force; Nicholson WK et al. Screening for osteoporosis to prevent fractures: US Preventive Services Task Force Recommendation Statement. JAMA. 2025;333:498. [PMID: 39808425]
Wei S et al. Priority interventions for the prevention of falls or fractures in patients with osteoporosis: a network meta-analysis. Arch Gerontol Geriatr. 2024;127:105558. [PMID: 39018968]

PREVENTION OF PHYSICAL INACTIVITY

Physical inactivity is an important cause of morbidity and mortality. The US Department of Health and Human Services, the CDC, and the WHO recommend that adults (including older adults) engage in 150 minutes of moderate-intensity (such as brisk walking) or 75 minutes of vigorous-intensity (such as jogging or running) aerobic activity or an equivalent mix of moderate- and vigorous-intensity aerobic activity each week. In addition to activity recommendations, the CDC recommends activities to strengthen all major muscle groups (abdomen, arms, back, chest, hips, legs, and shoulders) at least twice a week. However, one-third of adults worldwide are not meeting this level of activity.

Patients who engage in regular moderate to vigorous exercise have a lower risk of MI, stroke, hypertension, hyperlipidemia, type 2 diabetes mellitus, diverticular disease, and osteoporosis. Regular exercise may also have a positive effect on executive function in older adults.

In longitudinal cohort studies, individuals who report higher levels of leisure-time physical activity are less likely to gain weight or develop obesity. At least 60 minutes of daily moderate-intensity physical activity may be necessary to maximize weight loss and prevent significant weight regain when undertaking lifestyle-based weight management. For patients taking GLP-1 medications, aerobic physical activity (at recommended levels) combined with resistance training for 60–90 minutes per week may help preserve lean muscle mass and enhance weight loss and metabolic outcomes.

Systematic reviews have consistently found that more intensive counseling interventions are more effective than brief interventions.

Several factors influence physical activity behavior, including personal, social (eg, family and work), and environmental (eg, access to exercise facilities and well-lit parks) factors.

Mehrtash F et al. Integrating diet and physical activity when prescribing GLP-1s—lifestyle factors remain crucial. JAMA Intern Med. 2025;185:1151. [PMID: 40658434]
Patnode CD et al. Behavioral counseling interventions to promote a healthy diet and physical activity for cardiovascular disease prevention in adults without known cardiovascular disease risk factors: updated evidence report and systematic review for the US Preventive Services Task Force. JAMA. 2022;328:375. [PMID: 35881116]

Strain T et al; Country Data Author Group. National, regional, and global trends in insufficient physical activity among adults from 2000 to 2022: a pooled analysis of 507 population-based surveys with 5.7 million participants. Lancet Glob Health. 2024;12:e1232. [PMID: 38942042] Erratum in: Lancet Glob Health. 2025;13:e202. [PMID: 39653055]
US Preventive Services Task Force; Mangione CM et al. Behavioral counseling interventions to promote a healthy diet and physical activity for cardiovascular disease prevention in adults without cardiovascular disease risk factors: US Preventive Services Task Force Recommendation Statement. JAMA. 2022;328:367. [PMID: 35881115]
Zhu S et al. Effectiveness of behavioural interventions with motivational interviewing on physical activity outcomes in adults: systematic review and meta-analysis. BMJ. 2024;386:e078713. [PMID: 38986547]

PREVENTION OF OVERWEIGHT & OBESITY

Obesity is a true epidemic and public health crisis that both clinicians and patients must face. Obesity is associated with type 2 diabetes mellitus, hypertension, hyperlipidemia, cancer, osteoarthritis, CVD, obstructive sleep apnea, asthma, and (for more severe obesity) increased all-cause mortality. Risk assessment for overweight and obesity begins with determination of BMI, waist circumference for patients with a BMI of ≤ 35, presence of comorbid conditions, and a fasting blood glucose and lipid panel. Normal body weight is defined as a BMI of <25, overweight is defined as a BMI of 25.0–29.9, and obesity is defined as a BMI > 30. Persons with a BMI of ≥ 40 have death rates from cancers that are 52% higher for men and 62% higher for women than the rates in men and women of normal weight.

Primary, secondary, and tertiary prevention of overweight and obesity involves both increasing physical activity and dietary modification to reduce caloric intake. Adequate levels of physical activity appear to be important for the prevention of weight gain and the development of obesity. Physical activity programs consistent with public health recommendations may promote modest weight loss (about 2 kg); however, the amount of weight loss for any one individual is highly variable.

Clinicians can help prevent and treat obesity by intensive, multicomponent interventions, often best delivered by a trained nutritionist. Patients engaged in such interventions learn to develop personalized eating plans to reduce energy intake, particularly by recognizing the contributions of unhealthy fats, concentrated carbohydrates, and large portion sizes (see Chapter 33). Patients typically underestimate caloric content, especially when consuming food away from home. Providing patients with caloric and nutritional information may help limit caloric intake as part of a multicomponent intervention.

Other treatment options for obesity include pharmacotherapy and surgery (see Chapter 33). Recent evidence has demonstrated the effectiveness of GLP-1 agonists in producing sustained weight loss. However, the high cost of these medications has limited their access, especially for patients with low incomes and limited or no health insurance coverage. Effective use of GLP-1 medications also requires nutritional assessment and physical activity intervention to ensure preservation of muscle mass.

Weight loss strategies using dietary, physical activity, or behavioral interventions can produce modest improvements in weight among persons with prediabetes and a significant decrease in diabetes incidence. Intensive lifestyle interventions including diet combined with physical activity are effective in achieving weight loss and reducing cardiometabolic risk factors among patients with severe obesity.

Bariatric surgical procedures, eg, adjustable gastric band, sleeve gastrectomy, and Roux-en-Y gastric bypass, are reserved for patients with severe obesity in whom BMI exceeds 40 or for patients with less severe obesity (with BMIs between 35 and 40) and high-risk comorbid conditions, such as life-threatening cardiopulmonary problems (eg, sleep apnea, obesity-hypoventilation syndrome, and obesity-related HF) or diabetes mellitus. In selected patients, surgery can produce substantial weight loss (10–159 kg) over 1–5 years, with rare, but sometimes serious, complications. Surgery also appears to be successful in improving glycemic control and reducing diabetes. Nutritional deficiencies are one complication of bariatric surgical procedures and close monitoring of a patient's metabolic and nutritional status is essential. Further research is needed to best elucidate the optimal use of bariatric surgery in the era of effective GLP-1 agonists.

Lingvay I et al. Obesity in adults. Lancet. 2024;404:972. [PMID: 39159652]
Liu Y et al. The weight-loss effect of GLP-1RAs glucagon-like peptide-1 receptor agonists in non-diabetic individuals with overweight or obesity: a systematic review with meta-analysis and trial sequential analysis of randomized controlled trials. Am J Clin Nutr. 2023;118:614. [PMID: 37661106]

CANCER PREVENTION

Primary Prevention

Cancer mortality rates continue to decrease in the United States. Part of this decrease results from reductions in tobacco use, since cigarette smoking is the most important preventable cause of cancer; cancer incidence is also lower in persons with higher levels of physical activity and lower levels of obesity and alcohol use. Persons who engage in regular physical exercise, limit alcohol use, and avoid obesity have lower rates of breast and colon cancer.

Chemoprevention has been widely studied for primary cancer prevention without clear evidence of benefits (see earlier Chemoprevention section and Chapter 43). Use of tamoxifen, raloxifene, and aromatase inhibitors for breast cancer prevention is discussed in Chapters 19 and 43. Hepatitis B vaccination can prevent HCC. Screening and treatment of hepatitis C is another strategy to prevent HCC (see Chapter 18); new recommendations have extended the population eligible for screening.

HPV virus-like particle (VLP) vaccine is recommended to prevent cervical cancer (Table 1–2). HPV vaccines may also have a role in the prevention of HPV-related head and neck and possibly anal cancers.

Henschke N et al. Effects of human papillomavirus (HPV) vaccination programmes on community rates of HPV-related disease and harms from vaccination. Cochrane Database Syst Rev. 2025;11:CD015363. [PMID: 41276264]

Screening & Early Detection

Screening prevents death from cancers of the breast, colon, lung, and cervix. Current cancer screening recommendations from the USPSTF are available online at https://www.uspreventiveservicestaskforce.org/BrowseRec/Index/browse-recommendations.

Most guidelines are based on trial evidence from middle-aged adults, mostly of European ancestry. Cancer screening in adults over the age of 75 requires an individualized approach that considers differences in disease risk, differences in risk of adverse effects of diagnostic procedures and treatments and competing health issues.

Despite an increase in rates of screening for breast, cervical, lung, and colon cancer over the last decade, overall screening for these cancers is suboptimal. Interventions effective in promoting recommended cancer screening include group education, one-on-one education, patient reminders, reduction of structural barriers, reduction of out-of-pocket costs, and provider assessment and feedback. Multicomponent interventions are generally more effective than single-component ones.

Though breast cancer mortality is reduced with mammography screening, this screening has both benefits and downsides, including overdiagnosis (detecting cancers that would have never progressed to become clinically meaningful). Clinicians should discuss the risks and benefits with each patient and consider individual patient preferences and differences in risk when deciding when to begin screening (see Chapter 19).

Prostate cancer screening remains controversial: completed trials have not fully answered the question of whether early detection and treatment after screen detection produce sufficient benefits (in terms of cancer-specific mortality reduction) to outweigh harms of treatment and overdiagnosis. For men between the ages of 55 and 69, the decision to screen should be individualized and include a discussion of its risks and benefits with a clinician. The USPSTF recommends *against* PSA-based prostate cancer screening for men older than age 70 years (grade D recommendation).

The USPSTF recommends colorectal cancer screening for adults aged 45–75 years and selectively screening adults aged 76–85 years (considering the patient's preferences, overall health, and prior screening history). Choice of screening test is based on patient preferences. Screening colonoscopy every 10 years is one recommended screening option. Annual or biennial fecal occult blood testing reduces mortality from colorectal cancer and is also recommended, with fecal immunochemical tests (FIT) used most commonly. A combination of FIT and stool DNA testing has also shown good accuracy for colorectal cancer and advanced polyps. CT colonography (virtual colonoscopy) is another noninvasive option. It has been shown to have a high safety profile and accuracy similar to colonoscopy for large polyps and cancers.

The American Cancer Society recommends screening for persons aged 25–65 years with primary HPV testing every 5 years based on trial evidence showing it to be superior to other options. The USPSTF recommends screening for cervical cancer in women aged 21–65 years with a Papanicolaou smear (cytology) every 3 years or, for women aged 30–65 years who desire longer intervals, screening with cytology and HPV testing every 5 years. The USPSTF recommends against screening in women younger than 21 years of age and average-risk women over 65 with adequate negative prior screenings. Receipt of HPV vaccination does not yet affect recommended screening intervals, although it may in the future, as a greater proportion of persons are vaccinated.

The USPSTF recommends offering annual lung cancer screening with low-dose CT to current smokers aged 50 to 80 years and at least a 20-pack-year smoking history and to smokers who quit within the past 15 years. Updated American Cancer Society recommendations remove the restriction on the number of years since quitting. A person should stop screening when health problem that limits life expectancy to <5 years has developed or if the person cannot safely undergo treatment if lung cancer is detected. Screening should not be viewed as an alternative to smoking cessation but rather as a complementary approach.

US Preventive Services Task Force; Nicholson WK et al. Screening for breast cancer: US Preventive Services Task Force recommendation statement. JAMA. 2024;331:1918. [PMID: 38687503] Erratum in: JAMA. 2024;332:1396. [PMID: 38687503]
Wolf AMD et al. Screening for lung cancer: 2023 guideline update from the American Cancer Society. CA Cancer J Clin. 2024;74:50. [PMID: 37909877]

PREVENTION OF INJURIES & VIOLENCE

Injuries are an important cause of morbidity and mortality, particularly before age 65. Homicide and motor vehicle collisions are a major cause of injury-related deaths among young and middle-aged adults, and accidental falls are the most common cause of injury-related death in older adults.

Men, particularly those aged 16–35, are at especially high risk for serious injury and death from firearm-related violence, with Black men at greatest risk and Latino and American Indian men also at increased risk. Firearm suicide rates are highest for White men but have been increasing for other racial/ethnic groups. *Deaths from firearms have reached epidemic levels in the United States.* Having a gun in the home increases the likelihood of homicide nearly threefold and of suicide fivefold. Educating clinicians to recognize and treat depression, assess suicide risk, and restrict access to lethal methods in persons at risk has been found to reduce suicide rates.

Clinicians have a critical role in the detection, prevention, and management of intimate partner violence (IPV). The USPSTF recommends screening women of reproductive age for IPV and providing or referring women to intervention services when needed. Inclusion of a single question in the medical history—"At any time, has a partner ever hit you, kicked you, or otherwise physically hurt you?"—can increase identification of this common problem. Assessment for abuse and offering referrals to community resources create the potential to interrupt and prevent recurrence of IPV and associated trauma (and even mortality). Clinicians should take an active role in following up with patients whenever possible, since IPV screening with passive referrals to services may not be adequate to prevent recurrence and escalation.

Physical and psychological abuse, exploitation, and neglect of older adults are serious, underrecognized problems; they may occur in up to 10% of older adults. Risk factors for elder abuse include a culture of violence in the family; a demented, debilitated, or depressed and socially isolated victim; and a perpetrator profile of mental illness, alcohol or drug abuse, or emotional or financial dependence (or both) on the victim. Clues to elder mistreatment include the patient's ill-kempt appearance, recurrent urgent-care visits, missed appointments, suspicious physical findings, and implausible explanations for injuries. Currently, the USPSTF concludes that the evidence for routine screening in older or vulnerable adults is insufficient to determine the benefits and harms.

Curtin SC et al. Suicide rates for the three leading methods by race and ethnicity, 2000–2020. NCHS Data Brief, no 450. Hyattsville, MD: National Center for Health Statistics. 2022. [PMID: 36409535]

US Preventive Services Task Force; Silverstein M et al. Screening for intimate partner violence and caregiver abuse of older or vulnerable adults: US Preventive Services Task Force Recommendation Statement. JAMA. 2025;334:329. [PMID: 40553450]

PREVENTION OF SUBSTANCE USE DISORDERS: ALCOHOL & ILLICIT DRUGS

A. Alcohol

Unhealthy alcohol use is a major public health problem in the United States. The spectrum of alcohol use disorders (AUDs) includes alcohol dependence; harmful pattern use of alcohol; and entities such as alcohol intoxication, alcohol withdrawal, and several alcohol-induced mental disorders. The *ICD-11* includes a new category: *hazardous alcohol use*. Categorized as a risk factor, hazardous alcohol use is a pattern of alcohol use that appreciably increases the risk of harmful physical or mental health consequences to the user.

Underdiagnosis and undertreatment of alcohol misuse are substantial. As with cigarette use, clinician identification and counseling about unhealthy alcohol use are essential. The USPSTF recommends screening adults aged 18 years and older for unhealthy alcohol use. The National Institute on Alcohol Abuse and Alcoholism recommends the following single-question screening test (validated in primary care settings): "How many times in the past year have you had X or more drinks in a day?" ("X" is 5 for men and 4 for women, and a response of > 1 time is considered a positive screen.)

Persons who screen positive on the single-item questionnaire should complete the Alcohol Use Disorder Identification Test (AUDIT), which consists of questions on the quantity and frequency of alcohol consumption, on alcohol dependence symptoms, and on alcohol-related problems (Table 1–6).

Clinicians should provide persons who screen positive for hazardous or risky drinking with brief behavioral counseling interventions to reduce alcohol misuse. Use of screening procedures and brief intervention methods (see Chapter 47) can produce a 10–30% reduction in long-term alcohol use and alcohol-related problems. Those whose AUDIT scores suggest AUD (AUDIT > 12) should undergo more extensive evaluation and potential referral for treatment. Naltrexone and acamprosate are effective for treating AUD. However, <9% of eligible patients receive these effective medications.

B. Opioids

Deaths due to opioid overdose have increased dramatically since 2004, peaking in 2022, and somewhat declining since then. Opioid risk mitigation strategies for prescription opiate misuse include use of risk assessment tools, treatment agreements (contracts), and urine drug testing to limit diversion of prescription opiates. Additional strategies include establishing and strengthening prescription drug monitoring programs, regulating pain management facilities, and establishing dosage thresholds requiring consultation with pain specialists.

More recently, non-prescription opioid use has become predominant as a cause of opioid-related mortality. Harm reduction interventions are important, including strategies to prevent or treat overdose and strategies to reduce infectious complications of injection drug use. The US FDA supports greater access to naloxone and is exploring options to make naloxone more available to treat opioid overdose (see Chapters 5 and 47).

Medication-assisted treatment, the use of medications with counseling and behavioral therapy, is effective in the prevention of opioid overdose and substance abuse disorders. Methadone, buprenorphine, and naltrexone are FDA approved for use in medication-assisted treatment. Buprenorphine has potential as a medication to ameliorate the symptoms and signs of withdrawal from opioids and is effective in reducing concomitant cocaine and opioid abuse.

Use of non-opioid drugs—including cocaine, methamphetamine, and so-called designer drugs—either sporadically or episodically remains an important problem with or without concomitant use of opioids.

Clinical aspects of substance abuse are discussed in Chapter 47.

Garnett MF et al. Drug overdose deaths in the United States, 2003–2023. NCHS Data Brief, no 522. Hyattsville, MD: National Center for Health Statistics. 2024.

GBD 2021 US Burden of Disease Collaborators. The burden of diseases, injuries, and risk factors by state in the USA, 1990-2021: a systematic analysis for the Global Burden of Disease Study 2021. Lancet. 2024;404:2314. [PMID: 39645376]

Krist AH et al. Addressing alcohol use. N Engl J Med. 2025;392:1721. [PMID: 40305713]

McPheeters M et al. Pharmacotherapy for alcohol use disorder: a systematic review and meta-analysis. JAMA. 2023;330:1653. [PMID: 37934220]

Table 1–6. Screening for alcohol abuse using the Alcohol Use Disorder Identification Test (AUDIT).

(Scores for response categories are given in parentheses. Added together, Total Scores range from 0 to 40, with scores of 1 to 7 suggesting low-risk drinking; 8 to 14, hazardous or harmful drinking; and > 15, alcohol dependence.)				
1. How often do you have a drink containing alcohol?				
(0) Never	(1) Monthly or less	(2) Two to four times a month	(3) Two or three times a week	(4) Four or more times a week
2. How many drinks containing alcohol do you have on a typical day when you are drinking?				
(0) 1 or 2	(1) 3 or 4	(2) 5 or 6	(3) 7 to 9	(4) 10 or more
3. How often do you have six or more drinks on one occasion?				
(0) Never	(1) Less than monthly	(2) Monthly	(3) Weekly	(4) Daily or almost daily
4. How often during the past year have you found that you were not able to stop drinking once you had started?				
(0) Never	(1) Less than monthly	(2) Monthly	(3) Weekly	(4) Daily or almost daily
5. How often during the past year have you failed to do what was normally expected of you because of drinking?				
(0) Never	(1) Less than monthly	(2) Monthly	(3) Weekly	(4) Daily or almost daily
6. How often during the past year have you needed a first drink in the morning to get yourself going after a heavy drinking session?				
(0) Never	(1) Less than monthly	(2) Monthly	(3) Weekly	(4) Daily or almost daily
7. How often during the past year have you had a feeling of guilt or remorse after drinking?				
(0) Never	(1) Less than monthly	(2) Monthly	(3) Weekly	(4) Daily or almost daily
8. How often during the past year have you been unable to remember what happened the night before because you had been drinking?				
(0) Never	(1) Less than monthly	(2) Monthly	(3) Weekly	(4) Daily or almost daily
9. Have you or has someone else been injured as a result of your drinking?				
(0) No		(2) Yes, but not in the past year		(4) Yes, during the past year
10. Has a relative or friend or a doctor or other health worker been concerned about your drinking or suggested you cut down?				
(0) No		(2) Yes, but not in the past year		(4) Yes, during the past year

Reproduced with permission from Babor TF, Higgins-Biddle JC, Saunders JB, Montiero MG. *AUDIT. The Alcohol Use Disorders Identification Test. Guidelines for use of primary health care*, 2nd ed. Geneva, Switzerland: World Health Organization; 2001.

Common Symptoms

2

Paul L. Nadler, MD
Ralph Gonzales, MD, MSPH

COUGH

ESSENTIAL INQUIRIES

- Age, duration of cough, occupational history, environmental exposures, and risk of infection with SARS-CoV-2.
- Use of tobacco, cannabis, e-cigarettes (vaping).
- Dyspnea (at rest or with exertion).
- Vital signs (heart rate, respiratory rate, body temperature); pulse oximetry.
- Chest examination.
- CXR, especially when unexplained cough lasts > 3–6 weeks.

General Considerations

Cough is the most common symptom for which patients seek medical attention. Cough results from stimulation of mechanical or chemical afferent nerve receptors in the bronchial tree. Effective cough depends on an intact afferent–efferent reflex arc, adequate expiratory and chest wall muscle strength, and normal mucociliary production and clearance.

Clinical Findings

A. Symptoms

Distinguishing **acute** (< 3 weeks), **persistent** (3–8 weeks), and **chronic** (> 8 weeks) cough syndromes is a useful first step in evaluation. Postinfectious cough lasting 3–8 weeks is referred to as **subacute** cough to distinguish this common, distinct clinical entity from acute, persistent, and chronic cough.

1. Acute cough—In healthy adults, most acute cough syndromes are due to self-limited viral or bacterial or mixed respiratory tract infections. Cough duration is typically 1–3 weeks, yet patients frequently expect cough to last < 10 days. Additional features of infection such as fever, nasal congestion, and sore throat help confirm this diagnosis.

Dyspnea (at rest or with exertion) may signal a more serious condition and warrants further evaluation of oxygenation (pulse oximetry or ABG measurement), airflow (PEF or spirometry), and pulmonary parenchymal disease (CXR). The timing and character of the cough are not useful in establishing the cause of acute cough syndromes, although cough-variant asthma should be considered when there is prominent nocturnal cough. Loss of smell or dysgeusia accompanying a new cough illness is specific but not sensitive for COVID-19 infection. The presence of posttussive emesis or inspiratory whoop in adults modestly increases the likelihood of pertussis, and the absence of paroxysmal cough and the presence of fever decrease its likelihood. In a study of 115 patients with acute cough (1 week to 1 month), 3.5% had pertussis. All patients with pertussis reported paroxysmal cough with a mean duration of 20 days. Uncommon causes of acute cough include HF, hay fever (allergic rhinitis), and occupational exposures (such as farmworkers).

2. Persistent and chronic cough—Cough due to acute respiratory tract infection resolves within 3 weeks in > 90% of patients. Pertussis should be considered in adolescents and adults with persistent or severe cough lasting > 3 weeks who have not been adequately boosted with Tdap, and who have been exposed to a person with confirmed pertussis. It should also be considered in geographic areas where the prevalence of pertussis approaches 20% (although the prevalence is difficult to ascertain due to the limited sensitivity of diagnostic tests).

When ACE inhibitor use, acute respiratory tract infection, and CXR abnormalities are absent, most cases of persistent and chronic cough are related to postnasal drip (upper airway cough syndrome), cough-variant asthma, or GERD, or some combination of these three entities. A history of nasal or sinus congestion, wheezing, or heartburn should direct subsequent evaluation and treatment for these conditions, although these conditions can cause persistent cough in the absence of typical symptoms. Dyspnea at rest or with exertion is not commonly reported with persistent cough; dyspnea requires assessment for chronic lung disease, HF, anemia, PE, or pulmonary hypertension. Approximately 10% of cases of chronic cough are caused by nonasthmatic eosinophilic bronchitis.

Bronchogenic carcinoma is suspected when cough is accompanied by unexplained weight loss, hemoptysis, and fevers with night sweats, particularly in persons with significant tobacco or occupational exposures (asbestos, radon, diesel exhaust, and metals). Secondhand smoke is a risk factor for small airway dysfunction in patients with chronic cough who do not smoke cigarettes. Persistent and chronic cough with excessive phlegm increases the likelihood of COPD, particularly if there is a history of cigarette smoking, or of bronchiectasis if accompanied by recurrent or complicated pneumonia; CXRs are helpful in diagnosis. Chronic cough with dry eyes may represent Sjögren syndrome. A chronic dry cough may be the first symptom of idiopathic pulmonary fibrosis.

B. Physical Examination

Pneumonia is suspected when acute cough is accompanied by vital sign abnormalities (tachycardia, tachypnea, fever). Findings suggestive of airspace consolidation (crackles, decreased breath sounds, fremitus, egophony) are specific predictors of community-acquired pneumonia but are present in a minority of cases. Purulent sputum is associated with bacterial infections in patients with structural lung disease (eg, COPD, cystic fibrosis), but it is a poor predictor of pneumonia in the otherwise healthy adult. Wheezing and rhonchi are frequent findings with acute bronchitis and do not indicate consolidation or adult-onset asthma in most cases.

Examination of patients with persistent cough should include a search for chronic sinusitis, which may contribute to postnasal drip syndrome or to asthma. Physical examination may help distinguish COPD from HF. In patients with cough and dyspnea, a normal match test (ability to blow out a match from 25 cm away) and maximum laryngeal height > 4 cm (measured from the sternal notch to the cricoid cartilage at end-expiration) substantially decrease the likelihood of COPD. Similarly, normal jugular venous pressure and no hepatojugular reflux decrease the likelihood of biventricular HF.

C. Diagnostic Studies

1. Acute cough—CXR should be considered for any adult with acute cough whose vital signs are abnormal or whose chest examination suggests pneumonia. The relationship between specific clinical findings and the probability of pneumonia is shown in Table 2–1. A large, multicenter randomized study found that elevated serum CRP (> 20 mg/dL) improves diagnostic accuracy of clinical prediction rules for pneumonia in adults with acute cough; serum procalcitonin had only marginal utility in outpatient management of acute cough (in contrast to severe pneumonia requiring hospital care). A meta-analysis found that lung ultrasonography had better accuracy than CXR for diagnosing adult community-acquired pneumonia. In patients with dyspnea, pulse oximetry and PEF help exclude hypoxemia or obstructive airway disease.

Table 2–1. Positive and negative likelihood ratios of history, physical examination, and laboratory findings in the diagnosis of pneumonia (range).

Finding	Positive LR	Negative LR
Medical history		
Fever	1.7–2.1	0.6–0.7
Chills	1.3–1.7	0.7–0.9
Physical examination		
Tachypnea (respiratory rate > 25 breaths/min)	1.5–3.4	0.8
Tachycardia (> 100 beats/min or > 120 beats/min)[1]	1.6–2.3	0.5–0.7
Hyperthermia (> 37.8°C)	1.4–4.4	0.6–0.8
Chest examination		
Dullness to percussion	2.2–4.3	0.8–0.9
Decreased breath sounds	2.3–2.5	0.6–0.8
Crackles	1.6–2.7	0.6–0.9
Rhonchi	1.4–1.5	0.8–0.9
Egophony	2.0–8.6	0.8–1.0
Laboratory findings		
Leukocytosis (> 11,000/mcL [11×10^9/L] or ≥ 10,400/mcL [10.4×10^9/L])[1]	1.9–3.7	0.3–0.6
CRP > 20 mg/dL	3.8 (2.3–5.9)	0.5 (0.4–0.6)
Procalcitonin > 0.25 ng/mL	7.6 (3.3–15.1)	0.9 (0.8–0.9)

[1]Results from different studies.

However, a normal pulse oximetry value (eg, > 93%) does not rule out a significant alveolar-arterial (A–a) gradient when patients have effective respiratory compensation.

2. Persistent and chronic cough—CXR is indicated when ACE inhibitor therapy–related and postinfectious cough are excluded. If pertussis is suspected, PCR testing should be performed on a nasopharyngeal swab or nasal wash specimen—although the ability to detect pertussis decreases as the duration of cough increases. When the chest film is normal, postnasal drip, asthma, or GERD are the most likely causes. The presence of typical symptoms of these conditions directs further evaluation or empiric therapy, though typical symptoms are often absent. Definitive tests for determining the presence of each are available (Table 2–2). However, empiric therapy with a maximum-strength regimen for postnasal drip, asthma, or GERD for 2–4 weeks is one recommended approach since the presence of postnasal drip, asthma, or GERD does not mean they are the cause of the cough. Alternative approaches to identifying corticosteroid-responsive cough due to asthma include examining induced sputum for increased eosinophil counts

Table 2–2. Empiric therapy or definitive testing for persistent cough.

Suspected Condition	Step 1 (Empiric Therapy)	Step 2 (Definitive Testing)
Postnasal drip	Therapy for allergy or chronic sinusitis	Sinus CT scan; otolaryngologic referral
Asthma	β_2-Agonist	Spirometry; consider methacholine challenge if normal
GERD	Lifestyle and diet modifications with or without PPIs	Esophageal pH monitoring

(> 3%) or providing an empiric trial of prednisone, 30 mg daily orally for 2 weeks.

Nonasthmatic eosinophilic bronchitis can be diagnosed by finding eosinophils with induced sputum analysis after excluding other causes for chronic cough by clinical, radiologic, and lung function assessment.

Spirometry may help measure large airway obstruction (eg, foreign body or cancer) in patients who have persistent cough and wheezing and are not responding to asthma treatment. When empiric treatment trials are unsuccessful, additional evaluation with pH manometry, endoscopy, barium swallow, sinus CT, or HRCT of the chest may identify the cause.

Differential Diagnosis

A. Acute Cough

Acute cough may be a symptom of acute respiratory tract infection, COVID-19, asthma, allergic rhinitis, HF, and ACE inhibitor therapy, as well as less common causes.

When community influenza-like illness activity levels are high, clinical diagnosis of influenza (cough, fever, chills with or without sweats, myalgias, and acute onset) has a positive predictive value of approximately 70%; this usually obviates the need for rapid diagnostic tests to guide isolation and empiric treatment decisions. The CDC's FluView displays weekly updates of influenza surveillance data (https://www.cdc.gov/fluview/index.html).

B. Persistent and Chronic Cough

Causes of persistent cough include environmental exposures (cigarette smoke and e-cigarette use, air pollution), occupational exposures, pertussis, postnasal drip, asthma (including cough-variant asthma), GERD, COPD, chronic aspiration, bronchiectasis, nonasthmatic eosinophilic bronchitis, tuberculosis or other chronic infection, interstitial lung disease, bronchogenic carcinoma, and ACE inhibitor use. The prevalence of cough 1 year after hospitalization for COVID-19 is 2.5%. COPD is a common cause of persistent cough among patients aged > 50 years who have smoked cigarettes. Persistent cough may also be due to somatic cough syndrome or tic cough, or vocal fold dysfunction. When empiric treatment trials fail, consider other causes of chronic cough such as obstructive sleep apnea, tonsillar or uvular enlargement, and environmental fungi (see Chapter 40).

C. Cough in the Immunocompromised Patient

The evaluation of cough in immunocompromised patients is the same as in immunocompetent patients but with an increased concern for tuberculosis (regardless of radiographic findings), fungi, cytomegalovirus, varicella, herpesvirus, and *Pneumocystis jirovecii*.

Treatment

A. Acute Cough

Treatment of acute cough should target the underlying etiology of the illness, the cough reflex, and any additional factors that exacerbate the cough. An open randomized trial of adults with uncomplicated acute bronchitis (symptoms < 3 weeks) found no benefit compared with usual care with dextromethorphan 15 mg three times a day, ipratropium bromide inhaler 20 mcg 2 puffs three times a day, or 30 mg of honey three times a day for up to 14 days.

When influenza is diagnosed, oral oseltamivir or zanamivir or intravenous peramivir are equally effective (1 less day of illness) when initiated within 30–48 hours of illness onset; treatment is recommended regardless of illness duration when patients have severe, complicated, or progressive influenza and in patients requiring hospitalization. In *Chlamydophila*- or *Mycoplasma*-documented infection or outbreaks, first-line antibiotics include erythromycin (erythromycin 500 mg orally four times daily for 10–14 days) or doxycycline (doxycycline 100 mg orally twice daily for 7–14 days). Antibiotics do not otherwise improve cough severity or duration in patients with uncomplicated acute bronchitis. In patients with bronchitis and wheezing, inhaled β_2-agonists reduce severity and duration of cough. In patients with acute cough, treating the accompanying postnasal drip (with antihistamines, decongestants, saline nasal irrigation, or nasal corticosteroids) can be helpful. Two studies found codeine to be no more effective than placebo in reducing acute cough symptoms.

B. Subacute Cough

Most cases are postinfectious and self-limited. If upper airway symptoms (postnasal drip) are present, intranasal steroids and saline rinses may help. If there is concern for cough-variant asthma (history of asthma), a trial of inhaled bronchodilators and inhaled corticosteroids is reasonable. GERD symptoms should be treated.

C. Persistent and Chronic Cough

Evaluation and management of persistent cough often require multiple visits and therapeutic trials, which frequently lead to frustration, anger, and anxiety.

When pertussis infection is suspected early in its course, treatment with a macrolide antibiotic (see Chapter 37) is appropriate to reduce organism shedding and transmission. When pertussis has lasted > 7–10 days, antibiotic treatment does not affect the duration of cough, which can last up to 6 months. Early identification, revaccination with

Tdap, and treatment are encouraged for adult patients who work or live with persons at high risk for complications from pertussis (eg, pregnant women, infants younger than 1 year, and immunosuppressed individuals).

Table 2–2 outlines empiric treatments for persistent cough. There is no evidence to guide how long to continue treatment for persistent cough due to postnasal drip, asthma, or GERD. PPIs are not effective when used in isolation for treating chronic cough due to gastroesophageal reflux; most benefit appears to come from lifestyle modifications and weight reduction. Studies have not found a consistent benefit of inhaled corticosteroid therapy in adults with persistent cough, but cough from nonasthmatic eosinophilic bronchitis usually responds well to inhaled corticosteroids.

There is insufficient evidence to recommend routine pharmacologic treatments (antibiotics, bronchodilators, mucolytics) to relieve chronic cough due to stable chronic bronchitis.

Patients with idiopathic chronic cough should be managed in consultation with an otolaryngologist or a pulmonologist; consider an HRCT scan of the lungs. Treatment options include lidocaine throat spray, nebulized lidocaine therapy, and morphine sulfate, 5–10 mg orally twice daily. Sensory dysfunction of the laryngeal branches of the vagus nerve may contribute to persistent cough syndromes and may explain the effectiveness of gabapentin and baclofen in patients with chronic cough.

Speech pathology therapy combined with pregabalin has some benefit in chronic refractory cough. In patients with cough hypersensitivity syndrome, therapy aimed at shifting the patient's attentional focus from internal stimuli to external focal points can be helpful.

When to Refer

- Failure to control persistent or chronic cough following empiric treatment trials.
- Patients with recurrent symptoms should be referred to an otolaryngologist, pulmonologist, or gastroenterologist.

When to Admit

- Patients at high risk for tuberculosis for whom adherence to respiratory precautions is uncertain.
- Need for urgent bronchoscopy, such as suspected foreign body.
- Smoke or toxic fume inhalational injury.
- Gas exchange is impaired by cough.
- Patients at high risk for barotrauma (eg, recent pneumothorax).

Ebell MH et al. Acute cough in outpatients: what causes it, how long does it last, and how severe is it for different viruses and bacteria? Clin Microbiol Infect. 2024;30:1569. Erratum in: Clin Microbiol Infect. 2025;31:142. [PMID: 38977076]

Irwin RS et al. Unexplained or refractory chronic cough in adults. N Engl J Med. 2025;392:1203. [PMID: 40138554]

Mulhem E et al. Acute bronchitis: rapid evidence review. Am Fam Physician. 2025;111:214. [PMID: 40106287]

DYSPNEA

ESSENTIAL INQUIRIES

- Fever, cough, risk of COVID-19 infection, and chest pain.
- Vital sign measurements; pulse oximetry.
- Cardiac and chest examination.
- CXR and ABG measurement in selected patients.

General Considerations

Dyspnea is a subjective experience or perception of uncomfortable breathing. The relationship between the level of dyspnea and the severity of underlying disease varies widely. Dyspnea can result from conditions that increase the mechanical effort of breathing (eg, asthma, COPD, respiratory muscle weakness, pneumothorax, and pleural effusion [which impact gas exchange, as well]), alveolar lung disease (pulmonary edema, pneumonia, alveolar proteinosis), conditions that produce compensatory tachypnea (eg, hypoxemia, acidosis), primary pulmonary vasculopathy (pulmonary hypertension), or psychogenic conditions.

Clinical Findings

A. Symptoms

The duration, severity, and periodicity of dyspnea influence the tempo of the clinical evaluation. Rapid onset or severe dyspnea without other clinical features should raise concern for PE, increased LVEDP, or pneumothorax.

PE should always be suspected when a patient with new dyspnea reports a recent history (previous 4 weeks) of prolonged immobilization or surgery, estrogen therapy, or other risk factors for DVT (eg, previous history of thromboembolism, cancer, obesity, lower extremity trauma), but also when the cause of dyspnea is not apparent. Silent MI, which occurs more frequently in women and persons with diabetes, can result in increased LVEDP, acute HF, and dyspnea. Spontaneous pneumothorax is usually accompanied by chest pain and occurs most often in thin, young men and those with underlying lung disease.

Accompanying symptoms provide clues to causes of dyspnea. When cough and fever are present, pulmonary disease (particularly infection) is the primary concern; myocarditis, pericarditis, and septic emboli can also present in this manner. Chest pain should be further characterized as acute or chronic, pleuritic or exertional. Although acute pleuritic chest pain is the rule in acute pericarditis and pneumothorax, most patients with pleuritic chest pain in the outpatient clinic have pleurisy due to acute viral respiratory tract infection. Periodic chest pain that precedes the onset of dyspnea suggests myocardial ischemia or PE. Most cases of dyspnea associated with wheezing are due to acute bronchitis; however, other causes include new-onset asthma, foreign body, and vocal fold dysfunction. Interstitial lung disease and pulmonary hypertension should be considered in patients with symptoms (or history) of connective tissue disease, or in those who have ECG findings typical of pulmonary hypertension (RVH with strain, P pulmonale) and elevated (NT-pro-)BNP. Pulmonary lymphangitic carcinomatosis should be considered if a patient has a malignancy, especially breast, lung, or gastric cancer.

When a patient reports prominent dyspnea with mild or no accompanying features, consider chronic PE and noncardiopulmonary causes of impaired oxygen delivery (anemia, methemoglobinemia, cyanide ingestion, carbon monoxide poisoning), metabolic acidosis, panic disorder, and neuromuscular disorders.

The diagnosis of HFpEF as the cause of dyspnea is challenging in the absence of overt congestion; the diagnosis may be made by echocardiography.

Patients who recover from their initial COVID-19 infection may have persistent dyspnea as part of the "long COVID" syndrome. Platypnea-orthodeoxia syndrome is characterized by dyspnea and hypoxemia on sitting or standing that improves in the recumbent position. Hyperthyroidism can cause dyspnea from increased ventilatory drive, respiratory muscle weakness, or pulmonary hypertension.

B. Physical Examination

A focused physical examination should include evaluation of the head and neck, chest, heart, and lower extremities. Visual inspection of the patient can suggest obstructive airway disease (pursed-lip breathing, use of accessory respiratory muscles, barrel-shaped chest), pneumothorax (asymmetric excursion), or metabolic acidosis (Kussmaul respirations). Patients with impending upper airway obstruction (eg, epiglottitis, foreign body) or severe asthma sometimes assume a tripod position. Focal wheezing suggests a foreign body or other bronchial obstruction.

Maximum laryngeal height (the distance between the top of the thyroid cartilage and the suprasternal notch at end-expiration) is a measure of hyperinflation. Obstructive airway disease is virtually nonexistent when a nonsmoking patient < age 45 years has a maximum laryngeal height > 4 cm; factors increasing the likelihood of obstructive airway disease (in patients without known obstructive airway disease) include patient history of > 40 pack-years smoking (adjusted LR+ 11.6; LR– 0.9), patient age > 45 years (LR+ 1.4; LR– 0.5), and maximum laryngeal height ≤ 4 cm (LR+ 3.6; LR– 0.7). With all three of these factors present, the LR+ rises to 58.5, and the LR– falls to 0.3.

Absent breath sounds suggest a pneumothorax. An accentuated pulmonic component of the second heart sound (loud P_2) is a sign of pulmonary hypertension and PE.

Clinical predictors of increased LVEDP in dyspneic patients with no history of HF include tachycardia, systolic hypotension, jugular venous distention, hepatojugular reflux, bibasilar crackles, third heart sound, lower extremity edema, and chest film findings of pulmonary vascular redistribution or cardiomegaly. When none is present, there is a low probability (< 10%) of increased LVEDP, but when two or more are present, there is a high probability (> 90%) of increased LVEDP.

C. Diagnostic Studies

Causes of dyspnea that can be managed without CXR are few: anemia, carbon monoxide poisoning, and ingestions causing lactic acidosis and methemoglobinemia.

1. Chest radiography—The diagnosis of pneumonia should be confirmed by CXR in most patients, and elevated blood levels of procalcitonin or CRP can support the diagnosis of pneumonia in equivocal cases or in the presence of interstitial lung disease. Conversely, a low procalcitonin can help exclude pneumonia in dyspneic patients with HF. (See Table 2–1 for other diagnostic findings in pneumonia.)

CXR has a moderate sensitivity (53–75%) and a high specificity (86–96%) for new-onset HF (represented by redistribution of pulmonary venous circulation) and can help guide treatment of patients with other cardiac diseases. NT-proBNP can assist in diagnosing HF (see below). End-expiratory CXR enhances detection of small pneumothoraces. A normal CXR has substantial diagnostic value. When there is no physical examination evidence of COPD or HF and the CXR and ECG are normal, the major remaining causes of dyspnea include PE, *P jirovecii* infection (the initial radiograph may be normal in up to 25%), upper airway obstruction, foreign body, anemia, and metabolic acidosis. If a patient has tachycardia or dyspnea but a normal CXR and ECG, then tests to exclude pulmonary emboli, anemia, or metabolic acidosis are warranted.

2. Point-of-care ultrasonography (POCUS)—When added to a standard diagnostic pathway, studies have confirmed that using POCUS leads to a statistically significantly increase in correct diagnoses in patients with acute dyspnea than the standard diagnostic pathway alone. POCUS consistently improves the sensitivities and specificities of standard diagnostic pathways to detect HF, pneumonia, PE, pleural effusion, or pneumothorax.

3. High-resolution chest CT—This test is particularly useful in the evaluation of interstitial and alveolar lung disease. Helical ("spiral") CT is useful to diagnose PE since the images are high resolution and require only one breath hold by the patient. To minimize unnecessary testing and radiation exposure, however, the clinician should first employ a clinical decision rule for ruling out acute PE, such as the PERC (Pulmonary Embolism Rule-Out Criteria), the Wells score, the revised Geneva scores with fixed or adapted D-dimer thresholds, or the YEARS algorithm. It is appropriate to forego CT scanning in patients with low probability of pulmonary embolus when other causes of dyspnea are more likely (see Chapter 9).

4. Pulmonary function testing with diffusing capacity of the lungs for carbon monoxide—A low DLCO is associated with interstitial lung disease, emphysema, pulmonary vascular disease, chronic HF, and drug toxicity. A DLCO above the upper limit of normal (uncommon) may occur in individuals with asthma, obesity, or increased blood volume or hemoglobin (polycythemia, left-to-right cardiac shunt, pregnancy, pulmonary hemorrhage).

5. Cardiopulmonary exercise testing—A maximal exercise test with gas exchange analysis that provides minute ventilation, heart rate, oxygen uptake, and carbon dioxide output may identify the cause of exertional dyspnea, exercise intolerance, or exercise-induced hypoxemia.

6. Serum BNP and cardiac troponin—Laboratory findings suggesting increased LVEDP include elevated serum BNP or NT-proBNP levels. Acute decompensated HF is unlikely if NT-proBNP is < 300 pg/mL or BNP is < 100 pg/mL, and ECG is normal. High-sensitivity cardiac troponin T (hs-CTnT) may be a marker of HFpEF causing dyspnea.

7. Arterial blood gas—ABG measurement may be considered if clinical examination and routine diagnostic testing are equivocal. With two notable exceptions (carbon monoxide poisoning and cyanide toxicity), ABG measurement distinguishes increased mechanical effort dyspnea (respiratory acidosis with or without hypoxemia) from compensatory tachypnea (respiratory alkalosis with or without hypoxemia or metabolic acidosis) and from psychogenic dyspnea (respiratory alkalosis). Carbon monoxide and cyanide impair oxygen delivery with minimal alterations in PO_2; percent carboxyhemoglobin identifies carbon monoxide toxicity. Cyanide poisoning should be considered when profound lactic acidosis follows exposure to burning vinyl (eg, theater fire or industrial accident). Carbon monoxide poisoning or methemoglobinemia can be confirmed with venous carboxyhemoglobin or methemoglobin levels. Venous blood gas testing can assess acid-base and respiratory status by measuring venous pH and PCO_2 but is unable to provide information on oxygenation. To correlate with ABG values, venous pH is typically 0.03–0.05 units lower, and venous PCO_2 is typically 4–5 mm Hg higher than arterial samples.

8. Pulse oximetry—Because ABG testing is impractical in most outpatient settings, pulse oximetry is useful in the office evaluation of dyspnea. Oxygen saturation values > 96% almost always correspond with a PaO_2 > 70 mm Hg, whereas values < 94% may represent clinically significant hypoxemia. Important exceptions to this rule include carbon monoxide toxicity, which leads to normal oxygen and methemoglobinemia, which results in an oxygen saturation of about 85% that fails to increase with supplemental oxygen. Pulse oximetry to detect occult hypoxia is less accurate in Black patients (OR, 2.57) compared with White patients. A delirious or obtunded patient with obstructive lung disease warrants immediate measurement of ABGs to exclude hypercapnia and the need for intubation, regardless of the oxygen saturation. If a patient reports dyspnea with exertion but resting oximetry is normal, assessment of desaturation with ambulation (eg, a brisk walk around the clinic) can confirm impaired gas exchange. Persons with COVID-19 may have low oxygen saturation with minimal dyspnea and profound desaturation with minimal exertion.

For patients without known cardiac or pulmonary disease reporting dyspnea on exertion, spirometry, NT-proBNP, and CT imaging are the most informative tests.

Episodic dyspnea can be challenging if an evaluation cannot be performed during symptoms. Life-threatening causes include recurrent PE, myocardial ischemia, and reactive airway disease. When dyspnea follows an emotionally or physically stressful event, Takotsubo cardiomyopathy (stress cardiomyopathy or broken heart syndrome) should be considered. When associated with audible wheezing, vocal fold dysfunction should be considered, particularly in a young woman who does not respond to asthma therapy. Spirometry is helpful in further classifying patients with obstructive airway disease but is rarely needed in the initial or emergent evaluation of patients with acute dyspnea.

Differential Diagnosis

Urgent and emergent conditions causing acute dyspnea include pneumonia, COPD, asthma, pneumothorax, PE, cardiac disease (eg, HF, acute MI, valvular dysfunction, arrhythmia, intracardiac shunt), pleural effusion, COVID-19, diffuse alveolar hemorrhage, metabolic acidosis, cyanide toxicity, methemoglobinemia, and carbon monoxide poisoning. Chronic dyspnea may be caused by interstitial lung disease, pulmonary hypertension, or pulmonary alveolar proteinosis.

Treatment

Patients with hypoxemia should immediately be provided supplemental oxygen unless significant hypercapnia is strongly suspected pending ABG measurement. In managing acute respiratory failure, high-flow nasal oxygen may reduce all-cause mortality, rates of intubation, and hospital-acquired pneumonia compared with noninvasive ventilation.

Oxygen therapy is most beneficial to patients with significant hypoxemia (PaO_2 < 55 mm Hg) (see Chapter 5). In patients with severe COPD and hypoxemia, oxygen therapy improves exercise performance and mortality. Pulmonary rehabilitation programs are another therapeutic option for patients with moderate to severe COPD or interstitial pulmonary fibrosis. Noninvasive ventilation may be considered for patients with dyspnea caused by an acute COPD exacerbation.

Dyspnea frequently occurs in patients nearing the end of life. Oral opioid therapy, anxiolytics, and corticosteroids can provide substantial relief independent of the severity of hypoxemia. Inhaled opioids are not effective.

When to Refer

- Following acute stabilization, patients with advanced COPD should be referred to a pulmonologist, and patients with HF or valvular heart disease should be referred to a cardiologist.
- Cyanide toxicity or carbon monoxide poisoning should be managed in conjunction with a toxicologist.
- Lung transplantation can be considered for patients with advanced interstitial lung disease.

When to Admit

- Impaired gas exchange from any cause or high risk of PE pending definitive diagnosis.
- Suspected cyanide toxicity or carbon monoxide poisoning.

Ciumanghel I et al. Point-of-care lung ultrasound - a rapid and reliable diagnostic tool for emergency physicians treating patients with acute dyspnea in high-volume emergency departments. Emerg Radiol. 2025;32:329. [PMID: 40261500]
Keane R et al. Assessment of breathlessness: a pulmonologist's perspective - short of breath, but not short of answers. Breathe (Sheff). 2025;21:240096. [PMID: 40104257]
Laksono S et al. Dyspnea in emergency settings: up-to-date diagnosing and management in the emergency department. Current Medical Issues. 2024;22:37. doi: 10.4103/cmi.cmi_117_23
Stals MAM et al. Safety and efficiency of diagnostic strategies for ruling out pulmonary embolism in clinically relevant patient subgroups: a systematic review and individual-patient data meta-analysis. Ann Intern Med. 2022;175:244. [PMID: 34904857]
Valbuena VSM et al. Racial bias in pulse oximetry measurement among patients about to undergo ECMO in 2019–2020, a retrospective cohort study. Chest. 2022;161:971. [PMID: 34592317]

HEMOPTYSIS

ESSENTIAL INQUIRIES

- Fever, cough, and other symptoms of lower respiratory tract infection.
- Smoking history.
- Nasopharyngeal or GI bleeding.
- CXR and CBC (and, in some cases, INR).

General Considerations

Hemoptysis is the expectoration of blood that originates below the vocal folds. It is commonly classified as trivial, mild, or massive—the latter defined as > 200–600 mL (about 1–2 cups) in 24 hours. Massive hemoptysis can be usefully defined as any amount that is hemodynamically significant or threatens ventilation. Its in-hospital mortality was 6.5% in one study. The initial goal of management of massive hemoptysis is therapeutic, not diagnostic.

The causes of hemoptysis can be classified anatomically.

Upper airway bleeding may be from trauma, neoplasm, or foreign body.

Lower airway hemoptysis may arise from COPD, bronchiectasis, bronchial Dieulafoy disease, or bronchogenic carcinoma.

Pulmonary vasculature can be the source of hemoptysis in LV failure, mitral stenosis, PE, pulmonary arterial hypertension, telangiectasias, arteriovenous malformations, and multiple pulmonary artery aneurysms. Diffuse alveolar hemorrhage—manifested by alveolar infiltrates on CXR—is due to small vessel bleeding usually caused by autoimmune or hemostatic disorders, or rarely precipitated by hypertensive emergency, the antiplatelet medication tirofiban, anticoagulant therapy and infection.

Systemic circulation can be the source of hemoptysis when there is intralobar pulmonary sequestration or aortobronchial fistula.

Pulmonary parenchyma diseases due to pneumonia, fungal infections, inhalation of crack cocaine, granulomatosis with polyangiitis, or Takayasu arteritis with pulmonary arteritis can cause hemoptysis. Hemoptysis can also be caused by the parasitic diseases paragonimiasis (most common cause worldwide) and human echinococcosis.

Most outpatient cases of hemoptysis are due to infection (eg, acute or chronic bronchitis, pneumonia, tuberculosis, *Mycobacterium avium* complex, aspergillosis). Hemoptysis due to lung cancer increases with age, causing up to 20% of cases among older adults. Pulmonary venous hypertension (eg, mitral stenosis, PE) causes hemoptysis in < 10% of cases. Most cases of hemoptysis that have no visible cause on CT scan or bronchoscopy will resolve within 6 months without treatment, with the notable exception of patients at high risk for lung cancer (patients who smoke cigarettes and are > age 40). Iatrogenic hemorrhage may follow transbronchial lung biopsies, anticoagulation, or pulmonary artery rupture due to distal placement of a balloon-tipped catheter. Obstructive sleep apnea with elevated pulmonary arterial pressure may be a risk factor for hemoptysis. Amyloidosis of the lung can cause hemoptysis, as can endometriosis. No cause is identified in up to 15–30% of cases.

Clinical Findings

A. Symptoms

Blood-tinged sputum in the setting of an upper respiratory tract infection in an otherwise healthy, young (age < 40 years) nonsmoker does not warrant an extensive diagnostic evaluation if the hemoptysis subsides with resolution of the infection. However, hemoptysis is frequently a sign of serious disease, especially in patients with a high prior probability of underlying pulmonary pathology. Hemoptysis is the only symptom found to be a specific predictor of lung cancer. There is no value in distinguishing blood-streaked sputum and cough productive of blood during evaluation; the goal of the history is to identify patients at risk for one of the disorders listed earlier. Pertinent features include duration of symptoms, presence of respiratory infection, and past or current tobacco use. Nonpulmonary sources of hemorrhage—from the sinuses or the GI tract—must be excluded.

B. Physical Examination

Elevated pulse, hypotension, and decreased oxygen saturation suggest large-volume hemorrhage that warrants emergent evaluation and stabilization. The nares and oropharynx should be carefully inspected to identify a potential upper airway source of bleeding. Chest and cardiac examination may reveal evidence of HF or mitral stenosis.

C. Diagnostic Studies

Diagnostic evaluation should include a CXR and CBC. Kidney function tests, UA, and coagulation studies are appropriate in specific circumstances. Hematuria that accompanies hemoptysis may be a clue to anti-glomerular basement membrane antibody disease or vasculitis. Flexible bronchoscopy reveals endobronchial cancer in 3–6% of patients with hemoptysis who have a normal CXR. Nearly all these patients are > 40 years old and smoke cigarettes, and most will have had symptoms for > 1 week. HRCT of the chest complements bronchoscopy; it can visualize unsuspected bronchiectasis and arteriovenous malformations and will show central endobronchial cancers in many cases. It is the test of choice for suspected small peripheral malignancies. Helical pulmonary CT angiography is the initial test of choice for evaluating patients with suspected PE, although caution should be taken to avoid large contrast loads with even mild CKD (serum creatinine > 2.0 g/dL or rapidly rising creatinine in normal range). Helical CT scanning can be avoided in patients who are at "unlikely" risk for PE using the Wells score or PERC (Pulmonary Embolism Rule-Out Criteria) rule and the sensitive D-dimer test (see Chapter 9). Echocardiography may reveal evidence of HF or mitral stenosis. Multidetector CT angiography may help determine the location, etiology, and mechanism of the bleeding in mitral stenosis and HF.

Treatment

Mild hemoptysis management consists of identifying and treating the specific cause. One double-blind RCT compared treatment with inhalations of tranexamic acid (an antifibrinolytic drug) versus placebo (normal saline) in patients hospitalized with mild hemoptysis (< 200 mL of expectorated blood per 24 hours). The study findings included faster resolution of bleeding, shorter length of hospital stay, and fewer invasive procedures with tranexamic acid treatment; Decreased in-hospital mortality was observed in a separate randomized trial (11.5% mortality rate in control group versus 9.0% in patients who received tranexamic acid).

Massive hemoptysis is life-threatening. The airway should be protected with endotracheal intubation, ventilation ensured, and effective circulation maintained. If the location of the bleeding site is known, the patient should be placed in the decubitus position with the involved lung dependent. Uncontrollable hemorrhage warrants rigid bronchoscopy and surgical consultation. In stable patients, flexible bronchoscopy may localize the bleeding site, and angiography can embolize the involved bronchial arteries. Based on meta-analysis, BAE has a technical success rate of 97%, and is more effective than conservative treatment in controlling hemoptysis, but no difference in all-cause mortality. Hemoptysis recurrence and mortality rates after BAE were 25% and 2.3%, respectively. The anterior spinal artery arises from the bronchial artery in up to 5% of people, and paraplegia may result if it is inadvertently cannulated and embolized.

When to Refer

- Refer to a pulmonologist when bronchoscopy of the lower respiratory tract is needed.
- Refer to an otolaryngologist when an upper respiratory tract bleeding source is identified.
- Refer to a hematologist when severe coagulopathy complicates management.

When to Admit

- To stabilize bleeding in patients at risk for or experiencing massive hemoptysis.
- To correct disordered coagulation (using clotting factors or platelets, or both) or to reverse anticoagulation.
- To stabilize gas exchange.

Chandler JK et al. Evaluation & management of clinically significant hemoptysis—a clinical practice review. AME Med J. 2024;9:1. doi:10.21037/amj-23-99

Fujii H et al. Nationwide survey in Japan of the causative diseases of bloody sputum and hemoptysis in departments of respiratory medicine at university hospitals and core hospitals. Respir Investig. 2024;62:395. [PMID: 38484503]

Jaqua EE et al. Respiratory symptom evaluation in adults: hemoptysis. FP Essent. 2023;528:25. [PMID: 37220189]

Ye M et al. Nebulized tranexamic acid in the management of hemoptysis: an integrative review. Lung. 2025;203:28. [PMID: 39841268]

CHEST PAIN

ESSENTIAL INQUIRIES

- Pain onset, character, location/size, duration, periodicity, and exacerbators; shortness of breath.
- Vital signs; chest and cardiac examinations.
- ECG and biomarkers of myocardial necrosis in selected patients.

General Considerations

Chest pain (or chest discomfort) can occur as a result of cardiovascular, pulmonary, pleural, or musculoskeletal disease; esophageal or other GI disorders; herpes zoster; cocaine use; or anxiety states. The frequency and distribution of life-threatening causes of chest pain, such as ACS, pericarditis, aortic dissection, vasospastic angina, PE, pneumonia, and esophageal perforation, vary substantially between clinical settings.

SLE, rheumatoid arthritis, reduced eGFR, and HIV infection confer a strong risk of CAD. Precocious ACS (occurring in patients age < 35 years) may represent acute thrombosis independent of underlying atherosclerotic disease. Risk factors for precocious ACS are obesity, familial hypercholesterolemia, and cigarette use.

Although ACS presents with a broader range of symptoms in women than men, typical chest pain characteristics of acute MI do not differ in frequency or strength between men and women.

Because PE can present with a variety of symptoms, consideration of the diagnosis and rigorous risk factor assessment for VTE is critical. VTE risk factors include cancer, trauma, recent surgery, prolonged immobilization, pregnancy, oral contraceptives, family history, HF, COPD, and prior history of VTE. Sickle cell anemia can cause acute chest syndrome, often with chest pain, fever, and cough.

Clinical Findings

A. Symptoms

Myocardial ischemia is usually described as a dull, aching sensation of "pressure," "tightness," "squeezing," or "gas," rather than as sharp or spasmodic. Chest discomfort at rest is the most common presenting symptom of ACS, reported by 79% of men and 74% of women. Pain reaching maximum intensity in seconds is uncommon. Ischemic symptoms usually subside within 5–20 minutes but may last longer. Progressive symptoms or symptoms at rest may represent unstable angina. Up to one-third of patients with acute MI do not report chest pain. In patients who have a STEMI, chest pain is present in > 90% of persons aged < 65 years but in only 57% of those aged > 85 years.

Continuous chest pain lasting 24 hours or longer is unlikely to be due to an acute MI (LR, 0.15). However, chest pain lasting ≤ 1 minute does not exclude MI (LR, 0.95). When present, pain due to myocardial ischemia is commonly accompanied by a sense of anxiety or uneasiness. The location is usually retrosternal or left precordial, although a significant number of patients will report pain in the right shoulder, right arm and back. Because the heart lacks somatic innervation, precise localization of pain due to cardiac ischemia is difficult; the pain is commonly referred to the throat, lower jaw, shoulders, inner arms, upper abdomen, or back. Ischemic pain may be precipitated or exacerbated by exertion, cold temperature, meals, stress, or combinations of these factors and is usually relieved by rest. However, many episodes do not conform to these patterns, and a broader range of symptoms of ACS are more common in women, older adults, and persons with diabetes mellitus. Other symptoms that are associated with ACS include shortness of breath; dizziness; a feeling of impending doom; and vagal symptoms, such as nausea and diaphoresis. In older persons, unusual or unexplained fatigue is a common presenting symptom of ACS.

The presenting symptoms of acute MI in patients aged 18–55 (average age, 47) differ in men and women. The VIRGO study of this younger cohort hospitalized for MI found that women are more likely than men to present with three or more associated symptoms (eg, epigastric symptoms; palpitations; and pain or discomfort in the jaw, neck, arms, or between the shoulder blades; 61.9% for women versus 54.8% for men). In adjusted analyses, women with STEMI were more likely than men to present without chest pain (OR, 1.51). In comparison with men, women were more likely to perceive symptoms as stress/anxiety (20.9% versus 11.8%) but less likely to attribute symptoms to muscle pain (15.4% versus 21.2%).

One analysis found the following clinical features to be associated with MI: chest pain that radiates to the left, right, or both arms (LR, 2.3); diaphoresis (LR, 2.0); nausea and vomiting (LR, 1.9); third heart sound (LR, 3.2); systolic blood pressure < 80 mm Hg (LR, 3.1); pulmonary crackles (LR, 2.1); any ST-segment elevation ≥ 1 mm (LR, 11.2); any ST depression (LR, 3.2); any Q wave (LR, 3.9); any conduction defect (LR, 2.7); and new conduction defect (LR, 6.3).

A meta-analysis reported the clinical features and risk factors with highest positive LRs for ACS were prior abnormal stress test (specificity, 96%; LR, 3.1), peripheral arterial disease (specificity, 97%; LR, 2.7), and pain radiation to both arms (specificity, 96%; LR, 2.6), as well as the following ECG findings: ST-segment depression (specificity, 95%; LR, 5.3) and any evidence of ischemia (specificity, 91%; LR, 3.6). Risk scores derived from both the HEART trial (https://www.mdcalc.com/heart-score-major-cardiac-events) and TIMI trial (https://www.mdcalc.com/timi-risk-score-ua-nstemi#use-cases) performed well in detecting ACS (LR, 13 for HEART score of 7–10, and LR, 6.8 for TIMI score of 5–7).

Hypertrophy of either ventricle or aortic stenosis may give rise to chest pain with less typical features. Pericarditis produces pain that may be greater when supine than upright and increases with breathing, coughing, or swallowing. Pleuritic chest pain is usually not ischemic, and pain on palpation may indicate a musculoskeletal cause. Aortic dissection classically produces an abrupt onset of intense tearing pain that often radiates to the back; however, this classic presentation occurs in a small proportion of cases. Anterior aortic dissection can also lead to myocardial or cerebrovascular ischemia.

In PE, chest pain is present in about 75% of cases. The chief objective in evaluating suspected PE is to assess the clinical risk for VTE based on medical history and associated symptoms and signs (see above and Chapter 9). Rupture of the thoracic esophagus iatrogenically or from vomiting is another cause of chest pain.

B. Physical Examination

Findings on physical examination can occasionally yield important clues to the underlying cause of chest pain; however, a normal physical examination should never be used as the sole basis for ruling out most causes of chest pain, particularly ACS and aortic dissection. A normal physical examination is also compatible with panic/anxiety disorder and musculoskeletal disease. Vital signs (including pulse oximetry) and cardiopulmonary examination are the first steps for assessing the urgency and tempo of the subsequent examination and diagnostic workup. Although chest pain that is reproducible or worsened with palpation strongly suggests a musculoskeletal cause, up to 15% of patients with ACS will have reproducible chest wall tenderness. In one study, reproducible chest pain had a negative predictive value of 98%. A prominent xyphoid process painful to palpation may indicate xiphodynia. Slipping rib syndrome should be suspected if the chest pain is reproduced by the examiner pulling superiorly and anteriorly under the costal margin with their fingers. Pointing to the location of the pain with one finger has been shown to be highly correlated with nonischemic chest pain.

Aortic dissection can result in differential blood pressures between arms (> 20 mm Hg), pulse amplitude deficits, and new diastolic murmurs. Although hypertension is considered the rule in patients with aortic dissection, systolic blood pressure < 100 mm Hg is present in up to 25% of patients.

A cardiac friction rub represents pericarditis until proven otherwise. It can best be heard with the patient sitting forward at end-expiration. Tamponade should be excluded in all patients with a clinical diagnosis of pericarditis by assessing pulsus paradoxus (at least a 10 mm Hg decrease in systolic blood pressure during inspiration) and inspection of jugular venous pulsations. Subcutaneous emphysema is common following cervical esophageal perforation but present in only about one-third of thoracic perforations (ie, those most commonly presenting with chest pain).

The absence of abnormal physical examination findings in patients with suspected PE usually serves to *increase* its likelihood.

C. Diagnostic Studies

1. ECG—Unless a competing diagnosis can be confirmed, an ECG is warranted in the initial evaluation of most patients with acute chest pain to help exclude ACS. When compared with White patients, Black patients who came to the emergency department with chest pain were less likely to have an ECG ordered (adjusted OR, 0.82). In a study of 11 emergency departments in Italy, 67% of patients with confirmed ACS had new-onset alterations of the ECG (compared with only 6.2% among patients without ACS). ST-segment elevation is the ECG finding that is the strongest predictor of acute MI; however, up to 20% of patients with ACS can have a normal ECG.

In the emergency department, patients with suspected ACS can be safely removed from cardiac monitoring if pain-free at initial clinician assessment and have a normal or nonspecific ECG. This decision rule had 100% sensitivity for serious arrhythmia. Clinically stable patients with CVD risk factors, normal ECG, normal cardiac biomarkers, and no alternative diagnoses (such as typical GERD or costochondritis) should be followed up with an exercise stress test, ideally within 24–48 hours, that includes perfusion imaging. However, > 25% of patients with stable chest pain referred for noninvasive testing will have normal coronary arteries and no long-term clinical events. The ECG can also provide evidence for alternative diagnoses, such as pericarditis and PE.

2. Troponins—Diagnostic protocols using a single high-sensitivity troponin assay combined with a standardized clinical assessment are an efficient strategy to rapidly determine whether patients with chest pain are at low risk and may be discharged from the emergency department. A study of the modified HEART score using a single blood draw had a sensitivity of 100% for 30-day major adverse cardiac events if the results exceeded the threshold of either high-sensitivity troponin (3.9 ng/L), high-sensitivity troponin I (0.9 ng/L), or conventional troponin I (0.0 ng/L) at presentation.

Point-of-care conventional troponin testing (cut point of 0.080 ng/mL) for acute MI during ambulance transport to the emergency department has good specificity and positive predictive value (99.2% and 85.7%) but poor sensitivity (26.5%).

3. Risk scores—Six established risk scores for predicting acute MI are (1) the revised Goldman Risk Score (2) TIMI Risk Score (3) Global Registry of Acute Cardiac Events Risk Score (4) HEART Risk Score (5) Vancouver Chest Pain Rule and (6) the European Society of Cardiology (ESC) 0/1, 0/2, 0/3-h algorithm. A study comparing these risk scores (not including the ESC algorithm) for predicting acute MI within 30 days reported a sensitivity of 98% (which correlates with a negative predictive value of ≥ 99.5%) if patients had a modified Goldman score of < 1 with normal high-sensitivity troponin T, a TIMI score < 1 with normal high-sensitivity troponin T, TIMI score of 0 with normal high-sensitivity troponin T, or HEART score of ≤ 3 with normal high-sensitivity troponin I. In Black patients with average cardiovascular risk, HEART score better predicts 6-week major adverse cardiac events compared with TIMI score. Six-week major adverse cardiac events among patients with a low-risk HEART score (0–3) is 0.9–1.7%. However, the HEART score performs less accurately in stratifying risk from cocaine-associated chest pain and does not eliminate the potential for gender bias. A study found that female patients with high HEART scores were admitted to the hospital from the emergency room at lower rates than male patients with similar HEART scores, although the clinical decision pathway did not result in sex-based differences in risk stratification or noninvasive testing.

The 0/1-hour accelerated protocol for evaluation of MI compared with a 0/3-hour standard care protocol and application of a modified HEART score did not lead to safer ED discharges.

4. Chest radiography—CXR is often useful in evaluating chest pain and is always indicated when cough or shortness of breath accompanies chest pain. Findings of pneumomediastinum or new pleural effusion are consistent with esophageal perforation.

5. Stress echocardiography—Stress echocardiography is useful in risk stratifying patients with chest pain, even among those with significant obesity. Patients who arrive at the emergency department with chest pain of intermediate probability for ACS without electrocardiographic or biomarker evidence of an MI can be safely discharged from an observation unit after stress echocardiography if no wall motion abnormality is found.

6. Coronary CT angiography—Sixty-four–slice coronary CT angiography is an alternative to stress testing in the emergency department for detecting ACS among patients with normal or nonspecific ECG and normal biomarkers. A meta-analysis of nine studies found CT angiography had an estimated sensitivity of 95% for ACS and specificity of 87%, yielding a negative LR of 0.06 and a positive LR of 7.4.

7. Functional testing—Exercise ECG, nuclear stress testing, or stress echocardiography appear to be the best initial noninvasive tests in symptomatic patients with suspected CAD.

A minimal-risk model for discharging patients with suspected ACS for whom noninvasive testing may be deferred was developed by the PROMISE investigators, and includes 10 clinical variables that correlate with normal coronary CT angiography results and no clinical events: (1) younger age (mean 57.5); (2) female sex; (3) racial or ethnic minority; (4–6) no history of hypertension, diabetes, or dyslipidemia; (7) no family history of premature CAD; (8) never smoked cigarettes; (9) symptoms unrelated to physical or mental stress; and (10) higher HDL cholesterol level.

In the PROMISE trial, women had higher rates of normal noninvasive testing compared with men, but women with abnormalities on such testing were less likely to be referred for catheterization or to receive statin therapy.

In the evaluation of PE as the cause of chest pain, diagnostic test decisions and results must be interpreted in the context of the clinical likelihood of VTE. A negative D-dimer test helps exclude PE in patients with low clinical probability of VTE (3-month incidence, 0.5%); however, the 3-month risk of VTE among patients with intermediate and high risk of VTE is sufficiently high in the setting of a negative D-dimer test (3.5% and 21.4%, respectively) to warrant further imaging given the life-threatening nature of an untreated PE. CT angiography is the preferred initial diagnostic test, having approximately 90–95% sensitivity and 95% specificity for detecting PE (compared with pulmonary angiography). However, for patients with high clinical probability of VTE, lower extremity ultrasound or pulmonary angiogram may be indicated even with a normal helical CT.

Panic disorder is a common cause of chest pain, accounting for up to 25% of cases that present to emergency departments and a higher proportion of cases presenting in primary care office practices. Features that correlate with an increased likelihood of panic disorder include absence of CAD, atypical quality of chest pain, female sex, younger age, and a high level of self-reported anxiety. Depression is associated with recurrent chest pain with or without CAD (OR, 2.11).

Treatment

Treatment of chest pain should be guided by the underlying etiology. The term "noncardiac chest pain" is used when a diagnosis remains elusive after an extensive workup. Almost half of patients with noncardiac chest pain reported symptom improvement with high-dose PPI therapy. Relief of constipation may be therapeutic in PPI refractory noncardiac chest pain. A meta-analysis of 15 trials suggested modest to moderate benefit for psychological (especially cognitive-behavioral) interventions. It is unclear whether tricyclic or SSRI antidepressants have benefit in noncardiac chest pain. Hypnotherapy may offer some benefit.

When to Refer

- Refer patients with angina that is poorly controlled using maximal medical therapy to a cardiologist.
- Refer patients with poorly controlled, noncardiac chest pain to a pain specialist.
- Refer patients with sickle cell anemia to a hematologist.

When to Admit

- Failure to adequately exclude life-threatening causes of chest pain, particularly MI, dissecting aortic aneurysm, PE, and esophageal rupture.
- Patients with high risk of complications from PE, or when PE is likely despite negative spiral CT.
- TIMI score of 1 or more, HEART score > 3, abnormal ECG, and abnormal 0- and 2-hour troponin tests.
- Pain control for rib fracture that impairs gas exchange.

Dawson LP et al. Chest pain management using prehospital point-of-care troponin and paramedic risk assessment. JAMA Intern Med. 2023;183:203. [PMID: 36715993]

Irannejad K et al. Coronary CT angiography for acute chest pain in the emergency department: a systematic review of clinical utility. Emerg Care Med. 2025;2:46.

Mahler SA et al. Safety and effectiveness of the high-sensitivity cardiac troponin HEART pathway in patients with possible acute coronary syndrome. Circ Cardiovasc Qual Outcomes. 2024;17:e010270. [PMID: 38328912]

Rao SV et al. 2025 ACC/AHA/ACEP/NAEMSP/SCAI Guideline for the Management of Patients With Acute Coronary Syndromes: A Report of the American College of Cardiology/American Heart Association Joint Committee on Clinical Practice Guidelines. Circulation. 2025;151:e771. Erratum in: Circulation. 2025;151:e865. Erratum in: Circulation. 2025;151:e1098. Erratum in: Circulation. 2025;152:e402. [PMID: 40014670]

Rasmussen LD et al. The PROMISE minimal risk score improves risk classification of symptomatic patients with suspected CAD. JACC Cardiovasc Imaging. 2022;15:1442. [PMID: 35926903]

Spotts PH et al. Myocarditis and pericarditis. Prim Care. 2024;51:111. [PMID: 38278565]

Veasey CJ et al. The high-sensitivity HEART pathway safely reduces hospitalizations regardless of sex or race in a multisite prospective US cohort. Clin Cardiol. 2024;47:e70027. [PMID: 39417405]

PALPITATIONS

ESSENTIAL INQUIRIES

- Forceful, rapid, or irregular beating of the heart.
- Rate, duration, and degree of heartbeat regularity; age at first episode.
- Factors that precipitate or terminate episodes.
- Lightheadedness or syncope; neck pounding.
- Chest pain; history of MI or structural heart disease.

General Considerations

Palpitations are the reason that approximately 16% of patients with a cardiac symptom visit an outpatient clinic and represent 5.8 of every 1000 ED visits, with an admission rate of 24.6%. Palpitations are experienced in 3.3% to 11.5% of pregnancies. After ambulatory monitoring, most patients with palpitations are found to have benign atrial or ventricular ectopy or nonsustained ventricular tachycardia. In patients with structurally normal hearts, these arrhythmias are not associated with adverse outcomes. To avoid missing a dangerous cause of the patient's symptoms, clinicians sometimes pursue costly and invasive testing when a

Table 2–3. Palpitations: Patients at high risk for a cardiovascular cause.

Historical risk factors
Family history of significant arrhythmias
Personal or family history of syncope or resuscitated from sudden death
History of MI
Palpitations that occur during sleep
Anatomic abnormalities
Structural heart disease such as dilated or hypertrophic cardiomyopathies
Valvular disease (stenotic or regurgitant)
ECG findings
Long QT syndrome
Bradycardia
Second- or third-degree heart block
Sustained ventricular arrhythmias

conservative diagnostic evaluation is sufficient. The converse is also true.

Table 2–3 lists history, physical examination, and ECG findings suggesting a cardiovascular cause for the palpitations.

When assessing palpitations in an acute care setting, the clinician must ascertain whether the symptoms represent (1) significant CVD, (2) a cardiac manifestation of a systemic disease such as thyrotoxicosis, (3) an arrhythmia that is minor and transient, or (4) a benign somatic symptom that is amplified by the patient's underlying psychological state.

Etiology

Patients with palpitations who come to an emergency department instead of a medical clinic are more likely to have a cardiac cause (47% versus 21%), whereas psychogenic causes are more common among those who seek care in office practices (45% versus 27%). In a study of patients who went to a university medical clinic with the chief complaint of palpitations, the causes were cardiac in 43%, psychogenic in 31%, and miscellaneous in 10%.

Cardiac arrhythmias that can manifest as palpitations include sinus bradycardia; atrial fibrillation or flutter; sinus, supraventricular, and ventricular tachycardia; premature ventricular and atrial contractions; sick sinus syndrome; and advanced atrioventricular block.

Structural cardiac conditions that lead to palpitations due to cardiac arrhythmias include valvular heart diseases, such as aortic regurgitation or stenosis, atrial or ventricular septal defect, cardiomyopathy, congenital heart disease, pericarditis, arrhythmogenic RV cardiomyopathy, atrial myxoma, and rarely, left atrial appendage aneurysm, and primary cardiac angiosarcoma. The midsystolic click of mitral valve prolapse (MVP) does not diagnose a supraventricular arrhythmia (the association with MVP and supraventricular arrhythmia is epidemiologic). Ventricular arrhythmias are common in patients with mitral annulus disjunction.

Pericardial or myocardial infection with SARS-CoV-2 and other viruses, tuberculosis, and *Trypanosoma cruzi* (Chagas disease) can cause palpitations.

The most common psychogenic causes of palpitations are anxiety and panic disorder. The release of catecholamines during a significant stress or panic attack can trigger an arrhythmia. Asking a single question, "Have you experienced brief periods, for seconds or minutes, of an overwhelming panic or terror that was accompanied by racing heartbeats, shortness of breath, or dizziness?" can help identify patients with panic disorder.

Other causes of palpitations include fever, dehydration, hypoglycemia, hyperkalemia, anemia, thyrotoxicosis, mastocytosis, postural orthostatic tachycardia syndrome, and pheochromocytoma. Drugs (eg, cocaine, alcohol, caffeine, pseudoephedrine, cannabis, and illicit ephedra), prescription medications and drugs that prolong the QT interval (eg, digoxin, amitriptyline, erythromycin, methylphenidate, dofetilide), class 1 antiarrhythmics, dihydropyridine calcium channel blockers, acetylcholinesterase inhibitors, phenothiazines, theophylline, chemotherapeutic agents, and β-agonists can precipitate palpitations.

Pregnant patients are more prone to arrhythmias and ambulatory rhythm monitoring should be strongly considered.

Clinical Findings

A. Symptoms

Guiding patients through a careful description of their palpitations may indicate a mechanism and narrow the differential diagnosis. Pertinent questions include the age at first episode; precipitants; and rate, duration, and degree of regularity of the heartbeat during the subjective palpitations. Palpitations lasting < 5 minutes and a family history of panic disorder reduce the likelihood of an arrhythmic cause (LR+ = 0.38 and LR+ = 0.26, respectively). To better understand the symptom, ask patients to "tap out" the rhythm with their fingers. The circumstances associated with onset and termination can also help determine the cause. Palpitations that start and stop abruptly suggest supraventricular or ventricular tachycardias. Termination of palpitations using vagal maneuvers (eg, Valsalva maneuver or forced coughing) suggests supraventricular tachycardia.

Three common descriptions of palpitations are (1) "flip-flopping" (or "stop and start"), often caused by premature contraction of the atrium or ventricle, with the perceived "stop" from the pause following the contraction, and the "start" from the subsequent forceful contraction; (2) rapid "fluttering in the chest," with regular "fluttering" suggesting supraventricular or ventricular arrhythmias (including sinus tachycardia) and irregular "fluttering" suggesting atrial fibrillation, atrial flutter, or tachycardia with variable block; and (3) "pounding in the neck" or neck pulsations, often due to "cannon" A waves in the jugular venous pulsations that occur when the right atrium contracts against a closed tricuspid valve (common with premature ventricular contractions and atrial ventricular dissociation).

Palpitations associated with chest pain suggest ischemic heart disease, or if the chest pain is relieved by leaning forward, pericardial disease. Palpitations with lightheadedness, presyncope, or syncope suggest hypotension and may signify a life-threatening cardiac arrhythmia. Palpitations that occur regularly with exertion suggest silent ischemia, a rate-dependent bypass tract, hypertrophic cardiomyopathy, or arrhythmogenic RV cardiomyopathy. If a benign etiology cannot be determined at the initial visit, ambulatory monitoring or prolonged inpatient cardiac monitoring may be warranted.

Noncardiac symptoms should be elicited since palpitations may be caused by a normal heart responding to a metabolic or inflammatory condition. Weight loss suggests hyperthyroidism. Palpitations can be precipitated by vomiting or diarrhea causing electrolyte disorders and hypovolemia. Hyperventilation, hand tingling, and nervousness are common when anxiety or panic disorder is the cause of the palpitations. Palpitations associated with flushing, episodic hypertension, headaches, anxiety, and diaphoresis may be caused by a pheochromocytoma or paraganglioma.

A family history of palpitations or sudden death suggests an inherited etiology such as long QT syndrome or Brugada syndrome. Chagas disease may cause palpitations and acute myocarditis. Younger patients should be asked about consumption of "energy drinks." Dual use of cigarettes and e-cigarettes may cause palpitations.

B. Physical Examination

Cardiovascular examination can find abnormalities that increase the likelihood of specific cardiac arrhythmias. The presence of mitral valve prolapse (midsystolic click) is associated with the diagnosis of a supraventricular arrhythmia. The harsh holosystolic murmur of hypertrophic cardiomyopathy, which occurs along the left sternal border and increases with the Valsalva maneuver, suggests atrial fibrillation or ventricular tachycardia. A crescendo mid-diastolic murmur may be caused by an atrial myxoma. The presence of dilated cardiomyopathy, suggested by a displaced and enlarged cardiac point-of-maximal impulse, increases the likelihood of ventricular tachycardia and atrial fibrillation. In patients with chronic atrial fibrillation, in-office exercise (eg, a brisk walk in the hallway) may reveal an intermittent accelerated ventricular response. The clinician should look for signs of hyperthyroidism (eg, tremulousness, brisk deep tendon reflexes, or fine hand tremor) or signs of stimulant drug use (eg, dilated pupils or skin or nasal septal perforations). Visible neck pulsations (LR+, 2.68) in association with palpitations increase the likelihood of atrioventricular nodal reentry tachycardia.

C. Diagnostic Studies

1. ECG—A 12-lead ECG should be performed on all patients reporting palpitations; however, a specific arrhythmia will not be detected in most instances. Evidence of prior MI on ECG (eg, Q waves) increases the patient's risk of nonsustained or sustained ventricular tachycardia. Ventricular preexcitation (Wolff-Parkinson-White syndrome) is suggested by a short PR interval (< 0.20 ms) and δ-waves (upsloping PR segments). Left atrial enlargement (a terminal P-wave force in V1 more negative than 0.04 ms and notching in lead II) reflects an increased risk of atrial fibrillation. A prolonged QT interval and abnormal T-wave morphology suggest the long QT syndrome and an increased risk of ventricular tachycardia.

2. Monitoring devices—For high-risk patients (Table 2–3), further diagnostic studies are warranted. A stepwise approach has been suggested—starting with ambulatory monitoring devices (ambulatory ECG monitoring if the palpitations are expected to occur within the subsequent 72-hour period, event monitoring [see Zio Patch, below] if less frequent). An implantable loop recorder under the chest skin can be used for extended monitoring if clinical suspicion is high and symptom to rhythm correlation cannot be otherwise established. Although the use of an implantable loop recorder has traditionally been reserved for patients experiencing syncope, the diagnostic yield of this device may be cost-effective for a broader range of patients. In patients with recurrent unexplained palpitations, a single-lead, lightweight, continuously recording ambulatory adhesive patch monitor (Zio Patch) worn for 14–21 days increases diagnostic yield while reducing the cost of diagnosis. Symptom-rhythm correlation is 18% overall (highest for atrial fibrillation and isolated ectopic beats. Median time to actionable arrhythmia > 48 hours limiting utility of Holter monitor even with daily symptoms. Inpatient continuous monitoring is indicated if serious arrhythmias are strongly suspected despite normal findings on the ambulatory monitoring; invasive electrophysiologic testing should be done if the ambulatory or inpatient monitor records a worrisome arrhythmia.

An ambulatory cardiac monitoring or a signal-averaged ECG is an appropriate next step to help exclude ventricular tachycardia in patients with a prior MI. ECG exercise testing is appropriate in patients with suspected CAD and those with palpitations with physical exertion. Echocardiography is useful when physical examination or ECG suggests structural abnormalities or decreased ventricular function.

Treatment

Abstention from caffeine and tobacco may help. Often, reassurance suffices. If not, or in symptomatic patients, a trial of a β-blocker may be prescribed. A three-session course of cognitive-behavioral therapy that includes some physical activity has proven effective for patients with benign palpitations with or without chest pain. For treatment of specific atrial or ventricular arrhythmias, see Chapter 12.

When to Refer

- For electrophysiologic studies.
- For advice regarding treatment of atrial or ventricular arrhythmias.

When to Admit

- Palpitations associated with syncope or near-syncope, particularly for patients aged > 75 years with an abnormal ECG, hematocrit < 30%, shortness of breath, respiratory rate > 24/min, or a history of HF.
- Patients with risk factors for a serious arrhythmia.

Chua CE et al. Approach to palpitations in primary care. Singapore Med J. 2024;65:405. [PMID: 38973189]

De Backer J et al; ESC Scientific Document Group. 2025 ESC Guidelines for the management of cardiovascular disease and pregnancy. Eur Heart J. 2025;46:4462. [PMID: 40878294]
Mannhart D et al. Clinical validation of 5 direct-to-consumer wearable smart devices to detect atrial fibrillation: BASEL Wearable Study. JACC Clin Electrophysiol. 2023;9:232. [PMID: 36858690]

LOWER EXTREMITY EDEMA

ESSENTIAL INQUIRIES

- History of VTE.
- Symmetry of swelling.
- Pain.
- Change with dependence.
- Hyperpigmentation, stasis dermatitis, lipodermatosclerosis, ulceration.

General Considerations

Acute and chronic lower extremity edema present important diagnostic and treatment challenges.

Chronic venous insufficiency is by far the most common cause of lower extremity edema, affecting up to 2% of the population. Venous insufficiency is a common complication of DVT; however, only a small number of patients with chronic venous insufficiency report a history of this disorder. Venous ulceration commonly affects patients with chronic venous insufficiency, and its management is labor-intensive and expensive. Normal lower extremity venous pressure (in the erect position: 80 mm Hg in deep veins, 20–30 mm Hg in superficial veins) and cephalad venous blood flow require competent bicuspid venous valves, effective muscle contractions, normal ankle range of motion, and normal respirations. When one or more of these components fail, venous hypertension may result. The risk of cellulitis increases as the stage of chronic edema increases. Adults with unilateral or bilateral chronic edema have a 37–47% lifetime prevalence of cellulitis.

Clinical Findings

A. Symptoms and Signs

1. Unilateral lower extremity edema—Among common causes of unilateral lower extremity swelling, DVT is the most life-threatening. Clues suggesting DVT include a history of cancer, recent limb immobilization, or confinement to bed for at least 3 days following major surgery within the past month (Table 2–4). Adults with varicose veins have a significantly increased risk of DVT. Lower extremity swelling and inflammation in a limb recently affected by DVT could represent anticoagulation failure and thrombus recurrence but more often are caused by **postphlebitic syndrome** with valvular incompetence. Other causes of a painful, swollen calf include cellulitis, musculoskeletal disorders (Baker cyst rupture ["pseudothrombophlebitis"]), gastrocnemius tear or rupture, calf strain or trauma, and left common iliac vein compression (May-Thurner syndrome), complex regional pain syndrome, diabetic myonecrosis, as well as other sites of nonthrombotic venous outflow obstruction, such as the inguinal ligament, iliac bifurcation, and popliteal fossa.

Table 2–4. Risk stratification of adults referred for ultrasound to rule out DVT.

Step 1:		
Score 1 point for each		
Active cancer (treatment within the previous 6 months or current palliative care)		
Paralysis, paresis, or recent plaster immobilization of the lower extremities		
Recently bedridden for ≥ 3 days, or major surgery within the previous 12 weeks		
Localized tenderness along distribution of deep venous system		
Entire leg swelling		
Swelling of one calf ≥ 3 cm more than the other (measured 10 cm below the tibial tuberosity)		
Ipsilateral pitting edema		
Collateral superficial (nonvaricose) veins		
Previously documented DVT		
Step 2:		
Subtract 2 points if alternative diagnosis has equal or greater likelihood than DVT		
Step 3:		
Obtain sensitive D-dimer for score ≥ 0		
Score	**D-Dimer Positive[1]**	**D-Dimer Negative**
0–1	Obtain ultrasound	Ultrasound not required
≥ 2	Obtain ultrasound	

[1]"Positive" is above local laboratory threshold based on specific test and patient age.
Based on Wells PS et al. Evaluation of D-dimer in the diagnosis of suspected deep-vein thrombosis. N Engl J Med. 2003;349:1227. [PMID: 14507948]

2. Bilateral lower extremity edema—Bilateral involvement and significant improvement upon awakening favor systemic causes (eg, venous insufficiency) and can be presenting symptoms of volume overload (HF, cirrhosis, kidney disease [eg, nephrotic syndrome]). The most frequent symptom of chronic venous insufficiency is the sensation of "heavy legs," followed by itching. Chronic exposure to elevated venous pressure accounts for the brawny, fibrotic skin changes observed in patients with chronic venous insufficiency and the predisposition toward skin ulceration, particularly in the medial malleolar area. Pain, particularly if severe, is uncommon in uncomplicated venous insufficiency.

Lower extremity swelling is a familiar complication of therapy with calcium channel blockers (particularly felodipine and amlodipine), pioglitazone, gabapentin, and minoxidil. Airline flights longer than 10 hours are associated with edema even in the absence of DVT.

B. Physical Examination

Physical examination should include assessment of the heart, lungs, and abdomen for evidence of pulmonary hypertension (primary or secondary to chronic lung disease), HF, or cirrhosis. The skin findings related to chronic venous insufficiency depend on the severity and chronicity of the disease, ranging from hyperpigmentation and stasis dermatitis to abnormalities highly specific for chronic venous insufficiency: lipodermatosclerosis (thick, brawny skin; in advanced cases, the lower leg resembles an inverted champagne bottle) and atrophie blanche (small, depigmented macules within areas of heavy pigmentation). The size of both calves should be measured 10 cm below the tibial tuberosity and pitting and tenderness elicited. Swelling of the entire leg, or a leg that is ≥ 3 cm larger than the other, suggests deep venous obstruction. The left calf is normally slightly larger than the right due to the left common iliac vein coursing under the aorta.

A shallow, large, modestly painful ulcer located over the *medial* malleolus is a hallmark of chronic venous insufficiency, whereas small, deep, and more painful ulcers over the *lateral* malleolus are more apt to be due to arterial insufficiency, vasculitis, or infection. Diabetic vascular ulcers may be painless. When an ulcer is on the foot or above the mid-calf, causes other than venous insufficiency should be considered.

The physical examination is usually inadequate to distinguish lymphedema from venous insufficiency. Only the Kaposi-Stemmer sign (inability to pinch a fold of skin at the base of the second toe because of its thickness) is a significant predictor of lymphedema (OR, 7.9).

C. Diagnostic Studies

Patients without an obvious cause of acute unilateral lower extremity swelling (eg, calf strain) should have an ultrasound performed since DVT is difficult to exclude on clinical grounds. A prediction rule allows a clinician to exclude a lower extremity DVT in patients without an ultrasound if the patient has low pretest probability for DVT and a negative sensitive D-dimer test (the "Wells prediction rule") (https://www.mdcalc.com/wells-criteria-pulmonary-embolism) (Chapter 9). Previously unidentified lower extremity thrombi may be discovered in 21% of patients incompletely studied during the initial evaluation.

The diagnostic study of choice to detect chronic venous insufficiency due to venous incompetence is duplex ultrasonography. Assessment of the ankle-brachial pressure index is important in the management of chronic venous insufficiency since peripheral arterial disease may be exacerbated by compression therapy (see Chronic Venous Insufficiency, Chapter 14). Caution is required in interpreting the results of ankle-brachial pressure index in older patients and patients with diabetes due to the decreased compressibility of their arteries. A urine dipstick test that is strongly positive for protein can suggest nephrotic syndrome, and serum creatinine can estimate kidney function. Measuring serum albumin can further assess for nephrotic syndrome or chronic liver disease.

Lymphoscintigraphy can be confirm a clinical suspicion of lymphedema.

Treatment

See relevant chapters for treatment of edema in patients with HF (Chapter 11), nephrosis (Chapter 25), cirrhosis (Chapter 18), and lymphedema and venous stasis ulcers (Chapter 14). Edema resulting from calcium channel blocker therapy may respond to concomitant therapy with ACE inhibitors or ARBs.

A. Venous Insufficiency

In patients with chronic venous insufficiency without comorbid volume overload (eg, HF), it is best to avoid diuretic therapy since intravascular volume is relatively decreased. Instead, the most effective treatment involves (1) leg elevation, above the level of the heart, for 30 minutes three to four times daily and during sleep; (2) compression therapy; and (3) ambulatory exercise to increase venous return through calf muscle contractions.

A wide variety of stockings and devices are effective compression therapies to decrease swelling, prevent and heal venous leg ulcers, treat stasis dermatitis, and reduce the risk of cellulitis. They should be put on with awakening before hydrostatic forces result in edema. To control mild edema, 20–30 mm Hg compression is usually sufficient, whereas 30–40 mm Hg compression is usually required to control moderate to severe edema associated with ulcer formation. To maintain improvement, consider switching from an elastic stocking to one made of inelastic grosgrain material. Patients with decreased ankle-brachial pressure index should be managed in concert with a vascular surgeon. Compression stockings (12–18 mm Hg at the ankle) are effective in preventing edema and asymptomatic thrombosis associated with long airline flights in low- to medium-risk persons, and compression therapy decreases recurrence of cellulitis among patients with chronic venous insufficiency. Support stockings made of lighter material than compression stockings are recommended for pregnant patients during air travel.

A pilot study of neuromuscular stimulation in patients with chronic venous disease found less leg edema and improved blood supply to the skin and foot if worn 4–6 hours a day. A Cochrane review of 56 studies of the phlebotonics rutosides, hidrosmin, diosmine, calcium dobesilate, chromocarbe, Centella asiatica, disodium flavodate, French maritime pine bark extract, grape seed extract, and aminaftone found moderate-certainty evidence of slight edema reduction but little or no difference in quality of life and low-certainty evidence of no improvement in ulcer healing. Hydroxyethylrutoside and pycnogenol have shown some evidence of efficacy in reducing the pain of chronic venous insufficiency.

B. Lymphedema

For lymphedema, bandaging systems, such as the NOR-Band Short Stretch Compression Bandage or the Rosidal K

Short Stretch Bandage, applied twice weekly can be effective. Multicomponent compression bandaging may offer additional benefit. Short-term manual lymphatic drainage treatment may improve chronic venous insufficiency severity, symptoms, and quality of life. For patients with reduced mobility and leg edema, intermittent pneumatic compression treatment can reduce edema and improve ankle range of motion.

Liposuction, suction-assisted lipectomy, and subcutaneous drainage may have treatment benefit if conservative measures fail in treatment of lymphedema.

When to Refer

- Refer patients with chronic lower extremity ulcerations to wound care specialist.
- Refer patients with coexisting severe arterial insufficiency (claudication) that would complicate treatment with compression stockings to a vascular surgeon.

When to Admit

- Pending definitive diagnosis in patients at high risk for DVT despite normal lower extremity ultrasound.
- Severe, acute swelling, raising concern for an impending compartment syndrome.
- Severe edema impairing ability to ambulate or perform activities of daily living.

Hazim Alsararatee H et al. Assessing and managing lower limb oedema: a clinical review. Br J Nurs. 2024;33:S8. [PMID: 39506231]
Markarian B et al. Assessment modalities for lower extremity edema, lymphedema, and lipedema: a scoping review. Cureus. 2024;16:e55906. [PMID: 38601427]
Smith B et al. Chronic edema management of the lower extremities. Cureus. 2024;16:e63840. [PMID: 39099956]

FEVER & HYPERTHERMIA

ESSENTIAL INQUIRIES

- Age; injection substance use.
- Localizing symptoms of infection, weight loss; joint pain.
- Immunosuppression or neutropenia; history of cancer.
- Medications.
- Travel.

General Considerations

The average normal oral body temperature taken in midmorning is 36.7°C (range, 36–37.4°C). This range includes a mean and two standard deviations, thus encompassing 95% of a normal population (normal diurnal temperature variation is 0.5–1°C).

The normal rectal or vaginal temperature is 0.5°C higher than the oral temperature, and the axillary temperature is 0.5°C lower. However, a normal body temperature based on a peripheral thermometer (tympanic membrane, temporal artery, axillary, oral) does not always exclude the presence of a fever. To exclude a fever, a rectal temperature is more reliable than an oral temperature (particularly in patients who breathe through their mouth, are tachypneic, or are in an ICU setting where a rectal temperature probe can be placed to detect fever).

Fever is a regulated rise to a new "set point" of body temperature in the hypothalamus induced by pyrogenic cytokines. These cytokines include IL-1, TNF, interferon-γ, and IL-6. The elevation in temperature results from either increased heat production (eg, shivering) or decreased heat loss (eg, peripheral vasoconstriction).

Hyperthermia—not mediated by cytokines—occurs when body metabolic heat production (as in thyroid storm) or environmental heat load exceeds normal heat loss capacity or when there is impaired heat loss (eg, heat stroke).

Clinical Findings

A. Symptoms and Signs

1. Fever—Body temperature in cytokine-induced fever (38.0–41.0°C) seldom exceeds 41.0°C unless there is structural damage to hypothalamic regulatory centers. Fever in adult patients in the ICU is defined as ≥ 38.3°C (single measurement) and fever in patients who are neutropenic is defined as ≥ 38.3°C or ≥ 38.0°C (single oral temperature) sustained over at > 1 hour. Fever as a symptom provides important information about the presence of illness—particularly infections—and about changes in the clinical status of the patient. Fever may be more predictive of bacteremia in older patients. The fever pattern, however, is of marginal value for most specific diagnoses except for the relapsing fever of malaria, borreliosis, and occasional cases of lymphoma, especially Hodgkin disease. The degree of temperature elevation does not necessarily correspond to the severity of the illness. Fever with rash and eosinophilia defines the drug reaction with eosinophilia and systemic symptoms (DRESS) syndrome.

In general, the febrile response tends to be greater in children than adults. Older persons, neonates, and persons receiving certain medications (eg, NSAIDs, corticosteroids), rather than a fever, a normal temperature or even hypothermia may be observed. Markedly elevated body temperature may result in profound metabolic disturbances. Febrile patients admitted to a hospital with a body temperature above 39.5°C had higher mortality and AKI events compared to patients with less fever (38.0–38.1°C). High temperature during the first trimester of pregnancy may cause congenital disabilities, such as anencephaly. Fever increases insulin requirements and alters the metabolism and disposition of drugs used to treat the diverse diseases associated with fever.

The source of fever varies by population and setting. In patients who underwent shoulder arthroplasty and developed fever, an infectious cause was found in only six of 92 patients. In the neurologic ICU, fever can occur directly from brain injury ("central fever"). One model predicted "central fever" with 90% probability if a patient met all of the following criteria: (1) < 72 hours of neurologic ICU admission; (2) presence of subarachnoid hemorrhage, intraventricular hemorrhage, or brain tumor; (3) absence of infiltrate on CXR; and (4) negative cultures. For patients in the ICU, elevated procalcitonin and CRP levels favor infection, rather than central fever, as the cause of fever.

Spinal cord injury may cause fever by the loss of supraspinal control of the sympathetic nervous system and defective thermoregulation due to loss of sensation. Fever may also be more common in patients with other forms of trauma. In a study of 268 patients, including patients with multiple injuries (n = 59), isolated head injuries (n = 97), isolated body injuries (n = 100), and minor trauma (n = 12), the incidence of fever was similar in all groups irrespective of injury (11–24%). In all groups, there was a significant association between the presence of early fever and death in the hospital (6–18% versus 0–3%), as well as longer median ICU stays (3–7 days versus 2–3 days).

The prevalence of intrapartum fever of ≥ 38°C in pregnancies of 36 weeks' gestation or more is 6.8% (1 in 15 women in labor), but the neonatal sepsis rate among affected mothers is 0.24% (< 1 in 400 babies). This finding calls into question the need for universal laboratory work, cultures, and antibiotic treatment pending culture results for this newborn population.

Contrary to classical teaching, postoperative atelectasis probably does not cause fever. Febrile nonhemolytic transfusion reaction is common, occurring in about 1% of transfusion episodes, and is mediated by proinflammatory cytokines elaborated by donor leukocytes during storage.

2. Hyperthermia—Body temperature in life-threatening hyperthermia (core temperature ≥ 40°C) may rise to levels capable of producing irreversible protein denaturation and resultant brain damage; no diurnal variation is observed.

Malignant catatonia consists of catatonic symptoms, hyperthermia, autonomic instability, and altered mental status.

Neuroleptic malignant syndrome is a variant of malignant catatonia that is a rare and potentially lethal idiosyncratic reaction to neuroleptic medications, particularly haloperidol and fluphenazine. It has also been reported with atypical neuroleptics (such as olanzapine or risperidone) (see Chapter 28).

Serotonin syndrome resembles neuroleptic malignant syndrome but occurs within hours of ingestion of agents that increase levels of serotonin in the CNS, including SSRIs, MAOIs, tricyclic antidepressants, meperidine, dextromethorphan, bromocriptine, tramadol, lithium, and psychostimulants (such as cocaine, methamphetamine, and MDMA) (see Chapter 42).

Clonus and hyperreflexia are more common in serotonin syndrome, whereas "lead pipe" rigidity is more common in neuroleptic malignant syndrome.

Malignant hyperthermia of anesthesia (see Chapter 42) shares common clinical and pathophysiologic features with neuroleptic malignant and serotonin syndromes.

3. Fever of undetermined origin—See Fever of Unknown Origin, Chapter 34.

B. Laboratory Findings

Laboratory studies should include a CBC with differential, ESR or CRP, liver biochemical tests, UA, and blood and urine cultures.

Serum procalcitonin The utility of a serum procalcitonin level in determining the cause of a fever depends on the clinical setting. For patients in the emergency department who are being admitted with fever, procalcitonin may help differentiate infectious fever (elevated serum procalcitonin) and central fever (without significant elevation in serum procalcitonin). However, procalcitonin-on-admission has poor sensitivity in ruling out blood stream infections. In the ICU, elevated procalcitonin and CRP levels favor infection over central fever.

C. Imaging

Initial imaging studies include CXR, and possibly abdominal ultrasound, and chest and abdominal CT scan. A transesophageal echocardiogram can evaluate for endocarditis, as indicated.

D. Diagnostic Procedures

A temporal artery biopsy can diagnose temporal arteritis in a febrile patient aged ≥ 60 years who has an elevated ESR.

Treatment

Most fever is well tolerated. When the temperature is < 40°C, only symptomatic treatment is required. Although fever may be associated with poor clinical outcomes in patients with traumatic brain injury, cerebrovascular accident, and cardiac arrest, the treatment of fever with antipyretics does not appear to affect mortality of critically ill patients or the number of ICU-free days. *A temperature > 41°C is likely to be hyperthermia rather than cytokine-mediated fever, and emergent management is indicated.* (See Heat Stroke, Chapter 41.)

A. General Measures for Removal of Heat

Regardless of the cause of the fever, alcohol sponges, cold sponges, ice bags, ice-water enemas, and ice baths will lower body temperature (see Chapter 41). They are more useful in hyperthermia since in patients with fever, the cytokines can override these therapies.

B. Pharmacologic Treatment of Fever

1. Antipyretic drugs—Antipyretic therapy is only needed for patients with marginal hemodynamic status. It can, however, be used for symptomatic relief. Aspirin or acetaminophen, 325–650 mg orally every 4 hours, is effective in reducing fever. These drugs are best administered around the clock, rather than as needed, since "as needed" dosing results in periodic chills and sweats due to fluctuations in temperature caused by varying levels of drug.

2. Prophylactic antimicrobial therapy—Antibacterial and antifungal prophylactic regimens are recommended only for patients expected to have < 100 neutrophils/mcL for > 7 days, unless other factors increase risks for complications or mortality.

3. Empiric antimicrobial therapy—Empiric antibiotic therapy is sometimes warranted. Even before infection can be documented, prompt broad-spectrum antimicrobials are indicated for febrile patients who have hemodynamic instability, severe neutropenia (neutrophils < 500/mcL [0.5×10^9/L]), asplenia (surgical or from sickle cell disease), or immunosuppression (from HIV infection [see Chapter 35] or from medications such as systemic corticosteroids, azathioprine, cyclosporine) (Tables 34–1 and 34–5).

Fever with neutropenia requires that initial doses of empiric antibacterial therapy are received by patients within an hour of triage; patients should either be monitored for at least 4 hours to determine suitability for outpatient management or be admitted to the hospital (see Infections in the Immunocompromised Patient, Chapter Part 34). It is standard to admit patients to the hospital with febrile neutropenic episodes, although carefully selected patients may be managed as outpatients after systematic assessment beginning with a validated risk index (eg, Multinational Association for Supportive Care in Cancer [MASCC] score or Talcott rules). In the MASCC index calculation, low-risk factors include the following: age < 60 years (2 points), burden of illness (5 points for no or mild symptoms and 3 points for moderate symptoms), outpatient status (3 points), solid tumor or hematologic malignancy with no previous fungal infection (4 points), no COPD (4 points), no dehydration requiring parenteral fluids (3 points), and systolic blood pressure > 90 mm Hg (5 points). Patients with neutropenia and MASCC scores > 21 or in Talcott group 4 (presentation as an outpatient without significant comorbidity or uncontrolled cancer), and without other risk factors, can be managed safely as outpatients.

The carefully selected neutropenic outpatients determined to be at low risk by MASCC score (particularly in combination with a normal serum CRP level) or by Talcott rules can be managed with an oral fluoroquinolone plus amoxicillin/clavulanate (or clindamycin, if penicillin allergic), unless fluoroquinolone prophylaxis was used before fever developed. For treatment of fever during neutropenia following chemotherapy, outpatient parenteral antimicrobial therapy can be provided effectively and safely in low-risk patients with a single agent, such as cefepime, piperacillin/tazobactam, imipenem, meropenem, or doripenem. High-risk patients should be referred for inpatient management with combination parenteral antimicrobial therapy based on specific risk factors such as pneumonia-causing pathogens or central line–associated bloodstream infections (see Infections in the Immunocompromised Patient and Table 34–1 in Chapter 34 and see Infections in Chapter 43).

If a fungal infection is suspected in patients with prolonged fever and neutropenia, fluconazole is equally effective as amphotericin B but less toxic.

C. Treatment of Hyperthermia

Discontinuation of the offending agent is mandatory. Treatment of neuroleptic malignant syndrome includes dantrolene in combination with bromocriptine or levodopa (see Chapter 28). Treatment of serotonin syndrome includes a central serotonin receptor antagonist—cyproheptadine or chlorpromazine—alone or in combination with a benzodiazepine (see Chapter 42). In patients for whom it is difficult to distinguish which syndrome is present, treatment with a benzodiazepine may be the safest therapeutic option.

When to Admit

- For vital sign abnormalities or evidence of end-organ dysfunction when early sepsis is suspected.
- Patients with febrile neutropenia at high risk for clinical decompensation.
- For measures to control a temperature > 41°C or when fever is associated with seizure or other mental status changes.
- Heat stroke (see Chapter 41).
- Malignant catatonia; neuroleptic malignant syndrome; serotonin syndrome; malignant hyperthermia of anesthesia.

Alhazzani W et al. New fever in adults in the intensive care unit: current insights from the 2024 Society of Critical Care Medicine and Infectious Diseases Society of America guidelines. Pol Arch Intern Med. 2025;135:17121. [PMID: 40955858]

Barletta JF et al. Management of heat-related illness and injury in the ICU: a concise definitive review. Crit Care Med. 2024;52:362. [PMID: 38240487]

Holgersson J et al. Fever therapy in febrile adults: systematic review with meta-analyses and trial sequential analyses. BMJ. 2022;378:e069620. [PMID: 35820685]

Kwak H et al; SNUCARE investigator. Afebrile status at the time of emergency department visit is associated with delayed antibiotic therapy in patients with sepsis (revised). Am J Emerg Med. 2024;83:69. [PMID: 38976929]

O'Grady NP et al. Society of Critical Care Medicine and the Infectious Diseases Society of America Guidelines for Evaluating New Fever in Adult Patients in the ICU. Crit Care Med. 2023;51:1570. [PMID: 37902340]

Speaker SL et al. Relationship between oral temperature and bacteremia in hospitalized patients. J Gen Intern Med. 2023;38:2742. [PMID: 36997793]

INVOLUNTARY WEIGHT LOSS

ESSENTIAL INQUIRIES

- Age; caloric intake; secondary confirmation (eg, changes in clothing size).
- Fever; change in bowel habits.
- Substance use.
- Age-appropriate cancer screening history.

General Considerations

Body weight is determined by a person's caloric intake, absorptive capacity, metabolic rate, and energy losses. Body weight normally peaks by the fifth or sixth decade and then gradually declines at a rate of 1–2 kg per decade. In NHANES II, a national survey of community-dwelling older adults (aged 50–80 years), recent involuntary weight loss (IWL) (> 5% usual body weight) was reported by 7% of respondents, and this was associated with a 24% higher mortality. In postmenopausal women, unintentional weight loss was associated with increased rates of hip and vertebral fractures.

Etiology

IWL is clinically significant when it exceeds 5% or more of usual body weight over a 6- to 12-month period. While it often indicates serious physical or psychological illness, nonmalignant diseases more commonly cause unintentional weight loss than malignant causes. Physical causes are usually evident during the initial evaluation, but an easily identifiable cause is not found in 6–28% of cases. The most common causes are cancer (about 30%), GI disorders (about 15%), and dementia or depression (about 15%). At a university hospital in Thailand, the three most common causes of IWL were reduced appetite (20.1%), dementia (13.7%), and medications (11.0%). Nearly half of patients with Parkinson disease have weight loss associated with disease progression. When an adequately nourished–appearing patient reports weight loss, inquiry should be made about exact weight changes (with approximate dates) and changes in clothing size. Family members can confirm weight loss, as can old documents such as photographs from driver's licenses. A mild, gradual weight loss occurs in some older individuals because of decreased energy requirements. However, rapid IWL is predictive of morbidity and mortality.

In addition to various disease states, causes in older individuals include loss of teeth and consequent difficulty with chewing, medications interfering with taste or causing nausea, alcohol use disorder, and social isolation. Among Black persons at an adult day health center, 65% had a significant nutritional disorder: 48.5% reported IWL or weight gain, 21% ate fewer than two meals daily, and 41.2% had tooth loss or mouth pain.

Clinical Findings

Once the weight loss is established, the history, medication profile, physical examination, and conventional laboratory and radiologic investigations (eg, CBC, liver biochemical tests, kidney panel, serologic tests including HIV, TSH, UA, fecal occult blood test, and CXR) usually reveal the cause. Age-appropriate cancer screening should be completed as recommended by guidelines (eg, Papanicolaou smear, mammography, fecal occult blood test/screening colonoscopy/flexible sigmoidoscopy, possibly PSA) (Chapter 1). Whole-body CT imaging is increasingly used for diagnosis; one study found its diagnostic yield to be 33.5%. Another study found a low yield from CT scanning with contrast of the abdomen and pelvis for malignancy (2.3%) in patients whose only symptom was weight loss. When these tests are normal, a more definitive GI investigation (eg, tests for malabsorption, endoscopy) should be considered. However, one prospective case study in patients with IWL showed that colonoscopy did not find colorectal cancer if weight loss was the sole indication for the test. A low spot urinary creatinine may be a marker of muscle wasting in patients with new-onset or worsening HF as a cause of IWL.

If the initial evaluation is unrevealing, follow-up is preferable to further diagnostic testing. Death at 2-year follow-up was not nearly as common in patients with unexplained IWL (8%) as in those with weight loss due to malignant (79%) and established nonmalignant diseases (19%). Psychiatric consultation should be considered when there is evidence of depression, dementia, anorexia nervosa, or other emotional problems. Ultimately, in approximately 15–25% of cases, no cause for the weight loss can be found.

Differential Diagnosis

Malignancy, GI disorders (poorly fitting dentures, cavities, swallowing or malabsorption disorders, pancreatic insufficiency), HF, HIV, tuberculosis, psychological problems (dementia, depression, paranoia), endocrine disorders (hyper-, hypothyroidism, hyperparathyroidism, hypoadrenalism), Whipple disease, eating problems (dietary restrictions, lack of money for food, teeth problems), social issues (alcohol use disorder, social isolation), and medication side effects are all established causes.

Treatment

Weight stabilization occurs in most surviving patients with both established and unknown causes of weight loss through treatment of the underlying disorder and caloric supplementation. Nutrient intake goals are established in relation to the severity of weight loss, in general ranging from 30–40 kcal/kg/day. In order of preference, routes of administration include oral, temporary nasojejunal tube, or percutaneous gastric or jejunal tube. Parenteral nutrition is reserved for patients with serious associated problems. Various pharmacologic agents have been proposed for the treatment of weight loss. These can be categorized into appetite stimulants (corticosteroids, progestational agents, cannabinoids, and serotonin antagonists); anabolic agents (growth hormone, ghrelin, and testosterone derivatives); and anticatabolic agents (omega-3 fatty acids, pentoxifylline, hydrazine sulfate, and thalidomide). There is no evidence that appetite stimulants decrease mortality, and they may have severe adverse side effects. The anabolic agent nandrolone decanoate reversed weight and lean tissue loss in women with HIV, and human growth hormone temporarily increased weight and walking speed in undernourished older patients. However, studies have not consistently shown mortality benefit.

Exercise training may prevent or even reverse the process of muscle wasting in HF ("cardiac cachexia"). Protein or creatine supplementation combined with resistance exercise training and aerobic activity may prevent aging-related attenuation of muscle mass and functional performance. Some patients with cancer-associated weight loss may benefit from nutritional assessment and intervention as decreased food intake may be playing a role.

When to Refer

- Weight loss caused by malabsorption.
- Persistent nutritional deficiencies despite adequate supplementation.
- Weight loss as a result of anorexia or bulimia.

When to Admit

- Severe protein-energy malnutrition, including the syndromes of kwashiorkor and marasmus.
- Vitamin deficiency syndromes.
- Cachexia with anticipated progressive weight loss secondary to unmanageable psychiatric disease.
- Careful electrolyte and fluid replacement in protein-energy malnutrition and avoidance of "re-feeding syndrome."

Gay L et al. Things We Do for No Reason™: prescribing appetite stimulants to hospitalized older adults with unintentional weight loss. J Hosp Med. 2022;17:389. [PMID: 35585691]
Soo MRT et al. Approach to weight loss in adults. Singapore Med J. 2024;65:291. [PMID: 39075874]
Yao S et al. A metabolite score of unintentional weight loss explained a substantial proportion of associated mortality and mobility limitation risk in a biracial older cohort. Aging Cell. 2025;24:e70181. [PMID: 40767847]

FATIGUE

ESSENTIAL INQUIRIES

- Weight loss; fever.
- Sleep-disordered breathing.
- Medications; substance use.

General Considerations

Fatigue, as an isolated symptom, accounts for 1–3% of visits to generalists. Fatigue or lassitude and the closely related complaints of weakness, tiredness, and lethargy are often attributed to overexertion, poor physical conditioning, sleep disturbance, obesity, undernutrition, and emotional problems. A history of the patient's daily living and working habits may obviate the need for extensive and unproductive diagnostic studies.

Fatigue in older adults increases the development of negative health outcomes (mortality OR, 2.14), the development of disabilities in basic activities of daily living (OR, 3.22), or the occurrence of physical decline (OR, 1.42).

Chronic fatigue conditions have been classified using numerous approaches since 1986. The prevailing clinical criteria in use today for chronic fatigue conditions are those of the Institute of Medicine's (National Academy of Medicine) for **systemic exertion intolerance disease (SEID).** The CDC have adopted the SEID criteria but continue to use the term **myalgic encephalitis/chronic fatigue syndrome (ME/CFS)** to reference this disorder. Common to all definitions is the lack of a single pathogenic mechanism, and no single physical finding or laboratory test can confirm the diagnosis.

Clinical Findings

A. Fatigue

Clinically relevant fatigue is composed of three major components: generalized weakness (difficulty in initiating activities); easy fatigability (difficulty in completing activities); and mental fatigue (difficulty with concentration and memory). Important diseases that can cause fatigue include hyper- and hypothyroidism, hyperparathyroidism, HF, infections (endocarditis, hepatitis), COPD, asthma, interstitial lung disease, CKD stage 3 and 4 and ESKD, sleep apnea, anemia, autoimmune disorders, multiple sclerosis, IBD, irritable bowel syndrome, Parkinson disease, cerebral vascular accident, and cancer.

Alcohol use disorder, vitamin C deficiency (scurvy), side effects from medications (eg, sedatives and β-blockers), and psychological conditions (eg, insomnia, depression, anxiety, panic attacks, dysthymia, and somatic symptom disorder) may be the cause. Common outpatient infectious causes include mononucleosis and sinusitis. These conditions are usually associated with other characteristic signs, but patients may emphasize fatigue and not discuss their other symptoms unless directly asked. The lifetime prevalence of significant fatigue (present for ≥ 2 weeks) is about 25%. Fatigue of unknown cause or related to psychiatric illness exceeds that due to physical illness, injury, alcohol, or medications.

Although frequently associated with Lyme disease, severe fatigue as a long-term sequela is rare. Posttraumatic brain injury fatigue and sleep disturbance may respond to a light box and in-home dynamic light therapy.

B. Systemic Exertion Intolerance Disease or Myalgic Encephalitis/Chronic Fatigue Syndrome

Diagnosis of SEID or ME/CFS requires the presence of all three of the following symptoms:

1. Substantial reduction or impairment in the ability to engage in pre-illness levels of occupational, educational, social, or personal activities that persists for > 6 months and is accompanied by fatigue, which is often profound, is of new or definite onset (not lifelong), is not the result of ongoing excessive exertion, and is not substantially alleviated by rest.
2. Post-exertional malaise.
3. Unrefreshing sleep.

In addition, the patient must have at least one of the following two manifestations: (1) cognitive impairment or (2) orthostatic intolerance (lightheadedness, dizziness, and headache that worsen with upright posture and improve with recumbency).

The evaluation of SEID includes a history and physical examination as well as CBC; ESR; kidney function; serum electrolytes, glucose, creatinine, calcium; liver biochemical tests and thyroid function tests; UA; tuberculin skin test; and screening questionnaires for psychiatric disorders. Other tests to be performed as clinically indicated are serum cortisol, ANA, rheumatoid factor, immunoglobulin levels, Lyme serology in endemic areas (although rarely a long-term complication of this infection), and HIV antibody. More extensive testing is usually unhelpful, including antibody to Epstein-Barr virus. There may be an abnormally high rate of postural hypotension.

Treatment

A. Fatigue

Resistance training and aerobic exercise lessens fatigue and improves performance for several chronic conditions associated with a high prevalence of fatigue, including HF, COPD, arthritis, and cancer.

1. Fatigue from obstructive sleep apnea—Continuous positive airway pressure is an effective treatment for obstructive sleep apnea. Pitolisant, a selective histamine H_3-receptor antagonist with wake-promoting effect, may reduce daytime sleepiness in patients with moderate to severe obstructive sleep apnea who decline continuous positive airway pressure treatment.

2. Cancer-related fatigue—Psychostimulants such as methylphenidate have shown inconsistent results in randomized trials for cancer-related fatigue. Internet-based cognitive-behavioral therapy is effective in reducing severe fatigue in those who have experienced breast cancer. Therapeutic care (a complementary medicine modality that uses acupressure) reduced fatigue in some patients with breast cancer receiving chemotherapy, while moderate-intensity exercise did not. Six weeks of Swedish massage therapy reduced fatigue in women with breast cancer who had surgery plus radiation, chemotherapy/chemoprevention, or both. Oral melatonin does not improve fatigue in patients with advanced cancer.

3. Fatigue from nervous system disorders—Methylphenidate and cognitive-behavioral therapy may improve mental fatigue and cognitive function in patients with traumatic brain injury. There is limited and preliminary evidence that rasagiline, modafinil, and doxepin improve fatigue in Parkinson disease. Amantadine, modafinil, and methylphenidate were not found to be superior to placebo in improving fatigue in multiple sclerosis and caused more frequent adverse events.

4. Other causes of fatigue—Modafinil and armodafinil appear to be effective, well-tolerated agents in patients who have HIV with fatigue and as adjunctive agents in patients who have depression or bipolar disorder with fatigue. Testosterone replacement in hypoandrogenic men aged > 65 years had no significant benefits for walking distance or vitality, as assessed by the Functional Assessment of Chronic Illness Therapy-Fatigue scale. However, men receiving testosterone reported slightly better mood and lower severity of depressive symptoms than those receiving placebo. Exceeding the recommended dietary allowance for protein intake does not increase muscle or physical function, augment anabolic response to testosterone in older men, or reduce muscle soreness or fatigue after prolonged moderate-intensity walking exercise.

Vitamin D treatment significantly improved fatigue after kidney transplantation and in otherwise healthy persons with vitamin D deficiency. Solution-focused therapy has a significant initial beneficial effect on the severity of fatigue and quality of life in patients with quiescent IBD. There is insufficient evidence to make conclusions about the benefits or harms of pharmacological treatment of fatigue in primary brain tumor. Armodafinil showed no benefit, however, in fatigued patients with high-grade glioma.

The treatment of subclinical hypothyroidism is unlikely to benefit symptoms of fatigue.

B. Systemic Exertion Intolerance Disease or Myalgic Encephalitis/Chronic Fatigue Syndrome

A variety of agents and modalities have been tried for the treatment of SEID without improvement in symptoms.

Some patients with postural hypotension report response to increases in dietary sodium and fludrocortisone, 0.1 mg orally daily. The immunomodulator rintatolimod improved some measures of exercise performance compared with placebo in two trials (with low strength of evidence). Low-dose naltrexone is being used off-label with anecdotal reports of benefit. There is limited evidence that dietary modification is beneficial.

Patients with SEID have benefited from a comprehensive multidisciplinary intervention, including optimal medical management, treating any ongoing affective or anxiety disorder pharmacologically, and implementing a comprehensive cognitive-behavioral treatment program.

When to Refer

- Infections not responsive to standard treatment.
- Difficult-to-control hyper- or hypothyroidism.
- Severe psychological illness.
- Malignancy.

When to Admit

- Failure to thrive.
- Fatigue severe enough to impair activities of daily living.

Chapman EJ et al. Practice review: evidence-based and effective management of fatigue in patients with advanced cancer. Palliat Med. 2022;36:7. [PMID: 34903113]

Grach SL et al. Diagnosis and management of myalgic encephalomyelitis/chronic fatigue syndrome. Mayo Clin Proc. 2023;98:1544. [PMID: 37793728]

Latimer KM et al. Fatigue in adults: evaluation and management. Am Fam Physician. 2023;108:58. [PMID: 37440739]

White B et al. Underlying disease risk among patients with fatigue: a population-based cohort study in primary care. Br J Gen Pract. 2024;75:e57. [PMID: 39084871]

ACUTE HEADACHE

ESSENTIAL INQUIRIES

- Age > 40 years.
- Rapid onset and severe intensity (ie, "thunderclap" headache), trauma, onset during exertion.
- Fever, vision changes, neck stiffness.
- HIV infection.
- Current or past history of hypertension.
- Neurologic findings (mental status changes, motor or sensory deficits, loss of consciousness).

General Considerations

Approximately 90% of people in the United States experience a headache in their lifetime. A broad range of disorders can cause headache (see Chapter 27). This section deals only with acute nontraumatic headache in adults and adolescents; migraine headache is covered in Chapter 27. The challenge in the initial evaluation of acute headache is to identify which patients exhibit an uncommon but life-threatening condition; approximately 1% of patients seeking care in emergency department settings and considerably less in office practice settings fall into this category.

Diminution of headache in response to typical migraine therapies (such as serotonin receptor antagonists or ketorolac) does not rule out critical conditions such as subarachnoid hemorrhage or meningitis as the underlying cause. A "sentinel headache" before a subarachnoid hemorrhage is a sudden, intense, persistent headache different from previous headaches; it precedes subarachnoid hemorrhage by days or weeks and occurs in 15–60% of patients with spontaneous subarachnoid hemorrhage.

Clinical Findings

A. Symptoms

A careful history and physical examination should aim to identify causes of acute headache that require immediate treatment. These causes can be broadly classified as (1) imminent or completed vascular events (intracranial hemorrhage, thrombosis, cavernous sinus thrombosis, vasculitis, malignant hypertension, arterial dissection, cerebral venous thrombosis, reversible cerebral vasoconstriction syndrome, transient ischemic attack, or aneurysm); (2) infections (abscess, encephalitis, or meningitis), intracranial masses causing intracranial hypertension, preeclampsia; and (3) carbon monoxide poisoning and methemoglobinemia. Having the patient carefully describe the onset of headache can help diagnose a serious cause.

Report of a sudden-onset headache that reaches maximal and severe intensity within seconds or a few minutes is the classic description of a "thunderclap" headache; it should precipitate workup for subarachnoid hemorrhage, since the estimated prevalence of subarachnoid hemorrhage in patients with thunderclap headache is 43%.

Thunderclap headache during the postpartum period precipitated by the Valsalva maneuver or recumbent positioning may indicate reversible cerebral vasoconstriction syndrome or irreversible cerebral venous sinus thrombosis. Venous-specific imaging sequences may be needed for diagnosis. Other historical features that raise the need for diagnostic testing include headache brought on by cough, exertion, or sexual activity.

The medical history can guide the need for additional workup. Under most circumstances (including a normal neurologic examination), new headache in a patient aged > 50 years or with HIV infection warrants immediate neuroimaging (Table 2–5). When the patient has a history of hypertension—particularly uncontrolled hypertension—a complete search for other features of "malignant hypertension" is appropriate to determine the urgency of control of hypertension (see Chapter 13). Headache and hypertension associated with pregnancy may be due to preeclampsia. Episodic headache associated with the triad of hypertension, palpitations, and sweats is suggestive of pheochromocytoma. In the absence of thunderclap headache, advanced age, and HIV infection, a careful physical examination and detailed neurologic examination will usually determine acuity of the workup and need for further diagnostic testing. A history consistent with hypercoagulability is associated with an increased risk of cerebral venous thrombosis.

Findings in migraine headache are discussed in Chapter 27. A systematic list called the SNNOOP10 has been developed as a screening method for secondary causes of headache (Table 2–6).

B. Physical Examination

Critical components of the physical examination of a patient with acute headache include vital signs, neurologic examination, and vision testing with funduscopic examination. The

Table 2–5. Clinical features associated with acute headache that warrant urgent or emergent neuroimaging.

Indications for neuroimaging prior to lumbar puncture
Abnormal neurologic examination (particularly focal neurologic deficits)
Abnormal mental status
Abnormal funduscopic examination (papilledema; loss of venous pulsations)
Meningeal signs
Indications for emergent neuroimaging completed prior to leaving office or emergency department
Abnormal neurologic examination
Abnormal mental status
"Thunderclap" headache
Patients with HIV with new type of headache[1]
Indications for urgent neuroimaging scheduled prior to leaving office or emergency department
Age > 50 years (normal neurologic examination) with new type of headache

[1]Use CT with or without contrast or MRI if positive for HIV.

Data from American College of Emergency Physicians. Clinical policy: critical issues in the evaluation and management of patients presenting to the emergency department with acute headache. Ann Emerg Med. 2008;52:407.

Table 2–6. SNNOOP10 list of "red" flags for secondary causes of headache.

Sign or Symptom	Related Secondary Headaches
Systemic symptoms	Headache attributed to infection, nonvascular intracranial disorders, carcinoid, or pheochromocytoma (orange for isolated fever)
Neoplasm in history	Neoplasms of the brain; metastasis
Neurologic deficit/dysfunction	Headaches attributed to vascular, nonvascular intracranial disorders; brain abscess and other infections
Onset of headache is sudden or abrupt	Subarachnoid hemorrhage and other headache attributed to cranial or cervical vascular disorders
Older age (> 50 years)	Giant cell arteritis and other headache attributed to cranial or cervical vascular disorders; neoplasms and other nonvascular intracranial disorders
Pattern change or recent onset of headache	Neoplasms, headaches attributed to vascular, nonvascular intracranial disorders
Positional headache	Intracranial hypertension or hypotension
Precipitated by sneezing, coughing, or exercise	Posterior fossa malformations; Chiari malformation
Papilledema	Neoplasms and other nonvascular intracranial disorders; intracranial hypertension
Progressive headache and atypical presentations	Neoplasms and other nonvascular intracranial disorders
Pregnancy or puerperium	Headaches attributed to cranial or cervical vascular disorders; postdural puncture headache; hypertension-related disorders (eg, preeclampsia); cerebral sinus thrombosis; hypothyroidism; anemia; diabetes mellitus
Painful eye with autonomic features	Pathology in posterior fossa, pituitary region, or cavernous sinus; Tolosa-Hunt syndrome (severe, unilateral headaches with orbital pain and ophthalmoplegia due to extraocular palsies); other ophthalmic causes
Posttraumatic onset of headache	Acute and chronic posttraumatic headache; subdural hematoma and other headache attributed to vascular disorders
Immunosuppression, eg, HIV, immunosuppressive medications	Opportunistic infections
Painkiller overuse or new drug at onset of headache	Medication overuse headache; drug incompatibility

Reproduced with permission from Do TP et al. Red and orange flags for secondary headaches in clinical practice: SNNOOP10 list. Neurology. 2019;92(3):134. https://n.neurology.org/content/92/3/134.long

finding of fever with acute headache warrants additional maneuvers to elicit evidence of meningeal inflammation, such as a Kernig sign (a supine patient with hips flexed to 90 degrees who displays resistance or reports pain with passive extension of the knees) and Brudzinski sign (supine patient who reflexively flexes the hip and knees after the examiner passively flexes the neck). The absence of jolt accentuation of headache (patient rotates their head horizontally at 2–3 turns per second for several seconds) cannot accurately rule out meningitis. Patients aged > 60 years should be examined for scalp or temporal artery tenderness.

Careful assessment of visual acuity, ocular gaze, visual fields, pupillary defects, optic disks, and retinal vein pulsations is crucial. Diminished visual acuity suggests glaucoma, temporal arteritis, or optic neuritis. Ophthalmoplegia or visual field defects may be signs of venous sinus thrombosis, tumor, or aneurysm. Afferent pupillary defects can be due to intracranial masses or optic neuritis. Ipsilateral ptosis and miosis suggest Horner syndrome and in conjunction with acute headache may signify carotid artery dissection. Finally, papilledema or absent retinal venous pulsations are signs of elevated intracranial pressure—findings that should be followed by neuroimaging before performing lumbar puncture (Table 2–5). On nonmydriatic fundoscopy, up to 8.5% of patients who arrive at the emergency department reporting headache had abnormalities; although few had other significant physical examination findings, 59% of them had abnormal neuroimaging studies. In the setting of headache and hypertension, retinal cotton wool spots, flame hemorrhages, and disk swelling indicate acute severe hypertensive retinopathy.

Complete neurologic evaluations should include assessment of mental status, motor and sensory systems, reflexes, gait, cerebellar function, and pronator drift. Any abnormality on neurologic evaluation (especially mental status) warrants emergent neuroimaging (Table 2–5).

C. Diagnostic Studies

1. Neuroimaging indications—Indications for neuroimaging are listed in Table 2–5. Under most circumstances, a noncontrast head CT is sufficient to exclude intracranial hypertension with impending herniation, intracranial hemorrhage, and many types of intracranial masses (notable exceptions include lymphoma and toxoplasmosis in patients with HIV, herpes simplex encephalitis, and brain abscess). When needed, a contrast study can be ordered to follow a normal noncontrast study. A normal neuroimaging study does not exclude subarachnoid hemorrhage and should be followed by lumbar puncture. One study supported a change of practice wherein a lumbar puncture can be withheld when a head CT scan was performed < 6 hours after headache onset and showed no evidence of subarachnoid hemorrhage (negative predictive value of 99.9%).

In a prospective study of 1536 emergency department patients, the yield for acute findings on head CT differed based on the indications for imaging and were 27% for seizures, 20% for confusion, 19% for syncope, 16% for focal neurologic deficit, 15% for head injury, 12% for headache, and 8% for dizziness.

In patients for whom there is a high level of suspicion for subarachnoid hemorrhage or aneurysm, a normal CT and lumbar puncture should be followed by angiography within the next few days (provided the patient is medically stable).

MRI is the modality of choice for evaluation of headache in pregnant patients and supported as safe by the American College of Radiology. Gadolinium contrast should be avoided whenever possible.

2. Lumbar puncture—This test is indicated to exclude infectious causes of acute headache, particularly in patients with fever or meningeal signs. CSF tests should routinely include Gram stain, WBC count with differential, RBC count, glucose, total protein, and bacterial culture. In appropriate patients, also consider testing CSF for Venereal Disease Research Laboratory (syphilis), cryptococcal antigen (patients with HIV), acid-fast bacillus stain and culture, and complement fixation and culture for coccidioidomycosis. Storage of an extra tube with 5 mL of CSF is prudent for conducting unanticipated tests in the immediate future. PCR tests for specific infectious pathogens (eg, herpes simplex 2) should be considered in patients with evidence of CNS infection but no identifiable pathogen.

The Ottawa Subarachnoid Hemorrhage (SAH) Rule had 100% sensitivity (and 13–15% specificity in different studies) in predicting subarachnoid hemorrhage. According to it, patients who seek medical attention in an emergency department describing an acute nontraumatic headache that has reached maximal intensity within 1 hour should be evaluated for subarachnoid hemorrhage if they have one or more of the following factors: age > 40 years, neck pain or stiffness, witnessed loss of consciousness, onset during exertion, thunderclap headache (instantly peaking pain), or limited neck flexion on examination.

In addition to neuroimaging and lumbar puncture, additional diagnostic tests for exclusion of life-threatening causes of acute headache include ESR (temporal arteritis; endocarditis), UA (malignant hypertension; preeclampsia), and sinus CT (bacterial sinusitis, independently or as a cause of venous sinus thrombosis).

Treatment

The treatment of migraine headaches is discussed in Chapter 27. Table 5–4 lists common medications used to treat benign headaches. Severe benign headache treated in the emergency department responds to haloperidol (2.5 mg intravenously).

Galcanezumab is an approved treatment for episodic cluster headache. High-flow oxygen therapy may effectively treat all headache types in the emergency department setting (eg, benefiting older patients with cluster headaches).

Metoclopramide plus diphenhydramine was more effective than placebo for acute posttraumatic headache (with 43% of the patients who received metoclopramide reporting adverse events).

When to Admit

- Need for repeated doses of parenteral pain medication.
- To facilitate an expedited workup requiring a sequence of neuroimaging and procedures.
- To monitor for progression of symptoms and to obtain neurologic consultation when the initial emergency department workup is inconclusive.
- Pain severe enough to impair activities of daily living or impede follow-up appointments or consultations.
- Patients with subarachnoid hemorrhage, intracranial mass, or meningitis.

American College of Emergency Physicians Clinical Policies Subcommittee (Writing Committee) on Acute Headache; Godwin SA et al. Clinical policy: critical issues in the evaluation and management of adult patients presenting to the emergency department with acute headache. Ann Emerg Med. 2019;74:e41. [PMID: 31543134]

Greige T et al. Managing acute headache in pregnant and postpartum women. Ann Emerg Med. 2024;84:51. [PMID: 38597849]

Lebedeva ER. Diagnostic criteria for acute headache attributed to ischemic stroke and for sentinel headache before ischemic stroke. J Headache Pain. 2022;23:11. [PMID: 35057731]

Viera AJ et al. Acute headache in adults: a diagnostic approach. Am Fam Physician. 2022;106:260. [PMID: 36126007]

DYSURIA

ESSENTIAL INQUIRIES

- Fever; new back or flank pain; nausea or vomiting.
- Vaginal discharge.
- Pregnancy risk.
- Structural abnormalities.
- Instrumentation of urethra or bladder.

General Considerations

Dysuria (painful urination) is a common reason for adults and adolescents to seek urgent medical attention.

An inflammatory process (eg, bacterial UTI, herpes simplex, autoimmune disorder) underlies most causes of dysuria. In women, bacterial cystitis is diagnosed in up to 50–60% of cases of dysuria. Cystitis has an incidence of

0.5–0.7% per year in sexually active young women. The key objective in evaluating women with dysuria is to exclude serious upper urinary tract disease, such as acute pyelonephritis, and STIs. In older men, dysuria may be a symptom of prostatitis; in younger men, urethritis accounts for most cases of dysuria. Male cyclists have no worse sexual or urinary functions than swimmers or runners, but cyclists are more prone to urethral stricture.

Clinical Findings

A. Symptoms

Well-designed cohort studies have shown that some cases of uncomplicated bacterial cystitis can be reliably diagnosed without a physical examination or UA, and RCTs show that telephone management of uncomplicated cystitis is safe and effective. An increased likelihood of UTI is present when women report multiple irritative voiding symptoms (dysuria, urgency, frequency), fever, or back pain (positive LRs, 1.6–2.0). A cohort study found that dysuria most reliably predicted a culture-positive UTI, although older patients with cognitive impairment may not have local urinary tract symptoms. History of recurrent UTI is associated with a positive urine culture (recurrent UTI adjusted OR 2.45). Inquiring about symptoms of vulvovaginitis is imperative. When reproductive age women report dysuria and urinary frequency and deny vaginal discharge and irritation, the LR for culture-confirmed cystitis is 24.5. In contrast, when vaginal discharge or irritation is present, as well as dysuria or urinary frequency, the LR is 0.7. Gross hematuria in women with voiding symptoms usually represents hemorrhagic cystitis but can be a sign of bladder cancer (particularly in older patients) or upper tract disease. Failure of hematuria to resolve with antibiotic treatment should prompt further evaluation of the bladder and kidneys. Chlamydial infection should be strongly considered among women aged ≤ 25 years who are sexually active and seeking medical attention for a suspected UTI for the first time or who have a new sexual partner.

Fever, back pain, nausea, and vomiting are clinical criteria for acute pyelonephritis. Women with these symptoms should usually be examined before initiation of treatment to exclude coexistent urosepsis, hydronephrosis, or nephrolithiasis that would affect management decisions. Risk factors for acute pyelonephritis among women aged 18–49 years relate to sexual behaviors (frequent sexual intercourse [three times per week or more], new sexual partner in the previous year, recent spermicide use), as well as diabetes mellitus and recent UTI or incontinence.

Presence of UTI during pregnancy is strongly associated with preeclampsia (particularly UTI during the third trimester).

B. Physical Examination

Fever, tachycardia, or hypotension suggests urosepsis and potential need for hospitalization. In uncomplicated circumstances, a focused examination in women can be limited to ascertainment of costovertebral angle tenderness as a finding for pyelonephritis and to a lower abdominal and pelvic examination if the history suggests vulvovaginitis or cervicitis. Findings of vulvar atrophy, pale mucosa, and narrowing of the introitus is consistent with genitourinary syndrome of menopause.

C. Diagnostic Studies

1. Urinalysis—UA is probably overutilized in the evaluation of dysuria. The probability of culture-confirmed UTI among women with a history and physical examination compatible with uncomplicated cystitis is about 70–90%. UA is most helpful in atypical presentations of cystitis. Dipstick detection (> trace) of leukocytes, nitrites, or blood supports a diagnosis of cystitis; when both leukocyte and nitrite tests are positive, the LR is 4.2, and when both are negative, the LR is 0.3.

The negative predictive value of UA is not sufficient to exclude culture-confirmed UTI in women with multiple typical symptoms, and randomized trial evidence shows that antibiotic treatment is beneficial to women with typical symptoms and negative UA dipstick tests. Microscopy of unspun urine may also be helpful in diagnosis and reduces unnecessary use of antibiotics. The combination of urgency, dysuria, and pyuria assessed with the high-power (40×) objective for leukocytes (> 1 leukocyte/7 high-power fields) had a positive predictive value of 71 and LR of 2.97. Urine samples produced at home rarely meet diagnostic standards.

2. Urine culture—Urine culture should be considered for all women with upper urinary tract symptoms (before initiating antibiotic therapy), concern for complicated (structural or functional abnormality, immunosuppression) urinary tract infection, as well as those with dysuria and a negative urine dipstick test. In symptomatic women, a clean-catch urine culture is considered positive when 10^2–10^3 colony-forming U/mL of a uropathogenic organism are detected. While awaiting culture results in these women, it is reasonable to use NSAIDs for symptom relief and recommend cranberry (pure extract) while continuing close follow-up. Urine culture sensitivity decreases rapidly after empiric antibiotic administration (75% of cultures are negative 9 hours after antibiotic treatment). Multiplex PCR analysis is as beneficial as a urine culture.

3. Renal imaging—When severe flank or back pain is present, the possibility of complicated kidney infection (perinephric abscess, nephrolithiasis) or hydronephrosis should be considered. Renal ultrasound or CT scanning should be done to rule out abscess and hydronephrosis. To exclude nephrolithiasis, noncontrast helical CT scanning is more accurate than renal ultrasound and is the diagnostic test of choice. In a meta-analysis, the positive and negative LRs of helical CT scanning for diagnosis of nephrolithiasis were 23.2 and 0.05, respectively.

Differential Diagnosis

The differential diagnosis of dysuria in women includes acute cystitis, acute pyelonephritis, vaginitis (*Candida*, bacterial vaginosis, *Trichomonas*, herpes simplex), urethritis/cervicitis (*Chlamydia*, gonorrhea, *Mycoplasma genitalium*), and interstitial cystitis/painful bladder syndrome. Recurrent or chronic culture-negative dysuria may represent genitourinary syndrome of menopause. Pelvic congestion syndrome (dilated and refluxing pelvic veins) may also cause dysuria and pelvic pain.

Nucleic acid amplification tests from first-void urine or vaginal swab specimens are highly sensitive for detecting chlamydial infection in men and women. Other infectious pathogens associated with dysuria and urethritis in men include *Mycoplasma genitalium* and Enterobacteriaceae.

Treatment

An evidence-informed algorithm for managing suspected UTI in women is shown in Figure 2–1. This algorithm supports antibiotic treatment of most women with multiple and typical symptoms of UTI without performing UA or urine culture. Pregnancy, underlying structural factors (polycystic kidney disease, nephrolithiasis, neurogenic bladder), immunosuppression, diabetes mellitus, and a history of recent bladder or urethral instrumentation usually alter the treatment regimen (antibiotic choice or duration of treatment, or both) for cystitis.

Telemedicine may be an appropriate technology to assess and manage uncomplicated bacterial UTIs for average-risk patients who can self-diagnose. Antibiotic selection should be guided by local resistance patterns and expert-panel clinical practice guidelines; major options for uncomplicated cystitis include nitrofurantoin, fosfomycin, ciprofloxacin, and trimethoprim-sulfamethoxazole. Five days of nitrofurantoin results in a significantly greater likelihood of clinical and microbiologic resolution than single-dose fosfomycin.

According to the American Academy of Pediatrics Committee on Drugs, antibiotics that are usually acceptable when treating women who are breastfeeding include trimethoprim-sulfamethoxazole (unless G6PD deficiency is present), amoxicillin, nitrofurantoin, ciprofloxacin, and ofloxacin.

In men, prolonged treatment of UTIs (> 7 days) out of concern for delayed clearance of infection within the prostate does not appear to reduce early or late recurrences. A 5-day course of fluoroquinolones for outpatient men with UTI is as effective as a 10-day course. Another study found that among afebrile men with symptoms of UTI, treatment with ciprofloxacin or trimethoprim-sulfamethoxazole for 7 days was noninferior to 14 days regarding resolution of UTI symptoms.

Symptomatic relief can be provided with phenazopyridine, a urinary analgesic available over the counter; it is used in combination with antibiotic therapy (when a UTI has been confirmed) but for no more than 2 days. Patients should be informed that phenazopyridine will cause orange/red discoloration of their urine and other body fluids (eg, some contact lens wearers have reported discoloration of their lenses). Rare cases of methemoglobinemia and hemolytic anemia have been reported, usually with overdoses or underlying kidney dysfunction. NSAIDs have also been shown to be of symptomatic benefit, but less effective than antibiotic therapy. Although some women recover from uncomplicated UTI when treated with NSAIDs alone (53% in a Norwegian study), the rate of progression to pyelonephritis was substantial. Delayed antibiotic therapy in older patients with UTI leads to a substantially higher rate of urosepsis and all-cause mortality. If a broad-spectrum antibiotic was initially prescribed empirically for UTI and urine culture results return establishing efficacy of a narrow-spectrum antibiotic, treatment should be "de-escalated" to the narrow-spectrum antimicrobial. Among premenopausal women with recurrent UTIs, the group with increased daily water consumption (1500 mL per day) had a lower mean number of cystitis episodes over a 12-month period of 1.7 compared with 3.2 in the control group and reduced number of antibiotic prescriptions (1.9 and 3.6, respectively). A systematic review of six randomized controlled trials found methenamine hippurate to be as effective as antibiotic prophylaxis in reducing recurrent UTIs. A double-blind, randomized, placebo-controlled trial across 99 primary care centers examined the use of D-mannose for protection against recurrent UTIs and found no benefit. In patients with asymptomatic renal calculi and recurrent UTIs, stone extraction eliminated infections in 50% of women. Vaginal estrogen effectively relieves urinary urgency and frequency as well as recurrent UTIs associated with genitourinary syndrome of menopause.

In cases of interstitial cystitis/painful bladder syndrome (see Chapter 26), patients will often respond to a multimodal approach that may include urethral/vesicular dilation, biofeedback, cognitive-behavioral therapy, antidepressants, dietary changes, vaginal emollients, and other supportive measures.

Asymptomatic bacteriuria—Asymptomatic bacteriuria (ASB) is defined as > 10^5 CFU/mL in a voided urine specimen without signs or symptoms attributable to UTI, regardless of whether pyuria is present. The incidence of asymptomatic bacteriuria increases with age and may be > 15% in women aged > 80 years (50% for those who reside in long-term care facilities). A meta-analysis found that antibiotic treatment for most people with asymptomatic bacteriuria is not beneficial and may be harmful. Antibiotic treatment benefits pregnant patients with asymptomatic bacteriuria as well as persons about to undergo urologic surgery. The USPSTF recommends screening pregnant patients for asymptomatic bacteriuria by obtaining a urine culture (B recommendation). The USPSTF recommends against screening for asymptomatic bacteriuria in nonpregnant adults (D recommendation). Urine WBC count > 25 cells/high-power field was associated with a 53.8% rate of bacteriuria in a study of 46,127 adult inpatients and is suggested to be the optimal "cutoff" value.

There were no differences in the prevalence of postoperative UTI in women who had mixed flora on preoperative urine cultures compared to those with no growth on preoperative urine cultures.

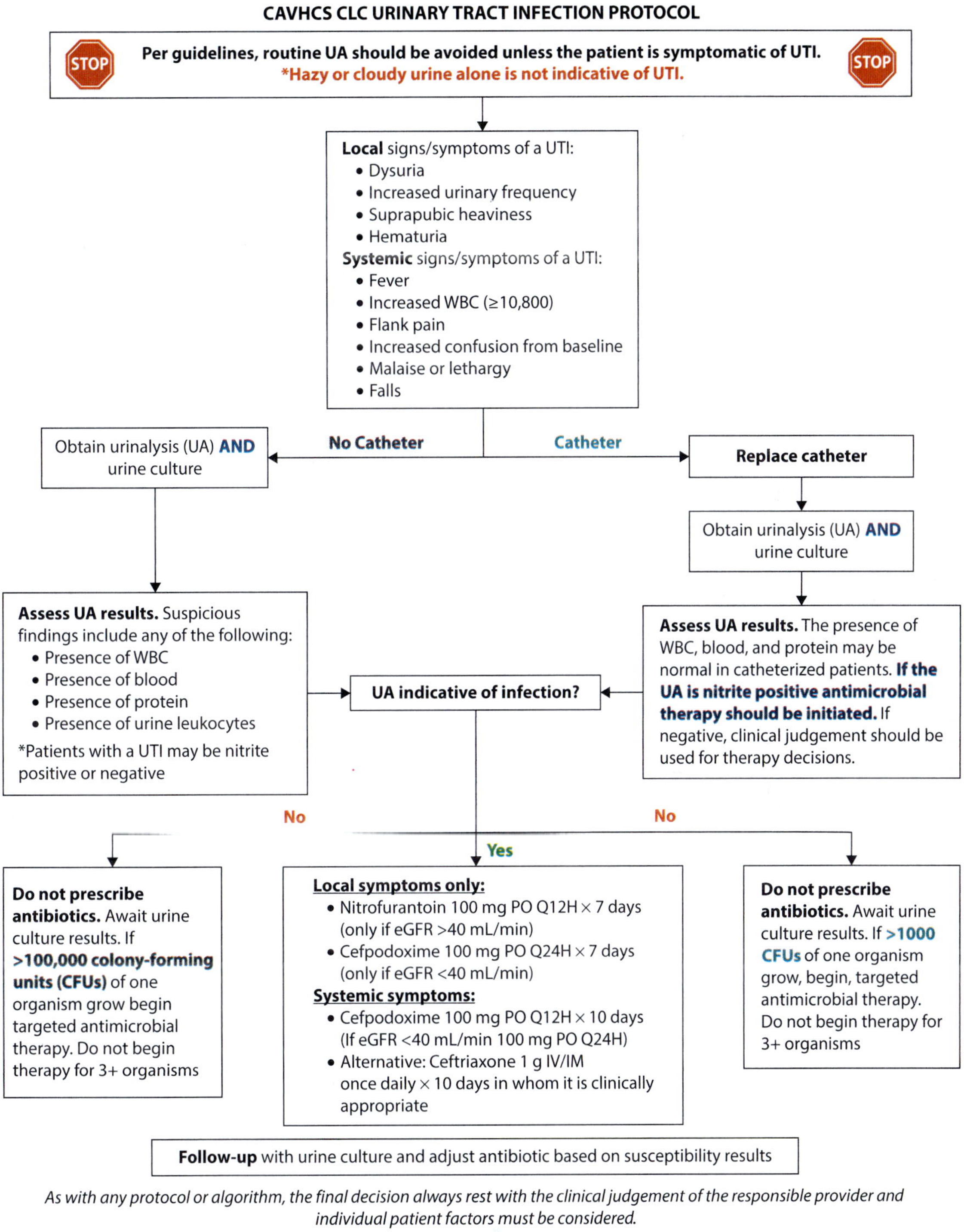

Figure 2–1. Algorithm outlining the Central Alabama Veterans Health Care System Community Living Center (CAVHCS CLC) protocol for evaluating UTI in women. (Reproduced with permission from Spencer H et al. Implementation of a urinary tract infection treatment protocol to improve prescribing practices in the long-term care facility of a veteran's healthcare system. Pharmacy (Basel). 2020;8:129. [PMID: 32722253])

When to Refer

- Anatomic abnormalities leading to repeated urinary infections.
- Infections associated with nephrolithiasis.
- Persistent interstitial cystitis/painful bladder syndrome.

When to Admit

- Severe pain requiring parenteral medication or impairing ambulation or urination (such as severe primary herpes simplex genitalis).
- Dysuria associated with urinary retention or obstruction.
- Pyelonephritis with ureteral obstruction.
- Symptoms and signs suggesting urosepsis.

Al Lawati H et al. Urinary tract infections: Core Curriculum 2024. Am J Kidney Dis. 2024;83:90. [PMID: 37906240]

Franco JVA et al. Advances in the diagnosis of urinary tract infection: a narrative review. Urogenit Tract Infect. 2025;20:17. doi:10.14777/uti.2550020010

Hayward G et al. d-Mannose for prevention of recurrent urinary tract infection among women: a randomized clinical trial. JAMA Intern Med. 2024;184:619. [PMID: 38587819]

Kurotschka PK et al. Acute uncomplicated UTIs in adults: rapid evidence review. Am Fam Physician. 2024;109:167. [PMID: 38393801]

Luu T et al. Asymptomatic bacteriuria: prevalence, diagnosis, management, and current antimicrobial stewardship implementations. Am J Med. 2022;135:e236. [PMID: 35367448]

Preoperative Evaluation & Perioperative Management

3

Hugo Q. Cheng, MD

EVALUATION OF THE ASYMPTOMATIC PATIENT

Patients without significant medical problems—especially those under age 50—are at very low risk for perioperative complications. Their preoperative evaluation should include a history and physical examination; emphasis should be on a pharmacologic history and assessment of functional status, exercise tolerance, and cardiopulmonary status to look for unrecognized disease that may require further evaluation before surgery. In addition, a directed bleeding history (Table 3–1) should be taken to uncover coagulopathy that could contribute to excessive surgical blood loss. Routine preoperative laboratory tests in asymptomatic healthy patients under age 50 have not been found to predict or prevent complications but adds a substantial unnecessary cost to surgical care. Even older patients undergoing minor or minimally invasive procedures (eg, cataract surgery) are unlikely to benefit from preoperative screening tests.

Mott NM et al. Right-size testing before elective surgery for patients with low risk. JAMA Netw Open. 2025;8:e2535750. [PMID: 41051774]

CARDIAC RISK ASSESSMENT & REDUCTION IN NONCARDIAC SURGERY

The most important perioperative cardiac complications are MI and cardiac death. Other complications include HF, arrhythmias, and need for urgent revascularization. The principal patient-specific risk factor for cardiac complications is the presence of end-organ CVD. This includes not only CAD and HF but also CKD and cerebrovascular disease. Diabetes mellitus, especially if treated with insulin, is considered a CVD equivalent that increases the risk of cardiac complications. Major abdominal, thoracic, and vascular surgical procedures carry a higher risk of postoperative cardiac complications. These six risk factors comprise the Revised Cardiac Risk Index (RCRI), a validated, multifactorial risk prediction tool (Table 3–2). Another widely used risk prediction tool comes from the American College of Surgeons' National Surgical Quality Improvement Program (NSQIP). This tool uses patient age, the type of operation, serum creatinine > 1.5 mg/dL (132.6 mcmol/L), dependency in activities of daily living, and the patient's American Society of Anesthesiologists physical status classification as predictors for postoperative MI or cardiac arrest. A risk calculator using the NSQIP tool can be found at https://qxmd.com/calculate/calculator_245/gupta-perioperative-cardiac-risk. The American College of Cardiology and American Heart Association endorse both prediction tools and define "elevated risk" as the presence of two or more RCRI predictors or a risk of perioperative MI or cardiac arrest > 1% as calculated by the NSQIP prediction tool.

Exercise capacity also predicts cardiac risk. Patients who are unable to exercise to four metabolic equivalents (METs), which is equivalent to walking two blocks on a flat surface at a normal pace or climbing one to two flights of stairs, have an elevated risk of cardiac complications. Patients with moderate to good exercise capacity can often forego further preoperative cardiac testing despite the presence of elevated risk based on a prediction tool.

Figure 3–1 shows an approach to preoperative cardiac risk assessment and management based on the 2024 American College of Cardiology and American Heart Association guideline and incorporating prediction tools, functional capacity, biomarkers, and noninvasive ischemia testing.

Table 3–1. Directed bleeding history: Findings suggestive of a bleeding disorder.

Unprovoked bruising on the trunk > 5 cm in diameter
Frequent unprovoked epistaxis or gingival bleeding
Menorrhagia with iron deficiency
Hemarthrosis with mild trauma
Prior excessive surgical blood loss or reoperation for bleeding
Family history of abnormal bleeding
Presence of severe kidney or liver disease
Use of medications that impair coagulation, including nutritional supplements and herbal remedies

Role of Preoperative Noninvasive Ischemia Testing

History and physical examination are sufficient to risk stratify most patients. A resting ECG should be obtained in patients with known or suspected heart or vascular disease before major surgery but generally omitted in asymptomatic

Table 3–2. Revised Cardiac Risk Index (RCRI).

Independent Predictors of Postoperative Cardiac Complications	
Intrathoracic, intraperitoneal, or suprainguinal vascular surgery	
History of ischemic heart disease	
History of HF	
Insulin treatment for diabetes mellitus	
Serum creatinine level > 2 mg/dL (> 176.8 mcmol/L)	
History of cerebrovascular disease	
Scoring (Number of Predictors Present)	**Risk of Major Cardiac Complications[1]**
0	0.4%
1	1%
2	2.4%
> 2	5.4%

[1]Cardiac death, MI, or nonfatal cardiac arrest.
Data from Devereaux PJ et al. Perioperative cardiac events in patients undergoing noncardiac surgery: a review of the magnitude of the problem, the pathophysiology of the events and methods to estimate and communicate risk. CMAJ. 2005;173:627.

patients undergoing minor operations. Additional noninvasive ischemia testing rarely improves risk stratification or management and should be avoided in patients without elevated risk based on a prediction tool, undergoing minor operations, or who have at least fair functional capacity. The 2024 American College of Cardiology and American Heart Association guideline emphasizes that stress testing or coronary CT angiography are primarily indicated to exclude high-risk coronary anatomy, such as left main coronary artery disease, rather than to identify undiagnosed CAD or assess risk. Prior to ordering these tests, providers should discuss their indication and how abnormal findings will be managed.

Role of Cardiac Biomarkers

Preoperative BNP or N-terminal fragment of proBNP (NT-proBNP) levels directly correlate with the risk for cardiac complications, and their measurement may improve risk assessment. The 2024 American College of Cardiology and American Heart Association guideline recommends measuring BNP or NT-proBNP in selected patients who have both elevated risk based on a prediction tool and limited functional capacity. Patients with normal biomarker measurements, defined as BNP < 92 ng/L or NT-proBNP < 300 ng/L, generally have acceptable cardiac risk and do not require additional risk stratification testing, even when clinical predictors indicate elevated risk.

Perioperative Management of Patients with Coronary Artery Disease

Patients with ACS require immediate management of cardiac disease before any preoperative evaluation (see Chapter 10).

A. Medications

1. Antianginal medications—Preoperative antianginal medications, including β-blockers, calcium channel blockers, and nitrates, should be continued throughout the perioperative period. Several trials have shown that initiation of β-blockers before major noncardiac surgery reduces the risk of nonfatal MI. However, in a 2008 trial, a high fixed-dose of metoprolol succinate *increased* total mortality and the risk of stroke. Because of the uncertain benefit-to-risk ratio, initiation of perioperative β-blockade should be considered only in patients with an indication that is independent of surgery. Initiation should be done far enough in advance of surgery (ideally > 1 week) to allow time to assess tolerability and titrate dosage. β-Blockers should not be started on the day of surgery.

2. Statins—Several randomized trials have found that HMG-CoA reductase inhibitors (statins) prevent MI in patients undergoing noncardiac surgery. Based on treatment protocols used in clinical trials, at least a moderate statin dose (eg, atorvastatin 20 mg or fluvastatin 80 mg orally daily) should be started in statin-naïve adults who meet criteria for long-term statin use and are scheduled for noncardiac surgery. Patients already taking statins should continue these agents during the perioperative period.

3. Aspirin—In patients without coronary stents, initiation of aspirin therapy before noncardiac surgery is not recommended because it did not reduce cardiac risk and caused increased bleeding in a large, randomized trial. Holding long-term prophylactic aspirin therapy in such patients does not increase cardiac risk.

B. Coronary Revascularization

A 2004 trial that randomly assigned over 500 patients with angiographically proven CAD to either coronary revascularization (with either coronary artery bypass grafting [CABG] or percutaneous coronary interventions [PCI]) or medical management alone before vascular surgery found no difference in postoperative MI, 30-day mortality, and long-term mortality. Thus, **preoperative CABG or PCI should be performed only when patients have guideline-concordant indications independent of the planned noncardiac operation.** Patients who have previously had CABG surgery or PCI have a relatively low risk of cardiac complications when undergoing subsequent noncardiac surgery.

Surgical patients who have undergone recent coronary stenting are at high risk for stent thrombosis, especially if antiplatelet therapy is stopped prematurely. **Elective surgery should be deferred for at least 30 days after placement of a bare-metal stent, for 6 months after placement of a drug-eluting stent for stable CAD, and for 12 months after drug-eluting stent placement for ACS.** If this delay poses significant risks, such as in patients undergoing an operation for cancer, surgery could be considered 3 months after drug-eluting stent implantation. Antiplatelet agents should be continued perioperatively if possible or resumed as soon as possible after surgery.

Step 1: Assess risk with the RCRI or NSQIP MICA calculator[1]
Are there ≥ 2 RCRI predictors or ≥ 1% risk of MICA?

No → Proceed to surgery

Yes ↓

Step 2: Assess functional capacity
Is functional capacity limited (eg, unable to perform at least 4 METs [eg, walk two blocks at normal pace or climb one to two flights of stairs]) or unknown?

No → Proceed to surgery

Yes ↓

Step 3: Consider whether BNP or NT-proBNP measurement will affect management[2]
If measured, is BNP > 92 ng/L or NT-proBNP > 300 ng/L?

No → Proceed to surgery

Yes ↓

Step 4: Multidisciplinary discussion on risks and benefits of delaying surgery for further testing and how test results will affect management[3]
If further testing is performed, are high-risk findings present (eg, indications of left main CAD or multivessel CAD with reduced EF)?

No → Proceed to surgery

Yes ↓

Step 5: Possible management options
- Select alternative invasive, noninvasive, or palliative management
- Re-evaluate after optimizing guideline-concordant heart disease treatment
- Perform invasive coronary angiography and revascularization if independent indications are present

[1]Regardless of prediction tool results, patients who have severe valve disease, severe pulmonary hypertension, cardiac implanted electronic devices, prior coronary revascularization, congenital heart disease, recent stroke, or severe frailty warrant condition-specific evaluation and management before surgery.
[2]If biomarker is not measured, consider deferral of planned operation, alternative invasive or noninvasive treatment, or palliation; or proceed to surgery with knowledge of elevated risk.
[3]Potential evaluation strategies include noninvasive stress testing, coronary CT angiography, and echocardiography. If further testing is not performed, consider deferral of planned operation, alternative invasive or noninvasive treatment, or palliation; or proceed to surgery with knowledge of elevated risk.

▲ **Figure 3–1.** Approach to cardiac evaluation in stable patients undergoing major elective surgery. METs, metabolic equivalents; NSQIP MICA, National Surgical Quality Improvement Program Myocardial Infarction and Cardiac Arrest; RCRI, Revised Cardiac Risk Index.

Postoperative MI

Postoperative MI (defined by a combination of ECG abnormality and cardiac enzyme elevation) typically occurs within 3 days of surgery and is usually not associated with chest pain. Clinical findings that should prompt its consideration include unexplained hypotension, hypoxemia, and delirium. An elevated postoperative troponin level is associated with higher mortality even in the absence of symptoms or signs of MI. Canadian and European cardiology society guidelines advocate routine postoperative screening of high-risk patients with troponin levels, whereas American guidelines remain equivocal about this strategy. It is unclear how to best manage postoperative type 2 MI (caused by ischemia from increased myocardial demand) or isolated troponin elevation, but optimizing cardiac risk reduction strategies is reasonable. Postoperative type 1 MI (caused by a primary coronary event, such as plaque rupture) should generally be managed in the same manner as in nonsurgical patients; however, recent surgery may impose limitations on diagnostic and treatment options, such as anticoagulation.

Heart Failure & LV Dysfunction

Elective surgery should be postponed until decompensated HF (manifested by an elevated jugular venous pressure, an audible third heart sound, or evidence of pulmonary edema) has been brought under control. In patients with compensated HF, the risk of perioperative cardiac complications is similar in patients with ischemic or nonischemic cardiomyopathy. HF with reduced EF likely confers more risk than HF with preserved EF. Guidelines recommend preoperative echocardiography to evaluate LV function in patients without known HF who have unexplained dyspnea and in patients with known HF with clinical deterioration. Routine evaluation of LV function should not be performed in asymptomatic and clinically stable patients.

Patients receiving diuretics should have serum electrolytes measured before surgery because abnormalities in these levels may increase the risk of perioperative arrhythmias. Clinicians must be cautious not to give too much diuretic since the volume-depleted patient will be much more susceptible to intraoperative hypotension. The surgeon and anesthesiologist should be made aware of the presence and severity of LV dysfunction so that appropriate decisions can be made regarding perioperative fluid management and intraoperative monitoring. Although most HF medications should be continued perioperatively in stable patients, SGLT-2 inhibitors should be stopped for 3–4 days before elective surgery to reduce the risk of euglycemic ketoacidosis.

Valvular Heart Disease

If the nature or severity of valvular lesions is unknown, or if there has been a recent change in clinical status, echocardiography should be performed before noncardiac surgery. In addition, patients with known or suspected moderate to severe stenotic or regurgitant valvular disease should undergo echocardiography within 1 year before surgery. Candidates for valvular intervention independent of elective noncardiac surgery should have the valve correction procedure performed first. Patients with uncorrected critical or symptomatic aortic stenosis are at particular risk for cardiac complications. They should undergo surgery only after consultation with a cardiologist and anesthesiologist. Patients with asymptomatic moderate or severe aortic stenosis and normal LV systolic function appear to be at lower risk than patients with symptomatic aortic stenosis and may be reasonable surgical candidates with appropriate intraoperative and postoperative monitoring at centers with experience operating on such patients. Patients with mitral stenosis require heart rate control to prolong diastolic filling time. Regurgitant valvular lesions are generally less problematic during surgery because the vasodilatory effect of anesthetics promotes forward flow. Patients with aortic or mitral regurgitation likely benefit from afterload reduction and careful attention to volume status; negative chronotropes may worsen the regurgitant volume and should be avoided.

Arrhythmias

The finding of a rhythm disturbance on preoperative evaluation should prompt consideration of further cardiac evaluation, particularly when the finding of structural heart disease would alter perioperative management. **Patients with adequately controlled rhythm disturbance without evidence of underlying heart disease are at low risk for perioperative cardiac complications.** While long-term antiarrhythmic medications should be continued perioperatively, there is no evidence that the use of medications to suppress an asymptomatic arrhythmia alters perioperative risk.

Patients with symptomatic arrhythmias should not undergo elective surgery until their cardiac condition has been addressed. Adequate rate control of atrial fibrillation or other supraventricular arrhythmias should be established before surgery. Symptomatic ventricular tachycardia must be thoroughly evaluated and controlled before surgery. Patients who have an independent indication for a permanent pacemaker or implanted defibrillator should have it placed before noncardiac surgery. **The surgical team must be notified that a patient has a cardiac implantable electronic device to prevent device malfunction from intraoperative electrocautery.**

After major surgery, previously undiagnosed atrial fibrillation develops in approximately 1% of patients. Although most episodes resolve spontaneously within hours to days, postoperative atrial fibrillation is associated with increased long-term risk of recurrent atrial fibrillation and stroke that may be similar to that of nonoperative cases. Whether the same criteria for anticoagulation therapy should be used for patients undergoing surgery as for patients not undergoing surgery is unclear. American cardiology guidelines advocate long-term anticoagulation for patients with postoperative atrial fibrillation using the same criteria as for patients with usual nonvalvular atrial fibrillation. Ambulatory rhythm monitoring also is reasonable for patients with postoperative atrial fibrillation that has resolved.

Hypertension

No evidence supports delaying surgery to control mild to moderate hypertension (systolic blood pressure < 180 mm Hg and diastolic blood pressure < 110 mm Hg). Severe hypertension (systolic pressure > 180 mm Hg or diastolic pressure > 110 mm Hg) appears to be an independent predictor of perioperative cardiac complications, including MI and HF. It is reasonable to consider delaying elective surgery in patients with such severe hypertension until blood pressure can be controlled, although it is not known whether the risk of cardiac complications is reduced with this approach.

Most medications for chronic hypertension should be continued up to and including the day of surgery. Continuation of ACE inhibitors and ARBs on the day of surgery increases the risk of intraoperative and postoperative hypotension; however, a 2024 trial found no difference in mortality or important complications, such as AKI or MI. One reasonable approach is to individualize management, favoring continuation in patients with HF or suboptimal hypertension control and holding them in patients with tight blood pressure control and no other indication for these drugs. Antihypertension medications held for surgery should be resumed postoperatively in clinically stable patients. Diuretic agents are sometimes held on the day of surgery to prevent hypovolemia and electrolyte disorders, although the benefit of this practice is uncertain.

Patients without chronic hypertension may manifest hypertension after surgery, and patients being treated for hypertension often experience decreased control of their blood pressure. Potential causes include elevated sympathetic tone due to injury or pain, volume overload from intravenous fluids, hypercarbia, urine retention, and withholding long-term antihypertensive medications. Before initiating postoperative medical management of hypertension, reversible contributors should be addressed. A 2023 trial found similar outcomes when blood pressure was tightly or loosely controlled during and after surgery.

Doherty JU et al. ACC/AHA/ASE/ASNC/HFSA/ HRS/SCAI/SCCT/SCMR/STS 2024 appropriate use criteria for multimodality imaging in cardiovascular evaluation of patients undergoing nonemergent, noncardiac surgery. JACC. 2024;84:1455. [PMID: 39207318]
Legrand M et al. Continuation vs discontinuation of renin-angiotensin system inhibitors before major noncardiac surgery. The Stop-or-Not randomized clinical trial. JAMA. 2024;332:970. [PMID: 39212270]
Lurati Buse GA et al. Risk assessment for major adverse cardiovascular events after noncardiac surgery using self-reported functional capacity: international prospective cohort study. Br J Anaesth. 2023;130:655. [PMID: 37012173]
Sahai SK et al. Preoperative management of medications: a Society for Perioperative Assessment and Quality Improvement (SPAQI) consensus statement. Mayo Clin Proc. 2022;97:1734. [PMID: 36058586]
Thompson A et al. AHA/ACC/ACS/ASNC/HRS/SCA/SCCT/SCMR/SVM guideline for perioperative cardiovascular management for noncardiac surgery: a report of the American College of Cardiology/American Heart Association Joint Committee on Clinical Practice Guidelines. Circulation. 2024;150:e351. [PMID: 39316661]

PULMONARY EVALUATION IN NON–LUNG RESECTION SURGERY

Pneumonia and respiratory failure requiring prolonged mechanical ventilation are the most important postoperative pulmonary complications. The occurrence of these complications has been associated with a significant increase in mortality and hospital length of stay. Pulmonary thromboembolism is another serious complication; prophylaxis against venous thromboembolic disease is detailed in Table 16–14.

Risk Factors for the Development of Postoperative Pulmonary Complications

Procedure-related risk factors for postoperative pulmonary complications include location of surgery (highest rates occur in cardiac, thoracic, and upper abdominal cases), prolonged anesthesia, and emergency cases. Operations not requiring general anesthesia tend to have lower rates of postoperative pulmonary complications; laparoscopic procedures tend to have lower risk than comparable open procedures.

A summary of patient-specific risk factors for pulmonary complications is presented in Table 3–3. The presence and severity of systemic disease of any type is associated with pulmonary complications. In particular, patients with COPD or HF have at least twice the risk of postoperative pulmonary complications compared with patients without these conditions. Advanced age, physical debility, malnutrition, and poor functional capacity also predict higher risk of postoperative pulmonary complications. An NSQIP risk calculator for predicting postoperative respiratory failure is available (https://qxmd.com/calculate/calculator_261/postoperative-respiratory-failure-risk-calculator).

Table 3–3. Clinical risk factors for postoperative pulmonary complications.

Upper abdominal or cardiothoracic surgery
Prolonged anesthesia time (> 4 hours)
Emergency surgery
Age > 60 years
COPD
HF
Severe systemic disease
Tobacco use (> 20 pack-years)
Impaired cognition or sensorium
Functional dependency or prior stroke
Preoperative sepsis
Low serum albumin level
Obstructive sleep apnea

Obstructive sleep apnea (OSA) is associated with both pulmonary and non-pulmonary surgical complications, including postoperative respiratory failure. The STOP-BANG screening questionnaire asks about **s**noring, **t**iredness during the day, **o**bserved apnea, high blood **p**ressure, **B**MI > 35, **a**ge > 50, **n**eck circumference > 17 inches (males) or 16 inches (female), and male **g**ender. Formal polysomnography to diagnose OSA before surgery is recommended for patients with evidence of impaired gas exchange or end-organ damage. Patients using positive airway pressure devices should continue to do so after surgery. Patients with OSA should be closely monitored for respiratory decompensation after surgery.

Pulmonary Function Testing & Laboratory Studies

The main role for preoperative PFTs is to identify pulmonary disease in patients with unexplained symptoms before major abdominal or cardiothoracic surgery. In patients with diagnosed lung disease, PFTs usually add little information above clinical assessment. CXRs in unselected patients also rarely add clinically useful information. ABG measurement is not routinely recommended except in patients with known lung disease and suspected hypoxemia or hypercapnia.

Preoperative Risk Reduction

Retrospective studies have shown that smoking cessation reduced the incidence of pulmonary complications, but only if it was initiated at least 1–2 months before surgery. A meta-analysis of randomized trials found that preoperative smoking cessation programs reduced both pulmonary and surgical wound complications, especially if smoking cessation was initiated at least 4 weeks before surgery. **The preoperative period may be an optimal time to initiate smoking cessation efforts.** A systematic review found that smoking cessation programs started in a preoperative evaluation clinic increased the odds of abstinence at 3–6 months by nearly 60%.

Elective surgery should not be scheduled within 2 weeks of SARS-CoV-2 infection, and risks and benefits should be assessed when infection occurred 2–7 weeks before scheduled surgery.

Postoperative Risk Reduction

Postoperative risk reduction strategies have centered on promoting lung expansion using incentive spirometry, deep breathing exercises, and in selected populations, continuous positive airway pressure (CPAP) or intermittent positive-pressure breathing (IPPB). Although trial results have been mixed, all these techniques reduce the incidence of postoperative atelectasis and, in a few studies, reduce the incidence of other postoperative pulmonary complications. In most comparative trials, these methods were equally effective. Given the higher cost of CPAP and IPPB, **incentive spirometry and deep breathing exercises are the preferred methods for most patients.** Multicomponent respiratory care programs may be beneficial. One program termed "I COUGH"—an acronym for *I*ncentive spirometry, *C*oughing and deep breathing, *O*ral care, *U*nderstanding (patient education), *G*et out of bed (early ambulation), and *H*ead of bed elevation—reduced the rates of pneumonia and unplanned intubation after general and vascular surgery.

Ceban F et al. Perioperative adverse events in adult patients with obstructive sleep apnea undergoing ambulatory surgery: An updated systematic review and meta-analysis. J Clin Anesth. 2024;96:111464. [PMID: 38718686]
Harrogate S et al. Peri-operative tobacco cessation interventions: a systematic review and meta-analysis. Anaesthesia. 2023;78:1393. [PMID: 37656151]
Palermo J et al. Evaluation and prevention of perioperative respiratory failure. J Clin Med. 2024;13:5083. [PMID: 39274295]

EVALUATION OF THE PATIENT WITH LIVER DISEASE

Risk Assessment in Surgical Patients with Liver Disease

Screening unselected patients with liver biochemical tests has a low yield and is not recommended. Patients with suspected or known liver disease based on history or physical examination, however, should have measurement of liver enzyme levels as well as tests of hepatic synthetic function performed before surgery.

Elective surgery in patients with acute viral or alcoholic hepatitis should be delayed until the acute episode has resolved. In three small series of patients with acute viral hepatitis who underwent abdominal surgery, the mortality rate was roughly 10%. Similarly, patients with undiagnosed alcoholic hepatitis had high mortality rates when undergoing abdominal surgery. In the absence of cirrhosis or synthetic dysfunction, chronic viral hepatitis is unlikely to increase risk significantly. Similarly, metabolic dysfunction-associated steatotic liver disease without cirrhosis probably does not pose a serious risk in surgical patients.

In patients with cirrhosis, postoperative complication rates correlate with the severity of liver dysfunction, and decompensated cirrhosis is associated with an extremely high perioperative mortality. Traditionally, severity of dysfunction has been assessed with the Child-Pugh score (see Chapter 18). A conservative approach would be to avoid elective surgery in patients with Child-Pugh class C cirrhosis and pursue it with great caution in class B patients. The Model for End-stage Liver Disease (MELD) score, based on serum bilirubin and creatinine levels, and the prothrombin time expressed as the INR, also predicted surgical mortality and outperformed the Child-Pugh classification in some studies. Generally, a MELD score < 10 predicts low risk, whereas a score > 16 portends high mortality after elective surgery. The VOCAL-Penn score also predicted mortality and risk of hepatic decompensation in surgical patients with cirrhosis and performed better than MELD-based prediction tools in an external validation study.

Ascites, encephalopathy, and coagulopathy should be controlled preoperatively. Ascites is a particular problem in abdominal operations, where it can lead to wound dehiscence and hernias. Great care should be taken when using analgesics and sedatives, since these can worsen hepatic encephalopathy; in general, short-acting agents and lower doses should be used. Postoperative constipation should be aggressively treated because it can precipitate encephalopathy. Kidney function and volume status need to be closely monitored to prevent AKI and volume overload, which are common complications in these patients. Patients with coagulopathy should receive vitamin K and may need fresh frozen plasma transfusion at the time of surgery; however, transfusing to a specific INR target for cirrhosis is discouraged.

Mahmoud N et al. ACG clinical guideline: perioperative risk assessment and management in patients with cirrhosis. Am J Gastroenterol. 2025;120:1968. [PMID: 40899690]

PERIOPERATIVE HEMATOLOGIC EVALUATION

Three common hematologic issues faced by the medical consultant are anemia, assessment of bleeding risk, and the perioperative management of long-term anticoagulation.

The main goals of the preoperative evaluation of patients with anemia are to determine the need for preoperative diagnostic evaluation and the need for transfusion. **When feasible, the diagnostic evaluation of the patient with previously unrecognized anemia should be done before surgery because certain types of anemia (particularly those due to sickle cell disease, hemolysis, and acute blood loss) have implications for perioperative management.** These types of anemia are typically associated with an elevated reticulocyte count. Given the prevalence of iron deficiency, excluding it as the cause of anemia is reasonable. Intravenous iron is more effective at raising preoperative hemoglobin levels than oral iron supplements; however, a beneficial effect on clinical outcomes or transfusion requirements is unproven. Although preoperative anemia is associated with higher postoperative morbidity and mortality, the impact of raising preoperative hemoglobin level to specific targets on postoperative outcomes is unknown. The clinician determining the need for preoperative transfusion in a patient must consider factors other than the absolute hemoglobin level, including the presence of cardiopulmonary disease, the type of surgery, and the likely severity of surgical blood loss. For most hemodynamically stable hospitalized patients, the AABB (formerly American Association of Blood Banks) recommends transfusion for a hemoglobin level < 7 g/dL (70 g/L); a threshold of 7.5 g/dL (75 g/L) may be considered for patients undergoing cardiac surgery and 8 g/dL (80 g/L) for patients who are undergoing orthopedic surgery or have underlying CVD.

Table 3–4. Recommendations for perioperative management of DOACs.

Drug and Kidney Function	Last Dose Before Procedure	Resume Medication
Dabigatran with normal creatinine clearance (> 50 mL/min [0.83 mL/s]); rivaroxaban, apixaban, edoxaban	2 days before procedure with low risk of bleeding or 3 days before procedure with high risk of bleeding	If hemostasis is adequate, resume 24 hours after procedure with low risk of bleeding or 48–72 hours after procedure with high risk of bleeding
Dabigatran with reduced creatinine clearance (30–50 mL/min [0.5–0.83 mL/s])	3 days before procedure with low risk of bleeding or 5 days before procedure with high risk of bleeding	

The most important component of the bleeding risk assessment is a directed bleeding history (see Table 3–1). Patients who provide a reliable history of no abnormal bleeding and have no suggestion of abnormal bleeding on physical examination are at very low risk for having an occult bleeding disorder. Laboratory tests of hemostatic parameters in these patients are generally not needed. When the directed bleeding history is unreliable or incomplete, or when abnormal bleeding is suggested, a formal evaluation of hemostasis should be done before surgery and include measurement of the prothrombin time, activated partial thromboplastin time, and platelet count (see Chapter 14).

Patients receiving long-term oral anticoagulation are at risk for thromboembolic complications when an operation requires interruption of this therapy. However, "bridging anticoagulation," where unfractionated or low-molecular-weight heparin is administered parenterally while oral anticoagulants are held, has not been shown to be beneficial and can increase bleeding. A cohort study found that DOACs could be safely held without bridging by using a protocol based on the patient's kidney function; the DOACs are withheld several days before surgery and restarted 24–48 hours after surgery if hemostasis appears adequate (Table 3–4). A 2015 randomized trial of bridging anticoagulation in surgical patients taking warfarin for atrial fibrillation demonstrated no difference in thromboembolism between those with and without bridging. Bleeding complications, however, were twice as common in patients who received bridging anticoagulation. A 2021 trial of postoperative bridging anticoagulation that included patients with atrial fibrillation or mechanical prosthetic heart valves also found no benefit for stroke prevention. **Most experts recommend bridging therapy only in patients at high risk for thromboembolism.** An approach to perioperative anticoagulation management with warfarin is shown in Table 3–5, but the recommendations must be considered in the context of patient preference and hemorrhagic risk.

Carson JL et al. Red blood cell transfusion: 2023 AABB international guidelines. JAMA. 2023;330:1892. [PMID: 37824153]
Douketis JD et al. Perioperative management of patients taking direct oral anticoagulants: a review. JAMA. 2024;332:825. [PMID: 39133476]

NEUROLOGIC EVALUATION

Delirium can occur after any major operation but is common after hip fracture repair and cardiovascular surgery, where the incidence is 30–60%. Postoperative delirium has been associated with higher rates of major postoperative

Table 3–5. Recommendations for management of perioperative anticoagulation with warfarin.

Thromboembolic Risk without Anticoagulation	Recommendation
Low Risk (eg, atrial fibrillation with CHA$_2$DS$_2$VASc score 0–6,[1] mechanical bileaflet aortic valve prosthesis, or single VTE > 3 months ago without hypercoagulability condition[2])	Stop warfarin 5 days before surgery Measure INR the day before surgery to confirm that it is acceptable (< 1.6 for most operations) Resume warfarin when hemostasis permits No bridging with parenteral anticoagulants before or after surgery
High Risk (eg, either atrial fibrillation or mechanical heart valve with stroke < 3 months prior, atrial fibrillation with CHA$_2$DS$_2$VASc score 7–9,[1] mechanical mitral valve prosthesis, caged-ball or tilting disk valve prosthesis, or VTE < 3 months ago or associated with hypercoagulability condition[2])	Stop warfarin 5 days before surgery Begin bridging with therapeutic dose UFH infusion or LMWH 2 days after stopping oral anticoagulation Administer last dose of LMWH 24 hours before surgery; discontinue UFH 4–6 hours before surgery Measure INR the day before surgery to confirm that it is acceptable (< 1.6 for most operations) Resume warfarin when hemostasis permits If hemostasis permits, consider bridging with therapeutic dose UFH infusion or LMWH beginning 48–72 hours after surgery and continuing until the INR is therapeutic

[1]See Table 12–2.
[2]Patients should receive VTE prophylaxis after surgery (see Chapter 16).
LMWH, low-molecular-weight heparin; UFH, unfractionated heparin.

cardiac and pulmonary complications, poor functional recovery, increased length of hospital stay, increased risk of subsequent dementia and functional decline, and increased mortality. The American Geriatrics Society recommends screening preoperative patients for these delirium risk factors: age > 65 years, chronic cognitive impairment or dementia, severe illness, poor vision or hearing, and the presence of infection. Patients with any of these risk factors should be enrolled in a multicomponent, nonpharmacologic delirium prevention program after surgery, which includes interventions such as reorientation, sleep hygiene, bowel and bladder care, mobilization and physical therapy, and the elimination of unnecessary medications. Moderate-quality evidence supports the use of these nonpharmacologic interventions.

Only a minority of patients with postoperative delirium will have a single, reversible etiology for their condition (see Delirium, Chapter 4). Evaluation of patients with delirium should exclude electrolyte derangements, occult UTI, and adverse effects from psychotropic medications, such as opioids, sedatives, anticholinergic agents, and antispasmodics. Conservative management includes reassuring and reorienting the patient; eliminating unneeded medications, intravenous lines, and urinary catheters; and keeping the patient active during the day while allowing uninterrupted sleep at night. Use of multimodal postoperative analgesic strategies can reduce or avoid the need for opioids. Scheduled administration of non-opioid analgesics such as acetaminophen or NSAID in the absence of contraindications often forms the core of these techniques. The analgesic effect of both opioid and non-opioid analgesics can be augmented by medications, such as gabapentin, which targets neuropathic pain; local or regional anesthetic agents; and nonpharmacologic approaches such as cognitive-behavioral therapy. When agitation jeopardizes patient or provider safety, neuroleptic agents given at the lowest effective dose for the shortest duration needed are preferred over the use of benzodiazepines or physical restraints (Table 28–1).

Stroke complicates < 1% of all surgical procedures but may occur in 1–6% of patients undergoing cardiac or carotid artery surgery. Most of the strokes in cardiac surgery patients are embolic in origin, and about half occur within the first postoperative day. Patients who had previously suffered a stroke had a high risk of MI, recurrent stroke, or cardiac death if they underwent noncardiac surgery within 3 months of the stroke. One retrospective study found that this risk declined over time and reached a nadir 9 months after the stroke, while another study found little additional risk reduction after 3 months. American cardiology and neurology societies suggest delaying elective surgery for 6–9 months after a stroke.

Symptomatic carotid artery stenosis is associated with a high risk of stroke in patients undergoing cardiac surgery. In general, patients with independent indications for correction of carotid stenosis should have the procedure done before elective surgery. In contrast, most studies suggest that asymptomatic carotid bruits and asymptomatic carotid stenosis are associated with little or no increased risk of stroke in surgical patients.

Hoogma DF et al. Postoperative delirium: identifying the patient at risk and altering the course. A narrative review. Eur J Anaesthesiol Intensive Care. 2023;2:e0022. [PMID: 39917289]
Shu L et al. Perioperative stroke: mechanisms, risk stratification, and management. Stroke. 2025;56:2798. [PMID: 40444359]

MANAGEMENT OF ENDOCRINE DISEASES

Diabetes Mellitus

The goal of management for all patients with diabetes is the prevention of severe hyper- or hypoglycemia in the perioperative period. In addition, patients with type 1 diabetes are at risk for developing ketoacidosis. Increased secretion of cortisol, epinephrine, glucagon, and growth hormone during and after surgery causes insulin resistance and hyperglycemia in patients with diabetes. Conversely, reduced caloric intake after surgery and frequent, unpredictable fasting periods increase hypoglycemia risk. Thus, all surgical patients with diabetes require frequent blood glucose monitoring. Ideally, such patients should undergo surgery early in the morning to avoid prolonged fasting. The specific pharmacologic management of diabetes during the perioperative period depends on the type of diabetes (insulin-dependent or not), the level of glycemic control, and the type and length of surgery.

Poor preoperative glycemic control, sometimes defined as a hemoglobin A_{1c} level > 8%, is associated with a greater risk of surgical complications, particularly infections. However, a strategy of delaying surgery until glycemic control improves has not been rigorously studied. The ideal postoperative blood glucose target is also unknown. Based on trials that showed increased mortality in hospitalized patients randomized to tight control, the American College of Physicians recommends maintaining serum glucose between 140 mg/dL and 200 mg/dL (7.8–11.1 mmol/L), whereas the British National Health Service guidelines recommend a range of 108–180 mg/dL (6–10 mmol/L).

A. Diabetes Controlled by Diet

For people with diabetes controlled with diet alone, no special precautions must be taken unless diabetic control is markedly disturbed by the procedure. If this occurs, small doses of short-acting insulin as needed will correct the hyperglycemia.

B. Diabetes Treated with Oral Hypoglycemic Agents

Most oral hypoglycemic agents should be held on the day of surgery. However, the SGLT-2 inhibitors (eg, canagliflozin) should be discontinued for 3–4 days before surgery due to their long half-life and associated risk of ketoacidosis. GLP-1 agonists delay gastric emptying and may increase the risk of aspiration during sedation and anesthesia. A multispecialty consensus statement recommends an individualized approach to determining how long to hold these agents before surgery. Oral hypoglycemic agents should not be restarted after surgery until patients are clinically stable and oral intake is adequate and unlikely to be interrupted.

A possible exception are dipeptidyl peptidase-4 inhibitors which have a low risk of causing hypoglycemia and might be continued perioperatively. Patients who experience significant hyperglycemia when oral agents are held should be treated in the same way as patients with type 2 diabetes who require insulin, as described below. Postoperative kidney function should be checked with a serum creatinine level before restarting metformin.

C. Diabetes Treated with Insulin

The protocol used to control glucose depends on (1) the kind of diabetes (type 1 or type 2); (2) whether it is minor surgery (lasting < 2 hours and patient able to eat afterward) or major surgery (lasting > 2 hours, with invasion of a body cavity, and patient not able to eat afterward); and (3) the preoperative insulin regimen (basal bolus or premixed insulin twice a day or premeal bolus only or regular insulin before meals and NPH at bedtime).

1. Preoperative insulin regimen—For patients with either type 1 or type 2 diabetes who are receiving insulin, a common practice is to reduce the last preoperative dose of long-acting, basal insulin (used to control fasting glucose levels) by 30–50% and hold rapid-onset, short-acting nutritional insulin (used to prevent hyperglycemia following meals).

2. Perioperative insulin regimen—Patients with type 1 diabetes must receive basal insulin to prevent the development of diabetic ketoacidosis. **Consultation with an endocrinologist or hospitalist should be strongly considered when a patient with type 1 diabetes mellitus undergoes major surgery.** Major surgical procedures in patients with type 1 diabetes lasting > 2 hours usually require an insulin infusion. Some patients with type 2 diabetes who are taking insulin will also need insulin infusion to maintain adequate glycemic control.

3. Postoperative insulin regimen—After surgery, when a patient with either type 1 or type 2 diabetes has resumed adequate oral intake, subcutaneous administration of insulin can be restarted. Intravenous administration of insulin and dextrose can be stopped 30 minutes after the first subcutaneous dose of long-acting insulin. Insulin needs may vary in the first several days after surgery because of continuing postoperative stresses and because of variable caloric intake. In this situation, multiple doses of short-acting insulin plus some long-acting basal insulin, guided by blood glucose determinations, can keep the patient in acceptable metabolic control. Use of correctional insulin only (without basal or nutritional insulin) after surgery is discouraged.

Glucocorticoid Replacement

Hypotension or shock resulting from primary or secondary adrenocortical insufficiency is rare, and the practice of administering supraphysiologic "stress-dose" glucocorticoid perioperatively is inadequately studied. A guideline from rheumatology and orthopedic surgery societies recommends that patients taking glucocorticoids continue their regimen when undergoing arthroplasty and not receive "stress-dose" glucocorticoids. Another approach is to administer stress-dose glucocorticoids to patients who have received the equivalent of at least 7.5 mg of prednisone daily for 3 weeks within the past year when they undergo major surgery. A commonly used stress-dose regimen is intravenous hydrocortisone succinate, 50 mg administered before anesthesia induction and 25 mg every 6–8 hours for 25 hours following surgery. Patients who have been taking < 5 mg of prednisone daily and those receiving alternate-day glucocorticoid dosing are unlikely to require supplemental coverage.

Thyroid Disease

Severe symptomatic hypothyroidism has been associated with perioperative complications, including intraoperative hypotension, HF, cardiac arrest, and death. Elective surgery should be delayed in patients with severe hypothyroidism until adequate thyroid hormone replacement can be achieved. It is not necessary to delay surgery to ensure adequate thyroid hormone replacement in patients with mild hypothyroidism (median TSH level 8.6 mIU/L). Patients with symptomatic hyperthyroidism are at risk for perioperative thyroid storm and should not undergo elective surgery until thyrotoxicosis is controlled; an endocrinologist should be consulted if emergency surgery is needed.

American Diabetes Association Professional Practice Committee. 16. Diabetes care in the hospital: standards of care in diabetes—2025. Diabetes Care. 2025;48(Suppl 1):S321. [PMID: 39651972]

Chen Cardenas SM et al. Perioperative evaluation and management of patients on glucocorticoids. J Endocr Soc. 2023;7: bvac185. [PMID: 36545644]

KIDNEY DISEASE

The development of AKI in patients undergoing general surgery is an independent predictor of mortality, even if mild or if kidney dysfunction resolves. The mortality associated with the development of perioperative AKI that requires dialysis exceeds 50%. Risk factors associated with postoperative deterioration in kidney function are shown in Table 3–6. Several medications,

Table 3–6. Risk factors for the development of AKI after noncardiac surgery.[1]

Age > 50 years
CKD
HF
Hepatic failure
Diabetes mellitus
Sepsis
Volume depletion
Crush injury

[1]Prowle JR et al. Postoperative acute kidney injury in adult noncardiac surgery: joint consensus report of the Acute Disease Quality Initiative and PeriOperative Quality Initiative. Nat Rev Nephrol. 2021;17:605.

including "renal-dose" dopamine, mannitol, *N*-acetylcysteine, and clonidine, failed to preserve kidney function during the perioperative period in clinical trials and should not be used for this indication. **Maintenance of adequate intravascular volume is likely to be the most effective method to reduce the risk of perioperative deterioration in kidney function.** Exposure to renal-toxic agents, such as NSAIDs and intravenous contrast, should be minimized or avoided.

Although the mortality rate for elective major surgery is low (1–4%) in patients with dialysis-dependent ESRD, the risk for perioperative complications, including postoperative hyperkalemia, pneumonia, fluid overload, and bleeding, is substantially increased. Patients should undergo dialysis preoperatively within 24 hours before surgery, and their serum electrolyte levels should be measured just before surgery and monitored closely during the postoperative period.

Douville NJ et al. Perioperative acute kidney injury: diagnosis, prediction, prevention, and treatment. Anesthesiology. 2025;142:180. [PMID: 39527650]

ANTIBIOTIC PROPHYLAXIS OF SURGICAL SITE INFECTIONS

Surgical site infection (SSI) is estimated to occur in roughly 4% of general or vascular operations. Although the type of procedure is the main factor determining the risk of developing a SSI, certain patient factors are associated with increased risk, including diabetes mellitus, older age, obesity, cigarette smoking, heavy alcohol consumption, admission from a long-term care facility, and multiple medical comorbidities. **For most major procedures, prophylactic antibiotics have been shown to reduce the incidence of SSIs.** Substantial evidence suggests that a single dose of an appropriate intravenous antibiotic—or combination of antibiotics—administered 30–60 minutes before skin incision is as effective as multiple-dose regimens that extend into the postoperative period. For most procedures, a first-generation cephalosporin (eg, cefazolin 2 g intravenously) is as effective as later-generation agents. In patients with nasal colonization by *Staphylococcus aureus,* treatment with 2% mupirocin ointment (twice daily for 5 days) before surgery reduces the risk of SSI by this organism.

Guidelines for antibiotic prophylaxis against infective endocarditis in patients undergoing invasive procedures are presented in Chapter 37. Given the lack of evidence for antibiotic prophylaxis before dental procedures to prevent prosthetic joint infection, guidelines from the American Academy of Orthopedic Surgeons and the American Dental Association recommend against this practice.

Seidelman JL et al. Surgical site infection prevention: a review. JAMA. 2023;329:244. [PMID: 36648463]
Smith M et al. Nasal decolonization: What antimicrobials and antiseptics are most effective before surgery and in the ICU. Am J Infect Control. 2023;51:A64. [PMID: 37890955]

Geriatric Disorders

Leah J. Witt, MD
Rossana Lau-Ng, MD
Tina R. Sadarangani, PhD, RN, ANP-C, GNP-BC, FAAN
G. Michael Harper, MD

4

GENERAL PRINCIPLES OF GERIATRIC CARE

The Geriatric 5Ms is a framework for optimizing care for the older adult, addressing Mind, Mobility, Medications, Multicomplexity, and what Matters Most. "Mind" relates to dementia, delirium, and depression. "Mobility" relates to function, balance, and fall prevention. "Medications" includes reviewing for polypharmacy and minimizing harm. "Multicomplexity" addresses the interplay of multiple comorbidities, functional status, prognosis, social factors, and patient preferences. What "Matters Most" centers care around individuals' goals, preferences, and priorities.

Along with the 5 Ms, the following principles help guide the care of older adults:

- Many disorders are multifactorial in origin and are best managed by multifactorial interventions.
- Diseases often present atypically or with nonspecific symptoms (eg, confusion, functional decline).
- Not all abnormalities require evaluation and treatment.
- Multiple chronic conditions and geriatric syndromes often coexist and should be managed in concert with one another.

COMPREHENSIVE ASSESSMENT OF THE OLDER ADULT

The *comprehensive geriatric assessment (CGA)* is a multidisciplinary evaluation of an older adult's medical conditions, functional limitations, and psychosocial risk factors. Its outcome is a goal-concordant care plan that maximizes the health and well-being of the individual being evaluated. CGAs incorporate an evaluation of the Geriatric 5M "multicomplexity," which (1) expands upon the conventional assessment of symptoms, diseases, and medications; (2) considers the biopsychosocial situation; and (3) includes an analysis of prognosis, values and preferences, and ability to function independently.

Assessment of Loneliness

Loneliness, the distressing feeling of being alone or separated, affects one in three older adults and is linked to conditions such as heart disease, depression, and cognitive decline, as well as mortality. Clinicians should routinely ask about loneliness and social connectedness using brief, validated tools such as the UCLA Loneliness Scale. Assessment should also explore changes in social networks, recent losses, and mobility restrictions, all of which can contribute to isolation.

Assessment of Prognosis

When an older person's life expectancy is > 10 years (ie, 50% of similar persons live > 10 years), it is reasonable to consider effective tests and treatments such as they are considered in younger persons. When life expectancy is < 10 years (and especially when it is much less), choices of tests and treatments should be made based on their ability to affect *a clinical outcome that is valued by the patient in the context of their estimated life expectancy* (Figure 4–1). The relative benefits and harms of tests and treatments often change as prognosis worsens and net benefit (benefits minus harms) diminishes.

A compilation of indices with online calculators that allow for estimating prognosis in multiple clinical settings can be found at ePrognosis (https://eprognosis.ucsf.edu).

Assessment of Values & Preferences

Although patients vary in their values and preferences, *many frail older adults prioritize maintaining their independence over prolonging survival.* Values and preferences, described by the Geriatric 5M what "Matters Most," are determined by speaking directly with a patient or, when the patient cannot express preferences reliably, with the patient's surrogate.

In assessing values and preferences, it is important to keep in mind the following:

1. Patients are experts about their preferences for outcomes and experiences; however, they may not have adequate information to make and express informed preferences for specific tests or treatments.
2. Patients' preferences often change over time. For example, some patients find living with a disability more acceptable than they thought before experiencing it.

Assessment of Function

People often lose function in multiple domains as they age, and as a result, they may not be able to do some activities as quickly or capably and may need assistance. Assessment

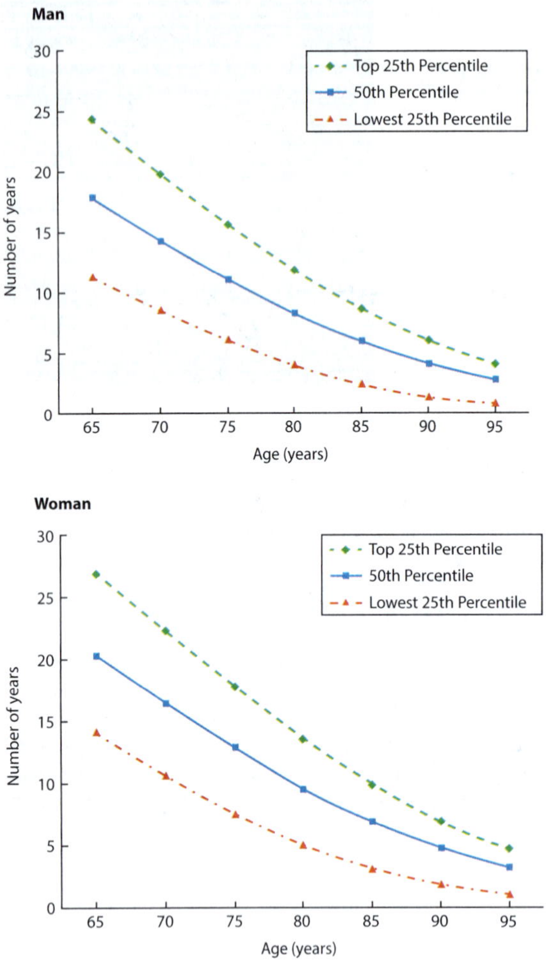

Figure 4–1. Median life expectancy of older men and women. (Data derived from Arias E. United States Life Tables, 2011. Natl Vital Stat Rep. 2015;64(11):1–63.)

of function improves prognostic estimates; it is also particularly important for determining an older adult's capacity to live independently and can guide care planning, caregiver involvement, and recommendations for supportive care or assistive technologies.

About one-fourth of patients over age 65 and half of persons older than 85 need help performing their basic activities of daily living (ADLs), such as bathing, dressing, eating, transferring from bed to chair, continence, and toileting. Assessment of ADLs provides crucial insight into functional status, care needs, and the necessary level of support on a daily basis. Declines in ADLs can signify disease progression, frailty, or the need for rehabilitation and support services. Regular monitoring of ADLs enables timely intervention to maintain function and independence. **Instrumental activities of daily living (IADLs)** include shopping, cooking, using the telephone, managing money, taking medications, housecleaning, or doing laundry and reflect a complex set of skills needed for community living. Evaluation of IADLs helps identify functional decline that may precede impairment in basic ADLs.

Functional screening should include assessment of ADLs and IADLs and questions to detect weight loss, falls, incontinence, depressed mood, self-neglect, fear for personal safety, and common serious impairments (eg, hearing, vision, cognition, and mobility). Two commonly used assessment tools for functional screening include the **Katz Index for ADLs** and **Lawton Scale for IADLs**. Functional screening may be assessed by interviewing the patient or caregiver. Standard functional screening measures may not be useful for capturing subtle impairments in highly functional independent older adults.

Frailty

Frailty is a syndrome characterized by loss of physiologic reserve and dysregulation across multiple systems, which heightens vulnerability to stressors, ultimately resulting in greater risk of poor health outcomes. Estimates of its prevalence in community-dwelling older adults range from 4.0% to 59.1%. Elements of frailty include **weakness (diminished grip strength)**, **slow gait speed**, **decreased physical activity**, **weight loss**, and **exhaustion or low energy**. Frailty can be assessed using a tool such as the Clinical Frailty Scale, but generally an individual is defined as frail when three or more of the above features are present. Persons with frailty are at increased risk for falls, hospitalization, functional decline, poorer outcomes associated with medical interventions (eg, surgery, dialysis), and death. *Exercise, particularly strength and resistance training, can increase walking speed and improve function.* Optimizing nutrition, especially with higher levels of protein intake, may be associated with reduced incidence of frailty. Medication review (focused on deprescribing) and management of underlying chronic conditions also play an essential role in the management of frailty. However, once frailty is established, the treatment is largely supportive, multifactorial, and individualized based on patient goals, life expectancy, and chronic conditions. A comfort-focused or hospice approach may be an appropriate intervention when irreversible complications from frailty develop.

Administration for Community Living. 2023 profile of older Americans. May 2024. https://acl.gov/sites/default/files/Profile%20of%20OA/ACL_ProfileOlderAmericans2023_508.pdf

Magnuson A et al. Geriatric assessment for the practicing clinician: the why, what, and how. CA Cancer J Clin. 2024;74:496. [PMID: 39207229]

MANAGEMENT OF COMMON GERIATRIC PROBLEMS

1. Dementia

ESSENTIALS OF DIAGNOSIS

- Progressive decline in one or more of six cognitive domains.
- Acquired cognitive deficits severe enough to impair function.
- Not due to delirium or another mental disorder.

General Considerations

Dementia, also called major neurocognitive disorder, is an acquired, persistent, and progressive impairment in mental processes, with compromise of one or more cognitive domains. The *DSM-5* identifies these domains (with example deficits) as: (1) **complex attention** (easily distracted, difficulty performing calculations), (2) **executive function** (poor organizing, mental flexibility, planning, and judgment), (3) **learning and memory** (difficulty recalling items from a list, forgetting recent events), (4) **language** (word finding and object naming difficulty), (5) **perceptual-motor function** (difficulty navigating in known environments, copying a drawing), and (6) **social cognition** (change in personality, trouble reading social cues). *The diagnosis of dementia requires a significant decline in function that is severe enough to result in the loss of independence in IADLs.* In comparison, **mild cognitive impairment (MCI)** is diagnosed when the deficits in cognitive abilities are not severe enough to result in a loss of independence of IADLs.

For more than two decades, age-specific prevalence of dementia among US adults 65 years or older has been declining. However, as the population ages, the absolute number of people living with dementia is projected to increase. (See Chapter 27 for further details about dementia in young people.) Alzheimer disease accounts for roughly two-thirds of dementia cases in the United States, with vascular dementia (either alone or combined with Alzheimer disease) and dementia with Lewy bodies accounting for much of the rest.

Depression and delirium are also common in older adults, may coexist with dementia, and may also present with cognitive impairment. Delirium, characterized by acute confusion, occurs much more commonly in patients with underlying dementia. Major depressive disorder may occur in up to 20–50% of patients with dementia, and because they share common features, distinguishing the two can prove difficult. Psychiatric disease sometimes leads to complaints of impaired cognition (**pseudodementia**). Impaired attention is usually to blame, and in some patients with depression or anxiety, poor focus and concentration may even be a primary complaint. The symptoms should improve with appropriate psychiatric treatment. Mood disorders are commonly seen in patients with neurodegenerative disease and in some cases are an early symptom. There is some evidence that a persistent, untreated mood disorder may predispose to the development of an age-related dementia, and psychiatric symptoms can exacerbate cognitive impairment in patients who already have dementia; therefore, suspicion of dementia should not distract from appropriate screening for and treatment of depression or anxiety. In persons diagnosed with depressive pseudodementia, ongoing surveillance for cognitive impairment is warranted because many will develop dementia over time.

Clinical Findings

A. Screening

1. Cognitive impairment—According to the USPSTF, there is insufficient evidence to recommend for or against screening all older adults for cognitive impairment. While there is logic in the argument that early detection may improve future planning and patient outcomes, empiric evidence that demonstrates a clear benefit for either patients or caregivers is lacking. For primary care clinicians, the Medicare Annual Wellness Visit mandates that clinicians assess patients for cognitive impairment based on the clinician's observations and reports from others.

Direct-to-consumer genetic testing for the Alzheimer disease susceptibility gene APOE-e4 is US FDA-approved and available to consumers. Although APOE-e4 carrier status influences the risk for developing Alzheimer disease, not all carriers will develop the dementia syndrome. Therefore, routine testing for screening purposes is *not* recommended, and for individuals who are considering it, genetic counseling should occur first.

When there is suspicion of cognitive impairment, a clinical evaluation should include a cognitive history and administration of a brief validated cognitive assessment instrument. An example is the **Mini-Cog**, a combination of a three-item word recall with a clock drawing task that can be completed in 3 minutes. When a patient fails this simple test, or there is a high index of suspicion for cognitive impairment despite a normal result, further evaluation is warranted. The **Montreal Cognitive Assessment (MoCA©)** is a 30-point test that takes about 10 minutes to administer and examines several areas of cognitive function. A score below 26 has a sensitivity of 0.94 or more and a specificity of 0.60 or less for detecting dementia. Free downloadable versions in multiple languages are available at https://www.mocacognition.com.

2. Decision-making capacity—Older adults with cognitive impairment commonly face serious medical decisions, and the clinicians involved in their care must ascertain whether the capacity exists to make those decisions. To determine capacity, the clinician should interview the patient using open-ended questions to assess the following four abilities: (1) **understanding** relevant information about the patient's condition, including the risks and benefits of the proposed intervention and the alternatives (including no intervention); (2) **expressing** a choice; (3) **appreciating** the relevant facts and how they relate to the patient's own situation; and (4) **reasoning** as demonstrated by comparing the consequences of the potential decisions.

Sensitivity must be used in applying these four components to people of various cultural backgrounds. *Decision-making capacity varies over time and is decision specific.*

B. Symptoms and Signs

Most patients with dementia can be identified by a primary care clinician after completion of a history (often requiring collateral information), a physical examination, and cognitive testing. The clinician can gather additional information about the type of dementia by asking about (1) the rate of progression of the deficits as well as their nature (including any personality or behavioral change); (2) the presence of other neurologic and psychiatric symptoms, particularly motor problems and psychotic symptoms; (3) risk factors for HIV; (4) family history of dementia; (5) substance use, particularly alcohol use disorder; and (6) medications, with particular attention to recent changes.

The time of symptom onset must be established, but subtle, early symptoms are often apparent only in retrospect. Another event, such as an illness or hospitalization, may lead to new recognition of existing symptoms. Symptoms often accumulate over time, and *the nature of the earliest symptom is most helpful in forming the differential diagnosis.* The history should establish risk factors for dementia, including family history, other chronic illnesses, and vascular disease risk factors. Finally, it is important to document the patient's current capacity to perform basic and instrumental activities of daily living and to note the extent of decline from the premorbid level of function. Indeed, *this functional assessment defines the presence and severity of dementia.*

Workup is directed at identifying any potentially *reversible* causes of dementia. However, such cases are rare. For a detailed description of the symptoms and signs of different forms of dementia, see Chapter 27.

C. Physical Examination

The neurologic examination emphasizes assessment of mental status but should also include evaluation for sensory deficits, previous strokes, parkinsonism, gait impairment, and peripheral neuropathy. The examination should focus on identifying comorbid conditions that may aggravate the individual's disability. A *neuropsychiatric evaluation* by a trained neuropsychologist or psychometrician is not required but may be helpful in cases with diagnostic uncertainty and to distinguish dementia from depression. The goals of such testing are to enhance localization by defining the cognitive domains that are impaired and to quantify the degree of impairment. There is no standard battery of tests, but several metrics are commonly used to assess the symptom types previously mentioned. Assessments are most accurate when a patient is well-rested, comfortable, and otherwise medically stable.

D. Laboratory Findings

For patients with dementia, laboratory studies should include a CBC and serum electrolytes, calcium, creatinine, glucose, TSH, and vitamin B_{12} levels. While hypothyroidism or vitamin B_{12} deficiency may contribute to cognitive impairment, treating these conditions typically does *not* reverse the dementia. HIV and rapid plasma reagin (RPR) tests, a heavy metal screen, and liver biochemical tests may be informative in selected patients but are not part of routine testing. The emergence of FDA-cleared and commercially available CSF and blood-based biomarkers for amyloid-β and τ proteins has significantly enhanced the diagnostic accuracy for Alzheimer disease. These biomarker tests are most useful for patients with MCI or early dementia who may be candidates for immunotherapy targeting amyloid-β to confirm a diagnosis of Alzheimer disease. *These tests are not recommended to screen for Alzheimer disease in asymptomatic individuals.* For a detailed description of laboratory findings, see Chapter 27.

E. Imaging

The American Academy of Neurology recommends neuroimaging (noncontrast MRI is preferred over CT when available and not contraindicated) in all patients with a new diagnosis of dementia to exclude a structural cause of dementia (eg, subdural hematoma, tumor, previous stroke, or hydrocephalus). In frail older patients with a typical picture of Alzheimer disease for whom neuroimaging would not alter management, it would be reasonable to consider foregoing MRI and CT.

For patients whose initial neuroimaging does not find a structural cause of cognitive impairment and who may be candidates for anti-amyloid therapy because of symptoms suggestive of MCI or early dementia due to Alzheimer disease, PET scans that detect amyloid-β in the brain can confirm a diagnosis of Alzheimer disease with a high degree of accuracy. Amyloid PET should not be used for individuals without cognitive impairment, and it should be noted that these scans are expensive and may only be available in specialized centers. For a detailed description of imaging, see Chapter 27.

Differential Diagnosis

Older individuals experience occasional difficulty retrieving items from memory (usually word-finding difficulty) and experience a slowing in their rate of information processing. In the **amnestic type of MCI**, a patient describes memory problems, demonstrates mild deficits (most commonly in short-term memory) on formal testing, but the impairment does not significantly impact function. Annual dementia conversion rates vary from 5–15%. An older patient with intact cognition but with severe impairments in vision or hearing may become confused in an unfamiliar medical setting and consequently may be falsely labeled as having dementia. See also Chapter 27 for more detail on differential diagnosis.

Treatment

Patients and families should be made aware of the Alzheimer's Association (http://www.alz.org) as well as the wealth of helpful community and online resources and publications available. *Caregiver support, education, and counseling* may prevent or delay nursing home placement. Education should include the manifestations and natural history of the different causes of dementia as well as the availability of local support services, such as respite care. Exercise should be a component of treatment since evidence suggests physical activity may have beneficial effects on cognition and physical function, while limited evidence has found that intellectual engagement through a variety of nonpharmacologic interventions may have a modest positive impact on cognitive function. Patients with hearing loss should be assessed for *hearing aids. Maintaining an active role in the family and community* as practically as possible is likely to be beneficial, emphasizing activities in which the patient feels confident. Evidence is emerging that computerized cognitive training may improve cognition and function in patients with MCI and mild-to-moderate dementia due to Alzheimer disease. These interventions can also introduce challenges for patients with dementia and may lead to frustration, particularly when problems arise from navigating unfamiliar technology.

A. Cognitive Impairment

1. Acetylcholinesterase inhibitors—Donepezil, galantamine, and rivastigmine are acetylcholinesterase inhibitors approved for the treatment of Alzheimer disease. These medications produce a modest improvement in cognitive function that is *not* likely to be detected in routine clinical encounters, and they have *not* convincingly been shown to delay clinically meaningful functional decline or institutionalization. Compared to patients with Alzheimer disease, acetylcholinesterase inhibitors may yield similarly modest cognitive benefits in patients with vascular dementia or dementia with Lewy bodies, but they should *not* be used in frontotemporal dementia because they may worsen behavioral problems. There is insufficient evidence to recommend their use in MCI to slow the progression toward dementia. See Chapter 27 for acetylcholinesterase inhibitor dosing details.

2. Memantine—In clinical trials, patients with moderate to severe Alzheimer disease have been shown to have statistical benefit from the use of memantine (5 mg orally daily to 10 mg twice daily), an *N*-methyl-D-aspartate (NMDA) antagonist, based on global assessment and behavioral scales. Long-term and meaningful functional outcomes are not well established, and evidence suggests *there is no clinically meaningful benefit to giving memantine in combination with an acetylcholinesterase inhibitor.* Evidence supporting the use of memantine in vascular dementia and dementia with Lewy bodies is similarly modest.

3. Immunotherapy targeting amyloid-β—Treatment with immunotherapy targeting amyloid-β should be done by or in consultation with dementia specialists. Lecanemab and donanemab are the two monoclonal anti-amyloid antibody treatments available in the United States that have FDA approval for MCI and mild dementia caused by Alzheimer disease. Both medications effectively remove amyloid-β from the brain and may modestly slow the progression of the disease, but uncertainty remains as to whether either medication will lead to meaningful clinical benefits (Table 4–1).

Amyloid-related imaging abnormalities (ARIA), subclassified as edema (ARIA-E), hemorrhage (ARIA-H), or both, are known class effects of these medications and occur commonly. While most cases are asymptomatic, treatment-related symptoms can include headache, nausea, confusion, dizziness, and seizures; these symptoms usually resolved after stopping the medication. A small number of treatment-related deaths were attributed to both medications. Another recognized phenomenon noted is that anti-amyloid antibodies cause accelerated brain volume loss, but the clinical impact is unknown. In the clinical trials of lecanemab and donanemab, the overall discontinuation rates due to adverse events were 6.9% and 13.1%, respectively, and adverse event rates were higher with both treatments compared to placebo.

Because of the lack of racial and ethnic diversity and limited data on the oldest patients in clinical trials for both lecanemab and donanemab, questions remain about generalizability of the results to more diverse populations. Any

Table 4–1. Anti-amyloid-β antibodies for Alzheimer disease treatment (listed in alphabetical order).

Medication	Relevant Clinical Trial Names	Dosing	Target Population	Primary Endpoint[1]	Outcomes	MRI Monitoring for ARIA[2]
Donanemab[3]	TRAILBLAZER-ALZ 2	700 mg intravenously every 4 weeks for three doses, then 1400 mg intravenously every 4 weeks	Patients with MCI or mild dementia due to AD	Change in the iADRS from baseline at 76 weeks	Slower decline in iADRS compared to placebo	Prior to initiation of treatment; at weeks 4, 12, 24, 52, and 76
Lecanemab[3]	Clarity AD	10 mg/kg intravenously every 2 weeks 360 mg subcutaneously weekly or 10 mg/kg intravenously every 4 weeks	Patients with MCI or mild dementia due to AD For maintenance in patients who have received 18 months of biweekly intravenous therapy[4]	Change in CDR-SB from baseline at 18 months	Slower decline in CDR-SB compared to placebo	Within 1 year prior to initiation of treatment; prior to fifth, seventh, and fourteenth infusions
Remternetug[5]	TRAILRUNNER-ALZ 1	Intravenous and subcutaneous formulations are being studied	Patients with MCI or mild dementia due to AD	Amyloid plaque clearance at 52 weeks	Study results expected in 2026 or later	Not available

AD, Alzheimer disease; ARIA, amyloid-related imaging abnormalities; CDR-SB, Clinical Dementia Rating Scale-Sum of Boxes; iADRS, integrated Alzheimer Disease Scale; MCI, mild cognitive impairment.
[1]For industry-sponsored clinical trials.
[2]APOE-e4 homozygotes have a higher incidence of ARIA.
[3]Fully FDA-approved for MCI and mild dementia due to AD.
[4]Clinical outcomes are being studied in an open-label extension of Clarity AD, and data are not yet available.
[5]Undergoing phase 3 clinical trials.

patient living with suspected Alzheimer disease under consideration for monoclonal antibody treatment requires a thorough evaluation performed by a dementia specialist to assess eligibility including confirming amyloid presence on a PET scan or detection of CSF or blood-based biomarkers and should be counseled about the known benefits and risks. Those that are chosen for treatment require regular monitoring for ARIA using MRI.

B. Behavioral Problems

1. Nonpharmacologic approaches—Behavioral problems in patients with dementia (eg, physical and verbal aggression, resisting care, sleep disturbances, disinhibition, wandering) are common and should first be addressed nonpharmacologically. The **DICE approach** provides an evidence-informed framework for assessing and managing behavioral problems. Specific nonpharmacologic interventions that are supported by evidence of variable quality include music therapy, massage, interprofessional team care, and multicomponent interventions (eg, caregiver training, environmental modifications, structured routines).

2. Pharmacologic approaches—Pharmacologic treatment should be reserved for those patients who pose an imminent danger to others or themselves or when symptoms are substantially distressing to the patient.

Despite evidence of harm and recommendations against their use because of limited effectiveness, antipsychotic medications have remained a mainstay for the treatment of behavioral disturbances, particularly agitation and aggression, largely because of the lack of alternatives. The atypical antipsychotic agents (eg, risperidone, olanzapine, quetiapine, aripiprazole, brexpiprazole) are usually the first choice because of an overall better side-effect profile compared to typical agents (eg, haloperidol) but should be used with caution in patients with vascular risk factors due to an increased risk of stroke; they can also cause weight gain, are associated with hyperglycemia in patients with diabetes. *Both typical and atypical antipsychotics increase the risk of mortality compared with placebo when used to treat older patients with dementia and behavioral disturbances.* Brexpiprazole was approved by the FDA in 2023 for agitation in Alzheimer disease. However, like all antipsychotic medications, it carries a boxed warning that older people treated with antipsychotics have a higher risk of death. Starting and target dosages should be much lower than those used in schizophrenia (eg, risperidone, 0.25–2 mg orally; quetiapine, 12.5–25 mg orally).

Citalopram at a dose of 30 mg daily may improve symptoms of agitation; however, the maximum recommended dose is 20 mg daily for patients older than 60 years because of the risk of QT prolongation and associated dysrhythmia. In the specific instance of patients living with dementia with Lewy bodies, treatment with acetylcholinesterase inhibitors has been shown to improve behavioral symptoms.

In small, short-term clinical trials of sleep disturbances in patients with Alzheimer disease and related dementias, the dual orexin receptor antagonists suvorexant and lemborexant modestly improved total sleep time, wakefulness after sleep onset, and sleep efficiency. While these studies showed a favorable side effect profile, patients should be monitored for falls, sedation, and other adverse effects associated with sedative-hypnotic agents. Cost is also a factor when considering this class of medications.

C. Driving

Although drivers with dementia are at an increased risk for motor vehicle accidents, many patients continue to drive safely well beyond the time of initial diagnosis, making the timing of when to recommend that a patient stop driving challenging.

There is no clear-cut evidence to suggest a single best approach to determining an individual patient's capability, and there is no accepted gold-standard test. The result is that clinicians must consider several factors upon which to base their judgment. For example, determining the severity of dementia can be useful. Patients with very mild or mild dementia according to the Clinical Dementia Rating Scale were able to pass formal road tests at rates of 88% and 69%, respectively. *Experts agree that patients with moderately severe or more advanced dementia should be counseled to stop driving.* Assessment of the ability to carry out IADLs may also assist in the determination of risk. Finally, in some cases of mild dementia, referral may be needed to a driver rehabilitation specialist for evaluation. Although not standardized, this evaluation often consists of both off- and on-road testing. Experts recommend such an evaluation for patients with mild dementia, for those with dementia whose driving skills are newly impaired, and for those with significant deficits in cognitive domains (such as attention, executive function, and visuospatial skills).

Clinicians must also be aware of the reporting requirements in their individual jurisdictions.

D. Advance Financial Planning

Difficulty in managing financial affairs often develops early in dementia. Although expertise is not expected, clinicians should have some proficiency to address financial concerns. Just as clinicians counsel patients and families about advance care planning, the same should be done to educate about the need for advance financial planning and to recommend that patients complete a **durable power of attorney for finance matters (DPOAF)** while the capacity to do so still exists.

No gold-standard test is available to identify when a patient with dementia no longer has financial capacity. However, the clinician should be on the lookout for signs that a patient is either at risk for or experiencing financial incapacity. Because financial impairment can occur when dementia is mild, making that diagnosis should alone be enough to warrant further investigation. Questioning patients and caregivers about late, missed, or repeated bill payments, unusual or uncharacteristic purchases or gifts, overdrawn bank accounts, or reports of missing funds can provide evidence of suspected financial impairment. *Patients with dementia are also at increased risk for becoming victims of financial abuse*, and some answers to these same questions might also be signs of potential exploitation. When financial abuse is suspected, clinicians should be aware of the reporting requirements in their local jurisdictions.

Prognosis

Median survival after a diagnosis of Alzheimer disease typically ranges from 4–8 years and can depend on several factors, including age at the time of diagnosis. Other neurodegenerative dementias, such as dementia with Lewy bodies, generally show more rapid decline. Hospice care is often appropriate for patients with end-stage dementia.

When to Refer

Referral for neuropsychological testing may be helpful to distinguish dementia from depression, to diagnose dementia in persons of poor education or high premorbid intellect, and to aid diagnosis when impairment is mild. For patients under consideration for treatment with novel anti-amyloid antibody therapy, clinicians should consult with a dementia specialist.

Alshiban A et al. Efficacy and safety of dual orexin receptor antagonist (DORA) for sleep disturbance in patients with Alzheimer's disease dementia. A review article. Am J Geriatr Psychiatry. 2025;33:209. [PMID: 39462720]

Expert Panel on Neurological Imaging; Soderlund KA et al. ACR Appropriateness Criteria® dementia: 2024 update. J Am Coll Radiol. 2025;22:S202. [PMID: 40409878]

Kim BH et al. Second-generation anti-amyloid monoclonal antibodies for Alzheimer's disease: current landscape and future perspectives. Transl Neurodegener. 2025;14:6. [PMID: 39865265]

Watt JA et al. Guideline recommendations on behavioral and psychological symptoms of dementia: a systematic review. J Am Med Dir Assoc. 2024;25:837. [PMID: 38640961]

2. Depression

ESSENTIALS OF DIAGNOSIS

- May manifest in older adults as physical symptoms (eg, fatigue, anhedonia) rather than symptoms of depressed mood.
- *Often undertreated in older adults.* Approximately one-third of those treated with an antidepressant will achieve remission, and two-thirds will need additional treatment.

General Considerations

Major depressive disorder has prevalence rates of approximately 2% among community-dwelling adults aged 55 years and older. Prevalence rises with increasing age as well as conditions such as chronic illness, multimorbidity, cognitive impairment, functional impairment, social isolation, and loneliness. The COVID-19 pandemic period also saw an increased prevalence of depression. Major depressive disorder is less common in older adults than in younger adults, but depressive symptoms (not meeting criteria for major depressive disorder) are common and present in up to 15% of older adults. Depression is more common among hospitalized and institutionalized elders. Older single men have the highest rate of completed suicides of any demographic group.

New incidence of depressive symptoms may be an early sign of cognitive impairment in older adults; therefore, evaluation of depression should include cognitive assessment. Older patients with depression and depressive symptoms who have comorbid conditions (eg, HF) are at higher risk for hospitalization, tend to have longer hospital stays, and have worse outcomes than patients without depression.

Clinical Findings

The **Patient Health Questionnaire-2 (PHQ-2)** is highly sensitive for detecting major depression in persons over age 65. Positive responses should be followed up with more comprehensive questionnaires, such as the PHQ-9 or the Geriatric Depression Scale.

Evaluation of depression should include a careful review of substances that can contribute to depressive symptoms, such as medications (eg, benzodiazepines) and alcohol/illicit drugs. A thorough evaluation of comorbidities is critical since many medical problems can cause fatigue, lethargy, or hypoactive delirium, all of which may be mistaken for depression.

Treatment

First-line treatment for major depressive disorder is the same for older adults as it is for younger adults. Psychotherapy and SSRI medications are the mainstays of treatment. Adjunctive treatment may include psychosocial interventions, increased physical activity, reduction of substance use (eg, alcohol), reduction of potentially contributing medications, or electroconvulsive therapy. In older patients with depressive symptoms who do not meet criteria for major depressive disorder, nonpharmacologic treatments are indicated. Among those with MCI or dementia, cognitive behavioral therapy (CBT) added to usual care probably increases depression remission and slightly reduces depression symptoms, based on a 2022 Cochrane review. Telehealth for mental health support is an important innovation in the field.

Choice of antidepressant agent is usually based on side-effect profile, cost, and patient-specific factors, such as presenting symptoms and comorbidities. SSRIs are used as first-line agents because they are relatively well-tolerated and have good evidence to support efficacy (see Table 28–6). Older adults are more susceptible to SSRI-induced hyponatremia, falls, and osteoporosis. SNRIs (eg, duloxetine and venlafaxine) lead to more adverse events versus placebo than do SSRIs. Regardless of the medication chosen, many experts recommend starting older adults at a relatively low dose, titrating to full dose slowly, and continuing for a longer trial (at least 8 weeks) before trying a different medication. Titration to full dose is critical to achieve efficacy of treatment.

One-third of older adults achieve remission after adequate treatment with first-line SSRI treatment. For the remainder, referral to a mental health specialist is indicated. For those who do not achieve remission, augmentation therapy (eg, with lithium, methylphenidate, or aripiprazole) can enhance clinical response. For patients with severe or catatonic depression, electroconvulsive therapy has high rates of efficacy (60–80%) and should be considered.

Pharmacologic treatment for the first episode of depression should continue for 1 year after remission. Clinicians and patients should share in decision-making regarding maintenance therapy for depression since risk of major depressive disorder recurrence is high. This decision should weigh how long-term pharmacotherapy may contribute to polypharmacy and adverse effects in the landscape of a patient's comorbidities and medication regimen.

When to Refer

- Any patient who might be considered for electroconvulsive therapy should be referred for psychiatric evaluation.
- Refer to psychiatry when patients have mania, psychosis, catatonia, or treatment-resistant depression.

When to Admit

Recommend urgent psychiatric evaluation and admission for patients who have psychosis, suicidality, homicidality, catatonia, grave disability, or self-neglect.

Orgeta V et al. Psychological treatments for depression and anxiety in dementia and mild cognitive impairment. Cochrane Database Syst Rev. 2022;4:CD009125. [PMID: 35466396]

Subramanian S et al. Treatment-resistant late-life depression: a review of clinical features, neuropsychology, neurobiology, and treatment. Psychiatr Clin North Am. 2023;46:371. [PMID: 37149351]

3. Delirium

ESSENTIALS OF DIAGNOSIS

- Rapid onset and fluctuating course.
- Primary deficit in attention rather than memory.
- May be hypo- or hyperactive.
- Dementia frequently coexists.

General Considerations

Delirium is described in the *DSM-5* as *a disturbance in attention and awareness of the environment that usually occurs acutely over a short period of time, represents a change from baseline, tends to fluctuate, and is accompanied by a change in cognition* (see also Chapter 28). It is often the pathophysiologic consequence of an underlying general medical condition (eg, infection, coronary ischemia, hypoxemia, metabolic derangement) or the adverse effect of a medication. Delirium occurs in 29–64% of hospitalized older adults, persists in 25% or more, and is associated with worse clinical outcomes (higher in-hospital and post-discharge mortality, longer lengths of stay, delayed and limited recovery of physical function, greater probability of placement in a nursing facility).

The acutely agitated older patient often comes to mind when imagining delirium. However, **hypoactive delirium** is more common than **hyperactive delirium** in hospitalized older adults, yet it is underrecognized and may be suspected only if the astute clinician notices new cognitive slowing or inattention.

Cognitive impairment is an important risk factor for delirium. Other risk factors include advanced age, functional impairment, severe illness, polypharmacy, use of psychoactive medications, sensory impairment, depression, volume depletion, and alcohol use disorder.

Clinical Findings

Several bedside instruments are available for the assessment of delirium. The **confusion assessment method (CAM)** requires (1) acute onset and fluctuating course and (2) inattention and *either* (3) disorganized thinking *or* (4) altered level of consciousness (https://oxfordmedicaleducation.com/geriatrics/cam/). The **3D CAM** (3-minute diagnostic CAM) is useful for clinical assessment of delirium in general medical and surgical patients (http://eddelirium.org/delirium-assessment/3d-cam/).

A key component of a delirium workup is review of medications because polypharmacy, the addition of a new medication, an increase in dose of a medication, or the discontinuation of a medication known to cause withdrawal symptoms are all associated with the development of delirium. Medications that are likely to increase the risk of delirium include sedative/hypnotics, anticholinergics, opioids, benzodiazepines, and H_1- and H_2-antihistamines.

Evaluation of most patients should include a CBC; BUN; serum electrolytes, creatinine, glucose, calcium, and liver biochemical tests; UA; and ECG. In selected cases, serum magnesium, medication levels, ABG measurements, blood cultures, CXR, urinary toxin screen, and lumbar puncture may be helpful. When delirium develops during a hospitalization in the absence of trauma or new localizing neurologic signs, a head CT is rarely revealing.

Prevention

The best evidence for prevention comes from nonpharmacologic multicomponent interventions. These components include improving cognition (frequent reorientation, activities, socialization with family and friends when possible), sleep (massage, noise reduction, minimizing interruptions at night), mobility (early initiation of rehabilitation services as appropriate), vision (visual aids and adaptive equipment), hearing (portable amplifiers or hearing aids, cerumen disimpaction), and hydration status (volume repletion). No medications have been consistently shown to prevent delirium or improve outcomes such as length of stay or mortality should delirium develop.

Treatment

Management of established episodes of delirium combines the elements of preventive interventions with reassurance and reorientation, treatment of underlying causes, eliminating unnecessary medications, and avoidance of indwelling catheters and restraints. *Antipsychotics offer little to no proven benefit and can cause harm.* For example, haloperidol and second-generation antipsychotics have not been found to reduce delirium severity or duration, hospital length of stay, or mortality when compared to placebo. QT interval prolongation can occur and is a potential risk for serious dysrhythmias. Benzodiazepines should be avoided except in the circumstance of alcohol or benzodiazepine withdrawal. In ventilated patients in the ICU setting, dexmedetomidine or propofol (or both) may also be useful alternatives to antipsychotic therapy in patients with delirium.

Most episodes of delirium clear in a matter of days to weeks after correction of the precipitant, but some patients suffer episodes of much longer duration, and a significant percentage never return to their former baseline level of functioning.

When to Refer

If an initial evaluation does not reveal the cause of delirium or if entities other than delirium are in the differential diagnosis, referral to a geriatrician, neuropsychologist, neurologist, or geropsychiatrist should be considered.

When to Admit

Patients with delirium of unknown cause should be admitted for an expedited workup if consistent with the patient's goals of care.

Fong TG et al. The inter-relationship between delirium and dementia: the importance of delirium prevention. Nat Rev Neurol. 2022;18:579. [PMID: 36028563]
LaHue SC et al. Approach to altered mental status and inpatient delirium. Neurol Clin. 2022;40:45. [PMID: 34798974]

4. Immobility

Mobility limitations are common in older adults and are associated with increased rates of morbidity, hospitalization, disability, and mortality. Hospital-associated bed rest is a common precipitant of immobility and functional decline. Among hospitalized medical patients over age 70, about 10% experience a decline in function, and those who experience critical illness are particularly at high risk.

The hazards of bed rest in older adults are multiple, serious, quick to develop, and slow to reverse. Within days of being confined to bed, deconditioning of the cardiovascular system occurs. This deconditioning causes fluid shifts, decreased cardiac output, decreased peak oxygen uptake, increased resting heart rate, and postural hypotension. More striking changes occur in skeletal muscle, resulting in loss of strength and function. Pressure injuries, VTE, and falls are additional serious complications of immobility and deconditioning.

Prevention & Treatment

Physical activity should be encouraged for all older adults, including during hospitalizations. Physical activity is associated with many health benefits in older adults. Structured physical activity programs may help reduce mobility-related disability among community-dwelling elders.

When immobilization cannot be avoided, several measures can be used to minimize its consequences. Avoiding restraints and discontinuing intravenous lines and urinary catheters will increase opportunities for early mobility. Graduated ambulation should begin as soon as it is feasible. Among hospitalized older adults, exercise protocols can improve functional outcomes. Prior to discharge, physical therapists can recommend appropriate exercises and assistive devices; after discharge, they can recommend home safety modifications and maintenance exercises. Severe functional disability impeding the patient's ability for independent self-care often leads to discharge to an acute or subacute rehabilitation facility. Recovery from illness-related deconditioning takes weeks to months, and in many cases, full recovery to the pre-illness physical condition does not occur. Evidence supports widespread implementation of **Acute Care for Elders units,** which protocolize delivery of the above preventive measures to prevent hospital-associated disability.

Myszenski AL et al. Risk categories for discharge planning using AM-PAC "6-clicks" basic mobility scores in non-surgical hospitalized adults. Cureus. 2024;16:e69670. [PMID: 39429401]

5. Falls & Gait Disorders

Annually, about one-third of people over age 65 fall, and the frequency of falls increases markedly with advancing age. About 10% of falls result in serious injuries. *Complications from falls (eg, hip fracture, subdural hematoma) are the leading cause of death from injury in persons over age 65, and fall-associated mortality is increasing.*

Every older person should be asked about falls. Fall assessments should include measurement of postural blood pressure and pulse; cardiac examination; cognitive assessment; evaluations of strength, range of motion, and proprioception; and examination of feet and footwear. A thorough gait assessment should be performed in all older people. Gait and balance can be readily assessed by the **"Timed Up and Go Test,"** in which the patient is asked to stand up from a sitting position without use of hands, walk 10 feet/3 meters, turn around, walk back, and sit down. An older adult who takes 12.5 seconds or greater is considered at increased risk for falling. The ability to recognize common patterns of gait disorders is an extremely useful clinical skill to develop.

Causes of Falls

Balance and ambulation require a complex interplay of cognitive, neuromuscular, and cardiovascular function. With age, balance can become compromised, reaction time slows, and postural sway increases. These changes predispose the older person to a fall when challenged by an additional insult to any of these systems.

Falls in older people are rarely due to a single cause, and effective intervention entails a comprehensive assessment of the patient's intrinsic factors (eg, diseases and medications),

Table 4–2. Fall risk factors, targeted interventions, and best evidence for fall prevention (fall risk factors listed in alphabetical order within sections).

To Consider for All Patients	
Exercise or physical therapy	Tai chi, gait training, balance training, strength training
Multifactorial intervention	Home safety assessment, medication review, review of specific conditions (below), advice on appropriate footwear, vision check, adaptive aids/devices as appropriate, physical therapy or exercise as appropriate
Condition	**Targeted Intervention**
Environmental hazards	Removal or mitigation of hazards; installation of safety equipment (eg, grab bars)
Gait impairment	Gait training, assistive devices, balance or strengthening exercises
High-risk footwear	Education on appropriate footwear (eg, avoid slippers, high heels)
Impairment in leg or arm muscle strength or limb range of motion	Exercise with resistance bands or putty, with graduated increases in resistance
Impairment in transfer or balance	Balance exercises, training in transfers, environmental alterations (eg, grab bars)
Inability to get up after a fall	Medical alert system, physical therapy training for fall-prevention strategies
Osteoporosis	Bisphosphonate treatment to prevent first or recurrent fractures
Postural hypotension (> 20 mm Hg drop in systolic blood pressure, or systolic blood pressure < 90 mm Hg)	Behavioral recommendations, such as hand clenching, elevation of head of bed; discontinuation or substitution of high-risk medications
Use of benzodiazepine or sedative/hypnotic agent	Education about sleep hygiene; discontinuation or substitution of medications
Use of multiple prescription medications	Review of medications with a focus on discontinuation (deprescribing)
Vision impairment	Cataract surgery or other interventions as appropriate (eg, corrective lenses)

the activity engaged in at the time of the fall, and environmental obstacles (Table 4–2).

Medication use is one of the most common, significant, and reversible causes of falling. Research shows that psychoactive medications such as sedative/hypnotics, antidepressants, and benzodiazepines were most likely to be associated with falling. Polypharmacy has also been associated with increased fall risk. Other often overlooked but treatable contributors include postural hypotension (including postprandial, which peaks 30–60 minutes after a meal), insomnia, use of multifocal lenses, and urinary urgency.

Since most falls occur in or around the home, a *home safety evaluation* by a visiting nurse, occupational therapist, or health care professional may be beneficial in identifying environmental obstacles.

Complications of Falls

The most common fall-related fractures are of the wrist, hip, and vertebrae. Osteoporosis significantly increases fracture risk and is undertreated in older adults. Following hip fracture, older women experience a high mortality rate (approximately 20% in 1 year), particularly if they had some functional or cognitive deficits prior to the time of the fracture. Fear of falling again is a common, serious, but treatable factor in the older person's loss of confidence and independence.

Chronic subdural hematoma is an easily overlooked complication of falls that must be considered in any older patient presenting with new neurologic symptoms or signs, including evidence of new cognitive impairment. Headache and known history of trauma may both be absent.

Prevention & Management

Exercise is the intervention that is most consistently reported to reduce the risk of falls. Balance focused exercises (eg, Tai Chi), gait, and strength training appear to be more effective for fall prevention than general exercise programs (Table 4–2). *Physical therapy* for gait training can help restore an individual's confidence and independence in ambulation, which can help prevent (and treat) falls.

Multifactorial interventions appear to have a small benefit in preventing falls. These interventions include an assessment of potentially modifiable risk factors and tailored interventions to reduce risk. Emphasis is placed on treating all contributory medical conditions, minimizing environmental hazards, and eliminating medications where the harms may outweigh the benefits (eg, sedative-hypnotics).

The USPSTF recommends *against* vitamin D supplementation to prevent falls in community-dwelling adults. Vitamin D supplementation might be considered for high-risk individuals (eg, institutionalized older adults) on a case-by-case basis.

Osteoporosis treatment (both preventive and postfracture) is essential to prevent first and recurrent fracture. First-line treatment with bisphosphonates is effective; for example, alendronate significantly reduces the risk of hip, vertebral and nonvertebral fracture in people with osteoporosis. Unfortunately, < 20% of people who sustain a fragility fracture receive osteoporosis treatment (this treatment failure is called the "osteoporosis care gap"; see Chapter 30 for more information).

Assistive devices, such as canes and walkers, are useful for many older adults but often are used incorrectly. Canes should be used on the "good" side. The height of walkers and canes should generally be at about the level of the wrist. Physical and occupational therapists are invaluable in assessing the need for an assistive device, selecting the best device, and training a patient in its correct use.

Eyeglasses, particularly bifocal or graduated lenses, may increase the risk of falls, especially in the early weeks of use. Patients should be counseled about the need to take extra care when new eyeglasses are being used.

Patients with repeated falls are often reassured by the availability of telephones at floor level, a mobile telephone on their person, a personalized fall detection system (eg, watch), or a lightweight radio call system.

When to Refer

Patients experiencing repeated falls should be referred for physical and occupational therapy, eye examination, and home safety evaluation.

When to Admit

Consider hospitalization for patients with new falls that are unexplained, particularly in combination with changes in the physical examination (eg, neurologic status) or with an injury/fracture requiring surgery.

Johari S et al. A systematic review and meta-analysis to examine the effectiveness of exercise training in people with osteoporosis or osteopenia compared to other rehabilitation interventions on fear of falling and the number of falls. J Geriatr Phys Ther. 2026;49:E1. [PMID: 40260904]

6. Urinary Incontinence

ESSENTIALS OF DIAGNOSIS

- Involuntary loss of urine.
- **Stress incontinence:** leakage of urine upon coughing, sneezing, or standing.
- **Urge incontinence:** urgency and inability to delay urination.
- **Overflow incontinence:** variable presentation.

General Considerations

Urinary incontinence in older adults is common, and interventions can greatly improve patients' quality of life. Many do not voluntarily disclose their experiences with urinary incontinence to their health care providers, possibly due to embarrassment or the belief that it is a normal part of aging. A simple question about involuntary leakage of urine is a reasonable annual screen: *"Do you have a problem with leaking urine or accidents?"*

Classification

A. Transient Causes

The mnemonic "DIAPPERS" represents categories of "transient" urinary incontinence.

1. Delirium—A clouded sensorium impedes recognition of both the need to void and the location of the nearest toilet. Delirium is the most common cause of incontinence in hospitalized patients.

2. Infection—Symptomatic UTIs can cause or contribute to urgency and incontinence. Asymptomatic bacteriuria does not.

3. Atrophic urethritis and vaginitis—Atrophic urethritis and vaginitis can usually be diagnosed by the presence of vaginal mucosal telangiectasia, petechiae, erosions, erythema, or friability.

4. Pharmaceuticals—Medications are one of the most common causes of transient incontinence. Typical offending agents include diuretics, anticholinergics, psychotropics, opioid analgesics, α-blockers (in women), α-agonists (in men), and calcium channel blockers.

5. Psychological factors—Severe depression with psychomotor retardation may impede the ability or motivation to reach a toilet.

6. Excess urinary output—Excess urinary output may overwhelm the ability of an older person to reach a toilet in time. In addition to diuretics, common causes include excess fluid intake; metabolic abnormalities (eg, hyperglycemia, hypercalcemia, diabetes insipidus); and peripheral edema.

7. Restricted mobility—If mobility cannot be improved, access to a urinal or bedside commode may improve continence.

8. Stool impaction—This is a common cause of urinary incontinence in hospitalized or immobile patients. A clinical clue to its presence is the onset of both urinary and fecal incontinence.

B. Established Causes

Causes of "established" incontinence should be addressed after any potential "transient" causes have been addressed.

1. Detrusor overactivity (urge incontinence)—Detrusor overactivity refers to uninhibited bladder contractions that cause leakage. It is the most common cause of established incontinence in older adults, accounting for two-thirds of cases. Women will report leakage associated with a strong and sudden urge to urinate that cannot be forestalled. In men, the symptoms are similar, but detrusor overactivity commonly coexists with urethral obstruction from benign prostatic hyperplasia. Because detrusor overactivity also may be due to bladder stones or tumor, the abrupt onset of unexplained urge incontinence should be investigated by urine cytology and cystoscopy.

2. Urethral incompetence (stress incontinence)—Urethral incompetence is the second most common cause of established urinary incontinence in older women. In men, it commonly occurs after radical prostatectomy. Stress incontinence is characterized by instantaneous leakage of urine in response to an increase in intra-abdominal pressure. It can coexist with detrusor overactivity causing "mixed" incontinence. Typically, urinary loss occurs with laughing, coughing, or lifting heavy objects. To test for stress incontinence, have the patient relax the perineum and cough vigorously (a single cough) while standing with a full bladder. Instantaneous leakage indicates stress incontinence.

3. Overflow incontinence—Urethral obstruction (due to prostatic enlargement, urethral stricture, bladder neck contracture, or prostatic cancer) is a more common cause of established incontinence in men than women. It can present as dribbling incontinence after voiding, urge incontinence due to detrusor overactivity, or overflow incontinence due to urinary retention. Detrusor underactivity is less common but can also cause overflow incontinence. It may be idiopathic or have an identifiable cause including medications and sacral lower motor nerve dysfunction. When it causes incontinence, detrusor underactivity is associated with urinary frequency, nocturia, and frequent leakage of small volumes.

Treatment

A. Transient Causes

Each identified transient cause should be treated regardless of whether an established cause coexists.

B. Established Causes

1. Detrusor overactivity—The cornerstone of treatment is *bladder training.* Patients start by voiding on a schedule based on the shortest interval recorded on a voiding diary. They then gradually lengthen the interval between voids by 30 minutes each week using relaxation techniques to postpone the urge to void. Lifestyle modifications, including weight loss and caffeine reduction, may also improve incontinence symptoms. *Pelvic floor muscle ("Kegel") exercises* can reduce the frequency of incontinence episodes when performed correctly and sustained. For cognitively impaired patients and nursing home residents who are unable to manage on their own, *timed and prompted voiding* initiated by caregivers is effective.

If behavioral approaches prove insufficient, pharmacotherapy with β_3-agonists or antimuscarinic agents can be considered. Efficiency and safety profiles are comparable in both groups, with fewer anticholinergic adverse drug effects reported in patients taking β_3-agonists. Mirabegron, at 20–50 mg by mouth daily, and vibegron, at 75 mg by mouth daily, are FDA-approved β_3-agonists for overactive bladder symptoms.

FDA-approved antimuscarinic agents include short-acting tolterodine, 1–2 mg orally twice daily; long-acting tolterodine, 2–4 mg orally daily; short-acting oxybutynin, 2.5–5 mg orally two or three times daily; long-acting oxybutynin, 5–15 mg orally daily; oxybutynin transdermal patch, 3.9 mg/day applied twice weekly; oxybutynin 10% topical gel, 100 mg applied daily; fesoterodine, 4–8 mg orally once daily; trospium chloride, 20 mg orally once or twice daily; long-acting trospium chloride, 60 mg orally daily; darifenacin, 7.5–15 mg orally daily; and solifenacin, 5–10 mg orally daily. They are commonly available, have low-cost generic options, come in short-acting and long-acting formulations, and can be combined with β_3-agonists for synergistic effects. Potential adverse drug effects to consider include cognitive impairment, dry mouth, constipation, and urinary retention.

Women who have persistent symptoms despite an adequate trial of initial treatment, or who are unable to tolerate pharmacotherapy options, may be referred to urologists or urogynecologists for alternative options. Other possible treatment approaches include percutaneous or transcutaneous tibial nerve stimulation and botulinum toxin type A injection into the detrusor muscle. Symptom relief from botulinum toxin injections has been reported to last 6–12 months; possible adverse effects include urinary retention and the need for self-catheterization.

In men with both benign prostatic hyperplasia and detrusor overactivity and with postvoid residual of 150 mL or less, an antimuscarinic agent added to an α-blocker may provide additional relief of lower urinary tract symptoms.

2. Urethral incompetence (stress incontinence)—*Lifestyle modifications* include limiting caffeine and fluid intake may be helpful for those with mixed stress/urge incontinence; strong evidence supports weight loss in women with BMI of 30 or more. *Pelvic floor therapy* is effective for women with mild to moderate stress incontinence. Instruct the patient to pull in the pelvic floor muscles and hold for 6–10 seconds and to perform three sets of 8–12 contractions daily. Benefits may not be seen for 6 weeks. *Pessaries* or *vaginal cones* may be helpful in some women but should be prescribed only by providers who are experienced with using these modalities. No medications are approved for the treatment of stress incontinence, and a clinical practice guideline from the American College of Physicians recommends against pharmacologic treatment. Patients experiencing symptoms despite initial approaches should be evaluated for *surgical treatments.* Midurethral sling procedures, with their rapid recovery times, high cure rates, and low risk of complications, have become the standard surgeries for stress incontinence in older women.

3. Overflow incontinence—Most men with overflow incontinence from obstructive uropathy will first undergo bladder decompression with intermittent or indwelling catheterization followed by initiation of α-blocking agents (eg, terazosin, 1–10 mg orally daily; prazosin, 1–5 mg orally twice daily; or tamsulosin, 0.4–0.8 mg orally daily taken 30 minutes after a meal). Finasteride, 5 mg orally daily, can provide additional benefit in men with an enlarged prostate. If medical therapy fails to allow for adequate bladder emptying, surgical decompression can be an option. For the nonoperative candidate with urinary retention, intermittent or indwelling catheterization are options. For the patient with a poorly contractile bladder, augmented voiding techniques (eg, double voiding, suprapubic pressure) can prove effective. If further emptying is needed, intermittent or indwelling catheterization is the only option. Antibiotics should be used only for symptomatic UTI or as prophylaxis against recurrent symptomatic infections in a patient using intermittent catheterization; they should not be used as prophylaxis in a patient with an indwelling catheter.

When to Refer

- Men with urinary obstruction who do not respond to medical therapy should be referred to a urologist.
- Women who do not respond to pelvic floor therapy, medical treatment, or both should be referred to a urogynecologist or urologist.

Lane GI et al. Treatment for urinary incontinence in women older than 65 years. Urogynecology (Phila). 2023;29:687. [PMID: 37490708]
Olagundoye O et al. A scoping review of risk factors for urinary incontinence in older men. BMC Geriatr. 2023;23:534. [PMID: 37660036]

7. Involuntary Weight Loss

General Considerations

Aging, even in the absence of disease, is associated with reduced appetite. Involuntary weight loss affects substantial numbers of older adults. Most studies of involuntary weight loss in community-dwelling older adults define it as the loss of 5% of body weight in 6 months or 10% of body weight in 1 year.

Clinical Findings

The many potential causes of involuntary weight loss include medical conditions (60–70%; eg, cancer, chronic HF) and psychiatric conditions (10–20%; eg, depression), but in up to 25%, the cause of weight loss cannot be identified. Social determinants of health factors, such as food insecurity and financial hardship, should be investigated. The clinical evaluation should search for symptoms and signs that could point to a potential cause (eg, abdominal pain to peptic ulcer disease; tachycardia to hyperthyroidism). When the history, physical examination, and basic laboratory studies do not suggest a possible diagnosis, additional evaluation (eg, total body CT scan) is usually low yield.

Treatment

Initial treatment should focus on identifying medical causes of involuntary weight loss while also addressing and improving social barriers, such as social isolation and lack of access to food. Social meals can improve intake and nutrition. Oral nutritional supplements of 200–1000 kcal/day can increase weight and improve outcomes in malnourished hospitalized older adults but have *not* been shown to have benefits in community-dwelling older adults. Megestrol acetate as an appetite stimulant has *not* been shown to increase lean body mass or lengthen life among elders and has significant side effects. Mirtazapine is often used for older adults with comorbid depression; however, effects on weight gain remain equivocal. For patients with advanced dementia, percutaneous liquid artificial nutrition ("tube feed") is *not* recommended, but rather assiduous hand feeding may allow maintenance of weight and provide more comfort.

Steiner L et al. A review of the efficacy of appetite stimulating medications in hospitalized adults. Nutr Clin Pract. 2023;38:80. [PMID: 35076955]

8. Pressure Injury

ESSENTIALS OF DIAGNOSIS

- Examine at-risk patients on admission to the hospital and routinely thereafter.
- Pressure injury is classified into one of six categories:
  - Stage 1: Non-blanchable erythema of intact skin
  - Stage 2: Partial-thickness skin loss with exposed dermis
  - Stage 3: Full-thickness skin loss
  - Stage 4: Full-thickness skin and tissue loss
  - Unstageable: Obscured full-thickness skin and tissue loss
  - Deep tissue: Persistent non-blanchable, deep red, maroon, or purple discoloration of intact skin

General Considerations

The National Pressure Injury Advisory Panel defines pressure injuries as damage to the skin and underlying tissue from pressure in combination with shear and friction forces, usually over a bony prominence, related to a medical device, or both. The term "pressure ulcer" was changed to "pressure injury" to more accurately reflect that the skin is intact in stage 1 and deep tissue injury, since the word "ulcer" implies that the skin has opened. Deep tissue and unstageable pressure injuries are included in the six pressure injury stages. An area of purple or maroon discolored intact skin or blood-filled blister is characteristic of deep tissue injury, sometimes preceded by tissue that is painful, firm, mushy, boggy, warmer, or cooler compared with adjacent tissue. Ulcers in which the base is covered by slough (yellow, tan, gray, green, or brown) or eschar (tan, brown, or black) are considered unstageable. Most pressure injuries develop during an acute illness. The primary risk factor for pressure injuries is immobility. Other contributing risk factors include reduced tissue perfusion, reduced sensory perception, increased moisture, and poor nutritional status.

Older adults should be assessed for their risk of developing pressure injuries, utilizing risk assessment instruments such as the *Braden Scale* and the *Norton score*. These tools should be used in conjunction with clinical judgment since each may cover a limited range of risk factors and results depend on the skills of the examiner.

Prevention

Using specialized support surfaces (eg mattresses, beds, and cushions), repositioning techniques, optimizing nutritional status, reducing shear and friction forces, and being mindful of skin integrity are strategies that have been shown to reduce pressure injuries. In general, advanced supportive surfaces are superior to standard hospital beds in preventing and managing pressure injuries, but there is no clear advantage of one support surface over another.

Evaluation

Evaluation of pressure injuries should include the patient's risk factors and goals of care; injury stage, size, and depth; absence or presence (and type) of exudate; appearance of the wound bed and possible infection; and any sinus tracking, undermining, or tunneling.

Treatment

High-quality evidence that rigorously examines the effectiveness of various treatments remains limited. Clinicians should therefore focus on the principles of wound care, including pressure reduction, removing necrotic debris, and maintaining a moist and clean wound bed to promote formation of granulation tissue and healing. The type of dressing recommended depends on the location and depth of the wound, whether necrotic tissue or dead space is present, and the amount of exudate (Table 4–3). Pressure-reducing devices (eg, air-fluid beds and low-air-loss beds) are associated with improved healing rates. Although poor nutritional status is a risk factor for the development of pressure injury, the evidence that nutritional supplementation helps correct pressure injury is limited.

Institutions should designate a wound care expert or team to select a streamlined wound care product line with simple guidelines. In a patient with end-stage disease who is receiving end-of-life care, appropriate treatment might be directed toward palliation only (including minimizing dressing changes and odors) rather than efforts directed at healing.

Complications

Bacteria contaminate all chronic pressure injuries with skin loss, and it can be difficult to identify those wounds that are infected. Suspicion for infection should rise if there is pain, increased or foul-smelling wound drainage, erythema of the skin around the wound, or if the wound will not heal. Fever and leukocytosis are other indicators of systemic infection but are not always present. Culture from a superficial swab adds little valuable diagnostic information. For nonhealing infected wounds without evidence of systemic involvement, topical antiseptics (eg, silver sulfadiazine) are recommended and may need to be accompanied by debridement of necrotic tissue. When systemic infections such as cellulitis and osteomyelitis are present, oral or parenteral antibiotics are warranted and medication choice should be guided by tissue culture, but obtaining this can be painful and it is not always readily available.

Table 4–3. Pressure injury dressings and other measures.

Injury Type	Dressing Type and Considerations
Stage 1	Barrier ointment Polyurethane film
Stage 2	Hydrocolloid dressings Semipermeable foam dressing Polyurethane film Hydrogel
Stages 3 and 4	For highly exudative wounds, use highly absorptive dressing or packing, such as calcium alginate; negative pressure wound therapy or vacuum-assisted wound closure also can be considered Wounds with necrotic debris should be debrided Debridement can be autolytic, enzymatic, mechanical, or surgical Shallow, clean wounds can be dressed with hydrocolloid wafers, semipermeable foam, hydrogels, or polyurethane film Deep wounds can be packed with gauze; if the wound is deep and highly exudative, an absorptive packing should be used
Heel injury	Do not remove eschar on heel pressure injury because it can help promote healing (eschar in other locations should be debrided)
Unstageable	Debride if appropriate before deciding on further therapy
Deep tissue injury	Offload pressure to the affected area Consider barrier ointment

When to Refer

- Pressure injuries that are large or nonhealing should be referred to a plastic or general surgeon or dermatologist for biopsy, debridement, and possible skin grafting.
- For hospitalized patients or residents of skilled nursing facilities in whom pressure injuries develop, early involvement of a wound care specialist is crucial.

When to Admit

Patients with pressure injury should be admitted if the primary residence is unable to provide adequate wound care or pressure reduction, or if the wound is infected or requires complex or surgical care.

Gould LJ et al. WHS guidelines for the treatment of pressure ulcers-2023 update. Wound Repair Regen. 2024;32:6. [PMID: 37970711]

9. Pharmacotherapy & Polypharmacy

ESSENTIALS OF DIAGNOSIS

- Older adults experience more adverse medication events than younger patients. Evaluate for dose reduction or medication avoidance based on kidney function, comorbidities, and other medication use.
- The **AGS Beers Criteria** list is useful for identifying high-risk medications for older adults. Particular caution/avoidance should be used in prescribing benzodiazepines and other sedative-hypnotic medications.

General Considerations

Polypharmacy refers to the condition of taking or being prescribed a multitude of prescription and nonprescription medications. More adverse drug events occur in older adults compared to younger patients for many reasons, including changing drug metabolism in the kidney or liver or both, drug interaction with comorbid conditions, and interactions between multiple medications. Polypharmacy itself is associated with adverse health outcomes, including falls, impaired cognition, hospitalizations, and death.

Medication metabolism is often impaired in older adults due to decreased GFR, reduced hepatic clearance, and changes in body composition (eg, lean body mass). Most emergency hospitalizations for adverse medication events among older adults result from commonly prescribed medications used alone or in combination.

Precautions in Prescribing Medications

Most medications prescribed for chronic disease management should be initiated at the low end of the usual adult dosage range, with slow increases in dosage until a therapeutic level is reached or intolerable side effects develop. At the same time, it is imperative that a medication's therapeutic dose be achieved, since older adults are at risk for undertreatment of conditions such as depression, if the starting dose is not increased with careful monitoring.

Optimal medication adherence is less likely with increasing numbers of pills and doses, high cost, and poor communication about medication changes as well as expected benefits and side effects; other factors affecting adherence include cognitive impairment, insurance issues, and psychosocial barriers. When possible, the clinician should simplify both dosing schedules with the fewest number of pills and doses (combination formulations can be useful in this regard, though perhaps complicate future dose adjustments) as well as modes of administration (eg, oral, ocular, transdermal, subcutaneous, inhalational). Other helpful medication management techniques include use of a single pharmacy, use of pillboxes or pharmacy-packaged medication sets, clarity about the prescriber of each medication (and ideally use of fewer prescribers), infrequent medication changes, and clear instructions about all medication changes using the "teach-back" method of patient communication. Clinicians should ask patients about their ability to afford their medications, and counsel patients about strategies for cost containment.

The patient or caregiver should bring in all medications at each visit for accurate **medication reconciliation** and instruction on medication use, dosage, frequency of administration, and possible adverse effects. Patients should also bring all supplements and over-the-counter medications used, including analgesics and sleep aids. Medication reconciliation is particularly important if the patient sees multiple clinicians. Clinicians should be aware of the "prescribing cascade" in which a medication is prescribed to counter the side effect of another medication.

The risk of toxicity goes up with the number of medications prescribed. Certain combinations of medications (eg, warfarin and many antibiotics, ACE inhibitors and NSAIDs, opioids and sedative-hypnotics) are likely to cause drug-drug interactions and should be monitored carefully.

Trials of medication discontinuation (deprescribing) should be considered when the original indication is unclear or the patient is having side effects. Medication discontinuation is particularly important in patients with limited life expectancy who may be experiencing increasing burdens from polypharmacy and modest, if any, benefits from the medication (eg, bisphosphonates, antilipemics). Clinical tools such as **"STOPP/START"** and the **AGS Beers Criteria** can inform safe medication prescribing for older adults.

When to Refer

- Refer patients with polypharmacy or poor medication adherence to a clinical pharmacist, when available.
- Refer homebound patients with poor medication adherence and suboptimal chronic disease management to a home health nurse for medication reconciliation and teaching.

2023 American Geriatrics Society Beers Criteria Update Expert Panel. American Geriatrics Society 2023 updated AGS Beers Criteria for potentially inappropriate medication use in older adults. J Am Geriatr Soc. 2023;71:2052. [PMID: 37139824]

10. Vision Impairment

Visual impairment due to age-related refractive error ("presbyopia"), macular degeneration, cataracts, glaucoma, or diabetic retinopathy is associated with several negative physical and mental health outcomes. These include falls, impaired mobility, and reduced quality of life. The 2022 USPSTF updated evidence report concluded that there was no direct evidence for better visual outcomes with screening in primary care. However, the American Academy of Ophthalmology recommends a complete eye examination every 1–2 years after age 65. Eye examinations should certainly be prioritized for patients with new or recurring falls, changes in vision, and conditions with risk of eye complications (eg, diabetes mellitus, thyroid disease). Patients with significant visual loss should be referred to low-vision community programs for support and assessment for assistive devices.

Jin H et al. Association between vision impairment and increased prevalence of falls in older US adults. J Am Geriatr Soc. 2024;72:1373. [PMID: 38514075]

11. Hearing Impairment

Hearing loss in older adults is common yet undertreated. *Over one-third of persons older than age 65 and half of those older than age 85 have some degree of hearing loss.* Hearing loss is associated with social isolation, depression, disability, frailty, dementia and accelerated cognitive decline, hospitalization, and nursing home placement. Hearing loss is undertreated because it is underrecognized by clinicians and hearing assistive devices are expensive and may not be covered by insurance.

Although the USPSTF found insufficient evidence for routine hearing screening, clinicians should periodically ask patients about hearing loss and refer them to audiology if hearing loss is suspected. A reasonable clinical screen is to ask patients if they have noticed any hearing impairment. Those who answer "yes" should be referred for audiometry. For those who answer "no" but in whom hearing loss is still suspected, further in-office screening can be performed using the **whispered voice test**. To determine the degree to which hearing impairment interferes with functioning, the provider may ask patients if they become frustrated when conversing with family members, have challenges understanding conversations, are embarrassed when meeting new people, or have difficulty watching television. Caregivers or family members can provide important collateral information regarding potential hearing loss and the impact of hearing loss on social interactions.

Hearing loss assistive devices and technology include hearing aids, cochlear implants, sound amplification for telephones and televisions, speech to text software, smart phone applications, hearing loops, and alerting devices to inform hearing-impaired people of an event such as a fire alarm. Hearing amplification and cochlear implantation improve hearing-related quality of life and reduce depressive symptoms. *Hearing aid use has been associated with lower dementia prevalence.* Compliance with hearing amplification can be a challenge because of the high device cost, dissatisfaction with performance, and stigma associated with hearing aid use. Newer digital devices may perform better but are considerably more expensive. In 2022, the FDA issued a new rule supporting over-the-counter sale of hearing aids for mild to moderate hearing loss without the need for a medical examination or prescription, in order to lower cost and expand access to such technology. For people with severe hearing loss, an audiologist and medical evaluation is recommended. Cochlear implantation is an underutilized treatment for profound hearing loss that improves understanding of speech and improves quality of life.

For those with milder hearing loss or who do not pursue hearing aids for a variety of reasons, portable sound amplifiers (eg, "pocket talkers") are useful over-the-counter and low-cost hand-held devices. Such devices are helpful in facilitating communication with hearing-impaired patients in clinical settings. Clinicians should develop skills in successful communication with people who have hearing impairment, such as facing toward patients when speaking, speaking at a moderate pace and in a low tone, and practicing the "teach-back" method to assess that information was adequately transmitted.

Lin FR et al. Hearing intervention versus health education control to reduce cognitive decline in older adults with hearing loss in the USA (ACHIEVE): a multicentre, randomised controlled trial. Lancet. 2023;402:786. [PMID: 37478886]
Ning H et al. Relationship of hearing impairment, social participation and depressive symptoms to the incidence of frailty in a community cohort. J Am Geriatr Soc. 2023;71:1167. [PMID: 36504135]

12. Elder Mistreatment & Self-Neglect

Elder abuse is an intentional or negligent act by any person that causes harm or a serious risk of harm to an older adult and includes abuse that is physical, sexual, emotional, or psychological; neglect; and financial abuse or exploitation. **Self-neglect** is the most common form of elder abuse and occurs among all demographic strata. Financial abuse is on the rise, and older adults with cognitive impairment are particularly vulnerable. Each year, at least 5% of older adults are victims of financial abuse or scams. Elder abuse and self-neglect can cause many health consequences, such as long-term care placement, anxiety, depression, and death.

Elder abuse risk factors include limited social support and poor physical health. Clues to the presence of elder mistreatment or self-neglect include physical signs on examination such as lacerations or bruises in unusual locations or that cannot be explained; fractures in sites other than the wrist, hip, or vertebrae; or dehydration or malnutrition. Carefully note behavior changes in the presence of the caregiver, delays between injury occurrence and treatment seeking, inconsistencies between an observed

Table 4–4. Phrases and actions that may be helpful in situations of suspected abuse or neglect.

Questions for the Older Patient
1. Has anyone hurt you?
2. Are you afraid of anybody?
3. Is anyone taking or using your money without your permission?
Questions for the Caregiver
1. Are your relative's needs more than you can handle?
2. Are you worried that you might hit your relative?
3. Have you hit your relative?
If abuse is suspected
Tell the patient that you are concerned, want to help, and will call Adult Protective Services for further assistance
Document any injuries
Document the patient's words
Document whether the patient has decision-making capacity using a tool such as "Aid to Capacity Evaluation"

injury and its associated explanation, lack of appropriate clothing or hygiene, and unfilled prescriptions.

The USPSTF has found no evidence that screening for abuse or neglect causes harm and does not recommend for or against screening. Clinicians caring for older adults should maintain a high index of suspicion and meet with patients without the presence of caregivers on occasion. In these encounters, clinicians can ask questions about the caregiver relationship, and directly question about possible mistreatment and neglect, if suspected (Table 4–4).

When self-neglect is suspected, it is critical to establish whether a patient has decision-making capacity regarding the suspected neglectful behavior. A patient who has full decision-making capacity should be provided help and support but can choose to live in conditions of self-neglect, providing that the public is not endangered by their actions. In contrast, more aggressive intervention is recommended for a patient who lacks decision-making capacity and lives in conditions of self-neglect.

When to Refer

- Refer older adults suffering from suspected elder abuse or self-neglect to **Adult Protective Services**, as required by law in most states (consult the National Adult Protective Services Association, https://www.napsa-now.org/)
- Refer to a mental health professional and neurologist for evaluation of those cases in which decision-making capacity is unclear, neuropsychiatric testing would be useful, or if untreated mental illness is suspected to play a role in self-neglect.

When to Admit

- Admit older adults who would be unsafe in the community when an alternative plan cannot be put into place in a timely manner. In cases of self-neglect, surrogate decision-makers need to be identified, and conservatorship may need to be pursued for safe discharge planning.

5 Palliative Care & Pain Management

Kara E. Bischoff, MD
Sarah Nouri, MD, MPH
J. Ben Arevalo, MD, MBA
Ann Cai Shah, MD
Karin Sinavsky, MD, MS

PALLIATIVE CARE

DEFINITION & SCOPE

Palliative care is medical care focused on improving quality of life for people living with serious illness. Serious illness is defined as "a condition that carries a high risk of mortality, negatively impacts quality of life and daily function, and/or is burdensome in symptoms, treatments or caregiver stress." Palliative care is an interdisciplinary practice that addresses physical and psychological symptoms, helps ensure that care aligns with patients' preferences and goals, and supports patients and their loved ones who are facing serious illness. Randomized studies have shown that palliative care provided alongside life-prolonging treatment throughout the course of a serious illness can reduce symptoms, improve quality of life, and even prolong life in some situations. Palliative care can be provided at any age or stage of serious illness, inpatient or outpatient, and alongside life-prolonging or curative treatment. On the other hand, hospice is a service provided near the end of life to patients with a prognosis of < 6 months who have chosen to forgo further life-prolonging treatments. Increasingly, outpatient palliative care is being tailored to specific populations and provided in close collaboration with disease-directed medical care.

All clinicians should have basic skills to care for people with serious illness, including routinely identifying and taking initial steps to manage symptoms, communicating about prognosis and eliciting patients' preferences for care, and helping identify and address sources of distress in patients and their care partners.

Khayal IS et al. What is in the palliative care 'syringe'? A systems perspective. Soc Sci Med. 2022;305:115069. [PMID: 35691210]

Temel JS et al. Stepped palliative care for patients with advanced lung cancer: a randomized clinical trial. JAMA. 2024;332:471. [PMID: 38824442]

Leiter RE et al. Top ten tips palliative care clinicians should know about delivering specialty-aligned palliative care. J Palliat Med. 2023;26:1401. [PMID: 37001173]

Yeh JC et al. Different associations between inpatient or outpatient palliative care and end-of-life outcomes for hospitalized patients with cancer. JCO Oncol Pract. 2022;18:e516. [PMID: 34914566]

PALLIATION OF COMMON NONPAIN SYMPTOMS

Many physical symptoms are common in the setting of serious illness, including pain, dyspnea, nausea and vomiting, constipation, fatigue, and delirium. Pain is discussed separately within this chapter. Treatment of depression and anxiety is discussed briefly in this chapter and extensively in Chapter 28. This chapter focuses primarily on the pharmacologic management of symptoms and also recognizes the benefits of many nonpharmacologic approaches to symptom management.

Dyspnea

Dyspnea is the subjective experience of difficulty breathing and may be characterized as shortness of breath, breathlessness, or tightness in the chest. Up to half of people at the end of life experience dyspnea.

Treatment of dyspnea is first directed at the underlying cause (see Chapter 9), assuming this care is consistent with a patient's goals. When disease-directed treatments for dyspnea (eg, diuresis, thoracentesis) are not sufficient or desired, dyspnea can be managed symptomatically with opioids. Starting doses are typically lower than what is necessary for the relief of pain. *Immediate-release* liquid morphine given orally (2–5 mg sublingually every 4 hours as needed) or intravenously (1–2 mg every 2 hours as needed) can treat dyspnea effectively. *Sustained-release* morphine given orally at a dose of 15 mg once or twice daily is safe and effective for most patients with frequent or chronic dyspnea. Supplemental oxygen may be useful for patients who are *hypoxic,* but oxygen is *not* helpful for dyspnea in patients who are not hypoxic. Noninvasive ventilation (eg, bilevel positive airway pressure [BIPAP]) can be helpful when ventilation is compromised, assuming there are no contraindications. Moving air from an open window or fan also can provide relief from dyspnea.

For patients with dyspnea and associated anxiety, nonpharmacologic relaxation techniques, such as mindfulness, meditation, and guided imagery, may be beneficial. Benzodiazepines may be useful adjuncts for treatment of dyspnea-related anxiety but should be used with caution, especially in combination with opioids, as they can increase risk of mortality.

Burge AT et al. Breathing techniques to reduce symptoms in people with serious respiratory illness: a systematic review. Eur Respir Rev. 2024;33:240012. [PMID: 39477355]
Simon ST et al; BETTER-B Consortium. Practice review: pharmacological management of severe chronic breathlessness in adults with advanced life-limiting diseases. Palliat Med. 2024;38:1079. [PMID: 39264397]

Nausea & Vomiting

Medications for nausea and vomiting are summarized in Table 5–1. Additionally, integrative medicine practices for treatment of nausea that are supported by evidence include ginger, inhaled isopropyl alcohol, acupuncture, and hypnosis. Medical cannabis and dronabinol (2.5–20 mg orally every 4–6 hours) can also be helpful in the management of nausea and can boost appetite. The management of severe, frequent nausea can require proactive dosing of medications (ie, scheduled around the clock rather than as needed) as well as multiple medications targeting more than one of the major mechanisms of nausea and vomiting (see Chapter 17).

Malignant bowel obstructions can cause nausea and vomiting that are particularly challenging to ameliorate. In those cases, suction via nasogastric tube may provide rapid relief, H_2-blocking medications (eg, famotidine 20–60 mg orally daily) can reduce gastric secretions, steroids (eg, dexamethasone 8 mg daily) can be used to decrease swelling associated with the tumor to relieve the obstruction, and somatostatin analogs (eg, octreotide 200 mcg every 8 hours) may be tried to decrease gastrointestinal secretions and motility, though evidence for their benefit is limited. Antipsychotics (ie, haloperidol, olanzapine) are the preferred antiemetic medications in the case of malignant bowel obstruction, while promotility agents (ie, metoclopramide) should be avoided in cases of complete obstruction. In refractory cases, a venting gastrostomy tube may be needed to provide symptomatic relief.

Table 5–1. Pharmacologic management of nausea and vomiting.

Medication Class	Medications and Dosing	Pathophysiologic Causes of Nausea, with Check Mark (√) Indicating Mechanisms of Each Medication Class				
		Toxins (eg, Chemotherapy, Infection)	Vestibular Disturbance	Gastrointestinal Dysmotility or Disturbance	Anticipation or Sensory Triggers	Increased Intracranial Pressure
5-HT3 antagonists	Ondansetron (4–8 mg orally or intravenously four times a day) Granisetron patch (3.1 mg transdermally daily) Mirtazapine (7.5–45 mg orally nightly)	√	√	√	√	√
Dopaminergic antagonists	Olanzapine (2.5–10 mg orally nightly) Prochlorperazine (5–10 mg orally or intravenously four times a day or 25 mg per rectum twice daily) Metoclopramide (5–10 mg orally or intravenously four times a day)	√		√		
Antihistaminic or anticholinergic	Diphenhydramine (12.5–25 mg orally or intravenously every 8 hours) Scopolamine (1.5-mg patch every 3 days)		√			
Neurokinin-1 receptor antagonists	Aprepitant (125 mg orally on day 1, 80 mg on days 2–3)	√				
Benzodiazepines	Lorazepam (0.5–1.0 mg orally every 6–8 hours)				√	
Corticosteroids	Dexamethasone (4 mg two to four times a day)			√		√
Acid suppressants	Famotidine (20–60 mg orally daily) Omeprazole (20 mg twice daily) (also available as orally dissolving tablet)			√		

Constipation

Constipation is a common problem in seriously ill patients, particularly given the frequent use of opioids, low intake of fluids and food, physical inactivity, and changes in strength and mobility that can affect toileting. Constipation is also a preventable and treatable cause of discomfort, so clinicians should be sure to inquire about hard, infrequent, and difficult-to-pass stools (see Chapter 17). Sometimes, mild constipation may be prevented or relieved if patients increase their activity and intake of fluids. Simple considerations, such as privacy, regular undisturbed toilet time, and a bedside commode rather than a bedpan, may be helpful.

Constipation from opioid use—*A prophylactic bowel regimen with a stimulant laxative (eg, senna or bisacodyl) should be offered whenever opioids are prescribed.* Table 17–4 lists other agents (including osmotic laxatives such as polyethylene glycol and lactulose) that can be added as needed, especially for firm or hard stools. Docusate, a stool softener, is *not* recommended because it does not add benefit beyond stimulant laxatives in seriously ill patients. In the setting of slowed peristalsis in opioid-induced constipation, bulk-forming laxatives, like psyllium, generally should be avoided. Peripherally acting mu-receptor antagonists (eg, naloxegol 12.5–25 mg orally daily and methylnaltrexone 8–12 mg subcutaneously every other day) are recommended to treat laxative-refractory opioid-induced constipation. Lubiprostone (8–24 mcg twice daily) and linaclotide (72–145 mcg daily) increase intestinal fluid secretion and also can be used. Suppositories (eg, bisacodyl 10 mg per rectum) and enemas (eg, tap water or saline) should be combined with oral medications in cases of severe constipation (eg, no bowel movement in > 3 days) or when use of oral medications is limited by vomiting. Patients who report being constipated and then have diarrhea may be passing liquid stool around impacted stool. Such patients should have a rectal examination to assess for impaction; if it is present, manual disimpaction can be the quickest way to provide relief.

PDQ Supportive and Palliative Care Editorial Board. PDQ Cancer Information Summaries. Table 1. Medical Agents for Constipation. Accessed January 2, 2026. https://www.ncbi.nlm.nih.gov/books/NBK65768/table/CDR0000062736__430/

Fatigue

Fatigue is the most common complaint among people with cancer, heart failure, and many other serious illnesses. Screening for and treating factors that contribute to fatigue is important (eg, insomnia, pain, depression, medication adverse effects, anemia, hypothyroidism, hypogonadism, and malnutrition). For nonspecific fatigue, a gradual increase of physical activity and physical rehabilitation may be most effective. There is strong evidence for exercise (eg, 150 minutes of aerobic exercise per week), yoga, and cognitive-behavioral therapy (CBT) to treat cancer-related fatigue. Psychostimulants (eg, methylphenidate 2.5–10 mg orally in the morning and mid-day as needed, modafinil 100–200 mg orally in the morning) and American ginseng (*Panax quinquefolius*) can be used to manage cancer-related fatigue, but evidence for their effectiveness is weaker. Corticosteroids can be beneficial but are most appropriate for patients with a short prognosis given their myriad side effects, which are most problematic with long-term use. Caffeine also can help some patients.

Robbins Welty GA et al. Top ten tips palliative care clinicians should know about diagnosing, categorizing, and addressing fatigue. J Palliat Med. 2025;28:389. [PMID: 39052494]
Stone P et al. Management of fatigue in patients with advanced cancer. Curr Treat Options Oncol. 2023;24:93. [PMID: 36656503]

Delirium & Agitation

Many seriously ill patients experience delirium—a waxing and waning in level of consciousness and cognition that develops over a short time course and is manifested by disorientation, sleep-wake cycle disruptions, psychomotor disturbances (eg, lethargy, restlessness), and mood disturbances (eg, fear, anxiety). Delirium may be hyperactive, hypoactive, or mixed. Hyperactive delirium at the end of life has also been called **terminal restlessness** and can be highly distressing.

Common reversible causes of delirium include infections, urinary retention, constipation, anticholinergic medications, pain, and sleep disruption; these should be addressed when they are found. There is no strong evidence that dehydration causes, or that hydration relieves, delirium. Nonpharmacologic measures—including modifying the environment to make it calming and safe, ensuring a clear distinction between day and night, and frequently reassuring and reorienting patients to where they are and what is happening—are the cornerstones of delirium treatment. Ramelteon, a melatonin agonist, 8 mg/day orally has been shown to prevent delirium in seriously ill, older, hospitalized patients. The use of scheduled antipsychotics (eg, haloperidol) in patients with moderate delirium has been shown to *increase* delirium and mortality compared to placebo. *Thus, antipsychotics generally should be avoided in this setting.* However, when agitated delirium is severe and poses a significant safety risk or quality of life concern, low-dose antipsychotics (eg, quetiapine 12.5–25 mg orally at bedtime or haloperidol 1–2 mg orally, subcutaneously, intramuscularly, or intravenously every 6 hours as needed) may be used to mildly sedate the patient. Although benzodiazepines can worsen delirium and generally should be avoided, they may be used when deeper sedation is needed to achieve comfort or relieve suffering near the end of life, including in the setting of terminal restlessness. Such sedation may be achieved with midazolam (0.5–5 mg/h subcutaneously or intravenously) or with barbiturates (eg, phenobarbital 200 mg orally or rectally).

Heijltjes MT et al. Physicians opinion and practice with the continuous use of sedatives in the last days of life. J Pain Symptom Manage. 2022;63:78. [PMID: 34333097]

Depression & Anxiety

The management of mood symptoms, such as depression and anxiety, is an important aspect of palliative care and is described in detail in Chapter 28. Feelings of hopelessness, worthlessness, or anhedonia help to distinguish depression from the low energy, changes in appetite, and other symptoms that are common in advanced illness. *Despite the significant sadness and grief that can be associated with facing a serious illness, clinical depression is not normal or inevitable and should be treated.* Coexisting depression can worsen outcomes in numerous serious illnesses.

SSRIs (eg, escitalopram starting at 10 mg daily) are the most common first-line treatment for depression and anxiety. However, in choosing a medication to treat depression or anxiety in a person with serious illness, it is prudent to consider whether it can also be beneficial for coexisting symptoms. For instance, serotonin norepinephrine reuptake inhibitors (SNRIs) are often preferred over SSRIs for patients with neuropathic pain in addition to depression because they can have secondary benefits for neuropathic pain. Mirtazapine can help with mood as well as with nausea and insomnia. When prognosis is short, it is important to use medications that render effects quickly. Therefore, for patients who have prominent fatigue in the setting of depression, a psychostimulant such as methylphenidate (2.5–10 mg orally at 8:00 AM and a second dose at 2:00 PM) or dextroamphetamine (2.5–7.5 mg orally at 8:00 AM and a second dose at 2:00 PM) can be started along with a traditional antidepressant medication to provide initial symptom relief while the benefits of SSRI or SNRI antidepressants take effect over 4–6 weeks. The stimulant can then be stopped or continued based on the patient's response to the stimulant, preferences, and prognosis. Similarly, for patients with prominent anxiety a benzodiazepine (eg, clonazepam 0.25 mg twice daily) can be used until SSRI or SNRIs take effect. There is also emerging evidence for the benefits of psychedelic-assisted therapy (eg, with psilocybin or ketamine) for depression and anxiety, including at the end of life.

Generally, best outcomes result from the combination of pharmacologic and behavioral treatments for depression and anxiety. **Cognitive behavioral therapy** and **acceptance and commitment therapy** are two evidence-based psychotherapeutic frameworks that are commonly used for people with depression, anxiety, or both. Additionally, there is good evidence for the benefits of mindfulness for depression and anxiety. A meta-analysis found that mindfulness-based interventions were associated with reductions in anxiety for at least 6 months. Many online and mobile applications can support people to develop and practice mindfulness skills.

Chammas D et al. Top ten tips palliative care clinicians should know about applying key psychotherapy concepts in practice. J Palliat Med. 2025;28:1108. [PMID: 39269882]

Gibson Watt T et al. Acceptance and Commitment Therapy (ACT) for people with advanced progressive illness, their caregivers and staff involved in their care: a scoping review. Palliat Med. 2023;37:1100. [PMID: 37489074]

Goodwin GM et al. Single-dose psilocybin for a treatment-resistant episode of major depression. N Engl J Med. 2022; 387:1637. [PMID: 36322843]

Whinkin E et al. Psilocybin in palliative care: an update. Curr Geriatr Rep. 2023;12:50. [PMID: 37305379]

COMMUNICATION

Prognostication

Most people with serious illness, and their loved ones, want accurate prognostic information. This information is necessary for people to be able to make informed decisions, typically influences the choices they make and how they spend their time, and—when delivered skillfully—does not negatively impact well-being.

However, determining and communicating prognosis is not easy. Studies have shown that clinicians' estimates of prognosis are often inaccurate and generally overly optimistic. Many people with cancer do not understand when the treatments they are on are palliative rather than curative. Other common causes of death—including heart disease, stroke, chronic lung disease, and dementia—have even more variable trajectories and difficult-to-predict prognoses than most cancers. Nonetheless, clinical experience, epidemiologic data, and prediction tools (eg, the Palliative Performance Scale, found with other prognostic tools at http://eprognosis.ucsf.edu) may be used in combination to offer patients more realistic estimates of prognosis. Clinicians can also ask themselves "Would I be surprised if this patient died in the next year?" If the answer is "no," then the clinician should plan for a discussion of goals of care. Recognizing that patients may have different preferences about when and how they receive prognostic information, clinicians should ask for permission before discussing prognosis, saying something like, *"I have information about what's likely to come with your illness. Would you like to talk about this?"* Additionally, it can be helpful to understand how patients want to receive this information with a statement such as, *"Some people prefer to hear information directly. Other people want information filtered through others, or don't want to hear certain information such as how much time they might have left to live. What are your preferences about receiving information about your illness and what is likely to come in the future?"* Palliative care communication resources, such as VitalTalk, offer detailed guidance around discussing prognosis (https://www.vitaltalk.org/guides/discussing-prognosis/).

Bischoff KE et al. Prognoses associated with palliative performance scale scores in modern palliative care practice. JAMA Netw Open. 2024;7:e2420472. [PMID: 38976269]

Canavan ME et al. Systemic anticancer therapy at the end of life—changes in usage pattern in the immunotherapy era. JAMA Oncol. 2022;8:1847. [PMID: 36264566]

Communication in the Care of Seriously Ill Patients

Communication skills are vitally important when caring for people with serious illness and can be improved through training. High-quality communication is associated with greater patient satisfaction and care that is more

Table 5–2. Suggested outline for the delivery of serious news.

Choose an appropriate place, time, and group of attendees.
Clinicians pre-meet and set an agenda for the conversation.
Introduce all attendees and ask permission to review the news.
Assess the patient and family's perspectives and what they already know or have been told.
Provide clinical information. Be brief and direct; avoid jargon and euphemisms. Pause frequently to check for understanding.
Leave space for silence and expression of emotions. Compassionately attend to emotions that arise.
Allow sufficient time for processing and collaborative decision-making, whenever possible.
Briefly summarize the conversation and next steps. Ensure a plan to address questions that arise.

often concordant with patients' wishes. Clinicians must be proficient at delivering sensitive information and supporting the people who hear it (Table 5–2). Resources are available to support clinicians around serious illness communication (https://www.vitaltalk.org/, https://www.ariadnelabs.org/serious-illness-care/), and evidence suggests that communication checklists and guides can be helpful. When the clinician and patient do not speak the same language fluently, the use of a professional interpreter is critical to facilitate clear communication.

Jacobsen J et al. Shifting to serious illness communication. JAMA. 2022;327:321. [PMID: 34994773]

Manz CR et al. Long-term effect of machine learning-triggered behavioral nudges on serious illness conversations and end-of-life outcomes among patients with cancer: a randomized clinical trial. JAMA Oncol. 2023;9:414. [PMID: 36633868]

Advance Care Planning & Advance Directives

Advance care planning is *"a process that supports adults at any age or stage of health in understanding and sharing their personal values, life goals, and preferences regarding future medical care."* Clinicians should encourage all patients—ideally well before the end of life—to consider their preferences, appoint a surrogate decision-maker, talk to that person and to their clinicians about their preferences for current and future care, and document their wishes. Most people with a serious illness have already thought about how they hope the end of their life will go, want to discuss their wishes with their clinicians, want clinicians to bring up the subject of advance care planning, and feel better for having had discussions. Patients who have such discussions with their clinicians are more satisfied with their clinicians, are less likely to die in a hospital, are more likely to utilize hospice care, and are perceived by their family as having a better quality of life at the end of life. The loved ones of people who engage in advance care planning discussions are also less likely to suffer from depression during bereavement.

Advance directives are written or oral statements made by patients when they are competent, which are intended to guide care should they lose the capacity to make and communicate their own decisions. While oral statements about these matters are ethically binding, they are not legally binding in all states. Through an advance directive, people can assign a **Durable Power of Attorney for Health Care (DPOA-HC)**, a surrogate decision-maker who is to use "substituted judgment" to decide *what a patient would have wanted* when the patient has become unable to make and communicate their own decisions. State-specific advance directive forms are available from a number of sources, including https://www.caringinfo.org/planning/advance-directives/, and online resources, such as https://prepareforyourcare.org, can guide people through the process of completing an advance directive.

Hickman SE et al. The care planning umbrella: the evolution of advance care planning. J Am Geriatr Soc. 2023;71:2350. [PMID: 36840690]

McMahan RD et al. What clinicians and researchers should know about the evolving field of advance care planning: a narrative review. J Gen Intern Med. 2024;39:652. [PMID: 38169025]

Resuscitation Preferences

Because the "default" in US hospitals is that patients will undergo cardiopulmonary resuscitation (CPR) in the event of cardiopulmonary arrest, as part of advance care planning, clinicians should elicit patient preferences about CPR upon hospital admission as well as at other times when cardiac arrest seems like a distinct possibility. Only about 17% of all patients who undergo CPR in the hospital survive to hospital discharge; among people with multisystem organ failure, metastatic cancer, and sepsis, the likelihood of survival to hospital discharge following CPR is much lower. Clinicians must describe CPR clearly, avoiding overly frightening or benign language that might unduly sway a patient's decision, and must inform patients about the possible sequelae of CPR if they do survive, including neurologic disability and need for other invasive interventions such as intubation and mechanical ventilation. Patients may ask their hospital clinician to write an order that CPR not be attempted should they experience cardiac arrest. Although this order initially was referred to as a **"DNR" (do not resuscitate)** order, some clinicians prefer the term **"DNAR" (do not attempt resuscitation)** to emphasize that resuscitation is not always successful or **"Allow Natural Death,"** which is particularly appropriate for situations in which death is imminent.

For patients with very short prognoses, decisions about CPR may be best understood as being about not *whether they will survive*, but about *how they will die*. Clinicians should correct the misconception that not doing CPR is tantamount to "withdrawing care" or "letting someone die." While respecting the patient's right to make the decision, clinicians should offer recommendations about DNAR orders that are grounded in their understanding of the patient's values and priorities, taking care to not be influenced by their own biases and prejudices. Providing such recommendations can protect dying patients and their families from feelings of guilt and from the added grief associated with having unrealistic hopes. When transitioning to a comfort-focused treatment plan, clinicians should also discuss which interventions will be continued and which started to promote comfort, rather than focusing only on which interventions will be stopped or withheld. For patients with an implanted cardioverter defibrillator, clinicians must also address turning off the defibrillator, while leaving the pacemaker function on, to prevent the distressing situation of the defibrillator discharging during the dying process.

Physician (or Medical) Orders for Life-Sustaining Treatment (POLST [or MOLST]) forms are active orders, including about resuscitation, that complement advance directives and can guide care for patients especially in the setting of an emergency. They document care preferences in a concise, standardized way that is transferrable across all care settings—home, hospital, and care facilities. They are available in most states within the United States and are appropriate for people with a serious illness, frailty, a short (roughly < 1 year) prognosis, or a combination of these conditions.

Cagino LM et al; American Heart Association's Get With The Guidelines-Resuscitation Investigators. Trends in return of spontaneous circulation and survival to hospital discharge for in-intensive care unit cardiac arrests. Ann Am Thorac Soc. 2023;20:1012. [PMID: 36939838]

Jang K et al. Factors affecting neurological outcomes of patients with sudden cardiac arrest in the emergency department. BMC Emerg Med. 2024;24:167. [PMID: 39271981]

Ethical Considerations

Clinicians' care of seriously ill patients is guided by the same ethical and legal principles that inform other types of medical care. Foremost among these are truth-telling, nonmaleficence, beneficence, autonomy, confidentiality, and procedural and distributive justice. *Important ethical principles may come into conflict when caring for patients with serious illness.* For example, many treatments that promote beneficence and autonomy, such as surgery or bone marrow transplantation, may end up violating clinicians' commitment to nonmaleficence; thus, balancing the benefits and risks of treatments is an important ethical responsibility in palliative care.

In most cases, clinicians, patients, and families agree on decisions to stop or forego life-sustaining interventions, and most disagreements between families and clinicians can be resolved with good communication and time for adaptation. However, when there is persistent disagreement between patients or family members and clinicians, it is recommended that the clinicians consult with an institutional ethics committee. In rare cases, clinicians may determine unilaterally that a particular intervention—such as CPR or dialysis in end-stage multisystem organ failure—offers no realistic possibility of benefit and thus need not be offered even when it is requested by a patient or family. Because such unilateral actions potentially violate the autonomy of the patient, clinicians should *rarely* resort to them. Clinicians must use caution in invoking "futility," since strict futility is rare and what constitutes futility is often a matter of controversy and subject to bias.

Psychological, Social, & Spiritual Aspects of Care

Illness and dying are not exclusively biomedical processes. They are human experiences with profound psychological, interpersonal, and existential meaning. For many people with serious illness, the prospect of impending death stimulates reassessment of their identity, relationships, values and priorities, the meaning and purpose of their life, and their legacy. Some individuals may grow through illness and, by offering presence, encouraging reflection, and providing support, clinicians may be a catalyst for this growth.

A. Psychological Considerations

Near the end of life, anticipatory grief is common. In 1969, Dr. Elisabeth Kübler-Ross identified five psychological reactions or patterns of emotions seen in grief: denial and isolation, anger, bargaining, depression, and acceptance. Many people will experience these reactions throughout the course of a serious illness, but generally not in an orderly progression. In addition to these five reactions are the challenges of anxiety and fear of the unknown. Providing information consistent with people's information preferences, attentive listening, reassurance when appropriate, and validation may help people with these psychological challenges. *Patients and families rank emotional support as one of the most important aspects of end-of-life care.* Meaning-centered psychotherapy is effective for treating emotional distress at the end of life. See above under "Palliation of Common Nonpain Symptoms" and Chapter 28 for a description of the pharmacologic treatment of pathologic depression and anxiety in the setting of serious illness.

Clinicians caring for seriously ill patients can also serve as catalysts for hope. While hope for a particular outcome such as cure may decline, hope can be refocused on *what is still possible.* Even if a patient hopes for a "miracle," clinicians can share that hope while simultaneously acknowledging their honest worries and encouraging more likely hopes, including for comfort, connection with loved ones, meaning-making, and spiritual growth. With such questions as, *"When you look to the future, what do you hope for?"* clinicians can explore meaningful and realistic goals and then develop plans to achieve them.

B. Social Considerations

In the face of serious illness, patients should be encouraged to attend to personal, professional, and logistical obligations. These tasks include completing important work or personal projects, distributing possessions, writing a will, and making funeral and burial arrangements, as desired. Some people find meaning in writing an "ethical will" that documents their wisdom and lessons learned (see also information about "legacy," below). The prospect of death often prompts people to examine the quality of their interpersonal relationships and to begin the process of saying goodbye. Concern about estranged relationships or "unfinished business" and interest in reconciliation may become paramount at this time. Financial concerns can be a significant source of distress, particularly given the rising costs of caregiving, which many people with serious illness require. Referrals to social workers can help identify potential resources or strategies to address these concerns.

C. Spiritual & Existential Considerations

As people near the end of life, spiritual and existential considerations often include attempts to understand the meaning of one's life, one's place in the universe, and one's legacy. Perhaps because of preoccupation with biologic aspects of treatment or lack of training, clinicians frequently ignore their patients' spiritual concerns or reflexively refer these important issues to chaplains or other spiritual care providers. However, existential considerations are central to the well-being of people with serious illness and should be the concern of all clinicians caring for them.

Unlike physical ailments, such as infections and fractures, which usually require a concrete intervention to be treated, a patient's spiritual and existential concerns are often best addressed through a clinician's devoted attention, active listening, and bearing witness, rather than attempts to "fix" problems. Clinicians can inquire about the patient's spiritual well-being and ask whether the patient wishes to discuss existential concerns. For example, asking, *"How are your spirits?"* or *"Are you at peace?"* communicates that the clinician is interested in the patient's whole experience and provides an opportunity for the patient to share perceptions about his or her inner life.

Legacy work and dignity therapy have been shown to be effective in improving spiritual well-being and quality of life. Clinicians can ask patients to recall what they are proudest of to promote a sense of value and dignity. Opportunities for storytelling give patients a chance to verbalize what is meaningful to them and to leave something of themselves behind, with the promise of being remembered by loved ones. Consider inviting patients to share their life stories with family members, make an audio or video recording, assemble a photo album or scrapbook, or write or dictate autobiographical vignettes.

Kluger BM et al. The total enjoyment of life: a framework for exploring and supporting the positive in palliative care. J Palliat Med. 2023;26:1322. [PMID: 37471240]
Tarbi EC et al. Top ten tips palliative care clinicians should know about attending to the existential experience. J Palliat Med. 2024;27:1379. [PMID: 38546453]
Wulandari BT et al. Effectiveness of dignity therapy on well-being among patients under palliative care: a systematic review and meta-analysis. Int J Nurs Stud. 2024;149:104624. [PMID: 37980718]

Cultural Considerations

Various religious, ethnic, and cultural traditions can influence a patient's style of communication, comfort in discussing particular topics, expectations about illness, dying, and medical interventions, and preferences about disposition of remains. While there are some differences in perspectives regarding advance care planning, withdrawal of life-sustaining interventions, autopsy, organ donation, and hospice care among patients of different demographic groups, clinicians should be careful not to make assumptions about any particular individual. Being curious about and respectful of each person's unique values, beliefs, and traditions are important responsibilities of the clinician caring for seriously ill patients. A clinician may ask, *"What do I need to know about you and your beliefs that will help me take the best care of you?"* and *"How do you make decisions in your family?"*

Clinicians must also appreciate that palliative care is susceptible to the same explicit and implicit biases documented in other medical specialties. Humility, self-reflection, and continual learning are key to the practice of palliative care. It is also imperative that palliative care practitioners work actively to identify and rectify injustice in the medical system, including racism, sexism, class discrimination, and homophobia.

Elbaum A et al. Decision-making across cultures. Cancer Treat Res. 2023;187:85. [PMID: 37851221]
Koffman J et al. Researching minoritised communities in palliative care: an agenda for change. Palliat Med. 2023;37:530. [PMID: 36271636]

Caring for the Family & Other Care Partners

In caring for seriously ill patients, clinicians must appreciate the central role played by family, friends, and other loved ones (sometimes called "caregivers" or "care partners"). Family and other informal care partners, most often women, provide the bulk of care for seriously ill patients, yet their work is often not adequately acknowledged, supported, or compensated. They can simultaneously struggle with physical caregiving responsibilities, care coordination challenges, and financial burdens. Care partners experience heightened rates of anxiety, depression, grief, chronic illness, and even mortality. However, palliative care has been shown to reduce depression, complicated grief, and posttraumatic stress disorder in care partners.

Clinicians treating people with serious illness should provide care not only for patients but also for care partners. It is important to hold family meetings so that all members can hear from clinicians, understand patients' values and preferences, and be heard. Acknowledging and respecting the role of care partners, and soliciting their perspectives, questions, and concerns, can be powerful. It is important to offer care partners an opportunity to meet with members of the medical team separately from the patient, which can be particularly meaningful when the informational preferences and needs of the care partner differ from those of the patient. Video telemedicine can allow care partners to participate in meetings even if they are unable to be physically present.

Fenton ATHR et al. Racial and ethnic disparities in cancer caregiver burden and potential sociocultural mediators. Support Care Cancer. 2022;30:9625. [PMID: 36190556]

CARING FOR PATIENTS AT THE END OF LIFE

Annually, > 3 million people die in the United States and approximately 61 million die worldwide. Caring for patients at the end of life is an important responsibility and can be deeply meaningful for clinicians. *The end of life is defined as the time when death is expected within hours to a few months and can no longer be significantly forestalled by medical intervention.* At the end of life, palliative care can do much to relieve distress and promote comfort and quality of life. For many patients at the end of life, palliative care becomes the primary or sole focus of care.

Counseling Patients Approaching the End of Life

Patients' experiences at the end of life are influenced by their expectations about how they will die and their sense of the meaning of death. Many fear *how* they will die more than death itself. Patients report fears of dying in pain or of suffocation, loss of control, indignity, isolation, and being a burden to their families. These anxieties may be ameliorated with attentive palliative care.

Death is often regarded by clinicians, patients, and families as a failure and an enemy to be battled rather than as an inevitability and a normal part of life. As a result, many people in the United States die in hospitals or long-term care facilities even though they may have wished otherwise. However, there has been a trend toward more deaths occurring at home and fewer deaths in hospitals, which was accelerated by the COVID-19 pandemic. In 2024, 39% of deaths in the United States occurred at home, 24% occurred in hospitals, and the remainder occurred in other care facilities.

Relieving suffering, providing support, and helping patients make the most of their final stage of life should be the foremost considerations, even when patients continue to pursue disease-directed treatment. People at the end of life and their care partners identify many factors as important to quality end-of-life care, including managing pain and other symptoms, avoiding unwanted invasive treatments, preserving dignity, having a sense of control, minimizing burdens on others, and strengthening relationships with loved ones. However, because there is a wide variation between people in terms of what they value most at the end of life, it is critical that clinicians ask patients about their priorities, preferences, and what matters most to them.

Additionally, it is important that clinicians caring for patients at the end of life pledge that they will care for the patient throughout the final stage of life, which can help curb the patients' fear and sense of isolation. *The promise of **nonabandonment** is a central principle of end-of-life care.* No matter what happens, clinicians can be a guide during uncertain times, a resource for practical problem-solving, and a witness to patients' experiences. Dying patients need their clinicians to offer their presence—not necessarily the ability to solve all problems but rather a commitment to witness and acknowledge the patients' experiences with respect and empathy. At its best, the patient–clinician relationship can be a covenant of compassion and affirmation of common humanity.

Chochinov HM. Intensive caring: reminding patients they matter. J Clin Oncol. 2023;41:2884. [PMID: 37075272]
Teasdale B et al. Place of death before and during the COVID-19 pandemic. JAMA Netw Open. 2024;7:e2350821. [PMID: 38190187]

Hospice

In the United States, hospice is a specific type of palliative care service that is available to patients with a prognosis of 6 months or less (a criterion for eligibility under the Medicare hospice benefit) who want to prioritize comfort and not pursue life-prolonging treatments. In the United States in 2024, nearly half (43–47%) of people who died use hospice, most at home where they were cared for by their family and other care partners with support from visiting hospice staff. Less often, hospice care is provided in residential facilities, nursing homes, and hospitals. As is true of all types of palliative care, hospice emphasizes individualized attention for patients and care partners, and uses an interdisciplinary team approach with nurses, social workers, chaplains, personal care attendants, physicians, and others working together. When patients enroll in hospice, the hospice team typically takes over their medical care, but patients can choose one medical provider (a preexisting provider or a hospice physician) to oversee their hospice care. Hospice is rated highly by families and has been shown to increase patient satisfaction and improve care partner bereavement. A study of bereaved family caregivers demonstrated higher opinions of end-of-life care provided by home hospice teams compared with end-of-life care provided in nursing homes, in hospitals, or at home without hospice care.

Despite evidence suggesting that hospice care does not shorten length of life, hospice care tends to be engaged late; in 2024 the median duration of hospice care was 18–19 days. Many people wait to enroll in hospice until they have decided with certainty that they no longer wish to pursue disease-directed treatments. Patients can be encouraged to enroll in hospice while they are still deciding about further life-prolonging treatment attempts (eg, upcoming clinical trials) and can disenroll from hospice if they decide to pursue them or other desired services not covered by hospice.

Nutrition & Hydration

People with serious illness often lose their appetite, and most stop eating and drinking in their final days. Clinicians should explain to families that people who are dying are not "starving to death." Rather, *the cessation of eating and drinking is a normal part of the dying process.* The ketonemia caused by not eating can produce a sense of mild euphoria and analgesia. However, carbohydrate intake even in small amounts (such as that provided by 5% dextrose intravenous solution) may block ketone production. The sensation of thirst can usually be reduced by moistening the mouth with ice chips, swabs, or popsicles.

Although the normal process of diminishing oral intake is very common in seriously ill people, it can be distressing to families who may associate the offering of food with loving care and lack of eating with starvation. In response, patients and families often ask about intravenous hydration or enteral or parenteral nutrition. *Artificial nutrition and hydration generally do not benefit those at the end of life (including patients with end-stage cancer or dementia) and rarely achieve patient and family goals.* Intravenous hydration may increase oropharyngeal secretions that can be difficult to manage, pulmonary edema, and third-spacing and thus is not indicated unless a patient has severe or symptomatic dehydration. Enteral feeding may cause nausea and diarrhea and increase risk of aspiration. Parenteral nutrition carries risks of line infection, electrolyte imbalance, and burden from blood draws used to monitor the treatment, in additional to the potential harms caused by the fluid delivered. Additionally, artificial hydration and nutrition for delirious patients may lead to the use of physical or chemical restraints to prevent lines or tubes from being dislodged.

Decisions about artificial nutrition and hydration are not simply medical and may have deep social and cultural significance for patients, care partners, and clinicians. Eliciting perceived goals of artificial nutrition and hydration, correcting misperceptions, offering comprehensive support to patients and care partners, and allowing sufficient time to make decisions can help patients and care partners make sound decisions. Care partners can be encouraged to express their love and care for patients in ways other than through artificial nutrition or hydration (eg, using ice chips or swabs to relieve symptomatic xerostomia). Individuals at the end of life have the right to voluntarily refuse nutrition and hydration.

Bower KL et al. Ethical implications of nutrition therapy at the end of life. Curr Gastroenterol Rep. 2023;25:69. [PMID: 36862286]

Withdrawal of Life-Prolonging Treatments

Informed and competent patients, or their surrogates, are allowed to refuse or stop life-sustaining treatments. The withdrawal of life-sustaining treatments, such as mechanical ventilation, must be done carefully to avoid patient suffering and distress for those in attendance. Clinicians should educate the patient and family about the expected course of events after withdrawal of life-sustaining treatments, and what can be expected regarding the approximate timing of death. Loved ones should be offered the opportunity to be at the bedside during the process of withdrawing life-sustaining interventions whenever possible. Sedating and analgesic agents should be administered to ensure patient comfort prior to any life-prolonging treatments being withdrawn, even if they contribute to respiratory depression or hypotension. The ethical **Principle of Double Effect** argues that hastening of an imminent death is acceptable if it comes as the known but unintended consequence of a primary intention to provide comfort and relieve suffering. When communicating with patients and their care partners, using language like "transitioning to comfort-focused care" and "stopping interventions that artificially sustain life" is preferred to using the phrase "withdrawing care," since the latter term may be perceived as entirely stopping the provision of care and attention.

Care of the Actively Dying Patient

Signs of approaching death (eg, alterations in breathing patterns, skin changes, and changes in mental status) should be recognized and shared with loved ones so they can be prepared. Loved ones can be encouraged to speak gently to and around the dying person, with the assumption that dying people might still have the ability to hear even when they cannot respond. Retained oropharyngeal and respiratory secretions are common in actively dying patients, and the sound caused by these can be distressing to families, but they are not thought to be uncomfortable to patients as they are not typically associated with other signs of distress. Turning the patient can decrease the sound and decreasing intravenous fluids also can help. There is no evidence that medications (eg, glycopyrolate, atropine) improve comfort, and deep suctioning should be avoided since it can cause discomfort.

Medical Aid in Dying

Medical aid in dying (MAID) is the legally sanctioned process in some regions by which seriously ill patients can request a lethal dose of medications for the purpose of ending their lives. While terminology for this process varies, the term "physician-assisted suicide" is discouraged because it is not considered suicide and patients who are actively suicidal from mental illness are *not* eligible for MAID in the United States.

Although support for MAID has grown over time, this remains an area of contention and debate. As of 2025, MAID has been legalized with careful restrictions and specific procedures for residents in 10 US states (Oregon, Washington, Montana, Vermont, California, Colorado, Hawaii, New Jersey, Maine, and New Mexico) as well as the District of Columbia. Internationally, MAID (and/or euthanasia, which is the administration of a lethal dose of medication by a clinician) is legal in a growing number of countries (the Netherlands, Belgium, Luxembourg, Switzerland, Austria, Spain, Colombia, Canada, Germany, New Zealand, and Australia). US laws permitting MAID require physician certification of a terminal illness with a prognosis of 6 months or less and require the patient to be competent to make and communicate their own health care decisions at that time, to be an adult resident of the state, and to be physically capable of self-administering the medication through an enteral route. Any clinician who hears a request for MAID should be familiar with the law governing it in their area.

Requests for MAID are relatively rare, and the use of these medications leads to about 0.3% of all deaths in the United States. *Requests for MAID are most often motivated by a desire to have control in the dying process and preserve dignity, rather than by intolerable pain or other symptoms.* In the United States, most patients who request MAID are male, white, college-educated, and receiving hospice care.

Each clinician must decide their personal approach to caring for patients who ask about MAID. Regardless of the clinician's feelings about MAID, the clinician should respond initially by *exploring the patient's reasons for making the inquiry*, as this could reveal important sources of distress or fears that might be mitigated. During the dialogue, the clinician should inform the patient about their comprehensive treatment options (including palliative care, hospice care, and psychosocial and spiritual support) and provide reassurance that people typically can be made comfortable around the end of life. For clinicians who object to MAID on moral or ethical grounds, documentation of the request and referral to another clinician to field the request is appropriate.

TASKS AFTER DEATH

After the death of a patient, the clinician is called upon to perform a number of tasks, both required and recommended. The clinician must do an examination to confirm the death, compassionately and directly inform the family of the death, inquire about preferences regarding autopsy, complete a death certificate, and contact an organ procurement organization, as indicated. Providing words of sympathy and support, time for questions, and, for people who die in the hospital or other health care facility, a quiet private room for the family to grieve is also important.

Pronouncement & Death Certificates

In the United States, statewide policies direct clinicians to confirm the death of a patient in a formal process called "pronouncement." The diagnosis of death is typically easy to make, and the clinician need only verify the absence of spontaneous respirations and cardiac activity by auscultating for each for 1 minute. In many states, when a patient whose death is expected dies outside of the hospital (eg, at home), nurses may be authorized to report the death over the telephone to a physician who assumes responsibility for signing the death certificate within 24 hours. While the pronouncement may sometimes seem like an awkward and unnecessary formality, both clinicians and families may use the ritual as an opportunity to begin to emotionally process the death of the patient. Clinicians may use this time to reassure the patient's loved ones at the bedside that the patient died peacefully and that all appropriate care had been given, when this is the case.

Physicians are legally required to accurately report the underlying cause of death on the death certificate and to report certain deaths to the coroner. The physician should be specific about the major cause of death being the condition without which the patient would not have died (eg, "decompensated cirrhosis") and its contributory cause (eg, "hepatitis B and hepatitis C infections") as well as any associated conditions (eg, "acute kidney injury"). It is not appropriate to write "cardiac arrest" as the cause of death. In cases where MAID is utilized, clinicians should document the patient's underlying terminal illness that qualified them for the prescription (eg, "metastatic pancreatic cancer"). "Medical aid in dying" should not be written anywhere on the death certificate.

Autopsy & Organ Donation

Discussing the options of autopsy and organ donation with patients prior to death is a good practice when possible, as it promotes patient autonomy and lessens the responsibilities of family members during the sensitive period immediately following the death. In the United States, federal regulations require that a designated representative of an organ procurement organization be the one to approach family members about organ donation because they are typically more experienced than treating clinicians at counseling family members about organ donation. While most people in the United States support organ donation, organ transplantation is severely limited by the availability of donor organs. Many families of donors feel it is gratifying to contribute so meaningfully to the lives of others, even through death.

Even with the use of sophisticated diagnostic tests, an autopsy can provide families important information about the cause of their loved one's illness and death, which can help with closure and can advance medical knowledge. Despite the benefits of autopsies, autopsy rates in US hospitals are only approximately 8%. Some families decline autopsies because of unwarranted fears about disfigurement of the body or delay of the funeral, and some say they were not asked. It is important to educate families that pathologists can perform autopsies without interfering with funeral plans and take care to limit the impact on the appearance of the deceased.

Scarl R et al. The hospital autopsy: the importance in keeping autopsy an option. Autops Case Rep. 2022;12:e2021333. [PMID: 35252044]

Bereavement Care

Comprehensive end-of-life care includes following up with surviving loved ones after the patient has died. Contacting loved ones provides clinicians with opportunities to express respect for deceased patients and their care partners, assuage guilt loved ones may have, assess how loved ones are coping including screening for complicated grief, provide education about the normal grieving process, and recommend bereavement groups and counseling as appropriate. Some clinical teams also send a card or make a telephone call months after patients' deaths or on anniversaries of deaths so that loved ones know that they and the deceased patient have not been forgotten and supportive services remain available to them.

After a patient dies, clinicians also grieve. Some deaths may cause feelings of grief, guilt, or remorse. A first step toward processing and ameliorating these feelings is recognizing them. *Each clinician should consider developing or participating in personal or communal practices to support them through difficult emotions.* Taking time for reflection, sharing stories and feelings with colleagues, engaging in rituals, and protecting time for other self-care practices may be helpful.

Lichtenthal WG et al. Investing in bereavement care as a public health priority. Lancet Public Health. 2024;9:e270. Erratum in: Lancet Public Health. 2024;9:e281. [PMID: 38492580]

Clinician Self-Care

Many clinicians find caring for patients with serious illness to be one of the most rewarding aspects of medical practice. However, working with this population is intense and can invoke difficult emotions. Clinicians must be able to tolerate uncertainty, ambiguity, powerlessness, and the limitations of modern medicine. They may even find themselves considering their own eventual mortality. Clinicians should strive to recognize and attend to their own needs, build and strengthen resiliency skills, and advocate for sustainable health care systems, in order to avoid being overburdened, overly distressed, or emotionally depleted by this work.

Bramati PS et al. Evaluation of a daily nine-item "Handbook for Self-Care at Work" for palliative care clinicians. J Palliat Med. 2023;26:622. [PMID: 36318801]

PAIN MANAGEMENT

TAXONOMY OF PAIN

The International Association for the Study of Pain (IASP) defines pain as "an unpleasant sensory and emotional experience associated with, or resembling that associated with, actual or potential tissue damage."

Acute pain resolves within the expected period of healing and is self-limited.

Chronic pain persists beyond the expected period of healing and is itself a disease state. In general, chronic pain is defined as extending beyond 3–6 months.

Cancer pain is in its own special category because of the unique ways neoplasia and its therapies (such as surgery, chemotherapy, immunotherapy, or radiation therapy) can lead to burdensome pain and can span acute and chronic pain.

Pain at the end of life entails measures to alleviate suffering that may take priority over promoting restoration of function.

Pain is a worldwide burden; across the globe, *one in five adults suffers from pain.* In 2010, members from 130 countries signed the Declaration of Montreal stating that *access to pain management is a fundamental human right.* The first CDC guidelines on opioid prescribing for chronic pain, including chronic noncancer pain, cancer pain, and pain at the end of life, were published in 2016, and continue to be updated. Notably, in 2022, the CDC opioid prescribing guidelines were revised with increased flexibility for opioid prescriptions.

Centers for Disease Control and Prevention (CDC). Opioid Prescribing Resources. 2022. Department of Health and Human Services. Pain Management Best Practices. Pain management best practices inter-agency task force report. 2022. Accessed August 25, 2025. https://www.cdc.gov/overdose-prevention/hcp/clinical-guidance/

Dowell D et al. CDC Clinical Practice Guideline for prescribing opioids for pain—United States, 2022. MMWR Recomm Rep. 2022;71:1. [PMID: 36327391]

Dowell D et al. Prescribing opioids for pain—the new CDC Clinical Practice Guideline. N Engl J Med. 2022;387:2011. [PMID: 36326116]

ACUTE PAIN

Management of acute pain depends on the underlying type of pain (**somatic, visceral,** or **neuropathic**) and on understanding the risks and benefits of potential therapies. At times, treating the underlying cause of the pain (eg, dental caries) may be all that is needed, and pharmacologic therapies may not be required for additional analgesia. Conversely, not relieving acute pain can have consequences beyond the immediate suffering. *Inadequately treated acute pain can develop into chronic pain in some patients.* This transition from acute to chronic pain ("chronification" of pain) depends on the pain's cause, type, and severity and on the patient's age, psychological status, and genetics, among other factors. Chronic pain leads to significant societal costs beyond the individual's experiences of suffering, helplessness, and depression. Increased intensity and duration of acute pain may be correlated with a higher incidence of chronic pain, and regional anesthesia, ketamine, and cyclooxygenase (COX) inhibitors may be helpful for prevention of chronic postsurgical pain. These approaches are particularly important given the concerns that exposure to opioids in the perioperative period can lead to chronic opioid dependence.

The *Oxford League Table of Analgesics* is a useful guide; it lists the number-needed-to-treat for specific doses of various medications to relieve acute pain. NSAIDs, including COX inhibitors, have the lowest number-needed-to-treat. Delivery routes for these medications include oral, intramuscular, intravenous, intranasal, rectal, and transdermal. The primary limitation in use of the COX inhibitors is their side effects of gastritis; kidney dysfunction; bleeding; and cardiovascular adverse events, such as hypertension, MI, and stroke. Like most pharmacologic therapies, COX inhibitors have a "ceiling" effect, meaning that beyond a certain dose, there is no additional benefit.

Acetaminophen (paracetamol) is effective as a sole agent, or in combination with an NSAID or an opioid in acute pain. When combined with other agents, it produces additive analgesic effects and can modestly improve the magnitude of pain relief compared with a single agent alone. Its mechanism of action remains undetermined but is thought to act centrally through mechanisms such as the prostaglandin, serotonergic, and opioid pathways. It is one of the most widely used and best tolerated analgesics; its primary limitation is hepatoxicity when given in high doses or to patients with underlying impaired liver function.

Patient-controlled analgesia (PCA) (including postoperatively) with intravenous opioids such as morphine and hydromorphone can achieve analgesia faster and with lower daily medication doses than with standard "as needed" or even scheduled intermittent dosing. PCA can also be used with oral analgesic opioid medications and with both opioids and local anesthetics via neuraxial delivery in the epidural and intrathecal spaces. The goal of PCA is to maintain a patient's plasma concentration of opioid in the "therapeutic window," between the minimum effective analgesic concentration and a toxic dose.

To prevent prolonged inappropriate opioid use and opioid use disorder, **multimodal analgesia** (including regional anesthesia) has been employed to decrease the need for postoperative opioids. Patients may undergo either neuraxial anesthesia with an epidural catheter, for example, or regional anesthesia with a nerve block with or without a catheter. These techniques are effective for management of both intraoperative pain and postoperative pain and can diminish the need for both intraoperative and postoperative opioids.

Macintyre PE et al. Current issues in the use of opioids for the management of postoperative pain. JAMA Surg. 2022;157:158. [PMID: 34878527]
Rech MA et al. Acute pain management in the emergency department: use of multimodal and non-opioid analgesic treatment strategies. Am J Emerg Med. 2022;58:57. [PMID: 35636044]

CHRONIC NONCANCER PAIN

Chronic noncancer pain may begin as acute pain that then fails to resolve and extends beyond the expected period of healing; it may also arise from a primary disease state, as opposed to the residual symptom from another condition. Common examples of chronic noncancer pain include chronic low-back pain and arthralgias (often somatic in origin), chronic abdominal pain and pelvic pain (often visceral in origin), chronic headaches, chronic (persistent) postoperative pain, peripheral neuropathy, and postherpetic neuralgia. Chronic noncancer pain is common, with both international and US estimates of prevalence of approximately 20% in adults.

Chronic noncancer pain requires interdisciplinary management. Generally, no one therapy by itself is sufficient to manage such chronic pain. Physical or functional therapy and cognitive behavioral therapy have been shown to be the most effective for treating chronic noncancer pain, but other modalities including pharmacologic therapy, interventional modalities, and complementary/integrative approaches are useful in caring for affected patients.

Chronic low-back pain, a common type of chronic noncancer pain, causes more disability globally than any other condition. Evidence-based practice does *not* support the use of prolonged opioid therapy for chronic low-back pain.

Andreoletti H et al. A systematic review and meta-analysis of three risk factors for chronic postsurgical pain: age, sex and preoperative pain. Minerva Anestesiol. 2022;88:827. [PMID: 35766955]
Yong RJ et al. Prevalence of chronic pain among adults in the United States. Pain. 2022;163:e328. [PMID: 33990113]

CANCER PAIN

Cancer pain is unique in cause and in therapies. Cancer pain consists of both acute pain and chronic pain from the neoplasm itself as well as from the therapies associated with it, including surgery, chemotherapy, radiation, and immunotherapy. In addition, patients with cancer pain may also have acute or chronic non–cancer-related pain, a possibility that should not be overlooked.

Cancer pain includes **somatic pain** (eg, neoplastic invasion of tissue), **visceral pain** (eg, painful hepatomegaly from liver metastases), **neuropathic pain** (eg, neoplastic invasion of sacral nerve roots), or **pain from a paraneoplastic syndrome** (eg, peripheral neuropathy). Chemotherapy can cause peripheral neuropathies, radiation can cause neuritis or skin allodynia, surgery can cause persistent postsurgical pain such as postmastectomy or post-thoracotomy pain syndromes, and immunotherapy can cause arthralgias.

Patients with cancer pain may have multiple reasons for pain and thus benefit from a comprehensive and multimodal strategy. The **WHO Analgesic Ladder** suggests starting medication treatment with nonopioid analgesics, then weak opioid agonists, followed by strong opioid agonists. While opioid therapy can be helpful for the majority of patients living with cancer pain, therapy must be individualized depending on the patient, their family, and the clinician. For example, if patients are experiencing sedation and cognitive dysfunction from opioids, interventional therapies such as nerve blocks and implantable devices may be an option, weighing their risks and costs against their potential benefits. Alternatively, in dying patients, provided there is careful documentation of continued, renewed, or accelerating pain, use of opioid doses exceeding those recommended as standard for acute (eg, postoperative) pain is acceptable and justified by the principle of double effect. Furthermore, for ongoing cancer pain, a long-acting opioid analgesic can be given around the clock with a short-acting opioid medication as needed for "breakthrough" pain.

One of the unique challenges in treating cancer pain is that it is often a "moving target," with disease progression and improvements or worsening pain directly stemming from chemotherapy, radiation, or immunotherapy. Therefore, *frequent adjustments may be required for any pharmacologic regimen.* Interventional approaches such as celiac plexus neurolysis and intrathecal therapy are well studied and may be appropriate for both analgesia and reduction of side effects from systemic medications. Radiation therapy (including single-fraction external beam treatments) may decrease the extent of both primary and metastatic disease and may treat the associated pain.

Aman MM et al. The American Society of Pain and Neuroscience (ASPN) best practices and guidelines for the interventional management of cancer-associated pain. J Pain Res. 2021;14:2139. [PMID: 34295184]
Zhang H. Cancer pain management—new therapies. Curr Oncol Rep. 2022;24:223. [PMID: 35080737]

PAIN AT THE END OF LIFE

Pain is what many people say they fear most about dying, and pain at the end of life is consistently undertreated. Up to 75% of patients dying of cancer, HF, COPD, AIDS, or other diseases experience pain. In the United States, the Joint Commission includes pain management standards in its reviews of health care organizations and mandates that each hospital have a designated leader in pain management.

The risk-to-benefit ratio changes in end-of-life pain management. Predictable but unintended harms from the use of opioid analgesics, including even death, eg, from respiratory depression (rare), are perhaps less of a concern in patients approaching the end of life. In all cases, clinicians must be prepared to use appropriate doses of opioids in order to relieve this distressing symptom for these patients. In the hospice setting, greater use of opioids is actually associated with decreased mortality.

PRINCIPLES OF PAIN MANAGEMENT

The experience of pain is unique to each person and influenced by many factors, including the patient's prior experiences with pain, meaning given to the pain, emotional stresses, and family and cultural influences. A brief means of assessing pain and evaluating the effectiveness of analgesia is to ask the patient to rate the degree of pain along a *numeric or visual pain scale* (Table 5–3), assessing trends over time. This should be complemented with discussions around function (or limitations thereof). Clinicians should ask about the nature, severity, timing, location, quality, and aggravating and relieving factors of the pain.

General guidelines for diagnosis and management of pain are recommended for the treatment of all patients with pain, but clinicians must comprehend that such guidelines may not be suited for every individual. Because pain is complex, it is important to understand the benefits and risks of treatment for each patient. *Distinguishing between nociceptive (somatic or visceral) and neuropathic pain is essential to proper management since therapies differ.*

In addition, while clinicians should seek to diagnose the underlying cause of pain and then treat it, they must balance the burden of diagnostic tests or therapeutic interventions with the patient's condition. For example, single-fraction radiation therapy for painful bone metastases or nerve blocks for neuropathic pain may obviate the need for ongoing treatment with analgesics and their side effects. Regardless of decisions about seeking and treating the underlying cause of pain, every patient should be offered *prompt* pain relief.

The aim of effective pain management is to meet specific goals, such as preservation or restoration of function or quality of life, and this aim must be discussed between clinician and patient, as well as their care partners. For example, some patients may wish to be completely free of pain even at the expense of significant sedation, while others will wish to prioritize maximal cognitive functioning at the expense of complete pain control.

Whenever possible, the *oral route of analgesic administration* is preferred because it is easier to manage at home, is not itself painful, and imposes no risk from needle exposure. In unique situations, or near the end of life, transdermal, subcutaneous, rectal, and intravenous routes of administration are used; intrathecal administration is used when necessary.

Finally, pain management does not automatically necessitate opioid therapy. While some individuals fare better with opioid therapy in specific situations, this does not mean that opioids are the answer for every patient. There are situations when opioids actually worsen the quality of life for individuals, due to a lack of adequate analgesic effect or due to their side effects.

Table 5–3. Pain assessment scales.

A. Numeric Rating Scale Verbal Intensity

No pain — Worst pain: 0 1 2 3 4 5 6 7 8 9 10	None, mild, moderate, severe (0), (1–4), (5–6), (7–10)

B. Numeric Rating Scale Translated into Word and Behavior Scales

Pain Intensity	Word Scale	Nonverbal Behaviors
0	No pain	Relaxed, calm expression
1–2	Least pain	Stressed, tense expression
3–4	Mild pain	Guarded movement, grimacing
5–6	Moderate pain	Moaning, restlessness
7–8	Severe pain	Crying out
9–10	Excruciating pain	Increased intensity of above

C. Wong-Baker FACES Pain Rating Scale[1]

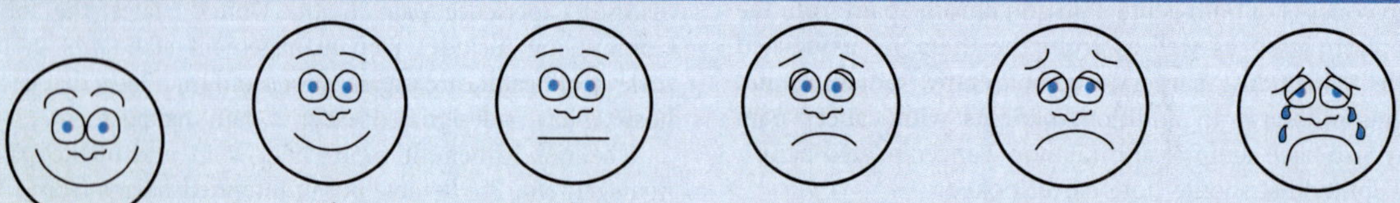

0	1	2	3	4	5
No hurt	Hurts Little Bit	Hurts Little More	Hurts Even More	Hurts Whole Lot	Hurts Worst

[1]Especially useful for patients who cannot read English (and for pediatric patients).
Wong-Baker FACES Foundation (2015). Wong-Baker FACES® Pain Rating Scale. Retrieved with permission from http://www.WongBakerFACES.org.

Barriers to Good Care

One barrier to good pain control is that many clinicians have limited training and clinical experience with pain management and thus are reluctant to attempt to manage severe pain. Lack of knowledge about the proper selection and dosing of analgesic medications carries with it attendant and typically exaggerated fears about the side effects of pain medications. Review of professional pain management guidelines (such as from the National Comprehensive Cancer Network) and consultation with a palliative care or pain management specialist may provide additional expertise.

Just as pain is a subjective experience of individual patients, its assessment and management by clinicians are likewise influenced by subjective perceptions that often reflect the same social biases and prejudices observed in broader society. Racial disparities in pain treatment span the entire continuum of care, from pediatric ED visits to the most advanced neuromodulation therapies. These disparities are often tied to false beliefs and implicit biases that begin during medical training and persist throughout practice. Remaining cognizant of individual and institutional sources of bias may enable providers to take appropriate corrective actions to safeguard the equitable treatment of all patients in pain.

Hildenbrand AK et al. Improving pain management for marginalized communities: educating the next generation of health care professionals. J Pain. 2025;37S:104683. [PMID: 39326721]

PHARMACOLOGIC PAIN MANAGEMENT STRATEGIES

Pain generally can be well controlled with nonopioid and opioid analgesic medications, complemented by nonpharmacologic adjunctive and interventional treatments. For mild to moderate pain, acetaminophen, aspirin, and NSAIDs (also known as COX inhibitors) may be sufficient. For moderate to severe pain, especially for those with acute pain, short courses of opioids are sometimes necessary; for those with cancer pain or pain from advanced, progressive, serious illness, opioids are generally required, and interventional modalities should be considered. In all cases, the choice of an analgesic medication must be guided by careful attention to the physiology of the pain, the patient's goals, and the benefits and risks of the particular analgesic being considered.

ACETAMINOPHEN & NSAIDS

Table 5–4 provides comparison information for acetaminophen, aspirin, the COX-2 inhibitor celecoxib, and other NSAIDs. At appropriate doses, acetaminophen may provide analgesic and antipyretic effects comparable to NSAIDs but without the associated risk of GI bleeding or ulceration. Acetaminophen can be given at a dosage of 500–1000 mg orally every 6 hours, not to exceed 4000 mg/day maximum for short-term use. Total acetaminophen doses should not exceed 3000 mg/day for long-term use or 2000 mg/day for older patients and those with liver disease. Hepatotoxicity is of particular concern given acetaminophen's presence in many common over-the-counter and prescription medications, which may lead to excessive doses of acetaminophen if there is a failure to account for the amount of acetaminophen ingested from *all* sources.

NSAIDs, including aspirin, are antipyretic, analgesic, and anti-inflammatory. Aspirin is dosed at 325–650 mg orally every 4 hours; GI irritation and bleeding are side effects that are lessened with enteric-coated formulations and by concomitant use of PPI medication. Bleeding, allergy, and an association with Reye syndrome in children and adolescents further limit its use.

Treatment with NSAIDs via COX-1 inhibition increases the risk of GI bleeding 1.5 times; the risks of bleeding and nephrotoxicity are both increased in elderly patients. Ketorolac is a COX-1 inhibitor with high analgesic potency. GI bleeding and ulceration may be prevented by the concurrent use of PPIs (eg, omeprazole, 20–40 mg orally daily). Alternatively, celecoxib (100 mg orally daily to 200 mg orally twice daily), the only COX-2 inhibitor available, may be chosen for fewer GI risks, but due to COX-2 inhibition, celecoxib is associated with higher risk of CVD. All NSAIDs can lead to fluid retention, kidney injury, and exacerbations of heart failure and should be used with caution in patients with these conditions. Topical formulations of NSAIDs (such as diclofenac 1.3% patch or 1% gel), placed over the painful body part for treatment of musculoskeletal pain, are associated with less systemic absorption and fewer side effects than oral administration and are likely underutilized in patients at risk for GI bleeding.

NOVEL NONOPIOID ANALGESICS

In 2025, the new nonopioid analgesic **suzetrigine** was approved. By blocking the Nav1.8 sodium channel, which is found primarily on peripheral nociceptors, suzetrigine decreases the perception of pain. It is approved for the short-term treatment of moderate to severe *acute* pain only and can reduce the need for opioid analgesics in the setting of recent surgery or injury. It is administered orally for up to 2 weeks and is generally well tolerated, with few serious side effects. Generally, it should be avoided in patients taking strong CYP3A inhibitors or with significant liver disease. Since it was only studied in the acute postsurgical setting, suzetrigine is not approved for chronic pain, and its long-term efficacy and safety remain unknown.

OPIOIDS

See also Chapter 47.

Opioid Mechanism of Action and Metabolism

Opioid medications mimic the pharmacologic properties of endogenous opioid peptides and activate the primary opioid receptors (μ, δ, and κ). Different opioid medications activate the different opioid receptors to varying degrees. Any substance that causes analgesia via binding an opioid receptor and is reversed by naloxone is referred to as an "opioid." This broad class of drugs includes alkaloids derived from the extract of a poppy plant (eg, codeine, morphine), semisynthetic opioids (eg, oxycodone, buprenorphine), and synthetic opioids (eg, methadone, fentanyl).

Table 5–4. Acetaminophen, aspirin, and useful NSAIDs and COX inhibitors. (Listed in alphabetical order.)

Medication (Proprietary)	Usual Dose for Adults Based on Total Body Weight	Comments[1]
Acetaminophen (Ofirmev)	≥ 50 kg: 1000 mg intravenously every 6–8 hours	
Acetaminophen or paracetamol[2] (Tylenol, Datril, etc)	≥ 50 kg: 325–500 mg orally every 4 hours or 500–1000 mg orally every 6 hours, up to 2000–4000 mg/day < 50 kg: 10–15 mg/kg every 4 hours orally; 15–20 mg/kg every 4 hours rectally, up to 2000–3000 mg/day	Not an NSAID because it lacks peripheral anti-inflammatory effects. Equivalent to aspirin as analgesic and antipyretic agent. Limit dose to 4000 mg/day in acute pain. Limit dose to 2000 mg/day in older patients and those with liver disease. Be mindful of multiple sources of acetaminophen from combination analgesics, cold remedies, and sleep aids.
Aspirin[3]	≥ 50 kg: 325–650 mg orally every 4 hours < 50 kg: 10–15 mg/kg every 4 hours orally; 15–20 mg/kg every 4 hours rectally	Available also in enteric-coated oral form that is more slowly absorbed but better tolerated.
Celecoxib[2] (Celebrex)	≥ 50 kg: 200 mg orally once daily (OA); 100–200 mg orally twice daily (RA) < 50 kg: 100 mg orally once or twice daily	COX-2 inhibitor. No antiplatelet effects. Lower doses for older adults who weigh < 50 kg. Lower incidence of endoscopic GI ulceration than NSAIDs. Not known if true lower incidence of GI bleeding. Celecoxib is contraindicated in sulfonamide allergy.
Diclofenac (Voltaren, Cataflam, Zorvolex, others)	≥ 50 kg: 50–75 mg orally two or three times daily; 1% gel 2–4 g four times daily	Increased risk of hepatotoxicity. Enteric-coated product; slow onset. Topical formulations may result in fewer side effects than oral formulations.
Diclofenac gel (Voltaren)	1% gel 2–4 g four times daily	Available OTC. Topical formulation may result in fewer side effects than oral formulations.
Diclofenac patch (Flector)	1.3% topical patch applied twice daily	Apply patch to most painful area.
Diclofenac sustained release (Voltaren-XR, others)	≥ 50 kg: 100–200 mg orally once daily	
Etodolac (Lodine, others)	≥ 50 kg: 200–400 mg orally every 6–8 hours	
Ibuprofen (Caldolor)	≥ 50 kg: 400–800 mg intravenously every 6 hours as needed (max 3.2 g/day)	
Ibuprofen (Motrin, Advil, Rufen, others)	≥ 50 kg: 400–800 mg orally every 6 hours as needed < 50 kg: 10 mg/kg orally every 6–8 hours	Relatively well tolerated and inexpensive. Consider coincident gastroprotection with a proton pump inhibitor.
Indomethacin (Indocin, Indometh, others)	≥ 50 kg: 25–50 mg orally two to four times daily	Increased risk of dose-related toxic effects, especially GI and bone marrow effects.
Ketorolac tromethamine	≥ 50 kg: 10 mg orally every 4–6 hours to a maximum of 40 mg/day orally	Short-term use (< 5 days) only; otherwise, increased risk of GI side effects.
Ketorolac tromethamine[4]	≥ 50 kg: 30–60 mg every 6 hours intramuscularly or intravenously as needed	Intramuscular or intravenous NSAID as alternative to opioid. Lower doses for elderly. Short-term use (< 5 days) only.
Magnesium salicylate (various)	≥ 50 kg: 325–650 mg orally every 6 hours	
Meloxicam (Mobic)	≥ 50 kg: 7.5 mg orally every 12 hours	Intermediate COX-2/COX-1 ratio similar to diclofenac.
Nabumetone (Relafen)	≥ 50 kg: 500–1000 mg orally once daily (max dose 2000 mg/day)	May be less ulcerogenic than ibuprofen, but overall side effects may not be less.
Naproxen (Naprosyn, Anaprox, Aleve [OTC], others)	≥ 50 kg: 250–500 mg orally every 6–8 hours < 50 kg: 5 mg/kg every 8 hours	Generally well tolerated. Lower doses for elderly.

COX, cyclooxygenase; OA, osteoarthritis; OTC, over the counter; RA, rheumatoid arthritis.

[1]The adverse effects of headache, tinnitus, dizziness, confusion, rashes, anorexia, nausea, vomiting, GI bleeding, diarrhea, nephrotoxicity, visual disturbances, etc, can occur with any of these drugs. Tolerance and efficacy are subject to great individual variations among patients. Note: All NSAIDs can increase serum lithium levels.

[2]Acetaminophen and celecoxib lack antiplatelet effects.

[3]May inhibit platelet aggregation for 1 week or more and may cause bleeding.

[4]Has the same GI toxicities as oral NSAIDs.

Opioids are primarily metabolized by the liver via phase I (cytochrome P450 isoenzyme 3A4 and 2D6) and phase II (glucuronidation) processes. Some opioid medications need to be metabolized to an active metabolite to produce analgesia (eg, codeine, a prodrug, metabolizes to morphine), while others are pharmacologically active and have active metabolites (eg, morphine metabolizes to morphine-6-glucuronide, an active metabolite). Cytochrome P450 allelic variants can predispose patients to being rapid or poor opioid metabolizers, affecting how they respond to various opioid medications. *Age-related changes in hepatic function predispose older individuals to adverse side effects from opioids, including delirium, falls, fractures, and respiratory depression.* Hepatic impairment will also affect plasma concentrations of opioids and their metabolites in a complex manner.

Most opioids are eliminated primarily in the urine, so opioid clearance is affected by kidney function. GFR typically decreases with age and can lead to an accumulation of active metabolites and consequent toxicity. For example, meperidine is metabolized to normeperidine and its accumulation can result in neurotoxicity (seizures) in older adults or those with renal impairment.

When initiating opioid therapy clinicians should "start low and go slow," particularly in patients with older age, liver disease, decreased kidney function, and higher total body fat. In addition, initially prescribing immediate-release opioid formulations is more desirable since these agents can be titrated down more rapidly in case of adverse reactions, and because long-acting formulations are associated with increased risk of overdose.

Aapro M et al. Opioid metabolism and drug-drug interaction in cancer. Oncologist. 2024;29:931. [PMID: 38780124]

Principles of Opioid Management & CDC Guidelines

Opioids, if prescribed, are just one component of a patient's pain management plan and are not appropriate for all pain situations. Nonpharmacologic treatments (eg, exercise, psychological intervention, other treatments) and nonopioid medications (eg, NSAIDs, SNRIs, gabapentinoids) are associated with improvements in pain and function that are comparable to improvements associated with opioid use for acute and chronic pain. In fact, a 12-month randomized trial of stepped therapy using opioid versus nonopioid medications for chronic musculoskeletal pain (SPACE trial) found increased pain intensity in the opioid treatment group. Observational studies suggest that *opioid use for acute pain is associated with subsequent long-term use, and there is a lack of robust evidence to support long-term opioid use for chronic noncancer pain.* Utilization of high dosages of opioids over time can result in **opioid-induced hyperalgesia** (enhanced pain to noxious stimuli) and **allodynia** (pain from stimuli that typically do not provoke pain), possibly secondary to upregulation and sensitization of NMDA (*N*-methyl-D-aspartate) receptors in the nervous system. Weaning opioids can be a difficult experience for patients and providers. An increase in suicidal ideation and risk of opioid overdose may occur around an opioid taper. Observational studies suggest opioid use is associated with increased risk of fracture and falls, OUD, overdose, mortality, and MI in a dose-dependent fashion. There is no known reliable way to predict who will experience harm from opioid use.

A. CDC Guidelines for Prescribing Opioids

In 2022, the CDC released updated guidelines for prescribing opioids for outpatients with pain. These guidelines are summarized in Table 5–5 and reviewed below. **Of note,** *the 2022 CDC guidelines are meant for outpatients with acute, subacute, and chronic noncancer pain. They are not meant to be applied to patients with pain related to cancer, sickle cell disease, or palliative or end-of-life care.*

Before starting opioid therapy, clinicians should have a frank conversation with the patient about the risks and realistic expected benefits of opioid use. Before prescribing and periodically during opioid therapy, clinicians should review the patient's prescribed controlled substance history in their *state prescription drug monitoring program.* When starting opioid therapy, providers should prescribe immediate-release opioids instead of extended-release opioids, since patients have a *higher risk of overdose with extended-release opioids* and no difference in pain or function is seen when using immediate-release versus extended-release opioids. When initiating opioids in opioid-naïve patients, the lowest effective dose should be used (Table 5–6). Caution should be used if prescribing opioids for a patient concurrently taking benzodiazepines or CNS depressant medications (eg, sedative hypnotics, muscle relaxants, gabapentinoids), since risk of respiratory depression may outweigh benefits. ***Naloxone*** *should be offered to patients prescribed opioids, especially those at increased risk of overdose (including patients prescribed > 50 morphine mg equivalents [MME]* [Table 5–7], *with concurrent benzodiazepine prescription, with loss of tolerance, or with history of sleep apnea, prior overdose, or substance use disorder).*

B. Acute Pain

The 2022 CDC guideline for prescribing opioids defines **acute pain** as lasting < 1 month. Nonopioid therapies are at least as effective as opioids for managing many types of acute pain. Thus, nonopioid treatments should be optimized, and opioids only considered if benefits will outweigh the risks of opioid use. If opioids are needed to treat acute pain, for example after a major surgery, providers should prescribe no more than the expected duration of pain severe enough to necessitate opioid use. If continuing opioids for acute pain, the provider should reassess the patient at least every 2 weeks and seriously weigh the benefit and risk before deciding to continue opioid therapy for longer than 1 month. The updated CDC guidelines no longer have a specific recommendation on duration of treatment. However, when considering duration of opioid treatment for acute pain, it is important to remember that opioid efficacy for pain management wanes over a short period of time, that opioid use for acute pain is associated with long-term use in observational studies, that there is *no*

Table 5–5. 2022 CDC clinical practice guideline for prescribing opioids for pain.

	Guideline
	Recommendations are for prescribing opioids for outpatients with pain, excluding pain related to sickle cell disease, cancer, palliative care, and end-of-life care.
Determining whether to initiate opioids	Acute pain: nonopioid therapies are at least as effective as opioids for many acute pain conditions. Maximize use of nonpharmacologic and nonopioid pharmacologic therapies, and only consider opioids if benefits are anticipated to outweigh risks. Subacute and chronic pain: nonopioid therapies are preferred. Maximize use of nonpharmacologic and nonopioid pharmacologic therapies, and only consider opioids if benefits to pain and function are anticipated to outweigh risks. Before initiating opioid therapy, clinicians should discuss realistic benefits and known risks of opioid therapy. Subacute and chronic pain: before starting opioid therapy, clinicians should work with patients to establish treatment goals for pain and function and consider how opioid therapy will be discontinued if benefits do not outweigh risks.
Opioid selection and dosage	When starting opioid therapy, clinicians should prescribe immediate-release opioids instead of extended-release/long-acting opioids. When starting opioids in opioid-naïve patients, prescribe the lowest effective opioid dose. If opioids are continued for subacute/chronic pain, clinicians should use caution when prescribing at any dosage, should carefully evaluate benefits and risks when considering dose increase, and should avoid increasing dose above levels likely to yield diminishing returns relative to risk. Patients already receiving opioid therapy: clinicians should carefully weigh benefits and risks and exercise care when changing opioid dosage. • If benefits outweigh risks—clinicians should work with patient to optimize nonopioid therapies while continuing opioid therapy. • If benefits do not outweigh risks—clinicians should optimize other therapies and work closely with patients to gradually taper to lower dosages or, if warranted, appropriately taper and discontinue opioids. • Unless there are indications of a life-threatening issue (eg, impending overdose), opioid therapy should not be discontinued abruptly or rapidly reduced from higher dosages.
Deciding duration of initial opioid prescription and conducting follow-up	For acute pain, prescribe no greater than quantity needed for expected duration of pain severe enough to require opioids. Evaluate benefits and risks within 1–4 weeks of starting opioids (for subacute or chronic pain) or of any dose escalation. Clinicians should regularly reevaluate benefits and risks of continued opioid therapy with patient.
Assessing risk and addressing potential harms of opioid use	Before starting and periodically during opioid therapy, clinicians should evaluate risk for opioid-related harms and discuss with the patient. Clinicians should work with the patient on a plan to mitigate risk including offering naloxone. Review the patient's history of controlled substance use through their state's prescription drug monitoring program before initiating and periodically during opioid therapy. Consider benefits and risks of urine toxicology testing when prescribing opioids for subacute or chronic pain (to assess for prescribed and non-prescribed controlled substances). Use particular caution when prescribing opioids and benzodiazepines (and other central nervous system depressants) concurrently. Manage or arrange treatment for opioid use disorder (OUD) with evidence-based medications. Detoxification without OUD medications is not recommended due to risk for resuming drug use, overdose, and overdose death.

Adapted from Dowell D, Ragan KR, Jones CM, Baldwin GT, Chou R. CDC Clinical Practice Guideline for Prescribing Opioids for Pain – United States, 2022. MMWR Recomm Rep 2022;71(No. RR-3):1-95. DOI: http://dx.doi.org/10.15585/mmwr.rr7103a1

Clinical practice guideline definition: Acute pain, duration < 1 month; Subacute pain, duration 1–3 months; Chronic pain, duration > 3 months.

robust evidence that long-term opioid use improves pain or function, and that long-term opioid use can increase the risk of OUD and overdose.

C. Subacute Pain and Chronic Pain

The 2022 CDC guideline for prescribing opioids defines **subacute** or **unresolved acute pain** as that persisting for 1–3 months, and **chronic pain** as that lasting > 3 months. Nonpharmacologic therapies and nonopioid medications should be optimized and are the preferred treatment for subacute and chronic pain. It is important to remember that opioids are *not* first-line treatment for chronic or subacute pain, and providers should utilize nonopioid treatments in most circumstances. If, after carefully weighing risks and benefits, a decision is made to start opioid therapy, providers should work with patients to determine treatment goals around pain and function and create a

Table 5–6. Opioids. (Listed in alphabetical order, within classes.)

Medication (Proprietary Name)	Routes of Administration and Available Doses	Approximate Equianalgesic Dose (compared to morphine 30 mg orally or 10 mg intravenously/subcutaneously)[1]	Usual Starting Dose in an Opioid-Naïve Patient Based on Weight
Opioid Agonists[2,3]			
Buprenorphine[4] *(not for long-term use)*	*Parenteral* (intravenous, intramuscular)	Not available	≥ 50 kg: 300 mcg intravenously slowly once, may be repeated after 30–60 minutes after initial dose; then 300 mcg every 6–8 hours as needed for acute pain
Buprenorphine (Belbuca)[4] *(note: buccal and sublingual formulations are associated with dental adverse events)*	*Buccal strips:* 75 mcg, 150 mcg, 300 mcg, 450 mcg, 600 mcg, 750 mcg, 900 mcg	Not available	≥ 50 kg: opioid-naïve patients or patients taking < 30 mg morphine equivalents/day–75 mcg buccally once daily or, if tolerated, every 12 hours for ≥ 4 days, then increase to 150 mcg every 12 hours Patients taking 30–89 mg of morphine equivalents/day – 150 mcg every 12 hours Patients taking 90–160 mg of morphine equivalents/day – 300 mcg every 12 hours Patients taking >160 mg of morphine equivalents/day – **may not provide adequate analgesia; consider use of an alternate analgesic** May titrate by 150 mcg every 12 hours no more frequently than every 4 days. Maximum: 900 mcg every 12 hours; 450 mcg every 12 hours in opioid naïve patients
Buprenorphine (Butrans)	*Transdermal:* 5 mcg/h, 7.5 mcg/h, 10 mcg/h, 15 mcg/h, 20 mcg/h	Not available	≥ 50 kg: opioid-naïve patients or patients taking < 30 mg morphine equivalents/day—5-mcg/h patch every 7 days Patients taking 30–80 mg morphine equivalents/day—consider 10 mcg/h every 7 days Patients taking > 80 mg morphine equivalents/day—could consider 20 mcg/h every 7 days, **but may not provide adequate analgesia; consider other analgesics** May increase by 5–10 mcg/h with a minimum titration interval of 72 hours Maximum: 20 mcg/h every 7 days (in the United States; higher doses available in some countries)
Fentanyl *(note: for use in ICU or closely monitored settings)*	*Parenteral* (intravenous, intramuscular): 50 mcg/mL	*Parenteral:* 50–100 mcg	≥ 50 kg: 12.5–50 mcg intravenously every 3–5 minutes until pain relieved, then every 30–60 minutes as needed for acute pain; 50–100 mcg intramuscularly every 1–2 hours as needed for acute pain < 50 kg: 0.5–1 mcg/kg intravenously every 1–2 hours as needed for acute pain; max 50-mcg/dose
Fentanyl (Actiq) *(not available in the United States)*	*Lozenge:* 200 mcg, 400 mcg, 600 mcg, 800 mcg, 1200 mcg, 1600 mcg	Not available	*Initial dose for breakthrough cancer pain:* ≥ 50 kg: 200 mcg consumed orally over 15 minutes; may repeat × 1 after 30 minutes if inadequate relief *(wait at least 4 hours before treating another episode; max 4 doses/day)*

(continued)

Table 5–6. Opioids. (Listed in alphabetical order, within classes.) (continued)

Medication (Proprietary Name)	Routes of Administration and Available Doses	Approximate Equianalgesic Dose (compared to morphine 30 mg orally or 10 mg intravenously/subcutaneously)[1]	Usual Starting Dose in an Opioid-Naïve Patient Based on Weight
Fentanyl (buccal: Fentora) (sublingual spray: Subsys – Not available in the United States) *(note: do not convert from other fentanyl formulations on a mcg-per-mcg basis)*	*Buccal:* 100 mcg, 200 mcg, 400 mcg, 600 mcg, 800 mcg	Not available	*Initial dose for breakthrough cancer pain:* ≥ 50 kg: 100-mcg buccal tab; may repeat × 1 after 30 minutes if inadequate relief *(wait at least 4 hours before another dose)*
Fentanyl[12] (Duragesic)	*Transdermal:* 12.5 mcg/h, 25 mcg/h, 37.5 mcg/h, 50 mcg/h, 62.5 mcg/h, 75 mcg/h, 87.5 mcg/h, 100 mcg/h	Initial doses: Conversion to fentanyl patch is based on total daily dose of oral morphine[2] (45 mg morphine/24 hours is approximately equivalent to 12-mcg/h fentanyl patch)	Note: it is safer to underestimate daily fentanyl requirement and provide break-through pain relief with immediate release opioid during initiation. Do not titrate fentanyl patch more frequently than every 3 days.
Hydromorphone[5] (Dilaudid)	*Oral:* 2 mg, 4 mg, 8 mg	*Oral:* 6 mg	*Oral:* ≥ 50 kg: 1–2 mg every 4–6 hours as needed < 50 kg: 0.03–0.06 mg/kg every 4–6 hours as needed
Hydromorphone[5] (Dilaudid)	*Parenteral* (intravenous, intramuscular, subcutaneous): 0.5 mg/0.5 mL, 1 mg/mL, 2 mg/mL, 4 mg/mL	*Parenteral:* 1 mg	*Parenteral:* ≥ 50 kg: 0.2 mg every 3–4 hours as needed < 50 kg: 0.015 mg/kg every 3–6 hours as needed
Hydromorphone extended release[12]	*Oral:* 8 mg ER, 12 mg ER, 16 mg ER, 32 mg ER	*Oral:* 6 mg	*Oral, initial dose:* ≥ 50 kg: Estimated total daily oral hydromorphone dose based on current daily short-acting opioid use. Once-daily administration. Not for use in opioid-naïve patients.
Levorphanol	*Oral:* 2 mg, 3mg	*Oral:* 2 mg	*Oral, initial dose:* 1–2 mg every 6–8 hours as needed
Meperidine[6] (Demerol)	*Oral:* 50 mg	*Oral:* 300 mg	*Oral:* Not recommended
Meperidine[6] (Demerol)	*Parenteral* (intravenous, intramuscular, subcutaneous): 25 mg/mL, 50 mg/mL, 75 mg/mL, 100 mg/mL	*Parenteral:* 100 mg	*Parenteral:* ≥ 50 kg: 50–100 mg every 3 hours; not to exceed 600 mg/24 hours < 50 kg: 0.8 mg/kg every 3–4 hours; not to exceed 50–75 mg/dose (*Note: NOT recommended for the treatment of acute pain due to potential for neurotoxicity, especially in older adults or patients with kidney disease*)
Methadone[7,12]	*Oral tab:* 5 mg, 10 mg *Soln:* 5 mg/5 mL, 10 mg/5 mL, 10 mg/mL	*Oral:* 7.5 mg *(Caution: conversion varies depending on magnitude of daily opioid use. See* Table 5–7.*)*	*Oral, initial dose:* ≥ 50 kg: 2.5 mg every 8–12 hours *(Increase dose not more frequently than every 3–5 days)*
Methadone[7,12]	*Parenteral:* 10 mg/mL	*Parenteral:* 4 mg *(Caution: conversion varies depending on magnitude of daily opioid use. See* Table 5–7.*)*	*Parenteral:* ≥ 50 kg: 1–2 mg every 8 hours < 50 kg: 0.1 mg/kg every 6–24 hours
Morphine[5] immediate release	*Oral:* 15 mg, 30 mg (tablets); 10 mg/5 mL, 20 mg/5 mL, 100 mg/5 mL (solution) *Rectal:* 5 mg, 10 mg, 20 mg, 30 mg (suppositories)	*Oral:* 30 mg	*Oral:* ≥ 50 kg: 4–8 mg every 3–4 hours as needed < 50 kg: 0.3 mg/kg every 3–4 hours as needed *Rectal:* 10 mg per rectum every 4 hours as needed

Morphine[5] immediate release (morphine sulfate, various)	*Intravenous:* varies	*Parenteral (intravenous):* 10 mg	*Parenteral (intravenous):* ≥ 50 kg: 1–4 mg every 3–4 hours < 50 kg: 0.05 mg/kg every 3–4 hours
Morphine controlled release, 12 hour[12] (MS Contin)	*Oral (tablets):* 15 mg ER, 30 mg ER, 60 mg ER, 100 mg ER, 200 mg ER	*Oral:* 30 mg	*Oral, initial dose:* ≥ 50 kg: Not for use in opioid-naïve patients. Initial dose should be based on current daily opioid use divided into dosing every 8–12 hours.
Morphine extended release, 24 hour[12] (Kadian)	*Oral (capsules):* 10 mg ER, 20 mg ER, 30 mg ER, 45 mg ER, 50 mg ER, 60 mg ER, 75 mg ER, 80 mg ER, 90 mg ER, 100 mg ER, 120 mg ER	*Oral:* 30 mg	*Oral, initial dose:* ≥ 50 kg: Not for use in opioid-naïve patients. Initial dose should be based on current daily opioid use. Dose given every 24 hours.
Oxycodone (Roxicodone, others)	*Oral:* *(capsules):* 5 mg *(tablets):* 5 mg, 10 mg, 15 mg, 20 mg, 30 mg *(solution):* 5 mg/5 mL, 100 mg/5 mL	*Oral:* 20 mg	*Oral, initial dose:* ≥ 50 kg: 5–10 mg every 4–6 hours as needed < 50 kg: 0.1–0.2 mg/kg every 4–6 hours as needed
Oxycodone controlled release[12] (OxyContin)	*Oral:* *(tablets):* 10 mg ER, 15 mg ER, 20 mg ER, 30 mg ER, 40 mg ER, 60 mg ER, 80 mg ER	*Oral:* 20 mg	Not for use in opioid-naïve patients. Dosing should be based on current daily opioid use. Dose given every 12 hours.
Oxycodone ER[12] tamper-resistant capsules (Xtampza ER)	*Oral (capsules):* 9 mg ER, 13.5 mg ER, 18 mg ER, 27 mg ER, 36 mg ER	Oral: 20 mg	Not for use in opioid-naïve patients. Dosing should be based on current daily opioid use. Dose given every 12 hours.
Oxymorphone[5,8] oral, immediate release	*Oral (tablets):* 5 mg, 10 mg	*Oral:* 10 mg	*Oral, initial dose:* ≥ 50 kg: 5–10 mg every 6 hours as needed
Oxymorphone[5,8,12] oral, extended release	*Oral (tablets):* 5 mg ER, 7.5 mg ER, 10 mg ER, 15 mg ER, 20 mg ER, 30 mg ER, 40 mg ER	*Oral:* 10 mg	Not for use in opioid-naïve patients. Dosing should be based on current daily opioid use. Dose given every 12 hours. May increase dose every 3–7+ days.
Combination Opioid Agonist–Nonopioid Preparations			
Codeine[9,10] (with acetaminophen; other combinations also available)	*Oral (tablets):* Acetaminophen/codeine: 300 mg/15 mg, 300 mg/30 mg, 300 mg/60 mg Codeine: 15 mg, 30 mg, 60 mg	*Oral:* 200 mg codeine	*Oral:* ≥ 50 kg: 15–60 mg codeine every 4–6 hours as needed; maximum total daily dose 360 mg/day < 50 kg: 0.5–1 mg/kg codeine every 6–12 hours *(Note: contraindicated in patients < 12 years old, and in patients 12–18 years old after tonsillectomy/adenoidectomy or at risk for respiratory depression)*
Codeine[9]	*Parenteral (not available in the United States)*		≥ 50 kg: 30–60 mg codeine phosphate every 4–6 hours intramuscularly/subcutaneously < 50 kg: Not recommended
Hydrocodone[8] (with acetaminophen)[11] (Hydrocodone also available as a tablet in combination with ibuprofen 200 mg)[11]	*Oral (solution):* 7.5 mg/325 mg per 15 mL, 10 mg/325 mg per 15 mL *Oral (tablets):* 5 mg/325 mg, 7.5 mg/325 mg, 10 mg/325 mg (various formulations)	30 mg hydrocodone	*Oral: Based on hydrocodone content* ≥ 50 kg: 5–10 mg every 4–6 hours as needed < 50 kg: 0.1–0.2 mg/kg hydrocodone every 4–6 hours as needed

(continued)

Table 5–6. Opioids. (Listed in alphabetical order, within classes.) (continued)

Medication (Proprietary Name)	Routes of Administration and Available Doses	Approximate Equianalgesic Dose (compared to morphine 30 mg orally or 10 mg intravenously/subcutaneously)[1]	Usual Starting Dose in an Opioid-Naïve Patient Based on Weight
Oxycodone (with acetaminophen)[10,11]	*Oral (tablets):* 2.5 mg/325 mg, 5 mg/325 mg, 7.5 mg/325 mg, 10 mg/325 mg *Oral (solution):* 5 mg/325 mg per 5 mL, 10 mg/300 mg per 5 mL	20 mg oxycodone	*Oral, initial dose:* ≥ 50 kg: 5–10 mg oxycodone every 4–6 hours as needed < 50 kg: 0.1–0.2 mg/kg oxycodone every 4–6 hours as needed
Combination Opioid Agonist–Norepinephrine Reuptake Inhibitor Preparations			
Tapentadol (Nucynta)	*Oral (tablets):* 50 mg, 75 mg, 100 mg	75 mg	*Oral, initial doses:* ≥ 50 kg: 50–100 mg every 4–6 hours as needed; maximum daily dose 600 mg
Tapentadol, extended release[12] (Nucynta ER)	*Oral:* 50 mg ER, 100 mg ER, 150 mg ER, 200 mg ER, 250 mg ER		*Oral:* ≥ 50 kg: 50 mg ER every 12 hours; can increase by 50-mg increments twice daily every 3+ days to dose of 100–250 mg ER twice daily; maximum total daily ER dose 500 mg/day
Tramadol (Ultram)	*Oral (tablets):* 50 mg, 100 mg *Oral (solution):* 5 mg/mL	150 mg	*Oral, initial dose:* ≥ 50 kg: Start 25–50 mg every 6 hours as needed; limit of 400 mg/day or 300 mg/day in patients > 75 years old
Tramadol extended release[12] (ConZip ER capsules)	*Oral (tablets):* 100 mg ER, 200 mg ER, 300 mg ER		*Extended release is for use in patients already taking tramadol IR for > 1 week.* Dosing should be based on current daily tramadol use. Dose given every 24 hours.

[1]Published tables vary in the suggested doses that are equianalgesic to morphine. Clinical response is the criterion that must be applied for each patient; titration to clinical efficacy is necessary. Because there is not complete cross-tolerance among these drugs, it is usually necessary to use a lower than equianalgesic dose initially when changing drugs and to retitrate to response.
[2]Conversion is conservative; therefore, do not use these equianalgesic doses for converting back from fentanyl patch to other opioids because they may lead to inadvertent overdose. Patients may require breakthrough doses of short-acting opioids during conversion to transdermal fentanyl.
[3]Several significantly more potent formulations of buprenorphine are available but generally reserved for the treatment of opioid use disorder with or without comorbid constant pain, most often by pain management or addiction specialists: a sublingual tablet or a sublingual film (Suboxone and others) in which the buprenorphine is combined with naloxone; a subdermal implant of buprenorphine alone (Probuphine); and a subcutaneous depot injection (Sublocade). Each of these is used in maintenance treatment to reduce problematic use of other opioids.
[4]Note, buprenorphine can precipitate withdrawal in patients already receiving opioids. In opioid-experienced patients, taper current opioids to 30 mg/day oral morphine equivalent prior to starting buccal buprenorphine. Thereafter, buprenorphine dosing schedule depends on prior current oral morphine equivalent:
<30 mg/day, 75 mcg buccally every 12 hours;
30–89 mg/day, 150 mcg buccally every 12 hours;
90–160 mg/day, 300 mcg buccally every 12 hours;
In all patients, use same dose escalation and maximum dose as shown for opioid-naïve patients.
[5]*Caution:* For morphine and hydromorphone, rectal administration is an alternative route for patients unable to take oral medications. Equianalgesic doses may differ from oral and parenteral doses. A short-acting opioid should normally be used for initial therapy.
[6]Not recommended for the treatment of pain due to potential neurotoxicity and availability of safer alternatives, especially in patients with kidney disease or older patients. Doses listed are for brief therapy of acute pain only.
[7]Methadone conversion varies depending on the equivalent total daily dose of morphine. Consult with a pain management or palliative care expert for conversion.
[8]*Caution:* Recommended doses do not apply to adult patients with kidney or liver impairment or other conditions affecting drug metabolism.
[9]*Caution:* Individual doses of codeine above 60 mg often are not appropriate because of diminishing incremental analgesia with increasing doses but continually increasing nausea, constipation, and other side effects.
[10]*Caution:* Doses of aspirin and acetaminophen in combination products must also be adjusted to the patient's body weight.
[11]*Caution:* Monitor total acetaminophen dose carefully, including any OTC use. Total acetaminophen dose maximum is 3 g/day. If liver impairment or heavy alcohol use, maximum is 2 g/day. Available dosing formulations of these combination medications are being adjusted to reflect increased caution about acetaminophen toxicity. Acetaminophen doses in a single combination tablet or capsule is limited to ≤ 325 mg.
[12]Extended-release opioid formulations are not recommended for use in opioid-naïve patients.

Table 5–7. Morphine milligram equivalent (MME) doses for commonly prescribed opioids. (Listed in alphabetical order, after morphine.)

Opioid	Conversion Factor
Morphine	1
Codeine	0.15
Fentanyl transdermal (in mcg/h)	2.4
Hydrocodone	1
Hydromorphone	4
Methadone[1]	
1–20 mg/day	4
21–40 mg/day	8
41–60 mg/day	10
≥ 61–80 mg/day	12
Oxycodone	1.5
Oxymorphone	3
Tapentadol[2]	0.4
Tramadol[2]	0.2

TO CALCULATE MMEs: Multiply the dose for each opioid by the conversion factor to determine the dose in MMEs. As an example: tablets containing hydrocodone 5 mg and acetaminophen 325 mg taken four times a day would contain a total of 20 mg of hydrocodone daily, equivalent to 20 × 1 = 20 MME daily. Or another example: Extended-release tablets containing oxycodone 10 mg taken twice a day contain a total of 20 mg of oxycodone daily, equivalent to 20 × 1.5 = 30 MME daily.

Note the following precautions: (1) All doses are in mg/day except for fentanyl, which is in mcg/hour. (2) Equianalgesic dose conversions are only estimates and cannot account for individual variability in genetics and pharmacokinetics. (3) Do not use the calculated dose in MMEs to determine the doses to use when converting one opioid to another; when converting opioids, the new opioid is typically dosed at a substantially lower dose than the calculated MME dose to avoid accidental overdose due to incomplete cross-tolerance and individual variability in opioid pharmacokinetics. (4) Use particular caution with methadone dose conversions because methadone has a long and variable half-life, and peak respiratory depressant effect occurs later and lasts longer than peak analgesic effect. (5) Use particular caution with fentanyl because it is dosed in mcg/hour instead of mg/day, and its absorption is affected by heat and other factors. (6) These conversion factors should not be applied to dosage decisions related to management of opioid use disorder.

[1]Methadone conversion uses different conversion ratios depending on dose.

[2]Tapentadol is a mu-receptor agonist and norepinephrine reuptake inhibitor. Tramadol is a mu-receptor agonist and norepinephrine and serotonin reuptake inhibitor. MMEs are based on degree of mu-receptor agonist activity; however, it is unknown whether tapentadol or tramadol is associated with overdose in the same dose-dependent manner as observed with medications that are sole mu-receptor agonists.

Adapted from Dowell D et al. CDC clinical practice guideline for prescribing opioids for chronic pain—United States, 2022. MMWR Recomm Rep. 2022;71(No. RR 3):31; by the CDC from Von Korff M et al. De Facto long-term opioid therapy for noncancer pain. Clin J Pain. 2008;24:521 and Nielsen S et al. Pharmacoepidemiol Drug Saf. 2016;25:733; Jutkiewicz EM et al. Table 23–4. Opioid Analgesics. In: Brunton LL et al, eds. *Goodman & Gilman's: The Pharmacological Basis of Therapeutics,* 14th ed. McGraw Hill Education; 2023. Accessed December 11, 2025. https://accessmedicine.mhmedical.com/content.aspx?bookid=3191&sectionid=269719481

strategy to discontinue opioid treatment if benefits no longer outweigh risks. Caution should be used when prescribing opioids at any dosage, and providers should avoid increasing the dose above levels likely to increase the risk to patients compared with the expected benefit. After initiating opioid treatment or any dose escalation, clinicians should reassess the benefits and risk to the patient within 1–4 weeks, and regularly thereafter. Before prescribing and at least annually, providers should consider **urine toxicology testing.** Test results should be used to increase patient safety and improve patient care (by assessing for prescribed or nonprescribed controlled substance use, or both, especially combinations that increase risk of overdose), not for punitive reasons.

D. Patients Already Receiving Opioid Therapy

Receiving and caring for a patient who has been started on opioids by another provider can be a complex and stressful situation for both patient and provider. The 2022 CDC guideline has a recommendation for this specific situation, starting with carefully considering the benefits and risks of continuing opioid therapy. If benefits outweigh risks, providers should optimize nonopioid therapies while continuing opioid therapy. If benefits do not outweigh risks, providers should optimize nonopioid therapies and work with the patient to gradually taper opioids to lower doses, with a goal to possibly discontinue opioids depending on the patient's circumstance. The CDC guideline recommends against rapidly tapering high-dose opioids or abruptly discontinuing opioids unless the patient has warning signs of an impending overdose (eg, confusion, sedation, slurred speech). Opioid taper or cessation is associated with increased nonprescribed heroin and other opioid use, increased emergency department and hospital visits, and higher rates of overdose, mental health crises, and overdose mortality (up to three times higher mortality in a 2019 retrospective study). *Opioid risk reduction practices* (eg, opioid consent process, prescription drug program monitoring, urine toxicology testing, overdose education, naloxone distribution, assessment of pain and function) should be considered and may be legally required in some jurisdictions while prescribing opioids.

E. Patients with Chronic Pain and OUD

Opioid use disorder (OUD) is characterized by a cluster of cognitive, behavioral, and physiologic symptoms indicating *continued use of opioids despite significant related problems*. Patients are diagnosed with OUD by meeting at least 2 of 11 symptoms outlined in the *DSM-5* that describe craving, loss of control, and drug use despite adverse consequences (Table 47–1). See Chapter 47, Substance Use Disorders, for details on diagnosis and treatment of OUD.

Managing patients with concomitant OUD and chronic pain can be complex. As with any patient with chronic pain, nonopioid and nonpharmacologic therapies should be optimized. Patients should be screened for OUD routinely. Per the 2022 CDC guideline, clinicians should provide or arrange *treatment of OUD with evidence-based medications (eg, buprenorphine usually with naloxone or methadone—both*

FDA approved medications for treatment of OUD). Buprenorphine has been associated with lower pain scores and higher quality of life in patients with OUD and chronic pain. Methadone and buprenorphine have long half-lives and have been shown to decrease withdrawal syndromes, opioid cravings, illicit drug use, overdose, overdose death, and all-cause mortality in patients with OUD even when used without psychosocial interventions. The CDC guideline recommends against detoxification without these medications. Providers should identify treatment resources for OUD in their community and obtain a waiver to prescribe buprenorphine for OUD (especially if working in communities with limited treatment capacity for OUD).

F. Cancer-related Pain

The 2022 CDC practice guideline for prescribing opioids is not meant to be applied to patients with cancer-related pain. Patients with cancer should be screened for pain at every clinic visit. Moderate to severe cancer-related pain can be treated with an opioid. Morphine is often used as first-line treatment; in an open-label RCT for moderate cancer pain, it produced more adequate analgesia than weak opioids (eg, codeine). Opioid switching (opioid rotation) may be appropriate when patients have inadequately managed pain or unacceptable side effects. A four-arm, phase 4 RCT reported improved pain relief and decreased side effects in 50% of patients who switched opioids after suboptimal response to initial opioid treatment. There is moderate evidence to support *epidural or intrathecal opioid administration* for cancer-related pain (eg, through an implanted intrathecal pump). This therapy requires access to a specialist pain management clinic. Nonpharmacologic pain interventions and self-management pain strategies also should be encouraged. Consider consulting with a palliative care team or pain management specialist early, especially for patients who may have more difficulty with pain management.

Opioid therapy in patients with concurrent cancer-related pain and OUD can be complicated. Both cancer-related pain and OUD should be treated as adequately as possible. Medications for treatment of OUD, such as methadone and buprenorphine-naloxone, should be continued. Depending on the individual patient's situation and prognosis, medications for treatment of OUDs could be administered in split dosing (rather than daily dosing), a full agonist opioid (eg, morphine) could be added in addition to the medications for treatment of OUD, or full agonist opioids could be switched to buprenorphine or methadone. Interdisciplinary management with addiction psychiatry, palliative care, chronic pain management, and primary care teams is often beneficial.

G. Pregnant Patients

Opioid use during pregnancy has been associated with stillbirth, poor fetal growth, and preterm delivery in observational studies and may lead to neonatal abstinence syndrome in some cases. However, the American College of Obstetricians and Gynecologists (ACOG) has emphasized that concern for **neonatal abstinence syndrome**, a treatable condition, should not be a reason to avoid treating acute pain in pregnant patients. For acute pain, the lowest effective opioid dose should be prescribed for no longer than the expected duration of pain requiring opioids. For pregnant patients with chronic pain, ACOG recommends employing strategies to minimize opioid use. The 2022 CDC guidelines recommend management by continuing medications for treatment of OUDs (buprenorphine, methadone) for pregnant patients with OUD rather than withdrawal of the opioid. If considering tapering opioids in a pregnant patient, providers should consult appropriate experts because of the risk to the patient and fetus if the patient develops withdrawal.

H. Neuropathic Pain

Currently, there is no high-level evidence that supports the use of opioids in the long-term management of neuropathic pain. Instead, opioids have been found to have significantly more adverse effects when compared to nonopioid, neuropathic medications (Table 5–8).

Coffin PO et al. Primary care management of long-term opioid therapy. Ann Med. 2022;54:2451. [PMID: 36111417]

Dowell D et al. CDC Clinical Practice Guideline for prescribing opioids for pain—United States, 2022. MMWR Recomm Rep. 2022;71:1. [PMID: 36327391]

Ganguly A et al. Cancer pain and opioid use disorder. Oncology (Williston Park). 2022;36:535. [PMID: 36107782]

Adverse Effects of Opioids

Common adverse effects of opioids include constipation, nausea, sedation, pruritus, physical dependence, opioid use disorder, hormonal disturbance and sexual dysfunction (especially hypogonadism in men), respiratory depression, and CNS depression. Core strategies to decrease adverse effects include dose reduction, opioid rotation, and symptom management. **Opioid-induced respiratory depression constitutes a medical emergency and must be managed appropriately.**

Although potentially fatal, respiratory depression can be rapidly reversed by the opioid receptor antagonist naloxone. There is moderate evidence that naloxone, when administered appropriately, can decrease opioid overdose–related mortality. *The CDC recommends coprescribing naloxone in patients who are receiving opioid doses of ≥ 50 MME/day, who have a respiratory condition, who are concomitantly prescribed benzodiazepines, who have a history of substance use disorder, or who are otherwise at high risk for overdose.* Prefilled nasal sprays (4-mg or 8-mg doses for intranasal administration) and syringe kits (2-mg or 5-mg doses for intramuscular injection) can be distributed to patients on opioid therapy. Naloxone kits may contain two doses, so a repeat dose can be given every 2–3 minutes until emergency help arrives. To avoid precipitating opioid withdrawal, the medication is titrated with the objective of improving the patient's respiratory function, rather than arousal. Naloxone-induced withdrawal can lead to cardiovascular events (increases in heart rate, mean arterial pressure, and cardiac index). Larger-dose naloxone kits have been created to combat overdose deaths related to the even more potent illicit synthetic opioids (eg, carfentanil), but their use is associated with a higher risk of opioid withdrawal.

Table 5–8. Pharmacologic management of neuropathic pain. (Listed in alphabetical order, within classes.)

Medication[1]	Starting Dose	Typical Dose	Number Needed to Treat[2]
Tricyclic Antidepressants[3,4]			
Amitriptyline	10–25 mg orally at bedtime	10–150 mg orally at bedtime	2.1
Desipramine	12.5 mg orally at bedtime	12.5–250 mg orally at bedtime (can be divided into two doses)	2.1
Nortriptyline	10–25 mg orally at bedtime	10–150 mg orally at bedtime	2.1
Calcium Channel $\alpha_2\delta$ Ligands			
Gabapentin[5]	100–300 mg orally once to three times daily	300–1200 mg orally three times daily	6.5
Pregabalin[6]	25 mg orally once daily	50–150 mg orally three times daily	4.5
Selective Serotonin Norepinephrine Reuptake Inhibitors[4]			
Duloxetine	60 mg orally daily	60–120 mg orally daily	5.1
Venlafaxine[7]	37.5–75 mg orally daily divided into two or three doses	150–225 mg orally daily divided into two or three doses	
Opioids	(see Table 5–6)	(see Table 5–6)	2.6
Topical and Other Medications			
Capsaicin	0.04% or 0.075% cream; 8% patch	0.04% or 0.075% cream applied three or four times daily or 8% patch applied twice daily	6.2
Diclofenac transdermal	1.3% patch or 1% gel	Patch applied twice daily or gel applied three times daily	
Lidocaine transdermal	4% patch applied for a maximum of 12 hours	4% or 5% patch 1–3 patches applied daily for a maximum of 12 hours; available OTC	
Tramadol hydrochloride[8]	50 mg orally four times daily	100 mg orally two to four times daily	4.9

[1]Begin at the starting dose and titrate up every 4 or 5 days. Within each category, drugs listed in order of prescribing preference.
[2]Data from Moulin D et al; Canadian Pain Society. Pharmacologic management of chronic neuropathic pain: revised consensus statement from the Canadian Pain Society. Pain Res Manag. 2014;19:328.
[3]Begin with a low dose. Use the lowest effective dose. Pain relief may be achieved at doses below antidepressant doses, thereby minimizing adverse side effects.
[4]Do not combine TCAs with SNRIs (or SSRIs) to avoid serotonin syndrome.
[5]Common side effects include nausea, somnolence, and dizziness. Must adjust dose for kidney impairment.
[6]Common side effects include dizziness, somnolence, peripheral edema, and weight gain. Must adjust dose for kidney impairment.
[7]*Caution:* Can cause hypertension and ECG changes. Consider obtaining baseline ECG and monitor.
[8]Tramadol is classified by the DEA as a Schedule IV controlled substance.

Opioid-induced constipation *is the most common adverse effect of opioids.* Opioids bind to mu receptors in the GI tract and decrease bowel motility and mucosal secretions in a dose-related fashion. Ideally, patients treated with opioids should have a bowel movement at least every 24–48 hours. Initial recommendations for management of opioid-induced constipation should include patient education, increased dietary fiber, adequate hydration, and regular physical activity. Additionally, osmotic laxatives (eg, Miralax) can be given with a stimulant laxative (eg, senna). Newer peripherally acting mu receptor antagonists (eg, naldemedine, naloxegol, methylnaltrexone) block the GI actions of opioids without decreasing the opioid's analgesic effects and are recommended if laxatives fail.

Opioid-induced nausea likely develops secondary to direct stimulation of the chemoreceptor trigger zone, to vestibular sensitivity, or to decreased GI motility. Management options include dopamine antagonists (eg, prochlorperazine), prokinetic agents (eg, metoclopramide), serotonin antagonists (eg, ondansetron), or antihistamines (eg, diphenhydramine, promethazine, meclizine). All of these agents have side effects that must be carefully monitored.

Sedation or decreased cognition most commonly occurs with initiation of opioid therapy or dose escalation. Dose reduction should be attempted first before pursuing pharmacologic intervention. Pharmacologic management options include methylphenidate; however, high-level evidence supporting its use for this indication is lacking.

Pruritus occurs in 2–10% of patients given opioids, possibly secondary to peripheral histamine release. Management options include an opioid rotation, dose reduction, diphenhydramine, and cool compresses.

Centers for Disease Control and Prevention (CDC). Stop overdose. Lifesaving naloxone. Accessed December 11, 2025. https://www.cdc.gov/stop-overdose/caring/naloxone.html

Payne ER et al. Comparison of administration of 8-milligram and 4-milligram intranasal naloxone by law enforcement during response to suspected opioid overdose—New York, March 2022–August 2023. MMWR Morb Mortal Wkly Rep 2024;73:110. [PMID: 38329911]

Basics of Opioid Monitoring

Prior to the initial opioid prescription, it is prudent to clearly define the underlying condition, diagnostic workup, nonopioid therapeutic management plan, and intended length of prescription. Ideally, the prescriber should determine how the opioid prescription fits into a broader comprehensive pain management plan.

The 2022 CDC guidelines for prescribing opioids recommend evaluating benefits and risks of opioid use within 1–4 weeks of initiating an opioid or escalating an opioid dose, as well as regularly during opioid therapy. Standardized assessments such as the **"PEG" scores** may be used at initial and follow-up visits to gauge the efficacy of treatment (Table 5–9). Meaningful improvement has been defined as 30% improvement in scores for both pain and function.

There is only weak to moderate evidence to support the efficacy of some risk management strategies when prescribing opioids such as urine toxicology testing, prescription drug monitoring programs, and treatment agreements or "contracts." The 2022 CDC guidelines recommend discussing realistic benefits and known risks of opioid therapy before initiating opioid treatment. Providers should create functional goals to evaluate treatment benefit. Additionally, before starting opioid treatment, an exit strategy should be developed and ready if opioid therapy is unsuccessful.

The 2022 CDC guidelines recommend checking *prescription drug monitoring program* data before initiating opioids for any patient, and at least every 3 months or more frequently for patients on long-term opioid therapy. Prescription drug monitoring program data can be used to determine if a patient is taking an opioid dosage or medication combination that puts them at risk for overdose. Prescription drug monitoring program information should be discussed with the patient and used to make decisions around patient safety and treatment.

Table 5–9. PEG score to gauge benefit from long-term opioid use.

During the past week:
1. What number best describes your *P*ain? 0 = no pain to 10 = worst pain imaginable
2. What number best describes how much your pain interfered with your *E*njoyment of life? 0 = no interference to 10 = complete interference
3. What number describes how much pain interfered with your *G*eneral activity? 0 = no interference to 10 = complete interference

To calculate PEG score, average scores from questions 1 through 3. Adapted from Krebs EE et al. Development and initial validation of the PEG, a three-item scale assessing pain intensity and interference. J Gen Intern Med. 2009;24:733. [PMID: 19418100]

The CDC recommends that all patients receiving long-term opioid therapy have urine toxicology tests before initiating opioids and at least annually. Patients should understand that urine drug tests may be conducted randomly and repeatedly during treatment. Toxicology tests should not be used in a punitive manner, and clinicians should not dismiss patients from their care on the basis of these results. Instead, providers should discuss unexpected results with the patient in a nonjudgmental manner.

Before initiating and periodically during opioid treatment, providers should *evaluate risk for opioid-related harms* (eg, assess alcohol and other substance use, screen for mental health and substance use disorder). **Naloxone** should be offered to patients taking opioids, especially those at increased risk for overdose. This includes patients with a history of overdose, substance use disorder, sleep apnea/sleep-disordered breathing, patients taking ≥ 50 MME/day, patients taking benzodiazepines or other CNS depressants, and patients who have lost tolerance and may return to higher opioid doses (eg, patients released from prison or undergoing opioid taper).

Dowell D et al. CDC Clinical Practice Guideline for prescribing opioids for pain—United States, 2022. MMWR Recomm Rep. 2022;71:1. [PMID: 36327391]

Manchikanti L et al. Comprehensive, evidence-based, consensus guidelines for prescription of opioids for chronic non-cancer pain from the American Society of Interventional Pain Physicians (ASIPP). Pain Physician. 2023;26:S7. [PMID: 38117465]

Weaning from Opioids

The goals during opioid tapers are to work with the patient to minimize symptoms and signs of withdrawal, and to mitigate risk of overdose and mental health crises during the wean. *Common symptoms and signs of withdrawal include anxiety, craving, tachycardia, vomiting, diarrhea, and mydriasis.* Opioid tapers may improve pain management and long-term patient safety, but they are precarious times when patients may be at higher risk for overdoses and mental health crises. A 2021 retrospective cohort study of patients originally prescribed at least 50 MME found an increased adjusted incident rate ratio (aIRR) of 1.28 for overdose events in patients during tapering periods compared with nontapering periods. Tapering was associated with an increased aIRR of 1.74 for mental health crises compared with nontapering periods.

Traditionally, a 10% decrease in opioid dosage *per week* was considered reasonable. However, a slower approximately 10% decrease in opioid dosage *per month* may be better tolerated and may result in an increased patient retention in the taper. Providers should work with patients during the taper to determine its speed, for example via smaller dosage decreases or a temporary taper pause. Some tapers may take months to years. Per the 2022 CDC guideline for opioid prescribing, a more rapid taper should only be considered if there is a life-threatening issue such as an impending overdose. Additional psychosocial support should be offered to the patient and nonopioid measures to manage pain (eg, physical therapy, cognitive behavioral therapy, adjuvant nonopioid analgesics) should be maximized during the period of weaning.

Fortuna RJ et al. Comprehensive approach to opioid management in a primary care network. Popul Health Manag. 2024;27:1. [PMID: 38237106]
Maharjan S et al. Opioid tapering and mental health crisis in older adults. Pharmacoepidemiol Drug Saf. 2024;33:e5698. [PMID: 37734725]

MEDICATIONS FOR NEUROPATHIC PAIN

When taking a patient's history, pain descriptions such as "burning," "shooting," "pins and needles," or "electricity" and pain associated with numbness suggest neuropathic pain. Studies are mixed regarding efficacy of opioids for neuropathic pain. There may be a theoretical advantage to methadone and buprenorphine over other opioids for neuropathic pain due to added NMDA and κ-receptor antagonism, respectively, but these are not first-line options and should be considered only in severe, refractory cases. However, a number of nonopioid medications have been found to be effective in randomized trials (Table 5–8). Successful management of neuropathic pain often requires the use of more than one effective medication. Since these medications bind to receptors on a large variety of neurons, they often have CNS side effects. These side effects often limit reaching therapeutic doses and may be the reason for higher numbers needed to treat (Table 5–8) compared with NSAIDs.

The calcium channel $\alpha_2\delta$ ligands gabapentin and pregabalin are first-line therapies for neuropathic pain. Neither medication has significant medication interactions. However, they can cause sedation, dizziness, ataxia, and GI side effects. Both gabapentin and pregabalin require dose adjustments in patients with kidney dysfunction. Gabapentin should be started at low dosages of 100–300 mg orally once daily and titrated upward by 100–300 mg/day every 4–7 days by adding additional doses throughout the day, with a typical effective dose of 1800–3600 mg/day in three divided doses. Pregabalin should be started at 50–150 mg/day in two or three divided doses. If necessary, the dose of pregabalin can be titrated upward to 300–600 mg/day in two or three divided doses. Both medications are relatively safe in accidental overdose and may be preferred over tricyclic antidepressants (TCAs) for a patient with a history of HF, arrhythmia, or risk of suicide.

The SNRIs duloxetine and venlafaxine also are first-line treatments for neuropathic pain. Duloxetine is usually titrated up to 60 mg once daily and is best taken with food due to the common side effect of nausea. SNRIs generally should not be combined with other serotonin or norepinephrine reuptake inhibitors, but they can be safely combined with gabapentin or pregabalin. Lower doses of venlafaxine have more serotonin than norepinephrine activity; therefore, higher doses may be required to treat neuropathic pain. Because venlafaxine can cause hypertension and induce ECG changes, patients with cardiovascular risk factors should be carefully monitored when starting this medication. Desvenlafaxine, the active metabolite of venlafaxine, also is available and may be tolerated better than venlafaxine.

TCAs are another class of medications for neuropathic pain that work through the norepinephrine and serotonin pathways. Among the TCAs that are effective for neuropathic pain, nortriptyline and desipramine are preferred over amitriptyline because they cause less orthostatic hypotension and have fewer anticholinergic side effects. Start with a low dosage (10–25 mg orally daily) and titrate upward in 10-mg increments every 4 or 5 days, aiming to use the lowest effective dose and to titrate up to a maximum of ≤ 50–100 mg daily. It may take several weeks for a TCA to have its full analgesic effect for neuropathic pain. Because TCAs and SNRIs both work through the serotonin and norepinephrine pathways, they generally should *not* be coprescribed due to concerns about the serotonin syndrome. For this reason, TCAs and SNRIs should be similarly avoided in patients already on an SSRI unless planning to cross-taper from an SSRI to one of these agents for improved pain control.

Topical medications, such as lidocaine 5% patch and capsaicin 8% patches, are considered second-line therapies. The lidocaine 5% patch is particularly effective in postherpetic neuralgia and may be effective in other types of localized neuropathic pain. Due to its relatively minimal adverse effects, it is commonly used despite being considered second-line. Topical lidocaine 4% patches and cream are available over the counter.

Medical cannabis strains high in cannabidiol have proven efficacy for some types of neuropathic pain.

ADJUVANT PAIN MEDICATIONS & TREATMENTS

While polypharmacy is generally avoided, it can be appropriate to combine lower doses of multiple pain medications to avoid intolerable medication side effects of one or two medications at higher doses.

For metastatic bone pain, the anti-inflammatory effect of NSAIDs can be helpful. Furthermore, bisphosphonates (such as pamidronate and zoledronic acid) and receptor activator of NF-κ-B ligand (RANKL) inhibitors (such as denosumab) may relieve such bone pain, although they are generally more useful for prevention of bone metastases than for analgesia.

Corticosteroids, such as dexamethasone, prednisone, and methylprednisolone, can be helpful for patients with headache due to increased intracranial pressure, pain from spinal cord compression, metastatic bone pain, and neuropathic pain due to invasion or infiltration of nerves by tumor. Because of the side effects of long-term corticosteroid administration, they are most appropriate for short-term use and in patients with end-stage disease. Low-dose intravenous, oral, buccal, and nasal ketamine has been used successfully for neuropathic and other pain syndromes refractory to opioids, although research data are limited.

PSYCHOLOGICAL, PHYSICAL, & INTEGRATIVE THERAPIES

Psychological Therapy

Nonpharmacologic and noninterventional therapies are valuable in treating pain. In fact, *cognitive behavioral therapy and physical or functional therapy have been shown to be the most effective for management of chronic pain.* In multiple randomized, controlled studies, cognitive behavioral therapy has been proven effective as a primary evidence-based treatment for chronic pain. Because mood and psychological issues play an important role in the patient's perception of and response to pain, psychotherapy, support groups, prayer, and pastoral counseling also can help in pain management. Other psychological approaches include biofeedback, meditation, framing, guided imagery, and cognitive distraction. Depression and anxiety, which may be instigated by chronic pain or may alter the response to pain, should be treated aggressively with antidepressants and anxiolytics.

Physical Therapy & Other Physical Interventions

Physical therapy is a mainstay of chronic pain management and encompasses several modalities, including strength training, manual therapy, and massage.

Physical therapy is useful for neuropathic pain and musculoskeletal pain. For example, if there is a cervical radiculopathy, the position and posture of individual neck muscles may exacerbate the narrowing of the neuroforamina or nerves may become entrapped within hypertrophied muscles, leading to neuropathic pain. Therefore, functional rehabilitation through physical therapy may address multiple types of pain.

Physical therapy for management of low-back pain may involve "core stabilization." Bounded by the diaphragm and the pelvic floor, the body's "core" is composed of the abdominal muscles and back and gluteal muscles. Exercises can help stabilize the entirety of the core, so that the low back does not need to exert as much effort for movement, lifting, bending, etc. "Core stabilization" can thereby decrease low-back pain.

Because physical therapy has minimal potential harms associated with it, it should be a key component in management of both acute and chronic pain. While physical therapy can be used on its own, it is often preferable to engage in it as part of a multidisciplinary approach to pain management (which may include psychological therapies).

For musculoskeletal pain, hot or cold packs, massage, and stretching (including traction), or the use of a TENS unit can be helpful.

Integrative Medicine Therapy

Integrative medicine therapies such as acupuncture, massage, reiki, cupping, tai chi/yoga, and music therapy may be helpful in treating pain. Studies have not shown strong evidence for integrative medicine for the treatment of chronic pain, but because these therapies are very low risk, they may be considered in appropriate patients.

SELECTED INTERVENTIONAL MODALITIES FOR PAIN RELIEF

Pain management specialists are physicians who have completed a residency in anesthesiology, physical medicine and rehabilitation, neurology, internal medicine, emergency medicine, or psychiatry followed by a fellowship in pain management to learn medication management and interventional techniques for acute, chronic, and cancer pain. Interventional pain management modalities performed by pain management specialists involve *neuromodulation* of specific targets to alleviate pain. The procedures they perform include percutaneous injection of local anesthetics or corticosteroids, radiofrequency (thermal) lesioning, cryotherapy, chemical neurolysis, or surgical implantation of intrathecal medication delivery pump systems or neurostimulation devices. *While invasive procedures have inherent risks such as bleeding or infection, they can drastically reduce or even obviate the need for conventional pharmacologic therapies that may be poorly tolerated or burdensome to the patient.*

For some patients, a nerve block, such as a celiac plexus block for pain from pancreatic cancer, can provide substantial relief. Intrathecal pumps may be most useful for patients with severe pain responsive to opioids but who experience intolerable side effects from systemic opioids (eg, sedation, urinary retention, constipation). In the palliative care setting, these pumps are appropriate when life expectancy is long enough to justify the discomfort and cost of surgical implantation.

Clinicians do not need to know all the details of interventional pain procedures but should consider referring their patients to pain management specialists if standard treatments are inadequate or associated with intolerable side effects. Ultimately, while the decision to pursue interventional management of pain hinges on the individualized assessment of the patient's goals, symptom trajectory, comorbidities, and prior response to therapy, primary clinicians should feel empowered to refer patients to a pain specialist when there is a need to expand the therapeutic options for patients whose pain remains inadequately controlled. Table 5–10 and Table 5–11 list the procedures and the agents typically used in interventional pain modalities.

INTRATHECAL DRUG DELIVERY

A. Indications

Intrathecal drug delivery therapy is indicated for patients with both malignant and nonmalignant pain and has been shown to be effective, cost-effective, and safe. It is generally accepted that intrathecal opioids have a 100- to 300-fold

Table 5–10. Interventional sites and techniques for chronic pain by anatomic location. (Listed in alphabetical order within general location.)

Anatomic sites for neurostimulation
Dorsal column stimulation (spinal cord stimulation)
Dorsal root ganglion stimulation
Peripheral nerve or field stimulation
Joints
Intra-articular injections
Joint denervation procedures
Neuraxial blockage (block in the CNS)
Noncontinuous
Epidural (caudal, lumbar, thoracic, cervical; interlaminar versus transforaminal)
Intrathecal
Continuous neuraxial drug delivery
Epidural (tunneled catheter, port)
Intrathecal (implanted intrathecal pump)
Paraneuraxial (planar blockade)
Paravertebral (intercostal)
Pectoralis and serratus anterior
Transversus abdominis plane/quadratus lumborum
Peripheral nerve (perineural blockade)
Brachial plexus and branches
Lumbar plexus and branches
Sympathetic ganglion
Celiac plexus
Cervical sympathetic blockade (stellate ganglion)
Ganglion impar
Gasserian ganglion
Lumbar sympathetic blockade
Sphenopalatine ganglion
Superior hypogastric plexus

Table 5–11. Agents used[1] in neuromodulatory therapies. (Listed in alphabetic order within classes.)

Adjuvants
Clonidine
Dexmedetomidine
Others
Chemical neurolysis
Alcohol
Phenol
Corticosteroids
Dexamethasone
Methylprednisolone
Triamcinolone
Neurostimulation
Various patterns, frequency, amplitude, pulse width
Opioids
Hydromorphone
Fentanyl
Morphine
Thermal neurolysis
Cryoanalgesia
Radiofrequency ablation
Voltage-gated sodium channel blockade—local anesthetics
Bupivacaine
Lidocaine
Mepivacaine
Ropivacaine

[1]Injected or applied.
List is not comprehensive but includes most commonly used agents.

efficacy compared with oral opioids; therefore, *the best candidates may be patients who obtain good analgesia from systemic opioids but experience intolerable side effects.* Common indications include cancer pain, chronic low-back pain (in particular, post-laminectomy syndrome), complex regional pain syndrome, and other causes of nociceptive or neuropathic pain. In a randomized controlled trial comparing intrathecal therapy with comprehensive medication management in cancer pain, intrathecal therapy was shown to provide superior analgesia with fewer side effects and longer life expectancy. Due to the cost of implanting the device and the recovery time required after surgical implantation, it is recommended that patients have a life expectancy of at least 2–3 months.

B. Procedure

Intrathecal drug delivery systems consist of a pump with a drug reservoir, typically implanted in the abdominal wall, connected to a catheter that delivers medications into the intrathecal space. A trial procedure—via epidural or intrathecal administration of a bolus or short infusion—is generally performed in patients with cancer and noncancer pain to assess expected analgesic benefit and tolerability before proceeding to full implantation. However, in select cancer patients, implantation may proceed without a formal trial to avoid treatment delays. The implantation of an intrathecal drug delivery system involves two incisions: one in the spine to accommodate the catheter and anchor, and another in the lower abdominal region to create a pocket to hold the pump. The catheter is tunneled through the lower abdominal and flank subcutaneous tissues to connect to the pump.

C. Medications Used

According to the Polyanalgesic Conference Consensus (PACC) guidelines for both malignant and nonmalignant pain, first-line intrathecal delivery medications include monotherapy with either morphine or ziconotide (a calcium channel inhibitor). However, the PACC guidelines also state that de facto practice includes combination therapy with opioids (eg, fentanyl, hydromorphone) and local anesthetic (eg, bupivacaine) and may include other medications (eg, baclofen or clonidine). Respiratory depression and sedation are two of the most concerning side effects of many intrathecal medications. Side effects of morphine and fentanyl include nausea, edema, constipation, urinary retention, and pruritus but at a much lower rate than these same medications administered systemically. While ziconotide is FDA-approved, its use is limited due to side effects including myositis and polyarthralgias as well as psychiatric and neurologic adverse effects (it is contraindicated in patients with preexisting psychosis).

D. Advantages and Disadvantages

The main advantage of intrathecal delivery therapy is targeted delivery of medication to the spinal cord with increased efficacy and diminished side effects compared with systemic analgesic medications. Intrathecal therapy has been found to be effective with decreased side effects and improved analgesia in 80% of patients with cancer. However, intrathecal therapy requires regular pump refills and may be complicated by rare adverse events including infections, catheter or pump malfunctions requiring surgical revision, or development of catheter tip granulomas, potentially leading to inadequate analgesia or neurologic deficits. Pump batteries may last from 5 years to 10 years depending on usage. Fatalities surrounding intrathecal therapy have been linked to respiratory depression when high doses and high cervical catheters are used or when combined with high systemic doses of medications; patients must be monitored for respiratory depression or sedation when initiating or increasing intrathecal therapeutic agents. Some intrathecal pumps need to be emptied prior to MRI; due to the magnetic forces of the MRI, the entirety of the drug reservoir could inadvertently open. Therefore, it is critical that the type of pump is known prior to placing the patient in an MRI machine. Additionally, anticoagulants and NSAIDs need to be stopped prior to pump implantation and need to be held briefly after the implantation as well; this temporary cessation imposes the risk of potentially causing blood clots.

E. Alternatives

For patients with limited life expectancy, continuous epidural drug delivery via an external pump or subcutaneous port may be more appropriate. Systemic medications delivered orally, intravenously, topically, or even by a subcutaneous infusion (as in palliative care settings) are alternatives to intrathecal therapy.

De Andres J et al. Intrathecal drug delivery: advances and applications in the management of chronic pain patient. Front Pain Res (Lausanne). 2022;3:900566. [PMID: 35782225]

Deer TR et al. The Polyanalgesic Consensus Conference (PACC)®: intrathecal drug delivery guidance on safety and therapy optimization when treating chronic noncancer pain. Neuromodulation. 2024;27:1107. [PMID: 38752946]

Perruchoud C et al. Management of cancer-related pain with intrathecal drug delivery: a systematic review and meta-analysis of clinical studies. Neuromodulation. 2022:S1094. [PMID: 35088743]

SPINAL STIMULATION

A. Indications

Spinal stimulation targets neuropathic pain in the trunk and limbs, such as from failed back surgery syndrome, complex regional pain syndrome, diabetic peripheral neuropathy, and radiculopathy, as well as neuropathic pain associated with cancer.

B. Procedure

Neurostimulation devices consist of an implantable pulse generator typically placed in the flank or abdomen just under the skin, and an array of electrical contacts on small cylindrical or paddle leads placed in the epidural space. *Neurostimulation devices transmit electrical pulses to the spinal cord or dorsal root ganglion to block pain transmission.* Paddle leads require neurosurgical implantation with laminotomy (and general anesthesia), while percutaneous wire leads may be implanted under sedation. Patients undergo a 3- to 7-day trial during which the leads are attached to an external battery source and undergo programming with different pulse waveforms to assess therapeutic efficacy prior to surgical implantation of permanent leads and implantable pulse generator.

C. Stimulation Parameters

Traditional neurostimulation resulted in paresthesias that were used to mask pain. It was presumed that these paresthesias were the result of stimulation of the dorsal column axons. Recent studies have revealed that analgesia can be obtained independent of paresthesias by altering a variety of spinal cord stimulation parameters, including constant high-frequency stimulation and burst high-frequency stimulation. Double-blind RCTs have shown that both functional status and pain scores can be significantly improved using spinal cord stimulation systems that adapt the output to the patient's individual neural response in a closed loop fashion, thereby providing long-term improvement in pain relief, sleep, mood, disability, and opioid reduction. For more focal neuropathic pain conditions such as postoperative inguinal nerve injuries or thoracic postherpetic neuralgias, stimulation of the dorsal root ganglion can provide focal analgesia.

D. Advantages and Disadvantages

Spinal cord stimulation is a reversible technology that may provide superior analgesic efficacy while eliminating the need for systemic medications. Literature suggests spinal cord stimulation is efficacious in 80–90% of well-selected patients, such as those with neuropathic low-back pain due to post-laminectomy syndrome. In fact, spinal cord stimulation has now advanced to a higher position in the treatment continuum; *it can be considered before using long-term moderate doses of systemic opioids.* On the other hand, because it is a surgical procedure, it may be associated with complications, such as infection, lead migration, device malfunction, or neurologic deficits. While MRIs were contraindicated with some older systems, most newer systems allow for limited MRI imaging. Batteries may require charging a few times a week but typically do not require replacement for 5–10 years. A psychological evaluation is typically performed prior to initiating therapy to rule out any severe untreated psychological comorbidities and assess expectation of treatment and appropriateness of implantation.

E. Alternatives

In addition to medication management for pain, two neuromodulatory techniques may serve as alternatives to dorsal horn and dorsal root ganglion stimulation. **Peripheral nerve stimulation** targets peripheral nerves using a similar system of a lead connected to a pulse generator. It may be most appropriate when there is a very specific neurologic target. **Transcutaneous electrical nerve stimulators (TENS)** and systemic pharmacologic therapies are also alternatives.

Kapural L ... Poree L et al. Durable multimodal and holistic response for physiologic closed-loop spinal cord stimulation supported by objective evidence from the EVOKE double-blind randomized controlled trial. Reg Anesth Pain Med. 2024;49:233. [PMID: 37491149]

Mekhail N ... Poree L et al; EVOKE Study Group. Durability of clinical and quality-of-life outcomes of closed-loop spinal cord stimulation for chronic back and leg pain: a secondary analysis of the Evoke randomized clinical trial. JAMA Neurol. 2022;79:251. Erratum in: JAMA Neurol. 2022;79:420. [PMID: 35156999]

Mekhail NA ... Poree L et al; EVOKE Study Group. ECAP-controlled closed-loop versus open-loop SCS for the treatment of chronic pain: 36-month results of the EVOKE blinded randomized clinical trial. Reg Anesth Pain Med. 2024;49:346. [PMID: 37640452]

CELIAC PLEXUS BLOCK & NEUROLYSIS

A. Indications

A celiac plexus block refers to injection of a long-acting anesthetic (eg, bupivacaine) with or without a corticosteroid (eg, methylprednisolone); with corticosteroids, the block can provide relief for a few weeks to months. ***Celiac plexus neurolysis*** involves injection of a neurolytic agent (eg, alcohol or phenol); it may provide pain relief more consistently for 2–6 months. The most common indication is pancreatic cancer pain, but it can be used for pain from other malignancies (eg, stomach, liver, spleen, kidney, and GI tract) or from chronic pancreatitis. Multiple randomized controlled trials and meta-analyses have shown superiority of celiac plexus neurolysis to medication management for pancreatic cancer, but evidence of its efficacy for chronic pancreatitis is more mixed.

B. Procedure

The most common approach is a percutaneous posterior approach under fluoroscopy guidance, with bilateral needles targeted to the celiac plexus at the level of T12–L1. Alternatively, ultrasound, CT, or endoscopic guidance can be used. Minimal sedation is required for the percutaneous approaches, while heavy sedation or general anesthesia may be required for endoscopic guidance.

C. Medications Used

Chemical neurolysis with alcohol or phenol is used to extend the duration of the analgesia to ≥ 2 months compared to a block with local anesthetic (eg, bupivacaine) and corticosteroid (eg, methylprednisolone), which produces an analgesic duration of weeks to months. For chemical neurolysis, ethanol is used most often because it does not require compounding and importantly has a lower chance of permanent neurologic damage compared with phenol; however, it is more painful on injection.

D. Advantages and Disadvantages

The primary advantage is improved analgesia without need for systemic medications and their untoward effects. Neurolytic celiac plexus blockade is effective in 70–80% of patients. Common side effects of celiac plexus interventions include transient hypotension and transient diarrhea. Transient or permanent spinal cord damage is rare (0–0.2%) with local anesthetic, but inadvertent peripheral nerve injury is increased with the use of alcohol or phenol.

E. Alternatives

Standard pain management is with oral or transdermal systemic analgesic (eg, opioid) medication. Intrathecal therapy is also an alternative, especially for cancer pain.

EPIDURAL CORTICOSTEROID INJECTION

A. Indications

Epidural corticosteroid injections are indicated for patients with chronic neck pain, low-back pain, and radicular pain resulting from central or neuroforaminal stenosis in the cervical, thoracic, or lumbosacral region. Both central and neuroforaminal stenosis may be caused by degenerative disk disease, disk herniation, or facet arthropathy. Epidural corticosteroid injections are relatively safe and are appropriate after conservative measures, such as physical therapy and analgesic medications, have been tried and found unsuccessful.

B. Procedure

Fluoroscopy is typically used to assist with visualizing bony landmarks; either an interlaminar or a transforaminal approach can be used. Interlaminar access is obtained by placing a needle between the lamina of adjacent vertebral levels, whereas transforaminal access is obtained by inserting a needle through the neuroforamen to access the epidural space. These needle insertion procedures can be performed with topical local anesthetic or with minimal sedation.

C. Medications Used

Typically, a particulate corticosteroid such as methylprednisolone is used alone or in combination with a local anesthetic. For the transforaminal approach, where inadvertent vascular access is more of a concern, a nonparticulate corticosteroid such as dexamethasone may be preferred.

D. Advantages and Disadvantages

Epidural corticosteroid injections are advantageous for patients who have not responded to conservative therapy, are not surgical candidates, or do not want surgery. The best evidence of the effectiveness of epidural corticosteroid injections is the short-term improvement of radiculopathy in both the lumbar and cervical regions. Disadvantages include possible post–dural puncture headache, transient weakness, and, rarely, permanent neurologic deficits. Patients receiving systemic anticoagulation may need to hold their anticoagulants before receiving corticosteroid injections, which could increase their risk of cardiovascular events; these cases should be discussed with the clinician managing the anticoagulation prior to performing any epidural corticosteroid injections.

E. Alternatives

Alternatives include conservative therapy, such as oral analgesic medication management, physical therapy, pain psychology, acupuncture, and surgery.

When to Refer

Patients should be referred to pain management specialists if they have:

- Pain that does not respond to low-dose systemic opioids at typical doses or the opioids cause major adverse effects at typical doses.
- Pain that cannot be controlled expeditiously or safely by other clinicians.
- Neuropathic pain that does not respond to first-line treatments.
- Complex medication management requiring high dose of medications, especially long-acting opioids such as buprenorphine or methadone.
- Severe pain from malignancy, including primary disease (eg, pancreatic cancer) or metastatic disease (eg, bony metastases).

When to Admit

- Severe exacerbation of pain not responsive to previous stable oral opioids given around-the-clock plus breakthrough doses.
- Severe pain that is uncontrollable at home.
- Uncontrollable side effects from opioids, including nausea, vomiting, myoclonus, and altered mental status.
- Need for a surgical procedure, such as implantation of an intrathecal drug delivery pump or neurostimulation device.

Dermatologic Disorders

Nathan W. Rojek, MD
Scott Worswick, MD

6

Dermatologic diseases are diagnosed by the types of lesions they cause. Identify the morphology of the lesion(s) to establish a differential diagnosis (Table 6–1), and obtain the elements of the history, physical examination, and appropriate laboratory and histopathologic tests to confirm the diagnosis. Specific clinical situations, such as immunocompromised or critically ill patients, lead to different diagnostic considerations.

PRINCIPLES OF DERMATOLOGIC THERAPY

Frequently Used Treatment Measures

A. Bathing

Soap should be used only in the axillae and groin and on the feet by persons with dry or inflamed skin. Soaking in water for 10–15 minutes before applying topical corticosteroids or emollients enhances their efficacy (Soak and Smear).

B. Topical Therapy

Nondermatologists should become familiar with a representative agent in each category for each indication (eg, topical corticosteroid, topical retinoid, etc).

1. Corticosteroids—Topical corticosteroid creams, lotions, ointments, gels, foams, and sprays are presented in Table 6–2. Topical corticosteroids are divided into classes based on potency. Agents within the same class are equivalent therapies; however, prices of topical corticosteroids vary dramatically. For a given agent, higher lipophilicity (greasiness) corresponds with increased potency, such that for the same compound and strength, an ointment formulation is more potent than a cream, which is more potent than a lotion. The potency of a topical corticosteroid may be dramatically increased by occlusion (covering with a water-impermeable barrier) for at least 4 hours. Depending on the location of the skin condition, gloves, plastic wrap, moist pajamas covered by dry pajamas (wet wraps), or plastic occlusive suits can be used. Caution should be used in applying topical corticosteroids to areas of thin skin (face, genitals, skin folds). Topical corticosteroid use on the eyelids may result in glaucoma or cataracts. The clinician may estimate the amount of topical corticosteroid needed by using the "rule of nines" (as in burn evaluation; see Figure 41–2). Approximately 20–30 g is necessary to cover the entire body surface of an adult. Systemic absorption does occur with topical corticosteroids, but complications of systemic corticosteroids are rare.

2. Emollients for dry skin ("moisturizers")—Dry skin is a result of abnormal function of the epidermis. Emollients restore the epidermis by promoting keratinocyte differentiation and by producing innate antimicrobials; some restore skin barrier lipids, including ceramides. Ointments and creams, rather than lotions, are the best moisturizers. **Emollients are most effective when applied to wet skin.** Plain petrolatum is allergen-free and can be used if allergic contact dermatitis to topical products is suspected.

The scaly appearance of dry skin may be improved by emollients with concomitant use of keratolytics, including urea, lactic acid, or glycolic acid–containing products, provided no inflammation (erythema or pruritus) is present.

3. Drying agents for weepy dermatoses—If the skin is weepy from infection or inflammation, drying agents may be beneficial. The best drying agent is water applied as repeated compresses for 15–30 minutes, alone or with aluminum salts (Burow solution, Domeboro tablets).

4. Topical antipruritics—Lotions that contain 0.5% each of camphor and menthol (Sarna) or pramoxine hydrochloride 1% (with or without 0.5% menthol, eg, Prax, PrameGel, Aveeno Anti-Itch lotion) are effective antipruritic agents. Hydrocortisone, 1% or 2.5%, may be incorporated for its anti-inflammatory effect (Pramosone cream, lotion, or ointment). Doxepin cream 5% reduces pruritus but may cause drowsiness. Pramoxine and doxepin are most effective when applied with topical corticosteroids. Topical capsaicin and lidocaine can be effective in some forms of neuropathic itch.

C. Systemic Antipruritic Drugs

H_1-blockers are the agents of choice for pruritus due to histamine, such as urticaria. Hydroxyzine 25–50 mg orally at night is a typical dose. Sedating and nonsedating antihistamines are of limited value for the treatment of pruritus

Table 6–1. Morphologic categorization of skin lesions and diseases.

Pigmented	Freckle, lentigo, seborrheic keratosis, nevus, blue nevus, halo nevus, melanoma
Scaly	Psoriasis, dermatitis (atopic, stasis, seborrheic, chronic allergic contact or irritant contact), xerosis (dry skin), lichen simplex chronicus, tinea pedis/cruris/corporis, tinea versicolor, secondary syphilis, pityriasis rosea, discoid lupus erythematosus, exfoliative dermatitis, drug eruption, actinic keratosis, Bowen disease
Vesicular	Herpes simplex, varicella, herpes zoster, pompholyx (vesicular dermatitis of palms and soles), vesicular tinea, autoeczematization, dermatitis herpetiformis, miliaria crystallina, scabies, photosensitivity, acute contact allergic dermatitis, drug eruption
Weepy or encrusted	Impetigo, acute contact allergic dermatitis, any vesicular dermatitis
Pustular	Acne vulgaris, acne rosacea, folliculitis, keratosis pilaris, candidiasis, miliaria pustulosa, pustular psoriasis, any vesicular dermatitis, drug eruption
Figurate ("shaped") erythema	Urticaria, erythema multiforme, erythema migrans, cellulitis, erysipelas, erysipeloid, arthropod bites, erythema annulare centrifigum, erythema marginatum, erythema chronicum migrans
Bullous	Impetigo, blistering dactylitis, pemphigus, pemphigoid, porphyria cutanea tarda, drug eruptions, erythema multiforme, toxic epidermal necrolysis
Papular	**Hyperkeratotic:** warts, corns, seborrheic keratoses **Purple-violet:** lichen planus, drug eruptions, Kaposi sarcoma, lymphoma cutis, Sweet syndrome **Flesh-colored, umbilicated:** molluscum contagiosum **Pearly:** basal cell carcinoma, intradermal nevi **Small, red, inflammatory:** acne, rosacea, miliaria rubra, candidiasis, scabies, folliculitis
Pruritus[1]	Xerosis, scabies, pediculosis, lichen planus, lichen simplex chronicus, bites, systemic causes, anogenital pruritus
Nodular, cystic	Erythema nodosum, furuncle, cystic acne, follicular (epidermal) inclusion cyst, metastatic tumor to skin
Photodermatitis	Drug eruption, polymorphic light eruption, lupus erythematosus, porphyria cutanea tarda
Morbilliform	Drug eruption, viral infection (classically measles), secondary syphilis
Erosive	Any vesicular dermatitis, impetigo, aphthae, lichen planus, erythema multiforme, intertrigo
Ulcerated	Decubiti, herpes simplex, skin cancers, parasitic infections, syphilis (chancre), chancroid, vasculitis, stasis, arterial disease, pyoderma gangrenosum

[1]Not a morphologic class but included because it is one of the most common dermatologic presentations.

Table 6–2. Useful topical dermatologic therapeutic agents.[1]

Agent	Formulations, Strengths	Frequency of Application	Potency Class	Common Indications	Comments
Corticosteroids (Listed in Order of Increasing Potency)					
Hydrocortisone acetate	Cream 1% Ointment 1% Solution 1%	Twice daily	Low	Seborrheic dermatitis Pruritus ani Intertrigo	Not the same as valerate or hydrocortisone butyrate Not for poison oak OTC lotion (Aquanil HC), OTC solution (Scalpicin)
	Cream 2.5% Ointment 2.5%			As for 1% hydrocortisone	Perhaps better for pruritus ani Not clearly better than 1% More expensive Not OTC
Alclometasone dipropionate (Aclovate)	Cream 0.05% Ointment 0.05%	Twice daily	Low	As for hydrocortisone	More efficacious than hydrocortisone Perhaps causes less atrophy
Desonide	Cream 0.05% Ointment 0.05% Lotion 0.05%	Twice daily	Low	As for hydrocortisone For lesions on face or body folds resistant to hydrocortisone	More efficacious than hydrocortisone Can cause rosacea or atrophy Not fluorinated

(continued)

Table 6–2. Useful topical dermatologic therapeutic agents.[1] (continued)

Agent	Formulations, Strengths	Frequency of Application	Potency Class	Common Indications	Comments
Clocortolone (Cloderm)	Cream 0.1%	Three times daily	Medium	Contact dermatitis Atopic dermatitis	Does not cross-react with other corticosteroids chemically and can be used in patients allergic to other corticosteroids
Prednicarbate (Dermatop)	Emollient cream 0.1% Ointment 0.1%	Twice daily	Medium	As for triamcinolone	May cause less atrophy No generic formulations Preservative-free
Triamcinolone acetonide	Cream 0.1% Ointment 0.1% Lotion 0.1%	Twice daily	Medium	Eczema on extensor areas Used for psoriasis with tar Seborrheic dermatitis and psoriasis on scalp	Caution in body folds, face Economical in 0.5-lb and 1-lb sizes for treatment of large body surfaces Economical as solution for scalp
	Cream 0.025% Ointment 0.025%	Twice daily	Medium	As for 0.1% strength	Possibly less efficacy and few advantages over 0.1% formulation
Fluocinolone acetonide	Cream 0.025% Ointment 0.025%	Twice daily	Medium	As for triamcinolone	
	Solution 0.01%	Twice daily	Medium	As for triamcinolone	
Mometasone furoate (Elocon)	Cream 0.1% Ointment 0.1% Lotion 0.1%	Once daily	Medium	As for triamcinolone	Often used inappropriately on the face or on children Not fluorinated
Desoximetasone	Cream 0.05% Cream 0.25% Gel 0.05% Ointment 0.25%	Twice daily	High	As for triamcinolone	Comparable potency to fluocinonide Suggested for use when allergic contact dermatitis to topical corticosteroid is suspected; ointment useful when allergic contact dermatitis to propylene glycol is suspected
Diflorasone diacetate	Cream 0.05% Ointment 0.05%	Twice daily	High	Nummular dermatitis Allergic contact dermatitis Lichen simplex chronicus	
Fluocinonide (Lidex)	Cream 0.05% Gel 0.05% Ointment 0.05% Solution 0.05%	Twice daily	High	As for betamethasone Gel useful for poison oak	Economical generics Lidex cream can cause stinging on eczema Lidex emollient cream preferred
Betamethasone dipropionate (Diprolene)	Cream 0.05% Ointment 0.05% Lotion 0.05%	Twice daily	Ultra-high	For lesions resistant to high-potency corticosteroids Lichen planus Insect bites	Economical generics available
Clobetasol propionate (Temovate)	Cream 0.05% Ointment 0.05% Lotion 0.05%	Twice daily	Ultra-high	As for betamethasone dipropionate	Somewhat more potent than diflorasone Limited to 2 continuous weeks of use Limited to 50 g or less per week Cream may cause stinging; use "emollient cream" formulation Generic available
Halobetasol propionate (Ultravate)	Cream 0.05% Ointment 0.05%	Twice daily	Ultra-high	As for clobetasol	Same restrictions as clobetasol Cream does not cause stinging Compatible with calcipotriene (Dovonex)
Flurandrenolide (Cordran)	Tape 3" roll Lotion 0.05%	Every 12 hours	Ultra-high	Lichen simplex chronicus	Tape version protects the skin and prevents scratching

(continued)

Table 6–2. Useful topical dermatologic therapeutic agents.[1] (continued)

Agent	Formulations, Strengths	Frequency of Application	Potency Class	Common Indications	Comments
Nonsteroidal Anti-inflammatory Agents Useful for Dermatitis (Listed Alphabetically)					
Crisaborole (Eucrisa)	Ointment 2%	Twice daily	N/A	Atopic dermatitis	Steroid substitute not causing atrophy or striae May sting or burn on initial application
Delgocitinib (Anzupgo)	Cream 2%	Twice daily	N/A	Chronic hand eczema	Steroid substitute not causing atrophy or striae Many potential systemic side effects including malignancy, infection and cardiovascular
Pimecrolimus[2] (Elidel)	Cream 1%	Twice daily	N/A	Atopic dermatitis	Steroid substitute not causing atrophy or striae
Ruxolitinib (Opzelura)	Cream 1.5%	Twice daily	N/A	Atopic dermatitis	Steroid substitute not causing atrophy or striae Many potential systemic side effects including malignancy, infection and cardiovascular
Roflumilast (Zoryve)	Cream 0.15%	Once daily	N/A	Atopic dermatitis Psoriasis Seborrheic dermatitis	Steroid substitute not causing atrophy or striae May cause diarrhea or headache
Tacrolimus[2] (Protopic)	Ointment 0.1% Ointment 0.03%	Twice daily	N/A	Atopic dermatitis	Steroid substitute not causing atrophy or striae Burns in ≥ 40% of patients with eczema May cause flushing with ingestion of alcohol
Tapinarof (Vtama)	Cream 1%	Once daily	N/A	Atopic dermatitis Psoriasis	Steroid substitute not causing atrophy or striae Common side effect is folliculitis
Antibiotics (for Acne) (Listed Alphabetically)					
Clindamycin phosphate	Solution 1% Gel 1% Lotion 1% Pledget 1%	Twice daily	N/A	Mild papular acne	Lotion is less drying than solution, gel, or pledgets for patients with sensitive skin Recommend use with benzoyl peroxide to avoid antibiotic resistance from monotherapy
Clindamycin/ Benzoyl peroxide (BenzaClin)	Gel	Twice daily	N/A	As for benzamycin	No generic More effective than either agent alone
Dapsone	Gel 5%	Once daily	N/A	Mild papulopustular acne	More expensive, well tolerated Recommend use with benzoyl peroxide to avoid antibiotic resistance from monotherapy
Erythromycin	Solution 2% Gel 2% Pledget 2%	Twice daily	N/A	As for clindamycin	Many different manufacturers Economical Recommend use with benzoyl peroxide to avoid antibiotic resistance from monotherapy
Erythromycin/ Benzoyl peroxide (Benzamycin)	Gel	Twice daily	N/A	As for clindamycin Can help treat comedonal acne	No generic More expensive More effective than other topical antibiotics Main jar requires refrigeration

(continued)

Table 6–2. Useful topical dermatologic therapeutic agents.[1] (continued)

Agent	Formulations, Strengths	Frequency of Application	Potency Class	Common Indications	Comments
Minocycline	Foam 4%	Once daily	N/A	As for clindamycin	No generic More expensive May cause skin yellowing (temporary, washes off)
Antibiotics (for Impetigo)					
Mupirocin (Bactroban)	Ointment 2% Cream 2%	Three times daily	N/A	Impetigo, folliculitis	Because of cost, use limited to tiny areas of impetigo Used in the nose twice daily for 5 days to reduce staphylococcal carriage
Retapamulin (Altabax)	Ointment 1%	Twice daily	N/A	Impetigo	For *Staphylococcus aureus* or *Streptococcus pyogenes* infection Typically reserved for mupirocin-resistant infections
Ozenoxacin (Ozanex)	Cream 1%	Twice daily (5 days)	N/A	Impetigo	Topical fluoroquinolone Activity against MRSA
Antifungals: Imidazoles (Listed Alphabetically)					
Clotrimazole	Cream 1% OTC Solution 1%	Twice daily	N/A	Dermatophyte and *Candida* infections	Available OTC Inexpensive generic cream available
Econazole (Spectazole)	Cream 1%	Once daily	N/A	As for clotrimazole	Somewhat more effective than clotrimazole and miconazole
Ketoconazole (Nizoral)	Cream 2% g	Once daily	N/A	As for clotrimazole	Somewhat more effective than clotrimazole and miconazole
Miconazole	Cream 2% OTC	Twice daily	N/A	As for clotrimazole	As for clotrimazole
Oxiconazole (Oxistat)	Cream 1% Lotion 1%	Twice daily	N/A	As for clotrimazole	
Sertaconazole (Ertaczo)	Cream 2%	Twice daily	N/A	Refractory tinea pedis	By prescription More expensive
Sulconazole (Exelderm)	Cream 1% Solution 1%	Twice daily	N/A	As for clotrimazole	No generic Somewhat more effective than clotrimazole and miconazole
Other Antifungals (Listed Alphabetically)					
Butenafine (Mentax)	Cream 1% OTC	Once daily	N/A	Dermatophytes	Fast response; high cure rate; expensive Available OTC
Ciclopirox (Loprox) (Penlac)	Cream 0.77% Lotion 0.77% Solution 8%	Twice daily	N/A	As for clotrimazole	No generic Somewhat more effective than clotrimazole and miconazole
Efinaconazole (Jublia)	Solution 10%	Once daily for 48 weeks	N/A	Onychomycosis	No generic; more effective than ciclopirox for nail disease
Naftifine (Naftin)	Cream 1% Gel 1%	Once daily	N/A	Dermatophytes	No generic Somewhat more effective than clotrimazole and miconazole
Tavaborole (Kerydin)	Solution 5%	Once daily for 48 weeks	N/A	Onychomycosis	No generic available
Terbinafine (Lamisil)	Cream 1% OTC	Once daily	N/A	Dermatophytes	Fast clinical response OTC
Antipruritics (Listed Alphabetically)					
Camphor/menthol (Sarna)	Lotion 0.5%/0.5%	Two to three times daily	N/A	Mild eczema, xerosis, mild contact dermatitis	

(continued)

Table 6–2. Useful topical dermatologic therapeutic agents.[1] (continued)

Agent	Formulations, Strengths	Frequency of Application	Potency Class	Common Indications	Comments
Capsaicin (various)	Cream 0.025% Cream 0.075%	Three to four times daily	N/A	Topical antipruritic, best used for neuropathic itching	Burning/stinging with initial application that subsides with consistent ongoing use
Doxepin (Zonalon)	Cream 5%	Four times daily	N/A	Topical antipruritic, best used in combination with appropriate topical corticosteroid to enhance efficacy	Can cause sedation
Pramoxine hydrochloride (Prax)	Lotion 1% OTC	Four times daily	N/A	Dry skin, varicella, mild eczema, pruritus ani	OTC formulations (Prax, Aveeno Anti-Itch Cream or Lotion; Itch-X Gel) By prescription mixed with 1% or 2% hydrocortisone

[1]For a given agent, higher lipophilicity (greasiness) corresponds with increased potency; for example, triamcinolone 0.1% ointment is more potent than triamcinolone 0.1% cream, which in turn is more potent than triamcinolone 0.1% lotion.
[2]Topical tacrolimus and pimecrolimus should be used only when other topical treatments are ineffective. Treatment should be limited to an area and duration be as brief as possible. Use of these agents should be avoided in persons with known immunosuppression, HIV infection, bone marrow and organ transplantation, or lymphoma; those at high risk for lymphoma; and those with a history of lymphoma.
MRSA, methicillin-resistant *Staphylococcus aureus;* N/A, not applicable; OTC, over-the-counter.

due to inflammatory skin disease. Preferred agents to antihistamines or systemic steroids include antidepressants (such as doxepin, mirtazapine, and paroxetine) and agents that act directly on the neurons that perceive or modulate pruritus (such as gabapentin, pregabalin, and duloxetine).

Lax SJ et al. Topical anti-inflammatory treatments for eczema: network meta-analysis. Cochrane Database Syst Rev. 2024;8:CD015064. [PMID: 39105474]

Mahmoud RH et al. Current and emerging drugs for the treatment of pruritus: an update of the literature. Expert Opin Pharmacother. 2024;6:655. [PMID: 38682595]

Zeidler C et al. Clinical aspects and management of chronic itch. J Allergy Clin Immunol. 2023;1:1. [PMID: 37178730]

Sunscreens

Protection from UV light reduces the incidence of sunburn, actinic keratoses, melanoma, and some nonmelanoma skin cancers when initiated at any age and in any skin type. The best protection is shade, but protective clothing, avoidance of direct sun exposure during the peak hours of the day, and daily use of sunscreens are important.

A broad-spectrum (protection against UVA and UVB) sunscreen should be used daily with a sun protective factor (SPF) of at least 30, and of at least 50 when high UV exposure activities such as skiing or swimming are being undertaken. Clinicians should reinforce regular sunscreen use and reapplication every few hours or more, depending on exercise level and exposure to water. Sunscreens with protection against UVA as well as UVB help manage photosensitivity disorders. Health implications of systemic absorption of chemical sunscreens are unknown.

Li E et al. Skin cancer, sunscreens, and prevention: discussions to have with patients. Gen Dent. 2023;71:57. [PMID: 37083615]

V Chałupczak N et al. Sunscreens: mechanisms and safety in depth. J Drugs Dermatol. 2025;24:142. [PMID: 39913224]

Complications of Topical Dermatologic Therapy

Complications of topical therapy include allergy, irritation, and other side effects. Reactions may result from the active or inactive ingredients, including fragrances and preservatives.

A. Allergy

Of the topical antibiotics, neomycin and bacitracin have the greatest potential for sensitization. Diphenhydramine, benzocaine, vitamin E, aromatic oils, preservatives, fragrances, tea tree oil, and even topical corticosteroids can cause allergic contact dermatitis.

B. Irritation

Preparations of tretinoin, benzoyl peroxide, and other acne medications should be applied sparingly to the skin.

C. Other Side Effects

Topical corticosteroids may induce acne-like lesions on the face (steroid rosacea) and atrophic striae in body folds.

Cruz S et al. Targeting inflammation in acne: current treatments and future prospects. Am J Clin Dermatol. 2023;24:681. [PMID: 37328614]

Lee J et al. Update on occupational dermatitis: reviewing toxic substances from OSHA standards. Int J Dermatol. 2025;64:72. [PMID: 39108222]

Ramani L et al. Allergens in common brands of clobetasol. J Drugs Dermatol. 2023;22:491. [PMID: 37133477]

NEOPLASTIC LESIONS

PIGMENTED NEOPLASMS

BENIGN PIGMENTED LESIONS

1. Melanocytic Nevi (Normal Moles)

In general, a benign mole (nevus) is a small (< 6 mm) macule or papule with a well-defined border and homogeneous beige or pink to dark brown pigment. They represent benign melanocytic growths.

Moles have a typical natural history. Early in life, moles often appear as flat, small, brown lesions and are termed "junctional nevi" because the nevus cells are at the junction of the epidermis and dermis. Over time, these moles enlarge and often become raised, reflecting the appearance of a dermal component, giving rise to "compound nevi" (Figure 6–1). Moles may darken and grow during pregnancy. As White patients enter their eighth decade, most moles have lost their junctional component and dark pigmentation because of normal senescence. At every stage of life, normal moles should be well demarcated, symmetric, and uniform in contour and color. Regular mole screening is not an evidence-based recommendation for all adults, although rates of screening continue to rise.

Henrikson NB et al. Skin cancer screening: updated evidence report and systematic review for the US Preventive Services Task Force. JAMA. 2023;329:1296. [PMID: 3707090]

Yeh I. Melanocytic naevi, melanocytomas and emerging concepts. Pathology. 2023;55:178. [PMID: 36642570]

Zhang Yet al. Nevi and melanoma. Hematol Oncol Clin North Am. 2024;38:939. [PMID: 38880666]

2. Atypical Nevi

The term "atypical nevus" is synonymous with the older term "dysplastic nevus." Dermoscopy by a trained clinician may be a useful tool in the evaluation of atypical nevi.

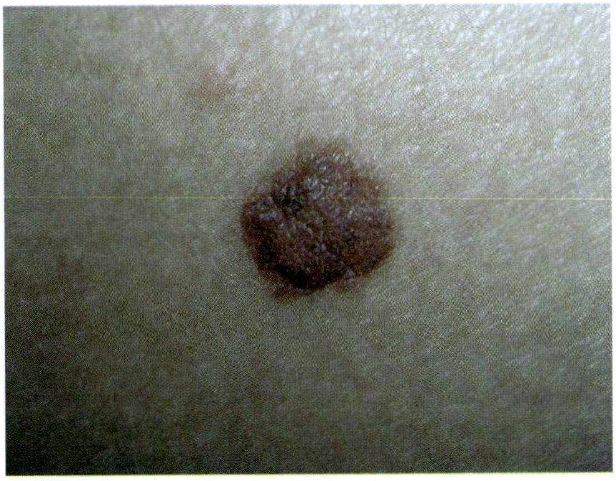

▲ **Figure 6–1.** Benign, compound nevus on the back. (Reproduced, with permission, from Richard P. Usatine, MD, in Usatine RP, Smith MA, Mayeaux EJ Jr, Chumley H. *The Color Atlas of Family Medicine*, 2nd ed. McGraw-Hill, 2013.)

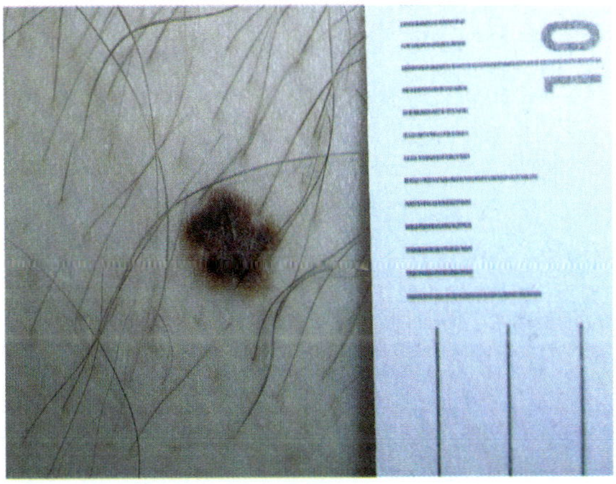

▲ **Figure 6–2.** Atypical (dysplastic) nevus on the chest. Note irregular border and variegation in color. (Reproduced, with permission, from Richard P. Usatine, MD, in Usatine RP, Smith MA, Mayeaux EJ Jr, Chumley H. *The Color Atlas of Family Medicine*, 2nd ed. McGraw-Hill, 2013.)

Clinically, these moles are large (6 mm or more in diameter), with an ill-defined, irregular border and irregularly distributed pigmentation (Figure 6–2). An estimated 5–10% of the White population in the United States has one or more atypical nevi, for which recreational sun exposure is the primary risk. There is an increased risk of melanoma in patients with 50 or more nevi, with one or more atypical moles, and one mole 8 mm or larger, and patients with any number of definitely atypical moles. These patients should be educated in how to recognize changes in moles and be monitored every 6–12 months by a clinician. Kindreds with familial melanoma (numerous atypical nevi and a family history of two first-degree relatives with melanoma) require closer attention since their risk of developing single or multiple melanomas approaches 50% by age 50. Moles should be removed only if they are suspected of being melanomas.

Drozdowski R et al. Dysplastic nevus part I: historical perspective, classification, and epidemiology. J Am Acad Dermatol. 2023;88:1. [PMID: 36038073]

Kashani-Sabet M et al. Early detection and prognostic assessment of cutaneous melanoma: consensus on optimal practice and the role of gene expression profile testing. JAMA Dermatol. 2023;159:545. [PMID: 36920356]

Lee J et al. Skin cancer screening recommendations by US cancer centers: inconsistency with national guidelines. J Med Screen. 2024;31:263. [PMID: 38863273]

3. Blue Nevi

Blue nevi are small, slightly elevated, blue-black lesions (Figure 6–3). They are common in persons of Asian descent and may be single or multiple. If the lesion has remained unchanged for years, it may be considered benign, since malignant blue nevi are rare. Blue-black papules and nodules that are new or growing must be evaluated to rule out nodular melanoma.

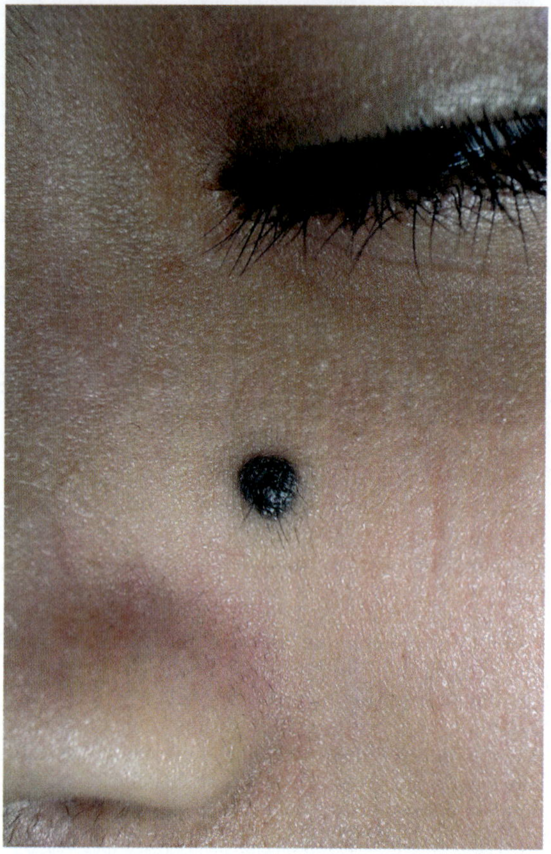

▲ **Figure 6–3.** Blue nevus on the left cheek, a darkly pigmented blue-black macule with some resemblance to a melanoma due to its dark pigmentation. (Reproduced, with permission, from Richard P. Usatine, MD, in Usatine RP, Smith MA, Mayeaux EJ Jr, Chumley H, Tysinger J. *The Color Atlas of Family Medicine*. McGraw-Hill, 2009.)

4. Freckles & Lentigines

Freckles (ephelides) and lentigines are flat brown macules, typically between 3 mm and 5 mm in diameter. Freckles first appear in young children, darken with UV exposure, and fade with cessation of sun exposure. They are determined by genetic factors. In adults, lentigines gradually appear in sun-exposed areas, particularly the face, dorsal hands, upper back, and upper chest, starting in the fourth to fifth decade of life, and are associated with photoaging as well as estrogen and progesterone use. They should be evaluated like all pigmented lesions: if the pigmentation is homogeneous and they are symmetric and flat, they are most likely benign. They can be treated with topical retinoids such as 0.1% tretinoin or 0.1% adapalene, hydroquinone, laser/light therapy, or cryotherapy.

5. Seborrheic Keratoses

Seborrheic keratoses are benign papules and plaques, beige to brown or even black, 3–20 mm in diameter, with a velvety or warty surface. They appear to be stuck or pasted onto the skin (Figure 6–4). They are extremely common—especially in older adults—and may be mistaken for melanomas or other types of cutaneous neoplasms. No treatment is needed. They may be frozen with liquid nitrogen or curetted if itchy or inflamed but usually recur after treatment.

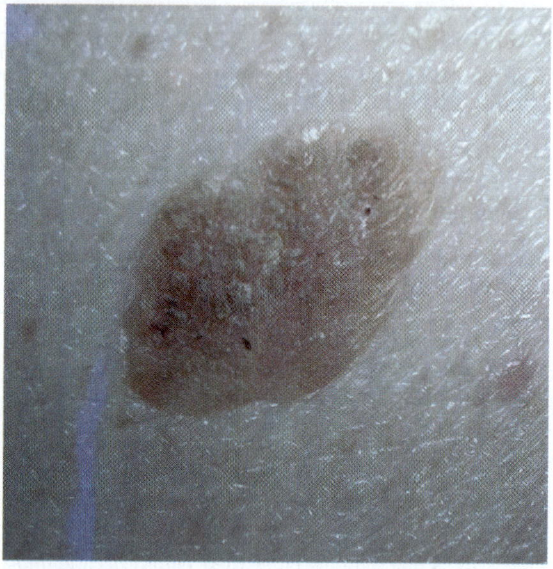

▲ **Figure 6–4.** Seborrheic keratosis with light pigmentation, with waxy, dry, "stuck-on" appearance. (Reproduced, with permission, from Richard P. Usatine, MD, in Usatine RP, Smith MA, Mayeaux EJ Jr, Chumley H. *The Color Atlas of Family Medicine*, 2nd ed. McGraw-Hill, 2013.)

Barthelmann S et al. Seborrheic keratosis. J Dtsch Dermatol Ges. 2023;21:265. [PMID: 36892019]
Natarelli N et al. Efficacy and safety of topical treatments for seborrheic keratoses: a systematic review. J Dermatolog Treat. 2023;34:2133532. [PMID: 36215682]
Wilson JL. Benign skin tumors. Prim Care. 2025;52:513. [PMID: 40835288]

MALIGNANT PIGMENTED LESIONS

1. Malignant Melanoma

ESSENTIALS OF DIAGNOSIS

- May be flat or raised with irregular borders.
- Examination may show varying colors, including brown, red, white, black, and blue.
- Should be suspected in any pigmented skin lesion with recent change in appearance.
- Less than 30% develop from existing moles.

General Considerations

Malignant melanoma, the fourth most common of all cancers in the United States, is the leading cause of death due to skin disease and has doubled in incidence over the past 30 years. In 2023, approximately 97,610 new invasive melanomas were diagnosed in the United States, leading to an estimated 7990 deaths (two-thirds in men). The lifetime risk of melanoma is 2% in White individuals and 0.1–0.5% in persons with skin of color. One in four cases occurs before age 40. Although the overall number of melanomas diagnosed each year continues to rise, there has simultaneously been a decrease in mortality (likely due to both earlier detection and availability of immunotherapy).

Melanoma thickness is the single most important prognostic factor. Ten-year survival rates historically were 95% if the thickness was < 1 mm; 80% for 1–2 mm; and 55% for 2–4 mm. Mortality rates have improved dramatically since the advent of immunotherapy. The 5-year survival rate for patients with lymph node involvement has increased from 62% to 75% and for patients with distant metastases from 16% to 35%.

Clinical Findings

Primary malignant melanomas may be classified into various clinicohistopathologic types, including superficial spreading melanoma (two-thirds of all melanomas arising on intermittently sun-exposed skin); lentigo melanoma (arising on chronically sun-exposed skin of older individuals); nodular melanoma; acral-lentiginous melanomas (arising on palms, soles, and nail beds); ocular melanoma; and melanomas on mucous membranes. Different types of melanomas appear to have distinct oncogenic mutations, which may be important in the treatment of patients with advanced disease. Clinical features of pigmented lesions suspicious for melanoma are an irregular, notched border where the pigment appears to be spreading into the normal surrounding skin and irregular surface topography (ie, partly raised and partly flat) (Figure 6–5). Color variation is present and is an important indication for referral. A helpful mnemonic is the ABCDE rule: Asymmetry, Border irregularity, Color variegation, Diameter > 6 mm, and Evolution. Less than 30% of melanomas develop from existing moles. **The history of a changing mole (evolution, including bleeding and ulceration) is the single most important historical reason for close evaluation and possible referral.** A mole that appears distinct from the patient's other moles deserves special scrutiny—the "ugly duckling sign."

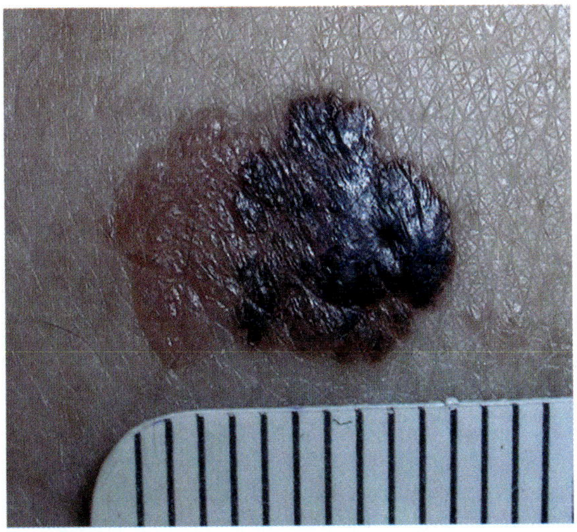

Figure 6–5. Malignant melanoma. Note the classic "ABCDE" features: asymmetry, irregular border, multiple colors, diameter > 6 mm, and evolution or change. (Reproduced, with permission, from Richard P. Usatine, MD, in Usatine RP, Smith MA, Mayeaux EJ Jr, Chumley H. *The Color Atlas of Family Medicine*, 2nd ed. McGraw-Hill, 2013.)

While superficial spreading melanoma is primarily a disease of White individuals, persons with darker skin pigmentation are at risk for this and other types of melanomas, particularly acral lentiginous melanomas, for which UV exposure may not be a significant association. These occur as dark, irregularly shaped lesions on the palms and soles and as new, often broad and solitary, darkly pigmented, longitudinal streaks in the nails, typically with involvement of the proximal nail fold. Acral lentiginous melanoma may be a difficult or delayed diagnosis because benign pigmented lesions of the hands, feet, and nails occur commonly in more darkly pigmented persons, and clinicians may hesitate to biopsy these sites. Clinicians should give special attention to new or changing lesions in these areas.

Treatment

Treatment starts with biopsy or excision of the melanoma to confirm the diagnosis and the tumor depth. After histologic diagnosis, re-excision is recommended with margins dictated by the thickness of the tumor. Recommended surgical margins are 0.5–1 cm for melanoma in situ, 1 cm for lesions < 1 mm in thickness, and 1–2 cm for lesions > 1 mm in thickness.

Sentinel lymph node biopsy using preoperative lymphoscintigraphy and intraoperative lymphatic mapping is effective for staging melanoma patients with intermediate risk (depth > 8–10 mm but without clinical adenopathy or metastasis or high-risk histologic features such as ulceration). This procedure may not confer a survival advantage.

Patients with melanomas with > 1 mm depth or spread to lymph nodes or other sites require multidisciplinary care from a dermatologist, surgical oncologist, and oncologist. First-line systemic therapy for patients with metastatic disease is with immunotherapy, most frequently with combined anti-PD-1 and anti-CTLA-4 therapies (pembrolizumab and ipilimumab most commonly). In some cases, identifying the oncogenic mutations in advanced melanomas may dictate targeted therapy. When specific BRAF mutation are present, combined therapy with a BRAF inhibitor and Mek inhibitor offer an additional option.

Lazaroff J et al. Targeted therapy and immunotherapy in melanoma. Dermatol Clin. 2023;41:65. [PMID: 36410984]

Long GV et al. Cutaneous melanoma. Lancet. 2023;402:450. [PMID: 37499671]

Rashid S et al. Melanoma classification and management in the era of molecular medicine. Dermatol Clin. 2023;4:49. [PMID: 36410983]

NONPIGMENTED NEOPLASMS

BENIGN LESIONS

1. Epidermal Inclusion Cyst

ESSENTIALS OF DIAGNOSIS

- Firm dermal papule or nodule.
- Overlying black comedone or "punctum."
- Expressible foul-smelling cheesy material.
- May become red and drain, mimicking an abscess.

General Considerations

Epidermal inclusion cysts (EICs) are common, benign growths of the upper portion of the hair follicle.

EICs favor the face and trunk and may complicate nodulocystic acne vulgaris. Individual lesions range in size from 0.3 cm to several centimeters. An overlying pore or punctum is characteristic. Dermoscopy can aid in observing a tiny punctum when not visible to the naked eye. Lateral pressure may lead to extrusion of a foul-smelling, cheesy material.

Differential Diagnosis

EICs are distinguished from lipomas by being more superficial (in the dermis, not the subcutaneous fat) and by their overlying punctum.

Complications

EICs may rupture, creating an acute inflammatory nodule very similar to an abscess. Cultures of the expressed material will be sterile.

Treatment

Treatment is not required if asymptomatic. Small (1–3 cm) lesions can be treated with a punch incision and removal of cystic contents. Inflamed lesions may be treated with incision and drainage or intralesional triamcinolone acetonide 5–10 mg/mL. For large or symptomatic cysts, surgical excision is usually curative.

Alexa AI et al. Therapeutic challenges in epidermal inclusion cysts with periocular localization: case reports. J Med Life. 2023;16:1575. [PMID: 38313165]

MALIGNANT & PREMALIGNANT LESIONS

1. Actinic Keratoses

Actinic keratoses are small (0.2–0.6 cm) papules—flesh-colored, pink, or slightly hyperpigmented—that feel like sandpaper and can be tender to palpation. They occur on sun-exposed parts of the body, mostly in persons of fair complexion. Actinic keratoses are considered premalignant; 1:1000 lesions per year progress to squamous cell carcinoma.

Application of liquid nitrogen provides rapid eradication of lesions, which crust and disappear after 10–14 days. "Field treatment" with a topical agent can be considered in patients with multiple lesions in one region (eg, forehead, dorsal hands, etc). Fluorouracil cream is the most effective topical agent used for field treatment; imiquimod and photodynamic therapy are also effective. Any lesions that persist or recur should be evaluated for possible biopsy.

Arcuri D et al. Pharmacological agents used in the prevention and treatment of actinic keratosis: a review. Int J Mol Sci. 2023;24:4989. [PMID: 36902419]
Lapidus AH et al. Topical calcipotriol plus 5-fluorouracil in the treatment of actinic keratosis, Bowen's disease, and squamous cell carcinoma: a systematic review. J Cutan Med Surg. 2024;28:375. [PMID: 38783539]
Worley B et al. Treatment of actinic keratosis: a systematic review. Arch Dermatol Res. 2023;31:1099. [PMID: 36454335]

2. Squamous Cell Carcinoma

ESSENTIALS OF DIAGNOSIS

- Nonhealing ulcer or warty nodule.
- Skin damage due to long-term sun exposure.
- Common in fair-skinned individuals and in organ transplant recipients.

Squamous cell carcinoma usually occurs after prolonged sun exposure on exposed parts in fair-skinned individuals who sunburn easily. It may arise from an actinic keratosis. The lesions appear as small red, conical, hard nodules that occasionally ulcerate (Figure 6–6). In actinically-induced squamous cell cancers, rates of metastasis are estimated to be 3–7%. Squamous cell carcinomas of the mucosal surfaces, ear, scalp, temple, and genitalia have much higher rates of recurrence or metastasis and require special management. Patients with multiple squamous cell carcinomas (especially > 10) have higher rates of local recurrence and nodal metastases. Nicotinamide, 500 mg orally twice daily, can decrease the rate of development of squamous cell carcinomas by 30% in high-risk groups.

Squamous cell carcinoma in situ can be treated with imiquimod or 5-fluorouracil (in similar dosing as for superficial basal cell carcinoma) or curettage and electrodessication. The preferred treatment for invasive squamous cell carcinoma is excision or Mohs micrographic surgery. Mohs micrographic surgery is recommended for higher-risk sites (lips, temples, ears, nose, genitalia), recurrent tumors, aggressive histologic subtypes (perineural or perivascular invasion), large lesions (> 1.0 cm on face, > 2.0 cm on trunk or extremities), immunosuppressed patients, lesions developing within a scar, and tumors arising in the setting of genetic diseases. Follow-up for squamous cell carcinoma should be performed at least yearly and include careful examination of lymph nodes. For patients with metastatic disease, advanced therapeutic options now exist including PD-1 blockade and use of cetuximab.

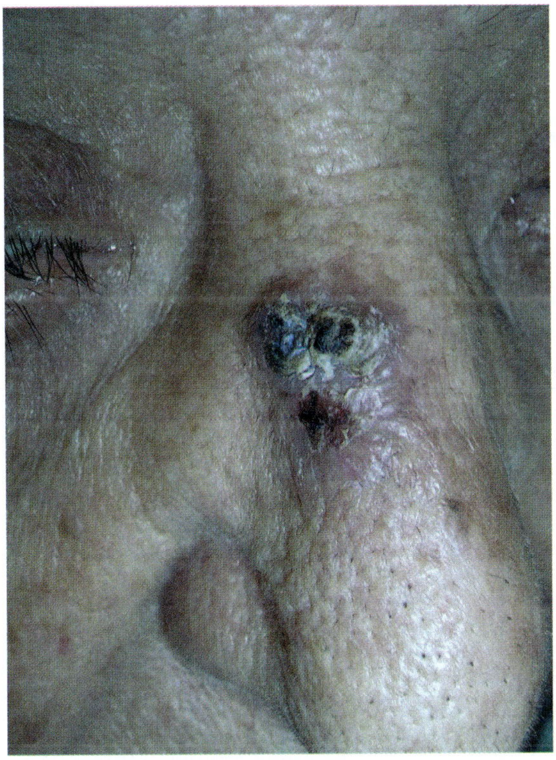

Figure 6–6. Squamous cell carcinoma: an irregular-shaped pink plaque with overlying hemorrhagic crust in a chronically sun-exposed area. (Reproduced, with permission, from Richard P. Usatine, MD, in Usatine RP, Smith MA, Mayeaux EJ Jr, Chumley H. *The Color Atlas of Family Medicine*, 2nd ed. McGraw-Hill, 2013.)

Multiple squamous cell carcinomas are common on the sun-exposed skin of organ transplant patients and typically begin to appear after 5 years of immunosuppression. Regular dermatologic evaluation in at-risk organ transplant recipients is recommended. Skin cancers in organ transplant recipients may be aggressive, and careful management is required. Other forms of immunosuppression, such as chronic lymphocytic leukemia, HIV/AIDS, and chronic iatrogenic immunosuppression, may also increase skin cancer risk and be associated with more aggressive skin cancer behavior.

Gross ND et al. Neoadjuvant cemiplimab and surgery for stage II-IV cutaneous squamous-cell carcinoma: follow-up and survival outcomes of a single-arm, multicentre, phase 2 study. Lancet Oncol. 2023;24:1196. [PMID: 37875144]
Wysong A. Squamous-cell carcinoma of the skin. N Engl J Med. 2023;388:2262. [PMID: 37314707]

3. Bowen Disease & Paget Disease

Bowen disease (intraepidermal squamous cell carcinoma) can develop on sun-exposed and non–sun-exposed skin. The lesion is usually a small (0.5–3 cm), well-demarcated, slightly raised, pink to red, scaly plaque and may resemble psoriasis or a large actinic keratosis. Lesions may progress to invasive squamous cell carcinoma. Excision or other definitive treatment, such as topical treatment (fluorouracil or imiquimod) or photodynamic therapy, is indicated.

Extramammary Paget disease, a manifestation of intraepidermal carcinoma or underlying genitourinary or GI cancer, resembles chronic eczema and usually involves apocrine areas such as the genitalia. Mammary Paget disease of the nipple is a unilateral, or rarely bilateral, red scaling plaque that may ooze and is associated with an underlying intraductal mammary carcinoma (see Figure 19–3). While these lesions appear as red patches and plaques in fair-skinned persons, hyperpigmentation may be prominent in darker-skinned individuals.

Ahmady S et al. Patient preferences for the treatment of Bowen disease. Br J Dermatol. 2025;192:653. [PMID: 39657744]
Pérez JC et al. Extramammary Paget disease: a therapeutic challenge, for a rare entity. Curr Oncol Rep. 2023;25:1081. [PMID: 37421583]
Shah RR et al. Extramammary Paget disease. Part II. Evidence-based approach to management. J Am Acad Dermatol. 2024;91:421. [PMID: 38588817]

4. Basal Cell Carcinoma

ESSENTIALS OF DIAGNOSIS

- Pearly papule, erythematous patch > 6 mm, or nonhealing ulcer.
- Usually in sun-exposed areas (face, trunk, lower legs).
- Common in fair-skinned persons with a history of sun exposure (often intense, intermittent).

General Considerations

Basal cell carcinomas are the most common form of cancer. They occur on sun-exposed skin in otherwise normal, fair-skinned individuals; UV light is the cause. Basal cell carcinomas can be divided into clinical and histologic subtypes, which determine both clinical behavior and treatment. The clinical subtypes include superficial, nodular, pigmented, and morpheaform. The histologic subtypes include superficial, nodular, micronodular, and infiltrative. Because a second basal cell carcinoma develops in up to half of patients, skin examination is required at least yearly to detect new or recurrent lesions. Nicotinamide, 500 mg orally twice daily, can decrease the rate of development of basal cell carcinomas by 20% in high-risk groups.

Clinical Findings

The most common presentation is a papule or nodule with a central erosion. Occasionally the nodules have stippled pigment (pigmented basal cell carcinoma). Basal cell carcinomas grow slowly, attaining a size of 1–2 cm or more in diameter, usually only after years of growth. There is a "pearly" appearance, with telangiectatic vessels easily visible (Figure 6–7). It is the pearly or translucent quality of these lesions that is most diagnostic, a feature best

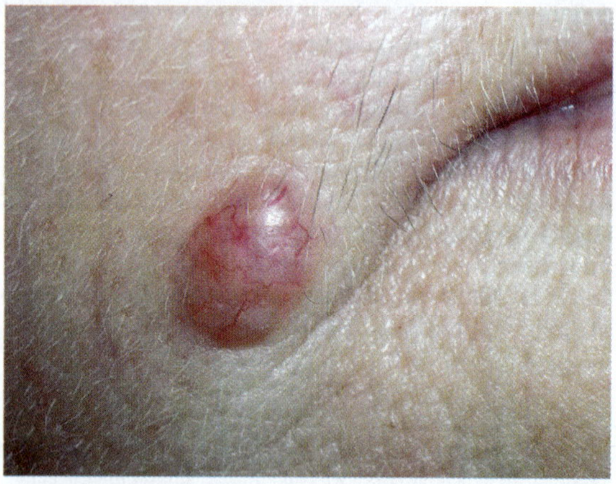

▲ **Figure 6–7.** Pearly nodular basal cell carcinoma on the face of a 52-year-old woman present for 5 years. (Reproduced, with permission, from Richard P. Usatine, MD, in Usatine RP, Smith MA, Mayeaux EJ Jr, Chumley H. *The Color Atlas of Family Medicine*, 2nd ed. McGraw-Hill, 2013.)

appreciated if the skin is stretched. On the back and chest, basal cell carcinomas appear as reddish, somewhat shiny, scaly thin papules or plaques. Morpheaform basal cell carcinomas are scar-like in appearance. Basal cell carcinomas are more common and more likely to recur in immunosuppressed patients, including those with non-Hodgkin lymphoma and those who have undergone solid organ or allogeneic hematopoietic stem cell transplantation.

▶ Treatment

Lesions suspected to be basal cell carcinomas should be biopsied by shave or punch biopsy. Therapy is then aimed at eradication with minimal cosmetic deformity. The histopathologic classification of basal cell carcinomas determines therapy. Imiquimod (applied topically 5 nights per week for 6–10 weeks, depending on patient reaction) and 5-fluorouracil (applied topically twice daily for up to 12 weeks) may be appropriate for select patients with superficial basal cell carcinomas, but the treated area must be observed for evidence of complete cure. Superficial or nodular type lesions can be treated with curettage and electrodesiccation, excision, or Mohs micrographic surgery. In patients with nodular lesions, combination treatment with superficial curettage followed by imiquimod yielded a 22% 5-year recurrence rate compared with 2% following surgical excision. Photodynamic therapy and topical application of a photosensitizing agent, followed by irradiation by a light source (typically blue or red), may be appropriate for some superficial and small nodular basal cell carcinomas.

Basal cell carcinomas classified as morpheaform, micronodular, or infiltrative should be treated with excision or Mohs micrographic surgery, depending on the size and location of the lesion. Mohs micrographic surgery—removal of the tumor followed by immediate frozen section histopathologic examination of margins with subsequent re-excision of tumor-positive areas and final closure of the defect—gives the highest cure rates (98%) and results in less tissue loss than a classic excision. It is an appropriate therapy for tumors of the eyelids, nasolabial folds, canthi, external ear, and temple; for recurrent lesions, where tissue sparing is needed for cosmesis; and for those with morpheaform, infiltrative, or micronodular histopathology in certain locations.

Radiotherapy is effective and sometimes appropriate for older individuals (over age 65), but recurrent tumors after radiation therapy are more difficult to treat and may be more aggressive. Radiation therapy is the most expensive method to treat basal cell carcinoma and should be used only if other treatment options are not appropriate.

Hedgehog pathway inhibitors (vismodegib, sonidegib) are reserved for the treatment of advanced or metastatic basal cell carcinoma or in patients with extensive tumor burden (eg, basal cell nevus syndrome).

Heath MS et al. Basal cell carcinoma. Dermatol Clin. 2023;41:13. [PMID: 36410973]
Kunstfeld R et al. New therapeutic developments for basal cell carcinoma. J Dtsch Dermatol Ges. 2023;21:382. [PMID: 37070499]
Peris K et al. European consensus-based interdisciplinary guideline for diagnosis and treatment of basal cell carcinoma—update 2023. Eur J Cancer. 2023;192:113254. [PMID: 37604067]
Verkouteren BJA et al. Imiquimod cream preceded by superficial curettage vs surgical excision for nodular basal cell carcinoma: a secondary analysis of a randomized clinical trial. JAMA Dermatol. 2025;161:299. [PMID: 39878970]

5. Kaposi Sarcoma

General Considerations

Human herpes virus 8 (HHV-8), or Kaposi sarcoma–associated herpes virus, is the cause of all forms of Kaposi sarcoma.

Red or purple plaques or nodules on cutaneous or mucosal surfaces are characteristic. Marked edema may occur with few or no skin lesions. Kaposi sarcoma commonly involves the GI tract. In asymptomatic patients, these lesions are not sought or treated. Pulmonary Kaposi sarcoma can present with shortness of breath, cough, hemoptysis, or chest pain; it may be asymptomatic, appearing only on CXR. Bronchoscopy may be indicated.

▶ Treatment

For Kaposi sarcoma in older adults, palliative local therapy with intralesional chemotherapy (vincristine, vinblastine, or bleomycin) or radiation is usually all that is required. In the setting of iatrogenic immunosuppression, the treatment of Kaposi sarcoma is primarily reduction of doses of immunosuppressive medications. In AIDS-associated Kaposi sarcoma, the patient should first be given ART. Other therapeutic options in these patients include cryotherapy or intralesional vinblastine (0.1–0.5 mg/mL); radiation therapy for accessible and space-occupying lesions; and laser surgery for certain intraoral and pharyngeal lesions. Systemic therapy is indicated in patients with skin disease that is cosmetically unacceptable or those with advanced cutaneous, oral, visceral, or nodal disease. ART plus chemotherapy appears to be more effective than ART alone (see Tables 43–5 and 43–6). First-line systemic therapies include liposomal doxorubicin and paclitaxel.

Aydin O et al. Comparison of clinical and prognostic characteristics of patients with classic and AIDS-related Kaposi sarcoma: a single-center experience. Medicine (Baltimore). 2025;104:e43576. [PMID: 40760592]
Bettuzzi T et al. Modern approach to manage patients with Kaposi sarcoma. J Med Virol. 2025;97:e70294. [PMID: 40119751]
Patel R et al. Clinical management of Kaposi sarcoma herpesvirus-associated diseases: an update on disease manifestations and treatment strategies. Expert Rev Anti Infect Ther. 2023;219:929. [PMID: 37578202]

6. Cutaneous T-Cell Lymphoma (Mycosis Fungoides)

ESSENTIALS OF DIAGNOSIS

- Localized or generalized erythematous patches that progress to scaly plaques and nodules.
- Sometimes associated with pruritus, lymphadenopathy.
- Distinctive histology.

General Considerations

Mycosis fungoides is a cutaneous T-cell lymphoma that begins on the skin and may remain there for years or decades. It may progress to systemic disease, including Sézary syndrome (erythroderma with circulating malignant T cells).

Clinical Findings

A. Symptoms and Signs

Localized or generalized erythematous patches or scaly plaques are usually present on the trunk. Plaques are frequently over 5 cm in diameter. Pruritus is common and can be severe. The lesions often begin as nondescript patches and may be present for more than a decade before the diagnosis is confirmed. Follicular involvement with hair loss is characteristic, and its presence should raise the suspicion of mycosis fungoides for any pruritic eruption. Tumors can appear early or late in the disease and are associated with a poorer prognosis, as is erythroderma and systemic disease. Local or diffuse lymphadenopathy may be due to benign expansion (dermatopathic lymphadenopathy) or involvement with mycosis fungoides.

B. Laboratory Findings

Diagnosis is based on a skin biopsy. Numerous biopsies may be required. In more advanced disease, circulating malignant T cells (Sézary cells) can be detected in the blood. Eosinophilia may be present.

Differential Diagnosis

Mycosis fungoides may be confused with psoriasis, drug eruption, photoallergy, eczematous dermatitis, syphilis, or tinea corporis but is distinguished by histologic examination.

Treatment

The treatment of mycosis fungoides is complex. Early and aggressive treatment has not been proven to cure or prevent disease progression. Skin-directed therapies, including topical corticosteroids, topical mechlorethamine, bexarotene gel, and UV phototherapy, are used initially. If the disease progresses, various treatments are employed, including psoralen and UVA (PUVA) plus retinoids, PUVA plus interferon, methotrexate, extracorporeal photopheresis, bexarotene, histone deacetylase inhibitors (romidepsin or vorinostat), targeted immunomodulators (brentuximab, mogamulizumab), and total skin electron beam treatment.

Prognosis

Mycosis fungoides is usually slowly progressive (over decades). Prognosis is much better with patch or plaque stage disease and worse with erythroderma, tumors, and lymphadenopathy. Overly aggressive treatment may lead to complications and premature demise.

Latzka et al. Mycosis fungoides and Sezary syndrome—review and outlook. J Dtsch Dermatol Ges. 2023;21:386. [PMID: 36971307]
Lee H. Mycosis fungoides and Sézary syndrome. Blood Res. 2023;58:66. [PMID: 37105561]
Miyashiro D et al. Mycosis fungoides and Sézary syndrome: clinical presentation, diagnosis, staging, and therapeutic management. Front Oncol. 2023;13:1141108. [PMID: 37124514]

CUTANEOUS INFECTIONS, INFESTATIONS, & BITES

FUNGAL INFECTIONS

The diagnosis of fungal infections of the skin is based on the location and characteristics of the lesions and on the following laboratory examinations: (1) Direct demonstration of fungi in 10% potassium hydroxide (KOH) evaluation of suspected lesions. **"If it's scaly, scrape it" is a time-honored maxim** (Figure 6–8). (2) Cultures of organisms from skin scrapings. (3) Histologic sections of biopsies stained with the periodic acid-Schiff technique may be diagnostic if scrapings and cultures are falsely negative.

Principles of Treatment

In general, fungal skin infections are treated topically (see Table 6–2). Oral agents (itraconazole, fluconazole, and terbinafine) may be useful for infections with extensive skin involvement or involvement of the nails or hair follicles, with special attention to their side effects and complications, including hepatic toxicity.

General Measures & Prevention

Since moist skin favors the growth of fungi, dry the skin carefully after perspiring heavily or after bathing. The use of a hair dryer on a low setting may be helpful. Antifungal or drying powders may be useful with the exception of powders containing corn starch (which may exacerbate

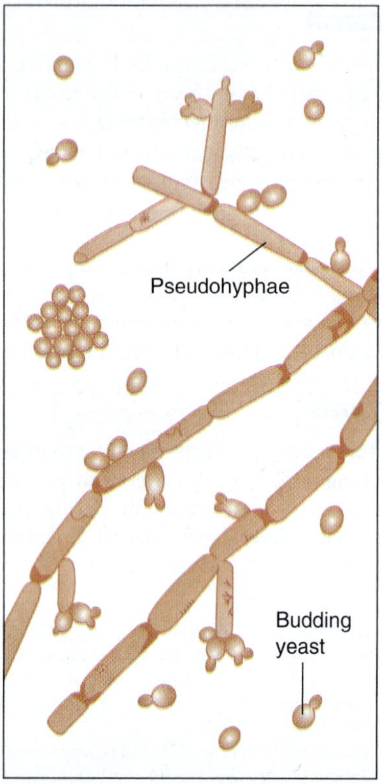

▲ **Figure 6–8.** KOH preparation of fungus demonstrating pseudohyphae and budding yeast forms. (Reproduced, with permission, from Nicoll D et al. *Guide to Diagnostic Tests*, 7th ed. McGraw-Hill, 2017.)

fungal infections) and talc powder (which has been shown to be a risk factor for ovarian carcinoma in women). The use of topical corticosteroids for other diseases may be complicated by intercurrent tinea or candidal infection, and topical antifungals are often used in intertriginous areas with corticosteroids to prevent this.

TINEA CORPORIS OR TINEA CIRCINATA

ESSENTIALS OF DIAGNOSIS

- Ring-shaped lesions with an advancing scaly border and central clearing, or scaly patches with a distinct border.
- Microscopic examination of scrapings or culture confirms the diagnosis.

General Considerations

The lesions are often on exposed areas of the body, such as the face and arms. A history of exposure to an infected pet (who may have a scaly rash or patches of alopecia) may occasionally be obtained, usually indicating *Microsporum* infection. *Trichophyton rubrum* is the most common pathogen, usually representing extension onto the trunk or extremities of tinea cruris, pedis, or manuum.

Clinical Findings

A. Symptoms and Signs

Itching may be present. In classic lesions, rings of erythema have an advancing scaly border and central clearing.

B. Laboratory Findings

The diagnosis should be confirmed by KOH preparation or culture.

Differential Diagnosis

Positive fungal studies distinguish tinea corporis from other skin lesions with annular configuration, such as annular lesions of psoriasis, lupus erythematosus, syphilis, granuloma annulare, or pityriasis rosea. Psoriasis typically involves the elbows, knees, scalp, and nails. Secondary syphilis is often manifested by characteristic palmar, plantar, and mucous membrane lesions. Tinea corporis rarely has the large number of symmetric lesions seen in pityriasis rosea. Granuloma annulare lacks scale.

Complications

Complications include extension of the disease down the hair follicles (which presents as papules and pustules and requires systemic antifungals to cure) and pyoderma.

Prevention

Treat infected household pets (*Microsporum* infections). To prevent recurrences, using foot powder and keeping feet dry by wearing sandals or changing socks can be helpful.

Treatment

A. Local Measures

Tinea corporis responds to most topical antifungals, including terbinafine, butenafine, econazole, miconazole, ciclopirox, and clotrimazole, many of which are available over the counter in the United States (see Table 6–2). Terbinafine and butenafine require shorter courses and lead to the most rapid response. **Treatment should be continued for 1–2 weeks after clinical clearing.** Betamethasone dipropionate with clotrimazole (Lotrisone) is not recommended. Long-term improper use may result in side effects from the high-potency corticosteroid component, especially in body folds.

B. Systemic Measures

Itraconazole as a single weeklong pulse of 200 mg orally daily is effective in tinea corporis. Terbinafine, 250 mg orally daily for 1 month, is an alternative.

Prognosis

Tinea corporis usually responds promptly to topical therapy or to an oral agent within 4 weeks. Exceptions include a variant of *Trichophyton indotineae* reported in travelers to southeast Asia, and *Trichophyton mentagrophytes* genotype VII, which is spread through sexual contact, mostly in men who have sex with men. These are more resistant to standard therapy.

Chanyachailert P et al. Cutaneous fungal infections caused by dermatophytes and non-dermatophytes: an updated comprehensive review of epidemiology, clinical presentations, and diagnostic testing. J Fungi (Basel). 2023;9:669. [PMID: 37367605]

Jabet A et al. *Trichophyton mentagrophytes* ITS genotype VII infections among men who have sex with men in France: an ongoing phenomenon. J Eur Acad Dermatol Venereol. 2025;39:407. [PMID: 39587983]

Khurana A et al. Therapeutic updates on the management of tinea corporis or cruris in the era of *Trichophyton indotineae*: separating evidence from hype—a narrative review. Indian J Dermatol. 2023;68:525. [PMID: 38099117]

Saed GM. Is there a link between talcum powder, oxidative stress, and ovarian cancer risk? Expert Rev Anticancer Ther. 2024;24:485. [PMID: 38712572]

TINEA CRURIS (Jock Itch)

ESSENTIALS OF DIAGNOSIS

- Marked itching in intertriginous areas, usually sparing the scrotum.
- Peripherally spreading, sharply demarcated, centrally clearing erythematous lesions.
- May have associated tinea infection of feet or toenails.
- Laboratory examination with microscope or culture confirms diagnosis.

General Considerations

Tinea cruris lesions are confined to the groin and gluteal cleft. Intractable pruritus ani may occasionally be caused by a tinea infection.

Clinical Findings

A. Symptoms and Signs

Itching may be severe, or the rash may be asymptomatic. The lesions have sharp margins, cleared centers, and active, spreading scaly peripheries. Follicular pustules are sometimes encountered. The area may be hyperpigmented on resolution.

B. Laboratory Findings

Hyphae can be demonstrated microscopically in KOH preparations or skin biopsy. The organism may be cultured.

Differential Diagnosis

Tinea cruris must be distinguished from other lesions involving the intertriginous areas, such as candidiasis, seborrheic dermatitis, intertrigo, psoriasis of body folds ("inverse psoriasis"), and erythrasma (corynebacterial infection of the intertriginous regions). Candidiasis is generally bright red and marked by satellite papules and pustules outside of the main border of the lesion. *Candida* typically involves the scrotum. Seborrheic dermatitis also often involves the face, sternum, axillae, and genitalia (but not the crural folds). Intertrigo tends to be less red, less scaly, and present in individuals with obesity in moist body folds with less extension onto the thigh. "Inverse psoriasis" is characterized by distinct plaques. Other areas of typical psoriatic involvement should be checked, and the KOH examination will be negative. Erythrasma is best diagnosed with Wood (UV) light—a brilliant coral-red fluorescence is seen.

Treatment

A. General Measures

Drying powder (eg, miconazole nitrate [Zeasorb-AF]) can be dusted into the involved area in patients with excessive perspiration or occlusion of skin due to obesity as a preventive measure but is less helpful for treatment.

B. Local Measures

Any of the topical antifungal preparations listed in Table 6–2 may be used. Terbinafine cream is curative in over 80% of cases after once-daily use for 7 days.

C. Systemic Measures

One week of either itraconazole, 200 mg orally daily, or terbinafine, 250 mg orally daily, can be effective.

Prognosis

Tinea cruris usually responds promptly to topical or systemic treatment but often recurs.

Lal N et al. Efficacy and safety of 250 mg versus 500 mg oral terbinafine in the treatment of tinea corporis and cruris: a randomized, assessor-blinded comparative study. Indian J Dermatol Venereol Leprol. 2023;89:665. [PMID: 36688883]

Nenoff P et al. Dermatomycoses: topical and systemic antifungal treatment. Dermatologie (Heidelb). 2024;8:655. [PMID: 38874607]

TINEA MANUUM & TINEA PEDIS (Tinea of Palms & Soles)

ESSENTIALS OF DIAGNOSIS

- Most often presents with asymptomatic scaling.
- May progress to fissuring or maceration in toe web spaces.
- May be a portal of entry for bacteria causing lower extremity cellulitis.
- Itching, burning, and stinging of interdigital web; scaling palms and soles; vesicles on soles in inflammatory cases.
- KOH preparation or fungal culture of skin scapings is usually positive.

General Considerations

Tinea of the hands and feet (athlete's foot) is a common acute or chronic dermatosis. Most infections are caused by *Trichophyton* species.

Clinical Findings

A. Symptoms and Signs

The presenting symptom may be itching, burning, or stinging. Pain may indicate secondary infection with complicating cellulitis. Interdigital tinea pedis is the most common predisposing cause of lower extremity cellulitis in healthy individuals. Regular examination of the feet of patients with diabetes for evidence of scaling and fissuring and treatment of any identified tinea pedis may prevent complications. Tinea pedis has several presentations that vary with the location. On the sole and heel, tinea may appear as chronic noninflammatory scaling, occasionally with thickening and fissuring. This may extend over the sides of the feet in a "moccasin" distribution (Figure 6–9). The KOH preparation is usually positive. Tinea pedis often appears as a scaling or fissuring of the toe webs, often with maceration (Figure 6–10). As the web spaces become more macerated, the KOH preparation and fungal culture are less often positive because bacterial species begin to dominate. Finally, there may also be vesicles, bullae, or generalized exfoliation of the skin of the soles, or nail involvement in the form of discoloration, friability, and thickening of the nail plate.

B. Laboratory Findings

KOH and culture do not always demonstrate pathogenic fungi from macerated areas.

Differential Diagnosis

Other skin conditions involving the same areas are interdigital erythrasma (which will be positive with Wood light), psoriasis (which may cause scaling on the palms or soles and nail changes), and contact dermatitis (often involving the dorsal surfaces). Vesicular lesions should be differentiated from pompholyx (dyshidrosis) and scabies by proper scraping of the roofs of individual vesicles. Rarely, gram-negative organisms may cause toe web infections, manifesting as an acute erosive flare of interdigital disease. *Candida* may also cause erosive interdigital disease.

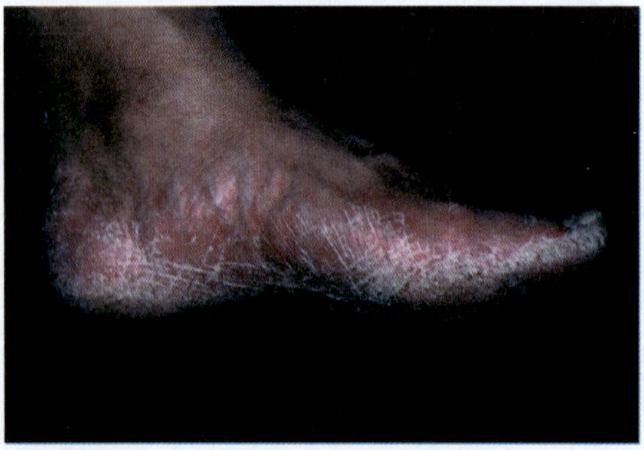

▲ **Figure 6–9.** Tinea pedis in the moccasin distribution. (Reproduced, with permission, from Richard P. Usatine, MD, in Usatine RP, Smith MA, Mayeaux EJ Jr, Chumley H. *The Color Atlas of Family Medicine*, 2nd ed. McGraw-Hill, 2013.)

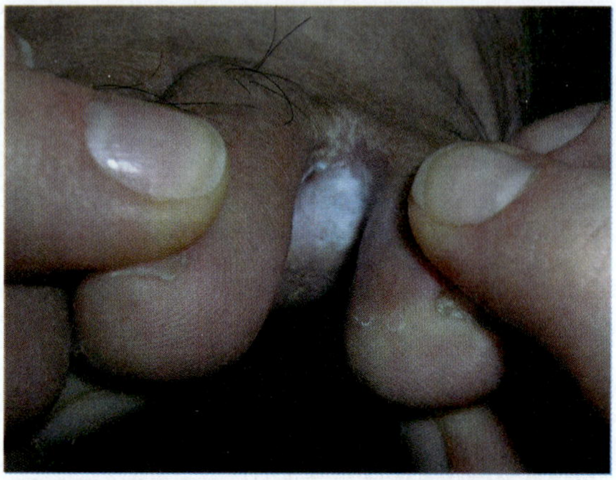

▲ **Figure 6–10.** Tinea pedis in the interdigital space between fourth and fifth digits. The differential diagnosis includes a bacterial primary or secondary infection with gram-negative organisms. (Reproduced, with permission, from Richard P. Usatine, MD, in Usatine RP, Smith MA, Mayeaux EJ Jr, Chumley HS. *The Color Atlas and Synopsis of Family Medicine*, 3rd ed. McGraw-Hill, 2019.)

Prevention

The essential factor in prevention is personal hygiene. Wear open-toed sandals if possible. Use of sandals in community showers and bathing places is often recommended, though the effectiveness of this practice has not been studied. Careful drying between the toes after showering is essential. A hair dryer used on cooler setting may be helpful. Socks should be changed frequently, and absorbent nonsynthetic socks are preferred. Apply dusting and drying powders as necessary. The use of powders containing antifungal agents (eg, Zeasorb-AF) or long-term use of antifungal creams may prevent recurrences of tinea pedis.

Treatment

A. Local Measures

1. Macerated stage—Treat with aluminum subacetate solution soaks for 20 minutes twice daily. Broad-spectrum antifungal creams and solutions (containing imidazoles or ciclopirox) (Table 6–2) will help combat diphtheroids and other gram-positive organisms present at this stage and alone may be adequate therapy. If topical imidazoles fail, 1 week of once-daily topical allylamine treatment (terbinafine or butenafine) will often result in clearing.

2. Dry and scaly stage—Use any of the antifungal agents listed in Table 6–2. The addition of urea 10–20% lotion or cream may increase the efficacy of topical treatments in thick ("moccasin") tinea of the soles.

B. Systemic Measures

Itraconazole, 200 mg orally daily for 2 weeks or 400 mg daily for 1 week, or terbinafine, 250 mg orally daily for 2–4 weeks, may be used in refractory cases. If the infection is cleared by systemic therapy, the patient should be encouraged to begin maintenance with topical therapy, since recurrence is common.

Prognosis

For many individuals, tinea pedis is a chronic affliction, temporarily cleared by therapy only to recur. Treatment of tinea pedis or manuum without systemic treatment of affected nails may result in recurrent skin disease.

Issa NT et al. Individual article: updated review of topical pharmaceuticals and complementary and alternative medications for the treatment of onychomycosis in both general and special populations in the United States. J Drugs Dermatol. 2023;22:SF378719 [PMID: 37683068]
Leung AK et al. Tinea pedis: an updated review. Drugs Context. 2023;12:2023-5-1. [PMID: 37415917]

TINEA VERSICOLOR (Pityriasis Versicolor)

ESSENTIALS OF DIAGNOSIS

- Velvety, tan, pink, or white macules, or white macules that do not tan with sun exposure.
- Fine scales that are not visible but are seen by scraping the lesion.
- Central upper trunk the most frequent site.
- Yeast and short hyphae observed on microscopic examination of scales.

General Considerations

Tinea versicolor is a mild, superficial *Malassezia* infection of the skin (usually of the upper trunk). This yeast is a colonizer of all humans, which accounts for the high recurrence rate after treatment. The eruption is often called to patients' attention by the fact that the involved areas will not tan, and the resulting hypopigmentation may be mistaken for vitiligo. A hyperpigmented form is not uncommon.

Clinical Findings

A. Symptoms and Signs

Lesions are asymptomatic, but a few patients note itching. The lesions are velvety, tan, pink, or white macules or thin papules that vary from 4 mm to 5 mm in diameter to large confluent areas. The lesions initially do not look scaly, but scales may be readily obtained by scraping the area. Lesions may appear on the trunk, upper arms, neck, and groin.

B. Laboratory Findings

Large, blunt hyphae and thick-walled budding spores ("spaghetti and meatballs") are seen on KOH. Fungal culture is not useful.

Differential Diagnosis

Vitiligo usually presents with larger periorificial and acral lesions and is also characterized by depigmentation rather than hypopigmentation (as is seen in tinea versicolor). Vitiligo does not scale. Pink and red-brown lesions on the chest are differentiated from seborrheic dermatitis of the same areas by the KOH preparation, though seborrheic dermatitis and tinea versicolor often co-exist in the same patient. Confluent and reticulated papillomatosis also occurs on the trunk but tends to be darker.

Treatment & Prognosis

A. Initial Treatment

Topical treatments include selenium sulfide lotion, which may be applied from neck to waist daily and left on for 5–15 minutes for 7 days followed by weekly treatment for a month. Weekly ketoconazole shampoo, 1% or 2%, lathered on the chest and back for 5 minutes and ketoconazole 2% cream applied daily for one month are other effective topical regimens.

Two doses of oral fluconazole (300 mg) given 14 days apart are highly effective and carries minimal risk of hepatitis. Additional doses may be required in severe cases or humid climates. Clinicians must stress to the patient that following treatment, the alterations in pigmentation may take months to resolve.

B. Maintenance Therapy

Topical treatments as described above can be used for maintenance therapy. Imidazole creams, solutions, and lotions (eg, clotrimazole or miconazole) are effective for localized areas but are too expensive for use over large areas, such as the chest and back. Without maintenance therapy, recurrences will occur in over 80% of "cured" cases.

Andersen PL et al. Pityriasis versicolor [Pityriasis versicolor]. Ugeskr Laeger. 2025;187:V10240670. [PMID: 40171908]
Genuino RNF et al. Systematic review and meta-analysis on synthetic antifungal versus keratolytic agents for topical treatment of pityriasis versicolor. Acta Med Philipp. 2024;58:64. [PMID: 38939846]
Labedz N et al. Pityriasis versicolor—a narrative review on the diagnosis and management. Life (Basel). 2023;13:2097. [PMID: 37895478]

MUCOCUTANEOUS CANDIDIASIS

ESSENTIALS OF DIAGNOSIS

- Severe pruritus of vulva, anus, or body folds.
- Superficial denuded, beefy-red areas with or without satellite vesicopustules.
- Whitish curd-like concretions on the oral and vaginal mucous membranes.
- Yeast and pseudohyphae on microscopic examination of scales or curd.

General Considerations

Mucocutaneous candidiasis is a superficial fungal infection that may involve almost any cutaneous or mucous surface.

It is most likely to occur in patients with diabetes, in persons with obesity, in the setting of immunosuppression, and during pregnancy. Systemic antibiotics, oral corticosteroids, hormone replacement therapy, and oral contraceptive agents may be contributory. Oral and interdigital candidiasis may be the first sign of HIV infection (see Chapter 35). Denture use predisposes to infection.

Clinical Findings

A. Symptoms and Signs

Itching may be intense. Burning is reported, particularly around the vulva and anus. The lesions consist of superficially denuded, beefy-red areas in the depths of the body folds, such as in the groin and the intergluteal cleft, beneath the breasts, at the angles of the mouth, in the webspaces of digits, and in the umbilicus. The peripheries of these denuded lesions are superficially undermined, and there may be satellite vesicopustules. Whitish, curd-like concretions may be present on mucosal lesions (Figure 6–11). Paronychia may occur.

B. Laboratory Findings

Clusters of budding yeast and pseudohyphae can be seen under high power (400×) when skin scales or curd-like lesions are mounted in 10% KOH. Culture can confirm the diagnosis.

Differential Diagnosis

Intertrigo, seborrheic dermatitis, tinea cruris, "inverse psoriasis," and erythrasma involving the same areas may mimic mucocutaneous candidiasis.

Complications

Systemic invasive candidiasis with candidemia may occur in patients who are immunosuppressed or receiving broad-spectrum antibiotic or intravenous hypertonic glucose solutions (eg, hyperalimentation) (Chapter 40). There may or may not be clinically evident mucocutaneous candidiasis.

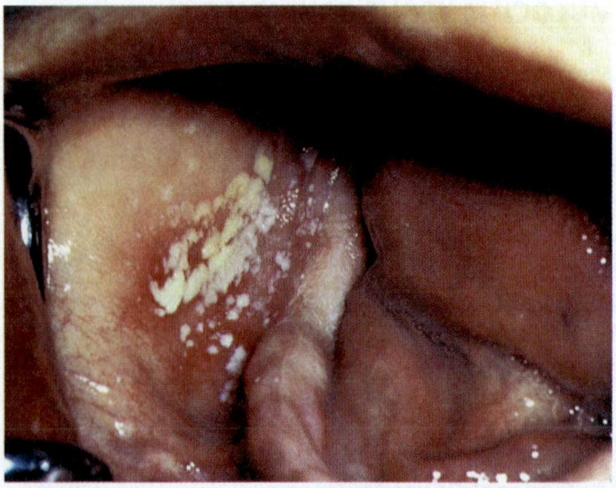

▲ **Figure 6–11.** Oral mucosal candidiasis. (From Sol Silverman, Jr., DDS/Centers for Disease Control and Prevention.)

Treatment

A. General Measures

Affected parts should be kept dry and exposed to air as much as possible. Water immersion should be minimized, and gloves should be worn for those with infected nails or digital skin. If possible, discontinue systemic antibiotics.

B. Local Measures

1. Nails and paronychia—Apply clotrimazole solution 1% twice daily. Thymol 4% in ethanol applied once daily is an alternative.

2. Skin—Apply nystatin ointment or clotrimazole cream 1% plus hydrocortisone cream 1–2.5%, twice daily. Gentian violet 0.5% solution is economical and highly effective in treating mucocutaneous candidiasis, but the purple discoloration may represent a cosmetic issue. Severe or widespread cutaneous disease responds to fluconazole, 100–200 mg orally daily, for 1 week.

3. Vulvar and anal mucous membranes—For vaginal candidiasis, single-dose fluconazole, 150 mg orally, is effective. Intravaginal clotrimazole, miconazole, terconazole, or nystatin may also be used. Long-term suppressive therapy may be required for recurrent or "intractable" cases. Non-albicans candidal species may be identified by culture in some refractory cases and may respond to oral itraconazole, 200 mg twice daily for 2–4 weeks.

4. Balanitis—This is most frequent in uncircumcised men and is usually caused by *Candida*. Topical nystatin ointment is the initial treatment if the lesions are mildly erythematous or superficially erosive. Soaking with dilute 5% aluminum acetate for 15 minutes twice daily may quickly relieve burning or itching. Chronicity and relapses, especially after sexual contact, suggest reinfection from a sexual partner who should be treated. Severe purulent balanitis is usually due to bacteria. If it is so severe that phimosis occurs, oral antibiotics—some with activity against anaerobes—are required; if rapid improvement does not occur, urologic consultation is indicated.

5. Mastitis—Lancinating breast pain and nipple dermatitis in breastfeeding women may be a manifestation of *Candida* colonization/infection of the breast ducts. Topical nystatin cream and clotrimazole 0.1% cream are safe during lactation. Topical gentian violet 0.5% daily for 7 days is also useful. Oral fluconazole, 200 mg daily for 2 weeks, is effective and safe during lactation.

Prognosis

Cases of cutaneous candidiasis range from the easily cured to the intractable and prolonged.

Hellier SD et al. Beyond fluconazole: a review of vulvovaginal candidiasis diagnosis and treatment. Nurse Pract. 2023;48:33. [PMID: 37643144]

Lu H et al. Candidiasis: from cutaneous to systemic, new perspectives of potential targets and therapeutic strategies. Adv Drug Deliv Rev. 2023;199:114960. [PMID: 37307922]

Shahabudin S et al. Candida albicans skin infection in diabetic patients: an updated review of pathogenesis and management. 2024;67:e13753. [PMID: 38877612]

INTERTRIGO

Intertrigo is caused by the macerating effect of heat, moisture, and friction. It is especially likely to occur in persons with obesity and in humid climates. The symptoms are itching, stinging, and burning. The body folds develop fissures, erythema, maceration, and superficial denudation. Candidiasis may complicate intertrigo, as can bacterial infections. "Inverse psoriasis," seborrheic dermatitis, tinea cruris, and erythrasma must be ruled out.

Maintaining hygiene and keeping the area dry are helpful. Compresses may be useful acutely. Hydrocortisone 1% cream combined with an imidazole or clotrimazole 1% cream is effective. Recurrences are common.

Romanelli M et al. The diagnosis, management and prevention of intertrigo in adults: a review. J Wound Care. 2023;32:411. [PMID: 37405940]

VIRAL INFECTIONS

HERPES SIMPLEX (Cold or Fever Sore; Genital Herpes)

ESSENTIALS OF DIAGNOSIS

- Recurrent small, grouped vesicles (especially orolabial and genital) on an erythematous base.
- May follow minor infections, trauma, stress, or sun exposure.
- Regional tender lymphadenopathy may occur.
- Direct fluorescent antibody or PCR tests are positive.

General Considerations

Over 85% of adults have serologic evidence of herpes simplex type 1 (HSV-1) infections, most often acquired asymptomatically in childhood. Occasionally, primary infections may be manifested as severe gingivostomatitis. Thereafter, the patient may have recurrent self-limited attacks, provoked by sun exposure, orofacial surgery, fever, viral infection, or immunosuppression.

About 25% of the US population has serologic evidence of infection with herpes simplex type 2 (HSV-2). HSV-2 causes lesions whose morphology and natural history are similar to those caused by HSV-1 but are typically located on the genitalia or buttocks. The infection is often acquired by sexual contact. In monogamous heterosexual couples where one partner has HSV-2 infection, seroconversion of the non-infected partner occurs in 10% over a 1-year period. Up to 70% of such infections appeared to be transmitted during periods of asymptomatic shedding. Genital herpes may also be due to HSV-1.

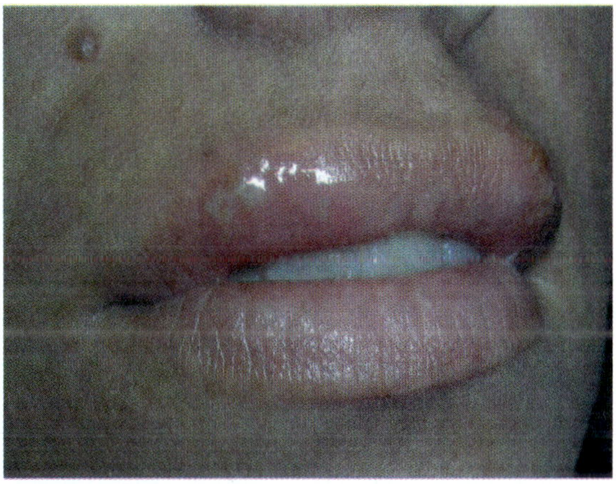

Figure 6–12. Orolabial herpes simplex showing deroofed blisters (ulcer). (Reproduced, with permission, from Richard P. Usatine, MD, in Usatine RP, Smith MA, Mayeaux EJ Jr, Chumley H. *The Color Atlas of Family Medicine*, 2nd ed. McGraw-Hill, 2013.)

Clinical Findings

A. Symptoms and Signs

The principal symptoms are burning and stinging. Neuralgia may precede or accompany attacks. The lesions consist of small, grouped vesicles on an erythematous base that can occur anywhere but that most often occur on the vermilion border of the lips (Figure 6–12), the oral cavity, penile shaft, the labia, the perianal skin, and the buttocks. Any erosion or fissure in the anogenital region can be due to herpes simplex. Regional lymph nodes may be swollen and tender. The lesions usually crust and heal in 1 week. Immunosuppressed patients may have unusual variants, including verrucous or nodular herpes lesions at typical sites of involvement. Lesions of herpes simplex must be distinguished from chancroid, syphilis, lymphogranuloma venereum, pyoderma gangrenosum, Behcet syndrome, or trauma.

B. Laboratory Findings

Direct fluorescent antibody slide tests offer rapid, sensitive diagnosis. Viral culture or PCR may also be helpful. Herpes serology is not used in the diagnosis of an acute genital ulcer. Specific HSV-2 serology can determine who is HSV-infected and potentially infectious, but the USPSTF does not recommend routine HSV-2 screening.

Complications

Complications include pyoderma, eczema herpeticum, herpetic whitlow, herpes gladiatorum (epidemic herpes transmitted by contact), proctitis, esophagitis, neonatal infection, keratitis, and encephalitis.

Treatment

A. Systemic Therapy

Three commonly used systemic agents are available for the treatment of acute herpes infections: acyclovir, valacyclovir, and famciclovir. All three agents are very effective, and when used properly, virtually nontoxic. Only acyclovir is available for intravenous administration.

1. For first clinical episode—Recommended treatment for the first clinical episodes of herpes simplex includes valacyclovir, 1000 mg orally twice daily; acyclovir, 400 mg orally five times daily (or 800 mg three times daily); or famciclovir, 250 mg orally three times daily. Treatment is for 7–10 days, depending on the severity and location of the outbreak.

2. For mild recurrences—Most cases do not require therapy. Pharmacotherapy of recurrent HSV is of limited benefit, reducing the average outbreak by only 12–24 hours. **To be effective, the treatment must be initiated by the patient at the first sign of recurrence**. If treatment is desired, recurrent genital herpes outbreaks may be treated with 3 days of valacyclovir, 500 mg orally twice daily, 5 days of acyclovir, 200 mg orally five times a day, or 5 days of famciclovir, 125 mg orally twice daily. Valacyclovir, 2 g twice daily for 1 day, and famciclovir, 1 g once or twice in 1 day, are equally effective short-course alternatives and can abort impending recurrences of both orolabial and genital herpes. The addition of a potent topical corticosteroid three times daily reduces the duration, size, and pain of orolabial herpes treated with an oral antiviral agent.

3. For frequent or severe recurrences—Suppressive treatment reduces recurrences by 85%, viral shedding by > 90%, and the risk of transmission by 50%. The recommended suppressive doses, taken continuously, are valacyclovir, 500 mg orally once daily; acyclovir, 400 mg orally twice daily; or famciclovir, 125–250 mg orally twice daily. Pritelivir, 100 mg orally once daily, may have a superior reduction of viral shedding in HSV-2 compared to valacyclovir, 500 mg orally once daily. Long-term suppression appears safe, and after 5–7 years, a substantial proportion of patients can discontinue treatment.

Sunscreens are useful adjuncts in preventing sun-induced orolabial recurrences. A preventive antiviral medication should be started beginning 24 hours before UV light exposure, dental surgery, or orolabial cosmetic surgery. The use of latex condoms and patient education has proved effective in reducing genital herpes transmission in some but not all studies. No single or combination intervention absolutely prevents transmission.

B. Local Measures

Topical therapy has limited efficacy and is generally not recommended because evidence shows that it minimally reduces skin healing time.

Prognosis

Aside from the complications described above, recurrent attacks last several days, and patients recover without sequelae.

Gopinath D et al. A comprehensive overview of epidemiology, pathogenesis and the management of herpes labialis. Viruses. 2023;15:225. [PMID: 36680265]

Meller N. Genital herpes simplex virus infections in women-a clinical update. Clin Obstet Gynecol. 2025;68:170. [PMID: 40008683]

HERPES ZOSTER (Shingles)

See Chapter 36.

MOLLUSCUM CONTAGIOSUM

Molluscum contagiosum, caused by a poxvirus, presents as single or multiple dome-shaped, waxy papules 2–5 mm in diameter that are umbilicated (Figure 6–13). Lesions at first are firm, solid, and flesh-colored but upon reaching maturity become soft, whitish, or pearly gray and may suppurate. The principal sites of involvement are the face, lower abdomen, and genitals.

The lesions are auto-inoculable and spread by wet skin-to-skin contact. In sexually active individuals, they may be confined to the penis, pubis, perianal area, and inner thighs and are considered an STI.

Molluscum contagiosum is common in patients with AIDS, usually with a helper T-cell count < 100/mcL (0.1×10^9/L). Extensive lesions tend to develop over the face and neck as well as in the genital area.

The diagnosis is easily established in most instances because of the distinctive central umbilication of the dome-shaped lesion. Estimated time to remission is 13 months. The best treatment is by curettage or applications of liquid nitrogen, as for warts, but more briefly. When lesions are frozen, the central umbilication often becomes more apparent. Light electrosurgery with a fine needle is also effective. Cantharidin (applied in the office and then washed off by the patient 4 hours later) is a safe and effective option. Another treatment option is 10% or 15% potassium hydroxide solution applied twice daily until lesions clear. Salicylic acid, podophyllotoxin, tretinoin, imiquimod, berdazimer 10.3% gel, and intralesional immunotherapy are additional treatment options. Physical destruction with a pulsed dye laser or via extraction of molluscum bodies with a comedone extractor or curette is also effective. Lesions are challenging to eradicate in patients with AIDS unless immunity improves; however,

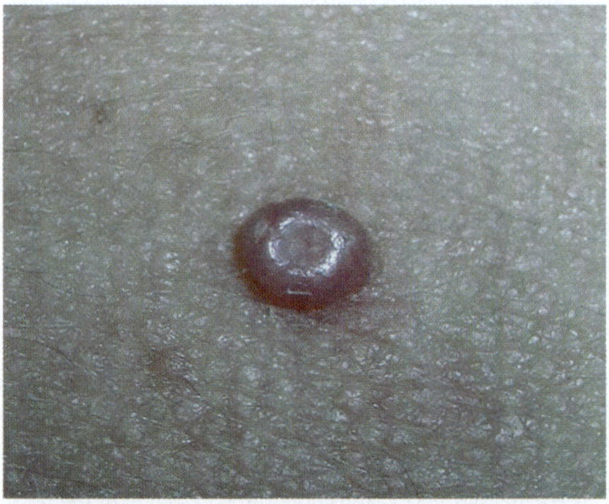

▲ **Figure 6–13.** Umbilicated—molluscum. (Reproduced, with permission, from Richard P. Usatine, MD, in Usatine RP, Smith MA, Mayeaux EJ Jr, Chumley H. *The Color Atlas of Family Medicine*, 3rd ed. McGraw-Hill, 2019.)

with antiretroviral treatment, molluscum usually spontaneously clears.

Chao YC et al. Comparative efficacy of treatments for molluscum contagiosum: a systematic review and network meta-analysis. J Dtsch Dermatol Ges. 2023;21:587. [PMID: 37199262]
Hebert AA et al. Molluscum contagiosum: epidemiology, considerations, treatment options, and therapeutic gaps. J Clin Aesthet Dermatol. 2023;16(Suppl 1):S4. [PMID: 37636018]
Silverberg NB. Latest breakthroughs in molluscum contagiosum therapy. Cutis. 2024;113:231. [PMID: 39082997]

WARTS

ESSENTIALS OF DIAGNOSIS

- Verrucous papules anywhere on the skin or mucous membranes, usually not > 1 cm in diameter.
- Prolonged incubation period (average 2–18 months).
- Spontaneous "cures" of common warts is 50% at 2 years.
- Recurrence and formation of new lesions are frequent.

General Considerations

Warts (common, plantar, and genital [condylomata acuminata]) are caused by HPV. Typing of HPV lesions is not a part of standard medical evaluation except in the case of anogenital dysplasia.

Clinical Findings

There are usually no symptoms. Tenderness on pressure occurs with plantar warts; itching occurs with anogenital warts (Figure 6–14). Flat warts are most evident under oblique illumination. Periungual warts may be dry, fissured, and hyperkeratotic and may resemble hangnails. Plantar warts resemble plantar corns or calluses.

Differential Diagnosis

Some warty-looking lesions are actually seborrheic keratosis, hypertrophic actinic keratoses or squamous cell carcinomas. Condylomata lata of secondary syphilis can resemble large warts. Molluscum contagiosum lesions are pearly with a central dell. In AIDS, wart-like lesions may be caused by herpes or varicella zoster virus.

Prevention

Administration of a vaccine against certain anogenital HPV types (Gardasil-9 is given in the United States and includes HPV 6, 11, 16, 18, 31, 33, 45, 52, and 58) can prevent infection with these wart types and reduce anogenital, oropharyngeal, and cervical cancer. It is recommended for all patients up to age 26, men who have sex with men, and immunocompromised patients (see Chapters 1 and 21).

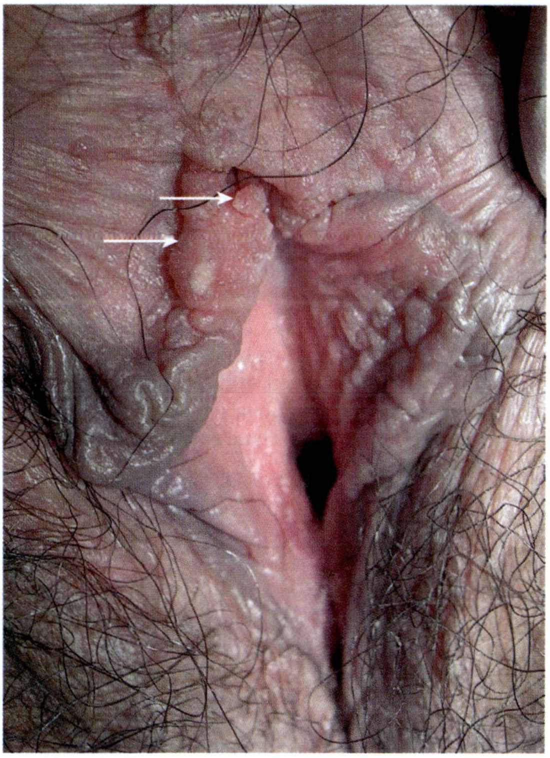

▲ **Figure 6–14.** Condylomata acuminata around the clitoris, labia minor, and opening of the vagina. (Reproduced, with permission, from Richard P. Usatine, MD, in Usatine RP, Smith MA, Mayeaux EJ Jr, Chumley H. *The Color Atlas of Family Medicine*, 2nd ed. McGraw-Hill, 2013.)

The FDA has approved the vaccine for all patients up to age 45. There may be a role for adjuvant vaccination in HPV-infected patients.

Treatment

Treatment is aimed at inducing "wart-free" intervals for as long as possible without scarring, since no treatment can guarantee a remission or prevent recurrences. In immunocompromised patients, the goal is to control the size and number of lesions present. Certain types (HPV 1) are more responsive to treatment than others (eg, HPV 2, HPV 27).

A. Treatment of Nongenital Warts

For common warts of the hands, patients are usually offered liquid nitrogen or keratolytic agents. The former may work in fewer treatments but requires office visits and is painful.

1. Liquid nitrogen—Liquid nitrogen cryotherapy is applied to achieve a thaw time of 30–45 seconds. Two freeze-thaw cycles are given every 2–4 weeks for several visits. Scarring and dyspigmentation can occur if it is performed incorrectly, particularly in individuals with darker skin pigmentation.

2. Keratolytic agents and occlusion—Salicylic acid products may be used against common warts or plantar warts. They are applied, then occluded. Plantar warts may be treated by applying a 40% salicylic acid plaster after paring.

The plaster may be left on for 5–6 days, then removed, the lesion pared down, and another plaster applied. Although it may take weeks or months to eradicate the wart, the method is safe and effective with almost no side effects. Chronic occlusion with water-impermeable tape (such as duct tape or adhesive tape) can work as well as cryotherapy.

3. Operative removal—Plantar warts may be removed by blunt dissection.

4. Laser therapy—The CO_2 laser can be effective for treating recurrent warts, periungual warts, plantar warts, and genital warts. It leaves open wounds that must fill in with granulation tissue over 4–6 weeks and is best reserved for warts resistant to all other modalities. Lasers with emissions of 585, 595, or 532 nm may also be used every 3–4 weeks to ablate common, plantar, facial, and anogenital warts.

5. Immunotherapy—Squaric acid dibutyl ester may be applied 1–5 times weekly in a concentration of 0.2–2% directly to the warts to induce a mild contact dermatitis. Between 60% and 80% of warts clear over 10–20 weeks. Injection of *Candida* antigen starting at 1:50 dilution and repeated every 3–4 weeks may be similarly effective in stimulating immunologic regression of common and plantar warts.

6. Other agents—Bleomycin (1 unit/mL), injected into common and plantar warts, has been shown to have a high cure rate. It should be used with caution on digital warts because of the potential complications of Raynaud phenomenon, nail loss, permanent scarring, and terminal digital necrosis. 5-Fluorouracil 5% cream applied once or twice daily, usually with occlusion, has similar efficacy to other treatment methods. Topical or intralesional cidofovir may be effective in treating recalcitrant lesions, especially in immunocompromised patients.

7. Physical modalities—Soaking warts in hot (42.2°C) water for 10–30 minutes daily for 6 weeks or application of heating pads for a few minutes each day may result in involution in some cases.

B. Treatment of Genital Warts

1. Liquid nitrogen—Cryotherapy is the first-line surgical treatment for genital warts. Liquid nitrogen cryotherapy is applied to achieve a thaw time of 30–45 seconds. Two freeze-thaw cycles are given every 2–4 weeks for several visits. Scarring will occur if it is used incorrectly.

2. Podophyllum resin—For genital warts, the purified active component of the podophyllum resin, podofilox, is applied by the patient twice daily, three consecutive days a week, for cycles of 4–6 weeks. It is less irritating and more effective than "clinician-applied" podophyllum resin. After a single 4-week cycle, 45% of patients are wart-free, but 60% relapse at 6 weeks. Thus, multiple cycles of treatment are often necessary. Patients unable to obtain the take-home podofilox may be treated in the clinician's office by painting each wart carefully (protecting normal skin) every 2–3 weeks with 25% podophyllum resin (podophyllin) in compound tincture of benzoin.

3. Imiquimod—A 5% cream of this local interferon inducer has moderate activity in clearing external genital warts. Treatment is once daily on three alternate days per week. Response may be slow.

4. Sinecatechins—Derived from green tea extract, sinecatechins (10% or 15%) are FDA-approved for the treatment of anogenital warts. Application three times daily for 16 weeks achieves clearance rates from 40% to 81%, with the 15% formulation resulting in higher efficacy.

5. Operative removal—For pedunculated or large genital warts, snip biopsy (scissors) removal is more effective than cryotherapy.

6. Laser therapy—See Treatment of Nongenital Warts, above. For genital warts, it has not been shown that laser therapy is more effective than electrosurgical removal. Both carry some risk of aerosolization of HPV with inoculation into the airway of the patient or provider. Photodynamic therapy can be considered for refractory genital warts.

Prognosis

There is a striking tendency to develop new lesions. Warts may disappear spontaneously or may be unresponsive to treatment. Combining therapies (eg, liquid nitrogen plus immunotherapy) may improve therapeutic response.

Kucharczyk E et al. Intralesional immunotherapy for non-genital viral warts: a review of current evidence and future perspectives. Int J Mol Sci. 2025;26:5644. [PMID: 40565110]

Le M et al. Energy-based devices for the treatment of cutaneous verrucae: a systematic review. Dermatol Surg. 2024;50:345. [PMID: 38551277]

Verma KK et al. Innovation in warts and molluscum: an updated comprehensive review. Dermatol Clin. 2025;43:95. [PMID: 39542567]

BACTERIAL INFECTIONS

IMPETIGO

ESSENTIALS OF DIAGNOSIS

- Superficial blisters filled with purulent material that rupture easily.
- Crusted superficial erosions.
- Positive Gram stain and bacterial culture.

General Considerations

Impetigo is a contagious and autoinoculable infection of the skin (epidermis) caused by staphylococci or streptococci.

Clinical Findings

A. Symptoms and Signs

The lesions consist of macules, vesicles, bullae, pustules, and honey-colored crusts that, when removed, leave denuded red areas (Figure 6–15). The face and other exposed parts are most often involved. Ecthyma is a deeper

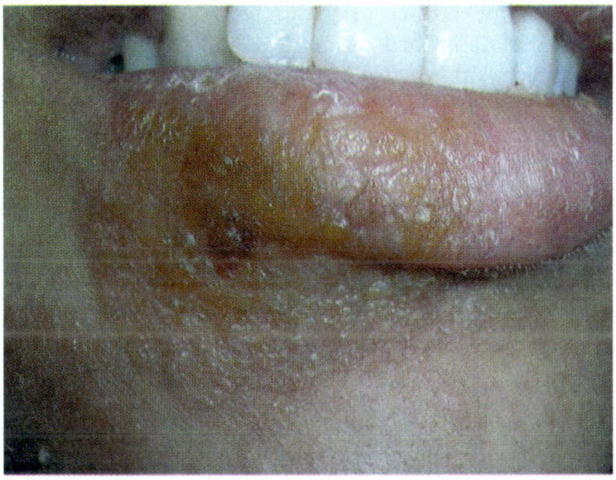

▲ **Figure 6–15.** Typical honey-crusted plaque on the lip of an adult with impetigo. (Reproduced, with permission, from Richard P. Usatine, MD, in Usatine RP, Smith MA, Mayeaux EJ Jr, Chumley HS. *The Color Atlas and Synopsis of Family Medicine*, 3rd ed. McGraw-Hill, 2019.)

form of impetigo caused by staphylococci or streptococci, with ulceration and scarring that occurs frequently on the extremities.

B. Laboratory Findings

Gram stain and culture confirm the diagnosis. In temperate climates, most cases are associated with *S aureus* infection. *Streptococcus* species are more common in tropical infections.

Differential Diagnosis

The primary differential diagnoses of honey-colored crusting are acute allergic contact dermatitis and herpes simplex. Contact dermatitis may be suggested by the history or by the linear distribution of the lesions, and culture should be negative for staphylococci and streptococci. Herpes simplex infection usually presents with grouped vesicles or discrete erosions and may be associated with a history of recurrences. Viral cultures are positive.

Treatment

Soaks and scrubbing can be beneficial, especially in unroofing lakes of pus under thick crusts. Topical agents, such as mupirocin, ozenoxacin, and retapamulin, are first-line treatment options for infections limited to small areas. In widespread cases or in immunosuppressed individuals, systemic antibiotics are indicated. Cephalexin, 250 mg orally four times daily, is usually effective. Community-associated methicillin-resistant *S aureus* (CA-MRSA) may cause impetigo, for which initial treatment may include doxycycline (100 mg orally twice daily) or trimethoprim-sulfamethoxazole (TMP-SMZ, double-strength tablet orally twice daily). Recurrent impetigo is associated with nasal carriage of *S aureus.* It can be treated with rifampin, 300 mg orally twice daily for 5 days, or with intranasal mupirocin ointment twice daily for 14 days.

Dallo M et al. Topical antibiotic treatment in dermatology. Antibiotics (Basel). 2023;12:188. [PMID: 36830098]

Zha M et al. Common skin conditions in children and adolescents: bacterial infections. FP Essent. 2024;541:14. [PMID: 38896828]

FOLLICULITIS

ESSENTIALS OF DIAGNOSIS

- Itching and burning in hairy areas.
- Pustule/papule surrounding and including the hair follicle.

General Considerations

Folliculitis has multiple causes. It is frequently caused by staphylococcal infection, followed by streptococcal and candida infections. When the lesion is deep-seated, chronic, and recalcitrant on the head and neck, it is called **sycosis**.

During antibiotic treatment of acne, gram-negative folliculitis may present as a flare of acne pustules or nodules. *Klebsiella, Enterobacter, Escherichia coli*, and *Proteus* have been isolated from these lesions.

Hot tub folliculitis (*Pseudomonas* folliculitis), caused by *Pseudomonas aeruginosa*, is characterized by pruritic or tender follicular, pustular lesions occurring within 1–4 days after bathing in a contaminated hot tub, whirlpool, or swimming pool. Flu-like symptoms may be present. Rarely, systemic infections may result.

Nonbacterial folliculitis may also be caused by friction and oils. Occlusion, perspiration, and chronic rubbing (eg, from tight-fitting clothing or heavy fabrics on the buttocks and thighs) can worsen this type of folliculitis.

Steroid acne may be seen during topical or systemic corticosteroid therapy and presents as eruptive monomorphous papules and papulopustules on the face and trunk. It responds to topical benzoyl peroxide.

Eosinophilic folliculitis is a sterile folliculitis that presents with urticarial papules with prominent eosinophilic infiltration. It is most common in immunosuppressed patients, especially those with AIDS. It may appear first with the institution of antiretroviral therapy (ART) and be mistaken for a drug eruption.

Pseudofolliculitis is caused by the ingrowth of tightly curled hairs in the beard area. In this entity, the papules and pustules are located at the side of and not in the follicles. It may be treated by growing a beard, by using chemical depilatories, or by shaving with a foil-guard razor. Laser hair removal is dramatically beneficial in patients with pseudofolliculitis.

Pityrosporum folliculitis (caused by *Malassezia*) presents as 1- to 2-mm pruritic pink papulopustules on the upper trunk, hairline, and arms. It is often pruritic and tends to develop during periods of excessive sweating. It can also occur in immunosuppressed patients.

Demodex folliculitis is caused by the mite *Demodex folliculorum*. It presents on the face as 1–2 mm papules and

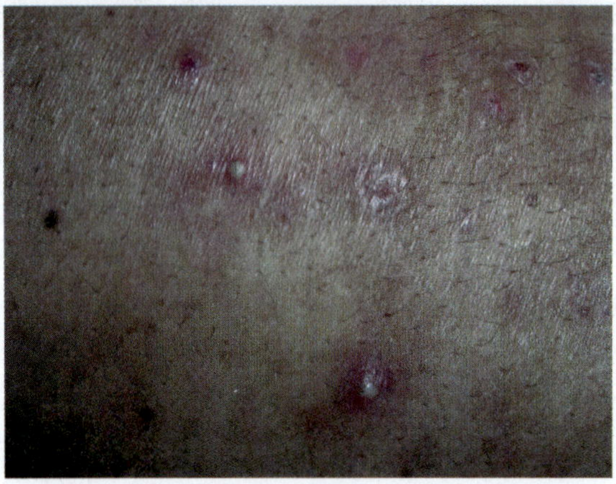

Figure 6–16. **Bacterial folliculitis. Hair emanating from the center of the pustule is the clinical hallmark of folliculitis.** (Reproduced, with permission, from Richard P. Usatine, MD, in Usatine RP, Smith MA, Mayeaux EJ Jr, Chumley H. *The Color Atlas of Family Medicine*, 2nd ed. McGraw-Hill, 2013.)

pustules on an erythematous base, often on the background of rosacea-like changes, in patients who have not responded to conventional treatment for rosacea. It is more common in immunosuppressed patients. KOH from the pustules will demonstrate *Demodex folliculorum* mites.

Clinical Findings

The symptoms range from slight burning and tenderness to intense itching. The lesions consist of papules or pustules centered around hair follicles (Figure 6–16).

Differential Diagnosis

It is important to differentiate bacterial from nonbacterial folliculitis. The history is essential for pinpointing the causes of nonbacterial folliculitis, and a Gram stain and culture are indispensable. One must differentiate bacterial folliculitis from acne vulgaris, pustular miliaria (heat rash), and other infections of the skin, such as impetigo or *Pityrosporum* folliculitis. Eosinophilic folliculitis in AIDS often requires biopsy for diagnosis.

Complications

Abscess formation is the major complication of bacterial folliculitis.

Prevention

Correct any predisposing local causes, such as oils or friction. Be sure that the water in hot tubs and spas is treated properly. If staphylococcal folliculitis is persistent, treatment of nasal or perineal carriage with rifampin, 600 mg daily for 5 days, or with topical mupirocin ointment 2% twice daily for 5 days, may help. Prolonged oral clindamycin, 150–300 mg/day for 4–6 weeks, or oral TMP-SMZ given 1 week per month for 6 months can be effective in preventing recurrent staphylococcal folliculitis and furunculosis. Bleach baths (¼–½ cup per 20 liters of bathwater for 15 minutes three to five times weekly) may reduce cutaneous staphylococcal carriage and not contribute to antibiotic resistance. Control of blood glucose in diabetes may reduce infections.

Treatment

A. Local Measures

Anhydrous ethyl alcohol containing 6.25% aluminum chloride, applied three to seven times weekly to lesions, may be helpful, especially for chronic frictional folliculitis of the buttocks. Topical antibiotics are generally ineffective if bacteria have invaded the hair follicle but may be prophylactic if used as an aftershave in patients with recurrent folliculitis after shaving.

B. Specific Measures

Pseudomonas folliculitis clears spontaneously in non-neutropenic patients if the lesions are superficial. It may be treated with ciprofloxacin, 500 mg orally twice daily for 5 days.

Systemic antibiotics are recommended for bacterial folliculitis due to other organisms. Extended periods of treatment (4–8 weeks or more) with antistaphylococcal antibiotics are required if infection involves the scalp or densely hairy areas, such as the axilla, beard, or groin (see Table 34–5).

Gram-negative folliculitis in acne patients may be treated with isotretinoin in compliance with all precautions discussed above.

Eosinophilic folliculitis may be treated initially by the combination of potent topical corticosteroids and oral antihistamines. In more severe cases, treatment is with one of the following: indomethacin, 50–75 mg orally daily; topical permethrin (application for 12 hours every other night for 6 weeks); itraconazole, 200–400 mg orally daily; cetirizine, 20–40 mg orally daily; UVB or PUVA phototherapy; or isotretinoin, 0.5 mg/kg/day orally for up to 5 months. Some of these therapies may induce remission, but long-term treatment may be required. In patients with HIV, initiation of ART can also help.

Pityrosporum folliculitis is treated with topical sulfacetamide lotion twice a day, alone or in combination with oral itraconazole or fluconazole.

Demodex folliculitis can be treated until cleared with topical 5% permethrin applied every other night; oral ivermectin, 200 mcg/kg once weekly; oral metronidazole, 500 mg once daily or 250 mg three times daily; or topical ivermectin or metronidazole.

Prognosis

Bacterial folliculitis usually resolves with appropriate treatment, but can be stubborn and persistent, requiring prolonged or intermittent courses of antibiotics.

Frazier WT et al. Common dermatologic conditions in skin of color. Am Fam Physician. 2023;107:26. [PMID: 36689965]

Green M et al. Clinical characteristics and treatment outcomes of *Pityrosporum folliculitis* in immunocompetent patients. Arch Dermatol Res. 2023;315:1497. [PMID: 36517586]

Zha M et al. Common skin conditions in children and adolescents: bacterial infections. FP Essent. 2024;541:14. [PMID: 38896826]

FURUNCULOSIS (Boils) & CARBUNCLES

ESSENTIALS OF DIAGNOSIS

- Extremely painful inflammatory abscess centered on a hair follicle.
- Coagulase-positive *S aureus* is the usual causative organism.
- Predisposing conditions (diabetes mellitus, HIV disease, injection drug use) are sometimes present.

General Considerations

A **furuncle (boil)** is a deep-seated infection (abscess), usually caused by *S aureus*, that involves the hair follicle and adjacent subcutaneous tissue. The most common sites of occurrence are the hairy parts exposed to irritation and friction, pressure, or moisture. Because the lesions are autoinoculable, they are often multiple. Diabetes mellitus (especially if using insulin injections), injection drug use, allergy injections, and HIV disease all increase the risk of staphylococcal infections by increasing the rate of carriage. Other specific exposures, such as hospitalization, athletic teams, prisons, military service, and lack of housing, may also increase the risk of infection.

A **carbuncle** consists of several furuncles developing in adjoining hair follicles and coalescing to form a conglomerate, deeply situated mass with multiple drainage points.

Recurrent furunculosis (three or more episodes in 12 months) tends to occur in those with direct contact with other infected individuals, especially family members.

Clinical Findings

A. Symptoms and Signs

Pain and tenderness may be prominent. The abscess is either rounded or conical. It gradually enlarges, becomes fluctuant, and then softens and opens spontaneously after a few days to 1–2 weeks to discharge a core of necrotic tissue and pus. The inflammation occasionally subsides before necrosis occurs.

B. Laboratory Findings

There may be slight leukocytosis. Pus can be cultured to rule out MRSA or other bacteria. Culture of the anterior nares and anogenital area (including the rectum to test for GI carriage) may identify chronic staphylococcal carriage in cases of recurrent cutaneous infection.

Differential Diagnosis

The most common entity in the differential is an inflamed **epidermal inclusion cyst** that suddenly becomes red, tender, and expands greatly in size over one to a few days. The history of a prior cyst in the exact location, the presence of a clearly visible cyst orifice, and the extrusion of malodorous cheesy material (rather than purulent material) help in making the diagnosis. Tinea profunda (deep dermatophyte infection of the hair follicle) may simulate recurrent furunculosis. Furunculosis is also to be distinguished from deep mycotic infections, such as sporotrichosis; from other bacterial infections, such as anthrax and tularemia (rare); from atypical mycobacterial infections; and from acne cysts. Hidradenitis suppurativa (acne inversa) presents with recurrent tender, sterile abscesses in the axillae and groin, on the buttocks, or below the breasts. The presence of old scars or sinus tracts, combined with negative cultures, suggests this diagnosis.

Complications

Serious and sometimes fatal complications of staphylococcal infection, such as septicemia, can occur.

Prevention

Identifying and eliminating the source of infection is critical to prevent recurrences after treatment. The source individual may have chronic dermatitis or be an asymptomatic carrier of MRSA. Nasal carriage of MRSA and the number of children in a household are risk factors for transmission between household members. Local measures, such as meticulous handwashing; no sharing of towels, clothing, and personal hygiene products; avoiding loofas or sponges in the bath or shower; changing underwear, sleepwear, towels, and washcloths daily; aggressive scrubbing of showers, bathrooms, and surfaces with bleach; bleach baths (¼–½ cup per 20 liters of bathwater for 15 minutes three to five times weekly), 4% chlorhexidine washes, and isolation of infected patients who reside in institutions to prevent spread are all effective measures.

Treatment

A. Specific Measures

Incision and drainage are recommended for all loculated suppurations and are the mainstay of therapy. Systemic antibiotics are given only if there are multiple lesions, evidence of surrounding cellulitis, or if the patient is immunosuppressed. Commonly prescribed antibiotics are TMP-SMZ (160/800 or 320/1600 mg orally twice a day for 10 days or 7 days, respectively) or clindamycin (300 mg orally three times daily for 10 days). Other oral antibiotic options include dicloxacillin or cephalexin, 1 g daily in divided doses for 10 days. For suspected MRSA, the following treatments are effective: doxycycline 100 mg twice daily, TMP-SMZ double-strength one tablet twice daily, clindamycin 150–300 mg twice daily, and linezolid 400 mg twice daily for 7–10 days. Recurrent furunculosis may be treated with a combination of cephalexin (250–500 mg orally four times daily) or doxycycline (100 mg orally twice daily) for 2–4 weeks plus either rifampin (300 mg orally twice daily for 5 days) or long-term clindamycin (150–300 mg orally daily for 1–2 months). Shorter courses of antibiotics (7–14 days) plus longer-term daily 4% chlorhexidine whole body washing and intranasal, axilla, and anogenital mupirocin or retapamulin may also cure recurrent furunculosis. Oral vancomycin (1 g twice daily for 5 days) can treat GI carriage of *S aureus*. Family members, pets, and intimate contacts may need evaluation for the staphylococcal carrier state and perhaps concomitant treatment. Stopping any high-risk behavior, such as injection drug use, can also prevent recurrence.

B. Local Measures

Avoid over manipulation of inflamed areas. Use moist heat to promote spontaneous lesion drainage. Use surgical incision and drainage for fluctuant, nondraining lesions.

Prognosis

Recurrent lesions may occur for months or years.

Long DR et al. Preventing surgical site infections in the era of escalating antibiotic resistance and antibiotic stewardship. JAMA Surg. 2024;159:949. [PMID: 38922606]

Zha M et al. Common skin conditions in children and adolescents: bacterial infections. FP Essent. 2024;541:14. [PMID: 38896826]

CELLULITIS

ESSENTIALS OF DIAGNOSIS

- Edematous, expanding, erythematous, warm plaque with or without vesicles or bullae.
- Lower leg is frequently involved.
- Pain, chills, and fever are commonly present.
- Septicemia may develop.

General Considerations

Cellulitis, a diffuse spreading infection of the dermis and subcutaneous tissue, is usually on the lower leg (Figure 6–17) and most commonly due to gram-positive cocci, especially group A β-hemolytic streptococci and *S aureus*. Rarely, gram-negative rods or even fungi can produce a similar picture. In otherwise healthy persons, the most common portal of entry for lower leg cellulitis is interdigital tinea pedis with fissuring. Prior episodes of cellulitis, chronic edema or lymphedema, chronic venous insufficiency, peripheral vascular disease, DVT, obesity, prior leg surgery, and any damage to the skin surface are associated with an increased risk of recurrent cellulitis. Bacterial cellulitis is almost never bilateral.

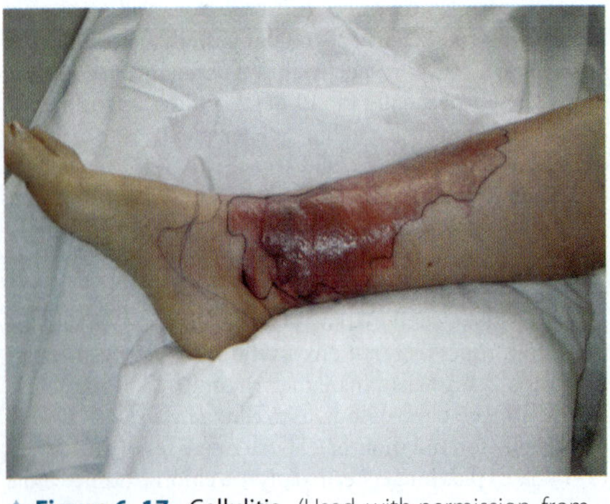

▲ **Figure 6–17.** Cellulitis. (Used, with permission, from Lindy Fox, MD.)

Clinical Findings

A. Symptoms and Signs

Cellulitis begins as a tender, small patch. Swelling, erythema, and pain are often present. The lesion expands over hours, so the time from onset to presentation is usually 6–36 hours. As the lesion grows, the patient becomes more ill with progressive chills, fever, and malaise. Lymphangitis and lymphadenopathy are often present. If septicemia develops, hypotension may develop, followed by shock.

B. Laboratory Findings

Leukocytosis or neutrophilia may be present early in the course. Blood cultures are variably positive. If a central ulceration, pustule, or abscess is present, culture may be of value. In immunosuppressed patients, or if an unusual organism is suspected and there is no loculated site to culture, a full-thickness skin biopsy should be sent for histologic evaluation and culture (bacterial, fungal, and mycobacterial). If a primary source for the infection is identified (wound, leg ulcer, toe web intertrigo), cultures from these sites isolate the causative pathogen in half of cases and can be used to guide antibiotic therapy.

Differential Diagnosis

DVT and necrotizing fasciitis are two potentially life-threatening entities that can mimic cellulitis (ie, present with a painful, red, swollen lower extremity). Necrotizing fasciitis should be suspected in a patient who has a toxic appearance, bullae, crepitus, or anesthesia of the involved skin, skin necrosis, and laboratory evidence of rhabdomyolysis (elevated creatine kinase) or disseminated intravascular coagulation. While these findings may be present with severe cellulitis and bacteremia, it is essential to rule out necrotizing fasciitis because rapid surgical debridement is necessary. Other noninfectious skin lesions that may resemble cellulitis are termed "pseudocellulitis." These include sclerosing panniculitis, an acute, exquisitely tender red plaque on the medial lower legs above the malleolus in patients with venous stasis or varicosities, and acute severe contact dermatitis on a limb, which produces erythema, vesiculation, and edema, as seen in cellulitis, but with itching instead of pain. Bilateral lower leg bacterial cellulitis is exceedingly rare, and other diagnoses, especially severe stasis dermatitis (see Figure 14–4), should be considered in this setting. In contrast to cellulitis, severe lower extremity stasis dermatitis usually develops over days to weeks (rather than hours) and is not as tender to palpation.

Cryptococcal cellulitis in the organ transplant recipient is often bilateral. The ALT-70 is a predictive model to diagnose cellulitis or a cellulitis mimic and to provide guidance about when a dermatology consultation is needed.

Treatment

Intravenous or parenteral antibiotics may be required for the first 2–5 days, with adequate coverage for *Streptococcus* and *Staphylococcus*. Methicillin-susceptible *S aureus* (MSSA) can be treated with nafcillin, cefazolin, clindamycin, dicloxacillin, cephalexin, doxycycline, or TMP-SMZ. If MRSA is suspected or proven, treatment options include vancomycin, linezolid, clindamycin, daptomycin, doxycycline, or TMP-SMZ. In mild cases or following the initial parenteral therapy, oral dicloxacillin or cephalexin, 250–500 mg four times daily for 5–10 days, is usually adequate. In patients in whom intravenous treatment is not instituted, the first dose of oral antibiotic can be doubled to achieve high blood levels rapidly. In patients with recurrent lower leg cellulitis (three to four episodes per year), oral penicillin 250 mg twice daily or oral erythromycin 250–500 mg twice daily can decrease the risk of recurrence. Additional measures to prevent recurrences include compression, treating toe web intertrigo and tinea pedis, and controlling venous insufficiency.

When to Admit

- Severe local symptoms and signs.
- Signs of sepsis.
- Elevated WBC count of 10,000/mcL (10×10^9/L) or more with marked left shift. Failure to respond to oral antibiotics.

Gunderson CG et al. Overdiagnosis of cellulitis. J Hosp Med. 2023;18:281. [PMID: 36510698]

Peghin M et al. Prevention and treatment of recurrent cellulitis. Curr Opin Infect Dis. 2023;36:95. [PMID: 36853755]

Pulia MS et al. Validation of thermal imaging and the ALT-70 prediction model to differentiate cellulitis from pseudocellulitis. JAMA Dermatol. 2024;160:511. [PMID: 38536160]

ERYSIPELAS

ESSENTIALS OF DIAGNOSIS

- Edematous, circumscribed, hot, erythematous area, with raised advancing border.
- The central face or lower extremity is frequently involved.
- Pain and systemic toxicity may be striking.

General Considerations

Erysipelas is a superficial form of cellulitis that is usually caused by β-hemolytic streptococci.

Clinical Findings

A. Symptoms and Signs

The symptoms are pain, malaise, chills, and moderate fever. A bright red patch appears and then spreads to form a tense, sharply demarcated, glistening, smooth, hot plaque. The sharp margin characteristically advances noticeably in days or even hours. The lesion has a raised edge and may pit slightly with finger pressure. Vesicles or bullae occasionally develop on the surface. The lesion does not usually become pustular or gangrenous and heals without scar formation. Breaks in the skin often provide a portal of entry for the organism. On the face, erysipelas begins near a fissure at the angle of the nose. On the lower extremity, tinea pedis with interdigital fissuring is a common portal of entry.

B. Laboratory Findings

Leukocytosis is almost invariably present; blood cultures may be positive.

Differential Diagnosis

Erysipeloid is a benign bacillary infection by *Erysipelothrix rhusiopathiae* that produces cellulitis of the skin of the fingers or the backs of the hands in fishermen and meat handlers.

Complications

Unless erysipelas is promptly treated, death may result from bacterial dissemination, particularly in older adults.

Treatment

Intravenous antibiotics effective against group A β-hemolytic streptococci and staphylococci should be considered, but outpatient treatment with oral antibiotics has demonstrated equal efficacy. Oral regimens include a 7-day course with penicillin VK (250 mg), dicloxacillin (250 mg), or a first-generation cephalosporin (250 mg) four times a day. Clindamycin (250 mg twice daily orally for 7–14 days) is an option for penicillin-allergic patients.

Prognosis

With appropriate treatment, rapid improvement is expected. The presence of lymphedema carries the greatest risk of recurrence.

Maciej S et al. Severe bullous erysipelas/cellulitis, atypically caused by *Escherichia coli*, in kidney transplant recipient—case report and review of the literature. Transplant Proc. 2024;56:976. [PMID: 38448250]

Shu Z et al. Efficacy and safety of first- and second-line antibiotics for cellulitis and erysipelas: a network meta-analysis of randomized controlled trials. Arch Dermatol Res. 2024;316:603. [PMID: 39240378]

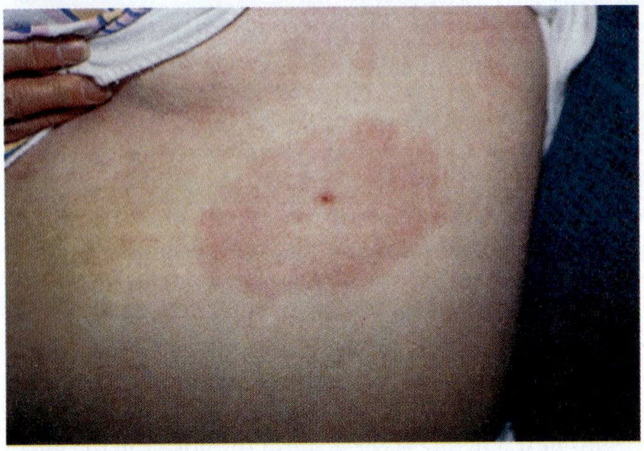

▲ **Figure 6–18.** Erythema migrans on trunk. Annular plaque with central clearing and central puncta from the bite. (Reproduced, with permission, from Soutor C, Hordinsky MK. *Clinical Dermatology.* The McGraw-Hill Companies; 2013.)

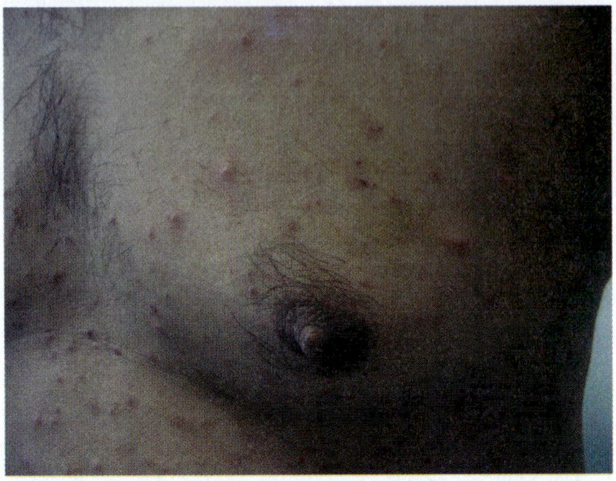

▲ **Figure 6–19.** Scabies. A polymorphic eruption of papulovesicles and excoriated papules scattered on the chest. (Used, with permission, from Kanade Shinkai, MD.)

ERYTHEMA MIGRANS

Erythema migrans is a unique cutaneous eruption that characterizes the localized or generalized early stage of Lyme disease (caused by *Borrelia burgdorferi*) (Figure 6–18) (see also Chapter 38).

Mahajan VK. Lyme disease: an overview. Indian Dermatol Online J. 2023;14:594. [PMID: 37727539]

PARASITIC INFESTATIONS

SCABIES

ESSENTIALS OF DIAGNOSIS

- Generalized very severe itching; infestation usually spares the head and neck.
- Burrows, vesicles, and pustules, especially on finger webs and in wrist creases.
- Mites, ova, and brown dots of feces (scybala) are visible microscopically.
- Red papules or nodules on the scrotum and on the penile glans and shaft are pathognomonic.

General Considerations

Scabies is caused by infestation with *Sarcoptes scabiei*, affecting over 200 million persons worldwide. Close physical contact for 15–20 minutes with an infected person is the typical mode of transmission. However, scabies may be acquired by contact with the bedding of an infested individual. Facility-associated scabies is common, primarily in long-term care facilities, and misdiagnosis is common. Index patients are usually older adults and immunosuppressed. When these patients are hospitalized, hospital-based epidemics can occur and are difficult to eradicate when health care workers become infected and spread the infestation to other patients.

Clinical Findings

A. Symptoms and Signs

Itching is almost always present and can be severe. The lesions consist of generalized excoriations with small pruritic vesicles, pustules, and "burrows" in the interdigital spaces of the hands and feet, on the heels of the palms, wrists, elbows, umbilicus, around the axillae, on or around the areolae (Figure 6–19), or on the penile shaft and scrotum in men. The burrow appears as a short, irregular mark, 2–3 mm long, and the width of a hair. Characteristic nodular lesions may occur on the scrotum or penis and along the posterior axillary line. The infestation usually spares the head and neck (though these areas may be involved in infants, older adults, and patients with AIDS).

Hyperkeratotic or crusted scabies presents as thick flaking scale. These areas contain millions of mites, and these patients are highly infectious. Pruritus is often absent. Patients with widespread hyperkeratotic scabies are at risk for superinfection with *S aureus*, which in some cases progresses to sepsis if left untreated. Crusted scabies is the cause of 83% of scabies outbreaks in institutions.

B. Laboratory Findings

The diagnosis should be confirmed by microscopic demonstration of the organism, ova, or feces in a mounted specimen, examined with tap water, mineral oil, or KOH. Best results are obtained when multiple lesions are scraped, choosing the best unexcoriated lesions from interdigital webs, wrists, elbows, or feet. A No. 15 blade is used to scrape each lesion until it is flat. Patients with crusted/hyperkeratotic scabies must be evaluated for immunosuppression (especially HIV and HTLV-1 infections) if no iatrogenic cause of immunosuppression is present.

Differential Diagnosis

Scabies must be distinguished from the various forms of pediculosis, from bedbug and flea bites, and from other causes of pruritus including dermatitis, nutritional dermatoses, and pruritus with excoriations. Crusted scabies must be distinguished from other causes of erythroderma (atopic dermatitis, drug reactions, psoriasis, mycosis fungoides, and others).

Treatment & Prognosis

Treatment is aimed at killing scabies mites and controlling the dermatitis, which can persist for months after effective eradication of the mites. Bedding and clothing should be laundered or set aside for 14 days in plastic bags while the patient is treated with prescription topical or oral agents. High heat (60°C) is required to kill the mites and ova. Treatment is aimed at all infected persons in a family or institutionalized group. Otherwise, reinfestations will likely occur, which is why scabies in nursing home patients, patients who are institutionalized, patients with a mental illness, and patients with AIDS may be much more difficult to treat.

1. Permethrin 5% cream—Treatment with permethrin, a highly effective and safe agent, consists of a single application from the neck down for 8–12 hours then washed off, repeated in 1 week. Patients often continue to itch for several weeks after treatment. Use of triamcinolone 0.1% cream helps resolve the dermatitis.

Pregnant patients should be treated only if they have documented scabies. Permethrin 5% cream once for 12 hours or 5% or 6% sulfur in petrolatum applied nightly for 3 nights from the neck down may be used.

Many failures in normal persons are related to incorrect use or incomplete treatment of the housing unit. In these cases, repeat treatment with permethrin once weekly for 2 weeks, with re-education regarding the method and extent of application, is suggested. In addition, there is a slowly increasing incidence of resistance to permethrin and other anti-scabetic agents.

2. Ivermectin—In immunocompetent individuals, 200 mcg/kg orally is effective in about 75% of cases with a single dose and in 95% of cases with two doses 2 weeks apart. Since the drug is not ovicidal, the second dose theoretically kills eggs that might have hatched after the first dose was given.

Ivermectin is often used in combination with permethrin. In immunosuppressed persons and those with crusted (hyperkeratotic) scabies, multiple doses of ivermectin (every 2 weeks for 2 or 3 doses) plus topical therapy with permethrin every 3 days to once weekly, depending on the degree of involvement, may be effective when topical treatment or oral therapy alone fail. A topical keratolytic (urea) should be used to help remove the scale of hyperkeratotic scabies, thereby decreasing the mite load.

Ivermectin can be beneficial in mass treatment to eradicate widespread infection. In endemic areas, mass intervention with ivermectin is effective in controlling both scabies and associated bacterial infections.

3. Spinosad—For treatment-resistant patients, 0.9% spinosad suspension, applied once over a time period longer than 6 hours, can be considered, though efficacy is lower than that for ivermectin or permethrin.

Al-Dabbagh J et al. The current available diagnostic tools and treatments of scabies and scabies variants: an updated narrative review. Medicine (Baltimore). 2023;102:e33805. [PMID: 37233429]

Amgarth-Duff I et al. Systematic review of the evidence for treatment and management of common skin conditions in resource-limited settings: an update. Trop Med Int Health. 2024;29:923. [PMID: 39396816]

Mbuagbaw L et al. Failure of scabies treatment: a systematic review and meta-analysis. Br J Dermatol. 2024;190:163. [PMID: 37625798]

PEDICULOSIS

ESSENTIALS OF DIAGNOSIS

- Pruritus with excoriation.
- Nits on hair shafts; lice on skin or clothes.
- Occasionally, sky-blue macules (maculae ceruleae) appear on the inner thighs or lower abdomen in pubic lice infestation.

General Considerations

Pediculosis is a parasitic infestation of the skin of the scalp, trunk, or pubic areas. Body lice usually occur among persons who live in overcrowded dwellings with inadequate hygiene facilities. Pubic lice may be sexually transmitted. Head lice may be transmitted by shared use of hats or combs. Adults in contact with children with head lice frequently acquire the infestation.

There are three different varieties: (1) **pediculosis capitis**, caused by *Pediculus humanus* var *capitis* (head louse); (2) **pediculosis corporis**, caused by *Pediculus humanus* var *corporis* (body louse); and (3) **pediculosis pubis**, caused by *Phthirus pubis* (pubic louse, "crabs").

Head and body lice are 3–4 mm long and similar in appearance. The "body louse" can seldom be found on the body because it comes onto the skin only to feed; it must be looked for in the seams of the clothing. Trench fever, relapsing fever, and typhus are transmitted by the body louse in countries where those diseases are endemic. In the United States, *Bartonella quintana* and *Rickettsia typhi*, the organisms that cause trench fever and typhus, have been found in lice infesting persons with housing instability.

Clinical Findings

In body lice infestations, itching may be very intense, and scratching may result in deep excoriations, especially over the upper shoulders, axillae, posterior flanks, and neck. In some cases, only itching is present, with few excoriations seen. Pyoderma (bacterial infection of the skin) may be the presenting sign. Diagnosis is made by examining the seams of clothing for nits and lice. Head lice present as scalp pruritus, often accompanied by erosions on the occipital scalp, posterior neck, and upper back. Diagnosis is made by finding lice on the scalp or small nits resembling pussy willow buds on the scalp hairs close to the skin. Nits are easiest to see above the ears and at the nape of the neck. Pubic lice infestations are occasionally generalized, particularly in hairy individuals; the lice may even be found on the eyelashes and in the scalp. Diagnosis is made by finding lice or nits on pubic hair, body hair, or eyelashes.

Differential Diagnosis

Head lice infestation must be distinguished from seborrheic dermatitis, body lice infestation from scabies and bedbug bites, and pubic lice infestation from anogenital pruritus and eczema.

Treatment

1. Pediculosis capitis—Permethrin 1% cream rinse (Nix) is a topical over-the-counter pediculicide and ovicide. Following application to the scalp and hair, it is left on for 8 hours and then rinsed off. Although it is the treatment of choice for head lice, permethrin resistance is common. Malathion lotion 1% (Ovide) is very effective but highly volatile and flammable, so application must be done in a well-ventilated room or outdoors. Topical ivermectin 0.5% lotion, benzyl alcohol 5%, Oxyphthirine® lotion, spinosad 0.9% suspension, dimethicone, and abametapir 0.74% lotion are additional agents that have efficacy against pediculosis capitis; of these, topical ivermectin is the most effective. All infested persons in a household, school, or other facility should ideally be treated at the same time. Other than topical ivermectin, topical therapies should be repeated 7–9 days after the initial treatment. For involvement of eyelashes, petrolatum is applied thickly twice daily for 8 days, and the remaining nits are plucked off. Systemic treatment options include oral ivermectin (200 mcg/kg orally, repeated in 7 days) (for children older than 5 years and > 15 kg), and oral TMP-SMZ (10 mg TMP/kg/day and 50 mg SMZ/kg/day divided twice daily for 10 days), which should be used in combination with a topical agent.

2. Pediculosis corporis—Body lice are treated by disposing of the infested clothing and addressing the patient's social situation.

3. Pediculosis pubis—Application of permethrin rinse 1% for 10 minutes or permethrin cream 5% for 8 hours to the pubis is effective. Sexual contacts should be treated. Clothes and bedclothes should be washed and dried at a high temperature.

Barbosa V et al. Scalp infection, inflammation, and infestation. Dermatol Clin. 2023;41:539. [PMID: 35619191]

Jordan KA et al. Lice: head, body, pubic. Pediatr Rev. 2024;45:57. [PMID: 38161152]

Strahan AG et al. Dermatologic care for refugees: effective management of scabies and pediculosis. 2024;113:e16. [PMID: 38820111]

SKIN LESIONS DUE TO OTHER ARTHROPODS

ESSENTIALS OF DIAGNOSIS

- Localized urticarial papules with pruritus.
- Lesions in linear groups of three ("breakfast, lunch, and dinner") are characteristic of bedbugs.
- Furuncle-like lesions containing live arthropods.
- Tender erythematous patches that migrate ("larva migrans").

General Considerations

Some arthropods (eg, mosquitoes and biting flies) are readily detected as they bite. Many others are not because they are too small, because there is no immediate reaction, or because they bite during sleep. Reactions are allergic and may be delayed for hours to days. Patients are most apt to consult a clinician when the lesions are multiple, and pruritus is intense.

Many persons react most severely to their earliest contacts with an arthropod, thus presenting with pruritic lesions when traveling, moving into new quarters, etc. Body lice, fleas, bedbugs, and mosquitoes should be considered. Bedbug exposure typically occurs in hotels and in housing with inadequate hygiene but also occurs in stable domiciles. Spiders are often incorrectly believed to be the source of bites, but they rarely attack humans. However, the brown recluse spider (*Loxosceles laeta*, *L reclusa*) may cause severe necrotic reactions and death due to intravascular hemolysis, and the black widow spider (*Latrodectus mactans*) may cause severe systemic symptoms and death. (See also Chapter 42.)

In addition to arthropod bites, the other most common causes of lesions due to exposures include venomous stings (wasps, hornets, bees, ants, scorpions) or bites (centipedes), furuncle-like lesions due to fly maggots or sand fleas in the skin, and a linear creeping eruption due to a migrating larva.

Clinical Findings

The diagnosis may be difficult when the patient has not noticed the initial attack but suffers a delayed reaction. Individual bites are often in clusters and tend to occur either on exposed parts (eg, midges and gnats) or under clothing, especially around the waist or at flexures (eg, small mites or insects in bedding or clothing). The reaction is often delayed for 1–24 hours or more. Pruritus is almost always present and may be all but intolerable once the patient starts to scratch. Secondary infection may follow scratching. Urticarial wheals are common. Papules may become vesicular. The diagnosis is aided by searching for exposure to arthropods and by considering the patient's occupation and recent activities.

The principal arthropods are as follows:

1. **Fleas:** Fleas are bloodsucking ectoparasites that feed on dogs, cats, humans, and other species. Flea saliva produces papular urticaria in sensitized individuals. To

break the life cycle of the flea, one must treat the home and pets, using quick-kill insecticides, residual insecticides, and a growth regulator.

2. **Bedbugs:** In crevices of beds or furniture; bites tend to occur in lines or clusters. Papular urticaria is a characteristic lesion of bedbug (*Cimex lectularius*) bites. Bedbugs are not restricted to any socioeconomic group and are a major health problem in some major metropolitan areas, especially in commercial and residential hotels.
3. **Ticks:** Usually picked up by brushing against low vegetation.
4. **Chiggers or red bugs:** These are larvae of trombiculid mites. A few species confined to particular regions and locally recognized habitats (eg, berry patches, woodland edges, lawns, brush turkey mounds in Australia, poultry farms) attack humans, often around the waist, on the ankles, or in flexures, raising intensely itching erythematous papules after a delay of many hours. The red chiggers may sometimes be seen in the center of papules that have not yet been scratched.
5. **Bird and rodent mites:** Larger than chiggers, bird mites infest birds and their nests. Bites are multiple anywhere on the body. Room air conditioning units may transmit outdoor bird mites to inhabitants of the room. Rodent mites from mice or rats may cause similar effects. If the domicile has evidence of rodent activity, then rodent mite dermatitis should be suspected, as the mites are rarely found. Pet rodents or birds may be infested with mites, maintaining the infestation.
6. **Mites in stored products:** These are white and almost invisible and infest products, such as copra, vanilla pods, sugar, straw, cottonseeds, and cereals. Persons who handle these products may be attacked, especially on the hands and forearms, and sometimes on the feet.
7. **Caterpillars of moths with urticating hairs:** The hairs are blown from cocoons or carried by emergent moths, causing severe and often seasonally recurrent outbreaks after mass emergence. The gypsy moth is a pest in the eastern United States.
8. **Tungiasis:** Tungiasis is due to the burrowing flea known as *Tunga penetrans* and is found in Africa, the West Indies, and South and Central America. The female burrows under the skin, sucks blood, swells to 0.5 cm, and then ejects her eggs onto the ground. Ulceration, lymphangitis, gangrene, and septicemia may result, in some cases with lethal effect. Simple surgical removal is usually performed.

Prevention

Arthropod infestations are best prevented by avoidance of contaminated areas, personal cleanliness, and disinfection of clothing, bedclothes, and furniture as indicated. Chiggers and mites can be repelled by permethrin applied to the head and clothing. (It is not necessary to remove clothing.) Bedbugs are no longer repelled by permethrin and can survive for up to 1 year without feeding. Aggressive cleaning, usually requiring removal of the affected occupant from the domicile, may be necessary to eradicate bedbug infestation in a residence.

Treatment

Living arthropods should be carefully removed with tweezers after alcohol application and preserved in alcohol for identification. In endemic Rocky Mountain spotted fever areas, ticks should not be removed with bare fingers.

Corticosteroid lotions or creams are helpful for the associated pruritus. Topical antibiotics may be applied if secondary infection is suspected. Localized persistent lesions may be treated with intralesional corticosteroids.

Stings produced by many arthropods may be alleviated by applying papain powder (Adolph's Meat Tenderizer) mixed with water, or aluminum chloride hexahydrate (Xerac AC).

Extracts from venom sacs of bees, wasps, yellow jackets, and hornets are available for immunotherapy of patients at risk for anaphylaxis.

Norton SA et al. Bed bugs. JAMA Dermatol 2024;160:1015. [PMID: 38985481]

Thomas C et al. Scabies, bedbug, and body lice infestations: a review. JAMA. 2024. [Epub ahead of print] [PMID: 39250129]

INFLAMMATORY NODULES

ERYTHEMA NODOSUM

ESSENTIALS OF DIAGNOSIS

- Painful nodules without ulceration on the anterior aspects of the legs.
- Slow regression over several weeks to resemble contusions.
- Women are predominantly affected by a ratio of 10:1 compared to men.
- Some cases are associated with infection, IBD, or medication exposure.
- Evaluation for the underlying cause is essential.

General Considerations

Erythema nodosum is a symptom complex of panniculitis characterized by tender, erythematous nodules that appear most commonly on the extensor surfaces of the lower legs. It usually lasts about 6 weeks and may recur. Most cases are idiopathic in nature. However, erythema nodosum can be a skin sign of systemic disease. Evaluation and management include making the diagnosis, treating the symptoms, and searching for an underlying cause. The disease may be associated with various infections—streptococcosis, primary coccidioidomycosis, other deep fungal infections, tuberculosis, *Yersinia pseudotuberculosis* and

Y enterocolitica infection, *Salmonella* and other GI pathogens, diverticulitis, or syphilis. It may accompany sarcoidosis, Behçet disease, and IBD. Erythema nodosum may be associated with pregnancy or with the use of oral contraceptives. It may occur secondary to medications or, more rarely, an underlying malignancy.

Clinical Findings

A. Symptoms and Signs

The subcutaneous swellings are exquisitely tender and may be preceded by fever, malaise, and arthralgia. They are most often located on the anterior surfaces of the legs below the knees, but may occur on the arms, trunk, and face. The lesions, 1–10 cm in diameter, are at first pink to red; with regression, all the various hues seen in a contusion can be observed (Figure 6–20), but, as a rule, the lesions do not ulcerate.

B. Laboratory Findings

Evaluation of patients presenting with acute erythema nodosum should include a careful history (including medication exposures) and physical examination. Significant findings include a history of prior upper respiratory infection, diarrheal illness, exposure to tuberculosis, or symptoms of any deep fungal infection endemic to the area. In patients lacking an obvious drug or medical cause, a CXR, a purified protein derivative, or blood interferon γ release assay (such as QuantiFERON) (see Pulmonary Tuberculosis in Chapter 9), and two consecutive ASO/DNAse B titers at 2- to 4-week intervals should be obtained. Coccidioidomycosis should be looked for in patients from endemic areas. If no underlying cause is found, only a small percentage of patients will go on to develop a significant underlying illness over the next year.

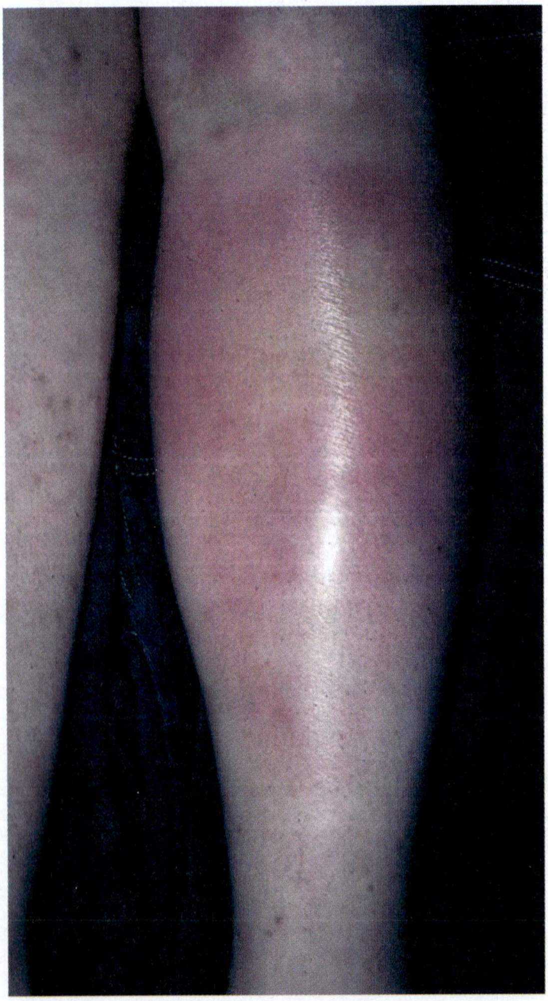

▲ Figure 6–20. Erythema nodosum. (Used, with permission, from TG Berger, MD, Dept Dermatology, UCSF.)

Differential Diagnosis

Unlike other forms of panniculitis, erythema nodosum rarely ulcerates. Erythema induratum from tuberculosis is seen on the posterior surfaces of the legs and may ulcerate. Lupus panniculitis presents as tender nodules in fatty areas of the buttocks and posterior arms and heals with depressed scars. In polyarteritis nodosa, the subcutaneous nodules are often associated with fixed livedo reticularis. In its late stages, erythema nodosum must be distinguished from simple bruises and contusions.

Treatment

The underlying cause should be identified and treated. Primary therapy is with NSAIDs in usual doses. Saturated solution of potassium iodide, 5–15 drops by mouth three times daily, results in prompt involution in many cases. Complete bed rest may be advisable if the lesions are painful. Systemic therapy directed against the lesions themselves may include corticosteroid therapy (see Chapter 30) (unless contraindicated by associated infection), dapsone, colchicine, or hydroxychloroquine.

Prognosis

The lesions usually disappear after about 6 weeks but may recur.

Lee B et al. Work-up and treatment for erythema nodosum. Skinmed. 2024;22:122. [PMID: 39089995]

SCALING DISORDERS

ATOPIC DERMATITIS

ESSENTIALS OF DIAGNOSIS

- Pruritic, xerotic, exudative, or lichenified eruption on face, neck, upper trunk, wrists, and hands, and in the antecubital and popliteal folds.
- Personal or family history of atopy (eg, asthma, allergic rhinitis, atopic dermatitis).
- Tendency to recur.
- Onset in childhood is most common; onset after age 30 is uncommon.

General Considerations

Atopic dermatitis (also known as eczema) has distinct presentations in persons of different ages and races. Diagnostic criteria for atopic dermatitis include pruritus, typical morphology and distribution (flexural lichenification, hand eczema, nipple eczema, and eyelid eczema in adults), onset in childhood, and chronicity. Also helpful are (1) a personal or family history of atopy (asthma, allergic rhinitis, atopic dermatitis), (2) xerosis-ichthyosis, (3) facial pallor with infraorbital darkening, (4) elevated serum IgE, and (5) repeated skin infections.

Clinical Findings

A. Symptoms and Signs

Itching is a key clinical feature and may be severe and prolonged. Ill-defined, scaly, red plaques affect the face, neck, and upper trunk. The flexural surfaces of elbows and knees are often involved. In chronic cases, the skin is dry and lichenified. In patients with darker skin with severe disease, pigmentation may be lost in lichenified areas. During acute flares, widespread redness with weeping, either diffusely or in discrete plaques, is common. Most patients with atopic dermatitis have skin disease before age 5; therefore, a new diagnosis of atopic dermatitis in an adult over age 30 should be made only after consultation with a dermatologist.

B. Laboratory Findings

Food allergy is an uncommon cause of flares of atopic dermatitis in adults. Eosinophilia and increased serum IgE levels may be present.

Differential Diagnosis

Atopic dermatitis must be distinguished from irritant or allergic contact dermatitis. Seborrheic dermatitis is less pruritic, with frequent scalp and central face involvement, greasy and scaly lesions, and responds quickly to therapy. Psoriasis is marked by sharply demarcated thickly scaled plaques on the elbows, knees, scalp, and intergluteal cleft. Secondary staphylococcal or herpetic infections may exacerbate atopic dermatitis and should be considered during hyperacute, weeping flares. An infra-auricular fissure is a cardinal sign of secondary staphylococcal infection.

Treatment

Patient education regarding gentle skin care and proper use of medications is critical to the successful management of atopic dermatitis.

A. General Measures

Atopic patients have hyperirritable skin. Anything that dries or irritates the skin may trigger dermatitis. Atopic individuals are sensitive to low humidity and often flare in the winter. Adults with atopic disorders should not bathe more than once daily. Soap should be confined to the armpits, groin, scalp, and feet. Washcloths and brushes should not be used. After rinsing, the skin should be patted dry (not rubbed) and then immediately—within minutes—covered with a thin film of an emollient or a corticosteroid as needed. Plain petrolatum can be used if contact dermatitis resulting from additives in medication is suspected. Skin may be irritated by rough fabrics, including wools and acrylics. Cottons are preferable, but synthetic blends are also tolerated. Other triggers may include sweating, ointments, and heat.

B. Local Treatment

Corticosteroids should be applied sparingly to the dermatitis once or twice daily. Their potency should be appropriate to the severity of the dermatitis. In general, for treatment of lesions on the body (excluding genitalia, axillary or crural folds), one should begin with triamcinolone 0.1% or a stronger corticosteroid, then taper to hydrocortisone or another slightly stronger mild corticosteroid (alclometasone, desonide). **It is vital that patients taper off corticosteroids and substitute emollients as the dermatitis clears to avoid the side effects of corticosteroids.** Tapering is also important to avoid dermatitis flares that may follow abrupt cessation. Tacrolimus ointment (Protopic 0.03% or 0.1%), pimecrolimus (Elidel 1%), crisaborole (Eucrisa 2%), ruxolitinib (Opzelura 1.5%), tapinarof (Vtama 1%), and roflumilast creams (Zoryve 15%) are nonsteroidal topical medications that may be effective in managing atopic dermatitis when applied daily or twice daily (see Table 6–2). These noncorticosteroid medications prevent complications of long-term corticosteroid use, including atrophy or striae. They are safe for application on the face and eyelids but are more expensive than generic topical corticosteroids.

There is a US FDA black box warning for both topical tacrolimus and pimecrolimus due to concerns about the development of T-cell lymphoma. A systematic review and meta-analysis found a weak association between topical calcineurin inhibitor use and lymphoma; however, the absolute risk is very low. The number needed to harm is estimated at 30,000 adults and 200,000 children.

The treatment of atopic dermatitis is dictated by the pattern of the dermatitis—acute/weepy, subacute/scaly, or chronic/lichenified.

1. Acute weeping lesions—Staphylococcal or herpetic superinfection should be excluded by bacterial and viral cultures. Aluminum subacetate solution (Domeboro or burow solution) or colloidal oatmeal can be used to bathe for 10–30 minutes two to four times daily. Lesions on extremities may be bandaged for protection at night. Use high-potency corticosteroids after soaking but spare the face and body folds. Tacrolimus is usually not tolerated at this stage. Systemic corticosteroids may be required. An allergic or irritating exposure should also be considered when acute weeping lesions are present since contact dermatitis is more likely to develop in atopic patients.

2. Subacute or scaly lesions—The lesions are dry but still red and pruritic. Mid- to high-potency corticosteroids in ointment form should be continued until skin lesions are cleared and itching is decreased substantially. At that point, patients should begin a 2- to 4-week taper from twice-daily to daily dosing with topical corticosteroids to reliance on emollients, with occasional use of corticosteroids only to inflamed areas. It is preferable to switch to daily use of a low-potency corticosteroid instead of further tapering the frequency of usage of a more potent corticosteroid. Tacrolimus and pimecrolimus may be substituted if corticosteroids cannot be stopped completely.

3. Chronic, dry, lichenified lesions—Thickened and usually well demarcated, they are best treated with high-potency to ultra–high-potency corticosteroid ointments. Nightly occlusion for 2–6 weeks may enhance the initial response. Adding tar preparations, such as liquor carbonis detergens 10% in Aquaphor or 2% crude coal tar, may be beneficial.

4. Maintenance treatment—Once symptoms have improved, constant application of effective moisturizers is recommended to prevent flares. In patients with moderate disease, use of topical anti-inflammatories only on weekends or three times weekly can prevent flares.

C. Systemic and Adjuvant Therapy

Increasingly, providers try to avoid the use of systemic steroids in the treatment of atopic dermatitis. Systemic corticosteroids are indicated only for severe acute exacerbations. Oral prednisone dosages should be high enough to suppress the dermatitis quickly, usually starting with 1 mg/kg daily and tapering off over a period of 2–4 weeks. Owing to the chronic nature of atopic dermatitis and the side effects of long-term systemic corticosteroids, **ongoing use of these agents is not recommended for maintenance therapy**. Bedtime doses of hydroxyzine, diphenhydramine, or doxepin may be helpful via their sedative properties to mitigate perceived pruritus, though multiple recent studies report no benefit from the use of non-sedating H_1-blockers in suppressing itch in patients with eczema. Dupilumab and the newer IL-13 inhibitors tralokinumab and lebrikizumab are targeted immunomodulators with minimal systemic adverse effects (hypersensitivity). Janus kinase (JAK) inhibitors (upadacitinib, abrocitinib), cyclosporine, mycophenolate mofetil, methotrexate, or azathioprine may also be used for the most severe and recalcitrant cases.

Complications of Treatment

The clinician should monitor for skin atrophy. Fissures, crusts, erosions, or pustules may indicate staphylococcal or herpetic infection clinically. Eczema herpeticum (herpes simplex superinfection) is manifested by monomorphic vesicles, crusts, or scalloped erosions superimposed on atopic dermatitis or other extensive eczematous processes and is treated with oral or intravenous acyclovir. Systemic anti-staphylococcal antibiotics should be given only if indicated and guided by bacterial culture. Cultures to exclude methicillin-resistant *S aureus* are recommended. In this setting, continuing and augmenting the topical anti-inflammatory treatment often improves the dermatitis despite the presence of infection.

Prognosis

Atopic dermatitis runs a chronic or intermittent course. Affected adults may have only hand dermatitis. Prognostic factors for persistence into adulthood include generalized disease or onset early in childhood and asthma. Only 40–60% of these patients have lasting remissions.

Chu AWL et al. Systemic treatments for atopic dermatitis (eczema): systematic review and network meta-analysis of randomized trials. J Allergy Clin Immunol. 2023;152:1470. [PMID: 37678577]
Clebak KT et al. Atopic dermatitis. Prim Care. 2023;50:191. [PMID: 37105601]
Schuler CF 4th et al. Novel insights into atopic dermatitis. J Allergy Clin Immunol. 2023;151:1145. [PMID: 36428114]

LICHEN SIMPLEX CHRONICUS (Circumscribed Neurodermatitis)

ESSENTIALS OF DIAGNOSIS

- Chronic itching and scratching.
- Lichenified lesions with exaggerated skin lines overlying a thickened, well-circumscribed, scaly plaque.
- Predilection for nape of neck, wrists, external surfaces of forearms, lower legs, and genitals.

General Considerations

Lichen simplex chronicus represents a self-perpetuating scratch-itch cycle that is hard to disrupt.

Clinical Findings

Intermittent itching incites the patient to scratch the lesions and may interfere with sleep. Dry, hypertrophic, lichenified plaques appear on the neck, wrists, ankles, or perineum (Figure 6–21). The patches are rectangular, thickened, and hyperpigmented. The skin lines are exaggerated.

Differential Diagnosis

This disorder can be differentiated from plaque-like lesions such as psoriasis (redder lesions having whiter scales on the elbows, knees, and scalp and nail findings) (Figure 6–22), lichen planus (violaceous, usually smaller polygonal

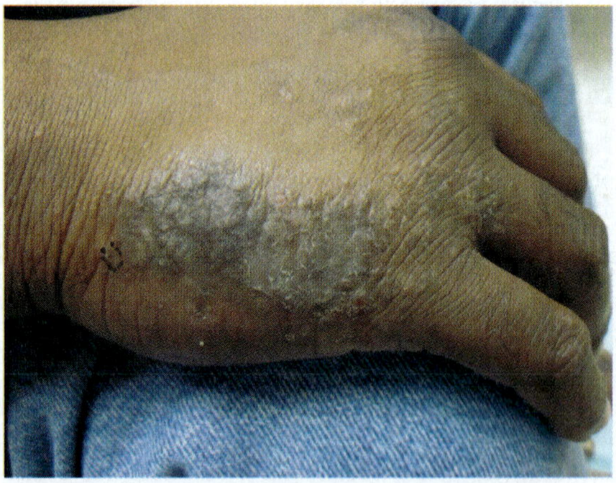

▲ **Figure 6–21.** Lichen simplex chronicus on the hand. (Used, with permission, from Lindy Fox, MD.)

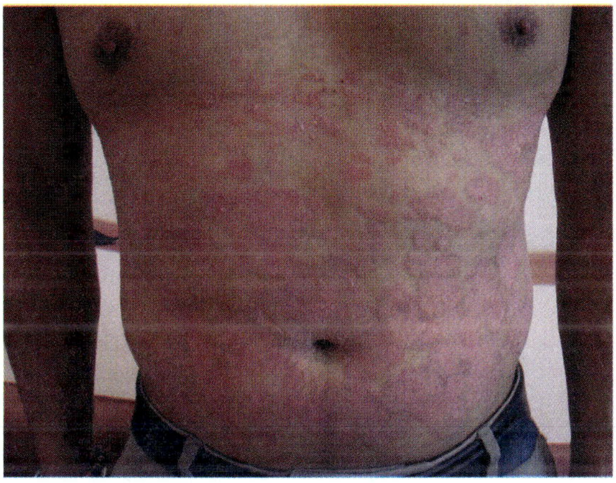

▲ **Figure 6–22.** Extensive plaque psoriasis involving trunk of person with dark skin type. (Used, with permission, from Kanade Shinkai, MD.)

papules), and nummular (coin-shaped) dermatitis. Lichen simplex chronicus may complicate chronic atopic dermatitis or scabetic infestation.

Treatment

For lesions in extragenital regions, ultra-high potency topical corticosteroids are effective, with or without occlusion, when used twice daily for several weeks (Table 6–2). In some patients, flurandrenolide (Cordran) tape may be effective since it prevents scratching and rubbing of the lesion. The injection of triamcinolone acetonide suspension (5–10 mg/mL) into the lesions may occasionally be curative. Continuous occlusion with a flexible hydrocolloid dressing for 7 days at a time for 1–2 months may also be helpful. For genital lesions, see the section Pruritus Ani.

Prognosis

The disease tends to remit during treatment but may recur or develop at another site.

Malhi K et al. Lichen simplex chronicus of the scalp: A clinical and trichoscopic perspective. Indian J Dermatol Venereol Leprol. 2024;90:819. [PMID: 39361858]

Moshkovich M et al. Lichen simplex chronicus: clinical perspectives and emerging therapeutic strategies. Am J Clin Dermatol. 2025;26:895. [PMID: 40855389]

PSORIASIS

ESSENTIALS OF DIAGNOSIS

- Silvery scales on bright red, well-demarcated plaques, usually on the knees, elbows, and scalp.
- Nails: pitting and onycholysis (separation of the nail plate from the bed).
- Mild itching is common.
- May be associated with psoriatic arthritis.
- Histopathology is helpful.

General Considerations

Psoriasis is a common benign, chronic inflammatory skin disease with both a genetic basis and known environmental triggers. Injury or irritation of normal skin tends to induce lesions of psoriasis at the site (Koebner phenomenon). Obesity worsens psoriasis, and significant weight loss may lead to substantial improvement. Psoriasis has several variants—the most common is the plaque type, and hand involvement is also common. Eruptive (guttate) psoriasis consisting of numerous, smaller lesions 3–10 mm in diameter occurs occasionally after streptococcal pharyngitis. Rarely, life-threatening forms (generalized pustular psoriasis and erythrodermic psoriasis) may occur.

Clinical Findings

There are often no symptoms, but itching may occur and be severe. Favored sites include the scalp, elbows, knees, palms and soles, and nails. The lesions are red, sharply defined plaques covered with silvery scale (Figure 6–22). The glans penis and vulva may be affected. Occasionally, only the flexures (axillae, inguinal areas) are involved (termed inverse psoriasis). Fine stippling ("pitting") in the nails is highly suggestive of psoriasis (Figure 6–23) as is onycholysis. The combination of red plaques with silvery scales on elbows and knees, with scaliness in the scalp or nail findings, is diagnostic. Patients with psoriasis often have a pink or red intergluteal fold. Not all patients have findings in all locations. Some patients have mainly hand or foot psoriasis with minimal findings elsewhere. There may be associated arthritis that is most commonly distal and oligoarticular, although polyarticular, axial, and arthritis mutilans involvement may occur. The psychosocial impact of psoriasis is a major factor in determining the treatment of the patient.

Differential Diagnosis

Psoriasis lesions are well demarcated and affect extensor surfaces—in contrast to atopic dermatitis, with poorly

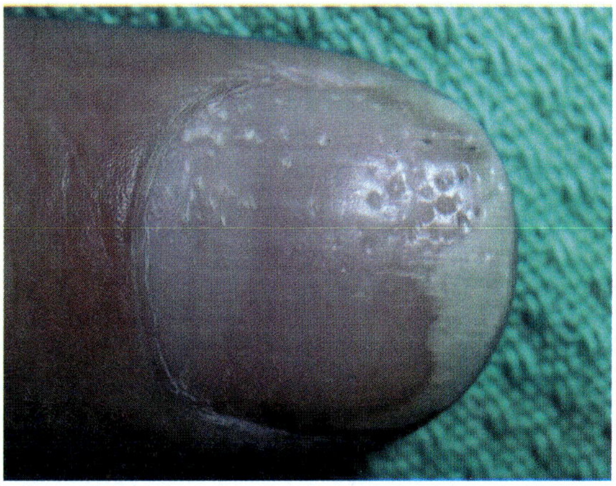

▲ **Figure 6–23.** Nail pitting due to psoriasis in a patient with dark skin. (Reproduced, with permission, from Richard P. Usatine, MD, in Usatine RP, Smith MA, Mayeaux EJ Jr, Chumley H. *The Color Atlas of Family Medicine*, 2nd ed. McGraw-Hill, 2013.)

demarcated plaques in flexural distribution. In body folds, scraping and culture for *Candida* and examination of scalp and nails will distinguish inverse psoriasis from intertrigo and candidiasis. Dystrophic changes in nails may mimic onychomycosis, and a KOH preparation or fungal culture is valuable in diagnosis. The cutaneous features of reactive arthritis, pityriasis rosea, SLE, and syphilis mimic psoriasis.

Treatment

There are many therapeutic options in psoriasis to be chosen according to the extent (body surface area [BSA] affected) and the presence of other findings (for example, arthritis). Certain medications, such as β-blockers, antimalarials, statins, lithium, and prednisone tapering, may flare or worsen psoriasis. Patients with moderate to severe psoriasis should be managed by or in conjunction with a dermatologist.

A. Limited Disease

For patients with large plaques and < 10% of the BSA involved, the easiest regimen is to use a high-potency to ultra–high-potency topical corticosteroid cream or ointment. It is best to restrict the ultra–high-potency corticosteroids to 2–3 weeks of twice-daily use and then use them in a pulse fashion three or four times on weekends or switch to a mid-potency corticosteroid. Topical corticosteroids rarely induce a lasting remission. Initially, patients may be treated with twice-daily topical corticosteroids plus a vitamin D analog (calcipotriene ointment 0.005% or calcitriol ointment 0.003%) twice daily. This rapidly clears the lesions; eventually, the topical corticosteroids are stopped, and once- or twice-daily application of the vitamin D analog is continued long-term. Calcipotriene usually cannot be applied to the groin or face because of irritation. Treatment of extensive psoriasis with vitamin D analogs may result in hypercalcemia so that the maximum dose for calcipotriene is 100 g/week and for calcitriol it is 200 g/week. Calcipotriene is incompatible with many topical corticosteroids (but not halobetasol), so if used concurrently, it must be applied at a different time. For patients with numerous small papules and plaques, such as guttate psoriasis, narrowband UVB phototherapy is the best therapy.

For thick plaques on the scalp, start with a daily tar shampoo. Additional treatments include 6% salicylic acid gel (eg, Keralyt), P & S solution (phenol, mineral oil, and glycerin), or fluocinolone acetonide 0.01% in oil (Derma-Smoothe/FS) under a shower cap at night, and shampoo in the morning. In order of increasing potency, triamcinolone 0.1%, fluocinolone, betamethasone dipropionate, amcinonide, and clobetasol are available in solution form for use on the scalp twice daily. Tacrolimus ointment 0.1% or 0.03% or pimecrolimus cream 1% may be effective in intertriginous, genital, and facial psoriasis, where potent corticosteroids are not recommended due to skin atrophy. Two additional nonsteroidal topical therapies approved to treat psoriasis are roflumilast cream 0.3% (phosphodiesterase-4 inhibitor) and tapinarof cream 1% (aryl hydrocarbon receptor agonist).

B. Moderate Disease

Psoriasis affecting 10–30% of the patient's BSA is frequently treated with narrowband UVB phototherapy, either in a medical office or via a home light unit. Systemic agents listed below may also be used.

C. Moderate to Severe Disease

If psoriasis in a given location is severe or involves > 30% of the body surface, it is difficult to treat with topical agents. These patients may be best managed in partnership with a dermatologist, especially when considering systemic therapy. The treatment of choice is outpatient narrowband UVB (NB-UVB) three times weekly. Clearing occurs in an average of 7 weeks, and maintenance may be required. Psoriatic arthritis may require distinct treatments and benefits from management in partnership with a rheumatologist or dermatologist.

Methotrexate is effective for severe psoriasis in doses up to 25 mg once weekly according to published protocols, however, its use largely has been supplanted by biologics and advanced oral systemic therapies (eg apremilast, deucravacitinib). Long-term methotrexate use may be associated with cirrhosis. After receiving a 3.5–4-g cumulative dose, the patient should be referred to a hepatologist for evaluation. Administration of folic acid, 1–2 mg daily, can eliminate nausea caused by methotrexate without compromising efficacy.

Acitretin, a synthetic retinoid, is most effective for pustular psoriasis in oral dosages of 0.5–0.75 mg/kg/day. Liver enzymes and serum lipids must be checked periodically. Because acitretin is a teratogen and persists for 2–3 years in fat, women of childbearing age must wait at least 3 years after completing acitretin treatment before considering pregnancy. When used as single agents, retinoids will flatten psoriatic plaques but will rarely result in complete clearing. Retinoids find their greatest use when combined with phototherapy—either UVB or PUVA, with which they are synergistic.

Among the systemic therapies for psoriasis, the IL-12/23 monoclonal antibodies (ustekinumab), IL-23 monoclonal antibodies (guselkumab, risankizumab, and tildrakizumab), oral tyrosine kinase 2 (TYK2) inhibitors (deucravacitinib), and IL-17 monoclonal antibodies (bimekizumab, secukinumab, brodalumab, and ixekizumab) are generally the most effective options. Although the TNF inhibitors etanercept, infliximab, certolizumab, and adalimumab are effective in pustular and chronic plaque psoriasis and for the associated arthritis, their use largely has been supplanted by IL-23 or IL-17 inhibitors due to their superior efficacy and safety profiles. Infliximab provides the most rapid response and can be used for severe pustular or erythrodermic flares. All TNF inhibitors can also induce or worsen psoriasis. The IL-36 receptor antibody spesolimab remains the only therapy approved specifically for generalized pustular psoriasis.

The oral phosphodiesterase-4 inhibitor apremilast is an approved option for psoriasis and psoriatic arthritis with minimal immunosuppressive effects and requires no laboratory monitoring. Deucravacitinib, an oral TYK2 inhibitor, is approved for moderate-to-severe plaque psoriasis and has the benefit of once-daily dosing. Cyclosporine dramatically improves psoriasis and may be used to control severe cases.

Prognosis

The course of psoriasis may be chronic and unpredictable, and it may be refractory to treatment. Patients (especially those older than 40 years) should be monitored for metabolic syndrome, which correlates with the severity of their skin disease. Complications of systemic therapy occur, and active monitoring for infection is needed.

Ferrara F et al. Current therapeutic overview and future perspectives regarding the treatment of psoriasis. Int Immunopharmacol. 2024;143:113388. [PMID: 39405929]
Ferrara F et al. Therapeutic advances in psoriasis: from biologics to emerging oral small molecules. Antibodies. 2024;13:76. [PMID: 39311381]
Lee H et al. Challenges and future trends in the treatment of psoriasis. Int J Mol Sci 2023;24:13313. [PMID: 37686119]
Wride AM et al. Biologics for psoriasis. Dermatol Clin 2024;42:339. [PMID: 38796266]

PITYRIASIS ROSEA

ESSENTIALS OF DIAGNOSIS

- Oval, fawn-colored, scaly eruption following cleavage lines of trunk.
- Herald patch precedes eruption by 1–2 weeks.
- Occasional pruritus.

General Considerations

Pityriasis rosea is a common mild, acute inflammatory disease that is 50% more common in females. Young adults are principally affected, mostly in the spring or fall. Concurrent household cases have been reported.

Clinical Findings

Itching is common but usually mild. The diagnosis is made by finding one or more classic lesions, such as oval, fawn-colored plaques up to 2 cm in diameter. The centers of a few lesions may have a characteristic crinkled or "cigarette paper" appearance and a collarette scale, ie, a thin bit of scale that is bound at the periphery and free in the center. Lesions follow cleavage lines on the trunk (so-called Christmas tree pattern, Figure 6–24), and the proximal portions of the extremities are often involved. A variant that affects the flexures (axillae and groin), so-called inverse pityriasis rosea, and a papular variant, especially in patients with more darkly pigmented skin types, also occur. An initial lesion ("herald patch") that is often larger than the later lesions often precedes the general eruption by 1–2 weeks. The eruption usually lasts 6–8 weeks and heals without scarring.

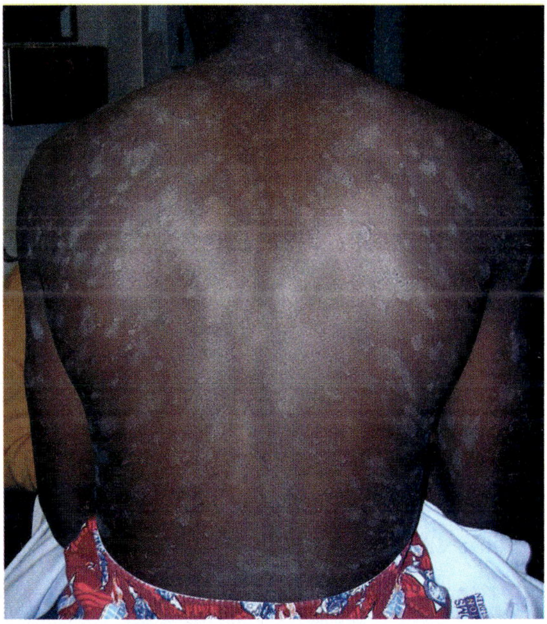

Figure 6–24. Pityriasis rosea with scaling lesions following skin lines and resembling a Christmas tree. (Used, with permission, from EJ Mayeaux, MD, in Usatine RP, Smith MA, Mayeaux EJ Jr, Chumley HS. *The Color Atlas and Synopsis of Family Medicine*, 3rd ed. McGraw-Hill, 2019.)

Differential Diagnosis

Serologic testing for syphilis should be performed if clinical risk factors are present. Palmar and plantar or mucous membrane lesions or adenopathy are features suggestive of secondary syphilis. Tinea corporis may present with a few red, slightly scaly plaques. Typically, the number of plaques of tinea corporis is significantly fewer than the number seen in pityriasis rosea. A KOH examination should be performed to exclude a fungal cause. Seborrheic dermatitis on occasion presents on the body with poorly demarcated patches over the sternum, in the pubic area, and in the axillae. Tinea versicolor lacks the typical collarette-rimmed lesions. Guttate or plaque psoriasis is an important diagnostic consideration and biopsy can help differentiate these from pityriasis rosea. Certain medications and immunizations rarely may induce a skin eruption mimicking pityriasis rosea. A pityriasis rosea–like eruption has been reported in association with SARS-CoV-2 infection and COVID-19 vaccination.

Treatment

Pityriasis rosea often requires no treatment unless patients are symptomatic. In darker-skinned individuals, more aggressive management may be indicated because dyspigmentation of lesions may result. While well-designed clinical trials have not demonstrated highly effective treatments, most dermatologists recommend UVB treatments or a short course of prednisone for severe or severely symptomatic cases. For mild to moderate cases, topical corticosteroids of medium strength (triamcinolone 0.1%) and oral antihistamines may be used if pruritus is bothersome. The role of macrolide antibiotics is not evidence-based.

Prognosis

Pityriasis rosea is usually an acute self-limiting illness that typically disappears in about 6 weeks, although prolonged variants have been reported.

Cao AL et al. From the Cochrane Library: interventions for pityriasis rosea. J Am Acad Dermatol. 2023;89:404. [PMID: 37062465]
Mashoudy KD et al. Beyond the herald patch: exploring the complex landscape of pityriasis rosea. Am J Clin Dermatol. 2025;26:237. [PMID: 39798062]
Mendez A et al. From the Cochrane Library: interventions for pityriasis rosea. JMIR Dermatol. 2023;6:e45388. [PMID: 37632939]

SEBORRHEIC DERMATITIS

ESSENTIALS OF DIAGNOSIS

- Dry scales and underlying erythema.
- Scalp, central face, presternal, interscapular areas, umbilicus, and body folds.

General Considerations

Seborrheic dermatitis is an acute or chronic dermatitis that often coexists with psoriasis and is associated with inflammation due to *Malassezia* species.

Clinical Findings

The scalp, face, chest, back, umbilicus, eyelid margins, genitalia, and body folds have dry scales (dandruff) or oily yellowish scurf (Figure 6–25). Pruritus is a variable finding. Patients with Parkinson disease, patients with HIV, and patients who become acutely ill often have seborrheic dermatitis.

Differential Diagnosis

There is a spectrum from seborrheic dermatitis to scalp psoriasis. Extensive seborrheic dermatitis may simulate intertrigo in flexural areas, but scalp, face, and sternal involvement suggests seborrheic dermatitis.

Treatment

A. Seborrhea of the Scalp

Shampoos that contain zinc pyrithione or selenium are used daily if possible. These may be alternated with ketoconazole shampoo (1% or 2%) used twice weekly. A combination of shampoos is used in refractory cases. Tar shampoos are also effective for milder cases and for scalp psoriasis. Topical corticosteroid solutions or lotions are then added if necessary and are used twice daily. (See treatment for scalp psoriasis, above.)

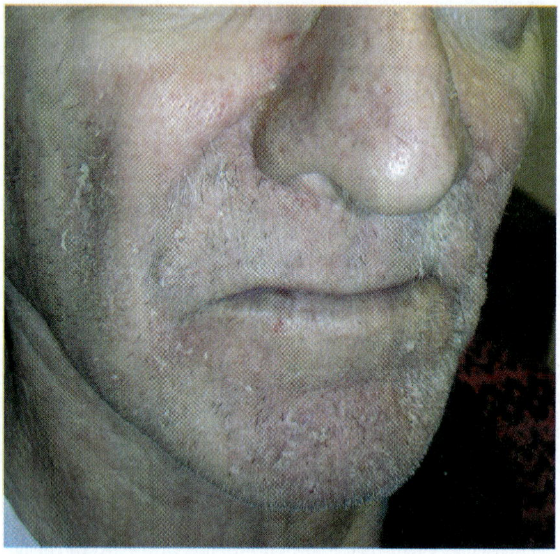

▲ **Figure 6–25.** **Close-up of seborrheic dermatitis showing flaking skin and erythema around the beard region.** (Reproduced, with permission, from Richard P. Usatine, MD, in Usatine RP, Smith MA, Mayeaux EJ Jr, Chumley H. *The Color Atlas of Family Medicine*, 2nd ed. McGraw-Hill, 2013.)

B. Facial Seborrheic Dermatitis

The mainstay of therapy is a mild corticosteroid (hydrocortisone 1%, alclometasone, desonide) used intermittently and not near the eyes. If the disorder cannot be controlled with intermittent use of a mild topical corticosteroid alone, ketoconazole 2% cream is added twice daily. Topical tacrolimus and pimecrolimus are steroid-sparing alternatives and may be more effective than antifungal therapy.

C. Seborrheic Dermatitis of Nonhairy or Intertriginous Areas

Low-potency corticosteroid creams (ie, 1% or 2.5% hydrocortisone, desonide, or alclometasone dipropionate) are highly effective when applied twice daily for 5–7 days and then once or twice weekly for maintenance as necessary. Selenium lotion, ketoconazole, or clotrimazole gel or cream may be a useful adjunct. Tacrolimus or pimecrolimus topically can obviate the use of corticosteroids in chronic cases. Roflumilast foam 0.3%, a topical (phosphodiesterase-4) PDE-4 inhibitor, was approved in 2023 for the treatment of seborrheic dermatitis in people aged 9 and older. It can be used on all affected areas of the body, including hair-bearing areas.

D. Involvement of Eyelid Margins

"Marginal blepharitis" usually responds to gentle cleaning of the lid margins nightly as needed, with undiluted baby shampoo or eyelid cleanser using a cotton swab.

Prognosis

The tendency is for lifelong recurrences. Individual outbreaks may last weeks, months, or years.

Blauvelt A et al. Roflumilast foam 0.3% for adolescent and adult patients with seborrheic dermatitis: a randomized, double-blinded, vehicle-controlled, phase 3 trial. J Am Acad Dermatol. 2024;90:986. [PMID: 38253129]
Turchin I et al. Current understanding of seborrheic dermatitis: epidemiology, burden of disease, and pathophysiology. J Cutan Med Surg. 2025;29(4_suppl):5S. [PMID: 40965103]
Turchin I et al. Current understanding of seborrheic dermatitis: treatment options. J Cutan Med Surg. 2025;29(4_suppl):24S. [PMID: 40965088]
Vano-Galvan S et al. A comprehensive literature review and an international expert consensus on the management of scalp seborrheic dermatitis in adults. Eur J Dermatol. 2024;34:4. [PMID: 38919137]

LICHEN PLANUS

ESSENTIALS OF DIAGNOSIS

- Pruritic, violaceous, flat-topped papules with fine white streaks and symmetric distribution.
- Lacy or erosive lesions of the buccal, vulvar, and vaginal mucosa; nail dystrophy.
- Commonly seen along linear scratch marks (Koebner phenomenon) on anterior wrists, penis, and legs.
- Diagnostic histopathology.

General Considerations

Lichen planus is an inflammatory pruritic disease of the skin and mucous membranes characterized by distinctive papules with a predilection for the flexor surfaces and trunk. The prevalence in the United States is 0.39%. The three cardinal findings are typical skin lesions, mucosal lesions, and histopathologic features of band-like infiltration of lymphocytes in the upper dermis. Allergy to mercury and other metal-containing amalgams can trigger oral lesions identical to lichen planus.

Clinical Findings

The lesions are violaceous, flat-topped, angulated papules, up to 1 cm in diameter, discrete or in clusters (Figure 6–26), with very fine white streaks (Wickham striae) on the flexor surfaces of the wrists and ankles; on lower back; and on mucous membranes, including the penis, lips, tongue, buccal, vulvar, vaginal, esophageal, and anorectal mucosa. Itching is mild to severe. The papules may become bullous or eroded. The disease may be generalized. Mucous membrane lesions have a lacy white network overlying them that may be confused with leukoplakia. The presence of oral and vulvovaginal lichen planus in the same patient is common. Patients with both these mucous membranes involved are at much higher risk for esophageal lichen planus. Lichen planus is also a cause of alopecia and nail dystrophy. The Koebner phenomenon (appearance of lesions in areas of trauma) may be seen.

A special form of lichen planus is the erosive or ulcerative variety, a major problem in the mouth or genitalia.

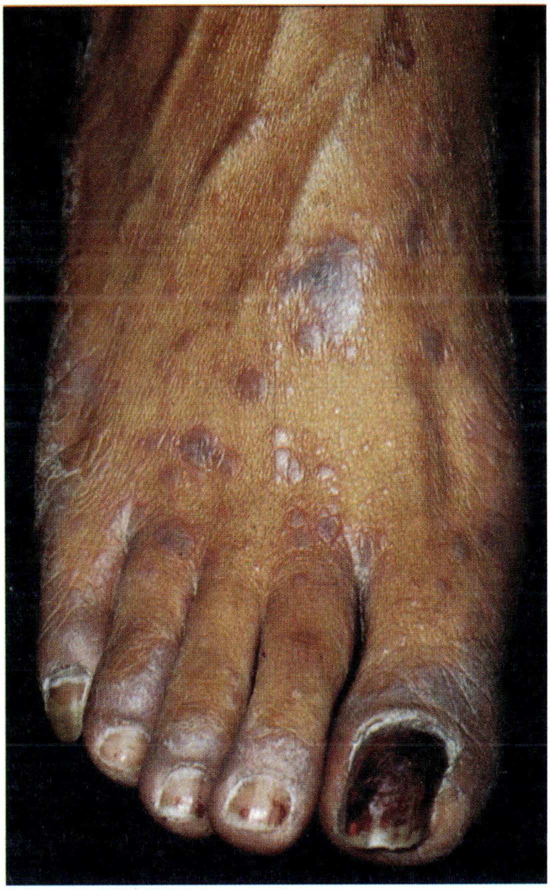

▲ **Figure 6–26.** Lichen planus. (Used, with permission, from TG Berger, MD, Dept Dermatology, UCSF.)

Squamous cell carcinoma develops in up to 5% of patients with erosive oral or genital lichen planus and may occur in esophageal lichen planus. There is also an increased risk of squamous cell carcinoma developing in lesions of hypertrophic lichen planus on the lower extremities.

Differential Diagnosis

Lichen planus must be distinguished from similar lesions produced by medications and other papular lesions, such as psoriasis, lichen simplex chronicus, graft-versus-host disease, and syphilis. Lichen planus on the mucous membranes must be differentiated from leukoplakia. Erosive oral lesions require biopsy and often direct immunofluorescence for diagnosis since lichen planus may simulate other erosive diseases, especially autoimmune blistering diseases that involve the oral mucosa.

Treatment

A. Topical Therapy

Superpotent topical corticosteroids applied twice daily are most helpful for localized disease in nonflexural areas. Alternatively, high-potency corticosteroid cream or ointment may be used nightly under thin, pliable plastic film.

Topical tacrolimus appears effective in oral and vaginal erosive lichen planus, but long-term therapy is required to prevent relapse. If tacrolimus is used, lesions must be observed carefully for development of squamous cell carcinoma. Since absorption can occur through mucous membranes, serum tacrolimus levels should be checked at least once if widespread mucosal application (> 5–10 cm^2) is used. If the erosive oral lichen planus lesions are adjacent to a metal-containing amalgam, removal of the amalgam may result in clearing of the erosions.

B. Systemic Therapy

NB-UVB, bath PUVA, oral PUVA, and the combination of an oral retinoid plus PUVA (re-PUVA) are all forms of phototherapy that can improve lichen planus. Hydroxychloroquine (5 mg/kg once daily), acitretin (10–25 mg orally daily), cyclosporine (3–5 mg/kg orally daily), and mycophenolate mofetil (1–3 g orally daily) can also be effective in mucosal and cutaneous lichen planus. Apremilast, oral JAK inhibitors, and anti-IL-12/23 and anti-IL-17 agents have been used with success in refractory cases. Systemic corticosteroids may be required in severe cases or in circumstances where the most rapid response to treatment is desired. Unfortunately, relapse almost always occurs as the corticosteroids are tapered, making this therapy an impractical option for the management of chronic lichen planus.

Prognosis

Lichen planus is a benign disease, but it may persist for months or years and may be recurrent. Hypertrophic lichen planus and oral lesions tend to be especially persistent, and neoplastic degeneration has been described in chronically eroded lesions.

Haigh C et al. Diagnosis and management of vulval lesions. Curr Opin Obstet Gynecol. 2025;37:317. [PMID: 40742979]
Louisy A et al. Oral lichen planus: an update on diagnosis and management. Am J Clin Dermatol. 2024;25:35. [PMID: 37713153]
Safari-Kish B et al. Treatment strategies for erosive genital lichen planus: a systematic review of therapeutic modalities and emerging breakthroughs. Health Sci Rep. 2024;7:e70129. [PMID: 39410948]

CUTANEOUS LUPUS ERYTHEMATOSUS

ESSENTIALS OF DIAGNOSIS

- Localized violaceous red plaques, usually on the head (discoid lupus erythematosus) or the trunk.
- Scaling, follicular plugging, atrophy, dyspigmentation, and telangiectasia of involved areas.
- Photosensitivity.
- Distinctive histology.

General Considerations

Common forms of cutaneous lupus include chronic cutaneous lupus erythematosus (CCLE), of which discoid lupus erythematosus (DLE) is the most common subtype, and erythematous nonscarring red plaques of subacute cutaneous lupus erythematosus (SCLE). All occur most frequently in photoexposed areas. Permanent hair loss and loss of pigmentation are common sequelae of discoid lesions.

SLE is discussed in Chapter 23. Patients with SLE frequently have acute cutaneous lupus erythematosus (ACLE) lesions but may also have CCLE or SCLE lesions. Ten percent of patients with SLE have discoid skin lesions, and 5% of patients with discoid lesions have SLE.

Clinical Findings

A. Symptoms and Signs

Symptoms are usually mild. In DLE, the lesions consist of violaceous-to-red, well-defined, single or multiple plaques, 5–20 mm in diameter, usually on the face, scalp, and external ears (conchal bowl). In discoid lesions, there is atrophy, telangiectasia, central depigmentation or scarring, a hyperpigmented rim, and follicular plugging. On the scalp, significant permanent hair loss may occur. In SCLE, the lesions are erythematous annular or psoriasiform plaques up to several centimeters in diameter and favor the upper chest and back.

B. Laboratory Findings

In patients with DLE, SLE should be considered if the following findings are present: positive ANA, or other serologic studies (eg, anti-double-stranded DNA or anti-Smith antibody), high ESR, proteinuria, hypocomplementemia, widespread lesions (not localized to the head), nail fold changes (dilated or thrombosed nail fold capillary loops), or arthralgias with or without arthritis. Patients with marked photosensitivity and symptoms otherwise suggestive of lupus may have negative ANA tests but are positive for antibodies against Ro/SSA or La/SSB (SCLE).

Differential Diagnosis

The diagnosis is based on the clinical appearance confirmed by skin biopsy in all cases. In DLE, the scale is dry and "thumbtack-like" and thus distinguished from that of seborrheic dermatitis and psoriasis. Older lesions have hyperpigmented borders, depigmented central scarring, or areas of hair loss that also differentiate lupus from these diseases. A number of medications may induce SCLE with a positive Ro/SSA.

Treatment

A. General Measures

Use photoprotective clothing and broad-spectrum sunblock of SPF of 30 or higher daily. UVA coverage is essential in photosensitive patients. Avoid radiation therapy or medications that are potentially photosensitizing when possible.

B. Local Treatment

For limited lesions, the following should be tried before systemic therapy: high-potency corticosteroid creams applied each night and covered with airtight, thin, pliable plastic film (eg, Saran Wrap); flurandrenolide (Cordran) tape; or ultra-high-potency corticosteroid cream or ointment applied twice daily without occlusion.

C. Local Infiltration

Triamcinolone acetonide suspension, 2.5–10 mg/mL, may be injected into DLE lesions once a month.

D. Systemic Treatment

1. Antimalarials—These medications should be used only when the diagnosis is secure because they have been associated with flares of psoriasis, which is in the differential diagnosis.

A. HYDROXYCHLOROQUINE SULFATE—Daily dose of no more than 5 mg/kg orally for several months may be effective and is often used prior to chloroquine. A minimum 3-month trial is recommended. Screening for ocular toxicity is needed.

B. CHLOROQUINE SULFATE—250 mg orally daily may be effective in some cases when hydroxychloroquine is not.

2. Isotretinoin—Isotretinoin, 1 mg/kg/day orally, is effective in hypertrophic DLE lesions.

3. Thalidomide—Thalidomide is effective in refractory cases in doses of 50–300 mg orally daily. Monitor for neuropathy. Lenalidomide (5–10 mg orally daily) may also be effective with less risk for neuropathy.

Isotretinoin, thalidomide, and lenalidomide are teratogens and should be used with appropriate contraception and monitoring in women of childbearing age.

Prognosis

The disease is persistent but not life-endangering unless systemic lupus is present. Treatment with one or more antimalarials is effective in more than half of cases. Patients with cutaneous lupus erythematosus should be examined and tested annually (CBC and UA) to screen for early signs of systemic involvement. Although the only morbidity may be cosmetic, this can have significant quality of life impact in more darkly pigmented patients with widespread disease. Scarring alopecia can be prevented or lessened with close attention and aggressive therapy. Over years, DLE tends to become inactive. Drug-induced SCLE usually resolves over months when the inciting medication is stopped.

Lee V et al. Collagen vascular diseases: a review of cutaneous and systemic lupus erythematosus, dermatomyositis, and distinguishing features in skin of color. Dermatol Clin. 2023;41:435. [PMID: 37236713]

Niebel D et al. Cutaneous lupus erythematosus: an update on pathogenesis and future therapeutic directions. Am J Clin Dermatol. 2023;24:521. [PMID: 37140884]

VESICULAR & BLISTERING DERMATOSES

CONTACT DERMATITIS

ESSENTIALS OF DIAGNOSIS

- Erythema and edema, with pruritus, vesicles, bullae, weeping, or crusting.
- **Irritant contact dermatitis:** occurs only in area of direct contact with irritant.
- **Allergic contact dermatitis:** extends beyond area of direct contact with allergen; positive patch test.

General Considerations

Contact dermatitis (irritant or allergic) is an acute or chronic dermatitis that results from direct skin contact with chemicals or allergens. Eighty percent of cases are due to excessive exposure to or additive effects of universal irritants (eg, soaps, detergents, organic solvents) and are called **irritant contact dermatitis**. The most common causes of **allergic contact dermatitis** are poison ivy or poison oak, topically applied antimicrobials (especially bacitracin and neomycin), anesthetics (benzocaine), preservatives, jewelry (nickel), rubber, essential oils, propolis (from bees), vitamin E, and adhesive tape. Occupational exposure is an important cause of allergic contact dermatitis.

Clinical Findings

A. Symptoms and Signs

1. Allergic contact dermatitis—The acute phase is characterized by intense pruritus, tiny vesicles, and weepy and crusted lesions (Figure 6–27). The lesions, distributed on exposed parts or in unusual asymmetric patterns, consist of erythematous macules, papules, and vesicles and may occur beyond the contact area, distinguishing it from irritant dermatitis. The affected area may also be edematous and warm with honey-colored crusting, simulating—and at times complicated by—bacterial or viral infection. The pattern of the eruption may be diagnostic (eg, typical linear streaked vesicles on the extremities in poison oak or ivy dermatitis). The location often suggests the cause: scalp involvement suggests hair dyes or shampoos; face involvement suggests creams, cosmetics, soaps, shaving materials, nail polish; and neck involvement suggests jewelry, hair dyes. Reactions may not develop for 48–72 hours after exposure.

2. Irritant contact dermatitis—The rash is erythematous and scaly (less likely vesicular) and occurs only in the direct sites of contact with the irritant. Resolving or chronic contact dermatitis presents with scaling, erythema, and possibly thickened skin. Itching, burning, and stinging may be severe in both allergic and irritant contact dermatitis. Reactions may develop within 24 hours of contact exposure.

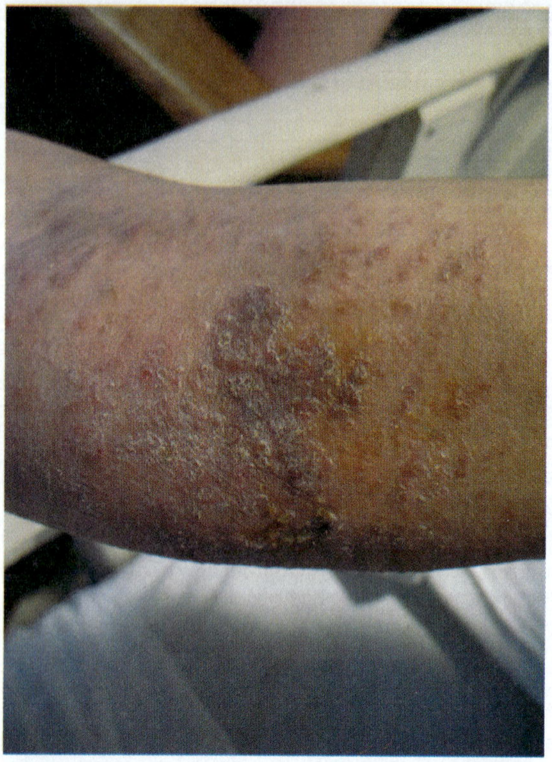

▲ **Figure 6–27.** Allergic contact dermatitis to an adhesive dressing in a patient with darker skin. Key features are erythematous papules with impetigo-like honey-colored crusting. (Used, with permission, from Kanade Shinkai, MD.)

B. Laboratory Findings

Gram stain and culture will rule out impetigo or secondary infection (impetiginization). After the episode of allergic contact dermatitis has cleared, patch testing may be useful if the triggering allergen is not known.

Differential Diagnosis

Asymmetric distribution, blotchy erythema around the face, linear lesions, and a history of exposure help distinguish acute contact dermatitis from other skin lesions. The most commonly mistaken diagnosis is impetigo, herpetic infection, or cellulitis. Chronic allergic contact dermatitis must be differentiated from scabies, particularly if itching is generalized, atopic dermatitis, and pompholyx.

Prevention

Removal of the causative oil by washing with liquid soap may be effective if done within 30 minutes after exposure to poison oak or ivy. Goop (oil remover) and Tecnu (chemical inactivator) have similar efficacy but are more expensive. Over-the-counter barrier creams may be effective when applied prior to exposure and prevent/reduce the severity of the dermatitis.

The mainstay of prevention is identification of the agent causing the dermatitis and strict avoidance of exposure or use of protective clothing and gloves. Some allergens will transmit through latex gloves. In industry-related cases, prevention may require special accommodations or retraining the worker.

Treatment

A. Overview

Localized involvement (except on the face) can often be managed solely with topical agents. While local measures are important, severe or widespread involvement is difficult to manage without systemic corticosteroids because even the highest-potency topical corticosteroids seem not to work well on vesicular and weepy lesions. **Irritant contact dermatitis** is treated by protection from the irritant and use of topical corticosteroids as for atopic dermatitis (described above). The treatment of **allergic contact dermatitis** is detailed below.

B. Local Measures

1. Acute weeping dermatitis—Gentle cleansing and drying compresses (such as Domeboro) are recommended. Calamine lotion or zinc oxide paste may be used between wet dressings, especially for involvement of intertriginous areas or when oozing is not marked. Lesions on the extremities may be bandaged with wet dressings for 30–60 minutes several times a day. High-potency topical corticosteroids in gel or cream form (eg, fluocinonide, clobetasol, or halobetasol) may help suppress acute contact dermatitis and relieve itching. This treatment should be followed by tapering of the number of applications per day or use of a mid-potency corticosteroid, such as triamcinolone 0.1% cream, to prevent rebound of the dermatitis. A soothing formulation is 2 oz of 0.1% triamcinolone acetonide cream in 7.5 oz Sarna lotion (0.5% camphor, 0.5% menthol, 0.5% phenol) mixed by the patient.

2. Subacute dermatitis (subsiding)—Mid-potency (triamcinolone 0.1%) to high-potency corticosteroids (clobetasol, fluocinonide, desoximetasone) are the mainstays of therapy.

3. Chronic dermatitis (dry and lichenified)—High-potency to superpotency corticosteroids are used in ointment form. Occlusion may be helpful on the hands.

C. Systemic Therapy

For acute severe cases, prednisone may be given orally for 12–21 days. Prednisone, 60 mg for 4–7 days, 40 mg for 4–7 days, and 20 mg for 4–7 days, without a further taper is one useful regimen. The key is to use enough corticosteroid (and as early as possible) to achieve a clinical effect and to taper slowly over 2–3 weeks to avoid rebound.

Prognosis

Allergic contact dermatitis is self-limited if re-exposure is prevented but often takes 2–3 weeks for full resolution. Removal of the causative agent is paramount to avoid recurrences.

Agrawal A. Artificial intelligence in contact dermatitis: current and future perspectives. Dermatitis. 2025. [Epub ahead of print] [PMID: 40916798]
Sullivan E et al. Atopic and contact dermatitis. Prim Care. 2025;52:553. [PMID: 40835290]
Tramontana M et al. Advancing the understanding of allergic contact dermatitis: from pathophysiology to novel therapeutic approaches. Front Med (Lausanne). 2023;10:1184289. [PMID: 37283623]

POMPHOLYX

ESSENTIALS OF DIAGNOSIS

- Pruritic "tapioca" vesicles of 1–2 mm on the palms, soles, and sides of fingers.
- Vesicles may coalesce to form multiloculated blisters.
- Scaling and fissuring may follow drying of the blisters.
- Appearance in the third decade, with lifelong recurrences.

General Considerations

Pompholyx, otherwise known as chronic hand eczema or vesiculobullous dermatitis of the palms and soles, is formerly known as dyshidrosis or dyshidrotic eczema. About half of patients have an atopic background, and many patients report flares with stress. Patients with widespread dermatitis due to any cause may develop pompholyx-like eruptions as a part of an autoeczematization response.

Clinical Findings

Small clear vesicles resembling grains of tapioca stud the skin at the sides of the fingers and on the palms (Figure 6–28) and may also affect the soles, albeit less frequently. They may be associated with intense itching. Later, the vesicles dry and the area becomes scaly and fissured.

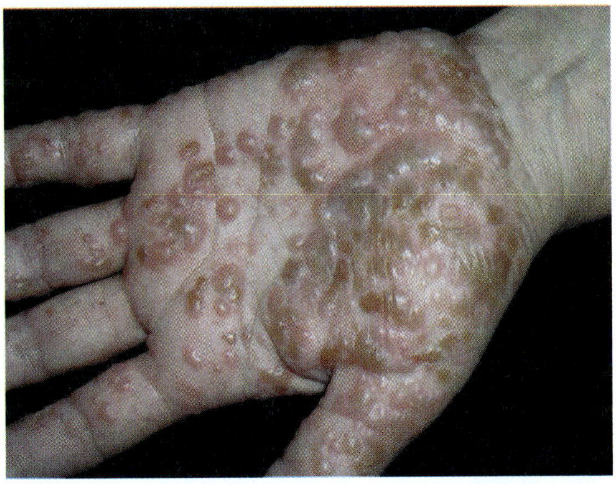

▲ **Figure 6–28.** Severe pompholyx. (Reproduced, with permission, from Richard P. Usatine, MD, in Usatine RP, Smith MA, Mayeaux EJ Jr, Chumley H. *The Color Atlas of Family Medicine*, 2nd ed. McGraw-Hill, 2013.)

Differential Diagnosis

Unroofing the vesicles and examining the blister roof with a KOH preparation will reveal hyphae in cases of bullous tinea. Patients with inflammatory tinea pedis may have a vesicular autoeczematization of the palms. NSAIDs may produce an eruption very similar to that of vesiculobullous dermatitis on the hands.

Prevention

There is no known way to prevent attacks if the condition is idiopathic. About one-third to one-half of patients with vesiculobullous hand dermatitis have a relevant contact allergen, especially nickel. Patch testing and avoidance of identified allergens can lead to improvement.

Treatment

Topical and systemic corticosteroids help some patients dramatically; however, systemic corticosteroids are generally not appropriate therapy. A high-potency topical corticosteroid used early may help abort the flare and ameliorate pruritus. Topical corticosteroids are also important in treating the scaling and fissuring that are seen after the vesicular phase. It is essential that patients avoid anything that irritates the skin; they should wear cotton gloves inside vinyl gloves when doing dishes or other wet chores and use a hand cream after washing the hands. Patients respond to UVB therapy and injection of botulinum toxin into the palms as for hyperhidrosis. In 2025, delgocitinib cream 2%, a topical JAK-inhibitor, became the first FDA-approved treatment for adults with moderate-to-severe chronic hand eczema.

Prognosis

For most patients, the disease is an inconvenience. For some, vesiculobullous hand eczema can be incapacitating.

Abdelhalim A et al. Topical delgocitinib for the treatment of chronic hand eczema. J Dermatolog Treat. 2025;36:2479126. [PMID: 40096745]
Bernier C et al. Assessment of practices in chronic hand eczema management from CHEMIN, a national Delphi survey. Contact Dermatitis. 2025;93:336. [PMID: 40641290]
Grada A et al. Demystifying hand eczema. J Invest Dermatol. 2023;143:1338. [PMID: 37115112]

PORPHYRIA CUTANEA TARDA

ESSENTIALS OF DIAGNOSIS

- Noninflammatory blisters on sun-exposed sites, especially the dorsal surfaces of the hands.
- Hypertrichosis, skin fragility.
- Associated liver disease.
- Elevated urine porphyrins.

General Considerations

Porphyria cutanea tarda is the most common type of porphyria. Cases are sporadic or hereditary. The disease is associated with ingestion of certain medications (eg, estrogens) and alcoholic liver disease, hemochromatosis, and hepatitis C.

Clinical Findings

A. Symptoms and Signs

Patients report painless blistering and fragility of the skin of the dorsal surfaces of the hands (Figure 6–29). Facial hypertrichosis and hyperpigmentation are common.

B. Laboratory Findings

Urinary uroporphyrins are elevated twofold to fivefold above coproporphyrins. Patients may also have abnormal liver biochemical tests, evidence of hepatitis C infection, increased liver iron stores, and hemochromatosis gene mutations.

Differential Diagnosis

Skin lesions identical to those of porphyria cutanea tarda may be seen in patients who undergo dialysis and in those who take certain medications (tetracyclines, voriconazole, and NSAIDs, especially naproxen). In this so-called pseudoporphyria, the biopsy results are the same as those associated with porphyria cutanea tarda, but urine porphyrins are normal.

Prevention

Photoprotective clothing is required. The lesions are triggered by sun exposure, but the wavelength of light triggering the lesions is beyond that absorbed by sunscreens.

Treatment

Stopping all triggering medications and reducing or stopping alcohol consumption may lead to improvement in most cases. Phlebotomy at a rate of 1 unit every 2–4 weeks will gradually lead to improvement. Very low-dose antimalarial medication (as low as 200 mg of hydroxychloroquine orally twice weekly), alone or in combination with phlebotomy, increases porphyrin excretion and improves the skin disease. Deferasirox, an iron chelator, can also be beneficial. Treatment is continued until the patient is asymptomatic. Urine porphyrins may be monitored.

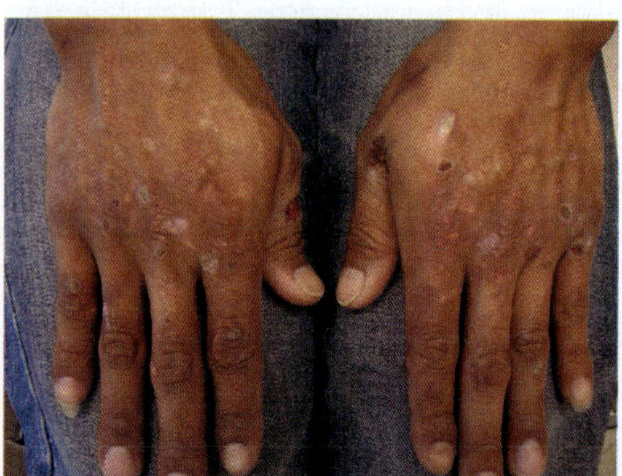

▲ **Figure 6–29.** Porphyria cutanea tarda of hands in a patient with darker skin. (Used, with permission, from Kanade Shinkai, MD.)

Prognosis

Most patients improve with treatment. Sclerodermoid skin lesions may develop on the trunk, scalp, and face.

Baltazar AM et al. Porphyria cutanea tarda: a multifactorial disease. Cureus. 2025;17:e87965. [PMID: 40821324]
Dickey AK et al. Update on the porphyrias. Annu Rev Med. 2024;75:321. [PMID: 37540847]
Sarkany RPE et al. The clinical management of porphyria cutanea tarda: an update. Liver Int. 2024;44:2191. [PMID: 38813949]

DERMATITIS HERPETIFORMIS

Dermatitis herpetiformis is an uncommon disease manifested by intensely pruritic papules, vesicles, and papulovesicles mainly on the elbows, knees, buttocks, posterior neck, and scalp. The histopathology is distinctive. Circulating antibodies to tissue transglutaminase are present in 90% of cases. Three-fourths of patients have gluten-sensitive enteropathy with villous atrophy on small bowel biopsy; however, GI symptoms are subclinical in most. Ingestion of gluten is the cause of dermatitis herpetiformis, and strict long-term avoidance of dietary gluten may eliminate the need for treatment or decrease the dose of dapsone (initial treatment dose is 100–200 mg orally daily) required to control the disease.

Didona D et al. Gluten-related skin disorders: clinical presentation, diagnostics and treatments. J Dtsch Dermatol Ges. 2025;23:857. [PMID: 40631603]
Lovell KK et al. Dapsone use in dermatology. Am J Clin Dermatol. 2024;25:811. [PMID: 39078587]
Shahid MA et al. Dermatitis herpetiformis, celiac disease and their impact on women and their families. Ital J Dermatol Venerol. 2025;160:501. [PMID: 40693943]

PEMPHIGUS

ESSENTIALS OF DIAGNOSIS

- Relapsing crops of bullae, often fragile and leading to erosions.
- Often preceded by mucous membrane bullae, erosions, and ulcerations.
- Superficial detachment of the skin after pressure or trauma variably present (Nikolsky sign).
- Acantholysis on biopsy.
- Immunofluorescence studies and serum ELISA for pathogenic antibodies are confirmatory.

General Considerations

Pemphigus is an uncommon intraepidermal blistering disease occurring on skin and mucous membranes. It is caused by autoantibodies to adhesion molecules expressed in the skin and mucous membranes. The bullae appear spontaneously and are tender and painful when they rupture. Drug-induced pemphigus has been reported. There are several forms of pemphigus: pemphigus vulgaris and its variant, pemphigus vegetans; and the more superficially blistering pemphigus foliaceus and its variant, pemphigus erythematosus. All forms may present at any age but most commonly in middle age. The vulgaris form begins in the mouth in over 50% of cases. The foliaceus form may be associated with other autoimmune diseases or may be drug-induced. Paraneoplastic pemphigus, a unique form of the disorder, is associated with numerous benign and malignant neoplasms, most frequently chronic lymphocytic leukemia, Castleman disease, B cell lymphoma, plasmacytoma, and thymoma. Associated bronchiolitis obliterans is characteristic.

Clinical Findings

A. Symptoms and Signs

Pemphigus is characterized by an insidious onset of flaccid bullae, crusts, and erosions in crops or waves (Figure 6–30). In pemphigus vulgaris, lesions often appear first on the oral mucous membranes. These rapidly become erosive. The scalp is another site of early involvement. Rubbing a cotton swab or finger laterally on the surface of uninvolved skin may cause easy separation of the epidermis (Nikolsky sign). Downward pressure on a fresh bulla may cause lateral spread (Asboe-Hansen sign). Pemphigus vegetans presents as erosive vegetating plaques, most often in intertriginous areas. Pemphigus foliaceus is a superficial form of pemphigus where cutaneous lesions present as flaccid bullae that quickly evolve into superficial erosions and thin pink plaques with overlying scale. Pemphigus erythematosus has overlapping features of pemphigus foliaceus and lupus erythematosus. It presents with flaccid bullae that develop overlying scale and crust in a photodistributed area. Mucosal lesions are rare with both pemphigus foliaceus and pemphigus erythematosus. Paraneoplastic pemphigus is histologically and immunologically distinct from other forms of the disease. Oral lesions predominate and cutaneous erythematous plaques resembling erythema multiforme are characteristic. Survival rates are low because of the underlying malignancy.

B. Laboratory Findings

The diagnosis is made by light microscopy, direct and indirect immunofluorescence (IIF) microscopy, and ELISA to detect autoantibodies to intercellular adhesion molecules (desmoglien 1 and 3).

Differential Diagnosis

Blistering diseases include erythema multiforme, Stevens-Johnson syndrome (SJS)/toxic epidermal necrolysis (TEN), drug eruptions, bullous impetigo, contact dermatitis, dermatitis herpetiformis, and bullous pemphigoid, but flaccid

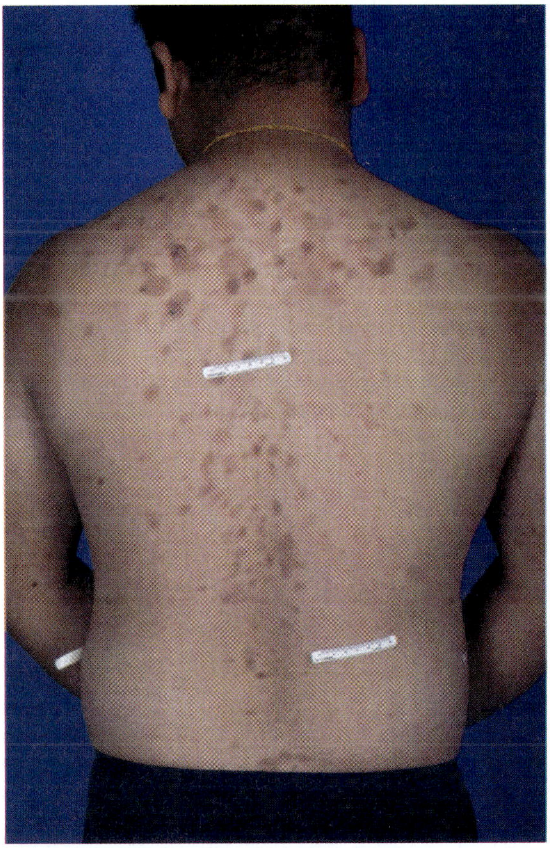

Figure 6–30. Pemphigus vulgaris on the back. (Reproduced, with permission, from Kelly AP, Taylor SC, Lim HW, Serrano AMA. *Taylor and Kelly's Dermatology for Skin of Color*, 2e. McGraw-Hill; 2016.)

blisters are not typical of these diseases, and acantholysis is not seen on biopsy. All these diseases have clinical characteristics and immunofluorescence test results that distinguish them from pemphigus. Pemphigus foliaceus must be distinguished from subacute cutaneous lupus erythematosus.

Complications

Secondary infection commonly occurs; this is a major cause of morbidity and mortality. Disturbances of fluid, electrolyte, and nutritional intake can occur as a result of painful oral ulcers.

Treatment

A. General Measures

Patients with severe disease should be hospitalized at bed rest and provided intravenous antibiotics and feedings as indicated. Anesthetic troches used before eating ease painful oral lesions.

B. Systemic Measures

Pemphigus requires systemic therapy as early in its course as possible. Initial therapy is with prednisone 1–2 mg/kg orally daily. In all but the mildest cases, a steroid-sparing agent is added from the beginning, since the disease course is long and the steroid-sparing agents take several weeks to exert their activity. Rituximab (1 g intravenously on days 1 and 15 as induction therapy followed by 500 mg intravenously every 6 months as maintenance therapy) is FDA approved for the treatment of pemphigus vulgaris, associated with induction of a complete remission, and considered by many experts to be first-line therapy. Repeated courses are efficacious and well tolerated in patients who do not achieve complete remission or relapse. Azathioprine (2–4 mg/kg orally daily) and mycophenolate mofetil (1–3 g orally daily) are other therapeutic options. In refractory cases, monthly intravenous immunoglobulin (IVIG) (2 g/kg intravenously over 3–4 days), pulse intravenous corticosteroids, cyclophosphamide, or plasmapheresis can be used.

C. Local Measures

In patients with limited disease, skin and mucous membrane lesions should be treated with topical corticosteroids. Secondary infection requires appropriate systemic and local antibiotic therapy.

Prognosis

Without antibiotic or corticosteroid treatment, the disease is fatal within 5 years. The course tends to be chronic in most patients; however, up to one-third experience remission. Infection is the most frequent cause of death, usually from *S aureus* septicemia.

Rahimi S et al. Desmoglein-driven dynamic signaling in pemphigus vulgaris: a systematic review of pathogenic pathways. NPJ Regen Med. 2025;10:39. [PMID: 40846710]
Vafaeian A et al. What is novel in the clinical management of pemphigus vulgaris? Expert Rev Clin Pharmacol. 2024;17:489. [PMID: 38712540]
Yamagami J. B-cell targeted therapy of pemphigus. J Dermatol. 2023;50:124. [PMID: 36478455]

BULLOUS PEMPHIGOID

Bullous pemphigoid is a relatively benign pruritic disease characterized by tense blisters in flexural areas, usually remitting in 5 or 6 years, with a course characterized by exacerbations and remissions. Most affected persons are over the age of 60 and men are affected twice as frequently as women. The appearance of blisters may be preceded by pruritic urticarial or edematous lesions for months. Oral lesions are present in one-third of cases. The disease may occur in various forms, including localized, vesicular, vegetating, erythematous, erythrodermic, and nodular. Drugs may induce bullous pemphigoid. The most common offender is furosemide. Immunotherapy for malignancies with PD-1 inhibitors can cause drug-induced bullous pemphigoid.

The diagnosis is made by biopsy with direct immunofluorescence examination and serum antibody testing. Light microscopy shows a subepidermal blister. With direct immunofluorescence, IgG and C3 are found at the dermal-epidermal junction. ELISA tests for bullous pemphigoid antibodies (BP 180 or BP 230) are 87% sensitive and 95% specific. If the patient has mild disease, ultrapotent topical corticosteroids may be adequate. Prednisone (0.5–1 mg/kg orally daily) is often used to achieve rapid control of more widespread disease. In 2025, dupilumab became the first targeted biologic to be FDA-approved to treat bullous pemphigoid and should be considered for first-line therapy. Doxycycline (100 mg orally twice a day), alone or combined with nicotinamide (500 mg orally three times daily)—not nicotinic acid or niacin—may control the disease in patients with mild to moderate disease who cannot use corticosteroids or may allow for decreasing or eliminating corticosteroids after control is achieved. Dapsone (50–200 mg orally daily) is particularly effective in mucous membrane pemphigoid. If these medications are not effective, methotrexate (5–25 mg orally weekly), azathioprine (2–4 mg/kg orally daily), or mycophenolate mofetil (1–3 g orally daily) may be used as steroid-sparing agents. Intravenous immunoglobulin, rituximab, and omalizumab have been used off-label with success in refractory cases.

Chen HC et al. Advancing treatment in bullous pemphigoid: a comprehensive review of novel therapeutic targets and approaches. Clin Rev Allergy Immunol. 2023;65:331. [PMID: 37897588]
Olbrich H et al. Emerging drugs for the treatment of bullous pemphigoid: what's new on the horizon? Expert Opin Emerg Drugs. 2025. [Epub ahead of print] [PMID: 40878514]
Singh S et al. Interventions for bullous pemphigoid. Cochrane Database Syst Rev. 2023;8:CD002292. [PMID: 37572360]

PUSTULAR DISORDERS

ACNE VULGARIS

ESSENTIALS OF DIAGNOSIS

- Almost universal in puberty; may begin in premenarchal girls and present or persist into the fourth or fifth decade.
- Comedones are the hallmark. Severity varies from comedonal to papular or pustular inflammatory acne to cysts or nodules.
- Face, neck, and upper trunk may be affected.
- Scarring may be a sequela of the disease or picking by the patient.

General Considerations

Acne vulgaris is polymorphic. Open and closed comedones, papules, pustules, and cysts are found.

In younger persons, acne vulgaris is more common and more severe in males. Acne may persist into adulthood. Twelve percent of women and 3% of men over age 25 have acne vulgaris. This rate does not decrease until the fourth or fifth decade of life. The skin lesions parallel sebaceous activity. Pathogenic events include plugging of the infundibulum of the follicles, retention of sebum, overgrowth of the acne bacillus (*Cutibacterium acnes*) with resultant release of and irritation by accumulated fatty acids, and foreign-body reaction to extrafollicular sebum. Antibiotics may help control acne because of their antibacterial or anti-inflammatory properties.

Hyperandrogenism may be a cause of acne in women and may be accompanied by hirsutism or irregular menses. Polycystic ovary syndrome (PCOS) is the most common identifiable cause. Acne may develop in patients who use systemic corticosteroids or topical fluorinated corticosteroids on the face. Acne may be exacerbated or caused by cosmetic creams or oils as well as androgenic supplements or masculinizing hormone therapy in transgender individuals.

Clinical Findings

There may be mild tenderness, pain, or itching. The lesions occur mainly over the face, neck, upper chest, back, and shoulders. Comedones (tiny, flesh-colored, white or black noninflamed superficial papules that give the skin a rough texture or appearance) are the hallmark of acne vulgaris. Inflammatory papules, pustules, ectatic pores, acne cysts, and scarring are also seen (Figure 6–31).

Acne may have different presentations at different ages. Preteens often present with comedones as their first lesions. Inflammatory lesions in young teenagers are often found in the middle of the face, extending outward as the patient becomes older. Adult females may present with comedonal or papular lesions especially on the chin and jawline.

Differential Diagnosis

In adults, rosacea presents with papules and pustules in the middle third of the face, but absence of truncal involvement, telangiectasia, flushing, and the absence of comedones distinguish rosacea from acne vulgaris. A pustular eruption on the face in patients receiving antibiotics or with otitis externa should be investigated with culture to rule out a gram-negative folliculitis. Pustules on the face can also be caused by dermatophytic or demodex infection. Lesions on the back are more problematic. When they occur alone, staphylococcal folliculitis, miliaria ("heat rash") or, uncommonly, *Pityrosporum* folliculitis should be suspected. Bacterial culture, trial of an antistaphylococcal antibiotic, and observing the response to therapy will help in the differential diagnosis. In patients with HIV infection, folliculitis is common and may be either staphylococcal folliculitis or eosinophilic folliculitis (typically pruritic tumid papules on the face and neck).

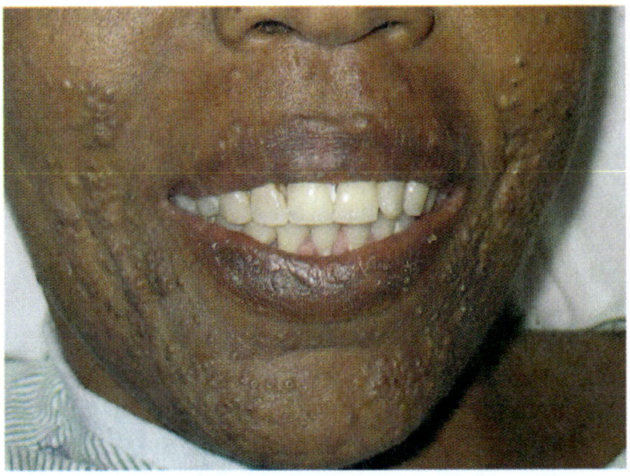

▲ **Figure 6–31.** Acne vulgaris. Extensive comedones and hyperpigmented macules are present in patient with dark skin. (Used, with permission, from Kanade Shinkai, MD.)

Complications

Cyst formation, pigmentary changes, scarring, and poor quality of life may result.

Treatment

A. General Measures

1. Education of the patient—Education on proper use of medications and cosmetics is paramount. Because lesions take 4–6 weeks to improve, clinical improvement should be measured by the number of new lesions forming after 6–8 weeks of therapy. Additional time (3–4 months) will be required to see improvement on the back and chest, as these areas are slowest to respond. Avoid topical exposure to oils, cocoa butter (theobroma oil), and greases in cosmetics, including hair products. Scarring may occur with or without the patient manipulating the lesions. It is essential that the patient be educated in a supportive way about this complication. Anxiety and depression are common in patients with excoriated acne.

2. Diet—A low glycemic diet has been associated with improvement and lower incidence of acne. This improvement was associated with a reduction in insulin resistance. Hyperinsulinemia has also been associated with acne in both eumenorrheic women and individuals with PCOS.

B. Comedonal Acne

Treatment of acne is based on the type and severity of lesions. Comedones require treatment different from that of pustules and cystic lesions. In assessing severity, take the sequelae of the lesions into account. An individual who gets only a few new lesions per month that scar or leave postinflammatory hyperpigmentation must be treated much more aggressively than a comparable patient whose lesions clear without sequelae. Hygiene plays little role in acne treatment, and a mild soap is almost always recommended. The agents effective in comedonal acne are listed below in the order in which they should be tried.

1. Topical retinoids—Tretinoin is very effective for comedonal and papular acne, but its usefulness is limited by irritation. Start with 0.025% cream (not gel) and have the patient use it at first twice weekly at night, increasing frequency to nightly as tolerated. A few patients cannot tolerate this low-strength preparation more than three times weekly, which may still promote improvement. A lentil-sized amount is sufficient to cover the entire face. To avoid irritation, have the patient wait 20 minutes after washing to apply. For patients irritated by standard tretinoin preparations, other options are adapalene gel 0.1% and reformulated tretinoin

(Renova, Retin A Micro, Avita). Although the absorption of tretinoin is minimal, its use during pregnancy is contraindicated. Patients should be warned that their acne may flare in the first 4 weeks of treatment.

2. Benzoyl peroxide—Benzoyl peroxide products are available in concentrations of 2.5%, 4%, 5%, 8%, and 10%, but 2.5% is as effective as 10% and less irritating. In general, water-based and not alcohol-based gels should be used to decrease irritation. Single formulations of benzoyl peroxide in combination with several other topical agents, including adapalene and topical antibiotics (erythromycin, clindamycin phosphate), are available.

C. Papular or Cystic Inflammatory Acne

Brief treatment (3 weeks to 3 months) with topical or oral antibiotics is the mainstay for treatment of inflammatory acne that does not respond to topical therapy with retinoids or benzoyl peroxide. Topical clindamycin phosphate and erythromycin are used only for mild papular acne or for patients who refuse or cannot tolerate oral antibiotics. To decrease resistance, benzoyl peroxide should be used in combination with the topical antibiotic.

1. Mild acne—The first choice of topical antibiotics in terms of efficacy and relative lack of induction of resistant *C acnes* is the combination of erythromycin or clindamycin with benzoyl peroxide topical gel or wash (Table 6–2). These may be used once or twice daily. The addition of tretinoin cream or gel at night, or topical clascoterone cream twice daily, may increase improvement since they work via a different mechanism. Topical retinoids should be used for long-term maintenance therapy.

2. Moderate acne—Common oral antibiotics used for acne include doxycycline (100 mg twice daily), minocycline (50–100 mg once or twice daily), TMP-SMZ (one double-strength tablet twice daily), or a cephalosporin (cefadroxil or cephalexin 500 mg twice daily), which should be used in combination with benzoyl peroxide to minimize development of antibiotic resistance. Sarecycline, a narrow-spectrum tetracycline-class antibiotic dosed by weight at 1.5 mg/kg once daily, is another option that is generally well-tolerated, but its high cost makes it less preferred compared to the aforementioned antibiotics. It may take 3 months or more for truncal acne to resolve with oral antibiotic treatment. In general, discontinuing antibiotics immediately without adjunctive topical therapy results in prompt recurrence. Topical retinoids are excellent for long-term maintenance following antibiotics. Subantimicrobial dosing of doxycycline (40–50 mg orally daily) can be used in patients who require long-term systemic therapy. Combination oral contraceptives or spironolactone (50–200 mg orally daily) are highly effective alternatives in women with treatment-resistant acne. Tetracycline, minocycline, and doxycycline are contraindicated in pregnancy, but certain oral erythromycins or cephalosporins may be used.

3. Severe acne—

A. ISOTRETINOIN—A vitamin A analog, isotretinoin is used for the treatment of severe acne that has not responded to conventional therapy. An oral dosage of 0.5–1 mg/kg/day for 20 weeks for a cumulative dose of at least 120 mg/kg is usually adequate for treating and preventing the recurrence of severe cystic acne. Patients should be offered isotretinoin therapy before they experience significant acne scarring. *Isotretinoin is absolutely contraindicated during pregnancy because of its teratogenicity.* Two forms of effective contraception must be used; abstinence is an acceptable alternative. Informed consent must be obtained before its use, and patients must be enrolled in a monitoring program (iPledge). In addition to its teratogenicity, isotretinoin has numerous side effects and should only be prescribed by clinicians well aware of these issues. Cheilitis, dry skin, and photosensitivity are almost universal side effects. Consider ordering laboratory tests, including triglyceride levels and liver enzyme tests (particularly ALT, which is the most liver-specific enzyme), in patients before treatment and after achieving therapeutic dosing; monitoring through the entire treatment may not be high value. Monthly pregnancy testing is required for individuals of childbearing potential.

Abnormal laboratory tests, especially elevated liver enzymes and triglyceride levels, return to normal quickly upon conclusion of therapy. The medication may induce long-term remissions in up to 70% of persons, or acne may recur that is more easily controlled with conventional therapy. Occasionally, a second course is needed if acne does not respond or recurs.

B. INTRALESIONAL INJECTION—Intralesional injection of dilute suspensions of triamcinolone acetonide (2.5 mg/mL, 0.05 mL per lesion) will often hasten the resolution of deeper papules and occasional cysts.

C. SCAR REVISION—Cosmetic improvement may be achieved by excision and punch-grafting of deep scars and by physical or chemical abrasion of inactive acne lesions, particularly flat, superficial scars.

Prognosis

Acne vulgaris eventually remits spontaneously, but when this will occur cannot be predicted. The condition may persist throughout adulthood and may lead to severe scarring if left untreated. Patients treated with antibiotics continue to improve for the first 3–6 months of therapy. Relapse during treatment may suggest the emergence of resistant *C acnes*. The disease is chronic and tends to flare intermittently despite treatment. Remissions following systemic treatment with isotretinoin may be lasting in up to 70% of cases. Relapses after isotretinoin usually occur within 3 years and require a second course in up to 20% of patients.

Huang CY et al. Comparative efficacy of pharmacological treatments for acne vulgaris: a network meta-analysis of 221 randomized controlled trials. Ann Fam Med. 2023;21:358. [PMID: 37487721]

Reynolds RV et al. Guidelines of care for the management of acne vulgaris. J Am Acad Dermatol. 2024;90:1006.e1. [PMID: 38300170]

Santer M et al. Managing acne vulgaris: an update. Drug Ther Bull. 2023;62:6. [PMID: 38154809]

ROSACEA

ESSENTIALS OF DIAGNOSIS

- A chronic disorder affecting the face.
- Neurovascular component: erythema and telangiectasis and a tendency to flush easily.
- Acneiform component: papules and pustules may be present.
- Glandular component: sebaceous hyperplasia and fibrosis of affected areas (eg, rhinophyma).

General Considerations

Rosacea is a common condition that presents in adulthood. The pathogenesis of this chronic disorder is not known. Topical corticosteroids applied to the face can induce rosacea-like conditions.

Clinical Findings

Patients frequently report flushing or exacerbation of their rosacea due to heat, hot drinks, spicy food, sunlight, exercise, alcohol, emotions, or menopausal flushing. The cheeks, nose, chin, and ears—at times the entire face—may be affected. No comedones are seen. In its mildest form, erythema and telangiectasias are seen on the cheeks. Inflammatory papules may be superimposed on this background and may evolve to pustules (Figure 6–32). Associated seborrhea may be found. Some patients describe burning or stinging with episodes of flushing and extremely cosmetic-intolerant skin. Patients may have associated ophthalmic disease, including blepharitis, keratitis, and chalazion, which often requires topical or systemic antibiotic or immunosuppressive therapy.

Differential Diagnosis

Rosacea is distinguished from acne by the presence of the neurovascular component and the absence of comedones. Lupus is often misdiagnosed, but the presence of pustules excludes that diagnosis.

Treatment

Educating patients to avoid the factors they know to produce exacerbations is important. Patients should wear a broad-spectrum mineral-based sunscreen; zinc- or titanium-based sunscreens are tolerated best. Medical management is most effective for the inflammatory papules and pustules and the erythema that surrounds them. Rosacea is usually a lifelong condition, so maintenance therapy is required. Most treatments target the papulopustular and cystic components. Only certain topical agents (brimonidine and oxymetazoline) and laser benefit erythema. Telangiectasias are benefited by laser therapy, and phymatous overgrowth of the nose can be treated by surgical reduction. Rhinophyma must be managed using surgical reduction.

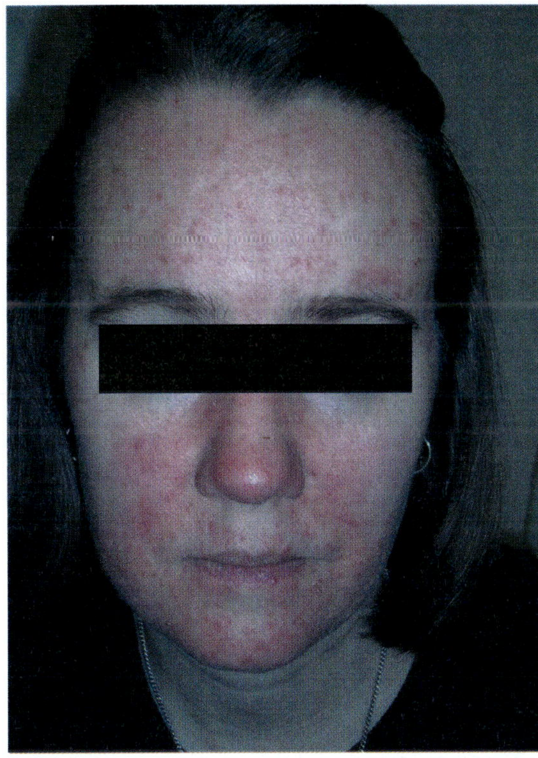

▲ **Figure 6–32.** Rosacea in a 34-year-old woman showing erythema, papules, and pustules covering much of the face. (Reproduced, with permission, from Richard P. Usatine, MD, in Usatine RP, Smith MA, Mayeaux EJ Jr, Chumley H. *The Color Atlas of Family Medicine*, 2nd ed. McGraw-Hill, 2013.)

A. Local Therapy

Avoidance of triggers (especially alcohol and spicy or hot foods) and drinking ice water may be effective in reducing facial erythema and flushing. Metronidazole (cream, gel, or lotion), 0.75% applied twice daily or 1% applied once daily, and ivermectin 1% cream applied once daily are effective topical treatments. Another effective treatment includes topical clindamycin (solution, gel, or lotion) 1% applied twice daily. Response is noted in 4–8 weeks. Sulfur-sodium sulfacetamide-containing topicals are helpful in patients only partially responsive to topical antibiotics. Topical retinoids or topical tacrolimus ointment (0.1%) can be carefully added for maintenance. Topical brimonidine tartrate gel 0.33% or oxymetazoline 1% cream can temporarily reduce the erythema, and laser treatment has longer-term benefit for erythema.

B. Systemic Therapy

Oral tetracyclines should be used when topical therapy is inadequate. Minocycline or doxycycline, 50–100 mg orally once or twice daily, is effective. Metronidazole or amoxicillin, 250–500 mg orally twice daily, or rifaximin, 400 mg orally three times daily (for 10 days), may be used in refractory cases. Side effects are few, although metronidazole may cause a disulfiram-like effect when the patient ingests alcohol and neuropathy with long-term use. Long-term maintenance with subantimicrobial dosing of minocycline or doxycycline is recommended once the initial flare of rosacea has resolved. Isotretinoin may succeed where other measures fail. A dosage of 0.5–1 mg/kg/day orally for 12–28 weeks is recommended, although very low-dose isotretinoin may also be effective. See precautions above.

Prognosis

Rosacea tends to be a persistent process. With the regimens described above, it can usually be controlled adequately.

Choe J et al. Emerging medical therapies in rosacea: a narrative review. Dermatol Ther (Heidelb). 2023;13:2933. [PMID: 37824060]

Nguyen C et al. Rosacea: practical guidance and challenges for clinical management. Clin Cosmet Investig Dermatol. 2024;17:175. [PMID: 38283794]

Volk K et al. Treatment management for rosacea: current pharmacological and non-pharmacological options. Expert Rev Clin Pharmacol. 2025;18:589. [PMID: 40836652]

HIDRADENITIS SUPPURATIVA

ESSENTIALS OF DIAGNOSIS

- Chronic, recurrent, painful deep-seated nodules, abscesses, draining sinus tracts, and scars.
- Lesions typically involve axillae, inguinal areas, submammary folds, and perianal area.
- Often associated with obesity.

General Considerations

Hidradenitis suppurativa (HS) is a chronic inflammatory skin condition that significantly impairs patients' quality of life. It is typified by recurrent painful nodules, abscesses, and draining sinus tracts primarily in intertriginous areas. Obesity is commonly associated with HS, and significant weight loss may lead to marked improvement. HS can produce disfigurement, embarrassment, mental health disorders, and work/social impairment.

Clinical Findings

Lesions include deep-seated nodules, abscesses, and sinus tracts that rupture and form scars. Pain is common and can be severe, disabling, or both. Lesions most frequently occur in the axillae and inguinal areas, but may also favor the submammary folds, perineal area, buttocks, mons pubis, scalp, postauricular area, and the back. A clinical diagnosis of HS is based upon three criteria: characteristic lesions, predilection for flexural sites, and lesion recurrence. There are multiple scoring systems used to assess disease severity, with the Hurley system most frequently used. The severity and psychosocial impact of HS are major factors in determining optimal treatment.

Differential Diagnosis

HS is commonly misdiagnosed as folliculitis, furunculosis/carbunculosis, or cutaneous abscess(es). As such, there is often a significant delay (average of 7 years) between symptom onset and the establishment of the correct diagnosis.

Treatment

The treatment of HS has been difficult because of continued uncertainty regarding the disease pathophysiology. Established successful therapies included anti-inflammatory agents, antibiotics, and surgery. New therapies that specifically target cytokines involved in HS pathogenesis have been recently identified. Weight loss and smoking cessation counseling should be recommended.

A. Mild Disease

For patients with mild disease (ie, Hurley stage 1), antibiotic monotherapy is often used as first-line treatment because HS lesions frequently are colonized with bacteria, and antibiotics have anti-inflammatory properties. Most commonly utilized are topical clindamycin 1% (applied twice daily) or oral doxycycline (100 mg twice daily). Therapy of up to 3 months is required to achieve maximal efficacy. Additionally, a combination of antibacterial soap, warm compresses, and sodium dusidate 2% ointment can decrease lesion size and symptoms.

Surgical and other procedural interventions are another treatment option. Deroofing or laser treatment can improve symptoms. Incision and drainage can be used in the acute setting for the treatment of painful, fluctuant abscesses.

B. Moderate to Severe Disease

Moderate to severe HS (Hurley stages 2 or 3) is difficult to treat with antibiotic monotherapy or surgical intervention alone. Such patients may be best managed with systemic therapies in partnership with a dermatologist. The TNF inhibitor adalimumab and the IL-17 inhibitors secukinumab and bimekizumab are approved by the FDA for treatment of moderate to severe HS. Maximal efficacy usually requires 3–6 months of continuous therapy. Additional non–FDA-approved systemic agents that can be considered include other TNF inhibitors (infliximab, etanercept, golimumab), IL-17 inhibitors (ixekizumab), IL-12/23 inhibitors (ustekinumab), the IL-1 inhibitor anakinra, and oral JAK inhibitors (eg, upadacitinib, abrocitinib, tofacitinib).

Non-biologic systemic therapies may be used alone or in conjunction with other treatments. These include combination oral clindamycin/rifampin 300 mg/300 mg twice daily for at least 10 weeks, intravenous ertapenem 1 g daily for about 2 months, intralesional or oral corticosteroids (or both), and oral retinoids (isotretinoin, acitretin). In women, hormonal agents can be considered, including spironolactone, oral contraceptives, finasteride, and dutasteride. Laser therapy and surgery can be helpful in the treatment of moderate to severe HS. Wide excision is the only treatment that is potentially curative.

Prognosis

The course of HS is generally chronic, unpredictable, and often refractory to treatment. Patients should be monitored for metabolic syndrome and other comorbidities (eg, IBD). Monitoring for infection, other adverse events, and complications of systemic therapy is required.

Jenkins T et al. Hidradenitis suppurativa. Dermatol Clin. 2023;41:471. [PMID: 37236715]
Snyder CL et al. Secuknimab in the treatment of hidradenitis suppurativa. Immunotherapy. 2023;15:1449. [PMID: 37840286]
Xue S et al. Progress of biologics and small molecule drugs in the treatment of hidradenitis suppurativa. J Dermatol. 2025;52:1337. [PMID: 40698757]

MILIARIA (Heat Rash)

ESSENTIALS OF DIAGNOSIS

- Burning, itching, superficial aggregated, small vesicles, papules, or pustules on covered areas of the skin, usually the trunk.
- More common in hot, moist climates.
- Rare forms associated with fever and even heat prostration.

General Considerations

Miliaria occurs most commonly on the trunk and intertriginous areas. A hot, moist environment is the most frequent cause. Occlusive clothing, fever while bedridden, and medications that enhance sweat gland function (eg, clonidine, β-blockers, opioids) may increase the risk. Plugging of the ostia of sweat ducts occurs, with ultimate rupture of the sweat duct, producing an irritating, stinging reaction.

Clinical Findings

The usual symptoms are burning and itching. The histologic depth of sweat gland obstruction determines the clinical presentation: miliaria crystallina in the superficial (subcorneal) epidermis, miliaria rubra in the deep epidermis, and miliaria profunda in the dermis. The lesions consist of small (1–3 mm) nonfollicular lesions. Subcorneal thin-walled, discrete clear fluid-filled vesicles are termed "miliaria crystallina." When fluid is turbid and lesions present as vesicopustules or pustules, they are called miliaria pustulosa. Miliaria rubra (prickly heat) presents as pink papules. Miliaria profunda presents as nonfollicular skin-colored papules that develop after multiple bouts of miliaria rubra. In a hospitalized patient, the reaction virtually always affects the back.

Differential Diagnosis

Miliaria is to be distinguished from a drug eruption and folliculitis.

Prevention

Use of a topical antibacterial preparation, such as chlorhexidine, prior to exposure to heat and humidity may help prevent the condition. Frequent turning or sitting of the hospitalized patient may reduce miliaria on the back.

Treatment

The patient should keep cool and wear light clothing. A mid-potency corticosteroid (triamcinolone acetonide, 0.1%) in a lotion or cream may be applied two to four times daily. Secondary infections (superficial pyoderma) are treated with appropriate antistaphylococcal antibiotics. Anticholinergic medications (eg, glycopyrrolate 1 mg orally twice a day or topically applied) may be helpful in severe cases.

Prognosis

Miliaria is usually a mild disorder, but severe forms (tropical anhidrosis and asthenia) result from interference with the heat-regulating mechanism.

Keller Goff G et al. Neonantal miliaria pustulosa–a case series. Pediatr Dermatol. 2025;42:278. [PMID: 39522544]
Palaniappan V et al. Miliaria crystallina. Clin Exp Dermatol. 2023;48:462. [PMID: 36692206]

ERYTHEMAS

REACTIVE ERYTHEMAS

URTICARIA & ANGIOEDEMA

ESSENTIALS OF DIAGNOSIS

- Evanescent wheals or hives with or without angioedema.
- Intense itching; very rarely, pruritus may be absent.
- Urticaria is divided into acute and chronic forms.
- Most episodes are acute and self-limited (1–2 weeks).
- Chronic urticaria (lasting > 6 weeks) may have an autoimmune basis.

General Considerations

Urticaria involves hives, angioedema, or both. It may be acute or chronic (more than 6-week duration). Chronic urticaria is further divided into chronic spontaneous urticaria and chronic inducible urticaria. Chronic inducible urticaria is reproducibly triggered by specific exposures. Examples include cholinergic urticaria, solar urticaria, cold urticaria, dermatographism, and delayed pressure urticaria. True urticaria should be differentiated from diseases that present with similar lesions that are not true urticaria (eg, adult-onset Still disease, urticarial vasculitis, and cryopyrin-associated periodic syndromes). Some patients with chronic spontaneous urticaria demonstrate autoantibodies directed against mast cell IgE receptors.

Clinical Findings

A. Symptoms and Signs

Lesions are itchy, red swellings of a few millimeters to many centimeters (Figure 6–33). The morphology of the lesions may vary over a period of minutes to hours, resulting in geographic or bizarre patterns. Individual lesions in true urticaria last < 24 hours and often only 2–4 hours. Angioedema is involvement of deeper subcutaneous tissue with swelling of the lips, eyelids, palms, soles, and genitalia. **Angioedema is no more likely than urticaria to be associated with systemic complications, such as laryngeal edema or hypotension.** Dermatographism is induced by scratching the skin and can be elicited during the clinic visit. The wheals of cholinergic urticaria are 2–3 mm in diameter with a large surrounding red flare.

B. Laboratory Findings

The most common causes of acute urticaria are foods, upper respiratory infections, and medications. The cause of chronic spontaneous urticaria is often not found. Although laboratory studies are not generally helpful in the evaluation of acute or chronic urticaria, a CBC with differential, ESR, CRP, TSH, and liver biochemical tests may be appropriate for some patients with chronic urticaria. Elevated inflammatory markers suggest an alternate diagnosis. In patients with individual lesions that persist past 24 hours, skin biopsy may confirm neutrophilic urticaria or urticarial vasculitis. A functional ELISA test looking for antibodies against the high-affinity receptor for IgE (Fc-Epislon RI) can identify those who may have an autoimmune basis for their chronic urticaria.

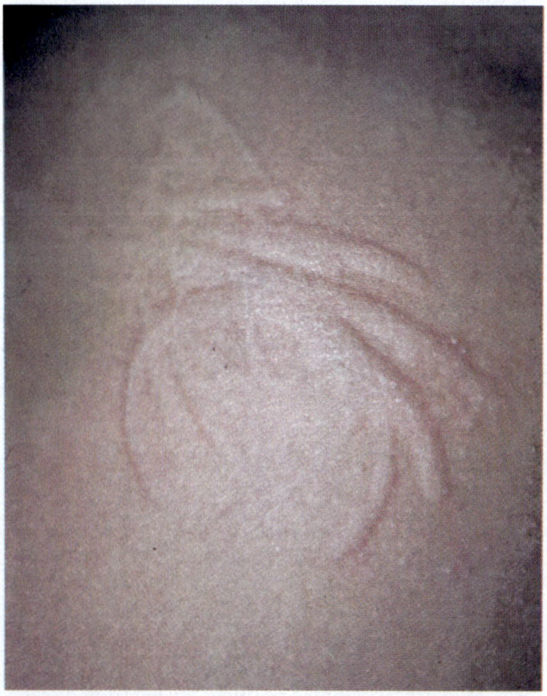

▲ **Figure 6–33.** Urticaria. (Used, with permission, from TG Berger, MD, Dept Dermatology, UCSF.)

Differential Diagnosis

Papular urticaria resulting from insect bites persists for days. A central punctum can usually be seen. Streaked urticarial lesions may be seen in the 24–48 hours before blisters appear in acute allergic plant dermatitis, eg, poison ivy, oak, or sumac. Urticarial responses to heat, sun, water, and pressure are quite rare. Urticarial vasculitis is defined as cutaneous vasculitis where the skin lesions clinically mimic urticaria. Lesions last longer than 24 hours and often sting or burn rather than itch. Patients do not respond to antihistamines. Urticarial vasculitis may be caused by viral hepatitis and may be seen as part of serum sickness. In hereditary angioedema, there is generally a positive family history and GI or respiratory symptoms. Wheals are not part of the syndrome, and the angioedema is not pruritic.

Treatment

A. General Measures

The etiology of acute urticaria is found in less than half of cases. The etiology of chronic urticaria is found in even fewer cases. In general, a careful history and physical examination are helpful, but extensive costly workups for chronic spontaneous urticaria are not indicated. Patients with chronic autoimmune urticaria may have other autoimmune diseases and be more difficult to treat. In cases of chronic inducible urticaria, exposure to physical factors, such as heat, cold, sunlight, pressure, heat induced by exercise, excitement, and hot showers, should be modulated.

B. Systemic Treatment

The mainstay of treatment initially includes H_1-antihistamines, often starting with second-generation antihistamines. Second-generation H_1-antihistamines include fexofenadine (180 mg orally once daily) or cetirizine or loratadine (10 mg orally daily). Less than 40% of chronic urticaria cases respond to standard H_1-blockade, and higher doses of second-generation antihistamines (up to four times the standard recommended dose) increase the likelihood of response to therapy to 60%. Combining antihistamines (eg, fexofenadine plus cetirizine) at these higher doses can be done safely to achieve remission in refractory cases. First-generation H_1-antihistamines such as hydroxyzine, 10–25 mg orally two or three times daily, or as a single nightly dose of 25–75 may be added to this regimen.

Cyproheptadine, 4 mg orally four times daily, may be especially useful for cold urticaria.

Doxepin (a tricyclic antidepressant with potent antihistaminic properties), 10–75 mg orally at bedtime, can be very effective in chronic urticaria. It has anticholinergic side effects and is sedating.

If a skin biopsy of a lesion of chronic urticaria identifies neutrophils as a significant component of the inflammatory infiltrate, dapsone or colchicine (or both) may be useful.

Although systemic corticosteroids will usually suppress acute and chronic urticaria, corticosteroids are rarely indicated and should be avoided if possible, as, once withdrawn, urticaria recurs. Omalizumab and dupilumab are approved for the treatment of refractory chronic urticaria and should be considered when severe chronic urticaria fails to respond to high-dose antihistamines. Cyclosporine (3–5 mg/kg/day), mycophenolate mofetil (1–3 g daily), and other immunosuppressives may be effective in severe cases of chronic urticaria.

C. Local Treatment

Local treatment is rarely rewarding.

Prognosis

Acute urticaria usually lasts only a few days to weeks. Half of patients whose urticaria persists for longer than 6 weeks will have it for years.

Badlow FMS et al. Treatment of acute urticaria: a systematic review. J Eur Acad Dermatol Venereol. 2024;38:2082. [PMID: 38420865]

Pathania YS. Treatment options in refractory chronic spontaneous urticaria. Curr Opin Allergy Clin Immunol. 2024;24:416. [PMID: 38920335]

Zuberbier T et al. Chronic urticaria: unmet needs, emerging drugs, and new perspectives on personalised treatment. Lancet. 2024;404:393. [PMID: 39004090]

ERYTHEMA MULTIFORME/STEVENS-JOHNSON SYNDROME/TOXIC EPIDERMAL NECROLYSIS

ESSENTIALS OF DIAGNOSIS

Erythema multiforme

- Herpes simplex is most common cause.
- Cutaneous lesions are true three-ring targets.
- Presents on the extensor surfaces, palms, soles, or mucous membranes.
- Disease remains localized.

Stevens-Johnson syndrome and toxic epidermal necrolysis

- Stevens-Johnson syndrome: < 10% body surface area (BSA) detachment.
- Stevens-Johnson syndrome/toxic epidermal necrolysis overlap: 10–30% BSA detachment.
- Toxic epidermal necrolysis: > 30% BSA detachment.
- Medications are most common cause.
- Cutaneous lesions are targetoid but often not true three-ring targets.
- Favors the trunk.
- Involves two or more mucous membranes.
- May progress to significant BSA involvement and may be life-threatening.

General Considerations

Erythema multiforme is an acute inflammatory skin disease that was traditionally divided into minor and major types based on the clinical findings. Approximately 90% of cases of erythema multiforme minor follow outbreaks of herpes simplex and are preferably termed "herpes-associated erythema multiforme." The term "erythema multiforme major" has largely been abandoned.

SJS is defined as atypical target lesions with < 10% BSA detachment; TEN is defined as lesions with > 30% BSA detachment; and patients with SJS/TEN overlap have between 10% and 30% BSA detachment. The abbreviation SJS/TEN is often used to refer to these three variants of what is considered one syndrome. SJS/TEN is characterized by toxicity and involvement of two or more mucosal surfaces (often oral and conjunctival but can involve any mucosal surface, including respiratory epithelium). SJS/TEN is most often caused by oral (rarely topical) medications, especially sulfonamides, NSAIDs, allopurinol, and anticonvulsants. In certain races, polymorphisms of antigen-presenting major histocompatibility (MHC) loci increase the risk for the development of SJS/TEN. *Mycoplasma pneumoniae* may trigger a mucocutaneous reaction with skin and oral lesions closely resembling SJS in children/young adults that tends not to progress to TEN-like disease and carries an overall good prognosis.

Clinical Findings

A. Symptoms and Signs

A classic target lesion, as in herpes-associated erythema multiforme, consists of three concentric zones of color change, predominantly on acral surfaces (hands, feet, elbows, and knees) (Figure 6–34). SJS/TEN presents with raised purpuric target-like lesions, with only two zones of color change and a central blister, or nondescript reddish or purpuric macules favoring the trunk and proximal upper

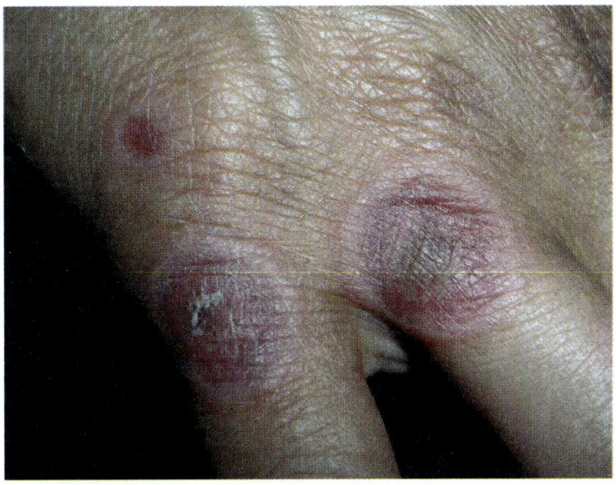

Figure 6–34. Erythema multiforme with classic target lesions. Note the three zones of color change. (Reproduced, with permission, from Richard P. Usatine, MD, in Usatine RP, Smith MA, Mayeaux EJ Jr, Chumley H. *The Color Atlas of Family Medicine*, 2nd ed. McGraw-Hill, 2013.)

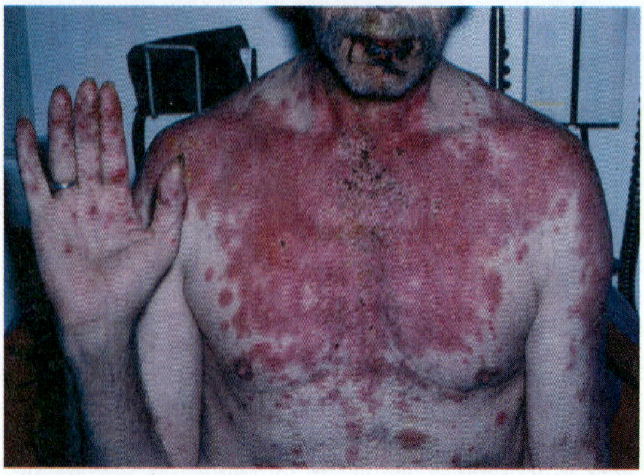

▲ **Figure 6–35.** Stevens-Johnson syndrome. (Used, with permission, from TG Berger, MD, Dept Dermatology, UCSF.)

extremities (Figure 6–35). Pain on eating, swallowing, and urination can occur if relevant mucosae are involved.

B. Laboratory Findings

Skin biopsy is diagnostic. Direct immunofluorescence studies are negative. Blood tests are not useful for diagnosis.

Differential Diagnosis

Urticaria and drug eruptions are the chief entities that must be differentiated from erythema multiforme. In true urticaria, lesions are not purpuric or bullous, last < 24 hours, and respond to antihistamines. The differential diagnosis of SJS/TEN includes autoimmune bullous diseases (eg, pemphigus vulgaris, bullous pemphigoid, and linear IgA bullous dermatosis), acute SLE, vasculitis, and Sweet syndrome. The presence of a blistering eruption requires biopsy and dermatologic consultation for appropriate diagnosis and treatment.

Complications

The tracheobronchial mucosa, conjunctiva, genital, and urethral mucosa may be involved and may result in scarring in severe cases.

Treatment

A. General Measures

Toxic epidermal necrolysis is best treated in an acute care environment, which may include an ICU or a burn unit. Patients should be admitted if mucosal involvement interferes with hydration and nutrition or extensive blistering develops. Open lesions should be managed like second-degree burns. Immediate discontinuation of the inciting medication (before blistering occurs) is a significant predictor of outcome. Delay in establishing the diagnosis and inadvertently continuing the offending medication results in higher morbidity and mortality.

B. Specific Measures

Oral and topical corticosteroids are useful in the oral variant of erythema multiforme. Oral acyclovir prophylaxis of herpes simplex infections may be effective in preventing recurrent herpes-associated erythema multiforme minor.

The most important aspect of treatment for SJS/TEN is to stop the offending medication and to move patients with > 25–30% BSA involvement to an appropriate acute care environment. Nutritional and fluid support and high vigilance for infection are the most important aspects of care. Reviews of systemic treatments for SJS and TEN have been conflicting. Some data support the use of corticosteroids. If corticosteroids are tried, they should be used early, before blistering occurs, and in high doses (prednisone 1–2 mg/kg/day). IVIG (3–4 g given over 3–4 days) used early in the course has resulted in decreased mortality in some studies. Cyclosporine (3–5 mg/kg/day for 7 days) may also be effective. Etanercept is the treatment of choice in some centers.

C. Local Measures

Topical corticosteroids are not very effective in this disease (except the oral variant).

Prognosis

Erythema multiforme minor usually lasts 2–6 weeks and may recur. SJS/TEN may be serious with a mortality of 30% in cases with > 30% BSA involvement. The ABCD-10 and SCORTEN are severity of illness scales that predict mortality in SJS/TEN.

When to Refer

- Refer to an ophthalmologist when ocular involvement is present because vision loss is a major consequence of SJS/TEN.
- Refer to a urologist, gynecologist, or both when genitourinary involvement is present.

Carr DF et al. Stevens-Johnson syndrome/toxic epidermal necrolysis: international consensus, advances and opportunities. Br J Dermatol. 2024;192:4. [PMID: 39283146]

Gungor T et al. Erythema multiforme: a retrospective study of etiologies, clinical manifestations, and treatments. J Dent Sci. 2024;19:2295. [PMID: 39347027]

Ogiji ED et al. Greater mechanistic understanding of the cutaneous pathogenesis of Stevens-Johnson syndrome/toxic epidermal necrolysis can shed light on novel therapeutic strategies: a comprehensive review. Curr Opin Allergy Clin Immunol. 2024;24:218. [PMID: 38753537]

EXFOLIATIVE DERMATITIS (Exfoliative Erythroderma)

ESSENTIALS OF DIAGNOSIS

- Desquamation and erythema over most of the body.
- Itching, malaise, fever, chills, weight loss.

General Considerations

Erythroderma describes generalized redness of > 90% of the skin surface. Erythroderma may be acute (presenting as erythema without scale) or subacute to chronic (presenting as widespread redness and scaling and referred to as exfoliative erythroderma). A preexisting dermatosis is the cause of exfoliative dermatitis in two-thirds of cases, including psoriasis, atopic dermatitis, contact dermatitis, pityriasis rubra pilaris, and seborrheic dermatitis. Reactions to topical or systemic medications account for 15% of cases, cancer 10% (most commonly cutaneous T-cell lymphoma), idiopathic 10%. Crusted scabies can present as an exfoliative erythroderma and is highly contagious. Without a clear-cut prior history of skin disease or medication exposure, it is often not possible to make a specific diagnosis of the underlying condition at the time of initial presentation. Definitive diagnosis may require continued observation.

Clinical Findings

A. Symptoms and Signs

Symptoms may include itching, weakness, malaise, fever, and weight loss. Chills are prominent. Erythema and desquamation are widespread. Loss of hair and nails can occur. Generalized lymphadenopathy may be due to lymphoma or leukemia or may be reactive. The mucosae are typically spared.

B. Laboratory Findings

A skin biopsy is required and may show changes of a specific inflammatory dermatitis or cutaneous T-cell lymphoma. In Sézary syndrome, helpful findings include peripheral leukocytes with clonal rearrangements of the T-cell receptor and flow cytometry demonstrating a CD4:CD8 ratio > 10:1 and loss of CD4 T cell markers such as CD7 and CD26. Skin biopsy is nonspecific in 50% of cases.

Complications

Protein and electrolyte loss as well as dehydration may develop in patients with generalized inflammatory exfoliative erythroderma; sepsis may occur.

Treatment

A. Topical Therapy

Home treatment is with cool to tepid baths and application of mid-potency corticosteroids under wet dressings or with occlusion with plastic wrap. If the condition becomes unmanageable in an outpatient setting, the patient should be hospitalized.

B. Specific Measures

Stop all medications, if possible. Systemic corticosteroids may provide marked improvement in severe or fulminant exfoliative dermatitis but should be avoided long-term (see Chapter 30). For cases of psoriatic erythroderma and pityriasis rubra pilaris, acitretin, methotrexate, cyclosporine, or a TNF inhibitor may be indicated. Erythroderma secondary to lymphoma or leukemia requires specific topical or systemic chemotherapy. Suitable antibiotic medications with coverage for *Staphylococcus* should be given when there is evidence of bacterial infection.

Prognosis

Careful follow-up may be necessary to identify the cause of exfoliative erythroderma. Most patients improve or recover completely, but some require long-term therapy. Deaths are rare in the absence of cutaneous T-cell lymphoma. A minority of patients will suffer from undiminished erythroderma for indefinite periods.

Kliniec K et al. Erythroderma: a retrospective study of 212 patients hospitalized in a tertiary center in lower Silesia, Poland. J Clin Med. 2024;13:645. [PMID: 38337339]

Pang Y et al. Deciphering the etiologies of adult erythroderma: an updated guide to presentations, diagnostic tools, pathophysiologies, and treatments. Am J Clin Dermatol. 2024;25:927. [PMID: 39348008]

PHOTODERMATITIS

ESSENTIALS OF DIAGNOSIS

- Painful or pruritic erythema, edema, or vesiculation on sun-exposed surfaces (face, neck, hands, and "V" of the chest).
- Inner upper eyelids and area under the chin are spared.

General Considerations

Photodermatitis is a cutaneous reaction to UV radiation. It comprises four groups: (1) primary, idiopathic immunologically mediated photodermatoses; (2) drug- or chemical-induced photodermatoses, (3) dermatoses that are worsened or aggravated by UV exposure; and (4) genetic diseases with mutations predisposing to photodermatitis.

Primary photodermatoses include polymorphic light eruption, chronic actinic dermatitis, and actinic prurigo. Drug- or chemical-induced photodermatitis may be either exogenous or endogenous in origin. Porphyria cutanea tarda and pellagra are examples of endogenous phototoxic dermatoses. Exogenous drug- or chemical-induced photodermatitis manifests either as phototoxicity (a nonimmunologic, UV-induced cytoxic injury presenting as a sunburn-like reaction) or as photoallergy (a true immunologic reaction that presents with dermatitis). There may be some clinical overlap between these two.

Drug-induced phototoxicity is triggered by UVA. The most common medications causing a phototoxic reaction are vemurafenib, NSAIDs, voriconazole, tetracyclines, quinolones, hydrochlorothiazide, amiodarone, and chlorpromazine. Other potent photosensitizers include TMP/SMZ, quinine or quinidine, griseofulvin, eculizumab, topical and systemic retinoids (tretinoin, isotretinoin, acitretin), and calcium channel blockers.

Contact photosensitivity may occur with plants, perfumes, and sunscreens. The sunscreen oxybenzone (a benzophenone) is a common cause of photoallergic dermatitis. Dermatoses that are worsened or aggravated by UV exposure include SLE and dermatomyositis. Three percent of persons with atopic dermatitis, especially middle-aged women, are photosensitive.

Clinical Findings

A. Symptoms and Signs

The acute inflammatory phase of phototoxicity, if severe enough, is accompanied by pain, fever, GI symptoms, malaise, and even prostration. Signs include erythema, edema, and possibly vesiculation and oozing on exposed surfaces. Peeling of the epidermis and pigmentary changes often result. The key to diagnosis is localization of the rash to photoexposed areas, though eruptions may become generalized with time to involve photoprotected areas. The lower lip may be affected.

B. Laboratory Findings

Blood and urine tests are generally not helpful unless porphyria cutanea tarda is suggested by the presence of blistering, scarring, milia (white cysts 1–2 mm in diameter) and skin fragility of the dorsal hands, and facial hypertrichosis. Eosinophilia may be present in chronic photoallergic responses.

Differential Diagnosis

The differential diagnosis is long. If a clear history of the use of a topical or systemic photosensitizer is not available, and if the eruption is persistent, then a workup including biopsy and light testing may be required. Photodermatitis must be differentiated from contact dermatitis that may develop from one of the many substances in sunscreens, as these may often have a similar distribution. Sensitivity to actinic rays may also be part of a more serious condition, such as porphyria cutanea tarda or lupus erythematosus. These disorders are diagnosed by appropriate blood or urine tests. Polymorphous light eruption (PMLE) is a common idiopathic photodermatitis and often has its onset in the third to fourth decades, except in American Indian persons and Latinas/Latinos, in whom it may present in childhood. PMLE is chronic in nature. Transitory periods of spontaneous remission do occur.

Complications

Some individuals continue to chronically react to light even when they are no longer exposed to photosensitizing medications.

Prevention

While sunscreens are useful agents in general and should be used by persons with photosensitivity, patients may react to such low amounts of energy that sunscreens alone may not be sufficient protection against photodermatoses. Sunscreens with an SPF of 30–60 and broad UVA coverage, containing dicamphor sulfonic acid (Mexoryl SX), avobenzone (Parasol 1789), titanium dioxide, and micronized zinc oxide, are especially useful in patients with photoallergic dermatitis. Photosensitivity due to porphyria is not prevented by sunscreens and requires barrier protection (clothing) to prevent outbreaks.

Treatment

A. Specific Measures

Medications should be suspected in cases of photosensitivity even if the particular medication (such as hydrochlorothiazide) has been used for months.

B. Local Measures

When the eruption is vesicular or weepy, treatment is similar to that of any acute dermatitis, using cooling and soothing wet dressings.

Sunscreens should be used as described above. Mid-potency to high-potency topical corticosteroids are of limited benefit in phototoxic reactions but may help in PMLE and photoallergic reactions. Since the face is often involved, close monitoring for corticosteroid side effects is recommended.

C. Systemic Measures

Aspirin may have some value for fever and pain of acute sunburn. Systemic corticosteroids in doses as described for acute contact dermatitis may be required for severe acute photosensitivity reactions. Otherwise, different photodermatoses are treated in specific ways.

Patients with chronic primary photodermatoses may require systemic treatment with hydroxychloroquine (5 mg/kg once daily), dupilumab, or immunosuppressives, such as azathioprine (50–300 mg once daily) or cyclosporine (3–5 mg/kg once daily).

Prognosis

The most common phototoxic sunburn reactions are usually benign and self-limited. PMLE and some cases of photoallergy can persist for years.

Holmes Z et al. Dupilumab for chronic actinic dermatitis: a case series and review of the literature. Australas J Dermatol. 2024;65:287. [PMID: 38629787]

Malekan M et al. JAK inhibitors as a promising therapy for immune-mediated photodermatoses. Drug Discov Today. 2025;30:104344. [PMID: 40157596]

DRUG ERUPTION (Dermatitis Medicamentosa)

ESSENTIALS OF DIAGNOSIS

- Usually, abrupt onset of widespread, symmetric erythematous eruption.
- May mimic any inflammatory skin condition.
- Constitutional symptoms (malaise, arthralgia, headache, and fever) may be present.

General Considerations

Rashes are among the most common adverse reactions to medications and occur in 2–3% of hospitalized patients. There are multiple different types of cutaneous reactions to medications. Penicillins, cephalosporins, and NSAIDs are the most common cause of urticarial drug eruptions. Antibiotics, anticonvulsants, allopurinol, and NSAIDs are common causes of maculopapular or morbilliform reactions. Drug-induced hypersensitivity reaction (DIHS) (also known as drug eruption with eosinophilia and systemic symptoms [DRESS] syndrome) is most often caused by anticonvulsants, allopurinol, and sulfonamides. SJS and TEN most commonly occur in response to antibiotics, sulfonamides, anticonvulsants, allopurinol, and NSAIDs. Phenolphthalein, pyrazolone derivatives, tetracyclines, NSAIDs, TMP-SMZ, and barbiturates are the major causes of fixed drug eruptions. Calcium channel blockers are a common cause of pruritus and eczemas in older adults. Immune checkpoint inhibitors and biologic agents can cause a variety of drug reactions.

Certain genetic polymorphisms of antigen-presenting MHC loci increase the risk for the development of severe drug eruptions, including SJS/TEN and DIHS. Pharmacogenetic testing can help predict who is at risk for and therefore should avoid certain medication exposures.

Clinical Findings

A. Symptoms and Signs

Drug eruptions are generally classified as "simple" or "complex," referring to the risk of morbidity and mortality associated with the specific eruption. Simple morbilliform or maculopapular drug eruptions involve an exanthem, usually appear in the second week of medication therapy, and have no associated constitutional symptoms or abnormal laboratory findings. Complex drug eruptions include DIHS and SJS/TEN.

DIHS occurs later than the simple morbilliform drug eruptions with signs and symptoms developing 2–6 weeks after the medication has been started and has associated constitutional symptoms and abnormal laboratory findings. These may include fevers, chills, hematologic abnormalities (especially eosinophilia and atypical lymphocytosis), and abnormal liver or kidney function. Coexistent reactivation of certain viruses, especially HHV-6, but also Epstein-Barr virus, cytomegalovirus, HHV-7, and parvovirus B19, may be present and may be important in the pathogenesis of these complex drug eruptions. Table 6–3 summarizes the types of skin reactions, their appearance and distribution, and the common offenders in each case.

B. Laboratory Findings

Routinely ordered blood work is of no value in the diagnosis of simple drug eruptions, except upon initial evaluation to ensure that there is no systemic involvement. In complex drug eruptions, the CBC, liver biochemical tests, and kidney function tests should be monitored. Skin biopsies may be helpful in making the diagnosis. Serum PCR for HHV-6, HHV-7, Epstein-Barr virus, cytomegalovirus, and parvovirus B19 is sometimes performed.

Differential Diagnosis

Observation after discontinuation, which may be a slow process, helps establish the diagnosis. Rechallenge, though of theoretical value, may pose a danger to the patient and is best avoided.

Complications

Some cutaneous drug reactions may be associated with visceral involvement. The organ systems involved depend on the individual medication or drug class. Most common is an infectious mononucleosis-like illness and hepatitis associated with administration of anticonvulsants. Myocarditis may be a serious complication of drug-induced hypersensitivity syndrome and may present acutely or months after initial rash onset. Months after recovering from DIHS, patients may suffer hypothyroidism or other autoimmune phenomena.

Treatment

A. General Measures

Systemic manifestations are treated as they arise (eg, anemia, icterus, purpura). Antihistamines may be of value in urticarial and angioneurotic reactions. Epinephrine 1:1000, 0.5–1 mL intravenously or subcutaneously, should be used as an emergency measure. In DIHS, corticosteroids are typically required; the most common regimen is oral prednisone, 1–1.5 mg/kg/day, which is tapered slowly over a minimum of 6 weeks, since rapid taper leads to rebound and more recalcitrant disease. In the case of allopurinol-induced DIHS, starting a steroid-sparing agent (eg, mycophenolate mofetil) at the time of prednisone initiation is recommended because allopurinol-induced DIHS tends to rebound after corticosteroid discontinuation. Treatment in this special case often takes up to 12 months.

B. Local Measures

SJS/TEN with extensive blistering eruptions resulting in erosions and superficial ulcerations demands hospitalization and nursing care in an acute care unit. See Erythema Multiforme/Stevens-Johnson Syndrome/Toxic Epidermal Necrolysis, above.

Prognosis

Drug rash usually disappears upon withdrawal of the medication and proper treatment. DIHS may be associated with autoimmune phenomena, including abnormal thyroid function. This can occur months after the hypersensitivity syndrome has resolved.

Calle AM et al. DRESS syndrome: a literature review and treatment algorithm. World Allergy Organ J. 2023;16:100673. [PMID: 37082745]

Wei BM et al. Drug-induced hypersensitivity syndrome/drug reaction with eosinophilia and systemic symptoms. Part II diagnosis and management. J Am Acad Dermatol. 2024;90:911. [PMID: 37516356]

Yan A et al. Morbilliform eruptions: differentiating low-risk drug eruptions, severe cutaneous adverse reactions, viral eruptions, and acute graft-versus-host disease. Am J Clin Dermatol. 2025;26:379. [PMID: 39888589]

Table 6–3. Skin reactions due to systemic medications.

Reaction	Appearance	Distribution and Comments	Common Offenders
Allergic vasculitis	The primary lesion is typically a 2–3 mm purpuric papule. Other morphologies include urticaria that lasts over 24 hours, vesicles, bullae, or necrotic ulcers.	Most severe on the legs.	Sulfonamides, phenytoin, propylthiouracil.
Drug exanthem	Morbilliform, maculopapular, exanthematous reactions.	The most common skin reaction to medications. Initially begins on trunk 7–10 days after the medication has been started. Spreads to extremities and begins to clear on the trunk over 3–5 days. In previously exposed patients, the rash may start in 2–3 days. Fever may be present.	Antibiotics (especially ampicillin and TMP-SMZ), sulfonamides and related compounds (including thiazide diuretics, furosemide, and sulfonylurea hypoglycemic agents), and barbiturates.
Drug-related subacute cutaneous lupus erythematosus (Drug-induced SLE rarely produces a skin reaction)	May present with a photosensitive rash, annular lesions, or psoriasis on upper trunk.	Less severe than SLE, sparing the kidneys and CNS. Recovery often follows medication withdrawal.	Diltiazem, etanercept, hydrochlorothiazide, infliximab, lisinopril, terbinafine.
Erythema nodosum	Inflammatory cutaneous nodules.	Usually limited to the extensor aspects of the legs. May be accompanied by fever, arthralgias, and pain.	Oral contraceptives.
Drug-induced hypersensitivity syndrome	Erythroderma	Entire skin surface. Typically associated with elevated liver biochemical tests, eosinophilia, and AKI. Eruption begins between 2 and 6 weeks after first dose of medication.	Allopurinol, sulfonamides, aromatic anticonvulsants, NSAID, dapsone, lamotrigine.
Fixed drug eruptions	Single or multiple demarcated, round, erythematous plaques that often become hyperpigmented.	Recur at the same site when the medication is repeated. Hyperpigmentation, if present, remains after healing.	Antimicrobials, analgesics (acetaminophen, ibuprofen, and naproxen), barbiturates, heavy metals, antiparasitic agents, antihistamines, phenolphthalein.
Acneiform eruptions	Papulopustular eruption resembling acne that may be pruritic or tender.	Face, chest, back.	Corticosteroids, isoniazid, lithium, phenytoin, EGFR inhibitors.
Lichenoid and lichen planus–like eruptions	Pruritic, erythematous to violaceous polygonal papules that coalesce or expand to form plaques.	May be in photo- or nonphotodistributed pattern.	Carbamazepine, furosemide, hydroxychloroquine, phenothiazines, β-blockers, quinidine, quinine, sulfonylureas, tetracyclines, thiazides, and triprolidine.
Photosensitivity: increased sensitivity to light, often of UVA wavelengths, but may be due to UVB or visible light as well	Sunburn, vesicles, papules in photodistributed pattern.	Exposed skin of the face, the neck, and the backs of the hands and, in women, the lower legs. Exaggerated response to UV light.	Sulfonamides and sulfonamide-related compounds (thiazide diuretics, furosemide, sulfonylureas), tetracyclines, phenothiazines, sulindac, amiodarone, voriconazole, and NSAIDs.
Pigmentary changes	Flat hyperpigmented areas.	Forehead and cheeks (chloasma, melasma). The most common pigmentary disorder associated with drug ingestion. Improvement is slow despite stopping the medication.	Oral contraceptives are the usual cause. Diltiazem causes facial hyperpigmentation that may be difficult to distinguish from melasma.

(*continued*)

Table 6–3. Skin reactions due to systemic medications. (continued)

Reaction	Appearance	Distribution and Comments	Common Offenders
	Blue-gray discoloration.	Light-exposed areas.	Chlorpromazine and related phenothiazines.
	Brown or blue-gray pigmentation.	Generalized.	Heavy metals (silver, gold, bismuth, and arsenic).
	Blue-black patches on the shins.		Minocycline, chloroquine.
	Blue-black pigmentation of the nails and palate and depigmentation of the hair.		Chloroquine.
	Slate-gray color.	Primarily in photoexposed areas.	Amiodarone.
	Brown discoloration of the nails.	Especially in more darkly pigmented patients.	Hydroxyurea.
Pityriasis rosea–like eruptions	Oval, red, slightly raised patches with central scale.	Mainly on the trunk.	Barbiturates, bismuth, captopril, clonidine, methopromazine, metoprolol, metronidazole, and tripelennamine.
Psoriasiform eruptions	Scaly red plaques.	May be located on trunk and extremities. Palms and soles may be hyperkeratotic. May cause psoriasiform eruption or worsen psoriasis.	Antimalarials, lithium, β-blockers, and TNF inhibitors.
SJS/TEN	Target-like lesions. Bullae may occur. Mucosal involvement. Nikolsky's sign.	Usually trunk and proximal extremities.	Sulfonamides, anticonvulsants, allopurinol, NSAIDs, lamotrigine.
Urticaria	Red, itchy wheals that vary in size from < 1 cm to many centimeters. May be accompanied by angioedema.	Chronic urticaria is rarely caused by medications.	Acute urticaria: penicillins, NSAIDs, sulfonamides, opioids, and salicylates. Angioedema is common in patients receiving ACE inhibitors and ARBs.

SJS/TEN, Stevens-Johnson syndrome/toxic epidermal necrolysis; TMP-SMZ, trimethoprim-sulfamethoxazole.

MISCELLANEOUS

PRURITUS

Pruritus is the sensation that provokes a desire to scratch. Pruritus as a medical complaint is 40% as common as low back pain. Older Asian men are most significantly affected, with 20% of all health care visits in Asian men over the age of 65 involving the complaint of itch. The quality of life of a patient with chronic pruritus is the same as a patient undergoing hemodialysis. Better understanding of the role of pruritogens (interleukins-31, -4, -13 and thymic stromal lymphopoietin) in the pathophysiology of itch has enabled recent therapeutic advances.

Dry skin is the first cause of itch that should be sought since it is common and easily treated. The next step is to determine whether a primary skin lesion with associated pruritus is present. Examples of primary cutaneous pruritic diseases include scabies, atopic dermatitis, insect bites, pediculosis, contact dermatitis, drug reactions, urticaria, psoriasis, lichen planus, bullous pemphigoid, and fiberglass dermatitis, all of which have recognizable morphologies. The treatment of an underlying primary skin condition usually results in control of the associated pruritus.

Persistent pruritus not explained by cutaneous disease or association with a primary skin eruption should prompt a staged workup for systemic causes. Common causes of pruritus associated with systemic diseases include endocrine disorders (eg, hypo- or hyperthyroidism or hyperparathyroidism), psychiatric disturbances, lymphoma, leukemia, internal malignant disorders, iron deficiency anemia, HIV, hypercalcemia, low vitamin D levels, cholestasis, and some neurologic disorders. Calcium channel blockers can cause pruritus with or without eczema, even years after they have been started, and it may take up to 1 year for pruritus to resolve after the calcium channel blocker has been stopped.

Treatment

The treatment of chronic pruritus can be frustrating. Most cases of pruritus are not mediated by histamine, hence the poor response of many patients to antihistamines. Emollients for dry skin are listed in Table 6–2. Emollient creams (preferred over lotions) should be generously applied from neck to toe immediately after towel drying and again one more time per day. Neuropathic pruritus responds to neurally acting agents, such as gabapentin (starting at 300 mg orally at around 4 PM and a second dose of 600 mg orally at bedtime) or pregabalin (150 mg orally daily). Combinations of antihistamines, doxepin, gabapentin, pregabalin, mirtazapine, and opioid antagonists can be attempted in refractory cases. In cancer-associated and other forms of pruritus, aprepitant 80 mg orally daily for several days can be dramatically effective. Pruritus in conjunction with uremia and hemodialysis and to a lesser degree the pruritus of liver disease may be helped by phototherapy with UVB or PUVA. Difelikefalin is currently the only treatment approved specifically for pruritus associated with CKD in those receiving hemodialysis. Other therapies that may relieve the pruritus of CKD include gabapentin or mirtazapine. Nemolizumab (IL-31 inhibitor) and dupilumab (IL-4/13 inhibitor) are each approved to treat prurigo nodularis.

Prognosis

Elimination of external factors and irritating agents may give complete relief. Pruritus accompanying a specific skin disease will subside when the skin disease is controlled. Pruritus accompanying serious internal disease may not respond to any type of therapy.

Butler DC et al. Chronic pruritus: a review. JAMA. 2024;331:2114. [PMID: 38809527]

Liao V et al. Prurigo nodularis: new insights into pathogenesis and novel therapeutics. Br J Dermatol. 2024;190:798. [PMID: 38345154]

Srihari S et al. Etiopathogenesis and current management of oncogenic pruritus–a narrative review. Indian J Dermatol. 2025;70:257. [PMID: 40918704]

ANOGENITAL PRURITUS

ESSENTIALS OF DIAGNOSIS

- Anogenital itching, chiefly nocturnal.
- Skin findings are highly variable, ranging from none to excoriations and inflammation of any degree, including lichenification.

General Considerations

Anogenital pruritus may be due to a primary inflammatory skin disease (intertrigo, psoriasis, lichen simplex chronicus, seborrheic dermatitis, lichen sclerosus), contact dermatitis (soaps, wipes, colognes, douches, and topical treatments), irritating secretions (diarrhea, leukorrhea, or trichomoniasis), infections (candidiasis, dermatophytosis, erythrasma), or oxyuriasis (pinworms). Erythrasma is diagnosed by coral-red fluorescence with Wood light and cured with erythromycin. Squamous cell carcinoma of the anus and extramammary Paget disease are rare causes of genital pruritus.

In pruritus ani, hemorrhoids are often found, and leakage of mucus and bacteria from the distal rectum onto the perianal skin may be important in cases in which no other skin abnormality is found.

Many women experience pruritus vulvae. Pruritus vulvae does not usually involve the anal area, though anal itching may spread to the vulva. In men, pruritus of the scrotum is most commonly seen in the absence of pruritus ani.

Up to one-third of unidentified causes of anogenital pruritus may be due to nerve impingements of the lumbosacral spine, so evaluation of lumbosacral spine disease is appropriate if no skin disorder is identified and topical therapy is ineffective.

Clinical Findings

A. Symptoms and Signs

The only symptom is itching. Physical findings are usually not present, but there may be erythema, fissuring, maceration, lichenification, excoriations, or changes suggestive of candidiasis or tinea.

B. Laboratory Findings

Microscopic examination or culture of tissue scrapings may reveal yeasts or fungi. Stool examination may show pinworms. Radiologic studies may demonstrate lumbarsacral spinal disease.

Differential Diagnosis

The etiologic differential diagnosis consists of *Candida* infection, parasitosis, local irritation from contactants or irritants, nerve impingement, and other primary skin disorders of the genital area, such as psoriasis, seborrhea, intertrigo, or lichen sclerosus.

Prevention

Instruct the patient in proper anogenital hygiene after treating systemic or local conditions.

Treatment

Treating constipation, preferably with high-fiber management (psyllium), may help. Instruct the patient to use very soft or moistened tissue or cotton after bowel movements and to clean the perianal area thoroughly with cool water if possible. Women should use similar precautions after urinating. Patch testing reveals clinically relevant allergy in about 20% of patients, often to methylchloroisothiazolinone or methylisothiazolinone, preservatives commonly found in "baby wipes" and other personal care products.

Pramoxine cream or lotion or hydrocortisone-pramoxine (Pramosone), 1% or 2.5% cream, lotion, or ointment, is helpful for anogenital pruritus and should be applied after a bowel movement. Topical doxepin cream 5% is similarly effective but may be sedating. Topical calcineurin inhibitors (tacrolimus 0.03%) improve pruritus ani in patients with atopic dermatitis. Underclothing should be changed daily, and in men, the seam of their "boxers" should not rub against or contact the scrotum. Balneol Perianal Cleansing Lotion or Tucks premoistened pads, ointment, or cream may be very useful for pruritus ani. About one-third of patients with scrotal or anal pruritus will respond to capsaicin cream 0.006%. Gabapentin or pregabalin may be helpful in cases where topical therapies have failed. The use of high-potency topical corticosteroids should be avoided in the genital area.

Prognosis

Although benign, anogenital pruritus is often persistent and recurrent.

Balfour A et al. Anogenital pruritus is associated with anxiety, depression, and other psychiatric disorders. Int J Womens Dermatol. 2024;10:e168. [PMID: 38989111]
Mashoudy KD et al. From compression to itch: exploring the link between nerve compression and neuropathic pruritus. Am J Clin Dermatol. 2025;26:23. [PMID: 39417971]

PIGMENTARY DISORDERS

Although the color of skin may be altered by many diseases and agents, the vast majority of patients have either an increase or decrease in pigment secondary to an inflammatory disease, such as acne or atopic dermatitis.

Other pigmentary disorders include those resulting from exposure to exogenous pigments, such as carotenemia, argyria, and tattooing. Other endogenous pigmentary disorders are attributable to metabolic substances (eg, hemosiderin [iron]) in purpuric processes, to homogentisic acid in ochronosis, and bile pigments.

Classification

Disorders of hyper- or hypopigmentation may be considered to be primary or secondary to other disorders. Depigmentation, the absence of all pigment, should be differentiated from hypopigmentation, in which the affected skin is lighter than baseline skin color, but not completely devoid of pigment.

The evaluation of pigmentary disorders is helped by Wood light, which accentuates epidermal pigmentation in hyperpigmented disorders and highlights complete loss of pigment in depigmentating disorders. Depigmentation, as seen in vitiligo, enhances with Wood light examination, whereas postinflammatory hypopigmentation does not.

A. Primary Pigmentary Disorders

1. Hyperpigmentation—The disorders in this category are nevoid, congenital, or acquired. Nevoid and congenital disorders include pigmented nevi, mosaic hyperpigmentation, ephelides (juvenile freckles), and lentigines (senile freckles). Hyperpigmentation due to systemic diseases may be seen in association with Addison disease, vitamin B_{12} deficiency, hemochromatosis, and Wilson disease. Melasma (chloasma) occurs as patterned hyperpigmentation of the face, most commonly as a direct effect of estrogens. It may occur during pregnancy, exposure to oral contraceptives, or be idiopathic. Although more common in women, melasma affects men and persons of all skin tones.

2. Hypopigmentation and depigmentation—Depigmenting disorders in this category are vitiligo, albinism, and piebaldism. In vitiligo, pigment cells (melanocytes) are destroyed

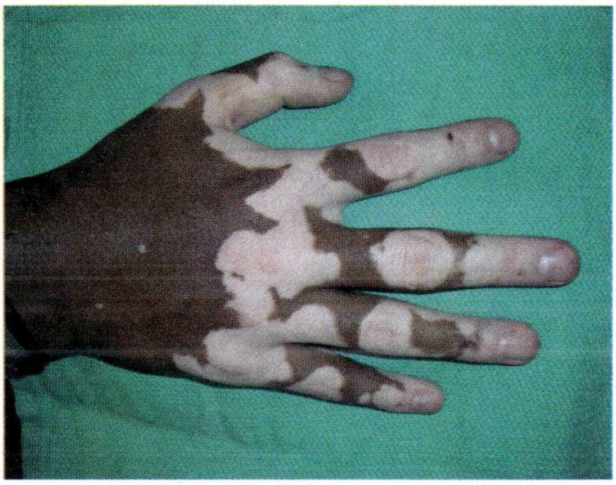

Figure 6–36. Depigmented—vitiligo. (Reproduced, with permission, from Richard P. Usatine, MD, in Usatine RP, Smith MA, Mayeaux EJ Jr, Chumley H. *The Color Atlas of Family Medicine*, 3rd ed. McGraw-Hill, 2019.)

(Figure 6–36). Vitiligo, present in approximately 1% of the population, may be associated with other autoimmune disorders, such as autoimmune thyroid disease, pernicious anemia, diabetes mellitus, and Addison disease.

B. Secondary Pigmentary Disorders

Any damage to the skin (irritation, allergy, infection, excoriation, burns, or dermatologic therapy, such as chemical peels and freezing with liquid nitrogen) may result in hyper- or hypopigmentation. Several disorders of clinical importance are described below.

1. Hyperpigmentation—The most common type of secondary hyperpigmentation occurs after another inflammatory dermatologic condition, such as acne, lichen planus, or eczema, and is most commonly seen in moderately pigmented skin tones. It is called post-inflammatory hyperpigmentation. Hemosiderin deposition, as in stasis dermatitis, may lead to hyperpigmentation that is red-brown in color.

Pigmentation may be produced by certain medications, eg, chloroquine, chlorpromazine, minocycline (Figure 6–37), and amiodarone. Fixed drug eruptions to phenolphthalein (in laxatives), TMP-SMZ, NSAIDs, and tetracyclines also lead to hyperpigmentation, typically in annular patches.

2. Hypopigmentation—Hypopigmentation may complicate atopic dermatitis, lichen planus, psoriasis, discoid lupus, and lichen simplex chronicus. It may also be post-traumatic or iatrogenic (eg, due to the use of superpotent topical corticosteroids) or both. *Clinicians must exercise special care in using liquid nitrogen on any patients with darker skin tones since doing so may result in hypopigmentation or depigmentation, at times permanent.* Intralesional or intra-articular injections of high concentrations of corticosteroids may also cause localized temporary hypopigmentation. Depigmentation indistinguishable from vitiligo is a known complication of immune checkpoint inhibitor therapy for melanoma.

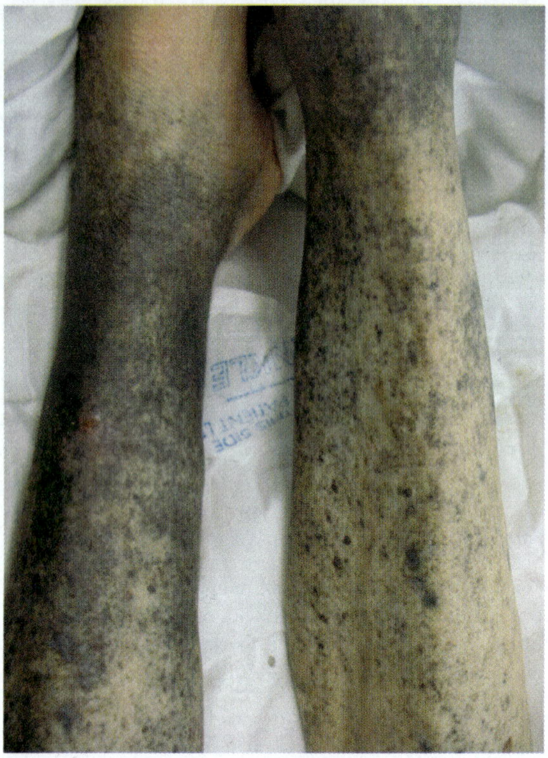

▲ **Figure 6–37.** Minocycline hyperpigmentation. (Used, with permission, from Lindy Fox, MD.)

Complications

Actinic keratoses and skin cancers are more likely to develop in persons with vitiligo. Severe emotional trauma may occur in extensive vitiligo or severe cases of hypo- and hyperpigmentation, particularly in persons with darker skin tones.

Treatment & Prognosis

A. Hyperpigmentation

Therapeutic bleaching preparations generally contain hydroquinone. Hydroquinone has occasionally caused unexpected hypo- or hyperpigmentation, or secondary ochronosis and pigmented milia with prolonged use.

The role of exposure to UV light cannot be overstressed as a factor promoting or contributing to most disorders of hyperpigmentation, and such exposure should be minimized. Melasma, ephelides, and postinflammatory hyperpigmentation may be treated with varying success with 4% hydroquinone and a sunscreen containing UVA photoprotectants (Avobenzone, Mexoryl, zinc oxide, titanium dioxide). Tretinoin cream, 0.025–0.1%, may be added. Adjuvant topical options for melasma include kojic acid, ascorbic acid, cysteamine, niacinamide, and azelaic acid. Superficial melasma responds well to topical therapy, but if there is predominantly dermal deposition of pigment (does not enhance with Wood light), the prognosis is poor. Response to therapy may take months and requires avoidance of sunlight. Hyperpigmentation often recurs after treatment if the skin is exposed to UV light. Tranexamic acid, 250 mg twice a day for 8–12 weeks, is an oral treatment for melasma. It should not be used in patients with hypercoagulability. Acne with postinflammatory hyperpigmentation responds well to azelaic acid and tretinoin since both address acne and hyperpigmentation. Solar lentigines respond to liquid nitrogen application. Tretinoin 0.1% cream or tazarotene 0.1% used over 10 months can fade solar lentigines, facial hyperpigmentation, and postinflammatory hyperpigmentation. Lasers are available for the removal of epidermal and dermal pigment and should be considered for patients whose responses to medical treatment are inadequate.

B. Hypopigmentation

In secondary hypopigmentation, repigmentation may occur spontaneously. Cosmetics such as Covermark and Dermablend are highly effective for concealing disfiguring patches. Therapy of vitiligo is long and tedious, and the patient must be strongly motivated. If < 20% of the skin is involved (most cases), topical tacrolimus 0.1% twice daily is the first-line therapy. A superpotent corticosteroid may also be used, but local skin atrophy from prolonged use may ensue. Topical ruxolitinib (JAK inhibitor) cream is FDA-approved for the treatment of vitiligo. With 20–25% involvement, narrowband UVB or oral PUVA is the best option. Severe phototoxic response (sunburn) may occur with PUVA. The face and upper chest respond best, and the fingertips and the genital areas do not respond as well to treatment. Years of treatment may be required.

Ali L et al. Pathogenesis of melasma explained. Int J Dermatol. 2025;64:1201. [PMID: 40022484]

Ko D et al. Disorders of hyperpigmentation. Part 2. Review of management and treatment options for hyperpigmentation. J Am Acad Dermatol. 2023;88:291. [PMID: 35158001]

Wang RF et al. Disorders of hyperpigmentation. Part 1. Pathogenesis and clinical features of common pigmentary disorders. J Am Acad Dermatol. 2023;88:271. [PMID: 35151757]

ALOPECIA

Classification

Alopecias are divided into scarring and nonscarring forms. When evaluating a patient who reports hair loss, it is most important to determine if follicular markings (the opening where hair exits the skin) are present or absent. Present follicular markings suggest a nonscarring alopecia; absent follicular markings suggest a scarring alopecia.

Nonscarring Alopecia

Nonscarring alopecia may occur in association with various systemic diseases, such as SLE, secondary syphilis, hyper- or hypothyroidism, iron deficiency anemia, vitamin D deficiency, and pituitary insufficiency. Prompt and adequate control of the underlying disorder usually leads to hair regrowth. Specific types of nonscarring alopecia are described below.

Androgenetic alopecia, the most common form of alopecia, is of genetic predetermination. In men, the earliest changes occur at the anterior portions of the calvarium on either side of the "widow's peak" and on the crown (vertex). The extent of hair loss is variable and unpredictable. Minoxidil 5% is available over the counter and can be recommended for persons with recent onset (< 5 years) and smaller areas of alopecia. Approximately 40% of patients treated twice daily for a year will have moderate to dense growth. Finasteride (Propecia), 1 mg orally daily, has similar efficacy and may be additive to minoxidil. Dutasteride, 0.5 mg orally daily, may be considered as an alternative to finasteride.

Androgenetic alopecia also occurs in women. Classically, there is retention of the anterior hairline while there is diffuse thinning of the vertex scalp hair and a widening of the part. Treatment includes topical minoxidil (5% once daily) and, in women not of childbearing potential, finasteride at doses up to 5 mg/day orally. Spironolactone 50–200 mg daily may be used in premenopausal women. Low-dose oral minoxidil (0.25–1 mg daily in women and 2.5–5 mg daily in men) is also safe and effective. A workup consisting of determination of serum testosterone, DHEAS, iron, total iron-binding capacity, ferritin, thyroid function tests, vitamin D level, and a CBC will identify most other causes of hair thinning in premenopausal women. Women who describe thin hair but show little evidence of alopecia need follow-up because > 50% of the scalp hair can be lost before the clinician can perceive it.

Telogen effluvium is a transitory increase in the number of hairs in the telogen (resting) phase of the hair growth cycle. This may occur spontaneously; appear at the termination of pregnancy; be precipitated by severe illness, "crash dieting," high fever, stress from surgery, shock, malnutrition, or iron deficiency; or be provoked by hormonal contraceptives. Whatever the cause, telogen effluvium usually has a latent period of 4 months. The prognosis is generally good. The condition is diagnosed by the presence of large numbers of hairs with white bulbs coming out upon gentle tugging of the hair. Patients will describe excessive shedding of hair without scalp itching or scaling. Counts of hairs lost by the patient on combing or shampooing often exceed 150 per day, compared to an average of 70–100. If iron deficiency is suspected, a serum ferritin should be obtained, and any value < 40 ng/mL followed with supplementation.

Alopecia areata is of unknown cause but is believed to be an immunologic process. It presents as hairless patches that are perfectly smooth and without scarring. Tiny hairs 2–3 mm in length, called "exclamation hairs," may be seen. Telogen hairs are easily dislodged from the periphery of active lesions. The beard, brows, and lashes may be involved. Involvement may extend to all of the scalp hair (**alopecia totalis**) or to all scalp and body hair (**alopecia universalis**). Alopecia areata is occasionally associated with autoimmune disorders, including Hashimoto thyroiditis, pernicious anemia, Addison disease, and vitiligo. Additional comorbidities may include SLE, atopy, and mental health disease.

Intralesional corticosteroids are first-line treatment for alopecia areata. Triamcinolone acetonide in a concentration of 2.5–10 mg/mL is injected in aliquots of 0.1 mL at approximately 1- to 2-cm intervals, not exceeding a total dose of 30 mg per month for adults. Alopecia areata is usually self-limiting, with complete regrowth of hair in up to 50% of patients with focal disease in the first year. Some mild cases are resistant to treatment, as are the extensive totalis and universalis types. Support groups for patients with extensive alopecia areata are beneficial. Oral JAK inhibitors (eg, baricitinib, ritlecitinib, and deuruxolitinib) are FDA-approved therapeutic options for patients with moderate-to-severe disease, although relapse is the rule once the medication has been stopped. Efficacy of topical JAK inhibitors for alopecia areata is under investigation.

In **trichotillomania** (the pulling out of one's own hair), the patches of hair loss are irregular, with short, growing hairs almost always present, since they cannot be pulled out until they are long enough. The patches are often unilateral, occurring on the same side as the patient's dominant hand. The patient may be unaware of the habit. *N*-acetylcysteine (1200–2400 mg orally per day for 12 weeks) may be effective.

Scarring (Cicatricial) Alopecia

Cicatricial alopecia may occur following any type of trauma or inflammation that may scar hair follicles. Examples include chemical or physical trauma, bacterial or fungal infections, severe herpes zoster, chronic discoid lupus erythematosus (DLE), systemic sclerosis (scleroderma), and excessive ionizing radiation. The specific cause is often suggested by the history, the distribution of hair loss, and the appearance of the skin, as in DLE. Specific dermatologic diseases of the scalp that result in scarring alopecia include lichen planopilaris, frontal fibrosing alopecia, dissecting cellulitis of the scalp, central centrifugal cicatrical alopecia, and folliculitis decalvans. Biopsy is useful in the diagnosis of scarring alopecia, but specimens must be taken from the active border and not from the scarred central zone. Scarring alopecias are irreversible and permanent. It is important to diagnose and treat the scarring process as early in its course as possible.

Dainichi T et al. Alopecia areata: what's new in the diagnosis and treatment with JAK inhibitors? J Dermatol. 2024;51:196. [PMID: 38087654]

Gao JL et al. Androgenetic alopecia in transgender and gender diverse populations: a review of therapeutics. J Am Acad Dermatol. 2023;89:774. [PMID: 34756934]

Sanchez K et al. Evaluating current and emergent JAK inhibitors for alopecia areata: a narrative review. Dermatol Ther (Heidelb). 2025;15:2749. [PMID: 40794245]

NAIL DISORDERS

1. Morphologic Nail Abnormalities

Classification

Acquired nail disorders may be classified as local or associated with systemic or generalized skin diseases.

A. Local Nail Disorders

1. Onycholysis (distal separation of the nail plate from the nail bed, usually of the fingers) is caused by excessive exposure to water, soaps, detergents, alkalies, and industrial cleaning agents. Candidal infection of the nail folds and subungual area, nail hardeners, drug-induced photosensitivity, hyper- or hypothyroidism, and psoriasis may cause onycholysis.
2. Distortion of the nail, including nail splitting, occurs as a result of chronic inflammation or infiltration of the nail matrix underlying the eponychial fold. Such changes may be caused by impingement on the nail matrix by inflammatory diseases (eg, psoriasis, lichen planus, eczema), warts, tumors, or cysts.
3. Discoloration and crumbly thickened nails are noted in dermatophyte infection and psoriasis.
4. Allergic reactions (to resins in undercoats and polishes or to nail glues) are characterized by onycholysis or by grossly distorted, hypertrophic, and misshapen nails.
5. Paronychia is inflammation of the lateral or proximal nail folds. Acute paronychia presents as a painful erythematous papulonodule or frank abscess of the nail fold and is most commonly due to infection with *S aureus* (Figure 6–38). Chronic paronychia is most often caused by irritation from water or chemicals with resultant inflammation and possible *Candida* superinfection.

B. Nail Changes Associated with Systemic or Generalized Skin Diseases

1. Beau lines (transverse furrows) affect all nails and classically develop after a serious systemic illness.
2. Atrophy of the nails may be related to trauma or to vascular or neurologic disease.
3. Clubbed fingers may be due to the prolonged hypoxemia associated with cardiopulmonary disorders (Figure 6–39) (see Chapter 9).

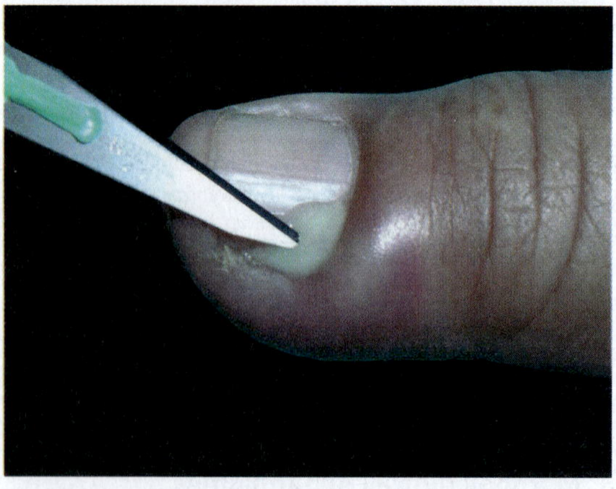

▲ **Figure 6–38.** Acute paronychia with incision and drainage. (Reproduced, with permission, from Richard P. Usatine, MD, in Usatine RP, Smith MA, Mayeaux EJ Jr, Chumley HS. *The Color Atlas and Synopsis of Family Medicine*, 3rd ed. McGraw-Hill, 2019.)

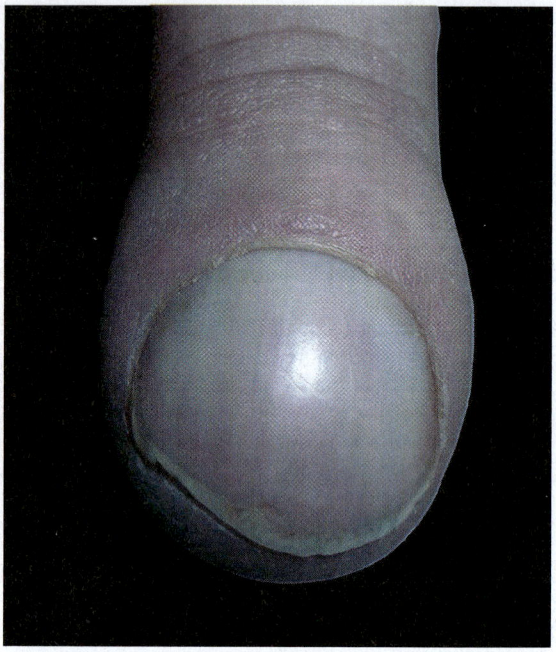

▲ **Figure 6–39.** Clubbing of the finger in a 31-year-old man with congenital heart disease. Note the thickening around the proximal nail folds. (Reproduced, with permission, from Richard P. Usatine, MD, in Usatine RP, Smith MA, Mayeaux EJ Jr, Chumley H. *The Color Atlas of Family Medicine*, 3rd ed. McGraw-Hill, 2019.)

4. Spoon nails may be seen in anemic patients.
5. Stippling or pitting of the nails is seen in psoriasis, alopecia areata, and hand eczema (see Figure 6–23).
6. Nail hyperpigmentation may be caused by many chemotherapeutic agents, but especially the taxanes.

Differential Diagnosis

Onychomycosis may cause nail changes identical to those seen in psoriasis. Careful examination for more characteristic lesions elsewhere on the body is essential to the diagnosis of the nail disorders. Cancer should be suspected (eg, Bowen disease or squamous cell carcinoma) as the cause of any persistent solitary subungual or periungual lesion.

Complications

Toenail changes may lead to an ingrown nail—in turn often complicated by bacterial infection and occasionally by exuberant granulation tissue. Poor manicuring and poorly fitting shoes may contribute to this complication. Cellulitis may result.

Treatment & Prognosis

Treatment consists usually of careful debridement and manicuring and, above all, reduction of exposure to irritants (soaps, detergents, alkali, bleaches, solvents, etc). Longitudinal grooving due to temporary lesions of the matrix, such as warts, synovial cysts, and other impingements, may be cured by removal of the offending lesion.

Acute paronychia is treated with topical antibiotics and drainage of the abscess, if present. To incise and drain an acute staphylococcal paronychia, insert a flat metal spatula or sharpened hardwood stick into the nail fold where it adjoins the nail. This will release pus from a mature lesion (Figure 6–38).

Treatment of chronic paronychia includes minimizing wetwork and toxic contactants, wearing gloves while performing tasks that expose the skin to water, minimizing trauma to the nail folds, and a combination of topical corticosteroids and an anticandidal twice daily to the affected area.

2. Tinea Unguium (Onychomycosis)

Tinea unguium is a trichophyton infection of one or more (but rarely all) fingernails or toenails. The species most commonly found is *T rubrum*. "Saprophytic" fungi may rarely cause onychomycosis (< 5% of cases). Evidence supporting a genetic defect in the innate and adaptive immune system may explain why some persons suffer from chronic tinea pedis and onychomycosis.

The nails are lusterless, brittle, and hypertrophic, and the substance of the nail is friable. Laboratory diagnosis is mandatory since only 50% of dystrophic nails are due to dermatophytosis. Portions of the nail should be clipped, digested with 10% KOH, and examined under the microscope for hyphae. Fungi may also be cultured from debris collected from underneath the nail plate. Periodic acid-Schiff stain of a histologic section of the nail plate also demonstrates the fungus readily. Each technique is positive in only 50% of cases so several different tests may need to be performed. Periodic acid-Schiff staining of nail plate coupled with fungal culture has a sensitivity of 96%.

Onychomycosis is difficult to treat because of the long duration of therapy required and the frequency of recurrences. Fingernails respond more readily than toenails. For toenails, treatment is indicated for patients with discomfort, inability to exercise, diabetes, and immune compromise.

In general, systemic therapy is required to effectively treat nail onychomycosis. Although historically topical therapy has had limited value, evidence suggests that efinaconazole 10% performs better than other topical treatment options like ciclopirox. Tavaborole 5% solution is also approved for the treatment of onychomycosis, but its clearance rates do not appear to be as good as those of efinaconazole. Adjunctive value of surgical procedures is unproven, and the efficacy of laser treatments is lacking, especially with regard to long-term cures.

Fingernails can virtually always be cured, and toenails are cured 35–50% of the time and are clinically improved about 75% of the time. In all cases, before treatment, the diagnosis should be confirmed. The costs of the various treatment options should be known and the most cost-effective treatment chosen. Medication interactions must be avoided. Ketoconazole, due to its higher risk for hepatotoxicity, is not recommended to treat any form of onychomycosis. For fingernails, ultramicronized griseofulvin 250 mg orally three times daily for 6 months can be effective. Alternative treatments are (in order of preference) oral terbinafine, 250 mg daily for 6 weeks; oral itraconazole, 200–400 mg daily for 7 days each month for 2 months; and oral itraconazole, 200 mg daily for 2 months. Off-label use of fluconazole, 150–400 mg once weekly for 6–9 months, can also be effective, but there is limited evidence for this option. Once clear, fingernails usually remain free of disease for some years.

Onychomycosis of the toenails does not respond to griseofulvin therapy. The best treatment, which is also FDA-approved, is oral terbinafine 250 mg daily for 12 weeks. Pulse terbinafine therapy with two cycles of 4 weeks on and 4 weeks off may be as efficacious as continuous oral therapy. Liver biochemical tests should be performed before oral terbinafine therapy. Because the risk of idiosyncratic liver injury is very low (transaminitis occurs in < 0.5% of patients) and the presentation of drug-induced liver injury is usually symptomatic (jaundice, malaise, abdominal pain), routine hepatic monitoring in healthy adults without known hepatic disease is not required. The dose might need adjustment in patients with reduced creatinine clearance. Itraconazole, 200 mg daily for 12 weeks, or pulse oral itraconazole, 200 mg twice daily for 1 week per month for 3 months, is inferior to standard terbinafine treatments, but it is an acceptable alternative for those unable to take terbinafine. The courses of terbinafine or itraconazole may need to be repeated 6 months after the first treatment cycle if fungal cultures of the nail are still positive. Fluconazole may be used off label at 150 mg weekly until the nail has grown out completely (12–18 month for toenails).

Treatment failures are multifactorial but may occur because of mixed infection with non-dermatophyte molds or reinfection. Culture of the nail to determine the organism responsible for infection is critical to choosing the correct therapy. In addition, part of the complete therapeutic regimen for onychomycosis should include replacing or sanitizing potential fungal reservoirs such as socks, shoes, and other textiles. Infected household members should also be treated. Shoes or sandals should be worn in high-risk areas (public showers or pools). Continued prophylactic therapy with topicals such as efinaconazole twice a week to nails and a topical antifungal cream to the feet should be continued for several years or longer after clearance of onychomycosis.

Yousefian F et al. Treatment options for onychomycosis: efficacy, side effects, adherence, financial considerations, and ethics. J Clin Aesthet Dermatol. 2024;17:24. [PMID: 38495549]

Zaraa I et al. Onychomycosis. Hand Surg Rehabili. 2024;43S:101638. [PMID: 38218374]

7 Disorders of the Eyes & Lids

Jacque L. Duncan, MD
Neeti B. Parikh, MD
Gerami D. Seitzman, MD

REFRACTIVE ERRORS

Refractive error is the most common cause of reduced clarity of vision (visual acuity).

Use of a pinhole will overcome most refractive errors and thus allows their identification as a cause of reduced visual acuity. Refractive error can be treated with glasses, contact lenses, or surgery.

Treatment

A. Contact Lenses

An estimated 45 million US adults wear contact lenses, mostly for correction of refractive errors, though decorative-colored contact lenses are used.

The major risk from contact lens wear is corneal infection, potentially a blinding condition. Such infections occur more often with soft lenses, particularly extended wear, for which there is at least a fivefold increase in risk of corneal infection compared with daily wear. Decorative contact lenses have a high prevalence of microbial contamination. Contact lens wearers should be made aware of the risks they face and ways to minimize them, such as avoiding overnight wear or use of lenses past their replacement date and maintaining meticulous lens hygiene, including not using tap water or saliva for lens cleaning. Contact lenses should be removed whenever there is ocular discomfort or redness.

Waghmare SV et al. A review of contact lens-related risk factors and complications. Cureus. 2022;14:e30118. [PMID: 36381898]

B. Surgery

Various surgical techniques can reduce refractive errors. Laser refractive surgery reshapes the middle layer (stroma) of the cornea with an excimer laser.

Other refractive surgery techniques are extraction of the crystalline lens with insertion of a single vision, multifocal, or accommodative intraocular lens as occurs after cataract extraction; insertion of an intraocular lens without removal of the crystalline lens (phakic intraocular lens); and intrastromal corneal ring segments.

C. Reduction of Rate of Progression of Nearsightedness

The rate at which nearsightedness progresses can be reduced by topical atropine rigid contact lens wear during sleep (orthokeratology); and various types of soft contact lenses and spectacles, but their long-term efficacy and safety are uncertain.

When to Refer

Any contact lens wearer with an acute painful red eye must be referred emergently for ophthalmologic evaluation.

DISORDERS OF THE LIDS & LACRIMAL APPARATUS

1. Hordeolum

Hordeolum is an acute infection that is commonly due to *Staphylococcus aureus.* It is characterized by a localized red, swollen, acutely tender area on the upper or lower lid.

Internal hordeolum is a meibomian gland abscess that usually points onto the conjunctival surface of the lid.

External hordeolum (or stye) is an abscess of the gland of Zeis. It is usually smaller than an internal hordeolum and on the lid margin.

Warm compresses are helpful. Incision may be indicated if resolution does not begin within 48 hours. An antibiotic ointment (ophthalmic bacitracin or erythromycin) applied to the lid every 3 hours may be beneficial during the acute stage. Internal hordeolum may lead to generalized cellulitis of the lid.

2. Chalazion

Chalazion is a common granulomatous inflammation of a meibomian gland that may follow an internal hordeolum. It is characterized by a hard, nontender swelling on the upper or lower lid with redness and swelling of the adjacent conjunctiva. Initial treatment is with warm compresses. If resolution has not occurred by 2–3 weeks, incision and curettage is indicated. Corticosteroid injection may also be effective.

3. Blepharitis

Blepharitis is an anterior or posterior eyelid inflammation. Anterior blepharitis is characterized by inflammatory debris on the eyelid skin and around the eyelashes and includes staphylococcal, seborrheic, and *Demodex* mite forms. Posterior blepharitis occurs with meibomian gland inflammation, which alters lipid secretion into the tear film and is a common etiology of dry eye syndrome. Clogged meibomian glands can lead to chalazia (swollen lumps in the eyelid). Ocular rosacea results in inflammation of meibomian glands and is a common cause of posterior blepharitis. Anterior and posterior blepharitis may appear singularly or together.

Clinical Findings

Symptoms are irritation, burning, and itching.

1. Anterior blepharitis—The eyes are "red-rimmed" and scales or collarettes can be seen clinging to the lashes.

2. Posterior blepharitis—The lid margins are hyperemic with telangiectasias, and the meibomian glands and their orifices are inflamed. The lid margin is frequently rolled inward to produce a mild entropion, and the tear film may be frothy or abnormally greasy.

Blepharitis is a common cause of recurrent conjunctivitis. Both anterior and, especially, posterior blepharitis may be complicated by hordeola or chalazia; abnormal lid or lash positions, producing trichiasis; epithelial keratitis of the lower third of the cornea; marginal corneal infiltrates; and inferior corneal vascularization and thinning.

Treatment

1. Anterior blepharitis—Eyelid hygiene is usually sufficient to control anterior blepharitis. Warm compresses help soften the scales and warm the meibomian gland secretions. Eyelid cleansing can be achieved by gentle eyelid massage and lid scrubs with baby shampoo or 0.01% hypochlorous acid. In acute exacerbations, an antibiotic eye ointment, such as bacitracin or erythromycin, is applied daily to the lid margins (Table 7–2).

2. Posterior blepharitis—Regular meibomian gland expression and warm compresses may be used to control mild posterior blepharitis. Inflammation of the conjunctiva and cornea is treated with long-term low-dose oral antibiotic therapy, eg, treat for 2–4 weeks with tetracycline (250 mg twice daily), doxycycline (100 mg daily), minocycline (50–100 mg daily), or erythromycin (250 mg three times daily), or treat with azithromycin (500 mg daily for 3 days in three cycles with 7-day intervals). These oral antibiotic therapies may be helpful in patients with rosacea. Short-term (5–7 days) topical corticosteroids, eg, prednisolone, 0.125% twice daily, may also be indicated. Topical therapy with antibiotics, such as ciprofloxacin 0.3% ophthalmic solution twice daily, may be helpful but should be restricted to short courses of 5–7 days (Table 7–2).

Lin A et al. American Academy of Ophthalmology Preferred Practice Pattern Cornea/External Disease Panel. Blepharitis Preferred Practice Pattern®. Ophthalmology. 2024;131:50. [PMID: 38349296]

4. Entropion & Ectropion

Entropion (inward turning of usually the lower lid) occurs occasionally in older people from degeneration of the lid fascia or may follow extensive scarring of the conjunctiva and tarsus. Surgery is indicated if the lashes rub on the cornea. Botulinum toxin injections may also be used for temporary correction of the involutional lower lid entropion of older people.

Ectropion (outward turning of the lower lid) is common with advanced age. Surgery is indicated if there is excessive tearing, exposure keratitis, or a cosmetic problem.

5. Tumors of the Lids

Lid tumors are usually benign. Basal cell carcinoma is the most common malignant tumor. Squamous cell carcinoma, meibomian gland carcinoma, and malignant melanoma also occur. Surgery for any lesion involving the lid margin should be performed by an ophthalmologist or suitably trained plastic surgeon to avoid deformity of the lid. Histopathologic examination of eyelid tumors should be routine, since 2% of lesions thought to be benign clinically are found to be malignant. Medications such as vismodegib, imiquimod, and 5-fluorouracil occasionally are used instead of or as an adjunct to surgery for some basal and squamous cell carcinomas.

6. Dacryocystitis

Dacryocystitis is infection of the lacrimal sac usually due to congenital or acquired obstruction of the nasolacrimal system. It may be acute or chronic and occurs most often in infants and in persons over 40 years. It is usually unilateral. Infection is typically with *S aureus* and streptococci in acute dacryocystitis and *Staphylococcus epidermidis*, streptococci, or gram-negative bacilli in chronic dacryocystitis.

Acute dacryocystitis is characterized by pain, swelling, tenderness, and redness in the tear sac area; purulent material may be expressed. In chronic dacryocystitis, tearing and discharge are the principal signs, and mucus or pus may also be expressed.

Acute dacryocystitis responds well to systemic oral antibiotics with gram-positive coverage, such as amoxicillin-clavulanate, cephalexin, ciprofloxacin, clindamycin, or trimethoprim-sulfamethoxazole; microbiologic culture is usually not necessary. To relieve the underlying obstruction, surgery is usually done electively but may be performed urgently in acute cases. The chronic form may be kept latent with systemic antibiotics, but relief of the obstruction is the only cure. In adults, the standard procedure is dacryocystorhinostomy, which involves surgical exploration of the lacrimal sac and formation of a fistula into the nasal cavity and, if necessary, supplemented by nasolacrimal intubation.

Congenital nasolacrimal duct obstruction is common and often resolves spontaneously. It can be treated by probing the nasolacrimal system, supplemented by nasolacrimal intubation or balloon catheter dilation, if necessary; dacryocystorhinostomy is rarely required.

CONJUNCTIVITIS

Conjunctivitis may be acute or chronic. Most cases are due to viral or bacterial (including gonococcal and chlamydial) infection. Other causes include keratoconjunctivitis sicca, allergy, chemical irritants, and trauma. The mode of transmission of infectious conjunctivitis is usually via direct contact of contaminated fingers or objects to the eye or to other persons. It may also be spread through respiratory secretions or contaminated eye drops.

Conjunctivitis must be differentiated from acute uveitis, acute glaucoma, and corneal disorders (Table 7–1).

Varu DM et al; American Academy of Ophthalmology Preferred Practice Pattern Cornea and External Disease Panel. Conjunctivitis Preferred Practice Pattern®. Ophthalmology. 2019;126:P94. [PMID: 30366797]

1. Viral Conjunctivitis

Viral conjunctivitis is a clinical diagnosis with etiology varying by location and rarely confirmed. Adenovirus is one common etiology. Often, there is sequential bilateral disease with copious watery discharge and a follicular conjunctivitis. Infection spreads easily. Epidemic keratoconjunctivitis, which may result in decreased vision from corneal subepithelial infiltrates, is usually caused by adenovirus types 8, 19, and 37. Active viral conjunctivitis lasts up to 2 weeks, with the immune-mediated keratitis occurring later. Infection with adenovirus types 3, 4, 7, and 11 can be associated with pharyngitis, fever, malaise, and preauricular adenopathy (pharyngoconjunctival fever). Contagious acute hemorrhagic conjunctivitis (see Chapter 36) may be caused by enterovirus 70 or coxsackievirus A24, though etiologies vary globally. Herpes simplex virus (HSV) conjunctivitis is typically unilateral and may be associated with lid vesicles. SARS-CoV-2 may present with conjunctivitis only. There are no clinical differentiating features between SARS-CoV-2 conjunctivitis and any other viral etiologies of conjunctivitis.

Except for HSV infection for which treatment with ophthalmic (eg, ganciclovir 0.15% gel) and/or systemic (eg, oral acyclovir, valacyclovir) antivirals is recommended (Table 36–1), there is no specific treatment for contagious viral conjunctivitis. Artificial tears and cold compresses may reduce discomfort. The use of ophthalmic antibiotics and corticosteroids in the acute viral infection is discouraged. Frequent hand and linen hygiene is encouraged to minimize spread. A single low-concentration ocular betadine wash commonly preceded by a drop of ophthalmic anesthesia (administered by an eye care specialist) may expedite recovery.

Tsui E ... Seitzman GD et al. Pathogen surveillance for acute infectious conjunctivitis. JAMA Ophthalmol. 2023;141:1140. [PMID: 37917077]

Vats S et al. One-time low concentration betadine eye wash: a novel treatment for epidemic viral conjunctivitis for accelerated recovery. Rom J Ophthalmol. 2024;68:268. [PMID: 39464754]

2. Bacterial Conjunctivitis

Common bacterial conjunctivitis pathogens are staphylococci, including methicillin-resistant *S aureus* (MRSA); streptococci, particularly *Streptococcus pneumoniae*; *Haemophilus* species; *Pseudomonas;* and *Moraxella*. All may produce purulent discharge and eyelid matting. Blurring of vision and discomfort are mild. In severe (hyperpurulent) cases, culture is recommended, particularly to identify gonococcal infection that requires emergent and systemic treatment.

The infection is usually self-limited, lasting about 10–14 days if untreated. Most ophthalmic antibiotics hasten clinical remission, and no ophthalmic antibiotic has proven superiority over another (Table 7–2).

A. Gonococcal Conjunctivitis

Gonococcal conjunctivitis, usually acquired through contact with infected genital secretions, typically causes copious purulent discharge. It is an ophthalmologic emergency because the cornea may perforate. The diagnosis should be

Table 7–1. The inflamed eye: differential diagnosis of common causes.

	Acute Conjunctivitis	Acute Anterior Uveitis (Iritis)	Acute Angle-Closure Glaucoma	Corneal Trauma or Infection
Incidence	Extremely common	Common	Uncommon	Common
Discharge	Moderate to copious	None	None	Watery or purulent
Vision	No effect on vision	Often blurred	Markedly blurred	Usually blurred
Pain	Mild	Moderate	Severe	Moderate to severe
Conjunctival injection	Diffuse	Mainly circumcorneal	Mainly circumcorneal	Mainly circumcorneal
Cornea	Clear	Usually clear	Cloudy	Clarity change related to cause
Pupil size	Normal	Small	Moderately dilated	Normal or small
Pupillary light response	Normal	Variable to poor	None	Normal
Intraocular pressure	Normal	Usually normal but may be elevated	Markedly elevated	Normal
Infectious	Commonly	Occasionally	No	Commonly

Table 7–2. Topical ophthalmic agents (selected list).

Agent	Recommended Regimen	Indications
Antibiotic Agents (ophthalmic)		
Azithromycin (AzaSite)	One drop two times daily for 2 days, then once daily for 5 days	Bacterial conjunctivitis
Bacitracin 500 U/g ointment (various)[1]	Apply 0.5 inch into lower conjunctival sac or to eyelids three to four times daily for 7–10 days	Bacterial conjunctivitis, blepharitis, stye
Bacitracin/Polymyxin ointment (Polysporin, AK-Poly)	Apply 0.5 inch into lower conjunctival sac or to eyelids three to four times daily for 7–10 days	Corneal abrasion Following corneal foreign body removal
Besifloxacin ophthalmic suspension, 0.6% (Besivance)	For bacterial conjunctivitis, typically one drop four times a day for 1 week For bacterial keratitis, depends on severity, often one drop every hour during the day and every 2 hours during the night for 48 hours, then gradually reduce	Bacterial conjunctivitis Bacterial keratitis
Ciprofloxacin HCl 0.3% solution (Ciloxan)	For bacterial conjunctivitis, typically one drop four times a day for 1 week For bacterial keratitis, depends on severity, often one drop every hour during the day and every 2 hours during the night for 48 hours, then gradually reduce	Bacterial conjunctivitis Bacterial keratitis
Ciprofloxacin HCl 0.3% ointment	Apply 0.5 inch into lower conjunctival sac or to eyelids three to four times daily for 7–10 days	Bacterial conjunctivitis
Erythromycin 0.5% ointment (various)	Apply 0.5 inch into lower conjunctival sac or to eyelids three to four times daily for 7–10 days	Bacterial infection of the conjunctiva or lid margin
Fusidic acid 1% gel (Fucithalmic) Not available in United States	One drop two times daily	Bacterial conjunctivitis, blepharitis, stye, keratitis
Gatifloxacin 0.5% solution (Zymaxid)	For bacterial conjunctivitis, typically one drop four times a day for 1 week For bacterial keratitis, depends on severity, often one drops every hour during the day and every 2 hours during the night for 48 hours, then gradually reduce	Bacterial conjunctivitis Bacterial keratitis
Gentamicin sulfate 0.3% solution (various)	One drop four times a day for bacterial conjunctivitis	Ocular surface infection
Gentamicin sulfate 0.3% ointment (various)	Apply 0.5 inch into lower conjunctival sac two to three times daily	Ocular surface infection
Gentamicin sulfate 1.5% (fortified preparation)	One drop every hour for 48 hours, then gradually reduce	Bacterial keratitis
Levofloxacin 0.5% solution (various)	For bacterial conjunctivitis, typically one drop four times a day for 1 week For bacterial keratitis, depends on severity, often one drop every hour during the day and every 2 hours during the night for 48 hours, then gradually reduce	Bacterial conjunctivitis Bacterial keratitis
Moxifloxacin 0.5% solution (Vigamox)	For bacterial conjunctivitis, typically one drop three times a day for 1 week For bacterial keratitis, depends on severity, often one drop every hour during the day and every 2 hours during the night for 48 hours, then gradually reduce	Bacterial conjunctivitis Bacterial keratitis
Neomycin/Polymyxin B/Gramicidin (Neosporin)	One drop three to four times a day for 1 week	Ocular surface infection
Norfloxacin 0.3% solution Not available in United States	For bacterial conjunctivitis, typically one drop four times a day for 1 week For bacterial keratitis, depends on severity, often one drop every hour during the day and every 2 hours during the night for 48 hours, then gradually reduce	Ocular surface infection Bacterial keratitis

(continued)

Table 7–2. Topical ophthalmic agents (selected list). (continued)

Agent	Recommended Regimen	Indications
Ofloxacin 0.3% solution (Ocuflox)	For bacterial conjunctivitis, typically one drop four times a day for 1 week For bacterial keratitis, depends on severity, often one drop every hour during the day and every 2 hours during the night for 48 hours, then gradually reduce	Bacterial conjunctivitis Bacterial keratitis
Polymyxin B 10,000 U/mL/Trimethoprim sulfate 1 mg/mL (Polytrim)[2]	For bacterial conjunctivitis, typically one drop four times a day for 1 week	Ocular surface infection
Sulfacetamide sodium 10% solution (various)	For bacterial conjunctivitis, typically one drop four times a day for 1 week	Bacterial infection of the conjunctiva or lid margin
Tobramycin 0.3% solution (various)	For bacterial conjunctivitis, typically one drop four times a day for 1 week For bacterial keratitis, depends on severity, often one drop every hour during the day and every 2 hours during the night for 48 hours, then gradually reduce	Bacterial conjunctivitis Bacterial keratitis
Tobramycin 1.5% (fortified) solution	One drop every hour during the day and every 2 hours during the night for 48 hours, then gradually reduce	Bacterial keratitis
Tobramycin 0.3% ointment (Tobrex)	Apply 0.5 inch into lower conjunctival sac or to eyelids three to four times daily for 7–10 days	Bacterial conjunctivitis
Antifungal Agents		
Amphotericin 0.1–0.5% solution	One drop every 1–2 hours initially, then reduce as dictated by the severity of the infection	Fungal blepharitis, conjunctivitis, keratitis
Natamycin 5% suspension (Natacyn)	One drop every 1–2 hours initially, then reduce as dictated by the severity of the infection	
Voriconazole 1% solution	One drop every 1–2 hours initially, then reduce as dictated by the severity of the infection	
Antiviral Agents		
Acyclovir 3% ointment (Zovirax) Not available in United States	Five times daily	Herpes simplex keratitis
Ganciclovir 0.15% gel (Zirgan)	Five times daily	
Trifluridine 1% solution (Viroptic)	One drop onto cornea every 2 hours while awake for a maximum daily dose of nine drops until resolution occurs; then an additional 7 days of one drop every 4 hours while awake (minimum five times daily)	
Antiparasitic Agents		
Lotilaner 0.25% solution	One drop applied twice daily for 6 weeks	*Demodex* mite blepharitis
Polyhexamethylene biguanide (PHMB) (0.02–0.8%)	One drop every 1–2 hours initially, then reduce as dictated by the severity of the infection	Acanthamoeba keratitis
Chlorhexidine (0.02–0.06%)	One drop every 1–2 hours initially, then reduce as dictated by the severity of the infection	Acanthamoeba keratitis
Anti-Inflammatory Agents		
Antihistamines[3] (ophthalmic)		
Emedastine difumarate 0.05% solution (Emadine) Not available in United States	One drop four times daily	Allergic eye disease
Levocabastine (Livostin) Not available in United States	One drop twice daily	
Mast cell stabilizers		
Cromolyn sodium 4% solution (Crolom)	One drop four times daily	
Lodoxamide tromethamine 0.1% solution (Alomide)	One or two drops twice a day	

(continued)

Table 7–2. Topical ophthalmic agents (selected list). (continued)

Agent	Recommended Regimen	Indications
Nedocromil sodium 2% solution (Alocril)	One drop twice daily	
Pemirolast potassium 0.1% solution (Alamast) Not available in United States	One drop four times daily	
Combined antihistamines and mast cell stabilizers		
Alcaftadine 0.25% ophthalmic solution (Lastacaft)	One drop once daily	
Azelastine HCl 0.05% ophthalmic solution (Optivar)	One drop two to four times daily	
Bepotastine besilate 1.5% solution (Bepreve)	One drop twice daily	
Epinastine hydrochloride 0.05% ophthalmic solution (Elestat)	One drop twice daily	
Ketotifen fumarate 0.025% solution (Zaditor)	One drop twice daily	
Ketotifen 0.025% preservative-free solution (Alaway)	One drop twice daily	
Olopatadine hydrochloride 0.1% solution (Patanol)	One drop twice daily	
Olopatadine hydrochloride 0.2% or 0.77% solution	One drop daily	
Nonsteroidal anti-inflammatory agents (ophthalmic)		
Bromfenac 0.09% solution (Xibrom)	One drop to operated eye twice daily beginning 24 hours after cataract surgery and continuing through 2 postoperative weeks	Treatment of postoperative inflammation following cataract extraction
Diclofenac sodium 0.1% solution (Voltaren)	One drop to operated eye four times daily beginning 24 hours after surgery and continuing through 2 postoperative weeks	Treatment of postoperative inflammation following cataract extraction and laser corneal surgery
Flurbiprofen sodium 0.03% solution (various)	One drop to operated eye four times daily beginning 24 hours after cataract surgery	Inhibition of intraoperative miosis, treatment of cystoid macular edema and inflammation after cataract extraction
Indomethacin 1% solution (Indocid) Not available in United States	One drop four times daily	Treatment of allergic eye disease, postoperative inflammation following cataract extraction and laser corneal surgery
Ketorolac tromethamine 0.5% solution (Acular)	One drop four times daily tapered with decreasing inflammation over 2 weeks, not to be used long term	Treatment of postoperative inflammation following cataract extraction
Nepafenac 0.1% suspension (Nevanac)	One drop to operated eye three times daily beginning 24 hours after cataract surgery and continuing through 2 postoperative weeks	Treatment of postoperative inflammation following cataract extraction
Corticosteroids[4]		
Dexamethasone sodium phosphate 0.1% solution (various)	One drop as often as indicated by severity; use every hour during the day and every 2 hours during the night in severe inflammation; taper off as inflammation decreases	Treatment of steroid-responsive inflammatory conditions
Difluprednate 0.05% suspension[5]	One drop four times daily beginning 24 hours after surgery and continuing throughout 2 postoperative weeks; then one drop twice daily for a week and then taper based on the response One drop four times daily for 2 weeks and then taper as clinically indicated	Treatment after ocular surgery and for non-infectious uveitis

(continued)

Table 7–2. Topical ophthalmic agents (selected list). (continued)

Agent	Recommended Regimen	Indications
Fluorometholone 0.1% suspension (various)[6]	One drop four times a day and tapered off as inflammation decreases	Treatment of ocular surface inflammatory conditions
Fluorometholone 0.25% suspension (FML Forte)[6]	One drop two to four times daily	
Fluorometholone 0.1% ointment (FML S.O.P.) Not available in United States	Apply thin coating on lower conjunctival sac three or four times daily	
Loteprednol etabonate 0.5% (Lotemax)	One drop twice daily for severe allergies. More frequently for intraocular inflammation, tapered off as inflammation decreases	Treatment of steroid-responsive ocular inflammatory conditions
Prednisolone acetate 0.12% suspension (Pred Mild)	One drop four times a day and tapered as inflammation decreases	Treatment of steroid-responsive ocular inflammatory conditions
Prednisolone acetate 1% suspension (various)	One drop as often as indicated by severity of inflammation; use every hour during the day and every 2 hours during the night in severe inflammation; taper off as inflammation decreases	Treatment of steroid-responsive ocular inflammatory conditions
Prednisolone sodium phosphate 1% solution (various)	One drop as often as indicated by severity of inflammation; use every hour during the day and every 2 hours during the night in severe inflammation; taper off as inflammation decreases	Treatment of steroid-responsive ocular inflammatory conditions
Immunomodulators		
Cyclosporine emulsion 0.05% (Restasis), 0.09%, 0.1% (commercial); 1%, 2% (compounded)	One drop twice daily	Dry eyes and severe allergic eye disease
Tacrolimus 0.03%, 0.1% ointment	Apply to lower conjunctival sac twice daily	Severe allergic eye disease (off-label)
Glaucoma and Ocular Hypertension Agents		
Sympathomimetics (ophthalmic)		
Apraclonidine HCl 0.5% solution (Iopidine)	One drop three times daily	Reduction of intraocular pressure; expensive; reserve for treatment of resistant cases
Apraclonidine HCl 1% solution (Iopidine)	One drop 1 hour before and immediately after anterior segment laser surgery	To control or prevent elevations of intraocular pressure after laser trabeculoplasty or iridotomy
Brimonidine tartrate 0.2% solution (Alphagan, Alphagan P [benzalkonium chloride-free])	One drop two or three times daily	Reduction of intraocular pressure
β-Adrenergic blocking agents (ophthalmic)		
Betaxolol HCl 0.5% solution (Betoptic) and 0.25% suspension (Betoptic S)[7]	One drop twice daily	Reduction of intraocular pressure
Carteolol HCl 1% and 2% solution (various, Teoptic)[8]	One drop twice daily	
Levobunolol HCl 0.25% and 0.5% solution (Betagan)[9]	One drop once or twice daily	
Metipranolol HCl 0.3% solution (OptiPranolol)[9]	One drop twice daily	
Timolol 0.25% and 0.5% solution (Betimol)[9]	One drop once or twice daily	
Timolol maleate 0.25% and 0.5% solution (Istalol, Ocudose [preservative-free], Timoptic) and 0.1%, 0.25%, and 0.5% gel (Timoptic-XE, Timoptic GFS)[9]	One drop once or twice daily	

(*continued*)

Table 7–2. Topical ophthalmic agents (selected list). (continued)

Agent	Recommended Regimen	Indications
Miotics (ophthalmic)		
Pilocarpine HCl 1–4% solution[10]	One drop up to four times daily for elevated intraocular pressure	Reduction of intraocular pressure, treatment of acute or chronic angle-closure glaucoma, and pupillary constriction
Carbonic anhydrase inhibitors (ophthalmic)		
Brinzolamide 1% suspension (Azopt)	One drop two to three times daily	Reduction of intraocular pressure
Dorzolamide HCl 2% solution (Trusopt)	One drop two to three times daily	
Prostaglandin analogs		
Bimatoprost 0.03% solution (Lumigan)	One drop once daily at night	Reduction of intraocular pressure
Latanoprost 0.005% solution (Xalatan, Monopost [preservative-free]) (Monopost not available in United States)	One drop once or twice daily at night	
Latanoprostene bunod 0.024% solution (Vyzulta)	One drop daily at night	
Tafluprost 0.0015% solution (Saflutan [preservative-free], Taflotan, Zioptan [preservative-free]) (Saflutan not available in United States)	One drop once daily at night	
Travoprost 0.004% solution (Travatan, Travatan Z [benzalkonium chloride-free])	One drop once daily at night	
Rho kinase inhibitor (ophthalmic)		
Netarsudil ophthalmic solution 0.02% (Rhopressa)	One drop daily in the evening	Reduction of intraocular pressure
Combined preparations (ophthalmic)		
Bimatoprost 0.03% and timolol 0.5% (Ganfort) Not available in United States	One drop daily in the morning	Reduction of intraocular pressure
Brimonidine 0.2% and timolol 0.5% (Combigan)	One drop twice daily	
Brimonidine 0.2% and brinzolamide 1% (Simbrinza)	One drop three times a day	
Brinzolamide 1% and timolol 0.5% (Azarga) Not available in United States	One drop twice daily	
Dorzolamide 2% and timolol 0.5% (Cosopt, Cosopt PF [preservative-free])	One drop twice daily	
Latanoprost 0.005% and timolol 0.5% (Xalacom) Not available in United States	One drop daily in the morning	
Tafluprost 0.0015% and timolol 0.5% (Taptiqom [preservative-free]) Not available in United States	One drop daily	
Travoprost 0.004% and timolol 0.5% (DuoTrav) Not available in United States	One drop daily	

(continued)

Table 7–2. Topical ophthalmic agents (selected list). (continued)

Agent	Recommended Regimen	Indications
Mydriatic Agents for Pupillary Dilation (ophthalmic)		
Tropicamide 1% and phenylephrine 2.5%	One drop	Shorter-acting mydriatic for eye examination
Cyclopentolate 1% and homatropine 5%	One drop twice daily	Long-acting cycloplegic for treatment of uveitis to prevent iris synechiae and relieve pain from ciliary spasm
Atropine 1%	One drop daily	

[1]Little efficacy against gram-negative organisms (except *Neisseria*).
[2]No gram-positive coverage.
[3]May produce rebound hyperemia and local reactions.
[4]Frequency of corticosteroid use is determined by the severity of the inflammation and is tapered as inflammation decreases. Long-term use may increase intraocular pressure (eye pressure should be monitored), may contribute to cataract development, and predisposes to bacterial, herpes simplex virus, and fungal keratitis.
[5]Because of its high potency, this is the corticosteroid most likely to cause increased intraocular pressure.
[6]Less likely to elevate intraocular pressure.
[7]Cardioselective (β-1) β-blocker.
[8]Teoptic is not available in the United States.
[9]Nonselective (β-1 and β-2) β-blocker. Monitor all patients for systemic side effects, particularly exacerbation of asthma.
[10]Decreased night vision and headaches possible.

confirmed by Gram stain and culture of the discharge. Systemic treatment is required with a single 500-mg dose of intramuscular ceftriaxone for patients < 150 kg or a 1-g dose for patients > 150 kg (see Chapter 37). Fluoroquinolone resistance is common. Eye irrigation with saline may promote resolution. Ophthalmic antibiotics such as erythromycin and bacitracin may be added. Other STIs, including chlamydiosis, syphilis, and HIV infection, should be considered. Standard treatment for chlamydial infection is recommended (see Chapter 37).

Alsoudi AF … Seitzman GD. Purulent conjunctivitis and progressive corneal stromal necrosis. JAMA Ophthalmol. 2021;139:908. [PMID: 34081098]

B. Chlamydial Keratoconjunctivitis

Inclusion conjunctivitis—This disease occurs after contact with chlamydia-infected secretions. Presentation closely resembles viral conjunctivitis with acute redness, discharge, irritation, and follicular conjunctivitis. A mild keratitis can develop. A nontender preauricular lymph node can often be palpated. Healing usually leaves no sequelae. Diagnosis can be rapidly confirmed by immunologic tests or PCR on conjunctival samples. Treatment is doxycycline, 100 mg orally twice daily for 7 days. All cases should be assessed for genital tract infection and other STIs.

3. Dry Eye

Dry eye is an umbrella term describing tear film instability and associated ocular and visual complaints. Dry eye is more common in women than men and increases with age. Aqueous deficient dry eye (keratoconjunctivitis sicca) arises from lacrimal gland hypofunction and may be secondary to a systemic disease (eg, Sjögren syndrome), aging, or systemic medications. Evaporative loss dry eye may be due to environmental factors (eg, excessive screen time, windy climate) or abnormalities of the lipid component of the tear film, as in blepharitis and ocular rosacea. Mucin deficiency leads to tear film instability and may be due to vitamin A deficiency or conjunctival scarring, Stevens-Johnson syndrome, mucous membrane pemphigoid, graft-versus-host disease, chemical burns, or ophthalmic drug toxicity.

Clinical Findings

The patient complains of dryness, redness, foreign body sensation, and variable vision. In severe cases, there is persistent marked discomfort, with photophobia, difficulty moving the lids, and excessive mucus secretion. Gross inspection often reveals no abnormality, but on slit-lamp examination there are abnormalities of tear film stability and reduced tear volume. In more severe cases, damaged corneal and conjunctival cells stain with fluorescein and lissamine green. In the most severe cases, there is marked conjunctival injection, mucoid discharge, loss of the normal conjunctival and corneal luster, and epithelial keratopathy that stains with fluorescein and may progress to frank ulceration. The Schirmer test, which measures the rate of production of the aqueous component of tears, may be helpful.

Treatment

Aqueous deficiency can be treated with artificial tears drops or ointments. Drop preparations containing a mucomimetic such as hydroxypropyl methylcellulose (HPMC) or carboxymethylcellulose (carmellose) provide more prolonged duration. Warm compresses to the eyelid can help unclog meibomian glands.

Artificial tear preparations are generally safe and, in most cases, are used three or four times a day. However, preservatives included in some preparations to maintain sterility are potentially toxic and allergenic and may cause ocular surface toxicity in frequent users. Such reactions may be misinterpreted as a worsening of the dry eye state requiring more frequent use of the artificial tears, leading to further deterioration, rather than being recognized as a need to change to a preservative-free preparation. Preservative-free preparations are recommended if use is more than four times a day. Eye drops claiming to "get the red out" are not recommended as they cause toxicity and rebound hyperemia with prolonged use.

Dry eye is considered an inflammatory ocular surface disease. Accordingly, disease modification may require episodic treatment with low potency anti-inflammatory drops. Ophthalmic corticosteroids should only be prescribed by eye specialists to monitor intraocular pressure for steroid-induced glaucoma and for cataracts. Corticosteroid-sparing anti-inflammatory drops such as cyclosporine 0.05% ophthalmic emulsion (Restasis) and lifitegrast 5% are commonly used with no universal consensus of efficacy.

Lacrimal punctal occlusion by canalicular plugs or cautery is useful in cases of severe aqueous deficiency.

McCann P et al. Interventions for dry eye: an overview of systematic reviews. JAMA Ophthalmol. 2024;142:58. [PMID: 38127364]

4. Allergic Eye Disease

Allergic eye disease is common. It may be environmental or an expression of atopy.

Clinical Findings

Symptoms include itching, tearing, redness, stringy discharge, and occasionally, photophobia and visual loss.

Allergic conjunctivitis is common. It may be seasonal (hay fever), often flaring during the spring, or perennial. Clinical signs include conjunctival hyperemia and edema (chemosis), the latter at times being marked and sudden in onset.

Vernal keratoconjunctivitis tends to occur in late childhood and early adulthood. It is usually seasonal, with a predilection for the spring. Large "cobblestone" papillae are noted on the upper tarsal conjunctiva.

Atopic keratoconjunctivitis is a more chronic disorder of adulthood. Both the upper and the lower tarsal conjunctivas exhibit a papillary conjunctivitis. Severe cases demonstrate conjunctival fibrosis, resulting in eyelid scarring, entropion, and trichiasis. Corneal involvement, including refractory ulceration, is frequent during exacerbations of both vernal and severe atopic keratoconjunctivitis. The latter may be complicated by herpes simplex keratitis.

Treatment

A. Mild and Moderately Severe Allergic Eye Disease

Ophthalmic anti-inflammatory agents include mast cell stabilizers and antihistamines (see Anti-Inflammatory Agents in Table 7–2). Mast cell stabilization takes longer to act than antihistamines but can be useful for prophylaxis. Ophthalmic vasoconstrictors, such as ephedrine, naphazoline, tetrahydrozoline, and phenylephrine, alone or in combination with antihistamines, are available as over-the-counter medications and not typically used because of limited efficacy, rebound hyperemia, and follicular conjunctivitis. Systemic antihistamines (eg, loratadine 10 mg orally daily) may be useful in prolonged atopic keratoconjunctivitis. In allergic conjunctivitis, specific allergens may be avoidable.

B. Acute Exacerbations and Severe Allergic Eye Disease

Ophthalmic corticosteroids (Table 7–2) may be required to control acute exacerbations of both vernal and atopic keratoconjunctivitis. The lowest-potency corticosteroid that controls ocular inflammation should be used. Corticosteroid-induced side effects should be monitored by eye care professionals and include cataracts, glaucoma, and exacerbation of herpes simplex keratitis. Ophthalmic cyclosporine or tacrolimus may be effective. Systemic corticosteroid or other immunosuppressant therapy may be required in severe atopic keratoconjunctivitis.

PINGUECULA & PTERYGIUM

Pinguecula is a yellowish, elevated conjunctival nodule adjacent to the cornea and in the palpebral fissure. It is common in persons over age 35 years. **Pterygium** is a fleshy, triangular encroachment of the conjunctiva onto the cornea and is usually associated with prolonged exposure to wind, sun, sand, and dust. Pinguecula and pterygium are often bilateral and occur more frequently on the nasal side of the conjunctiva.

Pingueculae rarely grow but may become inflamed (pingueculitis). Pterygia become inflamed and may enlarge. Treatment is rarely required for inflammation of pinguecula or pterygium, and artificial tears are often beneficial.

The indications for excision of pterygium are growth that threatens vision by encroaching on the cornea, marked induced astigmatism, or severe ocular irritation.

CORNEAL ULCER

Corneal ulcers are most commonly due to infection by bacteria, viruses, fungi, or amoebas. All persons wearing contact lenses should be counseled not to sleep, swim, or shower in lenses. Noninfectious causes—all of which may be complicated by infection—include neurotrophic keratitis (resulting from loss of corneal sensation), exposure keratitis (due to inadequate lid closure), severe dry eye, severe allergic eye disease, and systemic autoimmune disorders. Delayed or ineffective treatment of corneal ulceration may lead to devastating consequences and vision loss. Prompt referral is essential.

Patients complain of pain, photophobia, tearing, and reduced vision. The conjunctiva is injected, and there may be purulent or watery discharge. The corneal appearance varies according to the underlying cause.

When to Refer

Any patient with an acute painful red eye and corneal abnormality should be referred emergently to an ophthalmologist.

Contact lens wearers with acute eye pain, redness, and decreased vision should be referred immediately.

Ting DSJ ... Seitzman GD et al. Diagnostic armamentarium of infectious keratitis: a comprehensive review. Ocul Surf. 2022;23:27. [PMID: 34781020]

INFECTIOUS KERATITIS

1. Bacterial Keratitis

Risk factors for bacterial keratitis include contact lens wear—especially overnight wear—and corneal trauma, including surgery. The most common pathogens are staphylococci, including MRSA; streptococci; and *Pseudomonas aeruginosa, Moraxella* species, and other gram-negative bacilli. The cornea has an epithelial defect and an underlying opacity on slit-lamp examination, or may have a "white spot" on direct visualization. Hypopyon may be present. Ophthalmic fluoroquinolones, such as levofloxacin 0.5%, ofloxacin 0.3%, norfloxacin 0.3%, or ciprofloxacin 0.3%, are commonly used as first-line agents when the local prevalence of resistant organisms is low (Table 7–2). For severe central ulcers, diagnostic scrapings can be sent for Gram stain and culture. Treatment may include compounded high-concentration ophthalmic antibiotic drops applied hourly day and night for at least the first 48 hours. Fourth-generation ophthalmic fluoroquinolones (moxifloxacin 0.5% and gatifloxacin 0.3%) are also frequently used in this setting. Although early adjunctive ophthalmic corticosteroid therapy may improve visual outcome, it should be prescribed only by an ophthalmologist.

When to Refer

Any patient with suspected bacterial keratitis must be referred emergently to an ophthalmologist.

Lin A et al; American Academy of Ophthalmology Preferred Practice Pattern Cornea and External Disease Panel. Bacterial keratitis: Preferred Practice Pattern®. Ophthalmology. 2019;126:P1. [PMID: 30366799]

2. Herpes Simplex Keratitis

Primary ocular herpes simplex virus infection may manifest as lid, conjunctival, or corneal ulceration. Virus colonization of the trigeminal ganglion leads to recurrences that may be precipitated by fever, excessive exposure to sunlight, or immunodeficiency. Herpetic corneal disease is typically unilateral but can be bilateral with atopy or immunocompromise. The dendritic (branching) corneal ulcer is the most characteristic manifestation of herpetic corneal disease. More extensive "geographic" ulcers also occur, particularly if ophthalmic corticosteroids have been used. The corneal ulcers are most easily seen with a slit lamp after instillation of fluorescein and examination with a cobalt blue light. Treatment of corneal herpetic disease is with ophthalmic antiviral agents (eg, ganciclovir 0.15% gel, one drop five times daily until healing has occurred and then one drop three times daily for 1 more week, trifluoride drops, or acyclovir ointment) or oral antiviral agents (eg, acyclovir, 400–800 mg five times daily or valacyclovir 500–1000 mg three times daily for 7–14 days). Ophthalmic antiviral agents may cause corneal toxicity after 10–14 days of therapy and are not commonly used for long-term suppressive therapy.

Stromal herpes simplex keratitis produces increasingly severe corneal opacity with each recurrence. Antiviral agents alone are insufficient to control stromal disease; thus ophthalmic corticosteroids are also used, but they may enhance viral replication and steroid dependence frequently occurs. **Caution:** *For patients with known or possible herpetic disease, ophthalmic corticosteroids should be prescribed only with ophthalmologic consultation.* Severe stromal scarring may require corneal transplantation; recurrence in the new cornea is common and long-term oral antiviral agents are required.

The rate of recurrent corneal herpetic disease is reduced by using long-term oral acyclovir, 400 mg twice daily; famciclovir, 250 mg once daily; or valacyclovir, 500 mg once daily. Long-term oral antiviral dosing may be adjusted if the disease breaks through suppressive dosing or if kidney dysfunction is present.

When to Refer

Any patient with a history of herpes simplex keratitis and an acute red eye should be referred urgently to an ophthalmologist.

3. Herpes Zoster Ophthalmicus

Herpes zoster frequently involves the ophthalmic division of the trigeminal nerve. It presents with malaise, fever, headache, and periorbital burning and itching. These symptoms may precede the eruption by a day or more. The rash is initially vesicular, quickly becoming pustular and then crusting. Involvement of the tip of the nose or the lid margin predicts a higher risk of ocular involvement . Ocular signs include conjunctivitis, keratitis, episcleritis, and anterior uveitis, often with elevated intraocular pressure. If needed, PCR from aqueous or corneal pseudodendrites can confirm the clinical diagnosis. Recurrent anterior segment inflammation, neurotrophic keratitis, and posterior subcapsular cataract are long-term complications. Optic neuropathy, cranial nerve palsies, acute retinal necrosis, and cerebral angiitis occur infrequently. HIV infection is an important risk factor for herpes zoster ophthalmicus and increases the likelihood of complications.

High-dose oral acyclovir (800 mg five times a day), valacyclovir (1 g three times a day), or famciclovir (500 mg three times a day) for 7–10 days started within 72 hours after the rash appears reduces the incidence of ocular complications but not of postherpetic neuralgia. Treatment of keratitis is discussed above. Anterior uveitis requires additional treatment with ophthalmic corticosteroids and cycloplegic agents (eg, cyclopentolate). Ophthalmic corticosteroids, which promote viral replication, may have to be delayed until the keratitis has resolved. Neurotrophic keratitis is an important cause of long-term morbidity. Extending oral antiviral therapy for 12 months is recommended to reduce recurrence rates and duration of pain.

When to Refer

Any patient with herpes zoster ophthalmicus and ocular symptoms or signs should be referred urgently to an ophthalmologist.

Cohen EJ et al. Low-dose valacyclovir in herpes zoster ophthalmicus: the zoster eye disease randomized clinical trial. JAMA Ophthalmol. 2025;143:269. [PMID: 40048183]

4. Fungal Keratitis

Fungal keratitis tends to occur after corneal injury involving plant material or in agricultural settings, in eyes with chronic ocular surface disease, and in contact lens wearers. It may be an indolent process. The corneal infiltrate may have feathery edges and multiple "satellite" lesions. A hypopyon may be present. Unlike bacterial keratitis, an epithelial defect may or may not be present. Corneal scrapings should be cultured on media suitable for fungi. Diagnosis is often delayed, and treatment frequently requires ≥ 6 months for severe disease. Natamycin 5%, amphotericin 0.1–0.5%, and voriconazole 0.2–1% are commonly used ophthalmic agents (Table 7–2). Systemic azoles are probably not helpful unless there is scleritis or intraocular infection. Corneal grafting is often required.

Donovan C et al. Fungal keratitis: mechanisms of infection and management strategies. Surv Ophthalmol. 2022;67:758. [PMID: 34425126]

5. Amoebic Keratitis

Acanthamoeba keratitis is a painful, sight-threatening corneal infection. The two greatest risk factors in developed countries are contact lens wear and fresh-water or hot-tub exposure. Symptoms include severe eye pain, photophobia, tearing, and blurred vision. The keratitis progresses over months and can lead to corneal blindness. Although severe pain with perineural and ring infiltrates in the corneal stroma is characteristic, it is not specific and earlier forms with changes confined to the corneal epithelium are identifiable. Diagnostic techniques include corneal cultures, examination of stained specimens for cysts, PCR, and in vivo confocal microscopy. *Acanthamoeba* keratitis can be cured with aggressive and prolonged local therapy. Topical chlorhexidine digluconate (0.02–0.6%) or polyhexamethylene biguanide (0.2–0.8%) is commonly used for initial therapy. Oral miltefosine can be considered in severe cases with a deep cyst load. Corticosteroid therapy is controversial and should be initiated only after several weeks of adequate anti-*Acanthamoeba* treatment. Treatment duration depends on severity of the disease but commonly lasts many months. Corneal surgery is commonly required to help restore vision after the infection subsides.

Richardson QR ... Seitzman GD et al. Antiamoebic susceptibility in *Acanthamoeba keratitis*: comparison of isolates from South India and Northern California. Cornea. 2023;42:110. [PMID: 36036669]

ACUTE ANGLE-CLOSURE GLAUCOMA

ESSENTIALS OF DIAGNOSIS

- Older age group, particularly farsighted individuals.
- Rapid onset of severe pain and profound visual loss with "halos around lights."
- Red eye, cloudy cornea, dilated pupil.
- Hard eye on palpation.

General Considerations

Primary acute angle-closure glaucoma (acute angle-closure crisis) results from closure of a preexisting narrow anterior chamber angle. The predisposing factors are shallow anterior chamber, which may be associated with farsightedness or a small eye (short axial length); enlargement of the crystalline lens with age; and genetic inheritance, such as among persons of Inuit and Asian ancestry. Closure of the angle is precipitated by pupillary dilation and thus can occur from sitting in a darkened theater, during times of stress, following nonocular administration of anticholinergic or sympathomimetic agents (eg, nebulized bronchodilators, atropine, antidepressants, bowel or bladder antispasmodics, nasal decongestants, or tocolytics), or, rarely, from pharmacologic mydriasis (see Precautions in Management of Ocular Disorders, below). Subacute primary angle-closure glaucoma may present as recurrent headache.

Secondary acute angle-closure glaucoma does not require a preexisting narrow angle and the mechanism may differ between cases. It may occur in anterior uveitis, with dislocation of the lens, with hemodialysis, or due to various drugs (see Adverse Ophthalmic Effects of Systemic Drugs, below). The reduction in serum osmolarity that occurs with hemodialysis causes an osmotic gradient between the plasma and aqueous fluid, leading to a buildup of fluid in the aqueous compartment. Patients with a compromised outflow system (as with narrow angle) cannot accommodate the buildup and the intraocular pressure rises. Symptoms are the same as in primary acute angle-closure glaucoma, but differentiation is important for management.

Clinical Findings

Patients with acute glaucoma usually seek treatment immediately because of extreme pain and blurred vision, though there are subacute cases. Typically, the blurred vision is associated with halos around lights. Nausea and abdominal pain may occur. The eye is red, the cornea cloudy, and the pupil moderately dilated and nonreactive to light. Intraocular pressure is usually > 50 mm Hg, producing a hard eye on palpation.

Differential Diagnosis

Acute glaucoma must be differentiated from conjunctivitis, acute uveitis, and corneal disorders (Table 7–1).

Treatment

Initial treatment, regardless of mechanism, is reduction of intraocular pressure. A single 500-mg intravenous dose of acetazolamide, followed by 250 mg orally four times a day, together with topical medications such as timolol maleate (a β-blocker) that lower intraocular pressure (Table 7–2), is usually sufficient. Osmotic diuretics, such as oral glycerin and intravenous urea or mannitol—the dosage of all three being 1–2 g/kg—may be necessary if there is no response to acetazolamide. Definitive treatment depends on the mechanism.

A. Primary Angle-Closure Glaucoma

In primary acute angle-closure glaucoma, once the intraocular pressure has started to fall, topical 4% pilocarpine, 1 drop every 15 minutes for 1 hour and then four times a day, is used to reverse the underlying angle closure. The definitive treatment is cataract extraction. Laser peripheral iridotomy is also a first-line treatment.

All patients with primary acute angle closure should undergo prophylactic laser peripheral iridotomy to the unaffected eye, or early cataract extraction should be considered, unless that eye has already undergone cataract or glaucoma surgery.

B. Secondary Angle-Closure Glaucoma

In secondary acute angle-closure glaucoma, additional treatment is determined by the cause.

Prognosis

Untreated acute angle-closure glaucoma results in severe and permanent visual loss within 2–5 days after onset of symptoms. Affected patients need to be monitored for development of chronic glaucoma.

When to Refer

Any patient with suspected acute angle-closure glaucoma must be referred emergently to an ophthalmologist.

Gedde SJ et al. American Academy of Ophthalmology Preferred Practice Pattern Glaucoma Panel. Primary Angle-Closure Disease Preferred Practice Pattern®. Ophthalmology. 2021;128:30. [PMID: 34933744]

CHRONIC GLAUCOMA

ESSENTIALS OF DIAGNOSIS

- Three types of chronic glaucoma: open-angle glaucoma, angle-closure glaucoma, and normal-tension glaucoma.
- No symptoms in early stages.
- Insidious progressive bilateral loss of peripheral vision resulting in tunnel vision; visual acuities preserved until advanced disease.
- Pathologic cupping of the optic disks.
- Intraocular pressure is usually elevated.

General Considerations

Chronic glaucoma is characterized by gradually progressive excavation ("cupping") of the optic disk with loss of vision progressing from slight visual field loss to complete blindness.

Chronic open-angle glaucoma—intraocular pressure is elevated in either primary or secondary glaucoma due to reduced drainage of aqueous fluid through the trabecular meshwork.

Chronic angle-closure glaucoma—the flow of aqueous fluid into the anterior chamber angle is obstructed in this disorder, which is particularly common in persons of Inuit and eastern Asian ancestry.

Normal-tension glaucoma—intraocular pressure is not elevated in this form of open-angle glaucoma, but the same pattern of optic nerve damage occurs.

Primary chronic open-angle glaucoma is usually bilateral. There is an increased prevalence in first-degree relatives of affected individuals and in patients with diabetes. In Afro-Caribbean and African persons, and probably in Latino persons, it is more frequent, occurs at an earlier age, and results in more severe optic nerve damage. Secondary chronic open-angle glaucoma may result from ocular disease, eg, pigment dispersion, pseudoexfoliation, uveitis, or trauma; or corticosteroid therapy, whether it is intraocular, topical, inhaled, intranasal, or systemic.

It is estimated that 2% of Americans age > 40 have chronic glaucoma, affecting > 2.5 million individuals. At least 25% of cases are undetected. More than 90% of cases are of the open-angle type, within which the incidence of normal-tension glaucoma ranges from 10% to 50%. Worldwide, about 45 million people have open-angle glaucoma, of whom about 4.5 million are bilaterally blind. About 4 million people, of whom approximately 50% live in China, are bilaterally blind from chronic angle-closure glaucoma.

Clinical Findings

Because initially there are no symptoms, chronic glaucoma is often first suspected at a routine eye test. Diagnosis requires consistent and reproducible abnormalities in at least two of three parameters—optic disk or retinal nerve fiber layer (or both), visual field, and intraocular pressure.

1. Optic disk cupping—Optic disk cupping is identified as an absolute increase or an asymmetry between the two eyes of the ratio of the diameter of the optic cup to the diameter of the whole optic disk (cup-disk ratio). (Cup-disk ratio > 0.5 or asymmetry between eyes of ≥ 0.2 is suggestive.) Detection of optic disk cupping and associated abnormalities of the retinal nerve fiber layer is facilitated by optical coherence tomography scans.

2. Visual field abnormalities—Visual field abnormalities initially develop in the paracentral region, followed by constriction of the peripheral visual field. Central vision remains good until late in the disease.

3. Intraocular pressure—The normal range of intraocular pressure is 10–21 mm Hg. In many individuals, elevated intraocular pressure is not associated with optic disk or visual field abnormalities (ocular hypertension).

Monitoring for the development of glaucoma is required in all such cases; a significant proportion of eyes with primary open-angle glaucoma have initial normal intraocular pressure, and only repeated measurements identify the abnormally high pressure. In normal-tension glaucoma, intraocular pressure is always within the normal range.

Prevention

There are many causes of optic disk abnormalities or visual field changes that mimic glaucoma, and visual field testing may prove unreliable in some patients, particularly in the older age group. Although all persons age > 50 years may benefit from intraocular pressure measurement and optic disk examination every 3–5 years, screening for chronic open-angle glaucoma should be targeted at individuals with an affected first-degree relative, at persons who have diabetes mellitus, and at older individuals with African or Hispanic ancestry. Screening may also be warranted in patients taking long-term oral or combined intranasal and inhaled corticosteroid therapy. Screening for chronic angle-closure glaucoma should be targeted at persons with Inuit or Asian ancestry.

Treatment

A. Medications

Medical treatment is directed toward lowering intraocular pressure, even with normal-tension glaucoma. Prostaglandin analog eye drops are commonly used as first-line therapy because of their efficacy, lack of systemic side effects, and convenient once-daily dose (except unoprostone) (see Table 7–2). All may produce conjunctival hyperemia, permanent darkening of the iris and eyelash color, increased eyelash growth, and reduction of periorbital fat (prostaglandin-associated periorbitopathy). Latanoprostene bunod is metabolized into latanoprost and another component that releases nitric oxide, which increases trabecular outflow. Topical β-adrenergic blockers may be used alone or in combination with a prostaglandin analog. The use of topical β-adrenergic blockers may be contraindicated in patients with reactive airway disease or HF. Cardioselective betaxolol is theoretically safer in reactive airway disease but less effective at reducing intraocular pressure. Brimonidine 0.2%, a selective α_2-adrenoceptor agonist, and topical carbonic anhydrase inhibitors can be used in addition to a prostaglandin analog or a β-blocker or as initial therapy when prostaglandin analogs and β-blockers are contraindicated. All three are associated with allergic reactions. Brimonidine may cause uveitis. Apraclonidine, 0.5–1%, another α_2-adrenoceptor agonist, can be used to defer surgery in patients receiving maximal medical therapy, but long-term use is limited by adverse reactions. It is more commonly used to control acute rise in intraocular pressure, such as after laser therapy. The topical agent netarsudil ophthalmic solution 0.02% (a Rho kinase inhibitor) increases aqueous fluid outflow through the trabecular meshwork. Pilocarpine 1–4% is rarely used because of adverse effects. Oral carbonic anhydrase inhibitors (such as acetazolamide) may be used long-term if topical therapy is inadequate and surgical or laser therapy is inappropriate.

Various eye drop preparations combining two agents (eg, prostaglandin analogs, β-adrenergic blocking agents, brimonidine, and topical carbonic anhydrase inhibitors) are available to improve compliance when multiple medications are required. Formulations of one or two agents without preservative or not including benzalkonium chloride as the preservative are preferred to reduce adverse ocular effects for patients with allergies or severe dry eyes.

B. Laser Therapy and Surgery

1. Open-angle glaucoma—Laser trabeculoplasty is used as an adjunct to topical therapy to defer surgery for open-angle glaucoma; it is also advocated as primary treatment, especially when compliance with medications is an issue. Surgical trabeculectomy is generally undertaken when intraocular pressure is inadequately controlled by medical and laser therapy, but it may also be used as primary treatment in advanced cases. Trabeculectomy remains the standard procedure. Adjunctive treatment with subconjunctival mitomycin or fluorouracil is used perioperatively or postoperatively in worse prognosis cases. A variety of less invasive procedures that avoid a full-thickness incision into the eye, called microinvasive glaucoma surgery, are appropriate for moderate glaucoma and are associated with fewer complications but can be more difficult to perform.

2. Angle-closure glaucoma—In chronic angle-closure glaucoma, laser peripheral iridotomy, surgical peripheral iridectomy, or cataract extraction may be helpful. In patients with asymptomatic narrow anterior chamber angles, which includes about 10% of Chinese adults, prophylactic laser peripheral iridotomy can reduce the risk of acute and chronic angle-closure glaucoma. However, there are concerns about the efficacy of such treatment and the risk of cataract progression and corneal decompensation. In the United States, about 1% of people age > 35 years have narrow anterior chamber angles, but acute and chronic angle closure are sufficiently uncommon that prophylactic therapy is not generally advised.

3. Normal-tension glaucoma—The goal of treatment for normal-tension glaucoma is reduction in intraocular pressure by 30% (even if it is in the normal range) to prevent progression. As with open-angle glaucoma, if intraocular pressure is not lowered with medical therapy alone, laser trabeculoplasty is used as an adjunct. Trabeculectomy is the standard surgical procedure if medical and laser therapy are inadequate.

Prognosis

Untreated chronic glaucoma that begins at age 40–45 years will probably cause complete blindness by age 60–65. Early diagnosis and treatment can preserve useful vision throughout life. In primary open-angle glaucoma and if treatment is required in ocular hypertension, the aim is to reduce intraocular pressure to a level that will adequately reduce progression of visual field loss. In eyes with marked visual field or optic disk changes, intraocular pressure must be reduced to <16 mm Hg. In normal-tension glaucoma with progressive visual field loss, it is necessary to achieve even lower intraocular pressure such that surgery is often required.

When to Refer

All patients with suspected chronic glaucoma should be referred to an ophthalmologist or optometrist.

Gedde SJ et al. American Academy of Ophthalmology Preferred Practice Pattern Glaucoma Panel. Primary Open-Angle Glaucoma Preferred Practice Pattern®. Ophthalmology. 2021;128:71. [PMID: 34933745]

Gedde SJ et al. American Academy of Ophthalmology Preferred Practice Pattern Glaucoma Panel. Primary Open-Angle Glaucoma Suspect Preferred Practice Pattern®. Ophthalmology. 2021;128:151. [PMID: 34933743]

UVEITIS

ESSENTIALS OF DIAGNOSIS

- Usually immunologic but possibly infectious or neoplastic.
- Inflammation may be confined to the eye or may be systemic.
- **Acute anterior uveitis:** sudden redness and blurry vision, often with photophobia.
- **Posterior uveitis:** gradual loss of vision, commonly with floaters, in a variably inflamed eye.

General Considerations

Intraocular inflammation (uveitis) is clinically classified as acute or chronic and by which ocular anatomic locations are involved (anterior, intermediate, posterior, or all [panuveitis]).

In most cases the pathogenesis of uveitis is primarily immunologic, but infection may be the cause, particularly in immunodeficiency states. Most causes of uveitis can present in a variety of ocular anatomic locations.

1. Anterior uveitis—Systemic disorders associated with anterior uveitis include HLA-B27–related conditions (ankylosing spondylitis, reactive arthritis, psoriasis, ulcerative colitis, and Crohn disease). Sarcoidosis, toxoplasmosis, tuberculosis, syphilis, and Vogt-Koyanagi-Harada disease (bilateral uveitis associated with alopecia, poliosis [depigmented eyelashes, eyebrows, or hair], vitiligo, and hearing loss) can present as acute, chronic, anterior, and posterior uveitis. Behçet syndrome may present with chronic recurrent anterior uveitis, recurrent hypopyon, and posterior uveitis, characteristically with branch retinal vein occlusions. Sympathetic ophthalmia may present as anterior or posterior uveitis and occurs after penetrating ocular trauma. Chronic anterior uveitis occurs in juvenile idiopathic arthritis. Both herpes simplex and herpes zoster infections may cause acute anterior uveitis as well as retinitis (acute retinal necrosis).

2. Intermediate, posterior, and panuveitis—Intermediate uveitis generally manifests as peripheral retinal abnormalities (pars planitis). It is often idiopathic but can be due to multiple sclerosis or sarcoidosis. Retinal vasculitis predominantly manifests as posterior uveitis with central or peripheral retinal abnormalities. It can be caused by many infectious agents and noninfectious systemic conditions, including vasculitis, but may be idiopathic. With toxoplasmosis, there may be evidence of previous episodes of retinochoroiditis. Syphilis may induce a "salt and pepper" fundus but may present with a wide variety of clinical manifestations. Common pathogens resulting in ocular inflammation during HIV infection are cytomegalovirus (CMV), herpes simplex and herpes zoster viruses, mycobacteria, *Cryptococcus*, *Toxoplasma*, and *Candida*. Any etiology of uveitis that presents with anterior and posterior or intermediate and posterior uveitis is labeled panuveitis.

Clinical Findings

Anterior uveitis is characterized by inflammatory cells within the aqueous humor visualized with a slit lamp microscope. In severe cases, there may be hypopyon (layered collection of white cells) and fibrin within the anterior chamber. Cells may also be seen on the corneal endothelium as keratic precipitates. In granulomatous uveitis, there are large "mutton-fat" keratic precipitates, and sometimes iris nodules. In nongranulomatous uveitis, the keratic precipitates are smaller or absent with no iris nodules. The pupil may be irregularly shaped and poorly reactive if posterior synechiae (adhesions between the iris and anterior lens capsule) develop.

Anterior uveitis tends to present acutely with unilateral pain, redness, photophobia, and visual loss. However, the ocular inflammation associated with juvenile idiopathic arthritis is frequently indolent, commonly asymptomatic initially, and carries a high risk of sight-threatening complications. Chronic recurrent anterior uveitis may cause blurred vision in a variably inflamed eye. **Intermediate uveitis** presents with vitreous inflammation.

Posterior uveitis can occur with retinitis or choroiditis, with or without vasculitis or vitreous inflammation. New retinal lesions are yellow with indistinct margins, and there may be retinal hemorrhages. Older lesions have more defined margins and are commonly pigmented. Retinal vessel sheathing may occur adjacent to such lesions or more diffusely. In severe cases, vitreous opacity precludes visualization of retinal details.

Posterior uveitis can be unilateral or bilateral with symptoms of floaters and visual loss. Symptoms are commonly slower in onset, though acute presentations can occur. Visual loss may be due to vitreous haze and opacities, inflammatory lesions involving the macula, macular edema, retinal vein occlusion, or rarely, optic neuropathy.

Differential Diagnosis

Retinal detachment, intraocular tumors, and CNS lymphoma may all masquerade as uveitis.

Treatment

Anterior uveitis usually responds to ophthalmic corticosteroids (Table 7–2). Occasionally, periocular or intraocular corticosteroid injections or even systemic corticosteroids are required. Dilation of the pupil with a cycloplegic agent (eg, cyclopentolate, homatropine, atropine) (Table 7–2) is important to relieve discomfort and prevent permanent posterior synechiae. **Intermediate, posterior, and panuveitis** more commonly require systemic, periocular, or intravitreal corticosteroid therapy. In chronic cases, systemic corticosteroid-sparing immunomodulatory therapy with agents such as azathioprine, cyclosporine, mycophenolate, methotrexate, tacrolimus, or sirolimus is commonly required. Biologic therapies also are often used. Pupillary dilation is not usually necessary.

If an infectious cause is identified, specific antimicrobial therapy is often needed. In general, the prognosis for anterior uveitis is better than that for posterior uveitis.

When to Refer

- Any patient with suspected acute uveitis should be referred urgently to an ophthalmologist or emergently if there is visual loss or severe pain.
- Any patient with suspected chronic uveitis should be referred to an ophthalmologist, urgently if there is more than mild visual loss.

Al-Janabi A et al. Long-term outcomes of treatment with biological agents in eyes with refractory, active, noninfectious intermediate uveitis, posterior uveitis, or panuveitis. Ophthalmology. 2020;127:410. [PMID: 31607412]

CATARACT

ESSENTIALS OF DIAGNOSIS

- Gradually progressive blurred vision.
- No pain or redness.
- Lens opacities (may be grossly visible).

General Considerations

Cataracts are opacities of the crystalline lens and are usually bilateral. They are the leading cause of blindness worldwide. Age-related cataract is by far the most common cause. Other causes include (1) congenital (from intrauterine infections, such as rubella and CMV, or inborn errors of metabolism, such as galactosemia); (2) traumatic; (3) secondary to systemic disease (diabetes mellitus, myotonic dystrophy, atopic dermatitis); (4) topical, systemic, or inhaled corticosteroid treatment; (5) uveitis; (6) radiation exposure; and (7) increased exposure to UV light (eg, skiers). Most persons age > 60 have some degree of lens opacity. Cigarette smoking increases the risk of cataract formation. Multivitamin/mineral supplements and high dietary antioxidants may prevent the development of age-related cataract.

Clinical Findings

The predominant symptom is progressive blurring of vision. Glare, especially in bright light or with night driving; change of focusing, particularly development of nearsightedness; and monocular double vision may occur.

Even in its early stages, a cataract can be seen through a dilated pupil with an ophthalmoscope or slit lamp. As the cataract matures, the retina will become increasingly difficult to visualize, until finally the fundus reflection is absent and the pupil is white.

Treatment

Functional visual impairment, specifically its effect on daily activities and increased risk of falls, is the prime criterion for surgery. The cataract is usually removed by one of the techniques in which the posterior lens capsule remains (extracapsular), thus providing support for a prosthetic intraocular lens. Ultrasonic fragmentation (phacoemulsification) of the lens nucleus and foldable intraocular lenses allow cataract surgery to be performed through a small incision without the need for sutures, thus reducing the postoperative complication rate and accelerating visual rehabilitation. The standard monofocal prosthetic intraocular lens can correct near or far vision. Premium intraocular lenses (multifocal, extended depth of focus, and accommodative) reduce the need for both distance and near vision correction, although glasses may still be needed for activities such as night driving or reading in low light conditions in some individuals. The light-adjustable lens is a type of intraocular lens that can be adjusted to improve vision after cataract surgery. In the developing world, manual small-incision surgery, in which the lens nucleus is removed intact, is popular because less equipment is required. Additional laser treatment may be required subsequently (months to years after the initial cataract surgery) if the posterior capsule opacifies. The use of topical eye drops to dissolve or prevent cataracts has shown promising results in experimental models; surgery, however, is currently the only treatment option for a visually significant cataract.

Prognosis

Cataract surgery is cost-effective in improving survival and quality of life. In the developed world, it improves visual acuity in 95% of cases. In the other 5%, there is preexisting retinal damage or operative or postoperative complications. In less developed areas, the improvement in visual acuity is not as high, in part due to uncorrected refractive error postoperatively. Nasolacrimal duct obstruction increases the risk of intraocular infection (endophthalmitis).

A large number of drugs, such as α-adrenoreceptor antagonists for benign prostatic hyperplasia and antipsychotics, increase the risk of complications during surgery (floppy iris syndrome) and in the early postoperative period. The α-blocker tamsulosin has the greatest risk of floppy iris syndrome. There is no consensus about whether to stop α-blockers before surgery because the effects of the drug on the iris can persist for months to years. The surgeon must know if the patient is taking an α-blocker to prepare for iris issues during surgery. If the patient has not yet started an α-blocker and is planning to have cataract surgery shortly, it is best to wait until after surgery to begin the medication, if possible.

When to Refer

Patients with cataracts should be referred to an ophthalmologist when their visual impairment adversely affects their everyday activities.

Saad M et al. Alpha blocker-associated intraoperative floppy iris syndrome. Sr Care Pharm. 2022;37:227. [PMID: 35610768]
Miller KM et al. American Academy of Ophthalmology Preferred Practice Pattern Cataract/Anterior Segment Panel. Cataract in the Adult Eye Preferred Practice Pattern®. Ophthalmology. 2022;129:1. [PMID: 34780842]

RETINAL DETACHMENT

ESSENTIALS OF DIAGNOSIS

- Loss of vision in one eye that is usually rapid, possibly with "curtain" spreading across field of vision.
- No pain or redness.
- Detachment seen by ophthalmoscopy.

General Considerations

Most cases of retinal detachment are due to development of one or more peripheral retinal tears or holes (rhegmatogenous retinal detachment). This usually results from posterior vitreous detachment, related to degenerative changes in the vitreous, and often occurs in persons > 50 years of age. Nearsightedness and cataract extraction are the two most common predisposing causes. It may also be caused by penetrating or blunt ocular trauma and is more common in patients who previously have had cataract surgery, sometimes years earlier.

Tractional retinal detachment occurs when there is preretinal fibrosis, such as in proliferative retinopathy due to diabetic retinopathy or retinal vein occlusion, or as a complication of rhegmatogenous retinal detachment. Exudative retinal detachment results from accumulation of subretinal fluid, such as in neovascular age-related macular degeneration or secondary to choroidal tumor.

Clinical Findings

Rhegmatogenous retinal detachment usually starts in the peripheral retina, spreading rapidly to cause visual field loss. Symptoms of the predisposing posterior vitreous detachment with vitreoretinal traction include recent onset of or increase in floaters and photopsias (flashes of light). Central vision remains intact until the central macula becomes detached. On ophthalmoscopic examination, the retina may be elevated with an irregular surface (Figure 7–1). In tractional retinal detachment, there is irregular retinal elevation adherent to scar tissue on the retinal surface, sometimes extending into the vitreous. Exudative retinal detachments are dome-shaped and the subretinal fluid shifts position with changes in posture. Ocular ultrasonography assists in the detection and characterization of retinal detachment, especially if blood accompanies the retinal detachment.

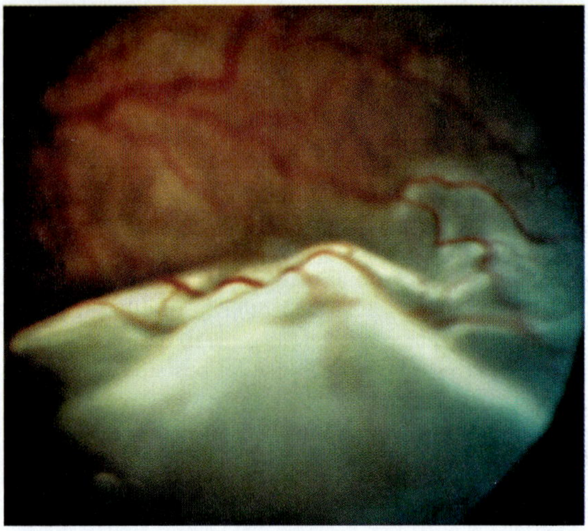

▲ **Figure 7–1.** Inferior retinal detachment as seen on direct or indirect ophthalmoscopy.

Treatment

Treatment of rhegmatogenous retinal detachments requires closing all the retinal tears and holes by forming a permanent adhesion with laser photocoagulation to the retinal pigment epithelium or with cryotherapy to the sclera. Certain types of uncomplicated retinal detachment may be treated by pneumatic retinopexy, in which an expansile gas is injected into the vitreous cavity and the patient's head is positioned to facilitate apposition between the gas and the hole, which permits reattachment of the retina. Once the retina is reattached, the retinal defects are surrounded by laser photocoagulation or cryotherapy scars; these two methods are also used to seal retinal defects without associated detachment.

In complicated retinal detachments, particularly tractional retinal detachments, retinal reattachment can be accomplished only by vitrectomy to enable direct manipulation of the retina or internal tamponade of the retina with air, expansile gas, or silicone oil. The presence of an expansile gas within the eye is a contraindication to air travel, mountaineering at high altitude, and nitrous oxide anesthesia, all of which can cause the gas to expand with severe increases in intraocular pressure. Such gases persist in the globe for weeks after surgery (see Chapter 41). Treatment of exudative retinal detachments is determined by the underlying cause.

Prognosis

About 90% of uncomplicated rhegmatogenous retinal detachments can be cured with one operation. The visual prognosis is worse if the macula is detached or if the detachment is of long duration.

When to Refer

All cases of retinal detachment must be referred urgently to an ophthalmologist, and emergently if central vision is good because this indicates that the macula has not yet detached. During transportation, the patient's head is positioned so that the retinal tear is placed at the lowest point of the eye to minimize extension of the detached retina. If the inferior retina is detached with superior visual field loss, the patient should keep the head upright so that the tear is located at the lowest point, whereas if the temporal retina is detached (visual field loss on the side by the nose), the patient should keep the temporal side of the head (ear side) down to reduce the chances that the fluid will extend beneath the central retina, causing the macula to detach. If vision is good and the macula is attached, patients should minimize eye motion; in some patients, patching both eyes can be helpful in preventing the eyes from moving until surgery can be performed to repair the retinal detachment.

Alshammari AJ et al. Retinal detachment following cataract surgery: a systematic review and meta-analysis of incidence, preoperative risk factors, and postoperative complications. Ophthalmic Surg Lasers Imaging Retina. 2024;55:668. [PMID: 39172224]

Lin JB et al. Retinal detachment. Nat Rev Dis Primers. 2024;10:18. [PMID: 38485969]

VITREOUS HEMORRHAGE

Patients with vitreous hemorrhage complain of sudden visual loss, abrupt onset of floaters that may progressively increase in severity, or occasionally, "bleeding within the eye." Visual acuity ranges from 20/20 (6/6) to light perception. The eye is not inflamed, red, or painful, and clues to diagnosis are inability to see fundus details or localized blood in the vitreous, in front of the retina. Causes of vitreous hemorrhage include retinal tear (with or without detachment), diabetic or sickle cell retinopathy, retinal vein occlusion, retinal vasculitis, neovascular age-related macular degeneration, retinal arterial macroaneurysm, blood dyscrasia, anticoagulation, trauma, subarachnoid hemorrhage, and severe straining (Valsalva retinopathy).

When to Refer

All patients with suspected vitreous hemorrhage must be referred urgently to an ophthalmologist to determine the etiology. If the vitreous hemorrhage is caused by a retinal tear or detachment, it must be repaired urgently to prevent permanent vision loss.

Strand E et al. Nondiabetic vitreous hemorrhage: a review of management strategy and outcomes. Ophthalmic Surg Lasers Imaging Retina. 2024;55:660. [PMID: 39172227]

AGE-RELATED MACULAR DEGENERATION

ESSENTIALS OF DIAGNOSIS

- Older age group.
- In one or both eyes; acute or chronic deterioration of central vision; distortion or abnormal size of images, sometimes developing acutely.
- No pain or redness.
- Classified as dry ("atrophic," "geographic") or wet ("neovascular," "exudative") macular degeneration.
- Macular abnormalities seen by ophthalmoscopy.

General Considerations

Age-related macular degeneration is the leading cause of permanent visual loss in the older population. Its prevalence progressively increases over age 50 years (to almost 30% by age 75). Its occurrence and response to treatment are likely influenced by genetically determined variations, many of which involve the complement pathway. Other associated factors include a slight female predominance, family history, hypertension, hypercholesterolemia, CVD, farsightedness, light iris color, and cigarette smoking (the most readily modifiable risk factor).

Although both dry and wet age-related macular degeneration are progressive and usually bilateral, a patient's eyes are often affected asymmetrically and manifestations, prognosis, and management may differ between the eyes.

Clinical Findings

Drusen are the hallmark of age-related macular degeneration. The macula can be visualized with the use of a direct ophthalmoscope, by fundus photographs, or with cross-sectional optical coherence tomography scans. Hard drusen appear as discrete yellow subretinal deposits. Soft drusen are paler and less distinct. Large, confluent soft drusen are risk factors for neovascular (wet) age-related macular degeneration. Vision loss in age-related macular degeneration involves the central vision or pericentral vision in most patients. Peripheral fields, and hence navigational vision, are maintained, except in patients with severe neovascular age-related macular degeneration or in patients with coincident optic nerve disease such as glaucoma. Although "dry" age-related macular degeneration is more common, untreated "wet" age-related macular degeneration accounts for about 90% of all cases of legal blindness due to age-related macular degeneration.

1. "Dry" age-related macular degeneration—There is gradual progressive bilateral visual loss due to geographic atrophy of the outer retina, the retinal pigment epithelium, and the choriocapillaris, which supplies blood to both the outer retina and the retinal pigment epithelium.

2. "Wet" age-related macular degeneration—Choroidal new vessels grow under either the retina or the retinal pigment epithelial cells, leading to accumulation of exudative fluid, hemorrhage, and fibrosis. The onset of visual loss is more rapid and more severe than in atrophic degeneration. The two eyes are frequently affected sequentially over a few years.

Treatment

No dietary modification has been shown to prevent the development of age-related macular degeneration, but its progression may be reduced by oral treatment with antioxidants (vitamins C and E), zinc, copper, and carotenoids (lutein and zeaxanthin, rather than vitamin A [β-carotene]). Oral omega-3 fatty acids do not provide additional benefit.

1. Dry age-related macular degeneration—Pegcetacoplan and avacincaptad pegol are FDA-approved agents for treatment of dry age-related macular degeneration with geographic atrophy of the outer retina extending toward the fovea. Both agents inhibit the complement pathway, are delivered by monthly or every-other-monthly injection into the vitreous, and slow the rate of growth of geographic atrophy lesions. However, both agents are associated with mildly increased risk of choroidal neovascularization, and intravitreal injection is associated with risks of infection (1/2000), retinal detachment (1/10,000), vitreous hemorrhage, and cataract. As with wet age-related macular degeneration, rehabilitation including low-vision aids is important. Patients should be advised to stop smoking cigarettes and to take vitamin supplements as described above, which are similarly effective to the complement inhibitor therapies in reducing rates of progression.

2. "Wet" age-related macular degeneration—Inhibitors of vascular endothelial growth factors (VEGF), such as ranibizumab, bevacizumab, aflibercept, faricimab, and biosimilar medications, such as ranibizumab-nuna and ranibizumab-eqrn, can cause regression of choroidal neovascularization with resorption of subretinal fluid and improvement or stabilization of vision. Long-term repeated intraocular injections are often required and must be administered in the eye clinic several times a year, if not monthly. Treatment is well tolerated with minimal adverse effects, but there is a risk of infection, retinal detachment, vitreous hemorrhage, and cataract with each injection. Some patients do not respond to anti-VEGF injections, and up to one-third of eyes lose vision despite regular treatment.

When to Refer

Older patients with sudden visual loss, particularly paracentral or central distortion or scotoma with preserved central acuity, should be referred urgently to an ophthalmologist.

Csaky KG et al. Drug approval for the treatment of geographic atrophy: how we got here and where we need to go. Am J Ophthalmol. 2024;263:231. [PMID: 38387826]

Fleckenstein M et al. Age-related macular degeneration: a review. JAMA. 2024;331:147. [PMID: 38193957]

Tzoumas N et al. Complement inhibitors for age-related macular degeneration. Cochrane Database Syst Rev. 2023;6:CD009300. [PMID: 37314061]

CENTRAL & BRANCH RETINAL VEIN OCCLUSIONS

ESSENTIALS OF DIAGNOSIS

- Sudden monocular loss of vision.
- No pain or redness.
- Widespread or sectoral retinal hemorrhages.

General Considerations

Central and branch retinal vein occlusion are common causes of acute vision loss, with branch vein occlusions being four times more common. The major predisposing factors are the etiologic factors associated with arteriosclerosis, but glaucoma is also a major risk factor.

Clinical Findings

A. Symptoms and Signs

1. Central retinal vein occlusion—Ophthalmoscopic signs include widespread retinal hemorrhages, retinal venous dilation and tortuosity, retinal cotton-wool spots, and optic disk swelling. Rarely, central retinal vein occlusion presents with severe vision loss and pain when neovascularization of the iris develops, usually about 90 days after a central retinal vein occlusion has caused severe retinal nonperfusion, release of vascular endothelial growth factor (VEGF), and growth of new blood vessels that block aqueous fluid from leaving the eye.

2. Branch retinal vein occlusion—Sudden loss of vision may occur at the time of occlusion if the fovea is involved, or some time afterward from vitreous hemorrhage due to retinal new vessels. More gradual visual loss may occur with development of macular edema. In acute branch retinal vein occlusion, the retinal abnormalities (hemorrhages, microaneurysms, venous dilation and tortuosity, and cotton-wool spots) are confined to the area drained by the obstructed vein.

To assess for possible reversible risk factors, check blood pressure and ask about tobacco smoking in all patients, and ask women about estrogen therapy (including combined oral contraceptives). Patients should be asked if they have glaucoma and should undergo a comprehensive eye examination to check intraocular pressure. A sleep study to assess for obstructive sleep apnea may be recommended.

B. Laboratory Findings

Obtain screening laboratory studies for diabetes mellitus, hyperlipidemia, and hyperviscosity (especially in simultaneous bilateral disease), including serum protein electrophoresis for paraproteinemia. Particularly in younger patients, consider obtaining antiphospholipid antibodies, lupus anticoagulant, tests for inherited thrombophilia, and plasma homocysteine levels.

Complications

If central retinal vein occlusion is associated with widespread retinal ischemia, manifesting as poor visual acuity (20/200 [6/60] or worse), extensive retinal hemorrhages, an afferent pupillary defect, and widespread capillary closure on fluorescein angiography, there is a high risk of development of neovascular (rubeotic) glaucoma, typically within the first 3 months after the occlusion. Branch retinal vein occlusion may be complicated by peripheral retinal neovascularization or chronic macular edema.

Treatment

A. Macular Edema

Intravitreal injection of VEGF inhibitors, including ranibizumab, bevacizumab, or aflibercept and biosimilar medications, is beneficial in macular edema due to either branch or central retinal vein occlusion.

B. Neovascularization

Eyes at risk for neovascular glaucoma following ischemic central retinal vein occlusion should be treated with panretinal laser photocoagulation prophylactically or as soon as there is evidence of neovascularization, with the latter approach necessitating frequent monitoring. Regression of retinal and iris neovascularization can be achieved with intravitreal injections of bevacizumab or other anti-VEGF agents, but panretinal laser photocoagulation is the definitive treatment and cannot be substituted by anti-VEGF agents. In branch retinal vein occlusion complicated by retinal neovascularization, the ischemic retina should be treated with laser photocoagulation.

Prognosis

In central retinal vein occlusion, severity of visual loss initially is a good guide to visual outcome. Initial visual acuity of 20/60 (6/18) or better indicates a good prognosis. Visual prognosis is poor for eyes with neovascular glaucoma. In branch retinal vein occlusion, visual outcome is determined by the severity of glaucoma and macular damage from hemorrhage, ischemia, or edema. Patients who experience retinal vein occlusion are at significantly increased risk of stroke and should be evaluated by their primary care provider.

When to Refer

All patients with retinal vein occlusion should be referred urgently to an ophthalmologist and should be evaluated by a primary care provider to assess and manage stroke risk.

Cornish EE et al. Management of macular oedema due to retinal vein occlusion: an evidence-based systematic review and meta-analysis. Clin Exp Ophthalmol. 2023;51:313. [PMID: 37060158]

CENTRAL & BRANCH RETINAL ARTERY OCCLUSIONS

ESSENTIALS OF DIAGNOSIS

- Sudden monocular loss of vision.
- No pain or redness.
- Widespread or sectoral pale retinal swelling.

General Considerations

Acute retinal arterial ischemia, including central and branch retinal artery occlusion, is a true ocular and medical emergency. In patients ≥ 50 years old with central retinal artery occlusion, giant cell arteritis must be considered (see Ischemic Optic Neuropathy and Chapter 23). Otherwise, even if no retinal emboli are identified on ophthalmoscopy, urgent investigation for carotid and cardiac sources of emboli must be undertaken in central and branch retinal artery occlusion for timely treatment to reduce the risk of stroke (see Chapters 14, 16, and 27). Diabetes mellitus, hyperlipidemia, and systemic hypertension are common etiologic factors. Migraine, oral contraceptives, systemic vasculitis, congenital or acquired thrombophilia, and hyperhomocysteinemia are also causes, particularly in young patients. Internal carotid artery dissection should be considered, especially when there is neck pain or a recent history of neck trauma.

Clinical Findings

A. Symptoms and Signs

1. Central retinal artery occlusion—This occlusion presents as sudden profound monocular visual loss. Visual acuity is usually reduced to counting fingers or worse, and visual field may be restricted to an island of vision in the temporal field. Ophthalmoscopy reveals pale swelling of the retina with a cherry-red spot at the fovea (Figure 7–2). Occasionally, emboli are seen in the central retinal artery or its branches. The retinal swelling subsides over a period of 4–6 weeks, leaving a pale optic disk with thinning of the inner retina on macular cross-sectional optical coherence tomography scans; these findings can help diagnose unexplained vision loss if the patient is examined after the acute occlusive event has resolved.

2. Branch retinal artery occlusion—This occlusion also may present with sudden loss of vision if the fovea is involved, but it more commonly presents with sudden loss of a discrete area in the visual field in one eye. Fundus signs of retinal swelling and sometimes adjacent cotton-wool spots are limited to the area of retina supplied by the occluded artery.

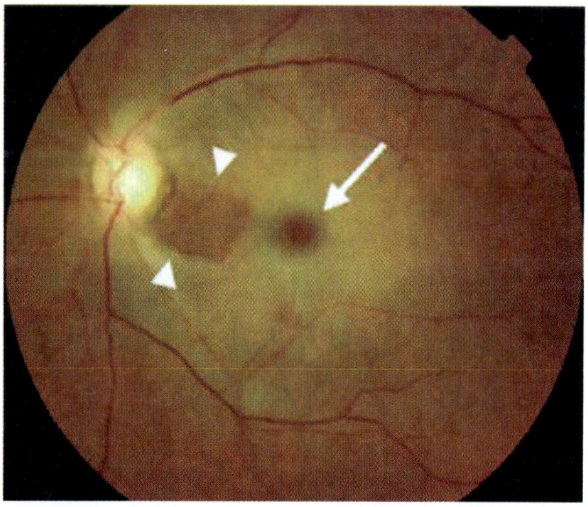

Figure 7–2. Acute central retinal artery occlusion with cherry-red spot (arrow) seen at the fovea centered in macular loss of retinal transparency, and preserved retinal perfusion (arrowheads) adjacent to the optic disk due to macular cilioretinal artery supply. (Reproduced, with permission, from Riordan-Eva P, Augsburger JJ. *Vaughan & Asbury's General Ophthalmology*, 19th ed. McGraw Hill, 2018.)

The clinician should identify risk factors for cardiac sources of emboli including arrhythmia, particularly atrial fibrillation, and cardiac valvular disease, and check the blood pressure. Clinical features of giant cell arteritis are age ≥ 50 years, headache, scalp tenderness, jaw claudication, general malaise, weight loss, symptoms of polymyalgia rheumatica, and tenderness, thickening, or absence of pulse of the superficial temporal arteries. Table 23–12 lists the clinical manifestations of vasculitis.

B. Laboratory Findings

Giant cell arteritis should be considered in cases of central retinal artery occlusion without visible emboli. ESR and CRP are usually elevated, but one or both may be normal (see Chapter 23). Consider screening for other types of vasculitis (see Table 23–11). Screen for diabetes mellitus and hyperlipidemia in all patients. Particularly in younger patients, consider testing for antiphospholipid antibodies, lupus anticoagulant, inherited thrombophilia, and elevated plasma homocysteine.

C. Imaging

A brain MRI with diffusion-weighted imaging sequences should be obtained urgently to look for cerebral infarction, which is present in up to 31% of patients with branch or central retinal artery occlusion. Obtain duplex ultrasonography of the carotid arteries, ECG, echocardiography with transesophageal studies to identify carotid and cardiac sources of emboli, and CT or MR studies for internal carotid artery dissection, if necessary.

Treatment

Retinal artery occlusions are a true emergency and require urgent referral to an emergency department, ideally with a stroke center, for imaging and clinical assessment to prevent subsequent stroke. If the patient is seen within a few hours after onset, emergency treatment, comprising laying the patient flat, ocular massage, high concentrations of inhaled oxygen, intravenous acetazolamide, and anterior chamber paracentesis, may influence the visual outcome. Early thrombolysis, particularly by local intra-arterial injection but also intravenously, has shown good results in central retinal artery occlusion not due to giant cell arteritis. However, local intra-arterial injection of thrombolytic agents has a high incidence of adverse effects and may be difficult to accomplish quickly enough to prevent permanent vision loss due to inner retinal ischemia, which may occur within 90 minutes of occlusion.

In giant cell arteritis, there is risk of involvement of the other eye without prompt treatment. Once giant cell arteritis is suspected, immediate treatment with intravenous methylprednisolone 1 g/day is recommended for 3 days. All patients require subsequent long-term corticosteroid therapy; concomitant administration of long-term low-dose aspirin therapy is controversial. Tocilizumab, a monoclonal antibody against the receptor for interleukin-6, is also approved to treat giant cell arteritis. (See Polymyalgia Rheumatica & Giant Cell Arteritis, Chapter 23, for further discussion of treatment.)

Patients with embolic retinal artery occlusion with 70–99% ipsilateral carotid artery stenosis, and possibly those with 50–69% stenosis, should be considered for carotid endarterectomy or possibly angioplasty within 2 weeks of the occlusion (see Chapters 14 and 27). Retinal embolization due to cardiac disease such as atrial fibrillation or a hypercoagulable state usually requires anticoagulation. Cardiac valvular disease and patent foramen ovale may require surgical treatment.

When to Refer

- Patients with retinal artery occlusions should be referred immediately to an emergency department, ideally with a stroke center, to evaluate for stroke manifestations.
- Patients with central retinal artery occlusion should be referred emergently to an ophthalmologist.
- Patients with branch retinal artery occlusion should be referred urgently for examination by an ophthalmologist.
- Patients with suspected giant cell arteritis should be referred to a rheumatologist to guide management.

When to Admit

Patients with visual loss due to giant cell arteritis may require emergency admission for high-dose corticosteroid therapy and close monitoring to ensure adequate treatment.

Bénard-Séguin É et al. Eye stroke protocol in the emergency department. J Stroke Cerebrovasc Dis. 2024;33:107895. [PMID: 39079617]
Chen C et al. Central retinal artery occlusion: a stroke of the eye. Eye (Lond). 2024;38:2319. [PMID: 38548943]
Webb Z. Intravenous thrombolysis for central retinal artery occlusion: a look at the literature for the emergency medicine physician. Cureus. 2023;15:e41878. [PMID: 37457612]

TRANSIENT MONOCULAR VISUAL LOSS

ESSENTIALS OF DIAGNOSIS

- Sudden-onset, monocular loss of vision usually lasting a few minutes with complete recovery.

Clinical Findings

A. Symptoms and Signs

Transient monocular visual loss ("ocular transient ischemic attack [TIA]") is usually caused by a retinal embolus from ipsilateral carotid disease or the heart. The visual loss is characteristically described as a curtain passing vertically across the visual field with complete monocular visual loss lasting a few minutes and a similar curtain effect as the episode passes (amaurosis fugax; also called "fleeting blindness"). An embolus is rarely seen on ophthalmoscopy. Other causes of transient, often recurrent, visual loss due to ocular ischemia are giant cell arteritis, hypercoagulable state (such as antiphospholipid syndrome), hyperviscosity, and severe occlusive carotid disease. More transient visual loss affecting one or both eyes, termed transient visual obscurations, lasts only a few seconds to 1 minute, usually is recurrent, and occurs in patients with optic disk swelling, such as in those with raised intracranial pressure or multiple sclerosis.

B. Diagnostic Studies

In most cases, clinical assessment and investigations are much the same as for retinal artery occlusion with emphasis on urgent neuroimaging to assess for cerebral infarction, and identification of a source of emboli, since patients with embolic transient vision loss are at increased risk for stroke, MI, and other vascular events. Optic disk swelling requires different investigations (see Optic Disk Swelling, below).

Treatment

All patients with possible embolic transient visual loss should be treated immediately with oral aspirin (at least 81 mg daily), or another antiplatelet drug, until the cause has been determined. Affected patients with 70–99% (and possibly those with 50–69%) ipsilateral carotid artery stenosis should be considered for urgent carotid endarterectomy or possibly angioplasty with stenting (see Chapters 14 and 27). In all patients, vascular risk factors (eg, hypertension) need to be controlled. Retinal embolization due to cardiac arrhythmia, such as atrial fibrillation, or a hypercoagulable state usually requires anticoagulation. Cardiac valvular disease and patent foramen ovale may require surgical treatment.

When to Refer

In all cases of episodic visual loss, early ophthalmologic consultation is advisable.

When to Admit

Referral to a stroke center or hospital admission is recommended in embolic transient visual loss if there have been two or more episodes in the preceding week ("crescendo TIA") or the underlying cause is cardiac or a hypercoagulable state.

Douglas VP et al. Transient monocular visual loss (amaurosis fugax): how does age impact diagnosis? Ophthalmol Ther. 2024;13:1417. [PMID: 38587773]

RETINAL DISORDERS ASSOCIATED WITH SYSTEMIC DISEASES

1. Diabetic Retinopathy

ESSENTIALS OF DIAGNOSIS

- By 20 years after diagnosis of diabetes, 99% of patients with type 1 diabetes and 60% of patients with type 2 diabetes will have diabetic retinopathy.
- **Nonproliferative retinopathy:** can be mild, moderate, or severe. Microvascular changes are limited to the retina.
- **Proliferative retinopathy:** new blood vessels grow on the surface of the retina, optic nerve, or iris.
- **Macular edema:** central retinal swelling; can occur with any severity level of diabetic retinopathy; can reduce visual acuity if the foveal center is involved.

General Considerations

Diabetic retinopathy is present in about one-third of patients in whom diabetes has been diagnosed, and about one-third of those have sight-threatening disease. In the United States, it affects about 4 million people; it is the leading cause of vision loss worldwide among adults age 25–74 years; and the number of affected individuals ≥ 65 years old is increasing. Retinopathy increases in prevalence and severity with increasing duration and poorer control of diabetes. In type 1 diabetes, retinopathy is not detectable for the first 5 years after diagnosis. In type 2 diabetes, about 20% of patients have retinopathy at diagnosis, likely because they had diabetes for many years before diagnosis. Macular involvement is the most common cause of legal blindness in type 2 diabetes.

There are two main categories of diabetic retinopathy: nonproliferative and proliferative. Diabetic macular edema can occur at any stage in both nonproliferative and proliferative retinopathy and is the most common reason for ophthalmic diabetic treatment.

Nonproliferative retinopathy (previously known as "background" retinopathy) is subclassified as mild, moderate, or severe. It represents the earliest stage of retinal involvement by diabetes. During this stage, the retinal capillaries leak proteins, lipids, or red cells into the retina. When this process occurs in the macula and causes clinically significant macular edema, visual acuity is affected; this is the most common cause of visual impairment in patients with type 2 diabetes.

Proliferative retinopathy is less common than nonproliferative retinopathy but causes more severe visual loss. It involves the growth of new vessels and fibrous tissue on the surface of the retina, extending into the vitreous chamber. It is a consequence of severe capillary occlusion, which causes retinal ischemia and release of VEGF; this, in turn, stimulates new vessel growth with vision loss from preretinal hemorrhage, fibrosis, and retinal traction.

Clinical Findings

Clinical assessment comprises visual acuity testing, stereoscopic examination of the retina, retinal imaging with optical coherence tomography, and sometimes fluorescein angiography.

Nonproliferative retinopathy manifests as microaneurysms, retinal hemorrhages, venous beading, retinal edema, and hard exudates. In mild nonproliferative diabetic retinopathy, there are mild retinal abnormalities without visual loss. Severe nonproliferative retinopathy is defined as having any one of the following: severe intraretinal hemorrhages and microaneurysms in four quadrants, venous beading in two or more quadrants, or intraretinal microvascular abnormalities in at least one quadrant.

Proliferative retinopathy is characterized by neovascularization, arising from either the optic disk or the retinal vascular arcades. Prior to proliferation of new capillaries, a preproliferative phase often occurs in which arteriolar ischemia is manifest as cotton-wool spots (small infarcted areas of retina). Vision is usually normal until macular edema, vitreous hemorrhage, or retinal detachment occurs. Proliferation into the vitreous of blood vessels, with associated fibrosis, may lead to vitreous hemorrhage and tractional retinal detachment.

Macular edema (focal or diffuse) is the most common reason for reduction in vision in diabetes. Macular ischemia is a separate entity from macular edema that can also impair vision in diabetic retinopathy. Macular ischemia is not treatable with anti-VEGF antibody therapies.

Diabetic retinopathy may worsen after bariatric surgery or in patients with long-standing hyperglycemia that is rapidly brought under tight control, such as after receiving an insulin pump or being treated with GLP-1 receptor agonists, SGLT-2 inhibitors, or dipeptidyl peptidase-4 inhibitors. It is believed that capillary endothelial cells retain "metabolic memory" of hyperglycemia and that epigenetic changes persist for several months after the hyperglycemia is corrected, sometimes causing retinopathy progression after intensive glycemic control is initiated; however, after the first 18–24 months, rates of progression are significantly lower in patients treated with intensive control compared to conventional regimens.

Screening

Visual symptoms and visual acuity are poor guides to the presence of diabetic retinopathy. Patients with diabetes mellitus should undergo regular fundus photography, which can be performed using telemedicine with computer detection software programs, or dilated examination of the retina. Ultrawide-field fluorescein angiography can identify peripheral retinal vascular lesions that predict disease worsening in eyes with nonproliferative diabetic retinopathy. Patients with type 1 diabetes mellitus should be screened 5 years after the diabetes is diagnosed. Patients with type 2 diabetes mellitus should be screened at or shortly after diagnosis of diabetes, since it is likely that hyperglycemia was present for some time before diagnosis. More frequent monitoring is required in women with type 1 or 2 diabetes during pregnancy and in those planning pregnancy, and for the first 2 years after intensive glycemic control is initiated.

Treatment

Treatment includes optimizing blood glucose, blood pressure, kidney function, and serum lipids. When patients are initially brought into intensive glycemic control, they should have an ophthalmologic examination every 3–4 months so they can be treated if retinopathy progresses. Glycemic control is the most important modifiable factor for diabetic retinopathy, but intensive blood pressure control and avoiding tobacco use also reduce retinopathy progression (see Chapter 31).

1. Nonproliferative retinopathy—VEGF inhibitor therapy improves diabetic retinopathy severity in eyes at all levels of nonproliferative diabetic retinopathy. In severe nonproliferative retinopathy, fluorescein angiography can demonstrate the extent of retinal ischemia, which can help determine whether panretinal laser photocoagulation should be performed prophylactically.

2. Proliferative retinopathy—This is usually treated by intravitreal injection of a VEGF inhibitor or panretinal laser photocoagulation, preferably before vitreous hemorrhage or tractional detachment has occurred. Proliferative diabetic retinopathy, especially after successful laser treatment, is not a contraindication to treatment with thrombolytic agents, aspirin, or warfarin unless there has been recent intraocular hemorrhage. Vitrectomy is necessary to remove persistent vitreous hemorrhage, improve vision, allow panretinal laser photocoagulation, treat tractional retinal detachment involving the macula, and manage rapidly progressive proliferative disease.

3. Macular edema—Intravitreal injection of a VEGF inhibitor (ranibizumab, bevacizumab, aflibercept, faricimab, and others) is the mainstay of treatment for diabetic macular edema. Macular edema and exudates, but not macular ischemia, may also respond to laser photocoagulation; to corticosteroid treatment (triamcinolone, dexamethasone implant, or fluocinolone implant); or to vitrectomy if there is traction from scarring on the retinal surface.

When to Refer

- All patients with sudden loss of vision or retinal detachment should be referred emergently to an ophthalmologist.
- Proliferative retinopathy or macular involvement requires urgent referral to an ophthalmologist.
- Severe nonproliferative retinopathy or unexplained reduction of visual acuity requires early referral to an ophthalmologist.

Garcia-Medina JJ et al. Novel antidiabetic drugs and the risk of diabetic retinopathy: a systematic review and meta-analysis of randomized controlled trials. J Clin Med 2024;13:1797. [PMID: 38542021]

Singh R et al. Diabetic retinopathy - pathophysiology to treatment: a review. Curr Diabetes Rev. 2025;21:58. [PMID: 38315658]

2. Hypertensive Retinochoroidopathy

Systemic hypertension affects both the retinal and choroidal circulations. The clinical manifestations vary according to the degree and rapidity of rise in blood pressure and the state of the ocular circulation. The most florid ocular changes occur in young patients with abrupt elevations of blood pressure, such as may occur in pheochromocytoma, hypertensive crisis with advanced bilateral retinopathy (malignant hypertension), or preeclampsia-eclampsia. Hypertensive retinopathy has been associated with increased risk of stroke; patients with hypertension should have routine retinal examinations for retinopathy.

Chronic hypertension accelerates the development of atherosclerosis. The retinal arterioles become more tortuous and narrower and develop abnormal light reflexes ("silver-wiring" and "copper-wiring") (Figure 13–2). There is increased venous compression at the retinal arteriovenous crossings ("arteriovenous nicking"), predisposing to branch retinal vein occlusions. Flame-shaped hemorrhages occur in the nerve fiber layer of the retina. Detection is aided by nonmydriatic fundus photography.

Acute elevations of blood pressure result in loss of autoregulation in the retinal circulation, leading to breakdown of endothelial integrity and occlusion of precapillary arterioles and capillaries that manifest as cotton-wool spots, retinal hemorrhages, retinal edema, and retinal exudates, often in a stellate appearance at the macula. Vasoconstriction and ischemia in the choroid result in exudative retinal detachments and retinal pigment epithelial infarcts that later develop into pigmented lesions that may be focal, linear, or wedge-shaped. The abnormalities in the choroidal circulation may also affect the optic nerve head, producing ischemic optic neuropathy with optic disk swelling. *Fundus abnormalities are the hallmark of hypertensive crisis with retinopathy (previously known as malignant hypertension) that requires emergency treatment* (see Chapter 13). Marked fundus abnormalities are likely to be associated with permanent retinal, choroidal, or optic nerve damage. Precipitous reduction of blood pressure may exacerbate such damage.

Sakuno G et al. Coronary artery and retinal vascularization by optical coherence tomography angiography: are eyes the window to the heart? Graefes Arch Clin Exp Ophthalmol. 2025;263:1503. [PMID: 39954049]

Wang Z et al. Hypertensive retinopathy can predict stroke: a systematic review and meta-analysis based on observational studies. J Stroke Cerebrovasc Dis. 2024;33:107953. [PMID: 39227002]

3. Blood Dyscrasias

Severe thrombocytopenia or anemia may result in retinal or choroidal hemorrhages, including white-centered retinal hemorrhages (Roth spots) that occur in leukemia and other situations (eg, bacterial endocarditis). Involvement of the macula may result in permanent visual loss.

Sickle cell retinopathy is particularly common in hemoglobin SC disease but may also occur with other hemoglobin S variants. Manifestations include "salmon-patch" preretinal/intraretinal hemorrhages, "black sunbursts" resulting from intraretinal hemorrhage, and new vessels. Severe visual loss is rare with sickle cell retinopathy but more common in patients with pulmonary hypertension. Retinal laser photocoagulation reduces the frequency of vitreous hemorrhage from new vessels. Surgery is occasionally needed for persistent vitreous hemorrhage or tractional retinal detachment. Yearly screening eye examinations are recommended for patients with hemoglobin SC disease, especially men, who are at high risk of retinopathy, and patients with hemoglobin SS disease.

Brandsen RP et al. Clinical and laboratory risk factors for sickle cell retinopathy and maculopathy: a scoping review of the current evidence. Haematologica. 2025;110:1092. [PMID: 39704162]

Nelson M et al. The clinical spectrum of HbSC sickle cell disease – not a benign condition. Br J Haematol. 2024;205:653. [PMID: 38898714]

4. HIV Infection/AIDS

See Chapter 35. **HIV retinopathy** causes cotton-wool spots, retinal hemorrhages, and microaneurysms but may also lead to reduced contrast sensitivity (diminished ability to delineate objects from their background) and retinal nerve fiber layer and outer retinal damage (HIV neuroretinal disorder).

CMV retinitis is less common since the availability of antiretroviral therapy (ART) but continues to be prevalent where resources are limited. It usually occurs when CD4 counts are <50/mcL (0.05×10^9/L) and is characterized by progressively enlarging yellowish-white patches of retinal opacification and retinal hemorrhages, usually beginning adjacent to the major retinal vascular arcades. Patients are often asymptomatic until there is involvement of the fovea or optic nerve, or until retinal detachment develops. See Table 35–3 for initial therapeutic recommendations. Maintenance therapy can be achieved with lower-dose systemic therapy. Systemic therapy has a greater risk of nonocular adverse effects but reduces the incidence of retinitis in the other eye and avoids intraocular complications of intravitreal administration. In all patients with CMV retinitis, ART needs to be instituted or adjusted. This may lead to immune reconstitution inflammatory syndrome (IRIS), which may lead to visual loss, predominantly due to cystoid macular edema. The likelihood of IRIS may be reduced by using immunomodulatory therapy to suppress the immune response causing the inflammation. If the CD4 count is maintained > 100/mcL (0.1×10^9/L), it may be possible to discontinue maintenance anti-CMV therapy.

Other ophthalmic manifestations of opportunistic infections occurring in patients with AIDS include herpes simplex retinitis, which usually manifests as acute retinal necrosis; toxoplasmic and candidal chorioretinitis, possibly progressing to endophthalmitis; herpes zoster ophthalmicus and herpes zoster retinitis, which can manifest as acute retinal necrosis or progressive outer retinal necrosis; and various entities due to syphilis, tuberculosis, or cryptococcosis. Kaposi sarcoma of the conjunctiva (see Chapter 35) and orbital lymphoma may also be seen on rare occasions.

Putera I et al. Antiviral therapy for cytomegalovirus retinitis: a systematic review and meta-analysis. Surv Ophthalmol. 2025;70:215. [PMID: 39549781]

Servillo A et al. Posterior herpetic uveitis: a comprehensive review. Ocul Immunol Inflamm. 2023:1. [PMID: 37364039]

Zhao Q et al. Clinical features of cytomegalovirus retinitis in patients with acquired immunodeficiency syndrome and efficacy of the current therapy. Front Cell Infect Microbiol. 2023;13:1107237. [PMID: 37305416]

5. Macular Telangiectasia

Macular telangiectasia type 2 (MacTel) is characterized by abnormal macular capillaries and neurodegeneration of the inner retinal layers and affects as many as 0.1% of people age > 40. It is diagnosed by features on examination, fundus photographs, and optical coherence tomography cross-sectional retinal images that may demonstrate loss of retinal transparency in the macula, telangiectatic capillaries, pigment figures, crystalline deposits, perifoveal atrophy, and, in some cases, new vessels that cause vision loss through bleeding, leakage, and subretinal fibrosis. MacTel is often associated with diabetes mellitus (28%), hypertension (52%), overweight (41% with BMI ≥ 25) or obesity (43% with BMI ≥ 30), and smoking history. The natural history of MacTel is asymmetric but bilateral slow progression of pericentral vision loss resulting from degeneration of the neural retina. The first US Food and Drug Administration–approved treatment for MacTel is revakinagene taroretcel. It is a cell-based implant containing retinal pigment epithelial cells that have been genetically modified to release a neuroprotective protein, ciliary neurotrophic factor, on a long-term basis. Patients with neovascular complications may benefit from treatment with anti–vascular endothelial growth factor (anti-VEGF) therapies that are approved for treatment of patients with neovascular age-related macular degeneration, diabetic retinopathy, and retinal vein occlusion.

Chew EY et al. Cell-based ciliary neurotrophic factor therapy for macular telangiectasia type 2. NEJM Evid. 2025;4:EVIDoa2400481. [PMID: 40693847]

Duncan JL. Ciliary neurotrophic factor—a promising new therapy for macular telangiectasia type 2. NEJM Evid. 2025;4.EVIDe2500127. [PMID: 40693849]

ISCHEMIC OPTIC NEUROPATHY

ESSENTIALS OF DIAGNOSIS

- Sudden painless visual loss with signs of optic nerve dysfunction.
- Optic disk swelling in anterior ischemic optic neuropathy.

Anterior ischemic optic neuropathy results from inadequate perfusion of the posterior ciliary arteries that supply the anterior portion of the optic nerve. Arteritic anterior ischemic optic neuropathy is caused by giant cell arteritis, while nonarteritic anterior ischemic optic neuropathy is seen in patients with congenitally crowded optic disk (compromising optic disk circulation), systemic hypertension, diabetes mellitus, hyperlipidemia, systemic vasculitis, inherited or acquired thrombophilia, interferon α therapy, and obstructive sleep apnea; hypotension and anemia during dialysis may also cause bilateral anterior ischemic optic neuropathy. Recent reports of nonarteritic anterior ischemic optic neuropathy have raised concern for an association with semaglutide, a GLP-1 receptor agonist.

Posterior ischemic optic neuropathy, involving the retrobulbar optic nerve without visible optic disk swelling, may occur with severe blood loss; nonocular surgery, particularly prolonged lumbar spine surgery in the prone position with increased orbital pressure; severe burns; or in association with dialysis, from profound hypotension and anemia. In all such situations, visual loss may be severe and irreversible.

Clinical Findings

Anterior ischemic optic neuropathy presents with sudden visual loss, usually with an altitudinal field defect, and optic disk swelling with pallor .

Posterior ischemic optic neuropathy does not cause any optic disk swelling, as the damage occurs behind the optic disc, but patients experience rapid-onset, severe vision loss with initially normal-appearing optic discs. Both anterior and posterior ischemic optic neuropathy that affect only one eye are associated with a relative afferent pupillary defect on the affected eye. Vision loss in patients with posterior ischemic optic neuropathy is more commonly bilateral and severe than in patients with anterior ischemic optic neuropathy.

Treatment

Arteritic anterior ischemic optic neuropathy necessitates emergent high-dose systemic corticosteroid treatment to prevent visual loss in the other eye. (See Central & Branch Retinal Artery Occlusions, above, and Polymyalgia Rheumatica & Giant Cell Arteritis, Chapter 23.) A systematic review of 32 studies found no evidence that treatment affects visual outcome in nonarteritic anterior ischemic optic neuropathy. In ischemic optic neuropathy after nonocular surgery or dialysis, treatment of anemia by blood transfusion may be beneficial.

When to Refer

Patients with ischemic optic neuropathy should be referred urgently to an ophthalmologist.

When to Admit

Patients with ischemic optic neuropathy due to giant cell arteritis or other vasculitis may require emergency admission for high-dose corticosteroid therapy and close monitoring to ensure that treatment is adequate.

Natividade GR et al. Ocular adverse events with semaglutide: a systematic review and meta-analysis. JAMA Ophthalmol. 2025;143:759. [PMID: 40810985]

Parthasarathi P et al. Review of evidence for treatments of acute non arteritic anterior ischemic optic neuropathy. Eye (Lond). 2024;38:2267. [PMID: 38778140]

OPTIC NEURITIS

ESSENTIALS OF DIAGNOSIS

- Subacute, usually unilateral, visual loss.
- Pain exacerbated by eye movements.
- Optic disk is usually normal in acute stages but subsequently develops pallor.

General Considerations

Inflammatory optic neuropathy is strongly associated with demyelinating disease (typical optic neuritis), particularly multiple sclerosis, but it also occurs in acute disseminated encephalomyelitis; sarcoidosis; neuromyelitis optica spectrum disorder, which is characterized by serum antibodies to aquaporin-4; in association with serum antibodies to myelin oligodendrocyte glycoprotein; following viral infection (usually in children); in varicella zoster virus infection; in autoimmune disorders, particularly SLE and Sjögren syndrome; during treatment with a biologic agent; and by spread of inflammation from the meninges, orbital tissues, or paranasal sinuses.

Clinical Findings

Optic neuritis in demyelinating disease is characterized by unilateral loss of vision developing over a few days. Visual acuity ranges from 20/30 (6/9) to no perception of light, with more severe visual loss being associated with low serum vitamin D. In almost all cases, there is pain behind the eye, exacerbated by eye movements, central visual field loss, color vision loss, and a relative afferent pupillary defect. In about two-thirds of cases, the optic nerve is normal during the acute stage (retrobulbar optic neuritis). In the remainder, the optic disk is swollen (papillitis) with occasional flame-shaped peripapillary hemorrhages. Visual acuity usually improves within 2–3 weeks and returns to 20/40 (6/12) or better in 95% of previously unaffected eyes. Optic atrophy subsequently develops if there has been extensive optic nerve fiber damage. Patients without a diagnosis of multiple sclerosis in whom visual recovery does not occur, or if there is continuing deterioration of vision, or pain persisting after 2 weeks, should undergo MRI of the head and orbits to look for periventricular white matter demyelination or a lesion compressing the optic nerve.

Treatment

In acute demyelinating optic neuritis, intravenous methylprednisolone (1 g daily for 3 days followed by a tapering course of oral prednisolone) has been shown to accelerate visual recovery, but not to improve final vision. However, in clinical practice, the oral taper is not often prescribed. Use in an individual patient is determined by the degree of visual loss, the state of the other eye, and the patient's visual requirements. Other therapies include monoclonal antibodies against immune cells and cell-based therapies to deplete or modulate T and B cell responses. Vitamin D may play immunoregulatory roles in cytokine production, immune cell development and differentiation, and antibody production and is often prescribed for optic neuritis.

Atypical optic neuritis due to sarcoidosis, neuromyelitis optica, herpes zoster, or SLE generally has a poorer prognosis, requires immediate and more prolonged corticosteroid therapy, may require plasma exchange, and may necessitate long-term immunosuppression.

Prognosis

Among patients with a first episode of clinically isolated optic neuritis, multiple sclerosis will develop in 50% within 15 years; however, the likelihood of developing multiple sclerosis ranges from 25% for patients without demyelinating lesions on brain MRI to 72% in patients with one or more demyelinating lesions. The major risk factors are female sex and multiple white matter lesions on brain MRI. Retinal nerve fiber layer optical coherence tomography quantifies axonal damage that can be used to monitor disease progression.

When to Refer

All patients with optic neuritis should be referred urgently for ophthalmologic or neurologic assessment.

Chaitanuwong P et al. Optic neuritis: a comprehensive review of current therapies and emerging treatment strategies. Front Neurol. 2025;16:1605075. [PMID: 40606143]

Tisavipat N et al. Acute optic neuropathy in older adults: differentiating between MOGAD optic neuritis and nonarteritic anterior ischemic optic neuropathy. Neurol Neuroimmunol Neuroinflamm. 2024;11:e200214. [PMID: 38547435]

OPTIC DISK SWELLING

Optic disk swelling may result from elevated intracranial pressure, orbital lesions, or intraocular lesions, including retinal and optic nerve lesions. Raised intracranial pressure usually causes bilateral disk swelling without reduced visual acuity and requires urgent imaging to exclude an intracranial mass, hemorrhage, infection, or cerebral venous sinus occlusion. Orbital lesions can cause optic nerve compression resulting in optic disk swelling. Intraocular causes of optic disk swelling include central retinal vein occlusion, posterior uveitis, and posterior scleritis. Optic nerve lesions causing disk swelling include anterior ischemic optic neuropathy; optic neuritis; optic nerve sheath meningioma; and infiltration by sarcoidosis, leukemia, or lymphoma.

Papilledema (optic disk swelling due to raised intracranial pressure) is usually bilateral and most commonly produces enlargement of the blind spot without loss of acuity. Severe acute papilledema or chronic papilledema, as in idiopathic intracranial hypertension and cerebral venous sinus occlusion, may be associated with visual field and occasionally with profound visual acuity loss. All patients with chronic papilledema must be monitored carefully—especially their visual fields—and CSF shunt or optic nerve sheath fenestration should be considered in those with progressive visual loss not controlled by medical therapy (weight loss where appropriate and usually acetazolamide in patients with idiopathic intracranial hypertension). In idiopathic intracranial hypertension, transverse venous sinus stenting is also an option for patients with progressive vision loss.

Bénard-Séguin É et al. Idiopathic intracranial hypertension with papilledema. Neurosurg Clin N Am. 2025;36:281. [PMID: 40054979]

Bouthour W et al. Diagnosis of optic disc oedema: fundus features, ocular imaging findings, and artificial intelligence. Neuroophthalmology. 2023;47:177. [PMID: 37434667]

CRANIAL NERVE PALSIES

A cranial nerve palsy of any of the three cranial nerves that supply the extraocular muscles can cause double vision.

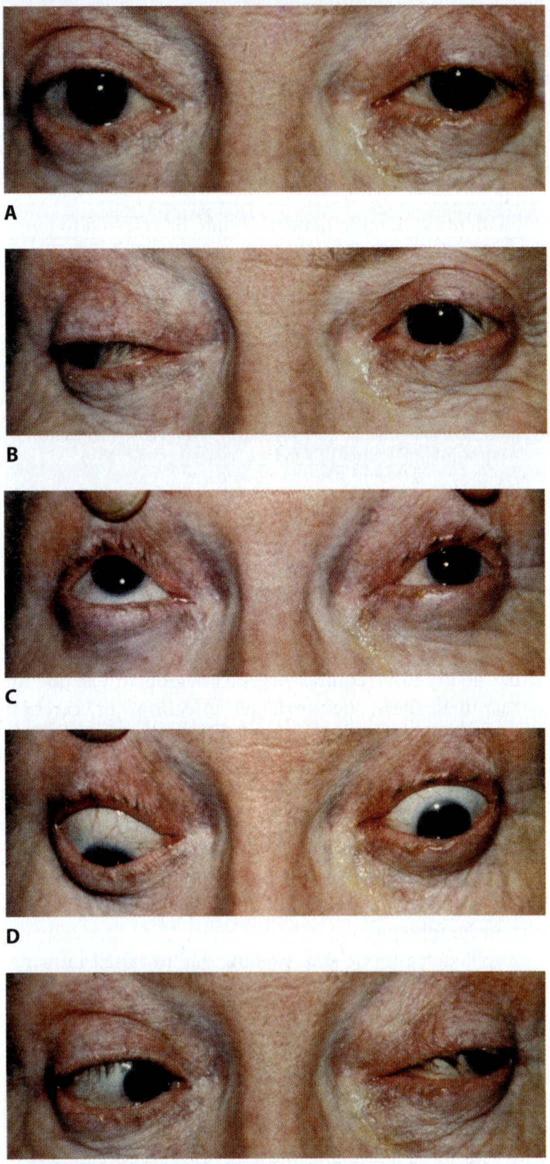

▲ **Figure 7–3.** Left partial third nerve palsy with ptosis **(A)**, reduced adduction **(B)**, reduced elevation **(C)**, and reduced depression **(D)** but normal abduction **(E)** of the left eye.

1. Third nerve palsy—In a complete third nerve palsy, there is ptosis with a divergent and slightly depressed eye (Figure 7–3). Extraocular movements are restricted in all directions except laterally (preserved lateral rectus function) (Figure 7–3E). Intact fourth nerve (superior oblique) function is detected by inward rotation on attempted depression of the eye. Pupillary involvement, manifesting as a relatively dilated pupil that does not constrict normally to light, usually means compression, which may be due to aneurysm of the posterior communicating artery or uncal herniation due to a supratentorial mass lesion. In acute painful isolated third nerve palsy with pupillary involvement, posterior communicating artery aneurysm must be excluded. Pituitary apoplexy is a rarer cause. Causes of isolated third nerve palsy without pupillary involvement include diabetes mellitus, hypertension, giant cell arteritis, and herpes zoster.

2. Fourth nerve palsy—There is upward deviation of the eye with failure of depression on adduction. In acquired cases, there is vertical and torsional diplopia that is most apparent on looking down. Trauma is a major cause of acquired—particularly bilateral—fourth nerve palsy, but posterior fossa tumor and medical causes, such as in third nerve palsy, should also be considered. Similar clinical features are seen in congenital cases due to developmental anomaly of the nerve, muscle, or tendon.

3. Sixth nerve palsy—There is convergent squint in the primary position with failure of abduction of the affected eye, producing horizontal diplopia that increases on gaze to the affected side and on looking into the distance. It is an important sign of raised intracranial pressure and may also be due to trauma, neoplasms, brainstem lesions, petrous apex lesions, or medical causes (such as diabetes mellitus, hypertension, giant cell arteritis, and herpes zoster).

In an isolated cranial nerve palsy presumed to be due a medical cause, brain MRI is not always required initially, but it is necessary if recovery has not begun within 3 months.

A cranial nerve palsy accompanied by other neurologic signs may be due to lesions in the brainstem, cavernous sinus, or orbit. Lesions around the cavernous sinus involve the first and second divisions of the trigeminal nerve, the third, fourth, and sixth cranial nerves, and occasionally the optic chiasm. Orbital apex lesions involve the optic nerve and the three cranial nerves supplying the extraocular muscles.

Myasthenia gravis and thyroid eye disease (see Graves Ophthalmopathy) should be considered in the differential diagnosis of disordered extraocular movements.

When to Refer

- In recent-onset isolated third nerve palsy, especially if there is pupillary involvement or pain, immediate referral is required for neurologic assessment and possibly CT, MRI, or catheter angiography for intracranial aneurysm.
- All patients with recent-onset double vision should be referred urgently to a neurologist or ophthalmologist, particularly if there are multiple cranial nerve dysfunctions or other neurologic abnormalities.

When to Admit

Patients with double vision due to giant cell arteritis may require emergency admission for high-dose corticosteroid therapy and close monitoring to ensure that treatment is adequate. (See Central & Branch Retinal Artery Occlusions and Chapter 23.)

Jain S. Diplopia: diagnosis and management. Clin Med (Lond). 2022;22:104. [PMID: 35304368]

THYROID EYE DISEASE (Graves Ophthalmopathy)

See Hyperthyroidism (Thyrotoxicosis) in Chapter 29.

ORBITAL CELLULITIS

Orbital cellulitis is characterized by fever, proptosis, restriction of extraocular movements, and swelling with redness of the lids. Immediate treatment with intravenous antibiotics is necessary to prevent optic nerve damage and spread of infection to the cavernous sinuses, meninges, and brain. Infection of the paranasal sinuses is the usual underlying cause; infecting organisms include *S pneumoniae*, the incidence of which has been reduced by the administration of pneumococcal vaccine; other streptococci, such as the anginosus group; *H influenzae*; and, less commonly, *S aureus* including MRSA. Broad-spectrum intravenous coverage with adjustments based on culture and local resistance patterns are recommended. Metronidazole or clindamycin are used to treat anaerobic infections. If trauma is the underlying cause, a cephalosporin, such as cefazolin or ceftriaxone, should be added to ensure coverage for *S aureus* and group A β-hemolytic streptococci. If MRSA infection is a concern, vancomycin or clindamycin may be required. For patients with penicillin hypersensitivity, vancomycin, levofloxacin, and metronidazole are recommended. The response to antibiotics is usually excellent, but surgery may be required to drain the paranasal sinuses or orbital abscess. In immunocompromised patients, mucormycosis must be considered.

When to Refer

Orbital cellulitis requires admission to the hospital and initiation of broad-spectrum intravenous antibiotics.

Miller JM et al. Guide to utilization of the microbiology laboratory for diagnosis of infectious diseases: 2024 Update by the Infectious Diseases Society of America (IDSA) and the American Society for Microbiology (ASM). Clin Infect Dis. 2024 Mar 5. [Epub ahead of print] [PMID: 38442248]
Tsirouki T et al. Orbital cellulitis. Surv Ophthalmol. 2018;63:534. [PMID: 29248536]

OCULAR TRAUMA

Ocular trauma is an important cause of avoidable severe visual impairment at all ages, and it is the leading cause of monocular blindness in young adult men in the United States. Thorough but safe clinical assessment, supplemented when necessary by imaging, is crucial to effective management. Ocular damage and the possible need for early assessment by an ophthalmologist need to be considered in the assessment of any patient with mid-facial injury.

Heath Jeffery RC et al. Eye injuries: understanding ocular trauma. Aust J Gen Pract. 2022;51:476. [PMID: 35773155]
Rho JY et al. Management of eye trauma for the primary care physician. J Am Board Fam Med. 2021;34:1018. [PMID: 34535529]

1. Conjunctival & Corneal Foreign Bodies

If a patient complains of "something in my eye" and gives a consistent history, a foreign body is usually present on the cornea or under the upper lid even though it may not be visible. Visual acuity should be tested before treatment is instituted to assess the severity of the injury and as a basis for comparison in the event of complications.

After a local anesthetic (eg, proparacaine, 0.5%) is instilled, the eye is examined with a slit lamp or with a hand flashlight, using oblique illumination, and loupe. The instillation of sterile fluorescein may make corneal foreign bodies more apparent, which are then removed with a sterile wet cotton-tipped applicator or hypodermic needle. Bacitracin-polymyxin ophthalmic ointment should be instilled. It is not necessary to patch the eye. All patients need to be advised to return promptly for reassessment if there is any increase in pain, redness, or impairment of vision.

Iron foreign bodies usually leave a diffuse rust ring. This requires excision and is best done under local anesthesia using a slit lamp. **Caution:** *Anesthetic drops should not be given to the patient for self-administration.*

If there is no infection, a layer of corneal epithelial cells will line the crater within 24 hours. While the epithelium is defective, the cornea is extremely susceptible to infection. Early infection is manifested by a white necrotic area around the crater and a small amount of gray exudate.

In the case of a foreign body under the upper lid, a local anesthetic is instilled and the lid is everted by grasping the lashes gently and exerting pressure on the mid portion of the outer surface of the upper lid with an applicator. If a foreign body is present, it can easily be removed by passing a wet sterile cotton-tipped applicator across the conjunctival surface.

When to Refer

Refer urgently to an ophthalmologist if a corneal foreign body cannot be removed or if there is suspicion of corneal infection.

Fraenkel A et al. Managing corneal foreign bodies in office-based general practice. Aust Fam Physician. 2017;46:89. [PMID: 28260265]

2. Intraocular Foreign Body

An intraocular foreign body requires emergency treatment by an ophthalmologist. Patients giving a history of "something hitting the eye"—particularly while hammering on metal or using grinding equipment—must be assessed for this possibility, especially when no corneal foreign body is seen, a corneal or scleral wound is apparent, or there is marked visual loss or media opacity. Such patients must be treated as for open globe injury and referred without delay. Intraocular foreign bodies significantly increase the risk of intraocular infection.

When to Refer

Patients with suspected intraocular foreign body must be referred emergently to an ophthalmologist.

3. Corneal Abrasions

A patient with a corneal abrasion complains of severe pain and photophobia. There is often a history of trauma to the eye, commonly involving a fingernail, piece of paper, or contact lens. Visual acuity is recorded, and the cornea and conjunctiva are examined with a light and loupe to rule out a foreign body. If an abrasion is suspected but cannot be seen, sterile fluorescein is instilled into the conjunctival sac: the area of corneal abrasion will stain because fluorescein stains areas that are devoid of epithelium.

Treatment includes bacitracin-polymyxin ophthalmic ointment or drops, or a fluoroquinolone topical antibiotic in contact lens wearers, as prophylaxis against infection. A mydriatic (cyclopentolate 1%) and either topical or oral NSAIDs can be used for pain control. Patching the eye is probably not helpful for small abrasions. Corneal abrasions heal more slowly in persons who smoke cigarettes. Recurrent corneal erosion may follow corneal abrasions.

Although treatment of pain from a corneal abrasion with topical tetracaine for 24 hours has been reported, there is a risk of delayed healing and severe corneal disease from misuse of topical anesthetics, so it is not recommended.

4. Contusions

Contusion injury of the eye (closed globe injury) and surrounding structures may cause ecchymosis ("black eye"), subconjunctival hemorrhage, edema of the cornea, hemorrhage into the anterior chamber (hyphema), rupture of the root of the iris (iridodialysis), paralysis of the pupillary sphincter, paralysis of the muscles of accommodation, cataract, dislocation of the lens, vitreous hemorrhage, retinal hemorrhage and edema (most common in the macular area), detachment of the retina, rupture of the choroid, fracture of the orbital floor ("blowout fracture"), or optic nerve injury. Many of these injuries are immediately obvious; others may not become apparent for days or weeks. The possibility of globe injury must always be considered in patients with facial injury, particularly if there is an orbital fracture. Patients with moderate to severe contusions should be seen by an ophthalmologist.

Any injury causing hyphema involves the danger of secondary hemorrhage, which may cause intractable glaucoma with permanent visual loss. The patient should be advised to rest until complete resolution has occurred. Frequent ophthalmologic assessment is essential. Aspirin and any drugs inhibiting coagulation increase the risk of secondary hemorrhage and are to be avoided. Sickle cell anemia or trait adversely affects outcome.

When to Refer

Patients with moderate or severe ocular contusion should be referred to an ophthalmologist, emergently if there is hyphema.

5. Lacerations

A. Lids

If the lid margin is lacerated, the patient should be referred for specialized care, since permanent notching may result. Lacerations of the lower eyelid near the inner canthus often sever the lower canaliculus, for which canalicular intubation is likely to be required. Lid lacerations not involving the margin may be sutured like any skin laceration.

B. Conjunctiva

In lacerations of the conjunctiva, sutures are not necessary. To prevent infection, topical sulfonamide or other antibiotic is used until the laceration is healed.

C. Cornea or Sclera

Patients with suspected corneal or scleral laceration or rupture (open globe injury) must be seen emergently by an ophthalmologist. Manipulation is kept to a minimum, since pressure may result in extrusion of intraocular contents. The eye is bandaged lightly and covered with a shield that rests on the orbital bones above and below. The patient should be instructed not to squeeze the eye shut and to remain still. If there may be a metallic intraocular foreign body, a radiograph or CT scan is obtained to identify and localize it. *MRI is contraindicated because of the risk of movement of any metallic foreign body but may be useful for non-metallic foreign body.* Endophthalmitis occurs in > 5% of open globe injuries.

When to Refer

Patients with suspected open globe injury must be referred emergently to an ophthalmologist.

CHEMICAL CONJUNCTIVITIS & KERATITIS

Chemical burns are treated by copious irrigation of the eyes as soon as possible after exposure. Saline solution or sterile eye wash solution is preferred. If not available, tap water can be used. Alkali injuries are more serious and require prolonged irrigation. It is important to remove any retained particulate matter, commonly present in injuries involving cement and building plaster. This often requires eversion of the upper lid. The pupil should be dilated with 1% cyclopentolate, 1 drop twice a day, to relieve discomfort, and prophylactic ophthalmic antibiotics should be started (Table 7–2). In moderate to severe injuries, intensive ophthalmic corticosteroids and systemic vitamin C are also necessary. Amniotic membrane transplants can promote corneal epithelial healing. Complications include mucus deficiency, scarring of the cornea and conjunctiva, symblepharon (adhesions between the tarsal and bulbar conjunctiva), tear duct obstruction, and secondary infection. A slit lamp examination is required to assess the severity of ocular surface chemical burns.

PRECAUTIONS IN MANAGEMENT OF OCULAR DISORDERS

1. Use of Local Anesthetics

Unsupervised self-administration of local anesthetics is dangerous because they are toxic to the corneal epithelium, delay healing, and the patient may further injure an anesthetized eye without realizing it.

Lee MD ... Seitzman GD. Cornea specialists do not recommend routine usage of ophthalmic anesthetics for corneal abrasions. Ann Emerg Med. 2019;74:463. [PMID: 31445551]

2. Pupillary Dilation

Dilating the pupil can very occasionally precipitate acute glaucoma if the patient has a narrow anterior chamber angle and should be undertaken with caution if the anterior chamber is obviously shallow (readily determined by oblique illumination of the anterior segment of the eye). A short-acting mydriatic (eg, tropicamide) should be used for diagnostic dilated eye examinations, while longer-acting cycloplegics are used therapeutically for uveitis. The patient should be warned to report immediately if ocular discomfort or redness develops. Angle closure is more likely to occur if pilocarpine is used to overcome pupillary dilation than if the pupil is allowed to constrict naturally.

3. Corticosteroid Therapy

Co-management with eye specialists is strongly recommended to monitor for ocular complications of corticosteroid therapy. Long-term use of local corticosteroids may be complicated by ocular hypertension leading to open-angle glaucoma; cataract formation; and exacerbation of ocular infections, such as herpes simplex (dendritic) and fungal keratitis. Furthermore, perforation of the cornea may occur when ophthalmic corticosteroids are used indiscriminately for infectious keratitis. The potential for causing or exacerbating systemic hypertension, diabetes mellitus, gastritis, osteoporosis, or glaucoma must always be borne in mind when systemic corticosteroids are prescribed.

4. Contaminated Eye Medications

Ophthalmic solutions are prepared with the same degree of care as fluids intended for intravenous administration.

Table 7–3. Adverse ophthalmic effects of systemic drugs (selected list).

Medications	Possible Ophthalmic Side Effects
Amebicides	
Diiodohydroxyquinoline	Optic neuropathy
Antibiotics	
Chloramphenicol	Optic neuropathy
Clofazimine	Crystalline deposits (conjunctiva, cornea, iris)
Ethambutol	Optic neuropathy
Fluoroquinolones	Diplopia, retinal detachment
Isoniazid	Optic neuropathy
Linezolid	Optic neuropathy
Rifabutin	Uveitis
Streptomycin	Optic neuropathy, epidermal necrolysis
Sulfonamides	Nearsightedness, angle-closure glaucoma due to ciliary body swelling
Tetracycline, doxycycline, minocycline	Papilledema
Antimalarial agents	
Chloroquine, hydroxychloroquine	Retinal degeneration principally involving the macula, vortex keratopathy
Quinine	Retinal toxicity, pupillary abnormalities
Antivirals	
Cidofovir	Uveitis
Bisphosphonates	
Alendronate, pamidronate	Scleritis, episcleritis, uveitis
Cardiovascular medications	
Amiodarone	Corneal deposits (vortex keratopathy), optic neuropathy, thyroid eye disease
Amlodipine	Chemosis (conjunctival edema)
Anticoagulants	Conjunctival, retinal, and vitreous hemorrhage
Carbonic anhydrase inhibitors (eg, acetazolamide, methazolamide)	Nearsightedness, angle-closure glaucoma due to ciliary body swelling

(continued)

Table 7–3. Adverse ophthalmic effects of systemic drugs (selected list). (continued)

Medications	Possible Ophthalmic Side Effects
Chlorthalidone	Angle-closure glaucoma due to ciliary body swelling
Digoxin	Disturbance of color vision, photopsia, optic neuropathy
Furosemide	Angle-closure glaucoma due to ciliary body swelling
Phosphodiesterase type 5 inhibitors (eg, sildenafil, tadalafil, vardenafil)	Color vision changes, nonarteritic anterior ischemic optic neuropathy
Statins	Extraocular muscle palsy (myasthenic syndrome)
Thiazides (eg, indapamide)	Angle-closure glaucoma, nearsightedness, xanthopsia (yellow vision), band keratopathy due to hypercalcemia, macular edema
Chelating agents	
Deferoxamine, deferasirox	Retinopathy, optic neuropathy, lens opacity
Penicillamine	Ocular pemphigoid, optic neuropathy, extraocular muscle palsy (myasthenic syndrome)
Chemotherapeutic agents	
Antibody–drug conjugates	Corneal pseudomicrocysts, conjunctivitis
Bortezomib	Chalazia
Chlorambucil	Optic neuropathy
Cisplatin	Optic neuropathy
Docetaxel	Lacrimal (canalicular) obstruction
Fluorouracil	Lacrimal (canalicular) obstruction
MEK inhibitors: trametinib, selumetinib, cobimetinib, pimasertib	Multifocal serous retinal detachment, retinal vein occlusion, cystoid macular edema
Vincristine	Optic neuropathy
CNS medications	
Amphetamines	Widening of palpebral fissure, blurring of vision due to mydriasis, elevated intraocular pressure
Anticholinergic agents including preoperative medications	Angle-closure glaucoma due to mydriasis, blurring of vision due to cycloplegia, dry eyes
Aripiprazole	Nearsightedness
Diazepam	Nystagmus
Haloperidol	Capsular cataract
Lithium carbonate	Proptosis, oculogyric crisis, nystagmus
MAO inhibitors	Nystagmus, visual hallucinations, diplopia, myasthenia gravis
Morphine/opioids	Miosis, visual hallucinations, diplopia, dry eye
Neostigmine	Nystagmus, miosis
Olanzapine	Angle-closure glaucoma due to mydriasis
Phenothiazines (eg, chlorpromazine)	Pigmentary deposits in conjunctiva, cornea, lens, and retina; oculogyric crisis Chlorpromazine causes floppy iris syndrome during intraocular surgery
Phenytoin	Nystagmus
Quetiapine	Floppy iris syndrome during intraocular surgery
Retigabine	Ocular pigmentation and retinopathy
Risperidone, paliperidone	Floppy iris syndrome during intraocular surgery
SNRIs (eg, venlafaxine)	Angle-closure glaucoma, mydriasis, dry eye
SSRIs (eg, paroxetine, sertraline)	Angle-closure glaucoma, ischemic optic neuropathy, cataract
Thioridazine	Corneal and lens deposits, retinopathy, oculogyric crisis

(*continued*)

Table 7–3. Adverse ophthalmic effects of systemic drugs (selected list). (continued)

Medications	Possible Ophthalmic Side Effects
Topiramate	Angle-closure glaucoma due to ciliary body swelling, nearsightedness, macular folds, anterior uveitis, corneal edema
Tricyclic agents (eg, imipramine)	Angle-closure glaucoma due to mydriasis, blurring of vision due to cycloplegia, dry eye
Triptans (eg, sumatriptan, zolmitriptan)	Angle-closure glaucoma due to ciliary body swelling, nearsightedness
Vigabatrin	Visual field constriction, cone dystrophy
Zonisamide	Angle-closure glaucoma due to ciliary body swelling, nearsightedness
Dermatologic agents	
Dupilumab	Conjunctivitis
Retinoids (eg, isotretinoin, tretinoin, acitretin, and etretinate)	Papilledema, blepharoconjunctivitis, corneal opacities, decreased contact lens tolerance, decreased dark adaptation, teratogenic ocular abnormalities, idiopathic intracranial hypertension, optic neuritis
Gastrointestinal medications	
Anticholinergic agents	Angle-closure glaucoma due to mydriasis, blurring of vision due to cycloplegia, dry eyes
H_2-blockers	Retinal vascular occlusion, optic neuropathy, retrobulbar optic neuritis
Hormonal agents	
Aromatase inhibitors (eg, anastrozole)	Dry eye, vitreoretinal traction, retinal hemorrhages
Cabergoline	Angle-closure glaucoma
Female sex hormones	Retinal artery occlusion, retinal vein occlusion, papilledema, cranial nerve palsies, ischemic optic neuropathy
Tamoxifen	Crystalline retinal and corneal deposits, altered color perception, cataract, optic neuropathy, macular edema, retinal pigmentary change
Hypoglycemic agents (oral)	
Chlorpropamide	Refractive error, epidermal necrolysis, optic neuropathy
Thiazolidinediones (glitazones)	Increase in diabetic macular edema
Immunomodulators	
Corticosteroids	Cataract (posterior subcapsular); susceptibility to viral (herpes simplex), bacterial, and fungal infections; steroid-induced glaucoma; idiopathic intracranial hypertension; central serous retinopathy
Cyclosporine	Posterior reversible leukoencephalopathy
Fingolimod	Macular edema, retinal vein occlusion
Interferon α	Retinopathy, keratoconjunctivitis, dry eyes, optic neuropathy
NSAIDs	Corneal opacity, vortex keratopathy, periorbital edema, dry eye
Tacrolimus	Optic neuropathy, posterior reversible leukoencephalopathy
Obstetric drugs	
Sympathomimetic tocolytics	Angle-closure glaucoma due to mydriasis
Respiratory medications	
Anticholinergic bronchodilators (eg, ipratropium)	Angle-closure glaucoma due to mydriasis, blurring of vision due to cycloplegia, dry eyes
Sympathomimetic bronchodilators (eg, salbutamol) and decongestants (eg, ephedrine)	Angle-closure glaucoma due to mydriasis
Rheumatologic agents	
Chloroquine, hydroxychloroquine	Retinal degeneration principally involving the macula, vortex keratopathy
Gold salts	Deposits in the cornea, conjunctiva, and lens
NSAIDs (eg, ibuprofen, naproxen, indomethacin)	Vortex keratopathy (ibuprofen, naproxen), corneal deposits (indomethacin), retinal degeneration principally involving the macula (indomethacin)

(*continued*)

Table 7–3. Adverse ophthalmic effects of systemic drugs (selected list). (continued)

Medications	Possible Ophthalmic Side Effects
Penicillamine	Ocular pemphigoid, optic neuropathy, extraocular muscle palsy (myasthenic syndrome)
Salicylates	Subconjunctival and retinal hemorrhages, nystagmus
Urinary tract medications	
α-Antagonists (eg, doxazosin, prazosin, tamsulosin, terazosin)	Intraoperative floppy iris syndrome
Anticholinergic agents	Angle-closure glaucoma due to mydriasis, blurring of vision due to cycloplegia, dry eyes
Finasteride	Floppy iris syndrome during intraocular surgery
Pentosan polysulfate sodium	Maculopathy
Phosphodiesterase type 5 inhibitors (eg, sildenafil, tadalafil, vardenafil)	Color vision changes, nonarteritic anterior ischemic optic neuropathy
Vitamins	
Vitamin A	Papilledema
Vitamin D	Band-shaped keratopathy from secondary hypercalcemia

Once ophthalmic solution bottles are opened, there is a risk of contamination, particularly with tetracaine, proparacaine, fluorescein, and any preservative-free preparations.

Four weeks after opening is the usual maximum time for use of an eye solution containing preservatives before discarding. Preservative-free preparations should be kept refrigerated and usually discarded within 1 week after opening.

If the eye has been injured by accident or by surgical trauma, it is important to use freshly opened bottles of sterile medications or single-use products.

5. Systemic Effects of Ocular Drugs

The systemic absorption of certain ophthalmic drugs must be considered when there is a systemic medical contraindication to the use of the drug (Table 7–3). Ophthalmic solutions of the nonselective β-blockers, eg, timolol, may worsen bradycardia, HF, or asthma. Phenylephrine eye drops may precipitate hypertensive crises and angina. Adverse interactions between systemically administered and ocular drugs also should be considered. Using only 1 or 2 drops at a time and a few minutes of nasolacrimal occlusion or eyelid closure ensures maximum ocular efficacy and decreases systemic side effects of ophthalmic agents.

Otolaryngology Disorders

Elliott D. Kozin, MD
Lawrence R. Lustig, MD

8

DISEASES OF THE EAR

HEARING LOSS

ESSENTIALS OF DIAGNOSIS

- Hearing loss is generally categorized as either conductive or sensorineural.
- Diagnostic evaluation routinely includes audiologic testing.

Classification & Epidemiology

Table 8–1 categorizes hearing loss as normal, mild, moderate, severe, or profound and outlines the vocal equivalent as well as the decibel range.

A. Conductive Hearing Loss

Conductive hearing loss results from a mechanical disruption of the external auditory canal or middle ear. Several mechanisms may result in impairment of the passage of sound vibrations to the inner ear, such as obstruction (eg, cerumen impaction), mass loading (eg, middle ear effusion), stiffness (eg, otosclerosis), and discontinuity (eg, ossicular disruption). Conductive losses in adults are most commonly due to cerumen impaction or transient eustachian tube dysfunction from upper respiratory tract infection. Persistent conductive losses usually result from chronic ear infection, trauma, or otosclerosis. Perforations of the tympanic membrane may also result in a conductive hearing loss. Conductive hearing loss is often correctable with medical (eg, use of a hearing aid) or surgical (eg, repair of tympanic membrane and ossicular chain) therapy, or both. CT of the temporal bone may be used as an adjunct to physical examination to determine the potential cause of conductive hearing loss.

B. Sensorineural Hearing Loss

Sensorineural hearing losses are common in adults and generally result from deficits of the inner ear or central (brain) auditory pathway. Sensory hearing loss results from deterioration of the cochlea, usually due to loss of sensory hair cells within the organ of Corti. The most common form of sensorineural hearing loss is **age-related hearing loss** that manifests as a gradually progressive, predominantly high-frequency hearing loss. Other causes of sensorineural hearing loss include excessive noise exposure; head trauma; ototoxic medications, such as cisplatin-based chemotherapy; and systemic diseases.

While most types of sensorineural hearing loss are gradual, sensorineural hearing loss may be sudden. ***Sudden* sensorineural hearing loss, often called idiopathic sudden sensorineural hearing loss, is considered an otologic emergency and may be treatable with oral or intratympanic corticosteroids if delivered within several weeks of onset.** Long-term severe to profound sensorineural hearing loss due to deficits at the level of the inner ear may be correctable with surgery, such as cochlear implantation. Sensorineural hearing loss may also be due to deficits at the level of the central auditory pathway, including lesions involving the eighth cranial nerve, auditory nuclei, ascending tracts, or auditory cortex. Examples of central causes of hearing loss include acoustic neuroma, multiple sclerosis, and auditory neuropathy. Treatment of hearing loss due to central causes are usually aimed at addressing the underlying pathology.

Evaluation of Hearing (Audiology)

In a quiet room, the hearing level may be estimated by having the patient repeat aloud words presented in a soft

Table 8–1. Hearing loss classification.

Classification	Vocal Equivalent	Decibel (dB) Range
Normal	Soft whisper	0–20 dB
Mild	Soft spoken voice	20–40 dB
Moderate	Normal spoken voice	40–60 dB
Severe	Loud spoken voice	60–80 dB
Profound	Shout	> 80 dB

whisper, a normal spoken voice, or a shout. Normal spoken voice is about 60 decibels. A 512-Hz tuning fork is useful in differentiating conductive from sensorineural hearing loss. In the **Weber test**, the tuning fork is placed directly on the forehead or front teeth. In conductive losses, the sound is heard as louder in the ear with *poorer hearing;* however, in sensorineural losses, the sound radiates to the ear that *hears better* than the other ear. In the **Rinne test**, the tuning fork is placed alternately on the mastoid bone (bone conduction) and in front of the ear canal (air conduction). In conductive losses > 25 dB, bone conduction sounds louder than air conduction.

Formal audiometric studies are performed in a soundproofed room. Pure-tone thresholds in decibels (dB) are obtained over the range of 250–8000 Hz. Conductive losses create a "gap" between the air and bone thresholds, whereas in sensorineural losses, both air and bone thresholds are equally diminished. Speech discrimination measures the clarity of hearing, reported as percentage correct (90–100% is normal). MRI scanning is the most sensitive and specific test to determine the possible location of a defect resulting in sensorineural hearing loss.

Every patient who reports hearing loss should be referred for audiologic evaluation unless the cause is easily remediable (eg, cerumen impaction, otitis media). Immediate audiometric referral is indicated for patients with idiopathic sudden sensorineural hearing loss because it requires treatment (corticosteroids) within a limited several-week time period.

Irace AL et al. Longitudinal associations of subclinical hearing loss with cognitive decline. J Gerontol A Biol Sci Med Sci. 2022;77:623. [PMID: 34516645]
Jiang F et al. A comprehensive evaluation on the associations between hearing and vision impairments and risk of all-cause and cause-specific dementia: results from cohort study, meta-analysis and Mendelian randomization study. BMC Med. 2024;22:518. [PMID: 39506811]
Kolo FB et al. Hearing loss, brain structure, cognition, and dementia risk in the Framingham Heart Study. JAMA Netw Open. 2025;8:e2539209. [PMID: 41191359]
Lin FR. Age-related hearing loss. N Engl J Med. 2024;390:1505. [PMID: 38657246]

Hearing Amplification

Patients with hearing loss not correctable by medical therapy may benefit from hearing amplification. Contemporary *hearing aids* are comparatively free of distortion and have been miniaturized to the point where they often may be contained entirely within the ear canal or lie inconspicuously behind the ear.

For patients with conductive loss or unilateral profound sensorineural loss, bone-conducting hearing aids directly stimulate the ipsilateral cochlea (for conductive losses) or contralateral ear (profound unilateral sensorineural loss). In most adults with severe to profound sensory hearing loss, the **cochlear implant**—an electronic device that is surgically implanted into the cochlea to stimulate the auditory nerve—offers socially beneficial auditory rehabilitation.

Daher GS et al. Cochlear implantation outcomes in adults with single-sided deafness: a systematic review and meta-analysis. Otol Neurotol. 2023;44:297. [PMID: 36791341]
Lindquist NR et al. Cochlear implants for single-sided deafness: quality of life, daily usage, and duration of deafness. Laryngoscope. 2023;133:2362. [PMID: 36254870]
Mammen L et al. Cochlear implantation in children with single-sided deafness under the age of 5 years: a review of current literature. Curr Opin Otolaryngol Head Neck Surg. 2024;32:324. [PMID: 39146020]
Romano DR et al. Academic outcomes with hearing amplification devices in children with unilateral hearing loss: a systematic review and narrative synthesis. Audiol Neurootol. 2024;29:429. [PMID: 38810609]
van Heteren JAA et al. Speech perception in noise after cochlear implantation for single-sided deafness: a randomized clinical trial. JAMA Otolaryngol Head Neck Surg. 2025;151:211. [PMID: 39820302]
Zeitler DM et al. American Cochlear Implant Alliance Task Force: Recommendations for determining cochlear implant candidacy in adults. Laryngoscope. 2024;134 (Suppl 3):S1. [PMID: 37435829]

DISEASES OF THE AURICLE

Disorders of the auricle include skin cancers due to sun exposure. Traumatic auricular hematoma must be drained to prevent significant cosmetic deformity "cauliflower ear" or canal blockage resulting from dissolution of supporting cartilage. Similarly, cellulitis of the auricle must be treated promptly to prevent perichondritis and resultant deformity. **Relapsing polychondritis** is characterized by recurrent, frequently bilateral, painful episodes of auricular erythema and edema and sometimes progressive involvement of the cartilaginous tracheobronchial tree. Treatment with corticosteroids may help forestall cartilage dissolution. Polychondritis and perichondritis may be differentiated from cellulitis by sparing of involvement of the lobule, which does not contain cartilage.

Hoshino K et al. Evaluation of semicircular canal function in relapsing polychondritis patients with dizziness and sensorineural hearing loss using video head impulse test. Otol Neurotol. 2024;45:1045. [PMID: 39186067]
Mertz P et al. Relapsing polychondritis: Best Practice & Clinical Rheumatology. Best Pract Res Clin Rheumatol. 2023;37:101867. [PMID: 37839908]

DISEASES OF THE EAR CANAL

1. Cerumen Impaction

Cerumen is a protective secretion produced by the outer portion of the ear canal. *In most persons, the ear canal is self-cleansing and no hygiene measures are recommended.* Cerumen impaction is most often self-induced through ill-advised cleansing attempts by entering the canal itself, eg, digital trauma or use of a cotton-tip applicator. It may be relieved by the patient using detergent ear drops (eg, 3% hydrogen peroxide; 6.5% carbamide peroxide) and irrigation, or by the clinician using mechanical removal, suction, or irrigation. Irrigation is performed with water at body temperature to avoid a vestibular caloric response. The stream should be directed at the posterior ear canal wall adjacent to the cerumen plug. Irrigation should be performed only when the tympanic membrane is known to be intact.

Use of jet irrigators (eg, WaterPik) should be avoided since they may result in tympanic membrane perforations. Following irrigation, the ear canal should be thoroughly dried (eg, by the patient using a hair blow-dryer on low-power setting or by the clinician instilling isopropyl alcohol) to reduce the likelihood of otitis externa. Specialty referral is indicated if impaction is frequently recurrent, if it has not responded to routine measures, or if there is tympanic membrane perforation or chronic otitis media.

2. Foreign Bodies

Foreign bodies in the ear canal are more frequent in children than in adults. Firm materials may be removed with a loop or a hook, taking care not to displace the object medially toward the tympanic membrane; microscopic guidance is helpful. Aqueous irrigation should *not* be performed for organic foreign bodies (eg, beans, insects), because water may cause them to swell. Living insects are best immobilized before removal by filling the ear canal with lidocaine or mineral oil. Lidocaine should *never* be used in a patient with a possible tympanic membrane perforation as this may result in a profound vestibular response.

3. Otitis Externa

ESSENTIALS OF DIAGNOSIS

- Otalgia.
- Erythema, edema, and purulence of the external auditory canal skin.
- Patients who are immunocompromised or have diabetes are at risk for "malignant" otitis externa (osteomyelitis of the skull base).

General Considerations

Otitis externa, often called "swimmer's ear," presents with otalgia with associated external auditory canal edema and purulent discharge. There is often a history of recent water exposure or mechanical trauma (eg, scratching, cotton applicators). Otitis externa is usually caused by gram-negative rods (eg, *Pseudomonas, Proteus*) or fungi (eg, *Aspergillus*), which grow in the presence of excessive moisture. In patients who are immunocompromised or have diabetes, persistent otitis externa may evolve into osteomyelitis of the skull base (so-called **malignant otitis externa**). Usually caused by *Pseudomonas aeruginosa*, osteomyelitis begins in the floor of the ear canal and may extend into the middle fossa floor, the clivus, and even the contralateral skull base.

Clinical Findings

Examination reveals erythema and edema of the ear canal skin, often with a purulent exudate (Figure 8–1), as well as surrounding periauricular cellulitis. Manipulation of the auricle elicits pain. The lateral surface of the tympanic membrane is often erythematous. When the canal skin is very edematous, it may be impossible to visualize the tympanic membrane. In immunocompromised patients, such as those with diabetes, malignant otitis externa typically presents with persistent otorrhea; granulation tissue in the ear canal; deep otalgia; and in advanced cases, progressive palsies of cranial nerves, such as cranial nerve VI, VII, IX, X, XI, or XII. Diagnosis of malignant otitis externa is confirmed by the demonstration of osseous erosion on CT scanning and laboratory testing showing high inflammatory markers, such as ESR and CRP. MRI scanning is often important to rule out abscesses that may result from malignant otitis externa.

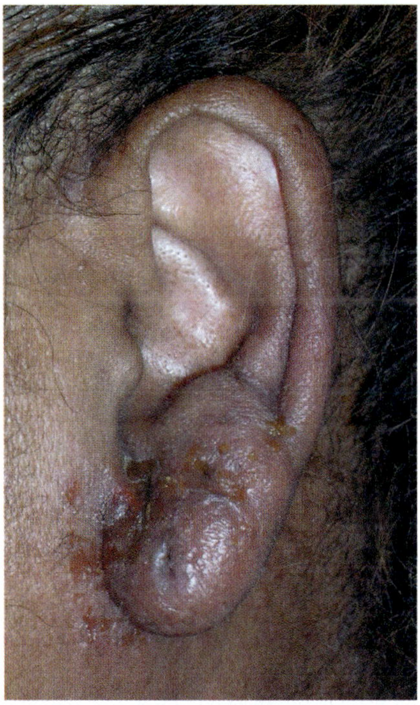

Figure 8–1. Malignant otitis externa in a 40-year-old woman with diabetes mellitus, with typical swelling and honey-colored crusting of the pinna. Both the external auditory canal and temporal bone were involved in the pseudomonal infection. (Used, with permission, from E.J. Mayeaux Jr, MD, in Usatine RP, Smith MA, Mayeaux EJ Jr, Chumley H. *The Color Atlas of Family Medicine*, 2nd ed. McGraw-Hill, 2013.)

Treatment

Treatment of otitis externa involves protection of the ear from additional moisture and avoidance of further mechanical injury by scratching. In cases of moisture in the ear (eg, swimmer's ear), acidification with a drying agent (ie, a 50/50 mixture of isopropyl alcohol/white vinegar) is often helpful. When infected, an otic antibiotic solution or suspension of an aminoglycoside (eg, neomycin/polymyxin B) or fluoroquinolone (eg, ciprofloxacin), with or without a corticosteroid (eg, hydrocortisone), is usually effective.

Purulent debris filling the ear canal should be gently removed to permit entry of the topical medication. Drops should be used abundantly (five or more drops three or four times a day) to penetrate the depths of the canal. When substantial edema of the canal wall prevents entry of drops into the ear canal, a wick is placed to facilitate their entry. In recalcitrant cases—particularly when cellulitis of the periauricular tissue has developed—oral fluoroquinolones (eg, ciprofloxacin, 500 mg twice daily for 1 week) are used because of their effectiveness against *Pseudomonas*. Newer medications that are ciprofloxacin suspensions hold promise to improve otitis externa outcomes. *Any case of persistent otitis externa in patients who are immunocompromised or have diabetes must be referred for specialty evaluation.*

Treatment of malignant otitis externa requires prolonged antipseudomonal antibiotic administration, often for several months. Although intravenous therapy is often required initially (eg, ciprofloxacin 200–400 mg every 12 hours), selected patients may be graduated to oral ciprofloxacin (500–1000 mg twice daily). To avoid relapse, antibiotic therapy should be continued, even in the asymptomatic patient, until gallium scanning indicates marked reduction or resolution of the inflammation. Surgical debridement of infected bone is reserved for cases of deterioration despite medical therapy.

Di Traglia R et al. Antibiotics versus non-antibiotic treatments for acute otitis externa: a systematic review and meta-analysis. Clin Otolaryngol. 2023;48:841. [PMID: 37550850]
Jackson EA et al. Acute otitis externa: rapid evidence review. Am Fam Physician. 2023;107:145. [PMID: 36791445]
Plum AW et al. An overview of acute otitis externa. Otolaryngol Clin North Am. 2023;56:891. [PMID: 37516653]

4. Pruritus

Pruritus of the external auditory canal, particularly at the meatus, is common. While it may be associated with otitis externa or with seborrheic dermatitis or psoriasis, most cases are self-induced from excoriation or overly zealous ear cleaning. To permit regeneration of the protective cerumen blanket, patients should be instructed to avoid use of soap and water or cotton swabs in the ear canal and avoid any scratching. Patients with excessively dry canal skin may benefit from application of mineral oil, which helps counteract dryness and repel moisture. When an inflammatory component is present, topical application of a corticosteroid (eg, 0.1% triamcinolone) may be beneficial.

5. Exostoses & Osteomas

Bony overgrowths of the ear canal are a frequent incidental finding and rarely have clinical significance. They present as skin-covered bony mounds in the medial ear canal obscuring the tympanic membrane to a variable degree. Solitary osteomas are of no significance as long as they do not cause obstruction or infection. Multiple exostoses, which are generally acquired from repeated exposure to cold water (eg, "surfer's ear"), may progress and require surgical removal if completely occluding the external auditory canal or resulting in frequent infections.

Wille AE et al. Prevention of external auditory canal exostosis in the Colorado whitewater community. J Osteopath Med. 2022;122:431. [PMID: 35355493]

6. Neoplasia

The most common neoplasm of the ear canal is squamous cell carcinoma. *When an apparent otitis externa does not resolve on therapy, a malignancy should be suspected and biopsy performed.* This disease carries a very high 5-year mortality rate because the tumor tends to invade the lymphatics of the cranial base and must be treated with wide surgical resection and radiation therapy. Adenomatous tumors, originating from the ceruminous glands, generally follow a more indolent course.

Dubray-Vautrin A et al. Squamous cell carcinoma of the temporal bone: the impact of local control on survival. Acta Otolaryngol. 2025;145:23. [PMID: 38343349]
Kang BC et al. Treatment outcomes and prognostic factors in external auditory canal squamous cell carcinoma. PLoS One. 2025;20:e0339860. [PMID: 41460837]
Sioufi K et al. Survival outcomes of temporal bone squamous cell carcinoma: a systematic review and meta-analysis. Otolaryngol Head Neck Surg. 2024;171:1. [PMID: 38341629]
Zhou P et al. The international expert consensus on management of external auditory canal carcinoma. Eur Arch Otorhinolaryngol. 2025;282:1677. [PMID: 39466369]

DISEASES OF THE EUSTACHIAN TUBE

1. Eustachian Tube Dysfunction

ESSENTIALS OF DIAGNOSIS

- Aural fullness.
- Discomfort with barometric pressure change.
- Retracted eardrum.

The tube that connects the middle ear to the nasopharynx—the eustachian tube—provides ventilation and drainage for the middle ear. It is normally closed, opening only during swallowing or yawning. When eustachian tube function is compromised, air trapped within the middle ear becomes absorbed and negative pressure results. The most common causes of eustachian tube dysfunction are diseases associated with edema of the tubal lining, such as viral upper respiratory tract infections and seasonal allergies. The patient usually reports a sense of fullness in the ear and mild to moderate impairment of hearing. When the tube is only partially blocked, swallowing or yawning may elicit a popping or crackling sound. Examination may reveal retraction of the tympanic membrane and decreased mobility on pneumatic otoscopy. Following a viral illness, this disorder is usually transient, lasting days to weeks. Treatment with systemic and intranasal decongestants (eg, pseudoephedrine, 60 mg orally every 4–6 hours; oxymetazoline, 0.05% spray every 8–12 hours), combined with **autoinsufflation** by forced exhalation against closed nostrils, may hasten relief. Autoinsufflation should not be recommended to patients with active intranasal infection since this maneuver may precipitate middle ear infection. Allergic patients may also benefit from intranasal corticosteroids (eg, beclomethasone dipropionate, two sprays in each nostril twice daily for 2–6 weeks). Air travel, rapid altitudinal change, and underwater diving should be avoided until resolution.

An overly patent eustachian tube (**"patulous eustachian tube"**) is a relatively uncommon, although quite distressing problem. Patients typically describe fullness in the ear and autophony (an exaggerated ability to hear oneself breathe and speak). A patulous eustachian tube may develop during rapid weight loss, such as following pregnancy, or it may be idiopathic. In contrast to eustachian tube dysfunction, the aural pressure is often made worse by exertion and may diminish during an upper respiratory tract infection. Although physical examination is usually normal, respiratory excursions of the tympanic membrane may occasionally be detected during vigorous breathing. Treatment includes avoidance of decongestant products and rarely surgery on the eustachian tube itself.

Alghamdi AS et al. Effect of balloon dilatation among adult population with eustachian tube dysfunction: a systematic review. Eur Arch Otorhinolaryngol. 2024;281:5363. [PMID: 38977475]
Kaderbay A et al. Balloon dilation for persistent unilateral chronic obstructive Eustachian tube dysfunction is effective: a prospective multicentre study. Eur Arch Otorhinolaryngol. 2023;280:1101. [PMID: 35932313]
Lin JT et al. Balloon dilation eustachian tuboplasty for dilatory dysfunction with and without effusion: a comprehensive outcome analysis. Otolaryngol Head Neck Surg. 2023;169:1179. [PMID: 37264984]
Mehta NK et al. Medical management for eustachian tube dysfunction in adults: a systematic review and meta-analysis. Laryngoscope. 2022;132:849. [PMID: 34606099]
Toivonen J et al. The case for balloon eustachian tuboplasty in children. Curr Opin Otolaryngol Head Neck Surg. 2024;32:346. [PMID: 39146019]
Yang HH et al. Clinical predictors of symptom improvement following eustachian tube balloon dilation. Ann Otol Rhinol Laryngol. 2023;132:1032. [PMID: 36226334]

2. Serous Otitis Media

ESSENTIALS OF DIAGNOSIS

- Negative pressure from eustachian tube obstruction causes transudation of fluid into the middle ear and stasis.
- Dull and hypomobile tympanic membrane.

Prolonged eustachian tube dysfunction with resultant negative middle ear pressure may cause a transudation of fluid. In adults, serous otitis media usually occurs with an upper respiratory tract infection, with barotrauma, or with chronic allergic rhinitis, but when persistent and unilateral, nasopharyngeal carcinoma must be excluded. The tympanic membrane is dull and hypomobile, occasionally accompanied by air bubbles in the middle ear and conductive hearing loss. The treatment of serous otitis media is similar to that for eustachian tube dysfunction. A short course of oral corticosteroids (eg, prednisone, 40 mg/day for 7 days) has been advocated by some clinicians, as have oral antibiotics (eg, amoxicillin, 250 mg three times daily for 7 days)—or even a combination of the two. The role of these regimens remains controversial, but they are probably of little lasting benefit. When medication fails to bring relief after several months, a **ventilating tube** placed through the tympanic membrane may restore hearing and alleviate the sense of aural fullness.

Mulvaney CA et al. Antibiotics for otitis media with effusion (OME) in children. Cochrane Database Syst Rev. 2023;10:CD015254. [PMID: 37870130]
Otteson T. Otitis media and tympanostomy tubes. Pediatr Clin North Am. 2022;69:203. [PMID: 35337534]
Paing A et al. Modifiable risk factors for developing otitis media with effusion in children under 12 years in high-income countries: a systematic review. Arch Dis Child. 2024;110:45. [PMID: 39304206]

3. Barotrauma

Persons with poor eustachian tube function (eg, congenital narrowness or acquired mucosal edema) may be unable to equalize the barometric stress exerted on the middle ear by air travel, rapid altitudinal change, or underwater diving. The problem is generally most acute during airplane descent, since the negative middle ear pressure tends to collapse and block the eustachian tube, causing pain. Several measures are useful to enhance eustachian tube function and avoid otic barotrauma. The patient should be advised to swallow, yawn, and autoinsufflate frequently during descent. Oral decongestants (eg, pseudoephedrine, 60–120 mg) should be taken several hours before anticipated arrival time so that they will be maximally effective during descent. Topical decongestants, such as 1% phenylephrine or oxymetazoline nasal spray, should be administered 1 hour before arrival.

For acute negative middle ear pressure that persists on the ground, treatment includes decongestants and attempts at autoinsufflation. **Myringotomy** with or without placement of a **tympanostomy tube** provides immediate relief and is appropriate for severe otalgia and hearing loss.

Underwater diving may represent an even greater barometric stress to the ear than flying. Patients should be warned to avoid diving when they have an upper respiratory infection or episode of nasal allergy. During the descent phase of the dive, if inflation of the middle ear via the eustachian tube has not occurred, pain will develop within the first 15 feet; the dive must be aborted. In all cases, divers must descend slowly and equilibrate in stages to avoid the development of severely negative pressures in the tympanum that may result in hemorrhage (hemotympanum) or in perilymphatic fistula. In the latter, the oval or round window ruptures, resulting in sensory hearing loss and acute vertigo. During the ascent phase of a saturation dive, sensory hearing loss or vertigo may develop as the first (or only) symptom of decompression sickness. Immediate recompression will return intravascular gas bubbles to solution and restore the inner ear microcirculation.

Tympanic membrane perforation is an absolute contraindication to diving, as the patient will experience an unbalanced thermal stimulus to the semicircular canals and may experience vertigo, disorientation, and even emesis.

DISEASES OF THE MIDDLE EAR

1. Acute Otitis Media

ESSENTIALS OF DIAGNOSIS

- Otalgia.
- Purulent fluid of the middle ear.
- Erythema and hypomobility of tympanic membrane.

General Considerations

Acute otitis media is a bacterial infection of the mucosally lined, air-containing spaces of the middle ear. Purulent material may extend to pneumatized mastoid air cells and petrous apex of the lateral skull base. *Acute otitis media is usually precipitated by a viral upper respiratory tract infection that causes eustachian tube obstruction.* This results in accumulation of fluid and mucus, which becomes secondarily infected by bacteria. The most common pathogens are *Streptococcus pneumoniae*, *Haemophilus influenzae*, and *Streptococcus pyogenes*.

Clinical Findings

Acute otitis media may occur at any age. Presenting symptoms and signs include otalgia, aural pressure, decreased hearing, and often fever. The typical physical findings are erythema and decreased mobility of the tympanic membrane (Figure 8–2). Occasionally, bullae will appear on the tympanic membrane.

Rarely, when middle ear empyema is severe, the tympanic membrane bulges outward. In such cases, tympanic membrane rupture is imminent. Rupture is accompanied by a sudden decrease in pain, followed by the onset of otorrhea. With appropriate therapy, spontaneous healing of the tympanic membrane occurs in most cases. Acute mastoiditis results from an infection extending from the middle ear to the mastoid air cells. It is diagnosed by pain, postauricular erythema, and occasionally proptosis of the auricle. Frank swelling over the mastoid bone or the association of cranial neuropathies or central findings indicates severe disease requiring urgent care. Evaluation includes imaging, such as CT, to determine presence of "coalescence" of air cells and associated soft-tissue abscess.

Treatment

The treatment of acute otitis media is specific antibiotic therapy, often combined with nasal decongestants. The first-choice antibiotic is amoxicillin 1 g orally every 8 hours for 5–7 days. Alternatives (useful in resistant cases) are amoxicillin-clavulanate 875/125 mg or 2 g/125 mg ER every 12 hours for 5–10 days; or cefuroxime 500 mg or cefpodoxime 200 mg orally every 12 hours for 5–7 days. Recurrent acute otitis media may be managed with long-term antibiotic prophylaxis. Single daily oral doses of sulfamethoxazole (500 mg) or amoxicillin (250 or 500 mg) are given over a period of 1–3 months. Failure of this regimen to control infection is an indication for insertion of ventilating tubes.

Surgical drainage of the middle ear (**myringotomy**), debridement of the mastoid (**mastoidectomy**), or both are reserved for patients with severe otalgia or when complications of otitis (eg, mastoiditis, meningitis) have occurred.

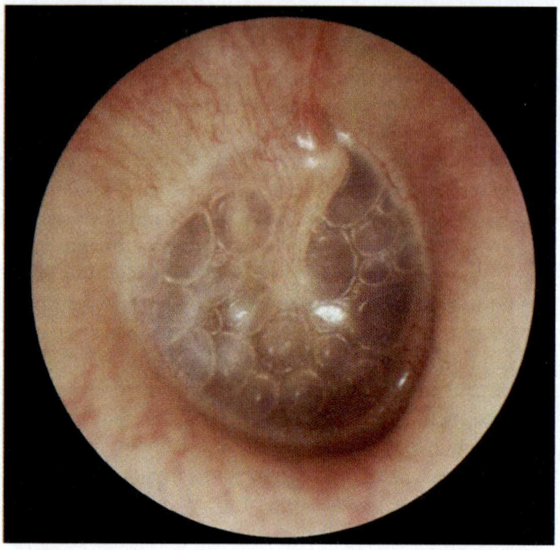

Figure 8–2. Acute otitis media with effusion of right ear, with multiple air-fluid levels visible through a translucent, slightly retracted, nonerythematous tympanic membrane. (Used, with permission, from Frank Miller, MD, in Usatine RP, Smith MA, Mayeaux EJ Jr, Chumley H. *The Color Atlas of Family Medicine,* 2nd ed. McGraw-Hill, 2013.)

Rosenfeld RM et al. Executive summary of clinical practice guideline on tympanostomy tubes in children (update). Otolaryngol Head Neck Surg. 2022;166:189. [PMID: 35138976]

Venekamp RP et al. Antibiotics for acute otitis media in children. Cochrane Database Syst Rev. 2023;11:CD000219. [PMID: 37965923]

Voigt A et al. Outcomes of in-office versus operating room insertion of tympanostomy tubes in children. Int J Pediatr Otorhinolaryngol. 2023;175:111772. [PMID: 37898011]

2. Chronic Otitis Media

ESSENTIALS OF DIAGNOSIS

- Chronic otorrhea with or without otalgia.
- Tympanic membrane perforation with conductive hearing loss.
- Often amenable to surgical correction.

General Considerations

Chronic infection of the middle ear and mastoid generally develops as a consequence of recurrent acute otitis media, although it may follow other diseases and trauma. Perforation or retraction of the tympanic membrane may be present. The bacteriology of chronic otitis media differs from that of acute otitis media. Common organisms include *P aeruginosa*, *Proteus* species, *Staphylococcus aureus*, and mixed anaerobic infections.

Clinical Findings

The clinical hallmark of chronic otitis media is purulent aural discharge. Drainage may be continuous or intermittent, with increased severity during upper respiratory tract infection or following water exposure. Pain is uncommon except during acute exacerbations. Conductive hearing loss results from destruction of the tympanic membrane or ossicular chain, or both.

Treatment

The medical treatment of chronic otitis media includes regular removal of infected debris, use of earplugs to protect against water exposure, and topical antibiotic drops (ofloxacin 0.3% or ciprofloxacin with dexamethasone) for exacerbations. Oral ciprofloxacin, active against *Pseudomonas*, 500 mg twice a day for 1–6 weeks, may help dry a chronically discharging ear.

In most cases, surgery is the definitive management of tympanic membrane perforations with or without association of ossicular disruption. Successful reconstruction of the tympanic membrane may be achieved with autologous tissue, such as temporalis fascia, in about 90% of cases, often with improvement in conductive hearing.

Hidaka H et al. Clinical practice guidelines for the diagnosis and management of otitis media with effusion (OME) in children in Japan – 2022 update. Auris Nasus Larynx. 2023;50:655. [PMID: 36577619]
Nokso-Koivisto J et al. Otitis media: Interactions between host and environment, immune and inflammatory responses. Int J Pediatr Otorhinolaryngol. 2024;176:111798. [PMID: 38041988]
Sainsbury E et al. Tissue engineering and regenerative medicine strategies for the repair of tympanic membrane perforations. Biomater Biosyst. 2022;6:100046. [PMID: 36824158]
Zahid A et al. Otitis media: recent advances in otitis media vaccine development and model systems. Front Microbiol. 2024;15:1345027. [PMID: 38328427]

Complications of Otitis Media

A. Cholesteatoma

Cholesteatoma is a special variety of chronic otitis media (Figure 8–3). The most common cause is prolonged eustachian tube dysfunction, with inward migration of the upper flaccid portion of the tympanic membrane. This creates a squamous epithelium-lined sac, which—when its neck becomes obstructed—may fill with desquamated keratin and become chronically infected. Cholesteatomas typically erode bone, including the ossicular chain with extension into the mastoid. Over time, cholesteatoma may erode into

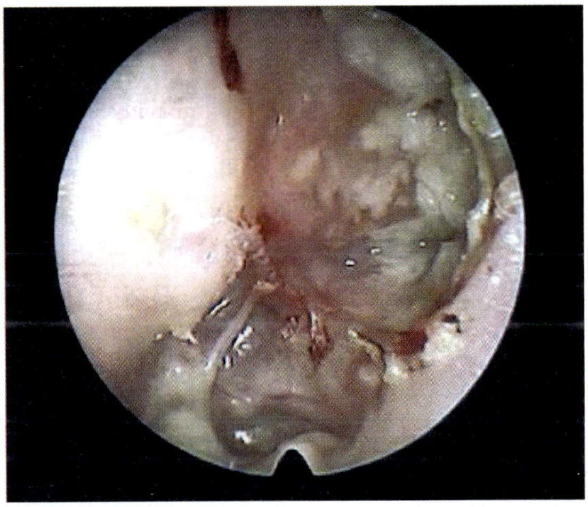

Figure 8–3. Cholesteatoma. (Used, with permission, from Vladimir Zlinsky, MD, in Roy F. Sullivan, PhD: Audiology Forum: Video Otoscopy, www.RCSullivan.com; from Usatine RP, Smith MA, Mayeaux EJ Jr, Chumley H. *The Color Atlas of Family Medicine*, 2nd ed. McGraw-Hill, 2013.)

the inner ear, involve the facial nerve and, on rare occasions, spread intracranially. Otoscopic examination may reveal a retraction pocket of the tympanic membrane or a marginal tympanic membrane perforation that exudes keratin debris or granulation tissue. The treatment of cholesteatoma is surgical, including marsupialization of the sac or its complete removal. This may require the creation of a "mastoid bowl" in which the ear canal and mastoid are joined into a large common cavity that must be periodically cleaned.

Chang AG et al. Key interventions related to middle ear cholesteatoma: a systematic umbrella review. Otol Neurotol. 2026;47:26. [PMID: 41220045]
Manzoor NF et al. Comparative analysis of recidivism after endoscopic and microscopic-based cholesteatoma resection. Otol Neurotol. 2022;43:466. [PMID: 35287152]
Popescu C et al. Comprehensive management of cholesteatoma in otitis media: diagnostic challenges, imaging advances, and surgical outcome. J Clin Med. 2024;13:6791. [PMID: 39597935]
Tan D et al. Outcomes with management of cholesteatoma. Otolaryngol Clin North Am. 2025;58:141. [PMID: 39322451]

B. Mastoiditis

Acute suppurative mastoiditis usually evolves following several weeks of inadequately treated acute otitis media. It is characterized by pain and postauricular cellulitis accompanied by a spiking fever. CT scan reveals coalescence of the mastoid air cells due to destruction of their bony septa. Initial treatment consists of intravenous antibiotics (eg, cefazolin 0.5–1.5 g every 6–8 hours) directed against the most common offending organisms (*S pneumoniae*, *H influenzae*, and *S pyogenes*), and myringotomy for culture and drainage. Failure of medical therapy indicates the need for surgical drainage, such as a mastoidectomy.

C. Petrous Apicitis

The medial portion of the petrous bone between the inner ear and clivus may become a site of persistent infection when the drainage of its pneumatic cell tracts becomes blocked. This may cause foul discharge, deep ear and retro-orbital pain, and sixth nerve palsy (**Gradenigo syndrome**); meningitis may be a complication. Treatment is with prolonged antibiotic therapy (based on culture results) or surgical drainage via petrous apicectomy or both.

Isaac H et al. Transmastoid and transtemporal drainage of petrous apicitis with otitis media. Ann Otol Rhinol Laryngol. 2021;130:314. [PMID: 32772562]

D. Facial Paralysis

Facial palsy may be associated with either acute or chronic otitis media. In the acute setting, it results from inflammation of the seventh nerve in its middle ear segment. Treatment consists of myringotomy for drainage and culture, followed by intravenous antibiotics (based on culture results). The use of corticosteroids is controversial. The prognosis is excellent, with complete recovery in most cases.

Facial palsy associated with chronic otitis media usually evolves slowly due to chronic pressure on the seventh nerve in the middle ear or mastoid by cholesteatoma. Treatment requires surgical correction of the underlying disease. The prognosis is less favorable than for facial palsy associated with acute otitis media.

Fichera P et al. Acute otitis media and facial paralysis in children: a systemic review and proposal of an operative algorithm. Audiol Res. 2023;13:889. [PMID: 37987335]
Freeman MH et al. Facial paralysis in skull base osteomyelitis - comparison of surgical and nonsurgical management. Laryngoscope. 2023;133:179. [PMID: 35546515]
Ibrahim NI et al. Complications of surgery: recognition and management. Otolaryngol Clin North Am. 2025;58:165. [PMID: 39266389]
Mohan S et al. Considerations in management of acute otitis media in the COVID-19 era. Ann Otol Rhinol Laryngol. 2021;130:520. [PMID: 32911957]

E. Sigmoid Sinus Thrombosis

Trapped infection within the mastoid air cells adjacent to the sigmoid sinus may cause septic thrombophlebitis. This is heralded by signs of systemic sepsis (spiking fevers, chills), at times accompanied by signs of increased intracranial pressure (headache, lethargy, nausea and vomiting, papilledema). Diagnosis can be made noninvasively by **magnetic resonance venography (MRV)**. Primary treatment is with intravenous antibiotics (based on culture results). Additional treatment, such as anticoagulation, surgical drainage, ligation of the internal jugular vein, or some combination thereof, may be indicated when embolization is suspected.

Ziv O et al. Post-operative clinical course in children undergoing mastoidectomy due to complicated acute mastoiditis. Eur Arch Otorhinolaryngol. 2022;279:3891. [PMID: 34714371]

F. Central Nervous System Infection

Otogenic meningitis is the most common intracranial complication of ear infection. In the setting of acute suppurative otitis media, it arises from hematogenous spread of bacteria, most commonly *H influenzae* and *S pneumoniae.* In chronic otitis media, it results either from passage of infection along preformed pathways, such as the petrosquamous suture line, or from direct extension of disease through the dural plates of the petrous pyramid.

Epidural abscesses arise from direct extension of disease in the setting of chronic infection. They are usually asymptomatic but may present with deep local pain, headache, and low-grade fever. They are often discovered as an incidental finding at surgery. **Brain abscess** may arise in the temporal lobe or cerebellum as a result of septic thrombophlebitis adjacent to an epidural abscess. The predominant causative organisms are *S aureus, S pyogenes,* and *S pneumoniae.* Rupture into the subarachnoid space results in meningitis and often death. (See Chapter 34.)

Antonelli PJ. Cochlear implant infections. Infect Dis Clin North Am. 2024;38:777. [PMID: 39277503]
Gkrinia E et al. Otogenic brain complications: a systematic review and meta-analysis. J Laryngol Otol. 2024;138:828. [PMID: 38440882]

3. Otosclerosis

Otosclerosis is a progressive disease with a marked familial tendency that affects the bony otic capsule. Lesions involving the footplate of the stapes result in increased impedance to the passage of sound through the ossicular chain, producing conductive hearing loss. This may be treated either through the use of a hearing aid or surgical replacement of the stapes with a prosthesis (stapedectomy). When otosclerotic lesions involve the cochlea ("cochlear otosclerosis"), permanent sensory hearing loss may occur.

Patel S et al. A systematic review of the effectiveness of bisphosphonates for otosclerosis. Otol Neurotol. 2022;43:530. [PMID: 35213475]
Teaima AA et al. Comparison of the efficacy of cochlear implantation and stapes surgery in far advanced otosclerosis: a meta-analysis study. Eur Arch Otorhinolaryngol. 2023;280:77. [PMID: 35687184]

4. Trauma to the Middle Ear

Tympanic membrane perforation may result from impact injury or explosive acoustic trauma (Figure 8–4). *Spontaneous healing occurs in most cases.* Persistent perforation may result from secondary infection brought on by exposure to water. During the healing period, patients should be advised to wear earplugs while swimming or bathing. Hemorrhage behind an intact tympanic membrane (**hemotympanum**) may follow blunt trauma or extreme barotrauma. Spontaneous resolution over several weeks is the usual course. When a conductive hearing loss > 30 dB persists for > 3 months following trauma, disruption of the ossicular chain should be suspected. Middle ear exploration with reconstruction of the ossicular chain, combined with repair of the tympanic membrane when required, will usually restore hearing.

Habarth-Morales TE et al. Incidence and epidemiology of traumatic tympanic membrane rupture: a national trauma data bank analysis. J Craniofac Surg. 2023;34:168. [PMID: 36190699]

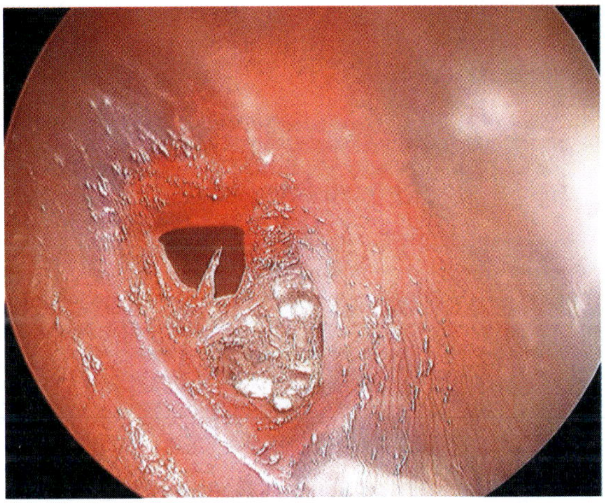

▲ **Figure 8–4.** Traumatic perforation of the left tympanic membrane. (Used, with permission, from William Clark, MD, in Usatine RP, Smith MA, Mayeaux EJ Jr, Chumley H. *The Color Atlas of Family Medicine,* 2nd ed. McGraw-Hill, 2013.)

Lubianca Neto JF et al. Comparison of inlay cartilage butterfly and underlay temporal fascia tympanoplasty. OTO Open. 2022;6:2473974X221108935. [PMID: 35836497]
Zhao X et al. The latest progress of tympanic membrane repair materials. Am J Otolaryngol. 2022;43:103408. [PMID: 36031699]

5. Middle Ear Neoplasia

Primary middle ear tumors are rare. **Glomus tumors** arise either in the middle ear (glomus tympanicum) or in the jugular bulb with upward erosion into the hypotympanum (glomus jugulare). They present clinically with pulsatile tinnitus and hearing loss. A vascular mass may be visible behind an intact tympanic membrane. Large glomus jugulare tumors are often associated with multiple cranial neuropathies, especially involving nerves VII, IX, X, XI, and XII. Treatment usually requires surgery, radiotherapy, or both. *Pulsatile tinnitus thus warrants* ***magnetic resonance angiography (MRA)*** *and MRV to rule out a vascular mass.*

Dharnipragada R et al. Modern management of complex tympanojugular paragangliomas: a systematic review and meta-analysis. World Neurosurg. 2023;170:149. [PMID: 36400356]
Fancello G et al. Tumor progression in tympanojugular paragangliomas: the role of radiotherapy and wait and scan. Eur Arch Otorhinolaryngol. 2024;281:2779. Erratum in: Eur Arch Otorhinolaryngol. 2024;281:2791. [PMID: 38184495]
Kunnath AJ et al. Endoscopic versus microscopic transcanal resection of glomus tympanicum: a retrospective comparative study. Otol Neurotol. 2024;45:426. [PMID: 38437815]
Natour A et al. Carbon dioxide (CO 2) laser glomus tympanicum resection: hearing outcomes and recurrence rates. Otol Neurotol. 2025;46:e399. [PMID: 40570318]
Radomska K et al. Algorithm of genetic diagnosis for patients with head and neck paraganglioma–update. Front Neurol. 2024;15:1437027. [PMID: 39268066]

EARACHE

Earache can be caused by a variety of otologic problems, but otitis externa and acute otitis media are the most common. Otitis externa and acute otitis media may be differentiated using history and physical examination, including pneumatic otoscopy. Pain out of proportion to the physical findings may be due to herpes zoster oticus, especially when vesicles appear in the ear canal or concha. Persistent pain and discharge from the ear suggest osteomyelitis of the skull base or cancer, and patients with these symptoms should be referred for specialty evaluation.

Nonotologic causes of otalgia are numerous. The sensory innervation of the ear is derived from the trigeminal, facial, glossopharyngeal, vagal, and upper cervical nerves. Because of this rich innervation, referred otalgia is quite frequent. Temporomandibular joint dysfunction is a common cause of referred ear pain. Pain is exacerbated by chewing or psychogenic grinding of the teeth (**bruxism**) and may be associated with dental malocclusion. Repeated episodes of severe lancinating otalgia may occur in glossopharyngeal neuralgia. Infections and neoplasia that involve the oropharynx, hypopharynx, and larynx frequently cause otalgia. Persistent earache demands specialty referral to exclude cancer of the upper aerodigestive tract.

Ramazani F et al. Referred otalgia: common causes and evidence-based strategies for assessment and management. Can Fam Physician. 2023;69:757. [PMID: 37963787]

DISEASES OF THE INNER EAR

1. Sensorineural Hearing Loss

Diseases of the cochlea and central auditory pathway result in hearing loss, a condition that is usually irreversible. The primary goals in the management of sensory hearing loss are prevention of further losses and functional improvement with auditory rehabilitation, such as with a hearing aid or cochlear implant.

A. Presbycusis

Presbycusis, or age-related hearing loss, is the most frequent cause of sensory hearing loss and is progressive, predominantly high-frequency, and symmetrical. Various etiologic factors (eg, prior noise trauma, drug exposure, genetic predisposition) may contribute to presbycusis. Most patients notice a loss of speech discrimination that is especially pronounced in noisy environments. *About 25% of people between the ages of 65 and 75 years and almost 50% of those over 75 experience hearing difficulties.* There is emerging evidence that conventional audiometry may not fully capture hearing loss (known as "hidden hearing loss"). Many patients may have subclinical hearing loss.

Diao T et al. Compensation in neuro-system related to age-related hearing loss. Acta Otolaryngol. 2024;144:30. [PMID: 38265951]
Lin FR. Age-related hearing loss. N Engl J Med. 2024;390:1505. [PMID: 38657246]

Tsai Do BS et al. Clinical practice guideline: age-related hearing loss executive summary. Otolaryngol Head Neck Surg. 2024;170:1209. [PMID: 38682789]
Yeo BSY et al. Association of hearing aids and cochlear implants with cognitive decline and dementia: a systematic review and meta-analysis. JAMA Neurol. 2023;80:134. [PMID: 36469314]
Zheng Z et al. Impact of hearing rehabilitation programs on presbycusis management: a systematic review and meta-analysis of randomized controlled trials. Front Aging. 2024;5:1299964. [PMID: 39497940]

B. Noise Trauma

Noise trauma is the second most common cause of sensorineural hearing loss. Sounds exceeding 85 dB for 8 hours or more are potentially injurious to the cochlea. The loss typically begins in the high frequencies (especially 4000 Hz) and, with continuing exposure, progresses to involve the speech frequencies. Among the more common sources of injurious noise are industrial machinery, weapons, and excessively loud music. Monitoring noise levels in the workplace by regulatory agencies has led to preventive programs that have reduced the frequency of occupational losses. Smartwatches have also recently gained capacity to measure environmental noise levels. *Individuals of all ages, especially those with existing hearing losses, should wear earplugs when exposed to moderately loud noises and specially designed earmuffs when exposed to explosive noises.*

Fischer T et al. Are smartwatches a suitable tool to monitor noise exposure for public health awareness and otoprotection? Front Neurol. 2022;13:856219. [PMID: 35432148]
Kitama T et al. Noise-induced hearing loss: overview and future prospects for research on oxidative stress. Int J Mol Sci. 2025;26:4927. [PMID: 40430068]
Makaruse N et al. Early identification of potential occupational noise-induced hearing loss: a systematic review. Int J Audiol. 2025;64:419. [PMID: 39468424]

C. Physical Trauma

Concussive head trauma has effects on the inner ear similar to those of severe acoustic trauma. Some degree of sensory hearing loss may occur following concussion and is frequent after lateral skull base fracture.

Harris M et al. Mild traumatic brain injury and the auditory system: an overview of the mechanisms, clinical presentations, and current diagnostic modalities. J Neurotrauma. 2024;41:1524. [PMID: 37742111]

D. Ototoxicity

Ototoxic substances may affect both the auditory and vestibular systems. The most commonly used ototoxic medications are aminoglycosides; loop diuretics; and several antineoplastic agents, notably cisplatin. *These medications may cause irreversible hearing loss even when administered in therapeutic doses.* When using these medications, it is important to identify high-risk patients, such as those with preexisting hearing losses or kidney disease. Patients simultaneously receiving multiple ototoxic agents are at particular risk owing to ototoxic synergy. Useful measures to reduce the risk of ototoxic injury include serial audiometry, monitoring of serum peak and trough levels, and substitution of equivalent nonototoxic medications whenever possible.

Correa-Morales JE et al. Prevention and treatment of cisplatin-induced ototoxicity in adults: a systematic review. Clin Otolaryngol. 2024;49:1. [PMID: 37818931]
Rose O et al. Cisplatin-induced hearing loss, oxidative stress, and antioxidants as a therapeutic strategy-a state-of-the-art review. Antioxidants (Basel). 2024;13:1578. [PMID: 39765905]
Tan WJT et al. Molecular characteristics of cisplatin-induced ototoxicity and therapeutic interventions. Int J Mol Sci. 2023;24:16545. [PMID: 38003734]
Zadrożniak M et al. Experimental and clinical approaches to preventing aminoglycoside-induced ototoxicity: a scoping review. Antioxidants (Basel). 2025;14:1467. [PMID: 41462666]

E. Idiopathic Sudden Sensory Hearing Loss

Idiopathic sudden loss of hearing in one ear may occur at any age, but typically it occurs in persons over age 20 years. In the setting a normal otologic physical examination, symptoms may include hearing loss, aural fullness, tinnitus, and dizziness. The cause is unknown; however, idiopathic sudden hearing loss may result from a viral infection or a sudden vascular occlusion of the internal auditory artery. Obtaining an MRI is essential after the diagnosis to rule out retrocochlear pathology (eg, tumors); however, this should not delay treatment. Prompt treatment with corticosteroids has been shown to improve the odds of recovery. Intratympanic administration of corticosteroids alone or in association with oral corticosteroids has been associated with an equal or more favorable prognosis. Because treatment appears to be most effective as close to the onset of the loss as possible, and appears not to be effective after 6 weeks, *a prompt audiogram should be obtained in all patients who present with sudden hearing loss without obvious middle ear pathology.* Prognosis is mixed, with many patients living with permanent deafness in the involved ear, while others have complete recovery.

Chaushu H et al. Spontaneous recovery rate of idiopathic sudden sensorineural hearing loss: a systematic review and meta-analysis. Clin Otolaryngol. 2023;48:395. [PMID: 36640119]
Chrysouli K et al. The effectiveness of intratympanic steroid injection in addition to systemic corticosteroids in the treatment of idiopathic sudden sensorineural hearing loss. Am J Otolaryngol. 2023;44:103872. [PMID: 37060782]
González-García M et al. Auditory prognosis of patients with sudden sensorineural hearing loss in relation to the presence of acute vestibular syndrome: a systematic literature review and meta-analysis. Ear Hear. 2025;46:8. [PMID: 39252156]
Meliante PG et al. Salvage treatment strategies for refractory sudden sensorineural hearing loss-a comprehensive review and meta-analysis with practical recommendations. Front Neurol. 2025;16:1627892. [PMID: 40734818]
Rodríguez-Izquierdo C et al. Current role of the nonsteroid treatment of idiopathic sudden sensorineural hearing loss (ISSNHL): a narrative review. J Clin Med. 2025;14:2811. [PMID: 40283640]

F. Autoimmune Hearing Loss

Sensorineural hearing loss that occurs in both ears simultaneously may be associated with a wide array of systemic autoimmune disorders, such as SLE, granulomatosis with polyangiitis, and Cogan syndrome (hearing loss, keratitis, aortitis). The loss is most often progressive. The hearing level often fluctuates, with periods of deterioration alternating with partial or even complete remission. Usually, there is the gradual evolution of permanent hearing loss, which often stabilizes with some remaining auditory function but occasionally proceeds to complete deafness. Vestibular dysfunction may accompany the auditory symptoms.

In many cases, the autoimmune pattern of audiovestibular dysfunction presents in the absence of recognized systemic autoimmune disease. Responsiveness to oral corticosteroid treatment is helpful in making the diagnosis and constitutes first-line therapy. If stabilization of hearing becomes dependent on long-term corticosteroid use, steroid-sparing immunosuppressive regimens may become necessary.

Balouch B et al. Use of biologics for treatment of autoimmune inner ear disease. Am J Otolaryngol. 2022;43:103576. [PMID: 35963108]
Creber N et al. Primary and secondary autoimmune disorders and hearing loss. Curr Opin Otolaryngol Head Neck Surg. 2025;33:286. [PMID: 40836789]
Gordis TM et al. Disease-modifying antirheumatic drugs in the treatment of autoimmune inner ear disease: a systematic review and meta-analysis of auditory and vestibular outcomes. Otol Neurotol. 2023;44:2. [PMID: 36509432]
Wang M et al. Investigating the process of autoimmune inner ear disease: unveiling the intricacies of pathogenesis and therapeutic strategies. Int J Med Sci. 2025;22:179. [PMID: 39744176]
Sharma N et al. A systematic review of the monogenic causes of non-syndromic hearing loss (NSHL) and discussion of current diagnosis and treatment options. Clin Genet. 2023;103:16. [PMID: 36089522]
Valayannopoulos V et al; CHORD Study Group. DB-OTO gene therapy for inherited deafness. N Engl J Med. 2025 Oct 12. [Epub ahead of print] [PMID: 41085057]

2. Tinnitus

ESSENTIALS OF DIAGNOSIS

- Phantom noise or sounds.
- Persistent tinnitus often, although not always, indicates the presence of hearing loss.
- Intermittent periods of mild, high-pitched tinnitus lasting seconds to minutes are common in normal-hearing persons.

General Considerations

Tinnitus is defined as the sensation of sound in the absence of an exogenous sound source. Tinnitus can accompany any form of hearing loss, and its presence provides no diagnostic value in determining the cause of a hearing loss. Approximately 15% of the general population experiences some type of tinnitus, with prevalence beyond 20% in aging populations.

Clinical Findings

A. Symptoms and Signs

Though tinnitus is commonly associated with hearing loss, tinnitus severity correlates poorly with the degree of hearing loss. About one in seven tinnitus sufferers experiences severe annoyance, and 4% are severely disabled. When severe and persistent, tinnitus may interfere with sleep and ability to concentrate, resulting in considerable psychological distress.

Pulsatile tinnitus—often described by the patient as listening to one's own heartbeat—should be distinguished from **tonal tinnitus**. Although often ascribed to conductive hearing loss, pulsatile tinnitus may be far more serious and may indicate a vascular abnormality, such as glomus tumor, venous sinus stenosis, carotid vaso-occlusive disease, arteriovenous malformation, or aneurysm.

A staccato **"clicking" tinnitus** may result from middle ear muscle spasm (middle ear myoclonus) or sometimes palatal myoclonus. The patient typically perceives a rapid series of popping noises, lasting seconds to a few minutes, accompanied by a fluttering feeling in the ear. Specialized forms of tympanometry may formally diagnose this condition, and it is typically treated surgically.

B. Diagnostic Testing

For routine, nonpulsatile tinnitus, audiometry should be ordered to rule out an associated hearing loss. For unilateral tinnitus, particularly associated with hearing loss in the absence of an obvious causative factor (ie, noise trauma), an MRI should be obtained to rule out a retrocochlear lesion, such as vestibular schwannoma. MRA and MRV and temporal bone CT should be considered for patients who have pulsatile tinnitus to exclude a causative vascular lesion or sigmoid sinus abnormality.

Treatment

The most important treatment of tinnitus is avoidance of exposure to excessive noise, ototoxic agents, and other factors that may cause cochlear damage. Masking the tinnitus with music or through amplification of normal sounds with a hearing aid may also bring some relief. In addition to masking techniques, habituation techniques, such as tinnitus retraining therapy and cognitive behavioral therapy, may prove beneficial in those with refractory symptoms. Among patients who have emotional distress due to tinnitus, numerous antidepressant and antipsychotic medications have been tried to allow the patient to cope with it better.

Conlon B et al. Different bimodal neuromodulation settings reduce tinnitus symptoms in a large randomized trial. Sci Rep. 2022;12:10845. [PMID: 35773272]
Hoare DJ et al. Neuromodulation treatments targeting pathological synchrony for tinnitus in adults: a systematic review. Brain Sci. 2024;14:748. [PMID: 39199443]
Perrotta MV et al. Bimodal stimulation for the reduction of tinnitus using vibration on the skin. Int Tinnitus J. 2023;27:1. [PMID: 38050877]
Sherlock LP et al. Clinical practice guideline for management of tinnitus: recommendations from the US VA/DOD Clinical Practice Guideline Work Group. JAMA Otolaryngol Head Neck Surg. 2025;151:513. [PMID: 40111327]

3. Hyperacusis

Excessive sensitivity to sound may occur following hearing loss, such as that due to noise trauma, in patients susceptible to migraines, or for psychological reasons. Patients with cochlear dysfunction commonly experience "recruitment," an abnormal sensitivity to loud sounds despite a reduced sensitivity to softer ones. Fitting hearing aids and other amplification devices to patients with recruitment requires use of compression circuitry to avoid uncomfortable overamplification.

Fernandez C et al. Quick hyperacusis screening and insights from extended high-frequency audiometry, speech-in-noise perception and natural sound evaluation. Hear Res. 2025;467:109436. [PMID: 41056620]
Savard MA et al. Toward cognitive models of misophonia. Hear Res. 2025;458:109184. [PMID: 39874936]

4. Vertigo

ESSENTIALS OF DIAGNOSIS

- Either a sensation of motion when there is no motion or an exaggerated sense of motion in response to movement.
- Duration of vertigo episodes with associated hearing loss or other neurologic issues are the keys to diagnosis.
- Evaluation includes audiogram, electronystagmography (ENG) or videonystagmography (VNG), and head MRI.

General Considerations

Vertigo can be caused by either a peripheral or central etiology, or both (Table 8–2).

Clinical Findings

A. Symptoms and Signs

Vertigo is the cardinal symptom of vestibular disease. Vertigo is typically experienced as a distinct "spinning" sensation or a sense of tumbling or of falling forward or backward. It should be distinguished from imbalance, light-headedness, and syncope, all of which are nonvestibular in origin (Table 8–3).

1. Peripheral vestibular disease—Peripheral vestibulopathy may cause vertigo of sudden onset, may be so severe that the patient is unable to walk or stand, and is frequently accompanied by nausea and vomiting. Tinnitus and hearing loss may be associated and provide strong support for a peripheral (ie, otologic) origin.

Critical elements of the history include the duration of the discrete vertiginous episodes (seconds, minutes to hours, or days) and associated symptoms (hearing loss). Triggers should be sought, including diet (eg, increased salt intake in the case of Ménière disease), stress, fatigue, and bright lights (eg, migraine-associated dizziness).

The physical examination of the patient with vertigo includes evaluation of the ears, observation of eye motion and nystagmus in response to head turning, cranial nerve examination, and Romberg testing. In acute peripheral lesions, nystagmus is usually horizontal with a rotatory component; the fast phase usually beats *away* from the diseased side. Visual fixation tends to inhibit nystagmus except in very acute peripheral lesions or with CNS disease. In benign paroxysmal positioning vertigo, **Dix-Hallpike**

Table 8–2. Causes of vertigo (listed in alphabetical order, within categories).

Peripheral causes
Benign paroxysmal positioning vertigo
Ethanol intoxication
Inner ear barotraumas
Ménière disease
Semicircular canal dehiscence
Vestibular neuritis/labyrinthitis
Central causes
Cerebellar ataxia syndromes
Chiari malformation
Multiple sclerosis
Seizure
Wernicke encephalopathy
Mixed central and peripheral causes
Cerebellopontine angle tumors
Meningioma
Vestibular schwannoma
Endocrinopathies
Hypothyroidism
Pendred syndrome
Hyperviscosity syndromes
Waldenström macroglobulinemia
Infections
Lyme disease
Syphilis
Migraine
Stroke and vascular insufficiency
Anterior inferior cerebellar artery stroke
Posterior inferior cerebellar artery stroke
Vasculitides
Behçet disease
Cogan syndrome
Granulomatosis with polyangiitis
Susac syndrome
Vertebral artery insufficiency
Vascular compression

Table 8–3. Common vestibular disorders: differential diagnosis based on classic presentations (listed by duration of episodes).

Duration of Typical Vertiginous Episodes	Auditory Symptoms Present	Auditory Symptoms Absent
Seconds	Perilymphatic fistula	Benign paroxysmal positioning vertigo (cupulolithiasis), vertebrobasilar insufficiency, migraine-associated vertigo
Hours	Ménière disease, syphilis	Migraine-associated vertigo
Days	Labyrinthitis, autoimmune inner ear disease, cerebellopontine angle tumor, ototoxicity	Vestibular neuronitis, migraine-associated vertigo, multiple sclerosis, cerebellar degeneration

testing (quickly lowering the patient to the supine position with the head extending over the edge and placed 30 degrees lower than the body, turned either to the left or right) will elicit a delayed-onset (~10 seconds) fatigable nystagmus. Nonfatigable nystagmus in this position indicates CNS disease.

Since visual fixation often suppresses observed nystagmus, many of these maneuvers are performed with **Frenzel goggles**, which prevent visual fixation, and often bring out subtle forms of nystagmus. The **Fukuda test** can demonstrate vestibular asymmetry when the patient steps in place with eyes closed and consistently rotates in one direction.

2. Central disease—Vertigo arising from CNS disease (Table 8–2) tends to develop gradually and then becomes progressively more severe and debilitating. Nystagmus is not always present but can occur in any direction, may be dissociated in the two eyes, and is often non fatigable, vertical rather than horizontal in orientation, without latency, and unsuppressed by visual fixation. ENG is useful in documenting these characteristics. Evaluation of audiovestibular dysfunction requires MRI of the brain.

Episodic vertigo can occur in patients with diplopia from external ophthalmoplegia and is maximal when the patient looks in the direction where the separation of images is greatest. Cerebral lesions involving the temporal cortex may also produce vertigo; it is sometimes the initial symptom of a seizure. Finally, vertigo may be a feature of a systemic disorder and can occur as a side effect of certain anticonvulsant, antibiotic, hypnotic, analgesic, and tranquilizer medications or of alcohol.

Arshad Q et al. What visuospatial perception has taught us about the pathophysiology of vestibular migraine. Curr Opin Neurol. 2024;37:32. [PMID: 38018799]
Lopez-Escamez JA et al. Update on the pathophysiology, diagnosis and management of Ménière's disease. Curr Opin Otolaryngol Head Neck Surg. 2024;32:306. [PMID: 39146194]
Mahmud M et al. Vestibular neurology for the generalist. J Neurol Neurosurg Psychiatry. 2024;95:1196. [PMID: 39313324]
Strupp M et al. World-wide survey on the treatment of peripheral vestibular disorders. Front Neurol. 2025;16:1540443. [PMID: 39968460]

B. Vestibular Testing

Vestibular investigations, such as audiologic evaluation, caloric stimulation, **electro- or videonystagmography (ENG or VNG)**, **vestibular-evoked myogenic potentials (VEMPs)**, and MRI, are indicated in patients with persistent vertigo or when CNS disease is suspected. These studies help distinguish between central and peripheral lesions and identify causes requiring specific therapy. ENG consists of objective recording of the nystagmus induced by head and body movements, gaze, and caloric stimulation. It is helpful in quantifying the degree of vestibular hypofunction.

Bery AK et al. Evaluation of acute dizziness and vertigo. Med Clin North Am. 2025;109:373. [PMID: 39893018]
Grove CR et al. Vestibular perceptual testing from lab to clinic: a review. Front Neurol. 2023;14:1265889. [PMID: 37859653]
Pastras CJ et al. Vestibular testing: new physiological results for the optimization of clinical VEMP stimuli. Audiol Res. 2023;13:910. [PMID: 37987337]
Rosengren SM et al. Vestibular function testing in the 21st century: video head impulse test, vestibular evoked myogenic potential, video nystagmography; which tests will provide answers? Curr Opin Neurol. 2022;35:64. [PMID: 34889807]

Vertigo Syndromes Due to Peripheral Lesions

A. Ménière Disease

The cause of Ménière disease is unknown. The classic syndrome consists of episodic vertigo, with discrete vertigo spells lasting 20 minutes to several hours in association with fluctuating, often low-frequency, sensorineural hearing loss, tinnitus (usually low-tone and "blowing" in quality), and a sensation of unilateral aural pressure (Table 8–3). These symptoms in presence of headaches or migraines may suggest migraine-associated dizziness. *Primary treatment is aimed at decreasing dizzy episodes. There are no treatments for reduction in hearing loss.* Treatment of Ménière disease typically involves preventive measures, including low-salt diet and daily diuretics (eg, acetazolamide). For symptomatic relief of acute vertigo attacks, lorazepam (0.5–1 mg) or diazepam (2–5 mg) can be used. Nausea may be treated with oral meclizine (25 mg). In refractory cases, patients may undergo intratympanic corticosteroid or gentamicin injections, endolymphatic sac decompression, or surgical or vestibular nerve section. There are increasing reports of imaging, such as CT or MRI, for evaluation of Ménière disease.

Bächinger D et al. Radiological feature heterogeneity supports etiological diversity among patient groups in Meniere's disease. Sci Rep. 2023;13:10303. [PMID: 37365255]

Lopez-Escamez JA et al. Update on the pathophysiology, diagnosis and management of Ménière's disease. Curr Opin Otolaryngol Head Neck Surg. 2024;32:306. [PMID: 39146194]
Tang M et al. Efficacy and safety of acupuncture in the treatment of Meniere's disease: a systematic review and meta-analysis. Front Med (Lausanne). 2024;11:1463821. [PMID: 39722819]

B. Labyrinthitis

Patients with labyrinthitis suffer from acute onset of continuous, usually severe vertigo lasting several days, accompanied by hearing loss and tinnitus. During a recovery period that lasts for several weeks, the vertigo gradually improves. Hearing may return to normal or remain permanently impaired in the involved ear. The cause of labyrinthitis is unknown. Treatment consists of antibiotics, if the patient is febrile or has symptoms of a bacterial infection, oral corticosteroids, and supportive care. Vestibular suppressants are useful during the acute phase of the attack (eg, diazepam) but should be discontinued as soon as feasible to avoid long-term dysequilibrium from inadequate compensation.

Cohen HS et al. Relationship between clinical measures of hearing and clinical measures of vestibular function. Am J Otolaryngol. 2024;45:104052. [PMID: 37801744]
Djian C et al. Infliximab for the treatment of inflammatory labyrinthitis: a retrospective cohort study. J Clin Med. 2023;12:4350. [PMID: 37445384]

C. Benign Paroxysmal Positioning Vertigo

Patients living with recurrent spells of vertigo, lasting a few (10–15) seconds per spell, associated with changes in head position (often provoked by rolling over in bed), usually have benign paroxysmal positioning vertigo (BPPV). The term "positioning vertigo" is more accurate than "positional vertigo" because it is *provoked by changes in head position* rather than by the maintenance of a particular posture.

The typical symptoms of BPPV occur in clusters that persist for several days. There is a brief (10–15 seconds) latency period following a head movement before symptoms develop, and the acute vertigo subsides within 10–60 seconds, although the patient may remain imbalanced for several hours. *Dizziness that lasts for more than a few seconds (that is several minutes or hours) is not BPPV.* Constant repetition of the positional change leads to habituation. Since some CNS disorders can mimic BPPV (eg, vertebrobasilar insufficiency), recurrent cases warrant head MRI/MRA. In central lesions, there is no latent period, fatigability, or habituation of the symptoms and signs. Treatment of BPPV involves physical therapy protocols (eg, the **Epley maneuver** or **Brandt-Daroff exercises**), based on the theory that it results from **cupulolithiasis** (free-floating statoconia, also known as otoconia) within a semicircular canal.

Gurberg J et al. Benign paroxysmal vertigo of childhood. Handb Clin Neurol. 2023;198:229. [PMID: 38043965]
Kim HJ et al. Effect of self-treatment of recurrent benign paroxysmal positional vertigo: a randomized clinical trial. JAMA Neurol. 2023;80:244. [PMID: 36648931]
Saishoji Y et al. Epley manoeuvre's efficacy for benign paroxysmal positional vertigo (BPPV) in primary-care and subspecialty settings: a systematic review and meta-analysis. BMC Prim Care. 2023;24:262. [PMID: 38042776]
Tarnutzer AA et al. Diagnostic errors in the acutely dizzy patient–lessons learned. Brain Sci. 2025;15:55. [PMID: 39851423]

D. Vestibular Neuronitis

In vestibular neuronitis, a paroxysmal, usually single attack of vertigo occurs without accompanying impairment of auditory function and will persist for several days before gradually abating. During the acute phase, examination reveals nystagmus and absent responses to caloric stimulation on one or both sides. The cause of the disorder is unclear though presumed to be viral. Treatment consists of supportive care; vestibular suppressants, such as diazepam 2–5 mg every 6–12 hours during the acute phases of the vertigo only; oral corticosteroids may potentially be used; and antiemetics, such as ondansetron and meclizine, followed by vestibular therapy if the patient does not completely compensate.

Chowdhury S et al. Association of vestibular neuritis following COVID-19 vaccination. Discoveries (Craiova). 2024;12:e195. [PMID: 39749143]
Farhat R et al. The "Vestibular Eye Sign"- "VES": a new radiological sign of vestibular neuronitis can help to determine the affected vestibule and support the diagnosis. J Neurol. 2023;270:4360. [PMID: 37219605]
Nham B et al. Modern vestibular tests can accurately separate stroke and vestibular neuritis. J Neurol. 2023;270:2031. [PMID: 36566345]

E. Traumatic Vertigo

Labyrinthine concussion is the most common cause of vertigo following head injury. Symptoms generally diminish within several days but may linger for a month or more. Basilar skull fractures that traverse the inner ear usually result in severe vertigo lasting several days to a week and deafness in the involved ear. Chronic posttraumatic vertigo may result from cupulolithiasis. This occurs when traumatically detached statoconia (otoconia) settle on the ampulla of the posterior semicircular canal and cause an excessive degree of cupular deflection in response to head motion. Clinically, this presents as episodic positioning vertigo. Treatment consists of supportive care and vestibular suppressant medication (diazepam) during the acute phase of the attack and vestibular therapy.

Aljabri A et al. The efficacy of vestibular rehabilitation therapy for mild traumatic brain injury: a systematic review and meta-analysis. J Head Trauma Rehabil. 2024;39:E59. [PMID: 37335202]
Harris M et al. Mild traumatic brain injury and the auditory system: an overview of the mechanisms, clinical presentations, and current diagnostic modalities. J Neurotrauma. 2024;41:1524. [PMID: 37742111]
Schlemmer E et al. Vestibular rehabilitation effectiveness for adults with mild traumatic brain injury/concussion: a mini-systematic review. Am J Audiol. 2022;31:228. [PMID: 35077655]

F. Perilymphatic Fistula

Leakage of perilymphatic fluid from the inner ear into the tympanic cavity via the round or oval window is a very rare cause of vertigo and sensory hearing loss. Most cases result from physical injury (eg, blunt head trauma, hand slap to ear); extreme barotrauma during airflight, scuba diving, etc; or vigorous Valsalva maneuvers (eg, during weight lifting).

Kitoh R et al; Research Group on Intractable Hearing Disorders and Japan Audiological Society. Clinical practice guidelines for the diagnosis and management of acute sensorineural hearing loss. Auris Nasus Larynx. 2024;51:811. [PMID: 38968877]

Sasaki A et al. Prevalence of perilymphatic fistula in patients with sudden-onset sensorineural hearing loss as diagnosed by Cochlin-tomoprotein (CTP) biomarker detection: its association with age, hearing severity, and treatment outcomes. Eur Arch Otorhinolaryngol. 2024;281:2373. [PMID: 38123733]

G. Cervicogenic Vertigo

Position receptors located in the facets of the cervical spine are important physiologically in the coordination of head and eye movements. Cervical proprioceptive dysfunction is a common cause of vertigo triggered by neck movements. This disturbance often commences after neck injury, particularly hyperextension; it is also associated with degenerative cervical spine disease. Although symptoms vary, vertigo may be triggered by assuming a particular head position as opposed to moving to a new head position (the latter typical of labyrinthine dysfunction). Cervical vertigo may often be confused with migraine-associated vertigo, which is also associated with head movement. Management consists of neck movement exercises to the extent permitted by orthopedic considerations.

Gill-Lussier J et al. Proprioceptive cervicogenic dizziness care trajectories in patient subpopulations: a scoping review. J Clin Med. 2023;12:1884. [PMID: 36902670]

Han E et al. Predictive model for diagnosing central lesions in emergency department patients with isolated dizziness who undergo diffusion-weighted magnetic resonance imaging. Acad Emerg Med. 2022;29:15. [PMID: 34414635]

Piromchai P et al. The efficacy of self-exercise in a patient with cervicogenic dizziness: a randomized controlled trial. Front Neurol. 2023;14:1121101. [PMID: 36864911]

H. Migrainous Vertigo

Episodic vertigo is frequently associated with migraine headache. Head trauma may also be a precipitating feature. The vertigo may be temporally related to the headache and last up to several hours, or it may also occur in the absence of any headache. Migrainous vertigo may resemble Ménière disease but without associated hearing loss or tinnitus. Accompanying symptoms may include head pressure; visual, motion, or auditory sensitivity; and photosensitivity. Symptoms typically worsen with lack of sleep and anxiety or stress. Food triggers include caffeine, chocolate, and alcohol, among others. There is often a history of motion intolerance (easily carsick as a child). Migrainous vertigo may be familial. Treatment includes dietary and lifestyle changes (improved sleep pattern, avoidance of stress) and antimigraine prophylactic medication.

Chu H et al. Prophylactic treatments for vestibular migraine: a systematic review and network meta-analysis of randomized clinical trials. Front Pharmacol. 2023;14:1332973. [PMID: 38186654]

Hac NEF et al. Advances in diagnosis and treatment of vestibular migraine and the vestibular disorders it mimics. Neurotherapeutics. 2024;21:e00381. [PMID: 38845250]

Mallampalli MP et al. Care gaps and recommendations in vestibular migraine: an expert panel summit. Front Neurol. 2022;12:812678. [PMID: 35046886]

Tu YH et al. Prevalence, clinical correlates, and functional implications of vestibular symptoms in patients with migraine. Neurology. 2025;105:e214248. [PMID: 41092249]

I. Superior Semicircular Canal Dehiscence

Deficiency in the bony covering of the superior semicircular canal may be associated with vertigo triggered by loud noise exposure, straining, and an apparent conductive hearing loss. **Autophony** is also a common feature. Diagnosis is with coronal HRCT scan and VEMP testing.

Eberhard KE et al. Transmastoid surgery for superior canal dehiscence: prospective longitudinal objective and patient-reported audiovestibular outcomes. Otol Neurotol. 2024;45:184. [PMID: 38206067]

Patel S et al. The history of superior semicircular canal dehiscence: a bibliometric analysis. World Neurosurg. 2024;185:e591. [PMID: 38395350]

Vertigo Syndromes Due to Central Lesions

CNS causes of vertigo include brainstem vascular disease, arteriovenous malformations, tumors of the brainstem and cerebellum, multiple sclerosis, and vertebrobasilar migraine (Table 8–2). Vertigo of central origin often becomes unremitting and disabling. The associated nystagmus is often nonfatigable, vertical rather than horizontal in orientation, without latency, and unsuppressed by visual fixation. ENG is useful in documenting these characteristics. There are commonly other signs of brainstem dysfunction (eg, cranial nerve palsies; motor, sensory, or cerebellar deficits in the limbs) or of increased intracranial pressure. Auditory function is generally spared.

Bassett A et al. Exploring vestibular assessment in patients with headache and dizziness. Otolaryngol Clin North Am. 2022;55:549. [PMID: 35490043]

Dieterich M et al. Central vestibular networking for sensorimotor control, cognition, and emotion. Curr Opin Neurol. 2024;37:74. [PMID: 38032266]

Rogers TS et al. Dizziness: evaluation and management. Am Fam Physician. 2023;107:514. [PMID: 37192077]

DISEASES OF THE CENTRAL AUDITORY & VESTIBULAR SYSTEMS

Lesions of the eighth cranial nerve and central audiovestibular pathways may produce hearing loss and dizziness (Table 8–3). One characteristic of neural hearing loss is deterioration of speech discrimination out of proportion to the decrease in pure-tone thresholds. Another is *auditory adaptation*, wherein a steady tone appears to the listener to decay and eventually disappear. Auditory evoked responses are useful in distinguishing cochlear from neural losses and may give insight into the site of lesion within the central pathways. The evaluation of central audiovestibular disorders usually requires imaging of the internal auditory canal, cerebellopontine angle, and brain with enhanced MRI.

1. Vestibular Schwannoma (Acoustic Neuroma)

Eighth cranial nerve schwannomas are among the most common intracranial tumors. Most are unilateral, but about 5% are associated with the hereditary syndrome neurofibromatosis type 2, in which bilateral eighth nerve tumors may be accompanied by meningiomas and other intracranial and spinal tumors. These benign lesions arise within the internal auditory canal and gradually grow to involve the cerebellopontine angle, eventually compressing the pons and resulting in hydrocephalus. Their typical auditory symptoms are unilateral hearing loss with a deterioration of speech discrimination exceeding that predicted by the degree of pure-tone loss. Nonclassic presentations, such as sudden unilateral hearing loss, are fairly common. *Any individual with a unilateral or asymmetric sensorineural hearing loss should be evaluated for an intracranial mass lesion.* Vestibular dysfunction more often takes the form of continuous dysequilibrium than episodic vertigo. Diagnosis is made by enhanced MRI. Treatment consists of observation, microsurgical excision, or stereotactic radiotherapy, depending on such factors as patient age, underlying health, and size of the tumor.

Barrett TF et al. Single-cell multi-omic analysis of the vestibular schwannoma ecosystem uncovers a nerve injury-like state. Nat Commun. 2024;15:478. [PMID: 38216553]

Gambacciani C et al. Surgical management of skull base meningiomas and vestibular schwannomas. Curr Opin Oncol. 2022;34:713. [PMID: 36093884]

2. Vascular Compromise

Vertebrobasilar insufficiency is a common cause of vertigo in the older adults. It is often triggered by changes in posture or extension of the neck. Reduced flow in the vertebrobasilar system may be demonstrated noninvasively through MRA. Empiric treatment is with vasodilators and aspirin.

Clark M et al. A review of carotid and vertebral artery dissection. Br J Hosp Med (Lond). 2022;83:1. [PMID: 35506728]

Nogueira RG et al. Endovascular therapy for acute vertebrobasilar occlusion (VERITAS): a systematic review and individual patient data meta-analysis. Lancet. 2025;405:61. [PMID: 39674187]

3. Multiple Sclerosis

Patients with multiple sclerosis may suffer from episodic vertigo and chronic imbalance. Hearing loss in this disease is most commonly unilateral and of rapid onset. Spontaneous recovery may occur.

Bissonnette JN et al. An investigation of auditory processing in relapsing-remitting multiple sclerosis. Exp Brain Res. 2023;241:1319. [PMID: 37004533]

OTOLOGIC MANIFESTATIONS OF AIDS

AIDS may result in many otologic signs and symptoms. The pinna and external auditory canal may be affected by Kaposi sarcoma and by persistent and potentially invasive fungal infections (particularly *Aspergillus fumigatus*). Serous otitis media due to eustachian tube dysfunction may arise from adenoidal hypertrophy (HIV lymphadenopathy), recurrent mucosal viral infections, or an obstructing nasopharyngeal tumor (eg, lymphoma). Unfortunately, ventilating tubes are seldom helpful and may trigger profuse watery otorrhea. Acute otitis media is usually caused by typical bacterial organisms, including *Proteus, Staphylococcus,* and *Pseudomonas,* and rarely, by *Pneumocystis jirovecii.* Sensorineural hearing loss is common and, in some cases, results from viral CNS infection. In cases of progressive hearing loss, cryptococcal meningitis and syphilis must be excluded. Acute facial paralysis due to herpes zoster infection (**Ramsay Hunt syndrome**) occurs commonly and follows a clinical course similar to that in nonimmunocompromised patients. Treatment is with high-dose acyclovir (see Chapter 36). Corticosteroids may also be effective as an adjunct.

Khoza-Shangase K. The association between HIV/AIDS, ototoxicity of its treatments, and occupational noise induced hearing loss: a narrative review mapping the existing literature and identifying research gaps. Int J Environ Res Public Health. 2025;22:487. [PMID: 40283716]

DISEASES OF THE NOSE & PARANASAL SINUSES

INFECTIONS OF THE NOSE & PARANASAL SINUSES

Rhinosinusitis may be classified by duration of symptoms. Rhinosinusitis is called **acute rhinosinusitis** if < 4 weeks' duration or as **chronic rhinosinusitis** if lasting > 12 weeks, with or without acute exacerbations. Acute rhinosinusitis may also be classified by presumed etiology, such as viral rhinosinusitis or acute bacterial rhinosinusitis.

1. Viral Rhinosinusitis (Common Cold)

ESSENTIALS OF DIAGNOSIS

- Associated malaise, headache, and cough.
- Nasal congestion, facial pressure, rhinorrhea, and hyposmia.
- Erythematous, engorged nasal mucosa without intranasal purulence.
- Symptoms are self-limited, lasting typically < 10 days.

Clinical Findings

Due to the numerous serologic types of rhinoviruses, adenoviruses, and other viruses, patients remain susceptible to the common cold throughout life. These infections, while generally quite benign and self-limited, have been implicated in the development or exacerbation of more serious conditions, such as acute bacterial sinusitis and acute otitis media, asthma, cystic fibrosis, and bronchitis. Nasal congestion, decreased sense of smell, rhinorrhea, and sneezing accompanied by general malaise, throat discomfort and, occasionally, headache, are typical in viral infections. Nasal examination usually shows erythematous, edematous mucosa and a watery discharge. The presence of purulent nasal discharge suggests bacterial rhinosinusitis.

Abdou EHE et al. Clinical and imaging evaluation of COVID-19-related olfactory dysfunction. Am J Rhinol Allergy. 2023;37:456. [PMID: 36945746]

Treatment

The main treatment for viral rhinitis is supportive care, including rest, hydration, and use of over-the-counter analgesics and decongestants. *There are no effective antiviral therapies for either the prevention or treatment of most viral rhinitis despite a common misperception among patients that antibiotics are helpful.* Buffered hypertonic saline (3–5%) nasal irrigation has been shown to improve symptoms and reduce the need for NSAIDs. Other supportive measures, such as oral decongestants (pseudoephedrine, 30–60 mg every 4–6 hours or 120 mg twice daily), may provide some relief of rhinorrhea and nasal obstruction.

Nasal sprays, such as oxymetazoline or phenylephrine, are rapidly effective but should *not* be used for more than a few days to prevent rebound congestion. Withdrawal of the medication after prolonged use leads to **rhinitis medicamentosa**, an almost addictive need for continuous usage. Topical intranasal corticosteroids (eg, flunisolide, 2 sprays in each nostril twice daily), intranasal anticholinergic (ipratropium 0.06% nasal spray, 2–3 sprays every 8 hours as needed), or a short tapering course of oral prednisone may help during the withdrawal process.

Complications

Other than mild eustachian tube dysfunction or transient middle ear effusion, complications of viral rhinitis are unusual. *Secondary acute bacterial rhinosinusitis is a well-accepted complication of acute viral rhinitis* and is suggested by persistence of symptoms beyond 10 days with purulent green or yellow nasal secretions and unilateral facial or dental pain.

2. Bacterial Rhinosinusitis

ESSENTIALS OF DIAGNOSIS

- Acute onset of symptoms.
- Purulent yellow-green nasal discharge or expectoration.
- Facial pain or pressure over the affected sinus or sinuses.
- Nasal obstruction.
- Associated cough, malaise, fever, and headache.

General Considerations

Compared with viral rhinitis, acute bacterial rhinosinusitis infections are uncommon, but they still affect nearly 20 million Americans annually and account for over 2 billion dollars in health care expenditures. Acute bacterial rhinosinusitis is believed to be the result of impaired mucociliary clearance, inflammation of the nasal cavity mucosa, and obstruction of the ostiomeatal complex. Edematous mucosa causes obstruction of the complex, resulting in the *accumulation of mucus in the sinus cavity that becomes secondarily infected by bacteria.* The largest of these ostiomeatal complexes is deep to the middle turbinate in the middle meatus. This complex is actually a confluence of complexes draining the maxillary, ethmoid, and frontal sinuses. The sphenoid drains from a separate complex between the septum and superior turbinate. The typical pathogens of bacterial rhinosinusitis are *S pneumoniae*, other streptococci, *H influenzae*, and less commonly, *S aureus* and *Moraxella catarrhalis*. Pathogens vary regionally in both prevalence and drug resistance; about 25% of healthy asymptomatic individuals may, if sinus aspirates are cultured, harbor such bacteria as well.

Clinical Findings

A. Symptoms and Signs

There are no agreed-upon criteria for the diagnosis of acute bacterial rhinosinusitis in adults. Major symptoms include purulent nasal drainage, nasal obstruction or congestion, facial pain/pressure, altered smell, cough, and fever. Minor symptoms include headache, otalgia, halitosis, dental pain, and fatigue. Many of the more specific symptoms and signs relate to the affected sinus(es). Bacterial rhinosinusitis can be distinguished from viral rhinitis by persistence of symptoms for > 10 days after onset or worsening of symptoms within 10 days after initial improvement. Acute rhinosinusitis is defined as lasting < 4 weeks and subacute rhinosinusitis, as lasting 4–12 weeks.

Acute maxillary sinusitis is the most common form of acute bacterial rhinosinusitis because the maxillary is the largest sinus with a single drainage pathway that is easily obstructed. Unilateral facial fullness, pressure, and tenderness over the cheek are common symptoms, but may not always be present. Pain may refer to the upper incisor and canine teeth via branches of the trigeminal nerve, which traverse the floor of the sinus. Purulent nasal drainage should be noted with nasal airway obstruction or facial pain (pressure). Maxillary sinusitis may result from dental infection, and teeth that are tender should be carefully examined for signs of abscess. Drainage of the periapical abscess or removal of the diseased tooth typically resolves the sinus infection.

Acute ethmoiditis in adults is often accompanied by maxillary sinusitis, and symptoms are similar to those described above. Localized ethmoid sinusitis may present with pain and pressure over the high lateral wall of the nose between the eyes that may radiate to the orbit.

Sphenoid sinusitis is usually seen in the setting of pansinusitis or infection of all the paranasal sinuses on at least one side. The patient may describe a headache "in the middle of the head" and often point to the vertex.

Acute frontal sinusitis may cause pain and tenderness of the forehead. This is most easily elicited by palpation of the orbital roof just below the medial end of the eyebrow.

Hospital-associated sinusitis is a form of acute bacterial rhinosinusitis that may present without the usual symptoms. Instead, it may be a cause of fever in critically ill patients. It is often associated with prolonged presence of a nasogastric or, rarely, nasotracheal tube causing nasal mucosal inflammation and ostiomeatal complex obstruction. Pansinusitis on the side of the tube is common on imaging studies.

B. Imaging

The diagnosis of acute bacterial rhinosinusitis can usually be made on clinical grounds alone. *Although more sensitive than clinical examination, routine radiographs are not cost-effective and are not recommended by the Agency for Health Care Policy and Research or American Association of Otolaryngology Guidelines.* Consensus guidelines recommend imaging when clinical criteria are difficult to evaluate, when the patient does not respond to appropriate therapy or has been treated repeatedly with antibiotics, when intracranial involvement or CSF rhinorrhea is suspected, when complicated dental infection is suspected, or when symptoms of more serious infection are noted.

When necessary, noncontrast screening coronal CT scans are more cost-effective and provide more information than conventional sinus films. CT provides a rapid and effective means to assess all of the paranasal sinuses, identify areas of greater concern (such as bony dehiscence, periosteal elevation, or maxillary tooth root exposure within the sinus), and direct appropriate therapy. CT scans are reasonably sensitive but are not specific. Swollen soft tissue and fluid may be difficult to distinguish when opacification of the sinus is due to other conditions, such as chronic rhinosinusitis, nasal polyposis, or mucus retention cysts. Sinus abnormalities can be seen in most patients with an upper respiratory infection, while bacterial rhinosinusitis develops in only 2%.

If malignancy, intracranial extension, or opportunistic infection is suspected, MRI with gadolinium should be ordered instead of, or in addition to, CT. MRI will distinguish tumor from fluid, inflammation, and inspissated mucus far better than CT, and will better delineate tumor extent (eg, involvement of adjacent structures, such as the orbit, skull base, and palate). Bone destruction can be demonstrated as well by MRI as by CT.

▶ Treatment

All patients with acute bacterial rhinosinusitis should have careful evaluation of pain. For symptom reduction in viral rhinitis and bacterial rhinosinusitis without complication, NSAIDs, saline nasal sprays, and nasal decongestants (pseudoephedrine, 30–60 mg every 6 hours, up to 240 mg/day; nasal oxymetazoline, 0.05% or oxymetazoline, 0.05–0.1%, one or two sprays in each nostril every 6–8 hours for up to 3 days) can be helpful. In cases of suspected bacterial rhinosinusitis, intranasal corticosteroids (eg, high-dose mometasone furoate 200 mcg each nostril twice daily for 21 days) can reduce nasal symptoms. Other medications, such as mucolytics, vitamin C, probiotics, and antihistamines, have *not* demonstrated efficacy in the management of acute rhinosinusitis.

Antibiotic therapy should be reserved for complicated or protracted acute bacterial rhinosinusitis. Between 40% and 69% of patients with acute bacterial rhinosinusitis improve symptomatically within 2 weeks without antibiotic therapy. Antibiotic treatment is controversial in uncomplicated cases of clinically diagnosed acute bacterial rhinosinusitis because only 5% of patients will note a shorter duration of illness with treatment, and antibiotic treatment is associated with nearly twice the number of adverse events compared with placebo. Antibiotics may be considered when symptoms last > 10 days or when symptoms (including fever, facial pain, and swelling of the face) are severe or when cases are complicated (such as immunodeficiency). In these patients, administration of antibiotics does reduce the incidence of clinical failure by 50% and represents the most cost-effective treatment strategy.

Selection of antibiotics is usually empiric and based on a number of factors, including regional patterns of antibiotic resistance, antibiotic allergy, cost, and patient tolerance. For adults younger than 65 years with mild to moderate acute bacterial rhinosinusitis, the recommended first-line therapy is amoxicillin-clavulanate (500 mg/125 mg orally three times daily or 875 mg/125 mg orally twice daily for 5–7 days), or in those with severe sinusitis, high-dose amoxicillin-clavulanate (2000 mg/125 mg extended-release orally twice daily for 7–10 days). In patients with a high risk for penicillin-resistant *S pneumoniae* (age over 65 years, hospitalization in the prior 5 days, antibiotic use in the prior month, immunocompromised status, multiple comorbidities, or severe sinus infection), the recommended first-line therapy is the high-dose amoxicillin-clavulanate option (2000 mg/125 mg extended-release orally twice daily for 7–10 days). For those with penicillin allergy or hepatic impairment, doxycycline (100 mg orally twice daily or 200 mg orally once daily for 5–7 days) or clindamycin (150–300 mg every 6 hours) plus a cephalosporin (cefixime 400 mg orally once daily or cefpodoxime proxetil 200 mg orally twice daily) for 10 days are options. Macrolides, trimethoprim-sulfamethoxazole, and second- or third-generation cephalosporins are not recommended for empiric therapy. Dupilumab, a monoclonal antibody with inhibition of IL-4 and IL-13, is approved for patients with chronic sinusitis with nasal polyposis.

Hospital-associated infections in critically ill patients are treated differently from community-acquired infections. Removal of a nasogastric tube and improved nasal hygiene (nasal saline sprays, humidification of supplemental nasal oxygen, and nasal decongestants) are critical interventions and often curative in mild cases without aggressive antibiotic use. Endoscopic or transantral cultures may help direct medical therapy in complicated cases. In addition, broad-spectrum antibiotic coverage directed at *P aeruginosa, S aureus* (including methicillin-resistant strains), and anaerobes may be required.

▶ Complications

Local complications of acute bacterial rhinosinusitis include orbital cellulitis and abscess, osteomyelitis, cavernous sinus thrombosis, and intracranial extension. Orbital complications typically occur by extension of ethmoid sinusitis through the lamina papyracea, a thin layer of bone that comprises the medial orbital wall. *Any change in the ocular examination necessitates immediate CT imaging.* Extension in this area may cause orbital cellulitis leading to proptosis, gaze restriction, and orbital pain. Select cases are responsive to intravenous antibiotics, with or without corticosteroids, and should be managed in close conjunction with an ophthalmologist or otolaryngologist, or both. Extension through the lamina papyracea can also lead to subperiosteal abscess formation (orbital abscess). Such abscesses cause marked proptosis, ophthalmoplegia, and pain with medial gaze. While some cases respond to antibiotics, such findings should prompt an immediate referral to a specialist for consideration of decompression and evacuation. Failure to intervene quickly may lead to permanent visual impairment and a "frozen globe."

Osteomyelitis requires prolonged antibiotics as well as removal of necrotic bone. The frontal sinus is most commonly affected, with bone involvement suggested by a tender swelling of the forehead (**Pott puffy tumor**). Following treatment, secondary cosmetic reconstructive procedures may be necessary.

Though rare, intracranial complications of sinusitis can occur either through hematogenous spread, as in cavernous sinus thrombosis and meningitis, or by direct extension, as in epidural and intraparenchymal brain abscesses. **Cavernous sinus thrombosis** is heralded by ophthalmoplegia, chemosis, and visual loss; the diagnosis is most commonly confirmed by MRI. When identified early, cavernous sinus thrombosis typically responds to intravenous antibiotics. Frontal epidural and intracranial abscesses are often clinically silent, but may present with altered mental status, persistent fever, or severe headache.

When to Refer

Failure of acute bacterial rhinosinusitis to resolve after an adequate course of oral antibiotics necessitates referral to an otolaryngologist for evaluation. Endoscopic cultures may direct further treatment choices. Nasal endoscopy and CT scan are indicated when symptoms persist longer than 4–12 weeks. Any patients with suspected extension of disease outside the sinuses should be evaluated urgently by an otolaryngologist and imaging should be obtained.

When to Admit

- Facial swelling and erythema indicative of facial cellulitis.
- Proptosis.
- Vision change or gaze abnormality indicative of orbital cellulitis.
- Abscess or cavernous sinus involvement.
- Mental status changes suggestive of intracranial extension.
- Failure to respond to appropriate first-line treatment or symptoms persisting longer than 4 weeks.

Cai S et al. Efficacy and safety of biologics for chronic rhinosinusitis with nasal polyps: a meta-analysis of real-world evidence. Allergy. 2025;80:1256. [PMID: 39985317]

Papacharalampous GX et al. Chronic rhinosinusitis with nasal polyps (CRSwNP) treated with omalizumab, dupilumab, or mepolizumab: a systematic review of the current knowledge towards an attempt to compare agents' efficacy. Int Forum Allergy Rhinol. 2024;14:96. [PMID: 37394893]

Poto R et al. Imaging of chronic rhinosinusitis with nasal polyps in the era of biological therapies. Curr Opin Allergy Clin Immunol. 2024;24:243. [PMID: 38205820]

Tănase MI et al. Biologic treatments for chronic rhinosinusitis with nasal polyps (CRSwNP): a comparative review of efficiency and risks. Cureus. 2025;17:e77804. [PMID: 39844880]

3. Nasal Vestibulitis & S aureus Nasal Colonization

Inflammation of the nasal vestibule may result from folliculitis of the hairs that line this orifice and is usually the result of nasal manipulation or hair trimming. Systemic antibiotics effective against *S aureus* (such as dicloxacillin, 250 mg orally four times daily for 7–10 days) are indicated. Topical mupirocin 2% nasal ointment (applied two or three times daily) also may be a helpful addition and may prevent future occurrences. If recurrent, the addition of rifampin (10 mg/kg orally twice daily for the last 4 days of dicloxacillin treatment) may eliminate the *S aureus* carrier state. If a furuncle exists, it should be incised and drained, preferably intranasally. Adequate treatment of these infections is important to prevent retrograde spread of infection through valveless veins into the cavernous sinus and intracranial structures.

S aureus is the leading nosocomial pathogen, and nasal carriage is a well-defined risk factor in the development and spread of nosocomial infections. Nasal and extranasal methicillin-resistant *S aureus* (MRSA) colonizations are associated with a 30% risk of developing an invasive MRSA infection during hospital stays. While the vast majority have no vestibulitis symptoms, screening by nasal swabs and PCR-based assays has demonstrated a 30% rate of *S aureus* colonization in hospital patients and an 11% rate of MRSA colonization in ICU patients. Elimination of the carrier state is challenging, but studies of mupirocin 2% nasal ointment application with chlorhexidine facial washing (40 mg/mL) twice daily for 5 days have demonstrated decolonization in 39% of patients.

Bessesen MT. Interventions targeting the nasal microbiome to eradicate methicillin-resistant *Staphylococcus*. Clin Microbiol Infect. 2025;31:190. [PMID: 39481681]

Ontario Health (Quality). Pre-surgical nasal decolonization of *Staphylococcus aureus*: a health technology assessment. Ont Health Technol Assess Ser. 2022;22:1. [PMID: 36160757]

Rigaill J et al. Staphylococcus aureus nasal colonization level and intracellular reservoir: a prospective cohort study. Eur J Clin Microbiol Infect Dis. 2023;42:621. [PMID: 36964269]

4. Invasive Fungal Sinusitis

Invasive fungal sinusitis is rare and includes both rhinocerebral mucormycosis (*Mucor, Absidia*, and *Rhizopus* spp.) and other invasive fungal infections, such as *Aspergillus*.

The fungus spreads rapidly through vascular channels and may be lethal if not detected early. Patients with mucormycosis almost invariably have some degree of immunocompromise, such as diabetes mellitus, long-term corticosteroid therapy, neutropenia associated with chemotherapy for hematologic malignancy, or end-stage renal disease. Occasional cases of sinonasal infection with *Aspergillus* spp. have been reported in patients with untreated HIV/AIDS. The initial symptoms may be similar to those of acute bacterial rhinosinusitis, although facial pain is often more severe. Nasal drainage is typically clear or straw-colored, rather than purulent, and visual symptoms may be noted at presentation in the absence of significant nasal findings. On examination, the classic finding of mucormycosis is a black eschar on the middle turbinate, but this finding is not universal and may not be apparent if the infection is deep or high within the nasal bones. Often the mucosa appears normal or simply pale and dry. This may be noted on the hard palate as well. Early diagnosis requires suspicion of the disease and nasal biopsy with silver stains, revealing broad nonseptate hyphae within tissues and necrosis with vascular occlusion. Imaging, such as CT or MRI, may initially show only soft tissue changes. Consequently, biopsy and ultimate debridement should be based on the clinical setting rather than radiographic demonstration of bony destruction or intracranial changes.

Invasive fungal sinusitis represents a medical and surgical emergency. Once recognized, voriconazole may be started by intravenous infusion, and prompt wide surgical debridement is indicated for patients with reversible immune deficiency (eg, poorly controlled hyperglycemia in diabetes). Other antifungals, including amphotericin or the less nephrotoxic lipid-based amphotericin B (Ambisome) and caspofungin, are alternatives to voriconazole and may be added to voriconazole depending on the fungus. Surgical management, while necessary for any possibility of cure, often results in tremendous disfigurement and functional deficits (eg, often resulting in the loss of at least one eye). Even with early diagnosis and immediate appropriate intervention, the prognosis is guarded. In persons with diabetes, the mortality rate is about 20%. If kidney disease is present or develops, mortality is over 50%; in the setting of AIDS or hematologic malignancy with neutropenia, mortality approaches 100%. Whether to undertake aggressive surgical management should be considered carefully because many patients are gravely ill at the time of diagnosis, and overall disease-specific survival is only about 57%.

Franzese C. Fungal sinusitis-invasive versus noninvasive. Med Clin North Am. 2026;110:45. [PMID: 41206202]

Gonzalez ML et al. Fungal infections of the sinonasal tract and their differential diagnoses. Surg Pathol Clin. 2024;17:533. [PMID: 39489547]

Luo YT et al. Diagnostic and therapeutic strategies of acute invasive fungal rhinosinusitis. Asian J Surg. 2023;46:58. [PMID: 35589479]

Tessler I et al. Impact of azole antifungal treatment on outcome in acute invasive fungal rhinosinusitis with orbitocranial involvement: a surgical perspective. Rhinology. 2023;61:561. [PMID: 37566791]

ALLERGIC RHINITIS

ESSENTIALS OF DIAGNOSIS

- Clear rhinorrhea, sneezing, tearing, eye irritation, and pruritus.
- Associated symptoms include cough, bronchospasm, and eczematous dermatitis.
- Environmental allergen exposure in the presence of allergen-specific IgE.

General Considerations

Allergic rhinitis is very common in the United States, with a prevalence of 20–30% of adults and up to 40% of children. Allergic rhinitis adversely affects school and work performance, costing about $6 billion annually in the United States through direct costs of therapy as well as the indirect costs of sleep deprivation, fatigue and reduced productivity, or absenteeism. Seasonal allergic rhinitis is most commonly caused by pollens and spores. Flowering shrub and tree pollens are most common in the spring, flowering plants and grasses in the summer, and ragweed and molds in the fall. *Climate change may have an impact on the occurrence of allergic rhinitis* since increased temperature and carbon dioxide exposure cause increased pollen production in ragweed plants and since the extended duration of summer correlates with longer periods of pollen production in these and other flowering weeds. Dust, household mites, air pollution, and pet dander may produce year-round symptoms, termed "**perennial rhinitis**."

Clinical Findings

The symptoms of "hay fever" are similar to those of viral rhinitis but are usually persistent and may show seasonal variation. Nasal symptoms are often accompanied by eye irritation, pruritus, conjunctival erythema, and excessive tearing. Many patients have a strong family history of atopy or allergy.

The clinician should be careful to distinguish allergic rhinitis from other types of nonallergic rhinitis. **Vasomotor rhinitis** (sometimes called **senile rhinitis**) is caused by increased sensitivity of the vidian nerve and is a common cause of clear rhinorrhea in older adults. Often patients will report that they have troubling rhinorrhea in response to numerous nasal stimuli, including warm or cold air, odors or scents, light, or particulate matter. Other types of rhinitis, including gustatory, atrophic, and drug-induced rhinorrhea, have also been described.

On physical examination, the mucosa of the turbinates is usually pale or violaceous because of venous engorgement. This is in contrast to the erythema of viral rhinitis. Nasal polyps, which are yellowish boggy masses of hypertrophic mucosa, are associated with long-standing allergic rhinitis.

Treatment

A. Intranasal Corticosteroids

Intranasal corticosteroid sprays remain the mainstay of treatment of allergic rhinitis. They are more effective and frequently less expensive than nonsedating antihistamines, though patients should be reminded that there may be a delay in onset of relief of 2 or more weeks. Corticosteroid sprays may also shrink hypertrophic nasal mucosa and nasal polyps, thereby providing an improved nasal airway and ostiomeatal complex drainage. Because of this effect, intranasal corticosteroids are critical in treating allergy in patients prone to recurrent acute bacterial rhinosinusitis or chronic rhinosinusitis. Available preparations include beclomethasone (42 mcg/spray twice daily per nostril), flunisolide (25 mcg/spray twice daily per nostril), mometasone furoate (200 mcg once daily per nostril), budesonide (100 mcg twice daily per nostril), and fluticasone propionate (200 mcg once daily per nostril). All are considered equally effective. Probably the most critical factors are compliance with regular use and proper introduction into the nasal cavity. In order to deliver medication to the region of the middle meatus, proper application involves *holding the bottle straight up with the head tilted forward and pointing the bottle toward the ipsilateral ear when spraying.*

B. Antihistamines

Antihistamines offer temporary, but immediate, control of many of the most troubling symptoms of allergic rhinitis. Effective oral antihistamines include nonsedating loratadine (10 mg once daily), desloratadine (5 mg once daily), and fexofenadine (60 mg twice daily or 120 mg once daily), and minimally sedating cetirizine (10 mg once daily). Brompheniramine or chlorpheniramine (4 mg orally every 6–8 hours, or 8–12 mg orally every 8–12 hours as a sustained-release tablet) and clemastine (1.34–2.68 mg orally twice daily) may be less expensive but are usually associated with some drowsiness. The safety and efficacy of the newer, less-sedating antihistamines is so compelling that one of them, the H_1-receptor antagonist nasal spray azelastine (1–2 sprays per nostril daily), is included in the treatment guidelines of many consensus statements; however, some patients object to its bitter taste. Other side effects of oral antihistamines besides sedation include xerostomia and antihistamine tolerance (with eventual return of allergy symptoms despite initial benefit after several months of use). In such patients, typically those with perennial allergy, alternating effective antihistamines periodically can control symptoms over the long term. A nasal spray containing the corticosteroid mometasone (25 mcg) and the H_1-inhibitor olopatadine hydrochloride (665 mcg) (Ryaltris) is approved for seasonal allergic rhinitis (2 sprays in each nostril daily).

C. Adjunctive Treatment Measures

Antileukotriene medications, such as montelukast (10 mg/day orally), alone or with cetirizine (10 mg/day orally) or loratadine (10 mg/day orally), may improve nasal rhinorrhea, sneezing, and congestion. Cromolyn sodium and sodium nedocromil may be useful adjunct agents for allergic rhinitis. They work by stabilizing mast cells and preventing proinflammatory mediator release. As topical agents, they have very few side effects, but they must be initiated *well before* allergen exposure (up to 4 weeks before). The most useful form of cromolyn is probably the ophthalmologic preparation placed dropwise into the nasal cavity. Intranasal cromolyn is cleared rapidly and must be administered four times daily for continued symptom relief. In practice, it is not nearly as effective as inhaled corticosteroid.

Intranasal anticholinergic agents, such as ipratropium bromide 0.03% or 0.06% sprays (42–84 mcg per nostril three times daily), may be helpful adjuncts when rhinorrhea is a major symptom. They are not as effective for treating allergic rhinitis but are more useful for treating vasomotor rhinitis.

Avoiding or reducing exposure to airborne allergens is the most effective means of alleviating symptoms of allergic rhinitis. Depending on the allergen, this can be extremely difficult. Maintaining an allergen-free environment by covering pillows and mattresses with plastic covers, substituting synthetic materials (foam mattress, acrylics) for animal products (wool, horsehair), and removing dust-collecting household fixtures (carpets, drapes, bedspreads, wicker) is worth the attempt to help more troubled patients. Air purifiers and dust filters may also aid in maintaining an allergen-free environment. Nasal saline irrigations are a useful adjunct in the treatment of allergic rhinitis to mechanically flush the allergens from the nasal cavity. When symptoms are extremely bothersome, a search for offending allergens may prove helpful. This can either be done by serum radioallergosorbent test (RAST) testing or skin testing by an allergist.

In some cases, allergic rhinitis symptoms are inadequately relieved by medication and avoidance measures. Often, such patients have a strong family history of atopy and may also have lower respiratory manifestations, such as allergic asthma. Referral to an otolaryngologist or allergist for **immunotherapy** may be appropriate. Such treatment involves proper identification of offending allergens, progressively increasing doses of allergen(s), and eventual maintenance dose administration over a period of 3–5 years. Immunotherapy has been proven to reduce circulating IgE levels in patients with allergic rhinitis and reduce the need for allergy medications. Both subcutaneous and topical immunotherapy have been shown to be effective in the long-term treatment of refractory allergic rhinitis.

Park M et al. Sublingual immunotherapy persistence and adherence in real-world settings: a systematic review. Int Forum Allergy Rhinol. 2023;13:924. [PMID: 36083179]

Pfaar O et al. Chronic rhinosinusitis with nasal polyps: key considerations in the multidisciplinary team approach. Clin Transl Allergy. 2025;15:e70010. [PMID: 39794887]

Wang H et al. A systematic review and meta-analysis of loratadine combined with montelukast for the treatment of allergic rhinitis. Front Pharmacol. 2023;14:1287320. [PMID: 37915414]

Wang Z et al. Efficacy and safety of sublingual immunotherapy for allergic rhinitis: an overview of systematic reviews and meta analyses. Eur Arch Otorhinolaryngol. 2025 Sep 11. [Epub ahead of print] [PMID: 40935870]

OLFACTORY DYSFUNCTION

ESSENTIALS OF DIAGNOSIS

- Subjective diminished smell or taste sensation.
- Lack of objective nasal obstruction.
- Objective decrease in olfaction demonstrated by testing.

General Considerations

Anatomic blockage of the nasal cavity with subsequent airflow disruption is the most common cause of olfactory dysfunction (hyposmia or anosmia). Polyps, septal deformities, and nasal tumors may be the cause. Due to localized inflammation, transient olfactory dysfunction often accompanies the common cold, nasal allergies, and perennial rhinitis through changes in the nasal and olfactory epithelium. About 20% of olfactory dysfunction is idiopathic, although it often follows a viral illness.

CNS neoplasms, especially those that involve the olfactory groove or temporal lobe, also may affect olfaction and should be considered in patients with no other explanation for their hyposmia. Head trauma is also a rare but severe cause of olfactory dysfunction due to shearing of the olfactory sensory cells. Head trauma accounts for < 5% of cases of hyposmia but is more commonly associated with anosmia than with hyposmia. Absent, diminished, or distorted smell has been reported in a wide variety of endocrine, nutritional, and nervous disorders.

Clinical Findings

Evaluation of olfactory dysfunction should include a thorough history of systemic illnesses and medication use as well as a physical examination focusing on the nose and nervous system. Nasal obstruction (from polyps, trauma, foreign bodies, or nasal masses) can cause functional hyposmia. Most clinical offices are not set up to test olfaction, but such tests may at times be worthwhile if only to assess whether a patient possesses any sense of smell at all.

Treatment

Olfactory dysfunction secondary to nasal polyposis, obstruction, and chronic rhinosinusitis may respond to surgically removing the anatomic blockage, as with endoscopic sinus surgery. Unfortunately, there is no specific treatment for primary disruption of olfaction; some disturbances spontaneously resolve. The degree of olfactory dysfunction is the greatest predictor of recovery, with less severe olfactory dysfunction recovering at a much higher rate. In permanent olfactory dysfunction, counseling should be offered about seasoning foods (such as using pepper that stimulates the trigeminal as well as olfactory chemoreceptors, rather than table salt) and safety issues (such as installing home smoke alarms and using electric rather than gas appliances).

De Cleene N et al. Olfactory dysfunction as potential biomarker in neurodegenerative diseases: a narrative review. Front Neurosci. 2025;18:1505029. [PMID: 39840019]
Krishnakumar HN et al. Pathogenesis and progression of anosmia and dysgeusia during the COVID-19 pandemic. Eur Arch Otorhinolaryngol. 2023;280:505. [PMID: 36209486]
O'Byrne L et al. Interventions for the treatment of persistent post-COVID-19 olfactory dysfunction. Cochrane Database Syst Rev. 2022;9:CD013876. [PMID: 36062970]
Schepens EJA et al. Diagnostic accuracy of the screenings Sniffin' Sticks Test (SST-12) in COVID-19 induced olfactory disorders. PLoS One. 2024;19:e0295911. [PMID: 38198490]
Zhang Z et al. Chronic sinusitis with nasal polyps and olfactory dysfunction: comparing olfactory training and glucocorticoid treatment. Laryngoscope. 2025;135:3824. [PMID: 40265744]

EPISTAXIS

ESSENTIALS OF DIAGNOSIS

- Bleeding from a unilateral anterior nasal cavity along the septum is most common.
- Most cases may be successfully treated by direct pressure on the bleeding site for 15 minutes. When this is inadequate, topical sympathomimetics and various nasal tamponade methods are usually effective.
- Posterior, bilateral, or large-volume epistaxis should be triaged immediately to a specialist in a critical care setting.

General Considerations

Epistaxis is an extremely common problem in the primary care setting. Bleeding is most common in the anterior septum where a confluence of veins creates a superficial venous plexus (**Kiesselbach plexus**). Predisposing factors include nasal trauma (nose picking, foreign bodies, forceful nose blowing), rhinitis, nasal mucosal drying from low humidity or supplemental nasal oxygen, deviation of the nasal septum, atherosclerotic disease, hereditary hemorrhagic telangiectasia (**Osler-Weber-Rendu syndrome**), inhaled nasal cocaine (or other drugs), and alcohol abuse. Poorly controlled hypertension is associated with epistaxis. Anticoagulation or antiplatelet medications may be associated with a higher incidence, more frequent recurrence, and greater difficulty in control of epistaxis, but they do not cause it.

Clinical Findings

Laboratory assessment of bleeding parameters may be indicated, especially in recurrent epistaxis. Once the acute episode has passed, careful examination of the nose and paranasal sinuses is indicated to rule out neoplasia and hereditary hemorrhagic telangiectasia. Repeated evaluation for diagnosis and treatment of clinically significant hypertension should be performed following control of epistaxis and removal of any packing.

Treatment

Most cases of anterior epistaxis may be successfully treated by direct pressure on the site by compression of the nares continuously for 15 minutes. Venous pressure is reduced in the sitting position, and slight leaning forward. Positioning the head backwards is *not* recommended because this may result in blood going toward the airway, resulting in possible aspiration. Similarly, pinching the bridge of the nose is generally ineffective as the origin of bleeding typically occurs at the tip. Short-acting topical nasal decongestants (eg, phenylephrine, 0.125–1% solution, one or two sprays or oxymetazoline), which act as vasoconstrictors, may also help. When the bleeding does not readily subside, the nose should be examined, using good illumination and suction, in an attempt to locate the bleeding site. When directly visible, the bleeding site may be cauterized with silver nitrate, diathermy, or electrocautery. A supplemental patch of Surgicel or Gelfoam may be helpful with a moisture barrier, such as petroleum-based ointment, to prevent drying and crusting.

Occasionally, a site of bleeding may be inaccessible to direct control, or attempts at direct control may be unsuccessful. In such cases, there are a number of alternatives. When the site of bleeding is anterior, a hemostatic sealant, pneumatic or other nasal tamponade, or anterior packing may suffice as the latter may be accomplished with several feet of lubricated iodoform packing systematically placed in the floor of the nose and then the vault of the nose.

About 5% of nasal bleeding originates in the posterior nasal cavity, commonly associated with atherosclerotic disease and hypertension. In such cases, it may be necessary to consult an otolaryngologist for a pack to occlude the choana before placing a pack anteriorly. In emergency settings, double balloon packs (Epistat) may facilitate rapid control of bleeding with little or no mucosal trauma. Because such packing is uncomfortable, bleeding may persist, and vasovagal syncope is possible, hospitalization for monitoring and stabilization is indicated. Posterior nasal packing is quite uncomfortable and may require an opioid analgesic for pain control.

Surgical management of epistaxis, through ligation of the nasal arterial supply (internal maxillary artery and ethmoid arteries) is indicated when direct pressure and nasal packing fail. The most common approach to surgical treatment is endoscopic sphenopalatine artery ligation. This method has a reported efficacy of 73–100% in studies; however, it may miss bleeds caused by the ethmoid arterial supply. Alternatively, endovascular epistaxis control is highly effective (75–92%) and can address all sources of intranasal bleeding except those from the anterior ethmoid artery. Its use may be reserved for when a surgical approach fails because it is associated with a 1.1–1.5% risk of stroke.

After control of epistaxis, the patient is advised to avoid straining and vigorous exercise for several days. Nasal saline should be applied to the packing frequently to keep the packing moist. Avoidance of hot or spicy foods and tobacco is also advisable, since these may cause nasal vasodilation. Avoiding nasal trauma, including nose picking, is an obvious necessity. Lubrication with petroleum jelly or bacitracin ointment and increased home humidity may also be useful ancillary measures. Finally, antistaphylococcal antibiotics (eg, cephalexin, 500 mg orally four times daily, or clindamycin, 150 mg orally four times daily) generally are indicated to reduce the risk of toxic shock syndrome developing while the packing remains in place (at least 5 days).

When to Refer

- Patients with recurrent epistaxis, large-volume epistaxis, and episodic epistaxis with associated nasal obstruction should be referred to an otolaryngologist for endoscopic evaluation and possible imaging.
- Those with ongoing bleeding beyond 15 minutes should be taken to a local emergency department if the clinician is not prepared to manage acute epistaxis.

Chitsuthipakorn W et al. Treatments of epistaxis in hereditary hemorrhagic telangiectasia: systematic review and network meta-analysis. Curr Allergy Asthma Rep. 2023;23:689. [PMID: 37995018]

Thiele B et al. Sclerotherapy for hereditary hemorrhagic telangiectasia-related epistaxis: a systematic review. Ann Otol Rhinol Laryngol. 2023;132:82. [PMID: 35152768]

NASAL TRAUMA

The nasal pyramid is the most frequently fractured bone in the body. Fracture is suggested by crepitance or palpably mobile bony segments. Epistaxis and pain are common, as are soft-tissue hematomas ("black eye"). It is important to make certain that there is no palpable step-off of the infraorbital rim, which would indicate the presence of a zygomatic complex fracture. Radiologic confirmation may at times be helpful but is not necessary in uncomplicated nasal fractures. It is also important to assess for possible concomitant additional facial, spine, pulmonary, or intracranial injuries when the circumstances of injury are suggestive, as in the case of automobile and motorcycle accidents.

Treatment is aimed at maintaining long-term nasal airway patency and cosmesis. Closed reduction can be performed under local or general anesthesia; closed reduction under general anesthesia appears to afford better patient satisfaction and decreased need for subsequent revision septoplasty or rhinoplasty.

Intranasal examination should be performed in all cases to rule out septal hematoma, which appears as a widening of the anterior septum, visible just posterior to the columella. The septal cartilage receives its only nutrition from its closely adherent mucoperichondrium. An untreated subperichondrial hematoma will result in loss of the nasal cartilage with resultant saddle nose deformity, septal perforation, or both. Septal hematomas may become infected, with *S aureus* most commonly, and should be drained with an incision in the inferior mucoperichondrium on both sides. The drained fluid should be sent for culture.

Packing for 2–5 days is often helpful to help prevent re-formation of the hematoma. Antibiotics with antistaphylococcal efficacy (eg, cephalexin, 500 mg four times daily, or clindamycin, 150 mg four times daily) should be given for 3–5 days or the duration of the packing to reduce the risk of toxic shock syndrome.

TUMORS & GRANULOMATOUS DISEASE

1. Benign Nasal Tumors

A. Nasal Polyps

Nasal polyps are pale, edematous, mucosally covered masses commonly seen in patients with allergic rhinitis. They may result in chronic nasal obstruction and a diminished sense of smell. In patients with nasal polyps and a history of asthma, aspirin should be avoided because it may precipitate a severe episode of bronchospasm, known as **triad asthma** ("Samter triad"). Such patients may have an immunologic salicylate sensitivity.

Use of topical intranasal corticosteroids improves the quality of life in patients with nasal polyposis and chronic rhinosinusitis. Initial treatment with topical nasal corticosteroids (see Allergic Rhinitis section for specific medications) for 1–3 months is usually successful for small polyps and may reduce the need for operation. A short course of oral corticosteroids (eg, prednisone, 6-day course using 21 [5 mg] tablets: 6 tablets [30 mg] on day 1 and tapering by 1 tablet [5 mg] each day) may also be of benefit, but when polyps are massive or medical management is unsuccessful obstructing polyps may be removed surgically. Polyps may readily be removed using endoscopic sinus surgery techniques. It may be necessary to remove polyps from the ethmoid, sphenoid, and maxillary sinuses to provide longer-lasting relief and open the affected sinuses. Intranasal corticosteroids should be continued following polyp removal to prevent recurrence, and the clinician should consider allergen testing to determine the offending allergen and avoidance measures. There are emerging treatments using biologics, such as dupilumab, for treatment of chronic rhinosinusitis with polyps.

Jin Z et al. Biological therapy in chronic rhinosinusitis with nasal polyps. Expert Rev Clin Immunol. 2025:1. [PMID: 39862235]
Lechien JR et al. Association between Helicobacter pylori, reflux and chronic rhinosinusitis: a systematic review. Eur Arch Otorhinolaryngol. 2025 Feb 2. [Epub ahead of print] [PMID: 39893593]
Papacharalampous GX et al. Chronic rhinosinusitis with nasal polyps (CRSwNP) treated with omalizumab, dupilumab, or mepolizumab: a systematic review of the current knowledge towards an attempt to compare agents' efficacy. Int Forum Allergy Rhinol. 2024;14:96. [PMID: 37394893]

B. Inverted Papillomas

Inverted papillomas are benign tumors caused by HPV that usually arise on the lateral nasal wall. They present with unilateral nasal obstruction and occasionally hemorrhage. They are often easily seen on anterior rhinoscopy as cauliflower-like growths in or around the middle meatus. *Because squamous cell carcinoma is seen in about 10% of inverted or schneiderian papillomas, complete excision is strongly recommended.* This usually requires an endoscopic medial maxillectomy. While rare, very extensive disease may require an open inferior or total maxillectomy for complete removal. Because recurrence rates for inverted papillomas are reported to be as high as 20%, subsequent clinical and radiologic follow-up is imperative. All excised tissue (not just a portion) should be carefully reviewed by the pathologist to be sure no carcinoma is present.

Alqudrah F et al. Human papilloma virus infection and sinonasal inverted papilloma recurrence: a meta-analysis. Otolaryngol Head Neck Surg. 2025;172:1155. [PMID: 39739414]
El-Adem D et al. The role of positron emission tomography for the management of sinonasal malignancies: a systematic review. Am J Rhinol Allergy. 2023;37:593. [PMID: 37229633]
Ferreli F et al. Association between human papillomavirus infection and malignant transformation of sinonasal inverted papilloma: a systematic review and meta-analysis. Am J Otolaryngol. 2022;43:103614. [PMID: 36113312]

2. Malignant Nasopharyngeal & Paranasal Sinus Tumors

Though rare, malignant tumors of the nose, nasopharynx, and paranasal sinuses are quite problematic because they tend to remain asymptomatic until late in their course. *Squamous cell carcinoma is the most common cancer found in the sinuses and nasopharynx.* It is especially common in the nasopharynx, where it obstructs the eustachian tube and results in serous otitis media. Nasopharyngeal carcinoma (nonkeratinizing squamous cell carcinoma or lymphoepithelioma) is usually associated with elevated IgA antibody to the viral capsid antigen of the Epstein-Barr virus (EBV). It is particularly common in patients of southern Chinese descent and has a weaker association with tobacco exposure than other head and neck squamous cell carcinomas. Adenocarcinomas, mucosal melanomas, sarcomas, and non-Hodgkin lymphomas are less commonly encountered neoplasms of this area.

Early symptoms are nonspecific, mimicking those of rhinitis or sinusitis. Unilateral nasal obstruction, otitis media, and discharge are common, with pain and recurrent hemorrhage often clues to the diagnosis of cancer. *All adults with persistent unilateral nasal symptoms or new otitis media should be thoroughly evaluated with nasal endoscopy and nasopharyngoscopy.* A high index of suspicion remains a key to early diagnosis of these tumors. Patients often present with advanced symptoms, such as proptosis, expansion of a cheek, or ill-fitting maxillary dentures. Malar hypesthesia, due to involvement of the infraorbital nerve, is common in maxillary sinus tumors. Biopsy is necessary for definitive diagnosis, and MRI is the best imaging study to delineate the extent of disease and plan appropriate surgery and radiation.

Treatment depends on the tumor type and the extent of disease. Early-stage disease may be treated with radiation therapy alone, but advanced nasopharyngeal carcinoma is best treated with concurrent radiation and chemotherapy. Chemoradiation therapy significantly decreases local, nodal, and distant failures and increases progression-free and overall survival in advanced disease. Locally recurrent nasopharyngeal carcinoma in selected cases may be treated with repeat irradiation protocols or surgery with moderate success and a high degree of concern about local wound healing. Other squamous cell carcinomas are best treated—when resectable—with a combination of surgery and irradiation. Cranial base surgery, which can be done endoscopically using image navigation, appears to be an effective modality in improving the overall prognosis in paranasal sinus malignancies eroding the ethmoid roof. Although the prognosis is poor for advanced tumors, the results of treating resectable tumors of paranasal sinus origin have improved with the wider use of skull base resections and intensity-modulated radiation therapy. Cure rates are often 45–60%.

Guven DC et al. Immunotherapy in the first-line treatment of advanced nasopharyngeal carcinoma: a systematic review and meta-analysis. Laryngoscope. 2024;134:7. [PMID: 37227161]
Luo J et al. Efficacy and safety of PD-1 inhibitors in recurrent or metastatic nasopharyngeal carcinoma patients after failure of platinum-containing regimens: a systematic review and meta-analysis. BMC Cancer. 2023;23:1172. [PMID: 38037076]

3. Sinonasal Inflammatory Disease (Granulomatosis with Polyangiitis & Sarcoidosis)

The nose and paranasal sinuses are involved in over 90% of cases of **granulomatosis with polyangiitis**. It is often not realized that involvement at these sites is *more common* than involvement of lungs or kidneys. Examination shows bloodstained crusts and friable mucosa. Biopsy, when positive, shows necrotizing granulomas and vasculitis. Other recognized sites of granulomatosis with polyangiitis in the head and neck include the subglottis and the middle ear. For treatment of granulomatosis with polyangiitis, see Chapter 23.

Sarcoidosis commonly involves the paranasal sinuses and is clinically similar to other chronic sinonasal inflammatory processes. Sinonasal symptoms, including rhinorrhea, nasal obstruction, and hyposmia or anosmia, may precede diagnosis of sarcoidosis in other organ systems. Clinically, the turbinates appear engorged with small white granulomas. Biopsy shows classic noncaseating granulomas. Notably, patients with sinonasal involvement generally have more trouble managing sarcoidosis in other organ systems.

Polymorphic reticulosis (midline malignant reticulosis, idiopathic midline destructive disease, lethal midline granuloma)—as the multitude of apt descriptive terms suggests—is not well understood but appears to be a nasal T-cell or NK-cell lymphoma. In contrast to granulomatosis with polyangiitis, involvement is limited to the mid-face, and there may be extensive bone destruction. Many destructive lesions of the mucosa and nasal structures labeled as polymorphic reticulosis are in fact non-Hodgkin lymphoma of either NK-cell or T-cell origin. Immunophenotyping, especially for CD56 expression, is essential in the histologic evaluation. Even when apparently localized, these lymphomas have a poor prognosis, with progression and death within a year the rule.

Almuhanna A et al. Current therapeutic approaches to subglottic stenosis in patients with GPA: a systematic review. Ear Nose Throat J. 2024;103:117. [PMID: 34392732]
Pavlidis P et al. Morphological changes in nasal mucosa in patients with sarcoidosis. Clin Otolaryngol. 2022;47:212. [PMID: 34555266]

DISEASES OF THE ORAL CAVITY & PHARYNX

LEUKOPLAKIA, ERYTHROPLAKIA, LICHEN PLANUS, & OROPHARYNGEAL CANCER

ESSENTIALS OF DIAGNOSIS

- **Leukoplakia:** A white plaque-like lesion that cannot be removed by rubbing the mucosal surface.
- **Erythroplakia:** Similar to leukoplakia except that it has a definite erythematous component.
- **Oral lichen planus:** Most commonly presents as lacy leukoplakia but may be erosive; definitive diagnosis requires biopsy.
- **Oral cancer:** Early lesions appear as leukoplakia or erythroplakia; more advanced lesions will be larger, painful, and can involve the tongue, gums, hard palate, inner lining of the lips or cheek. Ulceration may be present.
- **Oropharyngeal cancer:** Masses arising from the throat (tonsils, base of tongue, soft palate, or pharyngeal wall) typically presenting with painful swallowing, persistent ear pain, and weight loss.

Leukoplakic regions range from small to several centimeters in diameter (Figure 8–5). Histologically, they are often hyperkeratoses occurring in response to chronic irritation (eg, from dentures, tobacco, lichen planus); about 2–6%, however, represent either dysplasia or early invasive squamous cell carcinoma. *Distinguishing between **leukoplakia** and **erythroplakia** is important because about 90% of cases of erythroplakia are either dysplasia or carcinoma.* **Squamous cell carcinoma** accounts for 90% of oral cancer. Alcohol and tobacco use are the major epidemiologic risk factors.

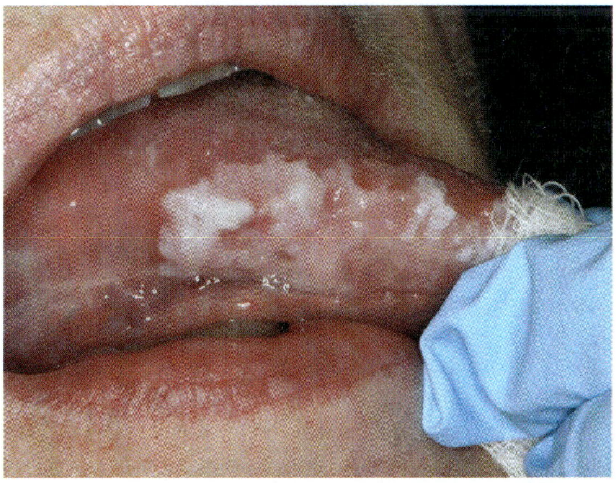

▲ **Figure 8–5.** Leukoplakia with moderate dysplasia on the lateral border of the tongue. (Used, with permission, from Ellen Eisenberg, DMD, in Usatine RP, Smith MA, Mayeaux EJ Jr, Chumley H. *The Color Atlas of Family Medicine*, 2nd ed. McGraw-Hill, 2013.)

The differential diagnosis may include oral candidiasis, necrotizing sialometaplasia, pseudoepitheliomatous hyperplasia, median rhomboid glossitis, and vesiculoerosive inflammatory disease, such as erosive lichen planus. This should not be confused with the brown-black gingival melanin pigmentation—diffuse or speckled—common in non-White persons, blue-black embedded fragments of dental amalgam, or other systemic disorders associated with general pigmentation (neurofibromatosis, familial polyposis, Addison disease). Intraoral melanoma is extremely rare and carries a dismal prognosis.

Any area of erythroplakia, enlarging area of leukoplakia, or a lesion that has submucosal depth on palpation or irregular appearance associated with pain or other symptoms should have an incisional biopsy. Ulcerative lesions are particularly suspicious and worrisome. Specialty referral should be sought early both for diagnosis and treatment. A systematic intraoral examination—including the lateral tongue, floor of the mouth, gingiva, buccal area, palate, and tonsillar fossae—and palpation of the neck for enlarged lymph nodes should be part of any general physical examination. Patients with current or former tobacco use or moderate alcohol drinking history are at higher risk of malignancy. Indirect or fiberoptic examination of the nasopharynx, oropharynx, hypopharynx, and larynx by an otolaryngologist, head and neck surgeon should be considered for such patients when there is unexplained or persistent throat or ear pain, oral or nasal bleeding, or oral erythroplakia. Fine-needle aspiration (FNA) biopsy may expedite the diagnosis if an enlarged lymph node is found.

To date, there remain no approved therapies for reversing or stabilizing leukoplakia or erythroplakia. The mainstays of management are surveillance following elimination of carcinogenic irritants (eg, smoking tobacco, chewing tobacco or betel nut, drinking alcohol) along with serial biopsies and excisions.

Oral lichen planus is a relatively common (0.5–2% of the population) chronic inflammatory autoimmune disease that may be difficult to diagnose clinically because of its numerous distinct phenotypic subtypes. For example, the reticular pattern may mimic candidiasis or hyperkeratosis, while the erosive pattern may mimic squamous cell carcinoma. Management begins with distinguishing it from other oral lesions. Exfoliative cytology or a small incisional or excisional biopsy is indicated, especially if squamous cell carcinoma is suspected. Therapy of lichen planus is aimed at managing pain and discomfort. Daily topical corticosteroid remains the most effective treatment for symptomatic lichen planus, but cyclosporine, retinoids, and tacrolimus have also been used. Many experts think there is a low rate (1%) of squamous cell carcinoma arising within lichen planus (in addition to the possibility of clinical misdiagnosis) and prevention of malignant transformation remains a goal of treatment.

Hairy leukoplakia occurs on the lateral border of the tongue and is a common early finding in HIV infection (see Chapter 35). It often develops quickly and appears as slightly raised leukoplakic areas with a corrugated or "hairy" surface (Figure 8–6). While much more prevalent in patients with HIV, hairy leukoplakia can occur following solid organ transplantation and is associated with EBV

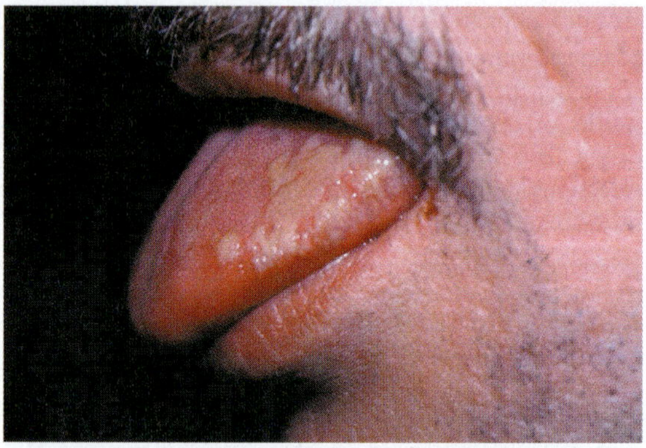

▲ **Figure 8–6.** Oral hairy leukoplakia on the side of the tongue in AIDS. (Reproduced, with permission, from Richard P. Usatine, MD, in Usatine RP, Smith MA, Mayeaux EJ Jr, Chumley H. *The Color Atlas of Family Medicine*, 2nd ed. McGraw-Hill, 2013.)

infection and long-term systemic corticosteroid use. Hairy leukoplakia waxes and wanes over time with generally modest irritative symptoms. Acyclovir, valacyclovir, and famciclovir have all been used for treatment but produce only temporary resolution of the condition. It does not appear to predispose to malignant transformation.

Oral cavity squamous cell carcinoma can be hard to distinguish from other oral lesions, but early detection is the key to successful management (Figure 8–7). Raised, firm, ulcerative lesions are highly suspicious and generally quite painful on even gentle palpation. Lesions < 3 mm in depth have a low propensity to metastasize. Most patients in whom the tumor is detected before it is 2 cm in diameter are cured by local resection. Radiation is reserved for patients with metastatic disease or tumors with adverse features, and chemotherapy is added if there are positive margins or if involved

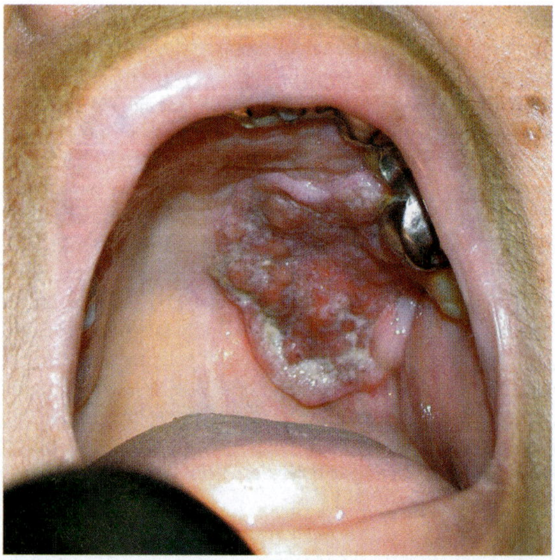

▲ **Figure 8–7.** Squamous cell carcinoma of the palate. (Used, with permission, from Frank Miller, MD, in Usatine RP, Smith MA, Mayeaux EJ Jr, Chumley H. *The Color Atlas of Family Medicine*, 2nd ed. McGraw-Hill, 2013.)

lymph nodes have extranodal extension. Large tumors are usually treated with a combination of resection, removal of lymph nodes from the neck (neck dissection), and external beam radiation. Reconstruction, if required, is done at the time of resection and can involve the use of myocutaneous flaps or vascularized free tissue transfer with or without bone. Novel fluorescence-guided surgeries are being developed to improve detection of margins and decrease recurrence.

Oropharyngeal squamous cell carcinoma generally presents later than oral cavity squamous cell carcinoma. The lesions tend to be larger and are often buried within the lymphoid tissue of the palatine or lingual tonsils. Most patients note only unilateral odynophagia and weight loss, but ipsilateral cervical lymphadenopathy is often identified by the careful clinician. While these tumors are typically associated with known carcinogens such as tobacco and alcohol, their epidemiology has changed dramatically over the past 25 years. Despite demonstrated reductions in tobacco and alcohol use within developed nations, the incidence of oropharyngeal squamous cell carcinoma has increased over this period. Known as a possible cause of head and neck cancer since 1983, *HPV—most commonly, type 16/18—is believed to be the cause of up to 70% of all oropharyngeal squamous cell carcinoma.* HPV-positive tumors are readily distinguished by immunostaining of primary tumor or FNA biopsy specimens for the p16 protein, a tumor suppressor protein that is highly correlated with the presence of HPV. These tumors often present in advanced stages of the disease with regional cervical lymph node metastases (stages III and IV) but have a better prognosis than similarly staged lesions in tobacco and alcohol users. This difference in disease control is so apparent in multicenter studies that, based on the presence or absence of the p16 protein, two distinct staging systems for oropharyngeal squamous cell carcinoma were introduced in 2018.

Auger S et al. Circulating tumor DNA in head and neck squamous cell carcinoma–current status and future prospects. Acad Oncol. 2024;1:10.20935/acadonco7456. [PMID: 39867572]

Pal R et al. Fluorescence lifetime of injected indocyanine green as a universal marker of solid tumours in patients. Nat Biomed Eng. 2023;7:1649. [PMID: 37845517]

Worthington HV et al. Interventions for the treatment of oral cavity and oropharyngeal cancers: surgical treatment. Cochrane Database Syst Rev. 2023;8:CD006205. [PMID: 37650478]

ORAL CANDIDIASIS

ESSENTIALS OF DIAGNOSIS

- Fluctuating throat or mouth discomfort.
- Associated with systemic or local immunosuppression, such as recent corticosteroid, chemotherapy, or antibiotic use.
- Erythema of the oral cavity or oropharynx with creamy-white, curd-like patches.
- Rapid resolution of symptoms with appropriate treatment.

Clinical Findings

A. Symptoms and Signs

Oral candidiasis (**thrush**) is usually painful and looks like creamy-white curd-like patches overlying erythematous mucosa (see Figure 6–11). Because these *white areas are easily rubbed off* (eg, by a tongue depressor)—unlike leukoplakia or lichen planus—only the underlying irregular erythema may be seen. Oral candidiasis is commonly associated with the following risk factors: (1) use of dentures, (2) debilitated state with poor oral hygiene, (3) diabetes mellitus, (4) anemia, (5) chemotherapy or local irradiation, (6) corticosteroid use (oral or systemic), or (7) broad-spectrum antibiotics. Another manifestation of candidiasis is **angular cheilitis** (also seen in nutritional deficiencies) (Figure 8–8).

B. Diagnostic Studies

The diagnosis is made clinically. A wet preparation using potassium hydroxide will reveal spores and may show nonseptate mycelia. Biopsy will show intraepithelial pseudomycelia of *Candida albicans*.

Candidiasis is often the first manifestation of HIV infection, and HIV testing should be considered in patients with no known predisposing cause for *Candida* overgrowth (see also Chapter 35). The US Department of Health Services Clinical Practice Guideline for Evaluation and Management of Early HIV Infection recommends examination of the oral mucosa with each clinician visit as well as at a dental examination every 6 months for individuals living with HIV.

Treatment

Effective antifungal therapy may be achieved with any of the following: fluconazole (100 mg orally daily for 7 days), ketoconazole (200–400 mg orally with breakfast [requires acidic gastric environment for absorption] for 7–14 days), clotrimazole troches (10 mg dissolved orally five times daily), or nystatin mouth rinses (500,000 units [5 mL of 100,000 units/mL] held in the mouth before swallowing three times daily). In patients with HIV infection, however, longer courses of therapy with fluconazole may be needed,

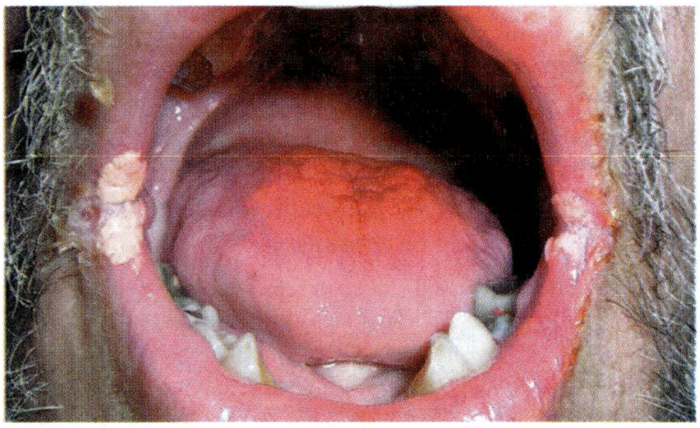

Figure 8–8. Severe angular cheilitis in a man with HIV with oral thrush. (Reproduced, with permission, from Richard P. Usatine, MD, in Usatine RP, Smith MA, Mayeaux EJ Jr, Chumley H. *The Color Atlas of Family Medicine,* 2nd ed. McGraw-Hill, 2013.)

and oral itraconazole (200 mg/day) may be indicated in fluconazole-refractory cases. Many of the *Candida* species in these patients are resistant to first-line azoles and may require newer medications, such as voriconazole. In addition, 0.12% chlorhexidine or half-strength hydrogen peroxide mouth rinses may provide local relief. Nystatin powder (100,000 units/g) applied to dentures three or four times daily and rinsed off for several weeks may help denture wearers.

Contaldo M et al. Oral candidiasis and novel therapeutic strategies: antifungals, phytotherapy, probiotics, and photodynamic therapy. Curr Drug Deliv. 2023;20:441. [PMID: 35440307].

Rossetti A et al. Efficacy of different therapeutic options for pain relief and treatment of burning mouth syndrome: a systematic review. Clin Oral Investig. 2025;29:551. [PMID: 41193828]

GLOSSITIS, GLOSSODYNIA, & BURNING MOUTH SYNDROME

Inflammation of the tongue with loss of filiform papillae leads to a red, smooth-surfaced tongue (**glossitis**). Rarely painful, it may be secondary to nutritional deficiencies (eg, niacin, riboflavin, iron, or vitamin E), drug reactions, dehydration, irritants, or foods and liquids, and possibly to autoimmune reactions or psoriasis. If the primary cause cannot be identified and corrected, empiric nutritional replacement therapy may be of value.

Glossodynia is burning and pain of the tongue, which may occur with or without glossitis. In the absence of any clinical findings, it has been termed **"burning mouth syndrome."** Glossodynia with glossitis has been associated with diabetes mellitus, medications (eg, diuretics), tobacco, xerostomia, and candidiasis as well as the listed causes of glossitis. The burning mouth syndrome typically has no identifiable associated risk factors and seems to be most common in postmenopausal women. Treating possible underlying causes, changing long-term medications to alternative ones, and smoking cessation may resolve symptoms of glossitis. Effective treatments for the burning mouth syndrome include α-lipoic acid and clonazepam. Clonazepam is most effective as a rapid-dissolving tablet placed on the tongue in doses from 0.25 mg to 0.5 mg every 8–12 hours. Both glossodynia and the burning mouth syndrome are benign, and reassurance that there is no infection or tumor is likely to be appreciated. Unilateral symptoms, symptoms that cannot be related to a specific medication, and symptoms and signs involving regions supplied by other cranial nerves all may suggest neuropathology, and imaging of the brain, brainstem, and skull base with MRI should be considered.

Alvarenga-Brant R et al. Treatments for burning mouth syndrome: a network meta-analysis. J Dent Res. 2023;102:135. [PMID: 36214096]

Castaño-Joaqui OG et al. Burning mouth syndrome underlying factors: a roadmap from a network perspective. Oral Dis. 2025;31:1861. [PMID: 39673150]

Ju HM et al. Distinctive salivary oral microbiome in patients with burning mouth syndrome depending on pain intensity compared to healthy subjects. J Dent Sci. 2025;20:462. [PMID: 39873084]

INTRAORAL ULCERATIVE LESIONS

1. Necrotizing Ulcerative Gingivitis (Trench Mouth, Vincent Angina)

Necrotizing ulcerative gingivitis, often caused by an infection with both spirochetes and fusiform bacilli, is common in young adults under stress (classically in students at examination time). Underlying systemic diseases may also predispose to this disorder. Clinically, there is painful acute gingival inflammation and necrosis, often with bleeding, halitosis, fever, and cervical lymphadenopathy. Warm half-strength peroxide rinses and oral penicillin (250 mg three times daily for 10 days) may help. Dental gingival curettage may prove necessary.

AlJoghaiman E. The relationship between mental health and periodontal disease: insights from NHANES data. F1000Res. 2024;13:709. [PMID: 39886649]

Schroeder FMM et al. Clinical and immunological features of chronic ulcerative stomatitis: a systematic review. J Oral Pathol Med. 2022;51:501. [PMID: 35092104]

2. Aphthous Ulcer (Canker Sore, Ulcerative Stomatitis)

Aphthous ulcers are very common and easy to recognize. Their cause remains uncertain, although an association with human herpesvirus 6 has been suggested. Found on freely moving, nonkeratinized mucosa (eg, buccal and labial mucosa and *not* attached gingiva or palate), they may be single or multiple, are usually recurrent, and appear as painful small round ulcerations with yellow-gray fibrinoid centers surrounded by red halos. Minor aphthous ulcers are < 1 cm in diameter and generally heal in 10–14 days. Major aphthous ulcers are > 1 cm in diameter and can be disabling due to the degree of associated oral pain. Stress seems to be a major predisposing factor to the eruptions of aphthous ulcers.

Treatment is challenging because no single systemic treatment has proven effective. Avoiding local irritants, such as certain toothpastes, may decrease symptoms and episodes. Topical corticosteroids (triamcinolone acetonide, 0.1%, or fluocinonide ointment, 0.05%) in an adhesive base (Orabase Plain) do appear to provide symptomatic relief in many patients. Other topical therapies shown to be effective in controlled studies include diclofenac 3% in hyaluronan 2.5%, doxymycine-cyanoacrylate, mouthwashes containing the enzymes amyloglucosidase and glucose oxidase, and amlexanox 5% oral paste. A 1-week tapering course of prednisone (40–60 mg/day) has also been used successfully. Cimetidine maintenance therapy may be useful in patients with recurrent aphthous ulcers. Thalidomide has been used selectively in recurrent aphthous ulcerations in patients with HIV.

Large or persistent areas of ulcerative stomatitis may be secondary to erythema multiforme or drug allergies, acute herpes simplex, pemphigus, pemphigoid, epidermolysis bullosa acquisita, bullous lichen planus, Behçet disease, or IBD. Squamous cell carcinoma may occasionally present in this fashion. When the diagnosis is not clear, incisional biopsy is indicated.

Abdelaziz A et al. Rebamipide for management of methotrexate-induced oral ulcers: a three-arm randomized clinical trial. Clin Oral Investig. 2025;29:106. [PMID: 39891768]
Ghalwash D et al. Efficacy of thyme honey in the management of oral aphthous ulcers: a randomized controlled clinical trial. Eur J Oral Sci. 2025;133:e13032. [PMID: 39723829]
Philipone EM et al. Ulcerative and inflammatory lesions of the oral mucosa. Oral Maxillofac Surg Clin North Am. 2023;35:219. [PMID: 36805903]

3. Herpes Stomatitis

Herpes gingivostomatitis is common, mild, and short-lived. Clinically, there is initial burning, followed by typical small vesicles that rupture and form scabs. Lesions are most commonly found on the attached gingiva and mucocutaneous junction of the lip, but lesions can also form on the tongue, buccal mucosa, and soft palate. In most adults, it requires no intervention. In immunocompromised persons, however, reactivation of herpes simplex virus infection is frequent and may be severe. Acyclovir (200–800 mg orally five times daily for 7–10 days) or valacyclovir (1000 mg orally twice daily for 7–10 days) may shorten the course and reduce postherpetic pain. *These treatments may be effective only when started within 24–48 hours of the onset of initial symptoms (pain, itching, burning) and are not effective once vesicles have erupted.* Differential diagnosis includes aphthous stomatitis, erythema multiforme, syphilitic chancre, and carcinoma.

Barros AWP et al. Is low-level laser therapy effective in the treatment of herpes labialis? Systematic review and meta-analysis. Lasers Med Sci. 2022;37:3393. [PMID: 36214942]
Coppola N et al. Supportive care and antiviral treatments in primary herpetic gingivostomatitis: a systematic review. Clin Oral Investig. 2023;27:6333. [PMID: 37733027]
Khalil M et al. Association of photodynamic therapy and photobiomodulation as a promising treatment of herpes labialis: a systematic review. Photobiomodul Photomed Laser Surg. 2022;40:299. [PMID: 35483089]

PHARYNGITIS & TONSILLITIS

ESSENTIALS OF DIAGNOSIS

- Centor criteria for streptococcal pharyngitis: exudate or swelling on tonsils, anterior cervical adenopathy, fever, lack of cough.
- Goal is to treat group A β-hemolytic streptococcal infection to prevent subsequent rheumatic fever (rash, arthralgias, myocarditis) and other sequelae (glomerulonephritis, posterior pharyngeal abscess).

General Considerations

Pharyngitis and tonsillitis account for over 10% of all office visits to primary care clinicians and 50% of outpatient antibiotic use. The main concern is determining who is likely to have a **group A β-hemolytic streptococcal (GABHS) infection**, since this can lead to subsequent complications, such as rheumatic fever and glomerulonephritis. A second public health policy concern is reducing the extraordinary cost (both in dollars and in the development of antibiotic-resistant *S pneumoniae*) associated with unnecessary antibiotic use.

Clinical Findings

A. Symptoms and Signs

The clinical features most suggestive of GABHS pharyngitis include fever over 38°C, tender anterior cervical adenopathy, lack of a cough, and pharyngotonsillar exudate (Figure 8–9). These four features (**the Centor criteria**), when present, strongly suggest GABHS. When two or three of the four are present, there is an intermediate likelihood of GABHS. When only one criterion is present, GABHS is unlikely. Sore throat may be severe, with odynophagia, tender adenopathy, and a scarlatiniform rash. An elevated white count and left shift are also possible. Hoarseness, cough, and coryza are not suggestive of this disease. It is also rare to have GABHS in individuals younger than 3 years old.

Marked lymphadenopathy and a shaggy, white-purple tonsillar exudate, often extending into the nasopharynx, suggest mononucleosis, especially if present in a young adult. With about 90% sensitivity, lymphocyte-to-white-blood-cell ratios of > 35% suggest EBV infection and not tonsillitis. Hepatosplenomegaly and a positive heterophile agglutination test or elevated anti-EBV titer are corroborative. However, about one-third of patients with infectious mononucleosis have secondary streptococcal tonsillitis, requiring treatment. *Ampicillin should routinely be avoided if mononucleosis is suspected* because it induces a rash that might be misinterpreted by the patient as a penicillin allergy. Diphtheria (extremely rare but described in persons with alcohol use disorder) presents with low-grade fever and an ill patient with a gray tonsillar pseudomembrane.

The most common pathogens other than GABHS in the differential diagnosis of "sore throat" are viruses, *Neisseria gonorrhoeae*, *Mycoplasma*, and *Chlamydia trachomatis*. Rhinorrhea and lack of exudate would suggest a virus, but

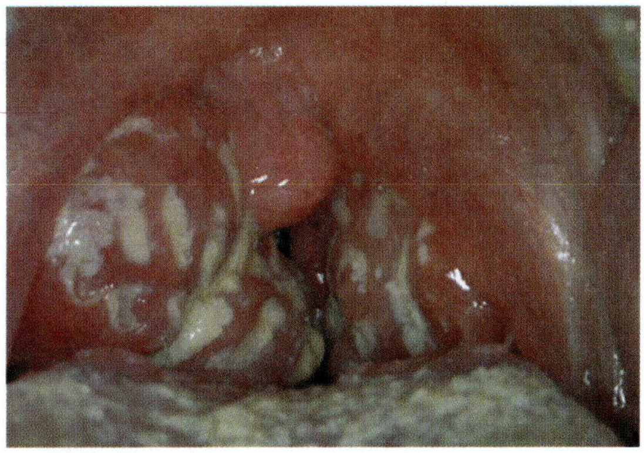

Figure 8–9. Marked exudative pharyngitis and tonsillitis due to group A β-hemolytic streptococci. (Used, with permission, from Lawrence B. Stack, MD, in Knoop KJ, Stack LB, Storrow AB, Thurman RJ. *The Atlas of Emergency Medicine,* 5th ed. McGraw Hill, 2021.)

in practice it is not possible to confidently distinguish viral upper respiratory infection from GABHS on clinical grounds alone. Infections with *Corynebacterium diphtheria*, anaerobic streptococci, and *Corynebacterium haemolyticum* (which responds better to erythromycin than penicillin) may also mimic pharyngitis due to GABHS. See also Chapter 37 for bacterial considerations.

B. Laboratory Findings

A single-swab throat culture is 90–95% sensitive and the **rapid antigen detection testing (RADT)** is 90–99% sensitive for GABHS. Results from the RADT are available in about 15 minutes. Routine throat culture in refractory cases may also be helpful to guide antibiotic selection or identify fewer common microbes associated with chronic infection.

Treatment

The Infectious Diseases Society of America recommends laboratory confirmation of the clinical diagnosis by means of either throat culture or RADT of the throat swab. The American College of Physicians–American Society of Internal Medicine (ACP-ASIM), in collaboration with the CDC, advocates use of a clinical algorithm alone—in lieu of microbiologic testing—for confirmation of the diagnosis in adults for whom the suspicion of streptococcal infection is high. Others examine the assumptions of the ACP-ASIM guideline for using a clinical algorithm alone and question whether those recommendations will achieve the stated objective of dramatically decreasing excess antibiotic use. A reasonable strategy to follow is that patients with zero or one Centor criterion are at very low risk for GABHS and therefore do not need throat cultures or RADT of the throat swab and should not receive antibiotics. Patients with two or three Centor criteria need throat cultures or RADT of the throat swab, since positive results would warrant antibiotic treatment. Patients who have all four Centor criteria are likely to have GABHS and can receive empiric therapy without throat culture or RADT.

Oral antibiotics are the preferred first-line therapy. Penicillin V potassium (250 mg orally three times daily or 500 mg twice daily for 10 days) and cefuroxime axetil (250 mg orally twice daily for 5–10 days) are both effective. The efficacy of a 5-day regimen of penicillin V potassium appears to be similar to that of a 10-day course, with a 94% clinical response rate and an 84% streptococcal eradication rate. Erythromycin (also active against *Mycoplasma* and *Chlamydia*) is a reasonable alternative to penicillin in allergic patients. Cephalosporins are somewhat more effective than penicillin in producing bacteriologic cures; 5-day courses of cefpodoxime and cefuroxime have been successful. The macrolide antibiotics have also been reported to be successful in shorter-duration regimens. Azithromycin (500 mg once daily), because of its long half-life, needs to be taken for only 3 days. For patients in whom adherence to medication is in question, or those unable to take oral medication, a single intramuscular injection of benzathine penicillin or procaine penicillin, 1.2 million units is an effective alternative.

Adequate antibiotic treatment usually avoids the streptococcal complications of scarlet fever, rheumatic myocarditis, glomerulonephritis, and local abscess formation.

Antibiotics for treatment failures are also somewhat controversial. Surprisingly, penicillin-tolerant strains are not isolated more frequently in those who fail treatment than in those treated successfully with penicillin. The reasons for failure appear to be complex, and a second course of treatment with the same medication is reasonable. Alternatives to penicillin include cefuroxime and other cephalosporins, dicloxacillin (which is β-lactamase-resistant), and amoxicillin with clavulanate. When there is a history of penicillin allergy, alternatives should be used, such as erythromycin. Erythromycin resistance—with failure rates of about 25%—is an increasing problem in many areas. In cases of severe penicillin allergy, cephalosporins should be avoided since cross-reaction occurs in > 8% of cases.

Ancillary treatment of pharyngitis includes analgesics and anti-inflammatory agents, such as aspirin, acetaminophen, and corticosteroids. In meta-analysis, corticosteroids increased the likelihood of complete pain resolution at 24 hours by threefold without an increase in recurrence or adverse events. Some patients find that salt water gargling is soothing. In severe cases, anesthetic gargles and lozenges (eg, benzocaine) may provide additional symptomatic relief. Occasionally, odynophagia is so intense that hospitalization for intravenous hydration and antibiotics is necessary. (See Chapter 37.)

Patients who have had rheumatic fever should be treated with a continuous course of antimicrobial prophylaxis (penicillin G, 500 mg once daily orally, or erythromycin, 250 mg twice daily orally) for at least 5 years.

Chow EPF et al. STI pathogens in the oropharynx: update on screening and treatment. Curr Opin Infect Dis. 2024;37:35. [PMID: 38112085]

Linder JA et al. 2025 clinical practice guideline update by the Infectious Diseases Society of America on group A streptococcal (GAS) pharyngitis: risk assessment using clinical scoring systems in children and adults. Clin Infect Dis. 2025 Dec 4. [Epub ahead of print] [PMID: 41343363]

Silva Veiga R et al. Acute rheumatic fever or post-streptococcal reactive arthritis: two different entities. Cureus. 2024;16:e72687. [PMID: 39618634]

Thacharodi A et al. The burden of group A *Streptococcus* (GAS) infections: the challenge continues in the twenty-first century. iScience. 2024;28:111677. [PMID: 39877071]

PERITONSILLAR ABSCESS & CELLULITIS

When infection penetrates the tonsillar capsule and involves the surrounding tissues, peritonsillar cellulitis results. Following therapy, peritonsillar cellulitis usually either resolves over several days or evolves into peritonsillar abscess. Peritonsillar abscess (**quinsy**) and cellulitis present with severe sore throat, odynophagia, trismus, medial deviation of the soft palate and peritonsillar fold, and an abnormal muffled ("hot potato") voice. CT may be a useful adjunct to clinical suspicion, but imaging is *not* required for the diagnosis. The existence of an abscess may be confirmed by aspirating pus from the peritonsillar fold just superior and medial to the upper pole of the tonsil. A 19-gauge or 21-gauge needle should be passed medial to the molar and no deeper than 1 cm, because the internal carotid artery may lie more medially than its usual location and pass posterior and deep to the tonsillar fossa. Most commonly, patients with peritonsillar abscess present to the emergency department and receive a dose of parenteral amoxicillin (1 g), amoxicillin-sulbactam (3 g), or clindamycin (600–900 mg). Less severe cases and patients who are able to tolerate oral intake may be treated for 7–10 days with oral antibiotics, including amoxicillin, 500 mg three times a day; amoxicillin-clavulanate, 875 mg twice a day; or clindamycin, 300 mg four times daily.

Although antibiotic treatment is generally undisputed, there is controversy regarding the surgical management of peritonsillar abscess. Methods include needle aspiration, incision and drainage, and tonsillectomy. Some clinicians incise and drain the area and continue with parenteral antibiotics, whereas others aspirate only and monitor as an outpatient. The data are largely equivocal for all three approaches. In patients with more severe or recurrent peritonsillar abscesses, it may be appropriate to consider immediate tonsillectomy (quinsy tonsillectomy) in the acutely infected setting, although practitioners have moved away from this approach because of the potential for complications. About 10% of patients with peritonsillar abscess exhibit relative indications for tonsillectomy after the infection has resolved. All three approaches are effective. Regardless of the method used, one must be sure the abscess is adequately treated, since complications such as extension to the retropharyngeal, deep neck, and posterior mediastinal spaces are possible. Bacteria may also be aspirated into the lungs, resulting in pneumonia. There is controversy about whether a single abscess is a sufficient indication for tonsillectomy; about 30% of patients aged 17–30 who do not undergo early planned tonsillectomy following peritonsillar abscess ultimately undergo surgery, and only about 13% of those over 30 have their tonsils removed. Recurrent or atypical peritonsillar abscesses in older adults should also be evaluated for an underlying head and neck malignancy.

Galluzzi F et al. Treatment of peritonsillar abscess in children: a systematic review. J Clin Med. 2024;13:7361. [PMID: 39685823]

Voruz F et al. Diagnosis of peritonsillar abscess–a prospective study comparing clinical with CT findings in 133 consecutive patients. Diagnostics (Basel). 2025;15:228. [PMID: 39857112]

DEEP NECK INFECTIONS

ESSENTIALS OF DIAGNOSIS

- Marked acute neck pain and swelling.
- Abscesses are emergencies because rapid airway compromise may occur.
- May spread to the mediastinum or cause sepsis.

General Considerations

Deep neck abscesses most commonly originate from odontogenic infections. Other causes include suppurative lymphadenitis; direct spread of pharyngeal infection; penetrating trauma; pharyngoesophageal foreign bodies; cervical osteomyelitis; and intravenous injection of the internal jugular vein, especially in people with substance use disorders. **Ludwig angina** is the most commonly encountered neck space infection. It is a cellulitis of the sublingual and submaxillary spaces, often arising from infection of the mandibular dentition. **Ludwig angina is an emergency as it may cause rapid upper airway compromise and necessitate creation of a surgical airway.** Recurrent deep neck infection may suggest an underlying congenital lesion, such as a branchial cleft cyst. Suppurative lymphadenopathy in middle-aged persons who smoke cigarettes and drink alcohol regularly should be considered a manifestation of malignancy (typically metastatic squamous cell carcinoma) until proven otherwise.

Clinical Findings

Patients with Ludwig angina have edema and erythema of the upper neck under the chin and often of the floor of the mouth. The tongue may be displaced upward and backward by the posterior spread of cellulitis, and coalescence of pus is often present in the floor of mouth. This may lead to occlusion of the airway. Microbiologic isolates include streptococci, staphylococci, *Bacteroides*, and *Fusobacterium*. Patients with diabetes may have different flora, including *Klebsiella*, and a more aggressive clinical course.

Patients with deep neck abscesses usually present with marked neck pain and swelling. Fever is common but not always present. *Deep neck abscesses are emergencies because they may rapidly compromise the airway.* Untreated or inadequately treated, they may spread to the mediastinum or cause sepsis.

Contrast-enhanced CT usually augments the clinical examination in defining the extent of the infection. It often will distinguish inflammation and phlegmon (requiring antibiotics) from abscess (requiring drainage) and define for the surgeon the extent of an abscess. CT with MRI may also identify thrombophlebitis of the internal jugular vein secondary to oropharyngeal inflammation. This condition, known as **Lemierre syndrome**, is rare and usually associated with severe headache. The presence of pulmonary infiltrates consistent with septic emboli in the setting of a neck abscess should lead one to suspect Lemierre syndrome or injection drug use, or both.

Treatment

Usual doses of penicillin plus metronidazole, ampicillin-sulbactam, clindamycin, or selective cephalosporins are good initial choices for treatment of Ludwig angina. Culture and sensitivity data are then used to refine the choice. Dental consultation is advisable to address the offending tooth or teeth. External drainage via bilateral submental incisions is required if the airway is threatened or when medical therapy has not reversed the process.

Treatment of deep neck abscesses includes securing the airway, intravenous antibiotics, and incision and drainage. When the infection involves the floor of the mouth, base of the tongue, or the supraglottic or paraglottic space, the airway may be secured either by intubation or tracheotomy. Tracheotomy is preferable in the patients with substantial pharyngeal edema, since attempts at intubation may precipitate acute airway obstruction. Bleeding in association with a deep neck abscess is very rare but suggests carotid artery or internal jugular vein involvement and requires prompt neck exploration both for drainage of pus and for vascular control.

Patients with Lemierre syndrome require prompt institution of antibiotics appropriate for *Fusobacterium necrophorum* as well as the more usual upper airway pathogens. The use of anticoagulation in treatment is of no proven benefit.

Meena Nandini R et al. Navigating the airway maze: challenges and strategies in deep neck space infections. Cureus. 2024;16:e72337. [PMID: 39583498]

Sheikh Z et al. The assessment and management of deep neck space infections in adults: a systematic review and qualitative evidence synthesis. Clin Otolaryngol. 2023;48:540. [PMID: 37147934]

Velhonoja J et al. Risk factors and preventive measures for severe orofacial and neck infections: a three-year observational study. BMC Oral Health. 2025;25:136. [PMID: 39856655]

SNORING

ESSENTIALS OF DIAGNOSIS

- Noise produced on inspiration due to upper aerodigestive tract blockage during sleep.
- Snoring is associated with obstructive sleep apnea (OSA) but may not alone disrupt sleep quality.

General Considerations

Ventilation disorders during sleep are extremely common. *While OSA occurs in 5–10% of Americans, clinically relevant snoring may occur in as many as 59%.* In general, sleep-disordered breathing problems are attributed to narrowing of the upper aerodigestive tract during sleep due to changes in position, muscle tone, and soft tissue hypertrophy or laxity. The most common sites of obstruction are the oropharynx and the base of the tongue. The spectrum of the problem ranges from simple snoring without cessation of airflow to OSA with long periods of apnea and life-threatening physiologic sequelae. OSA is discussed in Chapter 9. In contrast to OSA, snoring is almost exclusively *a social problem*, and despite its prevalence and association with OSA, there is comparatively little known about the management of this problem.

Clinical Findings

A. Symptoms and Signs

All patients who report snoring should be evaluated for OSA as discussed in Chapter 9. Symptoms of OSA (including snoring, excessive daytime somnolence, daytime headaches, and weight gain) may be present in as many as 30% of patients without demonstrable apnea or hypopnea on formal testing. Clinical examination should include examination of the nasal cavity, nasopharynx, oropharynx, and larynx to help exclude other causes of dynamic airway obstruction. In many cases of isolated snoring, the palate and uvula appear enlarged and elongated with excessive mucosa hanging below the muscular portion of the soft palate.

B. Imaging and Diagnostic Testing

Sleep examination with **polysomnography** is strongly advised in the evaluation of a patient who reports snoring. Radiographic imaging of the head or neck is generally not necessary. Additional testing may include sleep endoscopy.

Treatment

Expeditious and inexpensive management solutions for snoring are sought, often with little or no benefit. Diet modification and physical exercise can lead to improvement in snoring through the weight loss and improvement in pharyngeal tone that accompanies overall physical conditioning. Position change during sleep can be effective, and time-honored treatments, such as placing a golf or tennis ball into a pocket sewn on the back of the pajama top worn during sleep, may satisfactorily eliminate symptoms by ensuring recumbency on one side. Although numerous pharmacologic therapies have been endorsed, none demonstrate any significant utility when scrutinized.

Anatomic management of snoring can be challenging. As with OSA, snoring can come from a number of sites in the upper aerodigestive tract. While medical or surgical correction of nasal obstruction may help alleviate snoring problems, most interventions aim to improve airflow through the nasopharynx and oropharynx. Nonsurgical options include mandibular advancement appliances designed to pull the base of the tongue forward and continuous positive airway pressure via face or nasal mask. Adherence to both of these treatment options is problematic because snorers without OSA do not notice the physiologic benefits of these devices noted by patients with sleep apnea.

Surgical correction of snoring is most commonly directed at the soft palate and tongue base. Historical approaches involved resection of redundant mucosa and the uvula similar to uvulopalatopharyngoplasty that is used for OSA. Regardless of how limited the procedure or what technique was used, the postoperative pain, expense of general anesthesia, and high recurrence rates limit the utility of these procedures. Office-based approaches are more widely attempted because of these limitations. Most of these procedures aim to stiffen the palate to prevent vibration rather than remove it. A series of procedures, including injection snoreplasty, radiofrequency thermal fibrosis, and an implantable palatal device, have been used with variable success and patient tolerance. The techniques can be technically challenging. Persistent symptoms may occur following initial treatment necessitating costly (and sometimes painful) repeat procedures. The durability of these procedures in alleviating symptoms is also poorly understood, and late failures can lead to patient and clinician frustration. Newer approaches include hypoglossal nerve stimulation which directly stimulates movement of the tongue to increase space of the airway.

Correa EJ et al. Role of nasal surgery in adult obstructive sleep apnea: a systematic review. Sleep Sci. 2024;17:e310. [PMID: 39268344]
Kim DH et al. Hypoglossal nerve stimulation effects on obstructive sleep apnea over time: a systematic review and meta-analysis. Otolaryngol Head Neck Surg. 2024;170:736. [PMID: 38123511]
Yap YY. Evaluation and management of snoring. Sleep Med Clin. 2022;17:25. [PMID: 35216759]

DISEASES OF THE SALIVARY GLANDS

ACUTE INFLAMMATORY SALIVARY GLAND DISORDERS

1. Sialadenitis

Acute bacterial sialadenitis most commonly affects either the parotid or submandibular gland. It typically presents with acute swelling of the gland, increased pain and swelling with meals, and tenderness and erythema of the duct opening. Pus often can be massaged from the duct. Sialadenitis often occurs in the setting of dehydration or in association with chronic illness. Underlying Sjögren syndrome and chronic periodontitis may contribute. Ductal obstruction, often by an inspissated mucous plug, is followed by salivary stasis and secondary infection. The most common organism recovered from purulent draining saliva is *S aureus*. Treatment consists of intravenous antibiotics, such as nafcillin (1 g intravenously every 4–6 hours), and measures to increase salivary flow, including hydration, warm compresses, sialagogues (eg, lemon drops), and massage of the gland. Treatment can usually then be switched to an oral agent based on clinical improvement and microbiologic results to complete a 10-day treatment course. Less severe cases can often be treated with oral antibiotics with similar spectrum. Complete resolution of parotid swelling and pain can take 2–3 weeks. Failure of the process to improve and ultimately resolve on this regimen suggests abscess formation, ductal stricture, stone, or tumor causing obstruction. Ultrasound or CT scan may be helpful in establishing the diagnosis. In the setting of acute illness, a severe and potentially life-threatening form of sialadenitis, sometimes called suppurative sialadenitis, may develop. The causative organism is usually *S aureus*, but often no pus will drain from Stensen papilla. These patients often do not respond to rehydration and intravenous antibiotics and thus may require operative incision and drainage to resolve the infection. In patients with bilateral parotid sialadenitis, mumps should be considered.

2. Sialolithiasis

Calculus formation is more common in the **Wharton duct** (draining the submandibular glands) than in the **Stensen duct** (draining the parotid glands). Clinically, a patient may note postprandial pain and local swelling, often with a history of recurrent acute sialadenitis. Stones in the Wharton duct are usually large and radiopaque, whereas those in the Stensen duct are usually radiolucent and smaller. Those very close to the orifice of the Wharton duct may be palpated manually in the anterior floor of the mouth and removed intraorally by dilating or incising the distal duct. Those > 1.5–2 cm from the duct are too close to the lingual nerve to be removed safely in this manner. Similarly, dilation of the Stensen duct, located on the buccal surface opposite the second maxillary molar, may relieve distal stricture or allow a small stone to pass. Sialoendoscopy for the management of chronic sialolithiasis is superior to extracorporeal shock-wave lithotripsy and fluoroscopically guided basket retrieval. Repeated episodes of sialadenitis are usually associated with stricture and chronic infection. If the obstruction cannot be safely removed or dilated, excision of the gland may be necessary to relieve recurrent symptoms.

Aframian DJ et al. Integrated therapy of intraductal irrigations and sialoendoscopies of salivary glands to improve mouth dryness. Oral Dis. 2024;30:1198. [PMID: 36630587]
Soriano-Martín D et al. Sialendoscopy approach in treating juvenile recurrent parotitis: a systematic review. J Otolaryngol Head Neck Surg. 2023;52:53. [PMID: 37598195]

CHRONIC INFLAMMATORY & INFILTRATIVE DISORDERS OF THE SALIVARY GLANDS

Numerous infiltrative disorders may cause unilateral or bilateral parotid gland enlargement. Sjögren syndrome and sarcoidosis are examples of lymphoepithelial and granulomatous diseases that may affect the salivary glands. Metabolic disorders, including alcohol use disorder, diabetes mellitus, and vitamin deficiencies, may also cause diffuse enlargement. Several medications have been associated with parotid enlargement, including thioureas, iodine, and medications with cholinergic effects (eg, phenothiazines), which stimulate salivary flow and cause more viscous saliva.

SALIVARY GLAND TUMORS

A general rule of thumb is that the smaller the size of the salivary gland with a present mass, the more likely the possibility of malignancy. Approximately 80% of salivary gland tumors occur in the parotid gland. In adults, about 80% of these are benign. In the submandibular triangle, it is sometimes difficult to distinguish a primary submandibular gland tumor from a metastatic submandibular space node. Only 50–60% of primary submandibular tumors are benign. Tumors of the minor salivary glands are most likely to be malignant, with adenoid cystic carcinoma predominating, and may be found throughout the oral cavity or oropharynx.

Most parotid tumors present as an asymptomatic mass in the superficial part of the gland. Their presence may have been noted by the patient for months or years. Facial nerve involvement and pain correlate strongly with malignancy. Tumors may extend deep to the plane of the facial nerve or may originate in the parapharyngeal space. In such cases, medial deviation of the soft palate is visible on intraoral examination. MRI and CT scans have largely replaced sialography in defining the extent of tumor. At least one study demonstrates the potential benefit of enhanced MRI imaging in distinguishing among Warthin tumors and pleomorphic adenomas and malignant salivary gland tumors. Ultrasonography is a simple and effective initial test for identification of a suspected mass.

When the clinician encounters a patient with an otherwise asymptomatic salivary gland mass where tumor is the most likely diagnosis, the choice is whether to simply excise the mass via a parotidectomy with facial nerve dissection or submandibular gland excision or to first obtain an FNA biopsy. The **Milan System for Reporting Salivary Gland Cytopathology** is the accepted guide for diagnosis and management of salivary gland lesions based on biopsy results. In benign and small, low-grade malignant tumors, no additional treatment is needed. Postoperative irradiation is indicated for larger and high-grade cancers.

Di Santo D et al. Current evidence on diagnosis and treatment of parotid gland lymphomas: a systematic review. Eur Arch Otorhinolaryngol. 2023;280:5219. [PMID: 37638999]

Montenegro C et al. Treatment and outcomes of minor salivary gland cancers of the larynx and trachea: a systematic review. Acta Otorhinolaryngol Ital. 2023;43:365. [PMID: 37814980]

Szydłowski K et al. The impact of inflammation on the etiopathogenesis of benign salivary gland tumors: a scoping review. Int J Mol Sci. 2024;25:12558. [PMID: 39684268]

DISEASES OF THE LARYNX

HOARSENESS & STRIDOR

The primary symptoms of laryngeal disease are hoarseness and stridor. **Hoarseness** is caused by an abnormal vibration of the vocal folds. The voice is breathy when too much air passes incompletely apposed vocal folds, as in unilateral vocal fold paralysis or vocal fold mass. The voice is harsh when the vocal folds are stiff and vibrate irregularly, as is the case in laryngitis or malignancy. Heavy, edematous vocal folds produce a rough, low-pitched vocal quality. **Stridor** (a high-pitched, typically inspiratory, sound) is the result of turbulent airflow from a narrowed upper airway. Airway narrowing at or above the vocal folds produces inspiratory stridor. Airway narrowing below the vocal fold level produces either expiratory or biphasic stridor. The timing and rapidity of onset of stridor are critically important in determining the seriousness of the airway problem. **All cases of stridor should be evaluated by a specialist and rapid-onset stridor should be evaluated emergently.**

Evaluation of an abnormal voice begins with obtaining a history of the circumstances preceding its onset and an examination of the airway. *All patients with hoarseness that has persisted beyond 2 weeks should be evaluated by an otolaryngologist with laryngoscopy.* Especially when the patient has a history of tobacco use, laryngeal cancer or lung cancer (leading to paralysis of a recurrent laryngeal nerve), or concerns for cough and aspiration, must be strongly considered. In addition to structural causes of dysphonia, laryngoscopy can help identify functional problems with the voice, including vocal fold paralysis, muscle tension dysphonia, and spasmodic dysphonia.

Dewan K et al. Complementary and integrative medicine and the voice. Otolaryngol Clin North Am. 2022;55:1007. [PMID: 36088156]

Martins RHG et al. Dysphonia and COVID-19: a review. J Voice. 2025:S0892-1997(24)00419-3. [PMID: 39814621]

Saccente-Kennedy B et al. A systematic review of speech-language pathology interventions for presbyphonia using the rehabilitation treatment specification system. J Voice. 2024 Jan 8:S0892-1997(23)00396-X. [Epub ahead of print] [PMID: 38195333]

COMMON LARYNGEAL DISORDERS

1. Acute Laryngitis

Acute laryngitis is probably the most common cause of hoarseness, which may persist for a week or so after other symptoms of an upper respiratory infection have cleared. Supportive care includes resting the voice, drinking enough fluid to stay hydrated, and breathing humidified air. The patient should be warned to avoid vigorous use of the voice (singing, shouting) until their voice returns to normal, since persistent use may lead to the formation of traumatic vocal fold hemorrhage, polyps, and cysts. Although thought to be usually viral in origin, both *M catarrhalis* and *H influenzae* may be isolated from the nasopharynx at higher than expected frequencies. Despite this finding, *a meta-analysis has failed to demonstrate any convincing evidence that antibiotics significantly alter the natural resolution of acute laryngitis.* Erythromycin may speed improvement of hoarseness at 1 week and cough at 2 weeks when measured subjectively. Oral or intramuscular corticosteroids may be used in highly selected cases of professional vocalists to speed recovery and allow scheduled performances. Examination of the vocal folds and assessment of vocal technique are mandatory prior to corticosteroid initiation, since inflamed vocal folds are at greater risk for hemorrhage and the subsequent development of traumatic vocal fold pathology.

2. Laryngopharyngeal Reflux

ESSENTIALS OF DIAGNOSIS

- Commonly associated with hoarseness, throat irritation, heartburn, foreign body sensation, and chronic cough.
- Symptoms typically occur when upright, and many patients do not experience classic heartburn.
- Laryngoscopy is critical to exclude other causes of hoarseness.
- Diagnosis is often made based on response to PPI therapy.
- Treatment failure with PPIs is common and suggests other etiologies.

GERD has also been suggested as a contributing factor to other symptoms, such as throat clearing, throat discomfort, chronic cough, a sensation of postnasal drip, esophageal spasm, and some cases of asthma. Since less than half of patients with laryngeal acid exposure have typical symptoms of heartburn and regurgitation, the lack of such symptoms should not be construed as eliminating this cause. Indeed, *most patients with symptomatic laryngopharyngeal reflux, as it is now called, do not meet criteria for GERD by pH probe testing* and these entities must be considered separately. The prevalence of this condition is hotly debated in the literature, and laryngopharyngeal reflux may not be as common as once thought.

Evaluation should initially exclude other causes of dysphonia through laryngoscopy; consultation with an otolaryngologist is advisable. Many clinicians opt for an empiric trial of a PPI since no gold standard exists for diagnosing this condition. *Such an empiric trial should* not *precede visualization of the vocal folds to exclude other causes of hoarseness.* When used, the American Academy of Otolaryngology–Head and Neck Surgery recommends twice-daily therapy with full-strength PPI (eg, omeprazole 40 mg orally twice daily or equivalent) for a minimum of 3 months. Patients may note improvement in symptoms after 3 months, but the changes in the larynx often take 6 months to resolve. If symptoms improve and cessation of therapy leads to symptoms again, then a PPI is resumed at the lowest dose effective for remission, usually daily but at times on a demand basis. Although H_2-receptor antagonists are an alternative to PPIs, they are generally both less clinically effective and less cost-effective. Nonresponders should undergo pH testing and manometry. Twenty-four-hour pH monitoring of the pharynx should best document laryngopharyngeal reflux and is advocated by some as the initial management step, but it is costly, more difficult, and less available than lower esophageal monitoring alone. **Double pH probe** (proximal and distal esophageal probes) testing is the best option for evaluation, since lower esophageal pH monitoring alone does not correlate well with laryngopharyngeal reflux symptoms. Oropharyngeal pH probe testing is available, but its ability to predict response to reflux treatment in patients with laryngopharyngeal reflux is not known.

Lechien JR et al. Association between Helicobacter pylori, reflux and chronic rhinosinusitis: a systematic review. Eur Arch Otorhinolaryngol. 2025 Feb 2. [Epub ahead of print] [PMID: 39893593]

Lechien JR et al. Association between laryngopharyngeal reflux, gastroesophageal reflux and recalcitrant chronic rhinosinusitis: a systematic review. Clin Otolaryngol. 2023;48:501. [PMID: 36895147]

Sims HS et al. Dysphonia and laryngopharyngeal reflux. Otolaryngol Clin North Am. 2025 Jan 23:S0030-6665(24)00198-1. [Epub ahead of print] [PMID: 39855951]

3. Recurrent Respiratory Papillomatosis

Papillomas are common lesions of the larynx and other sites where ciliated and squamous epithelia meet. Unlike oral papillomas, recurrent respiratory papillomatosis typically becomes symptomatic, with hoarseness that occasionally progresses over weeks to months. These papillomas are almost always due to HPV types 6 and 11. Repeated laser vaporizations or cold knife resections via operative laryngoscopy are the mainstay of treatment. Severe cases can cause airway compromise in adults and may require treatment as often as every 6 weeks to maintain airway patency. Extension can occur into the trachea and lungs. Tracheotomy should be avoided, if possible, since it introduces an additional squamociliary junction for which papillomas appear to have an affinity. Interferon treatment has been under investigation for many years but is only indicated in severe cases with pulmonary involvement. Rarely, cases of malignant transformation have been reported (often in smokers), but recurrent respiratory papillomatosis should generally be thought of as a benign condition. Cidofovir (a cytosine nucleotide analog in use to treat cytomegalovirus retinitis) has been used with success as intralesional therapy for recurrent respiratory papillomatosis. Because cidofovir causes adenocarcinomas in laboratory animals, its potential for carcinogenesis is being monitored. The quadrivalent and new 9 serotype recombinant human HPV vaccines (Gardasil and Gardasil 9) offer hope for the eventual prevention of this benign, but terribly morbid, disease.

Ovcinnikova O et al. A systematic literature review of the epidemiology, clinical, economic and humanistic burden in recurrent respiratory papillomatosis. Respir Res. 2024;25:430. [PMID: 39696284]

Park I et al. Systematic review of the use of human papillomavirus vaccine as adjuvant therapy for juvenile-onset recurrent respiratory papillomatosis. Int J Pediatr Otorhinolaryngol. 2022;162:111314. [PMID: 36116179]

Zagzoog FH et al. Intralesional cidofovir vs. bevacizumab for recurrent respiratory papillomatosis: a systematic review and indirect meta-analysis. Eur Arch Otorhinolaryngol. 2024;281:601. [PMID: 37831132]

4. Epiglottitis

Epiglottitis (or, more correctly, ***supraglottitis****) should be suspected when a patient presents with a rapidly developing sore throat or when odynophagia (pain on swallowing) is out of proportion to apparently minimal oropharyngeal findings on examination.* It is more common in patients with diabetes and may be viral or bacterial in origin. Rarely in the era of *H influenzae* type b vaccine is this bacterium isolated in adults. Unlike in children, indirect laryngoscopy is generally safe and may demonstrate a swollen, erythematous epiglottis. Lateral plain radiographs may demonstrate an enlarged epiglottis (the epiglottis "thumb sign"). Initial treatment is hospitalization for intravenous antibiotics—eg, ceftizoxime, 1–2 g intravenously every 8–12 hours; or cefuroxime, 750–1500 mg intravenously every 8 hours; and dexamethasone, usually 4–10 mg as initial bolus, then 4 mg intravenously every 6 hours—and observation of the airway. Corticosteroids may be tapered as symptoms and signs resolve. Similarly, substitution of oral antibiotics may be appropriate to complete a 10-day course. Less than 10% of adults require intubation. Indications for intubation are dyspnea, rapid pace of sore throat (where progression to airway compromise may occur before the effects of corticosteroids and antibiotics), and endolaryngeal abscess noted on CT imaging. If the patient is not intubated, prudence suggests monitoring oxygen saturation with continuous pulse oximetry and initial admission to a monitored unit.

Adams CP et al. Airway watch: a rare case of adult epiglottitis. Cureus. 2024;16:e73160. [PMID: 39651013]
Bridwell RE et al. High risk and low prevalence diseases: adult epiglottitis. Am J Emerg Med. 2022;57:14. [PMID: 35489220]
Kravietz A et al. A large cohort analysis of epiglottic phenotypes and pharyngeal residue. Ann Otol Rhinol Laryngol. 2024;133:375. [PMID: 38197379]

MASSES OF THE LARYNX

1. Traumatic Lesions of the Vocal Folds

Vocal fold nodules are smooth, paired lesions that form at the junction of the anterior one-third and posterior two-thirds of the vocal folds. They are a common cause of hoarseness resulting from vocal abuse. In adults, they are referred to as "singer's nodules" and in children as "screamer's nodules." Treatment requires modification of voice habits, and referral to a speech therapist is indicated. While nearly all true nodules will resolve with behavior modification, recalcitrant nodules may require surgical excision. Often, additional pathology, such as a polyp or cyst, may be encountered.

Vocal fold polyps are unilateral masses that form within the superficial lamina propria of the vocal fold. They are related to vocal trauma and seem to follow resolution of vocal fold hemorrhage. Small, sessile polyps may resolve with conservative measures, such as voice rest and corticosteroids, but larger polyps are often irreversible and require operative removal to restore normal voice.

Vocal fold cysts are also considered traumatic lesions of the vocal folds and are either true cysts with an epithelial lining or pseudocysts. They typically form from mucus-secreting glands on the inferior aspect of the vocal folds. Cysts may fluctuate in size from week to week and cause a variable degree of hoarseness. They rarely, if ever, resolve completely and may leave behind a sulcus, or vocal fold scar, if they decompress or are marsupialized. Such scarring can be a frustrating cause of permanent dysphonia.

Polypoid corditis is different from vocal fold polyps and may form from loss of elastin fibers and loosening of the intracellular junctions within the lamina propria. This loss allows swelling of the gelatinous matrix of the superficial lamina propria (called **Reinke edema**). These changes in the vocal folds are strongly associated with smoking, but also with vocal abuse, chemical industrial irritants, and hypothyroidism. While this problem is common in both male and female smokers, women seem more troubled by the characteristic decline in modal pitch caused by the increased mass of the vocal folds. If the patient stops smoking or the lesions cause stridor and airway obstruction, surgical resection of the hyperplastic vocal fold mucosa may be indicated to improve the voice or airway, or both.

A common but often unrecognized cause of hoarseness and odynophonia are **contact ulcers** or their close relatives, **granulomas**. Both lesions form on the vocal processes of the arytenoid cartilages, and patients often can correctly inform the clinician which side is affected. The cause of these ulcers and granulomas is disputed, but they are clearly related to trauma and may be related to exposure of the underlying perichondrium. They are common following intubation and generally resolve quite quickly. Chronic ulceration or granuloma formation has been associated with gastroesophageal reflux but is also common in patients with muscle tension dysphonia. Treatment is often multimodal, and an inhaled corticosteroid (eg, fluticasone 440 mcg twice daily) may be the most effective pharmacologic therapy. Adjunctive treatment measures include PPI therapy (omeprazole 40 mg orally twice daily, or equivalent) and voice therapy with special attention to vocal hygiene. Rare cases can be quite stubborn and persistent without efficacious therapy. Surgical removal is rarely, if ever, required for nonobstructive lesions.

Adriaansen A et al. Short-term effects of semi-occluded vocal tract therapy on the phonation of children with vocal fold nodules: a randomized controlled trial. J Speech Lang Hear Res. 2025;68:456. [PMID: 39761117]
Bar R et al. Laryngeal office-based procedures: a safe approach. Am J Otolaryngol. 2023;45:104128. [PMID: 38039913]
Fan RS et al. Clinical voice outcomes for two voice rest protocols after phonomicrosurgery. Laryngoscope. 2024;134:2812. [PMID: 38217412]

2. Laryngeal Leukoplakia

Leukoplakia of the vocal folds is commonly *found in association with hoarseness in smokers*. Direct laryngoscopy with biopsy is advised in almost all cases. Histologic examination usually demonstrates mild, moderate, or severe dysplasia. In some cases, invasive squamous cell carcinoma is present in the initial biopsy specimen. Cessation of smoking may reverse or stabilize mild or moderate dysplasia. Some patients—estimated to be < 5% of those with mild dysplasia and about 35–60% of those with severe dysplasia—will subsequently develop squamous cell carcinoma. Treatment options include PPI therapy, close follow-up with laryngovideostroboscopy, serial resection, and external beam radiation therapy.

Klimza H et al. Vocal fold leukoplakia recurrence risk model. Sci Rep. 2024;14:266. [PMID: 38168150]
Sun K et al. Recurrence and malignant transformation of laryngeal leukoplakia treated with CO_2 laser: a systematic review and meta-analysis. Clin Otolaryngol. 2024;49:404. [PMID: 38558499]

3. Squamous Cell Carcinoma of the Larynx

ESSENTIALS OF DIAGNOSIS

- New and persistent (> 2 weeks' duration) voice changes and hoarseness, especially in a smoker.
- Persistent throat pain, especially with swallowing; weight loss; neck mass; hemoptysis.
- Stridor or other symptoms of a compromised airway.

General Considerations

Squamous cell carcinoma of the larynx, the most common malignancy of the larynx, occurs almost exclusively in patients with a history of significant tobacco use. Prevalence and mortality of laryngeal cancer are estimated at 2.76 cases/year per 100,000 individuals, 14.33 cases/year per 100,000 individuals, and 1.66 deaths/year per 100,000 individuals, respectively. The incidence and prevalence have increased by 12% and 24%, respectively, during the past three decades. Mortality has declined by ~5%. Squamous cell carcinoma is usually seen in men aged 50–70 years. There may be an association between laryngeal cancer and HPV type 16 or 18 infection, but this association is much less strong than that between HPV 16 or 18 and oropharyngeal cancer. In both cancer types, the association with HPV seems to be strongest in nonsmokers. Early detection is the key to maximizing posttreatment voice, swallowing, and breathing function.

Clinical Findings

A. Symptoms and Signs

A change in voice quality is most often the presenting symptom, although throat or ear pain, hemoptysis, dysphagia, weight loss, and airway compromise may occur. Because of their early impact on vocal quality, glottic cancers are among the smallest detectable human malignancies and treatment success is very high with early lesions. Neck metastases are not common in **early glottic (true vocal fold) cancer** in which the vocal folds are mobile, but a third of patients in whom there is impaired fold mobility will also have involved lymph nodes at neck dissection. **Supraglottic carcinoma** (false vocal folds, aryepiglottic folds, epiglottis), on the other hand, often metastasizes to both sides of the neck early in the disease. Complete head and neck examination, including laryngoscopy, is mandatory for any person with the concerning symptoms listed under Essentials of Diagnosis.

B. Imaging and Laboratory Studies

Radiologic evaluation by CT or MRI is helpful in assessing tumor extent. Imaging evaluates neck nodes, tumor volume, and cartilage sclerosis or destruction. A chest CT scan is almost always indicated to evaluate for a second primary lesion or metastases. Laboratory evaluation includes CBC and liver biochemical tests. Formal cardiopulmonary evaluation may be indicated, especially if partial laryngeal surgery is being considered. All partial laryngectomy candidates should have good to excellent lung function and exercise tolerance because chronic microaspiration may be expected following the procedure. A PET scan or CT-PET scan may be indicated to assess for distant metastases when there appears to be advanced local or regional disease.

C. Biopsy

Diagnosis is made by biopsy at the time of laryngoscopy when true fold mobility and arytenoid fixation, as well as surface tumor extent, can be evaluated. Most otolaryngologists recommend esophagoscopy and bronchoscopy at the same time to exclude synchronous primary tumor. Although an FNA biopsy of an enlarged neck node may have already been done, it is generally acceptable to assume radiographically enlarged neck nodes (> 1–1.5 cm) or nodes with necrotic centers are neck metastases. Open biopsies of nodal metastases should be *discouraged* because they may lead to higher rates of tumor treatment failure.

D. Tumor Staging

The American Joint Committee on Cancer (AJCC) staging of laryngeal cancers uses the TNM system to describe tumor extent and can be used for prognosis. Early laryngeal cancers, T1 and T2 (stage I and II) lesions, involve 1–2 laryngeal subsites locally with normal vocal fold mobility, and have no nodal metastases or profound functional abnormalities. T3 and T4 lesions may involve multiple laryngeal subsites with limitation of vocal fold mobility. These locally advanced lesions are stage III or IV cancers, and any size tumor with regional nodal metastases is at least a stage III tumor. Stage I and II lesions are generally treated with single-modality therapy (surgery or radiation), while multimodality therapy, usually including chemotherapy with radiation therapy, is reserved for more advanced stage III and IV lesions.

Treatment

Treatment of laryngeal carcinoma has four goals: cure, preservation of safe and effective swallowing, preservation of useful voice, and avoidance of a permanent tracheostoma. For early glottic and supraglottic cancers, radiation therapy is the standard of care since cure rates are > 95% and 80%, respectively. That said, radiation therapy carries substantial morbidity, and many early tumors (T1 and T2 lesions, without involved nodes) and selected advanced tumors (T3) may be treated with partial laryngectomy if at least one cricoarytenoid unit can be preserved. Five-year locoregional cure rates exceed 80–90% with surgery, and patient-reported satisfaction is excellent. In supraglottic tumors, even when clinically N0, elective limited neck dissection is indicated following surgical resection because of the high risk of neck node involvement.

Advanced stage III and IV tumors represent a challenging and ever-changing treatment dilemma. Twenty-five years ago, total laryngectomy was often recommended for such patients. However, the 1994 VA study (with induction cisplatin and 5-fluorouracil followed by irradiation alone in responders) demonstrated that two-thirds of patients could preserve their larynx. Subsequent studies have further defined **multimodal therapy**. Cisplatin-based chemotherapy concomitant with radiation therapy has been shown to be superior to either irradiation alone or induction chemotherapy followed by radiation. The same benefits have been demonstrated with the epidermal growth factor receptor blocker cetuximab with lower overall systemic toxicity and better patient tolerance. However, chemoradiation using either cetuximab or cisplatin is associated with prolonged gastrostomy-dependent dysphagia.

The high rate of dysphagia and morbidity associated with severe laryngeal stenosis following chemoradiation has prompted potential for **organ preservation therapy**. Organ preservation surgery should be considered and discussed as an alternative to chemoradiation but may require referral to an appropriate regional center where such techniques are offered. After thorough evaluation of candidacy and discussion of the treatment options, patient choice plays a critical role in the ultimate decision to pursue surgery or chemoradiation as a definitive treatment modality. The patient and treating clinicians must carefully consider different early and late side effects and complications associated with different treatment modalities.

The presence of malignant adenopathy in the neck affects the prognosis greatly. Supraglottic tumors metastasize early and bilaterally to the neck, and this must be included in the treatment plans even when the neck is apparently uninvolved. Glottic tumors in which the true vocal folds are mobile (T1 or T2) have a < 5% rate of nodal involvement; when a fold is immobile, the rate of ipsilateral nodal involvement climbs to about 30%. An involved neck is treated by surgery or chemoradiation, or both. This decision will depend on the treatment chosen for the larynx and the extent of neck involvement.

Total laryngectomy is largely reserved for patients with advanced resectable tumors with extralaryngeal spread or cartilage involvement, for those with persistent tumor following chemoradiation, and for patients with recurrent or second primary tumor following previous radiation therapy. In these cases, the larynx is entirely removed rendering a patient aphonic and with a permanent stoma in their neck through which they breathe. Voice rehabilitation via a primary or secondary tracheoesophageal puncture with voice prosthesis placement produces intelligible and serviceable speech in about 75–85% of patients. Indwelling prostheses that are changed every 3–6 months are a common alternative to patient-inserted prostheses, which need changing more frequently.

Long-term follow-up is critical in head and neck cancer patients. In addition to the 3–4% annual rate of second tumors and monitoring for recurrence, psychosocial aspects of treatment are common. Dysphagia, impaired communication, and altered appearance may result in patient difficulties adapting to the workplace and to social interactions. In addition, smoking cessation and alcohol abatement are common challenges. Nevertheless, about 65% of patients with larynx cancer are cured, most have useful speech, and many resume their prior livelihoods with adaptations.

When to Refer

- Specialty referral should be sought early for diagnosis and treatment.

When to Admit

- Airway compromise, hemorrhage, dehydration, significant weight loss.
- To determine an effective pain management regimen for severe pain.

Saba NF et al. Novel immunotherapeutic approaches to treating HPV-related head and neck cancer. Cancers. 2023;15:1959. [PMID: 37046621]

Scarini JF et al. Head and neck squamous cell carcinoma: exploring frontiers of combinatorial approaches with tyrosine kinase inhibitors and immune checkpoint therapy. Crit Rev Oncol Hematol. 2022;180:103863. [PMID: 36334881]

Wang W et al. Characterization of the immune cell function landscape in head and neck squamous carcinoma to assist in prognosis prediction and immunotherapy. Aging. 2023;15:12588. [PMID: 37955651]

VOCAL FOLD PARALYSIS

Vocal fold paralysis can result from a lesion or damage to either the vagus or recurrent laryngeal nerve. It may result in breathy dysphonia, effortful voicing, aspiration, and rarely airway compromise. Common causes of **unilateral recurrent laryngeal nerve** involvement include thyroid surgery (and occasionally thyroid cancer), other neck surgery (anterior discectomy and carotid endarterectomy), and mediastinal or apical involvement by lung cancer. Skull base tumors often involve or abut upon lower cranial nerves and may affect the **vagus nerve** directly, or the vagus nerve may be damaged during surgical management of the lesion. While iatrogenic injury is the most common cause of unilateral vocal fold paralysis, the second most common cause is idiopathic. However, before deciding whether the paralysis is due to iatrogenic injury or is idiopathic, the clinician must exclude other causes, such as malignancy. In the absence of other cranial neuropathies, a CT scan with contrast from the skull base to the aortopulmonary window (the span of the recurrent laryngeal nerve) should be performed. If other cranial nerve deficits or high vagal weakness with palate paralysis is noted, an MRI scan of the brain and brainstem is warranted.

Unilateral vocal fold paralysis is occasionally temporary and may take over a year to resolve spontaneously. Surgical management of persistent or irrecoverable symptomatic unilateral vocal fold paralysis has evolved over the last several decades. The primary goal is medialization of the paralyzed fold in order to create a stable platform for vocal fold vibration. Additional goals include advancing diet and improving pulmonary toilet by facilitating cough. Success has been reported for years with injection laryngoplasty using Teflon, Gelfoam, fat, and collagen. Once the paralysis is determined to be permanent, formal medialization thyroplasty may be performed by creating a small window in the thyroid cartilage and placing an implant between the thyroarytenoid muscle and inner table of the thyroid cartilage. This procedure moves the vocal fold medially and creates a stable platform for bilateral, symmetric mucosal vibration.

Unlike unilateral fold paralysis, **bilateral vocal fold paralysis** usually causes inspiratory stridor with deep inspiration and may cause rapid airway compromise. If the onset of bilateral fold paralysis is insidious, it may be asymptomatic at rest, and the patient may have a normal voice. However, **the acute onset of bilateral vocal fold paralysis with inspiratory stridor at rest should be managed by a specialist immediately in a critical care environment**. Causes of bilateral fold paralysis include thyroid surgery, esophageal cancer, and ventricular shunt malfunction. Unilateral or bilateral fold immobility may also be seen in trauma, cricoarytenoid arthritis secondary to advanced rheumatoid arthritis, intubation injuries, glottic and subglottic stenosis, and laryngeal cancer. The goal of intervention is the creation of a safe airway with minimal reduction in voice quality and airway protection from aspiration. A number of fold lateralization procedures for bilateral paralysis have been advocated as a means of removing the tracheotomy tube.

Bakkar S et al. Immediate repair of the recurrent laryngeal nerve during thyroid surgery via a tension-free end-to-side anastomosis with the vagus. Updates Surg. 2025;77:363. [PMID: 39808246]
Lee YJ et al. Ten-year outcomes of recurrent laryngeal nerve reinnervation for thyroidectomy-related unilateral vocal fold paralysis: a single-surgeon, prospective study. Am J Otolaryngol. 2024;45:104242. [PMID: 38479219]
Liao LJ et al. Management of unilateral vocal fold paralysis after thyroid surgery with injection laryngoplasty: state of art review. Front Surg. 2022;9:876228. [PMID: 35465431]

CRICOTHYROTOMY & TRACHEOSTOMY

The three main approaches to secure an airway include endotracheal intubation, cricothyrotomy, and tracheostomy. In an acute airway emergency where the airway above the trachea is blocked (ie, due to trauma, mass, or bleeding), cricothyrotomy secures an airway more rapidly than tracheotomy, with fewer potential immediate complications (eg, pneumothorax and hemorrhage). Depending on the airway emergency, a cricothyrotomy may need to be converted to a tracheostomy after the airway has been secured.

There are two primary indications for tracheotomy: airway obstruction at or above the level of the larynx and respiratory failure requiring prolonged mechanical ventilation. Tracheotomies may be performed via an open or percutaneous approach. In experienced hands, the various methods of percutaneous tracheotomy have been documented to be safe for carefully selected patients. Simultaneous videobronchoscopy can reduce the incidence of major complications. The major cost reduction comes from avoiding the operating room. Bedside tracheotomy (in the ICU) achieves similar cost reduction and is advocated by some experts as slightly less costly than the percutaneous procedures.

The most common indication for elective tracheotomy is the need for prolonged mechanical ventilation. There is no firm rule about how many days a patient must be intubated before conversion to tracheotomy should be advised. The incidence of serious complications, such as subglottic stenosis, increases with extended endotracheal intubation. *As soon as it is apparent that the patient will require protracted ventilatory support, tracheotomy should replace the endotracheal tube.* Less frequent indications for tracheostomy are life-threatening aspiration pneumonia, the need to improve pulmonary toilet to correct problems related to insufficient clearing of tracheobronchial secretions, and obstructive sleep apnea.

Posttracheotomy care requires humidified air to prevent secretions from crusting and occluding the inner cannula of the tracheotomy tube. The tracheotomy tube should be cleaned several times daily. The most frequent early complication of tracheotomy is dislodgment of the tracheotomy tube. Surgical creation of an inferiorly based tracheal flap sutured to the inferior neck skin may make reinsertion of a dislodged tube easier. It should be recalled that the act of swallowing requires elevation of the larynx, which is limited by tracheotomy. Therefore, frequent tracheal and bronchial suctioning is often required to clear the aspirated saliva as well as the increased tracheobronchial secretions. Care of the skin around the tracheostoma is important to prevent maceration and secondary infection.

Romem A et al. Percutaneous tracheostomy in the ICU: a review of the literature and recent updates. Curr Opin Pulm Med. 2023;29:47. [PMID: 36378112]
Rosario E et al. Coronavirus disease tracheostomy complications: a scoping review. J Laryngol Otol. 2023;137:7. [PMID: 36217670]
Szafran A et al. Early versus late tracheostomy in critically ill COVID-19 patients. Cochrane Database Syst Rev. 2023;11:CD015532. [PMID: 37982427]

FOREIGN BODIES IN THE UPPER AERODIGESTIVE TRACT

FOREIGN BODIES IN THE TRACHEA & BRONCHI

Aspiration of foreign bodies occurs much less frequently in adults than in children. Older adults and those who wear dentures appear to be at greatest risk. Wider familiarity with the **Heimlich maneuver** has reduced deaths. If the maneuver is unsuccessful, cricothyrotomy may be necessary in the acute setting.

If there is no airway compromise, a CXR may reveal a radiopaque foreign body. Detection of radiolucent foreign bodies may be aided by CT or inspiration-expiration films that demonstrate air trapping distal to the obstructed segment. Atelectasis and pneumonia may occur later. Tracheal and bronchial foreign bodies should be removed under general anesthesia with rigid or flexible bronchoscopy by a skilled endoscopist working with an experienced anesthesiologist.

FOREIGN BODIES IN THE ESOPHAGUS

Foreign bodies in the esophagus create are typically not life-threatening situations. However, the acuity may rise depending on the type of foreign body (eg, a button battery) or if the airway is compromised. **Button battery ingestion is a surgical emergency.** If there is no concern for caustic ingestion or airway compromise, there is typically time to consult an otolaryngologist for management. It is a useful diagnostic sign of complete obstruction if the patient is drooling or cannot handle secretions. Patients may often point to the exact level of the obstruction. Indirect laryngoscopy often shows pooling of saliva at the esophageal inlet. Plain films may detect radiopaque foreign bodies, such as chicken bones. Coins tend to align in the coronal plane in the esophagus and in the sagittal direction in the trachea. If a foreign body is suspected, a CT or barium swallow may also help make the diagnosis.

The treatment of an esophageal foreign body depends on identification of its cause. In children, swallowed nonfood objects are common. In adults, however, food foreign bodies are more common, and there is the greater possibility of underlying esophageal pathology. If there is nothing sharp, such as a bone, some clinicians advocate a hospitalized 24-hour observation period prior to esophagoscopy, noting that spontaneous passage of the foreign body will occur in 50% of adult patients. In the management of meat obstruction, the use of papain (meat tenderizer) should be discouraged because it can damage the esophageal mucosa and lead to stenosis or perforation. Esophageal foreign bodies that do not pass need to be removed surgically. Endoscopic removal and examination are usually best via flexible esophagoscopy or rigid laryngoscopy and esophagoscopy. Complications of penetrating or erosive esophageal foreign bodies may include mediastinitis or erosion in the trachea with associated tracheitis.

Philteos J et al. Airway complications resulting from pediatric esophageal button battery impaction: a systematic review. JAMA Otolaryngol Head Neck Surg. 2022;148:677. [PMID: 35616924]

Tambakis G et al. Management of foreign body ingestion in adults: time to STOP and rethink endoscopy. Endosc Int Open. 2023;11:E1161. [PMID: 38094028]

DISEASES PRESENTING AS NECK MASSES

The differential diagnosis of neck masses is heavily dependent on the location in the neck, the age of the patient, and the presence of associated disease processes. Rapid growth and tenderness suggest an inflammatory process, while firm, painless, and slowly enlarging masses are often neoplastic. In young adults, most neck masses are benign (branchial cleft cyst, thyroglossal duct cyst, reactive lymphadenitis), although malignancy should always be considered (lymphoma, metastatic thyroid carcinoma). Lymphadenopathy is common in persons with HIV, but a growing or dominant mass may well represent lymphoma. *In adults over age 40, cancer is the most common cause of persistent neck mass and should be definitively ruled out.* A metastasis from squamous cell carcinoma arising within the mouth, pharynx, larynx, or upper esophagus should be suspected. Risk factors for squamous cell carcinoma include smoking and HPV exposure. Especially among patients younger than 30 or older than 70, lymphoma also should be considered. In all cases, a comprehensive otolaryngologic examination is needed. Imaging and pathologic evaluation of the neck mass via FNA biopsy is likely to be the next step if a primary tumor is not obvious on physical examination.

CONGENITAL LESIONS PRESENTING AS NECK MASSES IN ADULTS

1. Branchial Cleft Cysts

Branchial cleft cysts usually present as a soft cystic mass along the anterior border of the sternocleidomastoid muscle. These lesions are usually recognized in the second or third decades of life, often when they suddenly swell or become infected. To prevent recurrent infection and possible carcinoma, they should be completely excised, along with their fistulous tracts.

First branchial cleft cysts present high in the neck, sometimes just below the ear. A fistulous connection with the floor of the external auditory canal may be present. Second branchial cleft cysts, which are far more common, may communicate with the tonsillar fossa. Third branchial cleft cysts, which may communicate with the piriform sinus, are rare and present low in the neck.

2. Thyroglossal Duct Cysts

Thyroglossal duct cysts occur along the embryologic course of the thyroid's descent from the tuberculum impar of the tongue base to its usual position in the low neck. Although they may occur at any age, they are most common before age 20. They present as a midline neck mass, often just below the hyoid bone, which moves with swallowing. Surgical excision is recommended to prevent recurrent infection and rare malignancy. This requires removal of the entire fistulous tract along with the middle portion of the hyoid bone through which many of the fistulas pass. CT or ultrasound or both are often obtained preoperatively to understand associated neck anatomy, including position of the thyroid.

INFECTIOUS & INFLAMMATORY NECK MASSES

1. Reactive Cervical Lymphadenopathy

Normal lymph nodes in the neck are usually < 1 cm in length. Infections involving the pharynx, salivary glands, and scalp often cause tender enlargement of neck nodes. Enlarged nodes are common in persons with HIV. Except for the occasional node that suppurates and requires incision and drainage, treatment is directed against the underlying infection. *An enlarged node (larger than 1.5 cm) or node with a necrotic center that is not associated with an obvious infection should be further evaluated, especially if the patient has a history of smoking, alcohol use, or prior cancer.* Other common indications for FNA biopsy of a node include its persistence or continued enlargement. Common causes of cervical adenopathy include cancer (eg, squamous cell carcinoma, lymphoma, occasional metastases from non-head and neck sites) and infection (eg, reactive nodes, mycobacteria, and cat-scratch disease). Rare causes of adenopathy include Kikuchi disease (histiocytic necrotizing lymphadenitis) and autoimmune adenopathy.

2. Tuberculous & Nontuberculous Mycobacterial Lymphadenitis

Granulomatous neck masses are uncommon in the United States unless there are specific risk factors for particular infectious exposures or granulomatous hereditary or autoimmune illness. The differential diagnosis includes mycobacterial adenitis, sarcoidosis, and cat-scratch disease due to *Bartonella henselae.* The incidence of mycobacterial lymphadenitis is on the rise both in immunocompromised and immunocompetent individuals. The usual presentation of granulomatous disease in the neck is simply single or matted nodes. Although mycobacterial adenitis can extend to the skin and drain externally (as described for atypical mycobacteria and referred to as scrofula), this late presentation is no longer common.

FNA biopsy is usually the best initial diagnostic approach: cytology, smear for acid-fast bacilli, mycobacterial culture, and a sensitivity test can all be done. PCR from FNA (or from excised tissue) is the most sensitive test and is particularly useful when conventional methods have not been diagnostic but clinical impression remains consistent for tuberculous infection. While FNA has a high sensitivity (about 88%), its specificity is low (49%); thus, an excisional biopsy is often required to confirm the diagnosis.

For atypical (nontuberculous) infection of the lymph nodes, treatment depends on the sensitivity results of culture, but antibiotics likely to be useful include 6 months of isoniazid and rifampin and, for at least the first 2 months, ethambutol—all in standard dosages. Some would totally excise the involved nodes prior to chemotherapy, depending on location and other factors, but this can lead to chronic draining fistulas.

Yadav V et al. Primary subglottic laryngeal tuberculosis mimicking as malignancy: a rare case report. Indian J Otolaryngol Head Neck Surg. 2024;76:6003. [PMID: 39559153]

3. Lyme Disease

Lyme disease, caused by the spirochete *Borrelia burgdorferi* and transmitted by ticks of the *Ixodes* genus, may have protean manifestations, but over 75% of patients have symptoms involving the head and neck. Facial paralysis, hearing loss, dysesthesias, dysgeusia, or other cranial neuropathies are most common. Headache, pain, and cervical lymphadenopathy may occur. It is essential to ask patients with cranial neuropathies about risk factors for Lyme disease. See Chapter 38 for a more detailed discussion.

Dersch R et al. Efficacy and safety of pharmacological treatments for Lyme neuroborreliosis: an updated systematic review. Eur J Neurol. 2023;30:3780. [PMID: 37565386]
Sébastien P et al. Diagnosis and treatment of "chronic Lyme": primum non nocere. BMC Infect Dis. 2023;23:642. [PMID: 37784031]

CANCER METASTASES

In older adults, 80% of firm, persistent, and enlarging neck masses are metastatic in origin. The majority of these arise from squamous cell carcinoma of the upper aerodigestive tract, such as nasopharynx, tonsils, tongue base, and larynx. A complete head and neck examination may reveal the cancer of origin, but often imaging and examination under anesthesia are necessary to detect the primary lesion. Detecting the primary lesion is essential since it may directly impact oncologic treatment modalities. Initial radiologic screening exams typically include a CT, MRI, or PET. After imaging, many patients require direct laryngoscopy, esophagoscopy, and tracheobronchoscopy to further elucidate the primary lesion. At this time, biopsies may be taken for suspicious lesions. FNA of neck masses are also routine and may help determine the diagnosis while evaluation of the primary malignancy is ongoing. *Open neck biopsy should only be performed by head and neck surgeons experienced in the management of head and neck cancer since complications from open biopsy may make subsequent formal neck dissections more challenging if cancer is detected.* With the exception of papillary thyroid carcinoma, non-squamous cell metastases to the neck are infrequent. While cancers that are not primary in the head or neck seldom metastasize to the cervical lymph nodes, the supraclavicular lymph nodes are quite often involved by lung, gastroesophageal, and breast cancers. Infradiaphragmatic cancers, with the exception of renal cell carcinoma and testicular cancer, rarely metastasize to the neck.

Chen AM. Management of unknown primary head and neck cancer with radiation therapy in the era of human papillomavirus (HPV): no longer cutting down the tree to get an apple. Radiother Oncol. 2023;189:109952. [PMID: 37844736]
Guarino P et al. A comprehensive systematic review on functional results, speech and swallowing outcomes after trans-oral robotic surgery for oropharyngeal squamous cell cancer. J Clin Med. 2024;13:6039. [PMID: 39457989]
Madani G et al. The radiological unknown primary of the head and neck: recommendations for imaging strategies based on a systematic review. Clin Otolaryngol. 2024;49:16. [PMID: 37846889]
Patel MR et al. The widespread application of trans-oral robotic surgery in HPV-related head and neck cancer: one size does not fit all. J Natl Cancer Inst. 2025;117:388. [PMID: 39699215]

LYMPHOMA

About 10% of lymphomas present in the head and neck. Multiple rubbery nodes, especially in young adults or in patients who have AIDS, are suggestive of lymphoma. A thorough physical examination may demonstrate other sites of nodal or organ involvement. FNA biopsy may be diagnostic, but open biopsy is often required to determine architecture and an appropriate treatment course.

Al-Khafaf AE et al. Lymphomas of the salivary glands: a systematic review. Acta Otolaryngol. 2023;143:610. [PMID: 37572309]
Danielson DT et al. Head and neck classic Hodgkin, T and NK lymphomas with eosinophilia. Head Neck Pathol. 2025;19:10. [PMID: 39873807]
Di Santo D et al. Current evidence on diagnosis and treatment of parotid gland lymphomas: a systematic review. Eur Arch Otorhinolaryngol. 2023;280:5219. [PMID: 37638999]

9 Pulmonary Disorders

Rime Abbas, MD
Meghan E. Fitzpatrick, MD
Belinda Rivera-Lebron, MD, MS, FCCP
Rachel Wojcik, MD, MS

DISORDERS OF THE AIRWAYS

Disorders of the airways can be classified as those that involve the upper airways—those above and including the vocal folds—and those that involve the lower airways.

DISORDERS OF THE UPPER AIRWAYS

Acute obstruction of the upper airway can be immediately life-threatening and must be relieved promptly to avoid asphyxia. Causes of acute upper airway obstruction include trauma to the larynx or pharynx, foreign body aspiration, laryngospasm, laryngeal edema or angioedema, infections (acute epiglottitis, Ludwig angina, pharyngeal or retropharyngeal abscess), and acute allergic laryngitis.

Chronic obstruction of the upper airway may be caused by goiter, carcinoma of the pharynx or larynx, laryngeal or subglottic stenosis, laryngeal granulomas or webs, or bilateral vocal fold paralysis. Laryngeal or subglottic stenosis may become evident weeks or months after endotracheal intubation. Laryngomalacia refers to the collapse of the supraglottic structures during inspiration. Inspiratory stridor, intercostal retractions on inspiration, a palpable inspiratory thrill over the larynx, and wheezing localized to the neck or trachea on auscultation are characteristic findings. Flow-volume loops may show characteristic flow limitations. Soft-tissue radiographs of the neck may show supraglottic or subglottic narrowing. CT and MRI scans can reveal exact sites of obstruction. Flexible endoscopy may be diagnostic, but caution is necessary to avoid exacerbating upper airway edema and precipitating critical airway narrowing.

Vocal fold dysfunction (also known as **inducible laryngeal obstruction [ILO]**) is characterized by transient, reversible narrowing of the larynx due to paradoxical vocal fold adduction during inspiration, expiration, or both. It presents as dyspnea and wheezing that may mimic asthma or exercise-induced asthma but may be distinguished by the lack of response to bronchodilator therapy, normal spirometry immediately after an attack, spirometric evidence of upper airway obstruction in a flow-volume loop, and a negative bronchial provocation test. However, vocal fold dysfunction may coexist with asthma or may be induced by exercise (exercise-induced laryngeal obstruction), inhalational irritant exposures (smoke, fumes, cleaning chemicals), laryngopharyngeal reflux of gastric contents, post-extubation or psychological stress. Definitive diagnosis requires direct visualization of adduction of the vocal folds on inspiration via laryngoscopy. Acute treatment consists of reassurance and supportive care until the episode spontaneously subsides; continuous positive airway pressure or helium-oxygen mixture (heliox) may also be used. For long-term prevention, strategies include avoiding precipitants (including psychogenic contributors), psychotherapy, and speech therapy. Botulinum toxin injections have been used in refractory cases to treat bilateral vocal fold hypomobility, laryngeal dystonia, and inducible laryngeal obstruction.

Gardner LS et al. Significance of inducible laryngeal obstruction phenotypes identified by latent class analysis. J Allergy Clin Immunol Pract. 2025;13:2817. [PMID: 40721159]

Koh J et al. A new paradigm for vocal cord dysfunction/inducible laryngeal obstruction: swift diagnosis and streamlined management pathways. Respirology. 2023;28:911. [PMID: 37612245]

Leong P et al. Diagnosis of vocal cord dysfunction/inducible laryngeal obstruction: an international Delphi consensus study. J Allergy Clin Immunol. 2023;152:899. [PMID: 37343843]

DISORDERS OF THE LOWER AIRWAYS

Tracheal obstruction may be intrathoracic (below the suprasternal notch) or extrathoracic. Fixed tracheal obstruction may be caused by acquired or congenital tracheal stenosis, primary or secondary tracheal neoplasms, extrinsic compression (tumors of the lung, thymus, or thyroid; lymphadenopathy; congenital vascular rings; aneurysms; etc), foreign body aspiration, tracheal granulomas and papillomas, tracheal trauma, or idiopathic subglottic stenosis. Variable or dynamic tracheal obstruction may be caused by tracheomalacia, foreign body aspiration, and retained secretions.

Acquired **tracheal stenosis** most commonly occurs post-endotracheal intubation or tracheostomy. Daily endotracheal tube (ETT) care including monitoring cuff pressure (ideally, 20–30 cm H_2O) to avoid overinflation, oral and endotracheal suctioning of secretions, and regular ETT rotation may help prevent tracheal stenosis. Onset of symptoms usually occurs weeks to months after tracheal decannulation or extubation. Symptoms may include dyspnea, dysphonia, dysphagia, cough, and inability to clear pulmonary secretions, but mild stenosis may be asymptomatic. Physical findings may be absent until tracheal diameter is reduced by ≥ 50%, when wheezing, a palpable tracheal thrill, and harsh breath sounds may be detected. When this diagnosis is suspected, CT of the neck and chest and PFT with flow-volume loop are initially performed, followed by bronchoscopic tracheal visualization. Management depends on stenosis location and severity. Options include balloon dilation, surgical resection with reconstruction, stent placement, or laser. Tracheostomy may be considered in those with refractory disease.

Bronchial obstruction may be caused by retained pulmonary secretions, aspiration, foreign bodies, bronchomalacia, bronchogenic carcinoma, compression by extrinsic masses, and tumors metastatic to the airway. Clinical and radiographic findings vary depending on the location of the obstruction and the degree of airway narrowing. Symptoms include dyspnea, cough, wheezing, and, if infection is present, fever and chills. A history of recurrent pneumonia in the same lobe or segment or slow resolution (> 3 months) of pneumonia on successive radiographs suggests the possibility of bronchial obstruction and the need for bronchoscopy. Radiographic findings include atelectasis (local parenchymal collapse), postobstructive infiltrates, and air trapping caused by unidirectional expiratory obstruction. CT scanning may demonstrate the nature and exact location of obstruction. Bronchoscopy is the definitive diagnostic study, particularly if tumor or foreign body aspiration is suspected. Management includes the use of bronchoscopic electrocautery, argon plasma coagulation, and laser and radiofrequency ablation.

Catano J et al. Presentation, diagnosis, and management of subglottic and tracheal stenosis during systemic inflammatory diseases. Chest. 2022;161:257. [PMID: 34324839]

Ravikumar N et al. The role of bronchoscopy in the multidisciplinary approach to benign tracheal stenosis. J Thorac Dis. 2023;15:3998. [PMID: 37559626]

Ulusan A et al. Long-term outcomes of surgical management in post-intubation tracheal stenosis: a retrospective analysis of tracheal resection and reconstruction. Updates Surg. 2025;77:533. [PMID: 39579255]

ASTHMA

ESSENTIALS OF DIAGNOSIS

- Respiratory symptoms, such as wheeze, dyspnea, or cough, possibly variable in time and severity.
- Variable expiratory airflow obstruction on PFT or positive bronchoprovocation challenge.

General Considerations

Asthma is a common disease, affecting approximately 5–10% of the population. It is more common in male than female children (7% versus 5.4%) and in female than male adults (10.8 versus 6.5%). There is a genetic predisposition to asthma, and rates vary by race and ethnicity. In the United States, Black persons are 44% more likely than White persons to have asthma. Prevalence, hospitalizations, and fatal asthma have all increased in the United States over the past 20 years. Each year, approximately 10 million office visits, 1.8 million emergency department visits, and > 3500 deaths in the United States are attributed to asthma. Hospitalization rates are highest among children and Black persons, and death rates are consistently highest among Black persons aged 15–24 years. The National Asthma Education and Prevention Program (NAEPP) and the Global Initiative for Asthma (GINA) report provide comprehensive and updated resources that address asthma diagnosis, assessment, management, and evidence-based recommendations.

Definition & Pathogenesis

Asthma is a chronic inflammatory disorder of the airways that results in an array of respiratory symptoms and signs and is characterized by variable levels of airway expiratory obstruction and hyperresponsiveness. The most common pathogeneses of asthma include airway inflammation with eosinophils, neutrophils, and lymphocytes (particularly T cells). Key features include goblet cell hyperplasia, plugging of small airways with mucus, collagen deposition beneath the basement membrane, bronchial smooth muscle hypertrophy, airway edema, mast cell activation, and denudation of airway epithelium.

The pathophysiology of asthma is heterogeneous, but a division into T2-high and T2-low endotypes (marked by high and low levels, respectively, of classic Th2 cytokines such as interleukin [IL]-4, IL-5, and IL-13) has been shown to be important in the selection of targeted biologic therapies and often correlates with specific clinical phenotypes. **Allergic asthma, late-onset T2-high asthma**, and **aspirin/NSAID-associated respiratory disease** are T2-high phenotypes. T2-low asthma phenotypes include **nonallergic asthma**, which tends to occur in adults and be marked by neutrophilic inflammation and variable response to standard therapies. **Asthma with persistent airflow limitation** is thought to be due to airway remodeling. **Asthma with obesity** refers to prominent respiratory symptoms in patients with obesity with little airway inflammation or eosinophilic involvement, but with an increasingly recognized role for adipokine-induced inflammation.

Many clinical phenotypes of asthma have been identified. The most common is **allergic asthma**, which usually begins in childhood and is associated with other allergic diseases (eg, eczema, allergic rhinitis, food allergy). Exposure of sensitive patients to inhaled allergens may cause symptoms immediately (early asthmatic response) or 4–6 hours after allergen exposure (late asthmatic response). Common allergens include house dust mites (often found in pillows, mattresses, upholstered furniture, carpets, and drapes), cockroaches, cat dander, and seasonal pollens. In response to inhaled triggers (eg, allergens, respiratory pathogens, particulate matter), epithelial-derived interleukins are produced which play a key role in activating downstream Th2 cells, group 2 innate lymphoid cells (ILC2s), and other immune effector cells.

Nonspecific precipitants of asthma include upper respiratory tract infections, rhinosinusitis, postnasal drip, aspiration, gastroesophageal reflux, changes in the weather, stress, and exercise. Exposure to **products of combustion** (eg, tobacco, methamphetamines, diesel fuel, and other agents) increases asthma symptoms and the need for medications and reduces lung function. **Air pollution** (increased air levels of respirable particles, ozone, SO_2, and NO_2) precipitates asthma symptoms and increases emergency department visits and hospitalizations. Selected individuals may experience asthma symptoms after exposure to aspirin (aspirin-exacerbated respiratory disease), NSAIDs, or tartrazine dyes. Other **medications** (eg, β-blockers, certain antibiotics) may precipitate asthma symptoms. **Occupational asthma** is triggered by various agents in the workplace and may occur weeks to years after initial exposure and sensitization. Women may experience **catamenial asthma** at predictable times during the menstrual cycle. **Exercise-induced bronchoconstriction** begins during exercise or within 3 minutes after its end, peaks within 10–15 minutes, and resolves within 20–30 minutes, though it may last up to 60 minutes in severe cases. This phenomenon is thought to result from airway warming and humidifying an increased volume of expired air during exercise. **Cough-variant asthma** has cough instead of wheezing as the predominant symptom of bronchial hyperreactivity.

Clinical Findings

Symptoms and signs vary widely among patients as well as within individuals over time. The level of asthma control is assessed by the frequency of day and nighttime symptoms and need for reliever medications as listed in Table 9–1.

A. Symptoms and Signs

Asthma symptoms include episodic wheezing, shortness of breath, chest tightness, and cough. Symptoms vary over time and in intensity and are often worse at night or in the early morning. Asthma symptoms may occur spontaneously or be precipitated or exacerbated by many different triggers, as discussed above.

Some physical examination findings increase the probability of asthma. Nasal mucosal swelling, increased secretions, and polyps are often seen in patients with allergic asthma. Eczema, atopic dermatitis, or other allergic skin disorders may also be present. Wheezing, a prolonged expiratory phase, or both during normal breathing are suggestive of airflow obstruction; wheezing during forced expiration does not. Chest examination may be normal between exacerbations in patients with mild asthma. During severe asthma exacerbations, airflow may be too limited to produce wheezing, and the only diagnostic clue on auscultation may be globally reduced breath sounds with prolonged expiration. Hunched shoulders and use of accessory muscles of respiration suggest an increased work of breathing.

B. Laboratory Findings

The T2-high phenotype of asthma is associated with eosinophilia. A blood eosinophil count > 150–300 cells/mcL is recommended for classifying the eosinophilic phenotype according to the European Respiratory Society and the American Thoracic Society and identifies persons with severe asthma who are candidates for targeted monoclonal antibody therapies. Serum IgE may also be helpful to guide selection of biologic therapy in persons with moderate to severe asthma or when allergic bronchopulmonary aspergillosis (ABPA) is suspected.

C. Pulmonary Function Testing

Pulmonary function testing with either spirometry or PEF measurements are important for the diagnosis and management of patients with asthma.

Important **spirometry measurements** include FEV_1, FVC, and FEV_1/FVC before and after the administration of a short-acting bronchodilator. These measurements help determine the presence and extent of airflow obstruction and whether it is immediately reversible. Airflow obstruction is indicated by a reduced FEV_1/FVC ratio, (< 0.7 or the lower limit of normal). Significant reversibility of airflow obstruction was previously defined by an increase of ≥ 12% and 200 mL in FEV_1 or FVC after inhaling a short-acting bronchodilator. Recommendations by the American Thoracic Society and the European Respiratory Society Technical Standards Committee define a bronchodilator response by an increase in FEV_1 or FVC of > 10% relative to the predicted value. A positive bronchodilator response

Table 9–1. Assessing asthma control.

Components of Asthma Control	Classification of Asthma Control		
	Well Controlled	Partly Controlled	Not Controlled
Daytime asthma symptoms > 2 ×/week Nighttime awakenings due to asthma Interference with normal activity due to asthma Reliever medication needed for asthma symptoms > 2 ×/week	None of these components within past 4 weeks	1 or 2 of these components within past 4 weeks	3 or 4 of these components within past 4 weeks

Adapted from National Asthma Education and Prevention Program. Expert Panel Report 3: Guidelines for the Diagnosis and Management of Asthma. National Institutes of Health Pub. No. 08-4051. Bethesda, MD, 2007, and Global Initiative for Asthma. Global Strategy for Asthma Management and Prevention 2022. Available at https://ginasthma.org

supports the diagnosis of asthma, but a lack of responsiveness does not exclude the diagnosis in a person who currently lacks obstruction. Severe airflow obstruction can result in air trapping, with an increase in residual volume and consequent reduction in FVC, mimicking a restrictive ventilatory defect pattern.

Bronchoprovocation testing with inhaled histamine or methacholine may be useful when asthma is suspected despite nondiagnostic spirometry. Bronchial provocation is not recommended if the FEV_1 is < 65% of predicted. A positive methacholine test is defined as a fall in the FEV_1 of ≥ 20% at exposure to a methacholine concentration of ≤ 8 mg/mL. A negative methacholine test has a negative predictive value for asthma of 95%. Exercise challenge testing may be useful in patients with symptoms of exercise-induced bronchospasm.

PEF meters are handheld devices designed as personal monitoring tools. PEF monitoring can establish peak flow variability, quantify asthma severity, and provide both patient and clinician with relatively objective measurements on which to base treatment titration decisions. Reliability of peak flow measurements may be affected by incorrect calibration and patient technique or effort. Comparison with reference values is less helpful than comparison with the patient's own baseline. PEF shows diurnal variation; it is generally lowest on first awakening and highest several hours before the midpoint of the waking day. PEF should be measured in the morning before the administration of a bronchodilator and in the afternoon after taking a bronchodilator. A 20% change in PEF values from morning to afternoon or from day to day suggests inadequately controlled asthma. PEF values < 200 L/min indicate severe airflow obstruction.

D. Additional Testing

Routine CXRs in patients with asthma are usually normal or only show hyperinflation. Chest imaging is indicated when pneumonia, which may mimic asthma, or a complication of asthma (eg, pneumothorax) is suspected.

Evaluations for paranasal sinus disease or gastroesophageal reflux should be considered in patients with persistent, severe, or refractory asthma symptoms.

Complications

Complications of asthma include exhaustion, dehydration, airway infection, tussive syncope, and, rarely, pneumothorax. Acute hypercapnic and hypoxemic respiratory failure occurs in severe disease.

Differential Diagnosis

Patients who have atypical symptoms or poor response to therapy may have one of several conditions that mimic asthma. **Upper airway disorders** that mimic asthma include vocal fold paralysis, vocal fold dysfunction syndrome, narrowing of the supraglottic airway, and laryngeal masses or dysfunction. **Lower airway disorders** include foreign body aspiration, tracheal masses or narrowing, tracheobronchomalacia, airway edema (eg, angioedema or inhalation injury), nonasthmatic COPD (chronic bronchitis or emphysema), bronchiectasis, ABPA (mycosis), cystic fibrosis (CF), eosinophilic pneumonia, hypersensitivity pneumonitis, sarcoidosis, and bronchiolitis obliterans. A **systemic vasculitis** with pulmonary involvement may have an asthmatic component, such as eosinophilic granulomatosis with polyangiitis. **Cardiac disorders** include HF ("cardiac asthma") and pulmonary hypertension. **Psychiatric causes** include conversion disorders ("functional" asthma), emotional laryngeal wheezing, or episodic laryngeal dyskinesis. Rarely, Münchausen syndrome or malingering may explain a patient's symptom presentation.

Approach to Management

Personalized asthma management is a continuous cycle that involves assessment, treatment adjustment, and periodic review with the goals of optimal symptom control; minimization of future risks, including exacerbations; and prevention of asthma-related deaths, as recommended in the updated 2024 GINA report. **Asthma assessment** includes the level of asthma control, risk factors for exacerbations, asthma severity, treatment adjustment, and periodic lung function testing.

1. Asthma control—Level of control is assessed by evaluating symptoms. Patients are asked about their past 4 weeks including frequency of symptoms (days per week), nocturnal symptoms (eg awakening from sleep), and use of reliever therapy (short-acting β-agonist [SABA], inhaled corticosteroid [ICS]-formoterol, or ICS-SABA) for symptom relief (Table 9–1). Patients should also be asked about activity limitations due to asthma.

2. Risk factors for exacerbations—Poor symptom control increases risk of exacerbations. Other risk factors include more than one exacerbation in the previous year; inadequate ICS use (due to under-treatment, poor adherence, or incorrect inhaler technique); and other comorbidities, such as chronic sinusitis, GERD, obesity, and smoking.

3. Asthma severity—Severity is evaluated retrospectively from the level of treatment needed to control symptoms and exacerbations. Table 9–2 describes the step therapy in a personalized asthma management plan. Typically, mild asthma responds to Step 1 or 2 treatments (low-dose ICS or low-dose combination therapies like ICS-formoterol), moderate asthma to Step 3 treatment (adding LABA or increasing ICS doses), and severe asthma to Step 4 or 5 treatments (high-dose ICS combinations with or without biologics). It is important to distinguish between uncontrolled and severe asthma in patients who are using Step 4 or Step 5 treatments. The clinician must assess inhaler technique, medication adherence, comorbidities (eg, obstructive sleep apnea, GERD), and ongoing exposure to allergens as causes of poor asthma control ("uncontrolled" asthma). If the patient still requires Step 4 or 5 therapy after these issues have been addressed, then the patient has "severe" asthma and should be referred to a pulmonary or asthma specialist. Serial lung function testing is beneficial at time of diagnosis, 3–6 months after treatment initiation, and periodically thereafter but is not necessarily needed at every visit.

Table 9–2. Step therapy in personalized asthma management plan.

	Preferred	Alternative
Steps 1 and 2	Low-dose ICS-formoterol as needed **or** Low-dose ICS daily and SABA as needed **or** Concomitant ICS and SABA as needed	LTRA daily and SABA as needed **or** Cromolyn **or** Nedocromil **or** Zileuton **or** Theophylline and SABA as needed
Step 3	Combination low-dose ICS plus formoterol daily and as needed	Medium-dose ICS daily and SABA as needed **or** Low-dose ICS-LABA daily **or** Low-dose ICS **plus** LAMA daily **or** Low-dose ICS **plus** LTRA and SABA as needed **or** Low-dose ICS daily **plus** theophylline or zileuton and SABA as needed
Step 4	Combination medium-dose ICS-formoterol daily and as needed	Medium-dose ICS-LABA daily **or** Medium-dose ICS **plus** LAMA daily and SABA as needed **or** Medium-dose ICS **plus** LTRA daily **or** Medium-dose ICS **plus** zileuton daily and SABA as needed **or** Medium-dose ICS **plus** theophylline daily
Step 5	Medium-high dose ICS-LABA plus LAMA and SABA as needed	Medium-high dose ICS-LABA daily **or** High-dose ICS **plus** LTRA and SABA as needed
Step 6	High-dose ICS-LABA plus oral systemic corticosteroids plus SABA as needed	

4. Treatment adjustment—The goals of asthma therapy are to minimize chronic symptoms that interfere with normal activity (including exercise), prevent recurrent exacerbations, reduce or eliminate the need for emergency department visits or hospitalizations, and maintain normal or near-normal pulmonary function. A multidisciplinary approach using pharmacologic and nonpharmacologic strategies is best to address disease pathogenesis and modifiable risk factors. Pharmacologic agents that satisfy the patient's expectations of asthma care with the fewest adverse events should be prescribed. Management should include **step-up** therapy if asthma remains uncontrolled despite adherence and good inhaler technique and **step-down** if asthma is well controlled to find the lowest effective therapeutic dose. Nonpharmacologic interventions include increasing physical activity and breathing exercises. Significant reduction in exposure to nonspecific airway irritants in all patients or to inhaled allergens in atopic patients may reduce symptoms and medication needs. Comorbid conditions that impair asthma management (eg, smoking, rhinosinusitis, GERD, obesity, obstructive sleep apnea) should be identified and treated. The asthma plan of care, level of symptom control, and patient satisfaction should be reviewed on a periodic basis and facilitated by guided patient self-management education and skills training. Self-management includes self-monitoring of symptoms or peak flow; a written action plan; and regular review of asthma control, treatment, and skills with a health care professional.

5. Periodic lung function testing—Serial spirometry is beneficial at time of diagnosis, 3–6 months after treatment initiation, and periodically thereafter to monitor the disease trajectory and response to therapy.

Treatment

A. Pharmacologic Agents

Asthma medications can be divided into three categories: (1) **long-term controller** medications (Table 9–3) used long term to reduce airway inflammation, symptoms, and risk of future exacerbations; (2) **reliever** medications for rapid onset relief (Table 9–4) used on an as-needed basis to relieve breakthrough symptoms; these include SABA, and more recently, ICS-SABA and ICS-formoterol combinations. The latter are gaining preference as both reliever medications and controller medications because formoterol is a LABA that has rapid onset (within 1–3 minutes), is longer acting than SABA, and provide increased therapeutic benefit in conjunction with an ICS; and (3) **add-on therapies** for severe asthma. See Table 9–2 for a personalized management plan for asthma to control symptoms and minimize future risk.

Most asthma medications are administered by inhalation or oral dosing. Inhalation of an appropriate agent results in a more rapid onset of pulmonary effects and fewer systemic effects compared with the oral dose required to achieve the same effect. Proper inhaler technique and the use of an inhalation chamber (a "spacer") with metered-dose inhalers (MDIs) decrease oropharyngeal drug deposition and improve drug delivery to the lung. Nebulizer therapy is reserved for patients who are acutely ill and those who cannot use inhalers because of difficulties with coordination, understanding, or cooperation.

1. Inhaled corticosteroids—ICSs are essential controller medications (Tables 9–4 and 9–5). Early initiation of ICS therapy after asthma diagnosis significantly improves lung function compared to delayed therapy. Prescribing ICS,

Table 9–3. Long-term controller medications for asthma.

Medication	Dosage Form	Adult Dose	Comments
Inhaled Corticosteroids (ICS)			**(See** Table 9–5)
Systemic Corticosteroids			**(Applies to all three corticosteroids)**
Methylprednisolone	2-, 4-, 6-, 8-, 16-, 32-mg tablets	40–60 mg	• Administer single dose in am either daily or on alternate days (alternate-day therapy may produce less adrenal suppression) as needed for control. • Short courses or "bursts" as single or two divided doses for 3–10 days are effective for establishing control when initiating therapy or during a period of gradual deterioration. • There is no evidence that tapering the dose following improvement in symptom control and pulmonary function prevents relapse.
Prednisolone	5-mg tablets; 5 mg/5 mL, 15 mg/5 mL oral solution	40–60 mg	
Prednisone	1-, 2.5-, 5-, 10-, 20-, 50-mg tablets; 5 mg/mL oral solution	7.5–60 mg	
Inhaled LABA			**Should not be used for symptom relief or exacerbations. Use with ICS.**
Formoterol	Inhalation: 20 mcg/2 mL nebulizer (DPI discontinued by US FDA)	20 mcg every 12 hours	• Additional doses should not be administered for at least 12 hours. • Agents should be used only with their specific inhaler and should not be taken orally. • Decreased duration of protection against EIB may occur with regular use.
Salmeterol	DPI: 50 mcg/actuation	1 blister every 12 hours	
Combined Medication			
Budesonide/formoterol	HFA MDI: 80 mcg/4.5 mcg 160 mcg/4.5 mcg	2 inhalations twice daily; dose depends on severity of asthma	• 80/4.5 mcg for asthma not controlled on low- to medium-dose ICS. • 160/4.5 mcg for asthma not controlled on medium- to high-dose ICS.
Fluticasone/salmeterol	DPI: 100 mcg/50 mcg 250 mcg/50 mcg 500 mcg/50 mcg HFA: 45 mcg/21 mcg 115 mcg/21 mcg 230 mcg/21 mcg	1 inhalation twice daily; dose depends on severity of asthma	• 100/50 mcg DPI or 45/21 mcg HFA for asthma not controlled on low- to medium-dose ICS. • 250/50 mcg DPI or 115/21 mcg HFA for asthma not controlled on medium- to high-dose ICS.
Fluticasone furoate/vilanterol	DPI: 100 mcg/25 mcg or 200 mcg/25 mcg per blister	1 puff inhaled daily	• Once-daily asthma maintenance.
Mometasone/formoterol	100 mcg/5 mcg/spray 200 mcg/5 mcg/spray	2 inhalations twice daily	
Cromolyn and Nedocromil			
Cromolyn	MDI: 0.8 mg/puff Nebulizer: 20 mg/ampule	2 puffs four times daily 1 ampule four times daily	• 4- to 6-week trial may be needed to determine maximum benefit. • Dose by MDI may be inadequate to affect hyperresponsiveness. • One dose before exercise or allergen exposure provides effective prophylaxis for 1–2 hours. Not as effective for EIB as SABA. • Once control is achieved, the frequency of dosing may be reduced.
Nedocromil	MDI: 1.75 mg/puff	2 puffs four times daily	
Inhaled Long-Acting Anticholinergic			**Should not be used for symptom relief or exacerbations. Use with ICS.**
Tiotropium	DPI: 18 mcg/blister	1 blister daily	
Leukotriene Receptor Antagonists			
Montelukast	4- or 5-mg chewable tablet; 10-mg tablet	10 mg daily at bedtime	• Exhibits a flat dose-response curve. Doses > 10 mg will not produce a greater response in adults.

(*continued*)

Table 9–3. Long-term controller medications for asthma. (continued)

Medication	Dosage Form	Adult Dose	Comments
Zafirlukast	10- or 20-mg tablet	20-mg tablet twice daily	• Administration with meals decreases bioavailability; take at least 1 hour before or 2 hours after meals. • Monitor for symptoms and signs of hepatic dysfunction.
5-Lipoxygenase Inhibitor			
Zileuton	600-mg tablet	600 mg four times daily	• Monitor hepatic enzyme (ALT).
Methylxanthines			
Theophylline	Liquids, sustained-release tablets, and capsules	Starting dose: 10 mg/kg/day up to 300 mg maximum Usual maximum dose: 800 mg/day	• Adjust dose to achieve serum concentration of 5–15 mcg/mL after at least 48 hours on same dose. • Due to wide interpatient variability in theophylline metabolic clearance, routine serum theophylline level monitoring is important.
Monoclonal Antibodies			
Omalizumab	Subcutaneous injection	Dependent on pretreatment IgE level; up to 375 mg every 2 weeks	• Binds to IgE; prevents interaction with IgE receptor on mast cells and basophils. • Carries black-box warning of anaphylaxis. • Suggested IgE level 30–1500 IU/mL.
Mepolizumab	Subcutaneous injection	100 mg every 4 weeks	• Binds to IL-5; prevents interaction with receptor. • Suggested AEC ≥ 150–300/mcL (0.15–0.3 × 10^9/L).
Reslizumab	Intravenous injection	3 mg/kg every 4 weeks	• Binds to IL-5; prevents interaction with receptor. • Carries black-box warning of anaphylaxis. • Suggested AEC ≥ 400/mcL (0.4 × 10^9/L).
Benralizumab	Subcutaneous injection	30 mg every 4 weeks for 3 doses, then every 8 weeks	• Binds to IL-5 receptor; blocks receptor-ligand interaction and also causes apoptosis of basophils and eosinophils. • Suggested AEC ≥ 300/mcL (0.3 × 10^9/L).
Dupilumab	Subcutaneous injection	200 or 300 mg every 2 weeks	• Binds to IL-4Rα; blocks IL-4 and IL-13 signaling. • Suggested AEC ≥ 150/mcL (0.15 × 10^9/L) or FENO ≥ 25 ppb, or both.

AEC, absolute eosinophil count; DPI, dry powder inhaler; EIB, exercise-induced bronchospasm; FENO, fractional exhaled nitric oxide; HFA, hydrofluoroalkane; LABA, long-acting β_2-agonist; MDI, metered-dose inhaler; SABA, short-acting β_2-agonist.

whether as needed or daily, underscores to the patient that both symptom control and risk reduction are fundamental to asthma treatment. The most important determinants of medication choice, device, and dose are a patient's symptoms and risk factors, along with practical issues (eg, cost, delivery mechanism). ICS dosages are classified as low-, medium-, and high-dose strengths. Dosages for ICS vary depending on the specific agent and delivery device (Table 9–5). For patients who require high-dose ICS to achieve adequate symptom control, the dose of ICS should be decreased after 3 months of good control to the lowest dose that preserves symptom control and minimizes exacerbation risk.

Concomitant use of an MDI and an inhalation chamber coupled with mouth washing after ICS use decreases systemic absorption and local side effects (cough, dysphonia, oropharyngeal candidiasis). Dry powder inhalers (DPIs) are not used with an inhalation chamber. Systemic effects (adrenal suppression, osteoporosis, skin thinning, easy bruising, and cataracts) may occur with high-dose ICS therapy. Combination inhalers with an ICS and a long-acting β_2-agonist (LABA) offer convenient treatment of asthma. The **GINA** 2024 guidelines recommend low-dose ICS-formoterol combination as a preferred long-term controller, based on strong clinical evidence, though cost and availability should be considered. Budesonide/formoterol is listed as an essential medicine by the **WHO**.

2. β-Agonists—β-Agonists are divided into SABAs and LABAs. **SABAs** (Table 9–4), including **albuterol, levalbuterol, bitolterol, pirbuterol,** and **terbutaline**, are mainstays of reliever or rescue therapy for patients with asthma. There is no convincing evidence to support the use of one agent over another. All patients with asthma should have immediate access to a reliever therapy with rapid onset bronchodilator containing a β-agonist; relievers can be SABA, ICS-SABA, or ICS-formoterol. Anti-inflammatory combination reliever medications, such as ICS-formoterol, when used as needed, may additionally reduce exacerbation rates. Administration before exercise effectively prevents exercise-induced bronchoconstriction. Of note, GINA guidelines discourage the use of SABA-only treatment in adults or adolescents due to the increased risk of asthma-related deaths or urgent healthcare visits, even if asthma symptoms are controlled.

Table 9–4. Reliever medications for asthma.

Medication	Dosage Form	Adult Dose	Comments
Inhaled Short-Acting β_2-Agonists (SABA)			
Albuterol CFC	MDI: 90 mcg/puff, 200 puffs/canister	2 puffs 5 minutes before exercise 2 puffs every 4–6 hours as needed	• An increasing use or lack of expected effect indicates diminished control of asthma. • Not recommended for long-term daily treatment. Regular use exceeding 2 days/week for symptom control (not prevention of EIB) indicates the need to step up therapy. • Differences in potency exist, but all products are essentially comparable on a per puff basis. • May double usual dose for mild exacerbations. • Prime the inhaler by releasing four actuations before use. • Periodically clean HFA activator, as drug may block/plug orifice.
Albuterol HFA	MDI: 90 mcg/puff, 200 puffs/canister	2 puffs 5 minutes before exercise 2 puffs every 4–6 hours as needed	
Pirbuterol CFC	MDI: 200 mcg/puff, 400 puffs/canister	2 puffs 5 minutes before exercise 2 puffs every 4–6 hours as needed	
Levalbuterol HFA	MDI: 45 mcg/puff, 200 puffs/canister	2 puffs 5 minutes before exercise 2 puffs every 4–6 hours as needed	
Albuterol	Nebulizer solution: 0.63 mg/3 mL 1.25 mg/3 mL 2.5 mg/3 mL 5 mg/mL (0.5%)	1.25–5 mg in 3 mL of saline every 4–8 hours as needed	• May mix with budesonide inhalant suspension, cromolyn, or ipratropium nebulizer solutions. • May double dose for severe exacerbations.
Levalbuterol (R-albuterol)	Nebulizer solution: 0.31 mg/3 mL 0.63 mg/3 mL 1.25 mg/0.5 mL 1.25 mg/3 mL	0.63–1.25 mg every 8 hours as needed	• Compatible with budesonide inhalant suspension. The product is a sterile-filled, preservative-free, unit dose vial.
Anticholinergics			
Ipratropium HFA	MDI: 17 mcg/puff, 200 puffs/canister	2–3 puffs every 6 hours	• Evidence is lacking for anticholinergics producing added benefit to β_2-agonists in long-term asthma control therapy.
	Nebulizer solution: 0.25 mg/mL (0.025%)	0.25 mg every 6 hours	
Ipratropium with albuterol	MDI: 18 mcg/puff of ipratropium bromide and 90 mcg/puff of albuterol, 200 puffs/canister	2–3 puffs every 6 hours	
	Nebulizer solution: 0.5 mg/3 mL ipratropium bromide and 2.5 mg/3 mL albuterol	3 mL every 4–6 hours	• Contains EDTA to prevent discolorations of the solution. This additive does not induce bronchospasm.
Anti-Inflammatory Relievers (Low-Dose ICS and Rapid Acting Bronchodilator)			
ICS-Albuterol	Albuterol/Budesonide MDI: 90 mcg/80 mcg per actuation	2 puffs every 4 hours as needed	Max 12 puffs/day
Budesonide/Formoterol	MDI: 80 mcg/4.5 mcg per actuation	1–2 puffs every 4 hours as needed	• Max 12 puffs/day including total maintenance plus as needed, delivering maximum 54 mcg of formoterol. • Should not be used as reliever if maintained on different ICS/LABA.
Beclomethasone/Formoterol	MDI: 100 mcg/6 mcg per actuation	1–2 puffs every 4 hours as needed	Max 8 inhalations per day
Systemic Corticosteroids			
Methylprednisolone	2-, 4-, 6-, 8-, 16-, 32-mg tablets	40–60 mg/day as single or 2 divided doses	• Short courses or "bursts" are effective for establishing control when initiating therapy or during a period of gradual deterioration. • The burst should be continued until symptoms resolve and the PEF is at least 80% of personal best. This usually requires 5–7 days but may require longer. There is no evidence that tapering the dose following improvements prevents relapse.

(continued)

Table 9–4. Reliever medications for asthma. (continued)

Medication	Dosage Form	Adult Dose	Comments
Prednisolone	5-mg tablets; 5 mg/5 mL, 15 mg/5 mL oral solution	40–60 mg/day as single or 2 divided doses	
Prednisone	1-, 2.5-, 5-, 10-, 20-, 50-mg tablets; 5 mg/mL oral solution	40–60 mg/day as single or 2 divided doses	
Methylprednisolone acetate	Repository injection: 40 mg/mL 80 mg/mL	240 mg intramuscularly once	• May be used in place of a short burst of oral corticosteroids in patients who are vomiting or if adherence is a problem.

CFC, chlorofluorocarbon; EIB, exercise-induced bronchospasm; HFA, hydrofluoroalkane; MDI, metered-dose inhaler.
Adapted from National Asthma Education and Prevention Program. Expert Panel Report 3: Guidelines for the Diagnosis and Management of Asthma. National Institutes of Health Pub. No. 08-4051. Bethesda, MD, 2007.

Inhaled SABA therapy is as effective as oral or parenteral β-agonist therapy in relaxing airway smooth muscle and improving acute asthma and offers the advantages of rapid onset of action (< 5 minutes) with fewer systemic side effects. Repetitive administration produces incremental bronchodilation. One or two inhalations of a SABA from an MDI are usually sufficient for mild to moderate symptoms. Severe exacerbations frequently require higher doses: 6–12 puffs every 30–60 minutes of albuterol by MDI with an inhalation chamber or 2.5 mg by nebulizer provide equivalent bronchodilation. Administration by nebulization does not offer more effective delivery than MDIs used correctly but does provide higher doses. With most SABAs, the recommended dose by nebulizer for acute asthma (albuterol, 2.5 mg) is 25–30 times that delivered by a single activation of the MDI (albuterol, 0.09 mg). This difference suggests that standard dosing of inhalations from an MDI may be insufficient in the setting of an acute exacerbation. Independent of dose, nebulizer therapy may be more effective in patients who are unable to coordinate inhalation of

Table 9–5. Estimated clinically comparable daily dosages for inhaled corticosteroids for adults with asthma.

Medication	Low Daily Dose	Medium Daily Dose	High Daily Dose
Beclomethasone dipropionate HFA 40 or 80 mcg/puff	80–240 mcg	> 240–480 mcg	> 480 mcg
Budesonide dipropionate DPI 90, 180, or 200 mcg/inhalation	180–400 mcg	> 400–800 mcg	> 800 mcg
Flunisolide 250 mcg/puff	500–1000 mcg	> 1000–2000 mcg	> 2000 mcg
Flunisolide HFA 80 mcg/puff	320 mcg	> 320–640 mcg	> 640 mcg
Fluticasone propionate **HFA/MDI:** 44, 110, or 220 mcg/puff **DPI:** 50, 100, or 250 mcg/inhalation	88–264 mcg 100–300 mcg	> 264–440 mcg > 300–500 mcg	> 440 mcg > 500 mcg
Mometasone furoate DPI 200 mcg/puff	200 mcg	400 mcg	> 400 mcg
Triamcinolone acetonide 75 mcg/puff	300–750 mcg	> 750–1500 mcg	> 1500 mcg

DPI, dry powder inhaler; HFA, hydrofluoroalkane; MDI, metered-dose inhaler.
Notes:

- The most important determinant of appropriate dosing is the clinician's judgment of the patient's response to therapy. Most of clinical benefit from inhaled corticosteroid therapy is seen at low doses; responsiveness varies among patients.
- Potential drug interactions: Several inhaled corticosteroids, including fluticasone, budesonide, and mometasone, are metabolized in the GI tract and liver by CYP 3A4 isoenzymes. Potent inhibitors of CYP 3A4, such as ritonavir and ketoconazole, have the potential for increasing systemic concentrations of these inhaled corticosteroids by increasing oral availability and decreasing systemic clearance. Some cases of clinically significant Cushing syndrome and secondary adrenal insufficiency have been reported.

Adapted from National Asthma Education and Prevention Program. Expert Panel Report 3: Guidelines for the Diagnosis and Management of Asthma. National Institutes of Health Pub. No. 08-4051. Bethesda, MD, 2007, and Global Initiative for Asthma. Global Strategy for Asthma Management and Prevention, 2019. (Available from: www.ginasthma.org.)

medication from an MDI because of age, agitation, or severity of the exacerbation.

LABAs provide bronchodilation for up to 12 hours after a single dose. **Salmeterol** and **formoterol** are LABAs available for asthma in the United States. In combination with an ICS, they are indicated for maintenance therapy of asthma. LABAs should never be used as monotherapy because they lack anti-inflammatory effect and because monotherapy has been associated with increased risk of severe or fatal asthma attacks in two large studies. Based on clinical trial data in patients with mild asthma, combination inhalers containing formoterol and low-dose budesonide are the preferred option, which have demonstrated a 64% reduction in severe exacerbations compared with SABA-only treatment and noninferiority for severe exacerbations compared to low-dose ICS alone.

3. Systemic corticosteroids—Systemic corticosteroids (oral prednisone or prednisolone or parenteral methylprednisolone) are most effective in achieving prompt control of asthma during acute exacerbations. Systemic corticosteroids are effective as primary treatments for patients with moderate to severe asthma exacerbations and for patients with exacerbations that do not respond promptly and completely to inhaled SABA therapy. These medications speed the resolution of airflow obstruction and reduce the rate of relapse. Delays in administering corticosteroids may result in progressive impairment. Therefore, patients with moderate to severe asthma should be prescribed oral corticosteroids so they are available for early, at-home administration, when needed. The minimal effective dose of systemic corticosteroids for patients with asthma has not been identified. Outpatient prednisone "burst" therapy of 0.5–1 mg/kg/day (typically 40–60 mg) in 1–2 doses for 5–7 days is commonly utilized. Severe exacerbations requiring hospitalization typically require 1 mg/kg of prednisone or methylprednisolone every 6–12 hours for 48 hours or until the FEV_1 (or PEF rate) returns to 50% of predicted (or 50% of baseline). The dose is then decreased to 0.5 mg/kg/day until the PEF reaches 70% of predicted or personal best. No clear advantage has been found for higher doses of corticosteroids. It may be prudent to administer corticosteroids intravenously to critically ill patients to avoid concerns about altered GI absorption.

In patients with refractory, poorly controlled asthma, or patients with frequent exacerbations despite optimized inhaler therapy, systemic corticosteroids may be required for the long-term suppression of symptoms. Repeated efforts should be made to reduce the dose to the minimum needed to control symptoms. Concurrent treatment with calcium supplements and vitamin D should be initiated to prevent corticosteroid-induced bone mineral loss with long-term administration. Bone mineral density testing after ≥ 3 months of cumulative systemic corticosteroid exposure can guide the use of bisphosphonates for treatment of steroid-induced osteoporosis. Rapid discontinuation of systemic corticosteroids after long-term use may precipitate adrenal insufficiency.

4. Anticholinergics—Anticholinergic agents reverse vagally mediated bronchospasm but not allergen- or exercise-induced bronchospasm. They may decrease mucous gland hypersecretion. Both **short-acting muscarinic antagonists** (SAMAs) and **long-acting muscarinic antagonists** (LAMAs) are available. Ipratropium bromide, a SAMA, is less effective than SABA for relief of acute bronchospasm but is the inhaled drug of choice for patients with intolerance to SABA or bronchospasm due to β-blocker medications. Ipratropium bromide reduces the rate of hospital admissions when added to inhaled SABAs in patients with moderate to severe asthma exacerbations. Studies have shown that the addition of tiotropium to medium-dose ICS and salmeterol improves lung function and reduces the frequency of asthma exacerbations.

5. Leukotriene modifiers—Leukotrienes are potent mediators that contribute to airway obstruction and asthma symptoms by contracting airway smooth muscle, increasing vascular permeability and mucous secretion, and attracting and activating airway inflammatory cells. **Zileuton** is a 5-lipoxygenase inhibitor that decreases leukotriene production, and **zafirlukast** and **montelukast** are cysteinyl leukotriene receptor antagonists. In RCTs, these agents caused modest improvements in lung function and reductions in asthma symptoms and lessened the need for SABA rescue therapy. These agents are less effective than ICS for exacerbation reduction or as first-line controller therapy but may be considered as alternatives in patients with asthma who are unable to take an ICS or who experience undesirable corticosteroid side effects.

6. Monoclonal antibody agents—Patients with asthma who require monoclonal antibody therapies should be evaluated by either a pulmonologist or allergist experienced in their use. **Omalizumab** is a recombinant antibody that binds IgE without activating mast cells. Clinical trials in patients with moderate to severe asthma and elevated serum IgE levels have found that omalizumab, when administered subcutaneously every 2–4 weeks, reduced the need for corticosteroids. Three IL-5 antagonist monoclonal antibodies (anti-IL-5/5R) are approved for the treatment of severe asthma with peripheral blood eosinophilia that has not responded to standard treatments: **reslizumab** (administered intravenously every 4 weeks), **mepolizumab** (administered subcutaneously every 4 weeks), and **benralizumab** (administered subcutaneously every 4–8 weeks). These treatments have been shown to reduce exacerbation rates and improve lung function in this patient population. **Dupilumab** is a monoclonal antibody (anti-IL-4Rα) that inhibits overactive signaling of IL-4 and IL-13 and is administered subcutaneously every 2 weeks. Dupilumab has been shown to improve asthma control, reduce exacerbations, and decrease the need for oral corticosteroids.

7. Phosphodiesterase inhibitor—Theophylline provides mild bronchodilation in patients with asthma. It also has anti-inflammatory and immunomodulatory properties, enhances mucociliary clearance, and strengthens diaphragmatic contractility. Sustained-release theophylline preparations are effective in controlling nocturnal symptoms and as added therapy in patients with moderate or severe persistent asthma whose symptoms are inadequately controlled by ICSs. Low-dose sustained-release theophylline is included as a less effective option in Step 3 treatment.

Neither theophylline nor aminophylline is recommended for therapy of acute asthma exacerbations.

8. Mediator inhibitors—Cromolyn sodium and **nedocromil** are long-term control medications that prevent asthma symptoms and improve airway function in patients with mild persistent or exercise-induced asthma.

B. Desensitization

Immunotherapy for specific allergens may be considered in selected patients with asthma who have exacerbations when exposed to allergens to which they are sensitive and when unresponsive to environmental control measures or other therapies. Studies show a reduction in asthma symptoms in patients treated with single-allergen immunotherapy. Because of the risk of immunotherapy-induced bronchoconstriction, it should be administered only in a setting where such complications can be immediately treated.

C. Vaccination

All adult patients with asthma should receive appropriate pneumococcal, influenza, and COVID-19 vaccination. (See Community Acquired Pneumonia: Prevention for full description.) The use of the intranasal live attenuated influenza vaccine may be associated with asthma exacerbations in young children.

Treatment of Asthma Exacerbations

Asthma expert panels, including GINA and National Asthma Education and Prevention Program, iterate the importance of patient education in early recognition and intervention of asthma exacerbations. An asthma action plan developed by care providers can assist the patient in their daily routine care and outline worsening signs or symptoms that suggest the need for health care evaluation. Symptoms of exacerbations include progressive breathlessness, increasing chest tightness, decreased peak flow, and lack of improvement after SABA therapy (Table 9–6). Most instances of uncontrolled asthma are mild and may be managed by patients at home with self-management plans. More severe exacerbations with persistent or worsening symptoms require evaluation and management by a health care provider who can assess the patient's exacerbation severity, respiratory status, and risk factors for asthma-related mortality and direct management accordingly (Figure 9–1).

A. Mild to Moderate Exacerbations

Mild asthma exacerbations are characterized by only minor changes in airway function (PEF or $FEV_1 \geq 70\%$ predicted or personal best) with minimal symptoms and signs of airway dysfunction. Many such patients respond quickly and fully to an inhaled SABA alone, or

Table 9–6. Evaluation and classification of severity of asthma exacerbations.

	Mild	Moderate	Severe	Respiratory Arrest Imminent
Symptoms				
Breathlessness	While walking	At rest, limits activity	At rest, interferes with conversation	While at rest, mute
Talks in	Sentences	Phrases	Words	Silent
Alertness	May be agitated	Usually agitated	Usually agitated	Drowsy or confused
Signs				
Respiratory rate	Increased	Increased	Often > 30/min	> 30/min
Body position	Can lie down	Prefers sitting	Sits upright	Unable to recline
Use of accessory muscles, suprasternal retractions	Usually not	Commonly	Usually	Paradoxical thoracoabdominal movement
Wheezing	Moderate, often only end-expiratory	Loud; throughout exhalation	Usually loud; throughout inhalation and exhalation	Absent
Pulse/minute	< 100	100–120	> 120	Bradycardia
Pulsus paradoxus	Absent < 10 mm Hg	May be present 10–25 mm Hg	Often present > 25 mm Hg	Absence suggests respiratory muscle fatigue
Functional Assessment				
PEF or FEV_1 % predicted or % personal best	≥ 70%	40–69%	< 40%	< 25%
PaO_2 (on air, mm Hg)	Normal[1]	≥ 60[1]	< 60: possible cyanosis	< 60: possible cyanosis
PCO_2 (mm Hg)	< 42[1]	< 42[1]	≥ 42[1]	≥ 42[1]
SaO_2 (on air)	> 95%[1]	90–95%[1]	< 90%[1]	< 90%[1]

[1]Test not usually necessary.
Adapted from National Asthma Education and Prevention Program. Expert Panel Report 3: Guidelines for the Diagnosis and Management of Asthma. National Institutes of Health Pub. No. 08-4051. Bethesda, MD, 2007.

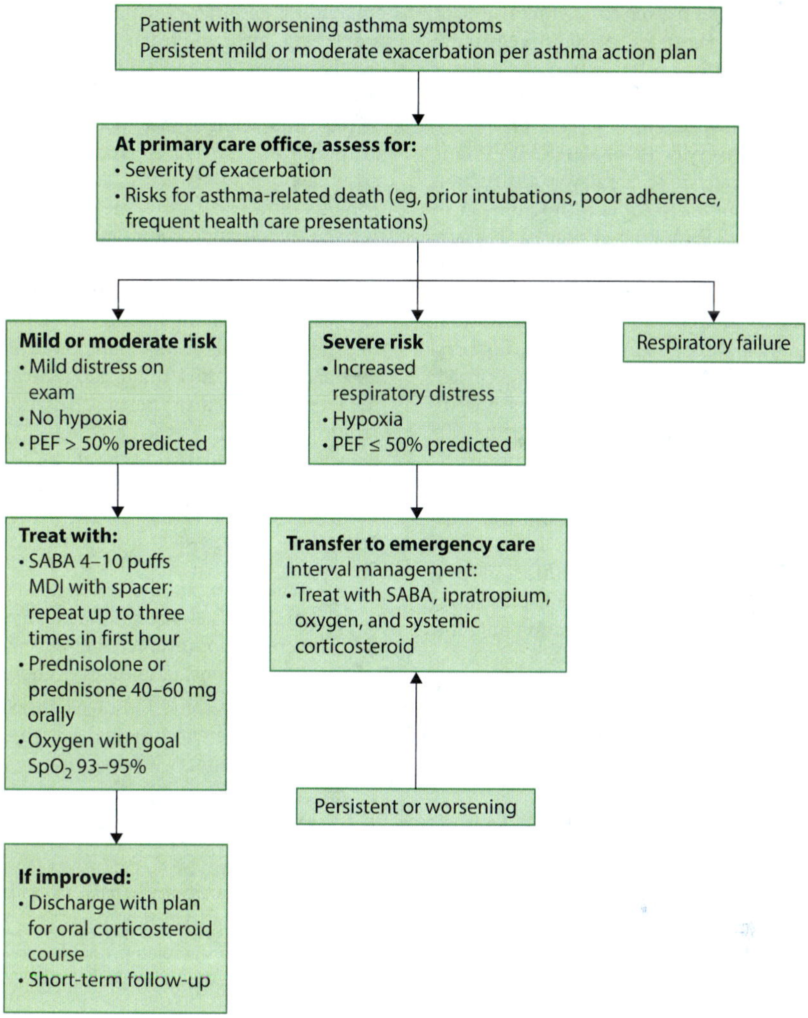

▲ **Figure 9–1.** Management of mild or moderate asthma exacerbations in primary care. MDI, metered-dose inhaler; SABA, short-acting β_2-agonist (doses are for salbutamol). (Used, from Rime Abbas, MD.)

combination glucocorticoid with a fast-acting β-agonist (budesonide-albuterol, budesonide-formoterol) which may need to be continued at increased doses (eg, every 3–4 hours for 24–48 hours). If SABA alone is being used, patients may also require a short-term increase in ICS to four times the usual dose. In patients not improving after 48 hours, a short course of oral corticosteroids (eg, prednisone 0.5–1.0 mg/kg/day for 5–7 days) may be necessary.

The principal goals for treating moderate asthma exacerbations are correcting hypoxemia, reversing airflow obstruction, and reducing the risk of relapse. Early intervention may lessen the severity and shorten the duration of an exacerbation. Airflow obstruction is treated with repeated or continuous administration of an **inhaled SABA** and the early administration of **systemic corticosteroids.** Systemic corticosteroids should be given to patients who have a peak flow < 70% of baseline or who do not respond to several treatments of SABA. Serial measurements of lung function to quantify the severity of airflow obstruction and its response to treatment are useful. The improvement in FEV_1 after 30–60 minutes of treatment correlates significantly with the severity of the asthma exacerbation. Serial measurement of airflow in the emergency department may reduce the rate of hospital admissions for asthma exacerbations. Postexacerbation care planning is important. All patients, regardless of severity, should be provided with (1) necessary medications and how to use them, (2) instruction in self-assessment, (3) a follow-up appointment, and (4) an action plan for managing recurrence.

B. Severe Exacerbations

Severe exacerbations of asthma can be life-threatening and require immediate treatment. Patients should immediately receive **oxygen**, a high dose **inhaled SABA**, and **systemic corticosteroids**. A focused history may be completed while therapy is initiated; detailed laboratory studies generally do not improve early decision making and can be deferred until after therapy is instituted. Correction of hypoxia and early initiation of **oxygen therapy** are paramount because asphyxia is a common cause of asthma deaths.

Supplemental oxygen should be given to maintain an SaO_2 ≥ 90% or a PaO_2 ≥ 60 mm Hg (and ≥ 95% in pregnancy). Oxygen-induced hypoventilation is extremely rare in patients with asthma, and concern for hypercapnia should never delay correction of hypoxemia.

Frequent high-dose delivery of an **inhaled SABA** is indicated and usually well tolerated in severe airway obstruction. At least three MDI or nebulizer treatments should be given in the first hour of therapy. Some studies suggest that continuous therapy is more effective than intermittent administration of these agents, but there is no clear consensus as long as similar doses are administered. After the first hour, the frequency of administration varies according to improvements in airflow and symptoms and occurrence of side effects. **Ipratropium bromide** reduces the rate of hospital admissions when added to inhaled SABAs in patients with moderate to severe asthma exacerbations.

Systemic corticosteroids are administered as detailed above. **Intravenous magnesium sulfate** (2 g intravenously over 20 minutes) is not recommended for routine use in asthma exacerbations. However, a 2 g infusion over 20 minutes may reduce hospitalization rates in acute severe asthma (FEV_1 < 25% of predicted on presentation or failure to respond to initial treatment).

Mucolytic agents (eg, acetylcysteine, potassium iodide) may worsen cough or airflow obstruction. Anxiolytic and hypnotic drugs are generally contraindicated in severe asthma exacerbations because of their potential respiratory depressant effects.

Multiple studies suggest that infections with viruses (rhinovirus) and bacteria (*Mycoplasma pneumoniae, Chlamydophila pneumoniae*) predispose to acute exacerbations of asthma and may underlie chronic, severe asthma. The use of empiric antibiotics is, however, not recommended in routine asthma exacerbations since there is no consistent evidence to show improved clinical outcomes. **Antibiotics** should be considered when there is a high likelihood of acute bacterial respiratory tract infection, such as when patients have fever or purulent sputum and evidence of pneumonia or bacterial sinusitis.

In the **emergency department setting**, repeat assessment of patients with severe exacerbations should be done after the initial dose of an inhaled SABA and again after three doses of an inhaled SABA (60–90 minutes after initiating treatment). The response to initial treatment is a better predictor of the need for hospitalization than is the severity of the exacerbation on presentation. The decision to hospitalize a patient should be based on the duration and severity of symptoms, severity of airflow obstruction, ABG results (if available), course and severity of prior exacerbations, medication use at the time of the exacerbation, access to medical care and medications, adequacy of social support and home conditions, and presence of psychiatric illness. In general, discharge to home is appropriate if the PEF or FEV_1 has returned to ≥ 60% of predicted or personal best and if symptoms are minimal or absent. Patients with a rapid response to treatment should be observed for 30 minutes after the most recent dose of bronchodilator to ensure stability of response before discharge.

In the **intensive care setting**, a small subset of patients will not respond to treatment and will progress to impending respiratory failure due to a combination of worsening airflow obstruction and respiratory muscle fatigue (Figure 9–2 and Table 9–6). Since such patients can deteriorate rapidly, they must be monitored in a critical care setting. Intubation of an acutely ill asthma patient is technically difficult and is best done semi-electively before the crisis of a respiratory arrest. At the time of intubation, the patient's intravascular volume should be closely monitored because hypotension commonly follows the administration of sedative medications and the initiation of positive-pressure ventilation; these patients are often dehydrated due to poor recent oral intake and high insensible losses.

The main goals of **mechanical ventilation** are to ensure adequate oxygenation and to avoid barotrauma. Controlled hypoventilation with permissive hypercapnia is often required to limit airway pressures. Frequent high-dose delivery of inhaled SABAs should be continued along with anti-inflammatory agents as discussed above.

When to Refer

- Atypical presentation or uncertain diagnosis of asthma, particularly if additional diagnostic testing is required (bronchoprovocation challenge, allergy skin testing, rhinoscopy, consideration of occupational exposure).
- Complicating comorbid problems, such as rhinosinusitis, multiple environmental allergies, suspected allergic bronchopulmonary aspergillosis.
- Occupational asthma.
- Uncontrolled symptoms despite a moderate-dose ICS and a LABA.
- Patient not meeting goals of asthma therapy after 3–6 months of treatment.
- Frequent asthma-related health care utilization.
- More than two courses of oral corticosteroid therapy in the past 12 months.
- Any life-threatening asthma exacerbation or exacerbation requiring hospitalization in the past 12 months.
- Presence of social or psychological issues interfering with asthma management.

Beasley R et al. The ICS/formoterol reliever therapy regimen in asthma. J Allergy Clin Immunol Pract. 2023;11:1015. [PMID: 36889609]

Dubin S et al. Update on asthma management guidelines. Cleve Clin J Med. 2024;91:389. [PMID: 38808037]

Global Initiative for Asthma. Global Strategy for Asthma Management and Prevention, 2024. https://ginasthma.org/2024-report

Hansen S et al. Clinical response and remission in patients with severe asthma treated with biologic therapies. Chest. 2024;165:253. [PMID: 37925144]

Levy ML et al. Key recommendations for primary care from the 2022–2023 update of the Global Initiative for Asthma. NPJ Prim Care Respir Med. 2023;33:15. [PMID: 37027574]

Papi A et al. European Respiratory Society short guidelines for the use of as-needed ICS/formoterol in mild Asthma. Eur Respir J. 2023;62:2300047. [PMID: 37678955]

Pleşca DA et al. Asthma prevention and recent advances in management. Adv Respir Med. 2024;92:226. [PMID: 39245573]

Rayner DG et al. Inhaled reliever therapies for asthma: Systematic review and network meta-analysis. J Clin Med. 2024;13:3251. [PMID: 38913977]

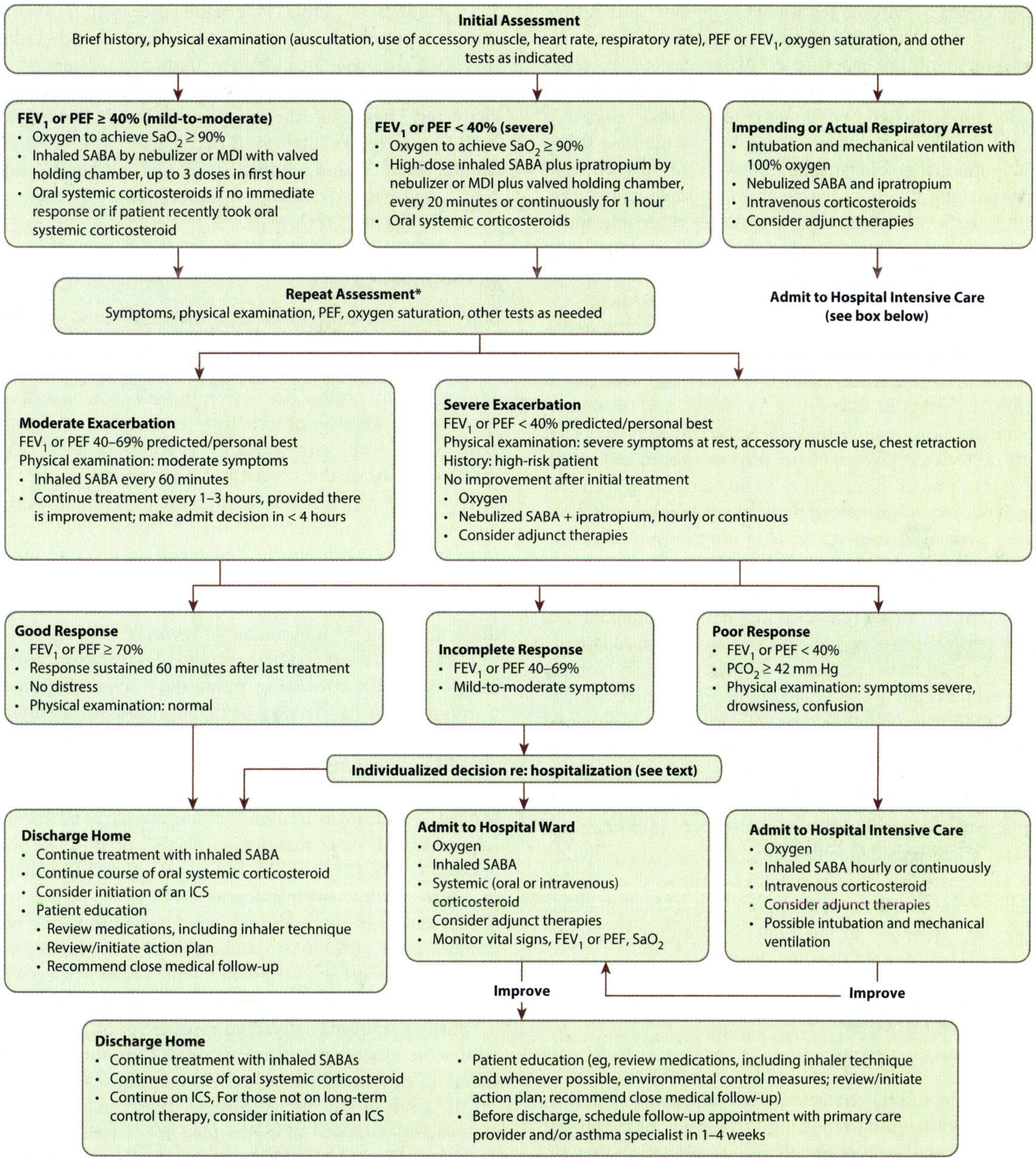

*Patients who have achieved ≥ 70% PEF or FEV_1 should go to the "Good Response" category.

Figure 9–2. Management of asthma exacerbations in acute care facility (eg, emergency department). ICS, inhaled corticosteroids; MDI, metered-dose inhaler; SABA, short-acting β_2-agonist. (Reproduced, with permission, from Hasegawa K, Craig SS, Teach SJ, Camargo CA Jr. Management of Asthma Exacerbations in the Emergency Department. J Allergy Clin Immunol Pract. 2021;9(7):2599-2610.)

CHRONIC OBSTRUCTIVE PULMONARY DISEASE

ESSENTIALS OF DIAGNOSIS

- History of cigarette smoking or other chronic inhalational exposure.
- Chronic cough, dyspnea, and sputum production.
- Rhonchi, decreased intensity of breath sounds, and prolonged expiration on physical examination.
- Airflow limitation on PFT that is not fully reversible and most often progressive.

General Considerations

The Global Initiative for Chronic Obstructive Lung Disease (GOLD) defines COPD as a heterogeneous lung condition characterized by chronic respiratory symptoms and airflow limitation due to airway and alveolar abnormalities usually caused by significant exposure to noxious particles or gases. The term "COPD" has evolved from an umbrella term for chronic bronchitis and emphysema to one that refers to a clinical syndrome of chronic respiratory symptoms, structural pulmonary abnormalities (airways or alveoli), and impaired lung function arising from multiple causes that result in airflow limitation that is not fully reversible and is often progressive. Symptoms include cough, dyspnea, and sputum production. COPD is a major cause of chronic morbidity and is the third leading cause of death worldwide.

The most important causes of COPD are cigarette smoking in the developed world and biomass fuel cooking in the developing world. Most smokers suffer an accelerated decline in lung function that is dose- and duration-dependent. One major study of active smokers reported yearly decreases in FEV_1 of 66 mL per year in men and 54 mL per year in women compared to 30 mL per year in men and 22 mL per year in women who sustained smoking cessation. Fifteen percent of smokers develop progressively disabling symptoms in their 40s and 50s. Approximately two-thirds of patients seen for COPD have significant exposure to tobacco smoke. The remaining one-third may have a combination of exposures to environmental tobacco smoke, occupational dusts and chemicals, and indoor air pollution from biomass fuel used for cooking and heating in poorly ventilated buildings. Outdoor air pollution, airway infection, environmental factors, and allergy have also been implicated, along with hereditary factors (most notably, deficiency of α_1-antitrypsin [α_1-antiprotease]). Atopy and bronchoconstriction in response to nonspecific airway stimuli may be important risk factors. There is evidence that lung exposures to pollution and allergens early in life, including antenatal and early childhood exposure, can lead to poor lung growth in childhood and expiratory airflow limitation, resulting in lower than predicted spirometric values in midlife.

Clinical Findings

A. Symptoms and Signs

Patients with COPD characteristically present in the fifth or sixth decade of life reporting excessive cough, sputum production, shortness of breath, or a combination thereof. Symptoms have often been present for ≥ 10 years, yet if diagnosed early, smoking cessation can reduce lung function decline. Dyspnea is noted initially on heavy exertion, but as the condition progresses, it occurs with mild activity. In severe disease, dyspnea occurs at rest. As the disease progresses, two symptom patterns tend to emerge, that were historically described as "pink puffers" and "blue bloaters"; however, the GOLD 2024 no longer recommends these labels. Most patients have overlapping features of emphysema and chronic bronchitis, and the clinical course and severity may involve other factors, such as central control of ventilation and concomitant sleep-disordered breathing. Symptom severity is better assessed using standardized tools, such as the COPD Assessment Test (CAT) or the modified Medical Research Council Dyspnea scale (mMRC) (Table 9–7).

A hallmark of COPD is the acute exacerbation of symptoms beyond normal day-to-day variation, often including increased dyspnea, an increased frequency or severity of cough, and increased sputum volume or change in sputum character. These exacerbations are commonly precipitated by infection (more often viral than bacterial) or environmental factors. Pneumonia, pulmonary hypertension, right-sided HF, and chronic respiratory failure characterize the late stage of COPD.

B. Diagnostic Tests

Spirometry is critical to the diagnosis and severity assessment of COPD. PFTs early in the course of COPD may reveal only abnormal closing volume and reduced mid-expiratory flow rates. Reduction in FEV_1 establishes the presence of airflow obstruction and reduction in the ratio of FEV_1 to vital capacity (FEV_1% or FEV_1/FVC ratio) establishes the severity of obstruction. Lung volume measurements reveal an increase in residual volume and in TLC, and an elevation of the RV/TLC ratio, indicative of air trapping and hyperinflation, common in patients with emphysema. In the setting of airflow obstruction, a reduction in the single-breath D_{LCO} predicts anatomic emphysema. A severely reduced D_{LCO} predicts exertional oxyhemoglobin desaturation and is associated with coexisting pulmonary hypertension. A 6-minute walking distance of < 350 m is associated with increased mortality.

ABG measurement characteristically shows no abnormalities early in COPD other than an increased A–a–DO_2. Indeed, ABG measurement is unnecessary unless (1) hypoxemia or hypercapnia is suspected, or in those with $SpO_2 \leq 92\%$ or (2) the FEV_1 or D_{LCO} is < 40% of predicted or severe airflow obstruction (GOLD 3–4). Hypoxemia occurs earlier in disease in which chronic bronchitis predominates. Hypercapnia and compensated respiratory acidosis occur as disease progresses, which may worsen with sleep and exercise, and during acute exacerbations.

Positive sputum bacterial cultures are poorly correlated with acute exacerbations, which more commonly are preceded by viral infections. The ECG may show sinus tachycardia, and in advanced disease there may be ECG abnormalities typical of right-sided HF. Supraventricular arrhythmias (multifocal atrial tachycardia, atrial flutter, and atrial fibrillation) and ventricular irritability also occur.

C. Imaging

Radiographs of patients with chronic bronchitis typically show only nonspecific peribronchial and perivascular markings. Plain radiographs are insensitive for the diagnosis of emphysema; hyperinflation with flattening of the diaphragm or peripheral arterial deficiency is seen in half of cases. Chest CT can identify and quantify the emphysema phenotype and detects airway narrowing and wall thickening characteristic of the bronchitic phenotype. In advanced disease, pulmonary hypertension may be suggested by enlargement of central pulmonary arteries on CXRs or chest CTs, and Doppler echocardiography

Table 9–7. Patterns of disease in advanced COPD.

	Type A: Pink Puffer (Emphysema Predominant)	Type B: Blue Bloater (Bronchitis Predominant)
History and physical examination	Major symptom is dyspnea, often severe, usually presenting after age 50. Cough is rare, with scant clear, mucoid sputum. Patients are thin, with recent weight loss common. They appear uncomfortable, with evident use of accessory muscles of respiration. Chest is very quiet without adventitious sounds. No peripheral edema.	Major symptom is chronic cough, productive of mucopurulent sputum, with frequent exacerbations due to chest infections. Often presents in late 30s and 40s. Dyspnea usually mild, though patients may note limitations to exercise. Patients frequently overweight and cyanotic but seem comfortable at rest. Peripheral edema is common. Chest is noisy, with rhonchi invariably present; wheezes are common.
Laboratory studies	Hemoglobin usually normal (12–15 g/dL). PaO_2 normal to slightly reduced (65–75 mm Hg) but SaO_2 normal at rest. $PaCO_2$ normal to slightly reduced (35–40 mm Hg). CXR shows hyperinflation with flattened diaphragms. Vascular markings are diminished, particularly at the apices.	Hemoglobin usually elevated (15–18 g/dL). PaO_2 reduced (45–60 mm Hg) and $PaCO_2$ slightly to markedly elevated (50–60 mm Hg). CXR shows increased interstitial markings ("dirty lungs"), especially at bases. Diaphragms are not flattened.
PFTs	Airflow obstruction ubiquitous. TLC increased, sometimes markedly so. D_{LCO} reduced. Static lung compliance increased.	Airflow obstruction ubiquitous. TLC generally normal but may be slightly increased. D_{LCO} normal. Static lung compliance normal.
Special Evaluations		
Ventilation-perfusion testing	Increased ventilation to high $\dot{V}/\dot{Q}$ areas, ie, high dead space ventilation.	Increased perfusion to low $\dot{V}/\dot{Q}$ areas.
Hemodynamics	Cardiac output normal to slightly low. Pulmonary artery pressures mildly elevated and increase with exercise.	Cardiac output normal. Pulmonary artery pressures elevated, sometimes markedly so, and worsen with exercise.
Nocturnal ventilation	Mild to moderate degree of oxygen desaturation not usually associated with obstructive sleep apnea.	Severe oxygen desaturation, frequently associated with obstructive sleep apnea.
Exercise ventilation	Increased minute ventilation for level of oxygen consumption; PaO_2 tends to fall; $PaCO_2$ rises slightly.	Decreased minute ventilation for level of oxygen consumption. PaO_2 may rise; $PaCO_2$ may rise significantly.

$\dot{V}/\dot{Q}$, ventilation-perfusion.

provides an estimate of pulmonary artery pressure. CT provides information in patients being considered for lung volume reduction surgery or endobronchial valve placement for underlying severe hyperinflation.

Differential Diagnosis

Clinical, imaging, and laboratory findings should enable the clinician to distinguish COPD from other obstructive pulmonary disorders, such as asthma, bronchiectasis, CF, bronchopulmonary aspergillosis, and central airflow obstruction. Asthma is characterized by complete or near-complete reversibility of airflow obstruction. Bronchiectasis is distinguished from COPD by recurrent pneumonia and hemoptysis, digital clubbing, and characteristic imaging abnormalities. CF occurs in children, adolescents, and young adults and has characteristic imaging as well as endocrine and hepatic abnormalities. Bronchopulmonary aspergillosis is characterized by eosinophilia; elevated levels of immunoglobulin E; and episodic worsening marked by fever, malaise, productive cough, and radiographic infiltrates. Mechanical obstruction of the central airways can be distinguished from COPD by flow-volume loops.

Complications

Acute bronchitis, pneumonia, pulmonary thromboembolism, atrial dysrhythmias (eg, atrial fibrillation, atrial flutter, multifocal atrial tachycardia), and concomitant LV failure may worsen otherwise stable COPD. PE is more common than previously thought and should be considered in patients with COPD exacerbations lacking clear infectious symptoms. Pulmonary hypertension, right-sided HF, and chronic respiratory failure are common in advanced COPD. Spontaneous pneumothorax occurs in a small fraction of patients with emphysema. Hemoptysis may result from chronic bronchitis, bronchiectasis or bronchogenic carcinoma and should prompt evaluation.

Prevention

COPD is largely preventable by eliminating long-term exposure to tobacco smoke, products of biomass fuels combustion, or other inhaled toxins. Smokers with early evidence of airflow limitation can significantly alter the course of their disease by smoking cessation. Influenza vaccination reduces the frequency and severity of influenza-like illness as well as the number of COPD exacerbations. Annual influenza vaccination is strongly recommended for all persons with COPD. Pneumococcal vaccination reduces both the frequency of community-acquired pneumonia and COPD exacerbations. Updated pneumococcal vaccine recommendations (ACIP 2023–2025) advise either PCV20 alone or PCV15 followed by PPSV23 for all adults with COPD. COVID-19 vaccination continues to reduce hospitalization and mortality in COPD. GOLD 2024 also recommends Tdap, shingles vaccination (Shingrix) for adults aged ≥ 50 years, and RSV vaccination for eligible older adults and those with chronic lung disease. In patients with COPD and diabetes, there is emerging evidence for possible benefit from GLP-1 receptor agonists and SGLT-2 inhibitors in reducing exacerbation rates.

Treatment

The treatment of COPD is guided by the severity of symptoms or the presence of an exacerbation of stable symptoms. Standards for the management of patients with stable COPD and COPD exacerbations from the American Thoracic Society and GOLD, a joint expert committee of the National Heart, Lung, and Blood Institute and the WHO, are incorporated in the recommendations below. Patients with COPD are classified into ABE groups based on symptom burden and exacerbation history: (1) Group A patients have few symptoms and one or no moderate exacerbations; (2) Group B patients have more symptoms (eg, high CAT or mMRC) and one or no moderate exacerbations; and (3) Group E are patients with at least two moderate exacerbations or at least one hospitalization in the previous year. This grouping guides the choice of initial and follow-up therapy.

A. Ambulatory Patients

1. Smoking cessation—The single most important intervention in smokers with COPD is to facilitate smoking cessation (see Chapter 1), which slows the accelerated decline in lung function caused by smoking. Simply telling a patient to quit succeeds 5% of the time. Behavioral approaches, ranging from clinician advice to intensive group programs, may improve cessation rates. Pharmacologic therapy includes bupropion, nicotine replacement (transdermal patch, gum, lozenge, inhaler, or nasal spray), and varenicline (a partial agonist of nicotinic acetylcholine receptors). Combined pharmacotherapies (two forms of nicotine replacement, or nicotine replacement and bupropion), with or without behavioral approaches, have been recommended. Varenicline is effective but use has been limited by concerns about neuropsychiatric side effect despite evidence negating such association. Electronic cigarettes are not recommended as a smoking cessation aid, due in part to concern for e-cigarette and vaping-associated lung injury (EVALI) (see below).

2. Oxygen therapy—Supplemental oxygen is indicated for patients with COPD with resting hypoxemia ($PaO_2 \le 55$ mm Hg or pulse oxygen saturation [SpO_2] ≤ 88%), or PaO_2 56–59 mm Hg with pulmonary hypertension. Long-term oxygen therapy improves survival in patient with severe resting hypoxemia; but a reduction in hospitalization has otherwise not been demonstrated in other groups. Survival in hypoxemic patients with COPD treated with supplemental oxygen therapy is directly proportional to the number of hours per day oxygen is administered: in hypoxemic patients with COPD treated with continuous oxygen for 24 hours daily, the survival after 36 months is about 65%—significantly better than the survival rate of about 45% in those treated with only nocturnal oxygen. Oxygen by nasal prongs must be given for at least 15 hours a day unless therapy is specifically intended only for exercise or sleep. However, several studies of supplemental oxygen therapy showed no survival benefit in patients with COPD and borderline low-normal resting oxygen levels (PaO_2 56–69 mm Hg). In a study of patients with stable COPD and resting or exercise-induced moderate desaturation, the prescription of long-term supplemental oxygen did not result in a longer time to first hospitalization or death than no long-term supplemental oxygen, nor did it provide sustained benefit in any other measured outcomes. Requirements for US Medicare coverage for a patient's home use of oxygen and oxygen equipment are listed in Table 9–8. ABG analysis is preferred over oximetry to guide initial oxygen therapy. Hypoxemic patients with pulmonary hypertension, chronic right-sided HF, erythrocytosis, impaired cognitive function, exercise intolerance, nocturnal restlessness, or morning headache are likely to benefit from home oxygen therapy.

Home oxygen may be supplied by liquid oxygen systems, compressed gas cylinders, or oxygen concentrators. Most patients benefit from having both stationary and portable systems. For most patients, a flow rate of 1–3 L/min achieves a $PaO_2 > 55$ mm Hg. Reservoir nasal cannulas or "pendants" and demand (pulse) oxygen delivery systems are available to conserve oxygen.

Table 9–8. Home oxygen therapy: requirements for Medicare coverage.[1]

Group I (any of the following):
$PaO_2 \le 55$ mm Hg or $SaO_2 \le 88\%$ taken while awake, at rest, breathing room air.
1. During sleep (prescription for nocturnal oxygen use only): $PaO_2 \le 55$ mm Hg or $SaO_2 \le 88\%$ for a patient who is awake, resting, room air PaO_2 is ≥ 56 mm Hg or $SaO_2 \ge 89\%$, *or* Decrease in $PaO_2 > 10$ mm Hg or decrease in $SaO_2 > 5\%$ associated with symptoms or signs reasonably attributed to hypoxemia (eg, impaired cognitive processes, nocturnal restlessness, insomnia).
2. During exercise (prescription for oxygen use only during exercise): $PaO_2 \le 55$ mg Hg or $SaO_2 \le 88\%$ taken during exercise for a patient who is awake, resting, room air PaO_2 is ≥ 56 mm Hg or $SaO_2 \ge 89\%$, *and* there is evidence that the use of supplemental oxygen during exercise improves the hypoxemia that was demonstrated during exercise while breathing room air.
Group II[2]:
PaO_2 = 56–59 mm Hg or SaO_2 = 89% if there is evidence of any of the following:
1. Dependent edema suggesting HF.
2. P pulmonale on ECG (P wave > 3 mm in standard leads II, III, or a).
3. Hematocrit > 56%.

[1]Centers for Medicare and Medicaid Services, Updated 2024 CMS Guidance.

[2]Patients in this group must have a second oxygen test 61–90 days after the initial oxygen setup.

3. Inhaled bronchodilators—Bronchodilators do not alter the inexorable decline in lung function that is a hallmark of COPD, but they improve symptoms, exercise tolerance, FEV_1, and overall health status. The bronchodilator regimen should be tailored to the clinical severity of the patient's disease. In patients who experience no symptomatic improvement, bronchodilators should be discontinued.

The initial drug of choice for patients with very mild disease and no exacerbations (Group A) is a LAMA. Per most recent recommendations and COPD treatment guidelines, LABAs are most effective when combined with a LAMA. Therefore, if the patient has more significant dyspnea and airflow obstruction (Group B/E), the 2024 GOLD update recommends early initiation of combination treatment with LABA-LAMA for stable COPD management, which leads to improved FEV_1 and reduced dyspnea burden and provides superior improvements in lung function, dyspnea, and exacerbation prevention over LABA alone. Combination ICS/LABA therapy is reserved for patients with eosinophils ≥ 300 cells/mcL, asthma-COPD clinical overlap, or exacerbations despite optimal bronchodilators.

The most commonly prescribed *short-acting* bronchodilators are the SAMA **ipratropium bromide** and the SABAs (eg, albuterol/salbutamol), delivered by MDI or as an inhalation solution by nebulizer. There has been no consistent difference in efficacy demonstrated between SABAs and SAMAs. Some clinicians prefer ipratropium as a first-line agent because of its longer duration of action and absence of sympathomimetic side effects. Furthermore, some studies have suggested that ipratropium achieves superior bronchodilation in patients with COPD. Typical doses are 2–4 puffs (36–72 mcg) every 6 hours. Other clinicians prefer SABAs because they are less expensive and have a more rapid onset of action, commonly leading to greater patient satisfaction. At maximal doses, β2-agonists have bronchodilator action equivalent to that of ipratropium but may cause tachycardia, tremor, or hypokalemia.

Although more expensive than short-acting agents, long-acting bronchodilators may have superior clinical efficacy in persons with advanced disease. LAMAs (eg, **tiotropium, aclidinium, umeclidinium, glycopyrrolate**) and LABAs (eg, **formoterol, salmeterol, indacaterol, arformoterol, vilanterol, ledazerol**) appear to achieve bronchodilation that is equivalent or superior to the SAMA ipratropium, in addition to similar improvements in health status. One RCT of long-term administration of **tiotropium** added to standard therapy reported fewer exacerbations or hospitalizations and improved dyspnea scores in the tiotropium group but no long-term effect on lung function.

The symptomatic benefits of long-acting bronchodilators are firmly established. The increased exacerbations and mortality reported in some patients with asthma treated with the LABA salmeterol have not been observed in patients with COPD, and some analyses suggest a nonsignificant trend toward lower mortality with salmeterol alone, compared with placebo. A 4-year trial with the LAMA tiotropium reported fewer cardiovascular events in the intervention group, and meta-analyses of LAMA that include the 4-year tiotropium trial did not find an increase in cardiovascular events. Most practitioners believe that the documented benefits of anticholinergic therapy outweigh any potential risks.

4. Corticosteroids—Multiple large clinical trials have reported a reduction in the frequency of COPD exacerbations and an increase in self-reported functional status in patients with COPD treated with ICSs. These same trials demonstrate no effect of ICS on mortality or the characteristic decline in lung function experienced by patients with COPD. The benefits of ICS must be weighed against the increased risk of cataracts, decreased bone densitometry, and bacterial pneumonia, especially in those with severe COPD. For these reasons, the updated 2024 GOLD guidelines do not encourage use of ICS in early stages of COPD and call for judicious use of ICS in patients with more severe COPD with frequent exacerbations, those with blood eosinophilia of ≥ 300 cells/mcL, concomitant asthma, or frequent exacerbations (≥ 2) despite optimal LABA+LAMA. Withdrawal of ICSs should be considered when patients have been stable for ≥ 1–2 years, especially if eosinophils are < 100 cells/mcL.

Apart from acute exacerbations, COPD is not generally responsive to oral corticosteroid therapy. Given the risks of adverse side effects, oral corticosteroids are not recommended for long-term treatment of COPD.

5. Theophylline—Low-dose oral theophylline is a fourth-line agent for treating patients with COPD who do not achieve adequate symptom control with inhaled anticholinergic, β_2-agonist, and corticosteroid therapies. Theophylline improves dyspnea ratings, exercise performance, and pulmonary function in many patients with stable COPD. Theophylline toxicity is a significant concern due to the medication's narrow therapeutic window, and long-term administration requires careful monitoring of serum levels. GOLD guidelines recommend theophylline only as a last resort if other bronchodilators are unavailable or unaffordable, with discontinuation if clinical improvement not seen.

6. Antibiotics—Antibiotics are commonly prescribed to outpatients with COPD for the following indications: (1) to treat an acute exacerbation, (2) to treat acute bronchitis, and (3) to prevent acute exacerbations of chronic bronchitis (prophylactic antibiotics). Antibiotics appear to improve outcomes slightly in all three situations, but those with a COPD exacerbation associated with increased sputum purulence accompanied by dyspnea or an increase in the quantity of sputum are thought to benefit most. The choice of antibiotic depends on local bacterial resistance patterns and individual risk of *Pseudomonas aeruginosa* infection (history of *Pseudomonas* isolation, FEV_1 < 50% of predicted, recent hospitalization [≥ 2 days in the past 3 months], more than three courses of antibiotics within the past year, use of systemic corticosteroids). Oral antibiotic options include doxycycline (100 mg every 12 hours), trimethoprim-sulfamethoxazole (160/800 mg every 12 hours), a cephalosporin (eg, cefpodoxime 200 mg every 12 hours or mepronil 500 mg every 12 hours), a macrolide (eg, azithromycin 500 mg followed by 250 mg daily for 5 days), a fluoroquinolone (eg, ciprofloxacin 500 mg every 12 hours), and amoxicillin-clavulanate (875/125 mg every 12 hours). Suggested duration of therapy is 3–5 days and depends on response to therapy. There are few controlled trials of antibiotics in severe COPD exacerbations, but prompt administration is appropriate, particularly in persons with risk factors for poor outcomes (eg, aged < 65 years, FEV_1 < 50% of predicted, three or more exacerbations in the past year, antibiotic therapy within the past 3 months, comorbid conditions, such as cardiac disease). In patients with COPD subject to frequent exacerbations despite optimal medical therapy, azithromycin (250 mg daily or 500 mg three times weekly) or moxifloxacin (a 5-day course 1 week in 8 over 48 weeks) are modestly effective in reducing the frequency of exacerbations; monitoring for hearing loss and QT prolongation is essential.

7. Pulmonary rehabilitation—Graded aerobic physical exercise programs (eg, walking 20 minutes three times weekly or bicycling) help prevent deterioration of physical condition and improve patients' ability to perform daily activities. Training of inspiratory muscles by inspiring against progressively larger resistive loads reduces dyspnea and improves exercise tolerance, health status, and respiratory muscle strength in some patients. Pursed-lip breathing to slow the rate of breathing and abdominal breathing exercises to relieve fatigue of accessory muscles of respiration may reduce dyspnea in some patients. Many patients undergo these exercise and educational interventions in a structured rehabilitation program. Pulmonary rehabilitation has been shown in multiple studies to improve exercise capacity, decrease hospitalizations, and enhance quality of life. Referral to a comprehensive rehabilitation program is recommended in patients who have severe dyspnea, reduced quality of life, or frequent hospitalizations despite optimal medical therapy.

8. Phosphodiesterase type 3 and 4 inhibitors—Roflumilast has been shown to reduce exacerbation frequency in patients who have moderate or severe (FEV_1 < 50% of predicted) COPD and chronic bronchitis, with frequent exacerbations, and who are taking LABA/ICS with or without a LAMA, or LAMA alone. **Ensifentrine**, a first-in-class inhaled dual PDE3/4 inhibitor, has demonstrated significant improvements in lung function, symptoms, and exacerbation reduction in COPD, offering a novel anti-inflammatory and bronchodilator option for patients with persistent symptoms despite standard therapy.

9. Other measures—In patients with chronic bronchitis, increased mobilization of secretions may be accomplished through adequate systemic hydration, effective cough training methods, or the use of a handheld flutter device and postural drainage, sometimes with chest percussion or vibration. Postural drainage and chest percussion should be used only in selected patients with excessive amounts of retained secretions that cannot be cleared by coughing and other methods; these measures are of no benefit in pure emphysema. Expectorant-mucolytic therapy has generally been regarded as unhelpful in patients with chronic bronchitis. Cough suppressants and sedatives should be avoided.

Human α_1-antitrypsin is available for replacement therapy in emphysema due to congenital deficiency (Piz or null genotype) of α_1-antitrypsin (α_1-antiprotease). Patients aged ≥ 18 years with airflow obstruction by spirometry and serum levels < 11 mmol/L (~50 mg/dL) are potential candidates for replacement therapy. α_1-Antitrypsin is administered intravenously in a dose of 60 mg/kg body weight once weekly.

Severe dyspnea despite optimal medical management may warrant a clinical trial of an **opioid** (eg, morphine 5–10 mg orally every 3–4 hours, oxycodone 5–10 mg orally every 4–6 hours, sustained-release morphine 10 mg orally once daily). Sedative-hypnotic drugs (eg, diazepam, 5 mg three times daily) marginally improve intractable dyspnea but cause significant drowsiness; they may benefit very anxious patients. Trans nasal positive-pressure ventilation at home to rest the respiratory muscles is an approach to improve respiratory muscle function and reduce dyspnea in patients with severe COPD.

See Chapter 41 for a discussion of air travel in patients with lung disease.

B. Hospitalized Patients

Management of patients hospitalized with an acute exacerbation of COPD includes (1) supplemental oxygen (titrated to maintain SaO_2 at 88–92% or PaO_2 at 60–70 mm Hg) (in order to avoid oxygen induced hypercapnia); (2) inhaled β_2-agonists (eg, albuterol 2.5 mg diluted with saline to a total of 3 mL by nebulizer, or MDI, 90 mcg per puff, four to eight puffs via spacer, every 1–4 hours as needed) with or without inhaled ipratropium bromide (500 mcg by nebulizer, or 36 mcg by MDI with spacer, every 4 hours as needed); (3) prednisone 40 mg orally once daily for 5 days (the current standard regimen); (4) antibiotics are recommended for patients with increased sputum expectoration and worsening dyspnea or the need for ventilatory support; and (5) chest physiotherapy in selected patients with significant mucus retention or bronchiectasis.

For patients without risk factors for *Pseudomonas*, antibiotic options include a fluoroquinolone (eg, levofloxacin 750 mg orally or intravenously per day, or moxifloxacin 400 mg orally or intravenously every 24 hours) or a third-generation cephalosporin (eg, ceftriaxone 1 g intravenously per day, or cefotaxime 1 g intravenously every 8 hours). Updated GOLD recommendations also include amoxicillin–clavulanate and doxycycline as first-line options for typical exacerbations.

For patients with risk factors for *Pseudomonas*, therapeutic options include piperacillin-tazobactam (4.5 g intravenously every 6 hours), ceftazidime (1 g intravenously every 8 hours), cefepime (1 g intravenously every 12 hours), or levofloxacin (750 mg orally or intravenously per day for 5–7 days).

Oxygen therapy should *not* be withheld for fear of worsening respiratory acidemia; hypoxemia is more detrimental than hypercapnia. Right-sided HF usually responds to measures that reduce pulmonary artery pressure, such as supplemental oxygen and correction of acidemia; bed rest, salt restriction, and diuretics may add some benefit. Cardiac dysrhythmias, particularly multifocal atrial tachycardia, usually respond to aggressive treatment of COPD itself. Atrial fibrillation and flutter may require DC cardioversion after initiation of the above therapy. Theophylline should not be initiated in the acute setting, but patients taking theophylline before acute hospitalization should have their theophylline serum levels measured and maintained in the therapeutic range. If progressive respiratory failure ensues, tracheal intubation and mechanical ventilation are necessary. For patients with hypercapnic acute respiratory failure, **noninvasive positive-pressure ventilation (NIPPV)** delivered via face mask may reduce the need for intubation, shorten lengths of stay in the ICU, and reduce the risk of nosocomial infections and antibiotic usage.

C. Procedures for COPD

1. Lung transplantation—Requirements for lung transplantation are severe lung disease, limited activities of daily living, exhaustion of medical therapy, ambulatory status, potential for pulmonary rehabilitation, limited life expectancy without transplantation, adequate function of other organ systems, and a good social support system. The 2-year survival rate after lung transplantation for COPD is 75%. Complications include acute rejection, opportunistic infection, and obliterative bronchiolitis. Substantial improvements in pulmonary function and exercise performance have been noted after transplantation.

2. Lung volume reduction surgery—Lung volume reduction surgery, or reduction pneumopathy, is a surgical approach to relieve dyspnea and improve exercise tolerance in patients with advanced diffuse emphysema and lung hyperinflation. Bilateral resection of 20–30% of lung volume in selected patients results in modest improvements in pulmonary function, exercise performance, and dyspnea. The duration of improvement as well as any mortality benefit remains uncertain. Prolonged air leaks occur in up to 50% of patients postoperatively. Mortality rates in centers with the largest experience with lung volume reduction surgery range from 4–10%.

The National Emphysema Treatment Trial compared lung volume reduction surgery with medical treatment in a randomized, multicenter clinical trial of 1218 patients with severe emphysema. Overall, surgery improved exercise capacity but not mortality when compared with medical therapy.

3. Bullectomy—Bullectomy is an older surgical procedure for palliation of dyspnea in patients with severe bullous emphysema. It is most commonly pursued when a single bulla occupies at least 30–50% of the hemithorax.

4. Endobronchial valves—In some patients with advanced heterogeneous emphysema and very severe air trapping, one-way valves may allow for flow out hyperinflated lung areas and thereby reduce hyperinflation. The US FDA has approved two endobronchial valves (Zephyr and Spiration) duckbill based on trials showing significant improvements in FEV_1, 6-minute walk distance, and respiratory symptoms in the treatment group compared with controls.

Prognosis

The outlook for patients with clinically significant COPD is poor. The degree of pulmonary dysfunction at the time the patient is first seen is an important predictor of survival: median survival of patients with FEV_1 of ≤ 1 L is about 4 years. A multidimensional index (the BODE index), which includes **B**MI, airway **O**bstruction (FEV_1), **D**yspnea (mMRC score), and **E**xercise capacity, is a tool that predicts death and hospitalization better than FEV_1 alone. Comprehensive care programs, cessation of smoking, and supplemental oxygen may reduce the rate of decline of pulmonary function, but therapy with bronchodilators and other approaches probably have little, if any, impact on the natural course of COPD.

Dyspnea at the end of life can be extremely uncomfortable and distressing to the patient and family. As patients near the end of life, meticulous attention to palliative care is essential to effectively manage dyspnea (see Chapter 5).

When to Refer

- COPD onset before the age of 40.
- Frequent exacerbations (two or more a year) despite optimal treatment.
- Severe or rapidly progressive COPD.
- Symptoms disproportionate to the severity of airflow obstruction.
- Need for long-term oxygen therapy.
- Onset of comorbid illnesses (eg, bronchiectasis, HF, or lung cancer).

When to Admit

- Severe symptoms or acute worsening that fails to respond to outpatient management.
- Acute or worsening hypoxemia, hypercapnia, peripheral edema, or change in mental status.
- Inadequate home care, or inability to sleep or maintain nutrition/hydration due to symptoms.
- The presence of high-risk comorbid conditions.

Foer D et al. Association of GLP-1 receptor agonists with chronic obstructive pulmonary disease exacerbations among patients with type 2 diabetes. Am J Respir Crit Care Med. 2023;208:1088. [PMID: 37647574]

Fortis S et al. COPD phenotypes: clinical relevance and treatment implications. Front Med. 2024;11:1375457. [PMID: 38601231]

GOLD Committee. Global Strategy for the Diagnosis, Management, and Prevention of COPD: 2025 Report. GOLD. 2025.

Patel N et al. An update on COPD prevention, diagnosis, and management: the 2024 GOLD Report. Respir Med. 2024;226:107478. [PMID: 38941078]

Singh D et al. Chronic obstructive pulmonary disease: recent advances in pharmacological treatment. Respir Res. 2025;26:14. [PMID: 39811275]

Waeijen-Smit E et al. Accuracy of the GOLD categories based on exacerbation history in COPD. JAMA Netw Open. 2024;7:e241234. [PMID: 38502127]

BRONCHIECTASIS

ESSENTIALS OF DIAGNOSIS

- Chronic productive cough with dyspnea and wheezing.
- Radiographic findings of dilated, thickened airways and scattered, irregular opacities.

General Considerations

Bronchiectasis is a congenital or acquired disorder of the large bronchi characterized by permanent, abnormal dilation and destruction of bronchial walls. It may be caused by recurrent inflammation or infection of the airways and may be localized or diffuse. Causes include CF, infections (tuberculosis and nontuberculous mycobacteria, fungal infections, lung abscess, recurrent pneumonia, including aspiration pneumonia), immunodeficiencies (congenital or acquired hypogammaglobulinemia; common variable immunodeficiency; selective IgA, IgM, and IgG subclass deficiencies; AIDS; lymphoma; plasma cell myeloma; leukemia), α_1-antitrypsin deficiency, primary ciliary dyskinesia, rheumatic diseases (rheumatoid arthritis, Sjögren syndrome), ABPA, and localized airway obstruction (foreign body aspiration, tumor, mucoid impaction).

Clinical Findings

A. Symptoms and Signs

Symptoms of bronchiectasis include chronic cough with production of copious amounts of purulent sputum, hemoptysis, pleuritic chest pain, dyspnea, and weight loss. Physical findings may include crackles at the lung bases and wheezing.

B. Laboratory Findings and Imaging

Laboratory tests include CBC with differential, immunoglobulin quantification (IgG, IgM, IgA); testing for CF with sweat chloride level, mutation analysis of *CFTR* gene, or both; and sputum culture for bacteria, nontuberculous mycobacteria, and fungi. Additional testing, if appropriate, may include aspergillus antibodies, IgE, α_1-antitrypsin level, and genotype, ciliary testing, autoimmune serologies, and swallow assessment. Obstructive lung disease is the most common finding on PFTs. HRCT is the diagnostic study of choice, which may show dilated and thickened bronchi that may appear as "tram tracks" or as "end-on ring" markings; mucus plugs in the airways, atelectasis, or focal consolidation.

C. Microbiology

Haemophilus influenzae, *Moraxella catarrhalis*, *P aeruginosa*, and *Staphylococcus aureus* are commonly identified. Nontuberculous mycobacteria, *Streptococcus pneumoniae*, and *Stenotrophomonas maltophilia* are seen less commonly. Chronic infection with *Pseudomonas* is a marker for disease severity, frequent exacerbation, accelerated course, and rapid decline in lung function.

Treatment

Treatment of acute exacerbations consists of antibiotics, airway clearance (postural drainage, chest percussion, hypertonic nebulization), and inhaled bronchodilators. Handheld flutter valve devices may be as effective as chest physiotherapy in clearing secretions. Routine use of ICS is not recommended. Antibiotic therapy should be considered in exacerbations. Empiric oral antibiotic therapy with amoxicillin or amoxicillin-clavulanate, ampicillin, a second- or third-generation cephalosporin, doxycycline, azithromycin, or a fluoroquinolone can be started and the antibiotics adjusted as necessary if a specific pathogen is identified by sputum culture, for a total 10–14 day course. For those with recurrent exacerbations (three or more per year), preventive macrolide (eg, azithromycin) or long-term inhaled antibiotics (colistin, gentamicin) has been found to decrease the frequency of exacerbations. Pulmonary rehabilitation is recommended in those with impaired exercise capacity.

Hemoptysis is the most common complication of bronchiectasis. Chest CT angiogram and bronchoscopy may help localize the bleeding site. Massive hemoptysis may require embolization of bronchial arteries, local bronchoscopic hemostasis techniques (balloon tamponade, topical vasoconstrictive agent, laser therapy) or surgical resection.

Following acute exacerbations most patients recover to their baseline, although irreversible worsening may occur. Patients with three or more exacerbations per year or *P aeruginosa* infection have increased mortality.

Barker AF et al. Non-cystic fibrosis bronchiectasis in adults: a review. JAMA. 2025;334:253. [PMID: 40293759]

Chalmers JD et al. European Respiratory Society Clinical Practice Guideline for the Management of Adult Bronchiectasis. Eur Respir J. 2025;66:2501126. [PMID: 41016738]

ALLERGIC BRONCHOPULMONARY ASPERGILLOSIS

ABPA is a pulmonary hypersensitivity disorder caused by allergy to *Aspergillus* fungal species that colonize the tracheobronchial trees. Criteria for the diagnosis of ABPA include (1) a clinical history of asthma or CF; (2) elevated serum total IgE levels (≥ 500 IU/mL); (3) elevated serum IgE levels specific to *Aspergillus fumigatus* ≥ 0.35 kU/L (preferred) or *Aspergillus* skin test positivity; and (4) at least two of the following: (a) e elevated serum *Aspergillus* IgG by immunoassay, (b) pulmonary radiographic abnormalities consistent with ABPA, or (c) peripheral blood eosinophil count ≥ 500 cells/mcL (0.5×10^9/L). Symptoms are similar to asthma (dyspnea, wheezing, cough, mucus production); and may include rhinosinusitis. Radiographic abnormalities include transient opacities, mucoid impaction, and proximal or central bronchiectasis. Asymptomatic patients should not be treated. Symptomatic acute ABPA (newly diagnosed or exacerbation) should receive high-dose corticosteroids (eg, prednisone 0.5–1 mg/kg orally per day) for at least 2 weeks followed by a gradual taper. Patients with corticosteroid-dependent disease may benefit from itraconazole or voriconazole. Relapses are frequent. For those who have frequent exacerbations or are unable to wean off steroids, the use of biologic agents, such as anti-IL-5 (mepolizumab, benralizumab), anti-IL4 receptor (dupilumab), or anti-IgE (omalizumab), has been shown to improve outcomes. Inhaled steroids and bronchodilators (see Table 9–4) may also be helpful in those with asthma. Complications include hemoptysis, severe bronchiectasis, and pulmonary fibrosis.

Agarwal R et al. Revised ISHAM-ABPA working group clinical practice guidelines for diagnosing, classifying and treating allergic bronchopulmonary aspergillosis/mycoses. Eur Respir J. 2024;63:2400061. [PMID: 38423624]

Chen X et al. Efficacy of biologics in patients with allergic bronchopulmonary aspergillosis: a systematic review and meta-analysis. Lung. 2024;202:367. [PMID: 38898129]

CYSTIC FIBROSIS

ESSENTIALS OF DIAGNOSIS

- Autosomal recessive disorder.
- Pulmonary disease: chronic or recurrent productive cough, dyspnea, and wheezing; recurrent infections or chronic colonization of the airways; bronchiectasis and scarring on imaging; airflow obstruction on spirometry.
- Extrapulmonary disease: sinuses (chronic sinusitis and nasal polyposis); GI (pancreatic insufficiency, recurrent pancreatitis, hepatobiliary disease, meconium ileus, and distal intestinal obstruction); genitourinary (absent vas deferens and male infertility).

General Considerations

CF is the most common chronic lung disease in young adults affecting approximately 40,000 people in the United States. It is an autosomal recessive disorder that is more common in White persons but may affect individuals of all racial and ethnic backgrounds. CF is caused by abnormalities in the CF transmembrane conductance regulator (CFTR) protein that results in altered chloride transport and water flux across the apical surface of epithelial cells. Over 2000 inherited variants of the *CFTR* gene have been identified with potential to cause disease. The most common mutation is ΔF508. Mutations of the *CFTR* gene are divided into five different classes: class I (defective protein production), class II (defective protein processing), class III (defective regulation), class IV (defective conduction), and class V (reduced amounts of functional CFTR protein).

Clinical Findings

A. Symptoms and Signs

Due to mandatory newborn screening for CF in many countries, more CF cases have been identified before symptoms develop. In infants and children, CF usually presents with meconium ileus, respiratory symptoms, or failure to thrive. In adults, respiratory symptoms, diabetes, recurrent pancreatitis, or infertility may be seen. Typical symptoms are cough, sputum production, decreased exercise tolerance, recurrent infections, chronic rhinosinusitis symptoms, steatorrhea, diarrhea, and abdominal pain. Patients with CF are often malnourished and have a low BMI. Physical examination findings include digital clubbing (see Figure 6–39), increased anteroposterior chest diameter, hyperresonance to percussion, and apical crackles. Nearly all men with CF have congenital bilateral absence of the vas deferens with azoospermia. Biliary cirrhosis and gallstones may occur.

B. Pulmonary Function Testing

Most patients with CF develop an obstructive pattern on PFTs. As the disease progresses, there is continued decline in FEV_1 and FEV_1/FVC, and there may be reduction in FVC and TLC. Air trapping (high ratio of residual volume to TLC) and reduction in pulmonary diffusing capacity are common.

C. Imaging

Hyperinflation is seen early in the disease process. Lung CT scans commonly reveal peribronchial cuffing, mucus plugging, bronchiectasis (ring shadows and cysts), increased interstitial markings, small, rounded peripheral opacities, and focal atelectasis.

D. Diagnosis

The following two criteria must be present: (1) One of the following: (a) clinical symptoms consistent with CF; (b) history of CF in sibling; (c) or a positive newborn screening test; and (2) one of the following: (a) elevated sweat chloride concentration (> 60 mEq/L); (b) presence of two *CFTR* mutations; (c) or abnormal nasal potential difference.

Treatment

Early recognition and comprehensive multidisciplinary therapy at a CF center improve symptom control and survival. CFTR modulators are a new class of medications that target underlying defects in the CFTR protein. Modulator therapy has been associated with improved lung function, BMI, rate of exacerbations and quality of life. All patients with CF should undergo CFTR genotyping to determine eligibility for modulator therapy. Selection of therapy depends on the mutation and patient age.

Airway clearance can be promoted by postural drainage, chest percussion or vibration techniques, positive expiratory pressure or flutter valve breathing devices, directed cough, inhaled recombinant human deoxyribonuclease (rhDNase, dornase-α) and hypertonic (7%) saline.

Short-term antibiotics are used to treat active exacerbations caused by airway infections based on results of culture and susceptibility testing of sputum. *S aureus* (including methicillin-resistant strains) and *P aeruginosa* are commonly present. *H influenzae*, *Stenotrophomonas maltophilia*, and *B cenocepacia* (a highly drug-resistant organism) are occasionally isolated. **Long-term antibiotic therapy**, such as azithromycin and various inhaled antibiotics (eg, tobramycin, aztreonam, colistin, and levofloxacin), helps slow disease progression and reduce exacerbations in patients with sputum cultures positive for *P aeruginosa*.

Inhaled bronchodilators (eg, albuterol) may be considered in patients who demonstrate an improvement of at least 12% in FEV_1 after an inhaled bronchodilator. An **ICS** should be added to the treatment regimen for patients who have CF with persistent asthma or ABPA.

Lung transplantation may be considered for advanced disease.

Vaccination against pneumococcal and coronavirus infections and annual influenza vaccination are advised.

Pancreatic enzyme replacement and nutritional support is also recommended (See Chapter 18).

Prognosis

The longevity of patients with CF is increasing. Death occurs from pulmonary complications (eg, pneumonia, pneumothorax, or hemoptysis) or from terminal chronic respiratory failure and right-sided HF.

Green DM et al. Cystic Fibrosis Foundation evidence-based guideline for the management of CRMS/CFSPID. Pediatrics. 2024;153:e2023064657. [PMID: 38577740]

Ong T et al. Cystic fibrosis: a review. JAMA. 2023;329:1859. [PMID: 37278811]

BRONCHIOLITIS

ESSENTIALS OF DIAGNOSIS

- Insidious onset of cough and dyspnea.
- Irreversible airflow obstruction and air trapping on PFTs.
- Minimal findings on CXR; air trapping on chest CT scan.
- Relevant exposure or risk factors: toxic fumes, viral infections, organ transplantation, connective tissue disease.

General Considerations

Bronchiolitis is a generic term applied to varied inflammatory processes that affect the bronchioles, which are small conducting airways < 2 mm in diameter. Although less common in adults than children, bronchiolitis is encountered in multiple clinical settings, such as postinfectious, inhalational injury (eg, vaping), organ transplantation, connective tissue diseases, and hypersensitivity pneumonitis.

The clinical approach to bronchiolitis divides patients into groups based on etiology, but different clinical syndromes may have identical histopathologic findings. As a result, no single classification scheme has been widely accepted, and there is an overlapping array of terms to describe these disorders from the viewpoints of the clinician, the pathologist, and the radiologist.

Clinical Findings

Acute bronchiolitis is rare in adults but may be present following viral infections.

Constrictive bronchiolitis (also referred to as obliterative bronchiolitis or bronchiolitis obliterans) may be caused by inhalation injury (ammonia, welding fumes, and heavy metals); rheumatoid arthritis; medication reactions (busulfan, gold, and penicillamine); and chronic rejection following heart-lung, lung, or hematopoietic stem cell transplantation (*bronchiolitis obliterans syndrome*). PFTs with airflow obstruction and air trapping; unremarkable CXRs, heterogeneous air trapping on chest CT scans.

Proliferative bronchiolitis (organizing pneumonia, previously called idiopathic bronchiolitis obliterans organizing pneumonia [BOOP]) is associated with diverse pulmonary disorders, including infection, aspiration, acute respiratory distress syndrome (ARDS), hypersensitivity pneumonitis, connective tissue diseases, and organ transplantation. PFTs typically reveal a restrictive ventilatory defect. It is more likely to have an abnormal CXR or chest CT scan with patchy consolidation, ground-glass opacities, or nodular appearance.

Follicular bronchiolitis is most commonly associated with connective tissue disease, especially rheumatoid arthritis and Sjögren syndrome, and with immunodeficiency states, such as HIV or common variable immunodeficiency. It may be seen in lymphoid interstitial pneumonia. Chest CT scan may show centrilobular and peribronchial nodules.

Respiratory bronchiolitis is the most common form of bronchiolitis in adults and is usually related to cigarette smoking. It usually occurs without symptoms or physiological evidence of lung impairment, but it may be seen with associated ILD (respiratory bronchiolitis-interstitial lung disease). PFTs may show mixed obstructive-restrictive pattern. Chest CT may show centrilobular nodules, patchy ground-glass opacities, air trapping, and "tree-in-bud" opacities.

Diffuse panbronchiolitis is most frequently diagnosed in Japan. Men are affected about twice as often as women, two-thirds are nonsmokers, and most patients have a history of chronic pansinusitis. PFTs reveal obstructive abnormalities, and the CXR shows a distinct pattern of diffuse, small, nodular shadows with hyperinflation.

Treatment

Therapy depends on the classification and etiology, however, evidence-based recommendations based on trials are limited. **Constrictive bronchiolitis** is relatively unresponsive to corticosteroids and frequently leads to progressive clinical deterioration. Azithromycin may slow progression of bronchiolitis obliterans syndrome in lung transplant recipients. In **proliferative bronchiolitis** corticosteroids are usually effective and provide prompt improvement. Initial therapy is prednisone 1 mg/kg/day orally for 1–3 months following by a slow tapering (as tolerated) to 20–40 mg/day, with weaning over the subsequent 3–6 months, as tolerated. Relapse is common if corticosteroids are stopped prematurely or tapered too quickly. In **follicular bronchiolitis,** treatment of underlying disease is recommended. Systemic steroids and azithromycin may be effective. Systemic steroids also may be utilized in **respiratory bronchiolitis**, although response is variable. Smoking cessation is recommended. Azithromycin is useful in the treatment of **diffuse bronchiolitis**.

Dalziel SR et al. Bronchiolitis. Lancet 2022;400:392. [PMID: 35785792]
Viskens K et al. Bronchiolitis in adults: etiology, diagnostic, and therapeutic approach. Respiration. 2025;104:445. [PMID: 39837285]

PULMONARY INFECTIONS

PNEUMONIA

Pneumonia has classically been considered in terms of the infecting organism (Table 9–9). This approach facilitates discussion of characteristic clinical presentations but is a limited guide to patient management since specific microbiologic information is usually not available at initial presentation. Classification schemes emphasize epidemiologic factors that predict etiology and guide initial therapy. Pneumonia may be classified as **community-acquired pneumonia (CAP)** or **nosocomial pneumonia** and, within the latter, as **hospital-acquired pneumonia (HAP)** or **ventilator-associated pneumonia (VAP).** These categories are based on differing settings and infectious agents and

Table 9–9. Characteristics of selected pneumonias.

Organism; Appearance on Smear of Sputum	Clinical Setting	Complications
Streptococcus pneumoniae (pneumococcus). Gram-positive diplococci.	Chronic cardiopulmonary disease; follows upper respiratory tract infection	Bacteremia, meningitis, endocarditis, pericarditis, empyema
Haemophilus influenzae. Pleomorphic gram-negative coccobacilli.	Chronic cardiopulmonary disease; follows upper respiratory tract infection	Empyema, endocarditis
Staphylococcus aureus. Plump gram-positive cocci in clumps.	Residence in long-term care facility, hospital-associated, influenza epidemics, cystic fibrosis, bronchiectasis, injection drug use	Empyema, cavitation
Klebsiella pneumoniae. Plump gram-negative encapsulated rods.	Alcohol abuse, diabetes mellitus; hospital-associated	Cavitation, empyema
Escherichia coli. Gram-negative rods.	Hospital-associated; rarely, community-acquired	Empyema
Pseudomonas aeruginosa. Gram-negative rods.	Hospital-associated; cystic fibrosis, bronchiectasis	Cavitation
Anaerobes. Mixed flora.	Aspiration, poor dental hygiene	Necrotizing pneumonia, abscess, empyema
Mycoplasma pneumoniae. PMNs and monocytes; no bacteria.	Young adults; summer and fall	Skin rashes, hemolytic anemia, encephalitis
Legionella species. Few PMNs; no bacteria.	Summer and fall; exposure to contaminated construction site, water source, air conditioner; community-acquired or hospital-associated	Empyema, cavitation, endocarditis, pericarditis
Chlamydophila pneumoniae. Nonspecific.	Clinically similar to *M pneumoniae*, but prodromal symptoms last longer (up to 2 weeks); sore throat with hoarseness common; mild pneumonia in teenagers and young adults	Reinfection in older adults with underlying COPD or HF may be severe or even fatal
Moraxella catarrhalis. Gram-negative diplococci.	Preexisting lung disease; older patients; corticosteroid or immunosuppressive therapy	Rarely, pleural effusions and bacteremia
Pneumocystis jirovecii. Nonspecific.	AIDS, immunosuppressive or cytotoxic drug therapy, cancer	Pneumothorax, respiratory failure, ARDS, death
SARS-CoV-2. Nonspecific.	Pandemic. Milder pneumonia (teenagers, young adults); more severe pneumonia (older, immunocompromised, multiple comorbidly ill adults)	Respiratory failure, ARDS, death

ARDS, acute respiratory distress syndrome; PMN, polymorphonuclear leukocyte; SARS-CoV-2, severe acute respiratory syndrome due to coronavirus-2 (see COVID-19 discussion, Chapter 37).

require different diagnostic and therapeutic interventions. **Anaerobic pneumonia** and **lung abscess** can occur in both hospital and community settings.

This section sets forth the evaluation and management of pulmonary infiltrates in immunocompetent persons separately from the approach to immunocompromised persons—defined as those with HIV disease, absolute neutrophil counts < 1000/mcL (1.0×10^9/L), or current or recent exposure to myelosuppressive or immunosuppressive medications.

1. Community-Acquired Pneumonia

ESSENTIALS OF DIAGNOSIS

- Fever or hypothermia, tachypnea, cough with or without sputum, dyspnea, chest discomfort.
- Bronchial breath sounds, rhonchi, or inspiratory crackles on chest auscultation.
- Airspace disease on chest imaging (occasionally not evident at presentation).
- Occurs outside of the hospital or within 48 hours of hospital admission.

General Considerations

CAP is a common disorder, with a high incidence rate among adults, approximately 25% of whom require hospitalization. It is the deadliest infectious disease in the United States and worldwide and is routinely among the top 10 causes of death; however, mortality among outpatients treated for milder disease is < 1%. Among patients hospitalized for CAP, in-hospital mortality is approximately 10–12% and 1-year mortality (in those over age 65) is > 40%; the majority of these mortalities occur among older adults. Risk factors for the development of CAP include older age; tobacco use; excessive alcohol use; comorbid medical conditions, especially COPD or other chronic lung disease; immunosuppression; and recent viral upper respiratory tract infection.

The patient's history, physical examination, and imaging studies are essential to establishing a diagnosis of CAP. For the identification of specific pathogen, sputum examination may be helpful, but 40% of patients cannot produce an evaluable sputum sample; additionally, test characteristics of sputum Gram stain and culture vary by organism and lack sensitivity for some of the most common causes of pneumonia. Since patient outcomes improve when the initial antibiotic choice is appropriate for the infecting organism, the American Thoracic Society and the Infectious Diseases Society of America recommend empiric treatment based on epidemiologic data (Table 9–10). Such treatment improves initial antibiotic coverage, reduces unnecessary hospitalization, and improves 30-day survival.

Definition & Pathogenesis

CAP is diagnosed outside of the hospital setting or within the first 48 hours of hospital admission. Pulmonary defense mechanisms (cough reflex, mucociliary clearance system, immune responses) normally prevent the development of lower respiratory tract infections following aspiration of oropharyngeal secretions containing bacteria or inhalation of infected aerosols. CAP occurs when there is a defect in one or more of these normal defense mechanisms or when a large infectious inoculum or a virulent pathogen overwhelms the immune response.

Prospective studies fail to identify the cause of CAP in 30–60% of cases; two or more causes are identified in up to one-third of cases. The most common bacterial pathogen identified in most studies of CAP is *S pneumoniae*, accounting for approximately two-thirds of bacterial isolates. Other common bacterial pathogens include *H influenzae*, *M pneumoniae*, *C pneumoniae*, *S aureus*, *Moraxella catarrhalis*, *Klebsiella pneumoniae*, other gram-negative rods, and *Legionella* species. Common viral causes of CAP include coronaviruses (SARS-CoV-2, MERS), influenza virus, RSV, adenovirus, and parainfluenza virus. A detailed assessment of epidemiologic risk factors may aid in diagnosing pneumonias due to the following uncommon causes: *Chlamydophila psittaci* (psittacosis); *Coxiella burnetii* (Q fever); *Francisella tularensis* (tularemia); *Blastomyces*, *Coccidioides*, *Histoplasma* (endemic fungi); and Sin Nombre virus (hantavirus pulmonary syndrome).

Clinical Findings

A. Symptoms and Signs

Most patients with CAP experience an acute or subacute onset of fever, cough with or without sputum production, and dyspnea. Other common symptoms include chills, rigors, pleurisy, fatigue, myalgias, anorexia, headache, and abdominal pain. Patients aged 80 years or older, however, may have an atypical presentation, including falls, delirium, lethargy, and anorexia.

Common physical findings include fever or hypothermia, tachypnea, and tachycardia. Many patients appear acutely ill. Chest examination often reveals inspiratory crackles, rhonchi, and bronchial breath sounds. Dullness to percussion may be observed if lobar consolidation or a parapneumonic pleural effusion is present. The clinical evaluation is < 50% sensitive compared to chest imaging for the diagnosis of CAP (see Imaging section below). In most patients, therefore, imaging is essential to the evaluation of suspected CAP.

B. Diagnostic Testing

Diagnostic testing for a specific infectious cause of CAP is not generally indicated in outpatients because empiric antibiotic therapy is almost always effective in this population. In ambulatory outpatients whose presentation (travel history, exposure) suggests an etiology not covered by standard therapy (eg, *Coccidioides*) or involves public health concerns (eg, SARS-CoV-2, *Mycobacterium tuberculosis*, influenza), diagnostic testing is appropriate. Diagnostic testing is recommended in hospitalized CAP patients for multiple reasons: the likelihood of an infectious cause unresponsive to standard therapy is higher in more severe illness, the inpatient setting allows narrowing of antibiotic

Table 9–10. Recommended empiric antibiotics for community-acquired bacterial pneumonia.

Outpatient management
1. For previously healthy patients with no risk factors for MRSA or *Pseudomonas*: a. Amoxicillin, 1 g orally three times daily, *or* b. Doxycycline, 100 mg orally twice a day, *or* c. In regions with a low rate (< 25%) of infection with high level (MIC ≥ 16 mcg/mL) macrolide-resistant *Streptococcus pneumoniae*, then a macrolide (clarithromycin, 500 mg orally twice a day; or azithromycin, 500 mg orally as a first dose and then 250 mg orally daily for 4 days, or 500 mg orally daily for 3 days).
2. For patients with comorbid medical conditions such as chronic heart, lung, liver, or kidney disease; diabetes mellitus; alcohol use disorder; malignancy; asplenia; immunosuppressant conditions or use of immunosuppressive drugs; or use of antibiotics within the previous 3 months (in which case an agent from a different antibiotic class should be selected): a. A macrolide *or* doxycycline (as above) *plus* an oral β-lactam (amoxicillin/clavulanate 500 mg/125 mg three times daily, amoxicillin/clavulanate 875 mg/125 mg twice daily, amoxicillin/clavulanate 2 g/125 mg twice daily; cefpodoxime, 200 mg twice daily; cefuroxime, 500 mg twice daily). b. Monotherapy with an oral fluoroquinolone (moxifloxacin, 400 mg daily; gemifloxacin, 320 mg daily; levofloxacin, 750 mg daily).
Inpatient management of nonsevere pneumonia (typically not requiring intensive care)
1. A respiratory fluoroquinolone. Oral and intravenous doses equivalent: moxifloxacin, 400 mg daily or levofloxacin, 500–750 mg daily *or*
2. A macrolide (see above for oral therapy) *plus* a β-lactam (see above for oral β-lactam therapy). For intravenous therapy: ampicillin/sulbactam, 1.5–3 g every 6 hours; cefotaxime, 1–2 g every 8 hours; ceftriaxone, 1–2 g every 12–24 hours; ceftaroline, 600 mg every 12 hours.
3. For patients with prior respiratory isolation of MRSA, strongly consider adding coverage for MRSA and obtain cultures or nasal PCR to confirm infection or to allow de-escalation of therapy: vancomycin, typically starting at 15 mg/kg intravenously every 12 hours with interval dosing based on kidney function to achieve serum trough concentration 15–20 mcg/mL *or* linezolid, 600 mg orally or intravenously every 12 hours.
4. For patients with prior respiratory isolation of *Pseudomonas aeruginosa*, strongly consider adding coverage for *P aeruginosa* and obtain cultures to confirm infection or to allow de-escalation of therapy. Intravenous therapy only: piperacillin-tazobactam, 3.375–4.5 g every 6 hours; cefepime, 1–2 g every 8 hours; imipenem, 0.5–1 g every 6 hours; meropenem, 1 g every 8 hours; or aztreonam 2 g every 8 hours.
Inpatient management of severe pneumonia (typically requiring intensive care). All agents administered intravenously, except as noted.
1. Azithromycin (500 mg orally as a first dose and then 250 mg orally daily for 4 days, *or* 500 mg orally daily for 3 days) or a respiratory fluoroquinolone (as above) plus an intravenous anti-pneumococcal β-lactam (as above).
2. For patients allergic to β-lactam antibiotics, a fluoroquinolone *plus* aztreonam (2 g every 8 hours).
3. For patients at risk for *P aeruginosa*, add coverage for *P aeruginosa* and obtain cultures to confirm infection or to allow de-escalation of therapy: piperacillin-tazobactam, 3.375–4.5 g every 6 hours; cefepime, 1–2 g every 8 hours; imipenem, 0.5–1 g every 6 hours; meropenem, 1 g every 8 hours; or aztreonam 2 g every 8 hours.
4. For patients at risk for *Pseudomonas* infection AND who are critically ill, at increased risk for drug resistance, or if local incidence of monotherapy-resistant *Pseudomonas* is > 10%, consider adding either an anti-pseudomonal fluoroquinolone (ciprofloxacin 400 mg every 8–12 hours or levofloxacin 750 mg daily) *or* an aminoglycoside (gentamicin, tobramycin, amikacin, all weight-based dosing administered daily adjusted to appropriate trough levels).
5. For patients at risk for MRSA infection, add coverage for MRSA and obtain cultures or nasal PCR, or both, to confirm infection or to allow de-escalation of therapy: vancomycin, typically starting at 15 mg/kg intravenously every 12 hours with interval dosing based on kidney function to achieve serum trough concentration 15–20 mcg/mL or linezolid, 600 mg every 12 hours.

MIC, minimum inhibitory concentration; MRSA, methicillin-resistant *Staphylococcus aureus*.
Recommendations assembled from Matley JP et al. Diagnosis and treatment of adults with community-acquired pneumonia. An official clinical practice guideline of the American Thoracic Society and Infectious Diseases Society of America. Am J Respir Crit Care Med. 2019;200(7):e45–e67.

coverage as specific diagnostic information is available, and the yield of testing is higher in more acutely ill patients.

Diagnostic tests are used to adjust empirically chosen therapy and to facilitate epidemiologic analysis. Three widely available diagnostic tests may guide therapy: the sputum Gram stain and culture, tests for viruses such as influenza and SARS-CoV-2, and urinary antigen tests. The usefulness of a sputum Gram stain lies in broadening initial coverage in patients hospitalized for CAP, most commonly to cover *S aureus* (including community-acquired methicillin-resistant *S aureus* [CA-MRSA] strains) or gram-negative rods (including *P aeruginosa* and Enterobacteriaceae). Urinary antigen assays for *Legionella pneumophila* and *S pneumoniae* are commonly available and do not rely on effective sputum expectoration. Urinary antigen assay for *L pneumophila* should be ordered for patients in an area with an outbreak, with recent travel, with severe disease, or in whom a high clinical index of suspicion exists. The utility of urinary antigen testing for *S pneumoniae* has been questioned due to its low sensitivity and predictive value. Rapid influenza and SARS-CoV-2 testing have intermediate sensitivity but high specificity, with sensitivity depending on the method of detection (nucleic acid or PCR-based tests have higher sensitivity than antigen-based detection). Positive tests for viruses may direct isolation of hospitalized patients but do not necessarily reduce the need for antibacterial therapy, since coinfection with bacterial and viral pathogens may occur, especially with influenza.

Rapid turnaround multiplex-PCR amplification from lower respiratory tract samples is increasingly available. Different commercial products can identify multiple strains of bacteria and viruses, in addition to genes that encode for antibiotic resistance. Early experience with multiplex-PCR shows improved overall diagnostic yield, particularly for viral infections, and a higher incidence of bacterial/viral coinfection than previously recognized. Limitations of multiplex-PCR include cost and availability, in addition to the challenge of interpreting potentially false-positive results from a highly sensitive test, since either viral or bacterial pathogens may colonize the airways. Studies in outpatients and hospitalized patients have failed to demonstrate benefit in antibiotic stewardship or outcome, despite the demonstrated improvement in diagnostic yield; further study will continue to inform its utility.

Additional microbiologic testing including pre-antibiotic sputum and blood cultures (at least two sets at separate sites) has been standard practice for patients with CAP who require hospitalization. The yield of blood and sputum cultures is low, as false-positive results are common, and the impact of culture results on patient outcomes is small. As a result, targeted testing is recommended for patients with severe disease and for those treated empirically for MRSA or *P aeruginosa* infection. The role of culture is to allow narrowing of initial empiric antibiotic coverage, adjustment of coverage based on specific antibiotic resistance patterns, to identify unsuspected pathogens not covered by initial therapy, and to provide information for epidemiologic analysis. Patients at risk for or treated empirically for MRSA should have an MRSA nasal screening test performed. A negative nasal screening test guides de-escalation of empiric MRSA coverage in patients who cannot expectorate a sputum sample.

Apart from microbiologic testing, hospitalized patients should undergo CBC with differential and a chemistry panel (including serum glucose, electrolytes, BUN, creatinine, bilirubin, and liver enzymes). Test results help assess severity of illness and guide evaluation and management. HIV testing should be considered in all adult patients and performed in those with risk factors.

C. Imaging

A pulmonary opacity on chest imaging is required to establish a diagnosis of CAP. Chest CT scan is more sensitive and specific than CXR and may be indicated in selected cases. Radiographic findings range from patchy airspace opacities to lobar consolidation with air bronchograms to diffuse alveolar or interstitial opacities. Additional findings can include pleural effusions and cavitation. Chest imaging cannot identify a specific microbiologic cause of CAP; no pattern of radiographic abnormalities is pathognomonic of any infectious cause. Chest ultrasound, which is more readily available in resource-constrained settings, has demonstrated variable sensitivity and specificity for pneumonia when compared to CT imaging, but is at least equivalent to CXR when performed and interpreted by experienced personnel. It is now recognized in some guidelines as an acceptable alternative to CXR.

Chest imaging may help assess severity and response to therapy over time. Progression of pulmonary opacities during antibiotic therapy or lack of radiographic improvement over time are poor prognostic signs and raise concerns about secondary or alternative pulmonary processes. Clearing of pulmonary opacities in patients with CAP can take 6 weeks or longer. Clearance is usually quickest in younger patients, nonsmokers, and those with single-lobe involvement.

D. Special Examinations

Patients with CAP who have significant pleural fluid collections may require diagnostic thoracentesis (with pleural fluid sent for glucose, LD, and total protein levels; leukocyte count with differential; pH determination; and Gram stain and culture). Positive pleural cultures or features of complex parapneumonic effusion indicate the need for tube thoracostomy drainage.

Patients with cavitary opacities should have sputum fungal and mycobacterial cultures.

Sputum induction or fiberoptic bronchoscopy to obtain samples of lower respiratory secretions are indicated in patients with a worsening clinical course who cannot provide expectorated sputum samples or who may have pneumonia caused by *M tuberculosis* infection or certain opportunistic infections, including *Pneumocystis jirovecii*.

Differential Diagnosis

The differential diagnosis of lower respiratory tract infection is extensive and includes upper respiratory tract infections, reactive airway diseases, HF, interstitial pneumonias, lung cancer, pulmonary vasculitis, pulmonary thromboembolic disease, malignancy, and atelectasis.

Treatment

Two general principles guide antibiotic therapy once the diagnosis of CAP is established: **prompt** initiation of a medication to which the etiologic pathogen is **susceptible**.

In patients who require specific diagnostic evaluation, sputum and blood culture specimens should be obtained before initiation of antibiotics. Since early administration of antibiotics to acutely ill patients is associated with improved outcomes, obtaining other diagnostic specimens or test results should not delay the initial dose of antibiotics.

Optimal antibiotic therapy would be pathogen directed, but a definitive microbiologic diagnosis is not typically available on presentation. A syndromic approach to therapy, based on clinical presentation and chest imaging, does not reliably predict the microbiology of CAP. Therefore, initial antibiotic choices are empiric, based on acuity (treatment as an outpatient, inpatient, or in the ICU), patient risk factors for specific pathogens, and local antibiotic resistance patterns (see Table 9–10).

Since *S pneumoniae* remains a common cause of CAP in all patient groups, local prevalence of drug-resistant *S pneumoniae* significantly affects initial antibiotic choice. Prior treatment with one antibiotic in a pharmacologic class (eg, β-lactam, macrolide, fluoroquinolone) predisposes to the emergence of drug-resistant *S pneumoniae*, with resistance developing against that class of antibiotics to which the pathogen was previously exposed. In vivo efficacy justifies maintaining macrolides as first-line therapy except in areas where there is a high prevalence of resistant strains. Macrolide resistance has increased (approximately one-third of *S pneumoniae* isolates show in vitro resistance); however, reported treatment failures remain rare compared to the number of patients treated. *S pneumoniae* resistance to fluoroquinolones is rare in the United States but is increasing.

CA-MRSA is genetically and phenotypically different from hospital-acquired MRSA strains and is more virulent. CA-MRSA is a rare cause of necrotizing pneumonia, empyema, respiratory failure, and shock; it appears to be associated with prior influenza infection. Linezolid may be preferred to vancomycin in treatment of CA-MRSA pulmonary infection due to bacterial toxin inhibition. Daptomycin should **not** be used in any MRSA pneumonia because it does not achieve adequate concentration in the lung. For expanded discussions of specific antibiotics, see Chapter 34.

A. Treatment of Outpatients

See Table 9–10 for specific medication dosages. The most common etiologies of CAP in outpatients who do not require hospitalization are *S pneumoniae*; *M pneumoniae*; *C pneumoniae*; and respiratory viruses, including influenza. For previously healthy patients with no recent (90 days) use of antibiotics, the recommended treatment is amoxicillin with or without a macrolide (clarithromycin or azithromycin), or doxycycline. In areas with a high incidence of macrolide-resistant *S pneumoniae*, initial therapy in patients with no comorbidities may include the combination of a β-lactam plus a macrolide, or a respiratory fluoroquinolone.

In outpatients with chronic heart, lung, liver, or kidney disease; diabetes mellitus; alcohol use disorder; malignancy; or asplenia or who received antibiotic therapy within the past 90 days, the recommended treatment is a macrolide or doxycycline plus a β-lactam (high-dose amoxicillin and amoxicillin-clavulanate are preferred to cefpodoxime and cefuroxime) or monotherapy with a respiratory fluoroquinolone (moxifloxacin, gemifloxacin, or levofloxacin).

The default duration of antibiotic therapy for CAP is 5 days; factors that may affect therapy duration are clinical stability, etiology (MRSA and *P aeruginosa* require minimum 7 days of therapy, for example), severity of illness, complications, and comorbid medical problems. New data suggest equal effectiveness of shorter duration of antibiotics (but not less than 3 days) in immunocompetent adult patients without comorbidities if they have reached clinical stability at day 3, but practical considerations may limit applicability in practice.

B. Treatment of Hospitalized and ICU Patients

1. Antibiotics—The most common etiologies of CAP in patients who require hospitalization but not intensive care are *S pneumoniae*, *M pneumoniae*, *C pneumoniae*, *H influenzae*, *Legionella* species, and respiratory viruses. Some patients have aspiration as an immediate precipitant to the CAP without a specific bacterial etiology. First-line therapy in hospitalized patients is the combination of a macrolide (clarithromycin or azithromycin) plus a β-lactam (cefotaxime, ceftriaxone, ceftaroline, or ampicillin-sulbactam) or monotherapy with a respiratory fluoroquinolone (eg, moxifloxacin, gemifloxacin, or levofloxacin) (Table 9–10).

Almost all patients admitted to a hospital for treatment of CAP receive intravenous antibiotics; however, no studies in hospitalized patients demonstrated superior outcomes with intravenous antibiotics compared with oral antibiotics, provided patients were able to tolerate oral therapy and the medication was well absorbed. Duration of inpatient antibiotic treatment is the same as for outpatients, with the clarification that durations of antibiotics < 5 days may be considered only for nonsevere cases that clearly demonstrate clinical improvement and stability between days 3–5 of antibiotic treatment.

The most common etiologies of CAP in patients who require admission to intensive care are *S pneumoniae*, *Legionella* species, *H influenzae*, Enterobacteriaceae species, *S aureus*, *Pseudomonas* species, and respiratory viruses. First-line antibacterial therapy in ICU patients with CAP is an anti-pneumococcal β-lactam (cefotaxime, ceftriaxone, ceftaroline, or ampicillin-sulbactam) plus either a macrolide or a respiratory fluoroquinolone.

Risk factors for *Pseudomonas*, Enterobacteriaceae, or MRSA infection must be considered when choosing empiric antibiotic therapy for inpatients with CAP. Specific risk factors for these organisms include (1) prior isolation of the pathogen, (2) inpatient hospitalization within the last 90 days, or (3) exposure to intravenous antibiotics within the last 90 days. In patients with specific risk factors for *Pseudomonas* infection, combine an anti-pneumococcal, anti-pseudomonal β-lactam (piperacillin-tazobactam, cefepime, imipenem, meropenem) with either azithromycin or a respiratory fluoroquinolone (moxifloxacin, gemifloxacin, or levofloxacin). In critically ill patients, in those at increased risk for drug resistance, or if the unit incidence of monotherapy-resistant *Pseudomonas* is > 10%, consider use of two agents with anti-pseudomonal efficacy: either ciprofloxacin or levofloxacin plus the above anti-pneumococcal, anti-pseudomonal β-lactam or an anti-pneumococcal, anti-pseudomonal β-lactam plus an aminoglycoside (gentamicin, tobramycin, amikacin) plus either azithromycin or a respiratory fluoroquinolone. Patients with specific risk factors for MRSA should be treated with vancomycin or linezolid. Patients with very severe disease (respiratory failure requiring mechanical ventilation or septic shock) should also be strongly considered for empiric MRSA therapy. Provided the patient is clinically improving, negative sputum and blood cultures obtained before initiation of antibiotics can support de-escalation of antibiotic therapy. Additionally, all patients prescribed vancomycin or linezolid should have nasal swabs for MRSA; if the swab results are negative, MRSA coverage can be safely de-escalated.

Patients with CAP in whom influenza is detected should be treated with the antiviral oseltamivir, whether influenza is identified as a single pathogen or as a coinfection along with a bacterial pathogen. Oseltamivir is most effective when begun within 2 days but may still be beneficial within several days after symptom onset, particularly in severe cases of CAP. Identification of a viral pathogen, especially influenza, does not obviate the need for antibacterials, as bacterial coinfection is common and bacterial pathogen testing is insensitive.

2. Adjunctive treatment: Corticosteroids—The role of corticosteroid therapy in the management of CAP has been controversial; however, a 2023 large RCT of adults with severe CAP hospitalized in an ICU identified a lower risk of mortality at 28 days in patients treated with hydrocortisone (200 mg/day for 4–7 days followed by tapering) than patients treated with placebo (6.2% versus 11.9%, respectively) and a lower requirement for mechanical ventilation. More recent meta-analyses including these data have added support for the role of corticosteroids in severe CAP, however in nonsevere CAP a benefit of steroids has not been demonstrated. Corticosteroid treatment of influenza pneumonia may be associated with higher mortality and should be avoided. Corticosteroid treatment is recommended for SARS-CoV-2 pneumonia when oxygen is required; see Chapter 36 for further discussion.

Prevention

Pneumococcal vaccines prevent or lessen the severity of pneumococcal infections in immunocompetent patients. Two classes of pneumococcal vaccines for adults are available and approved for use in the United States: polyconjugate vaccines (PCV)—including 20-valent (PCV20), 21-valent (PCV21), 15-valent (PCV15), and 13-valent (PCV13)—and polysaccharide vaccine, 23-valent (PPSV23).

The CDC Advisory Committee on Immunization Practices issued guidance in 2024, recommending routine pneumococcal vaccination for all adults age 50 and older, and adults aged 19–49 with certain medical comorbidities (diabetes, chronic lung disease, chronic liver disease), increased risk of meningitis (CSF leak, cochlear implant), or immunocompromising condition, including asplenia.

Approach to vaccination depends on prior history of pneumococcal vaccination. Most patients in the above categories who have *not* received previous vaccination with PCV21 or PCV20 should receive one of these vaccines, or a series of PCV15 followed by PPSV23. Recommendations are summarized in Table 9–11.

Influenza vaccine is effective in preventing severe disease due to influenza virus with a resulting positive impact

Table 9–11. Pneumococcal vaccination recommendations for adults with and without prior pneumococcal vaccination.

No Prior Vaccination		
Immunocompetent	Immunocompromised (Including Asplenia) or Increased Risk of Meningitis (Including Cochlear Implant or CSF Leak)	
PCV21 PCV20 (if PCV21 not available, or increased risk of serotype 4) PCV15, followed by PPSV23 12 months later (if PCV21/PCV20 not available)	PCV21 PCV20, followed by PPSV23 8 weeks later PCV15, followed by PPSV23 8 weeks later (if PCV20 not available)	
Prior Vaccination		
Prior PPSV23 Only	Prior PCV10 or PCV13 Only	Prior PCV10/PCV13 and PPSV23
All categories	All categories	Patients aged ≥ 50 years, received both vaccines before age 50
PCV21 or PCV20 at least 12 months after	PCV21 or PCV20 at least 12 months after PPSV23, if PCV21/PCV20 not available	PCV21 or PCV20 ≥ 5 years after last vaccine PPSV23, if PCV21/PCV20 not available
		Patients aged ≥ 50 years, received PPSV23 after age 50
		Consider PCV21 or PCV20 ≥ 5 years after last vaccine
		Patients aged 19–49 years with chronic conditions[1]
		PCV21 or PCV20 at age 50 (and ≥ 5 years after last vaccine) PPSV23, if PCV21/PCV20 not available
		Patients aged 19–49 years with immunocompromise
		PCV21 or PCV20 ≥ 5 years after last vaccine PPSV23, if PCV21/PCV20 not available, ≥ 8 weeks after PCV, and ≥ 5 years after last PPSV23
		Patients aged 19–49 years with increased meningitis risk
		PCV21 or PCV20 ≥ 5 years after last vaccine Consider PPSV23, if PCV21/PCV20 not available, ≥ 8 weeks after PCV, and ≥ 5 years after last PPSV23

[1]Chronic conditions include alcohol use disorder, chronic heart disease, chronic lung disease, chronic liver disease, diabetes, hemoglobinopathies, and tobacco smoking.

on both primary influenza pneumonia and secondary bacterial pneumonias. The seasonal influenza vaccine is recommended annually for all persons older than 6 months without contraindications, with priority given to persons at risk for complications of influenza infection (persons aged 50 years or older, immunocompromised persons, residents of long-term care facilities, patients with pulmonary or cardiovascular disorders, pregnant persons) as well as health care workers and others who may transmit influenza to high-risk patients. Higher dose or adjuvanted vaccination is recommended for adults 65 and older.

SARS-CoV-2 vaccinations are recommended for everyone older than 6 months without contraindications. Vaccinations (including boosters) reduce the likelihood of infection, pneumonia, hospitalization, and mortality (see COVID-19 discussion, Chapter 36).

RSV vaccination is recommended for persons at risk of developing severe disease, including age 75 or older, age 60 or older in congregate living (assisted living or skilled nursing), and adults with comorbidities including chronic pulmonary disease, heart disease, chronic renal disease, chronic liver disease, diabetes, hemoglobinopathies, neurological respiratory muscle weakness, severe obesity, and with immunocompromising conditions. Shared decision making is recommended for persons younger than 75, as an increased risk of Guillain-Barré syndrome has been reported in association with the adjuvanted and bivalent RSV vaccines. Pregnant persons who are 32–36 weeks' gestation during RSV season and have not previously been vaccinated are recommended to receive the vaccine, as a measure to prevent severe RSV disease in the infant.

When to Admit

Once a diagnosis of CAP is made, the first management decision is to determine the site of care: Is it safe to treat the patient at home or does he or she require hospital or ICU admission? When need for admission is not immediately apparent, there are two widely used clinical prediction rules available to guide admission and triage decisions, the **Pneumonia Severity Index (PSI)** and the **CURB-65**.

A. Hospital Admission Decision

The PSI is a validated prediction model that uses 20 items from demographics, medical history, physical examination, laboratory results, and imaging to stratify patients into five risk groups. In conjunction with clinical judgment, it facilitates safe decisions to treat CAP in the outpatient setting. An online PSI risk calculator is available at https://www.thecalculator.co/health/Pneumonia-Severity-Index-(PSI)-Calculator-977.html. The CURB-65 assesses five simple, independent predictors of increased mortality (**C**onfusion, **U**remia, **R**espiratory rate, **B**lood pressure, and age > **65**) to calculate a 30-day predicted mortality (https://www.mdcalc.com/curb-65-score-pneumonia-severity). Compared with the PSI, the simpler CURB-65 is less discriminating at low mortality but excellent at identifying patients with high mortality who may benefit from ICU-level care. A modified version (CRB-65) dispenses with BUN and eliminates the need for laboratory testing.

Hospital admission decision should also include circumstances of care independent of pneumonia severity, including comorbidities and the patient's ability to care for themselves effectively at home.

B. ICU Admission Decision

Expert opinion has defined major and minor criteria to identify patients at high risk for death. Major criteria are septic shock with need for vasopressor support and respiratory failure with need for mechanical ventilation. Minor criteria are respiratory rate of ≥ 30 breaths per minute, hypoxemia (defined as $PaO_2/FIO_2 \le 250$), hypothermia (core temperature < 36.0°C), hypotension requiring aggressive fluid resuscitation, confusion/disorientation, multilobar pulmonary opacities, leukopenia due to infection with WBC < 4000/mcL (< 4.0 × 10^9/L), thrombocytopenia with platelet count < 100,000/mcL (< 100 × 10^9/L), uremia with BUN of ≥ 20 mg/dL (≥ 7.1 mmol/L), metabolic acidosis, or elevated serum lactate level. Either one major criterion or three or more minor criteria of illness severity generally require ICU-level care.

Bergmann F et al. Efficacy and safety of corticosteroid therapy for community-acquired pneumonia: a meta-analysis and meta-regression of randomized, controlled trials. Clin Infect Dis. 2023;77:1704. [PMID: 37876267]

Britton A et al. Use of respiratory syncytial virus vaccines in adults aged ≥60 years: updated recommendations of the Advisory Committee on Immunization Practices – United States, 2024. MMWR Morb Mortal Wkly Report. 2024;73:696. [PMID: 39146277]

Dequin PF et al. Hydrocortisone in severe community-acquired pneumonia. N Engl J Med. 2023;388:1931. [PMID: 36942789]

Kobayashi M et al. Expanded recommendations for use of Pneumococcal conjugate vaccines among adults aged 50 years: recommendations of the Advisory Committee on Immunization Practices – United States, 2025. MMWR Morb Mortal Wkly Rep. 2025;74:1. [PMID: 39773952]

Martin-Loeches I et al. ERS/ESCIM/ESCMID/ALAT guidelines for the management of severe community-acquired pneumonia. Eur Respir J. 2023;61:2200735. [PMID: 37012080]

2. Nosocomial Pneumonia (Hospital-Acquired & Ventilator-Associated)

ESSENTIALS OF DIAGNOSIS

- **Hospital-acquired pneumonia (HAP)** is diagnosed in patients with clinical features and imaging consistent with pneumonia, occurring > 48 hours after admission to the hospital and excluding any infections present at the time of admission.
- **Ventilator-associated pneumonia (VAP)** requires clinical features concerning for new pneumonia with positive respiratory samples developing > 48 hours following tracheal intubation and mechanical ventilation.

General Considerations

Hospitalized patients carry different flora with different resistance patterns than healthy patients in the community, and their health status may place them at higher risk for more severe infection. The diagnostic approach and antibiotic treatment of patients with HAP is, therefore, different from patients with CAP. Similarly, management of patients in whom VAP develops following tracheal intubation and mechanical ventilation should address issues specific to this group of patients.

Considered together, nosocomial pneumonias (HAP or VAP) represent an important cause of morbidity and mortality despite widespread use of preventive measures, advances in diagnostic testing, and potent antimicrobial agents. HAP is one of the most common causes of infection among hospital inpatients and carries the highest burden of morbidity and mortality. Patients in ICUs and those who are being mechanically ventilated are at the highest risk for HAP (and VAP) and experience higher morbidity and mortality than other inpatients. Definitive identification of the infectious cause of a lower respiratory infection is rarely available on presentation; initial antibiotic treatment is therefore empiric and informed by epidemiologic and patient data rather than pathogen directed.

Definition & Pathogenesis

HAP develops > 48 hours after admission to the hospital, and VAP develops in a mechanically ventilated patient > 48 hours after tracheal intubation. Three factors distinguish nosocomial pneumonia from CAP: (1) different infectious causes; (2) different antibiotic susceptibility patterns, specifically, a higher incidence of drug resistance; and (3) poorer underlying health status of patients, putting them at risk for more severe infections. Since access to the lower respiratory tract occurs primarily through microaspiration, nosocomial pneumonia starts with a change in upper respiratory tract flora. Colonization is promoted by exogenous factors (eg, instrumentation of the upper airway with nasogastric and endotracheal tubes; contact with personnel, equipment, and contaminated aerosols; treatment with broad-spectrum antibiotics that promote the emergence of drug-resistant organisms); and patient factors (eg, malnutrition, advanced age, altered consciousness, swallowing disorders, and underlying pulmonary and systemic diseases). Impaired cellular and mechanical defense mechanisms in the lungs of hospitalized patients raise the risk of infection after aspiration has occurred.

Gastric acid may play a role in protection against nosocomial pneumonias. Observational studies have suggested that elevation of gastric pH due to antacids, H_2-receptor antagonists, PPIs, or enteral feeding is associated with gastric microbial overgrowth, tracheobronchial colonization, and HAP/VAP. Meta-analysis of RCTs suggested an increased risk of HAP among enterally fed patients receiving stress ulcer prophylaxis, but the findings are not universal. The IDSA and other professional organizations recommend that acid-suppressive medications (H_2-receptor antagonists and PPIs) be given only to patients at high risk for stress gastritis.

The microbiology of nosocomial pneumonias differs from CAP but is substantially the same among HAP and VAP. The most common organisms responsible for HAP and VAP include *S aureus* (both methicillin-sensitive *S aureus* and MRSA), *Streptococcus* species, *P aeruginosa*, other gram-negative rods, including extended spectrum β-lactamase (ESBL)–producing organisms (*Enterobacter* species, *K pneumoniae*, and *Escherichia coli*) and non-ESBL-producing organisms. VAP patients may be infected with *Acinetobacter* species and *S maltophilia*. Anaerobic organisms (*Bacteroides*, anaerobic streptococci, *Fusobacterium*) may also cause pneumonia in hospitalized patients; when these organisms are isolated, they are commonly part of a polymicrobial flora. VAP occurring before hospital day 4 in a previously healthy person with no antibiotic exposure is more likely to involve oral flora with minimal resistance profiles than multidrug-resistant pathogens. However, multidrug-resistant pathogens may complicate early-onset VAP in patients with antibiotic exposure in preceding 90 days, recent hospitalization, or prior colonization with multidrug-resistant pathogens.

Clinical Findings

A. Symptoms and Signs

The symptoms and signs associated with nosocomial pneumonias are nonspecific. However, two or more clinical findings (fever, leukocytosis, purulent sputum, worsening respiratory status) along with new or progressive pulmonary opacities on chest imaging are characteristic features of nosocomial pneumonia. Other findings include those listed above for CAP.

The differential diagnosis of new lower respiratory tract symptoms and signs in hospitalized patients includes HF, atelectasis, aspiration, ARDS, pulmonary thromboembolism, pulmonary hemorrhage, and medication reactions.

B. Laboratory Findings

Diagnostic evaluation for suspected nosocomial pneumonia includes blood cultures from two different sites. Blood cultures can identify the pathogen in 15–20% of patients with nosocomial pneumonias; positivity is associated with increased risk of complications and other sites of infection. Blood counts and clinical chemistry tests do not establish a specific diagnosis; however, they help define the severity of illness and identify complications. Thoracentesis for pleural fluid analysis should be considered in patients with pleural effusions.

Examination of lower respiratory tract secretions is attended by the same disadvantages as in CAP. Gram stains and cultures of sputum are neither sensitive nor specific in the diagnosis of nosocomial pneumonias; sensitivity of sputum decreases following antibiotic therapy, particularly after 72 hours of antibiotics. The identification of a bacterial organism by culture of lower respiratory tract secretions does not prove that the organism is a lower respiratory tract pathogen; however, it can be used to help identify bacterial antibiotic sensitivity patterns and as a guide to adjusting empiric therapy. Nasal swab for PCR detection of MRSA is recommended to guide de-escalation of broad-spectrum antibiotic therapy in patients with HAP and VAP.

C. Imaging

Radiographic findings in HAP/VAP are nonspecific and often confounded by other processes that led to hospitalization or ICU admission. (See CAP above.) Imaging may demonstrate complicating features including effusion, cavitation, or barotrauma.

D. Special Examinations

When HAP is suspected in a patient who subsequently requires mechanical ventilation, secretions may be obtained by spontaneous expectoration, sputum induction, nasotracheal suctioning, and endotracheal aspiration (qualitative or semiquantitative samples), or more invasively via bronchoscopic sampling of the lower airways (quantitative samples). The best approach remains a matter of debate, since qualitative or semiquantitative samples are more likely to return nonpathogenic organisms and are, thus, associated with higher antibiotic exposure (without improvement in mortality), while invasive quantitative sampling increases cost and patient risk. Invasive qualitative sampling is recommended when the patient does not improve during initial therapy directed at expected or isolated pathogens, or in immunocompromised persons in whom an opportunistic pathogen is suspected.

Treatment

The initial treatment of HAP and VAP is based on risk factors for MRSA and multiple drug-resistant pathogens (Table 9–12) as well as local antibiograms and mortality risk and is thus empiric (Table 9–13). The predictive capability of sets of risk factors for drug-resistant organisms in nosocomial pneumonia vary locally; strongest predictive factors include prior isolation of drug-resistant organisms, a high local prevalence of drug-resistant organisms, and antibiotic exposure within prior 90 days. Each hospital should generate antibiograms to guide the optimal choice of antibiotics with the goals of reducing exposure to unnecessary antibiotics and the development of antibiotic resistance. Because of the high mortality rate, therapy should be started as soon as HAP or VAP is suspected. After results of cultures are available, it may be possible to narrow initially broad therapy to more specific agents. Endotracheal aspiration cultures have significant negative predictive value but limited positive predictive value in the diagnosis of specific infectious causes of HAP/VAP. If an invasive diagnostic approach to suspected VAP using quantitative culture of bronchoalveolar lavage (BAL), protected specimen brush (PSB), or blind bronchial sampling (BBS) is used, antibiotics can be withheld when results are below a diagnostic threshold (BAL < 10^4 CFU/mL, PSB or BBS < 10^3 CFU/mL). Duration of antibiotic therapy is 7 days, consistent with clinical response, but should be individualized based on the pathogen, complications (empyema, necrotizing pneumonia), severity of illness, response to therapy, and comorbid conditions.

For expanded discussions of specific antibiotics, see Chapter 34.

Barbier F et al. Single-drug versus combination antimicrobial therapy in critically ill patients with hospital-acquired pneumonia and ventilator-associated pneumonia due to gram-negative pathogens: a multicenter retrospective cohort study. Crit Care. 2024;28:10. [PMID: 38172969]

Table 9–12. Risk factors for multidrug-resistant (MDR) pathogens, methicillin-resistant *Staphylococcus aureus* (MRSA), and *Pseudomonas* and other gram-negative bacilli in patients with hospital-acquired pneumonia (HAP) and ventilator-associated pneumonia (VAP).

Risk factors for MDR pathogens
Antibiotic therapy in the preceding 90 days
Septic shock
Acute respiratory distress syndrome preceding VAP
≥ 5 days in hospital before occurrence of HAP/VAP
Acute renal replacement therapy before HAP/VAP onset
Treatment in a unit where > 10% of gram-negative isolates are resistant to an agent being considered for monotherapy
Treatment in a unit where local antibiotic susceptibility rates are not known
Risk factors for MRSA
Antibiotic therapy in the preceding 90 days
Renal replacement therapy in the preceding 30 days
Use of gastric acid-suppressive agents
Positive culture or prior MRSA colonization, especially in the preceding 90 days
Hospitalization in a unit where > 20% of *S aureus* isolates are MRSA
Hospitalization in a unit where prevalence of MRSA is not known
Risk factors for *Pseudomonas aeruginosa* and other gram-negative bacilli
Antibiotic therapy in the preceding 90 days
Structural lung disease (COPD, especially with recurrent exacerbations; bronchiectasis; or cystic fibrosis)
Recent hospitalizations, especially with manipulation of the aerodigestive tract (Naso enteric nutrition, intubation)
High-quality Gram stain of respiratory secretions with numerous and predominant gram-negative bacilli
Positive culture for *P aeruginosa* in the past year

Data from Kalil AC et al. Management of adults with hospital-acquired and ventilator-associated pneumonia: 2016 Clinical Practice Guidelines by the Infectious Diseases Society of America and the American Thoracic Society. Clin Infect Dis. 2016;63:e61.

3. Anaerobic Pneumonia & Lung Abscess

ESSENTIALS OF DIAGNOSIS

- History of or predisposition to aspiration.
- Indolent symptoms, including fever, weight loss, and malaise.
- Poor dentition.
- Foul-smelling purulent sputum (in many patients).
- Infiltrate in dependent lung zone, with single or multiple areas of cavitation or pleural effusion.

General Considerations

Aspiration of small amounts of oropharyngeal secretions occurs during sleep in normal individuals but rarely causes disease. Sequelae of aspiration of larger amounts of

Table 9–13. Recommended initial empiric antibiotics for hospital-acquired pneumonia (HAP) and ventilator-associated pneumonia (VAP).

HAP not at high risk for mortality, or VAP with no risk factors for MRSA, MDR, or *Pseudomonas* and other gram-negative bacilli

USE **one** of the following:

- Piperacillin-tazobactam, 4.5 g intravenously every 6 hours[1]
- Cefepime, 2 g intravenously every 8 hours[1]
- Levofloxacin, 750 mg intravenously daily
- Imipenem, 500 mg intravenously every 6 hours[1]
- Meropenem, 1 g intravenously every 8 hours[1]

HAP or VAP with risk factors for MRSA but no risk factors for MDR, *Pseudomonas,* and other gram-negative bacilli

USE **one** of the following:

- Piperacillin-tazobactam, 4.5 g intravenously every 6 hours[1]
- Cefepime, 2 g intravenously every 8 hours[1]
- Ceftazidime, 2 g intravenously every 8 hours
- Levofloxacin, 750 mg intravenously daily
- Ciprofloxacin, 400 mg intravenously every 8 hours
- Imipenem, 500 mg intravenously every 6 hours[1]
- Meropenem, 1 g intravenously every 8 hours[1]
- Aztreonam, 2 g intravenously every 8 hours

PLUS **one** of the following:

- Vancomycin, 15 mg/kg intravenously every 8–12 hours with goal to target trough level = 15–20 mg/mL (consider a loading dose of 25–30 mg/kg once for severe illness)[2]
- Linezolid, 600 mg intravenously every 12 hours

HAP with risk factors for *Pseudomonas* and other gram-negative bacilli, but no risk factors for MRSA and not at high risk for mortality

USE **one** of the following:

- Piperacillin-tazobactam, 4.5 g intravenously every 6 hours[1]
- Cefepime, 2 g intravenously every 8 hours[1]
- Ceftazidime, 2 g intravenously every 8 hours
- Imipenem, 500 mg intravenously every 6 hours[1]
- Meropenem, 1 g intravenously every 8 hours[1]
- Aztreonam, 2 g intravenously every 8 hours

PLUS **one** of the following:

- Levofloxacin, 750 mg intravenously daily
- Ciprofloxacin, 400 mg intravenously every 8 hours
- Gentamicin, 5–7 mg/kg intravenously daily[2]
- Tobramycin, 5–7 mg/kg intravenously daily[2]
- Aztreonam, 2 g intravenously every 8 hours

HAP at high risk for mortality or VAP with risk factors for MRSA *and* risk factors for MDR, *Pseudomonas*, and other gram-negative bacilli

USE **one** of the following:

- Piperacillin-tazobactam, 4.5 g intravenously every 6 hours[1]
- Cefepime, 2 g intravenously every 8 hours[1]
- Ceftazidime, 2 g intravenously every 8 hours
- Imipenem, 500 mg intravenously every 6 hours[1]
- Meropenem, 1 g intravenously every 8 hours[1]
- Aztreonam, 2 g intravenously every 8 hours

PLUS **one** of the following:

- Levofloxacin, 750 mg intravenously daily
- Ciprofloxacin, 400 mg intravenously every 8 hours
- Amikacin, 15–20 mg/kg intravenously daily[2]
- Gentamicin, 5–7 mg/kg intravenously daily[2]
- Tobramycin, 5–7 mg/kg intravenously daily[2]
- Meropenem, 1 g intravenously every 8 hours[1]
- Polymyxin B, 2.5–3.0 mg/kg per day divided in 2 daily intravenous doses
- Colistin: consult clinical pharmacist for assistance with dosing

PLUS **one** of the following:

- Vancomycin, 15 mg/kg intravenously every 8–12 hours with goal to target trough level = 15–20 mg/mL (consider a loading dose of 25–30 mg/kg once for severe illness)[2]
- Linezolid, 600 mg intravenously every 12 hours

CrCl, creatinine clearance; MDR, multidrug-resistant; MRSA, methicillin-resistant *Staphylococcus aureus.*

[1]Extended infusions may be appropriate.

[2]Drug level monitoring and adjustment of dosing are required.

Data from Kalil AC et al. Management of adults with hospital-acquired and ventilator-associated pneumonia: 2016 Clinical Practice Guidelines by the Infectious Diseases Society of America and the American Thoracic Society. Clin Infect Dis. 2016;63:e61.

material include nocturnal asthma, chemical pneumonitis, mechanical obstruction of airways by particulate matter, bronchiectasis, and pleuropulmonary infection. Individuals predisposed to disease induced by aspiration include those with depressed levels of consciousness due to drug or alcohol use, seizures, general anesthesia, or CNS disease; those with impaired deglutition due to esophageal disease or neurologic disorders; and those with tracheal or nasogastric tubes, which disrupt the mechanical defenses of the airways.

Periodontal disease and poor dental hygiene, which increase the number of anaerobic bacteria in aspirated material, are associated with a greater likelihood of anaerobic pleuropulmonary infection. Aspiration of infected oropharyngeal contents initially leads to pneumonia in dependent lung zones. The onset of symptoms is insidious. By the time the patient seeks medical attention, necrotizing pneumonia, lung abscess, or empyema may be apparent.

In most cases of aspiration and necrotizing pneumonia, lung abscess, and empyema, multiple species of anaerobic bacteria are causing the infection. Most of the remaining cases are caused by infection with both anaerobic and aerobic bacteria. *Prevotella melaninogenica*, *Peptostreptococcus*, *Fusobacterium nucleatum*, and *Bacteroides* species are commonly isolated anaerobic bacteria. Lung abscess may occur independent of aspiration in syndromes including endovascular disease with septic embolization. In such cases, the organisms reflect those associated with the endovascular infection.

Clinical Findings

A. Symptoms and Signs

Patients with anaerobic pleuropulmonary infection usually present with constitutional symptoms, such as fever, weight loss, and malaise. Cough with expectoration of foul-smelling purulent sputum suggests anaerobic infection, though the absence of productive cough does not rule out such an infection. Dentition is often poor. Patients are rarely edentulous; if so, an obstructing bronchial lesion may be present.

B. Laboratory Findings

Expectorated sputum cultures may be difficult to interpret due to contaminating upper respiratory tract flora, but high colony count of a particular microorganism on Gram stain or in culture likely represents a true pathogen. Anaerobes and facultative anaerobes are difficult to recover on any culture, particularly following initiation of antibiotics; pleural fluid from empyema may be revealing.

C. Imaging

The different types of anaerobic pleuropulmonary infection are distinguished by their radiographic appearance. **Lung abscess** appears as a thick-walled solitary cavity surrounded by consolidation. An air-fluid level is usually present. Other causes of cavitary lung disease (tuberculosis, mycosis, cancer, infarction, necrobiotic nodules in rheumatoid arthritis, and pulmonary vasculitides) should be excluded. **Necrotizing pneumonia** is distinguished by multiple areas of cavitation within an area of consolidation. **Empyema** is characterized by the presence of purulent pleural fluid and may accompany either of the other two radiographic findings. Ultrasonography is of value in locating fluid and may also reveal pleural loculations.

Treatment

Medications of choice are directed at anaerobic organisms or facultative anaerobic streptococci and include a β-lactam/lactamase inhibitor combination, or a carbapenem. Second-line therapy includes a combination of third-generation cephalosporin and metronidazole, or a fluoroquinolone. Duration of antibiotic therapy for anaerobic pneumonia is controversial, but it is usually given for a minimum of 3 weeks, with some experts recommending treatment until the abscess cavity has resolved on imaging.

Peripheral lung abscess must be carefully distinguished from empyema because empyema requires tube thoracostomy; if tube thoracostomy is placed inadvertently into an abscess cavity, complications, such as a bronchopleural fistula, may result. Thoracic surgery consultation is recommended for large or nonresolving abscesses or for abscesses that rupture into the pleural space. Rarely, a large abscess requires surgical intervention (percutaneous drainage, segmentectomy, lobectomy, or pneumonectomy).

Pan D et al. Aspiration pneumonia. Semin Respir Crit Care Med. 2024;45:237. [PMID: 38211629]

PULMONARY INFILTRATES IN IMMUNOCOMPROMISED PATIENTS

Pulmonary infiltrates in immunocompromised patients (patients with HIV disease, absolute neutrophil counts < 1000/mcL [$< 1.0 \times 10^9/L$], current or recent exposure to myelosuppressive or immunosuppressive medications, or those taking > 20 mg/day of prednisone or equivalent for > 4 weeks) may arise from infectious or noninfectious causes. Infection may be due to bacterial, mycobacterial, fungal, protozoal, helminthic, or viral pathogens. Noninfectious processes, such as pulmonary edema, alveolar hemorrhage, medication reactions, pulmonary thromboembolic disease, malignancy, and radiation pneumonitis, may mimic infection.

Although almost any pathogen can cause pneumonia in an immunocompromised patient, two clinical tools help narrow the differential diagnosis. The first is knowledge of the underlying immunologic defect. Specific immunologic defects are associated with particular infections. Defects in humoral immunity predispose to bacterial infections; defects in cellular immunity lead to infections with viruses, fungi, mycobacteria, and protozoa. Neutropenia and impaired granulocyte function predispose to infections from *S aureus*, *Aspergillus*, gram-negative bacilli, and *Candida*. Second, the time course of infection also provides clues to the etiology of pneumonia in immunocompromised patients. A fulminant pneumonia is often caused by bacterial infection, whereas an insidious pneumonia is more apt to be caused by viral, fungal, protozoal, or mycobacterial infection. Pneumonia occurring within 2–4 weeks after organ transplantation is usually bacterial, whereas several months or more after transplantation, *P jirovecii*, viruses (eg, cytomegalovirus), and fungi (eg, *Aspergillus*) are encountered more often.

Clinical Findings

CXR is rarely helpful in narrowing the differential diagnosis. Examination of expectorated sputum for bacteria, fungi, mycobacteria, *Legionella*, and *P jirovecii* is important and may preclude the need for expensive, invasive diagnostic procedures. Sputum induction is often necessary for diagnosis. The sensitivity of induced sputum for detection of *P jirovecii* depends on institutional expertise, number of specimens analyzed, and detection methods.

Routine evaluation frequently fails to identify a causative organism. The clinician may begin empiric antimicrobial therapy before proceeding to invasive procedures, such as bronchoscopy, transthoracic needle aspiration, or open lung biopsy. The approach to management must be based on the severity of the pulmonary infection, the underlying disease, the risks of empiric therapy, and local expertise and experience with diagnostic procedures. BAL using flexible bronchoscopy is a safe and effective method for obtaining pulmonary secretions for microbiologic studies. It involves less risk of bleeding and other complications than transbronchial biopsy. Surgical lung biopsy, now often performed by video-assisted thoracoscopy, provides a definitive option for diagnosis of pulmonary infiltrates in immunocompromised patients; however, a specific diagnosis is obtained in only about two-thirds of cases, and the information obtained may not affect the outcome.

Arora S et al. Pneumonia in immunocompromised patients. Radiographics. 2025;45:e250021. [PMID: 41296608]

Epelbaum O et al. Treatment of invasive pulmonary Aspergillosis and preventive and empirical therapy for invasive Candidiasis in adult pulmonary and critical care patients: an official American Thoracic Society clinical practice guideline. Am J Respir Crit Care Med. 2025;211:34. [PMID: 39556361]

PULMONARY TUBERCULOSIS

ESSENTIALS OF DIAGNOSIS

- Fatigue, weight loss, fever, night sweats, and productive cough.
- Risk factors for acquisition of infection: household exposure, incarceration, drug use, travel to or residence in endemic area.
- CXR: pulmonary opacities, including nodular or cavitating.
- Acid-fast bacilli on smear of sputum, rapid molecular testing positive, or sputum culture positive for *M tuberculosis*.

General Considerations

Tuberculosis is one of the world's most widespread and deadly illnesses. *M tuberculosis*, the organism that causes tuberculosis infection and disease, infects one-quarter of the world's population, nearly 2 billion people. Based on WHO data, there were 10.7 million new cases of tuberculosis worldwide in 2024 and 1.23 million deaths. After having fallen from 2005 to 2019 due to disruption from the COVID-19 pandemic, the incidence increased since 2020 but started to stabilize in 2023. While most incident cases occur in low- and middle-income countries, tuberculosis is present in all regions of the world. Tuberculosis occurs disproportionately among disadvantaged populations, such as people with malnutrition and those living in overcrowded or substandard housing. There is an increased occurrence of tuberculosis among individuals with HIV.

Infection with *M tuberculosis* begins when a susceptible person inhales airborne droplet nuclei containing viable organisms. Tubercle bacilli that reach the alveoli are ingested by alveolar macrophages. Infection follows if the inoculum escapes alveolar macrophage microbicidal activity. Once infection is established, lymphatic and hematogenous dissemination of tuberculosis typically occurs before the development of an effective immune response. This stage of infection is usually clinically and radiographically silent. In most persons with intact cell-mediated immunity, T cells and macrophages surround the organisms in granulomas that limit their multiplication and spread. The infection is contained but not eradicated, since viable organisms may lie dormant within granulomas for years to decades.

Individuals with **tuberculosis infection** that is **latent** do not have active disease and cannot transmit the organism to others. However, reactivation of disease may occur if the patient's immune defenses are impaired. **Tuberculosis disease** (ie, **active tuberculosis, "reactivation disease"**) will develop in 5–15% of individuals with latent tuberculosis infection who are not given preventive therapy; half of these cases occur in the 2 years following primary infection. Diverse conditions such as gastrectomy, silicosis, diabetes mellitus, and an impaired immune response (eg, HIV infection; therapy with corticosteroids, TNF inhibitors, or other immunosuppressive drugs) are associated with an increased risk of reactivation disease.

In approximately 5% of cases, the cell-mediated immune response is inadequate to contain the primary infection, and **progressive primary tuberculosis** develops, accompanied by both pulmonary and constitutional symptoms. The clinical presentation does not definitively distinguish primary disease from reactivation of latent tuberculosis infection. Standard teaching has held that 90% of tuberculosis in adults represents activation of latent disease; however, as many as one-third of new cases in urban populations are primary infections resulting from person-to-person transmission.

The prevalence of drug-resistant strains is increasing worldwide, though in resourced countries including the United States, the rate of multidrug-resistant isolates has fallen to 1%. Incidence rates have decreased in most regions of the world. Risk factors for drug resistance include emigration from regions with a high prevalence of drug-resistant tuberculosis, close and prolonged contact with individuals with drug-resistant tuberculosis, unsuccessful or inappropriate initial therapy, and nonadherence to treatment. Drug resistance may be single or multiple. **Monoresistant tuberculosis** is resistant to one first-line antituberculous drug, either isoniazid (**isoniazid-resistant TB**) or rifampicin (**rifampicin-resistant TB [RR-TB]**). **Multidrug-resistant tuberculosis (MDR-TB)** is resistant to isoniazid and rifampicin. **Pre-extensively drug-resistant tuberculosis (pre-XDR-TB)** is resistant to rifampicin and any fluoroquinolone. **Extensively drug-resistant tuberculosis (XDR-TB)** is resistant to rifampicin, plus any fluoroquinolone, plus either bedaquiline or linezolid. Outcomes of drug-resistant tuberculosis treatment are worse than drug-sensitive tuberculosis organisms, and outcomes appear to vary with HIV status.

Clinical Findings

A. Symptoms and Signs

The patient with pulmonary tuberculosis typically presents with slowly progressive constitutional symptoms of malaise, anorexia, weight loss, fever, and night sweats. Chronic cough is the most common pulmonary symptom. It may be dry at first but typically becomes productive of purulent sputum as the disease progresses. Blood-streaked sputum is common, but significant hemoptysis is rarely a presenting symptom; life-threatening hemoptysis may occur in advanced disease. Dyspnea is unusual unless there is extensive disease. On physical examination, the patient appears chronically ill and malnourished and often has lymphadenopathy. On chest examination, there are no physical findings specific for tuberculosis infection. The examination may be normal or may reveal classic findings such as posttussive apical rales.

B. Laboratory Findings

Definitive diagnosis depends on recovery of *M tuberculosis* from cultures or identification of the organism by DNA or RNA amplification techniques (in concert with appropriate clinical context). At least three consecutive sputum specimens are advised, which should be collected 8 hours apart and include at least one early-morning sample. Acid-fast staining of a sputum smear is performed initially as a screening method, with sensitivity and negative predictive values that are low (50–80%) with a single smear but may improve to 90% with serial sampling. Smear sensitivity is lower in patients coinfected with HIV. Demonstration of acid-fast bacilli on sputum smear does not establish a diagnosis of *M tuberculosis* since nontuberculous mycobacteria may colonize the airways and are increasingly recognized to cause clinical illness in patients with underlying structural lung disease.

The slow rate of mycobacterial growth; the urgency to provide early, appropriate treatment to patients to improve their outcomes and limit community spread; and concerns about potential drug toxicities in patients treated empirically who do not have tuberculosis infection have fostered the use of rapid diagnostic techniques (Table 9–14). Molecular diagnostics offer multiple options and many advantages, though at increased expense. Nucleic acid amplification testing not only detects *M tuberculosis* (NAAT-TB) but also identifies resistance markers (NAAT-R). NAAT-TB can identify *M tuberculosis* within hours of sputum processing, allowing early isolation and treatment, though the negative predictive value is lower in smear-negative patients. In view of the rapidity of results in concert with rifampicin resistance identification, the WHO recommends initial rapid molecular testing for diagnosis and resistance profiling in persons in whom pulmonary or extrapulmonary tuberculosis is suspected.

Table 9–14. Essential laboratory tests for the detection of *Mycobacterium tuberculosis*.

Test	Time to Result	Test Characteristics
Acid-fast bacilli light microscopy	1 day	Three morning specimens recommended. Combined sensitivity of 70% (54% for the first specimen, 11% for the second specimen, and 5% for the third specimen). First morning specimen increased yield by 12% compared with spot specimen.
Nucleic acid amplification test, detection (NAAT-TB)	1 day	Sensitivity/specificity high for smear-positive specimens, 85–97% for both; sensitivity falls in smear-negative specimens to ~75–88%. A positive NAAT in smear-negative patients with intermediate to high (> 30%) pretest probability of *M tuberculosis* infection is helpful while a negative NAAT is not.
Nucleic acid amplification test, resistance markers (NAAT-R)	1–2 days	Multiple assays for rifampicin and isoniazid are available. Specificity uniformly high, > 98%. Sensitivity varies from ~84–96%.
Mycobacterial growth detection Liquid (broth based) medium Solid (agar or egg based) medium	Up to 6–8 weeks Avg 10–14 days Avg 3–4 weeks	Liquid culture methods are more sensitive than solid culture methods (~90% and 76%, respectively) with shorter time to detection but higher contamination with bacterial growth. Specificity exceeds 99% for all methods.
First-line drug susceptibility testing (liquid medium)	1–2 weeks[1]	Gold standard. Should be performed routinely on the initial isolate.

[1]Following detection of mycobacterial growth.

In patients who cannot produce satisfactory specimens or when the smear of the spontaneously expectorated sputum is negative for acid-fast bacilli, sputum induction with 3% hypertonic saline should be performed. Flexible bronchoscopy with bronchial washings has similar diagnostic yield to induced sputum; transbronchial lung biopsies do not increase the diagnostic yield but may lead to earlier diagnosis by identifying tissue granulomas. Post-bronchoscopy expectorated sputum specimens should be collected. Positive blood cultures for *M tuberculosis* are uncommon in patients with normal CD4 cell counts, but the organism may be cultured from blood in up to 50% of patients who are HIV seropositive with tuberculosis whose CD4 cell counts are < 100/mcL (< 0.1×10^9/L); mycobacterial blood and urine cultures should be obtained in such patients.

Tuberculous pleural effusions may be diagnosed on a clinical basis, without confirmatory testing, in patients with active pulmonary tuberculosis in whom there is no suspicion for an alternative cause. If tuberculous effusion is suspected in a patient without confirmed pulmonary tuberculosis, diagnostic thoracentesis is recommended. Pleural fluid cultures are positive for *M tuberculosis* in 23–58% of cases of pleural tuberculosis. Pleural fluid adenosine deaminase > 70 U/L has a 90% sensitivity and specificity for pleural tuberculosis. If thoracentesis is unrevealing, thoracoscopic or ultrasound-guided needle biopsy of the pleura reveals granulomatous inflammation or AFB with 60–90% sensitivity.

C. Imaging

Radiographic abnormalities in pulmonary tuberculosis do not reliably distinguish primary disease from reactivation of latent tuberculosis (Figure 9–3). The chest imaging pattern traditionally associated with primary disease includes small unilateral infiltrates, hilar and paratracheal lymph node enlargement, and segmental atelectasis. Pleural effusion is present in 30–40% of patients, sometimes as the sole radiographic abnormality. Reactivation tuberculosis traditionally has been associated with fibrocavitary apical disease, discrete nodules, and pneumonic infiltrates, usually in the apical or posterior segments of the upper lobes or in the superior segments of the lower lobes. Radiographic evidence of disease in other locations may be present in up to 30% of patients.

Patients with an impaired immune response are more likely to have atypical pattern on CXR—that is, disease that is not cavitary or associated with the upper lobe. In older patients, lower lobe infiltrates with or without pleural effusion are frequently encountered. A "miliary" pattern (diffuse small nodular densities) can be seen with hematologic or lymphatic dissemination of the organism. Immunocompromised patients—particularly those with late-stage HIV infection—often display lower lung zone, diffuse, or miliary infiltrates; pleural effusions; and involvement of hilar and mediastinal lymph nodes.

Resolution of active tuberculosis leaves characteristic radiographic findings. Dense nodules in the pulmonary hila, with or without obvious calcification, upper lobe fibronodular scarring, and bronchiectasis with volume loss are common findings. Ghon (calcified primary focus) and Ranke (calcified primary focus and calcified hilar lymph node) foci are seen in a minority of patients.

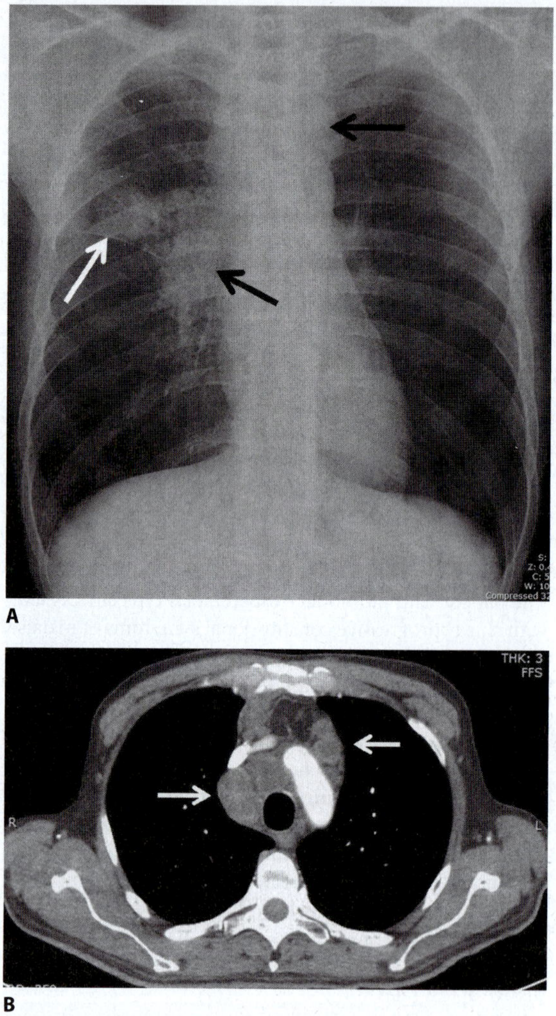

▲ **Figure 9–3.** Pulmonary tuberculosis. Primary pulmonary tuberculosis in a 20-year-old man with CXR **(A)** showing right upper lobe consolidation (white arrow) and right hilar and mediastinal lymphadenopathy (black arrows) and contrast-enhanced CT scan **(B)** showing mediastinal lymphadenopathy (arrows). (Used, with permission, from Carlos Santiago Restrepo, MD, in Usatine RP, Smith MA, Mayeaux EJ Jr, Chumley H. *The Color Atlas of Family Medicine*, 2nd ed. McGraw-Hill, 2013.)

D. Special Examinations

Testing for latent tuberculosis infection is used to evaluate an asymptomatic person in whom *M tuberculosis* infection is suspected (eg, following contact exposure) or to establish the prevalence of tuberculosis infection in a population. Testing may be used in a person with symptoms of active tuberculosis, but a positive test does not distinguish between active and latent infection, and a negative test does not rule out active disease. Routine testing of individuals at low risk for tuberculosis is not recommended. Empiric treatment of latent tuberculosis without testing is considered appropriate in persons with HIV or in young (< 5 years

Table 9–15. Classification of positive tuberculin skin test reactions.[1]

Induration Size	Group
≥ 5 mm	1. Persons with HIV. 2. Close contacts of a person with active tuberculosis disease 3. Persons with fibrotic changes on CXRs suggestive of prior tuberculosis. 4. Patients with organ transplants and other immunosuppressed patients (receiving the equivalent of > 15 mg/day of prednisone for ≥ 1 month, or those taking TNF α antagonists).
≥ 10 mm	1. People born in countries where TB disease is common. 2. Injection drug users without HIV. 3. Mycobacteriology laboratory personnel. 4. Residents of and employees in high-risk congregate settings: correctional institutions; long-term care facilities; hospitals and other health care facilities; residential facilities for patients with HIV/AIDS; and homeless shelters. 5. Persons with medical conditions that increase the risk of progression to tuberculosis disease: gastrectomy, weight loss to ≥ 10% below ideal body weight, jejunoileal bypass, diabetes mellitus, silicosis, advanced CKD, some hematologic disorders (eg, leukemias, lymphomas), and other specific malignancies (eg, carcinoma of the head or neck and lung). 6. Children aged < 5 years; children and adolescents exposed to adults at high risk.
≥ 15 mm	1. Persons with no known risk factors for tuberculosis.

[1]A tuberculin skin test reaction is considered positive if the transverse diameter of the *indurated* area reaches the size required for the specific group. All other reactions are considered negative.
Adapted from https://www.cdc.gov/tb/publications/factsheets/testing/Tuberculin_Skin_Testing_Information for_Health_Care_Providers.pdf

old) household contacts of persons with active tuberculosis in endemic areas.

The traditional approach to testing for latent tuberculosis infection is the **Mantoux tuberculin skin test**. The **transverse width in millimeters of induration** at the skin test site is measured after 48–72 hours. To optimize test performance, criteria for determining a positive reaction vary depending on the likelihood of infection. Table 9–15 summarizes the criteria established by the CDC for test interpretation. Skin test sensitivity and specificity are high: 77% and 97%, respectively. Specificity falls to 59% in populations previously vaccinated with bacillus Calmette-Guérin (BCG, an attenuated form of *M bovis*). False-negative tuberculin skin test reactions may result from improper testing technique; concurrent infections, including fulminant tuberculosis; malnutrition; advanced age; immunologic disorders; malignancy; corticosteroid therapy; CKD; and HIV infection. Some individuals with latent tuberculosis infection may have a negative tuberculin skin test when tested many years after exposure. Anergy testing is not recommended for routine use to distinguish a true-negative result from anergy. Interpretation of the tuberculin skin test in persons who have previously received BCG vaccination is the same as in those who have not had BCG.

Interferon-γ release assays are in vitro assays of CD4+ T-cell–mediated interferon-γ release in response to stimulation by specific *M tuberculosis* antigens. The antigens are absent from all BCG strains and most nontuberculous mycobacteria; therefore, the specificity of interferon-γ release assays is superior to the tuberculin skin test in BCG-vaccinated individuals. Sensitivity is comparable to the tuberculin skin test: 60–90% depending on the specific assay and study population. Sensitivity is reduced by HIV infection, particularly in patients with low CD4 counts. Specificity is > 95%. Potential advantages of interferon-γ release assay testing include fewer false-positive results from prior BCG vaccination, better discrimination of positive responses due to nontuberculous mycobacteria, and the requirement for only one patient contact. Disadvantages include the need for specialized laboratory equipment and personnel and the substantially increased cost compared to the tuberculin skin test. In endemic areas, interferon-γ release assays are no more sensitive than the tuberculin skin test in active tuberculosis (20–40% false-negative rate) and cannot distinguish active from latent disease.

In the diagnosis of latent infections, CDC guidelines allow interferon-γ release assays to be used interchangeably with the tuberculin skin testing. Interferon-γ release assays are preferred in patients with prior BCG vaccination. In individuals with a positive tuberculin skin test but a low prior probability of latent tuberculosis infection and low risk for progression to active disease, the interferon-γ release assay may be helpful as a confirmatory test to exclude a false-positive tuberculin skin test.

Treatment

A. General Measures

The goals of therapy are to cure the individual patient, minimize risk of morbidity and mortality related to treatment, reduce transmission of *M tuberculosis* to other persons, and prevent the emergence of clinically significant drug resistance in tubercle bacilli. The basic principles of antituberculous treatment are (1) to administer multiple medications to which the organisms are susceptible; (2) to provide the safest, most effective therapy for the shortest period of time; (3) to ensure adherence to therapy; and (4) to add at least two new antituberculous agents to a regimen when treatment failure is suspected.

All suspected and confirmed cases of tuberculosis should be reported promptly to local and state public health authorities. Patients with tuberculosis should be treated by clinicians who are skilled in the management of this infection. Clinical expertise is especially important in cases of drug-resistant tuberculosis.

Nonadherence to antituberculous treatment is a major cause of treatment failure, continued transmission of tuberculosis, and development of medication resistance. Adherence to treatment can be improved by providing detailed patient education about tuberculosis and its treatment in addition to a case manager who oversees all aspects of an individual patient's care. **Directly observed therapy (DOT)**, which requires that a health care worker physically observe the patient ingest antituberculous medications in the home, clinic, hospital, or elsewhere, also improves adherence to treatment. The CDC recommends DOT for all patients. Video DOT ("vDOT") and electronic DOT ("eDOT") are promising as more efficient care models in selected populations, and the CDC recommends it as equivalent to traditional DOT.

Hospitalization for initial therapy of tuberculosis is not necessary for most patients. It should be considered if a patient is incapable of self-care or is likely to expose new, susceptible individuals to tuberculosis. Hospitalized patients with active disease require a private room with appropriate environmental controls, including negative-pressure ventilation where available, until tubercle bacilli are no longer found in their sputum ("smear-negative") on three consecutive smears taken on separate days.

More complete information can be obtained from the CDC's website at https://www.cdc.gov/tb/hcp/treatment/ or the WHO tuberculosis website at https://www.who.int/health-topics/tuberculosis/.

B. Treatment of Tuberculosis Disease in Persons Without HIV

Most patients with previously untreated pulmonary tuberculosis can be effectively treated with either a 4-, 6-, or 9-month regimen.

In 2021, a 4-month regimen was added as an appropriate treatment option for many patients with drug-susceptible pulmonary TB. Professional societies now recommend the 4-month regimen in settings with the resources to support appropriate monitoring. The 4-month regimen includes 8 weeks of daily treatment with rifapentine, moxifloxacin, isoniazid, and pyrazinamide, followed by 9 weeks of daily rifapentine, moxifloxacin, and isoniazid.

The initial phase of a 6-month regimen consists of 2 months of daily isoniazid, rifampin, pyrazinamide, and ethambutol. Once the isolate is determined to be sensitive to isoniazid, rifampin, and pyrazinamide, ethambutol may be discontinued. If the *M tuberculosis* isolate is susceptible to isoniazid and rifampin, the second (continuation) phase of therapy consists of isoniazid and rifampin for a minimum of 4 additional months, guided by sputum AFB cultures and initial chest imaging. If no fibrocavitary disease was present on initial imaging and sputum AFB culture is negative at 2 months, the sputum AFB should be repeated at monthly intervals. If two consecutive negative cultures are obtained by 4 months, treatment may be considered completed at 6 months. If fibrocavitary disease is present on initial imaging and sputum culture is negative at 2 months, the same applies, but some experts extend the total duration of therapy to 9 months, as tolerated. If the sputum AFB culture remains positive at month 2 (irrespective of imaging at presentation), it should be repeated at month 3. If negative at month 3 and again at month 4, treatment may be completed after a total of 6 months (some experts extend to 9 months). If sputum AFB remains positive at month 3, susceptibility testing should be repeated, and if sputum AFB remains positive at month 4, this should be considered a treatment failure.

Patients who have contraindications to taking pyrazinamide (eg, pregnant persons; people with severe drug side effects such as hepatotoxicity) should receive daily isoniazid and rifampin along with ethambutol for 2 months. If susceptibility to isoniazid and rifampin is demonstrated or drug resistance is unlikely, ethambutol can be discontinued, and isoniazid and rifampin may be given for a total of 9 months of therapy. If drug resistance is a concern, patients should receive isoniazid, rifampin, and ethambutol for 9 months.

C. Treatment of Tuberculosis Disease in Persons with HIV

Management of tuberculosis is complex in patients with concomitant HIV disease. Experts in the management of both tuberculosis and HIV disease should be involved in the care of such patients. The CDC has published detailed recommendations for the treatment of tuberculosis in patients who test positive for HIV (https://www.cdc.gov/tb/hcp/clinical-care/hiv.html).

The basic approach to patients with HIV who have tuberculosis is similar to that detailed above for patients without HIV. Additional considerations in patients who test positive for HIV include (1) longer duration of therapy; (2) drug interactions between rifamycin derivatives such as rifampin and rifabutin used to treat tuberculosis and some of the protease inhibitors and nonnucleoside reverse transcriptase inhibitors (NNRTIs) used to treat HIV; (3) prevention of immune reconstitution inflammatory syndrome (IRIS) during treatment of patients with CD4 count < 100 or starting antiretroviral therapy. DOT is recommended for all patients with tuberculosis and HIV. Pyridoxine (vitamin B_6) should be given to all patients with HIV being treated with isoniazid to reduce central and peripheral nervous system side effects.

D. Treatment of Drug-Resistant Tuberculosis

Patients with drug-resistant *M tuberculosis* infection require careful supervision and management. Clinicians who are unfamiliar with the treatment of drug-resistant tuberculosis should seek expert advice. Tuberculosis resistant only to isoniazid can be successfully treated with a 6-month regimen of rifampin, pyrazinamide, ethambutol, and a fluoroquinolone or a 9–12-month regimen of rifampin, ethambutol, and a fluoroquinolone (provided susceptible). Tuberculosis resistant only to pyrazinamide can be treated with 9 months of isoniazid and ethambutol.

Rifampin-resistant TB, multidrug-resistant tuberculosis, pre-extensively drug-resistant tuberculosis, and extensively drug-resistant tuberculosis call for an individualized daily DOT plan under the supervision of an experienced clinician. Treatment regimens are based on the patient's overall status and the results of susceptibility studies; some guidelines now recommend a shorter (6 month) treatment regimen as equivalent to a 15-month regimen.

E. Treatment of Extrapulmonary Tuberculosis

In most cases, regimens that are effective for treating pulmonary tuberculosis are also effective for treating extrapulmonary disease. However, many experts recommend 9–12 months of therapy when miliary, meningeal, or bone and joint disease is present. Treatment of skeletal tuberculosis is enhanced by early surgical drainage and debridement of necrotic bone. Corticosteroid therapy has been shown to help prevent constrictive pericarditis from tuberculous pericarditis and to reduce neurologic complications from tuberculous meningitis (Chapter 37).

F. Treatment of Pregnant or Lactating Persons

Tuberculosis in pregnancy is usually treated with isoniazid, rifampin, and ethambutol for 2 months, followed by isoniazid and rifampin for an additional 7 months. Ethambutol can be stopped after the first month if isoniazid and rifampin susceptibility is confirmed. Since the risk of teratogenicity with pyrazinamide has not been clearly defined, pyrazinamide is often excluded from the regimen unless resistance to other drugs is documented. Streptomycin is contraindicated in pregnancy because it may cause congenital deafness. Pregnant persons taking isoniazid should receive pyridoxine to prevent peripheral neuropathy.

Small concentrations of antituberculous drugs are present in breast milk. First-line therapy is not known to be harmful to nursing newborns at these concentrations. Therefore, breastfeeding is not contraindicated while receiving first-line antituberculous therapy. If the regimen includes isoniazid, breastfed infants should receive pyridoxine supplementation. Lactating women receiving other agents should consult a tuberculosis expert.

G. Treatment Monitoring

Monthly follow-up of outpatients is recommended, including sputum smear and culture for *M tuberculosis* at monthly intervals until cultures are negative on two consecutive samples. Patients with negative sputum cultures after 2 months of treatment should have at least one additional sputum smear and culture performed at the end of therapy. Patients with drug-resistant isolates should have sputum cultures performed monthly during the entire course of treatment. A CXR at the end of therapy provides a useful baseline for any future comparison.

Patients whose cultures do not become negative or whose symptoms do not resolve despite 3 months of therapy should be evaluated for nonadherence to the regimen and for drug-resistant organisms. Positive sputum culture after 4 months of therapy should be considered treatment failure, and the addition of at least two drugs not previously given should be considered pending repeat drug susceptibility testing. The clinician should seek expert assistance if drug resistance is newly found, if the patient remains symptomatic, or if smears or cultures remain positive.

Patients with only a clinical diagnosis of pulmonary tuberculosis (smears and cultures negative for *M tuberculosis*) whose symptoms and radiographic abnormalities are unchanged after 3 months of treatment usually either have another process or have had tuberculosis in the past.

H. Treatment of Latent Tuberculosis Infection

Treatment of latent tuberculous infection is essential to controlling and eliminating tuberculosis and substantially reduces the risk that infection will progress to active disease. Targeted testing with the tuberculin skin test or interferon-γ release assay is used to identify persons who are at high risk for tuberculosis and benefit from treatment of latent infection. Table 9–15 gives the tuberculin skin test criteria for treatment of latent tuberculous infection. It is essential that each person who meets the criteria for treatment of latent tuberculous infection undergo a careful assessment to exclude active disease, including chest imaging. A history of past treatment for tuberculosis and contraindications to treatment should be sought. All patients at risk for HIV infection should have an HIV test. Patients suspected of having active tuberculosis disease should receive one of the recommended multidrug regimens for active disease until the diagnosis is confirmed or excluded.

Some close contacts of persons with active tuberculosis should be evaluated for treatment of latent tuberculous infection despite a negative tuberculin skin test reaction (< 5 mm of induration). These include immunosuppressed persons and those in whom disease may develop quickly after tuberculous infection. Close contacts who have a negative tuberculin skin test reaction on initial testing should be retested 10–12 weeks later.

Several treatment regimens for persons with and without HIV are available for the treatment of latent tuberculous infection. (1) **Isoniazid:** a 9-month oral regimen is preferable to 6 months of therapy. Persons at risk for developing isoniazid-associated peripheral neuropathy (those with diabetes mellitus, uremia, malnutrition, alcohol use disorder, HIV infection, pregnancy, or seizure disorder) may be given supplemental pyridoxine. (2) **Isoniazid and rifampin:** a 3-month oral regimen of daily isoniazid 5 mg/kg (maximum 300 mg/day) and rifampin 10 mg/kg (maximum 600 mg/dose). (3) **Isoniazid and rifapentine:** a 3-month oral regimen of once weekly isoniazid at 15 mg/kg (maximum 900 mg/dose) and weight-based rifapentine. (4) **Rifampin:** a 4-month oral regimen of rifampin at 10 mg/kg (maximum 600 mg/day). Of the regimens, WHO strongly recommends isoniazid (6 or 9 months), isoniazid plus rifampin (3 months), or isoniazid plus rifapentine (3 months), with alternative treatments of 4 months of rifampin. In contrast, CDC guidance recommends the three shorter-course rifamycin-containing regimens (options 2, 3 or 4) over isoniazid monotherapy, due to higher rates of completion of the shorter courses, Patients with HIV receiving protease inhibitors or NNRTIs who are given rifampin or rifapentine require management by experts in both tuberculosis and HIV disease (see Treatment of Tuberculosis in Persons with HIV, above).

Contacts of persons with isoniazid monoresistant tuberculosis should receive a 4-month regimen of daily rifampin. Contacts of persons with RR-TB should be treated with daily isoniazid for 9 months. Contacts of persons with MDR-TB that is sensitive to fluoroquinolones should receive 6 months of levofloxacin; however, if the MDR-TB of the contact is resistant to fluoroquinolone, the regimen should include two drugs to which the infecting organism has demonstrated susceptibility. Contacts who are HIV seronegative in whom the tuberculin skin test or interferon-γ release assay is negative may be observed without treatment or treated for 6 months. Contacts with HIV should be treated for 12 months. All contacts of persons with multidrug-resistant tuberculosis or extensively drug-resistant tuberculosis should have 2 years of follow-up regardless of type of treatment.

Persons with a positive tuberculin skin test (≥ 5 mm of induration) and fibrotic lesions suggestive of old tuberculosis on CXRs who have no evidence of active disease and no history of treatment for tuberculosis should receive 9 months of isoniazid or 4 months of rifampin (with or without isoniazid). Pregnant or breastfeeding persons with latent tuberculosis infection should receive either daily or twice-weekly isoniazid with pyridoxine.

Baseline laboratory testing is indicated for patients at risk for liver disease, patients with HIV infection, persons who are pregnant or within 3 months of delivery, and persons who use alcohol regularly. Patients receiving treatment for latent tuberculous infection should be evaluated once a month to assess for symptoms and signs of active tuberculosis and hepatitis and for adherence to their treatment regimen. Routine laboratory testing during treatment is indicated for those with abnormal baseline laboratory tests and for those at risk for developing liver disease.

BCG vaccine is an antimycobacterial vaccine developed from an attenuated strain of *M bovis*. Millions of individuals worldwide have been vaccinated with BCG. Vaccination is recommended in endemic areas (infancy) and regions with high prevalence (childhood), except in individuals with HIV infection or other immunodeficiency. The vaccine is not generally recommended in the United States because of the low prevalence of tuberculous infection, the vaccine's interference with the ability to determine latent tuberculous infection using tuberculin skin test reactivity, and its variable effectiveness in prophylaxis of pulmonary tuberculosis. Vaccination of health care workers should be considered individually in settings where a high percentage of patients with tuberculosis are infected with strains resistant to both isoniazid and rifampin, where transmission of such drug-resistant *M tuberculosis* and subsequent infection are likely, and where comprehensive tuberculous infection-control precautions have been implemented but not successful. The BCG vaccine is contraindicated in persons with impaired immune responses due to disease or medications.

Prognosis

Almost all properly treated immunocompetent patients with tuberculosis can be cured. Relapse rates are < 5% with current regimens. The main cause of treatment failure is nonadherence to therapy.

Clark RA et al. The potential impact of reductions in international donor funding on tuberculosis in low-income and middle-income countries: a modelling study. Lancet Glob Health. 2025;13:e1517. [PMID: 40659023]

Mangan JM et al. Recommendations for use of video directly observed therapy during tuberculosis treatment – United States, 2023. MMWR Morb Mortal Wkly Rep. 2023;72:313. [PMID: 36952279]

Motta I et al. Recent advances in the treatment of tuberculosis. Clin Microbiol Infect. 2024;30:1107. [PMID: 37482332]

Saukkonen JJ et al. Updates on the treatment of drug-susceptible and drug-resistant tuberculosis: an official ATS/CDC/ERS/IDSA clinical practice guideline. Am J Respir Crit Care Med. 2025;211:15. [PMID: 40693952]

Vasiliu A et al. Tuberculosis prevention: current strategies and future directions. Clin Microbiol Infect. 2024;30:1123. [PMID: 37918510]

PULMONARY DISEASE CAUSED BY NONTUBERCULOUS MYCOBACTERIA

ESSENTIALS OF DIAGNOSIS

- Chronic cough, sputum production, and fatigue; less commonly: malaise, dyspnea, fever, hemoptysis, and weight loss.
- Parenchymal opacities on CXR, most often thin-walled cavities or multiple small nodules associated with bronchiectasis.
- Isolation of nontuberculous mycobacteria in a sputum culture.

General Considerations

Nontuberculous mycobacteria (NTM), sometimes referred to as "atypical" mycobacteria—are ubiquitous in water and soil. Marked geographic variability exists, both in NTM species and in the prevalence of disease. These organisms are not considered communicable from person to person, although healthcare-associated transmissions have occurred in vulnerable patient groups (eg, CF). NTM have distinct laboratory characteristics and are often resistant to antituberculous medications (Chapter 37). Long-term epidemiologic data suggest that NTM disease has been increasing worldwide.

Definition & Pathogenesis

The diagnosis of lung disease caused by NTM is based on a combination of clinical, radiographic, and bacteriologic criteria and the exclusion of other diseases that can resemble the condition. Specific diagnostic criteria are discussed below. Complementary data are important for diagnosis because NTM organisms can colonize the airways without causing clinical disease.

Mycobacterium avium complex (MAC) is the most frequent cause of NTM pulmonary disease in the United States and worldwide. *M kansasii* and *M abscessus* are the next most frequent pulmonary pathogens. Other NTM causes of pulmonary disease include *M xenopi*, *M chelonae*, *M. fortuitum*, and *M malmoense* and other less common species. Most NTM cause a chronic pulmonary infection that resembles tuberculosis but tends to progress more slowly. Disseminated disease is rare in immunocompetent persons; however, disseminated MAC disease is common in patients with AIDS.

Clinical Findings

A. Symptoms and Signs

NTM infection among immunocompetent persons frequently presents in one of three prototypical patterns: cavitary, upper lobe lesions in older smokers that may mimic *M tuberculosis*; nodular bronchiectasis affecting the mid-lung zones in middle-aged women with chronic cough; and hypersensitivity pneumonitis following environmental exposure. Most patients with NTM infection experience a chronic cough, sputum production, and fatigue. Less common symptoms include malaise, dyspnea, fever, hemoptysis, and weight loss. Symptoms from coexisting lung disease (COPD, bronchiectasis, previous mycobacterial disease, CF, and pneumoconiosis) may confound the evaluation. In patients with bronchiectasis, coinfection with NTM and *Aspergillus* is a negative prognostic factor. New or worsening infiltrates as well as adenopathy or pleural effusion (or both) are described in patients with HIV and NTM infection as part of the IRIS following institution of antiretroviral therapy.

B. Laboratory Findings

The diagnosis of NTM infection rests on recovery of the pathogen from cultures. Sputum cultures positive for atypical mycobacteria do not prove infection, because NTM may colonize the airways or may be environmental contaminants. Bronchial washings are more sensitive than expectorated sputum samples; however, their specificity for clinical disease is not known.

Bacteriologic criteria have been proposed based on studies of patients with cavitary disease with MAC or *M kansasii*. Microbiologic criteria in immunocompetent persons include the following: positive culture results from at least two separate expectorated sputum samples; or positive culture from at least one bronchial wash or biopsy; or a positive culture from pleural fluid or any other normally sterile site. The diagnosis can also be established by demonstrating NTM cultured from a lung biopsy, bronchial wash, or sputum plus histopathologic changes, such as granulomatous inflammation in a lung biopsy. Microbiologic criteria must be combined with clinical and radiologic criteria. Rapid species identification of some NTM is possible using NAAT or a specialized mass spectrometry.

Diagnostic criteria are less stringent for patients with severe immunosuppression. Patients with HIV may show significant MAC growth on culture of bronchial washings without clinical infection; therefore, patients with HIV being evaluated for MAC infection must be considered individually.

Medication susceptibility testing on cultures of NTM is recommended for the following NTM: (1) *M avium intracellulare* to macrolides only (clarithromycin and azithromycin); (2) *M kansasii* to rifampin; and (3) rapid growers (eg, *M fortuitum, M chelonae, and M abscessus*) to amikacin, doxycycline, imipenem, fluoroquinolones, clarithromycin, cefoxitin, and sulfonamides.

C. Imaging

CXR findings include infiltrates that are progressive or persist for at least 2 months, cavitary lesions, and multiple nodular densities. The cavities are often thin-walled and have less surrounding parenchymal infiltrate than is commonly seen with MTB infections. Evidence of contiguous spread and pleural involvement is often present. HRCT of the chest may show multiple small nodules with or without multifocal bronchiectasis. Progression of pulmonary infiltrates during therapy or lack of radiographic improvement over time are poor prognostic signs and also raise concerns about secondary or alternative pulmonary processes. Clearing of pulmonary infiltrates due to NTM is slow.

Treatment

NTM infection does not mandate treatment in all cases, for two reasons. First, clinical disease may never develop in some patients, particularly asymptomatic patients with few organisms isolated from single specimens. Second, the spectrum of clinical disease severity is very wide; in patients with mild or slowly progressive symptoms, traditional antimicrobial regimens using a combination of agents may lead to drug-induced side effects worse than the disease itself. These features at least partly explain variability of adherence to treatment guidelines in practice.

Specific treatment regimens and responses to therapy vary with the species of NTM. Patients who are HIV seronegative with MAC pulmonary disease usually receive a combination of daily clarithromycin or azithromycin, rifampin or rifabutin, and ethambutol. For patients with severe fibrocavitary disease, streptomycin or amikacin is added for the first 2 months. The optimal duration of treatment is unknown, but therapy should be continued for 12 months after sputum conversion. Medical treatment is initially successful in about two-thirds of cases, but relapses after treatment are common; long-term benefit is demonstrated in about half of all patients. Those who do not respond favorably generally have active but stable disease. Surgical resection is an alternative for the patient with progressive disease that responds poorly to antimicrobials. Disease caused by *M kansasii* responds well to drug therapy. A daily regimen of rifampin, macrolide (alternatively, isoniazid), and ethambutol for at least 18 months with a minimum of 12 months of negative cultures is usually successful. Rapidly growing mycobacteria (*M abscessus*, *M fortuitum*, *M chelonae*) are generally resistant to standard antituberculous therapy.

Treatment recommendations for less common NTM (including *M chelonae*, *M fortuitum*, *M genavense*, *M gordonae*, *M malmoense*, *M simiae*, and *M szulgai*) are based primarily on case reports and case series; expert consultation should be sought to determine need for treatment.

When to Refer

Patients with rapidly growing mycobacteria or uncommon NTM should be referred for expert management.

Conyers L et al. Treatment of non-tuberculous mycobacteria: challenges and prospects. Front Microbiol. 2024;15:1394220. [PMID: 38887711]

Daley CL et al. Treatment of nontuberculous mycobacterial pulmonary disease: official ATS/ERS/ESCMID/IDSA clinical practice guideline. Eur Respir J. 2020;56:2000535. [PMID: 32636299]

Dhasmana D et al. A practical guide to the diagnosis and management of suspected non-tuberculous mycobacterial pulmonary disease (NTM-PD) in the United Kingdom. NPJ Prim Care Respir Med. 2024;34:45. [PMID: 39709516]

PULMONARY NEOPLASMS

See Chapter 43 for discussions of Lung Cancer, Secondary Lung Cancer, and Mesothelioma.

SCREENING FOR LUNG CANCER

Lung cancer remains the leading cause of cancer-related mortality, in large part secondary to advanced stage at diagnosis (Chapter 43). Annual low-dose CT (LDCT) screening is recommended for those at high risk by multiple organizations, including the USPSTF, the American Cancer Society, the American College of Chest Physicians, and the National Comprehensive Cancer Network. High-risk criteria for the USPSTF include age 50–80 years, at least a 20-pack-year smoking history, and either current smoking or quit date within past 15 years. Screening should be stopped once 15 years have elapsed since quitting smoking or if a comorbid condition renders the benefits of screening null. The updated 2023 American Cancer Society guidelines now recommend LDCT screening for adults ≥ 50 years with ≥ 20 pack-years, regardless of years since quitting. Simulation models have found yearly screening using these parameters to be the most efficient in reducing lung cancer-related deaths, though more false-positive test results are expected.

Annual CXRs are not recommended for lung cancer screening in current or former smokers as no mortality benefit has been demonstrated with serial exams in two large RCTs: the Prostate, Lung, Colorectal and Ovarian Randomized Trial (PLCO) and the National Lung Cancer Screening Trial (NLST). The NLST enrolled 53,454 current or former smokers who were randomly assigned to three annual posterior-anterior CXRs or three LDCT scans and monitored for an additional 6.5 years. Compared with CXR, LDCT detected more early-stage lung cancers and fewer advanced-stage lung cancers, indicating that LDCT screening systematically shifted the time of diagnosis to earlier stages, thereby providing more persons the opportunity for effective treatment. Furthermore, the cohort that received three annual LDCT scans had a significant mortality benefit, with reductions in both lung cancer deaths (20.0%) and all-cause mortality (6.7%).

Potential harms of LDCT screening include false-positive findings, overdiagnosis, radiation, and patient anxiety and distress, all of which should be discussed before the patient's referral for screening. Other concerns include **(1) Generalizability to practice:** NLST-participating institutions demonstrated a high level of expertise in imaging interpretation and diagnostic evaluation. Ninety-six percent of findings on CT were false-positives, but most patients were monitored with serial imaging. Invasive diagnostic evaluations were uncommon and were associated with a low complication rate (1.4%). **(2) Duration of screening:** The rate of detection of new lung cancers did not fall with subsequent annual screening over the 3-year trial. Since new lung cancers become detectable during each year-long screening interval, the optimal number of annual CT scans is unknown as is the optimal screening interval. **(3) Overdiagnosis:** After 6.4 years of post-screening observation, there were more lung cancers in the NLST CT cohort than the CXR cohort (1089 and 969, respectively). Since the groups were randomized and well matched, lung cancer incidence should have been identical. Therefore, 18.5% of the lung cancers detected by CT remained clinically silent and invisible on CXR for 6.4 years. Many, perhaps most, of these lung cancers would never cause clinical disease and represent overdiagnosis. **(4) Cost effectiveness:** Studies in the United States, Canada, and Europe suggest screening for lung cancer is cost effective; however, whether it is cost effective in all countries has not been determined. All patients participating in a screening program who still smoke should receive smoking cessation interventions.

Adams SJ et al. Lung cancer screening. Lancet. 2023;401:390. [PMID: 36563698]

Leiter A et al. The global burden of lung cancer: current status and future trends. Nat Rev Clin Oncol. 2023;20:624. [PMID: 37479810]

Wood DE et al. NCCN Guidelines® Insights: Lung cancer screening, Version 1.2024. J Natl Compr Canc Netw. 2024;22:500. [PMID: 38865774]

SOLITARY PULMONARY NODULE

A solitary pulmonary nodule, sometimes referred to as a "coin lesion," is a less-than-3-cm isolated, rounded opacity on chest imaging outlined by normal lung. Pulmonary nodules may be solid or subsolid with ground glass or mixed consistency. Most are asymptomatic and represent an incidental finding on CXR or CT scanning. Solitary nodules may be benign or malignant; the risk of malignancy varies depending on the patient population under study. Most benign nodules are infectious granulomas. Benign neoplasms, such as hamartomas, account for < 5% of solitary nodules. The probability of cancer in pulmonary nodules detected by LDCT is estimated at 1% of nodules. Malignant nodules are rare in persons under age 30. Above age 30, the likelihood of malignancy increases with age and smoking history. Patients with a prior malignancy have a higher likelihood of having a malignant solitary nodule.

The goals of evaluation are to identify and resect malignant tumors in patients who will benefit from resection while avoiding invasive procedures in benign disease. The task is to identify nodules with a sufficiently high probability of malignancy to warrant biopsy or resection or a sufficiently low probability of malignancy to justify observation. Clinical and imaging data can be used to assess the probability of malignancy. Comparison of prior and current imaging studies allows estimation of doubling time, which is an important marker for malignancy. Rapid progression (doubling time < 30 days) suggests infection, while long-term stability (doubling time > 465 days) suggests benignity. Radiographic features including size help in estimating the probability of malignancy. Chest CT is indicated for any suspicious solitary pulmonary nodule. Solitary nodules identified by CT scan showed a 1% malignancy rate in those measuring 2–5 mm, 24% in 6–10 mm, 33% in 11–20 mm, and 80% in 21–45 mm nodules. The appearance of a smooth, well-defined edge is characteristic of a benign process. Ill-defined margins or a lobular appearance suggest malignancy. A HRCT finding of spiculated margins and a peripheral halo are both highly associated with malignancy. Calcification and its pattern are also helpful clues. Benign lesions tend to have dense calcification in a central or laminated pattern. Malignant lesions are associated with sparser calcification that is typically stippled or eccentric. Cavitary lesions with thick (> 16 mm) walls are more likely to be malignant. HRCT offers better resolution of these characteristics than CXR and is more likely to detect lymphadenopathy or the presence of multiple lesions.

Treatment

Based on clinical and radiologic data, the clinician should assign a specific probability of malignancy to the lesion. The decision whether to recommend a biopsy or surgical excision depends on the probability of cancer, biopsy and surgical risk, and patient wishes and adherence to follow-up. Quantitative prediction models (Brock model, VA Cooperative model) are available to assess risk of malignancy. The probabilities in parentheses below represent guidelines only and should not be interpreted as definitive.

In the United States, follow-up of pulmonary nodules may be guided by either the Fleischner Society recommendations or Lung-RADS, depending on the clinical context. Incidental solitary pulmonary nodules are managed according to the Fleischner Society guidelines, which individualize surveillance based on nodule size, morphology, and patient risk factors. In contrast, nodules detected on low-dose CT as part of lung cancer screening are assessed using Lung-RADS, a structured risk-stratification system that assigns malignancy probability and specifies corresponding follow-up intervals and management pathways within the screening setting. The 2022–2023 Lung-RADS updates further refined criteria for subsolid nodules and introduced category modifiers to reduce unnecessary follow-up while maintaining cancer detection sensitivity.

In the case of solitary pulmonary nodules, a continuous probability function may be grouped into three categories. In patients with a **low probability (< 5%) of malignancy** (eg, age under 30, lesions stable for > 2 years, characteristic pattern of benign calcification), watchful waiting is appropriate. Management consists of serial imaging studies at intervals that could identify growth suggestive of malignancy. Three-dimensional reconstruction of HRCT images provides a more sensitive test for growth.

Patients with a **high probability (> 60%) of malignancy** should proceed directly to resection following staging, provided the surgical risk is acceptable. Biopsies rarely yield a specific benign diagnosis and are not indicated.

Optimal management of patients with an **intermediate probability of malignancy (5–60%)** remains controversial. The traditional approach is to obtain a diagnostic biopsy, either through bronchoscopy or transthoracic needle aspiration (TTNA). Bronchoscopy yields a diagnosis in 10–80% of procedures depending on the size of the nodule and its location. In general, the bronchoscopic yield for nodules that are < 2 cm and peripheral is low, although complications are generally rare. Robotic-assisted bronchoscopy has significantly improved access to peripheral lung lesions, with pooled diagnostic yields of ~77–88%, low complication rates, and enhanced success in assessment of nodules < 2 cm. TTNA has a diagnostic yield between 50% and 97%. The yield is strongly operator-dependent, however, and is affected by the location and size of the lesion. Complications are higher than bronchoscopy, with pneumothorax occurring in up to 30% of patients, possibly requiring chest tube placement.

Disappointing diagnostic yields and a high false-negative rate (up to 20–30% in TTNA) have prompted alternative approaches. Recent meta-analyses (2023–2024) confirm pooled PET-CT sensitivity of 89–92% and specificity 71–77% for solid nodules, though accuracy is significantly lower in subsolid nodules. A positive PET increases the likelihood of malignancy, and a negative PET excludes most cancers. False-negative PET scans can occur with tumors with low metabolic activity (most notably, carcinoid tumors and adenocarcinomas, particularly minimally invasive or in situ adenocarcinomas), so follow-up CT imaging is typically performed at discrete intervals to ensure absence of growth. PET has several other drawbacks: resolution below 1 cm is poor, the test is expensive, and availability remains limited.

Sputum cytology is highly specific but lacks sensitivity. It is used in central lesions and in patients who are poor candidates for invasive diagnostic procedures.

Some centers recommend **video-assisted thoracoscopic surgery (VATS)** resection of all solitary pulmonary nodules with intermediate probability of malignancy. In some cases, the surgeon will remove the nodule and evaluate it in the operating room with frozen section. If the nodule is malignant, he or she will proceed to lobectomy and lymph node sampling, either thoracoscopically or through conversion to standard thoracotomy. This approach is less common when preoperative PET scanning is available.

All patients should be provided with an estimate of the likelihood of malignancy and their preferences used to guide diagnostic and therapeutic decisions. A strategy that recommends observation may not be preferred by a patient who desires a definitive diagnosis. Similarly, a surgical approach may not be agreeable to all patients unless the presence of cancer is definitive. Patient preferences should be elicited, and patients should be well informed regarding the specific risks and benefits associated with the recommended approach as well as the alternative strategies.

Zhong D et al. Lung nodule management in low-dose CT screening for lung cancer: lessons from the NELSON trial. Radiology. 2024;313:e240535. [PMID: 39436294]

RIGHT MIDDLE LOBE SYNDROME

Right middle lobe syndrome is recurrent or persistent atelectasis of the right middle lobe. This collapse is related to the relatively long length and narrow diameter of the right middle lobe bronchus and the oval ("fish mouth") opening to the lobe, in the setting of impaired collateral ventilation. Fiberoptic bronchoscopy or CT scan is often necessary to rule out obstructing tumor. Foreign body or other benign causes are common.

BRONCHIAL CARCINOID TUMORS

Bronchial carcinoid tumors are malignant low- and intermediate-grade neuroendocrine tumors of the lung, with a favorable prognosis compared to high-grade neuroendocrine tumors such as small-cell lung cancer. Bronchial carcinoids typically occur as pedunculated or sessile growths in central bronchi. Common symptoms are hemoptysis, cough, focal wheezing, and recurrent postobstructive pneumonia. Peripherally located tumors are rare and present as asymptomatic solitary pulmonary nodules. **Carcinoid syndrome** (flushing, diarrhea, wheezing, hypotension) and paraneoplastic Cushing syndrome are rare. Fiberoptic bronchoscopy may reveal a pink or purple tumor in a central airway. These lesions have a well-vascularized stroma, and biopsy may be complicated by significant bleeding. CT scanning is helpful to localize the lesion and to follow its growth over time. Somatostatin receptor imaging with 68Ga-DOTATATE PET/CT has largely replaced traditional octreotide scintigraphy because of superior sensitivity for detecting primary tumors and metastatic disease.

Bronchial carcinoid tumors grow slowly; the aggressiveness is determined by the cell histology, with "typical carcinoid," a low-grade tumor, demonstrating a more indolent and favorable course than "atypical carcinoid," an intermediate-grade tumor. Bronchial carcinoid tumor staging follows the same TNM classification as other lung cancers. Surgical excision, including lymph node dissection and resection, is recommended for localized disease, and the prognosis is generally favorable. Most bronchial carcinoid tumors respond poorly to radiation and chemotherapy (see Chapter 43).

Adenomas, carcinomas, and other malignancies may rarely metastasize to the bronchi and present with endobronchial lesions. Hamartomas, myxomas, and amyloid are other rarer entities in the differential diagnosis of endobronchial mass lesions.

Callister ME et al. British Thoracic Society statement on the investigation and management of pulmonary nodules: 2023 update. Thorax. 2023;78:1210. [PMID: 37567053]

Fielding DIK et al. Robotic-assisted bronchoscopy for pulmonary lesions: an updated meta-analysis. Chest. 2024;165:1123. [PMID: 38241522]

Koehler K et al. Carcinoid tumors outside the abdomen. Cancer Med. 2023;12:7893. [PMID: 36560885]

McKee BJ et al. Lung-RADS 2022–2023 updates: impact on screening outcomes and nodule management. J Thorac Oncol. 2024;19:1023. [PMID: 38124577]

Nadig TR et al. Guided bronchoscopy for the evaluation of pulmonary lesions: an updated meta-analysis. Chest. 2023;163:1589. [PMID: 36640994]

Zhong D et al. Lung nodule management in low-dose CT screening for lung cancer: lessons from the NELSON trial. Radiology. 2024;313:e240535. [PMID: 39436294]

MEDIASTINAL MASSES

Various developmental, neoplastic, infectious, traumatic, and cardiovascular disorders may cause mediastinal masses. A useful convention arbitrarily divides the mediastinum into three compartments—anterior, middle, and posterior—in order to classify mediastinal masses and assist in differential diagnosis based on contents of these anatomic regions. The anterior compartment is bounded by the sternum anteriorly and the surface of the great vessels and pericardium posteriorly. The middle compartment extends from the anterior pericardium to the anterior surface of the thoracic spine. The posterior compartment is paravertebral. Specific mediastinal masses have a predilection for one or more of these compartments; most are located in the anterior or middle compartment.

The differential diagnosis of an **anterior mediastinal mass** includes tumors of the thymus, including thymoma and thymic carcinoma; teratoma; thyroid lesions; lymphoma; and mesenchymal tumors (lipoma, fibroma). The differential diagnosis of a **middle mediastinal mass** includes lymphadenopathy, pulmonary artery enlargement, aneurysm of the aorta or innominate artery, developmental cyst (bronchogenic, enteric, pleuropericardial), dilated azygous or hemiazygous vein, and foramen of Morgagni hernia. The differential diagnosis of a **posterior mediastinal mass** includes hiatal hernia, neurogenic tumor, meningocele, esophageal tumor, foramen of Bochdalek hernia, thoracic spine disease, and extramedullary hematopoiesis. The neurogenic tumor group includes neurilemmoma, neurofibroma, neurosarcoma, ganglioneuroma, and pheochromocytoma.

Symptoms and signs of mediastinal masses are nonspecific and are usually caused by the effects of the mass on surrounding structures. An insidious onset of retrosternal chest pain, dysphagia, or dyspnea is often an important clue to the presence of a mediastinal mass. In about half of cases, symptoms are absent, and the mass is detected on routine CXR. Physical findings vary depending on the nature and location of the mass.

CT scanning is helpful in management; additional radiographic studies of benefit include upper endoscopy if esophageal disease is suspected, Doppler sonography or venography of brachiocephalic veins and the superior vena cava, and angiography. MRI provides better delineation of cystic versus solid lesions, spinal canal involvement, neurogenic tumors, and vascular relationships and is increasingly used to complement CT in indeterminate cases. Tissue diagnosis via either needle or excisional biopsy is generally necessary when a neoplastic process is considered. Treatment and prognosis depend on the underlying cause of the mediastinal mass.

Ahuja J et al. Approach to imaging of mediastinal masses. Diagnostics (Basel). 2023;13:3171. [PMID: 37891992]
Taka M et al. Diagnostic approach for mediastinal masses with radiopathological correlation. Eur J Radiol. 2023;162:110767. [PMID: 36921376]

INTERSTITIAL LUNG DISEASE (Diffuse Parenchymal Lung Disease)

ESSENTIALS OF DIAGNOSIS

- Insidious onset of progressive dyspnea and nonproductive chronic cough.
- Tachypnea, bibasilar dry rales; digital clubbing and right HF with advanced disease.
- Lung CT scan with patchy distribution of ground glass, reticular, nodular, reticulonodular, or cystic opacities.
- PFTs with restrictive pattern with reduced lung volumes and diffusing capacity.
- Hypoxemia with exercise.

General Considerations

Interstitial lung disease (ILD) comprises a heterogeneous group of disorders that share common presentations (dyspnea), physical findings (late inspiratory crackles), and CXR findings (septal thickening and reticulonodular changes). Table 9–16 provides the extensive differential diagnosis of ILD, which includes disorders of known causes (eg, medications, environmental, infection, systemic disorders) and unknown causes (eg, idiopathic interstitial pneumonias).

Clinical Findings

The history, including associated comorbidities (including connective tissue disease), occupational exposures

Table 9–16. Differential diagnosis of interstitial lung disease (listed alphabetically within category).

Medication-related
Antiarrhythmic agents (amiodarone)
Antibacterial agents (nitrofurantoin, sulfonamides)
Antineoplastic agents (bleomycin, cyclophosphamide, methotrexate, nitrosoureas)
Antirheumatic agents (gold salts, penicillamine)
Phenytoin
Environmental and occupational (inhalation exposures)
Dust, inorganic (asbestos, beryllium, hard metals, silica)
Dust, organic (thermophilic actinomycetes, avian antigens, *Aspergillus* species)
Gases, fumes, and vapors (chlorine, isocyanates, paraquat, sulfur dioxide)
Ionizing radiation
Talc (injection drug users)
Infections
Fungus, disseminated (*Blastomyces dermatitidis, Coccidioides immitis, Histoplasma capsulatum*)
Mycobacteria, disseminated
Pneumocystis jirovecii
Viruses
Primary pulmonary disorders
Cryptogenic organizing pneumonia
Idiopathic interstitial pneumonia: acute interstitial pneumonia, desquamative interstitial pneumonia, nonspecific interstitial pneumonia, usual interstitial pneumonia, respiratory bronchiolitis–associated interstitial lung disease
Pulmonary alveolar proteinosis
Systemic disorders
Acute respiratory distress syndrome
Amyloidosis
Ankylosing spondylitis
Autoimmune disease: dermatomyositis, polymyositis, rheumatoid arthritis, SLE, systemic sclerosis (scleroderma)
Chronic eosinophilic pneumonia
Goodpasture syndrome
Granulomatosis polyangiitis
IBD
Idiopathic pulmonary hemosiderosis
Langerhans cell histiocytosis (eosinophilic granuloma)
Lymphangioleiomyomatosis
Lymphangitic spread of cancer (lymphangitic carcinomatosis)
Pulmonary edema
Pulmonary venous hypertension, chronic
Sarcoidosis

(smoking, radiation), and medications (amiodarone, nitrofurantoin, gold, among others), may provide evidence of a specific cause. Laboratory evaluation includes renal and liver function, CBC with differential to evaluate for anemia or eosinophilia, UA, creatine kinase for myositis, and serology for connective tissue diseases. Imaging commonly includes a HRCT, which may show reticular or linear opacities, airspace opacities, ground-glass opacities, honeycombing, or cysts. Typical PFTs show a restrictive defect, with decreased FVC and TLC.

Bronchoscopy with BAL may be indicated to diagnose (or rule out) cases of infection, particularly with *P jirovecii* or mycobacteria, or malignancy. BAL may be diagnostic of eosinophilic pneumonia, Langerhans cell histiocytosis, or alveolar proteinosis. Lung biopsy (by flexible bronchoscopy, VATS or thoracotomy) may be considered in those with atypical radiographic features. Transbronchial biopsy through the flexible bronchoscope can make a definitive diagnosis of sarcoidosis, lymphangitic spread of carcinoma, pulmonary alveolar proteinosis, miliary tuberculosis, and Langerhans cell histiocytosis. Surgical lung biopsy is the standard for diagnosis of diffuse ILD. Patients under age 60 without a specific diagnosis based on clinical and radiographic features should undergo surgical lung biopsy. In older and sicker patients, the risks and benefits must be weighed carefully, as (1) the morbidity of the procedure can be significant; (2) a definitive diagnosis may not be possible even with surgical lung biopsy; and (3) when a specific diagnosis is made, there may be no effective treatment. Empiric therapy or no treatment may be preferable to surgical lung biopsy in some patients.

Treatment

Treatment by a pulmonologist is recommended for ILD. Treatment varies depending on the cause. If associated with environmental or drug exposure, avoidance is advised. Oxygen supplementation in is provided to those with hypoxemia. Pulmonary rehabilitation is recommended to improve exercise capacity. Vaccination against respiratory infections is recommended.

For those with progressive pulmonary fibrosis (defined by worsening symptoms, lung function on PFTs, and radiographic fibrosis), a trial of high-dose corticosteroids utilized for acute exacerbations, followed by a taper. Consideration of anti-fibrotic therapy and lung transplant referral is discussed in the next section.

IDIOPATHIC INTERSTITIAL PNEUMONIA

ESSENTIALS OF DIAGNOSIS

- May be associated with connective tissue diseases or be idiopathic.
- Diagnosis commonly is made by HRCT scan with characteristic features or less commonly by lung biopsy.
- Accurate diagnosis identifies patients most likely to benefit from therapy.

General Considerations

Idiopathic interstitial pneumonias (IIP) is one of the categories of interstitial pneumonias. IIP may be further categorized by histopathology and radiographic criteria (Table 9–17). Only a small number of patients undergo surgical lung biopsy for diagnosis. Accurate diagnosis dictates treatment and prognosis.

Clinical Findings

The most common of the IIP is pulmonary fibrosis associated with the histopathologic pattern of **usual interstitial pneumonia (UIP).** Serologic studies should be obtained to rule out rheumatologic diseases associated with UIP, including ANA, RF, CCP, and, in selected cases, Jo1, SSA, SSB, dsDNA, and Scl70. When no associated cause is evident, it is classified as **idiopathic pulmonary fibrosis (IPF).** A diagnosis of IPF can be made in patients who have (1) idiopathic disease by history and inspiratory crackles on physical examination, (2) restrictive physiology on PFTs, and (3) characteristic UIP pattern on high-resolution chest CT (subpleural/peripheral, basilar reticular opacities associated with honeycombing and traction bronchiectasis) (Figure 9–4). Such patients do not need surgical lung biopsy. Assessment of pulmonary hypertension is recommended in advanced disease.

Treatment

There is no known cure for IPF. Long-term use of corticosteroid therapy is ineffective and not recommended. Nintedanib and pirfenidone are approved for the treatment of IPF based on reduction in rate of decline in lung function and longer time to first exacerbation, but neither agent improves survival. Nerandomilast, a phosphodiesterase 4B with antifibrotic and immunomodulatory properties, has recently been shown to slow the progression of IPF and has been approved by FDA. Early lung transplant evaluation should be considered. Supportive care is recommended with supplemental oxygen and pulmonary rehabilitation. Surveillance for pulmonary hypertension is advised.

When to Refer

- Patients with IIP should be referred early to a pulmonologist for expert diagnosis and management.
- Patients with IPF should be referred early to a lung transplant program for evaluation.

Maher TM. Interstitial lung disease: a review. JAMA. 2024;331:1655. [PMID: 38648021]

Newton CA et al. Performance characteristics for physiological measures of progressive pulmonary fibrosis. Am J Respir Crit Care Med. 2025;211:1867. [PMID: 40530983]

Raghu G et al. Idiopathic pulmonary fibrosis (an update) and progressive pulmonary fibrosis in adults: an official ATS/ERS/JRS/ALAT clinical practice guideline. Am J Respir Crit Care Med. 2022;205:e18. [PMID: 35486072]

Richeldi L et al. Nerandomilast in patients with idiopathic pulmonary fibrosis. N Engl J Med. 2025;392:2193. [PMID: 40387033]

Table 9–17. Idiopathic interstitial pneumonias.

Name and Clinical Presentation	Histopathology	Radiographic Pattern	Response to Therapy and Prognosis
Usual interstitial pneumonia (UIP) Age 55–60, slight male predominance. Insidious dry cough and dyspnea lasting months to years. Clubbing present at diagnosis in 25–50%. Diffuse fine late inspiratory crackles on lung auscultation. Restrictive ventilatory defect and reduced diffusing capacity on PFTs. ANA and RF positive in ~25% in the absence of documented collagen-vascular disease.	Patchy, temporally and geographically nonuniform distribution of fibrosis, honeycomb change, and normal lung. Type I pneumocytes are lost, and there is proliferation of alveolar type II cells. "Fibroblast foci" of actively proliferating fibroblasts and myofibroblasts. Inflammation is generally mild and consists of small lymphocytes. Intra-alveolar macrophage accumulation is present but is not a prominent feature.	Diminished lung volume. HRCT scanning shows increased linear or reticular bibasilar and subpleural opacities, with associated honeycombing. Unilateral disease is rare. Minimal ground-glass. Areas of normal lung may be adjacent to areas of advanced fibrosis.	No randomized study has demonstrated improved survival compared with untreated patients. Inexorably progressive. Median survival ~3 years, depending on stage at presentation. Nintedanib and pirfenidone reduce rate of decline in lung function. Refer early for lung transplantation evaluation.
Respiratory bronchiolitis–associated interstitial lung disease (RB-ILD)[1] Age 40–45. Presentation like that of UIP though in younger patients. Similar results on PFTs, but less severe abnormalities. Patients with respiratory bronchiolitis are invariably heavy smokers.	Increased numbers of macrophages evenly dispersed within the alveolar spaces. Rare fibroblast foci, little fibrosis, minimal honeycomb change. In RB-ILD the accumulation of macrophages is localized within the peribronchiolar air spaces; in DIP[1], it is diffuse. Alveolar architecture is preserved.	HRCT shows nodular or reticulonodular pattern, more likely to reveal diffuse ground-glass opacities. Honeycombing is rare. May also show upper lobe emphysema.	Spontaneous remission occurs in up to 20% of patients, so natural history unclear. Smoking cessation is essential. Prognosis clearly better than that of UIP: median survival > 10 years. Corticosteroids thought to be effective, but there are no randomized clinical trials to support this view.
Acute interstitial pneumonia (AIP) Clinically known as Hamman-Rich syndrome. Wide age range, many young patients. Acute onset of dyspnea followed by rapid development of respiratory failure. Half of patients report a viral syndrome preceding lung disease. Clinical course indistinguishable from that of idiopathic ARDS.	Pathologic changes reflect acute response to injury within days to weeks. Resembles organizing phase of diffuse alveolar damage. Fibrosis and minimal collagen deposition. May appear like UIP but more homogeneous and there is no honeycomb change—though this may appear if the process persists for > 1 month in a patient on mechanical ventilation.	Diffuse bilateral airspace consolidation with areas of ground-glass attenuation on HRCT scan.	Supportive care (mechanical ventilation) critical but effect of specific therapies unclear. High initial mortality: 50–90% die within 2 months after diagnosis. Not progressive if patient survives. Lung function may return to normal or may be permanently impaired.
Nonspecific interstitial pneumonia (NSIP) Age 45–55. Slight female predominance. Like UIP but onset of cough and dyspnea over months, not years.	Nonspecific in that histopathology does not fit into better-established categories. Varying degrees of inflammation and fibrosis, patchy in distribution but uniform in time, suggesting response to single injury. Most have lymphocytic and plasma cell inflammation without fibrosis. Honeycombing present but scant. Some have advocated division into cellular and fibrotic subtypes.	May be indistinguishable from UIP. Most typical picture is bilateral areas of ground-glass attenuation and fibrosis on HRCT. Honeycombing is rare.	Treatment with corticosteroids thought to be effective, but no prospective clinical studies have been published. Overall prognosis good but depends on the extent of fibrosis at diagnosis. Median survival > 10 years.
Cryptogenic organizing pneumonia (COP) Typically age 50–60 but wide variation. Abrupt onset, frequently weeks to a few months following a flu-like illness. Dyspnea and dry cough prominent, but constitutional symptoms are common: fatigue, fever, and weight loss. PFTs usually show restriction, but up to 25% show concomitant obstruction.	Included in the idiopathic interstitial pneumonias on clinical grounds. Buds of loose connective tissue (Masson bodies) and inflammatory cells fill alveoli and distal bronchioles.	Lung volumes normal. CXR typically shows interstitial and parenchymal disease with discrete, peripheral alveolar and ground-glass infiltrates. Nodular opacities common. HRCT shows subpleural consolidation and bronchial wall thickening and dilation.	Rapid response to corticosteroids in two-thirds of patients. Long-term prognosis generally good for those who respond. Relapses are common.

[1]Includes desquamative interstitial pneumonia.
ARDS, acute respiratory distress syndrome; RF, rheumatoid factor.

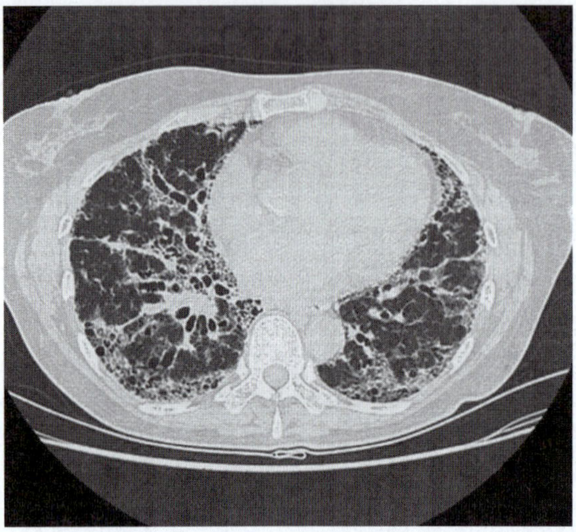

▲ **Figure 9–4.** Idiopathic pulmonary fibrosis. CT scan of the lungs showing the typical radiographic pattern of idiopathic pulmonary fibrosis, with a predominantly basilar, peripheral pattern of traction bronchiectasis, reticulation, and early honeycombing.

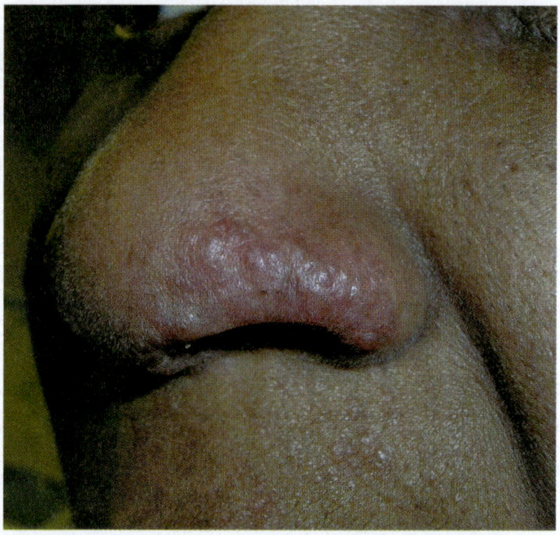

▲ **Figure 9–5.** Skin involvement in sarcoidosis (lupus pernio), here involving the nasal rim. (Reproduced, with permission, from Richard P. Usatine, MD, in Usatine RP, Smith MA, Mayeaux EJ Jr, Chumley HS. *The Color Atlas and Synopsis of Family Medicine*, 3rd ed. McGraw-Hill, 2019.)

SARCOIDOSIS

ESSENTIALS OF DIAGNOSIS

- Symptoms may involve the lung, skin, eyes, peripheral nerves, liver, kidney, heart.
- Diagnosis made by demonstration of noncaseating granulomas in a biopsy specimen.

General Considerations

Sarcoidosis is a systemic disease of unknown etiology characterized by granulomatous inflammation, primarily in the lungs. The incidence is highest in North American Black persons and northern European White persons. Among Black persons, women are more frequently affected than men. Onset of disease is usually in the third or fourth decade.

Clinical Findings

A. Symptoms and Signs

Patients may be asymptomatic. Dyspnea, cough, fatigue or chest pain are the most common symptoms. Lung or thoracic lymph node involvement occurs in > 90% of patients. Other systemic involvement include skin (erythema nodosum, lupus pernio [Figure 9–5]), iritis, peripheral neuropathy, arthritis (Chapter 23), cardiomyopathy or pulmonary hypertension. Physical findings of ILD with crackles are uncommon. Other findings may include parotid gland enlargement, hepatosplenomegaly, and lymphadenopathy. *Löfgren syndrome* involves sarcoidosis with acute fever onset, hilar adenopathy, erythema nodosum, and/or ankle arthritis.

B. Laboratory Findings

Laboratory tests are nonspecific and may show an elevated ESR, hypercalcemia (5%), or hypercalciuria (20%). ACE levels are elevated in 40–80% of patients with active disease, though this finding is neither sensitive nor specific. Physiologic testing may reveal evidence of airflow obstruction or restriction with decreased lung volumes and diffusing capacity, or both. ECG may show heart block and dysrhythmias.

C. Imaging

Radiographic findings are variable and include bilateral hilar adenopathy alone (radiographic stage I), hilar adenopathy and parenchymal involvement (radiographic stage II), parenchymal involvement alone (radiographic stage III), or advanced fibrotic changes principally in the upper lobes (radiographic stage IV). Parenchymal involvement is usually manifested radiographically by diffuse reticular infiltrates, but focal infiltrates, acinar shadows, nodules, and, rarely, cavitation may be seen. Echocardiogram may show signs of cardiomyopathy with HF or pulmonary hypertension.

D. Special Examinations

The diagnosis of sarcoidosis generally requires histologic demonstration of noncaseating granulomas in biopsies from a patient with other typical associated manifestations. Other granulomatous diseases (eg, berylliosis, tuberculosis), fungal infections, HIV, and lymphoma must be excluded. Biopsy of easily accessible sites (eg, palpable lymph nodes, skin lesions, or salivary glands) may be an initial step. Transbronchial lung biopsy has a high yield (75–90%) as well, especially in patients with radiographic evidence of parenchymal involvement. Some clinicians believe that tissue biopsy is not necessary when stage I radiographic findings are detected in a clinical situation that strongly favors the diagnosis of sarcoidosis. Biopsy is essential whenever clinical and radiographic findings suggest the possibility of an alternative diagnosis, such as lymphoma.

Patients require a yearly ophthalmologic evaluation, liver and renal function testing, PFTs, and an ECG. Cardiac MRI is favored over PET scan for patients with suspected cardiac involvement. Screening for pulmonary hypertension with echocardiogram is recommended in advanced disease.

Treatment

Oral corticosteroids have been utilized historically as first-line treatment for pulmonary sarcoidosis; however, a 2025 open-label trial comparing corticosteroids with methotrexate for 24 weeks in moderate to severe pulmonary sarcoidosis showed similar lung function improvement. Therefore, methotrexate now is preferred to avoid the long-term effects of steroid use. Other immunosuppressive medications(including azathioprine or infliximab) may be considered in patients who are intolerant or have refractory disease. A favorable response is defined by a decrease in symptoms, reduction of radiographic abnormalities, and improvement in PFTs.

Prognosis

The outlook is best for patients with hilar adenopathy alone or with erythema nodosum; radiographic involvement of the lung parenchyma is associated with a worse prognosis. About 20% of patients with lung involvement suffer irreversible lung impairment, characterized by progressive fibrosis, bronchiectasis, and cavitation. Pneumothorax, hemoptysis, mycetoma formation in lung cavities, pulmonary hypertension, and respiratory failure may often complicate this advanced stage. Myocardial sarcoidosis occurs in 5% of patients, sometimes leading to restrictive cardiomyopathy, cardiac dysrhythmias, and conduction disturbances. Death from respiratory insufficiency occurs in 5% of patients. Patients require long-term follow-up.

Fernández-Ramón R et al. Systemic treatment in sarcoidosis: experience over two decades. Eur J Intern Med. 2023;108:60. [PMID: 36446677]

Kahlmann V et al. First-line treatment of pulmonary sarcoidosis with prednisone or methotrexate. N Engl J Med. 2025;393:231. [PMID: 40387020]

PULMONARY ALVEOLAR PROTEINOSIS

Pulmonary alveolar proteinosis is a rare disease characterized by accumulation of lipoproteinaceous material within alveolar spaces. The condition may be primary (idiopathic) or secondary (occurring in immunodeficiency; hematologic malignancies; inhalation of mineral dusts; or following lung infections, including tuberculosis and viral infections). Progressive dyspnea is the usual presenting symptom. CXR shows bilateral alveolar infiltrates, and chest CT features a characteristic "crazy-paving" that refers to ground-glass opacities with superimposed interlobular and intralobular septal thickening. The diagnosis is based on demonstration of characteristic findings on BAL (milky appearance and periodic acid-Schiff [PAS]-positive lipoproteinaceous material) in association with clinical and radiographic features. In secondary disease, an elevated anti-GM-CSF (anti-granulocyte-macrophage colony-stimulating factor) titer in serum or BAL fluid is highly sensitive and specific.

The course of the disease varies. Some patients experience spontaneous remission; others develop progressive respiratory insufficiency. For patients with minimal symptoms, supportive care and oxygen evaluation is recommended. Therapy for advanced disease consists of periodic whole-lung lavage, inhalational or subcutaneous GM-CSF, or both. Pulmonary superinfection with *Nocardia* or fungi may occur.

Johnston JM et al. Pulmonary alveolar proteinosis: presentation, diagnostic challenges, and management. Br J Hosp Med (Lond). 2024;85:1. [PMID: 39347668]

Trapnell BC et al. Phase 3 trial of inhaled molgramostim in autoimmune pulmonary alveolar proteinosis. N Engl J Med. 2025;393:764. [PMID: 40834301]

EOSINOPHILIC PULMONARY SYNDROMES

Eosinophilic pulmonary syndromes are a diverse group of disorders typically characterized by peripheral blood eosinophilia (typically > 500 cells/mcL [0.5×10^9/L]), eosinophilic pulmonary infiltrates, dyspnea, and cough. Many patients have constitutional symptoms, including fever. Common causes include medications (nitrofurantoin, daptomycin, phenytoin, NSAIDs, acetaminophen, mesalamine, sulfasalazine) or infection with helminths (eg, *Ascaris*, hookworms, *Strongyloides*) or filariae (eg, *Wuchereria bancrofti*, *Brugia malayi*, tropical pulmonary eosinophilia). **Löffler syndrome** refers to acute eosinophilic pulmonary infiltrates in response to transpulmonary passage of helminth larvae. Pulmonary eosinophilia can also be a feature of other illnesses, including ABPA, eosinophilic granulomatosis with polyangiitis, systemic hypereosinophilic syndromes, eosinophilic granuloma of the lung (properly referred to as pulmonary Langerhans cell histiocytosis), neoplasms, and numerous interstitial lung diseases.

One-third of cases are idiopathic, and there are two common syndromes. **Acute eosinophilic pneumonia** is an acute, febrile illness characterized by cough and dyspnea, sometimes rapidly progressing to respiratory failure. The CXR is abnormal but nonspecific. BAL fluid frequently shows eosinophilia, but peripheral blood eosinophilia is rare at the onset of symptoms. **Chronic eosinophilic pneumonia** has a subacute-chronic presentation, characterized by fever, night sweats, weight loss, and dyspnea. Asthma or atopy is present in half of cases. Radiologic imaging often shows peripheral infiltrates, the "photographic negative" of pulmonary edema. BAL typically has a marked eosinophilia, and peripheral blood eosinophilia is present in > 80%.

Management depends on the underlying cause. Infectious causes require antimicrobials, while noninfectious causes usually are treated with steroids, which usually results in dramatic improvement. If an extrinsic cause is identified, therapy consists of removal of the offending medication.

Carbone RG et al. Acute and chronic eosinophilic pneumonia: an overview. Front Med (Lausanne). 2024;11:1355247. [PMID: 38711783]
Cottin V. Eosinophilic lung diseases. Immunol Allergy Clin North Am. 2023;43:289. [PMID: 37055090]
Rosenberg CE et al. Approach to eosinophilia presenting with pulmonary symptoms. Chest. 2021;159:507. [PMID: 33002503]

DISORDERS OF THE PULMONARY CIRCULATION

PULMONARY VENOUS THROMBOEMBOLISM

ESSENTIALS OF DIAGNOSIS

- Third most common cardiovascular cause of death in the United States.
- Dyspnea, pleuritic chest pain, hemoptysis, syncope, tachypnea, tachycardia, hypoxia may be present.
- Risk stratification with clinical scores, cardiac biomarkers, and RV imaging is key for management.

General Considerations

PE is a common, serious, and potentially fatal result of thrombus formation within the deep venous circulation that migrates to the pulmonary circulation. Management demands a vigilant systematic approach to diagnosis and an understanding of risk factors so that appropriate therapy can be initiated.

Many substances can embolize to the pulmonary circulation. Although thrombus is most common, others include air (during neurosurgery, from central venous catheters), amniotic fluid (during active labor), fat (long bone fractures), foreign bodies (talc in injection drug users), parasite eggs (schistosomiasis), septic emboli (acute infective endocarditis), and tumor cells (renal cell carcinoma). PE will develop in 50–60% of patients with proximal DVT; half of these embolic events will be asymptomatic. Approximately 50–70% of patients who have symptomatic PE will have lower extremity DVT when evaluated.

Risk factors include venous stasis, injury to the vessel wall, and hypercoagulability (Virchow triad). Venous stasis increases with immobility (obesity, stroke, bed rest—especially postoperative), injury to vessels (caused by orthopedic surgery or trauma), hypercoagulability (caused by medications [oral contraceptives, hormonal replacement therapy]), diseases (malignancy, surgery), inherited gene defects (factor V Leiden, prothrombin mutation), or acquired thrombophilias (protein C and protein S deficiency, antithrombin deficiency, antiphospholipid antibodies).

Pulmonary thrombus occlusion of > 20–25% of the pulmonary vascular bed causes RV dilation or dysfunction and increased pulmonary vascular resistance. Vascular obstruction increases physiologic dead space (wasted ventilation) and leads to hypoxemia through right-to-left shunting. This may cause decreased cardiac output with subsequent hypotension and cardiovascular collapse.

Clinical Findings

A. Symptoms and Signs

The clinical diagnosis of PE is notoriously challenging because the symptoms may be nonspecific. Dyspnea and chest pain on inspiration are common. Diagnosis primarily relies on clinical prediction scores to calculate the pretest probability of PE. Wells score is most commonly used and quantifies clinical risk assessment, allowing separation of patients into low, intermediate, or high probability groups, or PE-likely versus PE-unlikely groups (Table 9–18). The Pulmonary Embolism Rule-out Criteria (PERC) may be used to identify patients for whom no further testing is indicated (Table 9–19).

B. Laboratory Findings

The **ECG** is abnormal in 70% of patients with PE. However, the most common abnormalities are sinus tachycardia and nonspecific ST and T wave changes, nonspecific findings that are each seen in approximately 40% of patients. Less

Table 9–18. Clinical prediction rule for PE.

Variable	Points
Clinical symptoms and signs of DVT (leg swelling and pain with palpation of deep veins)	3.0
Alternative diagnosis less likely than PE	3.0
Heart rate > 100 beats/min	1.5
Immobilization for > 3 days or surgery in previous 4 weeks	1.5
Previous PE or DVT	1.5
Hemoptysis	1.0
Cancer (with treatment within past 6 months or palliative care)	1.0
Add **Points** *to determine* **Score**, *then refer to* **probability assessments** *below*:	
Three-tiered clinical probability assessment (Wells criteria)	**Score**
High	> 6.0
Moderate	2.0 to 6.0
Low	< 2.0
Dichotomous clinical probability assessment (Modified Wells criteria)	**Score**
PE likely	> 4.0
PE unlikely	≤ 4.0

Data from Wells PS et al. Derivation of a simple clinical model to categorize patients' probability of pulmonary embolism: increasing the models' utility with the Implied D-dimer. Throb Haemost. 2000;83:416.

Table 9–19. Pulmonary Embolism Rule-out Criteria (PERC) for low-risk patients.

For patients with a Modified Wells Score ≤ 4[1] who meet ALL of the following criteria, PE is excluded, monitor off anticoagulation, and search for alternative diagnoses. • Age < 50 years • Heart rate < 100 bpm • Oxyhemoglobin saturation on room air ≥ 95% • No prior history of VTE • No recent (within 4 weeks) trauma or surgery requiring hospitalization • No presenting hemoptysis • No estrogen therapy • No unilateral leg swelling

[1]See Table 9–18.

Data from Kline JA et al. Impact of a rapid rule-out protocol for pulmonary embolism on the rate of screening, missed cases, and pulmonary vascular imaging in an urban US emergency room. Ann Emerg Med. 2004;44:490.

than 5% of patients in the PIOPED I study had P pulmonale, RVH, right axis deviation, and right bundle branch block.

ABGs usually reveal acute respiratory alkalosis due to hyperventilation and may show hypoxemia.

Plasma levels of **D-dimer**, a degradation product of cross-linked fibrin, are elevated in the presence of thrombus. A normal D-dimer may be used to exclude the diagnosis of PE in those patients who have low pretest probability of PE or are PE-unlikely on Wells score. Additionally, an age-adjusted D-dimer value has increased specificity than the usually specified cutoff. Due to much higher false-positive rates, D-dimer is not useful for hospital inpatients.

Serum troponin I, troponin T, and plasma BNP levels are elevated in approximately 25% of patients with PE and are useful in the risk stratification of PE because they correlate with adverse outcomes, including mechanical ventilation, prolonged hospitalization, shock, and death.

C. Imaging and Special Examinations

1. CXR—A CXR in PE is usually normal but is nonetheless necessary to exclude other common lung diseases. Profound hypoxia with a normal CXR is highly suspicious for PE.

2. Pulmonary CT-angiography—Helical CT-PA with intravenous radiocontrast dye timed for the pulmonary artery is the gold standard diagnostic study for suspected PE due to its high sensitivity and specificity as well as wide availability. CT-PA usually is recommended for patients with low or intermediate pretest probability (or PE-unlikely) who have a positive D-dimer and those with high pretest probability (or PE-likely).

3. Ventilation-perfusion ($\dot{V}/\dot{Q}$) lung scanning—$\dot{V}/\dot{Q}$ scanning may be used as an alternative to CT-PA in patients in whom contrast is contraindicated, such as severe contrast-induced anaphylaxis or kidney dysfunction. A normal $\dot{V}/\dot{Q}$ scan excludes the diagnosis of clinically significant PE (negative predictive value of 91% in the PIOPED I study).

4. Venous thrombosis studies—**Venous ultrasonography** is the test of choice to detect DVT. Inability to compress the common femoral or popliteal veins in symptomatic patients is diagnostic (positive predictive value of 97%); full compressibility of both sites excludes proximal DVT (negative predictive value of 98%). A normal venous ultrasound does not rule out PE.

5. Pulmonary angiography—Although pulmonary angiography is the historical reference standard for the diagnosis of PE, it is now only used in the treatment of acute PE for catheter-directed thrombolysis or suction thrombectomy) or in chronic thromboembolic PE with pulmonary hypertension for balloon angioplasty.

Risk Stratification of Pulmonary Embolism

After a PE diagnosis is made, the next step is risk stratification since this will guide management. There are three categories based on mortality risk: high-risk PE, intermediate-risk PE, and low-risk PE. Patients with high-risk PE, also known as massive PE, have hemodynamic compromise, defined as systolic blood pressure < 90 mm Hg or a systolic blood pressure drop by ≥ 40 mm Hg for > 15 minutes, requiring a vasopressor, or causing a cardiac arrest. Patients with an intermediate-risk PE, also known as submassive PE, are hemodynamically stable but have signs of RV strain or dysfunction, either by imaging (CT-PA or echocardiogram) or elevated troponin. Patients with low-risk PE have normotension without signs of RV dysfunction.

PE severity scores, such as PE Severity Score Index (PESI) or the simplified PESI, compile useful patient characteristics that predict patient outcome. Such scores may also be used to decide which patients may be appropriate for outpatient PE treatment.

Prevention

Discussion of strategies for the prevention of VTE can be found in Chapter 16.

Treatment

A. Anticoagulation

Anticoagulation is the mainstay therapy for VTE. It impedes additional thrombus formation, allowing endogenous fibrinolytic mechanisms to lyse existing clot, thereby decreasing mortality and recurrence of PE. Initiation of anticoagulation should be considered even before a confirmed diagnosis when there is high clinical suspicion and low risk of bleeding.

In patients who require hospitalization, low-molecular-weight heparin (LMWH) are preferred, given their faster therapeutic activity compared to unfractionated heparin. For treatment of VTE in outpatients and after discharge from the hospital, DOACs are preferred over vitamin K antagonist (VKA or warfarin) as first-line anticoagulation due to their predictable pharmacokinetics and pharmacodynamics with fixed dosing, fewer drug interactions, and relatively short half-life.

The optimal duration of anticoagulation therapy for VTE depends on the risk factors for VTE recurrence.

Extended anticoagulation should be considered for patients with no identifiable risk factor for the index PE event, those with recurrent VTE, those with major persistent risk factors (malignancy), or those with a minor risk factor (such as immobility due to prolonged car or air travel, obesity, pregnancy, or increased age). However, those with major transient/reversible risk factors (such as fracture of lower limb; hip or knee surgery; or hospitalization for HF, atrial fibrillation, or MI) may be considered for discontinuation of anticoagulation after 3 months. Additionally, duration of therapy needs to take into consideration the patient's age, likelihood and potential consequences of hemorrhage, and preferences for continued therapy. In patients who continue taking extended anticoagulation, an annual risk-benefit assessment of continuing anticoagulation therapy should be done.

The major complication of anticoagulation is hemorrhage. Risk factors for hemorrhage include the intensity of the anticoagulation; duration of therapy; concomitant administration of medications, such as aspirin or NSAIDs, that interfere with platelet function; and patient characteristics, particularly increased age, previous GI hemorrhage, and coexistent kidney or liver disease.

B. Systemic Thrombolysis

Streptokinase, urokinase, and recombinant tissue plasminogen activator (rt-PA; alteplase) increase plasmin levels and thereby directly lyse intravascular thrombi accelerating resolution of emboli. Guidelines support systemic thrombolysis in patients with high-risk or massive PE (ie, hemodynamically unstable) who have a low risk of bleeding. Thrombolytic therapy is not routinely recommended in patients with intermediate-risk or submassive PE patients (ie, hemodynamically stable with evidence of right heart strain) due to a lack of mortality benefit (despite a decreased incidence of hemodynamic collapse) and an increased risk of major hemorrhagic complications (including intracranial hemorrhage). Absolute contraindications to thrombolytic therapy include active bleeding and stroke within the past 3 months. Relative contraindications include surgery or trauma within the past 4 weeks, thrombocytopenia, and renal or liver dysfunction, or both.

C. Additional Therapies

Catheter-directed thrombolysis delivers a low-dose of the thrombolytic agent directly into the pulmonary artery, and reverses RV dilation faster than anticoagulation alone. This procedure may be considered for patients with high-risk PE and selected intermediate-risk PE at increased risk of hemodynamic collapse with low risk of bleeding. Mechanical/suction embolectomy may be considered for patients with high-risk PE and selected patients with intermediate-risk (submassive) PE who have signs of clinical decompensation (such as severe hypoxemia, severe RV dysfunction, persistent tachycardia) or high-risk PE. The optimal catheter-directed therapy is unclear and the choice may be determined by local experience and resources. Although surgical embolectomy also may be considered in those with contraindications to or failed thrombolysis, there is decreased use due to increased availability of catheter therapies.

Inferior vena cava filters should be inserted in patients with contraindications to anticoagulation (active bleeding) and PE with lower extremity DVT. Consideration should be given for those with acute PE and presence of free-floating proximal DVT, since it carries an increased risk of embolization. Once placed, it must be assessed for removal at the earliest opportunity.

Prognosis

The outlook for most patients is generally good. However, mortality for intermediate-risk (submassive) PE or high-risk (massive) PE may be as high as 15% and 50%, respectively. Persons who have been impacted by PE may have long-term sequelae of PE, such as exercise intolerance, chronic thromboembolic disease, and chronic thromboembolic pulmonary hypertension. Therefore, follow-up care to assess whether patients have persistent or recurrent symptoms is very important.

When to Admit

The decision to admit patients with acute PE requires assessment of factors placing them at high risk, including their severity of illness (eg, severe hypoxemia), comorbidities (eg, DVT, cardiac dysfunction), educational needs (eg, lack of knowledge about PE and anticoagulation), and social situations (eg, prior nonadherence with therapy or follow-up care). Carefully selected patients with low-risk PE can be safely and effectively managed as outpatients with the aid of integrated clinical decision support systems.

Benavente K et al. A practical clinical approach to navigate pulmonary embolism management: a primer and narrative review of the evolving landscape. J Clin Med. 2024;13:7637. [PMID: 39768560]

Jaber WA et al. Large-bore mechanical thrombectomy versus catheter-directed thrombolysis in the management of intermediate-risk pulmonary embolism: primary results of the PEERLESS randomized controlled trial. Circulation. 2025;151:260. [PMID: 39470698]

Stevens SM et al. Antithrombotic therapy for VTE disease: compendium and review of CHEST guidelines 2012-2021. Chest. 2024;166:388. [PMID: 38458430]

PULMONARY HYPERTENSION

ESSENTIALS OF DIAGNOSIS

- Dyspnea, fatigue, chest pain, and syncope on exertion.
- Narrow splitting of second heart sound with loud pulmonary component; findings of RVH and HF in advanced disease.
- Echocardiographic evidence of RV dilation, dysfunction, or hypertrophy; right atrial enlargement; or elevated RV systolic pressure.
- Right heart catheterization required for confirmation of diagnosis.

General Considerations

Pulmonary hypertension is a complex problem characterized by pathologic elevation in pulmonary arterial pressure. Normal pulmonary artery systolic pressure at rest is 15–30 mm Hg, with a mean pressure < 20 mm Hg. The pulmonary circulation is a low-pressure, low-resistance system due to its large cross-sectional area, and it can accommodate significant increase in blood flow during exercise. The primary pathologic mechanism in pulmonary hypertension is an increase in pulmonary vascular resistance that leads to an increase in the pulmonary systolic pressure. Pulmonary hypertension is defined by a mean pulmonary arterial pressure > 20 mm Hg on a resting cardiac catheterization.

The World Symposium on Pulmonary Hypertension updated clinical classification includes five groups that are based on etiology and mechanism.

Group 1 (pulmonary arterial hypertension [PAH]): This group comprises diseases to the pulmonary arteries that lead to structural changes, smooth muscle hypertrophy, and endothelial dysfunction. It includes idiopathic (formerly primary) PAH; heritable PAH; drug- and toxin-induced PAH; PAH associated with HIV infection, portal hypertension, connective tissue disorders (most commonly scleroderma), congenital heart disease, and schistosomiasis; and PAH with features of veno-occlusive disease and pulmonary capillary hemangiomatosis.

Group 2 (pulmonary venous hypertension due to left heart disease): This group includes LV systolic or diastolic dysfunction and valvular heart disease.

Group 3 (pulmonary hypertension due to lung disease or hypoxemia): This group is caused by advanced lung disease, including COPD, ILD, pulmonary fibrosis, and high altitude exposure.

Group 4 (pulmonary hypertension due to pulmonary obstruction): This group primarily includes chronic thromboembolic pulmonary hypertension (CTEPH) but also other causes of pulmonary obstructions, such as sarcoma, metastatic malignancies, and congenital pulmonary artery stenosis.

Group 5 (pulmonary hypertension secondary to unclear or multifactorial mechanisms): These patients have pulmonary hypertension secondary to hematologic disorders (eg, chronic hemolytic anemia, sickle cell anemia, myeloproliferative disorders, splenectomy), systemic disorders (eg, sarcoidosis, vasculitis, pulmonary Langerhans cell histiocytosis, neurofibromatosis type 1), metabolic disorders (eg, glycogen storage disease, Gaucher disease, thyroid disease), and miscellaneous causes (eg, ESKD with or without hemodialysis, fibrosing mediastinitis).

The clinical severity of pulmonary hypertension is classified according to the NYHA/WHO classification system based primarily on symptoms and functional status. **Class I:** No limitation of physical activity; no dyspnea, fatigue, chest pain, or near syncope is present with exertion. **Class II:** Slight limitation of physical activity; no symptoms at rest, but ordinary physical activity causes dyspnea, fatigue, chest pain, or near syncope. **Class III:** Marked limitation of physical activity; no symptoms at rest, but less than ordinary activity causes dyspnea, fatigue, chest pain, or near syncope. **Class IV:** Inability to perform any physical activity without symptoms; dyspnea and fatigue are present at rest and symptoms worsen with any activity.

Clinical Findings

A. Symptoms and Signs

There are no specific symptoms or signs of pulmonary hypertension, which may delay its diagnosis and significantly affect its mortality. Typical symptoms include dyspnea with exertion. With advanced disease, there may be dyspnea at rest or syncope. Patients may have chest pain, nonproductive cough, and fatigue.

Findings on physical examination can include jugular venous distention, accentuated pulmonary valve component of the second heart sound, right-sided third heart sound, tricuspid regurgitation murmur, hepatomegaly, and lower extremity edema.

B. Laboratory Findings

BNP or pro-BNP is usually elevated. All patients should be evaluated for HIV, liver dysfunction, and connective tissue disorders.

The ECG is typically normal except in advanced disease, where RVH (right axis deviation, incomplete right bundle branch block) and right atrial enlargement (peaked P wave in the inferior and right-sided leads) can be noted.

C. Imaging and Special Examinations

Echocardiography is the best screening study. RV assessment is made by measuring RV size, function, and systolic pressure. Additionally, the echocardiogram is useful for assessing underlying cardiac disease (eg, pulmonary hypertension due to left heart disease).

Radiographs and CT scans of the chest are useful in diagnosis. Enlargement of the right and left main pulmonary arteries is common; RV and right atrial enlargement are seen in advanced disease. Chest CT scanning and PFTs are also useful in determining the cause of pulmonary hypertension for patients in Group 3 (pulmonary hypertension due to lung disease). In all patients, especially those with a history of PE or risk factors for thromboembolic disease, CTEPH (Group 4) should be excluded with $\dot{V}/\dot{Q}$ lung scanning before diagnosing idiopathic pulmonary hypertension. If abnormal, CT-PA or pulmonary angiography is the next step in confirming the diagnosis and establishing the distribution and extent of disease.

Right-sided cardiac catheterization is required for confirmation of diagnosis and assessment of disease severity and should be performed before initiation of vasodilator therapies. PAH is defined on a resting cardiac catheterization by a mean pulmonary arterial pressure > 20 mm Hg with a pulmonary capillary wedge pressure of ≤ 15 mm Hg, and a pulmonary vascular resistance of ≥ 2 Wood units. A vasodilator challenge can be performed during right heart catheterization; a significant acute vasodilator response consists of a drop in mean pulmonary pressure of > 10 mm Hg (or 20%) to < 40 mm Hg.

Treatment

Advanced therapies, such as pulmonary vasodilators, are available to treat pulmonary hypertension. Such therapies are chosen based on the patient's risk assessment which is based on a combination of clinical signs of right HF, functional status according to the NYHA/WHO classification, 6-minute walk distance, imaging, and hemodynamics. Their mechanisms of action follow four main pathways: (1) the nitric oxide pathway: phosphodiesterase inhibitors (PDE5I) (sildenafil, tadalafil) and soluble guanylate cyclase stimulators (sGCS) (riociguat); (2) the endothelin pathway: endothelin receptor antagonists (ERA) (bosentan, ambrisentan, macitentan); (3) the prostacyclin pathway: prostacyclin analogs (intravenous epoprostenol; intravenous, subcutaneous, inhaled, or oral treprostinil; inhaled iloprost) and prostacyclin receptor agonist (selexipag); and (4) the activin pathway (sotatercept). Sotatercept, the most recent drug approved in PAH, is a novel biologic agent targeting the transforming growth factor-β superfamily; it acts as a ligand trap for activins and related growth factors, which rebalances pro-and-anti-proliferative signaling.

Patients with Group 1 PAH and low/intermediate risk based on initial risk assessment, should be initiated on dual combination therapy with an ERA plus PDE5I. Following reassessment at 3–4 months, if the patient is not at low risk, additional therapy should be added, such as a prostacyclin or activin-signaling inhibitor or switching from PDE5I to sGCS. High-risk patients with Group 1 PAH should be started on combination therapy of continuous prostacyclin infusion (intravenous/subcutaneous) with ERA and PDE5I. Following a short-term interval reassessment if the risk is not improved, add an activin-signaling inhibitor and consider lung transplant referral. Oral calcium channel blockers may be used in patients with a significant vasodilator response during cardiac catheterization. Anticoagulation was commonly used in the past but has fallen out of favor due to lack of efficacy.

Treatment of patients with Group 2 PH (due to left HF) is discussed in Chapter 10. The main goal is to decrease pulmonary venous pressure by providing goal-directed therapy of HF and volume overload, primarily with the use of diuretics, ACEI, ARBs, and spironolactone.

Patients with Group 3 PH (due to lung disease) should be assessed for hypoxemia at rest or with physical activity and, if present, should receive supplemental oxygen. Patients with COPD, ILD, or obstructive sleep apnea should receive treatment for underlying disease. Inhaled treprostinil is the only pulmonary vasodilator approved for patients with PH due to ILD since it improved exercise capacity based on 6-minute walk assessment.

For patients with Group 4 PH (CTEPH), long-term anticoagulation is recommended. Additionally, patients with surgically accessible lesions and acceptable perioperative risk should undergo pulmonary thromboendarterectomy. For patients unable to undergo surgery or those with residual pulmonary hypertension postoperatively, medical therapy with riociguat, pulmonary artery balloon angioplasty, or both should be considered.

Lung transplantation is a treatment option for selected patients with pulmonary hypertension when medical therapy is no longer effective.

Prognosis

The prognosis of pulmonary hypertension varies by group. The prognosis of Group 1 patients has improved with the advent of pulmonary hypertension–specific therapy. Factors associated with poor prognosis include age older than 50 years, male sex, WHO/NYHA functional class III or IV, failure to improve to a lower functional class with therapy, and RV dysfunction.

When to Refer

Patients in whom pulmonary hypertension is suspected or has been diagnosed should be referred early to a specialized pulmonary hypertension center for expert management.

When to Admit

- Patients with pulmonary hypertension, severe symptoms, and evidence of decompensated right HF with volume overload should be admitted to the hospital for aggressive diuresis.
- Patients with Group 1 pulmonary hypertension and functional class IV symptoms should be admitted to a specialized center for initiation of advanced therapies, such as intravenous prostacyclins.

Chin KM et al. Treatment algorithm for pulmonary arterial hypertension. Eur Respir J. 2024;64:2401325. [PMID: 39209476]

Kovacs G et al. Definition, classification and diagnosis of pulmonary hypertension. Eur Respir J. 2024;64:2401324. [PMID: 39209475]

PULMONARY VASCULITIS

The pulmonary vasculature may be involved in several vasculitis syndromes. These include **antineutrophil cytoplasmic autoantibody (ANCA)–associated vasculitides, granulomatosis with polyangiitis, eosinophilic granulomatosis with polyangiitis, and anti-glomerular basement membrane (anti-GBM) antibody disease.** These are reviewed in Chapter 23.

ALVEOLAR HEMORRHAGE SYNDROMES

Diffuse alveolar hemorrhage may occur in a variety of immune and nonimmune disorders. Acute dyspnea, anemia, hemoptysis and, occasionally, fever are characteristic. CXR or CT chest with rapid clearing of diffuse lung infiltrates may be indicative of the diagnosis of diffuse alveolar hemorrhage. Sequential BAL on bronchoscopy is the preferred method for diagnosis with lavage aliquots becoming progressively more hemorrhagic.

Causes of diffuse **immune alveolar hemorrhage** include anti-basement membrane antibody disease (Goodpasture syndrome), granulomatosis with polyangiitis, systemic necrotizing vasculitis, pulmonary capillaritis associated with idiopathic rapidly progressive glomerulonephritis, SLE, and other vasculitic and collagen-vascular diseases (Chapter 23). **Nonimmune causes** of diffuse hemorrhage include coagulopathy, mitral stenosis, necrotizing pulmonary infection, drugs (penicillamine), toxins (trimellitic anhydride), and idiopathic pulmonary hemosiderosis.

Idiopathic pulmonary hemosiderosis is a disease of children or young adults characterized by recurrent pulmonary hemorrhage; iron deficiency is typical. It is frequently associated with celiac disease.

Treatment of massive pulmonary hemorrhage may require patient intubation and positioning of the lung with suspected hemorrhage in the dependent position. Tranexamic acid may be considered. Bronchoscopy with local iced saline lavage or injection of epinephrine can be used to achieve hemostasis. A bronchial blocker may be placed to apply pressure or isolate the bleeding lung. Embolization may be required for life-threatening bleeding.

Fan S et al. Bronchial artery embolization versus conservative treatment for hemoptysis: a systematic review and meta-analysis. BMC Pulm Med. 2024;24:428. [PMID: 39215233]

Gozzi L et al. Lung involvement in pulmonary vasculitis: a radiological review. Diagnostics (Basel). 2024;14:1416. [PMID: 39001306]

ENVIRONMENTAL & OCCUPATIONAL LUNG DISORDERS

SMOKE INHALATION

The inhalation of products of combustion may cause serious respiratory complications. As many as one-third of patients admitted to burn-treatment units have pulmonary injury from smoke inhalation. Morbidity and mortality due to smoke inhalation may exceed those attributed to the burns themselves. Pulmonary complications following burns and inhalation injury account for up to 77% of deaths.

All patients in whom significant smoke inhalation is suspected must be assessed for three consequences of smoke inhalation: impaired tissue oxygenation, thermal injury to the upper airway, and injury to the lower airways and lung parenchyma. Impaired tissue oxygenation may result from inhalation of a hypoxic gas mixture, carbon monoxide or cyanide, or from alterations in $\dot{V}/\dot{Q}$ matching, and is an immediate threat to life. Immediate treatment with 100% oxygen is essential. The management of patients with carbon monoxide and cyanide poisoning is discussed in Chapter 42.

Thermal injury to the mucosal surfaces of the upper airway occurs from inhalation of super-heated gases. Complications, including mucosal edema, upper airway obstruction, and impaired ability to clear oral secretions, usually become evident by 18–24 hours and produce inspiratory stridor. Respiratory failure occurs in severe cases. Early management (Chapter 41) includes the use of a high-humidity face mask with supplemental oxygen, gentle suctioning to evacuate oral secretions, elevation of the head 30 degrees to promote clearing of secretions, and topical epinephrine to reduce edema of the oropharyngeal mucous membrane. Helium-oxygen gas mixtures (Heliox) may reduce labored breathing due to critical upper airway narrowing. Close monitoring with ABGs and later with oximetry is important. Examination of the upper airway with a fiberoptic laryngoscope or bronchoscope is superior to routine physical examination. Endotracheal intubation is often necessary to maintain airway patency and is likely to be necessary in patients with deep facial burns or oropharyngeal or laryngeal edema. Tracheotomy should be avoided, if possible, because of an increased risk of pneumonia and death from sepsis.

Injury to the lower airways and lung parenchyma results from inhalation of toxic gases and products of combustion, including aldehydes and organic acids. The site of lung injury depends on the solubility of the gases inhaled, the duration of exposure, and the size of inhaled particles that transport noxious gases to distal lung units. Bronchorrhea and bronchospasm occur early after exposure along with dyspnea, tachypnea, and tachycardia. Labored breathing and cyanosis may follow. Physical examination at this stage reveals diffuse wheezing and rhonchi. Bronchiolar and alveolar edema (eg, ARDS) may develop within 1–2 days after exposure. Sloughing of the bronchiolar mucosa may occur within 2–3 days, leading to airway obstruction, atelectasis, and worsening hypoxemia. Bacterial colonization and pneumonia are common by 5–7 days after the exposure.

Treatment of smoke inhalation consists of supplemental oxygen, bronchodilators, suctioning of mucosal debris and mucopurulent secretions via an indwelling endotracheal tube, chest physical therapy to aid clearance of secretions, and adequate humidification of inspired gases. Positive end-expiratory pressure (PEEP) has been advocated to treat bronchiolar edema. Judicious fluid management and close monitoring for secondary bacterial infection round out the management protocol.

The routine use of corticosteroids for lung injury from smoke inhalation has been shown to be ineffective and may even be harmful. Routine or prophylactic use of antibiotics is not recommended.

Patients who survive should be watched for the late development of bronchiolitis obliterans.

Bittner E et al. Acute respiratory distress syndrome, mechanical ventilation, and inhalation injury in burn patients. Surg Clin North Am 2023;103:439. [PMID: 37149380]

Herdy Guerra Avila JE et al. Frequency, complications, and mortality of inhalation injury in burn patients: a systematic review and meta-analysis protocol. PLoS One. 2024;19:e0295318. [PMID: 38652713]

E-CIGARETTE OR VAPING PRODUCT–ASSOCIATED LUNG INJURY

General Considerations

E-cigarette or vaping product–associated lung injury (EVALI) began in the United States in 2019. Approximately 66% of patients have been male and 80% are under age 35. Over 95% of reported cases required hospitalization: 47% were admitted to intensive care, 22% were intubated, and many died. Based on the characteristics of these patients, the diagnosis of EVALI requires reported use of e-cigarette or vaping products within 3 months of symptom onset, compatible chest imaging findings, and an evaluation that excludes infectious etiologies.

No single causative agent has been identified. Most cases involved vaping products containing tetrahydrocannabinol (THC) or nicotine or both. Postulated factors contributing to the development of EVALI include e-cigarette flavorings, exposure to diacetyl (a popcorn flavoring that has been associated with lung injury), THC, adulteration of THC, adulteration of delivery devices, and vitamin E acetate (used as a thickening agent).

Clinical Findings

A. Symptoms and Signs

Patients with EVALI have respiratory symptoms (95%), including cough, shortness of breath, chest pain, and hemoptysis; GI symptoms (77%), including nausea, vomiting, and diarrhea; and constitutional symptoms (85%), including fever and chills. The illness is usually acute to subacute with patients having symptoms for days to weeks before seeking health care.

Tachycardia and tachypnea are present in 55% and 45% of patients, respectively, and 57% have a room air oxygen saturation of < 95%. Given the nonspecific nature of the presentation especially during influenza season and the COVID-19 pandemic, providers must have a high degree of clinical suspicion and ask patients specifically about vaping.

B. Laboratory Findings

There are no laboratory findings specific for the diagnosis of EVALI. There may be leukocytosis, elevated CRP, and elevated ESR. It is important to exclude other possible etiologies such as infectious or eosinophilic pneumonia.

C. Imaging

Imaging findings in EVALI show various patterns of lung injury. CXRs typically show bilateral diffuse pulmonary opacities. Chest CT scan findings are nonspecific and may show bilateral distribution with ground-glass densities with subpleural sparing.

Differential Diagnosis

The EVALI case definition requires a negative workup for infectious causes. Other diagnoses to consider include acute eosinophilic pneumonia, ARDS, hypersensitivity pneumonitis, lipoid pneumonia, and organizing pneumonia. Influenza testing should be done in season, and SARS-CoV-2 testing, as indicated.

Treatment

In published reports of hospitalized patients with EVALI who have received corticosteroids, rapid improvement has been described. Symptoms of fatigue, dyspnea, decreased exercise capacity, and cough may persist for months.

Ghuman A et al. A systematic literature review on the composition, health impacts, and regulatory dynamics of vaping. Cureus. 2024;16:e66068. [PMID: 39229398]

Rebuli ME et al. The e-cigarette or vaping product use-associated lung injury epidemic: pathogenesis, management, and future directions: an official American Thoracic Society workshop report. Ann Am Thorac Soc. 2023;20:1. [PMID: 36584985]

PULMONARY ASPIRATION SYNDROMES

1. Acute Aspiration of Gastric Contents

Acute aspiration of gastric contents may be catastrophic. The pulmonary response depends on the characteristics and amount of gastric contents aspirated. The more acidic the material, the greater the degree of chemical pneumonitis. Aspiration of pure gastric acid causes extensive desquamation of the bronchial epithelium, bronchiolitis, hemorrhage, and pulmonary edema and may lead to ARDS. The clinical picture is one of abrupt onset of respiratory distress, with cough, wheezing, fever, and tachypnea. Crackles may be audible at the bases of the lungs. Hypoxemia may be noted immediately after aspiration occurs. Radiographic abnormalities, consisting of patchy alveolar opacities in dependent lung zones, appear within a few hours. If particulate food matter has been aspirated along with gastric acid, radiographic features of bronchial obstruction may be observed. Fever and leukocytosis are common even in the absence of infection.

Recently, GLP-1 receptor agonists have been associated with reports of pulmonary aspiration due to delayed gastric emptying.

Treatment of acute aspiration of gastric contents consists of supplemental oxygen, measures to maintain the airway, and the usual measures for treatment of acute respiratory failure. There is no evidence to support the routine use of prophylactic antibiotics or corticosteroids, although use in critically ill patients is an area of uncertainty. Secondary pulmonary infection, which occurs in about one-fourth of patients, typically appears 2–3 days after aspiration. Hypotension or shock secondary to alveolar-capillary membrane injury and intravascular volume depletion may occur and is managed with typical supportive care.

2. Chronic Aspiration of Gastric Contents

Chronic aspiration of gastric contents may result from primary disorders of the larynx or the esophagus, such as achalasia, esophageal stricture, systemic sclerosis (scleroderma), esophageal carcinoma, esophagitis, and GERD. In GERD, relaxation of the tone of the lower esophageal sphincter allows reflux of gastric contents into the esophagus and predisposes to chronic pulmonary aspiration, especially when supine. Cigarette smoking, consumption of alcohol or caffeine, and certain medications (ie, anticholinergics, benzodiazepines, nitroglycerin) are all known to relax the lower esophageal sphincter. Pulmonary disorders linked to GERD and chronic aspiration include asthma, chronic cough, bronchiectasis, and pulmonary fibrosis. Even in the absence of aspiration, acid in the esophagus may trigger bronchospasm or bronchial hyperreactivity through reflex mechanisms.

The diagnosis and management of GERD and chronic aspiration are challenging. A discussion of strategies for the evaluation, prevention, and management of extraesophageal reflux manifestations can be found in Chapter 17.

3. Retention of an Aspirated Foreign Body

Retention of an aspirated foreign body in the tracheobronchial tree may produce both acute and chronic conditions, including atelectasis, postobstructive hyperinflation, acute or recurrent pneumonia, bronchiectasis, and lung abscess. Occasionally, a misdiagnosis of asthma, COPD, or lung cancer is made in adult patients who have aspirated a foreign body. CXR usually suggests the site of the foreign body. In some cases, an expiratory film, demonstrating regional hyperinflation due to a check-valve effect, is helpful. Bronchoscopy is usually necessary to establish the diagnosis and attempt removal of the foreign body.

4. Aspiration of Toxic Material

Aspiration of toxic material into the lung usually results in clinically evident pneumonia. **Hydrocarbon pneumonitis** is caused by aspiration of ingested petroleum distillates, eg, gasoline, kerosene, furniture polish, and other household petroleum products. Lung injury results mainly from vomiting of ingested products and secondary aspiration. Therapy is supportive. The lung should be protected from repeated aspiration with a cuffed endotracheal tube if necessary. **Lipoid pneumonia** is a chronic syndrome related to the repeated aspiration of oily materials, eg, mineral oil, cod liver oil, and oily nose drops; it usually occurs in older patients with impaired swallowing. Patchy opacities in dependent lung zones and lipid-laden macrophages in expectorated sputum are characteristic findings.

Santos LB et al. Effect of various perioperative semaglutide interruption intervals on residual gastric content assessed by esophagogastroduodenoscopy: a retrospective single center observational study. J Clin Anesth. 2024;99:111668. [PMID: 39476514]

Simpson AJ et al. BTS clinical statement on aspiration pneumonia. Thorax. 2023;78:s3. [PMID: 36863772]

Zhang D et al. Antibiotics versus non-antibiotic in the treatment of aspiration pneumonia: analysis of the MIMIC-IV database. BMC Pulm Med. 2024;24:621. [PMID: 39695560]

OCCUPATIONAL PULMONARY DISEASES

Many acute and chronic pulmonary diseases are related to inhalation of noxious substances encountered in the workplace. Disorders linked to occupational exposures may be classified as: (1) pneumoconioses, (2) hypersensitivity pneumonitis, (3) obstructive airway disorders, (4) toxic lung injury, (5) lung cancer, (6) pleural diseases, and (7) other.

1. Pneumoconioses

Pneumoconioses are chronic fibrotic lung diseases caused by the inhalation of inert inorganic dusts. Pneumoconioses range from asymptomatic disorders with diffuse nodular opacities on CXR to severe, symptomatic, life-shortening disorders. Clinically important pneumoconioses include coal worker's pneumoconiosis, silicosis, and asbestosis (Table 9–20). Treatment for each is supportive; pulmonary rehabilitation may be considered.

A. Coal Worker's Pneumoconiosis

In coal worker's pneumoconiosis, ingestion of inhaled coal dust by alveolar macrophages leads to the formation of coal macules, usually 2–5 mm in diameter, that appear on CXR as diffuse small opacities that are especially prominent in the upper lung. Simple coal worker's pneumoconiosis is usually asymptomatic with minimal impact on PFTs. In complicated coal worker's pneumoconiosis (**"progressive massive fibrosis"**), conglomeration and contraction in the upper lung zones occur, with radiographic features resembling complicated silicosis.

B. Silicosis

In silicosis, extensive or prolonged inhalation of free silica (silicon dioxide) particles (sandblasters, foundry, granite and stone cutting, molding, ceramics) in the respirable

Table 9–20. Selected pneumoconioses.

Disease	Agent	Occupations
Asbestosis	Asbestos	Mining, insulation, construction, shipbuilding
Baritosis	Barium salts	Glass and insecticide manufacturing
Coal worker's pneumoconiosis	Coal dust	Coal mining
Kaolin pneumoconiosis	Sand, mica, aluminum silicate	Mining of chine clay; pottery and cement work
Shaver disease	Aluminum powder	Manufacture of corundum
Siderosis	Metallic iron or iron oxide	Mining, welding, foundry work
Silicosis	Free silica (silicon dioxide)	Rock mining, quarrying, stone cutting, tunneling, sandblasting, pottery, diatomaceous earth
Stannosis	Tin, tin oxide	Mining, tin-working, smelting
Talcosis	Magnesium silicate	Mining, insulation, construction, shipbuilding

range (0.3–5 mcm) causes the formation of small, rounded opacities (silicotic nodules) throughout the lung. Calcification of the periphery of hilar lymph nodes ("egg-shell" calcification) is an unusual radiographic finding that strongly suggests silicosis. Simple silicosis is usually asymptomatic and without change on routine PFTs; in complicated silicosis, large conglomerate densities appear in the upper lung and are accompanied by dyspnea and obstructive and restrictive pulmonary dysfunction. The incidence of pulmonary tuberculosis is increased in patients with silicosis. All patients with silicosis should have a tuberculin skin test and a CXR to rule out tuberculosis.

C. Asbestosis

Asbestosis is a nodular interstitial fibrosis occurring in workers exposed to asbestos fibers (shipyard and construction workers, pipe fitters, insulators) over many years (typically 10–20 years). Patients with asbestosis usually first seek medical attention at least 15 years after exposure with the following symptoms and signs: progressive dyspnea, inspiratory crackles, and in some cases, clubbing and cyanosis. The radiographic features of asbestosis include linear streaking at the lung bases, opacities of various shapes and sizes, and honeycomb changes in advanced cases. The presence of pleural plaques may be a clue to diagnosis. HRCT scanning is the best imaging method for asbestosis because of its ability to detect parenchymal fibrosis and define the presence of coexisting pleural plaques. Cigarette smoking in asbestos workers increases the prevalence of radiographic pleural and parenchymal changes and markedly increases the incidence of lung carcinoma. It may also interfere with the clearance of short asbestos fibers from the lung. PFTs show restrictive dysfunction and reduced diffusing capacity. There is no specific treatment.

Hang W et al. Research progress on the pathogenesis and prediction of pneumoconiosis among coal miners. Environ Geochem Health. 2024;46:319. [PMID: 39012521]
Lee J et al. Computed tomography of contemporary occupational lung disease: a pictorial review. Diagnostics (Basel). 2024;14:1786. [PMID: 39202274]
Sun D et al. Candidate gene polymorphisms associated with silicosis and coal workers' pneumoconiosis: a systematic review and meta-analysis. BMC Pulm Med. 2024;24:580. [PMID: 39578762]

2. Hypersensitivity Pneumonitis

Hypersensitivity pneumonitis (also called extrinsic allergic alveolitis) is a nonatopic, nonasthmatic inflammatory pulmonary disease precipitated by exposure to an inhaled organic antigen such as microbial, avian, and animal antigens, and less commonly to an inorganic agent (Table 9–21). The immunologic hypersensitivity reaction leads to an acute illness. Prompt diagnosis is essential since symptoms are usually reversible if the offending antigen is removed from the patient's environment early in the course of illness. Continued exposure may lead to progressive fibrotic or nonfibrotic disease The histopathology of acute hypersensitivity pneumonitis is characterized by interstitial infiltrates of lymphocytes and plasma cells, with noncaseating granulomas in the interstitium and air spaces.

Table 9–21. Selected causes of hypersensitivity pneumonitis.

Disease	Antigen	Source
Farmer's lung	*Saccharopolyspora rectivirgula* (formerly, *Micropolyspora faeni*), *Thermoactinomyces vulgaris*	Moldy hay
"Humidifier" lung	Thermophilic actinomycetes	Contaminated humidifiers, heating systems, or air conditioners
Bird fancier's lung	Avian proteins	Bird serum and excreta
Bagassosis	*Thermoactinomyces sacchari* and *T vulgaris*	Moldy sugar cane fiber (bagasse)
Sequoiosis	*Graphium*, *Aureobasidium*, and other fungi	Moldy redwood sawdust
Maple bark stripper's disease	*Cryptostroma (Coniosporium) corticale*	Rotting maple tree logs or bark
Mushroom picker's disease	Same as farmer's lung	Moldy compost
Suberosis	*Penicillium frequentans*	Moldy cork dust
Detergent worker's lung	*Bacillus subtilis* enzyme	Enzyme additives

Clinical Findings

A. Acute Illness

Cough and dyspnea develop within days to weeks of exposure; constitutional symptoms such as low-grade fever, chills, and malaise are less common. Inspiratory squeaks on chest auscultation are characteristic when present. Small nodular densities sparing the apices and bases of the lungs are noted on CXR. Laboratory studies reveal an increase in the WBC count with a shift to the left, hypoxemia, and the presence in serum of precipitating antibodies to the offending agent. Hypersensitivity pneumonitis antibody panels against common offending antigens are available; positive results, while supportive, do not establish a definitive diagnosis. PFTs reveal restrictive dysfunction and reduced diffusing capacity.

B. Subacute and Chronic Illness

A subacute hypersensitivity pneumonitis syndrome (15% of cases) is characterized by the insidious onset of chronic cough and, with continued exposure, slowly progressive dyspnea, anorexia, and weight loss. Characteristic HRCT findings of nonfibrotic disease include upper- or mid-lung ground-glass or nodular opacities and signs of air trapping. Fibrotic disease is characterized by reticulation either in a random or mid-lung zone distribution. Surgical lung biopsy may be necessary for the diagnosis of subacute and chronic hypersensitivity pneumonitis, although the histopathologic patterns are nonspecific and overlap with several IIP.

Treatment

Treatment of acute hypersensitivity pneumonitis consists of identification of the offending agent and avoidance of further exposure. In severe acute or protracted cases, oral corticosteroids (prednisone, 0.5 mg/kg daily as a single morning dose for 2 weeks, tapered to nil over 4–6 weeks) may be given. Change in occupation is often required.

Barnes H et al. Diagnosis and management of hypersensitivity pneumonitis in adults: a position statement from the Thoracic Society of Australia and New Zealand. Respirology. 2024;29:1023. [PMID: 39467777]
Koster MA et al. Diagnosis of hypersensitivity pneumonitis in adults, 2020 clinical practice guideline: summary for clinicians. Ann Am Thorac Soc. 2021;18:559. [PMID: 33141595]

3. Obstructive Airway Disorders

Occupational pulmonary diseases manifested as obstructive airway disorders include occupational asthma and byssinosis.

A. Occupational Asthma

Asthma is one of the most common presentations of occupational lung disease. Approximately 25% of all cases of asthma are related to occupation. Offending agents in the workplace are numerous and classified into low- and high-molecular weight chemicals. High-molecular weight chemicals include animal proteins, flours, enzymes such as pancreatic extracts, and plant-based proteins such as wheat, grain dust, coffee beans, tobacco dust, and tobacco. Low-molecular weight inhaled agents include isocyanates, anhydrides, metals, pharmaceutical drugs, wood dust, dyes and bleaches, resins and glue, and various other agents. Treatment consists of avoidance of further exposure to the offending agent and bronchodilators, but symptoms may persist for years after workplace exposure has been terminated.

Barber CM et al. British Thoracic Society clinical statement on occupational asthma. Thorax. 2022;77:433. [PMID: 35314486]
Lantto J et al. Long-term clinical follow-up of irritant-induced occupational asthma. Occup Environ Med. 2024;81:588. [PMID: 39537354]

B. Byssinosis

Byssinosis is an asthma-like disorder in textile workers caused by inhalation of cotton dust. Repeated exposure leads to chronic bronchitis.

4. Lung Cancer

Many industrial pulmonary carcinogens have been identified, including asbestos, radon gas, arsenic, iron, chromium, nickel, coal tar fumes, petroleum oil mists, isopropyl oil, mustard gas, and printing ink. Cigarette smoking acts as a cocarcinogen with asbestos and radon gas to cause bronchogenic carcinoma. Asbestos alone causes malignant mesothelioma.

5. Other Occupational Pulmonary Diseases

Occupational diseases of the pleura may result from exposure to asbestos or talc. Inhalation of talc causes pleural plaques that are like those caused by asbestos. In some asbestos workers, benign asbestos pleural effusions (BAPE) occur, which are typically small, unilateral, and precede the onset of ILD. Pleural adhesions at the site of BAPE may cause a "rounded atelectasis" appearance on CXR. Occupational agents are also responsible for other pulmonary disorders, with a range of pathologies including occupational COPD, and ILDs. For this reason, it is important to obtain a thorough occupational history in any patient presenting with pulmonary symptoms.

Barnes H et al. Occupational interstitial lung diseases. Immunol Allergy Clin North Am. 2023;43:323. [PMID: 37055091]
Cohen RA et al. Global trends in occupational lung disease. Semin Respir Crit Care Med. 2023;44:317. [PMID: 37072021]

MEDICATION-INDUCED LUNG DISEASE

Typical patterns of pulmonary response to medications implicated in medication-induced respiratory disease are summarized in Table 9–22. Pulmonary injury due to medications occurs because of allergic reactions, idiosyncratic reactions, overdose, or undesirable side effects. In most patients, the mechanism of pulmonary injury is unknown.

Precise diagnosis of medication-induced pulmonary disease is often difficult because results of routine laboratory studies are not helpful and radiographic findings are not specific. A high index of suspicion and a thorough history of medication usage are critical to establishing the diagnosis of medication-induced lung disease. The clinical response to cessation of the suspected offending agent is also helpful. Acute episodes of medication-induced pulmonary disease may disappear 24–48 hours after the medication has been discontinued, but chronic syndromes may take longer to resolve. Challenge tests to confirm the diagnosis are risky and rarely performed.

Treatment of medication-induced lung disease consists of discontinuing the offending agent immediately, managing the pulmonary symptoms appropriately, and treating with corticosteroids if pulmonary toxicity is rapidly progressive. Observational data support the use of corticosteroids in severe cases; however, controlled data are lacking. Immune checkpoint inhibitors, commonly used treatments for a variety of malignant and nonmalignant conditions, are associated with a 5% risk of pneumonitis with up to 20% mortality when severe. Observational data support concurrent corticosteroid treatment in these cases.

Inhalation of crack cocaine may cause a spectrum of acute pulmonary syndromes, including pulmonary infiltration with eosinophilia, pneumothorax and pneumomediastinum, bronchiolitis obliterans, and acute respiratory failure associated with diffuse alveolar damage and alveolar hemorrhage. Corticosteroids have been used with variable success to treat alveolar hemorrhage.

Table 9–22. Pulmonary manifestations of selected medication toxicities (listed alphabetically within category).

Asthma	**Pulmonary edema**
Acetylcysteine	Cardiogenic
Aerosolized pentamidine	β-Blockers
Any nebulized medication	Noncardiogenic
Aspirin	Aspirin
β-Blockers	Chlordiazepoxide
Histamine	Cocaine
Methacholine	Ethchlorvynol
NSAIDs	Heroin/opiates
Chronic cough	**Pleural effusion**
ACE inhibitors	Any drug inducing SLE
Pulmonary infiltration	Bromocriptine
Without eosinophilia	Chemotherapeutic agents (eg, carmustine, cyclophosphamide, dasatinib, docetaxel, GM-CSF, methotrexate)
Amiodarone	Methysergide
Amitriptyline	Nitrofurantoin
Azathioprine	Tyrosine kinase inhibitors
With eosinophilia	**Mediastinal widening**
Crack cocaine	Corticosteroids
L-Tryptophan	Methotrexate
Methotrexate	Phenytoin
Nitrofurantoin	**Respiratory failure**
Penicillin	Neuromuscular blockade
Sulfonamides	Aminoglycosides
Drug-induced SLE	Paralytic agents
Chlorpromazine	CNS depression
Hydralazine	Alcohol
Isoniazid	Hypnotics
Phenytoin	Opioids
Procainamide	Sedatives
Interstitial pneumonitis/fibrosis	Tricyclic antidepressants
Bleomycin	
Busulfan	
Cyclophosphamide	
Immune checkpoint inhibitors	
Methysergide	
Nitrofurantoin	
Phenytoin	

GM-CSF, granulocyte-macrophage colony-stimulating factor.

Conte P et al. Drug-induced interstitial lung disease during cancer therapies: expert opinion on diagnosis and treatment. ESMO Open. 2022;7:100404. [PMID: 35219244]

Hu Q et al. Radiological assessment of immunotherapy effects and immune checkpoint-related pneumonitis for lung cancer. J Cell Mol Med. 2024;28:e17895. [PMID: 37525480]

RADIATION LUNG INJURY

The lung is an exquisitely radiosensitive organ that can be damaged by external beam radiation therapy. The degree of pulmonary injury is determined by the volume of lung irradiated, the dose and rate of exposure, and potentiating factors (eg, concurrent chemotherapy, previous radiation therapy in the same area, and simultaneous withdrawal of corticosteroid therapy). Symptomatic radiation lung injury occurs in about 10% of patients treated for carcinoma of the breast, 5–15% of patients treated for carcinoma of the lung, and 5–35% of patients treated for lymphoma. Two phases of the pulmonary response are apparent: an acute phase (radiation pneumonitis) and a chronic phase (radiation fibrosis).

1. Radiation Pneumonitis

Acute radiation pneumonitis usually occurs 4–12 weeks (range 1–6 months) after completion of radiotherapy and is characterized by insidious onset of dyspnea, intractable dry cough, chest fullness or pain, weakness, and fever. Late radiation pneumonitis may develop 6–12 months after completion of radiation. Occasionally, patients who are months to years removed from radiation therapy will experience "radiation recall" with an inflammatory reaction in the radiated region after treatment with a new round of chemotherapy; this phenomenon has also been reported with immune checkpoint inhibitors. Inspiratory crackles may be heard in the involved area. In severe disease, respiratory distress and cyanosis occur that are characteristic of ARDS. An increased WBC count and elevated ESR are common. PFTs reveal reduced lung volumes, reduced lung compliance, hypoxemia, reduced diffusing capacity, and reduced maximum voluntary ventilation. CXR, which correlates poorly with the presence of symptoms, usually demonstrates alveolar or nodular opacities limited to the irradiated area. Air bronchograms are often observed. Sharp borders of an opacity may help distinguish radiation pneumonitis from other conditions, such as infectious pneumonia, lymphangitic spread of carcinoma, and recurrent tumor; however, the opacity may extend beyond the radiation field.

No specific therapy is proven effective in radiation pneumonitis. Spontaneous resolution may occur in mild disease, but prednisone (1 mg/kg/day orally) is commonly given immediately to patients with a more severe presentation or pulmonary function decline; higher doses may be given in patients who are critically ill. After 1 week, the dose is reduced and maintained at 20–40 mg/day for several weeks, then slowly tapered. Radiation pneumonitis may improve in 2–3 weeks following onset of symptoms as the exudative phase resolves. Acute respiratory failure, if present, is treated supportively. Death from ARDS is unusual in radiation pneumonitis.

Chen F et al. Re-evaluating the risk factors for radiation pneumonitis in the era of immunotherapy. J Clin Med. 2023;12:1442. [PMID: 36835977]

Wang Y et al. Cytological changes in radiation-induced lung injury. Life Sci. 2024;358:123188. [PMID: 39481833]

2. Pulmonary Radiation Fibrosis

Radiation fibrosis may occur with or without antecedent radiation pneumonitis. Radiographic findings include obliteration of normal lung markings, dense interstitial and pleural fibrosis, reduced lung volumes, tenting of the diaphragm, and sharp delineation of the irradiated area. No specific therapy is proven effective, and corticosteroids have no value. Pulmonary fibrosis may develop after an intervening period (6–12 months) of well-being in patients who experience radiation pneumonitis. Pulmonary radiation fibrosis occurs in most patients who receive a full course of radiation therapy for cancer of the lung or breast. Most patients are asymptomatic, although slowly progressive dyspnea may occur.

Salem PP et al. Proton radiation therapy: a systematic review of treatment-related side effects and toxicities. Int J Mol Sci. 2024;25:10969. [PMID: 39456752]

PLEURAL DISEASES

PLEURITIS

Pleuritic pain or "pleurisy" is due to inflammation of the parietal pleura. It is typically well localized, sharp, fleeting, and made worse by coughing, sneezing, deep breathing, or movement. The pain, which is felt over the chest wall, is due to the cutaneous distribution of the intercostal nerves innervating the rib cage and lateral portion of each hemidiaphragm. Inflammation of the parietal pleura or central diaphragm, which are innervated by phrenic nerve fibers, may cause pain that is referred to the ipsilateral shoulder or neck. There are numerous causes of pleuritis. In young, otherwise healthy individuals, pleuritis is usually caused by viral respiratory infections or pneumonia (including tuberculosis in endemic regions). Other causes include PE, inflammatory disorders (serositis), malignancy, and drug reactions. The presence of pleural effusion, pleural thickening, or air in the pleural space requires further diagnostic and therapeutic measures, including pleural fluid sampling and analysis.

Treatment of pleuritis consists of treating the underlying condition. Anti-inflammatory analgesic medications are often helpful for pain relief.

Guo H et al. Pleural diseases in connective tissue diseases. Semin Respir Crit Care Med. 2024;45:305. [PMID: 38547917]

PLEURAL EFFUSION

ESSENTIALS OF DIAGNOSIS

- May be asymptomatic; chest pain frequently seen in the setting of pleuritis, trauma, or infection; dyspnea is common with large effusions.
- Dullness to percussion and decreased breath sounds over the effusion.
- Radiographic evidence of pleural effusion.
- Diagnostic findings on thoracentesis.

General Considerations

A pleural effusion is an abnormal accumulation of fluid in the pleural space. Pleural effusions may be classified by differential diagnosis (Table 9–23) or by underlying pathophysiology. Five pathophysiologic processes account for most effusions: increased production of fluid in the setting of normal capillaries due to increased hydrostatic or decreased oncotic pressures **(transudates)**; increased production of fluid due to abnormal capillary permeability **(exudates)**; decreased lymphatic clearance of fluid from the pleural space **(exudates)**; infection in the pleural space **(empyema)**; and bleeding into the pleural space **(hemothorax)**.

Table 9–23. Causes of pleural fluid transudates and exudates.

Transudates	Exudates
HF Cirrhosis with ascites Nephrotic syndrome Peritoneal dialysis Myxedema Atelectasis (acute) Constrictive pericarditis Superior vena cava obstruction PE Hypoalbuminemia Pulmonary arterial hypertension Urinothorax	Pneumonia (parapneumonic effusion, including empyema) Cancer PE Bacterial infection (including empyema) Tuberculosis Viral infection Fungal infection Rickettsial infection Parasitic infection Connective tissue disease Asbestos Meigs syndrome Pancreatic disease Uremia Chronic atelectasis Chylothorax Sarcoidosis Drug reaction Post–myocardial injury syndrome Esophageal perforation Chest radiation therapy

Diagnostic thoracentesis should be performed whenever there is a new pleural effusion and no clinically apparent cause. Observation is appropriate in some situations (eg, symmetric bilateral pleural effusions in the setting of HF), but an atypical presentation or failure of an effusion to resolve as expected warrants thoracentesis to identify the underlying process.

Clinical Findings

A. Symptoms and Signs

Patients with pleural effusions most often report dyspnea, cough, or respirophasic chest pain. Symptoms are more common in patients with existing cardiopulmonary disease. Small pleural effusions are less likely to be symptomatic than larger effusions. Physical findings are usually absent in small effusions. Larger effusions cause dullness to percussion and diminished or absent breath sounds over the effusion. Compressive atelectasis may cause bronchial breath sounds and egophony just above the effusion. A massive effusion with increased intrapleural pressure may cause contralateral shift of the trachea and bulging of the intercostal spaces. A pleural friction rub indicates pulmonary infarction or pleuritis.

B. Laboratory Findings

The gross appearance of pleural fluid helps identify several types of pleural effusion. Purulent fluid signifies empyema. Milky white pleural fluid should be centrifuged. A clear supernatant above a pellet of white cells indicates empyema, whereas a persistently turbid supernatant suggests a **chylous effusion;** analysis of this supernatant reveals chylomicrons and a high triglyceride level (> 100 mg/dL [1 mmol/L]), often from disruption of the thoracic duct. **Hemorrhagic pleural effusion** is a mixture of blood and pleural fluid. Ten thousand red cells per microliter create blood-tinged pleural fluid; 100,000 red cells/mcL (100×10^9/L) create grossly bloody pleural fluid. **Hemothorax** is the presence of gross blood in the pleural space, usually following chest trauma or instrumentation. It is defined as a ratio of pleural fluid hematocrit to peripheral blood hematocrit > 0.5, however a lower ratio may occur with chronic hemothorax due to secondary dilution.

Pleural fluid samples should be sent for measurement of protein, glucose, and LD in addition to total and differential WBC counts. Additional testing may be warranted, depending on the diagnostic considerations. Chemistry determinations are used to classify effusions as transudates or exudates. This classification is important because the differential diagnosis and subsequent evaluation for each entity varies (see Table 9–23). A **pleural exudate** (as defined by Light's criteria) has one or more of the following laboratory features: (1) ratio of pleural fluid protein to serum protein > 0.5; (2) ratio of pleural fluid LD to serum LD > 0.6; or (3) pleural fluid LD > two-thirds the upper limit of normal serum LD. Alternative diagnostic criteria that do not require the simultaneous sampling of serum but that perform similarly include the "two-test" (pleural fluid cholesterol > 40 mg/dL, pleural fluid LD > 0.6 times upper limit of normal serum LD) and the "three-test" (pleural fluid cholesterol > 55 mg/dL, pleural fluid LD > 0.67 times upper limit of normal serum LD, pleural fluid protein > 3.0 g/dL). **Pleural transudates** occur in the setting of normal capillary integrity and have none of the laboratory features of exudates. A transudate suggests the absence of local pleural disease; characteristic laboratory findings include a glucose near to serum glucose, pH between 7.40 and 7.55, and fewer than 1000 WBCs/mcL (1.0×10^9/L) with a predominance of mononuclear cells. Discrimination of exudate from transudate is less reliable near the cutoff values for any of the criteria. In conditions such as HF, effective diuresis may increase the protein or LD concentration in the transudative pleural fluid as water is reabsorbed, thus creating a borderline "pseudoexudative" chemistry.

HF accounts for most transudates. Bacterial pneumonia, cancer, and tuberculosis (in endemic regions) are the most common causes of exudative effusion. Other common causes of exudates with characteristic laboratory findings are summarized in Table 9–24.

Pleural fluid pH (normal = 7.60) is useful in the assessment of parapneumonic effusions, if it can be reliably measured, and is more useful than glucose measurement in determining need for drainage. Measurements of pH are affected by the presence of residual lidocaine, saline or heparin in the collecting syringe, or storage of pleural fluid at room temperature for > 1 hour. A pH < 7.20 suggests a complex parapneumonic pleural effusion that may require drainage; however, other causes include rheumatoid arthritis, lupus, malignancy, esophageal rupture, hemothorax, and pancreatic-pleural fistula. An elevated pleural fluid amylase suggests acute pancreatitis, pancreatic pseudocyst, adenocarcinoma of the lung or pancreas, or esophageal rupture.

Suspected tuberculous pleural effusion should be evaluated by thoracentesis with AFB smear and culture, although pleural fluid culture positivity for *M tuberculosis* is low. Tests for pleural fluid adenosine deaminase (approximately 90% sensitivity and specificity for pleural tuberculosis at levels > 60 U/L, tuberculosis rare if level is < 40 U/L) and interferon-γ (89% sensitivity, 97% specificity) can be helpful diagnostic aids, particularly in making decisions to pursue invasive testing in complex patients. NAAT is not recommended as a diagnostic test for pleural TB due to its suboptimal performance. Closed pleural biopsy is more sensitive than pleural fluid culture for diagnosis, revealing granulomatous inflammation in approximately 60% of patients; culture of three pleural biopsy specimens combined with histologic examination of a pleural biopsy for granulomas yields a diagnosis in up to 90% of patients.

Between 40% and 80% of exudative pleural effusions are malignant, while > 90% of malignant pleural effusions are exudative. Almost any form of cancer may cause effusions, but the most common are lung (one-third) and breast cancer. In 5–10% of malignant pleural effusions, no primary tumor is identified.

Pleural fluid specimens should be sent for cytologic examination in all cases of exudative effusions in patients suspected of harboring an underlying malignancy. The diagnostic yield depends on the nature and extent of the underlying malignancy. Sensitivity is 50–65% from one sample, but may increase with serial sampling. In a patient with a high prior probability of malignancy, a negative cytologic examination should be followed by one repeat thoracentesis. If that examination is negative, thoracoscopy (sensitivity 92–96%) is preferred to closed pleural biopsy.

C. Imaging

The lung is less dense than water and floats on pleural fluid that accumulates in dependent regions. On a standard upright CXR (Figure 9–6), approximately 75–100 mL of pleural fluid must accumulate in the posterior costophrenic sulcus to be visible on the lateral view and 175–200 mL in the lateral costophrenic sulcus to be visible on the frontal view. Ultrasonography increases the safety of thoracentesis and should be incorporated routinely by trained users. Chest CT scans may identify as little as 10 mL of fluid and allows assessment of the entire thorax.

Pleural fluid may become trapped (loculated) by pleural adhesions, thereby forming unusual collections along the lateral chest wall or within lung fissures. Round or oval fluid collections in fissures that resemble intraparenchymal masses are called pseudotumors.

Table 9–24. Characteristics of important exudative pleural effusions.

Etiology or Type of Effusion	Gross Appearance	WBC Count (cells/mcL)	RBC Count (cells/mcL)	Glucose	Comments
Malignancy	Turbid to bloody; occasionally serous	1000–100,000 (1.0–100 × 10^9/L) M	100 (0.1 × 10^9/L) to several hundred thousand	Equal to serum levels; < 60 mg/dL in 15% of cases	Eosinophilia uncommon; positive results on cytologic examination
Uncomplicated parapneumonic	Clear to turbid	5000–25,000 (5.0–25 × 10^9/L) P	< 5000 (5.0 × 10^9/L)	Equal to serum levels	Tube thoracostomy unnecessary
Empyema	Turbid to purulent	25,000–100,000 (25–100 × 10^9/L) P	< 5000 (5.0 × 10^9/L)	Less than serum levels; often very low	Drainage necessary; putrid odor suggests anaerobic infection
Tuberculosis	Serous to serosanguineous	5000–10,000 (5.0–10 × 10^9/L) M	< 10,000 (10 × 10^9/L)	Equal to serum levels; occasionally < 60 mg/dL	Protein > 4.0 g/dL (may exceed 5 g/dL); frequently lymphocyte predominant (> 50%); eosinophils (> 10%) or mesothelial cells (> 5%) make diagnosis unlikely; see text for additional diagnostic tests
Rheumatoid	Turbid; greenish yellow	1000–20,000 (1.0–20 × 10^9/L) M or P	< 1000 (1.0 × 10^9/L)	< 40 mg/dL	Secondary empyema common; high LD, low complement, high rheumatoid factor, cholesterol crystals are characteristic
Pulmonary infarction	Serous to grossly bloody	1000–50,000 (1.0–50 × 10^9/L) M or P	100 (0.1 × 10^9/L) to > 100,000 (100 × 10^9/L)	Equal to serum levels	Variable findings; no pathognomonic features
Esophageal rupture	Turbid to purulent; red-brown	< 5000 (5.0 × 10^9/L) to > 50,000 (50 × 10^9/L) P	1000–10,000 (1.0–10 × 10^9/L)	Usually low	High amylase level (salivary origin); pneumothorax in 25% of cases; effusion usually on left side; pH < 6.0 strongly suggests diagnosis
Pancreatitis	Turbid to serosanguineous	1000–50,000 (1.0–50 × 10^9/L) P	1000–10,000 (1.0–10 × 10^9/L)	Equal to serum levels	Usually left-sided; high amylase level

M, mononuclear cell predominance; P, polymorphonuclear leukocyte predominance.

Treatment

A. Transudative Pleural Effusion

Transudative pleural effusions characteristically occur in the absence of pleural disease. Therefore, treatment is directed at the underlying condition. Therapeutic thoracentesis for severe dyspnea typically offers only transient benefit. Pleurodesis or indwelling pleural catheters are rarely indicated but are appropriate for management of symptoms in selected patients whose symptoms respond to drainage and whose effusions are refractory to maximal medical therapy.

B. Malignant Pleural Effusion

Adopting a patient centered approach for management of a symptomatic malignant pleural effusion should include patient's life expectancy, performance status, risk for infections, the ability to re-expand the atelectatic lung, patient's preference, size or recurrence of the pleural effusion, and tumor chemosensitivity. Chemotherapy, radiation therapy, or both offer temporary control in some malignant effusions but are generally ineffective in lung cancer in the pleural space except for small-cell lung cancer. Asymptomatic malignant effusions usually do not require specific treatment. Symptomatic patients should be offered pleural drainage, either via initial therapeutic thoracentesis to determine symptomatic response to drainage, following which an indwelling pleural catheter can be placed, or via immediate placement of an indwelling pleural catheter. Indwelling pleural catheter placement is associated with shorter hospital stays than pleurodesis. The decision between indwelling pleural catheter versus pleurodesis is often dependent on multiple factors which include presence of expandable lung, rate of re-accumulation of the effusion, predicted response to chemotherapy, patient prognosis and functional status, patient preference, and institutional resources. Indwelling pleural catheters often effect a pleurodesis over time, at which point the catheter can be removed. Adverse effects of indwelling pleural catheters can include infections, metastases, and bleeding,

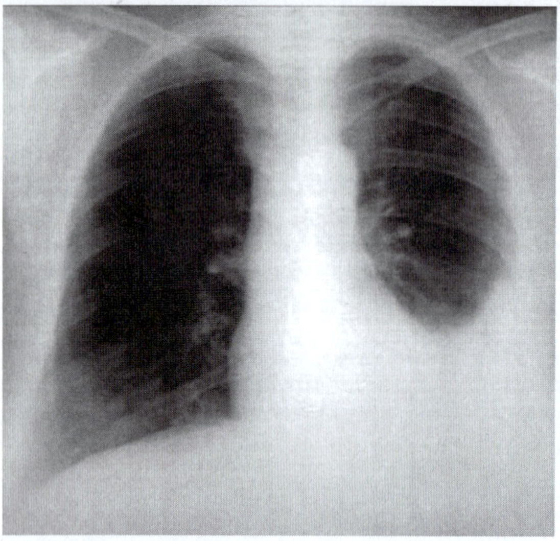

▲ **Figure 9–6.** Left pleural effusion. Frontal CXR showing a meniscus-shaped density at the left costophrenic angle sulcus indicative of a moderate-sized pleural effusion. (Reproduced, with permission, from Lechner AJ, Matuschak GM, Brink DS. *Respiratory: An Integrated Approach to Disease*. McGraw-Hill, 2012.)

while pleurodesis can cause post procedural pain and, in rare circumstances, acute respiratory complications.

C. Parapneumonic Pleural Effusion

Parapneumonic pleural effusions are divided into three categories, the classification of which can only be determined by sampling the fluid: uncomplicated (simple), complicated, and empyema. **Uncomplicated (simple) parapneumonic effusions** are free-flowing sterile exudates of modest size that resolve quickly with antibiotic treatment of pneumonia. They do not need drainage.

Complicated parapneumonic effusions present the most difficult management decisions. They tend to be larger than simple parapneumonic effusions and to show more evidence of inflammatory stimuli, such as low glucose level, low pH, or evidence of loculation. Tube thoracostomy usually is indicated when pleural fluid glucose is < 60 mg/dL (< 3.3 mmol/L) or the pH is < 7.2. The clinician may also consider drainage of a complicated effusion if the pleural fluid pH is between 7.2 and 7.3 or the LD is > 1000 U/L (> 20 mckat/L). Pleural fluid cell count and protein have little diagnostic value in this setting.

Empyema is gross infection of the pleural space indicated by positive Gram stain or culture. The patient should undergo drainage promptly and be referred to a thoracic specialist to determine whether tube thoracostomy versus decortication is needed to facilitate clearance of infection and reduce the probability of permanent fibrous encasement of the lung.

Tube thoracostomy drainage of empyema or complicated parapneumonic effusions is frequently complicated by loculation that prevents adequate drainage. Intrapleural instillation of fibrinolytic agents alone has not been shown in controlled trials to improve drainage. The combination of intrapleural tissue plasminogen activator and deoxyribonuclease (DNase) has been found to improve clinical outcome (increased drainage, decreased length of stay, and decreased surgical referral) compared with placebo or either agent alone, and should be considered when fever, leukocytosis, or anorexia persist despite antibiotics and tube thoracostomy, or when the lung fails to re-expand. Data suggest that tube thoracostomy with intrapleural enzyme treatment performs comparably to early surgical intervention.

D. Hemothorax

A small-volume hemothorax that is stable or improving on imaging may be managed by close observation. In all other cases, thoracic surgery consultation is indicated and immediate treatment rendered by insertion of a thoracostomy tube to (1) drain existing blood and clot and prevent lung entrapment, (2) quantify the amount of bleeding, (3) reduce the risk of fibrothorax, and (4) permit apposition of the pleural surfaces to reduce hemorrhage. Interventional radiology consultation and intervention may be indicated if the cause is intercostal bleeding. Thoracotomy may be required to control hemorrhage, remove clot, and treat complications.

Bedawi EO et al. Early video-assisted thoracoscopic surgery or intrapleural enzyme therapy in pleural infection: a feasibility randomized controlled trial. The third Multicenter Intrapleural Sepsis Trial – MIST-3. AJRCCM. 2023;12:1305. [PMID: 37820359]

Bedawi EO et al. ERS/ESTS statement on the management of pleural infection in adults. Eur Respir J. 2023;61:2201062. [PMID: 36229045]

Roberts ME et al. British Thoracic Society Guideline for pleural disease. Thorax. 2023;78(Suppl 3):s1. [PMID: 37433578]

Sundaralingam A et al. ERS statement on benign pleural effusion in adults. Eur Respir J. 2024;64:2302307. [PMID: 39060018]

PNEUMOTHORAX

ESSENTIALS OF DIAGNOSIS

- Acute onset of unilateral chest pain and dyspnea.
- Minimal physical findings in mild cases; unilateral chest expansion, decreased tactile fremitus, hyperresonance, diminished breath sounds, mediastinal shift, cyanosis, and hypotension in tension pneumothorax.
- Presence of pleural air on imaging.

General Considerations

Pneumothorax, or accumulation of air in the pleural space, is classified as spontaneous (primary or secondary), traumatic, or iatrogenic. **Primary spontaneous pneumothorax** occurs in the absence of an underlying lung disease, whereas **secondary spontaneous pneumothorax** is a complication of preexisting pulmonary disease. **Traumatic**

pneumothorax results from penetrating or blunt trauma and includes **iatrogenic pneumothorax** following procedures, such as thoracentesis, pleural biopsy, central venous catheter placement, percutaneous lung biopsy, bronchoscopy, and positive-pressure mechanical ventilation. **Tension pneumothorax** is an emergency that usually occurs in the setting of penetrating trauma, lung infection, CPR, or positive-pressure mechanical ventilation. In tension pneumothorax, the pressure of air in the pleural space exceeds alveolar and venous pressures throughout the respiratory cycle, resulting in compression of lung and reduction of venous return to the hemithorax; a check-valve mechanism may allow air to enter the pleural space on inspiration and to prevent egress of air on expiration.

Primary spontaneous pneumothorax is more likely among tall, thin, young (age < 45 years) individuals, more commonly men. It is thought to occur from rupture of subpleural apical blebs in response to high negative intrapleural pressures. Cigarette smoking is correlated with occurrence of primary spontaneous pneumothorax, as are connective tissue disorders such as Marfan and Ehlers-Danlos syndromes.

Secondary pneumothorax occurs as a complication of COPD, ILD, asthma, CF, tuberculosis, *Pneumocystis* pneumonia, necrotizing bacterial pneumonia, menstruation (catamenial pneumothorax), and a wide variety of cystic lung diseases, including lymphangioleiomyomatosis, tuberous sclerosis, Langerhans cell histiocytosis, and Birt-Hogg-Dube syndrome. Secondary pneumothorax, particularly in patients with underlying symptomatic lung disease, is more poorly tolerated due to the decreased respiratory reserve in this group.

Clinical Findings

A. Symptoms and Signs

Chest pain and dyspnea occur in nearly all patients, and cough is commonly reported. Pneumothorax may present with life-threatening respiratory failure if underlying lung disease is present or if tension pneumothorax physiology ensues.

If pneumothorax is small (< 15% of a hemithorax), physical findings, other than mild tachycardia, are normal. If pneumothorax is large, diminished breath sounds, decreased tactile fremitus, decreased movement of the chest, and hyper-resonant percussion note are often found. Tension pneumothorax should be suspected in the presence of marked tachycardia, hypotension, and mediastinal or tracheal shift.

B. Laboratory Findings

ABG analysis is often unnecessary but reveals hypoxemia and acute respiratory alkalosis in most patients. Left-sided primary pneumothorax may produce QRS axis and precordial T-wave changes on the ECG that may be misinterpreted as acute MI.

C. Imaging

Demonstration on CXR of lucency without lung markings between the chest wall and lung, and visualization of the visceral pleura (a "pleural line") is diagnostic. A few patients have secondary pleural effusion that demonstrates a characteristic air-fluid level on CXR. In supine patients, pneumothorax on a conventional CXR may appear as an abnormally radiolucent costophrenic sulcus (the "deep sulcus" sign). In patients with tension pneumothorax, CXRs show a large amount of air in the affected hemithorax and contralateral shift of the mediastinum.

Chest ultrasonography, performed at the bedside by experienced clinicians or technicians, demonstrates characteristic findings in the region of the pneumothorax. These findings include absent "lung sliding," or absent "lung pulse," or presence of a "lung point," all of which demonstrate a region of lung where the parietal and visceral pleural are not in normal apposition. Ultrasound may be more sensitive than supine CXR (supine positioning necessitated by clinical circumstance) for detecting pneumothorax in trauma patients and is frequently used in critical care, though comparisons of ultrasound to CXR or to CT scan report variable test characteristics.

Chest CT scan is more accurate than CXR for evaluating the size of a pneumothorax and identifying secondary pneumothorax etiologies such as cystic lung disease. However, its use as a first-line examination is limited due to higher costs, longer imaging times, and increased radiation exposure.

Differential Diagnosis

If the patient is young with typical clinical characteristics, the diagnosis of primary spontaneous pneumothorax is usually obvious and can be confirmed by CXR. In secondary pneumothorax, it is sometimes difficult to distinguish loculated pneumothorax from an emphysematous bleb. Occasionally, pneumothorax may mimic MI, PE, or pneumonia.

Complications

Tension pneumothorax may be life-threatening. Pneumomediastinum and subcutaneous emphysema may occur as complications of spontaneous pneumothorax. If pneumomediastinum is detected, rupture of the esophagus or a bronchus should be considered in the differential diagnosis.

Treatment

Treatment depends on the severity of the pneumothorax, based on size and symptoms, and the nature of the underlying disease. In a reliable patient with a stable, spontaneous primary pneumothorax, observation alone may be appropriate; many cases resolve spontaneously as air is absorbed from the pleural space. These patients should have no oxygen requirement, no limitation to ambulation, no increase in size of pneumothorax over 4 hours of monitoring, and be deemed reliable to return for care. Application of oxygen may hasten the resolution of the pneumothorax. Simple needle aspiration drainage of pleural air with a small-bore catheter (eg, 16-gauge angiocatheter or larger drainage catheter) can be performed for spontaneous primary pneumothoraxes that are large or progressive. Length of hospital stay appears to be shorter for conservative management (observation or needle aspiration) of primary spontaneous pneumothorax. Placement of a small-bore chest tube (7F to 14F) attached to a one-way Heimlich valve provides protection against development of tension pneumothorax and may permit observation from home. The patient should be treated symptomatically for cough and chest pain and monitored with serial CXRs every 24 hours.

Patients with secondary pneumothorax, tension pneumothorax, or severe symptoms; or those who have a pneumothorax on mechanical ventilation, should undergo chest tube placement (tube thoracostomy). The chest tube is placed under water-seal drainage, and suction is applied until the lung expands. The chest tube can be removed after the air leak subsides; prior to tube removal a clamping trial may first be performed, particularly in cases of secondary pneumothorax.

All patients who smoke should be advised to discontinue smoking and warned that the risk of recurrence is higher if cigarette smoking is continued.

Indications for surgical management (VATS) include recurrences of spontaneous pneumothorax, any occurrence of bilateral pneumothorax, and failure of tube thoracostomy for the first episode (failure of lung to re-expand or persistent air leak). Surgical intervention is also generally recommended for any patient with a secondary pneumothorax (presence of underlying lung disease) because the risk of recurrence is high, and the consequences of recurrences are greater. Surgery permits resection or repair of blebs or bullae responsible for the pneumothorax as well as mechanical or chemical pleurodesis. Patients who are not acceptable surgical candidates can be treated with chemical pleurodesis via a chest tube. Endobronchial valves may be considered for a persistent air leak.

Prognosis

About 30% of patients with spontaneous pneumothorax experience recurrence after either observation or tube thoracostomy for the first episode. Recurrence after surgical therapy is less frequent. Following successful therapy, there are no long-term complications. Secondary pneumothorax has up to a 50% likelihood of recurrence following the first event if surgical intervention is not undertaken.

Barton ED et al. The medical management of spontaneous pneumothorax: a concise review. Br J Hosp Med (Long) 2024;85:1. [PMID: 39347673]

Cheng HS et al. Management of spontaneous pneumothorax: a mini-review on its latest evidence. J Thorac Dis. 2024;16:4756. [PMID: 39144356]

Roberts ME et al. British Thoracic Society Guideline for pleural disease. Thorax. 2023;78(Suppl 3):s1. [PMID: 37433578]

DISORDERS OF CONTROL OF VENTILATION

The principal influences on ventilatory control are arterial PCO_2, pH, PO_2, and brainstem tissue pH. These variables are monitored by peripheral and central chemoreceptors. Under normal conditions, the ventilatory control system maintains arterial pH and PCO_2 within narrow limits; arterial PO_2 is more loosely controlled.

Abnormal control of ventilation can be seen with a variety of conditions ranging from rare disorders, such as primary alveolar hypoventilation, COVID-19, neuromuscular disorders, myxedema, starvation, and carotid body resection, to more common disorders, such as asthma, COPD, obesity, HF, and sleep-related breathing disorders. A few of these disorders will be discussed in this section.

HYPERVENTILATION SYNDROMES

Hyperventilation is an increase in alveolar minute ventilation that leads to hypocapnia. It may be caused by a variety of conditions, such as pregnancy, hypoxemia, obstructive and infiltrative lung diseases, sepsis, DKA, liver dysfunction, fever, and pain. Functional hyperventilation may be acute or chronic. **Acute hyperventilation** presents with hyperpnea, anxiety, paresthesia, carpopedal spasm, and tetany. Once organic causes of hyperventilation have been excluded, treatment of acute hyperventilation consists of breathing through pursed lips or through the nose with one nostril pinched or rebreathing expired gas from a paper bag held over the face to decrease respiratory alkalemia and its associated symptoms. Anxiolytic drugs may also be useful. **Chronic hyperventilation** may present with various nonspecific symptoms, including fatigue, dyspnea, anxiety, palpitations, and dizziness. The diagnosis of chronic hyperventilation syndrome is established if symptoms are reproduced during voluntary hyperventilation. When the symptoms are associated with paresthesia and dizziness, the diagnosis is often overlooked. Patients often report poor quality of life and most recently condition is described in post COVID syndrome and long COVID syndrome.

Genecand L et al. Dysfunctional breathing symptoms, functional impact and quality of life in patients with long COVD-19: a prospective case series. BMJ Open Respir Res. BMJ Open Respir Res. 2023;1:e001770. [PMID: 37433720]

Tavel ME. Hyperventilation syndrome: why is it regularly overlooked? Am J Med. 2021;134:13. [PMID: 32791056]

OBESITY-HYPOVENTILATION SYNDROME (Pickwickian Syndrome)

In obesity-hypoventilation syndrome, awake alveolar hypoventilation appears to result from a combination of blunted ventilatory drive and increased mechanical load imposed upon the chest by obesity. Diagnostic criteria include BMI > 30, an arterial partial pressure of carbon dioxide > 45 mm Hg, sleep disordered breathing, and exclusion of other causes of alveolar hypoventilation. Most patients with obesity-hypoventilation syndrome also suffer from obstructive sleep apnea (90% of patients with obesity-hypoventilation syndrome), which must be treated aggressively if identified as a comorbid disorder. Therapy of obesity-hypoventilation syndrome consists mainly of continuous positive airway pressure to treat the underlying obstructive sleep apnea or noninvasive ventilation when hypoventilation and hypercapnia predominates over obstructive sleep apnea. Lifestyle modification, including weight loss and rehabilitation strategies, in turn improves hypercapnia and hypoxemia as well as the ventilatory responses to hypoxia and hypercapnia; physiological responses described mostly in first year of bariatric surgery. Finally, targeting management of comorbidities, particularly during an exacerbation of respiratory failure, such as treatment of ACS, PE, pneumonia or decompensated HF should be managed aggressively. Avoidance of sedative-hypnotics, opioids, and alcohol is also recommended. The use of respiratory stimulants such as medroxyprogesterone and acetazolamide has been studied and improves $PaCO_2$ and PaO_2; however, they incur side effects and should only be used cautiously. Patients with obesity-hypoventilation syndrome have a higher risk of complications in the perioperative period, including respiratory failure, intubation, and HF. Recognition of these patients in the perioperative period is an important safety measure.

Orozco González BN et al. Obesity hypoventilation syndrome, literature review. Sleep Adv. 2024;5:zpae033 [PMID: 38966619]

SLEEP-RELATED BREATHING DISORDERS

Abnormal ventilation during sleep is manifested by apnea (breath cessation for at least 10 seconds) or hypopnea (decrement in airflow with drop in oxygen saturation of at least 4%). Episodes of apnea are **central** if ventilatory effort is absent for the duration of the apneic episode, **obstructive** if ventilatory effort persists throughout the apneic episode but no airflow occurs because of transient obstruction of the upper airway, or **mixed**. Obstructive and mixed sleep apneas are more common and may be associated with daytime somnolence that impacts quality of life and, in severe form, is associated with severe hypoxemia during sleep that may cause life-threatening cardiac arrhythmias, pulmonary hypertension, right-sided HF, systemic hypertension, and secondary erythrocytosis. Central sleep apnea is less prevalent in the general population. It may be an isolated finding or may occur in patients with HF, stroke with brainstem lesions, and opioid medication use.

Javaheri S et al. Central sleep apnea: pathophysiologic classification. Sleep. 2023;46:zsac113. [PMID: 35551411]

OBSTRUCTIVE SLEEP APNEA

ESSENTIALS OF DIAGNOSIS

- Daytime somnolence or fatigue.
- A history of loud snoring with witnessed apneic events.
- Overnight polysomnography demonstrating apneic episodes with hypoxemia.

General Considerations

Upper airway obstruction during sleep occurs when loss of normal pharyngeal muscle tone allows the pharynx to collapse passively during inspiration. Patients with anatomically narrowed upper airways (eg, micrognathia, macroglossia, obesity, tonsillar hypertrophy) are predisposed to the development of obstructive sleep apnea. Ingestion of alcohol or sedatives before sleeping or nasal obstruction of any type, including the common cold, may precipitate or worsen the condition. Hypothyroidism and cigarette smoking are additional risk factors for obstructive sleep apnea. Before making the diagnosis of obstructive sleep apnea, a drug history should be obtained; a seizure disorder, narcolepsy, and depression should be excluded.

Clinical Findings

A. Symptoms and Signs

Most patients with obstructive or mixed sleep apnea are middle-aged men with obesity. Arterial hypertension is common. Patients may report excessive daytime somnolence, morning sluggishness and headaches, daytime fatigue, cognitive impairment, recent weight gain, and impotence. Bed partners usually report loud cyclical snoring, breath cessation, witnessed apneas, restlessness, choking or gasping for air, and thrashing movements of the extremities during sleep. Personality changes, poor judgment, work-related problems, depression, and intellectual deterioration (memory impairment, inability to concentrate) may also be observed. The USPSTF does not recommend screening asymptomatic adults for sleep apnea.

Physical examination may be normal and includes a comprehensive assessment of BMI, neck circumference, and anatomy of craniofacial and upper airway structures. The patient may appear sleepy or even fall asleep during the evaluation. The oropharynx is frequently found to be narrowed by excessive soft tissue folds, large tonsils, elongated uvula, Mallampati class IV, or macroglossia. Nasal obstruction by a deviated nasal septum, poor nasal airflow, and a nasal twang to the speech may be observed. A "bull neck" appearance is common.

B. Laboratory Findings

Erythrocytosis is common. Thyroid function tests (serum TSH, FT_4) should be obtained to exclude hypothyroidism.

C. Other Studies

Observation of the sleeping patient may reveal loud snoring interrupted by episodes of increasingly strong respiratory effort that fail to produce airflow. A loud snort often accompanies the first breath following an apneic episode. Definitive diagnostic evaluation for suspected sleep apnea includes otorhinolaryngologic examination and overnight polysomnography (the monitoring of multiple physiologic factors during sleep). A complete **polysomnography** examination includes electroencephalography, electro-oculography, electromyography, ECG, pulse oximetry, and measurement of respiratory effort and airflow. Home sleep studies are best performed in patients without cardiorespiratory disease and a moderate to high pretest probability of obstructive sleep apnea. While some home studies cannot quantify the stages of sleep, they can provide a reliable index of respiratory and desaturation events. Obstructive sleep apnea is determined by the calculated apnea hypopnea index. Treatment is considered if the calculated apnea hypopnea index is above five events per hour with sleep symptoms or above 15 events per hour without symptoms.

Treatment

Weight loss with obesity management is an important strategy, recognized as part of the comprehensive management of obstructive sleep apnea. Incretins, hormones that regulate blood glucose levels, such as tirzepatide, a dual GLP-1 and glucose-dependent insulinotropic polypeptide (GIP) receptor agonist, resulted in approximately 16–17% weight loss compared with placebo and were accompanied by a reduction in apnea hypopnea index. **Continuous positive airway pressure (CPAP)** at night is curative in many patients. Auto-titrating airway pressure machines (APAP) allow a range of pressures (5–20 cm H_2O) that auto-adjust based on airflow obstruction. Unfortunately, CPAP adherence is suboptimal, and only 75% of patients continue to use nasal CPAP after 1 year. Supplemental oxygen may lessen the severity of nocturnal desaturation but may also lengthen apneas; it should not be routinely prescribed for treatment of obstructive sleep apnea. An **oral mandibular device** (mandibular repositioning device) at bedtime to hold the jaw forward and prevent pharyngeal occlusion is as effective as CPAP for treatment of mild to moderate obstructive sleep apnea.

Hypoglossal nerve stimulation can be an option for selected patients with moderate to severe obstructive sleep apnea (apnea hypopnea index between 15–100 events/hour) who do not tolerate or respond to CPAP. Patients are eligible who have absence of complete concentric collapse of the airway during drug-induced sleep endoscopy, BMI ≤ 35 (FDA recently approved for BMI < 40), and 25% respiratory events are due to central apneas.

Uvulopalatopharyngoplasty (UPPP), a procedure consisting of resection of pharyngeal soft tissue and amputation of approximately 15 mm of the free edge of the soft palate and uvula, is helpful in approximately 50% of selected patients. It is more effective in eliminating snoring than apneic episodes. **Nasal septoplasty** is performed if gross anatomic nasal septal deformity is present and may improve with adherence to CPAP therapy as opposed to improving apnea hypopnea index. **Tracheostomy** relieves upper airway obstruction and its physiologic consequences and represents the definitive treatment for obstructive sleep apnea. However, it has numerous adverse effects, including granuloma formation, difficulty with speech, and stoma and airway infection.

Chang JL et al. International Consensus Statement of Obstructive Sleep Apnea. Int Forum Allergy Rhinol. 2023;13:1061. [PMID: 36068685]

Malhotra A et al. Tirzepatide for the treatment of obstructive sleep apnea and obesity. N Engl J Med. 2024;391:1464. [PMID: 38912654]

ACUTE RESPIRATORY FAILURE

Respiratory failure is defined as respiratory dysfunction resulting in abnormalities of oxygenation or ventilation (CO_2 elimination) severe enough to threaten the function of vital organs. ABG criteria for respiratory failure are not absolute but may be arbitrarily established as a $PO_2 < 60$ mm Hg (7.8 kPa) or a $PCO_2 > 50$ mm Hg (6.5 kPa). Acute respiratory failure may occur in a variety of pulmonary and nonpulmonary disorders (Table 9–25). Only a few selected general principles of management will be reviewed here.

Table 9–25. Selected causes of acute respiratory failure in adults.

Airway disorders	**Neuromuscular and related disorders**
Asthma	Primary neuromuscular diseases
Acute exacerbation of chronic bronchitis or emphysema	Guillain-Barré syndrome
Obstruction of pharynx, larynx, trachea, mainstem bronchus, or lobar bronchus by edema, mucus, mass, or foreign body	Myasthenia gravis
Pulmonary edema	Poliomyelitis
Increased hydrostatic pressure	Polymyositis
LV dysfunction (eg, myocardial ischemia, HF)	Drug- or toxin-induced
Mitral regurgitation	Botulism
Left atrial outflow obstruction (eg, mitral stenosis)	Organophosphates
Volume overload states	Neuromuscular blocking agents
Increased pulmonary capillary permeability	Aminoglycosides
Acute respiratory distress syndrome	Spinal cord injury
Acute lung injury	Phrenic nerve injury or dysfunction
Unclear etiology	Electrolyte disturbances
Neurogenic	Hypokalemia
Negative pressure (inspiratory airway obstruction)	Hypophosphatemia
Re-expansion	Myxedema
Tocolytic-associated	**CNS disorders**
Parenchymal lung disorders	Drugs: sedatives, hypnotics, opioids, anesthetics
Pneumonia	Brainstem respiratory center disorders: trauma, tumor, vascular disorders, hypothyroidism
Interstitial lung diseases	Intracranial hypertension
Diffuse alveolar hemorrhage syndromes	CNS infections
Aspiration	**Increased CO_2 production**
Lung contusion	Fever
Pulmonary vascular disorders	Infection
Thromboembolism	Hyperalimentation with excess caloric and carbohydrate intake
Air embolism	Hyperthyroidism
Amniotic fluid embolism	Seizures
Chest wall, diaphragm, and pleural disorders	Rigors
Rib fracture	Drugs
Flail chest	
Pneumothorax	
Pleural effusion	
Massive ascites	
Abdominal distention and abdominal compartment syndrome	

Clinical Findings

Symptoms and signs of acute respiratory failure are those of the underlying disease combined with those of hypoxemia or hypercapnia. The chief symptom of hypoxemia is dyspnea, though profound hypoxemia may exist in the absence of symptoms. Signs of hypoxemia include cyanosis, restlessness, confusion, anxiety, delirium, tachypnea, bradycardia or tachycardia, hypotension or hypertension, cardiac dysrhythmias, and tremor. Dyspnea, headache, and confusion are the cardinal symptoms of hypercapnia. Signs of hypercapnia include peripheral and conjunctival hyperemia, hypertension, tachycardia, tachypnea, impaired consciousness, papilledema, myoclonus, and asterixis. The symptoms and signs of acute respiratory failure are both insensitive and nonspecific; therefore, the clinician must maintain a high index of suspicion and obtain blood gas analysis if respiratory failure is suspected.

Treatment

Treatment of the patient with acute respiratory failure consists of (1) specific therapy directed toward the underlying disease, (2) respiratory supportive care directed toward the maintenance of adequate gas exchange, and (3) general supportive care. Only the last two aspects are discussed below.

A. Respiratory Support

Respiratory support has both nonventilatory and ventilatory aspects.

1. Nonventilatory aspects—The main therapeutic goal in acute hypoxemic respiratory failure is to ensure adequate oxygenation of vital organs. Inspired oxygen concentration should be the lowest value that results in an arterial hemoglobin saturation of ≥ 90% (PaO_2 60 mm Hg). Higher arterial oxygen tensions have been studied with equivalent outcomes in adults. Restoration of normoxemia may rarely cause hypoventilation in patients with chronic hypercapnia; however, oxygen therapy should not be withheld for that concern. Hypoxemia in patients with obstructive airway disease is usually easily corrected by administering low-flow oxygen by nasal cannula (1–3 L/min) or Venturi mask (24–40%). Higher concentrations of oxygen are necessary to correct hypoxemia in patients with ARDS, pneumonia, and other parenchymal lung diseases. Humidified, high-flow nasal cannulae provide adjustable oxygen delivery and flow-dependent clearance of carbon dioxide from the upper airway, resulting in reduced work of breathing and better matching of respiratory demand during respiratory distress. In hypoxemia due to acute respiratory failure, oxygenation with use of humidified, high-flow nasal cannulae has been shown to be similar and, in some cases, superior to conventional low-flow oxygen supplementation and NIPPV; however, the use of high-flow nasal cannulae has no impact on mortality, and the impact on intubation rates, length of stay, dyspnea, and comfort are uncertain.

2. Ventilatory aspects—Ventilatory support consists of maintaining patency of the airway and ensuring adequate alveolar ventilation. Mechanical ventilation may be provided via mask (noninvasive) or through tracheal intubation.

A. Noninvasive positive-pressure ventilation—NIPPV delivered via a full-face mask or nasal mask is first-line therapy in patients with COPD with hypercapnic respiratory failure who can protect and maintain the patency of their airway, handle their own secretions, and tolerate the mask apparatus. Several studies have demonstrated the effectiveness of this therapy in reducing intubation rates and ICU stays in patients with ventilatory failure. A bilevel positive-pressure ventilation mode is preferred for most patients.

B. Tracheal intubation—Indications for tracheal intubation include (1) hypoxemia despite supplemental oxygen; (2) upper airway obstruction; (3) impaired airway protection; (4) inability to clear secretions; (5) respiratory acidosis; (6) progressive general fatigue, tachypnea, use of accessory respiratory muscles, or mental status deterioration; and (7) apnea. Patients in respiratory failure who undergo a trial of NIPPV and do not improve within 30–90 minutes should be intubated.

C. Mechanical ventilation—Indications for mechanical ventilation include (1) apnea, (2) acute hypercapnia that is not quickly reversed by appropriate specific therapy, (3) severe hypoxemia, and (4) progressive patient fatigue despite appropriate treatment.

Several modes of positive-pressure ventilation are available. Controlled mechanical ventilation is most appropriate for patients with acute respiratory failure. Modes of ventilation and specifics of ventilator management are beyond the scope of this text.

PEEP is useful in improving oxygenation in patients with diffuse parenchymal lung disease, such as ARDS. It should be used cautiously in patients with localized parenchymal disease, emphysema, hyperinflation, or very high airway pressure requirements during mechanical ventilation. Alveolar ventilation, which controls carbon dioxide exchange, is a function of the respiratory rate and tidal volume.

D. Complications of mechanical ventilation—Potential complications of mechanical ventilation are numerous. Migration of the tip of the endotracheal tube into a main bronchus can cause atelectasis of the contralateral lung and overdistention of the intubated lung. Barotrauma, (ie, loss of alveolar space integrity) may result from high transmural pressures applied during positive-pressure ventilation. It is manifested subcutaneous emphysema, pneumomediastinum, subpleural air cysts, pneumothorax, or systemic gas embolism. Volutrauma is sometimes used to refer to subtle parenchymal injury due to overdistention of alveoli from excessive tidal volumes without alveolar rupture, mediated through inflammatory rather than physical mechanisms. The principal strategy to avoid volutrauma is the use of low tidal volume ventilation.

Acute respiratory alkalosis caused by overventilation is common and best monitored by intermittent blood gas analysis. Hypotension induced by elevated intrathoracic pressure that results in decreased return of systemic venous blood to the heart may occur in patients treated with PEEP, particularly those with intravascular volume depletion, and in patients with severe airflow obstruction at high respiratory rates that promote dynamic hyperinflation ("breath stacking"). Ventilator-associated pneumonia is another serious complication of mechanical ventilation.

B. General Supportive Care

Hypokalemia and hypophosphatemia may worsen hypoventilation due to respiratory muscle weakness. Sedative-hypnotics and opioid analgesics should be titrated carefully to avoid oversedation and delirium, leading to prolongation of intubation. Temporary paralysis with a nondepolarizing neuromuscular blocking agent is used to facilitate mechanical ventilation and to lower oxygen consumption. Prolonged muscle weakness due to an acute myopathy is a potential complication of these agents.

Comprehensive care for patients with acute respiratory failure should include skin care and offloading to avoid pressure injuries, engagement in mobilization, meticulous avoidance of health care–associated infection and complications of endotracheal tubes, and psychological and emotional support for the patient and family.

Attention must also be paid to preventing complications associated with serious illness. Stress-ulcer prophylaxis is recommended for patients with acute respiratory failure requiring mechanical ventilation. The risk of DVT and PE may be reduced by subcutaneous administration of heparin or LMWH (see Table 16–14), or placement of sequential compression devices on the lower extremities.

Course & Prognosis

The course and prognosis of acute respiratory failure vary and depend on the underlying disease. The prognosis of acute respiratory failure caused by uncomplicated sedative or opioid overdose is excellent. Acute respiratory failure in patients with COPD who do not require intubation, and mechanical ventilation has a good immediate prognosis. On the other hand, ARDS and respiratory failure associated with sepsis have a worse prognosis.

Fujishima S. Guideline-based management of acute respiratory failure and acute respiratory distress syndrome. J Intensive Care. 2023;11:10. [PMID: 36895001]

Lagina M et al. Diagnosis and management of acute respiratory failure. Crit Care Clin. 2024;40:235. [PMID: 384432694]

Munshi L et al. Noninvasive respiratory support for adults with acute respiratory failure. N Engl J Med. 2022;387:1688. [PMID: 36322846]

ACUTE RESPIRATORY DISTRESS SYNDROME

ESSENTIALS OF DIAGNOSIS

- Onset of respiratory distress, often progressing to respiratory failure, within 7 days of a clinical insult.
- New, bilateral radiographic pulmonary opacities not explained by pleural effusion, atelectasis, or nodules.
- Respiratory failure not fully explained by HF or volume overload.
- Impaired oxygenation, with ratio of partial pressure of oxygen in arterial blood (PaO_2) to fractional concentration of inspired oxygen (FIO_2) < 300 mm Hg, or SaO_2:FIO_2 < 315.

General Considerations

ARDS as a clinical syndrome is based on three inclusion criteria plus one exclusion criterion, as detailed above. The severity of ARDS is based on the level of oxygenation impairment: **mild**, PaO_2/FIO_2 ratio of 200–300 mm Hg; **moderate**, PaO_2/FIO_2 ratio of 100–200 mm Hg; and **severe**, PaO_2/FIO_2 ratio < 100 mm Hg. An updated global definition of ARDS includes modifications that allow for diagnosis when PaO_2 cannot be measured and when patients are not mechanically ventilated, using an approximation equation for FIO_2.

ARDS may follow a wide variety of clinical events (Table 9–26). Common risk factors for ARDS include sepsis, aspiration of gastric contents, shock, infection, lung contusion, nonthoracic trauma, severe pancreatitis, burn, toxic inhalation, and near-drowning. About one-third of patients with ARDS initially have sepsis syndrome. Damage to capillary endothelial cells and alveolar epithelial cells is common to ARDS regardless of cause or mechanism of lung injury and results in increased vascular permeability and decreased production and activity of surfactant. These abnormalities in turn lead to interstitial and alveolar pulmonary edema, alveolar collapse, and hypoxemia.

Table 9–26. Selected disorders associated with ARDS.

Systemic Insults	Pulmonary Insults
Trauma	Aspiration of gastric contents
Sepsis	Embolism of thrombus, fat, air, or amniotic fluid
Pancreatitis	Diffuse pneumonia
Shock	Upper airway obstruction
Multiple transfusions	Free-base cocaine smoking
Disseminated intravascular coagulation	Near-drowning
Burns	Toxic gas inhalation
Drugs and drug overdose	Nitrogen dioxide
Opioids	Chlorine
Aspirin	Sulfur dioxide
Phenothiazines	Ammonia
Tricyclic antidepressants	Smoke
Amiodarone	Lung contusion
Chemotherapeutic agents	Radiation exposure
Nitrofurantoin	High-altitude exposure
Protamine	Lung re-expansion or reperfusion
Thrombotic thrombocytopenic purpura	
Cardiopulmonary bypass	
Head injury	

ARDS, acute respiratory distress syndrome; SARS, severe acute respiratory syndrome.

Clinical Findings

ARDS is marked by the rapid onset of profound dyspnea that usually occurs 12–48 hours after the initiating event. Labored breathing, tachypnea, intercostal retractions, and crackles are noted on physical examination. CXR shows diffuse or patchy bilateral infiltrates that rapidly become confluent. Air bronchograms occur in about 80% of cases. Heart size is usually normal, and pleural effusions are small or nonexistent. Marked hypoxemia occurs that is refractory to treatment with supplemental oxygen. Many patients with ARDS demonstrate multiple organ failure, particularly involving the kidneys, liver, gut, CNS, and cardiovascular system.

Differential Diagnosis

Since ARDS is a physiologic and radiographic syndrome rather than a specific disease, the concept of differential diagnosis does not strictly apply. Normal-permeability ("cardiogenic" or hydrostatic) pulmonary edema must be excluded because specific therapy is available for that disorder. Diffuse alveolar hemorrhage, inflammatory or autoimmune causes, and bilateral pneumonia without other ARDS characteristics should be excluded. Echocardiogram or measurement of pulmonary capillary wedge pressure may be required in selected patients with suspected cardiac dysfunction; however, routine use of the latter in ARDS is discouraged.

Prevention

No measures that effectively prevent ARDS have been identified, however lung-protective ventilation strategies in patients who are mechanically ventilated may be protective

Treatment

The first principle in management is to identify and treat the primary condition that has led to ARDS. Meticulous supportive care must then be provided to compensate for the severe dysfunction of the respiratory system associated with ARDS and to prevent complications.

Treatment of the hypoxemia seen in ARDS usually requires tracheal intubation and positive-pressure mechanical ventilation. The lowest levels of PEEP (used to recruit atelectatic alveoli) and supplemental oxygen required to maintain the PaO_2 > 60 mm Hg should be used. Efforts should be made to decrease FIO_2 as able. PEEP can be increased as needed if cardiac output and oxygen delivery do not decrease and airway pressures do not increase excessively (ie, plateau pressures remain below 30 cm H_2O). Prone positioning frequently improves oxygenation by helping recruit atelectatic alveoli and, when employed early, has been shown to provide a mortality benefit in moderate to severe ARDS. Routine use of neuromuscular blockade is controversial; one major trial showed improved mortality but a subsequent trial (intended to be confirmatory) did not.

A variety of mechanical ventilation strategies are available. The recognition of the potential for excessive alveolar stretch to cause lung injury has led to widespread adoption of low tidal volume ventilation, and lower mortality associated with constraint of ventilatory plateau and driving pressures. Varying ventilator modes have been used; conventional modes of ventilation are essentially equivalent, while high-frequency oscillatory ventilation should not be used.

Approaches to hemodynamic monitoring and fluid management in patients with acute lung injury have been carefully studied. Based on a prospective RCT comparing hemodynamic management guided either by a pulmonary artery catheter or a central venous catheter, a pulmonary artery catheter should not be routinely used for the management of acute lung injury. A subsequent randomized, prospective clinical study of restrictive fluid intake and diuresis as needed to maintain CVP < 4 mm Hg or pulmonary artery occlusion pressure < 8 mm Hg (conservative strategy group) versus a fluid management protocol to target a CVP of 10–14 mm Hg or a pulmonary artery occlusion pressure 14–18 mm Hg (liberal strategy group) showed that patients in the conservative strategy group experienced faster improvement in lung function and spent significantly fewer days on mechanical ventilation and in the ICU without an improvement in death by 60 days or worsening nonpulmonary organ failure at 28 days. Oxygen delivery can be increased in anemic patients by ensuring that the hemoglobin concentration is ≥ 7 g/dL (70 g/L); patients are not likely to benefit from higher levels.

Numerous innovative therapeutic interventions to improve outcomes in ARDS patients have been or are being investigated. Unfortunately, to date, none has consistently shown benefit in clinical trials. The 2024 American Thoracic Society (ATS) guidelines on ARDS recommend the use of corticosteroids for ARDS patients as a conditional recommendation with moderate certainty of evidence, highlighting their potential to reduce mortality and possibly reduce hospital stay and duration of mechanical ventilation while acknowledging the need for patient-specific considerations where corticosteroids are most effective in < 14 days of ARDS, in severe community-acquired pneumonia, or in COVID-19 patients.

Another therapeutic intervention is extracorporeal membrane oxygenation (ECMO). A 2018 trial comparing the early use of ECMO in very severe ARDS with conventional strategies built on low-tidal-volume ventilation failed to show a difference in 60-day mortality; however, 28% of the control group crossed over to receive ECMO. ECMO seems unlikely to become a standard first-line therapy but is likely to remain a salvage option for patients with very severe ARDS.

Course & Prognosis

ARDS mortality with low tidal volume ventilation is around 30%. The major causes of death are the primary illness and secondary complications, such as multiple organ system failure or sepsis.

Different clinical syndromes that lead to ARDS carry different prognoses. For example, patients with trauma-associated ARDS have better prognosis, with a mortality rate close to 20%, whereas those with end-stage liver disease have an 80% mortality rate. A hyperinflammatory phenotype associated with high levels of IL-6 and soluble TNF receptor in ARDS patients precipitated by sepsis is associated with more multiorgan dysfunction and higher mortality.

Failure to improve in the first week of treatment is a poor prognostic sign, although this may not be true of ARDS from certain etiologies, including COVID-19. Persons who have been impacted by ARDS tend to be young and pulmonary function generally recovers over 6–12 months, although residual abnormalities often remain, including restrictive or obstructive defects, low diffusion capacity, and impaired gas exchange with exercise. These persons also have diminished health-related and pulmonary disease–specific quality of life as well as systemic effects, such as muscle wasting, weakness, and fatigue.

Grasselli G et al. ESICM guidelines on acute respiratory distress syndrome: definition, phenotyping and respiratory support strategies. Intensive Care Med. 2023;49:727. [PMID: 37326646]

Latronico N et al. Improving management of ARDS: uniting acute management and long-term recovery. Crit Care. 2024;28:58. [PMID: 38395902]

Matthay M et al. A new global definition of acute respiratory distress syndrome. Am J Respir Crit Care Med. 2024;209:37. [PMID: 37487152]

Qadir N et al. An update on management of adult patients with acute respiratory distress syndrome: an official American Thoracic Society clinical practice guideline. Am J Respir Crit Care Med. 2024;209:24. [PMID: 38032683]

Wick KD et al. Acute respiratory distress syndrome. BMJ. 2024;387:e076612. [PMID: 39467606]

Coronary Artery Disease, Valvular Disease, & Other Key Topics in Cardiology

10

Zachary K. Wegermann, MD

CORONARY ARTERY DISEASE (Atherosclerotic or Ischemic Heart Disease)

Coronary artery disease (CAD) is the number one cause of death in the United States and worldwide. Every minute in the United States, a person dies of CAD. About 37% of people who experience an acute coronary event, either angina or MI, will die of it in the same year. Death rates of CAD have declined every year since 1968, with about half of the decline from 1980 to 2000 due to treatments and half due to improved risk factors. CAD is still responsible for 1 in 4 of all deaths in the United States. The prevalence rises steadily with age; thus, the aging of the US population promises to increase the overall burden of CAD.

Risk Factors for CAD

Most patients with CAD have an identifiable risk factor. These include a **positive family history** (the younger the onset in a first-degree relative, the greater the risk), **male sex, blood lipid abnormalities, diabetes mellitus, hypertension, physical inactivity, abdominal obesity, smoking,** and **psychosocial factors**. *Smoking remains the number one preventable cause of death and illness in the United States.* According to the WHO, 1 year after quitting, the risk of CAD decreases by 50%. Various interventions have been shown to increase the likelihood of successful smoking cessation (see Chapter 1) and should remain a target for risk reduction.

Hypercholesterolemia is an important modifiable risk factor for CAD. Risk increases with higher levels of LDL cholesterol and declines with higher levels of HDL cholesterol. Composite risk scores, such as the **Framingham score** and the **10-year atherosclerotic CVD risk calculator**, can provide estimates for the risk of developing CAD that can guide primary prevention strategies. The 2018 ACC/AHA Guideline on the Treatment of Blood Cholesterol to Reduce Atherosclerotic Cardiovascular Risk in Adults suggests statin therapy in four populations: patients with (1) clinical atherosclerotic disease, (2) LDL cholesterol 190 mg/dL or higher, (3) diabetes who are aged 40–75 years, and (4) an estimated 10-year atherosclerotic risk of 7.5% or more aged 40–75 years (Figure 10–1). Importantly, *the guidelines do not recommend treating to a target LDL cholesterol.* Patients in these categories should be treated with a moderate- or high-intensity statin, with high-intensity statin for populations with higher risk. The ACC/AHA atherosclerotic CVD estimator allows clinicians to determine the 10-year ASCVD risk to determine treatment decisions (http://tools.acc.org/ascvd-risk-estimator-plus). The 2022 USPSTF Lipid Recommendations suggest statin therapy for primary prevention of CVD in those 40 to 75 years of age with one or more risk factors and a 10-year estimated CVD risk of 10% or greater.

Metabolic syndrome is defined as a constellation of three or more of the following: abdominal obesity, triglycerides 150 mg/dL or higher, HDL cholesterol < 40 mg/dL for men or < 50 mg/dL for women, fasting glucose 110 mg/dL or higher, and hypertension, and is a growing risk factor for developing CAD.

Primary & Secondary Prevention of CAD

Although some risk factors for CAD are not modifiable, it is clear that interventions targeting modifiable risk factors (smoking cessation, treatment of dyslipidemia, and lowering of blood pressure [BP]) can both prevent coronary disease and delay its progression.

Lowering LDL levels delays the progression of atherosclerosis and in some cases may produce regression. With LDL-lowering therapy fewer new lesions develop, endothelial function may be restored, and cardiovascular event rates are markedly reduced in patients with clinical evidence of vascular disease.

Multiple clinical trials have demonstrated the efficacy of **hydroxymethylglutaryl coenzyme A (HMG-CoA) reductase inhibitors (statins)** in preventing death, coronary events, and strokes. Beneficial results have been found in patients who have already experienced coronary events (secondary prevention), those at particularly high risk for events (patients with diabetes and patients with peripheral artery disease), those with elevated cholesterol without multiple risk factors, and those without vascular disease or diabetes with elevated high-sensitivity CRP (hsCRP) with normal LDL levels. The benefits of statin therapy at moderate and high doses (see Risk Factors for CAD) are recommended by the cholesterol treatment guidelines. Benefits of statins occur regardless of age, race, baseline cholesterol levels, or the presence of hypertension. Evidence shows that

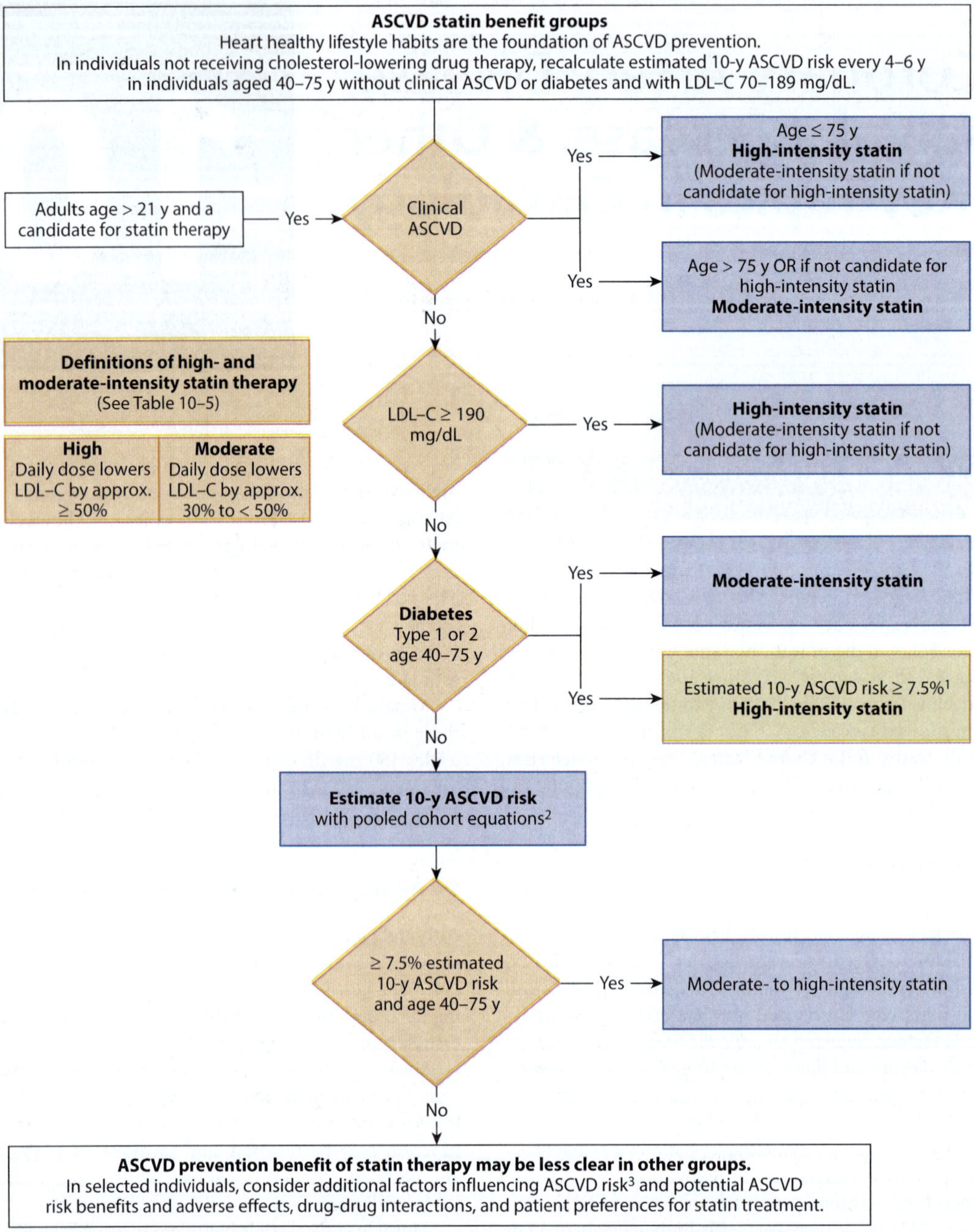

[1]Percent reduction in LDL–C can be used as an indication of response and adherence to therapy but is not in itself a treatment goal.

[2]The Pooled Cohort Equations can be used to estimate 10-year ASCVD risk in individuals with and without diabetes. A downloadable spreadsheet enabling estimation of 10-year and lifetime risk for ASCVD and a web-based calculator are available at http://my.americanheart.org/cvriskcalculator and http://www.cardiosource.org/science-and-quality/practice-guidelines-and-quality-standards/2013-prevention-guideline-tools.aspx.

[3]Primary LDL–C ≥ 160 mg/dL or other evidence of genetic hyperlipidemias, family history of premature ASCVD with onset < 55 years of age in a first-degree male relative or < 65 years of age in a first-degree female relative, high-sensitivity C-reactive protein > 2 mg/L, CAC score ≥ 300 Agatston units or ≥ 75 percentile for age, sex, and ethnicity, ankle-brachial index < 0.9, or elevated lifetime risk of ASCVD.

▲ **Figure 10–1.** Major recommendations for statin therapy for atherosclerotic CVD prevention. ASCVD, atherosclerotic CVD; CAC, coronary artery calcium; LDL–C, LDL cholesterol. (Adapted from Stone NJ et al. 2013 ACC/AHA guideline on the treatment of blood cholesterol to reduce atherosclerotic cardiovascular risk in adults: a report of the American College of Cardiology/American Heart Association Task Force on Practice Guidelines. Circulation. 2014;129:S1.)

for patients with vascular disease, statins provide benefit even with normal cholesterol levels, and that more aggressive statin use is associated with greater benefits. *All patients at significant risk for vascular events should receive a statin regardless of their cholesterol levels, and many experts recommend that with those who have prior cardiovascular events should have their LDL lowered below 70 mg/dL.*

The IMPROVE-IT study showed that **ezetimibe**, 10 mg daily, combined with simvastatin was modestly better than simvastatin alone in reducing the risk of MI and ischemic stroke, but *not* mortality, in stabilized patients following an ACS. This was associated with a reduction of LDL to 53.7 mg/dL compared with 69.7 mg/dL. With this data, ezetimibe can be used in combination with statin therapy in patients who are *not* at target cholesterol level for secondary prevention (for individuals at high risk for cardiovascular events with an LDL > 70 on maximal intensity statin therapy [IIa recommendation]) or cannot tolerate high-dose statin therapy.

Monoclonal antibodies that inhibit **proprotein convertase subtilisin/kexin type 9 (PCSK9)** reduce LDL cholesterol levels significantly beyond levels associated with statin therapy. PCSK9 inhibitors have been studied in randomized trials of patients with maximally tolerated statin therapy (and for patients with statin intolerance) and have lowered LDL with signals of improved cardiovascular outcomes. The FOURIER trial showed that the PCSK9 inhibitor evolocumab, added to a statin, reduced the composite of atherothrombotic outcomes by 20% but did *not* reduce mortality. The ODYSSEY Outcomes trial demonstrated alirocumab reduced cardiovascular events in patients with ACSs. *Alirocumab and evolocumab have been approved by the US Food and Drug Administration (FDA) for patients on maximally tolerated statin therapy with familial hypercholesterolemia and atherosclerotic vascular disease, or both, and who require additional lowering of LDL.* Alirocumab has also been approved by the FDA for secondary prevention of cardiovascular events. Inclisiran, a small interfering RNA that goes to the liver and prevents the production of PCSK9, has been studied as a twice-yearly injection showing reduction in LDL and was approved by the FDA in early 2022.

The placebo-controlled, double-blind CLEAR Outcomes trial randomized 13,970 patients with a history of or at high-risk of ASCVD and an LDL-C > 100 mg/dL to bempedoic acid therapy or placebo. Treatment with bempedoic acid, an ATP citrate lyase inhibitor, resulted in reduction in the composite primary endpoint of cardiovascular death, MI, stroke, or coronary revascularization procedure. This provides another option to reduce major adverse cardiac events in at-risk patients who cannot tolerate or prefer not to take statin therapy.

Fish oil supplements have *not* been shown consistently to provide benefit for reducing risk. As such, there is no guideline recommendation for their use. Icosapent ethyl, a concentrated eicosapentaenoic acid at a high dose, was shown to be beneficial in the REDUCE-IT trial. Patients with established CVD or with diabetes and other risk factors, with fasting triglyceride level of 135–499 mg/dL, who were on statins were randomized to 2 g of icosapent ethyl twice daily or placebo. There was a 26% relative risk reduction in cardiovascular death, MI, and stroke, as well as a 20% relative risk reduction in cardiovascular death. Icosapent ethyl is approved by the FDA as an adjunct to maximally tolerated statin therapy to reduce the risk of MI, stroke, coronary revascularization, or unstable angina requiring hospitalization in patients with triglycerides of 150 mg/dL or more and either established CVD or diabetes mellitus and two or more additional risk factors. The role of high-dose omega-3 fatty acids was studied compared with corn oil and not shown to reduce cardiovascular events, leading to increased interest in comparative studies.

Treatment to raise HDL levels has failed to show benefit. The AIM High trial found no benefit from the addition of niacin in patients with vascular disease and a serum LDL near 70 mg/dL who were receiving statin therapy. The HPS2-THRIVE trial found no benefit but rather substantial harm of extended-release niacin (2 g) plus laropiprant (an antiflushing agent) for preventing vascular events in a population of over 25,000 patients with vascular disease who were taking simvastatin.

For primary prevention, *aspirin has little overall benefit, including for patients with established diabetes, and is* not *recommended for most patients.* In 2022, the USPSTF issued guidance on the use of aspirin for primary prevention of cardiovascular events. The document recommended that patient aged 40–59 years with a 10-year ASCVD risk of 10% or greater should have a shared-decision making conversation regarding the potential risk and benefits of initiating aspirin therapy for primary prevention. In addition, the document recommended that patients 60 years of age and older should not initiate aspirin for primary prevention of CVD.

Antiplatelet therapy is a very effective measure for secondary prevention and patients with established vascular disease should be treated with aspirin. The exact dose of aspirin in chronic CAD (81 mg versus 325 mg) was evaluated in a large pragmatic trial (ADAPTABLE). The unique pragmatic clinical trial design demonstrated that 81 mg aspirin was associated with a favorable cardiovascular event risk and bleeding risk compared with 325 mg daily.

While clopidogrel was found to be effective at preventing vascular events for 9–12 months after ACSs, and there are some benefits in prolonging dual antiplatelet therapy after coronary stenting, clopidogrel was *not* found to be effective at preventing vascular events in combination with aspirin with longer-term treatment in the CHARISMA trial. This trial included patients with clinically evident stable atherothrombosis or with multiple risk factors; all were treated with aspirin and observed for a median of 28 months.

In the COMPASS trial, rivaroxaban, a direct factor Xa inhibitor, at a dose of 2.5 mg twice daily in addition to 100 mg of aspirin, was shown to reduce cardiovascular death, MI, and stroke by a relative risk reduction of 24% compared with 100 mg aspirin monotherapy in stable patients with CAD and peripheral artery disease. Bleeding was modestly increased. All-cause mortality was also reduced by 18%. This regimen is approved by the FDA and is used for long-term management of patients with CAD and peripheral artery disease, and should be considered in this group at high risk for adverse cardiac events with a low bleeding risk profile.

The HOPE and the EUROPA trials demonstrated that ACE inhibitors (ramipril 10 mg/day and perindopril 8 mg/day, respectively) reduced fatal and nonfatal vascular events (cardiovascular deaths, nonfatal MIs, and nonfatal strokes) by 20–25% in patients at high risk, including patients with diabetes with additional risk factors or patients with clinical coronary, cerebral, or peripheral arterial atherosclerotic disease. An overview of these trials has demonstrated that while low-risk patients may *not* derive substantial benefits from ACE inhibitors, *most patients with vascular disease, even in the absence of HF or LV dysfunction, should be treated with an ACE inhibitor.*

An interesting approach to secondary prevention of cardiovascular events was investigated in the SECURE trial. Utilizing a *polypill* (aspirin, ramipril, and atorvastatin) or standard medical therapy with multiple agents, 2499 patients with a history of an MI in the prior 6 months were randomized to polypill treatment or a standard approach with multiple agents and followed for 3 years. Medication adherence was statistically higher in the polypill cohort and this was associated with a statistically significant lower rate of major adverse cardiac events.

Over one-third of patients with vascular disease have type 2 diabetes. In addition to controlling risk factors, using high-intensity statins and ACE inhibitors or ARBs, *there is proven benefit to reduce cardiovascular events by using oral SGLT-2 inhibitors (specifically, empagliflozin, dapagliflozin, or canagliflozin) or injectable GLP-1–receptor agonists (liraglutide, semaglutide, dulaglutide).* The cardiovascular benefits appear to be independent from the glucose lowering effects, and SGLT-2 inhibitors have benefits for patients with HF regardless of whether they have diabetes (see Chapter 11). Importantly, the SELECT trial enrolled 17,604 patients with *a BMI > 27 and no history of diabetes mellitus* and showed a statistically significant decrease in the composite primary endpoint of cardiovascular death, MI, or stroke in the group treated with semaglutide.

Low-dose colchicine, at 0.5 mg daily, in addition to optimal medical therapy for CAD, has been shown to reduce major adverse cardiovascular events (MACE) in multiple RCTs. A study published in 2024 showed no significant reduction in MACE. However, meta-analyses of pooled data still suggest a significant reduction in MACE with colchicine in addition to optimal medical therapy. The European Society of Cardiology adopted colchicine into the secondary prevention guidelines in 2021. The FDA approved colchicine for secondary prevention in June 2023. Given the conflicting results of recent studies, further investigation in this area is likely warranted.

Castellano JM et al; SECURE Investigators. Polypill strategy in secondary cardiovascular prevention. N Engl J Med. 2022;387:967. [PMID: 36018037]

Jolly SS et al; CLEAR Investigators. Colchicine in acute myocardial infarction. N Engl J Med. 2025;392:633. [PMID: 39555823]

Lincoff AM et al; SELECT Trial Investigators. Semaglutide and cardiovascular outcomes in obesity without diabetes. N Engl J Med. 2023;389:2221. [PMID: 37952131]

Nissen SE et al; CLEAR Outcomes Investigators. Bempedoic acid and cardiovascular outcomes in statin-intolerant patients. N Engl J Med. 2023;388:1353. [PMID: 36876740]

US Preventive Services Task Force; Davidson KW et al. Aspirin use to prevent cardiovascular disease: US Preventive Services Task Force recommendation statement. JAMA. 2022;327:1577. [PMID: 35471505]

CHRONIC STABLE ANGINA PECTORIS (Chronic Coronary Syndromes)

ESSENTIALS OF DIAGNOSIS

- Chest pain precipitated by stress or exertion, relieved rapidly by rest or nitrates.
- ECG or imaging evidence of ischemia during pain or stress testing.
- Angiographic evidence of significant blockage of major coronary vessels.

General Considerations

Angina pectoris is the symptomatic manifestation of stable atherosclerotic heart disease. Coronary vasospasm may occur at the site of a lesion or, less frequently, in apparently normal vessels. Other unusual causes of coronary artery obstruction, such as congenital anomalies, emboli, arteritis, or dissection, may cause ischemia or infarction. Angina may also occur in the absence of coronary artery obstruction as a result of severe myocardial hypertrophy, severe aortic stenosis or regurgitation, or in response to increased metabolic demands, as in hyperthyroidism, marked anemia, or paroxysmal tachycardias with rapid ventricular rates. Angina may also occur in angiographically normal coronary arteries as the result of microvascular dysfunction.

Clinical Findings

A. Symptoms

The diagnosis of angina pectoris principally depends on the history, which should include the following information: circumstances that precipitate and relieve angina, characteristics of the discomfort, location and radiation, duration of attacks, and effect of nitroglycerin.

1. Circumstances that precipitate and relieve angina— Angina occurs most commonly during activity and is relieved by rest. Patients may prefer to remain upright rather than lie down, as increased preload in recumbency increases myocardial work. The amount of activity required to produce angina may be relatively consistent under comparable physical and emotional circumstances. The threshold for angina is usually lower after meals, during excitement, or on exposure to cold. It is often lower in the morning or after strong emotion; the latter can provoke attacks in the absence of exertion. In addition, discomfort may occur during sexual activity, at rest, or at night as the result of coronary spasm.

2. Characteristics of the discomfort—Patients often do not refer to angina as "pain" but as a sensation of tightness, squeezing, burning, pressure, aching, "gas," indigestion, or an ill-characterized discomfort. It is often characterized by *clenching a fist* over the mid chest. The distress of angina is rarely sharply localized and is not spasmodic.

3. Location and radiation—The distribution of the distress may vary widely in different patients but is usually the same for each patient. In most cases, the discomfort is typically substernal pressure. Although angina may radiate to any dermatome from C8 to T4, it radiates most often to the left shoulder and upper arm, frequently moving down the inner volar aspect of the arm to the elbow, forearm, wrist, or fourth and fifth fingers. It may also radiate to the right shoulder or arm, the lower jaw, the neck, or even the back.

4. Duration of attacks—Angina is generally of short duration and subsides completely without residual discomfort. If the attack is precipitated by exertion and the patient promptly stops to rest, it usually lasts under 3 minutes. Attacks following a heavy meal or brought on by anger can last longer. Attacks that do not resolve quickly with rest and/or sublingual nitroglycerin can suggest development of an acute coronary syndrome (ACS) and should prompt medical attention.

5. Effect of nitroglycerin—The diagnosis of angina pectoris is supported if sublingual nitroglycerin promptly and invariably shortens an attack and if prophylactic nitrates permit greater exertion or prevent angina entirely.

B. Signs

Examination during angina frequently reveals a significant elevation in systolic and diastolic BP, although hypotension may also occur, and may reflect more severe ischemia or inferior ischemia (especially with bradycardia) due to a **Bezold-Jarisch reflex**. Occasionally, a gallop rhythm and an apical systolic murmur due to transient mitral regurgitation from papillary muscle dysfunction are present during pain only. Supraventricular or ventricular arrhythmias may be present, either as the precipitating factor or as the result of ischemia.

It is important to detect signs of diseases that may contribute to or accompany atherosclerotic heart disease, eg, diabetes mellitus (retinopathy or neuropathy), xanthelasma tendinous xanthomas, hypertension, thyrotoxicosis, myxedema, or peripheral artery disease. Aortic stenosis or regurgitation, HCM, and mitral valve may also produce angina or other forms of chest pain.

C. Laboratory Findings

Blood tests are not helpful to diagnose chronic angina. However, in patients presenting with angina, laboratory tests (high sensitivity troponin assays) should be used to evaluate for ACS factors contributing to ischemia (such as anemia), and to screen for risk factors that may increase the probability of true CAD (such as hyperlipidemia and diabetes mellitus).

D. ECG

The resting ECG is often normal in patients with a history of angina. In the remainder, abnormalities include old MI, nonspecific ST changes, and LVH. During anginal episodes, as well as during asymptomatic ischemia, *the characteristic ECG change is horizontal or downsloping ST-segment depression that reverses after the ischemia resolves.* T wave flattening or inversion may also occur. Less frequently, transient ST-segment elevation is observed; this finding suggests severe (transmural) ischemia from coronary occlusion, and can occur with coronary spasm.

E. Pretest Probability

The history and personal risk factors, physical examination findings, and laboratory and ECG findings are used to develop a pretest probability of CAD as the cause of the clinical symptoms. Patients with a low to intermediate pretest probability for CAD should undergo noninvasive stress testing whereas patients with high pretest probability are generally referred for cardiac catheterization. National review of diagnostic cardiac catheterization findings in patients without known CAD undergoing angiography has shown that between 38% and 40% of patients do not have obstructive disease.

F. Exercise ECG

Exercise ECG testing is the most commonly used noninvasive procedure for evaluating inducible ischemia in the patient with angina. Exercise ECG testing is often combined with imaging studies (nuclear or echocardiography) to increase the sensitivity of testing, but in low-risk patients without baseline ST-segment abnormalities or in whom anatomic localization is not necessary, the exercise ECG remains the recommended initial procedure because of considerations of cost, convenience, and long-standing prognostic data.

Exercise testing can be done on a motorized treadmill or with a bicycle ergometer. A variety of exercise protocols are utilized, the most common being the **Bruce protocol**, which increases the treadmill speed and elevation every 3 minutes until limited by symptoms. At least two ECG leads should be monitored continuously.

1. Precautions and risks—The risk of exercise testing is about one infarction or death per 1000 tests, but individuals who have pain at rest or minimal activity are at higher risk and should not be tested. *Many of the traditional exclusions, such as recent MI or HF, are no longer used if the patient is stable and ambulatory, but symptomatic severe aortic stenosis remains a relative contraindication.*

2. Indications—Exercise testing is used to (1) confirm the diagnosis of angina; (2) determine the severity of limitation of activity due to angina; (3) assess prognosis in patients with known coronary disease, including those recovering from MI, by detecting groups at high or low risk; and (4) evaluate responses to therapy. Because false-positive tests often exceed true positives, leading to much patient anxiety and self-imposed or mandated disability, *exercise testing of asymptomatic individuals should be done only for those whose occupations place them or others at special risk (eg, airline pilots).*

3. Interpretation—The usual ECG criterion for a positive test is 1-mm (0.1-mV) *horizontal or downsloping ST-segment depression* (beyond baseline) measured 80 msec after the J point. By this criterion, 60–80% of patients with anatomically significant coronary disease will have a positive test, but 10–30% of those without significant disease will also be positive. False positives are uncommon when a 2-mm depression is present. Additional information is inferred from the time of onset and duration of the ECG changes, their magnitude and configuration, BP and heart rate changes, the duration of exercise, and the presence of associated symptoms. In general, patients exhibiting more severe ST-segment depression (> 2 mm) at low workloads (< 6 minutes on the Bruce protocol) or heart rates (< 70% of age-predicted maximum)—especially when the duration of exercise and rise in BP are limited or when hypotension occurs during the test—have more severe disease and a poorer prognosis. Depending on symptom status, age, and other factors, such patients should be referred for coronary angiography and possible revascularization. On the other hand, less impressive positive tests in asymptomatic patients can be false positives. Therefore, *exercise testing results that do not conform to the clinical suspicion should be confirmed by stress imaging.*

G. Myocardial Stress Imaging

Myocardial stress imaging (scintigraphy, echocardiography, or MRI) is indicated (1) when the resting ECG makes an exercise ECG difficult to interpret (eg, left bundle branch block, baseline ST–T changes, low voltage); (2) for confirmation of the results of the exercise ECG when they are contrary to the clinical impression (eg, a positive test in an asymptomatic patient); (3) to localize the region of ischemia; (4) to distinguish ischemic from infarcted myocardium; (5) to assess the completeness of revascularization following bypass surgery or coronary angioplasty; or (6) as a prognostic indicator in patients with known coronary disease.

1. Myocardial perfusion scintigraphy—This test, also known as **radionuclide imaging**, provides images in which radionuclide uptake is proportionate to blood flow at the time of injection.

Stress imaging is positive in about 75–90% of patients with anatomically significant coronary disease and in 20–30% of those without it. Occasionally, other conditions, including infiltrative diseases (sarcoidosis, amyloidosis), left bundle branch block, and dilated cardiomyopathy, may produce resting or persistent perfusion defects. False-positive radionuclide tests may occur as the result of diaphragmatic attenuation or, in women, breast attenuation artifact. Tomographic imaging (single-photon emission CT [SPECT]) can reduce the severity of artifacts.

2. Radionuclide angiography—This procedure, also known as **multi-gated acquisition scan**, or **MUGA scan**, uses radionuclide tracers to image the LV and measures its EF and wall motion. In coronary disease, resting abnormalities usually represent infarction, and those that occur only with exercise usually indicate stress-induced ischemia. Exercise radionuclide angiography has approximately the same sensitivity as myocardial perfusion scintigraphy, but it is less specific in older individuals and those with other forms of heart disease. In addition, because of the precision around LVEF, the test is also used for monitoring patients exposed to cardiotoxic therapies (such as some chemotherapeutic agents), although this is increasingly done using echocardiography.

3. Stress echocardiography—Echocardiograms performed during supine exercise or immediately following upright exercise may demonstrate exercise-induced *segmental wall motion abnormalities* as an indicator of ischemia. In experienced laboratories, the test accuracy is comparable to that obtained with scintigraphy—though a higher proportion of tests is technically inadequate. While exercise is the preferred stress because of other information derived, pharmacologic stress with **high-dose dobutamine** (20–40 mcg/kg/min) can be used as an alternative to exercise.

H. Other Imaging

1. PET—Increasingly, PET stress tests are used to evaluate for myocardial ischemia and can evaluate for viability of heart muscle in territories with known ischemic injury to help guide whether complex revascularization may be beneficial.

2. Coronary CT—*Multislice CT angiography can provide an anatomic assessment of coronary arteries without invasive angiography and, using flow modeling, can provide a functional assessment of flow reserve across detected stenoses.* Its use has been associated with lower 5-year mortality compared to standard care in patients with stable chest pain. In the PROMISE trial, patients with stable chest pain undergoing anatomic imaging with CT angiography had similar outcomes to patients undergoing functional testing (stress ECG, stress radionuclide, or stress echocardiography). CT angiography with noninvasive functional assessment of coronary stenosis (fractional flow reserve), termed **CT-FFR**, has also been evaluated in patients with low-intermediate likelihood of CAD. CT-FFR has been shown to reduce the number of patients without coronary disease requiring invasive angiography. CT-FFR has been approved for clinical use and is used in clinical practice in the United States and Europe. The use of CT-FFR has been endorsed with a level IIa recommendation for intermediate-risk patients with chest pain and no prior history of CAD with a 40–90% stenosis on CT imaging to guide need for revascularization in the 2021 ACC/AHA Guideline for the Evaluation and Diagnosis of Chest Pain.

Coronary calcium score by electron beam CT can quantify coronary artery calcification, which is highly correlated with atheromatous plaque and has high sensitivity, but low specificity, for obstructive coronary disease. This test has not traditionally been used in symptomatic patients. According to the AHA, persons who are at low risk (< 10% 10-year risk) or at high risk (> 20% 10-year risk) for obstructive coronary disease do not benefit from coronary calcium assessment (class III, level of evidence: B). However, in clinically selected, intermediate-risk patients (5–7.5% atherosclerotic CVD), it may be reasonable to determine the atherosclerosis burden using calcium score in order to refine clinical risk prediction and to select patients for more aggressive target values for lipid-lowering therapies (class IIb, level of evidence: B).

3. Cardiac MRI—**Cardiac MRI** provides high-resolution images of the heart and great vessels without radiation exposure or use of iodinated contrast media. Gadolinium contrast has been associated with a rare but fatal complication in patients with severe kidney disease, called **necrotizing systemic fibrosis**. Gadolinium can demonstrate perfusion using dobutamine or adenosine to produce a *pharmacologic stress test*. Advances have been made in imaging the proximal coronary arteries. Perhaps the most clinically used indication of cardiac MRI is for identification of **myocardial fibrosis**, either from MI or infiltration, done with gadolinium contrast. This allows high-resolution imaging of myocardial viability and infiltrative cardiomyopathies.

I. Coronary Angiography

Selective coronary angiography is the definitive diagnostic procedure for CAD. It can be performed with low mortality (about 0.1%) and morbidity (1–5%), but due to the invasive nature and cost, it is recommended only in patients with a high pretest probability of CAD.

Coronary angiography should be performed in the following circumstances if percutaneous transluminal coronary angioplasty or bypass surgery is a consideration:

1. Life-limiting stable angina despite an adequate medical regimen.
2. Clinical presentation (unstable angina, myocardial infarction, etc) or noninvasive testing suggests high-risk disease (see "Prevention of Further Attacks," section K, "Revascularization").
3. Concomitant aortic valve disease and angina pectoris, to determine whether the angina is due to accompanying coronary disease.
4. Asymptomatic older patients undergoing valve surgery so that concomitant bypass may be done if needed.
5. Recurrence of symptoms after coronary revascularization to determine whether bypass grafts or native vessels are occluded.
6. Cardiac failure where a surgically correctable lesion, such as LV aneurysm, valve disease, or reversible ischemic dysfunction, is suspected.
7. Persons who have experienced sudden death, symptomatic, or life-threatening arrhythmias when CAD may be a correctable cause.
8. Chest pain of uncertain cause or cardiomyopathy of unknown cause.
9. Emergently perform cardiac catheterization with intention to perform primary percutaneous coronary intervention (PCI) in patients with suspected acute MI.

A narrowing of > 50% of the luminal diameter is considered hemodynamically (and clinically) significant, although most lesions producing ischemia are associated with narrowing of > 70%. Intracoronary imaging with **intravascular ultrasound (IVUS)** or **optical coherence tomography (OCT)** is useful as an adjunct for both assessing lesions that are indeterminate by angiography alone. IVUS is the invasive diagnostic method of choice for assessing indeterminate proximal coronary lesions, such as left main lesions, and coronary dissections because it does not rely on washing out the blood pool with contrast. Additionally, outcomes are improved when intracoronary imaging is used to guide PCI.

Invasive fractional flow reserve (FFR) testing can be used as an adjunctive test of the hemodynamic significance of an indeterminate coronary lesion in the absence of stress testing data. At the time of invasive angiography a pressure wire is used to measure the relative change in pressure across a coronary lesion after adenosine-induced hyperemia. Similar modalities, such as **instantaneous wave-free ratio (iFR)** measurements facilitate similar testing without the use of adenosine and have become more common than FFR testing. Revascularization based on abnormal flow reserve improves clinical outcomes compared with revascularization of all angiographically stenotic lesions.

LV angiography can be performed at the same time as coronary arteriography if prior structural evaluation has not been performed with another modality, and it can assess for regional wall motion abnormalities, mitral regurgitation, and the presence of other mechanical complications of coronary artery disease. It is less commonly utilized in the current era given advances in noninvasive imaging of structural heart disease.

Differential Diagnosis

When atypical features are present, suspicion for noncardiac chest pain should be raised. However, it is important to recognize that atypical features do not exclude CAD as a cause of symptoms.

Anterior chest wall syndrome is characterized by a sharply localized tenderness of the intercostal muscles. Inflammation of the chondrocostal junctions may result in diffuse chest pain that is also reproduced by local pressure **(Tietze syndrome)**. Intercostal neuritis (due to herpes zoster or diabetes mellitus, for example) also mimics angina.

Cervical or thoracic spine disease involving the dorsal roots produces sudden sharp, severe chest pain suggesting angina in location and "radiation" but related to specific movements of the neck or spine, recumbency, and straining or lifting. Pain due to cervical or thoracic disk disease involves the outer or dorsal aspect of the arm and the thumb and index fingers rather than the ring and little fingers.

Reflux esophagitis, peptic ulcer, chronic cholecystitis, esophageal spasm, and functional GI disease may produce pain suggestive of angina pectoris. The picture may be especially confusing because ischemic pain may also be associated with upper GI symptoms, and esophageal motility disorders may be improved by nitrates and calcium channel blockers. Assessment of esophageal motility may be helpful.

Degenerative and inflammatory lesions of the left shoulder and thoracic outlet syndromes may cause chest pain due to nerve irritation or muscular compression; the symptoms are usually precipitated by movement of the arm and shoulder and are associated with paresthesias.

Pneumonia, PE, and spontaneous pneumothorax may cause chest pain as well as dyspnea. Dissection of the thoracic aorta can cause severe chest pain that is commonly felt in the back; it is sudden in onset, reaches maximum intensity immediately, and may be associated with changes in pulses. Other cardiac disorders, such as mitral valve prolapse, HCM, myocarditis, pericarditis, aortic valve disease, or RVH, may cause atypical chest pain or even myocardial ischemia.

Treatment

Sublingual nitroglycerin is the medication of choice for acute management; it acts in about 1–2 minutes. As soon as the attack begins, one fresh tablet is placed under the tongue. This may be repeated at 3- to 5-minute intervals, but if pain is not relieved or improving after 5 minutes, the patient should call 9-1-1; *pain not responding to three tablets or lasting > 20 minutes may represent evolving infarction*. The dosage and the number of tablets to be used before seeking further medical attention may be individualized. Nitroglycerin buccal spray is also available as a metered (0.4 mg) delivery system. It has the advantage of being more convenient for patients who have difficulty handling the pills and of being more stable.

Prevention of Further Attacks

A. Aggravating Factors

Angina may be aggravated by hypertension, LV failure, arrhythmia (usually tachycardias), strenuous activity, cold temperatures, and emotional states. These factors should be identified and treated when possible.

B. Nitroglycerin

Nitroglycerin, 0.3–0.6 mg sublingual or 0.4–0.8 mg translingual spray, can be taken 5 minutes before any activity likely to precipitate angina.

C. Long-Acting Nitrates

Longer-acting nitrate preparations include isosorbide dinitrate, 10–40 mg orally three times daily; isosorbide mononitrate, 10–40 mg orally twice daily or 60–120 mg once daily in a sustained-release preparation; oral sustained-release nitroglycerin preparations, 6.25–12.5 mg two to four times daily; nitroglycerin ointment, 2% ointment, 0.5–2 inches (7.5–30 mg in the morning and 6 hours later); and transdermal nitroglycerin patches that deliver nitroglycerin at rates of 0.2, 0.4, and 0.6 mg/hour rate (0.1–0.8 mg/hour), and should be taken off after 12–14 hours of use for a 10- to 12-hour patch-free interval daily. The main limitation to long-term nitrate therapy is *tolerance*, which can be limited by using a regimen that includes a minimum 8- to 10-hour period per day without nitrates. Isosorbide dinitrate can be given three times daily, with the last dose after dinner, or longer-acting isosorbide mononitrate once daily. Transdermal nitrate preparations should be removed overnight in most patients.

Nitrate therapy is often limited by headache. Other side effects include nausea, light-headedness, and hypotension. Importantly, phosphodiesterase inhibitors used commonly for erectile dysfunction should not be taken within 24 hours of nitrate use.

D. β-Blockers

β-Blockers are the only antianginal agents that have been demonstrated to prolong life in patients with coronary disease (post-MI). *β-Blockers should be considered for first-line therapy in most patients with chronic angina* and are recommended as such by the stable ischemic heart disease guidelines.

β-Blockers with intrinsic sympathomimetic activity, such as pindolol, are less desirable because they may exacerbate angina in some individuals and have not been effective in secondary prevention trials. Otherwise, despite differences in cardioselectivity, vasodilation, and lipid solubility all β-blockers seem to be equally efficacious in the treatment of stable ischemic heart disease. The pharmacology and side effects of the β-blockers are discussed in Chapter 13 (see Tables 13–10 and 13–11). The dosages of all these medications when given for angina are similar. The major contraindications are severe bronchospastic disease, bradyarrhythmias, and decompensated HF.

E. Ranolazine

Ranolazine has no effect on heart rate and BP, and it has been shown to prolong exercise duration and time to angina. It is safe to use with erectile dysfunction medications. The usual dose is 500 mg orally twice a day. Because it can cause QT prolongation, it is contraindicated in patients with existing QT prolongation; in patients taking QT prolonging medications, such as class I or III antiarrhythmics (eg, quinidine, dofetilide, sotalol); and in those taking potent and moderate CYP450 3A inhibitors (eg, clarithromycin and rifampin). Of interest, despite QT prolongation, there is a significantly lower rate of ventricular arrhythmias with its use following ACSs, as shown in the MERLIN trial.

F. Calcium Channel Blocking Agents

Calcium channel blockers have *not* been shown to reduce mortality postinfarction and in some cases have increased ischemia and mortality rates. This is the case with some dihydropyridines (eg, nifedipine) and with diltiazem and verapamil in patients with clinical HF or moderate to severe LV dysfunction. Meta-analyses have suggested that short-acting nifedipine in moderate to high doses causes an *increase* in mortality. It is uncertain whether these findings are relevant to longer-acting dihydropyridines. Nevertheless, considering the uncertainties and the lack of demonstrated favorable effect on outcomes, calcium channel blockers should be considered third-line anti-ischemic medications in the postinfarction patient. Similarly, these agents, with the exception of amlodipine (which proved safe in patients with HF in the PRAISE-2 trial), should be avoided in patients with HF or low EFs.

The pharmacologic effects and side effects of the calcium channel blockers are discussed in Chapter 13 and summarized in Table 13–8. Diltiazem, amlodipine, and verapamil are preferable because they produce less reflex tachycardia and because the former, at least, may cause fewer side effects. Nifedipine, nicardipine, and amlodipine are also approved agents for angina. Isradipine, felodipine, and nisoldipine are not approved for angina but probably are as effective as the other dihydropyridines.

G. Ivabradine

Ivabradine selectively blocks the I_f current and specifically lowers heart rate. It has been shown to reduce angina in patients with chronic stable angina and is approved in Europe. However, the SIGNIFY trial found no overall difference in clinical outcomes in patients without HF and angina and signal toward harm for patients with significant angina, including cardiovascular death and MI. It is not widely used as an antianginal.

H. Combination Therapies

Patients who do not respond to one class of antianginal medication often respond to another. *The stable ischemic heart disease guidelines recommend starting with a β-blocker as initial therapy, followed by long-acting nitrates, calcium channel blockers, or ranolazine.*

I. Platelet-Inhibiting Agents

Several studies have demonstrated the benefit of antiplatelet medications for patients with stable and unstable vascular disease. Therefore, *unless contraindicated,* ***aspirin*** *(81 mg orally daily) should be prescribed for all patients with angina.* A $P2Y_{12}$ inhibitor **clopidogrel**, 75 mg orally daily, reduces vascular events in patients with stable vascular disease (as an alternative to aspirin) and in patients with ACSs (in addition to aspirin). Thus, it is also a good alternative in aspirin-intolerant patients. Clopidogrel in addition to aspirin did not reduce MI, stroke, or cardiovascular death in the CHARISMA trial of patients with CVD or multiple risk factors, with about a 50% increase in bleeding. However, it might be reasonable to use combination clopidogrel and aspirin for certain high-risk patients with established coronary disease, as tested in the Dual Antiplatelet Therapy (DAPT) trial. Specifically, *prolonged use of dual antiplatelet therapy with aspirin and clopidogrel may be beneficial in patients after PCI with drug-eluting stents who have a low bleeding risk.* In patients with prior MI, long-term treatment with ticagrelor plus aspirin reduced cardiovascular events compared with aspirin alone. In patients with peripheral artery disease, ticagrelor monotherapy did *not* reduce cardiovascular events compared with clopidogrel.

Rivaroxaban, a direct factor Xa inhibitor, when used at a dose of 2.5 mg twice daily in addition to low-dose aspirin, was found to reduce cardiovascular events including cardiovascular death, MI, or stroke compared with aspirin monotherapy in patients with known CAD or peripheral artery disease. This provides another option for patients.

Guidelines recommend ***dual antiplatelet therapy*** *(aspirin and $P2Y_{12}$ therapy) in patients with recent MI (within 1 year) or recent stenting (within 6 months) and for prolonged therapy (> 1 year) in patients at high ischemic risk (multivessel coronary disease or polyvascular disease) and low bleeding risk.*

J. Risk Reduction

Patients with coronary disease should undergo aggressive **risk factor modification.** This approach, with a particular focus on statin treatment, treating hypertension, stopping smoking, and exercise and weight control (especially for patients with metabolic syndrome or at risk for diabetes), can improve outcomes. For patients with diabetes and CVD, antiglycemic medications should be re-evaluated and shifted to cardioprotective medications (SGLT-2 inhibitors, GLP-1 agonists) as appropriate. Aggressive BP control (target systolic BP < 120 mm Hg) in the ACCORD trial was *not* associated with reduction in CAD events despite reducing stroke. In contrast, the SPRINT trial, which did not include patients with diabetes, demonstrated a reduction in cardiovascular events in patients with a reduction in death from any cause and reduction in MI with a goal systolic BP of < 120 mm Hg versus of goal of < 140 mm Hg. Some increase in adverse events was noted. Based on this and the totality of results, *the AHA has recommended defining hypertension at the 130 mm Hg level.*

K. Revascularization

1. Indications—There is general agreement that otherwise healthy patients in the following groups should undergo revascularization: (1) patients with unacceptable symptoms despite medical therapy to its tolerable limits; (2) patients with left main coronary artery stenosis > 50% with or without symptoms; (3) patients with three-vessel disease with LV dysfunction (EF < 50% or previous transmural infarction); (4) patients with unstable angina who after symptom control by medical therapy continue to exhibit ischemia on exercise testing or monitoring; and (5) post-MI patients with continuing angina or severe ischemia on noninvasive testing. The use of revascularization for patients with ACSs and acute STEMI is discussed below.

Data from the COURAGE trial have shown that for patients with chronic angina and disease suitable for PCI, PCI in addition to stringent guideline-directed medical therapy aimed at both risk reduction and antianginal care offers no mortality benefit beyond excellent medical therapy alone, but improves long-term symptom burden. Therefore, *for patients with mild to moderate CAD and limited symptoms, revascularization may not provide significant quality-of-life benefit.* For patients with moderate to significant coronary stenosis, such as those who have two-vessel disease associated with underlying LV dysfunction, anatomically critical lesions (> 90% proximal stenoses, especially of the proximal left anterior descending artery), or physiologic evidence of severe ischemia (early positive exercise tests, large exercise-induced ischemic defects, or frequent episodes of ischemia), a heart team consisting of interventional cardiologists and cardiac surgeons should review cases and provide patients with the best revascularization options. A recent study examined the role of PCI plus optimal guideline-directed medical therapy versus optimal guideline-directed medical therapy alone in 700 randomized patients with ischemic cardiomyopathy (EF < 35%) and myocardial viability. Compared with optimal medical therapy alone, PCI did *not* improve mortality, rate of hospitalization for HF, or EF.

The ISCHEMIA trial found that for patients with moderate to severe ischemia on stress testing, coronary angiography and revascularization did not reduce the risk of cardiovascular death, MI, hospitalization for unstable angina, HF, or resuscitated cardiac arrest. Thus, in the context of optimal medical therapy to prevent cardiovascular events, a higher threshold for whom to evaluate with stress tests and coronary angiography may be reasonable.

2. Type of procedure—

A. Percutaneous coronary intervention—PCI, including balloon angioplasty and coronary stenting, can effectively open stenotic coronary artery lesions. Coronary stenting with drug-eluting stents has become the mainstay of percutaneous revascularization therapy to reduce the risk of restenosis, acute vessel closure, and periprocedural MI. Use of intracoronary imaging (IVUS, OCT) as an adjunct to angiography alone to guide PCI has improved outcomes through improved stent expansion and apposition, as well as coronary lesion preparation and treatment. Acute stent thrombosis largely can be avoided by appropriate antithrombotic therapy (adequate anticoagulation with bolus-dose heparin, loading aspirin, and a P2Y12 inhibitor before or at the time of angioplasty, and with the use of adjunctive antithrombotics such as glycoprotein IIb/IIIa inhibitors as needed). The risk of restenosis remains a challenge in coronary artery disease treated by PCI. Factors associated with higher restenosis rates include diabetes, small luminal diameter, longer and more complex lesions, and lesions with inadequate lesion preparation/stent expansion/lesion coverage. Cases of restenosis can be treated by repeat stenting, although the development of drug-coated balloons offers an alternative to further stenting at sites of stent restenosis. Stenting can also be used selectively for isolated left main coronary stenosis, particularly when CABG is contraindicated or deemed high risk. The rationale for many of the procedures performed in patients with stable angina should be for angina symptom reduction.

Although sometimes seen in practice, there is no role for routine functional stress testing following PCI. Stress testing following PCI was analyzed in a randomized study of 1706 patients, with no difference in all-cause death, MI, or hospitalization for unstable angina between the those assigned to surveillance stress testing at 1 year following PCI or those receiving standard care. Stress testing should be reserved for evaluating a change in symptom burden.

The COURAGE trial and the ORBITA sham-controlled trial have confirmed earlier studies in showing that, even for patients with moderate anginal symptoms and positive stress tests, PCI provides no benefit over medical therapy with respect to death or MI. PCI was more effective at relieving angina, although most patients in the medical group had improvement in symptoms. PCI was also not more effective than optimal medical therapy for exercise time in patients with one vessel coronary disease. Thus, *in patients with mild or moderate stable symptoms, aggressive lipid-lowering and antianginal therapy may be a preferable initial strategy, reserving PCI for patients with significant and refractory symptoms or for those who are unable to take the prescribed medicines.*

Several studies of PCI versus CABG in patients with multivessel disease have been reported. The SYNTAX trial as well other trials show comparable mortality and infarction rates over follow-up periods of 1–3 years but a high rates of reintervention following PCI. Stroke rates are higher with CABG. As a result, the choice of revascularization procedure may depend on details of coronary anatomy and is often a matter of patient preference. Outcomes with percutaneous revascularization in patients with diabetes and reduced LV ejection fraction have generally been inferior to those with CABG. The FREEDOM trial demonstrated that *CABG surgery was superior to PCI with regard to death, MI, and stroke for patients with diabetes and multivessel coronary disease* at 5 years across all subgroups of SYNTAX score.

B. Coronary artery bypass grafting—CABG can be accomplished with a low mortality rate (1–3%) in otherwise healthy patients with preserved cardiac function. However, the mortality rate of this procedure rises to 4–8% in older individuals, patients with multiple comorbidities, and patients who have had a prior CABG.

Grafts using one or both **internal mammary arteries** (usually to the left anterior descending artery or its branches) provide the best long-term results in terms of patency and flow. Segments of the **saphenous vein** (or, less optimally, other veins) or the **radial artery** interposed between the aorta and the coronary arteries distal to the obstructions are also used.

Minimally invasive surgical techniques may involve a limited sternotomy, lateral thoracotomy (MIDCAB), or thoracoscopy (port-access). They are more technically demanding, usually not suitable for more than two grafts, and do not have established durability. Bypass surgery can be performed both on circulatory support (on-pump) and without direct circulatory support (off-pump). Randomized trial data have *not* shown a benefit with off-pump bypass surgery, but minimally invasive surgical techniques may allow earlier postoperative mobilization and discharge.

The operative mortality rate is increased in patients with poor LV function (LVEF < 35%), multiple medical comorbidities, advanced age, frailty, or those requiring additional procedures (valve replacement). Thus, CABG should be used for symptomatic patients deemed to be appropriate surgical candidates. *Early (1–6 months) graft patency rates average 85–90% (higher for internal mammary grafts), and subsequent graft closure rates are about 4% annually.* Early graft failure is common in vessels with poor distal flow, while late closure is more frequent in patients who continue smoking and have undertreated risk factors. Antiplatelet therapy with aspirin improves graft patency rates. Repeat revascularization may be necessary because of recurrent symptoms due to progressive native vessel disease and graft occlusions. In addition, in patients with ischemic mitral regurgitation, mitral repair at the time of a CABG does *not* offer any clinical benefit.

L. Mechanical Extracorporeal Counterpulsation

Extracorporeal counterpulsation entails repetitive inflation of a high-pressure chamber surrounding the lower half of the body during the diastolic phase of the cardiac cycle for daily 1-hour sessions over a period of 7 weeks. Randomized trials have shown that extracorporeal counterpulsation reduces angina, thus it may be considered for relief of refractory angina in patients with stable coronary disease who have exhausted all other therapy options previously described.

M. Neuromodulation

Spinal cord stimulation can be used to relieve chronic refractory angina. Spinal cord stimulators are subcutaneously implantable via a minimally invasive procedure under local anesthesia. This is rarely used in practice and should be reserved for those with truly refractory angina despite all other therapies.

Prognosis

The prognosis of angina pectoris has improved with development of therapies aimed at secondary prevention. Mortality rates vary depending on the number of vessels diseased, the severity of obstruction, the status of LV function, and the presence of complex arrhythmias. *The outlook in individual patients is unpredictable, and nearly half of the deaths are sudden.* Therefore, risk stratification is important. Patients with accelerating symptoms have a poorer outlook. Among stable patients, those whose exercise tolerance is severely limited by ischemia (< 6 minutes on the Bruce treadmill protocol) and those with extensive ischemia by exercise ECG or scintigraphy have more severe anatomic disease and a poorer prognosis.

When to Refer

All patients with new or worsening symptoms believed to represent progressive angina or a positive stress test for myocardial ischemia with continued angina despite medical therapy (or both) should be referred to a cardiologist.

When to Admit

- Patients with elevated cardiac biomarkers, ischemic ECG findings, or hemodynamic instability.
- Patients with new or worsened symptoms, possibly thought to be ischemic, but who lack high-risk features can be observed with serial ECGs and biomarkers and discharged if stress testing shows low-risk findings.

Park DW et al; POST-PCI Investigators. Routine functional testing or standard care in high-risk patients after PCI. N Engl J Med. 2022;387:905. [PMID: 36036496]
Perera D et al; REVIVED-BCIS2 Investigators. Percutaneous revascularization for ischemic left ventricular dysfunction. N Engl J Med. 2022;387:1351. [PMID: 36027563]

CORONARY VASOSPASM & ANGINA OR MI WITH NORMAL CORONARY ARTERIOGRAMS

ESSENTIALS OF DIAGNOSIS

- Precordial chest pain, often occurring at rest during stress or without known precipitant, relieved rapidly by nitrates.
- ECG evidence of ischemia during pain, sometimes with ST-segment elevation.
- Angiographic demonstration of:
  - -No significant obstruction of major coronary vessels.
  - -Coronary spasm that responds to intracoronary nitroglycerin or calcium channel blockers.

General Considerations

Although most symptoms of myocardial ischemia result from a fixed stenosis, intraplaque hemorrhage, or thrombosis at the site of lesions, some ischemic events may be precipitated or exacerbated by coronary vasoconstriction.

Spasm of the coronary arteries with resulting decreased coronary blood flow may occur spontaneously or may be induced by exposure to cold, emotional stress, or vasoconstricting medications. Spasm may occur both in normal or stenosed coronary arteries. MI can occur as a result of spasm in the absence of visibly obstructive CAD.

Cocaine can induce myocardial ischemia and infarction by causing coronary artery vasoconstriction or by increasing myocardial energy requirements. It also may contribute to accelerated atherosclerosis and thrombosis. The ischemia in **Prinzmetal angina** usually results from coronary vasoconstriction. It tends to involve the right coronary artery and there may be no fixed stenoses. Myocardial ischemia may also occur in patients with normal coronary arteries as a result of disease of the coronary microcirculation or abnormal vascular reactivity. MI without obstructive coronary disease is more frequent in women and has been shown to be due to atherosclerosis or ruptured plaques in 80% of cases. The 2020 ESC guidelines recommend cardiac MRI to aid in determining the cause of MI without obstructive coronary disease.

Clinical Findings

Ischemia may be silent or result in angina pectoris. Prinzmetal angina is a clinical syndrome in which chest pain occurs without the usual precipitating factors and is associated with ST-segment elevation rather than depression. It often affects women < 50 years of age. It characteristically occurs in the early morning, awakening patients from sleep, and is apt to be associated with arrhythmias or conduction defects. It may be diagnosed by challenge with ergonovine (a vasoconstrictor), although the results of such provocation are not specific and it entails risk.

Treatment

Patients with chest pain associated with ST-segment elevation should undergo coronary arteriography to determine whether fixed stenotic lesions are present. If they are, aggressive medical therapy or revascularization is indicated, since the presence of these lesions may represent an unstable phase of the disease. If significant lesions are not seen, there may still be endothelial disruption and plaque rupture. If spasm is suspected, avoidance of precipitants, such as cigarette smoking and cocaine, is the top priority. Episodes of coronary spasm generally respond well to nitrates acutely, and both nitrates and calcium channel blockers (including long-acting nifedipine, diltiazem, or amlodipine [see Table 13–8]) are effective prophylactically. By allowing unopposed α_1-mediated vasoconstriction, β-blockers have exacerbated coronary vasospasm, but they may have a role in management of patients in whom spasm is associated with fixed stenoses.

When to Refer

All patients with persistent symptoms of chest pain that may represent spasm should be referred to a cardiologist.

ACUTE CORONARY SYNDROME WITHOUT ST-SEGMENT ELEVATION

ESSENTIALS OF DIAGNOSIS

- Distinction in ACS between patients with and without ST-segment elevation at presentation is essential to determine need for reperfusion therapy.
- nSTEMI does not require immediate angiography and invasive revascularization unless associated with refractory angina, HF, shock, or ventricular arrhythmia.
- Antiplatelet and anticoagulation therapies and coronary intervention are mainstays of treatment.

General Considerations

***ACS** comprises the spectrum of unstable cardiac ischemia from unstable angina to acute MI.* ACS is classified based on the presenting ECG as either **STEMI** or **nSTEMI**. This allows for immediate classification and guides determination of whether patients should be considered for acute reperfusion therapy. Serial cardiac biomarker testing is then used to determine if an MI occurred. ACS represents a *dynamic state* in which patients can shift from one category to another, as new ST elevation can develop after presentation and cardiac biomarkers can become abnormal with recurrent ischemic episodes.

Clinical Findings

A. Symptoms and Signs

Patients with ACS generally have symptoms and signs of myocardial ischemia either at rest or with minimal exertion. These symptoms and signs are similar to the chronic angina symptoms described above, consisting of substernal chest pain or discomfort that may radiate to the jaw, shoulder, or arm. Dyspnea, nausea, diaphoresis, or syncope either may accompany the chest discomfort or may be the only symptom of ACS. *About one-third of patients with MI do not describe chest pain—these patients tend to be older, be female, have diabetes, and be at higher risk for subsequent mortality.* Patients with ACS have signs of HF in about 10% of cases, and this is also associated with higher risk of death.

The advent of high-sensitivity troponin assays has allowed for more rapid diagnosis of ACS, decreasing the time to diagnosis with serial troponin testing to 3 hours. This allows for more rapid diagnosis of nSTEMI, and triage to admission versus further emergency department or outpatient testing.

B. Laboratory Findings

Depending on the time from symptom onset to presentation, initial laboratory findings may be normal. While all biomarkers of cardiac myocyte necrosis can be used to identify acute MI, *high-sensitivity troponin is the recommended biomarker to diagnose acute MI* (see Laboratory Findings, Acute Myocardial Infarction with ST-Segment Elevation). High-sensitivity troponin assays allow rapid assessment of possible MI in emergency departments by using 1- or 3-hour rule-out algorithms. The universal definition of MI is a rise of cardiac biomarkers with at least one value above the 99th percentile of the upper reference limit together with evidence of myocardial ischemia with at least one of the following: symptoms of ischemia, ECG changes of new ischemia or imaging evidence of new loss of viable myocardium or new wall motion abnormality.

C. ECG

Many patients with ACS will exhibit ECG changes during pain—either ST-segment elevation, ST-segment depression, or T wave flattening or inversion. Dynamic ST-segment shift is the most specific for ACS. ST-segment elevation in lead aVR can suggest left main or three-vessel disease.

Treatment

A. General Measures

Treatment of ACS without ST elevation should be multifaceted. Patients should be hospitalized, monitored, and treated with standard medical therapy in addition to further risk stratification and, in appropriate circumstances, undergo angiography and revascularization prior to discharge. Figure 10–2 provides an algorithm for initial management of nSTEMI.

B. Antiplatelet and Anticoagulation Therapy

Patients should receive a combination of antiplatelet and anticoagulant agents on presentation.

1. Antiplatelet therapy—

A. ASPIRIN—A 325-mg loading dose follow by 81 mg daily should be commenced immediately. Multiple studies of higher-dose aspirin over an extended time showed no benefit but a higher risk of bleeding. As such, 81 mg daily remains the recommended maintenance dose.

B. $P2Y_{12}$ INHIBITORS—ACC/AHA guidelines call for a $P2Y_{12}$ inhibitor (clopidogrel, prasugrel [at the time of PCI], or ticagrelor) as a class I recommendation. The ESC guidelines provide a stronger recommendation for a $P2Y_{12}$ inhibitor upfront (prior to angiography), as a class IA recommendation for all patients. Both sets of guidelines recommend postponing elective CABG surgery for at least 5 days after the last dose of clopidogrel or ticagrelor and at least 7 days after the last dose of prasugrel, due to risk of bleeding.

The ESC guidelines recommend ticagrelor for all patients at moderate to high risk for ACS (class I recommendation). Prasugrel is recommended for patients who have not yet received another $P2Y_{12}$ inhibitor, for whom a PCI is planned, and who are not at high risk for

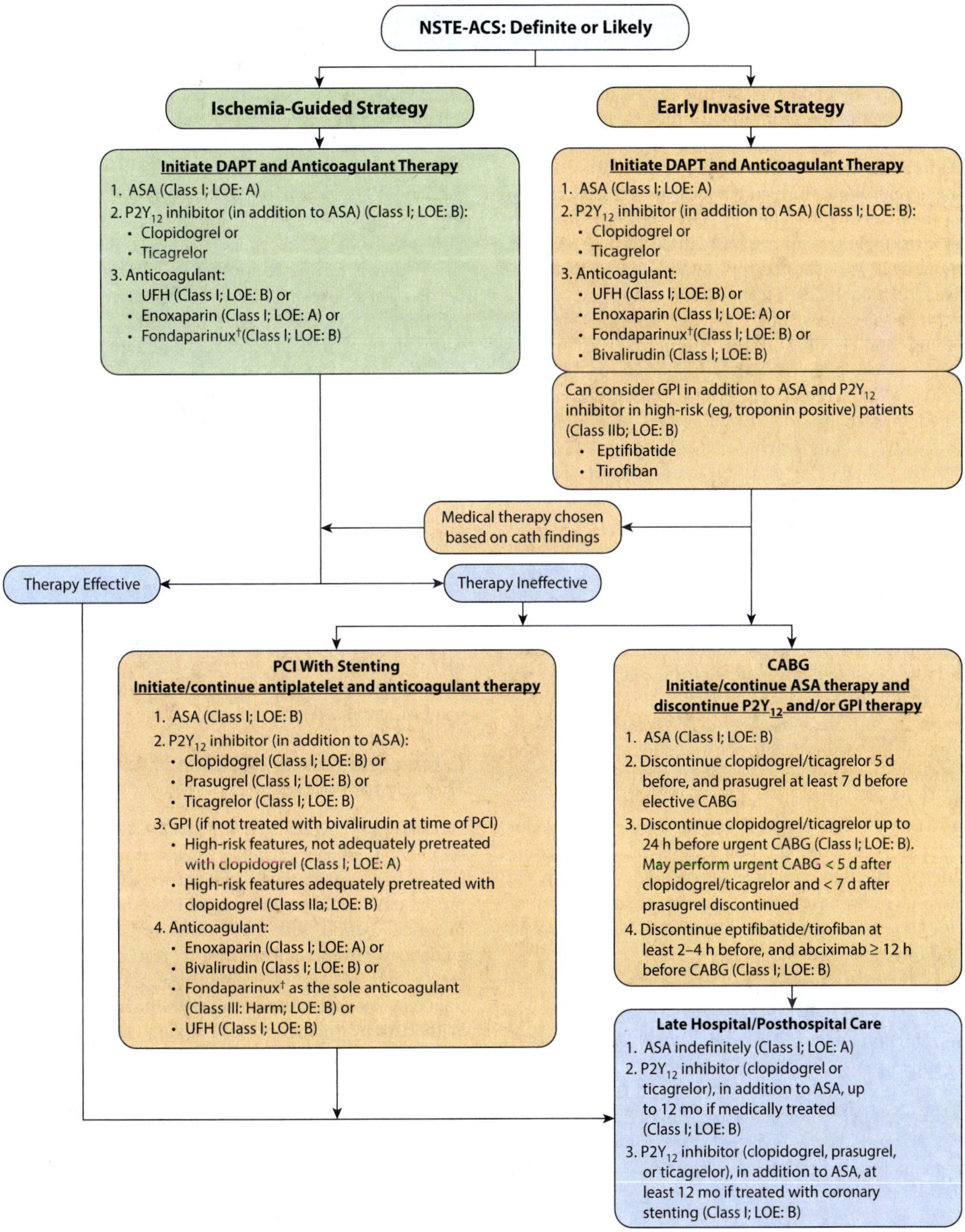

▲ **Figure 10–2.** Algorithm for management of patients with definite or likely NSTE-ACS. **See corresponding full-sentence recommendations and their explanatory footnotes. †In patients who have been treated with fondaparinux (as upfront therapy) who are undergoing PCI, an additional anticoagulant with anti-IIa activity should be administered at the time of PCI because of the risk of catheter thrombosis. ASA indicates aspirin; CABG, coronary artery bypass graft; cath, catheter; COR, Class of Recommendation; DAPT, dual antiplatelet therapy; GPI, glycoprotein IIb/IIIa inhibitor; LOE, Level of Evidence; NSTE-ACS, non–ST-elevation ACS; PCI, percutaneous coronary intervention; pts, patients; and UFH, unfractionated heparin. (Reproduced with permission from Amsterdam EA, Wenger NK, Brindis RG, et al. 2014 AHA/ACC Guideline for the Management of Patients with Non-ST-Elevation Acute Coronary Syndromes: a report of the American College of Cardiology/American Heart Association Task Force on Practice Guidelines [published correction appears in J Am Coll Cardiol. 2014;64(24):2713–2714.)

life-threatening bleeding. Clopidogrel is reserved for patients who cannot receive either ticagrelor or prasugrel. Some studies have shown an association between assays of residual platelet function and thrombotic risk during $P2Y_{12}$ inhibitor therapy, but both the European and the US guidelines do not recommend routine platelet function testing to guide therapy (class IIb recommendation).

Prasugrel is both more potent and has a faster onset of action than clopidogrel. The TRITON trial compared prasugrel with clopidogrel in patients with STEMI or nSTEMI in whom PCI was planned; prasugrel resulted in a 19% relative reduction in death from cardiovascular causes, MI, or stroke, at the expense of an increase in serious bleeding (including fatal bleeding). Stent thrombosis was reduced by half. Because patients with prior stroke or TIA had higher risk of intracranial hemorrhage, prasugrel is contraindicated in such patients. Bleeding was also higher in patients with low body weight (< 60 kg) and age ≥ 75 years, and caution should be used in these populations. For patients with STEMI treated with PCI, prasugrel appears to be especially effective (compared with clopidogrel) without a substantial increase in bleeding. For patients who will not receive revascularization, prasugrel, compared with clopidogrel, had no overall benefit in the TRILOGY trial (the dose of prasugrel was lowered for older adults).

Ticagrelor has a faster onset of action than clopidogrel and a more consistent and potent effect. The PLATO trial showed that when ticagrelor was started at the time of presentation in ACS patients (UA/nSTEMI and STEMI), it reduced cardiovascular death, MI, and stroke by 16% when compared with clopidogrel. In addition, there was a 22% relative risk reduction in mortality with ticagrelor. The overall rates of bleeding were similar between ticagrelor and clopidogrel, although non–CABG-related bleeding was higher. The finding of a lesser treatment effect in the United States may have been related to use of higher-dose aspirin, and thus when using ticagrelor, low-dose aspirin (81 mg/day) is recommended.

c. Glycoprotein IIb/IIIa inhibitors—Small-molecule inhibitors of the platelet glycoprotein IIb/IIIa receptor are useful adjuncts in high-risk patients with ACS, particularly at the time of PCI. Tirofiban, 25 mcg/kg over 3 minutes, followed by 0.15 mcg/kg/min, and eptifibatide, 180 mcg/kg bolus followed by a continuous infusion of 2 mcg/kg/min, have both been shown to be effective. Downward dose adjustments of the infusions are required in patients with reduced kidney function.

2. Anticoagulant therapy—

a. Heparin—Several trials have shown that LMWH (enoxaparin 1 mg/kg subcutaneously every 12 hours) is somewhat more effective than unfractionated heparin in preventing recurrent ischemic events in the setting of ACSs. However, the SYNERGY trial showed that unfractionated heparin and enoxaparin had similar rates of death or (re)infarction in the setting of frequent early coronary intervention. Additionally, enoxaparin is harder to manage with regard to bleeding. As such, *unfractionated IV heparin remains the initial anticoagulant of choice for patients presenting with ACS.*

b. Fondaparinux—Fondaparinux, a specific factor Xa inhibitor given in a dose of 2.5 mg subcutaneously once a day, was found in the OASIS-5 trial to be equally effective as enoxaparin among 20,000 patients at preventing early death, MI, and refractory ischemia, and resulted in a 50% reduction in major bleeding. This reduction in major bleeding translated into a significant reduction in mortality (and in death or MI) at 30 days. While catheter-related thrombosis was more common during coronary intervention procedures with fondaparinux, the FUTURA trial found that it can be controlled by adding unfractionated heparin (in a dose of 85 U/kg without glycoprotein IIb/IIIa inhibitors, and 60 U/kg with glycoprotein IIb/IIIa inhibitors) during the procedure. Guidelines recommend fondaparinux, describing it as especially favorable for patients who are initially treated medically and who are at high risk for bleeding, such as older adults.

c. Direct thrombin inhibitors—The ACUITY trial showed that bivalirudin appears to be a reasonable alternative to heparin (unfractionated heparin or enoxaparin) plus a glycoprotein IIb/IIIa antagonist for many patients with ACSs who are undergoing early coronary intervention. Bivalirudin (without routine glycoprotein IIb/IIIa inhibitor) is associated with substantially less bleeding than heparin plus glycoprotein IIb/IIIa inhibitor, although it may have numerically increased cardiovascular events. Bivalirudin does not have an FDA-approved indication for nSTEMI care.

C. Temporary Discontinuation of Antiplatelet Therapy for Procedures

Patients who have had recent coronary stents are at risk for thrombotic events, including stent thrombosis, if $P2Y_{12}$ inhibitors are discontinued prematurely. If possible, elective procedures should be delayed until the end of the necessary treatment period with $P2Y_{12}$ inhibitors. While treatment guidelines recommend at least 1 year of treatment with DAPT after ACS, more recent data suggest a 3-month duration may be safer (less bleeding) with improved survival. With current-generation drug-eluting stents, data suggest that DAPT can be discontinued after 1 month in high-bleeding-risk patients without an appreciable increase in mortality. If $P2Y_{12}$ inhibitors need to be stopped prior to guideline directed recommendations, it is prudent to consult a cardiologist for a shared decision-making assessment of the risks and benefits of early discontinuation. Aspirin should generally be continued throughout the period of the procedure.

D. Nitroglycerin

Nitrates are first-line therapy for patients with ACSs presenting with chest pain. Nonparenteral therapy with sublingual or oral agents is usually sufficient. If pain persists or recurs, intravenous nitroglycerin should be started. The usual initial dosage is 10 mcg/min. The dosage should be titrated upward by 10–20 mcg/min (to a maximum of 200 mcg/min) until angina disappears or mean arterial pressure drops by 10%. Careful BP monitoring is required when intravenous nitroglycerin is used. Avoid hypotension (systolic BP < 100 mm Hg). Tolerance to continuous nitrate infusion is common.

E. β-Blockers

β-Blockers are an important part of the initial treatment of ACS unless otherwise contraindicated. The pharmacology of these agents is discussed in Chapter 13 and summarized in Tables 13–10 and 13–11. Use of agents with intrinsic sympathomimetic activity should be avoided in this setting. Oral medication is adequate in most patients, but intravenous treatment with metoprolol, given as three 5-mg doses 5 minutes apart as tolerated and in the absence of HF, achieves a more rapid effect. Oral therapy should be titrated upward as BP permits.

F. Calcium Channel Blockers

Calcium channel blockers have *not* been shown to favorably affect outcome in ACS, and they should be used primarily as third-line therapy in patients with continuing angina who are taking nitrates and β-blockers or those who are not candidates for these medications. In the presence of nitrates and without accompanying β-blockers, diltiazem or verapamil is preferred, since nifedipine and the other dihydropyridines are more likely to cause reflex tachycardia or hypotension. The initial dosage should be low, but upward titration should proceed steadily (see Table 13–8).

G. Statins

The PROVE-IT trial provides evidence for starting a high-dose, high-intensity statin in the days immediately following an ACS. In this trial, more intensive therapy with atorvastatin 80 mg/day, regardless of total or LDL cholesterol level, improved outcome compared with pravastatin 40 mg/day, with the curves of major cardiovascular event separating as early as 3 months after starting therapy. *High-intensity statins are recommended for all patients with ACS.*

Indications for Coronary Angiography

For patients with ACS, including nSTEMI, risk stratification is important for determining intensity of care. Early invasive catheterization has the greatest benefit in higher-risk patients with ACS. As outlined in the ACC/AHA guidelines, patients with any high-risk feature (Table 10–1) generally warrant an early invasive strategy with catheterization and revascularization. For patients without these high-risk features, either an invasive or noninvasive approach, using exercise (or pharmacologic stress for patients unable to exercise) stress testing to identify patients who have residual ischemia, are at high risk, or both, can be used. Moreover, based on the ICTUS trial, a strategy based on selective coronary angiography and revascularization for instability or inducible ischemia is acceptable (ACC/AHA class IIb recommendation).

Two risk-stratification tools are available that can be used at the bedside, the **GRACE Risk Score** (https://www.mdcalc.com/calc/1099/grace-acs-risk-mortality-calculator) and the **TIMI Risk Score** (http://www.timi.org). The GRACE Risk Score, which applies to patients with or without ST elevation, was developed in a more generalizable registry population and has better discrimination of risk. It includes age (as a continuous variable), Killip class, BP,

Table 10–1. Indications for catheterization and percutaneous coronary intervention.[1]

	ACSs (unstable angina and nSTEMI)
Class I	Early invasive strategy for any of the following high-risk indicators:
	Recurrent angina/ischemia at rest or with low-level activity
	Elevated troponin
	ST-segment depression
	Recurrent ischemia with evidence of HF
	High-risk stress test result
	EF < 40%
	Hemodynamic instability
	Sustained ventricular tachycardia
	PCI within 6 months
	Prior CABG
	In the absence of these findings, either an early conservative or early invasive strategy
Class IIa	Early invasive strategy for patients with repeated presentations for ACS despite therapy
Class III	Extensive comorbidities in patients in whom benefits of revascularization are not likely to outweigh the risks
	Acute chest pain with low likelihood of ACS
	Acute MI after fibrinolytic therapy
Class I	Cardiogenic shock or acute severe HF that develops after initial presentation
	Intermediate- or high-risk findings on predischarge noninvasive ischemia testing
	Spontaneous or easily provoked myocardial ischemia
Class IIa	Failed reperfusion or reocclusion after fibrinolytic therapy
	Stable[2] patients after successful fibrinolysis, before discharge and ideally between 3 and 24 hours

[1]Class I indicates treatment is useful and effective, IIa indicates weight of evidence is in favor of usefulness/efficacy, class IIb indicates weight of evidence is less well established, and class III indicates intervention is not useful/effective and may be harmful. Level of evidence A recommendations are derived from large-scale randomized trials, and B recommendations are derived from smaller randomized trials or carefully conducted observational analyses.
[2]Although individual circumstances will vary, clinical stability is defined by the absence of low output, hypotension, persistent tachycardia, apparent shock, high-grade ventricular or symptomatic supraventricular tachyarrhythmias, and spontaneous recurrent ischemia.
ACCF/AHA, American College of Cardiology Foundation/American Heart Association; CABG, coronary artery bypass grafting; PCI, percutaneous coronary intervention.
Data from O'Gara PT et al. 2013 ACCF/AHA guideline for the management of ST-elevation myocardial infarction: a report of the American College of Cardiology Foundation/American Heart Association Task Force on Practice Guidelines. Circulation. 2013;127:e362–e425.

ST-segment deviation, cardiac arrest at presentation, serum creatinine, elevated creatine kinase (CK)-MB or troponin, and heart rate. The TIMI Risk Score was developed from a clinical trial population and includes seven variables: age 65 years or older, three or more cardiac risk factors, prior coronary stenosis of 50% or more, ST-segment deviation, two anginal events in prior 24 hours, aspirin in prior 7 days, and elevated cardiac markers.

When to Refer

- All patients with acute MI should be referred to a cardiologist.
- Patients who are taking a $P2Y_{12}$ inhibitor following coronary stenting should consult a cardiologist before discontinuing treatment.

Writing Committee Members; Lawton JS et al. 2021 ACC/AHA/SCAI Guideline for Coronary Artery Revascularization: a report of the American College of Cardiology/American Heart Association Joint Committee on Clinical Practice Guidelines. J Am Coll Cardiol. 2022;79:e21. Erratum in: J Am Coll Cardiol. 2022;79:1547. [PMID: 34895950]

ACUTE MI WITH ST-SEGMENT ELEVATION

ESSENTIALS OF DIAGNOSIS

- Sometimes painless, may masquerade as acute HF, syncope, stroke, or shock.
- ECG: ST-segment elevation or new left bundle branch block.
- Immediate reperfusion treatment with primary PCI is warranted.
- Primary PCI within 90 minutes of first medical contact is the goal and is superior to fibrinolytic therapy.
- Fibrinolytic therapy within 30 minutes of hospital presentation is the goal when primary PCI is not achievable within 120 minutes of presentation, and reduces mortality if given within 12 hours of onset of symptoms.

General Considerations

STEMI results, in most cases, from an occlusive coronary thrombus at the site of a preexisting (though not necessarily obstructive) atherosclerotic plaque. More rarely, infarction may result from prolonged vasospasm, inadequate myocardial blood flow (eg, hypotension), or excessive metabolic demand. Very rarely, MI may be caused by embolic occlusion, vasculitis, aortic root or coronary artery dissection, or aortitis. Cocaine, a cause of infarction, should be considered in young individuals without risk factors. A condition that may mimic STEMI is stress cardiomyopathy (also referred to as **takotsubo cardiomyopathy**). *ST elevation connotes an acute coronary occlusion and warrants immediate reperfusion therapy with activation of emergency services.*

Clinical Findings

A. Symptoms

1. Premonitory pain—There is usually a worsening in the patient's own pattern of angina preceding the onset of symptoms of MI; classically the onset of angina occurs with minimal exertion or at rest.

2. Pain of infarction—*Unlike anginal episodes, most infarctions occur at rest, and more commonly in the early morning.* The pain is similar to angina in location and radiation but it may be more severe, and it builds up rapidly or in waves to maximum intensity over a few minutes or longer. Nitroglycerin has little effect; opioids may not relieve the pain.

3. Associated symptoms—Patients may break out in a cold sweat, feel weak and apprehensive, and move about, seeking a position of comfort. They prefer not to lie quietly. Light-headedness, syncope, dyspnea, orthopnea, cough, wheezing, nausea and vomiting, or abdominal bloating may be present singly or in any combination.

4. Painless infarction—One-third of patients with acute MI present *without* chest "pain" per se, and these patients tend to be undertreated and have poor outcomes. Older patients, women, and patients with diabetes mellitus are more likely to present without chest pain. As many as 25% of ACSs are detected on routine ECG without any recallable acute episode.

5. Sudden death and early arrhythmias—Of all deaths from MI, about half occur before the patients arrive at the hospital, with death presumably caused by ventricular arrhythmias.

B. Signs

1. General—Patients may appear anxious and sometimes are sweating profusely. The heart rate may range from marked bradycardia (most commonly in inferior infarction) to tachycardia, low cardiac output, or arrhythmia. The BP may be high, especially in patients with previous hypertension, or low in patients with shock. Respiratory distress usually indicates HF. Fever, usually low grade, may appear after 12 hours and persist for several days.

2. Chest—The **Killip classification** is the standard way to classify HF in patients with acute MI and has powerful prognostic value. Killip class I is absence of rales and S_3, class II is rales that do not clear with coughing over one-third or less of the lung fields or presence of an S_3, class III is rales that do not clear with coughing over more than one-third of the lung fields, and class IV is cardiogenic shock (rales, hypotension, and signs of hypoperfusion).

3. Heart—The cardiac examination may be unimpressive or very abnormal. Jugular venous distention reflects RA hypertension, and a Kussmaul sign (failure of decrease of jugular venous pressure with inspiration) is suggestive of RV infarction. Soft heart sounds may indicate LV dysfunction. Atrial gallops (S_4) are the rule, whereas ventricular gallops (S_3) are less common and indicate significant LV dysfunction. Mitral regurgitation murmurs are not uncommon and may indicate papillary muscle dysfunction or, rarely, rupture. Pericardial friction rubs are uncommon in the first 24 hours but may appear later.

4. Extremities—Edema is usually not present. Cyanosis and cold temperature indicate a low-output shock state. The peripheral pulses should be noted, since later shock or emboli may alter the examination.

C. Laboratory Findings

Cardiac-specific markers of myocardial damage include quantitative determinations of **troponin I**, **troponin T**, and less commonly CK-MB. Troponins are more sensitive and specific than **CK-MB**. High-sensitivity troponin assays were approved in 2017. They are the standard assays in clinical practice, with a 10- to 100-fold lower limit of detection, allowing MI to be detected earlier, using the change in value over 3 hours.

Circulating levels of troponins may remain elevated for 5–7 days or longer and therefore are generally not useful for evaluating suspected early reinfarction. Elevated CK-MB generally normalizes within 24 hours, thus being more helpful for evaluation of reinfarction. Low-level elevations of troponin in patients with severe CKD may not be related to acute coronary disease but rather a function of the physiologic washout of the marker. While many conditions including chronic HF are associated with elevated levels of the high-sensitivity troponin assays, these assays may be especially useful when negative to exclude MI in patients reporting chest pain.

D. ECG

The extent of the ECG abnormalities, especially the sum of the total amount of *ST-segment deviation*, is a good indicator of the extent of acute infarction and risk of subsequent adverse events. The classic evolution of changes is from peaked ("hyperacute") T waves, to ST-segment elevation, to Q wave development, to T wave inversion. This may occur over a few hours to several days. *The evolution of new Q waves (longer than 30 msec in duration and 25% of the R wave amplitude) is diagnostic, but Q waves do not occur in 30–50% of acute infarctions* (**non–Q wave infarctions**, which are typically *not* associated with ST elevation). Left bundle branch block, especially when new (or not known to be old), in a patient with symptoms of an acute MI is considered to be a **"STEMI equivalent"**; reperfusion therapy is indicated for the affected patient. Concordant ST elevation (ie, ST elevation in leads with an overall positive QRS complex) with left bundle branch block is a specific finding indicating STEMI.

E. Chest Radiography

The CXR may demonstrate signs of HF, but these changes often lag behind clinical findings. Signs of aortic dissection, including mediastinal widening, should be sought as a possible alternative diagnosis.

F. Echocardiography

Echocardiography provides convenient *bedside assessment* of LV global and regional function. This can help with the diagnosis and management of infarction; echocardiography has been used successfully to make judgments about admission and management of patients with suspected infarction, including in patients with ST-segment elevation or left bundle branch block of uncertain significance, since normal wall motion makes an infarction unlikely. Doppler echocardiography is generally the most convenient procedure for diagnosing postinfarction mitral regurgitation or VSD.

G. Other Noninvasive Studies

Diagnosis of MI and extent of MI can be assessed by various imaging studies in addition to echocardiography. **MRI with gadolinium contrast enhancement** is the most sensitive test to detect and quantitate extent of infarction, with the ability to detect as little as 2 g of MI. **Technetium-99m pyrophosphate scintigraphy**, when injected at least 18 hours postinfarction, complexes with calcium in necrotic myocardium to provide a "hot spot" image of the infarction. This test is insensitive to small infarctions, and false-positive studies occur, so its use is limited to patients in whom the diagnosis by ECG and enzymes is not possible—principally those who present several days after the event or have intraoperative infarctions. **Scintigraphy with thallium-201** or **technetium-based perfusion tracers** will demonstrate "cold spots" in regions of diminished perfusion, which usually represent infarction when the radiotracer is administered at rest, but abnormalities do not distinguish recent from old damage. All of these tests may be considered after the patient has had revascularization.

H. Hemodynamic Measurements

Right heart catheterization measurements can be helpful in managing the patient with suspected cardiogenic shock. Use of PA catheters, however, has generally *not* been associated with better outcomes and should be limited to patients with severe hemodynamic compromise for whom the information would be anticipated to change management.

Treatment

A. Aspirin and $P2Y_{12}$ Inhibitors (Prasugrel, Ticagrelor, and Clopidogrel)

All patients with definite or suspected acute MI should receive aspirin at a dose of 324 mg at once regardless of whether the patient has been taking aspirin. Chewable aspirin provides more rapid blood levels. Patients with a definite aspirin allergy should be treated with a $P2Y_{12}$ inhibitor (clopidogrel, prasugrel, or ticagrelor) until aspirin desensitization can be safely performed.

$P2Y_{12}$ inhibitors, in combination with aspirin, have been shown to provide important benefits in patients with acute STEMI. Thus, guidelines call for a *$P2Y_{12}$ inhibitor to be added to aspirin for all patients with STEMI, regardless of whether reperfusion is given, and continued for at least 14 days, and generally for 1 year.* The preferred $P2Y_{12}$ inhibitors are prasugrel (60 mg orally on day 1, then 10 mg daily) or ticagrelor (180 mg orally on day 1, then 90 mg twice daily). Both of these medications demonstrated superior outcomes to clopidogrel in clinical studies of primary PCI. Clopidogrel should be administered as a loading dose of 600 mg orally for faster onset of action. Prasugrel is contraindicated in patients with a history of stroke or who are older than 75 years.

B. Reperfusion Therapy

Patients with STEMI who seek medical attention within 12 hours of the onset of symptoms should be treated with reperfusion therapy, preferentially with primary PCI when readily available.

1. Primary PCI—Immediate coronary angiography and primary PCI of the infarct-related artery are *superior* to thrombolysis when with rapid time from first medical contact to intervention ("door-to-balloon"). US and European guidelines call for *door-to-balloon times of 90 minutes or less.* Several trials have shown that if efficient transfer systems are in place, transfer of patients with acute MI from hospitals without primary PCI capability to hospitals with primary PCI capability with first door-to-device times of 120 minutes or less can improve outcome compared with fibrinolytic therapy at the presenting hospital, although this requires sophisticated systems to ensure rapid identification, transfer, and expertise in PCI.

Emergent PCI with stenting is standard for patients with acute ST-elevation MI.

"Facilitated" PCI, whereby a combination of medications (full- or reduced-dose fibrinolytic agents, with or without glycoprotein IIb/IIIa inhibitors) is given followed by immediate PCI, is *not* recommended. *Patients should be treated either with primary PCI or with fibrinolytic agents (and immediate rescue PCI for reperfusion failure), if it can be done promptly* as outlined in the ACC/AHA and European guidelines. Timely access to most appropriate reperfusion, including primary PCI, can be expanded with development of regional systems of care, including emergency medical systems and networks of hospitals. Patients treated with fibrinolytic therapy appear to have improved outcomes if transferred for routine coronary angiography and PCI within 24 hours. The AHA has a program called "Mission: Lifeline" to support the development of regional systems of care (https://www.heart.org/en/professional/quality-improvement/mission-lifeline).

2. Fibrinolytic therapy—

A. BENEFIT—Fibrinolytic therapy reduces mortality and limits infarct size in patients with STEMI. The greatest benefit occurs if treatment is initiated within the first 3 hours after the onset of presentation, when up to a 50% reduction in mortality rate can be achieved. The magnitude of benefit declines rapidly thereafter, but a 10% relative mortality reduction can be achieved up to 12 hours after the onset of chest pain. *Primary PCI of the infarct-related artery, however, is superior to thrombolysis when done by experienced operators with rapid time from first medical contact to intervention ("door-to-balloon").*

B. CONTRAINDICATIONS—Major bleeding complications occur in 0.5–5% of patients, the most serious of which is intracranial hemorrhage. The major risk factors for intracranial bleeding are age 75 years or older, hypertension at presentation (especially over 180/110 mm Hg), low body weight (< 70 kg), and the use of fibrin-specific fibrinolytic agents (alteplase, reteplase, tenecteplase). Although patients over age 75 years have a much higher mortality rate with acute MI and therefore may derive greater benefit, the risk of severe bleeding is also higher, particularly among patients with risk factors for intracranial hemorrhage, such as severe hypertension or recent stroke. Patients presenting > 12 hours after the onset of chest pain may also derive a small benefit, particularly if pain and ST-segment elevation persist, but rarely does this benefit outweigh the attendant risk.

Absolute contraindications to fibrinolytic therapy include previous hemorrhagic stroke, cerebrovascular events within 1 year, known intracranial neoplasm, recent head trauma (including minor trauma), active internal bleeding (excluding menstruation), or suspected aortic dissection. *Relative contraindications* are BP > 180/110 mm Hg at presentation, other intracerebral pathology not listed above as a contraindication, known bleeding diathesis, trauma within 2–4 weeks, major surgery within 3 weeks, prolonged (> 10 minutes) or traumatic CPR, recent (within 2–4 weeks) internal bleeding, noncompressible vascular punctures, active diabetic retinopathy, pregnancy, active peptic ulcer disease, a history of severe hypertension, current use of anticoagulants (INR > 2.0–3.0), and (for streptokinase) prior allergic reaction or exposure to streptokinase or anistreplase within 2 years.

C. FIBRINOLYTIC AGENTS—Four fibrinolytic agents are available for acute MI and are characterized in Table 10–2.

(1) Selection of a fibrinolytic agent—The differences in efficacy between agents are small compared with the potential benefit of treating a greater proportion of appropriate candidates in a prompt manner. The principal objective should be to administer a thrombolytic agent within 30 minutes of presentation—or even during transport. The ability to administer tenecteplase as a single bolus is an attractive feature that may facilitate earlier treatment. The combination of a reduced-dose thrombolytic given with a platelet glycoprotein IIb/IIIa inhibitor does not reduce mortality but does cause a modest increase in bleeding complications.

(2) Postfibrinolytic management—After completion of the fibrinolytic infusion, aspirin (81–325 mg/day) and anticoagulation should be continued until revascularization or for the duration of the hospital stay (or up to 8 days). Anticoagulation with LMWH (enoxaparin or fondaparinux) is preferable to unfractionated heparin.

(A) LOW-MOLECULAR-WEIGHT HEPARIN—In the EXTRACT trial, enoxaparin significantly reduced death and MI at day 30 (compared with unfractionated heparin), at the expense of a modest increase in bleeding. In patients younger than age 75, enoxaparin was given as a 30-mg intravenous bolus and 1 mg/kg subcutaneously every 12 hours; in patients aged 75 years and older, it was given with no bolus and 0.75 mg/kg subcutaneously every 12 hours. This appeared to attenuate the risk of intracranial hemorrhage in older adults that had been seen with full-dose enoxaparin. Another antithrombotic option is fondaparinux, given at a dose of 2.5 mg subcutaneously

Table 10–2. Fibrinolytic therapy for acute MI.

	Alteplase; Tissue Plasminogen Activator (t-PA)	Reteplase	Tenecteplase (TNK-t-PA)	Streptokinase
Source	Recombinant DNA	Recombinant DNA	Recombinant DNA	Group C *Streptococcus*
Half-life	5 minutes	15 minutes	20 minutes	20 minutes
Usual dose	100 mg	20 units	40 mg	1.5 million units
Administration	Initial bolus of 15 mg, followed by 50 mg infused over the next 30 minutes and 35 mg over the following 60 minutes	10 units as a bolus over 2 minutes, repeated after 30 minutes	Single weight-adjusted bolus, 0.5 mg/kg	750,000 units over 20 minutes followed by 750,000 units over 40 minutes
Anticoagulation after infusion	Aspirin, 325 mg daily; heparin, 5000 units as bolus, followed by 1000 units/hour infusion, subsequently adjusted to maintain PTT 1.5–2 times control	Aspirin, 325 mg; heparin as with t-PA	Aspirin, 325 mg daily	Aspirin, 325 mg daily; there is no evidence that adjunctive heparin improves outcome following streptokinase
Clot selectivity	High	High	High	Low
Fibrinogenolysis	+	+	+	+++
Bleeding	+	+	+	+
Hypotension	+	+	+	+++
Allergic reactions	+	+	+	++
Reocclusion	10–30%	—	5–20%	5–20%
Approximate cost[1]	$10,560.43	$5964.98	$7462.63	Not available in the United States

[1]Average wholesale price (AWP, for AB-rated generic when available) for quantity listed.
PTT, partial thromboplastin time.
Source: IBM Micromedex, Red Book (electronic version). IBM Watson Health, Greenwood Village, CO, USA. Available at https://www.micromedexsolutions.com (accessed April 8, 2020). AWP may not accurately represent the actual pharmacy cost because wide contractual variations exist among institutions.

once a day. There is no benefit of fondaparinux among patients undergoing primary PCI, and fondaparinux is *not* recommended as a sole anticoagulant during PCI due to risk of catheter thrombosis.

(b) Unfractionated heparin—Anticoagulation with intravenous heparin (initial dose of 60 U/kg bolus to a maximum of 4000 units, followed by an infusion of 12 U/kg/hour to a maximum of 1000 U/hour, then adjusted to maintain an aPTT of 50–75 seconds beginning with an aPTT drawn 3 hours after thrombolytic) is continued for at least 48 hours after alteplase, reteplase, or tenecteplase, and with continuation of an anticoagulant until revascularization (if performed) or until hospital discharge (or day 8). Unfractionated heparin remains the first-line anticoagulant after lytics due to its comparative safety profile with PCI.

(c) Prophylactic therapy against bleeding—For all patients with STEMI treated with intensive antithrombotic therapy, prophylactic treatment with PPIs, or antacids and an H_2-blocker, is advisable. However, certain PPIs, such as omeprazole and esomeprazole, may decrease the clinical effect of clopidogrel; in such cases, pantoprazole, lansoprazole, and dexlansoprazole may be better PPI options.

3. Assessment of myocardial reperfusion, recurrent ischemic pain, reinfarction—Myocardial reperfusion can be recognized clinically by the early cessation of pain and the resolution of ST-segment elevation. Although at least 50% resolution of ST-segment elevation by 90 minutes may occur without coronary reperfusion, *ST resolution is a strong predictor of better outcome.* Even with anticoagulation, 10–20% of reperfused vessels will reocclude during hospitalization, although reocclusion and reinfarction appear to be reduced following intervention. **Reinfarction**, indicated by recurrence of pain and ST-segment elevation, can be treated by readministration of a thrombolytic agent or immediate angiography and PCI.

C. General Measures

Cardiac care unit monitoring should be instituted as soon as possible. Patients without complications can be transferred to a telemetry unit after 24 hours. Early initiation of activity under supervision is beneficial. For patients without complications, discharge by day two is common and risk for subsequent ventricular arrhythmias is low.

D. Analgesia

An initial attempt should be made to relieve pain with sublingual nitroglycerin. However, if no response occurs after two or three tablets, intravenous opioids provide the most rapid and effective analgesia and may also reduce pulmonary congestion. Morphine sulfate, 4–8 mg, should be given. Subsequent small doses can be given every

15 minutes until pain abates. The best relief of pain will be delivered with primary PCI, which should not be delayed for pain control with other agents.

NSAIDs, other than aspirin, should be avoided during hospitalization for STEMI due to increased risk of mortality, myocardial rupture, hypertension, HF, and kidney injury with their use.

E. β-Adrenergic Blocking Agents

Aggressive β-blockade can increase shock, with overall harm in patients with HF. Thus, early β-blockade should be avoided in patients with any degree of HF, evidence of low-output state, increased risk of cardiogenic shock, or other relative contraindications to β-blockade. Carvedilol (beginning at 6.25 mg twice a day, titrated to 25 mg twice a day) was shown to be beneficial in the CAPRICORN trial following the acute phase of large MI. However, the more recent REDUCE-AMI trial found no long-term benefit from β-blockers in uncomplicated AMI patients with a normal LV ejection fraction.

F. Nitrates

Nitroglycerin is the agent of choice for continued or recurrent ischemic pain and is useful in lowering BP or relieving pulmonary congestion. However, routine nitrate administration is *not* recommended, since no improvement in outcome has been observed in the ISIS-4 or GISSI-3 trials. Nitrates should be avoided in patients who received phosphodiesterase inhibitors (sildenafil, vardenafil, and tadalafil) in the prior 24 hours.

G. ACE Inhibitors

Trials (SAVE, AIRE, SMILE, TRACE, GISSI-III, and ISIS-4) have shown short- and long-term improvement in survival with ACE inhibitor therapy. The benefits are greatest in patients with an EF of 40% or less, large infarctions, or clinical evidence of HF. Since substantial amounts of the survival benefit occur on the first day, ACE inhibitor treatment should be commenced early in patients without hypotension, especially patients with large or anterior MI. Given the benefits of ACE inhibitors for patients with vascular disease, it is reasonable to *use ACE inhibitors for all patients following STEMI who do not have contraindications.*

H. Angiotensin Receptor Blockers

Although there has been inconsistency in the effects of different ARBs on mortality for patients post-MI with HF, LV dysfunction, or both, the VALIANT trial showed that valsartan 160 mg orally twice a day is *equivalent* to captopril in reducing mortality. Thus, valsartan should be used for all patients with ACE inhibitor intolerance and is a reasonable alternative to captopril. *The combination of captopril and valsartan (at a reduced dose) was no better than either agent alone and resulted in more side effects.*

I. Aldosterone Antagonists

The EPHESUS trial showed a 15% relative risk reduction in mortality with eplerenone 25 mg daily for patients post-MI with LV dysfunction (LVEF of ≤ 40%) and either clinical HF or diabetes. Kidney dysfunction and hyperkalemia are contraindications, and patients must be monitored carefully for development of hyperkalemia.

J. Calcium Channel Blockers

There are no studies to support the routine use of calcium channel blockers in most patients with acute MI—and indeed, they have the potential to exacerbate ischemia and cause death from reflex tachycardia or myocardial depression. *Long-acting calcium channel blockers should generally be reserved for management of hypertension or ischemia as second- or third-line medications after β-blockers and nitrates.*

K. Long-Term Antithrombotic Therapy

Discharge on aspirin, 81 mg/day, is a key quality indicator of MI care. Patients who received a coronary stent should also receive a $P2Y_{12}$ inhibitor. However, many patients who undergo PCI also have an indication for long-term anticoagulation.

Patients who have received a coronary stent and who require warfarin anticoagulation present a particular challenge, since **triple therapy** with aspirin, $P2Y_{12}$ inhibitors, and an anticoagulant has a high risk of bleeding. The *consensus statements recommend that oral anticoagulation (with either warfarin or a DOAC) be combined with clopidogrel and with a relatively short duration of aspirin (1–4 weeks) for the typical patient with AF and coronary stents.* Dabigatran, 110 mg and 150 mg, also was studied in patients with who underwent PCI. Dual therapy with dabigatran and clopidogrel was shown to be beneficial for bleeding compared with triple therapy, with similar rates of thrombotic cardiovascular events. However, there were too few thrombotic events to be certain about efficacy of discontinuing the aspirin, and there was a suggestion that MI and stent thrombosis occurred more often with the 110-mg dose of dabigatran than with clopidogrel alone. The AUGUSTUS trial, which tested apixaban versus warfarin and aspirin versus placebo on top of a $P2Y_{12}$ inhibitor for all patients in a 2 × 2 factorial trial, found that apixaban resulted in 31% less major and clinically relevant nonmajor bleeding than warfarin for patients with AF and coronary stents or ACSs or both. Avoiding aspirin, after an average of 6 days after the PCI, resulted in less bleeding and a nonsignificant increase in stent thrombosis. It is reasonable to stop aspirin at hospital discharge or at day 7 for patients with AF who are taking apixaban or warfarin at the time of discharge, although continuing aspirin for 1 month may reduce stent thrombosis.

Given the trial evidence to date, for a typical patient, it is reasonable to use a DOAC and clopidogrel and to discontinue aspirin at the time of hospital discharge or 1 week after stenting.

L. Coronary Angiography

For patients who do not reperfuse based on lack of at least 50% resolution of ST elevation, **rescue angioplasty** should be performed and has been shown to reduce the composite risk of death, reinfarction, stroke, or severe HF. Patients treated with coronary angiography and PCI 3–24 hours after fibrinolytic therapy showed improved outcomes. Patients with recurrent ischemic pain prior to discharge should undergo catheterization and, if indicated, revascularization. PCI of a totally occluded infarct-related artery > 24 hours after STEMI should generally not be performed in asymptomatic patients with one- or two-vessel disease without evidence of severe ischemia.

When to Refer

All patients with acute STEMI should seek emergency medical care, including emergent consultation from a cardiologist.

Writing Committee Members; Lawton JS et al. 2021 ACC/AHA/SCAI Guideline for Coronary Artery Revascularization: a report of the American College of Cardiology/American Heart Association Joint Committee on Clinical Practice Guidelines. J Am Coll Cardiol. 2022;79:e21. Erratum in: J Am Coll Cardiol. 2022;79:1547. [PMID: 34895950]

Complications Post MI

Postinfarct ischemia indicates inadequate treatment. Most patients with postinfarction angina—and all who are refractory to medical therapy—should undergo early catheterization and revascularization by PCI or CABG. A variety of complications can occur after MI even when treatment is initiated promptly.

A. Arrhythmias

Abnormalities of rhythm and conduction are common.

1. Sinus bradycardia—This is most common in inferior infarctions or may be precipitated by medications. Observation or withdrawal of the offending agent is usually sufficient. If accompanied by signs of low cardiac output, atropine intravenously is usually effective. Temporary pacing is rarely required.

2. Supraventricular tachyarrhythmias—Sinus tachycardia is common and may reflect either increased adrenergic stimulation or hemodynamic compromise due to hypovolemia or pump failure. In the latter, β-blockade is contraindicated. Supraventricular premature beats are common and may be premonitory for AF. Electrolyte abnormalities and hypoxia should be corrected and causative agents stopped. *AF should be rapidly controlled or converted to sinus rhythm.* Intravenous β-blockers, such as metoprolol (2.5–5 mg intravenously every 2–5 minutes, maximum 15 mg over 10–minutes) or short-acting esmolol (50–200 mcg/kg/min), are the agents of choice if cardiac function is adequate. Intravenous diltiazem (5–15 mg/hour) may be used if β-blockers are contraindicated or ineffective. Electrical cardioversion may be necessary if AF is complicated by hypotension, HF, or ischemia, but the arrhythmia often recurs. Amiodarone (150 mg intravenous bolus and then 15–30 mg/hour intravenously, or rapid oral loading dose for cardioversion of 400 mg three times daily) may be helpful to restore or maintain sinus rhythm.

3. Ventricular arrhythmias—Ventricular arrhythmias are most common in the first few hours after infarction and are a marker of high risk. Ventricular premature beats may be premonitory for ventricular tachycardia or fibrillation, but generally should *not* be treated in the absence of frequent or sustained ventricular tachycardia. Lidocaine is *not* recommended as a prophylactic measure.

Sustained ventricular tachycardia should be treated with a 1mg/kg bolus of lidocaine if the patient is stable or by electrical cardioversion if not. If the arrhythmia cannot be suppressed with lidocaine, intravenous amiodarone (150 mg over 10 minutes, which may be repeated as needed, followed by 360 mg over 6 hours and then 540 mg over 18 hours) should be initiated, followed by an infusion of 0.5 mg/min (720 mg/24 hours). Ventricular fibrillation is treated by immediate defibrillation. All patients taking antiarrhythmics should be monitored with telemetry or ECGs during initiation. Unresponsive ventricular fibrillation should be treated with additional amiodarone and repeat cardioversion while CPR is administered.

Accelerated idioventricular rhythm is a regular, wide-complex rhythm at a rate of 60–120/min. It may occur with or without reperfusion and should *not* be treated with antiarrhythmics, which could cause asystole.

4. Conduction disturbances—All degrees of AV block may occur in the course of acute MI. Block at the level of the AV node is more common than infranodal block and occurs in approximately 20% of inferior MIs. First-degree block is the most common and requires no treatment. Second-degree block is usually of the Mobitz type I form (Wenckebach), is often transient, and requires treatment only if associated with a heart rate slow enough to cause symptoms. Complete AV block occurs in up to 5% of acute inferior infarctions, usually is preceded by Mobitz I second-degree block, and generally resolves spontaneously, though it may persist for hours to several weeks. The escape rhythm originates in the distal AV node or AV junction and hence has a narrow QRS complex and is reliable, albeit often slow (30–50 beats/min). Treatment is often necessary because of resulting hypotension. Intravenous atropine (1 mg) usually restores AV conduction temporarily, but if the escape complex is wide or if repeated atropine treatments are needed, temporary ventricular pacing is indicated. The prognosis for these patients is only slightly worse than for patients in whom AV block does not develop.

In anterior infarctions, the site of block is distal, below the AV node, and usually a result of extensive damage of the His-Purkinje system and bundle branches. New first-degree block (prolongation of the PR interval) is unusual in anterior infarction; Mobitz type II AV block or complete heart block may be preceded by intraventricular conduction defects or may occur abruptly. The escape rhythm, if present, is an unreliable wide-complex idioventricular rhythm. Urgent ventricular pacing is mandatory, but even with successful pacing, morbidity and mortality are high because of the extensive myocardial damage. New conduction abnormalities, such as right or left bundle branch block or fascicular blocks, may presage progression, often sudden, to second- or third-degree AV block. Temporary ventricular pacing is recommended for new-onset alternating bilateral bundle branch block, bifascicular block, or bundle branch block with worsening first-degree AV block. Patients with anterior infarction who progress to second- or third-degree block even transiently should be considered for insertion of a prophylactic permanent ventricular pacemaker before discharge.

B. Myocardial Dysfunction

Persons with hypotension not responsive to fluid resuscitation or refractory HF or cardiogenic shock should be considered for urgent echocardiography to assess left and right ventricular function and for mechanical complications, right heart catheterization, and continuous measurements of arterial pressure. These measurements permit the accurate assessment of volume status and may facilitate decisions about volume resuscitation, selective use of vasopressors and inotropes, and mechanical support.

1. Acute LV failure—Dyspnea, diffuse rales, and arterial hypoxemia usually indicate LV failure. General measures include supplemental oxygen to increase arterial saturation to above 95% and elevation of the trunk. Diuretics are usually the initial therapy unless RV infarction is present. Intravenous furosemide (10–40 mg) or bumetanide (0.5–1 mg) is preferred because of the reliably rapid onset and short duration of action of these medications. Higher dosages can be given if an inadequate response occurs. It is critical to exclude cardiogenic shock, as this necessitates prompt therapy that is different from systolic HF without shock. If a shock state is excluded, careful addition of medical therapy for systolic HF after successful revascularization is warranted (see Chapter 11).

Inotropic agents should be avoided if possible, because they often increase heart rate and myocardial oxygen requirements and worsen clinical outcomes. If inotropes or vasopressor medications are felt to be warranted, re-evaluation of shock state and appropriate treatment are necessary. Digoxin has not been helpful in acute infarction except to control the ventricular response in AF, but it may be beneficial if chronic HF persists.

2. Cardiogenic shock—*Patients with hypotension (systolic BP < 90 mm Hg, individualized depending on prior BP) and signs of diminished perfusion (low urinary output, confusion, cold extremities, lab evidence of end-organ dysfunction) that does not respond to fluid resuscitation should be presumed to have cardiogenic shock and should be considered for emergent catheterization and revascularization.* Recent data from the DanGer Shock study suggest that patients with cardiogenic shock in AMI (AMI-CS) benefit from use of an Impella (percutaneous ventricular assist device) compared with an intra-aortic balloon pump (IABP) and pressors/inotropes alone. Prior studies of IABPs have found no benefit in the setting of AMI-CS. Pericardial tamponade due to hemorrhagic pericarditis (especially after thrombolytic therapy or CPR) or ventricular rupture should be considered and excluded by echocardiography. RV infarction, characterized by a normal PCWP but elevated RA pressure, can produce hypotension. This is discussed below.

Norepinephrine (0.1–0.5 mcg/kg/min) is generally considered to be the most appropriate inotrope/vasopressor for cardiogenic shock based on limited randomized clinical trial evidence suggesting less arrhythmias and improved outcomes compared with dopamine. Dopamine is nonetheless also an option and can be initiated at a rate of 2–4 mcg/kg/min and increased at 5-minute intervals to the appropriate hemodynamic end point. At dosages lower than 5 mcg/kg/min, it improves renal blood flow; at intermediate dosages (2.5–10 mcg/kg/min), it stimulates myocardial contractility; at higher dosages (> 8 mcg/kg/min), it is a potent α_1-adrenergic agonist. In general, BP and cardiac index rise, but PCWP does not fall.

Patients with cardiogenic shock not due to hypovolemia have a poor prognosis, with 30-day mortality rates of 40–80%. Emergent cardiac catheterization and coronary angiography followed by percutaneous or surgical revascularization offer the best chance of survival. Additionally, revascularization in shock should be aimed at the culprit artery only, avoiding multivessel PCI.

C. RV Infarction

RV infarction is present in one-third of patients with inferior wall infarction but is clinically significant in < 50% of these. It presents as hypotension with relatively preserved LV function and *should be considered whenever patients with inferior infarction exhibit low BP, raised venous pressure, and clear lungs.* Hypotension is often exacerbated by medications that decrease intravascular volume or produce venodilation, such as diuretics, nitrates, and opioids. RA pressure and JVP are high, while PCWP is normal or low and the lungs are clear. The diagnosis is suggested by ST-segment elevation in right-sided anterior chest leads, particularly RV_4. The diagnosis can be confirmed by echocardiography or hemodynamic measurements. Treatment consists of fluid loading beginning with 500 mL of 0.9% saline over 2 hours to improve LV filling, and inotropic agents only if necessary.

D. Mechanical Defects

Partial or complete rupture of a papillary muscle or of the interventricular septum occurs in < 1% of acute MIs and carries a poor prognosis. These complications occur in both anterior and inferior infarctions, *usually 3–7 days after the acute event.* They are detected by the appearance of a new systolic murmur and clinical deterioration, often with pulmonary edema. The two lesions are distinguished by the location of the murmur (apical versus parasternal) and by echocardiography. Hemodynamic monitoring is essential for appropriate management and demonstrates an increase in oxygen saturation between the RA and PA in VSD and, often, a large *v* wave with mitral regurgitation. Treatment by nitroprusside and, preferably, **intra-aortic balloon counterpulsation (IABC)** reduces the regurgitation or shunt, but surgical correction is mandatory. In patients remaining hemodynamically unstable or requiring continuous parenteral pharmacologic treatment or counterpulsation, early surgery is recommended, though mortality rates are high (15% to nearly 100%, depending on residual ventricular function and clinical status). Patients who are stabilized medically can have delayed surgery with lower risks (10–25%), although this may be due to the death of sicker patients, some of whom may have been saved by earlier surgery.

E. Myocardial Rupture

Complete rupture of the LV free wall occurs in < 1% of patients and usually results in immediate death. It occurs 2–7 days postinfarction, usually involves the anterior wall, and is more frequent in older women. Incomplete or gradual rupture may be sealed off by the pericardium, creating a pseudoaneurysm. This may be recognized by echocardiography, radionuclide angiography, or LV angiography, often as an incidental finding. It demonstrates a narrow-neck connection to the LV. Early surgical repair is indicated, since delayed rupture is common.

F. LV Aneurysm

An LV aneurysm, a sharply delineated area of scar that bulges paradoxically during systole, develops in 10–20% of patients surviving an acute infarction. This usually follows anterior ST-segment elevation infarctions. Aneurysms are recognized by persistent ST-segment elevation (beyond 4–8 weeks), and a wide neck from the LV can be demonstrated by echocardiography, scintigraphy, or contrast angiography. They rarely rupture but may be associated with arterial emboli, ventricular arrhythmias, and HF. Surgical resection may be performed for these indications if other measures fail. The best results (mortality rates of 10–20%) are obtained when the residual myocardium contracts well and when significant coronary lesions supplying adjacent regions are bypassed.

G. Pericarditis

The pericardium is involved in approximately 50% of infarctions, but pericarditis is often not clinically significant. Twenty percent of patients with ST-segment elevation infarctions will have an audible friction rub if examined repetitively. Pericardial pain occurs in approximately the same proportion after 2–7 days and is recognized by its variation with respiration and position (improved by sitting). Often, no treatment is required, but aspirin (650 mg every 4–6 hours) will usually relieve the pain. Indomethacin and corticosteroids can cause impaired infarct healing and predispose to myocardial rupture and should generally be *avoided* in the early post-MI period. Anticoagulation should be used cautiously, since hemorrhagic pericarditis may result.

One week to 12 weeks after infarction, **Dressler syndrome** (post-MI syndrome) occurs in < 5% of patients. This is an autoimmune phenomenon and presents as pericarditis with associated fever, leukocytosis, and, occasionally, pericardial or pleural effusion. It may recur over months. Treatment is the same as for other forms of pericarditis. A short course of nonsteroidal agents or corticosteroids may help relieve symptoms, but the use of nonsteroidal agents in the first several weeks after MI may impair infarct healing.

H. Mural Thrombus

Mural thrombi are common in large anterior infarctions but not in infarctions at other locations. Arterial emboli occur in approximately 2% of patients with known infarction, usually within 6 weeks. Anticoagulation with heparin followed by short-term (3-month) warfarin or DOAC therapy results in clot resolution and prevents most emboli, and it should be considered in all patients with evidence of LV thrombi. Mural thrombi can be detected by echocardiography or cardiac MRI. If the thrombus is resolved at 3 months, then anticoagulation can be discontinued.

Postinfarction Management

After the first 24 hours, the focus of patient management is to prevent recurrent ischemia, improve infarct healing and prevent remodeling, and prevent recurrent vascular events. Patients with hemodynamic compromise, who are at high risk for death, need careful monitoring and management of volume status.

A. Risk Stratification

Risk stratification is important for the management of STEMI. GRACE and TIMI risk scores can be helpful tools. Patients with recurrent ischemia (spontaneous or provoked), hemodynamic instability, impaired LV function, HF, or serious ventricular arrhythmias should undergo cardiac catheterization (see Table 10–1). ACE inhibitor (or ARB) therapy is indicated in patients with clinical HF or LVEF of 40% or less. Aldosterone blockade is indicated for patients with an LVEF of 40% or less and either HF or diabetes mellitus.

For patients not undergoing cardiac catheterization, *submaximal* exercise (or pharmacologic stress testing for patients unable to exercise) before discharge or a *maximal* test after 3–6 weeks (the latter being more sensitive for ischemia) helps patients and clinicians plan the return to normal activity. Imaging in conjunction with stress testing adds additional sensitivity for ischemia and provides localizing information. Both exercise and pharmacologic stress imaging have successfully predicted subsequent outcomes. *One of these tests should be used prior to discharge in patients who have received thrombolytic therapy as a means of selecting appropriate candidates for coronary angiography.*

B. Secondary Prevention

Postinfarction management should begin with identification and modification of risk factors. Treatment of hyperlipidemia and smoking cessation both prevent recurrent infarction and death. Statin therapy should be started before the patient is discharged from the hospital to reduce recurrent atherothrombotic events. BP control as well as cardiac rehabilitation and exercise are also recommended. They can be of considerable psychological benefit and appear to improve prognosis.

While a variety of β-blockers have been shown to be beneficial, for patients with LV dysfunction managed with contemporary treatment, carvedilol titrated to 25 mg orally twice a day has been shown to reduce mortality. β-Blockers with intrinsic sympathomimetic activity have *not* proved beneficial in postinfarction patients.

Antiplatelet agents are beneficial; aspirin (75–100 mg daily, after the initial dose) and $P2Y_{12}$ inhibitor therapy for 1 year are recommended. Prasugrel provides further reduction in thrombotic outcomes compared with clopidogrel, at the cost of more bleeding, but is contraindicated for patients with prior stroke. Likewise, ticagrelor provides benefit over clopidogrel. Calcium channel blockers have *not* been shown to improve prognoses overall and should not be prescribed purely for secondary prevention. Antiarrhythmic therapy other than with β-blockers has *not* been shown to be effective except in patients with symptomatic arrhythmias. Amiodarone has been studied in several trials of postinfarct patients with either LV dysfunction or frequent ventricular ectopy. Although survival was not improved, amiodarone was not harmful—unlike other agents in this setting. Therefore, it is the *agent of choice for individuals with symptomatic postinfarction supraventricular arrhythmias.* While implantable defibrillators improve survival for patients with postinfarction LV dysfunction and HF, the DINAMIT trial found *no benefit to implantable defibrillators implanted in the 40 days following acute MI.*

C. ACE Inhibitors and ARBs in Patients with LV Dysfunction

Patients who sustain substantial myocardial damage often experience subsequent progressive LV dilation and dysfunction, leading to clinical HF and reduced long-term survival. In patients with EFs < 40%, long-term ACE inhibitor (or ARB) therapy prevents LV dilation and the onset of HF and prolongs survival. The HOPE trial, as well as an overview of trials of ACE inhibitors for secondary prevention, also demonstrated a reduction of approximately 20% in mortality rates and the occurrence of nonfatal MI and stroke with ramipril treatment of patients with coronary or peripheral vascular disease and without confirmed LV systolic dysfunction. Therefore, ACE inhibitor therapy should be strongly considered in this broader group of patients—and especially in patients with diabetes and those with even mild systolic hypertension, in whom the greatest benefit was observed (see Table 13–6).

D. Revascularization

The indications for CABG are similar to those for patients with chronic coronary syndromes, including left main stenosis and multivessel disease (particularly with type 2 diabetes or LV dysfunction, or both). For patients who have undergone primary PCI and have residual left main or multivessel disease, CABG may be appropriate, but the timing needs to take into account the high risk of stent thrombosis if $P2Y_{12}$ inhibitor therapy is interrupted. For patients with non-infarct-related CAD, stenting should generally be performed on these lesions prior to hospital discharge.

VALVULAR HEART DISEASE

The typical findings of each native valve lesion are described in Table 10–3. Table 10–4 outlines bedside maneuvers to distinguish among the various systolic murmurs.

The 2020 ACC/AHA valvular heart disease guidelines suggest all lesions may be classified clinically based on anatomy and symptoms.

Stage A: Patients at risk for valvular heart disease.

Stage B: Patients with progressive valvular heart disease (mild to moderate severity) and asymptomatic.

Stage C: Asymptomatic patients who have reached criteria for severe valvular heart disease.

- **C1:** Severe valve lesion. Asymptomatic. Normal LV function.
- **C2:** Severe valve lesion. Asymptomatic. Abnormal LV function.

Stage D: Symptomatic patients as a result of valvular heart disease.

Kronenberg F et al. Lipoprotein(a) in atherosclerotic cardiovascular disease and aortic stenosis: a European Atherosclerosis Society consensus statement. Eur Heart J. 2022;43:3925. [PMID: 36036785]

AORTIC STENOSIS

ESSENTIALS OF DIAGNOSIS

- Congenital bicuspid aortic valve (usually asymptomatic until middle or old age).
- "Degenerative" or calcific aortic stenosis; similar risk factors as atherosclerosis.
- Visual observation of immobile aortic valve plus a valve area of < 1.0 cm^2 define severe disease; low-flow low-gradient severe aortic stenosis occurs when the stroke volume is reduced.
- Echocardiography/Doppler is diagnostic.
- Transcatheter aortic valve replacement (TAVR) and surgical aortic valve replacement (SAVR) are equivalent at a population level, but the lifetime management of valve disease should be considered.

General Considerations

There are two common clinical scenarios in which aortic stenosis is prevalent. The first is due to a **congenitally abnormal valve,** often bicuspid rather than tricuspid. Symptoms can occur in young or adolescent individuals if the stenosis is severe, but they more often emerge at age ≥ 60 when calcification and degeneration of the valve become clinically apparent. A dilated ascending aorta, due to an intrinsic defect in the aortic root media and the hemodynamic effects of the eccentric aortic jet, may accompany a bicuspid valve in about half of these patients. Coarctation of the aorta is also seen in a number of patients with congenital aortic stenosis. Offspring of patients with a bicuspid valve have a much higher incidence of the disease in either the valve, the aorta, or both (up to 30% in some series), and screening for bicuspid valve disease is recommended for all first-degree relatives of patients with a bicuspid valve.

Degenerative or **calcific aortic stenosis** is thought to be related to calcium deposition due to processes similar to those that occur in atherosclerotic vascular disease,

Table 10–3. Differential diagnosis of valvular heart disease.

	Mitral Stenosis	Mitral Regurgitation	Aortic Stenosis	Aortic Regurgitation	Tricuspid Stenosis	Tricuspid Regurgitation
Inspection	Malar flush, precordial bulge, and diffuse pulsation in young patients.	Usually prominent and hyperdynamic apical impulse to left of MCL.	Sustained PMI, prominent atrial filling wave.	Hyperdynamic PMI to left of MCL and downward. Visible carotid pulsations. Pulsating nailbeds (Quincke sign), head bob (de Musset sign).	Giant *a* wave in jugular pulse with sinus rhythm. Peripheral edema or ascites, or both.	Large *v* wave in jugular pulse; time with carotid pulsation. Peripheral edema or ascites, or both.
Palpation	"Tapping" sensation over area of expected PMI. RV pulsation in left third to fifth ICS parasternally when pulmonary hypertension is present. P_2 may be palpable.	Forceful, brisk PMI; systolic thrill over PMI. Pulse normal, small, or slightly collapsing.	Powerful, heaving PMI to left and slightly below MCL. Systolic thrill over aortic area, sternal notch, or carotid arteries in severe disease. Small and slowly rising carotid pulse. If bicuspid AS, check for delay at femoral artery to exclude coarctation.	Apical impulse forceful and displaced significantly to left and downward. Prominent carotid pulses. Rapidly rising and collapsing pulses (Corrigan pulse).	Pulsating, enlarged liver in ventricular systole.	RV pulsation. Systolic pulsation of liver.
Heart sounds, rhythm, and blood pressure	S_1 loud if valve mobile. Opening snap following S_2. The worse the disease, the closer the S_2-opening snap interval.	S_1 normal or buried in early part of murmur (exception in mitral prolapse where murmur may be late). Prominent third heart sound when severe MR. Atrial fibrillation common. Blood pressure normal. Midsystolic clicks may be present and may be multiple.	A_2 normal, soft, or absent. Prominent S_4. Blood pressure normal, or systolic pressure normal with high diastolic pressure.	S_1 normal or reduced, A_2 loud. Wide pulse pressure with diastolic pressure < 60 mm Hg. When severe, gentle compression of femoral artery with diaphragm of stethoscope may reveal diastolic flow (Duroziez) and pressure in leg on palpation > 40 mm Hg than in arm (Hill).	S_1 often loud.	Atrial fibrillation may be present.
Murmurs						
Location and transmission	Localized at or near apex. Diastolic rumble best heard in left lateral position; may be accentuated by having patient do sit-ups. Rarely, short diastolic murmur along lower left sternal border (Graham Steell) in severe pulmonary hypertension.	Loudest over PMI; posteriorly directed jets (ie, anterior mitral prolapse) transmitted to left axilla left infrascapular area; anteriorly directed jets (ie, posterior mitral prolapse) heard over anterior precordium. Murmur unchanged after premature beat.	Right second ICS parasternally or at apex, heard in carotid arteries and occasionally in upper interscapular area. May sound like MR at apex (Gallavardin phenomenon), but murmur occurs after S_1 and stops before S_2.	Diastolic: louder along left sternal border in third to fourth interspace. Heard over aortic area and apex. May be associated with low-pitched mid-diastolic murmur at apex (Austin Flint) due to functional mitral stenosis. If due to an enlarged aorta, murmur may radiate to right sternal border.	Third to fifth ICS along left sternal border out to apex. Murmur increases with inspiration.	Third to fifth ICS along left sternal border. Murmur hard to hear but increases with inspiration. Sit-ups can increase cardiac output and accentuate murmur.

(*continued*)

Table 10–3. Differential diagnosis of valvular heart disease. (continued)

	Mitral Stenosis	Mitral Regurgitation	Aortic Stenosis	Aortic Regurgitation	Tricuspid Stenosis	Tricuspid Regurgitation
Timing	Relation of opening snap to A_2 important. The higher the LA pressure, the earlier the opening snap. Presystolic accentuation before S_1 if in sinus rhythm. Graham Steell begins with P_2 (early diastole) if associated pulmonary hypertension.	Pansystolic: begins with S_1 and ends at or after A_2. May be late systolic in mitral valve prolapse.	Begins after S_1, ends before A_2. The more severe the stenosis, the later the murmur peaks.	Begins immediately after aortic second sound and ends before first sound (blurring both); helps distinguish from MR.	Rumble often follows audible opening snap.	At times, hard to hear. Begins with S_1 and fills systole. Increases with inspiration.
Character	Low-pitched, rumbling; presystolic murmur merges with loud S_1.	Blowing, high-pitched; occasionally harsh or musical.	Harsh, rough.	Blowing, often faint.	As for mitral stenosis.	Blowing, coarse, or musical.
Optimum auscultatory conditions	After exercise, left lateral recumbency. Use stethoscope bell, lightly applied.	After exercise; use stethoscope diaphragm. In prolapse, findings may be more evident while standing.	Use stethoscope diaphragm. Patient resting, leaning forward, breath held in full expiration.	Use stethoscope diaphragm. Patient leaning forward, breath held in expiration.	Use stethoscope bell. Murmur usually louder and at peak during inspiration. Patient recumbent.	Use stethoscope diaphragm. Murmur usually becomes louder during inspiration.
Radiography	Straight left heart border from enlarged LA appendage. Elevation of left mainstem bronchus. Large RV and pulmonary artery if pulmonary hypertension is present. Calcification in mitral valve in rheumatic mitral stenosis or in annulus in calcific mitral stenosis.	Enlarged LV and LA.	Concentric LVH. Prominent ascending aorta. Calcified aortic valve common.	Moderate to severe LV enlargement. Aortic root often dilated.	Enlarged right atrium with prominent SVC and azygous shadow.	Enlarged right atrium and RV.
ECG	Broad P waves in standard leads; broad negative phase of diphasic P in V_1. If pulmonary hypertension is present, tall peaked P waves, right axis deviation, or RVH appears.	Left axis deviation or frank LVH. P waves broad, tall, or notched in standard leads. Broad negative phase of diphasic P in V_1.	LVH.	LVH.	Tall, peaked P waves. Possible RVH.	Right axis usual.

Echocardiography						
Two-dimensional echocardiography	Thickened, immobile mitral valve with anterior and posterior leaflets moving together. "Hockey stick" shape to opened anterior leaflet in rheumatic mitral stenosis. Annular calcium with thin leaflets in calcific mitral stenosis. LA enlargement, normal to small LV. Orifice can be traced to approximate mitral valve orifice area.	Thickened mitral valve in rheumatic disease; mitral valve prolapse; flail leaflet or vegetations may be seen. Dilated LV in volume overload. Operate for LV end-systolic dimension < 4.5 cm.	Dense persistent echoes from the aortic valve with poor leaflet excursion. LVH late in the disease. Bicuspid valve in younger patients.	Abnormal aortic valve or dilated aortic root. Diastolic vibrations of the anterior leaflet of the mitral valve and septum. In acute aortic regurgitation, premature closure of the mitral valve before the QRS. When severe, dilated LV with normal or decreased contractility. Operate when LV end-systolic dimension > 5.0 cm.	In rheumatic disease, tricuspid valve thickening, decreased early diastolic filling slope of the tricuspid valve. In carcinoid, leaflets fixed, but no significant thickening.	Enlarged RV with paradoxical septal motion. Tricuspid valve often pulled open by displaced chordae.
Continuous and color flow Doppler and TEE	Prolonged pressure half-time across mitral valve allows estimation of gradient. MVA estimated from pressure half-time. Indirect evidence of pulmonary hypertension by noting elevated RV systolic pressure measured from the tricuspid regurgitation jet.	Regurgitant flow mapped into LA. Use of PISA helps assess MR severity. TEE important in prosthetic mitral valve regurgitation.	Increased transvalvular flow velocity; severe AS when peak jet > 4 m/sec (64 mm Hg). Valve area estimate using continuity equation is poorly reproducible.	Demonstrates regurgitation and qualitatively estimates severity based on percentage of LV outflow filled with jet and distance jet penetrates into LV. TEE important in aortic valve endocarditis to exclude abscess. Mitral inflow pattern describes diastolic dysfunction.	Prolonged pressure half-time across tricuspid valve can be used to estimate mean gradient. Severe tricuspid stenosis present when mean gradient > 5 mm Hg.	Regurgitant flow mapped into right atrium and venae cavae. RV systolic pressure estimated by tricuspid regurgitation jet velocity.

A_2, aortic second sound; AS, aortic stenosis; ICS, intercostal space; LA, left atrial; MCL, midclavicular line; MR, mitral regurgitation; MVA, measured valve area; P_2, pulmonary second sound; PISA, proximal isovelocity surface area; PMI, point of maximal impulse; S_1, first heart sound; S_2, second heart sound; S_4, fourth heart sound; SVC, superior vena cava; TEE, transesophageal echocardiography; V_1, chest ECG lead 1.

Table 10–4. Effect of various interventions on systolic murmurs (listed in alphabetical order by intervention).

Intervention	Hypertrophic Cardiomyopathy	Aortic Stenosis	Mitral Regurgitation	Mitral Prolapse
Exercise	↑	↑ or ×	↓	↑
Handgrip or squatting	↓	↓ or ×	↑	↓
Standing	↑	↑ or ×	↓ or ×	↑
Supine position with legs elevated	↓	↑ or ×	×	↓
Valsalva	↑	↓	↓ or ×	↑ or ↓

↑, increased; ↓, decreased; ×, unchanged.
Reproduced with permission from Paraskos JA. Combined valvular disease. In: Dalen JE, Alpert JS, Rahimtoola SH (ed). *Valvular Heart Disease*, 3rd ed. Philadelphia: Lippincott Williams & Wilkins, 2000.

although the process is still poorly understood. Approximately 25% of patients over age 65 years and 35% of those over age 70 years have echocardiographic evidence of aortic valve thickening (**sclerosis**). About 10–20% of these will progress to hemodynamically significant aortic stenosis over a period of 10–15 years.

Aortic stenosis has become the most common valve lesion in developed countries, and most patients are older adults. The risk factors include hypertension, hypercholesterolemia, and smoking. Hypertrophic cardiomyopathy (with or without obstruction) may coexist with valvular aortic stenosis.

Clinical Findings

A. Symptoms and Signs

Slightly narrowed, thickened, or roughened valves (**aortic sclerosis**) or aortic dilation may contribute to the typical ejection murmur of aortic stenosis. In mild or moderate cases where the valve is still pliable, an ejection click may precede the murmur and the closure of the valve (S_2) is preserved. The characteristic systolic ejection murmur is heard at the aortic area and is usually transmitted to the neck and apex. In severe aortic stenosis, a palpable LV heave or thrill, a weak to absent aortic second sound, or reversed splitting of the second sound is present (see Table 10–3). In some cases, only the high-pitched components of the murmur are heard at the apex, and the murmur may sound like mitral regurgitation (the so-called **Gallavardin phenomenon**). When the valve area is < 1.0 cm^2 (normal, 3–4 cm^2), ventricular systole becomes prolonged and the typical carotid pulse pattern of delayed upstroke and low amplitude is present. A delayed upstroke, though, is an *unreliable* finding in older patients with extensive arteriosclerotic vascular disease and a stiff, noncompliant aorta. LVH increases progressively due to the pressure overload, eventually resulting in elevation of ventricular end-diastolic pressure. Cardiac output is maintained until the stenosis is severe. LV failure, angina pectoris, or syncope may be presenting symptoms of significant aortic stenosis; importantly, all symptoms tend to first occur with exertion.

B. Redefining Severe Aortic Stenosis

There are four measures used to define **severe aortic stenosis**: (a) peak velocity > 4 m/s, (b) mean gradient > 40 mm Hg, (c) aortic valve area (AVA) < 1 cm^2, and (d) dimensionless index < 0.25. Patients meeting one of these threshold measurements can be considered to have severe aortic stenosis in the appropriate clinical context. **Super-severe aortic stenosis** is defined as a mean gradient of > 55 mm Hg or peak velocity > 5 m/s by Doppler.

In some patients with an aortic valve area of < 1.0 cm^2 with a low cardiac output and stroke volume, the mean gradient may be < 40 mm Hg. This can occur when the LV systolic function is poor (**low-gradient severe aortic stenosis with low LVEF**) or when the LV systolic function is normal **(paradoxical low-flow severe aortic stenosis with a normal LVEF).** Low flow (low output) in these situations is defined by an echocardiographic stroke volume index of < 35 mL/min/m^2. Prognosis in patients with low gradient, low valve area, low output, and a normal LVEF aortic stenosis may be worse than in patients with the traditional high gradient, low valve area, normal output, and normal LVEF aortic stenosis. If low-flow severe aortic stenosis is present in the face of a low LVEF, provocative testing with dobutamine or nitroprusside is sometimes warranted to increase the stroke volume to discover if a mean aortic valve gradient of at least 40 mm Hg can be demonstrated without increasing the aortic valve area. If the aortic valve area can be made to increase and a mean gradient of > 40 mm Hg cannot be demonstrated by inotropic challenge, the presumption is that the low gradient is due to an associated cardiomyopathy and not the aortic valve stenosis. In this situation, intervention is not indicated. The guidelines acknowledge these four situations (Table 10–5). Intervention is indicated in super-severe aortic stenosis even without demonstrable symptoms (grade C) and in any of the other situations when symptoms are present: D1 defines the symptomatic high-gradient patient; D2 the symptomatic low-flow, low-gradient patient with low LVEF; and D3 the symptomatic low-flow, low-gradient patient with normal LVEF.

C. Diagnostic Studies

The echocardiogram provides useful data about aortic valve calcification and leaflet opening, the severity of LV wall thickness, and overall ventricular function, while Doppler can provide an excellent estimate of the aortic valve gradient. Cardiac catheterization can be used for an invasive hemodynamic assessment of the severity of AS, providing a direct measure of the peak to peak gradient, mean gradient, and

Table 10–5. Summary of AHA/ACC guideline definitions of symptomatic severe aortic stenosis.

Category of Severe Aortic Stenosis[1]	Properties
High Gradient	
High gradient	> 4.0 m/sec Doppler jet velocity > 40 mm Hg mean gradient
Super-severe	> 5.0 m/sec Doppler jet velocity > 55 mm Hg mean gradient
Low Gradient	
Low flow	Reduced LVEF (< 50%)
Low flow	Paradoxical with normal LVEF (> 50%)

[1]All categories of severe aortic stenosis have abnormal systolic opening of the aortic valve and an aortic valve area < 1.0 cm^2.

aortic valve area. Catheterization data can be important when there is a discrepancy between symptoms and the echocardiography/Doppler information of aortic stenosis severity, but is not required in the majority of cases. Stress testing can be done cautiously in patients in whom the aortic stenosis severity does not match the reported symptoms to confirm the reported clinical status. It should *not* be done in patients with super-severe aortic stenosis.

Prognosis & Treatment

*Valve intervention is warranted in all patients who have symptomatic severe aortic stenosis (*Figure 10–3*).* A recent clinical trial showed benefit for TAVR in asymptomatic severe aortic stenosis, mainly by reduction in HF hospitalizations when an Edwards SAPIEN valve was used. Additionally, asymptomatic patients with super-severe AS should undergo treatment regardless of symptoms. Following the onset of symptoms, the prognosis without intervention is poor (50% 3-year mortality rate). *There are no medical therapies currently available for treatment of aortic stenosis to prevent progression or cause regression of the degree of stenosis, and valve replacement with either surgery or transcatheter therapy is warranted.*

The surgical mortality rate for valve replacement is low, even in older adults, and ranges from 2% to 5%. This low risk is due to the dramatic hemodynamic improvement that occurs with relief of the increased afterload. Mortality rates are substantially higher when there is an associated ischemic cardiomyopathy. Severe coronary lesions are usually bypassed at the same time as aortic valve replacement (AVR), although there are few data to suggest this practice affects outcome. In some cases, a staged procedure with stenting of the coronaries prior to surgery may be considered, especially if a percutaneous AVR approach is being considered. Around one-third to one-half of all patients with aortic stenosis have significant CAD, so this is a common concern. With the success of TAVR, the treatment options have greatly expanded for many patients with severe aortic stenosis. For this reason, a **heart valve team** approach bringing together invasive and noninvasive cardiologists, radiologists, anesthesiologists, and cardiac surgeons is mandatory; clinical factors (such as frailty) and anatomic features (such as a calcified aorta, vascular access, etc) can affect the decision-making.

The interventional options in patients with aortic valve stenosis has expanded with the use of TAVR and depend on the patient's lifestyle and age. The algorithm to decide when an AVR is appropriate in various situations is outlined in Figure 10–4.

TAVR has been shown to be equivalent to SAVR in all the randomized trials of symptomatic patients, including those at low risk for surgery (STS risk of operative mortality < 4%). Surgery is recommended for patients younger than 65 years or with a life expectancy of > 20 years. TAVR is recommended for all patients older than 80 years. Either SAVR or TAVR can be considered for patients between 65 and 80 years. The decision about whether to perform SAVR or TAVR should be made by the Heart Team and account for patient specific considerations; anatomic issues (such as an enlarged aorta, a coronary that might be occluded by a leaflet when the valve is deployed, an annulus too large or too small, extensive LV outflow tract calcium, etc) are often the deciding factors for whether TAVR can be done.

Percutaneous balloon valvuloplasty has a limited role in the treatment of severe AS. Balloon valvuloplasty is associated with early restenosis in older adults and, thus, is rarely used except as a temporizing measure prior to a more permanent SAVR or TAVR.

The **Ross procedure** is considered a viable option in younger patients with a bicuspid valve, and it is performed by moving the patient's own pulmonary valve and a portion of its root to the aortic position and replacing the pulmonary valve with a homograft (or rarely a bioprosthetic valve). The coronaries require reimplantation. Guidelines suggest the Ross procedure should only be considered in those younger than 50 years. Middle-aged and younger adults generally can tolerate the anticoagulation therapy necessary for the use of mechanical aortic valves, so patients younger than 50 years generally undergo AVR with a bileaflet mechanical valve. In patients older than 50 years, bioprosthetic (either porcine or bovine pericardial) valves with a valve duration expectancy of about 10–15 years are routinely used instead of mechanical valves to avoid need for anticoagulation. Bioprosthetic valve degeneration can generally be treated by percutaneous valve-in-valve TAVR. Newer surgical aortic valve replacements can be placed quickly through a small incision and often require only three stitches to anchor (ie, the **Perceval** or **Intuity valve replacements**). These can shorten pump times at surgery.

Bicuspid aortic valve disease requiring surgery is associated with ascending aortic aneurysms in about half of cases. If there is an indication for AVR and the ascending aorta or aortic root is > 4.5 cm in diameter, treatment is recommended at the time of SAVR.

The use of mechanical versus bioprosthetic AVR has changed over time. A bioprosthetic valve is acceptable for patients at any age for whom anticoagulant therapy is contraindicated, not desired, or cannot be managed, and is preferred in patients over the age of 65. A mechanical valve should be used in patients younger than 50 years of age who can take warfarin. Shared decision making is key especially for patients 50–65 years old. ***Anticoagulation***

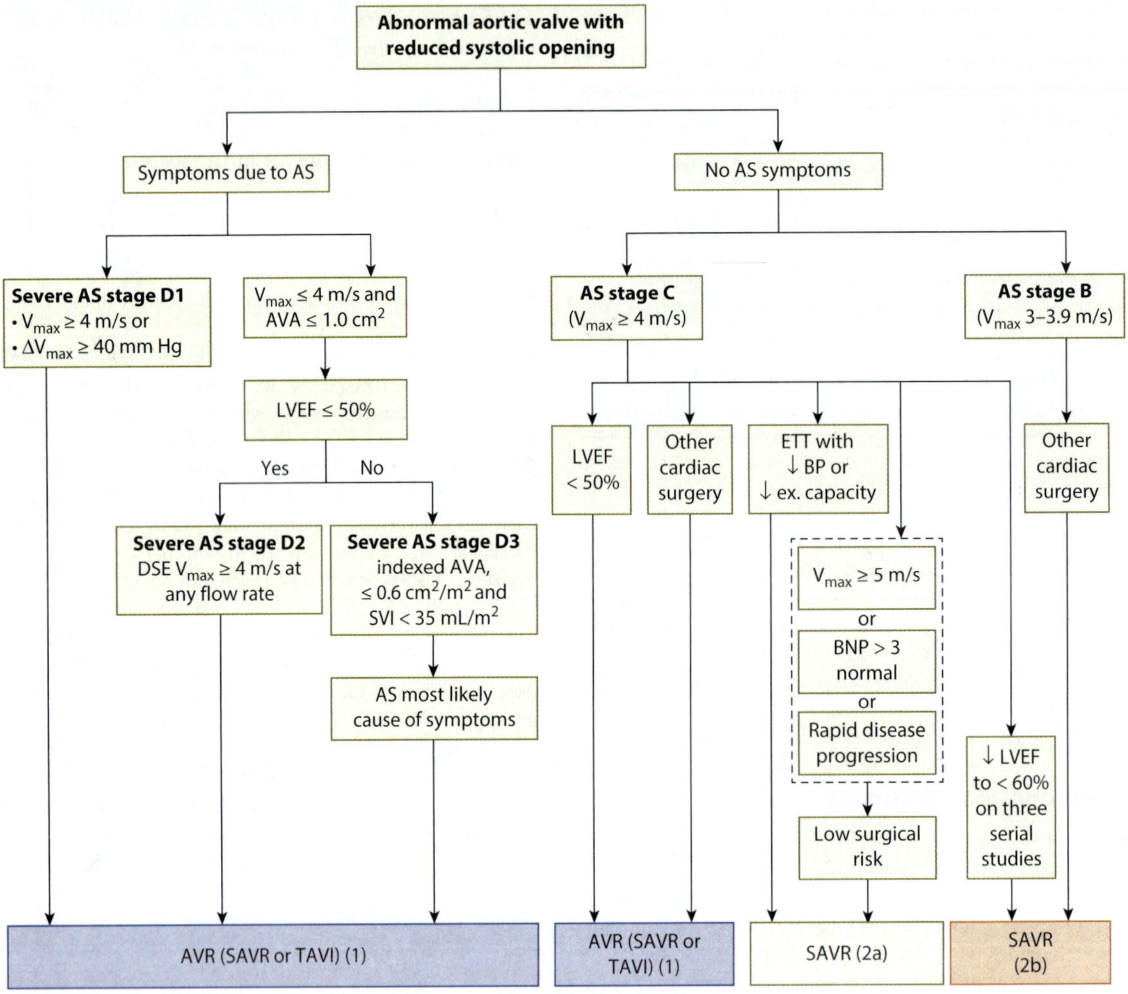

▲ **Figure 10–3.** Algorithm for the timing of intervention in aortic valve stenosis. AS, aortic stenosis; AVA, aortic valve area; AVAi, aortic valve area index; AVR, aortic valve replacement; BP, blood pressure; DSE, dobutamine stress echocardiography; ETT, exercise treadmill test; ΔP_{mean}, mean systolic pressure gradient between LV and aorta; SAVR, surgical aortic valve replacement; SVI, stroke volume index; TAVI, transcatheter aortic valve implantation; TAVR, transcatheter aortic valve replacement; V_{max}, maximum velocity. (Reproduced with permission from Otto CM et al. 2020 ACC/AHA guideline for the management of patients with valvular heart disease: a report of the American College of Cardiology. J Am Coll Cardiol. 2021;77: e25–e197.)

with warfarin is required with the use of mechanical aortic valves, and the INR should be maintained between 2.0 and 3.0. In general, mechanical aortic valves are less subject to thrombosis than mechanical mitral valves and do *not* require bridging with enoxaparin unless there are other thromboembolic risk factors or it is an older generation AVR. Low-dose aspirin (eg, 81 mg daily) is recommended if there is a low bleeding risk. Some newer bileaflet mechanical valves (On-X) allow for a lower INR range from 1.5 to 2.0. Aspirin monotherapy is recommended after TAVR, unless there is a separate indication for anticoagulation, in which case aspirin can be discontinued. DOACs are *contraindicated* for any mechanical valves but may be used in patients with a bioprosthetic AVR if treating AF or venous thrombosis.

TAVR is now the most common type of aortic valve replacement. The Edwards SAPIEN valve is a balloon-expandable valvular stent, while the CoreValve is a valvular stent that self-expands when pushed out of the catheter sheath. Other valves remain under study. Five-year outcome data comparing SAVR with TAVR show no difference in death or stroke with lower rates of AF and shorter length of procedure stay observed in patients undergoing TAVR. All professional societies stress the importance of a heart valve team when considering aortic stenosis intervention. Valve-in-valve TAVR is used frequently in bioprosthetic valve dysfunction, with both aortic stenosis and aortic regurgitation. While the results of TAVR in patients with bicuspid aortic valves (as opposed to tricuspid) have been less impressive, newer modifications have improved the success rates in these anatomic situations as well. This is supported by data from the TVT registry showing similar procedural and 1-year outcomes for patients with bicuspid or tricuspid aortic valve stenosis.

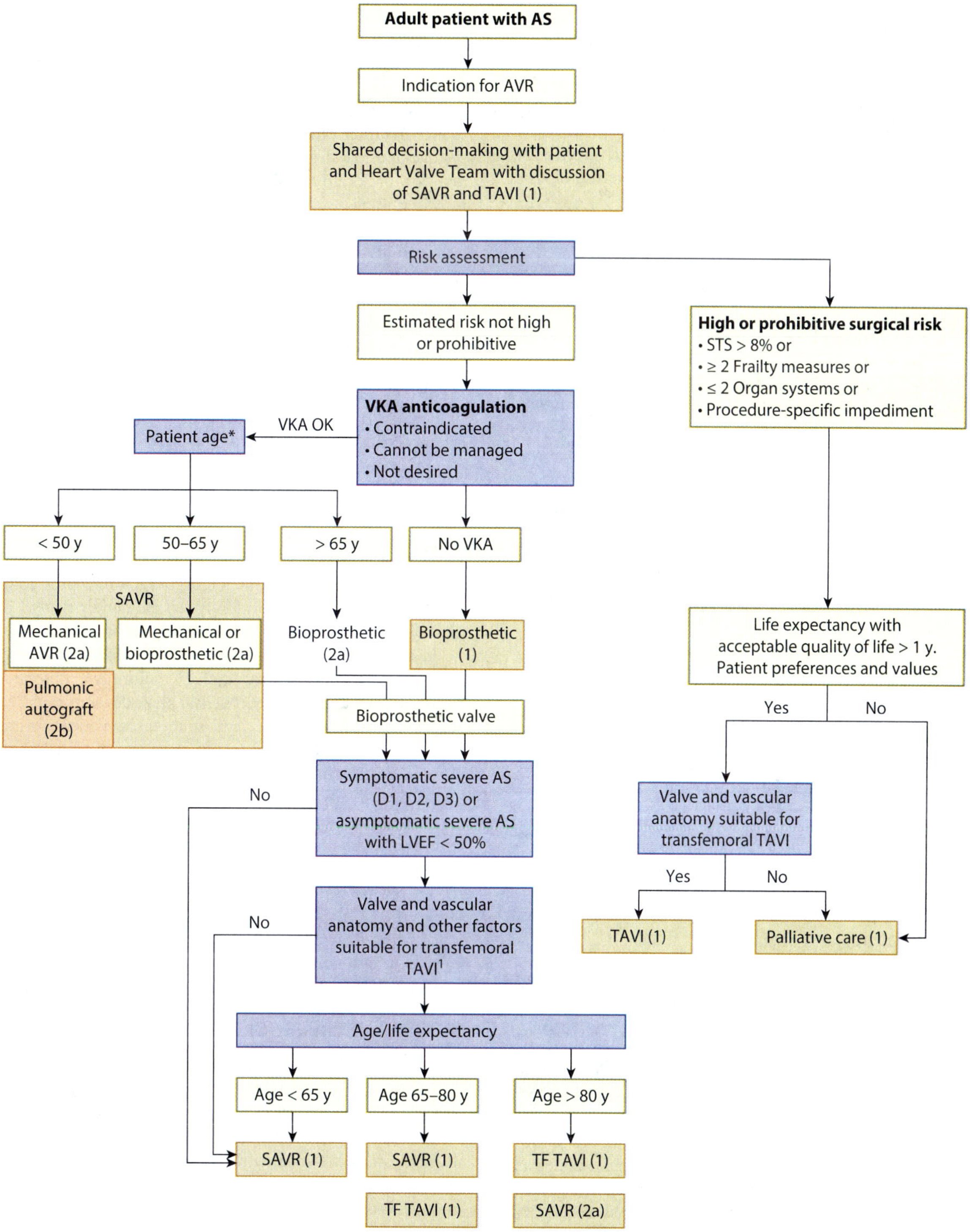

Figure 10–4. Algorithm for the type of valvular intervention in aortic valve stenosis. AS, aortic stenosis; AVR, aortic valve replacement; SAVR, surgical aortic valve replacement; STS, Society of Thoracic Surgeons; TAVI, transcatheter aortic valve implantation; TF, transfemoral; VKA, vitamin K antagonist. (Reproduced with permission from Otto CM et al. 2020 ACC/AHA guideline for the management of patients with valvular heart disease: a report of the American College of Cardiology. J Am Coll Cardiol. 2021; 77: e25–e197.)

When to Refer

- All patients with echocardiographic evidence for aortic stenosis should be referred to a cardiologist for evaluation and to determine the frequency of follow-up.
- Any patients with symptoms suggestive of aortic stenosis (ie, exertional symptoms of chest pressure, shortness of breath, or presyncope) should be seen by a cardiologist.

Mack MJ et al; PARTNER 3 Investigators. Transcatheter aortic-valve replacement in low-risk patients at five years. N Engl J Med. 2023;389:1949. [PMID: 37874020]

AORTIC REGURGITATION

ESSENTIALS OF DIAGNOSIS

- Usually asymptomatic until middle age; presents with left-sided failure or rarely chest pain.
- Echocardiography/Doppler is diagnostic.
- Surgery for symptoms, EF < 50%, LV end-systolic dimension > 50 mm, or LV end-diastolic dimension > 65 mm.

General Considerations

Rheumatic aortic regurgitation has become much less common than in the preantibiotic era; nonrheumatic causes now predominate. These include congenitally bicuspid valves, infective endocarditis, and hypertension. Many patients also have aortic regurgitation secondary to aortic root diseases, such as Marfan syndrome or aortic dissection. Rarely, inflammatory diseases, such as ankylosing spondylitis, may be implicated.

Clinical Findings

A. Symptoms and Signs

The clinical presentation is determined by the rapidity with which regurgitation develops. In **chronic aortic regurgitation**, the only sign for many years may be a soft aortic diastolic murmur. As the severity of the aortic regurgitation increases, diastolic BP falls, and the LV progressively enlarges. Most patients remain asymptomatic for long periods even at this point. LV failure is a late event and may be sudden in onset. Exertional dyspnea and fatigue are the most frequent symptoms, but paroxysmal nocturnal dyspnea and pulmonary edema may also occur. Angina pectoris or atypical chest pain may occasionally be present. Associated CAD and presyncope or syncope are less common than in aortic stenosis.

Hemodynamically, because of compensatory LV dilation, patients eject a large stroke volume, which is adequate to maintain forward cardiac output until late in the course of the disease. LV diastolic pressure may rise when HF occurs. Abnormal LV systolic function as manifested by reduced EF (< 50%) and increasing end-systolic LV volume (> 5.0 cm) are signs that surgical intervention is warranted.

The major physical findings in chronic aortic regurgitation relate to the high stroke volume being ejected into the systemic vascular system with rapid runoff as the regurgitation takes place (see Table 10–3). This results in a **wide arterial pulse pressure.** The pulse has a rapid rise and fall (**water-hammer pulse** or **Corrigan pulse**), with an elevated systolic and low diastolic pressure. The large stroke volume and flow back into the heart are also responsible for characteristic findings, such as **Quincke pulses** (nailbed capillary pulsations), **Duroziez sign** (to-and-fro murmur over a partially compressed femoral peripheral artery), and **Musset sign** (head bob with each pulse). In younger patients, the increased stroke volume may summate with the pressure wave reflected from the periphery and create a higher than expected systolic pressure in the lower extremities compared with the central aorta. Since the peripheral bed is much larger in the leg than the arm, the BP in the leg may be over 40 mm Hg higher than in the arm (**Hill sign**) in severe aortic regurgitation. The apical impulse is prominent, laterally displaced, usually hyperdynamic, and may be sustained. A systolic flow murmur is usually present and may be quite soft and localized; the aortic diastolic murmur is usually high-pitched and decrescendo. A mid or late diastolic low-pitched mitral murmur (**Austin Flint murmur**) may be heard in advanced aortic regurgitation, owing to relative obstruction of mitral inflow produced by partial closure of the mitral valve by the rapidly rising LV diastolic pressure due to the aortic regurgitation.

In **acute aortic regurgitation** (usually from aortic dissection or infective endocarditis), LV failure is manifested primarily as pulmonary edema and may develop rapidly; surgery is urgently required in such cases. Patients with acute aortic regurgitation do not have the dilated LV of chronic aortic regurgitation and the extra LV volume is handled poorly. For the same reason, the diastolic murmur is shorter, may be minimal in intensity, and the pulse pressure may not be widened—making clinical diagnosis difficult. The mitral valve may close prematurely even before LV systole has been initiated (**preclosure**) due to the rapid rise in the LV diastolic pressure, and the first heart sound is thus diminished or inaudible. Preclosure of the mitral valve can be readily detected on echocardiography and is considered an indication for urgent surgical intervention.

B. Diagnostic Studies

The ECG usually shows moderate to severe LVH. Radiographs show cardiomegaly with LV prominence and sometimes a dilated aorta.

Echocardiography demonstrates the major diagnostic features, including whether the lesion includes the proximal aortic root and what valvular pathology is present. *Annual assessments of LV size and function are critical in determining the timing for valve replacement when the aortic regurgitation is severe.* The 2020 ACC/AHA valvular guideline provides criteria for assessing the severity of aortic regurgitation. Cardiac MRI and CT can estimate aortic root size, particularly when there is concern for an ascending aneurysm. MRI can provide a regurgitant fraction to help confirm severity. Cardiac catheterization may be unnecessary in younger patients, particularly those with acute aortic regurgitation, but can help define hemodynamics, aortic root abnormalities, and associated CAD preoperatively in older patients. Increasing data are emerging that serum BNP or NT-proBNP may be an early sign of LV dysfunction, and it is possible that these data will be added to recommendations for surgical intervention in the future.

Treatment & Prognosis

Aortic regurgitation that appears or worsens during or after an episode of infective endocarditis or aortic dissection may lead to acute severe LV failure or subacute progression over weeks or months. The former usually presents as pulmonary edema; surgical replacement of the valve is indicated even during active infection. These patients may be transiently improved or stabilized by vasodilators.

Chronic aortic regurgitation may be tolerated for many years, but the prognosis without surgery becomes poor when symptoms occur. Since aortic regurgitation places both a preload (volume) and afterload increase on the LV, medications that decrease afterload can reduce regurgitation severity, although there are no convincing data that afterload reduction alters mortality. *Recommendations advocate afterload reduction in aortic regurgitation only when there is associated systolic hypertension (systolic BP > 130 mm Hg).* Afterload reduction in normotensive patients does not appear warranted. ARBs, rather than β-blockers, are the preferred additions to the medical therapy in patients with an enlarged aorta, such as in Marfan syndrome, because of the theoretical ability of an ARB to reduce aortic stiffness (by blocking TGF-β) and to slow the rate of aortic dilation. However, clinical trials evaluating the efficacy of ARBs to reduce aortic stiffness and slow the rate of aortic dilation have not yielded a positive outcome to support their use.

Surgery is indicated once symptoms emerge or for any evidence of LV dysfunction (as exhibited by a reduction in the LVEF to < 55% or increase in the LV end-systolic diameter to > 50 mm by echocardiography). In addition, it is suggested that surgery should be considered even when the LV becomes excessively enlarged (LV end-diastolic diameter > 65 mm). Guidelines also suggest it be considered (class IIb) if serial imaging reveals a progressive increase in the size of the LV (Figure 10–5).

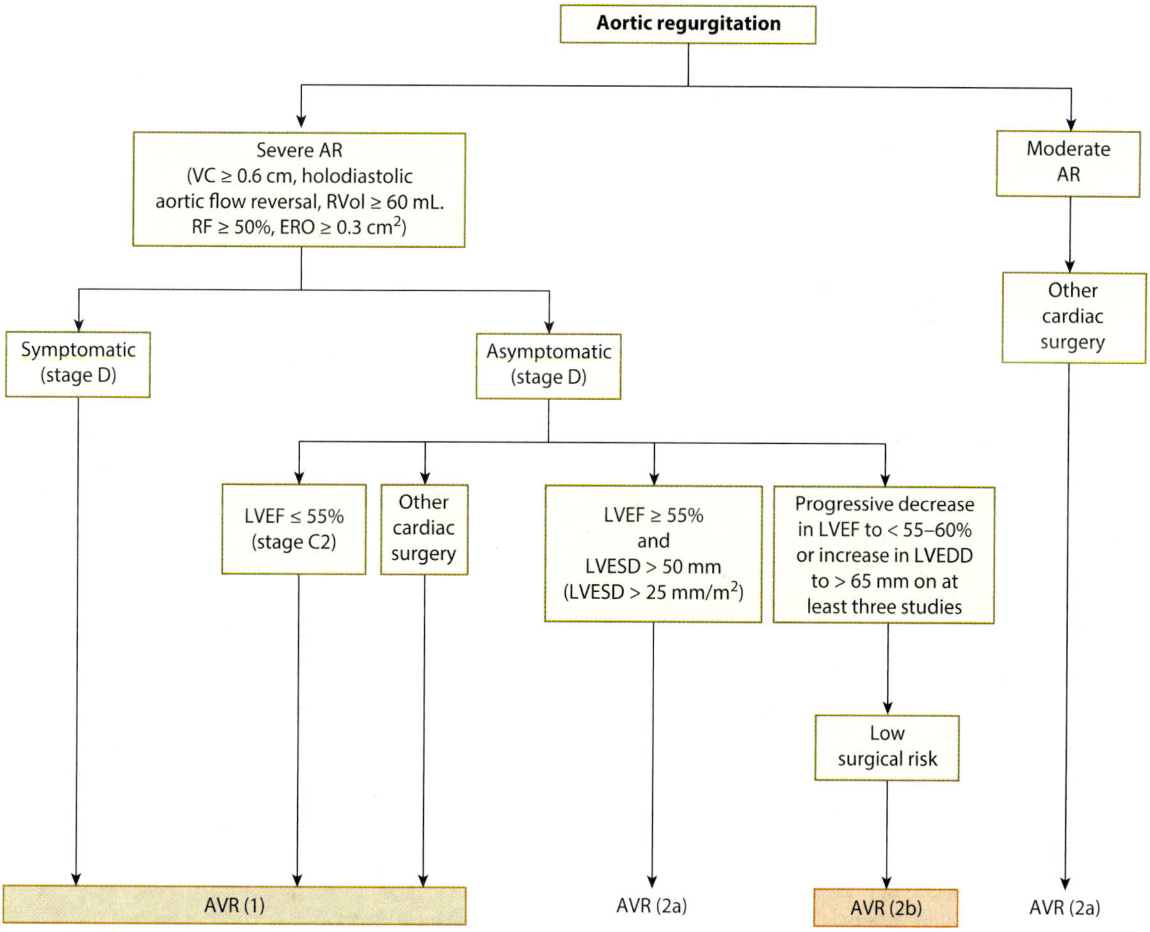

Figure 10–5. Algorithm for intervention in aortic regurgitation. AR, aortic regurgitation; AVR, aortic valve replacement; EDD, end-diastolic dimension; ERO, effective regurgitant orifice; LVESD, LV end-systolic dimension; RF, regurgitant fraction; RVol, regurgitant volume; VC, vena contracta. (Reproduced with permission from Otto CM et al. 2020 ACC/AHA guideline for the management of patients with valvular heart disease: a report of the American College of Cardiology. J Am Coll Cardiol. 2021;77: e25–e197.)

The issues with AVR covered in the above section concerning aortic stenosis pertain here. TAVR is less favorable in pure aortic regurgitation given the absence of degenerative calcification as an anchoring mechanism for the stent frame valve. The JenaValve has completed testing in pure aortic regurgitation but has yet to receive FDA approval.

Aortic regurgitation due to a paravalvular prosthetic valve defect can occasionally be occluded with percutaneous occluder devices. *The choice of prosthetic valve for AVR depends on the patient's age and compatibility with warfarin anticoagulation similar to the choices for AVR in aortic stenosis.*

Aortic regurgitation due to aortic root disease requires repair or replacement of the root as well as surgical treatment of the aortic valve. Although valve-sparing operations have improved recently, most patients with root replacement undergo valve replacement at the same time. Root replacement in association with valve replacement may require anastomosis of the coronary arteries, and thus the procedure is more complex than valve replacement alone. Following any aortic valve surgery, LV size usually decreases and LV function generally improves even when the baseline EF is depressed.

When to Refer

- Patients with audible aortic regurgitation should be seen, at least initially, by a cardiologist who can determine whether the patient needs follow-up.
- Patients with a dilated aortic root should be monitored by a cardiologist, since imaging studies other than the CXR or echocardiogram may be required to decide surgical timing.

MITRAL STENOSIS

ESSENTIALS OF DIAGNOSIS

- Fatigue, exertional dyspnea, and orthopnea when the stenosis becomes severe.
- Symptoms worsened by onset of AF or pregnancy.
- Intervention indicated for symptoms, AF, or evidence of pulmonary hypertension. Most symptomatic patients have a mitral valve area of < 1.5 cm^2.

General Considerations

Most patients with native valve mitral stenosis are presumed to have had rheumatic heart disease, although a history of rheumatic fever is noted in only about one-third. Rheumatic mitral stenosis results in thickening of the leaflets, fusion of the mitral commissures, retraction, thickening and fusion of the chordae, and calcium deposition in the valve. Mitral stenosis can also occur due to congenital disease with chordal fusion or papillary muscle malposition. The papillary muscles may be abnormally close together, sometimes so close that they merge into a single papillary muscle (the **"parachute mitral valve"**). In these patients, the chordae or valvular tissue (or both) may also be fused. In older patients and in those undergoing dialysis, mitral annular calcification may stiffen the mitral valve and reduce its motion to the point where a mitral gradient is present. Calcium in the mitral annulus virtually invades the mitral leaflet from the annulus inward as opposed to the calcium buildup in the leaflets and commissures as seen in rheumatic heart disease. Mitral valve obstruction may also develop in patients who have had mitral valve repair with a mitral annular ring that is too small, or in patients who have had a surgical valve replacement (patient–prosthesis mismatch or degeneration of the prosthetic valve over time).

Clinical Findings

A. Symptoms and Signs

Two clinical syndromes classically occur in patients with mitral stenosis. In mild to moderate mitral stenosis, LA pressure and cardiac output may be essentially normal, and the patient is either asymptomatic or symptomatic only with extreme exertion. The measured valve area is usually between 1.5 cm^2 and 1.0 cm^2. In severe mitral stenosis (valve area < 1.0 cm^2), severe pulmonary hypertension develops due to a "secondary stenosis" of the pulmonary vascular bed. In this condition, pulmonary edema is uncommon, but symptoms of low cardiac output and right HF predominate. Any measured valve area < 1.5 cm^2 should be considered significant.

A characteristic finding of rheumatic mitral stenosis is an **opening snap** following A_2 due to the stiff mitral valve. The interval between the opening snap and aortic closure sound is long when the LA pressure is low but shortens as the LA pressure rises and approaches the aortic diastolic pressure. As mitral stenosis worsens, there is a localized low-pitched diastolic murmur whose duration increases with the severity of the stenosis as the mitral gradient continues throughout more of diastole. The diastolic murmur is best heard at the apex with the patient in the left lateral position (see Table 10–3). Mitral regurgitation may be present as well.

Paroxysmal or chronic AF eventually develops in 50–80% of patients. Any increase in the heart rate reduces diastolic filling time and increases the mitral gradient. A sudden increase in heart rate may precipitate pulmonary edema. Therefore, *heart rate control is important*, with slow heart rates allowing for more diastolic filling of the LV.

B. Diagnostic Studies

Echocardiography is the most valuable technique for assessing mitral stenosis (see Table 10–3). LA size can also be determined by echocardiography; increased size denotes an increased likelihood of AF and thrombus formation. Because echocardiography and careful symptom evaluation provide most of the needed information, cardiac catheterization is used primarily to detect associated coronary or myocardial disease—usually after the decision to intervene has been made.

Treatment & Prognosis

In most cases, there is a long asymptomatic phase after the initial rheumatic infection, followed by subtle limitation of activity. Pregnancy and its associated increase in stroke volume and heart rate result in an increased transmitral pressure gradient and may precipitate symptoms. Toward the end of pregnancy, the cardiac output continues to be maintained by an increase in heart rate, increasing the mitral gradient by shortening diastolic time. Patients with moderate to severe mitral stenosis should have the condition corrected prior to becoming pregnant if possible (when the measured valve area is about 2.0 cm^2). Pregnant patients who become symptomatic can undergo successful surgery, preferably in the third trimester, although balloon valvuloplasty is the treatment of choice if the echocardiography valve score is appropriate.

The onset of AF often precipitates symptoms, which improve with rate control or restoration of sinus rhythm. Conversion to and subsequent maintenance of sinus rhythm is most successful when the duration of AF is brief (< 6–12 months) and the LA is not severely dilated (diameter < 4.5 cm). *Once AF occurs, the patient should receive warfarin even if sinus rhythm is restored,* since AF often recurs even with antiarrhythmic therapy and 20–30% of these patients will have systemic embolization if untreated. Systemic embolization in the presence of only mild to moderate disease is not an indication for surgery but should be treated with warfarin. DOACs (dabigatran, apixaban, rivaroxaban, edoxaban) are *not* recommended by the most recent guidelines, since patients with valvular AF (secondary to rheumatic mitral stenosis) were excluded from the approval trials. A randomized clinical trial published in 2022 supports this recommendation.

Indications for intervention focus on symptoms such as an episode of pulmonary edema, a decline in exercise capacity, or any evidence of pulmonary hypertension (peak systolic pulmonary pressure > 50 mm Hg). Some experts believe that the presence of AF should also be a consideration for an intervention. Most interventions are not pursued until the patient is symptomatic (stage D). In some patients, symptoms develop with calculated mitral valve areas between 1.5 cm^2 and 1.0 cm^2. Symptoms or evidence of pulmonary hypertension should drive the decision to intervene in these patients, not the estimated valve area (Table 10–6).

Open mitral commissurotomy is now rarely performed and has been replaced by percutaneous balloon valvuloplasty. Ten-year follow-up data comparing surgery to balloon valvuloplasty suggest no real difference in outcome between the two modalities. Replacement of the valve is indicated when combined stenosis and regurgitation are present or when the mitral valve echo score is much > 8–10. To determine the valve score, numbers 1 to 4 are assigned to four valve characteristics: mobility, calcification, thickening, and submitral scar, with a maximum score of 16. Percutaneous balloon valvuloplasty has a very low mortality rate (< 0.5%) and a low morbidity rate (3–5%). Operative mortality rates also are low (1–3%) in most institutions. Repeat balloon valvuloplasty can be done if the morphology of the valve remains suitable. At surgery, a **Maze procedure** may be done at the same time to reduce recurrent atrial arrhythmias. It involves a number of endocardial incisions across the right and left atria to disrupt the electrical activity that sustains atrial arrhythmias. In many institutions, the LA appendage is closed to help remove a potential future source for thrombosis.

Mechanical mitral prosthetic valves are more prone to thrombosis than mechanical aortic prosthetic valves. *The recommended INR range is thus higher (INR 2.5–3.5 or average of 3.0). Low-dose aspirin should be used in conjunction with warfarin if the bleeding risk is low. DOACs are* ***contraindicated*** *as anticoagulants.* It is a class IIa recommendation that warfarin be used for up to 6 months after implantation of a bioprosthetic mitral valve. Bioprosthetic valves tend to degenerate after about 10–15 years. Percutaneous balloon valvuloplasty is not effective when bioprosthetic valve stenosis occurs, but transcatheter valve-in-valve procedures have been successful with appropriate anatomy. Transcatheter valve-in-valve procedures are becoming more common in patients at high risk for repeat cardiac surgical valve replacement. Reported early outcomes have been positive in patients with bioprosthetic valves, certain ring annuloplasty, and in selected patients with calcific mitral stenosis. Younger patients and those with ESKD are generally believed to do the poorest with bioprosthetic heart valves, although data have questioned the role of CKD as a major risk factor. Endocarditis prophylaxis is indicated for patients with prosthetic heart valves but is not indicated in native valve disease. Mitral stenosis due to calcific encroachment of the leaflets from mitral annular calcium can progress to severe mitral stenosis at times. It does not lend itself to percutaneous valvuloplasty.

When to Refer

- Patients with mitral stenosis should be monitored with yearly examinations, and echocardiograms should be performed more frequently as the severity of the obstruction increases.
- All patients should initially be seen by a cardiologist, who can then decide how often the patient needs cardiology follow-up and whether intervention is indicated.

Connolly SJ et al; INVICTUS Investigators. Rivaroxaban in rheumatic heart disease-associated atrial fibrillation. N Engl J Med. 2022;387:978. [PMID: 36036525]

MITRAL REGURGITATION

ESSENTIALS OF DIAGNOSIS

- Severe mitral regurgitation may cause left-sided HF and lead to pulmonary hypertension and right-sided HF.
- For chronic primary mitral regurgitation, surgery is indicated for symptoms or when the LVEF is < 60% or the echocardiographic LV end-systolic dimension is > 4.0 cm. Surgery also indicated in patients who have a progressive increase in LV size or decline in LVEF.
- In patients with mitral prolapse and severe mitral regurgitation, earlier surgery is indicated if mitral repair can be performed successfully with a high degree of certainty.

Table 10–6. Management of rheumatic mitral stenosis.

Type of MS	Definition	Treatment
Progressive	Mitral valve area > 1.5 cm^2 Mean pressure gradient ≤ 5 mm Hg Half-life < 150 msec	Periodic monitoring when • Asymptomatic (stage B or C) *or* • Symptomatic with no other cause • PCWP ≤ 25 mm Hg; mean pressure gradient ≤ 15 mm Hg with exercise *or* • Symptomatic with no other cause • PCWP > 25 mm Hg; mean pressure gradient > 15 mm Hg with exercise • Unfavorable valve morphology,[1] left atrial clot, mitral regurgitation that is > mild PBMC (level IIb recommendation) when • Symptomatic with no other cause • PCWP > 25 mm Hg; mean pressure gradient > 15 mm Hg with exercise • Favorable valve morphology, no left atrial clot, mitral regurgitation is mild or absent
Severe	Mitral valve area ≤ 1.5 cm^2 Mean pressure gradient > 5 mm Hg Half-life ≥ 150 msec	Periodic monitoring when • Asymptomatic (stage B or C) *or* • New-onset AF and unfavorable valve morphology, left atrial clot, mitral regurgitation that is > mild PBMC (level IIb recommendation) when • New-onset AF and favorable valve morphology, no left atrial clot, mitral regurgitation that is mild or absent *or* • Symptomatic (stage D) • Unfavorable valve morphology, left atrial clot, mitral regurgitation that is > mild • NYHA class III/IV symptoms with high surgical risk PBMC (level I recommendation) when • Symptomatic (stage D) • Favorable valve morphology, no left atrial clot, no or mild mitral regurgitation Mitral valve replacement (level I recommendation) when • Symptomatic (stage D) • Unfavorable valve morphology, left atrial clot, mitral regurgitation that is > mild • Not NYHA class III/IV symptoms with high surgical risk
Very severe	Mitral valve area ≤ 1.0 cm^2 Mean pressure gradient > 10 mm Hg Half-life ≥ 220 msec	Periodic monitoring • Asymptomatic (stage C) • Unfavorable valve morphology, left atrial clot, mitral regurgitation that is > mild PBMC (level 1 recommendation) when • Asymptomatic (stage C) • Favorable valve morphology, no left atrial clot, no or mild mitral regurgitation *Or* • Symptomatic (stage D) • Favorable valve morphology, no left atrial clot, no or mild mitral regurgitation Mitral valve replacement (level 1 recommendation) when • Symptomatic (stage D) • Unfavorable valve morphology, left atrial clot, mitral regurgitation that is > mild • Not NYHA class III/IV symptoms with high surgical risk

[1]Unfavorable valve morphology: < 2+ mitral regurgitation, no left atrial clot, mitral leaflets without severe calcification, lack of severe subvalvular mitral calcification.
NYHA, New York Heart Association; PBMC, percutaneous balloon mitral commissurotomy; PCWP, pulmonary capillary wedge pressure.

- Transcatheter edge-to-edge repair, if possible, can be done in symptomatic patients at higher surgical risk regardless of whether the mitral regurgitation is primary or secondary.
- Patients with functional chronic mitral regurgitation may improve with biventricular pacing and guideline-directed management and therapy.

General Considerations

Mitral regurgitation results in a volume load on the heart (increases preload) and reduces afterload. The result is an enlarged LV with an increased EF. Over time, the stress of the volume overload reduces myocardial contractile function; when this occurs, there is a drop in EF and a rise in end-systolic volume.

Clinical Findings

A. Symptoms and Signs

In **acute mitral regurgitation**, the LA size is not large, and LA pressure rises abruptly, leading to pulmonary edema if severe. When **chronic**, the LA enlarges progressively and the increased volume can be handled without a major rise in the LA pressure; the pressure in pulmonary veins and capillaries may rise only during exertion. Exertional dyspnea and fatigue progress gradually.

Mitral regurgitation leads to chronic LA and LV enlargement and may result in subsequent AF and eventually LV dysfunction. Clinically, mitral regurgitation is characterized by a pansystolic murmur maximal at the apex, radiating to the axilla and occasionally to the base. The murmur does *not* change in intensity after a premature beat because the LV to LA gradient is unaffected. In addition, a hyperdynamic LV impulse and a brisk carotid upstroke may be present along with a prominent third heart sound due to the increased volume returning to the LV in early diastole. In acute mitral regurgitation, the murmur intensity may be modest due to little difference between the LA and LV systolic pressures during ventricular systole. The mitral regurgitation murmur due to mitral valve prolapse tends to radiate anteriorly in the presence of posterior leaflet prolapse and posteriorly when the prolapse is primarily of the anterior leaflet. Mitral regurgitation may not be pansystolic in these patients but occur only after the mitral click (until late in the disease process when it then becomes progressively more holosystolic).

B. Diagnostic Studies

Echocardiographic information demonstrating the underlying pathologic process (rheumatic, calcific, prolapse, flail leaflet, endocarditis, cardiomyopathy), LV size and function, LA size, PA pressure, and RV function can be invaluable in planning treatment as well as in recognizing associated lesions. The valvular heart disease guidelines provide details of the classification and measures of severity for primary and secondary mitral valve regurgitation. Doppler techniques provide qualitative and semiquantitative estimates of the severity of mitral regurgitation. TEE may help reveal the cause of regurgitation and is especially useful in patients who have had mitral valve replacement, in suspected endocarditis, and in identifying candidates for valvular repair. Echocardiographic dimensions and measures of systolic function are critical in deciding the timing of surgery. Asymptomatic patients with severe mitral regurgitation (stage C1) but preserved LV dimensions should undergo at least yearly echocardiography. Exercise hemodynamics with either Doppler echocardiography or cardiac catheterization may be useful when the symptoms do not fit the anatomic severity of mitral regurgitation. BNP or NT-proBNP is useful in the early identification of LV dysfunction in the presence of mitral regurgitation and asymptomatic patients, and values that trend upward over time appear to have prognostic importance.

Cardiac MRI is occasionally useful, especially if specific myocardial causes are being sought (such as amyloid or myocarditis) or if myocardial viability assessment is needed prior to deciding whether to add coronary artery bypass grafting to mitral valve surgery.

Cardiac catheterization provides a further assessment of regurgitation and its hemodynamic impact along with LV function, resting cardiac output, and PA pressure. *The guidelines recommend coronary angiography to determine the presence of incidental CAD prior to valve surgery in all men over age 40 years and in menopausal women with coronary risk factors.* In younger patients, no coronary angiography is needed unless there is a clinical suspicion of coronary disease. Cardiac multidetector coronary CT may be adequate to screen patients with valvular heart disease for asymptomatic CAD. A normal CT coronary angiogram has a high predictive value for patients with normal or insignificant disease.

Treatment & Prognosis

A. Primary Mitral Regurgitation

The degree of LV enlargement reflects the severity and chronicity of regurgitation. LV volume overload may ultimately lead to LV failure and reduced cardiac output. LA enlargement may be considerable in **chronic mitral regurgitation** and a large amount of mitral regurgitation regurgitant volume may be tolerated. Patients with chronic lesions may thus remain asymptomatic for many years. Surgery is necessary when symptoms develop or when there is evidence for LV dysfunction, since progressive and irreversible deterioration of LV function can occur prior to the onset of symptoms. Early surgery is indicated even in asymptomatic patients with a reduced EF (< 60%) or marked LV dilation with reduced contractility (end-systolic dimension > 4.0 cm) (Figure 10–6).

It is a class IIa indication for mitral valve surgery when the LVEF is > 60% and the LV end-systolic dimension is still < 4.0 cm but serial imaging reveals a progressive increase in the LV end-systolic dimension or a serial decrease in the EF. Pulmonary hypertension development suggests the mitral regurgitation is severe and should prompt intervention.

Acute mitral regurgitation may develop abruptly, as with papillary muscle dysfunction following MI, valve perforation in infective endocarditis, in patients with hypertrophic cardiomyopathy (HCM), or when there are ruptured chordae tendineae in patients with mitral valve prolapse. Emergency surgery may be required. In high- to extreme-risk surgical candidates, **transcatheter edge-to-edge repair of the mitral valve (M-TEER)** can be considered. Some patients may become hemodynamically unstable and require treatment with vasodilators or intra-aortic balloon counterpulsation that reduce the amount of retrograde regurgitant flow by lowering systemic vascular resistance and improving forward stroke volume.

B. Secondary Mitral Regurgitation

Mitral regurgitation commonly occurs from forces extrinsic to the valve itself, termed "secondary mitral regurgitation." This can occur due to annular dilation, as seen in cardiomyopathies causing LV enlargement, or in atrial functional MR, whereby atrial enlargement stretches the mitral valve annulus. Therapy should target the underlying cause of secondary mitral regurgitation, and if severe regurgitation and symptoms persist after medical therapy, a transcatheter or surgical correction should be considered.

When secondary MR occurs due to systolic HF, a HF cardiologist should be consulted for titration of guideline-directed medical therapy for systolic HF (see Chapter 11). Cardiac resynchronization therapy should be consider if the QRS duration is > 150 msec or left bundle branch block is present. If symptomatic severe MR persists thereafter, referral for either transcatheter or surgical treatment is appropriate.

M-TEER for secondary mitral regurgitation has been shown to improve survival in addition to guideline-directed medical therapy, as shown in the COAPT trial. This study showed improved survival and reduced HF hospitalizations in patients with symptomatic severe MR (3+ or 4+) and reduced EF compared with medical therapy alone. While another large, randomized control trial of M-TEER did not show benefit (MITRA-FR), this is thought to be due to the trial population including patients with a cardiomyopathy out of proportion to the degree of MR. As such, patients felt to benefit from M-TEER for secondary MR are those with an EF 20–50%, with a LV end-diastolic dimension < 7 mm, and with symptomatic MR that is refractory to maximal tolerated medical therapy. M-TEER is the recommended therapy for medically refractory secondary MR (IIa compared with IIb for surgery). Surgical treatment is the preferred strategy when performing CABG for revascularization in ischemic cardiomyopathy (IIa), but can be considered when M-TEER is not anatomically feasible. Transcatheter mitral valve replacement technologies remain experimental for secondary MR in native valve disease. Figure 10–7 outlines the recommendations for intervention in secondary mitral regurgitation.

When to Refer

- All patients with more than mild mitral regurgitation should be referred to a cardiologist for evaluation.
- Serial examinations and echocardiograms should be obtained and surgical referral made for primary MR if there is an increase in the LV end-systolic dimensions, a fall in the LVEF to < 60%, symptoms, evidence for pulmonary hypertension, or the new onset of AF.
- There is evidence that mitral valve repair should be done early in the course at Mitral Valve Centers of Excellence to improve mortality and morbidity.
- M-TEER should be considered for patients with symptomatic secondary MR refractory to optimal medical therapy

TRICUSPID STENOSIS

ESSENTIALS OF DIAGNOSIS

- Female predominance.
- Carcinoid disease and prosthetic valve degeneration are the most common etiologies in the United States.
- Echocardiography/Doppler is diagnostic.

General Considerations

Tricuspid stenosis is rare, affecting < 1% of the population in developed countries and < 3% worldwide. Native valve tricuspid valve stenosis is usually rheumatic in origin. In the United States, tricuspid stenosis is more commonly due to prior tricuspid valve repair or replacement or to the carcinoid syndrome. The incidence of tricuspid stenosis after tricuspid valve replacement increases considerably after 8 years post surgery. Tricuspid regurgitation frequently accompanies the lesion. It should be suspected when right HF appears in the course of mitral valve disease or in the postoperative period after tricuspid valve repair or replacement.

Clinical Findings

A. Symptoms and Signs

Tricuspid stenosis is characterized by right HF with hepatomegaly, ascites, and dependent edema. In sinus rhythm, a giant *a* wave is seen in the JVP, which is also elevated (see Table 10–3). The typical **diastolic rumble** along the lower left sternal border mimics mitral stenosis, though in tricuspid stenosis the rumble *increases with inspiration.* In sinus rhythm, a presystolic liver pulsation may be found. It should be considered when patients exhibit signs of carcinoid syndrome.

B. Diagnostic Studies

In the absence of AF, the ECG reveals RA enlargement. The CXR may show marked cardiomegaly with a normal PA size. A dilated superior vena cava and azygous vein may be evident.

The normal valve area of the tricuspid valve is 10 cm^2, so significant stenosis must be present to produce a gradient. Hemodynamically, a mean diastolic pressure gradient > 5 mm Hg is considered significant, although even a 2 mm Hg gradient can be considered abnormal. This can be demonstrated by echocardiography or cardiac catheterization. The 2017 update of the 2014 AHA/ACC guidelines suggests a tricuspid valve area of < 1.0 cm^2 and a pressure half-time longer than 190 msec should be defined as significant because the gradient may vary depending on the heart rate.

Treatment & Prognosis

Tricuspid stenosis may be progressive, eventually causing severe right-sided HF. Initial therapy is directed at reducing the fluid congestion, with diuretics the mainstay (see Chapter 11). When there is considerable bowel edema, torsemide or bumetanide may have an advantage over other loop diuretics, such as furosemide, because they are better absorbed from the gut. Aldosterone inhibitors also help, particularly if there is liver engorgement or ascites. Neither surgical nor percutaneous valvuloplasty is particularly effective for relief of tricuspid stenosis, as residual tricuspid regurgitation is common. Tricuspid valve replacement is the preferred surgical approach. Mechanical tricuspid valve replacement is rarely done because the low flow

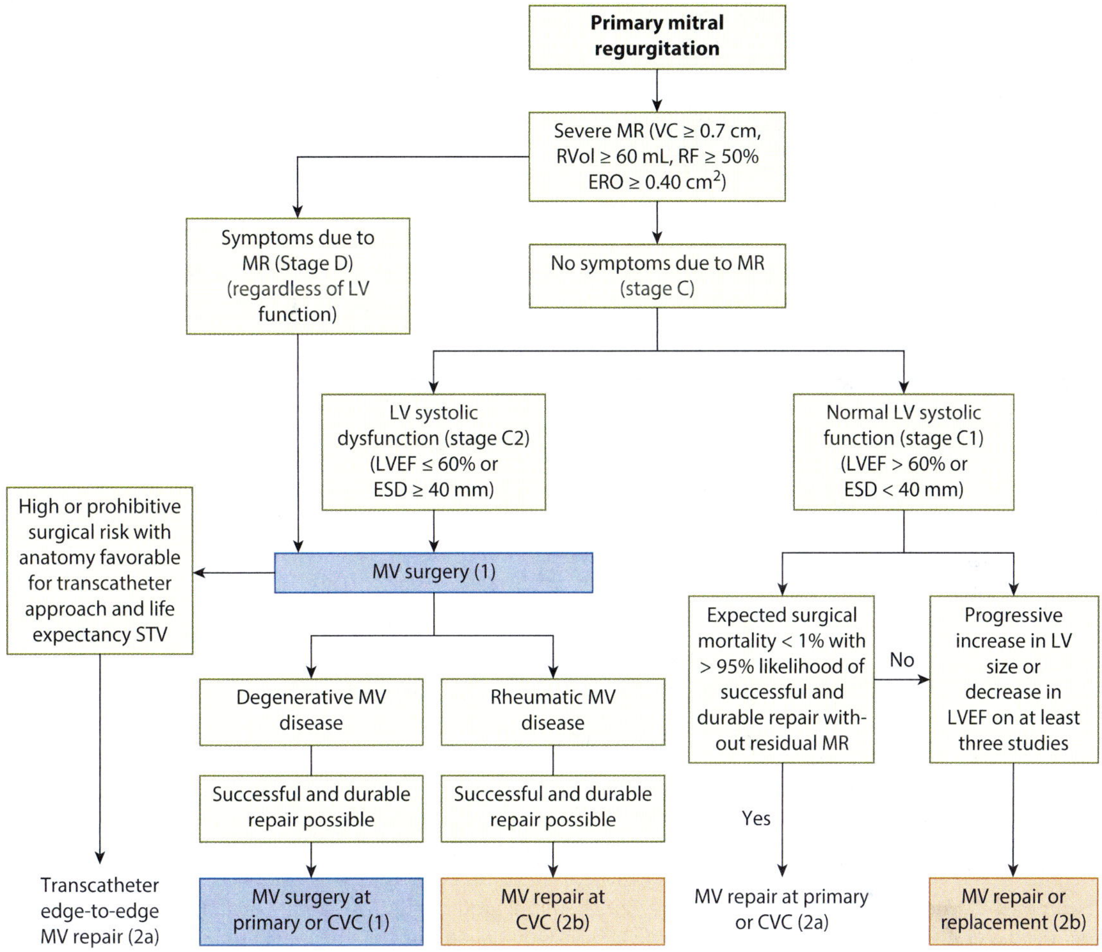

Figure 10–6. Algorithm for intervention in primary mitral regurgitation. CVC, comprehensive valve center; ERO, effective regurgitant orifice; ESD, end-systolic dimension; MR, mitral regurgitation; MV, mitral valve; MVR, mitral valve replacement; RF, regurgitant fraction; RVol, regurgitant volume; VC, vena contracta. (Reproduced with permission from Otto CM et al. 2020 ACC/AHA guideline for the management of patients with valvular heart disease: a report of the American College of Cardiology. J Am Coll Cardiol. 2021; 77: e25–e197.)

predisposes to thrombosis and because the mechanical valve cannot be crossed should the need arise for right heart catheterization or pacemaker implantation. Therefore, *bioprosthetic valves are almost always preferred.* Often tricuspid valve replacement is performed in conjunction with mitral valve replacement for rheumatic mitral stenosis or regurgitation. Percutaneous transcatheter valve replacement (stented valve) has been used in degenerative tricuspid prosthetic valve stenosis and a percutaneous tricuspid valve replacement device is being investigated. The indications for valve replacement in severe tricuspid stenosis are straightforward:

- **Class I** indication (LOE C): at time of operation for left-sided valve disease.
- **Class I** indication (LOE C): if symptomatic.
- **Class IIb** indication (LOE C): rarely percutaneous balloon commissurotomy for isolated tricuspid stenosis in high-risk patients with no significant tricuspid regurgitation.

When to Refer

All patients with any evidence for tricuspid stenosis on an echocardiogram should be seen and monitored by a cardiologist to assess when intervention may be required.

TRICUSPID REGURGITATION

ESSENTIALS OF DIAGNOSIS

- Frequently occurs in patients with pulmonary or cardiac disease with pressure or volume overload on the RV.
- Tricuspid valve regurgitation from pacemaker lead placement is becoming more common.
- Echocardiography useful in determining cause (low- or high-pressure tricuspid regurgitation).

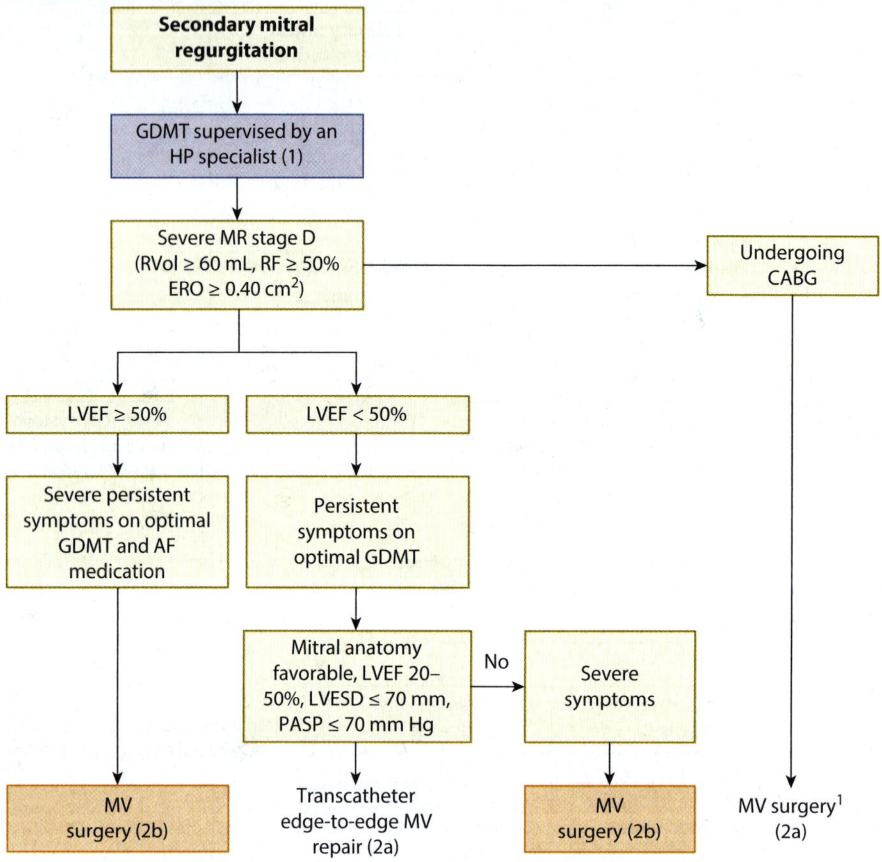

[1]Chordal-sparing MV replacement may be reasonable to choose over downsized annuloplasty repair.

Figure 10–7. Algorithm for intervention in secondary mitral regurgitation. AF, atrial fibrillation; CABG, coronary artery bypass graft; ERO, effective regurgitant orifice; GDMT, guideline-directed management and therapy; LVESD, LV end-systolic dimension; MR, mitral regurgitation; MV, mitral valve; PASP, pulmonary artery systolic pressure; RF, regurgitant fraction; RVol, regurgitant volume. (Reproduced with permission from Otto CM et al. 2020 ACC/AHA guideline for the management of patients with valvular heart disease: a report of the American College of Cardiology. J Am Coll Cardiol. 2021; 77: e25–e1.)

General Considerations

Tricuspid valvular regurgitation often occurs whenever there is RV dilation from any cause. As tricuspid regurgitation increases, the RV size increases further pulling the valve open due to chordal and papillary muscle displacement. This, in turn, worsens the severity of the tricuspid regurgitation. In addition, the tricuspid annulus is shaped like a horse's saddle. With RV failure, the annulus flattens and becomes elliptical, further distorting the relationship between the leaflets and chordal attachments. In most cases, the cause of the tricuspid regurgitation is the RV geometry (functional) and not primary tricuspid valve disease. An enlarged, dilated RV may be present if there is RV systolic hypertension from valvular or subvalvular pulmonary valve stenosis, pulmonary hypertension for any reason, in severe pulmonary valve regurgitation, or in cardiomyopathy. The RV may also be injured from an MI or may be inherently dilated due to infiltrative diseases (RV dysplasia or sarcoidosis). RV dilation often occurs secondary to left HF. Inherent abnormalities of the tricuspid valve include **Ebstein anomaly** (displacement of the septal and posterior, but not the anterior, leaflets into the RV), tricuspid valve prolapse, carcinoid plaque formation, collagen disease inflammation, valvular tumors, or tricuspid endocarditis. In addition, pacemaker lead valvular injury is an increasingly frequent iatrogenic cause.

Clinical Findings

A. Symptoms and Signs

The symptoms and signs of tricuspid regurgitation are identical to those resulting from RV failure due to any cause. As a generality, the diagnosis can be made by careful inspection of the JVP. The JVP waveform should decline during ventricular systole (the *x* descent). The timing of this decline can be observed by palpating the opposite carotid artery. As tricuspid regurgitation worsens, more and more of this *x* descent valley in the JVP is filled with the regurgitant wave until all of the *x* descent is obliterated and a positive systolic waveform will be noted in the JVP. An associated tricuspid regurgitation murmur may or may not be audible and can be distinguished from mitral regurgitation by the left parasternal location and an increase with inspiration (**Carvallo sign**). An S_3 may accompany the murmur and is related to the high flow returning to the RV from the RA. Cyanosis may be present if the increased RA pressure stretches the atrial septum and opens a PFO or there is a true ASD (eg, in about 50% of patients with Ebstein anomaly). Severe tricuspid regurgitation results in hepatomegaly, edema, and ascites.

B. Diagnostic Studies

The ECG is usually nonspecific, though atrial flutter or AF is common. The CXR may reveal evidence of an enlarged RA or dilated azygous vein and pleural effusion. The echocardiogram helps assess severity of tricuspid regurgitation (criteria available in the 2020 AHA/ACC valvular heart disease guidelines). In addition, echocardiography/Doppler provides RV systolic pressure as well as RV size and function. A paradoxically moving interventricular septum may be present due to the volume overload on the RV. Catheterization confirms the presence of the regurgitant wave in the RA and elevated RA pressures. If the PA or RV systolic pressure is < 40 mm Hg, primary valvular tricuspid regurgitation should be suspected. In addition, in patients with severe tricuspid regurgitation and ascites, a hepatic wedge pressure can be performed at the time of the right heart catheterization. If there is a high gradient between the mean RA pressure and mean hepatic wedge, then cirrhosis is likely present. Normally, the gradient across the liver is < 5 mm Hg. Mild cirrhosis is suspected if gradient is 5–10 mm Hg, moderate disease if 10–15 mm Hg, and significant cirrhosis if > 15 mm Hg.

Treatment & Prognosis

Mild tricuspid regurgitation is common and generally does not require treatment. When severe symptomatic tricuspid regurgitation is present, diuretics are the mainstay of therapy. Torsemide or bumetanide is better absorbed when gut edema is present. Aldosterone antagonists have a role as well, particularly if ascites is present. At times, the efficacy of loop diuretics can be enhanced by adding a thiazide diuretic (see Chapter 11).

Since most tricuspid regurgitation is secondary, definitive treatment usually requires elimination of the cause of the RV dysfunction. Surgical valve replacement in secondary (functional) tricuspid regurgitation is rarely if ever indicated until the cause of the RV dysfunction is resolved, and the mortality and morbidity of isolated tricuspid valve surgery remains high. Treatment for primary and secondary causes of pulmonary hypertension will generally reduce the tricuspid regurgitation. Guidelines suggest that tricuspid valve surgery may be considered when the tricuspid annular dilation at end-diastole exceeds 4.0 cm and the patient is symptomatic. It is a class I recommendation that tricuspid annuloplasty be performed when significant tricuspid regurgitation is present and mitral valve replacement or repair is being performed for mitral regurgitation. The valve leaflet itself can occasionally be primarily repaired in tricuspid valve endocarditis.

If there is an inherent defect in the tricuspid valve apparatus that cannot be repaired, then replacement of the tricuspid valve is warranted. A bioprosthetic valve, rather than a mechanical valve, is almost always used because the risk of mechanical valve thrombosis is increased if the INR is not stable. Anticoagulation is *not* required for bioprosthetic valves unless there is associated AF or flutter. Tricuspid regurgitation due to bioprosthetic degeneration has been shown to respond to transcatheter valve replacement.

Two transcatheter therapies are available for treatment of native tricuspid valve disease. **Transcatheter edge-to-edge repair of the tricuspid valve (T-TEER)** was recently shown to be safe and effective at reducing the degree of tricuspid regurgitation and improving quality of life in patients with severe tricuspid regurgitation. Transcatheter tricuspid valve replacement with the EVOQUE valve also demonstrated similar results. Both are options for treatment of medically refractory symptomatic tricuspid valve regurgitation.

When to Refer

- Anyone with moderate or severe tricuspid regurgitation should be seen at least once by a cardiologist to determine whether studies and intervention are needed.
- Severe tricuspid regurgitation requires regular follow-up by a cardiologist.

Hahn RT et al; TRISCEND II Trial Investigators. Transcatheter valve replacement in severe tricuspid regurgitation. N Engl J Med. 2025;392:115. [PMID: 39475399]

Sorajja P et al; TRILUMINATE Pivotal Investigators. Transcatheter repair for patients with tricuspid regurgitation. N Engl J Med. 2023;388:1833. [PMID: 36876753]

PULMONARY VALVE STENOSIS

ESSENTIALS OF DIAGNOSIS

- Severe cases may present with right-sided HF.
- P_2 delayed and soft or absent.
- Pulmonary ejection click often present and decreases with inspiration—the only right heart sound that *decreases* with inspiration; all other right heart sounds increase.
- Echocardiography/Doppler is diagnostic.
- Patients with peak pulmonic valve gradient > 64 mm Hg or a mean of 35 mm Hg by echocardiography/Doppler should undergo intervention regardless of symptoms. Otherwise, operate for symptoms or evidence for RV dysfunction.

General Considerations

Stenosis of the pulmonary valve or RV infundibulum increases the resistance to RV outflow, raises the RV pressure, and limits pulmonary blood flow. Pulmonic stenosis is often congenital and associated with other cardiac lesions. Pulmonary blood flow preferentially goes to the left lung in valvular pulmonic stenosis. In the absence of associated shunts, arterial saturation is normal. Peripheral pulmonic stenosis can accompany valvular pulmonic stenosis and may be part of a variety of clinical syndromes, including the congenital rubella syndrome. Patients who have had the **Ross procedure** for aortic valve disease (transfer of the pulmonary valve to the aortic position with a homograft pulmonary valve placed in the pulmonary position) may experience noncongenital postoperative pulmonic valvular or main pulmonary artery (PA) stenosis due to an immune response in the homograft. RV outflow obstructions can also occur when there is a conduit from the RV to the PA that becomes stenotic from degenerative changes over time or when there is degeneration of a bioprosthetic replacement pulmonary valve.

Clinical Findings

A. Symptoms and Signs

Mild cases of pulmonic stenosis are asymptomatic; moderate to severe pulmonic stenosis may cause symptoms of dyspnea on exertion, syncope, chest pain, and eventually RV failure.

On examination, there is often a palpable parasternal lift due to RVH and the pulmonary outflow tract may be palpable if the PA is enlarged. A loud, harsh systolic murmur and occasionally a prominent thrill are present in the left second and third interspaces parasternally. The murmur radiates toward the left shoulder due to the flow pattern within the main PA and increases with inspiration. In mild to moderate pulmonic stenosis, a loud ejection click can be heard to precede the murmur; this sound decreases with inspiration as the increased RV filling from inspiration prematurely opens the valve during atrial systole when inspiratory increased blood flow to the right heart occurs. The valve excursion during systole is thus less with inspiration than with expiration, and the click is therefore less audible with inspiration. *This is the only right-sided auscultatory event that decreases with inspiration.* All of the other auscultatory events increase with the increased right heart output that occurs with inspiration. In severe pulmonic stenosis, the second sound is obscured by the murmur and the pulmonary component of S_2 may be diminished, delayed, or absent. A right-sided S_4 and a prominent *a* wave in the venous pulse are present when there is RV diastolic dysfunction or a *c-v* wave may be observed in the jugular venous pressure if tricuspid regurgitation is present. Pulmonary valve regurgitation is relatively uncommon in primary pulmonic stenosis and may be very difficult to hear, as the gradient between the reduced PA diastolic pressure and the elevated RV diastolic pressure may be quite small (low-pressure pulmonary valve regurgitation).

B. ECG and Chest Radiography

Right axis deviation or RVH is noted; peaked P waves provide evidence of right atrial (RA) overload. Heart size may be normal on radiographs, or there may be a prominent RV and RA or gross cardiac enlargement, depending on the severity. There is often poststenotic dilation of the main and left pulmonary arteries. Pulmonary vascularity is usually normal, although there tends to be preferential flow to the left lung.

Table 10–7. Severity of pulmonary valve stenosis.

Mild	Moderate	Severe
Peak velocity < 3 m/sec Peak gradient < 36 mm Hg	Peak velocity 3–4 m/sec Peak gradient 36–64 mm Hg	Peak velocity > 4 m/sec Peak gradient > 64 mm Hg

Adapted from J Am Coll Cardiol. 2019;73:e81.

C. Diagnostic Studies

Echocardiography/Doppler is the diagnostic tool of choice, can provide evidence for a doming valve versus a dysplastic valve, can determine the gradient across the valve, and can provide information regarding subvalvular obstruction and the presence or absence of tricuspid or pulmonic valvular regurgitation. Grading the severity of pulmonic stenosis is based on the peak or mean gradient by echocardiography/Doppler (see Table 10–7). A lower gradient may be significant if there is RV dysfunction. Catheterization is usually unnecessary for the diagnosis; it should be used only if the data are unclear or in preparation for either percutaneous intervention or surgery.

Prognosis & Treatment

Patients with mild pulmonic stenosis have a normal life span with no intervention. Moderate stenosis may be asymptomatic in childhood and adolescence, but symptoms often appear as patients grow older. The degree of stenosis worsens with time, so serial follow-up is important. Severe stenosis is rarely associated with sudden death but can cause right HF in patients as early as in their 20s and 30s. Pregnancy and exercise tend to be well tolerated except in severe stenosis.

The AHA/ACC guidelines and the ESC guidelines generally agree, though the ESC suggests severe pulmonic stenosis should be considered if the RV systolic pressure is > 80 mm Hg. Class I (definitive) indications for intervention include all symptomatic patients and all those with a resting peak-to-peak gradient > 64 mm Hg or a mean > 35 mm Hg, regardless of symptoms. Symptoms can include cyanosis due to right-to-left shunting via a patent foramen ovale (PFO) or atrial septal defect (ASD). **Percutaneous balloon valvuloplasty** is highly successful in domed valve patients and is the treatment of choice. **Surgical commissurotomy** can also be done, or pulmonary **valve replacement** (with either a bioprosthetic valve or homograft) when pulmonary valve regurgitation is too severe or the valve is dysplastic. Pulmonary outflow tract obstruction due to RV to PA conduit obstruction or to homograft pulmonary valve stenosis can often be relieved with a percutaneously implanted pulmonary valve. Frequently the seating of these valves is facilitated by placing a stent within the PA first, then the transcatheter device within this stent. Because the new catheter valve may result in compression of the coronary artery, *it is a class I requirement to assess the effect of the device on the coronary by use of a temporary balloon inflation prior to delivery of the device.* Percutaneous pulmonary valve replacement is also FDA-approved for those with conduit stenosis or following the Ross procedure. Percutaneous valve replacements have also been performed off-label for patients with native pulmonary valve disease, including those who have had tetralogy of Fallot repair (assuming the PA root size is small enough to seat a percutaneous valve).

Endocarditis prophylaxis is unnecessary for native valves even after valvuloplasty unless there has been prior pulmonary valve endocarditis (an unusual occurrence). It should be used if surgical or percutaneous valve replacement has occurred. Research has shown infective endocarditis following transcatheter pulmonary valve replacement occurs in 9.5% of cases at 5 years and 16.9% of cases at 8 years. However, multivariate analysis did not show an association between infective endocarditis and specific transcatheter valve type.

When to Refer

All symptomatic patients (regardless of gradient) and all asymptomatic patients whose peak pulmonary valve gradient is > 64 mm Hg or whose mean gradient is > 35 mm Hg should be referred to a cardiologist with expertise in adult congenital heart disease. Patients also require intervention if cyanosis occurs due to a PFO or ASD or if there is exercise intolerance.

PULMONARY VALVE REGURGITATION

ESSENTIALS OF DIAGNOSIS

- Most cases are due to pulmonary hypertension resulting in high-pressure pulmonary valve regurgitation.
- Echocardiogram is definitive in high-pressure but may be less definitive in low-pressure pulmonary valve regurgitation.

General Considerations

Pulmonary valve regurgitation can be divided into **high-pressure causes** (due to pulmonary hypertension) and **low-pressure causes** (usually due to a dilated pulmonary annulus, a congenitally abnormal [bicuspid or dysplastic] pulmonary valve, carcinoid disease, surgical pulmonary valve replacement, or the residual physiology following a surgical transannular patch used to reduce the outflow gradient in tetralogy of Fallot). Because the RV tolerates a volume load better than a pressure load, it tends to tolerate low-pressure pulmonary valve regurgitation for long periods of time without dysfunction.

Clinical Findings

Most patients are asymptomatic. Those with marked pulmonary valve regurgitation may exhibit symptoms of right heart volume overload. On examination, a hyperdynamic RV can usually be palpated (**RV lift**). If the PA is enlarged, it also may be palpated along the left sternal border. P_2 will be palpable in pulmonary hypertension and both systolic and diastolic thrills are occasionally noted. On auscultation, the second heart sound may be widely split due to prolonged RV systole or an associated right bundle branch block. A pulmonary valve systolic click may be noted as well as a right-sided gallop. If pulmonic stenosis is also present, the ejection click may decline with inspiration, while any associated systolic pulmonary murmur will increase. In high-pressure pulmonary valve regurgitation, the pulmonary diastolic (**Graham Steell**) murmur is readily audible. It is often contributed to by a dilated pulmonary annulus. The murmur increases with inspiration and diminishes with the Valsalva maneuver. In low-pressure pulmonary valve regurgitation, the PA diastolic pressure may be only a few mm Hg higher than the RV diastolic pressure, and there is little diastolic gradient to produce a murmur or characteristic echocardiography/Doppler findings. At times, only contrast angiography or MRI of the main PA will show the free-flowing pulmonary valve regurgitation in low-pressure pulmonary valve regurgitation. This situation is common in patients following repair of tetralogy of Fallot where, despite little murmur, there may effectively be no pulmonary valve present. This can be suspected by noting an enlarging RV.

The ECG is generally of little value, although right bundle branch block is common, and there may be ECG criteria for RVH. The CXR may show only the enlarged RV and PA. Echocardiography may demonstrate evidence of RV volume overload (paradoxical septal motion and an enlarged RV), and Doppler can determine peak systolic RV pressure and reveal any associated tricuspid regurgitation. The interventricular septum may appear flattened if there is pulmonary hypertension. The size of the main PA can be determined and color flow Doppler can demonstrate the pulmonary valve regurgitation, particularly in the high-pressure situation. Cardiac MRI and CT can be useful for assessing the size of the PA, for estimating regurgitant flow, for excluding other causes of pulmonary hypertension (eg, thromboembolic disease, peripheral PA stenosis), and for evaluating RV function. Cardiac catheterization is confirmatory only.

Treatment & Prognosis

Pulmonary valve regurgitation rarely needs specific therapy other than treatment of the primary cause. In low-pressure pulmonary valve regurgitation due to surgical transannular patch repair of tetralogy of Fallot, pulmonary valve replacement may be indicated if RV enlargement or dysfunction is present. In tetralogy of Fallot, the QRS will widen as RV function declines (a QRS > 180 msec, among other features, suggests a higher risk for sudden death) and increasing RV volumes should trigger an evaluation for potential severe pulmonary valve regurgitation. In carcinoid heart disease, pulmonary valve replacement with a porcine bioprosthesis may be undertaken, though the plaque from this disorder eventually coats the prosthetic pulmonary valve, limiting the life span of these valves. In high-pressure pulmonary valve regurgitation, treatment to control the cause of the pulmonary hypertension is key. *High-pressure pulmonary valve regurgitation is poorly tolerated and is a serious condition that needs a thorough evaluation for cause and choice of therapy.* Pulmonary valve replacement requires a bioprosthetic valve in most cases. Pulmonary valve regurgitation due to an RV to PA conduit or due to a pulmonary autograft replacement as part of the Ross procedure can be repaired with a percutaneous pulmonary valve (Melody valve). Bioprosthetic pulmonary valve regurgitation has also been treated using a percutaneous valve (Edwards SAPIEN). When the pulmonary valve is replaced percutaneously, the PA is often stented open to provide a platform for the percutaneous valve.

When to Refer

- Patients with pulmonary valve regurgitation that results in RV enlargement should be referred to a cardiologist regardless of the estimated pulmonary pressures.

MANAGEMENT OF ANTICOAGULATION FOR PATIENTS WITH PROSTHETIC HEART VALVES

The risk of thromboembolism is much lower with bioprosthetic valves than mechanical prosthetic valves. Mechanical mitral valve prostheses pose a greater risk for thrombosis than mechanical aortic valves. For that reason, *the INR should be kept between 2.5 and 3.5 for mechanical mitral prosthetic valves but can be kept between 2.0 and 3.0 for most mechanical aortic prosthetic valves.* If there are additional risk factors in patients with a mechanical AVR (AF, previous thromboembolism, LV dysfunction, hypercoagulable state, or presence of older valve such as a ball-in-cage), then the INR for a mechanical AVR should be similar to a mechanical mitral valve replacement. Guidelines suggest the following as well: (1) a recommendation (class IIa) to expand the use of vitamin K antagonists (VKAs), such as warfarin, for up to 6 months after initial bioprosthetic valve replacement; (2) a lower target INR of 1.5–2.0 for a mechanical AVR using the On-X valve (class IIb); and (3) a consideration of VKA use with an INR of 2.5 for at least 3 months after TAVR (class IIa). It is acceptable, though, to use DOACs for the treatment of AF in patients with bioprosthetic valves. For patients with a TAVR valve, it is reasonable to use dual antiplatelet therapy (clopidogrel and aspirin) for 3–6 months after the procedure. After that, lifelong low-dose aspirin should be used. As noted earlier, using warfarin for at least 3 months after TAVR is reasonable (class IIb), although that practice is widely variable. Randomized trials have *not* shown a benefit with DOACs after TAVR.

The European Registry of Pregnancy and Cardiac Disease (ROPAC) reported on a registry that compared pregnant persons who had undergone mechanical and bioprosthetic valve replacement to pregnant persons who had not. Maternal mortality was similar between the mechanical and bioprosthetic valve patients (1.5% and 1.4%, respectively) but was much higher than those without an artificial valve (0.2%). When patients with either mechanical or bioprosthetic valves were further assessed, it was found that pregnant persons with mechanical valves were more likely to suffer adverse events than women with bioprosthetic valves. Hemorrhagic events occurred in 23.1% versus 9.2%, miscarriage on warfarin occurred in 28.6% versus 9.2%, and late fetal death was noted in 7.1% versus 0.7%, respectively. These data suggest *a high risk for morbidity and mortality for pregnant patients with mechanical heart valves,* and in the WHO Classification of Maternal Cardiac Risk, the presence of a mechanical valve is considered a class III (out of IV) risk for pregnancy complications.

Stoppage of warfarin for noncardiac surgery is likewise dependent on which mechanical valve is involved, the patient-specific risk factors, and the procedure contemplated. The risk of thromboembolism is highest in the first few months after valve replacement. While the interruption of warfarin therapy is generally safe, most cases of valve thrombosis occur during periods of inadequate anticoagulation, so the time interval without coverage should be kept as short as possible. High-risk features include AF, a prior history of thromboembolism, HF or low LVEF, a hypercoagulable state, a mechanical valve in the mitral position, a known high-risk valve (ball-in-cage), or concomitant hypercoagulable state (such as with an associated cancer). The use of *bridging VKAs,* unfractionated heparin, low-molecular-weight heparin (LMWH), and antifibrinolytics in various clinical situations in patients with valvular heart disease is summarized in Table 10–8. In general, low-risk procedures (eg, pacemaker implantation, cataract removal, and routine dental work) require no stoppage of VKAs, while in other situations the warfarin can be stopped 3 days ahead of the procedure and resumed the night after the procedure (ie, in patients with bileaflet aortic valves) without any bridging unfractionated heparin or LMWH. It is reasonable to consider bridging based on the CHA2DS2-VASc score in patients with bioprosthetic heart valves or annuloplasty rings who take anticoagulants for AF. In high-risk patients, principally just those with a mechanical mitral valve, the warfarin should be stopped and bridging with either unfractionated heparin or LMWH begun once the INR falls below therapeutic levels. Fresh frozen plasma or prothrombin complex concentrate is reasonable in an emergency situation for acute reversal if serious bleeding occurs. *Most patients with a mechanical valve should not have the warfarin reversed with vitamin K, if it can be avoided, because this can result in a transient hypercoagulable state, and it may take many days to reach a therapeutic INR again.*

Warfarin causes fetal skeletal abnormalities in up to 2% of patients who become pregnant while taking the medication, so every effort is made to defer mechanical valve replacement in women until after childbearing age. However, if an individual with a mechanical valve becomes pregnant while taking warfarin, the risk of stopping warfarin may be higher for the mother than the risk of continuing warfarin for the fetus. The risk of warfarin to the fetal skeleton is greatest during the first trimester and, remarkably, is more related to dose than to the INR level. Guidelines suggest it is reasonable to continue warfarin for the first trimester if the dose is 5 mg/day or less. If the dose is > 5 mg/day, it is appropriate to consider either LMWH (as long as the anti-Xa is being monitored [range: 0.8 U/mL to

Table 10–8. Recommendations for administering vitamin K antagonist (VKA) therapy in patients undergoing procedures or patients with certain clinical conditions (listed in alphabetical order, within categories).

Procedures	Recommendations
Bridging for mechanical heart valves	Required only for those at high risk for thromboembolism (generally only those with a mechanical mitral [not aortic] valve) Bridge with UFH or LMWH and stop UFH 4–6 hours before procedure or stop LMWH 24 hours before procedure Resume 48–72 hours after the procedure
General	Stop VKA 5 days prior and resume 12–24 hours after procedure
Clinical Situations	**Recommendations**
Aspirin use in patients with a bioprosthetic valve	
Bioprosthetic aortic or mitral valve replacement	Aspirin (50–100 mg) indefinitely. Reasonable to consider VKA to achieve INR 2.5 for first 3 months
Transcatheter valve replacement	Aspirin (50–100 mg) indefinitely
Mitral or aortic repair	Aspirin (50–100 mg) indefinitely
Atrial fibrillation and moderate or severe mitral stenosis	VKA (target INR 2.0–3.0) If patient prefers not to receive VKA, aspirin (50–100 mg) plus clopidogrel (75 mg)
Endocarditis	
Native valve or bioprosthetic valve endocarditis	No anticoagulation recommended
Mechanical valve endocarditis	Hold VKA until "safe to resume" (generally when mycotic aneurysm is ruled out or there is no need for urgent surgery)
Intermittent AF or history of systemic embolus and mitral stenosis	VKA (target INR 2.0–3.0)
Long-term anticoagulation after valve replacement	
Bioprosthetic valve in normal sinus rhythm	Aspirin (50–100 mg). Anticoagulation with a VKA to achieve an INR of 2.5 is reasonable for the first 3 months after surgical bioprosthetic MVR or AVR in patients at low risk for bleeding
Mechanical valve replacement	VKA (target INR 2.0–3.0 for mechanical aortic valve, target INR 1.5–2.5 for On-X aortic valve after the first 3 months with an initial target INR of 2.0–3.0, target INR 2.5–3.5 for mechanical mitral valve)
Pregnancy and a mechanical heart valve	Add aspirin (50–100 mg) for persons at high risk VKA may be used during first trimester and throughout pregnancy if dose of warfarin is ≤ 5 mg/day If VKA dosage normally > 5 mg/day, then adjusted dose LMWH twice daily throughout pregnancy (follow anti-Xa 4 hours after dose, with target of 0.8 U/mL to 1.2 U/mL) or LMWH may be used only during the first trimester, then resume VKA during second and third trimesters *or* Adjusted dose UFH every 12 hours throughout pregnancy (aPTT > 2 times control) or UFH may be used only during the first trimester, then resume VKA during second and third trimester Discontinuation of VKA with initiation of UFH (2 times normal PTT) recommended before planned vaginal delivery
Prosthetic valve thrombosis	
Right-sided valve	Slow-infusion fibrinolytic therapy or intravenous heparin
Left-sided valve	Early surgery if thrombus large (> 0.8 cm^2), symptomatic from valvular obstruction, high surgical risk, or LA thrombus. Thrombolysis with heparin or slow-infusion fibrinolytic therapy may be tried initially if patient is stable If thrombus evident on bioprosthetic valve creating increased gradient, use of VKA reasonable to assess whether obstructive gradient can be improved
Sinus rhythm and mitral stenosis	If left atrial size > 5.5 cm, then consider VKA (target 2.0–3.0)

aPTT, activated partial thromboplastin time; AVR, aortic valve replacement; LMWH, low-molecular-weight heparin; MVR, mitral valve replacement; PTT, partial thromboplastin time. UFH, unfractionated heparin.

Adapted from Nishimura RA et al. 2014 AHA/ACC guidelines for the management of patients with valvular heart disease: executive summary. Circulation. 2014;129:2440–92; and Nishimura RA et al. 2017 AHA/ACC focused update of the 2014 AHA/ACC guideline for the management of patients with valvular heart disease. J Am Coll Cardiol. 2017;70:252–289.

1.2 U/mL 4–6 hours post-dose]) or continuous intravenous unfractionated heparin (if the activated partial thromboplastin time [aPTT] can be monitored and is at least two times control). Guidelines suggest warfarin and low-dose aspirin are safe during the second and third trimester, and then should be stopped upon anticipation of delivery. At time of vaginal delivery, unfractionated intravenous heparin with aPTT at least two times control is desirable. DOACs (antithrombin or Xa inhibitors) should *not* be used in place of warfarin for mechanical prosthetic valves.

Management of suspected mechanical valve thrombosis depends on whether a left-sided or right-sided valve is involved, the size of the thrombus, and the patient's clinical condition. Simple fluoroscopy can help assess mechanical valve motion, although a TEE is indicated to assess thrombus size. *Therapeutic unfractionated heparin should be given to all patients with a thrombosed valve,* and this alone is generally effective. Fibrinolytic therapy is indicated if heparin therapy is ineffective and the clinical onset has been < 2 weeks, the thrombus is smaller than 0.8 cm^2, New York Heart Association (NYHA) class symptoms are mild (functional class I or II), or the valve is right-sided. Surgery is rarely indicated; it is reserved for those with left-sided mechanical valves in NYHA functional class III or IV HF or in whom TEE demonstrates a mobile thrombus larger than 0.8 cm^2. The use of urgent initial therapy for a thrombosed mechanical valve should include low-dose, slow-infusion fibrinolytic therapy or urgent surgery if the patient is symptomatic.

ADULT CONGENITAL HEART DISEASE

In the United States, there are many more adults with congenital heart disease than children, with an estimated 2 million adults in the United States surviving with congenital heart disease. As the number of patients with adult congenital heart disease has grown, there has been an increased appreciation of the need for more training and guidelines. In 2018, the ACC and AHA released updated guidelines for the assessment and treatment of patients with adult congenital heart disease. The ESC completed their update on the same topic in 2020.

COARCTATION OF THE AORTA

ESSENTIALS OF DIAGNOSIS

- Usual presentation is systemic hypertension.
- Echocardiography/Doppler is diagnostic; a peak gradient of > 20 mm Hg may be significant due to collaterals around the coarctation reducing gradient despite severe obstruction.
- Associated bicuspid aortic valve in 50–80% of patients.
- Delayed pulse in femoral artery compared with brachial artery.
- Systolic pressure is higher in upper extremities than in lower extremities; diastolic pressures are similar.

General Considerations

Coarctation of the aorta consists of localized narrowing of the aortic arch just distal to the origin of the left subclavian artery. If the stenosis is severe, collateral circulation develops around the coarctation site through the intercostal arteries and the branches of the subclavian arteries and can result in a lower trans-coarctation gradient by enabling blood flow to bypass the obstruction. *Coarctation is a cause of secondary hypertension and should be considered in young patients with elevated BP.* The renin-angiotensin system is often abnormal, however, and contributes to the hypertension occasionally seen even after coarctation repair. A **bicuspid valve** is seen in approximately 50–80% of the cases, and there is an increased incidence of cerebral berry aneurysms. Significant native or recurrent aortic coarctation has been defined as follows: upper extremity/lower extremity resting peak-to-peak gradient > 20 mm Hg or mean Doppler systolic gradient > 20 mm Hg; upper extremity/lower extremity gradient > 10 mm Hg or mean Doppler gradient > 10 mm Hg when there is either decreased LV systolic function or aortic regurgitation; or upper extremity/lower extremity gradient > 10 mm Hg or mean Doppler gradient > 10 mm Hg when there is evidence for collateral flow around the coarctation. This should be coupled with anatomic evidence for coarctation of the aorta, typically defined by advanced imaging (cardiac magnetic resonance, CT angiography). The ESC guidelines have expanded the severity criteria and suggest stenting is appropriate if the patient is normotensive but has a peak gradient of > 20 mm Hg (class IIa) or if the stenosis by angiography is > 50% (class IIb).

Clinical Findings

A. Symptoms and Signs

If cardiac failure does not occur in infancy, there are usually no symptoms until the hypertension produces LV failure. Cerebral hemorrhage, though rare, may occur. Approximately 10% of patients with coarctation of the aorta have intracranial aneurysms identified on magnetic resonance angiography or CT angiography. Increasing age has been identified as a risk factor. Strong arterial pulsations are seen in the neck and suprasternal notch. Hypertension is present in the arms, but the pressure is normal or low in the legs. This difference is exaggerated by exercise. Femoral pulsations are weak and are delayed in comparison with the brachial or radial pulse. A continuous murmur heard superiorly and midline in the back or over the left anterior chest may be present when large collaterals are present and is a clue that the coarctation is severe. The coarctation itself may result in systolic ejection murmurs heard in the left upper lung field anteriorly and near the spine on the left side posteriorly. There may be an aortic regurgitation or stenosis murmur due to an associated bicuspid aortic valve. Coarctation is associated with **Turner syndrome** (a sex chromosomal abnormality [XO]); a webbed neck may be present in these patients.

B. ECG and Chest Radiography

The ECG usually shows LVH. Radiography may show scalloping of the inferior portion of the ribs (**rib notching**) due to enlarged collateral intercostal arteries. Dilation of the left subclavian artery and poststenotic aortic dilation along with LV enlargement may be present. The coarctation region and the poststenotic dilation of the descending aorta may result in a **"3" sign** along the aortic shadow on the PA CXR (the notch in the "3" representing the area of coarctation).

C. Diagnostic Studies

Echocardiography/Doppler is usually diagnostic and may provide additional evidence for a bicuspid aortic valve. Both MRI and CT can provide excellent images of the coarctation anatomy, and one or the other should always be done to define the coarctation anatomic structure. MRI and echocardiography/Doppler can also provide estimates of the gradient across the lesion. Cardiac catheterization provides definitive gradient information and is obviously necessary if percutaneous stenting is to be considered.

Prognosis & Treatment

Cardiac failure is common in infancy and in older untreated patients when the coarctation is severe. Patients with a demonstrated peak gradient of > 20 mm Hg should be considered for intervention, especially if there is evidence of collateral blood vessels. As noted above, the ESC guidelines incorporate the stenosis severity (> 50%) as defining severe coarctation as well. Many untreated patients with severe coarctation die of hypertension, rupture of the aorta, infective endarteritis, or cerebral hemorrhage before the age of 50. Aortic dissection also occurs with increased frequency. Coarctation of any significance may be poorly tolerated in pregnancy because of the inability to support the placental flow.

Resection of the coarctation site has a surgical mortality rate of 1–4% and includes risk of spinal cord injury. The percutaneous interventional procedure of choice is **endovascular stenting;** when anatomically feasible, self-expanding and balloon-expandable covered stents have been shown to be advantageous over bare metal stents. These covered stents are FDA-approved. Most coarctation repair in adults is percutaneous. Otherwise, surgical resection (usually with end-to-end anastomosis) should be performed. About 25–50% of surgically corrected patients continue to be hypertensive years after surgery because of permanent changes in the renin-angiotensin system, endothelial dysfunction, aortic stiffness, altered arch morphology, and increased ventricular stiffness. Whether the repair was by balloon dilatation, stenting, or surgical resection may make a difference in the development of hypertension. Recurrence of the coarctation stenosis following intervention requires long-term follow-up.

When to Refer

All patients with aortic coarctation and any detectable gradient should be referred to a cardiologist with expertise in adult congenital heart disease.

ATRIAL SEPTAL DEFECT & PATENT FORAMEN OVALE

ESSENTIALS OF DIAGNOSIS

- Often asymptomatic and discovered on routine physical examination.
- With an ASD and left-to-right shunt: RV lift; S_2 widely split and fixed.
- Transesophageal echocardiography/Doppler is diagnostic.
- ASDs should be closed if there is evidence of an RV volume overload regardless of symptoms.
- A PFO, present in 20% of the population, rarely can lead to paradoxical emboli.

General Considerations

The most common form of ASD (80% of cases) is persistence of the ostium secundum in the mid-septum. A less common abnormality is persistence of the ostium primum (low in the septum). In most patients with an ostium primum defect, there are mitral or tricuspid valve "clefts" as well as a ventricular septal defect (VSD) as part of the atrioventricular (AV) septal defect. A sinus venosus defect is a hole, usually at the upper (or rarely the lower) part of the atrial septum, due to failure of the embryonic superior vena cava or the inferior vena cava to merge with the atria properly. The superior vena cava sinus venosus defect is usually associated with an anomalous connection of the right upper pulmonary vein into the superior vena cava. The coronary sinus ASD is rare and is basically an unroofed coronary sinus that results in shunting from the left atrium (LA) to the coronary sinus and then to the RA.

In all cases, *normally oxygenated blood from the higher-pressure LA shunts into the RA, increasing RV output and pulmonary blood flow.* In children, the degree of shunting across these defects may be quite large (pulmonary to systemic blood flow ratios of 3:1 or so). As the RV compliance worsens from the chronic volume overload, the RA pressure may rise and the degree of left-to-right shunting may decrease over time. Eventually, if the RA pressure exceeds the LA, the shunt may reverse and be primarily right-to-left. When this happens, systemic cyanosis appears. The major factor in the direction of shunt flow is thus the compliance of the respective atrial chambers.

The pulmonary pressures are modestly elevated in most patients with an ASD due to the high pulmonary blood flow, but severe pulmonary hypertension with cyanosis (**Eisenmenger physiology**) is actually unusual, occurring in only about 15% of the patients with an ASD alone. Increased pulmonary vascular resistance (PVR) and pulmonary hypertension secondary to pulmonary vascular disease rarely occur in childhood or young adult life in secundum defects and are more common in primum defects, especially if there is an associated VSD. Eventual RV failure may occur with any atrial shunt of significant size, and most shunts should be corrected unless they are quite small (< 1.5:1 left-to-right shunt). In adults, a large left-to-right shunt may have begun to reverse, so the absolute left-to-right shunt measurement (Qp/Qs, where Qp = pulmonary flow and Qs = systemic flow) at the time the patient is studied may underestimate the original shunt size. In addition, in most people the LV and LA compliance normally declines more over time than the RV and RA compliance; for this reason, the natural history of small atrial septal shunts is to increase the left-to-right shunting as the patient ages. There is generally only trivial shunting with a PFO compared with a true ASD. ASDs predispose to AF due to RA enlargement, and paradoxical right-to-left emboli do occur. If pulmonary hypertension does occur, the 2018 guidelines recommend that the shunt should still be closed as long as the left-to-right shunt is still > 1.5:1 and the systolic PA pressure is less than one-half the systemic arterial pressure and the PVR calculation is less than one-third systemic vascular resistance.

Interestingly, paradoxical emboli may be more common in patients with a PFO than a true ASD, especially when there is an atrial septal aneurysm. An aneurysm of the atrial septum is not a true aneurysm but rather simply a redundancy of the atrial septum that causes it to swing back and forth (> 10 mm). When present with a PFO, the back-and-forth swinging tends to pull open the PFO, encouraging shunting. This may help explain why more right-to-left shunting occurs in patients with an atrial septal aneurysm and PFO than in those with a PFO alone. This creates the anatomic substrate for the occurrence of paradoxical emboli. Other factors may distort the atrial septum (such as an enlarged aorta) and result in an increased shunting in patients with a PFO. Right-to-left PFO shunting may be more prominent upright than supine, creating orthostatic hypoxemia (**platypnea orthodeoxia**). There may also be increased shunting in patients with a PFO and sleep apnea as the RA compliance may worsen during apneic spells when pulmonary pressures increase.

Clinical Findings

A. Symptoms and Signs

Patients with a small or moderate ASD or with a PFO are asymptomatic unless a complication occurs. There is only trivial shunting in a PFO unless the RA pressure increases for some other reason or the atrial septum is distorted. With larger ASD shunts, exertional dyspnea or HF may develop, most commonly in the fourth decade of life or later. Prominent RV and PA pulsations are then readily visible and palpable. A moderately loud systolic ejection murmur can be heard in the second and third interspaces parasternally as a result of increased flow through the pulmonary valve. S_2 is widely split and does not vary with respiration. The left-to-right shunt across the defect decreases with inspiration (as the RA pressure increases) and then increases with expiration (as the RA pressure decreases), thus keeping the RV stroke volume relatively constant in inspiration and expiration. A **"fixed" splitting** of the second sound results. In very large left-to-right shunts, a tricuspid rumble may be heard due to the high flow across the tricuspid valve in diastole.

B. ECG and Chest Radiography

Right axis deviation or RVH may be present depending on the size of the RV volume overload. Incomplete or complete right bundle branch block is present in nearly all cases of ASD, and superior axis deviation (left anterior fascicular block) is noted in the complete AV septal defect, where complete heart block is often seen as well. With sinus venosus defects, the P axis is leftward of +15° due to abnormal atrial activation with loss of the upper RA tissue from around the sinus node. This creates the negative P waves in the inferior leads. The CXR shows large pulmonary arteries, increased pulmonary vascularity, and an enlarged RA and RV as with all pre-tricuspid valve cardiac left-to-right shunts. The LA is not traditionally enlarged due to an ASD shunt because the chamber is being decompressed.

C. Diagnostic Studies

Echocardiography demonstrates evidence of RA and RV volume overload. The atrial defect is usually observed by echocardiography, although sinus venosus defects may be elusive since they are high in the atrial septum. Many patients with a PFO also have an atrial septal aneurysm (defined as > 10-mm excursion of the septum from the static position). Echocardiography with saline injection **(bubble contrast)** can demonstrate the right-to-left component of the shunt, and both pulsed and color flow Doppler flow studies can demonstrate shunting in either direction. In platypnea orthodeoxia, the shunt may primarily result from inferior vena cava blood, and a femoral vein saline injection may be required to demonstrate the shunt. Transesophageal echocardiography (TEE) is helpful when transthoracic echocardiography quality is not optimal because it improves the sensitivity for detection of small shunts and provides a better assessment of PFO or ASD anatomy. Both CT and MRI can elucidate the atrial septal anatomy, better detect multiple fenestrations, and demonstrate associated lesions such as anomalous pulmonary venous connections. Atrial septal anatomy can be complex, and either MRI, TEE, or CT can reveal whether there is an adequate rim around the defect to allow for safe positioning of an atrial septal occluder device. These studies can also help identify any anomalous pulmonary venous connections. Cardiac catheterization can define the size and location of the shunt and determine the pulmonary pressure and PVR.

Prognosis & Treatment

Patients with small atrial shunts live a normal life span with no intervention. Large shunts usually cause disability by age 40 years. Because left-to-right shunts and RV overload tend to increase with normal age-related reduction in LV (and subsequently LA) compliance, both AHA/ACC and the ESC guidelines suggest that *closure of all left-to-right shunts > 1.5:1 should be accomplished either by a percutaneous device or by surgery if any right heart structures are enlarged at all.* If the pulmonary systolic pressure is more than two-thirds the systemic systolic pressure, then pulmonary hypertension may preclude ASD closure. The ESC guidelines add the pulmonary vascular resistance to the criteria and consider it a class IIa indication if the PVR is between 3 and 5 Wood units, and the guidelines preclude the use of closure if the PVR is ≥ 5 Wood units. Testing with transient balloon occlusion of the shunt, with pulmonary vasodilators, or with both may be required in the presence of pulmonary hypertension. Preservation of the cardiac output after transient balloon occlusion and evidence for preserved pulmonary vasoreactivity with pulmonary vasodilator testing all favor closure when pulmonary hypertension and at least a 1.5:1 left-to-right shunt are present. ESC guidelines favor bringing the patient back to the catheterization laboratory for retesting on pulmonary vasodilators, rather than using acute testing, to see if the PVR can be reduced below 5 Wood units. The ESC guidelines also suggest considering fenestrated closure in the face of pulmonary hypertension. The use of bosentan or sildenafil is recommended if the PVR is over 5 Wood units and there is a right-to-left shunt. After age 40 years, cardiac arrhythmias (especially AF) and HF occur with increased frequency due to the chronic right heart volume overload. Paradoxical systemic arterial embolization also becomes more of a concern as RV compliance is lost and the left-to-right shunt begins to reverse.

However, PFOs can be responsible for paradoxical emboli and are a possible cause of **cryptogenic strokes** in patients under age 55 years. Some shunting may occur with exercise if the right heart is enlarged or stiff. *Interestingly, the risk of recurrent paradoxical emboli is low regardless of whether the PFO is closed or not, and that observation has reduced the value of closing these defects in cryptogenic stroke.* Further confounding the advantage of PFO closure for cryptogenic stroke or transient ischemic attack (TIA) has been the discovery of frequent bouts of paroxysmal AF using **implantable loop recorders** for long-term heart rhythm monitoring in these patients, suggesting AF is actually the real stroke/TIA risk factor in some patients. Occasionally, a PFO that has not been pathologic may become responsible for cyanosis, especially if the RA pressure is elevated from pulmonary or RV hypertension or from severe tricuspid regurgitation.

Surgery involves stitching or patching of the foramen. For ostium secundum ASDs, percutaneous closure by use of a variety of devices is preferred over surgery when the anatomy is appropriate.

Patients who have hypoxemia (especially upon standing or with exercise) should have the PFO closed if no other cause for hypoxemia is evident and there is right-to-left shunting demonstrated through the PFO. *For patients with cryptogenic stroke or TIA, it remains uncertain whether closure of the PFO, either by open surgical or percutaneous techniques, has any advantage over anticoagulation with either warfarin, a DOAC, or aspirin.*

From a practical standpoint, *patients younger than 55 years with cryptogenic stroke/TIA and no other identifiable cause except for the presence of a PFO should still be considered for PFO closure.* A 2020 update from the guideline subcommittee of the American Academy of Neurology reaffirms no change in this overall policy. The presence of an atrial septal aneurysm (with the septum appearing "floppy" on echocardiogram) has been associated with a higher risk of recurrent stroke/TIA in patients with cryptogenic stroke/TIA. A workup for any causes for hypercoagulability and a 30-day monitor should be part of the clinical assessment to exclude other potential causes for cryptogenic stroke/TIA. In patients with risk factors for AF in which a 30-day heart rhythm monitor is negative, an implantable loop recorder should be considered for longer-term monitoring for AF. In meta-analysis of data in patients with cryptogenic stroke/TIA and PFO who have their PFO closed, ischemic stroke recurrence is less frequent compared with patients receiving medical treatment. Atrial fibrillation is more frequent but mostly transient in patients who have device closure. *There is no difference in TIA, all-cause mortality, or MI between those treated with medicine versus a closure device.* In a large, multicenter trial in France among patients who had had a recent cryptogenic stroke attributed to PFO with an associated atrial septal aneurysm or large interatrial shunt, the rate of stroke recurrence was lower among those assigned to PFO closure combined with antiplatelet therapy than among those assigned to antiplatelet therapy alone. PFO closure was associated with an increased risk of AF.

When to Refer

- All patients with an ASD should be evaluated by a cardiologist with expertise in adult congenital disease to ensure no other structural disease is present and to investigate whether the RV is enlarged.
- Patients younger than 55 years with cryptogenic stroke when no other source is identified except for a PFO with right-to-left shunting should be considered for PFO closure versus medical therapy.
- Patients with cyanosis and a PFO with evidence of a right-to-left shunt by agitated saline bubble contrast on echocardiography, especially if the cyanosis is worsened upon assuming the upright posture.

VENTRICULAR SEPTAL DEFECT

ESSENTIALS OF DIAGNOSIS

- A restrictive VSD is small and makes a louder murmur than an unrestricted one, often with an accompanying thrill. The higher the gradient across the septum, the smaller the left-to-right shunt.
- Small defects may be asymptomatic.
- Larger defects result in pulmonary hypertension (Eisenmenger physiology) if not repaired or if the pulmonary circuit is not protected by RV outflow tract obstruction.
- Echocardiography/Doppler is diagnostic.

General Considerations

Congenital VSDs occur in various parts of the ventricular septum. Membranous and muscular septal defects may spontaneously close in childhood as the septum grows and hypertrophies. A left-to-right shunt is present, with the degree depending on associated systolic RV pressure. The smaller the defect, the greater is the gradient from the LV to the RV and the louder the murmur. The presentation in adults depends on the size of the shunt and whether there is associated pulmonic or subpulmonic stenosis that has protected the lung from the systemic pressure and volume. Unprotected lungs with large shunts invariably lead to pulmonary vascular disease and severe pulmonary hypertension (Eisenmenger physiology). VSD sizes are defined by comparison to the aortic root size; a small or restrictive VSD diameter is < 25% of the aortic root diameter, a moderately restrictive VSD diameter is 25–75% of the aorta, and an unrestricted VSD size is > 75% of the aortic diameter. The size can also be quantitated based on the Qp/Qs (left-to-right shunt), with a restrictive lesion being < 1.5:1, moderately restrictive VSD being 1.5–2.2:1, and an unrestricted lesion being > 2.2:1. In rare cases of a VSD high in the ventricular septum, an aortic cusp (right coronary cusp) may prolapse into the VSD and reduce the VSD shunt but result in acute aortic regurgitation and acute HF.

Clinical Findings

A. Symptoms and Signs

The clinical features depend on the size of the defect and the presence or absence of RV outflow obstruction or increased PVR. Small shunts are associated with loud, harsh holosystolic murmurs in the left third and fourth interspaces along the sternum. A systolic thrill is common. Larger shunts may create both LV and RV volume and pressure overload. If pulmonary hypertension occurs, high-pressure pulmonary valve regurgitation may result. Right HF may gradually become evident late in the course, and the shunt will begin to balance or reverse as RV and LV systolic pressures equalize with the advent of pulmonary hypertension. Cyanosis from a developing right-to-left shunt may then occur. Cyanosis with pulmonary hypertension and an intracardiac shunt define the **Eisenmenger syndrome**.

B. ECG and Chest Radiography

The ECG may be normal or may show right, left, or biventricular hypertrophy, depending on the size of the defect and the PVR. With large shunts, the LV, the LA, and the pulmonary arteries are enlarged and pulmonary vascularity is increased on CXRs. The RV is often normal until late in the process. If an increased PVR (pulmonary hypertension) evolves, an enlarged PA with pruning of the distal pulmonary vascular bed is seen.

C. Diagnostic Studies

Echocardiography can demonstrate the size of the overloaded chambers and can usually define the defect anatomy. Doppler can qualitatively assess the magnitude of shunting by noting the gradient from LV to RV and, if some tricuspid regurgitation is present, the RV systolic pressure can be estimated. The septal leaflet of the tricuspid valve may be part of the VSD anatomy and the complex appears as a ventricular septal "aneurysm." These membranous septal aneurysms resemble a "windsock" and may fenestrate and result in a VSD shunt being present or they may remain intact. Color flow Doppler helps delineate the shunt severity and the presence of valvular regurgitation. MRI and cardiac CT can often visualize the defect and describe any other anatomic abnormalities. MRI can provide quantitative shunt data as well.

Cardiac catheterization is usually reserved for those with at least moderate shunting, to quantitate the PVR and the degree of pulmonary hypertension. The 2018 adult congenital heart disease guidelines suggest that if there is still at least a 1.5:1 left-to-right shunt and if the PVR is less than one-third that of the systemic vascular resistance, and the PA systolic pressure is more than one-half of the aortic systolic pressure, then the risk of VSD closure despite some pulmonary hypertension is acceptable and it should be done. If the PVR/systemic vascular resistance ratio or the systolic PA pressure/systolic aortic pressure ratio is greater than two-thirds or there is a net right-to-left shunt, then closure is contraindicated.

The vasoreactivity of the pulmonary circuit may be tested at catheterization using agents such as inhaled nitric oxide. The AHA/ACC guidelines suggest that if the pulmonary pressures can be lowered enough and the above ratios fall below the two-thirds value, then repair is reasonable as long as the left-to-right VSD shunt is > 1.5:1. The 2020 ESC guidelines focus not on the pulmonary to systemic systolic BP ratio, but on the pulmonary pressure and the PVR. A PVR of ≥ 5 Wood units is considered inoperable unless pulmonary vasodilators can reduce the PVR to below that value. Bosentan, an endothelial receptor blocker that reduces pulmonary pressure in Eisenmenger syndrome, has been given a class I indication in these patients in both guidelines.

Prognosis & Treatment

Patients with a small VSD have a normal life expectancy except for the small risk of infective endocarditis. *Antibiotic prophylaxis after dental work is recommended only when the VSD is residual from a prior patch closure or when there is associated pulmonary hypertension and cyanosis.* With large VSD shunts, HF may develop early in life, and survival beyond age 40 years is unusual without intervention.

Small shunts (Qp/Qs < 1.5) in asymptomatic patients do not require surgery or other intervention. The presence of RV infundibular stenosis or pulmonary valve stenosis may protect the pulmonary circuit such that some patients, even with a large VSD, may still be surgical candidates as adults if there is no pulmonary hypertension.

Surgical repair of a VSD is generally a low-risk procedure unless there is significant Eisenmenger physiology. Devices for nonsurgical closure of muscular VSDs are approved and those for membranous VSDs are being implanted with promising results; however, conduction disturbance is a major complication. Percutaneous devices are also approved for closure of a VSD related to acute MI, although the results in this very high-risk patient population have not been encouraging. In the acute MI setting, the devices have also been put across the ventricular septum at surgery to help provide a firm base on which to sew a pericardial patch, given the VSD in acute MI is often associated with widespread necrosis and multiple, serpiginous pathways. The medications used to treat pulmonary hypertension secondary to a VSD are similar to those used to treat idiopathic ("primary") pulmonary hypertension and at times can be quite effective in relieving symptoms and reducing the degree of cyanosis. *All patients who have a right-to-left shunt present should have filters placed on any intravenous lines to avoid any contamination or air bubbles from becoming systemic.*

When to Refer

All patients with a VSD should be referred to a cardiologist with expertise in adult congenital disease to decide if long-term follow-up or further studies are warranted.

TETRALOGY OF FALLOT

ESSENTIALS OF DIAGNOSIS

- Five features are characteristic:
  - VSD.
  - Concentric RVH.
  - RV outflow obstruction due to infundibular stenosis.
  - Septal overriding of the aorta in half the patients.
  - A right-sided aortic arch in 25%.
- Most adult patients with tetralogy of Fallot have been operated on, usually with an RV outflow patch and VSD closure. If patch overrides the pulmonary valve annulus, pulmonary regurgitation is common.
- Physical examination may be deceptive after classic tetralogy repair, with severe pulmonary valve regurgitation difficult to detect.
- Echocardiography/Doppler may underestimate significant pulmonary valve regurgitation. Be wary if the RV is enlarged or enlarging.
- Arrhythmias are common; periodic ambulatory monitoring is recommended.
- Serious arrhythmias and sudden death may occur if the QRS is wide, the RV enlarges, or both.

General Considerations

Patients with tetralogy of Fallot have a VSD, RV infundibular stenosis, RVH, and a dilated aorta (in about half of patients it overrides the septum). If there is an associated ASD, the complex is referred to as **pentalogy of Fallot**. The basic lesion is a large VSD with migration of the septum above the VSD and under the pulmonary valve. There may be pulmonary valve stenosis as well, usually due to either a bicuspid pulmonary valve or RV outflow hypoplasia. The aorta can be quite enlarged and aortic regurgitation may occur. If > 50% of the aorta overrides the ventricular septum, it is called **double outlet RV**. Two vascular abnormalities are common: a right-sided aortic arch (in 25%) and an anomalous left anterior descending coronary artery from the right cusp (7–9%). The latter is important in that surgical correction must avoid injuring the coronary artery when repairing the RV outflow obstruction. Pulmonary branch stenosis may also be present.

Most adult patients have undergone prior surgery. If significant RV outflow obstruction is present in the neonatal period, a systemic arterial to PA shunt may be the initial surgical procedure to improve pulmonary blood flow, though many infants undergo repair without this first step. Most adults will have had this initial palliative repair, however. The palliative procedure enables blood to reach the underperfused lung either by directly attaching one of the subclavian arteries to a main PA branch (**classic Blalock shunt**) or, more likely, by creating a conduit between the two (**modified Blalock shunt**). Total repair of the tetralogy of Fallot generally includes a VSD patch and usually an enlarging RV outflow tract patch, as well as a take-down of any prior arterial-PA shunt. If the RV outflow tract patch extends through the pulmonary valve into the PA (transannular patch), varying degrees of pulmonary valve regurgitation develop. Most surgeons approach the inside of the RV via the right atrium and through the tricuspid valve and try to avoid a transannular patch if possible. Over the years, the volume overload from residual severe pulmonary valve regurgitation becomes the major hemodynamic problem to deal with in adults. A large RV outflow patch contributes to a relative RV volume load. Ventricular arrhythmias can originate from the edge of either the VSD or outflow tract patch and tend to increase in frequency as the size of the RV increases.

Clinical Findings

Most adult patients in whom tetralogy of Fallot has been repaired are relatively asymptomatic unless right HF occurs or arrhythmias become an issue. Patients can be active and generally require no specific therapy.

A. Symptoms and Signs

Physical examination should include checking both arms for any loss of pulse from a prior shunt procedure in infancy. The jugular venous pulsations (JVP) may reveal an increased *a* wave from poor RV compliance or rarely a *c-v* wave due to tricuspid regurgitation. The right-sided arch has no consequence. The precordium may be active, often with a persistent pulmonary outflow murmur. P_2 may or may not be audible. A right-sided gallop may be heard. A residual VSD or an aortic regurgitation murmur may be present.

B. Diagnostic Studies

The ECG reveals RVH and right axis deviation; in repaired tetralogy, there is often a right bundle branch block pattern. The CXR shows a classic boot-shaped heart with prominence of the RV and a concavity in the RV outflow tract. This may be less impressive following repair. The aorta may be enlarged and right-sided. *Importantly, the width of the QRS on ECG should be examined yearly because a QRS width of > 180 msec is one of the risks for sudden death.* Most experts recommend ambulatory monitoring periodically (every 1–2 years) as well, especially if the patient experiences palpitations. Other identified risk factors for ventricular arrhythmias include having multiple prior cardiac surgeries, an elevated LVEDP, and older age at time of repair. In fact, it appears that the more the left side of the heart is involved, the higher the risk of sudden death.

Echocardiography/Doppler usually establishes the diagnosis by noting the unrestricted (large) VSD, the RV infundibular stenosis, and the enlarged aorta. In patients who have had tetralogy of Fallot repaired, echocardiography/Doppler also provides data regarding the amount of residual pulmonary valve regurgitation if a transannular patch is present, RV and LV function, and the presence of aortic regurgitation. Elevated N-terminal pro B-type natriuretic peptide (NT-proBNP) blood levels have also been correlated with increasing RV enlargement.

Cardiac MRI and CT can quantitate both the pulmonary regurgitation and the RV volumes. In addition, MRI and CT can identify whether there is either a native pulmonary arterial branch stenosis or a stenosis at the distal site of a prior arterial-to-PA shunt or other anomalies, such as an ASD. The ability of cardiac MRI to accurately quantitate the pulmonary regurgitation severity and provide more accurate RV volume measurements gives it an advantage over other imaging studies. Cardiac catheterization may be required to document the degree of pulmonary valve regurgitation because noninvasive studies depend on velocity gradients. Pulmonary angiography demonstrates the degree of pulmonary valve regurgitation, and RV angiography helps assess any postoperative outflow tract aneurysm.

The need for electrophysiologic studies with ventricular stimulation and potential ventricular tachycardia ablation has been suggested by some experts for patients who have had evidence for ventricular tachycardia, unexplained syncope, a wide QRS, are older, or who are about to undergo pulmonary valve replacement.

Prognosis & Treatment

A few patients with "just the right amount" of subpulmonic stenosis enter adulthood without having had surgical correction. However, most adult patients have had surgical repair, including VSD closure, resection of infundibular muscle, and insertion of an outflow tract patch to relieve the subpulmonic obstruction. Patients with pulmonary valve regurgitation should be monitored to ensure the RV volume does not progressively increase. In patients with tetralogy of Fallot, transthoracic echocardiogram monitoring of pulmonary valve regurgitation is recommended every 12–24 months based on the degree of regurgitation. Low-pressure pulmonary valve regurgitation is difficult to diagnose due to the fact that the RV diastolic pressures tend to be high and the pulmonary arterial diastolic pressure low. This means there is little gradient between the PA and the RV in diastole, so that there may be little murmur or evidence of turbulence on color flow Doppler. *If the RV begins to enlarge, it must be assumed that this is due to pulmonary valve regurgitation until proven otherwise.* Early surgical pulmonary valve replacement is increasingly being favored. The RV volumes from cardiac MRI are important in deciding when to intervene if the patient is not very symptomatic; an RV end-diastolic volume index of > 160 mm/m^2 or an RV end-systolic volume index of > 80 mm/m^2 is recommended as the cutoff. There are also a number of other triggers for intervention, details of which can be found in the AHA/ACC and ESC guidelines. A percutaneous approach to pulmonary valve regurgitation remains limited as the available percutaneous valve diameters are frequently too small for the size of the pulmonary annulus. The Melody valve is a bovine jugular vein prosthesis with the largest size being 22 mm in diameter. Percutaneous stented valves have been used successfully and can be used in patients with larger pulmonary root sizes. Often, a regular stent is placed within the PA first, with the stented valve then placed within this first stent. The expansion of the PA must not impede flow down any coronary artery; this is tested by a trial balloon expansion while imaging the coronary artery at the same time (class I requirement). There has been an increase in stented valve endocarditis noted after the placement of the Melody valve.

If an anomalous coronary artery is present, then an extracardiac conduit around it from the RV to the PA may be necessary as part of the tetralogy repair. By 20-year follow-up, reoperation of the common tetralogy repair is needed in about 10–15%, not only for severe pulmonary valve regurgitation but also for residual infundibular stenosis. Usually the pulmonary valve is replaced with a pulmonary homograft, although a porcine bioprosthetic valve is also suitable. Percutaneous valve-in-valve stented bioprosthetic valves have successfully been used when there is surgical bioprosthetic valve dysfunction. Cryoablation of the tissue giving rise to arrhythmias is sometimes performed at the time of reoperation. Branch pulmonary stenosis may be percutaneously opened by stenting. If a conduit has been used already for repair of the RV outflow obstruction, a percutaneous approach with a stented pulmonary valve may be possible. All patients require endocarditis prophylaxis. Most adults with stable hemodynamics can be quite active, and most women can carry a pregnancy adequately if RV function is preserved.

Atrial fibrillation, reentrant atrial arrhythmias, and ventricular ectopy are common, especially after the age of 45. Left heart disease appears to cause arrhythmias more often than right heart disease. Biventricular dysfunction is not an uncommon consequence as the patient ages. The cause of associated LV dysfunction is often multifactorial and frequently unclear. Similarly, the aorta may enlarge with accompanying aortic regurgitation, and these lesions can become severe enough to warrant surgical intervention. Patients with RV or LV dysfunction or with dysfunction of both ventricles may require a defibrillator.

When to Refer

All patients with tetralogy of Fallot should be referred to a cardiologist with expertise in adult congenital heart disease.

RHEUMATIC FEVER

ESSENTIALS OF DIAGNOSIS

- More common in developing countries (100 cases/100,000 population) than in the United States (~2 cases/100,000 population).
- Peak incidence between ages 5 and 15 years.
- Presence of two major Jones criteria or one major and two minor.
- May involve mitral and other valves acutely, rarely leading to HF.

General Considerations

Rheumatic fever is a systemic immune process that is a sequela of a β-hemolytic streptococcal infection of the pharynx. It is a major scourge in developing countries and responsible for 320,000 deaths in young people worldwide each year. Over 15 million people have evidence for rheumatic heart disease. Signs of **acute rheumatic fever** usually commence 2–3 weeks after infection but may appear as early as 1 week or as late as 5 weeks. The disease has become quite uncommon in the United States, except in immigrants, due to rapid detection and adequate treatment of infections in youth. The peak incidence is between ages 5 and 15 years; rheumatic fever is rare before age 4 years or after age 40 years. Rheumatic carditis and valvulitis may be self-limited or may lead to slowly progressive valvular deformity. The characteristic lesion is a perivascular granulomatous reaction with valvulitis. The mitral valve is acutely attacked in 75–80% of cases, the aortic valve in 30% (but rarely as the sole valve involved), and the tricuspid and pulmonary valves in under 5% of cases.

The clinical profile of the infection includes carditis in 50–70% and arthritis in 35–66%, followed by chorea (10–30%, predominantly in girls) then subcutaneous nodules (0–10%) and erythema marginatum (in < 6%). Echocardiography has been found to be superior to auscultation, and the 2015 guidelines introduced **subclinical carditis** to the Jones criteria to represent abnormal echocardiographic findings when auscultatory findings were either not present or not recognized.

Chronic rheumatic heart disease results from single or repeated attacks of rheumatic fever that produce rigidity and deformity of valve cusps, fusion of the commissures, or shortening and fusion of the chordae tendineae. Valvular stenosis or regurgitation results, and the two often coexist. In chronic rheumatic heart disease, the mitral valve alone is abnormal in 50–60% of cases; combined lesions of the aortic and mitral valves occur in 20%; pure aortic lesions are less common. Tricuspid involvement occurs in about 10% of cases, but only in association with mitral or aortic disease and is thought to be more common when recurrent infections have occurred. The pulmonary valve is rarely affected long term. *A history of rheumatic fever is obtainable in only 60% of patients with rheumatic heart disease.*

Clinical Findings

The presence of two major criteria—or one major and two minor criteria—establishes the diagnosis. While India, New Zealand, and Australia have all published revised guidelines since 2001, the 2015 recommendations have revised the **Jones criteria** in a scientific statement from the AHA where subclinical carditis is now recognized with the advent of echocardiography. The revised criteria also recognize that a lower threshold should be used to diagnosis acute rheumatic fever in populations with high risk.

A. Major Criteria

1. Carditis—Carditis is most likely to be evident in children and adolescents. Any of the following suggests the presence of carditis: (1) pericarditis; (2) cardiomegaly, detected by physical signs, radiography, or echocardiography; (3) HF, right- or left-sided—the former perhaps more prominent in children, with painful liver engorgement due to tricuspid regurgitation; and (4) mitral or aortic regurgitation murmurs, indicative of dilation of a valve ring with or without associated valvulitis or morphologic findings on echocardiography of rheumatic valvulitis. The **Carey-Coombs** short mid-diastolic mitral murmur may be present due to inflammation of the mitral valve. It is a class I (LOE B) indication to perform echocardiography/Doppler studies on all cases of suspected or confirmed acute rheumatic fever.

2. Erythema marginatum and subcutaneous nodules—Erythema marginatum begins as rapidly enlarging macules that may be less notable on darker skin tones and that assume the shape of rings or crescents with clear centers. They may be raised, confluent, and either transient or persistent and usually on the trunk or proximal extremities. Subcutaneous nodules are uncommon except in children. They are small (2 cm or less in diameter), firm, and nontender and are attached to fascia or tendon sheaths over bony prominences. They persist for days or weeks, are recurrent, and are indistinguishable from rheumatoid nodules. Neither the rash nor nodules ever occur as the sole manifestation of acute rheumatic fever.

3. Sydenham chorea—This is the most definitive manifestation of acute rheumatic fever. Defined as involuntary choreoathetoid movements primarily of the face, tongue, and upper extremities, Sydenham chorea may be the sole manifestation of rheumatic fever. Girls are more frequently affected than boys, and occurrence in adults is rare.

4. Polyarthritis—This is a migratory polyarthritis that involves the large joints sequentially. In adults and in certain populations with moderate to high risk, only a single joint may be affected. The arthritis lasts 1–5 weeks and subsides without residual deformity. Prompt response of arthritis to therapeutic doses of salicylates or nonsteroidal agents is characteristic.

B. Minor Criteria

These include fever, polyarthralgia, reversible prolongation of the PR interval, and an elevated ESR or CRP. A lower threshold is set for patients at high risk. The 2015 guidelines stipulate that evidence for a preceding streptococcal infection can be defined by an increase in or rising antistreptolysin O titer or streptococcal antibodies (anti-DNAase B), a positive throat culture for group A β-hemolytic *Streptococcus*, or a positive rapid group A streptococcal carbohydrate antigen test in a child with a high pretest probability of streptococcal pharyngitis.

Treatment

A. General Measures

The patient should be kept at strict bed rest until the temperature returns to normal (without the use of antipyretic medications) and the ESR, plus the resting pulse rate, and the ECG have all returned to baseline.

B. Medical Measures

1. Salicylates—The salicylates markedly reduce fever and relieve joint pain and swelling. They have no effect on the natural course of the disease. Adults may require large doses of aspirin, 0.6–0.9 g every 4 hours; children are treated with lower doses.

2. Penicillin—Penicillin (benzathine penicillin, 1.2 million units intramuscularly once, or procaine penicillin, 600,000 units intramuscularly daily for 10 days) is used to eradicate streptococcal infection if present. Erythromycin may be substituted (40 mg/kg/day). A 2022 randomized study demonstrated reduced progression of latent rheumatic heart disease with benzathine penicillin during 2 years of follow-up.

3. Corticosteroids—There is no proof that cardiac damage is prevented or minimized by corticosteroids. A short course of corticosteroids (prednisone, 40–60 mg orally daily, with tapering over 2 weeks) usually causes rapid improvement of the joint symptoms and is indicated when response to salicylates has been inadequate.

Prevention of Recurrent Rheumatic Fever

Improvements in socioeconomic conditions and public health are critical to reducing bouts of rheumatic fever. The initial episode of rheumatic fever can usually be prevented by early treatment of streptococcal pharyngitis with penicillin (see Chapter 36). Prevention of recurrent episodes of rheumatic fever is critical. Recurrences of rheumatic fever are most common in patients who have had carditis during their initial episode and in children, 20% of whom will have a second episode within 5 years. The preferred method of prophylaxis is with benzathine penicillin G, 1.2 million units intramuscularly every 4 weeks. Oral penicillin (250 mg twice daily) is less reliable.

If the patient is allergic to penicillin, sulfadiazine (or sulfisoxazole), 1 g daily, or erythromycin, 250 mg orally twice daily, may be substituted. The macrolide azithromycin is similarly effective against group A streptococcal infection. If the patient has not had an immediate hypersensitivity (anaphylactic-type) reaction to penicillin, then cephalosporin may also be used.

Recurrences are uncommon after 5 years following the first episode and in patients over 21 years of age. Prophylaxis is usually discontinued after these times except in groups with a high risk of streptococcal infection—parents or teachers of young children, nurses, military recruits, etc. Secondary prevention of rheumatic fever depends on whether carditis has occurred. Guidelines suggest that if there is no evidence for carditis, preventive therapy can be stopped at age 21 years. If carditis has occurred but there is no residual valvular disease, it can be stopped at 10 years after the acute rheumatic fever episode. If carditis has occurred with residual valvular involvement, it should be continued for 10 years after the last episode or until age 40 years if the patient is in a situation in which re-exposure would be expected.

Prognosis

Initial episodes of rheumatic fever may last months in children and weeks in adults. The immediate mortality rate is 1–2%. Persistent rheumatic carditis with cardiomegaly, HF, and pericarditis implies a poor prognosis; 30% of children thus affected die within 10 years after the initial attack. After 10 years, two-thirds of patients will have detectable valvular abnormalities (usually thickened valves with limited mobility), but significant symptomatic valvular heart disease or persistent cardiomyopathy occurs in < 10% of patients with a single episode. In developing countries, acute rheumatic fever occurs earlier in life and recurs more frequently; thus, the evolution to chronic valvular disease is both accelerated and more severe.

Beaton A et al. Secondary antibiotic prophylaxis for latent rheumatic heart disease. N Engl J Med. 2022;386:230. [PMID: 34767321]

DISEASES OF THE PERICARDIUM

ACUTE INFLAMMATORY PERICARDITIS

ESSENTIALS OF DIAGNOSIS

- Anterior pleuritic chest pain that is worse supine than upright.
- Pericardial rub.
- Fever common.
- ESR or inflammatory CRP usually elevated.
- ECG reveals diffuse ST-segment elevation with associated PR depression.

General Considerations

Acute (< 2 weeks) inflammation of the pericardium may be infectious in origin or may be due to systemic diseases (autoimmune syndromes, uremia), neoplasm, radiation, drug toxicity, hemopericardium, postcardiac surgery, or contiguous inflammatory processes in the myocardium or lung. In many of these conditions, the pathologic process involves both the pericardium and the myocardium. Overall pericarditis accounts for 0.2% of hospital admissions and about 5% of patients with nonischemic chest pain seen in the emergency department. The ESC in 2015 proposed four categories of pericarditis: acute, incessant, recurrent, and chronic. Each category has its own diagnostic criteria. In **acute pericarditis,** there are four criteria: (1) pericardial chest pain, (2) pericardial rub, (3) new widespread ST elevation or PR depression, and (4) new or worsening pericardial effusion. To establish the diagnosis of acute pericarditis, at least two of these four criteria must be present. **Incessant pericarditis** is defined by its duration; it lasts longer than 4–6 weeks but < 3 months without remission. **Recurrent pericarditis** can be diagnosed in a patient with one reported episode of pericarditis who has been symptom free for at least 4–6 weeks. Finally, **chronic pericarditis** is diagnosed when it persists for > 3 months.

Viral infections (especially infections with coxsackieviruses and echoviruses, but also influenza, Epstein-Barr, varicella, hepatitis, mumps, and HIV viruses) are the most common cause of acute pericarditis and probably are responsible for many cases classified as idiopathic. COVID-19 has been associated with both acute pericarditis and even cardiac tamponade. Males—usually under age 50 years—are most commonly affected. The differential diagnosis primarily requires exclusion of acute MI. Tuberculous pericarditis is rare in developed countries but remains common in certain areas of the world. It results from direct lymphatic or hematogenous spread; clinical pulmonary involvement may be absent or minor, although associated pleural effusions are common. Bacterial pericarditis is equally rare and usually results from direct extension from pulmonary infections. Pneumococci, though, can cause a primary pericardial infection. *Borrelia burgdorferi,* the organism responsible for Lyme disease, can also cause myopericarditis (and occasionally heart block). Uremic pericarditis is a common complication of advanced CKD. The pathogenesis is uncertain; it occurs both with untreated uremia and in otherwise stable dialysis patients. Spread of adjacent lung cancer as well as invasion by breast cancer, renal cell carcinoma, Hodgkin disease, and lymphomas are the most common neoplastic processes involving the pericardium and have become the most frequent causes of pericardial tamponade in many countries. Pericarditis may occur 2–7 days after infarction due to an inflammatory reaction to transmural myocardial necrosis (post-MI or postcardiotomy pericarditis [**Dressler syndrome**]). Radiation can initiate a fibrinous and fibrotic process in the pericardium, presenting as subacute pericarditis or constriction. Radiation pericarditis usually follows treatments of > 4000 cGy delivered to parts including > 30% of the heart.

Other causes of pericarditis include connective tissue diseases, such as SLE and rheumatoid arthritis, drug-induced pericarditis (minoxidil, penicillins, clozapine), and myxedema. In addition, pericarditis may result from pericardial injury from invasive cardiac procedures (such as coronary artery perforation, cardiac pacemaker/defibrillator lead perforation, and intracardiac ablation), and the implantation of intracardiac devices (such as PFO/ASD occluder devices).

Pericarditis and myocarditis may coexist in 20–30% of patients. Myocarditis is often suspected when there is an elevation of serum troponins, although there are no data that suggest troponin elevations are associated with a poor prognosis.

Clinical Findings

A. Symptoms and Signs

The presentation and course of inflammatory pericarditis depend on its cause, but most syndromes have associated chest pain, which is usually pleuritic and postural (relieved by sitting). The pain is substernal but may radiate to the neck, shoulders, back, or epigastrium. Dyspnea may also be present, and the patient is often febrile. A pericardial **friction rub** is characteristic, with or without evidence of fluid accumulation or constriction. The presentation of tuberculous pericarditis tends to be subacute, but nonspecific symptoms (fever, night sweats, fatigue) may be present for days to months. Pericardial involvement develops in 1–8% of patients with pulmonary tuberculosis. Symptoms and signs of bacterial pericarditis are similar to those of other types of inflammatory pericarditis, but patients appear toxic and are often critically ill. Uremic pericarditis can present with or without symptoms; fever is absent. Often neoplastic pericarditis is painless, and the presenting symptoms relate to hemodynamic compromise or the primary disease. At times the pericardial effusion is very large, consistent with its chronic nature. Post-MI or postcardiotomy pericarditis (Dressler syndrome) usually presents as a recurrence of pain with pleural-pericardial features. A rub is often audible, and repolarization changes on the ECG may be confused with ischemia. Large effusions are uncommon, and spontaneous resolution usually occurs in a few days. Dressler syndrome occurs days to weeks to several months after MI or open heart surgery, may be recurrent, and probably represents an autoimmune syndrome. Patients present with typical pain, fever, malaise, and leukocytosis. Rarely, other symptoms of an autoimmune disorder, such as joint pain and fever, may occur. *Tamponade is rare with Dressler syndrome after MI but not when it occurs postoperatively.* The clinical onset of radiation pericarditis is usually within the first year but may be delayed for many years; often a full decade or more may pass before constriction becomes evident.

B. Laboratory Findings and Diagnostic Studies

The diagnosis of viral pericarditis is usually clinical, and leukocytosis is often present. Rising viral titers in paired sera may be obtained for confirmation but are rarely done. Cardiac enzymes may be slightly elevated, reflecting an epicardial myocarditis component. The echocardiogram is often normal or reveals only a trivial amount of extra fluid during the acute inflammatory process. The diagnosis of tuberculous pericarditis can be inferred if acid-fast bacilli are found elsewhere. The tuberculous pericardial effusions are usually small or moderate but may be large when chronic. The yield of mycobacterial organisms by pericardiocentesis is low; pericardial biopsy has a higher yield but may also be negative, and pericardiectomy may be required. If bacterial pericarditis is suspected on clinical grounds, diagnostic pericardiocentesis can be confirmatory. In uremic patients not on dialysis, the incidence of pericarditis correlates roughly with the level of BUN and creatinine. The pericardium is characteristically "shaggy" in uremic pericarditis, and the effusion is hemorrhagic and exudative. The diagnosis of neoplastic pericarditis can occasionally be made by cytologic examination of the effusion or by pericardial biopsy, but it may be difficult to establish clinically if the patient has received mediastinal radiation within the previous year. Neoplastic pericardial effusions develop over a long period of time and may become quite huge (> 2 L). The ESR is high in post-MI or postcardiotomy pericarditis and can help confirm the diagnosis. Large pericardial effusions and accompanying pleural effusions are frequent. Myxedema pericardial effusions due to hypothyroidism usually are characterized by the presence of cholesterol crystals within the fluid.

C. Other Studies

The ECG usually shows generalized ST and T wave changes and may manifest a characteristic progression beginning with diffuse ST elevation, followed by a return to baseline and then to T wave inversion. Atrial injury is often present and manifested by PR depression, especially in the limb leads. The CXR is frequently normal but may show cardiac enlargement (if pericardial fluid is present), as well as signs of related pulmonary disease. Mass lesions and enlarged lymph nodes may suggest a neoplastic process. About 60% of patients have a pericardial effusion (usually mild) detectable by echocardiography. MRI and CT scan can visualize neighboring tumor in neoplastic pericarditis. A screening chest CT or MRI is often recommended to ensure there are no extracardiac diseases contiguous to the pericardium. A consensus statement from the American Society of Echocardiography proposes adding an elevated CRP and late gadolinium enhancement of the pericardium to confirmatory criteria for the diagnosis of pericarditis. There are data that the degree of quantitative delayed enhancement of the pericardium is associated with a higher rate of recurrent pericarditis. PET scanning can also be used to help define pericardial inflammation.

Treatment

For acute pericarditis, experts suggest a restriction in activity until symptom resolution. For athletes, the duration of exercise restriction should be until resolution of symptoms and normalization of all laboratory tests (generally 3 months). The 2015 ESC guidelines recommend aspirin 750–1000 mg every 8 hours for 1–2 weeks with a taper by decreasing the dose 250–500 mg every 1–2 weeks or ibuprofen 600 mg every 8 hours for 1–2 weeks with a taper by decreasing the dose by 200–400 mg every 1–2 weeks. Peptic ulcer prophylaxis should be included. Studies support initial treatment of the acute episode with colchicine to prevent recurrences. Colchicine should be added to the NSAID at 0.5–0.6 mg once (for patients < 70 kg) or twice (for patients > 70 kg) daily and continued for at least 3 months. Tapering of colchicine is not mandatory; however, in the last week of treatment, the dosage can be reduced every other day for patients < 70 kg or once a day for those > 70 kg. *Aspirin and colchicine should be used instead of NSAIDs in post-MI pericarditis (Dressler syndrome)*, since NSAIDs and corticosteroids may have an adverse effect on myocardial healing. Aspirin in doses of 750–1000 mg three times daily for 1–2 weeks plus 3 months of colchicine is the recommended treatment for Dressler syndrome. Despite initial treatment, recurrence has been reported in about 30%.

Colchicine should be used for at least 6 months as therapy in all refractory cases and in recurrent pericarditis. At times a longer duration of therapy is required. The CRP is used to assess the effectiveness of treatment, and once it is normalized, tapering is initiated. Indomethacin in doses of 25–50 mg every 8 hours can also be considered in recurrent pericarditis in place of ibuprofen. Systemic corticosteroids can be added in patients with severe symptoms, in refractory cases, or in patients with immune-mediated etiologies, but such therapy may entail a higher risk of recurrence and may actually prolong the illness. Colchicine is recommended in addition to corticosteroids, again for at least 3 months, to help prevent recurrences. Prednisone in doses of 0.25–0.5 mg/kg/day orally is generally suggested with tapering over a 4- to 6-week period. Studies have confirmed the advantage of adding anakinra, an interleukin-1 receptor antagonist, for the treatment of recurrent pericarditis, especially for corticosteroid-dependent and colchicine-resistant pericarditis.

As a rule, symptoms subside in several days to weeks. The major early complication is **tamponade**, which occurs in < 5% of patients. There may be recurrences in the first few weeks or months. Rarely, when colchicine therapy alone fails or cannot be tolerated (usually due to GI symptoms), the pericarditis may require more significant immunosuppression, such as cyclophosphamide, azathioprine, intravenous human immunoglobulins, interleukin-1 receptor antagonists (anakinra), or methotrexate. If colchicine plus more significant immunosuppression fails, surgical pericardial stripping may be considered in recurrent cases even without clinical evidence for constrictive pericarditis.

Standard antituberculous medication therapy is usually successful for tuberculous pericarditis (see Chapter 9), but constrictive pericarditis can occur. Uremic pericarditis usually resolves with the institution of—or with more aggressive—dialysis. Tamponade is somewhat common, and pericardiocentesis or partial pericardiectomy (**pericardial window**) may be necessary. Whereas anti-inflammatory agents may relieve the pain and fever associated with uremic pericarditis, indomethacin and systemic corticosteroids do *not* affect its natural history. The prognosis with neoplastic effusion is poor, with only a small minority surviving 1 year. If it is compromising the clinical comfort of the patient, the effusion is initially drained percutaneously. A pericardial window, either by a subxiphoid approach or via video-assisted thoracic surgery, allows for partial pericardiectomy and should be considered in recurrent effusions after pericardiocentesis. Installation of chemotherapeutic agents or tetracycline may be used to reduce the recurrence rate. Symptomatic therapy is the initial approach to radiation pericarditis, but recurrent effusions and constriction often require surgery.

Prognosis

Patients with acute pericarditis and any of the following criteria have the poorest prognosis: fever higher than 38°C, subacute onset, large effusion with or without tamponade, lack of response to anti-inflammatory medication after 1 week, myopericarditis, traumatic pericarditis, and those on oral anticoagulation. About 15% of patients have at least one of these high-risk findings.

When to Refer

Patients who do not respond initially to conservative management, who have recurrences, or who appear to be developing constrictive pericarditis should be referred to a cardiologist for further assessment.

PERICARDIAL EFFUSION & TAMPONADE

ESSENTIALS OF DIAGNOSIS

Pericardial effusion

- Clinical impact determined by the speed of accumulation.
- May or may not cause pain.

Tamponade

- Tachycardia with an elevated JVP and either hypotension or a paradoxical pulse.
- Low voltage or electrical alternans on ECG.
- Echocardiography is diagnostic.

Pericardial effusion can develop during any of the acute pericarditis processes. Because the pericardium covers the ascending aorta and arch, aortic dissection, rupture, or both can lead to tamponade. The *speed of accumulation* determines the physiologic importance of the effusion. Because of pericardial stretch, effusions larger than 1000 mL that develop slowly may produce no hemodynamic effects. Conversely, smaller effusions that appear rapidly can cause tamponade due to the curvilinear relationship between the volume of fluid and the intrapericardial pressure. *Tamponade is characterized by elevated intrapericardial pressure (> 15 mm Hg)*, which restricts venous return and ventricular filling. As a result, the stroke volume and arterial pulse pressure fall, and the heart rate and venous pressure rise. Shock and death may result.

Clinical Findings

A. Symptoms and Signs

Pericardial effusions may be associated with pain if they occur as part of an acute inflammatory process or may be painless, as is often the case with neoplastic or uremic effusion. Dyspnea and cough are common, especially with tamponade. Cardiac tamponade can be a life-threatening syndrome evidenced by tachycardia, hypotension, pulsus paradoxus, raised JVP, muffled heart sounds, and decreased ECG voltage or electrical alternans. Other symptoms may result from the primary disease. The prognosis is a function of the cause. Large idiopathic chronic effusions (over 3 months) have a 30–35% risk of progression to cardiac tamponade.

A pericardial friction rub may be present even with large effusions. In cardiac tamponade, tachycardia, tachypnea, a narrow pulse pressure, and a relatively preserved systolic pressure are characteristic. **Pulsus paradoxus** is defined as a decline of > 10 mm Hg in systolic pressure during inspiration. Since the RV and LV share the same pericardium, when there is significant pericardial effusion, as the RV enlarges with inspiratory filling, septal motion toward the LV chamber reduces LV filling and results in an accentuated drop in the stroke volume and systemic BP with inspiration (the **paradoxical pulse**). CVP is elevated and, since the intrapericardial, and thus intracardiac, pressures are high even at the initiation of diastole, there is no evident *y* descent in the RA, RV, or LV hemodynamic tracings because the pericardial pressure prevents early ventricular filling. This differs from constriction where most of the initial filling of the RV and LV occurs during early diastole (rapid *y* descent), and it is only in mid to late diastole that the ventricles can no longer fill. In tamponade, ventricular filling is inhibited throughout diastole. Edema or ascites are rarely present in tamponade; these signs favor a more chronic process.

B. Laboratory Findings

Laboratory tests tend to reflect the underlying processes (see causes of pericarditis under General Considerations above).

C. Diagnostic Studies

CXR can suggest chronic effusion by an enlarged flask shaped cardiac silhouette but may appear normal in acute situations. The ECG often reveals nonspecific T wave changes and reduced QRS voltage. **Electrical alternans** is present only occasionally but is pathognomonic and is believed to be due to the heart swinging within the effusion. Echocardiography is the primary method for demonstrating pericardial effusion and is quite sensitive. If tamponade is present, the high intrapericardial pressure may collapse lower pressure cardiac structures, such as the

RA and RV. Cardiac CT and MRI also demonstrate pericardial fluid, pericardial thickening, and any associated contiguous lesions within the chest. Diagnostic pericardiocentesis or biopsy may be indicated for microbiologic and cytologic studies; a pericardial biopsy may be performed relatively simply through a small subxiphoid incision or by use of a video-assisted thoracoscopic surgical procedure. Unfortunately, *the quality of the pericardial fluid itself rarely leads to a diagnosis*, and any type of fluid (serous, serosanguinous, bloody, etc) can be seen in most diseases. Pericardial fluid analysis is most useful in excluding a bacterial cause and is occasionally helpful in malignancies. Effusions due to hypothyroidism or lymphatic obstruction may contain cholesterol or be chylous in nature, respectively.

Treatment

Small effusions can be followed clinically by careful observations of the JVP and by testing for a change in the paradoxical pulse. The most common cause of a paradoxical pulse is severe pulmonary disease, where marked changes in intrapleural pressures occur with inspiration and expiration. Serial echocardiograms are indicated if no intervention is immediately contemplated. Vasodilators and diuretics should be avoided. **When tamponade is present, urgent pericardiocentesis or cardiac surgery is required.** Because the pressure–volume relationship in the pericardial fluid is curvilinear and upsloping, removal of even a small amount of fluid often produces a dramatic fall in the intrapericardial pressure and immediate hemodynamic benefit; but complete drainage with a catheter is preferable. Continued or repeat drainage may be indicated, especially in malignant effusions. Pericardial windows via video-assisted thoracoscopy have been particularly effective in preventing recurrences when the underlying cause of the effusion continues to be present and are more effective than needle pericardiocentesis, subxiphoid surgical windows, or percutaneous balloon pericardiotomy. Effusions related to recurrent inflammatory pericarditis can be treated as noted above (see Acute Inflammatory Pericarditis). The presence of pericardial fluid in patients with pulmonary hypertension is a poor prognostic sign.

When to Refer

- Any unexplained pericardial effusion should be referred to a cardiologist.
- Trivial pericardial effusions are common, especially in HF, and need not be referred unless symptoms of pericarditis are evident.
- Hypotension or a paradoxical pulse suggesting the pericardial effusion is hemodynamically compromising the patient is a medical emergency and requires immediate drainage.
- Any echocardiographic signs of tamponade.

Il'Giovine ZJ et al. Cardiac tamponade and pericardiocentesis: recognition, standard techniques, and modern advancements. Cardiol Clin. 2024;42:159. [PMID: 38631787]

CONSTRICTIVE PERICARDITIS

ESSENTIALS OF DIAGNOSIS

- Clinical evidence of right HF.
- No fall or an elevation of the JVP with inspiration (**Kussmaul sign**).
- Echocardiographic evidence for septal bounce and reduced mitral inflow velocities with inspiration.
- At times may be difficult to differentiate from restrictive cardiomyopathy.
- Cardiac catheterization may be necessary when clinical and echocardiographic features are equivocal.

General Considerations

Pericardial inflammation can lead to a thickened, fibrotic, adherent pericardium that restricts diastolic filling and produces chronically elevated venous pressures. In the past, tuberculosis was the most common cause of constrictive pericarditis, but while it remains so in underdeveloped countries, it is rare now in the rest of the world. Constrictive pericarditis rarely occurs following recurrent pericarditis. The risk of constrictive pericarditis due to viral or idiopathic pericarditis is < 1%. Its occurrence increases following immune-mediated or neoplastic pericarditis (2–5%) and is highest after purulent bacterial pericarditis (20–30%). Other causes include post cardiac surgery, radiation therapy, and connective tissue disorders. A small number of cases are drug-induced or secondary to trauma, asbestosis, sarcoidosis, or uremia. At times, both pericardial tamponade and constrictive pericarditis may coexist, a condition referred to as **effusive-constrictive pericarditis**. The only definitive way to diagnose this condition is to reveal the underlying constrictive physiology once the pericardial fluid is drained. *The differentiation of constrictive pericarditis from a restrictive cardiomyopathy may require cardiac catheterization and the utilization of all available noninvasive imaging methods.*

Clinical Findings

A. Symptoms and Signs

The principal symptoms are slowly progressive dyspnea, fatigue, and weakness. Chronic edema, hepatic congestion, and ascites are usually present. Ascites often seems out of proportion to the degree of peripheral edema. The examination reveals these signs and a characteristically elevated jugular venous pressure with a rapid *y* descent. This can be detected at bedside by careful observation of the jugular pulse and noting an apparent increased pulse wave at the end of ventricular systole (due to the relative accentuation of the *v* wave by the rapid *y* descent). **Kussmaul sign**—a failure of the JVP to fall with inspiration—is also a frequent finding. The apex may actually retract with systole and a pericardial "knock" may be heard in early diastole. Pulsus paradoxus is unusual. Atrial fibrillation is common.

B. Diagnostic Studies

At times, constrictive pericarditis is extremely difficult to differentiate from restrictive cardiomyopathy and the two may coexist. When unclear, the use of both noninvasive testing and cardiac catheterization is required to sort out the difference.

1. Radiographic findings—The CXR may show normal heart size or cardiomegaly. Pericardial calcification is best seen on the lateral view and is uncommon. It rarely involves the LV apex, and finding of calcification at the LV apex is more consistent with LV aneurysm.

2. Echocardiography—Echocardiography rarely demonstrates a thickened pericardium. A **septal "bounce"** reflecting the rapid early filling is common, though. RV/LV interaction may be demonstrated by an inspiratory reduction in the mitral inflow Doppler pattern of > 25%, much as in tamponade. Usually, the initial mitral inflow into the LV is very rapid, and this can be demonstrated as well by the Doppler inflow (E wave) pattern. Other echocardiographic features, such as the ratio of the medial and lateral mitral annular motion (e' velocity), the respiration-related septal shift, and hepatic vein expiratory diastolic reversal ratio, also suggest constrictive physiology.

3. Cardiac CT and MRI—These imaging tests are only occasionally helpful. Pericardial thickening of > 4 mm must be present to establish the diagnosis, but no pericardial thickening is demonstrable in 20–25% of patients with constrictive pericarditis. Some MRI techniques demonstrate the septal bounce and can provide further evidence for ventricular interaction.

4. Cardiac catheterization—This procedure is often confirmatory or can be diagnostic in difficult cases where the echocardiographic features are unclear or mixed. As a generality, the pulmonary pressure is low in constriction (as opposed to restrictive cardiomyopathy). In constrictive pericarditis, because of the need to demonstrate RV/LV interaction, cardiac catheterization should include simultaneous measurement of both the LV and RV pressure tracings with inspiration and expiration. This interaction can be demonstrated by cardiac MRI. Hemodynamically, patients with constriction have equalization of end-diastolic pressures throughout their cardiac chambers, there is rapid early filling then an abrupt increase in diastolic pressure (**"square-root" sign**), the RV end-diastolic pressure is more than one-third the systolic pressure, simultaneous measurements of RV and LV systolic pressure reveal a discordance with inspiration (the RV rises as the LV falls), and there is usually a Kussmaul sign (failure of the RA pressure to fall with inspiration). In restrictive cardiomyopathy, there is concordance of RV and LV systolic pressures with inspiration.

Treatment

Therapy should be aimed at the specific etiology initially. If there is laboratory evidence of ongoing inflammation, then anti-inflammatory medications may have a role. Once the hemodynamics are evident, the mainstay of treatment is diuresis. As in other disorders of right HF, the diuresis should be aggressive, using loop diuretics (oral torsemide or bumetanide if bowel edema is suspected or intravenous furosemide), thiazides, and aldosterone antagonists (especially in the presence of ascites and liver congestion). Surgical pericardiectomy should be recommended when diuretics are unable to control symptoms. Pericardiectomy removes only the pericardium between the phrenic nerve pathways, however, and most patients still require diuretics after the procedure, though symptoms are usually dramatically improved. Morbidity and mortality after pericardiectomy are high (up to 15%) and are greatest in those with the most disability prior to the procedure. Poor prognostic predictors include prior radiation, kidney dysfunction, higher pulmonary systolic pressures, abnormal LV systolic function, a lower serum sodium level, liver dysfunction, and older age. Pericardial calcium has no impact on survival.

When to Refer

If the diagnosis of constrictive pericarditis is unclear or the symptoms of fluid retention resist medical therapy, then referral to a cardiologist is warranted to both establish the diagnosis and recommend therapy.

PULMONARY HYPERTENSION

ESSENTIALS OF DIAGNOSIS

- Mean PA pressure ≥ 20 mm Hg or a pulmonary vascular resistance (PVR) > 2 Wood units.
- Echocardiography is a screening test only.
- Pressure measurements must be confirmed by right heart catheterization.

General Considerations

The normal pulmonary bed offers about one-tenth as much resistance to blood flow as the systemic arterial system. Based on the 2019 Sixth World Symposium on Pulmonary Hypertension and updated in 2022 to focus on early disease detection, the definition of pulmonary hypertension has changed. It is defined by a mean PA pressure of > 20 mm Hg with a PVR of > 2 Wood units. Three categories are defined:

1. **Precapillary pulmonary hypertension**: mean PA pressure > 20 mm Hg, PVR > 2.0 Wood units, PCWP ≤ 15 mm Hg
2. **Isolated post-capillary pulmonary hypertension**: mean PA pressure > 20 mm Hg, PVR ≤ 2.0 Wood units
3. **Combined pre- and post-pulmonary hypertension**: mean PA pressure > 20 mm Hg, PVR > 2.0 Wood units, PCWP > 15 mm Hg

The Sixth World Symposium on Pulmonary Hypertension developed a clinical classification of pulmonary hypertension.

Group I includes **pulmonary arterial hypertension (PAH)** related to an underlying pulmonary vasculopathy. It includes the former "primary pulmonary hypertension" under the term "idiopathic pulmonary hypertension" and is defined as pulmonary hypertension and elevated PVR in the absence of other disease of the lungs or heart. Its cause is unknown. About 6–10% have heritable PAH. Drug and toxic pulmonary hypertension have been described as associated with the use of anorexigenic agents that increase serotonin release and block its uptake. These include aminorex fumarate, fenfluramine, and dexfenfluramine. In some cases, there is epidemiologic linkage to ingestion of rapeseed oil or L-tryptophan and use of recreational drugs, such as amphetamines and cocaine. Pulmonary hypertension associated with connective tissue disease includes cases associated with systemic sclerosis—up to 8–12% of patients with systemic sclerosis may be affected. Pulmonary hypertension has also been associated with HIV infection, portal hypertension, congenital heart disease (Eisenmenger syndrome), schistosomiasis, and chronic hemolytic anemia (eg, sickle cell anemia). In rare instances, obstruction of the pulmonary venous circulation may occur (pulmonary veno-occlusive disease and capillary hemangiomatosis).

Group II includes all cases related to left heart disease. **Group III** includes cases due to parenchymal lung disease, impaired control of breathing, or living at high altitude. This group encompasses those with idiopathic pulmonary fibrosis and COPD. **Group IV** represents patients with chronic thromboembolic disease or other PA obstruction. **Group V** includes multifactorial causes such as hematologic, systemic, and metabolic disorders.

Clinical Findings

A. Symptoms and Signs

Early symptoms include dyspnea and fatigue, with progressive symptoms including syncope, abdominal distention, ascites, and peripheral edema as RV function worsens. *Chronic lung disease, especially sleep apnea, often is overlooked as a cause for pulmonary hypertension as is chronic thromboembolic disease (CTEPH).*

B. Diagnostic Studies

All patients with a high risk for PAH should undergo confirmatory right heart catheterization.

The laboratory evaluation of idiopathic pulmonary hypertension must exclude a secondary cause. A hypercoagulable state should be sought by measuring protein C and S levels, the presence of a lupus anticoagulant, the level of factor V Leiden, prothrombin gene mutations, and D-dimer. Chronic pulmonary emboli must be excluded (usually by ventilation-perfusion lung scan or contrast spiral CT); the ventilation-perfusion scan is the more sensitive test but not specific. If it is normal, then chronic thromboembolic pulmonary hypertension is very unlikely. The CXR helps exclude a primary pulmonary etiology—evidence for patchy pulmonary edema may raise the suspicion of pulmonary veno-occlusive disease due to localized obstruction in pulmonary venous drainage. A sleep study may be warranted if sleep apnea is suspected. The ECG is generally consistent with RVH and RA enlargement. Echocardiography with Doppler helps exclude an intracardiac shunt and usually demonstrates an enlarged RV and RA—at times they may be huge and hypocontractile. Severe pulmonic or tricuspid valve regurgitation may be present. Interventricular septal flattening seen on the echocardiogram is consistent with pulmonary hypertension. Doppler interrogation of the tricuspid regurgitation jet provides an estimate of RV systolic pressure. PFTs help exclude other disorders, though primary pulmonary hypertension may present with only a reduced carbon monoxide DLCO or severe desaturation (particularly if a PFO has been stretched open and a right-to-left shunt is present). A declining DLCO may precede the development of pulmonary hypertension in a patient with systemic sclerosis. Chest CT demonstrates enlarged pulmonary arteries and excludes other causes (such as emphysema or interstitial lung disease). Pulmonary angiography (or magnetic resonance angiography or CT angiography) reveals loss of the smaller acinar pulmonary vessels and tapering of the larger ones. Catheterization allows measurement of pulmonary pressures and testing for vasoreactivity using a variety of agents, but nitric oxide is the preferred testing agent due to its ease of use and short half-life. A positive response is defined as one that decreases the pulmonary mean pressure by > 10 mm Hg, with the final mean PA pressure < 40 mm Hg. Abdominal ultrasound is recommended to exclude portal hypertension. A lung biopsy is no longer suggested as relevant for the diagnosis.

Treatment & Prognosis

The treatment of PAH continues to evolve and depends on the etiology as well as the patient risk stratification. Risk stratification is performed on the basis of a patient's functional status, symptoms, exam findings of right HF, and imaging evidence of right heart dysfunction. For group I patients with a normal PCWP, treatment is related to the response to nitric oxide challenge with those responsive being initially treated with calcium channel blockers. The vast majority of patients, unfortunately, do not respond to the acute vasoreactivity testing. Specific PAH therapy is therefore recommended in this situation. This begins with monotherapy for low-risk patients but expands to the use of combination medication therapy when pulmonary pressures are not improved or risk stratification worsens. In critically ill hypotensive patients inotropic support may be required and lung transplantation candidacy should be considered in high-risk patients.

Medication monotherapy varies in effectiveness depending on the etiologic classification. Only those in class I who respond to nitric oxide should get calcium channel blockers. Medication therapies include endothelin-receptor blockers (ambrisentan, bosentan, macitentan), phosphodiesterase type-5 inhibitors (sildenafil, tadalafil, and vardenafil), a guanylate cyclase stimulator (riociguat), prostanoids (epoprostenol, iloprost, treprostinil, and beraprost), and an IP-receptor agonist (selexipag). Various medication combinations have been approved and, when ineffective, sequential medication therapies may be used.

Many medications interfere with HIV treatment, and this needs to be assessed if relevant. Due to inherent lung disease or left heart disease, there are no therapies that are specific to PAH. Bosentan, an endothelin-receptor blocker, has received a class I indication for patients with Eisenmenger syndrome. Anticoagulation is often recommended and is required lifelong in chronic thromboembolic pulmonary hypertension. The number of patients with inoperable chronic thromboembolic pulmonary hypertension being treated with balloon pulmonary angioplasty has increased dramatically since favorable results have been reported. Riociguat remains the only approved medical therapy for chronic thromboembolic pulmonary hypertension patients in this latter group.

Counseling and patient education are also important. Aerobic exercise is recommended. Routine immunizations are advised. Pregnancy should be strongly discouraged and preventive measures taken to ensure it does not occur. Maternal mortality in severe PAH may be up to 50%.

Diuretics are useful for the management of right-sided HF; clinical experience suggests loop diuretics (torsemide or bumetanide, which are absorbed even if bowel edema is present) plus spironolactone are preferable. Oxygen should be used to maintain oxygen saturation > 90%. Acute vasodilator testing (generally with nitric oxide) should be performed in all patients with idiopathic PAH who may be potential candidates for long-term therapy with calcium channel blockers. Patients with PAH caused by conditions other than idiopathic PAH respond poorly to oral calcium channel blockers, and there is little value of acute vasodilator testing in these patients.

When to Refer

All patients with suspected or confirmed pulmonary hypertension should be referred to either a cardiologist or pulmonologist who specializes in pulmonary hypertension.

Humbert M et al; ESC/ERS Scientific Document Group. 2022 ESC/ERS Guidelines for the diagnosis and treatment of pulmonary hypertension. Eur Respir J. 2023;61:2200879. [PMID: 36028254]

Maron BA. Revised definition of pulmonary hypertension and approach to management: a clinical primer. J Am Heart Assoc. 2023;12:e029024. [PMID: 37026538]

NEOPLASTIC DISEASES OF THE HEART

PRIMARY CARDIAC TUMORS

Primary cardiac tumors are rare and constitute only a small fraction of all tumors that involve the heart or pericardium. The most common primary tumor is **atrial myxoma**; it comprises about 50% of all tumors in adult case series. It is generally attached to the atrial septum and is more likely to grow on the LA side of the septum rather than the RA. Patients with myxoma can rarely present with the characteristics of a systemic illness, with obstruction of blood flow at the mitral valve level, or with signs of peripheral embolization. The syndrome includes fever, malaise, weight loss, leukocytosis, elevated ESR, and emboli (peripheral or pulmonary, depending on the location of the tumor). This is sometimes confused with infective endocarditis, lymphoma, other cancers, or autoimmune diseases. In most cases, the tumor may grow to considerable size and produce symptoms by simply obstructing mitral inflow. Episodic pulmonary edema (classically occurring when an upright posture is assumed) and signs of low output may result. Physical examination may reveal a diastolic sound related to motion of the tumor ("tumor plop") or a diastolic murmur similar to that of mitral stenosis. Right-sided myxomas may cause symptoms of right-sided failure. Familial myxomas occur as part of the Carney complex, which consists of myxomas, pigmented skin lesions, and endocrine neoplasia.

The diagnosis of atrial myxoma is established by echocardiography or by pathologic study of embolic material. Cardiac MRI is useful as an adjunct. Contrast angiography is frequently unnecessary, although it may demonstrate a "tumor blush" when the mass is vascular. Surgical excision is usually curative, though recurrences do occur and serial echocardiographic follow-up is recommended.

The second most common primary cardiac tumors are **valvular papillary fibroelastomas** and **atrial septal lipomas.** These tend to be benign and usually require no therapy. Papillary fibroelastomas are usually on the pulmonary or aortic valves, may embolize or cause valvular dysfunction, and should be removed if large and mobile. Other primary cardiac tumors include rhabdomyomas (that often appear multiple in both the RV and LV), fibrous histiocytomas, hemangiomas, and a variety of sarcomas. Some sarcomas may be of considerable size before discovery. Primary pericardial tumors, such as mesotheliomas related to asbestos exposure, may also occur. The diagnosis may be supported by an abnormal cardiac contour on radiograph. Echocardiography is usually helpful but may miss tumors infiltrating the ventricular wall. Cardiac MRI is the diagnostic procedure of choice along with gated CT imaging for all cardiac tumors.

SECONDARY CARDIAC TUMORS

Metastases from malignant tumors can also affect the heart. *Most often this occurs in malignant melanoma*, but other tumors that are known to metastasize to the heart include bronchogenic carcinoma; carcinoma of the breast; lymphoma; renal cell carcinoma; sarcomas; and, in patients with AIDS, Kaposi sarcoma. These are often clinically silent but may lead to pericardial tamponade, arrhythmias and conduction disturbances, HF, and peripheral emboli. The ECG may reveal regional Q waves. The diagnosis is often made by echocardiography, but cardiac MRI and CT scanning can often better delineate the extent of involvement. Metastatic tumors, especially lung or breast, may invade the pericardium and result in very large pericardial effusions as they result in slow accumulation of fluid. The prognosis is poor for all secondary cardiac tumors and treatment is generally palliative. On occasion, surgical resection for debulking or removal and chemotherapy may be effective in relieving symptoms.

Treatment

Many primary tumors may be resected. Atrial myxomas should be removed surgically due to the high incidence of embolization from these friable tumors. Recurrences require lifelong monitoring with echocardiography. Papillary fibroelastomas are usually benign but should be removed if they appear mobile and are larger than 10 mm in size or if there is evidence of embolization at the time of discovery. Large pericardial effusions from metastatic tumors may be drained for comfort, but the fluid invariably recurs. Rhabdomyomas may be surgically cured if the tumor is accessible and can be removed while still leaving enough functioning myocardium intact.

When to Refer

All patients with suspected cardiac tumors should be referred to a cardiologist or cardiac surgeon for evaluation and possible therapy.

TRAUMATIC HEART DISEASE

Trauma is the leading cause of death in patients aged 1–44 years; cardiac and vascular trauma is second only to neurologic injury as the reason for these deaths. Penetrating wounds to the heart are often lethal unless immediately surgically repaired. In a 20-year review of penetrating trauma at a single institution, it was found that gunshot wounds were fatal 13 times more often than stab wounds and that factors such as hypotension, Glasgow Coma Score < 8, Revised Trauma Score < 7.84, associated injuries, and the more severe the injuries (Injury Severity Score > 25) all added to the mortality and morbidity risk.

Blunt trauma is a more frequent cause of cardiac injuries. This type of injury is common in motor vehicle accidents and may occur with any form of chest trauma, including CPR efforts. The most common injuries are myocardial contusions or hematomas. The RV is particularly prone to contusion as it sits directly under the sternum. Other forms of nonischemic cardiac injury include metabolic injury due to burns, electrical current, or sepsis. These may be asymptomatic (particularly in the setting of more severe injuries) or may present with chest pain of a nonspecific nature or, not uncommonly, with a pericardial component. Elevations of cardiac enzymes are frequent, and can be quite high, but the levels do not correlate with prognosis. There are some data that the presence of certain other cardiac biomarkers, such as NT-proBNP, correlate better with significant myocardial injury. Echocardiography may reveal an akinetic myocardial segment or pericardial effusion. Cardiac MRI may also suggest acute injury. Coronary CT angiography or angiography can reveal a coronary dissection or acute occlusion if that is a concern. Pericardiocentesis is warranted if tamponade is evident. As noted above, takotsubo transient segmental myocardial dysfunction can occur due to the accompanying stress.

Severe trauma may also cause myocardial or valvular rupture. Cardiac rupture can involve any chamber, but survival is most likely if injury is to one of the atria or the RV. Hemopericardium or pericardial tamponade is the usual clinical presentation, and surgery is almost always necessary. Mitral and aortic valve rupture may occur during severe blunt trauma—the former presumably if the impact occurs during systole and the latter if during diastole. Patients reach the hospital in shock or severe HF. Immediate surgical repair is essential. The same types of injuries may result in transection of the aorta, either at the level of the arch or distal to the takeoff of the left subclavian artery at the ligamentum arteriosum. Transthoracic echocardiography and TEE are the most helpful and immediately available diagnostic techniques. CT and MRI may also be required to better define the injury before surgical intervention.

Blunt trauma may also result in damage to the coronary arteries. Acute or subacute coronary thrombosis is the most common presentation. The clinical syndrome is one of acute MI with attendant ECG, enzymatic, and contractile abnormalities. Emergent revascularization is sometimes feasible, either by the percutaneous route or by coronary artery bypass surgery. LV aneurysms are common outcomes of traumatic coronary occlusions, likely due to sudden occlusion with no collateral vascular support. Coronary artery dissection or rupture may also occur in the setting of blunt cardiac trauma.

As expected, patients with severe preexisting conditions fare the least well after cardiac trauma. Data from ReCONECT, a trauma consortium, reveal that mortality is linked to volume of cases seen at various centers, preexisting coronary disease or HF, intubation, age, and a severity scoring index.

HEART DISEASE & PREGNANCY

General principles to discuss with the patient include preconceptual counseling, pregnancy risk assessment, genetic risks, environmental risks, and pregnancy management. For some patients, it may also include a discussion regarding contraception, termination of a pregnancy, and a conversation about not only the delivery but what will happen post-pregnancy (including issues such as an eventual need for heart surgery or transplantation). In a review of 1315 pregnancies in patients with heart disease, 3.6% had serious cardiovascular complications and half were found to be preventable. Two-thirds of the complications occurred in the antepartum period. Adverse fetal and neonatal events, as expected, were much more common in those pregnancies with cardiovascular events.

The **Cardiac Disease in Pregnancy Investigation (CARPREG I)** scoring system for risk from cardiac events for women with heart disease noted four major risk factors: (1) NYHA FC III or IV HF, (2) prior cardiac events, (3) mitral or aortic obstruction, and (4) LVEF < 40%. One point is assigned to each. Patients with no points had a 5% risk, those with 1 point had a complication rate of 27%, while for those with 2 or more points, the risk was 74%. Other reviews have suggested that the major risk for adverse outcomes or death to either the mother or fetus include pulmonary hypertension (with pulmonary pressure greater than three-quarters of systemic pressure), maternal cyanosis, systemic ventricular dysfunction, poor maternal functional class, severe left-sided valvular obstruction, aortic coarctation, significantly dilated aortic root, significant unrepaired heart defects, and warfarin therapy in patients with mechanical valves. In 2018, this group reported the results from a follow-up study (**CARPREG II**). Cardiac complications occurred in 16% of pregnancies and were primarily related to arrhythmias and HF. Although the overall rates of cardiac complications during pregnancy did not change over the years, the frequency of pulmonary edema decreased (8% from 1994 to 2001 vs. 4% from 2001 to 2014). Ten predictors of maternal cardiac complications were identified: five general predictors (prior cardiac events or arrhythmias, poor functional class or cyanosis, high-risk valve disease/LV outflow tract obstruction, systemic ventricular dysfunction, no prior cardiac interventions); four lesion-specific predictors (mechanical valves, high-risk aortopathies, pulmonary hypertension, CAD); and one delivery of care predictor (late pregnancy assessment). These 10 predictors were incorporated into a new risk index (CARPREG II) shown in Figure 10–8.

The WHO offers guidelines for the management of pregnancy in patients with congenital heart disease. This 2011 guideline also outlines risks to the fetus. Table 10–9 summarizes the observations and recommendations. *Medication usage during pregnancy is always a difficult decision since most have not been studied.* ACE inhibitors and amiodarone are contraindicated. β-Blockers (including labetalol, metoprolol, and sotalol), digoxin, and calcium channel blockers are generally well tolerated (especially nifedipine, amlodipine, or verapamil, although there is controversy with diltiazem). There are concerns about the use of atenolol and premature birth, and it should not be used. Labetalol has been found to be particularly useful for treating hypertension as has methyldopa (though this is rarely used). Diuretics can generally be given safely. Pregnancy is a hypercoagulable state; the use of warfarin is discussed above under valvular disease and congenital heart disease, but fundamentally the risk is dose related (not INR related) and warfarin can be used during the first trimester if the dose is 5 mg or less. For many patients, the most common potential complication is an atrial arrhythmia or systemic hypertension (systemic BP > 140/90 mm Hg). Patients should be hospitalized if BP exceeds 170/110 mm Hg.

Patients with adult congenital heart disease are at risk not only for cardiovascular events but also for obstetric events such as hypertension, preeclampsia, placenta previa or abruption, and early delivery.

CARDIOVASCULAR COMPLICATIONS OF PREGNANCY

Pregnancy-related hypertension (eclampsia and preeclampsia) is discussed in Chapter 22.

1. Cardiomyopathy of Pregnancy (Peripartum Cardiomyopathy)

In approximately 1 in 3000 to 4000 live births, dilated cardiomyopathy develops in the mother in the final

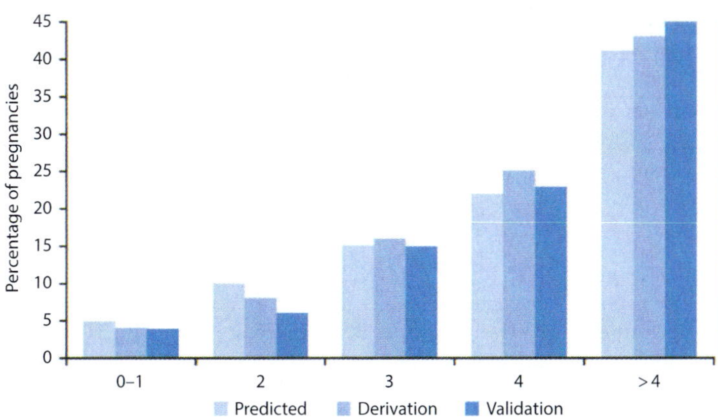

PREDICTOR	POINTS
Prior cardiac events or arrhythmias	3
Baseline NYHA III-IV or cyanosis	3
Mechanical valve	3
Ventricular dysfunction	2
High-risk left-sided valve disease/ left ventricular outflow tract obstruction	2
Pulmonary hypertension	2
Coronary artery disease	2
High-risk aortopathy	2
No prior cardiac intervention	1
Late pregnancy assessment	1

▲ **Figure 10–8.** Risk index for material cardiac complications in pregnancy (CARPREG II). The risk index is divided into five categories based on the sum of the points for a given pregnancy: 0 to 1 point; 2 points; 3 points; 4 points; and > 4 points. The predicted risks for primary cardiac events stratified according to point score were 0 to 1 point (5%), 2 points (10%), 3 points (15%), 4 points (22%), and > 4 points (41%). NYHA, New York Heart Association. (Reproduced with permission from Silversides CK, Grewal J, Mason J, et al. Pregnancy outcomes in women with heart disease: the CARPREG II Study. J Am Coll Cardiol. 2018;71(21):2419–2430.)

Table 10–9. Management strategies for women with valve disease, complex congenital heart disease, pulmonary hypertension, aortopathy, and dilated cardiomyopathy (in alphabetical order by disease).

High-Risk Heart Disease in Pregnancy
- Preconception counseling and pregnancy risk stratification for all women with high-risk heart disease of childbearing age
- In women considering pregnancy: Switch to safer cardiac medications and emphasize importance of close monitoring
- In women avoiding pregnancy: Discuss safe and effective contraception choices or termination in early pregnancy

	Management Strategy		
Disease	**Pregnancy Not Advised**	**Pregnancy Management**	**Delivery**
Aortopathy	***For some women*** • Marfan syndrome • Bicuspid aortic valve • Turner syndrome • Rapid growth of aortic diameter or family history of premature aortic dissection	• Treat hypertension • β-Blockers to reduce heart rate • Frequent echocardiographic assessment • Surgery during pregnancy or after C-section if large increase in aortic diameter	• C-section in cases of significant aortic dilation • Marfan syndrome: > 40 mm • Bicuspid aortic valve: > 45 mm • Turner syndrome: aortic size index > 20 mm/m^2
Complex congenital heart disease	• Significant ventricular dysfunction • Severe AV valve dysfunction • Falling Fontan circulation • Oxygen saturation < 85%	• Close follow-up	• Vaginal delivery preferred • C-section in case of fetal or maternal instability • Consider hemodynamic monitoring during labor and delivery
Dilated cardiomyopathy	• LVEF < 40% • History of peripartum cardiomyopathy	• Close follow-up • β-Blockers • Diuretic agents for volume overload • Vasodilators for hemodynamic and symptomatic improvement	• Vaginal delivery preferred • C-section in case of fetal or maternal instability • Consider hemodynamic monitoring during labor and delivery • Early delivery for clinical and hemodynamic deterioration
Pulmonary hypertension	• Established pulmonary arterial hypertension	• Close follow-up • Early institution of pulmonary vasodilators	• Vaginal delivery preferred • C-section in case of fetal or maternal instability • Timing of delivery depends on clinical and RV function • Early delivery advisable • Diuresis after delivery to prevent RV volume overload • Extended hospital stay after delivery
Valve disease	• Severe mitral and aortic valve disease • Mechanical prosthetic valves if effective anticoagulation not possible	• Close follow-up • Medication therapy for HF or arrhythmias • Balloon valvuloplasty or surgical valve replacement in refractory cases	• Vaginal delivery preferred • C-section in case of fetal or maternal instability • Early delivery for clinical and hemodynamic deterioration • Consider hemodynamic monitoring during labor and delivery

AV, atrioventricular; C-section, cesarean section.
Reproduced with permission from Elkayam U et al. High-risk cardiac disease in pregnancy: part I. J Am Coll Cardiol. 2016;68(4):396–410.

month of pregnancy or within 6 months after delivery. Risk factors include preeclampsia, twin pregnancies, and Black race (potentially via structural racism). The cause is slowly being elucidated. The vasculo-hormonal hypothesis requires two events. One is genetic, a reduction in a STAT3 transcription factor that results in cleavage of prolactin from the pituitary by cathepsin D. This results in a 16-kd fragment that increases microRNA 146a that results in myocardial apoptosis. The second is from the placenta, soluble tyrosine kinase that blocks VEGF (vascular endothelial growth factor). It appears both components may be necessary to effectively result in peripartum cardiomyopathy. The course of the disease is variable; most cases improve or resolve completely over several months, but others progress to refractory HF. About 60% of patients make a complete recovery. Serum BNP levels are routinely elevated in pregnancy, but serial values may be useful in predicting who may be at increased risk for a worse outcome. β-Blockers have been administered judiciously to these patients, with at least anecdotal success. Diuretics, hydralazine, and nitrates help treat the HF with minimal risk to the fetus. Sotalol is acceptable for ventricular or atrial arrhythmias if other β-blockers are ineffective. Some experts advocate anticoagulation because of an increased risk of thrombotic events, and both warfarin and heparin have their proponents. In severe cases, transient use of extracorporeal membrane oxygenation (ECMO) has been lifesaving. Recurrence in subsequent pregnancies is common, particularly if cardiac function has not completely recovered, and subsequent pregnancies are to be discouraged if the EF remains < 55%. The risk of recurrent HF in a subsequent pregnancy has been estimated to be 21%. Delivery of the baby is important, though the peak incidence of the problem is in the first week after delivery and a few cases appear up to 5 weeks after delivery. Since an anti-angiogenic cleaved prolactin fragment is considered causal for peripartum cardiomyopathy, bromocriptine (a prolactin release inhibitor) has been reported to be beneficial. A multicenter trial in Europe found LVEF improved to a greater extent in patients with peripartum cardiomyopathy who were given bromocriptine than those who were not given bromocriptine. In addition, bromocriptine treatment was associated with high rate of full LV recovery and low morbidity and mortality in peripartum cardiomyopathy patients compared with other peripartum cardiomyopathy cohorts not treated with bromocriptine.

2. Coronary Artery & Aortic Vascular Abnormalities During Pregnancy

ACS occurs in 2.8–8.1 per 1,000,000 pregnancies. Many are women over 35 years. It is known that pregnancy predisposes to dissection of the aorta and other arteries, perhaps because of the accompanying connective tissue changes. The risks are particularly high in patients with Marfan, Ehlers-Danlos, or Loeys-Dietz syndromes. The risk is highest in the third trimester, and coronary dissection, thrombosis, and atherosclerosis have about equal prevalence. The most frequent cause in one study was coronary dissection, and it has a peak incidence in the early postpartum period. Paradoxical emboli through a PFO to the coronary arteries have been implicated in a few instances. Clinical management is essentially similar to that of other patients with acute infarction, unless there is a connective tissue disorder. If nonatherosclerotic dissection is present, coronary intervention may be risky, as further dissection can be aggravated. In most instances, conservative management is warranted. At times, extensive aortic dissection requires surgical intervention. Marfan patients are particularly susceptible to further aortic expansion during pregnancy when the aortic diameter is > 4.5 cm ($\geq$ 27 mm/m^2), and pregnancy should be discouraged in these situations. Some data, however, suggest that there is an increased risk of dissection during pregnancy even when the elective repair is reasonable (ie, when the aortic root is > 4.0 cm in women with Marfan syndrome contemplating pregnancy). Acute infarction during pregnancy is associated with an 8% maternal mortality and 56% incidence of premature delivery. If PCI is required, it is recommended that a drug-eluting stent be placed. Medications that appear to be safe during pregnancy include aspirin, β-blockers, clopidogrel, heparin or enoxaparin, and nitrates. Medications that are not safe include aldosterone inhibitors, ACE inhibitors or ARBs, DOACs, and statins. If need be, fibrinolytics, GP IIb/IIIa inhibitors, bivalirudin, and calcium channel blockers can be used.

3. Management of Labor

Although vaginal delivery is usually well tolerated, unstable patients (including patients with severe hypertension and worsening HF) should have planned cesarean section. Spinal anesthesia results in a large drop in the systemic vascular resistance and can worsen right-to-left shunting. An increased risk of aortic rupture has been noted during delivery in patients with coarctation of the aorta and severe aortic root dilation with Marfan syndrome, and vaginal delivery should be avoided in these patients. For most patients, even those with complex congenital heart disease, vaginal delivery is the preferred method, however. Immediately following delivery, there are numerous fluid shifts that occur with the initial blood loss, reducing preload and accompanied by the loss of afterload reduction that had been provided by the placenta. Quickly, however, venous return increases as the uterus is no longer compressing the inferior vena cava and there is an infusion of fluid into the vascular system as the uterus quickly shrinks back toward its normal size. The sudden increase in preload and loss of afterload following delivery can result in HF during the first 48–72 hours after the delivery and that remains the high-risk time for susceptible patients.

CARDIOVASCULAR SCREENING OF ATHLETES

The sudden death of a competitive athlete inevitably becomes an occasion for local, if not national, publicity. On each occasion, the public and the medical community ask whether such events could be prevented by more careful or complete screening. Although each event is tragic, it must be appreciated that there are approximately 5 million competitive athletes at the high school level or above in any given year in the United States. The number of cardiac deaths occurring during athletic participation is unknown but estimates at the high school level range from one in 100,000 to one in 300,000 participants. Death rates among more mature athletes increase as the prevalence of CAD rises. These numbers highlight the problem of how best to screen individual participants. Even an inexpensive test such as an ECG would generate an enormous cost if required of all athletes, and it is likely that only a few individuals with high risk for sudden death would be detected. Echocardiography, either as a routine test or as a follow-up examination for abnormal ECGs, would be prohibitively expensive except for the elite professional athlete. Thus, *the most feasible approach is that of a careful medical history and cardiac examination performed by personnel aware of the conditions responsible for most sudden deaths in competitive athletes.*

It is important to point out that sudden death is much more common in the older than the younger athlete. Older athletes will generally seek advice regarding their fitness for participation. These individuals should recognize that strenuous exercise is associated with an increase in risk of sudden cardiac death and that appropriate training substantially reduces this risk. Preparticipation screening for risk of sudden death in the older athlete is a complex issue and at present is largely focused on identifying inducible ischemia due to significant coronary disease.

In a series of 158 athletic deaths in the United States between 1985 and 1995, *hypertrophic cardiomyopathy (36%) and coronary anomalies (19%) were by far the most frequent underlying conditions.* LVH was present in another 10%, ruptured aorta (presumably due to Marfan syndrome or cystic medial necrosis) in 6%, myocarditis or dilated cardiomyopathy in 6%, aortic stenosis in 4%, and arrhythmogenic RV dysplasia in 3%. In addition, commotio cordis, or sudden death due to direct myocardial injury, may occur. More common in children, ventricular tachycardia or ventricular fibrillation may occur even after a minor direct blow to the heart; it is thought to be due to the precipitation of a PVC just prior to the peak of the T wave on ECG.

A careful family and medical history and cardiovascular examination will identify most individuals at risk. An update in 2014 recommends that *all middle school and higher athletes undergo a medical screen questionnaire and examination.* The 12 elements in the examination are outlined in Table 10–10.

Table 10–10. 12-element AHA recommendations for preparticipation cardiovascular screening of competitive athletes.

Medical History
Personal History
1. Exertional chest pain/discomfort
2. Unexplained syncope/near-syncope
3. Excessive exertional and unexplained dyspnea/fatigue
4. Prior recognition of a heart murmur
5. Elevated systemic blood pressure
Family History
6. Premature death (sudden and unexpected, or otherwise) before age of 50 years due to heart disease in one or more relatives
7. Disability from heart disease in a close relative before age of 50 years
8. Specific knowledge of certain cardiac conditions in family members: hypertrophic cardiomyopathy, dilated cardiomyopathy, long QT syndrome or other ion channelopathies, Marfan syndrome, or other important arrhythmias
Physical Examination
9. Heart murmur
10. Diminished femoral pulse (to exclude coarctation)
11. Phenotype of Marfan syndrome
12. Brachial artery blood pressure (sitting position)

AHA, American Heart Association.

Reproduced with permission from Lawless CE, Asplund C, Asif IM, et al. Protecting the heart of the American athlete: proceedings of the American College of Cardiology Sports and Exercise Cardiology Think Tank October 18, 2012, Washington, DC. J Am Coll Cardiol. 2014;64(20):2146–2171.

A family history of premature sudden death or CVD, or of any of these predisposing conditions should mandate further workup, including an ECG and echocardiogram. Symptoms of unexplained fatigue or dyspnea, exertional chest pain, syncope, or near syncope also warrant further evaluation. A Marfan-like appearance, significant elevation of BP, abnormalities of heart rate or rhythm, and pathologic heart murmurs or heart sounds should also be investigated before clearance for athletic participation is given. Such an evaluation is recommended before participation at the high school and college levels and every 2 years during athletic competition.

Stress-induced syncope or chest pressure may be the first clue to an anomalous origin of a coronary artery. Anatomically, this lesion occurs most often when the left anterior descending artery or left main coronary arises from the right coronary cusp and traverses between the aorta and pulmonary trunks. The "slit-like" orifice that results from the angulation at the vessel origin is thought to cause ischemia when the aorta and pulmonary arteries enlarge during vigorous exercise and tension is placed on the coronary.

The toughest distinction may be in sorting out the healthy athlete with LVH from the athlete with hypertrophic cardiomyopathy. In general, the healthy athlete's heart is *less* likely to have an unusual pattern of LVH (such as asymmetric septal hypertrophy), or to have LA enlargement, an abnormal ECG, an LV cavity < 45 mm in diameter at end-diastole, an abnormal diastolic filling pattern, or a family history of hypertrophic cardiomyopathy. The athlete is more likely to be male than the individual with hypertrophic cardiomyopathy, where women are equally at risk. Cardiac MRI is emerging as a useful means to separate the athlete's heart from hypertrophic obstructive cardiomyopathy. Increased risk is also evident in patients with the WPW syndrome, a prolonged QTc interval, or those who demonstrate the abnormal ST changes in leads V_1 and V_2 consistent with the Brugada syndrome.

Selective use of routine ECG and stress testing is recommended in men above age 40 years and women above age 50 years who continue to participate in vigorous exercise and at earlier ages when there is a positive family history for premature CAD, hypertrophic cardiomyopathy, or multiple risk factors. Because at least some of the risk features (long QT, LVH, Brugada syndrome, WPW syndrome) may be evident on routine ECG screening, several cost-effectiveness studies have been done. Most suggest that preparticipation ECGs are of potential value, though what to do when the QTc is mildly increased is unclear. Many experts feel the high incidence of false-positive ECG studies makes it very ineffective as a screening tool. With the low prevalence of cardiac anomalies in the general public, it has been estimated that 200,000 individual athletes would need to be screened to identify the single individual who would die suddenly. A report from Canada reviewing 74 sudden cardiac arrests during sports activity noted that the vast majority occurred during noncompetitive sports.

The issue of routine screening, therefore, remains controversial. A report from the United Kingdom in 2018, screening adolescent soccer players from 1996 to 2016 (that included ECG and echocardiography), identified diseases associated with sudden death in only 0.38% of the 11,168 athletes screened for a total of 118,351 person-years. The incidence of sudden death was about 7 per 100,000 athletes and most were related to cardiomyopathies that had not been detected on the screening procedures.

In 2017, a position paper from a number of European societies presented arguments regarding the use of a number of preparticipation screening options. The manuscript also provided input from a number of international sports organizations. They concluded that there were data to support obtaining the clinical history, performing a physical examination, and performing a 12-lead ECG on all participants. They did *not* recommend echocardiography as a screening tool.

In 2017, a consensus statement from the American Medical Society for Sports Medicine was published summarizing the recommendations for the appropriate screening options in the various clinical scenarios. Once an individual with high risk has been identified, guidelines from the Bethesda conference and the ESC can be used to help determine whether the athlete may continue to participate in sporting events. Table 10–11 summarizes these recommendations.

Screening for return to play after myocardial/pericardial involvement with COVID-19 is an important issue (see Infectious Myocarditis in Chapter 11). An expert consensus statement from the ACC suggests the following:

1. In the athlete who has had COVID-19, the ECG and high-sensitivity troponin should be normal. If any clinical concerns remain, then a transthoracic echocardiogram should be obtained.
2. Point-of-care echocardiography is not recommended, as the most common echocardiogram abnormalities may be missed by point-of-care echocardiography. These include RV dysfunction, diastolic LV abnormalities, and early signs of LV dysfunction (including abnormal global longitudinal strain). These are "red flags."

Table 10–11. Recommendations for competitive sports participation among athletes with potential causes of SCD.

Condition	36th Bethesda Conference	European Society of Cardiology
Structural Cardiac Abnormalities		
HCM	Exclude athletes with a probable or definitive clinical diagnosis from all competitive sports. Genotype-positive/phenotype-negative athletes may still compete.	Exclude athletes with a probable or definitive clinical diagnosis from all competitive sports. Exclude genotype-positive/phenotype-negative individuals from competitive sports.
ARVC	Exclude athletes with a probable or definitive diagnosis from competitive sports.	Exclude athletes with a probable or definitive diagnosis from competitive sports.
CCAA	Exclude from competitive sports.	Not applicable.
	Participation in all sports 3 months after successful surgery would be permitted for an athlete with ischemia, ventricular arrhythmia or tachyarrhythmia, or LV dysfunction during maximal exercise testing.	
Electrical Cardiac Abnormalities		
WPW	Athletes without structural heart disease, without a history of palpitations, or without tachycardia can participate in all competitive sports. In athletes with symptoms, electrophysiological study and ablation are recommended. Return to competitive sports is allowed after corrective ablation, provided that the ECG has normalized.	Athletes without structural heart disease, without a history of palpitations, or without tachycardia can participate in all competitive sports. In athletes with symptoms, electrophysiological study and ablation are recommended. Return to competitive sports is allowed after corrective ablation, provided that the ECG has normalized.
LQTS	Exclude any athlete with a previous cardiac arrest or syncopal episode from competitive sports. Asymptomatic patients restricted to competitive low-intensity sports. Genotype-positive/phenotype-negative athletes may still compete.	Exclude any athlete with a clinical or genotype diagnosis from competitive sports.
BrS	Exclude from all competitive sports except those of low intensity.	Exclude from all competitive sports.
CPVT	Exclude all patients with a clinical diagnosis from competitive sports. Genotype-positive/phenotype-negative patients may still compete in low-intensity sports.	Exclude all patients with a clinical diagnosis from competitive sports. Genotype-positive/phenotype-negative patients are also excluded.

(*continued*)

Table 10–11. Recommendations for competitive sports participation among athletes with potential causes of SCD. (continued)

Condition	36th Bethesda Conference	European Society of Cardiology
Acquired Cardiac Abnormalities		
Commotio cordis	Eligibility for returning to competitive sport in survivors is a matter of individual clinical judgment. Survivors must undergo a thorough cardiovascular workup including 12-lead ECG, ambulatory ECG monitoring, and echocardiography.	Not applicable.
Myocarditis	Exclude from all competitive sports. Convalescent period of 6 months. Athletes may return to competition when test results normalize.	Exclude from all competitive sports. Convalescent period of 6 months. Athletes may return to competition when test results normalize.

ARVC, arrhythmogenic RV cardiomyopathy; BrS, Brugada syndrome; CCAA, congenital coronary artery anomalies; CPVT, catecholaminergic polymorphic ventricular tachycardia; HCM, hypertrophic cardiomyopathy; LQTS, long QT syndrome; SCD, sudden cardiac death; WPW, Wolff-Parkinson-White syndrome.

Reproduced with permission from Chandra N et al. Sudden cardiac death in young athletes: practical challenges and diagnostic dilemmas. J Am Coll Cardiol. 2013;61(10):1027–1040.

3. If any "red flags" from echocardiogram are present, then cardiac MRI should be obtained. MRI provides better assessment of RV function and abnormalities of myocardial edema (T2 imaging), intracellular and extracellular signaling (T1 imaging), and late gadolinium enhancement. The long-term significance of these findings is unknown.
4. Other imaging modalities can include coronary CT, chest CTA (looking for PE, given the hypercoagulable state COVID-19 creates), and rarely PET imaging.
5. Cardiopulmonary exercise testing is to be avoided during the acute phase but is valuable at 3–6 months after the illness if symptoms persist and as part of return to play guidelines.

Heart Failure & Cardiomyopathy

11

Christopher B. Granger, MD
Robert T. Short III, MD

HEART FAILURE

ESSENTIALS OF DIAGNOSIS

- LV failure: Often due to either systolic or diastolic dysfunction. Predominant symptoms are those of low cardiac output and congestion, including dyspnea.
- RV failure: Symptoms of fluid overload predominate; usually RV failure is due to LV failure.
- Echocardiographic assessment of LV, RV, and valvular function is a crucial part of diagnosis and management.
- Optimal management of chronic HF includes combination medical therapies, such as sacubitril-valsartan, mineralocorticoid receptor antagonists, β-blockers, and SGLT-2 inhibitors.

General Considerations

HF is a common disease that is increasing in incidence and prevalence. Approximately 7.7 million patients in the United States have HF, with ≥ 8 million patients projected to have HF by 2030. In 2022, in the United States, 1,215,174 patients were discharged from the hospital with a principal diagnosis of HF. Around 1 in 4 US adults will develop HF in their lifetime (24%). *It is primarily a disease of aging*, with > 75% of existing and new cases occurring in individuals > 65 years of age.

Classification

There are multiple ways to classify HF subtypes: laterality (ie, LV failure, RV failure, or both), ejection fraction, underlying etiology, myocardial morphology, American College of Cardiology/American Heart Association (ACC/AHA) stage, and New York Heart Association (NYHA) class.

A. Laterality

HF may be right-sided, left-sided, or both. Patients with **left HF** may have symptoms of low cardiac output and elevated pulmonary venous pressure; dyspnea is the predominant feature. **Right HF** manifests with signs of peripheral fluid retention. Most patients exhibit symptoms or signs of both right- and left-sided failure. LV dysfunction is the primary cause of RV failure.

B. Ejection Fraction

Patients with HF who have an LVEF ≤ 40% are given the diagnosis of HF with reduced EF (HFrEF), whereas those with EF ≥ 50% are deemed to have "preserved" EF (HFpEF). The term *HF with mildly reduced EF* (HFmrEF) is reserved for patients with an EF of 41–49%. Approximately half of patients with HF have HFrEF, whereas the other half have HFpEF, usually with some degree of **diastolic dysfunction**. *It is important to note that not all patients with signs and symptoms of HF and an EF > 50% are given the diagnosis of HFpEF. Rather, HFpEF is increasingly recognized as a distinct clinical entity.* According to expert consensus, conditions such as valvular HF, hypertrophic cardiomyopathy (HCM), restrictive cardiomyopathy, dilated cardiomyopathy, and high-output HF must be excluded in patients with HF and EF ≥ 50% before giving them the specific diagnosis of HFpEF. Instead, the terminology *HF due to valvular disease* or *HF due to restrictive cardiomyopathy* is preferred. Clinically, patients with HF—regardless of EF—may present with similar signs and symptoms.

C. Underlying Etiology

In developed countries, CAD leading to MI and loss of functioning myocardium (**ischemic cardiomyopathy**) is the most common cause of HFrEF. Hypertension also is a leading cause of HF and, even more commonly in the United States, an exacerbating factor in patients with cardiac dysfunction due to other causes, such as CAD. Cardiomyopathy may also arise from infiltrative diseases (eg, hemochromatosis, sarcoidosis, amyloidosis), infectious diseases (eg, viral myocarditis), metabolic disorders, cardiotoxins, and medication toxicity (eg, doxorubicin). **Valvular heart diseases**—particularly degenerative aortic stenosis and chronic aortic or mitral regurgitation—are not infrequent causes of HF. **Tachycardia-induced cardiomyopathies**, which arise from chronic, sustained arrhythmias (eg, uncontrolled AF), may also cause myocardial remodeling and LV systolic dysfunction. Diastolic cardiac dysfunction is associated with aging and related myocardial stiffening, as well as LVH, commonly resulting from hypertension.

D. Ventricular Morphology

Several processes may present with **dilated cardiomyopathy**, which is characterized by LV or biventricular dilation and generalized systolic dysfunction (LVEF < 50%). These are discussed elsewhere in this chapter, but the most common are alcohol-associated cardiomyopathy, viral myocarditis (including infections by HIV; see also the COVID-19 section in Chapter 36), and dilated cardiomyopathies with no obvious underlying cause (**idiopathic cardiomyopathy**). Conditions such as **hypertrophic** or **restrictive cardiomyopathy**, diabetes, and pericardial disease can produce similar clinical pictures.

E. ACC/AHA Staging

HF progression is often preventable through early detection and intervention. The importance of these approaches is emphasized by US guidelines that have incorporated a classification of HF that includes four stages. **Stage A** includes patients at risk for developing HF (such as patients with hypertension). In the majority of these patients, development of HF can be prevented with interventions such as aggressive treatment of hypertension, modification of coronary risk factors, and reduction of excessive alcohol intake. **Stage B** includes patients who have structural heart disease, increased filling pressures, risk factors, and elevated biomarkers, but no current or previously recognized symptoms of HF. Examples include patients with previous MI, other causes of reduced systolic function, LVH, or asymptomatic valvular disease. Both ACE inhibitors and β-blockers have been shown to decrease the risk of HF in the first two of these conditions, and more aggressive treatment of hypertension and early surgical intervention are effective in the latter two. **Stages C** and **D** include patients with clinical HF (current or previous) and the relatively small group of patients who have become refractory to the usual therapies, respectively.

F. NYHA Class

Finally, patients with HF are often categorized by their symptom severity, using the NYHA classification system: **class I** (asymptomatic), **class II** (symptomatic with mild activity), **class III** (symptomatic with moderate activity), or **class IV** (symptomatic at rest). This classification is important, as some treatments are indicated based on NYHA classification.

In summary, there are multiple ways to describe a particular patient's type of HF, and these are often used together to provide as much detail and specificity as possible when considering patient care.

▶ Clinical Findings

A. Symptoms

*The most common symptom of patients with **left HF** is shortness of breath. Exertional dyspnea often arises first, and then orthopnea, paroxysmal nocturnal dyspnea, and dyspnea at rest develop.* Nocturia due to excretion of fluid retained during the day and increased renal perfusion in the recumbent position is a common nonspecific symptom of HF, as are fatigue and exercise intolerance. *These symptoms correlate poorly with the degree of cardiac dysfunction. Patients with **right HF** have predominant signs of fluid retention, such as lower extremity swelling, abdominal fullness, and, on occasion, loss of appetite and nausea due to edema of the gut or impaired GI perfusion and ascites.*

Patients with HF may present with acute, chronic, or acute-on-chronic symptoms. Conditions such as acute MI or myocarditis may cause acute HF in a previously healthy patient. In contrast, patients with chronic, compensated HF may present with acute exacerbations. Exacerbations may be caused by alterations in therapy (or medication nonadherence), excessive salt or fluid intake, arrhythmias, infections, pulmonary embolism, or progression of the underlying disease.

B. Signs

Many patients with HF appear comfortable at rest. Others will become dyspneic with conversation or minor activity. Some patients with long-standing severe HF may appear cachectic. Vital signs may be normal, but tachycardia, hypotension, tachypnea, and narrow pulse pressure may be present. Important signs of HF can be detected by examination of the neck, the lungs, the abdomen, and the extremities.

1. Neck—*RA pressure may be estimated through the height of the pulsations in the jugular venous system.* With the patient at 45 degrees, measure the height of the pulsation about the sternal angle, and add 5 cm to estimate the height above the left atrium, with a pressure > 8 cm being abnormal. In addition to the height of the venous pressure, abnormal pulsations, such as regurgitant *v* waves, should be sought. Examination of the carotid pulse may allow estimation of pulse pressure as well as detection of aortic stenosis. Thyroid examination may reveal occult hyperthyroidism or hypothyroidism, which are readily treatable causes of HF.

2. Lungs—Crackles at the lung bases reflect transudation of fluid into the alveoli. Pleural effusions may cause bibasilar dullness to percussion. Expiratory wheezing and rhonchi also may be signs of HF.

3. Abdomen—Patients with severe right HF may have hepatic enlargement—tender or nontender—due to passive congestion. Sustained moderate pressure on the liver may increase jugular venous pressure (JVP) (a positive **hepatojugular reflux** is an increase of > 1 cm, which correlates with elevated pulmonary capillary wedge pressure [PCWP]). Ascites may also be present.

4. Extremities—Peripheral pitting edema is a common sign in patients with right HF and may extend into the hips (or sacrum in bed-bound or hospitalized patients) and abdominal wall. During times of HF decompensation, the extremities may feel cold due to peripheral vasoconstriction (activation of the renin-angiotensin-aldosterone system [RAAS]).

Cardinal cardiac examination signs are a parasternal lift, indicating pulmonary hypertension; an enlarged and sustained LV impulse, indicating LV dilation and hypertrophy; a diminished first heart sound, suggesting impaired contractility; and an S_3 gallop originating in the LV and sometimes the RV. An S_4 may be present in chronic hypertension causing HFpEF. Murmurs should be sought to exclude primary valvular disease; secondary mitral regurgitation and tricuspid regurgitation murmurs are common in patients with dilated ventricles.

C. Laboratory Findings

When a new diagnosis of HFrEF or HFpEF is suspected, clinicians should pursue additional workup to identify the underlying etiology. Careful history and physical should guide workup. *The ACC recommends standard laboratory testing including CBC, serum electrolytes and renal function, lipid panel, liver function tests, iron studies, and TSH. In addition, diagnostic workup for HFpEF should include targeted evaluation to exclude HFpEF "mimics" such as infiltrative/restrictive cardiomyopathies, HCM, and valvular disease.*

A blood count may reveal anemia and a high red-cell distribution width (RDW), both of which are associated with poor prognosis in chronic HF through poorly understood mechanisms. Renal function tests can reflect kidney impairment via poor arterial flow, venous congestion, or both. CKD is another poor prognostic factor in HF and may limit certain treatment options. Serum electrolytes analysis may show derangements in potassium (which increase risk of arrhythmias and may affect ability to use RAAS-inhibiting drugs) and hyponatremia (an indicator of marked RAAS activation and a poor prognostic sign). Thyroid function should be assessed to rule out occult thyrotoxicosis or myxedema. Iron studies should be checked to test for hemochromatosis. In the correct context, serum protein electrophoresis and advanced imaging (eg, cardiac MRI) may lead to a diagnosis of amyloidosis. When the diagnosis of a particular cardiomyopathy remains unclear despite imaging and serologic testing, endomyocardial biopsy may be helpful.

B-type natriuretic peptide is a powerful prognostic hormone in HF. Two serum tests—**BNP** and **NT-proBNP**—provide similar diagnostic and prognostic information. BNP is secreted primarily from the ventricles and is elevated when ventricular filling pressures are high. Serum BNP and NT-proBNP are quite sensitive for acute decompensated HF (sensitivity 90%, specificity 76%). However, compensated patients may have only slightly elevated or normal BNP or NT-proBNP levels. BNP and NT-proBNP are more sensitive in HFrEF compared with HFpEF. Sensitivity of BNP for HF is lower among individuals with obesity.

Studies have shown that BNP can aid in emergency department triage in the diagnosis of acute decompensated HF, such that an *NT-proBNP < 300 pg/mL or BNP < 100 pg/mL, combined with a normal ECG, makes HF unlikely.* BNP may be helpful in guiding the intensity of diuretic and a more consistent use of disease-modifying therapies, such as ACE inhibitors and β-blockers, for the management of chronic HF. BNP, but not NT-proBNP, is increased by neprilysin inhibitors, as neprilysin degrades BNP. Thus, while NT-proBNP is still reliable, BNP should *not* be used to monitor degree of HF when patients are treated with sacubitril/valsartan. Worsening shortness of breath or weight gain in the setting of a rising BNP (or both) might prompt increasing the dose of diuretics. However, *there is no proven value in using serial natriuretic peptide measurements to guide therapy*, as shown in the GUIDE-IT trial. Elevation of serum troponin, and especially of high-sensitivity troponin, is common in both chronic and acute HF, and it is associated with higher risk of adverse outcomes.

D. ECG and Chest Radiography

ECG may indicate an underlying or secondary arrhythmia, MI, or nonspecific changes that often include low voltage, intraventricular conduction defects, LVH, and nonspecific repolarization changes. CXRs provide information about the size and shape of the cardiac silhouette. Cardiomegaly is an important finding and is a poor prognostic sign. Evidence of pulmonary venous hypertension includes relative dilation of the upper lobe veins, perivascular edema (haziness of vessel outlines), interstitial edema, and alveolar fluid. In acute HF, these findings correlate moderately well with pulmonary venous pressure. However, patients with chronic HF may have relatively normal pulmonary vasculature despite markedly elevated pressures. Pleural effusions are common and tend to be bilateral or right-sided.

E. Echocardiography & Other Imaging

The most useful imaging test in HF is the ***transthoracic echocardiogram (TTE)****.* Echocardiography can define the size and function of both ventricles and atria and LVEF. LVEF is the most commonly used measurement to define systolic function, with a cut point of ≤ 40% used to characterize reduced EF. On a practical level, it is important that note that EF measurement is often not precise and thus many patients may be on the border of reduced EF, which may explain why patients with "mildly reduced" EF (ie, 41–49%) may derive benefit from treatments like sacubitril-valsartan. RV function is assessed by contractility and other measures, such as tricuspid annular plane systolic excursion. Additionally, echocardiography will also allow detection of pericardial disease, valvular abnormalities, intracardiac shunts, wall motion abnormalities, and myocardial deformities, all of which are considered when attempting to determine the etiology for a patient's HF.

Radionuclide angiography as well as cardiac MRI also measure LVEF and permit analysis of regional wall motion. These tests are especially useful when echocardiography is technically suboptimal, such as in patients with severe pulmonary disease and when contrast echocardiography is not available. MRI can further assess for presence of scar tissue and of infiltrative disease. When myocardial ischemia is suspected as a cause of LV dysfunction, as it should be unless there is another clear cause, stress testing, CT angiography or coronary angiography should be performed.

F. Cardiac Catheterization

In most patients with HF, clinical examination and noninvasive tests can determine LV size and function and valve function to support and refine the diagnosis. Invasive coronary angiography may be helpful to define the presence and extent of CAD, although CT angiography may also be appropriate. Evaluation for coronary disease is particularly important when LV dysfunction may be partially reversible by revascularization. The combination of angina or noninvasive evidence of significant myocardial ischemia with symptomatic HF is often an indication for coronary angiography if the patient is a potential candidate for revascularization. Right heart catheterization may be useful to select and monitor therapy among patients whose symptoms are refractory to standard therapy.

Treatment: Heart Failure with Reduced LVEF

The treatment of HF is aimed at relieving symptoms, improving functional status, and preventing hospitalizations and death. *The evidence of clinical benefit, including reducing death and hospitalization, as well as reducing sudden cardiac death, of most therapies is limited to patients with HF with reduced LVEF (≤ 40%).* ***Using angiotensin receptor–neprilysin inhibitors (ARNIs), β-blockers, mineralocorticoid receptor antagonists (MRAs), and SGLT-2 inhibitors in combination for HFrEF is estimated to reduce mortality by > 70%. Thus, this goal is as important as any in all of cardiology.*** It is now recognized that patients with mildly reduced EF (41–49%) may derive benefit from an MRA and ARNI (sacubitril/valsartan).

A. Correction of Reversible Causes

The major reversible causes of HFrEF, previously called *systolic HF*, include myocardial ischemia, uncontrolled hypertension, valvular disease, arrhythmias, alcohol- or drug-induced cardiomyopathy, hypothyroidism, intracardiac shunts, and high-output states. Calcium channel blockers with negative inotropy (specifically verapamil or diltiazem), antiarrhythmic medications, thiazolidinediones, and NSAIDs may be important contributors to worsening HF. Some metabolic and infiltrative cardiomyopathies may be partially reversible, or their progression may be slowed; these include hemochromatosis, sarcoidosis, and amyloidosis. Once possible reversible components are being addressed, the measures outlined below are appropriate.

B. Pharmacologic Treatment

See also the following section Acute Heart Failure & Pulmonary Edema.

While the all of following classes of medications may be useful in managing patients with HF, a 2025 meta-analysis showed that "quadruple therapy" (ARNI, β-blocker, MRA, and SGLT-2 inhibitor) provides the greatest mortality reduction in HFrEF. Therefore, *every effort should be made to ensure that patients with HFrEF receive maximally tolerated doses of these four medications, barring contraindications.* Renal insufficiency, hypotension, and medication cost are common reasons for lack of quadruple therapy for HFrEF patients.

1. Diuretic therapy—Diuretics are the most effective means of providing symptomatic relief to patients with moderate to severe HF with dyspnea and fluid overload. However, diuretics have *not* been shown to reduce mortality in HF, and excessive diuresis can lead to electrolyte imbalances and neurohormonal activation. *While a diuretic may be helpful in rapid relief of symptoms of volume overload, initiation of an SGLT-2 inhibitor and MRA (eg, eplerenone) also will reduce volume overload and, simultaneously, will improve major clinical outcomes for patients with HF and reduced LVEF.*

When fluid retention is mild, **thiazide diuretics** or a similar agent (hydrochlorothiazide, 25–100 mg; metolazone, 2.5–5 mg; chlorthalidone, 25–50 mg; etc) may be sufficient. Thiazides often provide better control of hypertension than short-acting loop agents. The thiazides are generally *ineffective* when the GFR falls below 30–40 mL/min/1.73 m^2—not an infrequent occurrence in patients with severe HF. *Metolazone maintains its efficacy down to a GFR of approximately 20–30 mL/min/1.73 m^2.* Adverse reactions include hypokalemia and intravascular volume depletion with resulting prerenal azotemia, as well as rashes, neutropenia, thrombocytopenia, hyperglycemia, hyperuricemia, and hepatic dysfunction.

Patients with more severe HF should be treated with one of the oral **loop diuretics.** These include furosemide (20–320 mg daily), bumetanide (1–8 mg daily), and torsemide (20–200 mg daily). These agents have a rapid onset and a relatively short duration of action. In patients with preserved kidney function, two or more daily doses are preferable to a single larger dose. In acute situations or when GI absorption is in doubt, they should be given intravenously. Higher doses may be required with severe renal impairment. The major adverse reactions include intravascular volume depletion, prerenal azotemia, and hypotension. Hypokalemia, particularly with accompanying digitalis therapy, is a major problem. Less common side effects include skin rashes, GI distress, and ototoxicity (the latter more common with ethacrynic acid and possibly less common with bumetanide).

The **potassium-sparing diuretics** (MRAs and epithelial sodium channel blockers) are often useful in combination with the loop diuretics and thiazides, with the superior choice being the MRAs spironolactone (12.5–100 mg daily) or eplerenone (25–100 mg daily), which also reduce mortality in HF. These medications spare loss of potassium and offer a modest diuretic effect (especially at higher doses). Their onsets of action are slower than the other potassium-sparing agents, and spironolactone's side effects include gynecomastia and hyperkalemia. Combinations of potassium supplements or ACE inhibitors/ARBs and potassium-sparing medications can increase the risk of hyperkalemia but have been used with success in patients with persistent hypokalemia. SGLT-2 inhibitors will modestly decrease potassium and thus may help in managing high potassium from inhibitors of the RAAS.

Patients with refractory edema may require a combination of a loop diuretic and thiazide-like agents. Metolazone, because of its maintained activity with CKD, is the most useful agent for such a combination. Extreme caution must be observed with this approach, as massive diuresis and electrolyte imbalances often occur; 2.5 mg of metolazone can be administered orally prior to the dosage of loop diuretic. In many cases this is necessary only once or twice a week, but dosages up to 10 mg daily have been used in some patients.

2. Inhibitors of the renin–angiotensin–aldosterone system—Inhibition of the RAAS with ACE inhibitors or ARBs should be part of the initial therapy of this syndrome based on their mortality benefits.

A. ACE INHIBITORS—At least seven ACE inhibitors have been shown to be effective for the treatment of HF or the related indication of postinfarction LV dysfunction (see Table 13–6). ACE inhibitors reduce mortality by approximately 20% in patients with symptomatic HF and have also been shown to prevent hospitalizations, increase exercise tolerance, and reduce symptoms in these patients. As a result, *ACE inhibitors are among first-line treatments of patients with symptomatic LV systolic dysfunction (EF < 40%), usually in combination with a diuretic. They are also indicated for the management of patients with reduced EFs without symptoms because they prevent the progression to clinical HF.*

Because ACE inhibitors may induce significant hypotension, particularly following the initial doses, they must be *started with caution.* Hypotension is most prominent in patients with pre-existing low-normal blood pressure (systolic pressure < 100 mm Hg), hypovolemia, prerenal azotemia (especially if it is diuretic-induced), and hyponatremia (an indicator of activation of the RAAS). These patients should generally be started at low dosages (eg, captopril 6.25 mg orally three times daily or enalapril 2.5 mg orally daily); however, other patients may be started at twice these dosages. Within several days (for those with the markers of higher risk), patients should be questioned about symptoms of hypotension, and both kidney function and potassium levels should be monitored.

ACE inhibitors should be titrated to the dosages proved effective in clinical trials (captopril 50 mg three times daily, enalapril 10 mg twice daily, ramipril 10 mg daily, lisinopril 20 mg daily, or the equivalent) over a period of 1–3 months. Most patients will tolerate these doses. *Asymptomatic hypotension is not a contraindication to up-titrating or continuing ACE inhibitors.* Some patients exhibit increases in serum creatinine or potassium, but they do *not* require discontinuation if the levels stabilize—even at values as high as 3 mg/dL and 5.5 mEq/L, respectively. Kidney dysfunction is more frequent in patients with diabetes, older patients, and those with low systolic pressures, and these groups should be monitored more closely. The most common side effects of ACE inhibitors in patients with HF are dizziness (often not related to the level of blood pressure) and cough, though the latter is more often due to HF or intercurrent pulmonary conditions. ACE inhibitor–induced cough is more common in women than in men.

B. ANGIOTENSIN II RECEPTOR BLOCKERS—Another approach to inhibiting the RAAS is the use of specific ARBs (see Table 13–6), which will decrease adverse effects of angiotensin II by blocking the AT_1 receptor.

However, these agents do *not* share the effects of ACE inhibitors on other potentially important pathways that produce increases in bradykinin, prostaglandins, and nitric oxide in the heart, blood vessels, and other tissues. ARBs, specifically candesartan or valsartan (but not losartan, which lacks evidence of benefit), provide important benefits as an alternative to ACE inhibitors in chronic HF with reduced LVEF. (A large trial of patients with chronic HF and preserved LVEF found no benefit from the ARB irbesartan.) While they have the same level of recommendation in the guidelines, *generally ACE inhibitors are preferred over ARBs for patients who tolerate them, although starting an ARB will avoid the need for a washout period when transitioning to sacubitril/valsartan.*

C. MINERALOCORTICOID RECEPTOR ANTAGONISTS—*Inhibiting aldosterone has become a mainstay of management of symptomatic HF with reduced LVEF, and it may also improve outcomes for patients with preserved EF.* The RALES trial compared spironolactone 25 mg daily with placebo in patients with advanced HF (current or recent class IV) already receiving ACE inhibitors and diuretics, and showed a 29% reduction in mortality, as well as similar decreases in other clinical endpoints. Based on the EMPHASIS-HF trial, the efficacy and safety of aldosterone antagonism—in the form of eplerenone, 25–50 mg orally daily—is established for patients with mild or moderate HF. Hyperkalemia was uncommon in severe HF clinical trial patients who received high doses of diuretic as maintenance therapy; however, hyperkalemia in patients taking spironolactone appears to be common in general practice. Potassium levels must be monitored closely during initiation of spironolactone (after 1 and 4 weeks of therapy) and periodically thereafter, particularly for patients with even mild degrees of kidney injury, and in patients receiving ACE inhibitors or ARBs.

Finally, the 2024 FINEARTS-HF trial showed that finerenone significantly reduces the risk of HF hospitalizations and death among patients with HFmrEF and HFpEF.

D. COMBINATION SACUBITRIL AND VALSARTAN—The combination of valsartan and sacubitril is called an **ARNI.** Compared with the ACE inhibitor enalapril, the ARNI was shown to further reduce cardiovascular death and hospitalization by 20% for patients with HF and reduced LVEF in a large randomized trial (PARADIGM-HF) of patients who had been taking an ACE inhibitor or ARB. Cardiovascular death itself was also reduced by 20%. This evidence led to a class I recommendation by the ACC/AHA and the European Society of Cardiology (ESC) guidelines for the use of *sacubitril/valsartan as a replacement for ACE inhibitors for patients with HF with reduced EF who remain symptomatic on an ACE inhibitor, β-blocker, and mineralocorticoid inhibitor.* Patients with baseline systolic blood pressure < 100 mm Hg were not included in the PARADIGM trial, and symptomatic hypotension is more common with sacubitril/valsartan than ACE inhibitor. Sacubitril/valsartan can be safely started in the hospital for patients admitted with decompensated failure, once they are stable with systolic blood pressure of at least 100 mm Hg and there has been a *36-hour washout period since the last dose of ACE inhibitor.*

While there was some evidence of benefit, sacubitril/valsartan did not result in significant improvement in the primary outcome of total HF hospitalizations and cardiovascular death in the PARAGON-HF trial studying a population of patients with HF and preserved LVEF (≥ 45%). However, the US Food and Drug Administration (FDA) has approved sacubitril/valsartan in this population, particularly for patients with EF "below normal" (HFmrEF: EF 41–49%).

3. β-Blockers—β-Blockers are a cornerstone in chronic HF management due to their life-saving benefits. The mechanism of this benefit remains unclear, but it is likely that chronic elevations of catecholamines and sympathetic nervous system activity cause progressive myocardial remodeling/damage, leading to worsening LV function and dilation. The primary evidence for this hypothesis is that over a period of 3–6 months, β-blockers produce consistent and substantial improvements in EF (averaging 10% absolute increase) and reductions in LV size and mass.

Three medications have strong evidence of reducing mortality: carvedilol (a nonselective β_1- and β_2-receptor blocker), metoprolol succinate (the β_1-selective extended-release agent), and bisoprolol (β_1-selective agent).

There is a strong recommendation that *stable patients (defined as having no recent deterioration or improving decompensation) with mild, moderate, and even severe HF should be treated with a β-blocker unless there is a noncardiac contraindication.* In the COPERNICUS trial, carvedilol was both well tolerated and highly effective in reducing mortality and HF hospitalizations in a group of patients with severe (NYHA class III or IV) symptoms, but care was taken to ensure that they were euvolemic at the time of initiation. In this study, one death was prevented for every 13 patients treated for 1 year—as dramatic an effect as has been seen with a pharmacologic therapy in the history of cardiovascular medicine.

Because even apparently stable patients may deteriorate when β-blockers are initiated, initiation must be done gradually and with great care. Carvedilol often is initiated at a dosage of 3.125 mg orally twice daily and may be increased to 6.25, 12.5, and 25 mg twice daily at intervals of approximately 2 weeks. The protocols for sustained-release metoprolol use were started at 12.5 or 25 mg orally daily and doubled at intervals of 2 weeks to a target dose of 200 mg daily (using the Toprol XL sustained-release preparation). Bisoprolol was administered at a dosage of 1.25, 2.5, 3.75, 5, 7.5, and 10 mg orally daily, with increments at 1- to 4-week intervals. More gradual up-titration is often more convenient and may be better tolerated. Patients on high doses of β-blockers should be monitored for bradycardia, dizziness, orthostasis, hypotension, and fatigue.

Patients should be instructed to monitor their weight at home as an indicator of fluid retention and to report any increase or change in symptoms immediately. Before each β-blocker dose increase, patients should be seen and examined to ensure that there has not been fluid retention or worsening of symptoms. If HF worsens, this can usually be managed by increasing diuretic doses and delaying further increases in β-blocker doses, though dose decrease or discontinuation is sometimes required.

4. SGLT-2 inhibitors—Two large clinical trials have shown that *SGLT-2 receptor inhibitors dapagliflozin and empagliflozin substantially reduce the risk of cardiovascular death and hospitalizations for HF among patients with EF < 50%, with or without diabetes.* Both medications are dosed at 10 mg daily and result in rapid benefits (within 2 weeks). SGLT-2 inhibitors are generally well tolerated with respect to blood pressure and renal function. SGLT-2 inhibitors also reduce kidney disease progression, and patients with eGFRs as low as 20 mL/min/1.73 m^2 have been included in these trials.

5. Digitalis glycosides—The efficacy of digitalis glycosides in reducing the symptoms of HF has been established in at least four multicenter trials. Digoxin has *not* been shown to reduce HF mortality, however. In the era of the favored "quadruple therapy," digoxin is rarely used for the sole indication of HF. Digoxin should be considered for (1) patients who remain symptomatic when on optimal guideline-directed medical therapy and (2) patients with HF who require additional rate control for AF. However, there is some uncertainty about the safety of digoxin in this population with atrial fibrillation, especially with higher digoxin concentrations.

Digoxin has a half-life of 24–36 hours and is eliminated almost entirely by the kidneys. The oral maintenance dose may range from 0.125 mg three times weekly to 0.5 mg daily. Dose requirements are lower in patients with kidney dysfunction, advanced age, or smaller lean body mass. Amiodarone, quinidine, propafenone, and verapamil are among the medications that may increase digoxin levels up to 100%. It is prudent to measure a serum digoxin level 7–14 days after starting (and at least 6 hours after the last dose was administered). Goal serum digoxin levels are 0.7–1.2 ng/mL. Digoxin may induce ventricular arrhythmias, especially when hypokalemia or myocardial ischemia is present. Digoxin toxicity is discussed in Chapter 42.

6. Nitrates and hydralazine—The combination of hydralazine and isosorbide dinitrate has been shown to *improve outcomes in self-identified Black persons.* ARBs or ARNIs have largely supplanted the use of the hydralazine–isosorbide dinitrate combination in patients with intolerance to ACE inhibitors.

A. Nitrates—Intravenous vasodilators (sodium nitroprusside or nitroglycerin) are used primarily for acute or severely decompensated chronic HF and cardiogenic shock, especially when accompanied by high afterload/narrow pulse pressure, hypertension or myocardial ischemia. The starting dosage for nitroglycerin is generally about 10 mcg/min, which is titrated upward by 10–20 mcg/min (to a maximum of 200 mcg/min) until mean arterial pressure drops by 10%. Hypotension (blood pressure < 100 mm Hg systolic) should be avoided. For sodium nitroprusside, the starting dosage is 5–10 mcg/min, with upward titration to a maximum dose of 400 mcg/min.

For the purposes of HF, oral isosorbide dinitrate, 20–40 mg orally three times daily, is used primarily for afterload reduction when weaning hospitalized patients with severe HF off of intravenous nitrate infusions. Nitrate therapy is generally well tolerated, but headaches and hypotension may limit the dose of all agents. The development of *tolerance* to long-term nitrate therapy occurs.

B. HYDRALAZINE—Oral hydralazine is a potent arteriolar dilator, often used primarily among hospitalized patients in conjunction with isosorbide dinitrate in order to liberate patients from intravenous nitrate infusions. When used as a single agent, it has *not* been shown to improve symptoms or exercise tolerance during long-term treatment.

7. Ivabradine—Ivabradine inhibits the I_f channel in the sinus node and has the specific effect of slowing heart rate. Ivabradine has *not* been shown to reduce mortality specifically. Ivabradine is approved by the FDA for use in stable/compensated patients with HF and sinus heart rate of 70 beats/min who are taking the maximally tolerated dose of β-blockers, or in patients in whom β-blockers are contraindicated. Both the US and the European guidelines assign ivabradine a class IIa recommendation for patients in sinus rhythm with a heart rate ≥ 70 beats/min with an EF ≤ 35%, and persisting symptoms despite treatment with an evidence-based dose of β-blocker (or a maximum tolerated dose below that), ACE inhibitor (or ARB), and an aldosterone antagonist.

8. Vericiguat (a soluble guanylate cyclase stimulator)—Vericiguat is FDA-approved to reduce the risk of cardiovascular death and HF hospitalization following a hospitalization for HF among patients with LVEF < 45%. The VICTORIA trial showed a modest but significant reduction in cardiovascular death and HF hospitalization with vericiguat when *added to other effective therapies* among high-risk patients. In contrast, the more recent VICTOR trial comprised stable outpatients and did not show reduction in HF hospitalizations of cardiovascular death, but it did show reduction in all-cause mortality. Pooled data across the two trials show a modest benefit of vericiguat.

9. Combination of medical therapies—Optimal management of chronic HF involves using combinations of proven life-saving therapies. *Patients with HFrEF should be treated with all four life-saving medications: β-blockers, MRAs, sacubitril/valsartan, and SGLT-2 inhibitors.* This combination, titrated to full tolerated doses, with careful monitoring of kidney function and potassium, provides the greatest pharmacologic benefit to most patients with HFrEF. Achieving this goal has been shown to be more effective using a systematic approach with established care pathways and frequent clinic visits. There are advantages to starting all of these medications before hospital discharge for patients hospitalized with HF, when possible.

10. Treatments that may cause harm in HF with reduced LVEF—Several therapies should be *avoided*, when possible, in patients with systolic HF. These include thiazolidinediones (glitazones), which cause worsening HF, nondihydropyridine calcium channel blockers, NSAIDs, and cyclooxygenase-2 inhibitors, which cause sodium and water retention and renal impairment.

11. Anticoagulation—Patients with LV failure and reduced EF are at somewhat increased risk for developing intracardiac thrombi and systemic arterial emboli. However, routine anticoagulation is *not* indicated for HFrEF alone Patients at risk of thromboembolic events are those with atrial fibrillation, known LV thrombus, or a history of prior thromboembolic phenomenon. DOACs appear to be as effective as warfarin for patients with LV thrombus

12. Antiarrhythmic therapy—Patients with moderate to severe HF have a high incidence of both symptomatic and asymptomatic arrhythmias. Although < 10% of patients have syncope or presyncope resulting from ventricular tachycardia, ambulatory monitoring reveals that up to 70% of patients have asymptomatic episodes of nonsustained ventricular tachycardia. These arrhythmias indicate a poor prognosis independent of the severity of LV dysfunction, but many of the deaths are probably not arrhythmia related. β-Blockers, because of their marked favorable effect on prognosis in general and on the incidence of sudden death specifically, should be initiated in these as well as all other patients with HF (see β-Blockers, above). *Other evidence-based therapies for HF, including ACE inhibitors, ARBs, MRAs, ARNIs, and SGLT-2 inhibitors, all appear to reduce sudden cardiac death.* Empiric antiarrhythmic therapy with amiodarone did not improve outcomes in the SCD-HeFT trial, and most other antiarrhythmic medications are contraindicated because of their proarrhythmic effects in this population and their adverse effect on cardiac function. *For patients with HFrEF and atrial fibrillation, a rhythm control strategy has not been shown to improve outcomes compared with a rate control strategy.*

13. Antihypertensives—The AHA and ACC recommend a systolic blood pressure of < 130 mm Hg in patients with HFrEF and hypertension. If blood pressure remains above goal despite quadruple therapy (ACE inhibitor/ARB/ARNI, β-blockers, SGLT2 inhibitors, and MRAs), additional agents should be added, such as a diuretic or dihydropyridine calcium channel blocker (eg, amlodipine).

14. Statin therapy—Even though vascular disease is present in many patients with chronic HF, the role of statins has not been well defined in patients with HF. The CORONA and the GISSI-HF trials showed no reduction in mortality or HF hospitalizations among patients with HFrEF, despite achieving lower LDL levels.

C. Nonpharmacologic Treatment

1. Implantable cardioverter defibrillators (ICDs)—Indications for ICDs include not only patients with symptomatic or asymptomatic arrhythmias but also patients with chronic HF and LV systolic dysfunction who are receiving contemporary HF treatments, including β-blockers. *The AHA/ACC recommend primary-prevention ICD implantation for the prevention of sudden cardiac death from ventricular arrhythmias for patients with ischemic or nonischemic HFrEF with LVEF ≤ 35% and NYHA II–III symptoms, after ≥ 3 months of maximally tolerated guideline-directed medical therapy, assuming > 1-year life expectancy.* In the second Multicenter Automatic Defibrillator Implantation Trial (MADIT II), 1232 patients with prior MI and an EF < 30% were randomized to an ICD or a control group. Mortality was 31% lower in the ICD group, which translated into 9 lives saved for each 100 patients who received a device and were monitored for 3 years. The Centers for Medicare and Medicaid Services provides reimbursement coverage to include patients with chronic HF and ischemic or nonischemic cardiomyopathy with an EF of ≤ 35%.

2. Biventricular pacing (resynchronization)—Many patients with HFrEF have abnormal intraventricular conduction that results in left and right ventricular dyssynchrony, and hence inefficient contractions. Patients with wide QRS complexes (generally ≥ 150 msec), reduced EFs, and moderate to severe symptoms have been studied to examine the potential benefits of pacing resynchronization. Several studies have evaluated the efficacy of "multisite" pacing, using leads that stimulate the RV from the apex and the LV from the lateral wall via the coronary sinus. Results from trials with up to 2 years of follow-up have shown an increase in EF, improvement in symptoms and exercise tolerance, and reduction in death and hospitalization. Therefore, the AHA/ACC/HRS recommend cardiac resynchronization therapy for patients with *LVEF ≤ 35% and NYHA class II–IV symptoms despite GDMT who are in sinus rhythm with LBBB and a QRS duration ≥ 150 msec*. The best responders to cardiac resynchronization therapy are patients with wider QRS, left bundle branch block, and nonischemic cardiomyopathy, and the lowest responders are those with narrow QRS and non–left bundle branch block pattern.

3. Case management, diet, exercise training, and integrative approaches—Thirty to 50 percent of HF patients who are hospitalized will be readmitted within 3–6 months. *Strategies to prevent clinical deterioration, such as* ***case management, home monitoring of weight and clinical status****, and* ***patient adjustment of diuretics****, can prevent rehospitalizations and should be part of the treatment regimen of advanced HF.* Involvement of a multidisciplinary team (rather than a single physician) and in-person (rather than just telephonic) communication appear to be important features of successful programs. Initiating life-saving medications during hospitalization for HF with rapid titration after discharge may improve outcomes.

Patients should routinely practice **moderate salt restriction** (2–2.5 g sodium or 5–6 g salt per day). More severe sodium restriction is usually difficult to achieve and unnecessary because of the availability of potent diuretic agents.

Exercise training improves activity tolerance by reversing the peripheral abnormalities associated with HF and deconditioning. In severe HF, restriction of activity may facilitate temporary recompensation. A large trial showed no significant benefit (nor harm) from a structured exercise training program on death or hospitalization, although functional status and symptoms were improved. *Thus, in stable patients, a prudent increase in activity or a regular exercise regimen can be encouraged.* Indeed, a gradual exercise program is associated with diminished symptoms and increases in exercise capacity and quality of life. Cardiac rehabilitation programs therefore are instrumental in the care for patients with HFrEF.

4. Coronary revascularization—As underlying CAD is the cause of HFrEF in the majority of patients, coronary revascularization has been thought to be able to both improve symptoms and prevent progression. While the STITCH trial failed to show an overall survival benefit from CABG among patients with HF and an LVEF of ≤ 35% and multivessel coronary disease at 5 years, there was indeed benefit at 10 years of follow-up. However, patients with left main CAD were excluded from this trial (an important group of patients). In contrast, data from the 2024 REVIVED-BCIS2 trial showed that revascularization with percutaneous coronary intervention did not improve survival or reduce HF hospitalizations among patients with ischemic HFrEF.

5. Cardiac transplantation—Because of the poor prognosis of advanced HF, cardiac transplantation is widely used. Many centers report 1-year survival rates exceeding 80–90% and 5-year survival rates above 70%. Infections, hypertension and renal dysfunction caused by immunosuppression, rapidly progressive coronary atherosclerosis, and immunosuppressant-related cancers constitute the major complications. The high cost and limited number of donor organs require careful patient selection and follow-up care.

6. Other surgical treatment options—Externally powered and implantable **ventricular assist devices** can be used in patients who require ventricular support, either to allow the heart to recover or as a bridge to transplantation. The latest generation devices are small enough to allow patients unrestricted mobility and even discharge from the hospital. *Continuous flow* devices appear to be more effective than *pulsatile flow* devices. However, complications are frequent, including bleeding, thromboembolism, and infection, and the cost is very high, exceeding $200,000 in the initial 1–3 months.

7. Palliative care—Despite the advances of recent years, many patients with chronic HF are older adults and have multiple comorbidities. *Many of them will not experience meaningful improvements in survival despite aggressive therapy.* The goal of management for these patients and all those with serious illness should include symptomatic improvement and palliative care as they approach the end of life (see Chapter 5).

Treatment: Heart Failure with Preserved LVEF

Although half of all HF occurs among patients with normal LVEF, often with diastolic dysfunction, *the only therapies clearly shown to reduce cardiovascular death or HF hospitalization in this population are SGLT-2 inhibitors and the nonsteroidal MRA finerenone.* Therefore, the mainstays of treating HF with preserved EF are SGLT-2 inhibitors, aldosterone antagonists, and diuretic therapy for fluid overload. *Achieving target (or maximally tolerated) dosing of these treatments is vital* (Table 11–1). Addressing comorbidities such as hypertension, diabetes, obesity, and arrhythmias (such as atrial fibrillation and high-burden premature ventricular complexes) also is important.

Table 11–1. Evidence-based doses of disease-modifying medications in key randomized trials in HFrEF or after MI (medications listed in alphabetical order within classes).

Medications	Starting Dose	Target Dose
ACE Inhibitors		
Captopril	6.25 mg three times daily	50 mg three times daily
Enalapril	2.5 mg twice daily	10–20 mg twice daily
Lisinopril	2.5–5.0 mg once daily	20–35 once daily
Ramipril	2.5 mg once daily	10 mg once daily
Trandolapril	0.5 mg once daily	4 mg once daily
β-Blockers		
Bisoprolol	1.25 mg once daily	10 mg once daily
Carvedilol	3.125 mg twice daily	25 mg twice daily
Metoprolol succinate (CR/XL)	12.5–25 mg once daily	200 mg once daily
Nebivolol	1.25 mg once daily	10 mg once daily
ARBs		
Candesartan	4–8 mg once daily	32 mg once daily
Losartan	50 mg once daily	150 mg once daily
Valsartan	40 mg twice daily	160 mg twice daily
Aldosterone Antagonists		
Eplerenone	25 mg once daily	50 mg once daily
Spironolactone	25 mg once daily	50 mg once daily
ARNI		
Sacubitril/valsartan	49/51 mg twice daily	97/103 mg twice daily
I_f Channel Blocker		
Ivabradine	5 mg twice daily	7.5 mg twice daily
SGLT-2 inhibitors		
Dapagliflozin	10 mg once daily	10 mg once daily
Empagliflozin	10 mg once daily	10 mg once daily

ARNI, angiotensin receptor–neprilysin inhibitor; HFrEF, HF with reduced EF.

A. Correction of Reversible Causes

Hypertension, pericardial disease, and atrial tachycardias are potentially reversible factors that can contribute to HF with preserved LVEF. Since tachycardia is associated with shorter overall diastolic filling time, controlling accelerated heart rate may be important. With effective treatment available for familial and wild type transthyretin amyloid cardiomyopathy, this diagnosis should be considered for patients with unexplained HFpEF, especially in older adults. Treating obesity, in particular with the **GLP-1 receptor agonist semaglutide** and **the dual-acting agonist of GLP-1 and glucose-dependent insulinotropic polypeptide receptor tirzepatide,** improves HF symptoms and exercise function.

B. Pharmacologic Treatment

1. Diuretic therapy—Diuretics are important to control symptoms of fluid overload in patients with HFpEF, which are similar to symptoms from systolic HF.

2. SGLT-2 inhibitors—Both empagliflozin and dapagliflozin have been shown to decrease cardiovascular mortality, heart failure hospitalizations, and worsening of HF of patients with HFpEF. They cause mild diuresis and mild reduction in blood pressure; thus care is needed during initiation for patients with hypovolemia or low blood pressure.

3. Inhibitors of the renin–angiotensin–aldosterone system—ACE inhibitors and ARBs have *not* been shown to improve outcome in patients with HFpEF, despite being excellent therapies for the comorbidity of hypertension. Sacubitril/valsartan does *not* substantially improve outcome in patients with HFpEF, although it does appear to improve outcome for patients with mildly reduced LVEF (41–49%). In 2025, the FINEARTS-HF trial was the first study to show definitive benefit of an MRA in HFpEF: finerenone was shown to reduce composite HF hospitalizations and cardiovascular death. In the TOPCAT trial, spironolactone was *not* shown to improve outcomes in a large trial of patients with HF and preserved LVEF, but there may have been some reduction in hospitalizations among patients enrolled in the Americas. Therefore, spironolactone should remain a therapeutic option, especially for HFpEF patients who also have hypertension.

4. Finerenone—the nonsteroidal mineralocorticoid receptor antagonist finerenone has been shown to reduce cardiovascular death and HF events in patients with mildly reduced or preserved EF (≥ 40% LVEF) in the FINEARTS-HF trial, and it is now FDA approved for this indication. A meta-analysis of trials of finerenone and spironolactone suggests there may be similar effects with these two mineralocorticoid receptor antagonists, with an advantage of fewer side effects with finerenone.

5. GLP receptor agonists—The GLP-1 receptor agonist semaglutide was recently shown to reduce HF symptoms and weight among patients with HFpEF and obesity, regardless of diabetes status. The dual-acting GLP-1 receptor agonist/ glucose-dependent insulinotropic polypeptide receptor agonist tirzepatide was shown to improve HF symptoms and exercise function and to reduce cardiovascular death among patients with HFpEF and obesity. Both agents are currently under FDA review.

C. Nonpharmacologic Treatment

Unlike in patients with HFrEF, ICD and resynchronization device treatments do *not* have a role in patients with preserved LVEF. Revascularization for patients with HF and preserved LVEF should be guided by the same considerations as for patients with HFrEF.

Prognosis

Once manifested, HF with reduced LVEF carries a poor prognosis. Even with appropriate treatment, the 5-year mortality is approximately 50%. Mortality rates vary from < 5% per year in those with no or few symptoms to > 30% per year in those with severe and refractory symptoms. These data emphasize the critical importance of early detection and intervention. Higher mortality is related to older age, lower LVEF, more severe symptoms, CKD, and diabetes. The prognosis of HF has improved in the past two decades, probably at least in part because of the more widespread use of quadruple therapy, which markedly improve survival in those with HFrEF.

When to Refer

Patients with new symptoms of HF not explained by an obvious cause should be referred to a cardiologist. Patients with continued symptoms of HF and reduced LVEF (≤ 35%) should be referred for consideration of placement of an ICD or cardiac resynchronization therapy (if QRS duration is ≥ 120 msec, especially with left bundle branch block pattern).

When to Admit

- Patients with unexplained new or worsened symptoms or positive cardiac biomarkers concerning for acute myocardial necrosis.
- Patients with hypoxia, gross fluid overload, or pulmonary edema not readily resolved in an outpatient setting.

Cannata A et al. Heart failure with preserved ejection fraction. N Engl J Med. 2025;392:173. [PMID: 39778171]

Chen SH et al. Comparative effectiveness of pharmacotherapy for heart failure with preserved ejection fraction: a systematic review and network meta-analysis. Diabetes Obes Metab. 2026 Jan 26. [Epub ahead of print] [PMID: 41588709]

Heidenreich PA et al. 2022 AHA/ACC/HFSA Guideline for the Management of Heart Failure: executive summary: a report of the American College of Cardiology/American Heart Association Joint Committee on Clinical Practice Guidelines. J Am Coll Cardiol. 2022;79:1757. [PMID: 35379504]

Jones DW et al; Peer Review Committee Members. 2025 AHA/ACC/AANP/AAPA/ABC/ACCP/ACPM/AGS/AMA/ASPC/NMA/PCNA/SGIM guideline for the prevention, detection, evaluation, and management of high blood pressure in adults: a report of the American College of Cardiology/American Heart Association Joint Committee on Clinical Practice Guidelines. J Am Coll Cardiol. 2025;86:1567. Erratum in: J Am Coll Cardiol. 2025;86:1679. [PMID: 40815242]

McDonagh TA et al. 2021 ESC Guidelines for the diagnosis and treatment of acute and chronic heart failure: developed by the Task Force for the diagnosis and treatment of acute and chronic heart failure of the European Society of Cardiology (ESC). With the special contribution of the Heart Failure Association (HFA) of the ESC. Eur J Heart Fail. 2022;24:4. [PMID: 35083827]

Packer M et al; SUMMIT Trial Study Group. Tirzepatide for heart failure with preserved ejection fraction and obesity. N Engl J Med. 2025;392:427. [PMID: 39555826]

Solomon SD et al. Finerenone in heart failure with mildly reduced or preserved ejection fraction. N Engl J Med. 2024;391:1475. [PMID: 39225278]

van Essen BJ et al. Pharmacologic treatment of heart failure with reduced ejection fraction: an updated systematic review and network meta-analysis. J Am Coll Cardiol. 2025;86:2513. [PMID: 40892608]

ACUTE HEART FAILURE & PULMONARY EDEMA

ESSENTIALS OF DIAGNOSIS

- Acute onset or worsening of dyspnea at rest.
- Tachycardia, diaphoresis, cyanosis.
- Pulmonary rales, rhonchi, expiratory wheezing.
- Radiograph shows interstitial and alveolar edema with or without cardiomegaly.
- Arterial hypoxemia.

General Considerations

Typical causes of acute cardiogenic pulmonary edema include acute MI or severe ischemia, exacerbation of chronic HF, acute severe hypertension, AKI, acute volume overload of the LV (aortic or mitral valvular regurgitation), and mitral stenosis. *By far the most common presentation in developed countries is one of acute or subacute deterioration of chronic HF, precipitated by discontinuation of medications, excessive salt intake, myocardial ischemia, tachyarrhythmias (especially rapid atrial fibrillation), or intercurrent infection.* Often in the latter group, there is preceding volume overload with worsening edema and progressive shortness of breath for which early intervention can avoid the need for hospital admission.

Clinical Findings

Acute pulmonary edema presents with a characteristic clinical picture of severe dyspnea, with or without the production of pink, frothy sputum, as well as diaphoresis and cyanosis. Rales are present in all lung fields, as are generalized wheezing and rhonchi. Pulmonary edema may appear acutely or subacutely in the setting of chronic HF or may be the first manifestation of cardiac disease, usually acute MI, which may be painful or silent. Less severe decompensations usually present with dyspnea at rest, rales, and other evidence of fluid retention but without severe hypoxia.

Noncardiac causes of pulmonary edema include pulmonary infections, acute respiratory distress syndrome, increased intracerebral pressure, high altitude, sepsis, medications, inhaled toxins, transfusion reactions, shock, and disseminated intravascular coagulation. These are distinguished from cardiogenic pulmonary edema by the clinical setting, history, and physical examination. Conversely, in most patients with cardiogenic pulmonary edema, an underlying cardiac abnormality can usually be detected clinically or by ECG, CXR, or echocardiogram.

The CXR reveals signs of pulmonary vascular redistribution, blurriness of vascular outlines, increased interstitial markings, and, characteristically, the butterfly pattern of distribution of alveolar edema. The heart may be enlarged or normal in size depending on whether HF was previously present. Assessment of cardiac function by echocardiography is important, as a substantial proportion of patients have normal EFs with elevated atrial pressures due to diastolic dysfunction. In cardiogenic pulmonary edema, BNP and PCWP are elevated. In noncardiogenic pulmonary edema, the wedge pressure may be normal or even low.

Treatment

Often, when patients with known HF are admitted for acute decompensations, they may exhibit AKI due to cardiorenal venous congestion or poor forward flow. Therefore, often most of their outpatient quadruple therapy should be temporarily held to prevent risk of further AKI. Oral β-blockers, though, should be continued, unless the initiation of the of β-blocker was thought to precipitate the decompensation or the patient has signs of severe HF/early cardiogenic shock (ie, lactic acidosis, severe AKI, hepatocellular injury, altered mental status).

In florid pulmonary edema, the patient should be placed in a sitting position with legs dangling over the side of the bed; this facilitates respiration and reduces venous return. **Oxygen** is delivered by mask to obtain an arterial PaO_2 > 60 mm Hg. Noninvasive pressure support ventilation may improve oxygenation and prevent severe CO_2 retention while pharmacologic interventions take effect. However, if respiratory distress remains severe, endotracheal intubation and mechanical ventilation may be necessary.

Intravenous diuretic therapy is the mainstay of treatment in acute decompensated HF and should be initiated promptly upon recognition of the condition. Intravenous loop diuretics produce venodilation prior to the onset of diuresis. The DOSE trial has shown that, for acute decompensated HF, bolus doses of furosemide are of similar efficacy as continuous intravenous infusion, and that higher-dose furosemide (2.5 times the patient's outpatient daily oral dose) resulted in more rapid fluid removal without a substantially higher risk of kidney impairment.

Narrow pulse pressure and cool extremities in patients presenting with acute decompensated HF suggest severe peripheral vasoconstriction, likely secondary to RAAS activation and high sympathetic tone in response to reduced cardiac output. In these patients, **intravenous nitrate therapy or nitroprusside** accelerates clinical improvement by reducing both blood pressure and LV filling pressures. These afterload-reducing agents will help reduce dyspnea rapidly prior to the onset of diuresis, as well as improve renal perfusion for superior diuresis. Finally, these agents are particularly valuable in patients with accompanying hypertension.

It is important to note that patients with HF exist on severity spectrum, ranging from asymptomatic, well-compensated outpatients, to mild decompensations requiring hospital admission for IV diuresis, to florid cardiogenic shock requiring intravenous inotropes, mechanical circulatory support, or extracorporeal membrane oxygenation (ECMO). Over the course of their lives, patients with HF may shift among these states.

Bronchospasm may occur in response to pulmonary edema and may itself exacerbate hypoxemia and dyspnea. Treatment with inhaled β-adrenergic agonists or intravenous aminophylline may be helpful, but both may also provoke tachycardia and supraventricular arrhythmias.

In most cases, pulmonary edema responds rapidly to therapy. When the patient has improved, the cause or precipitating factor should be ascertained. In patients without prior HF, evaluation should include echocardiography and, in many cases, cardiac catheterization with coronary angiography. Patients with acute decompensation of chronic HF should be treated to achieve an euvolemic state and have their medical regimen optimized. Ideally, an oral diuretic and quadruple therapy should be started, with efficacy and tolerability confirmed prior to discharge.

MYOCARDITIS & THE CARDIOMYOPATHIES

INFECTIOUS MYOCARDITIS

ESSENTIALS OF DIAGNOSIS

- Often follows an upper respiratory infection.
- May present with chest pain (pleuritic or nonspecific) or signs of HF.
- Echocardiogram may show global systolic dysfunction. Initial heart size is generally normal with thickened walls, with or without pericardial effusion.
- Myocardial biopsy, though not sensitive, may reveal a characteristic inflammatory pattern. MRI also has a role in diagnosis.

General Considerations

Myocarditis (inflammation of the myocardium) can be caused by a variety of different etiologies. Myocarditis is classified by etiology: infectious (eg, viral, bacterial, fungal), autoimmune (eg, SLE, vasculitis), drug-induced (eg, checkpoint inhibitors), inflammatory (eg, giant cell myocarditis), and toxic (eg, alcohol, cocaine). The clinical presentation of myocarditis is a spectrum: some patients may present with mild symptoms of dyspnea, whereas others may present with florid cardiogenic shock (ie, fulminant myocarditis). Additionally, the time course is variable, ranging from acute/fulminant to subclinical or chronic. Both cellular and humoral inflammatory processes contribute to the progression to myocardial injury, and there are subgroups that appear to benefit from immunosuppression.

Genetic predisposition is a likely factor in at least a few cases. Autoimmune myocarditis (eg, giant cell myocarditis) may occur with no identifiable viral infection. The heterogeneity of the clinical syndromes and the incomplete understanding of the immunopathology hinder a more complete understanding of the mechanisms involved.

Clinical Findings

A. Symptoms and Signs

Patients may present several days to a few weeks after the onset of an acute febrile illness or a respiratory infection or they may present with new HF without antecedent symptoms. The onset of HF may be gradual or may be abrupt and fulminant. In acute fulminant myocarditis, low output and shock may be present with severely depressed LV systolic function. The LV chamber size is typically not very enlarged. A pericardial friction rub may be present. In the European Study of Epidemiology and Treatment of Inflammatory Heart Disease, 72% of participants had dyspnea, 32% had chest pain, and 18% had arrhythmias. Pulmonary and systemic emboli may occur. Pleural-pericardial chest pain is common. Examination reveals tachycardia and other evidence of HF. At times, the presentation may mimic an acute MI with ST changes, positive cardiac markers, and regional wall motion abnormalities despite normal coronaries. Microaneurysms may also occur and may be associated with serious ventricular arrhythmias. It has been estimated that approximately 10% of all dilated cardiomyopathy patients have viral myocarditis as the cause.

B. ECG and Chest Radiography

ECG may show sinus tachycardia, other arrhythmias, nonspecific repolarization changes, and intraventricular conduction abnormalities. The presence of Q waves or left bundle branch block portends a higher rate of death or need for cardiac transplantation. Ventricular ectopy may be the initial and only clinical finding. The CXR is nonspecific, but cardiomegaly is frequent, though not universal. Evidence for pulmonary venous hypertension is common and frank pulmonary edema may be present.

C. Diagnostic Studies

No specific laboratory test exists to confirm or refute the diagnosis of myocarditis. WBC count, ESR, and CRP are often elevated but are nonspecific. Troponin levels are elevated in about one-third of patients, but creatine kinase-MB is elevated in only 10%. Other biomarkers, such as BNP and NT-proBNP, are usually elevated. Echocardiography provides the most convenient way of evaluating cardiac function and can exclude many other processes. MRI with gadolinium enhancement may reveal spotty areas of injury throughout the myocardium.

D. Endomyocardial Biopsy

Myocarditis can be confirmed with histologic evidence. The AHA/ACC/ESC class I recommendations for biopsy are (1) in patients with HF, a normal-sized or dilated LV < 2 weeks after onset of symptoms, and hemodynamic compromise; or (2) in patients with a dilated LV 2 weeks to 3 months after onset of symptoms, new ventricular arrhythmias or AV nodal block (Mobitz II or complete heart block) or who do not respond to usual care after 1–2 weeks. However, these recommendations are not based on high level of evidence and thus should only be considered after imaging, such as MRI, and judgement that a treatable cause is likely to be found. For example, identifying giant cell myocarditis will allow more targeted therapy. In some cases, the identification of inflammation without viral genomes by PCR suggests that immunosuppression might be useful. Because the cardiac involvement is often patchy, the diagnosis even with biopsy can be missed in up to one-half of cases.

Treatment & Prognosis

Treatment is directed toward the specific etiology for the myocarditis, if known. For example, patients with biopsy-confirmed giant cell myocarditis have been known to benefit from high-dose coricosteroids plus additional immunosuppression. Immune checkpoint inhibitor-associated myocarditis is treated by discontinuing the offending agent and using high-dose coricosteroids. Specific antimicrobial therapy is indicated if a specific infecting agent is identified. For patients who present with HFrEF or cardiogenic shock, quadruple therapy or supportive care, respectively, are indicated. Patients who present with concomitant pericarditis (ie, myopericarditis) should be treated with colchicine and likely NSAIDs.

Studies are lacking as to when to discontinue the chosen therapy if the patient improves. Patients with fulminant myocarditis require aggressive short-term support, including an IABP or other mechanical circulatory support. If severe pulmonary infiltrates accompany the fulminant myocarditis, extracorporeal membrane oxygenation (ECMO) support may be temporarily required and has had notable success.

Patients should be counseled to avoid exercise for 3–6 months after a diagnosis of myocarditis, as this may precipitate ventricular arrhythmias and sudden cardiac death (see Table 11–2).

Prognosis depends on etiology and illness severity. Patients with fulminant myocarditis may present with acute cardiogenic shock, with high mortality rates. Acute

Table 11–2. American College of Cardiology Sports and Exercise Section guidelines for athletes with COVID-19 myocarditis.

Myocarditis diagnosis if both of the following are present
• A clinical syndrome of < 3 months' duration
• Otherwise unexplained increase in serum troponin levels, ECG changes, arrhythmias, high-grade AV block, regional wall motion abnormalities, or pericardial effusion. MRI findings suggesting myocarditis including T1- or T2-weighted imaging or late gadolinium enhancement
Sports eligibility after myocarditis
• Must obtain a resting echocardiogram, 24-hour ambulatory ECG monitoring, and an exercise ECG no earlier than 3–6 months after the illness (class I, LOE C)
• Can resume exercise training if ALL of the following are met (class IIa, LOE C)
–Normal ventricular function
–Serum markers of myocardial injury, HF, and inflammation have returned to normal
–Clinically relevant arrhythmias on ambulatory ECG monitoring or exercise ECG are absent

AV, atrioventricular; LOE, level of evidence.

myocarditis has been implicated as a cause of sudden death in 5–22% of such cases in athletes younger than 35 years.

When to Refer

Patients in whom myocarditis is suspected should be seen by a cardiologist at a tertiary care center where facilities are available for diagnosis and therapies available should a fulminant course ensue. The facility should have cardiac catheterization capabilities, ventricular support devices, and transplantation options available.

Gluckman TJ et al. 2022 ACC expert consensus decision pathway on cardiovascular sequelae of COVID-19 in adults: myocarditis and other myocardial involvement, post-acute sequelae of sars-cov-2 infection, and return to play: a report of the American College of Cardiology Solution Set Oversight Committee. J Am Coll Cardiol. 2022;79:1717. [PMID: 35307156]

Shimabukuro TT. Update on myocarditis following mRNA COVID-19 vaccination. 2022 Jun 23. https://www.cdc.gov/vaccines/acip/meetings/downloads/slides-2022-06-22-23/03-covid-shimabukuro-508.pdf

NONINFECTIOUS MYOCARDITIS

Systemic disorders are also associated with myocarditis. These include giant cell myocarditis, eosinophilic myocarditis, celiac disease, granulomatosis with polyangiitis, and sarcoidosis. Giant cell myocarditis is typically rapid and severe in onset, often with ventricular arrhythmias, heart block, or both. Endomyocardial biopsy is important for diagnosis, since benefit from immunosuppressive therapy, especially in giant cell myocarditis, has been suggested in a number of observational studies, including those directed primarily at T cells (ie, using muromonab-CD3). Treatment of eosinophilic myocarditis includes the use of high-dose corticosteroids and removal of the offending medication or underlying trigger, if known. Most studies suggest that HIV is only indirectly responsible for HIV cardiomyopathy, and other factors, such as gp 120 protein, adverse reaction to antiretroviral therapy, and opportunistic infections have been implicated more often. Epstein-Barr and herpes simplex viruses have been identified in some patients' myocardium.

A wide range of medications, recreational drugs, and toxic substances can cause acute or chronic myocardial injury with highly variable clinical presentations, including ECG changes, arrhythmias, and HF. In addition, hypersensitivity reactions to medications such as sulfonamides, penicillins, and aminosalicylic acid can lead to cardiac dysfunction. Radiation can cause an acute inflammatory reaction as well as a chronic fibrosis of heart muscle, usually in conjunction with pericarditis.

The problem of cardiovascular side effects from cancer chemotherapy agents is an ever growing one and has spawned a new clinical area in cardiology called **cardio-oncology**. Anthracyclines (doxorubicin, daunorubicin, idarubicin, epirubicin, and mitoxantrone) remain the cornerstone of treatment of many malignancies but may result in cardiomyopathy. HF arises in 5% of patients treated with a cumulative dose of 400–450 mg/m^2, and this rate is doubled if the patient age is > 65. While symptoms and evidence for myocardial dysfunction usually appear within 1 year of starting therapy, late-onset manifestation of HF may appear up to a decade later. The major mechanism of cardiotoxicity is thought to be due to oxidative stress inducing myocyte apoptosis and necrosis, as well as sarcomere disruption. This pathologic understanding is the rationale behind the superoxide dismutase mimetic and iron-chelating agent, dexrazoxane, to protect from the injury. The use of trastuzumab in combination with anthracyclines increases the risk of cardiac dysfunction up to 28%; this has been an issue since combined use of these agents is particularly effective in *HER2*-positive breast cancer. Other risk factors for patients receiving anthracyclines include the use of paclitaxel, concurrent radiation, and preexisting CVD (including hypertension, peripheral vascular disease, CAD, and diabetes). Immune checkpoint point inhibitors also can cause myocarditis, which may be severe and may respond to steroids and immunomodulator therapy. A summary of cardiotoxic cancer therapeutic agents and their role may be found in the 2019 AHA statement on cardio-oncology.

In patients receiving chemotherapy, it is important to monitor for subtle signs of cardiovascular compromise. Serial echocardiography, cardiac MR, or both can provide concrete data regarding LV function. *Echo Doppler myocardial global strain abnormalities may be the first abnormality observed* (even prior to a drop in the LVEF); similarly, assessment of the T2 signal from cardiac MRI may also provide early detection of cardiotoxicity. Biomarkers such as BNP or NT-proBNP may be of some value when serial measures are obtained. Other biomarkers may appear early in the course of myocardial injury (especially troponin) and may allow for early detection of cardiotoxicity before other signs become evident. *There is some evidence that β-blocker therapy may reduce the negative effects on myocardial function.*

When to Refer

Many patients with myocardial injury from toxic agents can be monitored safely if ventricular function remains relatively preserved (EF > 40%) and no HF symptoms occur. Diastolic dysfunction may be subtle.

Once HF or a reduced LVEF becomes evident or significant conduction system disease arises, the patient should be evaluated and monitored by a cardiologist in case myocardial dysfunction worsens and further intervention becomes warranted.

DILATED CARDIOMYOPATHY

ESSENTIALS OF DIAGNOSIS

- Symptoms and signs of HF.
- Echocardiogram confirms LV dilation, thinning, and global dysfunction.
- Severity of RV dysfunction is critical in long-term prognosis.

General Considerations

Dilated cardiomyopathy is a primary myocardial disease that most often manifests as HFrEF but can present as HFmrEF or HFpEF early in its course or after partial recovery, highlighting that EF reflects phenotype rather than underlying pathology. Dilated cardiomyopathy is a large group of heterogeneous myocardial disorders characterized by reduced myocardial contractility in the absence of abnormal loading conditions such as with hypertension or valvular disease. The prevalence averages 59 cases/100,000 in the United States and accounts for at least 10,000 deaths annually. Black patients are affected three times as often as White patients. The prognosis is poor, with 50% mortality at 5 years once symptoms emerge.

Causes of dilated cardiomyopathy are multiple and diverse; up to 20–35% have a familial etiology. It is common for hereditary cases to first manifest with conduction system disease prior to a reduced LVEF. Endocrine, inflammatory, and metabolic causes include obesity, diabetes, thyroid disease, celiac disease, SLE, acromegaly, and growth hormone deficiency. While a large proportion of dilated cardiomyopathy causes are thought to be idiopathic, genetic variants may be responsible for many of these. Toxin-induced, drug-induced, and inflammatory causes are listed in the prior section. Nutritional diseases such as deficiency of thiamine, selenium, and carnitine have also been documented. Dilated cardiomyopathy may also be caused by prolonged tachycardia either from supraventricular arrhythmias, high PVC burden (> 15% of heart beats), or RV pacing. Dilated cardiomyopathy is also associated with HIV, Chagas disease, rheumatologic disorders, iron overload, sleep apnea, amyloidosis, sarcoidosis, chronic alcohol usage, ESKD, or cobalt exposure ("Quebec beer-drinkers' cardiomyopathy"). Peripartum cardiomyopathy also is a form of dilated cardiomyopathy, which will be discussed separately.

Clinical Findings

A. Symptoms and Signs

In most patients, symptoms of HF develop gradually. It is important to seek out a history of familial dilated cardiomyopathy and to identify behaviors that might predispose patients to the disease. The physical examination reveals rales, an elevated JVP, cardiomegaly, S_3 gallop rhythm, often the murmurs of functional mitral or tricuspid regurgitation, peripheral edema, or ascites. In severe HF, Cheyne-Stokes breathing, pulsus alternans, pallor, and cyanosis may be present.

B. ECG and Chest Radiography

The major findings are listed in Table 11–3. Sinus tachycardia is common. Other common abnormalities include left bundle branch block and ventricular or atrial arrhythmias.

Table 11–3. Classification of the cardiomyopathies by morphology.

	Dilated	Hypertrophic	Restrictive
Frequent causes	Idiopathic, alcoholic, major catecholamine discharge, myocarditis, postpartum, chemotherapy, endocrinopathies, genetic diseases, burnt out HOCM, CAD, tachycardia-induced, cocaine	Hereditary syndrome, possibly chronic hypertension in older adults	Amyloidosis, post-radiation, post–open heart surgery, diabetes, endomyocardial fibrosis, Fabry disease, sarcoidosis
Symptoms	Left or biventricular HF	Dyspnea, chest pain, syncope	Dyspnea, fatigue, right HF > left HF
Physical examination	Cardiomegaly, S_3, elevated jugular venous pressure, rales	Sustained point of maximal impulse, S_4, variable systolic murmur, bisferiens carotid pulse	Elevated jugular venous pressure
ECG	ST–T changes, conduction abnormalities, ventricular ectopy	LVH, exaggerated septal Q waves	ST–T changes, conduction abnormalities, low voltage
CXR	Enlarged heart, pulmonary congestion	Mild cardiomegaly	Mild to moderate cardiomegaly
Echocardiogram, nuclear studies, MRI, PET, CT	LV dilation and dysfunction	LVH, asymmetric septal or other myocardial wall thickness > 15 mm, small LV size, normal or supranormal function, systolic anterior mitral motion, diastolic dysfunction. May be nonobstructive or apical	Small or normal LV size, normal or mildly reduced LV function. Gadolinium hyperenhancement on MRI
Cardiac catheterization	LV dilation and dysfunction, high diastolic pressures, low cardiac output. Coronary angiography important to exclude ischemic cause	Small, hypercontractile LV, dynamic outflow gradient, diastolic dysfunction	High diastolic pressure, "square root" sign, normal or mildly reduced LV function

HOCM, hypertrophic obstructive cardiomyopathy.

The CXR reveals cardiomegaly, evidence for left and/or right HF, and pleural effusions (right more frequently than left).

C. Diagnostic Studies

Per the 2022 AHA/ACC/HFSA guidelines, patients with dyspnea should have a BNP or NT-proBNP measured to help establish prognosis and disease severity (class I, level of evidence [LOE] A).

An echocardiogram is indicated to exclude primary valvular or other lesions and confirm the presence of ventricular dilatation, reduced LV systolic function and associated RV systolic dysfunction, or pulmonary hypertension. Mitral Doppler inflow patterns also help in the diagnosis of concomitant diastolic dysfunction. Color flow Doppler can reveal valvular regurgitation, and continuous Doppler can estimate PA pressures. Intracavitary thrombosis is occasionally seen. Exercise or pharmacologic stress myocardial perfusion imaging may uncover underlying coronary disease. Radionuclide ventriculography provides a noninvasive measure of the EF and both RV and LV wall motion, though its use has been supplanted by cardiac MRI in most institutions. Cardiac MRI is particularly helpful in inflammatory or infiltrative processes, such as sarcoidosis or hemochromatosis, and is the diagnostic study of choice for RV dysplasia. MRI can also help define an ischemic etiology by noting gadolinium hyperenhancement consistent with myocardial scar from infarction or prior myocarditis. Coronary angiogram is seldom of specific value unless myocardial ischemia is suspected, although right heart catheterization should be considered to help guide therapy when the clinical syndrome is not clear cut (class I indication, LOE C). Myocardial biopsy is rarely useful in establishing the diagnosis, although occasionally the underlying cause (eg, sarcoidosis, hemochromatosis) can be discerned (class IIa indication with LOE of C), and it should not be used routinely.

Treatment

Patients with HFrEF due to dilated cardiomyopathy should be managed similarly to those with traditional HFrEF. Standard therapy includes control of blood pressure and of contributing factors such as obesity, excessive alcohol, smoking, diabetes, or potentially cardiotoxic agents. All patients with reduced LVEF should be given ACE inhibitors, ARBs, or ideally sacubitril/valsartan, as well as selected β-blockers, spironolactone, and SGLT-2 inhibitors. If congestive symptoms are present, diuretics should be added. Calcium channel blockers should be avoided except as necessary to control ventricular response in atrial fibrillation or flutter or hypertension after being on all guideline-directed treatments for the HF.

To help prevent sudden death, an ICD is reasonable (class IIa, LOE B) in asymptomatic ischemic cardiomyopathy patients with an LVEF of < 30% on appropriate medical therapy (at least 3 months post-MI). Many patients may be candidates for cardiac synchronization therapy with biventricular pacing if there is significant mitral regurgitation and the QRS width is > 150 msec. Cardiac rehabilitation and exercise training have consistently been found to improve clinical status.

Few cases of dilated cardiomyopathy are amenable to specific therapy for the underlying cause. Alcohol use should be discontinued, as there is often marked recovery of cardiac function following a period of abstinence in alcohol-associated cardiomyopathy. Endocrine causes (hyperthyroidism or hypothyroidism, acromegaly, and pheochromocytoma) should be treated. Empiric immunosuppressive therapy is not indicated in chronic dilated cardiomyopathy. There are some patients who may benefit from implantable LV assist devices either as a bridge to transplantation or as a temporary measure until cardiac function returns. LV assist devices can be considered as **destination therapy** in patients who are not candidates for cardiac transplantation. Arterial and pulmonary emboli are more common in dilated cardiomyopathy than in ischemic cardiomyopathy, and suitable candidates may benefit from long-term anticoagulation. *DOACs are preferred over warfarin unless there is associated moderate or severe mitral stenosis,* especially when a mobile LV thrombus is observed on the echocardiogram.

Prognosis

The prognosis of dilated cardiomyopathy without clinical HF is variable, with some patients remaining stable, some deteriorating gradually, and others declining rapidly. Once HF arises, the natural history is similar to that of other causes of HF, with an annual mortality rate of around 11–13%. The underlying cause of HF has prognostic value in patients with unexplained cardiomyopathy. Patients with peripartum cardiomyopathy or stress-induced cardiomyopathy appear to have a better prognosis than those with other forms of cardiomyopathy. Patients with cardiomyopathy due to infiltrative myocardial diseases, HIV infection, or doxorubicin therapy have an especially poor prognosis.

When to Refer

Patients with new or worsening symptoms of HF with dilated cardiomyopathy should be referred to a cardiologist. Patients with continued symptoms of HF and reduced LVEF (≤ 35%) should be referred for consideration of placement of an ICD or cardiac resynchronization therapy (if QRS duration is ≥ 150 msec, especially with a left bundle branch block pattern). Patients with advanced refractory symptoms should be referred to an advanced HF specialist for consideration of heart transplant or LV assist device therapy.

When to Admit

Patients with hypoxia, fluid overload, or pulmonary edema not readily resolved in an outpatient setting should be admitted.

Heidenreich PA et al. 2022 AHA/ACC/HFSA Guideline for the Management of Heart Failure: a report of the American College of Cardiology/American Heart Association Joint Committee on Clinical Practice Guidelines. J Am Coll Cardiol. 2022;79:e263. Erratum in: J Am Coll Cardiol. 2023;81:1551. [PMID: 35379503]

TAKOTSUBO CARDIOMYOPATHY

ESSENTIALS OF DIAGNOSIS

- Occurs after a major catecholamine surge.
- Acute chest pain or shortness of breath.
- Disproportionately affects postmenopausal women.
- Presentation is similar to acute anterior MI, but coronaries are often normal on angiography.
- Imaging reveals apical LV ballooning due to anteroapical stunning of the myocardium.
- Most patients recover completely, although there are complications similar to MI.

General Considerations

Takotsubo syndrome (also known as "stress-induced cardiomyopathy" or "stress cardiomyopathy") often follows a high catecholamine surge. The apical aspect of the LV takes a rounded ampulla form similar to a Japanese octopus pot (takotsubo). Mid-ventricular ballooning has also been described. The key feature is that the myocardial stunning does *not* follow the pattern suggestive of coronary ischemia (even though about 15% of patients will have coexisting CAD, and some may have concomitant plaque rupture MI). *More than two-thirds of patients report a prior stressful event,* either emotional or physical, including hypoglycemia, lightning strikes, earthquakes, ventricular tachycardia, alcohol withdrawal, recent surgery, hyperthyroidism, recent stroke, or recent emotional stress ("broken-heart syndrome"). *Virtually any event that triggers excess catecholamines has been implicated in a wide number of case reports.* Pericarditis and even tamponade have been described in isolated cases. Recurrences have also been described. In Western countries, the disease *predominantly affects women (up to 90%), primarily postmenopausal.* Compared to patients with isolated ACS, patients with stress cardiomyopathy are more likely to have concomitant neurologic and psychiatric disorders. Patients with COPD, migraines, or mood disorders who take β-agonists may have an increased risk of a poor outcome. The prognosis was previously thought to be benign, but subsequent studies have demonstrated that *both short- and long-term mortality are elevated;* mortality reported during the acute phase in hospitalized patients is approximately 4–5%, a figure comparable to that of STEMI in the era of primary percutaneous coronary interventions. Approximately 10% of patients will experience an adverse cardiac or neurologic event over the next year.

Stress-induced cardiomyopathy is mediated by the central and autonomic nervous systems. Acute stressors induce CNS activation, increasing bioavailability of cortisol and catecholamine. Both circulating epinephrine and norepinephrine released from adrenal medullary chromaffin cells, and norepinephrine released locally from sympathetic nerve terminals, are significantly increased. This catecholamine surge leads to myocardial damage through multiple mechanisms, including direct catecholamine toxicity, adrenoceptor-mediated damage, epicardial and microvascular coronary vasoconstriction and/or spasm, and increased cardiac workload. The relative preponderance among postmenopausal women suggests that estrogen deprivation may be facilitating, possibly via endothelial dysfunction.

Clinical Findings

A. Symptoms and Signs

The symptoms are similar to any ACS. Typical angina and dyspnea are usually present. Syncope is rare, although arrhythmias are not uncommon.

B. ECG and Chest Radiography

The ECG may reveal ST-segment elevation as well as deep anterior T-wave inversion. The dramatic T-wave inversions gradually resolve over time. The CXR is either normal or reveals pulmonary congestion.

C. Diagnostic Studies

The echocardiogram reveals LV apical dyskinesia and possible ballooning, usually not consistent with any particular coronary distribution, though distal LAD distribution may be present. The urgent cardiac catheterization will be negative for ACS (ie, coronaries without acute plaque rupture). Initial cardiac biomarkers, such as troponin and BNP, are usually positive but often taper quickly. In almost all cases, MRI hyperenhancement studies reveal no long-term scarring.

Treatment

Most patients are treated especially for ACS, given the similar clinical presentation, before an ischemic evaluation excludes ACS/ischemic cardiomyopathy. Treating clinicians should seek to identify and address the inciting stressor. If LVEF is < 50%, patients should be started on β-blockers and ACE inhibitors/ARBs until the LV recovers over subsequent weeks. See Treatment of Heart Failure with Reduced LVEF.

Prognosis

The rate of severe in-hospital complications, including shock and death, appears to be similar between patients with an ACS and Takotsubo cardiomyopathy. Overall, prognosis is good unless there is a serious complication (such as mitral regurgitation, ventricular rupture, or ventricular tachycardia). Recovery of the LVEF is expected in most cases after a period of days to weeks, especially with appropriate therapy. Echocardiogram should be repeated in 4–8 weeks.

When to Refer

All patients with an ACS should be seen urgently by a cardiologist for further evaluation and monitored until resolution of the ventricular dysfunction.

HYPERTROPHIC CARDIOMYOPATHY

ESSENTIALS OF DIAGNOSIS

- May manifest as dyspnea, chest pain, syncope.
- Though LV outflow tract (LVOT) gradient is classic, symptoms are primarily related to diastolic dysfunction.
- Echocardiogram is essential for diagnosis, with a hallmark LV wall thickness > 1.5 cm in the absence of chronically high afterload or infiltrative disease.
- Increased risk of sudden death.

General Considerations

In 2024, an ACC/AHA joint committee issued updated clinical practice guidelines for the diagnosis and treatment of HCM. The definition has evolved over time; while it traditionally was defined by LV outflow obstruction due to septal hypertrophy, currently it is considered present any time that *any portion of LV wall is measured at > 1.5 cm thick on an echocardiogram in the absence of elevated afterload (eg, chronic hypertension, aortic regurgitation) or myocardial infiltrative disease (eg, sarcoid, amyloid).* LVOT obstruction is not required for the diagnosis but may be present at rest or with maneuvers (eg, Valsalva). The increased wall thickness reduces LV systolic stress, increases the EF, and can result in "empty ventricle" at end systole. The interventricular septum may be disproportionately involved (**asymmetric septal hypertrophy**), but in some cases, the hypertrophy is localized to the midventricle or to the apex. In a normal heart, the LV apex may be paper thin; in HCM, the LVOT obstruction may trap blood just above the apex and the LV pressure may be very high there. This can result in the apex becoming aneurysmal. The LVOT is often narrowed during systole due to the hypertrophied septum. Systolic anterior motion of the mitral valve occurs as the anterior mitral valve leaflet is pulled into the LV outflow. The blood flow out of the LVOT is further worsened by factors that increase myocardial contractility (sympathetic stimulation, digoxin, and postextrasystolic beat) or that decrease LV filling (Valsalva maneuver, peripheral vasodilators). The amount of obstruction is preload and afterload dependent and can vary from day to day, and even moment to moment (eg, moving from sitting to standing). Apart from these systolic changes, *LV hypertrophy causes elevated diastolic pressures.* It is primarily this diastolic dysfunction that may cause symptoms of dyspnea and exercise intolerance. Rarely, systolic dysfunction develops late in the course of the disease. The LV is usually more involved than the RV, and the atria are frequently significantly enlarged.

HCM is most often inherited as an autosomal-dominant trait with variable penetrance and is caused by pathogenic variants in genes encoding sarcomeric proteins, most commonly β-myosin heavy chain (MYH7) or myosin-binding protein C (MYBPC 3). Prognosis can be influenced by the specific gene and phenotype. Clinical presentation is highly variable, but many patients are diagnosed in early adulthood. Elite athletes may demonstrate considerable hypertrophy that can be confused with HCM, but generally diastolic dysfunction is not present in the athlete and this finding helps separate pathologic disease from **athletic hypertrophy**. The apical variety is particularly common in those of Asian descent. *Older adults may exhibit LV hypertrophy that physiologically mimics true genetic HCM; this hypertrophy often involves a "sigmoid" interventricular septum, with a knob of cardiac muscle below the aortic valve, and is thought to be secondary to longstanding hypertension.* Mitral annular calcification also is often present. Mitral regurgitation is variable and often dynamic, depending on the degree of outflow tract obstruction.

Clinical Findings

A. Symptoms and Signs

The most frequent symptoms are dyspnea and chest pain. Syncope is also common and is typically postexertional, when diastolic filling diminishes due to tachycardia and fluid loss, increasing LV outflow tract obstruction. Residual circulating catecholamines accentuate these changes. Arrhythmias are an important problem. Atrial fibrillation is a long-term consequence of chronically elevated LA pressures and is a poor prognostic sign. Ventricular arrhythmias are also common, and sudden death may occur, often after extraordinary exertion.

Features on physical examination include a bisferiens carotid pulse, triple apical impulse (due to the prominent atrial filling wave and early and late systolic impulses), and a loud S_4. The JVP may reveal a prominent *a* wave due to reduced RV compliance. In cases with LV outflow obstruction, a loud systolic murmur is present along the left sternal border that increases with upright posture or Valsalva maneuver and decreases with squatting. These maneuvers help differentiate the murmur of HCM from that of aortic stenosis. In HCM, reducing the LV volume *increases* the outflow obstruction and the murmur intensity; whereas in valvular aortic stenosis, reducing the stroke volume across the valve *decreases* the murmur. Mitral regurgitation is frequently present as well.

B. ECG and Chest Radiography

LVH pattern is nearly universal in patients with HCM, though entirely normal ECGs are present in up to 25%, usually in those with localized hypertrophy. Exaggerated septal Q waves inferolaterally may mimic MI. The CXR is often unimpressive. Unlike with aortic stenosis, the ascending aorta is not dilated.

C. Diagnostic Studies

Echocardiogram is required for diagnosis, revealing LVH (involving the septum more commonly than the posterior walls), with or without systolic anterior motion of the mitral valve, early closing followed by reopening of the aortic valve, a small and hypercontractile LV, and delayed relaxation and filling of the LV during diastole. The septum can be 1.3–1.5 times the thickness of the posterior wall. Septal motion tends to be reduced. In hypertrophic obstructive cardiomyopathy, Doppler ultrasound reveals turbulent flow and a gradient in the LV outflow tract. Abnormalities in the diastolic filling pattern are present in 80% of patients. Mitral regurgitation often is seen as well. Echocardiography can usually differentiate HCM from **ventricular noncompaction**, a congenital myocardial disease pattern with marked trabeculation that partially fills the LV cavity.

Myocardial perfusion imaging may suggest septal ischemia in the presence of normal coronary arteries. Cardiac MRI confirms the hypertrophy and contrast enhancement frequently reveals evidence of scar at the junction of the RV attachment to the interventricular septum. Cardiac catheterization confirms the diagnosis and defines the presence or absence of CAD. Frequently, **coronary arterial milking** (squeezing of the coronary in systole) occurs, especially in the septal arteries. Exercise studies are recommended to assess for ventricular arrhythmias and to document the blood pressure response. Wearable patch monitors or longer-term implantable loop recorders are recommended for determination of ventricular ectopy.

Treatment

β-Blockers are the cornerstone of therapy for HCM, especially when dynamic outflow obstruction is noted on the echocardiogram. The resulting slower heart rates assist with diastolic filling of the stiff LV. β-Blockers also improve dyspnea, angina, and arrhythmias in about 50% of patients. Nondihydropyridine calcium channel blockers, especially verapamil, have also been effective in symptomatic patients and hold a class I recommendation. Their effect is due primarily to improved diastolic function; however, their vasodilating actions can also increase outflow obstruction and cause hypotension. Verapamil should not be used if there is hypotension or a resting gradient of > 100 mm Hg. Disopyramide is also effective because of its negative inotropic effects; it is usually used as an addition to the medical regimen rather than as primary therapy or to help control atrial arrhythmias. Oral diuretics are frequently necessary due to the high LV diastolic pressure and elevated LA pressures but should be used with caution to avoid dehydration that would increase obstruction. Digoxin is relatively contraindicated, except rarely for rate control in atrial fibrillation. For acute hypotension that does not respond to fluids, phenylephrine may be considered; pure α-receptor activity avoids β-adrenergic-mediated increases in HR and contractility, which can paradoxically reduce cardiac output in HCM. In a very small number of these patients, apical myomectomy may be considered.

The FDA has approved two novel agents for the treatment of symptomatic obstructive HCM: mavacamten (2022) and aficamten (2025). These medications are cardiac myosin inhibitors that decrease the number of active actin–myosin cross-bridges and thereby reduce cardiac hypercontractility. They have been shown to improve exercise capacity and symptoms.

HCM patients do best in sinus rhythm, and atrial fibrillation should be aggressively treated with antiarrhythmics or radiofrequency ablation. DOACs are preferred over warfarin if atrial fibrillation occurs. *Patients with HCM should anticoagulated regardless of their CHA_2DS_2-VASc score.*

The 2020 AHA/ACC guidelines recommend a preventive ICD for HCM patients with documented cardiac arrest or sustained ventricular tachycardia (class I). ICD placement holds a class IIa recommendation if any of the following risk factors are present: (1) sudden death in one or more first-degree or close relative 50 years of age or younger, (2) any LV wall ≥ 30 mm, (3) any recent syncope likely to have been arrhythmogenic, (4) LV apical aneurysm, or (5) LV systolic dysfunction (EF < 50%). It is a class IIb recommendation for an ICD if there is significant (> 15%) late gadolinium enhancement on cardiac MRI. In those who receive an ICD, antitachycardia pacing should be programmed to minimize defibrillator shocks. The use of an ICD is contraindicated, though, if the purpose is simply to allow for the patient to play competitive sports.

Excision of part of the outflow myocardial septum (**myotomy–myomectomy**) by experienced surgeons is successful in patients with symptoms unresponsive to medical therapy. A few surgeons advocate mitral valve replacement, since this results in resolution of the gradient and prevents associated mitral regurgitation. In some cases, myomectomy has been combined with an Alfieri stitch on the mitral valve (a stitch that binds the midportion of the anterior and posterior mitral valve leaflets together). Rare cases of progression to LV dilation or patients with intractable symptoms can be considered for cardiac transplantation. Nonsurgical septal ablation can be performed by injection of alcohol into septal branches of the left coronary artery to create a controlled myocardial infarct in the regions of greatest wall thickness. It is considered first-line therapy, if feasible, for those with LV outflow tract obstruction > 50 mm Hg who do not respond to medical therapy or who are not deemed surgical candidates. In "burnt out" HCM, the medical therapy is similar to that of dilated cardiomyopathy. In those with refractory arrhythmias or HF, cardiac transplantation is an option.

Pregnancy represents in an increased risk in patients with symptoms or outflow tract gradients of > 50 mm Hg. Genetic counseling is indicated before planned conception. In pregnant patients with HCM, continuation of β-blocker therapy is recommended. Further details on the impact of HCM on sport, activity, and occupation (such as driving commercially or piloting an aircraft) are outlined in the 2024 AHA/ACC guidelines.

When to Refer

Patients should be referred to a cardiologist to establish care, consider genetic testing, review the presence of any high-risk features, and discuss medications or the need for any intervention. This is particularly important if any symptoms are present.

Ommen SR et al; Peer Review Committee Members. 2024 AHA/ACC/AMSSM/HRS/PACES/SCMR guideline for the management of hypertrophic cardiomyopathy: a report of the American Heart Association/American College of Cardiology Joint Committee on Clinical Practice Guidelines. Circulation. 2024;149:e1239. Erratum in: Circulation. 2024;150:e198. [PMID: 38718139]

RESTRICTIVE CARDIOMYOPATHY

ESSENTIALS OF DIAGNOSIS

- Right HF tends to dominate over left HF.
- Pulmonary hypertension is often present.
- Echocardiography is required for diagnosis.
- Amyloidosis is the most common cause.

General Considerations

Restrictive cardiomyopathy is characterized by *impaired diastolic function due to stiffened ventricles. A variety of processes can lead to restrictive cardiomyopathy, such as infiltrative diseases (eg, amyloidosis), storage diseases (eg, Fabry disease), fibrotic processes (eg, post-radiation), medications (eg, chemotherapies), and idiopathic processes.* Unlike HCM and dilated cardiomyopathy, the ventricles are typically non-hypertrophied and non-dilated. The condition is relatively uncommon, with the most frequent cause being amyloidosis. HF due to restrictive cardiomyopathy often presents with a preserved EF (≥ 50%). However, as discussed previously, it is inappropriate to give these patients the diagnostic label of HFpEF, which is its own clinical entity. Rather, the terminology *HF due to restrictive cardiomyopathy* is preferred.

The diagnosis of **cardiac amyloidosis** has dramatically increased in the last few years as diagnostic testing has improved and there is a greater awareness of its prevalence. The prevalence of **AL amyloid** (immunoglobulin light chain) is approximately 12 cases per million; the prevalence of **variant or hereditary ATTR amyloid** is about 0.3 cases per million; and the prevalence of **wild type ATTR amyloid** is 155–191 cases per million. Many experts believe the actual prevalence of wild-type ATTR is much higher. While light-chain amyloid proteins can be toxic to cardiomyocytes, they may also internalize into many cell types, further leading to cardiac dysfunction. ATTR refers to *transthyretin*, a protein normally found in the liver that helps transport thyroid hormones and vitamin A. TTR is a tetramer that can dissociate into four monomers and aggregate as amyloid fibrils. Wild type (normal protein) occurs more commonly in older adults and in men, and previously was referred to as "senile systemic amyloidosis." Hereditary or variant ATTR is genetically transmitted; deposition occurs at an earlier age and the disease has an associated neurologic impact.

Clinical Findings

A. Symptoms and Signs

Traditional HF symptoms are often present. Other symptoms may include angina, syncope, stroke, and peripheral neuropathy. Periorbital purpura, a thickened tongue, and hepatomegaly are all suggestive physical findings of amyloidosis specifically.

B. Diagnostic Studies

When clinicians encounter new HF due to diastolic dysfunction, they should consider the broad differential diagnosis of restrictive cardiomyopathy (as above). Careful history and physical may guide raise suspicion for a particular underlying etiology and guide serologic workup.

Of note, restrictive cardiomyopathy must be distinguished from constrictive pericarditis (see Table 11–3).

Evaluation for cardiac amyloidosis itself includes assessment for a monoclonal protein using serum free light chain assay in combination with serum and urine immunofixation electrophoresis. If negative, primary or light chain amyloidosis are ruled out. Conduction disturbances are frequently present. Low voltage on the ECG combined with ventricular hypertrophy on the echocardiogram is suggestive of the disease. **Technetium-99 pyrophosphate imaging (bone scan imaging)** can also identify amyloid deposition in the myocardium, and it has become the noninvasive imaging modality of choice for diagnosing transthyretin (ATTR) amyloidosis. With typical scintigraphic findings in patients without a monoclonal gammopathy, biopsy is no longer necessary for diagnosis. Cardiac MRI is helpful when technetium-99 pyrophosphate scan is negative but a high suspicion remains for another type of cardiac amyloidosis (eg, AL amyloid); it will show a distinctive pattern of diffuse hyperenhancement of the gadolinium. A high degree of late gadolinium enhancement suggests more extensive cardiac involvement. The echocardiogram reveals a small, thickened LV with bright myocardium (speckled), rapid early diastolic filling revealed by the mitral inflow Doppler, and biatrial enlargement. Characteristic longitudinal strain patterns may help identify cardiac amyloidosis. The LV chamber size is usually normal with a reduced LVEF. Atrial septal thickening may be evident and an amyloid variant that primarily affects the atria has been described. Rectal, abdominal fat, or gingival biopsies can confirm systemic involvement, but myocardial involvement may still be present if these are negative and requires endomyocardial biopsy for the confirmation that cardiac amyloid is present. Demonstration of tissue infiltration on biopsy specimens using special stains followed by immunohistochemical studies and genetic testing are essential to define which specific protein is involved. TTR gene sequencing in patients in whom the TTR wild type or TTR variant is suspected and mass spectroscopy on all tissue in question are recommended highly. BNP and NT-proBNP are traditionally elevated and have been used to help distinguish constrictive pericarditis from a restrictive cardiomyopathy.

Treatment

Treatment for restrictive cardiomyopathy is not the same as "garden-variety" HFpEF. SGLT2 inhibitors and MRAs have *not* been shown to confer benefit. Rather, treatment should be directed at the disease process underlying the restrictive physiology.

In acute HF in restrictive cardiomyopathy, diuretics can help, but excessive diuresis can produce worsening kidney dysfunction. Atrial thrombi are not uncommon, although the role of anticoagulation in amyloidosis remains ill defined. Digoxin may precipitate arrhythmias and should *not* be used. β-Blockers help slow heart rates and improve filling by increasing diastolic time. Verapamil presumably works by improving myocardial relaxation and increasing diastolic filling time. Slower heart rates are desired to allow for increased diastolic filling time. ACE inhibition or angiotensin II receptor blockade may improve diastolic relaxation and filling at times and can be tried with caution if the systemic blood pressure is adequate. Corticosteroids may be helpful in sarcoidosis. Restrictive cardiomyopathy due to hemochromatosis is treated with phlebotomy, chelation, or both.

AL amyloidosis includes alkylator-based chemotherapy or high-dose melphalan followed by autologous stem cell transplantation. In immunoglobin light-chain amyloidosis, standard- or high-dose chemotherapy with stem cell rescue is often pursued. Treatment of ATTR amyloid is undergoing an evolution. Two medications that stabilize transthyretin—tafamidis and acoramidis—are approved by the FDA to treat ATTR cardiomyopathy. They both reduced the composite of all-cause mortality and cardiovascular hospitalizations in clinical trials. An amyloid RNA interference therapeutic, vutrisiran, that reduces liver production of the amyloid protein, also has been approved by the FDA to treat cardiac amyloid.

When to Refer

All patients with the diagnosis of a restrictive cardiomyopathy should be referred to a cardiologist to discern etiology and plan appropriate treatment. Unexplained LVH with relatively preserved LVEF, low voltage on ECG, and symptoms of HF should raise prompt consideration of cardiac amyloid, particularly now that there are effective targeted treatments.

Kittleson MM et al. 2023 ACC Expert Consensus Decision Pathway on Management of Heart Failure With Preserved Ejection Fraction: a report of the American College of Cardiology Solution Set Oversight Committee. J Am Coll Cardiol. 2023;81:1835. [PMID: 37137593]

Writing Committee; Kittleson MM et al. 2023 ACC Expert Consensus Decision Pathway on Comprehensive Multidisciplinary Care for the Patient With Cardiac Amyloidosis: a report of the American College of Cardiology Solution Set Oversight Committee. J Am Coll Cardiol. 2023;81:1076. Erratum in: J Am Coll Cardiol. 2023;81:1135. [PMID: 36697326]

Disorders of Cardiac Rhythm

12

Kevin P. Jackson, MD

DISORDERS OF RATE & RHYTHM

Abnormalities of cardiac rhythm and conduction can be symptomatic (syncope, near syncope, dizziness, fatigue, or palpitations) or asymptomatic. In addition, they can be lethal (sudden cardiac death [SCD]) or dangerous to the extent that they reduce cardiac output, so that perfusion of the brain and myocardium is impaired. Stable supraventricular tachycardia (SVT) is generally well tolerated in patients without underlying heart disease but may lead to myocardial ischemia or HF in patients with coronary disease, valvular abnormalities, and systolic or diastolic myocardial dysfunction. Ventricular tachycardia, if prolonged, often results in hemodynamic compromise and may deteriorate into ventricular fibrillation if left untreated.

Whether slow heart rates produce symptoms at rest or with exertion depends on whether cerebral and peripheral perfusion can be maintained, which is generally a function of whether the patient is upright or supine and whether LV function is adequate to maintain stroke volume. If the heart rate abruptly slows, as with the onset of complete heart block or sinus arrest, syncope or convulsions (or both) may result. *Unless a clear, reversible cause is found, most symptomatic patients require implantation of a permanent pacemaker.*

The diagnosis of an abnormal tachyarrhythmia often can be made via cardiac monitoring, including in-hospital and ambulatory ECG monitoring, event recorders, continuous mobile cardiac telemetry, or implantable loop recorders. Additionally, optic sensors on wearable devices, such as smartwatches, utilize a passive irregular pulse notification algorithm to identify possible arrhythmia, with a positive predictive value for detection of atrial fibrillation of approximately 85%. Devices, such as Apple Watch, Fitbit, and the AliveCor device, can record ECGs of the rhythm that can be transmitted to health care providers. More invasive testing, including catheter-based electrophysiologic studies (to assess sinus node function, atrioventricular [AV] conduction, and inducibility of arrhythmias), and tests of autonomic nervous system function (tilt-table testing) can also be performed.

Treatment of tachyarrhythmias varies and can include modalities such as antiarrhythmic medications and more invasive techniques such as catheter ablation.

Antiarrhythmic Medications

Antiarrhythmic medications are frequently used to treat arrhythmias but have variable efficacy and produce frequent side effects (Table 12–1). They are often divided into classes based on their electropharmacologic actions and many of these medications have multiple actions. The most frequently used classification scheme is the **Vaughan-Williams**, which consists of four classes.

Class I agents block membrane sodium channels. Three subclasses are further defined by the effect of the agents on the Purkinje fiber action potential. **Class Ia** medications (ie, quinidine, procainamide, disopyramide) slow the rate of rise of the action potential (V_{max}) and prolong its duration, thus slowing conduction and increasing refractoriness. **Class Ib** agents (ie, lidocaine, mexiletine) shorten action potential duration; they do not affect conduction or refractoriness. **Class Ic** agents (ie, flecainide, propafenone) prolong V_{max} and slow repolarization, thus slowing conduction and prolonging refractoriness, but more so than class Ia medications.

Class II agents are the β-blockers, which decrease automaticity, prolong AV conduction, and prolong refractoriness.

Class III agents (ie, amiodarone, dronedarone, sotalol, dofetilide, ibutilide) block potassium channels and prolong repolarization, prolonging the QT interval. Drug-induced torsade de pointes occurs in up to 3% of patients on sotalol and dofetilide and these agents require careful monitoring.

Class IV agents are the calcium channel blockers, which decrease automaticity and AV conduction.

There are some antiarrhythmic agents that do not fall into one of these categories. Ivabradine affects the spontaneous depolarization ("funny current") of the sinoatrial node and slows the sinus rate. Digoxin inhibits the Na^+, K^+-ATPase pump, which prolongs AV nodal conduction and the AV nodal refractory period. Adenosine can block AV nodal conduction and shortens atrial refractoriness. Ranolazine is an antianginal medication that prolongs atrial and ventricular action potential duration and may treat refractory atrial and ventricular arrhythmias when used in combination with other agents (ie, amiodarone or dronedarone).

Table 12–1. Antiarrhythmic medications (listed in alphabetical order within classes).

Agent	Intravenous Dosage	Oral Dosage	Therapeutic Plasma Level	Route of Elimination	Side Effects
Class Ia: Action: Sodium channel blockers: Depress phase 0 depolarization; slow conduction; prolong repolarization.					
Indications: Supraventricular tachycardia, ventricular tachycardia, symptomatic ventricular premature beats.					
Disopyramide		Immediate release: 100–200 mg every 6 hours Sustained release: 200–400 mg every 12 hours	2–8 mg/mL	Renal	Urinary retention, dry mouth, markedly ↓ LVF, QT prolongation
Procainamide	Loading: 10–17 mg/kg at 20–50 mg/min Maintenance: 1–4 mg/min	50 mg/kg/day in divided doses every 4 hours (short-acting)	4–10 mg/mL; NAPA (active metabolite), 10–20 mcg/mL	Renal	
Quinidine	6–10 mg/kg (intramuscularly or intravenously) over 20 minutes (rarely used parenterally)	324–648 mg every 8 hours	2–5 mg/mL	Hepatic	GI, ↓ LVF, ↑ Dig
Class Ib: Action: Shorten repolarization.					
Indications: Ventricular tachycardia, prevention of ventricular fibrillation, symptomatic ventricular premature beats.					
Lidocaine	Loading: 1 mg/kg Maintenance: 1–4 mg/min		1–5 mg/mL	Hepatic	CNS, GI, ↓ LVF
Mexiletine		100–300 mg every 8–12 hours; maximum: 1200 mg/day	0.5–2 mg/mL	Hepatic	CNS, GI, leukopenia
Class Ic: Action: Depress phase 0 repolarization; slow conduction. (Propafenone is a weak calcium channel blocker and β-blocker and prolongs action potential and refractoriness.)					
Indications: Ventricular tachycardia (in the absence of structural heart disease), refractory supraventricular tachycardia.					
Flecainide		50–150 mg twice daily	0.2–1 mg/mL	Hepatic	CNS, GI, AFL with 1:1 conduction, ventricular proarrhythmia
Propafenone		150–300 mg every 8–12 hours	Note: Active metabolites	Hepatic	CNS, GI, AFL with 1:1 conduction, ventricular proarrhythmia
Class II: Action: β-blockers, slow AV conduction.					
Indications: Supraventricular tachycardia, ventricular tachycardia, symptomatic ventricular premature beats, long QT syndrome.					
Esmolol	Loading: 500 mcg/kg over 1–2 minutes Maintenance: 50–300 mcg/kg/min	Other β-blockers may be used concomitantly	Not established	Hepatic	↓ LVF, bradycardia, AV block
Metoprolol	5 mg every 5 minutes up to 3 doses	25–200 mg daily	Not established	Hepatic	↓ LVF, bradycardia, AV block, fatigue
Propranolol	1–3 mg every 5 minutes up to total of 5 mg	40–320 mg in 1–4 doses daily (depending on preparation)	Not established	Hepatic	↓ LVF, bradycardia, AV block, bronchospasm
Class III: Action: Prolong action potential.					
Indications: *Amiodarone:* refractory ventricular tachycardia, supraventricular tachycardia, prevention of ventricular tachycardia, atrial fibrillation, ventricular fibrillation; *Dofetilide:* atrial fibrillation and flutter; *Dronedarone:* atrial fibrillation (not persistent); *Ibutilide:* conversion of atrial fibrillation and flutter; *Sotalol:* ventricular tachycardia, atrial fibrillation.					
Amiodarone	150–300 mg infused rapidly, followed by 1 mg/min infusion for 6 hours and then 0.5 mg/min for 18 hours	800–1600 mg/day for 7–14 days; maintain at 100–400 mg/day	1–5 mg/mL	Hepatic	Pulmonary fibrosis, hypothyroidism, hyperthyroidism, photosensitivity, corneal and skin deposits, hepatitis, neurotoxicity, GI

(*continued*)

Table 12–1. Antiarrhythmic medications (listed in alphabetical order within classes). (continued)

Agent	Intravenous Dosage	Oral Dosage	Therapeutic Plasma Level	Route of Elimination	Side Effects
Dofetilide		125–500 mcg every 12 hours		Renal (dose must be reduced with kidney dysfunction)	Torsades de pointes in 3%; interaction with cytochrome P-450 inhibitors
Dronedarone		400 mg twice daily		Hepatic (contra-indicated in severe impairment)	Contraindicated in HF (NYHA class IV or recent decompensa-tion), persistent AF
Ibutilide	1 mg over 10 minutes, followed by a second infusion of 0.5–1 mg over 10 minutes			Hepatic and renal	Torsades de pointes in up to 3% of patients within 3 hours after administration; patients must be monitored with defibrillator nearby
Sotalol	75 mg every 12 hours	80–160 mg every 12 hours (maximum 320 mg daily)		Renal (dosing interval should be extended if creatinine clearance is < 60 mL/min)	Torsades de pointes in 1%; ↓ LVF, bradycardia, fatigue (and other side effects associated with β-blockers)
Class IV: Action: Calcium channel blockers.					
Indications: Supraventricular tachycardia, ventricular tachycardia (outflow tract, idiopathic).					
Diltiazem	0.25 mg/kg over 2 minutes; second 0.35-mg/kg bolus after 15 minutes if response is inadequate; infusion rate, 5–15 mg/hour	120–360 mg daily in 1–3 doses depending on preparation		Hepatic metabo-lism, renal excretion	Hypotension, ↓ LVF, bradycardia
Etripamil	70 mg administered as two nasal sprays; may be repeated after 10 minutes			Renal and fecal	Nasal discomfort, throat irritation, hypotension
Verapamil	2.5-mg bolus followed by additional boluses of 2.5–5 mg every 1–3 minutes; total 20 mg over 20 minutes; main-tain at 5 mg/kg/min	80–120 mg every 6–8 hours; 240–480 mg once daily with sustained-release preparation	0.1–0.15 mg/mL	Hepatic	Hypotension, ↓ LVF, constipation
Miscellaneous					
Adenosine	6-mg bolus followed by rapid saline flush; may repeat with 12-mg bolus after 1–2 minutes if needed			Adenosine recep-tor stimula-tion, metabolized in blood	Transient flushing, dyspnea, chest pain, AV block, sinus bradycardia; effect ↓ by theophylline, ↑ by dipyridamole
Digoxin	0.5 mg over 20 minutes followed by increment of 0.25 or 0.125 mg to 1–1.5 mg over 24 hours	1–1.5 mg over 24–36 hours in 3 or 4 doses; maintenance, 0.125–0.5 mg/day	0.7–2 mg/mL	Renal	AV block, arrhythmias, GI, visual changes
Ivabradine		5–7.5 mg every 12 hours		Renal and fecal	Bradycardia, phosphenes (visual brightness)
Ranolazine		500–750 mg every 12 hours		Renal and fecal	Dizziness, nausea

AF, atrial fibrillation; AV, atrioventricular; Dig, elevation of serum digoxin level; ↓LVF, reduced LV function; NAPA, *N*-acetylprocainamide; NYHA, New York Heart Association.

Although the in vitro electrophysiologic effects of most of these agents have been defined, their use remains largely empiric. *Many can exacerbate arrhythmias (**proarrhythmic effect**), and some depress LV function.*

The risk of antiarrhythmic agents has been highlighted by many studies, most notably the Coronary Arrhythmia Suppression Trial (CAST), in which two class Ic agents (flecainide, encainide) and a class Ia agent (moricizine) *increased* mortality rates in patients with asymptomatic ventricular ectopy after MI. Class Ic antiarrhythmic agents should therefore *not* be used in patients with prior MI or structural heart disease.

The use of antiarrhythmic agents for specific arrhythmias is discussed below.

Catheter Ablation for Cardiac Arrhythmias

Catheter ablation has become the primary modality of therapy for many symptomatic supraventricular arrhythmias, including AV nodal reentrant tachycardia, tachycardias involving accessory pathways, paroxysmal atrial tachycardia, and atrial flutter. Catheter ablation of atrial fibrillation is more complex and involves complete electrical isolation of the pulmonary veins (which are often the sites of initiation of atrial fibrillation) and at times placing linear lesions within the atria to prevent propagation throughout the atrial chamber. This technique is considered a reasonable therapy for symptomatic patients with medication-refractory atrial fibrillation or as an alternative to long-term antiarrhythmic medication treatment. In younger patients, catheter ablation of atrial fibrillation may be first-line therapy to improve symptoms and prevent progression to persistent atrial fibrillation. Catheter ablation of ventricular arrhythmias has proved more difficult, but experienced centers have demonstrated reasonable success with all types of ventricular tachycardias including bundle branch reentry, tachycardia originating in the ventricular outflow tract or papillary muscles, tachycardias originating in the specialized conduction system (fascicular ventricular tachycardia), and ventricular tachycardias occurring in patients with ischemic or dilated cardiomyopathy. Ablation of many of these arrhythmias can be performed from the endocardial surface via endovascular catheter placement or on the epicardial surface of the heart via a percutaneous subxiphoid approach.

Catheter ablation has also been successfully performed for the treatment of ventricular fibrillation when a uniform premature ventricular contraction (PVC) can be identified. In addition, patients with symptomatic PVCs or PVCs occurring at a high enough burden to result in a cardiomyopathy (usually > 10,000/day) may be considered for catheter ablation as well.

Catheter ablation procedures are generally safe, with an overall major complication rate ranging from 1% to 5%. Major vascular damage during catheter insertion occurs in < 2% of patients. There is a low incidence of perforation of the myocardial wall resulting in pericardial tamponade. Inadvertent damage to the AV node requiring permanent cardiac pacing occurs in < 1% of patients. When transseptal access through the interatrial septum or retrograde LV catheterization is required, additional potential complications include damage to the heart valves, damage to a coronary artery, or systemic emboli.

Merino J et al. Practical compendium of antiarrhythmic drugs: a clinical consensus statement of the European Heart Rhythm Association of the European Society of Cardiology. Europace. 2025;27;euaf076. [PMID: 40159403]

SINUS ARRHYTHMIA, BRADYCARDIA, & TACHYCARDIA

ESSENTIALS OF DIAGNOSIS

- Wide variation in sinus rate is common in young, healthy individuals and generally not pathologic.
- Symptomatic bradycardia may require permanent pacemaker implantation, especially in older adults or patients with underlying heart disease.
- Sinus tachycardia is usually secondary to another underlying process (ie, fever, pain, anemia, alcohol withdrawal).
- Sick sinus syndrome manifests as sinus bradycardia, pauses, or inadequate heart rate response to physiologic demands (chronotropic incompetence).

General Considerations

Sinus arrhythmia is an irregularity of the normal heart rate defined as variation in the PP interval of > 120 msec. This occurs commonly in young, healthy people due to changes in vagal influence on the sinus node during respiration (phasic) or independent of respiration (nonphasic). This is generally *not* a pathologic arrhythmia and requires no specific cardiac evaluation.

Sinus bradycardia is defined as a heart rate slower than 60 beats/min and may be due to increased vagal influence on the normal sinoatrial pacemaker or organic disease of the sinus node. In healthy individuals, and particularly in well-trained athletes, sinus bradycardia to rates of 50 beats/min or lower especially during sleep is a normal finding. However, in older adult patients and individuals with heart disease, sinus bradycardia may be an indication of true sinus node pathology. *When the sinus rate slows severely, the atrial-nodal junction or the nodal-His bundle junction may assume pacemaker activity for the heart, usually at a rate of 35–60 beats/min.*

Sinus tachycardia is defined as a heart rate faster than 100 beats/min that is caused by rapid impulse formation from the sinoatrial node. It is a normal physiologic response to exercise or other conditions in which catecholamine release is increased. *The onset and termination are usually gradual, in contrast to paroxysmal supraventricular tachycardia (PSVT) due to reentry.* In rare instances, otherwise healthy individuals may present with "inappropriate" sinus tachycardia where persistently elevated basal heart rates are not in-line with physiologic demands. Long-term consequences of this disorder are few.

Sick sinus syndrome is a broad diagnosis applied to patients with sinus arrest, sinoatrial exit block (recognized by a pause equal to a multiple of the underlying PP interval or progressive shortening of the PP interval prior to a pause), or persistent sinus bradycardia. A common presentation in older adult patients is of recurrent SVT (often atrial fibrillation) accompanied by bradyarrhythmias (**"tachy-brady syndrome"**). The long pauses that often follow the termination of tachycardia cause the associated symptoms. Sick sinus syndrome may also manifest as **chronotropic incompetence**, defined as an inappropriate heart rate response to the physiologic demands of exercise or stress, and is an underrecognized cause of poor exercise tolerance.

Clinical Findings

In most patients, sinus arrhythmia (bradycardia or tachycardia) does not cause symptoms in the absence of underlying cardiac disease or other comorbidities. When severe sinus bradycardia results in low cardiac output, however, patients may report weakness, confusion, or syncope if cerebral perfusion is impaired. Sinus bradycardia is often exacerbated by medications (digitalis, calcium channel blockers, β-blockers, sympatholytic agents, antiarrhythmics), and nonessential agents that may be responsible should be withdrawn prior to making the diagnosis.

Sinus tachycardia is most often a normal response to conditions that require an increase in cardiac output, including fever, pain, anxiety, anemia, HF, hypovolemia, or thyrotoxicosis. Alcohol and alcohol withdrawal are common causes of sinus tachycardia and other supraventricular arrhythmias. In patients with underlying cardiac disease, sinus tachycardia may cause dyspnea or chest pain due to increased myocardial oxygen demand or reduced coronary artery blood flow.

Symptoms from sinus node dysfunction are nonspecific and may be due to other causes. It is therefore essential that symptoms be demonstrated to coincide temporally with arrhythmias. This may require prolonged ambulatory monitoring or the use of an event recorder.

Treatment

Asymptomatic patients generally do not *require treatment. For symptomatic patients with bradycardia or sick sinus syndrome, implantation of a permanent pacemaker is usually indicated.* In patients without evidence of AV nodal or bundle branch conduction abnormality, a single chamber atrial pacemaker is reasonable. *Atrial-based pacing (single or dual chamber) is superior to ventricular-only pacing for patients with sinus node dysfunction.* When a dual-chamber pacemaker is implanted for sinus node dysfunction with intact AV conduction, unnecessary ventricular pacing should be avoided because it may exacerbate HF, especially in patients with preexisting LV dysfunction. In most situations, sinus tachycardia will improve or resolve with treatment of the underlying cause. Inappropriate sinus tachycardia in the presence of symptoms (palpitations, dizziness, exertional intolerance) can be treated with a trial of β-blockers or calcium channel blockers although treatment is often challenging. Ivabradine (5–7.5 mg twice daily), a selective inhibitor of the sinoatrial node "funny current" (I_f), may be an effective treatment option.

When to Refer

Patients with symptoms related to bradycardia or tachycardia when reversible etiologies have been excluded.

AV BLOCK

ESSENTIALS OF DIAGNOSIS

- Conduction disturbance between the atrium and ventricle that can be physiologic (due to enhanced vagal tone) or pathologic.
- Block occurs in the AV node (**first-degree, second-degree Mobitz type I**) or below the AV node (**second-degree Mobitz type II, third-degree**).
- Symptomatic AV block or block below the AV node in the absence of a reversible cause usually warrants permanent pacemaker implantation.

General Considerations

AV block can be physiologic (due to increased vagal tone) or pathologic (due to underlying heart disease such as ischemia, myocarditis, fibrosis of the conduction system, or after cardiac surgery). AV block is categorized as **first-degree** (PR interval > 200 msec with all atrial impulses conducted), **second-degree** (intermittent blocked beats), or **third-degree** (complete heart block, in which no atrial impulses are conducted to the ventricles). Second-degree AV block is further subclassified into **Mobitz type I (Wenckebach)**, in which the AV conduction time (PR interval) progressively lengthens before the blocked beat, and **Mobitz type II**, in which there are intermittently nonconducted atrial beats not preceded by lengthening AV conduction. When only 2:1 AV block is present on the ECG, the differentiation between Mobitz type I or Mobitz type II is more difficult. If the baseline PR interval is prolonged (> 200 msec) or the width of the QRS complex is narrow (< 120 msec), the block is usually nodal (Mobitz type I); if the QRS complex is wide (≥ 120 msec), the block is more likely infranodal (Mobitz type II).

AV dissociation occurs when an intrinsic ventricular pacemaker (accelerated idioventricular rhythm, ventricular premature beats, or ventricular tachycardia) is firing at a rate faster than or close to the sinus rate, such that atrial impulses arriving at the AV node when it is refractory may not be conducted. This phenomenon does not necessarily indicate AV block. No treatment is required aside from management of the causative arrhythmia.

Clinical Findings

The clinical presentation of first-degree and Mobitz type I block is typically benign and rarely produces symptoms. Normal, physiologic block of this type occurs in response to increases in parasympathetic output. This is commonly seen during sleep, with carotid sinus massage, or in well-trained athletes. It may also occur as a medication effect (calcium channel blockers, β-blockers, digitalis, or antiarrhythmics). Pathologic causes, including myocardial ischemia or infarction, inflammatory processes (ie, Lyme disease), fibrosis, calcification, or infiltration (ie, amyloidosis or sarcoidosis), should be considered.

Mobitz type II block and complete (third-degree) heart block are almost always due to pathologic disease involving the infranodal conduction system, and symptoms including fatigue, dyspnea, presyncope or syncope are common. With complete heart block, where no atrial impulses reach the ventricle, the ventricular escape rate is usually slow (< 50 beats/min) and severity of symptoms may vary depending on the rate and stability of the escape rhythm. As for lesser degrees of AV block, pathologic causes should be explored.

Intraventricular conduction block is relatively common and may be transient (ie, related to increases in heart rate) or permanent. **Right bundle branch block** is often seen in patients with structurally normal hearts. The left bundle is composed of two components (anterior and posterior fascicles) and **left bundle branch block** is more often a marker of underlying cardiac disease, including ischemic heart disease, inflammatory or infiltrative disease, cardiomyopathy, and valvular heart disease. In asymptomatic patients with bifascicular block (block in two of three infranodal components—right bundle, left anterior, and left posterior fascicle), the incidence of occult complete heart block or progression to it is low (1% annually).

Treatment

Asymptomatic patients with first- or second-degree Mobitz type I AV block do *not* require any specific therapy. Patients should undergo treatment of any potentially reversible cause (ie, myocardial ischemia or medication effect). Asymptomatic AV block from high vagal tone (ie, during sleep) does not require pacemaker implantation. *Symptomatic patients with any degree of heart block should be treated* urgently *with atropine (initial dose 0.5 mg given intravenously), infusion of a β-adrenergic agonist (ie, isoproterenol, dopamine, or epinephrine), or temporary pacing (transcutaneous or transvenous).* The indications for permanent pacing are symptomatic bradyarrhythmias with any degree of AV block or asymptomatic high-degree AV block (second-degree Mobitz type II or third-degree heart block) not attributable to a reversible or physiologic cause. Patients with presumed cardiac syncope with normal heart rates and rhythm but bifascicular or trifascicular block on ECG should also be considered for permanent pacing.

A **standardized nomenclature for pacemaker generators** is used, usually consisting of four letters. The first letter refers to the chamber that is paced (A, atrium; V, ventricle; D, dual [for both]). The second letter refers to the chamber that is sensed (also A, V, or D). An additional option (O) indicates absence of sensing. The third letter refers to how the pacemaker responds to a sensed event (I, inhibition by a sensed impulse; T, triggering by a sensed impulse; D, dual modes of response; O, no response to sensed impulse). The fourth letter refers to the programmability or rate response capacity (R, rate modulation), a function that can increase the pacing rate in response to motion or respiratory rate when the intrinsic heart rate is inappropriately low.

A dual-chamber pacemaker that senses and paces in both chambers is the most physiologic approach to pacing patients who remain in sinus rhythm. **AV synchrony** is particularly important in patients in whom atrial contraction produces a substantial augmentation of stroke volume. For patients in permanent atrial fibrillation who require pacing for symptomatic bradycardia or pauses, catheter-based implantation of a leadless pacemaker directly to the RV endocardium may be considered. In patients with complete heart block with LV systolic dysfunction, implantation of a pacemaker capable of direct capture of the native specialized conduction system (His bundle or left bundle) or simultaneous LV and RV pacing (biventricular) may be indicated. Complications from pacemaker implantation include infection, hematoma, cardiac perforation, pneumothorax, and lead dislodgement.

When to Refer

Patients with symptomatic AV block (any degree) or asymptomatic high-degree (second-degree Mobitz type II or third-degree) AV block after reversible causes have been excluded.

PAROXYSMAL SUPRAVENTRICULAR TACHYCARDIA

ESSENTIALS OF DIAGNOSIS

- Rapid, regular tachycardia most commonly seen in young adults and characterized by abrupt onset and offset.
- QRS duration narrow (< 120 msec) except in the presence of bundle branch block or accessory pathway.
- Often responsive to vagal maneuvers, AV nodal blockers, or adenosine. Cardioversion rarely required.

General Considerations

PSVT is an intermittent arrhythmia that is characterized by a sudden onset and offset and a regular ventricular response. Episodes may last from a few seconds to several hours or longer. PSVT often occurs in patients without structural heart disease. The most common mechanism for PSVT is *reentry*, which may be initiated or terminated by a fortuitously timed atrial or ventricular premature beat. The reentrant circuit usually involves dual pathways (a slow and a fast pathway) within the AV node; this is referred to as **AV nodal reentrant tachycardia** and accounts for 60% of cases of PSVT. Less commonly (30% of cases), reentry is due to an *accessory pathway* between the atria and ventricles, referred to as **AV reciprocating tachycardia (AVRT)**. The pathophysiology and management of arrhythmias due to accessory pathways differ in important ways and are discussed separately below.

Clinical Findings

A. Symptoms and Signs

Symptoms of PSVT can be quite variable depending on the degree of heart rate elevation, resultant hypotension, or presence of other comorbidities. Symptoms may include palpitations, diaphoresis, dyspnea, dizziness, and mild chest pain (even in the absence of associated CHD). Syncope is rare.

B. ECG

Obtaining a 12-lead ECG when feasible is important to help determine the tachycardia mechanism. The QRS duration will be narrow (< 120 ms) except in cases of PSVT with aberrant conduction (left bundle branch block, right bundle branch block, or antegrade conducting accessory pathway). The heart rate is regular and is usually 160–220 beats/min but may be > 250 beats/min. The P wave usually differs in contour from sinus beats and is often simultaneous with or just after the QRS complex.

Treatment

In the absence of structural heart disease, serious effects are rare, and most episodes resolve spontaneously. Particular effort should be made to terminate the episode quickly if HF, syncope, or anginal pain develops or if there is underlying cardiac or (particularly) coronary disease. Because reentry is the most common mechanism for PSVT, effective therapy requires that conduction be interrupted at some point in the reentry circuit and the vast majority of these circuits involve the AV node.

A. Mechanical Measures

A variety of maneuvers have been used to interrupt episodes, and *patients may learn to perform these themselves.* These maneuvers result in an acute increase in vagal tone and include the Valsalva maneuver, lowering the head between the knees, coughing, splashing cold water on the face, and breath holding. The **Valsalva maneuver** is performed with the patient semirecumbent (45 degrees), exerting around 40 mm Hg of intrathoracic pressure (by blowing through a 10 mL syringe) for at least 15 seconds. Moving the patient supine immediately following the strain maneuver and passively raising their legs for an additional 15 seconds may increase effectiveness of the maneuver. **Carotid sinus massage** is an additional technique often performed by clinicians but *should be avoided if the patient has a carotid bruit.* Firm but gentle pressure and massage are applied first over the right carotid sinus for 10–20 seconds and, if unsuccessful, then over the left carotid sinus. Pressure should not be exerted on both sides at the same time. **Facial contact with cold water** may cause transient bradycardia and termination of PSVT, a phenomenon known as the *diving reflex.* When performed properly, these maneuvers result in abrupt termination of the arrhythmia in 20–50% of cases.

B. Medication Therapy

If mechanical measures fail to terminate the arrhythmia, pharmacologic agents should be tried. **Intravenous adenosine** is recommended as the first-line agent due to its brief duration of action and minimal negative inotropic activity (see Table 12–1). Because the half-life of adenosine is < 10 seconds, the medication is given rapidly (in 1–2 seconds) as a 6-mg bolus followed by 20 mL of fluid. If this regimen is unsuccessful at terminating the arrhythmia, a second higher dose (12 mg) may be given. Adenosine causes block of electrical conduction through the AV node and results in termination of PSVT in approximately 90% of cases. Minor side effects are common and include transient flushing, chest discomfort, nausea, and headache. Adenosine may excite both atrial and ventricular tissue causing atrial fibrillation (in up to 12% of patients) or rarely ventricular arrhythmias, and therefore, administration should be performed with continuous cardiac monitoring and availability of an external defibrillator. Etripamil is a novel self-administered intranasal calcium channel blocker approved for termination of PSVT. The medication has rapid pharmacokinetics with peak plasma concentration by 8 minutes and 60% of patients converting to sinus rhythm by 30 minutes.

When acute measures or medications fail to terminate the arrhythmia, **intravenous calcium channel blockers**, including verapamil and diltiazem, may be used (see Table 12–1). Verapamil in particular has been shown to be as effective at terminating PSVT in the acute setting (approximately 90%) as adenosine. Calcium channel blockers should be used with caution in patients with HF due to their negative inotropic effects. Their longer half-life compared with adenosine may result in prolonged hypotension despite restoration of normal rhythm.

Intravenous β-blockers include esmolol (a very short-acting β-blocker), propranolol, and metoprolol. While β-blockers cause less myocardial depression than calcium channel blockers, the evidence of their effectiveness to terminate PSVT is limited. Although **intravenous amiodarone** is safe, it is usually not required and often ineffective for treatment of these arrhythmias.

C. Cardioversion

If the patient is hemodynamically unstable or if adenosine, β-blockers, and calcium channel blockers are contraindicated or ineffective, synchronized electrical cardioversion (beginning at 100 J) should be performed.

Prevention

A. Catheter Ablation

Because of concerns about the safety and the intolerability of antiarrhythmic medications, *radiofrequency ablation is the preferred approach in patients with recurrent symptomatic reentrant PSVT*, whether it is due to dual pathways within the AV node or to accessory pathways.

B. Medications

AV nodal blocking agents are the medications of choice as first-line medical therapy (see Table 12–1). β-Blockers or nondihydropyridine calcium channel blockers, such as diltiazem and verapamil, are typically used first. Patients who do not respond to agents that increase refractoriness of the AV node may be treated with antiarrhythmics. The class Ic agents (flecainide, propafenone) can be used in patients without underlying structural or CHD. In patients with evidence of structural heart disease, class III agents, such as sotalol or amiodarone, should be used because of the lower incidence of ventricular proarrhythmia during long-term therapy.

When to Refer

All patients with sustained or symptomatic PSVT should be referred to a cardiologist or cardiac electrophysiologist for long-term treatment options (including observation, pharmacotherapy, or ablation).

PSVT DUE TO ACCESSORY AV PATHWAYS (Preexcitation Syndromes)

ESSENTIALS OF DIAGNOSIS

- Two classic features of **Wolff-Parkinson-White (WPW)** pattern on ECG are short PR interval and wide, slurred QRS complex due to manifest preexcitation (δ wave).
- Most patients with WPW pattern do not have clinical history of arrhythmia but have a higher risk of SCD due to the possibility of rapidly conducted atrial fibrillation through the accessory pathway.
- Risk factors for SCD with WPW include age younger than 20, history of tachycardia, and rapid conduction properties at electrophysiologic testing.

General Considerations

Accessory pathways or bypass tracts between the atrium and the ventricle bypass the compact AV node and can predispose to reentrant arrhythmias, such as AVRT and atrial fibrillation. When direct AV connections conduct antegrade (manifest preexcitation), they produce a classic **WPW pattern** on the baseline ECG consisting of a short PR interval and a wide, slurred QRS complex **(δ wave)** owing to early ventricular depolarization of the region adjacent to the pathway. Although the morphology and polarity of the δ wave can suggest the location of the pathway, mapping by intracardiac recordings is required for precise anatomic localization.

Accessory pathways occur in 0.1–0.3% of the population and facilitate reentrant arrhythmias owing to the disparity in refractory periods of the AV node and accessory pathway. **WPW syndrome** refers to a patient with baseline WPW pattern on ECG with associated SVT. Whether the tachycardia is associated with a narrow or wide QRS complex is frequently determined by whether antegrade conduction is through the node (narrow) or the bypass tract (wide). Some bypass tracts only conduct in a retrograde direction. In these cases, the bypass tract is termed "concealed" because it is not readily apparent on a baseline (sinus) ECG. **Orthodromic reentrant tachycardia** accounts for approximately 90% of AVRT episodes and is characterized by conduction antegrade down the AV node and retrograde up the accessory pathway, resulting in a narrow QRS complex (unless an underlying bundle branch block or interventricular conduction delay is present). **Antidromic reentrant tachycardia** conducts antegrade down the accessory pathway and retrograde through the AV node, resulting in a wide and often bizarre-appearing QRS complex that may be mistaken for ventricular tachycardia. Accessory pathways often have shorter refractory periods than specialized conduction tissue and thus tachycardias involving accessory pathways have the potential to be more rapid.

Clinical Findings

Patients with WPW in whom arrhythmia develops often have palpitations, dizziness, or mild chest pain. Most patients that have a δ wave found incidentally on ECG (WPW pattern) do *not* have a clinical history of arrhythmia and are therefore asymptomatic. However, these patients are still at higher risk for SCD than the general population. Atrial fibrillation with antegrade conduction down the accessory pathway and a rapid ventricular response will develop in up to 30% of patients with WPW. If this conduction is very rapid, it can potentially degenerate to ventricular fibrillation. The 10-year risk of SCD in patients with WPW syndrome ranges from 0.15% to 0.24%. Risk factors include age younger than 20, a history of symptomatic tachycardia, and multiple accessory pathways.

Multiple risk stratification strategies have been proposed to identify asymptomatic patients with WPW pattern ECG who may be at higher risk for lethal cardiac arrhythmias. A sudden loss of preexcitation during ambulatory monitoring or exercise testing likely indicates an accessory pathway with poor conduction properties and therefore low risk for rapid anterograde conduction. In the absence of this finding, patients may be referred for invasive electrophysiology testing. During the study, patients found to have the shortest preexcited R-R interval during atrial fibrillation of 250 msec or less or inducible SVT are at increased risk for SCD and should undergo catheter ablation.

Treatment

A. Pharmacotherapy

Initial treatment of narrow-complex reentrant rhythms involving a bypass tract (orthodromic AVRT) is similar to other forms of PSVT and includes vagal maneuvers, intravenous adenosine, or verapamil. Treatment of wide-complex tachycardia in the presence of an accessory pathway, be it reentrant-type (antidromic AVRT) or atrial fibrillation with antegrade conduction down the bypass tract, must be managed differently. Agents such as calcium channel blockers and β-blockers may increase the refractoriness of the AV node with minimal or no effect on the accessory pathway, often leading to faster ventricular rates and increasing the risk of ventricular fibrillation. Therefore, these agents should be *avoided*. Intravenous class Ia (procainamide) and class III (ibutilide) antiarrhythmic agents will increase the refractoriness of the bypass tract and are the medications of choice for wide-complex tachycardias involving accessory pathways. If hemodynamic compromise is present, electrical cardioversion is warranted.

B. Catheter Ablation

For long-term management, catheter ablation is the procedure of choice in patients with accessory pathways and recurrent symptoms or asymptomatic patients with WPW pattern on ECG and high-risk features at baseline or during electrophysiology study. Success rates for ablation of accessory pathways with radiofrequency catheters exceed 95% in appropriate patients. Major complications from catheter ablation are rare but include AV block, cardiac tamponade, and thromboembolic events. Minor complications, including hematoma at the catheter access site, occur in 1–2% of procedures. For patients who are not candidates for catheter ablation, class Ic or class III antiarrhythmic medication may be considered.

When to Refer

- Asymptomatic patients with an incidental finding of WPW pattern on ECG with high-risk features.
- Patients with recurrent or prolonged tachycardia episodes despite treatment with AV nodal blocking agents.
- Patients with preexcitation and a history of atrial fibrillation or syncope.

ATRIAL FIBRILLATION

ESSENTIALS OF DIAGNOSIS

- Presents as an irregularly irregular heart rhythm on examination and ECG.
- Prevention of stroke should be considered in all patients with risk factors for stroke (those with HF, hypertension, age 65 or older, diabetes mellitus, prior history of stroke or transient ischemic attack [TIA], or vascular disease).
- Heart rate control with β-blocker or calcium channel blockers generally required. Restoration of sinus rhythm with cardioversion, antiarrhythmic medications, or catheter ablation in symptomatic patients.

General Considerations

Atrial fibrillation is the most common chronic arrhythmia, with an estimated global prevalence of 59 million individuals. It occurs in rheumatic and other forms of valvular heart disease, dilated cardiomyopathy, and CHD as well as in patients with no apparent cardiac disease. Modifiable risk factors include obesity, hypertension, obstructive sleep apnea, diabetes mellitus, physical inactivity, and alcohol consumption. Acute alcohol excess and alcohol withdrawal (termed **holiday heart**) may precipitate atrial fibrillation. For regular, moderate drinkers, abstinence from alcohol reduces recurrences of atrial fibrillation by about 50%. Atrial fibrillation often appears in a **paroxysmal** fashion before becoming a more persistent rhythm.

Atrial fibrillation is associated with a 2-fold increased risk of death, a 2.4-fold risk of stroke, and a 5-fold risk of HF. Atrial fibrillation increases the propensity for thrombus formation due to circulatory stasis in the left atrial appendage and consequent embolization, most devastatingly to the cerebral circulation. *Untreated, the rate of stroke is approximately 5% per year.* However, patients with significant obstructive valvular disease, chronic HF or LV dysfunction, diabetes mellitus, hypertension, or age > 75 years and those with a history of prior stroke or other embolic events are at substantially higher risk (up to nearly 20% per year in patients with multiple risk factors). In patients presenting with embolic stroke of unknown source (cryptogenic stroke), a substantial portion will have **asymptomatic** or **"subclinical"** atrial fibrillation detected with implantable loop recorders, allowing initiation of oral anticoagulation.

Clinical Findings

A. Symptoms and Signs

Atrial fibrillation itself is rarely life-threatening; however, it can have serious consequences if the ventricular rate is sufficiently rapid to precipitate hypotension, myocardial ischemia, or tachycardia-induced myocardial dysfunction. Moreover, *particularly in patients with risk factors, atrial fibrillation is a major preventable cause of stroke.* Although some patients—particularly with advanced age or an inactive lifestyle—have relatively few symptoms if the rate is controlled, many patients are aware of the irregular rhythm. Most patients will report fatigue whether they experience other symptoms or not. The heart rate may range from quite slow to extremely rapid but is uniformly irregular unless underlying complete heart block with junctional escape rhythm or a permanent ventricular pacemaker is in place. *Atrial fibrillation is the only common arrhythmia in which the ventricular rate is rapid and the rhythm very irregular.*

B. ECG

The surface ECG typically demonstrates erratic, disorganized atrial activity between discrete QRS complexes occurring in an irregular pattern. The atrial activity may be very fine and difficult to detect on the ECG, or quite coarse and often mistaken for atrial flutter.

C. Echocardiography

Echocardiography provides assessment of chamber volumes, LV size and function, or the presence of concomitant valvular heart disease and should be performed in all patients with a new diagnosis of atrial fibrillation. TEE is the most sensitive imaging modality to identify thrombi in the left atrium or left atrial appendage prior to any attempt at chemical or electrical cardioversion.

Treatment

A. Newly Diagnosed Atrial Fibrillation

1. Initial management—

A. HEMODYNAMICALLY UNSTABLE PATIENT—If the patient is hemodynamically unstable, usually as a result of a rapid ventricular rate or associated cardiac or noncardiac conditions, hospitalization and immediate treatment of atrial fibrillation are required. Intravenous β-blockers (esmolol, propranolol, and metoprolol) or calcium channel blockers (diltiazem and verapamil) are usually effective at rate control in the acute setting. Urgent electrical cardioversion is only indicated in patients with shock or severe hypotension, pulmonary edema, or ongoing MI or ischemia. *There is a potential risk of thromboembolism in patients undergoing cardioversion who have not received anticoagulation therapy if atrial fibrillation has been present for > 48 hours or is of unknown duration*; however, in hemodynamically unstable patients the need for immediate rate control outweighs that risk. An initial biphasic shock with at least 200 J is administered in synchrony with the R wave. If sinus rhythm is not restored, an additional attempt with 360 J is indicated. If this fails, cardioversion may be successful after loading with intravenous ibutilide (1 mg over 10 minutes, repeated in 10 minutes if necessary).

B. HEMODYNAMICALLY STABLE PATIENT—If the patient has no symptoms, hemodynamic instability, or evidence of important precipitating conditions (such as silent MI or ischemia, decompensated HF, or hemodynamically significant valvular disease), hospitalization is usually *not* necessary. In most of these cases, atrial fibrillation is an unrecognized chronic or paroxysmal condition and should be managed accordingly (see Subsequent Management, below). For new-onset atrial fibrillation, basic blood tests (CBC, metabolic panel, and thyroid function) and echocardiography to assess for occult valvular or myocardial disease should be performed.

In stable patients with atrial fibrillation, an initial strategy of rate control and anticoagulation is often suitable. The choice of agent is guided by the hemodynamic status of the patient, associated conditions, and the urgency of achieving rate control. In the stable patient with atrial fibrillation, a nondihydropyridine calcium channel blocker or β-blocker (orally or intravenously) is the first-line agent for ventricular rate control. In the setting of MI or ischemia, β-blockers are the preferred agent. The most frequently used agents are either metoprolol (2.5- to 5-mg intravenous bolus, repeated up to three times at intervals of 5 minutes and then given orally at total daily doses of 25–200 mg) or, in unstable patients, esmolol (0.5-mg/kg intravenous bolus, followed by a titrated infusion of 0.05–0.3 mg/kg/min). If β-blockers are contraindicated, calcium channel blockers are rapidly effective. Diltiazem (10- to 20-mg bolus, repeated after 15 minutes if necessary, followed by a maintenance infusion of 5–15 mg/hour) is the preferred calcium channel blocker if hypotension is present. Otherwise, verapamil (5–10 mg intravenously over 2–3 minutes, repeated after 30 minutes if necessary) may be used. Rate control using digoxin is relatively slow (onset of action > 1 hour with peak effect at 6 hours); however, it may be useful as an adjunct when rate control with the previously cited agents is incomplete. Similarly, amiodarone, even when administered intravenously, has a relatively slow onset and is most useful when cardioversion is planned in the near future. Care should be taken in patients with hypotension or HF because the rapid intravenous administration of amiodarone may worsen hemodynamics.

Up to two-thirds of patients experiencing acute onset (shorter than 36 hours) of atrial fibrillation will spontaneously revert to sinus rhythm without the need for cardioversion. *If atrial fibrillation has been present for > 1 week, spontaneous conversion is unlikely* and cardioversion may be considered for symptomatic patients. Importantly, *if the onset of atrial fibrillation was > 48 hours prior to presentation (or unknown), a transesophageal echocardiogram should be performed prior to cardioversion to exclude left atrial thrombus.* If thrombus is present, the cardioversion is delayed until after a 3–6-week period of therapeutic anticoagulation and repeated imaging. Because atrial contractile activity may not recover for several weeks after restoration of sinus rhythm in patients who have been in atrial fibrillation for > 48 hours, *therapeutic anticoagulation should be established pre-cardioversion and continued without interruption for at least 1 month afterwards.* Younger patients without HF, diabetes, hypertension, or other risk factors for stroke may not require long-term anticoagulation.

2. Subsequent management—If immediate cardioversion is not performed, adequate long-term rate control can usually be achieved with β-blockers or nondihydropyridine calcium channel blockers. Choice of the initial rate control medication is best based on the presence of accompanying conditions: Patients with hypertension can be given β-blockers or calcium blockers (see Tables 13–8, 13–10, and 13–11). Patients with CHD or HF should receive a β-blocker (carvedilol, long-acting metoprolol or bisoprolol) preferentially, whereas β-blockers should be avoided in patients with severe COPD or asthma. Digoxin may be used as a second agent when rate-control is inadequate with β-blocker or calcium channel blocker alone (target serum concentration 0.5–1.2 ng/mL). In symptomatic patients, *a resting heart rate of < 80 beats/min is targeted.* In asymptomatic patients without LV dysfunction, a more lenient resting heart rate of 85–110 beats/min is reasonable. *Ambulatory monitoring to assess heart rate during exercise should be considered in all patients with a goal not to exceed* ***maximum predicted heart rate*** *(220 – age).*

A. ANTICOAGULATION—*For patients with atrial fibrillation, even when it is paroxysmal or occurs rarely, the need for oral anticoagulation should be evaluated and treatment initiated for those without strong contraindication.* Patients under the age of 65 years with atrial fibrillation in the absence of associated heart disease, hypertension, atherosclerotic vascular disease, diabetes mellitus, or history of stroke or TIA do not require antithrombotic treatment. Patients with **transient atrial fibrillation**, such as in the setting of acute MI or pneumonia, but no prior history of arrhythmia, are at high risk for future development of atrial fibrillation and appropriate anticoagulation should be initiated based on risk factors. If the cause is reversible, such as after coronary artery bypass surgery or associated with hyperthyroidism, then long-term anticoagulation may not be necessary.

Table 12–2. CHA_2DS_2-VASc Risk Score for assessing risk of stroke and for selecting anticoagulant therapy for patients with atrial fibrillation.

CHA_2DS_2-VASc Risk Score	
HF or LVEF ≤ 40%	1
Hypertension	1
Age ≥ 75 years	2
Diabetes mellitus	1
Stroke, transient ischemic attack, or thromboembolism	2
Vascular disease (previous MI, peripheral artery disease, or aortic plaque)	1
Age 65–74 years	1
Female sex (but not a risk factor if female sex is the only factor)	1
CHA_2DS_2-VASc score 0 (men) or 1 (women): No anticoagulation recommended	
CHA_2DS_2-VASc score 1 (men) or 2 (women): Anticoagulation is reasonable; shared-decision making recommended	
CHA_2DS_2-VASc score ≥ 2 (men) or ≥ 3 (women): Oral anticoagulation recommended; DOACs preferred over warfarin	

Data from Camm AJ et al. 2012 focused update of the ESC Guidelines for the management of atrial fibrillation: an update of the 2010 ESC Guidelines for the management of atrial fibrillation. Developed with the special contribution of the European Heart Rhythm Association. *Eur Heart J*. 2012 Nov;33(21):2719–47.

The **CHA_2DS_2-VASc** score is considered the most validated risk score to guide anticoagulant use in patients with atrial fibrillation and includes the traditional five risk factors that comprise the **$CHADS_2$** score (HF, hypertension, age 75 years or older, diabetes mellitus, and [2 points for] history of stroke or TIA), with three additional factors (age 65–74 years, female sex, and presence of vascular disease) (Table 12–2). *If the CHA_2DS_2-VASc score is ≥ 2 in men or ≥ 3 in women, oral anticoagulation is recommended.* For patients at low-moderate risk (CHA_2DS_2-VASc score 1 in men, 2 in women), oral anticoagulation can be considered, taking into account risk, benefit, and patient preferences.In patients with atrial fibrillation and no clinical risk factors (CHA_2DS_2-VASc score 0), there is no indication for anticoagulant or antithrombotic therapy. *In general, unless there is an indication for antiplatelet therapy (CHD, peripheral vascular disease), patients with atrial fibrillation should not be prescribed aspirin for stroke prevention.*

Warfarin and other vitamin K antagonists (VKAs) have historically been first-line agents for stroke prevention in patients with atrial fibrillation. Their narrow therapeutic window, multiple drug interactions, dietary restrictions, requirement for frequent monitoring, and low safety profile affected routine use of VKAs in practice. *Four DOACs—dabigatran, rivaroxaban, apixaban, and edoxaban—have been shown to be at least as effective as warfarin for stroke prevention in patients with atrial fibrillation, with improved safety profiles and ease of use, and are therefore recommended as first-line therapy over warfarin in patients with atrial fibrillation* (Table 12–3). *Importantly, the DOACs have not been studied in patients with moderate or severe mitral stenosis, and they should not be used for patients with mechanical prosthetic valves.*

Dabigatran (studied in the RE-LY trial) is superior to warfarin at preventing stroke at the 150-mg twice-daily dose, and it is noninferior at the 110-mg twice-daily dose, although this dose is not approved for treatment of atrial fibrillation in the United States. Both doses result in *less* intracranial hemorrhage than warfarin but also in *more* GI bleeding than warfarin. Neither dabigatran nor any of the DOACs should be used in patients with mechanical prosthetic heart valves where the medications are less effective and riskier.

Rivaroxaban is noninferior to warfarin for stroke prevention in atrial fibrillation (in the ROCKET-AF trial). Rivaroxaban is dosed at 20 mg once daily, with a reduced dose (15 mg/day) for patients with creatinine clearances between 15 and 50 mL/min. It should be *administered with*

Table 12–3. DOACs for stroke prevention in patients with atrial fibrillation (DOACs listed in alphabetical order).

	Apixaban	Dabigatran	Edoxaban	Rivaroxaban
Class	Factor Xa inhibitor	Antithrombin	Factor Xa inhibitor	Factor Xa inhibitor
Bleeding risk compared with warfarin	Substantially lower risk of major bleeding Less intracranial bleeding	Less intracranial bleeding Higher incidence of GI bleeding	Lower risk of major bleeding Less intracranial bleeding	Less intracranial bleeding Higher incidence of GI bleeding
Dosage	5 mg twice daily	150 mg twice daily	60 mg once daily	20 mg once daily
Dosage adjustments	2.5 mg twice daily for patients with at least two of three risk factors: 1. Age ≥ 80 years 2. Body weight ≤ 60 kg 3. Serum creatinine ≥ 1.5 mg/dL	75 mg twice daily for creatinine clearance[1] 15–30 mL/min	30 mg once daily for creatinine clearance[1] ≤ 50 mL/min FDA recommends not to use if creatinine clearance[1] > 95 mL/min	15 mg once daily for creatinine clearance[1] < 50 mL/min

[1]Creatinine clearance calculated by Cockcroft-Gault equation.
Data from Nishimura RA et al. 2014 AHA/ACC Guideline for the Management of Patients With Valvular Heart Disease: A Report of the American College of Cardiology/American Heart Association Task Force on Practice Guidelines. *Circulation*. 2014 Jun 10;129(23):e521–643.

food, since that results in a 40% higher drug absorption. As with dabigatran, there is substantially less risk of intracranial hemorrhage with rivaroxaban than warfarin.

Apixaban is more effective than warfarin at stroke prevention while having a substantially lower risk of major bleeding (in the ARISTOTLE trial) and a lower risk of all-cause mortality. The apixaban dosage is 5 mg twice daily or 2.5 mg twice daily for patients with two of three high-risk criteria (age 80 years or older, body weight 60 kg or less, and serum creatinine of 1.5 mg/dL or more). Apixaban is associated with less intracranial hemorrhage and is well tolerated.

Edoxaban, 60 mg once a day, is noninferior to warfarin for stroke prevention with lower rates of major bleeding and lower rates of hemorrhagic stroke (studied in the ENGAGE-AF trial). Edoxaban carries a boxed warning in FDA labeling that it should *not* be used in patients whose creatinine clearance is > 95 mL/min because it is less effective in this population. The dose is decreased to 30 mg/day for patients whose creatinine clearance is ≤ 50 mL/min.

In part because of lower rates of intracerebral hemorrhage, *DOACs have particular advantage over warfarin in older adults and frail patients, including patients with history of falls.* For patients who fall, shared-decision making weighing risks and benefits should be incorporated. However, oral anticoagulation should generally be continued.

Warfarin remains first-line therapy in patients who have mechanical prosthetic valves, moderate or severe mitral stenosis, and those who cannot afford DOACs. Patients who have been stable while receiving warfarin for a long time, with a high time in target INR range, and who are at lower risk for intracranial hemorrhage will have relatively less benefit with a switch to a DOAC. One way to reduce bleeding for patients taking oral anticoagulants is to avoid concurrent aspirin, unless there is a clear indication, like recent MI or coronary stent. Even then, use of oral anticoagulant plus clopidogrel without aspirin, or with only a brief period of "triple" therapy and then discontinuation of aspirin, may be a reasonable approach.

There are some important practical issues with using the DOACs. *It is important to monitor blood counts and kidney function at baseline and at least twice a year, or more often for those with impaired kidney function.* Each of the DOACs interacts with other medications affecting the P-glycoprotein pathway, such as oral ketoconazole, verapamil, dronedarone, and phenytoin. To transition patients from warfarin to a DOAC, wait until the INR decreases to about 2.0. Each of the medications has a half-life of about 10–12 hours for patients with normal kidney function. *For elective procedures, stop the medications two to three half-lives (usually 24–48 hours) before procedures with low to moderate bleeding risk (ie, colonoscopy, dental extraction, cardiac catheterization), and five half-lives before major surgery.* Discontinuation times should be extended in patients with impaired renal function, particularly with dabigatran. For patients discontinuing DOAC periprocedurally, there is no need for bridging anticoagulation.

Approximately 2–4% of patients on oral anticoagulation have major bleeding which may require intervention. For bleeding, standard measures (ie, diagnosing and controlling the source, stopping antithrombotic agents, and replacing blood products) should be taken. If the DOAC was taken in the prior 6–8 hours, activated oral charcoal may be used to reduce absorption. If the patient is taking aspirin, consider platelet transfusion. Due to the short half-life of the DOACs (10–12 hours with normal kidney function), supportive measures (local control, packed RBCs, platelets) may suffice until the medication has cleared. Antidotes should be considered for life-threatening bleeding or for patients with need for immediate surgery. A patient with severe bleeding while taking dabigatran may be treated with the reversal agent **idarucizumab** (given as 5 g intravenous infusion over 5 minutes), a humanized monoclonal antibody that binds the medication resulting in rapid reversal of its anticoagulation effect. For life-threatening bleeding with warfarin or other VKAs, **four-factor prothrombin complex concentrate** in addition to intravenous vitamin K may partially reverse the anticoagulant effect and is preferred over fresh frozen plasma.

In patients who are unsuitable for long-term anticoagulation due to excessive bleeding risk, **left atrial appendage occluders** (including the Watchman and Amulet devices) have been shown to protect against stroke, although they may not be as effective as warfarin in preventing ischemic stroke. Occlusion of the left atrial appendage during cardiac surgery provides further protection against ischemic stroke over and above ongoing oral anticoagulant use.

B. Rate control or rhythm control—After assessing stroke risk and initiating anticoagulation where appropriate, two main treatment strategies for long-term management of atrial fibrillation exist: rate control or rhythm control, although they are not mutually exclusive. *Rate control should be considered background treatment in nearly all patients with atrial fibrillation, regardless of whether rhythm restoration is eventually pursued, and may be considered the primary treatment in patients with minimal to no symptoms related to long-standing atrial fibrillation.* In patients with recent-onset atrial fibrillation (< 1 year), rhythm control with antiarrhythmic medication or catheter ablation is associated with a lower risk of death from cardiovascular causes, stroke, or hospitalization for HF.

The decision to pursue rhythm control is often individualized, based on symptoms, the type of atrial fibrillation (paroxysmal or persistent), comorbidities (such as HF), as well as general health status. As first treatment, elective cardioversion (200 J or more, biphasic energy) is recommended in patients in whom atrial fibrillation is thought to be of recent onset (< 48 hours) or when there is an identifiable precipitating factor. Similarly, cardioversion is appropriate in patients who remain symptomatic from the rhythm despite efforts to achieve rate control. In patients with atrial fibrillation duration of > 48 hours (or unknown), a minimum of 3 weeks of anticoagulation or exclusion of left atrial thrombus by TEE pre-cardioversion is required. Anticoagulation should be continued for at least 4 weeks in all patients following cardioversion to prevent thromboembolism. In patients with prior left atrial appendage occlusion, data on peri-cardioversion stroke risk and anticoagulation strategies are lacking. However, TEE is recommended to exclude device-related thrombus or peri-device leak, which may prompt anticoagulant initiation.

In cases in which elective cardioversion is required, it may be accomplished pharmacologically or electrically. Pharmacologic cardioversion with intravenous ibutilide (1 mg over

10 minutes, repeated in 10 minutes if necessary) or procainamide (15 mg/kg over 30 minutes) may be used in a setting in which the patient can undergo continuous ECG monitoring for at least 4–6 hours following administration. Pretreatment with intravenous magnesium (1–2 g) may prevent rare episodes of torsades de pointes associated with ibutilide administration. Given significant prolongation of the QT interval with ibutilide, patients should have continuous ECG monitoring during infusion and for 4 hours after completion. In patients in whom a decision has been made to continue antiarrhythmic therapy to maintain sinus rhythm (see next paragraph), cardioversion can be attempted with an agent that is being considered for long-term use. For instance, after therapeutic anticoagulation has been established, amiodarone can be initiated on an outpatient basis (400 mg twice daily for 2 weeks, followed by 200 mg twice daily for at least 2–4 weeks and then a maintenance dose of 200 mg daily). Because amiodarone increases the prothrombin time in patients taking warfarin and increases digoxin levels, careful monitoring of anticoagulation and medication levels is required.

Other antiarrhythmic medications that can be used for long-term maintenance therapy include propafenone, flecainide, dronedarone, dofetilide, and sotalol. Dofetilide (125–500 mcg twice daily orally) must be initiated in hospital due to the potential risk of torsades de pointes and the downward dose adjustment that is required for patients with significant QT interval prolongation. Propafenone (150–300 mg orally every 8 hours) and flecainide (50–150 mg orally twice daily) should be avoided in patients with structural heart disease (CHD, systolic dysfunction, or significant LVH) and should be used in conjunction with an AV nodal blocking medication, especially if there is a history of atrial flutter. Sotalol (80–160 mg orally twice daily) should be initiated in the hospital in patients with structural heart disease due to a risk of torsades de pointes; it is not very effective for converting atrial fibrillation but can be used to maintain sinus rhythm following cardioversion. Dronedarone should not be used in patients with recent decompensated HF or when atrial fibrillation has become persistent.

In patients treated long-term with an antiarrhythmic agent, sinus rhythm will persist in 30–50%. Given this high rate of arrhythmia recurrence, the decision to maintain long-term anticoagulation should be based on risk factors (CHA_2DS_2-VASc score, Table 12–2) and not on the perceived presence or absence of atrial fibrillation, since future episodes may be asymptomatic.

B. Recurrent and Refractory Atrial Fibrillation

1. Recurrent paroxysmal atrial fibrillation—For select patients with symptomatic but rare (a few times a year) episodes of atrial fibrillation, an effective treatment strategy is on-demand pharmacologic cardioversion, termed **pill-in-the-pocket treatment**. Patients without coronary or structural heart disease may be given flecainide (200–300 mg) or propafenone (450–600 mg) in addition to a β-blocker or nondihydropyridine calcium channel blocker as a single dose at the onset of symptoms. It is recommended that the first such treatment take place in a monitored setting (eg, the emergency department or hospital) to evaluate safety and effectiveness. For more frequent, symptomatic arrhythmic episodes, daily antiarrhythmic agents are first-line therapy; however, they are not often successful in preventing all paroxysmal atrial fibrillation episodes and long-term tolerability is poor.

2. Refractory atrial fibrillation—Atrial fibrillation should be considered refractory if it causes persistent symptoms or limits activity despite attempts at rate or rhythm control. If antiarrhythmic or rate control medications fail to improve symptoms, **catheter ablation** around the pulmonary veins to isolate the triggers that initiate and maintain atrial fibrillation may be considered. It is a reasonable therapy for individuals with symptomatic paroxysmal or persistent atrial fibrillation that is refractory to pharmacologic therapy and for select patients (younger than 65 years or with concurrent HF) as first-line therapy. *The primary benefit of catheter ablation is an improvement in quality of life.* Current evidence has not consistently demonstrated reductions in hard endpoints such as stroke or death. Ablation is successful about 50–70% of the time but repeat ablation may be required in up to 20% of patients. The procedure is routinely performed in the electrophysiology laboratory using a catheter-based approach and adverse event rates are low when performed by experienced operators. **Surgical ablation** can also be performed via a subxiphoid approach, thoracoscopically via thoracotomy, or via median sternotomy in the operating room as a standalone or adjunct procedure. Finally, in symptomatic patients with poor rate control and deemed inappropriate for pulmonary vein isolation, **radiofrequency ablation** of the AV node and **permanent pacing** ensure rate control and may facilitate a more physiologic rate response to activity, but this is usually performed only after other therapies have failed.

When to Refer

- Symptomatic atrial fibrillation with or without adequate rate control.
- Asymptomatic atrial fibrillation with poor rate control despite AV nodal blockers.
- Patients at risk for stroke who have not tolerated oral anticoagulants.

Wolfes J et al. Comparison of the latest ESC, ACC/AHA/ACCP/HRS, and CCS guidelines on the management of atrial fibrillation. JACC Clin Electrophysiol. 2025;11:836. [PMID: 39985521]

ATRIAL FLUTTER

ESSENTIALS OF DIAGNOSIS

- Rapid, regular tachycardia presenting classically with 2 to 1 block in the AV node and ventricular heart rate of 150 beats/min.
- ECG shows "sawtooth" pattern of atrial activity (rate 300 beats/min).
- Stroke risk should be considered *equivalent* to that with atrial fibrillation.
- Catheter ablation is highly successful and is considered the definitive treatment for typical atrial flutter.

General Considerations

Atrial flutter is less common than fibrillation. It may occur in patients with structurally normal hearts but is more commonly seen in patients with COPD, valvular or structural heart disease, atrial septal defects, or surgically repaired congenital heart disease.

Clinical Findings

Patients typically present with reports of palpitations, fatigue, or mild dizziness. In situations where the arrhythmia is unrecognized for a prolonged period of time, symptoms and signs of HF (dyspnea, exertional intolerance, edema) due to tachycardia-induced cardiomyopathy may develop. The ECG typically demonstrates a **"sawtooth" pattern** of atrial activity in the inferior leads (II, III, and AVF). The reentrant circuit generates atrial rates of 250–350 beats/min, usually with transmission of every second, third, or fourth impulse through the AV node to the ventricles.

Treatment

Ventricular rate control is accomplished using the same agents used in atrial fibrillation, but it is generally more difficult. Conversion of atrial flutter to sinus rhythm with class I antiarrhythmic agents is also difficult to achieve, and administration of these medications has been associated with slowing of the atrial flutter rate to the point at which 1:1 AV conduction can occur at rates in excess of 200 beats/min, with subsequent hemodynamic collapse. The intravenous class III antiarrhythmic agent ibutilide has been significantly more successful in converting atrial flutter (see Table 12–1). About 50–70% of patients return to sinus rhythm within 60–90 minutes following the infusion of this agent. Electrical cardioversion also is very effective for atrial flutter, with approximately 90% of patients converting following synchronized shocks of 100–200 J.

Although the organization of atrial contractile function in this arrhythmia may provide some protection against thrombus formation, *the risk of thromboembolism should be considered equivalent to that with atrial fibrillation* due to the common coexistence of these arrhythmias. As with atrial fibrillation, anticoagulation should be established for at least 3 weeks or thrombus excluded with TEE pre-cardioversion for atrial flutter of > 48 hours or of unknown duration. Anticoagulation should be continued for at least 4 weeks after electrical or chemical cardioversion and chronically in patients with risk factors for thromboembolism.

Catheter ablation is the treatment of choice for long-term management of atrial flutter owing to the high success rate and safety of the procedure. The anatomy of the typical circuit is well defined and catheter ablation within the right atrium results in immediate and permanent elimination of atrial flutter in > 90% of patients. Due to the frequent coexistence of atrial flutter with atrial fibrillation, however, some patients may require catheter ablation of both arrhythmias. If pharmacologic therapy is chosen, class III antiarrhythmics (amiodarone or dofetilide) are generally preferred (see Table 12–1).

When to Refer

All patients with atrial flutter should be referred to a cardiologist or cardiac electrophysiologist for consideration of definitive treatment with catheter ablation.

ATRIAL TACHYCARDIA

ESSENTIALS OF DIAGNOSIS

- Characterized by bursts of rapid, regular tachycardia.
- Multifocal atrial tachycardia commonly seen with severe COPD and presents with three or more distinct P wave morphologies on ECG, often confused for atrial fibrillation.
- Treatment of the underlying lung disease is most effective therapy.

General Considerations

Atrial tachycardia is an uncommon form of PSVT characterized by paroxysms or bursts of rapid, regular arrhythmia due to focal atrial impulses originating outside of the normal sinus node. Common sites include the tricuspid annulus, the crista terminalis of the right atrium, and the coronary sinus. **Multifocal atrial tachycardia** is a particular subtype seen in patients with severe COPD and characterized by varying P wave morphology (by definition, three or more foci) and markedly irregular PP intervals. The rate is typically > 100 beats/min, and the rhythm is often confused for atrial fibrillation. **Solitary atrial premature beats** are benign and generally not associated with underlying cardiac disease. They occur when an ectopic focus in the atria fires before the next sinus node impulse. The contour of the P wave usually differs from the patient's normal complex, unless the ectopic focus is near the sinus node. Acceleration of the heart rate by any means usually abolishes most premature beats.

Clinical Findings

Focal atrial tachycardias are usually intermittent and self-limiting although incessant forms do exist and may present with signs and symptoms of HF due to tachycardia-induced cardiomyopathy. Most patients report palpitations with an abrupt onset, similar to other forms of PSVT. Patients with underlying cardiac pathology (eg, CHD) can present with dyspnea or angina. Close inspection of the P wave on 12-lead ECG suggests a focus away from the sinus node, although certain locations (eg, high right atrial crista terminalis) may mimic sinus tachycardia. In this situation, the abrupt onset and offset of the arrhythmia are helpful in distinguishing atrial from sinus tachycardia, although electrophysiologic study is sometimes necessary.

Treatment

Initial management of atrial tachycardia is similar to other types of PSVT; however, vagal maneuvers and intravenous adenosine are generally less effective. Intravenous β-blockers or calcium channel blockers can be given in the hemodynamically stable patient with a transition to oral formulations for long-term management. Antiarrhythmic medications or catheter ablation should be considered in patients who continue to have symptomatic episodes. Long-term anticoagulation is not indicated in the absence of coexistent atrial fibrillation or atrial flutter.

For patients with multifocal atrial tachycardia, treatment of the underlying condition (eg, COPD) is paramount; verapamil, 240–480 mg orally daily in divided doses, may be effective in some patients.

When to Refer

All patients with atrial tachycardia in whom initial medical management fails should be referred to a cardiologist or cardiac electrophysiologist.

PREMATURE VENTRICULAR CONTRACTIONS

ESSENTIALS OF DIAGNOSIS

- Common but rarely symptomatic.
- Ambulatory ECG monitoring to quantify daily burden of PVCs.
- Asymptomatic patients with > 10% PVC burden should have periodic echocardiogram to exclude development of LV dysfunction.

General Considerations

Premature ventricular contractions, or **PVCs**, are isolated beats typically originating from the outflow tract or His-Purkinje regions of ventricular tissue. In most patients, the presence of PVCs is a benign finding; however, they rarely may trigger ventricular tachycardia or ventricular fibrillation, especially in patients with underlying heart disease.

Clinical Findings

Patients may be asymptomatic or experience palpitations, dizziness, or vague chest pain. Some patients feel the irregular beat; however, *symptoms can often be secondary to post-PVC augmentation of contractility or a post-PVC compensatory pause.* Increase in the sinus rate with exercise generally abolishes premature beats in normal hearts. PVCs are characterized by wide QRS complexes that differ in morphology from the patient's normal beats. They are usually not preceded by a P wave, although retrograde ventriculoatrial conduction may occur. **Bigeminy** and **trigeminy** are arrhythmias in which every second or third beat is premature. Ambulatory ECG monitoring may reveal more frequent and complex PVCs than occur in a single routine ECG. An increased frequency of PVCs during exercise is associated with a higher risk of cardiovascular mortality and should be investigated further.

Treatment

If no associated cardiac disease is present and if the ectopic beats are asymptomatic, no therapy is indicated. Mild symptoms or anxiety from palpitations may be allayed with reassurance to the patient of the benign nature of this arrhythmia. A substantial decrease or resolution of PVCs occurs spontaneously in nearly half of patients without treatment. If PVCs are frequent (bigeminal or trigeminal pattern) or multifocal, electrolyte abnormalities (ie, hypo- or hyperkalemia and hypomagnesemia) and occult cardiac disease (eg, ischemic heart disease or LV dysfunction) should be excluded. In addition, an echocardiogram should be performed in patients in whom a burden of PVCs of > 10,000 per day has been documented by ambulatory ECG monitoring. Pharmacologic treatment is indicated only for patients who are symptomatic or who develop cardiomyopathy thought to be due to a high burden of PVCs (generally > 10% of daily heart beats). β-Blockers or nondihydropyridine calcium channel blockers are appropriate as first-line therapy. The class I and III antiarrhythmic agents (see Table 12–1) may be effective in reducing PVCs but are often poorly tolerated and can be proarrhythmic in up to 5% of patients. Catheter ablation is a well-established therapy for symptomatic individuals who do not respond to medication or for those patients whose burden of ectopic beats has resulted in a cardiomyopathy.

When to Refer

Patients with symptomatic PVCs who do not respond to initial medical management or asymptomatic patients with daily PVC burden > 10% on ambulatory ECG monitoring should be referred to a cardiologist or cardiac electrophysiologist.

Shoureshi P et al. Arrhythmia-induced cardiomyopathy: JACC State-of-the-Art Review. J Am Coll Cardiol. 2024;83:2214. [PMID: 38811098]

VENTRICULAR TACHYCARDIA

ESSENTIALS OF DIAGNOSIS

- Fast, wide QRS complex on ECG.
- Associated with ischemic heart disease, particularly in older patients.
- In the absence of reversible cause, implantable cardioverter defibrillator (ICD) is recommended if meaningful life expectancy is > 1 year.

General Considerations

Ventricular tachycardia is defined as three or more consecutive ventricular premature beats. It is classified as either **nonsustained** (lasting < 30 seconds and terminating spontaneously) or **sustained** with a heart rate > 100 beats/min. In individuals without heart disease, nonsustained ventricular tachycardia is generally associated with a benign prognosis. In patients with structural heart disease, nonsustained ventricular tachycardia is associated with an increased risk of subsequent symptomatic ventricular tachycardia and sudden death, especially when seen > 48 hours after MI.

Ventricular tachycardia is a frequent complication of acute MI and dilated cardiomyopathy but may occur in chronic coronary disease, hypertrophic cardiomyopathy (HCM), myocarditis, and in most other forms of myocardial disease. It can also be a consequence of rarer forms of cardiomyopathies, such as arrhythmogenic RV cardiomyopathy. However, idiopathic ventricular tachycardia can also occur in patients with structurally normal hearts. **Accelerated idioventricular rhythm** is a regular wide-complex rhythm with a rate of 60–120 beats/min, usually with a gradual onset. It occurs commonly in acute infarction and following reperfusion with thrombolytic medications. Treatment is not indicated unless there is hemodynamic compromise or more serious arrhythmias. **Torsades de pointes**, a form of ventricular tachycardia in which the QRS morphology twists around the baseline, may occur in the setting of severe hypokalemia, hypomagnesemia, or in the setting of a prolonged QT interval (inherited or medication-induced).

Clinical Findings

A. Symptoms and Signs

Patients commonly experience palpitations, dyspnea, or lightheadedness, but on rare occasion may be asymptomatic. Syncope or cardiac arrest can be presenting symptoms in patients with underlying cardiac disease or other severe comorbidities. Episodes may be triggered by exercise or emotional stress.

B. Diagnostic Studies

Comprehensive blood laboratory work should be performed because ventricular tachycardia *can occur in the setting of hypokalemia and hypomagnesemia*. Cardiac markers may be elevated when ventricular tachycardia presents in the setting of acute MI or as a consequence of underlying CAD and demand ischemia. In patients with sustained, hemodynamically tolerated ventricular tachycardia, a 12-lead ECG during tachycardia should be obtained. Cardiac evaluation with echocardiography or cardiac MRI, ambulatory ECG monitoring, and exercise testing may be warranted depending on the clinical situation. Survivors of cardiac arrest or life-threatening ventricular arrhythmia should be evaluated for ischemic heart disease (CT or invasive coronary angiography) and undergo revascularization when appropriate.

There is generally no role for invasive electrophysiologic study in patients with sustained ventricular tachycardia who otherwise meet criteria for ICD. In patients with structural heart disease and syncope of unknown cause, or in situations in which the mechanism of wide-complex tachycardia is uncertain, electrophysiologic study may provide important information.

C. Differentiation of Aberrantly Conducted Supraventricular Beats from Ventricular Beats

The distinction on 12-lead ECG of ventricular tachycardia from SVT with aberrant conduction may be difficult in patients with a wide-complex tachycardia; it is important because of the differing prognostic and therapeutic implications of each type. Findings favoring a **ventricular origin** include: (1) AV dissociation; (2) a QRS duration exceeding 0.14 second; (3) sinus capture or fusion beats; (4) left axis deviation with right bundle branch block morphology; (5) monophasic (R) or biphasic (qR, QR, or RS) complexes in V_1; and (6) a qR or QS complex in V_6. **Supraventricular origin** is favored by: (1) typical right or left bundle branch block morphology; (2) QRS duration < 0.14 second; and (3) the presence of preexcitation syndrome by history or on prior ECG. *Patients with a wide-complex tachycardia, especially those with known cardiac disease, should be presumed to have ventricular tachycardia if the diagnosis is unclear.*

Treatment

A. Initial Management

The treatment of acute ventricular tachycardia is determined by the degree of hemodynamic compromise and the duration of the arrhythmia. In patients with structurally normal hearts, the prognosis is generally benign and syncope is uncommon. The etiology is often triggered activity from the RV or LV outflow tract or from the His-Purkinje fibers, and immediate treatment with a short-acting intravenous β-blocker or verapamil may terminate the episode.

In the presence of known or suspected structural heart disease, assessment of hemodynamic stability determines the need for urgent direct current cardioversion. When ventricular tachycardia causes hypotension, HF, or myocardial ischemia, immediate synchronized direct current cardioversion with 100–200 J should be performed. If ventricular tachycardia recurs, intravenous amiodarone (150-mg bolus followed by 1-mg/min infusion for 6 hours and then 0.5 mg/min for 18 hours) should be administered to achieve a stable rhythm with further attempts at cardioversion as necessary. Significant hypotension can occur with rapid infusions of amiodarone.

In patients with sustained ventricular tachycardia who are hemodynamically stable, medical treatment with intravenous amiodarone, lidocaine, or procainamide can be used; however, direct current cardioversion should be performed if the ventricular tachycardia fails to terminate or symptoms worsen. Empiric magnesium replacement (1–2 g intravenously) may help, especially for polymorphic ventricular tachycardia. If polymorphic ventricular tachycardia recurs, increasing the heart rate with isoproterenol infusion (up to 20 mcg/min) or atrial pacing with a temporary pacemaker (at 90–120 beats/min) will effectively shorten the QT interval to prevent further episodes. In patients with polymorphic ventricular tachycardia in the setting of a normal QT interval, myocardial ischemia should be considered with prompt evaluation and coronary revascularization performed as indicated.

B. Long-Term Management

Patients with symptomatic or sustained ventricular tachycardia in the absence of a reversible precipitating cause (acute MI or ischemia, electrolyte imbalance, medication toxicity, etc) are at high risk for recurrence. In patients with structurally normal hearts and ventricular tachycardia with typical outflow tract (left bundle branch block with inferior axis) or left posterior fascicle (right bundle branch block with superior axis) appearance on ECG, suppressive treatment with β-blocker or a nondihydropyridine calcium channel blocker may be tried. Catheter ablation has a high success rate in these patients who fail initial medical treatment. In patients with significant LV dysfunction, subsequent sudden death is common and ICD implantation is recommended if meaningful survival is expected to be longer than 1 year. β-Blockers are the mainstay for medical treatment of ventricular tachycardia in patients with structural heart disease. Antiarrhythmic medications (eg, amiodarone or sotalol) have *not* been shown to lower mortality in these patients but may decrease subsequent episodes and reduce the number of ICD shocks. Catheter ablation is an important treatment option for those patients with recurrent tachycardia who do not respond to or are intolerant of medical therapy. Owing to the potential side effects from long-term antiarrhythmic use, catheter ablation may be considered as a first-line treatment especially for patients with ischemic cardiomyopathy.

When to Refer

Any patient with sustained ventricular tachycardia or syncope of unknown cause in the presence of underlying structural cardiac disease.

Russo A et al. ACC/AHA/ASE/HFSA/HRS/SCAI/SCCT/SCMR 2025 appropriate use criteria for implantable cardioverter-defibrillators, cardiac resynchronization therapy, and pacing. J Am Coll Cardiol. 2025;85:1213. [PMID: 39808105]

VENTRICULAR FIBRILLATION & SUDDEN DEATH

ESSENTIALS OF DIAGNOSIS

- Most patients with SCD have underlying CHD.
- In the absence of reversible cause, ICD is recommended.

General Considerations

SCD is defined as unexpected nontraumatic death in clinically well or stable patients who die within 1 hour after onset of symptoms. *The causative rhythm in most cases is ventricular fibrillation.* **Sudden cardiac arrest** is a term reserved for the successful resuscitation of patients with ventricular fibrillation, either spontaneously or via intervention (defibrillation).

Clinical Findings

Approximately 70% of cases of SCD are attributable to underlying CHD; in up to 40% of patients, SCD may be the initial manifestation of CHD. In patients younger than 35, most cases of SCD are caused by inherited heart disease (long QT syndrome, catecholaminergic polymorphic ventricular tachycardia, Brugada syndrome, HCM, arrhythmogenic RV cardiomyopathy, dilated cardiomyopathy). *Over the age of 35, CHD is the most common cause of SCD, although inherited causes are common up until the age of 50.* Non-inherited forms of heart disease can also lead to SCD, including valvular heart disease (aortic stenosis, pulmonic stenosis), congenital heart disease, and myocarditis. Prompt evaluation to exclude reversible causes of sudden cardiac arrest should begin immediately following resuscitation. Laboratory testing should be performed to exclude severe electrolyte abnormalities (particularly hypokalemia and hypomagnesemia) and acidosis and to evaluate cardiac biomarkers. Caution should be taken in attributing cardiac arrest solely to an electrolyte disturbance, however, because laboratory abnormalities may be secondary to resuscitation and not causative of the event. A 12-lead ECG should be performed to evaluate for ongoing ischemia or conduction system disease. Ventricular function should be evaluated with echocardiography. Evaluation for ischemic heart disease (CT or coronary angiography) should be performed to exclude coronary disease as the underlying cause, since revascularization may prevent recurrence. In the absence of coronary disease, contrast-enhanced cardiac MRI may be used to evaluate for the presence of myocardial scar, which is a strong predictor of recurrent ventricular tachycardia/ventricular fibrillation in patients with nonischemic cardiomyopathy.

Treatment

Unless ventricular fibrillation occurs shortly after MI, is associated with ischemia, or is seen with a correctable process (such as an electrolyte abnormality or medication toxicity), surviving patients require intervention since recurrences are frequent. Survivors of cardiac arrest have improved long-term outcomes if a **targeted temperature management protocol** is rapidly initiated and continued for 24–36 hours after cardiac arrest.

*Patients who survive sudden cardiac arrest have a high incidence of recurrence, so an **ICD** is generally indicated.* Sudden cardiac arrest in the setting of acute ischemia or infarct should be managed with prompt coronary revascularization. However, implantation of a prophylactic ICD in patients immediately after MI is associated with *worse* outcomes. High-risk patients (ie, EF ≤ 35%) may be managed with a **wearable cardioverter defibrillator** until recovery of ventricular function can be assessed by echocardiogram at a later date (6–12 weeks following MI or coronary intervention). In patients in whom ventricular function remains low (EF ≤ 35%), a permanent subcutaneous ICD (when pacing is not required) or transvenous ICD should be implanted.

When to Refer

All survivors of sudden cardiac arrest should be referred to a cardiologist or cardiac electrophysiologist.

INHERITED ARRHYTHMIA SYNDROMES

ESSENTIALS OF DIAGNOSIS

- Includes long QT syndrome, Brugada syndrome, arrhythmogenic RV cardiomyopathy, and catecholaminergic polymorphic ventricular tachycardia.
- Genetic testing for patients with suspected congenital long QT syndrome based on family history, ECG or exercise testing, or severely prolonged QT interval (> 500 msec) on serial ECGs.
- Patients with long QT syndrome or catecholaminergic polymorphic ventricular tachycardia should be treated long term with an oral β-blocker (nadolol or propranolol).
- ICD is indicated for patients with ventricular arrhythmia or syncope despite medical treatment.

General Considerations

Inherited arrhythmia syndromes may result in life-threatening ventricular arrhythmias due to gene mutations in cardiac channels resulting in abnormal electrolyte regulation across the cardiac cell membrane. **Congenital long QT syndrome** is an uncommon disease (1 in 2500 live births) that is characterized by a long QT interval (usually > 470 msec) and ventricular arrhythmia, typically polymorphic ventricular tachycardia. **Acquired long QT syndrome** is usually secondary to use of antiarrhythmic agents (sotalol, dofetilide), methadone, antidepressant medications, or certain antibiotics; electrolyte abnormalities; myocardial ischemia; or significant bradycardia. **Brugada syndrome** accounts for up to 20% of SCD in patients with structurally normal hearts and is often due to a defect in a sodium channel gene. **Arrhythmogenic RV cardiomyopathy** is an inherited cardiomyopathy that predominantly affects the RV and is characterized by areas of myocardial replacement with fibrosis and adipose tissue that frequently causes ventricular arrhythmia. **Catecholaminergic polymorphic ventricular tachycardia** is a rare but important cause of SCD associated with exercise.

Clinical Findings

Patients with an inherited arrhythmia syndrome have a variable clinical presentation; they may be asymptomatic or have palpitations, sustained tachyarrhythmia, syncope, or sudden cardiac arrest. In young patients, syncopal episodes may be misdiagnosed as a primary seizure disorder. Personal and family history should be thoroughly reviewed in all patients. A 12-lead ECG should be performed with careful attention to any abnormality in the ST segment, T wave, and QT interval. A corrected QT interval longer than 500 msec on serial ECGs in the absence of a secondary cause (medication or electrolyte abnormality) identifies a high-risk subset of patients with long QT syndrome. Ambulatory ECG monitoring may be used to evaluate for ventricular arrhythmias as well as dynamic changes to the QT interval or T wave. Exercise ECG testing should be performed in patients with suspected long QT syndrome to assess for lack of appropriate QT interval shortening with higher heart rates. In cases where the cause of sudden cardiac arrest is suspected to be heritable, genetic testing under the guidance of a multidisciplinary genetics team is recommended to both determine the diagnosis and to facilitate the identification of first-degree family members at risk for developing the same disease.

Treatment

Management of polymorphic ventricular tachycardia (torsades de pointes) that occurs in the setting of a long QT interval differs from that of other forms of ventricular tachycardia. *Class Ia or III antiarrhythmics, which prolong the QT interval, should be avoided—or withdrawn immediately if being used in patients with long QT syndrome.* Intravenous β-blockers may be effective in treating electrical storm due to long QT syndrome or catecholaminergic polymorphic ventricular tachycardia. Increasing the heart rate, whether by infusion of β-agonist (dopamine or isoproterenol) or temporary atrial or ventricular pacing, is an effective approach that can both break and prevent the rhythm.

Long-term treatment of patients with inherited arrhythmia syndromes depends on the presence of high-risk features. Use of β-blockers (particularly propranolol or nadolol) is the mainstay of treatment for patients with long QT syndrome or catecholaminergic polymorphic ventricular tachycardia. Surgical left cardiac sympathetic denervation should be considered for patients who do not respond to or are intolerant of β-blockers. For patients with Brugada syndrome, prevention of arrhythmias focuses on prompt treatment of exacerbating triggers, particularly fever. Quinidine may be used to prevent ventricular tachycardia and ICD shocks, but initiation and management of antiarrhythmic medications should always be done under the direction of a specialist. ICD implantation is recommended for patients with an inherited arrhythmia syndrome in whom sudden cardiac arrest is the initial presentation. An ICD should be considered in patients with recurrent sustained ventricular arrhythmias or syncope despite medical therapy.

When to Refer

Any patient with known or suspected inherited arrhythmia syndrome or with severe corrected QT interval prolongation (> 500 msec on serial ECGs) should be referred to a cardiologist or cardiac electrophysiologist.

SYNCOPE

ESSENTIALS OF DIAGNOSIS

- Transient loss of consciousness and postural tone from vasodepressor or cardiogenic causes with prompt recovery without resuscitative measures.
- High-risk features include history of structural heart disease, abnormal ECG, and age > 60 years.

General Considerations

Syncope is a symptom defined as a transient, self-limited loss of consciousness, usually leading to a fall. Thirty percent of the adult population will experience at least one episode of syncope. It accounts for approximately 3% of emergency department visits. *A specific cause of syncope is identified in about half of cases during the initial evaluation.* The prognosis is relatively favorable except when accompanying cardiac disease is present. In many patients with recurrent syncope or near syncope, arrhythmias are not the cause. This is particularly true when the patient has no evidence of associated heart disease by history, examination, standard ECG, or noninvasive testing.

Reflex (neurally mediated) syncope may be due to excessive vagal tone or impaired reflex control of the peripheral circulation. The most frequent type is **vasovagal syncope** or the "common faint," which is often initiated by a stressful, painful, or claustrophobic experience. Enhanced vagal tone with resulting hypotension is the cause of syncope in **carotid sinus hypersensitivity** and **postmicturition syncope**; vagal-induced sinus bradycardia, sinus arrest, and AV block are common accompaniments and may themselves be the cause of syncope.

Orthostatic (postural) hypotension is another common cause of vasodepressor syncope, especially in older adult patients; in patients with diabetes or others with autonomic neuropathy; in patients with blood loss or hypovolemia; and in patients taking vasodilators, diuretics, and adrenergic-blocking medications. In addition, a syndrome of **chronic idiopathic orthostatic hypotension** exists primarily in older men. In most of these conditions, the normal vasoconstrictive response to assuming upright posture, which compensates for the abrupt decrease in venous return, is impaired.

Cardiogenic syncope can occur on a mechanical or arrhythmic basis. There is usually no prodrome; thus, injury secondary to falling is common. Mechanical problems that can cause syncope include aortic stenosis (where syncope may occur due to the inability of the heart to adequately increase stroke volume in circumstances of increased peripheral demand), pulmonary stenosis, HCM, congenital heart disease associated with pulmonary hypertension or right-to-left shunting, and left atrial myxoma obstructing the mitral valve. Episodes are commonly exertional or postexertional. Additionally, cardiac syncope may be due to disorders of automaticity (sick sinus syndrome), conduction disorders (AV block), or tachyarrhythmias (especially ventricular tachycardia).

Clinical Findings

A. Symptoms and Signs

Vasovagal syncope often has a prodrome of **vasodepressor premonitory symptoms**, such as nausea, diaphoresis, tachycardia, and pallor. Episodes can be aborted by lying down or removing the inciting stimulus. Cardiogenic syncope by contrast is characteristically abrupt in onset, often resulting in injury, transient (lasting for seconds to a few minutes), and followed by prompt recovery of full consciousness. In orthostatic (postural) hypotension, a greater than normal decline (20 mm Hg) in BP immediately upon arising from the supine to the standing position is observed, with or without tachycardia depending on the status of autonomic (baroreceptor) function.

B. Diagnostic Tests

The evaluation for syncope depends on findings from the history and physical examination (especially orthostatic BP evaluation, auscultation of carotid arteries, and cardiac examination).

1. ECG—A resting ECG is recommended for all patients undergoing evaluation for syncope. High-risk findings on ECG include non-sinus rhythm, complete or partial left bundle branch block, and voltage criteria indicating LVH. Patients with a normal initial evaluation, including unremarkable history and physical, absence of cardiac disease or significant comorbidities and normal baseline ECG may not need further testing. When initial evaluation suggests a possible cardiac arrhythmia, continuous ambulatory ECG monitoring, event recorder (for infrequent episodes), or a wearable or implantable cardiac monitor can be considered. *Caution is required before attributing a patient's syncopal event to rhythm or conduction abnormalities observed during monitoring without concomitant symptoms.* For instance, dizziness or syncope in older patients may be unrelated to incidentally observed bradycardia, sinus node abnormalities, or ventricular ectopy.

2. Autonomic testing—Tilt-table testing may be useful in patients with suspected vasovagal syncope where the diagnosis is unclear after initial evaluation, especially when syncope is recurrent. The hemodynamic response to tilting determines whether there is a *cardioinhibitory*, *vasodepressor*, or *mixed* response. The overall utility of the test is improved when there is a high pretest probability of neurally mediated syncope, since the sensitivity and specificity of the test in the general population are only moderate.

3. Electrophysiologic studies—Electrophysiologic study has limited role in the evaluation of syncope, particularly in patients without structural heart disease or when there is a low suspicion for arrhythmic etiology. In patients with ischemic heart disease, LV dysfunction, known conduction disease, or arrhythmia, electrophysiologic study may help elucidate the mechanism of syncope and guide treatment decisions. The diagnostic yield in patients with structural heart disease is approximately 50%.

Treatment

In patients with vasovagal syncope, treatment consists largely of education on the benign nature of the condition and counseling to avoid predisposing situations. **Counterpressure maneuvers** (squatting, leg-crossing, abdominal contraction) can be helpful in limiting or terminating episodes. Medical therapy is reserved for patients with symptoms despite these measures. Midodrine is an α-agonist that can increase peripheral vasoconstriction and decrease venous pooling during vasovagal episodes and has been shown to reduce the frequency of syncopal episodes in small randomized trials. Fludrocortisone and β-blockers have also been used but generally provide minimal benefit. SSRIs have shown some benefit in select patients. For patients with orthostatic hypotension, medications including midodrine and droxidopa (a norepinephrine precursor) may be considered when nonpharmacologic measures are insufficient. There is generally no role for permanent pacemaker implantation in patients with vasovagal syncope, with the possible exception of patients older than age 40 years with prolonged (longer than 3 seconds), symptomatic episodes of asystole documented on ambulatory monitoring. Pacemaker implantation based solely upon tilt-table–induced asystolic (cardioinhibitory) response is rarely indicated. Catheter ablation of ganglionated plexi (cardioneuroablation) in patients with vasovagal syncope with profound cardioinhibitory response significantly decreased recurrent syncope compared with medical therapy in a small RCT. Ongoing randomized controlled studies comparing cardioneuroablation with midodrine, pacemaker implantation, or sham procedure will help clarify the effectiveness and safety of this catheter ablation procedure in the broader management of vasovagal syncope.

If symptomatic bradyarrhythmias or supraventricular tachyarrhythmias are detected and felt to be the cause of syncope, therapy can usually be initiated without additional diagnostic studies. **Permanent pacing** is indicated in patients with cardiogenic syncope and documented severe pauses (> 3 seconds), bradycardia, or high-degree AV block (second-degree Mobitz type II or complete heart block) when symptoms are correlated to the arrhythmia.

An important consideration in patients who have experienced syncope, symptomatic ventricular tachycardia, or aborted sudden death is to provide recommendations concerning **automobile driving restrictions**. Patients with syncope thought to be due to temporary factors (acute MI, bradyarrhythmias subsequently treated with permanent pacing, medication effect, electrolyte imbalance) should be advised after recovery not to drive for at least 1 week. Patients with symptomatic ventricular tachycardia or aborted sudden death, whether treated pharmacologically, with an ICD, or with ablation therapy, warrant longer driving restriction (3–6 months).

When to Refer

- Patients with syncope and underlying structural heart disease, documented arrhythmia, or conduction disturbance.
- Unclear etiology of syncope with high-risk features (HF, abnormal ECG findings, advanced age, multiple unexplained episodes).

Aksu T et al. Cardioneuroablation for the treatment of reflex syncope and functional bradyarrhythmias: a scientific statement of the European Heart Rhythm Association (EHRA) of the ESC, the Heart Rhythm Society (HRS), the Asia Pacific Heart Rhythm Society (APHRS) and the Latin American Heart Rhythm Society (LAHRS). Europace. 2024;26:euae206. [PMID: 39082698]

Systemic Hypertension

Michael Sutters, MD, MRCP (UK)

13

INTRODUCTION

Based on data from the 2017–2020 National Health and Nutrition Examination Survey, 32.9% of adults in the United States meet the traditional criteria of having hypertension (blood pressure > 140/90 mm Hg or being treated for hypertension). An estimated 79% of people with hypertension defined in this way are aware of the diagnosis. Ninety-one percent of those aware of the diagnosis are receiving antihypertensive treatment. Blood pressure is controlled < 140/90 mm Hg in only 48% of those receiving antihypertensive therapy. Cardiovascular morbidity and mortality increase as both systolic and diastolic blood pressures rise, but in individuals aged > 50 years, the systolic pressure and pulse pressure better predict complications than diastolic pressure. The prevalence of hypertension increases with age. Adequate blood pressure control reduces the incidence of ACS by 20–25%, stroke by 30–35%, and HF by 50%.

HOW IS BLOOD PRESSURE MEASURED & HYPERTENSION DIAGNOSED?

Blood pressure should be measured with a well-calibrated sphygmomanometer. The bladder width within the cuff should encircle ≥ 80% of the arm circumference. Readings should be taken after the patient has been resting comfortably, with the back supported in the sitting or supine position, for ≥ 5 minutes and ≥ 30 minutes after smoking cigarettes or drinking coffee. Office blood pressure readings obtained with devices that permit multiple automated measurements after a programmed rest period produce data independently of digit-preference bias (ie, the tendency to favor numbers ending in zero or five) and avoid the "white coat" phenomenon (elevated blood pressure readings in the clinic that are normal at home). Blood pressure measurements taken outside the clinic, either with intermittent self-monitoring (home blood pressure) or an automated device programmed to take measurements at regular intervals (ambulatory blood pressure), are stronger predictors of outcomes and are recommended in clinical guidelines. Numerous cuffless and wearable devices can measure blood pressure using pulse wave analysis or applanation tonometry. These technologies facilitate home measurement and integrated assessment of 24-hour blood pressure burden. However, standardization and calibration protocols are needed before national guidelines can widely recommend these devices for the management of hypertension.

A single elevated blood pressure reading is not sufficient to establish the diagnosis of hypertension. The major exceptions to this rule are hypertension presenting with unequivocal evidence of life-threatening end-organ damage, as seen in hypertensive emergency, or without life-threatening end-organ injury, when blood pressure is > 220/125 mm Hg. In less severe cases, the diagnosis of hypertension depends on a series of measurements of blood pressure since readings can vary and tend to regress toward the mean with time. Patients whose initial blood pressure is in the hypertensive range exhibit the greatest fall toward the normal range between the first and second encounters. However, the concern for diagnostic precision needs to be balanced by an appreciation of the importance of establishing the diagnosis of hypertension as quickly as possible since a 3-month delay in treatment of hypertension in high-risk patients is associated with a twofold increase in cardiovascular morbidity and mortality. The 2025 guidelines from the American College of Cardiology and American Heart Association (ACC/AHA) (based on conventional office-based measurements) contain the following definitions:

Normal blood pressure < 120/80 mm Hg
Elevated blood pressure 120–129/< 80 mm Hg
Stage 1 hypertension 130–139/80–89 mm Hg
Stage 2 hypertension ≥ 140/90 mm Hg.

As exemplified by Hypertension Canada's 2025 guidelines (Figure 13–1), automated and home blood pressure measurements have assumed greater prominence in the diagnostic algorithms published by many national hypertension workgroups. Equivalent blood pressures for these different modes of measurement are described in Table 13–1.

Blood pressure is normally lowest at night; the loss of this nocturnal dip is a dominant predictor of cardiovascular risk, particularly risk of thrombotic stroke. An accentuation of the normal morning increase in blood pressure is associated with increased likelihood of cerebral hemorrhage.

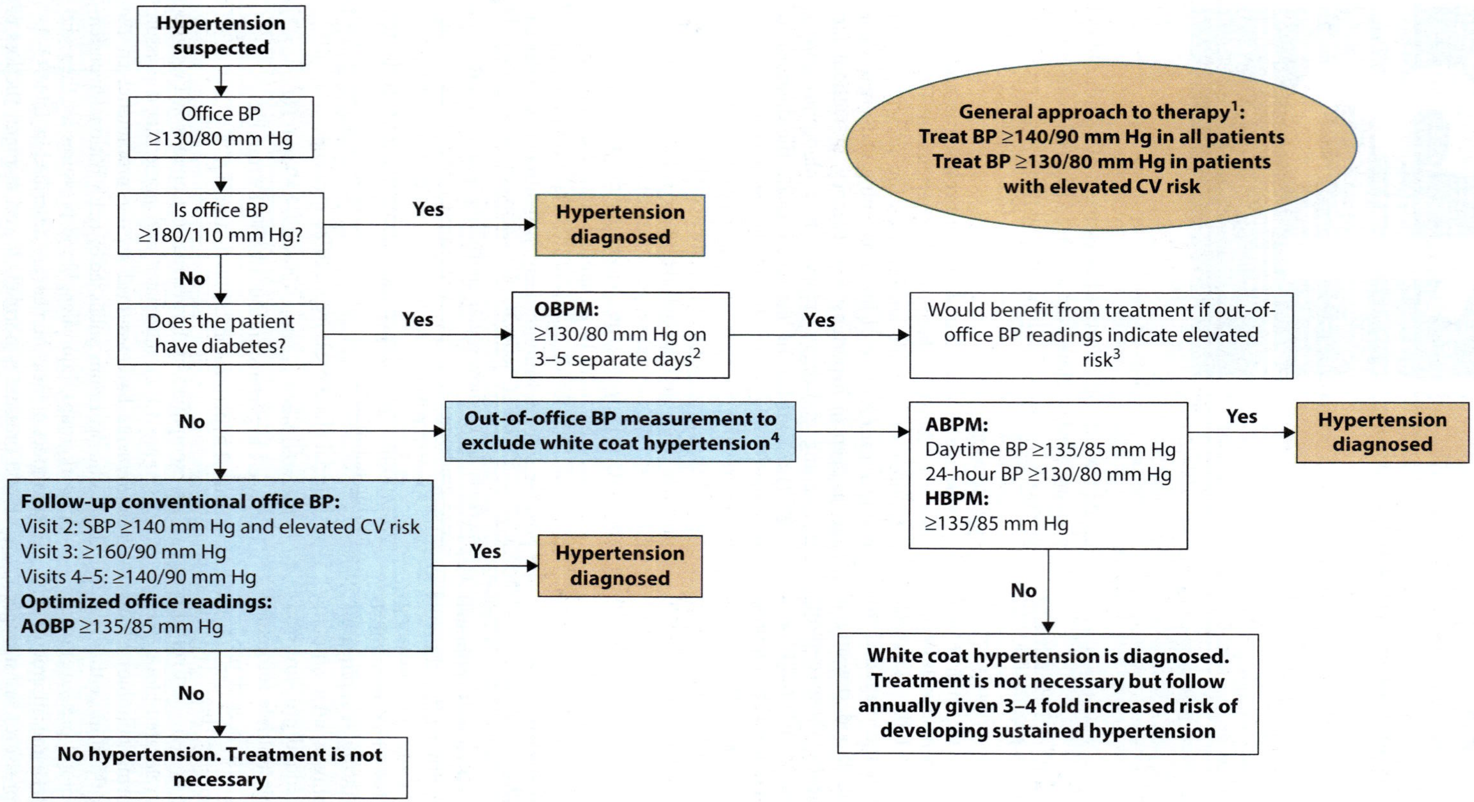

Notes:

1. Hypertension Canada introduced a generalizable recommendation for a typical primary care population to simplify the decision-making process. These guidelines do not specify the BP measurement technique or location for these threshold values for treatment, but they likely reflect optimized office-based data.
2. Outcomes data based on conventional office measurement support the treatment of hypertension at a lower BP threshold in patients with diabetes. Treatment thresholds for AOBP and home-based BP measurements in patients with diabetes have not been established in controlled trials.
3. Consider white coat effect in patients with diabetes who have elevated office BP. However, there are no controlled trials to establish out-of-office thresholds for treating BP in patients with diabetes; clinical judgement is required.
4. White coat hypertension is not associated with increased risk and should be excluded by home-based BP measurements to avoid unnecessary treatment. Masked hypertension is associated with increased risk, requires treatment, and is diagnosed also by home-based BP measurements.

▲ **Figure 13–1.** Hypertension Canada 2025 guidelines for the prevention, diagnosis, risk assessment, and treatment of hypertension. ABPM, ambulatory blood pressure measurement; AOBP, automated office blood pressure; BP, blood pressure; CV, cardiovascular; HBPM, home blood pressure measurements; OBPM, office blood pressure measurements; SBP, systolic blood pressure. (Data abstracted from Goupil R, Tsuyuki RT, Santesso N, et al. Hypertension Canada guideline for the diagnosis and treatment of hypertension in adults in primary care. CMAJ. 2025;197:E549.)

Table 13–1. Corresponding blood pressure values across a range of blood pressure measurement methods.

Manual Measurement in Clinic[1]	Home Blood Pressure Measurement	Ambulatory Blood Pressure Measurement (Daytime)	Ambulatory Blood Pressure Measurement (Nighttime)	Ambulatory Blood Pressure Measurement (24-Hour)
120/80 mm Hg	120/80 mm Hg	120/80 mm Hg	100/65 mm Hg	115/75 mm Hg
130/80 mm Hg	130/80 mm Hg	130/80 mm Hg	110/65 mm Hg	125/75 mm Hg
140/90 mm Hg	135/85 mm Hg	135/85 mm Hg	120/70 mm Hg	130/80 mm Hg
160/100 mm Hg	145/90 mm Hg	145/90 mm Hg	140/85 mm Hg	145/90 mm Hg

[1]Clinic manual blood pressures are critically dependent on technique. The use of automated devices in an unattended setting typically result in systolic blood pressures 9–13 mm Hg lower than clinic manual pressures. Data abstracted from Greenland P et al. The New 2017 ACC/AHA Guidelines "up the pressure" on diagnosis and treatment of hypertension. JAMA. 2017;318:2083.

It is important to recognize that patients in whom hypertension is diagnosed do not automatically require drug treatment, as this decision depends on the clinical setting and evaluation of cardiovascular risk.

White Coat, Masked, & Labile Hypertension

Cardiovascular risk in white coat hypertension (see above) is elevated but much less so than in established hypertension. Lifestyle changes are recommended. However, individuals with white coat hypertension have a three-to-fourfold higher risk of developing sustained hypertension over 10 years; the modest increase in cardiovascular risk associated with white coat hypertension likely reflects the three-to-fourfold risk of progression to sustained hypertension in these patients. "Masked" hypertension describes the opposite situation, where blood pressure is normal in the office setting but elevated at home. Masked hypertension is associated with a cardiovascular risk at least as high as in established hypertension. Variability of systolic blood pressure, often described as labile hypertension, predicts cardiovascular events independently of mean systolic blood pressure.

Filippone EJ et al. Controversies in hypertension I: the optimal assessment of blood pressure load and implications for treatment. Am J Med. 2022;135:1043. [PMID: 35636476]

Goupil R et al. Hypertension Canada guideline for the diagnosis and treatment of hypertension in adults in primary care. CMAJ. 2025;197:E549. [PMID: 40419299]

Jones DW et al. 2025 AHA/ACC/AANP/AAPA/ABC/ACCP/ACPM/AGS/AMA/ASPC/NMA/PCNA/SGIM Guideline for the Prevention, Detection, Evaluation and Management of High Blood Pressure in Adults: A Report of the American College of Cardiology/American Heart Association Joint Committee on Clinical Practice Guidelines. Hypertension. 2025;82:e212. [PMID: 40811516]

Raymond R et al. White coat hypertension & cardiovascular outcomes. Curr Hypertens Rep. 2024;26:399. [PMID: 38761349]

APPROACH TO HYPERTENSION

Etiology & Classification

A. Primary Essential Hypertension

"Essential hypertension" is the term applied to the 95% of hypertensive patients in whom elevated blood pressure results from complex interactions between multiple genetic and environmental factors. The onset is usually between ages 25 and 50 years; it is uncommon before age 20 years. The best understood pathways underlying hypertension include overactivation of the sympathetic nervous and renin-angiotensin-aldosterone systems (RAAS), blunting of the pressure-natriuresis relationship, variation in cardiovascular and renal development, and elevated intracellular sodium and calcium levels.

Exacerbating factors include obesity, sleep apnea, increased salt intake, excessive alcohol use, cigarette smoking, polycythemia, NSAID therapy, and low potassium intake. Drinking 1–3 cups of coffee daily does not cause a sustained increase in blood pressure and might reduce the risk of death from any cause. Obesity is associated with an increase in intravascular volume; elevated cardiac output; activation of the renin-angiotensin system; and, probably, increased sympathetic outflow. Lifestyle-driven weight reduction lowers blood pressure modestly, but the more significant weight reduction following bariatric surgery or treatment with GLP-1 agonists results in improved blood pressure in most patients, and actual remission of hypertension in 20–40% of cases. In patients with sleep apnea, treatment with continuous positive airway pressure (CPAP) has been associated with improvements in blood pressure. Increased salt intake probably elevates blood pressure in some individuals, so dietary salt restriction is recommended in patients with hypertension. Excessive use of alcohol also raises blood pressure, perhaps by increasing plasma catecholamines. Hypertension can be difficult to control in patients who consume > 40 g of ethanol daily or drink in "binges." The National Institute on Alcohol and Alcoholism defines a "standard" drink as one that contains 14 g/drink, however the actual amount contained is dependent upon the drink volume and alcohol percentage. Drinks containing approximately 14 g of alcohol include:

- 12 oz beer with 5% alcohol by volume
- 5 oz wine with 12% alcohol by volume
- 1.5-oz shot glass of distilled spirits with 40% alcohol by volume

Cigarette smoking raises blood pressure by increasing plasma norepinephrine. Although the long-term effect of smoking on blood pressure is less clear, the synergistic effects of smoking and high blood pressure on cardiovascular risk are well documented. The relationship of exercise to hypertension is variable. Aerobic exercise lowers blood pressure in previously sedentary individuals, but increasingly strenuous exercise in already active subjects has less effect. The relationship between stress and hypertension is not established. Polycythemia, whether primary, drug-induced, or due to diminished plasma volume, increases blood viscosity and may raise blood pressure. NSAIDs raise blood pressure by an average of 5 mm Hg and should be avoided in patients with borderline or elevated blood pressures. Low potassium intake is associated with higher blood pressure in some patients; a daily intake of 90 mmol is recommended.

The complex of abnormalities termed the **"metabolic syndrome"** (upper body obesity, insulin resistance, and hypertriglyceridemia) is associated with both the development of hypertension and an increased risk of adverse cardiovascular outcomes. Affected patients usually also have low HDL cholesterol levels and elevated catecholamines and inflammatory markers, such as CRP.

B. Secondary Hypertension

Approximately 5% of patients have hypertension secondary to identifiable specific causes (Table 13–2). Secondary hypertension should be suspected in patients in whom hypertension develops at an early age or after the age of 50 years, and in those previously well controlled who become refractory to treatment. Hypertension resistant to maximum doses of three medications is another clue, although multiple medications are usually required to control hypertension in persons with diabetes.

Table 13–2. Causes of secondary hypertension.

Renal
Parenchymal kidney disease
Polycystic kidney disease
Systemic sclerosis (scleroderma)
Page kidney (subcapsular compression of the kidney)
Mutations in genes encoding ion transport proteins
Vascular
Renal artery stenosis
Coarctation
Endocrine
Conn syndrome (hyperaldosteronism)
Licorice
Cushing syndrome (hypercortisolism)
Thyroid disease
Pheochromocytoma
Acromegaly
Mutations in steroid gene regulatory domains
Hypercalcemia
Autonomic
Neurogenic
Medications
NSAIDs
Corticosteroids
Calcineurin inhibitors
Stimulants
Decongestants
Angiogenesis inhibitors
Tyrosine kinase inhibitors
Estrogen
Erythropoietin
Alcohol, cocaine
Gemcitabine
Atypical antipsychotics
MAO inhibitors
Other
Obstructive sleep apnea
Pregnancy

1. Genetic causes—Hypertension can be caused by mutations in single genes, inherited on a Mendelian basis. Although rare, these conditions provide important insight into blood pressure regulation and possibly the genetic basis of essential hypertension. Glucocorticoid remediable aldosteronism is an autosomal dominant cause of early-onset hypertension with normal or high aldosterone and low renin levels. The syndrome of hypertension exacerbated in pregnancy is inherited as an autosomal dominant trait. In these patients, a mutation in the mineralocorticoid receptor makes it abnormally responsive to progesterone and, paradoxically, to spironolactone. Liddle syndrome is an autosomal dominant condition characterized by early-onset hypertension, hypokalemic alkalosis, low renin, and low aldosterone levels. Gordon syndrome, or pseudohypoaldosteronism type II, is most often transmitted in an autosomal dominant pattern and presents with early-onset hypertension associated with hyperkalemia, metabolic acidosis, and relative suppression of aldosterone.

2. Kidney disease—Renal parenchymal disease is a common cause of secondary hypertension, which results from increased intravascular volume and increased activity of the RAAS. Increased sympathetic nerve activity may also contribute.

3. Renal vascular hypertension—Renal artery stenosis is present in 1–2% of hypertensive patients. The most common cause is atherosclerosis, but fibromuscular dysplasia should be suspected in women younger than 50 years of age. Excessive renin release occurs due to reduction in renal perfusion pressure, while attenuation of pressure natriuresis contributes to hypertension in patients with a single kidney or bilateral lesions.

Renal vascular hypertension should be suspected in the following circumstances: (1) documented onset is before age 20 or after age 50 years, (2) hypertension is resistant to three or more drugs, (3) there are epigastric or renal artery bruits, (4) there is atherosclerotic disease of the aorta or peripheral arteries (15–25% of patients with symptomatic lower limb atherosclerotic vascular disease have renal artery stenosis), (5) there is an abrupt increase (> 25%) in the serum creatinine after administration of ACE inhibitors, or (6) episodes of pulmonary edema are associated with abrupt surges in blood pressure. (See Renal Artery Stenosis, Chapter 25.)

4. Primary hyperaldosteronism—Increased aldosterone secretion from an adrenal adenoma or bilateral adrenal hyperplasia is the most common cause of secondary hypertension.

Hyperaldosteronism should be considered in patients with resistant hypertension, blood pressures consistently > 150/100 mm Hg, hypokalemia (although this is often absent), or adrenal incidentaloma, and in those with a family history of hyperaldosteronism. Obstructive sleep apnea and atrial fibrillation are also linked to hyperaldosteronism. Mild hypernatremia and metabolic alkalosis may occur. Hypersecretion of aldosterone is estimated to be present in 5–10% of hypertensive patients and, besides noncompliance, is the most common cause of resistant hypertension. The initial screening step is the simultaneous measurement of aldosterone and renin in blood in a morning sample collected after 30 minutes quietly seated. Hyperaldosteronism is suggested when the plasma aldosterone concentration is elevated (normal: 1–16 ng/dL) in association with suppression of plasma renin activity (normal: 1–2.5 ng/mL/hour). However, the plasma aldosterone/renin ratio (normal < 30) is not highly specific as a screening test. This is because renin levels may approach zero, which leads to exponential increases in the plasma aldosterone/renin ratio even when aldosterone levels are normal. Hence, an elevated plasma aldosterone/renin ratio should probably not be taken as evidence of hyperaldosteronism unless the aldosterone level is actually elevated.

During the workup for hyperaldosteronism, an initial plasma aldosterone/renin ratio can be measured while the patient continues taking usual medications. If under these circumstances the ratio proves normal or equivocal, medications that alter renin and aldosterone levels, including ACE inhibitors, ARBs, diuretics, β-blockers, and clonidine, should be discontinued for 2 weeks before repeating the plasma aldosterone/renin ratio; spironolactone and eplerenone should be held for 4 weeks. Slow-release verapamil and α-blockers can be used to control blood pressure during this drug washout period. Patients with a plasma aldosterone level > 16 ng/dL and an aldosterone/renin ratio of 30 or more might require further evaluation for primary hyperaldosteronism.

5. Cushing syndrome—Hypertension occurs in about 80% of patients with spontaneous Cushing syndrome. Excess glucocorticoid may act through salt and water retention (via mineralocorticoid effects), increased angiotensinogen levels, or permissive effects in the regulation of vascular tone. Diagnosis and treatment of Cushing syndrome are discussed in Chapter 29.

6. Pheochromocytoma—Pheochromocytomas are discussed in Chapter 29. They are found in < 0.1% of all patients with hypertension and in approximately two individuals per million population. Chronic vasoconstriction of the arterial and venous beds leads to a reduction in plasma volume and predisposes to postural hypotension. Glucose intolerance develops in some patients. Hypertensive crisis in pheochromocytoma may be precipitated by a variety of drugs, including tricyclic antidepressants, antidopaminergic agents, metoclopramide, and naloxone.

7. Coarctation of the aorta—This uncommon cause of hypertension is discussed in Chapter 10. Evidence of radial-femoral delay should be sought in all younger patients with hypertension.

8. Hypertension associated with pregnancy—Hypertension occurring de novo or worsening during pregnancy, including preeclampsia and eclampsia, is one of the most common causes of maternal and fetal morbidity and mortality (see Chapter 21). Autoantibodies with the potential to activate the angiotensin II type 1 receptor have been causally implicated in preeclampsia, in resistant hypertension, and in progressive systemic sclerosis.

9. Estrogen use—A small increase in blood pressure occurs in most women taking oral contraceptives. A more significant increase of 8/6 mm Hg in systolic/diastolic is noted in about 5% of women, mostly in individuals with obesity aged > 35 years who have been treated for > 5 years. This is caused by increased hepatic synthesis of angiotensinogen. The lower dose of postmenopausal estrogen does not generally cause hypertension but rather maintains endothelium-mediated vasodilation.

10. Other causes of secondary hypertension—Hypertension has been associated with hypercalcemia, acromegaly, hyperthyroidism, hypothyroidism, baroreceptor dysfunction (sometimes seen after treatment of head and neck cancer), compression of the ventrolateral medulla and increased intracranial pressure. Certain medications may cause or exacerbate hypertension—most importantly cyclosporine, tacrolimus, angiogenesis inhibitors, and erythrocyte-stimulating agents (such as erythropoietin). Decongestants, NSAIDs, cocaine, and alcohol should also be considered. Over-the-counter products should not be overlooked.

When to Refer

Referral to a hypertension specialist should be considered in cases of severe, resistant, or early- or late-onset hypertension or when secondary hypertension is suggested by screening.

Byrd JB et al. Primary aldosteronism. Circulation. 2018;138:823. [PMID: 30359120]
Herrmann SM et al. Renovascular hypertension. Endocrinol Metab Clin North Am. 2019;48:765. [PMID: 31655775]

Complications of Untreated Hypertension

Many adverse outcomes in hypertension are associated with thrombosis rather than bleeding, possibly because increased vascular shear stress converts the normally anticoagulant endothelium to a prothrombotic state. Increases in systolic blood pressure have the greatest impact on cardiovascular risk, but diastolic pressure also increases risk independently of systolic pressure. Target-organ damage varies markedly between individuals with similar levels of office hypertension; home and ambulatory pressures are superior to office readings in the prediction of end-organ damage (Table 13–1).

A. Hypertensive Cardiovascular Disease

Cardiac complications are the major sequelae of hypertension. For any level of blood pressure, LVH is associated with incremental cardiovascular risk in association with HF (through systolic or diastolic dysfunction), ventricular arrhythmias, myocardial ischemia, and sudden death.

The occurrence of HF is reduced by 50% with antihypertensive therapy. Hypertensive LVH regresses with therapy and is most closely related to the degree of systolic blood pressure reduction. Diuretics have produced equal or greater reductions of LV mass when compared with other drug classes. Conventional β-blockers are less effective in reducing LVH but play a specific role in patients with established CAD or impaired LV function.

B. Hypertensive Cerebrovascular Disease and Dementia

Hypertension is the major predisposing cause of hemorrhagic and ischemic stroke. Cerebrovascular complications are more closely correlated with systolic than diastolic blood pressure. The incidence of these complications is markedly reduced by antihypertensive therapy. Preceding hypertension is associated with a higher incidence of subsequent dementia of both vascular and Alzheimer types. Home and ambulatory blood pressure may be a better predictor of cognitive decline than office readings in older people. Effective blood pressure control reduces the risk of cognitive dysfunction developing later in life.

C. Hypertensive Kidney Disease

Chronic hypertension is associated with injury to vascular, glomerular, and tubulointerstitial compartments within the kidney, accounting for about 25% of ESKD. Nephrosclerosis is particularly prevalent in persons of sub-Saharan African ancestry, in whom susceptibility is linked to *APOL1* variants and hypertension results from kidney disease rather than causing it.

D. Aortic Dissection

Hypertension is a contributing factor in many patients with dissection of the aorta. Its diagnosis and treatment are discussed in Chapter 14.

E. Atherosclerotic Complications

Most Americans with hypertension die of complications of atherosclerosis, but the impact of antihypertensive therapy on atherosclerotic complications is less clear than that seen in the prevention of HF, stroke, and kidney disease. Prevention of cardiovascular outcomes related to atherosclerosis probably requires control of multiple risk factors, of which hypertension is only one.

Flint AC et al. Effect of systolic and diastolic blood pressure on cardiovascular outcomes. N Engl J Med. 2019;381:243. [PMID 31314968]

Supiano MA et al. New guidelines and SPRINT results: implications for geriatric hypertension. Circulation. 2019;140:976. [PMID: 31525101]

Clinical Findings

The clinical and laboratory findings of hypertension arise from involvement of the target organs: heart, brain, kidneys, eyes, and peripheral arteries.

A. Symptoms

Mild to moderate primary (essential) hypertension is largely asymptomatic for many years. The most frequent symptom, headache, is nonspecific. Without concrete symptoms associated with actual end-organ injury, there is no evidence that patients can predict their blood pressure by how they feel.

The classification of the more urgent presentations of hypertension have been reduced to two categories, uncontrolled hypertension and hypertensive emergency.

Uncontrolled hypertension is usually asymptomatic and typically presents as an incidental finding.

Hypertensive emergencies are defined as events where uncontrolled hypertension results in end-organ damage. Presenting symptoms will depend on the profile of the organ injury. Hypertensive encephalopathy is characterized by headache, somnolence, and vomiting that usually improve with prompt control of hypertension. The symptom complex associated with posterior reversible encephalopathy syndrome includes headache, seizures, altered consciousness, and disturbance of vision. Focal neurologic deficits indicate cerebral infarction or hemorrhage. Intracranial hemorrhage may be intraparenchymal, ventricular, or subarachnoid and is often felt as an abrupt onset of the worst headache ever experienced. Subarachnoid hemorrhage may cause loss of consciousness and neck stiffness.

Symptoms associated with acute elevation of LV afterload include angina and dyspnea. Aortic dissection or rupture causes chest or abdominal pain that is usually severe.

Hypertension in patients with pheochromocytomas that secrete predominantly norepinephrine is usually sustained but may be episodic. The typical attack lasts from minutes to hours and is associated with headache, anxiety, palpitation, profuse perspiration, pallor, tremor, and nausea and vomiting. Blood pressure is markedly elevated, and angina or acute pulmonary edema may occur. In primary aldosteronism, patients may have muscular weakness, and polyuria and nocturia due to hypokalemia; hypertensive emergency is rare. Chronic hypertension often leads to LVH and diastolic dysfunction, which can present with exertional and paroxysmal nocturnal dyspnea. Cerebral involvement in chronic hypertension causes stroke due to thrombosis or hemorrhage from microaneurysms of small penetrating intracranial arteries.

B. Signs

Like symptoms, physical findings depend on the cause of hypertension, its duration and severity, and the degree of effect on target organs.

1. Blood pressure—Blood pressure is taken in both arms and, if lower extremity pulses are diminished or delayed, in the legs to exclude coarctation of the aorta. If blood pressure differs between right and left arms, the higher reading should be recorded as the actual blood pressure and subclavian stenosis suspected in the other arm. An orthostatic drop of at least 20/10 mm Hg is often present in pheochromocytoma. Older patients may have falsely elevated readings by sphygmomanometry because of noncompressible vessels. This may be suspected in the presence of

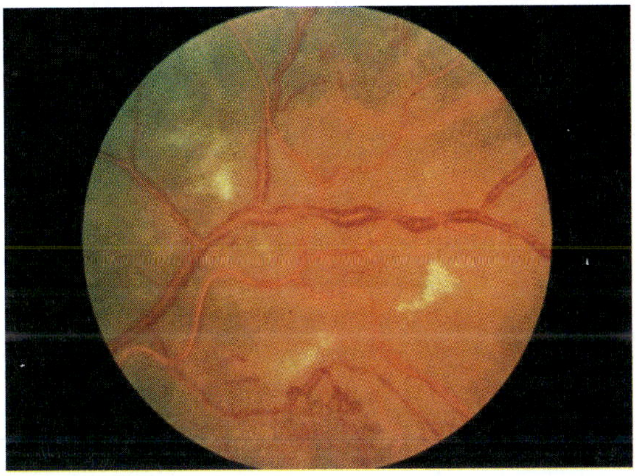

Figure 13–2. Severe, chronic hypertensive retinopathy with hard exudates, increased vessel light reflexes, and sausage-shaped veins. (Used, with permission, from Richard E. Wyszynski, MD, in Knoop KJ, Stack LB, Storrow AB, Thurman RJ. *The Atlas of Emergency Medicine*, 4th ed. McGraw-Hill, 2016.)

Osler sign—a palpable brachial or radial artery when the cuff is inflated above systolic pressure. Occasionally, it may be necessary to make direct measurements of intra-arterial pressure, especially in patients with apparent severe hypertension who do not tolerate therapy.

2. Retinas—Narrowing of arterial diameter to < 50% of venous diameter, copper or silver wire appearance, exudates, hemorrhages, and hypertensive retinopathy are associated with a worse prognosis. The typical changes of severe hypertensive retinopathy are shown in Figure 13–2 (see Chapter 7).

3. Heart—An LV heave indicates severe hypertrophy. Aortic regurgitation may be auscultated in up to 5% of patients, and hemodynamically insignificant aortic regurgitation can be detected by Doppler echocardiography in 10–20%. A presystolic (S_4) gallop due to decreased compliance of the LV is quite common in patients in sinus rhythm.

4. Pulses—Radial-femoral delay suggests coarctation of the aorta; loss of peripheral pulses occurs due to atherosclerosis, less commonly aortic dissection, and rarely Takayasu arteritis, all of which can involve the renal arteries.

C. Laboratory Findings

Recommended testing includes hemoglobin; serum electrolytes and serum creatinine; fasting blood sugar level (hypertension is a risk factor for the development of diabetes, and hyperglycemia can be a presenting feature of pheochromocytoma); plasma lipids (necessary to calculate cardiovascular risk and as a modifiable risk factor); serum uric acid (hyperuricemia is a relative contraindication to diuretic therapy); and UA.

D. ECG and Chest Radiographs

Electrocardiographic criteria are highly specific but not sensitive for LVH. The "strain" pattern of ST–T-wave changes is a sign of more advanced disease and is associated with a poor prognosis. A CXR is not necessary in the workup of uncomplicated hypertension.

E. Echocardiography

The primary role of echocardiography should be to evaluate clinical symptoms or signs of cardiac disease.

F. Diagnostic Studies

Additional diagnostic studies are indicated only if the clinical presentation or routine tests suggest secondary or complicated hypertension. These may include 24-hour urine-free cortisol, urine or plasma metanephrines, and plasma aldosterone and renin concentrations to screen for endocrine causes of hypertension. Renal ultrasound will detect structural changes (such as polycystic kidneys, asymmetry, and hydronephrosis); increased echogenicity and reduced cortical volume are reliable indicators of advanced CKD. Evaluation for renal artery stenosis should be undertaken in consultation with a subspecialist.

G. Summary

Since most hypertension is essential or primary, few studies are necessary beyond those listed above. If conventional therapy is unsuccessful or if secondary hypertension is suspected, further studies and perhaps referral to a hypertension specialist are indicated.

Nonpharmacologic Therapy

Lifestyle modification is recommended for all patients with elevated blood pressure. In a study from China of persons aged > 60 years or who had a history of stroke and hypertension, study participants were randomly assigned to consume ordinary salt or a salt substitute containing 75% sodium chloride and 25% potassium chloride (by mass). Those using the salt substitute had a 14% decline in the rate of the primary endpoint of stroke, and a roughly 12% decline in the secondary endpoints of cardiovascular events and all-cause mortality. A diet rich in fruits, vegetables, and low-fat dairy foods and low in saturated and total fats (DASH diet) has been shown to lower blood pressure. Increased dietary fiber lowers blood pressure. For every 7 g of dietary fiber ingested, cardiovascular risk could be lowered by 9%. The effect of diet on blood pressure may be mediated by shifts in the microbial species in the gut, the intestinal microbiota. Hand squeezing exercises three times a week can lower systolic blood pressure by 6 mm Hg. The protocol comprises four repeats of 2 minutes at 30% of maximum force (using a handheld dynamometer) with 1- to 3-minute rest intervals between squeezes. The use of cell phone applications to support behavioral changes to lower blood pressure has shown efficacy in randomized studies. There is limited evidence on the long-term benefit of stress reduction strategies such as biofeedback, yoga, and mindfulness. The impact of a variety of dietary supplements (such as garlic extract and fish oil) upon long-term blood pressure control also is uncertain. The effects of a range of lifestyle changes upon blood pressure are listed in Table 13–3.

Table 13–3. The impact of lifestyle modifications.

Modification	Intervention	Resulting Decrease in Blood Pressure
Weight loss	Target BMI 18.5–24.9	5–20 mm Hg/ 10-kg loss
DASH diet	Fruit, vegetables, low-fat dairy	8–14 mm Hg
Sodium intake	< 100 mmol/day (< 6 g salt)	2–8 mm Hg
Alcohol intake	Male ≤ 2 drinks/day Female ≤ 1 drink/day	4 mm Hg
Exercise	Aerobic 30 minutes/day Dynamic 90–150 minutes/week Isometric (hand grip 4 repetitions 3 times/week)	5–10 mm Hg
Mindfulness	Meditation and breathing control	5 mm Hg

DASH, Dietary Approaches to Stop Hypertension.

Kario K et al. Digital therapeutics in hypertension: evidence and perspectives. Hypertension. 2022;79:2148. [PMID: 35726619]
Maniero C et al. Non-pharmacological factors for hypertension management: a systematic review of international guidelines. Eur J Prev Cardiol. 2023;30:17. [PMID: 35947982]

Neal B et al. Effect of salt substitution on cardiovascular events and death. N Engl J Med. 2021;385:1067. [PMID: 34459569]
Rodrigues GD et al. Are home-based exercises effective to reduce blood pressure in hypertensive adults? A systematic review. Clin Hypertens. 2022;28:28. [PMID: 36104807]

Who Should Be Treated With Medications?

Treatment should be offered to all persons in whom blood pressure reduction, irrespective of initial blood pressure levels, will reduce cardiovascular risk with an acceptably low rate of medication-associated adverse effects. The ACC/AHA, Hypertension Canada, and the European Society of Hypertension and European Society of Cardiology (ESH/ESC) have developed independent guidelines for the evaluation and management of hypertension. There is a broad consensus in these guidelines that, in most cases, antihypertensive therapy should be started when blood pressure consistently exceeds 140/90 mm Hg, with a goal blood pressure of < 130/80 mm Hg (Table 13-4). Since evaluation of total cardiovascular risk (Table 13–5) is important in deciding who to treat with antihypertensive medications, risk calculators are essential clinical tools. The AHA "Prevent" online risk calculator incorporates cardiovascular, renal, and metabolic parameters to estimate 10 year and 30 year total cardiovascular risk with separate breakdowns for atherosclerotic and HF events (https://professional.heart.org/en/guidelines-and-statements/prevent-calculator). Using this algorithm, the cutoff point for elevated risk is 7.5% at 10 years. The interaction

Table 13–4. Comparison of treatment thresholds and target blood pressure published by the ACC/AHA, Hypertension Canada, and ESH/ESC.[1]

Guidelines	Cardiovascular Risk	Threshold for Pharmacotherapy (mm Hg)	Target BP (mm Hg)
ACC/AHA	Not increased	140/90[2]	< 130/80[3]
	Increased	130/80	< 130/80[4]
	Due to age > 80 yr	130/80	< 130/80[5]
Hypertension Canada	Not increased	140/90[2]	SBP < 130
	Increased	130/80	SBP < 130[6]
	Age > 75 yr[7]	Not specified	Not specified
ESH/ESC	Not increased	140/90[8]	< 130/80[8]
	Increased	130/80	< 130/80
	Due to age 65–80 yr	140/90	Not specified
	Due to age > 80 yr	SBP >160	SBP 130–140 while keeping DBP > 70

[1]In all three sets of guidelines, BP values are based on nonautomated office BP readings.
[2]Consider treating if BP remains >130/80 mm Hg after 3–6 months of lifestyle modification.
[3]Target of <120 mm Hg is *considered reasonable* if tolerated.
[4]Target of <120 mm Hg is *encouraged* if tolerated.
[5]Age alone has no impact on thresholds or goals until aged > 80 years.
[6]Despite elevated risk, the Canadian guidelines do not suggest a more aggressive BP target since conventional office SBP < 130 mm Hg is considered equivalent to study SBP < 120 mm Hg.
[7]Recommendations for older adult patients are not explicitly specified, but age >75 years is considered an elevated risk category.
[8]These guidelines diverge from others by not recommending more aggressive thresholds and targets in patients with diabetes.
ACC, American College of Cardiology; AHA, American Heart Association; BP, blood pressure; DBP, diastolic blood pressure; ESC, European Society of Cardiology; ESH, European Society of Hypertension; SBP, systolic blood pressure.

Table 13–5. Cardiovascular risk factors.

Major risk factors
Hypertension[1]
Cigarette smoking
Obesity (BMI ≥ 30)[1]
Physical inactivity
Dyslipidemia[1]
Diabetes mellitus[1]
Microalbuminuria or estimated GFR < 60 mL/min/1.73 m^2
Age (> 55 years for men, > 65 years for women)
Family history of premature CVD (< 55 years for men, < 65 years for women)
Target-organ damage
Heart
LVH
Angina or prior MI
Prior coronary revascularization
HF
Brain
Stroke or transient ischemic attack
CKD
Peripheral arterial disease
Retinopathy

[1]Components of the metabolic syndrome.
Data from Chobanian AV et al. The Seventh Report of the Joint National Committee on Prevention, Detection, Evaluation, and Treatment of High Blood Pressure: the JNC 7 report. JAMA. 2003;289:2560.

between risk and age deserves careful attention. At any given level of calculated risk, treatment is likely to have a greater impact in young versus older adults. Consequently, setting absolute risk thresholds for treatment might lead to undertreatment of young adults and overtreatment of older adults.

Goals of Treatment

Observational studies of untreated individuals suggest that there does not seem to be a naturally occurring blood pressure level below which decrements in cardiovascular risk taper off, and several RCTs have suggested that treatment to blood pressure targets considerably < 140 mm Hg may benefit certain patient groups.

The SPRINT study suggests that outcomes improve in nondiabetic patients with considerably elevated cardiovascular risk when treatment lowers systolic pressure to < 120 mm Hg compared to < 140 mm Hg. On the other hand, in the HOPE3 study of largely nondiabetic patients at somewhat lower risk than those in SPRINT, reducing blood pressure by an average of 6/3 mm Hg systolic/diastolic from a baseline of 138/82 mm Hg provided no significant outcomes benefits. Accordingly, guidelines recommend that blood pressure targets should be lower in people at greater estimated cardiovascular risk. Some experts note that manual office measurements of approximately 130/80 mm Hg are likely to approximate the lower blood pressure targets specified in the SPRINT study, which used automated office blood pressure measuring devices that have been demonstrated to read as much as 16/7 mm Hg lower than manual office readings. Table 13–4 compares the treatment thresholds and target recommendations laid out in the American, Canadian, and European guidelines. Treatment to blood pressures < 130 mm Hg systolic seems especially important in stroke prevention. In the ACCORD study of patients with diabetes, reduction in blood pressure < 130-135 mm Hg significantly reduced the risk of stroke. In the 2013 SPS3 trial, the treatment of nondiabetic patients with a recent lacunar stroke to a systolic blood pressure < 130 mm Hg (mean systolic blood pressure of 127 mm Hg among treated versus mean systolic blood pressure 138 mm Hg among untreated patients) probably reduced the risk of recurrent stroke. Blood pressure management in acute stroke is discussed below.

How Low to Go?

Although observational studies indicate that the blood pressure–risk relationship holds up at levels considerably below a naturally occurring systolic pressure of 120 mm Hg, there has been uncertainty about whether this relationship is true for treated blood pressure. This question was addressed in a secondary analysis of data from the ONTARGET and TRANSCEND studies in which participants with elevated cardiovascular risk but no history of stroke were treated with telmisartan (plus or minus ramipril) or placebo. The risk of the composite cardiovascular endpoint was lowest at a treated systolic blood pressure range of 120–140 mm Hg. Increased risk was observed at blood pressures below and above this range. The risk of stroke was the only exception, with incremental benefit observed below a treated systolic pressure of 120 mm Hg. With respect to diastolic blood pressure on treatment, composite risk began to increase at levels < 70 mm Hg. This suggests that the blood pressure–cardiovascular risk relationship evident in observational studies of untreated hypertension may not hold in the case of treated blood pressure and that there are grounds for a degree of caution in treating below a systolic pressure of 120 mm Hg.

In seeking to simplify decision making in the treatment of hypertension, some authors have suggested that a systolic blood pressure goal in the 120–130 mm Hg range would be safe and effective in high-risk patients, and a systolic blood pressure of around 130 mm Hg would be reasonable in lower-risk patients, irrespective of diastolic pressures. Diastolic blood pressure will track with systolic blood pressure; the main concern about diastolic blood pressure is that treatment will lower it too much in patients who have wider pulse pressures. However, it seems that a lower diastolic blood pressure because of treatment does not negate the benefits of systolic blood pressure control, even though wider pulse pressures at baseline are associated with cardiovascular mortality. Medications with preferential effects on systolic pressure, such as calcium channel blockers and diuretics, may minimize the impact of antihypertensive therapy on diastolic pressure.

Treatment of Other Cardiovascular Risk Factors

Data from multiple studies indicate that statins should be part of the strategy to reduce overall cardiovascular risk. The HOPE3 study of persons at intermediate cardiovascular risk showed that 10 mg of rosuvastatin reduced average LDL cholesterol from 130 mg/dL to 90 mg/dL (3.36–2.33 mmol/L) and significantly reduced the risk of multiple cardiovascular events, including MI and coronary revascularization. Low-dose aspirin (81 mg/day) is no longer recommended in the primary prevention of MI or stroke. Low-dose aspirin is effective in prevention of recurrent cardiovascular events, but blood pressure should first be controlled to minimize the risk of cerebral hemorrhage.

Jones DW et al; American Heart Association Council on Hypertension; Council on the Kidney in Cardiovascular Disease; Council on Arteriosclerosis, Thrombosis and Vascular Biology; Council on Cardiovascular Radiology and Intervention; Council on Lifelong Congenital Heart Disease and Heart Health in the Young; and Stroke Council. Management of stage 1 hypertension in adults with a low 10-year risk for cardiovascular disease: filling a guidance gap: a scientific statement from the American Heart Association. Hypertension. 2021;77:e58. [PMID: 33910363]

Lauder L et al. European guidelines for hypertension in 2024: a comparison of key recommendations for clinical practice. Nat Rev Cardiol. 2025;22:675. [PMID 40691360]

Visseren FLJ et al; ESC Scientific Document Group. 2021 ESC Guidelines on cardiovascular disease prevention in clinical practice. Eur J Prev Cardiol. 2022;29:5. [PMID: 34558602]

DRUG THERAPY: CURRENT ANTIHYPERTENSIVE AGENTS

There are many classes of antihypertensive agents of which six (ACE inhibitors, ARBs, renin inhibitors, calcium channel blockers, diuretics, and β-blockers) are suitable for initial therapy based on efficacy and tolerability. The specific classes of antihypertensive medications are discussed below.

A. Angiotensin-Converting Enzyme Inhibitors

ACE inhibitors are commonly used as the initial medication in mild to moderate hypertension (Table 13–6). Their primary mode of action is inhibition of the RAAS, but they also inhibit bradykinin degradation, stimulate the synthesis of vasodilating prostaglandins, and can reduce sympathetic nervous system activity. ACE inhibitors appear to be more effective in younger White patients. They are relatively less effective in Black and older persons and in predominantly systolic hypertension. Although as single therapy they achieve adequate antihypertensive control in only about 40–50% of patients, the combination of an ACE inhibitor and a diuretic or calcium channel blocker is potent.

ACE inhibitors are the agents of choice in persons with type 1 diabetes with frank proteinuria or evidence of kidney dysfunction because they delay the progression to ESKD. Many authorities have expanded this indication to include persons with type 1 and type 2 diabetes mellitus with microalbuminuria who do not meet the usual criteria for antihypertensive therapy. ACE inhibitors may also delay the progression of nondiabetic kidney disease. The Heart Outcomes Prevention Evaluation (HOPE) trial demonstrated that the ACE inhibitor ramipril reduced the number of cardiovascular deaths, nonfatal myocardial infarctions, and nonfatal strokes and also reduced the incidence of new-onset HF, kidney dysfunction, and new-onset diabetes in a population of patients at high risk for vascular events. Although this was not specifically a hypertensive population, the benefits were associated with a modest reduction in blood pressure, and the results inferentially support the use of ACE inhibitors in similar patients with hypertension. ACE inhibitors are a drug of choice (usually in conjunction with a diuretic and a β-blocker) in patients with HF with reduced EF and are indicated also in asymptomatic patients with reduced EF.

How to initiate therapy—Baseline serum potassium and creatinine levels should be measured prior to starting medications that interfere with the RAAS, and repeated 1–2 weeks after initiation of therapy to detect hyperkalemia or disproportionate elevation of creatinine. Minor dose adjustments of these medications rarely trigger significant shifts in these values.

Side effects—An advantage of the ACE inhibitors is their relative freedom from troublesome side effects (Table 13–6). Severe hypotension can occur in patients with bilateral renal artery stenosis. An increase in serum creatinine > 25% from baseline suggests volume contraction or renovascular disease and is usually reversible with discontinuation of the ACE inhibitor. Hyperkalemia may develop in patients with kidney disease and type IV renal tubular acidosis (commonly seen in patients with diabetes) and in older adults. A chronic dry cough is common, seen in 10% of patients or more, and may require stopping the drug. Skin rashes are observed with any ACE inhibitor. Angioedema is an uncommon but potentially dangerous side effect of all agents of this class because of their inhibition of kininase. Exposure of the fetus to ACE inhibitors during the second and third trimesters of pregnancy has been associated with a variety of defects due to hypotension and reduced renal blood flow.

B. Angiotensin II Receptor Blockers

ARBs can improve cardiovascular outcomes in patients with hypertension as well as in patients with related conditions, such as HF and type 2 diabetes with nephropathy. ARBs have not been compared with ACE inhibitors in RCTs in patients with hypertension, but two trials comparing losartan with captopril in HF and post–MI LV dysfunction showed trends toward worse outcomes in the losartan group. By contrast, valsartan seems as effective as ACE inhibitors in these settings. Within group heterogeneity of antihypertensive potency and duration of action might explain such observations. The Losartan Intervention for Endpoints (LIFE) trial in nearly 9000 patients with hypertension and electrocardiographic evidence of LVH—comparing losartan with the β-blocker atenolol as initial therapy—demonstrated a significant reduction in stroke with losartan. Of note is that in patients with diabetes, death and MI were also reduced, and there was a lower occurrence of new-onset diabetes. In a subgroup analysis from the LIFE trial, atenolol appeared to be superior to losartan in African-American persons, while the opposite was the case in non–African-American persons. A similar reduced efficacy of lisinopril compared to diuretics and calcium channel blockers was observed in

Table 13–6. Antihypertensive drugs: renin and ACE inhibitors and ARBs.

Medication (Proprietary Name)	Oral Dosage	Adverse Effects	Comments
Renin Inhibitors			
Aliskiren (Tekturna)	*Initial:* 150 mg once daily *Range:* 150–300 mg once daily	Angioedema, hypotension, hyperkalemia. Contraindicated in pregnancy.	Probably metabolized by CYP3A4. Absorption is inhibited by high-fat meal.
Aliskiren and HCTZ (Tekturna HCT)	*Initial:* 150 mg/12.5 mg once daily *Range:* 150 mg/12.5 mg–300 mg/25 mg once daily		
ACE Inhibitors			
Benazepril (Lotensin)	*Initial:* 10 mg once daily *Range:* 5–40 mg in 1 or 2 doses	Cough, hypotension, dizziness, hyperkalemia, kidney dysfunction, angioedema; taste alteration and rash (may be more frequent with captopril); rarely, proteinuria, blood dyscrasia. Contraindicated in pregnancy.	More fosinopril is excreted by the liver in patients with kidney dysfunction (dose reduction may or may not be necessary). Captopril and lisinopril are active without metabolism. Captopril, enalapril, lisinopril, and quinapril are approved for HF.
Benazepril and HCTZ (Lotensin HCT)	*Initial:* 5 mg/6.25 mg once daily *Range:* 5 mg/6.25 mg–20 mg/25 mg		
Benazepril and amlodipine (Lotrel)	*Initial:* 10 mg/2.5 mg once daily *Range:* 10 mg/2.5 mg–40 mg/10 mg		
Captopril (Capoten)	*Initial:* 6.25–25 mg two to three times daily *Range:* 50–150 mg in 2 or 3 doses		
Captopril and HCTZ (Capozide)	*Initial:* 25 mg/15 mg twice daily *Range:* 25 mg/15 mg–50 mg/25 mg		
Enalapril (Vasotec)	*Initial:* 5 mg once daily *Range:* 5–40 mg in 1 or 2 doses		
Enalapril and HCTZ (Vaseretic)	*Initial:* 5 mg/12.5 mg once daily *Range:* 5 mg/12.5 mg–20 mg/50 mg		
Fosinopril (Monopril)	*Initial:* 10 mg once daily *Range:* 10–80 mg once daily		
Fosinopril and HCTZ (Monopril-HCT)	*Initial:* 10 mg/12.5 mg once daily *Range:* 10 mg/12.5 mg–80 mg/50 mg		
Lisinopril (Prinivil, Zestril)	*Initial:* 5–10 mg once daily *Range:* 5–40 mg once daily		
Lisinopril and HCTZ (Prinzide or Zestoretic)	*Initial:* 10 mg/12.5 mg once daily *Range:* 10 mg/12.5 mg–80 mg/50 mg		
Moexipril (Univasc)	*Initial:* 3.75–7.5 mg once daily *Range:* 7.5–30 mg in 1 or 2 doses		
Perindopril (Aceon)	*Initial:* 4 mg once daily *Range:* 4–16 mg once daily		
Perindopril and amlodipine (Prestalia)	*Initial:* 3.5 mg/2.5 mg once daily *Range:* 3.5 mg/2.5–14 mg/10 mg once daily		
Quinapril (Accupril)	*Initial:* 10–20 mg once daily *Range:* 10–80 mg in 1 or 2 doses		
Quinapril and HCTZ (Accuretic)	*Initial:* 10 mg/12.5 mg once daily *Range:* 10 mg/12.5 mg–20 mg/25 mg		
Ramipril (Altace)	*Initial:* 2.5 mg once daily *Range:* 2.5–20 mg in 1 or 2 doses		
Trandolapril (Mavik)	*Initial:* 1 mg once daily *Range:* 1–4 mg once daily		
Trandolapril and verapamil (Tarka)	*Initial:* 2 mg/180 mg SR once daily *Range:* 2 mg/180 mg SR–4 mg/240 mg SR		

(continued)

Table 13–6. Antihypertensive drugs: renin and ACE inhibitors and ARBs. (continued)

Medication (Proprietary Name)	Oral Dosage	Adverse Effects	Comments
ARBs			
Azilsartan (Edarbi)	*Initial:* 40 mg once daily *Range:* 40–80 mg once daily	Hyperkalemia, kidney dysfunction, rare angioedema. Combinations have additional side effects. Contraindicated in pregnancy.	Losartan has a flat dose-response curve. Valsartan and irbesartan have wider dose-response ranges and longer durations of action. Addition of low-dose diuretic (separately or as combination pills) increases the response.
Azilsartan and chlorthalidone (Edarbychlor)	*Initial:* 40 mg/12.5 mg once daily *Range:* 40 mg/12.5–40 mg/25 mg once daily		
Candesartan cilexetil (Atacand)	*Initial:* 8 mg once daily *Range:* 8–32 mg once daily		
Candesartan cilexetil and HCTZ (Atacand HCT)	*Initial:* 16 mg/12.5 mg once daily *Range:* 32 mg/12.5 mg once daily		
Eprosartan (Teveten)	*Initial:* 600 mg once daily *Range:* 400–800 mg in 1–2 doses		
Irbesartan (Avapro)	*Initial:* 150 mg once daily *Range:* 150–300 mg once daily		
Irbesartan and HCTZ (Avalide)	*Initial:* 150 mg/12.5 mg once daily *Range:* 150 mg/12.5 mg–300 mg/25 mg once daily		
Losartan and HCTZ (Hyzaar)	*Initial:* 50 mg/12.5 mg once daily *Range:* 50 mg/12.5 mg–100 mg/25 mg once daily		
Olmesartan (Benicar)	*Initial:* 20 mg once daily *Range:* 20–40 mg once daily		
Olmesartan and HCTZ (Benicar HCT)	*Initial:* 20 mg/12.5 mg once daily *Range:* 20 mg/12.5 mg–40 mg/25 mg once daily		
Olmesartan and amlodipine (Azor)	*Initial:* 20 mg/5 mg once daily *Range:* 20 mg/5 mg–40 mg/10 mg		
Olmesartan and amlodipine and HCTZ (Tribenzor)	*Initial:* 20 mg/5 mg/12.5 mg once daily *Range:* 20 mg/5 mg/12.5 mg–40 mg/10 mg/25 mg once daily		
Telmisartan (Micardis)	*Initial:* 20–40 mg once daily *Range:* 20–80 mg once daily		
Telmisartan and HCTZ (Micardis HCT)	*Initial:* 40 mg/12.5 mg once daily *Range:* 40 mg/12.5 mg–80 mg/25 mg once daily		
Telmisartan and amlodipine (Twynsta)	*Initial:* 40 mg/5 mg once daily *Range:* 40 mg/5 mg–80 mg/10 mg once daily		
Valsartan (Diovan)	*Initial:* 80 mg once daily *Range:* 80–320 mg once daily		
Valsartan and HCTZ (Diovan HCT)	*Initial:* 80 mg/12.5 mg once daily *Range:* 80 mg/12.5 mg–320 mg/25 mg once daily		
Valsartan and amlodipine (Exforge)	*Initial:* 160 mg/5 mg once daily *Range:* 160 mg/5 mg–320 mg/10 mg once daily		
Other Combination Products			
Amlodipine and valsartan and HCTZ (Exforge HCT)	*Initial:* 5 mg/160 mg/12.5 mg once daily *Range:* 5 mg/160 mg/12.5 mg–10 mg/320 mg/25 mg once daily		

HCTZ, hydrochlorothiazide; SR, sustained release.

Black persons in the Antihypertensive and Lipid-Lowering Treatment to Prevent Heart Attach Trial (ALLHAT), suggesting that ACE inhibitors and ARBs may not be the preferred agents in Black patients (see Table 13–12). In the treatment of hypertension, combination therapy with an ACE inhibitor and an ARB is not advised because it generally offers no advantage over monotherapy at maximum dose with addition of a complementary class where necessary, and increases the risk of hyperkalemia and renal dysfunction.

Side effects—Unlike ACE inhibitors, the ARBs rarely cause cough and are less likely to be associated with skin rashes or angioedema (Table 13–6). However, as seen with ACE inhibitors, problematic hyperkalemia can occur, and patients with bilateral renal artery stenosis may exhibit hypotension and worsened kidney function. Olmesartan has been linked to a sprue-like syndrome, presenting with abdominal pain, weight loss, and nausea, which subsides upon drug discontinuation. An observational study suggests that ARBs and ACE inhibitors are less likely to be associated with depression than calcium channel blockers and β-blockers.

C. Renin Inhibitors

Since renin cleavage of angiotensinogen is the rate-limiting step in the renin-angiotensin cascade, the most efficient inactivation of this system would be expected with renin inhibition. Conventional ACE inhibitors and ARBs probably offer incomplete blockade, even in combination. Aliskiren, a renin inhibitor, binds the proteolytic site of renin, thereby preventing cleavage of angiotensinogen. Aliskiren effectively lowers blood pressure, reduces albuminuria, and limits LVH, but it has yet to be established as a first-line drug since large-scale prospective trial data are lacking. The combination of aliskiren with ACE inhibitors or ARBs in persons with type 2 diabetes mellitus offers no advantage and might even increase the risk of adverse cardiac or renal consequences.

D. Calcium Channel Blocking Agents

These agents act by causing peripheral vasodilation but with less reflex tachycardia and fluid retention than other vasodilators. They are effective as single-drug therapy in approximately 60% of patients in all demographic groups and all grades of hypertension (Table 13–7). For these reasons, they may be preferable to β-blockers and ACE inhibitors in Black and older persons. Verapamil and diltiazem should be combined cautiously with β-blockers because of their potential for depressing atrioventricular (AV) conduction and sinus node automaticity as well as contractility.

Calcium channel blockers are equivalent to ACE inhibitors and thiazide diuretics in prevention of CHD, major cardiovascular events, cardiovascular death, and total mortality. A protective effect against stroke with calcium channel blockers is well established, and in two trials (ALLHAT and the Systolic Hypertension in Europe trial), these agents appeared to be more effective than diuretic-based therapy.

Side effects—The most common side effects of calcium channel blockers are headache, peripheral edema, bradycardia, and constipation (especially with verapamil in older adults) (Table 13–7). The dihydropyridine agents—nifedipine, nicardipine, isradipine, felodipine, nisoldipine, and amlodipine—are more likely to produce symptoms of vasodilation, such as headache, flushing, palpitations, and peripheral edema. Edema is minimized by coadministration of an ACE inhibitor or ARB. Calcium channel blockers have negative inotropic effects and should be used cautiously in patients with cardiac dysfunction. Amlodipine is the only calcium channel blocker with established safety in patients with severe HF.

E. Diuretics

Thiazide diuretics (Table 13–8) are the antihypertensives that have been most extensively studied and most consistently effective in clinical trials. They lower blood pressure initially by decreasing plasma volume, but during long-term therapy, their major hemodynamic effect is reduction of peripheral vascular resistance. Most of the antihypertensive effect of these agents is achieved at lower dosages (typically, 12.5 mg of hydrochlorothiazide or equivalent), but their biochemical and metabolic effects are dose related. Thiazides may be used at higher doses if plasma potassium is above 4.5 mmol/L. The loop diuretics (such as furosemide) may lead to electrolyte and volume depletion more readily than the thiazides and have short durations of action. Because of these adverse effects, loop diuretics should be reserved for use in patients with kidney dysfunction (serum creatinine > 2.5 mg/dL [208.3 mcmol/L]; estimated eGFR < 30 mL/min/1.73 m^2) in which case they are more effective than thiazides. Relative to β-blockers and ACE inhibitors, diuretics are more potent in persons who are Black, older, or have obesity, and other subgroups with increased plasma volume or low plasma renin activity (or both). They are relatively more effective in persons who smoke cigarettes than in those who do not smoke. Long-term thiazide administration also mitigates the loss of bone mineral content in older women at risk for osteoporosis.

Overall, diuretics administered alone control blood pressure in 50% of patients with mild to moderate hypertension and can be used effectively in combination with all other agents. They are also useful for lowering isolated or predominantly systolic hypertension.

Side effects—The adverse effects of diuretics relate primarily to the metabolic changes listed in Table 13–8. Erectile dysfunction, skin rashes, and photosensitivity are less frequent. Hypokalemia has been a concern but is uncommon at the recommended dosages. The risk can be minimized by limiting dietary salt or increasing dietary potassium; potassium replacement is not usually required to maintain serum K^+ at > 3.5 mmol/L. Higher serum K^+ levels are prudent in patients at special risk from intracellular potassium depletion, such as those taking digoxin or with a history of ventricular arrhythmias, in which case a potassium-sparing agent could be used. Compared with ACE inhibitors and ARBs, diuretic therapy is associated with a slightly higher incidence of mild new-onset diabetes. Diuretics of all types can cause hyponatremia, but this side effect occurs most commonly with thiazides; the pathophysiology is complex and incompletely understood. Diuretics also increase serum uric acid and may precipitate gout. Increases in blood glucose, triglycerides, and LDL cholesterol may occur but are relatively minor during long-term low-dose therapy. The potential for worsening of diabetes is outweighed by the advantages of blood pressure control, and diuretics should not be withheld from patients with diabetes.

Table 13–7. Antihypertensive drugs: calcium channel blocking agents.

Medication (Proprietary Name)	Oral Dosages	Special Properties			Adverse Effects	Comments
		Peripheral Vasodilation	Cardiac Automaticity and Conduction	Contractility		
Nondihydropyridine Agents						
Diltiazem						
(Cardizem SR)	*Initial:* 90 mg SR twice daily *Range:* 180–360 mg SR in 2 doses	++	↓↓	↓↓	Edema, headache, bradycardia, bloating and constipation, dizziness, AV block, HF, urinary frequency.	Also approved for angina.
(Cardizem CD)	*Initial:* 180 mg ER once daily *Range:* 180–360 mg ER once daily					
(Cartia XT)	*Initial:* 180 or 240 mg ER once daily *Range:* 180–480 mg ER once daily					
(Dilt-XR)	*Initial:* 180 or 240 mg ER once daily *Range:* 180–540 mg ER once daily					
(Taztia XT)	*Initial:* 120 or 180 mg ER once daily *Range:* 120–540 mg ER once daily					
(Tiazac)	*Initial:* 120 or 240 mg ER once daily *Range:* 120–540 mg ER once daily					
Verapamil						
(Calan)	*Initial:* 40 mg three times daily *Range:* 120–480 mg in 3 divided doses	++	↓↓↓	↓↓↓	Same as diltiazem but more likely to cause constipation and HF.	Also approved for angina and arrhythmias.
(Calan SR)	*Initial:* 120 mg ER once daily *Range:* 120–480 mg ER in 1 or 2 doses					
(Verelan)	*Initial:* 120 or 240 mg ER once daily *Range:* 240–480 mg ER once daily					
(Verelan PM)	*Initial:* 100 or 200 mg ER once daily at bedtime *Range:* 100–400 mg ER once daily at bedtime					

(*continued*)

Table 13–7. Antihypertensive drugs: calcium channel blocking agents. (continued)

Medication (Proprietary Name)	Oral Dosages	Special Properties			Adverse Effects	Comments
		Peripheral Vasodilation	Cardiac Automaticity and Conduction	Contractility		
Dihydropyridines						
Amlodipine (Norvasc)	*Initial:* 2.5 mg once daily *Range:* 2.5–10 mg once daily	+++	↓/0	↓/0	Edema, dizziness, palpitations, flushing, headache, hypotension, tachycardia, bloating and constipation, urinary frequency.	
Amlodipine and atorvastatin (Caduet)	*Initial:* 2.5 mg/10 mg once daily *Range:* 10 mg/80 mg once daily	+++	↓/0	↓/0	Edema (amlodipine), myopathy and hepatotoxicity (atorvastatin).	Amlodipine, nicardipine, and nifedipine also approved for angina.
Felodipine (Plendil)	*Initial:* 5 mg ER once daily *Range:* 5–10 mg ER once daily	+++	↓/0	↓/0		
Isradipine (DynaCirc)	*Initial:* 2.5 mg twice daily *Range:* 2.5–5 mg twice daily	+++	↓/0	↓		
Nicardipine (Cardene)	*Initial:* 20 mg three times daily *Range:* 20–40 mg three times daily	+++	↓/0	↓		
Nifedipine (Procardia XL)	*Initial:* 30 or 60 mg ER once daily *Range:* 30–120 mg ER once daily					
Nisoldipine (Sular)	*Initial:* 17 mg daily *Range:* 17–34 mg daily	+++	↓/0	↓		

AV, atrioventricular; ER, extended release; SR, sustained release.

F. Aldosterone Receptor Blockers and Aldosterone Synthase Inhibitors

The aldosterone receptor blockers spironolactone and eplerenone have reemerged in the treatment of hypertension, particularly in resistant hypertension, and are helpful additions to most other antihypertensive medications. Consistent with the importance of aldosterone in essential hypertension, the aldosterone receptor blockers are effective at lowering blood pressure in Black persons and all other patients with hypertension regardless of renin level. Aldosterone plays a central role in target-organ damage, including the development of ventricular and vascular hypertrophy and renal and myocardial fibrosis. Aldosterone receptor antagonists ameliorate these consequences of hypertension, to some extent independently of effects on blood pressure. Amiloride blocks aldosterone-mediated activation of the epithelial sodium channel, is useful in preventing diuretic associated hypokalemia, and lowers blood pressure in patients with hyperaldosteronism and resistant hypertension. Aldosterone receptor blockers, and to a lesser extent amiloride, offer an alternative to adrenalectomy in primary hyperaldosteronism. However, long-term outcomes with medical treatment of primary hyperaldosteronism are inferior to those following surgical adrenalectomy.

Aldosterone synthase inhibitors such as lorundrostat and baxdrostat are in late phase clinical trials (and not yet FDA-approved), and seem safe, well tolerated, and effective. The risk of hyperkalemia seems comparable to that with mineralocorticoid receptor antagonists. It remains to be seen whether aldosterone synthase inhibitors are as effective as surgical adrenalectomy.

Table 13–8. Antihypertensive drugs: diuretics (in descending order of preference).

Drugs	Proprietary Names	Oral Doses	Adverse Effects	Comments
Thiazides and Related Diuretics				
Chlorthalidone	Thalitone	*Initial:* 12.5 or 25 mg once daily *Range:* 12.5–50 mg once daily	↓K^+, ↓Mg^{2+}, ↑Ca^{2+}, ↓Na+, ↑uric acid, ↑glucose, ↑LDL cholesterol, ↑triglycerides; rash, erectile dysfunction.	Better 24-hour blood pressure control than HCTZ because of longer half-life but outcomes are no different and metabolic profile is worse.
Hydrochlorothiazide (HCTZ)	Esidrix, Microzide	*Initial:* 12.5 or 25 mg once daily *Range:* 12.5–50 mg once daily		Low dosages are effective in many patients without associated metabolic abnormalities
Metolazone	Zaroxolyn	*Initial:* 2.5–5 mg once daily *Range:* 1.25–20 mg in 1 or 2 divided doses		More effective with concurrent kidney disease
Indapamide	Lozol	*Initial:* 2.5 mg once daily *Range:* 2.5–5 mg once daily		Does not alter serum lipid levels
Bendroflumethiazide	Aprinox Neo-Naclex	*Initial:* 2.5 mg once daily		Not available in United States
Loop Diuretics				
Furosemide	Lasix	*Initial:* 20 mg twice daily *Range:* 40–320 mg in 2 or 3 doses	Same as thiazides, but with higher risk of excessive diuresis and electrolyte imbalance. Increases calcium excretion.	Short duration of action a disadvantage; should be reserved for patients with kidney disease or fluid retention. Poor antihypertensive.
Ethacrynic acid	Edecrin	*Initial:* 25–50 mg once daily *Range:* 50–400 mg once or twice daily		
Bumetanide	Bumex	*Initial:* 0.25 mg twice daily *Range:* 0.5–10 mg in 2 or 3 doses		
Torsemide	Demadex	*Initial:* 10–20 mg once daily *Range:* 10–100 mg once or twice daily		Effective blood pressure medication at low dosage.
Aldosterone Receptor Blockers				
Spironolactone	Aldactone	*Initial:* 12.5 or 25 mg once daily *Range:* 12.5–100 mg once daily	Hyperkalemia, metabolic acidosis, gynecomastia.	Can be useful add-on therapy in patients with refractory hypertension.
Amiloride	(generic)	*Initial:* 5 mg once daily *Range:* 5–10 mg in 1 or 2 divided doses		
Eplerenone	Inspra	*Initial:* 25 mg once daily *Range:* 25–100 mg once daily		
Combination Products				
HCTZ and triamterene	Dyazide, Maxzide-25 (25/37.5 mg)	*Initial:* 25 mg/37.5 mg once daily *Range:* 25 mg/37.5 mg–50 mg/75 mg once daily	Same as thiazides plus GI disturbances, hyperkalemia rather than hypokalemia, headache; triamterene can cause kidney stones and kidney dysfunction; spironolactone causes gynecomastia. Hyperkalemia can occur if this combination is used in patients with advanced kidney disease or those taking ACE inhibitors.	Use should be limited to patients with demonstrable need for a potassium-sparing agent.

(*continued*)

Table 13–8. Antihypertensive drugs: diuretics (in descending order of preference). (continued)

Drugs	Proprietary Names	Oral Doses	Adverse Effects	Comments
HCTZ and amiloride	(generic) (50/5 mg)	*Initial:* 25 mg/2.5 mg once daily *Range:* 50 mg/5 mg–100 mg/10 mg once daily		
HCTZ and spironolactone	Aldactazide (25/25 mg; 50/50 mg)	*Initial:* 25 mg/25 mg once daily *Range:* 25 mg/25 mg–100 mg/100 mg once daily		

Side effects—Spironolactone can cause breast pain and gynecomastia in men through activity at the progesterone receptor, an effect not seen with the more specific eplerenone. Hyperkalemia is a problem with agents that block the effects of aldosterone, chiefly in patients with CKD. Hyperkalemia is more likely if the pretreatment plasma potassium exceeds 4.5 mmol/L.

Flack JM et al. Efficacy and safety of baxdrostat in uncontrolled and resistant hypertension. N Engl J Med. 2025;393:1363. [PMID: 40888730]
Goh JS et al. Efficacy and safety of aldosterone synthase inhibitors in hypertension: a systematic review and meta-analysis. Endocrinol Diabetes Metab. 2025;8:e70094.[PMID: 40944342].

G. β-Blocking Agents

These drugs are effective in hypertension because they decrease the heart rate and cardiac output. The β-blockers also decrease renin release and are more efficacious in populations with elevated plasma renin activity, such as younger White patients. β-Blockers neutralize the reflex tachycardia caused by vasodilators and are useful in patients with associated conditions that benefit from the cardioprotective effects of these agents. These include individuals with angina pectoris, previous myocardial infarction, persistent sinus tachycardia and stable HF as well as those with migraine headaches and somatic manifestations of anxiety.

Although all β-blockers appear to be similar in antihypertensive potency, they differ in pharmacologic properties (these differences are summarized in Table 13–9), including specificity to the cardiac β-1-receptors (cardioselectivity) and whether they block the β-2-receptors in the bronchi and vasculature; *at higher dosages, however, all agents are nonselective.* The β-blockers also differ in their pharmacokinetics, lipid solubility—which determines whether they cross the blood-brain barrier predisposing to CNS side effects—and route of metabolism. Metoprolol succinate reduces mortality and morbidity in patients with chronic stable HF with reduced EF (see Chapter 11). Carvedilol and nebivolol maintain cardiac output and are also beneficial in these patients. Carvedilol and nebivolol may reduce peripheral vascular resistance by concomitant α-blockade (carvedilol) and increased nitric oxide release (nebivolol). Because of the lack of efficacy in primary prevention of MI and inferiority compared with other drugs in prevention of stroke and LVH, traditional β-blockers should not be used as first-line agents in the treatment of hypertension without specific compelling indications (eg, active CAD).

Side effects—The side effects of β-blockers include inducing or exacerbating bronchospasm in predisposed patients; sinus node dysfunction and AV conduction depression (resulting in bradycardia or AV block); nasal congestion; Raynaud phenomenon; and CNS symptoms with nightmares, excitement, depression, and confusion. Fatigue, lethargy, and erectile dysfunction may occur. The traditional β-blockers (but not the vasodilator β-blockers carvedilol and nebivolol) have an adverse effect on lipids and glucose metabolism. β-Blockers are used cautiously in patients with type 1 diabetes since they can mask the symptoms of hypoglycemia and prolong these episodes by inhibiting gluconeogenesis. These drugs should also be used with caution in patients with advanced peripheral vascular disease associated with rest pain or nonhealing ulcers, but they are generally well tolerated in patients with mild claudication. Nebivolol can be safely used in patients with stage II claudication (claudication at 200 m).

In treatment of pheochromocytoma, β-blockers should not be administered until α-blockade (eg, phentolamine) has been established. Otherwise, blockade of vasodilatory β-2-adrenergic receptors will allow unopposed vasoconstrictor α-adrenergic–receptor activation with worsening of hypertension. *For the same reason, β-blockers should not be used to treat hypertension arising from cocaine use.*

Great care should be exercised if the decision is made, without compelling indications, to remove β-blockers from the treatment regimen because abrupt withdrawal can precipitate acute coronary events and severe increases in blood pressure.

Esler M et al. Diverse pharmacological properties, trial results, comorbidity prescribing and neural pathophysiology suggest European hypertension guideline downgrading of beta-blockers is not justified. Blood Press. 2022;31:210. [PMID: 36029011]

H. α-Antagonists

Prazosin, terazosin, and doxazosin (Table 13–10) block postsynaptic α-receptors, relax smooth muscle, and reduce blood pressure by lowering peripheral vascular resistance. These agents are effective as single-drug therapy in some individuals, but tachyphylaxis may appear during long-term therapy. Unlike some β-blockers and diuretics,

Table 13–9. Antihypertensive drugs: β-blocking agents.

Medication (Proprietary Name)	Oral Dosage	Special Properties: β-1 Selectivity[1]	ISA[2]	MSA[3]	Lipid Solubility	Renal Versus Hepatic Elimination	Comments[4]
Acebutolol (Sectral)	*Initial:* 200–400 mg once daily *Range:* 200–1200 mg in 2 doses	+	+	+	+	H > R	Positive ANA; rare LE syndrome; also indicated for arrhythmias. Doses > 800 mg have β-1 and β-2 effects.
Atenolol (Tenormin)	*Initial:* 25 mg once daily *Range:* 25–100 mg in 1 or 2 doses	+	0	0	0	R	Also indicated for angina and post-MI. Doses > 100 mg have β-1 and β-2 effects.
Atenolol/chlorthalidone (Tenoretic)	*Initial:* 50 mg/25 mg once daily *Range:* 50 mg/25 mg–100 mg/25 mg once daily	+	0	0	0	R	
Betaxolol (Kerlone)	*Initial:* 5–10 mg once daily *Range:* 10–20 mg once daily	+	0	0	+	H > R	
Bisoprolol (Zebeta)	*Initial:* 2.5–5 mg once daily *Range:* 5–20 mg once daily	+	0	0	0	R = H	Also effective for HF.
Bisoprolol and HCTZ (Ziac)	*Initial:* 2.5 mg/6.25 mg once daily *Range:* 2.5 mg/6.25 mg–10 mg/6.25 mg once daily	+	0	0	0	R = H	Low-dose combination approved for initial therapy.
Carvedilol (Coreg)	*Initial:* 6.25 mg twice daily *Range:* 12.5–25 mg twice daily	0	0	0	+++	H > R	α: β-blocking activity 1:9; may cause orthostatic symptoms; effective for HF. Nitric oxide potentiating vasodilatory activity.[5]
Carvedilol (Coreg CR)	*Initial:* 20 mg ER once daily *Range:* 20–80 mg ER once daily	0	0	0	+++	H > R	
Labetalol (Trandate)	*Initial:* 100 mg twice daily *Range:* 200–2400 mg in 2 doses	0	0/+	0	++	H	α: β-blocking activity 1:3; more orthostatic hypotension, fever, hepatotoxicity.
Metoprolol tartrate (Lopressor)	*Initial:* 50 mg twice daily *Range:* 50–200 mg twice daily	+	0	+	+++	H	Also indicated for angina and post-MI. Approved for HF. Doses > 100 mg have β-1 and β-2 effects.
Metoprolol succinate (Toprol-XL [SR preparation])	*Initial:* 25 mg once daily *Range:* 25–400 mg once daily						
Metoprolol and HCTZ (Lopressor HCT)	*Initial:* 50 mg/12.5 mg twice daily *Range:* 50 mg/25 mg–200 mg/50 mg in single or divided doses	+	0	+	+++	H	

(*continued*)

Table 13–9. Antihypertensive drugs: β-blocking agents. (continued)

Medication (Proprietary Name)	Oral Dosage	Special Properties					Comments[4]
		β-1 Selectivity[1]	ISA[2]	MSA[3]	Lipid Solubility	Renal Versus Hepatic Elimination	
Nadolol (Corgard)	*Initial:* 20 mg once daily *Range:* 20–320 mg once daily	0	0	0	0	R	
Nebivolol (Bystolic)	*Initial:* 5 mg once daily *Range:* 40 mg once daily	+	0	0	++	H	Nitric oxide potentiating vasodilatory activity.[5]
Pindolol (Visken)	*Initial:* 5 mg twice daily *Range:* 10–60 mg in 2 doses	0	++	+	+	H > R	In adults, 35% renal clearance.
Propranolol							
(Inderal)	*Initial:* 20 mg twice daily *Range:* 40–320 mg in 2 doses	0	0	++	+++	H	Also indicated for angina and post-MI.
(Inderal LA)	*Initial:* 80 mg ER once daily *Range:* 120–320 mg ER once daily						
(InnoPran XL)	*Initial:* 80 mg ER once nightly *Range:* 80–120 mg ER once nightly						
Propranolol and HCTZ (generic)	*Initial:* 40 mg/25 mg twice daily *Range:* 40 mg/25 mg–80 mg/25 mg twice daily	0	0	++	+++	H	
Timolol (generic)	*Initial:* 10 mg twice daily *Range:* 10–60 mg in 2 doses	0	0	0	++	H > R	Also indicated for post-MI; 80% hepatic clearance.

[1]Agents with β-1 selectivity are less likely to precipitate bronchospasm and decrease peripheral blood flow in low doses, but selectivity is only relative.
[2]Agents with ISA cause less resting bradycardia and lipid changes.
[3]MSA generally occurs at concentrations greater than those necessary for β-blockade. The clinical importance of MSA by β-blockers has not been defined.
[4]Adverse effects of all β-blockers: bronchospasm, fatigue, sleep disturbance and nightmares, bradycardia and atrioventricular block, worsening of HF, cold extremities, GI disturbances, erectile dysfunction, ↑ triglycerides, ↓ HDL cholesterol, rare blood dyscrasias.
[5]Carvedilol and nebivolol stimulate release of nitric oxide by vascular endothelium, which may augment the vasodilatory effects of drugs such as hydralazine and prazosin.
ANA, antinuclear antibody; ER, extended release; HCTZ, hydrochlorothiazide; ISA, intrinsic sympathomimetic activity; LE, lupus erythematosus; MSA, membrane-stabilizing activity; SR, sustained release; 0, no effect; +, some effect; ++, moderate effect; +++, most effect.

α-blockers have no adverse effect on serum lipid levels. In fact, α-blockers increase HDL cholesterol while reducing total cholesterol; whether this is beneficial in the long term has not been established.

Side effects—Side effects are relatively common (Table 13–10). These include marked hypotension after the first dose which, therefore, should be small and given at bedtime. Post-dosing palpitations, headache, and nervousness may continue to occur during long-term therapy; these symptoms may be less frequent or severe with doxazosin because of its more gradual onset of action. In ALLHAT, however, persons receiving doxazosin as initial therapy had a significant increase in HF hospitalizations and a higher incidence of stroke relative to those receiving diuretics, prompting discontinuation of this arm of the study. Cataractectomy in patients exposed to α-blockers can be complicated by the floppy iris syndrome, even after discontinuation of the drug, so the ophthalmologist should be alerted that the patient has been taking the drug prior to surgery.

To summarize, α-blockers should generally not be used as initial agents to treat hypertension—except perhaps in men with symptomatic prostatism or nightmares linked to PTSD.

Table 13–10. α-Blocking agents, sympatholytics, and vasodilators.

Medication (Proprietary Names)	Oral Dosage	Adverse Effects	Comments
α-Blockers			
Doxazosin (Cardura)	*Initial:* 1 mg at bedtime *Range:* 1–16 mg once daily	Syncope with first dose; postural hypotension, dizziness, palpitations, headache, weakness, drowsiness, sexual dysfunction, anticholinergic effects, urinary incontinence; first-dose effects may be less with doxazosin.	May ↑ HDL and ↓ LDL cholesterol. May provide short-term relief of obstructive prostatic symptoms. Less effective in preventing cardiovascular events than diuretics.
Doxazosin (Cardura XL)	*Initial:* 4 mg ER once daily *Range:* 4–8 mg ER once daily		
Prazosin (Minipress)	*Initial:* 1 mg two or three times daily; take first dose at bedtime *Range:* 2–20 mg in 2 or 3 doses		
Terazosin (Hytrin)	*Initial:* 1 mg at bedtime *Range:* 1–20 mg in 1 or 2 doses		
Endothelin Receptor Antagonists			
Aprocitentan	12.5 mg daily	Fluid retention, anemia, teratogenicity in pregnancy.	Likely useful in resistant hypertension. Verify negative pregnancy status at baseline, monthly during treatment, and one month after stopping therapy when indicated.
Central Sympatholytics			
Clonidine (Catapres)	*Initial:* 0.1 mg twice daily *Range:* 0.2–0.6 mg in 2 doses	Sedation, dry mouth, sexual dysfunction, headache, bradyarrhythmias; side effects may be less with guanfacine. Contact dermatitis with clonidine patch.	"Rebound" hypertension may occur even after gradual withdrawal.
Clonidine (Catapres TTS [transdermal patch])	*Initial:* 0.1 mg/day patch weekly *Range:* 0.1–0.3 mg/day patch weekly		
Clonidine and chlorthalidone (Clorpres)	*Initial:* 0.1 mg/15 mg one to three times daily *Range:* 0.1 mg/15 mg–0.6 mg/30 mg in single or divided doses		
Guanfacine (Tenex)	*Initial:* 0.5–1 mg once daily at bedtime *Range:* 1–3 mg once daily		
Methyldopa (Aldochlor)	*Initial:* 250 mg two or three times daily *Range:* 500–3000 mg in 2 doses	Hepatitis, hemolytic anemia, fever.	Avoid in favor of safer agents.
Peripheral Neuronal Antagonists			
Reserpine (not available in the United States)	*Initial:* 0.1 mg once daily *Range:* 0.05–0.25 mg once daily	Depression (less likely at dosages < 0.25 mg), night terrors, nasal stuffiness, drowsiness, peptic disease, GI disturbances, bradycardia.	
Direct Vasodilators			
Hydralazine (Apresoline)	*Initial:* 10 mg four times daily *Range:* 50–300 mg in 2–4 doses	GI disturbances, tachycardia, headache, nasal congestion, rash, LE-like syndrome.	May worsen or precipitate angina.
Minoxidil (generic)	*Initial:* 5 mg once daily *Range:* 10–40 mg in 1–3 divided doses	Tachycardia, fluid retention, headache, hirsutism, pericardial effusion, thrombocytopenia.	Should be used in combination with β-blocker and diuretic.

ER, extended release; LE, lupus erythematosus.

I. Endothelin Receptor Antagonists

The endothelins are 21 amino acid peptides that have pleiotropic actions on vascular biology. Endothelin 1, the predominant isopeptide, is a potent vasoconstrictor with additional activity in promoting vascular remodeling and inflammation. In the phase 3 Precision trial, aprocitentan, a dual antagonist at type A and B endothelin receptors, reduced 24-hour ambulatory systolic blood pressure by around 5 mm Hg when added as a fourth medication in patients with resistant hypertension. Aprocitentan appears to be well tolerated and is FDA-approved for treatment of resistant hypertension.

Schlaich MP et al; PRECISION Investigators. Dual endothelin antagonist aprocitentan for resistant hypertension (PRECISION): a multicentre, blinded, randomised, parallel-group, phase 3 trial. Lancet. 2022;400:1927. [PMID: 36356632]

J. Drugs With Central Sympatholytic Action

Methyldopa, clonidine, guanabenz, and guanfacine (Table 13–10) lower blood pressure by stimulating α-adrenergic receptors in the CNS, thus reducing efferent peripheral sympathetic outflow. There is considerable experience with methyldopa in pregnant persons, and it is still used for this population. Clonidine is available as patches, which may have particular value in noncompliant patients. All of these central sympatholytic agents are effective as single therapy in some patients, but they are usually used as second- or third-line agents because of the high frequency of drug intolerance.

Side effects—Side effects include sedation, fatigue, dry mouth, postural hypotension, and erectile dysfunction. An important concern is rebound hypertension following withdrawal. Methyldopa also causes hepatitis and hemolytic anemia and should be restricted to individuals who have already tolerated long-term therapy.

K. Peripheral Sympathetic Inhibitors

These agents are usually used only in refractory hypertension. Reserpine remains a cost-effective antihypertensive agent (Table 13–10). Its reputation for inducing mental depression and its other side effects—sedation, nasal stuffiness, sleep disturbances, and peptic ulcers—has made it unpopular, though these problems are uncommon at low dosages. Guanethidine and guanadrel inhibit catecholamine release from peripheral neurons but frequently cause orthostatic hypotension (especially in the morning or after exercise), diarrhea, and fluid retention.

L. Arteriolar Dilators

Hydralazine and minoxidil (Table 13–10) relax vascular smooth muscle and produce peripheral vasodilation. When given alone, they stimulate reflex tachycardia; increase myocardial contractility; and cause headache, palpitations, and fluid retention. To counteract these effects, the agents are usually given in combination with diuretics and β-blockers in resistant patients. Hydralazine produces frequent GI disturbances and may induce a lupus-like syndrome. Minoxidil causes hirsutism and marked fluid retention; this very potent agent is reserved for the most refractory of cases.

Antihypertensive Medications & the Risk of Cancer

Several observational studies have examined the association between long-term exposure to antihypertensive medications and cancer. Weak associations have been suggested by some of these studies, but results have been mixed. Without large-scale prospective studies with cancer as a prespecified outcome measure, the effect of antihypertensive drugs on the risk of cancer remains uncertain. By contrast, the beneficial effect of these drugs on cardiovascular outcomes has been clearly established. Concern about increased risk of cancer should not be minimized, but at present there are no compelling data to prompt a change in prescribing patterns.

Kidoguchi S et al. Antihypertensive drugs and cancer risk. Am J Hypertens. 2022;35:767. [PMID: 35595533]

Procedures That Modulate the Activity of the Autonomic Nervous System

Before the advent of antihypertensive medications, lumbar sympathectomy was used to lower blood pressure. In a more specific and less invasive approach to modulate the activity of the autonomic nervous system, the renal sympathetic nerves can be ablated using radiofrequency or ultrasound energy applied to the luminal surface of the renal arteries. The SPYRAL HTN-OFF MED study, using an intensive and closely controlled ablation strategy, demonstrated a modest but clinically meaningful blood pressure reduction compared to a control group who received a sham intervention. This effect on blood pressure has been confirmed by several subsequent studies and is equivalent to the effect of adding spironolactone as a fourth agent in the treatment of resistant hypertension. Studies of sympathetic nerve ablation have demonstrated a 20–30% nonresponse rate. Renal denervation is FDA-approved but should be reserved for patients with uncontrolled hypertension from drug intolerance. Resistant hypertension, the other indication for renal denervation, is often pseudoresistant from unrecognized noncompliance, which should be addressed once identified. Secondary hypertension should be carefully excluded before considering renal nerve ablation. Several concerns arise when considering more widespread or less discriminating use of this technology: The impact on blood pressure is unpredictable on an individual basis, results are likely to be operator dependent, and there is a risk of developing renal artery stenosis (0.2% per year) or dissection. In addition, the magnitude of effect on blood pressure lowering is rather modest and may not be durable, there are no cardiovascular outcomes data to support the procedure, and the cost is substantial.

Messerli FH et al. Renal denervation in the antihypertensive arsenal—knowns and known unknowns. J Hypertens. 2022:40;1859. [PMID: 36052518]

Developing an Antihypertensive Regimen

Historically, data from large placebo-controlled trials supported the overall conclusion that antihypertensive therapy with diuretics and β-blockers had a major beneficial effect on a broad spectrum of cardiovascular outcomes, reducing the incidence of stroke by 30–50% and of HF by 40–50%, and halting progression to accelerated hypertension syndromes. The decrease in fatal and nonfatal CHD and cardiovascular and total mortality were less dramatic, ranging from 10% to 15%. Similar placebo-controlled data pertaining to the newer agents are generally lacking, except for stroke reduction with the calcium channel blocker nitrendipine in the Systolic Hypertension in Europe trial. However, there is substantial evidence that ACE inhibitors, and to a lesser extent ARBs, reduce adverse cardiovascular outcomes in other related populations (eg, patients with diabetic nephropathy, HF, or post-MI and individuals at high risk for cardiovascular events). Most large clinical trials that have compared outcomes in relatively unselected patients have failed to show a difference between newer agents—such as ACE inhibitors, calcium channel blockers, and ARBs—and the older diuretic-based regimens with regard to survival, myocardial infarction, and stroke. Where differences have been observed, they have mostly been attributable to subtle asymmetries in blood pressure control rather than to any inherent advantages of one agent over another. Recommendations for initial treatment identify ACE inhibitors, ARBs, and calcium channel blockers as valid choices. Because of their adverse metabolic profile, initial therapy with thiazides might best be restricted to older patients. Thiazides are acceptable as first-line therapy in Black persons because of specific efficacy in this group.

As discussed above, β-blockers are not ideal first-line drugs in the treatment of hypertension without compelling indications for their use (such as active CAD and HF). Vasodilator β-blockers (such as carvedilol and nebivolol) may produce better outcomes than traditional β-blockers; however, this possibility remains speculative.

Theoretically, restoration of nocturnal dipping by dosing some antihypertensive medications at the end of the day seems desirable. However, the impact of nocturnal dosing of antihypertensive medications on hypertension control and clinical outcomes remains unresolved. The HYGIA study reported significant benefits of evening compared to morning dosing. However, because of the risk of ischemic events from profound nocturnal hypotension and because clinical benefits remain uncertain, many experts have criticized this study and urged caution before general acceptance of nocturnal dosing.

Medications that interrupt the renin-angiotensin cascade are more effective in young White persons, in whom renin tends to be higher. Calcium channel blockers and diuretics are more effective in Black or older persons, in whom renin levels are generally lower. Many patients require two or more medications and even then a substantial proportion fail to achieve the goal blood pressure. A stepped care approach to the drug treatment of hypertension is outlined in Table 13–11. In patients with diabetes, three or four drugs are usually required to reduce systolic blood pressure to goal. In many patients, blood pressure cannot be adequately controlled with any combination. As a result, debating the appropriate first-line agent is less relevant than determining the most appropriate combinations of agents.

The mnemonic ABCD can be used to remember four classes of antihypertensive medications. These four classes can be divided into two categories: AB and CD. AB refers to drugs that block the RAAS (**A**CE/ARB and β-blockers). CD refers to those that work in other pathways (**c**alcium channel blockers and **d**iuretics). Combinations of drugs between the two categories are more potent than combinations from within a category. Many experts recommend the use of a fixed-dose combination (between two categories) of antihypertensive agents as first-line therapy. Because of the unwanted metabolic effects of thiazides, calcium channel blockers may be the preferred second agent in the younger patient who is already taking an ACE inhibitor or ARB. However, studies have repeatedly confirmed the effectiveness of thiazide diuretics as first-line agents in prevention of multiple clinical endpoints. Based on the results from the ACCOMPLISH trial, a combination of ACE inhibitor and calcium channel blocker may prove optimal for patients at high risk for cardiovascular events. The initial use of low-dose combinations allows faster blood pressure reduction without substantially higher intolerance rates and is likely to be better accepted by patients. Data from the ALTITUDE study (in patients with type 2 diabetes and CKD or CVD or both) indicate that the addition of aliskiren to either ARB or ACE inhibitor was associated with worse outcomes and cannot be recommended, at least in this population. A suggested approach to treatment, tailored to patient demographics, is outlined in Table 13–12.

In sum, as a prelude to treatment, the patient should be informed of common side effects and the need for diligent

Table 13–11. A stepped care approach to the initiation and titration of antihypertension medications.[1,2]

Step 1	ACE inhibitor/ARB **or**[3] Calcium channel blocker **or** Thiazide diuretic[4]
Step 2	ACE inhibitor/ARB **plus** Calcium channel blocker **or** thiazide diuretic[5]
Step 3	ACE inhibitor/ARB **plus** calcium channel blocker **plus** thiazide diuretic
Step 4	ACE inhibitor/ARB **plus** calcium channel blocker **plus** thiazide diuretic **plus** spironolactone[6]

[1]Allow 2 weeks to reach full effect of each drug. Proceed through steps until target blood pressure is attained.
[2]β-Blockers can be used at any stage if specifically indicated, eg, HF or angina.
[3]Initiation with combination therapy should be considered in patients with higher levels of blood pressure and higher cardiovascular risk.
[4]Thiazide or calcium channel blocker is more effective initial therapy in Blacks and older people.
[5]If required, add a calcium channel blocker rather than diuretic in younger patients to avoid long-term exposure to metabolic side effects of diuretics.
[6]Alternatives to spironolactone include eplerenone, amiloride, or triamterene. Watch for hyperkalemia, especially if also receiving ACE inhibitor/ARB. Avoid potassium-sparing diuretics in advanced CKD. If more than three drugs are required at maximum dose, consider specialist referral.

Table 13–12. Choice of antihypertensive agent based on demographic considerations.[1,2]

	Black Persons, All Ages[3]	All Others, Age < 55 Years	All Others, Age > 55 Years
First-line	CCB or diuretic[4,5]	ACE inhibitor or ARB[6] or CCB or diuretic[4,5]	CCB or diuretic[4,5]
Second-line	ARB[6] or ACE inhibitor[6,7] or vasodilating β-blocker[8]	Vasodilating β-blocker[8]	ACE inhibitor[6] or ARB[6] or vasodilating β-blocker[8]
Resistant hypertension	Aldosterone receptor blocker	Aldosterone receptor blocker	Aldosterone receptor blocker
Additional options	Centrally acting α-agonist or peripheral α-antagonist[9]	Centrally acting α-agonist or peripheral α-antagonist[9]	Centrally acting α-agonist or peripheral α-antagonist[9]

[1]Compelling indications may alter the selection of an antihypertensive drug.
[2]Start with full dose of one agent, or lower doses of combination therapy. In more severe hypertension (≥ 140/90 mm Hg), consider initiating therapy with a fixed-dose combination.
[3]The reasons why the responses to some medications tend to differ in Black patients are complex and poorly understood. Observations such as these should not be taken as evidence of biological differences based on racial categories.
[4]For patients with significant kidney dysfunction, use loop diuretic instead of thiazide.
[5]The adverse metabolic effects of thiazide diuretics and β-blockers should be considered in younger patients but may be less important in the older patient.
[6]Women of childbearing age should avoid ACE inhibitors and ARBs or discontinue as soon as pregnancy is diagnosed.
[7]Despite the elevated risk of angioedema and cough in Black patients, ACE inhibitors are generally well tolerated and are a useful adjunct.
[8]There are theoretical advantages in the use of vasodilating β-blockers such as carvedilol and nebivolol.
[9]α-Antagonists may precipitate or exacerbate orthostatic hypotension in older adults.
CCB, calcium channel blocker.

compliance. In patients with blood pressure < 160/90 mm Hg in whom pharmacotherapy is indicated, treatment should start with a single agent or two-drug combination at a low dose. Follow-up visits usually should be at 4- to 6-week intervals to allow for full medication effects to be established (especially with diuretics) before further titration or adjustment. If, after titration to well-tolerated doses, the patient has shown a discernible but incomplete response, another medication should be added. See Goals of Treatment, above. As a rule of thumb, a blood pressure reduction of 10 mm Hg can be expected for each antihypertensive agent added to the regimen and titrated to the optimum dose. In those with more severe hypertension, or with comorbidities (such as diabetes) that are likely to render them resistant to treatment, initiation with combination therapy is advised and more frequent follow-up is indicated. Most guidelines recommend the use of home blood pressure monitors in the diagnosis and management of hypertension. Web based technology makes it possible to monitor the patient's self-measured response to therapy with direct transmission of oscillometric blood pressure readings to the clinic. The availability of blood pressure profiles generated from multiple home-gathered data points over continuous intervals allows more precise control of the overall hypertensive burden.

Evaluation for secondary hypertension should be considered for patients compliant with their medications who do not respond to conventional combination regimens.

Medication Nonadherence

Adherence to antihypertensive treatment is alarmingly poor. In one European study of antihypertensive medication compliance, only 39% of patients were found to be taking their medications continuously over a 10-year period. Collaborative care, employing clinicians, pharmacists, social workers, and nurses to encourage compliance, has had a variable and often rather modest effect on blood pressure control. Adherence is enhanced by patient education and by use of home blood pressure measurement. The choice of antihypertensive medication is important. Better compliance has been reported for patients whose medications could be taken once daily or as combination pills. Adherence is best with ACE inhibitors and ARBs, and worse with β-blockers and diuretics.

Sex-Specific Considerations in Hypertension

Because of the preponderance of male recruitment into large-scale clinical trials, the impact of a patient's sex on the evaluation and management of hypertension remains uncertain. The limited data that exist suggest a steeper relationship in women between 24-hour ambulatory and nighttime systolic blood pressure and the risk of cardiovascular events. There are many sex-specific effects on the mechanisms and end-organ impact of hypertension. In younger adults, men are more likely to be hypertensive than women, a relationship that reverses in later life. Regression of LVH in response to ACE inhibitors is less pronounced in women. Women are more likely to have isolated systolic hypertension, probably because they develop more active LV systolic function and greater vascular stiffness than men. Fibromuscular dysplasia of the renal artery is much more common in women than men. The side effects of many antihypertensive drugs are more pronounced in women than men, including ACE inhibitor–associated cough and hyponatremia and hypokalemia in response to diuretics. Conversely, thiazides can help preserve bone density. Dependent edema due to amlodipine is more likely in women, and women are more sensitive to β-blockers. There are no data to support a different blood pressure target in women, but this question has not been examined in dedicated clinical trials.

Treatment of Hypertension in Diabetes

Patients with hypertension and diabetes are at particularly high risk for cardiovascular events. Data from the ACCORD study of patients with diabetes demonstrated that most of the benefits of blood pressure lowering were seen with a systolic target of < 140 mm Hg. Although there was a reduction in stroke risk at a systolic target < 120/70 mm Hg, treatment to this lower target was associated with an *increased* risk of serious adverse effects. US and Canadian guidelines recommend a blood pressure goal of < 130/80 mm Hg in patients with diabetes. Because of the beneficial effects of ACE inhibitors in diabetic nephropathy, they should be part of the initial treatment regimen. ARBs or perhaps renin inhibitors may be substituted in those who cannot tolerate ACE inhibitors. While the ONTARGET study showed that combinations of ACE inhibitors and ARBs in persons with atherosclerosis or type 2 diabetes with end-organ damage appeared to minimize proteinuria, this strategy slightly increased the risks of progression to dialysis and of death; thus, it is not recommended. Most patients with diabetes require combinations of three to five agents to achieve target blood pressure, usually including a diuretic and a calcium channel blocker or β-blocker. Patients with diabetes can be treated with agents that are not considered traditional antihypertensive drugs yet probably improve cardiovascular outcomes independent of their rather modest effects to lower blood pressure. Inhibitors of sodium-glucose transport protein 2 (SGLT-2) are widely employed in clinical practice. In the CREDENCE trial of patients with diabetic nephropathy, canagliflozin, an SGLT-2 inhibitor, improved glycemic control, generally modestly lowered blood pressure by 3–4 mm Hg, improved renal outcomes, and reduced cardiovascular risk. Finerenone, a nonsteroidal mineralocorticoid receptor antagonist that blocks the effects of aldosterone, has a risk of hyperkalemia that is about half that of spironolactone. In the FIGARO-DKD study of patients with diabetes and CKD stage 2–4, finerenone lowered blood pressure by a modest 3 mm Hg but showed significant benefits in prevention of cardiovascular outcomes and possible benefit in retarding the progression of kidney disease. GLP-1 agonists also provide significant benefit with modest blood pressure lowering. In addition to rigorous blood pressure control, treatment of persons with diabetes should include aggressive treatment of other risk factors.

Treatment of Hypertension in Chronic Kidney Disease

Hypertension is present in 40% of patients with a GFR of 60–90 mL/min/1.73 m^2 and 75% of patients with a GFR < 30 mL/min/1.73 m^2. The rate of progression of CKD is markedly slowed by the treatment of hypertension. In the SPRINT trial, the reduction in cardiovascular risk associated with lower blood pressure targets was also observed in the subgroup with a GFR of < 60 mL/min/1.73 m^2. However, an effect of *lower* blood pressure targets on the slowing of CKD progression appears to be restricted to those with pronounced proteinuria. In the SPRINT trial, the lower blood pressure goal was associated with increased risk of AKI, but this was generally reversible and not associated with elevated biomarkers for ischemic injury. Most experts recommend a blood pressure target of < 130/80 mm Hg in patients with CKD, with consideration of more intensive lowering if proteinuria > 1 g per 24 hours is present. Medications that interrupt the renin-angiotensin cascade can slow the progression of kidney disease and are preferred for initial therapy, especially in those with albuminuria of > 300 mg/g creatinine. Transition from thiazide to loop diuretic is often necessary to control volume expansion as the eGFR falls below 30 mL/min/1.73 m^2, but thiazide diuretics maintain antihypertensive efficacy in advanced CKD. ACE inhibitors remain protective and safe in kidney disease associated with significant proteinuria and serum creatinine as high as 5 mg/dL (380 mcmol/L). However, the use of drugs blocking the RAAS cascade in patients with advanced CKD should be supervised by a nephrologist. Kidney function and electrolytes should be measured 1 week after initiating treatment and subsequently monitored carefully in patients with kidney disease. An increase in creatinine of 20–30% is acceptable and expected; more exaggerated responses suggest the possibility of renal artery stenosis or pre-renal states. Although lower blood pressure levels are associated with acute decreases in GFR, this appears not to translate into an increased risk of developing ESKD in the long term. Persistence with ACE inhibitor or ARB therapy as the serum potassium level > 5.5 mEq/L is probably not warranted, since other antihypertensive medications are renoprotective as long as goal blood pressures are maintained. However, diuretics and SGLT2 inhibitors can help control mild hyperkalemia, and there are novel cation exchange polymers (such as patiromer) that sequester potassium in the gut and are more effective and better tolerated than sodium polystyrene sulfonate.

Treatment of Hypertension in Black Patients

Substantial evidence indicates that Black Americans are not only more likely to become hypertensive and more susceptible to the cardiovascular and renal complications of hypertension but also respond differently to many antihypertensive medications. The REGARDS study illustrates these differences. At systolic blood pressures < 120 mm Hg, Black and White Americans aged 45–64 years had equal risk of stroke. For a 10-mm Hg increase in systolic blood pressure, the risk of stroke was threefold higher in Black participants. At levels > 140–159/90–99 mm Hg, the hazard ratio for stroke in Black compared to White participants aged 45–64 years was 2.35. This increased susceptibility may reflect environmental factors, such as structural racism, diet, activity, stress, or access to health care services, differences in occurrence of comorbid conditions such as diabetes or obesity, or genetic ancestry and epigenetics. More studies are needed to determine the source of these differences, and it should be noted that racial disparities are not synonymous with inherent biologic differences based on race. In all persons with hypertension, a multifaceted program of education and lifestyle modification is warranted. Early introduction of combination therapy has been advocated, but there are no clinical trial data to support a lower than usual blood pressure goal in Black patients. Because ACE inhibitors and ARBs without concomitant diuretics—appear less effective in Black than in White patients, initial therapy should generally be a diuretic or a diuretic in combination with a calcium channel blocker. However, RAAS inhibitors lower blood pressure in Black patients, are useful adjuncts to the recommended diuretic and calcium channel blockers, and should be used in patients with hypertension and compelling indications, such as HF and kidney disease, especially with proteinuria (Table 13–13). *Black patients have an elevated risk of ACE inhibitor–associated angioedema and cough, so ARBs would be the preferred choice.*

Treatment of Hypertension in Older Adults

Several studies in persons aged > 60 years have confirmed that antihypertensive therapy prevents fatal and nonfatal MI and reduces overall cardiovascular mortality. Updated guidelines suggest that blood pressure goals should not generally be influenced by age alone. A subgroup analysis of the SPRINT study found that people aged > 75 years showed benefit at the 120 mm Hg systolic treatment target. Importantly, these benefits were also evident in patients classified as frail. This more aggressive approach was, however, associated with greater risk of falls and worsening kidney function, indicating that close monitoring is required in older adult patients treated to lower blood pressure goals. It is also important to note that the SPRINT study did not include patients with diabetes mellitus, stroke, or orthostatic hypotension.

Blood pressure treatment goals should be individualized in older adults. In the SPRINT MIND study, the lower systolic blood pressure target of 120 mm Hg was associated with a 15% reduction in the incidence of mild cognitive impairment and probable all-cause dementia compared to 140 mm Hg in the target group. Based upon this data, aggressive control of hypertension in high-risk individuals would have a significant impact on the prevalence of dementia. As discussed above, it is important to note that blood pressure measurements in the SPRINT study were made by automated devices, which are known to read lower than conventional office measurements.

How to initiate antihypertensive therapy in older patients—The same medications are used in older patients but at 50% lower doses. Pressure should be reduced more gradually with a safe intermediate systolic blood pressure goal of 160 mm Hg. As treatment is initiated, older patients should be carefully monitored for orthostasis, altered cognition, and electrolyte disturbances. Older adults are especially susceptible to problems associated with polypharmacy, including drug interactions and dosing errors.

Management of Supine Hypertension in Patients With Orthostatic Hypotension

Supine hypertension is common in patients with orthostatic hypotension and is associated with increased cardiovascular risk. Treatment of orthostasis can exacerbate supine hypertension and vice versa. Life expectancy is often reduced in patients with profound autonomic nervous system dysfunction. Treatment of nocturnal hypertension might be considered with the use of shorter acting agents (eg, captopril, hydralazine, losartan, or quick-release nifedipine). In patients with supine hypertension, medications used to increase blood pressure during the day should not be given within 5 hours of bedtime.

Follow-Up of Patients Receiving Hypertension Therapy

Once blood pressure is controlled on a well-tolerated regimen, follow-up visits can be infrequent and laboratory testing limited to those appropriate for the patient and the medications used. Yearly monitoring of blood lipids is recommended, and an ECG could be repeated at 2- to 4-year intervals depending on whether initial abnormalities are present and on the presence of coronary risk factors. Patients who have had excellent blood pressure control for several years, especially if they have lost weight and initiated favorable lifestyle modifications, might be considered for a trial of reduced antihypertensive medications.

Table 13–13. Recommended antihypertensive medications for coexisting indications.

	Antihypertensive Medication					
Indication	**Diuretic**	**β-Blocker**	**ACE Inhibitor**	**ARB**	**Calcium Channel Blocker**	**Aldosterone Antagonist**
HF	√	√	√	√		√
Following MI		√	√			√
High coronary disease risk	√	√	√		√	
Diabetes	√	√	√	√	√	
CKD			√	√		
Recurrent stroke prevention	√		√			

Deere BP et al. Hypertension and race/ethnicity. Curr Opin Cardiol. 2020;35:342. [PMID: 32398604]
Milani RV et al. New aspects in the management of hypertension in the digital era. Curr Opin Cardiol. 2021;36:398. [PMID: 33871402]
Suchard MA et al. Comprehensive comparative effectiveness and safety of first-line antihypertensive drug classes: a systematic, multinational, large-scale analysis. Lancet. 2019;394:1816. [PMID: 31668726]
Supiano MA et al. New guidelines and SPRINT results: implications for geriatric hypertension. Circulation. 2019;140:976. [PMID: 31525101]
Vogel B et al. The Lancet Women and Cardiovascular Disease Commission: reducing the global burden by 2030. Lancet. 2021;397:2385. [PMID: 34010613]

RESISTANT HYPERTENSION

Resistant hypertension is defined as the failure to reach blood pressure control in patients who are adherent to full doses of an appropriate three-drug regimen (including a diuretic). Adherence is a major issue: the rate of partial or complete noncompliance probably approaches 50% in this group of patients. In the approach to resistant hypertension, the clinician should first confirm compliance and rule out "white coat hypertension," ideally using ambulatory or home-based measurement of blood pressure. Exacerbating factors should be considered (as outlined above). Finally, identifiable causes of resistant hypertension should be sought (Table 13–14). The clinician should pay particular attention to the type of diuretic being used in relation to the patient's kidney function. Aldosterone may play an important role in resistant hypertension and aldosterone receptor blockers and amiloride can be very useful. If goal blood pressure cannot be achieved following completion of these steps, consultation with a hypertension specialist should be considered. Renal sympathetic nerve ablation is a consideration for patients who have failed or are intolerant to maximal medical therapy but requires referral to a specialist center for evaluation and intervention. Aprocitentan, an FDA-approved dual endothelin receptor antagonist for treatment of resistant hypertension, is an option in patients uncontrolled on three drugs, including a diuretic.

Table 13–14. Causes of resistant hypertension.

Improper blood pressure measurement
Nonadherence
Volume overload and pseudotolerance[1]
Excess sodium intake
Volume retention from kidney disease
Inadequate diuretic therapy
Drug induced or other causes
Inadequate doses
Inappropriate combinations
NSAIDs; cyclooxygenase-2 inhibitors
Cocaine, amphetamines, other illicit drugs
Sympathomimetics (decongestants, anorectics)
Oral contraceptives
Adrenal steroids
Cyclosporine and tacrolimus
Erythropoietin
Licorice (including some chewing tobacco)
Selected over-the-counter dietary supplements and medicines (eg, ephedra, ma huang, bitter orange)
Associated conditions
Obesity
Excess alcohol intake
Identifiable causes of hypertension (see Table 13–2)

[1]Pseudotolerance is blunting of the antihypertensive action of vasodilators because they promote salt retention.
Data from Chobanian AV et al. The Seventh Report of the Joint National Committee on Prevention, Detection, Evaluation, and Treatment of High Blood Pressure: the JNC 7 report. JAMA. 2003;289:2560.

Zeng W et al. Options for patients with out-of-control blood pressure: after all avenues have been exhausted. Expert Rev Cardiovasc Ther. 2024;22:459. [PMID: 39258872]

UNCONTROLLED HYPERTENSION & HYPERTENSIVE EMERGENCY

General Considerations

A. Emergency Department/Urgent Care Setting

Historically there has been a profusion of terms describing various forms of acute hypertensive presentations including hypertensive crisis, accelerated hypertension, hypertensive emergency, malignant hypertension, hypertensive encephalopathy, posterior reversible encephalopathy syndrome, hypertensive urgency, and uncontrolled hypertension. Some expert guidelines have condensed this profusion of terms into two categories, uncontrolled hypertension and hypertensive emergency, which are based on the presence (hypertensive emergency) or absence (uncontrolled hypertension) of acute hypertension-mediated end-organ injury.

The diagnosis of hypertensive emergency is made when significant hypertension (usually but not always exceeding 180/120 mm Hg) is the cause of injury to the heart, retina, brain, kidneys, large arteries, or microcirculation. Preeclampsia is a special case discussed in Chapter 21. Acute elevation of blood pressure without evidence of end-organ injury is described as uncontrolled hypertension. This scheme distinguishes patients whose blood pressure must be controlled immediately from those whose blood pressure control may safely be secured over hours to days. In hypertensive emergency, hospital admission is required to manage the consequences of organ injury and to closely monitor the blood pressure response to intravenous blood pressure–lowering therapy. By contrast, uncontrolled hypertension can be managed with conventional oral hypotensive therapy with a limited period of observation and ambulatory follow-up; hospital admission is unnecessary. In a hypertensive emergency, the profile of organ injury will determine the choice of antihypertensive agent, the rate at which blood pressure should be reduced, and the interval and final blood pressure goals in response to therapy.

B. Inpatient Setting

Management of hypertensive emergency in inpatients should not differ from the strategy outlined above for patients presenting to urgent care or emergency room facilities. Aggressive treatment of asymptomatic uncontrolled hypertension, however, should generally be avoided in inpatients. Observational studies that adjust for confounding variables or propensity analysis suggest that in the inpatient setting, escalation of oral antihypertensive therapy or the addition of intravenous medications increases the risk of mortality, stroke, troponin release and transfer to the ICU. Blood pressure elevations during hospitalization may be spurious because of inappropriate technique, or arise from reversible causes such as pain, anxiety, expanded fluid volumes, or alcohol withdrawal. If blood pressures were controlled out of hospital, patients should be placed back on their usual home medications. As-needed antihypertensives prescribed during hospital admission carry a high risk of hypotensive organ injury and are best avoided.

Clinical Findings

How to Detect End-Organ Injury in Hypertensive Emergency

Often, the presence of end-organ injury is apparent from the history and physical examination with an obvious focal or global neurologic deficit, abnormal retinal examination, absent pulses, asymmetric blood pressure readings, severe chest pain, back pain, or frank pulmonary edema. Blood tests should be selected to screen for thrombotic microangiopathy, AKI, and myocardial damage. Urine is examined for blood and protein, and for screening for substances of abuse (typically cocaine or ecstasy). Where clinically indicated, various imaging modalities may confirm pulmonary edema, myocardial dysfunction, aortic dissection, or acute intracranial bleed, thrombosis, or cerebral microvascular injury (eg, posterior reversible encephalopathy syndrome).

Acute hypertensive microangiopathy—The complex of elevated blood pressure associated with retinopathy (retinal hemorrhages, cotton-wool spots, or papilledema), AKI, and thrombotic microangiopathy has been termed malignant hypertension. Approximately 10% of patients will also have evidence of hypertensive encephalopathy (seizures, lethargy, cortical blindness, or coma) that is not always accompanied by classic hypertensive retinopathy. The susceptibility of the posterior cerebrum to hypertensive injury arises from the sparsity of sympathetic innervation in this region and consequently limited autoregulatory capacity. The microangiopathic changes of thrombocytopenia, schistocytes, and elevated LDH also occur in hemolytic uremic syndrome (HUS) and thrombotic thrombocytopenic purpura (TTP), thereby presenting a diagnostic challenge. However, the presence of advanced retinal changes indicates that the likely primary cause is hypertension, whereas the hematologic abnormalities associated with TTP or HUS are typically more dramatic.

Treatment

A. Management of Hypertensive Emergency Based on Type of End-Organ Damage

1. Acute hypertensive microangiopathy—In general, the initial goal is to reduce mean arterial pressure by no more than 25% (within minutes to 1–2 hours) and then toward a level of 160/100 mm Hg within 2–6 hours. The risk of organ ischemia from excessive reductions in pressure is minimized by using agents that have a predictable, dose-dependent, transient, and progressive antihypertensive effect (Table 13–15). *In that regard, the use of sublingual or oral fast-acting nifedipine preparations is best avoided.*

2. Acute ischemic stroke—This is often associated with marked elevation of blood pressure, which will usually fall spontaneously. In such cases, antihypertensives should only be used if the systolic blood pressure exceeds 180–200 mm Hg, and blood pressure should be reduced cautiously by 10–15% over 24 hours (Table 13–15). If thrombolytics are to be given, blood pressure should be maintained at < 185/110 mm Hg during treatment and for 24 hours following treatment.

3. Intracerebral hemorrhage—The aim of therapy for intracerebral hemorrhage is to minimize bleeding by reducing the systolic blood pressure in most patients to 140 mm Hg within the first 6 hours. In acute subarachnoid hemorrhage, as long as the bleeding source remains uncorrected, a compromise must be struck between preventing further bleeding and maintaining cerebral perfusion in the face of cerebral vasospasm. In this situation, blood pressure goals depend on the patient's usual blood pressure. In previously normotensive patients, the target should be a systolic blood pressure of 110–120 mm Hg; in patients with hypertension, blood pressure should be reduced to 20% below baseline pressure. In the treatment of hypertensive emergencies complicated by (or precipitated by) CNS injury, labetalol and nicardipine are good choices since they are nonsedating and do not appear to cause significant increases in cerebral blood flow or intracranial pressure. Patients with subarachnoid hemorrhage should receive nimodipine for 3 weeks following presentation to minimize cerebral vasospasm. *In hypertensive emergencies arising from catecholaminergic mechanisms, such as pheochromocytoma or cocaine use, β-blockers can worsen the hypertension because of unopposed peripheral vasoconstriction; nicardipine, clevidipine, or phentolamine is preferred.* Labetalol is useful in these patients if the heart rate must be controlled but should not be used as first-line therapy because it exhibits more β- than α-blockade.

4. Acute aortic dissection—Systolic blood pressure and heart rate should be reduced within 30 minutes to < 120 mm Hg and < 60 beats per minute, using a combination of vasodilation and β-blockade.

Therapeutic strategies for specific end-organ damage profiles, including those associated with cardiac injury, preeclampsia, scleroderma renal crisis, and hyperadrenergic states, are outlined in Table 13–15.

Table 13–15. Treatment of hypertensive emergency depending on primary site of end-organ damage. See Table 13–16 for dosages.

Type of Hypertensive Emergency	Recommended Drug Options and Combinations	Drugs to Avoid
Acute hypertensive microangiopathy	Labetolol Nicardipine	
Hypertensive encephalopathy and posterior reversible encephalopathy syndrome	Labetalol Nicardipine	Nitroprusside, methyldopa, clonidine, nitroglycerin
Myocardial ischemia and infarction	Nicardipine plus esmolol[1] Nitroglycerin plus labetalol Nitroglycerin plus esmolol[1]	Hydralazine, diazoxide, minoxidil, nitroprusside
AKI	Fenoldopam Nicardipine Clevidipine	
Aortic dissection	Esmolol plus nicardipine Esmolol plus clevidipine Labetalol Esmolol plus nitroprusside	Hydralazine, diazoxide, minoxidil
Acute pulmonary edema from LV systolic dysfunction	Nicardipine plus nitroglycerin[2] plus a loop diuretic Clevidipine plus nitroglycerin[2] plus a loop diuretic	Hydralazine, diazoxide, β-blockers
Acute pulmonary edema from LV diastoliic dysfunction	Esmolol plus low-dose nitroglycerin plus a loop diuretic Labetalol plus low-dose nitroglycerin plus a loop diuretic	
Ischemic stroke (systolic blood pressure > 180–200 mm Hg)	Nicardipine Clevidipine Labetalol	Nitroprusside, methyldopa, clonidine, nitroglycerin
Intracerebral hemorrhage (systolic blood pressure > 140–160 mm Hg)	Nicardipine Clevidipine Labetalol	Nitroprusside, methyldopa, clonidine, nitroglycerin
Hyperadrenergic states, including cocaine use	Nicardipine plus a benzodiazepine Clevidipine plus a benzodiazepine Phentolamine Labetalol	β-Blockers
Preeclampsia, eclampsia	Labetalol Nicardipine	Diuretics, ACE inhibitors
Scleroderma renal crisis	Captopril or intravenous enalaprilat	

[1]Avoid if there is LV systolic dysfunction.
[2]Drug of choice if LV systolic dysfunction is associated with ischemia.

B. Pharmacologic Management

1. Parenteral agents—In most situations, appropriate control of blood pressure is best achieved using combinations of nicardipine or clevidipine plus labetalol or esmolol; sodium nitroprusside is no longer the treatment of choice for acute hypertensive problems. (Table 13–16 lists drugs, dosages, and adverse effects.)

A. NICARDIPINE—Intravenous nicardipine is the most potent and longest acting parenteral calcium channel blocker. As a primarily arterial vasodilator, it has the potential to precipitate reflex tachycardia, and for that reason, it should be used with a β-blocker in patients with CAD.

B. CLEVIDIPINE—Intravenous clevidipine is an L-type calcium channel blocker with a 1-minute half-life, which facilitates swift and tight control of severe hypertension. It acts on arterial resistance vessels and is devoid of venodilatory or cardiodepressant effects.

C. LABETALOL—This combined β- and α-blocking agent is the most potent adrenergic blocker for rapid blood pressure reduction. Other β-blockers are far less potent. Excessive blood pressure drops are unusual. Experience with this agent in hypertensive syndromes associated with pregnancy has been favorable.

D. ESMOLOL—This rapidly acting β-blocker is approved only for treatment of supraventricular tachycardia but is often used for lowering blood pressure. It is less potent than labetalol and should be reserved for patients in whom there is particular concern about serious adverse events related to β-blockers.

E. FENOLDOPAM—Fenoldopam is a peripheral dopamine-1 (DA_1) receptor agonist that causes a dose-dependent

Table 13–16. Drugs for hypertensive emergencies and urgencies (in descending order of preference).

Agent	Action	Dosage	Onset	Duration	Adverse Effects	Comments
Hypertensive Emergencies						
Nicardipine (Cardene)	Calcium channel blocker	5 mg/hour intravenously; may increase by 1–2.5 mg/hour every 15 minutes to 15 mg/hour	1–5 minutes	3–6 hours	Hypotension, tachycardia, headache.	May precipitate myocardial ischemia.
Clevidipine (Cleviprex)	Calcium channel blocker	1–2 mg/hour intravenously initially; double rate every 90 seconds until near goal, then by smaller amounts every 5–10 minutes to a maximum of 32 mg/hour	2–4 minutes	5–15 minutes	Headache, nausea, vomiting.	Lipid emulsion: contraindicated in patients with allergy to soy or egg.
Labetalol (Trandate)	β- and α-blocker	20–40 mg intravenously every 10 minutes to 300 mg; 2 mg/min infusion	5–10 minutes	3–6 hours	Nausea, hypotension, bronchospasm, bradycardia, heart block.	Avoid in acute LV systolic dysfunction, asthma. May be continued orally.
Esmolol (Brevibloc)	β-blocker	Loading dose 500 mcg/kg intravenously over 1 minute; maintenance, 25–200 mcg/kg/min	1–2 minutes	10–30 minutes	Bradycardia, nausea.	Avoid in acute LV systolic dysfunction, asthma. Weak antihypertensive.
Fenoldopam (Corlopam)	Dopamine receptor agonist	0.1–1.6 mcg/kg/min intravenously	4–5 minutes	< 10 minutes	Reflex tachycardia, hypotension, increased intraocular pressure.	May protect kidney function.
Enalaprilat (Vasotec)	ACE inhibitor	1.25 mg intravenously every 6 hours	15 minutes	6 hours or more	Excessive hypotension.	Additive with diuretics; may be continued orally.
Furosemide (Lasix)	Diuretic	10–80 mg orally or intravenously	15 minutes	4 hours	Hypokalemia, hypotension.	Adjunct to vasodilator.
Hydralazine (Apresoline)	Vasodilator	5–20 mg intravenously; may repeat after 20 minutes	10–30 minutes	2–6 hours	Tachycardia, headache, vomiting, diarrhea	Avoid in CAD, dissection. Rarely used except in pregnancy.
Nitroglycerin	Vasodilator	0.25–5 mcg/kg/min intravenously	2–5 minutes	3–5 minutes	Headache, nausea, hypotension, bradycardia.	Tolerance may develop. Useful primarily with myocardial ischemia.
Nitroprusside (Nitropress)	Vasodilator	0.25–10 mcg/kg/min intravenously	Seconds	3–5 minutes	Anxiety, increased intracranial pressure, vomiting, bowel obstruction; thiocyanate and cyanide toxicity, especially with kidney and liver dysfunction; hypotension. Coronary steal, decreased cerebral blood flow, increased intracranial pressure.	No longer the first-line agent.
Hypertensive Urgencies						
Clonidine (Catapres)	Central sympatholytic	0.1–0.2 mg orally initially; then 0.1 mg every hour to 0.8 mg orally	30–60 minutes	6–8 hours	Sedation.	Rebound may occur.
Captopril (Capoten)	ACE inhibitor	12.5–25 mg orally	15–30 minutes	4–6 hours	Excessive hypotension.	

reduction in arterial pressure without evidence of tolerance, rebound, withdrawal, or deterioration of kidney function. In higher dosage ranges, tachycardia may occur. This drug is natriuretic, which may simplify volume management in AKI.

F. Enalaprilat—This is the active form of the ACE inhibitor enalapril. The onset of action is usually within 15 minutes, but the peak effect may be delayed for up to 6 hours. Thus, enalaprilat is used primarily as an adjunctive agent.

G. Diuretics—Intravenous loop diuretics can be helpful when the patient has signs of HF or fluid retention, but the onset of their hypotensive response is slow, making them an adjunct rather than a primary agent for hypertensive emergencies. Low dosages should be used initially (furosemide, 20 mg, or bumetanide, 0.5 mg). They facilitate the response to vasodilators, which often stimulate fluid retention.

H. Hydralazine—Hydralazine can be given intravenously or intramuscularly, but its effect is less predictable than that of other drugs in this group. It produces reflex tachycardia and should not be given without β-blockers in patients with possible coronary disease or aortic dissection. Hydralazine is used primarily in pregnancy and in children, but even in these situations, it is not a first-line drug.

I. Nitroglycerin, intravenous—This agent should be reserved for patients with accompanying acute coronary ischemic syndromes.

J. Nitroprusside sodium—This agent is given by controlled intravenous infusion gradually titrated to the desired effect. It lowers the blood pressure within seconds by direct arteriolar and venous dilation. Monitoring with an intra-arterial line avoids hypotension. Nitroprusside—in combination with a β-blocker—is useful in patients with aortic dissection.

2. Oral agents—Patients with less severe acute hypertensive syndromes can often be treated with oral therapy. Suitable drugs will reduce the blood pressure over hours. In those presenting because of noncompliance, it is usually sufficient to restore the patient's previously established oral regimen.

A. Clonidine—Clonidine, 0.2 mg orally initially, followed by 0.1 mg every hour to a total of 0.8 mg, will usually lower blood pressure over several hours. Sedation is frequent, and rebound hypertension may occur if the drug is stopped.

B. Captopril—Captopril, 12.5–25 mg orally, will lower blood pressure in 15–30 minutes. The response is variable and may be excessive. Captopril is the drug of choice in the management of systemic sclerosis hypertensive crisis.

C. Nifedipine—The effect of fast-acting nifedipine capsules is unpredictable and may be excessive, resulting in hypotension and reflex tachycardia. Because MI and stroke have been reported in this setting, the use of sublingual nifedipine is not advised.

3. Subsequent therapy—When the blood pressure has been brought under control, combinations of oral antihypertensive agents can be added as parenteral drugs are tapered off over a period of 2–3 days.

Bress AP et al; American Heart Association Council on Hypertension; Council on Cardiovascular and Stroke Nursing; and Council on Clinical Cardiology. The management of elevated blood pressure in the acute care setting: a scientific statement from the American Heart Association. Hypertension. 2024;81:e94. [PMID: 38804130]

Miller JB et al. Evaluation and management of hypertensive emergency. BMJ. 2024386:e077205. [PMID: 39059997]

Blood Vessel & Lymphatic Disorders

14

Warren J. Gasper, MD
James C. Iannuzzi, MD, MPH
Meshell D. Johnson, MD

ATHEROSCLEROTIC PERIPHERAL VASCULAR DISEASE

Occlusive atherosclerotic lesions in the extremities, or peripheral artery disease (PAD), is evidence of a systemic atherosclerotic process. The prevalence of PAD is 30% in patients who are 70 years old without other risk factors, or 50 years old with risk factors such as diabetes mellitus or tobacco use. Pathologic changes of atherosclerosis may be diffuse, but flow-limiting stenoses occur segmentally. In the lower extremities, stenoses classically occur in three anatomic segments: the aortoiliac segment, femoral-popliteal segment, and the infrapopliteal or tibial segment of the arterial tree.

CHRONIC OCCLUSIVE DISEASE: AORTA & ILIAC ARTERIES

ESSENTIALS OF DIAGNOSIS

- Claudication: cramping pain or tiredness in the calf, thigh, or hip while walking.
- Diminished femoral pulses.
- Tissue loss (ulceration, gangrene) or rest pain.

General Considerations

Lesions in the distal aorta and proximal common iliac arteries classically occur in men aged 50–60 years who smoke cigarettes. Disease progression may lead to complete occlusion of one or both common iliac arteries, which can precipitate occlusion of the entire abdominal aorta to the level of the renal arteries.

Clinical Findings

A. Symptoms and Signs

The pain from aortoiliac lesions may extend into the thigh and buttocks; erectile dysfunction may occur with bilateral common iliac disease. Rarely, patients experience only leg weakness when walking, or extreme limb fatigue. The symptoms are relieved with rest and are reproducible when the patient walks again. Femoral pulses and distal pulses are absent or very weak. Bruits may be heard over the aorta, iliac, and femoral arteries.

B. Doppler and Vascular Findings

By Doppler examination, the ratio of systolic blood pressure at the ankle compared with the brachial artery (ankle-brachial index [ABI]) is reduced to < 0.9 (normal ratio is 0.9–1.2); this difference is exaggerated by exercise. Both the dorsalis pedis and the posterior tibial arteries are measured and the higher of the two artery pressures is used for calculation. Segmental waveforms or pulse volume recordings obtained through blood pressure cuffs demonstrate blunting of the arterial waveform throughout the lower extremity.

C. Imaging

CT angiography (CTA) and magnetic resonance angiography (MRA) can identify the anatomic location of disease. Due to overlying bowel gas, duplex ultrasonography has limited utility for aortoiliac imaging. Imaging is required only when symptoms necessitate intervention, since a history and physical examination with vascular testing can locate the involved levels of the arterial tree.

Treatment

A. Medical and Exercise Therapy

The cornerstones of aortoiliac disease treatment are cardiovascular risk factor reduction and an exercise program.

1. Risk factor reduction—Essential elements include cigarette smoking cessation, antiplatelet therapy, weight loss, and lipid and blood pressure management. Nicotine replacement therapy, bupropion, varenicline, and counseling have established benefits in cigarette smoking cessation (see Chapter 1). While not recommended for primary prevention of CVD, antiplatelet agents (aspirin [81 mg orally daily] or clopidogrel [75 mg orally daily]) are important for secondary prevention of cardiovascular events in those with PAD and to reduce peripheral vascular morbidity. Dual treatment with low-dose rivaroxaban (2.5 mg orally twice daily) and aspirin 81 mg orally daily further reduces major cardiovascular and limb-related adverse events in symptomatic patients. All patients with PAD should receive a high-dose statin (eg, atorvastatin 80 mg daily if tolerated) to treat hypercholesterolemia and arterial inflammation. Cilostazol, 100 mg orally twice a day, a phosphodiesterase III inhibitor that is an arterial vasodilator with antiplatelet activity, improves walking distance in approximately two-thirds of patients but may take 2–4 weeks to be effective and 12 weeks until it reaches full effect.

2. Exercise programs—Supervised exercise programs for PAD provide significant improvements in pain, walking distance, and quality of life and may be more effective than endovascular treatment alone. A minimum training goal is a walking session of 30–45 minutes at least 3 days per week for a minimum of 12 weeks. Structured community or home-based exercise programs as well as alternative exercises (cycling, upper-body ergometry) may also be effective. Programs that include behavior modification have demonstrated improvements in sustained walking distance and patients' ability to cope with their disease.

B. Endovascular Therapy

Focal atherosclerotic lesions in the aorta or iliac arteries can be effectively treated with angioplasty and stenting, matching the results of surgery for single stenoses, but effectiveness and durability decrease with longer or multiple stenoses.

C. Surgical Intervention

A prosthetic aortofemoral bypass graft that bypasses the diseased aorta or iliac artery segments is a highly effective and durable treatment. Patients may also be treated with a graft from the axillary artery to the femoral arteries (axillofemoral bypass graft) or with a graft from the contralateral femoral artery (femoral–femoral bypass) if iliac disease is unilateral. The operative risk of axillofemoral and femoral–femoral bypass grafts is lower because the abdominal cavity is not entered and the aorta is not cross-clamped, but the grafts are less durable.

Complications

The complications of aortofemoral bypass are those of any major abdominal surgery in a patient population with a high prevalence of CVD. Mortality is low (2–3%), but morbidity is higher and includes a 5–10% rate of MI. While endovascular approaches are safer and the complication rate is 1–3%, they are less durable with extensive disease.

Prognosis

Patients with isolated aortoiliac disease may have further reduction in walking distance without intervention, but symptoms rarely progress to rest pain or limb threat. Life expectancy is limited by attendant CVD, with 5-year mortality of 25–40%.

Symptomatic relief is generally excellent with supervised exercise or after intervention. Aortofemoral bypass 5-year patency is 90%. In short stenoses, endovascular patency and symptom relief also are good, with 80% of patients symptom free at 3 years. In more extensive disease, recurrence rates increase to 30–50%.

When to Refer

Patients with progressive reduction in walking distance despite risk factor modification, consistent exercise, or limitations that interfere with activities of daily living should be referred for vascular surgical evaluation.

When to Admit

- Patients with acute limb ischemia need urgent treatment with intravenous anticoagulation, pain control, and surgical evaluation.
- Patients with evidence of chronic limb-threatening ischemia, including lower extremity rest pain and tissue loss, since these may quickly progress to amputation of the foot or leg.

Canonico ME et al. Medical therapy for peripheral artery disease. Curr Cardiol Rep. 2024;26:651. [PMID: 38696099]

Conte MS et al. Society for Vascular Surgery Clinical Practice Guideline on the management of intermittent claudication: focused update. J Vasc Surg. 2025;82:303. [PMID: 40316185]

Thangada ND et al. Exercise therapy for peripheral artery disease. Curr Cardiol Rep. 2024;26:405. [PMID: 38722492]

CHRONIC OCCLUSIVE DISEASE: FEMORAL & POPLITEAL ARTERIES

ESSENTIALS OF DIAGNOSIS

- Cramping pain or tiredness in the calf with exercise.
- Reduced popliteal and pedal pulses.
- Foot pain at rest, relieved by dependency.
- Foot gangrene or ischemic ulcers.

General Considerations

The superficial femoral artery is the peripheral artery most commonly occluded by atherosclerosis. Atherosclerosis of the femoral-popliteal segment usually occurs about a decade after the development of aortoiliac disease, has an even gender distribution, and commonly affects Black and Latino/Latina patients. The disease frequently occurs where the superficial femoral artery passes through the abductor magnus tendon in the distal thigh (Hunter canal). The common femoral artery and the popliteal artery are less often diseased but lesions in these vessels are debilitating, resulting in short-distance claudication.

Clinical Findings

A. Symptoms and Signs

Symptoms of intermittent claudication caused by lesions of the common femoral artery, superficial femoral artery, and popliteal artery are confined to the calf. Claudication occurs when there is occlusion or stenosis of the superficial femoral artery at the adductor canal, provided good collateral vessels from the profunda femoris are maintained. However, with concomitant disease of the profunda femoris or the popliteal artery, shorter distances may trigger symptoms. With short-distance claudication, dependent rubor of the foot may be present; pallor on elevation distinguishes rubor from erythema. Chronic low blood flow states will also cause atrophic changes in the lower leg and foot with loss of hair, thinning of the skin and subcutaneous tissues, and disuse atrophy of the muscles. With segmental occlusive disease of the superficial femoral artery, the common femoral pulsation is normal, but the popliteal and pedal pulses are reduced.

B. Doppler and Vascular Findings

ABI values < 0.9 are diagnostic of PAD and levels < 0.4 coincide with chronic limb-threatening ischemia. ABI readings depend on arterial compression; since vessels may be calcified in patients with diabetes mellitus, CKD, and in older adults, ABIs can be misleading. In such patients, the toe-brachial index is usually reliable with a value < 0.7 considered diagnostic of PAD. Pulse volume recordings with cuffs placed at the high thigh, mid-thigh, calf, and ankle will delineate the levels of obstruction with reduced pressures and blunted waveforms.

C. Imaging

Duplex ultrasonography, CTA, and MRA all adequately show the anatomic location of the obstructive lesions and are performed only if revascularization is planned. After revascularization, patients should be monitored with annual ultrasonograms.

Treatment

A. Medical and Exercise Therapy

As with aortoiliac disease, risk factor reduction, medical optimization with an antiplatelet agent, high-dose statin, and exercise treatment are the cornerstone of therapy and can reduce 5-year mortality by two-thirds. Dual treatment with rivaroxaban (2.5 mg orally twice daily) and aspirin (81 mg orally daily) reduces limb-related events, major amputation, and cardiovascular events. Cilostazol, 100 mg orally twice a day, may improve intermittent claudication symptoms.

B. Surgical Intervention

Intervention is indicated if claudication is progressive, is incapacitating, or interferes significantly with activities of daily living, employment, or quality of life. Intervention is critical if there is ischemic rest pain or if ischemic ulcers threaten the foot.

1. Bypass surgery—The most effective and durable treatment for superficial femoral artery lesions is a femoral-popliteal bypass with autologous saphenous vein. Synthetic material, usually polytetrafluoroethylene, can be used, but these grafts do not have the durability of single segment vein bypass.

2. Endovascular techniques—Endovascular techniques, such as angioplasty and stenting, are often used for lesions in the superficial femoral artery. These techniques have lower morbidity than bypass surgery but also have decreased durability and may limit future options for bypass.

Endovascular therapy is most effective in patients undergoing aggressive risk factor modification in whom lesions measure < 10 cm long. Paclitaxel-eluting stents or paclitaxel-coated balloons offer modest improvement over bare metal stents and noncoated balloons. The 1-year patency rate is 50% for balloon angioplasty, 70% for drug-coated balloons, 80% for bare metal stents, and 90% for drug-eluting stents. However, by 3 years, patency is significantly worse than bypass for all four techniques and reintervention for restenosis is common. Paclitaxel-coated devices remain controversial when considering outcomes beyond artery patency. The SWEDEPAD 2 clinical trial and meta-analyses of device-approval clinical trials found significantly increased mortality at 5 years in patients with intermittent claudication treated with paclitaxel-coated devices. Analyses of large claims databases and retrospective analyses of single-center data have not demonstrated a difference in survival with paclitaxel-coated devices.

3. Thromboendarterectomy—Removal of the atherosclerotic plaque is limited to common femoral and profunda femoris artery lesions where endovascular techniques have limited efficacy.

Complications

Open surgical procedures of the lower extremities, particularly long bypasses with vein harvest, have a risk of wound infection that is higher than in other areas of the body. Wound infection or seroma can occur in as many as 10–15% of cases. After open surgery, MI rates are 5–10%, and mortality 1–4%. Complication rates of endovascular surgery are 1–5%, making these therapies attractive despite their lower durability.

Prognosis

The prognosis for motivated patients with isolated superficial femoral artery disease is excellent, and surgery is not recommended for mild or moderate claudication. However, when claudication significantly limits daily activity and cardiovascular health, intervention may be warranted. All interventions require close postprocedure follow-up with repeated ultrasound surveillance so that recurrent narrowing can be detected and treated promptly with angioplasty or bypass to prevent complete occlusion. The reported 3-year patency rate of bypass grafts of the femoral artery, superficial femoral artery, and popliteal artery is 65–70%, whereas the patency of angioplasty is < 50%.

Because of extensive atherosclerotic disease, including coronary lesions, 5-year survival with lower extremity PAD is 70% and decreases to 50% when there is involvement of the tibial arteries. However, with aggressive risk factor modification, substantial improvement in longevity has been reported.

When to Refer

Patients with progressive symptoms, short-distance claudication, rest pain, or any ulceration should be referred to a peripheral vascular specialist.

When to Admit

Individuals with chronic limb-threatening ischemia (eg, ischemic rest pain, tissue loss) warrant admission because of a high risk for rapid progression to limb loss. If there is concern for a foot infection, particularly in patients with diabetes, admit for broad-spectrum antibiotics. Emergent surgical debridement may be necessary to prevent ascending infections that could be limb- and life-threatening.

Falkenber M et al. Paclitaxel-coated versus uncoated devices for infrainguinal endovascular revascularisation in chronic limb-threatening ischaemia (SWEDEPAD 1): a multicentre, participant-masked, registry-based, randomised controlled trial. Lancet. 2025;406:1103. [PMID: 40902617]

Nordanstig J et al. Paclitaxel-coated versus uncoated devices for infrainguinal endovascular revascularisation in patients with intermittent claudication (SWEDEPAD 2): a multicentre, participant-masked, registry-based, randomised controlled trial. Lancet. 2025;406:1115. [PMID:40902614]

CHRONIC OCCLUSIVE DISEASE: TIBIAL & PEDAL ARTERIES

ESSENTIALS OF DIAGNOSIS

- Severe pain of the forefoot that is relieved by dependency (ischemic rest pain).
- Pain or numbness of the foot with walking.
- Ulcer or gangrene, and not claudication, is a frequent initial manifestation.
- Rubor when the foot is dependent and pallor when the foot is elevated.

General Considerations

Occlusive processes of the tibial arteries of the lower leg and pedal arteries in the foot occur primarily in patients with diabetes. There often is extensive calcification of the artery wall.

Clinical Findings

A. Symptoms and Signs

Isolated tibial disease will manifest as rest pain, an ulcer, or gangrene rather than claudication. Chronic limb-threatening ischemia is defined as the presence of ischemic rest pain or ulcers and is associated with the highest rate of amputation. Classically, ischemic rest pain is confined to the dorsum of the forefoot and is relieved with dependency: the pain does not occur with standing, sitting, or dangling the leg over the edge of the bed. It is severe and burning in character and experienced when recumbent, possibly awakening the patient.

On examination, femoral and popliteal pulses may or may not be present depending on disease extent, but palpable pedal pulses will be absent. Dependent rubor may be prominent with pallor on elevation. The skin of the foot is generally cool, atrophic, and hairless. Risk for transfemoral or transtibial amputation can be calculated using the wound, ischemia, and foot infection classification system.

B. Doppler and Vascular Findings

The ABI is often < 0.4; however, the ABI may be falsely elevated due to calcification of the arterial media layer from diabetes or CKD (Mönckeberg medial calcific sclerosis) and may not be compressible. Toe-brachial indices are preferred for assessing perfusion and predicting wound healing.

C. Imaging

Digital subtraction angiography is the gold standard method to delineate the anatomy of the tibial-popliteal segment. MRA or CTA is less helpful for detection of lesions in this location due to the small vasculature and other technical issues related to image resolution.

Differential Diagnosis

It is important to differentiate rest pain from diabetic neuropathic dysesthesia. Neuropathic pain is often described as plantar surface burning and is not relieved with leg dependency. Similarly, leg night cramps should not be confused with ischemic rest pain. Dependent rubor in the presence of a toe wound can often be mistaken for cellulitis; pallor on elevation helps confirm the diagnosis of rubor.

Treatment

Good foot care may prevent ulcers, and most patients with diabetes will do well with a conservative regimen and podiatric care. However, if ulcerations appear and there is no significant healing within 2–3 weeks, blood flow studies (ankle-brachial index/toe-brachial index) are indicated. Poor blood flow and a foot ulcer or nightly ischemic rest pain requires expeditious revascularization to avoid a major amputation.

A. Bypass and Endovascular Techniques

Bypass with a single segment saphenous vein to treat rest pain and heal ischemic foot ulcers provides significantly better survival and limb preservation rates than endovascular therapies. However, an endovascular therapy–first strategy has similar survival and limb preservation rates compared to bypass with a conduit other than a single segment saphenous vein.

B. Amputation

Patients with ischemic rest pain or ulcers have a 30–40% 1-year risk for major amputation. Patients with diabetes and tibial disease can be asymptomatic due to peripheral neuropathy, presenting more frequently with tissue loss. Patients with diabetes and PAD have a 4-fold risk of chronic limb-threatening ischemia compared with nondiabetic patients with PAD and have a risk of amputation up to 20-fold when compared to an age-matched population. Tibial artery disease is a major risk factor for amputation and is included as a factor in the Global Limb Anatomic Staging System (GLASS) vascular guidelines.

Complications

The complications of intervention are similar to those listed for superficial femoral artery disease; the overall cardiovascular risk of intervention increases with decreasing ABI. Patients with chronic limb-threatening ischemia require aggressive risk factor modification. Wound infection risk after bypass is higher if there is an open foot wound.

Prognosis

Patients with tibial atherosclerosis have extensive atherosclerotic burden and a high prevalence of diabetes. Their prognosis without intervention is poor and complicated by the risk of amputation.

When to Refer

Patients with diabetes and foot ulcers should be referred for a formal vascular evaluation and podiatric care.

When to Admit

Any patient with diabetes and a foot ulcer and foot infection should be evaluated for an emergent operative incision and drainage. Empiric broad-spectrum intravenous antibiotics should be given (eg, vancomycin for methicillin-resistant *Staphylococcus aureus* [MRSA] plus either ertapenem or piperacillin/tazobactam for gram-negative and anaerobic organisms). Multidisciplinary limb preservation centers, staffed with vascular surgeons, podiatrists, plastic and orthopedic surgeons, prosthetics and orthotic specialists, and diabetes specialists, have improved limb salvage rates.

Farber A et al. Surgery or endovascular therapy for chronic limb-threatening ischemia. N Engl J Med. 2022;387:2305. [PMID: 36342173]

Gallagher KA et al. Current status and principles for the treatment and prevention of diabetic foot ulcers in the cardiovascular patient population: a scientific statement from the American Heart Association. Circulation. 2024;149:e232. [PMID: 38095068]

ACUTE OCCLUSIVE DISEASE: LIMB ARTERIES

ESSENTIALS OF DIAGNOSIS

- Sudden pain in a limb with absent limb pulses.
- Usually some neurologic dysfunction with numbness, weakness, or complete paralysis.
- Loss of light touch sensation requires revascularization within 3 hours for limb viability.
- Unlike chronic limb ischemia, acute limb ischemia is a surgical emergency.

General Considerations

Acute occlusion may be due to an embolus or to thrombosis of a diseased atherosclerotic segment. Emboli large enough to occlude proximal arteries in the lower extremities are almost always cardiac in origin. Atrial fibrillation is the most common cause of embolism; other causes are valvular disease or thrombus formation on the ventricular surface of a large anterior myocardial infarct.

Emboli from arterial sources such as endoluminal ulcerations or calcified excrescences are usually small and go to the distal arterial tree (toes).

Typically, a patient with primary thrombosis will have a history of claudication and an abrupt worsening of symptoms. If the stenosis is chronic, collateral blood vessels will develop, and the resulting occlusion may cause only a minimal increase in symptoms.

Clinical Findings

A. Symptoms and Signs

The sudden onset of extremity pain, with loss or reduction in pulses, is diagnostic of acute arterial occlusion. This often will be accompanied by neurologic dysfunction, such as numbness or paralysis in extreme cases. With popliteal occlusion, symptoms may affect only the foot. With proximal occlusions, the whole leg may be affected. Signs of severe arterial ischemia include pallor, coolness of the extremity, and mottling. Impaired neurologic function progressing to anesthesia with paralysis indicates irreversible injury requiring amputation.

B. Doppler and Laboratory Findings

There will be little or no flow on Doppler examination of the distal vessels. Imaging, if done, may show an abrupt cutoff of contrast with embolic occlusion. Blood work may show myoglobinemia and metabolic acidosis.

C. Imaging

Whenever possible, imaging should be done in the operating room because obtaining angiography, MRA, or CTA may delay revascularization and jeopardize the viability of the extremity. However, in cases with only modest symptoms and where light touch of the extremity is maintained, imaging may be helpful in planning revascularization.

Treatment

Immediate revascularization is required in all cases of symptomatic acute arterial thrombosis. *Evidence of neurologic injury, including loss of light touch sensation, indicates that collateral flow is inadequate to maintain limb viability and revascularization should be accomplished within 3 hours.* Longer delays carry a significant risk of irreversible tissue damage approaching 100% at 6 hours.

A. Heparin

As soon as the diagnosis is made, an initial intravenous bolus of unfractionated heparin (80 U/kg) should be given followed by a continuous heparin infusion (12–18 U/kg/hour) to maintain the activated partial thromboplastin time (aPTT) in the therapeutic range (60–85 seconds). This helps prevent clot propagation and may also relieve associated vessel spasm. Other intravenous anticoagulation agents should be considered in cases of possible heparin-induced thrombocytopenia (eg, bivalirudin or argatroban) (see Heparin-Induced Thrombocytopenia). Intravenous anticoagulation may improve symptoms, but revascularization will still be required.

B. Endovascular Techniques

Pharmacomechanical thrombectomy catheters can achieve rapid revascularization and are most effective for the smaller arteries of the lower leg. Catheter-directed chemical thrombolysis into the clot with a tissue plasminogen activator (TPA) (alteplase or tenecteplase) may be done but often requires 24 hours or longer to fully lyse the thrombus. TPA can only be used in patients with mild ischemia, as determined by an intact neurologic examination. Patients with moderate to severe ischemia require immediate revascularization. Absolute contraindications for TPA include bleeding diathesis, GI bleeding, intracranial trauma, or neurosurgery within the past 3 months. Heparin is administered systemically to prevent thrombus formation around the sheath. Frequent vascular and access site examinations are required during the thrombolytic procedure to guard against the development of a hematoma.

C. Surgical Intervention

General anesthesia is usually indicated for surgical exploration of an acute arterial occlusion of a limb; local anesthesia may be used in high-risk patients if the exploration is limited to the common femoral artery. In extreme cases, it may be necessary to perform thrombo-embolectomy from the femoral, popliteal, and even the pedal vessels to revascularize the limb. The combined use of devices that pulverize and aspirate clot and intraoperative thrombolysis with TPA improves outcomes.

Complications

Complications of revascularization of an acutely ischemic limb include severe metabolic acidosis, hyperkalemia, AKI, and cardiac arrest. When several hours have elapsed but recovery of viable tissue may still be possible, significant levels of lactic acid, potassium, and other harmful agents such as myoglobin may be released into the circulation during revascularization. Administering sodium bicarbonate (150 mEq $NaHCO_3$ in 1 L of dextrose 5% in water at a rate of 1–1.5 L in the first hour and then adjust the rate to manage acidosis) before reestablishing arterial flow is required. Surgery in the presence of thrombolytic agents and heparin carries a high risk of postoperative wound hematoma.

Prognosis

There is a 10–25% risk of amputation with an acute arterial embolic occlusion, and a ≥ 25% in-hospital mortality rate. Prognosis for acute thrombotic occlusion of an atherosclerotic segment is generally better because the collateral flow can maintain extremity viability. The longer-term survival reflects the overall condition of the patient. In high-risk patients, an acute arterial occlusion is associated with a dismal prognosis.

King EG et al. What is the best treatment for acute limb ischemia? Adv Surg. 2022;56:287. [PMID: 36096573]

OCCLUSIVE CEREBROVASCULAR DISEASE

ESSENTIALS OF DIAGNOSIS

- Sudden onset of weakness and numbness of an extremity or the face, aphasia, dysarthria, or unilateral blindness (amaurosis fugax).
- Bruit heard loudest in the mid neck.

General Considerations

Unlike the other vascular territories, symptoms of ischemic cerebrovascular disease are predominantly due to emboli. When collateral flow reestablishes perfusion, ischemia reverses (transient ischemic attacks [TIAs]) but signals a high risk for additional emboli and stroke. The origins of emboli that cause ischemic strokes are the heart (approximately half) and an arterial source (20%). Approximately 90% of emboli from an arterial source originate from the proximal internal carotid artery, an area uniquely prone to the development of atherosclerosis. The aortic arch may also be an atheroembolic source. Intracranial atherosclerotic lesions are uncommon in western populations but are the most frequent location of cerebrovascular disease in Asian populations.

Clinical Findings

A. Symptoms and Signs

Generally, the symptoms of a TIA last only a few seconds to minutes (but may continue up to 24 hours) while a stroke is defined as persistent symptoms beyond 24 hours. The most common lesions associated with carotid disease involve the middle cerebral artery and anterior cerebral artery territories, frequently causing both motor and sensory deficits. Emboli to the retinal artery cause unilateral blindness; transient monocular blindness is termed "amaurosis fugax." Posterior circulation symptoms referable to the brainstem, cerebellum, and visual regions of the brain may be due to atherosclerosis of the vertebral basilar systems and are much less common.

Signs of cerebrovascular disease may include carotid artery bruits. However, there is poor correlation between the degree of stenosis and the presence of the bruit. Furthermore, the presence of a bruit does not correlate with stroke risk. Nonfocal symptoms, such as dizziness and unsteadiness, seldom are related to cerebrovascular atherosclerosis.

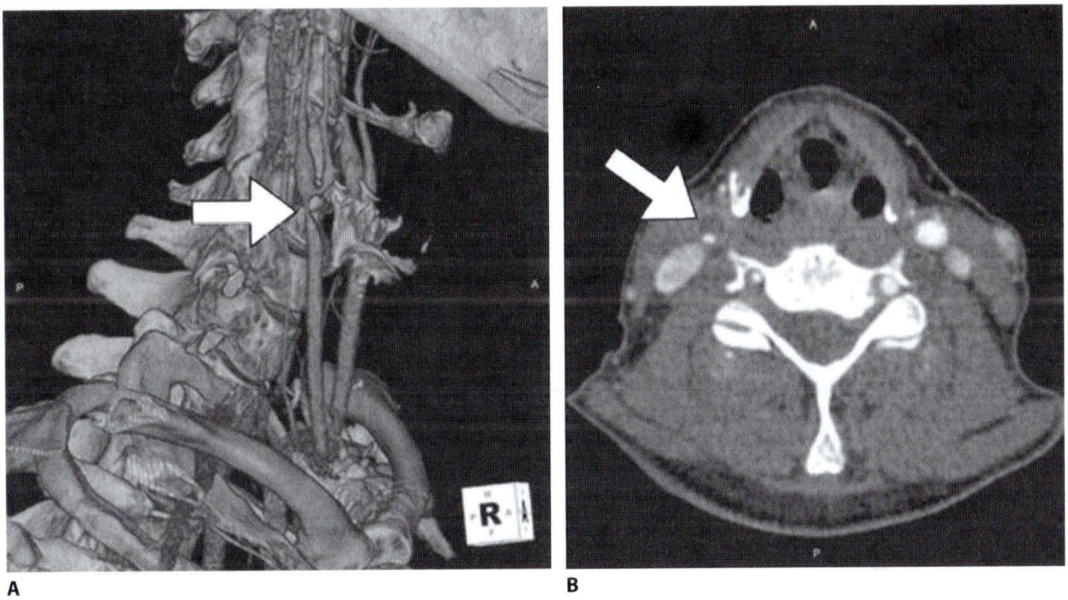

Figure 14–1. Carotid bifurcation occlusive disease. **A:** Three-dimensional CT angiogram of neck demonstrating carotid bifurcation stenosis. **B:** Axial CT view demonstrating the lesion. (Reproduced, with permission, from Doherty GM. *Current Diagnosis & Treatment: Surgery*, 15e. McGraw-Hill 2020.)

B. Imaging

Duplex ultrasonography is the imaging modality of choice with high specificity and sensitivity for detecting and grading the degree of stenosis at the carotid bifurcation (see Chapter 27).

Excellent depiction of the full anatomy of the cerebrovascular circulation from aortic arch to cranium can be obtained with MRA or CTA (Figure 14–1). Each of the modalities may have false-positive or false-negative findings. Since the decision to intervene in cases of carotid stenosis depends on an accurate assessment of the degree of stenosis, it is recommended that at least two modalities be used to confirm the degree of stenosis. Diagnostic cerebral angiography is reserved when carotid artery stenting is planned or other imaging modalities are contraindicated.

Treatment

See Chapter 27 for a discussion of the medical management of occlusive cerebrovascular disease.

A. Asymptomatic Patients

Large studies have shown a 5-year reduction in stroke rate with surgical treatment of asymptomatic carotid stenosis that is > 70%; these patients may benefit from carotid intervention if their risk from intervention is low and their expected survival is longer than 5 years. The CREST-2 trial demonstrated that healthy patients with asymptomatic carotid stenosis > 70% treated with aggressive medical therapy had an approximately 1% annual risk of stroke. A durable reduction in the rate of stroke was seen at 4 years in patients treated with medical therapy plus carotid stent (2.8%) versus medical therapy (6.0%) and in patients treated with medical therapy plus carotid endarterectomy (3.7%) versus medical therapy (5.3%). Mild to moderate disease (30–50% stenosis) indicates the need for ongoing monitoring and aggressive risk factor modification. Patients with carotid stenosis that suddenly worsens likely have an unstable plaque and are at particularly high risk for embolic stroke.

B. Symptomatic Patients

Large randomized trials have shown that patients with TIAs or strokes from which they have completely or nearly completely recovered will benefit from carotid intervention if the ipsilateral carotid artery has a stenosis of > 70%, and intervention should be considered for 50–69% stenoses due to potential benefit. In these situations, carotid endarterectomy (CEA) and, in selected cases, carotid artery stenting, have a durable effect in preventing further events. In symptomatic patients, intervention should ideally be planned within 2 weeks since delays increase the risk of a second event.

Complications

The most common complication from carotid intervention is cranial nerve injury, while the most dreaded complication is stroke from embolization or carotid occlusion. Major cardiovascular societies recommend 3% as the upper limit of acceptable combined morbidity and mortality rates for patients with asymptomatic carotid stenosis and 6% for patients with symptomatic carotid stenosis. Higher rates of morbidity and mortality negate the therapeutic benefit of carotid intervention.

A. Carotid Endarterectomy

The stroke risk for CEA is 1–2%. CEA also carries a 1–2% risk of permanent cranial nerve injury (usually the vagus nerve). A postoperative neck hematoma can cause acute airway compromise. CAD is a comorbidity in most of these patients, and MI rates after CEA are approximately 2–6%.

B. Carotid Angioplasty and Stenting

Carotid artery stenting is performed from a transcervical or transfemoral approach with reported stroke risks of 1–2% and 2–3%, respectively. Transfemoral stenting has worse outcomes for women or patients ≥ age 70. The approach should be dictated by patient anatomy and risk factors. The risk of MI is lower with carotid artery stenting compared to CEA (1.1% versus 2.3%). Carotid artery stenting is indicated for reoperative cases, prior neck radiation, and high carotid bifurcations not otherwise accessible surgically. Nonetheless, emboli are more common during transfemoral carotid artery stenting in spite of embolic protection devices, especially when the carotid artery is heavily calcified. Transcervical carotid stenting, performed through a small incision at the base of the neck, avoids the aortic arch, uses cerebral protective flow reversal, and has lower reported embolization rates than transfemoral carotid stenting.

Prognosis

Twenty-five percent of patients with carotid stenosis and a TIA or small stroke will have further brain ischemia within 18 months with most of the events occurring within the first 6 months. Historically, patients with asymptomatic carotid stenosis likely had an annual stroke rate of just over 2%; however, recent clinical trials with aggressive, protocol-driven medical management have demonstrated annual stroke rates of 1–1.5%. Prospective ultrasound screening at least annually is recommended in asymptomatic patients with known carotid stenosis to identify plaque progression, which increases stroke risk. Concomitant CAD is common and is an important factor both for perioperative risk and long-term prognosis. Aggressive risk factor modification should be prescribed for patients with cerebrovascular disease regardless of planned intervention (see Chapter 27).

When to Refer

Both asymptomatic and symptomatic patients with a carotid stenosis of ≥ 70% by ultrasound criteria and patients with carotid stenosis of ≥ 50% with symptoms of a TIA or stroke should be referred to a vascular specialist for consultation.

When to Admit

Hospitalization should be considered for patients within a week of a TIA or when there is an increased risk for early recurrence. Patients with an acute stroke should be hospitalized.

Brott TG et al; CREST-2 Investigators. Medical management and revascularization for asymptomatic carotid stenosis . N Engl J Med. 2026;394:219. [PMID: 41269206]

Columbo JA et al. Appropriateness of care: asymptomatic carotid stenosis including transcarotid artery revascularization. Semin Vasc Surg. 2024;37:179. [PMID: 39151997]

Evans NR et al. Management of carotid atherosclerosis in stroke. Pract Neurol. 2024;24:382. [PMID: 38589215]

VISCERAL ARTERY INSUFFICIENCY (Intestinal Angina)

ESSENTIALS OF DIAGNOSIS

- Severe postprandial abdominal pain.
- Weight loss with a "fear of eating."
- **Acute mesenteric ischemia:** severe abdominal pain yet minimal findings on physical examination.

General Considerations

Acute mesenteric ischemia results from occlusive mesenteric arterial disease, either embolic occlusion or primary thrombosis of at least one major mesenteric artery.

Nonocclusive mesenteric ischemia can occur with low-flow states, such as severe HF, sepsis, or hypotension.

Chronic mesenteric ischemia, also called intestinal angina, occurs when increased flow demands during feeding are not met resulting in abdominal pain. Because of the rich collateral mesenteric network, generally at least two of the three major visceral vessels (celiac, superior mesenteric, inferior mesenteric arteries) must be affected before symptoms develop.

Ischemic colitis is a variant of mesenteric ischemia and usually develops in the distribution of the inferior mesenteric artery. The intestinal mucosa is the most sensitive to ischemia and will slough if underperfused.

Clinical Findings

A. Symptoms and Signs

1. Acute mesenteric ischemia—Visceral arterial embolism presents acutely with severe abdominal pain. In contrast, patients with primary visceral arterial thrombosis often have an antecedent history consistent with chronic mesenteric ischemia. The key finding with acute mesenteric ischemia is severe, steady, diffuse abdominal pain without focal tenderness or distention. This "pain out of proportion" to physical examination findings occurs because ischemia initially is mucosal and does not impact the peritoneum until transmural ischemia inflames the peritoneal lining. Late findings include a high WBC count, lactic acidosis, hypotension, and abdominal distention.

2. Nonocclusive mesenteric ischemia—This variant of acute mesenteric ischemia presents with severe abdominal pain in seriously ill patients who have required high dose vasopressor therapy for hypotension, thus reducing arterial flow to the visceral arteries. As with visceral artery occlusion, there will be "pain out of proportion" to physical examination findings; late occurrences of high WBC count, lactic acidosis, and abdominal distension are ominous.

3. Chronic mesenteric ischemia—Patients are generally > age 45 and may have evidence of atherosclerosis in other vascular beds. Symptoms consist of epigastric or periumbilical postprandial pain lasting 1–3 hours. To avoid the pain, patients limit food intake and may develop a fear of eating. Weight loss is universal. In severe cases of intestinal angina, patients may become dehydrated, which can cause hypotension and acute thrombosis.

4. Ischemic colitis—Characteristic symptoms are left lower quadrant pain and tenderness, abdominal cramping, and mild diarrhea (non-bloody or bloody). Rectal discharge will appear mucus-like or bloody.

B. Imaging and Colonoscopy

Contrast-enhanced CT is accurate at identifying the presence of ischemic intestine. In acute or chronic mesenteric ischemia, a CTA or MRA can demonstrate narrowing of the proximal visceral vessels. In nonocclusive mesenteric ischemia from a low-flow state, angiography is needed to display a typical "pruned tree" appearance of the distal visceral vascular bed. Ultrasound scanning of the mesenteric vessels can show elevated flow velocities in severe stenosis and proximal obstructing lesions.

In patients with ischemic colitis, flexible sigmoidoscopy is necessary to assess the grade of ischemia that occurs most often in watershed areas, such as the rectal sigmoid and splenic flexure.

Differential Diagnosis

Patients with acute mesenteric ischemia develop acute severe abdominal pain similar to abdominal catastrophes such as small bowel obstruction, bowel perforation, and intra-abdominal abscess. Chronic mesenteric ischemia typically presents as weight loss in an older patient and evaluation for malignancy is paramount. Patients with ischemic colitis need an evaluation for inflammatory, malignant, and peptic sources of GI tract bleeding.

Treatment

1. Acute mesenteric ischemia—A high suspicion of acute mesenteric ischemia dictates immediate exploration to assess bowel viability. If the bowel remains viable, arterial bypass using a prosthetic conduit can be done either from the supra-celiac aorta or common iliac artery to the celiac and the superior mesentery artery. Angioplasty and stenting of the arteries can be used, but an open surgical evaluation of bowel viability is often necessary.

2. Nonocclusive mesenteric ischemia—As with occlusive acute mesenteric ischemia, surgical assessment of bowel viability is necessary. Minimizing vasopressor therapy and initiating vasodilator treatment, either with systemic prostaglandin or intra-arterial papaverine, can improve visceral artery flow. Ultimately, treatment of the patient's underlying illness is needed to resolve the condition.

3. Chronic mesenteric ischemia—Angioplasty and stenting of the proximal vessel may be beneficial depending on the anatomy of the stenosis. Should an endovascular solution not be available, an aorto-visceral artery bypass is the preferred management. The long-term results are highly durable.

4. Ischemic colitis—The mainstay of treatment is maintenance of blood pressure and perfusion until collateral circulation becomes well established. The patient must be monitored closely for evidence of perforation necessitating resection.

Prognosis

The combined morbidity and mortality rates from surgical intervention of acute mesenteric ischemia is 50–69%, and only 25% of patients will survive 1 year. Survival is poor with nonocclusive mesenteric ischemia, often driven by the underlying severe illness that caused the condition. The combined morbidity and mortality are 10–15% from surgical intervention of chronic mesenteric ischemia, in part due to patients' malnutrition and frailty. Without intervention, acute, nonocclusive, and chronic mesenteric ischemia are uniformly fatal. Adequate collateral circulation usually develops in those who have ischemic colitis, and the prognosis for this entity is better than for chronic mesenteric ischemia.

When to Refer

Any patient in whom there is a suspicion of mesenteric ischemia should be urgently referred for imaging and possible intervention. When there is "pain out of proportion to examination," a high index of suspicion is warranted to expedite the diagnosis.

When to Admit

Indications for admission include the presence of abdominal pain out of proportion to abnormal physical findings (there are no findings of peritonitis and the abdomen is soft) or a history of worsening intestinal angina with inability to tolerate a diet.

Andraska EA et al. Contemporary management of acute and chronic mesenteric ischemia: 10-year experience from a multihospital healthcare system. J Vasc Surg. 2022;75:1624. [PMID: 34788652]

Huber TS et al. Chronic mesenteric ischemia: clinical practice guidelines from the Society for Vascular Surgery. J Vasc Surg. 2021;73:87S. [PMID: 33171195]

Lehane DJ et al. Survival, reintervention, and value of open and endovascular repair for chronic mesenteric ischemia. Ann Vasc Surg. 2023:97:203. [PMID: 37659648]

ACUTE MESENTERIC VEIN OCCLUSION

The hallmarks of acute mesenteric vein occlusion are postprandial pain and evidence of a hypercoagulable state. Acute mesenteric vein occlusion presents similarly to the arterial occlusive syndromes but is much less common. Patients at risk include those with paroxysmal nocturnal hemoglobinuria; protein C, protein S, or antithrombin deficiencies; or the *JAK2* mutation. Thrombolysis is the mainstay of therapy. Aggressive long-term anticoagulation is required.

NONATHEROSCLEROTIC VASCULAR DISEASE

THROMBOANGIITIS OBLITERANS (Buerger Disease)

ESSENTIALS OF DIAGNOSIS

- Typically occurs in men who smoke cigarettes.
- Distal extremities involved with severe ischemia, progressing to tissue loss.
- Thrombosis of the superficial veins may occur.
- Smoking cessation is essential to stop disease progression.

General Considerations

Thromboangiitis obliterans (Buerger disease) is a segmental, inflammatory, and thrombotic process of the distal-most arteries and occasionally veins of the extremities. Pathologic examination reveals arteritis in the affected vessels. The cause is not known but it is rarely seen in patients who do not smoke cigarettes. Arteries most commonly affected are the plantar and digital vessels of the foot and lower leg. In advanced stages, the fingers and hands may become involved. The incidence of thromboangiitis obliterans has decreased dramatically.

Clinical Findings

A. Symptoms and Signs

Thromboangiitis obliterans may be initially difficult to differentiate from atherosclerotic peripheral vascular disease, but in most cases, the lesions are on the toes and the patient is younger than 40 years. The observation of superficial thrombophlebitis may aid the diagnosis. Because the distal vessels are usually affected, intermittent claudication is not common, but rest pain, particularly pain in the distal most part of the extremity (ie, toes), is frequent. This pain often progresses to tissue loss and amputation unless the patient stops smoking cigarettes. The progression of the disease seems to be intermittent with acute and dramatic episodes followed by some periods of remission.

B. Imaging

MRA or invasive angiography can demonstrate the obliteration of the distal arterial tree typical of thromboangiitis obliterans.

Differential Diagnosis

In atherosclerotic peripheral vascular disease, the onset of tissue ischemia tends to be less dramatic than in thromboangiitis obliterans, and symptoms of proximal arterial involvement, such as claudication, predominate.

Symptoms of Raynaud disease may be difficult to differentiate from thromboangiitis obliterans and may coexist in 40% of patients. Repetitive atheroemboli may also mimic thromboangiitis obliterans. It may be necessary to image the aorta and leg arteries to rule out sources of microemboli.

Treatment

Cessation of cigarette smoking is the mainstay of therapy and will halt the disease in most cases. As the distal arterial tree is occluded, revascularization is often not possible. Intra-arterial infusion of prostacyclin analogs (eg, iloprost) can improve ulcer healing in select cases. Sympathectomy is rarely effective.

Prognosis

With abstinence from smoking tobacco, the outlook for thromboangiitis obliterans may be better than with premature peripheral vascular disease. If tobacco smoking continues, then the prognosis is generally poor, with possible need for both upper and lower extremity amputation.

Cacione DG et al. Pharmacological treatment for Buerger's disease. Cochrane Database Syst Rev. 2020;5:CD011033. [PMID: 32364620]

Evans NS et al. Vascular disease patient information page: thromboangiitis obliterans (Buerger disease). Vasc Med. 2024;29:565. [PMID: 39239807]

ARTERIAL ANEURYSMS

ABDOMINAL AORTIC ANEURYSM

ESSENTIALS OF DIAGNOSIS

- Most aortic aneurysms are asymptomatic until rupture.
- 80% of AAAs measuring 5 cm are palpable; the usual treatment threshold is 5.5 cm in men and 5.0 cm in women.
- Back or abdominal pain with aneurysmal tenderness may precede rupture.
- Rupture is catastrophic: excruciating abdominal pain that radiates to the back; hypotension.

General Considerations

Dilatation of the infrarenal aorta is a normal part of aging. The aorta of a healthy young man measures approximately 2 cm. An aneurysm is present when the aortic diameter > 3 cm, but aneurysms rarely rupture until their diameter > 5 cm. AAAs are found in 2% of men > 55 years of age; the male to female ratio is 4:1. Ninety percent of abdominal atherosclerotic aneurysms originate below the renal arteries. The aneurysms usually involve the aortic bifurcation and often involve the common iliac arteries.

Aortic inflammation is uncommon with atherosclerotic aneurysms and may be due to inflammation from aortic vasculitis, as in Takayasu disease or Behçet disease. Rarely, inflammatory aortitis is due to infections, including *Salmonella*, tuberculosis, and syphilis. Periaortic inflammation without vasculitis or infection (inflammatory aneurysm) is due to retroperitoneal fibrosis, either idiopathic or secondary (IgG_4-related disease).

Clinical Findings

Patients often have concomitant CAD, carotid disease, kidney disease, and emphysema, typically seen in older men who smoke cigarettes. Aortic aneurysms are less common in patients with diabetes mellitus.

A. Symptoms and Signs

1. Asymptomatic—Although 80% of 5-cm infrarenal aneurysms are palpable on routine physical examination, most aneurysms are discovered on ultrasound or CT imaging as part of a screening program or incidentally. Most aneurysms have a thick layer of thrombus lining the aneurysmal sac, but embolization to the lower extremities occurs rarely.

2. Symptomatic—

A. PAIN—Aneurysmal expansion may be accompanied by mild to severe midabdominal discomfort often radiating to the lower back. The pain may be constant or intermittent and is exacerbated by even gentle pressure on the aneurysm sack. Pain may also accompany inflammatory aneurysms.

B. RUPTURE—The sudden escape of blood into the retroperitoneal space causes severe pain and hypotension. Free rupture into the peritoneal cavity is lethal.

B. Laboratory Findings

In acute cases of a contained retroperitoneal rupture, the hematocrit may be normal, since there has been no opportunity for hemodilution.

C. Imaging

Abdominal ultrasonography is the diagnostic study of choice for initial screening for aneurysm. In approximately three-quarters of patients with aneurysms, curvilinear calcifications outlining portions of the aneurysm wall may be visible on plain radiographs of the abdomen or back. CT scans provide a more reliable assessment of aneurysm diameter and should be done when the aneurysm nears the diameter threshold (5.5 cm in men or 5.0 cm in women) for treatment. Contrast-enhanced CT scans show the arteries above and below the aneurysm. CT imaging will often demonstrate mural thrombus within the aneurysm and is not an indication for anticoagulation.

Once an aneurysm is identified, routine follow-up with ultrasound will determine size and growth rate. The frequency of imaging depends on aneurysm size: every 3 years for aneurysms 3–3.9 cm, every 12 months for aneurysms 4–4.9 cm, and every 6 months for aneurysms ≥ 5 cm. When an aneurysm measures approximately 5 cm, a CTA with contrast should be performed to define arterial anatomy and more accurately assess aneurysm size.

Screening

Guidelines recommend abdominal ultrasound screening in men 65–75 years old who have ever smoked tobacco but conflict on whether women with the same exposure should be screened. While patients are monitored, smoking cessation and treatment of underlying hypertension, hyperlipidemia, and diabetes are recommended.

Differential Diagnosis

Conditions that can mimic a symptomatic AAA include a perforated viscus (peptic ulcer, appendix, gallbladder, diverticulitis), pancreatitis, intestinal ischemia, urinary calculi, bowel obstruction, and descending aortic dissection.

Treatment

A. Elective Repair

The risk of rupture increases with aneurysm diameter. In general, elective repair is indicated for an AAA ≥ 5.5 cm in diameter in men or 5 cm in women. Other indications for repair are aneurysm growth (> 0.5 cm in 6 months) or saccular morphology. Symptoms such as pain or tenderness may indicate impending rupture and require urgent repair regardless of the aneurysm's diameter. Pharmacologic therapies do not prevent aneurysm rupture, although clinical trials are testing the use of instilled elastin cross linking agents to prevent aneurysmal growth.

B. Aneurysmal Rupture

A ruptured aneurysm is a lethal event. Approximately half the patients exsanguinate before reaching a hospital. In the remainder, bleeding may be temporarily contained in the retroperitoneum (contained rupture), allowing the patient to undergo emergent surgery. However, only half of those patients survive. Endovascular repair is recommended for ruptured aneurysm treatment due to lower perioperative mortality compared to open repair.

C. Aortic Inflammation/Inflammatory Aneurysm

Aortic or periaortic inflammation requires medical treatment for the underlying cause (vasculitis, infection, or retroperitoneal fibrosis). Indications for surgical treatment are based on the size of the aneurysm (5.5 cm or larger), associated compression of retroperitoneal structures (such as the ureter), or pain upon palpation of the aneurysm. Inflammation encasing an inflammatory aneurysm recedes after repair.

D. Assessment of Operative Risk

Aneurysms are a variant of systemic atherosclerosis, and patients with aneurysms have a high rate of coronary disease; trial data, though, demonstrate minimal value in addressing stable CAD prior to aneurysm resection. In patients with symptomatic CAD, however, the CAD should be treated first. Aneurysm repair should follow shortly thereafter due to a slightly increased aneurysm rupture risk after the coronary procedures.

E. Open Surgical Resection Versus Endovascular Repair

In open surgical aneurysm repair, a graft is sutured to healthy nondilated vessels above and below the aneurysm. This involves an abdominal incision, extensive dissection, and interruption of aortic blood flow. The mortality rate is low (2–5%) in centers that have a high volume for this procedure and when it is performed in good-risk patients. Older, sicker patients may not tolerate the cardiopulmonary stresses of the operation. With endovascular aortic repair (EVAR), a stent-graft is introduced through small incisions over the femoral arteries and positioned within the aorta under fluoroscopic guidance. The stent must seal securely against the wall of the aorta above and below the aneurysm, thereby excluding blood from flowing into the aneurysm sac. The anatomic requirements for endovascular repairs are more precise than for open repairs. Most studies have found that EVAR offers patients reduced operative morbidity and mortality as well as shorter recovery periods. Long-term survival is equivalent between the two techniques. After endovascular repair, patients need lifelong monitoring because of a 10–15% incidence of continued aneurysm growth.

Complications

The most common complication after open repair is MI, occurring in up to 10% of patients. The incidence of MI is substantially lower with endovascular repair. For routine infrarenal aneurysms, kidney injury is unusual; however, when it does occur, or if there is baseline kidney injury, it can be a postoperative complication. Respiratory complications are similar to those seen in most major abdominal surgeries. GI hemorrhage, even years after aortic surgery, suggests a **graft enteric fistula**, most commonly between the aorta and the distal duodenum; the incidence of this complication is higher when the initial surgery is performed emergently.

Prognosis

Mortality for an open elective surgical resection is 2–5%, and mortality for endovascular therapy is 0.5–2%. Among those who survive surgery, approximately 60% are alive at 5 years; MI is the leading cause of death. The long-term survival (5 years or more) after open and endovascular repairs is equivalent.

Mortality of untreated aneurysms varies with aneurysm diameter: 12% annual risk of rupture with an aneurysm > 6 cm in diameter and a 25% annual risk of rupture in aneurysms of > 7 cm diameter. In general, a patient with an aortic aneurysm > 5.5 cm has a threefold greater chance of dying due to aneurysm rupture than of dying due to the surgical resection.

Endovascular aneurysm repair may be less definitive than open surgical repair and requires close follow up with an imaging procedure. Device migration, component separation, and graft limb thrombosis or kinking are common reasons for repeat intervention. With complete exclusion of blood from the aneurysm sac, the pressure is lowered causing the aneurysm to shrink. An "endoleak" from the top or bottom seal zone (type 1) or through a graft defect (type 3) is associated with a persistent risk of rupture. Indirect leakage of blood through lumbar and inferior mesenteric branches of the aneurysm (type 2) produces an intermediate picture with somewhat reduced pressure in the sac, slow shrinkage, and low rupture risk. Lack of aneurysm sack regression after EVAR is associated with lower long-term survival.

When to Refer

- Any patient with a ≥ 4.5-cm aortic aneurysm should be referred to a vascular specialist for observation and assessment.
- Urgent referrals should be made if the patient complains of pain and gentle palpation of the aneurysm confirms that it is the source, regardless of the aneurysmal size.

When to Admit

- Patients with a tender aneurysm to palpation or signs of aortic rupture require emergent hospital admission.
- Evidence of infection after repair.

Baman JR et al. What is an abdominal aortic aneurysm? JAMA Patient Page. 2022;328:2280. [PMID: 36511924]
Golledge J et al. Pathogenesis and management of abdominal aortic aneurysm. Eur Heart J. 2023;44:2682. [PMID: 37387260]
LeFevre N et al. How best to diagnose and manage abdominal aortic aneurysms. J Fam Pract. 2023;72:325. [PMID: 37862627]
Schanzer A et al. Management of abdominal aortic aneurysms. N Engl J Med. 2021;385:1690. [PMID: 34706173]

THORACIC AORTIC ANEURYSMS

ESSENTIALS OF DIAGNOSIS

- Widened mediastinum on CXR.
- With rupture, sudden onset of chest pain radiating to the back.

General Considerations

Most thoracic aortic aneurysms are due to atherosclerosis; syphilis is a rare cause. Disorders of connective tissue and Ehlers-Danlos and Marfan syndromes also are rare causes but have important therapeutic implications. Traumatic, false aneurysms, caused by partial tearing of the aortic wall with deceleration injuries, may occur just beyond the origin of the left subclavian artery. Less than 10% of aortic aneurysms occur in the thoracic aorta.

Clinical Findings

A. Symptoms and Signs

Most thoracic aneurysms are asymptomatic. When symptoms occur, they depend largely on the size and the position of the aneurysm and its rate of growth. Substernal back or neck pain may occur. Pressure on the trachea, esophagus, or superior vena cava can result in the following symptoms and signs: dyspnea, stridor or brassy cough, dysphagia, and edema in the neck and arms as well as distended neck veins. Stretching of the left recurrent laryngeal nerve causes hoarseness. With aneurysms of the ascending aorta, aortic regurgitation may be present due to dilation of the aortic valve annulus. Rupture of a thoracic aneurysm is catastrophic because bleeding is rarely contained, allowing no time for emergent repair.

B. Imaging

The aneurysm may be diagnosed on CXR by the calcified outline of the dilated aorta. CT scanning with contrast enhancement is the modality of choice, but MRA can be used to demonstrate the anatomy and aneurysmal size and to exclude lesions that can mimic aneurysms, such as neoplasms or substernal goiter. There is no low-cost alternative (eg, ultrasonography) for screening or surveillance. Cardiac catheterization and echocardiography may be required to describe the relationship of the coronary vessels to an aneurysm of the ascending aorta.

Treatment

Indications for repair depend on the location of dilation, rate of growth, associated symptoms, and overall condition of the patient. Aneurysms that involve the proximal aortic arch or ascending aorta represent particularly challenging problems and may be considered for repair when they measure 5.5 cm. Open surgery is usually required, carrying substantial risk of morbidity (including stroke, diffuse neurologic injury, and intellectual impairment) because interruption of arch blood flow is required. Repair of aortic arch aneurysms should be undertaken only if there is a skilled surgical team with an acceptable record of outcomes for these complex procedures. The availability of thoracic aortic endograft techniques using complex branched endovascular reconstructions for aneurysms involving the arch or visceral aorta (custom-made grafts with branches to the vessels involved in the aneurysm) does not change the indications for aneurysm repair. Descending thoracic aneurysms measuring ≥ 5.5 cm should be considered for repair, since the 5-year survival is 54% in untreated patients. Aneurysms of the descending thoracic aorta are treated routinely by endovascular grafting.

Complications

With the exception of endovascular repair for discrete saccular aneurysms of the descending thoracic aorta, the morbidity and mortality of thoracic aneurysm repair are higher than for infrarenal AAA repair. Paraplegia remains a devastating complication. Most large series report approximately 4–10% rate of paraplegia following endovascular repair of thoracic aortic aneurysms. The spinal arterial supply is segmental through intercostal branches of the aorta with variable degrees of intersegmental connection. Therefore, the more extensive the aneurysm, the greater is the risk of paraplegia with repair. Prior infrarenal abdominal aortic surgery, subclavian or internal iliac artery occlusion, and hypotension all increase the paraplegia risk. Involvement of the aortic arch also increases the risk of stroke, even when the aneurysm does not directly affect the carotid artery.

Prognosis

Generally, degenerative aneurysms of the thoracic aorta will enlarge (on average 0.1 cm/year) and require repair to prevent death from rupture. Endovascular repair of saccular aneurysms, particularly those distal to the left subclavian artery and the descending thoracic aorta, have good results. Branched/fenestrated endovascular grafting technology has reduced morbidity and mortality and expanded eligibility for repair.

When to Refer

- Ascending aortic aneurysms ≥ 4.5 cm should be referred to a cardiac surgeon for observation and assessment and considered for repair at 5.5 cm.
- Descending thoracic aortic aneurysm should be referred to a vascular specialist when they reach 5 cm for observation and assessment and considered for repair at 5.5 cm.

When to Admit

- Any patient with chest or back pain with a known or suspected thoracic aorta aneurysm must be brought to the hospital and undergo urgent imaging studies to rule out the aneurysm as a cause of the pain.

Oderich GS et al. Early and late aortic-related mortality and rupture after fenestrated-branched endovascular aortic repair of thoracoabdominal aortic aneurysms: a prospective multicenter cohort study. Circulation. 2024;150:1343. [PMID: 38989575]

Upchurch GR et al. Society for Vascular Surgery clinical practice guidelines of thoracic endovascular aortic repair for descending thoracic aortic aneurysms. J Vasc Surg. 2021;73:55S. [PMID: 32628988]

PERIPHERAL ARTERY ANEURYSMS

ESSENTIALS OF DIAGNOSIS

- Widened, prominent pulses.
- Acute leg or foot pain and paresthesias with loss of distal pulses.
- High association of popliteal aneurysm with AAA.

General Considerations

The normal diameter of a popliteal artery is 4–5 mm and aneurysms are > 10 mm. Like aortic aneurysms, peripheral artery aneurysms are silent until critically symptomatic. However, unlike aortic aneurysms, the presenting manifestations are due to peripheral embolization and thrombosis. Popliteal artery aneurysms account for 70% of peripheral arterial aneurysms. Popliteal aneurysms may embolize repetitively over time and occlude distal arteries. Due to the redundant parallel arterial supply to the foot, ischemia does not occur until a final embolus occludes flow.

Primary femoral artery aneurysms are much less common than popliteal aneurysms. However, the incidence of pseudoaneurysms of the femoral artery following arterial punctures for arteriography and cardiac catheterization ranges from 0.05% to 6%.

Clinical Findings

A. Symptoms and Signs

The patient may be aware of a pulsatile mass when the aneurysm is in the groin, but popliteal aneurysms are often undetected by the patient and clinician. Rarely, peripheral aneurysms may produce symptoms by compressing the local vein or nerve. The first symptom may be due to ischemia of acute arterial occlusion. The symptoms range from sudden-onset pain and paralysis to short-distance claudication that slowly lessens as collateral circulation develops. Symptoms from recurrent embolization to the leg are often transient, if they occur at all. Sudden ischemia may appear in a toe or part of the foot, followed by slow resolution, and the true diagnosis may be elusive. The onset of recurrent episodes of pain in the foot, particularly if accompanied by cyanosis, suggests embolization and requires investigation of the heart and proximal arterial tree.

Because popliteal pulses are somewhat difficult to palpate even in normal individuals, a particularly prominent or easily felt pulse is suggestive of aneurysm and should be investigated by ultrasound. Since popliteal aneurysms are bilateral in 60% of cases, the diagnosis of thrombosis of a popliteal aneurysm is often aided by the palpation of a pulsatile aneurysm in the contralateral popliteal space. Approximately 50% of patients with popliteal aneurysms have an aneurysmal abdominal aorta.

B. Imaging Studies

Duplex color ultrasound is the most efficient investigation to confirm the diagnosis of peripheral aneurysm, measure its size and configuration, and demonstrate mural thrombus. MRA or CTA is required to define the aneurysm and local arterial anatomy for reconstruction. Arteriography is not recommended because mural thrombus reduces the apparent diameter of the lumen on angiography. Patients with popliteal aneurysms should undergo abdominal ultrasonography to determine whether an AAA is also present.

Treatment

Open surgical bypass is indicated when a popliteal or femoral aneurysm is associated with any peripheral embolization, the aneurysm is > 2 cm, or a mural thrombus is present. Endovascular exclusion of the aneurysm can be done but has anatomic constraints and is reserved for high-risk patients. To prevent limb loss, immediate or urgent surgery is indicated when acute embolization or thrombosis has caused acute leg ischemia. Intra-arterial thrombolysis for acute ischemia may be done if examination (light touch) remains intact, suggesting that immediate surgery is not imperative. Acute pseudoaneurysms of the femoral artery due to arterial punctures can be successfully treated using ultrasound-guided compression or thrombin injection.

Prognosis

In untreated patients, symptoms will develop in approximately one-third within 1 year and in two-thirds within 5 years. The long-term patency of bypass grafts for femoral and popliteal aneurysms is generally excellent but depends on the adequacy of the outflow tract. Late graft occlusion is less common than in similar surgeries for occlusive disease.

When to Refer

- Peripheral arterial aneurysms measuring 2 cm or with ultrasound evidence of thrombus within the aneurysm should be referred to a vascular specialist.

When to Admit

- Patients with symptoms of ischemia or any signs of embolization should be admitted.

Farber A et al. The Society for Vascular Surgery clinical practice guidelines on popliteal artery aneurysms. J Vasc Surg. 2022;75:109S. [PMID: 34023430]

AORTIC DISSECTION

ESSENTIALS OF DIAGNOSIS

- Sudden searing chest pain with radiation to the back, abdomen, or neck in a hypertensive patient.
- Widened mediastinum on CXR.
- Pulse discrepancy in the extremities.
- Acute aortic regurgitation may develop.

General Considerations

Aortic dissection occurs when a spontaneous intimal tear develops and blood dissects into the media of the aorta. The tear can result from repetitive torque to the ascending and proximal descending aorta during the cardiac cycle; hypertension is an important component of this disease process. Dissections are classified by the entry point and distal extent. **Type A dissection** involves the arch proximal to the left subclavian artery, and **type B dissection** occurs in the proximal descending thoracic aorta typically just beyond the left subclavian artery. Dissections may occur in the absence of hypertension but abnormalities of smooth muscle, elastic tissue, or collagen should be considered in these cases. Pregnancy, bicuspid aortic valve, bovine arch, and coarctation are associated with increased risk of dissection.

Blood entering the intimal tear may extend the dissection into the abdominal aorta, the lower extremities, the carotid arteries, or less commonly, the subclavian arteries. Both absolute blood pressure and pulse pressure are important in propagation of dissection. *Aortic dissection is a true emergency and requires immediate control of blood pressure to limit the extent of the dissection.* Type A dissection has the worse prognosis; death may occur within hours due to rupture of the dissection into the pericardial sac or dissection into the coronary arteries, resulting in MI. Rupture into the pleural cavity is also possible. The intimal/medial flap of the aortic wall created by the dissection may occlude major aortic branches, resulting in ischemia of the brain, intestines, kidney, or extremities.

Clinical Findings

A. Symptoms and Signs

Severe persistent chest pain of sudden onset radiating down the back, neck, or possibly into the anterior chest is characteristic. The patient is usually hypertensive. Syncope, hemiplegia, or paralysis of the lower extremities may occur. Mesenteric ischemia or kidney injury may develop. Peripheral pulses may be diminished or unequal. Branch vessel occlusion can be static or dynamic with variable ischemia due to mobility of the intimal flap during the cardiac cycle. A diastolic murmur may result from dissection in the ascending aorta close to the aortic valve, causing valvular regurgitation, HF, or cardiac tamponade.

B. Electrocardiographic Findings

LVH from long-standing hypertension is often present. Acute changes suggesting myocardial ischemia develop when the dissection involves the coronary artery ostium. Classically, inferior wall abnormalities predominate since dissection leads to compromise of the right rather than the left coronary artery. In some patients, the ECG may be normal.

C. Imaging

A multiplanar CT scan with contrast is the diagnostic imaging modality of choice; clinicians should have a low threshold for obtaining a CT scan in any hypertensive patient with chest pain and equivocal findings on ECG. The CT scan should include the chest, abdomen, and pelvis to fully delineate the extent of the dissected aorta. MRA is an excellent imaging modality for chronic dissections, but in the acute situation, the longer imaging time and the difficulty of monitoring patients in the MRI scanner make CT scan preferable. CXRs may reveal an abnormal aortic contour or widened superior mediastinum. Although transesophageal echocardiography (TEE) is an excellent diagnostic imaging method, it is generally not readily available in the acute setting.

Differential Diagnosis

Aortic dissection is most commonly misdiagnosed as MI or pulmonary embolization. Dissections may occur with minimal pain; branch vessel occlusion of the lower extremity can mimic arterial embolus.

Treatment

A. Medical

When an aortic dissection is suspected, aggressive measures to lower blood pressure and heart rate should be initiated, even before a definitive diagnosis is made. Treatment requires a simultaneous reduction of the systolic blood pressure to 100–120 mm Hg and heart rate to 60–70 beats/min. β-Blockers are first-line therapy because they reduce the LV ejection force that weakens the arterial wall. Labetalol, both an α- and β-blocker, lowers heart rate and achieves rapid blood pressure control. Give 20 mg over 2 minutes by intravenous injection. Additional doses of 40–80 mg intravenously can be given every 10 minutes (maximum dose 300 mg) until the desired blood pressure has been reached. Alternatively, 2 mg/min may be given by intravenous infusion, titrated to the desired effect. The short half-life of esmolol allows for rapid titration and for testing a patient's reaction to a β-blocker if there are concerns about asthma or bradycardia. Give a loading dose of esmolol, 0.5 mg/kg intravenously over 1 minute, followed by an infusion of 0.0025–0.02 mg/kg/min. Titrate the infusion to a goal heart rate of 60–70 beats/min. For patients who cannot tolerate a β-blocker or who need a second agent to control the hypertension, intravenous calcium channel blocker infusions, such as nicardipine, are an alternative. Start nicardipine 5 mg/hour intravenously and titrate the infusion to the desired effect. If an additional agent is needed to control the hypertension, nitroprusside may be added as follows: 50 mg of nitroprusside in 1000 mL of 5% dextrose and water, infused at a rate of 0.5 mL/min for a 70-kg person (0.3 mcg/kg/min); the infusion rate is increased by 0.5 mL every 5 minutes until adequate control of the pressure has been achieved. Morphine sulfate is the appropriate drug to use for pain relief. Long-term medical care of patients should include β-blockers in their antihypertensive regimen.

B. Surgical Intervention

1. Type A dissection—*Urgent surgical intervention is required for all type A dissections.* If a skilled cardiovascular team is not available, the patient should be transferred to an appropriate facility. The procedure involves replacing the diseased portion of the arch with a graft and brachiocephalic vessel bypass as necessary. Replacement of the aortic valve may be required with reattachment of the coronary arteries.

2. Type B dissection with malperfusion—*Urgent surgery is required for type B dissections if there is aortic branch compromise resulting in malperfusion of the renal, visceral, or extremity vessels.* The immediate goal of surgery is to restore flow to the ischemic tissue. Endovascular stenting of the entry tear at the level of the subclavian artery may result in obliteration of the false lumen and restoration of flow into the branch vessel from the true lumen.

3. Type B dissection without malperfusion—For acute type B dissections without malperfusion, blood pressure control is the primary treatment. Long-term aortic-specific survival and late aneurysm formation rates are improved with early repair using thoracic stent grafts, especially in healthy patients with high-risk anatomic features (aortic diameter > 4 cm or partial false lumen thrombosis).

Prognosis & Follow-Up

The mortality rate for untreated type A dissections is approximately 1% per hour for 72 hours and over 90% at 3 months. Mortality is also extremely high for untreated type B dissections with malperfusion or rupture. The surgical and endovascular therapies for aortic dissections are technically demanding and require an experienced team to achieve perioperative mortalities of < 10%. Aneurysmal enlargement of the residual false lumen may develop despite adequate antihypertensive therapy. Yearly CT scans are required to monitor for aneurysm development. Indications for late aneurysm repair are determined by aneurysm size (6 cm or larger), similar to undissected thoracic aneurysms.

When to Admit

- All patients with an acute dissection should be hospitalized for blood pressure management and observation.
- Urgent surgical repair is indicated for all type A dissections and for complicated type B dissections with malperfusion, rupture, persistent symptoms, or uncontrolled hypertension.

Carrel T et al. Acute aortic dissection. Lancet. 2023;401:773. [PMID: 36640801]

VENOUS DISEASES

VARICOSE VEINS

ESSENTIALS OF DIAGNOSIS

- Dilated, tortuous superficial veins in the legs.
- Asymptomatic or aching discomfort or pain.
- Often hereditary.
- Increased frequency after pregnancy.

General Considerations

Varicose veins develop in the lower extremities. Periods of high venous pressure related to prolonged standing or heavy lifting are contributing factors, but the highest incidence occurs in women after pregnancy. Varicosities develop in over 20% of all adults.

The combination of progressive venous reflux and venous hypertension is the hallmark of chronic venous disease. The superficial veins are involved, typically the great saphenous vein and its tributaries, but the short saphenous vein (posterior lower leg) may also be affected. Distention of the vein prevents the valve leaflets from coapting, creating incompetence and reflux of blood toward the foot.

Secondary varicosities can develop due to obstructive changes and valve damage in the deep venous system following thrombophlebitis, or rarely as a result of proximal venous occlusion due to neoplasm or fibrosis. Congenital or acquired arteriovenous fistulas or venous malformations are also associated with varicosities and should be considered in young patients with varicosities.

Clinical Findings

A. Symptoms and Signs

Symptom severity is not correlated with the number and size of the varicosities; extensive varicose veins may produce no subjective symptoms, whereas minimal varicosities may produce many symptoms. Dull, aching heaviness or a feeling of fatigue of the legs brought on by periods of standing is the most common complaint. Itching from venous eczema may occur either above the ankle or directly overlying large varicosities.

Dilated, tortuous veins of the thigh and calf are visible and palpable when the patient is standing and can be tender to palpation. Longstanding varicose veins may progress to chronic venous insufficiency with associated ankle edema, brownish skin hyperpigmentation (venous stasis dermatitis), and chronic skin induration or fibrosis (lipodermatosclerosis). A bruit or thrill is not consistent with primary varicose veins and signals the presence of an arteriovenous fistula or malformation.

B. Imaging

The identification of the source of venous reflux that feeds the symptomatic veins is necessary for effective surgical treatment. Duplex ultrasonography by a technician experienced in the diagnosis and localization of venous reflux is the test of choice for planning therapy. In most cases, reflux will arise from the greater saphenous vein.

Differential Diagnosis

Varicose veins due to primary superficial venous reflux should be differentiated from those secondary to previous or ongoing obstruction of the deep veins (post-thrombotic syndrome). Pain or discomfort from neuropathy should be distinguished from symptoms associated with coexistent varicose veins. Similarly, vein symptoms should be distinguished from pain due to intermittent claudication that occurs after a predictable amount of exercise and resolves with rest. In adolescent patients with varicose veins, imaging of the deep venous system is obligatory to exclude a congenital malformation or atresia of the deep veins. *Surgical treatment of varicose veins in these patients is contraindicated because the varicosities may play a significant role in venous drainage of the limb.*

Complications

Superficial thrombophlebitis of varicose veins is uncommon. The typical presentation is acute localized pain with tender, firm veins. The process is usually self-limiting, resolving within several weeks. The risk of DVT or embolization is very low unless the thrombophlebitis extends into the great saphenous vein in the upper medial thigh. Predisposing conditions include pregnancy, local trauma, or immobility. Superimposed infection leading to septic thrombophlebitis requires antibiotics; suppurative thrombophlebitis requires surgical incision and drainage.

In older patients, superficial varicosities may bleed with even minor trauma. The amount of bleeding can be alarming as the pressure in the varicosity is high.

Treatment

A. Nonsurgical Measures

Nonsurgical treatment is effective. Elastic graduated compression stockings (20–30 mm Hg pressure) reduce the venous pressure in the leg and may prevent the progression of disease. Good control of symptoms can be achieved when stockings are worn daily during waking hours and legs are elevated, especially at night. Compression stockings are well-suited for older patients or patients who do not want surgery. Wire frames (Donner) are useful devices to put on the stockings, which can be a difficult task for frail patients. If patients are unable to reach their feet, a compressive leg wrap can be used.

B. Varicose Vein Sclerotherapy

Direct injection of a sclerosing agent induces permanent fibrosis and obliteration of the target veins. Chemical irritants (eg, glycerin) or hypertonic saline are often used for small, < 4-mm reticular veins or telangiectasias. Foam sclerotherapy is used to treat the great saphenous vein, varicose veins > 4 mm, and perforating veins. *Sclerotherapy of varicose veins without treatment of underlying saphenous vein reflux is associated with varicosity recurrence rates > 50% as uncorrected reflux progressively dilates adjacent veins.* Complications such as phlebitis, tissue necrosis, or infection may occur with any sclerosing agent.

C. Surgical Reflux Treatment

Treatment for reflux from the great saphenous vein obliterates the vein surgically (vein stripping), or endovenously with thermal energy (laser or radiofrequency catheter), or injection with cyanoacrylate glue or a foam sclerosant.

Endovenous treatments can often be performed with local anesthesia alone and the early success is equal to vein stripping. Long-term success is highest with vein stripping and thermal treatments while the long-term durability of cyanoacrylate glue and foam is unknown. One major complication is ablation-related thrombus extension requiring prolonged anticoagulation. Less common sources of reflux include the small saphenous vein (for varicosities in the posterior calf) and incompetent perforator veins arising directly from the deep venous system. Correction of reflux is performed at the same time as excision of the symptomatic varicose veins. When superficial venous reflux is present, concomitant reflux in the deep venous system is often secondary to volume overload, which will resolve with correction of the superficial reflux.

Prognosis

Surgical treatment of superficial vein reflux and excision of varicose veins provide excellent results. The 5-year success rate (defined as lack of pain and recurrent varicosities) is 85–90%. Even after adequate treatment, secondary tissue changes may persist.

When to Refer

- Absolute indications for referral for saphenous varicose vein ablation include thrombophlebitis and bleeding.
- Pain and cosmetic concerns are responsible for most referrals for ablation.

Gloviczki P et al. The 2023 Society for Vascular Surgery, American Venous Forum, and American Vein and Lymphatic Society clinical practice guidelines for the management of varicose veins of the lower extremities. Part II: Endorsed by the Society of Interventional Radiology and the Society for Vascular Medicine. J Vasc Surg Venous Lymphat Disord. 2024;12:101670. [PMID: 37652254]

SUPERFICIAL VENOUS THROMBOPHLEBITIS

ESSENTIALS OF DIAGNOSIS

- Red, painful induration along a superficial vein, usually at the site of a recent intravenous line.
- Marked swelling of the extremity may not occur.

General Considerations

Short-term venous catheterization of superficial arm veins as well as the use of longer-term peripherally inserted central catheter (PICC) lines are the most common cause of superficial thrombophlebitis. Intravenous catheter sites should be observed daily for signs of local inflammation and should be removed if a local reaction develops in the vein. Serious thrombotic or septic complications can occur if this policy is not followed; *S aureus* is the most common pathogen. Other organisms, including fungi, may be responsible.

Superficial thrombophlebitis may occur spontaneously, often in pregnant or postpartum women or in individuals with varicose veins, or it may be associated with trauma, as with a blow to the leg or following intravenous therapy with irritating solutions. It also may be a manifestation of systemic hypercoagulability from abdominal cancer such as carcinoma of the pancreas and may be the earliest sign of the condition. Superficial thrombophlebitis related to a PICC may be associated with occult DVT in about 20% of cases, but occult DVT is much less commonly associated with spontaneous superficial thrombophlebitis of the saphenous vein (about 5% of cases). Pulmonary emboli are exceedingly rare and occur from an associated DVT (see Chapters 9 and 16).

Clinical Findings

A. Symptoms and Signs

In spontaneous superficial thrombophlebitis, the great saphenous vein is most often involved. The patient usually experiences a dull pain in the region of the involved vein. Local findings consist of induration, redness, and tenderness along the course of a vein. The process may be localized, or it may involve most of the great saphenous vein and its tributaries. The inflammatory reaction generally subsides in 1–2 weeks; a firm cord may remain for a much longer period. Edema of the extremity is uncommon.

Localized redness and induration at the site of a recent intravenous line require urgent attention. Proximal extension of the induration and pain with chills and high fever suggest septic phlebitis and require urgent treatment.

B. Imaging

Duplex ultrasound of the involved extremity is the standard of care to establish the extent of superficial thrombophlebitis and detect the presence of DVT.

Differential Diagnosis

The linear rather than circular nature of the lesion and the distribution along the course of a superficial vein differentiate superficial phlebitis from cellulitis, erythema nodosum, erythema induratum, panniculitis, and fibrositis. Lymphangitis and deep thrombophlebitis must also be considered.

Treatment

For focal, spontaneous thrombophlebitis not near the saphenofemoral junction, local heat and NSAIDs are usually effective in limiting the process. Prophylactic dose fondaparinux or rivaroxaban is recommended for ≥ 5 cm superficial thrombophlebitis of the great saphenous vein that is above the knee and > 3 cm from the saphenofemoral junction (see Table 16–14) and full anticoagulation is reserved for disease that is rapidly progressing or if there is concern for extension into the deep system (closer than 3 cm from the saphenofemoral junction) (see Table 16–16). Active malignancy, a history of VTE, and known thrombophilia are also indications for full dose anticoagulation. The usual course of treatment of superficial thrombophlebitis is 6 weeks. When the lower extremity superficial thrombosis is < 5 cm but the patient has risk factors such as hospitalization, immobilization, or recent surgery, prophylactic dose anticoagulation may be deferred unless there is extension of the thrombus on repeat ultrasonography 7–10 days later. If the induration is extensive or is progressing toward the saphenofemoral junction (leg) or cephalo-axillary junction (arm) despite anticoagulation, ligation and division of the vein at the junction of the deep and superficial veins is indicated. If venous reflux persists after the inflammation has resolved, ablation should be considered.

Septic superficial thrombophlebitis is an intravascular infection or abscess and requires urgent treatment with heparin or fondaparinux to limit further thrombus formation (see Table 16–16), and removal of the offending catheter in catheter-related infections (see Chapter 34). Treat with antibiotics (eg, vancomycin, 15 mg/kg intravenously every 12 hours, plus ceftriaxone, 1 g intravenously every 24 hours). If blood cultures are positive, therapy should be continued for 7–10 days or for 4–6 weeks if complicating endocarditis cannot be excluded. Surgical excision of the involved vein may be necessary to control the infection.

Prognosis

With spontaneous thrombophlebitis, the course is generally benign and brief. In patients with phlebitis secondary to varicose veins, recurrent episodes are likely unless correction of the underlying venous reflux and excision of varicosities is done. In contrast, the mortality from septic thrombophlebitis is ≥ 20% and requires aggressive treatment. However, if the involvement is localized, the mortality is low and prognosis is excellent with early treatment.

Piazza G et al. Superficial vein thrombosis: a review. JAMA. 2025;334:2020. [PMID: 40952730]

CHRONIC VENOUS INSUFFICIENCY

ESSENTIALS OF DIAGNOSIS

- History of prior DVT or leg injury.
- Edema, (brawny) skin hyperpigmentation, subcutaneous lipodermatosclerosis in the lower leg.
- Venous ulcers: large ulcerations at or above the medial ankle.

General Considerations

Chronic venous insufficiency is a severe manifestation of venous hypertension. One of the most common etiologies is prior deep venous thrombophlebitis, although about 25% of patients do not have a known history of DVT. In these cases, there may be a history of leg trauma or surgery; obesity is often a complicating factor. Progressive superficial venous reflux is also a common cause. Other causes include congenital or neoplastic obstruction of the pelvic veins or a congenital or acquired arteriovenous fistula.

The basic pathology is vein valve leaflets that do not coapt because they are either thickened and scarred (postthrombotic syndrome) or in a dilated vein and are therefore functionally inadequate. With the valves unable to stop venous blood from returning to the foot (venous reflux), the leg develops venous hypertension and an abnormally high hydrostatic force is transmitted to the subcutaneous veins and tissues of the lower leg. The resulting edema leads to dramatic and deleterious secondary changes. The stigmata of chronic venous insufficiency include sclerosis due to fibrosis of the subcutaneous tissue and skin, pigmentation of skin (hemosiderin taken up by the dermal macrophages) and, later, ulceration, which is extremely slow to heal. Itching may precipitate the formation of ulceration or local wound cellulitis. Dilation of the superficial veins may occur, leading to varicosities. Although surgical treatment for venous reflux can improve symptoms, controlling edema and the secondary skin changes usually require lifelong compression therapy.

Clinical Findings

A. Symptoms and Signs

Progressive pitting edema of the leg (particularly the lower leg) is the primary presenting symptom, often with a dull discomfort made worse by periods of standing. Dermatitis, often pruritic, commonly occurs. Secondary changes in the skin and subcutaneous tissues develop over time. The skin at the ankle is usually shiny and taut from swelling. A brownish pigmentation (hemosiderin) often develops (venous stasis dermatitis). If the condition is longstanding, the subcutaneous tissues become thick and sclerotic (lipodermatosclerosis).

1. Ulceration—Venous insufficiency (venous stasis) ulcers may develop, usually just above the ankle on the medial or anterior aspect of the leg and are generally painful. The typical ulcer has a clean base with fibrinous exudate and may have copious serous drainage (Figure 14–2).

Healing results in a thin scar on a fibrotic base that often breaks down with minor trauma or further bouts of leg swelling. Varicosities may appear that are associated with incompetent perforating veins.

2. Cellulitis—Blanching erythema with pain may help distinguish cellulitis that occurs with venous insufficiency from hemosiderin pigmentation (Figure 14–3). The diagnosis of cellulitis in the setting of a venous insufficiency ulcer can be difficult. Surface cultures are of limited value. Cellulitis should be considered when there is expanding warmth and erythema surrounding the ulceration with or without increasing pain of the ulceration.

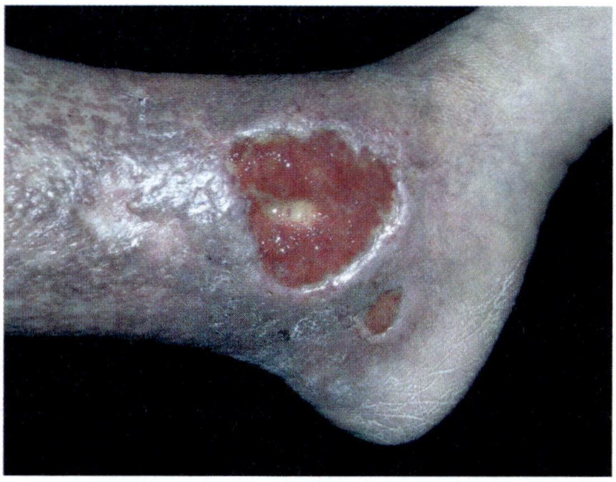

Figure 14–2. Ulcer—venous stasis ulcer. (Reproduced, with permission, from Richard P. Usatine, MD, in Usatine RP, Smith MA, Mayeaux EJ Jr, Chumley H. *The Color Atlas of Family Medicine*, 3rd ed. McGraw-Hill, 2019.)

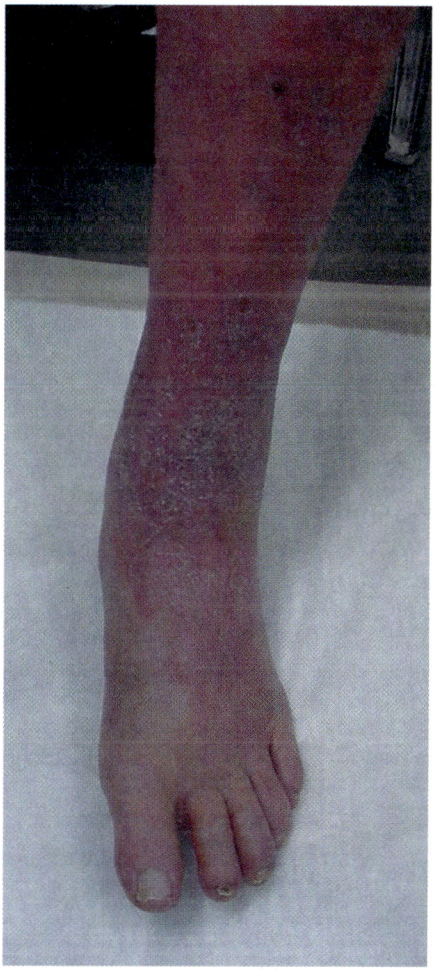

Figure 14–3. Cellulitis in an older man with venous stasis dermatitis. (Used, with permission, from Richard P. Usatine, MD, in Usatine RP, Smith MA, Mayeaux EJ Jr, Chumley HS. *The Color Atlas of Family Medicine*, 3rd ed. McGraw-Hill, 2019.)

B. Imaging

Patients with post-thrombotic syndrome or signs of chronic venous insufficiency should undergo duplex ultrasonography to determine whether superficial reflux is present and to evaluate the degree of deep reflux and obstruction. Evaluation for coexisting arterial insufficiency with an ankle-brachial index is recommended for older patients and for venous ulcers.

Differential Diagnosis

Patients with HF, CKD, or decompensated liver disease may have bilateral edema of the lower extremities. Many medications can cause edema (eg, calcium channel blockers, NSAIDs, thiazolidinediones). Swelling from lymphedema involves the feet and may be unilateral, but varicosities are absent. Edema from these causes pit easily and brawny discoloration is rare. Lipedema is a disorder of adipose tissue that occurs almost exclusively in women, is bilateral and symmetric, and is characterized by stopping at a distinct line just above the ankles.

Primary varicose veins may be difficult to differentiate from the secondary varicosities of post-thrombotic syndrome or venous obstruction.

Other conditions associated with chronic ulcers of the leg include diabetic neuropathic ulcers, arterial insufficiency (often manifests as painful *lateral* ankle ulcers with absent pulses; conversely, *medial* ankle ulcers are usually due to venous insufficiency), autoimmune diseases (eg, vasculitis, Felty syndrome), sickle cell anemia, erythema induratum (bilateral and usually on the posterior aspect of the lower part of the leg), pyoderma gangrenosum, and fungal infections. Other diagnoses should be considered for ulcers that appear on the feet, on the toes, or above the knees. When the diagnosis is uncertain, a punch biopsy from the border (not base) of the lesion may be helpful.

Prevention

Irreversible tissue changes and associated complications in the lower legs can be reduced through early and aggressive anticoagulation of acute DVT to minimize the valve damages. If edema develops from venous insufficiency, compression stockings are the most important means of prevention of complications (see below). Treatment of acute iliofemoral DVT with catheter-directed thrombolysis or mechanical thrombectomy does not reduce post-thrombotic syndrome and chronic venous insufficiency.

Treatment

A. General Measures

Fitted, graduated compression stockings (≥ 20–30 mm Hg pressure) worn from the foot to just below the knee during the day and evening are the mainstays of treatment and are usually sufficient, but they should not be used with arterial insufficiency and an ABI < 0.7. When compression stockings are insufficient, avoidance of long periods of sitting or standing, intermittent elevations of the involved leg, and sleeping with the legs kept above the level of the heart, may be necessary to control the swelling. Pneumatic compression of the leg, which can pump the fluid out of the leg, is used in refractory cases but many patients have severe pain with the "milking" action of the pump device.

B. Cellulitis

Oral antibiotics are recommended when cellulitis is present. Cephalexin, 500 mg three times daily, or clindamycin, 300 mg three times daily, for 1 week is usually adequate.

C. Ulceration

As the primary pathology is edema and venous hypertension, healing of the ulcer will not occur until the edema is controlled and compression is applied. Circumferential nonelastic bandages on the lower leg enhance the pumping action of the calf muscles on venous blood flow out of the calf. A lesion can often be treated on an ambulatory basis by means of a semi-rigid gauze boot made with Unna paste (Gelocast, Medicopaste) or a multilayer compression dressing (eg, Profore). Initially, the ulcer needs to be debrided and the boot changed every 2–3 days to control ulcer drainage. As the edema and drainage subside, the boot is changed every 5–7 days until the ulcer heals. The ulcer, tendons, and bony prominences must be adequately padded. Alternatively, knee-high graduated compression stockings with an absorbent dressing may be used, if wound drainage is minimal.

Pentoxifylline, 400 mg orally three times daily administered with compression dressings, is beneficial in accelerating healing of venous insufficiency leg ulcers. There is little evidence to support the use of topical antibiotics. If cellulitis accompanies the ulcer, oral antibiotics are recommended (see B. Cellulitis, above). Some patients will require hospital admission for complete bed rest and leg elevation to achieve ulcer healing. The ulcer should begin to heal within weeks, and healing should be complete within 4–6 months. Failure of the ulcer to heal or persistent drainage should prompt reevaluation for arterial insufficiency, underlying osteomyelitis, or nonvenous etiologies. After the ulcer has healed, daily graduated compression stocking therapy is mandatory to prevent ulcer recurrence.

D. Vein Treatment (Reflux or Obstruction)

Treatment of superficial vein reflux (see Varicose Veins, above) has been shown to decrease the recurrence rate of venous ulcers. Where there is substantial obstruction of the femoral or popliteal deep venous system, superficial varicosities supply the venous return and should not be removed.

Venous stents as treatment of chronic iliac deep vein stenosis or obstruction may improve venous ulcer healing and reduce the ulcer recurrence rate in severe cases.

Prognosis

Edema often recurs, particularly if support stockings that have at least 20–30 mm Hg compression are not worn consistently. Failure of venous insufficiency ulcerations to heal is most often due to inconsistent use of first-line treatment methods. Ongoing control of edema is essential to prevent recurrent ulceration; the use of compression stockings following ulcer healing is critical, with recurrence rates 2–20 times higher if compression stockings are not used.

When to Refer

- Patients with significant saphenous reflux should be evaluated for ablation.
- Patients with ulcers should be monitored by an interdisciplinary wound care team so that these challenging wounds receive aggressive care.

Ozsvath K. Delayed diagnosis of chronic venous insufficiency in patients with a darker complexion. J Vasc Surg Venous Lymphat Disord. 2023;11:895. [PMID: 37591600]

Raffetto JD et al. Why venous leg ulcers have difficulty healing: overview on pathophysiology, clinical consequences, and treatment. J Clin Med. 2020;10:29. [PMID: 33374372]

Wasan S. Chronic venous insufficiency evaluation and medical management. Curr Cardiol Rep. 2024;26:1241. [PMID: 39215951]

SUPERIOR VENA CAVAL OBSTRUCTION

ESSENTIALS OF DIAGNOSIS

- Swelling of the neck, face, and upper extremities.
- Dilated veins over the upper chest and neck.

General Considerations

Partial or complete obstruction of the superior vena cava is a relatively rare condition that is usually secondary to neoplastic or inflammatory processes in the superior mediastinum. The most frequent causes are (1) neoplasms, such as carcinoma of the lung with direct extension (> 80%), lymphomas, or primary malignant mediastinal tumors; (2) chronic fibrotic mediastinitis, either of unknown origin or secondary to tuberculosis, histoplasmosis, pyogenic infections, or drugs (especially methysergide); (3) DVT, often by extension of the process from the axillary or subclavian vein into the innominate vein and vena cava associated with catheterization of these veins for dialysis or for hyperalimentation; (4) aneurysm of the aortic arch; and (5) constrictive pericarditis.

Clinical Findings

A. Symptoms and Signs

The onset of symptoms is acute or subacute. Symptoms include swelling of the neck and face and upper extremities. Symptoms are often perceived as congestion and present as headache, dizziness, visual disturbances, stupor, syncope, or cough. There is progressive obstruction of the venous drainage of the head, neck, and upper extremities. The cutaneous veins of the upper chest and lower neck become dilated, and flushing of the face and neck develops. Brawny edema of the face, neck, and arms occurs later, and cyanosis of these areas then appears. Cerebral and laryngeal edema ultimately result in impaired function of the brain as well as respiratory insufficiency. Bending over or lying down accentuates the symptoms; sitting quietly is generally preferred. The manifestations are more severe if the obstruction develops rapidly and if the azygos junction or the vena cava between that vein and the heart is obstructed.

B. Laboratory Findings

The venous pressure is elevated (often > 20 cm of water) in the arm and is normal in the leg. Since lung cancer is a common cause, bronchoscopy is often performed; transbronchial biopsy, however, is relatively contraindicated because of venous hypertension and the risk of bleeding.

C. Imaging

CXR and CT scan can define the location and often the nature of the obstructive process, and contrast venography or magnetic resonance venography will map out the extent and degree of the venous obstruction and the collateral circulation. Brachial venography or radionuclide scanning following intravenous injection of technetium (Tc-99m) pertechnetate demonstrates a block to the flow of contrast material into the right heart and enlarged collateral veins. These techniques also allow estimation of blood flow around the occlusion as well as serial evaluation of the response to therapy.

Treatment

Conservative measures, such as elevation of the head of the bed and lifestyle modification to avoid bending over, are useful. Balloon angioplasty of the obstructed caval segment combined with stent placement provides prompt relief of symptoms and is the procedure of choice for all etiologies. Occasionally, anticoagulation is needed, while thrombolysis is rarely needed.

Urgent treatment for neoplasm consists of (1) cautious use of intravenous diuretics and (2) mediastinal irradiation, starting within 24 hours, with a treatment plan designed to give a high daily dose of radiation but a short total course of therapy to rapidly shrink the local tumor. Intensive radiation therapy combined with chemotherapy will palliate the process in up to 90% of patients. In patients with a subacute presentation, radiation therapy alone usually suffices; chemotherapy is added if lymphoma or small-cell carcinoma is diagnosed.

Urgent treatment for acute central airway obstruction or cerebral edema with endovascular angioplasty/stenting and thrombolysis may be indicated. In cases where the thrombosis is secondary to an indwelling catheter, thrombolysis may be attempted. Clinical judgment is required since a long-standing clot may be fibrotic and the risk of bleeding can outweigh the potential benefit. Long-term outcomes are complicated by the risk of re-occlusion from either thrombosis or neoplasm growth. Surgical procedures to bypass the obstruction are complicated by bleeding from high venous pressure.

Prognosis

The prognosis depends on the nature and degree of obstruction and its speed of onset. Slowly developing forms secondary to fibrosis may be tolerated for years. A high degree of obstruction of rapid onset secondary to cancer is often fatal in a few days or weeks because of increased intracranial pressure and cerebral hemorrhage, but treatment of the tumor with radiation and chemotherapeutic drugs may result in significant palliation. Balloon angioplasty and stenting provide good relief but may require re-treatment for recurrent symptoms due to thrombosis or restenosis.

When to Refer

- Any patient with progressive head and neck swelling should be referred to a vascular specialist to rule out superior vena cava syndrome.

When to Admit

- Any patient with acute edema of the head and neck or with signs and symptoms of airway compromise, such as hoarseness or stridor, should be admitted.

Azizi AH et al. Superior vena cava syndrome. JACC Cardiovasc Interv. 2020;13:2896. [PMID: 33357528]
Chow R et al. Management of malignant superior vena cava syndrome. Ann Palliat Med. 2024;13:620. [PMID: 38600814]

DISEASES OF THE LYMPHATIC CHANNELS

LYMPHANGITIS & LYMPHADENITIS

ESSENTIALS OF DIAGNOSIS

- Red streak from wound or cellulitis toward regional lymph nodes, which are usually enlarged and tender.
- Chills, fever, and malaise may be present.

General Considerations

Lymphangitis and lymphadenitis are common manifestations of a bacterial infection that is usually caused by hemolytic streptococci or *S aureus* (or by both organisms) and becomes invasive, generally from an infected wound, cellulitis, or an abscess. The wound may be very small or superficial, or an established abscess may be present, feeding bacteria into the lymphatics. The involvement of the lymphatics is often manifested by a red streak in the skin extending in the direction of the regional lymph nodes.

Clinical Findings

A. Symptoms and Signs

Throbbing pain is usually present at the site of bacterial invasion from a wound, cellulitis, or abscess. Malaise, sweating, chills, and fever of 38–40°C develop quickly, often with a rapid pulse. The red streak, when present, may be definite or may be faint and easily missed, especially in dark-skinned patients (Figure 14–4). The involved regional lymph nodes may be significantly enlarged and are usually tender. The infection may progress rapidly, often in a matter of hours, and may lead to septicemia and death.

B. Laboratory Findings

Leukocytosis with a left shift is usually present. Blood cultures may be positive, most often for staphylococcal or streptococcal species. Culture and sensitivity studies of the wound exudate or pus may be helpful in treatment of the more severe or refractory infections but are often difficult to interpret because of skin contaminants.

Differential Diagnosis

The erythema and induration of superficial thrombophlebitis are localized in and around the thrombosed vein. Venous thrombosis is not associated with lymphadenitis, and an entrance wound with secondary cellulitis is generally absent.

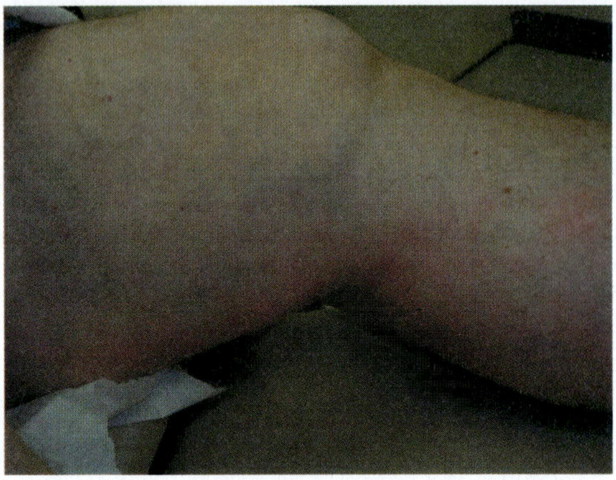

Figure 14–4. Ascending lymphangitis characterized by lymphatic streaking up the leg in a 55-year-old man with cellulitis. (Used, with permission, from Richard P. Usatine, MD, in Usatine RP, Smith MA, Mayeaux EJ Jr, Chumley HS. *The Color Atlas of Family Medicine*, 3rd ed. McGraw-Hill, 2019.)

Cat-scratch fever *(Bartonella henselae)* is a cause of lymphadenitis; the nodes, though often very large, are relatively nontender. Exposure to cats is common, but the patient may have forgotten about the scratch.

It is extremely important to differentiate cellulitis as the origin of lymphangitis from acute streptococcal hemolytic gangrene or a necrotizing soft tissue infection. These are deeper infections that may be extensive and are potentially lethal. Patients are more seriously ill; there may be redness due to leakage of red cells, creating a non-blanching erythema; subcutaneous crepitus, a late finding, may be palpated or auscultated; and subcutaneous air may be present on radiography or CT scan. Immediate surgical consultation is needed for wide debridement of all involved deep tissues if a necrotizing infection is suspected.

Treatment

A. General Measures

Prompt treatment should include heat (hot, moist compresses or heating pad), elevation when feasible, and immobilization of the infected area. Analgesics may be prescribed for pain.

B. Specific Measures

Empiric antibiotic therapy for hemolytic streptococci or *S aureus* (or both organisms) should always be instituted. Cephalosporins or extended-spectrum penicillins are commonly used (eg, cephalexin, 0.5 g orally four times daily for 7–10 days; see Table 34–6). Trimethoprim-sulfamethoxazole (two double-strength tablets orally twice daily for 7–10 days) should be considered when there is concern that the pathogen is MRSA (see Tables 34–5 and 34–6). Vancomycin, 15 mg/kg intravenously every 12 hours, is used for patients with signs of a systemic inflammatory response.

C. Wound Care

Any wound that is the initiating site of lymphangitis should be treated aggressively. Any necrotic tissue must be debrided and loculated pus drained.

Prognosis

With proper therapy including an antibiotic effective against the invading bacteria, control of the infection can usually be achieved in a few days. Delayed or inadequate therapy can lead to overwhelming infection with septicemia.

When to Admit

- Infections causing lymphangitis should be treated in the hospital with intravenous antibiotics.
- Debridement may be required and prompt surgical consultation is prudent.

LYMPHEDEMA

ESSENTIALS OF DIAGNOSIS

- Painless persistent edema of one or both lower extremities, primarily in young women.
- Pitting edema without ulceration, varicosities, or stasis pigmentation.
- Lymphangitis and cellulitis may occur.

General Considerations

The **primary form** of lymphedema is caused by congenital hypo- or hyperplastic proximal or distal lymphatics. The obstruction may be in the pelvic or lumbar lymph channels and nodes when the disease is extensive and progressive. The **secondary form** of lymphedema involves inflammatory or mechanical lymphatic obstruction from trauma, regional lymph node resection or irradiation, or extensive involvement of regional nodes by malignant disease or filariasis. Lymphedema may occur following surgical removal of the lymph nodes in the groin or axillae. Episodes of acute and chronic inflammation may be superimposed, with further stasis and secondary fibrosis.

Clinical Findings

Hypertrophy of the limb results, with markedly thickened and fibrotic skin and subcutaneous tissue in very advanced cases.

T_2-weighted MRI has been used to identify lymphatics and proximal obstructing masses. Lymphangiography and radioactive isotope studies may identify focal defects in lymph flow but are of little value in planning therapy.

Treatment

There is no effective cure for lymphedema; treatment strategies can control the lymphedema and allow normal function. Most patients can be treated with some of the following measures: (1) Aid the flow of lymph out of the extremity through intermittent elevation, especially during the sleeping hours (foot of bed elevated 15–20 degrees, achieved by placing pillows beneath the mattress); constant use of graduated elastic compression stockings; and massage toward the trunk—either by hand or by means of pneumatic pressure devices designed to milk edema out of an extremity. Wound care centers specializing in the care of patients with lymphedema may be helpful. (2) Avoid secondary infection by means of good hygiene and treatment of any trichophytosis of the toes. Once an infection starts, it should be treated by periods of elevation and antibiotic therapy that covers *Staphylococcus* and *Streptococcus* organisms (see Table 34–6). Infections can be a serious and recurring problem and are often difficult to control. Prophylactic antibiotics have not been shown to be of benefit. (3) Intermittent courses of diuretic therapy, especially in those with premenstrual or seasonal exacerbations, are rarely helpful. (4) Amputation is used only for the rare complication of lymphangiosarcoma in the extremity.

Conservative management is the primary approach to the treatment of lymphedema. Surgical management may be indicated to restore lymphatic flow using lymphatic bypass techniques or to perform reductive procedures to remove the lymphedematous fibrotic tissue.

Prognosis

With aggressive treatment, including pneumatic compression devices, good relief of symptoms can be achieved. The long-term outlook is dictated by the associated conditions and avoidance of recurrent cellulitis.

Chen K et al. Surgical management of postmastectomy lymphedema and review of the literature. Ann Plast Surg. 2021;86:S173. [PMID: 33346539]

Manrique OJ et al. Overview of lymphedema for physicians and other clinicians: a review of fundamental concepts. Mayo Clin Proc. 2022;97:1920. [PMID: 32829905]

SHOCK

ESSENTIALS OF DIAGNOSIS

- Hypotension, tachycardia, oliguria, altered mental status.
- Peripheral hypoperfusion and impaired oxygen delivery.
- Four classifications: hypovolemic, cardiogenic, obstructive, or distributive.

General Considerations

Shock occurs when the rate of arterial blood flow is inadequate to meet tissue metabolic needs. This results in regional hypoxia and subsequent lactic acidosis from anaerobic metabolism in peripheral tissues as well as eventual end-organ damage and failure.

Classification

Table 14–1 outlines common causes and mechanisms associated with each type of shock.

A. Hypovolemic Shock

Hypovolemic shock results from decreased intravascular volume due to loss of blood or fluids and electrolytes. The etiology may be suggested by the clinical setting (eg, trauma) or by signs and symptoms of blood loss (eg, GI bleeding) or dehydration (eg, vomiting or diarrhea). Compensatory vasoconstriction may transiently maintain the blood pressure but unreplaced losses of > 15% of the intravascular volume can result in hypotension and progressive tissue hypoxia.

Table 14–1. Classification of shock by mechanism and common causes.

Hypovolemic shock			
	Blood loss		
		Traumatic hemorrhage	
			Exsanguination
			Hemothorax
			Hemoperitoneum
			Fracture (femur and pelvis)
		Nontraumatic hemorrhage	
			GI bleed
			AAA rupture
			Ectopic pregnancy rupture
	Volume loss		
		Burns	
		Skin integrity loss (toxic epidermal necrolysis)	
		Vomiting	
		Diarrhea	
		Hyperosmolar states (eg, hyperosmolar hyperglycemic state)	
		Third spacing (eg, ascites, pancreatitis)	
		Decreased intake	
Cardiogenic shock			
	Myocardial disease		
		Left or right ventricular infarction	
		Dilated cardiomyopathy	
	Mechanical		
		Valvular	
			Aortic regurgitation from dissection
			Papillary muscle rupture from ischemia
			Acute valvular rupture from abscess
		Ventricular aneurysm rupture	
		Ventricular septum rupture	
		Ventricular free wall rupture	
	Dysrhythmia		
		Bradycardias and blocks	
		Tachycardias	
Obstructive shock			
	Pericardial disease		
		Pericardial tamponade	
		Constrictive pericarditis	
	Tension pneumothorax		
	High-risk (massive) PE		
	Severe pulmonary hypertension		
	Auto PEEP from mechanical ventilation		
Distributive (vasodilatory) shock			
	Septic shock		
	Anaphylactic shock		
	Neurogenic shock		
	Drug-induced vasodilation		
	Adrenal insufficiency		

Reproduced with permission from Stone CK, Humphries RL (editors). *Current Emergency Diagnosis & Treatment*, 7th ed. NY: McGraw-Hill, 2011.
PEEP, positive end expiratory pressure.

B. Cardiogenic Shock

Cardiogenic shock results from failure of the heart to pump enough blood to maintain adequate tissue perfusion. The clinical definition of cardiogenic shock is evidence of tissue hypoxia from decreased cardiac output (cardiac index $\leq$ 2.2 L/min/m^2) in the presence of adequate intravascular volume. This is most often caused by MI but can also be due to cardiomyopathy, myocardial contusion, valvular incompetence or stenosis, or arrhythmias. See Chapters 10, 11, and 12.

C. Obstructive Shock

Pericardial tamponade, tension pneumothorax, and massive PE can acutely decrease cardiac output, resulting in shock. These are medical emergencies requiring prompt diagnosis and treatment.

D. Distributive Shock

Distributive or vasodilatory shock has many causes including sepsis, anaphylaxis, traumatic spinal cord injury, or acute adrenal insufficiency. The reduction in systemic vascular resistance (SVR) results in inadequate cardiac output and tissue hypoperfusion despite normal circulatory volume.

1. Septic shock—Sepsis is the most common cause of distributive shock and carries a mortality rate of 20–50%. The Society of Critical Care Medicine and the European Society of Intensive Care Medicine's 2016 definition for **sepsis** is life-threatening organ dysfunction caused by a dysregulated host response to infection from any organism (bacterial, viral, or fungal). **Septic shock** is clinically defined as sepsis with fluid-unresponsive hypotension (systolic blood pressure < 100 mm Hg), serum lactate level > 2 mmol/L, and a need for vasopressors to keep mean arterial pressure (MAP) > 65 mm Hg. The most common cause of septic shock in hospitalized patients is bacterial infection from pneumonia and intra-abdominal infection. Sepsis from multidrug resistant and fungal organisms is increasing but remain less than that for bacterial infections. Risk factors for septic shock include bacteremia, extremes of age, diabetes mellitus, cancer, immunosuppression, and history of a recent invasive procedure.

CLINICAL TOOLS TO IDENTIFY SEPSIS AND SEPTIC SHOCK—Multiple tools exist to screen for sepsis. The Third International Consensus Definitions for Sepsis and Septic Shock (SEPSIS-3) recommend using the Sequential Organ Failure Assessment (SOFA) score to define sepsis (https://en.wikipedia.org/wiki/SOFA_score); an increase of $\geq$ 2 SOFA score points in a patient with infection is diagnostic of sepsis with a predicted 10% mortality.

Systemic inflammatory response syndrome (SIRS) criteria is another screening tool. SIRS is defined as a systemic response to a nonspecific infectious or noninfectious insult resulting in at least two of the following findings: (1) body temperature > 38°C (100.4°F) or < 36°C (96.8°F), (2) heart rate > 90 beats per minute, (3) respiratory rate > 20 breaths per minute or hyperventilation with an arterial carbon dioxide tension ($Paco_2$) < 32 mm Hg, or (4) abnormal WBC count (> 12,000/mcL or < 4000/mcL or > 10% immature [band] forms). Vasodilatory shock from SIRS is often due to burns; pancreatitis; autoimmune disorders, such as vasculitis or inflammatory colitis; air or amniotic fluid embolus; ischemia; or trauma.

2. Anaphylactic shock—Anaphylactic shock is a life-threatening acute hypersensitivity reaction to an allergen, most often insect venom, food, or medication. Immediate identification and treatment with epinephrine and fluids can be lifesaving.

3. Neurogenic shock—Neurogenic shock is caused by traumatic spinal cord injury or effects of an epidural or spinal anesthetic. This results in loss of sympathetic tone with a reduction in SVR and hypotension without a compensatory tachycardia. Reflex vagal parasympathetic stimulation evoked by pain, gastric dilation, or fright may simulate neurogenic shock, producing hypotension, bradycardia, and syncope.

4. Endocrine shock—Endocrine shock can arise from hyper- or hypothyroidism or adrenal insufficiency (either primary adrenal crisis from Addison disease or secondary adrenal insufficiency [see Chapter 29]). Adrenal insufficiency most often occurs with abrupt cessation of long-term corticosteroid use, but it can also be precipitated by infection, trauma, surgery, or pituitary injury. In addition to hypotension, symptoms include weakness, nausea, abdominal pain, and confusion. Hypothyroidism can lead to myxedema coma, presenting with vasodilation and depressed cardiac output. Shock from hyperthyroidism most often produces high-output cardiac failure.

Clinical Findings

A. Symptoms and Signs

Hypotension is defined as a systolic blood pressure of ≤ 90 mm Hg or a MAP of < 60–65 mm Hg but must be evaluated relative to the patient's normal blood pressure. A drop in systolic pressure of > 10–20 mm Hg or an increase in pulse of > 15 beats per minute with positional change suggests depleted intravascular volume. Blood pressure may not be the best indicator of end-organ perfusion because compensatory mechanisms, such as increased heart rate, increased cardiac contractility, and vasoconstriction can prevent hypotension. Patients with hypotension often have cool or mottled extremities and weak or thready peripheral pulses. Splanchnic vasoconstriction may lead to oliguria, bowel ischemia, and liver dysfunction, which can ultimately result in multiorgan failure. Patients may become restless, agitated, confused, lethargic, or comatose as a result of inadequate perfusion of the brain.

Hypovolemic shock is evident when signs of hypoperfusion, such as oliguria, altered mental status, and cool extremities, are present. Jugular venous pressure is low, and there is a narrow pulse pressure indicative of reduced stroke volume. Rapid replacement of fluids can restore tissue perfusion.

Cardiogenic shock manifests by signs of global hypoperfusion with oliguria, altered mental status, and cool extremities. Jugular venous pressure is elevated and there may be evidence of pulmonary edema with respiratory compromise in the setting of left-sided HF. *A transthoracic echocardiogram (TTE) or a transesophageal echocardiogram (TEE) is an effective diagnostic tool to differentiate hypovolemic from cardiogenic shock.* In hypovolemic shock, the LV will be small because of decreased filling, but contractility is often preserved. In cardiogenic shock, there is a decrease in LV contractility. The LV may appear dilated and full because of its inability to eject a sufficient stroke volume.

Obstructive shock is suggested when the CVP is elevated but the TTE or TEE shows reduced LV filling, a pericardial effusion in the case of tamponade, thickened pericardium in the case of pericarditis, or RV dysfunction in the case of massive PE. Pericardiocentesis or pericardial window for pericardial tamponade, chest tube placement for tension pneumothorax, or catheter-directed thrombolytic therapy or mechanical thrombectomy for massive PE can be lifesaving in cases of obstructive shock.

Distributive shock signs include hyperdynamic heart sounds, warm extremities initially, and a wide pulse pressure indicative of large stroke volume. The echocardiogram may show a hyperdynamic LV. **Septic shock** is diagnosed when there is clinical evidence of infection in the setting of persistent hypotension and evidence of organ hypoperfusion, such as lactic acidosis, decreased urinary output, or altered mental status despite adequate volume resuscitation (see Clinical Tools to Identify Sepsis and Septic Shock, above). **Anaphylactic shock** typically presents with hives, edema of the lips, tongue, and throat, bronchospasm, and hypotension. **Neurogenic shock** is diagnosed when there is evidence of CNS injury and persistent hypotension despite adequate volume resuscitation. A history of long-term corticosteroid use or thyroid disease can increase the likelihood of **endocrine shock.**

B. Laboratory Findings and Imaging

Blood tests should include CBC, electrolytes, glucose, ABG determinations, coagulation parameters, and lactate levels. Based on clinical reasoning and initial laboratory test results, additional studies may include typing and cross-matching for concerns of bleeding, bacterial blood, urine, and sputum cultures, and nasal PCR swabs for respiratory pathogens including COVID-19, influenza, and RSV for concerns for sepsis. An ECG and CXR should be part of the initial assessment. Point-of-care ultrasonography can rapidly assess global cardiac function, presence of pericardial effusion, and intravascular volume status via inferior vena cava inspection in cases of undifferentiated hypotension. A TTE can more formally assess right- and left-sided filling pressures and cardiac output.

Treatment

A. General Measures

Initial management consists of basic life support with an assessment of the patient's circulation, airway, and breathing. This may entail airway intubation and mechanical ventilation. Mechanical ventilation along with sedation can decrease respiratory muscle oxygen demand, allowing improved oxygen delivery to hypoperfused tissues. Ventilatory failure should be anticipated in patients with severe metabolic acidosis due to shock. Intravenous access and fluid resuscitation should be instituted along with cardiac monitoring and assessment of hemodynamic parameters such as blood pressure and heart rate. Cardiac monitoring can detect myocardial ischemia or malignant arrhythmias, which can be treated by standard advanced cardiac life support (ACLS) protocols (https://hospitalhandbook.ucsf.edu/content/20-advanced-cardiac-life-support).

Unresponsive or minimally responsive patients should have their glucose levels checked immediately, and if low, 1 ampule of 50% dextrose should be given intravenously; if the glucose level is normal and the Glasgow Coma Score (GCS) is < 8, they should undergo intubation for airway protection. An arterial line should be placed for continuous blood pressure measurement, and an indwelling urinary catheter should be inserted to monitor urinary output.

B. Hemodynamic Measurements

Early consideration is given to placement of a central venous catheter (CVC) (also known as a central line) for infusion of fluids and medications and for hemodynamic measurements. A CVC can provide measurements of the CVP and the central venous oxygen saturation ($ScvO_2$), both of which can be used to manage septic and cardiogenic shock. Pulmonary artery catheters (PACs) allow measurement of the pulmonary artery pressure, left-sided filling pressure or the pulmonary capillary wedge pressure (PCWP), the mixed venous oxygen saturation (SvO_2), and cardiac output. Studies suggest that PACs do not increase overall mortality or length of hospital stay but are associated with higher use of inotropes and intravenous vasodilators in select groups of critically ill patients. The attendant risks associated with PACs (infection, arrhythmias, vein thrombosis, and pulmonary artery rupture) can be as high as 4–9%; thus, the routine use of PACs is not recommended. However, in complex situations, PACs may be useful in distinguishing between cardiogenic and septic shock, so their use must be carefully weighed for each patient. TTE is a noninvasive alternative to the PAC. TTE can measure cardiac function and cardiac output. The $ScvO_2$, obtained through the CVC, can be used as a surrogate for the SvO_2. Pulse pressure variation, as determined by arterial line waveform analysis or stroke volume variation, is useful as dynamic measures of fluid responsiveness in volume resuscitation, but these measurements have only been validated in patients who are mechanically ventilated with tidal volumes of 8 mL/kg, not triggering the ventilator, and in normal sinus rhythm. Point-of-care ultrasound measurements of the inferior vena cava (IVC) can suggest intravascular volume status and guide fluid replacement. The IVC diameter is ~ 2.1 cm in adults and typically does not dilate unless the patient is receiving positive pressure ventilation. If the patient is mechanically ventilated and the IVC does not dilate with inspiration, the patient is likely fluid replete. If the IVC dilates to > 2.5 cm while on mechanical ventilation, the patient is likely to respond to fluid repletion. If the patient is spontaneously breathing, they may be fluid-responsive if their IVC is < 2 cm in diameter and collapses by > 50% with each inspiration.

A CVP < 5 mm Hg suggests hypovolemia and > 18 mm Hg suggests volume overload, cardiac failure, tamponade, or pulmonary hypertension. A cardiac index lower than 2 $L/min/m^2$ indicates a need for inotropic support. A cardiac index > 4 $L/min/m^2$ in a hypotensive patient is consistent with early septic shock. The SVR is low (< 800 dynes · s/cm^{-5}) in sepsis and neurogenic and anaphylactic shock; SVR is high (> 1500 dynes · s/cm^{-5}) in hypovolemic and cardiogenic shock. Treatment is directed at maintaining a CVP of 8–12 mm Hg, a MAP of ≥ 65 mm Hg, a cardiac index of 2–4 $L/min/m^2$, and a $ScvO_2$ > 70%.

C. Volume Replacement

Volume replacement is critical in the initial management of shock.

Hemorrhagic shock is treated with immediate efforts to achieve hemostasis and rapid infusions of blood substitutes, such as type-specific or type O negative packed RBCs (PRBCs) or whole blood, which provides extra volume and clotting factors. Each unit of PRBCs or whole blood raises the hematocrit by 3%.

Hypovolemic shock secondary to dehydration is managed with rapid boluses of isotonic crystalloid solutions, usually in 1-L increments.

Cardiogenic shock in the absence of fluid overload requires smaller boluses of crystalloid fluid challenges, usually in increments of 250 mL.

Septic shock usually requires larger volumes of fluid for resuscitation (typically 30 mL/kg) as the associated capillary leak releases fluid into the extravascular space. Typically, 2–3 L of crystalloid solutions are administered, but less should be given in patients with HF or CKD. *Caution must be used in cases of large-volume resuscitation with unwarmed fluids because this can produce hypothermia, which can lead to hypothermia-induced coagulopathy.* Warming of fluids before administration can avoid this complication.

Choice of resuscitation fluid—Recent studies have demonstrated no difference in incidence of death or hospital readmission within 90 days for patients receiving balanced (lactated Ringer solution or Plasma-Lyte) or unbalanced (0.9% saline) crystalloid solutions. Comparisons of 0.9% saline and colloid (albumin) solutions in critically ill patients found no difference in outcome except in patients with traumatic brain injury, where albumin resuscitation led to higher mortality. Regardless of fluid choice, prompt fluid resuscitation is crucial. If the patient does not respond to fluid resuscitation, early use of vasopressors should be considered.

D. Early Goal-Directed Therapy

Compensated shock can occur in the setting of normalized hemodynamic parameters with ongoing global tissue hypoxia. Traditional endpoints of resuscitation such as blood pressure, heart rate, urinary output, mental status, and skin perfusion can therefore be misleading. Following set protocols for the treatment of septic shock by adjusting the use of fluids, vasopressors, and inotropes to meet hemodynamic targets (MAP ≥ 65 mm Hg, CVP 8–12 mm Hg, $ScvO_2$ > 70%) is termed **early goal-directed therapy (EGDT).** Lactate clearance (a decline of lactate levels) of > 10% can be used as a substitute for $ScvO_2$ criteria if $ScvO_2$ monitoring is not available.

The 2021 Surviving Sepsis Campaign recommendations for patients with sepsis or septic shock are to measure lactate level; obtain blood cultures prior to administration of broad-spectrum antibiotics, *which should occur within 1 hour of sepsis diagnosis;* and administer 30 mL/kg crystalloid solution (0.9 normal saline, lactated Ringer solution, or Plasma-Lyte) for hypotension or lactate > 4 mmol/L within the first 3 hours of presentation. Smaller resuscitation volumes may be appropriate for patients with HF, cirrhosis, or advanced kidney disease. Vasopressors should be administered for hypotension not responsive to initial fluid resuscitation to maintain MAP at ≥ 65 mm Hg. Remeasure lactate if the initial level was high and reassess volume status and tissue perfusion frequently. A meta-analysis of hemodynamic optimization trials suggests that early treatment before the development of organ failure results in improved survival, and patients who respond well to initial efforts demonstrate a survival advantage over nonresponders.

E. Medications

1. Vasoactive therapy—Vasopressors and inotropic agents are administered only after adequate fluid resuscitation. Choice of vasoactive therapy depends on the presumed etiology of shock and cardiac output. If there is continued hypotension with high cardiac output after adequate volume resuscitation (as in septic shock), then vasopressor support is needed to improve vasomotor tone. If there is low cardiac output with high filling pressures, inotropic support is needed to improve contractility.

A. DISTRIBUTIVE (VASODILATORY) SHOCK—When increased vasoconstriction is required to maintain an adequate perfusion pressure, α-adrenergic catecholamine agonists (such as norepinephrine and phenylephrine) are generally used. Although norepinephrine is both an α-adrenergic and β-adrenergic agonist, it preferentially increases MAP over cardiac output. The initial dose is 1–2 mcg/min as an intravenous infusion, titrated to maintain MAP at ≥ 65 mm Hg. The usual maintenance dose is 2–4 mcg/min intravenously (maximum dose is 30 mcg/min). Patients with refractory shock may require dosages of 10–30 mcg/min intravenously. Epinephrine, also with both α- and β-adrenergic effects, may be used in severe shock and during acute resuscitation. It is the vasopressor of choice for anaphylactic shock. For severe shock, give epinephrine 1 mcg/min as a continuous intravenous infusion initially and titrate to hemodynamic response; the usual dosage range is 1–10 mcg/min intravenously. The preferred delivery of vasopressors is via a CVC, but peripheral access can be safely used up to 24 hours while awaiting central line placement.

There is no evidence documenting a survival benefit from, or the superiority of, a particular vasopressor in septic shock. Norepinephrine is the initial vasopressor of choice in septic shock to maintain the MAP at ≥ 65 mm Hg. Phenylephrine can be used for hyperdynamic septic shock if dysrhythmias or tachycardias prevent the use of agents with β-adrenergic activity.

Vasopressin (ADH) is often used as an *adjunctive therapy* to catecholamine vasopressors in the treatment of distributive shock. Vasopressin causes peripheral vasoconstriction via V1 receptors located on smooth muscle cells. Vasopressin also potentiates the effects of catecholamines on the vasculature and stimulates cortisol production. Intravenous infusion of vasopressin at a low dose (0.01–0.04 units/min) as a second agent to norepinephrine has been beneficial in patients with sepsis and hypotension refractory to fluid resuscitation and conventional catecholamine vasopressors. Higher doses of vasopressin decrease cardiac output and may put patients at greater risk for splanchnic and coronary artery ischemia. Studies do not favor the use of vasopressin as first-line therapy.

Angiotensin II, a component of the renin-angiotensin-aldosterone system axis, is a potent direct vasoconstrictor that acts on the arteries and veins to increase blood pressure. Angiotensin II (Giapreza) is an *additional agent* for vasodilatory shock that is refractory to catecholamines and vasopressin. The recommended starting dose is 20 ng/kg/min via continuous intravenous infusion through a CVC. It can be titrated every 5 minutes by increments of up to 15 ng/kg/min as needed to achieve MAP goals, but not to exceed 80 ng/kg/min during the first 3 hours of use. Maintenance doses should not exceed 40 ng/kg/min. Concurrent VTE prophylaxis is indicated as studies revealed a higher incidence of VTE with angiotensin II use.

B. CARDIOGENIC SHOCK—Given meta-analyses documenting decreased mortality, norepinephrine should be the first-line vasopressor for cardiogenic shock (see doses in Distributive (Vasodilatory) Shock, above). Dobutamine, a predominantly β-adrenergic agonist, increases contractility and decreases afterload. It is used for patients with low cardiac output and high PCWP but who do not have hypotension. Dobutamine can be added to a vasopressor if there is reduced myocardial function (decreased cardiac output and elevated PCWP), or if there are signs of hypoperfusion despite adequate volume resuscitation and an adequate MAP. The initial dose is 0.1–0.5 mcg/kg/min intravenous infusion, which can be titrated every few minutes to hemodynamic effect; the usual dosage range is 2–20 mcg/kg/min intravenously. Tachyphylaxis can occur after 48 hours from the downregulation of β-adrenergic receptors. Milrinone is a phosphodiesterase inhibitor that can be substituted for dobutamine. A 2021 study of patients with cardiogenic shock found no significant difference in mortality when comparing milrinone to dobutamine.

2. Antibiotics—Definitive therapy for septic shock includes early initiation of empiric broad-spectrum antibiotics (see Table 34–1) after appropriate cultures have been obtained and within 1 hour of recognition of septic shock. Imaging studies may prove useful to localize sources of infection. Surgical management may also be necessary if necrotic tissue or loculated infections are present in attempts to control the source of infection.

3. Corticosteroids—Corticosteroids are the treatment of choice in patients with shock secondary to adrenal insufficiency, defined as a cortisol response of ≤ 9 mcg/dL after one injection of 250 mcg of corticotropin. Studies supporting corticosteroid use in patients with shock from sepsis or other etiologies are mixed, but meta-analyses slightly favor their use. In a 2023 phase 3 multicenter RCT, patients hospitalized in the ICU with severe CAP treated with low-dose corticosteroids had reduced 28- and 90-day mortality compared to placebo. The 2018 APROCCHSS study demonstrated lower 90-day all-cause mortality for patients receiving hydrocortisone plus fludrocortisone for any etiology of septic shock. Subgroup analysis of the APROCCHSS trial in 2024 showed a significant reduction in 90-day mortality in patients with septic shock from community-acquired pneumonia (39% versus 51%) who were administered low-dose corticosteroids. A 2025 large systematic review and meta-analysis measured the efficacy of corticosteroids in the critically ill. This study analyzed 43 RCTs with > 10,000 patients and found that early initiation (within 72 hours of ICU admission) of low dose corticosteroids (≤ 400 mg/day hydrocortisone equivalent) for a prolonged period (> 7 days) reduced short term mortality by nearly 15% without increasing the incidence of secondary infections or GI bleeding. Hyperglycemia was higher in the corticosteroid group. Thus, for ICU patients with refractory septic shock, not responding to vasopressors, the recommended dosing is hydrocortisone 50 mg intravenously every 6 hours or 200 mg/day continuous intravenous infusion (10 mg/hour), plus fludrocortisone 50 mcg by mouth or nasogastric tube daily for 7 days or until vasopressors are no longer needed. Hydrocortisone can be tapered off over 2–3 days.

F. Other Treatment Modalities

Cardiac failure may require placement of an intra-arterial balloon pump, a microaxial flow pump (Impella), LV assist device, or institution of extracorporeal life support. Emergent revascularization by percutaneous angioplasty or coronary artery bypass surgery appears to improve long-term outcome with increased survival compared with initial medical stabilization for patients with myocardial ischemia leading to cardiogenic shock (see Chapter 10). Urgent renal replacement therapy may be indicated for maintenance of fluid and electrolyte balance during AKI resulting in shock from multiple modalities. Studies do not support the use of intravenous vitamin C, thiamine, methylene blue, or vitamin B_{12} as treatments for sepsis.

Bosch NA et al. Comparative effectiveness of fludrocortisone and hydrocortisone vs hydrocortisone alone among patients with septic shock. JAMA Intern Med. 2023;183:451. [PMID: 36972033]

Cao L et al. Efficacy and safety of corticosteroids in critically ill patients: a systematic review and meta-analysis. BMC Anesthesiol. 2025;25:319. [PMID: 40597594]

Dequin et al; CRICS-TriGGERSep Network. Hydrocortisone in severe community-acquired pneumonia. N Engl J Med. 2023;388:1931. [PMID: 36942789]

Evans L et al. Surviving sepsis campaign: international guidelines for management of sepsis and septic shock 2021. Intensive Care Med. 2021;47:1181. [PMID: 34599691]

Heming N et al. Hydrocortisone plus fludrocortisone for community acquired pneumonia-related septic shock: a subgroup analysis of the APROCCHSS phase 3 randomised trial; Lancet Respir Med. 2024;12:366. [PMID: 38310918]

McIntyre L et al; Canadian Critical Care Trials Group. A crossover trial of hospital-wide lactated ringer's solution versus normal saline. N Engl J Med. 2025;393:660. [PMID: 40503714]

Blood Disorders

15

Lloyd E. Damon, MD
Charalambos Babis Andreadis, MD, MSCE

ANEMIAS

General Approach to Anemias

Anemia is present in adults if the hematocrit is < 41% (hemoglobin < 13.6 g/dL [135 g/L]) in males or < 36% (hemoglobin < 12 g/dL [120 g/L]) in females. Congenital anemia is suggested by the patient's personal and family history. *The most common cause of anemia is iron deficiency.* Poor diet may result in folic acid deficiency and contribute to iron deficiency, but *bleeding is the most common cause of iron deficiency in adults.* Physical examination demonstrates pallor. Attention to physical signs of primary (mostly malignant) hematologic diseases (lymphadenopathy; hepatosplenomegaly; or bone tenderness, especially in the sternum or anterior tibia) is important. Mucosal changes such as a smooth tongue suggest megaloblastic anemia.

Anemias are classified according to their pathophysiologic basis, ie, whether related to diminished production (relative or absolute reticulocytopenia) or to increased production due to accelerated loss of RBCs (reticulocytosis) (Table 15–1), and according to RBC size (Table 15–2). **Reticulocytosis** occurs in one of three pathophysiologic states: acute blood loss, recent replacement of a missing erythropoietic nutrient, or reduced RBC survival (ie, hemolysis). A severely microcytic anemia (mean corpuscular volume [MCV] < 70 fL) is due either to iron deficiency or thalassemia, while a severely macrocytic anemia (MCV > 120 fL) is almost always due to either megaloblastic anemia or to cold agglutinins in blood analyzed at room temperature. A **bone marrow biopsy** is generally needed to complete the evaluation of anemia when the blood laboratory evaluation fails to reveal an etiology, when additional cytopenias are present, or when an underlying primary or secondary bone marrow process is suspected.

IRON DEFICIENCY ANEMIA

ESSENTIALS OF DIAGNOSIS

- Iron deficiency: serum ferritin is < 12 ng/mL (27 pmol/L) or < 30 ng/mL (67 pmol/L) if also anemic.
- Caused by bleeding in adults unless proven otherwise.
- Responds to iron therapy.

General Considerations

Iron deficiency is the most common cause of anemia worldwide. The causes are listed in Table 15–3. Aside from circulating RBCs, the major location of iron in the body is the storage pool as ferritin or hemosiderin in macrophages.

The average American diet contains 10–15 mg of iron per day. About 10% of this amount is absorbed in the stomach, duodenum, and upper jejunum under acidic conditions. Dietary iron present as heme is efficiently absorbed (10–20%) but nonheme iron less so (1–5%), mainly because of interference by phosphates, tannins, and other food constituents. The major iron transporter from the diet across the intestinal lumen is ferroportin, which also facilitates the transport of iron to apotransferrin in macrophages for delivery to erythroid progenitor cells in the bone marrow prepared to synthesize hemoglobin. Hepcidin, which is increasingly produced during inflammation, negatively regulates iron transport by promoting the degradation of ferroportin. Small amounts of iron—approximately 1 mg/day—are normally lost through exfoliation of skin and GI mucosal cells.

Menstrual blood loss plays a major role in iron metabolism. The average monthly menstrual blood loss is approximately 50 mL but may be five times greater in some individuals. People with heavy menstrual losses must absorb 3–4 mg of iron from the diet each day to maintain adequate iron stores, which is not commonly achieved. People with menorrhagia of this degree will almost always become iron-deficient without iron supplementation.

In general, iron metabolism is balanced between GI absorption and GI loss of 1 mg/day. Pregnancy and lactation upset the iron balance since requirements increase to 2–5 mg of iron per day. Normal dietary iron cannot supply these requirements, and *medicinal iron is needed during pregnancy and lactation.* Decreased iron absorption can also cause iron deficiency, as seen in people with celiac disease (gluten enteropathy) and is common after gastric resection or jejunal bypass surgery.

Table 15–1. Classification of anemia by RBC pathophysiology (in alphabetical order, within categories).

Decreased RBC production (relative or absolute reticulocytopenia)
Bone marrow infiltration: carcinoma, lymphoma, fibrosis, sarcoidosis, Gaucher disease, others
DNA synthesis lesion: megaloblastic anemia (vitamin B_{12} deficiency or folic acid deficiency), DNA synthesis inhibitor medications
Hematopoietic stem cell lesion: aplastic anemia (short telomere syndrome, others), leukemia
Hemoglobin synthesis lesion: iron deficiency, thalassemia, anemia of chronic disease (inflammation or various organ failure), hypoerythropoietinemia, lead toxicity
Immune-mediated inhibition: aplastic anemia, pure RBC aplasia
Increased RBC destruction or accelerated RBC loss (reticulocytosis)
Acute blood loss
Hemolysis (extrinsic)
Immune: warm antibody, cold antibody
Hemolysis (intrinsic)
Membrane lesion: hereditary spherocytosis, elliptocytosis
Hemoglobin lesion: sickle cell, thalassemia, unstable hemoglobin
Glycolysis lesion: pyruvate kinase deficiency
Oxidation lesion: glucose-6-phosphate dehydrogenase deficiency
Hypersplenism
Infection: *Clostridium perfringens*, malaria
Maldistribution of RBC
Hypersplenism
Microangiopathic: disseminated intravascular coagulation, thrombotic thrombocytopenic purpura, hemolytic-uremic syndrome, mechanical cardiac valve, paravalvular leak

Table 15–2. Classification of anemia by mean RBC volume (MCV) (in alphabetical order, within categories).

Microcytic
Anemia of chronic disease
Iron deficiency
Lead toxicity
Thalassemia
Zinc deficiency
Normocytic
Copper deficiency
Kidney disease
Mild form of most acquired microcytic or macrocytic etiologies of anemia
Non-thyroid endocrine gland failure
Macrocytic (megaloblastic)
DNA synthesis inhibitors
Folate deficiency
Vitamin B_{12} deficiency
Macrocytic (nonmegaloblastic)
Aplastic anemia
Bone marrow failure state (eg, pure RBC aplasia, marrow infiltrative disorder, etc)
Copper deficiency
Hemolysis
Hypothyroidism
Liver disease
Myelodysplasia
Reticulocytosis

Table 15–3. Causes of iron deficiency (in alphabetical order, within categories).

Blood loss (chronic)
Blood donation
GI
Hemoglobinuria
Menstruation
Decreased absorption
Autoimmune gastritis
Celiac disease
Helicobacter pylori gastritis
Hereditary iron-refractory iron deficiency anemia
Zinc deficiency
Deficient diet
Idiopathic
Increased iron requirements
Lactation
Pregnancy
Iron sequestration
Pulmonary hemosiderosis

The most important cause of iron deficiency anemia in adults is chronic blood loss. *Iron deficiency demands a search for a source of GI bleeding if other sites of blood loss (excess uterine bleeding, hematuria, and repeated blood donations) are excluded.* Prolonged aspirin or NSAID use may cause it without a documented structural lesion. Celiac disease, even when asymptomatic, can cause iron deficiency through poor absorption in the GI tract. Zinc deficiency is another cause of poor iron absorption. Chronic hemoglobinuria may lead to iron deficiency, but this is uncommon. Traumatic hemolysis due to a prosthetic cardiac valve and other causes of intravascular hemolysis (eg, paroxysmal nocturnal hemoglobinuria) should also be considered. The cause of iron deficiency is not found in up to 5% of cases.

Pure iron deficiency might prove refractory to oral iron replacement. Refractoriness is defined as a hemoglobin increment of < 1 g/dL (10 g/L) after 4–6 weeks of 100 mg/day of elemental oral iron. The differential diagnosis in these cases (Table 15–3) includes malabsorption from autoimmune gastritis, *Helicobacter pylori* gastric infection, celiac disease, and hereditary iron-refractory iron deficiency anemia.

Clinical Findings

A. Symptoms and Signs

The primary symptoms of iron deficiency anemia are those of the anemia itself (easy fatigability, tachycardia, palpitations, and dyspnea on exertion). Severe deficiency causes skin and mucosal changes, including a smooth tongue, brittle nails, spooning of nails (koilonychia), and cheilosis. Dysphagia due to esophageal web formation (**Plummer-Vinson syndrome**) may occur in severe iron deficiency. **Pica** (ie, craving for specific foods [ice chips, etc] not rich in iron) develops in many iron-deficient patients.

B. Laboratory Findings

Iron deficiency develops in stages. The first is depletion of iron stores without anemia followed by anemia with a normal RBC size (normal MCV) followed by anemia with reduced RBC size (low MCV). The reticulocyte count is low or inappropriately normal. ***Ferritin** is a measure of total body iron stores.* A ferritin value < 12 ng/mL (27 pmol/L) (in the absence of scurvy) is a highly reliable indicator of reduced iron stores. Note that the lower limit of normal for ferritin is often < 12 ng/mL (27 pmol/L) in women because the normal ferritin range is generated by including healthy menstruating people who are iron deficient but not anemic. However, because serum ferritin levels may rise in response to inflammation or other stimuli, a normal or elevated ferritin level does not exclude a diagnosis of iron deficiency. A ferritin level < 30 ng/mL (67 pmol/L) almost always indicates iron deficiency in anyone who is anemic. As iron deficiency progresses, serum iron values decline to < 30 mcg/dL (67 pmol/L) and **transferrin** (the iron transport protein) levels rise to compensate, leading to transferrin saturations of < 15%. Low transferrin saturation is also seen in anemia of inflammation, so caution in interpreting this test is warranted. Isolated iron deficiency anemia has a low hepcidin level (not yet a universally clinically available test). As the MCV falls (ie, microcytosis), the blood smear shows hypochromic microcytic cells. With further progression, **anisocytosis** (variations in RBC size) and **poikilocytosis** (variation in shape of RBCs) develop. Severe iron deficiency will produce a bizarre peripheral blood smear, with severely hypochromic cells, target cells, pencil-shaped, cigar-shaped cells, or a combination of these. Bone marrow biopsy for evaluation of iron stores is rarely performed. If the biopsy is done, it shows the absence of iron in erythroid progenitor cells by Prussian blue staining. The platelet count is commonly increased, but it usually remains under 800,000/mcL (800×10^9/L).

Differential Diagnosis

Other causes of microcytic anemia include anemia of chronic disease (specifically, anemia of inflammation), thalassemia, lead poisoning, zinc deficiency, and congenital X-linked sideroblastic anemia. Anemia of chronic disease is characterized by normal or increased iron stores in bone marrow macrophages and a normal or elevated ferritin level; the serum iron and transferrin saturation are low, often drastically so, and the **total iron-binding capacity (TIBC)** (the blood's capacity for iron to bind to transferrin) and transferrin are either normal or low. Thalassemia produces a greater degree of microcytosis for any given level of hemoglobin than does iron deficiency and, unlike virtually every other cause of anemia, has a normal or elevated (rather than a low) RBC count and a reticulocytosis. In thalassemia, RBC morphology on the peripheral smear resembles severe iron deficiency.

Treatment

The diagnosis of iron deficiency anemia can be made either by the laboratory demonstration of an iron-deficient state or by evaluating the response to a *therapeutic trial* of iron replacement. Since the anemia itself is rarely life-threatening, the most important part of management is identifying the cause—especially a source of occult blood loss.

A. Oral Iron

Ferrous sulfate, 325 mg once daily or every other day on an empty stomach, is a standard approach for replenishing iron stores. As oral iron stimulates hepcidin production, once daily or every other day dosing maximizes iron absorption compared to multiple daily doses, and with fewer side effects. Nausea and constipation limit compliance with ferrous sulfate. Taking ferrous sulfate with food reduces side effects but also its absorption. An appropriate response to oral iron is a return of the hematocrit level halfway toward normal within 3 weeks with full return to baseline after 2 months. *Iron therapy should continue for 3–6 months after restoration of normal hematologic values to replenish iron stores.* Failure to respond to iron therapy is usually due to noncompliance, although some patients may absorb iron poorly, particularly if the stomach is achlorhydric. Such patients may benefit from concomitant administration of oral ascorbic acid. Other reasons for failure to respond include incorrect diagnosis (anemia of chronic disease, thalassemia), celiac disease, and ongoing blood loss that exceeds the rate of new erythropoiesis. Treatment of *H pylori* infection, in appropriate cases, can improve oral iron absorption.

B. Parenteral Iron

The indications are intolerance of or refractoriness to oral iron, GI disease (usually IBD) precluding the use of oral iron, and continued blood loss that cannot be corrected, such as chronic hemodialysis. Historical parenteral iron preparations, such as high-molecular-weight iron dextran, were problematic due to long infusion times (hours), polyarthralgia, and hypersensitivity reactions, including anaphylaxis. Current parenteral iron preparations coat the iron in protective carbohydrate shells or contain low-molecular-weight iron dextran, are safe, and can be administered over 15 minutes to 1 hour. Most iron-deficient patients need 1–1.5 g of parenteral iron; this dose corrects for the iron deficit and replenishes iron stores for the future.

When to Refer

Patients should be referred to a hematologist if the suspected diagnosis is not confirmed or if they are not responsive to oral iron therapy.

Fertrin KY. Diagnosis and management of iron deficiency in chronic inflammatory conditions (CIC): is too little iron making your patient sick? Hematol Am Soc Hematol Educ Program. 2020;2020:478. [PMID: 33275757]

Kumar A et al. Iron deficiency anaemia: pathophysiology, assessment, practical management. BMJ Open Gastroenterol. 2022;9:e000759. [PMID: 34996762]

Talamo G et al. Platelet levels before and after iron replacement therapy in patients with iron deficiency anemia. Hematology. 2025;30:2458358. [PMID: 39918288]

Van Doren L et al. Expert consensus guidelines: intravenous iron uses, formulations, administration, and management of reactions. Am J Hematol. 2024;99:1338. [PMID: 38282557]

ANEMIA OF CHRONIC DISEASE

ESSENTIALS OF DIAGNOSIS

- Mild or moderate normocytic or microcytic anemia.
- Normal or increased ferritin and normal or reduced transferrin.
- Underlying chronic disease.

General Considerations

Many chronic systemic diseases are associated with mild or moderate anemia. The anemias of chronic disease are characterized according to etiology and pathophysiology. First, the **anemia of inflammation** is associated with chronic inflammatory states (such as IBD, rheumatologic disorders, chronic infections, and malignancy) and is mediated through hepcidin (a negative regulator of ferroportin) primarily via elevated IL-6, resulting in reduced iron uptake in the gut and reduced iron transfer from macrophages to erythroid progenitor cells in the bone marrow. This is referred to as **iron-restricted erythropoiesis** since the patient is iron replete. There is also reduced responsiveness to erythropoietin, the elaboration of hemolysins that shorten RBC survival, and the production of other inflammatory cytokines that dampen RBC production. Second, the **anemia of organ failure** can occur with kidney disease, liver failure, and endocrine gland failure. Erythropoietin production is reduced and the RBC mass decreases in response to the diminished signal for RBC production. Third, the **anemia of older adults** is present in up to 20% of individuals over age 85 years in whom a thorough evaluation for an explanation of anemia is negative. This anemia is a consequence of (1) a relative resistance to RBC production in response to erythropoietin, (2) a decrease in erythropoietin production relative to the nephron mass, (3) a dampening of erythropoiesis due to high levels of chronic inflammatory cytokines in older adults, and/or (4) the presence of various somatic pathogenic variants in myeloid genes typically associated with myeloid neoplasms. The latter condition is now referred to as **clonal cytopenias of undetermined significance**, which has a 15–20% per-year rate of transformation to a myeloid neoplasm, such as a myelodysplastic syndrome (MDS).

Clinical Findings

A. Symptoms and Signs

The clinical features are those of the causative condition and anemia. The diagnosis should be suspected in patients with known chronic diseases. *In cases of significant anemia, coexistent iron, folic acid, or vitamin B_{12} deficiency should be suspected.* Decreased dietary intake of iron or folic acid is common in chronically ill patients, many of whom will also have ongoing GI blood losses. Patients undergoing hemodialysis regularly lose both iron and folic acid during dialysis.

B. Laboratory Findings

The hematocrit rarely falls < 60% of baseline (except in kidney failure). The MCV is usually normal or slightly reduced. RBC morphology is usually normal, and the reticulocyte count is mildly decreased or normal.

1. Anemia of inflammation—In the anemia of inflammation, serum iron and transferrin values are low, and the transferrin saturation may be extremely low, leading to an erroneous diagnosis of iron deficiency. In contrast to iron deficiency, serum ferritin values should be normal or increased. A serum ferritin value < 30 ng/mL (67 pmol/L) indicates coexistent iron deficiency. Anemia of inflammation has elevated hepcidin levels; however, no universal clinical test is yet available. A particular challenge is diagnosing iron deficiency in the setting of anemia of inflammation, in which serum ferritin can be as high as 200–500 ng/mL (450–1125 pmol/L). The diagnosis is established by a bone marrow biopsy with iron stain (although rarely done for this purpose). Absent iron staining indicates iron deficiency, whereas iron localized in marrow macrophages indicates primarily anemia of inflammation. Another test supporting iron deficiency in the setting of inflammation is a reticulocyte hemoglobin concentration of < 28 pg. A functional test is hemoglobin response to oral or parenteral iron in the setting of inflammation when iron deficiency is suspected. A note of caution: certain circumstances of iron-restricted erythropoiesis (such as malignancy) will partially respond to parenteral iron infusion even when the iron stores are replete due to the immediate distribution of iron to erythropoietic progenitor cells after the infusion.

2. Other anemias of chronic disease—In the anemias of organ failure and of older adults, the iron studies are generally normal. The anemia of older persons is a diagnosis of exclusion. Clonal cytopenias of undetermined significance are diagnosed by sending a blood or bone marrow aspirate sample for karyotype, myeloid gene sequencing, or both.

Treatment

In most cases, no treatment of the anemia of chronic disease is necessary and the primary management is to address the condition causing the anemia. When the anemia is severe or is adversely affecting the quality of life or functional status, then treatment involves either RBC transfusions or parenteral **recombinant erythropoietin** (epoetin-α or darbepoetin). The FDA-approved indications for recombinant erythropoietin are hemoglobin < 10 g/dL and anemia due to rheumatoid arthritis, IBD, hepatitis C, zidovudine therapy in HIV-infected patients, myelosuppressive chemotherapy of solid malignancy (treated with palliative intent only), or CKD (eGFR of < 60 mL/min/1.73 m^2). The dosing and schedule of recombinant erythropoietin are individualized to maintain the hemoglobin between 10 g/dL (100 g/L) and 12 g/dL (120 g/L). Recombinant erythropoietin is associated with an increased risk of venous thromboembolism and arterial thrombotic episodes, especially if the hemoglobin rises to > 12 g/dL (120 g/L). *There is concern that recombinant erythropoietin is associated with reduced survival in patients with solid malignancies.*

When to Refer

Referral to a hematologist is not usually necessary.

Diez SC et al. Anemia of inflammation and iron metabolism in chronic diseases. Rev Clin Esp (Barc). 2024;224:598. [PMID: 39236980]

Fertrin KY. Diagnosis and management of iron deficiency in chronic inflammatory conditions (CIC): is too little iron making your patient sick? Hematol Am Soc Hematol Educ Program. 2020;2020:478. [PMID: 33275757]

Weeks LD et al. Prediction of risk for myeloid malignancy in clonal hematopoiesis. NEJM Evid. 2023;2:10.10566. [PMID: 37483562]

THE THALASSEMIAS

ESSENTIALS OF DIAGNOSIS

- Microcytosis disproportionate to the degree of anemia.
- Positive family history.
- Lifelong personal history of microcytic anemia.
- Normal or elevated RBC count.
- Abnormal RBC morphology with microcytes, hypochromia, acanthocytes, and target cells.
- In β-thalassemia, elevated levels of hemoglobin A_2 and F.

General Considerations

The thalassemias are hereditary disorders characterized by reduced synthesis of globin chains (α or β). Reduced globin chain synthesis causes reduced hemoglobin synthesis and a hypochromic microcytic anemia because of insufficient hemoglobinization of RBCs. Thalassemias can be considered among the hyperproliferative hemolytic anemias, the anemias related to abnormal hemoglobin, and the hypoproliferative anemias, since all of these factors play a role in their pathophysiology. *The hallmark laboratory features are small (low MCV) and pale (low mean corpuscular hemoglobin [MCH]) RBCs, anemia, and a normal to elevated RBC count (ie, a large number of the small and pale RBCs are being produced).* Although patients often exhibit an elevated reticulocyte count, generally the degree of reticulocyte output is inadequate to meet the degree of RBC destruction (hemolysis) occurring in the bone marrow and the patients remain anemic (ie, a relative hypoproliferative state).

Normal adult hemoglobin is primarily hemoglobin A, representing approximately 98% of circulating hemoglobin. **Hemoglobin A** is formed from a tetramer of two α-globin chains and two β-globin chains—and is designated α2β2. Two copies of the α-globin gene are located on each chromosome 16, and there is no substitute for α-globin in the formation of adult hemoglobin. One copy of the β-globin gene resides on each chromosome 11 adjacent to genes encoding the β-like globins δ and γ (the so-called β-globin gene cluster region). The tetramer of α2δ2 forms **hemoglobin A_2**, which normally composes 1–3% of adult hemoglobin. The tetramer α2γ2 forms **hemoglobin F**, which is the major hemoglobin of fetal life and which composes < 1% of normal adult hemoglobin.

Table 15–4. α-Thalassemia syndromes.

Number of α-Globin Genes Transcribed	Syndrome	Hematocrit	MCV
4	Normal	Normal	Normal
3	Silent carrier	Normal	Normal
2	Thalassemia minor (or trait)	28–40%	60–75 fL
1	Hemoglobin H[1] disease	22–32%	60–70 fL
0	Hydrops fetalis[2]	< 18%	< 60 fL

[1]β4
[2]Hemoglobin Barts (γ4)
MCV, mean corpuscular volume.

The thalassemias are described as **thalassemia trait** when there are laboratory features without significant clinical impact, **thalassemia intermedia** when there is an occasional RBC transfusion requirement or other moderate clinical impact, and **thalassemia major** when the disorder is life-threatening and the patient is transfusion-dependent. Most patients with thalassemia major die of the consequences of iron overload from RBC transfusions despite modern iron chelation therapy.

α-Thalassemia is due primarily to gene deletions causing reduced α-globin chain synthesis (Table 15–4). Each α-globin gene produces one-quarter of the total α-globin quantity, so there is a predictable proportionate decrease in α-globin output with each lost α-globin gene. Since all adult hemoglobins are α containing, *α-thalassemia produces no change in the proportions of hemoglobins A, A_2, and F* on hemoglobin electrophoresis. In severe forms of α-thalassemia, excess β chains may form a β-4 tetramer called **hemoglobin H.** In the presence of reduced α chains, the excess β chains are unstable and precipitate, causing damage to RBC membranes. This leads to both intramedullary (bone marrow) and peripheral blood hemolysis.

β-Thalassemias are usually caused by point mutations rather than deletions (Table 15–5). These mutations result in premature chain termination or in problems with transcription of RNA and ultimately cause reduced or absent β-globin chain synthesis. The molecular defects leading to β-thalassemia are numerous and heterogeneous. Defects that result in absent β-globin chain expression are termed β^0, whereas those causing reduced but not absent synthesis are termed β^+. In β^+ thalassemia, the degree of reduction of β-globin synthesis is consistent within families but is quite variable between families. The reduced β-globin chain synthesis in β-thalassemia results in a relative increase in the proportions of hemoglobins A_2 and F compared to hemoglobin A on hemoglobin electrophoresis, as the β-like globins (δ and γ) substitute for the missing β

Table 15–5. β-Thalassemia syndromes.

	β-Globin Genes Transcribed	Hb A	Hb A_2	Hb F	Transfusions
Normal	Homozygous β	97–99%	1–3%	< 1%	None
Thalassemia minor	Heterozygous $β^0$	80–95%	4–8%	1–5%	None
	Heterozygous $β^+$	80–95%	4–8%	1–5%	None
Thalassemia intermedia	Homozygous $β^+$ (mild)	0–40%	4–8%	6–50%	Occasional
Thalassemia major	Homozygous $β^0$	0%	4–10%	90–96%	Dependent
	Homozygous $β^+$ (severe)	0–10%	4–10%	90–96%	Dependent

Hb, hemoglobin; $β^0$, no β-globin produced; $β^+$, some β-globin produced.

chains. In the presence of reduced β chains, excess α chains are unstable and precipitate, causing damage to RBC membranes. This leads to both intramedullary (bone marrow) and peripheral blood hemolysis. The bone marrow aspirate and biopsy demonstrate erythroid hyperplasia under the stimulus of anemia due to ineffective erythropoiesis (intramedullary destruction of the developing erythroid cells). In cases of severe β-thalassemia, the marked expansion of the erythroid compartment in the bone marrow may cause severe bony deformities, osteopenia, and pathologic bone fractures as well as extramedullary hematopoiesis (ie, hematopoiesis outside of the bone marrow).

Clinical Findings

A. Symptoms and Signs

The **α-thalassemia** syndromes are seen primarily in persons from Southeast Asia and China and, less commonly, in Black persons and persons of Mediterranean origin (Table 15–4). Normally, adults have four copies of the α-globin chain. When three α-globin genes are present, the patient is hematologically normal (**silent carrier**). When two α-globin genes are present, the patient is said to have **α-thalassemia trait**, a form of thalassemia minor. In α-thalassemia-1 trait, the α gene deletion is heterozygous (α –/α –) and affects mainly those of Asian descent. In α-thalassemia-2 trait, the α gene deletion is homozygous (α α/– –) and affects mainly Black persons. These patients are clinically normal and have a normal life expectancy and performance status, with a mild microcytic anemia. When only one α-globin chain is present (α –/– –), the patient has **hemoglobin H disease** (α-thalassemia-3). This is a chronic hemolytic anemia of variable severity (thalassemia minor or intermedia). Physical examination might reveal pallor and splenomegaly. Affected individuals usually do not need transfusions; however, transfusions may be required during transient periods of hemolytic exacerbation caused by infection or other stressors or during periods of erythropoietic shutdown caused by certain viruses ("aplastic crisis"). When all four α-globin genes are deleted, no normal adult hemoglobin is produced and the affected fetus is stillborn (**hydrops fetalis**), whereby the only hemoglobin species made is γ and is called **hemoglobin Bart's** (γ4).

β-Thalassemia primarily affects persons of Mediterranean origin (Italian, Greek) and to a lesser extent Asian and Black persons (Table 15–5). Patients homozygous for β-thalassemia ($β^0/β^0$ or some with $β^+/β^+$) have **β-thalassemia major** (Cooley anemia). Affected children are normal at birth, but after 6 months, when hemoglobin synthesis switches from hemoglobin F to hemoglobin A, severe anemia develops that requires transfusion. Numerous clinical problems ensue, including stunted growth, bony deformities (abnormal facial structure, pathologic bone fractures), hepatosplenomegaly, jaundice (due to hemolysis, gallstones, hepatitis-related cirrhosis, or any combination), and thrombophilia. The clinical course is modified significantly by transfusion therapy, but **transfusional iron overload (hemosiderosis)** results in a clinical picture similar to hemochromatosis, with HF, cardiac arrhythmias, cirrhosis, endocrinopathies, and pseudoxanthoma elasticum (calcification and fragmentation of the elastic fibers of the skin, retina, and cardiovascular system), usually after more than 100 units of RBCs have been transfused. Iron overloading occurs because the human body has no active iron excretory mechanism. Before the application of allogeneic stem cell transplantation and the development of more effective forms of iron chelation, death from iron overload usually occurred between the ages of 20 and 30 years.

Patients homozygous for a milder form of β-thalassemia ($β^+/β^+$ but allowing a higher rate of β-globin synthesis) have **β-thalassemia intermedia**. These patients have chronic hemolytic anemia but do not require transfusions except under periods of stress or during aplastic crises. They also may develop iron overload because of periodic transfusion. They survive into adult life but often with hepatosplenomegaly and bony deformities. Patients heterozygous for β-thalassemia ($β/β^0$ or $β/β^+$) have **β-thalassemia minor** and a clinically insignificant microcytic anemia.

Prenatal diagnosis is available, and genetic counseling should be offered and the opportunity for prenatal diagnosis discussed.

B. Laboratory Findings

1. α-Thalassemia trait—These patients have mild or no anemia, with hematocrits between 28% and 40%. The MCV is strikingly low (60–75 fL) despite the modest anemia, and the RBC is normal or increased. The peripheral blood smear shows microcytes, hypochromia, occasional target cells, and acanthocytes (cells with irregularly spaced spiked projections). The reticulocyte count is normal or mildly increased. Hemoglobin electrophoresis is normal. Genetic testing to demonstrate α-globin gene deletion is available.

2. Hemoglobin H disease—These patients have a more marked anemia, with hematocrits between 22% and 32%. The MCV is remarkably low (60–70 fL) and the peripheral blood smear is markedly abnormal, with hypochromia, microcytosis, target cells, and poikilocytosis. The reticulocyte count is elevated, and the RBC count is normal or elevated. Hemoglobin electrophoresis will show a fast-migrating hemoglobin (hemoglobin H), which comprises 10–40% of the hemoglobin. A peripheral blood smear can be stained with supravital dyes to demonstrate the presence of hemoglobin H.

3. β-Thalassemia minor—These patients have a modest anemia with hematocrit between 28% and 40%. The MCV ranges from 55 fL to 75 fL, and the RBC count is normal or increased. The reticulocyte count is normal or slightly elevated. The peripheral blood smear is mildly abnormal, with hypochromia, microcytosis, and target cells. In contrast to α-thalassemia, basophilic stippling is present. Hemoglobin electrophoresis shows an elevation of hemoglobin A_2 to 4–8% and occasional elevations of hemoglobin F to 1–5%.

4. β-Thalassemia intermedia—These patients have a moderate anemia with hematocrit between 17% and 33%. The MCV ranges from 55 fL to 75 fL, and the RBC count is normal or increased. The reticulocyte count is elevated. The peripheral blood smear is abnormal with hypochromia, microcytosis, basophilic stippling, and target cells. Hemoglobin electrophoresis shows up to 40% hemoglobin A, an elevation of hemoglobin A_2 up to 10%, and elevation of hemoglobin F from 6% to 50%.

5. β-Thalassemia major—These patients have severe anemia, and without transfusion the hematocrit may fall to < 10%. The peripheral blood smear is bizarre, showing severe poikilocytosis, hypochromia, microcytosis, target cells, basophilic stippling, and nucleated RBCs. Little or no hemoglobin A is present. Variable amounts of hemoglobin A_2 are seen, and the predominant hemoglobin present is hemoglobin F.

Differential Diagnosis

Mild forms of thalassemia must be differentiated from iron deficiency. Compared to iron deficiency anemia, patients with thalassemia have a lower MCV, a normal or elevated RBC count (rather than low), a more abnormal peripheral blood smear even at modest levels of anemia, and usually a reticulocytosis. Iron studies are normal, or the transferrin saturation or ferritin (or both) are elevated. The diagnosis of β-thalassemia is made by the above findings and hemoglobin electrophoresis showing elevated levels of hemoglobins A_2 and F (provided the patient is replete in iron), or by β-globin gene sequencing. The diagnosis of α-thalassemia is made by exclusion since there is no change in the proportion of the normal adult hemoglobin species or confirmed by α gene deletion studies. *The only other microcytic anemia with a normal or elevated RBC count is iron deficiency in a patient with polycythemia vera.*

Treatment

Patients with mild thalassemia (α-thalassemia trait or β-thalassemia minor) require no treatment and should be identified to avoid repeated evaluations and mistaken treatment for iron deficiency. Patients with hemoglobin H disease should take folic acid supplementation (1 mg/day orally) and avoid medicinal iron and oxidative drugs such as sulfonamides. Patients with severe thalassemia are maintained on a regular RBC transfusion schedule (in part to suppress endogenous erythropoiesis and therefore suppress bone marrow expansion) and receive folic acid supplementation. Splenectomy is performed if hypersplenism causes a marked increase in the transfusion requirement or refractory symptoms. Patients with regular transfusion requirements should be treated with iron chelation (oral, parenteral, or both) to prevent or delay life-limiting organ damage from iron overload. Luspatercept is FDA approved for adults with transfusion-dependent β-thalassemia. It is a TGF-β ligand trap that promotes erythroid maturation and reduces transfusion needs.

Allogeneic stem cell transplantation is the treatment of choice for children with β-thalassemia major. Children who have not yet experienced organ damage from iron overload do well, with long-term survival in > 80% of cases. Autologous hematopoietic stem cell gene therapy is now available (betibeglogene autotemcel contains a $\beta^{A\text{-}T87Q}$ gene and exagamglogene autoleucel enhances the production of gamma globin to increase hemoglobin F) for transfusion-dependent β-thalassemia in children.

When to Refer

All patients with thalassemia intermedia or major should be referred to a hematologist. Any patient with an unexplained microcytic anemia should be referred to help establish a diagnosis. Patients with thalassemia minor or intermedia should be offered genetic counseling because offspring of thalassemic couples are at risk for inheriting thalassemia major.

Hokland P et al. Thalassaemia-a global view. Br J Haematol. 2023;201:199. [PMID: 36799486]

Locatelli F et al. Betibeglogene autotemcel gene therapy for non-β^0/β^0 genotype β-thalassemia. N Engl J Med. 2022;386:415. [PMID: 34891223]

Musallam KM et al. Alpha-thalassemia: a practical overview. Blood Rev. 2024;64:101165. [PMID: 38182489]

Soteriades ES et al. The disease burden of β-thalassemia. Hematol. 2025;30:2551450. [PMID: 40916705]

VITAMIN B_{12} DEFICIENCY

ESSENTIALS OF DIAGNOSIS

- Macrocytic anemia.
- Megaloblastic blood smear (macro-ovalocytes and hypersegmented neutrophils).
- Low serum vitamin B_{12} level.

General Considerations

Vitamin B_{12} belongs to the family of cobalamins and serves as a cofactor for two important reactions in humans. As methylcobalamin, it is a cofactor for methionine synthetase in the conversion of homocysteine to methionine, and as adenosylcobalamin for the conversion of methylmalonyl-coenzyme A (CoA) to succinyl-CoA. Vitamin B_{12} comes from the diet and is present in all foods of animal origin. The daily dietary absorption of vitamin B_{12} is 5 mcg.

After being ingested, vitamin B_{12} is bound to intrinsic factor, a protein secreted by gastric parietal cells in an acid environment. The vitamin B_{12}–intrinsic factor complex travels through the intestine and is absorbed in the terminal ileum by cells with specific receptors for the complex. It is then transported through plasma and stored in the liver.

The liver contains 2–5 mg of stored vitamin B_{12}. Since daily utilization is 3–5 mcg, the body usually has sufficient stores of vitamin B_{12} so that it takes > 3 years for vitamin B_{12} deficiency to occur if all intake or absorption immediately ceases.

Since vitamin B_{12} is present in foods of animal origin, dietary vitamin B_{12} deficiency is rare but is seen in vegans—strict vegetarians who avoid all dairy products, meat, fish, and vitamin supplementation (Table 15–6). **Pernicious anemia** is an autoimmune illness whereby autoantibodies destroy gastric parietal cells (that produce intrinsic factor) and cause atrophic gastritis, or bind to and neutralize intrinsic factor, or both. Abdominal surgery may lead to vitamin B_{12} deficiency in several ways. Gastrectomy will eliminate the site of intrinsic factor production; blind loop syndrome will cause competition for vitamin B_{12} by bacterial overgrowth in the intestinal lumen; and surgical resection of the ileum will eliminate the GI site of vitamin B_{12} absorption. Metformin can cause B_{12} deficiency. Rare causes of vitamin B_{12} deficiency include fish tapeworm (*Diphyllobothrium latum*) infection, in which the parasite uses luminal vitamin B_{12}; pancreatic insufficiency (with failure to inactivate competing cobalamin-binding proteins [R-factors]); severe Crohn disease, causing sufficient destruction of the ileum to impair vitamin B_{12} absorption; and perhaps prolonged use of PPIs.

Table 15–6. Causes of vitamin B_{12} deficiency (in alphabetical order within categories).

Competition for vitamin B_{12} in the gut
Blind loop syndrome
Fish tapeworm (rare)
Decreased ileal absorption of vitamin B_{12}
Crohn disease
Surgical resection
Decreased production or availability of intrinsic factor
Gastrectomy
Pernicious anemia (autoimmune)
Dietary deficiency
Helicobacter pylori infection
Metformin
Pancreatic insufficiency
PPIs
Transcobalamin II deficiency (rare)

Clinical Findings

A. Symptoms and Signs

Vitamin B_{12} deficiency causes a moderate to severe anemia of slow onset; patients may have few symptoms relative to the degree of anemia. In advanced cases, the anemia may be severe (with hematocrits as low as 10–15%) and may be accompanied by leukopenia and thrombocytopenia. The deficiency also produces changes in mucosal cells, leading to glossitis, as well as other vague GI disturbances such as anorexia and diarrhea. Vitamin B_{12} deficiency also leads to a complex neurologic syndrome. Peripheral nerves are usually affected first, and patients initially report paresthesias. As the posterior columns of the spinal cord become impaired, patients report difficulty with balance or proprioception, or both. In more advanced cases, cerebral function may be altered as well, and on occasion, dementia and other neuropsychiatric abnormalities may be present. *It is critical to recognize that the nonhematologic manifestations of vitamin B_{12} deficiency can be manifest despite a completely normal CBC.*

Patients are usually pale and may be mildly icteric or sallow. Typically, later in the disease course, neurologic examination may reveal any combination of decreased vibration sense, position sense, or memory disturbance.

B. Laboratory Findings

The diagnosis of vitamin B_{12} deficiency is made by finding a low serum vitamin B_{12} (cobalamin) level. Whereas the normal vitamin B_{12} level is > 300 pg/mL (221 pmol/L), most patients with overt vitamin B_{12} deficiency have serum levels < 200 pg/mL (148 pmol/L), with symptomatic patients often having levels < 100 pg/mL (74 pmol/L). The diagnosis of vitamin B_{12} deficiency in low or low-normal values (level of 200–300 pg/mL [147.6–221.3 pmol/L]) is best confirmed by finding an elevated level of serum methylmalonic acid (MMA), homocysteine, or both. Of note, elevated levels of serum MMA can be due to kidney disease.

The anemia of vitamin B_{12} deficiency is typically moderate to severe with the MCV quite elevated (110–140 fL). However, it is possible to have vitamin B_{12} deficiency with a normal MCV from coexistent thalassemia or iron deficiency; in other cases, the reason is obscure. *Patients with neurologic symptoms and signs that suggest possible vitamin B_{12} deficiency should be evaluated for that deficiency despite a normal MCV or the absence of anemia.* In typical cases, the peripheral blood smear is megaloblastic, defined as RBCs that appear as macro-ovalocytes and neutrophils that are hypersegmented (six [or greater]-lobed neutrophils or mean neutrophil lobe counts > four). The reticulocyte count is reduced and the WBC count and the platelet count are reduced in severe cases. Other laboratory abnormalities include elevated serum LD and a modest increase in indirect bilirubin. These two findings reflect the intramedullary destruction of developing but disturbed erythroid cells.

Bone marrow aspirate and biopsy morphology are characteristically abnormal. Marked erythroid hyperplasia is present as a response to defective RBC production (ineffective erythropoiesis). Megaloblastic changes in the erythroid series include abnormally large cell size and asynchronous maturation of the nucleus and cytoplasm—ie, cytoplasmic maturation continues while impaired DNA synthesis causes retarded nuclear development. In the myeloid series, giant bands and meta-myelocytes are characteristically seen.

Differential Diagnosis

Vitamin B_{12} deficiency should be differentiated from folic acid deficiency, the other common cause of megaloblastic anemia, in which RBC folic acid is low while serum vitamin B_{12} levels are normal. The bone marrow findings of vitamin B_{12} deficiency are sometimes mistaken for a MDS or even acute erythrocytic leukemia. The distinction between vitamin B_{12} deficiency and myelodysplasia is based on the characteristic morphology and the low vitamin B_{12} and elevated MMA levels.

Treatment

Initially, patients with severe vitamin B_{12} deficiency are usually treated with parenteral therapy. Intramuscular or subcutaneous injections of 100–1000 mcg of vitamin B_{12} are adequate for each dose (with the higher dose recommended initially). Replacement is usually given daily for the first week, weekly for the next month, and then monthly. Oral or sublingual methylcobalamin or cyanocobalamin (1 mg/day) may be used instead of parenteral therapy once initial correction of the deficiency has occurred. Oral or sublingual replacement is effective, even in pernicious anemia, since approximately 1% of the dose is absorbed in the intestine via passive diffusion in the absence of active transport. It must be continued indefinitely and serum vitamin B_{12} levels must be monitored to ensure adequate replacement. The vitamin deficiency will recur if patients discontinue their therapy. For patients with neurologic symptoms due to vitamin B_{12} deficiency, long-term parenteral vitamin B_{12} therapy is often recommended, though its superiority over oral therapy has not been proven. Because some patients are concurrently folic acid deficient from intestinal mucosal atrophy, simultaneous folic acid replacement (1 mg daily) is advised for at least the first several months of vitamin B_{12} replacement.

Patients respond to therapy with rapid improvement in their sense of well-being. Hypokalemia may complicate the first several days of therapy, particularly if the anemia is severe. A brisk reticulocytosis occurs in 5–7 days, and the hematologic picture normalizes in 2 months. CNS symptoms and signs are potentially reversible if they have been present for < 6 months. RBC transfusions are rarely needed despite the severity of anemia.

When to Refer

Referral to a hematologist is not usually necessary.

Abdelwahab OA et al. Efficacy of different routes of vitamin B12 supplementation in the treatment of patients with vitamin B12 deficiency: a systematic review and network meta-analysis. Ir J Med Sci. 2024;193:1621. [PMID: 38231320]

Obeid R et al. Diagnosis, treatment and long-term management pf vitamin B12 deficiency in adults: a Delphi expert consensus. J Clin Med. 2024;13:2176. [PMID: 38673453]

Patel M et al. Vitamin B12 deficiency: common questions and answers. Am Fam Physician. 2025;112:249. [PMID: 40961307]

Sahu P et al. Neuropsychiatric manifestations in vitamin B12 deficiency. Vitam Horm. 2022;119:457. [PMID: 35337631]

FOLIC ACID DEFICIENCY

ESSENTIALS OF DIAGNOSIS

- Macrocytic anemia.
- Megaloblastic blood smear (macro-ovalocytes and hypersegmented neutrophils).
- Reduced folic acid levels in RBCs or serum.
- Normal serum vitamin B_{12} level.

General Considerations

"Folic acid" is the term commonly used for pteroylmonoglutamic acid (vitamin B_9). Folic acid is present in most fruits and vegetables (especially citrus fruits and green leafy vegetables). Daily dietary requirements are 50–100 mcg. Total body stores of folic acid are approximately 5 mg, enough to supply requirements for 2–3 months.

The most common cause of folic acid deficiency is inadequate dietary intake (Table 15–7). Alcohol abuse or anorectic patients, persons who do not eat fresh fruits and vegetables, and those who overcook their food are candidates for folic acid deficiency. Reduced folic acid absorption is rarely seen, since absorption occurs from the entire GI tract. However, medications such as phenytoin, trimethoprim-sulfamethoxazole, or sulfasalazine may interfere with its absorption. *Folic acid absorption is poor in some patients with vitamin B_{12} deficiency due to GI mucosal atrophy.* Folic acid requirements are increased in pregnancy, hemolytic anemia, and exfoliative skin disease, and in these cases the increased requirements (5–10 times normal) may not be met by a normal diet.

Table 15–7. Causes of folic acid deficiency (in alphabetical order within categories).

Decreased absorption
Celiac disease
Concurrent vitamin B_{12} deficiency
Medications: phenytoin, sulfasalazine, trimethoprim-sulfamethoxazole
Dietary deficiency
Excess loss: hemodialysis
Increased requirement
Chronic hemolytic anemia
Exfoliative skin disease
Pregnancy/lactation
Inhibition of reduction to active form
Methotrexate

Clinical Findings

A. Symptoms and Signs

The clinical features are similar to those of vitamin B_{12} deficiency. However, isolated folic acid deficiency does *not* result in neurologic abnormalities. Hospitalized patients with folic acid deficiency have a higher hospital mortality than those replete in folic acid.

B. Laboratory Findings

Megaloblastic anemia is identical to anemia resulting from vitamin B_{12} deficiency. An RBC folic acid level < 150 ng/mL (340 nmol/L) is diagnostic of folic acid deficiency. Whether to order a serum or an RBC folate level remains unsettled since there are few, if any, data to support one test over the other (presumably the latter is a better assessment of long-term folic acid levels).

Differential Diagnosis

The megaloblastic anemia of folic acid deficiency should be differentiated from vitamin B_{12} deficiency by the finding of a normal vitamin B_{12} level and a reduced RBC (or serum) folic acid level. Patients who abuse alcohol, who often have nutritional deficiency, may also have anemia of liver disease. Pure anemia of liver disease causes a macrocytic anemia but does not produce megaloblastic morphologic changes in the peripheral blood; rather, target cells are often present. Hypothyroidism is associated with mild macrocytosis and also with pernicious anemia.

Treatment

Folic acid deficiency is treated with daily oral folic acid (1 mg). The response is similar to that seen in the treatment of vitamin B_{12} deficiency, with rapid improvement and a sense of well-being, reticulocytosis in 5–7 days, and total correction of hematologic abnormalities within 2 months. Large doses of folic acid may produce initial hematologic responses in cases of vitamin B_{12} deficiency, but permit neurologic damage to progress; hence, obtaining a serum vitamin B_{12} level in suspected folic acid deficiency is paramount.

When to Refer

Referral to a hematologist is not usually necessary.

Skorochod R et al. Incidence of inpatient folate deficiency and effect on overall in-hospital mortality. Am J Med. 2021;134:e235. [PMID: 33637191]

Torrez M et al. How I investigate acquired megaloblastic anemia. Int J Lab Hematol. 2022;44:236. [PMID: 34981651]

HEMOLYTIC ANEMIAS

The hemolytic anemias are a group of disorders in which RBC survival is reduced, either episodically or continuously. The bone marrow has the ability to increase erythroid production up to eightfold in response to reduced RBC survival, so anemia will be present only when the ability of the bone marrow to compensate is outstripped. This will occur when RBC survival is extremely short or when the ability of the bone marrow to compensate is impaired.

Table 15–8. Classification of hemolytic anemias (in alphabetical order within categories).

Extrinsic
Burns
Hypersplenism
Immune: autoimmune, lymphoproliferative disease, drug-induced, idiopathic
Infection: *Plasmodium, Clostridium, Babesia*
Microangiopathic: thrombotic thrombocytopenic purpura, hemolytic-uremic syndrome, disseminated intravascular coagulation, valve hemolysis, pregnancy, familial, metastatic adenocarcinoma, vasculitis, copper overload
Intrinsic
Glycolytic defects: pyruvate kinase deficiency, severe hypophosphatemia
Hemoglobinopathies: sickle cell syndromes, thalassemia, unstable hemoglobins
Membrane defects: hereditary spherocytosis, hereditary elliptocytosis, paroxysmal nocturnal hemoglobinuria
Oxidation vulnerability: glucose-6-phosphate dehydrogenase deficiency, methemoglobinemia

Hemolytic disorders are generally classified according to whether the defect is intrinsic to the RBC or due to some external factor (Table 15–8). **Intrinsic defects** have been described in all components of the RBC, including the membrane, enzyme systems, and hemoglobin; most of these disorders are hereditary. Hemolytic anemias due to **external factors** are classified as immune, microangiopathic, drug-induced, RBC infection, and burn injury–related.

Certain laboratory features are common to all hemolytic anemias. **Haptoglobin**, a normal plasma protein that binds and clears free hemoglobin released into plasma, is depressed in hemolytic disorders. However, the haptoglobin level is influenced by many factors and is not always a reliable indicator of hemolysis, particularly in end-stage liver disease (its site of synthesis). When intravascular hemolysis occurs, transient hemoglobinemia ensues. Hemoglobin is filtered through the renal glomerulus and is usually reabsorbed by tubular cells. Hemoglobinuria will be present only when the capacity for reabsorption of hemoglobin by renal tubular cells is exceeded. In the absence of hemoglobinuria, evidence for prior intravascular hemolysis is the presence of hemosiderin in shed renal tubular cells (positive urine hemosiderin). With severe intravascular hemolysis, hemoglobinemia and methemoglobinemia (hemoglobin in the Fe+3, rather than the Fe+2, state) may be present. Hemolysis increases the indirect bilirubin, and the total bilirubin may rise to 4 mg/dL (68 mcmol/L) or more. Bilirubin levels higher than this may indicate some degree of hepatic dysfunction. Serum LD levels are strikingly elevated in cases of microangiopathic hemolysis (thrombotic thrombocytopenic purpura, hemolytic-uremic syndrome) and may be elevated in other hemolytic anemias.

PAROXYSMAL NOCTURNAL HEMOGLOBINURIA

ESSENTIALS OF DIAGNOSIS

- Episodic hemoglobinuria.
- Thrombosis is common.
- Suspect in confusing cases of hemolytic anemia with or without pancytopenia.
- Flow cytometry demonstrates deficiencies of CD55 and CD59.

General Considerations

Paroxysmal nocturnal hemoglobinuria (PNH) is a rare acquired clonal hematopoietic stem cell disorder that results in abnormal sensitivity of the RBC membrane to lysis by complement and therefore hemolysis. Free hemoglobin is released into the blood that scavenges nitric oxide and promotes esophageal spasms, male erectile dysfunction, kidney damage, and thrombosis in addition to episodic hemolysis. Patients with significant PNH have shortened survival; thrombosis is the primary cause of death.

Clinical Findings

A. Symptoms and Signs

Classically, patients report episodic hemoglobinuria resulting in reddish-brown urine. Hemoglobinuria is most often noticed in the first morning urine void due to the fall in blood pH while sleeping (hypoventilation) that facilitates this hemolysis. Besides anemia, these patients are prone to thrombosis, especially within mesenteric and hepatic veins, CNS veins (sagittal vein), and skin vessels (with formation of painful nodules). As this is a hematopoietic stem cell disorder, PNH may appear de novo or arise in the setting of aplastic anemia or myelodysplasia with rare progression to acute myeloid leukemia (AML). It is common that patients with idiopathic aplastic anemia have a small PNH clone (< 2%) on blood or bone marrow analysis; this should not be considered true PNH per se, especially in the absence of a reticulocytosis or thrombosis.

B. Laboratory Findings

Anemia is of variable severity and frequency, so reticulocytosis may or may not be present at any given time. Abnormalities on the blood smear are nondiagnostic but may include macro-ovalocytes and polychromasia. Since the episodic hemolysis is mainly intravascular, **urine hemosiderin** is a useful test. Serum LD is characteristically quite elevated. Iron deficiency is commonly present due to chronic iron loss from hemoglobinuria.

The WBC count and platelet count may be decreased and are always decreased in the setting of aplastic anemia. The best screening test is **flow cytometry** of blood erythrocytes, granulocytes, and monocytes to demonstrate deficiency of CD55 and CD59. The proportion of erythrocytes deficient in these proteins might be low compared to granulocytes and monocytes due to the ongoing destruction of affected erythrocytes. The **FLAER assay** (fluorescein-labeled proaerolysin) by flow cytometry is more sensitive. Bone marrow aspirate and biopsy morphology are variable and may show either generalized hypoplasia or erythroid hyperplasia or both. The bone marrow karyotype may be either normal or demonstrate a clonal abnormality.

Treatment

Many patients with PNH have mild disease not requiring intervention. In severe cases and in those occurring in the setting of myelodysplasia or aplastic anemia, allogeneic hematopoietic stem cell transplantation may prove curative. In patients with severe hemolysis (usually requiring RBC transfusions), thrombosis, or both, treatment with complement blockers is warranted. Eculizumab is a humanized monoclonal antibody against complement protein C5 given every 2 weeks. Binding of eculizumab to C5 prevents its cleavage so the membrane attack complex cannot assemble. Eculizumab improves quality of life and reduces hemolysis, transfusion requirements, fatigue, and thrombosis rate. Eculizumab increases the risk of *Neisseria meningitidis* infections, so patients receiving the antibody should undergo meningococcal vaccination (including vaccines for serogroup ACWY and also B) and take oral penicillin (or equivalent) as meningococcal prophylaxis. Ravulizumab is a longer-acting version of eculizumab; it is given every 8 weeks and demonstrates fewer breakthrough hemolytic episodes than eculizumab. A third C5 inhibitor is crovalimab-akkz. A C3 inhibitor, pegcetacoplan, is also available for PNH and blocks both intra- and extravascular hemolysis pathways, resulting in higher hemoglobins than C5 blockade. An oral complement factor B inhibitor (iptacopan) is also now FDA approved as well as a complement factor D inhibitor (danicopan; as an add-on to those with an inadequate response to eculizumuab or ravulizumab). Iron replacement is indicated for treatment of iron deficiency when present, which may improve the anemia while also causing a transient increase in hemolysis.

When to Refer

Most patients with PNH should be under the care of a hematologist.

Szlendak U et al. Paroxysmal nocturnal hemoglobinuria: advances in the understanding of pathophysiology, diagnosis, and treatment. Pol Arch Intern Med. 2022;132:16271. [PMID: 35699625]

Versino F et al. Progress in the use of biological therapies to treat paroxysmal nocturnal hemoglobinuria: focus on patient profiling. Expert Opin Biol Ther. 2025;25:1071. [PMID: 41082261]

Waheed A et al. Paroxysmal nocturnal hemoglobinuria: review of the patient experience and treatment landscape. Blood Rev. 2024;64:101158. [PMID: 38071133]

GLUCOSE-6-PHOSPHATE DEHYDROGENASE DEFICIENCY

ESSENTIALS OF DIAGNOSIS

- X-linked recessive disorder common in American Black men.
- Episodic hemolysis in response to oxidant medications or infection.
- Bite cells and blister cells on the peripheral blood smear.
- Reduced levels of glucose-6-phosphate dehydrogenase between hemolytic episodes.

General Considerations

Glucose-6-phosphate dehydrogenase (G6PD) deficiency is a hereditary enzyme defect that causes episodic hemolytic anemia because of the decreased ability of RBCs to manage oxidative stress. G6PD deficiency leads to excess oxidized glutathione that forces hemoglobin to denature and form precipitants called **Heinz bodies.** Heinz bodies cause RBC membrane damage, leading to premature removal of these RBCs by reticuloendothelial cells within the spleen (ie, extravascular hemolysis).

Numerous G6PD isoenzymes have been described. The usual isoenzyme found in American Black persons is designated G6PD-A and that found in White persons is designated G6PD-B, both of which have normal function and stability and therefore no hemolytic anemia. Ten to 15 percent of American Black persons have the variant G6PD isoenzyme, designated A–, in which there is both a reduction in normal enzyme activity and a reduction in its stability. The A-isoenzyme activity declines rapidly as the RBC ages past 40 days, a fact that explains the clinical findings in this disorder. More than 150 G6PD isoenzyme variants have been described, including some Mediterranean, Ashkenazi Jewish, and Asian variants with very low enzyme activity, episodic hemolysis, and exacerbations due to oxidizing substances including fava beans. Patients with G6PD deficiency seem to be protected from malaria parasitic infection, have more CAD, and possibly have fewer cancers and greater longevity.

Clinical Findings

G6PD deficiency is an X-linked disorder affecting 10–15% of American hemizygous Black males and rare female homozygotes. Female carriers are rarely affected—only when an unusually high percentage of cells producing the normal enzyme are X-inactivated.

A. Symptoms and Signs

Patients are usually healthy, without chronic hemolytic anemia or splenomegaly. Hemolysis occurs episodically due to oxidative stress on the RBCs, generated either by infection or exposure to certain medications. Medications initiating hemolysis that should be avoided include dapsone, methylene blue, phenazopyridine, primaquine, rasburicase, toluidine blue, nitrofurantoin, trimethoprim/sulfamethoxazole, sulfadiazine, pegloticase, and quinolones. Other medications, such as chloramphenicol, chloroquine, colchicine, diaminophenyl sulfone, diphenhydramine, glyburide, quinine, high-dose aspirin, NSAIDs, and isoniazid, have been implicated but are less certain as offenders since they are often given during infections. Even with continuous use of the offending medication, the hemolytic episode is self-limited because older RBCs (with low enzyme activity) are removed and replaced with a population of young RBCs (reticulocytes) with adequate functional levels of G6PD. Severe G6PD deficiency (as in Mediterranean variants) may produce a chronic hemolytic anemia.

B. Laboratory Findings

Between hemolytic episodes, the blood is normal. During episodes of hemolysis, the hemoglobin rarely falls < 8 g/dL (80 g/L), and there is a reticulocytosis and increased serum indirect bilirubin. The peripheral blood cell smear often reveals a small number of **"bite" cells**—cells that appear to have had a bite taken out of their periphery, or "blister" cells. This indicates pitting of precipitated membrane hemoglobin aggregates (ie, Heinz bodies) by the splenic macrophages. Heinz bodies can be demonstrated by staining a peripheral blood smear with cresyl violet; they are not visible on the usual Wright-Giemsa–stained blood smear. Specific enzyme assays for G6PD reveal a low level but may be falsely normal if performed during or shortly after a hemolytic episode during the period of reticulocytosis. In these cases, the enzyme assays should be repeated weeks after hemolysis has resolved. In severe cases of G6PD deficiency, enzyme levels are always low.

Treatment

No treatment is necessary except to avoid known oxidant medications.

Andrews PH et al. Clinical associations and potential cellular mechanism linking G6PD deficiency and atherosclerotic cardiovascular disease. NPJ Metab Health Dis. 2025;3:16. [PMID: 40292229]

Nannelli C et al. Genetic variants causing G6PD deficiency: clinical and biochemical data support new WHO classification. Br J Haematol. 2023;202:1024. [PMID: 37415281]

Shah SS et al. The global role of G6PD in infection and immunity. Front Immunol. 2024;15:1393213. [PMID: 38938571]

SICKLE CELL ANEMIA & RELATED SYNDROMES

ESSENTIALS OF DIAGNOSIS

- Recurrent pain episodes.
- Positive family history and lifelong history of hemolytic anemia.
- Irreversibly sickled cells on peripheral blood smear.
- Hemoglobin S is the major hemoglobin seen on electrophoresis.

General Considerations

Sickle cell anemia is an autosomal recessive disorder in which an abnormal hemoglobin leads to chronic hemolytic anemia with numerous clinical consequences. A single DNA base change leads to an amino acid substitution of valine for glutamate in the sixth position on the β-globin chain. The abnormal β chain is designated β^s and the tetramer of α-$2\beta^s$-2 is designated **hemoglobin SS. Hemoglobin S** is unstable and polymerizes in the setting of various stressors, including hypoxemia and acidosis, leading to the formation of sickled RBCs. Sickled cells result in hemolysis. The free hemoglobin from hemolysis scavenges nitric oxide causing endothelial dysfunction, vascular injury, and pulmonary hypertension.

The rate of sickling is influenced by the intracellular concentration of hemoglobin S and by the presence of other hemoglobins within the cell. Hemoglobin F cannot participate in polymer formation, and its presence markedly retards sickling. Factors that increase sickling are RBC dehydration and conditions that lead to formation of deoxyhemoglobin S (eg, acidosis and hypoxemia), either systemic or local in tissues. Hemolytic crises may be related to splenic sequestration of sickled cells (primarily in childhood before the spleen has been infarcted as a result of repeated sickling) or with coexistent disorders such as G6PD deficiency.

The β^S gene is carried in 8% of American Black persons, and 1 of 400 American Black children will be born with sickle cell anemia; prenatal diagnosis is available when sickle cell anemia is suspected. Genetic counseling should be made available to patients.

Clinical Findings

A. Symptoms and Signs

The disorder has its onset during the first year of life, when hemoglobin F levels fall as a signal is sent to switch from production of γ-globin to β-globin. Chronic hemolytic anemia produces jaundice, pigment gallstones (calcium bilirubinate), splenomegaly (early in life), and poorly healing skin ulcers over the lower tibia. Life-threatening severe anemia can occur during hemolytic or aplastic crises, the latter generally associated with viral or other infection caused by immunoincompetence from hyposplenism, or by folic acid deficiency causing reduced erythropoiesis.

Acute painful episodes due to acute **vaso-occlusion** from clusters of sickled RBCs may occur spontaneously or be provoked by infection, dehydration, or hypoxia. Common sites of acute painful episodes include the spine and long appendicular bones. These episodes last hours to days and may produce low-grade fever. Acute vaso-occlusion may cause strokes due to sagittal sinus venous thrombosis or to bland or hemorrhagic CNS arterial ischemia. Vaso-occlusion may also cause priapism. Vaso-occlusive episodes are not associated with increased hemolysis.

Repeated episodes of vascular occlusion especially affect the heart, lungs, and liver. **Acute chest syndrome** is characterized by acute chest pain, hypoxemia, and pulmonary infiltrates on a CXR and must be distinguished from an infectious pneumonia. Ischemic necrosis of bones may occur, rendering the bone susceptible to osteomyelitis due to salmonellae and (somewhat less commonly) staphylococci. Infarction of the papillae of the renal medulla causes renal tubular concentrating defects and gross hematuria, more often encountered in sickle cell trait (**hemoglobin AS**) than in sickle cell anemia. Retinopathy is often present and may lead to visual impairment. Pulmonary hypertension may develop and is associated with a poor prognosis. These patients are prone to delayed puberty. An increased incidence of infection is related to hyposplenism as well as to defects in the alternate complement pathway.

On examination, patients are often chronically ill and jaundiced. There is often hepatomegaly, but the spleen is not palpable in adult life. The heart may be enlarged with a hyperdynamic precordium and systolic murmurs and, in some cases, a pronounced increase in P2. Nonhealing cutaneous ulcers of the lower leg and retinopathy may be present.

B. Laboratory Findings

Chronic hemolytic anemia is present. The hematocrit is usually 20–30%. The peripheral blood smear is characteristically abnormal, with sickled cells comprising 5–50% of RBCs. Other findings include reticulocytosis (10–25%), nucleated RBCs, and hallmarks of hyposplenism such as Howell-Jolly bodies and target cells. The WBC count is characteristically elevated to 12,000–15,000/mcL ($12–15 \times 10^9$/L), and reactive thrombocytosis may occur. Indirect bilirubin levels are high.

The diagnosis of sickle cell anemia is confirmed by hemoglobin electrophoresis (Table 15–9). Hemoglobin S will usually comprise 85–98% of hemoglobin. In homozygous S disease, no hemoglobin A will be present. Hemoglobin F levels are sometimes increased, and high hemoglobin F levels (15–20%) are associated with a more benign clinical course. Patients with S-β^+-thalassemia and SS α-thalassemia also have a more benign clinical course than straight sickle cell anemia (SS) patients.

Treatment

Supportive care is the mainstay of treatment for sickle cell anemia. Patients are maintained on folic acid supplementation (1 mg orally daily) and given transfusions for aplastic or hemolytic crises. When acute painful episodes occur, precipitating factors should be identified and infections treated if present. The patient should be kept well hydrated, given generous analgesics, supplied oxygen if hypoxic, and given VTE prophylaxis if hospitalized. Pneumococcal vaccination reduces the incidence of infections with this pathogen while hydroxyurea and L-glutamine reduce hospitalizations for acute pain. ACE inhibitors are recommended in patients with microalbuminuria.

Exchange transfusions are indicated for the treatment of severe or intractable acute vaso-occlusive crises, acute chest syndrome, prolonged priapism, and stroke. Long-term transfusion therapy is effective in reducing the risk of recurrent stroke in children. Phenotypically matched transfused RBCs are recommended to reduce the risk of RBC alloimmunization. It has been recommended that children with SS who are aged 2–16 years have annual transcranial ultrasounds and, if the Doppler velocity is abnormal (≥ 200 cm/s), the clinician should strongly consider beginning

Table 15–9. Hemoglobin distribution in sickle cell syndromes.

Genotype	Clinical Diagnosis	Hb A	Hb S	Hb A_2	Hb F
AA	Normal	97–99%	0%	1–2%	< 1%
AS	Sickle trait	60%	40%	1–2%	< 1%
AS, α-thalassemia	Sickle trait, α-thalassemia	70–75%	25–30%	1–2%	< 1%
SS	Sickle cell anemia	0%	86–98%	1–3%	5–15%
SS, α-thalassemia (3 genes)	SS α-thalassemia (silent)	0%	90%	3%	7–9%
SS, α-thalassemia (2 genes)	SS α-thalassemia (trait)	0%	80%	3%	11–21%
S, β^0-thalassemia	Sickle β^0-thalassemia	0%	70–80%	3–5%	10–20%
S, β^+-thalassemia	Sickle β^+-thalassemia	10–20%	60–75%	3–5%	10–20%

Hb, hemoglobin; β^0, no β-globin produced; β^+, some β-globin produced.

transfusions to prevent stroke. Iron chelation is needed for those on chronic transfusion therapy.

Existing pharmacologic options modulate disease severity: hydroxyurea increases hemoglobin F levels epigenetically. Oral hydroxyurea (15–35 mg/kg/day) reduces the frequency of painful crises in patients whose quality of life is disrupted by frequent vaso-occlusive pain episodes (three or more per year). Long-term follow-up of patients taking hydroxyurea demonstrates it improves overall survival and quality of life with little evidence for secondary malignancy. Omega-3 (n-3) fatty acid supplementation may also reduce vaso-occlusive episodes and reduce transfusion needs in patients with sickle cell anemia. L-glutamine has been shown to favorably modulate sickle pain crises and acute chest syndrome. A monoclonal antibody (crizanlizumab-tmca) reduces vaso-occlusive episodes by 50%. It blocks P-selectin on activated endothelial cells and thus disrupts the adverse interactions of platelets, RBCs, and leukocytes with the endothelial wall.

Two genetically engineered stem cell products used with autologous transplantation are approved in the United States for patients 12 years or older with severe disease and offer the potential for long-term disease control. These are lovotibeglogene autotemcel, which produces an anti-sickling Hgb (HgA^{T87Q}), and exagamglogene autotemcel, that uses clustered regularly interspaced short palindromic repeats (CRISPR) gene-editing therapy to disrupt the *BCL11A* gene and increase hemoglobin F levels. Allogeneic hematopoietic cell transplant (ie, from another person as the donor) is potentially curative in younger patient with SS disease but with treatment-related morbidity and mortality as competing considerations.

Prognosis

Sickle cell anemia becomes a chronic multisystem disease, leading to organ failure and shortened survival. With improved supportive care, average life expectancy is now between 40 and 50 years of age.

When to Refer

Patients with sickle cell anemia should have their care coordinated with a hematologist and should be referred to a Comprehensive Sickle Cell Center, if available.

When to Admit

Patients should be admitted for management of acute chest syndrome, for aplastic crisis, or for painful episodes that do not respond to outpatient interventions.

Ball J et al. Hematopoietic stem cell therapy with gene modification to treat sickle cell disease. Stem Cells Transl Med. 2025;14:szaf042. [PMID: 40966451]

Bhalla N et al. Allogeneic hematopoietic stem cell transplantation to cure sickle cell disease: a review. Front Med (Lusanne). 2023;10:1036939. [PMID: 36910492]

Dassap AM et al. Guidelines for the management of emergencies and critical illness in pediatric and adult patients with sickle cell disease. Ann Intensive Care. 2025;15:74. [PMID: 40439782]

Kanter J et al. Biologic and clinical efficacy of LentiGlobin for sickle cell disease. N Engl J Med. 2022;386:617. [PMID: 34898139]

Youssry I et al. Sickle cell disease: combination new therapies vs. CRISPR-Cas9 potential and challenges—review article. Ann Hematol. 2024;103:2623. [PMID: 37867187]

SICKLE THALASSEMIA

Patients with **homozygous sickle cell anemia and α-thalassemia** have less vigorous hemolysis and run higher hemoglobins than SS patients. This is due to reduced RBC sickling related to a lower hemoglobin concentration within the RBC and higher hemoglobin F levels (Table 15–9). The MCV is low, and the RBCs are hypochromic.

Patients who **are compound heterozygotes for β^s and β-thalassemia** are clinically affected with sickle cell syndromes. **Sickle β^0-thalassemia** is clinically very similar to homozygous SS disease. Vaso-occlusive crises may be somewhat less severe, and the spleen is not always infarcted. The MCV is low unlike the normal MCV of sickle cell anemia. Hemoglobin electrophoresis reveals no hemoglobin A but will show an increase in hemoglobins A_2 and F (Table 15–9).

Sickle β^+-thalassemia is a milder disorder than homozygous SS disease, with fewer pain episodes but more acute chest syndrome than sickle β^0-thalassemia. The spleen is usually palpable. The hemolytic anemia is less severe, and the hematocrit is usually 30–38%, with reticulocytes of 5–10%. Hemoglobin electrophoresis shows some hemoglobin A and elevated hemoglobins A_2 and F (Table 15–9). The MCV is low.

Kirkham JK et al. Genetic variation and sickle cell disease severity: a systematic review and meta-analysis. JAMA Netw Open. 2023;6:e2337484. [PMID: 37851445]

WARM AUTOIMMUNE HEMOLYTIC ANEMIA

ESSENTIALS OF DIAGNOSIS

- Acquired hemolytic anemia caused by IgG autoantibody.
- Spherocytes and reticulocytosis on peripheral blood smear.
- Positive antiglobulin (Coombs) test.

General Considerations

Warm autoimmune hemolytic anemia is an acquired disorder in which an IgG autoantibody is formed that binds to an RBC membrane protein and does so most avidly at body temperature (ie, a "warm" autoantibody). The antibody is most commonly directed against a basic component of the Rh system present on RBCs. When IgG antibodies coat the RBC, the Fc portion of the antibody is recognized by macrophages present in the spleen and other portions of the reticuloendothelial system. The interaction between splenic macrophages and the antibody-coated RBC results in removal of RBC membrane and the formation of a spherocyte due to the decrease in surface-to-volume ratio of the surviving RBC. These spherocytic cells have decreased deformability and are unable to squeeze through the 2-mcm fenestrations of splenic sinusoids and become trapped in the red pulp of the spleen. When large amounts of IgG are present on RBCs, complement may also be fixed. Direct complement lysis of cells is rare, but the presence of C3b on the surface of RBCs allows Kupffer cells in the liver to participate in the hemolytic process via C3b receptors. *The destruction of RBCs in the spleen and liver indicates extravascular hemolysis.* The clinical distinction between extra- and intravascular hemolysis is not always straightforward.

Approximately one-half of all cases of autoimmune hemolytic anemia are idiopathic. The disorder may also be seen in association with SLE, other rheumatic disorders, chronic lymphocytic leukemia (CLL), or lymphomas. It must be distinguished from drug-induced hemolytic anemia. When penicillin (or other medications, especially cefotetan, ceftriaxone, and piperacillin) coats the RBC membrane, the autoantibody is directed against the membrane-drug complex (ie, the hemolysis is hapten-mediated). Fludarabine, an antineoplastic, causes autoimmune hemolytic anemia through immune dysregulation: there is defective self- versus non–self-immune surveillance permitting the escape of a B-cell clone, which produces the offending autoantibody.

Clinical Findings

A. Symptoms and Signs

Autoimmune hemolytic anemia typically produces an anemia of rapid onset that may be life-threatening. Patients report fatigue and dyspnea and may present with angina pectoris or HF or CNS ischemic symptoms. On examination, jaundice and splenomegaly are often present.

B. Laboratory Findings

The anemia is of variable degree but may be very severe, sometimes with a hematocrit of < 10%. Reticulocytosis is present, and spherocytes are seen on the peripheral blood smear. In cases of severe hemolysis, the stressed bone marrow may also release nucleated RBCs. As with other hemolytic disorders, the serum indirect bilirubin is increased and the haptoglobin is low. Approximately 10% of patients with autoimmune hemolytic anemia have coincident immune thrombocytopenia (**Evans syndrome**).

The antiglobulin (Coombs) test forms the basis for diagnosis. The Coombs reagent is a rabbit IgM antibody raised against human IgG or human complement. The **direct antiglobulin (Coombs) test (DAT)** is performed by mixing the patient's RBCs with the Coombs reagent and looking for agglutination, which indicates the presence of IgG or both IgG and complement on the RBC surface. The **indirect antiglobulin (Coombs) test** is performed by mixing the patient's serum with a panel of type O RBCs. After incubation of the test serum and panel RBCs, the Coombs reagent is added. Agglutination in this system indicates the presence of free antibody (autoantibody or alloantibody) in the patient's serum.

The direct antiglobulin test is positive (for IgG or both IgG and complement) in about 90% of patients with autoimmune hemolytic anemia. The more sensitive "super-Coombs" test might be positive in some of the 10% negative group. The indirect antiglobulin test may or may not be positive. A positive indirect antiglobulin test indicates the presence of a large amount of autoantibody that has saturated binding sites on the RBC and consequently appears in the serum. Because the patient's serum usually contains the autoantibody, it may be difficult to obtain a "compatible" cross-match with homologous RBCs for transfusions since the cross-match indicates the possible presence (true or false) of an RBC "alloantibody."

Treatment

Initial treatment consists of oral prednisone, 1–2 mg/kg/day for several weeks, followed by a slow taper. Patients with DAT-positive and DAT-negative warm autoimmune hemolysis respond equally well to corticosteroids. Transfused RBCs will survive similarly as the patient's own RBCs (ie, shortened survival). Because of difficulty in performing the cross-match, often "incompatible" blood may need to be given. Decisions regarding transfusions should be made in consultation with a hematologist and a blood bank specialist. Death from cardiovascular collapse can occur in the setting of very rapid hemolysis. In such patients, therapeutic plasmapheresis should be performed early in management to remove autoantibodies.

Patients with warm autoimmune hemolytic anemia refractory to prednisone may also be treated with a variety of agents. Treatment with rituximab, a monoclonal antibody against the B-cell antigen CD20, is effective in many cases. The suggested dose is 375 mg/m^2 intravenously weekly for 4 weeks. Rituximab is used in conjunction with corticosteroids as initial therapy in some patients with severe disease. In patients receiving rituximab with past hepatitis B virus (HBV) infection, an anti-HBV agent should be used since HBV reactivation, fulminant hepatitis and, rarely, death can otherwise occur. Immunosuppressive agents, including cyclophosphamide, vincristine, azathioprine, mycophenolate mofetil, alemtuzumab (an anti-CD52 antibody), or cyclosporine, may also be used. High-dose intravenous immune globulin (1 g/kg daily for 2 days) may be effective in controlling hemolysis, but the benefit is short-lived (1–3 weeks) and immune globulin is very expensive. If prednisone or other medical therapies are ineffective, splenectomy can be considered, which may cure the disorder. The long-term prognosis for patients with this disorder is good, especially if there is no other underlying autoimmune disorder or lymphoproliferative disorder. Treatment of an associated lymphoproliferative disorder will also treat the hemolytic anemia. Bruton tyrosine kinase (BTK) inhibitors have proven effective in treating autoimmune hemolysis in conjunction with CLL, and there is some evidence that these agents can work in idiopathic cases (particularly rilzabrutinib).

When to Refer

Patients with autoimmune hemolytic anemia should be referred to a hematologist for confirmation of the diagnosis and subsequent care.

When to Admit

Patients should be hospitalized for symptomatic anemia or rapidly falling hemoglobin levels.

Loriamini M et al. Autoimmune hemolytic anemias: classifications, pathophysiology, diagnoses and management. Int J Mol Sci. 2024;25:4296. [PMID: 38673882]

Mukherjee D et al. Advancements in autoimmune hemolytic anemia (AIHA) treatment: exploring emerging therapies. Leuk Res. 2025;156:107910. [PMID: 40669399]

Robak E et al. Bruton's kinase inhibitors for the treatment of immunological diseases: current status and perspectives. J Clin Med. 2022;11:2807. [PMID: 35628931]

COLD AGGLUTININ DISEASE

ESSENTIALS OF DIAGNOSIS

- Increased reticulocytes on peripheral blood smear.
- Antiglobulin (Coombs) test positive only for complement.
- Positive cold agglutinin titer.

General Considerations

Cold agglutinin disease is an acquired hemolytic anemia due to an *IgM autoantibody (called a "cold agglutinin") usually directed against the I/i antigen on RBCs.* These IgM autoantibodies characteristically will react poorly with cells at 37°C but avidly at lower temperatures, usually at 0–4°C (ie, "cold" autoantibody). Since the blood temperature (even in the most peripheral parts of the body) rarely goes lower than 20°C, only cold autoantibodies reactive at relatively higher temperatures will produce clinical effects. Hemolysis results indirectly from attachment of IgM, which in the cooler parts of the circulation (fingers, nose, ears) binds and fixes complement. When the RBC returns to a warmer temperature, the IgM antibody dissociates, leaving complement on the cell. Complement lysis of RBCs rarely occurs. Rather, C3b, present on the RBCs, is recognized by liver Kupffer cells (which have receptors for C3b) and RBC sequestration and destruction in the liver ensues (extravascular hemolysis). However, in some cases, the complement membrane attacks complex forms, lysing the RBCs (intravascular hemolysis).

Most cases of chronic cold agglutinin disease are idiopathic. Others occur in association with Waldenström macroglobulinemia, lymphoma, or CLL, in which a monoclonal IgM paraprotein is produced. Acute postinfectious cold agglutinin disease can occur following mycoplasma pneumonia or viral infection (infectious mononucleosis, measles, mumps, or cytomegalovirus [CMV] with autoantibody directed against antigen i rather than I).

Clinical Findings

A. Symptoms and Signs

In chronic cold agglutinin disease, symptoms related to RBC agglutination occur on exposure to cold temperatures, and patients may report mottled or numb fingers or toes, acrocyanosis, episodic low back pain, and dark-colored urine. Hemolytic anemia is occasionally severe. Episodic hemoglobinuria may occur on exposure to cold. Hemolytic anemia in acute postinfectious syndromes is usually nonexistent or mild.

B. Laboratory Findings

Mild anemia is present with reticulocytosis and rarely spherocytes. The blood smear made at room temperature shows agglutinated RBCs (there is no agglutination on a blood smear made at body temperature). *The direct antiglobulin (Coombs) test will be positive for complement only.* Serum cold agglutinin titer will semi-quantitate the autoantibody. A monoclonal IgM is often found on serum protein electrophoresis and confirmed by serum immunoelectrophoresis. There is indirect hyperbilirubinemia and the haptoglobin is low during periods of hemolysis. Serum free hemoglobin is often elevated, and hemoglobinuria is present when intravascular hemolysis is occurring.

Treatment

Treatment is largely symptomatic, based on avoiding exposure to cold. Splenectomy and prednisone are usually ineffective (except when associated with a lymphoproliferative disorder) since hemolysis takes place in the liver and bloodstream. Rituximab is the treatment of choice, but in patients with past HBV infection, it must be used with anti-HBV prophylaxis. The suggested rituximab dose is 375 mg/m^2 intravenously weekly for 4 weeks. Relapses may be effectively re-treated. High-dose intravenous immunoglobulin (2 g/kg) may be temporarily effective, but it is rarely used because of the high cost and short duration of benefit. Patients with severe disease may be treated with cytotoxic agents, such as bendamustine (plus rituximab), cyclophosphamide, fludarabine, or bortezomib, or with immunosuppressive agents, such as cyclosporine. Complement blockade of the C1s protein with sutimlimab (a monoclonal protein) is now FDA approved for cold agglutinin hemolysis. As in warm IgG-mediated autoimmune hemolysis, it may be difficult to find compatible blood for transfusion. RBCs should be transfused through an in-line blood warmer.

Loriamini M et al. Autoimmune hemolytic anemias: classifications, pathophysiology, diagnoses and management. Int J Mol Sci. 2024;25:4296. [PMID: 38673882]
Röth A et al. Sutimlimab in cold agglutinin disease. N Engl J Med. 2021;384:1323. [PMID: 33826820]

APLASTIC ANEMIA

ESSENTIALS OF DIAGNOSIS

- Pancytopenia.
- No abnormal hematopoietic cells seen in blood or bone marrow.
- Hypocellular bone marrow.

General Considerations

Aplastic anemia is a condition of bone marrow failure that arises from suppression of, and/or injury to, the hematopoietic stem cell. The bone marrow becomes hypoplastic, fails to produce mature blood cells, and pancytopenia develops.

There are a number of causes of aplastic anemia (Table 15–10). Direct hematopoietic stem cell injury may be caused by radiation, chemotherapy, toxins, or pharmacologic agents. SLE may rarely cause suppression of the hematopoietic stem cell by an IgG autoantibody directed against it. However, the most common pathogenesis of aplastic anemia appears to be autoimmune suppression of hematopoiesis by a T-cell-mediated cellular mechanism, so-called **idiopathic aplastic anemia.** In some cases of idiopathic aplastic anemia, defects in maintenance of the hematopoietic stem cell telomere length (eg, dyskeratosis congenita) or in DNA repair pathways (eg, Fanconi anemia) have been identified and are likely linked to both the initiation of bone marrow failure and the propensity to later progress to myelodysplasia, PNH, or AML. Complex detrimental immune responses to viruses can also cause aplastic anemia.

Table 15–10. Causes of aplastic anemia (in alphabetical order).

Autoimmune: idiopathic, SLE
Chemotherapy, radiotherapy
Congenital: defects in telomere length maintenance or DNA repair (dyskeratosis congenita, Fanconi anemia, etc)
Malignancy: T cell large granular lymphocytic leukemia (T-LGL)
Medications: chloramphenicol, gold salts, sulfonamides, phenytoin, carbamazepine, quinacrine, tolbutamide
Non-hepatitis viruses (EBV, parvovirus, CMV, echovirus 3, others)
Paroxysmal nocturnal hemoglobinuria
Post-viral hepatitis (viral agent known or unknown)
Pregnancy
Toxins: benzene, toluene, insecticides

CMV, cytomegalovirus; EBV, Epstein-Barr virus.

Clinical Findings

A. Symptoms and Signs

Patients come to medical attention because of the consequences of bone marrow failure. Anemia leads to symptoms of weakness and fatigue, neutropenia causes vulnerability to bacterial or fungal infections, and thrombocytopenia results in mucosal and skin bleeding. Physical examination may reveal signs of pallor, purpura, and petechiae. Other abnormalities, such as hepatosplenomegaly, lymphadenopathy, or bone tenderness, should *not* be present, and their presence should prompt questioning of the diagnosis.

B. Laboratory Findings

The hallmark of aplastic anemia is **pancytopenia (neutropenia, anemia, and thrombocytopenia)**. However, early in the evolution of aplastic anemia, only one or two cell lines may be reduced.

Anemia may be severe and is always associated with reticulocytopenia. RBC morphology is unremarkable, but there may be mild macrocytosis (increased MCV). Neutrophils and platelets are reduced in number, and no immature or abnormal forms are seen on the blood smear. The bone marrow aspirate and the bone marrow biopsy appear hypocellular, with only scant amounts of morphologically normal hematopoietic progenitors. The prior dictum that the bone marrow karyotype should be normal (or germline if normal variant) has evolved and *some clonal abnormalities or other genetic aberrations may be present even in the setting of idiopathic aplastic anemia.*

Differential Diagnosis

Aplastic anemia must be differentiated from other causes of pancytopenia (Table 15–11). Hypocellular forms of myelodysplasia or acute leukemia may occasionally be confused with aplastic anemia. These are differentiated by the presence of cellular morphologic abnormalities, increased percentage of blasts, or abnormal karyotype in bone marrow cells typical of MDS or acute leukemia. Hypocellular hairy cell leukemia has been misdiagnosed as aplastic anemia and

Table 15–11. Causes of pancytopenia (in alphabetical order within categories).

Bone marrow disorders
Acute leukemia
Aplastic anemia
Chronic idiopathic myelofibrosis
Infiltrative disease: lymphoma, myeloma, carcinoma, hairy cell leukemia, etc
Myelodysplasia
Non–bone marrow disorders
Cytotoxic chemotherapy
Hypersplenism (with or without portal hypertension)
Infection: tuberculosis, HIV, leishmaniasis, brucellosis, CMV, parvovirus B19
Ionizing radiation
Nutritional deficiency (megaloblastic anemia)
Medications
SLE

CMV, cytomegalovirus.

should be recognized by the presence of splenomegaly and by abnormal "hairy" lymphoid cells in a hypocellular bone marrow biopsy. Pancytopenia with a normocellular bone marrow may be due to SLE, disseminated infection, hypersplenism, nutritional (eg, vitamin B_{12} or folate) deficiency, or myelodysplasia. Isolated thrombocytopenia may occur early as aplastic anemia develops and may be confused with immune thrombocytopenia.

Treatment

Mild cases of idiopathic aplastic anemia may be treated with supportive care, including erythropoietic (epoetin or darbepoetin or biosimilars) or myeloid (filgrastim or sargramostim or other biosimilars) growth factors, or both. RBC transfusions and platelet transfusions are given as necessary, and antibiotics are used to treat or prevent infections.

Severe aplastic anemia is defined by a neutrophil count of < 500/mcL (0.5×10^9/L), platelets < 20,000/mcL (20×10^9/L), reticulocytes < 1%, and bone marrow cellularity < 20%. The treatment of choice for young adults (under age 40 years) with severe idiopathic aplastic anemia who have an HLA-matched sibling or unrelated donor is allogeneic bone marrow transplantation. Because of the increased risks associated with unrelated donor allogeneic bone marrow transplantation compared to sibling donors, this treatment is sometimes reserved for patients who have not responded to immunosuppressive therapy.

For adults over age 40 years or those without HLA-matched hematopoietic bone marrow donors, the treatment of choice for severe idiopathic aplastic anemia is immunosuppression with equine antithymocyte globulin (ATG) plus cyclosporine and hematopoietic stimulation with eltrombopag (a thrombopoietin mimetic) (response rates approaching 90%). Equine ATG is given in the hospital in conjunction with transfusion and antibiotic support. An established regimen is equine ATG 40 mg/kg/day intravenously for 4 days in combination with cyclosporine, 6 mg/kg orally twice daily, and eltrombopag, 150 mg orally daily. Equine ATG is superior to rabbit ATG, resulting in a higher response rate and better survival. ATG should be used in combination with corticosteroids (prednisone or methylprednisolone 1–2 mg/kg/day orally for 1 week, followed by a taper over 2 weeks) to avoid ATG infusion reactions and serum sickness. Responses usually occur within 1–3 months and are usually only partial, but the blood counts rise high enough to give patients a safe and transfusion-free life. The full benefit of immunosuppression is generally assessed at 4 months post-equine ATG. Eltrombopag is maintained at full doses for 6 months and then stopped in responding patients, with cyclosporine generally continued for 2 years.

Course & Prognosis

Patients with severe aplastic anemia have a rapidly fatal illness if left untreated. Allogeneic bone marrow transplant from an HLA-matched sibling donor produces survival rates of over 90% in recipients under 20 years old and of about 85% in those 20–50 years old. Respective survival rates drop by about 5% when the donor is HLA-matched but unrelated. Equine ATG-cyclosporine immunosuppressive treatment leads to a response in approximately 70% of patients (including those with hepatitis virus–associated aplastic anemia) and in up to 90% of patients with the addition of eltrombopag. Up to one-third of patients will relapse with aplastic anemia after ATG-based therapy. Clonal hematologic disorders, such as PNH, AML, or myelodysplasia, may develop in one-quarter of patients treated with immunosuppressive therapy after 10 years of follow-up. Factors that predict response to ATG-cyclosporine therapy are patient's age, reticulocyte count, lymphocyte count, and age-adjusted telomere length of leukocytes at the time of diagnosis.

When to Refer

All patients should be referred to a hematologist.

When to Admit

Admission is necessary for treatment of neutropenic infection, the administration of ATG, or allogeneic bone marrow transplantation.

Guo H et al. Safety and efficacy of eltrombopag in patients with aplastic anemia: a systematic review and meta-analysis of randomized clinical trials. Hematology. 2024;29:2335419. [PMID: 38553907]

Hong Y et al. Efficacy and safety of hematopoietic stem cell transplantation vs. immunosuppressive therapy in patients with hepatitis-associated aplastic anemia: a systematic review and meta-analysis. Hematology. 2025;30:2548990. [PMID: 40922718]

Pan P et al. Autoimmune pathogenesis, immunosuppressive therapy and pharmacological mechanism in aplastic anemia. Int Immunopharmacol. 2023;117:110036. [PMID: 36940553]

Piekarska A et al. The state of the art in the treatment of severe aplastic anemia: immunotherapy and hematopoietic cell transplantation in children and adults. Front Immunol. 2024;15:1378432. [PMID: 38646536]

NEUTROPENIA

ESSENTIALS OF DIAGNOSIS

- Neutrophils < 1800/mcL (1.8 × 10^9/L).
- Severe if neutrophils < 500/mcL (0.5 × 10^9/L).

General Considerations

Neutropenia is present when the absolute neutrophil count is < 1800/mcL (1.8 × 10^9/L), although *Black, South Asian, and other persons in specific ethnic groups may have normal neutrophil counts as low as 800–1200/mcL (0.8–1.2 × 10^9/L) or even less.* Africans with isolated neutropenia usually have a Duffy-null (Fy(a) and Fy(b) negative) RBC phenotype (protective against malaria), now referred to as DNAC (Duffy Null associated neutrophil count). The non-DNAC neutropenic patient is increasingly vulnerable to infection by gram-positive and gram-negative bacteria and by fungi. The risk of infection is related to the severity of neutropenia. The risk of serious infection rises sharply with neutrophil counts < 500/mcL (0.5 × 10^9/L), and a high risk of infection within days occurs with neutrophil counts < 100/mcL (0.1 × 10^9/L) ("**profound neutropenia**"). The classification of neutropenic syndromes is unsatisfactory as the pathophysiology and natural history of different syndromes overlap. Patients with DNAC are free of infection despite very low stable neutrophil counts; they respond adequately to infections and inflammatory stimuli with an appropriate neutrophil release from the bone marrow. In contrast, the neutrophil count of patients with **cyclic neutropenia** periodically oscillates (usually in 21-day cycles) between normal and low, with infections and oral ulcers occurring during the nadirs. Congenital neutropenia is lifelong neutropenia punctuated with bouts of infection.

A variety of bone marrow disorders and non-marrow conditions may cause neutropenia (Table 15–12). All the causes of aplastic anemia (Table 15–10) and pancytopenia (Table 15–11) may cause neutropenia. The **new** onset of an **isolated** neutropenia is most often due to an idiosyncratic reaction to a medication, and **agranulocytosis** (complete absence of neutrophils in the peripheral blood) is almost always due to a drug reaction. In these cases, bone marrow examination shows a nearly complete absence of granulocyte precursors, with other cell lines undisturbed. Neutropenia in the presence of a normal bone marrow may be due to immunologic peripheral destruction (**autoimmune neutropenia**), sepsis, or hypersplenism. The presence in the serum of antineutrophil antibodies supports the diagnosis of autoimmune neutropenia but does not prove this as the pathophysiologic reason for neutropenia. **Felty syndrome** is an immune neutropenia associated with seropositive nodular rheumatoid arthritis and splenomegaly. Severe neutropenia may be associated with clonal disorders of T lymphocytes, often with the morphology of large granular lymphocytes, referred to as CD3-positive T-cell large granular lymphoproliferative disorder. Isolated neutropenia is an uncommon presentation of hairy cell leukemia or MDS. By its nature, myelosuppressive cytotoxic chemotherapy causes neutropenia in a predictable manner.

Table 15–12. Causes of neutropenia (in alphabetical order within categories).

Bone marrow disorders
Congenital
Dyskeratosis congenita
Fanconi anemia
Other
Congenital neutropenia
Cyclic neutropenia
Hairy cell leukemia
Large granular lymphoproliferative disorder
Myelodysplasia
Non–bone marrow disorders
Aplastic anemia
Benign chronic neutropenia
DNAC
Hypersplenism
Medications: antiretroviral medications, cephalosporins, chlorpromazine, chlorpropamide, cimetidine, methimazole, myelosuppressive cytotoxic chemotherapy, penicillin, phenytoin, procainamide, rituximab, sulfonamides
Other immune
Autoimmune (idiopathic)
Felty syndrome
HIV infection
SLE
Pure WBC aplasia
Sepsis

DNAC, Duffy Null associated neutrophil count.

Clinical Findings

Neutropenia results in stomatitis and in infections due to gram-positive or gram-negative aerobic bacteria or to fungi such as *Candida* or *Aspergillus*. The most common infectious syndromes are sinusitis, cellulitis, pneumonia, septicemia, and neutropenic fever of unknown origin. *Fever in neutropenic patients should always be initially assumed to be of infectious origin until proven otherwise* (Chapter 34).

Treatment

Treatment of neutropenia depends on its cause. Potential causative medications (especially cephalosporin antibiotics, chloramphenicol, or neuroleptics) should be discontinued and replaced as feasible. Myeloid growth factors (filgrastim or sargramostim or biosimilar myeloid growth factors) help facilitate neutrophil recovery after offending medications are stopped. Chronic myeloid growth factor administration (daily or other interval) is effective at dampening the neutropenia seen in cyclic or congenital neutropenia. Novel treatments are being explored (inhibitors of CXCR4, neutrophil elastase, and SGLT-2). When Felty syndrome leads to repeated bacterial infections, splenectomy has been the treatment of choice, but sustained use of myeloid growth factors is effective and provides a nonsurgical alternative. Patients with autoimmune neutropenia respond in the short term to immunosuppression with corticosteroids but are best managed long term with intermittent doses of myeloid growth factors. The neutropenia associated with large granular lymphoproliferative disorder may respond to therapy with oral methotrexate, cyclophosphamide, or cyclosporine as well as other fourth-line treatments.

Fevers during neutropenia should be considered as infectious until proven otherwise and can be life-threatening. Enteric gram-negative bacteria are of primary concern and often empirically treated with fluoroquinolones or third- or fourth-generation cephalosporins (see Infections in the Immunocompromised Patient, Chapter 34). For protracted neutropenia, fungal infections are problematic and empiric coverage with azoles (fluconazole for yeast and voriconazole, itraconazole, posaconazole, or isavuconazole for molds) or echinocandins is recommended. The neutropenia following myelosuppressive chemotherapy is predictable and is partially ameliorated with myeloid growth factors. For patients with acute leukemia undergoing intense chemotherapy or patients with solid cancer undergoing high-dose chemotherapy, the prophylactic use of antimicrobial agents and myeloid growth factors is recommended.

When to Refer

Refer to a hematologist if neutrophils are persistently and unexplainably < 1000/mcL (1.0×10^9/L) or if continued therapy is needed.

When to Admit

Neutropenia by itself is not an indication for hospitalization. However, many patients with severe neutropenia may have a serious underlying disease that may require inpatient treatment. Many patients with febrile neutropenia require hospitalization to treat infection.

Cossey J et al. Evaluation and management of febrile neutropenia in patients with cancer. JAAPA. 2024;37:16. [PMID: 38980295]
Dale DC et al. Outcomes for patients with severe chronic neutropenia treated with granulocyte colony-stimulating factor. Blood Adv. 2022;6:3861. [PMID: 35476051]
Dale DC et al. The promise of novel treatments for severe chronic neutropenia. Expert Rev Hematol. 2023;16:1025. [PMID: 37978893]

Table 15–13. WHO classification of myeloid neoplasms (modified).

Myeloproliferative neoplasms
Chronic myeloid leukemia
Chronic neutrophilic leukemia
Polycythemia vera
Primary myelofibrosis (PMF)
Essential thrombocythemia
Chronic eosinophilic leukemia
Myeloproliferative neoplasm, not otherwise specified
Juvenile myelomonocytic leukemia
Mastocytosis
Myelodysplastic/myeloproliferative neoplasms (MDS/MPN)
Myelodysplastic neoplasms
Acute myeloid leukemia and related neoplasms
Acute myeloid leukemia with defining genetic abnormalities
Acute myeloid leukemia defined by differentiation
Acute myeloid leukemia, myelodysplasia-related
Myeloid sarcoma
Myeloid neoplasms associated with germline predisposition
Myeloid neoplasms post cytotoxic therapy
Acute leukemias of ambiguous lineage
B lymphoblastic leukemia/lymphoma
T lymphoblastic leukemia/lymphoma

LEUKEMIAS & OTHER MYELOPROLIFERATIVE NEOPLASMS

Myeloproliferative disorders are due to *acquired clonal abnormalities of the hematopoietic stem cell.* Since the stem cell gives rise to myeloid, erythroid, and platelet cells, qualitative and quantitative changes are seen in all of these cell lines. Classically, the myeloproliferative disorders produce characteristic syndromes with well-defined clinical and laboratory features (Tables 15–13 and 15–14). However, these disorders are grouped together because they may evolve from one into another and because hybrid disorders are commonly seen. All of the myeloproliferative disorders may progress to AML.

The Philadelphia chromosome seen in chronic myeloid leukemia (CML) was the first recurrent cytogenetic abnormality to be described in a human malignancy. Since that time, there has been tremendous progress in elucidating the genetic nature of these disorders, with identification of pathogenic variants of *JAK2, MPL, CALR, CSF3R,* and other genes.

Table 15–14. Laboratory features of myeloproliferative neoplasms (listed in alphabetical order).

	White Count	Hematocrit	Platelet Count	RBC Morphology
Chronic myeloid leukemia	↑↑	N or ↓	N or ↑ or ↓	N
Essential thrombocytosis	N or ↑	N	↑↑	N
Polycythemia vera	N or ↑	↑↑	N or ↑	N
Primary myelofibrosis	N or ↓ or ↑	↓	↓ or N or ↑	Abn

Abn, abnormal; N, normal.

Loscocco GG et al. Mutation profiling of chronic myeloproliferative neoplasms: improving clinical-molecular prognostic models. Expert Rev Mol Diagn. 2025;25:775. [PMID: 41074259]
Prakash S et al. Diagnostic approach to myeloproliferative neoplasms and myelodysplastic/myeloproliferative neoplasms. Adv Anat Pathol. 2025;32:284. [PMID: 40243206]

POLYCYTHEMIA VERA

ESSENTIALS OF DIAGNOSIS

- Pathogenic variant of *JAK2 (V617F)*.
- Splenomegaly.
- Normal arterial oxygen saturation.
- Usually elevated WBC and platelet count.

General Considerations

Polycythemia vera is an acquired myeloproliferative disorder that causes overproduction of all three hematopoietic cell lines, most prominently the RBCs. Sixty percent of patients are men, and the median age at presentation is 60 years. Polycythemia vera rarely occurs in persons under age 40 years. Erythroid production is independent of erythropoietin, and the serum erythropoietin level is low. True erythrocytosis, with an elevated RBC mass, should be distinguished from spurious erythrocytosis caused by a constricted plasma volume.

A pathogenic variant in exon 14 of *JAK2 (V617F)*, a signaling molecule, has been demonstrated in 95% of cases. Additional *JAK2* variants have been identified (exon 12) and suggest that *JAK2* is involved in the pathogenesis of this disease and is a therapeutic target.

Clinical Findings

A. Symptoms and Signs

Headache, dizziness, tinnitus, blurred vision, and fatigue are common complaints related to expanded blood volume and increased blood viscosity. Generalized pruritus, especially following a warm shower or bath, is related to histamine release from the basophilia. Epistaxis is related to engorgement of mucosal blood vessels in combination with abnormal hemostasis.

Physical examination reveals plethora and engorged retinal veins. The spleen is palpable in 75% of cases but is nearly always enlarged when imaged. Thrombosis is the most common complication of polycythemia vera and the major cause of morbidity and death in this disorder. Thrombosis appears to be related both to increased blood viscosity and abnormal platelet function. Uncontrolled polycythemia leads to a very high incidence of thrombotic complications of surgery, and elective surgery should be deferred until the condition has been treated. Paradoxically, in addition to thrombosis, increased bleeding can occur. There is also a high incidence of peptic ulcer disease.

B. Laboratory Findings

According to the ICC and revised WHO criteria, the hallmark of polycythemia vera is a *hematocrit (at sea level) that exceeds 49% in males or 48% in females*. RBC morphology is normal (Table 15–14). The WBC is usually elevated to 10,000–20,000/mcL ($10–20 \times 10^9$/L), and the platelet count is variably increased, sometimes to counts exceeding 1,000,000/mcL (1000×10^9/L). Basophilia and eosinophilia are frequently present. Erythropoietin is suppressed and serum levels are usually low. The diagnosis should be confirmed with screening for a *JAK2* pathogenic variant. The absence of a variant in either exon 14 (most common) or 12 should lead the clinician to question the diagnosis.

The bone marrow is hypercellular, with hyperplasia of all hematopoietic elements, but bone marrow examination is not necessary to establish the diagnosis. Iron stores are usually absent from the bone marrow, having been transferred to the increased circulating RBC mass. Iron deficiency may also result from chronic GI blood loss. Bleeding may lower the hematocrit to the normal range (or lower), creating diagnostic confusion, and may lead to a situation with significant microcytosis yet a normal hematocrit.

Vitamin B_{12} levels are strikingly elevated because of increased levels of transcobalamin III (secreted by WBCs). Overproduction of uric acid may lead to hyperuricemia.

Although RBC morphology is usually normal at presentation, microcytosis, hypochromia, and poikilocytosis may result from iron deficiency following treatment by phlebotomy. Progressive hypersplenism may also lead to elliptocytosis (eg, with RBCs the size and shape of those in hereditary elliptocytosis).

Differential Diagnosis

Spurious polycythemia, in which an elevated hematocrit is due to contracted plasma volume rather than increased RBC mass, may be related to diuretic use or may occur without obvious cause.

A **secondary cause of polycythemia** should be suspected if splenomegaly is absent and the high hematocrit is not accompanied by increases in other cell lines. Secondary causes of polycythemia include hypoxia and smoking; carboxyhemoglobin levels may be elevated in smokers (Table 15–15). A renal CT scan or sonogram may be considered to look for an erythropoietin-secreting cyst or tumor. A positive family history should lead to investigation for a congenital high-oxygen-affinity hemoglobin. An absence of a pathogenic variant in *JAK2* suggests a different

Table 15–15. Causes of polycythemia (in alphabetical order within categories).

Polycythemia vera
Secondary polycythemia
Abnormal hemoglobins (rare)
Carboxyhemoglobin: smoking
Erythropoietin-secreting tumors, eg, kidney lesions (rare)
Hypoxia: cardiac disease, pulmonary disease, high altitude
Spurious polycythemia

diagnosis. However, *JAK2* variants are also commonly found in other myeloproliferative disorders, essential thrombocytosis, and myelofibrosis.

Polycythemia vera should be differentiated from other myeloproliferative disorders (Table 15–14). Marked elevation of the WBC (> 30,000/mcL [30 × 10^9/L]) suggests CML. Abnormal RBC morphology and nucleated RBCs in the peripheral blood are seen in myelofibrosis. Essential thrombocytosis is suggested when the platelet count is strikingly elevated.

Treatment

The treatment of choice is phlebotomy. One unit of blood (approximately 500 mL) is removed weekly until the hematocrit is < 45%; the hematocrit is maintained at < 45% by repeated phlebotomy as necessary. Because repeated phlebotomy intentionally produces iron deficiency, the requirement for phlebotomy should gradually decrease. It is important to avoid medicinal iron supplementation, as this can thwart the goals of a phlebotomy program. A diet low in iron is not necessary but will increase the intervals between phlebotomies. Maintaining the hematocrit at normal levels has been shown to decrease the incidence of thrombotic complications.

Occasionally, myelosuppressive therapy is indicated. Indications include a high phlebotomy requirement, thrombocytosis, and intractable pruritus. There is evidence that reducing the platelet count to < 600,000/mcL (600 × 10^9/L) reduces the risk of thrombotic complications. Hydroxyurea has historically been used when myelosuppressive therapy is indicated. The usual dose is 500–1500 mg/day orally, adjusted to keep platelets < 500,000/mcL (500 × 10^9/L) without reducing the neutrophil count to < 2000/mcL (2.0 × 10^9/L).

Ropeginterferon α-2b, a novel interferon, is approved as first-line therapy for patients without symptomatic splenomegaly, with 53% of patients achieving a complete hematologic response and with improved disease burden at 3 years' follow-up. Toxicity includes abnormal liver biochemical tests. The JAK1/2 inhibitor ruxolitinib, dosed at 10 mg twice a day, is the second-line therapy of choice for patients with refractory hematocrit without splenomegaly; it has a durable 22% improvement in control of the hematocrit. A novel hepcidin mimetic peptide, rusfertide, has shown great promise as another adjunctive treatment to phlebotomy with 60% of patients reaching the target hemoglobin level compared to 17% on placebo. Only 13% of the patients experienced an adverse event, with the most common being an injection site reaction.

Low-dose aspirin (75–81 mg/day orally) has been shown to reduce the risk of thrombosis without excessive bleeding and should be part of therapy for all patients without contraindications to aspirin. Aspirin should be used with caution in patients with extreme thrombocytosis due to the likelihood of acquired von Willebrand disease. Allopurinol 300 mg orally daily may be indicated for hyperuricemia. Antihistamine therapy with diphenhydramine or other H_1-blockers and, rarely, SSRIs are used to manage pruritus.

Prognosis

Polycythemia is an indolent disease with median survival of over 15 years. The major cause of morbidity and mortality is arterial thrombosis. Over time, polycythemia vera may convert to myelofibrosis. In approximately 5% of cases, the disorder progresses to AML, which is usually refractory to therapy.

When to Refer

Patients with polycythemia vera should be referred to a hematologist.

When to Admit

Inpatient care is rarely required.

Kremyanskaya M et al. Rusfertide, a hepcidin mimetic, for control of erythrocytosis in polycythemia vera. N Engl J Med. 2024;390:723. [PMID: 38381675]

Massarova L et al. Ten years of experience with ruxolitinib since approval for polycythemia vera: a review of clinical efficacy and safety. Cancer. 2025;131:e35661. [PMID: 39616447]

Tremblay D et al. Diagnosis and treatment of polycythemia vera: a review. JAMA. 2025;333:153. [PMID: 39556352]

ESSENTIAL THROMBOCYTOSIS

ESSENTIALS OF DIAGNOSIS

- Elevated platelet count in absence of other causes.
- Normal RBC mass.
- Absence of *bcr/abl* gene (Philadelphia chromosome).

General Considerations

Essential thrombocytosis is an uncommon myeloproliferative disorder in which marked proliferation of the megakaryocytes in the bone marrow leads to elevation of the platelet count.

Clinical Findings

A. Symptoms and Signs

The median age at presentation is over 60 years, and there is a slightly increased incidence in women. The disorder is often suspected when an elevated platelet count is found. Less frequently, the first sign is thrombosis, which is the most common clinical problem. The risk of thrombosis rises with age. Venous thromboses may occur in unusual sites such as the mesenteric, hepatic, or portal vein. Some patients experience erythromelalgia, painful burning of the hands accompanied by erythema; this symptom is reliably relieved by aspirin. Bleeding, typically mucosal, is less common and is related to a concomitant qualitative platelet defect. Splenomegaly is present in at least 25% of patients.

B. Laboratory Findings

An elevated platelet count is the hallmark of this disorder and may be over 2,000,000/mcL (2000 × 10^9/L) (see Table 15–14). The WBC count is often mildly elevated, usually not above 30,000/mcL (30 × 10^9/L), with some immature myeloid forms. The hematocrit is normal. The peripheral blood smear reveals large platelets, but giant degranulated forms seen in myelofibrosis are not observed. RBC morphology is normal.

The bone marrow shows increased numbers of megakaryocytes but no other morphologic abnormalities. The peripheral blood should be tested for the *bcr/abl* fusion gene (**Philadelphia chromosome**) since it can differentiate CML, where it is present, from essential thrombocytosis, where it is absent.

Differential Diagnosis

Essential thrombocytosis must be distinguished from secondary causes of an elevated platelet count. In reactive thrombocytosis, the platelet count seldom exceeds 1,000,000/mcL (1000 × 10^9/L). Inflammatory disorders such as rheumatoid arthritis and ulcerative colitis cause significant elevations of the platelet count, as may chronic infection. The thrombocytosis of iron deficiency is observed only when anemia is significant. The platelet count is temporarily elevated after a splenectomy. Regarding other myeloproliferative disorders, the lack of erythrocytosis distinguishes it from polycythemia vera. Unlike myelofibrosis, RBC morphology is normal, nucleated RBCs are absent, and giant degranulated platelets are not seen. In CML, the Philadelphia chromosome (or *bcr/abl* by molecular testing) establishes the diagnosis.

Approximately 80% of patients express driver mutations in JAK2, CALR, or MPL; about 50% harbor other mutations, the most frequent being TET2 (9–11%), ASXL1 (7–20%), DNMT3A (7%), and SF3B1 (5%). Abnormal karyotype is seen in < 10% of patients and includes +9/20q–/13q-.

Treatment

Patients are considered at high risk for thrombosis if they are older than 60 years, have a *JAK2* pathogenic variant, and have a previous history of thrombosis. They also have a higher risk for bleeding. The risk of thrombosis can be reduced by control of the platelet count, which should be kept under 500,000/mcL (500 × 10^9/L). The current treatment of choice is oral hydroxyurea in a dose of 500–1000 mg/day. In rare cases in which hydroxyurea is poorly tolerated due to anemia, low-dose anagrelide (1–2 mg/day orally) may be added. Higher doses of anagrelide can be complicated by headache, peripheral edema, and HF. Pegylated interferon α2 can induce significant hematologic responses and can potentially target the malignant clone in *CALR*-variant cases. Newer approaches to therapy include the orally available lysine-specific demethylase 1 (LSD1) inhibitor bomedemstat, which has shown promise in early clinical trials and is now being compared to first line treatment with hydroxyurea. Moreover, an antibody targeting the mutant calreticulin molecule on the cell surface in patients with type 1 CALR mutations, INCA033989, showed promise in early trials with rapid, durable hematological responses and a favorable safety profile and has received breakthrough designation by the FDA.

Vasomotor symptoms such as erythromelalgia and paresthesias respond rapidly to aspirin. Historically, low-dose aspirin (81 mg/day orally) has been used to reduce the risk of thrombotic complications in low-risk patients, but once daily dosing is not as effective as an every 12-hour regimen. In the unusual event of severe bleeding, the platelet count can be lowered rapidly with plateletpheresis. In cases of marked thrombocytosis (≥ 1,000,000/mcL [1000 × 10^9/L]) or of any evidence of bleeding, **acquired von Willebrand syndrome** must be excluded before starting low-dose aspirin. Strict control of coexistent cardiovascular risk factors is mandatory for all patients.

Course & Prognosis

Essential thrombocytosis is an indolent disorder that allows long-term survival. Average survival is longer than 18 years from diagnosis, and the survival of patients younger than age 50 years does not appear different from matched controls. The major source of morbidity—thrombosis—can be reduced by appropriate platelet control. Late in the disease course, the bone marrow may become fibrotic, and massive splenomegaly may occur, sometimes with splenic infarction. There is a 10–15% risk of progression to myelofibrosis after 15 years, and a 1–5% risk of transformation to acute leukemia over 20 years.

When to Refer

Patients with essential thrombocytosis should be referred to a hematologist.

Guy A et al. How I approach the treatment of thrombotic complications in patients with myeloproliferative neoplasms. Blood. 2025;145:1769. [PMID: 39541574]

Mazza GL et al; Myeloproliferative Neoplasms Research Consortium (MPN-RC) 111 and 112 trial teams. Symptom burden and quality of life in patients with high-risk essential thrombocythaemia and polycythaemia vera receiving hydroxyurea or pegylated interferon alfa-2a: a post-hoc analysis of the MPN-RC 111 and 112 trials. Lancet Haematol. 2022;9:e38. [PMID: 34971581]

Rocca B et al. A randomized double-blind trial of 3 aspirin regimens to optimize antiplatelet therapy in essential thrombocythemia. Blood. 2020;136:171. [PMID: 32266380]

Tefferi A et al. Essential thrombocythemia: a review. JAMA. 2025;333:701. [PMID: 39869325]

PRIMARY MYELOFIBROSIS

ESSENTIALS OF DIAGNOSIS

- Striking splenomegaly.
- Teardrop poikilocytosis on peripheral smear (misshapen RBCs).
- Leukoerythroblastic blood picture (abnormal white and red cell precursors in peripheral blood).
- Presence of giant abnormal platelets.

General Considerations

Primary myelofibrosis (PMF) is a myeloproliferative disorder characterized by clonal hematopoiesis that is often accompanied by pathogenic variants of *JAK2*, *CALR*, or *MPL* genes; bone marrow fibrosis; anemia; splenomegaly; and a leukoerythroblastic peripheral blood picture with **teardrop poikilocytosis**. In response to bone marrow fibrosis, extramedullary hematopoiesis takes place in the liver, spleen, and lymph nodes. According to the WHO and ICC classifications, "prefibrotic" primary myelofibrosis is distinguished from "overtly fibrotic" primary myelofibrosis; the former might mimic essential thrombocytosis in its presentation, and it is prognostically relevant to distinguish the two. The latter also can *occur as a secondary process following the other myeloproliferative disorders (eg, polycythemia vera, essential thrombocytosis).*

Clinical Findings

A. Symptoms and Signs

Primary myelofibrosis develops in adults over age 50 years and is usually insidious in onset. Patients most commonly present with fatigue due to anemia or with abdominal fullness related to splenomegaly. Uncommon presentations include bleeding and bone pain. On examination, splenomegaly is almost invariably present and is commonly massive. The liver is enlarged in > 50% of cases.

Later in the course of the disease, progressive bone marrow failure takes place as it becomes increasingly more fibrotic. Progressive thrombocytopenia leads to bleeding. The spleen continues to enlarge, which leads to early satiety. Painful episodes of splenic infarction may occur. The patient becomes cachectic and may experience severe bone pain, especially in the upper legs. Hematopoiesis in the liver leads to portal hypertension with ascites and esophageal varices, and occasionally myelopoiesis in the epidural space causes transverse myelitis.

B. Laboratory Findings

Patients are almost invariably anemic at presentation. The WBC is variable—either low, normal, or elevated—and may be increased to 50,000/mcL (50×10^9/L). The platelet count is variable. The peripheral blood smear is dramatic, with significant poikilocytosis and numerous teardrop forms in the RBC line. Nucleated RBCs are present, and the myeloid series is shifted, with immature forms including a small percentage of promyelocytes or myeloblasts. Platelet morphology may be bizarre, and giant degranulated platelet forms (megakaryocyte fragments) may be seen. *The triad of teardrop poikilocytosis, leukoerythroblastic blood, and giant abnormal platelets is highly suggestive of myelofibrosis.*

The bone marrow usually cannot be aspirated (dry tap), though early in the course of the disease, biopsy shows it to be hypercellular, with a marked increase in megakaryocytes. Fibrosis at this stage is detected by a silver stain demonstrating increased reticulin fibers. Later, biopsy reveals more severe fibrosis, with eventual replacement of hematopoietic precursors by collagen. There is no characteristic chromosomal abnormality. *JAK2* is mutated in ~65% of cases, and *MPL* and *CALR* are mutated in the majority of the remaining cases.

Differential Diagnosis

A leukoerythroblastic blood picture from other causes may be seen in response to severe infection, inflammation, or infiltrative bone marrow processes. However, teardrop poikilocytosis and giant abnormal platelet forms will not be present. Bone marrow fibrosis may be seen in metastatic carcinoma, Hodgkin lymphoma, and hairy cell leukemia. These disorders are diagnosed by characteristic morphology of involved tissues.

Of the other myeloproliferative disorders, CML is diagnosed when there is marked leukocytosis, normal RBC morphology, and the presence of the *bcr/abl* fusion gene. Polycythemia vera is characterized by an elevated hematocrit. Essential thrombocytosis shows predominant platelet count elevation.

Treatment

Prognostic scoring systems (detailed below) are used to designate patients as being at lower or higher risk. The primary goal of treatment is to reduce spleen size and minimize disease-related symptoms. Observation with supportive care is a reasonable treatment strategy for asymptomatic patients with low-risk disease in the absence of high-risk pathogenic gene variants. For patients at higher risk who are eligible for transplant, allogeneic transplant is a potentially curative approach, with a bridge of a JAK inhibitor; patients who are not eligible for transplant are usually offered long-term therapy with a JAK inhibitor. Ruxolitinib, the first-in-class JAK2 inhibitor, results in reduction of spleen size and improvement of constitutional symptoms but does not induce complete clinical or cytogenetic remissions. Moreover, ruxolitinib can exacerbate cytopenias. Another selective JAK2 inhibitor, fedratinib, can lead to sustained reduction in spleen size and improvement in disease-associated symptoms for patients with advanced-stage myelofibrosis. However, it carries a significant risk of serious and fatal encephalopathy, including Wernicke encephalopathy, and providers should regularly assess thiamine levels in all patients. The newer JAK2 inhibitor pacritinib is an option for patients with a platelet count < 50,000/mcL (50×10^9/L). Momelotinib is the first inhibitor of JAK1 and JAK2 shown to also inhibit activin A receptor type 1 (ACVR1), a key regulator of iron homeostasis, and has demonstrated improvements in splenomegaly, constitutional symptoms, and anemia in myelofibrosis.

In terms of supportive therapy, anemia can be controlled with transfusion, androgens, prednisone, or lenalidomide. Splenectomy is not routinely performed but is indicated for medication-refractory splenic enlargement causing recurrent painful episodes, severe thrombocytopenia, or an unacceptable transfusion requirement. Perioperative complications can occur in 28% of patients and include infections, abdominal vein thrombosis, and bleeding. Radiation therapy has a role for painful sites of extramedullary hematopoiesis, pulmonary hypertension, or severe bone pain. Transjugular intrahepatic portosystemic shunt might also be considered to alleviate symptoms of portal hypertension.

Course & Prognosis

The median survival from time of diagnosis is approximately 5 years. Therapies with biologic agents and reduced-intensity allogeneic stem cell transplantation appear to offer the potential to improve outcomes for many patients. End-stage myelofibrosis is characterized by generalized asthenia, liver failure, and bleeding from thrombocytopenia, with some cases terminating in AML. Two new prognostic systems for primary myelofibrosis have recently been introduced: **GIPSS** (genetically inspired prognostic scoring system) and **MIPSS70+ version 2.0** (MIPSSv2; mutation- and karyotype-enhanced international prognostic scoring system). GIPSS is based exclusively on mutations and karyotype. MIPSSv2 includes, in addition to genetic and karyotypic variants, clinical risk factors. Patients with certain pathogenic variants, including the SRSF2, ASXL1, and U2AF1-Q157 mutations, have an adverse prognosis regardless of clinical features. By contrast, patients with type 1/like *CALR* variants, compared to their counterparts with other driver mutations, experience significantly better survival. Lastly, RAS/CBL mutations predict resistance to ruxolitinib therapy.

When to Refer

Patients in whom myelofibrosis is suspected should be referred to a hematologist.

When to Admit

Admission is not usually necessary.

Gagelmann N et al. Allogeneic stem cell transplant for myelofibrosis and myelodysplastic syndromes: a contemporary review. Am J Hematol. 2025;100 Suppl 4(Suppl 4):16. [PMID: 40079242]

Jain AG et al. How I treat anemia in myelofibrosis. Blood. 2025;145:1738. [PMID: 39808793]

Verstovsek S et al. Momelotinib long-term safety and survival in myelofibrosis: integrated analysis of phase 3 randomized controlled trials. Blood Adv. 2023;7:3582. [PMID: 37042865]

Waksal JA et al. Novel therapies in myelofibrosis: beyond JAK inhibitors. Curr Hematol Malig Rep. 2022;17:140. [PMID: 35984598]

CHRONIC MYELOID LEUKEMIA

ESSENTIALS OF DIAGNOSIS

- Elevated WBC count.
- Markedly left-shifted myeloid series but with a low percentage of promyelocytes and blasts.
- Presence of *bcr/abl* gene (Philadelphia chromosome).

General Considerations

CML is a myeloproliferative disorder characterized by overproduction of myeloid cells. These myeloid cells continue to differentiate and circulate in increased numbers in the peripheral blood.

CML is characterized by a specific chromosomal abnormality and a specific molecular abnormality. The **Philadelphia chromosome** is a reciprocal translocation between the long arms of chromosomes 9 and 22. The fusion gene *bcr/abl* produces a novel protein that possesses tyrosine kinase activity.

Early CML ("chronic phase") does not behave like a malignant disease. Normal bone marrow function is retained, WBCs differentiate, and despite some qualitative abnormalities, the neutrophils combat infections normally. However, untreated CML is inherently unstable, and without treatment, the disease can progress to an "acute blast" phase, which is morphologically indistinguishable from acute leukemia.

Clinical Findings

A. Symptoms and Signs

CML is a disorder of middle age (median age at presentation is 55 years). Patients usually report fatigue, night sweats, and low-grade fevers related to the hypermetabolic state caused by overproduction of WBCs. Patients may also report abdominal fullness related to splenomegaly. In some cases, an elevated WBC is discovered incidentally. Rarely, the patient will present with a clinical syndrome related to leukostasis with blurred vision, respiratory distress, or priapism. The WBC in these cases is usually > 100,000/mcL (100×10^9/L) but < 500,000/mcL (500×10^9/L). On examination, the spleen is enlarged (often markedly so), and sternal tenderness may be present as a sign of marrow overexpansion. In cases discovered during routine laboratory monitoring, these findings are often absent. Acceleration of the disease is often associated with fever (in the absence of infection), bone pain, and splenomegaly.

B. Laboratory Findings

CML is characterized by an elevated WBC count; the median WBC count at diagnosis is 150,000/mcL (150×10^9/L), although in some cases the WBC count is only modestly increased (see Table 15–14). The peripheral blood is characteristic. The myeloid series is left shifted, with mature forms dominating and with cells usually present in proportion to their degree of maturation. Blasts are usually < 5%. Basophilia and eosinophilia may be present. At presentation, the patient is usually not anemic. RBC morphology is normal, and nucleated RBCs are rarely seen. The platelet count may be normal or elevated (sometimes to strikingly high levels). *A bone marrow biopsy is essential to ensure sufficient material for a complete karyotype and for morphologic evaluation to confirm the phase of disease.* The bone marrow is hypercellular, with left-shifted myelopoiesis. Myeloblasts compose < 5% of marrow cells. The hallmark of the disease is the *bcr/abl* gene that is detected by PCR testing of the peripheral blood and bone marrow.

With progression to the blast phase, progressive anemia and thrombocytopenia occur, and the percentage of blasts in the blood and bone marrow increases. Blast-phase CML is diagnosed when blasts comprise > 20% of bone marrow cells.

Differential Diagnosis

Early CML must be differentiated from the reactive leukocytosis associated with infection. In such cases, the WBC count is usually < 50,000/mcL (50×10^9/L), splenomegaly is absent, and the *bcr/abl* gene is not present.

CML must be distinguished from other myeloproliferative disease (see Table 15–14). The hematocrit should not be elevated, the RBC morphology is normal, and nucleated RBCs are rare or absent. Definitive diagnosis is made by finding the *bcr/abl* gene.

Treatment

Treatment is usually not emergent even with WBC counts > 200,000/mcL (200×10^9/L), since the majority of circulating cells are mature myeloid cells that are smaller and more deformable than primitive leukemic blasts. In the rare instances in which symptoms result from extreme hyperleukocytosis (priapism, respiratory distress, visual blurring, altered mental status), emergent leukapheresis is performed in conjunction with myelosuppressive therapy.

In chronic-phase CML, the goal of therapy is normalization of the hematologic abnormalities and suppression of the malignant *bcr/abl*-expressing clone. The treatment of choice consists of a **tyrosine kinase inhibitor** (eg, imatinib, nilotinib, dasatinib, bosutinib, or asciminib) targeting the aberrantly active abl kinase. Imatinib mesylate was the first tyrosine kinase inhibitor to be approved and it results in nearly universal (98%) hematologic control of chronic-phase disease at a dose of 400 mg/day. The rate of a major molecular response with imatinib in chronic-phase disease is ~30% at 1 year. The second-generation tyrosine kinase inhibitors nilotinib, dasatinib, and bosutinib are also used as front-line therapy especially for patients with intermediate- or high-risk disease. They can significantly increase the rate of a major molecular response compared to imatinib and result in a lower rate of progression to advanced-stage disease. However, these agents are associated with additional toxicity.

Patients taking tyrosine kinase inhibitors should be monitored with a quantitative PCR assay. It is expected that a hematologic complete remission, with normalization of blood counts and splenomegaly will occur within 3 months of treatment initiation. Second, a reduction of *bcr/abl* transcripts to < 10% on the international scale should be achieved, ideally within 3 months but certainly within 6 months. Finally, a major molecular response (≤ 0.1% transcripts) is desired within 12 months. Patients who achieve this level of molecular response have an excellent prognosis, with overall survival approaching 100% since disease progression is uncommon.

Patients with a consistent increase in *bcr/abl* transcript or those with a suboptimal molecular response as defined above should undergo testing for a pathogenic variant of *abl* and then be switched to an alternative tyrosine kinase inhibitor. The *T315I* variant of *abl* is specifically resistant to therapy with imatinib, dasatinib, nilotinib, and bosutinib but appears to be sensitive to the third-generation agent ponatinib or the allosteric inhibitor asciminib. Notably, ponatinib is associated with a high rate of vascular thrombotic complications. Asciminib dose-limiting toxicity includes asymptomatic elevations in the lipase level and clinical pancreatitis. Olverembatinib is another oral, third-generation tyrosine kinase inhibitor with activity against the *T315I* variant. Patients in whom a good molecular response to any of these agents cannot be achieved or in whom disease progresses despite therapy should be considered for allogeneic stem cell transplantation.

Patients with myeloid or lymphoid blast crisis should be treated with a tyrosine kinase inhibitor alone or in combination with myelosuppressive chemotherapy. The doses of tyrosine kinase inhibitors in that setting are usually higher than those appropriate for chronic-phase disease. Since the duration of response to tyrosine kinase inhibitors in this setting is limited, patients who have accelerated or blast-phase disease should ultimately be considered for allogeneic stem cell transplantation.

Course & Prognosis

Patients with good molecular responses to tyrosine kinase inhibitor therapy have an excellent prognosis, with essentially 100% survival at last follow-up. Studies suggest that tyrosine kinase inhibitor therapy may be safely discontinued after 2 years in patients who achieve a sustained major molecular response, with ~50% of patients remaining in molecular remission at least 1 year posttreatment. Of importance, > 80% of recurrences occur within the first 6–8 months after stopping therapy, and loss of major molecular response is uncommon after 1 year. About 90–95% of patients who experience molecular recurrence regain their initial molecular level after restarting tyrosine kinase inhibitor therapy.

When to Refer

All patients with CML should be referred to a hematologist.

When to Admit

Hospitalization is rarely necessary and should be reserved for symptoms of leukostasis at diagnosis or for transformation to acute leukemia.

Cruz-Rodriguez N et al. Novel treatment strategies for chronic myeloid leukemia. Blood. 2025;145:931. [PMID: 39729529]

García-Gutiérrez V et al. A clinician perspective on the treatment of chronic myeloid leukemia in the chronic phase. J Hematol Oncol. 2022;15:90. [PMID: 35818053]

Guilhot F et al. Long-term outcomes of tyrosine kinase inhibitors in chronic myeloid leukemia. Blood. 2025;145:910. [PMID: 39486043]

Laganà A et al. Understanding and overcoming resistance to tyrosine kinase inhibitors (TKIs) in chronic myeloid leukemia (CML). Expert Rev Hematol. 2025;18:65. [PMID: 39647915]

Oehler VG et al. Dose modifications in the management of chronic phase chronic myeloid leukemia: who, what, and when. J Natl Compr Canc Netw. 2024;22:e247044. [PMID: 39536447]

MYELODYSPLASTIC NEOPLASMS

ESSENTIALS OF DIAGNOSIS

- Cytopenias with a hypercellular bone marrow.
- Morphologic abnormalities in one or more hematopoietic cell lines.

General Considerations

The **myelodysplastic syndrome (MDS)** consists of a group of acquired clonal neoplasms of the hematopoietic stem cell. They are characterized by the constellation of cytopenias, a usually hypercellular marrow, morphologic dysplasia, and genetic abnormalities. The disorders are usually idiopathic but may be caused by prior exposure to cytotoxic chemotherapy, radiation, or both. In addition to cytogenetics, sequencing can detect genetic pathogenic variants in 80–90% of MDS patients. Importantly, acquired clonal variants identical to those seen in MDS can occur in the hematopoietic cells of ~10% of apparently healthy older individuals, defining the disorder of **clonal hematopoiesis (CH).**

MDS encompasses several heterogeneous neoplasms. A key distinction is whether there is an increase in bone marrow blasts (> 5% of marrow elements). The category of **MDS with increased blasts** represents a more aggressive form of the disease, often leading to AML. Those without increased blasts are characterized by the presence of defining genetic alterations, eg, *SF3B1* or *TP53* mutations. Patients with **isolated 5q loss**, constitute an important subgroup of patients with a different natural history. Lastly, a proliferative syndrome including sustained peripheral blood monocytosis > 1000/mcL (1.0×10^9/L) is termed **chronic myelomonocytic leukemia (CMML)**, a disorder that shares features of myelodysplastic and myeloproliferative neoplasms. An **International Prognostic Scoring System (IPSS)** classifies patients by risk status based on the percentage of bone marrow blasts, cytogenetics, and severity of cytopenias. The IPSS is associated with the rate of progression to AML and with overall survival, which can range from a median of 6 years for the low-risk group to 5 months for the high-risk patients.

Clinical Findings

A. Symptoms and Signs

Patients are usually over age 60 years. Many patients are asymptomatic when the diagnosis is made because of the finding of abnormal blood counts. Fatigue, infection, and bleeding related to bone marrow failure are usually the presenting symptoms and signs. The course may be indolent, and the disease may present as a wasting illness with fever, weight loss, and general debility. On examination, splenomegaly may be present, along with pallor, bleeding, and various signs of infection. MDS can also be accompanied by a variety of paraneoplastic syndromes before or following this diagnosis.

B. Laboratory Findings

Anemia may be marked with the MCV normal or increased, and transfusion support may be required. On the peripheral blood smear, macro-ovalocytes may be seen. The WBC count is usually normal or reduced, and neutropenia is common. The neutrophils may exhibit morphologic abnormalities, including deficient numbers of granules or deficient segmentation of the nucleus, even a bilobed nucleus (the so-called **Pelger-Huët abnormality**). The myeloid series may be left shifted, and small numbers of promyelocytes or blasts may be seen. The platelet count is normal or reduced, and hypogranular platelets may be present.

The bone marrow is characteristically hypercellular but occasionally may be hypocellular. Erythroid hyperplasia is common, and can be accompanied by signs of abnormal erythropoiesis. The Prussian blue stain may demonstrate ringed sideroblasts. In the marrow, too, the myeloid series is often left shifted, with variable increases in blasts. Deficient or abnormal granules may be seen. A characteristic abnormality is the presence of **dwarf megakaryocytes with a unilobed nucleus.** Genetic abnormalities define MDS; there are frequent cytogenetic abnormalities involving chromosomes 5 and 7. Some patients with an indolent form have an isolated partial deletion of chromosome 5 (MDS with isolated del[5q]). Aside from cytogenetic abnormalities, the most common genes with pathogenic variants are *SF3B1*, *TET2*, *SRSF2*, *ASXL1*, *DNMT3A*, *RUNX1*, *U2AF1*, *TP53*, and *EZH2*. Mutations in the *UBA1* gene can cause the recently identified VEXAS syndrome (Vacuoles, E1 enzyme, X-linked, Autoinflammatory, Somatic), a severe inflammatory condition primarily affecting older men, and leading to fevers, rashes, chondritis, and importantly myelodysplasia and other hematologic abnormalities.

Differential Diagnosis

MDS should be distinguished from megaloblastic anemia, aplastic anemia, myelofibrosis, HIV-associated cytopenias, and acute or chronic drug effect. In subtle cases, cytogenetic evaluation of the bone marrow may help distinguish this clonal disorder from other causes of cytopenias. As the number of blasts increases in the bone marrow, myelodysplasia is arbitrarily separated from AML by the presence of < 20% blasts.

Treatment

Myelodysplasia is a heterogeneous disease, and the appropriate treatment depends on a number of factors. For patients with anemia who have a low serum erythropoietin level (≤ 500 U/L), erythropoiesis-stimulating agents may raise the hematocrit and reduce the RBC transfusion requirement in 40%. Addition of intermittent granulocyte colony-stimulating factor (G-CSF) therapy may augment the erythroid response to epoetin. Unfortunately, the patients with the highest transfusion requirements and those with erythropoietin levels > 200 U/L are the least likely to respond. Patients who are dependent on RBC transfusion and can tolerate it should receive iron chelation in order to prevent serious iron overload; the oral agent deferasirox is given as 20 mg/kg/day in divided doses. Patients affected primarily with severe neutropenia may benefit from myeloid growth factors such as filgrastim. Oral thrombopoietin analogs, such as romiplostim and eltrombopag, have shown effectiveness in raising the platelet count in myelodysplasia. Finally, occasional patients can benefit from immunosuppressive therapy including ATG. Predictors of response to ATG include age younger than 60 years, absence of 5q–, and presence of HLA DR15.

For patients who do not respond to these interventions, several therapeutic options are available. Lenalidomide is the treatment of choice in patients with MDS with isolated del(5q) with significant responses in 70% of patients, and responses typically lasting longer than 2 years. In addition, nearly half of these patients enter a cytogenetic remission with clearing of the abnormal 5q– clone. The recommended initial dose of lenalidomide is 10 mg/day orally. The most common side effects are neutropenia and thrombocytopenia, but venous thrombosis occurs and warrants prophylaxis with aspirin, 81 mg/day orally. Luspatercept targets signaling via the SMAD2–SMAD3 pathway, which is constitutively increased in the bone marrow cells of patients with MDS and ineffective erythropoiesis. For patients who do not respond to or are not candidates for erythropoiesis-stimulating agents, luspatercept can induce transfusion independence in 38% of lower-risk MDS patients. The most common adverse events included fatigue, diarrhea, asthenia, nausea, and dizziness. The novel telomerase inhibitor imetelstat has been approved to treat adults with low- to intermediate-1 risk MDS with transfusion-dependent anemia and erythropoietin levels > 500 U/L. Imetelstat can result in > 24 weeks of freedom from RBC transfusions or anemia symptoms in 28% of patients and is generally well tolerated, except for manageable cytopenias and liver abnormalities.

For patients with high-risk MDS, hypomethylating agents are the treatment of choice. Azacitidine can improve both symptoms and blood counts and prolong overall survival and time to conversion to acute leukemia. It is used at a dose of 75 mg/m^2 daily for 5–7 days every 28 days and up to six cycles of therapy may be required to achieve a response. Decitabine, a related hypomethylating agent, given at 20 mg/m^2 daily for 5 days every 28 days, can produce similar hematologic responses but has not demonstrated a benefit in overall survival compared to supportive care alone. Oral therapy with decitabine (35 mg) and cedazuridine (100 mg) daily for 5 days of every 28 days can provide more convenient dosing for patients. The addition of the BCL2 inhibitor venetoclax to 5-azacytidine or decitabine has been shown to be well tolerated and may lead to higher response rates, especially for patients who are headed to allogeneic stem cell transplant. Lastly, the IDH1 inhibitors ivosidenib and olutasidenib have been approved in combination with 5-azacytidine for patients with the IDH1 mutation.

Allogeneic stem cell transplantation is the only curative therapy for myelodysplasia, but its role is limited by the advanced age of many patients and the variably indolent course of the disease.

Course & Prognosis

Myelodysplasia is an ultimately fatal disease, and allogeneic transplantation is the only curative therapy, with cure rates of 30–60% depending primarily on the risk status of the disease. Patients most commonly die of infections or bleeding. Patients with MDS with isolated del(5q) have a favorable prognosis, with 5-year survival over 90%. Other patients with low-risk disease (with absence of both excess blasts and adverse cytogenetics) may also do well, with similar survival. Those with increased blasts or CMML have a higher (30–50%) risk of developing acute leukemia, and short survival (< 2 years) without allogeneic transplantation.

When to Refer

All patients with myelodysplasia should be referred to a hematologist.

When to Admit

Hospitalization is needed only for specific complications, such as severe infection.

Feurstein S et al. Germline predisposition variants occur in myelodysplastic syndrome patients of all ages. Blood. 2022;140:2533. [PMID: 35969835]

Gattermann N. Iron overload in acquired sideroblastic anemias and MDS: pathophysiology and role of chelation and luspatercept. Hematology Am Soc Hematol Educ Program. 2024;2024:443. [PMID: 39644054]

Lennox AL et al. Imetelstat, a novel, first-in-class telomerase inhibitor: mechanism of action, clinical, and translational science. Clin Transl Sci. 2024;17:e70076. [PMID: 39555853]

Nakajima H et al. VEXAS syndrome. Int J Hematol. 2025;122:341. [PMID: 38819628]

Stomper J et al. Hypomethylating agents (HMA) for the treatment of acute myeloid leukemia and myelodysplastic syndromes: mechanisms of resistance and novel HMA-based therapies. Leukemia. 2021;35:1873. [PMID: 33958699]

Tefferi A et al. Chronic myelomonocytic leukaemia. Br J Haematol. 2025;207:2280. [PMID: 41177945]

ACUTE LEUKEMIA

ESSENTIALS OF DIAGNOSIS

- Short duration of symptoms, including fatigue, fever, and bleeding.
- Cytopenias or pancytopenia.
- Blasts in peripheral blood in 90% of patients.
- More than 20% blasts in the bone marrow.

General Considerations

Acute leukemia is a malignancy of the hematopoietic progenitor cell. Malignant immature cells proliferate in an uncontrolled fashion and replace normal bone marrow elements. Most cases arise without a clear cause. However, radiation and some toxins (benzene) are leukemogenic. In addition, a number of chemotherapeutic agents (especially cyclophosphamide, melphalan, other alkylating agents, and etoposide) may cause leukemia. The leukemias seen after toxin or chemotherapy exposure often develop from a myelodysplastic prodrome and are often associated with abnormalities in chromosomes 5 and 7. Those related to etoposide or anthracyclines may have abnormalities in chromosome 11q23 (MLL locus).

Most of the clinical findings in acute leukemia are due to replacement of normal bone marrow elements by the malignant cells. Less common manifestations result from organ infiltration (skin, GI tract, meninges). Acute leukemia is potentially curable with combination chemotherapy.

The myeloblastic subtype, AML, is primarily an adult disease with a median age at presentation of 60 years and an increasing incidence with advanced age. The lymphoblastic subtype of acute leukemia, ALL, comprises 80% of the acute leukemias of childhood. The peak incidence is between 3 and 7 years of age. It is also seen in adults, causing approximately 20% of adult acute leukemias.

Classification of the Leukemias

A. Acute Myeloid Leukemia (AML)

AML is primarily categorized based on recurrent structural chromosomal and molecular abnormalities. The cytogenetic abnormalities can be identified on traditional **karyotyping** or metaphase **fluorescence in situ hybridization (FISH)** and the molecular abnormalities are identified by either targeted or genome-wide sequencing of tumor DNA. Favorable cytogenetics such as t(8;21) producing a chimeric RUNX1/RUNX1T1 protein and inv(16)(p13;q22) are seen in 15% of cases and are termed the **"core-binding factor" leukemias**. These patients have a higher chance of achieving both short- and long-term disease control. Unfavorable cytogenetics confer a very poor prognosis. These consist of chromosomal translocations [t(6;9), t(3;3) or inv (3), t(v;11q23)], isolated monosomy 5 or 7, the presence of two or more other monosomies, or three or more separate cytogenetic abnormalities and account for 25% of the cases. The majority of cases of AML are of intermediate risk by traditional cytogenetics and have either a normal karyotype or chromosomal abnormalities that do not confer strong prognostic significance. However, there are several recurrent gene pathogenic variants with prognostic significance in this subgroup. On the one hand, internal tandem duplication in the gene *FLT3* occurs in ~30% of AML and is conditionally associated with a poor prognosis in the setting of wild type *NPM1*. Other pathogenic variants conferring a poor prognosis occur in *RUNX1, ASXL1*, and *TP53*. On the other hand, a relatively favorable group of patients has been identified that lacks *FLT3-ITD* pathogenic variants and includes variants of nucleophosmin 1 (*NPM1*) or carries *CEBPA* biallelic variants.

B. Acute Promyelocytic Leukemia (APL)

In considering the various types of AML, APL is discussed separately because of its unique biologic features and response to non-chemotherapy treatments. APL is characterized by the cytogenetic finding of t(15;17) and the fusion gene *PML-RAR*-α. It is a highly curable form of leukemia (< 90%) with integration of all-trans-retinoic acid (ATRA) and arsenic trioxide (ATO) in induction, consolidation, and maintenance regimens.

C. Acute Lymphoblastic Leukemia (ALL)

ALL is best classified as follows: **B cell (Philadelphia chromosome positive or negative)** and **T cell**. Hyperdiploidy (with > 50 chromosomes), especially of chromosomes 4, 10, and 17, and translocation t(12;21) (TEL-AML1), is associated with a better prognosis. Unfavorable cytogenetics are hypodiploidy (< 44 chromosomes), the Philadelphia chromosome t(9;22), the t(4;11) translocation (which has fusion genes involving the *MLL* gene at 11q23), and a complex karyotype with more than five chromosomal abnormalities.

D. Acute Leukemia of Ambiguous Lineage (ALAL)

These leukemias consist of blasts that lack differentiation along the lymphoid or myeloid lineage or blasts that express both myeloid and lymphoid lineage-specific antigens. This group is considered very high risk and has a poor prognosis. The limited available data suggest that an "acute lymphoblastic leukemia–like" regimen followed by allogeneic stem cell transplant may be advisable; addition of a tyrosine kinase inhibitor in patients with t(9;22) translocation is recommended.

Clinical Findings

A. Symptoms and Signs

Most patients have been ill only for days or weeks. Bleeding (usually due to thrombocytopenia) occurs in the skin and mucosal surfaces, with gingival bleeding, epistaxis, or menorrhagia. Less commonly, widespread bleeding is seen in patients with disseminated intravascular coagulation (DIC) (in APL and monocytic leukemia). Infection is due to neutropenia, with the risk of infection rising as the neutrophil count falls < 500/mcL (0.5×10^9/L). Common presentations include cellulitis, pneumonia, and perirectal infections; death within a few hours may occur if treatment with appropriate antibiotics is delayed. Fungal infections are also commonly seen.

Patients may also seek medical attention because of gum hypertrophy and bone and joint pain. The most dramatic presentation is hyperleukocytosis, in which a markedly elevated circulating blast count (total WBC count > 100,000/mcL [100×10^9/L]) leads to impaired circulation, presenting as headache, confusion, and dyspnea. *Such patients require emergent chemotherapy with adjunctive leukapheresis* since mortality approaches 40% in the first 48 hours.

On examination, patients appear pale and have purpura and petechiae; signs of infection may not be present. Stomatitis and gum hypertrophy may be seen in patients with monocytic leukemia, as may rectal fissures. There is variable enlargement of the liver, spleen, and lymph nodes. Bone tenderness may be present, particularly in the sternum, tibia, and femur.

B. Laboratory Findings

The hallmark of leukemia is the presence of increased numbers of circulating white cells. In acute leukemia, these cells are circulating blasts. However, blasts may be absent from the peripheral smear in as many as 10% of cases (**"aleukemic leukemia"**). The bone marrow is usually hypercellular and dominated by blasts (> 20%).

Hyperuricemia may be seen. If DIC is present, the fibrinogen level will be reduced, the prothrombin time prolonged, and fibrin degradation products or fibrin D-dimers present. Patients with ALL (especially T cell) may have a mediastinal mass visible on CXR. Meningeal leukemia will have blasts present in the spinal fluid, seen in approximately 5% of cases at diagnosis; it is more common in monocytic types of AML and can be seen with ALL.

The **Auer rod**, an eosinophilic needle-like inclusion in the cytoplasm, is a characteristic of AML (though sometimes seen in APL, high-grade MDS, and myeloproliferative disorders). The phenotype of leukemia cells is usually demonstrated by flow cytometry or immunohistochemistry. AML cells usually express myeloid antigens such as CD13 or CD33 and myeloperoxidase. ALL cells of B lineage will express CD19, and most cases will express CD10, formerly known as the "common ALL antigen." ALL cells of T lineage will usually not express mature T-cell markers, such as CD3, CD4, or CD8, but will express some combination of CD2, CD5, and CD7 and will not express surface immunoglobulin. Almost all cells express terminal deoxynucleotidyl transferase (TdT).

Differential Diagnosis

AML must be distinguished from other myeloproliferative disorders, CML, and MDS. Acute leukemia may also resemble a left-shifted bone marrow recovering from a previous toxic insult. If the diagnosis is in doubt, a bone marrow study should be repeated in several days to see if maturation has taken place. ALL must be separated from other lymphoproliferative disease such as CLL, lymphomas, and hairy cell leukemia. It may also be confused with the atypical lymphocytosis of mononucleosis and pertussis.

Treatment

Acute leukemia is considered a curable disease, especially among younger patients without significant comorbidities. The first step in treatment is to obtain complete remission, defined as normal peripheral blood with resolution of cytopenias, normal bone marrow with no excess blasts, and normal clinical status. The type of initial chemotherapy depends on the subtype of leukemia.

1. AML—Most patients with AML who are treated with curative intent receive a combination of an anthracycline (daunorubicin or idarubicin) plus cytarabine, either alone or in combination with other agents (eg, gemtuzumab ozogamicin). This therapy will produce complete remissions in 80–90% of patients under age 60 years and in 50–60% of older patients (see Table 43–2). Patients with secondary AML (evolved from prior myelodysplastic or myeloproliferative disorders) or treatment-associated AML benefit from the drug Vyxeos (a liposomal formulation of daunorubicin and cytarabine). Patients with a pathogenic variant of *FLT3* benefit from the addition of a FLT3 kinase inhibitor to their regimen (midostaurin or quizartinib). More recent data suggest that lower intensity therapy with the combination of a hypomethylating agent (5-azacitidine) and the bcl2 inhibitor venetoclax may achieve improved response rates and survival outcomes compared to these chemotherapy approaches for many patients with AML. This approach leads to fewer serious infectious complications and improved quality of life and hospitalizations. Post-remission therapy options include additional chemotherapy and/or allogeneic stem cell transplantation depending on the genetic risk profile and response to induction therapy.

Newer therapies are changing the treatment landscape of AML. These include: venetoclax (bcl2 inhibitor), ivosidenib (targeting IDH1 mutations), enasidenib (targeting IDH2 mutations), gilteritinib (targeting FLT3 mutations) and revumenib or ziftomenib (menin inhibitors). These agents are being incorporated in the care of patients in the relapsed/refractory setting but also increasingly being studied in front line combinations.

2. ALL—Adults with ALL are treated with combination chemotherapy, including daunorubicin, vincristine, prednisone, and asparaginase. This treatment produces complete remissions in 90% of patients. Those patients with Philadelphia chromosome-positive ALL (or *bcr-abl*-positive ALL) should receive a tyrosine kinase inhibitor, such as dasatinib or ponatinib, added to their initial chemotherapy. Remission induction therapy for ALL is less myelosuppressive than treatment for AML and does not necessarily produce prolonged marrow aplasia. Patients should also receive CNS prophylaxis so that meningeal sequestration of leukemic cells does not develop.

After achieving complete remission, patients may be treated with either additional cycles of chemotherapy or high-dose chemotherapy and allogeneic stem cell transplantation. Treatment decisions are made based on patient age and disease risk factors. Adults younger than 39 years have uniformly better outcomes when treated under pediatric protocols. For older patients, minimal residual disease testing early on can identify high-risk patients who will not be cured with chemotherapy alone and who will do better with allogeneic transplantation. For patients with relapsed disease, the bispecific antibody blinatumomab targeting CD19 and the antibody-drug conjugate inotuzumab ozogamicin targeting CD22 have shown remarkable activity and are considered superior to traditional chemotherapy options. Based on its activity, blinatumomab has moved to front-line therapy of ALL for older patients and as a consolidation approach for all disease subgroups. Chimeric antigen receptor T-cell therapy targeting CD19 is approved for patients with relapsed or refractory B-ALL but is mostly used as a bridge to allogeneic transplantation.

Prognosis

Approximately 70–80% of adults with AML under age 60 years achieve complete remission and ~50% are cured using risk-adapted post-remission therapy. Older adults with AML achieve complete remission in up to 50% of instances. The cure rates for older patients with AML have been very low (approximately 20%) even if they achieve remission and are able to receive post-remission chemotherapy.

Patients younger than 39 years with ALL have excellent outcomes after undergoing chemotherapy followed by risk-adapted intensification and transplantation (cure rates of 60–80%). Patients with adverse cytogenetics, poor response to chemotherapy, or older age have a much lower chance of cure (cure rates of 20–40%).

When to Refer

All patients should be referred to a hematologist.

When to Admit

Most patients with acute leukemia will be admitted for treatment.

Chen EC et al. Biology and management of acute myeloid leukemia with mutated NPM1. Am J Hematol. 2025;100:652. [PMID: 39901865]

Curran E et al. Innovative approaches to the management of acute lymphoblastic leukemia across the age spectrum. Am Soc Clin Oncol Educ Book. 2022;42:1. [PMID: 35503981]

Dholaria B et al. The evolving role of allogeneic haematopoietic cell transplantation in the era of chimaeric antigen receptor T-cell therapy. Br J Haematol. 2021;193:1060. [PMID: 33928630]

Gupta S et al. Determinants of outcomes and advances in CD19-directed chimeric antigen receptor therapy for B-cell acute lymphoblastic leukemia. Eur J Haematol. 2024;112:51. [PMID: 38105391]

Sabakhtarishvili G et al. Maintenance therapy in acute myeloid leukemia. Am J Clin Oncol. 2025;48:38. [PMID: 39238120]

Shimony S et al. Acute myeloid leukemia: 2025 update on diagnosis, risk-stratification, and management. Am J Hematol. 2025;100:860. [PMID: 39936576]

Passet M et al Genetic subtypes of B-cell acute lymphoblastic leukemia in adults. Blood. 2025;145:1451. [PMID: 39786374]

CHRONIC LYMPHOCYTIC LEUKEMIA

ESSENTIALS OF DIAGNOSIS

- B-cell lymphocytosis with CD19 expression > 5000/mcL (> 5.0 × 10^9/L).
- Coexpression of CD19, CD5 on lymphocytes.

General Considerations

CLL is a clonal malignancy of B lymphocytes. The disease is usually indolent, with slowly progressive accumulation of long-lived small lymphocytes. These cells are immune-incompetent and respond poorly to antigenic stimulation.

CLL is manifested clinically by immunosuppression, bone marrow failure, and organ infiltration with lymphocytes. Immunodeficiency is also related to inadequate antibody production by the abnormal B cells. With advanced disease, CLL may cause damage by direct tissue infiltration.

CLL usually pursues an indolent course. In 5–10% of cases, CLL may be complicated by autoimmune hemolytic anemia or autoimmune thrombocytopenia. In approximately 5% of cases an aggressive large-cell lymphoma (**Richter syndrome**) can develop.

Clinical Findings

A. Symptoms and Signs

CLL is a disease of older patients, with 90% of cases occurring after age 50 years and a median age at presentation of 70 years. Many patients will be incidentally discovered to have lymphocytosis. Others present with fatigue or lymphadenopathy. On examination, 80% of patients will have diffuse lymphadenopathy and 50% will have enlargement of the liver or spleen. Some patients present with a predominantly nodal form of the disease without circulating lymphocytosis (Small Lymphocytic Lymphoma).

The long-standing **Rai classification system** remains prognostically useful: stage 0, lymphocytosis only; stage I, lymphocytosis plus lymphadenopathy; stage II, organomegaly (spleen, liver); stage III, anemia; stage IV, thrombocytopenia. These stages can be collapsed into low risk (stages 0–I), intermediate risk (stage II), and high risk (stages III–IV).

B. Laboratory Findings

The hallmark of CLL is isolated lymphocytosis. The WBC count is elevated and may be markedly abnormal (elevated to several hundred thousand). Usually 75–98% of the circulating cells are lymphocytes. Lymphocytes appear small and mature, with condensed nuclear chromatin, and are morphologically indistinguishable from normal lymphocytes, but smaller numbers of larger and activated lymphocytes may be seen. The hematocrit and platelet count are usually normal at presentation. The bone marrow is variably infiltrated with small lymphocytes. The immunophenotype of CLL demonstrates co-expression of the B lymphocyte lineage marker CD19 with the T lymphocyte marker CD5; this finding is commonly observed only in CLL and mantle cell lymphoma. CLL is distinguished from mantle cell lymphoma by the expression of CD23, CD200, and LEF-1, low expression of surface immunoglobulin and CD20, and the absence of a translocation or overexpression of cyclin D1. Patients whose CLL cells have pathogenic variants of the immunoglobulin gene (IgVH somatic mutation) have a more indolent form of disease; conversely, patients whose cells have non-variant IgVH genes do less well and require treatment sooner. The assessment of genomic changes by FISH provides important prognostic information as well. The finding of deletion of chromosome 17p (TP53) confers the worst prognosis, while deletion of 11q (ATM) confers an inferior prognosis to the average genotype, and isolated deletion of 13q has a more favorable outcome. Hypogammaglobulinemia is present in 50% of patients and becomes more common with advanced disease. In some, a small amount of IgM paraprotein is present in the serum.

Differential Diagnosis

Few syndromes can be confused with CLL. Viral infections producing lymphocytosis should be obvious from the presence of fever and other clinical findings; however, fever may occur in CLL from concomitant infection. Pertussis may cause a particularly high total lymphocyte count. Other lymphoproliferative diseases such as Waldenström macroglobulinemia, hairy cell leukemia, or non-Hodgkin lymphoma (especially mantle cell lymphoma) in the leukemic phase are distinguished based on the morphology and immunophenotype of circulating lymphocytes and bone marrow. Monoclonal B-cell lymphocytosis is a disorder characterized by < 5000/mcL (5.0×10^9/L) B cells and is considered a precursor to B-CLL.

Treatment

The treatment of CLL is evolving as several active targeted agents are now available. Most cases of early indolent CLL require no specific therapy, and the standard of care for early-stage disease has been observation. Indications for treatment include progressive fatigue, symptomatic lymphadenopathy, anemia, or thrombocytopenia. These patients have either symptomatic and progressive Rai stage II disease or stage III/IV disease. Initial treatment for patients with CLL consists of targeted biologic therapy in most cases. Options include a BTK inhibitor as a single agent (ibrutinib, acalabrutinib, or zanubrutinib) or venetoclax (a bcl2 inhibitor resulting in apoptosis) in combination with a BTK inhibitor or with anti-CD20 antibody therapy. Choice between these agents is based on toxicity as well as patient preference. BTK inhibitors are oral agents that require continuous dosing to be effective; they are well-tolerated but can be associated with hypertension, atrial fibrillation, and bleeding. Caution should be exercised when these agents are used in conjunction with anticoagulants (DOACs) and in the pre- and postoperative setting. Venetoclax (slowly titrated up to 400 mg daily) is usually given in combination for a self-limited course of therapy and is associated with tumor lysis syndrome and neutropenia; some patients may require hospitalization for initial therapy. For older patients, chlorambucil, 0.6–1 mg/kg orally every 4 weeks, in combination with obinutuzumab is another therapy option.

Patients who relapse while taking a BTK inhibitor should undergo testing to identify recurrent BTK pathogenic variants (eg, *C481S*) that may respond to the novel agent pirtobrutinib. Alternatively, they can be treated with a combination of venetoclax and an anti-CD20 antibody. For patients who relapse following venetoclax-based therapy, a BTK inhibitor is often used. Chimeric antigen receptor T-cell therapy targeting CD19 is another option for refractory patients with CLL and can result in long-lasting remissions. Lastly, allogeneic transplantation can offer a potentially curative treatment for patients with CLL, but it should be used only in patients whose disease cannot be controlled by the available therapies due to the high morbidity and mortality associated with this therapy.

Of note, BTK inhibitors initially can be associated with marked lymphocytosis due to release of tumor cells from the lymph nodes into the peripheral blood. This results in a significant early reduction in lymphadenopathy but a potentially misleading, more delayed clearance of lymphocytes from peripheral blood and bone marrow.

Associated autoimmune hemolytic anemia or immune thrombocytopenia may require treatment with rituximab, prednisone, or splenectomy. Rituximab should be used with anti-HBV agent prophylaxis in patients with past HBV infection. Patients with recurrent bacterial infections and hypogammaglobulinemia benefit from prophylactic infusions of γ globulin (0.4 g/kg/month), but this treatment is cumbersome and expensive, justified only when these infections are severe.

Prognosis

Targeted therapies have changed the prognosis of CLL. Patients with stage 0 or stage I disease have a median survival of 10–15 years, and these patients may be reassured that they can live a normal life. Patients with stage III or IV disease had a median survival of < 2 years in the past, but with current therapies, 5-year survival is > 70% and the long-term outlook appears substantially improved. For patients with high-risk and resistant forms of CLL, there is evidence that allogeneic transplantation can overcome risk factors and lead to long-term disease control.

When to Refer

All patients with CLL should be referred to a hematologist.

When to Admit

Hospitalization is rarely needed.

Brown JR et al. Fixed-duration acalabrutinib combinations in untreated chronic lymphocytic leukemia. N Engl J Med. 2025;392:748. [PMID: 39976417]

Davids MS et al. Measurable residual disease-driven treatment in first-line chronic lymphocytic leukaemia. Br J Haematol. 2025;206:33. [PMID: 39538975]

Kittai AS et al. International consensus statement on diagnosis, evaluation, and research of Richter transformation: the ERIC recommendations. Blood. 2025;146:291. [PMID: 40239121]

Tam CS et al. Novel mechanisms of resistance in CLL: variant BTK mutations in second-generation and noncovalent BTK inhibitors. Blood. 2025;145:1005. [PMID: 39808800]

Tausch E et al. Risk-stratification in frontline CLL therapy: standard of care. Hematology Am Soc Hematol Educ Program. 2024;2024:457. [PMID: 39644006]

HAIRY CELL LEUKEMIA

ESSENTIALS OF DIAGNOSIS

- Pancytopenia.
- Splenomegaly, often massive.
- Hairy cells present on blood smear and especially in bone marrow biopsy.

General Considerations

Hairy cell leukemia is a rare malignancy of hematopoietic stem cells differentiated as mature B lymphocytes with hairy cytoplasmic projections. The V600E pathogenic variant in the *BRAF* gene is recognized as the causal genetic event of hairy cell leukemia since it is detectable in almost all cases at diagnosis and is present at relapse.

Clinical Findings

A. Symptoms and Signs

The disease characteristically presents in middle-aged men. The median age at presentation is 55 years, and there is a striking *5:1 male predominance*. Most patients present with gradual onset of fatigue, others describe symptoms related to markedly enlarged spleen, and some come to attention because of infection.

Splenomegaly is almost invariably present and may be massive. The liver is enlarged in 50% of cases; lymphadenopathy is uncommon.

Hairy cell leukemia is usually an indolent disorder whose course is dominated by pancytopenia and recurrent infections, including mycobacterial infections.

B. Laboratory Findings

The hallmark of hairy cell leukemia is pancytopenia. Anemia is nearly universal, and 75% of patients have thrombocytopenia and neutropenia. The **"hairy cells"** are usually present in small numbers on the peripheral blood smear and have a characteristic appearance with numerous cytoplasmic projections. The bone marrow is usually inaspirable (dry tap), and the diagnosis is made by characteristic morphology on bone marrow biopsy. Adequate immunophenotyping is essential for establishing the diagnosis and for distinguishing between classical hairy cell leukemia and the hairy cell variant. On immunophenotyping, the cells coexpress the antigens CD11c, CD20, CD22, CD25, CD103, and CD123. Pathologic examination of the spleen shows marked infiltration of the red pulp with hairy cells. This is in contrast to the usual predilection of lymphomas to involve the white pulp of the spleen.

Differential Diagnosis

Hairy cell leukemia should be distinguished from other lymphoproliferative diseases that involve the bone marrow. It also may be confused with other causes of pancytopenia, including hypersplenism due to any cause, aplastic anemia, and paroxysmal nocturnal hemoglobinuria.

Treatment

Treatment is indicated for symptomatic disease, eg, splenic discomfort, recurrent infections, or significant cytopenias. The treatment of choice is a nucleoside analog, specifically pentostatin or cladribine for a single course, producing a complete remission in 70–95% of patients. Treatment is associated with infectious complications, and patients should be closely monitored. The median duration of response is over 8 years and patients who relapse a year or more after initial therapy can be treated again with one of these agents. Rituximab can be used in the relapsed setting either as a single agent or in combination with a nucleoside analog. The BRAF inhibitor vemurafenib exhibits ~100% overall response rate in patients with refractory/relapsed hairy cell leukemia, with 35–40% complete remissions. The median relapse-free survival is ~19 months in patients who achieved complete remission and 6 months in those who obtained a partial response. Vemurafenib in combination with an anti-CD20 antibody can be used as initial therapy for patients who are frail or have active infections. The next generation BRAF inhibitor dabrafenib in combination with trametinib can be used for patients refractory to initial nucleoside analogue–based therapy. Lastly, the BTK inhibitors ibrutinib and zanubrutinib and the bcl2 inhibitor venetoclax have activity in patients with refractory disease.

Course & Prognosis

More than 95% of patients with hairy cell leukemia live longer than 10 years.

Falini B et al. How I treat refractory/relapsed hairy cell leukemia with BRAF inhibitors. Blood. 2022;139:2294. [PMID: 35143639]

Kreitman R et al. Dabrafenib plus trametinib in patients with relapsed/refractory BRAF V600E mutation-positive hairy cell leukemia. Blood. 2023;141:996. [PMID: 36108341]

Levy Yurkovski I et al. Approach to hairy-cell leukemia in the new therapeutic era with special emphasis on age and comorbidities. Acta Haematol. 2025 Aug 4. [Epub ahead of print] [PMID: 40759084]

Tiacci E et al. Vemurafenib plus rituximab in refractory or relapsed hairy-cell leukemia. N Engl J Med. 2021;384:1810. [PMID: 33979489]

LYMPHOMAS

NON-HODGKIN LYMPHOMAS

ESSENTIALS OF DIAGNOSIS

- Often present with painless lymphadenopathy.
- Diagnosis is made by tissue biopsy.

General Considerations

The non-Hodgkin lymphomas are a heterogeneous group of cancers of lymphocytes usually presenting as enlarged lymph nodes. The disorders vary in clinical presentation and course from indolent to rapidly progressive.

Lymphomas often harbor characteristic molecular alterations, eg, balanced chromosomal translocations whereby *an oncogene becomes juxtaposed next to either an immunoglobulin gene (B-cell lymphoma) or the T-cell receptor gene or related gene (T-cell lymphoma)*. The best-studied example is **Burkitt lymphoma**, in which a characteristic translocation between the long arms of chromosomes 8 and 14 places the protooncogene c-*myc* on chromosome 8

Table 15–16. WHO classification of lymphomas (modified from 2022 version).

Precursor B-cell lymphoblastic lymphoma
Mature B-cell lymphomas
Chronic lymphocytic leukemia/small lymphocytic lymphoma
Monoclonal B-cell lymphocytosis
Hairy cell leukemia
Diffuse large B-cell lymphoma
Primary diffuse large B-cell lymphoma of the CNS
High-grade B-cell lymphoma, with *MYC* and *BCL2* and/or *BCL6* rearrangements
Mediastinal (thymic) large B-cell lymphoma
Follicular lymphoma
Lymphoplasmacytic lymphoma (Waldenström macroglobulinemia)
Mantle cell lymphoma
Burkitt lymphoma
Marginal zone lymphoma
KSHV/HHV8-associated B-cell lymphoid proliferations and lymphomas
Mature T- (and NK-) cell lymphomas
Anaplastic large-cell lymphoma
Angioimmunoblastic T-cell lymphoma
Peripheral T-cell lymphoma, NOS
Cutaneous T-cell lymphoma (mycosis fungoides, Sézary syndrome)
Extranodal NK-/T-cell lymphoma, nasal type
Adult T-cell leukemia/lymphoma
T-cell large granular lymphocytic leukemia
Hodgkin lymphoma
Nodular lymphocyte predominant Hodgkin lymphoma
Classic Hodgkin lymphoma
Posttransplant lymphoproliferative disorders
Histiocytic and dendritic cell neoplasms

KSHV, Kaposi sarcoma–associated herpes virus; HHV8, human herpesvirus-8 (also known as Kaposi sarcoma herpes virus); NOS, not otherwise specified.

next to the immunoglobulin heavy chain locus on chromosome 14. Overexpression of c-*myc* is related to malignant transformation through excess B-cell proliferation. In follicular lymphoma, the t(14;18) translocation is characteristic and *bcl-2* is overexpressed, resulting in protection against apoptosis, the usual mechanism of B-cell death.

Classification of the lymphomas is a dynamic area still undergoing evolution. The **2022 grouping** (Table 15–16) separates diseases based on both clinical and pathologic features. Eighty-five percent of non-Hodgkin lymphomas are B-cell and 15% are T-cell or NK-cell in origin. Even though non-Hodgkin lymphomas represent a diverse group of diseases, they are historically divided in two categories based on clinical behavior and pathology: the **indolent** (low-grade) and the **aggressive** (intermediate- or high-grade).

Clinical Findings

A. Symptoms and Signs

Patients with non-Hodgkin lymphomas usually present with lymphadenopathy. Involved lymph nodes may be present peripherally (cervical, axillary or inguinal stations), centrally (in the retroperitoneum, mesentery, and pelvic side wall), or both. The indolent lymphomas are usually disseminated at the time of diagnosis, and bone marrow involvement is frequent. Many patients with lymphoma have constitutional symptoms such as fever, drenching night sweats, and weight loss of > 10% of prior body weight (referred to as **"B symptoms"**).

On examination, lymphadenopathy may be isolated or diffuse, and extranodal sites of disease (such as the skin, GI tract, liver, and bone marrow) may be found. Patients with Burkitt lymphoma are noted to have abdominal pain or abdominal fullness because of the predilection of the disease for the abdomen.

Once a pathologic diagnosis is established, staging is done using a whole-body PET/CT scan, a bone marrow biopsy (in selected cases), and, in patients with high-grade lymphoma or intermediate-grade lymphoma with high-risk features, brain imaging and a lumbar puncture.

B. Laboratory Findings

The peripheral blood is usually normal even with extensive bone marrow involvement by lymphoma. Circulating lymphoma cells in the blood are not commonly seen.

Bone marrow involvement is manifested as paratrabecular monoclonal lymphoid aggregates. In some high-grade lymphomas, the meninges are involved and malignant cells are found with CSF cytology. The serum LD, a useful prognostic marker, is incorporated in risk stratification of treatment.

The diagnosis of lymphoma is made by tissue biopsy. Needle aspiration may yield evidence for non-Hodgkin lymphoma, but an excisional or core needle biopsy is required for accurate diagnosis and classification.

Treatment

A. Indolent Lymphomas

The most common lymphomas in this group are **follicular lymphoma, marginal zone lymphomas**, and **small lymphocytic lymphoma (SLL)**. The treatment of indolent lymphomas depends on the stage of disease and the patient's clinical status. A small number of patients have limited disease with only one or two contiguous abnormal lymph node groups and may be treated with localized irradiation with curative intent. However, most patients (85%) with indolent lymphoma have disseminated disease at the time of diagnosis and are not considered curable. *Historically, treatment of these patients has not affected overall survival; therefore, treatment is offered only when symptoms develop or for high tumor bulk.* Even though not considered curable, most patients can expect a normal lifespan. Some patients will have temporary spontaneous remissions (8%). There are an increasing number of reasonable treatment options for indolent lymphomas, but no consensus exists on the best strategy. Treatment with rituximab (375 mg/m^2 intravenously weekly for 4 weeks) is commonly used either alone or in combination with chemotherapy and may be the only agent to affect overall survival in these disorders. Patients should be screened for hepatitis B because rare cases of fatal fulminant hepatitis have been described with the use of anti-CD20 monoclonal therapies without anti-HBV agent prophylaxis. Rituximab is added to chemotherapy regimens including bendamustine; cyclophosphamide, vincristine, and prednisone (R-CVP); and cyclophosphamide, doxorubicin, vincristine, and prednisone (R-CHOP) (see Table 43–2). The immunomodulatory agent lenalidomide in combination with anti-CD20 therapy is an alternative option with similar outcomes to chemotherapy. The regimens mentioned above can also be used for patients with relapsed disease. The CD20:CD3 bispecific antibodies mosunetuzumab and epcoritamab are highly active in patients who have progressed after two lines of therapy; they can result in an overall response in 80% of patients for a median duration of ~2 years. Chimeric antigen receptor T-cell therapy targeting CD19 is also available for patients with at least two relapses. Stem cell transplantation (either allogeneic or autologous) is another option for these patients.

Patients with **mucosa-associated lymphoid tissue (MALT)** lymphomas may benefit from pathogen eradication therapy. MALT lymphomas of the stomach may be appropriately treated with combination antibiotics directed against *H pylori* and with acid blockade but require frequent endoscopic monitoring. MALT lymphomas of the spleen are usually associated with hepatitis C and may remit following hepatitis C eradication therapy.

B. Aggressive Lymphomas

Patients with **diffuse large B-cell lymphoma** are treated with curative intent. Most patients are treated with four to six cycles of immunochemotherapy such as R-CHOP (see Table 43–2). Involved nodal radiotherapy may be added for patients with bulky or extranodal disease. **High-grade lymphoma** with chromosomal translocations affecting *MYC*, such as t(8;14), and *BCL2*, such as t(14;18), also called "double-hit lymphoma," has a very aggressive course. Patients with this disease may do better with dose-adjusted R-EPOCH as front-line therapy.

Patients with diffuse large B-cell lymphoma or high-grade lymphoma who relapse after initial chemotherapy can still be cured with chimeric antigen receptor T-cell therapy targeting CD19, which produces durable complete response rates of ~40%. High-dose chemotherapy with autologous hematopoietic stem cell transplantation is another potentially curable option but is used less frequently at this time. The CD20:CD3 bispecific antibodies epcoritamab and glofitamab have shown clinical activity in patients who have progressed after two lines of therapy.

Mantle cell lymphoma is not effectively treated with standard immunochemotherapy regimens as it tends to recur years following initial therapy. Intensive initial immunochemotherapy, followed by maintenance therapy, can lead to long-lasting remission in patients without TP53 mutations. The BTK inhibitors ibrutinib, acalabrutinib, zanubrutinib, and pirtobrutinib are active in relapsed or refractory patients with mantle cell lymphoma. They are increasingly used in front-line therapy for patients who harbor TP53 mutations. Chimeric antigen receptor T-cell therapy targeting CD19 (CART19) shows promising activity in patients whose disease progresses after treatment with chemotherapy and BTK inhibitors. Reduced-intensity allogeneic stem cell transplantation offers curative potential for selected patients. For **primary CNS lymphoma**, high-dose intravenous methotrexate–containing regimens can produce long term remissions in about 50% of patients.

Patients with **highly aggressive lymphomas** (Burkitt or lymphoblastic) require urgent, intense, cyclic chemotherapy in the hospital similar to that given for ALL, and they also require intrathecal chemotherapy as CNS prophylaxis.

Patients with **peripheral T-cell lymphomas** usually have advanced-stage nodal and extranodal disease and typically have inferior response rates to therapy compared to patients with aggressive B-cell lymphomas. Autologous stem cell transplantation is often incorporated in first-line therapy. The antibody–drug conjugate brentuximab vedotin has significant activity in patients with CD30-positive peripheral T-cell lymphomas, such as anaplastic large-cell lymphoma. The combination of brentuximab vedotin with cyclophosphamide, doxorubicin, and prednisone is the initial treatment of choice for CD30-positive peripheral T-cell lymphomas.

Prognosis

About 80% of patients with **indolent lymphoma** will have a normal lifespan. Patients who progress within 2 years after their first treatment are considered high-risk and have inferior survival. Some patients with indolent lymphomas can present with or progress to an aggressive lymphoma (transformation) and need to be treated accordingly.

The **International Prognostic Index** is widely used to categorize patients with **aggressive lymphoma** into risk groups. Factors that confer adverse prognosis are age over 60 years, elevated serum LD, stage III or stage IV disease, more than one extranodal site of disease, and poor performance status. Cure rates after primary therapy range from > 80% for low-risk patients (zero risk factors) to < 50% for high-risk patients (four or more risk factors). For patients who relapse after initial chemotherapy, chimeric antigen receptor T-cell therapy or autologous hematopoietic stem cell transplantation can offer a 40–50% chance of long-term lymphoma-free survival. The treatment of older patients with aggressive lymphoma has been difficult because of poorer tolerance of aggressive chemotherapy. The use of reduced-intensity regimens (eg, R-miniCHOP) with myeloid growth factors and prophylactic antibiotics are preferred.

When to Refer

All patients with lymphoma should be referred to a hematologist or an oncologist.

When to Admit

Admission is necessary only for specific complications of lymphoma or its treatment and for the treatment of all high-grade lymphomas.

Armitage JO et al. Mantle-cell lymphoma. N Engl J Med. 2022;386:2495. [PMID: 35767440]
Bock AM et al. Therapeutic landscape of primary refractory and relapsed diffuse large B-cell lymphoma: recent advances and emerging therapies. J Hematol Oncol. 2025;18:68. [PMID: 40597378]
Minson AG et al. New bispecific antibodies in diffuse large B-cell lymphoma. Haematologica. 2025;110:1483. [PMID: 39911111]
Nastoupil LJ et al. Management of aggressive lymphoma after CAR T-cell therapy failure. Hematology Am Soc Hematol Educ Program. 2023;2023:364. [PMID: 38066908]
Rossi D et al. Marginal-zone lymphomas. N Engl J Med. 2022;386:5681. [PMID: 35139275]
Sehn LH et al. Diffuse large B-cell lymphoma. N Engl J Med. 2021;384:842. [PMID: 33657296]
Tavares A et al. Diffuse large B-cell lymphoma in very elderly patients: towards best tailored treatment—a systematic review. Crit Rev Oncol Hematol. 2021;160:103294. [PMID: 33675907]

HODGKIN LYMPHOMA

ESSENTIALS OF DIAGNOSIS

- Often painless lymphadenopathy.
- Constitutional symptoms may or may not be present.
- Pathologic diagnosis by lymph node biopsy.

General Considerations

Hodgkin lymphoma is characterized by lymph node biopsy showing **Reed-Sternberg cells** in an appropriate reactive cellular background. The malignant cell is derived from B lymphocytes of germinal center origin.

Clinical Findings

There is a bimodal age distribution, with one peak in the 20s and a second over age 50 years. Most patients seek medical attention because of a painless mass, commonly in the neck. Others may seek medical attention for constitutional symptoms such as fever, weight loss, or drenching night sweats, or for generalized pruritus. An unusual symptom of Hodgkin lymphoma is pain in an involved lymph node following alcohol ingestion.

An important feature of Hodgkin lymphoma is its tendency to arise within single lymph node areas and spread in an orderly fashion to contiguous areas of lymph nodes. Late in the course of the disease, vascular invasion leads to widespread hematogenous dissemination.

Hodgkin lymphoma is divided into two subtypes: **classic Hodgkin** (nodular sclerosis, mixed cellularity, lymphocyte rich, and lymphocyte depleted) and **non-classic Hodgkin** (nodular lymphocyte predominant). Hodgkin lymphoma should be distinguished pathologically from other malignant lymphomas and may occasionally be confused with reactive lymph nodes seen in infectious mononucleosis, cat-scratch disease, or drug reactions (eg, phenytoin).

Patients undergo a staging evaluation to determine the extent of disease, including serum chemistries, whole-body PET/CT scan, and, occasionally, a bone marrow biopsy.

Treatment

Chemotherapy is the mainstay of treatment for Hodgkin lymphoma and is dosed based on disease risk. Low-risk patients are those with stage I or II disease without bulky lymphadenopathy or evidence of excess systemic inflammation. They traditionally receive a combination of short-course chemotherapy with involved nodal radiotherapy, but involved nodal radiotherapy can be eliminated for those with an early negative PET/CT scan without a significant change in outcomes (see Table 43–3). ABVD (doxorubicin, bleomycin, vinblastine, dacarbazine) remains the standard first-line regimen for these patients due to its manageable toxicity.

High-risk patients are those with stage III or IV disease or with stage II disease and a large mediastinal or other bulky mass or systemic inflammation. These patients are treated with a full course of chemotherapy. The substitution of the antibody–drug conjugate brentuximab vedotin for bleomycin in ABVD (called A-AVD) has demonstrated somewhat superior progression-free and overall survival and is frequently used for patients with higher-risk stage III or IV disease. It requires growth factor support due to the higher risk of infectious complications. The checkpoint inhibitor nivolumab, when added to AVD (Nivo-AVD), can produce superior response rates to A-AVD and is being increasingly used for these patients. Lastly, the response-adapted combination regimen BrECADD (Brentuximab Vedotin, Etoposide, Cyclophosphamide, Doxorubicin, Dacarbazine, Dexamethasone) has shown promise as a shorter regimen for these patients.

If using ABVD, attention must be paid to pulmonary function as bleomycin can be associated with significant pulmonary toxicity, including fibrosis and death. An interim PET scan is advisable after two cycles of ABVD chemotherapy. Patients with a negative scan can have bleomycin eliminated from their treatment without a detriment to efficacy.

Classic Hodgkin lymphoma relapsing after initial treatment is treatable with high-dose chemotherapy and autologous hematopoietic stem cell transplantation. This offers upwards of 50% chance of cure when disease is still chemotherapy responsive. Immune checkpoint inhibition by PD1 blockade with nivolumab or pembrolizumab has shown remarkable activity in patients with relapsed or refractory disease (overall response rate [ORR], 65%). These agents as well as brentuximab vedotin are increasingly incorporated in second-line regimens prior to or, for ineligible patients, in lieu of stem cell transplantation.

Prognosis

All patients should be treated with curative intent. Prognosis in advanced-stage Hodgkin lymphoma is influenced by seven features: stage, age, gender, hemoglobin, albumin, WBC count, and lymphocyte count. The cure rate is 75% if zero to two risk features are present and 55% when three or more risk features are present. The prognosis of patients with stage IA or IIA disease is excellent, with 10-year survival rates in excess of 90%. Patients with advanced disease (stage III or IV) have 10-year survival rates of 50–60%. Inferior results are seen in patients who are older, those who have bulky disease, and those with lymphocyte depletion or mixed cellularity on histologic examination. Nodular lymphocyte-predominant Hodgkin lymphoma is highly curable with radiotherapy alone for early-stage disease; however, for high-stage disease, it is characterized by long survival with repetitive relapses after chemotherapy or monoclonal anti-CD20 antibody therapy.

When to Refer

- All patients should be sent to an oncologist or hematologist.
- Secondary referral to a radiation oncologist might be appropriate.

When to Admit

Patients should be admitted for complications of the disease or its treatment.

Ansell SM et al; ECHELON-1 Study Group. Overall survival with brentuximab vedotin in stage III or IV Hodgkin's lymphoma. N Engl J Med. 2022;387:310. [PMID: 35830649]

Borchmann P et al. Assessing the efficacy and tolerability of PET-guided BrECADD versus eBEACOPP in advanced-stage, classical Hodgkin lymphoma (HD21): a randomised, multicentre, parallel, open-label, phase 3 trial. Lancet. 2024;404:341. [PMID: 38971175]

Herrera AF et al. Nivolumab+AVD in advanced-stage classic Hodgkin's lymphoma. N Engl J Med. 2024;391:1379. [PMID: 39413375]

Zhang Y et al. Novel agents for relapsed and refractory classical Hodgkin lymphoma: a review. Front Oncol. 2022;12:929012. [PMID: 35928877]

PLASMA CELL MYELOMA

ESSENTIALS OF DIAGNOSIS

- Bone pain, often in the spine, ribs, or proximal long bones.
- Monoclonal immunoglobulin (ie, paraprotein) in the serum or urine.
- Clonal plasma cells in the bone marrow or in a tissue biopsy, or both.
- Organ damage due to plasma cells (eg, bones, kidneys, hypercalcemia, anemia) or other defined criteria.

General Considerations

Plasma cell myeloma (previously called "multiple myeloma") is a malignancy of hematopoietic stem cells terminally differentiated as plasma cells. It is characterized by infiltration of the bone marrow, bone destruction, and paraprotein production. The diagnosis is established when monoclonal plasma cells (either kappa or lambda light chain restricted) are found in the bone marrow (any percentage) or in a tumor (plasmacytoma). This is associated with end-organ damage (such as bone disease [lytic lesions seen on bone radiographs, MRI, or PET/CT scan], anemia [hemoglobin < 10 g/dL {100 g/L}], hypercalcemia [calcium > 11 mg/dL {2.75 mmol/L}], or kidney injury [creatinine > 2 mg/dL {176.8 mcmol/L} or creatinine clearance < 40 mL/min]) with or without paraprotein elaboration. Sixty percent or more clonal plasma cells in the bone marrow, or a serum free kappa to lambda ratio of > 100 or < 0.01 (both criteria regardless of end-organ damage), are also diagnostic of plasma cell myeloma. Smoldering myeloma is defined as 10–59% clonal plasma cells in the bone marrow, a serum paraprotein level of 3 g/dL (30 g/L) or higher, or both, without plasma cell–related end-organ damage.

Malignant plasma cells can form tumors (**plasmacytomas**) that may cause spinal cord compression or other soft-tissue–related problems. Bone disease is common and due to excessive osteoclast activation mediated largely by the interaction of the receptor activator of NF-kappa-B (RANK) with its ligand (RANKL). In plasma cell myeloma, osteoprotegerin (a decoy receptor for RANKL) is underproduced, thus promoting the binding of RANK with RANKL with consequent excessive bone resorption.

The **paraproteins (monoclonal immunoglobulins)** secreted by the malignant plasma cells may cause additional problems. Very high paraprotein levels (either IgG or IgA) may cause **hyperviscosity**, although this is more common with the IgM paraprotein as in Waldenström macroglobulinemia. The light chain component of the immunoglobulin, when produced in excess, often leads to kidney injury (frequently aggravated by hypercalcemia or hyperuricemia, or both). Light chain components may be deposited in tissues as amyloid, resulting in kidney failure with albuminuria and a vast array of other systemic syndromes (restrictive cardiomyopathy, autonomic and peripheral neuropathy, enlarged tongue, etc).

Myeloma patients are prone to recurrent infections for a number of reasons, including neutropenia, the underproduction of normal immunoglobulins (so-called **immunoparesis**), and the immunosuppressive effects of chemotherapy. Myeloma patients are especially prone to infections with encapsulated organisms such as *Streptococcus pneumoniae* and *Haemophilus influenzae* and should receive vaccinations against them.

Clinical Findings

A. Symptoms and Signs

Myeloma is a disease of older adults (median age 65 years). The most common presenting complaints are those related to anemia, bone pain, kidney disease, and infection. Bone pain is most common in the back, hips, or ribs or may present as a pathologic fracture, especially of the femoral neck or vertebrae. Patients may also come to medical attention because of spinal cord compression from a plasmacytoma or the hyperviscosity syndrome (mucosal bleeding, vertigo, nausea, visual disturbances, alterations in mental status, hypoxia). Many patients are diagnosed because of laboratory findings of elevated total protein, hypercalcemia, proteinuria, elevated ESR, or abnormalities on serum protein electrophoresis obtained for symptoms or in routine screening studies. A few patients come to medical attention because of organ dysfunction due to amyloidosis.

Examination may reveal pallor, bone tenderness, or soft tissue masses. Patients may have neurologic signs related to neuropathy or spinal cord compression. Fever occurs mainly with infection. Acute oliguric or nonoliguric kidney injury may be present due to hypercalcemia, hyperuricemia, light chain cast injury, or primary amyloidosis.

B. Laboratory Findings

Anemia is nearly universal. RBC morphology is normal, but rouleaux formation is common and may be marked. The absence of rouleaux formation, however, excludes neither plasma cell myeloma nor the presence of a serum paraprotein. The neutrophil and platelet counts are usually normal at presentation. Only rarely will plasma cells be visible on peripheral blood smear (plasma cell leukemia if > 20%).

The hallmark of myeloma is the finding of a paraprotein on serum or urine **protein electrophoresis (PEP)** or **immunofixation electrophoresis (IFE)**. Most patients will have a monoclonal spike visible in the γ- or β-globulin region of the PEP. The semi-quantification of the paraprotein on the PEP is referred to as the M-protein, and IFE will reveal this to be a monoclonal immunoglobulin. Approximately 15% of patients will have no demonstrable paraprotein in the serum on PEP because their myeloma cells produce only light chains and not intact immunoglobulin (but often seen on serum IFE), and the light chains pass rapidly through the glomerulus into the urine. Urine PEP and IFE usually demonstrate the light chain paraprotein in this setting. The **free light chain assay** will sometimes demonstrate excess monoclonal light chains in serum and urine, and in a small proportion of patients, will be the only means to identify and quantify the paraprotein being produced. Overall, the paraprotein is IgG (60%), IgA (20%), or light chain only (15%) in plasma cell myeloma, with the remainder being rare cases of IgD, IgM, or biclonal gammopathy. In sporadic cases, no paraprotein is present (**"nonsecretory myeloma"**); these patients have particularly aggressive disease.

The bone marrow will be infiltrated by variable numbers of monoclonal plasma cells. The plasma cells may be morphologically abnormal often demonstrating multinucleation and vacuolization. The plasma cells will display marked skewing of the normal kappa-to-lambda light chain ratio, which will indicate their clonality. Many benign inflammatory processes can result in bone marrow plasmacytosis, but without clonality and morphologic atypia.

C. Imaging

Bone radiographs are important in establishing the diagnosis of myeloma. Lytic lesions are most commonly seen in the axial skeleton: skull, spine, proximal long bones, and ribs. At other times, only generalized osteoporosis is seen. The radionuclide bone scan is not useful in detecting bone lesions in myeloma since there is little osteoblastic component. In the evaluation of patients with known or suspected plasma cell myeloma, MRI and PET/CT scans are more sensitive to detect bone disease than plain radiographs and are now preferred.

Differential Diagnosis

When a patient is discovered to have a paraprotein, the distinction between plasma cell myeloma or another lymphoproliferative malignancy with a paraprotein (CLL/SLL, Waldenström macroglobulinemia, non-Hodgkin lymphoma, primary amyloid, cryoglobulinemia) or monoclonal gammopathy of undetermined significance (MGUS) must be made. Plasma cell myeloma, smoldering plasma cell myeloma, and MGUS must be distinguished from reactive (benign) polyclonal hypergammaglobulinemia (which is commonly seen in cirrhosis or chronic inflammation).

Treatment

Patients with low-risk smoldering myeloma are observed. Those with high-risk smoldering disease may be treated with lenalidomide (an immunomodulatory agent) and dexamethasone since this therapy prolongs the time to symptomatic myeloma and may prolong survival compared to no treatment though at the expense of treatment-related side effects.

Most patients with plasma cell myeloma require treatment at diagnosis because of bone pain or other symptoms and complications related to the disease. The initial treatment currently involves quadruple therapy with an immunomodulatory agent, such as lenalidomide; a proteasome inhibitor, such as bortezomib or carfilzomib; an anti-CD38 monoclonal antibody, eg, daratumumab; and moderate- or high-dose dexamethasone. An immunomodulatory agent is sometimes replaced with an alkylating agent, cyclophosphamide, in the setting of kidney injury. The major side effects of lenalidomide are neutropenia and thrombocytopenia, skin rash, VTE, peripheral neuropathy, and possibly congenital disabilities. Bortezomib and carfilzomib have the advantages of producing rapid responses and of being effective in poor-prognosis myeloma. The major side effect of bortezomib is neuropathy (both peripheral and autonomic), which is largely ameliorated when given subcutaneously rather than intravenously. Carfilzomib rarely causes neuropathy but sometimes causes acute pulmonary hypertension or cardiac systolic dysfunction that is usually reversible. Daratumumab (1800 mg) plus hyaluronidase-fihj (30,000 units) is administered subcutaneously into the abdomen over 3–5 minutes and can cause local infusion reactions, infusion-related reactions.

An oral proteasome inhibitor, ixazomib, is available for relapsed disease. Pomalidomide, an immunomodulatory agent, is effective as salvage therapy after relapse. Other salvage agents include daratumumab or isatuximab (anti-CD38 antibodies), elotuzumab (an anti-SLAMF7 monoclonal antibody), and selinexor (causes cell cycle arrest and apoptosis) as part of combination therapy.

For patients with multi-agent refractory disease, chimeric antigen receptor T-cell therapy targeting the early plasma cell antigen BCMA has shown remarkable activity with response rates exceeding 70% and approaching 100%. Most of these patients though will eventually relapse. The T-cell engaging antibodies targeting BCMA (like teclistamab) or GPRC5D (like talquetamab) have shown significant activity after 3 lines of therapy and are being studied earlier in the disease course. Lastly, belantamab mafodotin (an anti-BCMA antibody conjugated to a cytotoxic agent) has activity after 4 prior lines of therapy.

After initial therapy, many patients under age 80 years are consolidated with autologous hematopoietic stem cell transplantation following high-dose melphalan (an alkylating chemotherapeutic agent). Autologous stem cell transplantation prolongs both duration of remission and overall survival, but these studies were done prior to the availability of T-cell engager therapies. Lenalidomide prolongs remission and survival when given as posttransplant maintenance therapy but at the expense of an elevated rate of second malignancies. Proteasome inhibitors prolong remissions in high-risk patients after autologous stem cell transplantation.

Localized radiotherapy may be useful for palliation of bone pain or for eradicating tumor at the site of pathologic fracture. Vertebral collapse with its attendant pain and mechanical disturbance can be treated with vertebroplasty or kyphoplasty. Hypercalcemia and hyperuricemia should be treated aggressively with immobilization and hydration. The bisphosphonates (pamidronate or zoledronic acid) or the RANKL-inhibitor (denosumab) given intravenously monthly reduces pathologic fractures in patients with bone disease. These medications are important adjuncts in this subset of patients. The bisphosphonates are also used to treat myeloma-related hypercalcemia. However, long-term bisphosphonates have been associated with a risk of osteonecrosis of the jaw and other bony areas, so their use is limited to 1–2 years after definitive initial therapy in most patients. Myeloma patients with oliguric or anuric kidney disease at diagnosis due to high free light chain levels should be treated aggressively with chemotherapy and considered for therapeutic plasma exchange (to reduce the paraprotein burden) because return of kidney function can sometimes occur.

Prognosis

The outlook for patients with myeloma has been steadily improving. The median survival of patients is > 7 years. Patients with low-stage disease who lack high-risk genomic changes respond very well to treatment and derive significant benefit from autologous hematopoietic stem cell transplantation with survival approaching a decade. The International Staging System for myeloma relies on two factors: β_2-microglobulin and albumin. Stage 1 patients have both β_2-microglobulin < 3.5 mg/L and albumin > 3.5 g/dL (survival > 5 years). Stage 3 is established when β_2-microglobulin is > 5.5 mg/L (survival < 2 years). Stage 2 is established with values in between stage 1 and 3. Other adverse prognostic findings are an elevated serum LD or bone marrow genetic abnormalities established by FISH involving the immunoglobulin heavy chain locus at chromosome 14q32, multiple copies of the 1q21-23 locus, or 17p chromosome abnormalities (causing the loss or mutation of *TP53*).

When to Refer

All patients with plasma cell myeloma should be referred to a hematologist or an oncologist.

When to Admit

Hospitalization is indicated for treatment of AKI, hypercalcemia, or suspicion of spinal cord compression, for certain chemotherapy regimens, or for autologous hematopoietic stem cell transplantation.

Costa LJ et al. International myeloma working group immunotherapy committee recommendation on sequencing immunotherapy for treatment of multiple myeloma. Leukemia. 2025;39:543. [PMID: 39870767]

Cowan AJ et al. Diagnosis and management of multiple myeloma: a review. JAMA. 2022;327:464. [PMID: 35103762]

Perrot A. Transplant in myeloma: who, when, and why? Hematology Am Soc Hematol Educ Program. 2024;2024:561. [PMID: 39643987]

Zanwar S et al. Risk-adapted treatment for multiple myeloma: assessing the current potential and a roadmap for the future. Leuk Lymphoma. 2025;66:573. [PMID: 39709634]

MONOCLONAL GAMMOPATHY OF UNDETERMINED SIGNIFICANCE

ESSENTIALS OF DIAGNOSIS

- Monoclonal immunoglobulin (ie, paraprotein) in the serum (< 3 g/dL [< 30 g/L]) or urine or both.
- Clonal plasma cells in the bone marrow < 10%.
- No symptoms and no organ damage from the paraprotein.

General Considerations

MGUS is present in 1% of all adults (5% of those over age 50 years and > 8% of those over age 70 years). Among all patients with paraproteins, *MGUS is far more common than plasma cell myeloma.* MGUS is defined as bone marrow clonal plasma cells < 10% in the setting of a paraprotein in the serum or urine or both (serum M-protein < 3 g/dL [30 g/L]) and the absence of plasma cell–related end-organ damage. If an excess of serum free light chains (kappa or lambda) is established, the kappa to lambda ratio is < 100 and > 0.01 (otherwise, this is diagnostic of plasma cell myeloma). In approximately one-quarter of cases, MGUS progresses to overt malignant disease in a median of one decade. *The transformation of MGUS to plasma cell myeloma is approximately 1% per year.* Two adverse risk factors for progression of MGUS to a plasma cell or lymphoid malignancy are an abnormal serum free kappa to lambda free light chain ratio or a serum monoclonal protein (M-protein) level ≥ 1.5 g/dL. Patients with MGUS have shortened survival (median 8.1 years versus 12.4 years for age- and sex-matched controls). In addition, 12% of patients with MGUS will convert to primary amyloidosis in a median of 9 years. Plasma cell myeloma, smoldering plasma cell myeloma, and MGUS must be distinguished from reactive (benign) polyclonal hypergammaglobulinemia (common in cirrhosis or chronic inflammation).

Laboratory Findings

To establish the diagnosis, serum and urine should be sent for PEP and IFE to search for a monoclonal protein; serum should be sent for free light chain analysis and quantitative immunoglobulins. Additional tests include a hemoglobin and serum albumin, calcium, and creatinine. If these additional tests are normal (or if abnormal but otherwise explained), then a bone marrow biopsy is usually deferred provided the serum M-protein is < 3 g/dL (< 30 g/L). In asymptomatic individuals, a skeletal survey (radiographs) is performed, but if there are some bone complaints or a question regarding bone disease, MRI or PET/CT imaging is preferred. MGUS is diagnosed if patients do not meet the criteria for smoldering plasma cell myeloma, plasma cell myeloma, or other lymphoproliferative neoplasm.

Treatment

Patients with MGUS are observed without treatment. Annual monitoring of the serum PEP, serum free light chains, CBC, and serum chemistries is recommended.

Rajkumar SV et al. Monoclonal gammopathy of undetermined significance. N Engl J Med. 2025;393:1315. [PMID: 41032708]
Schmidt T et al. SOHO state of the art updates and next questions: diagnosis and management of monoclonal gammopathy of undetermined significance and smoldering multiple myeloma. Clin Lymphoma Myeloma Leuk. 2024;24:653. [PMID: 38641486]

WALDENSTRÖM MACROGLOBULINEMIA

ESSENTIALS OF DIAGNOSIS

- Monoclonal IgM paraprotein.
- Infiltration of bone marrow by plasmacytic lymphocytes.
- Absence of lytic bone disease.
- *L265P* pathogenic variant in the gene *MYD88*.

General Considerations

Waldenström macroglobulinemia is a syndrome of *IgM hypergammaglobulinemia* that occurs in the setting of a low-grade non-Hodgkin lymphoma (lymphoplasmacytic lymphoma) characterized by B cells that are morphologically a hybrid of lymphocytes and plasma cells. These cells characteristically secrete the IgM paraprotein, and many clinical manifestations of the disease are related to this macroglobulin.

Clinical Findings

A. Symptoms and Signs

This disease characteristically develops insidiously in patients in their 60s or 70s. Patients usually present with fatigue related to anemia. Hyperviscosity of serum may manifest in a number of ways. Mucosal and GI bleeding is related to engorged blood vessels and platelet dysfunction. Other complaints include nausea, vertigo, and visual disturbances. Alterations in consciousness vary from mild lethargy to stupor and coma. The IgM paraprotein may also cause symptoms of cold agglutinin disease (hemolysis) or chronic demyelinating peripheral neuropathy.

On examination, there may be hepatosplenomegaly or lymphadenopathy. The retinal veins are engorged. Purpura may be present. There should be no bone tenderness.

B. Laboratory Findings

Anemia is nearly universal, and rouleaux formation is common, although the RBCs are agglutinated when the blood smear is prepared at room temperature. The anemia is related in part to expansion of the plasma volume by 50–100% due to the presence of the paraprotein. Other blood counts are usually normal. The abnormal plasmacytic lymphocytes may appear in small numbers on the peripheral blood smear. The bone marrow is characteristically infiltrated by the plasmacytic lymphocytes. The *L265P* pathogenic variant in *MYD88* is detectable in about 95% of patients. Additionally, CXCR4 mutations are found in 30–40% of patients and are associated with have higher bone marrow disease burden, higher serum immunoglobulin M levels, and incidence of symptomatic hyperviscosity.

The hallmark of macroglobulinemia is the presence of a monoclonal IgM spike seen on serum PEP in the β-globulin region. The serum viscosity is usually increased above the normal of 1.4–1.8 times that of water. Symptoms of hyperviscosity usually develop when the serum viscosity is over four times that of water, and marked symptoms usually arise when the viscosity is over six times that of water. Because paraproteins vary in their physicochemical properties, there is no strict correlation between the concentration of paraprotein and serum viscosity.

The IgM paraprotein may cause a positive antiglobulin (Coombs) test for complement and have cold agglutinin or cryoglobulin properties. If macroglobulinemia is suspected but the serum PEP shows only hypogammaglobulinemia, the test should be repeated while taking special measures to maintain the blood at 37°C, since the paraprotein may precipitate out at room temperature. Bone radiographs are normal, and there is no evidence of kidney injury.

Differential Diagnosis

Waldenström macroglobulinemia is differentiated from MGUS by the finding of bone marrow infiltration with monoclonal malignant cells. It is distinguished from CLL by bone marrow morphology, the absence of CD5 expression, and the absence of lymphocytosis, and it is distinguished from plasma cell myeloma by bone marrow morphology, the finding of the characteristic IgM paraprotein, and the absence of lytic bone disease.

Treatment

Patients with marked hyperviscosity syndrome (stupor, coma, pulmonary edema) should be treated on an emergency basis with plasmapheresis. When treatment is required for symptoms of hyperviscosity, neurologic complications, cytopenias, or the presence of amyloidosis, combination therapy with rituximab and bendamustine has been historically used (see Table 43–3). *Rituximab use alone is contraindicated for patients with hyperviscosity as the IgM often rises first after rituximab therapy before it falls.* The oral BTK inhibitors ibrutinib (420 mg daily) and zanubrutinib (160 mg twice daily) have shown significant activity in the front-line setting with a 90% response rate and a 73% major response rate that can result in durable remissions. Nonsense CXCR4 variants may confer resistance to BTK inhibitors. Proteasome inhibitors (bortezomib, carfilzomib), the bcl2 inhibitor venetoclax, and lenalidomide also have been shown to have activity in this disease. Autologous hematopoietic stem cell transplantation is reserved for relapsed or refractory patients.

Prognosis

Waldenström macroglobulinemia is an indolent disease with a median survival rate of 5 years, and 10% of patients are alive at 15 years.

When to Refer

All patients should be referred to a hematologist or an oncologist.

When to Admit

Patients should be admitted for treatment of hyperviscosity syndrome.

Castillo JJ et al. Venetoclax in previously treated Waldenström macroglobulinemia. J Clin Oncol. 2022;40:63. [PMID: 34793256]

Gertz MA. Waldenström macroglobulinemia: 2025 update on diagnosis, risk stratification, and management. Am J Hematol. 2025;100:1061. [PMID: 40095219]

Treon SP et al. How I use genomics and BTK inhibitors in the treatment of Waldenström macroglobulinemia. Blood. 2024;143:1702. [PMID: 38211337]

AMYLOIDOSIS

ESSENTIALS OF DIAGNOSIS

- Congo red positive amyloid protein on tissue biopsy.
- Primary amyloid protein is kappa or lambda immunoglobulin light chain.
- In primary amyloidosis, there is usually a serum or urine (or both) light chain paraprotein.

General Considerations

Amyloidosis is a rare condition whereby a protein abnormally deposits in tissue resulting in organ dysfunction. The propensity of a protein to be amyloidogenic is a consequence of disturbed translational or posttranslational protein folding and lack of consequential water solubility. The input of amyloid protein into tissues far exceeds its output, so amyloid build up inexorably proceeds to organ dysfunction and ultimately organ failure and premature death.

Amyloidosis is classified according to the type of amyloid protein deposited. The six main categories are **primary** (immunoglobulin light chain [AL]), **secondary** (serum protein A, produced in inflammatory conditions [AA]), **hereditary** (mutated transthyretin [TTR]; many others), **senile** (wild-type TTR; atrial natriuretic peptide; others), **dialysis-related** (β_2-microglobulin, not filtered out by dialysis membranes [Aβ-2M]), and **LECT2** (associated with Latina/Latino ethnicity). Amyloidosis is further classified as **localized** (amyloid deposits only in a single tissue type or organ) or, most commonly, **systemic** (widespread amyloid deposition).

Clinical Findings

A. Symptoms and Signs

Patients with **localized amyloidosis** have symptoms and signs related to the affected single organ, such as hoarseness (vocal folds) or proptosis and visual disturbance (orbits). Patients with **systemic amyloidosis** have symptoms and signs of unexplained medical syndromes, including HF (infiltrative/restrictive cardiomyopathy), nephrotic syndrome, malabsorption and weight loss, hepatic dysfunction, autonomic insufficiency, carpal tunnel syndrome (often bilateral), and sensorimotor peripheral neuropathy. Other symptoms and signs include an enlarged tongue; waxy, rough plaques on skin; contusions (including the periorbital areas); cough or dyspnea; and disturbed deglutition. These symptoms and signs arise insidiously, and the diagnosis of amyloidosis is generally made late in the disease process.

B. Laboratory Findings

The diagnosis of amyloid protein requires a tissue biopsy that demonstrates deposition of a pink interstitial substance in the tissue with the hematoxylin and eosin stain. This protein stains red with Congo red and becomes an apple-green color when the light is polarized. In primary amyloidosis, the amyloid protein is either the kappa or lambda immunoglobulin light chain.

When systemic amyloidosis is suspected, a blind aspiration of the abdominal fat pad will reveal amyloid two-thirds of the time. If the fat pad aspiration is unrevealing, then the affected organ needs biopsy. In 90% of patients with primary amyloidosis, analysis of the serum and urine will reveal a kappa or lambda light chain paraprotein by PEP, IFE, or free light chain assay; in the remainder, mass spectroscopy demonstrates light chain in the tissue biopsy. Lambda amyloid is more common than kappa amyloid, a relative proportion opposite from normal B-cell stoichiometry. Most patients with primary amyloidosis have a small amount of kappa- or lambda-restricted plasma cells in the bone marrow (but < 10%). The bone marrow may or may not demonstrate interstitial amyloid deposition or amyloid in the blood vessels.

Patients with ***primary cardiac amyloidosis*** have an infiltrative cardiomyopathy with thick ventricular walls on echocardiogram that sometimes shows a specific speckling pattern. Paradoxically, QRS voltages are low on ECG. Cardiac MRI has a distinctive delayed enhancement of gadolinium that is virtually diagnostic. With renal amyloid, albuminuria is present, which can be in the nephrotic range. Later in renal involvement, kidney function decreases (see Chapter 25, Renal Amyloidosis).

Differential Diagnosis

Amyloidosis must be distinguished from MGUS and plasma cell myeloma or other malignant lymphoproliferative disorders with an associated paraprotein. Of note, 12% of patients with MGUS will convert to primary amyloidosis in a median of 9 years. One-fifth of patients who have primary amyloidosis will meet the diagnostic criteria for plasma cell myeloma; conversely, 5% of patients with plasma cell myeloma will have amyloid deposition.

Treatment

The treatment approach to primary amyloidosis closely resembles that of plasma cell myeloma. The goal is reduction of light chain production and thus tissue deposition as a means to arrest progressive end-organ dysfunction. Active agents in primary amyloidosis include melphalan, cyclophosphamide, dexamethasone, lenalidomide, bortezomib, and daratumumab (see Table 43–3). As in plasma cell myeloma, autologous hematopoietic stem cell transplantation after high-dose melphalan is used in patients with reasonable organ function and a good performance status. The treatment-related mortality, however, is higher in patients with primary amyloidosis than in plasma cell myeloma (6% versus 1%). After transplant, the median survival is a decade with one-third alive at 20 years. Some patients will demonstrate end-organ improvement after therapy. Agents are being developed that facilitate amyloid dissolution or correct protein folding abnormalities in the amyloid protein. Treatment of AA amyloid is treatment of the underlying cause of inflammation. Treatment of familial TTR is liver transplantation. Treatment of acquired TTR are tetramer stabilizers (tafamidis or acoramidis) or antisense oligonucleotides (patisiran).

Prognosis

Untreated primary amyloidosis is associated with progressive end-organ failure and premature death. There is no known cure for primary amyloidosis. Although virtually every tissue examined at autopsy will contain amyloid, patients with primary amyloidosis usually have one or two primary failing organs that clinically drive the presentation and prognosis. The cardiac biomarkers BNP, N-terminal pro-BNP, and troponins T and I are prognostic in this disease regardless of overt clinical cardiac involvement. Historically, patients with predominantly cardiac or autonomic nerve presentations had survivals of 3–9 months, those with carpal tunnel syndrome or nephrosis had survivals of 1.5–3 years, and those with peripheral neuropathy had survivals of 5 years. *These survivals are roughly doubled with plasma cell myeloma-like treatment.* In those patients able to undergo autologous hematopoietic stem cell transplantation, the median survival is about 5 years (and approaches 10 years for those achieving a complete hematologic remission).

When to Refer

- All patients who have primary amyloidosis or in whom it is suspected should be referred to a hematologist or oncologist.
- Patients with hereditary TTR amyloidosis should be referred to a hepatologist for consideration of liver transplantation.

When to Admit

- Patients with systemic amyloidosis require hospitalization to treat exacerbations of end-organ failure, including the heart, liver, or kidneys.
- Patients with primary amyloidosis require hospitalization to undergo autologous hematopoietic stem cell transplantation.

Gertz MA. Immunoglobulin light chain amyloidosis: 2024 update on diagnosis, prognosis, and treatment. Am H Hematol. 2024;99:309. [PMID: 38095141]

Parmar H et al. Role of autologous stem cell transplantation in systemic light chain amyloidosis. Clin Lymphoma Myeloma Leuk. 2024;24:770. [PMID: 39122638]

Sanchorawala V. Systemic light chain amyloidosis. N Engl J Med. 2024;390:2295. [PMID: 38924733]

Tschope C et al. Transthyretin amyloid cardiomyopathy–2025 update: diagnostic approaches and emerging therapeutic options. J Ckin Med. 2025;14:4785. [PMID: 40649158]

BLOOD TRANSFUSIONS

Most blood products are leukoreduced in-line during acquisition and are thus prospectively leukocyte-poor. Leukoreduced blood products reduce the incidence of leukoagglutination reactions, platelet alloimmunization, transfusion-related acute lung injury, and CMV exposure.

RBC TRANSFUSIONS

RBC transfusions are given to raise the hemoglobin levels in patients with clinically significant anemia or to replace losses after acute bleeding episodes.

Preparations of RBCs for Transfusion

Several types of preparations containing RBCs are available (whole blood, packed RBCs, frozen RBCs, or autologous non-frozen RBCs).

A. Fresh Whole Blood

The advantage of whole blood for transfusion is the simultaneous presence of RBCs, plasma, and fresh platelets.

Fresh whole blood is not absolutely necessary, since all the above components are available separately. The major indications for use of whole blood are cardiac surgery with hemorrhage or massive hemorrhage when more than 10 units of blood is required in a 24-hour period.

B. Packed RBCs

Packed RBCs are the component most commonly used to raise the hemoglobin. Each unit has a volume of about 300 mL, of which approximately 200 mL consists of RBCs. One unit of packed RBCs will usually raise the hemoglobin by approximately 1 g/dL. Current guidelines recommend a transfusion "trigger" hemoglobin threshold of 7–8 g/dL (70–80 g/L) for hospitalized patients, including those who are critically ill, those undergoing cardiothoracic surgery or repair of a hip fracture, those with upper GI bleeding, and those with hematologic malignancy undergoing chemotherapy or hematopoietic cell transplant.

C. Autologous Packed RBCs

Patients scheduled for elective surgery may donate blood for autologous transfusion. These units may be stored for up to 35 days before freezing is necessary.

Compatibility Testing

Before transfusion, the recipient's and the donor's blood are typed and cross-matched to avoid **hemolytic transfusion reactions**. Although many antigen systems are present on RBCs, only the ABO and Rh systems are specifically tested prior to all transfusions. The A and B antigens are the most important because everyone who lacks one or both RBC antigens has IgM isoantibodies (called isoagglutinins) in his or her plasma against the missing antigen(s). The isoagglutinins activate complement and can cause rapid intravascular lysis of the incompatible RBCs. In emergencies, *type O/Rh-negative blood can be given to any recipient*, but usually packed RBCs are given to minimize transfusion of donor plasma containing anti-A and anti-B antibodies with the use of whole blood.

The other important antigen routinely tested for is the D antigen of the Rh system. Approximately 15% of the population lacks this antigen. In patients lacking the antigen, anti-D antibodies are not naturally present, but the D antigen is highly immunogenic. A recipient whose RBCs lack D and who receives D-positive blood often develop anti-D antibodies that can cause severe lysis of subsequent transfusions of D-positive RBCs or abort a D-positive fetus.

Blood typing includes a cross-match assay of recipient serum for alloantibodies directed against donor RBCs by mixing recipient serum with panels of RBCs representing commonly occurring minor RBC antigens. The screening is particularly important if the recipient has had previous transfusions or pregnancy.

Hemolytic Transfusion Reactions

The most severe hemolytic transfusion reactions are **acute** (temporally related to the transfusion), involving incompatible mismatches in the ABO system that are isoagglutinin-mediated. Most of these cases are due to clerical errors and mislabeled specimens. With current compatibility testing and double-check clerical systems, the risk of an acute hemolytic reaction is 1 in 76,000 transfused units of RBCs. Death from acute hemolytic reaction occurs in 1 in 1.8 million transfused units. When hemolysis occurs, it is rapid and intravascular, releasing free hemoglobin into the plasma causing acute DIC and acute renal injury. The severity of these reactions depends on the dose of RBCs given. The most severe reactions are those seen in surgical patients under anesthesia.

Delayed hemolytic transfusion reactions are caused by minor RBC antigen discrepancies and are typically less severe. The hemolysis usually takes place at a slower rate and is mediated by IgG alloantibodies causing extravascular RBC destruction. These transfusion reactions may be delayed for 5–10 days after transfusion. In such cases, the recipient has received RBCs containing an immunogenic antigen, and in the time since transfusion, a new alloantibody has formed. The most common antigens involved in such reactions are Duffy, Kidd, Kell, and C and E loci of the Rh system. The current risk of a delayed hemolytic transfusion reaction is 1 in 6000 transfused units of RBCs.

A. Symptoms and Signs

Major acute hemolytic transfusion reactions cause fever and chills, with backache and headache. In severe cases, there may be apprehension, dyspnea, hypotension, and cardiovascular collapse. Patients under general anesthesia will not manifest such symptoms, and the first indication may be tachycardia, generalized bleeding, or oliguria. *The transfusion must be stopped immediately*. In severe cases, acute DIC, AKI from tubular necrosis, or both can occur. Death occurs in 4% of acute hemolytic reactions due to ABO incompatibility. Delayed hemolytic transfusion reactions are usually without any or only mild symptoms or signs.

B. Laboratory Findings

When an acute hemolytic transfusion episode is suspected, the identification of the recipient and of the transfusion product bag label should be rechecked. The transfusion product bag with its pilot tube must be returned to the blood bank, and a fresh sample of the recipient's blood must accompany the bag for retyping and re-cross-matching of donor and recipient blood samples. The hemoglobin will fail to rise by the expected amount after a transfusion. Chemistries and coagulation studies may reveal evidence of acute DIC, AKI, or both. The recipient's plasma-free hemoglobin will be elevated, resulting in hemoglobinuria.

In cases of delayed hemolytic reactions, there will be an unexpected drop in hemoglobin and an increase in the total and indirect bilirubins. The new offending alloantibody is easily detected in the patient's serum.

C. Treatment

If an acute hemolytic transfusion reaction is suspected, the transfusion should be stopped at once. The patient should be vigorously hydrated to prevent ATN. Forced diuresis with mannitol may help prevent or minimize AKI.

Leukoagglutinin Reactions

Many transfusion reactions are not hemolytic but represent reactions to antigens present on transfused passenger leukocytes in patients sensitized to leukocyte antigens through previous transfusions or pregnancy. Transfusion products relatively rich in leukocyte-rich plasma, especially platelets, are most likely to cause this. Moderate to severe **leukoagglutinin reactions** occur in 1% of RBC transfusions and 2% of platelet transfusions. The risk of a leukoagglutination reaction is minimal if the transfused blood product is leukoreduced in-line upon collection. Most commonly, fever and chills develop within 12 hours after transfusion. In severe cases, cough and dyspnea may occur and the CXR may show transient pulmonary infiltrates. Because no hemolysis is involved, the hemoglobin rises by the expected amount despite the reaction.

Leukoagglutinin reactions may respond to acetaminophen (500–650 mg orally) and diphenhydramine (25 mg orally or intravenously); corticosteroids, such as hydrocortisone (1 mg/kg intravenously), are also of value. Overall, leukoagglutination reactions are diminishing through the routine use of in-line leukotrapping during blood donation (ie, leukoreduced blood). Patients experiencing severe leukoagglutination episodes despite receiving leukoreduced blood transfusions should receive leukopoor or washed blood products.

Hypersensitivity Reactions

Urticaria or bronchospasm may develop during or soon after a transfusion. These reactions are almost always due to exposure to allogeneic plasma proteins rather than to leukocytes. The risk is low enough that the routine use of antihistamine premedications has been eliminated before packed RBC transfusions. However, a hypersensitivity reaction, including anaphylactic shock, may develop in patients who are IgA deficient because of antibodies to IgA in the patient's plasma directed against the IgA in the transfused blood product. Patients with such reactions may require transfusion of washed or even frozen RBCs to avoid future severe reactions.

Contaminated Blood

Blood products can be contaminated with bacteria. Platelets are especially prone to bacterial contamination because they cannot be refrigerated. Bacterial contamination occurs in 1 of every 30,000 RBC donations and 1 of every 5000 platelet donations. Receipt of a blood product contaminated with gram-positive bacteria will cause fever and bacteremia but rarely causes a sepsis syndrome. Receipt of a blood product contaminated with gram-negative bacteria often causes septic shock, acute DIC, and AKI due to the transfused endotoxin and is usually fatal. Strategies to reduce bacterial contamination include enhanced venipuncture site skin cleansing, diverting of the first few milliliters of donated blood, use of single-donor blood products (as opposed to pooled-donor products), and point-of-care rapid bacterial screening in order to discard questionable units. Blood products infused with psoralen and then exposed to UVA light will have no living organisms in them but add cost to acquisition of the blood product. The current risk of a septic transfusion reaction from a culture-negative unit of single-donor platelets (not psoralen treated) is 1 in 60,000. In any patient who may have received contaminated blood, the recipient and the donor blood bag should both be cultured, and antibiotics should be given immediately to the recipient.

Infectious Diseases Transmitted Through Transfusion

Despite the use of only volunteer blood donors and the routine screening of blood, transfusion-associated viral diseases remain a problem. *All blood products (RBCs, platelets, plasma, cryoprecipitate) can transmit viral diseases.* All blood donors are screened with questionnaires designed to detect (and therefore reject) donors at high risk for transmitting infectious diseases. For example, the American Red Cross does not accept blood donation from persons with SARS-CoV-2 virus or from contacts of persons who have or are suspected to have the causal SARS-CoV-2 virus. All blood is screened for hepatitis B surface antigen, antibody to hepatitis B core antigen, antibody to syphilis, antibodies to HIV-1 and HIV-2 and NAT (nucleic acid amplification) for HIV, antibody to hepatitis C virus (HCV) and NAT for hepatitis C, antibody to human T-cell lymphotropic/leukemia virus (HTLV), and NAT for West Nile virus. Zika virus contamination is screened for by donor questionnaire, but the routine use of an FDA-approved detection test has not been uniformly adopted to screen donated blood. It is recommended that blood donors get screened once for antibodies against *Trypanosoma cruzi*, the infectious agent that causes Chagas disease (and if negative, no further screening for additional blood donations).

With improved screening, the risk of posttransfusion hepatitis has steadily decreased after the receipt of screened "negative" blood products. The risk of acquiring hepatitis B is about 0.8 in 1 million transfused units in the United Kingdom. The risk of hepatitis C acquisition is 0.02 in 1 million transfused units in the United Kingdom. The risk of HIV acquisition is 0.4 in 1 million transfused units in the United Kingdom. Unscreened but leukoreduced blood products appear to be equivalent to CMV screened-negative blood products in terms of the risk of CMV transmission to a CMV-seronegative recipient.

Transfusion Graft-Versus-Host Disease

Allogeneic passenger lymphocytes in transfused blood products will engraft in some recipients and mount an alloimmune attack against tissues expressing discrepant HLA antigens causing graft-versus-host disease (GVHD). The symptoms and signs of transfusion-associated GVHD include fever, rash, diarrhea, hepatitis, lymphadenopathy, and severe pancytopenia. The outcome is usually fatal. Transfusion-associated GVHD occurs most often in recipients with immune defects, malignant lymphoproliferative disorders, solid tumors being treated with chemotherapy or immunotherapy, treatment with immunosuppressive medications (especially purine analogs such as fludarabine), older patients undergoing cardiac surgery, or use of family donor-designated blood. HIV infection alone does not increase the risk. The use of leukoreduced blood products is inadequate to prevent transfusion-associated GVHD. This complication can be avoided by irradiating blood products (25 Gy or more) to prevent lymphocyte proliferation in blood products given to recipients at high risk for transfusion-associated GVHD.

Transfusion-Related Acute Lung Injury

Transfusion-related acute lung injury (TRALI) occurs in 1 in every 5000 transfused units of blood products. TRALI is clinically defined as noncardiogenic pulmonary edema after a blood product transfusion without other explanation. Transfused surgical and critically ill patients seem most susceptible. It has been associated with allogeneic antibodies in the donor plasma component that bind to recipient leukocyte antigens, including HLA antigens and other granulocyte- and monocyte-specific antigens (such as human neutrophil antigen [HNA]-1a, -1b, -2a, and -3a). In 20% of cases, no antileukocyte antibodies are identified, raising the concern that bioactive lipids or other substances that accumulate while the blood product is in storage can also mediate TRALI in susceptible recipients. Ten to 20% of female blood donors and 1–5% of male blood donors have antileukocyte antibodies in their serum. The risk of TRALI is reduced by using male-only plasma donors when possible. There is no specific treatment for TRALI, only supportive care.

PLATELET TRANSFUSIONS

Platelet transfusions are indicated in cases of thrombocytopenia due to decreased platelet production. They are of some use in immune thrombocytopenia when active bleeding is evident, but the clearance of transfused platelets is rapid as they are exposed to the same pathophysiologic forces experienced by the recipient's endogenous platelets. The risk of bleeding rises when the platelet count falls to < 80,000/mcL (80×10^9/L), and the risk of life-threatening spontaneous bleeding increases when the platelet count is < 5000/mcL (5×10^9/L). Because of this, *prophylactic platelet transfusions are often given at these very low levels, usually when < 10,000/mcL (10×10^9/L).* Platelet transfusions are also given before invasive procedures or surgery in thrombocytopenic patients, and the goal is often to raise the platelet count to 20,000–50,000/mcL ($20–50 \times 10^9$/L), procedure-dependent. Attempting to transfuse to 100,000/mcL (100×10^9/L) is advised for nonoperative intracranial hemorrhage.

Platelets for transfusion are most commonly derived from single-donor apheresis collections (roughly the equivalent to the platelets recovered from six donations of whole blood). A single donor unit of platelets should raise the platelet count by 50,000 to 60,000 platelets per mcL ($50–60 \times 10^9$/L) in a transfusion-naïve recipient without hypersplenism or ongoing platelet consumptive disorder. Transfused platelets typically last for 2 or 3 days. Platelet transfusion responses may be suboptimal with poor platelet increments and short platelet survival times. Poor platelet transfusion response may be due to one of several causes, including fever, sepsis, hypersplenism, DIC, large body habitus, low platelet dose in the transfusion unit, or platelet alloimmunization (from prior transfusions, prior pregnancy, or prior organ transplantation). Many, but not all, alloantibodies causing platelet destruction are directed at HLA antigens. Patients requiring long periods of platelet transfusion support should be monitored to document adequate responses to transfusions so that the most appropriate product can be used. If random platelet transfusions prove inadequate, then the patient should be cross-matched with potential donors who might prove better able to provide adequate platelet-transfusion increments and platelet survival. Patients requiring ongoing platelet transfusions who become alloimmunized may benefit from HLA-matched platelets derived from either volunteer donors or family members.

TRANSFUSION OF PLASMA COMPONENTS

Fresh frozen plasma (FFP) is available in units of approximately 200 mL. FFP contains normal levels of all coagulation factors (about 1 unit/mL of each factor). FFP is used to correct coagulation factor deficiencies (such as in liver disease) and to treat idiopathic thrombotic thrombocytopenic purpura. FFP is also used to correct or prevent coagulopathy in trauma patients receiving massive transfusion of packed RBC (PRBC). *An FFP:PRBC ratio of 1:2 or more is associated with improved survival in trauma patients receiving massive transfusions, regardless of the presence of a coagulopathy. Recommended massive transfusion protocols are 1:1:1 (1 unit RBC, 1 unit FFP, 1 unit of random donor platelets) or 4:4:1.* The **prothrombinase complex concentrate (PCC)** contains the vitamin K-dependent factors (II, VII, IX, X, protein C, and protein S) and is used to correct clinically important warfarin overdoses (see Table 16–21).

Cryoprecipitate is made from fresh plasma by cooling the plasma to 4°C and collecting the precipitate. One unit of cryoprecipitate has a volume of approximately 15–20 mL and contains approximately 250 mg of fibrinogen and between 80 and 100 units of factor VIII and von Willebrand factor as well as 40–60 IU of factor XIII. Cryoprecipitate is most commonly used to supplement fibrinogen in cases of acquired hypofibrinogenemia (eg, acute DIC) or in rare instances of congenital hypofibrinogenemia. One unit of cryoprecipitate will raise the fibrinogen level by about 8 mg/dL (0.24 mcmol/L). Cryoprecipitate is sometimes used to temporarily correct the acquired qualitative platelet dysfunction associated with kidney disease.

Carson JL et al. Red blood cell transfusion: 2023 AABB International Guidelines. JAMA. 2023;330:1892. [PMID: 37824153]

Dutra VF et al. Infectious diseases and the impact on transfusion medicine: a historical review and lessons for the future. Transfus Clin Biol. 2023;30:376. [PMID: 37328129]

Lier H et al. Massive transfusion in trauma. Curr Opin Anaesthesiol. 2024;37:117. [PMID: 38390985]

Metcalf RA et al. Platelets transfusion: 2025 AABB and ICTMG international clinical practice guidelines. JAMA. 2025;334:606. [PMID: 40440268]

White SK et al. The incidence of transfusion-related acute lung injury using active surveillance: a systematic review and meta-analysis. Transfusion. 2024;64:289. [PMID: 38116828]

16 Disorders of Hemostasis, Thrombosis, & Antithrombotic Therapy

Andrew D. Leavitt, MD
Erika Leemann Price, MD, MPH

To evaluate patients for defects of hemostasis, the clinical context must be considered carefully (Table 16–1). **Heritable defects** are suggested by bleeding that begins in infancy or childhood, affects family members, is recurrent, and occurs at multiple anatomic sites, although other patterns of presentation are possible. **Acquired disorders** of hemostasis typically are associated with bleeding that begins later in life and may relate to introduction of medications (eg, agents that affect platelet activity) or to onset of underlying medical conditions (eg, kidney disease, liver disease, aortic stenosis, prosthetic aortic valve, myeloproliferative neoplasms), or may be idiopathic (acquired hemophilia A, acquired von Willebrand disease). Importantly, a sufficient hemostatic challenge, such as major trauma, may produce excessive bleeding even in individuals with normal hemostasis. Obtaining a personal history of hemostatic challenges (eg, circumcision, trauma, injury during youth sports, tooth extractions, prior surgery, pregnancy and delivery) and a family history of bleeding is essential.

PLATELET DISORDERS

THROMBOCYTOPENIA

Selected causes of thrombocytopenia are shown in Table 16–2. The age of the patient and presence of comorbid conditions can help direct the diagnostic workup.

The risk of clinically relevant spontaneous bleeding (including petechial hemorrhage and bruising) does not typically increase appreciably until the platelet count falls below ~20,000/mcL (~20×10^9/L), although patients with dysfunctional platelets or local vascular defects can bleed with higher platelet counts. Suggested platelet counts to prevent spontaneous bleeding or to provide adequate hemostasis around the time of invasive procedures are found in Table 16–3. However, most medical centers develop their own guidelines to have a consistent approach to such complex situations.

DECREASED PLATELET PRODUCTION

1. Bone Marrow Failure

ESSENTIALS OF DIAGNOSIS

- Determine if bone marrow failure is congenital or acquired.
- Most congenital marrow failure disorders present in childhood.

General Considerations

Congenital conditions that cause thrombocytopenia usually feature isolated thrombocytopenia. The exceptions are Fanconi anemia and dyskeratosis congenita, which typically have cytopenias in other blood cell lineages (Table 16–2). Pathogenic variants associated with inherited thrombocytopenia include *FLI1*, *MYH9*, *GATA1*, *ETV6*, and *RUNX1*.

Acquired causes of bone marrow failure (see Chapter 15) leading to thrombocytopenia include acquired aplastic anemia, myelodysplastic syndrome (MDS), alcohol, drugs, and splenomegaly (Table 16–2). Unlike aplastic anemia, MDS is more common among older patients.

Clinical Findings

See Chapter 15 for symptoms and signs of aplastic anemia. Acquired aplastic anemia typically presents with pancytopenia (anemia, thrombocytopenia, and neutropenia). A bone marrow biopsy is required for diagnosis and reveals marked hypocellularity. MDS also presents as cytopenias and can have pancytopenia, but the marrow typically demonstrates hypercellularity and dysplastic features. The presence of macrocytosis, ringed sideroblasts on iron staining of the bone marrow aspirate, dysplasia of hematopoietic elements, or cytogenetic abnormalities (especially monosomy 5 or 7 and trisomy 8) is more suggestive of MDS.

Table 16–1. Evaluation of the bleeding patient.

Necessary Component of Evaluation	Diagnostic Correlate
Location	
Mucocutaneous (bruises, petechiae, gingivae, nosebleeds, GI, GU)	Suggests qualitative/quantitative platelet defects; vWD; HHT
Joints, soft tissue	Suggests disorders of coagulation factors
Onset	
Infancy/childhood	Suggests heritable condition
Adulthood	Suggests milder heritable condition or acquired defect of hemostasis (eg, ITP, medication, acquired factor VIII deficiency; acquired vWD)
Clinical Context	
Postsurgical	Anatomic/surgical defect must be ruled out
Pregnancy	Consider vWD, HELLP syndrome, ITP, acquired factor VIII inhibitor
Sepsis	May indicate DIC
Exposure to anticoagulants	Rule out excessive anticoagulation
Personal History[1]	
Absent	Suggests acquired rather than congenital defect, or anatomic/surgical defect (if applicable)
Present	Suggests established acquired defect or congenital disorder
Family History	
Absent	Suggests acquired defect or no defect of hemostasis
Present	May signify hemophilia A or B, vWD, other heritable bleeding disorders such as HHT

[1]Prior spontaneous bleeding and excessive bleeding with circumcision, menses, dental extractions, trauma, minor procedures (eg, endoscopy, biopsies), and major procedures (surgery).
DIC, disseminated intravascular coagulation; GU, genitourinary; HELLP, hemolysis, elevated liver enzymes, low platelets; HHT, hereditary hemorrhagic telangiectasia; ITP, immune thrombocytopenia; vWD, von Willebrand disease.

Differential Diagnosis

Adult patients with acquired amegakaryocytic thrombocytopenia (rare) have isolated thrombocytopenia, reduced or absent megakaryocytes in the bone marrow, and elevated thrombopoietin levels, which along with failure to respond to immunomodulatory regimens typically administered in immune thrombocytopenia (ITP), distinguishes them from patients with ITP. Bone marrow

Table 16–2. Selected causes of thrombocytopenia.

Decreased production of platelets
- Congenital bone marrow failure
  - Amegakaryocytic thrombocytopenia, Wiskott-Aldrich syndrome, Fanconi anemia, thrombocytopenia-absent radius syndrome, dyskeratosis congenita
- Acquired bone marrow failure
  - Aplastic anemia, myelodysplastic syndrome, leukemia
  - Exposure to chemotherapy, irradiation, medications (https://ouhsc.edu/platelets/ditp.html)
  - Marrow infiltration (neoplastic, infectious)
  - Nutritional (deficiency of vitamin B_{12}, folate)
  - Other: HIV, alcohol
- Other inherited thrombocytopenias
  - Bernard-Soulier syndrome, gray platelet syndrome, May-Hegglin anomaly, Hermansky Pudlak syndrome, *MYH9* mutations, and others

Increased destruction of platelets
- Immune thrombocytopenia (primary)
- Immune thrombocytopenia (secondary), including drug-induced, lymphoproliferative disorders (eg, CLL) or viral infections (eg, hepatitis C virus, Epstein-Barr virus, or HIV), vaccines
- Heparin-induced thrombocytopenia
- Thrombotic microangiopathy/microangiopathic hemolytic anemias
- Disseminated intravascular coagulation
- Posttransfusion purpura
- Mechanical (aortic valvular dysfunction; extracorporeal bypass)
- von Willebrand disease, type 2B
- Hemophagocytosis (hemophagocytic lymphohistiocytosis)

Increased sequestration of platelets
- Hypersplenism (eg, cirrhosis, myeloproliferative disorders, lymphoma)

Other conditions causing thrombocytopenia
- Gestational thrombocytopenia
- Pseudothrombocytopenia
- *Helicobacter pylori*

CLL, chronic lymphocytic leukemia.

Table 16–3. Desired platelet count ranges.

Clinical Scenario	Platelet Count/mcL (× 10^9/L)
Prevention of spontaneous mucocutaneous bleeding	> 10,000–20,000 (> 10–20)
Insertion of central venous catheters	> 20,000–50,000[1] (> 20–50)
Administration of therapeutic anticoagulation	> 30,000–50,000 (> 30–50)
Minor surgery and selected invasive procedures[2]	> 50,000–80,000 (> 50–80)
Major surgery	> 80,000–100,000 (> 80–100)

[1]A platelet target within the higher reference range is required for tunneled catheters.
[2]Such as endoscopy with biopsy.

biopsy and genetic testing are often required to establish a diagnosis.

Treatment

A. Congenital Conditions

Treatment is varied but may include blood product support, blood cell growth factors, androgens and, in some cases, allogeneic hematopoietic stem cell transplantation.

B. Acquired Conditions

Patients with severe aplastic anemia are treated with immunosuppressive therapy or allogeneic hematopoietic stem cell transplantation (see Chapter 15).

Treatment of thrombocytopenia due to MDS, if clinically significant bleeding is present or if the risk of bleeding is high, is limited to chronic transfusion of platelets in most instances (Table 16–3). Additional treatment is discussed in Chapter 15.

Warren JT et al. Genetics of inherited thrombocytopenias. Blood. 2022;139:3264. [PMID: 35167650]

2. Bone Marrow Infiltration

Replacement of the normal bone marrow elements by leukemic cells, plasma cell myeloma, lymphoma, or nonhematologic tumors or by infections (such as mycobacterial disease or ehrlichiosis) may cause thrombocytopenia; however, abnormalities in other blood cell lines are usually present. These entities are easily diagnosed after examining the bone marrow biopsy and aspirate or determining the infecting organism from an aspirate specimen, and they often lead to a leukoerythroblastic peripheral blood smear (left-shifted myeloid lineage cells, nucleated RBCs, and teardrop-shaped RBCs). Treatment of thrombocytopenia is directed at eradication of the underlying infiltrative disorder, but platelet transfusion may be required if clinically significant bleeding is present (Table 16–3).

3. Chemotherapy & Irradiation

Chemotherapeutic agents and irradiation may lead to thrombocytopenia by direct toxicity to megakaryocytes, hematopoietic progenitor cells, or both. The severity and duration of chemotherapy-induced depressions in the platelet count are determined by the specific agent and regimen used, although the platelet count typically resolves more slowly following a chemotherapeutic insult than does neutropenia or anemia, especially if multiple cycles of treatment have been given. Until recovery occurs, patients may be supported with transfused platelets if bleeding is present or the risk of bleeding is high (Table 16–3). Studies suggest that platelet growth factors, such as eltrombopag and romiplostim, may help prevent chemotherapy-induced thrombocytopenia and allow patients to receive their full chemotherapy doses on schedule. Checkpoint inhibitors can also lead to thrombocytopenia that mimics immune thrombocytopenic purpura.

Kuter DJ. Treatment of chemotherapy-induced thrombocytopenia in patients with non-hematologic malignancies. Haematologica. 2022;107:1243. [PMID: 35642485]

4. Nutritional Deficiencies

Thrombocytopenia, typically in concert with anemia, may be observed with a deficiency of folate (that may accompany alcohol use disorder) or vitamin B_{12} (concomitant neurologic findings may be manifest). In addition, thrombocytopenia can occur in very severe iron deficiency, albeit rarely, whereas thrombocytosis is far more common. Replacing the deficient vitamin or mineral results in improvement in the platelet count.

5. Cyclic Thrombocytopenia

Cyclic thrombocytopenia is a rare disorder that produces cyclic oscillations of the platelet count, usually with a periodicity of 3–6 weeks. The pathophysiologic mechanism of the condition is unclear. Severe thrombocytopenia can occur, and bleeding may occur at the platelet nadir. Oral contraceptive medications, androgens, azathioprine, and thrombopoietic growth factors have been used successfully in the management of cyclic thrombocytopenia.

INCREASED PLATELET DESTRUCTION

1. Immune Thrombocytopenia

ESSENTIALS OF DIAGNOSIS

- Isolated thrombocytopenia (rule out pseudothrombocytopenia by review of peripheral smear).
- Assess for new causative medications, HIV, hepatitis B, hepatitis C, and *Helicobacter pylori* infections.
- Immune thrombocytopenia (ITP) is a diagnosis of exclusion.

General Considerations

ITP is an autoimmune condition in which pathogenic antibodies bind platelets, accelerating their clearance from the circulation; additional pathophysiologic mechanisms include T cells. Many patients with ITP also lack appropriate compensatory platelet production, which may, in part, reflect the antibody's effect on megakaryocytopoiesis and thrombopoiesis. ITP is primary (idiopathic) in most adult patients, although it can be secondary (ie, associated with autoimmune disease, such as SLE; lymphoproliferative disease, such as lymphoma; medications; and infections caused by hepatitis C virus, HIV, and *H pylori*), and ITP can be exacerbated by SARS-CoV-2 vaccination. Nonetheless, patients with ITP should be encouraged to receive a

SARS-CoV-2 vaccine. The provider may wish to obtain a baseline CBC prior to the vaccine and a CBC 5–7 days post vaccine. The decision to monitor a CBC regarding a SARS-CoV-2 vaccine is subjective and depends on the length of time since ITP has been clinically active. Antiplatelet antibody targets include glycoproteins IIb/IIIa and Ib/IX on the platelet membrane, although antibodies are demonstrable in only two-thirds of patients; testing for such antibodies is not standard of care given the significant false-positive and false-negative results. In addition to production of antiplatelet antibodies, HIV and hepatitis C virus may lead to thrombocytopenia through additional mechanisms (eg, direct suppression of platelet production [HIV] and cirrhosis-related decreased thrombopoietin [TPO] production and secondary splenomegaly [hepatitis C virus]).

Clinical Findings

A. Symptoms and Signs

Mucocutaneous bleeding may be present, depending on the platelet count. Clinically relevant spontaneous bruising, epistaxis, gingival bleeding, or other types of hemorrhage generally do not occur until the platelet count is < 20,000/mcL (20×10^9/L). Individuals with secondary ITP (see above) may have additional disease-specific findings.

B. Laboratory Findings

Typically, patients have isolated thrombocytopenia. If substantial bleeding has occurred, anemia may also be present. Hepatitis B and C viruses and HIV infections should be excluded by serologic testing. A urea breath test and fecal antigen test are noninvasive tests for *H pylori* infections. Bone marrow biopsy should be obtained in patients with unexplained cytopenias in two or more lineages, in patients aged > 40 years with isolated thrombocytopenia, or in those who do not respond to primary ITP-specific therapy. A bone marrow biopsy is not necessary in all cases to make an ITP diagnosis in younger patients. Megakaryocyte morphologic abnormalities and hypocellularity or hypercellularity are not characteristic of ITP. Patients with ITP often have increased numbers of bone marrow megakaryocytes. If there are clinical findings suggestive of a lymphoproliferative malignancy, chest/abdomen/pelvic CT scan should be performed. In the absence of such findings, otherwise asymptomatic patients aged < 40 years with unexplained isolated thrombocytopenia of recent onset lacking both the above infections and lacking concerns for rheumatologic disorders (eg, SLE), may be considered to have ITP.

Treatment

Individuals with platelet counts < 25,000–30,000/mcL ($25–30 \times 10^9$/L) or those with significant bleeding should be treated; those with higher platelet counts may be monitored serially for progression, but the platelet cutoff is a patient-specific decision. The mainstay of initial treatment is a short course of prednisone (1mg/kg orally) with or without intravenous immunoglobulin (IVIG) or anti-D (WinRho) (Figure 16–1). A short course of high-dose dexamethasone (typically, 40 mg orally daily for 4 days) is also an option for initial treatment. Response to corticosteroids is generally seen within 3–7 days of initiating treatment, with response to IVIG typically seen in 24–36 hours. Platelet transfusions may be given concomitantly if active bleeding is present. Adding the anti–B-cell (anti-CD20) monoclonal antibody rituximab to corticosteroids as first-line treatment may improve the initial response rate, but it is associated with increased toxicity and is not regarded as first-line therapy in many centers.

Although over two-thirds of patients with ITP respond to initial treatment with oral corticosteroids, most relapse following reduction of the corticosteroid dose. Patients with a persistent platelet count < 30,000/mcL (30×10^9/L) or clinically significant bleeding are appropriate candidates for second-line treatments (Figure 16–1). These treatments are chosen empirically, bearing in mind potential toxicities and patient preference. IVIG or anti-D (WinRho) temporarily increases platelet counts (duration, up to 3 weeks, rarely longer). Serial IVIG or anti-D treatment is an option for some adult patients while alternate safe treatment is pursued. Rituximab and other biosimilar anti-CD20 antibody therapeutics lead to clinical responses in about 50% of patients with corticosteroid-refractory chronic ITP, which decreases to about 20% at 5 years. The TPO mimetics romiplostim (subcutaneously; weekly), eltrombopag (oral; daily), and avatrombopag (oral; daily) are used in adult patients with chronic ITP who have not responded durably to corticosteroids. Romiplostim, eltrombopag, or avatrombopag can be taken indefinitely to maintain the platelet response and can be used as second-line therapy, but many patients can ultimately discontinue taking these agents and maintain an adequate platelet count (> 30,000/mcL [30×10^9/L]). The decision to use an anti-CD20 antibody before or after a TPO mimetic is patient-specific. The Syk inhibitor fostamatinib can treat ITP that has not responded to corticosteroids, TPO mimetics, or rituximab. Splenectomy is used infrequently but still has a role in selected patients; it has a durable response rate of > 50% and may be considered for cases of severe ITP that fail to respond durably to initial treatment or are refractory to second-line agents. Patients should receive pneumococcal, *Haemophilus influenzae* type b, and meningococcal vaccination at least 2 weeks before therapeutic splenectomy. If available, laparoscopic splenectomy is preferred. Additional treatments for ITP are found in Figure 16–1. Rilzabrutinib, a bruton tyrosine kinase inhibitor, is a treatment option for refractory disease.

For thrombocytopenia associated with HIV or hepatitis C virus, effective treatment of either infection leads to an amelioration of thrombocytopenia in most cases; refractory thrombocytopenia may require the use of IVIG, splenectomy, TPO mimetic, or anti-CD20 therapy. Occasionally, ITP treatment response is impaired due to *H pylori* infection, which should be ruled out in the appropriate situation. For ITP associated with SARS-CoV-2 vaccine, most cases require only monitoring for progression. If treatment is indicated (see above), corticosteroids or a TPO-mimetic are typically used.

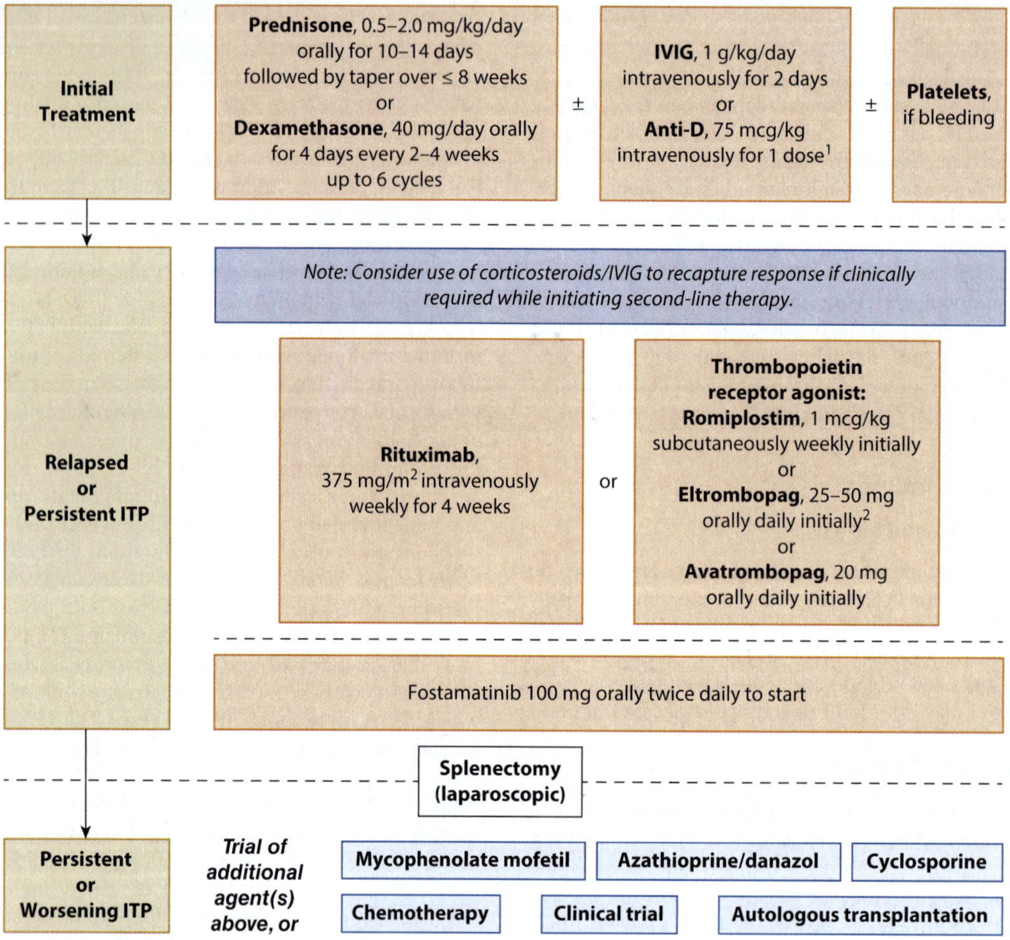

[1]Use in non-splenectomized, Rh blood type–positive, non-anemic patients only.
[2]Recommended starting dose in Asian patients is 25 mg daily.

Figure 16–1. Management of immune thrombocytopenia (ITP), a simplified overview.

Pregnancy-associated ITP—Management goals are a platelet count of ≥ 30,000/mcL (30×10^9/L) during gestation, and ≥ 50,000/mcL (50×10^9/L) prior to cesarean section or vaginal delivery. Moderate-dose oral prednisone or intermittent IVIG infusions are standard treatment options. Splenectomy is reserved for failure to respond to these therapies and may be performed in the first or second trimester. Management requires close interaction between the obstetrician and the hematologist. TPO mimetics are not approved for use during pregnancy.

When to Refer

All patients with ITP need to be managed by a hematologist because of the complexity of the therapy.

When to Admit

Patients with major hemorrhage or severe thrombocytopenia with bleeding should be admitted and monitored in-hospital until the platelet count is consistently > 20,000–30,000/mcL ($20–30 \times 10^9$/L) and hemodynamic stability has been achieved.

Al-Samkari H et al. Novel therapeutics and future directions for refractory immune thrombocytopenia. Br J Haematol. 2023;203:65. [PMID: 37735554]

Kuter DJ et al. Safety and efficacy of rilzabrutinib vs placebo in adults with immune thrombocytopenia: the phase 3 LUNA3 study. Blood. 2025;145:2914. [PMID: 40090011]

Lee EJ...Leavitt AD et al. SARS-CoV-2 vaccination and immune thrombocytopenia in de novo and pre-existing ITP patients. Blood. 2022;139:1564. [PMID: 34587251]

Neunert C et al. American Society of Hematology 2019 guidelines for immune thrombocytopenia. Blood Adv. 2019;3:3829. [PMID: 31794604]

2. Thrombotic Microangiopathy

ESSENTIALS OF DIAGNOSIS

- Microangiopathic hemolytic anemia and thrombocytopenia, without another plausible explanation, are sufficient for a presumptive diagnosis of thrombotic microangiopathy (TMA).

- Fever, neurologic impairment, and kidney disease may occur but are not required for diagnosis.
- Kidney injury is more common and more severe in hemolytic-uremic syndrome (HUS).

General Considerations

The TMAs include, but are not limited to, thrombotic thrombocytopenic purpura (TTP) and HUS. These disorders are characterized by thrombocytopenia due to the incorporation of platelets into fibrin thrombi in the microvasculature, and microangiopathic hemolytic anemia, which results from shearing of erythrocytes in fibrin networks in the microcirculation.

In idiopathic TTP, autoantibodies against ADAMTS-13, also known as the von Willebrand factor (vWF) cleaving protease (vWFCP), lead to accumulation of ultra-large vWF multimers. The ultra-large multimers aggregate platelets in the absence of hemostatic triggers, which leads to the vessel obstruction and various organ dysfunctions in TTP. In some cases of pregnancy-associated TMA, an antibody to ADAMTS-13 is present. In contrast, the activity of ADAMTS-13 in congenital TTP is decreased due to a pathogenic variant in the gene encoding the molecule.

Classic HUS, called Shiga toxin–mediated HUS, is thought to be secondary to toxin-mediated endothelial damage and is often contracted through the ingestion of undercooked ground beef contaminated with *Escherichia coli* (especially types O157:H7 or O145). Complement-mediated HUS (formerly called atypical HUS) is not related to Shiga toxin. Patients with complement-mediated HUS often have genetic defects in proteins that regulate complement activity. Damage to endothelial cells, hematopoietic stem cell transplantation in the setting of cancer, or HIV infection may also lead to TMA. Certain medications (eg, cyclosporine, quinine, ticlopidine, clopidogrel, mitomycin C, and bleomycin) are associated with the development of TMA, possibly by promoting injury to endothelial cells, although inhibitory antibodies to ADAMTS-13 have been demonstrated in some cases.

Clinical Findings

A. Symptoms and Signs

Microangiopathic hemolytic anemia, schistocytes on blood smear, and thrombocytopenia are presenting signs in all patients with TTP and most patients with HUS; in a subset of patients with HUS, the platelet count remains in the normal range. Only about 25% of patients with TTP manifest all components of the original pentad of findings (microangiopathic hemolytic anemia, thrombocytopenia, fever, kidney disease, and neurologic abnormalities) (Table 16–4). Most patients (especially children) with HUS have a recent or current diarrheal illness, often bloody. Neurologic manifestations, including headache, somnolence, delirium, seizures, paresis, and coma, may result

Table 16–4. Presentation and management of thrombotic microangiopathies.

	TTP	Complement-Mediated HUS	Shiga Toxin–Mediated HUS
Patient population	Adults	Children (occasionally adults)	Usually children, often following bloody diarrhea
Pathogenesis	Acquired autoantibody to ADAMTS-13	Some cases: heritable deficiency in function of complement regulatory proteins	Bacterial (such as enterotoxigenic *Escherichia coli*; Shiga toxin)
Thrombocytopenia	Typically severe, except in very early clinical course	Variable	May be mild/absent in a minority of patients
Fever	Typical	Variable	Atypical
Kidney disease	Typical, but may be mild	Typical	Typical
Neurologic impairment	Variable	Less than half of cases	Less than half of cases
Laboratory investigation	Decreased activity of ADAMTS-13; inhibitor usually identified	Defects in complement regulatory proteins	Typically normal ADAMTS-13 activity Positive stool culture for *E coli* o157:H7 or detectable antibody to Shiga toxin
Management	Immediate TPE in most cases Hemodialysis for severe kidney disease Caplacizumab (selected patients) Platelet transfusions contraindicated unless TPE underway	Immediate TPE initially in most cases Eculizumab Supportive care Hemodialysis for severe kidney disease	Hemodialysis for severe kidney disease Supportive care TPE rarely beneficial (exception: selected cases in adults)

ADAMTS-13, a disintegrin and metalloproteinase with a thrombospondin type 1 motif, member 13; HUS, hemolytic-uremic syndrome; TPE, therapeutic plasma exchange; TTP, thrombotic thrombocytopenic purpura.

from deposition of microthrombi in the cerebral vasculature. The plasmic score may help identify patients with schistocytes who have TTP (https://www.mdcalc.com/calc/10200/plasmic-score-ttp).

B. Laboratory Findings

Laboratory features of TMA include thrombocytopenia; abnormalities associated with microangiopathic hemolytic anemia (anemia, elevated reticulocyte count, LD, and indirect bilirubin, decreased haptoglobin, schistocytes on the blood smear, and a negative direct antiglobulin test); elevated creatinine; positive stool culture for *E coli* O157:H7 or stool assays for Shiga toxin (HUS); reductions in ADAMTS-13 activity with the presence (acquired TTP) or absence (inherited TTP) of ADAMTS-13 inhibitor; and pathogenic variants of genes encoding complement proteins (complement-mediated HUS; specialized laboratory assessment). Routine coagulation studies (prothrombin time [PT], activated partial thromboplastin time [aPTT], fibrinogen) are within the normal range in most patients with TTP or HUS.

Treatment

With the exception of children or adults with endemic diarrhea-associated HUS, who generally recover with supportive care only, plasma exchange is initiated in all cases of suspected or confirmed TTP. *Immediate administration of plasma exchange is essential in TTP because the mortality rate without treatment is over 95%.* Plasma exchange usually is administered once daily until the platelet count is > 150,000/mcL (150×10^9/L) for at least 2 days, after which the frequency of treatments may be tapered or stopped while the platelet count and LD are monitored for relapse. In cases of insufficient response to once-daily plasma exchange, twice-daily treatments can be considered. In cases of TTP relapse following initial treatment, plasma exchange should be reinstituted. Fresh frozen plasma (FFP) may be administered if immediate access to plasma exchange is not available or in cases of familial TMA. *Platelet transfusions are rarely used* in the treatment of TMA due to reports of worsening TMA, possibly due to propagation of platelet-rich microthrombi. In cases of documented life-threatening bleeding, however, platelet transfusions may be given slowly and preferably after plasma exchange is underway. RBC transfusions may be administered in cases of clinically significant anemia. Hemodialysis should be considered for patients with significant kidney injury. Caplacizumab, a bi-specific antibody that prevents vWF interaction with the platelet glycoprotein Ib-IX-V receptor, can reduce the time to platelet count normalization and 30-day mortality. The use of caplacizumab for treating TTP remains somewhat controversial given its high cost, despite its inclusion in 2020 vWD guidelines.

In addition to plasma exchange, immunosuppression with corticosteroids is initiated at the start of TTP treatment. Rituximab, an anti-CD20 antibody, is often given to provide extended immunosuppression and to minimize corticosteroid use. In refractory cases, repeat rituximab, vincristine, cyclophosphamide, and splenectomy are considered.

In idiopathic TTP, careful monitoring of the ADAMTS-13 activity and inhibitor status are required. Subsequent immunosuppression with an anti-CD20 antibody can prevent dangerous relapses.

Complement-mediated HUS may respond to plasma infusion/exchange initially; however, once this diagnosis is strongly suspected, the plasma-based treatment is typically stopped and serial infusions of an anti–complement C5 antibody such as eculizumab or ravulizumab are given, which can produce sustained remissions in some patients. Hemodialysis or kidney transplantation may be necessary for irreversible kidney injury.

When to Refer

Consultation by a hematologist or transfusion medicine specialist familiar with plasma exchange is required at the time of presentation. Patients with TMA and TTP require ongoing care by a hematologist.

When to Admit

All patients with newly suspected or diagnosed TMA should be hospitalized immediately.

Yassin M et al. An updated systematic review and meta-analysis of caplacizumab for immune thrombotic thrombocytopenic purpura: insights into efficacy and safety. Blood Rev. 2025 Dec 20. [Epub ahead of print] [PMID: 41478741]

Zheng XL et al; International Society on Thrombosis and Haemostasis. 2025 focused update of the 2020 ISTH guidelines for management of thrombotic thrombocytopenic purpura. J Thromb Haemost. 2025;23:3711. [PMID: 40533296]

3. Heparin-Induced Thrombocytopenia

ESSENTIALS OF DIAGNOSIS

- Thrombocytopenia within 5–14 days of exposure to heparin.
- Decline in baseline platelet count of ≥ 50%.
- Thrombosis occurs in up to 50% of cases; bleeding is uncommon.

General Considerations

Heparin-induced thrombocytopenia (HIT) is an acquired disorder that affects about 3% of patients exposed to unfractionated heparin and ~0.3–0.6% of patients exposed to low-molecular-weight heparin (LMWH). The condition results from formation of IgG antibodies to heparin-platelet factor 4 (PF4) complexes; the antibody:heparin-PF4 complex binds to and activates platelets independent of physiologic hemostasis, which leads to thrombocytopenia and thromboses. vWF has been postulated to play a role in the thrombotic events that take place long after heparin is cleared from the patient's system.

Clinical Findings

A. Symptoms and Signs

Patients are often asymptomatic, and due to the prothrombotic nature of HIT, bleeding usually does not occur. Thrombosis (at any venous or arterial site), however, may be detected in up to 50% of patients, up to 30 days post diagnosis. If thrombosis has not already been detected, the use of duplex Doppler ultrasound of the lower extremities should be considered to rule out subclinical DVT.

B. Laboratory Findings

A presumptive diagnosis of HIT is made when new-onset thrombocytopenia is detected in a patient (typically a hospitalized patient) within 5–14 days of initial exposure to heparin; other presentations (eg, rapid-onset HIT) are less common and reflect recent prior heparin exposure. A decline of ≥ 50% from the baseline platelet count is typical. The 4T score (http://www.qxmd.com/calculate) is a clinical prediction rule for assessing pretest probability for HIT. Low 4T scores have been shown to be more predictive of excluding HIT than are intermediate or high scores of predicting its presence. Once HIT is clinically suspected, the clinician must establish the diagnosis by performing a screening PF4-heparin antibody ELISA. If the PF4-heparin antibody ELISA is positive, the diagnosis must be confirmed using a functional assay (such as serotonin release assay). The magnitude of a positive ELISA result correlates with the clinical probability of HIT, but even high ELISA values may be falsely positive. The confirmatory functional assay is essential.

Treatment

Treatment should be initiated as soon as HIT is suspected, before confirmatory laboratory test results are available.

Management of HIT (Table 16–5) involves the immediate discontinuation of all forms of heparin. Despite thrombocytopenia, platelet transfusions are rarely necessary and should be avoided. Due to the substantial frequency of thrombosis among HIT patients, an alternative anticoagulant should be administered immediately while awaiting confirmatory testing. The use of the subcutaneous indirect anti-Xa inhibitor fondaparinux for initial treatment of HIT is a reasonable option in clinically stable patients. A parenteral direct thrombin inhibitor (DTI), such as argatroban or bivalirudin, is preferred in critical illness because of the shorter duration of action. For confirmed HIT, the DTI or fondaparinux should be continued until the platelet count has recovered to at least 100,000/mcL (100×10^9/L), at which point treatment with a vitamin K antagonist (warfarin) or an oral anti-Xa agent may be initiated. If using a vitamin K antagonist, the parenteral DTI should be continued until therapeutic anticoagulation has been achieved (ie, INR 2.0–3.0); the infusion of argatroban must be temporarily discontinued for 4–5 hours before the INR is obtained so that it reflects the anticoagulant effect of warfarin alone. In all patients with HIT, some form of anticoagulation (warfarin, fondaparinux, or an oral anti-Xa agent) should be continued for at least 30 days, due to a persistent risk of thrombosis even after the platelet count has recovered; in patients in whom thrombosis has been documented (heparin-induced thrombocytopenia and thrombosis; HITT), anticoagulation should continue for 3–6 months.

Subsequent exposure to heparin should be avoided in all patients with a prior history of HIT, if possible. If its use is regarded as necessary for a procedure, it should be withheld until PF4-heparin antibodies are no longer detectable by ELISA (usually 100 days following an episode of HIT), and exposure should be limited to the shortest time period possible. A common example is a cardiac catheterization. The heparin is gone before the antibody returns, so HIT is avoided. However, the HIT antibody does not recur in most patients when re-exposed to heparin.

Table 16–5. Management of suspected or proven HIT.

I. Discontinue all forms of heparin. Send PF4-heparin ELISA. Send confirmatory serotonin release assay if positive ELISA.		
II. Begin treatment with direct thrombin inhibitor, or in some circumstances, fondaparinux.		
Agent	**Indication**	**Dosing**
Argatroban	Prophylaxis or treatment of HIT	Continuous intravenous infusion of 0.5–1.2 mcg/kg/min, titrate to aPTT = 1.5 to 3 × the baseline value.[1] Max infusion rate is 10 mcg/kg/min.
Bivalirudin	Percutaneous coronary intervention[2]	Bolus of 0.75 mg/kg intravenously followed by initial continuous intravenous infusion of 1.75 mg/kg/hour. Manufacturer indicates monitoring should be by ACT.
Fondaparinux	Treatment of HIT	5–10 mg subcutaneously (weight based)
III. Perform Doppler ultrasound of lower extremities to rule out subclinical thrombosis (if indicated).		
IV. Follow platelet counts daily until recovery occurs.		
V. When platelet count has recovered, transition anticoagulation to warfarin, fondaparinux, or an oral anti-Xa agent; treat for 30 days (HIT) or 3–6 months (HITT).		
VI. Document heparin allergy in medical record (confirmed cases).		

[1]Liver insufficiency: initial infusion rate = 0.5 mcg/kg/min.
[2]Not approved for HIT/HITT.
ACT, activated clotting time; aPTT, activated partial thromboplastin time; HIT, heparin-induced thrombocytopenia; HITT, heparin-induced thrombocytopenia and thrombosis; PF4, platelet factor 4.

When to Refer

Due to the tremendous thrombotic potential of the disorder and the complexity of use of the DTI, all patients with HIT should be evaluated by a hematologist.

When to Admit

Most patients with HIT are hospitalized at the time of detection of thrombocytopenia. Admission is a clinical decision for an outpatient in whom HIT is suspected and who is a candidate for subcutaneous fondaparinux or an oral anti-Xa agent. Other outpatients may need admission for intravenous DTIs. Regardless, a hematologist needs to be involved as soon as the diagnosis is suspected or treatment is indicated.

Choi PY et al; SSC Platelet Immunology of the ISTH. Results of an international survey of opinions on the definitions and treatments for heparin-induced thrombocytopenia: communication from the ISTH SSC Subcommittee on Platelet Immunology. J Thromb Haemost. 2024;22:1772. [PMID: 38301999]

Warkentin TE et al. Laboratory testing for heparin-induced thrombocytopenia and vaccine-induced immune thrombotic thrombocytopenia antibodies: a narrative review. Semin Thromb Hemost. 2023;49:621. [PMID: 36455619]

4. Disseminated Intravascular Coagulation

ESSENTIALS OF DIAGNOSIS

- Associated with cancer, sepsis, trauma, and pregnancy-associated complications.
- Prolonged PT and aPTT, and low/declining fibrinogen.
- Thrombocytopenia.

General Considerations

Disseminated intravascular coagulation (DIC) is caused by uncontrolled local or systemic activation of coagulation, which leads to depletion of coagulation factors and fibrinogen, and often results in thrombocytopenia as platelets are activated and consumed.

Numerous disorders are associated with DIC, including sepsis (in which coagulation is activated by presence of lipopolysaccharide), cancer, trauma, burns, and pregnancy-associated complications (in which tissue factor is released). Aortic aneurysm and cavernous hemangiomas may promote localized intravascular coagulation, and snake bites may result in DIC due to exogenous toxins. The HELLP syndrome (hemolysis, elevated liver enzymes, low platelets) is a severe form of DIC with a particularly high mortality rate that occurs in peripartum women.

Clinical Findings

A. Symptoms and Signs

Bleeding in DIC usually occurs at multiple sites, such as at intravenous catheters or incisions, and may be widespread (purpura fulminans). Malignancy-related DIC may manifest principally as thrombosis (Trousseau syndrome).

B. Laboratory Findings

In early DIC, the platelet count and fibrinogen levels often remain within the normal range, albeit reduced from baseline levels. There is progressive thrombocytopenia (rarely severe), prolongation of the PT, decrease in fibrinogen levels, and eventually elevation in the aPTT. D-dimer levels typically are elevated due to the activation of coagulation and diffuse cross-linking of fibrin followed by fibrinolysis. Schistocytes on the blood smear, due to shearing of red cells through the microvasculature, are present in 10–20% of patients. Laboratory abnormalities in the HELLP syndrome include elevated liver transaminases and kidney injury due to gross hemoglobinuria and pigment nephropathy. Malignancy-related DIC may initially feature normal platelet counts and coagulation studies, followed by a dropping platelet count and fibrinogen, with a rising INR, highlighting the importance of serial laboratory values to make the diagnosis.

Treatment

The underlying causative disorder must be treated (eg, antimicrobials, chemotherapy, surgery, or delivery of conceptus).

Blood products are administered if clinically significant hemorrhage has occurred or is thought likely to occur without intervention based on progressively increasing PT and PTT and decreasing fibrinogen and platelets levels (Table 16–6). The goal of platelet therapy for most cases is > 20,000/mcL (20×10^9/L) or > 50,000/mcL (50×10^9/L) for serious bleeding, such as intracranial bleeding. FFP is typically given only to patients with a prolonged aPTT and PT as well as bleeding. Cryoprecipitate or fibrinogen concentrates (eg, RiaSTAP) is given for hypofibrinogenemia < 100 mg/dL, or higher if decline is active. The clinician should correct the fibrinogen level prior to giving FFP for prolonged PT and aPTT to see if the fibrinogen replacement alone corrects the PT and aPTT. The PT, aPTT, fibrinogen, and platelet count should be monitored at least every 6–8 hours in acutely ill patients with DIC.

In some cases of refractory bleeding despite replacement of blood products, administration of low doses of heparin is considered. Since DIC is primarily a disorder of excessive clotting with secondary fibrinolysis, heparin can interfere with thrombin generation, which leads to less consumption of coagulation proteins and platelets. An infusion of 5 units/kg/hour (no bolus) may be used with appropriate clinical judgement, up-titrated as clinically indicated. *Heparin may be relatively contraindicated if the platelet count cannot be maintained above 20,000–30,000/mcL (20–30 × 10^9/L) and in cases of CNS hemorrhage, GI bleeding, placental abruption, and a condition likely to require imminent surgery.* Fibrinolysis inhibitors may be considered in select patients who have DIC with bleeding, but their use can promote dangerous clotting and requires great caution and only in consultation with a hematologist.

Table 16–6. Management of DIC.

I. Assess for underlying cause of DIC and treat.	
II. Establish baseline platelet count, PT, aPTT, fibrinogen, D-dimer.	
III. Transfuse blood products only if ongoing bleeding or high risk of bleeding.	**Platelets:** goal > 20,000/mcL (20×10^9/L) (most patients) or > 50,000/mcL (50×10^9/L) (serious bleeding, eg, intracranial hemorrhage)
	Cryoprecipitate: goal fibrinogen > 80–100 mg/dL
	Fresh frozen plasma: goal PT and aPTT < 1.5 × normal
	Packed RBCs: goal hemoglobin > 8 g/dL or improvement in symptomatic anemia
IV. Follow platelets, aPTT, PT, fibrinogen every 4–12 hours as clinically indicated.	
V. If persistent bleeding due to severe consumption or consumption that requires excessive blood product use, consider cautious use of heparin[1] (initial infusion, 5 units/kg/hour) and titrate to desired clinical goals; do not administer bolus.	
VI. Follow laboratory parameters every 4–12 hours as clinically indicated until DIC resolves	

[1]Heparin may be relatively contraindicated if the platelet count cannot be maintained above 20,000-30,000 mcL (20-30 × 10^9/L) and in cases of CNS hemorrhage, GI bleeding, placental abruption, and a condition likely to require immediate surgery.
aPTT, activated partial thromboplastin time; DIC, disseminated intravascular coagulation; PT, prothrombin time.

1. HELLP syndrome—The treatment must include evacuation of the uterus (eg, delivery of a term or near-term infant or removal of retained placental or fetal fragments).

2. Trousseau syndrome—Patients require treatment of the underlying malignancy and administration of unfractionated heparin or subcutaneous therapeutic-dose LMWH as treatment of thrombosis, since warfarin typically is less effective at secondary prevention of thromboembolism in the disorder. Typically, the heparin or LMWH treatment will gradually return the fibrinogen, PT (INR), aPTT, and platelet count back to normal, but it can take weeks. Oral anti-Xa agents or oral DTIs can be considered once the patient is stabilized with parenteral heparin or LMWH, but extended LMWH is often used in this setting.

Immediate initiation of medical treatment (usually within 24 hours of diagnosis) is required for acute promyelocytic leukemia (APL)–associated DIC, along with administration of blood products as clinically indicated.

When to Refer

- Diffuse bleeding unresponsive to administration of blood products should be evaluated by a hematologist.
- All patients with DIC should be cared for by a hematologist before starting treatment with heparin or LMWH.

When to Admit

Most patients with DIC are hospitalized when DIC is detected.

Cuker A et al. American Society of Hematology 2018 guidelines for management of venous thromboembolism: heparin-induced thrombocytopenia. Blood Adv. 2018;2:3360. [PMID: 30482768]
Iba T et al. Disseminated intravascular coagulation: the past, present, and future consideration. Semin Thromb Hemost. 2022;48:978. [PMID: 36100234]
Scarlatescu E et al. Disseminated intravascular coagulation and cirrhotic coagulopathy: overlap and differences. The current state of knowledge. Communication from the SSC of the ISTH. J Thromb Haemost. 2025;23:1085. [PMID: 39662873]

OTHER CONDITIONS CAUSING THROMBOCYTOPENIA

1. Drug-Induced Thrombocytopenia

Drug-induced thrombocytopenia is often immune-mediated but can also be due to marrow suppression. The University of Oklahoma Health Sciences center maintains a useful website for drug-induced thrombocytopenia (https://ouhsc.edu/platelets/Thrombocytopenia/DITP). The typical presentation of drug-induced, antibody-mediated thrombocytopenia is severe thrombocytopenia and mucocutaneous bleeding 5–14 days after exposure to a new drug, although a range of presentations is possible. Discontinuation of the offending agent leads to resolution of thrombocytopenia within 3–7 days in most cases, but recovery kinetics depend on rate of drug clearance, which can be affected by liver and kidney function. Patients with severe thrombocytopenia should be given platelet transfusions with or without IVIG.

2. Posttransfusion Purpura

Posttransfusion purpura (PTP) is a rare disorder of sudden-onset severe thrombocytopenia that occurs within 1 week after transfusion of red cells, platelets, or plasma. Antibodies against the human platelet antigen PL^{A1} are detected in most individuals with PTP. Patients with PTP often are either multiparous women or persons who have received transfusions previously. Severe thrombocytopenia and bleeding are typical. Initial treatment consists of administration of IVIG (1 g/kg/day for 2 days), which should be administered as soon as the diagnosis is suspected. Platelets are not indicated unless severe bleeding is present, but if they are to be administered, HLA-matched PL^{A1}-negative platelets are preferred. A second course or IVIG, plasma exchange, corticosteroids, TPO-mimetics, or splenectomy may be required in case of refractoriness. PL^{A1}-negative or washed blood products are preferred for subsequent transfusions, but data supporting various treatment options are limited.

Vu K, Leavitt AD. Posttransfusion purpura with antibodies against human platelet antigen-4a following checkpoint inhibitor therapy: a case report and review of the literature. Transfusion. 2018;58:2265. [PMID: 30222869]

3. von Willebrand Disease Type 2B

vWD type 2B leads to chronic, characteristically mild to moderate thrombocytopenia due to an abnormal vWF molecule that binds platelets with increased affinity, resulting in aggregation and clearance (see von Willebrand Disease, below).

4. Platelet Sequestration

One-third of the normal platelet mass is typically sequestered in the spleen. Splenomegaly, due to a variety of conditions, may lead to thrombocytopenia of variable severity. When possible, treatment of the underlying disorder should be pursued, but splenectomy, splenic embolization, or splenic irradiation may be considered in selected cases.

5. Pregnancy

Gestational thrombocytopenia is mild and of uncertain mechanism, but hemodilution and increased clearance are thought to contribute. Cytopenias result even though blood cell production is normal or increased. Platelet counts < 100,000/mcL (100×10^9/L), however, are observed in < 10% of pregnant women in the third trimester; decreases to < 70,000/mcL (70×10^9/L) should prompt consideration of pregnancy-related ITP as well as preeclampsia or pregnancy-related thrombotic microangiopathy.

6. Infection or Sepsis

The exact mechanism underlying sepsis-related thrombocytopenia remains ill-defined. Immune-mediated destruction and enhanced clearance by the liver are possible explanations, and there may be significant overlap with concomitant DIC. Regardless, the platelet count typically improves with effective antimicrobial treatment or after the infection has resolved. Hemophagocytosis may occur in some critically ill patients; a defect in immunomodulation may lead to bone marrow macrophages (histiocytes) engulfing cellular components of the marrow. The phenomenon typically resolves with resolution of the infection, but with certain infections (Epstein-Barr virus) immunosuppression may be required. Hemophagocytosis also may occur with malignancy, in which case the disorder is usually unresponsive to treatment with immunosuppression and requires treatment of the malignancy.

7. Pseudothrombocytopenia

Pseudothrombocytopenia results from ethylenediaminetetraacetic acid (EDTA) anticoagulant-induced platelet clumping. It typically disappears when blood is collected in a tube containing citrate anticoagulant. Pseudothrombocytopenia diagnosis requires review of the peripheral blood smear and is not associated with bleeding.

Ghimire S et al. Current understanding and future implications of sepsis-induced thrombocytopenia. Eur J Haematol. 2021;106:301. [PMID: 33191517]

QUALITATIVE PLATELET DISORDERS

CONGENITAL DISORDERS OF PLATELET FUNCTION

ESSENTIALS OF DIAGNOSIS

- Usually diagnosed in childhood.
- Family history usually is positive.
- May be diagnosed in adulthood when there is excessive bleeding.

General Considerations

Heritable qualitative platelet disorders are far less common than acquired platelet function disorders and lead to variably severe bleeding, often beginning in childhood. Occasionally, disorders of platelet function may go undetected until later in life when excessive bleeding occurs following a sufficient hemostatic challenge. Thus, the true incidence of hereditary qualitative platelet disorders is unknown.

Bernard-Soulier syndrome is a rare, autosomal recessive bleeding disorder due to reduced or abnormal platelet membrane expression of glycoprotein Ib/IX (vWF receptor).

Glanzmann thrombasthenia results from an abnormality in the platelet glycoprotein IIb/IIIa receptor on the platelet membrane. Glycoprotein IIb/IIIa is the fibrinogen receptor critical for linking platelets during initial platelet aggregation/platelet plug formation. Inheritance is autosomal recessive.

Gray platelet syndrome gets its name from the appearance of platelets that lack granules on a blood smear. The most common cause is a biallelic mutation in NBEAL2, which encodes BEACH domain protein critical for platelet α-granule biogenesis.

Under normal circumstances, activated platelets release the contents of platelet granules to reinforce the aggregatory response. Storage pool disease includes a spectrum of defects in release of α or dense (δ) platelet granules, or both (α-δ storage pool disease).

Clinical Findings

A. Symptoms and Signs

Bleeding due to defective platelets is generally mucocutaneous, but it is not limited to these surfaces. Patients with Bernard-Soulier syndrome and gray platelet syndrome bruise easily, and have prolonged bleeding and frequent nosebleeds. The onset of bleeding with Glanzmann thrombasthenia is usually in infancy or childhood, but some milder forms present later in life. The degree of deficiency in IIb/IIIa may not correlate well with bleeding symptoms. Patients with storage pool disease are affected by variable bleeding, ranging from mild and trauma-related to spontaneous.

B. Laboratory Findings

Patients with Bernard-Soulier syndrome have abnormally large platelets (approaching the size of red cells), moderate thrombocytopenia, and a prolonged bleeding time. Platelet aggregation studies show a marked defect in response to ristocetin, whereas aggregation in response to other agonists is normal; the addition of normal platelets corrects the abnormal aggregation. The diagnosis can be confirmed by platelet flow cytometry.

In Glanzmann thrombasthenia, platelet aggregation studies show marked impairment of aggregation in response to stimulation with various agonists, which reflects the critical role of the fibrinogen receptor in platelet plug formation.

Storage pool disease includes defects in the number, content, or function of platelet α or dense granules, or both. The gray platelet syndrome comprises abnormalities of platelet α granules, thrombocytopenia, and marrow fibrosis. The blood smear shows agranular platelets, and the diagnosis is confirmed with electron microscopy.

▶ Treatment

The mainstay of treatment (including periprocedural prophylaxis) is transfusion of normal platelets, although desmopressin acetate (DDAVP), antifibrinolytic agents, and recombinant human activated factor VII each have a role in selected clinical situations, all of which should be under the direction of a hematologist.

Al-Huniti A et al. Inherited platelet disorders: diagnosis and management. Transfus Med Rev. 2020;34:277. [PMID: 33082057]

Hayward CPM et al. When it's not Glanzmann thrombasthenia or Bernard-Soulier syndrome: diagnosing other qualitative platelet disorders. Hematology Am Soc Hematol Educ Program. 2025;2025:137. [PMID: 41348029]

Lee RH et al. Platelet transfusion for patients with platelet dysfunction: effectiveness, mechanisms, and unanswered questions. Curr Opin Hematol. 2020;27:378. [PMID: 32868672]

ACQUIRED DISORDERS OF PLATELET FUNCTION

Platelet dysfunction is more commonly acquired than inherited; the widespread use of platelet-altering medications accounts for most of the cases of qualitative defects. In cases where platelet function is irreversibly altered (eg, aspirin), platelet inhibition typically recovers within 7–9 days following discontinuation of the drug, which is the time it takes to replace all the impaired platelets with newly produced platelets. In cases where platelet function is non-irreversibly affected (eg, NSAIDs), platelet inhibition recovers with clearance of the drug from the system. Transfusion of platelets may be required for clinically significant bleeding.

DISORDERS OF COAGULATION

CONGENITAL DISORDERS OF COAGULATION

1. Hemophilia A & B

ESSENTIALS OF DIAGNOSIS

- **Hemophilia A:** congenital deficiency of coagulation factor VIII.
- **Hemophilia B:** congenital deficiency of coagulation factor IX.
- Recurrent hemarthroses and arthropathy.
- Risk of development of inhibitory antibodies to factor VIII or factor IX.
- Many older patients received blood products contaminated with HIV or hepatitis C virus.

▶ General Considerations

Hemophilia A occurs in ~1 per 5000 live male births, whereas hemophilia B occurs in ~1 in 25,000 live male births. Inheritance is X-linked recessive for both, leading to affected males and carrier (affected) females with variable bleeding tendencies. Daughters of all affected males are obligate carriers. There is no race predilection. Factor activity testing is indicated for male infants with a hemophilic maternal pedigree who are asymptomatic or who experience excessive bleeding, for all daughters of affected males (100% chance of being affected) and carrier mothers (50% chance of being affected), and for otherwise asymptomatic adolescents or adults who experience unexpected excessive bleeding with trauma or invasive procedures.

Inhibitors to factor VIII develop in approximately 20–25% of patients with severe hemophilia A; inhibitors to factor IX develop in < 5% of patients with severe hemophilia B. Risk of inhibitor formation exists for both plasma-derived and recombinant factor products.

A substantial proportion of older patients with hemophilia acquired infection with HIV or HCV or both in the 1980s due to exposure to contaminated factor concentrates and blood products.

▶ Clinical Findings

A. Symptoms and Signs

Severe hemophilia (factor VIII activity < 1%) presents in infancy or early childhood with spontaneous bleeding into joints, soft tissues, or other locations. Spontaneous bleeding is much less common in patients with mild hemophilia (factor VIII activity > 5%), but bleeding is common with provoked bleeding (eg, surgery, trauma). Intermediate clinical symptoms are seen in patients with moderate hemophilia (factor VIII activity 1–5%). Female carriers of hemophilia can have a wide range of factor VIII activity and therefore have variable bleeding tendencies.

Significant hemophilic arthropathy can be minimized in patients who receive long-term regular prophylaxis with factor concentrate or non-factor products (eg, emicizumab for hemophilia A) starting in early childhood, whereas destructive joint disease is common in adults who have experienced recurrent hemarthroses. Patients tend to have one or two "target" joints into which they bleed most often.

Inhibitor development to factor VIII or factor IX is characterized by new or atypical bleeding and by bleeding episodes that are resistant to treatment with clotting factor VIII or IX concentrate.

B. Laboratory Findings

Hemophilia A or B is diagnosed by an isolated reproducibly low factor VIII or factor IX activity level, in the absence of other conditions. If the aPTT is prolonged, it typically corrects upon mixing with normal plasma. Depending on the level of residual factor VIII or factor IX activity, and the sensitivity of the thromboplastin used in the aPTT coagulation reaction, the aPTT may or may not be prolonged, although it typically is markedly prolonged in severe hemophilia. Hemophilia is classified according to the level of factor activity in the plasma:

Mild hemophilia has > 5% to ~50% factor activity

Moderate hemophilia has 1% to 5% factor activity

Severe hemophilia has < 1% factor activity

Female carriers may be symptomatic if lyonization (where one of two X chromosomes is inactivated in utero) has occurred favoring the defective factor VIII or factor IX gene, leading to factor VIII or factor IX activity level < 50%. Typically, a clinical bleeding diathesis occurs once the factor activity is < 20–30%, but this appears to be patient-specific, and bleeding can occur in trauma, surgery, and delivery if the factor activity is < 50% and heavy menstrual bleeding at levels below normal. In the presence of an inhibitor to factor VIII or factor IX, there is accelerated clearance of and suboptimal or absent rise in measured activity of infused factor, and the aPTT does not correct on mixing. The Bethesda assay measures the potency of the inhibitor.

Treatment

A. Factor VIII or IX Products

Plasma-derived or recombinant factor VIII or IX products have been the mainstay of therapy before the advent of non-factor treatment and gene therapy. The optimal care for individuals with severe hemophilia is primary prophylaxis: by the age of 2, most children with severe hemophilia receive regular infusions of factor to prevent the recurrent joint bleeding that otherwise would characterize the disorder and lead to severe musculoskeletal morbidity. In less severe hemophilia, or as an adjunct to prophylaxis in severe hemophilia, treatment with factor products is given periprocedurally, prior to high-risk activities (such as sports), or as needed for bleeding episodes (Table 16–7). Recombinant factor VIII and factor IX molecules that are bioengineered to have an extended half-life may allow for extended dosing intervals in patients who are treated prophylactically. EHL factor IX and some EHL factor VIII products have clear added value in reducing frequency of factor injections often to weekly or less often. Patients with mild hemophilia A may respond to as-needed (on demand) intravenous or intranasal DDAVP. Antifibrinolytic agents (eg, tranexamic acid or ε-aminocaproic acid) may be useful in cases of mucosal bleeding and are commonly used adjunctively, such as following dental procedures.

B. Non-factor Treatments

Emicizumab is a novel bi-specific antibody that brings activated factor IX and factor X together, effectively replacing the cofactor function of factor VIII in the clotting cascade, providing a major therapeutic advance for patients with hemophilia A and inhibitors. Emicizumab has also been demonstrated to be effective for patients without inhibitors. It is given subcutaneously weekly, every other week, or every 4 weeks, making it easier to administer than intravenous factor products. For severe hemophilia A, many children start on emicizumab well before age 1 year. Over half of patients with severe hemophilia A receive emicizumab, rather than factor products. Higher-potency versions of bispecific antibodies (Mim8 and NXT007) that bring together factor IXa and factor X (similar to emicizumab) are in phase 3 clinical trials.

Nonfactor products (rebalancing agents) for treatment of hemophilia A and B with and without inhibitors include fitusiran, an siRNA therapeutic that reduces antithrombin expression, and two tissue factor pathway inhibitors, marstacimab and concizumab. The rebalancing agents are disease agnostic and are effective with hemophilia A or B. A rebalancing agent that impairs protein S activity to reduce bleeding in patients with von Willibrand disease (vWD) is in clinical trial.

Mahlangu J et al. Concizumab in hemophilia with inhibitors: longer-term efficacy and safety results from the phase 3 explorer7 study. Blood Adv. 2026;10:1854. [PMID: 41499759]

Matino D et al. Efficacy and safety of marstacimab prophylaxis in hemophilia A/B with inhibitors: results from the phase 3 BASIS trial. Blood. 2026;147:920. [PMID: 41351884]

Young G et al. Safety and efficacy of a fitusiran antithrombin-based dose regimen in people with hemophilia A or B: the ATLAS-OLE study. Blood. 2025;145:2966. [PMID: 40053895]

C. Gene Therapy

Gene therapy clinical trials for hemophilia A and B have shown great promise for patients with severe hemophilia A and B. For most patients, gene therapy has eliminated spontaneous bleeding as well as the need for factor replacement. Importantly, patients are freed from the daily tasks of managing their hemophilia. The clinical trials have been restricted to patients aged > 18 years without a history of factor inhibitors and extensive prior exposure to an exogenous factor. The first gene therapy product for

Table 16–7. Treatment of bleeding in selected inherited disorders of hemostasis.

Disorder	Subtype	Treatment for Minor Bleeding	Treatment for Major Bleeding	Comment
Hemophilia A	Mild Moderate or severe	DDAVP[1] Factor VIII product	DDAVP[1] or factor VIII product Factor VIII product	Treat for 3–10 days for major bleeding or following surgery, keeping factor activity level 50–80% initially. Adjunctive EACA or TXA may be useful for mucosal bleeding or procedures
Hemophilia B	Mild, moderate, or severe	Factor IX product	Factor IX product	
von Willebrand disease	Type 1 Type 2 Type 3	DDAVP[1] DDAVP,[1] vWF product vWF product	DDAVP,[1] vWF product vWF product vWF product	
Factor XI deficiency	—	FFP or EACA	FFP	Adjunctive EACA or TXA should be used for mucosal bleeding or procedures

[1]Mild hemophilia A and type 2A or 2B vWD patients: therapeutic trial must have previously confirmed an adequate response (ie, elevation of factor VIII or vWF activity level into the normal range) and (for type 2B) no exacerbation of thrombocytopenia. DDAVP is not typically effective for type 2M vWD. A vWF-containing factor VIII concentrate is preferred for treatment of type 2N vWD.

Notes:

DDAVP dose is 0.3 mcg/kg intravenously in 50 mL saline over 20 minutes, or nasal spray 300 mcg for weight > 50 kg or 150 mcg for < 50 kg, every 24 hours, maximum of three doses in a 72-hour period. If more than two doses are used in a 48-hour period, free water restriction and monitoring for hyponatremia are essential.

EACA dose is 50 mg/kg orally four times daily for 3–5 days; maximum 24 g/day, useful for mucosal bleeding/dental procedures.

Factor VIII product dose is 50 units/kg for severe hemophilia A intravenously initially followed by 25 units/kg every 8 hours followed by lesser doses at longer intervals once hemostasis has been established.

Factor IX product dose is 100 units/kg (120 units/kg if using Benefix) intravenously initially for severe hemophilia B followed by 50 units/kg (60 units/kg if using Benefix) every 8 hours followed by lesser doses at longer intervals once hemostasis has been established.

vWF-containing factor VIII product dose is 60–80 RCoF units/kg intravenously every 12 hours initially followed by lesser doses at longer intervals once hemostasis has been established.

FFP is typically administered in 4-unit boluses and may not need to be re-bolused after the initial administration due to the long half-life of factor XI.

DDAVP, desmopressin acetate; EACA, epsilon-aminocaproic acid; FFP, fresh frozen plasma; TXA, tranexamic acid; vWF, von Willebrand factor.

hemophilia B was FDA approved in 2022 and for hemophilia A in 2023.

D. Factor VIII or IX Inhibitors

Factor inhibitors (antibodies that interfere with activity or half-life) are a major clinical problem for patients with hemophilia. It may be possible to overcome low-titer inhibitors (< 5 Bethesda units [BU]) by giving larger doses of factor, whereas treatment of bleeding in the presence of a high-titer inhibitor (> 5 BU) requires infusion of an activated prothrombin complex concentrate (such as FEIBA [factor eight inhibitor bypassing activity]) or recombinant activated factor VII. Recombinant porcine factor VIII also is an option but is reserved for selective circumstances because of its cost. Inhibitor tolerance induction, achieved by giving large doses (50–300 units/kg intravenously of factor VIII daily) for 6–18 months, succeeds in eradicating the inhibitor in 70% of patients with hemophilia A and in 30% of patients with hemophilia B. Patients with hemophilia B who receive inhibitor tolerance induction, however, are at risk for development of nephrotic syndrome and anaphylactic reactions, making eradication of their inhibitors more problematic. Additional immunomodulation may allow for eradication of the inhibitor in selected patients who are refractory to inhibitor tolerance induction. Emicizumab is used for prophylaxis in patients who have hemophilia A with inhibitors. The new rebalancing agents will provide prophylaxis for patients with hemophilia B and inhibitors (see B. Non-factor Treatments).

When to Refer

All patients with hemophilia should be seen regularly in a comprehensive hemophilia treatment center.

When to Admit

- Bleeding that is unresponsive to outpatient treatment.

Cuker A...Leavitt AD et al; BENEGENE-2 Trial Investigators. Gene therapy with fidanacogene elaparvovec in adults with hemophilia B. N Engl J Med. 2024;391:1108. [PMID: 39321362]

Leavitt AD et al. Efficacy, safety, and quality of life 4 years after valoctocogene roxaparvovec gene transfer for severe hemophilia A in the phase 3 GENEr8-1 trial. Res Pract Thromb Haemost. 2024;8:102615. [PMID: 39687929]

Pasi KJ et al. Multiyear follow-up of AAV5-hFVIII-SQ gene therapy for hemophilia A. N Engl J Med. 2020;382:29. [PMID: 31893514]
Pipe SW et al. Gene therapy with etranacogene dezaparvovec for hemophilia B. N Engl J Med. 2023;388:706. [PMID: 36812434]

2. von Willebrand Disease

ESSENTIALS OF DIAGNOSIS

- The most common inherited bleeding disorder.
- vWF binds platelets to subendothelial surfaces, aggregates platelets, and prolongs the half-life of factor VIII.

General Considerations

vWF is an unusually large multimeric glycoprotein that binds to subendothelial collagen and its platelet receptor, glycoprotein Ib, bridging platelets to the subendothelial matrix at the site of vascular injury and contributing to linking them together in the platelet plug. vWF also has a binding site for factor VIII, prolonging factor VIII half-life in the circulation.

Between 75% and 80% of patients with vWD have type 1, a *quantitative abnormality* of the vWF molecule that usually does not feature an identifiable causal mutation in the vWF gene.

Type 2 vWD is seen in 15–20% of patients with vWD. In type 2A or 2B vWD, a *qualitative defect* in the vWF molecule is causative. Types 2N and 2M vWD are due to defects in vWF that decrease binding to factor VIII or to platelets, respectively. Type 2M vWD features a normal multimer pattern. Importantly, type 2N vWD can clinically resemble hemophilia A because factor VIII activity levels are decreased, and vWF activity and antigen (Ag) are normal. Type 3 vWD is rare, and like type 1, is a quantitative defect, with mutational homozygosity or compound heterozygosity yielding very low levels of vWF and severe bleeding in infancy or childhood. Due to its factor VIII carrier function, a severely low vWF level leads to low factor VIII activity and prolonged aPTT.

Clinical Findings

A. Symptoms and Signs

Patients with type 1 vWD usually have mild or moderate platelet-type bleeding (mucocutaneous) that may be evident in childhood. Heavier bleeding may occur with menses, surgery, or following delivery. Patients with type 2 vWD usually have moderate to severe bleeding that presents in childhood or adolescence. Patients with type 3 vWD demonstrate a severe bleeding phenotype that typically manifests in childhood or infancy.

B. Laboratory Findings

In type 1 vWD, the vWF activity (ristocetin co-factor or VWF:GPIbM assay) and the vWF Ag are mildly depressed, whereas the vWF multimer pattern is normal (Table 16–8). Laboratory testing of type 2A or 2B vWD typically shows a ratio of vWF Ag:vWF activity of approximately 2:1 and a multimer pattern that lacks the highest molecular weight multimers. Thrombocytopenia is common in type 2B vWD due to a gain-of-function mutation of the vWF molecule, which leads to increased vWF binding to its receptor on platelets, resulting in platelet clearance; a ristocetin-induced platelet aggregation (RIPA) study shows an increase in platelet aggregation in response to low concentrations of ristocetin. Except in the more severe forms of vWD that feature a significantly decreased factor VIII activity, aPTT is most commonly normal in patients with vWD. The PT is not affected by vWD. vWD type 2N has normal vWF antigen and activity but a low factor VIII due to impaired vWF binding to factor VIII.

Treatment

The treatment of vWD is outlined in Table 16–7. DDAVP can treat mild bleeding in most cases of type 1 and some cases of type 2 vWD. DDAVP causes release of vWF and factor VIII from storage sites (endothelial cells), leading to a two- to sevenfold increase in vWF and factor VIII. A therapeutic DDAVP trial to document sufficient rise in vWF level is critical prior to relying on DDAVP as a treatment option. Due to tachyphylaxis and the risk of significant hyponatremia from fluid retention, DDAVP treatment should be limited to one dose per 24 hours and no more than three doses over 5 days. vWF-containing factor VIII

Table 16–8. Laboratory diagnosis of von Willebrand disease.

Type		vWF Activity	vWF Antigen	Factor VIII	RIPA	Multimer Pattern
1		↓	↓	Nl or ↓	↓	Normal pattern; uniform ↓ intensity of bands
2	A	↓↓	↓	↓	↓	Large and intermediate multimers decreased or absent
	B	↓↓	↓	↓	↑	Large multimers decreased or absent
	M	↓	↓	↓	↓	Normal pattern; uniform ↓ intensity of bands
	N	Nl	Nl	↓↓	Nl	Nl
3		↓↓↓	↓↓↓	↓↓↓	↓↓↓	Multimers absent

Nl, normal; RIPA, ristocetin-induced platelet aggregation; vWF, von Willebrand factor.

concentrates or recombinant VWF products are used in all other clinical scenarios, and when bleeding is not controlled with DDAVP. Antifibrinolytic agents (eg, aminocaproic acid or tranexamic acid) may be used adjunctively for mucosal bleeding or procedures. Cryoprecipitate is no longer used as a source of vWD. Pregnant patients with type 1 vWD often do not require treatment at the time of delivery because of the physiologic increase in vWF levels (up to threefold that of baseline) that are observed by parturition. However, vWF levels need to be confirmed in late pregnancy, and if they are low or if excessive bleeding is encountered, vWF products should be given. Moreover, patients are at risk for significant bleeding 1–2 weeks postpartum when vWF levels fall secondary to the fall in estrogen levels and return to baseline vWF levels.

Connell NT et al. ASH ISTH NHF WFH 2021 guidelines on the management of von Willebrand disease. Blood Adv. 2021; 5:301. [PMID: 33570647]

James PD et al. ASH ISTH NHF WFH 2021 guidelines on the diagnosis of von Willebrand disease. Blood Adv. 2021;5:280. [PMID: 33570651]

3. Factor XI Deficiency

Factor XI deficiency (also called hemophilia C) is inherited in an autosomal recessive manner, leading to heterozygous, compound heterozygous, or homozygous defects. It is most prevalent among individuals of Ashkenazi Jewish descent but is in the differential diagnosis of any unexplained prolonged aPTT. In contrast to hemophilia A and B, factor XI levels do not correlate well with bleeding symptoms. Mild bleeding is most common, and diagnosis is often made after unexpected, excessive bleeding following surgery or trauma. Importantly, factor XI deficiency that can lead to provoked excessive bleeding does not always prolong the aPTT. FFP is the mainstay of treatment when plasma-derived factor XI concentrate is not available. Adjunctive aminocaproic acid or tranexamic acid is administered for procedures or bleeding episodes involving the mucosa (Table 16–7).

4. Less Common Heritable Disorders of Coagulation

Congenital deficiencies of clotting factors II, V, VII, and X are rare and typically inherited in an autosomal recessive pattern. A prolongation in the PT (and aPTT for factor X, factor V, and factor II deficiency) that corrects upon mixing with normal plasma is typical. Definitive diagnosis requires testing for specific factor activity. The treatment of factor II deficiency is with a prothrombin complex concentrate; factor V deficiency is treated with infusions of FFP or platelets (which contain factor V in α granules); factor VII deficiency is treated with recombinant human activated factor VII. Factor X deficiency is treated with an FDA-approved plasma-derived factor X product (Coagadex).

Deficiency of factor XIII characteristically leads to delayed bleeding that occurs hours to days after a hemostatic challenge, such as surgery or trauma. The condition is usually life-long, and spontaneous intracranial hemorrhages and recurrent pregnancy loss appear to occur with increased frequency in these patients compared with other congenital deficiencies. Cryoprecipitate can be used to provide factor XIII, but if available, plasma-derived factor XIII concentrate (Corifact) is preferred to treat bleeding or for surgical prophylaxis. Regular prophylactic factor XIII replacement is indicated for severe factor XIII deficiency. Factor XIII has an A and B subunit. Recombinant factor XIII A-subunit (Tretten) is an option for patients deficient in the factor XIII A subunit. Factor XIII deficiency does not cause a prolongation of the PT or aPTT.

Congenital deficiencies of factor XII, prekallikrein, and high-molecular-weight kininogen may lead to a prolonged aPTT that corrects with extended incubation but do not lead to bleeding.

National Hemophilia Foundation. Products Licensed in the US. https://www.hemophilia.org/healthcare-professionals/guidelines-on-care/products-licensed-in-the-us8

ACQUIRED DISORDERS OF COAGULATION

1. Acquired Antibodies to Factor II

Patients with antiphospholipid antibodies occasionally have antibody specificity to coagulation factor II (prothrombin) that accelerates factor II clearances and can lead to severe hypoprothrombinemia and bleeding. Mixing studies may or may not reveal the presence of an inhibitor, as the antibody typically binds to a non-enzymatically active portion of the molecule leading to accelerated clearance, but characteristically the PT is prolonged and levels of factor II are low. FFP should be administered to treat bleeding. Treatment is immunosuppressive.

2. Acquired Antibodies to Factor V

Products containing bovine factor V (such as topical thrombin or fibrin glue, frequently used in surgical procedures) can lead to formation of an anti–factor V antibody that cross-reacts with human factor V. Clinicopathologic manifestations range from a prolonged PT in an otherwise asymptomatic individual to severe bleeding. Mixing studies suggest the presence of an inhibitor, and the factor V activity level is low. In cases of serious or life-threatening bleeding, IVIG or platelet transfusions, or both, should be administered, and immunosuppression (as for acquired inhibitors to factor VIII) may be offered.

3. Acquired Antibodies to Factor VIII

Acquired hemophilia A due to factor VIII inhibitors is the most common acquired factor-specific bleeding disorder. Spontaneous antibodies to factor VIII can occur in adults without a prior history of hemophilia; older adults and patients with lymphoproliferative malignancy or autoimmune disease and those who are postpartum or postsurgical are at highest risk. The clinical presentation, which should be viewed as a medical emergency, typically includes extensive soft tissue ecchymoses, hematomas, and mucosal bleeding, as opposed to hemarthrosis characteristic of congenital hemophilia A. The aPTT is typically prolonged and does not correct upon mixing; factor VIII activity is low and a Bethesda assay reveals the titer of the inhibitor. Inhibitors of low titer (< 5 BU) may sometimes be overcome by infusion of high doses of factor VIII concentrates, whereas high-titer inhibitors (> 5 BU) must be treated with serial infusions of activated prothrombin complex concentrates, recombinant human activated factor VII, or recombinant porcine factor VIII. Emicizumab is an excellent treatment option to prevent bleeding. Along with establishment of hemostasis by one of these measures, immunosuppressive treatment with corticosteroids with or without oral cyclophosphamide or rituximab must be instituted to eradicate the autoantibody. Treatment with IVIG and plasmapheresis can be considered in refractory cases. Unlike in congenital factor VIII deficiency of hemophilia A, the patient's bleeding does not correlate well with the factor VIII activity level, so the clinician must be concerned with any elevation of aPTT secondary to acquired factor VIII inhibitor. All such patients require immediate referral to a hematologist.

Poston JN et al. Real-world impact of emicizumab and immunosuppression on acquired hemophilia A: a multicenter US cohort. Blood Adv. 2024;8:5896. [PMID: 39361769]
Thomas VM et al. Off-label use of emicizumab in persons with acquired haemophilia A and von Willebrand disease: a scoping review of the literature. Haemophilia. 2022;28:4. [PMID: 34820989]

4. Vitamin K Deficiency

Vitamin K deficiency may occur because of deficient dietary intake of vitamin K (from green leafy vegetables, soybeans, and other sources), malabsorption, or decreased production by intestinal bacteria (due to treatment with chemotherapy or antibiotics). Vitamin K is required for normal function of vitamin K epoxide reductase that assists in posttranslational γ-carboxylation of the coagulation factors II, VII, IX, and X, which is necessary for their activity. Thus, mild to moderate vitamin K deficiency typically features a prolonged PT that corrects upon mixing; aPTT is prolonged if the deficiency is more severe, and activity levels of individual clotting factors II, VII, IX, and X typically are low. Importantly, a concomitantly low factor V activity level is not indicative of isolated vitamin K deficiency and may indicate an underlying defect in liver synthetic function. Hospitalized patients on broad-spectrum antibiotics and with poor or no oral intake are at high risk for vitamin K deficiency.

For treatment, vitamin K_1 (phytonadione) may be administered via intravenous or oral routes; the subcutaneous route is not recommended due to erratic absorption. The oral dose is 5–10 mg/day and absorption is typically excellent; at least partial improvement in the PT should be observed within 18–24 hours of administration. Intravenous administration (2–10 mg) results in faster normalization of a prolonged PT than oral administration; due to infrequent reported hypersensitivity/anaphylactoid reactions, parenteral doses should be administered slowly (eg, over 30 minutes) with concomitant monitoring.

5. Coagulopathy of Liver Disease

Impaired liver function due to cirrhosis or other causes leads to decreased synthesis of clotting factors, including factors II, V, VII, IX, X, and fibrinogen; factor VIII levels, largely made in endothelial cells, may be elevated despite depressed levels of other coagulation factors. The PT (and with advanced disease, the aPTT) is typically prolonged and usually corrects on mixing with normal plasma. A normal factor V level, with decreased activity of factors II, VII, IX, and X, suggests vitamin K deficiency rather than liver disease. Qualitative and quantitative deficiencies of fibrinogen also are prevalent among patients with advanced liver disease, typically leading to a prolonged PT, thrombin time, and reptilase time.

The coagulopathy of liver disease usually does not require hemostatic treatment unless bleeding occurs. Infusion of FFP may be considered if active bleeding is present and the aPTT and PT are prolonged; however, the effect is transient and concern for volume overload may limit infusions. Patients with bleeding and a fibrinogen level consistently below 80–100 mg/dL should receive cryoprecipitate or a fibrinogen product (RiaSTAP). Liver transplantation, if feasible, results in production of coagulation factors at normal levels. The use of recombinant human activated factor VII in patients with bleeding varices is controversial, although some patient subgroups may benefit. The coagulopathy of liver disease can predispose to bleeding or thrombosis, so caution and experience are needed for optimal management.

Roberts LN. How to manage hemostasis in patients with liver disease during interventions. Am Soc Hematol Educ Program. 2023;2023:274. [PMID: 38066857]

6. Warfarin Ingestion

See Antithrombotic Therapy section, below.

7. Disseminated Intravascular Coagulation

See Disseminated Intravascular Coagulation, above.

8. Heparin/Fondaparinux/Direct-Acting Oral Anticoagulant Use

See Classes of Anticoagulants, below.

9. Lupus Anticoagulants

Lupus anticoagulants prolong the aPTT by interfering with interactions between the clotting cascade and the phospholipid surface on which they function, but they do not lead to bleeding. Rather, they predispose to thrombosis. Lupus anticoagulants were so named because of their early identification in patients with autoimmune disease, although they also occur with increased frequency in individuals with underlying infection, inflammation, or malignancy, and in some asymptomatic individuals in the general population. A prolongation in the aPTT is observed that does not correct completely on mixing but that normalizes with excessive phospholipid. Specialized testing such as a positive hexagonal phase phospholipid neutralization assay, a prolonged dilute Russell viper venom time, and positive platelet neutralization assays can confirm the presence of a lupus anticoagulant. Rarely, the antibodies also interfere with factor II activity, and that tiny subset of patients with lupus anticoagulant are at risk for bleeding.

Müller-Calleja N et al. Tissue factor pathway inhibitor primes monocytes for antiphospholipid antibody-induced thrombosis. Blood. 2019;134:1119. [PMID: 31434703]

OTHER CAUSES OF BLEEDING

Occasionally, abnormalities of the vasculature and integument may lead to bleeding despite normal hemostasis; congenital or acquired disorders may be causative. Congenital abnormalities include Ehlers-Danlos syndrome, osteogenesis imperfecta, hereditary hemorrhagic telangiectasia (HHT; Osler-Weber-Rendu disease) (see Chapter 44), and Marfan syndrome. Acquired disorders include integument thinning due to prolonged corticosteroid administration or normal aging, amyloidosis, vasculitis, and scurvy. The bleeding time often is prolonged. If possible, treatment of the underlying condition should be pursued, but if this is not possible or feasible (ie, congenital syndromes), globally hemostatic agents such as antifibrinolytic agents or DDAVP can be considered for treatment of bleeding.

ANTITHROMBOTIC THERAPY

The currently available anticoagulants include unfractionated heparin, low-molecular-weight heparins (LMWHs), fondaparinux, vitamin K antagonists (ie, warfarin), and DOACs (ie, dabigatran, rivaroxaban, apixaban, edoxaban). For discussion of injectable direct thrombin inhibitors, see Heparin-Induced Thrombocytopenia, above.

Classes of Anticoagulants

A. Unfractionated Heparin and LMWHs

The heparins function by inducing a conformational change in antithrombin that leads to inactivation of activated factor Xa; unfractionated heparin inactivates thrombin as well. The pharmacokinetics of unfractionated heparin are unpredictable, so therapeutic dosing is monitored by aPTT or anti-Xa levels. Heparin is minimally metabolized by the kidneys, making it safe to use in most patients with significant kidney disease.

LMWHs (eg, enoxaparin, dalteparin) have more predictable pharmacokinetics than unfractionated heparin, due to less protein and cellular binding allowing for fixed weight-based dosing. LMWHs have a longer half-life than unfractionated heparin, which allows for once- or twice-daily subcutaneous dosing with greater convenience and outpatient therapy in selected cases. *All LMWHs are principally renally cleared and must be avoided in individuals with creatinine clearance < 30 mL/min.* Most patients do not require monitoring, although monitoring using the anti-Xa activity level is appropriate for patients with moderate kidney disease, those with elevated BMI or low weight, and selected pregnant patients. LMWHs are associated with a lower frequency of heparin-induced thrombocytopenia and thrombosis (HITT) (approximately 0.6%) than unfractionated heparin (3%).

B. Fondaparinux

Fondaparinux is a synthetic molecule consisting of the highly active pentasaccharide sequence found in LMWHs. It exerts almost no thrombin inhibition and inhibits factor Xa by binding to antithrombin. *Fondaparinux, like the LMWHs, is almost exclusively metabolized by the kidneys and should be avoided in patients with creatinine clearance < 30 mL/min.* Predictable pharmacokinetics allow for weight-based dosing.

C. Vitamin K Antagonist (Warfarin)

The oral vitamin K antagonist warfarin inhibits the vitamin K–dependent carboxylase responsible for post-translational modification of coagulation factors II, VII, IX, and X. Individual differences in nutritional status, comorbid diseases, concomitant medications, and genetic polymorphisms lead to a poorly predictable anticoagulant response. Individuals taking warfarin must undergo periodic monitoring to verify the intensity of the anticoagulant effect, reported as the INR.[1]

D. Direct-Acting Oral Anticoagulants

Unlike warfarin, the DOACs act directly against coagulation factors. Dabigatran is a direct thrombin inhibitor (DTI); rivaroxaban, apixaban, and edoxaban are direct factor Xa inhibitors. DOACs (1) have a predictable dose effect and do not require laboratory monitoring, (2) have anticoagulant activity independent of vitamin K with no need for dietary stasis, and (3) are renally metabolized to varying degrees, requiring restrictions or dose reductions related to kidney function (Table 16–9). While the DOACs have fewer drug interactions than warfarin, if DOACs are given with potentially interacting medications, there is no reliable way to measure the impact of the interaction on anticoagulant activity. There is also no reliable way to measure adherence. DOAC levels are affected by medications that modify P-glycoprotein (P-gp) transport in the gut; apixaban and rivaroxaban are also affected by medications that modify hepatic CYP4A4 metabolism. Medications that decrease DOAC metabolism may increase patients' bleeding risk, while medications that increase DOAC metabolism may increase thrombotic risk. Concomitant medications should be carefully reviewed; antiepileptic, antifungal, antiarrhythmic, and antiviral medications are categories with frequent interactions. DOACs should not be used with strong CYP3A4 inducers such as rifampin, carbamazepine, and St John's wort. Nirmatrelvir/ritonavir (Paxlovid) contains a strong combined P-gp and CYP3A4 inhibitor, and patients receiving acute VTE dosages of DOACs will need to hold, reduce dose, or transition to LMWH if given Paxlovid

[1]Importantly, because the INR is not standardized for abnormalities of factor V and fibrinogen, the INR should be used only in reference to anticoagulation in patients who are receiving warfarin.

Table 16–9. DOACs for VTE prophylaxis and treatment. See Table 12–3 for dosing of anticoagulation in atrial fibrillation.

	Dabigatran	Rivaroxaban	Apixaban	Edoxaban
Mechanism	Oral direct thrombin inhibitor	Oral direct factor Xa inhibitor	Oral direct factor Xa inhibitor	Oral direct factor Xa inhibitor
Approved uses for VTE	VTE treatment and secondary prevention VTE prophylaxis post-hip replacement	VTE treatment and secondary prevention VTE prophylaxis post-hip or knee replacement VTE prophylaxis in select adult patients hospitalized for acute medical illness	VTE treatment and secondary prevention VTE prophylaxis post-hip or knee replacement	VTE treatment and secondary prevention
Dosing for VTE	Acute VTE: 150 mg twice daily following 5–10 day parenteral lead-in for acute VTE Postsurgical prophylaxis after hip replacement: 110 mg first day, then 220 mg once daily for 28–35 days CrCl < 30 mL/min; avoid use No guidance for hepatic impairment	Acute VTE: 15 mg daily with food for first 21 days of acute VTE therapy, then 20 mg daily Postsurgical prophylaxis or secondary prevention: 10 mg daily with or without food CrCl < 15 mL/min: avoid use Hepatic impairment: no dose adjustment for Child-Pugh Class A; avoid use in Child-Pugh Class B and Child-Pugh Class C[1]	Acute VTE: 10 mg twice daily for first 7 days of acute VTE therapy, then 5 mg twice daily Postsurgical prophylaxis or secondary prevention: 2.5 mg twice daily Limited data for patients with CrCl < 15 mL/min Hepatic impairment: no dose adjustment for Child-Pugh Class A; caution advised for Child-Pugh class B due to limited data; not recommended in Child-Pugh Class C	Acute VTE: 60 mg once daily following 5–10 day parenteral lead-in for acute VTE CrCl 15–50 mL/min, or weight ≤ 60 kg, or if certain P-gp inhibitors are present: 30 mg once daily CrCl < 15 mL/min: avoid use Hepatic impairment: no dose adjustment for Child-Pugh Class A; not recommended for Child-Pugh class B or Child-Pugh Class C[1]
Food	With or without food	With food (for 15- and 20-mg tablets)	With or without food	With or without food
Crushable?	No	Can crush; do not administer via J tube	Can crush and administer orally or via NG tube	No data
Renal clearance	80%	30–60%	25%	50%
Kinetics (with normal renal function; half-lives are prolonged in renal impairment)	t ½ = 12–17 hours; tmax = 2 hours	t ½ = 5–9 hours (11–13 hours in elderly); tmax = 3 hours	t ½ = 12 hours; tmax = 3 hours	t ½ = 10–14 hours; tmax = 2 hours

Impact on INR	↑ (or →)	↑↑ (or → at low concentrations)	↑ (or →)	↑
Impact on aPTT	↑↑	↑	↑	↑
Drug interactions[2] (list not comprehensive; dosing guidance refers to VTE indication only; recommend checking with updated drug reference)	**Avoid** P-gp inducers: apalutamide, carbamazepine, rifampin, St John's wort, and possibly carbamazepine **Caution** with P-gp inhibitors: amiodarone, clarithromycin, dronedarone, ketoconazole, quinidine, verapamil; avoid if CrCl < 50 No dose adjustment if CrCl > 50 mL/min **Reduce dose** to 75 mg orally twice daily if CrCl 30–50 mL/min and concurrent use of dronedarone or ketoconazole	**Avoid** P-gp and strong CYP3A4 inducers: apalutamide, carbamazepine, conivaptan, indinavir/ritonavir, itraconazole, ketoconazole, lopinavir/ritonavir, phenytoin, rifampin, ritonavir, St John's wort **Caution** with the concurrent use of combined P-gp inhibitors and/or weak or moderate inhibitors of CYP3A4 (eg, amiodarone, azithromycin, diltiazem, dronedarone, erythromycin, felodipine, quinidine, ranolazine, verapamil) particularly in patients with impaired kidney function	**Avoid** P-gp and strong CYP3A4 inducers: apalutamide, carbamazepine, phenytoin, rifampin, St John's wort. **Caution** with concurrent use of P-gp and CYP3A4 inhibitors; consider dose reduction when starting itraconazole, ketoconazole, or ritonavir: If on apixaban 5 mg twice daily, decrease to 2.5 mg twice daily if starting itraconazole, ketoconazole, or ritonavir. If already on decreased dose of apixaban, avoid co-administration. **Caution** with clarithromycin	**Avoid** rifampin **Reduce dose** from 60 mg daily to 30 mg daily with certain P-gp inhibitors (eg, amiodarone, azithromycin, verapamil, ketoconazole, clarithromycin). Use has not been studied with many other P-gp inhibitors and inducers. Some experts recommend avoiding concurrent use altogether
Considerations	Dyspepsia is common Higher GI bleeding risk vs warfarin	Higher GI bleeding risk vs warfarin	Lowest bleeding risk	

[1]Child-Pugh Class A is mild impairment
Child-Pugh Class B is moderate impairment
Child-Pugh Class C is severe impairment or hepatic disease associated with coagulopathy
[2]Guidance adapted from: AC Forum Direct Oral Anticoagulant (DOAC) Drug-Drug Interaction Guidance, updated 9/2024, available at https://acforum.org/web/resource_files/1729293731-1600.pdf; Mar PL, Gopinathannair R, Gengler BE, et al. Drug interactions affecting oral anticoagulant use. Circ Arrhythm Electrophysiol. 2022;15(6); Hellfritzsch M, Henriksen JN, Holt MI, Grove EL. Drug-drug interactions in the treatment of cancer-associated venous thromboembolism with direct oral anticoagulants. Semin Thromb Hemost. 2024;50:489.
All DOACs: caution regarding increased bleeding risk with concurrent use of antiplatelet agents.
CrCl, creatinine clearance.

Table 16–10. Transitioning between therapeutic dosing of DOACs and other anticoagulants.

	Dabigatran	Rivaroxaban	Apixaban	Edoxaban
From DOAC to warfarin	Start warfarin and overlap with dabigatran; CrCl > 50 mL/min, overlap 3 days CrCl 30–50 mL/min, overlap 2 days CrCl 15–30 mL/min, overlap 1 day	Stop DOAC; start warfarin and LMWH at time of next scheduled DOAC dose and bridge with LMWH or other parenteral agent until INR ≥ 2.0	Stop DOAC; start warfarin and LMWH at time of next scheduled DOAC dose and bridge with LMWH or other parenteral agent until INR ≥ 2.0	For 60-mg dose, reduce dose to 30 mg and start warfarin concomitantly For 30-mg dose, reduce dose to 15 mg and start warfarin concomitantly Stop edoxaban when INR ≥ 2.0
From warfarin to DOAC	Start when INR < 2.0	Start when INR < 3.0	Start when INR < 2.0	Start when INR ≤ 2.5
From DOAC to unfractionated heparin infusion	Discontinue DOAC and start heparin at the time when next DOAC dose would be due. For patients at high bleeding risk, consider omitting initial bolus. For patients with renal failure, especially those taking dabigatran, a longer washout period may be appropriate.			
From unfractionated heparin infusion to DOAC	Stop heparin infusion and start DOAC within two hours after heparin discontinuation.			
From DOAC to low-molecular-weight heparin	Stop DOAC and initiate LMWH at the time when next DOAC dose would be given For patients at high bleeding risk or with renal impairment, especially those taking dabigatran, a longer washout period may be appropriate.			
From low-molecular-weight heparin to DOAC	Stop LMWH and initiate DOAC at time when next LMWH dose would be given.			

(Table 16–10). Clinicians must consider kidney function, concomitant medications, indication, candidacy for lead-in parenteral therapy (as required for acute VTE treatment with edoxaban and dabigatran only), weight, and anticipated adherence. (See Table 16–9 for details.) For patients who are morbidly obese (> 120 kg or BMI ≥ 40), standard doses of apixaban or rivaroxaban should be chosen rather than dabigatran or edoxaban. Data for DOAC use in patients who weigh > 140 kg are limited. DOACs are not recommended for VTE treatment in the acute setting following bariatric surgery due to concerns about absorption but can be considered for ongoing treatment after the initial 4 weeks of therapy; when available, apixaban or rivaroxaban trough levels can be checked to ensure they are within expected ranges.

Reversal agents are available for dabigatran, apixaban, rivaroxaban, and edoxaban. Idarucizamab is a specific reversal agent licensed for reversal of dabigatran in major bleeding or when reversal is needed for emergent procedures; dabigatran is the only DOAC that has a specific reversal agent. When idarucizamab is not available or when reversal is needed for patients taking oral factor Xa inhibitors (apixaban, rivaroxaban, and edoxaban), nonspecific reversal agents (prothrombin complex concentrates, or PCCs) may be used (Table 16–11). As use of nonspecific reversal agents is off-label, dosing guidelines are not available in the manufacturer's prescribing information, and institutional practices may vary. Andexanet alfa, previously licensed for reversal of rivaroxaban or apixaban in major bleeding, was removed from the US market in 2025. **Routine monitoring** is not recommended for patients taking DOACs. However, there are clinical scenarios where assessing anticoagulant activity may be helpful, including active bleeding, pending urgent surgery, suspected therapeutic failure, or concern for accumulation. Drug-specific anti-Xa levels are not widely available, and guidance is lacking regarding clinical approach to the results. However, a drug level < 30 ng/mL is usually considered negligible for all the DOACs. DOACs have varying effects on the PT and aPTT. A normal dilute thrombin time excludes the presence of clinically relevant dabigatran levels. An elevated aPTT suggests clinically relevant levels of dabigatran, while an elevated PT suggests clinically relevant levels of rivaroxaban. However, a normal aPTT or normal PT does not rule out clinically significant amounts of dabigatran or rivaroxaban, respectively. An undetectable LMWH anti-Xa level indicates that there is no clinically significant drug level of an oral Xa inhibitor.

Levy HJ et al. Reversal of direct oral anticoagulants: guidance from the SSC of the ISTH. J Thromb Haemost. 2024;22:2889. [PMID: 39029742]

Prevention of Venous Thromboembolic Disease

In the United States, an estimated 900,000 people have VTE events each year, leading to 100,000 premature deaths. About 50% of these VTE cases occur during or after hospitalization, with especially high incidence among critical care patients and high-risk surgical patients.

Avoidance of fatal PE is a major goal of pharmacologic prophylaxis. Tables 16–12 and 16–13 provide risk stratification for DVT/VTE among hospitalized surgical and medical inpatients. Standard pharmacologic prophylactic

Table 16–11. Medications to consider for reversing anticoagulant effect during life-threatening bleeding.[1]

Anticoagulants	Guidance
Parenteral	
Heparins	Protamine provides total (for unfractionated heparin) or partial (for LMWHs) reversal of anticoagulant effect. • Administration: Very slow infusion • Maximum dose: 50 mg intravenously • Caution: risk of anaphylactoid reactions and true hypersensitivity reactions, especially if allergy to other protamine-containing medications (such as NPH insulin) or to fish (black box warning) • Dosing depends on dose given and time elapsed • Dosing calculator at https://clincalc.com/Protamine/
Unfractionated heparin	Protamine (100% neutralization) • 1 mg protamine neutralizes approximately 100 units of heparin sulfate • Monitor drug activity with aPTT and/or heparin anti-Xa activity
LMWH (enoxaparin, dalteparin)	Protamine (approximately 60% neutralization) • Last dose < 8 hours ago: 1 mg protamine for each 100 units of dalteparin or 1 mg enoxaparin • Last dose > 8 hours ago: 0.5 mg protamine for each 100 units of dalteparin or 1 mg enoxaparin • Degree of reversal can be assessed with LMWH anti-Xa activity
Oral	
DOACs	Guidance for all DOAC-associated major bleeding: • Supportive measures recommended for all patients • If ingested within 2 hours, administer activated charcoal • Reversal agent is recommended ONLY if bleeding is life-threatening or into a critical organ; for dabigatran, idarucizamab can be considered if reversal is required for an urgent procedural intervention that cannot be delayed • Reversal agent is not recommended for DOAC overdose without bleeding
Dabigatran	Idarucizumab 5 g intravenously once If idarucizumab is not available: administer APCC or four-factor PCC 50 units/kg intravenously
Apixaban	Administer four-factor PCC 2000 units or 25–50 IU/kg (max, 5000 units); use higher dose for life-threatening bleeding
Rivaroxaban	Administer four-factor PCC 2000 units or 25–50 IU/kg (max, 5000 units); use higher dose for life-threatening bleeding
Warfarin	See Table 16–21

[1]Guidance adopted from Anticoagulation Forum and American Society of Hematology 2019 guidelines; Van Es N et al. Reversal agents for current and forthcoming direct oral anticoagulants. European Heart Journal. 2023;44:1795; Anticoagulation Forum Rapid Resource "Reversal and Treatment Strategies for DOAC-Related Bleeding": https://acforum.org/r/FWmLZf8oo3uAUMuCDH

APCC, three-factor prothrombin complex concentrate; FFP, fresh frozen plasma; LMWH, low-molecular-weight heparin; PCC, four-factor prothrombin complex concentrate.

regimens are listed in Table 16–14. Prophylactic strategies should be guided by individual risk stratification, with all moderate- and high-risk patients receiving pharmacologic prophylaxis, unless contraindicated. Contraindications to VTE prophylaxis for hospital inpatients at high risk for VTE are listed in Table 16–15. In patients at high risk for VTE with absolute contraindications to pharmacologic prophylaxis, mechanical devices such as intermittent pneumatic compression devices should be used, ideally in portable form with at least an 18-hour daily wear time.

1. Primary VTE prophylaxis for medical patients—VTE prophylaxis should be used judiciously in hospitalized medical patients who are not critically ill since evidence suggests harm from bleeding in low-risk patients given low-dose heparin, and skin necrosis from compression stockings in stroke patients. Risk assessment models like the Padua Risk Score (Table 16–13) and the IMPROVE risk score can help identify patients who may benefit from DVT prophylaxis. The IMPROVE investigators also developed a bleeding risk model that may aid in identifying acutely ill medical inpatients at increased risk for bleeding: https://www.outcomes-umassmed.org/IMPROVE/risk_score/index.html. Rivaroxaban has been approved for extended-duration prophylaxis after discharge for medically ill patients; how to identify those who will have clinical benefit from this practice is unclear. For VTE prophylaxis in severe COVID-19, see below.

2. Primary VTE prophylaxis for surgical patients—The Caprini score may help guide VTE prophylaxis in surgical patients (https://www.mdcalc.com/caprini-score-venous-thromboembolism-2005). Certain high-risk surgical patients should also be considered for extended-duration prophylaxis of up to 1 month, including those undergoing total hip replacement, hip fracture repair, and abdominal and pelvic cancer surgery. For surgical patients at high risk for VTE who also have active bleeding or high perceived

Table 16–12. Risk stratification for incurring DVT/VTE among surgical inpatients.

High risk[1]
Recent major orthopedic surgery/arthroplasty/fracture
Abdominal/pelvic cancer undergoing surgery
Spinal cord injury[2] or major trauma within 90 days
More than three of the intermediate risk factors (see below)
Intermediate risk
Not ambulating independently outside of room at least twice daily
Active infectious or inflammatory process
Active malignancy
Major surgery (nonorthopedic)
History of VTE
Stroke
Central venous access or PICC line
IBD
Prior immobilization (> 72 hours) preoperatively
Obesity (BMI > 30)
Patient age > 50 years
Hormone replacement or oral contraceptive therapy
Hypercoagulable state
Nephrotic syndrome
Burns
Cellulitis
Varicose veins
Paresis
HF (systolic dysfunction)
COPD exacerbation
Low risk
Minor procedure and age < 40 years with no additional risk factors
Ambulatory with expected length of stay of < 24 hours or minor surgery

[1]Risk is highest in first month and persists for up to 90 days.
[2]Direct spinal cord trauma is a contraindication to VTE prophylaxis in the immediate post-injury period; consult with neurosurgical experts regarding timing of initiation.
PICC, peripherally inserted central catheter.

bleeding risk (Table 16–12), mechanical devices such as intermittent pneumatic compression devices and graduated compression stockings provide some measure of thromboprophylaxis, although pharmacologic prophylaxis should be started as soon as it is safe. Patients undergoing surgery for abdominal or pelvic cancer may transition to prophylactic doses of rivaroxaban or apixaban after an initial 7- to 10-day period of LMWH or unfractionated heparin. Prophylaxis should be considered for up to 4 weeks in patients undergoing major open or laparoscopic abdominal or pelvic cancer surgery with risk factors such as limited mobility, obesity, or history of VTE.

Table 16–13. Padua Risk Assessment Model for VTE prophylaxis in hospitalized medical patients.

Condition	Points[1]
Active cancer, history of VTE, immobility, laboratory thrombophilia	3 points each
Recent (≤ 1 month) trauma and/or surgery	2 points each
Age ≥ 70; acute MI or ischemic stroke; acute infection or rheumatologic disorder; BMI ≥ 30; hormonal therapy	1 point each

[1]A score ≥ 4 connotes high risk of VTE in the noncritically ill medical patients and pharmacologic prophylaxis is indicated, absent absolute contraindications.
CVA, cerebrovascular accident.

3. Primary VTE prophylaxis for ambulatory patients with cancer—Some ambulatory patients with cancer undergoing chemotherapy who are at moderate to high risk of VTE (Khorana risk score ≥ 2) (https://www.mdcalc.com/khorana-risk-score-venous-thromboembolism-cancer-patients) may benefit from pharmacologic DVT prophylaxis, although bleeding risk is increased and caution should be taken, particularly in patients with GI or intracranial malignancy, and other risk factors for anticoagulant-related bleeding such as thrombocytopenia and kidney dysfunction. DOACs should be avoided when there are possible interactions with chemotherapeutic agents.

Key NS et al. Venous thromboembolism prophylaxis and treatment in patients with cancer: ASCO Guideline Update. J Clin Oncol. 2023;41:3063. [PMID: 37075273]

Treatment of VTE Disease

A. Anticoagulant Therapy for VTE

Treatment for VTE should be offered to patients with objectively confirmed DVT or PE, or to those in whom the clinical suspicion is high for the disorder but who have not yet undergone diagnostic testing (see Chapter 9). Management of VTE primarily involves administration of anticoagulant to prevent thrombosis recurrence, extension, or embolization, and to reduce the risk of post-thrombotic syndrome. Suggested regimens are found in Table 16–16.

B. Risk Stratification for Appropriate Initial Anticoagulant Therapy for VTE

1. DVT without PE—Most such patients may be treated as outpatients, provided that their risk of bleeding is low and they have good follow-up. Table 16–17 outlines proposed selection criteria for outpatient treatment of DVT.

2. Low-risk patients with PE—These patients have a PE-related mortality rate < 3%. The simplified PE severity index (PESI) and the Bova score (https://www.mdcalc.com/bova-score-pulmonary-embolism-complications) accurately identify patients at low risk for 30-day PE-related mortality (Table 16–18) and provide further risk stratification. For patients with 0 points on the simplified PESI and Bova scores, the Hestia criteria (https://www.mdcalc.com/calc/3918/hestia-criteria-outpatient-pulmonary-embolism-treatment) can help identify patients suitable for expedited discharge or outpatient treatment by incorporating additional considerations such as kidney or liver dysfunction, need for symptom control, and pregnancy.

3. Isolated subsegmental PE—PE that is limited to the subsegmental branches of the pulmonary arteries should prompt assessment for DVT. Risk factors for progression or decompensation include hospitalization, need for oxygen,

Table 16–14. Pharmacologic prophylaxis of VTE in selected clinical scenarios.[1]

Anticoagulant	Dose	Frequency	Clinical Scenario	Comment
LMWH and Fondaparinux				
Enoxaparin	40 mg subcutaneously	Once daily	Medical inpatients at high risk for VTE and most critical care patients[2]	—
			Surgical patients (moderate risk for VTE)	—
			Abdominal/pelvic cancer surgery	Consider continuing for 4 weeks total duration after abdominal/pelvic cancer surgery.
		Twice daily	Bariatric surgery	Higher doses may be required.
	30 mg subcutaneously	Twice daily	Orthopedic surgery[3]	Give for at least 10 days. For THR, TKR, or HFS, consider continuing up to 35 days after surgery in high-risk patients.
			Major trauma	Not applicable to patients with isolated lower extremity trauma.
			Spinal cord injury[4]	—
Dalteparin	2500 units subcutaneously	Once daily	Medical inpatients at high risk for VTE[2]	—
			Abdominal surgery (moderate risk for VTE)	Give for 5–10 days.
	5000 units subcutaneously	Once daily	Orthopedic surgery[3]	First dose = 2500 units. Give for at least 10 days. For THR, TKR, or HFS, consider continuing up to 35 days after surgery in high-risk patients.
			Abdominal surgery (higher risk for VTE)	Give for 5–10 days. Consider continuing for 4 weeks total duration after abdominal/pelvic cancer surgery.
			Medical inpatients	—
Fondaparinux	2.5 mg subcutaneously	Once daily	Orthopedic surgery[3]	Give for at least 10 days. For THR, TKR, or HFS, consider continuing up to 35 days after surgery in high-risk patients.
Direct-Acting Oral Anticoagulants				
Rivaroxaban	10 mg orally	Once daily	Orthopedic surgery: THR, TKR	Give for 12 days following TKR; give for 35 days following THR.
Apixaban	2.5 mg orally	Twice daily	Following THR or TKR	Give for 12 days following TKR; give for 35 days following THR.
Dabigatran	110 mg orally first day, then 220 mg	Once daily	Following THR	For patients with CrCl > 30 mL/min. Consider continuing up to 1 month after surgery in high-risk patients.
Unfractionated Heparin				
Unfractionated heparin	5000 units subcutaneously	Three times daily	Higher VTE risk with low bleeding risk	Includes gynecologic and urologic cancer surgery and medical patients with multiple risk factors for VTE.
	5000 units subcutaneously	Twice daily	Hospitalized patients at intermediate risk for VTE	Includes gynecologic surgery (moderate risk).
			Patients with epidural catheters	LMWH is usually avoided due to risk of spinal hematoma (catheter should not be removed within 4 hours of last heparin dose).
			Patients with CrCl < 30 mL/min	LMWH is contraindicated.

(*continued*)

Table 16–14. Pharmacologic prophylaxis of VTE in selected clinical scenarios.[1] (continued)

Anticoagulant	Dose	Frequency	Clinical Scenario	Comment
Warfarin and Aspirin				
Warfarin	(Variable) oral	Once daily	Orthopedic surgery[3]	Titrate to goal INR = 2.5. Give for at least 10 days. For high-risk patients undergoing THR, TKR, or HFS, consider continuing up to 1 month after surgery.
Aspirin	81 mg orally	Twice daily	TKR, THR	For patients at otherwise low VTE risk following major orthopedic surgery. Give for at least 14 days.

[1]See Table 16–15 for contraindications.
[2]See Prevention of Venous Thromboembolic Disease text, above, for definition of high-risk patients.
[3]Includes TKR, THR, and HFS.
[4]Direct spinal cord trauma is a contraindication to VTE prophylaxis in the immediate post-injury period; consult with neurosurgical experts regarding timing of initiation.
CrCl, creatinine clearance; HFS, hip fracture surgery; LMWH, low-molecular-weight heparin; P-gp, P-glycoprotein; THR, total hip replacement; TKR, total knee replacement.

active cancer, a prior history of VTE, and known thrombophilia. For patients with incidentally discovered or asymptomatic subsegmental PE who are at low risk for progression or recurrence and who do not have DVT, anticoagulation can be deferred in favor of close observation, especially when the bleeding risk is high. In these scenarios, however, repeat lower extremity ultrasonography should be obtained after 5–7 days. Even for low-risk patients with subsegmental PE and absence of DVT on serial lower extremity ultrasonography, the risk for recurrent PE remains higher than in the general population, especially in older patients and those with multiple subsegmental PEs noted on initial diagnosis.

Table 16–15. Contraindications to VTE prophylaxis for medical or surgical hospital inpatients at high risk for VTE.

Absolute contraindications
Acute hemorrhage from wounds or drains or lesions
Intracranial hemorrhage within prior 24 hours
Heparin-induced thrombocytopenia (HIT): consider using fondaparinux
Severe trauma to head or spinal cord or extremities
Epidural anesthesia/spinal block within 12 hours of initiation of anticoagulation (concurrent use of an epidural catheter and anticoagulation other than low prophylactic doses of unfractionated heparin requires review and approval by service who performed the epidural or spinal procedure, eg, anesthesia/pain service, and in many cases, should be avoided entirely)
Currently receiving warfarin or heparin or LMWH or direct thrombin inhibitor for other indications
Relative contraindications
Coagulopathy (INR > 1.5)
Intracranial lesion or neoplasm
Severe thrombocytopenia (platelet count < 50,000/mcL [50×10^9/L])
Intracranial hemorrhage within past 6 months
GI or genitourinary hemorrhage within past 6 months

LMWH, low-molecular-weight heparin.
Adapted from guidelines used at the Veterans Affairs Medical Center, San Francisco, CA.

4. Intermediate-risk patients with PE—For hemodynamically stable PE patients not definitively classified as low-risk, additional assessment is warranted to stratify risk for PE-associated cardiovascular collapse. Because the Bova score includes serum troponin and evidence of RV dysfunction (by CT or echocardiography), it identifies those patients with high-intermediate risk ("submassive") PE who warrant close monitoring and should be admitted to a higher level of inpatient care. Echocardiography provides better assessment of RV dysfunction than CT when there is concern. Serum biomarkers such as BNP and troponin are most useful for their negative predictive value, and mainly in combination with other predictors. High-intermediate-risk patients have a mortality rate of up to 15%, and there should be case-by-case consideration of thrombolysis. Catheter-directed techniques may be an option for patients who are poor candidates for systemic thrombolysis in centers with expertise.

5. High-risk patients with PE—Patients with persistent hemodynamic instability are classified as high-risk patients (previously referred to as having "massive PE") and have an early PE-related mortality of > 15%. These patients should be admitted to an ICU and generally receive thrombolysis and anticoagulation with intravenous heparin.

Selection of an initial anticoagulant should be determined by patient characteristics (kidney function, immediate bleeding risk, weight) and the clinical scenario (eg, whether thrombolysis is being considered, active cancer, thrombosis location) as described in Table 16–16.

C. Parenteral and Oral Anticoagulants for VTE

1. Parenteral anticoagulants for VTE—

Heparins—In patients in whom parenteral anticoagulation is being considered, LMWHs are often preferred over

Table 16–16. Initial anticoagulation for VTE.[1]

Anticoagulant	Dose/Frequency	Clinical Scenario: DVT of the Upper or Lower Extremity or PE	VTE with Concomitant Severe Kidney Disease[2]	VTE, Cancer-Related	Comment
Unfractionated Heparin					
Unfractionated heparin	80 units/kg intravenous bolus, then continuous intravenous infusion of 18 units/kg/hour	×	×	× (anticoagulant of choice when bleeding risk is high since it is reversible)	Bolus may be omitted if risk of bleeding is elevated. Maximum bolus, 10,000 units. Requires aPTT or heparin anti-Xa monitoring. Most patients: begin warfarin at time of initiation of heparin.
	330 units/kg subcutaneously × 1, then 250 units/kg subcutaneously every 12 hours	×			Fixed-dose; no aPTT monitoring required
LMWH and Fondaparinux					
Enoxaparin[3]	1 mg/kg subcutaneously every 12 hours **or** 1.5 mg/kg subcutaneously daily	×			Most patients: begin warfarin at time of initiation of LMWH
Dalteparin[3]	200 units/kg subcutaneously once daily for first month, then 150 units/kg/day	×		×	Preferred LMWH for patients with cancer; administer for at least 3–6 months (warfarin not preferred but may transition to DOAC)
Fondaparinux	5 mg subcutaneously once daily for body weight < 50 kg; 7.5 mg for body weight 50–100 kg; 10 mg for body weight > 100 kg	×			
Direct-Acting Oral Anticoagulants (DOACs)					
Rivaroxaban	15 mg orally twice daily with food for 21 days, then 20 mg orally daily with food	×		×	Contraindicated if CrCl < 15 mL/min Monotherapy without need for initial parenteral therapy Caution in luminal GI or genitourinary cancer
Apixaban	10 mg orally twice daily for first 7 days, then 5 mg twice daily	×		×	Limited data for CrCl < 15 mL/min Lowest bleeding risk of DOACs Monotherapy without need for initial parenteral therapy
Edoxaban	5–10 days of parenteral anticoagulation, then 60 mg orally once daily; 30 mg once daily recommended if CrCl is 15–50 mL/min, if weight ≤ 60 kg, or if certain P-gp inhibitors are present	×		×	Contraindicated if CrCl < 15 mL/min Initial need for parenteral therapy Caution in luminal GI or genitourinary cancer
Dabigatran	5–10 days of parenteral anticoagulation, then begin 150 mg orally twice daily	×			Contraindicated if CrCl < 30 mL/min Initial need for parenteral therapy

[1]Obtain baseline hemoglobin, platelet count, aPTT, PT/INR, and creatinine prior to initiation of anticoagulation. *Anticoagulation is contraindicated in the setting of active bleeding (See text for other contraindications).*
[2]Defined as creatinine clearance < 30 mL/min.
[3]If body weight < 50 kg, reduce dose and monitor anti-Xa levels.
CrCl, creatinine clearance; P-gp, P-glycoprotein.
Note: An "×" denotes appropriate use of the anticoagulant.

Table 16–17. Patient selection for outpatient treatment of DVT.

Patients considered appropriate for outpatient treatment
No clinical signs or symptoms of PE and pain is controlled
Confirmed ability to pay for medication (either by insurance or out-of-pocket)
Capable and willing to comply with frequent follow-up
Initially, patients may need to be seen daily to weekly
Potential contraindications for outpatient treatment
DVT involving inferior vena cava, iliac, common femoral, or upper extremity vein (these patients might benefit from vascular intervention)
Comorbid conditions requiring inpatient management
Active peptic ulcer disease, GI bleeding in past 14 days, liver synthetic dysfunction
Brain metastases, current or recent CNS or spinal cord injury/surgery in the last 10 days, CVA ≤ 4–6 weeks
Familial bleeding diathesis
Active bleeding from source other than GI
Thrombocytopenia
Creatinine clearance < 30 mL/min
Weight < 55 kg (male) or < 45 kg (female)
Recent surgery, spinal or epidural anesthesia in the past 3 days
History of heparin-induced thrombocytopenia
Inability to reliably take medication at home, recognize changes in health status, or understand or follow directions

CVA, cerebrovascular accident.

unfractionated heparin as initial treatment because of predictable pharmacokinetics, which allow for subcutaneous, once- or twice-daily dosing with no requirement for monitoring in most patients. LMWHs also may be more effective than unfractionated heparin in immediate treatment of VTE and carry lower risk of HIT. Scenarios that warrant intravenous unfractionated heparin as immediate VTE treatment include severe kidney disease (creatinine clearance < 30 mL/min), which carries a bleeding risk due to accumulation of LMWH, and other situations where there is a higher risk of bleeding (recent bleeding, postoperative state, thrombocytopenia), given the shorter half-life and reversibility of unfractionated heparin. Unfractionated heparin is also preferred when concomitant thrombolysis is being considered. Unfractionated heparin can be neutralized with protamine sulfate, while protamine may only have partial reversal effect on LMWH. Use of unfractionated heparin leads to HIT and thrombosis in approximately 3% of patients, so daily CBCs are recommended during the initial 10–14 days of exposure.

Table 16–18. Simplified Pulmonary Embolism Severity Index (PESI).

		Points
Age > 80 years old		1
Cancer		1
Chronic cardiopulmonary disease		1
Systolic blood pressure < 100 mm Hg		1
Oxygen saturation ≤ 90%		1
Severity Class	**Points**	**30-Day Mortality**
Low risk	0	1%
High risk	≥ 1	10%

Data from Jiménez D et al; RIETE Investigators. Simplification of the pulmonary embolism severity index for prognostication in patients with acute symptomatic pulmonary embolism. Arch Intern Med. 2010;170:1383.

Weight-based, fixed-dose daily subcutaneous fondaparinux may also be used for the initial treatment of DVT and PE, with no increase in bleeding over that observed with LMWH. Its lack of reversibility, long half-life, and renal clearance limit its use in patients with an increased risk of bleeding or kidney disease.

2. Oral anticoagulants for VTE—

A. **Direct-acting oral anticoagulants**—DOACs have a predictable dose effect, few drug-drug interactions, rapid onset of action, and freedom from laboratory monitoring (Table 16–10). Dabigatran, rivaroxaban, apixaban, and edoxaban are approved for treatment of acute DVT and PE. While rivaroxaban and apixaban can be used as monotherapy, patients treated with dabigatran or edoxaban must first receive 5–10 days of parenteral anticoagulation and then be transitioned to the oral agent per prescribing information. Unlike warfarin, DOACs do not require an overlap since these agents are immediately active; the DOAC is started when the parenteral agent is stopped (Table 16–10). Compared to warfarin and LMWH, the DOACs are all noninferior with respect to prevention of recurrent VTE; both rivaroxaban and apixaban have a lower bleeding risk than warfarin with LMWH bridging. Apixaban is associated with less bleeding risk than other DOACs. While DOACs are recommended as first-line therapy for acute VTE, agent selection should be individualized with consideration of kidney function, concomitant medication use, indication, cost, and adherence. Heparins may be preferable as initial therapy when hospitalized patients have clinical instability and fluctuating renal or hepatic function; when bleeding risk is high; or when thrombolysis may be required.

B. **Warfarin**—If warfarin is chosen as the oral anticoagulant, it should be initiated along with the parenteral anticoagulant, which is continued until INR is in therapeutic range. Most patients require 5 mg of warfarin daily for initial treatment, but lower doses (2.5 mg daily) should be considered for older adults and those with hyperthyroidism, HF, liver disease, recent major surgery, malnutrition, or certain polymorphisms for the *CYP2C9* or *VKORC1* genes, as well as those who are receiving concurrent medications that increase sensitivity to warfarin. Conversely, patients with larger BMI or hypothyroidism, or those who are receiving medications that increase warfarin metabolism (eg, rifampin), may require higher initial doses (7.5 mg daily). Daily INR results should guide dosing adjustments in the hospitalized patient, while at least biweekly INR results guide dosing in the outpatient during the initial period of therapy (Table 16–19). Web-based warfarin dosing calculators incorporating clinical and genetic factors

Table 16–19. Warfarin dosing adjustment guidelines for initiation of warfarin therapy.

Measurement Day	INR	Action
For Hospitalized Patients Newly Starting Therapy		
Day 1		5 mg (2.5 or 7.5 mg in select populations[1])
Day 2	< 1.5	Continue dose
	≥ 1.5	Decrease or hold dose[2]
Day 3	≤ 1.2	Increase dose[2]
	> 1.2 and < 1.7	Continue dose
	≥ 1.7	Decrease dose[2]
Day 4 until therapeutic	Daily increase < 0.2 units	Increase dose[2]
	Daily increase 0.2–0.3 units	Continue dose
	Daily increase 0.4–0.6 units	Decrease dose[2]
	Daily increase ≥ 0.7 units	Hold dose
For Outpatients Newly Starting Therapy		
Measure PT/INR on Day 1	Baseline	Start treatment with 2–7.5 mg
Measure PT/INR on Day 3–4	< 1.5	Increase weekly dose by 5–25%
	1.5–1.9	No dosage change
	2.0–2.5	Decrease weekly dose by 25–50%
	> 2.5	Decrease weekly dose by 50% or HOLD dose
Measure PT/INR on Day 5–7	< 1.5	Increase weekly dose by 10–25%
	1.5–1.9	Increase weekly dose by 0–20%
	2.0–3.0	No dosage change
	> 3.0	Decrease weekly dose by 10–25% or HOLD dose
Measure PT/INR on Day 8–10	< 1.5	Increase weekly dose by 15–35%
	1.5–1.9	Increase weekly dose by 5–20%
	2.0–3.0	No dosage change
	> 3.0	Decrease weekly dose by 10–25% or HOLD dose
Measure PT/INR on Day 11–14	< 1.6	Increase weekly dose by 15–35%
	1.6–1.9	Increase weekly dose by 5–20%
	2.0–3.0	No dosage change
	> 3.0	Decrease weekly dose by 5–20% or HOLD dose

[1]See text.
[2]In general, dosage adjustments should not exceed 2.5 mg or 50%.
Data from Kim YK et al. J Thromb Haemost. 2010;8:101. From Center for Health Quality, Outcomes, and Economic Research, VA Medical Center, Bedford, MA.

are available to help clinicians choose appropriate starting doses (eg, see http://www.warfarindosing.org). Because an average of 5 days is required to achieve a steady-state reduction in the activity of vitamin K–dependent coagulation factors, the parenteral anticoagulant should be continued for at least 5 days from warfarin initiation and until the INR is > 2.0. Meticulous follow-up should be arranged for all patients taking warfarin because of the bleeding risk associated with initiation of therapy. Once stabilized, the INR should be checked at least every 6 weeks and warfarin dosing should be adjusted by guidelines (Table 16–20); this strategy has been shown to improve the time patients spend in the therapeutic range and their clinical outcomes. Supratherapeutic INRs should be managed according to evidence-based guidelines (Table 16–21).

D. Duration of Anticoagulation Therapy for VTE

The clinical scenario in which thrombosis occurred is the strongest predictor of recurrence and, in most cases, guides duration of anticoagulation (Table 16–22). In the first year after discontinuation of anticoagulation therapy, the frequency of recurrent VTE when thrombosis occurred in the setting of a transient, major, reversible risk factor (such as surgery) is approximately 3% after completion of 3 months of anticoagulation, compared with at least 8% for

Table 16–20. Warfarin-dosing adjustment guidelines for patients receiving long-term therapy, with target INR 2–3.

Patient INR	Weekly Dosing Change	
	Dose Change	Follow-Up INR
≤ 1.5	Increase by 10–15%	Within 1 week
1.51–1.79	If falling or low on two or more occasions, increase weekly dose by 5–10%.	7–14 days
1.80–2.29	Consider not changing the dose unless a consistent pattern has been observed.	7–14 days
2.3–3.0 (in range)	No change in dosage.	28 days (42 days if INR in range three times consecutively)
3.01–3.20	Consider not changing the dose unless a consistent pattern has been observed.	7–14 days
3.21–3.69	Do not hold warfarin. If rising or high on two or more occasions, decrease weekly dose by 5–10%.	7–14 days
3.70–4.99	Hold warfarin for 1 day and decrease weekly dose by 5–10%.	Within 1 week, sooner if clinically indicated
5.0–8.99	Hold warfarin. Clinical evaluation for bleeding. When INR is therapeutic, restart at lower dose (decrease weekly dose by 10–15%). Check INR at least weekly until stable. Consider vitamin K if bleeding risk is high (see Table 16–21).	Within 1 week, sooner if clinically indicated, then weekly until stabilized
≥ 9	See Table 16–21.	

From Center for Health Quality, Outcomes, and Economic Research, VA Medical Center, Bedford, MA. Data from Kim YK et al. J Thromb Haemost. 2010;8:101. See also Van Spall HE et al. Variation in warfarin dose adjustment practice is responsible for differences in the quality of anticoagulation control between centers and countries: an analysis of patients receiving warfarin in the randomized evaluation of long-term anticoagulation therapy (RE-LY) trial. Circulation. 2012;126:2309.

individuals whose thrombosis was unprovoked, and > 20% in patients with cancer. Men have > twofold higher risk of recurrent VTE compared to women; recurrent PE is more likely to develop in patients with clinically apparent PE than in those with DVT alone and has a case fatality rate of nearly 10%; and proximal DVT has a higher recurrence risk than distal DVT.

1. Role of provoking factors for VTE—Patients with VTE with major transient provoking factors are generally treated

Table 16–21. American College of Chest Physicians evidence-based clinical practice guidelines for the management of supratherapeutic INR.

Clinical Situation	INR	Recommendations
No significant bleed	Above therapeutic range but < 5.0	• Lower dose or omit dose (see Table 16–20) • Monitor more frequently and resume at lower dose when INR falls within therapeutic range (if INR only slightly above range, may not be necessary to decrease dose)
	≥ 5.0 but < 9.0	• Hold next 1–2 doses • Monitor more frequently and resume therapy at lower dose (see Table 16–20) when INR falls within therapeutic range • *Patients at high risk for bleeding*[1]: Hold warfarin and consider giving vitamin K_1 1–2.5 mg orally; check INR in 24–48 hours to ensure response to therapy
	≥ 9.0	• Hold warfarin • Vitamin K_1 2.5–5 mg orally • Monitor frequently and resume therapy at lower dose when INR within therapeutic range
Serious/life-threatening bleed		• Hold warfarin and give 10 mg vitamin K by slow intravenous infusion supplemented by FFP, PCC, or recombinant factor VIIa (PCC preferred)

[1]Patients at higher risk for bleeding include elderly people, and conditions that increase the risk of bleeding include kidney disease, hypertension, falls, liver disease, and history of GI or genitourinary bleeding.
FFP, fresh frozen plasma; PCC, prothrombin complex concentrate.

Table 16–22. Duration of treatment of VTE.

Scenario	Suggested Duration of Therapy	Comments
Provoked by major transient risk factor (eg, major surgery, major trauma, major hospitalization)	3 months; consider up to 6 months if major event and bleeding risk allows	VTE prophylaxis upon future exposure to transient risk factor
Unprovoked	At least 3 months; consider indefinite if bleeding risk allows	May individually risk-stratify for recurrence with D-dimer, clinical risk scores, and clinical presentation Consider transition to DOAC secondary prevention dose after initial treatment period
Recurrent unprovoked	Indefinite	If recurrent despite therapeutic anticoagulation, consider hematology consultation for further evaluation and guidance
Cancer-related	≥ 3–6 months or as long as cancer is active, whichever is longer	LMWH or carefully selected DOAC recommended for initial treatment (see Table 16–16)
Underlying significant thrombophilia (eg, antiphospholipid antibody syndrome, antithrombin deficiency, protein C deficiency, protein S deficiency, ≥ two concomitant thrombophilic conditions)	Indefinite	To avoid false positives, consider delaying investigation for laboratory thrombophilia until 3 months after event

LMWH, low-molecular-weight heparin.

with a minimum of 3 to 6 months of anticoagulation. VTE without clear strong provoking factors, or with persistent (non-transient) risk factors, should prompt consideration of indefinite anticoagulation provided the patient is not at high risk for bleeding, since unprovoked VTE carries a recurrence risk of > 30% at 10 years (with 4% of recurrences resulting in death). Extending duration of anticoagulation beyond 3 months for unprovoked PE will not reduce risk of recurrence once anticoagulation is stopped. Individual risk stratification may help identify patients most likely to suffer recurrent disease and thus most likely to benefit from ongoing anticoagulation therapy (see below). Normal D-dimer levels 1 month after cessation of anticoagulation are associated with lower recurrence risk, although some would argue not low enough to consider stopping anticoagulant therapy, particularly in men.

2. Risk scoring systems to guide therapy duration—The HERDOO2 risk scoring system uses BMI, age, D-dimer, and postphlebitic symptoms to identify women at lower risk for recurrence after unprovoked VTE (https://www.mdcalc.com/herdoo2-rule-discontinuing-anticoagulation-unprovoked-vte). The Vienna Prediction Model, a simple scoring system based on age, sex, D-dimer, and location of thrombosis, can help estimate an individual's recurrence risk to guide duration of therapy decisions.

3. Cancer-related VTE—Cancer-associated VTE may be treated with parenteral agents (LMWH, unfractionated heparin, fondaparinux) or DOACs. Warfarin is not recommended as it is associated with higher VTE recurrence rates in patients with malignancy. Apixaban carries the lowest bleeding risk of the DOACs. For patients with intracranial malignancy and VTE, bleeding risk depends on tumor type; generally metastatic tumors, such as melanoma, renal cell carcinoma, HCC, thyroid cancer, and choriocarcinoma, have a higher risk of bleeding than primary tumors. For patients with high-risk malignancies and VTE, brain imaging to search for metastatic disease is recommended, along with interdisciplinary consultation (eg, with oncology and neurosurgery), to help determine risk of initiating anticoagulation and individualize the clinical decision. DOACs do not appear to confer higher bleeding risk compared to LMWH in patients with brain tumors. Clinicians must be aware that chemotherapeutic agents may interact with DOACs, and their use should be avoided in cases of potential interactions because there is no reliable way to measure the anticoagulant effect of DOACs.

4. Thrombophilia workup in determining duration—Laboratory workup for thrombophilia is not recommended routinely for determining duration of therapy because clinical presentation is a much stronger predictor of recurrence risk. Evaluation may be pursued in patients < age 50, with a strong family history, with thrombosis in unusual locations, or with recurrent thromboses (Table 16–23). In addition, thrombophilia evaluation may be considered in women of childbearing age in whom results may influence fertility and pregnancy outcomes and management or in those patients in whom results will influence duration of therapy. The American Society of Hematology suggests consideration of thrombophilia testing in patients with VTE provoked by a nonsurgical transient risk factor, in patients who had VTE associated with pregnancy or the postpartum period, and in patients with VTE associated with oral contraceptives, when negative results might lead to consideration of stopping treatment. Patients should be informed that negative thrombophilia testing does not

Table 16–23. Candidates for thrombophilia workup if results will influence management.

Patients < 50 years of age
Strong family history of VTE
Clot in unusual locations
Recurrent thromboses
Women of childbearing age
Suspicion for APS (avoid DOACs if APS is strongly suspected or confirmed)
VTE provoked by transient nonmajor risk factor
VTE associated with pregnancy or the postpartum period
VTE associated with oral contraceptives

APS, antiphospholipid syndrome.

imply absence of risk for VTE recurrence. An important hypercoagulable state to identify is antiphospholipid syndrome because these patients have a marked increase in recurrence rates, are at risk for both arterial and venous thrombosis, generally should receive bridge therapy during any interruption of anticoagulation and should not receive DOACs as first-line antithrombotic therapy due to increased arterial events compared to warfarin. Due to effects of anticoagulants and acute thrombosis on many of the tests, the thrombophilia workup should be delayed in most cases until at least 3 months after the acute event, if indicated at all (Table 16–24). The benefit of anticoagulation must be weighed against the bleeding risks posed, and the benefit-risk ratio should be assessed at the initiation of therapy, at 3 months, and then at least annually in any patient receiving prolonged anticoagulant therapy. Bleeding risk scores, such as the Riete score (https://www.mdcalc.com/riete-score-risk-hemorrhage-pulmonary-embolism-treatment) have been developed to estimate risk of these complications. Their performance, however, may not offer any advantage over a clinician's subjective assessment, particularly in older individuals. Consideration of bleeding risk is of particular importance when identifying candidates for extended duration therapy for treatment of unprovoked VTE; defined courses should be considered for patients at high bleeding risk.

E. Secondary Prevention

Antithrombotic therapy for secondary prevention offered after the initial 3–6 months of treatment should be considered in patients with VTE that is not majorly provoked; it is most compelling for those with unprovoked VTE. For most

Table 16–24. Laboratory evaluation of thrombophilia.

Hypercoagulable State	When to Suspect	Laboratory Workup	Influence of Anticoagulation and Acute Thrombosis
Antiphospholipid antibody syndrome	Unexplained DVT/PE CVA/TIA before age 50 years Recurrent thrombosis (despite anticoagulation) Thrombosis at an unusual site Arterial and venous thrombosis Livedo reticularis, Raynaud phenomenon, thrombocytopenia, recurrent early pregnancy loss	Anti-cardiolipin IgG and/or IgM medium or high titer (ie, > 40 GPL or MPL, or > the 99th percentile)[1] Anti-β_2 glycoprotein I IgG and/or IgM medium or high titer (> the 99th percentile)[1] Lupus anticoagulant[1]	Lupus anticoagulant can be falsely positive or falsely negative on any anticoagulant (eg, heparins, warfarin, DOACs) Antibody levels (anti-cardiolipin; anti-β_2 glycoprotein) are not influenced by anticoagulation
Protein C, S, antithrombin deficiencies	Thrombosis < 50 years of age with family history of VTE	Screen with protein C activity, free protein S, antithrombin activity[2]; if free protein S is normal, check protein S activity	Acute thrombosis can result in decreased protein C, S, and antithrombin activity. Warfarin can decrease protein C and S activity; heparin can decrease antithrombin activity. DOACs can increase protein C, S, and antithrombin activity Where available, genetic testing may enable identification of specific mutations leading to hereditary (but not acquired) protein C, S, or antithrombin deficiency without interruption of anticoagulation
Factor V Leiden, prothrombin gene mutation	Thrombosis on OCPs, cerebral vein thrombosis, DVT/PE in White patients	PCR for factor V Leiden or prothrombin gene mutation	No influence
Hyperhomocysteinemia		Fasting homocysteine	No influence

[1]Detected on two occasions not < 12 weeks apart.
[2]Nephrotic syndrome and liver disease can reduce protein C, protein S, and antithrombin; pregnancy causes decreased free protein S.
CVA/TIA, cerebrovascular accident/transient ischemic attack; OCPs, oral contraceptives.

patients on apixaban or rivaroxaban who continue medication to prevent recurrence, the dose can be reduced to prophylactic intensity after the initial 6 months of therapy (Table 16–14). For patients with cancer, dose-reduced apixaban (2.5 mg twice daily rather than 5 mg twice daily) after an initial 6 months of therapeutic anticoagulation carries a similar risk of recurrence of VTE but with a lower bleeding risk. In patients without cancer deemed poor candidates for ongoing DOAC or warfarin use but who warrant some secondary prevention, low-dose (81–100 mg) aspirin may be used; however, this will provide far less reduction in risk of recurrent VTE with similar bleeding risk.

Perioperative management of anticoagulation is reviewed in Chapter 3.

Key NS et al. Venous thromboembolism prophylaxis and treatment in patients with cancer: ASCO Guideline Update. J Clin Oncol. 2023;41:3063. [PMID: 37075273]

Le Gal G et al. Risk for recurrent venous thromboembolism in patients with subsegmental pulmonary embolism managed without anticoagulation: a multicenter prospective cohort study. Ann Intern Med. 2022;175:29. [PMID: 34807722]

Mahé I et al. Extended reduced-dose apixaban for cancer-associated venous thromboembolism. N Engl J Med. 2025;392:1363. [PMID: 40162636]

Middeldorp S et al. American Society of Hematology 2023 guidelines for management of venous thromboembolism: thrombophilia testing. Blood Adv. 2023;7:7101. [PMID: 37195076]

Piazza G et al. Apixaban for extended treatment of provoked venous thromboembolism. N Engl J Med. 2025;393:1166. [PMID: 40888734]

Stevens SM et al. Antithrombotic therapy for VTE disease: second update of the CHEST Guideline and Expert Panel Report. Chest. 2021;160:e545. [PMID: 34352278]

F. Thrombolytic Therapy

1. Thrombolytic therapy for high-risk, massive PE— Anticoagulation alone is appropriate treatment for most patients with PE. However, patients with high-risk, massive PE (defined as PE causing sustained hypotension [systolic blood pressure < 90 mm Hg]) or requirement for inotropic support) have an in-hospital mortality rate that approaches 30% and, absent contraindications (Table 16–25), require immediate thrombolysis in combination with anticoagulation (Table 16–26).

2. Thrombolytic therapy for intermediate-risk, submassive PE—Systemic thrombolytic therapy has been used in carefully selected patients with intermediate-risk, submassive PE (defined as PE without hemodynamic instability but with evidence of RV compromise and myocardial injury). Thrombolysis in this cohort decreases risk of hemodynamic compromise but increases the risk of major hemorrhage and stroke. A lower dose of alteplase (tPA) than commonly used for PE treatment (50 mg rather than 100 mg) has been evaluated in small trials; findings suggested similar hemodynamic improvement and lower bleeding risk with the lower dose, but dosing protocols varied across studies and there are no standard guidelines for systemic use of low-dose tPA. Catheter-directed therapy for acute PE may be considered for high-risk or intermediate-risk PE when systemic thrombolysis has failed or as an alternative to systemic thrombolytic therapy when local expertise is available.

3. Thrombolytic therapy for other indications—In patients with large proximal iliofemoral DVT, data from RCTs are limited on the benefit of catheter-directed thrombolysis in addition to treatment with anticoagulation but do show increased risk of major bleeding. Thrombolytic therapy should be reserved for patients at the highest risk for limb ischemia from extensive acute thrombosis.

Kahn SR et al. Pulmonary embolism. N Engl J Med. 2022;387:45. [PMID: 35793208]

G. Nonpharmacologic Therapy

1. Graduated compression stockings—Graduated compressions stockings may provide symptomatic relief to selected patients with ongoing swelling but do not reduce risk of postthrombotic syndrome at 6 months. They are contraindicated in patients with peripheral vascular disease.

2. Inferior vena caval (IVC) filters—There is a paucity of data to support the use of permanent or retrievable IVC filters for the prevention of PE in any clinical scenario. There are two randomized, controlled trials of IVC filters for prevention of PE. In the first study, patients with documented DVT received full-intensity, time-limited anticoagulation with or without placement of a permanent IVC filter. Patients with permanent IVC filters had a lower rate of nonfatal asymptomatic PE at 12 days but an increased rate of DVT at 2 years. In the second study, patients with symptomatic PE and residual proximal DVT plus at least one additional risk factor for PE severity received full-intensity anticoagulation with or without a retrievable IVC filter. IVC filter use did not reduce the risk of symptomatic recurrent PE at 3 months. While IVC filters were once commonly used to prevent VTE recurrence in the setting of anticoagulation failure, many experts now recommend switching to an alternative agent or increasing the intensity of the current anticoagulant regimen instead. Most experts agree with placement of a retrievable IVC filter in patients with acute proximal DVT or PE and an absolute contraindication to anticoagulation; evidence to support this practice, however, is lacking. The remainder of the indications (submassive/intermediate-risk PE, free-floating iliofemoral DVT, perioperative risk reduction) are controversial. If a device is placed, whenever possible, it should be removed once anticoagulation has been started and has been shown to be tolerated. Rates of IVC filter retrieval are very low, often due to failure to arrange for removal. Removal of the device should be arranged at the time of device placement.

Complications of IVC filters include local thrombosis, tilting, migration, fracture, and inability to retrieve the device. When considering placement of an IVC filter, it is best to consider both short- and long-term complications, since devices intended for removal may become permanent. To improve patient safety, institutions should develop systems that guide appropriate patient selection for IVC filter placement, tracking, and removal.

3. Mechanical embolectomy—Patients with high-risk VTE and very high bleeding risk may be considered for mechanical embolectomy if local expertise and resources are available.

Table 16–25. Contraindications to thrombolytic therapy for PE.

	Contraindication		
	Absolute	**Major**	**Relative**
American Heart Association	Previous intracranial hemorrhage Structural intracranial disease Ischemic stroke within 3 months Suspected aortic dissection Active bleeding or bleeding diathesis Recent surgery encroaching on the spinal canal or brain Recent closed-head or facial trauma with radiographic evidence of bony fracture or brain injury		Age > 75 years Anticoagulant therapy Pregnancy Noncompressible vascular punctures Traumatic or prolonged CPR (> 10 minutes) Recent internal bleeding (within 2–4 weeks) Chronic, poorly controlled hypertension Systolic BP > 180 mm Hg or diastolic BP > 110 mm Hg Dementia Ischemic stroke > 3 months ago Major surgery within 3 weeks
European Society of Cardiology	Previous hemorrhagic stroke or stroke of unknown origin CNS damage or neoplasms Ischemic stroke within 6 months GI bleeding within 1 month Recent major trauma, surgery, or head injury in the preceding 3 weeks Known bleeding risk		TIA in preceding 6 months Anticoagulant therapy Pregnancy Noncompressible puncture site Traumatic resuscitation Active peptic ulcer disease Infective endocarditis Refractory hypertension (systolic BP > 180 mm Hg) Advanced liver disease
American College of Chest Physicians		Previous intracranial hemorrhage Structural intracranial disease Ischemic stroke within 3 months Active bleeding Bleeding diathesis Recent brain or spinal surgery Recent head trauma with fracture or brain injury	Age > 75 years Anticoagulant therapy Pregnancy Recent invasive procedure Traumatic CPR Recent non-intracranial bleeding Pericarditis or pericardial fluid Systolic BP > 180 mm Hg or diastolic BP > 110 mm Hg Weight < 60 kg Ischemic stroke > 3 months ago Recent surgery Diabetic retinopathy Female Black race

Reproduced with permission from Kaplovitch E, Shaw JR, Douketis J. Thrombolysis in pulmonary embolism: an evidence-based approach to treating life-threatening pulmonary emboli. Crit Care Clin. 2020;36(3):465–480.

When to Refer

- History of HIT, prolonged PTT, or kidney failure for alternative anticoagulation regimens.
- Consideration of IVC filter placement.
- Clots in unusual locations (eg, renal, hepatic, or cerebral vein), or simultaneous arterial and venous thrombosis, to assess possibility of a hypercoagulable state.
- Recurrent VTE while receiving therapeutic anticoagulation.

When to Admit

- High-risk PE for urgent embolectomy or catheter-directed therapies.
- Intermediate-risk PE if considering thrombolysis.
- Documented or suspected PE at high risk for bleeding or poor candidate for outpatient treatment.
- DVT with poorly controlled pain, high bleeding risk, or concerns about follow-up.
- Presence of large iliofemoral VTE, unprovoked upper extremity DVT, IVC thrombosis, portal vein thrombosis, or Budd-Chiari syndrome for consideration of catheter-directed thrombolysis.
- Hospitalization according to the Hestia criteria.
- Acute PE/DVT and absolute contraindication to anticoagulation for IVC filter placement.
- Venous thrombosis despite therapeutic anticoagulation.
- Suspected Paget-Schroetter syndrome (spontaneous upper extremity thrombosis related to thoracic outlet syndrome).

Table 16–26. Thrombolytic regimens for acute PE.

Alteplase[1]		Streptokinase[1]		Urokinase[1]		Reteplase	Tenecteplase
Classical Regimen	Accelerated Regimen	Classical Regimen	Accelerated Regimen	Classical Regimen	Accelerated Regimen		
100 mg infusion over 2 hours	0.6 mg/kg (up to 50 mg) bolus over 15 minutes	250,000 IU bolus over 30 minutes, followed by 100,000 IU/hour over 12–24 hours	1.5 million IU infusion over 2 hours	4400 IU/kg bolus followed by 4400 IU/kg/hour infusion over 12–24 hours	3 million IU infusion over 2 hours	Two boluses of 10 units given 30 minutes apart	Weight-based bolus over 5 seconds: < 60 kg: 30 mg ≥ 60 to < 70 kg: 35 mg ≥ 70 to < 80 kg: 40 mg ≥ 80 to < 90 kg: 45 mg ≥ 90 kg: 50 mg

[1]FDA approved thrombolytic for PE.

Reproduced with permission from Kaplovitch E, Shaw JR, Douketis J. Thrombolysis in pulmonary embolism: an evidence-based approach to treating life-threatening pulmonary emboli. Crit Care Clin. 2020;36(3):465–480.

Benedetti R et al. Inferior vena cava filters: a clinical review and future perspectives. J Clin Med. 2024;13:1761. [PMID: 38541986]

PRIMARY VTE PREVENTION & TREATMENT IN SEVERE COVID-19

Patients hospitalized with severe COVID-19 have an increased incidence of thrombotic complications, including venous (DVT, PE) and arterial (stroke, limb occlusion) events.

Clinical Findings

While the hypercoagulability in COVID-19 resembles DIC, laboratory and clinical findings are somewhat different. Laboratory findings in patients with severe COVID-19 may include markedly elevated D-dimer and modestly prolonged prothrombin time. However, patients with COVID-19 tend to have elevated fibrinogen levels; thrombocytopenia is rare and nonsevere; and bleeding complications are unusual. Thrombosis in patients with COVID-19 is associated with a poor prognosis and often occurs despite standard pharmacologic prophylaxis.

Risk Stratification & Initial Prognostication in Severe COVID-19

Given the prevalence and prognostic value of abnormal laboratory findings at presentation, patients hospitalized due to severe COVID-19 should have PT/INR, PTT, D-dimers, and fibrinogen measured at presentation. Serial monitoring should be considered even in patients who are otherwise clinically stable. Worsening laboratory parameters during hospitalization should prompt consideration of transfer to a higher level of care and heightened clinical suspicion for thrombosis.

VTE Prophylaxis for Severe COVID-19

In the absence of strong contraindications, all patients hospitalized with COVID-19 should receive pharmacologic VTE prophylaxis. LMWH is preferred over unfractionated heparin to minimize staff exposure and the chance of HIT.

For patients with prior VTE who take an oral anticoagulant for secondary prevention at the time of admission, transition to LMWH may be considered due to its shorter half-life and potential anti-inflammatory properties.

Some patients who are hospitalized due to COVID-19, who have very elevated D-dimer values (> 4 times the upper limit of normal) and require supplemental oxygen, and who have *low* bleeding risk may benefit from therapeutic dosing of anticoagulation using LMWH or unfractionated heparin (Table 16–16). Patients who are critically ill in ICUs have not been shown to benefit from therapeutic dosing of anticoagulation. There is also no clear benefit from VTE prophylaxis for patients with COVID-19 who do not require hospitalization. For select patients hospitalized for COVID-19 who have an increased risk of thromboembolism (IMPROVE VTE score ≥ 4 or score 2–3 with elevated D-dimer) (https://www.mdcalc.com/calc/10349/improve-risk-score-venous-thromboembolism-vte) and do not have an increased risk of bleeding, extended prophylaxis after hospital discharge with rivaroxaban 10 mg orally daily for 35 days may be considered.

Schulman S et al. 2023 ISTH update of the 2022 ISTH guidelines for antithrombotic treatment in COVID-19. J Thromb Haemost. 2024;22:1779. [PMID: 38503600]

17

Gastrointestinal Disorders

Kenneth R. McQuaid, MD

SYMPTOMS & SIGNS OF GI DISEASE

DYSPEPSIA

ESSENTIALS OF DIAGNOSIS

- Predominant epigastric pain or discomfort.
- Heartburn, nausea, postprandial fullness, or vomiting may occur
- Endoscopy is warranted in all patients aged ≥ 60 years and selected younger patients with "alarm" features.
- In all other patients, testing for *Helicobacter pylori* is recommended; if positive, antibacterial treatment is given.
- Patients who test *H pylori* negative or do not improve after *H pylori* eradication should be prescribed a trial of empiric PPI therapy.
- Patients with persistent symptoms should be offered a trial of a tricyclic antidepressant.

General Considerations

Dyspepsia refers to acute, chronic, or recurrent epigastric pain, burning or discomfort, early satiety, or postprandial fullness. These symptoms may also be associated with nausea, bloating, or vomiting. Dyspepsia symptoms that are present for at least 1 month are clinically relevant. Dyspepsia occurs in 10–20% of the adult population and accounts for 3% of general medical office visits. Heartburn (retrosternal burning) should be distinguished from dyspepsia. When heartburn is the dominant complaint, GERD is nearly always present. Functional dyspepsia refers to dyspepsia for which no organic, systemic, or metabolic etiology has been determined by endoscopy or other testing. This is the most common cause of *chronic* dyspepsia, accounting for up to 75% of patients.

Etiology

Acute, self-limited dyspepsia ("indigestion") may be caused by overeating, eating too quickly, eating high-fat foods, eating during stressful situations, or drinking too much alcohol or coffee. Prescription and nonprescription medications should be carefully reviewed since many may cause dyspepsia.

Peptic ulcer disease is present in 5–15% and GERD is present in up to 20% of patients with dyspepsia, even without significant heartburn. Chronic gastric infection with *H pylori* is an important cause of peptic ulcer disease and may cause dyspepsia in a subset of patients in the absence of peptic ulcer disease. Gastric or esophageal cancer is identified in < 1%; cancer is extremely rare in persons aged < 60 years with uncomplicated dyspepsia. Diabetes mellitus, thyroid disease, CKD, myocardial ischemia, intra-abdominal malignancy, gastroparesis, gastric volvulus or paraesophageal hernia, chronic gastric or intestinal ischemia, and pregnancy are sometimes accompanied by acute or chronic epigastric pain or discomfort. Pancreatic carcinoma and chronic pancreatitis may cause chronic epigastric pain, but usually it is more severe, and is associated with anorexia, rapid weight loss, steatorrhea, or jaundice. Other causes of dyspepsia include parasitic infection (*Giardia, Strongyloides, Anisakis*).

Clinical Findings

A. Symptoms and Signs

Given the nonspecific nature of dyspeptic symptoms, the history has limited diagnostic utility. It should clarify the chronicity, location, and quality of the epigastric pain, and its relationship to meals. Concomitant weight loss, persistent vomiting, constant or severe pain, progressive dysphagia, hematemesis, melena, or unexplained iron deficiency anemia are "alarm" symptoms for serious organic disease. Potentially offending medications and excessive alcohol use should be identified and discontinued if possible. The patient should be asked about a family history of upper GI cancer. The patient's reason for seeking care should be determined. Recent changes in employment, marital discord, physical and sexual abuse, anxiety, depression, and fear of serious disease may all contribute to the development and reporting of symptoms.

Functional dyspepsia—Patients with functional dyspepsia often are younger, report a variety of abdominal and extragastrointestinal complaints, show signs of anxiety or depression, or have used psychotropic medications. The symptom profile alone does not differentiate between functional dyspepsia and organic GI disorders. Primary care clinicians therefore misdiagnose nearly half of patients with peptic ulcers or gastroesophageal reflux.

The physical examination is rarely helpful. Signs of serious organic disease such as weight loss, organomegaly, abdominal mass, or fecal occult blood must be further evaluated.

B. Laboratory Findings

In patients aged < 60 years with uncomplicated dyspepsia (in whom gastric cancer is rare), a noninvasive test for *H pylori* (fecal antigen test, urea breath test) should be performed first—both of which have 95% accuracy. Serologic tests for *H pylori* antibodies are not recommended due to their poor performance characteristics. If *H pylori* fecal antigen test or breath test results are negative in a patient not taking NSAIDs, peptic ulcer disease is virtually excluded. In patients aged > 60 years, initial laboratory work should include a CBC, serum electrolytes, liver enzymes, calcium, and thyroid function tests but the cost-effectiveness of such studies is uncertain.

C. Upper Endoscopy

Upper endoscopy is mainly indicated to look for upper gastric or esophageal malignancy in *all* patients aged > 60 years with new-onset dyspepsia (in whom there is increased malignancy risk). In patients aged < 60 years, the risk of malignancy is < 1% so guidelines recommend against routine endoscopy for most younger patients—except those with prominent "alarm" features, such as progressive weight loss, progressive dysphagia, persistent vomiting, evidence of bleeding or iron deficiency anemia, palpable abdominal mass, or a family history of upper GI cancer. For patients born in regions in which there is a higher incidence of gastric cancer, such as Central or South America, China and Southeast Asia, or Africa, an age threshold of 45 years may be more appropriate.

Endoscopy may also be warranted when symptoms fail to respond to initial empiric management or when frequent symptom relapse occurs after discontinuation of empiric therapy.

D. Other Tests

In patients with refractory symptoms or progressive weight loss, antibodies for celiac disease or stool testing for ova and parasites or *Giardia* antigen, fat, or elastase (for exocrine pancreatic insufficiency) may be considered. Abdominal imaging (ultrasonography or CT) is performed only when pancreatic, biliary tract, vascular disease, or volvulus is suspected. Gastric emptying studies may be useful in patients with recurrent nausea and vomiting who have not responded to empiric therapies.

Treatment

Initial empiric treatment is recommended for patients aged < 60 years who lack severe or worrisome "alarm" features that warrant further testing with endoscopy or abdominal imaging. Those whose symptoms do not respond to or relapse after empiric treatment should undergo upper endoscopy with subsequent treatment directed at the specific disorder identified (eg, peptic ulcer, GERD, cancer). When endoscopy is performed, gastric biopsies should be obtained to test for *H pylori* infection. If infection is present, antibacterial treatment should be given.

A. Empiric Therapy

Patients aged < 60 years should be tested for *H pylori* and, if positive, treated with an effective regimen (see Table 17–10). *H pylori* eradication therapy proves definitive for patients with underlying peptic ulcers and may improve symptoms in a small subset (< 10%) of patients infected with *H pylori* who have functional dyspepsia.

Patients who test *H pylori*–negative and patients with persistent dyspepsia after *H pylori* eradication most likely have functional dyspepsia or atypical GERD and should be treated with a PPI for 4 weeks. Symptom improvement occurs in up to 50% of patients treated with a PPI. For patients who have symptom relapse after discontinuation of the PPI, intermittent or long-term PPI therapy may be considered.

B. Treatment of Functional Dyspepsia

Patients who have no significant findings on endoscopy as well as patients aged < 60 years who do not respond to *H pylori* eradication or empiric PPI therapy are presumed to have functional dyspepsia. Patients with mild, intermittent symptoms may respond to reassurance and lifestyle or dietary changes. A food diary, where patients record their food intake, symptoms, and daily events, may reveal dietary or psychosocial precipitants of pain. Herbal therapies (peppermint, caraway) may offer benefit with little risk of adverse effects. In a 2022 RCT, cannabidiol (CBD) was not more effective than placebo in relief of functional dyspepsia.

Antisecretory drugs (PPIs or H_2-receptor antagonists) have demonstrated limited efficacy in the treatment of functional dyspepsia. Low doses of tricyclic antidepressants (eg, desipramine or nortriptyline, 25–50 mg orally at bedtime) benefit some patients, possibly by moderating visceral afferent sensitivity. Doses should be increased slowly to minimize side effects. SSRIs do not appear to be beneficial. Mirtazapine (15 mg orally once daily) also has demonstrated benefit in limited studies. Although some prokinetics have demonstrated modest improvement in global symptoms compared with placebo in controlled trials, the more effective agents are either not available in the United States (domperidone) or were removed from the market due to rare but serious adverse events (cisapride). Metoclopramide (5–10 mg orally three times daily) may improve symptoms but cannot be recommended for long-term use due to the risk of tardive dyskinesia.

Oshima T. Functional dyspepsia: current understanding and future perspective. Digestion. 2024;105:26. [PMID: 37598673]
Sanayei AM et al. Burden and treatment of chronic upper GI symptoms and diagnoses: a nationwide study. Clin Gastroenterol Hepatol. 2024;22:1307. [PMID: 38278192]
Sarnelli G et al. Italian guidelines for the diagnosis and treatment of functional dyspepsia – joint consensus from the Italian societies of gastroenterology and endoscopy (SIGE), Neurogastroenterology and motility (SINGEM), hospital gastroenterologists and endoscopists (AIGO), digestive endoscopy (SIED) and general medicine (SIMG). Dig Liver Dis 2025;57:1730. [PMID: 40628573]

NAUSEA & VOMITING

Nausea is a vague, intensely disagreeable sensation of sickness or "queasiness" and is distinguished from anorexia. Vomiting or retching often follow. Vomiting should be distinguished from regurgitation, the effortless reflux of liquid or food stomach contents; and from rumination, the chewing and swallowing of food that is regurgitated volitionally after meals.

The brainstem vomiting center is composed of a group of neuronal areas within the medulla that coordinate emesis. It may be stimulated by four sources of afferent input: (1) Visceral afferent stimulation: Afferent vagal fibers from the GI viscera, which are rich in serotonin 5-HT_3 receptors, may be stimulated by biliary or GI distention, mucosal or peritoneal irritation, or infections. (2) Vestibular disorders: Fibers of the vestibular system have high concentrations of histamine H_1 and muscarinic cholinergic receptors. (3) CNS disorders (amygdala): Certain sights, smells, or emotional experiences may induce vomiting. (4) Irritation of chemoreceptor trigger zone: This trigger zone, located outside the blood-brain barrier in the medulla, is rich in opioid, serotonin 5-HT_3, neurokinin 1 (NK_1), and dopamine D_2 receptors. This region may be stimulated by drugs and chemotherapeutic agents, toxins, hypoxia, uremia, acidosis, and radiation therapy. Although the causes of nausea and vomiting are many, a simplified list is provided in Table 17–1.

Clinical Findings

A. Symptoms and Signs

Acute nausea and vomiting without abdominal pain are typically caused by food poisoning, infectious gastroenteritis, drugs, or systemic illness. Inquiry should be made into recent changes in medications, diet, other intestinal symptoms, or similar illnesses in family members. COVID-19 infection may be associated with nausea, vomiting, or abdominal pain. The acute onset of severe pain and vomiting suggests peritoneal irritation, acute gastric or intestinal obstruction, or pancreaticobiliary disease. Persistent vomiting suggests pregnancy, gastric outlet obstruction, gastroparesis, intestinal dysmotility, psychogenic disorders, and CNS or systemic disorders. Vomiting that occurs in the morning before breakfast is common with pregnancy, uremia, alcohol intake, and increased intracranial pressure. Inquiry should be made into use of cannabis products. Suspect cannabinoid hyperemesis syndrome in patients with prolonged use, especially in those who report compulsive showering or bathing. Vomiting immediately after meals strongly suggests bulimia or psychogenic causes. Vomiting of undigested food one to several hours after meals is characteristic of gastroparesis or a gastric outlet obstruction; physical examination may reveal a succussion splash. Patients with acute or chronic symptoms should be asked about neurologic symptoms (eg, headache, stiff neck, vertigo, and focal paresthesias or weakness) that suggest a CNS cause. Episodic bouts of repetitive vomiting (lasting < 7 days) interspersed with episode-free periods for weeks to months may suggest cyclic vomiting syndrome.

B. Laboratory Findings

With vomiting that is severe or protracted, serum electrolytes should be obtained to look for hypokalemia, azotemia, or metabolic alkalosis resulting from loss of gastric contents. Serum glucose, creatinine, and TSH can exclude diabetes, kidney disease, or hypothyroidism. A pregnancy test should be obtained in premenopausal women. Abnormal liver biochemical tests or elevated amylase or lipase suggest pancreaticobiliary disease, which may be investigated with an abdominal sonogram or CT scan.

C. Imaging and Diagnostic Studies

Flat and upright abdominal radiographs or abdominal CT are obtained in patients with severe pain or suspicion of mechanical obstruction to look for free intraperitoneal air or dilated loops of small bowel. The cause of gastric outlet obstruction is best demonstrated by upper endoscopy, and the cause of small intestinal obstruction is best demonstrated by abdominal CT. Gastroparesis is confirmed by nuclear scintigraphic studies or ^{13}C-octanoic acid breath tests, which show delayed gastric emptying, and either upper endoscopy or barium upper GI series showing no evidence of mechanical gastric outlet obstruction. CNS causes are best evaluated with either head CT or MRI.

Complications

Complications include dehydration, hypokalemia, metabolic alkalosis, aspiration, rupture of the esophagus (Boerhaave syndrome), and bleeding secondary to a mucosal tear at the gastroesophageal junction (Mallory-Weiss syndrome).

Treatment

A. General Measures

Most causes of acute vomiting are mild, self-limited, and require no specific treatment. Patients should ingest clear liquids (broths, tea, soups, noncaffeinated carbonated beverages) and small quantities of dry foods (soda crackers). Ginger may be an effective nonpharmacologic treatment. For more severe acute vomiting, hospitalization may be required. Intravenous 0.45% saline solution with 20 mEq/L of potassium chloride is given in most cases to maintain hydration. A nasogastric suction tube for gastric or mechanical small bowel obstruction improves patient comfort and permits monitoring of fluid loss.

Table 17–1. Causes of nausea and vomiting.

Visceral afferent stimulation	**Mechanical obstruction** Gastric outlet obstruction: peptic ulcer disease, malignancy, gastric volvulus Small intestinal obstruction: adhesions, hernias, volvulus, Crohn disease, carcinomatosis **Dysmotility** Gastroparesis: diabetes, postviral, postvagotomy Small intestine: systemic sclerosis (scleroderma), amyloidosis, chronic intestinal pseudo-obstruction, familial myoneuropathies GLP-1 and gastric inhibitory polypeptide agonists **Peritoneal irritation** Peritonitis: perforated viscus, appendicitis, spontaneous bacterial peritonitis **Infections** Viral gastroenteritis: norovirus, rotavirus, SARS-CoV-2 "Food poisoning": toxins from *Bacillus cereus*, *Staphylococcus aureus*, *Clostridium perfringens* Acute systemic infections **Hepatobiliary or pancreatic disorders** Acute or chronic pancreatitis Cholecystitis or choledocholithiasis **Topical GI irritants** Alcohol, NSAIDs, oral antibiotics **Postoperative** **Other** Cardiac disease: acute MI, HF Urologic disease: stones, pyelonephritis Vascular disease: chronic mesenteric ischemia, superior mesenteric artery syndrome
Vestibular disorders	Labyrinthitis, Ménière disease, motion sickness
CNS disorders	**Increased intracranial pressure** CNS tumors, subdural or subarachnoid hemorrhage **Migraine** **Cyclical vomiting syndrome** **Infections** Meningitis, encephalitis **Psychogenic** Anticipatory vomiting, anorexia nervosa and bulimia, psychiatric disorders
Irritation of chemoreceptor trigger zone	**Antitumor chemotherapy** **Medications and drugs** Opioids Marijuana Anticonvulsants Antiparkinsonism medications β-Blockers, antiarrhythmics, digoxin Oral contraceptives Cholinesterase inhibitors Diabetes medications (metformin, acarbose, pramlintide, exenatide) **Radiation therapy** **Systemic conditions** Diabetic ketoacidosis Uremia Adrenocortical crisis Parathyroid disease Hypothyroidism Pregnancy Paraneoplastic syndrome

B. Antiemetic Medications

Medications may be given either to prevent or to control vomiting. Combinations of drugs from different classes may provide better control of symptoms with less toxicity in some patients. Table 17–2 outlines common antiemetic dosing regimens.

1. Serotonin 5-HT_3-receptor antagonists—Ondansetron, granisetron, and palonosetron are effective in preventing chemotherapy- and radiation-induced emesis when initiated prior to treatment. Due to its prolonged mode of action, palonosetron is superior to other serotonin 5-HT_3-receptor antagonists for the prevention of acute and delayed chemotherapy-induced emesis from moderately or highly

Table 17–2. Common antiemetic dosing regimens.

	Dosage	Route
Serotonin 5-HT_3 Antagonists		
Ondansetron	Doses vary: 4–8 mg for postoperative nausea and vomiting 8 mg once intravenously or 8 mg twice daily orally for moderately or highly emetogenic chemotherapy	Intravenously, orally Intravenously, orally
Granisetron	1 mg once daily 1–2 mg once daily	Intravenously Orally
Palonosetron	0.25 mg once as a single dose 30 minutes before start of chemotherapy 0.5 mg once as single dose	Intravenously Orally
Corticosteroids		
Dexamethasone	4–12 mg once pre-induction for prevention of postoperative nausea and vomiting 8 mg once daily for chemotherapy	Intravenously, orally Intravenously, orally
Neurokinin Receptor Antagonists[1]		
Aprepitant	125 mg once before chemotherapy; then 80 mg on days 1 and 2 after chemotherapy	Orally
Fosaprepitant	150 mg once 30 minutes before chemotherapy	Intravenously
Rolapitant	180 mg once before chemotherapy	Orally
Netupitant/palonosetron	Netupitant 300 mg/palonosetron 0.50 mg once before chemotherapy	Orally
Dopamine Receptor Antagonists		
Metoclopramide	10–20 mg or 0.5 mg/kg every 6–8 hours 10–20 mg every 6–8 hours	Intravenously Orally
Prochlorperazine	5–10 mg every 4–6 hours 25 mg suppository every 12 hours	Intravenously, intramuscularly, orally Per rectum
Promethazine	12.5–25 mg every 6–8 hours 25 mg every 6–8 hours	Intravenously, orally Per rectum
Trimethobenzamide	200 mg every 6–8 hours 250–300 mg every 6–8 hours	Orally Intravenously, orally
Olanzapine	5–10 mg once daily on days 1–4 for chemotherapy	

[1]Neurokinin receptor antagonists are used solely for highly emetogenic chemotherapy regimens in combination with 5-HT_3 antagonists or dexamethasone or both.

emetogenic chemotherapeutic regimens. Although serotonin 5-HT_3-receptor antagonists are effective as single agents for the prevention of chemotherapy-induced nausea and vomiting, their efficacy is enhanced by combination therapy with a corticosteroid (dexamethasone) and an NK_1-receptor antagonist. Serotonin antagonists also are used for the prevention of postoperative nausea and vomiting.

2. Corticosteroids—Corticosteroids (eg, dexamethasone) have antiemetic properties, but the basis for these effects is unknown. These agents enhance the efficacy of serotonin receptor antagonists for preventing acute and delayed nausea and vomiting in patients receiving moderately to highly emetogenic chemotherapy regimens.

3. Neurokinin receptor antagonists—Aprepitant, fosaprepitant, and rolapitant are highly selective antagonists for NK_1-receptors in the area postrema. They are used in combination with corticosteroids and serotonin antagonists for the prevention of acute and delayed nausea and vomiting with highly emetogenic chemotherapy regimens. Netupitant, another oral NK_1-receptor antagonist, is administered in a fixed-dose combination with palonosetron. Combined therapy with an NK_1-receptor antagonist prevents acute and delayed emesis in 70–90% of patients treated with highly emetogenic regimens.

4. Dopamine antagonists—The atypical antipsychotic agent olanzapine has potent antiemetic properties that may be mediated by blockade of both dopamine and serotonin neurotransmitters. In patients receiving highly emetogenic chemotherapy, the addition of olanzapine to a standard regimen (dexamethasone, serotonin-5-HT_3 receptor antagonist, and NK_1-receptor antagonist) significantly reduces the risk of acute and delayed nausea and vomiting. The phenothiazines, butyrophenones, and substituted benzamides (eg, prochlorperazine, promethazine) have antiemetic properties.

High doses of these agents are associated with antidopaminergic side effects, including extrapyramidal reactions and depression. With the advent of more effective and safer antiemetics, these agents are infrequently used, mainly in outpatients with minor, self-limited symptoms.

5. Antihistamines and anticholinergics—These drugs (eg, meclizine, dimenhydrinate, transdermal scopolamine) may be valuable in the prevention of vomiting arising from stimulation of the labyrinth, ie, motion sickness, vertigo, and migraines. They may induce drowsiness. A combination of oral vitamin B_6 and doxylamine is recommended by the American College of Obstetricians and Gynecologists as first-line therapy for nausea and vomiting during pregnancy.

6. Cannabinoids—Marijuana has been used widely as an appetite stimulant and antiemetic. Some states allow the use of medical marijuana with a clinician's certification. Strains of medical marijuana with different proportions of various naturally occurring cannabinoids (primarily THC and cannabidiol [CBD]) can be chosen to minimize its psychoactive effects. Excessive cannabinoid may cause nausea, vomiting, and abdominal pain (cannabinoid hyperemesis syndrome), which may be temporarily relieved with hot showers or bathing.

Camilleri M et al. Cannabinoids and the gastrointestinal tract. Clin Gastroenterol Hepatol. 2023;21:3217. [PMID: 36778488]
Levinthal DJ et al. AGA clinical practice update on diagnosis and management of cyclic vomiting syndrome: commentary. Gastroenterology. 2024;167:804. [PMID: 39023502]
Malagelada C et al. European guideline on chronic nausea and vomiting – a UEG and ESNM consensus for management. United European Gastroenterol J. 2025;13:427. [PMID: 39754724]

HICCUPS

Though usually a benign and self-limited annoyance, hiccups may be persistent and a sign of serious underlying illness. In patients on mechanical ventilation, hiccups can trigger a full respiratory cycle and result in respiratory alkalosis.

Causes of benign, self-limited hiccups include gastric distention (carbonated beverages, air swallowing, overeating), sudden temperature changes (hot then cold liquids, hot then cold shower), alcohol ingestion, and states of heightened emotion (excitement, stress, laughing). There are over 100 causes of recurrent or persistent hiccups due to GI, CNS, cardiovascular, and thoracic disorders. Persistent hiccups may be an atypical presentation of COVID-19.

Clinical Findings

Evaluation of the patient with persistent hiccups should include a detailed neurologic examination, serum creatinine, liver chemistry tests, and a CXR. When the cause remains unclear, CT or MRI of the head, chest, and abdomen; upper endoscopy; and echocardiography may help.

Treatment

Some simple remedies may be helpful in patients with acute benign hiccups. (1) Irritation of the nasopharynx by tongue traction, lifting the uvula with a spoon, catheter stimulation of the nasopharynx, or eating 1 teaspoon (tsp) (7 g) of dry granulated sugar. (2) Interruption of the respiratory cycle by breath holding, Valsalva maneuver, sneezing, gasping (fright stimulus), or rebreathing into a paper bag. (3) Stimulation of the vagus by carotid massage. (4) Irritation of the diaphragm by holding knees to chest or by continuous positive airway pressure during mechanical ventilation. (5) Relief of gastric distention by belching or insertion of a nasogastric tube.

Several drugs have been promoted as being useful in the treatment of hiccups. Chlorpromazine, 25–50 mg orally or intramuscularly, is most commonly used. Other agents include anticonvulsants (valproic acid, carbamazepine), benzodiazepines (lorazepam, midazolam), metoclopramide, baclofen, and gabapentin. For severe, intractable hiccups, phrenic nerve block, vagal nerve stimulation and, occasionally, general anesthesia have been used with variable efficacy.

He J et al. Pathogenesis and treatment of perioperative hiccups: a narrative review. Ann Med. 2025;57:2474173. [PMID: 40055925]

CONSTIPATION

Constipation occurs in 10% of adults and up to one-third of older adults, more commonly in women. Older individuals are predisposed due to comorbid medical conditions, medications, poor eating habits, decreased mobility, and in some cases, inability to sit on a toilet (bed-bound patients). The first step in the evaluation is to determine what is meant by "constipation." Patients may define constipation as infrequent stools (fewer than three in a week), hard or lumpy stools, excessive straining, or a sense of incomplete evacuation. Table 17–3 summarizes the many causes of constipation, which are discussed below.

Etiology

A. Primary Constipation

Most patients have constipation that is not attributed to any structural abnormalities or systemic disease. These patients may be further categorized as having normal colonic transit time, slow transit, or defecatory disorders (with or without slow colonic transit). Normal colonic transit time is about 35 hours; > 72 hours is significantly abnormal. Slow colonic transit is commonly idiopathic (due to dysfunction of the enteric nervous system) but may be part of a generalized GI dysmotility syndrome. Normal defecation requires coordination between relaxation of the anal sphincter and pelvic floor musculature while abdominal pressure is increased. Patients with defecatory disorders (also known as dyssynergic defecation)—women more often than men—have impaired relaxation or paradoxical contraction of the anal sphincter and/or pelvic floor muscles during attempted defecation that impedes the bowel movement. This problem may be acquired during childhood or adulthood. Patients may describe excessive straining, sense of incomplete evacuation, need for digital manipulation, or adoption of a

Table 17–3. Causes of constipation in adults.

Most common
Inadequate fiber or fluid intake
Poor bowel habits
Irritable bowel syndrome
Systemic disease
Endocrine: hypothyroidism, hyperparathyroidism, diabetes
Metabolic: hypokalemia, hypercalcemia, uremia, porphyria
Neurologic: Parkinson disease, multiple sclerosis, sacral nerve damage (prior pelvic surgery, tumor), paraplegia, autonomic neuropathy
Medications
Opioids
Diuretics
Calcium channel blockers
GLP-1 agonists
Anticholinergics
Psychotropics
Calcium and iron supplements
Clonidine
Cholestyramine
Structural abnormalities
Anorectal: rectal prolapse, rectocele, rectal intussusception, anorectal stricture, anal fissure, solitary rectal ulcer syndrome
Perineal descent
Colonic mass with obstruction: adenocarcinoma
Colonic stricture: radiation, ischemia, diverticulosis
Hirschsprung disease
Idiopathic megarectum
Slow colonic transit
Idiopathic: slow transit isolated to colon
Psychogenic
Eating disorders
Chronic intestinal pseudo-obstruction
Pelvic floor dyssynergia

non-sitting (eg, standing) position during defecation. Patients with predominant complaints of abdominal pain or bloating with chronic idiopathic constipation are more appropriately given a diagnosis of irritable bowel syndrome (IBS) with constipation.

B. Secondary Constipation

Constipation may be caused by systemic disorders, medications, or obstructing colonic lesions. Systemic disorders include neurologic gut dysfunction, myopathies, endocrine disorders, or electrolyte abnormalities (eg, hypercalcemia or hypokalemia); medication side effects are often responsible (eg, anticholinergics or opioids). Colonic lesions that obstruct fecal passage, such as neoplasms and strictures, are an uncommon cause but important in new-onset constipation. Such lesions should be excluded in patients aged > 45 years, in patients with "alarm" symptoms or signs (hematochezia, weight loss, anemia, or positive fecal occult blood tests [FOBT] or fecal immunochemical tests [FIT]), and in patients with a family history of colon cancer or IBD. Defecatory difficulties also can be due to a variety of anorectal problems that impede or obstruct flow (perineal descent, rectal prolapse, rectocele), some of which may require surgery, and to Hirschsprung disease (usually suggested by lifelong constipation).

Clinical Findings

A. Symptoms and Signs

All patients should undergo a history and physical examination to distinguish primary from secondary causes of constipation. Physical examination should include digital rectal examination with assessment for anatomic abnormalities, such as anal stricture, rectocele, rectal prolapse, or perineal descent during straining as well as assessment of pelvic floor motion during simulated defecation (ie, the patient's ability to "expel the examiner's finger"). Patients with fecal impaction may have decreased appetite, nausea and vomiting, abdominal pain, and distention. There may be paradoxical "diarrhea" as liquid stool leaks around the impacted feces. Firm feces are palpable on digital examination of the rectal vault.

B. Laboratory and Diagnostic Studies

Additional tests should be performed in patients with any of the following: signs of systemic disease, recent onset of constipation without apparent cause, "alarm" symptoms (hematochezia, weight loss, anemia, positive FOBT or FIT), family history of colon cancer or IBD, and aged > 45 years with no prior colonoscopy screening. These tests should include CBC; serum electrolytes, calcium, glucose, and TSH; and a colonoscopy.

C. Special Examinations

Patients with refractory constipation not responding to routine medical management warrant further diagnostic studies. Anorectal manometry including a balloon expulsion test should be performed first to evaluate for defecatory disorders. Inability to expel a balloon (attached to a 16F indwelling urinary catheter) filled with 50 mL of warm water within 1–2 minutes while sitting on a toilet is strongly suggestive of pelvic floor dyssynergia. Defecography to further assess pelvic floor function may be considered in selected patients. Subsequent colon transit studies are recommended only after defecatory disorders have been excluded. Colon transit time may be assessed by radiopaque markers, scintigraphy, or wireless motility capsule.

Treatment

A. Chronic Constipation

1. Dietary and lifestyle measures—Patients should be instructed on normal defecatory function and optimal toileting habits, including regular timing, proper positioning, and abdominal pressure. Adequate dietary fluid and fiber intake should be emphasized. Increased dietary fiber may cause distention or flatulence, which often diminishes over several days. Soluble fiber supplements (eg, psyllium, methylcellulose) are a convenient, well-tolerated way to increase dietary fiber (Table 17–4). Response to fiber therapy is not immediate and increases in dosage should be made gradually over 7–10 days. Fiber is most likely to benefit patients with normal colonic transit. However, fiber may not benefit patients with symptoms due to delayed colonic transit (colonic inertia), defecatory disorders, opioid-induced constipation, or IBS; it may even exacerbate

Table 17–4. Pharmacologic management of constipation (in descending order of recommendation within each class of agents).

Agent	Dosage	Onset of Action	Comments
Fiber Laxatives			
Psyllium	1 tbs (3.5 g fiber) once or twice daily	Days	(Metamucil; Perdiem)
Methylcellulose	1 tbs (2 g fiber) once or twice daily	Days	(Citrucel) Less gas, flatulence
Calcium polycarbophil	1 or 2 tablets once or twice daily	12–24 hours	(FiberCon) Does not cause gas; pill form
Wheat dextrin	1 tbsp once or twice daily	Days	(Benefiber) Non-gritty, tasteless, less gas
Stool Surfactants			
Docusate sodium	100 mg once or twice daily	12–72 hours	(Colace) Marginal benefit
Mineral oil	15–45 mL once or twice daily	6–8 hours	May cause lipoid pneumonia if aspirated
Osmotic Laxatives			
Polyethylene glycol (PEG) 3350	17 g in 8 oz liquid once or twice daily	6–24 hours	(MiraLAX) More effective, less bloating than lactulose, sorbitol
Magnesium hydroxide	15–30 mL orally once or twice daily	6–24 hours	(Milk of magnesia) May cause hypermagnesemia if CKD
Stimulant Laxatives			
Bisacodyl	5–10 mg orally as needed	6–8 hours	May cause cramps; avoid daily use if possible
Bisacodyl suppository	10 mg per rectum as needed	1 hour	
Senna	17.2–34.4 mg orally	8–12 hours	(ex-lax; Senokot; Senna-S) May cause cramps; avoid daily use if possible
Secretagogues			
Lubiprostone	24 mcg orally twice daily	12–48 hours	Expensive; may cause nausea; contraindicated in pregnancy
Linaclotide	72–145 mcg orally once daily	1 week	Expensive; contraindicated in pediatric patients
Plecanatide	3 mg orally once daily	1 week	Expensive; contraindicated in pediatric patients
Prucalopride	1–2 mg orally once daily	2–6 hours	Expensive
Enemas			
Tap water	500 mL per rectum	5–15 minutes	
Sodium phosphate enema	120 mL per rectum	5–15 minutes	Commonly used for acute constipation or to induce movement prior to medical procedures
Mineral oil enema	100–250 mL per rectum	5–15 minutes	To soften and lubricate fecal impaction
Acute Purgative Agents or to Clean Bowel Prior to Medical Procedures			
Magnesium citrate	10 oz orally	3–6 hours	Lemon-flavored
Polyethylene glycol (PEG) 3350	4 L orally administered over 2–4 hours	< 4 hours	(GoLYTELY; CoLyte; NuLyte, MoviPrep) Used to cleanse bowel before colonoscopy

these symptoms. Regular exercise is associated with a decreased risk of constipation. When possible, discontinue medications that may be causing or contributing to constipation. Meta-analysis of limited RCTs suggests probiotics may improve stool frequency and consistency.

2. Laxatives—Laxatives may be given on an intermittent or chronic basis for constipation that does not respond to dietary and lifestyle changes (Table 17–4). In a 2020 survey of US adults with constipation symptoms, 45% were taking fiber supplements or nonprescription laxatives; only 3% were taking prescription laxatives. There is no evidence that long-term use of these agents is harmful to intestinal motility.

A. Osmotic laxatives—Treatment usually is initiated with regular (daily) use of an osmotic laxative. Nonabsorbable osmotic agents promote defecation by increased retention of water in the intestinal lumen, leading to softening of the stool and secondary stimulation of colonic peristalsis. Polyethylene glycol 3350 (MiraLAX) should be the first-line agent in most situations due to its established efficacy in controlled clinical trials and low incidence of adverse events. MiraLAX 17 g once daily has demonstrated superiority to placebo, lactulose, and prucalopride. Nondigestible carbohydrates (sorbitol, lactulose) are efficacious but less preferred because they may cause bloating, cramps, and flatulence. Magnesium-containing laxatives (magnesium hydroxide [milk of magnesia], magnesium oxide, magnesium sulfate) may be suitable for intermittent therapy but should not be given to patients with CKD. When used in conventional doses, the onset of action of osmotic agents is generally within 24 hours. For more rapid treatment of acute constipation, purgative laxatives may be used, such as magnesium citrate (8–10 oz) or large-volume polyethylene glycol solutions (2–4 L, administered over 2–4 hours). Magnesium citrate may cause hypermagnesemia.

B. Stimulant laxatives—For patients with incomplete response to osmotic agents, stimulant laxatives may be prescribed as needed as a "rescue" agent or on a regular basis (daily or alternate days). These agents stimulate fluid secretion and colonic contraction, resulting in a bowel movement within 6–12 hours after oral ingestion or 15–60 minutes after rectal administration. Oral agents are usually administered once daily at bedtime. Common nonprescription preparations include bisacodyl and senna (Table 17–4).

C. Secretagogues—Several agents stimulate intestinal chloride secretion either through activation of chloride channels (lubiprostone) or guanylate cyclase C (linaclotide and plecanatide), resulting in increased intestinal fluid and accelerated colonic transit. In controlled trials, oral lubiprostone 24 mcg twice daily, linaclotide 145 mcg once daily, or plecanatide 3 mg once daily increased the number of bowel movements compared with placebo. Because these agents are expensive, they should be reserved for patients who have suboptimal response or side effects with less expensive agents.

D. Serotonin 5-HT$_4$-receptor agonist—Prucalopride is a high-affinity 5-HT$_4$-agonist that is approved in the United States for the treatment of chronic constipation (2 mg once daily). In clinical trials, 19–38% of patients treated with prucalopride experienced at least three spontaneous bowel movements per week, which was 5–23% more than with placebo.

E. Opioid-receptor antagonists—Long-term use of opioids can cause constipation by increasing tonic, nonpropulsive colonic contractions that lead to increased intestinal fluid absorption and dry, hard stools. Methylnaltrexone (450 mg orally once daily), naloxegol (12.5–25 mg orally once daily), and naldemedine (0.2 mg orally once daily) are μ-opioid receptor antagonists that block peripheral opioid receptors (including in the GI tract) without affecting central analgesia. These medications are recommended for the treatment of opioid-induced constipation in patients receiving prolonged opioid therapy who have not had an adequate laxative response with an osmotic agent (usually PEG-3300) and a stimulant laxative (usually bisacodyl or senna) (see Chapter 5). A subcutaneous formulation of methylnaltrexone is approved for patients receiving palliative care for advanced illness who have not responded to conventional laxative regimens.

B. Fecal Impaction

Severe impaction of stool in the rectal vault may result in obstruction to further fecal flow, leading to partial or complete large bowel obstruction. Predisposing factors include medications (eg, opioids), severe psychiatric disease, prolonged bed rest, neurogenic disorders of the colon, and spinal cord disorders. Initial treatment is directed at relieving the impaction with enemas (saline, mineral oil, or diatrizoate) or digital disruption of the impacted fecal material. Long-term care is directed at maintaining soft stools and regular bowel movements (as above).

When to Refer

- Patients with "alarm" symptoms or aged > 45 years should be referred for colonoscopy.
- Patients with refractory constipation should be considered for anorectal manometry, balloon expulsion test, and colonic transit study.
- Patients with defecatory disorders may benefit from biofeedback therapy.
- Rarely, surgery (subtotal colectomy) is required for patients with severe colonic inertia.

Chang L et al. American Gastroenterological Association-American College of Gastroenterology clinical practice guideline: pharmacological management of chronic idiopathic constipation. Am J Gastroenterol. 2023;118:936. [PMID: 37211280]

Naito T et al. Effects of bowel training and defecation posture on chronic constipation in older adults with dementia: a randomized controlled trial. Am J Gastroenterol. 2023;118:531. [PMID: 36066478]

Sharma A et al. Parkinson disease and the gut: a primer for gastroenterologists. Am J Gastroenterol 2025;120:2510. [PMID: 40298214]

Van Der Schoot A et al. Systematic review and meta-analysis: foods, drinks and diets and their effect on chronic constipation in adults. Aliment Pharmacol Ther. 2024;59:157. [PMID: 37905980]

GASTROINTESTINAL GAS

1. Belching

Belching (eructation) is the involuntary or voluntary release of gas from the stomach or esophagus. It occurs most frequently after meals, when gastric distention results in transient lower esophageal sphincter (LES) relaxation. Belching is a normal reflex and does not itself denote GI dysfunction. Virtually all stomach gas comes from swallowed air. With each swallow, 2–5 mL of air is ingested, and excessive amounts may result in distention, flatulence, and abdominal pain. This may occur with rapid eating, gum chewing, smoking, and the ingestion of carbonated beverages. Evaluation should be restricted to patients with additional complaints such as dysphagia, heartburn, early satiety, or vomiting.

Chronic excessive belching is almost always caused by supragastric belching (voluntary diaphragmatic contraction, followed by upper esophageal relaxation with air inflow to the esophagus) or true air swallowing (aerophagia), both of which are behavioral disorders that are more common in patients with anxiety or psychiatric disorders. These patients may benefit from referral to a behavioral or speech therapist.

2. Bloating & Flatus

Bloating is a complaint of increased abdominal pressure that may or may not be accompanied by visible distention. Organic causes of acute bloating with distention, vomiting, and/or pain include ascites, celiac disease, gastroparesis, small intestine bacterial overgrowth, GI obstruction (gastric fundoplication, gastric outlet obstruction, small intestine or colon obstruction), and constipation. Reports of chronic abdominal distention or bloating are common. Some patients swallow excess air (aerophagia, poorly fitting dentures, sleep apnea, and rapid eating) or produce excess gas from malabsorption. Others have impaired gas propulsion or expulsion, increased bowel wall tension, enhanced visceral sensitivity, or altered viscerosomatic reflexes leading to abdominal protrusion. Many of these patients have an underlying functional GI disorder such as IBS or functional dyspepsia. Constipation should be treated, and exercise (which accelerates gas propulsion) is recommended. Medications that inhibit GI motility should be avoided (eg, opioids and calcium channel blockers).

Healthy adults pass flatus up to 20 times daily and excrete up to 750 mL. Flatus is derived from two sources: swallowed air (primarily nitrogen) and bacterial fermentation of undigested carbohydrate (which produces H_2, CO_2, and methane). Bloating and gas commonly arise from ingestion of fermentable oligosaccharides, disaccharides, monosaccharides, and polyols (FODMAPs), which are foods containing various short-chain carbohydrates that are incompletely absorbed in the small intestine and pass into the colon, where their metabolism may release gas. These include lactose (dairy products); fructose (fruits, corn syrups, and some sweeteners); polyols (stone-fruits, mushrooms, and some sweeteners); and oligosaccharides (legumes, lentils, cruciferous vegetables, garlic, onion, pasta, and whole grains). Less common causes of abnormal gas production are conditions causing malabsorption, including celiac disease, small intestinal bacterial overgrowth, pancreatic insufficiency, and Crohn disease. Flatulence that has a foul odor may be caused by garlic, onion, eggplant, mushrooms, and certain herbs and spices.

Determining abnormal from normal amounts of flatus is difficult. Patients who report excess flatus may also describe bloating, cramping, and altered stool habits (diarrhea or constipation). Treatment of organic causes is based on the underlying condition. Patients with a long-standing history of flatulence and no other symptoms or signs of malabsorption disorders can be treated conservatively. Gum chewing and carbonated beverages should be avoided to reduce air swallowing. Lactose intolerance may be assessed by a 2-week trial of a lactose-free diet or by a hydrogen breath test. A list of foods containing FODMAPs should be provided and high FODMAP foods eliminated for 2–4 weeks. If symptoms improve, FODMAP groups may be sequentially introduced to identify triggers. Multiple low-FODMAP dietary guides are available; however, referral to a knowledgeable dietician may be helpful.

Nonprescription Beano (α-galactosidase enzyme) reduces gas caused by foods containing galacto-oligosaccharides (legumes, chickpeas, lentils) but no other FODMAPs. Activated charcoal may afford relief. Simethicone has no proven benefit.

Gibson PR et al. Diet as a therapeutic tool in chronic gastrointestinal disorders: lessons from the FODMAP journey. J Gastroenterol Hepatol. 2022;37:644. [PMID: 34994019]

Melchior C et al. European consensus on functional bloating and abdominal distention – an ESNM/UEG recommendations for clinical management. United European Gastroenterol J. 2025;13:1613. [PMID: 40844856]

Moshiree B et al. AGA Clinical Practice update on evaluation and management of belching, abdominal bloating, and distention: expert review. Gastroenterology. 2023;165:791. [PMID: 37452811]

DIARRHEA

Diarrhea can range in severity from an acute self-limited episode to a severe, life-threatening illness. To properly evaluate the complaint, the clinician must determine the patient's normal bowel pattern and the nature of the current symptoms.

Approximately 10 L/day of fluid enter the duodenum of which all but 1.5 L/day are absorbed by the small intestine. The colon absorbs most of the remaining fluid, with < 200 mL/day lost in the stool. Although diarrhea sometimes is defined as stool weight of > 200–300 g/24 hours, quantification of stool weight is necessary only in some patients with chronic diarrhea. In most cases, the clinician's working definition of diarrhea is increased stool frequency (more than three bowel movements per day) or liquidity of feces.

The causes of diarrhea are myriad. In clinical practice, it is helpful to distinguish acute from chronic diarrhea, as the evaluation and treatment are different (Tables 17–5 and 17–6).

1. Acute Diarrhea

ESSENTIALS OF DIAGNOSIS

- Diarrhea of < 2 weeks' duration is most commonly caused by invasive or noninvasive pathogens and their enterotoxins.

Acute noninflammatory diarrhea

- Watery, nonbloody.
- Usually mild, self-limited.
- Caused by a virus; noninvasive, toxin-producing bacterium; or parasite.
- Diagnostic evaluation is limited to patients with diarrhea that is severe or persists beyond 7 days.

Acute inflammatory diarrhea

- Blood or pus, fever.
- Usually caused by an invasive or toxin-producing bacterium.
- Diagnostic evaluation requires routine stool bacterial testing (including *E coli* O157:H5 and O157:H7) in all patients and testing as clinically indicated in others for *Clostridioides difficile* and parasites.

Table 17–5. Causes of acute infectious diarrhea.

Noninflammatory Diarrhea	Inflammatory Diarrhea
Viral Noroviruses, astrovirus, adenovirus, rotavirus, sapovirus, SARS-CoV-2	**Viral** Cytomegalovirus
Protozoal *Giardia lamblia* *Cryptosporidium* *Cyclospora*	**Protozoal** *Entamoeba histolytica*
Bacterial Preformed enterotoxin production *Staphylococcus aureus* *Bacillus cereus* *Clostridium perfringens* Enterotoxin production Enterotoxigenic *Escherichia coli* (ETEC) *Vibrio cholerae, Vibrio vulnificus*	**Bacterial** Cytotoxin production Shiga toxin–producing *E coli* (STEC) *Vibrio parahaemolyticus* *Clostridioides difficile* Mucosal invasion *Shigella* *Campylobacter jejuni* *Salmonella* Enteroinvasive *E coli* (EIEC) *Listeria monocytogenes* *Aeromonas* *Yersinia enterocolitica* Infectious proctitis *Chlamydia* *Neisseria gonorrhoeae*

General Considerations

Diarrhea acute in onset and persisting for < 2 weeks is most commonly caused by infectious agents, bacterial toxins (either preformed or produced in the gut), parasites, or medications. Community outbreaks (including norovirus and SARS-CoV-2 in nursing homes, schools, cruise ships) suggest a viral etiology or a common food source. Similar recent illnesses in family members suggest an infectious origin. Ingestion of improperly stored or prepared food implicates "food poisoning" due to bacterial toxins that are either present in the ingested food (preformed) or produced within the GI tract after ingestion. Pregnant individuals have an increased risk of developing listeriosis. Day care attendance or exposure to unpurified water (camping, swimming) may result in infection with *Giardia* or *Cryptosporidium*. Large *Cyclospora* outbreaks have been traced to contaminated produce. Recent travel abroad suggests "traveler's diarrhea" (see Chapter 34). Antibiotic administration within the preceding several weeks increases the likelihood of *C difficile* colitis. Risk factors for HIV infection or STIs should be determined. (AIDS-associated diarrhea is discussed in Chapter 35; infectious proctitis is discussed below under Anorectal Infections.) Persons engaging in anal intercourse or oral-anal sexual activities are at risk for a variety of infections that cause proctitis, including gonorrhea, syphilis, lymphogranuloma venereum, and herpes simplex.

The nature of the diarrhea helps distinguish among different infectious causes (Table 17–5 and Table 34–4).

Table 17–6. Causes of chronic diarrhea.

Medications Common offenders: SSRIs, GLP-1 agonists, cholinesterase inhibitors, NSAIDs, PPIs, ARBs, metformin, allopurinol **Osmotic diarrhea** CLUES: Stool volume decreases with fasting; increased stool osmotic gap Medications: antacids, lactulose, sorbitol Disaccharidase deficiency: lactose intolerance Factitious diarrhea: magnesium (antacids, laxatives) **Secretory diarrhea** CLUES: Large volume (> 1 L/day); little change with fasting; normal stool osmotic gap Hormonally mediated: VIPoma, carcinoid, medullary carcinoma of thyroid (calcitonin), Zollinger-Ellison syndrome (gastrin) Factitious diarrhea (laxative abuse); phenolphthalein, senna Villous adenoma Bile salt malabsorption (idiopathic, ileal resection; Crohn ileitis; postcholecystectomy) Medications **Inflammatory conditions** CLUES: Fever, hematochezia, abdominal pain Ulcerative colitis Crohn disease Microscopic colitis Malignancy: lymphoma, adenocarcinoma (with obstruction and pseudodiarrhea) Radiation enteritis	**Malabsorption syndromes** CLUES: Weight loss, abnormal laboratory values; fecal fat > 10 g/24 hours Small bowel mucosal disorders: celiac disease, tropical sprue, Whipple disease, eosinophilic gastroenteritis, small bowel resection (short bowel syndrome), Crohn disease Pancreatic disease: chronic pancreatitis, pancreatic carcinoma Bacterial overgrowth: motility disorders (diabetes, vagotomy), systemic sclerosis (scleroderma), fistulas, small intestinal diverticula Lymphatic obstruction: lymphoma, carcinoid, infectious (tuberculosis, MAI), Kaposi sarcoma, sarcoidosis, retroperitoneal fibrosis **Motility disorders** CLUES: Prior abdominal surgery or systemic disease Irritable bowel syndrome Postsurgical: vagotomy, partial gastrectomy, blind loop with bacterial overgrowth Systemic disorders: systemic sclerosis (scleroderma), diabetes mellitus, hyperthyroidism **Chronic infections** Parasites: *Giardia lamblia, Cryptosporidium, Entamoeba histolytica, Strongyloides stercoralis, Capillaria philippinensis* AIDS-related: Viral: cytomegalovirus Bacterial: *Clostridioides difficile*, MAI Protozoal: microsporidia (*Enterocytozoon bieneusi*), *Cryptosporidium, Cystoisospora belli* (formerly *Isospora belli*) **Systemic disorders**

MAI, *Mycobacterium avium-intracellulare.*

A. Noninflammatory Diarrhea

Watery, nonbloody diarrhea associated with periumbilical cramps, bloating, nausea, or vomiting suggests a small bowel source caused by either a virus (rotavirus, norovirus, adenovirus, astrovirus, coronavirus), a toxin-producing bacterium (enterotoxigenic *E coli* [ETEC], *Staphylococcus aureus*, *Bacillus cereus*, *Clostridium perfringens*), or a parasite (*Giardia*, *Cryptosporidium*) that disrupts normal absorption and secretory process in the small intestine. Prominent vomiting suggests viral enteritis or food poisoning due to a preformed toxin (*S aureus*, *B cereus*). Although typically mild, the diarrhea (which originates in the small intestine) can be voluminous and result in dehydration with hypokalemia and metabolic acidosis (eg, cholera). Because tissue invasion does not occur, fecal leukocytes are not present.

B. Inflammatory Diarrhea

The presence of fever and bloody diarrhea (dysentery) indicates colonic tissue damage caused by invasion (shigellosis, salmonellosis, *Campylobacter* or *Yersinia* infection, amebiasis) or a toxin (*C difficile*, Shiga-toxin–producing *E coli* [STEC; also known as enterohemorrhagic *E coli*]). Because these organisms predominantly involve the colon, the diarrhea is small in volume (< 1 L/day) and associated with left lower quadrant cramps, urgency, and tenesmus. Fecal leukocytes or lactoferrin usually are present in infections with invasive organisms. STEC is a Shiga toxin–producing noninvasive organism most commonly acquired from contaminated meat that has resulted in several outbreaks of an acute, often severe hemorrhagic colitis. A major complication of STEC is hemolytic-uremic syndrome, which develops in 6–22% of cases. In immunocompromised patients and those with HIV, cytomegalovirus (CMV) can cause intestinal ulceration with watery or bloody diarrhea. *Listeria monocytogenes* has been implicated in several outbreaks of foodborne gastroenteritis, which have been characterized by fever (60–100%), watery diarrhea, and nausea or vomiting.

Clinical Findings

A. Symptoms and Signs

The goal of initial evaluation of acute diarrhea is to distinguish mild disease from more serious illness. In > 90% of patients with acute noninflammatory diarrhea, the illness is mild and self-limited. Prompt medical evaluation is indicated in the following situations (Figure 17–1): (1) signs of inflammatory diarrhea manifested by any of the following: fever (> 38.5°C), WBC ≥15,000/mcL (15×10^9/L), bloody diarrhea, or severe abdominal pain; (2) the passage of ≥ 6 unformed stools in 24 hours; (3) profuse watery diarrhea and dehydration; (4) frail older patients or nursing home residents; (5) immunocompromised patients (AIDS,

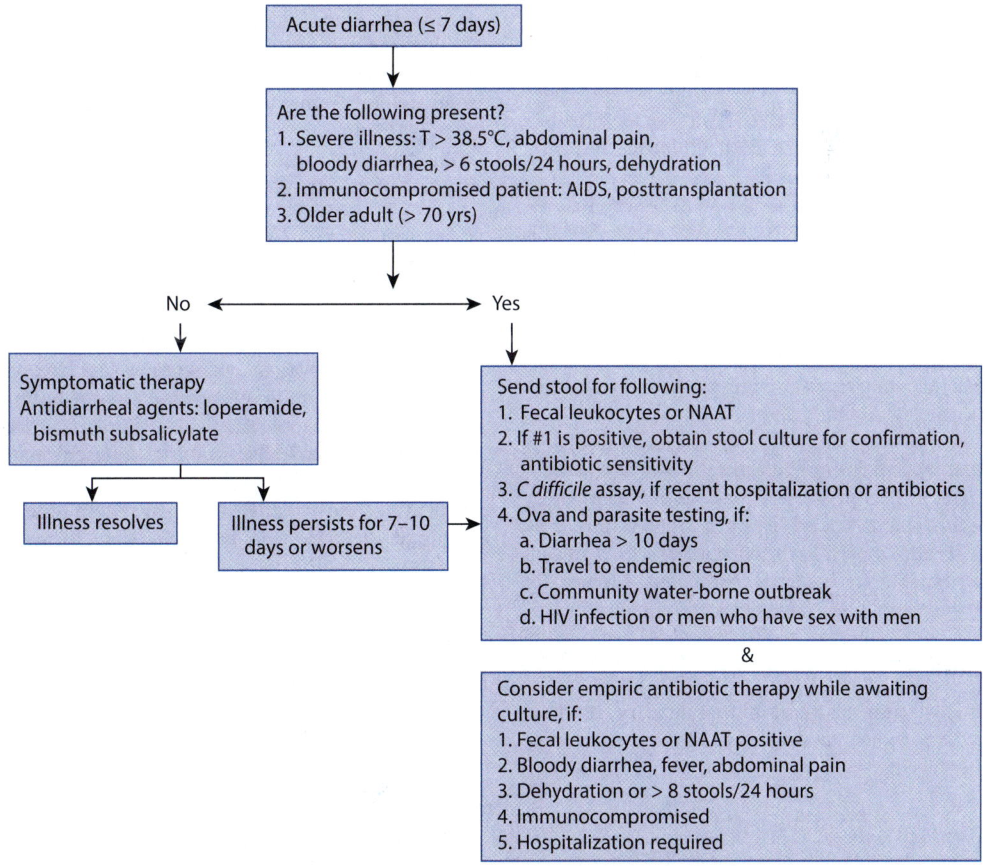

Figure 17–1. Evaluation of acute diarrhea. NAAT, nucleic acid amplification test.

posttransplantation); (6) exposure to antibiotics; (7) hospital-acquired diarrhea (onset following at least 3 days of hospitalization); or (8) systemic illness.

Physical examination pays note to the patient's level of hydration, mental status, and the presence of abdominal tenderness or peritonitis. Peritoneal findings may be present in infection with *C difficile* or STEC.

B. Laboratory Findings

The isolation rate of bacterial pathogens from stool cultures in patients with acute noninflammatory diarrhea is < 3%; therefore, diagnostic investigation is unnecessary except in suspected outbreaks or in patients at high risk for spreading infection to others. Stool should be sent for microbial assessment when patients have dysentery (bloody stools), severe illness, or persistent diarrhea beyond 7 days. Until recently, stool specimens were sent for microscopy (to assess for fecal white cells and protozoa) and bacterial cultures. These traditional methods provided a positive diagnosis in 60–75% of patients with dysenteric diarrhea but required 48–72 hours. Currently, many centers perform microbial assessment using multiplex molecular techniques with nucleic acid amplification (eg, PCR assays) that screen for a panel of pathogens, including viruses, protozoa, and bacteria, within 1–5 hours. If the PCR assay detects a bacterial pathogen, stool culture is recommended for confirmation and antibiotic sensitivity testing. In patients who are hospitalized or who have a history of antibiotic exposure, a stool sample should be tested for *C difficile* (eg, enzyme immunoassay [EIA] for glutamate dehydrogenase or PCR test for *C difficile* toxin gene) (see Antibiotic-Associated Colitis, below). Patients with severe diarrhea or dysentery and a known history of IBD or prior immune checkpoint inhibitor therapy require expedited evaluation with stool studies and possible sigmoidoscopy or colonoscopy with biopsy to exclude infection (*C difficile*, other bacteria, CMV) prior to therapy with intravenous corticosteroids.

Differential Diagnosis

Infectious dysentery must be distinguished from acute ulcerative colitis, which may also present acutely with fever, abdominal pain, and bloody diarrhea. Immune checkpoint inhibitor therapy may cause GI side effects in 8–27% of patients that range from mild diarrhea to severe enterocolitis characterized by abdominal pain and inflammatory diarrhea with mucus, blood, elevated stool calprotectin, and colitis at endoscopy. Diarrhea that persists for > 14 days is not attributable to bacterial pathogens (except for *C difficile*) and should be evaluated as chronic diarrhea.

Treatment

Most patients with acute noninflammatory diarrhea respond within 5 days to simple rehydration therapy or antidiarrheal agents.

A. Diet

Most mild diarrhea will not lead to dehydration provided the patient takes adequate oral fluids containing carbohydrates and electrolytes. Patients find it more comfortable to rest the bowel by avoiding high-fiber foods, fats, milk products, caffeine, and alcohol. Drinking tea and "flat" carbonated beverages and eating soft, easily digested foods (eg, soups, crackers, bananas, applesauce, rice, toast) are encouraged.

B. Rehydration

In more severe diarrhea, dehydration can occur quickly, especially in children and frail older adults. Oral rehydration with fluids containing glucose, Na^+, K^+, Cl^-, and bicarbonate or citrate is preferred when feasible. A convenient mixture is ½ tsp salt (3.5 g), 1 tsp baking soda (2.5 g $NaHCO_3$), 8 tsp sugar (40 g), and 8 oz orange juice (1.5 g KCl), diluted to 1 L with water. Alternatively, oral electrolyte solutions (eg, Pedialyte, Gatorade) are readily available. Oral fluids should be given at rates of 50–100 mL/kg/24 hours depending on the hydration status. Intravenous fluids (lactated Ringer injection) are preferred in patients with severe dehydration.

C. Antidiarrheal Agents

Antidiarrheal agents may be used safely with mild to moderate noninflammatory diarrheal illnesses to improve patient comfort. Opioid agents help decrease the stool number and liquidity and control fecal urgency. However, they should not be used in patients with bloody diarrhea, high fever, or systemic toxicity and should be discontinued in patients whose diarrhea is worsening despite therapy. With these provisos, such drugs provide excellent symptomatic relief. Loperamide 4 mg orally initially is preferred followed by 2 mg after each loose stool (maximum: 8 mg/24 hours). Anticholinergic agents (eg, diphenoxylate with atropine) are contraindicated in acute diarrhea because of the rare precipitation of toxic megacolon.

D. Antibiotic Therapy

1. Empiric treatment—Empiric antibiotic treatment of patients with acute, community-acquired diarrhea generally is not indicated. Even patients with inflammatory diarrhea caused by invasive pathogens usually have symptoms that will resolve within several days without antimicrobials. In centers where stool microbial testing with rapid molecular assays is not available, empiric treatment may be considered for 1–3 days while the stool bacterial culture is incubating, particularly in patients with non–hospital-acquired diarrhea who have moderate to severe fever, tenesmus, or bloody stools and no suspicion of infection with STEC. It should also be considered in patients who are immunocompromised or who have significant dehydration. The oral medications of choice for 1- to 3-day empiric treatment are the fluoroquinolones (eg, ciprofloxacin 500 mg twice daily, ofloxacin 400 mg, or levofloxacin 500 mg once daily) or azithromycin (eg, 1 g single dose or 500 mg daily for 3 days). Empiric treatment of noninflammatory traveler's diarrhea is discussed in Chapter 34.

2. Specific antimicrobial treatment—Antibiotics are not recommended in patients with nontyphoid *Salmonella*, *Campylobacter*, or *Yersinia*, except in severe disease, because they do not hasten recovery or reduce the period of fecal bacterial excretion. STEC infection should not be treated with antibiotics due to an increased risk of hemolytic-uremic syndrome, especially in children. The infectious bacterial diarrheas for which treatment is recommended are shigellosis, cholera, extraintestinal salmonellosis, listeriosis, and *C difficile*. The parasitic infections for which treatment is indicated are amebiasis, giardiasis, cryptosporidiosis, cyclosporiasis, and *Enterocytozoon bieneusi* infection. Therapy for traveler's diarrhea, infectious (sexually transmitted) proctitis, and AIDS-related diarrhea is presented in Chapters 34 and 35.

When to Admit

- Severe dehydration for intravenous fluids, especially if the patient is vomiting or unable to maintain sufficient oral fluid intake.
- Bloody diarrhea that is severe or worsening in order to distinguish infectious versus noninfectious cause.
- Severe abdominal pain, worrisome for toxic colitis, IBD, intestinal ischemia, or surgical abdomen.
- Signs of severe infection or sepsis (temperature > 39.5°C, leukocytosis, rash); altered mental status
- Severe or worsening diarrhea in patients who are older than 70 years or immunocompromised.
- Signs of hemolytic-uremic syndrome (AKI, thrombocytopenia, hemolytic anemia).

Camilleri M. When and what to test for diarrhea: focus on stool testing Am J Gastroenterol. 2025;120:778. [PMID: 39480027]
Marx T et al. A systematic review of tools for predicting complications in patients with acute infectious diarrhea. Am J Emerg Med. 2023;64:78. [PMID: 36469970]

2. Chronic Diarrhea

ESSENTIALS OF DIAGNOSIS

- Diarrhea present for > 4 weeks.
- Before embarking on extensive workup, common causes should be excluded, including medications, chronic infections, and IBS.

General Considerations

The causes of chronic diarrhea may be grouped into the following major pathophysiologic categories: osmotic diarrheas, secretory diarrheas, inflammatory conditions, medications, malabsorptive syndromes, motility disorders, chronic infections, and systemic disorders (Table 17–6).

A. Medications

Numerous medications can cause diarrhea. All medications should be carefully reviewed, and discontinuation of potential culprits should be considered.

B. Osmotic Diarrheas

As stool leaves the colon, fecal osmolality is equal to the serum osmolality, ie, approximately 290 mOsm/kg. Under normal circumstances, the major osmoles are Na^+, K^+, Cl^-, and HCO_3^-. The stool osmolality may be estimated by multiplying the stool (Na^+ + K^+) × 2. The **osmotic gap** is the difference between the *measured* stool and serum osmolality and is normally < 50 mOsm/kg. An increased osmotic gap (> 75 mOsm/kg) implies that the diarrhea is caused by ingestion or malabsorption of an osmotically active substance. The most common causes are carbohydrate malabsorption (lactose, fructose, sorbitol), laxative abuse, and malabsorption syndromes. Osmotic diarrheas resolve during fasting. Those caused by malabsorbed carbohydrates are characterized by abdominal distention, bloating, and flatulence due to increased colonic gas production.

Carbohydrate malabsorption is common and should be considered in all patients with chronic, postprandial diarrhea. Patients should be asked about their intake of dairy products (lactose), fruits and artificial sweeteners (fructose and sorbitol), processed foods and soft drinks (high-fructose corn syrup), and alcohol. The diagnosis of carbohydrate malabsorption may be established by an elimination trial for 2–3 weeks or by hydrogen breath tests.

Ingestion of magnesium- or phosphate-containing compounds (laxatives, antacids) should be considered in enigmatic chronic diarrhea.

C. Secretory Conditions

Increased intestinal secretion or decreased absorption results in a high-volume watery diarrhea with a normal osmotic gap. There is little change in stool output during the fasting state, and dehydration and electrolyte imbalance may develop. Causes include endocrine tumors (stimulating intestinal or pancreatic secretion), bile salt malabsorption (stimulating colonic secretion), and microscopic colitis. Microscopic colitis is a common cause of chronic watery diarrhea in older adults (see Inflammatory Bowel Disease, below).

D. Inflammatory Conditions

Diarrhea is present in most patients with IBD (ulcerative colitis, Crohn disease). A variety of other symptoms may be present, including abdominal pain, fever, weight loss, and hematochezia.

E. Malabsorptive Conditions

The major causes of malabsorption are small intestinal mucosal diseases, intestinal resections, lymphatic obstruction, small intestinal bacterial overgrowth, and pancreatic insufficiency. Its characteristics are weight loss, osmotic diarrhea, steatorrhea, and nutritional deficiencies. Significant diarrhea in the absence of weight loss is not likely to be due to malabsorption. The physical and laboratory abnormalities related to deficiencies of vitamins or minerals are discussed in Chapter 33.

F. Motility Disorders (Including IBS)

IBS is the most common cause of chronic diarrhea in young adults (see Irritable Bowel Syndrome, below). It should be considered in patients with lower abdominal pain and altered bowel habits who have no other evidence of serious organic disease (weight loss, nocturnal diarrhea, anemia, or GI bleeding). Abnormal intestinal motility secondary to systemic disorders, radiation enteritis, or surgery may result in diarrhea due to rapid transit or to stasis of intestinal contents with bacterial overgrowth, resulting in malabsorption.

G. Chronic Infections

Chronic parasitic infections may cause diarrhea through a number of mechanisms. Pathogens most commonly associated with diarrhea include the protozoans *Giardia*, *Entamoeba histolytica*, *Cryptosporidium*, and *Cyclospora* as well as the intestinal nematodes. Strongyloidiasis and capillariasis should be excluded in patients from endemic regions, especially in the presence of eosinophilia. Bacterial infections with *C difficile* and, uncommonly, *Aeromonas* and *Plesiomonas* may cause chronic diarrhea.

Immunocompromised patients are susceptible to infectious organisms that can cause acute or chronic diarrhea (see Chapter 36), including microsporidia, *Cryptosporidium*, CMV, *Cystoisospora belli* (formerly *Isospora belli*), *Cyclospora*, and *Mycobacterium avium* complex.

H. Systemic Conditions

Chronic systemic conditions, such as thyroid disease, diabetes, and collagen vascular disorders, may cause diarrhea through alterations in motility or intestinal absorption.

Clinical Findings

A. Symptoms and Signs

The history and physical examination commonly suggest the pathophysiology that guides the subsequent diagnostic workup (Figure 17–2). The clinician should establish whether the diarrhea is continuous or intermittent, whether it has a relationship to meals, and whether it occurs at night or during fasting. The stool appearance may suggest a malabsorption disorder (greasy or malodorous), inflammatory

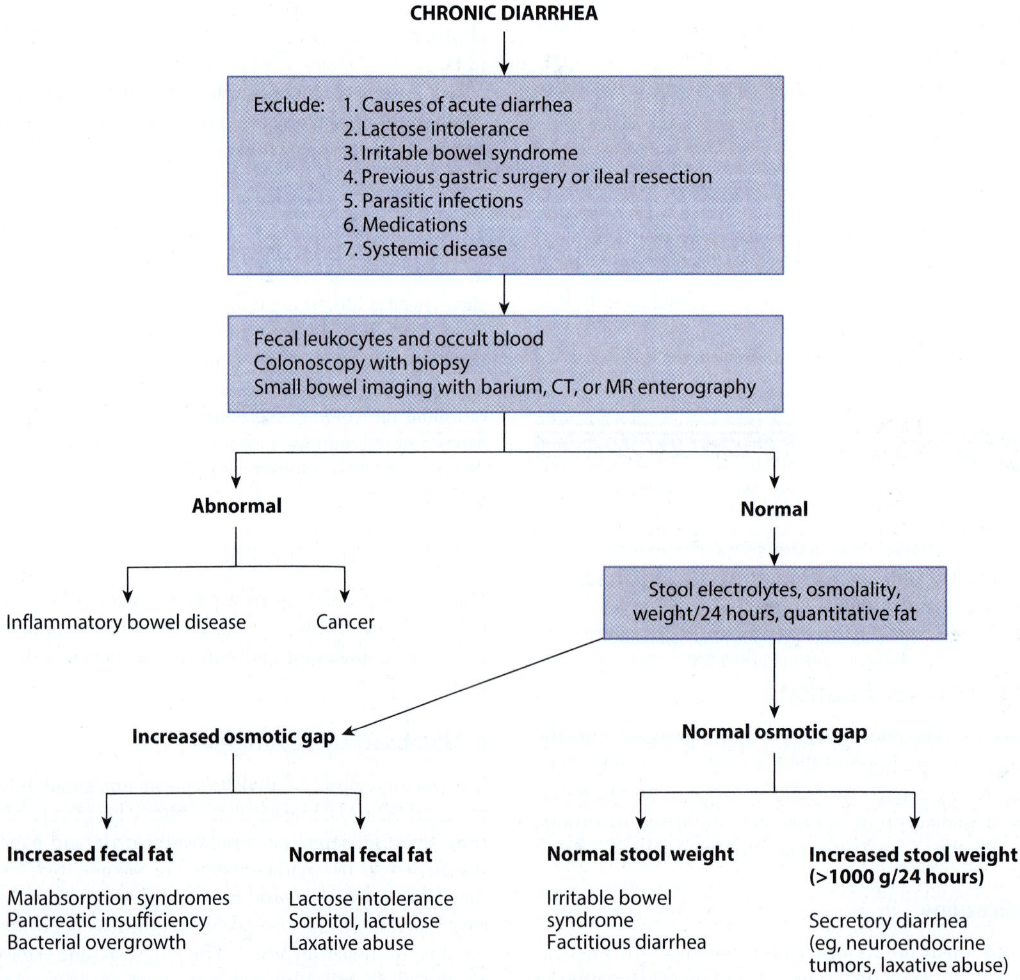

Figure 17–2. Decision diagram for diagnosis of causes of chronic diarrhea.

disorder (containing blood or pus), or a secretory process (watery). Work in daycare centers or exposure to contaminated water (camping, swimming pools) increases the risk for acquiring *Giardia* and *Cryptosporidia*. The presence of abdominal pain suggests IBS or IBD. Medications, diet, and recent psychosocial stressors should be reviewed. Physical examination should assess for signs of malnutrition, dehydration, and IBD.

Because chronic diarrhea is caused by many conditions, the subsequent diagnostic approach is guided by the relative suspicion for the underlying cause, and no specific algorithm can be followed in all patients. Prior to embarking on an extensive evaluation, the most common causes of chronic diarrhea should be considered, including medications, IBS, and lactose intolerance. The presence of nocturnal diarrhea, weight loss, anemia, or positive results on FOBT are inconsistent with these disorders and warrant further evaluation. AIDS-associated diarrhea is discussed in Chapter 35.

B. Initial Diagnostic Studies

1. Routine laboratory tests—CBC, serum electrolytes, liver chemistries, calcium, phosphorus, albumin, TSH, vitamin A and D levels, prothrombin time with INR, ESR, and CRP should be obtained in most patients. Serologic testing for celiac disease with an IgA tissue transglutaminase (IgA anti-tTG) test is recommended in the evaluation of most patients with chronic diarrhea even in the absence of signs of malabsorption. Anemia occurs in malabsorption syndromes (folate, iron, or vitamin B_{12} deficiency) as well as in inflammatory conditions. Hypoalbuminemia is present in malabsorption, protein-losing enteropathies, and inflammatory diseases. Hyponatremia and non–anion gap metabolic acidosis occur in secretory diarrheas. Increased ESR or CRP suggests IBD. Elevated serum fasting levels (> 48 ng/mL) of the bile acid precursor 7αC4 are strongly predictive of bile acid diarrhea.

2. Routine stool studies—Stool samples should be analyzed for ova and parasites, electrolytes (to calculate osmotic gap), qualitative staining for fat (Sudan stain), occult blood, and either leukocytes or fecal calprotectin or lactoferrin. Parasitic infections (*Giardia*, *E histolytica*, *Cryptosporidia*, and *Cyclospora*) may be diagnosed with stool multiplex PCR assays that test for a panel of pathogens within 1–5 hours, or, where PCR is unavailable, by microscopy with special stains. As discussed above, an increased osmotic gap suggests an osmotic diarrhea or disorder of malabsorption. A positive fecal fat stain suggests a disorder of malabsorption. In patients with positive fecal fat or suspicion for chronic pancreatitis, a stool sample should be sent for measurement of pancreatic elastase, which is low with pancreatic insufficiency. The presence of fecal leukocytes or elevated fecal calprotectin may suggest IBD. Measurement in a single stool specimen of total bile acid concentration >1.88 μmol/g with > 4.6% primary bile acids is strongly suggestive of bile acid diarrhea.

3. Endoscopic examination and mucosal biopsy—Most patients with chronic persistent diarrhea undergo colonoscopy with mucosal biopsy to exclude IBD (including Crohn disease and ulcerative colitis), microscopic colitis, and colonic neoplasia. Upper endoscopy with small bowel biopsy is performed when a small intestinal malabsorptive disorder is suspected (celiac disease, Whipple disease) from abnormal laboratory studies or a positive fecal fat stain. It may also be done in patients with advanced AIDS to document *Cryptosporidium*, microsporidia, and *M avium-intracellulare* infection.

C. Further Studies

If the cause of diarrhea is still not apparent, further studies may be warranted.

1. 24- to 48-hour stool collection quantification of total weight and fat—A stool weight of < 300 g/24 hours excludes diarrhea and suggests a functional disorder such as IBS. A weight > 1000–1500 g suggests a significant secretory process, including neuroendocrine tumors. A fecal fat determination > 14 g/24 hours confirms a malabsorptive disorder. Fecal elastase < 100 mcg/g suggests that malabsorption is caused by pancreatic insufficiency. (See Celiac Disease and specific tests for malabsorption [Table 17–11], below.)

2. Other imaging studies—Calcification on a plain abdominal radiograph confirms a diagnosis of chronic pancreatitis, although abdominal CT and endoscopic ultrasonography are more sensitive for the diagnosis of chronic pancreatitis as well as pancreatic cancer. Small intestinal imaging with CT or MRI enterography is helpful in the diagnosis of Crohn disease, small bowel lymphoma, carcinoid, and jejunal diverticula. Neuroendocrine tumors may be localized using CT, and metastases may be detected using somatostatin receptor PET scanning. Retention of < 11% at 7 days of intravenous 75Se-homotaurocholate on scintigraphy suggests bile salt malabsorption; however, this test is unavailable in the United States.

3. Laboratory tests—

A. SEROLOGIC TESTS FOR NEUROENDOCRINE TUMORS—Secretory diarrheas due to neuroendocrine tumors are rare but should be considered in patients with chronic, high-volume watery diarrhea (> 1 L/day) with a normal osmotic gap that persists during fasting. Secretagogues of various neuroendocrine tumors may be assayed, including serum chromogranin A (pancreatic neuroendocrine tumors), vasoactive intestinal peptide (VIP) (VIPoma), calcitonin (medullary thyroid carcinoma), gastrin (Zollinger-Ellison syndrome), and urinary 5-hydroxyindoleacetic acid (5-HIAA) (carcinoid).

B. BREATH TEST—The diagnosis of small bowel bacterial overgrowth is suggested by a noninvasive breath test (glucose or lactulose); however, a high rate of false-positive test results limits its utility. A definitive diagnosis of bacterial overgrowth requires aspiration of small intestinal contents for quantitative aerobic and anaerobic bacterial culture; however, this procedure is not available at most centers.

Treatment

A number of antidiarrheal agents may be used in certain patients with chronic diarrheal conditions and are listed below.

Loperamide: 4 mg orally initially, then 2 mg after each loose stool (maximum: 16 mg/day).

Diphenoxylate with atropine: One tablet orally three or four times daily as needed.

Clonidine: α_2-Adrenergic agonists inhibit intestinal electrolyte secretion. Clonidine, 0.1–0.3 mg orally twice daily, or a clonidine patch, 0.1–0.2 mg/day, may help in some patients with secretory diarrheas, diabetic diarrhea, or cryptosporidiosis.

Octreotide: This somatostatin analog stimulates intestinal fluid and electrolyte absorption and inhibits intestinal fluid secretion and the release of GI peptides. It is given for secretory diarrheas due to neuroendocrine tumors (VIPomas, carcinoid). Effective doses are 50 mcg to 250 mcg subcutaneously three times daily.

Bile salt binders: Cholestyramine 2–4 g or colestipol (1–2 g once to three times daily) or colesevelam (625 mg, 1–3 tablets once or twice daily) may be useful in patients with bile salt-induced diarrhea, which may be idiopathic or secondary to intestinal resection or ileal disease.

Camilleri M. When and what to test for diarrhea: focus on stool testing. Am J Gastroenterol. 2025;120:778. [PMID: 39480027]

Dilmaghani S et al. Simplifying diagnosis of bile acid diarrhea with clinical and biochemical measurements on blood and single stool sample. Clin Gastroenterol Hepatol. 2025;23:2318. [PMID: 40378992]

Ferris A et al. Approach to diarrhea. Prim Care. 2023;50:447. [PMID: 37516513]

Leite G et al. Defining small intestinal bacterial overgrowth by culture through high throughput sequencing. Clin Gastroenterol Hepatol. 2024;22:259. [PMID: 37315761]

GI BLEEDING

1. Acute Upper GI Bleeding

ESSENTIALS OF DIAGNOSIS

- Hematemesis (bright red blood or "coffee grounds").
- Melena in most cases; hematochezia in massive upper GI bleeds.
- Volume status to determine severity of blood loss; hematocrit is a poor early indicator of blood loss.
- Endoscopy diagnostic and may be therapeutic.

General Considerations

In the United States there are > 250,000 hospitalizations a year for acute upper GI bleeding with a mortality rate for nonvariceal upper GI bleeding of 2.1%; however, the rate may be increasing due to the widespread use of antiplatelet and anticoagulant therapies. Mortality is higher in patients aged > 60 years and in patients in whom bleeding develops during hospitalization. Patients seldom die of exsanguination but rather of complications from an underlying disease.

The most common presentation of upper GI bleeding is hematemesis or melena. Hematemesis may be either bright red blood or brown "coffee grounds" material. Melena develops after as little as 50–100 mL of blood loss in the upper GI tract, whereas hematochezia requires a loss of > 1000 mL. Although hematochezia generally suggests a lower bleeding source (eg, colonic), severe upper GI bleeding may present with hematochezia in 10% of cases.

Upper GI bleeding is self-limited in 80% of patients; urgent medical therapy and endoscopic evaluation are obligatory in the rest. Patients with bleeding > 48 hours prior to presentation have a low risk of recurrent bleeding.

Etiology

Peptic ulcers account for 40% of major upper GI bleeding with an overall mortality rate of < 5%. In North America, the incidence of bleeding from ulcers is declining due to eradication of *H pylori* and prophylaxis with PPIs in high-risk patients.

Portal hypertension accounts for 10–20% of upper GI bleeding. Bleeding usually arises from esophageal varices and less commonly from gastric or duodenal varices or portal hypertensive gastropathy. Approximately 25% of patients with cirrhosis have medium to large esophageal varices, of whom 30% experience acute variceal bleeding within a 2-year period. Due to improved care, the hospital mortality rate has declined from 40% to 15%. Nevertheless, a mortality rate of 60–80% is expected at 1–4 years due to recurrent bleeding or other complications of chronic liver disease.

Lacerations of the gastroesophageal junction (Mallory Weiss tear) cause 5–10% of cases of upper GI bleeding. Many patients report a history of heavy alcohol use or retching. Less than 10% have continued or recurrent bleeding.

Vascular anomalies are found throughout the GI tract and may be the source of chronic or acute GI bleeding. They account for 7% of cases of acute upper tract bleeding. The most common are **angioectasias** (angiodysplasias), which are 1–10 mm distorted, aberrant submucosal vessels caused by chronic, intermittent obstruction of submucosal veins. They have a bright red stellate appearance and occur throughout the GI tract but most commonly in the right colon. **GAVE** (Gastric Antral Vascular Ectasias) are dilated mucosal capillaries (often associated with portal hypertension) that appear in the gastric antrum as diffuse or striped red lesions. **Telangiectasias** are small, cherry red lesions caused by dilation of venules that may be part of systemic conditions (hereditary hemorrhagic telangiectasia, CREST syndrome) or occur sporadically. The **Dieulafoy lesion** is an aberrant, large-caliber submucosal artery, most commonly in the proximal stomach that causes recurrent, intermittent bleeding.

Gastric neoplasms cause about 1% of upper GI hemorrhages.

Erosive gastritis is superficial, so it is a relatively unusual cause of severe GI bleeding (< 5% of cases) and more commonly results in chronic blood loss. Gastric mucosal erosions are due to NSAIDs, alcohol, or severe medical or surgical illness (stress-related mucosal disease).

Severe erosive esophagitis due to chronic gastroesophageal reflux may rarely cause significant upper GI bleeding, especially in patients who are bedbound long-term.

An **aortoenteric fistula** complicates 2% of abdominal aortic grafts or, rarely, can occur as the initial presentation of a previously untreated aneurysm. **Unusual causes** of upper GI bleeding include hemobilia (from hepatic tumor, angioma, penetrating trauma), and pancreatic malignancy and pseudoaneurysm (hemosuccus pancreaticus).

Initial Evaluation & Treatment

A. Stabilization

The initial step is assessment of the hemodynamic status. A systolic blood pressure < 100 mm Hg identifies a high-risk patient with severe acute bleeding. A heart rate > 100 beats/min with a systolic blood pressure > 100 mm Hg signifies moderate acute blood loss. A normal systolic blood pressure and heart rate suggest relatively minor hemorrhage. Postural hypotension and tachycardia are useful when present but may be due to causes other than blood loss. Because the hematocrit may take 24–72 hours to equilibrate with the extravascular fluid, it is not a reliable indicator of the severity of acute bleeding.

In patients with significant bleeding, two 18-gauge or larger intravenous lines should be started prior to further diagnostic tests. Blood is sent for CBC, prothrombin time with INR, serum creatinine, liver biochemical enzymes, and blood typing and screening (in anticipation of the possible need for transfusion). In patients without hemodynamic compromise or overt active bleeding, aggressive fluid repletion can be delayed until the extent of the bleeding is further clarified. Patients with evidence of hemodynamic compromise are given 0.9% saline or lactated Ringer infusion and cross-matched for 2–4 units of packed RBCs (see below). It is rarely necessary to administer type-specific or O-negative blood. CVP monitoring is desirable in some cases, but line placement should not interfere with rapid volume resuscitation.

Placement of a nasogastric tube is not routinely recommended in clinical guidelines but may be helpful in the initial assessment and triage of selected patients with suspected active upper tract bleeding. The aspiration of red blood or "coffee grounds" confirms an upper GI source of bleeding, though up to 18% of patients with confirmed upper tract sources of bleeding have nonbloody aspirates—especially when bleeding originates in the duodenum. Erythromycin (250 mg) administered intravenously 30 minutes prior to upper endoscopy promotes gastric emptying and may improve the quality of endoscopic evaluation when substantial amounts of blood or clot in the stomach is suspected. Efforts to stop or slow bleeding by gastric lavage with large volumes of fluid are of no benefit and expose the patient to an increased risk of aspiration.

B. Blood Replacement

The amount of fluid and blood products required is based on assessment of vital signs, evidence of active bleeding from nasogastric aspirate, and laboratory tests.

1. RBC transfusion—In patients who are hemodynamically stable, a restrictive policy for RBC transfusion is recommended utilizing a threshold of < 7 g/dL in most patients but < 8 g/dL in patients with known CVD. In the absence of continued bleeding, the hemoglobin should rise approximately 1 g/dL for each unit of transfused packed RBCs. Sufficient packed RBCs should be given to maintain a hemoglobin of 7–9 g/dL. In patients with severe GI bleeding, it is desirable to transfuse blood before the hemoglobin reaches 7 g/dL to prevent decreases below that level occurring from hemodilution with fluid resuscitation. Transfusion of blood should not be withheld from patients with massive active bleeding regardless of the hemoglobin value.

2. Platelet transfusion—In actively bleeding patients, platelets are transfused (eg, six units of whole blood–derived platelets or one apheresis unit) if the platelet count is < 50,000/mcL (50×10^9/L). Guidelines recommend against platelet transfusion for impaired platelet function due to aspirin or clopidogrel. Patients with uremia (who also have dysfunctional platelets) with active bleeding are given three doses of desmopressin (DDAVP), 0.3 mcg/kg intravenously, at 12-hour intervals.

3. Reversal of anticoagulation—In patients with active bleeding who have been taking anticoagulants, the benefits of reversal of the anticoagulation (reduced bleeding and reduced need for blood products) must be weighed against the risks (thromboembolism, ischemia). In patients taking warfarin, endoscopy may be performed safely and effective hemostasis treatment applied if the INR is < 2.5. In patients with massive bleeding and/or a supratherapeutic INR, administration of four factor prothrombin complex concentrates is preferred (rather than fresh frozen plasma) because it is more rapid and effective at correcting the INR and requires a smaller volume. In patients taking the direct thrombin inhibitor (dabigatran) or factor Xa inhibitors (rivaroxaban, apixaban, edoxaban), restoration of normal anticoagulation usually requires 24–48 hours (presuming normal kidney and liver function). Therefore, reversal should only be considered in patients with life-threatening bleeding. Idarucizumab (an intravenous monoclonal antibody) is approved for the reversal of dabigatran. Andexanet alfa (a modified factor Xa decoy protein) was previously approved by the FDA for the reversal of apixaban and rivaroxaban but removed from the market in 2025 by the manufacturer due to an increased risk of thromboembolic events. For management of coagulation abnormalities in patients with cirrhosis and upper GI bleeding, see Esophageal Varices.

C. Initial Triage

A preliminary assessment of risk based on several clinical factors aids in the resuscitation as well as the rational triage of the patient. Clinical predictors of increased risk of further bleeding and death include liver disease, HF, syncope, systolic blood pressure < 100 mm Hg, pulse > 100 beats/min, bright red blood in the nasogastric aspirate or on rectal examination, and initial hemoglobin < 13 g/dL (in men) or < 12 g/dL (in women).

1. High risk—Patients with active bleeding manifested by hematemesis or bright red blood on nasogastric aspirate, shock, persistent hemodynamic derangement despite fluid resuscitation, serious comorbid medical illness, or evidence of advanced liver disease require admission to an ICU. Endoscopy should be performed within 12–24 hours in most patients, but only after adequate hemodynamic resuscitation and management of other active comorbidities (eg, ACS). In a large RCT of patients with acute upper GI bleeding at high risk for recurrent bleeding or death, there was no difference in 30-day mortality among patients in whom endoscopy was performed within 6 hours versus within 6–24 hours.

2. Low to moderate risk—All other patients are admitted to an observation unit, medical ward, or step-down unit after appropriate stabilization for further evaluation and treatment. Patients without evidence of active bleeding undergo nonemergent endoscopy, usually within 24 hours.

Subsequent Evaluation & Treatment

Specific treatment of the various causes of upper GI bleeding is discussed elsewhere in this chapter. The following general comments apply to most patients with bleeding.

The clinician's impression of the bleeding source is correct in only 40% of cases. Signs of chronic liver disease implicate bleeding due to portal hypertension, but a different lesion is identified in 25% of patients with cirrhosis. A history of dyspepsia, NSAID use, or peptic ulcer disease suggests peptic ulcer. Acute bleeding preceded by heavy alcohol ingestion or retching suggests a Mallory-Weiss tear, though most patients with Mallory-Weiss tears have neither.

A. Upper Endoscopy

Virtually all patients with upper tract bleeding should undergo upper endoscopy within 24 hours of arriving in the emergency department. The benefits of endoscopy in this setting are threefold.

1. To identify the source of bleeding—The appropriate acute and long-term medical therapy is determined by the cause of bleeding. Patients with portal hypertension will be treated differently from those with ulcer disease. If surgery or radiologic interventional therapy is required for uncontrolled bleeding, the source of bleeding identified at endoscopy will determine the approach.

2. To determine the risk of rebleeding and guide triage—Patients with a nonbleeding Mallory-Weiss tear, esophagitis, gastritis, and ulcers that have a clean, white base have a very low risk (< 5%) of rebleeding. Patients with one of these findings who are aged < 60 years, without hemodynamic instability or transfusion requirement, without serious coexisting illness, and who have stable social support may be discharged from the emergency department or medical ward after endoscopy with outpatient follow-up. All others with one of these low-risk lesions should be observed on a medical ward for 24–48 hours. Patients with ulcers that are actively bleeding or have a visible vessel or adherent clot, or who have variceal bleeding usually require at least a 3-day hospitalization with closer initial observation in an ICU or step-down unit.

3. To render endoscopic therapy—Hemostasis can be achieved in actively bleeding lesions with endoscopic modalities such as cautery, injection, endoclips, over-the-scope clips, or topical hemostatic powder. About 90% of bleeding or nonbleeding varices can be effectively treated immediately with application of rubber bands to the varices. Similarly, 90% of bleeding ulcers, angiomas, or Mallory-Weiss tears can be controlled with either endoscopic injection of epinephrine, direct cauterization of the vessel by a heater probe or multipolar electrocautery probe, clips, or application of a hemostatic powder spray. Certain nonbleeding lesions, such as ulcers with visible blood vessels, and angioectasias are also treated with these therapies. Specific endoscopic therapy of varices, peptic ulcers, and Mallory-Weiss tears is dealt with elsewhere in this chapter.

B. Acute Pharmacologic Therapies

1. Acid inhibitory therapy—**Intravenous PPIs** (esomeprazole or pantoprazole, 80 mg bolus, followed by 8 mg/hour continuous infusion for 72 hours) reduce the risk of rebleeding in patients with peptic ulcers with high-risk features (active bleeding, visible vessel, or adherent clot) after endoscopic treatment. **Oral PPIs** (omeprazole, esomeprazole, or pantoprazole 40 mg; lansoprazole or dexlansoprazole 30–60 mg) once or twice daily are sufficient for lesions at low risk for rebleeding (eg, esophagitis, gastritis, clean-based ulcers, and Mallory-Weiss tears).

Administration of continuous intravenous PPI *before* endoscopy results in a decreased number of ulcers with lesions that require endoscopic therapy. It therefore is standard clinical practice at many institutions to administer either an intravenous or a high-dose oral PPI prior to endoscopy in patients with significant upper GI bleeding. Based on the findings during endoscopy, the intravenous PPI may be continued or discontinued.

2. Octreotide—Continuous intravenous infusion of octreotide (100-mcg bolus, followed by 50–100 mcg/hour) reduces splanchnic blood flow and portal blood pressures and is effective in the initial control of bleeding related to portal hypertension. It is administered promptly to all patients with active upper GI bleeding and evidence of liver disease or portal hypertension until the source of bleeding can be determined by endoscopy. In countries where it is available, terlipressin may be preferred to octreotide for the treatment of bleeding related to portal hypertension because of its sustained reduction of portal and variceal pressures and its proven reduction in mortality. Terlipressin is FDA-approved for the treatment of hepatorenal syndrome.

C. Other Treatment

1. Intra-arterial embolization—Angiographic treatment is used in patients with persistent bleeding from ulcers, angiomas, or Mallory-Weiss tears who have failed endoscopic therapy and are poor operative risks. Compared with surgical intervention for recurrent or refractory bleeding, embolization achieves equivalent clinical success rates with lower mortality.

2. Transvenous intrahepatic portosystemic shunts (TIPS)—Placement of a wire stent from the hepatic vein through the liver to the portal vein provides effective decompression of the portal venous system and control of acute variceal bleeding. It is indicated in patients in whom endoscopic modalities have failed to control acute variceal bleeding.

Alali AA et al. Assessment, resuscitation and medical management of variceal and nonvariceal bleeding. Gastrointest Endosc Clin N Am. 2024;34:189. [PMID: 38395478]
Barkun A et al. Canadian Association of Gastroenterology clinical practice guideline for the endoscopic management of nonvariceal nonpeptic ulcer upper gastrointestinal bleeding. Gastroenterology. 2025;169:863. [PMID: 40778886]
D'Amore K et al. Patient blood management guideline for adults with critical bleeding. Emerg Med Clin North Am. 2020;38:871. [PMID: 32981623]
Liu K et al. Efficacy of hemostatic powder monotherapy versus conventional endoscopic treatment for nonvariceal GI bleeding: a meta-analysis and trial sequential analysis. Gastrointest Endosc 2025;101:539. [PMID: 39265743]
Metcalf RA et al. Platelet Transfusion: 2025 AABB and ICTMG International Clinical Practice Guidelines. JAMA. 2025;334:606. [PMID: 40440268]
Mitra B et al; Clinical and Consumer Reference group for the update of Patient Blood Management Guidelines (Module 1: Critical Bleeding/Massive Transfusion). Patient blood management guideline for adults with critical bleeding. Med J Aust. 2024;220:211. [PMID: 38282333]

2. Acute Lower GI Bleeding

ESSENTIALS OF DIAGNOSIS

- Hematochezia usually present.
- Ten percent of cases of hematochezia, however, are due to upper GI source.
- Evaluation with colonoscopy in stable patients.
- Massive active bleeding evaluated with CT angiography, followed by angiography or endoscopy.

General Considerations

Lower GI bleeding is defined as that arising below the ligament of Treitz, ie, the small intestine or colon; however, up to 95% of cases arise from the colon. The severity of lower GI bleeding ranges from mild anorectal bleeding to massive, large-volume hematochezia. Bright red blood that drips into the bowl after a bowel movement or is mixed with solid brown stool signifies mild bleeding, usually from an anorectosigmoid source, and can be evaluated in the outpatient setting. In patients hospitalized with GI bleeding, lower tract bleeding is one-third as common as upper GI hemorrhage and tends to have a more benign course. Patients hospitalized with lower GI tract bleeding are less likely to present with shock or orthostasis (< 5%) or to require transfusions (< 40%). Spontaneous cessation of bleeding occurs in > 75% of cases, and hospital mortality is approximately 1%.

Etiology

The likely cause of lower GI bleeding depends on both the age of the patient and the severity of the bleeding. In patients aged < 50 years, the most common causes are infectious colitis, anorectal disease, and IBD. In older patients, significant hematochezia is most often seen with diverticulosis, angioectasias, malignancy, or ischemia. There is an increased risk of lower GI bleeding in patients taking aspirin, nonaspirin antiplatelet agents, anticoagulants, NSAIDs, and SSRIs.

A. Diverticulosis

Hemorrhage occurs in 3–5% of all patients with diverticulosis and is the most common cause of major lower tract bleeding, accounting for > 60% of cases. Diverticular bleeding usually presents as acute, painless, large-volume maroon or bright red hematochezia in patients aged > 50 years. More than 95% of cases require < 4 units of blood transfusion. Bleeding subsides spontaneously in 80% but may recur in up to 25% of patients.

B. Angioectasias

Angioectasias (angiodysplasias) occur throughout the upper and lower intestinal tracts and cause painless bleeding ranging from melena or hematochezia to occult blood loss. They are responsible for 2–5% of cases of lower GI bleeding, where they are most often seen in the cecum and ascending colon. They are flat, red lesions (2–10 mm) with ectatic peripheral vessels radiating from a central vessel and are most common in patients aged > 70 years and in those with CKD. Bleeding in younger patients more commonly arises from the small intestine.

Ectasias can be identified in up to 6% of persons aged > 60 years, so the mere presence of ectasias does not prove that the lesion is the source of bleeding, since active bleeding is seldom seen.

C. Neoplasms

Benign polyps and malignant carcinomas are associated with chronic occult blood loss or intermittent anorectal hematochezia and cause up to 3% of acute lower GI hemorrhage.

After endoscopic removal of colonic polyps, important bleeding may occur up to 2 weeks later in 0.1–1% of patients overall but in 3–10% following mucosal resection of large (> 2 cm) polyps. In up to one-half of cases, colonoscopy is required to treat postpolypectomy hemorrhage and minimize the need for transfusions.

D. Inflammatory Bowel Disease

Patients with IBD (especially ulcerative colitis) often have diarrhea with variable amounts of hematochezia. Bleeding varies from occult blood loss to recurrent hematochezia mixed with stool. Symptoms of abdominal pain, tenesmus, and urgency are often present.

E. Anorectal Disease

Anorectal disease (hemorrhoids, fissures) usually results in small amounts of bright red blood noted on the toilet paper, streaking of the stool, or dripping into the toilet bowl; clinically significant blood loss can sometimes occur. Hemorrhoids are the source in 2–10% of patients admitted with lower bleeding. Rectal ulcers may account for up to 8% of lower bleeding, usually in older adults or debilitated patients with constipation.

F. Ischemic Colitis

This condition is seen commonly in older patients, most of whom have atherosclerotic disease. Most cases occur spontaneously due to transient episodes of nonocclusive ischemia. Ischemic colitis may also occur in 5% of patients after surgery for ileoaortic aneurysm or an AAA. In younger patients, colonic ischemia may develop due to vasculitis, coagulation disorders, estrogen therapy, and long-distance running. Ischemic colitis results in hematochezia or bloody diarrhea associated with mild cramps. In most patients, the bleeding is mild and self-limited.

G. Others

Chronic radiation-induced changes in the rectum may cause anorectal bleeding that develops months to years after pelvic radiation of urologic, gynecologic, or anorectal malignancies. Endoscopy reveals multiple rectal vascular ectasias ("radiation proctopathy"). Acute infectious colitis (see Acute Diarrhea, above) commonly causes bloody diarrhea. Rare causes of lower tract bleeding include vasculitic ischemia, solitary rectal ulcer, NSAID-induced ulcers in the small bowel or right colon, small bowel diverticula, and colonic varices.

Clinical Findings

A. Symptoms and Signs

The color of the stool helps distinguish upper from lower GI bleeding, especially when observed by the clinician. Brown stools mixed or streaked with blood predict a source in the rectosigmoid or anus. Large volumes of bright red blood suggest a colonic source; maroon stools imply a lesion in the right colon or small intestine; and black stools (melena) predict a source proximal to the ligament of Treitz. Although 10% of patients admitted with self-reported hematochezia have an upper GI source of bleeding (eg, peptic ulcer), this almost always occurs in the setting of massive hemorrhage with hemodynamic instability. Painless large-volume bleeding usually suggests diverticular bleeding. Bloody diarrhea associated with cramping abdominal pain, urgency, or tenesmus is characteristic of IBD, infectious colitis, or ischemic colitis.

B. Diagnostic Tests

Important considerations in management include exclusion of an upper tract source and visualizing the lower tract bleeding source (eg, anoscopy and sigmoidoscopy, colonoscopy, CT angiography and angiography, and small intestine enteroscopy or capsule imaging). The studies selected depend on the severity of bleeding at presentation and the presence of hemodynamic instability with suspected ongoing, active bleeding.

1. Anoscopy and sigmoidoscopy—In otherwise healthy patients without anemia aged < 45 years with small-volume bleeding, anoscopy and sigmoidoscopy are performed to look for evidence of anorectal disease, IBD, or infectious colitis. If a lesion is found, no further evaluation is needed immediately unless the bleeding persists or is recurrent. In patients aged > 45 years with small-volume hematochezia, the entire colon must be evaluated with colonoscopy to exclude tumor.

2. Colonoscopy—In patients with acute, large-volume bleeding requiring hospitalization, colonoscopy is the preferred initial study in most cases. For patients with stable vital signs and whose lower GI bleeding appears to have stopped (> 75% of patients), colonoscopy can be performed electively during the hospital stay after appropriate resuscitation and bowel cleansing. For patients who are resuscitated and hemodynamically stable but have signs of continued active bleeding (< 25% of patients), earlier colonoscopy (within 12–24 hours) can be considered after oral administration of colonic lavage solution (4–8 L of GoLYTELY, CoLyte, or NuLyte) over 2–5 hours to clear the bowel of clots. The probable site of bleeding can be identified in 70–85% of patients, and a high-risk lesion can be identified and treated in up to 25%.

3. CT angiography—In patients with massive lower GI bleeding, hemodynamic instability, and suspected active bleeding, urgent radiographic imaging is warranted. Multidetector CT angiography is recommended to detect active arterial bleeding and to help localize bleeding to the stomach, upper GI tract, small intestine, right colon, or left colon. In patients with active bleeding demonstrated at CT angiography, urgent angiography with selective transcatheter embolization therapy is performed.

4. Exclusion of an upper tract source—To exclude an upper GI source of hematochezia, upper endoscopy should be considered in patients who have risk factors for an upper GI source (eg, prior peptic ulcer, decompensated liver disease, or an elevated BUN to creatinine ratio [BUN/Cr > 30]), and in patients with hematochezia and hemodynamic instability, unless prior CT angiography has demonstrated a bleeding site in the lower GI tract.

Treatment

Initial stabilization, blood replacement, and triage are managed in the same manner as described above in Acute Upper GI Bleeding. In patients with ongoing bleeding, consideration should be given to temporary discontinuation of antiplatelet agents and anticoagulants for up to 7 days. After cessation of the bleeding, resumption of antiplatelet agents or anticoagulants (if clinically indicated) is recommended to reduce the risk of serious cardiovascular and thromboembolic events, although the risk of recurrent hemorrhage is increased.

A. Therapeutic Colonoscopy

High-risk lesions (eg, angioectasia or diverticulum, rectal ulcer with active bleeding or a visible vessel) may be treated endoscopically with epinephrine injection, cautery (bipolar or heater probe), application of metallic endoclips or bands, or application of a hemostatic powder. Radiation-associated vascular ectasias are effectively treated with cautery.

B. Intra-arterial Embolization

When a bleeding lesion is identified, angiography with selective embolization achieves immediate hemostasis in > 95% of patients. Major complications occur in 5% (mainly ischemic colitis) and rebleeding occurs in up to 25%.

C. Surgical Treatment

Emergency surgery is rarely required with acute lower GI bleeding due to the efficacy of colonoscopic and angiographic therapies.

Surgery may be considered in patients with recurrent diverticular hemorrhage depending on the severity of bleeding and the patient's other comorbid conditions.

Sengupta N et al. Management of patients with acute lower gastrointestinal bleeding: an updated ACG guideline. Am J Gastroenterol. 2023;118:208. [PMID: 36735555]
Wan DW et al. Management of lower gastrointestinal bleeding. Am J Gastroenterol. 2024;119:10. [PMID: 37725688]

3. Suspected Small Bowel Bleeding

Bleeding from the small intestine can be overt or occult. *Overt* small bowel bleeding manifests as melena, maroon stools, or bright red blood per rectum. Up to 5–10% of patients admitted to hospitals with clinically overt GI bleeding do not have a cause identified on upper endoscopy or colonoscopy and may be suspected to have a small bowel source. *Occult* small bowel bleeding refers to bleeding that is manifested by recurrent positive FOBTs or FITs or recurrent iron deficiency anemia, or both in the absence of visible blood loss.

Evaluation of Overt Bleeding from Suspected Small Bowel Site

The most common causes of small intestinal bleeding in patients younger than 40 years are neoplasms (stromal tumors, lymphomas, adenocarcinomas, carcinoids), Crohn disease, celiac disease, and Meckel diverticulum. These disorders also occur in patients aged > 40 years; however, angioectasias (also called angiodysplasia or vascular ectasia) and NSAID-induced ulcers are far more common.

The evaluation of overt suspected small bowel bleeding depends on the age and overall health status of the patient, associated symptoms, and severity of the bleeding. Before pursuing evaluation of the small intestine, upper endoscopy and colonoscopy are often repeated to ascertain that a lesion in these regions has not been overlooked. If these studies are unrevealing and the patient is hemodynamically stable, capsule endoscopy should be performed to evaluate the small intestine. Further management depends on the capsule endoscopic findings, most commonly, angioectasias (25%), ulcers (10–25%), and neoplasms (1–10%). Multiphasic CT enterography may be considered if capsule endoscopy is unrevealing, since it is more sensitive for the detection of small bowel neoplasms and can exclude hepatic or pancreatic sources of bleeding. Laparotomy is warranted if a small bowel tumor is identified by capsule endoscopy or radiographic studies.

Most other lesions identified by capsule imaging can be further evaluated with enteroscopes that use overtubes with balloons to advance the scope through most of the small intestine (device-assisted enteroscopy). Neoplasms can be biopsied or resected. Angioectasias may be cauterized; however, recurrent occult or overt bleeding may recur, requiring iron supplementation or red blood cell transfusions. For bleeding attributed to angioectasias that persists, treatment with long-acting octreotide may be considered. In a 2024 multicenter randomized trial of patients with transfusion-dependent anemia from angioectasias previously treated endoscopically (when possible), those who received long-acting octreotide (40 mg intramuscular) every 28 days required fewer transfusions (11.0 at 1 year) than patients who received standard care (21.2 at 1 year).

For active, hemodynamically significant acute bleeding, CT angiography may be useful to identify and localize active small bowel bleeding and guide subsequent urgent angiography with embolization. A nuclear scan for Meckel diverticulum should be obtained in patients under age 30. With the advent of capsule imaging and advanced endoscopic technologies for evaluating and treating bleeding lesions in the small intestine, intraoperative enteroscopy of the small bowel is seldom required.

Goltstein LC et al. Standard of care versus octreotide in angiodysplasia-related bleeding (the OCEAN study): a multicenter randomized controlled trial. Gastroenterology. 2024;166:690. [PMID: 38158089]
Wild D et al. Small bowel bleeding. Clin Gastroenterol Hepatol 2025;23:24. [PMID: 39278261]

4. Occult GI Bleeding

Occult GI bleeding refers to bleeding that is not apparent to the patient. Chronic GI blood loss of < 100 mL/day may cause no appreciable change in stool appearance. Thus, occult bleeding in an adult is identified by a positive FOBT, FIT, or iron deficiency anemia in the absence of visible blood loss. FOBT or FIT may be performed in patients with GI symptoms or as a screening test for colorectal neoplasia (see Chapter 43). From 2% to 6% of patients in screening programs have a positive FOBT or FIT.

In the United States, 2% of men and 5% of women have iron deficiency anemia (serum ferritin < 30–45 mcg/L). In premenopausal women, iron deficiency anemia is most commonly attributable to menstrual and pregnancy-associated iron loss; however, a GI source of chronic blood loss is present in 10%. Occult blood loss may arise from anywhere in the GI tract. Among men and postmenopausal women, a potential GI cause of blood loss can be identified in the colon in 15–30% and in the upper GI tract in 35–55%; a malignancy is present in the lower GI tract in 8.9% and upper tract in 2.0%. Iron deficiency on rare occasions is caused by malabsorption (especially celiac disease) or malnutrition. The most common causes of occult bleeding with iron deficiency are (1) neoplasms; (2) vascular abnormalities (angioectasias); (3) acid-peptic lesions (esophagitis, peptic ulcer disease, erosions in hiatal hernia); (4) infections (nematodes, especially hookworm; tuberculosis); (5) medications (especially NSAIDs or aspirin); and (6) other causes such as IBD.

Evaluation of Occult Bleeding

Asymptomatic adults with positive FOBTs or FITs that are performed for routine colorectal cancer screening should undergo colonoscopy (see Chapter 43). *Symptomatic adults* with positive FOBTs or FITs or iron deficiency anemia should undergo evaluation of the lower and upper GI tract with colonoscopy and upper endoscopy, unless the anemia can be definitively ascribed to a nongastrointestinal source (eg, menstruation, blood donation, or recent surgery). Patients in whom upper and lower endoscopy did not reveal a bleeding source should be evaluated for possible celiac disease with either IgA anti-tTG or duodenal biopsy. After these evaluations, the origin of occult bleeding remains unexplained in 30–50% of patients.

For patients with iron deficiency anemia who have no significant findings on upper endoscopy or colonoscopy and who are without symptoms of small intestinal disease, an initial trial of empiric iron therapy is recommended. Once daily administration of oral formulations containing 150 mg of elemental iron are commonly recommended, but lower daily doses (60–100 mg) or alternate day dosing may be equally efficacious and better tolerated. A sustained rise in ferritin and hemoglobin with 1–2 months of iron therapy may obviate the need for further studies.

In patients who have anemia that responds poorly to empiric iron supplementation, who have signs of ongoing bleeding (fecal occult blood), or who have worrisome symptoms (abdominal pain, weight loss), further investigation of the small intestine is recommended. Capsule endoscopy is recommended as the initial study in most of these patients to look for vascular ectasias and to exclude a small intestinal neoplasia or IBD. If a small intestine source is identified, device-assisted enteroscopy, abdominal CT, or laparotomy is pursued, as indicated. When possible, antiplatelet agents (aspirin, NSAIDs, clopidogrel) should be discontinued. Patients with occult bleeding without a bleeding source identified after upper endoscopy, colonoscopy, and capsule endoscopy have a low risk of recurrent bleeding and usually can be managed with close observation.

DeLoughery TG et al. AGA Clinical Practice Guideline on management of iron deficiency anemia: expert review. Clin Gastroenterol Hepatol. 2024;22:1575. [PMID: 38864796]
Singh S et al. Management of obscure gastrointestinal bleeding. Am J Gastroenterol. 2025;120:500. [PMID: 39051790]

DISEASES OF THE PERITONEUM

ASSESSMENT OF THE PATIENT WITH ASCITES

Etiology of Ascites

The term "ascites" denotes the pathologic accumulation of fluid in the peritoneal cavity. The causes of ascites may be classified into two broad pathophysiologic categories: that which is associated with a normal peritoneum and that which occurs due to a diseased peritoneum (Table 17–7). The most common cause of ascites is portal hypertension secondary to chronic liver disease, which accounts for > 80% of patients with ascites. The management of portal hypertensive ascites is discussed in Chapter 18. The most common causes of nonportal hypertensive ascites include infections (tuberculous peritonitis), intra-abdominal malignancy, inflammatory disorders of the peritoneum, and ductal disruptions (chylous, pancreatic, biliary).

Table 17–7. Causes of ascites.

Normal Peritoneum
Portal hypertension (SAAG ≥ 1.1 g/dL)
Hepatic congestion[1]
HF
Constrictive pericarditis
Tricuspid insufficiency
Budd-Chiari syndrome
Veno-occlusive disease
Liver disease[2]
Cirrhosis
Alcoholic hepatitis
Fulminant hepatic failure
Massive hepatic metastases
Hepatic fibrosis
Acute fatty liver of pregnancy
Portal vein occlusion
Myxedema
Hypoalbuminemia (SAAG < 1.1 g/dL)
Nephrotic syndrome
Protein-losing enteropathy
Severe malnutrition with anasarca
Miscellaneous conditions (SAAG < 1.1 g/dL)
Chylous ascites
Pancreatic ascites
Bile ascites
Nephrogenic ascites
Urine ascites
Ovarian disease
Diseased Peritoneum
Infections (SAAG < 1.1 g/dL)[2]
Bacterial peritonitis
Tuberculous peritonitis
Fungal peritonitis
HIV-associated peritonitis
Malignant conditions (SAAG < 1.1 g/dL)
Peritoneal carcinomatosis
Primary mesothelioma
Pseudomyxoma peritonei
Massive hepatic metastases
HCC
Other conditions (SAAG < 1.1 g/dL)
Familial Mediterranean fever
Vasculitis
Granulomatous peritonitis
Eosinophilic peritonitis

[1]Hepatic congestion is usually associated with SAAG ≥ 1.1 g/dL and ascitic fluid total protein > 2.5 g/dL.
[2]There may be cases of "mixed ascites" in which portal hypertensive ascites is complicated by a secondary process such as infection. In these cases, the SAAG is ≥ 1.1 g/dL.
SAAG, serum-ascites albumin gradient = serum albumin minus ascitic fluid albumin.

Clinical Findings

A. Symptoms and Signs

The history usually is one of increasing abdominal girth, with the presence of abdominal pain depending on the cause. Because most ascites is secondary to chronic liver disease with portal hypertension, patients should be asked about risk factors for liver disease, especially alcohol consumption, transfusions, tattoos, injection drug use, a history of viral hepatitis or jaundice, and birth in an area endemic for hepatitis. A history of cancer or marked weight loss arouses suspicion of malignant ascites. Fevers may suggest infected peritoneal fluid, including bacterial peritonitis (spontaneous or secondary). Patients with chronic liver disease and ascites are at greatest risk for developing spontaneous bacterial peritonitis. In immigrants from regions of high infectivity, immunocompromised hosts, or severely malnourished persons with alcohol use disorder, tuberculous peritonitis should be considered.

Physical examination should look for signs of portal hypertension and chronic liver disease. Elevated jugular venous pressure may suggest right-sided HF or constrictive pericarditis. A large tender liver is characteristic of acute alcoholic hepatitis or Budd-Chiari syndrome (thrombosis of the hepatic veins). Large abdominal wall veins with cephalad flow suggest portal hypertension; inferiorly directed flow implies hepatic vein obstruction. Signs of chronic liver disease include palmar erythema, cutaneous spider angiomas, gynecomastia, muscle wasting, and asterixis from hepatic encephalopathy. Anasarca results from HF or nephrotic syndrome with hypoalbuminemia. Finally, firm lymph nodes in the left supraclavicular region or umbilicus suggest intra-abdominal malignancy.

The physical examination is relatively insensitive for detecting ascitic fluid. Even the experienced clinician may find it difficult to distinguish between obesity and small-volume ascites. Abdominal ultrasound establishes the presence of fluid.

B. Laboratory Testing

1. Abdominal paracentesis—Abdominal paracentesis is performed as part of the diagnostic evaluation in all patients with new onset of ascites. It also is recommended for patients admitted to the hospital with cirrhosis and ascites (in whom the prevalence of bacterial peritonitis is 10–20%) and when patients with known ascites deteriorate clinically (with fever, abdominal pain, worsened hepatic encephalopathy or worsened kidney function) to exclude bacterial peritonitis.

A. INSPECTION—Cloudy ascitic fluid is seen with infection. Milky fluid indicates chylous ascites (due to hypertriglyceridemia). Bloody fluid suggests either a traumatic paracentesis or malignant ascites (in up to 20% of cases).

B. ROUTINE STUDIES—

(1) Cell count—An ascitic WBC count with differential is the most important test. Normal ascitic fluid contains < 500 leukocytes/mcL (0.5×10^9/L) and < 250 polymorphonuclear neutrophils (PMNs)/mcL. Any inflammatory condition can cause an elevated ascitic WBC count. A PMN count of > 250/mcL (0.25×10^9/L) (neutrocytic ascites) with a PMN percentage of > 75% of all white cells is highly suggestive of bacterial peritonitis, either spontaneous primary peritonitis or secondary peritonitis (due to an intra-abdominal source of infection, eg, a perforated viscus or appendicitis). An elevated ascitic WBC with a predominance of lymphocytes arouses suspicion of tuberculosis or peritoneal carcinomatosis.

(2) Albumin and total protein—The serum-ascites albumin gradient (SAAG) is the best single test for the classification of ascites into portal hypertensive and nonportal hypertensive causes (Table 17–7). Calculated by subtracting the ascitic fluid albumin from the serum albumin, the gradient correlates directly with the portal pressure. A SAAG ≥ 1.1 g/dL suggests underlying portal hypertension, while gradients < 1.1 g/dL implicate nonportal hypertensive causes.

The accuracy of the SAAG exceeds 95% in classifying ascites. It should be recognized, however, that approximately 4% of patients have "mixed ascites," ie, underlying cirrhosis with portal hypertension complicated by a second cause for ascites formation (such as malignancy or tuberculosis). Thus, a high SAAG is indicative of portal hypertension but does not exclude concomitant malignancy.

The ascitic fluid total protein provides some additional clues to the cause. An elevated SAAG and a high protein level (> 2.5 g/dL) are seen in most cases of hepatic congestion secondary to cardiac disease or Budd-Chiari syndrome. However, a high ascitic fluid protein is also found in up to 20% of cases of uncomplicated cirrhosis and in two-thirds of patients with malignant ascites.

(3) Culture and Gram stain—The best technique consists of the inoculation of aerobic and anaerobic blood culture bottles with 5–10 mL of ascitic fluid at the patient's bedside, which increases the sensitivity for detecting bacterial peritonitis to over 85% in patients with neutrocytic ascites (> 250 PMNs/mcL [0.25×10^9/L]), compared with approximately 50% sensitivity by conventional agar plate or broth cultures.

C. OPTIONAL STUDIES—Other useful ascitic fluid laboratory tests include glucose and LD (helpful in distinguishing spontaneous from secondary bacterial peritonitis); amylase (elevation suggests pancreatic ascites or perforation of the GI tract with leakage of pancreatic secretions); creatinine (elevation suggests leakage of urine from the bladder or ureters); bilirubin (elevation suggests perforation of the biliary tree. Ascitic fluid cytologic examination is ordered if peritoneal carcinomatosis is suspected. Adenosine deaminase may be useful for the diagnosis of tuberculous peritonitis.

C. Imaging

Abdominal ultrasound is useful in confirming the presence of ascites and in guiding paracentesis. Both ultrasound and CT imaging can aid in distinguishing between causes of portal and nonportal hypertensive ascites. Doppler ultrasound and CT can detect Budd-Chiari syndrome. In nonportal hypertensive ascites, these studies can detect lymphadenopathy and masses in the mesentery, liver, ovaries, and pancreas. Furthermore, they permit directed percutaneous needle biopsies of these lesions. However, ultrasound and CT are not useful for detecting peritoneal carcinomatosis; the role of PET imaging is unclear.

D. Laparoscopy

In evaluating some patients with nonportal hypertensive ascites (low SAAG) or mixed ascites, laparoscopy permits direct visualization and biopsy of the peritoneum, liver, and some intra-abdominal lymph nodes. Cases of suspected peritoneal tuberculosis or suspected malignancy with nondiagnostic CT imaging and ascitic fluid cytology are best evaluated by laparoscopy.

Du L et al. Differential diagnosis of ascites: etiologies, ascitic fluid analysis, diagnostic algorithm. Clin Chem Lab Med. 2023;62:1266. [PMID: 38112289]

ASCITES COMPLICATED BY BACTERIAL INFECTION

"Spontaneous" bacterial infection of ascitic fluid occurs in the absence of an apparent intra-abdominal source of infection. (See Spontaneous Bacterial Peritonitis in Chapter 18.) It is seen with few exceptions in patients with ascites caused by chronic liver disease. Approximately 20–30% of patients with cirrhosis and ascites develop spontaneous peritonitis; however, the incidence is > 40% in patients with ascitic fluid total protein < 1 g/dL. The most important diagnostic test is abdominal paracentesis. Ascitic fluid should be sent for cell count with differential, and blood culture bottles should be inoculated at the bedside; in the proper clinical setting, an ascitic fluid PMN count > 250 cells/mcL (neutrocytic ascites) is presumptive evidence of bacterial peritonitis. Virtually all cases of spontaneous bacterial peritonitis are caused by a monomicrobial infection. The most common pathogens are enteric gram-negative bacteria (*E coli*, *Klebsiella pneumoniae*) or gram-positive bacteria (*Streptococcus pneumoniae*, viridans streptococci, *Enterococcus* species). Anaerobic bacteria are not associated with spontaneous bacterial peritonitis.

Secondary bacterial peritonitis must be distinguished from spontaneous bacterial peritonitis; in secondary bacterial peritonitis, ascitic fluid has become secondarily infected by an intra-abdominal infection and accounts for 3% of cases of infected ascitic fluid. Causes include appendicitis, diverticulitis, perforated peptic ulcer, and perforated gallbladder. Even with perforation, clinical symptoms and signs of peritonitis may be lacking owing to the separation of the visceral and parietal peritoneum by the ascitic fluid. Up to two-thirds of patients with secondary bacterial peritonitis have at least two of the following ascitic fluid findings: decreased glucose level (< 50 mg/dL), elevated LD level (greater than serum), and elevated total protein (> 1 g/dL). The presence of multiple organisms on ascitic fluid Gram stain or culture is diagnostic of secondary peritonitis. If secondary bacterial peritonitis is suspected, abdominal CT imaging of the upper and lower GI tracts should be obtained to look for evidence of an intra-abdominal source of infection. If these studies are negative and secondary peritonitis still is suspected, repeat paracentesis should be performed after 48 hours of antibiotic therapy to see if the PMN count is decreasing. In secondary bacterial peritonitis, the PMN count is not below the pretreatment value at 48 hours.

MALIGNANT ASCITES

Two-thirds of cases of malignant ascites are caused by peritoneal carcinomatosis. The most common causes are primary adenocarcinomas of the ovary, uterus, pancreas, stomach, colon, lung, or breast. The remaining one-third is due to lymphatic obstruction or portal hypertension due to HCC or diffuse hepatic metastases. Patients present with nonspecific abdominal discomfort and weight loss associated with increased abdominal girth. Nausea or vomiting may be caused by partial or complete intestinal obstruction. Abdominal CT may be useful to demonstrate the primary malignancy or hepatic metastases but seldom confirms the diagnosis of peritoneal carcinomatosis. In patients with carcinomatosis, paracentesis demonstrates a low serum ascites-albumin gradient (< 1.1 mg/dL), an increased total protein (> 2.5 g/dL), and an elevated WBC (often both neutrophils and mononuclear cells) but with a lymphocyte predominance. Cytology is positive in over 95%, but laparoscopy may be required in patients with negative cytology to confirm the diagnosis and to exclude tuberculous peritonitis, with which it may be confused. Malignant ascites attributable to portal hypertension usually is associated with an increased serum ascites-albumin gradient (> 1.1 g/dL), a variable total protein, and negative ascitic cytology. Ascites caused by peritoneal carcinomatosis does not respond to diuretics.

Patients may be treated with periodic large-volume paracentesis for symptomatic relief. Indwelling catheters can be left in place for patients approaching the end of life who require periodic paracentesis for symptomatic relief. Intraperitoneal chemotherapy is sometimes used to shrink the tumor, but the overall prognosis is extremely poor, with only 10% survival at 6 months. Ovarian cancers represent an exception to this rule. With newer treatments consisting of surgical debulking and intraperitoneal chemotherapy, long-term survival from ovarian cancer is possible.

Vierra MA et al. Novel therapies for palliation of malignant ascites. J Surr Res 2025;307:157. [PMID: 40037156]

FAMILIAL MEDITERRANEAN FEVER

This is a rare autosomal recessive disorder of unknown pathogenesis that almost exclusively affects people of Mediterranean ancestry, especially those of Sephardic Jewish, Armenian, Turkish, and Arab ancestry. Patients lack a protease in serosal fluids that normally inactivates interleukin (IL)-8 and the chemotactic complement factor 5A. Symptoms present in most patients before the age of 20 years. It is characterized by episodic bouts of acute peritonitis that may be associated with serositis involving the joints and pleura. Peritoneal attacks are marked by the sudden onset of fever, severe abdominal pain, and abdominal tenderness with guarding or rebound tenderness. If left untreated, attacks resolve within 24–48 hours. Because symptoms resemble those of surgical peritonitis, patients may undergo unnecessary exploratory laparotomy. Colchicine, 0.6 mg orally two or three times daily, has been shown to decrease the frequency and severity of attacks.

Ruscitti P et al. The clinical management of adult patients with Familial Mediterranean Fever. Expert Rev Clin Immunol. 2025;21:1503. [PMID: 41176687]

MESOTHELIOMA

(See Chapter 43.)

DISEASES OF THE ESOPHAGUS

(See Chapter 43 for Esophageal Cancer.)

Symptoms

Heartburn, dysphagia, and odynophagia almost always indicate a primary esophageal disorder.

A. Heartburn

Heartburn (pyrosis) is the feeling of substernal burning, often radiating to the neck. Most commonly caused by the reflux of acidic (or, rarely, alkaline) material into the esophagus, heartburn is highly suggestive of GERD.

B. Dysphagia

Dysphagia is defined as difficulty swallowing food or liquid due to the sensation of it sticking in the throat or chest, with a discomfort, or a choking sensation. Up to 15% of adults report dysphagia that requires compensatory maneuvers (avoiding certain foods or cutting into smaller pieces; eating more slowly; drinking liquids). Difficulties in swallowing may arise from problems in transferring the food bolus from the oropharynx to the upper esophagus (oropharyngeal dysphagia) or from impaired transport of the bolus through the body of the esophagus (esophageal dysphagia). The history often suggests the correct diagnosis.

1. Oropharyngeal dysphagia—The oropharyngeal phase of swallowing is a complex process requiring elevation of the tongue, closure of the nasopharynx, relaxation of the upper esophageal sphincter, closure of the airway, and pharyngeal peristalsis. A variety of mechanical and neuromuscular conditions can disrupt this process (Table 17–8). Problems with the oral phase of swallowing cause drooling or spillage of food from the mouth, inability to chew or initiate swallowing, or dry mouth. Oropharyngeal dysphagia is characterized by an immediate sense of the bolus catching in the neck, the need to swallow repeatedly to clear food from the pharynx, or coughing or choking during meals. There may be associated dysphonia, dysarthria, or other neurologic symptoms.

Table 17–8. Causes of oropharyngeal dysphagia.

Neurologic disorders
Brainstem cerebrovascular accident, mass lesion
Amyotrophic lateral sclerosis, multiple sclerosis, pseudobulbar palsy, post-polio syndrome, Guillain-Barré syndrome
Parkinson disease, Huntington disease, dementia
Tardive dyskinesia
Muscular and rheumatologic disorders
Myopathies, polymyositis
Oculopharyngeal dystrophy
Sjögren syndrome
Metabolic disorders
Thyrotoxicosis, amyloidosis, Cushing disease, Wilson disease
Medication side effects
Anticholinergics, phenothiazines
Infectious diseases
Polio, diphtheria, botulism, Lyme disease, syphilis, mucositis (*Candida*, herpes)
Structural disorders
Zenker diverticulum
Cervical osteophytes, cricopharyngeal bar, proximal esophageal webs
Oropharyngeal tumors
Postsurgical or radiation changes
Pill-induced injury
Motility disorders
Upper esophageal sphincter dysfunction

2. Esophageal dysphagia—Esophageal dysphagia may be caused by **mechanical obstructions** of the esophagus or by **motility disorders** (Table 17–9). Patients with **mechanical obstruction** experience dysphagia, primarily for solids. This is recurrent, predictable, and, if the lesion progresses, will worsen as the lumen narrows. Patients with **motility disorders** have dysphagia for both solids and liquids. It is episodic, unpredictable, and can be progressive.

Table 17–9. Causes of esophageal dysphagia.

Cause	Clues
Mechanical obstruction	**Solid foods worse than liquids**
Schatzki ring	Intermittent dysphagia; not progressive
Peptic stricture	Chronic heartburn; progressive dysphagia
Gastroesophageal reflux	Most with heartburn or regurgitation
Esophageal cancer	Progressive dysphagia; age > 50 years
Eosinophilic esophagitis	Young adults; small-caliber lumen, proximal stricture, corrugated rings, or white papules
Motility disorder	**Solid and liquid foods**
Achalasia	Progressive dysphagia
Spastic esophageal disorders	Intermittent; not progressive; may have chest pain
Systemic sclerosis (scleroderma)	Chronic heartburn; Raynaud phenomenon
Ineffective esophageal motility	Intermittent; not progressive; commonly associated with GERD

C. Odynophagia

Odynophagia is sharp substernal pain on swallowing that may limit oral intake. It usually reflects severe erosive disease most commonly from infectious esophagitis due to *Candida*, herpesviruses, or CMV, especially in immunocompromised patients. It may also be caused by corrosive injury due to caustic ingestions and by pill-induced ulcers.

Diagnostic Studies

A. Upper Endoscopy

Endoscopy is the study of choice for evaluating persistent heartburn, dysphagia, odynophagia, and structural abnormalities detected on barium esophagography. In addition to direct visualization, it allows for biopsy of mucosal abnormalities and of normal mucosa (to evaluate for eosinophilic esophagitis) as well as for dilation of strictures.

B. Videoesophagography

Oropharyngeal dysphagia is best evaluated with rapid-sequence videoesophagography.

C. Barium Esophagography

Patients with esophageal dysphagia often are evaluated first with a barium esophagography to differentiate between mechanical lesions and motility disorders, providing important information about the latter in particular. In patients in whom there is a high suspicion of a mechanical lesion, many clinicians will proceed first to endoscopic evaluation because it better identifies mucosal lesions (eg, erosions) and permits mucosal biopsy and dilation. However, barium study is more sensitive for detecting subtle esophageal narrowing due to rings, achalasia, and proximal esophageal lesions.

D. Esophageal Manometry

Esophageal motility may be best assessed using high-resolution manometry with multiple, closely spaced sensors. Manometry is indicated (1) to determine the location of the LES to allow precise placement of a conventional electrode pH probe; (2) to establish the etiology of dysphagia when a mechanical obstruction cannot be found, especially if a diagnosis of achalasia is suspected by endoscopy or barium study; and (3) during the preoperative assessment of for antireflux surgery to exclude an alternative diagnosis (eg, achalasia) or possibly to assess peristaltic function in the esophageal body.

Functional lumen imaging probe (FLIP) is an FDA-approved device that can be used during upper endoscopy to assess the diameter and distensibility of the GE junction (using a fluid-filled balloon) and the contractile response of the esophageal body (using pressure impedance sensors). Although high-resolution manometry remains the gold standard for motility testing, FLIP is useful to screen for a motility disorder in patients with dysphagia in whom endoscopic evaluation reveals no apparent structural or mechanical cause. It also is useful for further assessment of the GE junction when manometry detects elevated GE junction relaxation pressures (to distinguish achalasia from esophagogastric junction outflow obstruction) and following surgical or endoscopic treatment of achalasia.

E. Esophageal pH Recording and Impedance Testing

The pH within the esophageal lumen may be monitored continuously for 24–96 hours. Catheter-based systems use a long transnasal catheter that is connected directly to the recording device. With wireless systems, a capsule is attached directly to the esophageal mucosa under endoscopic visualization and data are transmitted by radiotelemetry to the recording device. The recording provides information about the amount of esophageal acid reflux and the temporal correlations between symptoms and reflux.

Wireless pH monitoring devices provide information about the amount of esophageal acid reflux but not nonacid reflux. Transnasal catheters using combined pH and multichannel intraluminal impedance allow assessment of acid and nonacid liquid reflux. They may be useful in the evaluation of atypical reflux symptoms or persistent symptoms despite therapy with PPIs to diagnose hypersensitivity, functional symptoms, and symptoms caused by nonacid reflux.

Gregor J et al. Comprehensive multidisciplinary evaluation of dysphagia. Clin Gastroenterol Hepatol. 2025;23:707. [PMID: 39855630]

Nguyen A et al. AGA clinical practice update on incorporating functional lumen imaging probe into esophageal clinical practice. Gastroenterology. 2025;169:726. [PMID: 40679455]

GASTROESOPHAGEAL REFLUX DISEASE

ESSENTIALS OF DIAGNOSIS

- Heartburn; may be exacerbated by meals, bending, or recumbency.
- Typical uncomplicated cases do not require diagnostic studies.
- Endoscopy demonstrates abnormalities in one-third of patients.

General Considerations

GERD is a condition that develops when the reflux of stomach contents causes troublesome symptoms or complications. Approximately 30% of adults experience GERD symptoms at least weekly. The two most common symptoms are heartburn and regurgitation. Other symptoms of GERD include dyspepsia, dysphagia, belching, chest pain, cough, hoarseness, and impaired sleep. Although most patients have mild disease, esophageal mucosal damage (reflux esophagitis) develops in up to one-third and more serious complications develop in a few others. Several factors may contribute to GERD.

A. Dysfunction of the Gastroesophageal Junction

The antireflux barrier at the gastroesophageal junction depends on LES pressure, the intra-abdominal location of the sphincter, and the extrinsic compression of the sphincter by the crural diaphragm. Although most patients with GERD have normal LES pressures, a subset has an incompetent LES that results in increased acid reflux, especially when supine or when intra-abdominal pressures are increased by lifting or bending. A hypotensive sphincter is present in up to 50% of patients with severe erosive GERD.

Hiatal hernias are found in one-fourth of patients with nonerosive GERD, three-fourths of patients with severe erosive esophagitis, and over 90% of patients with Barrett esophagus. They are caused by movement of the LES above the diaphragm, resulting in dysfunction of the gastroesophageal junction reflux barrier. Hiatal hernias are common and may cause no symptoms; however, in patients with gastroesophageal reflux, they are associated with higher amounts of acid reflux and delayed esophageal acid clearance, leading to more severe esophagitis and Barrett esophagus. Increased reflux episodes occur during normal swallowing-induced relaxation, transient LES relaxations, and straining due to reflux of acid from the hiatal hernia sac into the esophagus.

Truncal obesity may contribute to GERD, presumably due to an increased intra-abdominal pressure, which contributes to dysfunction of the gastroesophageal junction and increased likelihood of hiatal hernia.

B. Irritant Effects of Refluxate

Esophageal mucosal damage is related to the potency of the refluxate and the amount of time it is in contact with the mucosa. Acidic gastric fluid (pH < 4.0) is extremely caustic to the esophageal mucosa and is the major injurious agent in the majority of cases. In some patients, reflux of bile or alkaline pancreatic secretions may be contributory.

C. Abnormal Esophageal Clearance

Acid refluxate normally is cleared and neutralized by esophageal peristalsis and salivary bicarbonate. Patients with severe GERD may have diminished clearance due to weak, ineffective peristaltic contractions. Certain medical conditions such as systemic sclerosis (scleroderma) are associated with diminished peristalsis. Sjögren syndrome, anticholinergic medications, and oral radiation therapy may exacerbate GERD due to impaired salivation.

D. Delayed Gastric Emptying

Impaired gastric emptying due to gastroparesis or partial gastric outlet obstruction potentiates GERD.

E. Esophageal Hypersensitivity

Patients with reflux hypersensitivity experience reflux symptoms that correlate with some acid reflux events but have normal total levels of measured esophageal acid reflux over a 24-hour period of esophageal pH recording. This heightened sensitivity may be exacerbated by stress or anxiety.

Clinical Findings

A. Symptoms and Signs

The typical symptom is heartburn. This most often occurs 30–60 minutes after meals and upon reclining. Patients often report relief from taking antacids or baking soda. Many patients, however, have less specific dyspeptic symptoms with or without heartburn. Heartburn severity is not correlated with the presence or severity of tissue damage. In fact, some patients with severe esophagitis are only mildly symptomatic. Patients may report regurgitation—the spontaneous reflux of sour or bitter gastric contents into the mouth. Dysphagia occurs in one-third of patients and may be due to erosive esophagitis, abnormal esophageal peristalsis, or the development of an esophageal stricture. Overall, a clinical diagnosis of GERD has a sensitivity and specificity of only 65%.

"Atypical" or "extraesophageal" manifestations of GERD may occur, including asthma, chronic cough, chronic laryngitis, sore throat, noncardiac chest pain, and sleep disturbances. In the absence of heartburn or regurgitation, atypical symptoms are unlikely to be related to gastroesophageal reflux.

Physical examination and laboratory data are normal in uncomplicated disease.

B. Special Examinations

Upper endoscopy is recommended for patients with "alarm" symptoms (dysphagia, odynophagia, iron deficiency anemia, weight loss) to identify complications of reflux disease and for patients at increased risk for Barrett esophagus (ie, chronic reflux for > 5 years with three or more risk factors: age > 50 years, obesity, White race, male sex, tobacco use, and family history). Initial diagnostic studies are not warranted for typical GERD symptoms that suggest uncomplicated reflux disease and no "alarm" symptoms. Such patients should be treated empirically with a once-daily PPI for 4–8 weeks. Further investigation with upper endoscopy, ambulatory esophageal pH monitoring, or both is warranted in patients with symptoms that persist despite empiric acid inhibitory therapy.

1. Upper endoscopy—Upper endoscopy is excellent for documenting the type and extent of tissue damage in GERD; for detecting other gastroesophageal lesions that may mimic GERD; and for detecting GERD complications, including esophageal stricture, Barrett metaplasia, and esophageal adenocarcinoma. In the absence of prior antisecretory therapy, up to one-third of patients with GERD have visible mucosal damage (known as reflux esophagitis), characterized by single or multiple erosions or ulcers in the distal esophagus at the squamocolumnar junction. In patients treated with a PPI prior to endoscopy, preexisting reflux esophagitis may be partially or completely healed. The Los Angeles (LA) classification grades reflux esophagitis on a scale of A (one or more isolated mucosal breaks ≤ 5 mm that do not extend between the tops of two mucosal folds) to D (one or more mucosal breaks that involve at least 75% of the esophageal circumference).

2. Barium esophagography—This study should not be routinely performed to diagnose GERD; for severe dysphagia, it is sometimes obtained prior to endoscopy to identify a stricture. It is also performed prior to antireflux surgery to assess hiatal hernia size.

3. Esophageal pH or combined esophageal pH-impedance testing—Esophageal pH monitoring measures the amount of esophageal acid reflux, whereas combined pH-impedance testing measures both acidic and nonacidic reflux. Both tests may be useful to establish whether there is a temporal relationship between reflux events and symptoms. They are the most accurate studies for documenting gastroesophageal reflux but are unnecessary in most patients who have typical symptoms and satisfactory response to empiric antisecretory therapy. They are indicated in patients with typical symptoms who have unsatisfactory response to empiric antisecretory therapy, for atypical or extraesophageal symptoms, and for those who are being considered for antireflux surgery.

Differential Diagnosis

Symptoms of GERD may be similar to those of other diseases such as angina pectoris, eosinophilic esophagitis, esophageal motility disorders, dyspepsia, peptic ulcer, or functional disorders. Reflux erosive esophagitis may be confused with pill-induced damage, eosinophilic esophagitis, or infections (CMV, herpes, *Candida*).

Complications

A. Barrett Esophagus

This is a condition in which the squamous epithelium of the esophagus is replaced by metaplastic columnar epithelium containing goblet and columnar cells (specialized intestinal metaplasia). Present in 1–5% of the general population and 7–11% of patients with chronic reflux, Barrett esophagus is believed to arise from chronic reflux-induced injury to the esophageal squamous epithelium; however, it is also increased in patients with truncal obesity independent of GERD. Barrett esophagus is suspected at endoscopy from the presence of orange, gastric type epithelium that extends upward > 1 cm from the gastroesophageal junction into the distal tubular esophagus in a tongue-like or circumferential fashion. Biopsies obtained at endoscopy confirm the diagnosis. Three types of columnar epithelium may be identified: gastric cardiac, gastric fundic, and specialized intestinal metaplasia. It is the latter that carries an increased risk of dysplasia.

The most serious complication of Barrett esophagus is esophageal adenocarcinoma. Most adenocarcinomas of the esophagus and many such tumors of the gastric cardia likely arise from dysplastic epithelium in Barrett esophagus. The incidence of adenocarcinoma in patients with Barrett esophagus is estimated at 0.2–0.5% per year. Although this is an 11-fold increased risk compared with patients without Barrett esophagus, adenocarcinoma of the esophagus remains a relatively uncommon malignancy in the United States (9000 cases/year). The prognosis for adenocarcinomas of the esophagus that are diagnosed after the onset of symptoms (eg, dysphagia, pain, anemia) is poor. Therefore, several professional societies advocate for endoscopic screening of patients with chronic GERD to detect intestinal metaplasia of the esophagus (Barrett esophagus), esophageal dysplasia, or early-stage adenocarcinoma. Given the large number of adults with chronic GERD relative to the small number in whom adenocarcinoma develops and the costs and risks of upper endoscopy, 2022 American College of Gastroenterology guidelines recommend endoscopic screening only in adults who have had at least weekly GERD symptoms for 5 or more years with three or more risk factors for adenocarcinoma (age > 50 years, male sex, White race, truncal obesity, current or prior history of smoking, or a family history of esophageal adenocarcinoma). Using high-definition endoscopes, any visualized columnar epithelium extending into the esophagus > 1 cm above the gastroesophageal junction should be carefully examined and undergo multiple forceps biopsies to determine the presence of specialized intestinal metaplasia (Barrett esophagus) with or without dysplasia. As an alternative to endoscopic screening, the 2022 ACG guideline also endorses a swallowable capsule-sponge to obtain esophageal cytology for the assessment of biomarkers that predict the presence of Barrett esophagus.

In patients known to have nondysplastic Barrett esophagus, surveillance endoscopy every 3–5 years (depending on the length of the Barrett change in the esophagus) is recommended to look for low- or high-grade dysplasia or adenocarcinoma. A 2025 AGA guideline recommends that surveillance be performed using a combination of high-definition white light endoscopy and enhanced imaging with chromoendoscopy. Biopsies are obtained from nodular or irregular mucosa (which have an increased risk of high-grade dysplasia or cancer) as well as randomly from the esophagus every 1–2 cm. In patients with nondysplastic Barrett esophagus, the risk of progression to high-grade dysplasia or cancer is related to the length of Barrett epithelium. This risk is 0.29%/year for those with columnar epithelium lengths of 1–3 cm (short-segment) and 0.91%/year in those with lengths > 3 cm (long-segment). The finding of dysplasia should be confirmed by a second, expert pathologist.

Endoscopic therapy is the standard of care for patients who have Barrett esophagus with high-grade dysplasia or well-differentiated mucosal adenocarcinoma (Tis or T1a). Patients with low-grade dysplasia may be recommended for either endoscopic therapy or close endoscopic surveillance every 6–12 months. Therapy should be performed by endoscopists with expertise in advanced resection and ablation techniques. All nodules should be removed to assess for the presence and depth of cancer. Following resection, ablation of any remaining Barrett mucosa is performed with radiofrequency wave electrocautery. The efficacy of endoscopic ablation therapies in patients with Barrett dysplasia is supported by several studies. When high-dose PPIs are administered to normalize intraesophageal pH, radiofrequency wave ablation and electrocautery eradication of Barrett columnar epithelium is followed by complete healing with normal squamous epithelium in > 78% of patients and elimination of dysplasia in 91%.

Endoscopic ablation techniques have a risk of complications (bleeding, perforation, strictures). Therefore, endoscopic eradication therapy is not recommended for patients with nondysplastic Barrett esophagus for whom the risk of developing esophageal cancer is low and treatment does not appear to be cost-effective.

B. Peptic Stricture

Stricture formation occurs in up to 5% of patients with esophagitis. Gradual progressive solid food dysphagia develops over months to years. Most strictures are located at the gastroesophageal junction. Endoscopy with biopsy is mandatory in all cases to differentiate peptic stricture from stricture by esophageal carcinoma. Active erosive esophagitis is often present. Up to 90% of symptomatic patients are effectively treated by dilation at the time of endoscopy or fluoroscopically. Dilation is continued over one to several sessions. A luminal diameter of 15–18 mm is usually sufficient to relieve dysphagia. Long-term therapy with a PPI is required to decrease the likelihood of stricture recurrence.

Treatment

A. Medical Treatment

The goal of treatment is to provide symptomatic relief, to heal esophagitis (if present), and to prevent complications. In the majority of patients with uncomplicated disease, empiric treatment is initiated based on a compatible history without the need for further confirmatory studies. Patients not responding and those with suspected complications undergo further evaluation with upper endoscopy or ambulatory esophageal pH recording.

1. Mild, intermittent symptoms—Patients with mild or intermittent symptoms that do not impact adversely on quality of life may benefit from lifestyle modifications with medical interventions taken as needed. Eating smaller meals and elimination of acidic foods (citrus, tomatoes, coffee, spicy foods), foods that precipitate reflux (fatty foods, chocolate, peppermint, alcohol), and cigarettes may reduce symptoms. Weight loss should be recommended for patients who are overweight or have had recent weight gain. All patients should be advised to avoid lying down within 3 hours after meals (the period of greatest reflux). Patients with nocturnal symptoms should also elevate the head of the bed on 6-inch blocks or a foam wedge to reduce reflux and enhance esophageal clearance. Sleeping on the left side significantly reduces nighttime esophageal acid exposure compared with the right side and supine positions.

Infrequent heartburn (less than once weekly) may be treated on demand with antacids or oral H_2-receptor antagonists. Antacids provide rapid relief of heartburn; however, their duration of action is < 2 hours. Many are available over the counter. Alginate-containing formulations (eg, Gaviscon Double Action liquid) may be superior to other antacids in reducing postprandial symptoms. Antacids containing magnesium or aluminum should not be used for patients with kidney disease.

The oral H_2-receptor antagonists may be used on demand for intermittent heartburn symptoms or taken prophylactically before meals known to provoke symptoms. They come in a variety of strengths: cimetidine 200 mg; famotidine 10 mg and 20 mg; and nizatidine 75 mg and 150 mg. Most of these drug strengths are available over the counter. When taken for active heartburn, these agents have a delay in onset of at least 30 minutes. However, once these agents take effect, they provide heartburn relief for up to 8 hours.

2. Troublesome symptoms—

A. INITIAL THERAPY—More frequent or troublesome symptoms should be treated with a once-daily oral PPI for 4–8 weeks. Following daily, preprandial dosing (30–60 minutes before breakfast), they achieve significant acid suppression, which wanes during the nocturnal period. Available compounds include omeprazole or immediate-release omeprazole, 20 mg; rabeprazole, 20 mg; lansoprazole, 30 mg; dexlansoprazole, 30–60 mg; esomeprazole, 20–40 mg; or pantoprazole, 40 mg. Because there is little difference between these agents in efficacy or side-effect profiles, the choice of agent is determined by cost. For patients with an inadequate symptom response, dosing may be increased to twice daily (30 minutes before breakfast and dinner) or changed to another PPI. Once-daily PPIs achieve adequate control of heartburn in 70–80% of patients, complete heartburn resolution in > 50%, and healing of erosive esophagitis (when present) in 75–85%. In contrast, PPIs are less effective in reducing bothersome regurgitation. Because of their superior efficacy and ease of use, PPIs are preferred to H_2-receptor antagonists for the initial treatment of troublesome acute and chronic GERD.

B. LONG-TERM THERAPY—In those who achieve good symptomatic relief with a course of empiric once- or twice-daily PPI, therapy may be discontinued after 4–8 weeks. More than 80% of patients will experience relapse of GERD symptoms, usually within 3 months. Patients whose symptoms relapse may be treated with either continuous PPI therapy (prescribed at the lowest effective dose), alternative day therapy, intermittent 2- to 4-week courses, or "on-demand" therapy (ie, drug taken until symptoms abate) depending on symptom frequency and patient preference. Patients who require twice-daily PPI therapy for initial symptom control and patients with complications of GERD, including severe erosive esophagitis, Barrett esophagus, or peptic stricture, should be maintained on long-term therapy with a once- or twice-daily PPI titrated to the lowest effective dose to achieve satisfactory symptom control.

PPIs are considered to be extremely safe. Although a number of safety concerns have been raised in retrospective observational studies, it is difficult to determine whether the modest associations identified are due to a causal relationship. Long-term use of PPIs likely does have a small increased risk of infectious gastroenteritis (including *C difficile*) and small intestinal bacterial overgrowth, as well as micronutrient deficiencies (iron, vitamin B_{12}, magnesium). High-quality studies have not found an increased risk of other previously reported adverse events, including micronutrient deficiency (iron, magnesium, B_{12}), osteoporosis, and CKD (due to interstitial nephritis); however, a small risk cannot be excluded with certainty. Long-term PPI therapy should be prescribed to patients with appropriate indications and at the lowest effective dose.

3. Unresponsive disease—Up to one-third of patients report inadequate relief of heartburn or regurgitation with once-daily PPI therapy. Patients unresponsive to once-daily therapy should undergo endoscopy for detection of inadequately treated erosive reflux esophagitis and for other gastroesophageal conditions (including eosinophilic esophagitis and achalasia) that may mimic GERD. Refractory erosive esophagitis may be caused by medical nonadherence, resistance to PPIs, or gastrinoma with gastric acid hypersecretion (Zollinger-Ellison syndrome). Patients with persistent erosive esophagitis may respond to an increase in PPI therapy to twice daily (30 minutes before breakfast or dinner).

Vonoprazan is a novel, reversible, potassium-competitive acid blocker of the proton pump (P-CAB) that is FDA-approved for the treatment of non-erosive and erosive esophagitis. In contrast to standard PPIs, vonoprazan may be given with meals and achieves potent, sustained acid suppression both daytime and nighttime that begins on the first day of therapy. In an RCT of patients with erosive esophagitis, vonoprazan (20 mg orally once daily) achieved higher healing than lansoprazole (30 mg orally once daily) among patients with severe erosive esophagitis (LA grades C and D): 92% versus 72%, respectively. The efficacy of vonoprazan versus a PPI twice daily (commonly prescribed for severe esophagitis) for treatment of severe erosive esophagitis has not been established. In the United States, vonoprazan is more expensive than a single- or double-dose PPI. The risk of long-term use of vonoprazan likely is similar to that of PPIs. Based on higher costs and fewer long-term safety data than PPIs, vonoprazan may be considered in patients with persistent heartburn or erosive esophagitis that is unresponsive to twice-daily PPI therapy.

For patients with refractory symptoms without clear evidence of reflux disease, ambulatory esophageal pH testing is recommended after stopping PPI therapy for 96 hours to determine if significant esophageal acid reflux is present and if the symptoms are associated with reflux episodes. Approximately 30% of patients with unresponsive symptoms do not have increased reflux or a significant symptom correlation with reflux episodes and are diagnosed with "functional heartburn," a functional disorder. Cognitive behavioral therapy, instruction on diaphragmatic breathing, or treatment with a low-dose tricyclic antidepressant (eg, imipramine or nortriptyline 25 mg orally at bedtime) may be beneficial.

4. Extraesophageal reflux manifestations—Establishing a causal relationship between gastroesophageal reflux and extraesophageal symptoms (eg, asthma, hoarseness, cough, sleep disturbances) is difficult. Gastroesophageal reflux seldom is the sole cause of extraesophageal disorders but may be a contributory factor. Although ambulatory esophageal pH testing can document the presence of increased acid esophageal reflux, it does not prove a causative connection. Guidelines recommend that a trial of a twice-daily PPI be administered for 2–3 months in patients with suspected extraesophageal GERD syndromes who also have typical GERD symptoms. Improvement of extraesophageal symptoms suggests but does not prove that acid reflux is the causative factor. Esophageal impedance-pH testing may be performed in patients whose extraesophageal symptoms persist after 3 months of PPI therapy and may be considered before PPI therapy in patients without typical GERD symptoms in whom other causes of extraesophageal symptoms have been excluded.

B. Surgical Treatment

Surgical fundoplication affords good to excellent relief of symptoms and healing of esophagitis in over 85% of properly selected patients and can be performed laparoscopically with low complication rates in most instances. Although patient satisfaction is high, typical reflux symptoms recur in 10–30% of patients. Furthermore, new symptoms of dysphagia, bloating, increased flatulence, dyspepsia, or diarrhea develop in > 30% of patients. In a 2019 RCT of patients with refractory heartburn and confirmed reflux (acid or nonacid) despite twice-daily PPI therapy, fundoplication resulted in 67% adequate symptom relief at 1 year compared with 12–28% with continued medical therapy. Surgical treatment is not recommended for patients who are well controlled with medical therapies but should be considered for those with severe reflux disease who do not accept lifelong medical therapy due to its expense, inconvenience, or theoretical risks as well as for patients with proven refractory GERD symptoms or bothersome regurgitation despite PPI therapy. Gastric bypass (rather than fundoplication) should be considered for patients with obesity who also have GERD.

A minimally invasive magnetic artificial sphincter is FDA approved for the treatment of GERD in patients with hiatal hernias < 3 cm in size. In prospective clinical trials with up to 5 years of follow-up, magnetic sphincter augmentation has demonstrated GERD symptom relief equivalent to laparoscopic fundoplication but with far fewer side effects (long-term dysphagia 4–10%, bloating 8%, diarrhea 2%, nausea/vomiting 2%). In patients with moderate to severe regurgitation, magnetic sphincter augmentation led to significant improvement of regurgitation in 96% of patients compared with 19% treated with twice-daily PPIs. Given the excellent safety and efficacy data demonstrated with this device to date, it should be considered as an alternative to fundoplication surgery for patients with GERD, especially those with troublesome regurgitation, and hiatal hernias < 3 cm in size.

Several endoscopic procedures have been developed to treat GERD; however, none have found wide acceptance, largely due to limited long-term efficacy.

When to Refer

- Patients with typical GERD whose symptoms do not resolve with empiric management with a twice-daily PPI.
- Patients with suspected extraesophageal GERD symptoms that do not resolve with 3 months of twice-daily PPI therapy.

- Patients with significant dysphagia or other "alarm" symptoms for upper endoscopy.
- Patients with Barrett esophagus for endoscopic surveillance.
- Patients who have Barrett esophagus with dysplasia or early mucosal cancer.
- Surgical therapy is considered.

Kamboj AK et al. Long-term proton pump inhibitor use: review of indications and special considerations. Clin Gastroenterol Hepatol. 2024;22:1373. [PMID: 38471653]
Patel A et al. AGA clinical practice update on integrating potassium-competitive acid blockers into clinical practice: expert review. Gastroenterology. 2024;167:1226. [PMID: 39269391]
Rubenstein JH et al. AGA clinical practice guideline on endoscopic eradication therapy of Barrett's esophagus and related neoplasia. Gastroenterology. 2024;166:1020. [PMID: 38763697]
Saha B et al. Prevalence of Barrett's esophagus and esophageal adenocarcinoma with and without gastroesophageal reflux: a systematic review and meta-analysis. Clin Gastroenterol Hepatol. 2024;22:1381. [PMID: 37879525]
Wani S et al. AGA clinical practice guideline on surveillance of Barrett's esophagus. Gastroenterology. 2025;169:1184. [PMID: 41125322]
Zhuang Q et al. Comparative efficacy of P-CAB vs proton pump inhibitors for grade C/D esophagitis: a systematic review and network meta-analysis. Am J Gastroenterol. 2024;119:803. [PMID: 38345252]

INFECTIOUS ESOPHAGITIS

ESSENTIALS OF DIAGNOSIS

- Immunosuppressed patient.
- Odynophagia, dysphagia, and chest pain.
- Endoscopy with biopsy establishes diagnosis.

General Considerations

Infectious esophagitis occurs most commonly in immunosuppressed patients. Patients with AIDS, solid organ transplants, leukemia, lymphoma, and those receiving immunosuppressive drugs are at particular risk for opportunistic infections. *Candida albicans*, herpes simplex, and CMV are the most common pathogens. *Candida* infection may occur also in patients who have uncontrolled diabetes and those being treated with systemic corticosteroids, radiation therapy, or systemic antibiotic therapy. Herpes simplex can affect normal hosts, in which case the infection is generally self-limited.

Clinical Findings

A. Symptoms and Signs

The most common symptoms are odynophagia and dysphagia. Substernal chest pain occurs in some patients. Patients with candidal esophagitis are sometimes asymptomatic. Oral thrush is present in only 75% of patients with candidal esophagitis but also occurs in 25–50% of patients with viral esophagitis and is therefore an unreliable indicator of the cause of esophageal infection. Patients with esophageal CMV infection may have infection at other sites such as the colon and retina. Oral ulcers (herpes labialis) are often associated with herpes simplex esophagitis.

B. Special Examinations

Treatment may be empiric. For diagnostic certainty, endoscopy with biopsy and brushings (for microbiologic and histopathologic analysis) is preferred because of its high diagnostic accuracy. The endoscopic signs of candidal esophagitis are diffuse, linear, yellow-white plaques adherent to the mucosa. CMV esophagitis is characterized by one to several large, shallow, superficial ulcerations. Herpes esophagitis results in multiple small, deep ulcerations.

Treatment

A. Candidal Esophagitis

Systemic therapy is required for esophageal candidiasis. An empiric trial of antifungal therapy is often administered without performing diagnostic endoscopy. Initial therapy is generally with fluconazole, 400 mg orally on day 1, then 200–400 mg/day for 14–21 days. Patients not responding to empiric therapy within 3–5 days should undergo endoscopy with brushings, biopsy, and culture to distinguish resistant fungal infection from other infections (eg, CMV, herpes). Esophageal candidiasis not responding to fluconazole therapy may be treated with itraconazole suspension (not capsules), 200 mg/day orally, or voriconazole, 200 mg orally twice daily. Refractory infection may be treated intravenously with micafungin 150 mg daily or caspofungin 50 mg daily for 28 days. Consultation with an infectious disease specialist is advised.

B. Cytomegalovirus Esophagitis

In patients with HIV infection, immune restoration with antiretroviral therapy is the most effective means of controlling CMV disease. Initial therapy is with ganciclovir, 5 mg/kg intravenously every 12 hours for 3–6 weeks. Neutropenia is a frequent dose-limiting side effect. Once resolution of symptoms occurs, it may be possible to complete the course of therapy with oral valganciclovir, 900 mg once daily. Patients who either do not respond to or cannot tolerate ganciclovir are treated acutely with foscarnet, 90 mg/kg intravenously every 12 hours for 3–6 weeks. The principal toxicities are AKI, hypocalcemia, and hypomagnesemia.

C. Herpetic Esophagitis

Immunocompetent patients may be treated symptomatically and generally do not require specific antiviral therapy. Immunosuppressed patients may be treated with oral acyclovir, 400 mg orally five times daily, or 250 mg/m^2 intravenously every 8–12 hours, usually for 14–21 days. Oral famciclovir, 500 mg orally three times daily, or valacyclovir, 1 g twice daily, are also effective but more expensive than generic acyclovir. Patients who do not respond require therapy with foscarnet, 40 mg/kg intravenously every 8 hours for 21 days.

Prognosis

Most patients with infectious esophagitis can be effectively treated with complete symptom resolution. Depending on the patient's underlying immunodeficiency, relapse of symptoms off therapy can raise difficulties. Long-term suppressive therapy is sometimes required.

Hasoda K et al. Herpetic esophagitis in healthy young adult. J Clin Gastroenterol. 2023;16:803. [PMID: 37713095]

Hirai T et al. Pharmacological management of oral and esophageal candidiasis: a clinical pharmacotherapy perspective. J Clin Med. 2025;14:7537. [PMID: 41226935]

PILL-INDUCED ESOPHAGITIS

A number of different medications may injure the esophagus. The most commonly implicated are NSAIDs, bisphosphonates, potassium chloride, quinidine, zalcitabine, zidovudine, alendronate and risedronate, emepronium bromide, iron, vitamin C, and antibiotics (doxycycline, tetracycline, clindamycin, trimethoprim-sulfamethoxazole). Because injury is most likely to occur if pills are swallowed without water or while supine, hospitalized or bed-bound patients are at greater risk. Symptoms include severe retrosternal chest pain, odynophagia, and dysphagia, often beginning several hours after taking a pill. These may occur suddenly and persist for days. Some patients (especially older patients) have relatively little pain, presenting with dysphagia. Endoscopy may reveal one to several discrete ulcers that may be shallow or deep. Chronic injury may result in severe esophagitis with stricture, hemorrhage, or perforation. Healing occurs rapidly when the offending agent is eliminated. To prevent pill-induced damage, patients should take pills with 4 oz of water and remain upright for 30 minutes after ingestion. Known offending agents should not be given to patients with esophageal dysmotility, dysphagia, or strictures.

Angelette AL et al. Tetracycline-, doxycycline-, minocycline-induced pseudotumor cerebri and esophageal perforation. Adv Ther. 2023;40:1366. [PMID: 36763302]

Hourany G et al. Isotretinoin-induced pill esophagitis. ACG Case Rep J. 2025;12:e01596. [PMID: 39925793]

BENIGN ESOPHAGEAL LESIONS

1. Mallory-Weiss Syndrome (Mucosal Laceration of Gastroesophageal Junction)

ESSENTIALS OF DIAGNOSIS

- Hematemesis; usually self-limited.
- Prior history of vomiting, retching in 50%.
- Endoscopy establishes diagnosis.

General Considerations

Mallory-Weiss syndrome is characterized by a nonpenetrating mucosal tear at the gastroesophageal junction that arises from events that suddenly raise transabdominal pressure, such as lifting, retching, or vomiting. Alcohol use disorder is a strong predisposing factor. Mallory-Weiss tears are responsible for approximately 5% of cases of upper GI bleeding.

Clinical Findings

A. Symptoms and Signs

Patients usually present with hematemesis with or without melena. A history of retching, vomiting, or straining is obtained in about 50% of cases.

B. Laboratory Findings

Blood is sent for CBC, INR, serum creatinine, liver enzymes, and blood typing and screening (in anticipation of the possible need for transfusion).

C. Special Examinations

As with other causes of upper GI hemorrhage, upper endoscopy should be performed after the patient has been appropriately resuscitated. The diagnosis is established by identification of a 0.5- to 4-cm linear mucosal tear usually located either at the gastroesophageal junction or, more commonly, just below the junction in the gastric mucosa.

Differential Diagnosis

At endoscopy, other potential causes of upper GI hemorrhage are found in over 35% of patients with Mallory-Weiss tears, including peptic ulcer disease, erosive gastritis, arteriovenous malformations, and esophageal varices. Patients with underlying portal hypertension are at higher risk for continued or recurrent bleeding.

Treatment

Patients are initially treated as needed with fluid resuscitation and blood transfusions (see Acute Upper GI Bleeding, above). Most patients stop bleeding spontaneously and require no therapy. Endoscopic hemostatic therapy is employed in patients who have continuing active bleeding. Injection with epinephrine (1:10,000), cautery with a bipolar or heater probe coagulation device, or mechanical compression of the artery by application of an endoclip or band is effective in 90–95% of cases. Angiographic arterial embolization or operative intervention is required in patients who do not respond to endoscopic therapy. Oral PPIs generally are administered to promote mucosal healing (pantoprazole 40 mg, omeprazole or esomeprazole 40 mg, lansoprazole 30 mg, once daily for 8 weeks).

Barkun A et al. Canadian Association of Gastroenterology clinical practice guideline for the endoscopic management of nonvariceal nonpeptic ulcer upper gastrointestinal bleeding. Gastroenterology. 2025;169:863: [PMID: 40778886]

2. Eosinophilic Esophagitis

General Considerations

Eosinophilic esophagitis (EE) is a disorder in which food, environmental antigens or gastroesophageal reflux are thought to stimulate an esophageal eosinophilic-predominant inflammatory response. Ongoing inflammation may lead to the development of strictures and rings. It occurs most commonly in children and young or middle-aged adults (estimated prevalence 43/100,000). A history of allergies or atopic conditions (asthma, eczema, hay fever) is present in over half of patients. Other disorders that may cause increased esophageal eosinophils include hypereosinophilic syndrome, eosinophilic gastroenteritis, celiac disease, achalasia, pemphigus, connective tissue disorders, drug hypersensitivity, and Crohn disease.

Clinical Findings

Most adults have a long history of dysphagia for solid-foods or an episode of food impaction. Heartburn or chest pain may be present. Symptom severity may increase with anxiety or hypervigilance. On laboratory tests, a few have eosinophilia or elevated IgE levels. Barium swallow studies may demonstrate a small-caliber esophagus; focal or long, tapered strictures; or multiple concentric rings. However, endoscopy with esophageal biopsy and histologic evaluation is required to establish the diagnosis. Endoscopic appearances include **E**dema, concentric **R**ings ("trachealization"), **E**xudates (white plaques), **F**urrows (vertical lines), and **S**trictures (EREFS); however, the esophagus is grossly normal in up to 5% of patients. Several biopsies (6–8) from both the mid/proximal and distal esophagus should be obtained to demonstrate multiple (> 15/high-powered field) eosinophils in the mucosa. Skin testing for food allergies may be helpful to identify causative factors.

Treatment

The goals of therapy are improvement of symptoms, reduction of inflammation, and prevention and treatment of esophageal strictures. Treatment options include PPIs, topical corticosteroids, food elimination diets, and esophageal dilation. First-line therapy for most adults is a standard-dose PPI (eg, omeprazole 20 mg) orally twice daily for 2–3 months followed by repeat endoscopy and mucosal biopsy. Approximately one-half of patients have clinical and histologic improvement (< 15 eosinophils/high-power field) with PPI treatment. PPI therapy should be discontinued in patients with persistent symptoms and inflammation.

In patients with continued symptoms, optimal treatment is uncertain. Referral to an allergist for evaluation of coexisting atopic disorders and for testing for food and environmental allergens may be considered. The two most common allergenic foods are dairy and wheat followed by egg, soy, peanuts, and shellfish. Guided by an experienced dietician, empiric elimination of suspected dietary allergens leads to clinical improvement in 80% and histologic remission in up to 60% of adults.

Topical corticosteroids lead to symptomatic and histologic improvement in > 60–70% of adults. Either FDA-approved topical budesonide suspension (2 mg/10 mL orally) or powdered fluticasone, 880 mcg (from foil-lined inhaler Diskus orally), is administered twice daily for 8–12 weeks with similar efficacy. In Europe, budesonide orodispersible tablets 0.5 or 1.0 mg twice daily are approved for initial and maintenance therapy of EE. Symptomatic relapse is common after discontinuation of therapy and may require once or twice-daily maintenance topical corticosteroid therapy. Oral and esophageal candidiasis occurs in up to 20% of treated patients and adrenal suppression in < 5%.

Dupilumab (300 mg subcutaneous weekly) is FDA-approved for the treatment of EE. In clinical trials, histologic remission after 24 weeks of treatment was achieved in 60% of patients treated with dupilumab versus 6% with placebo. Dupilumab may be considered in patients with EE who have other allergic conditions or have not responded to or are intolerant of other therapies.

Graduated esophageal dilation of strictures or narrow-caliber esophagus may improve dysphagia in up to 95% of patients; it should be performed cautiously because there is an increased risk of perforation (0.4%) and postprocedural chest pain.

Dellon E et al. ACG Clinical Guideline: diagnosis and management of eosinophilic esophagitis. Am J Gastroenterol. 2025;120:31. [PMID: 39745304]

Dellon E et al. Long-term safety and efficacy of budesonide oral suspension for eosinophilic esophagitis: a 4-year, phase 3, open-label study. Clin Gastroenterol Hepatol. 2025;23:2155. [PMID: 39954913]

Von Arnim U et al. Monitoring patients with eosinophilic esophagitis in routine clinical practice – international expert recommendations. Clin Gastroenterol Hepatol. 2023;21:2526. [PMID: 36572109]

3. Esophageal Webs & Rings

Esophageal webs are thin, diaphragm-like membranes of squamous mucosa that typically occur in the mid or upper esophagus and may be multiple. They may be congenital but also occur with eosinophilic esophagitis, graft-versus-host disease, pemphigoid, epidermolysis bullosa, pemphigus vulgaris, and, rarely, in association with iron deficiency anemia (Plummer-Vinson syndrome). Esophageal "Schatzki" rings are smooth, circumferential, thin (< 4 mm in thickness) mucosal structures located in the distal esophagus at the squamocolumnar junction. Their pathogenesis is controversial. They are associated in nearly all cases with a hiatal hernia, and reflux symptoms are common, suggesting that acid gastroesophageal reflux may be contributory in many cases. Most webs and rings are over 20 mm in diameter and are asymptomatic. Solid food dysphagia most often occurs with rings < 13 mm in diameter. Characteristically, dysphagia is intermittent and not progressive. Large poorly chewed food boluses are most likely to cause symptoms. Obstructing boluses may pass by drinking extra liquids or after regurgitation. In some cases, an impacted bolus must be extracted endoscopically. Esophageal webs and rings may be visualized using a barium esophagogram or with upper endoscopy.

The majority of symptomatic patients with a single ring or web can be effectively treated with the passage of bougie or endoscopic balloon dilators to disrupt the lesion or with endoscopic electrosurgical incision of the ring. A minimum lumen diameter of 15–18 mm achieves symptom remission in most patients. A single dilation may suffice, but repeat dilations are required in many patients. Patients who have heartburn or who require repeated dilation should receive long-term acid suppressive therapy with a PPI.

Rodrigues-Pinto E et al. How to prevent and treat the most adverse events related to luminal dilation and stenting in benign disease. Am J Gastroenterol. 2023;118:1521. [PMID: 36946679]

4. Zenker Diverticulum

Zenker diverticulum is a protrusion of pharyngeal mucosa that develops at the pharyngoesophageal junction between the inferior pharyngeal constrictor and the cricopharyngeus. The cause is believed to be loss of elasticity of the upper esophageal sphincter, resulting in restricted opening during swallowing. Symptoms of dysphagia and regurgitation tend to develop insidiously over years in older, predominantly male patients. Initial symptoms include vague oropharyngeal dysphagia with coughing or throat discomfort. As the diverticulum enlarges and retains food, patients may note halitosis, spontaneous regurgitation of undigested food, nocturnal choking, gurgling in the throat, or a protrusion in the neck. Complications include aspiration pneumonia, bronchiectasis, and lung abscess. The diagnosis is best established by a videoesophagography.

Symptomatic patients require cricopharyngeal myotomy with incision of the septum between the diverticulum and esophagus. Minimally invasive intraluminal approaches that use endoscopes are preferred. Significant improvement occurs in over 90% of patients with a recurrence rate of 11%. Small asymptomatic diverticula may be observed.

Delgado LM et al. Endoscopic submucosal tunneling techniques versus flexible endoscopic septotomy for Zenker's diverticulum: a systematic review and meta-analysis. Gastrointest Endosc. 2025;101:751. [PMID: 39603545]

Fair L et al. Modern approaches to treating Zenker's diverticulum. Curr Opin Gastroenterol. 2023;39:333. [PMID: 37278290]

Fayyaz F et al. Open Zenker's peroral endoscopic myotomy: technical and clinical outcomes of a novel technique (with videos). Gastrointest Endosc. 2025;102:550. [PMID: 40024287]

5. Esophageal Varices

ESSENTIALS OF DIAGNOSIS

- Develop secondary to portal hypertension.
- Found in 50% of patients with cirrhosis.
- One-third of patients with varices develop upper GI bleeding.
- Diagnosis established by upper endoscopy.

General Considerations

Esophageal varices are dilated submucosal veins that develop in patients with underlying portal hypertension and that may result in serious upper GI bleeding. The causes of portal hypertension are discussed in Chapter 18. Under normal circumstances, there is a 2–6 mm Hg pressure gradient between the portal vein and the inferior vena cava. When the gradient exceeds 10–12 mm Hg, significant portal hypertension exists. Esophageal varices are the most common cause of GI bleeding due to portal hypertension, though bleeding may also be caused by portal hypertensive gastropathy, GAVE, gastric varices and, rarely, intestinal varices. Bleeding from esophageal varices most commonly occurs in the distal 5 cm of the esophagus.

The most common cause of portal hypertension is cirrhosis. Approximately 50% of patients with cirrhosis have esophageal varices. Bleeding from varices occurs in 30% of patients with esophageal varices. However, 20% of patients with chronic liver disease in whom bleeding develops have a nonvariceal source of bleeding. With current therapies, the 6-week mortality rate associated with bleeding esophageal varices is 15–20%.

A number of factors have been identified that may portend an increased risk of bleeding from esophageal varices. The most important factors that portend an increased risk of bleeding from esophageal varices are (1) the size of the varices (increased risk with varices that are > 5 mm); (2) the presence at endoscopy of red wale markings (longitudinal dilated venules on the varix surface); (3) the severity of liver disease (as assessed by Child scoring); and (4) active alcohol use—patients with cirrhosis who continue to drink have an extremely high risk of variceal bleeding.

Clinical Findings

A. Symptoms and Signs

Bleeding esophageal varices present with symptoms and signs of acute GI hemorrhage. (See Acute Upper GI Bleeding, above.) In some cases, there may be preceding retching or dyspepsia attributable to alcoholic gastritis or withdrawal. Varices per se do not cause symptoms of dyspepsia, dysphagia, or retching. Variceal bleeding usually is severe, resulting in hypovolemia manifested by postural vital signs or shock.

B. Laboratory Findings

These are identical to those listed above in the section on Acute Upper GI Bleeding.

Initial Management

A. Acute Resuscitation

Variceal hemorrhage is life-threatening; rapid assessment and resuscitation with fluids or blood products are essential. The initial management of patients with acute variceal bleeding is discussed in the section on Acute Upper GI Bleeding. Overtransfusion should be avoided because it leads to increased central and portal venous pressures, increasing the risk of rebleeding. Most patients with bleeding esophageal varices have advanced liver disease with coagulopathy due to thrombocytopenia; deficiencies of liver-derived clotting factors I (fibrinogen), II, VII, IX, and X; and accelerated intravascular fibrinolysis. The INR does not accurately reflect the coagulopathy in advanced liver disease. Fresh frozen plasma should *not* be administered routinely in patients with an elevated INR because it has no proven benefit but does have potential harms, including increased portal pressures and risk of thrombotic complications including DVT or portal vein thrombosis. Likewise, recombinant factor VIIa, prothrombin complex concentrates, and cryoprecipitate have not demonstrated efficacy and are not generally recommended in patients with bleeding varices. In patients with decompensated cirrhosis and active severe upper GI bleeding, platelet transfusion is recommended for platelet counts below 50,000/mcL (50×10^9/L). Patients with advanced liver disease are at high risk for poor outcome regardless of the bleeding source and should be in an ICU. After acute resuscitation, abdominal ultrasound with Doppler is commonly performed to exclude portal vein thrombosis.

B. Pharmacologic Therapy

1. Antibiotic prophylaxis—Patients with cirrhosis admitted with upper GI bleeding have a > 50% chance of developing a severe bacterial infection during hospitalization—such as bacterial peritonitis, pneumonia, or UTI. Most infections are caused by gram-negative organisms of gut origin. Prophylactic administration of intravenous third-generation cephalosporins (eg, ceftriaxone, 1 g/day) for 5–7 days reduces the risk of serious infection to 10–20% as well as hospital mortality, especially in patients with Child-Pugh class C cirrhosis.

2. Vasoactive drugs—Octreotide and somatostatin infusions reduce portal pressures in ways that are poorly understood. Octreotide (50-mcg intravenous bolus followed by 50 mcg/hour) or somatostatin (250 mcg/hour)—reduces splanchnic and hepatic blood flow and portal pressures in cirrhotic patients. Both agents appear to provide acute control of variceal bleeding in up to 80% of patients although neither has been shown to reduce mortality. Somatostatin infusion is not available in the United States. Combined treatment with octreotide or somatostatin infusion and endoscopic therapy with band ligation is superior to either modality alone in controlling acute bleeding and early rebleeding, and it may improve survival. For upper GI hemorrhage with advanced liver disease, it is reasonable to initiate therapy with octreotide on admission and continue for 3–5 days if varices are confirmed by endoscopy. If bleeding is determined by endoscopy not to be secondary to portal hypertension, the infusion can be discontinued.

Terlipressin is a synthetic vasopressin analog that causes a significant and sustained reduction in portal and variceal pressures while preserving renal perfusion. Outside the United States, terlipressin often is preferred to somatostatin or octreotide for the treatment of esophageal variceal hemorrhage. In the United States, terlipressin is FDA-approved for the treatment of hepatorenal syndrome with an acute decline in renal function that has not responded to an albumin infusion, but the appropriate role and dosing in patients with acute variceal hemorrhage awaits guidance. Terlipressin is contraindicated in patients with significant coronary, cerebral, or peripheral vascular disease.

3. Vitamin K—In patients with cirrhosis and an abnormal prothrombin time, vitamin K (10 mg intravenously) should be administered.

4. Lactulose—Encephalopathy may complicate an episode of GI bleeding with severe liver disease. In patients with encephalopathy, lactulose should be administered in a dosage of 30 mL orally every 1–2 hours until evacuation occurs then reduced to 15–45 mL/hour every 8–12 hours as needed to promote two or three bowel movements daily. (See Chapter 18.)

C. Emergent Endoscopy

Emergent endoscopy is performed after the patient's hemodynamic status has been appropriately stabilized (usually within 12–24 hours). In patients with active bleeding, endotracheal intubation is commonly used to protect against aspiration during endoscopy. An endoscopic examination is performed to confirm esophageal varices are the likely source of GI bleeding and to exclude other or associated causes. In many patients, variceal bleeding has stopped spontaneously by the time of endoscopy, and the diagnosis of variceal bleeding is made presumptively. Immediate endoscopic treatment of the varices generally is performed with banding. Banding arrests active bleeding in 80–90% of patients and reduces the chance of in-hospital recurrent bleeding to about 20%.

D. Balloon Tube Tamponade

In patients with massive variceal GI bleeding, mechanical tamponade with specially designed nasogastric tubes containing large gastric and esophageal balloons (Minnesota or Sengstaken-Blakemore tubes) may provide initial control of hemorrhage in 60–90% of patients. Balloon tamponade is used as a temporizing measure only in patients with bleeding that cannot be controlled with pharmacologic or endoscopic techniques until more definitive decompressive therapy (eg, TIPS) can be provided.

E. Emergency Transvenous Intrahepatic Portosystemic Shunt (TIPS)

In the 10–20% of patients with variceal bleeding that cannot be controlled with pharmacologic or endoscopic therapy, emergency portal decompression with TIPS may be considered.

In this procedure, an expandable wire mesh stent (8–12 mm in diameter) is passed through the liver parenchyma via a catheter and wire that are inserted in the jugular vein creating a portosystemic shunt from the portal vein to the hepatic vein. TIPS can control acute hemorrhage in > 90% of patients actively bleeding from gastric or esophageal varices. However, when TIPS is performed in the actively bleeding patient, the mortality approaches 40%, especially in patients requiring ventilatory support or blood pressure support and patients with kidney disease, bilirubin > 3 mg/dL, or encephalopathy. Therefore, TIPS should be considered in the 10–20% of patients with acute variceal bleeding that cannot be controlled with pharmacologic and endoscopic therapy, but it may not be warranted in patients with a particularly poor prognosis.

Prevention of Rebleeding

Once the initial bleeding episode has been controlled, therapy is needed to reduce the high risk (60%) of rebleeding that occurs in the absence of treatment. Optimized therapy has reduced rebleeding rates from 20% to 12%.

A. Combination β-Blockers and Variceal Band Ligation

Nonselective β-adrenergic blockers (carvedilol, propranolol, nadolol) alone reduce the risk of rebleeding from esophageal varices to about 40%. The Baveno VII international consensus group favors carvedilol over other nonselective β-blockers due to its anti-α-adrenergic effects, which promote vasodilation and a greater reduction in portal pressures. Likewise, long-term treatment with endoscopic band ligation reduces the incidence of rebleeding to about 30%. In most patients, two to six treatment sessions of band ligation (performed at 2- to 4-week intervals) are needed to eradicate the varices.

Meta-analyses of RCTs suggest that a *combination* of band ligation plus β-blockers is superior to either variceal band ligation alone or β-blockers alone. Therefore, combination therapy is recommended for patients without contraindications to β-blockers. Over the past 20 years, 1-year bleeding related mortality has fallen to 12%, reflecting improved long-term management. Recommended starting doses of β-blockers are carvedilol (6.25 mg orally once daily), propranolol (20 mg orally twice daily), long-acting propranolol (60 mg orally once daily), or nadolol (20–40 mg orally once daily), with gradual increases in the dosage every 1–2 weeks until the heart rate falls by 25% or reaches 55–60 beats/min, provided the systolic blood pressure remains above 90 mm Hg and the patient has no side effects. The average dosage of carvedilol is 12.5 mg once daily, long-acting propranolol is 120 mg once daily, and nadolol is 80 mg once daily. One-third of patients with cirrhosis have contraindications or are intolerant of β-blockers, experiencing fatigue or hypotension. In such patients, variceal ligation alone is recommended.

B. Transvenous Intrahepatic Portosystemic Shunt

TIPS has resulted in a significant reduction in recurrent bleeding and mortality rate compared with band ligation. At 1 year, rebleeding rates in patients treated with TIPS versus various endoscopic therapies average 20% and 40%, respectively. However, TIPS is associated with a higher incidence of encephalopathy (35% versus 15%), and stenosis and thrombosis of the stents occur in the majority of patients over time with a consequent risk of rebleeding. Given these problems, TIPS should be reserved for patients who have recurrent (two or more) episodes of variceal bleeding that have failed endoscopic or pharmacologic therapies. TIPS is also useful in patients with recurrent bleeding from gastric varices or portal hypertensive gastropathy (for which endoscopic therapies cannot be used). TIPS is likewise considered in patients who are noncompliant with other therapies or who live in remote locations (without access to emergency care).

C. Liver Transplantation

Candidacy for orthotopic liver transplantation should be assessed in all patients with chronic liver disease and bleeding due to portal hypertension. Transplant candidates should be treated with band ligation or TIPS to control bleeding pretransplant.

Prevention of First Episodes of Variceal Bleeding

Bleeding occurs each year in 12% of patients with varices that have not previously bled, with a lifetime risk of 30%. Because of the high mortality rate associated with variceal hemorrhage, prevention of the initial bleeding episode is desirable. Therefore, it is recommended that patients with chronic liver disease with compensated cirrhosis or suspected cirrhosis should undergo diagnostic endoscopy or capsule endoscopy to determine whether varices are present. Transient elastography (FibroScan) is a noninvasive ultrasonographic method for assessing liver stiffness and fibrosis that may be used to stratify patients at high risk for varices (who may benefit from endoscopy) versus those at low risk (in whom endoscopy is not needed). Varices are present in 40% of patients with Child-Pugh class A cirrhosis and in 85% with Child-Pugh class C cirrhosis. In patients without varices on screening endoscopy, a repeat endoscopy is recommended in 3 years since varices develop in 8% of patients per year. Patients with varices have a higher risk of bleeding if they have varices > 5 mm, varices with red wale markings, or Child-Pugh class B or C cirrhosis. The risk of bleeding with varices < 5 mm is 5% per year and with large varices is 15–20% per year. Patients with small varices without red wale marks and compensated (Child-Pugh class A) cirrhosis have a low risk of bleeding; hence, prophylaxis is unnecessary, but endoscopy should be repeated in 1–2 years to reassess size.

Nonselective β-adrenergic blockers (carvedilol, nadolol, or propranolol) are recommended to reduce the risk of first variceal hemorrhage in patients without contraindications to these agents who have medium/large varices or have small varices with advanced cirrhosis (Child-Pugh class B or C). (See Combination β-Blockers and Variceal Band Ligation, above.) For patients with compensated cirrhosis, 2022 guidelines favor the use of carvedilol for primary prevention of variceal bleeding. Carvedilol is initiated at a dose of 6.25 mg orally once daily and increased, as tolerated, to a maximum of 12.5 mg once daily provided the systolic blood pressure remains > 90 mm Hg. Compared with other nonselective β-blockers, carvedilol (which causes vasodilation due to mild α-adrenergic inhibition), achieves greater reductions in portal pressures and lower rates of variceal bleeding. Carvedilol is not recommended for patients with decompensated cirrhosis. Prophylactic band ligation may be preferred over β-blockers for patients at higher risk for bleeding, especially patients with medium/large varices with red wale markings or with advanced cirrhosis (Child-Pugh class B or C) as well as patients with contraindications to or intolerance of β-blockers. Band ligation is not recommended for small varices due to technical difficulties in band application.

When to Refer

- All patients with upper GI bleeding and suspected varices should be evaluated by a physician skilled in therapeutic endoscopy.
- Patients being considered for TIPS procedures or liver transplantation.
- Patients with cirrhosis for endoscopic evaluation for varices.

When to Admit

All patients with acute upper GI bleeding and suspected cirrhosis should be admitted to an ICU.

Pfisterer N et al. Improved clinical outcomes of patients with cirrhosis and acute variceal bleeding over the past 2 decades. Gastrointest Endosc. 2025;102:733. [PMID: 40324727]
Pierre-Emmanuel R et al. Bleeding and thrombotic complications in patients with cirrhosis: a state-of-the-art appraisal. Clin Gastroenterol Hepatol. 2023;21:2110. [PMID: 37121529]
Tapper EB et al. Diagnosis and management of cirrhosis and its complications: a review. JAMA. 2023;329:1589. [PMID: 37159031]
Zuckerman MJ et al. Endoscopic treatment of esophageal varices. Clin Liver Dis. 2022;26:21. [PMID: 34802661]

ESOPHAGEAL MOTILITY DISORDERS

1. Achalasia

ESSENTIALS OF DIAGNOSIS

- Gradual, progressive dysphagia for solids and liquids.
- Regurgitation of undigested food.
- Barium esophagogram with "bird's beak" distal esophagus.
- Esophageal manometry confirms diagnosis.

General Considerations

Achalasia is an idiopathic motility disorder characterized by loss of peristalsis in the distal two-thirds (smooth muscle) of the esophagus and impaired relaxation of the LES.

Clinical Findings

A. Symptoms and Signs

The incidence of achalasia increases with age; however, it can be seen in individuals as young as 25 years. Patients report the gradual onset of dysphagia for solid foods and, in the majority, for liquids also. Symptoms at presentation may have persisted for months to years. Substernal discomfort or fullness may be noted after eating. Many patients eat more slowly and adopt specific maneuvers such as lifting the neck or throwing the shoulders back to enhance esophageal emptying. Regurgitation of undigested food is common and may occur during meals or up to several hours later. Nocturnal regurgitation can provoke coughing or aspiration. Up to 50% of patients report substernal chest pain that is unrelated to meals or exercise and may last up to hours. Weight loss is common. Physical examination is unrevealing.

B. Imaging

CXRs may show an air-fluid level in the enlarged, fluid-filled esophagus. Barium esophagography discloses characteristic findings, including esophageal dilation, loss of esophageal peristalsis, poor esophageal emptying, and a smooth, symmetric "bird's beak" tapering of the distal esophagus. Five minutes after ingestion of 8 oz of barium, a column height of > 2 cm has a sensitivity and specificity of > 85% in differentiating achalasia from other causes of dysphagia. Without treatment, the esophagus may become markedly dilated ("sigmoid esophagus").

C. Special Examinations

After esophagography, endoscopy is always performed to evaluate the distal esophagus and gastroesophageal junction to exclude a distal stricture or a submucosal infiltrating carcinoma. The diagnosis is confirmed by high-resolution esophageal manometry demonstrating absence of normal peristalsis and impaired esophagogastric junction relaxation after swallowing. An integrated post-swallow relaxation pressure > 15 mm Hg has a diagnostic sensitivity of 97%. Three achalasia subtypes are recognized based on esophageal contractility and pressure patterns: types I and II (both with 100% failed peristalsis) and type III (failed peristalsis with 20% or more distal premature "spastic" contractions).

Differential Diagnosis

Chagas disease is associated with esophageal dysfunction that is indistinguishable from idiopathic achalasia and should be considered in patients from endemic regions (Central and South America); it is becoming more common in the southern United States. Primary or metastatic tumors can invade the gastroesophageal junction, resulting in a picture resembling that of achalasia, or "pseudoachalasia." Endoscopic ultrasonography and chest CT may be required to examine the distal esophagus in suspicious cases.

Treatment

Several effective treatment options are available, all of which promote improved esophageal emptying by lowering distal esophageal pressure either through endoscopic injection with botulinum toxin or disruption of the LES by pneumatic balloon dilation or cardioesophageal myotomy (surgical or endoscopic).

A. Botulinum Toxin Injection

Endoscopically guided injection of botulinum toxin directly into the LES results in a marked reduction in LES pressure with initial improvement in symptoms in 65–85% of patients. However, symptoms recur in over 50% of patients within 6–9 months and in all patients within 2 years. This therapy is most appropriate for patients who are poor candidates for more invasive procedures.

B. Pneumatic Dilation

Over 80% of patients derive good to excellent relief of dysphagia after one to three sessions of pneumatic dilation of the LES. Dilation is less effective in patients who are aged < 45 years, have the type III variant, or have a dilated esophagus. Perforations occur in < 3% of dilations but infrequently require operative repair. In a meta-analysis of RCTs, laparoscopic Heller myotomy and per oral endoscopic myotomy (POEM) were not significantly different in treatment success but both were superior to pneumatic dilation. Patients who do not respond to initial treatment with pneumatic dilation may be treated with cardiomyotomy (Heller or POEM) (see below).

C. Surgical Heller Cardiomyotomy

A Heller cardiomyotomy of the LES and cardia (usually performed with a laparoscopic approach) results in symptomatic improvement in approximately 90% of patients. Because gastroesophageal reflux develops in up to 20% of patients after myotomy, most surgeons also perform an antireflux procedure (fundoplication), and most patients are prescribed a once-daily PPI. Symptoms recur in > 5–15% of cases within 10 years but usually respond to pneumatic dilation.

D. Per Oral Endoscopic Myotomy

POEM is a less invasive endoscopic procedure than surgery in which the endoscope dissects through the submucosal space to the LES, where the circular muscle fibers of the cardia and distal esophagus are incised. Because a fundoplication is not performed, long-term antisecretory therapy for gastroesophageal reflux with a PPI is required in most patients. POEM may be the preferred treatment modality for type III achalasia (where a longer myotomy of the distal esophagus is indicated). A RCT of 221 patients with achalasia showed that satisfactory symptom improvement was equivalent both in patients treated with POEM (83%) and in those treated with surgical myotomy (81.7%) 2 years after treatment. Serious adverse events occurred in 2.7% of patients treated with POEM and 7.3% with surgical myotomy, but postoperative reflux esophagitis was higher with POEM (44%) than with surgical myotomy (29%).

In summary, optimal treatment of achalasia depends on the patient's age, achalasia subtype, provider's expertise, and patient's preferences or concerns regarding surgery or posttreatment gastroesophageal reflux.

Management of Refractory Achalasia

Complete esophagectomy or percutaneous gastrostomy is required in the 1% of patients in whom massive dilation of the esophagus (megaesophagus) develops despite dilation or myotomy. In megaesophagus, dysphagia, food retention, and regurgitation may decrease nutrition and quality of life and increase risk of aspiration.

Geeratragool T et al. Long-term outcomes of pneumatic balloon dilation versus peroral endoscopic myotomy in type I and II achalasia patients: a propensity score-matched analysis. Gastrointest Endosc. 2025;101:558. [PMID: 39477022]

Provenza CG et al. Achalasia: diagnosis and management. Surg Clin North Am. 2025;105:143. [PMID: 39523069]

Ramchandani M et al. Recent advancements and future perspectives of per oral endoscopic myotomy. Clin Gastroenterol Hepatol. 2024;22:1983. [PMID: 38759824]

2. Other Primary Esophageal Motility Disorders

Clinical Findings

A. Symptoms and Signs

Abnormalities in esophageal motility besides achalasia may cause dysphagia or chest pain. Dysphagia for liquids as well as solids tends to be intermittent and nonprogressive. Periods of normal swallowing may alternate with periods of dysphagia, which usually is mild though bothersome—rarely severe enough to result in significant alterations in lifestyle or weight loss. Dysphagia may be provoked by stress, large boluses of food, or hot or cold liquids. Some patients may experience anterior chest pain that may be confused with angina pectoris but usually is nonexertional. The pain generally is unrelated to eating.

B. Diagnostic Tests

The evaluation of suspected esophageal motility disorders includes barium esophagography, upper endoscopy, and, in some cases, esophageal manometry. Barium esophagography is useful to exclude mechanical obstruction and to evaluate esophageal motility. The presence of simultaneous contractions (spasm), disordered or failed peristalsis, or delayed emptying supports a diagnosis of esophageal dysmotility. Upper endoscopy also is performed to exclude a mechanical obstruction (as a cause of dysphagia) and to look for evidence of erosive reflux esophagitis (a common cause of chest pain) or eosinophilic esophagitis (confirmed by esophageal biopsy).

Manometry is not routinely used for mild to moderate symptoms because the findings seldom influence medical management, but it may be useful in patients with persistent, disabling dysphagia to exclude achalasia and to look for other disorders of esophageal motility. These include esophagogastric junction outflow obstruction, spastic esophageal disorders (distal esophageal spasm and hypercontractile ["jackhammer"] esophagus), and esophageal hypomotility (ineffective or failed peristalsis).

Treatment

For patients with mild symptoms of dysphagia, therapy is directed at symptom reduction and reassurance. Patients should be instructed to chew carefully, eat more slowly, and take smaller bites of food with liquids. Because unrecognized gastroesophageal reflux may cause dysphagia, a trial of a PPI (esomeprazole 40 mg, pantoprazole 40 mg) orally once daily should be administered for 4–8 weeks. Opioids may exacerbate esophageal dysmotility and should be discontinued, if possible. No medications have been shown to improve symptoms in patients with esophageal hypomotility. Treatment of patients with severe dysphagia or chest pain attributed to spastic disorders is empiric. Uncontrolled studies report benefit with (1) smooth muscle relaxants (isosorbide [10–20 mg orally four times daily] or nitroglycerin [0.4 mg sublingually as needed]); (2) calcium channel blockers (nifedipine [10 mg] or diltiazem [60–90 mg] orally 30–45 minutes before meals); (3) phosphodiesterase type 5 inhibitors (eg, sildenafil); (4) botulinum toxin injection into the lower esophagus; (5) esophageal dilation; or (6) POEM.

Kamboj AK et al. A practical approach to ineffective esophageal motility. Neurogastroenterol Motil. 2024;36:e14839. [PMID: 38837280]
Patel DA et al. Esophageal motility disorders: current approach to diagnostics and therapeutics. Gastroenterology. 2022;162:1617. [PMID: 35227779]

DISEASES OF THE STOMACH & DUODENUM

(See Chapter 43 for Gastric Cancers.)

GASTRITIS & GASTROPATHY

The term "gastropathy" should be used to denote conditions in which there is epithelial or endothelial damage without inflammation, and "gastritis" should be used to denote conditions in which there is histologic evidence of inflammation. In clinical practice, the term "gastritis" is commonly applied to three categories: (1) erosive and hemorrhagic "gastritis" (gastropathy); (2) nonerosive, nonspecific (histologic) gastritis; and (3) other specific types of gastritis, characterized by distinctive histologic and endoscopic features diagnostic of specific disorders.

1. Erosive & Hemorrhagic "Gastritis" (Gastropathy)

ESSENTIALS OF DIAGNOSIS

- Most commonly seen in alcohol use disorder, critically ill patients, or patients taking NSAIDs.
- Often asymptomatic; may cause epigastric pain, nausea, and vomiting.
- May cause hematemesis; usually insignificant bleeding.

General Considerations

The most common causes of erosive gastropathy are medications (especially NSAIDs), alcohol, stress due to severe medical or surgical illness, and portal hypertension ("portal gastropathy"). Uncommon causes of erosive gastropathy include ischemia, caustic ingestion, and radiation. Erosive and hemorrhagic gastropathy typically are diagnosed at endoscopy, often being performed because of dyspepsia or upper GI bleeding. Endoscopic findings include subepithelial hemorrhages, petechiae, and erosions. These lesions are superficial, vary in size and number, and may be focal or diffuse. There typically is no significant inflammation on histologic examination.

Clinical Findings

A. Symptoms and Signs

Erosive gastropathy is usually asymptomatic. Symptoms, when they occur, include anorexia, epigastric pain, nausea, and vomiting. There is poor correlation between symptoms and the number or severity of endoscopic abnormalities. The most common clinical manifestation of erosive gastritis is upper GI bleeding, which presents as hematemesis, "coffee grounds" emesis, or bloody aspirate in a patient receiving nasogastric suction, or as melena. Because erosive gastritis is superficial, hemodynamically significant bleeding is rare.

B. Laboratory Findings

The laboratory findings are nonspecific. The hematocrit is low if significant bleeding has occurred; iron deficiency may be found.

C. Special Examinations

Upper endoscopy is the most sensitive method of diagnosis. Although bleeding from gastritis is usually insignificant, it cannot be distinguished on clinical grounds from more serious lesions such as peptic ulcers or esophageal varices. Hence, endoscopy is generally performed within 24 hours for upper GI bleeding to identify the source.

Differential Diagnosis

Epigastric pain may be due to peptic ulcer, GERD, gastric cancer, biliary tract disease, food poisoning, viral gastroenteritis, and functional dyspepsia. With severe pain, one should consider a perforated or penetrating ulcer, pancreatic disease, esophageal rupture, ruptured aortic aneurysm, gastric volvulus, GI ischemia, and myocardial ischemia. Causes of upper GI bleeding include peptic ulcer disease, esophageal varices, Mallory-Weiss tear, and angioectasias.

Specific Causes & Treatment

A. Stress Gastritis

1. Prophylaxis—Stress-related mucosal erosions and subepithelial hemorrhages may develop within 72 hours in critically ill patients. Clinically overt bleeding occurs in 6% of ICU patients, but clinically important bleeding occurs in < 1.5%. Bleeding is associated with a higher mortality rate but is seldom the cause of death. Major risk factors for stress gastritis include coagulopathy, shock, trauma, burns, liver failure, multiorgan failure, and need for mechanical ventilation or renal replacement therapy. When these risk factors are absent, the risk of significant bleeding is only 0.1%.

Prophylaxis should be considered in critically ill patients with risk factors for significant bleeding upon admission. Prophylactic suppression of gastric acid with H_2-receptor antagonists (intravenous) or PPIs (oral or intravenous) have both been shown to reduce the incidence of clinically overt and significant bleeding. In a 2024 trial of 4821 critically ill patients undergoing mechanical ventilation, clinically significant bleeding occurred in 1% of patients who received an intravenous PPI (pantoprazole 40 mg daily) versus 3.5% who received placebo. Meta-analyses of RCTs suggest that PPIs are more effective than H_2-receptor antagonists in reducing clinically significant bleeding; however, these analyses are conflicting as to whether PPIs decrease or increase mortality compared with H_2-receptor antagonists.

The optimal, cost-effective prophylactic regimen remains uncertain; hence, clinical practices vary. For patients with nasoenteric tubes, immediate-release omeprazole (40 mg at 1 and 6 hours on day 1; then 40 mg once daily beginning on day 2) may be preferred because of lower cost and ease of administration. For intravenous administration, continuous intravenous infusions of H_2-receptor antagonists provide adequate control of intragastric pH in most patients in the following doses over 24 hours: cimetidine (900–1200 mg) or famotidine (20 mg). The optimal dosing of intravenous PPIs is uncertain; however, in clinical trials pantoprazole doses ranging from 40 mg to 80 mg and administered every 8–24 hours appear equally effective.

2. Treatment—Once bleeding occurs, patients should receive continuous infusions of a PPI (esomeprazole or pantoprazole, 80 mg intravenous bolus, followed by 8 mg/hour continuous infusion) as well as sucralfate suspension, 1 g orally every 4–6 hours. Endoscopy should be performed for clinically significant bleeding to look for treatable causes, especially stress-related peptic ulcers with active bleeding or visible vessels. When bleeding arises from diffuse gastritis, endoscopic hemostasis techniques are not helpful.

B. NSAID Gastritis

Of patients receiving NSAIDs in clinical trials, 25–50% have gastritis and 10–20% have ulcers at endoscopy; however, symptoms of significant dyspepsia develop in about 5%. NSAIDs that are more selective for the cyclooxygenase (COX)-2 enzyme ("coxibs"), such as celecoxib, etodolac, and meloxicam, decrease the incidence of endoscopically visible ulcers by approximately 75% and significant ulcer complications by up to 50% compared with nonselective NSAIDs (nsNSAIDs). COX-2 selective NSAIDs are associated with increased risk of cardiovascular complications and therefore should be used with caution in patients with cardiovascular risk factors (see Peptic Ulcer Disease: NSAID-Induced Ulcers).

Dyspepsia is increased 1.5- to 2-fold with both nsNSAID and coxib use. However, dyspeptic symptoms correlate poorly with mucosal abnormalities (erosions or ulcers) or the development of adverse clinical events (ulcer bleeding or perforation). Patients with "alarm" symptoms or signs, such as severe pain, weight loss, vomiting, GI bleeding, or anemia, should undergo diagnostic upper endoscopy. For other patients, symptoms may improve with discontinuation of the agent, reduction to the lowest effective dose, or administration with meals. PPIs have demonstrated efficacy in controlled trials for the treatment of NSAID-related dyspepsia and superiority to H_2-receptor antagonists for healing of NSAID-related ulcers even in the setting of continued NSAID use. Therefore, an empiric 2- to 4-week trial of an oral PPI (omeprazole, rabeprazole, or esomeprazole, 20–40 mg/day; lansoprazole or dexlansoprazole, 30 mg/day; pantoprazole, 40 mg/day) is recommended for NSAID-related dyspepsia, especially if continued NSAID treatment is required. If symptoms do not improve, diagnostic upper endoscopy should be conducted.

C. Alcohol-induced Gastritis

Excessive alcohol consumption may lead to dyspepsia, nausea, emesis, and minor hematemesis—a condition sometimes labeled "alcoholic gastritis." However, it is not proven that alcohol alone causes significant erosive gastritis. Therapy with H_2-receptor antagonists, PPIs, or sucralfate for 2–4 weeks often is empirically prescribed.

D. Portal Hypertensive Gastropathy

Portal hypertension commonly results in gastric mucosal and submucosal congestion of capillaries and venules, which is correlated with the severity of the portal hypertension and underlying liver disease. Usually asymptomatic, it may cause chronic GI bleeding in 10% of patients and, less commonly, clinically significant bleeding with hematemesis. Treatment with nonselective β-blockers (nadolol, propranolol, carvedilol) reduces the incidence of recurrent acute bleeding by lowering portal pressures. Initial oral doses (nadolol 20 mg once daily; propranolol 20 mg twice daily; carvedilol 6.25 mg daily) are titrated upward every 1–2 weeks until the resting heart rate declines by 25% (or reaches 55–60 beats per minute), provided the patient has no symptoms and systolic blood pressure remains above 90 mmHg. Carvedilol is not recommended in patients with decompensated cirrhosis. Patients who fail propranolol therapy may be successfully treated with portal decompressive procedures (see section above on treatment of esophageal varices).

When to Refer

- NSAID gastritis with persistent dyspepsia despite discontinuation of NSAIDs or empiric PPI therapy.
- Upper GI hemorrhage.

When to Admit

- Acute upper GI hemorrhage.
- Severe dyspepsia with concern for complicated peptic ulcer disease or alternative diagnosis.
- Alcoholic gastritis with protracted vomiting and/or acute upper GI hemorrhage or signs of alcohol withdrawal

Cook D et al. Stress ulcer prophylaxis during invasive mechanical ventilation. N Engl J Med. 2024;391:20. [PMID: 38875111]
Khalifa A et al. Role of endoscopy in the diagnosis, grading, and treatment of portal hypertensive gastropathy and gastric antral vascular ectasia. Gastrointest Clin N Am. 2024;34:263. [PMID: 38395483]

2. Nonerosive Gastritis & Intestinal Metaplasia

A. *Helicobacter pylori* Gastritis

H pylori is a spiral gram-negative rod that resides beneath the gastric mucous layer adjacent to gastric epithelial cells. Although not invasive, it causes gastric mucosal inflammation with PMNs and lymphocytes.

In developed countries, the prevalence of *H pylori* is rapidly declining. In the United States, the prevalence rises in non-immigrants from < 10% under age 30 years to > 40% in those over age 60 years. The prevalence is higher in Black and Latino/Latina individuals and immigrants from developing countries and is correlated inversely with socioeconomic status. Transmission is from person to person, mainly during infancy and childhood; however, the mode of transmission is unknown.

Acute infection with *H pylori* may cause a transient clinical illness characterized by nausea and abdominal pain that may last for several days and is associated with acute histologic gastritis with PMNs. After these symptoms resolve, the majority progress to chronic infection with chronic, diffuse mucosal inflammation (gastritis) characterized by PMNs and lymphocytes. Most persons are asymptomatic and suffer no sequelae. Many patients have inflammation that predominates in the gastric antrum but spares the gastric body (where acid is secreted). People with this phenotype tend to have increased gastrin; increased acid production; and increased risk of developing peptic ulcers, especially duodenal ulcers. Over time, inflammation may become more diffuse, involving the gastric body. In some patients, this may lead to destruction of acid-secreting glands with resultant mucosal atrophy, decreased acid secretion, and intestinal metaplasia. This phenotype is associated with an increased risk of gastric ulcers and gastric cancer. Chronic *H pylori* gastritis leads to the development of duodenal or gastric ulcers in up to 10%, gastric cancer in 0.1–3%, and low-grade B cell gastric lymphoma (mucosa-associated lymphoid tissue lymphoma; MALToma) in < 0.01%. *H pylori* is estimated to account for 80–89% of non-cardia gastric cancers.

Eradication of *H pylori* may be achieved with antibiotics in > 85% of patients, leads to resolution of the chronic gastritis, and may arrest the progression to gastric metaplasia and atrophic gastritis (see Table 17–10). Testing for *H pylori* is indicated for patients with either active or a past history of documented peptic ulcer disease, gastric metaplasia (see above), gastric MALToma, or a personal or family history of gastric carcinoma. Testing and empiric treatment are cost-effective in patients aged < 60 years with uncomplicated dyspepsia prior to further medical evaluation. Testing for and treating *H pylori* in patients with functional dyspepsia is generally recommended (see Dyspepsia, above). In addition, to reduce the risk of ulcer-related bleeding, testing for (and, if positive, treating) *H pylori* infection is recommended in patients > 65 years of age taking dual antiplatelet therapy or NSAIDs long-term. Some groups recommend population-based screening of all asymptomatic persons in regions in which there is a high prevalence of *H pylori* and gastric cancer (such as Japan, Korea, and China) to prevent the progression to atrophic gastritis and reduce the incidence of gastric cancer. In a RCT conducted in *H pylori*–infected adults in China who were followed for 26.5 years, participants with successful *H pylori* eradication had a 54% reduction in gastric cancer incidence compared with participants in the placebo group. Population-based screening of asymptomatic individuals currently has not been recommended in western countries, in which the incidence of gastric cancer is low; however, a 2023 retrospective study of Northern California Kaiser Permanente patients with *H pylori* infection reported that patients treated for *H pylori* infection had a marked reduction in developing gastric cancer within 8 years (HR 0.37) compared with those who did not undergo treatment. Pending further guidelines for *H pylori* screening and treatment in the general population of western countries, screening is recommended for persons who immigrated from high-prevalence regions.

1. Noninvasive testing for *H pylori*—The recommended noninvasive tests for *H pylori* are the stool-based immunoassay for antigen or PCR assay and urea breath tests, both of which have excellent sensitivity and specificity (> 95%). Recent PPIs or antibiotics significantly reduce the sensitivity of fecal antigen assays. Prior to testing, PPIs should be discontinued for 14 days and antibiotics for at least 28 days. Due to lower sensitivity and specificity for active infections, clinical guidelines no longer endorse the use of serologic testing for *H pylori* infection.

2. Endoscopic testing for *H pylori*—When upper endoscopy is performed in patients with symptoms suggestive of upper GI disease (dyspepsia, dysphagia, vomiting, weight loss, GI bleeding), gastric biopsy specimens can be obtained for histology and detection of *H pylori* with a sensitivity and specificity of > 95%. Molecular-based testing of biopsy specimens for antibiotic susceptibility is commercially available.

Table 17–10. Treatment options for peptic ulcer disease.

Active *Helicobacter pylori*–associated ulcer

1. Treat with anti–*H pylori* regimen for 14 days. Best empiric treatment options:

   Optimized Bismuth Quadruple Therapy[1]
   - PPI orally twice daily[2]
   - Bismuth subsalicylate 262 mg (Pepto Bismol; two tablets orally) or bismuth subcitrate[3] (560 mg) orally four times daily
   - Tetracycline 500 mg orally four times daily
   - Metronidazole 500 mg three or four times daily

   Rifabutin-Based Triple Therapy (Talicia)[4]
   - Omeprazole 40 mg orally every 8 hours
   - Rifabutin 50 mg orally every 8 hours
   - Amoxicillin 1000 mg orally every 8 hours

   Vonoprazan Triple Therapy (Voquezna Triple Pak[5])
   - Vonoprazan 20 mg orally, twice daily
   - Amoxicillin 1 g orally, twice daily
   - Clarithromycin 500 mg orally, twice daily

   Vonoprazan Dual Therapy (Voquezna Dual Pak[5])
   - Vonoprazan 20 mg orally, twice daily
   - Amoxicillin 1 g orally, three times daily

   Standard Clarithromycin Triple Therapy No Longer Recommended (except in locales where clarithromycin resistance is < 15% or antibiotic sensitivity testing performed)
   - PPI orally twice daily
   - Clarithromycin 500 mg orally twice daily
   - Amoxicillin 1 g orally twice daily (or, if penicillin allergic, metronidazole 500 mg orally twice daily)
2. After completion of course of *H pylori* eradication therapy, continue treatment with PPI[2] once daily or vonoprazan 20 mg once daily for additional 4–6 weeks if ulcer is large (> 1 cm) or complicated.
3. Confirm successful eradication of *H pylori* with fecal antigen or PCR test, or endoscopy with biopsy at least 4 weeks after completion of antibiotic treatment and 2 weeks after completion of PPI treatment.

Active ulcer not attributable to *H pylori*

Consider other causes: NSAIDs, Zollinger-Ellison syndrome, gastric malignancy, vasculitis.

Treatment options:
- PPIs:[2]
  Uncomplicated duodenal ulcer: treat for 4 weeks
  Uncomplicated gastric ulcer: treat for 8 weeks
- H_2-receptor antagonists: no longer recommended due to lower efficacy than PPIs

Prophylaxis of ulcer disease in high-risk patients

1. High-risk patients
   NSAID use with other risk factors: age > 65 years, prior peptic ulcer disease, or concomitant aspirin, antiplatelet agents, or anticoagulants
   Combination aspirin and antiplatelet agent with other risk factors: age > 65 years, prior peptic ulcer disease, or concomitant anticoagulants
   Oral anticoagulants and concomitant NSAIDs or antiplatelet agents
2. Prophylactic measures
   Test and treat for *H pylori*
   Administer PPI once daily[2]
   If NSAID prescribed, use a COX-2 selective inhibitor (eg, celecoxib, meloxicam)

[1]2024 American College of Gastroenterology (ACG) *H pylori* infection treatment guideline provides strong recommendation for optimized bismuth quadruple therapy (BQT) as first-line therapy for treatment-naïve patients and for treatment of patients with persistent infection who did not previously receive BQT.

[2]Oral PPIs: omeprazole 40 mg, rabeprazole 20 mg, lansoprazole 30 mg, dexlansoprazole 30–60 mg, pantoprazole 40 mg, esomeprazole 40 mg. PPIs are administered 30 minutes before meals.

[3]Pylera is an FDA-approved formulation containing bismuth subcitrate 140 mg/tetracycline 125 mg/metronidazole 125 mg per capsule. Take four tablets of each agent orally, four times daily, and PPI twice daily. Packaged for a 10-day course, but a 14-day treatment is recommended.[1]

[4]Talicia is an FDA-approved, rifabutin-based, triple-combination formulation, with each capsule containing omeprazole 10 mg/rifabutin 12.5 mg/amoxicillin 250 mg. Four capsules orally, three times daily for 14 days, are recommended. Rifabutin-based triple therapy is recommended for patients with persistent *H pylori* infection who previously received BQT.

[5]Voquenza Triple Pak is an FDA-approved co-packaged product containing vonoprazan 20 mg, amoxicillin 500 mg, and clarithromycin 500 mg. Voquezna Dual Pak contains vonoprazan 20 mg and amoxicillin 500 mg only. These regimens received a conditional recommendation for treatment-naïve patients.

Chey WD et al. ACG clinical guideline: treatment of *Helicobacter pylori* infection. Am J Gastroenterol. 2024;119:1730. [PMID: 39626064]

Shah S et al. *Helicobacter pylori* burden in the United States according to individual demographics and geography: a nationwide analysis of the Veterans Healthcare System. Clin Gastroenterol Hepatol. 2024;22:42. [PMID: 37245717]

B. Autoimmune (Pernicious Anemia) Gastritis

Autoimmune gastritis (AIG) is an autoimmune disorder in which autoantibodies targeting the parietal cells results in chronic inflammation with gradual destruction of the oxyntic glands (located in the gastric corpus (body and fundus)) with resultant achlorhydria and decreased iron absorption, and decreased intrinsic factor secretion (resulting in vitamin B_{12} malabsorption with macrocytic anemia). Of patients with B_{12} deficiency, only a small number have AIG. AIG histology is characterized by severe atrophy of the gastric body and fundus and replacement of the glands by fibrous and metaplastic tissue. The gastric antrum (which does not contain oxyntic glands) is spared unless concomitant *H pylori* infection is present. Anti-intrinsic factor antibodies are present in 30–60% but are highly specific (> 95%) for AIG. Anti–parietal cell antibodies are present in 70% of patients but may also be positive in patients with *H pylori*–associated gastritis. Patients may have other associated autoimmune conditions, including autoimmune thyroiditis and type 1 diabetes mellitus.

With the development of atrophic gastritis, the risk of gastric adenocarcinoma is increased threefold (with a prevalence of 1–3%), but recent data suggest this risk is primarily in those with concomitant *H pylori* infection. Patients with AIG should undergo testing for *H pylori* infection and treatment, if positive. Achlorhydria leads to pronounced hypergastrinemia (> 1000 pg/mL) that may induce hyperplasia of gastric enterochromaffin-like cells and the development of type 1 gastric carcinoids in 5% of patients that usually are small (< 1 cm) and indolent.

In light of the risk of gastric adenocarcinoma and carcinoid tumors, endoscopy with biopsy currently is recommended in patients with pernicious anemia at the time of diagnosis. Carcinoids < 2 cm should undergo endoscopic resection; lesions > 2 cm have a greater risk of metastatic spread and should be referred for surgical resection. Subsequent endoscopic surveillance every 3 years may be considered in those with severe atrophic gastritis or carcinoid tumors. Pernicious anemia is discussed in detail in Chapter 15.

Morgan D et al. ACG Guideline: diagnosis and management of gastric premalignant conditions. Am J Gastroenterol. 2025;120:709. [PMID: 40072510]

C. Atrophic Gastritis with Intestinal Metaplasia

Ongoing inflammation and glandular destruction may lead to patchy or diffuse atrophy of the gastric antrum, incisura, or body (corpus) with subsequent development of gastric intestinal metaplasia, which is the most important precursor to the development of noncardia gastric adenocarcinoma. Approximately 80% of noncardia gastric cancer is attributable to atrophy and metaplasia that is due to chronic *H pylori* infection.

The diagnosis of atrophic gastritis and intestinal metaplasia is based on histologic assessment of mucosal biopsies obtained at endoscopy. Although difficult to visualize with older "standard definition" endoscopes, atrophic gastritis and intestinal metaplasia can be accurately identified with use of high-definition endoscopes and electronic or dye-based image enhancement. The presence, extent, and severity of mucosal atrophy and intestinal metaplasia requires histologic assessment from at least five random biopsies of the antrum, incisura, and body as well as targeted biopsies of abnormal areas. Assessment for *H pylori* should be performed and followed (if positive) by eradication treatment, which results in a 36% relative risk reduction for future gastric cancer.

Because most gastric cancer develops in patients with gastric intestinal metaplasia, endoscopic screening for gastric metaplasia and early gastric cancer is recommended in high-risk populations. Gastric cancer is the fifth most common cancer worldwide with the highest incidence in Asia, Latin America, and Eastern Europe. In Japan and South Korea, where population-based endoscopic screening is widely practiced, 60% of gastric cancers are detected at an early, curable stage and overall survival is > 60–70%. In the United States, < 20% of gastric cancers are diagnosed at an early stage and overall survival is 32%. American professional guidelines do not endorse population-based endoscopic screening due to the overall low gastric cancer incidence and lack of cost-effectiveness; however, a 2025 AGA guideline recommends that screening be *considered* in high-risk groups, including non-White racial and ethnic groups, first-generation immigrants from high-incidence regions, and those with a family history of gastric cancer in first-degree relatives.

Endoscopic surveillance with biopsy every 3 years is recommended for patients with severe atrophic gastritis or gastric intestinal metaplasia that is multifocal or incomplete. Lesions with low- or high-grade dysplasia should be endoscopically resected.

Morgan DR et al. ACG clinical guideline: diagnosis and management of gastric premalignant conditions. Am J Gastroenterol. 2025;120:709. [PMID: 40072510]
Shah S et al. AGA Clinical Practice update on screening and surveillance in individuals at increased risk for gastric cancer in the United States: expert review. Gastroenterology. 2025;168:405. [PMID: 39718517]

3. Other Specific Types of Gastritis

Infectious Gastritis

Acute bacterial infection of the gastric submucosa and muscularis with a variety of aerobic or anaerobic organisms produces a rare, rapidly progressive, life-threatening condition known as phlegmonous or necrotizing gastritis, which requires broad-spectrum antibiotic therapy and, in many cases, emergency gastric resection. Viral infection with CMV is seen in patients with AIDS and after bone marrow or solid organ transplantation. Endoscopic findings include thickened gastric folds and ulcerations. Fungal infection with mucormycosis and *Candida* may occur in immunocompromised and patients with diabetes. Larvae of *Anisakis marina* ingested in raw fish or sushi may become embedded in the gastric mucosa, producing severe abdominal pain. Pain persists for several days until the larvae die. Endoscopic removal of the larvae provides rapid symptomatic relief.

PEPTIC ULCER DISEASE

ESSENTIALS OF DIAGNOSIS

- History of dyspepsia in 80–90% of patients with variable relationship to meals.
- Ulcer complications present without antecedent symptoms in 10–20% of patients.
- Most NSAID-induced ulcers are asymptomatic.
- Upper endoscopy with gastric biopsy for *H pylori* is the diagnostic procedure of choice in most patients.
- Gastric ulcer biopsy or documentation of complete healing necessary to exclude gastric malignancy.

General Considerations

Peptic ulcer is a break in the gastric or duodenal mucosa that arises when the normal mucosal defensive factors are impaired or are overwhelmed by aggressive luminal factors such as acid and pepsin. In the United States, there are about 500,000 new cases per year of peptic ulcer and 4 million ulcer recurrences. Ulcers occur either in the duodenum, where over 95% are in the bulb or pyloric channel, or in the stomach, where benign ulcers are located most commonly in the antrum (60%) or at the junction of the antrum and body on the lesser curvature (25%).

The incidence of duodenal ulcer disease has been declining dramatically for the past 30 years (due to the eradication of *H pylori*), but the incidence of gastric ulcers has not declined (due to the widespread use of NSAIDs and low-dose aspirin).

Etiology

Two major factors account for 75% of peptic ulcers: NSAIDs and chronic *H pylori* infection. Evidence of *H pylori* infection or NSAID ingestion therefore should be sought in all patients with peptic ulcer. Less than 5% of ulcers are caused by other conditions, including acid hypersecretory states (such as Zollinger-Ellison syndrome or systemic mastocytosis), CMV (especially in transplant recipients), Crohn disease, vasculitis, lymphoma, or chronic medical illness (cirrhosis or CKD). Approximately 20% of peptic ulcers are idiopathic. Alcohol, dietary factors, and stress do not appear to cause ulcer disease.

A. *H pylori*–Associated Ulcers

H pylori infection with associated gastritis appears to be a necessary cofactor for the majority of duodenal and gastric ulcers not associated with NSAIDs. Ulcer disease will develop in an estimated 10% of infected patients. The prevalence of *H pylori* infection in patients with duodenal ulcers is 70–90%. The association with gastric ulcers is lower, but *H pylori* is found in most patients in whom NSAIDs cannot be implicated.

In the absence of specific antibiotic treatment to eradicate *H pylori*, 85% of patients will have an endoscopically visible ulcer recurrence within 1 year. Half of these will be symptomatic. After successful eradication of *H pylori* with antibiotics, ulcer recurrence rates are reduced dramatically to 5–20% at 1 year. Most of these ulcer recurrences are due to NSAID use or, rarely, reinfection with *H pylori*.

B. NSAID-Induced Ulcers

Approximately 2–5%/year of long-term NSAID users will have a gastric or duodenal ulcer that causes clinically significant dyspepsia or a serious complication. The incidence of serious GI complications (hospitalization, bleeding, perforation) is 0.2–1.9%/year. Meta-analyses of clinical trials detected an increased risk of upper GI bleeding in patients taking low-dose aspirin (1 of 1000), coxibs (2 of 1000), and nsNSAIDs (4–6 of 1000). The risk of NSAID complications is greater within the first 3 months of therapy and in patients who are older than 65 years; who have a prior history of ulcer disease; or who take NSAIDs in combination with aspirin, corticosteroids, or anticoagulants.

Traditional nsNSAIDs and aspirin inhibit prostaglandins through inhibition of both COX-1 and COX-2 enzymes. Coxibs (or selective NSAIDs) preferentially inhibit COX-2—the principal enzyme involved in prostaglandin production at sites of inflammation—while providing relative sparing of COX-1, the principal enzyme involved with mucosal cytoprotection in the stomach and duodenum. Celecoxib is the only coxib currently available in the United States, although other older NSAIDs (etodolac, meloxicam) may have similar COX-2/COX-1 selectivity.

Compared with nsNSAIDs, coxibs decrease the incidence of endoscopically visible ulcers by approximately 75% and the risk of significant clinical events (obstruction, perforation, bleeding) by up to 50%. Some coxibs (rofecoxib, valdecoxib) were removed from the market due to an increased risk of cardiovascular complications. A review by an FDA panel suggested that all NSAIDs (other than aspirin and, possibly, naproxen) may be associated with an increased risk of cardiovascular complications, but concluded that celecoxib, which has less COX-2 selectivity than rofecoxib and valdecoxib, does not have higher risk than other nsNSAIDs when used in recommended doses (200 mg/day). In a large, randomized trial comparing ibuprofen, naproxen, and celecoxib in patients with arthritis who have increased cardiovascular risk, no difference was found in cardiovascular safety between the three drugs over 3 years. However, celecoxib was associated with a 30% reduction in serious GI events.

Use of even low-dose aspirin (81–325 mg/day) leads to a twofold increased risk of GI bleeding complications (1.2% per year). However, patients with a prior history of peptic ulcers or GI bleeding have a markedly increased risk of complications on low-dose aspirin. It should be noted that low-dose aspirin in combination with NSAIDs or coxibs increases the risk of ulcer complications by up to tenfold compared with NSAIDs or low-dose aspirin alone. Dual antiplatelet therapy with aspirin and a thienopyridine (eg, clopidogrel) incurs a twofold to threefold increased risk of bleeding compared with aspirin alone.

H pylori infection increases the risk of ulcer disease and complications over threefold in patients taking NSAIDs or low-dose aspirin. It is hypothesized that NSAID initiation may potentiate or aggravate ulcer disease in susceptible infected individuals.

Clinical Findings

A. Symptoms and Signs

Epigastric pain (dyspepsia), the hallmark of peptic ulcer disease, is present in 80–90% of patients. However, this complaint is not sensitive or specific enough to serve as a reliable diagnostic criterion for peptic ulcer disease. Less than 10% of patients with dyspepsia have ulcer disease at endoscopy. Twenty percent of patients with ulcer complications such as bleeding have no antecedent symptoms ("silent ulcers"). Nearly 60% of patients with NSAID-related ulcer complications do not have prior symptoms.

Pain is typically well localized to the epigastrium and not severe. It is described as gnawing, dull, aching, or "hunger-like." Other symptoms may include nausea, substernal chest discomfort, or early satiety. Approximately 50% of patients report relief of pain with food or antacids. However, many patients deny any relationship to meals or report worsening of pain. Nausea and anorexia may occur. Two-thirds of duodenal ulcers and one-third of gastric ulcers cause nocturnal pain that awakens the patient. A change from a patient's typical rhythmic discomfort to constant or radiating pain may reflect ulcer penetration or perforation. Significant vomiting and weight loss are unusual with uncomplicated ulcer disease and suggest gastric outlet obstruction or gastric malignancy. Most patients have symptomatic periods lasting up to several weeks with intervals of months to years in which they are pain free (periodicity).

The physical examination is often normal in uncomplicated peptic ulcer disease. Mild, localized epigastric tenderness to deep palpation may be present. FOBT or FIT is positive in one-third of patients.

B. Laboratory Findings

Laboratory tests are normal in uncomplicated peptic ulcer disease but are ordered to exclude ulcer complications or confounding disease entities. Anemia may occur with acute blood loss from a bleeding ulcer or less commonly from chronic blood loss. Leukocytosis suggests ulcer penetration or perforation. An elevated serum amylase in a patient with severe epigastric pain suggests ulcer penetration into the pancreas. A fasting serum gastrin level to screen for gastrinoma (Zollinger-Ellison syndrome) is obtained in patients with ulcers that are recurrent or refractory to standard medical treatment.

C. Endoscopy

Upper endoscopy is the procedure of choice for the diagnosis of duodenal and gastric ulcers. Duodenal ulcers are virtually never malignant and do not require biopsy. Three to 5 percent of benign-appearing gastric ulcers prove to be malignant. Hence, biopsies of the ulcer margin are almost always performed. Provided that the gastric ulcer appears benign to the endoscopist and adequate biopsy specimens reveal no evidence of cancer, dysplasia, or atypia, the patient may be monitored without further endoscopy. If these conditions are not fulfilled, follow-up endoscopy should be performed 8–12 weeks after the start of therapy to document complete healing; nonhealing ulcers are suspicious for malignancy.

D. Imaging

Abdominal CT imaging is obtained in patients with suspected complications of peptic ulcer disease (perforation, penetration, or obstruction). Barium upper GI series is no longer recommended.

E. Testing for *H pylori*

In patients in whom an ulcer is diagnosed by endoscopy, gastric mucosal biopsies should be obtained for histologic evaluation. Noninvasive assessment for *H pylori* with fecal antigen, fecal PCR assay, or urea breath testing may be done in patients with a history of peptic ulcer disease to diagnose active infection or in patients following its treatment to confirm successful eradication with a sensitivity and specificity for infection of 95%. PPIs may cause false-negative fecal antigen tests and should be withheld for at least 14 days before testing. Because of its lower sensitivity (85%) and specificity (79%), serologic testing should not be performed unless fecal testing is unavailable.

Differential Diagnosis

Peptic ulcer disease must be distinguished from other causes of epigastric distress (dyspepsia). Over 50% of patients with dyspepsia have no obvious organic explanation for their symptoms and are classified as having functional dyspepsia (see sections above on Dyspepsia). Atypical gastroesophageal reflux may be manifested by epigastric symptoms. Biliary tract disease is characterized by discrete, intermittent episodes of pain that should not be confused with other causes of dyspepsia. Severe epigastric pain is atypical for peptic ulcer disease unless complicated by a perforation or penetration. Other causes include acute pancreatitis, acute cholecystitis or choledocholithiasis, esophageal rupture, gastric volvulus, gastric or intestinal ischemia, and ruptured aortic aneurysm.

Pharmacologic Agents

Agents that enhance the healing of peptic ulcers are acid-antisecretory agents and agents that promote healing through eradication of *H pylori*.

A. Acid-Antisecretory Agents

1. PPIs—PPIs covalently bind the acid-secreting enzyme H^+-K^+-ATPase, or "proton pump," permanently inactivating it.

Six oral PPIs are available: omeprazole, rabeprazole, esomeprazole, lansoprazole, dexlansoprazole, and pantoprazole. Despite minor differences in their pharmacology, they are equally efficacious in the treatment of peptic ulcer disease. Treatment with oral PPIs results in over 90%

healing of duodenal ulcers after 4 weeks and 90% of gastric ulcers after 8 weeks when given once daily (30 minutes before breakfast) at the following recommended doses: omeprazole, 20–40 mg; esomeprazole, 40 mg; rabeprazole, 20 mg; lansoprazole, 30 mg; dexlansoprazole, 30–60 mg; and pantoprazole, 40 mg. Compared with H_2-receptor antagonists, PPIs provide faster pain relief and more rapid ulcer healing. The PPIs are remarkably safe for short-term therapy. (For potential long-term risks, see Gastroesophageal Reflux Disease.)

2. H_2-receptor antagonists—Although H_2-receptor antagonists are effective in the treatment of peptic ulcer disease, PPIs are the preferred agents because of their ease of use and superior efficacy. Three H_2-receptor antagonists are available: cimetidine, famotidine, and nizatidine. For uncomplicated peptic ulcers, H_2-receptor antagonists may be administered once daily at bedtime as follows: nizatidine 300 mg, famotidine 40 mg, and cimetidine 800 mg. Duodenal and gastric ulcer healing rates of 85–90% are obtained within 6 weeks and 8 weeks, respectively.

B. *H pylori* Eradication Therapy

Eradication of *H pylori* has proved difficult. Combination regimens that use two or three antibiotics with a PPI or bismuth are required to achieve adequate rates of eradication and to reduce the number of failures due to antibiotic resistance. In the United States, approximately 30% of strains are resistant to metronidazole or levofloxacin, and 50% are resistant to clarithromycin. Resistance to tetracycline and amoxicillin remains low.

Commercial laboratories offer molecular-based (PCR) testing of stool or biopsy specimens with next-generation sequencing for *H pylori* genes associated with antibiotic resistance. At present, PCR with next-generation sequencing is recommended for patients with persistent *H pylori* infection after initial empiric therapy to determine the optimal regimen for subsequent treatment.

Recommended treatment regimens are listed in Table 17–10. Updated 2024 American College of Gastroenterology (ACG) treatment guidelines recommend that triple therapy with a PPI, clarithromycin, and amoxicillin no longer be used (due to increasing clarithromycin resistance) except in areas with known low-level clarithromycin resistance (< 15%) or when susceptibility has been confirmed by molecular-based tests. In most settings, empiric treatment for 14 days is recommended with either a bismuth-based quadruple therapy (BQT) regimen or a rifabutin-based triple therapy regimen. Both achieve a > 85% eradication rate. The ACG treatment guideline provides a strong recommendation for use of the BQT regimen as the preferred first-line empiric therapy. BQT consists of bismuth, tetracycline, metronidazole, and a PPI. It is effective even for metronidazole-resistant strains. The rifabutin-based regimen contains omeprazole, rifabutin, and amoxicillin (Talicia). Four capsules are taken orally every 8 hours. Rifabutin-resistant strains are rare.

FDA-approved vonoprazan-based *H pylori* eradication regimens are another option. (These combination regimens consist of vonoprazan 20 mg, amoxicillin 1000 mg, and clarithromycin 500 mg, all taken twice daily for 14 days; or vonoprazan 20 mg twice daily and amoxicillin 1000 mg three times daily for 14 days [Voquezna Triple Pak and Dual Pak].) In phase 3 RCTs in Europe and the United States, *H pylori* eradication following 14-day treatment was compared with vonoprazan triple therapy, vonoprazan dual therapy, and standard triple therapy with a PPI (lansoprazole), amoxicillin, and clarithromycin (LAC). Eradication rates for patients with nonresistant *H pylori* infections were vonoprazan triple therapy, 84.7%; vonoprazan dual therapy, 78.5%; and lansoprazole–clarithromycin triple therapy, 78.8%. Eradication rates for clarithromycin-resistant strains were vonoprazan triple therapy, 65.8%; vonoprazan dual therapy, 69.6%; and lansoprazole triple therapy, 37.7%. The ACG provides a conditional recommendation for vonoprazan–amoxicillin dual therapy as empiric therapy for treatment-naïve patients and advises against use of the vonoprazan–clarithromycin triple therapy unless infection with a clarithromycin-sensitive *H pylori* strain is confirmed.

For patients with persistent infection following an initial course of empiric treatment, the optimal treatment regimens should be determined by antibiotic resistance patterns based on individual fecal PCR tests. If antibiotic sensitivity testing is unavailable, the ACG guideline favors empiric use of the BQT regimen for persistent infection following clarithromycin-based triple therapy and rifabutin-based triple therapy for persistent infection following BQT.

Medical Treatment

Patients should be encouraged to eat balanced meals at regular intervals. There is no justification for bland or restrictive diets. Moderate alcohol intake is not harmful. Cigarette smoking retards the rate of ulcer healing and increases the frequency of recurrences and should cease.

A. Treatment of *H pylori*–Associated Ulcers

1. Treatment of active ulcer—The goals of treatment of active *H pylori*–associated ulcers are to relieve dyspeptic symptoms, to promote ulcer healing, and to eradicate *H pylori* infection. Uncomplicated *H pylori*–associated ulcers should be treated for 14 days with one of the PPI-based or vonoprazan-based *H pylori* eradication regimens listed in Table 17–10. At that point, no further antisecretory therapy is needed, provided the ulcer was small (< 1 cm) and dyspeptic symptoms have resolved. For patients with large or complicated ulcers, treatment with a once-daily PPI should be continued for an additional 2–4 weeks (duodenal ulcer) or 4–6 weeks (gastric ulcer) after completion of the antibiotic regimen to ensure complete ulcer healing (as listed in Table 17–10). Confirmation of *H pylori* eradication is recommended for all patients > 4 weeks after completion of antibiotic therapy and > 2 weeks after discontinuation of the PPI with either a fecal antigen test or endoscopy with biopsy for histology.

2. Therapy to prevent recurrence—Successful eradication reduces ulcer recurrences to < 20% after 1–2 years. The most common cause of recurrence after antibiotic therapy is failure to achieve successful eradication. Once cure has been achieved, reinfection rates are < 0.5% per year. In all patients with recurrent ulcers, persistent *H pylori* infection, NSAID usage (unintentional or surreptitious) and hypersecretory states (including gastrinoma) should be excluded.

B. Treatment of NSAID-Induced Ulcers

1. Treatment of active ulcers—In patients with NSAID-induced ulcers, the offending agent should be discontinued whenever possible. Both gastric and duodenal ulcers respond rapidly to therapy with PPIs (Table 17–10) once NSAIDs are eliminated. All patients with NSAID-associated ulcers should undergo testing for *H pylori* infection. Antibiotic eradication therapy should be given if *H pylori* tests are positive.

2. Prevention of NSAID-induced ulcers—Clinicians should carefully weigh the benefits of NSAID therapy with the risks of cardiovascular and GI complications. Ulcer complications occur in up to 2% of all nsNSAID-treated patients per year, but in up to 10–20% per year of patients with multiple risk factors. These include age > 65 years, history of ulcer disease or complications, concurrent use of antiplatelet therapy (low-dose aspirin or clopidogrel, or both), concurrent therapy with anticoagulants or corticosteroids, and serious underlying medical illness. After considering the patient's risk of cardiovascular and GI complications due to NSAID use, the clinician can decide what type of NSAID (oral nsNSAID, coxib, or topical NSAID) is appropriate and what strategies should be used to reduce the risk of such complications. To minimize cardiovascular and GI risks, all NSAIDs should be used at the lowest effective dose and for the shortest time necessary.

A. TEST FOR AND TREAT H PYLORI INFECTION—All patients with a known history of peptic ulcer disease who are treated with NSAIDs or antiplatelet agents (aspirin, clopidogrel) should be tested for *H pylori* infection (see above) and treated, if positive. Although *H pylori* eradication may decrease the risk of NSAID-related complications, co-therapy with a PPI is still required in high-risk patients.

B. PPI—Treatment with an oral PPI given once daily (rabeprazole 20 mg, omeprazole 20–40 mg, lansoprazole 30 mg, dexlansoprazole 30–60 mg, pantoprazole 40 mg, or esomeprazole 40 mg) is effective in the prevention of NSAID-induced gastric and duodenal ulcers and is approved by the FDA for this indication. Nonetheless, PPIs are not fully protective in high-risk patients in preventing NSAID-related complications. In prospective, controlled trials of patients with a prior history of NSAID-related ulcer complications, the incidence of recurrent bleeding was almost 5% after 6 months in patients taking nsNSAIDs and a PPI. In prospective, controlled trials of patients with a prior history of ulcer complications related to low-dose aspirin, the incidence of recurrent ulcer bleeding in patients taking low-dose aspirin alone was approximately 15% per year compared with 0–2% per year in patients taking low-dose aspirin and PPI. Thus, PPIs are highly effective in preventing complications related to low-dose aspirin, even in high-risk patients. Enteric coating of aspirin may reduce direct topical damage to the stomach but does not reduce its other complications.

C. RECOMMENDATIONS TO REDUCE RISK OF ULCER COMPLICATIONS FROM NSNSAIDS AND COXIBS—For patients with a low risk of CVD who have no risk factors for GI complications, an nsNSAID alone may be given. For patients with one or two GI risk factors, a coxib alone, a topical NSAID (diclofenac), or an nsNSAID should be given with a PPI once daily to reduce the risk of GI complications. NSAIDs should be avoided, if possible, in patients with multiple risk factors; if required, however, combination therapy of celecoxib or a partially COX-2 selective nsNSAID (etodolac, meloxicam) with a PPI once daily is recommended. For patients with an increased risk of cardiovascular complications, it is preferable to avoid NSAIDs, if possible.

D. RECOMMENDATIONS TO REDUCE RISK OF ULCER COMPLICATIONS WITH USE OF ANTIPLATELET AGENTS—The risk of significant GI complications in persons taking low-dose aspirin (81–325 mg/day) or clopidogrel, or both, for cardiovascular prophylaxis is 0.5%/year. Aspirin, 81 mg/day, is recommended in most patients because it has a lower risk of GI complications but equivalent cardiovascular protection compared with higher aspirin doses. Complications are increased with combinations of aspirin and clopidogrel or aspirin and anticoagulants. Patients with dyspepsia or prior ulcer disease should be tested for *H pylori* infection and treated, if positive. Patients younger than 65–70 years who have no other risk factors for GI complications may be treated with low-dose aspirin or dual antiplatelet therapy without a PPI. Virtually all other patients who require low-dose aspirin or aspirin plus anticoagulant therapy should receive a PPI once daily.

Clopidogrel is a prodrug that is activated by the cytochrome P450 CYP2C19 enzyme. All PPIs inhibit CYP2C19 to varying degrees, with omeprazole and esomeprazole having the highest level of inhibition. The FDA has issued a warning that patients should avoid using clopidogrel with omeprazole and esomeprazole. Once-daily treatment with other oral PPI (pantoprazole 40 mg; rabeprazole 20 mg; lansoprazole or dexlansoprazole 30 mg) may be recommended for patients who have an increased risk of upper GI bleeding (prior history of peptic ulcer disease or GI bleeding; concomitant NSAIDs).

C. Refractory Ulcers

Ulcers that are truly refractory to medical therapy are now uncommon. Less than 5% of ulcers are unhealed after 8 weeks of once daily therapy with PPIs, and almost all benign ulcers heal with twice-daily therapy. Thus, nonadherence is the most common cause of ulcer nonhealing. NSAID and aspirin use, sometimes surreptitious, are commonly implicated in refractory ulcers and must be stopped. Single or multiple linear gastric ulcers may occur in large hiatal hernias where the stomach slides back and forth through the diaphragmatic hiatus ("Cameron lesions"); this may be a cause of iron deficiency anemia. Other causes of nonhealing ulcers include acid hypersecretion due to gastrinoma (Zollinger-Ellison syndrome), unrecognized malignancy (adenocarcinoma or lymphoma), medications causing GI ulceration (eg, iron or bisphosphonates), Crohn disease, vasculitis, and unusual infections (*H heilmannii*, CMV, mucormycosis). Fasting serum gastrin levels should be obtained to exclude gastrinoma with acid hypersecretion (Zollinger-Ellison syndrome). Repeat ulcer biopsies are mandatory after 2–3 months of therapy in all nonhealed ulcers to look for malignancy or infection. Patients with persistent nonhealing ulcers are referred for surgical therapy after exclusion of NSAID use and persistent *H pylori* infection.

Almadi MA et al. Peptic ulcer disease. Lancet. 2024;404:68. [PMID: 38885678]

Chey WD et al. ACG clinical guideline: treatment of *Helicobacter pylori* infection. Am J Gastroenterol. 2024;119:1730. [PMID: 39626064]

Moss SF et al. Evolving concepts in *Helicobacter pylori* management. Gastroenterology. 2024;166:267. [PMID: 37806461]

Patel A et al. AGA clinical practice update on integrating potassium-competitive acid blockers into clinical practice: expert review. Gastroenterology. 2024;167:1128. [PMID: 39269391]

COMPLICATIONS OF PEPTIC ULCER DISEASE

1. Upper GI Hemorrhage

ESSENTIALS OF DIAGNOSIS

- "Coffee grounds" emesis, hematemesis, melena, or hematochezia.
- Emergent upper endoscopy is diagnostic and therapeutic.

General Considerations

Approximately 50% of all episodes of upper GI bleeding are due to peptic ulcer. Clinically significant bleeding occurs in 10% of ulcer patients. About 80% of patients stop bleeding spontaneously and generally have an uneventful recovery; the remaining 20% have more severe bleeding. The overall mortality rate for ulcer bleeding is 7%, but it is higher in older patients, in patients with comorbid medical problems, and in patients with hospital-associated bleeding. Mortality is also higher in patients who present with persistent hypotension or shock, bright red blood in the vomitus or nasogastric lavage fluid, or severe coagulopathy.

Clinical Findings

A. Symptoms and Signs

Up to 20% of patients have no antecedent pain; this is particularly true of patients receiving NSAIDs. Common presenting signs include melena and hematemesis. Massive upper GI bleeding or rapid GI transit may result in hematochezia rather than melena; this may be misinterpreted as signifying a lower tract bleeding source.

B. Laboratory Findings

The hematocrit may fall as a result of bleeding or expansion of the intravascular volume with intravenous fluids. The BUN may rise as a result of absorption of blood nitrogen from the small intestine and from prerenal azotemia.

Treatment

A. Medical Therapy

1. Antisecretory agents—Intravenous PPIs have been associated with a reduction in rebleeding, transfusions, need for further endoscopic therapy, and surgery in the subset of patients with high-risk ulcers, ie, an ulcer with active bleeding, visible vessel, or adherent clot. Therefore, intravenous PPIs should be administered to all patients admitted with upper GI bleeding until upper endoscopy is performed. Either esomeprazole or pantoprazole is given 40 mg intravenously every 12 hours. After endoscopy, continuous high-dose PPI infusions are administered for 72 hours to patients who have undergone endoscopic treatment of high-risk ulcers (omeprazole, esomeprazole, or pantoprazole, all dosed at 80-mg bolus injection, followed by 8 mg/hour). Patients with nonbleeding, low-risk ulcers may be treated with a once-daily PPI for 4–6 weeks to promote ulcer healing (see Table 17–10). Intravenous H_2-receptor antagonists have not been demonstrated to be of any benefit in the treatment of acute ulcer bleeding.

2. Long-term prevention of rebleeding—Recurrent ulcer bleeding develops within 3 years in one-third of patients if no specific therapy is given. In patients with bleeding ulcers who are *H pylori*–positive, successful eradication effectively prevents recurrent ulcer bleeding in almost all cases. It is therefore recommended that all patients with bleeding ulcers be tested for *H pylori* infection and treated if positive. (See Treatment of *H pylori*–Associated Ulcers.) Four weeks after completion of antibiotic therapy, a urea breath or fecal antigen test for *H pylori* should be administered or endoscopy performed with biopsy and histology for confirmation of successful eradication. In patients with NSAID-induced bleeding ulcers, NSAIDS should be discontinued whenever possible. When not possible, topical diclofenac or combination therapy of a COX-2–selective inhibitor (eg, celecoxib, etodolac, meloxicam) with a PPI once daily is recommended (see Table 17–10).

B. Endoscopy

Endoscopy is the preferred diagnostic procedure in almost all cases of upper GI bleeding because of its high diagnostic accuracy, its ability to predict the likelihood of recurrent bleeding, and its availability for therapeutic intervention in high-risk lesions. Endoscopy should be performed within 24 hours in most cases. In cases of severe active bleeding, endoscopy should be performed after patients have been appropriately resuscitated and are hemodynamically stable.

On the basis of clinical and endoscopic criteria, it is possible to predict which patients are at a higher risk of rebleeding and therefore to make more rational use of hospital resources. Nonbleeding ulcers under 2 cm in size with a base that is clean have a $< 5\%$ chance of rebleeding. Most otherwise healthy patients under age 60 years with clean-based ulcers may be safely discharged from the emergency department or hospital after endoscopy. Ulcers that have a flat red or black spot have a < 10% chance of significant rebleeding. Patients who are hemodynamically stable with these findings should be admitted to a hospital ward for 24–72 hours and may begin immediate oral feedings and antiulcer (or anti–*H pylori*) medication.

By contrast, the risk of rebleeding or continued bleeding in ulcers with a nonbleeding visible vessel is 50%, and with active bleeding, it is 80–90%. Endoscopic therapy with thermocoagulation (bipolar or heater probes) or application of endoscopic clips (akin to a staple) is the standard of care for such lesions because it reduces the risk of rebleeding, the number of transfusions, and the need for subsequent surgery. The optimal treatment of ulcers with a dense clot that adheres despite vigorous washing is controversial; removal of the clot followed by endoscopic treatment of an underlying vessel may be considered in selected high-risk patients. For actively bleeding ulcers, a combination of epinephrine injection followed by thermocoagulation or clip application commonly is used. These techniques achieve successful hemostasis of actively bleeding lesions in 90% of patients. After endoscopic therapy followed by an intravenous PPI, significant rebleeding occurs in < 10% of cases, of which over 70% can be managed successfully with repeat endoscopic treatment. After endoscopic treatment, patients should remain hospitalized for at least 72 hours, when the risk of rebleeding falls to below 3%.

To the present, endoscopic application of topical hemostatic powder has been restricted in most clinical settings as an adjunctive therapy to provide temporary hemostasis for massive bleeding that interferes with effective application of thermocoagulation or endoclip placement, for treatment of lesions located in areas that are difficult to treat with conventional endoscopic modalities, and for treatment of diffuse mucosal bleeding from malignancies. A 2025 meta-analysis of eight RCTs reported similar rates of initial hemostasis and recurrent bleeding between topical hemostatic powder and conventional endoscopic therapies for non-malignancy-related GI bleeding. The 2021 ACG guideline has provided a conditional recommendation for use of topical hemostatic powder for actively bleeding ulcers.

C. Recurrent Bleeding

Less than 5% of patients have persistent or recurrent bleeding that cannot be controlled with endoscopic techniques. The availability of newer, larger over-the-scope clips has further reduced the risk of persistent bleeding requiring other more aggressive interventions. For patients in whom endoscopic therapy is unsuccessful, percutaneous radiologic embolization or surgery should be considered. Overall surgical mortality for emergency ulcer bleeding is < 6%. The prognosis is poorer for patients over age 60 years, those with serious underlying medical illnesses or CKD, and those who require > 10 units of blood transfusion.

2. Ulcer Perforation

Perforations develop in < 5% of ulcers, usually from ulcers on the anterior wall of the stomach or duodenum. Perforation results in a chemical peritonitis that causes sudden, severe generalized abdominal pain that prompts most patients to seek immediate attention. Older adults or debilitated patients and those receiving long-term corticosteroid therapy may experience minimal initial symptoms, presenting late with bacterial peritonitis, sepsis, and shock. On physical examination, patients appear ill, with a rigid, quiet abdomen and rebound tenderness. Hypotension develops later after bacterial peritonitis has developed. If hypotension is present early with the onset of pain, other abdominal emergencies should be considered such as a ruptured aortic aneurysm, mesenteric infarction, or acute pancreatitis. Leukocytosis is almost always present. A mildly elevated serum amylase (less than twice normal) is sometimes seen with ulcer perforation. Abdominal CT usually establishes the diagnosis without need for further studies. The absence of free air may lead to a misdiagnosis of pancreatitis, cholecystitis, or appendicitis.

Laparoscopic closure of perforations can be performed in many centers, significantly reducing operative morbidity compared with open laparotomy.

3. Ulcer Penetration

An ulcer located along the posterior wall of the duodenum or stomach may perforate and penetrate into contiguous structures such as the pancreas, liver, or biliary tree. Patients report a change in the intensity and rhythmicity of their ulcer symptoms. The pain becomes more severe and constant, may radiate to the back, and is unresponsive to antacids or food. Physical examination and laboratory tests are nonspecific. Mild amylase elevations may sometimes occur. Endoscopy confirms the ulceration and abdominal CT imaging demonstrates the penetration. Patients should be given intravenous PPIs and monitored closely. Those who do not improve should be considered for surgery.

4. Gastric Outlet Obstruction

Gastric outlet obstruction occurs in < 2% of ulcers and is due to edema or cicatricial narrowing of the pylorus or duodenal bulb. With the advent of potent antisecretory therapy with PPIs and the eradication of *H pylori*, obstruction is less commonly caused by peptic ulcers than by gastric neoplasms or extrinsic duodenal obstruction by intra-abdominal neoplasms. The most common symptoms are early satiety, vomiting, and weight loss. Patients may develop dehydration, metabolic alkalosis, and hypokalemia. On physical examination, a succussion splash may be heard in the epigastrium. In most cases, nasogastric aspiration will result in evacuation of a large amount (> 200 mL) of foul-smelling fluid, which establishes the diagnosis. Patients are treated initially with intravenous isotonic saline and KCl to correct fluid and electrolyte disorders, an intravenous PPI, and nasogastric decompression of the stomach. Upper endoscopy is performed after 24–72 hours to define the nature of the obstruction, to exclude gastric neoplasm, and to perform balloon dilation of pyloric stenosis when caused by peptic ulcer disease.

Arshad S et al. Management of perforated peptic ulcer: a review. JAMA Surg. 2025;160:450. [PMID: 39937493]
Liu K et al. Efficacy of hemostatic powder monotherapy versus conventional endoscopic treatment for nonvariceal GI bleeding: a meta-analysis and trial sequential analysis. Gastrointest Endosc. 2025;101:539. [PMID: 39265743

ZOLLINGER-ELLISON SYNDROME (Gastrinoma)

ESSENTIALS OF DIAGNOSIS

- Peptic ulcer disease; may be severe and atypical.
- Gastric acid hypersecretion.
- Diarrhea common, relieved by nasogastric suction.
- Most cases are sporadic; 25% occur with multiple endocrine neoplasia type 1 (MEN 1).

General Considerations

Zollinger-Ellison syndrome is caused by gastrin-secreting gut neuroendocrine tumors (gastrinomas), which result in hypergastrinemia and acid hypersecretion. Less than 1% of peptic ulcer disease is caused by gastrinomas. Primary gastrinomas may arise in the pancreas (25%), duodenal wall (45%), or lymph nodes (5–15%), and in other locations including unknown primary sites (20%). Approximately 80% arise within the "gastrinoma triangle" bounded by the porta hepatis, the neck of the pancreas, and the third portion of the duodenum. Most gastrinomas are solitary or multifocal nodules that are potentially resectable. Approximately 25% of patients have small multicentric gastrinomas associated with MEN 1 that are more difficult to resect. Over two-thirds of gastrinomas are malignant, and one-third have already metastasized to the liver at initial presentation.

Clinical Findings

A. Symptoms and Signs

Over 90% of patients with Zollinger-Ellison syndrome develop peptic ulcers. In most cases, the symptoms are indistinguishable from other causes of peptic ulcer disease, and therefore, the syndrome may go undetected for years. Ulcers usually are solitary and located in the duodenal bulb, but they may be multiple or occur more distally in the duodenum. Isolated gastric ulcers do not occur. Gastroesophageal reflux symptoms occur often. Gastric acid hypersecretion can cause direct intestinal mucosal injury and pancreatic enzyme inactivation, resulting in diarrhea, steatorrhea, and weight loss; nasogastric aspiration of stomach acid stops the diarrhea. Screening for Zollinger-Ellison syndrome with fasting gastrin levels should be done in patients with ulcers that are refractory to standard therapies, giant ulcers (> 2 cm), ulcers located distal to the duodenal bulb, multiple duodenal ulcers, frequent ulcer recurrences, ulcers associated with diarrhea, ulcers occurring after ulcer surgery, and ulcers with complications. Patients with ulcers and hypercalcemia or family histories of ulcers (suggesting MEN 1) should also be screened. Finally, patients with peptic ulcers who are *H pylori* negative and who are not taking NSAIDs should be screened.

B. Laboratory Findings

The most sensitive and specific method for identifying Zollinger-Ellison syndrome is demonstration of an increased fasting serum gastrin concentration (> 150 pg/mL [150 ng/L]). If possible, levels should be obtained with patients not taking H_2-receptor antagonists for 24 hours or PPIs for 6 days; however, withdrawal of the PPI may result in marked gastric hypersecretion with serious consequences and patients should be closely monitored. The median gastrin level in Zollinger-Ellison syndrome is 500–700 pg/mL (500–700 ng/L), and 60% of patients have levels < 1000 pg/mL (1000 ng/L). Hypochlorhydria with increased gastric pH is a much more common cause of hypergastrinemia than is gastrinoma. Therefore, a measurement of gastric pH is performed in patients with fasting hypergastrinemia. A gastric pH > 3.0 implies hypochlorhydria and excludes gastrinoma. In a patient with a serum gastrin level > 1000 pg/mL (1000 ng/L) and gastric pH < 2, the diagnosis of Zollinger-Ellison syndrome is established. With lower gastrin levels (150–1000 pg/mL [150–1000 ng/L]) and acid secretion, a secretin stimulation test may be performed to distinguish Zollinger-Ellison syndrome from other causes of hypergastrinemia. In all patients with Zollinger-Ellison syndrome, serum parathyroid hormone (PTH), prolactin, LH-FSH, and growth hormone (GH) levels should be obtained to exclude MEN 1.

C. Imaging

Imaging studies are obtained in an attempt to determine whether there is metastatic disease and, if not, to identify the site of the primary tumor. CT and MRI scans are commonly obtained first to look for large hepatic metastases and primary lesions, but they have low sensitivity for small lesions. Full body ^{68}Ga-PET scans (preferably combined with CT) have a sensitivity of > 90% for detection of primary tumor in the pancreas, duodenum, and lymph nodes as well as for detection of metastatic disease in liver and bone. Where available, ^{68}Ga-PET/CT has supplanted somatostatin receptor scintigraphy with single PET. In patients with negative ^{68}Ga-PET/CT or somatostatin receptor scintigraphy, endoscopic ultrasonography may be useful to detect small gastrinomas in the duodenal wall, pancreas, or peripancreatic lymph nodes.

Differential Diagnosis

Gastrinomas are one of several gut neuroendocrine tumors that have similar histopathologic features and arise either from the gut or pancreas. These include carcinoid, insulinoma, VIPoma, glucagonoma, and somatostatinoma.

These tumors usually are differentiated by the gut peptides that they secrete; however, poorly differentiated neuroendocrine tumors may not secrete any hormones. Patients may present with symptoms caused by tumor metastases (jaundice, hepatomegaly) rather than functional symptoms. Once a diagnosis of a neuroendocrine tumor is established from the liver biopsy, the specific type of tumor can subsequently be determined. Both carcinoid and gastrinoma tumors may be detected incidentally during endoscopy after biopsy of a submucosal nodule and must be distinguished by subsequent studies.

Hypergastrinemia due to gastrinoma must be distinguished from other causes of hypergastrinemia. Atrophic gastritis with decreased acid secretion is detected by gastric secretory analysis. Other conditions associated with hypergastrinemia (eg, gastric outlet obstruction, vagotomy, CKD) are associated with a negative secretin stimulation test.

Treatment

A. Metastatic Disease

The most important predictor of survival is the presence of metastases (liver or bone). In patients with multiple metastases, initial therapy should be directed at controlling hypersecretion. Oral PPIs (omeprazole, esomeprazole, rabeprazole, pantoprazole, lansoprazole, dexlansoprazole) are given at a dose of 40–120 mg/day, titrated to achieve a basal acid output < 10 mEq/hour. At this level, there is complete symptomatic relief and ulcer healing. Systemic therapies include long-acting somatostatin analogs (octreotide LAR, lanreotide), tyrosine kinase inhibitors, and peptide receptor radionucleotide therapy. Owing to the slow growth of these tumors, 30% of patients with hepatic metastases have a survival of 10 years.

B. Localized Disease

Cure can be achieved only if the gastrinoma can be resected before hepatic metastatic spread has occurred. Lymph node metastases do not adversely affect prognosis. Laparotomy should be considered in all patients in whom preoperative studies fail to demonstrate hepatic or other distant metastases. A combination of preoperative studies, duodenotomy with careful duodenal inspection, and intraoperative palpation and sonography allows successful localization and resection in the majority of cases. The 15-year survival of patients who do not have liver metastases at initial presentation is over 95%. Surgery usually is not recommended in patients with MEN 1 due to the presence of multifocal tumors and long-term survival in the absence of surgery in most patients.

Chatzipanagiotou O et al. All you need to know about gastrinoma today – gastrinoma and Zollinger Ellison syndrome: a thorough update. J Neuroendocrinol. 2023;35:e13267. [PMID: 37042078]

DISEASES OF THE SMALL INTESTINE

MALABSORPTION

The term "malabsorption" denotes disorders in which there is a disruption of digestion and nutrient absorption. The clinical and laboratory manifestations of malabsorption are summarized in Table 17–11.

Table 17–11. Clinical manifestations and laboratory findings in malabsorption of various nutrients.

Manifestations	Laboratory Findings	Malabsorbed Nutrients
Steatorrhea (bulky, light-colored stools)	Increased fecal fat; decreased serum cholesterol; decreased serum carotene, vitamin A, vitamin D	Triglycerides, fatty acids, phospholipids, cholesterol. Fat-soluble vitamins: A, D, E, K
Diarrhea (increased fecal water)	Increased stool volume and weight; increased fecal fat; increased stool osmolality gap	Fats, carbohydrates
Weight loss; muscle wasting	Increased fecal fat; decreased carbohydrate (D-xylose) absorption	Fat, protein, carbohydrates
Microcytic anemia	Low serum iron	Iron
Macrocytic anemia	Decreased serum vitamin B_{12} or RBC folate	Vitamin B_{12} or folic acid
Paresthesia; tetany; positive Trousseau and Chvostek signs	Decreased serum calcium or magnesium	Calcium, vitamin D, magnesium
Bone pain; pathologic fractures; skeletal deformities	Osteopenia on radiograph; osteoporosis (adults); osteomalacia (children)	Calcium, vitamin D
Bleeding tendency (ecchymoses, epistaxis)	Prolonged prothrombin time or INR	Vitamin K
Edema	Decreased serum total protein and albumin; increased fecal loss of α_1-antitrypsin	Protein
Milk intolerance (cramps, bloating, diarrhea)	Abnormal lactose tolerance test	Lactose

1. Celiac Disease

ESSENTIALS OF DIAGNOSIS

- *Typical symptoms*: bloating, chronic diarrhea, weight loss, growth retardation.
- *Atypical symptoms*: dermatitis herpetiformis, iron deficiency anemia, osteoporosis.
- Abnormal serologic test results.
- Abnormal small bowel biopsy.
- Clinical improvement on gluten-free diet.

General Considerations

Celiac disease (also called sprue, celiac sprue, and gluten enteropathy) is a permanent dietary disorder caused by an immunologic response to gluten, a storage protein found in certain grains, that results in diffuse damage to the proximal small intestinal mucosa with malabsorption of nutrients. Although symptoms may manifest between 6 months and 24 months of age after the introduction of weaning foods, most cases present in childhood or adulthood. Population screening with serologic tests suggests that the global prevalence of this disease is 1.4%. In North America, the prevalence of biopsy-confirmed disease is 0.7%. Although the precise pathogenesis is unclear, celiac disease arises in a small subset of genetically susceptible (-DQ2 or -DQ8) individuals when dietary gluten stimulates a pathologic immunologic response.

Clinical Findings

The most important step in diagnosing celiac disease is to consider the diagnosis. Because of its protean manifestations, celiac disease is underdiagnosed in adults.

A. Symptoms and Signs

The GI symptoms and signs of celiac disease depend on the length of small intestine involved and the patient's age when the disease presents. "Classic" symptoms of malabsorption, including diarrhea, steatorrhea, weight loss, abdominal distention, weakness, muscle wasting, or growth retardation, more commonly present in infants (aged < 2 years). Older children and adults are less likely to manifest signs of serious malabsorption. They may report bloating, chronic diarrhea, or flatulence due to colonic bacterial digestion of malabsorbed nutrients, but the severity of weight loss is variable. Many adults have minimal or no GI symptoms but present with extraintestinal "atypical" manifestations, including fatigue, depression, iron deficiency anemia, abnormal liver tests, osteoporosis, short stature, delayed puberty, amenorrhea, or reduced fertility. Approximately 40% of patients with positive serologic tests consistent with disease have no symptoms of disease; the natural history of these patients with "silent" disease is unclear.

Physical examination may be normal in mild cases or may reveal signs of malabsorption such as loss of muscle mass or subcutaneous fat, pallor due to anemia, easy bruising due to vitamin K deficiency, hyperkeratosis due to vitamin A deficiency, bone pain due to osteomalacia, or neurologic signs (peripheral neuropathy, ataxia) due to vitamin B_{12} or vitamin E deficiency (Table 17–11). Abdominal examination may reveal distention with hyperactive bowel sounds.

Dermatitis herpetiformis is regarded as a cutaneous variant of celiac disease. It is a characteristic skin rash consisting of pruritic papulovesicles over the extensor surfaces of the extremities and over the trunk, scalp, and neck. Dermatitis herpetiformis occurs in < 10% of patients with celiac disease; however, almost all patients who present with dermatitis herpetiformis have evidence of celiac disease on intestinal mucosal biopsy, though it may not be clinically evident.

B. Laboratory Findings

1. Routine laboratory tests—Depending on the severity of illness and the extent of intestinal involvement, nonspecific laboratory abnormalities may be present that may raise the suspicion of malabsorption and celiac disease (Table 17–11). Limited proximal involvement may result only in microcytic anemia due to iron deficiency. Up to 3% of adults with iron deficiency not due to GI blood loss have undiagnosed celiac disease. Megaloblastic anemia may be due to folate or vitamin B_{12} deficiency (due to terminal ileal involvement or associated autoimmune gastritis). Low serum calcium or elevated alkaline phosphatase may reflect impaired calcium or vitamin D absorption with osteomalacia or osteoporosis. Elevations of prothrombin time, or decreased vitamin A or D levels reflect impaired fat-soluble vitamin absorption. A low serum albumin may reflect small intestine protein loss or poor nutrition. Other deficiencies may include zinc and vitamin B_6. Mild elevations of aminotransferases are found in up to 40%. Dual-energy x-ray densitometry scanning is recommended for all patients with celiac disease to screen for osteoporosis.

2. Serologic tests—Serologic tests should be performed in all patients in whom there is a suspicion of celiac disease. Patient self-elimination of gluten before serologic testing may result in false-negative test results. The recommended test is the IgA tissue transglutaminase-2 antibody (IgA anti-tTG2), which has a 98% sensitivity and 98% specificity for the diagnosis of celiac disease. Antigliadin antibodies are not recommended because of their lower sensitivity and specificity. An IgA level should be obtained in patients with a negative IgA anti-TG2 when celiac disease is strongly suspected because up to 3% of patients with celiac disease have IgA deficiency. In patients with IgA deficiency, tests that measures IgG antibodies to tissue transglutaminase (IgG tTG) or to deamidated gliadin peptides (anti-DGP) have excellent sensitivity and specificity.

C. Mucosal Biopsy

Endoscopic mucosal biopsy of the proximal duodenum (bulb) and distal duodenum is the standard method for confirmation of the diagnosis in patients with a positive serologic test for celiac disease. At endoscopy, atrophy or scalloping of the duodenal folds may be observed. Histology abnormalities include intraepithelial lymphocytosis, hypertrophy of the intestinal crypts, and blunting or complete loss of intestinal villi. In patients in whom celiac disease is first suspected on intestinal biopsies, celiac serologic tests should be obtained to confirm the diagnosis. Repeat upper endoscopy with duodenal biopsies are recommended after 2–3 years in patients who have had good clinical improvement on the gluten-free diet to confirm complete histologic healing and other patients whose symptoms have persisted or recurred despite good dietary adherence.

Differential Diagnosis

Many patients with chronic diarrhea or flatulence are erroneously diagnosed as having IBS. Celiac disease must be distinguished from other causes of malabsorption, as outlined above. Severe panmalabsorption of multiple nutrients is almost always caused by mucosal disease. The visual or histologic appearance of celiac disease may resemble other mucosal diseases such as tropical sprue, bacterial overgrowth, eosinophilic enteritis, autoimmune enteropathy, common variable immunodeficiency, and mucosal damage caused by acid hypersecretion associated with gastrinoma.

Over the past several years, a growing proportion (now 10%) of the population has reported symptoms after gluten ingestion who do not have serologic or histologic evidence of celiac disease. This has led to increases in gluten-free offerings from the restaurant and food industry. Foods with gluten often contain a number of other FODMAPs. Blinded clinical trials suggest that self-reported wheat sensitivity is not due to gluten intolerance and that the symptom improvement reported by patients with gluten restriction is due to broader FODMAP elimination.

Treatment

Removal of all gluten (wheat, rye, and barley) from the diet is essential to therapy but strict adherence can be difficult to achieve. Even among patients who report adherence to the gluten-free diet, gluten peptides can be detected in almost 40% of stool and urine specimens over a 4-week period. Although oats are safe for patients, commercial oat products may be contaminated with wheat or barley during processing. Because of the pervasive use of gluten products in manufactured foods and additives, in medications, and by restaurants, it is imperative that patients and their families confer with a knowledgeable dietitian to comply satisfactorily with this lifelong diet. Several excellent dietary guides and patient support groups are available. Most patients with celiac disease also have lactose intolerance either temporarily or permanently and should avoid dairy products until the intestinal symptoms have improved on the gluten-free diet. Dietary supplements (folate, iron, zinc, calcium, and vitamins A, B_6, B_{12}, D, and E) should be provided in the initial stages of therapy but usually are not required long-term with a gluten-free diet. Patients with confirmed osteoporosis may require long-term calcium, vitamin D, and bisphosphonate therapy.

Improvement in symptoms should be evident within a few weeks on the gluten-free diet. The most common reason for treatment failure is incomplete removal of gluten.

Prognosis & Complications

If appropriately diagnosed and treated, patients with celiac disease have an excellent prognosis. After a patient is placed on a gluten-free diet, symptoms improve in the majority (80%) within 2–6 months and the serologic tests decrease (and usually normalize) within 1–2 years. Celiac disease may be associated with other autoimmune disorders, including Hashimoto thyroiditis and Graves disease, type 1 diabetes mellitus, primary biliary cholangitis, autoimmune atrophic gastritis, Sjögren syndrome, and idiopathic pancreatitis. In some patients, celiac disease may evolve and become refractory to the gluten-free diet. The most common cause is intentional or unintentional dietary nonadherence, which may be suggested by positive serologic tests. Celiac disease that is truly refractory to gluten withdrawal occurs in 0.5–1.5% and generally carries a poor prognosis. There are two types of refractory disease, which are distinguished by their intraepithelial lymphocyte phenotype.

Corticosteroid therapy with oral open-capsule budesonide or prednisone is effective in the treatment of both type I and II refractory celiac disease. Type I has a normal (polyclonal) lymphocyte population, and most cases respond to corticosteroids (prednisone or budesonide); however, long-term therapy is usually required. Type II disease has an aberrant population characterized by loss of surface expression of CD3 and CD8 and monoclonal rearrangement of the surface T-cell receptor by PCR. It is less responsive to corticosteroid therapy. Type II disease has a high risk of progression to T-cell lymphoma (50% at 5 years), which carries a poor prognosis with either chemotherapy or autologous bone marrow transplantation. This diagnosis should be considered in patients previously responsive to the gluten-free diet in whom new weight loss, abdominal pain, and malabsorption develop. All patients with type II disease therefore should undergo capsule endoscopy and either MR or CT enterography at the time of diagnosis.

Celiac Disease Foundation, 20350 Ventura Blvd, Suite #240, Woodland Hills, CA 91364. https://celiac.org

Malamut G et al. Advances in nonresponsive and refractory celiac disease. Gastroenterology. 2024;167:132. [PMID: 38556189]

Rubio-Tapia A et al. American College of Gastroenterology guidelines update: diagnosis and management of celiac disease. Am J Gastroenterol. 2023;118:59. [PMID: 36602836]

Sharma R et al. Evaluating for celiac disease in patients on a gluten-free diet: a practical approach. Am J Gastroenterol. 2025;120:1676. [PMID: 40146033]

2. Whipple Disease

ESSENTIALS OF DIAGNOSIS

- Multisystem disease.
- Fever, lymphadenopathy, arthralgias.
- Weight loss, malabsorption, chronic diarrhea.
- Duodenal biopsy with periodic acid-Schiff (PAS)-positive macrophages with characteristic bacillus.

General Considerations

Whipple disease is a rare multisystem illness with an estimated prevalence of 1 per 100,000 caused by infection with the bacillus *Tropheryma whipplei*. It may occur at any age but most commonly affects White men in the fourth to sixth decades. The source of infection is unknown, but no cases of human-to-human spread have been documented.

Clinical Findings

A. Symptoms and Signs

The clinical manifestations are protean; however, the most common are arthralgias, diarrhea, abdominal pain, and weight loss. Arthralgias or a migratory, nondeforming arthritis occurs in 80% and is typically the first symptom experienced. GI symptoms occur in approximately 75% of cases. They include abdominal pain, diarrhea, and some degree of malabsorption with distention, flatulence, and steatorrhea. Weight loss is the most common presenting symptom—seen in almost all patients. Loss of protein due to intestinal or lymphatic involvement may result in protein-losing enteropathy with hypoalbuminemia and edema. In the absence of GI symptoms, the diagnosis often is delayed for several years. Intermittent low-grade fever occurs in over 50% of cases.

Physical examination may reveal hypotension (a late finding), low-grade fever, and evidence of malabsorption (see Table 17–11). Lymphadenopathy is present in 50%. Heart murmurs due to valvular involvement may be evident. Peripheral joints may be enlarged or warm, and peripheral edema may be present. Neurologic findings are protean, and include ophthalmoplegia, dementia (confusion, memory loss), cerebellar ataxia, chronic meningitis, myelopathy, and seizures. Hyperpigmentation on sun-exposed areas is evident in up to 40%.

B. Laboratory Findings

If significant malabsorption is present, patients may have laboratory abnormalities as outlined in Table 17–11. There may be steatorrhea.

C. Histologic Evaluation

The diagnosis of Whipple disease is established in 90% of cases by endoscopic biopsy of the duodenum with histologic evaluation, which demonstrates infiltration of the lamina propria with PAS-positive macrophages that contain gram-positive bacilli (which are not acid-fast) and dilation of the lacteals. The remainder of cases are diagnosed by *T whipplei*–specific PCR or immunohistochemistry of duodenal biopsies or extraintestinal fluids (cerebrospinal, synovial) or tissue (lymph nodes, synovium, endocardium). Because asymptomatic CNS infection occurs in 40% of patients, examination of the CSF by PCR for *T whipplei* should be performed routinely.

Differential Diagnosis

Whipple disease should be considered in patients who present with signs of malabsorption, fever of unknown origin, lymphadenopathy, seronegative arthritis, culture-negative endocarditis, or multisystem disease. Small bowel biopsy readily distinguishes Whipple disease from other mucosal malabsorptive disorders, such as celiac disease.

Treatment

Antibiotic therapy results in a dramatic clinical improvement within several weeks, even in some patients with neurologic involvement. The optimal regimen is unknown. Drugs that cross the blood-brain barrier are preferred. Effective treatment regimens include ceftriaxone 1 g intravenously twice daily or meropenem 1 g intravenously three times daily for 2 weeks, followed by trimethoprim-sulfamethoxazole 160/800 mg twice daily for at least 12 months. An alternative regimen is doxycycline 100 mg orally twice daily and hydroxychloroquine 200 mg orally twice daily for 12 months. After treatment, repeat duodenal biopsies for histologic analysis every 6 months for at least 1 year. In patients with CNS involvement, extended treatment for several years may be required as guided by close CSF monitoring for at least 2 years to confirm eradication. The absence of PAS-positive material predicts a low likelihood of clinical relapse.

Prognosis

If untreated, the disease is fatal. Because some neurologic signs may be permanent, the goal of treatment is to prevent this progression. Patients must be followed closely after treatment for signs of symptom recurrence.

Cappellini A et al. Whipple's disease: a rare disease that can be spotted by many doctors. Eur J Intern Med. 2024;121:25. [PMID: 38105122]

Moos V et al. Oral treatment of Whipple's disease with doxycycline and hydroxychloroquine versus intravenous therapy with ceftriaxone followed by oral trimethoprim-sulfamethoxazole in German: a phase 2/3, prospective, open-label, randomised, controlled, non-inferiority trial. Lancet Infect Dis. 2025;25:788. [PMID: 39978372]

3. Bacterial Overgrowth

ESSENTIALS OF DIAGNOSIS

- Symptoms of diarrhea, bloating, and flatulence.
- Advanced cases associated with weight loss, steatorrhea, and deficiencies of iron or vitamins A, D, and B_{12}.
- Diagnosis suggested by breath tests using glucose or lactulose.
- Diagnosis confirmed by jejunal aspiration with quantitative bacterial cultures.

General Considerations

The small intestine normally contains a small number of bacteria. Bacterial overgrowth in the small intestine of whatever cause may result in malabsorption via several mechanisms. Passage of malabsorbed bile acids and carbohydrates into the colon leads to an osmotic and secretory diarrhea and increased flatulence.

Causes of bacterial overgrowth include (1) gastric achlorhydria (including PPI therapy); (2) anatomic abnormalities of the small intestine with stagnation (afferent limb of Billroth II gastrojejunostomy, resection of ileocecal valve, small intestine diverticula, obstruction, blind loop); (3) small intestine motility disorders (vagotomy, systemic sclerosis, diabetic enteropathy, chronic intestinal pseudo-obstruction); (4) gastrocolic or coloenteric fistula (Crohn disease, malignancy, surgical resection); and (5) miscellaneous disorders. Bacterial overgrowth is an important cause of diarrhea in older patients, perhaps because of decreased gastric acidity or impaired intestinal motility. It may also be present in a subset of patients with IBS.

Clinical Findings

Many patients with bacterial overgrowth are asymptomatic. Symptoms are nonspecific and include diarrhea, bloating, flatulence, and sometimes steatorrhea with weight loss. Bacterial overgrowth should be considered in any patient with these symptoms, especially patients with a predisposing cause (such as prior GI surgery) and older adults with unexplained diarrhea and weight loss. Bacterial synthesis of folic acid and consumption of cobalamin may cause elevated serum folate and decreased vitamin B_{12} levels. Severe cases may result in clinically significant vitamin and mineral deficiencies, including fat-soluble vitamins A or D, and low serum albumin (Table 17–11). A specific diagnosis can be established firmly only by an aspirate and culture of distal duodenal secretion that demonstrates over 10^3 organisms/mL. However, this is an invasive and laborious test that requires careful collection and culturing techniques and therefore is not available in most clinical settings. Noninvasive breath hydrogen and methane tests with glucose or lactulose as substrates are generally preferred because of their ease of use. Following ingestion of glucose 75 g or lactulose 10 g, a rise in exhaled breath hydrogen of 20 ppm or methane of 10 ppm or more within 90 minutes is suggestive of bacterial overgrowth. A small bowel study (CT or MR enterography, barium radiography) may be obtained to look for mechanical factors predisposing to intestinal stasis.

A 2020 American College of Gastroenterology guideline suggests breath testing when bacterial overgrowth is suspected. However, many clinicians prefer to use an empiric antibiotic trial as a diagnostic and therapeutic strategy.

Treatment

Where possible, the anatomic defect that has potentiated bacterial overgrowth should be corrected. Otherwise, treatment for 7–10 days with oral broad-spectrum antibiotics improves symptoms in up to 90% of patients for weeks to months. Recommended regimens include ciprofloxacin, 250 mg twice daily; amoxicillin clavulanate, 875 mg twice daily; trimethoprim-sulfamethoxazole (one double-strength tablet) twice daily; rifaximin, 400–550 mg three times daily; or a combination of neomycin, 500 mg twice daily, plus metronidazole, 250 mg three times daily.

Within 6 months of completing antibiotic therapy, symptoms recur in over 25% of patients. In patients with more frequent symptomatic relapse, cyclic antibiotic therapy (eg, 1 week out of 4) may be sufficient. Continuous antibiotics should be avoided, if possible, to prevent development of bacterial antibiotic resistance.

Barlow GM et al. Modern concepts of small intestinal bacterial overgrowth. Curr Opin Gastroenterol. 2025;41:399. [PMID: 40960427]

Rangan V et al. Small intestinal bacterial overgrowth breath testing in gastroenterology: clinical utility and pitfalls. Clin Gastroenterol Hepatol. 2022;20:1450. [PMID: 35301986]

4. Short Bowel Syndrome

Short bowel syndrome is the malabsorptive condition that arises from removal of significant segments of the small intestine. The most common causes in adults are Crohn disease, mesenteric infarction, radiation enteritis, volvulus, tumor resection, and trauma. The type and degree of malabsorption depend on the length and site of the resection and the degree of adaptation of the remaining bowel.

Terminal Ileal Resection

Resection of the terminal ileum results in malabsorption of bile salts and vitamin B_{12}, which are normally absorbed in this region. Patients with low serum vitamin B_{12} levels or resection of over 50 cm of ileum require monthly subcutaneous or intramuscular vitamin B_{12} injections. In patients with < 100 cm of ileal resection, bile salt malabsorption stimulates fluid secretion from the colon, resulting in watery diarrhea. This may be treated with administration of bile salt-binding resins one to three times daily with meals (cholestyramine, 2–4 g/day orally, colestipol tablets, 2 g orally, or colesevelam, 625 mg orally). Resection of over 100 cm of ileum leads to a reduction in the bile salt pool that results in steatorrhea and malabsorption of fat-soluble vitamins. Treatment is with a low-fat diet and vitamins supplemented with medium-chain triglycerides, which do not require micellar solubilization. Cholesterol gallstones due to decreased bile salts are common also. In patients with resection of the ileocolonic valve, bacterial overgrowth may occur in the small intestine, further complicating malabsorption.

Extensive Small Bowel Resection

Resection of up to 40–50% of the total length of small intestine usually is well tolerated. A more massive resection may result in "short bowel syndrome," characterized by weight loss and diarrhea due to nutrient, water, and electrolyte malabsorption. If the colon is preserved, 100 cm of proximal jejunum may be sufficient to maintain adequate oral nutrition with a low-fat, high-complex carbohydrate diet, though fluid and electrolyte losses may still be significant. In patients in whom the colon has been removed, at least 200 cm of proximal jejunum is typically required to maintain oral nutrition. Antidiarrheal agents (loperamide,

2–4 mg orally three times daily) slow transit and reduce diarrheal volume. Octreotide reduces intestinal transit time and fluid and electrolyte secretion. Gastric hypersecretion initially complicates intestinal resection and should be treated with PPIs.

Patients with < 100–200 cm of proximal jejunum remaining almost always require parenteral nutrition. Teduglutide (recombinant) is a glucagon-like peptide-2 analogue that stimulates small bowel growth and absorption and is FDA approved for the treatment of short bowel syndrome. In clinical trials, it resulted in a reduced need for parenteral nutrition. Small intestine transplantation has a reported 5-year graft survival rate of 40%. It is performed chiefly in patients in whom serious problems develop due to parenteral nutrition.

Jeppesen P et al. Glepaglutide, a long-acting glucagon-like peptide-2 analogue, reduces parenteral support in patients with short-bowel syndrome: a phase 3 randomized controlled trial. Gastroenterology. 2025;168:701. [PMID: 39708985]

5. Lactase Deficiency

ESSENTIALS OF DIAGNOSIS

- Diarrhea, bloating, flatulence, and abdominal pain after ingestion of milk-containing products.
- Diagnosis supported by symptomatic improvement on lactose-free diet.
- Diagnosis confirmed by hydrogen breath test.

General Considerations

Lactase is a brush border enzyme that hydrolyzes the disaccharide lactose into glucose and galactose. The concentration of lactase enzyme levels is high at birth but declines steadily in most people of non-European White ancestry during childhood and adolescence and into adulthood. In the United States the prevalence of lactose intolerance is 15% among White adults and > 50% among Asian Americans, African Americans, Native Americans, and Latino Americans. Lactase deficiency may also arise secondary to other GI disorders that affect the proximal small intestinal mucosa. These include Crohn disease, celiac disease, viral gastroenteritis, giardiasis, short bowel syndrome, and malnutrition. Malabsorbed lactose is fermented by intestinal bacteria, producing gas and organic acids. The nonmetabolized lactose and organic acids result in an increased stool osmotic load with an obligatory fluid loss.

Clinical Findings

A. Symptoms and Signs

Patients have great variability in clinical symptoms, depending both on the severity of lactase deficiency and the amount of lactose ingested. Because of the nonspecific nature of these symptoms, there is a tendency for both lactose-intolerant and lactose-tolerant individuals to mistakenly attribute a variety of abdominal symptoms to lactose intolerance. Most patients with lactose intolerance can drink at least one 8-oz serving of milk daily (12 g of lactose) without symptoms, though rare patients have almost complete intolerance. With mild to moderate amounts of lactose malabsorption, patients may experience bloating, abdominal cramps, and flatulence. With higher lactose ingestions, an osmotic diarrhea will result. Isolated lactase deficiency does not result in other signs of malabsorption or weight loss. If these findings are present, other GI disorders should be pursued.

B. Laboratory Findings

The most widely available test for the diagnosis of lactase deficiency is the hydrogen breath test. After ingestion of 50 g of lactose, a rise in breath hydrogen of > 20 ppm within 90 minutes is a positive test, indicative of bacterial carbohydrate metabolism. In clinical practice, many clinicians prescribe an empiric trial of a lactose-free diet for 2 weeks. Resolution of symptoms (bloating, flatulence, diarrhea) is suggestive of lactase deficiency (though a placebo response cannot be excluded) and may be confirmed, if necessary, with a hydrogen breath test.

Differential Diagnosis

The symptoms of late-onset lactose intolerance are nonspecific and may mimic several GI disorders, such as IBD, mucosal malabsorptive disorders, IBS, and pancreatic insufficiency. Furthermore, lactase deficiency frequently develops secondary to other GI disorders (as listed above).

Treatment

The goal of treatment of isolated lactase deficiency is patient comfort. Patients usually find their "threshold" of intake at which symptoms will occur. Foods that are high in lactose include milk (12 g/cup), ice cream (9 g/cup), and cottage cheese (8 g/cup). Aged cheeses have a lower lactose content (0.5 g/oz). Unpasteurized yogurt contains bacteria that produce lactase and is generally well tolerated.

By spreading dairy product intake throughout the day in quantities of < 12 g of lactose (one cup of milk), most patients can take dairy products without symptoms and do not require lactase supplements. Most food markets provide milk that has been pretreated with lactase, rendering it 100% lactose free (Fairlife). Lactase enzyme replacement is commercially available as nonprescription formulations (Lactaid, Lactrase, Dairy Ease). Caplets or drops of lactase may be taken with milk products, improving lactose absorption and eliminating symptoms. The number of caplets ingested depends on the degree of lactose intolerance. Patients who choose to restrict or eliminate milk products should consider calcium supplementation (calcium citrate 650 mg 2 tablets orally two times daily) to meet calcium intake needs and reduce risk of osteoporosis.

Gallo A et al. Lactose malabsorption and intolerance in older adults. Curr Opin Clin Nutr Metab Care. 2024;27:333. [PMID: 38836813]

INTESTINAL MOTILITY DISORDERS

1. Acute Paralytic Ileus

ESSENTIALS OF DIAGNOSIS

- Precipitating factors: surgery, peritonitis, electrolyte abnormalities, medications, severe medical illness.
- Nausea, vomiting, obstipation, distention.
- Minimal abdominal tenderness; decreased bowel sounds.
- Plain abdominal radiography with gas and fluid distention in small and large bowel.

General Considerations

Ileus is a condition in which there is neurogenic failure or loss of peristalsis in the intestine in the absence of any mechanical obstruction. It is commonly seen in hospitalized patients as a result of (1) intra-abdominal processes such as recent GI or abdominal surgery or peritoneal irritation (peritonitis, pancreatitis, ruptured viscus, hemorrhage); (2) severe medical illness such as pneumonia, respiratory failure requiring intubation, sepsis or severe infections, uremia, diabetic ketoacidosis, and electrolyte abnormalities (hypokalemia, hypercalcemia, hypomagnesemia, hypophosphatemia); and (3) medications that affect intestinal motility (opioids, anticholinergics, phenothiazines). Following surgery, small intestinal motility usually normalizes first (often within hours), followed by the stomach (24–48 hours), and the colon (48–72 hours). Postoperative ileus is reduced with minimally invasive (eg, laparoscopic) surgery, by the use of patient-controlled or epidural analgesia, and by avoidance of intravenous opioids as well as early ambulation, coffee consumption, gum chewing, and early initiation of a clear liquid diet.

Clinical Findings

A. Symptoms and Signs

Patients report mild diffuse, continuous abdominal discomfort with nausea and vomiting. Generalized abdominal distention is present with minimal abdominal tenderness but no signs of peritoneal irritation (unless due to the primary disease). Bowel sounds are diminished to absent.

B. Laboratory Findings

The laboratory abnormalities are attributable to the underlying condition. Serum electrolytes (sodium, potassium), magnesium, phosphorus, and calcium should be obtained to exclude abnormalities as contributing factors.

C. Imaging

Plain film radiography of the abdomen demonstrates distended gas-filled loops of the small and large intestine. Air-fluid levels may be seen. It may be difficult to distinguish ileus from partial small bowel obstruction. A CT scan may be useful in such instances to exclude mechanical obstruction, especially in postoperative patients.

Differential Diagnosis

Pain from small bowel mechanical obstruction is usually intermittent, cramping, and associated initially with profuse vomiting. Acute gastroenteritis, acute appendicitis, and acute pancreatitis may all present with ileus.

Treatment

The primary medical or surgical illness that has precipitated adynamic ileus should be treated. Most cases of ileus respond to restriction of oral intake with gradual liberalization of diet as bowel function returns. Severe or prolonged ileus requires nasogastric suction and parenteral administration of fluids and electrolytes. Alvimopan is a peripherally acting μ-opioid receptor antagonist with limited absorption or systemic activity that reverses opioid-induced inhibition of intestinal motility.

When to Refer

- Persistent ileus lasting > 3–5 days warrants further evaluation for underlying cause and to exclude mechanical obstruction.

When to Admit

- All patients with ileus require admission for intravenous fluids.

Chatterjee A et al. Mechanisms and management of ileus. Am J Gastroenterol. 2026;121:573. [PMID: 40980931]

2. Acute Colonic Pseudo-Obstruction (Ogilvie Syndrome)

ESSENTIALS OF DIAGNOSIS

- Severe abdominal distention.
- Occurs postoperatively or with severe medical illness.
- May be precipitated by electrolyte imbalances, medications.
- Absent to mild abdominal pain; minimal tenderness.
- Massive dilation of cecum or right colon.

General Considerations

Spontaneous massive dilation of the cecum and proximal colon may occur in many different settings in hospitalized patients. Progressive cecal dilation may lead to ischemia and spontaneous perforation with dire consequences. The risk of perforation increases with duration of distention beyond 6 days but correlates poorly with absolute cecal size. Early detection and management are important to reduce morbidity and mortality. Colonic pseudo-obstruction is most commonly detected in postsurgical patients (mean 3–5 days), after trauma, and in medical patients with respiratory failure, metabolic imbalance, malignancy, MI, HF, pancreatitis, or a recent neurologic event (stroke, subarachnoid hemorrhage, trauma). Liberal use of opioids or anticholinergic agents may precipitate colonic pseudo-obstruction in susceptible patients.

Clinical Findings

A. Symptoms and Signs

Many patients are on ventilatory support or are unable to report symptoms due to altered mental status. Abdominal distention is frequently noted by the clinician as the first sign, often leading to a plain film radiograph that demonstrates colonic dilation. Some patients are asymptomatic, although most report constant but mild abdominal pain. Nausea and vomiting may be present. Bowel movements may be absent, but up to 40% of patients continue to pass flatus or stool. Abdominal tenderness with some degree of guarding or rebound tenderness may be detected; however, signs of peritonitis are absent unless perforation has occurred. Bowel sounds may be normal or decreased.

B. Laboratory Findings

Laboratory findings reflect the underlying medical or surgical problems. Serum sodium, potassium, magnesium, phosphorus, and calcium should be obtained to exclude abnormalities as contributing factors. Significant fever or leukocytosis raises concern for colonic ischemia or perforation.

C. Imaging

Radiographs demonstrate colonic dilation, usually confined to the cecum and proximal colon. The upper limit of normal for cecal size is 9 cm. A cecal diameter > 10–12 cm is associated with an increased risk of colonic perforation. Varying amounts of small intestinal dilation and air-fluid levels due to adynamic ileus may be seen. Generally, a CT scan should be obtained to exclude a distal colonic mechanical obstruction due to malignancy, volvulus, or fecal impaction.

Differential Diagnosis

Colonic pseudo-obstruction should be distinguished from distal colonic mechanical obstruction (as above) and toxic megacolon, which is acute dilation of the colon due to inflammation (IBD) or infection (*C difficile*–associated colitis, CMV). Patients with toxic megacolon manifest fever; dehydration; significant abdominal pain; leukocytosis; and diarrhea, which is often bloody.

Treatment

Conservative treatment is the appropriate first step for patients with no or minimal abdominal tenderness, no fever, no leukocytosis, and a cecal diameter smaller than 12 cm. The underlying illness is treated appropriately. A nasogastric tube and a rectal tube should be placed. Patients should be ambulated or periodically rolled from side to side and to the knee-chest position in an effort to promote expulsion of colonic gas. All drugs that reduce intestinal motility, such as opioids, anticholinergics, and calcium channel blockers, should be discontinued if possible. Enemas may be administered judiciously if large amounts of stool are evident on radiography. *Oral laxatives are not helpful and may cause perforation, pain, or electrolyte abnormalities.*

Conservative treatment is successful in > 80% of cases within 1–2 days. Patients must be watched for signs of worsening distention or abdominal tenderness. Cecal size should be assessed by abdominal radiographs every 12 hours. Intervention should be considered in patients with any of the following: (1) no improvement or clinical deterioration after 24–48 hours of conservative therapy; (2) cecal dilation > 10 cm for a prolonged period (> 3–4 days); or (3) patients with cecal dilation > 12 cm. Neostigmine injection should be given unless contraindicated. A single dose (2 mg intravenously) results in rapid (within 30 minutes) colonic decompression in 75–90% of patients. Cardiac monitoring during neostigmine infusion is indicated for possible bradycardia that may require atropine administration. Colonoscopic decompression is indicated in patients who fail to respond to neostigmine. In patients in whom colonoscopy is unsuccessful, a tube cecostomy can be created through a small laparotomy or with percutaneous radiologically guided placement.

Prognosis

In most cases, the prognosis is related to the underlying illness. The risk of perforation or ischemia is increased with cecal diameter > 12 cm and when distention has been present for > 6 days. With aggressive therapy, the development of perforation is unusual.

Sen A et al. Update on the diagnosis and management of acute colonic pseudo-obstruction (ACPO). Curr Gastroenterol Rep. 2023;25:191. [PMID: 37486594]

3. Gastroparesis

Chronic gastroparesis is due to an impairment in gastric emptying that occurs in the absence of mechanical obstruction and leads to a host of upper GI symptoms. Most commonly caused by diabetes, it may also be idiopathic or attributable to prior infections (viral, food poisoning), neurologic disorders (Parkinson disease), rheumatologic disease (scleroderma), thyroid disease, prior gastrointestinal surgery (vagotomy), or medications (GLP-1 receptor agonists, opiates, anticholinergic agents). Functional dyspepsia has similar symptoms but has normal gastric emptying, which distinguishes it from gastroparesis.

Clinical Findings

A. Symptoms and Signs

Symptoms of gastroparesis may be chronic or intermittent and include with early satiety, nausea, vomiting (1–3 hours after meals), bloating, lack of appetite, and epigastric pain. These symptoms correlate poorly with the severity of gastric emptying

B. Imaging

Plain film radiography may demonstrate dilation of stomach. Mechanical obstruction of the stomach must be excluded with endoscopy. Gastric scintigraphy with a low-fat solid meal and wireless motility capsule are the preferred methods for assessing gastric emptying; gastric retention on scintigraphy of > 10% after 4 hours or of the wireless capsule for > 5 hours is abnormal.

Treatment

Patients should eat small, frequent meals that are low in fiber, milk, gas-forming foods, and fat. Foods that are well tolerated include tea, ginger ale, soup, white rice, potatoes and sweet potatoes, fish, gluten-free foods, and applesauce. Some patients may require liquid enteral supplements. Agents that reduce GI motility (opioids, anticholinergics, GLP-1 receptor agonists) should be avoided. In patients with diabetes, glucose levels should be maintained below 200 mg/dL since hyperglycemia may slow gastric emptying even in the absence of diabetic neuropathy, and amylin and GLP-1 analogs should be discontinued.

Prokinetic agents have shown limited improvement of gastric emptying or upper GI symptoms in patients with gastroparesis. Metoclopramide (5–10 mg orally or 15 mg intranasally, given 30 minutes before meals three times daily) may enhance gastric emptying and reduce upper GI symptoms. The use of metoclopramide for > 3 months is associated with a small risk (2.5 per 100,000 patient-years) of tardive dyskinesia; patients are advised to discontinue the medication if neuromuscular side effects, particularly involuntary movements, develop. For patients who require chronic therapy, some recommend discontinuation every 3 months for 10–14 days. Low-dose erythromycin (40–150 mg orally, given 30 minutes before meals) is a motilin agonist that has strong prokinetic activity that improves early satiety and postprandial fullness but may not improve nausea or vomiting. Due to the development of tachyphylaxis with continued use, 3 weeks of therapy followed by 1 week off therapy is recommended. Antiemetics (eg, serotonin 5-HT3 and dopamine-receptor antagonists) may be used as needed (Table 17–2).

For patients who fail these measures, other agents may be useful but are not recommended as first-line therapies in 2025 AGA guidelines. Domperidone (10–20 mg orally three times daily) is an antidopaminergic agent that enhances gastric emptying and has efficacy as an antiemetic agent. Although unavailable in the United States, it is available in most other countries, where its use is preferred to metoclopramide. Some experts endorse the use of pyridostigmine (60 mg orally before each meal), an acetylcholinesterase inhibitor, as beneficial for some patients with diabetic gastroparesis. Prucalopride (2 mg orally daily), is a prokinetic serotonin 5-HT_4-receptor agonist that may be useful in patients with gastroparesis and constipation. Low-dose SSRIs (eg, nortriptyline 25–50 mg once daily at bedtime) may promote symptom improvement through modulation of visceral afferent pathways.

Optimal management of severe, refractory symptoms requires a multidisciplinary team that includes the primary care provider, dietician, endocrinologist, and gastroenterologist. Selected patients may be considered for advanced therapies, including pyloric botulinum injection, endoscopic pyloromyotomy, gastric electrical stimulation, enteral feedings and, rarely, parenteral nutrition.

Hasler WL et al. Benefits of prokinetics, gastroparesis diet, or neuromodulators alone or in combination for symptoms of gastroparesis. Clin Gastroenterol Hepatol 2024;22:867. [PMID: 37913936]

Liu J et al. The management of gastroparesis symptoms. Am J Gastroenterol. 2025;120:2213. [PMID: 39882788]

Staller K et al. AGA Clinical Practice Guideline on management of gastroparesis. Gastroenterology. 2025;169:828. [PMID: 39023502]

APPENDICITIS

ESSENTIALS OF DIAGNOSIS

- *Early:* periumbilical pain; *later:* right lower quadrant pain and tenderness.
- Anorexia, nausea and vomiting, obstipation.
- Tenderness or localized rigidity at McBurney point.
- Low-grade fever and leukocytosis.

General Considerations

Appendicitis is the most common abdominal surgical emergency, affecting approximately 10% of the population. It occurs most commonly between the ages of 10 and 30 years. It is initiated by obstruction of the appendix by a fecalith, inflammation, foreign body, or neoplasm. Obstruction leads to increased intraluminal pressure, venous congestion, infection, and thrombosis of intramural vessels. If untreated, gangrene and perforation develop within 36 hours.

Clinical Findings

A. Symptoms and Signs

Appendicitis usually begins with vague, often colicky periumbilical or epigastric pain. Within 12 hours the pain shifts to the right lower quadrant, manifested as a steady ache that is worsened by walking or coughing. Almost all patients have nausea with one or two episodes of vomiting. Protracted vomiting or vomiting that begins before the onset of pain suggests another diagnosis. A sense of constipation is typical, and some patients administer cathartics in an effort to relieve their symptoms—though some report diarrhea. Low-grade fever (below 38°C) is typical; high fever or rigors suggest another diagnosis or appendiceal perforation.

On physical examination, localized tenderness with guarding in the right lower quadrant can be elicited with gentle palpation with one finger. When asked to cough, patients may be able to precisely localize the painful area, a sign of peritoneal irritation. Light percussion may also elicit pain. Although rebound tenderness is also present, it is unnecessary to elicit this finding if the above signs are present. The psoas sign (pain on passive extension of the right hip) and the obturator sign (pain with passive flexion and internal rotation of the right hip) are indicative of adjacent inflammation and strongly suggestive of appendicitis.

B. Atypical Presentations of Appendicitis

Owing to the variable location of the appendix, there are a number of "atypical" presentations. When the retrocecal appendix does not touch the anterior abdominal wall, the pain remains less intense and poorly localized; abdominal tenderness is minimal and may be elicited in the right flank. The psoas sign may be positive. With pelvic appendicitis, there is pain in the lower abdomen, often on the left, with an urge to urinate or defecate. Abdominal tenderness is absent, but tenderness is evident on pelvic or rectal examination; the obturator sign may be present. In older adult patients, the diagnosis of appendicitis is often delayed because patients present with minimal, vague symptoms and mild abdominal tenderness.

C. Laboratory Findings

Moderate leukocytosis (10,000–20,000/mcL [$10–20 \times 10^9$/L]) with neutrophilia is common. Microscopic hematuria and pyuria are present in 25% of patients, presumed due to an inflammation of the right ureter from the adjacent appendicitis.

D. Imaging

Both abdominal ultrasound and CT are useful in diagnosing appendicitis as well as excluding other diseases presenting with similar symptoms, including adnexal disease in younger women. However, CT appears to be more accurate (sensitivity 94%, specificity 95%, positive LR 13.3, negative LR 0.09). Abdominal CT is also useful in cases of suspected appendiceal perforation to diagnose a periappendiceal abscess. In patients in whom there is a clinically high suspicion of appendicitis, some surgeons feel that preoperative diagnostic imaging is unnecessary. However, studies suggest that even in this group, imaging studies suggest an alternative diagnosis in up to 15%.

Differential Diagnosis

Given its frequency and myriad presentations, appendicitis should be considered in the differential diagnosis of all patients with abdominal pain. A several-hour period of close observation with reassessment usually clarifies the diagnosis. The diagnosis is more commonly missed in women, patients with comorbidities, and patients who experienced abdominal pain with constipation. Absence of classic migration of pain (from epigastrium to right lower abdomen); right lower quadrant pain; fever; or guarding each makes appendicitis less likely. Widespread use of ultrasonography and CT has reduced the number of incorrect diagnoses to < 2%. Still, in some cases, diagnostic laparotomy or laparoscopy is required.

The most common causes of diagnostic confusion are gastroenteritis and gynecologic disorders. Viral gastroenteritis presents with nausea, vomiting, low-grade fever, and diarrhea and can be difficult to distinguish from appendicitis. The onset of vomiting before pain makes appendicitis less likely. As a rule, the pain of gastroenteritis is more generalized and the tenderness less well localized. Acute salpingitis or tubo-ovarian abscess should be considered in young, sexually active women with fever and bilateral abdominal or pelvic tenderness. A twisted ovarian cyst may also cause sudden severe pain. The sudden onset of lower abdominal pain in the middle of the menstrual cycle suggests mittelschmerz. Sudden severe abdominal pain with diffuse pelvic tenderness and shock suggests a ruptured ectopic pregnancy. A positive pregnancy test and pelvic ultrasonography are diagnostic. Retrocecal or retroileal appendicitis (often associated with pyuria or hematuria) may be confused with ureteral colic or pyelonephritis. Other conditions that may resemble appendicitis are diverticulitis, carcinoid of the appendix, perforated colonic cancer, Crohn ileitis, perforated peptic ulcer, cholecystitis, and mesenteric adenitis. It is virtually impossible to distinguish appendicitis from Meckel diverticulitis, but both require surgical treatment.

Complications

Perforation occurs in 20% of patients and should be suspected in patients with pain persisting for > 36 hours, high fever, diffuse abdominal tenderness or peritoneal findings, a palpable abdominal mass, or marked leukocytosis. Localized perforation results in a contained abscess, usually in the pelvis. A free perforation leads to suppurative peritonitis with toxicity. Septic thrombophlebitis (pylephlebitis) of the portal venous system is rare and suggested by high fever, chills, bacteremia, and jaundice.

Treatment

A. Surgical Appendectomy

The treatment of early, uncomplicated appendicitis is surgical appendectomy in most patients. When possible, a laparoscopic approach is preferred to open laparotomy. Prior to surgery, patients should be given broad-spectrum antibiotics with gram-negative and anaerobic coverage to reduce the incidence of postoperative infections. Recommended preoperative intravenous regimens include cefoxitin, cefotetan, or cefazolin 2 g and metronidazole 500 mg.

B. Conservative Management

Management with antibiotics alone may be considered in patients with a nonperforated appendicitis with surgical contraindications or with a strong preference to avoid surgery; however, appendectomy generally still is recommended in most patients to prevent recurrent appendicitis (20–35% within 1 year). Up to 80–90% of patients with uncomplicated appendicitis treated with antibiotics alone for 7–10 days have resolution of symptoms and signs. Treatment is with intravenous antibiotics for 1–3 days (piperacillin–tazobactam 3.375 g every 6 hours or metronidazole 500 mg every 8 hours plus a cephalosporin every 8 hours [eg, cefazolin 2 g, ceftriaxone 2g, or cefotaxime 2 g]), followed in those with improvement by oral antibiotics for an additional 7–10 days (eg, amoxicillin–clavulanic acid [875/125-mg tablet] every 8–12 hours or a combination of metronidazole 500 mg every 8 hours and levofloxacin 750 mg once daily).

C. Perforated Appendicitis

Emergency appendectomy is required in patients with perforated appendicitis with generalized peritonitis. The optimal treatment of stable patients with perforated appendicitis and a contained abscess is controversial. Surgery in this setting can be difficult. Many recommend percutaneous CT-guided drainage of the abscess with intravenous fluids and empiric broad-spectrum antibiotics with coverage against gram-negative and anerobic organisms to allow the inflammation to subside. An interval appendectomy may be performed after 6 weeks to prevent recurrent appendicitis.

Prognosis

The mortality rate from uncomplicated appendicitis is extremely low. Even with perforated appendicitis, the mortality rate in most groups is only 0.2%, though it approaches 15% in older adults.

Kumar SS et al. SAGES guideline for the diagnosis and treatment of appendicitis. Surg Endosc. 2024;38:2974. [PMID: 38740595]
Zagales I et al. Comparing outcomes of appendectomy versus non-operative antibiotic therapy for acute appendicitis: a systematic review and meta-analysis of randomized clinical trials. Am Surg. 2023;89:2644. [PMID: 35818927]

INTESTINAL TUBERCULOSIS

Intestinal tuberculosis (TB) is common in underdeveloped countries but rare in the United States except in immigrant groups or in patients with untreated AIDS. It is caused by both *Mycobacterium tuberculosis* and *M bovis*. Active pulmonary disease is present in < 50% of patients. The most frequent site of involvement is the ileocecal region; however, any region of the GI tract may be involved. Patients may be without symptoms or describe chronic abdominal pain, obstructive symptoms, weight loss, and diarrhea. An abdominal mass may be palpable. Complications include intestinal obstruction, hemorrhage, and fistula formation. The purified protein derivative (PPD) skin test may be negative, especially in patients with weight loss or AIDS. Abdominal CT may show thickening of the cecum and ileocecal valve and massive lymphadenopathy. Colonoscopy may demonstrate an ulcerated mass, multiple ulcers with steep edges and adjacent small sessile polyps, small ulcers or erosions, or small diverticula, most commonly in the ileocecal region. The differential diagnosis includes Crohn disease, carcinoma, lymphoma, and intestinal amebiasis. The diagnosis is established by either endoscopic or surgical biopsy revealing acid-fast bacilli, caseating granuloma, or positive cultures, or PCR for the organism; however, the sensitivity of these tests for intestinal TB is low (< 25%). Due to their similar symptoms, signs, and endoscopic findings, it may be particularly difficult to distinguish intestinal TB from Crohn disease in regions in which TB is endemic. When there is diagnostic uncertainty, an empiric trial of anti-TB therapy should be administered for 4–8 weeks (followed by clinical and endoscopic reassessment) before considering immunosuppressive therapy for possible Crohn disease.

Mouli V et al. Navigating the differential diagnosis of intestinal tuberculosis and Crohn's disease. Gastroenterology. 2025;169:1139. [PMID: 40840713]

PROTEIN-LOSING ENTEROPATHY

Protein-losing enteropathy comprises a number of conditions that result in excessive loss of serum proteins into the GI tract. In most cases, protein-losing enteropathy is a sequela of a known GI mucosal disorder or by diseases that obstruct the intestinal lymphatic drainage. In patients in whom the cause is unclear, evaluation is indicated and is guided by the clinical suspicion.

Hypoalbuminemia is the sine qua non of protein-losing enteropathy. However, other serum proteins such as α_1-antitrypsin also are lost from the gut epithelium. In protein-losing enteropathy caused by lymphatic obstruction, loss of lymphatic fluid commonly results in lymphocytopenia (< 1000/mcL), hypoglobulinemia, and hypocholesterolemia.

Protein-losing enteropathy must be distinguished from other causes of hypoalbuminemia, which include liver disease and nephrotic syndrome, and from HF.

Laboratory evaluation of protein-losing enteropathy includes serum protein electrophoresis, lymphocyte count, and serum cholesterol to look for evidence of lymphatic obstruction. Serum ANA and C3 levels are useful to screen for autoimmune disorders. Stool samples should be examined for ova and parasites. Evidence of malabsorption is evaluated by means of a stool qualitative fecal fat determination. Protein-losing enteropathy is confirmed by determining the gut α_1-antitrypsin clearance (24-hour volume of feces × stool concentration of α_1-antitrypsin ÷ serum α_1-antitrypsin concentration). A clearance > 27 mL/24 hours is abnormal. Intestinal imaging is obtained with small bowel enteroscopy, CT enterography, or wireless capsule endoscopy of the small intestine. Colonic diseases are excluded with colonoscopy. CT of the abdomen is performed to look for evidence of neoplasms or lymphatic obstruction. Rarely, lymphangiography is helpful. In some situations, laparotomy with full-thickness intestinal biopsy is required to establish a diagnosis.

Treatment is directed at the underlying cause.

Ozen A et al. Protein-losing enteropathy. N Engl J Med. 2023;389:733. [PMID: 37611123]

DISEASES OF THE COLON & RECTUM

(See Chapter 43 for Colorectal Cancer.)

IRRITABLE BOWEL SYNDROME

ESSENTIALS OF DIAGNOSIS

- Chronic functional disorder characterized by abdominal pain with alterations in bowel habits.
- Symptoms usually begin in late teens to early twenties.
- Limited evaluation to exclude organic causes of symptoms.

General Considerations

IBS can be defined as an idiopathic clinical entity characterized by chronic (> 3 months) abdominal pain that occurs in association with altered bowel habits. These symptoms may be continuous or intermittent. The Rome IV consensus definition of IBS is recurrent abdominal pain that occurs an average of at least 1 day/week and is associated with two or more of the following three features: (1) related to defecation (relief or worsening), (2) associated with a change in frequency of stool, or (3) associated with a change in form (appearance) of stool. Other symptoms supporting the diagnosis include abnormal stool frequency; abnormal stool form (lumpy or hard; loose or watery); abnormal stool passage (straining, urgency, or feeling of incomplete evacuation); and abdominal bloating or a feeling of abdominal distention.

Patients may have other somatic or psychological complaints such as dyspepsia, heartburn, chest pain, headaches, fatigue, myalgias, urologic dysfunction, gynecologic symptoms, anxiety, or depression.

The disorder is a common problem presenting to both gastroenterologists and primary care physicians. Up to 5% of adults have symptoms compatible with the diagnosis, but most never seek medical attention. Approximately two-thirds of patients with IBS are women.

Pathogenesis

A. Abnormal Motility

A variety of abnormal myoelectrical and motor abnormalities have been identified in the colon and small intestine. In some cases, these are temporally correlated with episodes of abdominal pain or emotional stress. Differences between patients with constipation-predominant (slow intestinal transit or pelvic floor dyssynergia) and diarrhea-predominant (rapid intestinal transit, bile acid malabsorption) syndromes are reported.

B. Visceral Hypersensitivity

Patients often have a lower visceral pain threshold, reporting abdominal pain at lower volumes of colonic gas insufflation or colonic balloon inflation than controls. Many patients report bloating and distention, which may be due to increased visceral sensitivity, increased gas production, impaired gas transit through the intestine, or impaired rectal expulsion. Many patients also report rectal urgency despite small rectal volumes of stool.

C. Intestinal Inflammation

It is postulated that dietary factors, medications (antibiotics), or infections may increase intestinal permeability, leading to intestinal inflammation that may contribute to alterations in intestinal motility or visceral hypersensitivity.

Symptoms compatible with IBS develop within 1 year in > 10% of patients after an episode of bacterial gastroenteritis compared with < 2% of controls. Women and patients with antibiotic exposure or psychological stress at the onset of gastroenteritis appear to be at increased risk for developing "postinfectious" IBS.

Alterations in the intestinal microbiome composition may cause increased postprandial gas as well as bloating and distention due to degradation of undigested, fermentable carbohydrates in the small intestine or colon. A subset of patients with IBS appear to have small intestinal bacterial overgrowth. However, estimates of the proportions of patients affected vary widely in part due to the different methods used to diagnose bacterial overgrowth. In a 2020 meta-analysis of 25 studies of patients with IBS who underwent testing for bacterial overgrowth, an increase in breath hydrogen or methane excretion was reported in 62% following lactulose ingestion but in 21% following glucose ingestion, and only 14% using the "gold standard" of jejunal aspirates and bacterial cultures.

D. Psychosocial Abnormalities

More than 50% of patients with irritable bowel who seek medical attention have underlying depression, anxiety, or somatization. Psychological abnormalities may influence how the patient perceives or reacts to illness and minor visceral sensations. Chronic stress may alter intestinal motility or modulate pathways that affect central and spinal processing of visceral afferent sensation.

Clinical Findings

A. Symptoms and Signs

Irritable bowel is a chronic condition. Symptoms usually begin in the late teens to twenties. The diagnosis is established in the presence of compatible symptoms and the judicious use of tests to exclude organic disease.

Abdominal pain usually is intermittent, crampy, and in the lower abdominal region. Pain is typically associated with a change in stool frequency or form and may be improved or worsened by defecation. It does not usually occur at night or interfere with sleep. Patients with IBS may be classified into one of four categories based on the predominant stool habits and stool form: IBS with diarrhea, IBS with constipation, IBS with mixed constipation and diarrhea, or IBS that is not subtyped. It is important to clarify what the patient means by these complaints. Patients with irritable bowel and constipation report infrequent bowel movements (less than three per week), hard or lumpy stools, or straining. Patients with IBS with diarrhea refer to loose or watery stools, frequent stools (more than three per day), urgency, or fecal incontinence. Many patients report that they have a firm stool in the morning followed by progressively looser movements. Complaints of visible distention and bloating are common, though these are not always clinically evident.

The patient should be asked about "alarm" symptoms that suggest a diagnosis other than IBS and warrant further investigation. The acute onset of symptoms raises the likelihood of organic disease, especially in patients older than 45 years. Nocturnal diarrhea, severe constipation or diarrhea, hematochezia, weight loss, and fever are incompatible with a diagnosis of IBS and warrant investigation for underlying disease. Patients who have a family history of cancer, IBD, or celiac disease should undergo additional evaluation. Eating habits and nutrient intake should be evaluated to screen for eating disorders.

A physical examination is indicated to look for evidence of organic disease and to allay the patient's anxieties. The physical examination usually is normal. Abdominal tenderness, especially in the lower abdomen, is common but not pronounced. A digital rectal examination should be performed in patients with constipation to screen for paradoxical anal squeezing during attempted straining that may suggest pelvic floor dyssynergia. A pelvic examination is recommended for postmenopausal women with recent-onset constipation and lower abdominal pain to screen for gynecologic malignancy.

B. Laboratory Findings and Special Examinations

Although the vague nature of symptoms and patient anxiety may prompt clinicians to consider a variety of diagnostic studies, overtesting should be avoided, since the likelihood of serious organic disease is low. Nonetheless, AGA and ACG practice guidelines recommend selected laboratory tests in patients with chronic diarrhea to exclude other diagnoses. A CBC should be obtained to screen for iron deficiency anemia and CRP to screen for inflammation. A fecal calprotectin level is recommended to screen for IBD; a value of > 50 mcg/g may warrant further endoscopic evaluation. Serologic testing for celiac disease (IgA anti-tTG2) should be performed. Stool specimen examinations should be obtained in patients with increased likelihood of parasitic infection (eg, day care workers, campers, foreign travelers) for *Giardia* antigen or for multiple organisms (*Giardia, Cryptosporidium, Cyclospora, Entamoeba histolytica*) using nucleic acid amplification (PCR) tests. If these tests are negative, further testing is not necessary in most patients and education, reassurance, and initial empiric treatment is recommended. Routine sigmoidoscopy or colonoscopy is not recommended in patients aged < 45 years with symptoms of IBS without "alarm" symptoms but should be considered along with further laboratory testing in patients who do not improve with conservative management. In all patients aged ≥ 45 years who have not had a previous evaluation, colonoscopy should be obtained to exclude malignancy. When colonoscopy is performed, random mucosal biopsies should be obtained to look for evidence of microscopic colitis (which may have similar symptoms). Patients with symptoms or signs of pelvic floor disorder (dyssynergic defecation) should be referred for anorectal physiology testing (manometry and balloon expulsion test). Routine testing for bacterial overgrowth with hydrogen breath tests is not recommended.

Differential Diagnosis

A number of disorders may present with similar symptoms. Examples include colonic neoplasia, IBD (ulcerative colitis, Crohn disease, microscopic colitis), bile-acid diarrhea, hyper- or hypothyroidism, parasites, malabsorption (especially celiac disease, bacterial overgrowth, lactase deficiency), causes of chronic secretory diarrhea (carcinoid), and gynecologic disorders (endometriosis, ovarian cancer). Psychiatric disorders such as depression, panic disorder, and anxiety must be considered as well. Women with refractory symptoms have an increased incidence of prior sexual and physical abuse. These diagnoses should be excluded in patients with presumed IBS who do not improve within 2–4 weeks of empiric treatment or in whom subsequent "alarm" symptoms develop.

Treatment

A. General Measures

As with other functional disorders, the most important interventions the clinician can offer are reassurance, education, and support. This includes identifying and responding to the patient's concerns in a sensitive, nonjudgmental manner, careful explanation of the pathophysiology and natural history of the disorder, setting realistic treatment goals, and involving the patient in the treatment process. Because irritable bowel symptoms are chronic, the patient's reasons for seeking consultation at this time should be determined. These may include major life events or recent psychosocial stressors, dietary or medication changes, concerns about serious underlying disease, or reduced quality of life and impairment of daily activities. In discussing with the patient the importance of the mind-gut interaction, it may be helpful to explain that alterations in visceral motility and sensitivity may be exacerbated by environmental, social, or psychological factors such as foods, medications, hormones, and stress. Symptoms such as pain, bloating, and altered bowel habits may lead to anxiety and distress, which in turn may further exacerbate bowel disturbances due to disordered communication between the gut and the CNS. Fears that the symptoms will progress, require surgery, or degenerate into serious illness should be allayed. The patient should understand that IBS is a chronic disorder characterized by periods of exacerbation and quiescence. The emphasis should be shifted from finding the cause of the symptoms to finding a way to cope with them. Moderate exercise is beneficial. Clinicians must resist the temptation to chase chronic complaints with new or repeated diagnostic studies.

B. Dietary Therapy

Patients commonly report dietary intolerances. Proposed mechanisms for dietary intolerance include food allergy, hypersensitivity, effects of gut hormones, changes in bacterial flora, increased bacterial gas production (arising in the small or large intestine), and direct chemical irritation. Fatty foods, alcohol, caffeine, spicy foods, and grains are poorly tolerated by many patients with IBS. In patients with diarrhea, bloating, and flatulence, lactose intolerance should be excluded with a hydrogen breath test or a trial of a lactose-free diet. A host of poorly absorbed, fermentable, monosaccharides and short-chain carbohydrates (FODMAPs) may exacerbate bloating, flatulence, and diarrhea in some patients. These include six food groups: fructose (corn syrups, apples, pears, honey, watermelon, raisins), lactose, fructans (garlic, onions, leeks, asparagus, artichokes), wheat-based products (breads, pasta, cereals, cakes), sorbitol (stone fruits), and galacto-oligosaccharides (legumes, lentils, Brussels sprouts, soybeans, cabbage). Of these, studies suggest fructans and galacto-oligosaccharides may be primarily responsible. Dietary restriction of these fermentable carbohydrates for 2–4 weeks may improve symptoms (especially abdominal pain and bloating) in 50–65% of patients. Responders should gradually reintroduce different FODMAPs to identify food triggers. Ingestion of α-galactosidase supplement ("Beano") with meals containing foods with high galactoside content (eg, beans, peas, lentils, soy) may improve bowel symptoms. Gluten has not been demonstrated to increase bowel symptoms independent of other FODMAPs, and a gluten-free diet is not recommended.

Poorly fermentable soluble fiber (psyllium, methylcellulose, oatmeal, flesh of fruits and vegetables) may improve global symptoms, especially constipation, and such fiber is recommended by the 2021 American College of Gastroenterology guideline and the 2022 American Gastroenterological Association Clinical Practice update. Fermentable or insoluble fiber (bran, whole grains, skins of fruits and vegetables) may increase gas and bloating.

C. Pharmacologic Measures

More than two-thirds of patients with IBS have mild symptoms that respond readily to education, reassurance, and dietary interventions. Drug therapy should be reserved for patients with moderate to severe symptoms that do not respond to conservative measures. These agents should be viewed as being adjunctive rather than curative. Given the wide spectrum of symptoms, no single agent is expected to provide relief in all or even most patients. Nevertheless, therapy targeted at the specific dominant symptom (pain, constipation, or diarrhea) may be beneficial.

1. Antispasmodic agents—Over-the-counter, enteric-coated peppermint oil formulations (thought to relax smooth intestine) are widely available. The 2021 ACG guideline has suggested that peppermint oil may be useful to relieve global IBS symptoms and abdominal pain.

Despite a lack of well-designed trials demonstrating efficacy, anticholinergic agents are also recommended by current guidelines to treat pain and bloating. Available agents include hyoscyamine, 0.125 mg orally or sublingually, 3–4 times daily as needed or sustained-release, 0.037 mg or 0.75 mg orally twice daily; dicyclomine, 10–20 mg orally 3–4 times daily; or methscopolamine, 2.5–5 mg orally before meals and at bedtime. Anticholinergic side effects are common, including urinary retention, constipation, tachycardia, and dry mouth. Hence, these agents should be used with caution in older patients and in patients with constipation.

2. Antidiarrheal agents—Loperamide (2 mg orally three or four times daily) is effective for the treatment of patients with diarrhea, reducing stool frequency, liquidity, and urgency although it does not improve abdominal pain. It may best be used "prophylactically" in situations in which diarrhea is anticipated (such as stressful situations) or would be inconvenient (social engagements). Increased intracolonic bile acids due to alterations in enterohepatic circulation may contribute to diarrhea in a subset of patients with diarrhea. An empiric trial of bile salt–binding agents (cholestyramine, 2–4 g orally one to three times daily with meals; colesevelam, 625 mg, 1–3 tablets twice daily) may be considered. In patients with persistent severe symptoms, eluxadoline or alosetron may be considered. Eluxadoline (75–100 mg twice daily) is a mixed υ- and κ-opioid receptor agonist and δ-opioid antagonist that is approved for treatment of IBS with diarrhea. In phase 3 trials, it decreased abdominal pain and improved stool consistency in approximately 25% of patients versus 16–19% with placebo. Due to a small risk of pancreatitis and sphincter of Oddi spasm, it is contraindicated in patients without a gallbladder or with increased alcohol intake. Alosetron (0.5–1.0 mg orally twice daily) is a selective 5-HT_3 antagonist. Due to a small risk of ischemic colitis (1.03 cases/1000 patient-years), its use is restricted to women with severe IBS with diarrhea under a risk-management program.

3. Anticonstipation agents—Treatment with oral osmotic laxatives such as polyethylene glycol 3350 (MiraLAX, 17–34 g/day) may increase stool frequency, improve stool consistency, and reduce straining but do not improve abdominal pain. Lactulose and sorbitol produce increased flatus and distention and should be avoided in patients with IBS. For patients with inadequate response to polyethylene glycol, several agents are available that may yield modest improvement in stool frequency and form, abdominal pain, and global IBS symptoms. The secretagogues lubiprostone (8 mcg orally twice daily), linaclotide (290 mcg orally once daily), plecanatide (3 mg orally once daily), and tenapanor (50 mg orally twice daily) are FDA approved for treatment of IBS with constipation based on modest demonstrated efficacy and are recommended in the 2021 ACG and 2022 AGA guidelines. Through different mechanisms, these agents stimulate increased fluid secretion, resulting in accelerated colonic transit. Tenapanor is FDA-approved for the treatment of IBS with constipation. It is a locally acting small molecule that inhibits the Na^+/H^+ exchange pump on the apical surface of the small and large intestine, increasing fluid secretion into the intestinal lumen.

In phase 3 clinical trials, 34.7% of patients treated with tenapanor met the FDA-approved endpoint versus 21.7% treated with placebo. Diarrhea led to tenapanor discontinuation in 6.5%. Tegaserod is a 5-HT_4-receptor agonist that stimulates peristalsis; it was voluntarily withdrawn from the market in 2007 because of cardiovascular safety concerns. In 2019, after evaluation of clinical and safety data from 29 placebo-controlled trials and newer treatment outcome data, tegaserod (6 mg orally twice daily) was reapproved by the FDA for women aged < 65 years with IBS and constipation. It may be considered for treatment of women age younger than 65 years with one or fewer cardiovascular risk factors whose IBS with constipation has not improved with secretagogue therapy. Patients with intractable constipation should undergo further assessment for slow colonic transit and pelvic floor dysfunction (see Constipation, above).

4. Psychotropic agents—Patients with predominant symptoms of pain or bloating may benefit from low doses of tricyclic antidepressants, which are believed to have effects on motility, visceral sensitivity, and central pain perception that are independent of their psychotropic effects. Because of their anticholinergic effects, these agents may be more useful in patients with diarrhea-predominant than constipation-predominant symptoms. Oral nortriptyline, desipramine, or imipramine may be started at a low dosage of 10 mg at bedtime and increased gradually to a maximum of 30–50 mg as tolerated. Response rates do not correlate with dosage, and many patients respond to doses of ≤ 50 mg daily. Higher doses used in treatment of depression (150–300 mg daily) are not needed for treatment of GI symptoms. Side effects are common, and lack of efficacy with one agent does not preclude benefit from another. Agents with higher anticholinergic activity may improve diarrhea but worsen constipation. Improvement should be evident within 4 weeks. The oral SSRIs (sertraline, 25–100 mg daily; citalopram, 10–20 mg; paroxetine, 20–50 mg daily; or fluoxetine, 10–40 mg daily) may be used to treat irritable bowel symptoms as well as treat mood disorders. SSRIs may accelerate GI transit and improve constipation. Anxiolytics should not be used chronically in IBS because of their habituation potential. Patients with major depression or anxiety disorders should be identified and treated with therapeutic doses of appropriate agents.

5. Nonabsorbable antibiotics—Rifaximin (550 mg orally three times daily for 14 days) may be considered in patients with refractory symptoms, especially bloating. A 2012 meta-analysis identified a 9.9% greater improvement in bloating with rifaximin compared with placebo, a modest gain that is similar to other less expensive therapies. Symptom improvement may be attributable to suppression of bacteria in either the small intestine or colon, resulting in decreased bacterial carbohydrate fermentation, diarrhea, and bloating.

6. Probiotics—Meta-analyses of small controlled clinical trials of probiotics report improved symptoms of pain, bloating, and flatulence in some patients; however, there is no proven benefit. Probiotics are not recommended for IBS treatment in the 2020 AGA and 2021 ACG guidelines.

D. Psychological Therapies

Cognitive-behavioral therapies, relaxation techniques, yoga, and hypnotherapy appear to be beneficial in some patients. Patients with underlying psychological abnormalities may benefit from evaluation by a psychiatrist or psychologist. Patients with severe disability should be referred to a pain management center.

Prognosis

Most patients with IBS learn to cope with their symptoms and lead productive lives.

Cuffe M et al. Efficacy of dietary interventions in irritable bowel syndrome: a systematic review and network meta-analysis. Lancet Gastroenterol Hepatol. 2025;10:520. [PMID: 40258374]

Eswaran S et al. All FODMAPs aren't created equal: results of a randomized reintroduction trial in patients with irritable bowel syndrome. Clin Gastroenterol Hepatol. 2025;23:351. [PMID: 387294234]

Goodoory VC et al. Effect of brain-gut behavioral treatments on abdominal pain irritable bowel syndrome: systematic review and network meta-analysis. Gastroenterology. 2024;167:934. [PMID: 38777133]

Hanna-Jairala I et al. Central neuromodulators in irritable bowel syndrome: why, how, and when. Am J Gastroenterol. 2024;119:1272. [PMID: 38595149]

ANTIBIOTIC-ASSOCIATED COLITIS

ESSENTIALS OF DIAGNOSIS

- Most cases of antibiotic-associated diarrhea are not attributable to *C difficile* and are usually mild and self-limited.
- Symptoms of antibiotic-associated colitis vary from mild to fulminant; almost all colitis is attributable to *C difficile*.
- Diagnosis in most cases established by stool assay.

General Considerations

Antibiotic-associated diarrhea is a common clinical occurrence. Characteristically, the diarrhea occurs during the period of antibiotic exposure, is dose related, and resolves spontaneously after discontinuation of the antibiotic. In most cases, this diarrhea is mild, self-limited, and does not require any specific laboratory evaluation or treatment. Stool examination usually reveals no fecal leukocytes, and stool cultures reveal no pathogens. Although *C difficile* is identified in the stool of 15–25% of cases of antibiotic-associated diarrhea, it is also identified in 5–10% of patients treated with antibiotics who do not have diarrhea. Most cases of antibiotic-associated diarrhea are due to changes in colonic bacterial fermentation of carbohydrates and are not due to *C difficile*.

Antibiotic-associated colitis is a significant clinical problem almost always caused by *C difficile* infection that colonizes the colon and releases two toxins: TcdA and

TcdB. A more virulent strain of *C difficile* (NAP1) results in higher toxin A and B production. This hypervirulent strain is more prevalent among hospital-associated infections and is associated with outbreaks of severe disease but appears to be declining in incidence.

Found throughout hospitals in patient rooms and bathrooms, *C difficile* is readily transmitted from patient to patient by hospital personnel. Fastidious hand washing and use of disposable gloves are helpful in minimizing transmission and reducing infections in hospitalized patients. In hospitalized patients, *C difficile* colitis occurs in approximately 20% of those who are colonized at admission and 3.5% of those not colonized. In both hospital-associated and community infections, most episodes of colitis occur in people who have received antibiotics that disrupt the normal bowel flora and thus allow the bacteria to flourish. Although almost all antibiotics have been implicated, colitis most commonly develops after use of ampicillin, clindamycin, third-generation cephalosporins, and fluoroquinolones. Symptoms usually begin during or shortly after antibiotic therapy but may be delayed for up to 8 weeks. All patients with acute diarrhea should be asked about recent antibiotic exposure. Patients who are older; debilitated; immunocompromised; receiving multiple antibiotics or prolonged (> 10 days) antibiotic therapy; receiving enteral tube feedings, PPIs , or chemotherapy; or who have IBD have a higher risk of acquiring *C difficile* and developing *C difficile*–associated diarrhea.

Clinical Findings

A. Symptoms and Signs

Most patients report mild to moderate greenish, foul-smelling watery diarrhea 3–15 times per day with lower abdominal cramps. Physical examination is normal or reveals mild left lower quadrant tenderness. The stools may have mucus but seldom gross blood. Over half of hospitalized patients diagnosed with *C difficile* colitis have severe disease as defined by a white blood count > 15,000/mcL (15×10^9/L) or serum creatinine > 1.5 g/dL. Fever is uncommon. Fulminant disease occurs in up to 10% of patients. It is characterized severe disease with hypotension or shock, ileus, or megacolon.

B. Special Examinations

1. Stool studies—Stool testing for *C difficile* is recommended in hospitalized patients with dysentery or three or more liquid stools within 24 hours or outpatients with diarrhea persisting longer than 1 week. As the initial diagnostic test, most laboratories screen for *C difficile* with one of two tests: (1) the most commonly used is an enzyme immunoassay (EIA) for glutamate dehydrogenase (GDH) protein, which has high sensitivity and negative predictive value (95%) for the detection of toxigenic and nontoxigenic *C difficile* but does not distinguish active infection with toxin secretion from colonization; (2) an alternative is a PCR test that amplifies one of the *C difficile* toxin genes (usually *TcdB*)—these have extremely high sensitivity (97–99%) for detection of *C difficile* and the ability to detect the hypervirulent NAP1 strain but, like the GDH assay, cannot distinguish active infection from colonization. A negative GDH assay or PCR effectively excludes infection; however, a positive GDH or PCR test requires secondary laboratory testing with an EIA for the presence of *C difficile* toxins TcdA and TcdB to distinguish colonization from active toxin-producing infection.

2. Flexible sigmoidoscopy—Flexible sigmoidoscopy is not needed in patients who have typical symptoms and a positive stool test for *C difficile*. It may clarify the diagnosis in patients with positive *C difficile* toxin assays who have atypical symptoms or who have persistent diarrhea despite appropriate therapy. In patients with mild to moderate symptoms, there may be no abnormalities or only patchy or diffuse, nonspecific colitis indistinguishable from other causes. **Pseudomembranous colitis** may be seen in some patients with severe illness.

3. Imaging studies—Abdominal radiographs or noncontrast abdominal CTs are obtained in patients with severe or fulminant symptoms to look for evidence of colonic dilation and wall thickening. Abdominal CT also is useful in the evaluation of hospitalized patients with abdominal pain or ileus without significant diarrhea, in whom the presence of colonic wall thickening suggests unsuspected *C difficile* colitis. CT is also useful in the detection of possible perforation.

Differential Diagnosis

In the hospitalized patient in whom acute diarrhea develops after admission, the differential diagnosis includes simple antibiotic-associated diarrhea (not related to *C difficile*), enteral feedings, medications, and ischemic colitis. Other infectious causes are unusual in hospitalized patients in whom diarrhea develops > 72 hours after admission, and it is not cost-effective to obtain stool cultures unless tests for *C difficile* are negative. *Klebsiella oxytoca* may cause a distinct form of antibiotic-associated hemorrhagic colitis that is segmental (usually in the right or transverse colon); spares the rectum; and is more common in younger, healthier outpatients.

Complications

Severe colitis may progress quickly to fulminant disease, resulting in hemodynamic instability, respiratory failure, metabolic acidosis, megacolon (> 7-cm diameter), perforation, and death. Chronic untreated colitis may result in weight loss and protein-losing enteropathy.

Treatment

A. Initial Treatment

To reduce transmission within health care facilities, patients with suspected or proven *C difficile* infection should be placed on strict contact precautions and health care workers should apply careful handwashing before and after contact. If possible, therapy with the inciting antibiotic should be discontinued as soon as possible. The treatment of an initial episode of *C difficile* colitis is determined by the severity of disease. For patients with nonsevere disease, oral fidaxomicin

(200 mg orally two times daily) and vancomycin (125 mg orally four times daily) are equally effective for initial treatment, but recurrence rates are lower with fidaxomicin than vancomycin (15% versus 25%). Fidaxomicin may be preferred as first-line treatment for patients believed to be at higher risk for recurrent disease. Recommended treatment duration is 10 days in most situations but is extended in patients requiring prolonged antibiotic therapy for other infections. Metronidazole (500 mg orally three times daily) is no longer recommended for initial therapy except in mild disease when vancomycin or fidaxomicin is unavailable. Symptomatic improvement occurs in most patients within 72 hours. Following treatment, stool assays may remain positive for several weeks after symptom resolution.

For patients with severe or fulminant disease, vancomycin 500 mg orally four times daily along with metronidazole 500 mg intravenously every 8 hours are recommended. In patients with ileus, vancomycin may be administered by nasoenteric tube and by rectal enema (500 mg in 100 mL normal saline by enema every 6 hours). The efficacy of fidaxomicin for severe or fulminant disease requires further investigation. Early surgical consultation is recommended for all patients with severe or fulminant disease. Total abdominal colectomy or loop ileostomy with colonic lavage may be required in patients with toxic megacolon, perforation, sepsis, or hemorrhage. Poor surgical candidates should be considered for **fecal microbiota transplantation (FMT)** administered by colonoscopy at 3- to 5-day intervals (see below).

B. Treatment of Relapse

Up to 20% of patients have a relapse of diarrhea from *C difficile* within 8 weeks after stopping initial therapy. This may be due to reinfection or failure to eradicate the organism. Guidelines recommend that the first recurrence be treated with fidaxomicin 200 mg orally twice daily for 10 days or with a prolonged tapering regimen of vancomycin 125 mg orally four times daily for 14 days; twice daily for 7 days; once daily for 7 days; then every other 2 or 3 days for 2–8 weeks. Second recurrence should be treated with an additional vancomycin tapering regimen, as above.

For patients with two or more relapses, guidelines recommend consideration of FMT, in which a suspension or capsule formulation of fecal microbiota specimens derived from healthy donors is given to the patient following treatment with vancomycin or fidaxomicin. There are two FDA-approved formulations to prevent *C difficile* recurrence following antibacterial treatment. VOWST is an oral capsule formulation administered as 4 capsules orally, once daily for 3 days. In clinical trials, *C difficile* recurrence rates at 8 weeks were 12.4% in treated patients versus 38.8% in those given placebo. Rebyota is administered once as a rectal enema (150 mL). In clinical trials, *C difficile* recurrence rates at 8 weeks were 29% in treated patients versus 42% given placebo enemas.

When to Refer

- Lack of improvement after 3–5 days of therapy
- Fulminant colitis or toxic megacolon
- Multiple relapses
- Early surgical consultation for all patients with severe or fulminant disease

When to Admit

- Severe colitis: pain, diarrhea, dehydration, fever (temperature > 40.0°C), abdominal tenderness, leukocytosis

Di Bella S et al. *Clostridioides difficile* infection: history, epidemiology, risk factors, prevention, clinical manifestations, treatment and future options. Clin Microbiol Rev. 2024;37:e0013523. [PMID: 38421181]

Feuerstadt P et al. Practical use of RBX2660 for the prevention of recurrent *Clostridioides difficile* infection. Am J Gastroenterol. 2023;118:1303. [PMID: 36695753]

Gulati A et al. Fecal microbiota transplantation across the lifespan: balancing efficacy, safety, and innovation. Am J Gastroenterol. 2023;118:435. [PMID: 36580630]

Peery A et al. AGA Clinical Practice Guideline on fecal microbiota-based therapies for select gastrointestinal diseases. Gastroenterology. 2024;166:409. [PMID: 38395525]

Vaughn B et al. Effectiveness and safety of colonic and capsule fecal microbiota transplantation for *Clostridioides difficile* infection. Clin Gastroenterol Hepatol. 2023;21:1330. [PMID: 36126907]

INFLAMMATORY BOWEL DISEASE

The term *inflammatory bowel disease* includes ulcerative colitis and Crohn disease. The diagnosis and management of each will be reviewed in the sections below. After a marked (up to 4-fold) increase over the past 40 years in northern European countries and the United States, the incidence in these regions may have stabilized. In the United States, there are approximately 2.4 million people with IBD (0.7%) with an adjusted annual incidence of 10.9 cases/100,000 person-years. The prevalence of ulcerative colitis is slightly higher than Crohn disease. These diseases can occur at any age but most commonly begin in adolescents and adults aged < 40 years. The natural history of both varies from mild, often intermittent disease symptoms to severe disease characterized by elevated inflammatory markers and mucosal ulcerations that may lead to intestinal complications (bleeding, strictures, fistulas, surgery), nutritional deficiencies, and impaired quality of life. Both diseases may be associated with several extraintestinal manifestations, including oral ulcers, oligoarticular or polyarticular nondeforming peripheral arthritis, spondylitis or sacroiliitis, episcleritis or uveitis, erythema nodosum, pyoderma gangrenosum, hepatitis and sclerosing cholangitis, and thromboembolic events.

Pharmacologic Therapy

Although ulcerative colitis and Crohn disease appear to be distinct entities, several pharmacologic agents are used to treat both. For many years, the primary therapeutic options were 5-aminosalicylic acid agents, corticosteroids, and immunomodulating drugs (thiopurines and methotrexate). The therapeutic options today have greatly expanded to include other small-molecule agents (Janus kinase [JAK] inhibitors and sphingosine 1-phosphate receptor modulators) and biologic therapies (tumor necrosis factor [TNF] antagonists, IL-12/23 antibodies, and anti-integrins). See Table 17–13.

A. 5-Aminosalicylic Acid (5-ASA)

5-ASA is a topically active agent that has a variety of anti-inflammatory effects. Several oral and topical compounds have been designed to target delivery of 5-ASA to the colon or distal small intestine.

1. Oral formulations—Mesalamine compounds are oral 5-ASA formulations that are either coated in various pH-sensitive resins (Asacol, Apriso, and Lialda) or timed-release capsules (Pentasa). Side effects of these compounds are uncommon but include nausea, rash, diarrhea, pancreatitis, and acute interstitial nephritis. Sulfasalazine and balsalazide are oral formulations that contain 5-ASA linked by an azo bond to another agent (sulfapyridine or an inert peptide, respectively) to prevent small intestine absorption. Following cleavage of the azo bond by colonic bacteria, 5-ASA is released in the colon. The sulfapyridine group is absorbed and may cause side effects in 15–30% of patients, including nausea, oligospermia, leukopenia, agranulocytosis, impaired folate metabolism, and hypersensitivity (fever, rash, hemolytic anemia, pneumonitis). Because of its side effects, sulfasalazine is used less frequently than balsalazide and other 5-ASA agents.

2. Topical mesalamine—5-ASA is provided in the form of suppositories (Canasa; 1000 mg) and enemas (Rowasa; 4 g/60 mL). These formulations can deliver much higher concentrations of 5-ASA to the distal colon than oral compounds. Side effects are uncommon.

B. Corticosteroids

A variety of intravenous, oral, and topical corticosteroid formulations have utility in the short-term treatment of moderate to severe IBD. However, long-term use is associated with serious, potentially irreversible side effects and is to be avoided. The agents, route of administration, duration of use, and tapering regimens used are based more on personal bias and experience than on data from rigorous clinical trials. Oral formulations include prednisone or methylprednisolone. Budesonide, another oral corticosteroid, has high topical anti-inflammatory activity but low systemic activity due to high first-pass hepatic metabolism; the enteric-coated formulation (Entocort) targets delivery to the terminal ileum and proximal colon, and a multimatrix, delayed-release formulation (budesonide multimatrix [MMX] formulation [Uceris]) releases budesonide throughout the colon. Topical preparations are provided as hydrocortisone suppositories (25 mg and 30 mg), foam (10%, 80 mg), and enemas (100 mg) and as budesonide foam (2 mg).

C. Immunomodulating Drugs and Other Small Molecules

1. Thiopurines (mercaptopurine and azathioprine)—These drugs are mainly used in combination with anti-TNF agents (see section D.1. below) in patients with moderate to severe Crohn disease and ulcerative colitis to reduce antibody formation against the biologic agent and to increase the likelihood of clinical remission through increased anti-TNF drug levels and possible synergistic effects. In some settings, they continue to be used as monotherapy to maintain remission in patients with quiescent disease. Side effects of mercaptopurine and azathioprine, including allergic reactions (fever, rash, or arthralgias) and nonallergic reactions (nausea, vomiting, pancreatitis, hepatotoxicity, bone marrow suppression, infections), occur in 15% of patients. Thiopurines are associated with up to a 2.5-fold increased risk of non-Hodgkin lymphomas (0.5/1000 patient-years). The risk rises after 1–2 years of exposure and is higher in men aged < 30 years and patients aged > 50 years. Thiopurines also are associated with a risk of HPV-related cervical dysplasia and with an increased risk of non-melanoma skin cancer. Younger patients also are at risk for severe primary Epstein-Barr virus (EBV) infection, if not previously exposed.

About 1 person in 300 has a homozygous pathogenic variant of one of the enzymes that metabolizes thiopurine methyltransferase (TPMT), placing them at risk for profound immunosuppression; 1 person in 9 is heterozygous for TPMT, resulting in intermediate enzyme activity. *Measurement of TPMT functional activity is recommended prior to initiation of thiopurine therapy.* Treatment should be withheld in patients with absent TPMT activity. The most effective dose of mercaptopurine is 1–1.5 mg/kg orally and for azathioprine, is 2–3 mg/kg orally daily. For patients with normal TPMT activity, both drugs may be initiated at the weight-calculated dose. A CBC should be obtained weekly for 4 weeks, biweekly for 4 weeks, and then every 1–3 months for the duration of therapy. Liver biochemical tests should be measured periodically. Some clinicians prefer gradual dose escalation, especially for patients with intermediate TPMT activity or for whom TPMT measurement is not available; both drugs may be started at 25 mg/day and increased by 25 mg every 1–2 weeks while monitoring for myelosuppression until the target dose is reached. If the WBC count falls < 4000/mcL (4.0×10^9/L) or the platelet count falls < 100,000/mcL (100×10^9/L), the medication should be held for at least 1 week before reducing the daily dose by 25–50 mg. Measurement of thiopurine metabolites (6-TG and 6-MMP) is of unproved value in most patients but is recommended in patients who have not responded to standard, weight-based dosing or in whom adverse effects develop.

2. Methotrexate—Low-dose oral methotrexate (12.5 mg once weekly) is used in combination with anti-TNF agents to prevent immunogenicity. Side effects of methotrexate include nausea, vomiting, stomatitis, infections, bone marrow suppression, hepatic fibrosis, and life-threatening pneumonitis. A CBC and liver chemistries should be monitored every 3 months. Folate supplementation (1 mg/day orally) should be administered. Because methotrexate is teratogenic, it should be discontinued in men and women at least 6 months before conception and during pregnancy.

3. Janus kinase inhibitors—Tofacitinib and upadacitinib are nonbiologic small molecules that inhibit Janus kinase, which is involved through the JAK-STAT pathway in modulation of multiple interleukins. Tofacitinib has greater inhibition of JAK1/3, whereas upadacitinib has greater selectivity for JAK1. Due to an increased risk of herpes zoster (up to 5% of patients), vaccination with inactivated (not live) recombinant zoster (Shingrix) is recommended for all patients. Other adverse events include acne, URIs, nonmelanoma skin cancers, lymphoma, and GI perforations. Opportunistic infections, including TB, occur rarely. Laboratory abnormalities include lymphopenia, neutropenia, elevated CK, and elevated lipids. There is an FDA black box warning for an increased risk of thrombosis, including MI, stroke, arterial thrombosis, DVT, PE, and death. They therefore should not be prescribed to patients deemed at higher risk for thrombosis.

4. Sphingosine 1-phosphate receptor modulators— Ozanimod and etrasimod are oral agents that bind to lymphocyte sphingosine 1-phosphate (S1P) receptors, thereby blocking their ability to leave lymph tissue, including the GI tract. They lead to a mean 45% reduction of peripheral lymphocyte count that may last for up to 4 weeks after drug discontinuation. Liver chemistries and CBC should be obtained 3–6 months after drug initiation. Severe lymphopenia $< 200 \times 10^9$/L ($< 0.2 \times 10^9$/L) should prompt drug dosage reduction or discontinuation. Other serious adverse events includes hypertension, liver transaminase elevation, and macular edema. Due to a low risk of bradycardia and AV conduction delays, an ECG should be obtained prior to initiating therapy to exclude conduction abnormalities; a cardiology consultation should be considered for patients with heart or cerebrovascular disease, arrhythmias, or AV block. Herpes simplex reactivation or herpes zoster may occur; inactivated recombinant zoster (Shingrix) vaccination is recommended.

D. Biologic Therapies

1. Anti-TNF therapies—Four monoclonal antibodies to TNF are available for subcutaneous administration for the treatment of IBD: infliximab, adalimumab, golimumab, and certolizumab. All four agents bind and neutralize soluble as well as membrane-bound TNF on macrophages and activated T lymphocytes, thereby preventing TNF stimulation of effector cells.

Infliximab is a chimeric (75% human/25% mouse) IgG_1 antibody that is administered by intravenous infusion or subcutaneous injection. Acute infusion reactions occur in 5–10% of infusions but are uncommon in patients receiving regularly scheduled infusions or concomitant immunomodulators (ie, azathioprine or methotrexate). Most reactions are mild and can be treated by slowing the infusion rate and administering acetaminophen and diphenhydramine. Severe reactions (hypotension, severe shortness of breath, rigors, severe chest discomfort) occur in < 1% and may require oxygen, diphenhydramine, hydrocortisone, and epinephrine. With repeated, intermittent intravenous injections, antibodies to infliximab develop in up to 40% of patients, which are associated with a shortened duration or loss of response and increased risk of acute or delayed infusion reactions. Giving infliximab in a regularly scheduled maintenance therapy (eg, every 8 weeks) or in combination with other immunomodulating agents (azathioprine, mercaptopurine, or methotrexate) significantly reduces the development of antibodies to < 10%.

Adalimumab and golimumab are fully human IgG_1 antibodies. Certolizumab is a chimeric compound in which the TNF antibody (95% human/5% mouse) is bound to polyethylene glycol in order to prolong the drug half-life. However, certolizumab is infrequently used due to lower clinical efficacy. Hypersensitivity reactions are rare with subcutaneous anti-TNF therapies. Injection-site reactions (burning, pain, redness, itching) are relatively common but usually mild and self-limited. Antibodies to adalimumab or golimumab develop in 5% of patients and to certolizumab in 10%, which may lead to shortened duration or loss of response to the drug.

Serious infections with anti-TNF therapies may occur in 2–5% of patients, including sepsis, pneumonia, abscess, and cellulitis; however, the increased risk is partially attributable to increased severity of disease and concomitant use of corticosteroids or immunomodulators. Patients treated with anti-TNF therapies are at increased risk for the development of opportunistic infections with intracellular bacterial pathogens including tuberculosis, mycoses (candidiasis, histoplasmosis, coccidioidomycosis, nocardiosis), and listeriosis, and with reactivation of viral infections, including hepatitis B, herpes simplex, varicella zoster, and EBV. Prior to use of these agents, patients should be screened for latent tuberculosis with PPD testing and a CXR. ANA and anti-DNA antibodies occur in a large percentage of patients; however, the development of drug-induced lupus is rare. All agents may cause severe hepatic reactions leading to acute hepatic failure; liver biochemical tests should be monitored routinely during therapy. Anti-TNF therapies may increase the risk of skin cancer, hence annual dermatologic examinations are recommended. There may be a small risk of non-Hodgkin lymphoma in patients taking anti-TNF monotherapy; however, the risk is much higher in patients receiving a combination of anti-TNF and a thiopurine. Rare cases of optic neuritis and demyelinating diseases, including multiple sclerosis, have been reported. Anti-TNF therapies may worsen HF in patients with cardiac disease.

In patients with active IBD, monitoring of anti-TNF trough levels and any anti-drug antibodies is useful to optimize drug levels and guide therapy. Maintenance of drug trough levels above specified thresholds is associated with higher clinical response rates and decreased risk of formation of neutralizing antibodies. Therapeutic drug monitoring is indicated in patients who have poor clinical response or who have lost clinical response. Patients with high titers of anti-drug antibodies should be switched to a different anti-TNF agent. Anti-TNF therapy has failed when patients have a poor response despite adequate anti-TNF trough concentrations; another class of drugs should be tried. Increasingly, experts recommend proactive measurement of drug and antibody concentrations in all patients to optimize clinical response and minimize drug antibody formation (more common at low drug levels). At present, recommended trough concentrations during maintenance therapy are > 7 mcg/mL for infliximab, > 7–10 mcg/mL for adalimumab, and > 1 mcg/mL for golimumab.

2. Anti-integrins—Anti-integrins decrease the trafficking of circulating leukocytes through the vasculature, reducing chronic inflammation. Vedolizumab is an anti-integrin that blocks the $\alpha_4\beta_7$ heterodimer, selectively blocking gut, but not brain, lymphocyte trafficking. It is approved for administration as both an intravenous and subcutaneous formulation. Vedolizumab is not associated with an increased risk of serious infections or malignancy. Infusion reactions are uncommon. Antibodies develop in 3.7% but may not interfere with drug efficacy. Combination therapy with immunomodulators does not appear to increase rates of clinical response or remission. Therapeutic drug monitoring is of uncertain utility.

3. Anti-IL-12/23p40 and anti-IL-23p19 antibodies—Ustekinumab is a human IgG_1 monoclonal antibody that binds the p40 subunit of IL-12 and IL-23, interfering with their receptor binding on T cells, NK cells, and antigen presenting cells. Risankizumab, mirikizumab, and guselkumab are IgG monoclonal antibodies that bind to the p19 subunit of IL-23, selectively inhibiting the IL-23 (but not the IL-12) receptor. All four IL antibodies are available as an intravenous formulation for induction therapy and subcutaneous formulations for maintenance therapy. Adverse effects include infusion- and injection-site reactions, arthralgias, an increased risk for URIs, nasopharyngitis, and herpes simplex and zoster infections. There has been no demonstrated increase in severe infections or malignancy with these agents, although prescribing information cites an increased risk for tuberculosis. Other serious events are rare. Antibodies to these agents develop in < 4% of patients and their impact on treatment efficacy is uncertain. Combination therapy with immunomodulators does not appear to increase rates of clinical response or remission. Therapeutic drug monitoring is of uncertain utility.

Bourgonje A et al. Targeting the interleukin 23 pathway in inflammatory bowel disease. Gastroenterology. 2025;168:29. [PMID: 371700220]

Hanauer SB et al. Subcutaneous infliximab (CT-P13 SC) as maintenance therapy for inflammatory bowel disease: two randomized phase 3 trials (LIBERTY). Gastroenterology. 2024;167:919. [PMID: 38788861]

Khan N et al. Incidence of thiopurine-induced severe myelosuppression in a nationwide cohort of patients with inflammatory bowel disease. Am J Gastroenterol. 2025;120:667. [PMID: 39436267]

Lim SH et al. Safety, effectiveness, and treatment persistence of subcutaneous vedolizumab in IBD: a multicenter study from the United Kingdom. Inflamm Bowel Dis. 2024;30:1284. [PMID: 37603730]

Solitano V et al. Comparative risk of serious infections with biologic agents and small molecules in inflammatory bowel disease: a systematic review and meta-analysis. Clin Gastroenterol Hepatol. 2023;21:907. [PMID: 35944832]

Weiss A et al. A practical guide to the use of upadacitinib in ulcerative colitis and Crohn's disease. Am J Gastroenterol. 2024;119:1211. [PMID: 38047577]

Immunizations & Preventive Care

Due to increased risk of vaccine-preventable infections, vaccination status should be confirmed in *all* patients with IBD and vaccination initiated if not immune. When possible, vaccines should be administered before initiation of immune-modifying agents. Live virus vaccines (MMR, varicella) should *not* be administered to patients taking immunosuppressive agents. Inactivated vaccines—hepatitis A and B, HPV and DTaP (tetanus, diphtheria, pertussis) vaccines—may be safely administered in patients receiving immunosuppressive agents; however, efficacy may be attenuated. Recombinant herpes zoster (Shingrix) and pneumococcal vaccine are recommended for patients with IBD aged > 50 years and patients aged 19–49 years who are receiving immunosuppressive agents. All adult patients should receive annual influenza vaccination and vaccination against SARS-CoV-2 per national guidelines.

Due to an increased risk of melanoma and nonmelanoma skin cancer, all patients with IBD should adopt measures for sun protection (eg, sunscreen, protective clothing) and undergo annual dermatologic screening. Women receiving immune-modifying therapies should undergo cervical cancer screening every 1–3 years. Dual-energy x-ray absorptiometry (DEXA) testing for bone mineral density is recommended at the time of IBD diagnosis and in patients with a history of corticosteroid use, fractures, or cigarette smoking, and in postmenopausal women.

Farraye F et al. ACG Clinical Guideline update: preventive care in inflammatory bowel disease. Am J Gastroenterol. 2025;120:447. [PMID: 40701559]

Lifestyle & Social Support for Patients

IBD is a lifelong illness that can have profound physical, psychological, and social impacts on the individual and their family. A therapeutic relationship between the patient and clinician that involves trust, open communication, and shared decision-making is critical to achieving optimal outcomes. Adherence to a healthy lifestyle is associated with improved outcomes, including reduced mortality. Smoking is associated with more severe disease and decreased response to therapy; all patients should be counseled to quit. Patients may be encouraged to limit to no or only light alcohol consumption and to engage in moderate to vigorous physical activity. Patients should be screened for anxiety and depression, and psychological support (including cognitive behavioral therapy) offered when appropriate. Patients should be encouraged to become involved in the Crohn's and Colitis Foundation of America (CCFA) for patient-centered educational materials and local support groups (https://www.crohnscolitisfoundation.org/).

Figueroa E et al. Practical guide to diet and IBD. Am J Gastroenterol. 2024;120:1941. [PMID: 39787366]

Hashash JG et al. AGA Clinical Practice update in diet and nutritional therapies in patients with inflammatory bowel disease: expert review. Gastroenterology. 2024;166:521. [PMID: 38276922]

Issokson K et al. The role of diet in inflammatory bowel disease onset, disease management, and surgical optimization. Am J Gastroenterol. 2025;120:98. [PMID: 39298569]

1. Crohn Disease

ESSENTIALS OF DIAGNOSIS

- Insidious onset.
- Intermittent bouts of low-grade fever, diarrhea, and right lower quadrant pain.
- Right lower quadrant mass and tenderness.
- Perianal disease with abscess, fistulas.
- Radiographic or endoscopic evidence of ulceration, stricturing, or fistulas of the small intestine or colon.

General Considerations

Crohn disease is a *transmural* process that may involve *any* segment of the GI tract, unlike ulcerative colitis. One-third of cases of Crohn disease involve the small bowel only, most commonly the terminal ileum (ileitis). Half of all cases involve the small bowel and colon, most often the terminal ileum and adjacent proximal ascending colon (ileocolitis). In 20% of cases, the colon alone is affected. One-third of patients have associated perianal disease (fistulas, fissures, abscesses). Less than 5% of patients have symptomatic involvement of the upper intestinal tract. Crohn disease results in mucosal inflammation and ulceration, stricturing, fistula development, and abscess formation. Cigarette smoking is strongly associated with the development of Crohn disease, resistance to medical therapy, and early disease relapse.

Clinical Findings

A. Symptoms and Signs

Because of the variable location of involvement and severity of inflammation, Crohn disease may present with a variety of symptoms and signs. In eliciting the history, the clinician should take particular note of fevers, weight loss, ability to tolerate oral intake, abdominal pain, number of liquid bowel movements per day, general sense of well-being, and prior surgical resections. Physical examination should focus on the patient's temperature, weight, and nutritional status, abdominal tenderness or mass, rectal examination, and extraintestinal manifestations. Approximately 20–30% of patients have an indolent, nonprogressive course. Most commonly, there is one or a combination of the following clinical constellations.

1. Luminal inflammatory disease—This is the most common presentation at diagnosis (60–80%). Patients report malaise, weight loss, and loss of energy. With ileitis or ileocolitis, there may be diarrhea, usually nonbloody and often intermittent. With colitis involving the rectum or left colon, there may be bloody diarrhea and fecal urgency, mimicking the symptoms of ulcerative colitis. Cramping or steady right lower quadrant or periumbilical pain is common. Physical examination reveals focal tenderness, usually in the right lower quadrant. A palpable, tender mass that represents thickened or matted loops of inflamed intestine may be present in the lower abdomen.

2. Intestinal stricture—Narrowing of the small bowel may occur as a result of inflammation or fibrotic stenosis (stricture). Patients report postprandial bloating, cramping pains, and loud borborygmi. This may occur in patients with active inflammatory symptoms or later in the disease from chronic fibrosis without other systemic symptoms or signs of inflammation.

3. Penetrating disease and fistulae—Within 20 years of diagnosis, up to one-half of patients will develop an intestinal stricture, fistula, or abscess. Sinus tracts may penetrate through the bowel (sometimes developing within or proximal to a stricture), where they may be contained, form fistulae to adjacent structures, or form an abscess or phlegmon. Fistulae between the small intestine and colon commonly are asymptomatic but can result in diarrhea, weight loss, bacterial overgrowth, and malnutrition. Fistulae to the bladder produce recurrent infections. Fistulae to the vagina result in malodorous drainage and problems with personal hygiene. Fistulae to the skin usually occur at the site of surgical scars. An intra-abdominal or retroperitoneal phlegmon or abscess is manifested by fevers, chills, a tender abdominal mass, and leukocytosis.

4. Perianal disease—One-third of patients with either large or small bowel involvement develop perianal disease manifested by large painful skin tags, anal fissures, perianal abscesses, and fistulas.

5. Extraintestinal manifestations—Extraintestinal manifestations may include oral aphthous ulcers, arthralgias and arthritis (peripheral, spine, ankylosing spondylitis), ocular findings (iritis, episcleritis or uveitis), skin findings (pyoderma gangrenosum or erythema nodosum), primary sclerosing cholangitis, thromboembolic complications, and other immune-mediated disorders.

B. Laboratory Findings

Laboratory values may reflect inflammatory activity or nutritional complications of disease. A CBC and serum albumin should be obtained in all patients. Anemia may reflect chronic inflammation, mucosal blood loss, iron deficiency, or vitamin B_{12} malabsorption secondary to terminal ileal inflammation or resection. Leukocytosis may reflect inflammation or abscess formation or may be secondary to corticosteroid therapy. Hypoalbuminemia may be due to intestinal protein loss, malabsorption, bacterial overgrowth, or chronic inflammation. The CRP level is elevated (> 5 mg/L) in many patients during active inflammation; however, 15% have a normal CRP level. Fecal calprotectin is an excellent noninvasive test. Elevated fecal calprotectin levels (> 50–100 mcg/g) are correlated with active inflammation as demonstrated by ileocolonoscopy or CT or MR enterography. Stool specimens are sent for examination for routine pathogens and *C difficile* toxin by microscopy, culture, and toxin assay or by rapid multiplex PCR diagnostic assessment.

C. Special Diagnostic Studies

In most patients, the initial diagnosis of Crohn disease is based on a compatible clinical picture with supporting endoscopic, pathologic, and radiographic findings. Colonoscopy usually is performed first to evaluate the colon and terminal ileum and to obtain mucosal biopsies. Typical endoscopic findings include aphthoid, linear or stellate ulcers, strictures, and segmental involvement with areas of normal-appearing mucosa adjacent to inflamed mucosa. Large or deep mucosal ulcers portend a higher risk for progressive disease. In 10% of cases, it may be difficult to distinguish ulcerative colitis from Crohn disease. CT or MR enterography is obtained in patients with suspected small bowel involvement. Suggestive findings include ulcerations, strictures, and fistulas; in addition, CT or MR enterography may identify bowel wall thickening and vascularity, mucosal enhancement, and fat stranding. MR enterography, where available, may be preferred due to its lack of radiation exposure. Capsule imaging may help establish a diagnosis when clinical suspicion for small bowel involvement is high but radiographs are normal or nondiagnostic. Point-of-care intestinal ultrasound is increasingly used to assess intestinal inflammation and transmural healing as evaluated by bowel wall thickness and layer stratification, vascularity, and mesenteric fat hypertrophy. Barium upper GI series with small bowel follow-through should no longer be performed.

Complications

A. Abscess

The presence of a tender abdominal mass with fever and leukocytosis suggests an abscess. Emergent CT or MR of the abdomen is necessary to confirm the diagnosis. Patients should be given broad-spectrum antibiotics. Suggested regimens include metronidazole 500 mg intravenously every 8 hours plus cefepime 2 g or ceftazidime 2 g intravenously every 8 hours; or piperacillin–tazobactam 3.375 g intravenously every 6 hours. Smaller abscesses (< 3 cm) respond to antibiotic therapy, but larger abscesses usually require percutaneous or surgical drainage.

B. Obstruction

Small bowel obstruction may develop secondary to active inflammation or chronic fibrotic stricturing and is often acutely precipitated by dietary indiscretion. Patients should be given intravenous fluids with nasogastric suction. Systemic corticosteroids are indicated for symptoms or signs of active inflammation but are unhelpful in patients with inactive, fixed disease. Patients unimproved on medical management require endoscopic dilation or surgical resection or stricturoplasty.

C. Abdominal and Rectovaginal Fistulas

Many fistulas are asymptomatic and require no specific therapy. For symptomatic fistulas, medical therapy is effective in a subset of patients and is usually tried first in outpatients who otherwise are stable. Anti-TNF agents may promote closure in up to 60% within 10 weeks; however, relapse occurs in over one-half of patients within 1 year despite continued therapy. Surgical therapy is required for symptomatic fistulas that do not respond to medical therapy. Fistulas that arise above (proximal to) areas of intestinal stricturing commonly require surgical treatment.

D. Perianal Disease

Patients with fissures, fistulas, and skin tags commonly have perianal discomfort. Patients should be instructed on proper perianal skin care, including gentle wiping with a premoistened pad (baby wipes) followed by drying with a cool hair dryer, daily cleansing with sitz baths or a water wash, and use of perianal cotton balls or pads to absorb drainage. Successful treatment of active intestinal disease may improve coexisting perianal disease. Specific treatment of perianal disease can be difficult and is best approached jointly with a surgeon with an expertise in colorectal disorders.

Anorectal abscesses should be suspected in patients with severe, constant perianal pain, or perianal pain in association with fever. Superficial abscesses are evident on perianal examination, but deep perirectal abscesses may require digital examination or pelvic CT or MR scan. Depending on the abscess location, surgical drainage may be achieved by incision, or catheter or seton placement. Pelvic MRI is the best noninvasive study for evaluating perianal fistulas. Oral antibiotics (metronidazole, 250 mg three times daily, or ciprofloxacin, 500 mg twice daily) may promote symptom improvement or healing in patients with uncomplicated fistulas; however, recurrent symptoms are common. For complex fistulas, surgical evaluation with either fistulotomy or seton placement should be performed before initiation of immunosuppressive therapies. Combining seton drainage with anti-TNF agents (often combined with oral antibiotics), vedolizumab, anti-IL23 antibodies, or upadacitinib may promote symptomatic improvement in > 75% of patients with anal fistulas and with complete closure in some patients up to 50%; however, recurrence may occur.

E. Carcinoma

Patients with colonic Crohn disease are at increased risk for developing colon carcinoma; hence, annual screening colonoscopy to detect dysplasia or cancer is recommended for patients with a history of ≥ 8 years of Crohn colitis. Patients with Crohn disease also have an increased risk of lymphoma and small bowel adenocarcinoma; however, both are rare.

F. Hemorrhage

Unlike ulcerative colitis, severe hemorrhage is unusual in Crohn disease.

G. Malabsorption

Malabsorption may arise after extensive surgical resections of the small intestine and from bacterial overgrowth in patients with enterocolonic fistulas, strictures, and stasis. Serum levels of vitamins A, D, and B_{12} should be obtained at diagnosis and monitored periodically in patients with ileal inflammation or resection.

Differential Diagnosis

Chronic cramping abdominal pain and diarrhea are typical of both IBS and Crohn disease, but radiographic examinations are normal in the former. Celiac disease may cause diarrhea with malabsorption. Acute fever and right lower quadrant pain may resemble appendicitis or *Yersinia enterocolitica* enteritis. Intestinal lymphoma causes fever, pain, weight loss, and abnormal small bowel radiographs that may mimic Crohn disease. Patients with undiagnosed AIDS may present with fever and diarrhea. Segmental colitis may be caused by tuberculosis, *E histolytica, Chlamydia*, or ischemic colitis. *C difficile* or CMV infection may develop in patients with IBD, mimicking disease recurrence. In patients from tuberculosis-endemic countries, it can be extremely difficult to distinguish active intestinal tuberculosis from Crohn disease, even with biopsies and PCR analyses. Diverticulitis or appendicitis with abscess formation may be difficult to distinguish acutely from Crohn disease. NSAIDs may exacerbate IBD and may also cause NSAID-induced colitis characterized by small bowel or colonic ulcers, erosions, or strictures, often most severe in the terminal ileum and right colon.

Treatment of Active Disease

Crohn disease is a chronic lifelong illness characterized by exacerbations and remissions. Although no specific therapy exists, early treatment that successfully achieves endoscopic and histologic remission is associated with a reduced risk of disease complications, including fistulas, abscesses, and surgeries. Risk stratification is therefore appropriate to guide selection of the optimal treatment. Risk factors for an aggressive disease course include (1) young age at disease onset; (2) early need for corticosteroids; (3) perianal disease, fistulizing or stricturing disease, or upper GI involvement; (4) laboratory markers of severe inflammation, including low albumin or hemoglobin, elevated CRP, or elevated fecal calprotectin; or (5) endoscopic findings of deep ulcerations. Approximately 20–30% of patients have mild, intermittent disease with a nonprogressive course. Most patients have moderate to severe disease for which early use of biologic therapies is warranted to control inflammation and to slow or arrest disease progression. Hospitalization is warranted in some patients with symptoms or signs of severe disease, especially those with high fever, persistent vomiting, evidence of intestinal obstruction, severe weight loss, severe abdominal tenderness, or for suspicion of an abscess.

A. Mild/Low-Risk Disease

Patients may be characterized as having mild disease with a low risk of disease progression if they have mild symptoms, no significant weight loss, no systemic symptoms or signs, normal hemoglobin, normal or only mildly elevated inflammatory markers (CRP, fecal calprotectin, serum albumin), absence of intestinal complications (stricturing, abscess, fistula, perianal disease), and limited intestinal involvement with only aphthous lesions or superficial mucosal ulcers.

1. Nutrition—Patients should eat a well-balanced diet with as few restrictions as possible. Eating smaller but more frequent meals may be helpful. Patients with diarrhea should be encouraged to drink fluids to avoid dehydration. Many patients report that certain foods worsen symptoms, especially fried or greasy foods. Because lactose intolerance is common, a trial off dairy products is warranted if flatulence or diarrhea is a prominent complaint. Probiotics have not proven beneficial for Crohn disease.

2. Symptomatic therapy—Loperamide (2–4 mg orally) may be given for diarrhea as needed up to four times daily.

3. Drug therapy—It is recommended that therapy for mild, low-risk Crohn disease begin with medications that are less potent but have a lower risk of adverse effects. Recommended drug treatment depends on the location of disease involvement.

A. TERMINAL ILEUM OR ASCENDING COLON DISEASE—For patients with mild disease involving the terminal ileum or ascending colon, initial treatment is recommended with extended-release budesonide (Entocort), 9 mg orally once daily for 8 weeks, which induces remission in 50–70% of patients. If disease remission is achieved, budesonide is tapered over 2–4 weeks in 3 mg increments and the patient observed. For treatment of mild ileocolonic Crohn disease, oral mesalamine is *not* recommended by current guidelines but remains in widespread clinical use despite an absence of clinical trial data supporting its efficacy.

B. LEFT-SIDED OR DIFFUSE COLITIS—For patients with mild colitis that is diffuse or involves only the left side of the colon, oral corticosteroids (prednisone or prednisolone) are recommended. The initial dose of either agent is 40 mg once daily for 1–2 weeks, followed in those who respond by gradual tapering of 5–10 mg/week over 4–8 weeks. Sulfasalazine (1.5–3 g orally twice daily) appears effective in improving symptoms and inducing remission in patients with mild Crohn disease involving the colon (not small intestine) and is recommended in some treatment guidelines. For patients who respond, sulfasalazine 2–4 g/day may be continued as long-term maintenance. Because of sulfasalazine's side effects (see Inflammatory Bowel Disease: Pharmacologic Therapy), many clinicians prescribe other oral 5-ASA agents for mild Crohn colitis despite a lack of clinical data supporting efficacy. Such agents include those that release 5-ASA throughout the colon: delayed-release mesalamine (Lialda or Asacol 2.4–4.8 g/day; Apriso 2.25–4.5 g/day) and balsalazide (2.25 g three times daily).

C. LONG-TERM FOLLOW-UP—In patients with mild Crohn disease who respond to initial therapy with budesonide or prednisone, treatment should be discontinued and the patient monitored periodically for disease recurrence (symptoms, CRP, fecal calprotectin, or endoscopy every 1–2 years). Patients who respond to treatment with sulfasalazine or other 5-ASA formulations should continue long-term maintenance therapy. Patients with mild disease who either do not respond to initial therapy or those who experience symptom relapse more than once every 1–2 years following tapering of corticosteroids should be reclassified as moderate to high risk for disease progression and "stepped up" to more potent therapies (oral corticosteroids, immunomodulators, or biologic agents).

B. Moderate to Severe/High-Risk Crohn Disease

Moderate to severe disease may be characterized by frequent diarrhea, weight loss, daily abdominal pain, abdominal tenderness, and perianal disease. Evidence of significant inflammation includes elevated CRP, anemia, low serum albumin, elevated fecal calprotectin, or the findings of deep ulceration, stricture, or penetrating disease on endoscopy or radiologic imaging. Patients characterized as having moderate to severe Crohn disease warrant early treatment with biologic agents (with or without immunomodulators) to promote sustained clinical remission and intestinal mucosal healing ("endoscopic remission"). The choice of therapies depends on patient age and comorbidities, patient preference, and the presence of extraintestinal manifestations. Third-party payers often limit access to preferred biologic agents by requiring prior authorizations and step therapy through less effective (but less expensive) agents. Sustained clinical remission with intestinal mucosal healing should be the therapeutic goal in most patients; however, this cannot always be achieved.

1. Nutrition—Patients with obstructive symptoms should be placed on a low-roughage diet, ie, no raw fruits or vegetables, popcorn, nuts, etc. High intake of processed foods, which are associated with increased risk of IBD, should be curtailed. TPN sometimes is used short term in patients with active disease and progressive weight loss, especially those awaiting surgery who have malnutrition but cannot tolerate enteral feedings because of high-grade obstruction, high-output fistulas, severe diarrhea, or abdominal pain. Parenteral vitamin B_{12} (1000 mcg subcutaneously per month) and oral vitamin D supplementation (2000 IU/day) are commonly needed for patients with previous ileal resection or extensive terminal ileal disease.

2. Symptomatic therapy—Involvement of the terminal ileum with Crohn disease or prior ileal resection may lead to reduced absorption of bile acids that may induce secretory diarrhea from the colon. Secretory diarrhea responds to agents that bind the malabsorbed bile salts: cholestyramine 2–4 g or colestipol 1–2 g one to three times daily with meals; or colesevelam, 625 mg, one to three tablets twice daily. Patients with extensive ileal disease (requiring > 100 cm of ileal resection) have severe bile salt malabsorption causing steatorrhea. Such patients may benefit from a low-fat diet; bile salt–binding agents exacerbate the diarrhea and should not be given. Patients with Crohn disease are at risk for the development of small intestinal bacterial overgrowth due to enteral fistulas, ileal resection, and impaired motility and may benefit from a course of broad-spectrum antibiotics (see Bacterial Overgrowth, above). Other causes of diarrhea include lactase deficiency and short bowel syndrome. Use of oral antidiarrheal agents may provide benefit in some patients.

3. Drug therapy—The goal of drug treatment for moderate to severe, high-risk Crohn disease is to induce and maintain clinical disease remission, including mucosal healing..

A. CORTICOSTEROIDS—Corticosteroids dramatically suppress the acute clinical symptoms and signs in most patients with both small and large bowel disease; however, they do not alter the natural history of the underlying disease. Because of their rapidity of onset, corticosteroids commonly are used in patients with moderate to severe disease to promote early symptomatic improvement while other disease-modifying agents with slower onset of action are initiated. In patients with a tender, palpable inflammatory abdominal mass, CT of the abdomen should be obtained prior to administering corticosteroids to rule out an abscess. If no abscess is identified, hospitalized patients may be treated with parenteral corticosteroids (methylprednisolone 40–60 mg daily). Outpatients may be treated with oral prednisone or methylprednisolone, 40 mg/day for 1–2 weeks followed by slow tapering of 5–10 mg/week over 4–8 weeks. Remission or significant improvement occurs in > 80% of patients after 8–16 weeks of therapy. It is recommended in most patients that a biologic agent be initiated as the corticosteroid is tapered and withdrawn. Use of long-term low corticosteroid doses should be avoided because of associated complications. If a decision is made not to initiate a biologic agent, long-term treatment with an immunomodulator (azathioprine, mercaptopurine, or methotrexate) is recommended to attempt to provide a steroid-free disease maintenance. However, approximately 20% of patients cannot be completely withdrawn from corticosteroids without experiencing a symptomatic flare-up.

B. BIOLOGIC THERAPIES—*Induction therapy with a biologic agent is recommended for almost all patients with moderate to severe Crohn disease;* those with a favorable clinical response to induction treatment should be maintained on long-term therapy with a goal of achieving clinical and endoscopic remission. Treatment options include anti-TNF monoclonal antibodies (infliximab, adalimumab, certolizumab), anti-integrin monoclonal antibody (vedolizumab), and anti-IL monoclonal antibodies (ustekinumab, risankizumab). (See Inflammatory Bowel Disease: Pharmacologic Therapy, above.) In the absence of head-to-head comparative trials of these agents, relative differences in efficacy and safety are suggested by network meta-analyses. The choice of biologic agent depends on the disease severity, patient age and comorbidities, patient preference, and drug cost/pharmacy tiering. For most patients, anti-TNF antibodies or anti-IL23 antibodies are the preferred first-line agents due to their efficacy and known safety profiles.

(1) Anti-TNF therapies—For patients with moderate to severe Crohn disease, three anti-TNF therapies (infliximab, adalimumab, certolizumab) are recommended as first-line agents to induce remission either as monotherapy or in combination with immunomodulating agents (azathioprine, mercaptopurine, or methotrexate). Up to two-thirds of patients have significant clinical improvement during acute induction therapy (see Inflammatory Bowel Disease: Pharmacologic Therapy and Table 17–13 for dosing). Although direct comparisons of these anti-TNF agents are unavailable, indirect evidence suggests that intravenous, weight-based infliximab infusion may be preferred to subcutaneous, fixed-dose adalimumab or certolizumab for patients with severe disease, extraintestinal manifestations, perianal disease, or obesity. Compared with anti-TNF monotherapy, clinical trials suggest that combination of an anti-TNF agent (infliximab or adalimumab) with an immunomodulator (azathioprine, mercaptopurine, or methotrexate) achieves higher rates of clinical and mucosal healing. Despite these benefits, the role of combination therapy versus monotherapy is controversial due to an increased risk of adverse events, including myelosuppression, infections, and malignancies (lymphoma, skin cancer). Because of the complexity and higher risks of combination therapy, many clinicians prefer monotherapy with drug monitoring to optimize anti-TNF trough levels and reduce the risk of developing anti-drug antibodies. Retrospective clinical trial data suggest that remission rates are similar between combination therapy and anti-TNF monotherapy when adjusted for trough levels. Combination therapy is favored for patients at higher risk for disease progression or who previously developed antibodies to a biologic agent.

After initial clinical response, symptom relapse occurs in > 80% of patients within 1 year in the absence of further maintenance therapy. Therefore, scheduled maintenance therapy is strongly recommended (see Table 17–13). With long-term maintenance therapy, approximately two-thirds of patients have continued clinical response and up to one-half have complete symptom remission. Therapeutic drug monitoring with serum anti-TNF trough levels and drug antibody levels may guide therapy in patients who have lost response. Patients with low serum anti-TNF trough levels and absent drug antibodies should receive increased anti-TNF dosing (intravenous infliximab 10 mg/kg; adalimumab 80 mg) or decreased dosing intervals (intravenous infliximab every 6 weeks; adalimumab every week). Patients with high antibodies to the anti-TNF agent and low anti-TNF trough levels should be switched to another agent (either a different anti-TNF agent or alternative biologic or small molecule agent). Patients with inadequate response despite adequate anti-TNF trough levels should be changed to an anti-IL23 antibody (risankizumab, mirikizumab, or guselkumab), vedolizumab, or upadacitinib. In patients receiving combination therapy with an anti-TNF agent and immunomodulating agent (eg, azathioprine, mercaptopurine), consideration should be given to stopping or reducing the dose of the immunomodulating agent after 6–12 months for patients in remission, most especially men aged < 30 years who have a higher risk of hepatosplenic T-cell lymphoma and for adults aged > 50–60 years in whom there is a higher risk of lymphoma and of infectious complications.

(2) Anti-IL-23 antibodies—The anti–IL-23p19 formulations (risankizumab, mirikizumab, guselkumab) and anti–IL-12/23p40 formulation (ustekinumab) are appropriate as first-line induction therapy for patients with moderate to severe Crohn disease, especially those at increased risk for complications of anti-TNF therapy. They are also recommended in patients who did not respond to or lost response to prior anti-TNF therapy. In phase 3 clinical trials, 50–65% of patients with moderate to severe Crohn disease achieve significant clinical improvement during induction therapy at 12 weeks during and clinical remission at 1 year with long-term maintenance therapy (see Table 17–13).

The anti–IL-23p19 antibodies risankizumab and guselkumab have demonstrated superiority to ustekinumab (an anti–IL-12/23p40 antibody) in prospective, head-to-head treatment trials. In two phase 3 48-week studies of patients with moderate to severe Crohn disease, guselkumab was superior to ustekinumab for endoscopic remission (33–37% versus 25%) and for a composite endpoint of clinical remission and endoscopic response (42–47% versus 34%). In a 48-week open label trial of patients with moderate to severe Crohn disease who had not responded or lost response to prior biologic agents, treatment with risankizumab versus ustekinumab achieved higher clinical remission (61% versus 40%) and endoscopic remission (32% versus 16%). In another 52-week trial, mirikizumab versus ustekinumab demonstrated nonsignificant but numerically higher clinical remission (51% versus 42%) and endoscopic response (45% versus 40%). Based on these data, risankizumab and guselkumab are preferred to ustekinumab in patients with moderate to severe Crohn disease who have failed or lost response to prior biologic agents.

(3) Anti-integrins—Due to its relative lack of systemic immunologic suppression vedolizumab may be chosen as a first-line agent for induction therapy in patients with moderate Crohn disease at increased risk for complications from anti-TNF or other biologic agents due to advanced age, multiple comorbidities, or prior malignancy. For patients who have not responded or lost response to anti-TNF agents, vedolizumab appears to be less effective than anti-IL agents (risankizumab or ustekinumab). Vedolizumab may be less effective than anti-TNF or ustekinumab in the treatment of extraintestinal manifestations and fistulous disease.

C. Oral small molecules—The oral JAK inhibitor upadacitinib is FDA-approved for the induction and maintenance therapy for Crohn disease. In two phase 3 induction trials, clinical remission rates after 12 weeks were 39–50% among patients treated with oral upadacitinib 45 mg once daily versus 21–29% with placebo. After 52 weeks, remission rates were higher with upadacitinib 15 mg once daily (37%) and 30 mg once daily (48%) than placebo (15%). Network meta-analyses suggest upadacitinib may be equivalent to biologic agents in the treatment of Crohn disease and offers the convenience of oral therapy. However, in light of the uncertain risks of JAK inhibitors for serious complications (including thrombosis, cardiovascular events, and malignancy), upadacitinib should be reserved for patients who have failed biologic therapies.

Indications for Surgery

Over 50% of patients will require at least one surgical procedure. The main indications for surgery are intractability to medical therapy, intra-abdominal abscess, massive bleeding, symptomatic refractory internal or perianal fistulas, and intestinal obstruction. Patients with chronic obstructive symptoms due to a short segment of ileal stenosis are best treated with resection or stricturoplasty (rather than long-term medical therapy), which promotes rapid return of well-being and elimination of corticosteroids. After surgery, endoscopic evidence of recurrence occurs in 60% within 1 year. Endoscopic recurrence precedes clinical recurrence by months to years; clinical recurrence occurs in 20% of patients within 1 year and 80% within 10–15 years. In a controlled trial of 297 patients undergoing ileocolonic resection, endoscopic recurrence occurred in 30% of patients treated with infliximab every 8 weeks compared with 60% treated with placebo. It may be reasonable to initiate empiric infliximab postoperatively for patients at high risk for disease recurrence and to perform endoscopy in low-risk patients 6 months after surgery in order to identify patients with early endoscopic recurrence who may benefit from biologic therapy.

Prognosis

With proper medical and surgical treatment, the majority of patients are able to cope with this chronic disease and its complications and lead productive lives. Few patients die as a direct consequence of the disease.

When to Refer

- For endoscopic procedures or capsule endoscopy.
- For follow-up of any patient requiring hospitalization.
- Patients with moderate to severe disease for whom therapy with immunomodulators or biologic agents is being considered.
- When surgery may be necessary.

When to Admit

- An intestinal obstruction is suspected.
- An intra-abdominal or perirectal abscess is suspected.
- A serious infectious complication is suspected, especially in patients who are immunocompromised due to concomitant use of corticosteroids, immunomodulators, or anti-TNF agents.
- Patients with severe symptoms of diarrhea, dehydration, weight loss, or abdominal pain.
- Patients with severe or persisting symptoms despite treatment with corticosteroids.

Ananthakrishnan AN et al. AGA Clinical Practice guideline on the role of biomarkers for the management of Crohn's disease. Gastroenterology. 2023;165:1367. [PMID: 37981354]

Elmasry S et al. Evidence-based approach to the management of mild Crohn's disease. Clin Gastroenterol Hepatol. 2024;22:480. [PMID: 38141661]

Ferrante M et al. Efficacy and safety of mirikizumab in patients with moderately-to-severely active Crohn's disease: a phase 3, multicentre, randomized, double-blind, placebo-controlled, and active controlled, treat-through study. Lancet. 2024;404:2423. [PMID: 39581202]

Loftus EV et al. Upadacitinib induction and maintenance therapy for Crohn's disease. N Engl J Med. 2023;388:1966. [PMID: 37224198]

Lichtenstein G et al. ACG Clinical Guideline: management of Crohn's disease. Am J Gastroenterol. 2025;120:1225. [PMID: 29610508]

Panaccione R et al. Efficacy and safety of intravenous induction and subcutaneous maintenance therapy with guselkumab for patients with Crohn's disease (GALAXI-2 and GALAXI-3): 48-week results from two phase 3, randomized, placebo and active comparator, double-blind, triple-dummy trials. Lancet. 2025;406:358. [PMID: 40684778]

Peyrin-Biroulet L et al. Risankizumab versus ustekinumab for moderate-to-severe Crohn's disease. N Engl J Med. 2024;391:213. [PMID: 390185321]

2. Ulcerative Colitis

ESSENTIALS OF DIAGNOSIS

- Bloody diarrhea.
- Lower abdominal cramps and fecal urgency.
- Anemia, low serum albumin.
- Negative stool studies for pathogens.
- Sigmoidoscopy is the key to diagnosis.

General Considerations

Ulcerative colitis is a chronic, recurrent disease involving only the colon. It is characterized by diffuse mucosal inflammation that results in friability, erosions, and ulcers with bleeding. Ulcerative colitis invariably involves the rectum and may extend proximally in a continuous fashion to involve part or all of the colon. Approximately 30% of patients have disease confined to the rectum (proctitis), 40% have disease that extends to the splenic flexure (left-sided colitis), and 30% have disease that extends more proximally (extensive colitis). With distal colitis, the disease progresses with time to more extensive involvement in 25%. There is some correlation between disease extent and symptom severity. In most patients, the disease is characterized by periods of symptomatic flare-ups and periods of mild activity or remission. Approximately 15% of patients may have an aggressive course with increased risk of hospitalization or surgery. Of patients hospitalized with severe colitis, colectomy is required in up to 30% for unresponsive or "fulminant" disease. Ulcerative colitis is more common in persons who do not smoke or who smoked in the past. Disease severity may be lower in persons who actively smoke and may worsen in patients who stop smoking.

Clinical Findings

A. Symptoms and Signs

The clinical profile in ulcerative colitis is highly variable. Bloody diarrhea is the hallmark. Several clinical and laboratory parameters help classify patients as having mild, moderate, or severe disease (Table 17–12). Patients should

Table 17–12. Ulcerative colitis: assessment of disease activity.

	Mild	Moderate	Severe
Stool frequency (per day)	< 4	4–6	> 6–10
Blood in stools	Intermittent	Frequent	Continuous
Hematocrit (%)	Normal	30–40	< 30
CRP	Normal or elevated	Elevated	Elevated
ESR (mm/hour)	< 30	> 30	> 30
Endoscopy (Mayo subscore)	1	2–3	3

be asked about stool frequency, the presence and amount of rectal bleeding, cramps, abdominal pain, fecal urgency, tenesmus, and extraintestinal symptoms. Physical examination should focus on the patient's volume status as determined by orthostatic blood pressure and pulse measurements and by nutritional status. On abdominal examination, the clinician should look for tenderness and evidence of peritoneal inflammation. Red blood may be present on digital rectal examination.

1. Mild to moderate disease—Patients with mild to moderate disease have fewer than four to six bowel movements per day, mild to moderate rectal bleeding, and no constitutional symptoms. Stools may be formed or loose in consistency. Because of rectal inflammation, there is fecal urgency and tenesmus. Left lower quadrant cramps relieved by defecation are common, but there is no significant abdominal pain or tenderness. There may be mild anemia and hypoalbuminemia.

2. Severe disease—Patients with severe disease have more than six bloody bowel movements per day, resulting in severe anemia, hypovolemia, and impaired nutrition with hypoalbuminemia. Abdominal pain and tenderness are present. "Fulminant colitis" is a subset of severe disease characterized by rapidly worsening symptoms with signs of toxicity.

B. Laboratory Findings

The degree of abnormality of the hematocrit, serum albumin, and inflammatory markers (ESR and CRP) reflects disease severity (Table 17–12). For patients with ulcerative colitis previously in disease remission, acute symptom relapse with a CRP > 5 mg/L or fecal calprotectin > 50–100 mcg/g is highly suggestive of disease relapse.

C. Endoscopy

In acute colitis, the diagnosis is readily established by sigmoidoscopy. The mucosal appearance is characterized by edema, friability, mucopus, and erosions. The "Mayo" endoscopic scoring system is commonly used in clinical practice and therapeutic trials. A score of 0 indicates normal or inactive colitis; 1 indicates erythema, decreased vascularity; 2 indicates friability, marked erythema, erosions; and 3 indicates ulcerations, severe friability, spontaneous bleeding. Mayo endoscopic scores 1–2 are consistent with mild to moderate disease clinical activity, and Mayo scores 2–3 are usually seen with moderate to severe clinical activity. Colonoscopy should not be performed in patients with fulminant disease because of the risk of perforation. After patients have demonstrated improvement on therapy, colonoscopy is performed to determine the extent of disease.

D. Imaging

Abdominal imaging with plain radiographs or CT is obtained in patients with severe colitis to look for significant colonic dilation. Barium enemas are of little utility and may precipitate toxic megacolon.

Differential Diagnosis

The initial presentation of ulcerative colitis is indistinguishable from other causes of colitis, clinically as well as endoscopically. Thus, the diagnosis of idiopathic ulcerative colitis is reached after excluding other known causes of colitis. Infectious colitis should be excluded by testing stool specimens for *Salmonella*, *Shigella*, *Campylobacter*, Shiga toxin–producing *E coli*, *C difficile*, and amebiasis. Where available, microbial assessment using multiplex molecular techniques provides results within 1–4 hours with excellent sensitivity and is preferred to conventional labor-intensive stool microscopy, culture, and toxin testing. CMV colitis occurs in immunocompromised patients, including patients receiving prolonged corticosteroid therapy, and is diagnosed on mucosal biopsy. Gonorrhea, chlamydial infection, herpes, mpox, and syphilis are considerations in sexually active patients with proctitis. In older adult patients with CVD, ischemic colitis may involve the rectosigmoid. A history of radiation to the pelvic region can result in proctitis months to years later. Crohn disease involving the colon but not the small intestine may be confused with ulcerative colitis. In 10% of patients, a distinction between Crohn disease and ulcerative colitis may not be possible.

Treatment

There are three main treatment objectives: (1) to terminate the acute, symptomatic attack; (2) to achieve complete remission of clinical and endoscopic disease activity; and (3) to prevent recurrence of attacks. The treatment of acute ulcerative colitis depends on the extent of colonic involvement and the severity of illness. Patients with systemic signs of inflammation (ie, anemia, low serum albumin, elevated CRP or ESR levels) and ulcerations with extensive disease on colonoscopy are at increased risk for hospitalization or surgery, and early aggressive therapy with biologic agents is warranted.

A. Proctitis

Patients with disease confined to the rectum (distal 18 cm) generally have mild to moderate but distressing symptoms. Patients may be treated with topical mesalamine, topical corticosteroids, or oral aminosalicylates (5-ASA) according to patient preference and cost considerations. Topical mesalamine is the drug of choice and is superior to topical corticosteroids and oral 5-ASA. Mesalamine is administered as a suppository, 1000 mg once daily at bedtime for proctitis, or as an enema, 4 g at bedtime for proctosigmoiditis, for 4–8 weeks, with 75% of patients improving. In patients achieving clinical remission, topical 5-ASA (1 g/day) should be maintained long-term. Patients who are nonresponsive to topical 5-ASA may be treated with a topical corticosteroid (budesonide foam, 2 mg twice daily for 2 weeks, then once daily) or hydrocortisone foam (80–100 mg once daily) for 6–8 weeks followed by tapering. Systemic effects from short-term use of topical corticosteroids are very slight.

Patients with proctitis or proctosigmoiditis who achieve complete remission with oral or rectal 5-ASA should continue indefinitely on the same therapy to reduce the likelihood of symptomatic relapse. Maintenance treatment with 5-ASA reduces the 12-month relapse rate from 75% to < 40%. Some patients, however, may prefer intermittent therapy for symptomatic relapse. Long-term topical corticosteroids are ineffective for maintaining remission of distal colitis and not recommended.

B. Mild to Moderate Colitis

1. 5-ASA agents—Disease extending above the rectum is best treated with both an oral and rectal 5-ASA agent. For induction of remission, the optimal dose of oral 5-ASA (mesalamine) is 2–4.8 g once daily in combination with 5-ASA 1 g suppository at bedtime. Most patients improve within 4–8 weeks. Some patients prefer to initiate therapy with oral 5-ASA, adding topical therapy if initial response is inadequate. These agents achieve clinical improvement in 75% of patients and remission in 20–30%. For patients who achieve clinical remission, long-term, low-dose oral 5-ASA therapy (1.5–2.4 g/day) should be administered. Oral sulfasalazine (1.5–2 g twice daily) is uncommonly used due to its side effects.

2. Corticosteroids—Patients with mild to moderate colitis who do not improve within 4–8 weeks of 5-ASA therapy should have an oral corticosteroid therapy added with budesonide MMX or prednisone. Budesonide MMX (Uceris) 9 mg/day orally for 4–8 weeks may be preferred in mild to moderate colitis due to its low incidence of corticosteroid-associated side effects, especially in those for whom other systemic corticosteroids are deemed high risk. Dosing of oral prednisone is detailed below. For patients who require more than one course of corticosteroid therapy every 1–2 years for symptomatic relapse, treatment should be "stepped up" to include a thiopurine (azathioprine or mercaptopurine) or a biologic agent, as described below for Moderate to Severe Colitis.

C. Moderate to Severe Colitis

1. Corticosteroids—An oral corticosteroid (prednisone or methylprednisolone) is commonly prescribed as the first-line agent for nonhospitalized patients with moderate to severe colitis. The initial oral dose of prednisone is 40 mg daily. Rapid improvement is observed in most patients within 2 weeks. Thereafter, tapering of prednisone should proceed by 5 mg/week. After tapering to 20 mg/day, slower tapering (2.5 mg/week) is sometimes required. Complete tapering of prednisone without symptomatic flare-ups is possible in the majority of patients. Corticosteroids should not be continued long-term to control symptoms because of an unacceptable risk of adverse side effects. Up to 30% of patients either do not respond to prednisone or have symptomatic flares during tapering that prevent its complete withdrawal. Biologic agents or small molecules are recommended for patients in whom corticosteroids cannot be completely withdrawn or who require more than one course of corticosteroids every 1–2 years. The addition of a thiopurine (azathioprine or mercaptopurine) is sometimes used to promote complete corticosteroid withdrawal and maintain long-term remission.

2. Biologic agents and small molecules—Anti-TNF antibodies (infliximab, adalimumab, golimumab), anti-integrin antibody (vedolizumab), anti–IL-12/23p40 antibody (ustekinumab), anti–IL23p19 antibodies (guselkumab, mirikizumab, risankizumab), JAK inhibitors (tofacitinib, upadacitinib), and S1P receptor modulators (ozanimod, etrasimod) all have demonstrated efficacy for treatment of moderate to severe colitis. See Inflammatory Bowel Disease: Pharmacologic Therapy for a description of their mechanism of action, adverse effects, and monitoring. The preferred agent depends on several considerations: prior exposure and response to biologic agents; disease severity; patient comorbidities; preferred mode of administration (intravenous, subcutaneous, oral); and insurance company tiering. Few head-to-head trials comparing therapies exist; hence network meta-analyses are used to gauge their relative efficacy. See Table 17–13 for dosing and adverse events.

a. Treatment of patients naïve to prior biologic therapy—**Infliximab** or **vedolizumab** is often administered as first-line therapies for moderate to severe colitis based on their efficacy and safety profiles. These two agents have had the highest rankings of all biologic agents for induction of clinical remission in a network meta-analysis among patients who have not previously been treated with other biologic therapies.

Infliximab may be the more effective agent—especially for patients with severe disease or extraintestinal manifestations (Table 17–13). An induction regimen of infliximab results in clinical response in 65% of patients. When initiating induction therapy with anti-TNF agents, many clinicians add an immunomodulator (azathioprine, mercaptopurine, or methotrexate) for the first year to increase the likelihood of disease remission and to reduce the development of antibodies that may result in secondary loss of response to anti-TNF therapies. If anti-TNF monotherapy is preferred, proactive drug monitoring of serum trough levels and anti-drug antibody titers should be obtained during induction and maintenance therapy in order to optimize drug dosing. During long-term maintenance treatment with infliximab, clinical improvement or remission is achieved in approximately 50% of patients. Network meta-analyses suggest superiority of infliximab (weight-based, intravenous infusion) over the other

Table 17–13. Biologic agents for treatment of IBD.

	Disease Indications	Induction Doses	Maintenance Doses	Comments	Adverse Events
TNF Antagonists					
Infliximab	Ulcerative colitis Crohn disease	5 mg/kg intravenously at 0, 2, and 6 weeks	5–10 mg/kg intravenously every 8 weeks 120 mg subcutaneously every 2 weeks	May be used in combination with thiopurines to enhance efficacy; may be used with thiopurine or low-dose methotrexate to reduce development of antidrug antibodies	Hypersensitivity, infusion- or injection-site reactions, hypersensitivity, opportunistic infections, (tuberculosis, fungal), bacterial sepsis, hepatitis B reactivation, lymphoma, non-melanoma skin cancer, psoriasis, demyelinating disorders, autoimmunity, HF
Adalimumab	Ulcerative colitis Crohn disease	160 mg subcutaneously at week 0, then 80 mg subcutaneously at week 2	40 mg subcutaneously every 2 weeks		
Golimumab	Ulcerative colitis	200 mg subcutaneously at week 0, then 100 mg at week 2	100 mg subcutaneously every 4 weeks		
Certolizumab	Crohn disease	400 mg subcutaneously at weeks 0, 2 and 4	400 mg subcutaneously every 4 weeks		
Interleukin Antagonists					
Risankizumab (anti-IL-23)	Ulcerative colitis Crohn disease	1200 mg intravenously at weeks 0, 4, and 8 600 mg intravenously at weeks 0, 4 and 8	180 or 360 mg subcutaneously at week 12 and every 8 weeks thereafter		Hypersensitivity, infusion- or injection-site reactions, URI, herpes infections (herpes simplex, herpes zoster), tuberculosis
Mirikizumab (anti-IL-23)	Ulcerative colitis Crohn disease	300 mg intravenously at weeks 0, 4, and 8 900 mg intravenously at weeks 0, 4, and 8	200 mg subcutaneously at week 12 and every 4 weeks thereafter 300 mg subcutaneously at week 12, then every 4 weeks thereafter		
Guselkumab (anti-IL-23)	Ulcerative colitis Crohn disease	200 mg intravenously at weeks 0, 4, and 8 200 mg intravenously at weeks 0, 4, and 8 OR 400 mg subcutaneously on weeks 0, 4, and 8	100 mg subcutaneously at week 16 and every 8 weeks thereafter; or 200 mg subcutaneously at week 12 and every 4 weeks thereafter (use lowest effective dose)		
Ustekinumab (anti-IL-12/23)	Ulcerative colitis Crohn disease	6 mg/kg intravenously at week 0	90 mg subcutaneously every 8 weeks		

(continued)

Table 17–13. Biologic agents for treatment of IBD. (continued)

	Disease Indications	Induction Doses	Maintenance Doses	Comments	Adverse Events
Anti-Integrins					
Vedolizumab	Ulcerative colitis Crohn disease	300 mg intravenously at weeks 0, 2, and 6	300 mg intravenously every 8 weeks 108 mg subcutaneously every 2 weeks		Hypersensitivity, infusion or injection site reactions, nasopharyngitis, URI, arthralgias
Janus Kinase Inhibitors					
Upadacitinib (JAK1)	Ulcerative colitis Crohn disease	45 mg orally daily for 8 weeks 45 mg orally daily for 12 weeks	15–30 mg orally daily	Due to concerns for increased CV events with tofacitinib, this class is currently restricted to patients with inadequate response to TNF blockers; higher maintenance doses associated with increased risks of OI and CV event	Hypersensitivity, thrombosis, CV events (MI, stroke), URI, opportunistic infections, herpes (zoster, simplex), lymphoma, non-melanoma skin cancers, GI perforations, lymphopenia, neutropenia, elevated cholesterol and CK, acne
Tofacitinib (JAK1,2,3)	Ulcerative colitis	10 mg orally twice daily for 8–16 weeks	5–10 mg orally twice daily		
Tofacitinib XR (JAK1,2,3)	Ulcerative colitis	22 mg orally daily for 8–16 weeks	11–22 mg orally daily		
Sphingosine 1-phosphate Receptor Modulators					
Ozanimod	Ulcerative colitis	Days 1–4: 0.23 mg orally daily Days 5–7: 0.46 mg orally daily Thereafter: 0.92 mg orally daily	0.92 mg orally daily		Lymphopenia, HTN, macular edema, bradycardia, AV conduction delay, herpes reactivation (simplex, zoster), PML
Etrasimod	Ulcerative colitis	2 mg orally daily	2 mg orally daily		

AV, atrioventricular; CK, creatine kinase; CV, cardiovascular; HTN, hypertension; OI, opportunistic infections; PML, progressive multifocal leukoencephalopathy; URI, upper respiratory tract infection.

anti-TNF agents, adalimumab and golimumab (fixed-dose, subcutaneous injection). Treatment with adalimumab or golimumab may nonetheless be selected in patients with moderate (not severe) disease who prefer the convenience of subcutaneous, self-injection. Subcutaneous infliximab is available for maintenance therapy but not approved for induction therapy.

Vedolizumab intravenous induction therapy led to clinical improvement in 47% of patients compared with 25% who were given placebo. Among patients who demonstrated initial clinical improvement, 42% of those given long-term maintenance treatment with vedolizumab were in clinical remission at 1 year compared with 16% of those given placebo. Due to its efficacy and superior safety profile, vedolizumab (with its gut-selectivity) may be the preferred first-line biologic agent for older patients or those with increased risks from systemic immunosuppression. In one of the only head-to-head trials comparing biologic therapies, intravenous vedolizumab was superior to adalimumab for induction and maintenance treatment of moderate to severe ulcerative colitis. Subcutaneous vedolizumab is available for maintenance therapy but not approved for induction therapy.

B. Second-line treatment for patients who have not responded to anti-TNF agents or vedolizumab— In patients with moderate to severe colitis who have not responded to or lost response to first-line biologic therapy, injectable IL-23 antibodies (guselkumab, mirikizumab, risankizumab, or ustekinumab) or oral small molecules (JAK inhibitors and S1P receptor modulators) are favored as second- or third-line therapy. See Table 17–13 for dosing and adverse events. In the absence of head-to-head comparative trials, it is difficult to determine their relative efficacy. Despite the convenience and rapid symptom response of oral small molecules, the injectable interleukin antibodies offer a superior safety profile, especially in patients who are older or have an increased risk of cardiovascular or thrombosis events.

(1) IL-23 antibodies—Among patients who failed prior treatment with biologic agents, the clinical response rates at 12 weeks following intravenous **guselkumab** versus placebo were 62% and 28%, respectively; following **mirikizumab** versus placebo were 56% and 31%, respectively; following intravenous risankizumab (180 or 360 mg) versus placebo were 65% and 36%, respectively; and following intravenous **ustekinumab** versus placebo at 8 weeks were 52% and 26%, respectively. Among all treatment responders who entered long-term maintenance treatment with subcutaneous injections every 8 weeks, clinical remission at 1 year was significantly higher with guselkumab (45–50%), ustekinumab (45%), mirikizumab (51%), risankizumab (57–61%), and ustekinumab (45%) compared with placebo (14–27%).

(2) Oral small molecules—The small model JAK inhibitors (**upadacitinib** and **tofacitinib**) offer the convenience of oral administration and rapid symptom improvement within 3 days. Furthermore, network meta-analyses suggest these agents are highly effective in achieving disease remission in patients who have failed therapy with biologic agents. However, both agents carry an FDA black box warning for a potential increased risk of thrombosis, cardiovascular events, malignancy, and serious infections. Pending further clinical experience, safety data, and guideline development, they are likely to remain relegated to second- or third-line therapy, particularly in patients who are older, have known CVD, or at an increased risk for thrombotic events. In phase 3 trials of patients with moderate to severe ulcerative colitis, induction treatment with oral upadacitinib for 8 weeks led to clinical improvement in 73% of patients versus 26% of those who received placebo. In a continued maintenance study, the rate of clinical remission at 52 weeks in subjects who received oral upadacitinib 15 mg once daily was 42%; 30 mg once daily was 52%; and placebo was 12%. Induction therapy with oral tofacitinib for 8 weeks led to clinical improvement in 57% of patients with ulcerative colitis versus 31% of those who received placebo. Among clinical responders, the remission rate at 52 weeks with oral tofacitinib 5 mg once daily was 34%; 10 mg once daily was 41%; and placebo was 11%.

The small-molecule S1P receptor modulators **ozanimod** and **etrasimod** are once-daily oral agents that are FDA-approved for the treatment of moderate to severe ulcerative colitis. Ozanimod, but not etrasimod, requires dosage escalation (Table 17–13). In phase 3 trials of patients with moderate to severe ulcerative colitis, both agents resulted in higher clinical remission rates than placebo following 10–12 weeks of induction therapy (ozanimod 18% versus placebo 6%; etrasimod 27% versus placebo 7%) and after 52 weeks of maintenance therapy (ozanimod 37% versus placebo 19%; etrasimod 32% versus placebo 7%). Remission rates were lower among patients who had not previously responded to anti-TNF agents. Given possible risks of bradycardia and heart block with this class of agents, caution is recommended in prescribing ozanimod in patients with heart disease and cerebrovascular disease until further clinical experience and safety data are available.

D. Severe and Fulminant Colitis

About 15% of patients with ulcerative colitis have a more severe course. Of these, a small subset has a fulminant course with rapid progression of symptoms over 1–2 weeks and signs of severe toxicity. These patients appear quite ill, with fever, prominent hypovolemia, hemorrhage requiring transfusion, and abdominal distention with tenderness. Toxic megacolon develops in < 2% of cases of ulcerative colitis. It is characterized by colonic dilation of > 6 cm on plain films with signs of toxicity.

1. General measures—Discontinue all oral intake for 24–48 hours or until the patient demonstrates clinical improvement. TPN is indicated only in patients with poor nutritional status or if feedings cannot be reinstituted within 7–10 days. All opioid or anticholinergic agents should be discontinued. Restore circulating volume with fluids, correct electrolyte abnormalities, and consider transfusion for significant anemia (hematocrit < 25–28%). A plain abdominal radiograph or CT scan should be ordered on admission to look for evidence of colonic dilation. Send stools for assessment of bacterial pathogens,

C difficile and parasites, either by conventional bacterial culture, *C difficile* toxin assay, and ova and parasite examinations or by rapid, multiplex PCR assay. CMV superinfection should be considered in patients receiving long-term immunosuppressive therapy who are unresponsive to corticosteroid therapy. Due to a high risk of VTE disease, VTE prophylaxis should be administered to all hospitalized patients with IBD. Surgical consultation should be sought for all patients with severe disease.

Patients with fulminant disease are at higher risk for toxic megacolon or perforation and must be monitored closely. Abdominal examinations should be repeated to look for evidence of worsening distention or pain. Empiric broad-spectrum antibiotics in the absence of confirmed infection are not recommended. Nasogastric suction should be initiated. Patients with toxic megacolon should be instructed to roll from side to side and onto the abdomen in an effort to decompress the distended colon. Serial abdominal plain films should be obtained to look for worsening dilation or signs of ischemia. Patients with fulminant disease or toxic megacolon who worsen or do not improve within 48–72 hours should undergo surgery to prevent perforation. If the operation is performed before perforation, the mortality rate should be low.

2. Corticosteroid therapy—Methylprednisolone, 40–60 mg, is administered intravenously. There appears to be no difference in efficacy between single-dose, divided-dose, or continuous-infusion regimens. Hydrocortisone enemas (100 mg) may also be administered twice daily for treatment of urgency or tenesmus. Clinical improvement with systemic corticosteroids should be evident within 3 days. Once symptomatic improvement has occurred, oral fluids are reinstituted. If these fluids are well tolerated, intravenous corticosteroids are discontinued and oral prednisone (as described for moderate disease) is started. Patients without significant improvement within 3 days of intravenous corticosteroid therapy should be referred for surgery or considered for anti-TNF or other therapies. Criteria indicative of nonresponse include > 8 stools/day or 3–8 stools/day with a CRP > 45 mg/L.

3. Anti-TNF therapies—Intravenous infusion of infliximab (5–10 mg/kg) is the most commonly used agent for treatment of patients with severe ulcerative colitis who have not improved within 3 days of intravenous corticosteroid therapy. In a controlled study of patients hospitalized for ulcerative colitis, colectomy was required within 3 months in 69% who received placebo therapy, compared with 47% who received infliximab.

4. Janus kinase inhibitors—Uncontrolled studies suggest tofacitinib (given as 10 mg, three times daily for 3 days, followed by two times daily) or upadacitinib (45 mg once daily) is an effective salvage regimen.

5. Cyclosporine—Intravenous cyclosporine (2–4 mg/kg/day as a continuous infusion) benefits 60–75% of patients with severe colitis who have not improved after corticosteroids, but it is associated with significant toxicity (nephrotoxicity, seizures, infection, hypertension). Studies suggest similar efficacy (85%) with cyclosporine and infliximab (85%) therapy.

6. Surgical therapy—Patients with severe disease who do not improve after corticosteroid, infliximab, or other salvage therapies are unlikely to respond to further medical therapy, and surgery is recommended.

Monitoring of Patients in Disease Remission

For all patients with acute ulcerative colitis, a primary goal of therapy, is to achieve complete remission of clinical symptoms and complete mucosal healing, whenever possible. Disease activity is assessed by clinical symptoms (stool frequency, consistency, and rectal bleeding), laboratory data (hemoglobin, albumin), inflammatory markers (CRP), fecal calprotectin, and proctoscopy. In patients with recurrence of mild symptoms, a CRP > 5 mg/L or fecal calprotectin > 150 mcg/g, suggests possible disease relapse and warrants endoscopic evaluation for confirmation. Empiric treatment adjustment (rather than endoscopic evaluation), may be preferred for patients with moderate to severe symptoms and elevated inflammatory markers. The possibility of intercurrent enteric infections (including ***C difficile***) should be excluded. Among patients with disease relapse who are adherent to the prescribed medication regimen, a change in therapy usually is required—either an escalation in drug dosing or a change in drug treatment class. For patients receiving anti-TNF agents, therapeutic monitoring with measurement of drug trough levels and drug antibodies is useful to determine whether drug escalation may be useful or switching to an alternative anti-TNF agent (presence of antidrug antibodies) or another therapeutic class is preferred. The role of therapeutic monitoring for other biologic agents is uncertain.

Risk of Colon Cancer

In patients with ulcerative colitis with disease proximal to the rectum and in patients with Crohn colitis, there is an increased risk of developing colon carcinoma. This risk has decreased over time due to improved medical therapies and endoscopic surveillance. Recent studies suggest a cumulative risk of colon cancer of 0.02–1%, 3–4.8%, and 7–13.9% after 10, 20, and 30 years, respectively. Colonoscopies are recommended beginning 8 years after disease diagnosis. The use of high-definition colonoscopes with electronic enhancement or spray application of dilute blue dye (chromoendoscopy) enhances the detection of subtle mucosal lesions, thereby significantly increasing the detection of dysplasia compared with standard colonoscopy. At colonoscopy, all polypoid and nonpolypoid lesions should be resected, when possible, and biopsies obtained of endoscopically unresectable lesions. Subsequent surveillance colonoscopies are performed every 1–5 years, depending on ulcerative colitis extent and activity, and presence of colonic scarring, pseudopolyps, or dysplasia.

Surgery in Ulcerative Colitis

With the advent of more effective medical therapies, the requirement for surgical colectomy has decreased. Current 1-, 5-, and 10-year risks are 2.8%, 7%, and 9.6%, respectively. Severe hemorrhage, perforation, and documented carcinoma are absolute indications for surgery. Surgery is indicated also in patients with fulminant colitis or toxic megacolon that does not improve within 48–72 hours, in patients with invisible flat dysplasia or non-endoscopically resectable dysplastic lesions on surveillance colonoscopy, and in patients with refractory disease requiring long-term corticosteroids to control symptoms.

Although total proctocolectomy (with placement of an ileostomy) provides complete cure of the disease, most patients seek to avoid it out of concern for the impact it may have on their bowel function, their self-image, and their social interactions. After complete colectomy, patients may have a standard ileostomy with an external appliance or an internal ileal pouch that is anastomosed to the anal canal (ileal pouch–anal anastomosis). The latter maintains intestinal continuity, thereby obviating an ostomy. Under optimal circumstances, patients have five to seven loose bowel movements per day without incontinence. Endoscopic or histologic inflammation in the ileal pouch ("pouchitis") develops in > 40% of patients within 1 year and in up to 80% over the long term, resulting in increased stool frequency, fecal urgency, cramping, and bleeding, but usually resolves with a 2-week course of oral metronidazole (250–500 mg three times daily) or ciprofloxacin (500 mg twice daily). Patients with frequently relapsing pouchitis may need continuous antibiotics. Probiotics do not appear to be of benefit.

Prognosis

Ulcerative colitis is a lifelong disease characterized by exacerbations and remissions. For most patients, the disease is readily controlled by medical therapy without need for surgery. The majority never require hospitalization. A subset of patients with more severe disease will require surgery, which results in complete cure of the disease. Properly managed, most patients with ulcerative colitis lead close to normal productive lives.

When to Refer

- For colonoscopy to evaluate activity and extent of active disease and to undertake surveillance for neoplasia in patients with quiescent disease for > 8 years.
- For follow-up of any patient requiring hospitalization.

When to Admit

- Patients with severe disease manifested by frequent bloody stools, anemia, weight loss, and fever.
- Patients with fulminant disease manifested by rapid progression of symptoms, worsening abdominal pain, distention, high fever, and tachycardia.
- Patients in whom surgical colectomy is indicated.

Barnes E et al. AGA Clinical Practice Guideline on the management of pouchitis and inflammatory pouch disorders. Gastroenterology. 2024;166:59. [PMID: 38128971]

Berinstein JA et al. Effectiveness of upadacitinib for patients with severe ulcerative colitis: a multicenter experience. Am J Gastroenterol. 2024;119:1421. [PMID: 38275248]

Rubin D et al. ACG Clinical Guideline update: ulcerative colitis in adults. Am J Gastroenterol. 2025;120:1187. [PMID: 40701556]

Singh S et al. AGA living clinical practice guideline on pharmacologic management of moderate-to-severe ulcerative colitis. Gastroenterology. 2024;167:1307. [PMID: 39572132]

Sofia MA et al. White paper: American Gastroenterological Association position statement: the future of IBD care in the United States – removing barriers and embracing opportunities. Clin Gastroenterol Hepatol. 2024;22:944. [PMID: 38428707]

3. Microscopic Colitis

Microscopic colitis is an idiopathic condition that is found in up to 15% of patients who have chronic or intermittent watery diarrhea with normal-appearing mucosa at endoscopy. There are two major subtypes—collagenous colitis and lymphocytic colitis. In both, histologic evaluation of mucosal biopsies reveals chronic inflammation (lymphocytes, plasma cells) in the lamina propria and increased intraepithelial lymphocytes. Collagenous colitis is further characterized by the presence of a thickened band (> 10 mcm) of subepithelial collagen. Both forms occur more commonly in women, especially in the fifth to sixth decades. Symptoms tend to be chronic or recurrent but may remit in most patients after several years. A more severe illness characterized by abdominal pain, fatigue, dehydration, and weight loss may develop in a subset of patients. The cause of microscopic colitis usually is unknown. Several medications have been implicated as etiologic agents, including NSAIDs, PPIs, low-dose aspirin, SSRIs, ACE inhibitors, β-blockers, and menopausal estrogen hormonal therapy. Diarrhea usually abates within 30 days of stopping the offending medication. Celiac disease may be present in 2–9% of patients and should be excluded with serologic testing (IgA anti-tTG). Treatment is largely empiric since there are few well-designed, controlled treatment trials. Antidiarrheal therapy with loperamide is the first-line treatment for mild symptoms, providing symptom improvement in up to 70%. The next option is delayed-release budesonide 9 mg orally daily for 6–8 weeks. Budesonide induces clinical remission in > 80% of patients; however, relapse occurs in two-thirds after stopping therapy. Remission is maintained in 75% of patients treated long-term with low doses of budesonide. In clinical practice, budesonide is tapered to the lowest effective dose for suppressing symptoms (3 mg every other day to 6 mg daily). For patients who do not respond to budesonide, uncontrolled studies report that treatment with bile-salt binding agents (cholestyramine, colestipol) or 5-ASAs (sulfasalazine, mesalamine) may be effective in some patients. Less than 3% of patients have refractory or severe symptoms, which may be treated with immunosuppressive agents (azathioprine or methotrexate) or anti-TNF agents (infliximab, adalimumab).

Peery A et al. Update on the epidemiology and management of microscopic colitis. Clin Gastroenterol Hepatol. 2025;23;490. [PMID: 392270919]

Zhang SW et al. Drug exposure and risk of microscopic colitis: a systematic review and meta-analysis. Dig Dis. 2023;41:217. [PMID: 36067746]

DIVERTICULAR DISEASE OF THE COLON

Colonic diverticulosis increases with age, ranging from a prevalence of 5% in those under age 40 to > 50% by age 60 years in Western societies.

Colonic diverticula may vary in size from a few millimeters to several centimeters and in number from one to several dozen. Almost all patients with diverticulosis have involvement in the sigmoid and descending colon; however, only 15% have proximal colonic disease.

For > 40 years, it has been believed that diverticulosis arises after many years of a diet deficient in fiber. However, epidemiologic studies have identified no association between the prevalence of asymptomatic diverticulosis and low dietary fiber intake or constipation. Thus, the etiology of diverticulosis is uncertain. The extent to which abnormal motility and hereditary factors contribute to diverticular disease is unknown. Patients with abnormal connective tissue are also disposed to development of diverticulosis, including Ehlers-Danlos syndrome, Marfan syndrome, and systemic sclerosis.

1. Uncomplicated Diverticulosis

More than 90% of patients with diverticulosis have uncomplicated disease and no specific symptoms. In most, diverticulosis is an incidental finding detected during colonoscopy. Some patients have nonspecific complaints of chronic constipation, abdominal pain, or fluctuating bowel habits. Physical examination is usually normal but may reveal mild left lower quadrant tenderness with a thickened, palpable sigmoid and descending colon. Screening laboratory studies should be normal in uncomplicated diverticulosis.

There is no reason to perform imaging studies for the purpose of diagnosing asymptomatic, uncomplicated disease. Diverticula are well seen on colonoscopy and CT. Involved segments of colon may also be narrowed and deformed.

Patients in whom diverticulosis is discovered should be encouraged to increase dietary fiber either through diet (fruits, vegetables, whole grains) or fiber supplements (psyllium, methylcellulose), which is associated with a lower risk of diverticulitis in prospective cohort studies. Studies suggest that the risk of diverticulitis may be further reduced with exercise and avoidance of red meats and NSAIDs.

2. Diverticular Bleeding

Half of all cases of acute lower GI bleeding are attributable to diverticulosis (see Acute Lower GI Bleeding, above).

3. Diverticulitis

ESSENTIALS OF DIAGNOSIS

- Acute abdominal pain and fever.
- Left lower abdominal tenderness and mass.
- Leukocytosis.

Clinical Findings

A. Symptoms and Signs

Diverticulitis is defined as macroscopic inflammation of a diverticulum that may reflect a spectrum from inflammation to microperforation with localized paracolic inflammation, to macroperforation with either abscess or generalized peritonitis. Thus, there is a range from mild to severe disease. Most patients with localized inflammation or infection report mild to moderate aching abdominal pain, usually in the left lower quadrant. Constipation or loose stools may be present. Nausea and vomiting are frequent. In many cases, symptoms are so mild that the patient may not seek medical attention until several days after onset. Physical findings include a low-grade fever, left lower quadrant tenderness, and a palpable mass. Stool occult blood is common, but hematochezia is rare. Leukocytosis is mild to moderate. Patients with free perforation present with a more dramatic picture of generalized abdominal pain and peritoneal signs.

B. Imaging

In those presenting for the first time with mild symptoms, an abdominal CT is obtained to look for evidence of diverticulitis (colonic diverticula, wall thickening, pericolic fat infiltration) and to exclude other causes of abdominal pain. An abdominal CT is also indicated in patients with fever, leukocytosis, and sepsis or peritonitis or in those who are immunocompromised to look for evidence of complicated disease (abscess, phlegmon, perforation, fistula). Patients who respond to acute medical management should undergo complete colonic evaluation with colonoscopy or CT colonography 6–8 weeks after resolution of clinical symptoms to exclude colorectal cancer (which may mimic diverticulitis). Cancer is identified in 1% and 8% of patients following a diagnosis of uncomplicated or complicated diverticulitis, respectively. Endoscopy and colonography are contraindicated during the initial stages of an acute attack because of the risk of free perforation.

Differential Diagnosis

Diverticulitis must be distinguished from other causes of lower abdominal pain, including perforated colonic carcinoma, Crohn disease, appendicitis, ischemic colitis, *C difficile*–associated colitis, and gynecologic disorders (ectopic pregnancy, ovarian cyst or torsion), by abdominal CT scan, pelvic ultrasonography, or radiographic studies of the distal colon that use water-soluble contrast enemas.

Complications

Complications, such as phlegmon, abscess, perforation, peritonitis, or sepsis, develop in approximately 12% of patients with acute diverticulitis. Chronic inflammation or an untreated abscess may lead to smoldering disease (ongoing pain, leukocytosis); formation of fistulas to the bladder, ureter, vagina, uterus, bowel, and abdominal wall; or stricturing of the colon with partial or complete obstruction.

Treatment

A. Medical Management

Most patients with uncomplicated disease can be managed with conservative measures. Patients with mild symptoms and no peritoneal signs may be managed initially as outpatients on a clear liquid diet for 2–3 days. Although broad-spectrum oral antibiotics with anaerobic activity commonly are prescribed, large clinical trials confirm that antibiotics are not beneficial in uncomplicated disease. Antibiotics should be used selectively for uncomplicated disease, including patients who are immunocompromised, have significant comorbid disease, or have small pericolonic abscesses (< 3–4 cm). Reasonable oral regimens include amoxicillin and clavulanate potassium (875 mg/125 mg) twice daily; or metronidazole, 500 mg three times daily plus either ciprofloxacin, 500 mg twice daily, or trimethoprim-sulfamethoxazole, 160/800 mg twice daily, for 7–10 days or until the patient is afebrile for 3–5 days. Symptomatic improvement usually occurs within 3 days, at which time the diet may be advanced. Once the acute episode has resolved, a high-fiber diet is recommended.

Patients with increasing pain, fever, or inability to tolerate oral fluids require hospitalization. Hospitalization is also required in patients who are immunocompromised, have significant comorbid illness, have abscesses > 3–4 cm, or have signs of severe diverticulitis (high fevers, leukocytosis, or peritoneal signs). Patients should be given nothing by mouth and should receive intravenous fluids. Intravenous antibiotics should be given to cover anaerobic and gram-negative bacteria. Regimens may include piperacillin-tazobactam 3.375 g every 6 hours, or ertapenem 1 g once daily or a combination of metronidazole 500 mg every 8 hours plus either a second- or third-generation cephalosporin every 8 hours (cefuroxime 1.5 g, ceftriaxone 2 g, or cefotaxime 2 g). Symptomatic improvement should be evident within 2–3 days. Intravenous antibiotics should be continued for 5–7 days, before changing to oral antibiotics.

B. Surgical Management

Surgical consultation and repeat abdominal CT should be obtained on all patients with severe disease or those who do not improve after 72 hours of medical management. Patients with a localized abdominal abscess ≥ 4 cm are usually treated urgently with a percutaneous catheter drain placed by an interventional radiologist. This permits control of the infection and resolution of the immediate infectious inflammatory process. Indications for emergent surgical management include generalized peritonitis, large undrainable abscesses, and clinical deterioration despite medical management and percutaneous drainage. Following recovery from complicated diverticulitis, a subsequent elective one-stage surgical resection has generally been recommended to reduce recurrent episodes of complicated disease; however, a conservative approach may be selected for some patients. Patients with chronic disease resulting in fistulas or colonic obstruction will require elective surgical resection.

Prognosis

Diverticulitis recurs in 15–20% of patients treated with medical management over 10–20 years. However, < 5% have more than two recurrences. Among patients who have an episode of uncomplicated diverticulitis, < 5% later develop complicated disease. Therefore, elective surgical resection is no longer routinely recommended in patients with recurrent bouts of uncomplicated disease but is individualized based on patient preference, age, comorbid disease, and frequency and severity of attacks. Diverticulosis is not associated with an increased risk of colorectal cancer.

When to Refer

- Failure to improve within 72 hours of medical management.
- Presence of significant peridiverticular abscesses (≥ 4 cm) requiring possible percutaneous or surgical drainage.
- Generalized peritonitis or sepsis.
- Recurrent attacks.
- Chronic complications, including colonic strictures or fistulas.

When to Admit

- Severe pain or inability to tolerate oral intake.
- Signs of sepsis or peritonitis.
- CT showing signs of complicated disease (abscess, perforation, obstruction).
- Failure to improve with outpatient management.
- Immunocompromised or frail, older patient.

Long B et al. Emergency medicine updates: acute diverticulitis. Am J Emerg Med. 2023;76:1. [PMID: 37956503]
Morris AM et al. Recurrent lower abdominal pain, altered bowel habits, and malaise: conservative or surgical approach to a common disorder. Gastroenterology. 2023;164:541. [PMID: 36657527]
Strate L et al. Tips for the medical management of diverticulitis. Am J Gastroenterol. 2023;118:585. [PMID: 36434810]

POLYPS OF THE COLON

Polyps are discrete mass lesions that protrude into the intestinal lumen. Although most commonly sporadic, they may be inherited as part of a familial polyposis syndrome. Polyps may be divided into four major pathologic groups: mucosal adenomatous polyps (tubular, tubulovillous, and villous), mucosal serrated polyps (hyperplastic, sessile serrated polyps, and traditional serrated adenoma), mucosal nonneoplastic polyps (juvenile polyps, hamartomas, inflammatory polyps), and submucosal lesions (lipomas, lymphoid aggregates, carcinoids, pneumatosis cystoides intestinalis). Of polyps removed at colonoscopy, > 70% are adenomatous; most of the remainder are serrated.

NONFAMILIAL ADENOMATOUS & SERRATED POLYPS

Adenomatous polyps (adenomas) and serrated polyps may be non-polypoid (flat, slightly elevated, or depressed), sessile, or pedunculated (containing a stalk). Their significance is that > 95% of cases of adenocarcinoma of the colon are believed to arise from these lesions. Early detection and removal of these precancerous lesions through screening programs has resulted in a 34% reduction in deaths from colorectal cancer since 2000. It is proposed that there is a polyp → carcinoma sequence whereby nonfamilial colorectal cancer develops through a continuous process from normal mucosa to adenomatous or serrated polyp and later to carcinoma. An estimated 75% of cancers arise in adenomas after inactivation of the *APC* gene leads to chromosomal instability and inactivation or loss of other tumor suppressor genes. The remaining 25% of cancers arise through the serrated pathway in which hyperplastic polyps develop *Kras* mutations (forming traditional serrated adenomas) or *BRAF* oncogene activation (forming sessile serrated lesions) with widespread methylation of CpG-rich promoter regions that leads to inactivation of tumor suppressor genes or mismatch repair genes (*MLH1*) with microsatellite instability.

A. Adenomas

Adenomas are present in > 30% of men and 20% of women over the age of 50. Most adenomas are < 5 mm and have a low risk of becoming malignant. Adenomas are classified as "advanced" if they are ≥ 1 cm or contain villous features or high-grade dysplasia. In the general population, the prevalence of advanced adenomas is 6%. Advanced lesions are believed to have a higher risk of harboring or progressing to malignancy. It has been estimated from longitudinal studies that it takes an average of 5 years for a medium-sized polyp to develop from normal-appearing mucosa and 10 years for a gross cancer to arise.

B. Serrated Polyps

There are three types of serrated polyps: hyperplastic polyps, sessile serrated lesions, and traditional serrated adenomas. It is believed that sessile serrated lesions (prevalence 5–12%) and traditional serrated adenomas (prevalence < 1%) entail an increased risk of colorectal cancer similar or greater to that of adenomas and account for up to 20–30% of colorectal cancers. Many pathologists cannot reliably distinguish between hyperplastic polyps and sessile serrated lesions. Diminutive hyperplastic polyps (< 5 mm) are extremely common (prevalence 20–30%), especially in the rectum, and believed to be without significant risk.

Serrated polyposis syndrome is characterized by a large number of serrated polyps and an increased risk of colorectal cancer. The estimated prevalence is 0.4–0.9% of patients undergoing screening colonoscopy with a 20% risk of developing colorectal cancer. A genetic defect has not been identified. Surveillance colonoscopy is recommended every 1–2 years with removal of serrated lesions larger than 3–5 mm.

Clinical Findings

A. Symptoms and Signs

Most patients with adenomatous and serrated polyps are asymptomatic. Chronic occult blood loss may lead to iron deficiency anemia. Large polyps may ulcerate, resulting in intermittent hematochezia.

B. Fecal Occult Blood or Multitarget DNA Tests

FOBT, FIT, and fecal DNA tests are available as part of colorectal cancer screening programs (see Chapter 43). FIT is a fecal immunochemical test for hemoglobin with a single specimen having a sensitivity of approximately 80% for colorectal cancer and 20–30% for advanced adenomas but a much lower sensitivity for serrated lesions. FIT is more sensitive than guaiac-based tests for the detection of colorectal cancer and advanced adenomas. Cologuard is a test combining a fecal DNA test with a fecal immunochemical test for stool hemoglobin. In a prospective comparative trial conducted in persons at average risk for colorectal cancer undergoing colonoscopy, the sensitivity for colorectal cancer for Cologuard was 92.3% compared with 73.8% for FIT and the sensitivity for large (> 1 cm) adenomas or serrated polyps for Cologuard was 42.4% compared with 23.8% for FIT.

C. Radiologic Tests

CT colonography ("virtual colonoscopy") uses data from helical CT with computer-enabled luminal image reconstruction to generate two-dimensional and three-dimensional images of the colon. Using optimal imaging software with multidetector helical CT scanners, several studies report a sensitivity of 90% or more for the detection of polyps > 10 mm in size. However, the accuracy for detection of polyps 5–9 mm in size is significantly lower (sensitivity 50%). A small proportion of these diminutive polyps harbor advanced histology (up to 1.2%) or carcinoma (< 1%). Abdominal CT also results in a radiation exposure that may lead to a small risk of cancer.

D. Endoscopic Tests

Colonoscopy allows evaluation of the entire colon and is the best means of detecting and removing adenomatous and serrated polyps. It should be performed in all patients who have positive FOBT, FIT, or fecal DNA tests or iron deficiency anemia (see Occult GI Bleeding, above) since the prevalence of colonic neoplasms is increased in these patients. Colonoscopy should also be performed in patients with polyps detected on CT colonography or adenomas detected on flexible sigmoidoscopy to remove these polyps and to fully evaluate the entire colon. Capsule endoscopy may be considered in patients who are unsuitable or unwilling to undergo colonoscopy or who have an incomplete colonoscopy.

Treatment

A. Colonoscopic Polypectomy

Most adenomatous and serrated polyps are < 2 cm in size and are readily amenable to colonoscopic removal; this can be done with biopsy forceps or cold snare excision for those

< 3 mm; with cold snare excision for those < 10 mm; or with cold snare or hot snare cautery for those 10–20 mm. Sessile polyps larger than 2 cm may be removed by appropriately trained physicians using a variety of endoscopic techniques (eg, saline-lift mucosal resection or dissection) or infrequently may require surgical resection. Patients with large sessile polyps removed in piecemeal fashion should undergo repeated colonoscopy in 6 months to verify complete polyp removal. Complications after colonoscopic polypectomy include perforation in 0.2% and clinically significant bleeding in 0.3–1.0% of all patients, but in 4–8% following mucosal resection of large lesions.

B. Postpolypectomy Surveillance

Adenomas and serrated polyps can be found in 30–40% of patients when another colonoscopy is performed within 3–5 years after the initial examination and polyp removal. Periodic colonoscopic surveillance is therefore recommended to detect these "metachronous" lesions, which either may be new or may have been overlooked during the initial examination. Most of these polyps are small, without high-risk features, and of little immediate clinical significance. The probability of detecting advanced neoplasms at surveillance colonoscopy depends on the number, size, and histologic features of the polyps removed on initial (index) colonoscopy. The US Multi-Society Task Force Guideline provides the following recommendations for repeat colonoscopy that depend on the findings at baseline colonoscopy: (1) **10 years:** normal colonoscopy or fewer than 20 hyperplastic polyps < 10 mm in the distal colon or rectum; (2) **7–10 years:** 1–2 adenomas < 10 mm; (3) **5–10 years:** 1–2 sessile serrated polyps < 10 mm; (4): **3–5 years:** 3–4 adenomas or sessile serrated polyps < 10 mm; (5) **3 years:** 5–10 adenomas *or* sessile serrated polyps < 10 mm; *or* 1 or more adenomas or sessile serrated polyp 10 mm or larger *or* an adenoma containing villous features or high-grade dysplasia *or* a sessile serrated polyp with dysplasia. Patients with > 10 adenomas should have a repeat colonoscopy at 1 year and may be considered for evaluation for a familial polyposis syndrome.

Copland AP et al. AGA clinical practice update on appropriate and tailored polypectomy: expert review. Clin Gastroenterol Hepatol. 2024;22:470. [PMID: 38032585]
Issaka R et al. AGA Clinical Practice Update on risk stratification for colorectal cancer screening and post-polypectomy surveillance: expert review. Gastroenterology. 2023;165:1280. [PMID: 37737817]
Pilonis N et al. Adenoma detection rates by physicians and subsequent colorectal cancer risk. JAMA. 2025;333:400. [PMID: 39680377]

HEREDITARY COLORECTAL CANCER & POLYPOSIS SYNDROMES

Up to 4% of all colorectal cancers are caused by germline genetic pathogenic variants that impose on carriers a high lifetime risk of developing colorectal cancer (see Chapter 43). Because the diagnosis of these disorders has important implications for treatment of affected patients and for screening of family members, it is important to consider these disorders in patients with a family history of colorectal cancer that has affected more than one family member, those with a personal or family history of colorectal cancer developing at an early age (aged ≤ 50 years), those with a personal or family history of multiple polyps (> 10), and those with a personal or family history of multiple extracolonic malignancies.

1. Familial Adenomatous Polyposis

ESSENTIALS OF DIAGNOSIS

- Inherited condition characterized by early development of hundreds to thousands of colonic adenomatous polyps.
- Variety of extracolonic manifestations (eg, duodenal adenomas, desmoid tumors, and osteomas) and extracolonic cancers (stomach, duodenum, thyroid).
- Attenuated variant with < 100 (average 25) colonic adenomas.
- Genetic testing confirms pathogenic variant of *APC* gene (90%) or *MUTYH* gene (8%).
- Prophylactic colectomy recommended to prevent otherwise inevitable colorectal cancer (adenocarcinoma).

General Considerations

Familial adenomatous polyposis (FAP) is a syndrome affecting 1:10,000 people and accounts for approximately 0.5% of colorectal cancers. The classic form of FAP is characterized by the development of hundreds to thousands of colonic adenomatous polyps and a variety of extracolonic manifestations. Of patients with classic FAP, approximately 90% have a pathogenic variant of the *APC* gene that is inherited in an autosomal dominant fashion and 8% have pathogenic variants in the *MUTYH* gene that are inherited in an autosomal recessive fashion. FAP arises de novo in 25% of patients in the absence of pathogenic gene variants in the parents. An attenuated variant of FAP also has been recognized in which an average of only 25 polyps (range of 1–100) develop.

Clinical Findings

A. Symptoms and Signs

In classic FAP, colorectal polyps develop by a mean age of 15 years and cancer often by age 40 years. Unless prophylactic colectomy is performed, colorectal cancer is inevitable by age 50 years. In attenuated FAP, the mean age for development of cancer is about 56 years.

Adenomatous polyps of the duodenum and periampullary area develop in > 90% of patients, resulting in a 5–8% lifetime risk of adenocarcinoma. Adenomas occur less frequently in the gastric antrum and small bowel and, in those locations, have a lower risk of malignant transformation.

Gastric fundus gland polyps occur in > 50% but have an extremely low (0.6%) malignant potential.

A variety of other benign extraintestinal manifestations, including soft tissue tumors of the skin, desmoid tumors, osteomas, and congenital hypertrophy of the retinal pigment, develop in some patients with FAP. These extraintestinal manifestations vary among families, depending in part on the type or site of mutation in the *APC* gene. Desmoid tumors are locally invasive fibromas, most commonly intra-abdominal, that may cause bowel obstruction, ischemia, or hemorrhage. They occur in 15% of patients and are the second leading cause of death in FAP. Malignancies of the CNS (Turcot syndrome) and tumors of the thyroid and liver (hepatoblastomas) may also develop in patients with FAP.

B. Genetic Testing

Genetic counseling and testing should be offered to patients found to have multiple adenomatous polyps at endoscopy and to first-degree family members of patients with FAP. Most centers perform genetic testing using a multigene panel of 14–67 hereditary cancer genes, including *APC* and *MUTYH*. Pathogenic *APC* gene variants are identified in 80% of patients with > 1000, and 56% with 100–1000 polyps (ie, the classic phenotype of FAP). Guidelines recommend that genetic testing be considered in individuals with as few as 10 adenomas to exclude a diagnosis of attenuated disease, most especially in patients aged < 50–60 years.

Treatment

Once the diagnosis has been established, complete proctocolectomy with ileoanal anastomosis or colectomy with ileorectal anastomosis is recommended in most patients, usually before age 20 years. Colonoscopy every 1–2 years with polypectomy may be considered for patients with attenuated FAP and a low number of polyps. Upper endoscopic evaluation of the stomach, duodenum, and periampullary area should be performed every 1–3 years to look for adenomas or carcinomas with resection of duodenal or ampullary polyps > 10 mm, increasing in size, or suspicious for high-grade dysplasia or cancer. Sulindac and celecoxib have been shown to decrease the number and size of polyps in the rectal stump but not the duodenum.

Beck S et al. Cancer risks in attenuated and classical familial adenomatous polyposis: a nationwide cohort with matched, nonexposed individuals. Am J Gastroenterol. 2025;120:1345. [PMID: 39471488]

2. Hamartomatous Polyposis Syndromes

Hamartomatous polyposis syndromes are rare and account for < 0.1% of colorectal cancers. They include Peutz-Jeghers syndrome, familial juvenile polyposis, and Cowden disease.

Boland RC et al. Diagnosis and management of cancer risk in gastrointestinal hamartomatous polyposis syndromes: recommendations from the US Multi-Society Task Force on Colorectal Cancer. Am J Gastroenterol. 2022;117:846. [PMID: 35487791]

3. Lynch Syndrome

ESSENTIALS OF DIAGNOSIS

- Autosomal dominant inherited condition.
- Caused by pathogenic variants in a gene that detects and repairs DNA base-pair mismatches, resulting in DNA microsatellite instability and inactivation of tumor suppressor genes.
- Increased lifetime risk of colorectal cancer (22–75%), endometrial cancer (30–60%), and other cancers; they may develop at young ages.
- Evaluation warranted in patients with personal history of early-onset colorectal cancer or family history of colorectal, endometrial, or other Lynch syndrome–related cancers at young age or in multiple family members.
- Diagnosis suspected by tumor tissue immunohistochemical staining for mismatch repair proteins or by testing for microsatellite instability.
- Diagnosis confirmed by genetic testing.

General Considerations

Lynch syndrome (also known as hereditary nonpolyposis colon cancer [HNPCC]) is an autosomal dominant condition in which there is a markedly increased risk of developing colorectal cancer as well as a host of other cancers, including endometrial, ovarian, kidney, bladder, hepatobiliary, prostate, brain, gastric, and small intestinal cancers. It is estimated to account for up to 3% of all colorectal cancers. Affected individuals have a 22–75% lifetime risk of developing colorectal carcinoma and a 30–60% lifetime risk of endometrial cancer, depending on the variant gene. Unlike individuals with familial adenomatous polyposis, patients with Lynch syndrome develop only a few adenomas, which may be flat and more often contain villous features or high-grade dysplasia. In contrast to the traditional polyp → cancer progression (which may take > 10 years), these polyps are believed to undergo rapid transformation over 1–2 years from normal tissue → adenoma → cancer. Colon and endometrial cancer tend to develop at an earlier age (mean age 45–50 years) than sporadic, nonhereditary cancers. A germline pathogenic variant is identified in 20% of patients in whom colon cancer was diagnosed before age 50. Compared to patients with sporadic tumors of similar pathologic stage, those with Lynch syndrome tumors have improved survival. However, synchronous or metachronous cancers occur within 10 years in up to 45% of patients.

Lynch syndrome is caused by a defect in one of several genes that are important in the detection and repair of DNA base-pair mismatches: *MLH1, MSH2, MSH6,* and *PMS2* or EPCAM, a promoter for *MSH2*. Germline pathogenic variants in *MLH1* and *MSH2* account for almost 90% of the known variants in families with Lynch syndrome. Variants in any of these mismatch repair genes result in a characteristic phenotypic DNA abnormality known as microsatellite instability.

Clinical Findings

A thorough family cancer history is essential to identify families that may be affected by the Lynch syndrome so that appropriate genetic and colonoscopic screening can be offered. The National Colorectal Cancer Roundtable recommends a simple three-question tool for identifying increased risk and meriting more detailed assessment: (1) Have you had colorectal cancer or polyps diagnosed before age 50? (2) Do you have three or more relatives with colorectal cancer? and (3) Do you have a first-degree relative with colorectal cancer or another Lynch syndrome–related cancer diagnosed before age 50? The PREMM5 probability model is available for calculating the likelihood of Lynch syndrome based on family and personal history (https://premm.dfci.harvard.edu/). Genetic evaluation is recommended for those with a personal or family history of colorectal cancer under age 50, a history of multiple family members with cancer, or a > 5% PREMM5 model-predicted chance of Lynch syndrome. Genetic testing can be performed with multigene panels that test for germline cancer genes (ie, Lynch, familial adenomatous polyposis, and hamartomatous syndromes) as well as others of uncertain significance. Referral to a genetic counselor is recommended.

Personal and family history alone are insufficient to identify a significant proportion of patients with Lynch syndrome. For this reason, the National Comprehensive Cancer Network recommend that *all* colorectal cancers should undergo testing for Lynch syndrome with either immunohistochemistry or microsatellite instability. Universal testing has the greatest sensitivity for the diagnosis of Lynch syndrome and is cost-effective. Individuals whose tumors have normal immunohistochemical staining or do not have microsatellite instability are unlikely to have germline pathogenic variants in mismatch repair genes, do not require further genetic testing, and do not require intensive cancer surveillance. Up to 15% of sporadic (noninherited) tumors have microsatellite instability or absent *MLH1* staining due to somatic (noninherited) methylation of the *MLH1* gene promoter and somatic *BRAF* pathogenic variants, which must be excluded before further genetic testing is considered. Germline testing for genetic variants is positive in > 90% of individuals whose tumors show absent histochemical staining of one of the mismatch repair genes or high level of microsatellite instability without a *BRAF* gene variant.

Screening & Treatment

If a pathogenic variant is detected in a patient with cancer in one of the known mismatch genes, genetic testing of other first-degree family members is indicated. If genetic testing documents a Lynch syndrome gene variant, affected relatives should be screened with colonoscopy every 1–2 years beginning at age 25 (or at age 5 years younger than the age at diagnosis of the youngest affected family member). If cancer is found, subtotal colectomy with ileorectal anastomosis (followed by annual surveillance of the rectal stump) should be performed. Women should undergo screening for endometrial and ovarian cancer beginning at age 30–35 years with pelvic examination, transvaginal ultrasound, and endometrial sampling. Prophylactic hysterectomy and oophorectomy are recommended to women at age 40 or once they have finished childbearing. Screening for gastric cancer with upper endoscopy should be considered every 2–3 years beginning at age 30–35 years.

Ito S et al. Cost-effectiveness of Lynch syndrome screening in colorectal cancer: universal germline vs sequential screening. Clin Gastroenterol Hepatol. 2025;23:2328. [PMID: 40315972]

ANORECTAL DISEASES

(See Chapter 43 for Carcinoma of the Anus.)

HEMORRHOIDS

ESSENTIALS OF DIAGNOSIS

- Bright red blood per rectum.
- Protrusion, discomfort.
- Characteristic findings on external anal inspection and anoscopic examination.

General Considerations

Internal hemorrhoids are subepithelial vascular cushions consisting of connective tissue, smooth muscle fibers, and arteriovenous communications between terminal branches of the superior rectal artery and rectal veins. They are a normal anatomic entity, occurring in all adults, that contribute to normal anal pressures and ensure a water-tight closure of the anal canal. They commonly occur in three primary locations—right anterior, right posterior, and left lateral. External hemorrhoids arise from the inferior hemorrhoidal veins located below the dentate line and are covered with squamous epithelium of the anal canal or perianal region.

Hemorrhoids may become symptomatic as a result of activities that increase venous pressure, resulting in distention and engorgement. Straining at stool, diarrhea, constipation, prolonged sitting, pregnancy, obesity, and low-fiber diets all may contribute. With time, redundancy and enlargement of the venous cushions may develop and result in bleeding or protrusion.

Clinical Findings

A. Symptoms and Signs

Patients often attribute a variety of perianal complaints to "hemorrhoids." However, the principal problems attributable to internal hemorrhoids are bleeding, prolapse, and mucoid discharge. Bleeding is manifested by bright red blood that may range from streaks of blood visible on toilet paper or stool to bright red blood that drips into the toilet bowl after a bowel movement. Uncommonly, bleeding is severe and prolonged enough to result in anemia. Initially, internal hemorrhoids are confined to the anal canal (stage I). Over time, the internal hemorrhoids may gradually enlarge and protrude from the anal opening. At first, this mucosal prolapse occurs during straining and reduces spontaneously (stage II). With progression over time, the prolapsed hemorrhoids may require manual reduction after bowel movements (stage III) or may remain chronically protruding (stage IV). Chronically prolapsed hemorrhoids may result in a sense of fullness or discomfort and mucoid discharge, resulting in irritation of perianal skin and soiling of underclothes. Pain is unusual with internal hemorrhoids, occurring only when there is extensive inflammation and thrombosis of irreducible tissue or with thrombosis of an external hemorrhoid.

B. Examination

External hemorrhoids are readily visible on perianal inspection. Nonprolapsed internal hemorrhoids are not visible but may protrude through the anus with gentle straining while the clinician spreads the buttocks. Prolapsed hemorrhoids are visible as protuberant purple nodules covered by mucosa. The perianal region should also be examined for other signs of disease such as fistulas, fissures, skin tags, condyloma, anal cancer, or dermatitis. On digital examination, uncomplicated internal hemorrhoids are neither palpable nor painful. Anoscopic evaluation, best performed in the prone jackknife position, provides optimal visualization of internal hemorrhoids.

Differential Diagnosis

Small volume rectal bleeding may be caused by an anal fissure or fistula, neoplasms of the distal colon or rectum, ulcerative colitis or Crohn colitis, infectious proctitis, or rectal ulcers. Rectal prolapse, in which a full thickness of rectum protrudes concentrically from the anus, is readily distinguished from mucosal hemorrhoidal prolapse. Proctosigmoidoscopy or colonoscopy should be performed in all patients with hematochezia to exclude disease in the rectum or sigmoid colon that could be misinterpreted in the presence of hemorrhoidal bleeding.

Treatment

A. Conservative Measures

Most patients with early (stage I and stage II) disease can be managed with conservative treatment. To decrease straining with defecation, patients should be given instructions for a high-fiber diet and told to increase fluid intake with meals, avoid straining, and limit sitting time on the toilet to < 5 minutes. Dietary fiber may be supplemented with bran powder (1–2 tbsp twice daily added to food or in 8 oz of liquid) or with commercial bulk laxatives (eg, Benefiber, Metamucil, Citrucel). Suppositories and rectal ointments have no demonstrated utility in the management of mild disease. Mucoid discharge may be treated effectively by the local application of a cotton ball tucked next to the anal opening after bowel movements.

B. Medical Treatment

Patients with stage I, stage II, and stage III hemorrhoids and recurrent bleeding despite conservative measures may be treated without anesthesia with rubber band ligation, injection sclerotherapy, or application of electrocoagulation (bipolar cautery or infrared photocoagulation). The choice of therapy is dictated by operator preference, but rubber band ligation is preferred due to its ease of use and high rate of efficacy. Major complications occur in < 2%, including pelvic sepsis, pelvic abscess, urinary retention, and bleeding. Recurrence is common unless patients alter their dietary habits. Edematous, prolapsed (stage IV) internal hemorrhoids may be treated acutely with topical creams, foams, or suppositories containing various combinations of emollients, topical anesthetics, (eg, pramoxine, dibucaine), vasoconstrictors (eg, phenylephrine), astringents (witch hazel), and corticosteroids. Common preparations include Preparation H (several formulations), Anusol HC, Proctofoam, Nupercainal, Tucks, and Doloproct (not available in the United States).

C. Surgical Treatment

Surgical excision (traditional hemorrhoidectomy or stapled hemorrhoidopexy) is reserved for < 5–10% of patients with chronic severe bleeding due to stage III or stage IV hemorrhoids or patients with acute thrombosed stage IV hemorrhoids with necrosis. Complications of surgical hemorrhoidectomy include postoperative pain (which may persist for 2–4 weeks) and impaired continence.

Thrombosed External Hemorrhoid

Thrombosis of the external hemorrhoidal plexus results in a perianal hematoma. It most commonly occurs in otherwise healthy young adults and may be precipitated by coughing, heavy lifting, or straining at stool. The condition is characterized by the relatively acute onset of an exquisitely painful, tense and bluish perianal nodule covered with skin that may be up to several centimeters in size. Pain is most severe within the first few hours but gradually eases over 2–3 days as edema subsides. Symptoms may be relieved with warm sitz baths, analgesics, and ointments. With symptom resolution, a perianal skin tag may persist, which can be a source of irritation. If the patient is evaluated in the first 24–48 hours, removal of the clot may hasten symptomatic relief. With the patient in the lateral position, the skin around and over the lump is injected subcutaneously with 1% lidocaine using a tuberculin syringe with a 30-gauge needle. An ellipse of skin is then excised and the clot evacuated. A dry gauze dressing is applied for 12–24 hours, and then daily sitz baths are begun.

When to Refer

- Stage I, II, or III: When conservative measures fail and expertise in medical procedures is needed (injection, banding, thermocoagulation).
- Stage IV: When surgical therapy is required.

When to Admit

- Severe bleeding with anemia (rare).
- Incarcerated, thrombosed grade IV internal hemorrhoids.
- Pelvic cellulitis after banding or sclerotherapy.

Akinmoladun O et al. Management of hemorrhoids and anal fissures. Surg Clin North Am. 2024;104:473. [PMID: 38677814]

ANORECTAL INFECTIONS

A number of organisms can cause inflammation of the anal and rectal mucosa. Proctitis is characterized by anorectal discomfort, tenesmus, constipation, and mucus or bloody discharge. Most cases of proctitis are sexually transmitted, especially by anal-receptive intercourse. Infectious proctitis must be distinguished from noninfectious causes of anorectal symptoms, including anal fissures or fistulae, perirectal abscesses, anorectal carcinomas, and IBD (ulcerative colitis or Crohn disease).

Etiology & Management

Several organisms may cause infectious proctitis.

A. *Neisseria gonorrhoeae*

Gonorrhea may cause itching, burning, tenesmus, and a mucopurulent discharge, although many anorectal infections are asymptomatic. Nucleic acid amplification testing for gonorrhea and chlamydia has excellent sensitivity and specificity and is preferred in most clinical settings due to ease of transport and laboratory processing; rectal swab specimens should be taken during anoscopy. Swabs should also be taken from the pharynx and urethra in men and from the pharynx and cervix in women because rectal swabs may have lower sensitivity than other sites. Culture with sensitivity testing may be required in patients with suspected infection recurrence. Complications of untreated infections include strictures, fissures, fistulas, and perirectal abscesses. (For treatment, see Chapter 37.)

B. *Treponema pallidum*

Anal syphilis may be asymptomatic or may lead to perianal pain and discharge. With primary syphilis, the chancre may be at the anal margin or within the anal canal and may mimic a fissure, fistula, or ulcer. Proctitis or inguinal lymphadenopathy may be present. With secondary syphilis, condylomata lata (pale-brown, flat verrucous lesions) may be seen, with secretion of foul-smelling mucus. Although the diagnosis may be established with dark-field microscopy or fluorescent antibody testing of scrapings from the chancre or condylomas, this requires proper equipment and trained personnel. The serum VDRL or RPR test is positive in 75% of primary cases and in 99% of secondary cases. (For treatment, see Chapter 38.)

C. *Chlamydia trachomatis*

Chlamydial infection may cause proctitis similar to gonorrheal proctitis; however, some infections are asymptomatic. It also may cause lymphogranuloma venereum, characterized by proctocolitis with fever and bloody diarrhea, painful perianal ulcerations, anorectal strictures and fistulas, and inguinal adenopathy (buboes). An increasing number of infections have been identified among men who have sex with men. The diagnosis is established by PCR-based testing of rectal discharge or rectal biopsy. Recommended treatment is doxycycline 100 mg orally twice daily for 21 days.

D. Herpes Simplex Type 2

Herpes simplex type 2 virus is a common cause of anorectal infection. Symptoms occur 4–21 days after exposure and include severe pain, itching, constipation, tenesmus, urinary retention, and radicular pain from involvement of lumbar or sacral nerve roots. Small vesicles or ulcers may be seen in the perianal area or anal canal. Sigmoidoscopy is not usually necessary but may reveal vesicular or ulcerative lesions in the distal rectum. Diagnosis is established by viral culture, PCR, or antigen detection assays of vesicular fluid. Symptoms resolve within 2 weeks, but viral shedding may continue for several weeks. Patients may remain asymptomatic with or without viral shedding or may have recurrent mild relapses. Treatment of acute infection for 7–10 days with oral acyclovir, 400 mg three times daily, famciclovir, 250 mg orally three times daily, or valacyclovir, 1 g orally twice daily, has been shown to reduce the duration of symptoms and viral shedding. Patients with AIDS and recurrent relapses may benefit from long-term suppressive therapy (see Chapter 35).

E. Condylomata Acuminata

Condylomata acuminata (warts) are a significant cause of anorectal symptoms. Caused by the HPV, they may occur on the perianal area, in the anal canal, or on the genitals. Perianal or anal warts are seen in up to 25% of men who have sex with men. Individuals with HIV and condylomas have a higher relapse rate after therapy and a higher rate of progression to high-grade dysplasia or anal cancer. The warts are located on the perianal skin and extend within the anal canal up to 2 cm above the dentate line. Patients may have no symptoms or may report itching, bleeding, and pain. The warts may be small and flat or verrucous, or may form a confluent mass that may obscure the anal opening. Warts must be distinguished from condyloma lata (secondary syphilis) or anal cancer. Biopsies should be obtained from large or suspicious lesions. Treatment can be difficult. Sexual partners should also be examined and treated. The treatment of anogenital warts is discussed in Chapter 6. The HPV vaccine, Gardasil-9 valent, has demonstrated efficacy in preventing anogenital warts and is now recommended for all persons aged 9–14 (two or three doses) and persons aged 15–45 (three doses), as well as all men of any age who have sex with men (see Chapters 1 and 34). Individuals with HIV and condylomas who have detectable serum HIV RNA levels should have anoscopic surveillance for anal cancer every 3–6 months.

Quilter LA et al. The management of gonorrhea in the era of emerging antimicrobial resistance: what primary care clinicians should know. Med Clin North Am. 2024;108:279. [PMID: 38331480]

Wolf J et al. Human papillomavirus infection: epidemiology biology, host interactions, cancer development, prevention, and therapeutics. Rev Med Virol. 2024;34:e2537. [PMID: 38666757]

FECAL INCONTINENCE

The prevalence of fecal incontinence is 8%. It is higher in persons aged ≥ 60 years (9.3%) than in younger persons (4.95) and higher in women (9.1%) than in men (7.4%). There are five general requirements for bowel continence: (1) solid or semisolid stool (even healthy young adults have difficulty maintaining continence with liquid rectal contents); (2) a distensible rectal reservoir (as sigmoid contents empty into the rectum, the vault must expand to accommodate); (3) a sensation of rectal fullness (if the patient cannot sense this, overflow may occur before the patient can take appropriate action); (4) intact pelvic nerves and muscles; and (5) the ability to reach a toilet in a timely fashion.

Minor Incontinence

Many patients describe an inability to control flatus or slight soilage of undergarments that tends to occur after bowel movements or with straining or coughing. This may be due to local anal problems such as prolapsed hemorrhoids that make it difficult to form a tight anal seal or isolated weakness of the internal anal sphincter, especially if stools are somewhat loose. Patients should be treated with fiber supplements to provide greater stool bulk. Coffee and other caffeinated beverages should be eliminated. The perianal skin should be cleansed with moist, lanolin-coated tissue (baby wipes) to reduce excoriation and infection. After wiping, loose application of a cotton ball near the anal opening may absorb small amounts of fecal leakage. Prolapsing hemorrhoids may be treated with band ligation or surgical hemorrhoidectomy. Control of flatus and seepage may be improved by Kegel perineal exercises. Conditions such as ulcerative proctitis that cause tenesmus and urgency, chronic diarrheal conditions, and IBS may result in difficulty in maintaining complete continence, especially if a toilet is not readily available. Loperamide 2 mg orally may be helpful to reduce urge incontinence in patients with loose stools and may be taken in anticipation of situations in which a toilet may not be readily available. Older patients may require more time or assistance to reach a toilet, which may lead to incontinence. Scheduled toileting and the availability of a bedside commode are helpful. Older adult patients with chronic constipation may develop stool impaction leading to "overflow" incontinence.

Major Incontinence

Complete uncontrolled loss of stool reflects a significant problem with central perception or neuromuscular function. Incontinence that occurs without awareness suggests a loss of central awareness (eg, dementia, cerebrovascular accident, multiple sclerosis) or peripheral nerve injury (eg, spinal cord injury, cauda equina syndrome, pudendal nerve damage due to obstetric trauma or pelvic floor prolapse, aging, or diabetes mellitus). Incontinence that occurs despite awareness and active efforts to retain stool suggests sphincteric damage, which may be caused by traumatic childbirth (especially forceps delivery), episiotomy, prolapse, prior anal surgery, and physical trauma.

Physical examination should include careful inspection of the perianal area for hemorrhoids, rectal prolapse, fissures, fistulas, and either gaping or a keyhole defect of the anal sphincter (indicating severe sphincteric injury or neurologic disorder). The perianal skin should be stimulated to confirm an intact anocutaneous reflex. Digital examination during relaxation gives valuable information about resting tone (due mainly to the internal sphincter) and contraction of the external sphincter and pelvic floor during squeezing. It also excludes fecal impaction. Anoscopy is required to evaluate for hemorrhoids, fissures, and fistulas. Proctosigmoidoscopy is useful to exclude rectal carcinoma or proctitis. Anal ultrasonography or pelvic MRI is the most reliable test for definition of anatomic defects in the external and internal anal sphincters. Anal manometry may also be useful to define the severity of weakness, to assess sensation, and to predict response to biofeedback training.

Patients who are incontinent only of loose or liquid stools are treated with bulking agents and oral antidiarrheal drugs (eg, loperamide, 2 mg before meals and prophylactically before social engagements, shopping trips, etc). Patients with incontinence of solid stool benefit from scheduled toilet use after glycerin suppositories or tap water enemas. Biofeedback training with pelvic floor strengthening (Kegel) exercises (alternating 5-second squeeze and 10-second rest for 10 minutes twice daily) may be helpful in motivated patients to lower the threshold for awareness of rectal filling, strengthen the pelvic floor, and improve continence. In a 2019 RCT, global incontinence symptom improvement occurred in 38% of patients instructed on daily pelvic floor contraction exercises (three sets of 10 contractions sustained for up to 10 seconds and two sets of 3 contractions sustained for up to 30 seconds) compared with 18% who did not perform these exercises. Operative management is seldom needed but should be considered in patients with major incontinence due to prior injury to the anal sphincter who have not responded to medical therapy.

When to Refer

- Conservative measures fail.
- Anorectal tests are deemed necessary (manometry, ultrasonography, electromyography).
- A surgically correctable lesion is suspected.

Blackett J et al. Fecal incontinence in adults: new therapies. Am J Gastroenterol. 2025;120:2027. [PMID: 40079456]

Frye J et al. Anorectal manometry: when, how to perform and interpret, and is it useful? Am J Gastroenterol. 2024;119:1449. [PMID: 38275246]

OTHER ANAL CONDITIONS

Anal Fissures

Anal fissures are linear or rocket-shaped ulcers that are usually < 5 mm in length. Most fissures are believed to arise from trauma to the anal canal during defecation, perhaps caused by straining, constipation, or high internal sphincter tone. They occur most commonly in the posterior midline, but 10% occur anteriorly. Fissures that occur off the midline should raise suspicion for Crohn disease, HIV/AIDS, tuberculosis, syphilis, or anal carcinoma. Patients report severe, tearing pain during defecation followed by throbbing discomfort that may lead to constipation due to fear of recurrent pain. There may be mild associated hematochezia, with blood on the stool or toilet paper. Anal fissures are confirmed by visual inspection of the anal verge while gently separating the buttocks. Acute fissures look like cracks in the epithelium. Chronic fissures result in fibrosis and the development of a skin tag at the outermost edge (sentinel pile). Digital and anoscopic examinations may cause severe pain and may not be possible. Medical management is directed at promoting effortless, painless bowel movements. Fiber supplements and sitz baths should be prescribed. Topical anesthetics (5% lidocaine; 2.5% lidocaine plus 2.5% prilocaine) may provide temporary relief. Healing occurs within 2 months in up to 45% of patients with conservative management. Chronic fissures may be treated with topical 0.125–0.4% nitroglycerin, diltiazem 2% ointment, or nifedipine 0.5% (1 cm of ointment) applied 2–3 times daily just inside the anus with the tip of a finger for 4–8 weeks, or injection of botulinum toxin (20 units) into the internal anal sphincter. All these treatments result in healing in 60–90% of patients with chronic anal fissure, but headaches occur in up to 40% of patients treated with nitroglycerin. Botulinum toxin may cause transient anal incontinence. Fissures recur in up to 40% of patients after treatment. Chronic or recurrent fissures benefit from lateral internal sphincterotomy; however, minor incontinence may complicate this procedure.

Akinmoladun O et al. Management of hemorrhoids and anal fissures. Surg Clin North Am. 2024;104:473. [PMID: 38677814]

Lunsford TN et al. A pain in the butt: hemorrhoids, fissures, fistulas, and other anorectal syndromes. Gastroenterol Clin North Am. 2022;51:123. [PMID: 35135658]

Perianal Abscess & Fistula

The anal glands located at the base of the anal crypts at the dentate line may become infected, leading to abscess formation. Other causes of abscess include anal fissure and Crohn disease. Abscesses may extend upward or downward through the intersphincteric plane. Symptoms of perianal abscess are throbbing, continuous perianal pain. Erythema, fluctuance, and swelling may be found in the perianal region on external examination or in the ischiorectal fossa on digital rectal examination. Perianal abscesses are treated with local incision and drainage, while ischiorectal abscesses require drainage in the operating room. After drainage of an abscess, most patients are found to have a fistula in ano.

Fistula in ano most often arises in an anal crypt and is usually preceded by an anal abscess. In patients with fistulas that connect to the rectum, other disorders such as Crohn disease, lymphogranuloma venereum, rectal tuberculosis, and cancer should be considered. Fistulas are associated with purulent discharge that may lead to itching, tenderness, and pain. The treatment of Crohn-related fistula is discussed elsewhere in this chapter. Treatment of simple idiopathic fistula in ano is by surgical incision or excision under anesthesia. Care must be taken to preserve the anal sphincters. Surgical fistulotomy for treatment of complex (high, transsphincteric) anal fissures carries a high risk of incontinence. Techniques for healing the fistula while preserving the sphincter include an endoanal advancement flap over the internal opening and insertion of a bioprosthetic plug into the fistula opening.

Reza L et al. European Society of Coloproctology: guidelines for the diagnosis and treatment of cryptoglandular anal fissure. Colorectal Dis. 2024;26:145. [PMID: 38050857]

Perianal Pruritus

Perianal pruritus is characterized by perianal itching and discomfort. It may be caused by poor anal hygiene associated with fistulas, fissures, prolapsed hemorrhoids, skin tags, and minor incontinence. Conversely, overzealous cleansing with soaps may contribute to local irritation or contact dermatitis. Contact dermatitis, atopic dermatitis, bacterial infections (*Staphylococcus* or *Streptococcus*), parasites (pinworms, scabies), candidal infection (especially in patients with diabetes), STIs (condylomata acuminata, herpes, syphilis, molluscum contagiosum), and other skin conditions (psoriasis, Paget disease, lichen sclerosis) must be excluded. In patients with idiopathic perianal pruritus, examination may reveal erythema, excoriations, or lichenified, eczematous skin. Education is vital to successful therapy. Spicy foods, coffee, chocolate, and tomatoes may cause irritation and should be eliminated. After bowel movements, the perianal area should be cleansed with non-scented wipes premoistened with lanolin followed by gentle drying. A piece of cotton ball should be tucked next to the anal opening to absorb perspiration or fecal seepage. Anal ointments and lotions may exacerbate the condition and should be avoided. A short course of high-potency topical corticosteroid may be tried, although efficacy has not been demonstrated. Diluted capsaicin cream (0.006%) led to symptomatic relief in 75% of patients in a double-blind crossover study.

Albuquerque A. Anal pruritus: don't look away. World J Gastrointest Endosc. 2024;16:112. [PMID: 38577644]

18 Liver, Biliary Tract, & Pancreas Disorders

Elliot B. Tapper, MD, FAASLD
James Buxbaum, MD

EVALUATION OF ABNORMAL LIVER BIOCHEMICAL TESTS

ESSENTIALS OF DIAGNOSIS

- Persistent mild elevations of aminotransferase levels are common in clinical practice and caused most often by metabolic dysfunction–associated steatotic liver disease (MASLD) (formerly nonalcoholic fatty liver disease, NAFLD).
- Severe elevations in aminotransferase levels are most commonly caused by acute viral hepatitis, ischemic hepatitis, drug-induced liver injury, and acute biliary obstruction.
- Evaluation of obstructive jaundice begins with ultrasonography and is usually followed by cholangiography.
- Jaundice results from accumulation of bilirubin in serum (hyperbilirubinemia) and body tissues; the cause may be hepatic or nonhepatic.
- Hyperbilirubinemia may be due to abnormalities in the formation, transport, metabolism, or excretion of bilirubin.

General Considerations

The upper limit of normal for ALT is 29–33 U/L in men and 19–25 U/L in women. Elevated aminotransferases have multiple etiologies (see Table 18–4). Persistent mild elevations (< 5 times normal) have myriad causes but are caused most often by metabolic dysfunction–associated steatotic liver disease (MASLD) (formerly non-alcoholic fatty liver disease, NAFLD). Severe elevations (> 15 times normal and often > 1000 U/L [20 mckat/L]) are the hallmark of hepatocellular necrosis or inflammation caused by a different spectrum of disorders. Cholestasis is defined by an elevated alkaline phosphatase level (> 120 IU/L) most commonly caused by biliary obstruction or cholestatic liver disease. Total serum bilirubin is normally 0.2–1.2 mg/dL (3.42–20.52 mcmol/L) with higher mean levels in men than women. Jaundice (icterus) may be caused by increases in serum unconjugated or conjugated bilirubin in the serum and body tissues (Table 18–1). Jaundice may not be clinically recognizable until serum bilirubin levels are ≥ 3 mg/dL (51.3 mcmol/L).

Clinical Findings

A. Elevated Aminotransferases

Most patients with mildly elevated ALT or AST (< 5 times normal) **are asymptomatic.** MASLD is by far the most common cause of persistent mildly to moderately elevated aminotransferase levels and should be considered in patients with metabolic syndrome and/or obesity. The next most common cause is excess alcohol consumption. Alcohol-related injury may be suspected when the rise in AST exceeds the rise in ALT, especially if the AST/ALT ratio is > 2:1. Chronic hepatitis B or C are less frequent but important causes. Drug or herbal induced liver injury must also be considered and excluded. Occasionally, mild elevations can be caused by systemic infections and muscle injury. Other causes of mildly elevated aminotransferases are listed in Table 18–4.

Severe aminotransferase elevations (> 15 times normal (sometimes exceeding 1000 U/L) reflect hepatocellular inflammation or necrosis. The most common causes include ischemic hepatitis, acute bile duct obstruction, drug-induced liver injury, acute viral hepatitis (A–E, herpes), and toxins (eg, mushroom poisoning) (see Table 18–4). Moderate aminotransferase elevations (5–15 times normal) can be caused by almost any liver disease.

B. Elevated Alkaline Phosphatase

An elevated alkaline phosphatase often reflects cholestasis, which may be due to medications, obstruction of bile flow through the intra- or extrahepatic bile ducts (eg, choledocholithiasis, cholangiocarcinoma, pancreatic neoplasms) or infiltrative liver disease (eg, tumor granulomatous disease, or amyloidosis) (see Figure 18–1 and Table 18–1). Increases in alkaline phosphatase also may occur with disorders causing hepatocellular inflammation or injury. A predominant rise in alkaline phosphatase should prompt initial evaluation that includes imaging of the liver and biliary tract and exclusion of drug induced liver injury.

Table 18–1. Classification of jaundice.

Type of Hyperbilirubinemia	Location and Cause
Unconjugated hyperbilirubinemia (predominantly indirect bilirubin)	Increased bilirubin production (eg, hemolytic anemias, hemolytic reactions, hematoma, pulmonary infarction) Impaired bilirubin uptake and storage (eg, posthepatitis hyperbilirubinemia, Gilbert syndrome, Crigler-Najjar syndrome, drug reactions)
Conjugated hyperbilirubinemia (predominantly direct bilirubin)	**Hereditary Cholestatic Syndromes** (see also Table 18–2)
	Faulty excretion of bilirubin conjugates (eg, Dubin-Johnson syndrome, Rotor syndrome) or pathogenic variant in genes coding for bile salt transport proteins (eg, progressive familial intrahepatic cholestasis syndromes, benign recurrent intrahepatic cholestasis, and some cases of intrahepatic cholestasis of pregnancy)
	Hepatocellular Injury
	Biliary epithelial and hepatocyte damage (eg, hepatitis, hepatic cirrhosis) Intrahepatic cholestasis (eg, certain drugs, biliary cirrhosis, sepsis, postoperative jaundice) Hepatocellular damage or intrahepatic cholestasis resulting from miscellaneous causes (eg, spirochetal infections, infectious mononucleosis, cholangitis, sarcoidosis, lymphomas, hyperthyroidism, industrial toxins)
	Biliary Obstruction
	Choledocholithiasis, biliary atresia, carcinoma of biliary duct, sclerosing cholangitis, IgG_4-related cholangitis, ischemic cholangiopathy, COVID cholangiopathy, choledochal cyst, external pressure on bile duct, pancreatitis, pancreatic neoplasms

Ig, immunoglobulin.

C. Hyperbilirubinemia

Unconjugated hyperbilirubinemia may result from overproduction of bilirubin because of hemolysis; impaired hepatic uptake of bilirubin due to certain drugs; or impaired conjugation of bilirubin by glucuronide, due to mild decreases in uridine diphosphate (UDP) glucuronyl transferase (Gilbert syndrome), or moderate decreases (type II) or absence (type I) of UDP glucuronyl transferase (Crigler-Najjar syndrome) (Table 18–2). Hemolysis alone rarely elevates the serum bilirubin level to more than 7 mg/dL (119.7 mcmol/L). Stool and urine color are normal. There is mild jaundice and increased serum indirect (unconjugated) bilirubin, but bilirubin is not present in the urine. Splenomegaly occurs with chronic hemolytic disorders except sickle disease.

Conjugated hyperbilirubinemia in conjunction with abnormalities in other liver enzymes is usually caused by conditions causing hepatocellular injury (associated with increased aminotransferases), intrahepatic cholestasis, or extrahepatic biliary obstruction (associated with increased alkaline phosphatase), drugs, or sepsis (Table 18–2). Common intrahepatic causes include cirrhosis, alcohol-associated hepatitis, and chronic biliary diseases such as primary sclerosing cholangitis. Common extrahepatic causes include pancreatic or ampullary masses and obstructive disorders of the common bile duct such as stones, strictures, cholangiocarcinoma, and biliary malformations. Conjugated hyperbilirubinemia due to hepatocellular injury is often accompanied by jaundice, dark urine, light-colored stools, and pruritus. Malaise, anorexia, low-grade fever, and right upper quadrant discomfort are frequent, although the patient may be asymptomatic. An enlarged tender liver, spider telangiectasias, palmar erythema, ascites, gynecomastia, sparse body hair, fetor hepaticus, and asterixis may be present, depending on the cause, severity, and chronicity of liver dysfunction. Fever and chills are more common in benign biliary obstruction with associated cholangitis. Predominantly conjugated hyperbilirubinemia without significant elevations in other liver enzymes may result from impaired excretion of bilirubin from the liver due to hereditary hepatocanalicular transport defects (such as Dubin-Johnson syndrome, progressive familial intrahepatic cholestasis syndromes, and intrahepatic cholestasis of pregnancy).

Diagnostic Studies

(See Figure 18–1, Table 18–3, and Table 18–4.)

A. Laboratory Findings

The initial evaluation of **mildly elevated aminotransferases** should include both etiologic and prognostic investigations. Evaluation should assess the level of alcohol use and include serum testing for hepatitis B and C. Phosphatidylethanol (PEth) testing is a sensitive indicator of alcohol consumption over the prior 2–4 weeks. Where PEth is unavailable, standardized alcohol screening surveys such as AUDIT-C should be performed. The most common cause of mildly elevated liver enzymes is MASLD which should be suspected (but not limited to) persons with metabolic syndrome (eg, obesity, diabetes mellitus). If initial evaluation and management is unrevealing, serum tests for other less common and rare diseases should be considered, including serum ferritin and transferrin iron saturation for iron

Table 18–2. Hyperbilirubinemic disorders.

	Nature of Defect	Type of Hyperbilirubinemia	Clinical and Pathologic Characteristics
Gilbert syndrome[1]	Reduced activity of uridine diphosphate glucuronyl transferase	Unconjugated (indirect) bilirubin	Benign, asymptomatic hereditary jaundice. Hyperbilirubinemia increased by 24- to 36-hour fast. No treatment required. Associated with reduced mortality from CVD.
Dubin-Johnson syndrome[2]	Reduced excretory function of hepatocytes	Conjugated (direct) bilirubin	Benign, asymptomatic hereditary jaundice. Gallbladder does not visualize on oral cholecystography. Liver darkly pigmented on gross examination. Biopsy shows centrilobular brown pigment. Prognosis excellent.
Rotor syndrome[3]	Reduced hepatic reuptake of bilirubin conjugates	Conjugated (direct) bilirubin	Similar to Dubin-Johnson syndrome, but the liver is not pigmented, and the gallbladder is visualized on oral cholecystography. Prognosis excellent.
Recurrent or progressive intrahepatic cholestasis[4]	Cholestasis, often on a familial basis	Predominantly conjugated (direct) bilirubin	Episodic attacks or progressive jaundice, itching, and malaise. Onset in early life; may persist for a lifetime. Alkaline phosphatase increased. Cholestasis found on liver biopsy. (Biopsy may be normal during remission.) Prognosis is generally excellent for "benign" recurrent intrahepatic cholestasis but may not be for familial forms.
Intrahepatic cholestasis of pregnancy[5]	Cholestasis	Predominantly conjugated (direct) bilirubin	Benign cholestatic jaundice, usually occurring in the third trimester of pregnancy. Itching, GI symptoms, abnormal liver excretory function tests, and elevated serum bile acid levels (> 10 mcmol/L). Cholestasis noted on liver biopsy. Prognosis excellent, but recurrence with subsequent pregnancies or use of oral contraceptives is characteristic.

[1]Gilbert syndrome generally results from the addition of extra dinucleotide(s) TA sequences to the TATA promoter of the conjugating enzyme *UGT1A1*.
[2]Dubin-Johnson syndrome is caused by a pathogenic variant in the *ABCC2* gene coding for organic anion transporter multidrug resistance protein 2 in bile canaliculi on chromosome 10q24.
[3]Rotor syndrome is caused by pathogenic variants in the genes coding for organic anion transporting polypeptides OATP1B1 and OATP1B3 on chromosome 12p.
[4]Pathogenic variants in genes that control hepatocellular transport systems that are involved in the formation of bile and inherited as autosomal recessive traits are on chromosomes 18q21–22, 2q24, 7q21, and others in families with progressive familial intrahepatic cholestasis. Pathogenic variants of genes on chromosome 18q21–22 alter a P-type ATPase expressed in the small intestine and liver and those on chromosome 2q24 alter the bile acid export pump and also cause benign recurrent intrahepatic cholestasis. Pathogenic variants in the *ABCB4* gene on chromosome 7 that encodes multidrug resistance protein 3 account for progressive familial intrahepatic cholestasis type 3. Less common causes of progressive familial intrahepatic cholestasis are pathogenic variants in genes that encode TJP2, FXR, MY05B, and others.
[5]Pathogenic variants in genes (especially *ABCB4* and *ABCB11*) that encode biliary canalicular transporters account for many cases of intrahepatic cholestasis of pregnancy.

Table 18–3. Liver biochemical tests: normal values and changes in hepatocellular and obstructive jaundice.

Tests	Normal Values	Hepatocellular Jaundice	Obstructive Jaundice
Bilirubin[1]			
Direct	0.1–0.3 mg/dL (1.71–5.13 mcmol/L)	Increased	Increased
Indirect	0.2–0.7 mg/dL (3.42–11.97 mcmol/L)	Increased	Increased
Urine bilirubin	None	Increased	Increased
Serum albumin	3.5–5.5 g/dL (35–55 g/L)	Decreased	Generally unchanged
Alkaline phosphatase	30–115 U/L (0.6–2.3 mkat/L)	Mildly increased (+)	Markedly increased (++++)
Prothrombin time	INR of 1.0–1.4. After vitamin K, 10% decrease in 24 hours	Prolonged if damage is severe; does not respond to parenteral vitamin K	Prolonged if obstruction is marked; generally responds to parenteral vitamin K
ALT, AST	ALT, ≤ 30 U/L (0.6 mkat/L) (men), ≤ 19 U/L (0.38 mkat/L) (women); AST, 5–40 U/L (0.1–0.8 mkat/L)	Increased, as in viral hepatitis	Minimally increased

[1]Measured by the van den Bergh reaction, which overestimates direct bilirubin in normal persons.

Table 18–4. Causes of serum aminotransferase elevations.[1]

Mild Elevations (< 5 × normal)	Severe Elevations (> 15 × normal)
Hepatic: ALT-predominant	Acute viral hepatitis (A–E, herpes)
Metabolic dysfunction–associated steatotic liver disease (MASLD)	Medications/toxins
Chronic hepatitis B, C, and D	Ischemic hepatitis
Acute viral hepatitis (A-E, EBV, CMV, others)	Autoimmune hepatitis
Hemochromatosis	Wilson disease
Medications/toxins	Acute bile duct obstruction
Autoimmune hepatitis	Acute Budd-Chiari syndrome
α_1-Antitrypsin (α_1-antiprotease) deficiency	Hepatic artery ligation
Wilson disease	
Celiac disease	
Glycogenic hepatopathy	
Hepatic: AST-predominant	
Alcohol-related liver injury (AST:ALT > 2:1)	
Cirrhosis	
COVID-19	
Nonhepatic	
Strenuous exercise	
Hemolysis	
Myopathy	
Thyroid disease	
Macro-AST	

[1]Almost any liver disease can cause moderate aminotransferase elevations (5–15 × normal).

CMV, cytomegalovirus; EBV, Epstein-Barr virus.

Reproduced with permission from Green RM et al. AGA technical review on the evaluation of liver chemistry tests. *Gastroenterology*. 2002;123(4):1367–1384.

overload (ie, hemachromatosis). Understanding the risk of advanced liver disease is important. To screen for possible underlying hepatic fibrosis or cirrhosis, the Fibrosis-4 Index (a composite calculator based on age, ALT, AST, and platelet count) should be performed. Values > 1.3 (or > 2 for people ≥ 55 years old) are considered abnormal and could prompt additional evaluation including elastography.

For patients with **severely elevated aminotransferases**, an initial serological evaluation tailored to the epidemiology of the condition may include acetaminophen levels, testing for acute viral hepatitis (A, B, and C), and consideration of serum testing for ANA, immunoglobulin G levels, and smooth muscle antibodies.

In patients with **increased alkaline phosphatase** from suspected intrahepatic cholestasis, serum antimitochondrial antibody is obtained. In patients with an isolated alkaline phosphatase elevation (with normal aminotransferases and bilirubin), hepatic origin of the alkaline phosphatase (rather than bone, intestine, or placenta) is supported by fractionation of the alkaline phosphatase isoenzymes. Although commonly performed, elevated γ-glutamylpeptidase (GGT) levels do not confirm cholestatic injury as these also can be elevated from hepatocellular injury.

B. Imaging

Ultrasonography is frequently performed for patients with mildly elevated aminotransferases. This can be helpful in identifying steatosis and suggesting the presence of cirrhosis (80% sensitivity and specificity). Elastography is the preferred imaging test for assessment of advanced liver disease. Magnetic resonance elastography can be considered if elastography fails or when the BMI is > 40.

In patients with severely elevated aminotransferases, abdominal imaging with ultrasound or CT scan may identify acute biliary obstruction (usually caused by choledocholithiasis), but magnetic resonance cholangiopancreatography (MRCP) may be required. MRCP has 85% sensitivity for choledocholithiasis. In patients with suspected ischemic hepatitis, echocardiography may be helpful to identify acute HF.

In patients with cholestasis and jaundice, various imaging studies may be obtained to distinguish causes of extrahepatic biliary obstruction and intrahepatic cholestasis. Demonstration of dilated bile ducts by ultrasonography, or CT, indicates extrahepatic biliary obstruction (90–95% sensitivity). MRCP is a sensitive, noninvasive method of detecting bile duct stones, strictures, and dilatation; however, it is less reliable than endoscopic retrograde cholangiopancreatography (ERCP) for distinguishing malignant from benign strictures. ERCP requires a skilled endoscopist and may be used to demonstrate pancreatic or ampullary causes of jaundice, carry out sphincterotomy and stone extraction, insert a stent through an obstructing lesion, or facilitate direct cholangiopancreatoscopy. Complications of ERCP include pancreatitis (5% or less) and, less commonly, cholangitis, bleeding, or duodenal perforation after sphincterotomy. Percutaneous transhepatic cholangiography is an alternative approach to evaluating the anatomy of the biliary tract when endoscopic access is limited by post-surgical anatomy. Serious complications of PTC occur in 3% and include fever, bacteremia, bile peritonitis, and intraperitoneal hemorrhage. Endoscopic ultrasonography (EUS) is highly sensitive for detecting or excluding bile duct stones and therefore is commonly performed immediately before ERCP. It also is used to evaluate small lesions of the ampulla or pancreatic head, to detect portal vein invasion by pancreatic cancer, and to guide fine-needle aspiration and biopsy of possible pancreatic tumors. In patients with suspected intrahepatic cholestasis (ie, nondilated bile ducts) ultrasonography, CT, and MRI may demonstrate hepatomegaly, intrahepatic tumors, and portal hypertension. MRI is the most accurate technique for identifying hepatic malignancy and metastases, and iron overload.

C. Liver Biopsy

Percutaneous liver biopsy can be used to determine the cause and histologic severity of hepatocellular dysfunction or infiltrative liver disease, although it is subject to sampling error. It is generally performed under ultrasound or, when targeting an hepatic mass or suspected metastatic disease, under CT guidance. A transjugular route can be used in patients with ascites. In selected cases endoscopic

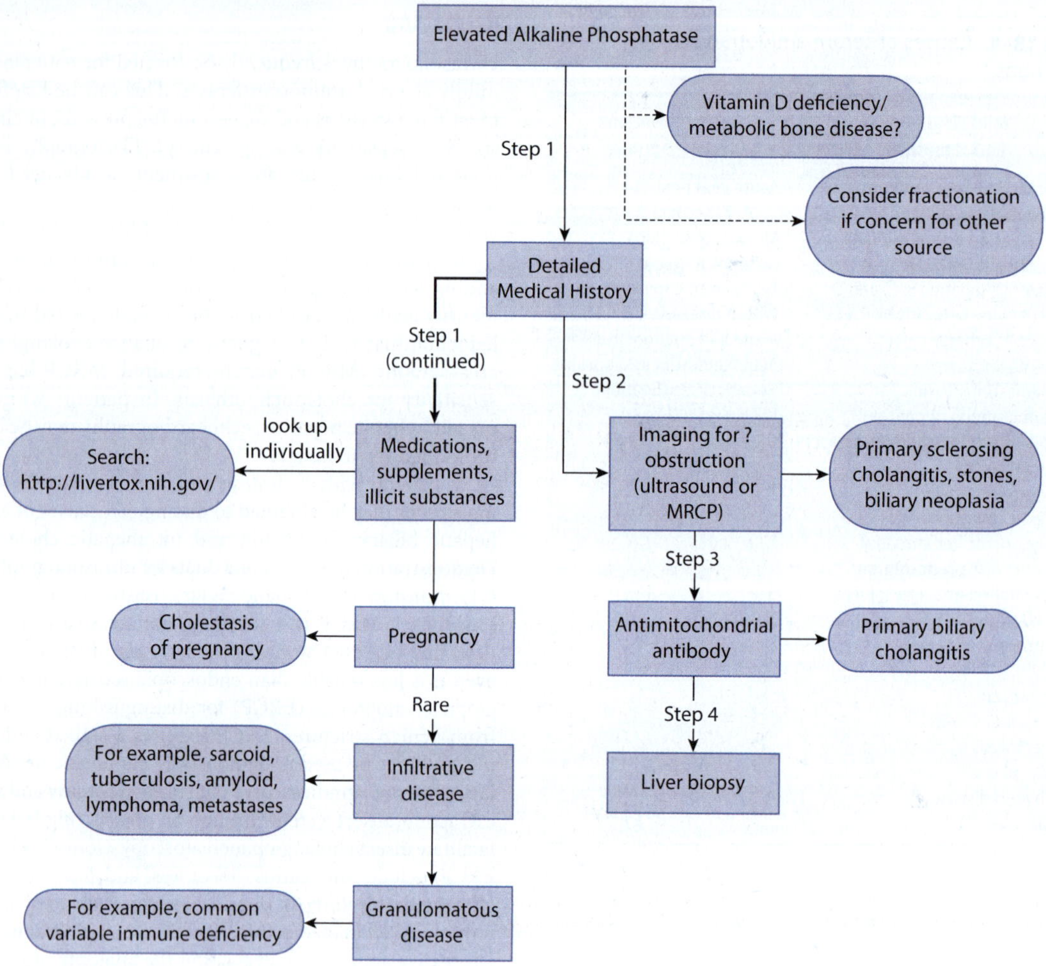

▲ **Figure 18–1.** Evaluation of elevated alkaline phosphatase.

ultrasound-guided liver biopsy may be advantageous. The risk of major bleeding after a percutaneous liver biopsy is approximately 0.5% but is increased in persons with a platelet count of 50,000/mcL (50×10^9/L) or less. The risk of death is 0.01%.

When to Refer

Patients with or at high risk for cirrhosis should be referred for subspecialty consultation. Obstructive jaundice should be referred for diagnostic procedures and possible therapy.

When to Admit

Patients with acute cholangitis or liver failure should be hospitalized.

Mohamed MF et al. Choledocholithiasis can present with marked transaminases elevation: systematic review and meta-analysis. Dig Dis Sci. 2023;68:3428. [PMID: 37269372]
Mohamed MF et al. Etiologies and outcomes of transaminase elevation > 1000 IU/L: a systematic review and meta-analysis. Dig Dis Sci. 2023;68:2843. [PMID: 37184617]
Poynard T et al. Clinical and genetic definition of serum bilirubin levels for the diagnosis of Gilbert syndrome and hypobilirubinemia. Hepatol Commun. 2023;7:e0245. [PMID: 37738404]
Thiele M et al. Population screening for cirrhosis. Hepatol Commun. 2024;8:e0512. [PMID: 39185917]

DISEASES OF THE LIVER

See Chapter 43 for HCC.

ACUTE HEPATITIS A

ESSENTIALS OF DIAGNOSIS

- Prodrome of anorexia, nausea, vomiting, malaise, aversion to smoking.
- Fever, enlarged and tender liver, jaundice.
- Markedly elevated aminotransferases.
- Antibody to hepatitis A virus (anti-HAV) appears early in the course of the illness

General Considerations

Hepatitis A virus (HAV) is a 27-nm RNA hepatovirus (in the picornavirus family) that causes epidemics or sporadic cases of hepatitis. HAV infection is hyperendemic in developing countries. Globally, over 1.5 million people are infected with HAV annually. The virus is transmitted by the fecal-oral route by either person-to-person contact or ingestion of contaminated food or water, and its spread is favored by crowding and poor sanitation. In the United States, about 30% of the population have serologic evidence of previous HAV infection (IgG anti-HAV). Since introduction of the HAV vaccine in the United States in 1995, the incidence rate of HAV infection has declined from 14 to 0.4 per 100,000 population, with a corresponding decline in the mortality rate from 0.1 to 0.02 deaths per 100,000 population and an increase in the mean ages of infection and death. Nevertheless, the majority of persons aged 25 years or older in the United States are unvaccinated and still susceptible to HAV, and vulnerable populations are especially at risk. Common source outbreaks resulting from contaminated food, including inadequately cooked shellfish, or untreated ground water from wells continue to occur, although no drinking water–associated outbreaks have occurred in the United States since 2009. At-risk groups include homeless persons, people who inject drugs, unvaccinated residents living in institutions, men who have sex with men, and international adoptees and their contacts.

The incubation period averages 30 days. HAV is excreted in feces for up to 2 weeks before clinical illness but rarely after the first week of illness. The mortality rate for hepatitis A is low, and acute liver failure due to hepatitis A is uncommon. There is no chronic carrier state.

Clinical Findings

A. Symptoms and Signs

Figure 18–2 shows the typical course of acute hepatitis A. Clinical illness is more severe in adults than in children, in whom it is usually asymptomatic. The onset may be abrupt or insidious, with malaise, myalgia, arthralgia, easy fatigability, upper respiratory symptoms, and anorexia. A distaste for smoking, paralleling anorexia, may occur early. Nausea and vomiting are frequent, and diarrhea or constipation may occur. Fever is generally present but is low-grade except in occasional cases in which systemic toxicity may occur. Defervescence and a fall in pulse rate often coincide with the onset of jaundice.

Abdominal pain is usually mild and constant in the right upper quadrant or epigastrium, often aggravated by jarring or exertion, and rarely may be severe enough to simulate cholecystitis. Jaundice occurs after 5–10 days but may appear at the same time as the initial symptoms. In many patients, jaundice never develops. With the onset of jaundice, prodromal symptoms often worsen, followed by progressive clinical improvement. Stools may be acholic during this phase. Hepatomegaly—rarely marked—is present in over half of cases. Liver tenderness is usually present. Splenomegaly is reported in 15% of patients, and soft, enlarged lymph nodes—especially in the cervical or epitrochlear areas—may be noted.

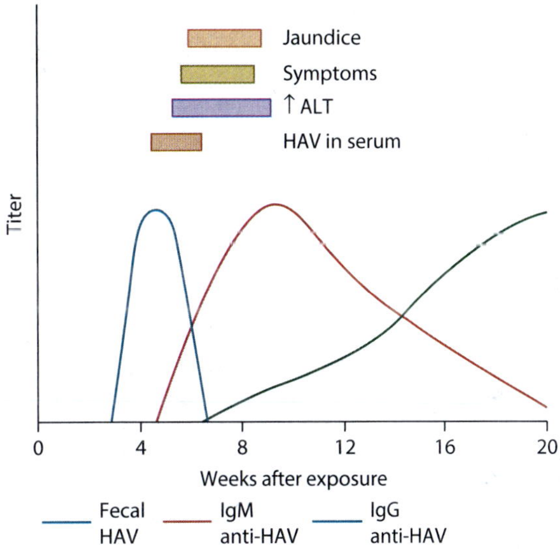

Figure 18–2. The typical course of acute type A hepatitis. Anti-HAV, antibody to hepatitis A virus; HAV, hepatitis A virus. (Reproduced with permission from Koff RS. Acute viral hepatitis. In: Friedman LS, Keeffe EB. *Handbook of Liver Disease*, 4th ed. Philadelphia: Saunders Elsevier, 2018.)

The acute illness usually subsides over 2–3 weeks with complete clinical and laboratory recovery by 9 weeks. In some cases, clinical, biochemical, and serologic recovery may be followed by one or two relapses, but recovery is the rule. Occasional extrahepatic complications include AKI, arthritis, vasculitis, acute pancreatitis, aplastic anemia, and a variety of neurologic manifestations.

B. Laboratory Findings

The WBC count is normal to low, especially in the preicteric phase. Large atypical lymphocytes may occasionally be seen. Mild proteinuria is common, and bilirubinuria often precedes the appearance of jaundice. Strikingly elevated ALT or AST levels occur early, followed by elevations of bilirubin and alkaline phosphatase; in a minority of patients, the latter persist after aminotransferase levels have normalized. Cholestasis is occasionally marked. Both IgM and IgG anti-HAV are detectable in serum soon after the illness onset (Figure 18–2). Peak titers of IgM anti-HAV occur during the first week of clinical disease and usually disappear within 3–6 months. Detection of IgM anti-HAV is an excellent test for diagnosing acute hepatitis A. Titers of IgG anti-HAV rise after 1 month of the disease and may persist for years. IgG anti-HAV (in the absence of IgM anti-HAV) indicates previous exposure to HAV, noninfectivity, and immunity.

Differential Diagnosis

The differential diagnosis includes other viruses that cause acute hepatitis, particularly hepatitis B (HBV) and C (HCV) viruses, and diseases such as infectious mononucleosis, cytomegalovirus infection, herpes simplex virus infection, influenza, Ebola virus, and SARS-CoV-2; spirochetal diseases such as leptospirosis and secondary syphilis; brucellosis; rickettsial diseases such as Q fever; drug-induced liver injury; and ischemic hepatitis (shock liver). Rarely, metastatic cancer of the liver, lymphoma, or leukemia may present as a hepatitis-like picture.

Prevention

Strict isolation of patients is not necessary, but hand washing after bowel movements is required. Unvaccinated persons who are exposed to HAV are advised to receive postexposure prophylaxis with a single dose of HAV vaccine or immune globulin (0.01 mL/kg), or both, within 2 weeks of exposure. The vaccine is preferred in healthy persons aged 1 year to 40 years, whereas immune globulin plus the vaccine is preferred in those who are younger than 1 year or older than 40 years, are immunocompromised, or have chronic liver disease.

Vaccination with one of two effective inactivated hepatitis A vaccines available in the United States provides long-term immunity and is recommended for persons living in or traveling to endemic areas), persons over age 40, patients with chronic liver disease upon diagnosis after prescreening for immunity, men who have sex with men, persons with HIV infection, animal handlers, persons who use injection or noninjection drugs, persons experiencing homelessness, persons who are incarcerated, close personal contacts of international adoptees, persons living in group settings for those with developmental disabilities, and persons who request protection against HAV. For healthy travelers, a single dose of vaccine at any time before departure can provide adequate protection. Routine vaccination is advised by the Advisory Committee on Immunization Practices of the CDC for all children aged 12–23 months in the United States, with catch-up vaccination for children and adolescents aged 2–18 years who have not previously received the HAV vaccine. HAV vaccine is also effective in the prevention of secondary spread to household contacts of primary cases. The recommended dose for adults is 1 mL (1440 ELISA units) of Havrix (GlaxoSmithKline) or 1 mL (50 units) of Vaqta (Merck) intramuscularly, followed by a booster dose at 6–18 months. A combined hepatitis A and B vaccine (Twinrix, GlaxoSmithKline) is available.

Treatment

Most symptoms respond to supportive care. Dietary management consists of palatable meals as tolerated, without overfeeding. Fluid replacement may be necessary if nausea and vomiting are pronounced. Strenuous physical exertion, alcohol, and hepatotoxic agents should be avoided.

Prognosis

In most patients, clinical recovery is generally complete within 3 months. Laboratory evidence of liver dysfunction may persist for a longer period, but most patients recover completely. Hepatitis A does not cause chronic liver disease, although it may persist for up to 1 year, and clinical and biochemical relapses may occur before full recovery. The mortality rate is < 1.0%, with a higher rate in older adults than in younger persons.

When to Admit

- Encephalopathy is present.
- INR > 1.6.
- The patient is unable to maintain hydration.

Gabrielli F et al. Treatment options for hepatitis A and E: a nonsystematic review. Viruses. 2023;15:1080. [PMID: 37243166]

Van Damme P et al. Hepatitis A virus infection. Nat Rev Dis Primers. 2023;9:51. [PMID: 37770459]

ACUTE HEPATITIS B

ESSENTIALS OF DIAGNOSIS

- Prodrome of anorexia, nausea, vomiting, malaise, aversion to smoking.
- Fever, enlarged and tender liver, jaundice.
- Normal to low WBC count; markedly elevated aminotransferases early in the course.
- Elevation of HBsAg or hepatitis B virus DNA.

General Considerations

HBV is a 42-nm hepadnavirus with a partially double-stranded DNA genome, inner core protein (hepatitis B core antigen, HBcAg), and outer surface coat (hepatitis B surface antigen, HBsAg). There are 10 different genotypes (A–J). HBV is usually transmitted by inoculation of infected blood or blood products or by sexual contact, and it is present in saliva, semen, and vaginal secretions. HBsAg-positive mothers may transmit HBV at delivery.

Since 1990, the incidence of HBV infection in the United States has decreased from 8.5 to 1.5 cases per 100,000 population. The prevalence is 0.27% in persons aged 6 or older. Because of universal vaccination since 1992, exposure to HBV is low among persons aged 18 or younger. HBV is prevalent in men who have sex with men and in people who inject drugs (about 7% of HIV-infected persons are coinfected with HBV), but the greatest number of cases result from heterosexual transmission. Other groups at risk include patients and staff at hemodialysis centers, physicians, dentists, nurses, and personnel working in clinical and pathology laboratories and blood banks. Half of all patients with acute hepatitis B in the United States have previously been incarcerated or treated for an STI. Screening for HBV infection is recommended for high-risk groups by the CDC, which includes persons incarcerated or formerly incarcerated in a jail, prison, or other detention setting; persons with a history of sexually transmitted infections or multiple sex partners; and persons with a history of hepatitis C virus infection. Testing also is recommended in all who request HBV testing as some may be reluctant to disclose stigmatizing risks.

The incubation period of HBV is 6 weeks to 6 months (average 12–14 weeks), and symptom onset is often insidious. Acute liver failure occurs in < 1%, with a mortality rate of up to 60%. Following acute hepatitis B, HBV infection persists in 1–2% of immunocompetent adults, but in a higher percentage of children and immunocompromised adults. There are an estimated 2.4 million persons (including an estimated 1.47 million foreign-born persons from endemic areas) with chronic hepatitis B in the United States and 296 million worldwide. Compared with the general population, the prevalence of chronic HBV infection is increased two- to threefold in non-Latina/Latino Black persons and tenfold in Asian persons. Those with chronic HBV, particularly when HBV infection is acquired early in life and viral replication persists, are at substantial risk for cirrhosis and HCC (up to 25–40%); men are at greater risk than women. Chronic hepatitis with low levels of viral replication as well as previously cleared HBV (as evidenced by the presence of core IgG) can "reactivate," especially following the use of immunosuppressants, causing acute hepatitis B infection. The risk of reactivation is highest with B-cell depleting agents (such as rituximab).

Clinical Findings

A. Symptoms and Signs

The clinical picture of HBV hepatitis is extremely variable, ranging from asymptomatic infection without jaundice to acute liver failure and death within days to weeks. Figure 18–3 shows the typical course of acute HBV infection. The onset may be abrupt or insidious, and the clinical features are similar to those for acute hepatitis A. Serum sickness may be seen early in acute HBV infection. Fever is generally present and is low-grade. Defervescence and a fall in pulse rate often coincide with the onset of jaundice.

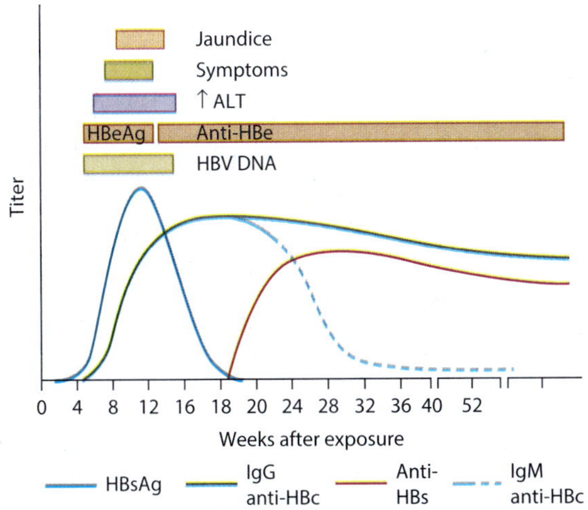

Figure 18–3. The typical course of acute type B hepatitis. Anti-HBe, antibody to HBeAg; anti-HBc, antibody to hepatitis B core antigen; anti-HBs, antibody to HBsAg; HBeAg, hepatitis Be antigen; HBsAg, hepatitis B surface antigen. (Reproduced with permission from Koff RS. Acute viral hepatitis. In: Friedman LS, Keeffe EB. *Handbook of Liver Disease*, 3rd ed. Philadelphia: Saunders Elsevier, 2012.)

Infection caused by HBV may be associated with glomerulonephritis, polyarteritis nodosa, and Guillain-Barré syndrome.

The acute illness usually subsides over 2–3 weeks with complete clinical and laboratory recovery by 16 weeks. In 5–10% of cases, the course may be more protracted, but < 1% will develop acute liver failure. HBV infection may become chronic.

B. Laboratory Findings

The laboratory features are similar to those for acute hepatitis A, although serum aminotransferase levels are higher on average in acute hepatitis B, and marked cholestasis is not a feature. Marked prolongation of the prothrombin time in severe hepatitis correlates with increased mortality.

The different states of HBV infections are characterized by HBV DNA levels and various viral antigens and antibodies that are useful in diagnosis. Interpretation of common serologic patterns is shown in Table 18–5.

1. HBsAg—The appearance of HBsAg in serum is the first evidence of infection, appearing before biochemical evidence of liver disease, and persisting throughout the clinical illness. Persistence of HBsAg more than 6 months after the acute illness signifies the development of chronic hepatitis B.

2. Anti-HBs—Specific antibody to HBsAg (anti-HBs) appears in most individuals after clearance of HBsAg and after successful vaccination against hepatitis B. Disappearance of HBsAg and the appearance of anti-HBs signal recovery from HBV infection, noninfectivity, and immunity.

3. Anti-HBc—IgM anti-HBc appears shortly after HBsAg is detected. In the setting of acute hepatitis, the presence of IgM anti-HBc indicates a diagnosis of acute hepatitis B and is useful in the serologic "gap" in rare patients who have cleared HBsAg but do not yet have detectable anti-HBs. IgM anti-HBc can persist for 3–6 months, sometimes longer, and may reappear during flares of previously inactive chronic hepatitis B. IgG anti-HBc also appears during acute hepatitis B but persists indefinitely, whether the patient recovers (with the appearance of anti-HBs in serum) or develops chronic hepatitis B (with persistence of HBsAg). In asymptomatic persons such as blood donors, an isolated anti-HBc with no other positive HBV serologic results may represent a falsely positive result or latent infection in which HBV DNA is detectable in serum only by PCR testing.

4. HBeAg—HBeAg is a secretory form of HBcAg that appears in serum during the incubation period shortly after the detection of HBsAg. HBeAg indicates viral replication and infectivity. Persistence of HBeAg beyond 3 months indicates an increased likelihood of chronic hepatitis B. Its disappearance is often followed by the appearance of anti-HBe, generally signifying diminished viral replication and decreased infectivity.

5. HBV DNA—The presence of HBV DNA in serum generally parallels the presence of HBeAg, although HBV DNA

Table 18–5. Common serologic patterns in hepatitis B virus (HBV) infection and their interpretation.

HBsAg	Anti-HBs	Anti-HBc	HBeAg	Anti-HBe	Interpretation
+	–	IgM	+	–	Acute hepatitis B
+	–	IgG[1]	+	–	Chronic hepatitis B with active viral replication
+	–	IgG	–	+	Inactive HBV carrier state (low HBV DNA level) or HBeAg-negative chronic hepatitis B with active viral replication (high HBV DNA level)
+	+	IgG	+ or –	+ or –	Chronic hepatitis B with heterotypic anti-HBs (about 10% of cases)
–	–	IgM	+ or –	–	Acute hepatitis B
–	+	IgG	–	+ or –	Recovery from hepatitis B (immunity)
–	+	–	–	–	Vaccination (immunity)
–	–	IgG	–	–	Infection in remote past; but often false positive

[1]Low levels of IgM anti-HBc may also be detected.

is a more sensitive and precise marker of viral replication and infectivity. In some patients with chronic hepatitis B, HBV DNA is present at high levels without HBeAg in serum because of development of a pathogenic variant in the core promoter or pre-core region of the gene that codes HBcAg; these variants prevent synthesis of HBeAg in infected hepatocytes. When additional variants in the core gene are also present, the severity of HBV infection is enhanced and the risk of cirrhosis is increased.

Differential Diagnosis

The differential diagnosis includes hepatitis A and the same disorders listed for the differential diagnosis of acute hepatitis A. In addition, coinfection with hepatitis D virus (HDV) must be considered.

Prevention

Strict isolation of patients is not necessary. Thorough hand washing by medical staff who may contact contaminated utensils, bedding, or clothing is essential. Medical staff should handle disposable needles carefully and not recap them. Screening of donated blood for HBsAg, anti-HBc, and anti-HCV has reduced the risk of transfusion-associated hepatitis markedly. All pregnant women should undergo testing for HBsAg. HBV-infected persons should practice safe sex. Immunoprophylaxis of the neonate reduces the risk of perinatal transmission of HBV infection; when the mother's serum HBV DNA level is 200,000 IU/mL or higher, antiviral treatment of the mother should also be initiated in the third trimester (see Chronic Hepatitis B & Chronic Hepatitis D). Health care workers infected with HBV are not precluded from practicing medicine or dentistry if they follow CDC guidelines.

Hepatitis B immune globulin (HBIG) may be protective—or may attenuate the severity of illness—if given within 7 days after exposure (adult dose is 0.06 mL/kg body weight) followed by initiation of the HBV vaccine series. This approach is recommended for unvaccinated persons exposed to HBsAg-contaminated material via mucous membranes or through breaks in the skin and for individuals who have had sexual contact with a person with HBV infection (irrespective of the presence or absence of HBeAg in the source). HBIG is also indicated for newborn infants of HBsAg-positive mothers, with initiation of the vaccine series at the same time, both within 12 hours of birth (administered at different injection sites).

The CDC recommends HBV vaccination of all infants and children in the United States and, as of 2022, all adults under age 60 years, as well as those aged 60 and older with risk factors for HBV infection. Over 90% of recipients of the vaccine mount protective antibody to hepatitis B; immunocompromised persons, including patients receiving dialysis (especially those with diabetes mellitus), respond poorly (see Table 34–7). The standard regimen for adults is 10–20 mcg (depending on the formulation) repeated again at 1 and 6 months, but alternative schedules have been approved, including accelerated schedules of 0, 1, 2, and 12 months and of 0, 7, and 21 days plus 12 months. For greatest reliability of absorption, the deltoid muscle is the preferred site of inoculation. A newer vaccine, Heplisav-B, which uses a novel immune system–stimulating ingredient, was approved by the FDA for only adults in 2017. Immunization requires only two injections, and Heplisav-B appears to be more effective than previous HBV vaccines. When documentation of seroconversion is considered desirable, postimmunization anti-HBs titers may be checked. Protection appears to be excellent even if the titer wanes—persisting for at least 20 years—and booster reimmunization is not routinely recommended but is advised for immunocompromised persons in whom anti-HBs titers fall below 10 mIU/mL. For vaccine nonresponders, three additional vaccine doses may elicit seroprotective anti-HBs levels in 30–50% of persons. Doubling of the standard dose or use of Heplisav-B may also be effective. Universal vaccination of neonates in countries endemic for HBV has reduced the incidence of HCC. Incomplete immunization is the most important predictor of liver disease among vaccinees. Unfortunately, approximately 64 million high-risk adults in the United States remain susceptible to HBV.

Treatment

Treatment of acute hepatitis B is the same as that for acute hepatitis A. Encephalopathy or severe coagulopathy indicates acute liver failure, and hospitalization at a liver transplant center is mandatory. Antiviral therapy is generally unnecessary in patients with acute hepatitis B but is usually prescribed in cases of acute liver failure caused by HBV as well as in spontaneous reactivation of chronic hepatitis B presenting as acute-on-chronic liver failure (see Acute Liver Failure).

Prognosis

In most patients, clinical recovery is complete in 3–6 months. Laboratory evidence of liver dysfunction may persist for a longer period, but most patients recover completely. The mortality rate for acute hepatitis B is 0.1–1% but is higher with superimposed hepatitis D. Chronic hepatitis B, characterized by elevated aminotransferase levels for more than 3–6 months, develops in 1–2% of immunocompetent adults with acute hepatitis B, but in as many as 90% of infected neonates and infants and a substantial proportion of immunocompromised adults (see Chronic Hepatitis B & Chronic Hepatitis D).

When to Refer

Refer patients with acute hepatitis who require liver biopsy for diagnosis.

When to Admit

- Encephalopathy is present.
- INR > 1.6.
- The patient is unable to maintain hydration.

Conners EE et al. Screening and testing for hepatitis B virus infection: CDC recommendations - United States, 2023. MMWR Recomm Rep. 2023;72:1. [PMID: 36893044]

Jeng WJ et al. Hepatitis B. Lancet. 2023;401:1039. [PMID: 36774930]

Jeng WJ et al. What will it take to cure hepatitis B? Hepatol Commun. 2023;24:e0084. [PMID: 36972391]

So S et al. Universal adult hepatitis B screening and vaccination as the path to elimination. JAMA. 2023;329:1639. [PMID: 36897598]

ACUTE HEPATITIS C & OTHER CAUSES OF ACUTE VIRAL HEPATITIS

Viruses other than HAV and HBV that can cause acute hepatitis are hepatitis C virus (HCV), HDV, and hepatitis E virus (HEV) (an enterically transmitted hepatitis seen in epidemic form in Asia, the Middle East, and North Africa and sporadically in Western countries). Human pegivirus (formerly hepatitis G virus [HGV]) rarely, if ever, causes frank hepatitis. In immunocompromised and rare immunocompetent persons, cytomegalovirus, Epstein-Barr virus, and herpes simplex virus should be considered in the differential diagnosis of hepatitis. Middle East respiratory syndrome (MERS), severe acute respiratory syndrome (SARS), SARS coronavirus infection (SARS-CoV-2), Ebola virus infection, and influenza may be associated with elevated serum aminotransferase levels (occasionally marked). Unidentified and other rare pathogens account for a small percentage of cases of acute viral hepatitis.

1. Hepatitis C

HCV is a single-stranded RNA virus (hepacivirus) with properties similar to those of flaviviruses. Eight genotypes of HCV have been identified. Testing of donated blood for HCV has reduced the risk of transfusion-associated hepatitis C from 10% in 1990 to about 1 case per 2 million units in 2011. Over 60% of cases of HCV infection are transmitted by injection drug use, and both reinfection and superinfection of HCV are common in people who actively inject drugs. Body piercing, tattoos, and hemodialysis are risk factors. The risk of sexual and maternal–neonatal transmission is low. Having multiple sexual partners, unprotected receptive anal intercourse with ejaculation, and HIV coinfection increase the risk of HCV transmission. Transmission via breastfeeding has not been documented. Hospital- and outpatient facility–acquired transmission has occurred via multidose vials of saline used to flush portacaths; through reuse of disposable syringes; and through drug "diversion" and tampering with injectable opioids by an infected health care worker. Incarceration in prison is a risk factor, with a seroprevalence of 17% in Louisiana, for example. According to the CDC in 2023, the incidence of acute HCV continues to rise, from 0.3 to 1/100,000 in women and from 0.3 to 2/100,000 in men. Globally, about 1.5 million new infections occur per year.

Clinical Findings

A. Symptoms and Signs

Figure 18–4 shows the typical course of HCV infection. The incubation period for hepatitis C averages 6–7 weeks. Clinical illness is asymptomatic in 70% or mild and characterized by waxing and waning aminotransferase elevations and a high rate (> 80%) of chronic hepatitis.

B. Laboratory Findings

Diagnosis of hepatitis C is based on an enzyme immunoassay (EIA) that detects antibodies to HCV or HCV RNA PCR. Anti-HCV is not protective, but in patients with acute or chronic hepatitis, its presence in serum generally signifies that HCV is the cause. A diagnosis of hepatitis C must be confirmed by using an assay for HCV RNA.

Treatment

Many people will clear hepatitis C spontaneously following acute hepatitis; however, antiviral treatment may be cost-effective. A 6–8-week course of direct acting antivirals has been shown to prevent chronic hepatitis in patients with acute hepatitis C who have not had spontaneous clearance after 3 months (see Chronic Viral Hepatitis).

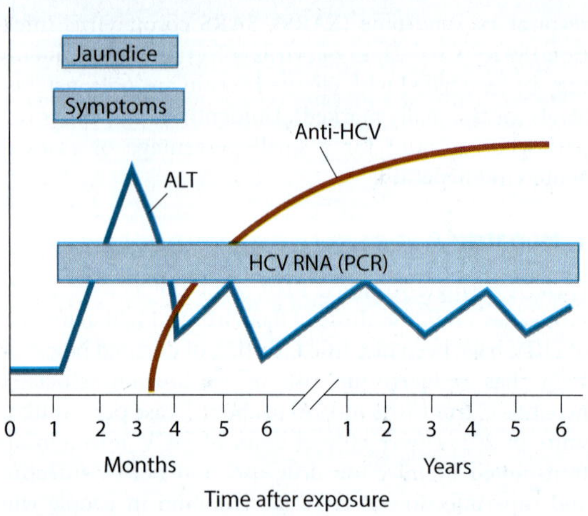

▲ **Figure 18–4.** The typical course of acute and chronic hepatitis C. Anti-HCV, antibody to hepatitis C virus by enzyme immunoassay; HCV RNA PCR, hepatitis C viral RNA by PCR.

Prognosis

In most patients, clinical recovery is complete in 3–6 months. Laboratory evidence of liver dysfunction may persist for a longer period. Acute liver failure or mortality due to acute HCV is vanishingly rare. Chronic hepatitis, which progresses slowly in many cases, develops in as many as 85% of all persons with acute hepatitis C. Ultimately, cirrhosis develops in up to 30% of those with chronic hepatitis C; the risk of cirrhosis and hepatic decompensation is higher in patients coinfected with both HCV and HBV or HIV.

Bhattacharya D et al. Hepatitis C Guidance 2023 Update: AASLD-IDSA recommendations for testing, managing, and treating hepatitis C virus infection. Clin Infect Dis. 2023 May 25. [Epub ahead of print] [PMID: 37229695]

Chen P-H et al. Trends in the prevalence of hepatitis C infection during pregnancy and maternal-infant outcomes in the US, 1998 to 2018. JAMA Netw Open. 2023;6:e2324770. [PMID: 37477918]

Martinello M et al. Hepatitis C. Lancet. 2023;402:1085. [PMID: 37741678]

2. Hepatitis D

HDV is a defective RNA virus that causes hepatitis only in association with HBV infection and specifically only in the presence of HBsAg; it is cleared when the latter is cleared.

HDV may coinfect with HBV or may superinfect a person with chronic hepatitis B, usually by percutaneous exposure. When acute hepatitis D is coincident with acute HBV infection, the infection is generally similar in severity to acute hepatitis B alone, and both viruses usually clear. In chronic hepatitis B, superinfection by HDV carries a worse short-term prognosis, often resulting in acute liver failure or severe chronic hepatitis that progresses rapidly to cirrhosis, although 50% of patients have a more indolent course.

Twelve to 72 million persons are infected with HDV worldwide. New cases of hepatitis D are infrequent in the United States primarily because of the control of HBV infection, and cases seen today are usually from cohorts infected years ago who survived the initial impact of hepatitis D and now have cirrhosis. These patients are at risk for decompensation and have a threefold increased risk of HCC. HDV is estimated to cause 18% of cases of cirrhosis and 20% of cases of HCC associated with HBV infection. New cases are seen primarily in immigrants from endemic areas, including Africa, central Asia, Eastern Europe, and the Amazon region of Brazil. As many as 13% of HBV carriers are infected with HDV worldwide; principal risk factors are injecting drug use, high-risk sexual behavior, and HIV and HCV coinfections. The diagnosis of hepatitis D is made by detection of antibody to hepatitis D antigen (anti-HDV) and, where available, hepatitis D antigen (HDAg) or HDV RNA in serum.

Asselah T et al. Hepatitis D virus infection. N Engl J Med. 2023;389:58. [PMID: 37407002]

Negro F et al. Hepatitis D: a review. JAMA. 2023;330:2376. [PMID: 37943548]

3. Hepatitis E

HEV is a 27- to 34-nm RNA hepevirus and is the most common cause of acute viral hepatitis worldwide. HEV genotypes 1 and 2 cause acute hepatitis by fecal-oral transmission throughout Central and Southeast Asia. HEV infection should be considered in patients with acute hepatitis after a trip to an endemic area. Although uncommon in the United States, as many as 20% of the population have antibodies to HEV. In industrialized countries, HEV genotypes 3 and 4 may be spread zoonotically, as by swine, and having a pet in the home and consuming undercooked organ meats or infected cow's milk are risk factors. The risk appears to be increased in patients undergoing hemodialysis.

Illness generally is self-limited (no carrier state), but instances of chronic hepatitis with rapid progression to cirrhosis attributed to HEV genotype 3 have been reported in transplant recipients on tacrolimus and, rarely, in persons with HIV infection, preexisting liver disease, or cancer undergoing chemotherapy.

Reported extrahepatic manifestations include arthritis; pancreatitis; thyroiditis; myocarditis; glomerulonephritis; monoclonal gammopathy; thrombocytopenia; aplastic anemia; a variety of neurologic complications, including Guillain-Barré syndrome and neuralgic amyotrophy (which involves the brachial plexuses bilaterally); and hemophagocytic lymphohistiocytosis. In endemic regions, the mortality rate is high (15–25%) in pregnant women.

The diagnosis of acute hepatitis E is made by testing for IgM anti-HEV in serum, although available tests may not be reliable and are not FDA approved. A 3-month course of treatment with oral ribavirin has been reported to induce sustained clearance of HEV RNA from the serum in 78% of patients with persistent HEV infection and may be considered in patients with severe acute hepatitis E. Improved public hygiene reduces the risk of HEV infection in endemic areas. Recombinant vaccines against HEV have shown promise in clinical trials, and one (Hecolin) is approved in China.

Ouyang G et al. Global burden of acute hepatitis E between 1990 and 2019 and projections until 2030. Liver Int. 2024;44:1329. [PMID: 38426633]
Willauer AN et al. Hepatitis E virus: has anything changed? Curr Opin Gastroenterol. 2023;39:169. [PMID: 36976855]

ACUTE LIVER FAILURE

ESSENTIALS OF DIAGNOSIS

- May be fulminant or subfulminant; both forms carry a poor prognosis.
- Acetaminophen and idiosyncratic drug reactions are the most common causes.

General Considerations

Acute liver failure may be fulminant or subfulminant. Fulminant hepatic failure is characterized by the development of hepatic encephalopathy within 8 weeks after the onset of acute liver injury. Coagulopathy (INR 1.5 or higher) is invariably present. Subfulminant hepatic failure occurs when these findings appear between 8 weeks and 6 months after the onset of acute liver injury and carries an equally poor prognosis. This is distinguished from acute-on-chronic liver failure, which refers to acute deterioration in liver function in a person with preexisting liver disease (often caused by infection or alcohol).

An estimated 1600 cases of acute liver failure occur each year in the United States. Toxicity caused by acetaminophen (a direct hepatotoxin) is the most common cause, accounting for at least 45% of cases. Suicide attempts account for almost half of cases of acetaminophen-induced hepatic failure, and unintentional acetaminophen overdoses ("therapeutic misadventures") account for the remainder (often as a result of a decrease in the threshold toxic dose due to chronic alcohol use, fasting, or weight loss surgery). Idiosyncratic drug reactions are the second most common cause of acute liver failure due most commonly to antibiotics, antituberculosis drugs, and antiepileptics, herbal and dietary supplements. Other causes include acute viral hepatitis, poisonous mushrooms (*Amanita phalloides*), shock, heat stroke, Budd-Chiari syndrome, malignancy (most commonly lymphomas), autoimmune hepatitis, Wilson disease, Reye syndrome, and acute fatty liver of pregnancy. The cause is indeterminate in approximately 5% of cases.

Clinical Findings

GI symptoms, systemic inflammatory response, and kidney dysfunction are common. Clinically significant bleeding is uncommon and reflects severe systemic inflammation rather than coagulopathy. Adrenal insufficiency and subclinical myocardial injury (manifesting as an elevated serum troponin I level) often complicate acute liver failure. Jaundice may be absent or minimal early in the course, but laboratory tests show severe hepatocellular damage. In acetaminophen toxicity, serum aminotransferase elevations are often towering (> 5000 U/L); however, acetaminophen is undetectable in plasma in 50% of cases, particularly if patients present in liver failure. In acute liver failure due to microvesicular steatosis (eg, fatty liver of pregnancy), serum aminotransferase elevations may be modest (< 300 U/L). The blood ammonia level is typically elevated and correlates (along with the Model for End-Stage Liver Disease [MELD] score) with the development of encephalopathy and intracranial hypertension; intracranial hypertension rarely develops when the blood ammonia level is < 75 mcmol/L but is more likely when > 200 mcmol/L. The severity of extrahepatic organ dysfunction (as assessed by the Sequential Organ Failure Assessment [SOFA]) also correlates with the likelihood of intracranial hypertension. AKI frequently complicates acute-on-chronic liver failure, which may also be complicated by lung, circulatory, and brain failure.

Treatment

The treatment of acute liver failure is directed toward achieving metabolic and hemodynamic stability. Intravascular volume should be preserved, but large-volume infusions of hypotonic fluids should be avoided. Norepinephrine is the preferred vasopressor; vasopressin may be added for persistent hypotension. Hypoglycemia should be prevented. Continuous renal replacement therapy may be required. To preserve muscle mass and immune function, enteral administration of protein, 1–1.5 g/kg/day, is advised if the patient cannot resume oral intake within 5–7 days. Coagulopathy should generally not be corrected.

Cerebral edema and sepsis are the leading causes of death. Prophylactic antibiotic therapy may decrease the risk of infection but has no effect on survival and is not routinely recommended. Microbiological screening cultures should be obtained for patients admitted to hospital. For suspected sepsis, broad coverage is indicated. Despite a high rate of adrenal insufficiency, corticosteroids do not reduce mortality and may lower overall survival in patients with a high MELD score, although they may reduce vasopressor requirements. Stress gastropathy prophylaxis with an H_2-receptor blocker or PPI is recommended. Administration of N-acetylcysteine (NAC; 140 mg/kg orally followed by 70 mg/kg orally every 4 hours for an additional 17 doses or 150 mg/kg in 5% dextrose intravenously over 15 minutes followed by 50 mg/kg over 4 hours and then 100 mg/kg over 16 hours) prevents acetaminophen toxicity if administered within 12 hours of ingestion and may be beneficial when given up to 72 hours after ingestion. For massive acetaminophen overdoses, treatment with intravenous NAC may need to be extended in duration until the serum aminotransferase levels are declining and serum acetaminophen levels are undetectable. NAC may be helpful in non-acetaminophen related causes. Penicillin G (300,000 to 1 million U/kg/day) or silibinin (silymarin or milk thistle), which is not licensed in the United States, is administered to patients with mushroom poisoning. Nucleoside analogs are recommended for patients with acute liver failure caused by HBV (see Chronic Viral Hepatitis), and intravenous acyclovir is beneficial for herpes simplex virus hepatitis. Acute liver failure due to Wilson disease should prompt transplant evaluation.

Early transfer to a liver transplantation center is essential. The head of the patient's bed should be elevated to 30 degrees. Patients with stage 3 or 4 encephalopathy should be intubated. In some centers, extradural sensors are placed in patients at high risk for intracranial hypertension to monitor intracranial pressure for impending cerebral edema. The goal is to maintain the intracranial pressure below 20 mm Hg and the cerebral perfusion pressure above 70 mm Hg, but sensor placement may be associated with complications. Lactulose and rifaximin are of uncertain value and should not be used routinely. Mannitol, 0.5 g/kg, or 100–200 mL of a 20% solution by intravenous infusion over 10 minutes, may decrease cerebral edema but should be used with caution in patients with advanced CKD. Intravenously administered hypertonic saline to induce hypernatremia (serum sodium concentration of 145–155 mEq/L [145–155 mmol/L]) also may reduce intracranial hypertension. The value of hyperventilation is uncertain. A short-acting barbiturate, propofol, or intravenous boluses of indomethacin, 25 mg, are considered for refractory intracranial hypertension. Hemodialysis raises intracranial pressure and should be avoided, but continuous renal replacement therapy may be used, if necessary, in patients with AKI.

Prognosis

Survival has improved steadily since the 1970s to as high as 75% due to earlier recognition and treatment of acute liver failure with a decline in the frequency of cerebral edema. However, the survival rate in acute liver failure with severe encephalopathy is as low as 20%. The cause of liver injury is the most important determinant of transplant-free survival. In acetaminophen hepatotoxicity, the transplant-free survival is 75%, and no more than 8% of patients undergo liver transplantation. Survival rates are also favorable for hepatitis A, ischemic hepatitis, and pregnancy-related liver disease. For patients with acute liver failure not due to acetaminophen, the outlook is poor in patients younger than 10 and older than 40 years of age and in those with an idiosyncratic drug reaction but appears to be improved when acetylcysteine is administered to patients with stage 1 or 2 encephalopathy. Other adverse prognostic factors are a serum bilirubin level > 18 mg/dL (307.8 mcmol/L), INR > 6.5, onset of encephalopathy more than 7 days after the onset of jaundice, and a low factor V level. For acetaminophen-induced acute liver failure, indicators of a poor outcome are acidosis (pH < 7.3), INR > 6.5, and azotemia (serum creatinine ≥ 3.4 mg/dL [283.22 mcmol/L]), whereas a rising serum α-fetoprotein level predicts a favorable outcome. Other predictors of poor survival in patients with acute liver failure are an elevated blood lactate level (> 3.5 mEq/L [3.5 mmol/L]), elevated blood ammonia level (> 211 mcg/dL [124 mcmol/L]), and possibly hyperphosphatemia (> 3.7 mg/dL [1.2 mmol/L]).

A number of prognostic indices have been proposed: the "BiLE" score, based on the serum bilirubin, serum lactate, and etiology; the Acute Liver Failure Early Dynamic (ALFED) model, based on the arterial ammonia level, serum bilirubin, INR, and hepatic encephalopathy; and the Acute Liver Failure Study Group (ALFSG) index, based on coma grade, INR, serum bilirubin and phosphorous levels, and serum levels of M30, a cleavage product of cytokeratin-18 caspase. The likelihood of transplant-free survival on admission has been reported to be predicted by a regression model that incorporates the grade of hepatic encephalopathy, etiology, vasopressor use, and log transformations of the serum bilirubin and INR. For acetaminophen-induced acute liver failure, a model that incorporates hepatic encephalopathy grade ≥ 3, Glasgow coma score, cardiovascular failure, mean arterial pressure, INR, serum bilirubin, serum AST, serum creatinine, arterial pH, and arterial lactate has shown good discrimination.

In general, emergency liver transplantation is considered for patients with stage 2 to stage 3 encephalopathy or a MELD score of 30.5 or higher (see Cirrhosis) and is associated with a 70% survival rate at 5 years. For mushroom poisoning, liver transplantation should be considered when the interval between ingestion and the onset of diarrhea is < 8 hours or the INR is ≥ 6.0, even in the absence of encephalopathy.

When to Admit

All patients with acute liver failure should be hospitalized.

European Association for the Study of the Liver. EASL Clinical Practice Guidelines on acute-on-chronic liver failure. J Hepatol. 2023;79:461. [PMID: 37364789]

Maiwall R et al. Acute liver failure. Lancet. 2024;404:789. [PMID: 39098320]

Shingina A et al. Acute liver failure guidelines. Am J Gastroenterol. 2023;118:1128. [PMID: 37377263]

CHRONIC VIRAL HEPATITIS

ESSENTIALS OF DIAGNOSIS

- Defined by chronic infection (HBV, HCV, HDV) for longer than 3–6 months.
- Diagnosis is usually made by antibody tests and viral nucleic acid in serum.

General Considerations

Chronic hepatitis is defined as chronic necroinflammation of the liver of more than 3–6 months' duration, demonstrated by persistently elevated serum aminotransferase levels or characteristic histologic findings, often in the absence of symptoms. In many cases, the diagnosis of chronic hepatitis may be made on initial presentation. The causes of chronic hepatitis include viruses (HBV, HCV, and HDV). Chronic hepatitis is categorized based on etiology grade of portal, periportal, and lobular inflammation (minimal, mild, moderate, or severe); and stage of fibrosis (none, mild, moderate, severe, cirrhosis). In the absence of advanced cirrhosis, patients are often asymptomatic or have mild nonspecific symptoms. The WHO has outlined an ambitious strategy for eliminating chronic viral hepatitis by 2030 (by vaccinating against hepatitis B, ensuring blood safety and injection safety, timely birth dosing of hepatitis B vaccine, harm reduction from injecting drug use, and testing and treating persons coinfected with hepatitis viruses and HIV).

1. Chronic Hepatitis B & Chronic Hepatitis D

Clinical Findings & Diagnosis

Chronic hepatitis B afflicts 296 million people worldwide (2 billion overall have been infected; endemic areas include Asia and sub-Saharan Africa) and an estimated 2.4 million (predominantly males) in the United States. It may be identified during the continued follow up of a patient with acute hepatitis B or diagnosed by repeated detection of serum HBsAg, often done in the evaluation of a patient with elevated aminotransferase levels.

Five phases of chronic HBV infection are recognized: immune tolerant phase, immune active (or immune clearance) phase, inactive HBsAg carrier state, reactivated chronic hepatitis B phase, and the HBsAg-negative phase (see Table 18–5). In the *immune tolerant phase* **(HBeAg-positive chronic HBV infection)**, HBeAg and HBV DNA are present in serum and are indicative of active viral replication; however, the serum aminotransferase levels are normal and there is little necroinflammation in the liver. This phase is common in infants and young children whose immature immune system fails to mount an immune response to HBV.

Persons in the immune tolerant phase and those who acquire HBV infection later in life may enter an *immune active phase* **(HBeAg-positive chronic hepatitis B)**, in which aminotransferase and HBV DNA levels *are* elevated and necroinflammation *is* present in the liver. Patients in this phase have a risk of progression to cirrhosis (at a rate of 2–5.5% per year) and of HCC (at a rate of more than 2% per year in those with cirrhosis); low-level IgM anti-HBc is present in serum in about 70%.

Patients enter the *inactive HBsAg carrier state* **(HBeAg-negative chronic HBV infection)** when biochemical improvement follows immune clearance. This improvement coincides with disappearance of HBeAg, the appearance of anti-HbE, reduced HBV DNA levels (< 10^5 copies/mL, or < 20,000 IU/mL) in serum, and integration of the HBV genome into the host hepatocyte genome. Patients in this phase are at a low risk for cirrhosis (if it has not already developed) and for HCC. Those with persistently normal serum aminotransferase levels infrequently have histologically significant liver disease, especially if the HBsAg level is low.

The *reactivated chronic hepatitis B phase* **(HBeAg-negative chronic hepatitis B)** may result from infection by a pre-core mutant of HBV or from spontaneous mutation of the pre-core or core promoter region of the HBV genome during the course of chronic hepatitis caused by wild-type HBV. HBeAg-negative chronic hepatitis B accounts for < 10% of cases of chronic hepatitis B in the United States, up to 50% in southeast Asia, and up to 90% in Mediterranean countries, reflecting in part differences in the frequencies of HBV genotypes. In reactivated chronic hepatitis B, there is a rise in serum HBV DNA levels and possible progression to cirrhosis (at a rate of 8–10% per year), particularly when additional pathogenic variants in the core gene of HBV are present.

In patients with either HBeAg-positive or HBeAg-negative chronic hepatitis B, the risk of cirrhosis and of HCC correlates with the serum HBV DNA level. Other risk factors include advanced age, male sex, alcohol use, cigarette smoking, HBV genotype C, and coinfection with HCV or HDV. HIV coinfection is also associated with an increased frequency of cirrhosis when the CD4 count is low.

Only 1% of treated and untreated patients per year reach the *HBsAg-negative phase*, in which anti-HBe may remain detectable, serum ALT levels are normal, and HBV DNA is undetectable in serum but remains present in the liver. This phase is also referred to as a "**functional cure**." In some cases, anti-HBs appears in serum.

Acute **hepatitis D** infection superimposed on chronic HBV infection may result in severe chronic hepatitis, which may progress rapidly to cirrhosis and may be fatal. Patients with long-standing chronic hepatitis D and B often have inactive cirrhosis and are at risk for decompensation and HCC. The diagnosis is confirmed by detection of anti-HDV or HDAg (or HDV RNA) in serum.

Treatment

Patients with cirrhosis should be treated irrespective of the viral load. Patients with active viral replication (HBeAg and HBV DNA [≥ 10^5 copies/mL, or ≥ 20,000 IU/mL] in serum) and elevated aminotransferase levels (> 2 times the upper limit of normal) may be treated with a nucleoside or nucleotide analog or with pegylated interferon. For patients with ALT < 2 times the upper limit of normal, shared decision-making regarding treatment is suggested and treatment considered for those with fibrosis (≥ F2). Nucleoside and nucleotide analogs are preferred because they are better tolerated and can be taken orally.

For patients who are HBeAg-negative, treatment is considered if HBV DNA level is detectable **or** the serum ALT level is elevated. The threshold for treatment is a serum HBV DNA level of ≥ 10^4 copies/mL, or ≥ 2000 IU/mL. For patients with DNA < 2,000 IU/ml and ALT < 2 times the upper limit of normal, shared decision-making regarding treatment is indicated; treatment may be recommended if there is concern for cirrhosis, age > 40 years, male sex, or the presence of other risk factors for HCC (eg, family history). Therapy is aimed at reducing and maintaining the serum HBV DNA level to the lowest possible levels and normalization of the ALT level, which may lead to histologic improvement.

Patients who wish to discontinue antiviral therapy should meet all of the following criteria: no cirrhosis, HBeAg-negative and anti-HBe positive for ≥ 1 year (if HBeAg-positive at start of treatment), HBV DNA undetectable ≥ 2 years, no HIV or HDV co-infection, and agreement to participate in frequent laboratory monitoring. ALT with HBV DNA levels should be monitored monthly for 6 months, every 3 months for a year and then every 3–6 months thereafter with treatment reinitiated if an increase of the ALT or DNA > 10,000 IU/mL

The available nucleoside and nucleotide analogs—entecavir, tenofovir, lamivudine, adefovir, and telbivudine—differ in efficacy and rates of resistance; however, in HBeAg-positive patients, all achieve an HBeAg-to-anti-HBe seroconversion rate of about 20% at 1 year, with higher rates after more prolonged therapy. The preferred first-line oral agents are entecavir (0.5 mg orally once daily) and tenofovir disoproxil fumarate (300 mg orally once daily). Entecavir is rarely associated with resistance but should not be administered to patients who previously became resistant to lamivudine. Suppression of HBV DNA in serum occurs in nearly all patients treated with entecavir and histologic improvement in 70%. It has caused lactic acidosis when used in patients with decompensated cirrhosis. Tenofovir disoproxil fumarate is equally effective as entacavir and has been used as a first-line agent or when resistance to a nucleoside analog (eg, lamivudine) has developed. Like entecavir, it has a low rate of resistance when used as initial therapy. Long-term use of tenofovir disoproxil fumarate may lead to an elevated serum creatinine level and reduced serum phosphate level (Fanconi-like syndrome) that is reversible with discontinuation of the drug. Tenofovir alafenamide, 25 mg orally daily, is a newer formulation of tenofovir that is associated with a lower rate of renal and bone toxicity than tenofovir disoproxil fumarate and is increasingly preferred over tenofovir disoproxil fumarate. Nucleoside and nucleotide analogs are well tolerated even in patients with decompensated cirrhosis.

Nucleoside analogs are also recommended to prevent reactivation in both inactive HBV carriers and those positive only for anti-HBc prior to the initiation of immunosuppressive therapy (especially B-cell–depleting agents, such as rituximab or moderate- or high-dose corticosteroid therapy) or cancer chemotherapy. In patients infected with both HBV and HIV, antiretroviral therapy, including two drugs active against both viruses (eg, tenofovir plus lamivudine or emtricitabine), has been recommended when treatment of HIV infection is indicated. Tenofovir, telbivudine, and lamivudine have been shown to be safe in pregnant women. Antiviral therapy has been recommended, beginning in the third trimester, when the mother's serum HBV DNA level is 200,000 IU/mL or higher to reduce levels at the time of delivery.

In **chronic hepatitis D**, peginterferon α-2b (1.5 mcg/kg/week for 48 weeks) may lead to normalization of serum aminotransferase levels, histologic improvement, and elimination of HDV RNA from serum in 20–50% of patients, but relapse may occur, and tolerance is poor. Nucleoside and nucleotide analogs are generally not effective in treating chronic hepatitis D.

Prognosis

The sequelae of chronic hepatitis secondary to hepatitis B include cirrhosis, liver failure, and HCC. The 5-year mortality rate is 0–2% in those without cirrhosis, 14–20% in those with compensated cirrhosis, and 70–86% following decompensation. The risk of cirrhosis and HCC correlates with serum HBV DNA levels, and a focus of therapy is to suppress HBV DNA levels < 300 copies/mL (60 IU/mL). In patients with cirrhosis, even low levels of HBV DNA in serum increase the risk of HCC compared with undetectable levels. A risk score (PAGE-B) based on a patient's age, sex, and platelet count has been reported to predict the 5-year risk of HCC in White patients taking entecavir or tenofovir.

Ghany MG et al. AASLD/IDSA Practice Guideline on treatment of chronic hepatitis B. Hepatology. 2026;83:974. [PMID: 41186418]
Pan C et al. Diagnosis and management of hepatitis delta virus infection. Dig Dis Sci. 2023;68:3237. [PMID: 37338616]
Su F et al. Chronic hepatitis B: treat all who are viremic? Clin Liver Dis. 2023;27:791. [PMID: 37778770]
Yardeni D et al. Current best practice in hepatitis B management and understanding long-term prospects for cure. Gastroenterology. 2023;164:42. [PMID: 36243037]

2. Chronic Hepatitis C

Clinical Findings & Diagnosis

Chronic hepatitis C develops in up to 85% of patients with acute hepatitis C. It is clinically indistinguishable from chronic hepatitis due to other causes. Worldwide, 57 million people are infected with HCV, with 1.8% of the US population infected. Peak prevalence in the United States (about 4%) is in persons born between 1945 and 1964. In approximately 40% of cases, serum aminotransferase levels are persistently normal. The diagnosis is confirmed by detection of anti-HCV by EIA. In rare cases of suspected chronic hepatitis C but a negative EIA, HCV RNA is detected by PCR testing. Progression to cirrhosis occurs in 20% of affected patients after 20 years, with an increased risk in men, those who drink more than 50 g of alcohol daily, and those who acquire HCV infection after age 40 years. Persons with chronic hepatitis C and persistently normal serum aminotransferase levels usually have mild chronic hepatitis with slow or absent progression to cirrhosis; however, cirrhosis is present in 10% of these patients. Serum fibrosis testing (eg, FibroSure, FIB-4) or elastography may be used to identify the absence of fibrosis or presence of cirrhosis but is less helpful for determining reversal of fibrosis following treatment.

Treatment

Treatment can be offered to all persons with HCV infection with the goal of achieving a cure. The introduction of direct-acting antiviral agents has rapidly expanded the therapeutic armamentarium (Table 18–6). With the availability of all-oral regimens, the criterion for a sustained virologic response was shortened from 24 weeks to 12 weeks following the completion of treatment. The definition of clearance of HCV RNA requires use of a sensitive

Table 18–6. Direct-acting antiviral agents for HCV infection (in alphabetical order within class).[1]

Agent	Genotype(s)	Dose[2]	Comment
NS3/4A Protease Inhibitors			
Glecaprevir	1–6	300 mg orally once daily	Used in combination with pibrentasvir[3] with or without ribavirin
Grazoprevir	1 and 4	100 mg orally once daily	Used in combination with elbasvir[4]
Voxilaprevir	1–6	100 mg orally once daily	Used in combination with sofosbuvir and velpatasvir[5]
NS5A Inhibitors			
Elbasvir	1 and 4	50 mg orally once daily	Used in combination with grazoprevir (see above)[4]
Ledipasvir	1, 4–6	90 mg orally once daily	Used in combination with sofosbuvir[6]
Pibrentasvir	1–6	120 mg orally once daily	Used in combination with glecaprevir[3] with or without ribavirin
Velpatasvir	1–6	100 mg orally once daily	Used in combination with sofosbuvir,[7] may be used with sofosbuvir and voxilaprevir
NS5B Nucleos(t)ide Polymerase Inhibitor			
Sofosbuvir	1–6	400 mg orally once daily	Used in combination with ribavirin (genotypes 2 and 3) or with simeprevir (genotypes 1 and 4) or with daclatasvir (all genotypes) or with ledipasvir (genotypes 1, 3, and 4) or with velpatasvir (all genotypes) or with velpatasvir and voxilaprevir (all genotypes)

[1]Regimens approved by the FDA as of early 2022.
[2]The preferred regimen and duration of treatment may vary depending on HCV genotype, presence or absence of cirrhosis or CKD, or nonresponse to prior therapy for HCV infection. In selected cases, testing for resistance-associated substitutions may be considered.
[3]Marketed as Mavyret.
[4]Marketed as Zepatier (Merck) for HCV genotypes 1 and 4 infection.
[5]Marketed as Vosevi (Gilead Sciences).
[6]Marketed as Harvoni (Gilead Sciences).
[7]Marketed as Epclusa (Gilead Sciences).

real-time reverse transcriptase-PCR assay to monitor HCV RNA during treatment (the lower limit of quantification should be 25 IU/mL or less, and the limit of detection should be 10–15 IU/mL).

Several types of direct-acting antiviral agents have been developed (Tables 18–6 and 18–7). HCV protease inhibitors ("...previrs") generally have high antiviral potency but differ with respect to the development of resistance (although resistance-associated substitutions in the HCV genome tend not to persist after therapy with these agents is stopped). Examples include glecaprevir and voxilaprevir. Medications in this class are contraindicated in patients with decompensated cirrhosis.

NS5A inhibitors ("...asvirs"), such as ledipasvir and velpatasvir, are characterized by high antiviral potency at picomolar doses. The cross-genotype efficacy of these agents varies.

HCV polymerase inhibitors ("...buvirs") are categorized as nucleoside or nucleotide analog and nonnucleoside polymerase inhibitors. Nucleos(t)ide analogs are active against all HCV genotypes and have a high barrier to resistance. Sofosbuvir has been the sole available agent in this category.

The American Association for the Study of Liver Diseases and the Infectious Diseases Society of America recommended two preferred and highly effective combination

Table 18–7. Preferred FDA-approved oral direct-acting antiviral (DAA) treatment regimens for HCV infection.[1]

Regimen	Indication	Duration of Treatment in Noncirrhotic Treatment-Naïve Patients (weeks)
Glecaprevir and pibrentasvir	Genotypes 1–6 and DAA-experienced genotype 1	8
Sofosbuvir and velpatasvir	Genotypes 1–6, and DAA-experienced genotypes 1b and 2	12
Sofosbuvir, velpatasvir, and voxilaprevir	DAA-experienced genotypes 1–6	–

[1]Based on the American Association for the Study of Liver Diseases/Infectious Diseases Society of America 2018 Guidance. In late 2019, two preferred regimens were proposed: glecaprevir and pibrentasvir for 8 weeks (genotypes 1–6) and sofosbuvir and velpatasvir for 12 weeks (genotypes 1, 2, 4, 5, 6). See HCV Guidance: Recommendation for testing, managing, and treating hepatitis C. http://www.hcvguidelines.org, accessed December 17, 2021.

regimens for genotypes 1–6: glecaprevir plus pibrentasvir for 8–12 weeks and sofosbuvir plus velpatasvir for 12 weeks (Table 18–7). The combination of glecaprevir and pibrentasvir is approved for 8 weeks in treatment-naïve, noncirrhotic or compensated cirrhotic and treatment-experienced noncirrhotic patients, including those coinfected with HIV, and for 12 weeks in treatment-experienced, compensated cirrhotic patients. Sofosbuvir and velpatasvir should also be administered for 12 weeks in treatment-experienced compensated cirrhotic patients. In patients with decompensated cirrhosis, treatment with sofosbuvir, velpatasvir, and ribavirin is recommended for 12 weeks, or for 24 weeks if ribavirin cannot be taken. The combination of glecaprevir and pibrentasvir is also a pangenotypic option for patients with CKD, including those receiving dialysis. The combination of sofosbuvir, velpatasvir, and voxilaprevir for 12 weeks can be used as "rescue" therapy in patients with nonresponse or relapse following treatment with an NS5A-containing regimen. Use of any regimen containing a protease inhibitor is contraindicated in patients with decompensated cirrhosis.

HCV infection is easy to cure with oral direct-acting agents, with expected sustained virologic response rates well above 90%. Treatment failure is infrequent and most likely in patients with hepatocellular carcinoma. Certain cytochrome P450/P-glycoprotein inducing medications, such as carbamazepine, phenytoin, and phenobarbital, contraindicate the use of all HCV direct-acting antiviral regimens.

Prognosis

Chronic hepatitis C is an indolent, often subclinical disease that may lead to cirrhosis and HCC after decades; however, mortality or transplantation rates rise to 5% per year once cirrhosis develops. FIB-4, a risk score combining age, platelet count, and AST-to-ALT ratio, has been proposed as the first test to evaluate the possible presence of cirrhosis, followed by confirmatory elastography. Antiviral therapy has a beneficial effect on mortality, cardiovascular events, type 2 diabetes mellitus, and quality of life, is cost effective, appears to retard and even reverse fibrosis, and reduces (but does not eliminate) the risk of decompensated cirrhosis and HCC in responders with advanced fibrosis. Although mortality from cirrhosis and HCC due to hepatitis C is still substantial, the need for liver transplantation for chronic hepatitis C has declined, and survival after transplantation has improved. The risk of mortality from drug addiction is higher than that for liver disease in patients with chronic hepatitis C. HCV infection appears to be associated with increased cardiovascular mortality, especially in persons with diabetes mellitus and hypertension. Statin use has been reported to be associated with improved virologic response to antiviral therapy and decreased progression of liver fibrosis and frequency of HCC.

When to Refer

- For liver biopsy.
- For antiviral therapy.

When to Admit

For complications of decompensated cirrhosis.

American Association for the Study of Liver Diseases and the Infectious Diseases Society of America. HCV guidance: recommendations for testing, managing, and treatment hepatitis C. Hepatitis C Guidelines. https://www.hcvguidelines.org

Hamill V et al. Mortality rates among patients successfully treated for hepatitis C in the era of interferon-free antivirals: population based cohort study. BMJ. 2023;382:e074001. [PMID: 37532284]

Ogawa E et al. Association of direct-acting antiviral therapy with liver and nonliver complications and long-term mortality in patients with chronic hepatitis C. JAMA Intern Med. 2023;183:97. [PMID: 36508196]

AUTOIMMUNE HEPATITIS

ESSENTIALS OF DIAGNOSIS

- Incidence peaks in fourth to sixth decade of life.
- Chronic hepatitis with high serum globulins and characteristic liver histology.
- Positive ANA or smooth muscle antibody, or both, in most cases in the United States.
- Responds to corticosteroids.

General Considerations

The incidence of autoimmune hepatitis (which is rising) is 2–4 per 100,000 and the prevalence is 26–31 per 100,000. Autoimmune hepatitis can occur in either sex at any age; however, there are bimodal incidence peaks among young and older women. The risk of autoimmune hepatitis is increased in first-degree relatives of affected patients. The cause remains unknown. Patients with autoimmune hepatitis are at increased risk for cirrhosis with an increased risk of HCC.

Clinical Findings

A. Symptoms and Signs

The onset is usually insidious. About 25% of cases present with acute severe hepatitis (and occasionally acute liver failure), and some cases follow a viral illness (such as hepatitis A, Epstein-Barr infection, or measles) or exposure to a drug or toxin (such as nitrofurantoin, minocycline, hydralazine, methyldopa, infliximab, or an immune checkpoint inhibitor). Exacerbations may occur postpartum. Amenorrhea may be a presenting feature, and the frequency of depression appears to be increased. Thirty-four percent of patients, and particularly older patients, are asymptomatic. Examination may reveal a healthy-appearing young person (commonly a woman) with multiple spider telangiectasias, cutaneous striae, acne, hirsutism, and hepatomegaly. Cirrhosis is present in 28–33% of adults at presentation. Extrahepatic features may include arthritis, Sjögren syndrome, thyroiditis, nephritis, and Coombs-positive hemolytic anemia. Concurrent primary biliary cholangitis (PBC) or primary sclerosing cholangitis ("overlap syndrome") may occur in 7–13% and 6–11% of patients, respectively.

B. Laboratory Findings

In acute cases, serum aminotransferase levels may be > 1000 U/L, and the total bilirubin is usually increased. Autoimmune hepatitis has been classified as type I or type II, although the clinical features and response to treatment are similar between the two types. In type I (classic) autoimmune hepatitis, ANA or smooth muscle antibodies (either or both) are often detected in serum. Serum γ-globulin levels are typically elevated (up to 5–6 g/dL [0.05–0.06 g/L]) In acute severe autoimmune hepatitis, ANA is absent and serum IgG is normal, each in up to 39% of cases. Antibodies to soluble liver antigen (anti-SLA) characterize a variant of type I that is marked by severe disease, a high relapse rate after treatment, and absence of the usual antibodies (ANA and smooth muscle antibodies). Type II, seen more often in girls under age 14 in Europe, is characterized by circulating antibodies to liver-kidney microsome type 1 (anti-LKM1) without smooth muscle antibodies or ANA. In some cases, antibodies to liver cytosol type 1 are detected. Type II autoimmune hepatitis can be seen in patients with autoimmune polyglandular syndrome type 1. Of note, elevated levels of ANA or smooth muscle antibodies are not specific for the diagnosis of autoimmune hepatitis, occurring more commonly in other conditions. Liver biopsy is indicated to help establish the diagnosis (interface hepatitis is the diagnostic hallmark) as well as to evaluate disease severity, stage of fibrosis, and to determine the need for treatment.

Simplified diagnostic criteria based on the detection of autoantibodies (1 point for a titer of > 1:40 or 2 points for a titer of > 1:80), elevated IgG levels (1 point for IgG level greater than or equal to upper limit of normal or 2 points for level greater than or equal to 1.1 times upper limit of normal), characteristic histologic features (1 or 2 points depending on how typical the features are), and exclusion of viral hepatitis (2 points) can be useful for diagnosis; a total score of 6 indicates probable and a score of 7 indicates definite autoimmune hepatitis with a high degree of specificity but moderate sensitivity.

Treatment

Prednisone with or without azathioprine improves symptoms; decreases the serum bilirubin, aminotransferase, and γ-globulin levels; and reduces hepatic inflammation. Symptomatic patients with aminotransferase levels elevated tenfold (or fivefold if the serum globulins are elevated at least twofold) are optimal candidates for therapy. Asymptomatic patients with modest enzyme elevations may be considered for therapy depending on the clinical circumstances and histologic severity; however, they usually remain asymptomatic, have either mild hepatitis or inactive cirrhosis on liver biopsy specimens, and have a good long-term prognosis without therapy.

Prednisone is given initially in a dose of 20–40 mg orally daily. Azathioprine, 50 mg orally daily, is generally initiated with prednisone or after 2 weeks of prednisone therapy and is usually well tolerated. A decrease in serum AST levels by 80% after 8 weeks predicts normalization of AST levels at 1 year. For patients with severe autoimmune hepatitis, intravenous corticosteroids or prednisone, 40–60 mg orally daily, is recommended; azathioprine is often started 2 weeks later. In patients with noncirrhotic autoimmune hepatitis, budesonide, 3 mg orally two or three times daily, may be effective for those intolerant of prednisone.

Patients should undergo testing for the genotype of thiopurine methyltransferase prior to treatment with azathioprine to detect those with increased risk of toxicity due to genetic variants. Adjusting the dose of azathioprine based on thiopurine metabolite levels, as in IBD, has been suggested. An alternative to azathioprine is mycophenolate mofetile (1000–2000 mg daily in divided doses). Blood counts are monitored weekly for the first 2 months of therapy and monthly thereafter because of the small risk of bone marrow suppression.

Based on treatment response, the dosage of prednisone is lowered in a stepwise fashion with frequent evaluations of the liver enzymes to confirm stability. Although many patients can remain corticosteroid free, many others require a maintenance dosage of 5–10 mg/day. While symptomatic improvement is often prompt, biochemical improvement is more gradual, with normalization of serum aminotransferase levels after an average of 22 months. Histologic resolution of inflammation lags biochemical remission by 3–6 months. Repeat liver biopsy should be considered in persons with at least 2 years of biochemical remission. Failure of aminotransferase levels to return to normal invariably predicts lack of histologic resolution.

The response rate to therapy with prednisone and azathioprine is 80%, with remission in 65% by 3 years. Older patients are more likely to respond than younger patients and those with hyperbilirubinemia or a high MELD score (12 or higher, see Cirrhosis). Fibrosis may reverse with therapy and rarely progresses after apparent biochemical and histologic remission. Once complete remission is achieved, therapy may be withdrawn, but the subsequent relapse rate is 90% by 3 years. Relapses may be treated in the same manner as the initial episode, with the same remission rate. After successful treatment of a relapse, the patient may continue taking azathioprine (up to 2 mg/kg) or the lowest dose of prednisone (with or without azathioprine [50 mg/day]) needed to maintain aminotransferase levels as close to normal as possible. Another attempt at withdrawing therapy may be considered in patients remaining in long-term remission (≥ 4 years). During pregnancy, hepatitis flares can be treated with prednisone, and maintenance azathioprine does not have to be discontinued. Bone density should be monitored—particularly in patients receiving maintenance corticosteroid therapy—and measures undertaken to prevent or treat osteoporosis (see Chapter 30).

Nonresponses to corticosteroids and azathioprine is reflected by failure of serum aminotransferase levels to decrease by 50% within 4 weeks of prednisone and azathioprine therapy. Nonresponders may be considered for a trial of cyclosporine, tacrolimus, rituximab, or infliximab. Mycophenolate mofetil may be effective in up to 60% of patients refractory to or intolerant of standard therapy but is a known teratogen and must be withdrawn prior to conception. Liver transplantation may be required for treatment failures, in patients with a severe acute presentation with lack of improvement after 2 weeks of corticosteroids, or immediately with acute liver failure.

Prognosis

Long-term mortality of patients with autoimmune hepatitis and cirrhosis is twofold higher than that of the general population despite response to immunosuppressive therapy. Factors that predict the need for liver transplantation or liver-related death include (1) age at presentation ≤ age 20 or ≥ age 60 years, (2) low serum albumin at diagnosis, (3) evidence of cirrhosis at diagnosis, (4) the presence of anti-SLA, or (5) incomplete normalization of the serum AST level after 6 months of treatment. The disease appears to be more aggressive in Black patients than White patients.

When to Refer

- For liver biopsy.
- For immunosuppressive therapy.

When to Admit

- Hepatic encephalopathy.
- INR > 1.6.

European Association for the Study of the Liver. EASL Clinical Practice Guidelines on the management of autoimmune hepatitis. J Hepatol. 2025;83:453. [PMID: 40348684]

Muratori L et al. Diagnosis and management of autoimmune hepatitis. BMJ. 2023;380:e070201. [PMID: 36746473]

Snijders RJALM et al. An open-label randomised-controlled trial of azathioprine vs. mycophenolate mofetil for the induction of remission in treatment-naive autoimmune hepatitis. J Hepatol. 2024;80:576. [PMID: 38101756]

ALCOHOL-ASSOCIATED LIVER DISEASE

ESSENTIALS OF DIAGNOSIS

- Chronic alcohol intake usually exceeds 80 g/day in men and 30–40 g/day in women with alcohol-associated hepatitis or cirrhosis.
- Hepatic steatosis is often asymptomatic.
- Fever, right upper quadrant pain, tender hepatomegaly, and jaundice characterize alcohol-associated hepatitis, but the patient may be asymptomatic.
- AST is usually elevated but infrequently > 300 U/L (6 mckat/L); AST is > ALT, often by a factor of two or more.
- Alcohol-associated hepatitis is the most common precursor of cirrhosis in the United States; however, it is often reversible with abstinence from alcohol.

General Considerations

Excessive alcohol intake can lead to steatosis, hepatitis, and cirrhosis. Validated tools, such as the Alcohol Use Disorders Inventory Test (AUDIT), can be used to identify persons with alcohol abuse and dependence (see Table 1–6). Alcohol-associated hepatitis is characterized by acute or chronic inflammation and parenchymal necrosis of the liver induced by alcohol. It is often a reversible disease but is the most common precursor of cirrhosis in the United States. It is associated with 4–5 times the number of hospitalizations and deaths as hepatitis C. Mortality from alcohol-associated liver disease has been increasing since 1999.

The frequency of alcohol-associated cirrhosis is estimated to be 10–15% among persons who consume over 50 g of alcohol (15 oz wine, 36 oz beer, or 4.5 oz of whiskey) daily for more than 10 years. Women appear to be more susceptible than men, in part because of lower gastric mucosal alcohol dehydrogenase levels, as are patients with bariatric surgery. Over 80% of patients with alcohol-associated hepatitis have been drinking ≥ 5 years before symptoms attributable to liver disease develop; the longer the duration of drinking (10–15 or more years) and the larger the alcohol consumption, the greater the probability of developing alcohol-associated hepatitis and cirrhosis. In individuals who drink alcohol excessively, the rate of ethanol metabolism can be sufficiently high to permit the consumption of large quantities without raising the blood alcohol level > 80 mg/dL.

Clinical Findings

A. Symptoms and Signs

The clinical presentation of alcohol-associated liver disease can vary from asymptomatic hepatomegaly to a rapidly fatal acute illness (acute-on-chronic liver failure) or end-stage cirrhosis. A recent period of heavy drinking, complaints of anorexia and nausea, and the demonstration of hepatomegaly and jaundice strongly suggest the diagnosis. Abdominal pain and tenderness, splenomegaly, ascites, fever, and encephalopathy may be present. Infection, including invasive aspergillosis, is common in patients with severe alcohol-associated hepatitis.

B. Laboratory Findings

In patients with steatosis, mild liver enzyme elevations may be the only laboratory abnormality. In order to accurately differentiate alcohol from other causes, alcohol biomarkers such as serum phosphatidylethanol (PEth) and urine ethylglucoronide are helpful. Anemia (usually macrocytic) may be present. Leukocytosis with a shift to the left is common in patients with severe alcohol-associated hepatitis. Leukopenia is occasionally seen and resolves after cessation of drinking. About 10% of patients have thrombocytopenia related to a direct toxic effect of alcohol on megakaryocyte production or to hypersplenism. AST is usually elevated but infrequently above 400 U/L (6 mckat/L). AST is classically greater than ALT, usually by a factor of two or more; however, this is not always the case. Serum alkaline phosphatase is generally elevated, but seldom more than three times the normal value. Serum bilirubin levels > 10 mg/dL

(171 mcmol/L) and marked prolongation of the prothrombin time (6 seconds or more above control) indicate severe alcohol-associated hepatitis with a mortality rate above 20%. Increased ferritin, transferrin saturation, hepatic iron stores, and sideroblastic anemia are found in many patients with alcohol use disorder. Folic acid deficiency may coexist.

C. Imaging

Imaging studies can detect moderate to severe hepatic steatosis reliably but not inflammation or fibrosis. Ultrasonography helps exclude biliary obstruction and identifies subclinical ascites. CT with intravenous contrast or MRI may be indicated in selected cases to evaluate patients for collateral vessels, space-occupying lesions of the liver, or concomitant disease of the pancreas.

D. Liver Biopsy

Liver biopsy, if done, demonstrates macrovesicular fat and, in patients with alcohol-associated hepatitis, polymorphonuclear infiltration with hepatic necrosis, Mallory (or Mallory-Denk) bodies (alcoholic hyaline), and perivenular and perisinusoidal fibrosis. Micronodular cirrhosis may be present as well. The findings are similar to those of metabolic dysfunction–associated steatohepatitis (MASLD).

Differential Diagnosis

Alcohol-associated hepatitis may be closely mimicked by cholecystitis, choledocholithiasis, and drug toxicity. Other causes of hepatitis or chronic liver disease may be excluded by serologic or biochemical testing, imaging studies, or liver biopsy. Alcohol biomarkers such as PEth are strongly recommended to screen for recent alcohol use.

Treatment

A. General Measures

Abstinence from alcohol is essential. Hospitalized patients should be monitored for alcohol withdrawal; the Clinical Institute Withdrawal Assessment for Alcohol-Revised (CIWA-Ar) is often used in practice. Medications to treat alcohol use disorder should be considered (Chapter 47). Hepatic steatosis is quickly reversible with abstinence. Every effort should be made to provide sufficient amounts of carbohydrates and calories in anorectic patients to reduce endogenous protein catabolism, promote gluconeogenesis, and prevent hypoglycemia. Nutritional support (30–40 [and not < 21.5] kcal/kg with 1.0–1.5 g/kg as protein) improves liver disease, but not necessarily survival, in patients with malnutrition. Intensive enteral nutrition is difficult to implement. The administration of micronutrients—particularly folic acid, thiamine, and zinc—is indicated, especially when deficiencies are noted; glucose administration increases the thiamine requirement and can precipitate Wernicke-Korsakoff syndrome if thiamine is not coadministered.

B. Pharmacologic Measures

Corticosteroids (eg, prednisone up to 40 mg daily or the equivalent) can be considered for up to 1 month. They may reduce short-term (1-month, but not 6-month) mortality in patients with alcohol-associated hepatitis but should be reserved for patients with elevated bilirubin and MELD score between 25 and 39 (see Cirrhosis). Combination with N-acetylcysteine has been reported to further improve 1-month, but not 6-month, survival and reduce the risk of hepatorenal syndrome and infections; the combination may be superior to corticosteroids alone, but more data are needed. Response to corticosteroids should be evaluated by examining the rate of change in the total bilirubin or the Lille score (which includes age, serum creatinine, serum albumin, prothrombin time [or INR], serum bilirubin on admission, and serum bilirubin) at day 4–7, discontinuing therapy in those who are non-responders. For patients who respond, prednisone should be tapered by 10 mg per week without reductions in effectiveness. Medications to treat alcohol use disorder should be considered.

Prognosis

A. Short-Term

The 28-day overall mortality rate for alcohol-associated hepatitis is 20%; however, for patients with compensated cirrhosis, short-term mortality is excellent. For those with decompensated cirrhosis, 90-day mortality is best estimated with the MELD score and long-term mortality with the Child-Pugh score. Unfavorable prognostic factors are older age, a serum bilirubin > 10 mg/dL (171 mcmol/L), hepatic encephalopathy, coagulopathy, azotemia, leukocytosis, sepsis, pneumonia, and other infections, systematic inflammatory response syndrome (which is associated with multiorgan failure), lack of response to corticosteroid therapy, a low serum transferrin level, and, possibly, a paucity of steatosis on a liver biopsy specimen and reversal of portal blood flow by Doppler ultrasonography.

Failure of the serum bilirubin level to decline after 7 (and probably 4) days of treatment with corticosteroids predicts nonresponse and poor long-term survival, as does the Lille model). The MELD score used for cirrhosis and the Glasgow alcohol-associated hepatitis score (based on age, WBC count, BUN, prothrombin time ratio, and bilirubin level) also correlate with mortality from alcohol-associated hepatitis and have higher specificities than the discriminant function and Lille score. For patients admitted to an ICU, the "50% rule" is a useful mnemonic: 50% mortality rate; 50% chance of readmission to the hospital in survivors; and 50% chance of delisting if the patient is listed for liver transplantation.

B. Long-Term

The most important long-term prognostic factor in alcohol-associated liver disease is continued excessive drinking. The overall 10-year survival among all persons with alcohol-associated liver disease is 88% among those who are abstinent compared with 73% in those who experience a relapse in drinking. There is no safe level of drinking in persons with alcohol-associated liver disease or other liver diseases. In many countries, ethyl glucuronide (an ethanol metabolite) in urine or serum PEth is used as a direct marker of continued alcohol consumption.

The 3-year mortality rate of persons who recover from acute alcohol-associated hepatitis is 10 times greater than that of control individuals of comparable age, with a 5-year mortality as high as 85%. Histologically severe disease is associated with continued excessive mortality rates after 3 years, whereas the 3-year death rate is not increased in those with only mild alcohol-associated hepatitis. Complications of portal hypertension (ascites, variceal bleeding, hepatorenal syndrome), coagulopathy, and severe jaundice following recovery from acute alcohol-associated hepatitis also suggest a poor long-term prognosis. Alcohol-associated cirrhosis is a risk factor for bone fractures and HCC.

Liver transplantation can improve outcomes for patients with decompensated cirrhosis, HCC, and alcohol-associated hepatitis. Optimal transplantation candidates have adequate social support, do not smoke, have no psychosis or personality disorder, are adherent to therapy, and have regular appointments with a psychiatrist or psychologist who specializes in addiction treatment. Patients with alcohol-associated liver disease are at higher risk for post-transplant malignancy than those with other types of liver disease because of alcohol and tobacco use.

When to Refer

Refer patients with alcohol-associated hepatitis who require liver biopsy for diagnosis.

When to Admit

- Hepatic encephalopathy.
- INR > 1.6.
- Total bilirubin ≥ 10 mg/dL.
- Inability to maintain hydration.

Amonker S et al. Prevalence of alcohol-associated liver disease: a systematic review and meta-analysis. Hepatol Commun. 2023;7:e0133. [PMID: 37102767]

Hofer BS et al. Alcohol abstinence improves prognosis across all stages of portal hypertension in alcohol-related cirrhosis. Clin Gastroenterol Hepatol. 2023;21:2308. [PMID: 36481475]

Kulkarni AV, et al. Infections in standard or tapered dose of prednisolone for alcohol-associated hepatitis: a randomized trial (STASH Trial). Am J Gastroenterol. 2025;120:2821. [PMID: 40079479]

Mellinger JL et al. Management of alcohol use disorder in patients with chronic liver disease. Hepatol Commun. 2023;7:e00145. [PMID: 37314739]

DRUG- & TOXIN-INDUCED LIVER INJURY

ESSENTIALS OF DIAGNOSIS

- Drug-induced liver injury can mimic viral hepatitis, biliary tract obstruction, or other types of liver disease.
- Clinicians must inquire about the use of many therapeutic agents, including over-the-counter "natural" and herbal and dietary supplements, in any patient with liver disease.

General Considerations

Many therapeutic agents may cause drug-induced liver injury, with jaundice occurring in 30% of cases and up to 10% of patients dying or undergoing liver transplantation within 6 months of onset. In any patient with liver disease, the clinician must inquire carefully about the use of potentially hepatotoxic drugs or exposure to hepatotoxins, including over-the-counter herbal and dietary supplements. A useful resource is the **NIH LiverTox website**; several causality assessment tools are also available. The medications most commonly implicated are antibiotics because of their widespread use. In some cases, coadministration of a second agent may increase the toxicity of the first (eg, isoniazid and rifampin, acetaminophen and alcohol, combinations of immune checkpoint inhibitors). The diagnosis often depends on exclusion of other causes of liver disease. A relationship between increased serum ALT levels in premarketing clinical trials and postmarketing reports of hepatotoxicity has been identified. Except for drugs used to treat tuberculosis and HIV infection, and possibly azithromycin, the risk of hepatotoxicity is not increased in patients with preexisting cirrhosis, but hepatotoxicity may be more severe and the outcome worse when it does occur. Older persons may be at higher risk for hepatotoxicity from certain agents, such as amoxicillin-clavulanic acid, isoniazid, and nitrofurantoin, and more likely to have persistent and cholestatic, rather than hepatocellular, injury compared with younger persons. Drug toxicity may be categorized based on pathogenesis or predominant histologic appearance (although a liver biopsy is often unnecessary). The **R value** (R = ALT/ULN divided by Alkaline phosphatase/ULN) is used to categorize idiosyncratic drug hepatotoxicity as hepatocellular (R value 5 or higher), mixed (R value between 2 and 5), or cholestatic (R value < 2). Drug-induced liver injury can mimic viral hepatitis, biliary tract obstruction, vanishing bile duct syndrome, or other types of liver disease (and vice versa). The development of jaundice in a patient with serum aminotransferase levels at least three times the upper limit of normal predicts a mortality rate of at least 10% ("Hy's Law"). A model based on the presence of comorbidities, the MELD score, and serum albumin has been reported to predict 6-month mortality. Patients with jaundice or an INR ≥ 1.5 should be referred for subspecialty care.

Categorization by Pathogenesis

A. Direct Hepatotoxicity

Liver toxicity caused by this group of drugs is characterized by dose-related severity, a latent period following exposure, and individual susceptibility. One example is acetaminophen (the toxicity of which may be estimated by the Rumack-Matthew nomogram), which is enhanced by fasting-induced depletion of glutathione and long-term alcohol use–induced depletion of glutathione and induction of P450 2E1; in contrast, acetaminophen toxicity may be reduced by statins, fibrates, NSAIDs, and acetylcysteine treatment. Other examples include alcohol, *Amanita phalloides* mushrooms, carbon tetrachloride, chloroform, heavy metals, mercaptopurine, niacin, plant alkaloids, phosphorus, pyrazinamide, tetracyclines, tipranavir, valproic acid, and vitamin A.

B. Idiosyncratic Reactions

Except for acetaminophen, most severe hepatotoxicity is idiosyncratic. Reactions of this type are (1) sporadic, (2) not related to dose above a general threshold of 100 mg/day, and (3) occasionally associated with features suggesting an allergic reaction, such as fever and eosinophilia (including drug rash with eosinophilia and systemic symptoms [DRESS] syndrome), which may be associated with a favorable outcome. Drug-induced liver injury may be observed during postmarketing surveillance but not during preclinical trials. Examples include abacavir, abeparvovec, alemtuzumab, atabecestat, amiodarone, aspirin, carbamazepine, chloramphenicol, dapsone, diclofenac, disulfiram, duloxetine, ezetimibe, flavocoxid (a "medical food"), fluoroquinolones, flutamide, halothane, isoniazid, ketoconazole, lamotrigine, methyldopa, natalizumab, nevirapine, oxacillin, phenytoin, pyrazinamide, quinidine, remdesivir, rivaroxaban, streptomycin, temozolomide, thiazolidinediones, tolvaptan, and perhaps tacrine. Statins, like all cholesterol-lowering agents, may cause serum aminotransferase elevations but rarely cause true hepatitis, and even more rarely cause acute liver failure, and are not contraindicated in patients with liver disease. Most acute idiosyncratic drug-induced liver injury is reversible with discontinuation of the offending agent. Risk factors for chronicity (longer than 1 year) are older age, dyslipidemia, and severe acute injury.

C. Indirect Hepatotoxicity

Indirect hepatotoxicity refers to liver injury that results when use of a drug leads to exacerbation of preexisting liver disease. An example is a flare of HBV infection in the setting of immunosuppressive therapy for a nonhepatic autoimmune disease.

Categorization by Histopathology

A. Cholestatic Injury

1. Noninflammatory—Drug-induced cholestasis results from inhibition or genetic deficiency of various hepatobiliary transporter systems. The following drugs cause cholestasis: anabolic steroids containing an alkyl or ethinyl group at carbon 17, azathioprine, cetirizine, cyclosporine, diclofenac, estrogens, febuxostat, indinavir (increased risk of indirect hyperbilirubinemia in patients with Gilbert syndrome), mercaptopurine, methyltestosterone, tamoxifen, temozolomide, and ticlopidine.

2. Inflammatory—The following drugs cause inflammation of portal areas with bile duct injury (cholangitis [and, in some cases, bile duct loss or predominantly large-duct injury]), often with allergic features such as eosinophilia: amoxicillin-clavulanic acid (among the most common causes of drug-induced liver injury), azathioprine, azithromycin, captopril, celecoxib, cephalosporins, chlorothiazide, chlorpromazine, erythromycin, mercaptopurine, pazopanib, penicillamine, prochlorperazine, semisynthetic penicillins (eg, cloxacillin), sulfadiazine, and temozolomide. Ketamine abuse may cause secondary biliary cirrhosis. Cholestatic and mixed cholestatic-hepatocellular toxicity is more likely than pure hepatocellular toxicity to lead to chronic liver disease.

B. Hepatocellular Injury

Medications that may result in acute or chronic hepatitis that is histologically and, in some cases, clinically similar to autoimmune hepatitis include minocycline and nitrofurantoin, most commonly, as well as aspirin, isoniazid (increased risk in HBV and HCV carriers), methyldopa, NSAIDs, propylthiouracil, terbinafine, TNF inhibitors, and varenicline. Histologic features that favor a drug cause include portal tract neutrophils and hepatocellular cholestasis. Hepatitis also can occur in patients taking cocaine, diclofenac, dimethyl fumarate, efavirenz, imatinib mesylate, ipilimumab, nivolumab, and other checkpoint inhibitors, which may also cause cholangitis, methylenedioxymethamphetamine (MDMA; ecstasy), nefazodone (has a black box warning for a potential to cause liver failure), nevirapine (like other HIV protease inhibitors, increased risk in HBV and HCV carriers), pioglitazone, ritonavir (greater rate than other HIV protease inhibitors), rosiglitazone, saquinavir, sulfonamides, telithromycin, tocilizumab, and zafirlukast. A variety of alternative remedies (eg, black cohosh, chaparral, garcinia cambogia, germander, green tea extract, Herbalife products, Hydroxycut, jin bu huan, kava, saw palmetto, skullcap, turmeric [particularly when packaged with piperine or black pepper], usnic acid, and other Chinese herbal preparations), in addition to dietary supplements (eg, 1,3-dimethylamylamine in OxyELITE Pro, a weight loss supplement withdrawn from the US market) may also cause hepatocellular injury.

C. Other Reactions

1. Fatty liver—

A. MACROVESICULAR—This type of liver injury may be produced by alcohol, amiodarone, corticosteroids, haloperidol, irinotecan, lomitapide, mipomersen, tamoxifen, vinyl chloride (in exposed workers), zalcitabine, and possibly oxaliplatin.

B. MICROVESICULAR—Often resulting from mitochondrial injury, microvesicular steatosis is associated with aspirin (Reye syndrome), didanosine, linezolid, stavudine, tetracyclines, valproic acid, and zidovudine.

2. Granulomas—Allopurinol, hydralazine, pembrolizumab and other immune checkpoint inhibitors, phenytoin, pyrazinamide, quinidine, quinine, sulfasalazine, and vemurafenib can lead to granulomas and, in some cases, granulomatous hepatitis.

3. Sinusoidal obstruction syndrome (veno-occlusive disease)—This disorder may result from treatment with antineoplastic agents (eg, pre–bone marrow transplant, busulfan, gemtuzumab ozogamicin, inotuzumab ozogamicin, oxaliplatin), mycophenolate mofetil, and pyrrolizidine alkaloids (eg, comfrey).

4. Peliosis hepatis (blood-filled cavities)—Peliosis hepatis may be caused by anabolic steroids and oral contraceptive steroids as well as azathioprine and mercaptopurine, which may also cause nodular regenerative hyperplasia and other forms of liver injury.

5. Nodular regenerative hyperplasia—regenerative hyperplasia may be caused by many therapies, most notably azathioprine (or thioguanine), 5-fluorouracil, and oxaliplatin.

6. Neoplasms—Neoplasms may result from therapy with oral contraceptive steroids, including estrogens (hepatic adenoma but not focal nodular hyperplasia) and vinyl chloride (angiosarcoma).

When to Refer

Refer patients with drug- and toxin-induced hepatitis who have severe disease or synthetic dysfunction, or those who require liver biopsy for diagnosis.

When to Admit

Patients with liver failure should be hospitalized.

Andrade RJ et al. Nomenclature, diagnosis and management of drug-induced autoimmune-like hepatitis (DI-ALH): an expert opinion meeting report. J Hepatol. 2023;79:853. [PMID: 37164270]

Atallah E et al. Risk of liver fibrosis associated with long-term methotrexate therapy may be overestimated. J Hepatol. 2023;78:989. [PMID: 36702175]

Dart RC et al. Management of acetaminophen poisoning in the US and Canada: a consensus statement. JAMA Netw Open. 2023;6:e2327739. [PMID: 37552484]

Fontana RJ et al. AASLD practice guidance on drug, herbal, and dietary supplement-induced liver injury. Hepatology. 2023;77:1036. [PMID: 35899384]

LiverTox. National Institute of Diabetes and Digestive and Kidney Diseases. Updated January 21, 2026. https://www.ncbi.nlm.nih.gov/books/NBK547852/

METABOLIC DYSFUNCTION–ASSOCIATED STEATOTIC LIVER DISEASE

ESSENTIALS OF DIAGNOSIS

- Often asymptomatic.
- Elevated aminotransferase levels, hepatomegaly, or steatosis on ultrasonography.
- Predominantly macrovesicular steatosis with or without inflammation and fibrosis on liver biopsy.

General Considerations

Steatotic liver disease (**SLD**) is the umbrella term for excess hepatic fat. **MASLD** indicates the presence of at least one component of the metabolic syndrome in the setting of SLD: overweight or obesity, type 2 diabetes mellitus, impaired glucose regulation, hypertension, and dyslipidemia (generally reduced HDL). MASLD (formerly NAFLD) is estimated to affect 36% of the US adult population and has increased in incidence at least fivefold since the late 1990s. Even adolescents and young adults may be affected. The principal causes of MASLD are obesity and insulin resistance (including diabetes mellitus) as part of the metabolic syndrome. When women and men with MASLD consume moderate amounts of alcohol (20–50 g/day and 30–60 g/day, respectively), the term **metabolic and alcohol-associated liver disease (MetALD)** is used for this group of patients. The risk of MASLD in persons with metabolic syndrome is 4 to 11 times higher than that of persons without insulin resistance. Nonobese persons (more frequently Asian persons) account for 7–20% of persons with NAFLD and have metabolic profiles characteristic of insulin resistance. Other causes of fatty liver include corticosteroids, amiodarone, diltiazem, tamoxifen, irinotecan, oxaliplatin, antiretroviral therapy, toxins (vinyl chloride, carbon tetrachloride, yellow phosphorus), endocrinopathies such as Cushing syndrome and hypopituitarism, polycystic ovary syndrome, hypothyroidism, hypobetalipoproteinemia and other metabolic disorders, obstructive sleep apnea (with chronic intermittent hypoxia), excessive dietary fructose consumption, malnutrition, starvation and refeeding syndrome, and total parenteral nutrition. The risk of MASLD is increased in persons with psoriasis and appears to correlate with its activity. Soft drink consumption is strongly associated with MASLD. Physical activity protects against the development of MASLD.

In addition to macrovesicular steatosis, histologic features may include focal infiltration by polymorphonuclear neutrophils and Mallory hyalin, a picture indistinguishable from that of alcohol-associated hepatitis and referred to as metabolic dysfunction–associated steatohepatitis (**MASH**), which affects 3–6% of the US population and leads to cirrhosis in approximately 20% of affected persons. In patients with MASLD, older age, obesity, and diabetes mellitus are risk factors for advanced hepatic fibrosis and cirrhosis, whereas coffee consumption reduces the risk. The frequency and severity of MASLD is greater in men than in women during reproductive age, but after menopause the frequency is higher in women than men, suggesting that estrogen is protective. However, in women, synthetic hormone use (oral contraceptives and hormone replacement therapy) increases the histologic severity of MASH. Persons with MASLD are at increased risk for CVD, CKD, and colorectal cancer.

Clinical Findings

A. Symptoms and Signs

Most patients with MASLD are asymptomatic or have mild right upper quadrant discomfort. Hepatomegaly is present in up to 75% of patients, but stigmata of chronic liver disease are uncommon. Signs of portal hypertension generally signify advanced liver fibrosis or cirrhosis.

B. Laboratory Findings

Laboratory studies may show mildly elevated aminotransferase and alkaline phosphatase levels; however, laboratory values may be normal in up to 80% of persons with hepatic steatosis. In contrast to alcohol-associated liver disease, the ratio of ALT to AST is almost always > 1.0 in MASLD, but it decreases, often to < 1.0, as advanced fibrosis and cirrhosis develop. ANA or smooth muscle antibodies and an elevated serum ferritin level may each be detected in 30% of patients with MASH.

For the assessment of fibrosis, noninvasive clinical scoring systems now are generally preferred to liver biopsy. Because of its simplicity, the FIB-4 score is often used. It is based on age, platelet count, and serum AST and ALT levels, and it should be repeated every 1–2 years. When the FIB-4 score is elevated, elastography to assess fibrosis stage may be indicated. Other risk scores include the SAFE (steatosis-associated fibrosis estimator), based on age, BMI, diabetes, platelets, AST, ALT, and globulins and LiverRisk. The Enhanced Liver Fibrosis (ELF) score, consisting of tissue inhibitor of metalloproteinase 1, amino-terminal propeptide of type III procollagen, and hyaluronic acid, shows good correlation with fibrosis stage.

C. Imaging

Macrovascular steatosis may be demonstrated on ultrasonography, CT, or MRI. However, imaging does not distinguish steatosis from steatohepatitis or detect fibrosis. Where available, the controlled attenuation parameter measured during transient elastography or MRI-proton density fat fraction allows hepatic fat content to be quantitated. Fibrosis can be estimated using elastography; results may be less accurate in obese than in nonobese persons.

D. Liver Biopsy

Percutaneous liver biopsy has been the standard approach to assessing the degree of inflammation and fibrosis. The histologic spectrum of MASLD includes fatty liver, isolated portal fibrosis, steatohepatitis, and cirrhosis. The risks of the procedure must be balanced against the impact of the added information on management decisions and assessment of prognosis. In most patients, noninvasive approaches to the assessment of fibrosis are now preferred, with liver biopsy reserved for when noninvasive measures are discordant or require confirmation. In addition, when aminotransferase levels are higher than typical for MASLD (ie, ALT > 200 IU/L), noninvasive testing is less reliable, and biopsy may be needed to exclude other causes of liver disease. Liver biopsy is generally not recommended in asymptomatic persons with unsuspected hepatic steatosis detected on imaging but normal liver biochemistry test results.

Treatment

Treatment consists of lifestyle changes to remove or modify the offending factors often in the context of a multidisciplinary clinic. Weight loss, dietary caloric and fructose restriction, increased dietary fiber, and moderate exercise often lead to improvement in liver biochemical tests and steatosis in obese patients with MASLD. A useful rule is that loss of 5% body weight leads to reduced steatosis; of 7.5% leads to reduced inflammation; and of 10% leads to reduced fibrosis. Exercise may reduce liver fat with minimal or no weight loss and no reduction in ALT levels. Resistance training and aerobic exercise are equally effective in reducing hepatic fat content in patients with MASLD and type 2 diabetes mellitus. Avoidance of alcohol is recommended.

Various drugs for the treatment of MASH are under study. In 2024, the FDA granted accelerated approval to resmetirom, a thyroid hormone receptor-β-agonist, for patients with MASH and fibrosis. In 2025, semaglutide, a glucagon-like protein-1 analogs, was approved for MASH based on its ability to improve the resolution of MASH and fibrosis. Vitamin E 800 IU/day (to reduce oxidative stress) appears to be of benefit in patients who do not have diabetes mellitus. There is controversy as to whether vitamin E increases the risk of prostate cancer in men and hemorrhagic stroke; moreover, the benefit is often not sustained. Statins are not contraindicated in persons with MASLD and may protect against histologic progression in some patients. Bariatric surgery may be considered in patients with a BMI > 35 and leads to histologic regression of MASH in most patients. Liver transplantation is indicated in appropriate candidates with advanced cirrhosis caused by MASH.

Prognosis

Hepatic steatosis often has a benign or slowly progressive course and is readily reversible with discontinuation of alcohol and treatment of other underlying conditions. If untreated, fibrosis progresses at an average rate of one stage every 14 years, with 20% of patients progressing more rapidly. MASH may be associated with hepatic fibrosis in 40% of cases with progression at a rate of one stage every 7 years; cirrhosis develops in 9–25%; and decompensated cirrhosis occurs in 30–50% of cirrhotic patients over 10 years. The course may be more aggressive in diabetic persons than in nondiabetic persons. In the United States, MASLD is associated with 8% of all-cause mortality and more than one-third of deaths associated with liver disease and with diabetes mellitus. Mortality is increased in patients with MASLD, correlates with fibrosis stage, and is most often the result of CVD. In the general population, both excess adiposity and reduced activity are significant predictors of liver-related mortality. Obesity is an independent risk factor for death from cirrhosis of any cause. HCC is a complication of cirrhosis caused by MASH, as it is for other causes of cirrhosis, and has been reported even in the absence of cirrhosis. MASH accounts for a substantial percentage of cases labeled as cryptogenic cirrhosis and can recur following liver transplantation.

When to Refer

Refer patients with MASLD who require liver biopsy for diagnosis and those with evidence of advanced fibrosis for management.

Harrison SA et al. A phase 3, randomized, controlled trial of resmetirom in NASH with liver fibrosis. N Engl J Med. 2024; 390:497. [PMID: 38324483]

Noureddin M et al. Efruxifermin in compensated liver cirrhosis caused by MASH. N Engl J Med. 2025;392:2413. [PMID: 40341827]

Rinella ME et al. AASLD Practice Guidance on the clinical assessment and management of nonalcoholic fatty liver disease. Hepatology. 2023;77:1797. [PMID: 36727674]

Sanyal Aj et al. Phase 3 Trial of semaglutide in metabolic dysfunction-associated steatohepatitis. N Engl J Med. 2025; 392:2089. [PMID: 40305708]

Verrastro O et al. Bariatric-metabolic surgery versus lifestyle intervention plus best medical care in non-alcoholic steatohepatitis (BRAVES): a multicentre, open-label, randomised trial. Lancet. 2023;401:1786. [PMID: 37088093]

Wattacheril JJ et al. AGA Clinical Practice Update on the role of noninvasive biomarkers in the evaluation and management of nonalcoholic fatty liver disease: expert review. Gastroenterology. 2023;165:1080. [PMID: 37542503]

CIRRHOSIS

ESSENTIALS OF DIAGNOSIS

- Result of injury that leads to both fibrosis and regenerative nodules.
- May be reversible if cause is removed.
- The clinical features result from hepatic cell dysfunction, portosystemic shunting, and portal hypertension.

General Considerations

Cirrhosis is the result of hepatocellular injury with inflammation that leads to both fibrosis and regenerative nodules throughout the liver. The prevalence is 0.27%, with an estimated 1.5 billion persons having chronic liver disease and 2.14 million liver-related deaths worldwide (11th leading cause). Hospitalization rates for cirrhosis and portal hypertension are rising in the United States, and patients with chronic liver disease have longer hospital stays, more readmissions, and less access to post-acute care than patients with other chronic diseases. Causes include alcohol; MASLD; chronic viral hepatitis; drug toxicity; autoimmune and metabolic liver diseases; and miscellaneous disorders. Celiac disease appears to be associated with an increased risk of cirrhosis. Many patients have more than one risk factor (eg, chronic hepatitis and alcohol use) and likely genetic predisposition. Clinically, cirrhosis is considered to progress through three stages that correlate with the thickness of fibrous septa: compensated, compensated with portal hypertension, and decompensated (ascites, variceal bleeding, encephalopathy, or jaundice).

A diagnosis of acute-on-chronic liver failure should be made in a patient with cirrhosis and acute decompensation (new or worsening ascites, GI hemorrhage, overt encephalopathy, worsening nonobstructive jaundice, or bacterial infection associated with other organ failure). Precipitating factors include infections, hemodynamic instability, heavy alcohol use, and drug hepatotoxicity.

Clinical Findings

A. Symptoms and Signs

The clinical features of cirrhosis result from hepatocyte dysfunction, portosystemic shunting, and portal hypertension. Patients may have no symptoms for long periods. The onset of symptoms may be insidious or, less often, abrupt. Fatigue, disturbed sleep, muscle cramps, and weight loss are common. In advanced cirrhosis, anorexia is usually present and may be extreme, with associated nausea and occasional vomiting, as well as reduced muscle strength and exercise capacity. Abdominal pain may be present and is related either to hepatic enlargement and stretching of Glisson capsule or to the presence of ascites. Abdominal wall hernias occur in 20% of persons with cirrhosis. Menstrual abnormalities (usually amenorrhea), erectile dysfunction, loss of libido, sterility, and gynecomastia may occur. Hematemesis is the presenting symptom in 15–25%. The risk of falls is increased in patients with cirrhosis, and the falls are associated with mortality.

Skin manifestations consist of spider telangiectasias (invariably on the upper half of the body), palmar erythema (mottled redness of the thenar and hypothenar eminences), Dupuytren contractures, and Terry nails. Evidence of vitamin deficiencies (glossitis and cheilosis) is common. Weight loss, wasting (due to sarcopenia), and the appearance of chronic illness are present in advanced cirrhosis. Jaundice—usually not an initial sign—is mild at first, increasing in severity during the later stages of the disease. In 70% of cases, the liver is enlarged, palpable, and firm if not hard and has a sharp or nodular edge; the left lobe may predominate. Splenomegaly is present in 35–50% of cases and is associated with an increased risk of complications of portal hypertension. The superficial veins of the abdomen and thorax are dilated, reflecting the intrahepatic obstruction to portal blood flow, as do rectal varices. The abdominal wall veins fill from below when compressed. Ascites, pleural effusions, peripheral edema, and ecchymoses are late findings. Ascites is classified as grade 1, or mild, when it is detectable only by ultrasound; grade 2, or moderate, when associated with symmetrical abdominal distention; and grade 3, or gross, when associated with marked abdominal distention. Encephalopathy is graded as covert (poor sleep, loss of balance, and deficits in executive function) and overt (asterixis, tremor, dysarthria, delirium, drowsiness, and, ultimately, coma).

B. Laboratory Findings

Laboratory abnormalities are either absent or minimal in early or compensated cirrhosis. Anemia, a frequent finding, is often macrocytic; causes include suppression of erythropoiesis by alcohol as well as folate deficiency, hemolysis, hypersplenism, and occult or overt blood loss from the GI tract. The WBC count may be low, reflecting hypersplenism, or high, suggesting infection. Thrombocytopenia, the most common cytopenia in cirrhotic patients, is secondary to alcohol-induced marrow suppression, sepsis, folate deficiency, or splenic sequestration. Prolongation of the prothrombin time may result from reduced levels of hepatically synthesized clotting factors. However, bleeding risk correlates poorly with the prothrombin time because of concomitant increases in factor VIII and von Willebrand factor, varying degrees of platelet activation, and abnormalities of fibrinolysis. In general, patients with compensated cirrhosis are more likely to experience spontaneous thrombotic events than bleeding.

Blood chemistries reflect hepatocellular injury and dysfunction, manifested by modest elevations of AST and alkaline phosphatase and progressive elevation of the bilirubin. Serum albumin decreases as the disease progresses; γ-globulin levels are increased and may be as high as in autoimmune hepatitis. In cirrhosis of all causes, the following are common: (1) blunted cardiac inotropic and chronotropic responses to exercise, stress, and drugs, (2) prolongation of the QT interval in the setting of a hyperkinetic circulation, and (3) systolic and diastolic ventricular dysfunction in the absence of other known causes of cardiac disease ("cirrhotic cardiomyopathy"). Relative adrenal insufficiency appears to be common in patients with advanced cirrhosis, even in the absence of sepsis, and in those with acute-on-chronic liver failure.

C. Imaging

Ultrasonography is helpful for assessing liver size and detecting ascites or hepatic nodules, including small HCCs. Together with a Doppler study, it may establish patency of the splenic, portal, and hepatic veins. Hepatic nodules are characterized further by contrast-enhanced CT or MRI. Nodules indeterminant for malignancy may be biopsied under ultrasound or CT guidance.

The most important imaging modality for establishing the presence of cirrhosis and further stratifying the risk of progression is elastography. Using mechanical (vibration) or sound-based shear waves, modified ultrasounds can calculate the stiffness of the liver in kilopascals (kPa). The most widely validated method is called 'vibration-controlled transient elastography'; it measures stiffness at a fixed depth from the probe when placed over the liver between the ribs. A helpful rule to interpret the stiffness is 'the rule of 5': 5 kPa is normal, < 10 rules out cirrhosis, 15 generally indicates cirrhosis, and values > 20 may indicate cirrhosis with portal hypertension. Importantly, liver stiffness derived from MRI (magnetic resonance elastography, MRE) uses a *different* scale in which 5 kPa is strongly suggestive of cirrhosis. MRE is not as widely validated but can be considered when elastography fails to obtain a reliable estimate. All forms of elastography can yield false positive results in the setting of inflammation (eg, ALT > 120 IU/L) and central venous congestion.

D. Liver Biopsy

Liver biopsy may be useful to diagnose cirrhosis and to suggest the likely underlying cause. Liver biopsy commonly is performed by percutaneous US-guided technique but may be performed by US-guided endoscopy or laparoscopy. In patients with severe coagulopathy, a transjugular approach may be used, which can simultaneously assess for the presence of portal hypertension. Biopsy is not needed when the history (eg, long term alcohol use) and imaging (eg, nodular liver with intra-abdominal varices) are consistent with a diagnosis of cirrhosis.

In clinical practice, noninvasive clinical scoring systems for fibrosis, such as the FIB-4 index (based on age, platelet count, and serum AST and ALT levels) and elastography, have generally replaced biopsy for the diagnosis or exclusion of cirrhosis. The combination of increased liver stiffness (on transient elastography) and a platelet count < 150,000/mcL (150 × 109/L) is an indicator of clinically significant portal hypertension and an indication to initiate β-blockers or screen for esophageal varices; conversely, low liver stiffness and high platelets can be used to forego endoscopic screening.

E. Other Tests

Esophagogastroduodenoscopy confirms the presence of varices and detects specific causes of bleeding in the esophagus, stomach, and proximal duodenum. In selected cases, wedged hepatic vein pressure measurement may establish the presence and cause of portal hypertension.

Differential Diagnosis

The most common causes of cirrhosis are alcohol, chronic HCV or HBV infection, and MASLD. Hemochromatosis is the most commonly identified genetic disorder. Other diseases associated with cirrhosis include Wilson disease, α_1-antitrypsin (α_1-antiprotease) deficiency, and celiac disease. PBC occurs more frequently in women than men. Secondary biliary cirrhosis may result from chronic biliary obstruction due to a stone, stricture, or neoplasm. HF and constrictive pericarditis may lead to hepatic fibrosis ("cardiac cirrhosis") complicated by ascites. Hereditary hemorrhagic telangiectasia can lead to portal hypertension because of portosystemic shunting and nodular transformation of the liver as well as high-output HF. Many cases of cirrhosis are "cryptogenic," in which unrecognized MASLD may play a role. Some patients may have "non-cirrhotic portal hypertension" due to disorders of hepatic architecture and vasculature caused by genetic mutations, hematological conditions, or medication exposures.

Complications

Varices, ascites, and encephalopathy may arise when there is clinically significant portal hypertension (hepatic venous pressure gradient > 10 mm Hg). Upper GI tract bleeding may occur from varices, gastric antral vascular ectasias, portal hypertensive gastropathy, or gastroduodenal ulcer (see Chapter 17). Portal vein thrombosis is common in cirrhosis and it may result in variceal bleeding or intestinal infarction. Infections are common in cirrhosis. These include nosocomial infections, which may include spontaneous bloodstream infections, UTIs, pulmonary infections, spontaneous bacterial peritonitis, *Clostridioides difficile* infection, and intervention-related infections. Osteoporosis occurs in 12–55% of patients with cirrhosis.

The risk of HCC is increased greatly in persons with cirrhosis (see Chapter 43).

Treatment

A. General Measures

Most important is abstinence from alcohol. The diet should be palatable, with adequate calories (20–40 kcal/kg body weight per day depending on the patient's BMI and the presence or absence of malnutrition) and protein (1.2–1.5 g/kg ideal body weight/day) and, if there is fluid retention, no added sodium. If hepatic decompensation is present, prolonged fasting must be avoided with provision of late-night snacks and breakfast on awakening that include ≥ 200 kcal and protein. In the presence of hepatic encephalopathy, protein needs should be monitored and protein intake maintained at 60–80 g/day (ie, not restricted). Vitamin supplementation is desirable. Muscle cramps may be helped by sips of pickle juice (at cramp onset), taurine (1000 mg twice daily), or intravenous albumin. In patients with clinically significant portal hypertension, carvedilol, a nonselective β-receptor antagonist with α_1-blocking activity, appears to reduce the frequency of decompensating events, although it may lead to hypotension, particularly in patients with decompensated cirrhosis. Patients with cirrhosis should receive the HAV, HBV, pneumococcal, COVID-19, and influenza vaccines. Liver transplantation in appropriate candidates is curative. Care coordination and palliative care, when appropriate, have been shown to improve outcomes and reduce readmission rates.

B. Treatment of Complications

1. Ascites and edema—Ascites in patients with cirrhosis results from portal hypertension (increased hydrostatic pressure), hypoalbuminemia (decreased oncotic pressure), and peripheral vasodilatation with resulting increases in renin and angiotensin levels and sodium retention by the kidneys and increased aldosterone secretion.

Diagnostic paracentesis is indicated for patients who have new ascites or who have been hospitalized for a complication of cirrhosis to diagnose possible bacterial peritonitis. When performed within 12 hours of admission, it reduces mortality. Even in asymptomatic outpatient cirrhotic patients with ascites, the frequency of bacterial peritonitis is 2%. Serious complications of paracentesis, including bleeding, infection, or bowel perforation, occur in 1.6% of procedures. Nonetheless, pre-paracentesis prophylactic transfusions are not indicated in patients with high INR or low platelets. Complications occur more commonly in those with therapeutic (versus diagnostic) paracentesis and those with Child-Pugh class C cirrhosis or acute kidney injury. In addition to a cell count and culture, the ascitic albumin level should be determined: a serum-ascites albumin gradient (serum albumin minus ascitic fluid albumin) ≥ 1.1 suggests portal hypertension; total protein levels < 2.5 g/dL suggest that cardiac causes of ascites are less likely. An elevated ascitic adenosine deaminase level is suggestive of tuberculous peritonitis, but the sensitivity of the test is reduced in patients with portal hypertension. Occasionally, cirrhotic ascites is chylous (rich in triglycerides); other causes of chylous ascites are malignancy, tuberculosis, and recent abdominal surgery or trauma.

In patients with cirrhotic ascites, the urinary sodium concentration is often < 10 mEq/L (10 mmol/L). Free water excretion is impaired in cirrhosis, and hyponatremia may develop. Dietary sodium intake may initially be restricted to 2000 mg/day but liberalized slightly after diuresis ensues. Many who restrict sodium, also miss their calorie and protein targets, which must be avoided. NSAIDs, ACE inhibitors, and angiotensin II antagonists reduce renal perfusion and should be avoided. In patients with significant hyponatremia (< 125 mEq/L [125 mmol/L]) despite adjustments in diuretics, fluid intake is often restricted to 1000 mL/day. Treatment of severe hyponatremia (< 120 mEq/L [120 mmol/L]) with vasopressin receptor antagonists (eg, tolvaptan) can be considered, but is expensive, causes thirst, and does not improve survival. Oral tolvaptan has a black box warning for potential hepatotoxicity.

A. Diuretics—Spironolactone, generally in combination with furosemide, should be used. The dose of spironolactone is initially 100 mg orally daily and may be increased by 100 mg every 3–5 days (up to a maximal conventional daily dose of 400 mg/day, although higher doses have been used) until diuresis is achieved, typically preceded by a rise in the urinary sodium concentration. Monitoring for hyperkalemia is important. In patients who cannot tolerate spironolactone because of side effects, such as painful gynecomastia, amiloride (another potassium-sparing diuretic) may be used in a starting dose of 5–10 mg orally daily. Another reasonable alternative is eplerenone (starting dose 50–100 mg twice daily), which has a shorter half-life and lower potency than spironolactone. Hypokalemia is avoided and diuresis is augmented by the addition of a loop diuretic such as furosemide in an initial dose of 40 mg daily. This potent diuretic will maintain its effect even with a falling GFR with resulting prerenal azotemia. The dose of oral furosemide is increased in concert with spironolactone and ranges from 40 mg/day to 160 mg/day; blood pressure, urinary output, mental status, and serum electrolytes (especially potassium) should be monitored in patients taking these drugs. The goal of weight loss in the ascitic patient without associated peripheral edema should be no more than 1–1.5 lb/day (0.5–0.7 kg/day).

B. Large-volume paracentesis—In patients with massive ascites and respiratory compromise or ascites that is refractory to diuretics ("diuretic resistant") or that produces intolerable diuretic side effects ("diuretic intractable") (affecting 5–10% of patients with cirrhosis and ascites), large-volume paracentesis (> 5 L) is effective. Intravenous albumin concomitantly at a dosage of 6–8 g/L of ascites fluid removed protects the intravascular volume and may prevent post-paracentesis circulatory dysfunction, although the usefulness of this costly practice is debated. If possible, diuretics should be continued in the hope of preventing recurrent ascites.

C. Transjugular intrahepatic portosystemic shunt (TIPS)—TIPS is an effective treatment of variceal bleeding refractory to standard therapy (eg, endoscopic band ligation) and has shown benefit in the treatment of severe refractory ascites, specifically in patients on maximum diuretic therapy who require at least three large-volume paracenteses per year. The technique involves insertion of an expandable metal stent between a branch of the hepatic vein and the portal vein over a catheter inserted via the internal jugular vein. Increased renal sodium excretion and control of ascites refractory to diuretics can be achieved in about 75% of selected cases. The success rate is lower in patients with underlying CKD and diastolic dysfunction. TIPS may be considered for refractory hepatic hydrothorax (translocation of ascites across the diaphragm to the pleural space); video-assisted thoracoscopy with pleurodesis using talc may be effective when TIPS is contraindicated. Complications of TIPS include hepatic encephalopathy in 20–30% of cases, infection, shunt stenosis in up to 60% of cases, and shunt occlusion in up to 30% of cases when bare stents are used; polytetrafluoroethylene-covered stents are associated with long-term patency rates of 80–90%. Long-term patency often requires periodic shunt revisions. In most cases, patency can be maintained by balloon dilation, local thrombolysis, or placement of an additional stent. TIPS is particularly useful in patients who require short-term control of variceal bleeding or ascites until liver transplantation can be performed. In patients with refractory ascites, TIPS results in lower rates of ascites recurrence and hepatorenal syndrome but a higher rate of hepatic encephalopathy (the frequency of which is reduced with prophylactic rifaximin) than occurs with repeated large-volume paracentesis; benefits to sarcopenia and to survival have been demonstrated. CKD, diastolic cardiac dysfunction, refractory encephalopathy, and hyperbilirubinemia (> 5 mg/dL [85.5 mcmol/L]) are associated with increased mortality after TIPS. Patients with a serum bilirubin > 3 mg/dL (50 mcmol/L), platelets < 75,000/mcL (75 × 10^9/L), active infection, severe HF, or severe pulmonary hypertension may not benefit from TIPS. Well-controlled encephalopathy is not a contraindication to TIPS.

2. Spontaneous bacterial peritonitis—Spontaneous bacterial peritonitis may be heralded by abdominal pain, increasing ascites, fever, and progressive encephalopathy in a patient with cirrhotic ascites, although symptoms are typically mild. Up to 25% are asymptomatic at diagnosis. Paracentesis reveals an ascitic fluid with, most commonly a high polymorphonuclear (PMN) cell count (250/mcL [0.25 × 109/L] or more). Cultures of ascites give the highest yield—80–90% positive—when specialized culture bottles are inoculated at the bedside. Common isolates are *Escherichia coli* and *Streptococcus spp*. Gram-positive cocci and resistant organisms are more common among patients with recent healthcare contacts. The frequency of enterococcal isolates is increasing. Anaerobes are uncommon. Pending culture results, if there are 250 or more PMNs/mcL or symptoms or signs of infection, intravenous antibiotic therapy should be initiated with cefotaxime, 2 g every 8–12 hours for at least 5 days. Alternative choices include ceftriaxone 2 g daily, amoxicillin-clavulanic acid, and levofloxacin (in patients not receiving fluoroquinolone prophylaxis). Piperacillin-tazobactam or meropenem is recommended for patients with risk factors for multidrug-resistant organisms, including hospital-acquired spontaneous bacterial peritonitis, and specific therapy should be guided by local resistance patterns. Vancomycin should be added in patients with prior bacterial peritonitis or a positive surveillance swab for methicillin-resistant *Staphylococcus aureus*. Daptomycin should be added in patients with a positive surveillance swab for vancomycin-resistant enterococcus. In patients with spontaneous bacterial peritonitis diagnosed during hospitalization, or in the setting of recent hospitalization, or in the setting acute-on-chronic liver failure, treatment with meropenem and daptomycin is recommended. Supplemental administration of intravenous albumin, 1.5 g/kg at diagnosis and 1 g/kg on day 3, prevents further renal impairment and reduces mortality. This schedule and dosing, however, is arbitrary. Nonselective β-blockers should be held in patients who develop hypotension (mean arterial pressure < 65 mm Hg) or AKI. Given the increasing failure of initial empiric antibiotic therapy, response to therapy should be documented by a decrease in the PMN count of at least 75% on repeat paracentesis 48 hours after initiation of therapy. The overall mortality rate is high—up to 30% during hospitalization and up to 70% by 1 year.

In survivors of bacterial peritonitis, the risk of recurrent peritonitis may be decreased by long-term ciprofloxacin (eg, 500 mg orally once per day), norfloxacin (400 mg orally daily; no longer available in the United States), or trimethoprim-sulfamethoxazole (eg, one double-strength tablet once per day). In cases of recurrent peritonitis, the causative organism is often resistant to fluoroquinolones and may become multidrug resistant in some cases.

In patients with ascites who have not had bacterial peritonitis, primary prophylaxis with antibiotics is controversial and should be avoided. Results of the 2025 UK ASEPTIC trial demonstrated no benefit from primary prophylaxis using trimethoprim-sulfamethoxazole. In patients hospitalized for acute variceal bleeding, intravenous ceftriaxone (1 g per day) reduces the risk of infections including bacterial peritonitis but benefit is uncertain for otherwise compensated patients. Antibiotics should be continued for no longer than 5 days.

3. Hepatorenal syndrome—Hepatorenal syndrome occurs in up to 10% of patients with advanced cirrhosis and ascites. It is characterized by azotemia (increase in serum creatinine level of > 0.3 mg/dL [26.5 mcmol/L]) within 48 hours or increase by 50% or more from baseline within the previous 7 days or a urine volume < 0.5 mL/kg/hour for 6 hours or longer in the absence of (1) current or recent nephrotoxic drug use, (2) macroscopic signs of structural kidney injury, or (3) shock and failure of kidney function to improve following 2 days of diuretic withdrawal and volume expansion with albumin, 1 g/kg up to a maximum of 100 g/day. Oliguria, hyponatremia, and a low urinary sodium concentration are typical features. Hepatorenal syndrome is diagnosed only when other causes of AKI (including prerenal azotemia and ATN) have been excluded. AKI-hepatorenal syndrome (formerly type 1 hepatorenal syndrome) is typically associated with at least doubling of the serum creatinine to a level > 2.5 mg/dL (208.25 mcmol/L) or by halving of the creatinine clearance to < 20 mL/minute (0.34 mL/s/1.73 m^2 BSA) in < 2 weeks. CKD (or non-AKI)-hepatorenal syndrome (formerly type 2 hepatorenal syndrome) is more slowly progressive and chronic. The pathogenesis involves intense renal vasoconstriction, possibly because of impaired synthesis of renal vasodilators such as prostaglandin E2 and decreased total renal blood flow; histologically, the kidneys are normal. An acute decrease in cardiac output is often the precipitant.

For initial treatment of hepatorenal syndrome, diuretics should be discontinued and intravenous albumin provided (1 g/kg on day 1). Albumin therapy thereafter must be used with caution and repeated assessments of volume status to avoid pulmonary edema. Two medical regimens may also lead to clinical improvement and an increase in short-term survival: (1) intravenous terlipressin (FDA approved); (2) intravenous norepinephrine. These regimens are administered for 7–14 days until 24 hours following the return of serum creatinine to within 0.3 mg/dL of baseline for 2 consecutive days. Terlipressin therapy is preferred and is more effective than midodrine. Terlipressin is administered intravenously as 0.85 mg every 6 hours for 3 days; at that point, it is discontinued if the serum creatine is unchanged or increased from day 1 baseline; continued at the same dose if the serum creatinine has decreased by > 30%; and increased to 1.7 mg every 6 hours if the serum creatinine has decreased by < 30%. Complications include abdominal pain, nausea, diarrhea, dyspnea, and respiratory failure. Combination therapy of octreotide and midodrine may not be effective and should only be used if vasoconstrictor therapy is contraindicated or unavailable. Midodrine should be increased until the mean arterial pressure rises by 10 mm Hg, beginning at 10 mg three times daily and increasing as needed.

Continuous venovenous hemofiltration and hemodialysis are of uncertain value in hepatorenal syndrome. Liver transplantation is the ultimate treatment of choice, but many patients die before a donor liver can be obtained. Mortality correlates with the MELD score and presence of a systemic inflammatory response. AKI-hepatorenal syndrome is often irreversible in patients with a systemic infection. The 3-month probability of survival in cirrhotic patients with hepatorenal syndrome (15%) is lower than that for renal failure associated with infections (31%), hypovolemia (46%), and parenchymal kidney disease (73%).

4. Hepatic encephalopathy—Hepatic encephalopathy (HE) is a state of disordered CNS function resulting from failure of the liver to detoxify noxious agents of gut origin because of hepatocellular dysfunction and portosystemic shunting. The clinical spectrum ranges from day–night reversal and mild intellectual impairment to coma. Patients with covert (formerly minimal) HE have no recognizable clinical symptoms but demonstrate mild cognitive, psychomotor, and attention deficits on standardized psychometric tests and an increased rate of traffic accidents. The stages of overt encephalopathy are (1) mild confusion, (2) drowsiness, (3) stupor, and (4) coma. A revised staging system known as SONIC (Spectrum Of Neurocognitive Impairment in Cirrhosis) encompasses absent, covert, and stage 2 to 4 encephalopathy. Ammonia is the most readily identified and measurable toxin but is not solely responsible for the disturbed mental status. Bleeding into the intestinal tract delivers albumin and glutamine-rich hemoglobin to gut bacteria, which may precipitate encephalopathy. Other precipitants include infection, constipation, dehydration, potassium deficiency, hypnotics, and sedatives. Encephalopathy is increased in patients with portosystemic shunts (including TIPS). The diagnosis is based primarily on detection of characteristic symptoms and signs, including asterixis. The animal naming test (number of unique animals named in 1 minute) and a smartphone app called EncephalApp using the "Stroop test" (asking the patient to name the color of a written word rather than the word itself, even when the word is the name of a different color) has proved useful for detecting covert hepatic encephalopathy.

When HE is triggered by GI bleeding, blood should be purged from the GI tract (after hemostasis is achieved). This can be accomplished with 120 mL of magnesium citrate by mouth or nasogastric tube (or comparable bowel preparation) every 3–4 hours until the stool is free of gross blood or by administration of lactulose.

Lactulose, a nonabsorbable synthetic disaccharide syrup, is first line therapy for HE. When given orally, the initial dose of lactulose for acute hepatic encephalopathy is 30–60 mL every 2 hours until improved mental status or a first bowel movement. Thereafter, the dose should be titrated in 2–3 daily doses so that the patient produces 2–3 soft stools per day. If the patient is unable to take medicines orally, it may be administered as a rectal retention enema (200 g/300 mL) given as a solution of lactulose in saline or sorbitol; it may be repeated every 4–6 hours. Continued use of lactulose after an episode of acute encephalopathy reduces the frequency of recurrences.

The nonabsorbable agent rifaximin, 550 mg orally twice daily, has been shown as well to maintain remission of and reduce the risk of rehospitalization for hepatic encephalopathy over a 24-month period, with or without the concomitant use of lactulose. Metronidazole, 250 mg orally three times daily, may also help.

Adequate protein intake must be confirmed. Opioids should be used sparingly and with careful attention to the risk of constipation. Zinc can be provided with care to avoid overdose (which can cause copper deficiency).

5. Coagulopathy—Bleeding risk does not correlate with the INR. Plasma infusions generally are not recommended, either before invasive procedures (including paracentesis) or for active bleeding, because they fail to correct hemostatic function while raising portal pressure. Recombinant activated factor VIIa does correct INR, but did not improve re-bleeding in randomized trial of patients with variceal hemorrhage.

In patients with active bleeding, blood product replacement should be judicious with a target hemoglobin of 7g/dL. Generally, platelet counts > 20,000/mcL (20 × 10^9/L) are sufficient for most procedures.

6. Hemorrhage from esophageal varices—See Chapter 17.

7. Hepatopulmonary syndrome and portopulmonary hypertension—Shortness of breath in patients with cirrhosis may result from pulmonary restriction and atelectasis caused by massive ascites or hepatic hydrothorax. The hepatopulmonary syndrome—the triad of chronic liver disease, an increased alveolar-arterial gradient while the patient is breathing room air, and intrapulmonary vascular dilatations or arteriovenous communications that result in a right-to-left intrapulmonary shunt—occurs in 5–32% of patients with cirrhosis. Patients often have greater dyspnea (platypnea) and arterial deoxygenation (orthodeoxia) in the upright than in the recumbent position. The diagnosis should be suspected in a cirrhotic patient with a pulse oximetry level of 96% or lower.

Contrast-enhanced echocardiography is a sensitive screening test for detecting pulmonary vascular dilatations. HRCT may be useful for detecting dilated pulmonary vessels that may be amenable to embolization in patients with severe hypoxemia (PO_2 < 60 mm Hg [7.8 kPa]) who respond poorly to supplemental oxygen.

Medical therapy has been disappointing. Long-term oxygen therapy is recommended for severely hypoxemic patients. The syndrome may reverse with liver transplantation, although postoperative morbidity and mortality from severe hypoxemic respiratory failure are increased in patients with a preoperative arterial PO_2 < 44 mm Hg (5.9 kPa) or with substantial intrapulmonary shunting.

Portopulmonary hypertension occurs in 0.7% of patients with cirrhosis. Female sex, autoimmune hepatitis, and genetic variation in aromatase have been reported to be risk factors. Large spontaneous portosystemic shunts are present in many affected patients and are associated with a lack of response to treatment. In cases confirmed by right-sided heart catheterization, several treatments may reduce pulmonary hypertension and thereby facilitate liver transplantation. These include the prostaglandins epoprostenol, iloprost, or treprostinil (the latter two are easier to administer); the endothelin-receptor antagonists ambrisentan and macitentan (bosentan is no longer used because of potential hepatotoxicity); the phosphodiesterase-5 inhibitors sildenafil, tadalafil, or vardenafil; the oral prostacyclin receptor agonist selexipag; or the direct cyclic GMP analog riociguat. β-Blockers worsen exercise capacity and are contraindicated, and calcium channel blockers should be used with caution because they may worsen portal hypertension. Liver transplantation is contraindicated in patients with moderate to severe pulmonary hypertension (mean pulmonary pressure > 35 mm Hg or, if pulmonary vascular resistance is low, > 45 mm Hg).

C. Liver Transplantation

Liver transplantation is indicated in selected cases of irreversible, progressive chronic liver disease, acute-on-chronic liver failure, acute liver failure, hepatocellular carcinoma, and certain metabolic diseases in which the metabolic defect is in the liver. Patients with alcohol use disorder should generally be abstinent prior to transplantation and must be engaged in multidisciplinary care. Prioritization in the United States is now based on the MELD-3.0 score. Combined liver-kidney transplantation is indicated in patients with associated kidney failure presumed to be irreversible. Adult living donor liver transplantation is an option for some patients and extended-criteria donors are used. Five-year survival rates over 80% are now reported. HCC, hepatitis B and C, Budd-Chiari syndrome, and autoimmune liver disease may recur in the transplanted liver. The incidence of recurrence of hepatitis B can be reduced by preoperative and postoperative treatment with a nucleoside or nucleotide analog and perioperative administration of HBIG, and hepatitis C can be treated with direct-acting antiviral agents. Immunosuppression is achieved with combinations of cyclosporine, tacrolimus, sirolimus, corticosteroids, azathioprine, and mycophenolate mofetil. It may be complicated by infections, advanced CKD, neurologic disorders, and drug toxicity, as well as graft rejection, vascular occlusion, or bile leaks. Patients taking these drugs are at risk for obesity, diabetes mellitus, and hyperlipidemia and may develop recurrent or de novo MASLD following transplantation.

Prognosis

Prognostic scoring systems for cirrhosis include the Child-Pugh and MELD scores (Table 18–8). The MELD-3.0 score, which incorporates gender and the serum bilirubin, creatinine, sodium levels, INR, and albumin, is also a measure of mortality risk in patients with decompensated

Table 18–8. Child-Pugh and Model for End-Stage Liver Disease (MELD) scoring systems for staging cirrhosis.

Child-Pugh Scoring System			
	Numerical Score		
Parameter	1	2	3
Ascites	None	Slight	Moderate to severe
Encephalopathy	None	Slight to moderate	Moderate to severe
Bilirubin, mg/dL (mcmol/L)	< 2.0 (34.2)	2–3 (34.2–51.3)	> 3.0 (51.3)
Albumin, g/dL (g/L)	> 3.5 (35)	2.8–3.5 (28–35)	< 2.8 (28)
Prothrombin time (seconds increased)	1–3	4–6	> 6.0
	Total Numerical Score and Corresponding Child-Pugh Class		
	Score		Class
	5–6		A
	7–9		B
	10–15		C

MELD Scoring Systems

Original MELD score = 11.2 $\log_e$ (INR) + 3.78 $\log_e$ (bilirubin [mg/dL]) + 9.57 $\log_e$ (creatinine [mg/dL]) + 6.43. (Range 6–40.)

MELD-Na score = MELD + (140 – Na) × (1 – 0.025 × MELD).

cirrhosis and is particularly useful for predicting short- and intermediate-term survival and complications of cirrhosis (eg, bacterial peritonitis) as well as determining allocation priorities for donor livers. Additional (MELD-exception) points are given for patients with conditions such as hepatopulmonary syndrome and HCC that may benefit from liver transplantation.

The risk of death from compensated cirrhosis is 4.7 times that of the risk in the general population, and the risk from decompensated cirrhosis is 9.7 times higher. Use of statins appears to decrease the risk of decompensation in patients with compensated cirrhosis. Obesity and diabetes mellitus appear to be risk factors for clinical deterioration and cirrhosis-related mortality, as is continued alcohol use in patients with alcohol-associated cirrhosis. The use of β-blockers for portal hypertension is beneficial early in the course; patients with cirrhosis, with or without ascites, who respond to treatment with a β-blocker based on a reduction in the hepatic venous pressure gradient have a reduced risk of death or need for liver transplantation. However, β-blockers may become ineffective and may be associated with reduced survival in patients with refractory ascites, spontaneous bacterial peritonitis, sepsis, or severe alcohol-associated hepatitis because of their negative effect on cardiac compensatory reserve. In general, β-blockers should be discontinued when the systolic blood pressure is < 90 mm Hg, the serum sodium level is < 130 mEq/L, or AKI has developed, although results of some studies have challenged these guidelines.

Only 50% of patients with severe hepatic dysfunction (serum albumin < 3 g/dL [30 g/L], bilirubin > 3 mg/dL [51.3 mcmol/L], ascites, encephalopathy, cachexia, and upper GI bleeding) survive 6 months without transplantation. The risk of death in this subgroup of patients with advanced cirrhosis is associated with muscle wasting or frailty, age 65 years or older, mean arterial pressure ≤ 82 mm Hg, severe kidney dysfunction, cognitive dysfunction, ventilatory insufficiency, prothrombin time 16 seconds or longer, delayed and suboptimal treatment of sepsis, and second infections.

In-hospital mortality from cirrhosis declined from 9.1% in 2002 to 5.4% in 2010, and that from variceal bleeding in patients with cirrhosis declined from over 40% in 1980 to 15% in 2000. Rates and costs of hospital admissions, however, increased substantially between 2005 and 2015, primarily because of increases in the rates of cirrhosis caused by MASLD. Severe kidney dysfunction increases mortality up to sevenfold in patients with cirrhosis, and at least 25% of patients who survive an episode of AKI develop CKD. Patients hospitalized with cirrhosis and an infection are at high risk for subsequent infections, particularly if they are older, taking a PPI, or receiving antibiotic prophylaxis for spontaneous bacterial peritonitis. For patients with cirrhosis admitted with acute decompensations, the MELD score and presence of extrahepatic organ failures known as 'acute-on-chronic liver failure' (ACLF) predict mortality. The definition of ACLF organ failures varies according to different expert consortia but invariably includes severe hepatic encephalopathy (grade III-IV), kidney failure, circulatory failure or shock, and respiratory failure (hypoxia or need for mechanical ventilation); the ACLF grading is dependent on the number of failures.

Patients with cirrhosis are at risk for the development of HCC, which are highest for untreated viral hepatitis and lowest for MASH cirrhosis. Liver transplantation has markedly improved the outlook for patients with cirrhosis who are candidates and are referred for evaluation early in the course. Patients with compensated cirrhosis are given additional priority for liver transplantation if they are found to have a lesion consistent with HCC that is > 2 cm.

When to Refer

- For liver biopsy.
- When the MELD score is 14 or higher.
- For upper endoscopy to screen for gastroesophageal varices.

When to Admit

- GI bleeding.
- Stage 3–4 hepatic encephalopathy.
- Worsening kidney function.
- Severe hyponatremia.
- Serious infection.
- Profound hypoxia.

Bajaj JS et al. Role of oral health, frailty, and minimal hepatic encephalopathy in the risk of hospitalization: a prospective multi-center cohort of outpatients with cirrhosis. Clin Gastroenterol Hepatol. 2023;21:1864. [PMID: 36328307]

Karvellas CJ et al. AASLD practice guidance on acute-on-chronic liver failure and the management of critically ill patients with cirrhosis. Hepatology. 2024;79:1463. [PMID: 37939273]

Lucey MR et al. Liver transplantation. N Engl J Med. 2023;389:1888. [PMID: 37966287]

Nadim MK et al. Acute kidney injury in patients with cirrhosis. N Engl J Med. 2023;388:733. [PMID: 36812435]

Tapper EB et al. Diagnosis and management of cirrhosis and its complications: a review. JAMA. 2023;329:1589. [PMID: 37159031]

Zanetto A et al. Haemostasis in cirrhosis: understanding destabilising factors during acute decompensation. J Hepatol. 2023;78:1037. [PMID: 36708812]

PRIMARY BILIARY CHOLANGITIS

ESSENTIALS OF DIAGNOSIS

- Most common in middle-aged women.
- Often asymptomatic.
- Elevation of alkaline phosphatase, positive antimitochondrial antibodies, increased cholesterol.
- Characteristic liver biopsy.
- In later stages, can present with fatigue, jaundice, features of cirrhosis, xanthelasmas, xanthomas, steatorrhea.

General Considerations

PBC is a chronic disease of the liver characterized by autoimmune destruction of small intrahepatic bile ducts and cholestasis. The designation "primary biliary cholangitis" has replaced "primary biliary cirrhosis" because many patients do not have cirrhosis. The disease is insidious in onset, occurs usually in women aged 40–60 years, and is often detected by the chance finding of elevated alkaline phosphatase levels. Estimated incidence and prevalence rates in the United States are 4.5 and 65.4 per 100,000, respectively, in women, and 0.7 and 12.1 per 100,000, respectively, in men. These rates may be increasing. The frequency of the disease among first-degree relatives of affected persons is 1.3–6%, the risk is increased in second- and third-degree relatives, and the concordance rate in identical twins is high. PBC is associated with HLA *DRB1*08* and *DQB1*. The disease may be associated with Sjögren syndrome, autoimmune thyroid disease, Raynaud syndrome, systemic sclerosis (scleroderma), hypothyroidism, and celiac disease; all patients with PBC should be screened for these conditions. Infection with *Novosphingobium aromaticivorans* or *Chlamydophila pneumoniae* may trigger or cause PBC. A history of UTIs (caused by *E coli* or *Lactobacillus delbrueckii*), smoking, and possibly use of hormone replacement therapy and hair dye, are risk factors. A clustering of cases in time and space also argues for a causative role of environmental agents.

Clinical Findings

A. Symptoms and Signs

Many patients are asymptomatic for years. The onset of clinical illness is insidious and is heralded by fatigue (excessive daytime somnolence) and pruritus. With progression, physical examination reveals hepatosplenomegaly. Xanthomatous lesions may occur in the skin and tendons and around the eyelids. Jaundice, steatorrhea, and signs of portal hypertension are late findings, although occasional patients have esophageal varices despite an early histologic stage. Autonomic dysfunction, including orthostatic hypotension and associated fatigue and cognitive dysfunction, appear to be common. The risk of low bone density, osteoporosis, and fractures is increased in patients with PBC possibly due in part to polymorphisms of the vitamin D receptor.

B. Laboratory Findings

Blood counts are normal early in the disease. Liver biochemical tests reflect cholestasis with elevation of alkaline phosphatase, cholesterol, and, in later stages, bilirubin. Antimitochondrial antibodies are present in 90% of patients, and serum IgM levels are often elevated.

Diagnosis

The diagnosis of PBC is based on the detection of cholestatic liver chemistries (often initially an isolated elevation of the alkaline phosphatase) and antimitochondrial antibodies in a titer > 1:40 in serum. Baseline hepatobiliary ultrasonography should be obtained. Liver biopsy is not necessary for diagnosis unless antimitochondrial antibodies are absent but permits histologic staging: I, portal inflammation with granulomas; II, bile duct proliferation, periportal inflammation; III, interlobular fibrous septa; and IV, cirrhosis. Histologic stage may be estimated noninvasively by elastography.

Differential Diagnosis

PBC must be differentiated from chronic biliary tract obstruction (eg, stone or stricture), carcinoma of the bile ducts, primary sclerosing cholangitis, sarcoidosis, cholestatic drug toxicity, and (in some cases) chronic hepatitis. Patients with a clinical and histologic picture of PBC but no antimitochondrial antibodies are said to have antimitochondrial antibody-negative PBC (previously termed "autoimmune cholangitis"), which has been associated with lower serum IgM levels and a greater frequency of smooth muscle antibodies and ANA. Some patients have overlapping features of PBC and autoimmune hepatitis.

Treatment

Ursodeoxycholic acid (13–15 mg/kg/day, generally in two doses) is the preferred medical treatment for PBC. It has been shown to slow the progression of disease (particularly in early-stage disease), stabilize histology, improve long-term survival, reduce the risk of developing esophageal varices, and delay (and possibly prevent) the need for liver transplantation, even in the absence of liver biochemical improvement. Complete normalization of liver biochemical tests occurs in 20% of treated patients within 2 years and 40% within 5 years, and survival is similar to that of healthy controls when the drug is given to patients with stage 1 or 2 PBC. The rate of improvement in the alkaline phosphatase to normal or near-normal levels has been reported to be lower in men than women (72% versus 80%) and higher in women whose disease is diagnosed after age 70 than before age 30 (90% versus 50%). Side effects include weight gain and rarely loose stools. The drug can be continued during pregnancy.

Agents that activate peroxisome proliferator-activated receptors (PPARs) inhibit bile acid synthesis and improve symptoms (including pruritus), liver biochemical tests, and fibrosis in clinical trials. Seladelpar (10 mg orally once daily), a PPAR-δ agonist, and elafibranor (80 mg orally once daily), PPAR-α/δ agonist, are approved for use in patients without response to or intolerance of ursodiol with biochemical response rates in RCTs of 42–47% higher than placebo. Fibrates also activate these receptors. Bezafibrate (not available in the United States) and fenofibrate also have shown promise as second-line agents. Use of these agents should be avoided in decompensated cirrhosis. For patients with advanced disease, liver transplantation is the treatment of choice.

Cholestyramine (4 g) in water or juice three times daily may be beneficial for pruritus; colestipol and colesevelam may be better tolerated but have not been shown to reduce pruritus. Second line agents include rifampin, naltrexone, sertraline, gabapentin, and fibrates (as above). Deficiencies of vitamins A, D, and K may occur if steatorrhea is present and are aggravated when cholestyramine is administered.

Prognosis

Without liver transplantation, survival averages 7–10 years once symptoms develop but has improved since the introduction of ursodeoxycholic acid. Patients with early-stage disease in whom the alkaline phosphatase and AST are < 1.5 times normal and bilirubin is ≤ 1 mg/dL (17.1 mcmol/L) after 1 year of therapy with ursodeoxycholic acid (Paris II criteria) are at low long-term risk for cirrhosis and have a life expectancy similar to that of the healthy population. Attainment of a serum bilirubin level < 0.6 times the upper limit of normal or a normal alkaline phosphatase level is associated with the lowest risk for liver transplantation or death. Pregnancy is well tolerated.

In advanced disease, an adverse prognosis is indicated by a high Mayo risk score that includes older age, high serum bilirubin, edema, low serum albumin, and prolonged prothrombin time as well as by variceal hemorrhage. Other prognostic models include the Globe index, which is based on age, serum bilirubin, serum albumin, serum alkaline phosphatase, and platelet count and, in treated patients, the UK-PBC score, which is based on the baseline serum albumin and platelet count and the serum bilirubin, aminotransferases, and alkaline phosphatase after 12 months of ursodeoxycholic acid. Using elastography, an increase in liver stiffness of more than 2.1 kPa per year indicates an adverse prognosis. Liver transplantation should be considered when the MELD-3.0 score is at least 15 or in the presence of cirrhotic decompensations. A reduced risk of recurrence, graft loss, and death is associated with preventive treatment with ursodeoxycholic acid in combination with cyclosporine (rather than tacrolimus).

When to Refer

- For liver biopsy.
- For liver transplant evaluation.

When to Admit

- GI bleeding.
- Stage 3–4 hepatic encephalopathy.
- Worsening kidney function.
- Severe hyponatremia.
- Profound hypoxia.

Abbas N et al. UK-wide multicenter evaluation of second-line therapies in primary biliary cholangitis. Clin Gastroenterol Hepatol. 2023;21:1561. [PMID: 35961518]

Hirschfield GM et al. A phase 3 trial of seladelpar in primary biliary cholangitis. N Engl J Med. 2024;390:783. [PMID: 38381664]

Khakoo NS et al. Efficacy and safety of bezafibrate alone or in combination with ursodeoxycholic acid in primary biliary cholangitis: systematic review and meta-analysis. Dig Dis Sci. 2023;68:1559. [PMID: 36180756]

Kowdley KV et al. Application of the latest advances in evidence-based medicine in primary biliary cholangitis. Am J Gastroenterol. 2023;118:232. [PMID: 36729104]

Kowdley KV et al. Efficacy and safety of elafibranor in primary biliary cholangitis. N Engl J Med. 2024;390:795. [PMID: 37962077]

Trivella J et al. Primary biliary cholangitis: epidemiology, prognosis, and treatment. Hepatol Commun. 2023;7:e0179. [PMID: 37267215]

HEMOCHROMATOSIS

ESSENTIALS OF DIAGNOSIS

- Usually suspected because of a family history or an elevated iron saturation or serum ferritin.
- Most patients are asymptomatic; the disease is rarely recognized clinically before the fifth decade.
- Hepatic abnormalities and cirrhosis, HF, hypogonadism, and arthritis.
- Pathogenic variant of *HFE* gene (usually C282Y/C282Y) is found in most cases.

General Considerations

Hemochromatosis is characterized by increased accumulation of iron as hemosiderin in the liver, pancreas, heart, adrenals, testes, pituitary, and kidneys. Eventually, hepatic and pancreatic insufficiency, HF, and hypogonadism may develop. Hemochromatosis is an autosomal recessive disease caused in most cases by a pathogenic variant in the *HFE* gene on chromosome 6. The HFE protein is thought to play an important role in the process by which duodenal crypt cells sense body iron stores, and the variant gene leads to increased iron absorption from the duodenum. A decrease in the synthesis or expression of hepcidin, the principal iron regulatory hormone, is thought to be a key pathogenic factor in all forms of hemochromatosis. About 95% of persons with well-established hemochromatosis are homozygous for the C282Y variant (type 1a hemochromatosis). The frequency of the C282Y variant is 1 in 7 persons in Northern European and North American White populations, resulting in a 0.5% frequency of homozygotes, of whom roughly 10% will develop biochemical evidence of iron overload. Environmental factors influence the risk of iron overload, particularly alcohol consumption and metabolic syndrome. Among persons with the pathogenic HFE variant, phenotypic expression including iron overload and severe liver disease is often highly dependent on these environmental factors. The C282Y gene variant and hemochromatosis are uncommon in Black and Asian American populations. A second pathogenic gene variant (H63D) may contribute to the development of iron overload in a small percentage (1.5%) of persons who are compound heterozygotes for C282Y and H63D (type 1b); iron overload–related disease develops in only a few patients (particularly those who have a comorbidity such as diabetes mellitus and fatty liver). A third gene variant (S65C) may lead to increased serum iron and ferritin levels without clinical significance (type 1c).

Clinical Findings

A. Symptoms and Signs

The onset of clinical disease is usually after age 50 years—earlier in men than in women; however, because of widespread liver biochemical testing and iron screening, the diagnosis is usually made long before symptoms develop. Early symptoms are nonspecific (eg, fatigue, arthralgia). Later clinical manifestations include a symmetric arthropathy that is similar to osteoarthritis and calcium pyrophosphate deposition disease (and ultimately the need for joint replacement surgery in some cases) and hepatomegaly and evidence of hepatic dysfunction. Other manifestations may include skin pigmentation (combination of slate-gray due to iron and brown due to melanin, sometimes resulting in a bronze color), cardiac enlargement with or without HF or conduction defects, diabetes mellitus (especially in those with cirrhosis), and erectile dysfunction and osteoporosis in men. In patients in whom cirrhosis develops, the risk of decompensation and HCC can be high without treatment. Affected patients are at increased risk of infection with *Vibrio vulnificus, Listeria monocytogenes, Yersinia enterocolitica*, and other siderophilic organisms.

B. Laboratory Findings

Laboratory findings include mildly abnormal liver tests (AST, alkaline phosphatase), an elevated plasma iron with > 45% transferrin saturation, a low unsaturated iron-binding capacity, and an elevated serum ferritin (> 200 mcg/L in premenopausal women and 300 mcg/L in men and postmenopausal women). Affected men are more likely than affected women to have an elevated ferritin level. Testing for *HFE* variants is most indicated when elevated transferrin saturation and ferritin are detected; however, elevated ferritin more commonly is attributable to other causes (eg, alcohol use or the metabolic syndrome).

C. Imaging

MRI and CT may show changes consistent with iron overload of the liver, and MRI-based techniques (eg, T2 spin echo and T2* gradient-recalled echo MRI) can quantitate hepatic iron stores, distinguish primary from secondary iron overload (eg, when iron is observed in lymphatic tissue like the spleen), and assess the degree of hepatic fibrosis.

D. Liver Biopsy

In patients who are homozygous for the C282Y variant, liver biopsy was indicated in the past to determine whether cirrhosis is present. However, serum biomarkers of fibrosis and elastography now are preferred to liver biopsy for identifying advanced fibrosis. Risk factors for advanced fibrosis include male sex, excess alcohol consumption, and diabetes mellitus. In patients with hemochromatosis, liver biopsy characteristically shows extensive iron deposition in hepatocytes and in bile ducts, and the hepatic iron index—hepatic iron content per gram of liver converted to micromoles and divided by the patient's age—is generally higher than 1.9 (though no longer used for diagnosis). Secondary hemochromatosis will generally yield iron deposition that is also in the Kupffer cells. Only 5% of patients with hereditary hemochromatosis identified by screening in a primary care setting have cirrhosis.

Screening

Iron studies are recommended for all first-degree family members of a proband; children of an affected person (C282Y homozygote) need to be screened only if the patient's spouse carries the C282Y or H63D mutation. General population screening for hemochromatosis is not recommended because the clinical penetrance of C282Y homozygosity and morbidity and mortality from hemochromatosis are low. Patients with otherwise unexplained chronic liver disease, chondrocalcinosis, erectile dysfunction, and type 1 diabetes mellitus (especially late-onset) should be screened for iron overload.

Treatment

Affected persons are advised to avoid foods rich in iron (such as red meat), alcohol, vitamin C, raw shellfish, and supplemental iron, although dietary restrictions may not be necessary in those undergoing phlebotomy. Weekly phlebotomies of 1 or 2 units (250–500 mL) of blood (each containing about 250 mg of iron) are indicated in all symptomatic patients, and those with a serum ferritin level of at least 300 mcg/L (men) or 200 mcg/L (women) with an increased fasting iron saturation (≥ 45%); these phlebotomies should be continued for up to 2–3 years to achieve depletion of iron stores. The hematocrit and serum iron values should be monitored. When iron store depletion is achieved (iron saturation < 50% and serum ferritin level 50–100 mcg/L), phlebotomies (every 3–4 months) to maintain serum ferritin levels between 50 mcg/L and 100 mcg/L are continued, although compliance has been reported to decrease with time. Administration of a PPI, which reduces intestinal iron absorption, decreases the maintenance phlebotomy volume requirement. In C282Y homozygous women, a BMI > 28 is associated with a lower phlebotomy requirement, possibly because hepcidin levels are increased by overweight. Complications of hemochromatosis—arthropathy, diabetes mellitus, heart disease, portal hypertension, and hypopituitarism—also require treatment.

The chelating agent deferoxamine is indicated for patients with hemochromatosis and anemia or in those with secondary iron overload due to thalassemia who cannot tolerate phlebotomies. The drug is administered intravenously or subcutaneously in a dosage of 20–40 mg/kg/day infused over 24 hours and can mobilize 30 mg of iron per day; however, treatment is painful and time-consuming. Two oral chelators, deferasirox, 20 mg/kg once daily, and deferiprone, 25 mg/kg three times daily, have been approved for treatment of iron overload due to blood transfusions and used in persons with hemochromatosis who cannot tolerate phlebotomy but have a number of side effects and drug-drug interactions that limit their usefulness.

Prognosis

The course of hemochromatosis appears to be favorably altered by phlebotomy therapy; hepatic fibrosis may regress and cirrhosis may be prevented in precirrhotic patients. In patients with cirrhosis, varices may reverse, the risk of variceal bleeding declines, and the risk of HCC may be reduced. Cardiac conduction defects may improve with treatment; however, joint disease, diabetes mellitus, and hypogonadism may not reverse. More severe joint symptoms are associated with persistent increases in the transferrin saturation, even if the serum ferritin level is maintained below 50 mcg/L. In those with an initial serum ferritin level > 1000 mcg/L (2247 pmol/L), the risk of death is fivefold greater than in those with a serum ferritin of ≤ 1000 mcg/L (2247 pmol/L). In treated patients, only those with a serum ferritin > 2000 mcg/L (4494 pmol/L) are reported to have increased mortality, mainly related to liver disease. Following liver transplantation, serum iron studies and hepcidin levels are normal, and phlebotomy is not required.

When to Refer

- For liver biopsy.
- For initiation of therapy.

Adams PC et al. Haemochromatosis. Lancet. 2023;401:1811. [PMID: 37121243]

Cathcart J et al. European Association for Study of the Liver (EASL) clinical practice guidelines on haemochromatosis. Frontline Gastroenterol. 2023;14:282. [PMID: 37409332]

Sohal A et al. Association between pattern of hepatic iron deposition and severity of MASH among patients enrolled in the NASH Clinical Research Network. Hepatology Communications. 2025;9:e0847. [PMID: 41264906]

WILSON DISEASE

ESSENTIALS OF DIAGNOSIS

- Rare autosomal recessive disorder that usually occurs in persons under age 40.
- Excessive deposition of copper in the liver and brain.
- Serum ceruloplasmin, the plasma copper-carrying protein, is low.
- Urinary excretion of copper and hepatic copper concentration are high.

General Considerations

Wilson disease (hepatolenticular degeneration) is a rare autosomal recessive disorder that usually occurs in persons between 3 and 55 years of age. The worldwide prevalence is about 30 per million population, but the frequency of the allele is greater than implied by this estimate. The condition is characterized by excessive deposition of copper in the liver and brain. The genetic defect, localized to chromosome 13 (*ATP7B*), has been shown to affect a copper-transporting adenosine triphosphatase in the liver and leads to copper accumulation in the liver and oxidative damage of hepatic mitochondria. Most patients are compound heterozygotes (ie, carry two different pathogenic variants). Over 600 variants in the Wilson disease gene have been identified. The H1069Q variant accounts for 37–63% of disease alleles in populations of Northern European descent. The major physiologic aberration in Wilson disease is excessive absorption of copper from the small intestine and decreased excretion of copper by the liver, resulting in increased tissue deposition, especially in the liver, brain, cornea, and kidney.

Clinical Findings

Wilson disease tends to present as liver disease in adolescents (more common in females) and neuropsychiatric disease in young adults (more common in males), but there is great variability, and onset of symptoms after age 40 is more common than previously thought. The diagnosis should be considered in any child or young adult with hepatitis, splenomegaly with hypersplenism, Coombs-negative hemolytic anemia, portal hypertension, and neurologic or psychiatric abnormalities. Wilson disease should also be considered in persons under 40 years of age with chronic hepatitis or acute liver failure.

Hepatic involvement may range from elevated liver biochemical tests (although the alkaline phosphatase may be *low*, particularly in patients with acute severe liver disease) to cirrhosis and portal hypertension. The neurologic manifestations of Wilson disease are related to basal ganglia dysfunction and include an akinetic-rigid syndrome similar to parkinsonism, pseudosclerosis with tremor, ataxia, and a dystonic syndrome. Dysarthria, dysphagia, incoordination, and spasticity are common. Migraines, insomnia, and seizures have been reported. Psychiatric features include behavioral and personality changes and emotional lability and may precede characteristic neurologic features. The risk of depression is increased. The pathognomonic sign of the condition is the brownish or gray-green Kayser-Fleischer ring, which represents fine pigmented granular deposits in Descemet membrane in the cornea (Figure 18–5). The ring is usually most marked at the superior and inferior poles of the cornea. It is sometimes seen with the naked eye and is readily detected by slit-lamp examination. It may be absent in patients with hepatic manifestations only but is usually present in those with neuropsychiatric disease. Renal calculi, aminoaciduria, renal tubular acidosis, hypoparathyroidism, infertility, hemolytic anemia, and subcutaneous lipomas may occur.

Diagnosis

The diagnosis can be challenging, even with the use of scoring systems (eg, the Leipzig criteria, New Wilson

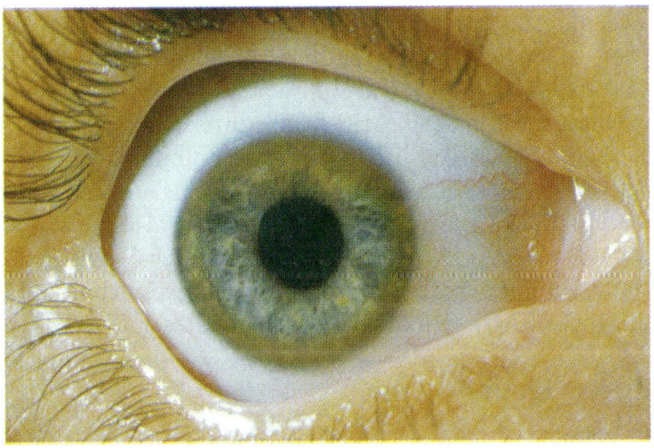

▲ **Figure 18–5.** Brownish Kayser-Fleischer ring at the rim of the cornea in a patient with Wilson disease. (Used, with permission, from Mediscan/Alamy Stock Photo.)

Index), and is generally based on demonstration of increased urinary copper excretion (> 40 mcg/24 hours and usually > 100 mcg/24 hours), low serum ceruloplasmin levels (< 14 mg/dL [140 mg/L]), and elevated hepatic copper concentration (> 250 mcg/g of dry liver). Increased urinary copper and a low serum ceruloplasmin level, while useful, are neither completely sensitive nor specific for Wilson disease. A ratio of serum exchangeable copper to total copper ("relative exchangeable copper") over 18.5% has been reported to be a reliable test for the diagnosis of Wilson disease. Other supportive features are the presence of Kayser-Fleischer rings, neurologic symptoms, and Coombs-negative hemolytic anemia. Liver biopsy may show acute or chronic hepatitis or cirrhosis. MRI of the brain may show evidence of increased basal ganglia, brainstem, and cerebellar copper even early in the course of the disease. Cerebellar atrophy may be seen in patients with hepatic manifestations only. The absence of Kayser-Fleischer rings in a patient with MRI abnormalities of the brain makes a diagnosis of Wilson disease unlikely. Molecular analysis of *ATP7B* pathogenic variants can be diagnostic and should be performed when clinical and biochemical testing is inconclusive. Direct measurement of ATP7B peptide concentrations in dried blood specimens has been reported to identify most patients with Wilson disease.

Treatment

Early treatment to remove excess copper before it can produce hepatic or neurologic damage is essential. Restriction of dietary copper (shellfish, organ meats, nuts, mushrooms, soy-based products, and chocolate) may be of value but is not sufficient. Oral D-penicillamine (0.75–2 g/day in divided doses taken 1 hour before or 2 hours after food) has traditionally been the drug of choice and enhances urinary excretion of chelated copper. Oral pyridoxine, 50 mg per week, is added because D-penicillamine is an antimetabolite of this vitamin. If D-penicillamine treatment cannot be tolerated because of GI intolerance, hypersensitivity, autoimmune reactions, nephrotoxicity, or bone marrow toxicity, trientine hydrochloride, 250–500 mg three times a day, a chelating agent as effective as D-penicillamine but with a lower rate of adverse effects, is used. Trientine is increasingly prescribed as a first-line and maintenance agent, although its cost has been high. Trientine tetrahydrochloride reduces serum non-ceruloplasmin copper levels without increasing copper excretion and is associated with fewer side effects; it is approved by the FDA for maintenance therapy in previously treated, D-penicillamine–tolerant patients. Oral zinc acetate or zinc gluconate, 50 mg of elemental zinc three times a day taken 30 minutes before or 2 hours after a meal, interferes with intestinal absorption of copper, promotes fecal copper excretion, and has been used as first-line therapy in asymptomatic or pregnant patients and those with neurologic disease, in combination with a chelating agent, or as maintenance therapy after decoppering with a chelating agent; however, adverse GI effects often lead to discontinuation and its long-term efficacy and safety (including a risk of hepatotoxicity) have been questioned.

Treatment should continue indefinitely, and adherence (without overtreatment) is critical. The doses of penicillamine and trientine should be reduced during pregnancy. Once the serum nonceruloplasmin copper level is within the normal range (50–150 mcg/L), the dose of chelating agent can be reduced to the minimum necessary for maintaining that level. The prognosis is good in patients who are effectively treated before liver or brain damage has occurred, but long-term survival is reduced in patients with cirrhosis at diagnosis (84% after 20 years). Liver transplantation is indicated for acute liver failure (often after plasma exchange or dialysis with MARS as a stabilizing measure) and decompensated cirrhosis (with excellent outcomes). Liver transplantation is generally not recommended for intractable isolated neuropsychiatric disease. All first-degree relatives, especially siblings, require screening with serum ceruloplasmin, liver biochemical tests, and slit-lamp examination or, if the causative pathogenic gene variant is known, with variant analysis.

When to Refer

All patients with Wilson disease should be referred for diagnosis and treatment.

When to Admit

- Acute liver failure.
- GI bleeding.
- Stage 3–4 hepatic encephalopathy.
- Worsening kidney function.
- Severe hyponatremia.
- Profound hypoxia.

Alkhouri N et al. Wilson disease: a summary of the updated AASLD Practice Guidance. Hepatol Commun. 2023;7:e0150. [PMID: 37184530]

Roberts EA et al. Current and emerging issues in Wilson's disease. N Engl J Med. 2023;389:922. [PMID: 37672695]

Schilsky M et al. A multidisciplinary approach to the diagnosis and management of Wilson disease: 2022 practice guidance on Wilson disease from the American Association for the Study of Liver Diseases. Hepatology. 2025;82:E41. [PMID: 36151586]

HEPATIC VENOUS OUTFLOW OBSTRUCTION (Budd-Chiari Syndrome)

ESSENTIALS OF DIAGNOSIS

- Right upper quadrant pain and tenderness.
- Ascites.
- Imaging studies show occlusion/absence of flow in the hepatic vein(s) or inferior vena cava.
- Clinical picture is similar in sinusoidal obstruction syndrome, but major hepatic veins are patent.

General Considerations

The prevalence of primary hepatic venous outflow obstruction, or Budd-Chiari syndrome, is 1 case per million persons per year. Predisposing factors, including hereditary and acquired hypercoagulable states, can be identified in up to 75% of affected patients. Up to 50% of cases are associated with polycythemia vera or other myeloproliferative neoplasms (which entail a 1% risk of Budd-Chiari syndrome). These cases are often associated with a specific pathogenic variant (*V617F*) in the gene that codes for JAK2 tyrosine kinase and may otherwise be subclinical. Hepatic vein obstruction may be associated with caval webs, right-sided HF or constrictive pericarditis, neoplasms that cause hepatic vein occlusion, paroxysmal nocturnal hemoglobinuria, hyperhomocysteinemia, Behçet syndrome, vasculitis, sarcoidosis, IBD, celiac disease, blunt abdominal trauma, use of oral contraceptives, and pregnancy. Some cytotoxic agents and pyrrolizidine alkaloids (comfrey or "bush teas") may cause **sinusoidal obstruction syndrome** (previously known as veno-occlusive disease because the terminal venules are often occluded), which mimics Budd-Chiari syndrome clinically. Sinusoidal obstruction syndrome may occur in patients who have undergone hematopoietic stem cell transplantation, particularly those with pretransplant serum aminotransferase elevations or fever during cytoreductive therapy with cyclophosphamide, azathioprine, carmustine, busulfan, etoposide, or gemtuzumab ozogamicin or those receiving high-dose cytoreductive therapy or high-dose total body irradiation.

Clinical Findings

A. Symptoms and Signs

The presentation is most commonly subacute but may be fulminant, acute, or chronic; it may present as acute-on-chronic liver failure (see Cirrhosis). Clinical manifestations generally include ascites, painful hepatic enlargement, jaundice, splenomegaly, and AKI. With chronic disease, bleeding varices and hepatic encephalopathy may be evident; hepatopulmonary syndrome may occur.

B. Imaging

Hepatic imaging studies may show a prominent caudate lobe since its venous drainage may be occluded. The screening test of choice is contrast-enhanced, color, or pulsed-Doppler ultrasonography, which has a sensitivity of 85% for detecting evidence of hepatic venous or inferior vena caval thrombosis. MRI with spin-echo and gradient-echo sequences and intravenous gadolinium injection allows visualization of the obstructed veins and collateral vessels. Direct venography can delineate caval webs and occluded hepatic veins ("spider-web" pattern) most precisely but is rarely required. Concomitant splanchnic vein thrombosis may be found in 4–21% of cases.

C. Liver Biopsy

Percutaneous or transjugular liver biopsy in Budd-Chiari syndrome may be considered when the results of noninvasive imaging are inconclusive. The biopsy frequently shows characteristic centrilobular congestion and fibrosis and often multiple large regenerative nodules. Biopsy is rarely required, however, and is often contraindicated in sinusoidal obstruction syndrome because of thrombocytopenia, and the diagnosis is based on clinical findings.

Treatment

Ascites should be treated with diuretics. Treatable causes of Budd-Chiari syndrome should be sought. Prompt recognition and treatment of an underlying hematologic disorder may avoid the need for surgery; however, the optimal anticoagulation regimen is uncertain, and anticoagulation is associated with a high risk of bleeding, particularly in patients with portal hypertension and those undergoing invasive procedures. Low-molecular-weight heparins are preferred over unfractionated heparin because of a high rate of heparin-induced thrombocytopenia with the latter. Warfarin and DOACs seem to have comparable efficacy. Infusion of a thrombolytic agent into recently occluded veins has been attempted with success. Defibrotide, an adenosine receptor agonist that increases endogenous tissue plasminogen activator levels, has been approved by the FDA for the prevention and treatment of the sinusoidal obstruction syndrome. The drug is given as an intravenous infusion every 6 hours for a minimum of 21 days. Serious adverse effects include hypotension and hemorrhage; the drug is expensive and has no benefit in severe sinusoidal obstruction syndrome.

Balloon angioplasty, often with placement of an intravascular metallic stent, is preferred in patients with an inferior vena caval web and is performed commonly in patients with hepatic vein thrombosis. TIPS placement may be attempted in patients with Budd-Chiari syndrome and persistent hepatic congestion or failed thrombolytic therapy and possibly in those with sinusoidal obstruction syndrome. TIPS is preferred over surgical decompression (side-to-side portacaval, mesocaval, or mesoatrial shunt), which is associated with higher early morbidity and mortality. Older age, a higher serum bilirubin level, and a greater INR predict a poor outcome with TIPS. When TIPS is technically not feasible because of complete hepatic vein obstruction, ultrasound-guided direct intrahepatic portosystemic shunt is an alternative approach. Liver transplantation can be considered in patients with acute liver failure, cirrhosis with hepatocellular dysfunction, and failure of other treatments. Patients with Budd-Chiari syndrome often require lifelong anticoagulation, including treatment of any underlying myeloproliferative disease; antiplatelet therapy with aspirin and hydroxyurea has been suggested as an alternative to warfarin in patients with a myeloproliferative disorder.

Prognosis

The overall 5-year survival rate is 50–90% with treatment (but < 10% without intervention). Adverse prognostic factors in patients with Budd-Chiari syndrome are older age, high Child-Pugh score, ascites, encephalopathy, sepsis, elevated total bilirubin, prolonged prothrombin time, elevated serum creatinine, acute respiratory failure, concomitant portal vein thrombosis, cancer, and histologic features of acute liver disease superimposed on chronic liver injury. The 3-month mortality may be predicted by the Rotterdam score, which is based on encephalopathy, ascites, prothrombin time, and bilirubin. A serum ALT level at least fivefold above the upper limit of normal on presentation indicates hepatic ischemia and predicts a poor outcome, particularly when the ALT level decreases slowly. Patients with chronic Budd-Chiari syndrome should undergo surveillance for HCC with abdominal ultrasonography and serum α-fetoprotein levels every 6 months, but the risk is low in the absence of cirrhosis; other risk factors include combined hepatic vein and inferior vena cava obstruction and a long-segment inferior vena cava blockage.

When to Admit

All patients with hepatic vein obstruction should be hospitalized.

Åberg F et al. Three-fold increased risk of death in Budd-Chiari syndrome compared to matched controls: a population-based cohort study. Clin Gastroenterol Hepatol. 2023;21:995. [PMID: 35569740]

Garcia-Pagán JC et al. Primary Budd-Chiari syndrome. N Engl J Med. 2023;388:1307. [PMID: 37018494]

THE LIVER IN HEART FAILURE

Ischemic hepatitis, also called **ischemic hepatopathy, hypoxic hepatitis, shock liver**, or **acute cardiogenic liver injury**, results from an acute fall in cardiac output due to acute MI, arrhythmia, or septic or hemorrhagic shock, usually in a patient with passive congestion of the liver. Almost all cases involve dysfunction of the right ventricle. When heart failure is due to diastolic dysfunction, echocardiography is often insensitive. Clinical hypotension may be absent (or unwitnessed). In some cases, the precipitating event is arterial hypoxemia due to respiratory failure, sleep apnea, severe anemia, heat stroke, carbon monoxide poisoning, cocaine use, or bacterial endocarditis. More than one precipitant is common.

The hallmark of ischemic hepatitis is a rapid and striking elevation of serum aminotransferase levels (often > 1000 U/L). Elevations of serum alkaline phosphatase and bilirubin are usually mild, but jaundice is associated with worse outcomes. Mortality due to the underlying disease is high (particularly in patients receiving vasopressor therapy or with septic shock, acute kidney disease, or coagulopathy), but in patients who recover, the aminotransferase levels return to normal quickly, usually within 1 week—in contrast to viral hepatitis.

In patients with **passive congestion of the liver** ("nutmeg liver") due to right-sided HF, the serum bilirubin level may be elevated, occasionally as high as 40 mg/dL (684 mcmol/L), due in part to hypoxia of perivenular hepatocytes. Its level is a predictor of mortality and morbidity. Serum alkaline phosphatase levels are normal or slightly elevated, and, in the absence of superimposed ischemia, aminotransferase levels are only mildly elevated. Hepatojugular reflux is present, and with tricuspid regurgitation the liver may be pulsatile. Ascites may be out of proportion to peripheral edema, with a high serum-ascites albumin gradient (≥ 1.1) and an ascitic fluid protein level of > 2.5 g/dL (25 g/L). A markedly elevated serum N-terminal-proBNP or BNP level (> 364 pg/mL [364 ng/L]) has been reported to distinguish ascites due to HF from ascites due to cirrhosis in the absence of renal insufficiency. In severe cases, signs of encephalopathy may develop. Liver stiffness measurement by elastography is increased even in the absence of fibrosis. Mortality is generally attributable to the underlying heart disease but has also been reported to correlate with a noninvasive measure of liver stiffness. The MELD score excluding the INR (MELD-XI) predicts the clinical outcome.

Brankovic M et al. Cardiac syndromes in liver disease: a clinical conundrum. J Clin Transl Hepatol. 2023;11:975. [PMID: 37408802]

NONCIRRHOTIC PORTAL HYPERTENSION

ESSENTIALS OF DIAGNOSIS

- Splenomegaly or upper GI bleeding from esophageal or gastric varices in patients without liver disease.
- Portal vein thrombosis complicating cirrhosis.

General Considerations

Causes of noncirrhotic portal hypertension include extrahepatic portal vein obstruction (portal vein thrombosis often with cavernous transformation [portal cavernoma]), splenic vein obstruction (presenting as gastric varices without esophageal varices), schistosomiasis, nodular regenerative hyperplasia, and arterial-portal vein fistula. Idiopathic noncirrhotic portal hypertension is common in India and has been attributed to chronic infections, exposure to medications or toxins, prothrombotic disorders, immunologic disorders, and genetic disorders that result in obliterative vascular lesions in the liver. It is rare in Western countries, where increased mortality is attributable to associated disorders and older age; the term *portosinusoidal vascular disease* has been proposed and includes nodular regenerative hyperplasia, obliterative portal venopathy/portal vein stenosis, hepatoportal sclerosis, and incomplete septal fibrosis/cirrhosis on liver biopsy.

Portal vein thrombosis may occur in 10–25% of patients with cirrhosis. It is associated with the severity of the liver disease and portal hypertension (resulting in stagnant portal venous blood flow). It may be associated with HCC and possibly clinical deterioration but not with increased mortality. Risk factors for portal vein thrombosis in patients without cirrhosis are oral contraceptive use, pregnancy, chronic inflammatory diseases (including pancreatitis), and injury to the portal venous system (including surgery). In the absence of an apparent precipitating cause, an underlying hypercoagulable conditions or myeloproliferative neoplasms (eg, polycythemia vera, essential thrombocytosis) is found in many patients, the latter of which is often associated with a specific pathogenic variant (*V617F*) in the gene coding for JAK2 tyrosine kinase. In many cases, hypercoagulability is a secondary phenomenon due to portosystemic shunting and reduced hepatic blood flow. Portal vein thrombosis may be classified as type 1, involving the main portal vein; type 2, involving one (2a) or both (2b) branches of the portal vein; or type 3, involving the trunk and branches of the portal vein. Additional descriptors are occlusive or nonocclusive, recent or chronic, and extension (into the mesenteric vein) as well as the nature of any underlying liver disease. **Splenic vein thrombosis** may complicate pancreatitis or pancreatic cancer. **Pylephlebitis** (septic thrombophlebitis of the portal vein) may complicate intra-abdominal inflammatory disorders such as appendicitis or diverticulitis, particularly when anaerobic organisms (especially *Bacteroides* species) are involved.

Nodular regenerative hyperplasia results from altered hepatic perfusion and can be associated with collagen vascular diseases; myeloproliferative disorders; and drugs, including azathioprine, 5-fluorouracil, oxaliplatin, and thioguanine. In patients infected with HIV, long-term use of didanosine and use of a combination of didanosine and stavudine have been reported to account for some cases of noncirrhotic portal hypertension often due to nodular regenerative hyperplasia; genetic factors may play a role. The term **obliterative portal venopathy** is used to describe primary occlusion of intrahepatic portal veins in the absence of cirrhosis, inflammation, or hepatic neoplasia. Incomplete septal fibrosis/cirrhosis may represent regressing cirrhosis.

Clinical Findings

A. Symptoms and Signs

Acute portal vein thrombosis usually causes abdominal pain. Aside from splenomegaly, the physical findings are not remarkable, although hepatic decompensation can follow severe GI bleeding, and intestinal infarction may occur when portal vein thrombosis is associated with mesenteric venous thrombosis. Ascites may occur in 25% of persons with noncirrhotic portal hypertension. Covert hepatic encephalopathy is reported to be common in patients with noncirrhotic portal vein thrombosis.

B. Laboratory Findings

Liver biochemical test levels are usually normal or minimally elevated, but there may be findings of hypersplenism (ie, thrombocytopenia and leukopenia).

C. Imaging

Color Doppler ultrasonography is usually the initial diagnostic test for portal vein thrombosis. Contrast-enhanced CT or magnetic resonance angiography (MRA) of the portal system is generally confirmatory and can assess extension of thrombus into the mesenteric veins and exclude tumor thrombus in patients with cirrhosis. Absence of liver surface nodularity on CT favors noncirrhotic rather than cirrhotic portal hypertension but nodularity is not uncommon. In patients with jaundice, magnetic resonance cholangiography may demonstrate compression of the bile duct by a large portal cavernoma (portal biliopathy), a finding that may be more common in patients with an underlying hypercoagulable state than in those without one. In patients with pylephlebitis, CT may demonstrate an intra-abdominal source of infection, thrombosis or gas in the portal venous system, or a hepatic abscess.

D. Other Studies

Endoscopy shows esophageal or gastric varices. Liver biopsy may be indicated to diagnose schistosomiasis, nodular regenerative hyperplasia, and noncirrhotic portal fibrosis and may demonstrate sinusoidal dilatation. A low liver stiffness measurement by elastography may help distinguish noncirrhotic portal hypertension from cirrhosis.

Treatment

Anticoagulation, particularly with low-molecular-weight or unfractionated heparin, or thrombolytic therapy may be indicated for isolated acute portal vein thrombosis and possibly for acute splenic vein thrombosis. Anticoagulation leads to partial recanalization in up to 75% of patients with isolated portal vein thrombosis when started within 6 months of thrombosis. An oral anticoagulant is continued long-term if a hypercoagulable disorder is identified or if an acute portal vein thrombosis extends into the mesenteric veins. In selected cases, TIPS may be considered. Rarely, progressive liver dysfunction requires liver transplantation.

The decision to prescribe an anticoagulant for a patient with cirrhosis and portal vein thrombosis depends on the presence of ascites, the patient's fall risk, the extent and progression of the clot, and the patient's candidacy for liver transplantation. Partial portal vein thrombosis may resolve in 30–50% of cases. Data on the use of DOACs, like all anticoagulants, is low quality in patients with cirrhosis and portal vein thrombosis.

In cases of noncirrhotic portal hypertension with variceal bleeding, band ligation followed by β-blockers to reduce portal pressure is initiated, with portosystemic shunting (including TIPS) reserved for failures of endoscopic therapy. If splenic vein thrombosis is the cause of variceal bleeding, splenectomy or spleen embolization is helpful.

When to Refer

All patients with noncirrhotic portal hypertension should be referred.

Chaudhry H et al. Incidence and factors associated with portal vein thrombosis in patients with acute pancreatitis: a United States national retrospective study. Pancreatology. 2023;23:350. [PMID: 37012176]

Guerrero A et al. Anticoagulation improves survival in patients with cirrhosis and portal vein thrombosis: the IMPORTAL competing-risk meta-analysis. J Hepatol. 2023;79:69. [PMID: 36858157]

Magaz M et al. Porto-sinusoidal vascular liver disorder with portal hypertension: natural history and long-term outcome. J Hepatol. 2025;82:72. [PMID: 39181213]

Mironova M et al. Granulomatous liver diseases. Hepatology Communications. 2024;8:e0392. [PMID: 38497932]

Mukund A et al. Safety and efficacy of transjugular intrahepatic portosystemic shunt for non-tumoral cirrhotic portal vein thrombosis not responding to anticoagulation therapy. Dig Dis Sci. 2023;68:3174. [PMID: 37169934]

PYOGENIC HEPATIC ABSCESS

ESSENTIALS OF DIAGNOSIS

- Fever, right upper quadrant pain, jaundice.
- Often occur in setting of biliary disease, but up to 40% are "cryptogenic" in origin.
- Detected by imaging studies.

General Considerations

The incidence of liver abscess is 3.6 per 100,000 population in the United States and has increased since the 1990s. The liver can be invaded by bacteria via (1) the bile duct (acute "suppurative" [formerly ascending] cholangitis); (2) the portal vein (pylephlebitis); (3) the hepatic artery, secondary to bacteremia; (4) direct extension from an infectious process; and (5) traumatic implantation of bacteria through the abdominal wall or GI tract (eg, a fish or chicken bone). Predisposing conditions and factors include older age, male sex, and the presence of malignancy, diabetes mellitus, IBD, and cirrhosis; necessity for liver transplantation; and endoscopic sphincterotomy.

Acute cholangitis resulting from biliary obstruction due to a stone, stricture, or neoplasm is the most common identifiable cause of hepatic abscess in the United States. In 10% of cases, liver abscess is secondary to appendicitis or diverticulitis. At least 40% of abscesses have no demonstrable cause and are classified as cryptogenic; a dental source is identified in some cases. The most frequently encountered organisms are *E coli, Klebsiella pneumoniae, Proteus vulgaris, Enterobacter aerogenes*, and multiple microaerophilic and anaerobic species (eg, *Streptococcus anginosus* [also known as *S milleri*]); 25% are polymicrobial. Liver abscess caused by hypervirulent strains of *K pneumoniae* may be associated with thrombophlebitis of the portal or hepatic veins and hematogenously spread septic ocular or CNS complications; the abscess may be gas-forming, associated with diabetes mellitus, and result in a high mortality rate. Hepatic candidiasis, tuberculosis, and actinomycosis are seen in immunocompromised patients and those with hematologic malignancies. Rarely, HCC can present as a pyogenic abscess because of tumor necrosis, biliary obstruction, and superimposed bacterial infection (see Chapter 43). The possibility of an amoebic liver abscess must always be considered (see Chapter 39).

Clinical Findings

A. Symptoms and Signs

The presentation is often insidious. Fever (either steady or spiking fever) is almost always present and may antedate other symptoms or signs. Pain may be a prominent complaint and is localized to the right upper quadrant or epigastric area. Jaundice and tenderness in the right upper abdomen are the chief physical findings. The risk of AKI is increased.

B. Laboratory Findings

Laboratory examination reveals leukocytosis with a shift to the left. Liver biochemical tests are nonspecifically abnormal. Blood cultures are positive in 50–100% of cases.

C. Imaging

Chest films may reveal elevation of the diaphragm if the abscess is in the right lobe of the liver. Ultrasonography, CT, or MRI may reveal the presence of intrahepatic lesions. On MRI, characteristic findings include high signal intensity on T2-weighted images and rim enhancement. The characteristic CT appearance of hepatic candidiasis, usually seen in the setting of systemic candidiasis, is that of multiple "bull's-eyes," but imaging studies may be negative in neutropenic patients.

Treatment

Treatment should consist of antimicrobial agents (generally a third-generation cephalosporin such as ceftriaxone 2 g intravenously every 24 hours and metronidazole 500 mg intravenously every 6 hours) that are effective against coliform organisms and anaerobes; if an extended-spectrum β-lactamase–producing organism is suspected, a carbapenem such as meropenem 500 mg intravenously every 6 hours is recommended. The frequency of abscesses caused by multidrug-resistant organisms is increasing. Antibiotics are administered for 2–3 weeks, and sometimes for up to 6 weeks. In selected cases, oral antibiotics may be considered. If the abscess is at least 5 cm in diameter or the response to antibiotic therapy is not rapid, intermittent needle aspiration, percutaneous or EUS-guided catheter drainage or stent placement, or surgical drainage should be done. Other suggested indications for abscess drainage are patient age of at least 55 years, symptom duration of at least 7 days, and involvement of two lobes of the liver. The underlying source (eg, biliary disease, dental infection) should be identified and treated. The mortality rate is substantial (at least 5% in most studies) and is highest in patients with underlying biliary malignancy or severe multiorgan dysfunction. Other risk factors for mortality include older age, cirrhosis, CKD, and other cancers. Fungal abscesses (eg, candidiasis) are associated with mortality rates of up to 50% and are treated with intravenous amphotericin B and drainage.

When to Admit

Nearly all patients with pyogenic hepatic abscess should be hospitalized.

Lam JC et al. Management of pyogenic liver abscesses: contemporary strategies and challenges. J Clin Gastroenterol. 2023;57:774. [PMID: 37249909]

BENIGN LIVER NEOPLASMS

Benign neoplasms of the liver must be distinguished from HCC, intrahepatic cholangiocarcinoma, and metastases (see Chapter 43). The most common benign neoplasm of the liver is the **cavernous hemangioma**, often an incidental finding on ultrasonography or CT. This lesion may enlarge in women who take hormonal therapy and must be differentiated from other space-occupying intrahepatic lesions, usually by contrast-enhanced MRI, CT, or ultrasonography.

Distinct benign lesions with characteristic clinical, radiologic, and histopathologic features include focal nodular hyperplasia, hepatocellular adenoma, and rare instances of sinusoidal dilatation and peliosis hepatis. **Focal nodular hyperplasia** occurs at all ages and in both sexes. In women it is not caused by contraceptives. It is often asymptomatic and appears as a hypervascular mass, often with a central hypodense "stellate" scar on contrast-enhanced ultrasonography, CT, or MRI. Focal nodular hyperplasia may also occur in patients with cirrhosis, with exposure to certain drugs such as azathioprine, and with antiphospholipid syndrome. The prevalence of hepatic hemangiomas is increased in patients with focal nodular hyperplasia.

Hepatocellular adenoma occurs most commonly in women in the third and fourth decades of life and is usually caused by oral contraceptives but also occurs as a result of obesity and metabolic syndrome or use of anabolic steroids. Acute abdominal pain may occur if the tumor undergoes necrosis or hemorrhage. The tumor may be associated with pathogenic variants in a variety of genes, some of which are associated with an increased risk of malignant transformation. The most important of these mutations are the hepatocyte nuclear factor 1 α (NHF1α) gene, β-catenin gene, exon 3 mutations in the catenin-1 gene (CTNNB1), and genes involved in the JAK/STAT pathway activation. Unclassified adenomas account for up to 7% of adenomas. As seen microscopically, the hepatocellular adenoma consists of sheets of hepatocytes without portal tracts or central veins.

Mucinous cystic neoplasms of the liver (previously termed cystadenoma and cystadenocarcinoma) must be distinguished from simple and echinococcal cysts, Von Meyenburg complexes (hamartomas), and polycystic liver disease.

Clinical Findings

The only physical finding in focal nodular hyperplasia or hepatocellular adenoma is a palpable abdominal mass in a minority of cases. Liver biochemistries are usually normal. Contrast-enhanced ultrasonography, arterial phase helical CT, and especially multiphase dynamic MRI with contrast can distinguish an adenoma from focal nodular hyperplasia without the need for biopsy in 80–90% of cases and may suggest a specific subtype of adenoma.

Treatment

In women with focal nodular hyperplasia, oral contraceptives should not be discontinued. The prognosis is excellent. Hepatocellular adenoma may undergo bleeding, necrosis, and rupture in women, often after hormone therapy or in the third trimester of pregnancy, or in men, in whom the rate of malignant transformation is high. Resection is advised in all affected men and in women in whom the tumor causes symptoms or is ≥ 5 cm in diameter, even in the absence of symptoms. Pregnant women should undergo ultrasonography during each trimester and 12 weeks postpartum; a lesion < 5 cm in diameter usually poses little risk of complications. However, if an adenoma is < 5 cm in size, resection is recommended if a biopsy confirms a β-catenin gene pathogenic variant. In selected cases, laparoscopic resection or percutaneous radiofrequency ablation may be feasible. Rarely, liver transplantation is required. Regression of benign hepatic tumors may follow cessation of oral contraceptives and weight loss. Transarterial embolization is the initial treatment for adenomas complicated by hemorrhage or rupture.

When to Refer

- Diagnostic uncertainty.
- For surgery.

When to Admit

- Severe pain.
- Rupture.

Demory A et al. Body weight changes and duration of estrogen exposure modulate the evolution of hepatocellular adenomas after contraception discontinuation. Hepatology. 2023;77:430. [PMID: 35980227]

Reguram R et al. Practical approach to diagnose and manage benign liver masses. Hepatol Commun. 2024;8:e0560. [PMID: 39470338]

DISEASES OF THE BILIARY TRACT

See Chapter 43 for Carcinoma of the Biliary Tract.

CHOLELITHIASIS (Gallstones)

ESSENTIALS OF DIAGNOSIS

- Often asymptomatic.
- Classic biliary pain ("episodic gallbladder pain") characterized by infrequent episodes of steady severe pain in epigastrium or right upper quadrant with radiation to right scapula.
- Gallstones detected on ultrasonography.

General Considerations

Gallstones are more common in women than in men and increase in incidence in both sexes and all races with age. In the United States, the prevalence of gallstones is 8.6% in women and 5.5% in men; rates have doubled since 1988. The highest rates are in persons over age 60, and rates are higher in Latino/Latina persons than in non-Latino/Latina White and Black persons. As many as 75% of Pima and other American Indian women over 25 years of age have cholesterol cholelithiasis. Obesity is a risk factor for gallstones, especially in women. Rapid weight loss, as occurs after bariatric surgery or use of weight loss medications, also increases the risk of symptomatic gallstone formation. Diabetes mellitus, glucose intolerance, insulin resistance, and tobacco use are risk factors for gallstones, and a high intake of carbohydrate and high dietary glycemic load increase the risk of cholecystectomy in women. The prevalence of gallbladder disease is increased in men (but not women) with cirrhosis and HCV infection. Moreover, cholecystectomy has been reported to be associated with an increased risk of MASLD and cirrhosis, possibly because gallstones and liver disease share risk factors. Gallstone disease is associated with increased overall, cardiovascular, and cancer mortality.

The incidence of gallstones is high in individuals with Crohn disease; approximately one-third of those with inflammatory involvement of the terminal ileum have gallstones due to disruption of bile salt resorption that results in decreased solubility of the bile. Drugs such as clofibrate, octreotide, and ceftriaxone can cause gallstones, and the risk is increased with use of glucagon-like peptide-1 receptor agonists. Prolonged fasting (over 5–10 days) can lead to formation of biliary "sludge" or microlithiasis, which usually resolves with refeeding but can lead to gallstones or biliary symptoms. Pregnancy, particularly in obese women and those with insulin resistance, is associated with an increased risk of gallstones and of symptomatic gallbladder disease. Hormone replacement therapy appears to increase the risk of gallbladder disease and need for cholecystectomy; the risk is lower with transdermal than oral therapy. A low-carbohydrate diet and a Mediterranean diet as well as physical activity and cardiorespiratory fitness may help prevent gallstones. Consumption of caffeinated coffee appears to protect against gallstones in women, and a high intake of magnesium and of polyunsaturated and monounsaturated fats reduces the risk of gallstones in men. A diet high in fiber and rich in fruits and vegetables and statin use reduce the risk of cholecystectomy, particularly in women.

Gallstones are classified according to their predominant chemical composition as cholesterol or calcium bilirubinate stones. The latter comprise < 20% of the gallstones found in patients in the United States or Europe but 30–40% of gallstones found in patients in Japan. Calcium bilirubinate stones attributable to hemolysis occurs in over a third of individuals with sickle cell disease.

Clinical Findings

Table 18–9 lists the clinical and laboratory features of several diseases of the biliary tract as well as their treatment. Cholelithiasis is frequently asymptomatic and is discovered during a routine imaging study, surgery, or autopsy. Symptoms (biliary [or "episodic gallbladder"] pain) develop in 10–25% of patients (1–4% annually), and acute cholecystitis develops in 20% of these symptomatic persons over time. Risk factors for the development of symptoms or complications include female sex; young age; awareness of having gallstones; large, multiple, and older stones; gallbladder polyps; and chronic hemolytic anemia.

Treatment

Laparoscopic cholecystectomy is the treatment of choice for symptomatic gallbladder disease. Pain relief after cholecystectomy is most likely in patients with episodic pain (generally once a month or less), pain lasting 30 minutes to 24 hours, pain in the evening or at night, and the onset of symptoms 1 year or less before presentation. The procedure is often performed on an outpatient basis and is suitable for most patients, including those with acute cholecystitis. Conversion to a conventional open cholecystectomy may be necessary in 2–8% of cases (higher for acute cholecystitis than for uncomplicated cholelithiasis). Bile duct injuries occur in 0.1% of cases done by experienced surgeons. The overall complication rate is 11% and correlates with the patient's comorbidities, duration of surgery, and emergency admissions for gallbladder disease prior to cholecystectomy. There is generally no need for prophylactic cholecystectomy in an asymptomatic person unless the gallbladder is calcified, gallstones are ≥ 3 cm in diameter, large (> 1 cm) or rapidly growing gallbladder polyps are found, or the patient is a candidate for bariatric surgery or cardiac transplantation. In pregnant patients, a conservative approach to biliary pain is advised, but for patients with repeated attacks of biliary pain or acute cholecystitis, cholecystectomy can be performed—even by the laparoscopic route—preferably in the second trimester.

When to Refer

Patients should be referred when they require surgery.

Table 18–9. Diseases of the biliary tract.

Disease	Clinical Features	Laboratory Features	Diagnosis	Treatment
Asymptomatic gallstones	Asymptomatic	Normal	Ultrasonography	None
Symptomatic gallstones	Biliary pain	Normal	Ultrasonography	Laparoscopic cholecystectomy
Cholesterolosis of gallbladder	Usually asymptomatic	Normal	Oral cholecystography	None
Adenomyomatosis	May cause biliary pain	Normal	Oral cholecystography	Laparoscopic cholecystectomy if symptomatic
Porcelain gallbladder	Usually asymptomatic; high risk of gallbladder cancer	Normal	Radiograph or CT	Laparoscopic cholecystectomy
Limey bile	Usually asymptomatic; may cause biliary pain or cholecystitis or obstructive jaundice if the bile migrates to the bile duct	Normal	Plain film (incidental finding) or found at cholecystectomy	None in absence of symptoms
Acute cholecystitis	Epigastric or right upper quadrant pain, nausea, vomiting, fever, Murphy sign	Leukocytosis	Ultrasonography, HIDA scan	Antibiotics, laparoscopic cholecystectomy
Chronic cholecystitis	Biliary pain, constant epigastric or right upper quadrant pain, nausea	Normal	Ultrasonography (stones), oral cholecystography (nonfunctioning gallbladder)	Laparoscopic cholecystectomy
Choledocholithiasis	Asymptomatic or biliary pain, jaundice, fever; gallstone pancreatitis	Cholestatic liver biochemical tests; leukocytosis and positive blood cultures in cholangitis; elevated amylase and lipase in pancreatitis	Ultrasonography (dilated ducts), EUS, MRCP, ERCP	Endoscopic sphincterotomy and stone extraction; antibiotics for cholangitis

ERCP, endoscopic retrograde cholangiopancreatography; EUS, endoscopic ultrasonography; HIDA, hepatic iminodiacetic acid; MRCP, magnetic resonance cholangiopancreatography.

Chiang et al. Glucagon-like peptide 1 receptor agonists and gastrointestinal adverse events: a systematic review and meta-analysis. Gastroenterology. 2025;169:1268. [PMID: 40499378]

Konyn P et al. Gallstone disease and its association with nonalcoholic fatty liver disease, all-cause and cause-specific mortality. Clin Gastroenterol Hepatol. 2023;21:940. [PMID: 35643414]

Morris-Stiff G et al. The natural history of asymptomatic gallstones: a longitudinal study and prediction model. Clin Gastroenterol Hepatol. 2023;21:319. [PMID: 35513234]

ACUTE CHOLECYSTITIS

ESSENTIALS OF DIAGNOSIS

- Steady, severe pain and tenderness in the right hypochondrium or epigastrium.
- Nausea and vomiting.
- Fever and leukocytosis.

General Considerations

Cholecystitis is associated with gallstones in 90–95% of cases. It occurs when a stone becomes impacted in the cystic duct and inflammation develops behind the obstruction. Acalculous cholecystitis should be considered when unexplained fever or right upper quadrant pain occurs within 2–4 weeks of major surgery or in a critically ill patient who has had no oral intake for a prolonged period; multiorgan failure is often present. Acute cholecystitis rarely may be caused by infectious agents (eg, cytomegalovirus, cryptosporidiosis, microsporidiosis) in patients with AIDS and by vasculitis (eg, polyarteritis nodosa, Henoch-Schönlein purpura).

Clinical Findings

A. Symptoms and Signs

The acute attack is often precipitated by a large, fatty meal and is characterized by the sudden appearance of steady pain localized to the epigastrium or right hypochondrium, which may gradually subside over a period of 12–18 hours. Vomiting occurs in about 75% of patients and in half of instances affords variable relief. Fever is typical. Right upper quadrant abdominal tenderness (often with a Murphy sign, ie, inhibition of inspiration by pain on palpation of the right upper quadrant) is almost always present and is usually associated with muscle guarding and rebound tenderness (Table 18–9). A palpable gallbladder is present in about 15% of cases. Jaundice is present in about 25% of cases and, when persistent or severe, suggests the possibility of choledocholithiasis.

B. Laboratory Findings

The WBC count is usually elevated (often 12,000–15,000/mcL [12–15 × 10^9/L]). There may be elevations in total serum bilirubin level (1–4 mg/dL [17.1–68.4 mcmol/L]) as well as aminotransferase even in the absence of bile duct obstruction due to inflammation of liver parenchyma adjacent to the inflamed gallbladder. Laboratory findings that may suggest the presence of concomitant choledocholithiasis include a bilirubin ≥ 1.8 mg/dL, serum aminotransferase levels > 3 times the upper limit of normal, or an elevated alkaline phosphatase level.

C. Imaging

Plain films of the abdomen may show radiopaque gallstones in 15% of cases. Right upper quadrant abdominal ultrasonography, which is often performed first, may show gallstones but is not as sensitive for acute cholecystitis (sensitivity 81%, specificity 83%); findings suggestive of acute cholecystitis are gallbladder wall thickening, pericholecystic fluid, and a sonographic Murphy sign. ^{99m}Tc hepatobiliary imaging (using iminodiacetic acid compounds), also known as the hepatic iminodiacetic acid (HIDA) scan, is useful in demonstrating an obstructed cystic duct, which is the cause of acute cholecystitis in most patients. This test is reliable if the bilirubin is under 5 mg/dL (85.5 mcmol/L) (96% sensitivity and 90% specificity for acute cholecystitis). False-positive results can occur with prolonged fasting, liver disease, and chronic cholecystitis, and the specificity can be improved by intravenous administration of morphine, which induces spasm of the sphincter of Oddi. MRI has a sensitivity of 88% and specificity of 89% for acute cholecystitis. CT may show complications of acute cholecystitis, such as perforation or gangrene. Above all, however, it is important to not anchor on "negative" imaging as patients with initial unremarkable imaging tests can progress to gangrene or perforation.

Differential Diagnosis

The disorders most likely to be confused with acute cholecystitis are myocardial ischemia, choledocholithiasis (with or without cholangitis), peptic ulcer disease (including perforations), acute pancreatitis, liver abscess, hepatitis, pneumonia with pleurisy, appendicitis, diverticulitis near the hepatic flexure, and perforated colonic carcinoma. Localization of pain and tenderness in the right upper quadrant, with radiation of pain around to the infrascapular area, strongly favors the diagnosis of acute cholecystitis. True cholecystitis without stones suggests acalculous cholecystitis, which typically occurs in the context of critical illness.

Complications

A. Gangrene of the Gallbladder

Continuation or progression of right upper quadrant abdominal pain, tenderness, muscle guarding, fever, and leukocytosis after 24–48 hours suggests severe inflammation and possible gangrene of the gallbladder, resulting from ischemia due to splanchnic vasoconstriction and intravascular coagulation. Necrosis may occasionally develop without specific signs particularly in persons who are obese, older, immunosuppressed, or have diabetes. Gangrene may lead to gallbladder perforation, usually with formation of a pericholecystic abscess, and rarely to generalized peritonitis. Other serious acute complications include emphysematous cholecystitis (secondary infection with a gas-forming organism) and empyema.

B. Chronic Cholecystitis and Other Complications

Chronic cholecystitis results from repeated episodes of acute cholecystitis or chronic irritation of the gallbladder wall by stones and is characterized pathologically by varying degrees of chronic inflammation of the gallbladder. Calculi are usually present. In about 4–5% of cases, the villi of the gallbladder undergo polypoid enlargement due to deposition of cholesterol that may be visible to the naked eye ("strawberry gallbladder," "scalloping," or cholesterolosis). In other instances, hyperplasia of all or part of the gallbladder wall may be so marked as to give the appearance of a myoma (adenomyomatosis). Hydrops of the gallbladder results when acute cholecystitis subsides but cystic duct obstruction persists, producing distention of the gallbladder with a clear mucoid fluid. Occasionally, a stone in the neck of the gallbladder may compress the common hepatic duct and cause jaundice (Mirizzi syndrome).

Cholelithiasis with chronic cholecystitis may be associated with acute exacerbations of gallbladder inflammation, bile duct stones, pancreatitis and, rarely, carcinoma of the gallbladder. Fistulization to the stomach, duodenum, or small intestine may lead to intestinal obstruction ("gallstone ileus") or Bouveret syndrome (pylorus or duodenum obstruction), which rarely may be the initial manifestation of cholelithiasis. Calcified (porcelain) gallbladder is associated with gallbladder carcinoma and is generally an indication for cholecystectomy; the risk of gallbladder cancer may be higher when calcification is mucosal rather than intramural.

Treatment

Acute cholecystitis usually subsides on a conservative regimen, including withholding oral feedings, intravenous fluids, analgesics, and intravenous antibiotics for 4–7 days (generally a second- or third-generation cephalosporin such as ceftriaxone 1 g intravenously every 24 hours, with the addition of metronidazole, 500 mg intravenously every 6 hours), although they may be stopped 24 hours after cholecystectomy in selected cases without complications. In severe cases, a fluoroquinolone such as ciprofloxacin, 400 mg intravenously every 12 hours, plus metronidazole, may be given. Morphine or meperidine may be administered for pain.

Because of the high risk of recurrent attacks (up to 10% by 1 month and over 20% by 1 year), cholecystectomy generally is performed laparoscopically within 24 hours of admission to the hospital for acute cholecystitis. Conversion to an open cholecystectomy is required in 2–15% of laparoscopic cholecystectomies. Compared with delayed surgery, surgery within 72 hours is associated with a shorter length of stay, lower costs, and greater patient satisfaction, although possibly a higher rate of operative adverse outcomes.

In a patient who is older or has severe comorbidities (especially diabetes) initial non-surgical management may be elected, followed by deferred, elective cholecystectomy if the acute episode resolves. Patients must be watched carefully for recurrent symptoms, evidence of gangrene of the gallbladder, or cholangitis. In patients with high surgical risk, percutaneous cholecystostomy tube placement or endoscopic approaches to gallbladder drainage (such as ultrasound guided cholecystoduodenostomy or retrograde placement of transpapillary stents into the gallbladder) may be considered. Percutaneous drainage may also be considered if gallbladder perforation has occurred. Surgical treatment of chronic cholecystitis is the same as for acute cholecystitis.

Prognosis

The overall mortality rate of cholecystectomy is < 0.2%, but mortality rates are higher in patients who are older or have diabetes or cirrhosis. In appropriately selected patients, the surgical procedure is generally followed by complete resolution of symptoms. Complications of cholecystectomy are reviewed in "Cholelithiasis," above.

When to Admit

All patients with acute cholecystitis should be hospitalized.

ASGE Standards of Practice Committee; Pawa S et al. American Society for Gastrointestinal Endoscopy guideline on the role of therapeutic EUS in the management of biliary tract disorders: summary and recommendations. Gastrointest Endosc. 2024;100:967. [PMID: 39078360]

Bang J et al. EUS-guided gallbladder drainage in acute cholecystitis: long-term problems with surgical approach. Gut. 2024;73:395. [PMID: 38050116]

Hudson JL et al. Endoscopic approaches to cholecystitis. Am J Gastroenterol. 2023;118:1711. [PMID: 37272848]

Inoue T et al. Comparison of the long-term outcomes of EUS-guided gallbladder drainage and endoscopic transpapillary gallbladder drainage for calculous cholecystitis in poor surgical candidates: a multicenter propensity score-matched analysis. Gastrointest Endosc. 2023;98:362. [PMID: 37059367]

Irani SS et al. AGA Clinical Practice Update on role of EUS-guided gallbladder drainage in acute cholecystitis: commentary. Clin Gastroenterol Hepatol. 2023;21:1141. [PMID: 36967319]

PRE- & POSTCHOLECYSTECTOMY SYNDROMES

1. Precholecystectomy

In a small group of patients (mostly women) with biliary pain, conventional radiographic studies of the upper GI tract and gallbladder—initially transabdominal ultrasound—are unremarkable. Persistent symptoms despite negative first line imaging should prompt HIDA scan with cholecystokinin to assess for reduced emptying of the gallbladder. Endoscopic ultrasound may reveal sludge in enigmatic cases in which cross sectional imaging is negative. Cholecystectomy may be curative in such cases. Histologic examination of the resected gallbladder may show chronic cholecystitis or microlithiasis.

2. Postcholecystectomy

Following cholecystectomy, some patients complain of continuing symptoms, ie, right upper quadrant pain, flatulence, and fatty food intolerance. The persistence of symptoms in this group of patients suggests the possibility of an incorrect diagnosis prior to cholecystectomy, eg, esophagitis, pancreatitis, radiculopathy, or functional bowel disease. Pain may also be associated with dilatation of the cystic duct remnant, neuroma formation in the ductal wall, foreign body granuloma, anterior cutaneous nerve entrapment syndrome, or traction on the bile duct by a long cystic duct. Bile-acid diarrhea can present for the first time following cholecystectomy, which can be treated with bile-salt binding agents (colestipol, cholestyramine, colesevelam) (see Chapter 17).

The clinical presentation of right upper quadrant pain, chills, fever, or jaundice suggests biliary tract disease with cholangitis. Choledocholithiasis or bile duct stricture should be ruled out with MRCP or EUS (see Bile Duct stones). Biliary pain associated with elevated liver biochemical tests or a dilated bile duct in the absence of an obstructing stone or lesion may suggest sphincter of Oddi dysfunction. When *both* elevated biochemical tests and bile duct dilation are present, sphincter or papillary stenosis is likely (formerly called type I sphincter of Oddi dysfunction), and endoscopic sphincterotomy may relieve symptoms. In the absence of either elevated liver biochemical tests or a dilated bile duct ("functional pain," formerly type III sphincter of Oddi dysfunction), a nonbiliary source of symptoms should be suspected; sphincterotomy does *not* benefit this group and is associated with a high rate of pancreatitis. When biliary pain is associated with either elevated liver biochemical tests or a dilated bile duct, referral to a specialized center for consideration of biliary manometry to assess for elevated baseline sphincter of Oddi pressures ("sphincter disorder," formerly called type II sphincter of Oddi dysfunction) and multidisciplinary treatment is suggested. In refractory cases, surgical sphincteroplasty or removal of the cystic duct remnant may be considered.

When to Refer

Patients with suspected sphincter of Oddi dysfunction should be referred to tertiary care centers for multidisciplinary diagnostic evaluation and treatment.

Beran A et al. Predictors of post-endoscopic retrograde pancreatitis: a comprehensive systematic review and meta-analysis. Clin Gastroenterol Hepatol. 2025;23:1905. [PMID: 39694210]

Beyer G et al. Definition of age-dependent reference values for the diameter of the common bile duct and pancreatic duct on MRCP: a population-based, cross-sectional cohort study. Gut. 2023;72:1738. [PMID: 36828626]

Coté GA et al. Characteristics of patients undergoing endoscopic retrograde cholangiopancreatography for sphincter of Oddi disorders. Clin Gastroenterol Hepatol. 2022;20:e627. [PMID: 33716141]

Coté GA et al. Sphincterotomy for biliary for biliary sphincter of Oddi disorder and idiopathic acute recurrent pancreatitis: then RESPOnD longitudinal cohort. Gut. 2024;74:58. [PMID 39244217]

CHOLEDOCHOLITHIASIS & CHOLANGITIS

ESSENTIALS OF DIAGNOSIS

- Often a history of biliary pain, which may be accompanied by jaundice.
- Occasional patients present with painless jaundice.
- Nausea and vomiting.
- Cholangitis should be suspected with right upper quadrant pain, jaundice, shock, and leukocytosis.
- Stones in bile duct most reliably detected by MRCP, EUS, or ERCP.

General Considerations

Bile duct stones usually originate in the gallbladder but may also form spontaneously in the bile duct (primary duct stones), particularly if there is biliary stasis, a history of prior biliary injury, or juxtapapillary duodenal diverticuli. Symptoms and possible cholangitis result if the bile duct stone leads to biliary obstruction. About 15% of patients with gallstones in the gallbladder have choledocholithiasis (bile duct stones) though the prevalence is higher in older adults. Compared with cholesterol stones that originate in the gallbladder, primary bile duct stones tend to have higher calcium content and are more commonly associated with cholangitis.

Clinical Findings

A. Symptoms and Signs

A history of biliary pain or jaundice may be obtained. Characteristic features that suggest the presence of a bile duct stone are recurring attacks of right upper abdominal pain that is severe and persists for hours and jaundice. Biliary pain results from rapid increases in bile duct pressure due to obstructed bile flow (see Table 18–9). Tenderness is usually present on examination of the right upper quadrant or epigastrium.

The combination of jaundice, chills, and fever associated with right upper quadrant pain represents **Charcot triad** and denotes the classic picture of acute cholangitis, although one that has a low diagnostic sensitivity. The addition of altered mental status and hypotension (**Reynolds pentad**) signifies acute suppurative cholangitis and is an endoscopic emergency. According to the Tokyo guidelines (revised in 2018), the diagnosis of acute cholangitis is established by an elevated WBC (signifying systemic inflammation) with either elevated liver biochemical test levels, imaging evidence of biliary dilatation, or both. The BILE criteria have also been proposed for the diagnosis of acute cholangitis: *b*iliary imaging abnormalities, *i*nflammatory test abnormalities, *l*iver test abnormalities, and *e*xclusion of cholecystitis and acute pancreatitis.

B. Laboratory Findings

Acute obstruction of the bile duct (most commonly causes by a stone) typically produces a transient but substantial increase in serum aminotransferase levels (sometimes > 1000 U/L [20 mckat/L]). Elevation of the serum bilirubin is present if the bile duct remains obstructed, and levels commonly fluctuate. Serum alkaline phosphatase levels rise more slowly and, if elevated, typically indicate chronic obstruction. Leukocytosis is present in patients with acute cholangitis. Not uncommonly, serum amylase elevations are present because of secondary pancreatitis. When extrahepatic obstruction persists for more than a few weeks, differentiation of obstruction from chronic cholestatic liver disease becomes more difficult. Prolongation of the prothrombin time can result from the obstructed flow of bile to the intestine. In contrast to hepatocellular dysfunction, hypoprothrombinemia due to obstructive jaundice will respond to intravenous vitamin K, 10 mg, or water-soluble oral vitamin K (phytonadione), 5 mg, within 24–36 hours.

In patients with acute calculous cholecystitis, predictors of concomitant choledocholithiasis are serum aminotransferase levels over three times the upper limit of normal, an alkaline phosphatase level above normal, a serum lipase over three times the upper limit of normal, a bilirubin ≥ 1.8 mg/dL, and a bile duct diameter > 6 mm.

C. Imaging

Ultrasonography and CT may demonstrate dilated bile ducts but have poor sensitivity for detecting bile duct stones. Magnetic resonance cholangiography (MRCP) and EUS have higher sensitivity for detecting bile duct stones and are most useful diagnostically in patients thought to be at intermediate risk for choledocholithiasis prior to ERCP (ie, age > 55 years, elevated serum bilirubin 1.8–4 mg/dL [30.78–68.4 mcmol/L], other elevated liver enzymes, or bile duct diameter > 6 mm on ultrasonography). A decision analysis has suggested that magnetic resonance cholangiography is preferable when the risk of bile duct stones is low (< 40%), and EUS is preferable when the risk is intermediate (40–91%).

In patients undergoing cholecystectomy for acute or chronic cholecystitis, patients deemed at low risk of having concomitant choledocholithiasis (ie, age < 55 years without liver tests abnormalities or ductal dilation), may proceed directly to cholecystectomy without further presurgical evaluation biliary evaluation with MRCP, EUS, or ERCP. In those deemed at intermediate risk for choledocholithiasis, intraoperative cholangiography is an alternative to preoperative ERCP and may require fewer bile duct investigations than performing a preoperative ERCP that is triggered by a positive MRCP or EUS.

If the likelihood is high that biliary obstruction is caused by a stone (serum bilirubin > 4 mg/dL [68.4 mcmol/L]; acute cholangitis with dilated bile duct seen on cross sectional imaging; a bile duct stone seen on ultrasonography, cross sectional imaging, MRCP or EUS), ERCP usually provides the most direct means for diagnosing and treating the cause of biliary obstruction.

Bile duct obstruction lasting more than 30 days results in liver damage leading to cirrhosis. Hepatic failure with portal hypertension occurs in untreated cases of biliary obstruction.

Differential Diagnosis

The most common cause of obstructive jaundice is a bile duct stone. Next in frequency are neoplasms of the pancreas, ampulla of Vater, or bile duct, an obstructed stent placed previously for decompression of an obstructing tumor, or a benign stricture. Extrinsic compression of the bile duct may result from metastatic carcinoma (usually from the GI tract or breast) involving porta hepatis lymph nodes or, rarely, from a large duodenal diverticulum. Gallbladder cancer extending into the bile duct often presents as obstructive jaundice. Chronic cholestatic liver diseases (PBC, sclerosing cholangitis, drug-induced) must be considered. Hepatocellular jaundice can usually be differentiated by the history, clinical findings, and liver biochemical tests, but liver biopsy is necessary on occasion. Recurrent pyogenic cholangitis should be considered in persons from Asia (and occasionally elsewhere) with intrahepatic biliary stones (particularly in the left ductal system) and recurrent cholangitis.

Treatment

In general, bile duct stones, even small ones, should be removed. A bile duct stone in a patient with cholelithiasis or cholecystitis is usually treated by ERCP with endoscopic sphincterotomy and stone removal using an extraction balloon or basket. Subsequent laparoscopic cholecystectomy ideally is performed during the same hospitalization for inpatients or as soon as possible for outpatients.

Choledocholithiasis discovered at laparoscopic cholecystectomy by intraoperative palpation, cholangiography, or ultrasonography may be managed via laparoscopic bile duct exploration, postoperative ERCP with endoscopic sphincterotomy, or, less commonly, open bile duct exploration. In selected cases, laparoscopic cholecystectomy and ERCP can be performed in a single session with lower morbidity and a shorter hospital stay.

In patients with cholangitis, intravenous fluids and antibiotics should be administered as soon as possible. Pressors should be considered in those who remain hypotensive despite resuscitation with 2 L of intravenous fluid. For mild-to-moderately severe community-acquired acute cholangitis, ciprofloxacin (400 mg intravenously every 12 hours) penetrates well into bile and is effective treatment, with metronidazole (500 mg intravenously every 6–8 hours) for anaerobic coverage. An alternative regimen is ampicillin-sulbactam (3 g intravenously every 6 hours). Regimens for patients with severe or hospital-acquired acute cholangitis, and those potentially infected with an antibiotic-resistant pathogen, include intravenous piperacillin-tazobactam (3.375 or 4 g every 6 hours) or a carbapenem such as meropenem (1 g intravenously every 8 hours).

Following antibiotic administration and patient stabilization, ERCP with sphincterotomy, biliary drainage, and stone removal or stent placement, should be performed generally within 48 hours and before cholecystectomy in patients with jaundice (serum total bilirubin > 4 mg/dL [68.4 mcmol/L]), a dilated bile duct (> 6 mm), or stones in the bile duct seen on ultrasonography or CT. Conversely, in patients whose symptoms, fever, WBC, and abnormal liver chemistries rapidly improve (suggesting possible passage of the duct stone), ERCP may not be necessary if cholecystectomy with intraoperative cholangiography is planned or if MRCP or EUS do not demonstrate a bile duct stone. Emergent decompression of the bile duct, generally by ERCP, is required for patients with choledocholithiasis and cholangitis who are septic or fail to improve on antibiotics within 12–24 hours. EUS-guided medical therapy alone is most likely to fail in patients with tachycardia, a serum albumin < 3 g/dL (30 g/L), marked hyperbilirubinemia, a high serum ALT level, a high WBC count, and a prothrombin time > 14 seconds on admission.

Choledocholithiasis may ultimately recur in up to 12% of patients, particularly in older patients, when the bile duct diameter is ≥ 15 mm or when brown pigment stones (suggesting primary choledocholithiasis) are found at the time of the initial sphincterotomy.

When to Refer

All symptomatic patients with choledocholithiasis should be referred.

When to Admit

All patients with acute cholangitis should be hospitalized.

Facciorusso A et al. Endoscopic treatment of large bile duct stones: a systematic review and network meta-analysis. Clin Gastroenterol Hepatol. 2023;21:33. [PMID: 34666153]

Srinu et al. Conventional vs short duration of antibiotics in patients with moderate or severe cholangitis: noninferiority randomized trial. Am J Gastroenterol. 2024;119:176. [PMID: 37732816]

BILIARY STRICTURE

Biliary strictures may be caused by benign disease or malignancy (most commonly pancreatic carcinoma, ampullary carcinoma, cholangiocarcinoma, or gallbladder carcinoma). Benign biliary strictures occur in 95% of cases at the site of surgical anastomosis (including liver transplantation) or at the site of surgical bile duct injury. The remainder of cases are caused by blunt external injury to the abdomen, pancreatitis, primary sclerosing cholangitis, erosion of the duct by a gallstone, or prior endoscopic sphincterotomy. Strictures caused by IgG_4-related disease are sometimes difficult to distinguish from primary sclerosing cholangitis or cholangiocarcinoma.

Signs of injury to the duct may or may not be recognized in the immediate postoperative period. If complete occlusion has occurred, jaundice will develop rapidly. More often, a tear has been made accidentally in the duct, from which the earliest manifestation of injury may be excessive or prolonged loss of bile from the surgical drains. Bile leakage resulting in a bile collection (biloma) may predispose to localized infection, which in turn accentuates scar formation and the ultimate development of a fibrous stricture.

Cholangitis is the most common complication of stricture. Typically, the patient experiences episodes of pain, fever, chills, and jaundice within a few weeks to months after cholecystectomy. Physical findings may include jaundice during an acute attack of cholangitis and right upper quadrant abdominal tenderness. Serum alkaline phosphatase is usually elevated. Hyperbilirubinemia is variable, fluctuating during exacerbations and usually remaining in the range of 5–10 mg/dL (85.5–171 mcmol/L). Blood cultures may be positive during an acute episode of cholangitis. Secondary biliary cirrhosis may develop if a stricture is not treated.

MRCP is most valuable in demonstrating the stricture and outlining the anatomy. ERCP is the first-line interventional approach and permits sphincterotomy (to allow a bile leak to close), stricture biopsy or EUS-guided fine needle aspiration (to exclude malignancy), stricture dilation (often repeated), and stent placement (to maintain bile duct patency and drainage). When ERCP is unsuccessful, dilation of a stricture may be accomplished by PTC or under EUS guidance. EUS (often with ERCP) is the preferred initial approach for evaluation of a pancreatic mass.

Placement of multiple plastic biliary stents appears to be more effective than placement of a single stent. The use of fully covered self-expanding metal stents, which are more easily removed endoscopically than uncovered metal stents are generally preferable to use of plastic stents and requires fewer ERCPs to achieve stricture resolution including those occurring post–liver transplantation; stent migration may occur in 10% of cases. Following liver transplantation, endoscopic management is more successful for anastomotic than for nonanastomotic strictures. Results for nonanastomotic strictures may be improved with repeated dilations or the use of multiple plastic stents.

Endoscopic ultrasound can usually differentiate malignant from benign distal biliary strictures. For hilar strictures, this differentiation often is more challenging. Initial approaches to evaluation of biliary strictures include ERCP with fluoroscopically guided brushing and biopsy. When malignancy cannot be excluded with certainty, additional diagnostic approaches include intraductal ultrasonography and direct peroral cholangioscopy in conjunction with various enhanced imaging modalities. Differentiation from cholangiocarcinoma may ultimately require surgical exploration in 20% of cases. Operative treatment of a stricture frequently necessitates performance of an end-to-end ductal repair, choledochojejunostomy, or hepaticojejunostomy to reestablish bile flow into the intestine.

When to Refer

All patients with biliary stricture should be referred.

When to Admit

Patients with acute cholangitis should be hospitalized.

Bardhi O et al. Next-generation sequencing improves the detection of malignant biliary strictures and changes management. Gastrointest Endosc. 2025;102:56. [PMID 39716538]

Elmunzer BJ et al. ACG clinical guideline: diagnosis and management of biliary strictures. Am J Gastroenterol. 2023;118:405. [PMID: 36863037]

Fujii-Lau LL et al. American Society for Gastrointestinal Endoscopy guideline on the role of endoscopy in the diagnosis of malignancy in biliary strictures of undetermined etiology: summary and recommendations. Gastrointest Endosc. 2023;98:685. [PMID: 37307900]

Kohli DR et al. American Society for Gastrointestinal Endoscopy guideline on management of post-liver transplant biliary strictures: summary and recommendations. Gastrointest Endosc. 2023;97:607. [PMID: 36797162]

PRIMARY SCLEROSING CHOLANGITIS

ESSENTIALS OF DIAGNOSIS

- Most common in men aged 20–50 years.
- Often associated with ulcerative colitis.
- Progressive jaundice, itching, and other features of cholestasis.
- Diagnosis based on characteristic cholangiographic findings.
- At least 10% risk of cholangiocarcinoma.

General Considerations

Primary sclerosing cholangitis is an uncommon disease thought to result from an increased immune response to intestinal endotoxins and characterized by diffuse inflammation of the biliary tract leading to fibrosis and strictures of the biliary system. From 60% to 70% of affected persons are male, usually 20–50 years of age (median age 41). It has a prevalence of 16.2 per 100,000 population (21 per 100,000 men and 6 per 100,000 women) in the United States.

Primary sclerosing cholangitis is closely associated with IBD (more commonly ulcerative colitis than Crohn colitis), which is present in approximately two-thirds of patients; however, clinically significant sclerosing cholangitis develops in only 1–4% of patients with ulcerative colitis. The diagnosis of primary sclerosing cholangitis may be difficult to make after biliary surgery.

Clinical Findings

A. Symptoms and Signs

Primary sclerosing cholangitis presents as progressive obstructive jaundice, frequently associated with fatigue, pruritus, anorexia, and indigestion. A patient's disease may be diagnosed in the presymptomatic phase because of an elevated alkaline phosphatase level or a subclinical phase based on abnormalities on magnetic resonance cholangiography despite normal liver enzyme levels. Complications of chronic cholestasis, such as osteoporosis, malabsorption of fat-soluble vitamins, and malnutrition, may occur late in the course. Risk factors for osteoporosis include older age, lower BMI, and longer duration of IBD. Esophageal varices on initial endoscopy are most likely in patients with a higher Mayo risk score based on age, bilirubin, albumin, and AST and a higher AST/ALT ratio, and new varices are likely to develop in those with a lower platelet count and higher bilirubin at 2 years. In patients with primary sclerosing cholangitis, ulcerative colitis is frequently characterized by rectal sparing and backwash ileitis.

B. Diagnostic Findings

The diagnosis of primary sclerosing cholangitis is generally made by MRCP, the sensitivity of which approaches that of ERCP. ERCP should be avoided, if possible, to reduce the risk of bacterial cholangitis. Characteristic cholangiographic findings are segmental fibrosis of bile ducts with saccular dilatations between strictures. Biliary obstruction by a stone or tumor should be excluded. Liver biopsy is not necessary for diagnosis when cholangiographic findings are characteristic. The disease may be confined to small intrahepatic bile ducts in about 15% of cases, in which case MRCP and ERCP are normal, and the diagnosis is suggested by liver biopsy findings. These patients have a longer survival than patients with involvement of the large ducts and do not appear to be at increased risk for cholangiocarcinoma unless large-duct sclerosing cholangitis develops (which occurs in about 20% over 7–10 years). Liver biopsy may show characteristic periductal fibrosis ("onion-skinning") and allows staging, which is based on the degree of fibrosis and which correlates with liver stiffness as measured by elastography.

Differential Diagnosis

Occasional patients have clinical and histologic features of both sclerosing cholangitis and autoimmune hepatitis. Cholangitis in IgG_4-related disease is sometimes difficult to distinguish from primary sclerosing cholangitis (and even cholangiocarcinoma). IgG_4-related sclerosing cholangitis is associated with autoimmune pancreatitis (see Chronic Pancreatitis) and is responsive to corticosteroids. A serum IgG_4 level more than four times the upper limit of normal or an IgG_4:IgG_1 ratio of more than 0.24 strongly suggests IgG_4-related sclerosing cholangitis, but in up to one-third of cases, the serum IgG_4 level is normal. In IgG_4-related cholangiopathy, EUS reveals symmetric ductal thickening and ERCP reveals a band-like stricture due to dense inflammatory infiltrate of the duct wall. Primary sclerosing cholangitis must also be distinguished from idiopathic adulthood ductopenia (a rare disorder that affects young to middle-aged adults who develop cholestasis due to loss of interlobular and septal bile ducts. Other conditions that can resemble primary sclerosing cholangitis are cystic fibrosis liver disease, AIDS cholangiopathy, graft-versus-host disease, and ischemic cholangiopathy caused by hepatic artery thrombosis, shock, or respiratory failure.

Complications

Cholangiocarcinoma may complicate the course of primary sclerosing cholangitis in up to 20% of cases (1.2% per year) and may be difficult to diagnose by cytologic examination or biopsy because of false-negative results. A serum CA 19-9 level above 100 U/mL is suggestive but not diagnostic of cholangiocarcinoma. Semiannual MRI with MRCP or right upper quadrant US (or alternating MRI and US), and, by some guidelines, serum CA 19-9 testing are recommended for surveillance. MRCP is more sensitive than US. If the results of screening are suggestive of malignancy, ERCP is performed with biliary cytology and biopsy, FISH, and increasingly next-generation sequencing. MRI with MRCP every 3–5 years is recommended in patients with small-duct disease. Serum fibrosis tests and/or elastography can be done every 2–3 years to monitor for advanced fibrosis. The risks of gallstones, cholecystitis, gallbladder polyps, and gallbladder carcinoma appear to be increased in patients with primary sclerosing cholangitis.

Patients with ulcerative colitis and primary sclerosing cholangitis are at a 10-fold higher risk for colorectal neoplasia compared with other ulcerative colitis patients, especially in the right colon. Strict adherence to a colonoscopic surveillance program is recommended: yearly for those with ulcerative colitis and every 5 years for those without ulcerative colitis.

Treatment

Episodes of acute bacterial cholangitis may be treated with appropriate antibiotics selected on the basis of culture data or empirically using fluoroquinolones (eg, ciprofloxacin) or broad-spectrum penicillin (eg, ampicillin-sulbactam). Ursodeoxycholic acid in standard doses (10–15 mg/kg/day orally) may improve liver biochemical test results but does not appear to alter the natural history. However, withdrawal of ursodeoxycholic acid may result in worsening of liver biochemical test levels and increased pruritus.

Careful endoscopic evaluation of the biliary tract may permit endoscopic balloon dilation of localized strictures. Repeated dilation of a dominant stricture may improve survival, although such patients have reduced survival compared with patients who do not have a dominant stricture. Short-term (2–3 weeks) placement of a stent in a major stricture also may relieve symptoms and improve biochemical abnormalities, with sustained improvement after the stent is removed, but may not be superior to balloon dilation alone; long-term stenting may increase the rate of complications such as cholangitis and is not recommended.

Cholecystectomy is indicated in patients with primary sclerosing cholangitis and a gallbladder polyp > 8 mm in diameter. In patients without cirrhosis, surgical resection of a dominant bile duct stricture may lead to longer survival than endoscopic therapy by decreasing the subsequent risk of cholangiocarcinoma. When feasible, extensive surgical resection of cholangiocarcinoma complicating primary sclerosing cholangitis may result in 5-year survival rates of > 50%. For patients with cirrhosis and clinical decompensation, liver transplantation is the treatment of choice; primary sclerosing cholangitis recurs in the graft in 30% of cases, with a possible reduction in the risk of recurrence when colectomy has been performed for ulcerative colitis before transplantation.

Prognosis

Transplant-free survival of patients with primary sclerosing cholangitis averages 9–17 years, and up to 21 years in population-based studies. Adverse prognostic markers are older age, hepatosplenomegaly, higher serum bilirubin and AST levels, lower albumin levels, a history of variceal bleeding, a dominant bile duct stricture, extrahepatic duct changes, and bile duct colonization with *Enterococci*. Patients in whom serum alkaline phosphatase levels decline by 40% or more (spontaneously, with ursodeoxycholic acid therapy, or after treatment of a dominant stricture) have longer transplant-free survival times than those in whom the alkaline phosphatase does not decline. Moreover, improvement in the serum alkaline phosphatase to < 1.5 times the upper limit of normal is associated with a reduced risk of cholangiocarcinoma; however, use of the serum alkaline phosphatase alone to predict outcomes is not recommended. Risk of progression can be predicted by three findings on MRI and MRCP: a cirrhotic appearance to the liver, portal hypertension, and enlarged perihepatic lymph nodes.

Several models are proposed to predict transplant-free survival in patients with primary sclerosing cholangitis. These include the Amsterdam-Oxford model, the UK-PSC risk score, and the PSC risk estimate tool (PREsTo). Transplant-free survival can also be predicted by serum levels of markers of liver fibrosis—hyaluronic acid, tissue inhibitor of metalloproteinase-1, and propeptide of type III procollagen. Anti integrin αvβ6 antibodies are higher in those with PSC and IBD and correlate with disease severity. Reduced quality of life is associated with older age, large-duct disease, and systemic symptoms. Interestingly, patients with milder ulcerative colitis tend to have more severe primary cholangitis and a higher rate of liver transplantation.

Actuarial survival rates with liver transplantation are as high as 72% at 5 years, but rates are much lower once cholangiocarcinoma has developed. Following transplantation, the disease recurs in 30%. Post-transplant patients have an increased risk of nonanastomotic biliary strictures and—in those with ulcerative colitis—colon cancer. The retransplantation rate is higher than that for PBC. Patients who are unable to undergo liver transplantation will ultimately require high-quality palliative care (see Chapter 5).

Assis DN et al. Recent advances in the management of primary sclerosing cholangitis. Clin Gastroenterol Hepatol. 2023;21:2065. [PMID: 37084929]

Bloeman H. Anti-integrin αvβ6 autoantibodies ae increased in primary sclerosing cholangitis patients with concomitant inflammatory bowel disease and correlate with liver disease severity. Clin Gastroenterol Hepatol. 2025;23:1612. [PMID 39490950]

Bowlus CL et al. AASLD practice guidance on primary sclerosing cholangitis and cholangiocarcinoma. Hepatology. 2023;77:659. [PMID: 36083140]

European Association for the Study of the Liver. EASL Clinical Practice Guidelines on sclerosing cholangitis. J Hepatol. 2022;77:761. [PMID: 35738507]

Kamp EJCA et al. Next-generation sequencing mutation analysis on biliary brush cytology for differentiation of benign and malignant strictures in primary sclerosing cholangitis. Gastrointest Endosc. 2023;97:456. [PMID: 36252869]

Wentworth BJ et al. The many faces of primary sclerosing cholangitis: controversy abounds. Dig Dis Sci. 2023;68:3514. [PMID: 37358638]

Yang H et al. Current status of pharmacotherapy for primary sclerosing cholangitis. Front Med. 2025;12:1544601. [PMID: 40655103]

DISEASES OF THE PANCREAS

See Chapter 43 for Carcinoma of the Pancreas and Periampullary Area.

ACUTE PANCREATITIS

ESSENTIALS OF DIAGNOSIS

- Abrupt onset of deep epigastric pain, often with radiation to the back.
- History of previous episodes, often related to alcohol intake.
- Nausea, vomiting, sweating, weakness.
- Abdominal tenderness and distention and fever.
- Leukocytosis, elevated serum amylase and serum lipase.

General Considerations

The annual incidence of acute pancreatitis ranges from 110 to 140 per 100,000 population and has increased since 1990. Most cases of acute pancreatitis are related to biliary tract disease (40–70%) (due to a passed gallstone, usually 5 mm or less in diameter) or heavy alcohol intake (20–30%), with worldwide variations. Among the numerous other causes or associations are hyperlipidemias (chylomicronemia, hypertriglyceridemia, or both), hypercalcemia, abdominal trauma (including surgery), ERCP (overall risk 5–15%), EUS, single- or double-balloon enteroscopy, and medications (including azathioprine, mercaptopurine, asparaginase, pentamidine, didanosine, valproic acid, tetracyclines, dapsone, isoniazid, estrogen and tamoxifen [by raising serum triglycerides], sulfonamides, mesalamine, celecoxib, sulindac, leflunomide, thiazides, simvastatin, fenofibrate, enalapril, sitagliptin, GLP-1 receptor agonists, and others). Unusual causes include vasculitis, infections (eg, hepatitis viruses, mumps, cytomegalovirus, *M avium intracellulare* complex, SARS-CoV-2), peritoneal dialysis, cardiopulmonary bypass, and scorpion bite (rare). In patients with pancreas divisum, a congenital anomaly in which the dorsal and ventral pancreatic ducts fail to fuse, acute pancreatitis may result from stenosis of the minor papilla with obstruction to flow from the accessory pancreatic duct, although concomitant gene variants, particularly in the cystic fibrosis transmembrane conductance regulator (*CFTR*) gene, may account for acute pancreatitis in these patients. Acute pancreatitis may also result from an anomalous junction of the pancreaticobiliary duct (pancreaticobiliary malunion). Rarely, acute pancreatitis may be the presenting manifestation of a pancreatic or ampullary neoplasm or pancreatic cyst. Apparently "idiopathic" acute pancreatitis is often caused by occult biliary microlithiasis or rarely by sphincter of Oddi dysfunction involving the pancreatic duct. Between 15% and 25% of cases are truly idiopathic. Smoking, high dietary glycemic load, and abdominal adiposity increase the risk of pancreatitis, and older age and obesity increase the risk of a severe course.

Clinical Findings

A. Symptoms and Signs

Epigastric abdominal pain, generally abrupt in onset, is steady, boring, and severe. It may be made worse by walking or lying supine and improved by sitting and leaning forward. The pain usually radiates into the back but may radiate to the right or left. Nausea and vomiting are usually present. Weakness, sweating, and anxiety are noted in severe attacks. There may be a history of alcohol intake or a heavy meal immediately preceding the attack or a history of milder similar episodes or biliary pain in the past.

The upper abdomen is tender, most often without guarding, rebound, or rigidity. The abdomen may be distended, and bowel sounds may be absent with associated ileus. Fever of 38.4–39°C, tachycardia, hypotension (even shock), pallor, and cool clammy skin are present in severe cases. Jaundice may be seen. Occasionally, an upper abdominal mass due to the inflamed pancreas or a pseudocyst may be palpated. AKI (usually prerenal azotemia) may occur early in the course of acute pancreatitis.

B. Laboratory Findings

Serum lipase and amylase are elevated—usually more than three times the upper limit of normal—within 24 hours in 90% of cases; their return to normal is variable depending on the severity of disease. Lipase remains elevated longer than amylase and is slightly more accurate for the diagnosis of acute pancreatitis. Leukocytosis (10,000–30,000/mcL [10–30 × 10^9/L]), proteinuria, granular casts, glycosuria (10–20% of cases), hyperglycemia, and elevated serum bilirubin may be present. BUN and serum alkaline phosphatase may be elevated and coagulation tests abnormal. An elevated serum creatinine level (> 1.8 mg/dL [149.94 mcmol/L]), hematocrit (> 47%), or BUN (> 20 mg/dL) are associated with the development of pancreatic necrosis. In patients with clear evidence of acute pancreatitis, a serum ALT level > 150 U/L (3 mkat/L) suggests biliary (gallstone-induced) pancreatitis. A decrease in serum calcium may reflect saponification and correlates with severity of the disease. Levels < 7 mg/dL (1.75 mmol/L) (when serum albumin is normal) are associated with tetany and an unfavorable prognosis. Patients with acute pancreatitis caused by hypertriglyceridemia generally have fasting triglyceride levels > 1000 mg/dL (10 mmol/L) and often have other risk factors for pancreatitis. In patients in whom ascites or a left pleural effusion develops, fluid amylase content is high. ECG may show ST–T wave changes.

C. Assessment of Severity

In addition to the individual laboratory parameters noted above, the severity of acute alcohol-associated pancreatitis can be assessed using several scoring systems (none of which has been shown to have high prognostic accuracy), including the **Ranson criteria** (Table 18–10). The **revised Atlanta classification** of the severity of acute pancreatitis uses the following three categories: (1) **mild** disease is defined as the absence of organ failure (renal, cardiovascular, respiratory) and local ([peri]pancreatic necrosis or fluid collections) or systemic complications; (2) **moderate** disease is the presence of transient (under 48 hours) organ failure, and local (necrosis, fluid collections) or systemic (eg, exacerbation of comorbidity) complications; and (3) **severe** disease is the presence of persistent (48 hours or more) organ failure. The severity of acute pancreatitis can also be predicted by the **Pancreatitis Activity Scoring System (PASS)** based on organ failure, intolerance to a

Table 18–10. Ranson criteria for assessing the severity of acute pancreatitis.

Three or more of the following predict a severe course complicated by pancreatic necrosis with a sensitivity of 60–80%
- Age > 55 years
- WBC count > 16 × 10^3/mcL (> 16 × 10^9/L)
- Blood glucose > 200 mg/dL (> 11 mmol/L)
- Serum LD > 350 U/L (> 7 mkat/L)
- AST > 250 U/L (> 5 mkat/L)

Development of the following in the first 48 hours indicates a worsening prognosis
- Hematocrit drop of > 10 percentage points
- BUN rise > 5 mg/dL (> 1.8 mmol/L)
- Arterial PO_2 of < 60 mm Hg (< 7.8 kPa)
- Serum calcium of < 8 mg/dL (< 0.2 mmol/L)
- Base deficit over 4 mEq/L
- Estimated fluid sequestration of > 6 L

Mortality rates correlate with the number of criteria present

Number of Criteria	Mortality Rate
0–2	1%
3–4	16%
5–6	40%
7–8	100%

solid diet, systemic inflammatory response syndrome, abdominal pain, and dose of intravenous morphine (or its equivalent) required to control pain. PanPROMISE is a patient reported outcome scale with domains including pain, distension, difficulty eating, constipation, nausea, thirst, and weakness. Another simple 5-point clinical scoring system (the **Bedside Index for Severity in Acute Pancreatitis**, or **BISAP**) based on **B**UN above 25 mg/dL (9 mmol/L), **I**mpaired mental status, **S**ystemic inflammatory response syndrome, **A**ge older than 60 years, and **P**leural effusion during the first 24 hours (before the onset of organ failure) identifies patients at increased risk for mortality. More simply, the presence of a systemic inflammatory response alone and an elevated BUN level on admission as well as a rise in BUN within the first 24 hours of hospitalization are independently associated with increased mortality; the greater the rise in BUN after admission, the greater the mortality rate. An elevated CRP concentration (> 150 mg/L [1500 mg/L]) at 48 hours suggests severe disease.

Several tools used in medicine more broadly can also be used to determine pancreatitis severity. These include the **Sequential Organ Failure Assessment (SOFA)** score or **modified Marshall scoring system** and the **Acute Physiology and Chronic Health Evaluation (APACHE II)** score. Recently artificial intelligence and machine learning techniques have been used to develop sophisticated prediction systems which utilize numerous physiologic and clinical parameters to predict disease course and guide therapy.

D. Imaging

Ultrasonography is often not helpful in diagnosing acute pancreatitis because of intervening bowel gas but may identify gallstones in the gallbladder. Unenhanced CT is useful for demonstrating an enlarged pancreas when the diagnosis of pancreatitis is uncertain, differentiating pancreatitis from other possible intra-abdominal catastrophes, and providing an initial assessment of prognosis but is often unnecessary early in the course (Table 18–11). Rapid-bolus intravenous contrast-enhanced CT is of particular value after the first 3 days of severe acute pancreatitis for identifying areas of necrotizing pancreatitis and assessing the degree of necrosis (although the use of intravenous contrast may increase the risk of complications of pancreatitis and of AKI and should be avoided when the serum creatinine level is above 1.5 mg/dL [124.95 mcmol/L]). MRI appears to be a suitable alternative to CT. Perfusion CT on day 3 demonstrating areas of ischemia in the pancreas has been reported to predict the development of pancreatic necrosis. Identification of local complications on imaging signifies at least moderately severe disease by the Revised Atlanta Classification with increased risk of mortality; they are further classified as to whether they are acute (< 4 weeks after onset of pancreatitis) or chronic (> 4 weeks after onset) and whether they are associated with interstitial disease (acute inflammation with an absence of necrosis) or necrotizing disease (inflammation with parenchymal or peripancreatic necrosis).

With **interstitial pancreatitis,** acute peripancreatic fluid collections (APFC) occur around the pancreas. With **necrotizing pancreatitis**, acute necrotic collections (ANC), defined as fluid and necrosis, occur within or around the pancreas. After approximately 4 weeks, peripancreatic fluid collections from interstitial pancreatitis may evolve into **chronic pancreatic pseudocysts** (homogenous, encapsuled fluid collections with minimal or no necrosis); in contrast, necrotic collections associated with necrotizing pancreatitis may evolve into **walled-off necrosis (WON),** which is an encapsulated collection of solid necrosis and liquid. CT-guided needle aspiration of areas of necrotizing pancreatitis after the third day may disclose infection, usually by enteric organisms, which typically requires debridement; however, the false-negative rate is 25%. In current practice, this is rarely performed. The presence of gas bubbles on CT implies infection by gas-forming organisms.

Following a single attack of idiopathic acute pancreatitis, a negative EUS examination predicts a low risk of relapse. ERCP is generally not indicated for diagnostic evaluation after acute pancreatitis and is reserved for therapeutic objectives such as removal of bile duct stones following gallstone pancreatitis. EUS and MRCP should be considered especially after repeated attacks of idiopathic acute pancreatitis. They are useful in identifying occult biliary disease (eg, small stones, sludge, microlithiasis),

Table 18–11. Estimated mortality rates of pancreatitis based on severity.

Point Value for Appearance of Pancreas Based on CT scan		Additional Points for Percentage of Pancreatic Necrosis		Estimated Mortality Rate Based on Total Points Sum	
Condition of Pancreas	Points	Percentage of Necrosis	Points	Total Points	Estimated Mortality Rate
Normal pancreas	0	0%	0	0	0%
Enlargement of pancreas	1 point	0%	0	1	0%
Inflammation of the pancreas or peripancreatic fat or both	2 points	< 30%	2 points	4	< 3%
Single new peripancreatic fluid collection	3 points	30–50%	4 points	7	> 6%
Two or more new peripancreatic fluid collections or retroperitoneal air	4 points	> 50%	6 points	10	~17%

which is present in many patients with apparently 'idiopathic' acute pancreatitis and are indicated in persons over age 40 to exclude malignancy.

Differential Diagnosis

Acute pancreatitis must be differentiated from an acutely perforated duodenal ulcer, acute cholecystitis, acute intestinal obstruction, leaking aortic aneurysm, renal colic, and acute mesenteric ischemia. Serum amylase may also be elevated in proximal intestinal obstruction, gastroenteritis, mumps not involving the pancreas (salivary amylase), and ectopic pregnancy and after administration of opioids and abdominal surgery. Serum lipase may also be elevated in many of these conditions.

Complications

A. Local Complications

Approximately one-third of patients with interstitial pancreatitis and APFC will develop **pseudocysts** which are encapsulated fluid collections with high amylase content and minimal or no necrosis. They most commonly are located within or adjacent to the pancreas but can develop almost anywhere (eg, mediastinum, retrorectal) by extension along anatomic planes. Multiple pseudocysts are seen in 14% of cases. The great majority of pseudocysts do not require drainage and will resolve spontaneously. Drainage of pseudocysts may be indicated to relieve symptoms caused by cyst compression of adjacent structures (eg, nausea and vomiting due to gastric outlet compression; jaundice and pruritus due to bile duct compression). Pseudocysts also may require drainage after becoming secondarily infected (ie, pancreatic abscess). Pancreatic abscess is characterized by rising fever, an epigastric mass and localized tenderness, and leukocytosis that typically develops > 6 weeks after pancreatitis onset. It may be associated with a left-sided pleural effusion or an enlarging spleen secondary to splenic vein thrombosis. In contrast to infected necrosis, the mortality rate is low following drainage.

Sterile or infected necrotizing pancreatitis may complicate the course in 5–10% of cases of acute pancreatitis and accounts for most of the deaths. The risk of infection does not correlate with the extent of necrosis. Pancreatic necrosis is often associated with fever, leukocytosis, and, in some cases, shock and is associated with organ failure (eg, GI bleeding, respiratory failure, AKI) in 50% of cases. It may lead to complete transection of the pancreatic duct (disconnected pancreatic duct syndrome), which may result in recurrent fluid collections or persistent fistulae months or years after necrosis has resolved. Necrotizing pancreatic collections mature into **walled-off necrosis** 3–4 weeks after pancreatitis onset. While a greater proportion of WON collections require intervention, 40–60% may be managed conservatively. Akin to pseudocysts, indications for drainage of WON include symptoms due to mass effect causing anorexia or jaundice and infection.

Pancreatic ascites may present after recovery from acute pancreatitis as a gradual increase in abdominal girth and persistent elevation of the serum amylase level in the absence of frank abdominal pain. Marked elevations in ascitic protein (> 3 g/dL) and amylase (> 1000 U/L [20 mkat/L]) concentrations are typical. The condition results from disruption of the pancreatic duct or drainage of a pseudocyst into the peritoneal cavity.

Rare local complications of acute pancreatitis include hemorrhage caused by erosion into a blood vessel to form a pseudoaneurysm and colonic necrosis. Porto-splenomesenteric venous thrombosis frequently develops; anticoagulation may be considered for acute thrombosis of the portal vein. Other local complications of acute pancreatitis include abdominal compartment syndrome and intestinal ischemia. Chronic pancreatitis (with associated exocrine insufficiency or diabetes mellitus) may develop after acute (especially recurrent) pancreatitis. Statin use may reduce the risk of diabetes.

B. Systemic Complications

Renal, pulmonary, and cardiovascular complications occur transiently in moderately severe pancreatitis; if they persist for more than 48 hours, they are diagnostic of severe pancreatitis which carries substantial risk of mortality. Intravascular volume depletion secondary to leakage of fluids into the pancreatic bed and to ileus with fluid-filled loops of bowel may result in prerenal azotemia and ATN. Systemic complications usually occur within 24 hours of the onset of acute pancreatitis and lasts 8–9 days. Some patients require renal replacement therapy.

Pulmonary complications of acute pancreatitis include pulmonary edema, pleural effusions, and acute respiratory distress syndrome (ARDS); cardiac dysfunction may be superimposed. These usually occur 3–7 days after the onset of pancreatitis in patients who have required large volumes of fluid and colloid to maintain blood pressure and urinary output. Most patients with ARDS require intubation, mechanical ventilation, and supplemental oxygen.

Treatment

A. Treatment of Acute Disease

1. Mild disease—In most patients, acute pancreatitis is a mild disease ("non-severe acute pancreatitis") that subsides spontaneously within several days. Goal-directed therapy with moderate fluid resuscitation (a bolus of 10 mL/kg in patients with signs of hypovolemia followed by no more than 1.5 mL/kg per hour) may reduce the frequency of systemic inflammatory response syndrome and organ failure in this group of patients and appears to have the greatest benefit in patients with acute pancreatitis predicted to be mild in severity when started within 4 hours of the patient's arrival at the hospital. Lactated Ringer solution may be preferable to normal saline. Overly aggressive fluid resuscitation may lead to fluid overload, respiratory compromise, and increased abdominal pressure and may require diuretic therapy. Careful re-evaluation of the patient's volume status after early phase resuscitation is critical and may result in reduction, pause, or discontinuation in fluid administration.

Pain is controlled with NSAIDs or acetaminophen and, when necessary, meperidine, up to 100–150 mg intramuscularly every 3–4 hours as necessary. In those with severe liver or kidney dysfunction, the dose may need to be reduced. Morphine had been thought to cause sphincter of Oddi spasm but is now considered an acceptable alternative and, given the potential side effects of meperidine, may even be preferable. Oral intake of fluid and solid foods can be resumed early in the disease course when the patient expresses an appetite (even if the serum amylase is still elevated) and has been demonstrated to shorten length of hospitalization. Pain may recur on refeeding in 20% of patients requiring a more conservative approach with clear liquids or short-term bowel rest.

Following recovery from acute biliary pancreatitis, laparoscopic cholecystectomy is performed (often during the same hospital admission). It is associated with a reduced rate of recurrent gallstone-related complications compared with *delayed* cholecystectomy, except in frail older patients or those with local or systemic pancreatitis complications.

2. Severe disease—In more severe pancreatitis—particularly necrotizing pancreatitis—there may be considerable leakage of fluids, that may necessitate large amounts of intravenous fluids. However, care must be taken to monitor for and avoid fluid overload. Risk factors for high levels of fluid sequestration include younger age, alcohol etiology, higher hematocrit value, higher serum glucose, and systemic inflammatory response syndrome in the first 48 hours of hospital admission. Hemodynamic monitoring in an ICU is required, and the goals should be adequate urinary output, stabilization of blood pressure and heart rate, restoration of central venous pressure, and a modest decrease in hematocrit value while avoiding fluid overload. Calcium gluconate must be given intravenously if there is evidence of hypocalcemia with tetany. With colloid solutions, the risk of ARDS may be increased. If shock persists after adequate volume replacement (including packed red cells), vasopressors may be required. For the patient requiring a large volume of parenteral fluids, central venous pressure and blood gases should be monitored at regular intervals.

Enteral nutrition via a nasojejunal or possibly nasogastric feeding tube is preferable to parenteral nutrition in patients who will otherwise be without oral nutrition for at least 7–10 days and reduces the risk of multiorgan failure and mortality when started within 48 hours of admission. However, it is not tolerated in some patients (eg, those with an ileus) and may not reduce the rates of infection and death compared with resumption of oral feeding after 72 hours. Parenteral nutrition (including lipids) should be considered in patients who have severe pancreatitis and ileus; glutamine supplementation appears to reduce the risk of infectious complications and mortality.

The routine use of antibiotics to prevent conversion of sterile necrotizing pancreatitis to infected necrosis is of no benefit and generally is not indicated in patients with < 30% pancreatic necrosis. Imipenem (500 mg intravenously every 6 hours) or possibly cefuroxime (1.5 g intravenously three times daily, then 250 mg orally twice daily) administered for no more than 14 days to patients with sterile necrotizing pancreatitis has been reported in some studies to reduce the risk of pancreatic infection and mortality, but in general, prophylactic antibiotics are not recommended; meropenem and the combination of ciprofloxacin and metronidazole do not appear to reduce the frequency of infected necrosis, multiorgan failure, or mortality. Serum procalcitonin, which is elevated in infection, may help to guide antibiotic therapy and reduce unnecessary use. When infected necrotizing pancreatitis is confirmed, imipenem or meropenem should be continued. Drug-resistant organisms are increasingly prevalent. In occasional cases, a fungal infection is found, and appropriate antifungal therapy should be prescribed.

NSAIDs (eg, indomethacin or diclofenac administered rectally) and aggressive hydration with lactated Ringer solution have been reported to reduce the frequency (by 50%) and, possibly, severity of post-ERCP pancreatitis in persons at high risk; they may also to reduce the frequency by 50% in unselected persons. Rectal indomethacin is widely used. Ample periprocedural hydration also is recommended though benefits may be less significant in the setting of rectal NSAID use. Placement of a stent across the pancreatic duct or orifice has been shown to reduce the risk of post-ERCP pancreatitis in high-risk patients; a combination of pancreatic stent and NSAIDs provides more protection than NSAIDs alone and is recommended.

B. Treatment of Complications and Follow-Up

A surgeon should be consulted in all cases of severe acute pancreatitis. If the diagnosis is in doubt and investigation indicates a strong possibility of a serious surgically correctable lesion (eg, perforated peptic ulcer), exploratory laparotomy is indicated. When acute pancreatitis is found unexpectedly at laparotomy, it is usually wise to close without additional intervention. If the pancreatitis appears mild and cholelithiasis or microlithiasis is present, cholecystectomy or cholecystostomy may be justified.

When severe pancreatitis results from choledocholithiasis and jaundice (serum total bilirubin > 5 mg/dL [85.5 mcmol/L]) or cholangitis is present, ERCP with endoscopic sphincterotomy and stone extraction is indicated. Endoscopic sphincterotomy does not appear to improve the outcome of severe pancreatitis in the absence of cholangitis or jaundice.

Most pseudocysts do not require therapy, but if symptoms arise due to mechanical compression (see Local Complications above), endoscopy with EUS-guided drainage approaches are favored to traditional surgical drainage due to a reduced length of hospital stay. EUS guidance reduces the risk of adverse events from drainage, particularly bleeding relative to "blind" endoscopic approaches using a needle knife or cystotome.

In patients with necrotizing pancreatitis, necrosectomy may improve survival in patients with clinical deterioration due to multiorgan failure or lack of resolution by 4 weeks. It also is performed for infected necrosis, although a substantial proportion (40–60%) of relatively stable patients with infected pancreatic necrosis may be managed with antibiotics alone. Outcomes are best if necrosectomy is delayed until the necrosis has organized, usually about 4 weeks after disease onset, which enables better differentiation of those who need drainage and debridement versus those who respond to conservative therapy.

A "step-up" approach to treatment of walled-off pancreatic necrosis increasingly is used in which nonsurgical catheter drainage by either endoscopic transluminal (transgastric or transduodenal) or percutaneous placement under radiologic guidance (possibly performed < 4 weeks after development) reduces major complications and mortality relative to traditional open surgical approaches. While endoscopic and percutaneous approaches are both efficacious, the latter is associated with more pancreaticocutaneous fistula A combination of both approaches is needed for extensive necrosis. Treatment is labor intensive, and multiple procedures are often required; however, costs and complication rates are lower than for surgical necrosectomy. Surgical necrosectomy has a crucial role for necrotic collections that are too extensive or solid in consistency. In some cases, laparoscopic guidance (video-assisted retroperitoneal debridement) is an additional option, depending on local expertise. Endoscopic or surgical interventions may be required for chronic disconnected pancreatic duct syndrome, pancreatic duct leaks and fistulas.

Prognosis

Overall mortality rates for acute pancreatitis have declined from at least 10% to around 5% since the 1980s. The mortality rate for severe acute pancreatitis (more than three Ranson criteria; see Table 18–10) remains at least 20%, with rates of 10% and 25% in those with sterile and infected necrosis, respectively. Severe acute pancreatitis is predicted by features of the systemic inflammatory response on admission; a transient inflammatory response is associated with a mortality rate of 8% and a persistent systemic inflammatory response with a mortality rate of 25%. Half of these deaths occur within the first 2 weeks, usually from multiorgan failure. The mortality rate associated with multiorgan failure is at least 30%, but it is over 50% if it persists beyond the first 48 hours. Later deaths usually occur because of complications of infected necrosis. The risk of death doubles when both organ failure and infected necrosis are present. Moreover, hospital-acquired infections increase the mortality of acute pancreatitis, independent of severity. Readmission to the hospital for acute pancreatitis within 30 days may be predicted by a scoring system based on five factors during the index admission: eating less than a solid diet at discharge; nausea, vomiting, or diarrhea at discharge; pancreatic necrosis; use of antibiotics at discharge; and pain at discharge. Male sex, an alcohol etiology, and severe acute disease are risk factors. Recurrences are common (24%) in alcohol-associated pancreatitis, particularly in patients who smoke (40%), but can be reduced by repeated, regularly scheduled interventions to eliminate alcohol consumption and smoking after discharge from the hospital. A severe initial attack also increases the risk of subsequent exocrine pancreatic insufficiency. The risk of chronic pancreatitis following an episode of acute alcohol-associated pancreatitis is 8% in 5 years, 13% in 10 years, and 16% in 20 years, and the risk of diabetes mellitus is increased more than twofold over 5 years. Overall, chronic pancreatitis develops in 36% of patients with recurrent acute pancreatitis; alcohol use and smoking are principal risk factors. An association between a diagnosis of acute pancreatitis and long-term risk of pancreatic cancer has been reported.

When to Admit

While nearly all patients with acute pancreatitis should be hospitalized, several paradigms are being developed to identify those who might not require admission or may be discharged early. The absence of rebound abdominal tenderness or guarding with a normal hematocrit value and serum creatinine level (the "**harmless acute pancreatitis score**," or **HAPS**) predict a non-severe course with 98% accuracy.

Akshintala VS. Incidence, severity, and mortality of post-ERCP pancreatitis: an updated systematic review and meta-analysis of 145 randomized controlled trials. Gastrointest Endosc. 2023;98:1. [PMID: 37004815]

Bang J et al. Upfront endoscopic necrosectomy or step-up endoscopic approach for infected necrotising pancreatitis (DESTIN): a single-blinded, multicentre, randomised trial. Lancet Gastroenterol Hepatol. 2024;9:22. [PMID: 37980922]

Czapári D et al. Detailed characteristics of post-discharge mortality in acute pancreatitis. Gastroenterology. 2023;165:682. [PMID: 37247642]

Di Martino M et al. Timing of cholecystectomy after moderate and severe acute biliary pancreatitis. JAMA Surg. 2023;158:e233660. [PMID: 37610760]

Elmunzer BJ et al. Indomethacin with or without prophylactic pancreatic stent placement to prevent pancreatitis after ERCP: a randomised non-inferiority trial. Lancet. 2024;403:450. [PMID: 38219767]

Guilabert L et al. Evaluation of the PAN-PROMISE symptom scale in a randomized controlled trial of fluid resuscitation in acute pancreatitis. Am J Gastroenterol. 2025;120:1852 [PMID: 40471836]

IAP/APA/EPC/IPC/JPS Working Group. International Association of Pancreatology revised guidelines on acute pancreatitis 2025: supported and endorsed by the American Pancreatic Association, European Pancreatic Club, Indian Pancreas Club, and Japan Pancreas Society. Pancreatology. 2025;25:770. [PMID: 40651900]

Thiruvengadam NR et al. Association of statin usage and the development of diabetes mellitus after acute pancreatitis. Clin Gastroenterol Hepatol. 2023;21:1214. [PMID: 35750248]

CHRONIC PANCREATITIS

ESSENTIALS OF DIAGNOSIS

- Chronic or intermittent epigastric pain, steatorrhea, weight loss, abnormal pancreatic imaging.
- A mnemonic for the predisposing factors of chronic pancreatitis is TIGAR-O: toxic-metabolic, idiopathic, genetic, autoimmune, recurrent and severe acute pancreatitis, or obstructive.

General Considerations

The incidence and prevalence of chronic pancreatitis in the United States are 5–8 and 42–73 per 100,000 population, respectively, with a peak in persons aged 46–55 years.

A useful mnemonic for the predisposing factors to chronic pancreatitis is **TIGAR-O**: **T**oxic-metabolic, **I**diopathic, **G**enetic, **A**utoimmune, **R**ecurrent and severe acute pancreatitis, or **O**bstructive.

Chronic pancreatitis occurs most often in patients with alcohol use disorder (45–80% of all cases). The risk of chronic pancreatitis increases with the duration and amount of alcohol consumed, but pancreatitis develops in only 5–10% of heavy drinkers. Tobacco smoking is a risk factor for idiopathic chronic pancreatitis and accelerates progression of alcohol-associated chronic pancreatitis. About 2% of patients with hyperparathyroidism develop pancreatitis. In tropical Africa and Asia, tropical pancreatitis, related in part to malnutrition, is the most common cause of chronic pancreatitis. By contrast, in Western societies, obesity can lead to pancreatic steatosis, which may lead ultimately to pancreatic exocrine and endocrine insufficiency and an increased risk of pancreatic cancer. A stricture, stone, or tumor obstructing the pancreas can lead to obstructive chronic pancreatitis.

Autoimmune pancreatitis is associated with hypergammaglobulinemia (IgG_4 in particular), often with autoantibodies and other autoimmune diseases, and is often responsive to corticosteroids. Affected persons are at increased risk for various cancers. Type 1 autoimmune pancreatitis (lymphoplasmacytic sclerosing pancreatitis, or simply autoimmune pancreatitis) is a multisystem disease, typically in a patient over age 60, characterized by lymphoplasmacytic infiltration and fibrosis on biopsy, associated bile duct strictures, retroperitoneal fibrosis, renal and salivary gland lesions, and a high rate of relapse after treatment. It is the pancreatic manifestation of IgG_4-related disease. Type 2 ("idiopathic duct-centric chronic pancreatitis") affects the pancreas alone, typically in a patient aged 40–50 years, and is characterized by intense duct-centric lymphoplasmacytic infiltration on biopsy, lack of systemic IgG_4 involvement, an association with IBD in 25% of cases, often a tumor-like mass, and a low rate of relapse after treatment. Type 3 autoimmune pancreatitis is a relatively infrequent complication of immune checkpoint inhibitor therapy; it is often asymptomatic but causes rapid pancreatic atrophy.

Between 10% and 30% of cases of chronic pancreatitis are idiopathic, with either early onset (median age 20) or late onset (median age 58). Genetic factors may predispose to chronic pancreatitis in nearly half of the early-onset cases and a quarter of the late-onset cases and include pathogenic variants of the *CFTR* gene, the pancreatic secretory trypsin inhibitory gene (*PSTI*, also known as the serine protease inhibitor, *SPINK1*), the chymotrypsin-C (*CTRC*) gene, and the genes for carboxypeptidase A1 (*CPA1*) and possibly uridine 5′-diphosphate glucuronosyltransferase (*UGT1A7*). A variant of the cationic trypsinogen gene on chromosome 7 (serine protease 1, *PRSS1*) is associated with hereditary pancreatitis, transmitted as an autosomal dominant trait with variable penetrance. Younger patients with family history of pancreatitis are more likely to test positive for pancreatitis-related genetic variants.

Chronic pancreatitis following a first (sentinel) acute pancreatitis event initiates an inflammatory process that results in injury and later fibrosis ("necrosis-fibrosis"). In many cases, chronic pancreatitis is a self-perpetuating disease characterized by chronic pain or recurrent episodes of acute pancreatitis and ultimately by pancreatic exocrine or endocrine insufficiency (sooner in alcohol-associated pancreatitis than in other types). After many years, chronic pain may resolve spontaneously or following surgery tailored to the cause of pain. Over 80% of adults develop diabetes mellitus within 25 years after the clinical onset of chronic pancreatitis.

Clinical Findings

A. Symptoms and Signs

Persistent or recurrent episodes of epigastric and left upper quadrant pain are typical. Anorexia, nausea, vomiting, constipation, flatulence, and weight loss are common. During attacks, tenderness over the pancreas, mild muscle guarding, and ileus may be noted. Attacks may last for only a few hours or for as long as 2 weeks; pain may eventually be almost continuous. Steatorrhea (as indicated by bulky, foul, fatty stools) may occur late in the course.

B. Laboratory Findings

Serum amylase and lipase may be elevated during acute attacks; however, normal values do not exclude the diagnosis. Serum alkaline phosphatase and bilirubin may be elevated owing to compression of the bile duct. Glycosuria may be present. Excess fecal fat may be demonstrated on chemical analysis of the stool. Exocrine pancreatic insufficiency generally is confirmed by a fecal elastase level < 100 mcg/g stool and subsequent response to therapy with pancreatic enzyme supplements; the secretin stimulation test can be used if available (and has a high negative predictive value for ruling out early acute chronic pancreatitis), as can detection of decreased fecal chymotrypsin levels, although the latter test lacks sensitivity and specificity. Vitamin B_{12} malabsorption is detectable in about 40% of patients, but clinical deficiency of vitamin B_{12} and fat-soluble vitamins is rare.

Accurate diagnostic tests are available for the major trypsinogen gene pathogenic variants, but because of uncertainty about the mechanisms linking heterozygous *CFTR* and *PSTI* variants with pancreatitis, genetic testing for mutations in these two genes is recommended primarily in younger patients in whom the etiology of chronic pancreatitis is unclear.

Elevated IgG_4 levels, ANA, antibodies to lactoferrin and carbonic anhydrase II, and other autoantibodies are often found in patients with autoimmune pancreatitis (especially type 1). Pancreatic biopsy in autoimmune pancreatitis, if necessary, shows a lymphoplasmacytic inflammatory infiltrate with characteristic IgG_4 immunostaining, which is also found in biopsy specimens of the major papilla, bile duct, and salivary glands, in type 1 autoimmune pancreatitis.

C. Imaging

Contrast-enhanced CT is recommended as initial testing for diagnosis of chronic pancreatitis, although plain films show calcifications due to pancreatolithiasis in 30% of affected patients. CT may show calcifications not seen on plain films as well as ductal dilatation and heterogeneity or atrophy of the gland. Occasionally, the findings raise suspicion of pancreatic cancer ("tumefactive chronic pancreatitis"). MRI with magnetic resonance cholangiopancreatography provides enhanced visualization of parenchymal changes and ductal abnormalities including strictures. Secretin-enhanced MRCP may be considered in selected cases. When CT or MRI is inconclusive, EUS may be helpful but has an increased false positive rate particularly in the setting of dyspepsia and chronic abdominal pain. ERCP now is primarily used for therapeutic procedures but reveals dilated ducts, intraductal stones, strictures, and leaks. Histology is the gold standard for diagnosis when clinical suspicion is strong, but imaging studies are inconclusive.

Characteristic imaging features of autoimmune pancreatitis include diffuse enlargement of the pancreas, a peripheral rim of hypoattenuation, and irregular narrowing of the main pancreatic duct. In the United States, the diagnosis of autoimmune pancreatitis is based on the **HISORt** criteria: **H**istology, **I**maging, **S**erology, other **O**rgan involvement, and **R**esponse to corticosteroid **T**herapy.

Complications

Opioid addiction is common. Other frequent complications include brittle diabetes mellitus, recurrent acute attacks with local and systemic complications, bile duct stricture resulting in cholestatic liver enzymes (with or without jaundice), exocrine pancreatic insufficiency, malnutrition, osteoporosis, and peptic ulcer. Pancreatic cancer develops in 5% of patients after 20 years although surveillance for pancreatic cancer is not recommended in asymptomatic patients; the risk may relate to tobacco and alcohol use. In patients with hereditary pancreatitis, the risk of pancreatic cancer rises after 50 years of age and reaches 19% by age 70 (see Chapter 43).

Treatment

A. Medical Measures

A low-fat diet should be prescribed. Smoking cessation is strongly recommended and abstinence from alcohol is imperative. Preferred agents for pain are acetaminophen, NSAIDs, and, if an opioid is necessary, tramadol, along with pain-modifying agents such as tricyclic antidepressants, SSRIs, and gabapentin or pregabalin. Strong opioids are sometimes necessary for those with more severe or frequent pain patterns. Exocrine pancreatic insufficiency is treated with pancreatic enzyme replacement therapy selected based on high lipase activity (Table 18–12). A total dose of at least 500–1000 USP units/kg of lipase in capsules is given with each meal. Doses of 90,000 USP units (30,000 IU) or more of lipase per meal may be required in some cases. The tablets should be taken at the start of, during, and at the end of a meal. Concurrent administration of an H_2-receptor antagonist (eg, famotidine, 20 mg orally twice daily), a PPI (eg, omeprazole, 20–60 mg orally daily), or sodium bicarbonate (650 mg orally before and after meals) decreases the inactivation of lipase by acid and may thereby further decrease steatorrhea. In selected cases of alcohol-associated pancreatitis and in cystic fibrosis, enteric-coated microencapsulated preparations may offer an advantage; however, in patients with cystic fibrosis, high-dose pancreatic enzyme replacement therapy has been associated with strictures of the ascending colon. Associated diabetes mellitus should be treated (see Chapter 31).

Autoimmune pancreatitis is treated with prednisone 40 mg/day orally for 1–2 months, followed by a taper of

Table 18–12. FDA-approved pancreatic enzyme (pancrelipase) preparations.

Product	Enzyme Content/Unit Dose, USP Units		
	Lipase	Amylase	Protease
Immediate-Release Capsules			
Non-enteric–coated			
Viokace 10,440	10,440	39,150	39,150
Viokace 20,880	20,880	78,300	78,300
Delayed-Release Capsules			
Enteric-coated minimicrospheres			
Creon 3000	3000	15,000	9500
Creon 6000	6000	30,000	19,000
Creon 12,000	12,000	60,000	38,000
Creon 24,000	24,000	120,000	76,000
Creon 36,000	36,000	180,000	114,000
Enteric-coated minitablets			
Ultresa 13,800	13,800	27,600	27,600
Ultresa 20,700	20,700	46,000	41,400
Ultresa 23,000	23,000	46,000	41,400
Enteric-coated beads			
Zenpep 3000	3000	16,000	10,000
Zenpep 5000	5000	27,000	17,000
Zenpep 10,000	10,000	55,000	34,000
Zenpep 15,000	15,000	82,000	51,000
Zenpep 20,000	20,000	109,000	68,000
Zenpep 25,000	25,000	136,000	85,000
Enteric-coated microtablets			
Pancreaze 4200	4200	17,500	10,000
Pancreaze 10,500	10,500	43,750	25,000
Pancreaze 16,800	16,800	70,000	40,000
Pancreaze 21,000	21,000	61,000	37,000
Bicarbonate-buffered enteric-coated microspheres			
Pertzye 8000	8000	30,250	28,750
Pertzye + 16,000	16,000	60,500	57,500

USP, US Pharmacopeia.

5 mg every 2–4 weeks. Nonresponse or relapse occurs in 45% of type 1 cases (particularly in those with concomitant IgG_4-associated cholangitis); rituximab is an effective induction and maintenance agent, and azathioprine or long-term low-dose corticosteroid use appears to reduce the risk of relapse. Targeted immunotherapy with monoclonal antibodies to immunoglobulin G components shows promise for systemic IgG_4-associated associated disease.

B. Endoscopic and Surgical Treatment

Endoscopic therapy or surgery may be indicated in chronic pancreatitis to treat underlying biliary tract disease, ensure free flow of bile into the duodenum, drain persistent pseudocysts, treat other complications, eliminate obstruction of the pancreatic duct, attempt to relieve pain, or exclude pancreatic cancer. Liver fibrosis may regress after biliary drainage. Distal bile duct obstruction may be relieved by endoscopic placement of multiple plastic stents or a fully covered self-expandable metal stent in the bile duct. When obstruction of the duodenal end of the pancreatic duct can be demonstrated by ERCP, dilation, placement of a stent in the duct, pancreatic duct stone lithotripsy, or surgical resection of the tail of the pancreas with implantation of the distal end of the duct by pancreaticojejunostomy may be performed. Endoscopic therapy is successful in about 50% of cases.

In patients who do not respond to endoscopic therapy, surgery is successful in about 50%. When the pancreatic duct is diffusely dilated, anastomosis between the duct after it is split longitudinally and a defunctionalized limb of jejunum (modified Puestow procedure), in some cases combined with resection of the head of the pancreas (Beger or Frey procedure), is associated with relief of pain in 80% of cases. In advanced cases, subtotal or total pancreatectomy with islet autotransplantation may be considered as a last resort but has variable efficacy and causes pancreatic insufficiency and diabetes mellitus.

Endoscopic or surgical (including laparoscopic) drainage is indicated for symptomatic pseudocysts (see Acute Pancreatitis Complications). For patients with evidence of ductal obstruction (dilation, stricture, stones), surgical approaches appear to be more efficacious that endoscopic therapies. Most patients nonetheless opt for an initial attempt at less invasive endoscopic therapy. Pancreatic sphincterotomy with fragmentation of stones in the pancreatic duct by pancreatoscopy or fluoroscopy-guided electrohydraulic or laser lithotripsy and endoscopic stone removal may relieve pain in selected patients. Extracorporeal shock wave lithotripsy in combination with endoscopic therapy or alone also may be helpful. Patients who step up from endoscopic to surgical therapy may be less likely to exhibit long-term complete pain relief than those who start with operative therapy and should be counseled about both options at the outset of treatment. For patients with chronic pain and nondilated ducts, a percutaneous celiac plexus nerve block may be considered under either CT or EUS guidance, with pain relief (albeit often short-lived) in approximately 50% of patients (see Chapter 5).

Prognosis

Chronic pancreatitis often leads to disability and reduced quality of life. The prognosis is best in patients with recurrent acute pancreatitis caused by a remediable condition, such as hyperparathyroidism, hyperlipidemia, or autoimmune pancreatitis. The Chronic Pancreatitis Prognosis Score based on pain, hemoglobin A_{1c} level, CRP level, BMI, and platelet count has been shown to correlate with hospital admissions and number of hospital days. In alcohol-associated pancreatitis, pain relief is most likely when a dilated pancreatic duct can be decompressed. In patients with disease not amenable to decompressive surgery, addiction to opioids is a frequent outcome of treatment. A poorer quality of life is associated with constant rather than intermittent pain, pain-related disability or unemployment, current smoking, and comorbidities.

When to Refer

All patients with chronic pancreatitis should be referred for diagnostic and therapeutic procedures.

When to Admit

- Severe pain.
- New jaundice.
- New fever.

AGSE Standards of Practice Committee; Sheth S et al. American Society for Gastrointestinal Endoscopy guideline on the role of endoscopy in the management of chronic pancreatitis: summary and recommendations. Gastrointest Endosc. 2025;100:584. [PMID: 39115496]

Cohen SM et al. Etiology, diagnosis, and modern management of chronic pancreatitis: a systematic review. JAMA Surg. 2023;158:652. [PMID: 37074693]

Phillips AE et al. Prevalence and patterns of opioid use in chronic pancreatitis. Clin Transl Gastroenterol. 2025;16: e00807. [PMID 39907252]

Ramsey M et al. Germline multigene panel testing in acute and chronic pancreatitis. PLoS One. 2024;19:e0307076. [PMID: 39172977]

Stone JH et al. Inebilizumab for treatment of IgG_4-related disease. N Engl J Med. 2025;392:1168. [PMID: 39541094]

van-Veldhuisen CL et al. Long-term outcomes of early surgery vs endoscopy first in chronic pancreatitis: follow-up analysis of the ESCAPE randomized clinical trial. JAMA Surg. 2025;160:126. [PMID: 39565607]

Whitcomb DC et al. AGA Clinical Practice Update on the epidemiology, evaluation, and management of exocrine pancreatic insufficiency: expert review. Gastroenterology. 2023;165:1292. [PMID: 37737818]

ASYMPTOMATIC PANCREATIC CYSTS

Cross sectional imaging studies and autopsy studies reveal asymptomatic pancreatic cysts in 3–20% of adults. Previously it was felt these cysts were benign. It is now recognized that a proportion of these cysts are mucinous and have a variable pre-malignant potential. Most pancreatic cysts may be classified according to whether they connect to the pancreatic ductal system and whether they are mucinous or non-mucinous in nature. Connection to the ductal system is demonstrated radiographically or by evidence of elevated amylase in cyst fluid. Mucinous etiology is suggested by the presence of elevated cyst carcinoembryonic antigen (CEA) or low glucose levels.

Non-Mucinous Cysts

Post-inflammatory collections, including **pancreatic pseudocysts,** have an elevated cyst amylase (due to ductal connection) but minimal CEA levels. **Serous cystadenoma** have a negligible cyst amylase level (due to absence of ductal connection) and a low cyst CEA. They often exhibit a pathognomonic microcystic honeycombed morphology with a central stellate scar. Given their low malignant potential, cyst FNA sampling often is not required. When it is performed, cells containing abundant glycogen rich cytoplasm are identified. Von-Hippel Lindau (VHL) is associated with serous cystadenoma as well as neoplastic neuroendocrine lesions.

Mucinous Pancreatic Cysts

The most common asymptomatic pancreatic cysts are **intraductal mucinous neoplasms (IMPN)** which are mucinous cysts that arise from pancreatic duct side-branches. These lesions exhibit high cyst amylase (given their ductal connection) and elevated CEA. Most have low malignant potential; therefore, surveillance imaging is the preferred management approach in most patients. **Mucinous cystic neoplasms (MCN)** are mucin-rich cysts with elevated CEA but normal cyst amylase given the absence of ductal connection. They have ovarian-type stroma. They are frequently found in young and middle-aged women in the body or tail of the pancreas. While they were initially thought to have higher neoplastic potential than branch duct IPMN, they are now thought to have comparable risk and are managed similarly. IPMN involving the main pancreatic duct often exhibit a patulous "fish eye" duct orifice due to chronic extrusion of mucin from the main pancreatic duct. Due to their high malignant potential, surgical resection of *main duct* IPMN involved portions of the pancreas usually is recommended.

Recent studies indicated that most cases of neoplastic progression or IPMN and MCN occur within the first-year following detection. It is therefore recommended that repeat cross sectional (CT or MRI) be performed at 6 months for suspected *side-branch* IPMN and MCN. If cyst morphology and size remain stable, most guidelines recommend increasingly long surveillance imaging intervals. The neoplastic risk of small, stable mucinous cysts is very low and cessation of surveillance imaging in select cases may be considered.

Rapid growth of cysts or the development of high-risk features such as mural nodularity, solid component, duct dilation, or size > 3 cm should prompt EUS-guided cyst needle aspiration and biopsy and potentially a surgical resection. In patient at very high risk for surgery, EUS-guided ablation with alcohol or radiofrequency ablation may be used with mixed results.

Other Asymptomatic Pancreatic Cysts

A non-mucinous cyst of clinical importance is the solid pseudopapillary tumor, which is found in young women and may resemble neuroendocrine tumors. Given their substantial malignant potential, they should be removed operatively. Lymphoepithelial cysts are unilocular or multilocular cysts lined by squamous epithelium; they are typically found in men and do not require resection. Autosomal dominant polycystic kidney disease is associated with simple benign pancreatic cysts lesions which require therapy only if symptomatic.

Gardner T et al. Diagnosis and management of pancreatic cysts. Gastroenterology. 2024;167:454. [PMID 38442782]

Gonda T et al. Pancreatic cysts. N Engl J Med. 2024;391:832. [PMID 39231345]

Han Y et al. Optimal surveillance interval of branch duct intraductal papillary mucinous neoplasm of the pancreas. JAMA Surg. 2024;159:389. [PMID 38231494]

Machicado J et al. Structured training program on confocal laser endomicroscopy for pancreatic cystic lesions: a multicenter prospective study among early-career endosonographers. Gastrointest Endosc. 2023;98:953. [PMID 37473969]

Paniccia A et al. Prospective, multi-institutional, real-time next-generation sequencing of pancreatic cyst fluid reveals diverse genomic alterations that improve the clinical management of pancreatic cysts. Gastroenterology. 2023;164:117. [PMID: 36209796]

Breast Disorders

19

Armando E. Giuliano, MD, FACS, FRCSEd
Sara A. Hurvitz, MD

BENIGN BREAST DISORDERS

FIBROCYSTIC CONDITION

ESSENTIALS OF DIAGNOSIS

- Painful breast masses; often multiple and bilateral.
- Rapid fluctuation in mass size is common.
- Pain often worsens during premenstrual phase of cycle.
- Most common age is 30–50 years. Rare in postmenopausal women not receiving hormonal replacement.

General Considerations

Fibrocystic condition is the most frequent lesion of the breast. Although commonly referred to as "fibrocystic disease," it does not, in fact, represent a pathologic or anatomic disorder. It encompasses a wide variety of benign histologic changes in the breast epithelium, some of which are so common in normal breasts that they are probably variants of normal but have nonetheless been termed a "condition" or "disease." Fibrocystic condition is common in women 30–50 years of age but rare in postmenopausal women who are not taking hormonal replacement. Estrogen is considered a causative factor. There may be an increased risk in women who drink alcohol.

The microscopic findings of fibrocystic condition include cysts (gross and microscopic), papillomatosis, adenosis, fibrosis, and ductal epithelial hyperplasia. Although it has been thought that a fibrocystic condition increases the risk of breast cancer, *only the variants with a component of epithelial proliferation (especially with atypia), papillomatosis, or increased breast density on mammogram represent true risk factors.*

Clinical Findings

A. Symptoms and Signs

Fibrocystic condition may produce an asymptomatic breast mass that is discovered by accident, but pain and tenderness are often symptoms. Discomfort frequently occurs or worsens during the premenstrual phase of the cycle when the cysts tend to enlarge. Fluctuations in size and rapid appearance or disappearance of a breast mass are common, as are multiple or bilateral masses and serous nipple discharge. Patients describe a transient lump in the breast or cyclic breast pain.

B. Diagnostic Tests

Mammography and ultrasonography should be used to evaluate a mass in a patient with fibrocystic condition. Ultrasonography alone may be used in women aged < 30 years; mammography may be helpful, but the breast tissue in young women is usually too radiodense to permit a worthwhile study. Ultrasonography is useful in differentiating a cystic mass from a solid mass, especially in women with dense breasts. Simple cysts are not worrisome and require no treatment or follow-up unless they are symptomatic and cause pain, in which case they may be aspirated. Ultrasonography can reliably distinguish fibroadenoma from carcinoma but not from a phyllodes tumor. Because a mass due to fibrocystic condition may nonetheless be difficult to distinguish from carcinoma on the basis of clinical findings and imaging studies, *suspicious lesions should be biopsied.* Core needle biopsy, rather than fine-needle aspiration (FNA), is the preferable technique. If the lesion is cystic, needle aspiration will suffice. Excisional biopsy is rarely necessary but should be done for lesions with atypia or where imaging and biopsy results are discordant. Surgery should be conservative since the primary objective is to exclude cancer. Simple mastectomy or extensive removal of breast tissue is rarely, if ever, indicated for fibrocystic condition.

Differential Diagnosis

Pain, fluctuation in size, and multiplicity of lesions in fibrocystic condition are most helpful factors in differentiating it from carcinoma. If a dominant mass is present, the diagnosis of cancer should be assumed until disproven by imaging or biopsy. Final diagnosis depends on biopsy.

Treatment

When the diagnosis of fibrocystic condition has been established by previous biopsy or is likely because the history is classic, aspiration of a discrete mass suggestive of a cyst is indicated to alleviate pain and, importantly, to confirm the cystic nature of the mass. The patient is reexamined at intervals thereafter. If no fluid is obtained by aspiration, if fluid is bloody, if a mass persists after aspiration, or if at any time during follow-up a persistent or recurrent mass is noted, biopsy should be performed.

Breast pain associated with generalized fibrocystic condition is best treated by avoiding trauma and by wearing a supportive brassiere during the night and day. Most hormone therapies are not advisable because they do not cure the condition and have undesirable side effects; danazol (100–200 mg orally twice daily), a synthetic androgen, is the only FDA-approved treatment for patients with severe pain. Danazol suppresses pituitary gonadotropins, but androgenic effects (acne, edema, hirsutism) usually make this treatment intolerable; in practice, it is rarely used. Similarly, tamoxifen reduces some symptoms of fibrocystic condition, but because of its side effects, it is not useful for young women unless it is given to reduce the risk of cancer. Postmenopausal women receiving hormone replacement therapy may stop or change doses of hormones to reduce pain. Oil of evening primrose (3 g orally daily), a natural form of gamolenic acid, has been shown to decrease pain in 44–58% of users. Studies have also demonstrated that a low-fat diet or decreasing dietary fat intake may reduce the painful symptoms of fibrocystic condition. Topical treatments are rarely of value.

The role of caffeine consumption in the development and treatment of fibrocystic condition is controversial.

Prognosis

Exacerbations of pain, tenderness, and cyst formation may occur at any time until menopause, when symptoms usually subside, except in patients receiving hormonal replacement. The risk of breast cancer developing in women with fibrocystic condition with a proliferative or atypical epithelial hyperplasia or papillomatosis is higher than that of the general population. These women should be monitored carefully with physical examinations and imaging studies.

Athanasiou A et al. ESR Essentials: diagnostic work-up in patients with symptomatic breast disease-practice recommendations by the European Society of Breast Imaging. Eur Radiol. 2025;35:723. [PMID: 39085641]

ElSherif A et al. Management of mastalgia. Surg Clin North Am. 2022;102:929. [PMID: 36335929]

Malherbe K et al. Fibrocystic breast disease. In: StatPearls [Internet]. Treasure Island (FL): StatPearls Publishing; 2025 Jan. [PMID: 31869073]

FIBROADENOMA OF THE BREAST

1. Fibroadenoma—This common benign neoplasm occurs most frequently in young women, usually within 20 years after puberty. It is more frequent and occurs at an earlier age in Black women. Multiple tumors are found in 10–15% of patients. The typical fibroadenoma is a round or ovoid, rubbery, discrete, relatively movable, nontender mass 1–5 cm that is usually discovered accidentally. Clinical diagnosis in young patients is generally not difficult. In women aged > 30 years, fibrocystic condition of the breast, phyllodes tumors, and carcinoma of the breast must be considered. Cysts can be identified by aspiration or ultrasonography. Fibroadenoma does not normally occur after menopause but may occasionally develop after administration of hormones.

No treatment is usually necessary if the diagnosis of fibroadenoma can be made by core needle biopsy. Excision with pathologic examination of the specimen is performed if the diagnosis is uncertain or the lesion grows significantly. Cryoablation, or freezing of the fibroadenoma, appears to be a safe procedure if the lesion is a biopsy-proven fibroadenoma prior to ablation. Cryoablation is not appropriate for all fibroadenomas because some are too large to freeze or the diagnosis may not be certain. There is no clinical advantage to cryoablation of a histologically proven fibroadenoma beyond the relief that some patients experience when the mass is gone. At times, a mass of scar or fat necrosis may replace the mass of the fibroadenoma after cryoablation. Reassurance seems preferable to treatment. Distinguishing a large fibroadenoma from a phyllodes tumor based on needle biopsy results or imaging alone is usually not possible; histologic examination after excision is usually required. Presumed fibroadenomas larger than 3–4 cm should be excised to rule out phyllodes tumors, which may be malignant.

2. Phyllodes tumor—This fibroadenoma-like tumor with cellular stroma grows rapidly. It may reach a large size and, if inadequately excised, will recur locally. The lesion can be benign or malignant. If benign, phyllodes tumor is treated by local excision. The treatment of malignant phyllodes tumor is more controversial, but complete removal of the tumor with a margin of normal tissue avoids recurrence. Because these tumors may be large, total mastectomy is sometimes necessary. Lymph node dissection is not performed, since the sarcomatous portion of the tumor metastasizes to the lungs and not the lymph nodes.

Del Calvo H et al. Margin width and local recurrence in patients with phyllodes tumors of the breast. Ann Surg Oncol. 2024;31:8048. [PMID: 39085546]

Valenza C et al. Primary malignant phyllodes tumors of the breast: a retrospective analysis from a referral center. Eur J Cancer. 2024;196:113423. [PMID: 37977104]

NIPPLE DISCHARGE

In order of decreasing frequency, the following are the most common causes of nipple discharge in the nonlactating breast: duct ectasia, intraductal papilloma, and

Table 19–1. Characteristics of nipple discharge in the nonpregnant, nonlactating woman.

Finding	Significance
Serous	Most likely benign FCC (ie, duct ectasia)
Bloody	More likely neoplastic (eg, papilloma, carcinoma)
Associated mass	More likely neoplastic
Unilateral	Either neoplastic or non-neoplastic
Bilateral	Most likely non-neoplastic
Single duct	More likely neoplastic
Multiple ducts	More likely FCC
Milky	Endocrine disorders, medications
Spontaneous	Either neoplastic or non-neoplastic
Produced by pressure at single site	Either neoplastic or non-neoplastic
Persistent	Either neoplastic or non-neoplastic
Intermittent	Either neoplastic or non-neoplastic
Related to menses	More likely FCC
Premenopausal	More likely FCC
Taking hormones	More likely FCC

FCC, fibrocystic condition.

carcinoma. The important characteristics of the discharge and other factors to be evaluated are listed in Table 19–1.

1. Discharge from a single duct—Spontaneous, unilateral, serous, or serosanguineous discharge from a single duct is usually caused by an ectatic duct or an intraductal papilloma or, rarely, by an intraductal cancer. A mass may not be palpable. The involved duct may be identified by pressure at different sites around the nipple at the margin of the areola. Bloody discharge is suggestive of cancer but is more often caused by a benign papilloma in the duct. Cytologic examination may identify malignant cells, but negative findings do not rule out cancer, which is more likely in older women. In any case, the involved bloody duct—and a mass if present—should be excised. A ductogram (a mammogram of a duct after radiopaque dye has been injected), like cytology, is of limited value since excision of the suspicious ductal system is indicated regardless of findings. Ductoscopy, evaluation of the ductal system with a small scope inserted through the nipple, is not effective management.

2. Discharge from multiple ducts—In premenopausal women, spontaneous multiple duct discharge, unilateral or bilateral, most noticeable just before menstruation, is often due to fibrocystic condition. Discharge may be green or brownish. Papillomatosis and ductal ectasia are usually detected only by biopsy. If a mass is present, it should be removed.

A milky discharge from multiple ducts in the nonlactating breast may occur from hyperprolactinemia. Serum prolactin levels should be obtained to search for a pituitary tumor. TSH helps exclude causative hypothyroidism. Numerous antipsychotic medications and other medications may also cause a milky discharge that ceases on discontinuance of the medication.

Oral contraceptives or estrogen replacement therapy may cause clear, serous, or milky discharge from a single duct, but multiple duct discharge is more common. In the premenopausal woman, the discharge is more evident just before menstruation and disappears on stopping the medication. If it does not stop, is from a single duct, and is copious, exploration should be performed since this may be a sign of cancer.

A purulent discharge may originate in a subareolar abscess and requires drainage of the abscess and removal of the related lactiferous sinus.

When localization of the discharge is not possible, no mass is palpable, and the discharge is nonbloody, the patient should be reexamined every 3 or 4 months for a year, and a mammogram and an ultrasound should be performed. Although most discharge is from a benign process, patients may find it annoying or disconcerting. To eliminate the discharge, proximal duct excision can be performed both for treatment and diagnosis.

Gulati M et al. Nipple discharge: when is it worrisome? Curr Probl Diagn Radiol. 2023;52:560. [PMID: 37460358]

Pleasant V. Management of breast complaints and high-risk lesions. Best Pract Res Clin Obstet Gynaecol. 2022:83:46. [PMID: 35570155]

FAT NECROSIS

Fat necrosis is a rare lesion of the breast but is of clinical importance because it produces a mass (often accompanied by skin or nipple retraction) that is usually indistinguishable from carcinoma, even with imaging studies. Fat necrosis can occur after trauma; after fat injections to augment breast size or fill defects after breast surgery; and after segmental resection, radiation therapy, or flap reconstruction following mastectomy. If untreated, the mass gradually disappears. If imaging is not typical of fat necrosis, the safest course is to obtain a biopsy. Core needle biopsy is usually adequate.

BREAST ABSCESS

During nursing, an area of redness, tenderness, and induration may develop in the breast. The organism most commonly found in these abscesses is *Staphylococcus aureus* (see Puerperal Mastitis, Chapter 22).

Infection in the nonlactating breast is rare. A subareolar abscess may develop in young or middle-aged women who are not lactating. Often needle or catheter drainage is adequate to treat an abscess, but surgical incision and drainage may be necessary; these infections tend to recur after incision and drainage unless the area is explored during a quiescent interval, with excision of the involved lactiferous duct or ducts at the base of the nipple. In the nonlactating breast, inflammatory carcinoma must always be considered. Thus, incision and biopsy of any indurated tissue with a small piece of erythematous skin is indicated when suspected abscess or cellulitis in the nonlactating breast does not resolve promptly with antibiotics.

Ammann AM et al. Breast infections: a review of current literature. Am J Surg. 2024;228:78. [PMID: 37949727]

DISORDERS OF THE AUGMENTED BREAST

At least 4 million American women have had breast implants. Breast augmentation is performed by placing implants under the pectoralis muscle or, less desirably, in the subcutaneous tissue of the breast. Most implants are made of an outer silicone shell filled with a silicone gel, saline, or some combination of the two. Capsule contraction or scarring around the implant develops in about 15–25% of patients, leading to a firmness and distortion of the breast that can be painful. Some require removal of the implant and surrounding capsule.

Implant rupture may occur in as many as 5–10% of women, and bleeding of gel through the capsule is noted even more commonly. The FDA has advised symptomatic women with ruptured silicone implants to discuss possible surgical removal with their clinicians. However, women who are asymptomatic and have no evidence of rupture of a silicone gel prosthesis do not require removal of the implant. Although silicone gel may be an immunologic stimulant, there is *no increase* in autoimmune disorders in patients with such implants. Women with symptoms of autoimmune illnesses often undergo removal, but no benefit has been shown.

Studies have failed to show any association between implants and an increased incidence of breast cancer. However, breast cancer may develop in a patient with an augmentation prosthesis, as it does in women without them. Detection in patients with implants may be more difficult because mammography is less able to detect early lesions. Mammography has better detection capabilities if the implant is subpectoral rather than subcutaneous. Local recurrence is usually cutaneous or subcutaneous and is easily detected by palpation. Rarely, lymphoma of the breast with silicone implants has been reported.

If a cancer develops in a patient with implants, it should be treated in the same manner as in women without implants. Such women should be offered the option of mastectomy or breast-conserving therapy, which may require removal or replacement of the implant. Radiotherapy of the augmented breast often results in marked capsular contracture. Adjuvant treatments should be given for the same indications as for women who have no implants.

Boyd CJ et al. Systematic review of capsular contracture management following breast augmentation: an update. Plast Reconstr Surg. 2024;153:303e. [PMID: 36877620]

Clemens MW et al. American Association of Plastic Surgeons consensus on breast implant-associated anaplastic large-cell lymphoma. Plast Reconstr Surg. 2024;154:473. [PMID: 38412359]

CARCINOMA OF THE FEMALE BREAST

ESSENTIALS OF DIAGNOSIS

- Risk factors: Age, nulliparity, childbirth after age 30, family history of breast cancer or deleterious mutations (*BRCA1*, *BRCA2*, or others), and personal history of breast cancer or some types of proliferative conditions.
- Early findings: Mammographic abnormalities and no palpable mass, or single, nontender, firm to hard mass with ill-defined margins.
- Later findings: Skin or nipple retraction; axillary lymphadenopathy; breast enlargement, edema, erythema, pain; fixation of mass to skin or chest wall.

Incidence & Risk Factors

In the United States, breast cancer will develop in *one of eight* women. Next to skin cancer, breast cancer is the most common cancer in American women. It is second only to lung cancer as a cause of cancer death except in Black and Latina women for whom breast cancer is the leading cause of cancer death. In 2025, ~317,000 new cases of invasive breast cancer were diagnosed and an estimated 42,000 women died of breast cancer. Additionally, about 59,000 new cases of ductal carcinoma in situ (DCIS) were diagnosed in women.

Worldwide, breast cancer is diagnosed in ~2.3 million women, and about 665,000 die of breast cancer each year. Globally, breast cancer has surpassed lung cancer as the most commonly diagnosed non-skin cancer among women.

The most significant risk factor for the development of breast cancer is age. A woman's risk of breast cancer rises rapidly until her early 60s, peaks in her 70s, and then declines. A significant family history of breast or ovarian cancer imparts a high risk of developing breast cancer. Germline mutations in the *BRCA* family of tumor suppressor genes or other breast cancer susceptibility genes account for ~5–10% of breast cancer diagnoses and tend to cluster in certain ethnic groups, including women of Ashkenazi Jewish descent. Women with a mutation in the *BRCA1* gene, located on chromosome 17, have an estimated 85% chance of developing breast cancer in their lifetime. Other genes associated with an increased risk of breast and other cancers include *BRCA2* (associated with a gene on chromosome 13); ataxia-telangiectasia mutation (*ATM*), *BARD1*, *CHEK2*, *PALB2*, *RAD51D*; and mutation of the tumor suppressor gene *p53*. Primary care clinicians should assess a woman's personal and family history for breast, ovarian, tubal, or peritoneal cancer (as family history of ovarian and peritoneal cancers increases a woman's risk of breast cancer) using a familial risk assessment tool (eg, https://www.uspreventiveservicestaskforce.org/uspstf/document/

RecommendationStatementFinal/brca-related-cancer-risk-assessment-genetic-counseling-and-genetic-testing#tab1). Those with a positive result should receive genetic counseling to decide whether genetic testing is indicated.

Even when genetic testing fails to reveal a predisposing genetic mutation, women with a strong family history of breast cancer are at higher risk for development of breast cancer. Compared with a woman with no affected family members, a woman who has one first-degree relative with breast cancer has double the risk of developing breast cancer and a woman with two first-degree relatives with breast cancer has triple the risk of developing breast cancer. The risk is further increased for a woman whose affected family member was premenopausal at the time of diagnosis or had bilateral breast cancer. Lifestyle and reproductive factors also contribute to the risk of breast cancer. Nulliparous women and women whose first full-term pregnancy occurred after the age of 30 have an elevated risk. Early menarche (under age 12) and late natural menopause (after age 55) are associated with an increase in risk, especially for hormone receptor–positive (estrogen receptor [ER]–positive or progesterone receptor [PR]–positive or both) breast cancer. Combined oral contraceptive pills also appear to increase the risk of breast cancer, with longer use associated with higher risk. Several studies show that, in postmenopausal women, concomitant administration of progesterone and estrogen may increase the incidence of breast cancer, compared with the use of estrogen alone or with no hormone replacement treatment. A prior history of chest wall radiation (eg, for Hodgkin lymphoma) increases the risk of breast cancer years later. Alcohol consumption, high dietary intake of fat, and lack of exercise may also increase the risk of breast cancer. Fibrocystic condition is associated with an increased incidence of cancer only when it is accompanied by proliferative changes, papillomatosis, atypical epithelial hyperplasia, or increased breast density on mammogram. A woman who had cancer in one breast is at increased risk for cancer developing in the other breast. In these women, a contralateral cancer develops at rate of ~1% per year. Women with cancer of the uterine corpus have a risk of breast cancer significantly higher than that of the general population, and women with breast cancer have a comparably increased risk of endometrial cancer. Breast cancer tends to be diagnosed more frequently in women of higher socioeconomic status.

Women at greater than average risk for developing breast cancer (Table 19–2) should be identified by their clinicians and monitored carefully. Several risk assessment models have been validated to estimate a woman's risk of developing cancer. Women with genetic mutations in whom breast cancer develops may be treated in the same way as women who do not have mutations (ie, lumpectomy), though there is an increased risk of ipsilateral and contralateral breast cancer after lumpectomy for these women.

Goddard KAB et al. Estimation of cancer deaths averted from prevention, screening and treatment efforts, 1975-2020. JAMA Oncol. 2025;11:162. [PMID: 39636625]

Table 19–2. Factors associated with increased risk of breast cancer (listed in alphabetical order).

Age	Older
Family history	Breast cancer in parent, sibling, or child (especially bilateral or premenopausal)
Genetics	*BRCA1*, *BRCA2*, or other unknown mutations
Menstrual history	Early menarche (under age 12) Late menopause (after age 55)
Previous medical history	Endometrial cancer Proliferative forms of fibrocystic disease Cancer in other breast
Race	White
Reproductive history	Nulliparous or first pregnancy after age 30 years

Kim J et al. Estrogens and breast cancer. Ann Oncol. 2025;36:134. [PMID: 39522613]
Kim J et al. Global patterns and trends in breast cancer incidence and mortality across 185 countries. Nat Med. 2025;31:1154. [PMID: 39994475]
Kurian AW et al. Germline genetic testing after cancer diagnosis. JAMA. 2023;330:43. [PMID: 37276540]
Zhang Y et al. Genetic risk, health-associated lifestyle, and risk of early-onset total cancer and breast cancer. J Natl Cancer Inst. 2025;117:40. [PMID: 39189966]

Prevention

Multiple clinical trials have evaluated the use of selective ER modulators (SERMs), including tamoxifen and raloxifene, or aromatase inhibitors (eg, anastrozole) for prevention of breast cancer in women with no personal history of breast cancer but at high risk for developing the disease. A meta-analysis of six of these studies including 50,927 women demonstrated a 32% reduction in breast cancer incidence with the use of tamoxifen (generally 20 mg) compared to placebo and a 47% reduction in risk of breast cancer with the use of an aromatase inhibitor compared with placebo. An increased risk of endometrial cancer, cataracts, and venous thromboembolic events has been associated with tamoxifen and a higher rate of fractures and musculoskeletal side effects are associated with aromatase inhibitors. Use of this intervention by women has been relatively low, possibly due to the perceived risks and side effects of therapy. Ten-year follow-up from the TAM-01 trial showed that low-dose tamoxifen (5 mg daily for 3 years) is an effective risk-reducing strategy in women with proliferative atypia or carcinoma in situ, providing women with a better tolerated alternative.

Some women at high risk may consider prophylactic mastectomy or oophorectomy.

Bennett A et al. Screening for breast cancer: a systematic review update to inform the Canadian Task Force on Preventive Health Care guideline. Syst Rev. 2024;13:304. [PMID: 39702409]

Laws A et al. Endocrine therapy for primary and secondary prevention after diagnosis of high-risk breast lesions or preinvasive breast cancer. J Clin Oncol. 2023;41:3092. [PMID: 37126767]

Lazzeroni M et al. Randomized placebo controlled trial of low-dose tamoxifen to prevent recurrence in breast noninvasive neoplasia: a 10-year follow-up of TAM-01 study. J Clin Oncol. 2023;41:3116. [PMID: 36917758]

Early Detection of Breast Cancer

A. Screening Programs

Substantial evidence supports the use of routine screening mammography; however, recommendations relating to timing and frequency vary by different agencies and countries. About one-third of the abnormalities detected on screening mammograms will be found to be malignant when biopsy is performed. The probability of cancer on a screening mammogram is directly related to the Breast Imaging Reporting and Data System (BIRADS) assessment, and workup should be performed based on this classification. The sensitivity of mammography varies from approximately 60–90%. This sensitivity depends on several factors, including patient age, breast density, tumor size, tumor histology (lobular versus ductal), location, and mammographic appearance. In young women with dense breasts, mammography is less sensitive than in older women with fatty breasts, in whom mammography can detect at least 90% of malignancies. Smaller tumors, particularly those without calcifications, are more difficult to detect, especially in dense breasts. The lack of sensitivity and the low incidence of breast cancer in young women have led to questions concerning the value of mammography for screening in women 40–50 years of age. The specificity of mammography in women under 50 years varies from about 30% to 40% for nonpalpable mammographic abnormalities to 85% to 90% for clinically evident malignancies. Guidelines from at least six separate organizations exist in the United States and each differs slightly, making it complex for clinicians and patients to navigate. The American College of Radiology, American Medical Association, USPSTF, and National Comprehensive Cancer Network (NCCN) recommend starting mammography screening at age 40. Most guidelines recommend annual screening; however, the American Cancer Society recommends decreasing the frequency of screening to every 1–2 years starting at age 55 years and the USPSTF recommends screening mammography every other year beginning at age 40 years. It is generally agreed that mammography should continue until life expectancy is shorter than 7–10 years. The USPSTF has concluded that there is insufficient evidence to guide use of screening mammography in women after age 74 (https://www.uspreventiveservicestaskforce.org/uspstf/draft-recommendation/breast-cancer-screening-adults#bcei-recommendation-title-area). Thus, clinicians should have an informed discussion with patients about screening mammography regarding its potential risks (eg, false positives, overdiagnosis, radiation exposure) and benefits (eg, early diagnosis), taking into consideration a patient's individual risk factors.

B. Imaging

1. Mammography—Mammography is the most reliable means of detecting breast cancer before a mass can be palpated. Most slowly growing cancers can be identified by mammography at least 2 years before reaching a size detectable by palpation.

Indications for mammography are as follows: (1) screening at regular intervals in asymptomatic women at risk for developing breast cancer; (2) evaluating each breast when a diagnosis of potentially curable breast cancer has been made, and at regular intervals thereafter; (3) evaluating a questionable or ill-defined breast mass or other suspicious change in the breast; (4) searching for an occult breast cancer in women with metastatic disease in axillary nodes or elsewhere from an unknown primary; (5) screening women prior to cosmetic operations or prior to biopsy of a mass, to examine for an unsuspected cancer; (6) monitoring women with breast cancer who have been treated with breast-conserving surgery and radiation; and (7) monitoring the contralateral breast in women with breast cancer treated with mastectomy.

Calcifications are the most easily recognized mammographic abnormality. The most common findings associated with carcinoma of the breast are clustered pleomorphic microcalcifications. Such calcifications are usually at least five to eight in number, aggregated in one part of the breast and differing from each other in size and shape, often including branched or V- or Y-shaped configurations. There may be an associated mammographic mass density or, at times, only a mass density with no calcifications. Such a density usually has irregular or ill-defined borders and may lead to architectural distortion within the breast but may be subtle and difficult to detect.

Patients with a dominant or suspicious mass on examination must undergo biopsy despite mammographic findings. The mammogram should be obtained prior to biopsy so that other suspicious areas can be noted and the contralateral breast can be evaluated. *Mammography is never a substitute for biopsy* because it may not reveal clinical cancer, especially in a very dense breast.

Communication and documentation among the patient, the referring clinician, and the interpreting physician are critical for high-quality screening and diagnostic mammography. The patient should be told about *how* she will receive timely results of her mammogram; that mammography does not "rule out" cancer; and that she may receive a correlative examination such as ultrasound at the mammography facility if referred for a suspicious lesion. She should also be aware of the technique and need for breast compression and that this may be uncomfortable. The mammography facility should be informed in writing by the clinician of abnormal physical examination findings. The Agency for Health Care Policy and Research Clinical Practice Guidelines strongly recommend that all mammography reports be communicated in writing to the patient and referring clinician. In the United States, legislation exists in a number of states that requires imaging facilities to report to patients the density of their breasts. This may prompt women with dense breasts to discuss with their clinician whether or not additional screening options would be appropriate in addition to mammogram.

2. MRI—MRI may be useful for screening women at high risk for breast cancer but not for the general population. The *sensitivity* of MRI is much higher than mammography; however, the *specificity* is significantly lower, and this results in multiple unnecessary biopsies. The increased sensitivity despite decreased specificity may be considered a reasonable trade-off for those at increased risk for breast cancer but not for normal-risk population. The NCCN guidelines recommend MRI in addition to screening mammography for high-risk women, including those with deleterious mutations, those who have a lifetime risk of breast cancer of at least 20%, and those with a personal history of lobular carcinoma in situ (LCIS).

Women who received radiation therapy to the chest in their teens or twenties are at high risk for developing breast cancer and screening MRI may be considered in addition to mammography. A Netherlands study (Dense Tissue and Early Breast Neoplasm Screening "DENSE") involving > 40,000 women with extremely dense breast tissue demonstrated that the addition of annual MRI to screening mammography was associated with a lower rate of cancers being diagnosed in 2 years. MRI is useful in women with breast implants to determine the character of a breast lesion, to search for implant rupture, and may be helpful in patients with prior lumpectomy and radiation.

Kenealy BP et al. Cancer screening in women. Prim Care. 2025;52:233. [PMID: 40412903]
US Preventive Services Task Force et al. Screening for breast cancer: US Preventive Services Task Force recommendation statement. JAMA. 2024;331:1918. [PMID: 38687503]

C. Clinical Breast Examination and Self-Examination

Breast self-examination has *not* been shown to improve survival. Because of the lack of strong evidence demonstrating value, the American Cancer Society no longer recommends monthly breast self-examination. Nonetheless, patients should recognize and report any breast changes to their clinicians as it remains an important facet of proactive care.

Clinical Findings Associated with Early Detection of Breast Cancer

A. Symptoms and Signs

The presenting complaint in about 70% of patients with breast cancer is a lump (usually painless) in the breast. About 90% of these breast masses are discovered by the patient. Less frequent symptoms are breast pain; nipple discharge; erosion, retraction, enlargement, or itching of the nipple; and redness, generalized hardness, enlargement, or shrinking of the breast. Rarely, an axillary mass or swelling of the arm may be the first symptom. Back or bone pain, jaundice, or weight loss may be the result of systemic metastases, but these symptoms are rarely seen on initial presentation.

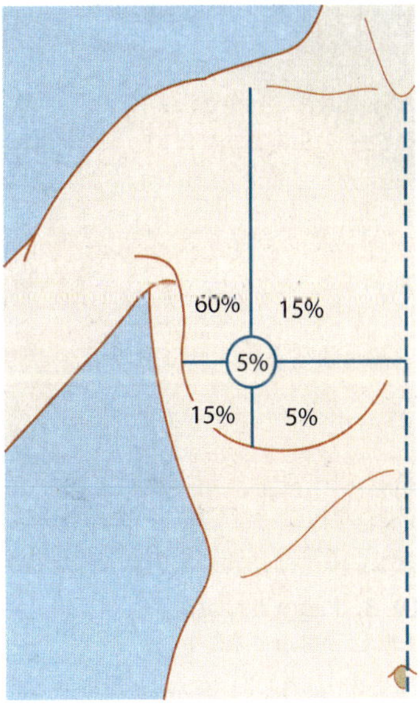

Figure 19–1. Frequency of breast carcinoma at various anatomic sites.

The relative frequency of carcinoma in various anatomic sites in the breast is shown in Figure 19–1.

Inspection of the breast is the first step in the physical examination and should be carried out with the patient sitting, arms at her sides and then overhead. Abnormal variations in breast size and contour, minimal nipple retraction, and slight edema, redness, or retraction of the skin (dimpling) can be identified (Figure 19–2). Asymmetry of the breasts and retraction or dimpling of the skin can often be accentuated by having the patient raise her arms overhead or press her hands on her hips to contract the pectoralis muscles. Axillary and supraclavicular areas should be thoroughly palpated for enlarged nodes with the patient sitting. Palpation of the breast for masses or other changes should be performed with the patient both seated and supine with the arm abducted. Palpation with a rotary motion of the examiner's fingers as well as horizontal pressure and movement has been recommended.

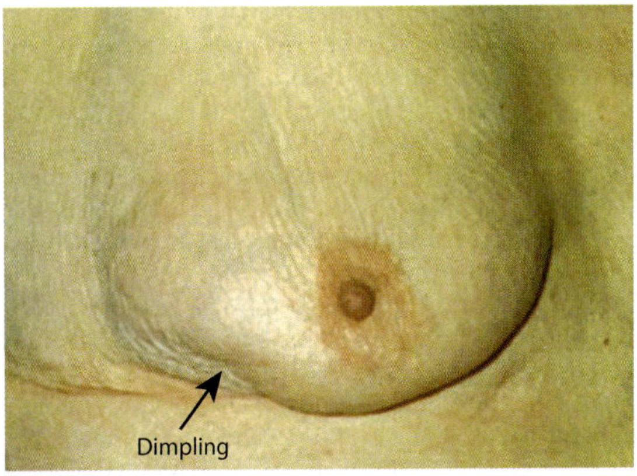

Figure 19–2. Skin dimpling. (Used, with permission, from Armando E. Giuliano, MD.)

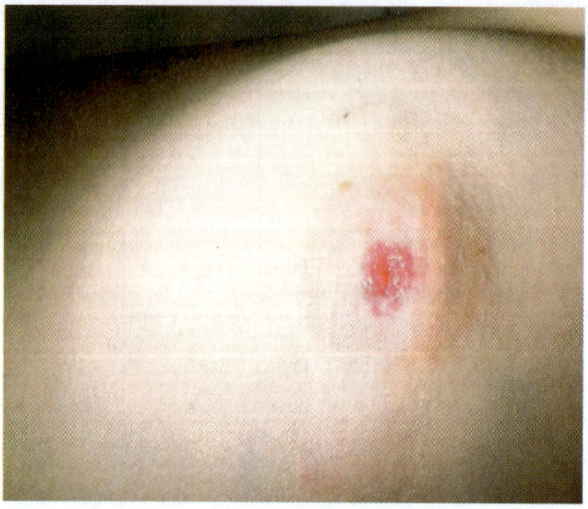

▲ **Figure 19–3.** Paget disease. (Used, with permission, from Armando E. Giuliano, MD.)

Breast cancer usually consists of a nontender, firm or hard mass with poorly delineated margins (caused by local infiltration). Small (1–2 mm) erosions of the nipple epithelium may be the only manifestation of Paget disease of the breast (Figure 19–3). Watery, serous, or bloody discharge from the nipple is an occasional early sign but is more often associated with benign disease.

A lesion < 1 cm in diameter may be difficult or impossible for the examiner to feel but may be discovered by the patient. The patient should always be asked to demonstrate the location of the mass. If the clinician fails to confirm the patient's suspicions and imaging studies are normal, the examination should be repeated in 2–3 months, preferably 1–2 weeks after the onset of menses. During the premenstrual phase of the cycle, increased innocuous nodularity may suggest neoplasm or may obscure an underlying lesion. If there is any question regarding the nature of an abnormality under these circumstances, the patient should be asked to return after her menses.

Metastases tend to first involve regional lymph nodes, which may be palpable. One or two movable, nontender, not particularly firm axillary lymph nodes ≤ 5 mm in diameter are frequently present and are generally not significant. Firm or hard nodes ≥ 1 cm are typical of metastases. Axillary nodes that are matted or fixed to skin or deep structures indicate advanced disease (at least stage III). The incidence of positive axillary nodes increases with the size of the primary tumor. Metastases in node(s) are present in about 30% of patients with clinically negative nodes.

In most cases, no nodes are palpable in the supraclavicular fossa. Firm or hard nodes of any size in this location or just beneath the clavicle should be biopsied. Ipsilateral supraclavicular or infraclavicular nodes containing cancer indicate that the tumor is in an advanced stage (stage III or IV). Edema of the ipsilateral breast or arm, commonly caused by metastatic infiltration of regional lymphatics, is also a sign of advanced cancer.

B. Laboratory Findings

Liver or bone metastases may be associated with elevation of serum alkaline phosphatase. Hypercalcemia is an occasional important finding in advanced breast cancer. Serum tumor markers such as carcinoembryonic antigen and CA 15-3 or CA 27-29 are *not* recommended for diagnosis of early lesions or for routine surveillance for recurrence after a breast cancer diagnosis.

C. Imaging

1. For lesions felt only by the patient—Ultrasonography is often valuable and mammography essential when an area is felt by the patient to be abnormal but the clinician feels no mass. MRI is more sensitive than other imaging modalities but more costly and has a high false-positive rate. A negative MRI cannot entirely rule out cancer because MRI has a false-negative rate of about 3–5%. Although lower than mammography, this false-negative rate cannot permit safe elimination of the possibility of cancer and a biopsy should still be considered. False-negative results with imaging are more likely seen in infiltrating lobular carcinoma, DCIS, and low-grade invasive ductal carcinoma than in higher-grade invasive carcinoma.

2. For metastatic lesions—For patients with suspicious symptoms or signs (bone pain, abdominal symptoms, elevated liver biochemical tests) or locally advanced disease (clinically abnormal lymph nodes or large primary tumors), staging scans are indicated before surgery or systemic therapy. Chest imaging with CT or radiographs may be done to evaluate for pulmonary metastases. Abdominal imaging with CT or ultrasound may be obtained to evaluate for liver metastases. Bone scans using ^{99m}Tc-labeled phosphates or phosphonates are more sensitive than skeletal radiographs in detecting metastatic breast cancer. Bone scanning has not proved to be of clinical value as a routine preoperative test in the absence of symptoms, physical findings, or abnormal alkaline phosphatase or calcium levels. The frequency of abnormal findings on bone scan parallels the status of the axillary lymph nodes on pathologic examination. PET scanning alone or combined with CT (PET-CT) may also be used for detecting soft tissue or visceral metastases in patients with locally advanced disease or with symptoms or signs of metastatic disease.

D. Diagnostic Tests

1. Aspiration—If a tumor is palpable and feels like a cyst, an 18-gauge needle can be used to aspirate the fluid and make the diagnosis of cyst. If a cyst is aspirated and the fluid is nonbloody, it does not have to be examined cytologically. If the mass does not recur, no further diagnostic test is necessary.

2. Biopsy—The diagnosis of breast cancer depends on examination of tissue or cells removed by biopsy. Treatment should never be undertaken without an unequivocal histologic or cytologic diagnosis of cancer. About 60% of lesions clinically thought to be cancer prove on biopsy to be benign, while about 30% of clinically benign lesions are found to be malignant. These findings demonstrate the fallibility of clinical judgment and the necessity for biopsy. *The safest course is biopsy examination of all suspicious lesions found on physical examination or imaging, or both.*

There is only one probable exception to the need for a histologic diagnosis of a breast mass: a nonsuspicious, presumably fibrocystic mass, in a premenopausal woman. Rather, these masses can be observed through one or two menstrual cycles. However, the mass must be biopsied if it does not completely resolve during this time and ultrasonographic findings show that it is not cystic or benign appearing (like a fibroadenoma or intramammary lymph node). Figures 19–4 and 19–5 present algorithms for management of breast masses in premenopausal and postmenopausal patients.

The simplest biopsy method is needle biopsy, either by obtaining a small core of tissue with a large hollow needle (core needle biopsy) or aspiration of tumor cells (FNA cytology).

A. Core needle biopsy—A core of tissue is removed with a large cutting needle for histologic examination and *is the diagnostic procedure of choice* for both palpable and image-detected abnormalities. Handheld biopsy devices make large-core needle (14-gauge) biopsy of a palpable mass easy and cost effective in the office with local anesthesia. As in

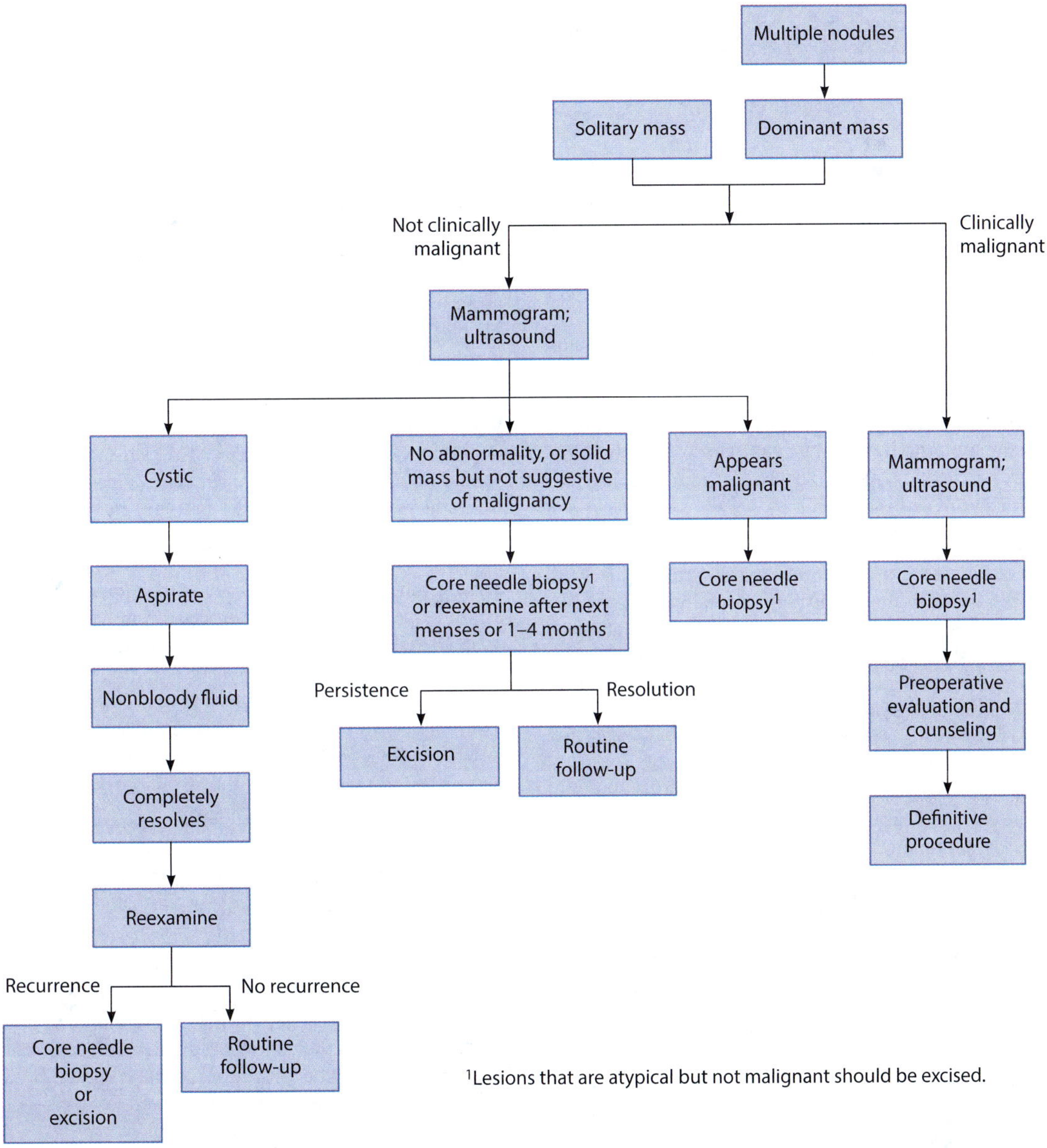

Figure 19–4. Evaluation of breast masses in *premenopausal* women. (Reproduced with permission from Giuliano AE, Srour MK. Breast disease. In: Berek JS, Hacker NF [editors]. *Berek & Hacker's, Gynecologic Oncology*. 7th ed. Philadelphia: Wolters Kluwer, 2021.)

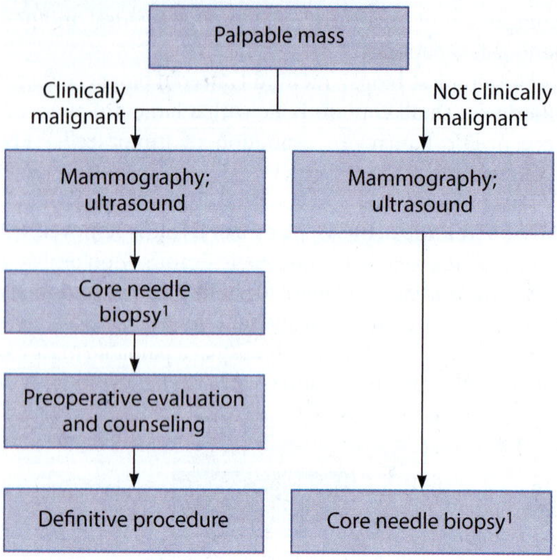

[1]Lesions that are atypical but not malignant should be excised.

Figure 19–5. Evaluation of breast masses in *postmenopausal* women. (Reproduced with permission from Giuliano AE, Srour MK. Breast disease. In: Berek JS, Hacker NF [editors]. *Berek & Hacker's, Gynecologic Oncology*. 7th ed. Philadelphia: Wolters Kluwer, 2021.)

the case of any needle biopsy, the main problem is sampling error due to improper positioning of the needle, giving rise to a false-negative test result. This is extremely unusual with image-guided biopsies. Core needle biopsy allows the tumor to be tested for the expression of biologic markers, such as ER, PR, and HER2 (human epidermal growth factor receptor 2).

B. FNA cytology—In this technique, cells are aspirated with a small needle and examined cytologically. This technique can be performed easily with virtually no morbidity and is much less expensive than excisional or open biopsy. The main disadvantages are that it requires a pathologist skilled in the cytologic diagnosis of breast cancer and it is subject to sampling problems. Furthermore, noninvasive cancers usually cannot be distinguished from invasive cancers. The incidence of false-positive diagnoses is extremely low, perhaps 1–2%. The false-negative rate is as high as 10%. Most experienced clinicians would not leave a suspicious dominant mass in the breast even when FNA cytology is negative unless the clinical diagnosis, breast imaging studies, and cytologic studies were all in agreement, such as for a fibrocystic lesion or fibroadenoma. Given the stated limitations, *core needle biopsy, rather than FNA, is the modality of choice for sampling an abnormal breast mass.* FNA can be useful for biopsy of suspicious lymph nodes near the axillary vein.

C. Open excisional biopsy—This separate procedure, which is done under local anesthesia before deciding on definitive therapy, is less common with the increased use of core needle biopsy. Core needle biopsy, when positive, offers a more rapid approach with less expense and morbidity, but when nondiagnostic it must be followed by open biopsy. It generally consists of an excisional biopsy, which is done through an incision with the intent to remove the entire abnormality, not simply a sample. Intraoperative frozen section examination of a breast biopsy has generally been abandoned unless there is a high clinical suspicion of malignancy in a patient well prepared for the diagnosis of cancer and its treatment options.

In general, the two-step approach—outpatient core needle biopsy followed by definitive operation at a later date—is preferred in the diagnosis and treatment of breast cancer because patients can be given time to adjust to the diagnosis of cancer, can consider alternative forms of therapy, and can seek a second opinion if they wish. *There is no adverse effect on the cancer from the few weeks' delay of the two-step procedure.*

3. Biopsy with ultrasound guidance—Ultrasonography may show signs suggestive of carcinoma, such as an irregular mass or a mass within a cyst in the rare case of intracystic carcinoma. Nonpalpable mammographic densities that appear benign should be investigated with ultrasound to determine whether the lesions are cystic or solid or have features suggestive of a malignancy. These may even be needle biopsied with ultrasound guidance.

4. Biopsy with mammographic guidance—When a suspicious abnormality is identified by mammography alone and cannot be palpated by the clinician, the lesion should be biopsied under mammographic guidance. Mammographic guidance can be used for core needle biopsies or excisional biopsies.

5. Other imaging modalities—Automated breast ultrasonography can help distinguish cystic from solid lesions but should be used only as a supplement to physical examination and mammography. MRI is useful in differentiating scar from recurrence post-lumpectomy. It may also examine for multicentricity when there is a known primary cancer; examine the contralateral breast in women with cancer; examine the extent of cancer, especially lobular carcinomas; or determine the response to neoadjuvant chemotherapy. Moreover, MRI-detected suspicious findings that are not seen on mammogram or ultrasound may be biopsied under MRI guidance. PET scanning does not appear useful in evaluating the breast itself but is useful to examine for distant metastases.

6. Cytology—Cytologic examination of nipple discharge or cyst fluid may be helpful on rare occasions. As a rule, mammography (or ductography) and breast biopsy are required when nipple discharge or cyst fluid is bloody or cytologically questionable.

Differential Diagnosis

The most common lesions in the differential diagnosis of breast cancer are the following, in descending order of frequency: fibrocystic condition of the breast, fibroadenoma, intraductal papilloma, lipoma, and fat necrosis.

Staging

The American Joint Committee on Cancer and the International Union Against Cancer have a joint TNM (tumor, regional lymph nodes, distant metastases) staging system for breast cancer. All patients are assigned an anatomic stage based on TNM (T0, carcinoma in situ; T1, tumor ≤ 2 cm; T2, tumor > 2 cm and ≤ 5 cm with or without spread to regional lymph nodes; T3, tumor > 5 cm; T4, tumor of any size that has invaded the chest wall or skin). The eighth edition is a landmark change because it adds biologic markers (ER, PR, HER2, histologic grade, and 21-gene recurrence score) to modify the anatomic staging. Thus, each patient is assigned not only an anatomic stage but also a prognostic stage, incorporating these biologic factors. The *clinical* prognostic stage, in which TNM grade and HER2 and hormone receptor status are incorporated, is assigned to all breast cancer patients and is the only prognostic staging classification appropriate for patients who receive neoadjuvant (presurgical) systemic therapy or who do not undergo surgery. The *pathologic* prognostic stage is assigned to those patients who undergo surgery as their initial breast cancer treatment. This is based on T, N, M, grade, HER2, hormone receptor status, and in some patients with small ER-positive, HER2-negative, node-negative tumors, 21-gene recurrence score.

Pathologic Types

Numerous pathologic subtypes of breast cancer can be identified histologically (Table 19–3).

Except for the in situ cancers, the histologic subtypes have only a slight bearing on prognosis when outcomes are compared after accurate staging. The noninvasive cancers by definition are confined by the basement membrane of the ducts and lack the ability to spread. Histologic parameters for invasive cancers, including lymphovascular invasion and tumor grade, have been shown to be of prognostic value. Immunohistochemical analysis for expression of hormone receptors and for overexpression of HER2 in the primary tumor offers prognostic and therapeutic information.

Table 19–3. Histologic types of breast cancer.[1]

Invasive Type (~322,000 cases in the United States in 2026, ~84%)	Frequency of Occurrence
Invasive ductal	80–90%
Infiltrating ductal (not otherwise specified)	~80%
Medullary	3–5%
Colloid (mucinous)	1–7%
Tubular	1–4%
Papillary	1–2%
Invasive lobular	10–15%
Rare cancers	< 1%
Juvenile (secretory)	
Adenoid cystic	
Epidermoid	
Sudoriferous	
Noninvasive Type (~61,000 cases in the United States in 2026, 15–20%)	**Frequency of Occurrence**
Noninvasive (ductal carcinoma in situ)	~1 in 5 cancers

[1]American Cancer Society estimates of frequencies (https://www.cancer.org/cancer/types/breast-cancer/about/how-common-is-breast-cancer.html).

Special Clinical Forms of Breast Cancer

A. Paget Carcinoma

Paget carcinoma is uncommon (about 1% of all breast cancers). Over 85% of cases are associated with an underlying invasive or noninvasive cancer, usually a well-differentiated infiltrating ductal carcinoma or a DCIS. Gross nipple changes are often minimal, and a tumor mass may not be palpable.

Because the nipple changes appear innocuous, the diagnosis is frequently missed. The first symptom is often itching or burning of the nipple, with superficial erosion or ulceration. These are often treated as dermatitis or bacterial infection, leading to delay or failure in detection. The diagnosis is established by biopsy of the erosion. When the lesion consists of nipple changes only or an associated DCIS, the incidence of axillary metastases is extremely low, and the prognosis is excellent. When a breast mass or invasive cancer is also present, the incidence of axillary metastases rises, with an associated marked decrease in rates of cure by surgical or other treatment.

B. Inflammatory Carcinoma

This is the most malignant form of breast cancer and constitutes < 3% of all cases. The clinical findings consist of a rapidly growing, sometimes painful mass that enlarges the breast. The overlying skin becomes erythematous, edematous, and warm. Often there is no distinct mass since the tumor diffusely infiltrates the involved breast. The inflammatory changes, often mistaken for an infection, are caused by carcinomatous invasion of the subdermal lymphatics, with resulting edema and hyperemia. *If the clinician suspects infection but the lesion does not respond to antibiotics within 1–2 weeks, biopsy should be performed.* The diagnosis should be made when the redness involves more than one-third of the skin over the breast and biopsy shows infiltrating carcinoma, often with invasion of the subdermal lymphatics. Metastases tend to occur early and widely; while rarely deemed curable in the past, anti-HER2 therapy (if HER2 overexpressing or amplified), surgery, and chemotherapy have resulted in some long-term cures. Mastectomy is indicated when chemotherapy has resulted in clinical remission with no evidence of distant metastases. In these cases, residual disease in the breast may be eradicated. Sentinel node biopsy is not indicated due to the high false-negative rate.

Breast Cancer Occurring During Pregnancy or Lactation

Pregnancy-associated breast cancer (diagnosed within 1 year of giving birth) and postpartum-associated pregnancy (diagnosed up to 10 years after pregnancy) are associated with a poor prognosis.

Breast cancer complicates up to one in 3000 pregnancies. Its incidence is increasing as women are having children at an older age. The diagnosis is frequently delayed because physiologic changes in the breast may obscure the lesion and screening mammography is not done in young or pregnant women. Termination of pregnancy has not been shown to improve maternal prognosis. The decision whether to terminate the pregnancy must be made on an individual basis, taking into account the patient's wishes, the clinical stage of the cancer and overall prognosis, the gestational age of the fetus, and the potential for premature ovarian failure in the future with systemic therapy. Clinicians need to be aware of laws regarding availability of abortion in the jurisdiction of their practice.

It is important for primary care and reproductive specialists to aggressively work up any breast abnormality discovered in a pregnant woman. Pregnancy (or lactation) is not a contraindication to operation or treatment, and therapy should be based on the stage of the disease as in the nonpregnant (or nonlactating) woman. Women with early-stage gestational breast cancer who choose to continue their pregnancy should undergo surgery to remove the tumor and receive systemic therapy if indicated. Often neoadjuvant systemic therapy may be given during pregnancy and the operation and radiation therapy delayed. Retrospective reviews of patients treated with anthracycline-containing regimens for gestational cancers (including leukemia and lymphomas) have established the relative safety of these regimens during pregnancy for both the patient and the fetus. Taxane-based regimens have not been evaluated extensively; however, data suggest they may be safe. Trastuzumab should not be given during pregnancy. Radiation therapy should be delayed until after delivery.

Bilateral Breast Cancer

Bilateral breast cancer occurs in < 5% of cases, but there is a 20–25% incidence of later occurrence of cancer in the second breast. Bilaterality occurs more often in familial breast cancer, in women aged < 50 years, and when there is a deleterious germline mutation. The incidence of second breast cancers increases directly with the length of time the patient is alive after her first cancer—about 1–2% per year. Tamoxifen or aromatase inhibitors decrease the risk of a contralateral hormone receptor–positive cancer.

In patients with breast cancer, mammography should be performed before primary treatment and at regular intervals thereafter to search for occult cancer in the opposite breast or conserved ipsilateral breast.

Lobular Carcinoma In Situ & Noninvasive Cancer

Noninvasive cancer within the ducts, or DCIS, tends to be unilateral and is believed to progress to invasive cancer if untreated. Invasive cancer will develop in the same breast in ~40–60% of women who have unresected DCIS. In the eighth edition of the American Joint Committee on Cancer (AJCC) Cancer Staging Manual, LCIS is no longer considered a cancer. *LCIS is generally agreed to be a marker of an increased risk of breast cancer rather than a direct precursor of breast cancer itself.* The probability of breast cancer (DCIS or invasive cancer in either breast) in a woman in whom LCIS has been diagnosed is estimated to be 1% per year. If LCIS is detected on core needle biopsy, an excisional biopsy without lymph node sampling may be performed to rule out DCIS or invasive cancer, but NCCN guidelines suggest observation alone is satisfactory. The incidence of LCIS is rising, likely due to increased use of screening mammography. In addition, the rate of mastectomy after the diagnosis of LCIS is increasing even though mastectomy is only recommended in those patients who otherwise have an increased risk of breast cancer through family history, genetic mutation, or past exposure to thoracic radiation. Pleomorphic LCIS may behave more like DCIS and may be associated with invasive carcinoma. For this reason, pleomorphic LCIS should be surgically removed with clear margins.

The treatment of intraductal lesions is controversial. DCIS can be treated by wide excision with or without radiation therapy or with total mastectomy. Conservative management is advised in patients with small lesions amenable to lumpectomy. Patients in whom LCIS is diagnosed or who have received lumpectomy for DCIS may discuss chemoprevention (with hormonal blockade therapy such as low-dose tamoxifen) with their clinician, which is effective in reducing the risk of developing breast cancer. Axillary metastases from in situ cancers should not occur unless there is an occult invasive cancer. Because a sentinel lymph node biopsy after mastectomy cannot be performed, it should be performed in a patient undergoing mastectomy for DCIS in case an invasive component is discovered. The COMET trial (NCT02926911) examined the nonoperative management of patients with low-risk DCIS (grade 1 or 2, hormone receptor–positive). With almost 1000 patients randomized to either active monitoring or surgery (with or without radiation), 2-year follow-up demonstrated no difference in the risk of ipsilateral invasive breast cancer recurrence.

Giuliano AE et al. Eighth edition of the AJCC Cancer Staging Manual: breast cancer. Ann Surg Oncol. 2018;25:1783. [PMID: 29671136]

Hwang ES et al; COMET Study Investigators. Active monitoring with or without endocrine therapy for low-risk ductal carcinoma in situ: the COMET randomized clinical trial. JAMA. 2025;333:972. [PMID: 39665585]

Li C et al. Time for detailed clinical management of Paget's disease of the breast. Int J Surg. 2024;110:1266. [PMID: 37889547]

Loibl S et al. ESMO expert consensus statements on the management of breast cancer during pregnancy (PrBC). Ann Oncol. 2023;34:849. [PMID: 37572987]

Roesch E et al. Multidisciplinary management of pregnancy-associated breast cancer. JCO Oncol Pract. 2025;21:313. [PMID: 39383485]

Tumor Biomarkers & Gene Expression Profiling

Hormone receptor–positive tumors are ER-positive or PR-positive, or both. Treatment with a hormonally targeted agent (anti-estrogen or anti-ER) is an essential therapy for hormone receptor–positive breast cancer. Hormone receptor–negative cancers do not respond to endocrine treatments. Patients whose tumors are hormone receptor–positive tend to have a more indolent disease course than those whose tumors are hormone receptor–negative.

The *HER2* gene is an oncogene; breast cancer cells with amplification of the *HER2* gene ("HER2-positive" cancers) overproduce the growth-promoting protein HER2. HER2-positive breast cancer is generally more aggressive than breast cancer with normal HER2 expression (HER2-negative breast cancer). Targeted therapies that block HER2 signaling have been shown to significantly improve outcomes for patients with HER2-positive disease. "HER2-low" breast cancer occurs when HER2 proteins are present but expressed less than in "HER2-positive" breast cancers. HER2-low breast cancers were classified as HER2-negative in the past. This does not represent a distinct molecular subtype of breast cancer with unique behavior, but rather denotes that the cancer may be targeted with a novel antibody-drug conjugate, trastuzumab deruxtecan, which has demonstrated efficacy in metastatic "HER2-low" breast cancer. An antibody-drug conjugate combines a monoclonal antibody (in this case, trastuzumab) targeted to a protein expressed on the cancer cell (in this case, HER2) with a cytotoxic drug (deruxtecan) to deliver the drug (cytotoxic payload) directly to the cancer.

Determining the ER, PR, and HER2 status of the tumor at the time early breast cancer is diagnosed and, if possible, at the time of recurrence is critical, both to gauge a patient's prognosis and to determine the best treatment regimen. In addition to ER, PR, and HER2 status, other important prognostic factors include the rate at which the tumor divides (assessed by an immunohistochemical stain for Ki67) and the grade and differentiation of the cells. These markers may be obtained on core biopsy or surgical specimens, but not reliably on FNA cytology. Individually these biomarkers are predictive and thus provide insight to guide appropriate therapy. Moreover, when combined, they provide useful information regarding risk of recurrence and prognosis in the curative setting.

"Triple-negative" tumors, which lack expression of ER and PR and do not have an overexpression of HER2, generally have a higher risk of early recurrence and metastases and are associated with a worse survival compared with other types. Endocrine therapy is not useful for this type of breast cancer. Chemotherapy has been the primary treatment option for triple-negative breast cancer. In contrast, patients with early-stage, hormone receptor–positive breast cancer may not benefit from the addition of chemotherapy to hormonally targeted treatments. Several molecular tests can assess risk of recurrence and predict which patients are most likely to benefit from chemotherapy for early-stage disease. Oncotype DX (Genomic Health/Exact Sciences) evaluates the expression of 21 genes relating to ER, HER2, and proliferation in a tumor specimen and categorizes a patient's risk of recurrence (recurrence score, "RS") as high, intermediate, or low. Patients in low- or intermediate-risk categories do not benefit from chemotherapy, especially when aged ≥ 50. This test is primarily indicated for ER-positive, lymph node-negative tumors, but results from the RxPONDER trial suggest that postmenopausal women with 1–3 positive lymph nodes with a recurrence score of < 26 may not benefit from the use of chemotherapy.

MammaPrint (Agendia) is an FDA-approved 70-gene signature assay to evaluate prognosis. This test classifies patients into good and poor prognostic groups to predict clinical outcome and may be used on patients with hormone receptor–positive or hormone receptor–negative breast cancer. The American Society of Clinical Oncology (ASCO) does not recommend using this assay in hormone receptor–negative or HER2-positive breast cancer. The eighth edition of the AJCC staging system incorporates genomic assays to provide a prognostic stage. Patients with low-risk genomic assays may be downstaged from their TNM stage.

Berton Giachetti PPM et al. Current controversies in the use of Oncotype DX in early breast cancer. Cancer Treat Rev. 2025;135:102887. [PMID: 40048856]
Kang S et al. HER2-low breast cancer: now and in the future. Cancer Res Treat. 2024;56:700. [PMID: 38291745]
Shaaban AM et al. HER2-low breast cancer-current knowledge and future directions. Medicina (Kaunas). 2025;61:644. [PMID: 40282933]

Curative Treatment

Most patients with early breast cancer can be cured. Treatment with a curative intent is advised for clinical stage I, II, and III disease (see Table 43–2). Patients with locally advanced (T3, T4) and even inflammatory tumors may be cured with multimodality therapy. When distant metastatic disease (outside the breast or regional lymph nodes) is diagnosed, palliation becomes the goal of therapy. Treatment with palliative intent is appropriate for all patients with stage IV disease and for patients with unresectable local cancers. Some patients with metastatic disease treated with immunotherapy or targeted therapy can achieve long-term remission.

A. Choice and Timing of Primary Therapy

The extent of disease and its biologic aggressiveness are the principal determinants of the outcome of primary therapy. Clinical and pathologic staging help in assessing extent of disease, but each is imprecise. Other factors such as tumor grade, hormone receptor status, *HER2* amplification, and genomic assays are of prognostic and predictive value for benefits from systemic therapy but are not as relevant in determining the type of local therapy. In contrast, the presence of a germline deleterious mutation in *BRCA1* or *BRCA2* may have implications for both local and systemic therapy options; thus, genetic testing of patients with newly diagnosed breast cancer should be considered.

Traditionally, the standard of care for stage I, stage II, and most stage III cancer has been surgical resection followed by adjuvant (postoperative) radiation or systemic therapy, or both, when indicated. Administering chemotherapy before surgery (neoadjuvant) may shrink large tumors, making some patients who require mastectomy candidates for lumpectomy. In addition, the response to neoadjuvant therapy may determine the need for additional postoperative systemic therapy, which may result in improved survival for some tumor types. It is important for patients to understand all the surgical options, including reconstructive options, prior to having surgery. Patients with large primary tumors, inflammatory cancer, or palpably enlarged lymph nodes should have staging scans performed to rule out distant metastatic disease prior to definitive surgery. In general, adjuvant systemic therapy is started when the breast has adequately healed, ideally within 4–8 weeks after surgery. While no prospective studies have defined the appropriate timing of adjuvant chemotherapy, a single-institution study of over 6800 patients suggests that *systemic therapy should be started within 60 days of surgery*, especially in women with stage II or III breast cancer, triple-negative breast cancer, or HER2-positive disease.

B. Surgical Resection

1. Breast-conserving therapy—Multiple, large, randomized studies including the Milan and NSABP trials show that disease-free and overall survival rates are similar for patients with stage I and stage II breast cancer treated with partial mastectomy (breast-conserving lumpectomy or "breast conservation") plus axillary dissection followed by radiation therapy and for those treated by modified radical mastectomy (total mastectomy plus axillary dissection).

Tumor size is a major consideration in determining the feasibility of breast conservation. The NSABP lumpectomy trial randomized patients with tumors as large as 4 cm. To achieve an acceptable cosmetic result, the patient must have a breast of sufficient size to enable excision of a 4-cm tumor without considerable deformity. Therefore, large tumor size is only a relative contraindication. Subareolar tumors, also difficult to excise without deformity, are not contraindications to breast conservation. Oncoplastic techniques combining principles of plastic and reconstructive surgery with surgical oncologic principles enable resection of large tumors with excellent cosmetic results. Clinically detectable multifocality is a relative contraindication to breast-conserving surgery, as is fixation to the chest wall or skin or involvement of the nipple or overlying skin. While multiple primary tumors in the same breast are typically treated with mastectomy, research suggests that it may be appropriate to treat multiple tumors or even recurrent tumors in the same breast with breast-conserving therapy. The patient—not the surgeon—should be the judge of what is cosmetically acceptable. A history of prior therapeutic radiation to the ipsilateral breast or chest wall (or both) is also generally a contraindication for breast conservation, although accelerated partial breast irradiation may permit a second breast irradiation.

Axillary dissection has been used to properly stage cancer and plan radiation and systemic therapy. Intraoperative lymphatic mapping identifies lymph nodes most likely to harbor metastases if present. Sentinel node biopsy is a proven alternative to axillary dissection in patients without clinical evidence of axillary lymph node metastases. If sentinel node biopsy reveals no evidence of axillary metastases, it is highly likely that the remaining lymph nodes are free of disease and axillary dissection may be omitted. An important study from the American College of Surgeons Oncology Group randomized women with sentinel node metastases to undergo completion of axillary dissection or to receive no further axillary-specific treatment after lumpectomy; no difference in 10-year survival was found. Omission of axillary dissection is acceptable for women with tumor-free sentinel nodes or those with involvement of one or two sentinel nodes who are treated with lumpectomy, whole breast irradiation, and adjuvant systemic therapy. One phase 3 study showed that omission of lymph node sampling is noninferior to sentinel node biopsy in patients with T1 tumors and negative axillary ultrasound, thus further supporting surgical de-escalation in select cases. The SOUND and INSEMA randomized trials showed that sentinel node biopsy may be omitted in postmenopausal women who have low-grade primary tumors and no ultrasonographic sign of axillary metastases; recurrence and overall survival was noninferior compared with women who had a sentinel node biopsy. These results have not yet been widely adopted; questions are being addressed about the use of adjuvant systemic therapy and radiation in women whose nodal status is unproven. *Breast-conserving surgery with sentinel node biopsy and radiation is the preferred form of treatment for patients with early-stage breast cancer.* Further surgical de-escalation is possible. ASCO guidelines state that clinicians should not recommend routine sentinel lymph node biopsy in postmenopausal patients aged ≥ 50 years who have grade 1–2, small (≤ 2 cm), hormone receptor–positive, HER2-negative breast cancer and negative findings on preoperative axillary ultrasonography who undergo breast-conserving therapy. Despite numerous randomized trials showing no survival benefit of mastectomy over breast-conserving partial mastectomy with irradiation or of axillary dissection over sentinel node biopsy, these conservative procedures still appear to be underutilized.

2. Mastectomy—Modified radical mastectomy was previously the standard therapy for early-stage breast cancer. This operation removes the entire breast, overlying skin, nipple, and areolar complex usually with underlying pectoralis fascia with the axillary lymph nodes in continuity. The major advantage of modified radical mastectomy is that radiation therapy may not be necessary, although radiation may be used when lymph nodes are involved with cancer or when the primary tumor is ≥ 5 cm. The disadvantage of mastectomy is the cosmetic and psychological impact associated with breast loss. Radical mastectomy, which removes the underlying pectoralis muscle, should be performed rarely, if at all. Axillary node dissection is not indicated for noninvasive cancers because nodal metastases are rarely present. Skin-sparing mastectomies, including those with preservation of the nipple-areolar complex, provide excellent cosmetic and oncologic results. Skin-sparing and nipple-sparing mastectomies, however, are not appropriate for all patients such as those whose tumor is in close proximity to or directly involves the skin or is directly under the nipple-areolar complex. Breast reconstruction, immediate or delayed, should be discussed with patients who choose or require mastectomy. Patients should have an interview with a reconstructive plastic surgeon to discuss options prior to making a decision regarding reconstruction. Time is well spent preoperatively in educating the patient and family about these matters.

Gentilini OD et al. Sentinel lymph node biopsy vs no axillary surgery in patients with small breast cancer and negative results on ultrasonography of axillary lymph nodes: the SOUND randomized clinical trial. JAMA Oncol. 2023;9:1557. [PMID: 37733364]

Giuliano AE et al. Effect of axillary dissection vs no axillary dissection on 10-year overall survival among women with invasive breast cancer and sentinel node metastasis: The ACOSOG Z0011 (Alliance) Randomized Clinical Trial. JAMA. 2017;318:918. [PMID: 28898379]

Park KU et al. Sentinel lymph node biopsy in early-stage breast cancer: ASCO Guideline Update. J Clin Oncol. 2025;43:1720. [PMID: 40209128]

Reimer T et al. Axillary surgery in breast cancer – primary results of the INSEMA trial. N Engl J Med. 2025;392:1051. [PMID: 39665649]

C. Radiotherapy

Radiotherapy after breast-conserving surgery has traditionally consisted of 5–7 weeks of radiation for a total dose of 50–60 Gy but has been shortened to as little as 5 days for select patients. Most radiation oncologists use a boost dose (10–14 Gy) to the cancer location, though omission of a boost may be considered in women aged > 60 years with stage I biologically low risk tumors. These shorter fractionation schedules may be reasonable for women with low-risk, early-stage breast cancer. Guidelines by the American Society of Radiation Oncology and the European Society for Radiotherapy indicate that it is appropriate to discuss accelerated partial breast radiation for women aged > 50 years with node-negative, hormone receptor–positive, small (T1) tumors with surgical margins of at least 2 mm free of disease. Moreover, in women aged > 70 years with small (< 2 cm), lymph node-negative, hormone receptor–positive cancers, radiation therapy may be avoided. Studies suggest that even younger women with favorable lesions may avoid post-lumpectomy radiation. Radiation alone may be preferable to the combination of radiation and hormone therapy in older women with low-risk breast cancer. Radiation may be avoided in women who have complete disappearance of their cancer after neoadjuvant systemic therapy. The recurrence rates after intraoperative radiation, while low, appear significantly higher than postoperative whole breast radiation therapy. However, in all these situations, a balanced discussion with a radiation oncologist is warranted to weigh the risks and benefits of each approach.

Post-mastectomy radiotherapy has traditionally been given to women with one to three involved axillary nodes; a large, randomized trial (SUPREMO), however, showed that this was unnecessary for women with these intermediate risk factors who receive adjuvant systemic therapy.

Ghannam Y et al. Radiotherapy of breast cancer: 2025 update. Cancer Radiother. 2025;29:104767. [PMID: 41270649]

Kunkler IH et al; SUPREMO Trial Investigators. Ten-year survival after postmastectomy chest-wall irradiation in breast cancer. N Engl J Med. 2025;393:1771. [PMID: 41191939]

Mamounas EP et al. Omitting regional nodal irradiation after response to neoadjuvant chemotherapy. N Engl J Med. 2025;392:2113. [PMID: 40466065]

Meattini I et al; EUROPA Trial Investigators. Single-modality endocrine therapy versus radiotherapy after breast-conserving surgery in women aged 70 years and older with luminal A-like early breast cancer (EUROPA): a preplanned interim analysis of a phase 3, non-inferiority, randomised trial. Lancet Oncol. 2025;26:37. [PMID: 39675376]

D. Systemic Therapy

The goal of systemic therapy, including hormone-modulating medications (endocrine therapy), cytotoxic chemotherapy, HER2-targeted agents (such as trastuzumab, pertuzumab, the antibody-drug conjugate trastuzumab emtansine [T-DM1], neratinib), immune checkpoint inhibition (pembrolizumab), cyclin dependent kinase (CDK) 4/6 inhibitors (abemaciclib, ribociclib), and therapies that target DNA repair in *BRCA1/2* mutation carriers (olaparib), is to kill cancer cells that have escaped the breast and axillary lymph nodes as micrometastases before they become macrometastases (ie, stage IV cancer).

1. Neoadjuvant therapy—The use of systemic therapy prior to resection of the primary tumor (neoadjuvant) is a standard option that should be considered and discussed with patients who have triple-negative or HER2-positive breast cancer. These patients are more likely to have a pathologic complete response (meaning no residual invasive cancer in the breast and sampled nodes at the time of surgery) to neoadjuvant chemotherapy than those with hormone receptor–positive, HER2-negative breast cancer. A pathologic complete response at the time of surgery, especially in hormone receptor–negative tumors, is associated with improvement in event-free and overall survival. Neoadjuvant chemotherapy also increases the chance of breast conservation by shrinking the primary tumor in women who would otherwise need mastectomy for local control. Survival after neoadjuvant chemotherapy is similar to that seen with postoperative adjuvant chemotherapy.

A. HER2-POSITIVE BREAST CANCER—In the neoadjuvant setting, two six-cycle regimens are preferred: (1) TCH, which is docetaxel (T), carboplatin (C), and trastuzumab (H), or (2) TCHP, which is TCH plus pertuzumab (P, a HER2-targeted monoclonal antibody that is synergistic in combination with trastuzumab) (NCCN Guidelines Version 5.2025 BINV-M, 4). After completing a surgical resection, patients should resume HER2-targeted therapy. If residual disease is found at surgery, the standard of care is to give 14 cycles of T-DM1 based on the KATHERINE trial that showed T-DM1 is associated with a significantly improved invasive disease-free survival and overall survival for patients who had residual disease after standard neoadjuvant treatment. In the case of pathologic complete response, trastuzumab with (ie, if node-positive) or without pertuzumab is given to complete 1 year of total therapy with consideration for the use of neratinib as extended adjuvant therapy for high-risk (lymph node–positive, hormone receptor–positive) disease. The 2025 findings of the DESTINY-Breast11 trial, which evaluated the neoadjuvant use of trastuzumab deruxtecan (T-DXd) followed by taxane, trastuzumab, and pertuzumab, might change practice with the use of this antibody-drug conjugate for neoadjuvant treatment of high-risk, early-stage HER2-positive breast cancer.

B. Hormone receptor–positive, HER2-negative breast cancer—Patients with hormone receptor–positive breast cancer have a lower chance of experiencing a pathologic complete response with neoadjuvant therapy than those patients with triple-negative or HER2-positive breast cancers. Studies indicate similar clinical response rates with neoadjuvant endocrine therapy compared to neoadjuvant chemotherapy. Typically, responses are not appreciated unless 6 or more months of therapy are given. Outside of the clinical trial setting, the use of neoadjuvant hormonal therapy is generally restricted to postmenopausal patients who are unable or unwilling to undergo chemotherapy. Preliminary evidence from two trials suggests that adding an immune checkpoint inhibitor to chemotherapy improves the pCR rate in high-grade hormone receptor–positive cancers. Long-term outcome data are awaited before this can become a standard strategy.

C. Triple-negative breast cancer—The anti–PD-1 immune checkpoint inhibitor pembrolizumab is FDA-approved for treatment of triple-negative breast cancer in the neoadjuvant setting in combination with chemotherapy (a taxane, platinum, anthracycline-based regimen), followed by adjuvant single-agent pembrolizumab to complete a year. The addition of pembrolizumab to this chemotherapy was shown to improve the event-free survival and overall survival for patients with stage II or greater triple-negative breast cancer regardless of tumor PD-L1 expression. It is not clear whether use of pembrolizumab solely in the adjuvant setting (without use in neoadjuvant setting) benefits patients and one study indicated the use of adjuvant atezolizumab, a different immune checkpoint inhibitor, did not improve outcomes for patients; thus, the use of postoperative immune therapy for patients who did not receive it prior to surgery is not recommended.

Questions remain regarding optimal adjuvant treatment of patients with residual triple-negative disease after neoadjuvant therapy. A standard option based on the CREATE-X study is to use eight cycles of adjuvant capecitabine after neoadjuvant therapy. It is not known whether adding adjuvant capecitabine to pembrolizumab benefits patients who have received neoadjuvant pembrolizumab plus chemotherapy and have residual disease at the time of definitive breast surgery. An ongoing phase 3 trial (NCT05633654) is evaluating whether adjuvant treatment with the trophoblastic cell surface antigen-2 (Trop2)-directed antibody-drug conjugate sacituzumab govitecan plus pembrolizumab improves outcomes compared with the treating physician's choice of pembrolizumab with or without capecitabine for early-stage tumor-negative breast cancer with residual disease after standard neoadjuvant therapy.

For patients with a *BRCA1* or *BRCA2* mutation and residual triple-negative breast cancer at the time of definitive breast surgery, the use of adjuvant olaparib is an option that has been shown to improve overall survival. The combination or sequencing of olaparib and pembrolizumab is untested in this setting.

D. Timing of sentinel lymph node biopsy in neoadjuvant setting—Sentinel node biopsy should be performed after neoadjuvant chemotherapy since the presence of residual disease in the breast or in the nodes is of prognostic and therapeutic importance. Large multicenter studies such as ACOSOG 1071, SENTINA, and others showed sentinel node biopsies after neoadjuvant chemotherapy have high false-negative rates. However, the use of both dye and radioisotope and removal of at least three nodes and, when possible, resection of a prior biopsied cancer-containing node can lower the false-negative rate to acceptable levels. Targeted axillary dissection involves placement of a clip in a previously biopsied cancer-containing node and then resecting that node after the receipt of neoadjuvant chemotherapy. False-negative rates on the order of ≤ 5% can be readily achieved with targeted dissection.

Mamounas EP et al. Omitting regional nodal irradiation after response to neoadjuvant chemotherapy. N Engl J Med. 2025;392:2113. [PMID: 40466065]

Schmid P et al; KEYNOTE-522 Investigators. Overall survival with pembrolizumab in early-stage triple-negative breast cancer. N Engl J Med. 2024;391:1981. [PMID: 39282906]

2. Adjuvant systemic therapy—Adjuvant (post-surgery) systemic therapy improves survival and is advocated for most patients with curable breast cancer. In practice, most medical oncologists use chemotherapy for patients with either node-positive or higher-risk (eg, hormone receptor–negative or HER2-positive) node-negative breast cancer and use endocrine therapy for all hormone receptor–positive invasive breast cancer unless contraindicated. Prognostic factors other than nodal status that determine the patient's risks of recurrence are tumor size, ER and PR status, nuclear grade, histologic type, proliferative rate (Ki-67), oncogene expression (Table 19–4), and patient's age and menopausal status. In general, systemic chemotherapy decreases the chance of recurrence by about 30%, hormonal modulation decreases the relative risk of recurrence by 40–50% (for hormone receptor–positive cancer), and HER2-targeted therapy decreases the relative risk of recurrence by ~40% (for HER2-positive cancer). Systemic chemotherapy is usually given sequentially, rather than concurrently, with radiation. Typically, chemotherapy is given before radiation while endocrine therapy is started concurrent with or after radiation therapy.

The long-term advantage of systemic therapy is well established. All patients with invasive hormone receptor–positive tumors should consider the use of hormone-modulating therapy. Almost all patients with HER2-positive tumors should receive trastuzumab-containing chemotherapy regimens. In general, adjuvant systemic chemotherapy should not be given to women who have small node-negative breast cancers with favorable histologic

Table 19–4. Prognostic factors for recurrence in node-negative breast cancer.

Prognostic Factors	Increased Recurrence	Decreased Recurrence
Size[1]	T3, T2	T1, T0
Hormone receptors (ER, PR)	Negative	Positive
Histologic grade	High	Low
S phase fraction	> 5%	< 5%
Lymphatic or vascular invasion	Present	Absent
HER2 oncogene amplification	High	Low
Epidermal growth factor receptor	High	Low
High Oncotype DX Recurrence Score or other genomic prognostic assays	High score	Low score

ER, estrogen receptor; PR, progesterone receptor.
[1]See text for description of tumor node metastasis stages.

findings and tumor biomarkers. Prognostic validated tools such as Oncotype DX and MammaPrint (see Biomarkers and Gene Expression Profiling above) enable clinicians to better select patients with HER2-negative, hormone receptor–positive, lymph node-negative tumors who can safely omit chemotherapy.

A. Chemotherapy—The Early Breast Cancer Trialists' Collaborative Group (EBCTCG) meta-analysis involving over 28,000 women enrolled in 60 trials of adjuvant polychemotherapy versus no chemotherapy demonstrated a significant benefit of chemotherapy on clinical outcome in stage I–III breast cancer. This study showed that *adjuvant chemotherapy reduces the risk of recurrence and breast cancer–specific mortality in all women and women aged < 50 years derived the greatest benefit.*

(1) Anthracycline- and cyclophosphamide-containing regimens—Studies comparing the anthracycline Adriamycin (doxorubicin) and cyclophosphamide (AC) or the anthracycline epirubicin and cyclophosphamide (EC) to cyclophosphamide-methotrexate-5-fluorouracil (CMF) have shown that treatments with anthracycline-containing regimens in the adjuvant setting are at least as effective as treatment with CMF. Given this, for HER2-negative, node-negative breast cancer, four cycles of AC or six cycles of CMF are probably equally effective. *Data do not support the routine use of anthracyclines for HER2-positive or node-negative hormone receptor–positive disease.*

(2) Taxanes—Multiple trials of taxanes (paclitaxel and docetaxel) have been conducted to evaluate their use in combination with anthracycline-based regimens. The majority of these trials showed an improvement in disease-free survival and at least one showed an improvement in overall survival with the taxane-based regimen. It is generally agreed that *taxanes should be used for most patients receiving chemotherapy for early breast cancer.*

(3) Duration, dose, and side effects of chemotherapy—The ideal duration of adjuvant chemotherapy remains uncertain. However, based on the meta-analysis performed in the Oxford Overview (EBCTCG), the recommendation is for 3–6 months of the commonly used regimens.

Chemotherapy side effects, which are discussed in Chapter 43, are generally well controlled.

B. Targeted therapy—Targeted therapy refers to agents that are directed specifically against a protein or molecule expressed uniquely on tumor cells or in the tumor microenvironment.

(1) HER2-targeted therapy—Approximately 20% of breast cancers are characterized by amplification of the *HER2* oncogene leading to overexpression of the HER2 oncoprotein ("HER2-positive"). The poor prognosis associated with HER2 overexpression has been drastically improved with the development of HER2-targeted therapy. Trastuzumab (Herceptin [H]), a monoclonal antibody that binds to HER2, is effective in combination with chemotherapy (AC-TH or TCH [docetaxel, carboplatin, trastuzumab]) in patients with HER2-overexpressing early breast cancer. Both AC-TH and TCH are FDA-approved for nonmetastatic, HER2-positive breast cancer. In these regimens, trastuzumab is given with chemotherapy and then continued beyond the course of chemotherapy with a goal, in general, to complete a full year. Studies have indicated improved safety and similar efficacy with non-anthracycline based therapy (TCH or TCHP), making them the preferred regimens based on National Comprehensive Cancer Center guidelines. Adjuvant trastuzumab with pertuzumab is primarily restricted to patients with high-risk, node-positive disease. Neratinib, an orally bioavailable dual HER1 (EGFR), HER2 tyrosine kinase inhibitor, is FDA-approved as extended adjuvant therapy (to be given after completion of 1 year of trastuzumab). The phase 3 placebo-controlled EXTENET study demonstrated that neratinib improves invasive disease-free survival when given for 1 year after completion of a year of standard adjuvant trastuzumab-based therapy (median follow-up 5.2 years, stratified HR 0.73, $P = 0.0083$). The benefit of neratinib appears to be restricted to those with tumor co-expression of hormone receptor(s). Neratinib is associated with GI toxicity (especially diarrhea).

Patients who undergo neoadjuvant trastuzumab-based chemotherapy and have residual disease remaining at the time of surgery have a poor outcome. In the phase 3 randomized KATHERINE trial, 1486 patients with residual disease after standard neoadjuvant trastuzumab/taxane therapy (18% of whom also received neoadjuvant pertuzumab) were randomized to receive the antibody-drug conjugate T-DM1 or standard trastuzumab for 14 cycles after surgery. Patients treated with T-DM1 had a statistically significantly improved 7-year invasive disease-free survival (81% versus 67%), and 34% relative reduction in risk of death (89% overall survival versus 84% at 7 years). Adjuvant T-DM1 is FDA-approved for patients with residual disease after standard trastuzumab-containing neoadjuvant therapy. The 2025 DESTINY-Breast05 study demonstrated a significant improvement in invasive disease-free survival with adjuvant T-DXd compared with T-DM1 in high-risk patients who have residual disease after standard neoadjuvant therapy. This treatment may soon become standard of care for select patients.

Retrospective studies have shown that even small (stage T1a,b) *HER2*-positive tumors have a worse prognosis compared with same-sized *HER2*-negative tumors and may thus be appropriate for trastuzumab-based regimens. The use of a de-escalated approach with trastuzumab plus weekly paclitaxel is an appropriate option for node-negative smaller HER2-positive tumors based on the phase 2 adjuvant paclitaxel and trastuzumab (APT) trial.

Cardiomyopathy develops in a small but significant percentage (0.4–4%) of patients who receive trastuzumab-based regimens. For this reason, anthracyclines, if they are being used, and trastuzumab should not be given concurrently and cardiac function is monitored periodically throughout HER2-targeted therapy.

(2) Endocrine therapy—Adjuvant hormone modulation therapy is highly effective in decreasing relative risk of recurrence by 40–50% and mortality by 25% in women with hormone receptor–positive tumors regardless of menopausal status.

(A) TAMOXIFEN—Disease-free and overall survival are significantly improved in women who received 10 years of adjuvant tamoxifen, particularly after year 10. The clinical application of long-term tamoxifen use must be discussed with patients individually, taking into consideration risks of tamoxifen (such as secondary uterine cancers, venous thromboembolic events, and side effects that impact quality of life). Ovarian suppression in addition to tamoxifen has been shown to significantly improve 12-year disease-free survival (71.9% versus 76.1%) and 12-year overall survival (86.8% versus 89.0%) compared to tamoxifen alone in the randomized Suppression of Ovarian Function Trial (SOFT) study, though the benefits appeared to be seen primarily in chemotherapy-treated patients with higher-risk disease.

(B) AROMATASE INHIBITORS FOR POSTMENOPAUSAL WOMEN—AIs, including anastrozole, letrozole, and exemestane, reduce estrogen production and are also effective in the adjuvant setting for postmenopausal women. At least seven large, randomized trials enrolling > 24,000 postmenopausal patients with hormone receptor–positive nonmetastatic breast cancer have compared the use of AIs with tamoxifen or placebo as adjuvant therapy. All these studies have shown small but statistically significant improvements in disease-free survival (absolute benefits of 2–6%) with the use of AIs. In addition, AIs reduce the risk of contralateral breast cancers and have fewer associated serious side effects (such as endometrial cancers and thromboembolic events) than tamoxifen. However, they are associated with accelerated bone loss and an increased risk of fractures as well as a musculoskeletal syndrome characterized by arthralgias or myalgias (or both) in the majority of patients. The ASCO and the NCCN have recommended that *postmenopausal women with hormone receptor–positive breast cancer be offered an AI either initially or after tamoxifen therapy.* HER2 status should not affect the use or choice of hormone therapy. In general, AIs are given for 5 years. However, extended adjuvant therapy for 7–10 years total may provide additional benefit. The use of extended adjuvant AIs is reserved for high-risk patients after a balanced discussion regarding potential risks versus benefits.

(C) AROMATASE INHIBITORS FOR PREMENOPAUSAL WOMEN—AIs should not be used in a patient with functioning (premenopausal) ovaries since they do not block ovarian production of estrogen. However, a combined analysis of the SOFT and Tamoxifen and Exemestane Trial (TEXT) studies showed that exemestane plus ovarian suppression with triptorelin was associated with a reduced risk of relapse compared to tamoxifen, making this a viable adjuvant therapy option for premenopausal women with high-risk ER-positive breast cancers.

(3) Bisphosphonates and other bone-modifying agents—Multiple randomized studies have evaluated the use of adjuvant bisphosphonates in addition to standard local and systemic therapy for early-stage breast cancer and have shown, in addition to improvement in bone density, a consistent reduction in the risk of metastatic recurrence in postmenopausal patients. Side effects associated with bisphosphonate therapy include bone pain, fever, osteonecrosis of the jaw, esophagitis or ulcers (for oral bisphosphonates), and kidney injury. The jointly published guidelines of the Cancer Care Ontario and ASCO recommend that bisphosphonate use (zoledronic acid or clodronate) be considered as adjuvant therapy for postmenopausal breast cancer patients. Denosumab, an antibody directed against receptor activator of nuclear factor κ B ligand (RANK-L) that blocks osteoclastic activity, may reduce the risk of breast cancer recurrence, though evidence is conflicting, and it is not recommended as a breast cancer risk-reducing strategy.

(4) Cyclin dependent kinase 4/6 inhibitors—Hormonally driven breast cancer may be particularly sensitive to inhibition of cell cycle regulatory proteins, called CDK4/6. Three oral CDK4/6 inhibitors, palbociclib, abemaciclib, and ribociclib, are FDA-approved for treatment of hormone receptor–positive, HER2-negative metastatic breast cancer.

Trials evaluating the use of adjuvant palbociclib (PENELOPE-B and PALLAS) in high-risk curable breast cancer failed to demonstrate improved outcomes for patients. Abemaciclib and ribociclib, however, did show significant benefits and are both FDA-approved. Adjuvant abemaciclib for 2 years significantly improved the 7-year invasive disease-free survival rate by 6.5% and the overall survival rate by 1.8% (hazard ratio, 0.842) for those with high-risk, node-positive, HR-positive/HER2-negative disease. In the NATALEE trial, the addition of ribociclib for 3 years to adjuvant aromatase inhibitor therapy also significantly improved the 4-year invasive disease-free survival rate from 83.6% to 88.5% for patients with stage IIA or greater breast cancer; overall survival from this trial is still immature but is trending toward an improvement.

(5) PARP inhibitors—*BRCA*-mutation–associated cancers are deficient in double-strand DNA repair mechanisms and become reliant on an alternative enzyme, poly (adenosine diphosphate-ribose) polymerase (PARP), for DNA repair and survival. Thus, targeting PARP selectively kills breast cancer cells in patients who carry a germline mutation in *BRCA1* or *BRCA2*. Two PARP inhibitors (olaparib and talazoparib) are FDA-approved for the

treatment of *BRCA*-associated metastatic breast cancer. In the curative setting, olaparib has been shown to reduce the relative risk of an invasive recurrency for *BRCA1/2* carriers with high-risk disease by just over 40% and significantly improves overall survival. The NCCN guidelines include adjuvant olaparib for select patients and recommend germline genetic testing for any patient who may be a candidate for adjuvant olaparib.

While olaparib should be given in combination with standard adjuvant endocrine therapy for hormone receptor–positive disease, the use of olaparib in combination with a CDK4/6 inhibitor has not been studied and is not recommended given the potential side effects. Thus, if a patient is a candidate for both agents, decisions regarding which agent to use must be made on a case-by-case basis in discussion with the patient. The use of olaparib has also not been studied in combination with capecitabine (see CREATE-X trial); thus, there are no data to guide selection between these agents in triple-negative *BRCA*-mutation–associated breast cancer with residual disease after neoadjuvant chemotherapy.

c. Adjuvant therapy in older women—Data relating to the optimal use of adjuvant systemic treatment for women aged > 65 years are limited. Results from the EBCTCG overview indicate that while adjuvant chemotherapy yields a smaller benefit for older women compared with younger women, it still improves clinical outcomes. Moreover, individual studies show that older women with higher-risk disease derive benefits from chemotherapy. The benefits of endocrine therapy for hormone receptor–positive disease appear to be independent of age. In general, decisions relating to the use of systemic therapy should consider a patient's comorbidities and physiological age, more so than chronologic age.

Brunner C et al. Incidence of medication-related osteonecrosis of the jaw in patients with breast cancer during a 20-year follow up: a population-based multicenter retrospective study. J Clin Oncol. 2025;43:180. [PMID: 39163561]

Early Breast Cancer Trialists' Collaborative Group (EBCTCG). Anthracycline-containing and taxane-containing chemotherapy for early-stage operable breast cancer: a patient-level meta-analysis of 100 000 women from 86 randomised trials. Lancet. 2023;401:1277. [PMID: 37061269]

Fasching PA et al. Ribociclib plus endocrine therapy in hormone receptor-positive/ERBB2-negative early breast cancer: 4-year outcomes form the NATALEE randomized clinical trial. JAMA Oncol. 2025;11:1364. [PMID: 40996773]

Francis PA et al. Adjuvant endocrine therapy in premenopausal breast cancer: 12-year results from SOFT. J Clin Oncol. 2023;41:1370. [PMID: 36493334]

Geyer CE et al; KATHERINE Study Group. Survival with trastuzumab emtansine in residual HER2-positive breast cancer. N Engl J Med. 2025;392:249. [PMID: 39813643]

Johnson S et al. Overall survival with abemaciclib in early breast cancer. Ann Oncol. 2026;37:155. [PMID: 41110697]

Loibl S et al; DESTINY-Breast05 Trial Investigators. Trastuzumab deruxtecan in residual HER2-positive early breast cancer. N Engl J Med. 2026;394:845. [PMID: 41370739]

Slamon D et al. Ribociclib plus endocrine therapy in early breast cancer. N Engl J Med. 2024;390:1080. [PMID: 38507751]

Palliative Treatment

Palliative treatments are aimed to manage symptoms, improve quality of life, and even prolong survival, without the expectation of achieving cure. Even when cure of the disease is not expected, palliative treatments are appropriate for breast cancer metastatic to distant sites. In the United States, it is uncommon to have distant metastases at the time of diagnosis (de novo metastases). However, most patients who have a breast cancer recurrence after initial local and adjuvant therapy have metastatic rather than local (in breast) disease. Breast cancer most commonly metastasizes to the liver, lungs, and bone, causing symptoms such as fatigue, change in appetite, abdominal pain, cough, dyspnea, or bone pain. Headaches, imbalance, vision changes, vertigo, and other neurologic symptoms may be signs of brain metastases. Triple-negative (ER-, PR-, HER2-negative) and HER2-positive tumors have a higher rate of brain metastases than hormone receptor–positive, HER2-negative tumors.

A. Radiotherapy and Bisphosphonates

Palliative radiotherapy may be advised for primary treatment of locally advanced cancers with distant metastases to control ulceration, pain, and other manifestations in the breast and regional nodes. Irradiation of the breast and chest wall and the axillary, internal mammary, and supraclavicular nodes should be undertaken in an attempt to cure locally advanced and inoperable lesions when there is no evidence of distant metastases. A small number of patients in this group are cured despite extensive breast and regional node involvement.

Palliative irradiation is of value also in the treatment of bone or soft tissue metastases to control pain or avoid fracture. Radiotherapy is especially useful in the treatment of isolated bony metastases, chest wall recurrences, and brain metastases and, sometimes, in lieu of the preferred option of orthopedic surgery for acute spinal cord compression.

In addition to radiotherapy, bisphosphonate therapy has shown excellent results in delaying and reducing skeletal events in women with bony metastases. Pamidronate and zoledronic acid are FDA-approved intravenous bisphosphonates for bone metastases or hypercalcemia of malignancy from breast cancer. Denosumab is also FDA-approved for the treatment of bone metastases from breast cancer.

Caution should be exercised when combining radiation therapy with chemotherapy because toxicity of either or both may be augmented by their concurrent administration. In general, *only one type of therapy should be given at a time* unless it is necessary to irradiate a destructive lesion of weight-bearing bone while the patient is receiving chemotherapy. Systemic therapy should be changed only if the disease is clearly progressing or if intolerable side effects have developed. This is especially difficult to determine for patients with destructive bone metastases, since changes in the status of these lesions are difficult to determine radiographically.

B. Targeted Therapy for Metastatic Disease

1. Hormonally based therapy for metastatic disease— The following therapies have all been shown to be effective in hormone receptor–positive metastatic breast cancer:

medications that block ERs (such as tamoxifen) or downregulate ERs (such as fulvestrant, elacestrant, and imlunestrant) or medications that block the synthesis of hormones (such as AIs); ablation of the ovaries, adrenal, or pituitary glands; and hormones (eg, estrogens, androgens, progestins); see Table 19–5. Because only 5–10% of women with ER-negative tumors respond, they should not receive endocrine therapy. Women within 1 year of their last menstrual period are arbitrarily considered to be premenopausal and should have surgical (bilateral oophorectomy) or chemical ovarian ablation (using a gonadotropin-releasing hormone [GnRH] analog such as leuprolide [Lupron], goserelin [Zoladex], or triptorelin). Premenopausal women who have had chemical or surgical ovarian ablation are then eligible to receive the same hormonally targeted therapies that are available to postmenopausal women. Guidelines indicate that sequential hormonal therapy (Table 19–5) is the preferred treatment for hormone receptor–positive metastatic breast cancer except in the rare case when disease is immediately threatening visceral organs.

A. First-line treatment options—

(1) Hormonally targeted agents—Single-agent hormonally targeted therapy options include the selective estrogen receptor degrader (SERD) fulvestrant, tamoxifen, or an AI (anastrozole, letrozole, or exemestane) (Table 19–5). The side effect profile of AIs differs from tamoxifen. The main side effects of tamoxifen are nausea, skin rash, and hot flushes. Rarely, tamoxifen induces hypercalcemia in patients with bony metastases. Tamoxifen also increases the risk of venous thromboembolic events and uterine hyperplasia and cancer. The main side effects of AIs include hot flushes, vaginal dryness, and joint stiffness; however, osteoporosis and bone fractures are significantly higher than with tamoxifen. Fulvestrant is associated with slightly improved progression-free survival compared to an AI, but it requires a monthly intramuscular injection.

(2) Hormonally targeted therapy plus cyclin dependent kinase inhibition—**Clinical trials support the use of a CDK4/6 inhibitor plus an AI as the gold standard treatment in the first-line setting of hormone receptor–positive metastatic breast cancer.**

Hormonally driven breast cancer is particularly sensitive to inhibition of the cell cycle regulatory proteins CDK4/6. Studies of three CDK4/6 inhibitors (palbociclib, ribociclib, and abemaciclib) combined with an endocrine agent (AI or fulvestrant) all demonstrated a median progression-free survival of > 2 years; the longest median progression-free survival (length of time after starting treatment when the cancer does not worsen) reported in metastatic ER-positive breast cancer to date. Importantly, these therapies yield objective response rates as good as or better than that seen with chemotherapy. All three CDK4/6 inhibitors are FDA-approved in the first-line setting in combination with endocrine therapy. Thus far, ribociclib is the only CDK4/6 inhibitor to report an overall survival benefit (in MONALEESA-2, MONALEESA-3, and MONALEESA-7) when added to endocrine therapy in patients who previously have not received endocrine

Table 19–5. Hormonally targeted agents commonly used for management of metastatic breast cancer (listed in alphabetical order).

Medications	Action	Dose, Route, Frequency	Major Side Effects
Anastrozole (Arimidex)	AI	1 mg orally daily	Hot flushes, skin rashes, nausea and vomiting, bone loss
Elacestrant (Orserdu)	Estrogen receptor antagonist	345 mg orally daily	Hypercholesterolemia and hypertriglyceridemia Fetal harm if given during pregnancy
Exemestane (Aromasin)	AI	25 mg orally daily	Hot flushes, increased arthralgia/arthritis, myalgia, bone loss
Fulvestrant (Faslodex)	Steroidal estrogen receptor antagonist	500 mg intramuscularly days 1, 15, 29 and then monthly	GI upset, headache, back pain, hot flushes, pharyngitis, injection site pain
Goserelin (Zoladex)	Synthetic LH-releasing analog	3.6 mg subcutaneously monthly	Arthralgias, blood pressure changes, hot flushes, headaches, vaginal dryness, bone loss
Letrozole (Femara)	AI	2.5 mg orally daily	Hot flushes, arthralgia/arthritis, myalgia, bone loss
Leuprolide (Lupron)	Synthetic LH-releasing analog	3.75 or 7.5 mg subcutaneously monthly	Arthralgias, blood pressure changes, hot flushes, headaches, vaginal dryness, bone loss
Megestrol acetate (Megace)	Progestin	40 mg orally four times daily	Fluid retention, venous thromboembolic events; rarely used except in late-stage, treatment-refractory disease
Tamoxifen citrate (Nolvadex)	SERM	20 mg orally daily	Hot flushes, uterine bleeding, thrombophlebitis, rash
Toremifene citrate (Fareston)	SERM	60 mg orally daily	Hot flushes, sweating, nausea, vaginal discharge, dry eyes, dizziness

AI, aromatase inhibitor; SERM, selective estrogen receptor modulator.

therapy for metastatic disease (first-line setting). In general, CDK4/6 inhibitors are well tolerated, though monitoring patients for neutropenia (especially with ribociclib and palbociclib) and management of diarrhea (especially with abemaciclib) are necessary. Febrile neutropenia and infections are rare, and use of growth factors is not required; however, palbociclib and ribociclib are given for 3 consecutive weeks, stopping for 1 week to allow white cell count to recover. Abemaciclib is given twice daily continuously (28-day cycles). A phase 3 trial (SONIA), which randomized patients to receive a CDK4/6 inhibitor in the first- or second-line setting, demonstrated no difference in the time to second progression event. Thus, in select patients, it may be appropriate to start with single-agent endocrine therapy and defer use of the CDK4/6 inhibitor to the second-line setting.

B. Treatment options when disease progresses after hormonal-based therapy—

(1) Fulvestrant plus CDK4/6 inhibitor—**The combination of fulvestrant with palbociclib, ribociclib, or abemaciclib is FDA-approved for treatment of disease that has progressed on prior endocrine therapy and is the gold standard second-line regimen for patients who have not received a CDK4/6 inhibitor in the first-line setting.**

In clinical trials in patients whose disease has progressed on prior endocrine therapy, palbociclib, ribociclib, and abemaciclib have all shown a significant improvement in median progression-free survival (PALOMA-3, MONALEESA-3, MONARCH-2, respectively); ribociclib and abemaciclib have also shown a significant improvement in overall survival when added to fulvestrant. Abemaciclib is also FDA-approved as a single agent (200 mg orally twice daily) for patients with advanced ER-positive breast cancer who have received prior endocrine therapy and chemotherapy.

(2) Secondary or tertiary single-agent hormonal therapy—Patients who have disease progression following first-line endocrine-based therapy may be offered a different form of endocrine therapy. In the pivotal phase 3 EMERALD trial, the oral SERD elacestrant (Orserdu) was associated with a significantly improved progression-free survival compared with standard single-agent endocrine therapy (fulvestrant or an AI) for metastatic breast cancer after disease progression on a CDK4/6 inhibitor. Elacestrant is the first oral SERD that is FDA-approved for the treatment of breast cancer. Subsequently, another oral SERD, imlunestrant, received regulatory approval based on the phase 3 EMBER-3 trial, which showed improved progression-free survival compared with standard endocrine therapy. Because both elacestrant and imlunestrant demonstrated greater benefit in patients with tumor mutations in the gene for estrogen receptor (*ESR1*), their regulatory approvals are restricted to patients with a tumor *ESR1* mutation.

(3) Phosphatidylinositol-3-kinase (PI3K) pathway inhibitors plus endocrine therapy

Everolimus plus endocrine therapy—Everolimus (Afinitor) is an oral inhibitor of the mammalian target of rapamycin (MTOR)—a protein in the PI3K pathway whose activation has been associated with the development of endocrine resistance. The BOLERO-2 trial evaluated the AI exemestane with or without everolimus in 724 patients with AI-resistant, hormone receptor–positive metastatic breast cancer and found that patients treated with everolimus had a significantly improved progression-free survival but no significant difference in overall survival. The main side effect of everolimus is stomatitis (mouth sores). This can be avoided, almost completely, by the prophylactic use of oral steroid mouthwash starting with cycle 1. The phase 3 evERA trial evaluated the combination of everolimus with either an oral SERD, giredestrant, or standard-of-care endocrine therapy in patients with disease progression on CDK4/6 inhibitor therapy; a significant improvement in progression-free survival has been reported in the giredestrant arm.

Gedatolisib plus endocrine therapy with or without palbociclib—Gedatolisib is an IV-delivered inhibitor of PI3K and mTOR. The VIKTORIA-1 trial evaluated the combination of giredestrant plus fulvestrant, with or without palbociclib, compared with single-agent fulvestrant in patients who had received a prior CDK4/6 inhibitor and did not have a mutation in the gene encoding PI3K, *PIK3CA*. The progression-free survival was improved with both the triplet and doublet compared with fulvestrant alone.

PI3K pathway inhibitors plus endocrine therapy for PI3K pathway-altered breast cancer—Approximately 40% of hormone receptor–positive breast cancers have activation of the PI3K-AKT-mTOR pathway, most commonly due to an activating mutation of PI3K on the *PIK3CA* gene. Alpelisib is an oral α-isoform selective inhibitor of PI3K that is FDA-approved for *PIK3CA*-mutated hormone receptor–positive breast cancer. Side effects include hyperglycemia, diarrhea, rash, and transaminitis. The oral AKT inhibitor capivasertib is also approved for patients with hormone receptor–positive metastatic breast cancer and a tumor *PIK3CA*, *AKT1*, or *PTEN* alteration. Inavolisib, a selective inhibitor of the α isoform of the p110 subunit of PI3K, was shown to improve progression-free and overall survival when combined with fulvestrant and palbociclib in patients with *PIK3CA*-mutated breast cancer that relapsed during or within 12 months of completion of adjuvant hormonally targeted therapy. All three FDA-approved therapies are associated with significant side effects, thus careful patient selection and monitoring are indicated. There is no evidence that these agents can be used sequentially.

Bardia A et al. Elacestrant in ER+, HER2– metastatic breast cancer with ESR1-mutated tumors: subgroup analyses from the phase III EMERALD trial by prior duration of endocrine therapy plus CDK4/6 inhibitor and in clinical subgroups. Clin Cancer Res. 2024;30:4299. [PMID: 39087959]

Hurvitz SA et al. Gedatolisib (geda) + fulvestrant ± palbociclib (palbo) vs fulvestrant in patients with HR+/HER2-/PIK3CA wild-type (WT) advanced breast cancer (ABC): first results from VIKTORIA-1. Ann Oncol. 2025;36:S1562.

Jhaveri KL et al; EMBER-3 Study Group. Imlunestrant with or without abemaciclib in advanced breast cancer. N Engl J Med. 2025;392:1189. [PMID: 39660834]

Jhaveri KL et al. Overall survival with inavolisib in *PIK3CA*-mutated advanced breast cancer. N Engl J Med. 2025;393:151. [PMID: 40454641]

Mayer EL et al. Giredestrant (GIRE), an oral selective oestrogen receptor (ER) antagonist and degrader, + everolimus (E) in patients with ER-positive, HER2-negative advanced breast cancer (ER+, HER2–, aBC) previously treated with a CDK4/6 inhibitor (i): primary results of the phase III evERA BC trial. Ann Oncol. 2025;36(suppl_2):S1.

Sonke GS et al; SONIA Study Consortium. Early versus deferred use of CDK4/6 inhibitors in advanced breast cancer. Nature. 2024;636:474. [PMID: 39604725]

2. HER2-targeted agents—

A. Monoclonal antibodies—Trastuzumab, a monoclonal antibody, targets HER2. FDA-approved for metastatic HER2-positive disease, trastuzumab plus chemotherapy significantly improves clinical outcomes, including survival, compared to chemotherapy alone. Pertuzumab is also an FDA-approved monoclonal antibody that targets the extracellular domain of HER2 at a different epitope than targeted by trastuzumab. It acts synergistically when combined with trastuzumab. Margetuximab is another antibody that is similar to trastuzumab but designed to improve the antibody-dependent cellular cytotoxicity mechanism of action.

B. Antibody drug conjugates—T-DM1 is an FDA-approved antibody-drug conjugate in which trastuzumab is stably linked to a chemotherapy (derivative of maytansine), enabling targeted delivery of the cytotoxic chemotherapy to HER2-overexpressing cells. T-DM1 had been the second-line gold standard for HER2-positive metastatic breast cancer but has been replaced by another antibody-drug conjugate.

C. Tyrosine kinase inhibitors—In addition to pertuzumab, trastuzumab, margetuximab, T-DM1, and trastuzumab deruxtecan, three other HER2-targeted therapies that target the intracellular portion of HER2 are FDA-approved for patients who have received two or more prior lines of therapy for advanced-stage disease. One of these is tucatinib, a HER2-selective oral tyrosine kinase inhibitor that penetrates the blood-brain barrier. A large, randomized trial (HER2CLIMB) compared capecitabine plus trastuzumab plus either tucatinib or placebo in patients with pretreated, HER2-positive advanced disease and demonstrated an improved progression-free survival in the overall population, improved progression-free survival in those with CNS metastases, and importantly, a significantly improved overall survival. Other agents are neratinib (in combination with capecitabine) and lapatinib (in combination with capecitabine or trastuzumab).

D. Sequencing of therapies for HER2-positive disease—There are eight FDA-approved HER2-directed therapies for metastatic HER2-positive breast cancer. Advances in systemic therapy have led to substantial improvements in long-term outcomes, and many patients now receive multiple sequential lines of therapy, with median overall survival likely exceeding 5 years. From 2012 through 2025, the standard first-line regimen was pertuzumab, trastuzumab, and docetaxel (THP) based on the CLEOPATRA trial. Patients typically receive 4–8 cycles of THP, after which the taxane is discontinued and maintenance therapy with trastuzumab and pertuzumab (HP) is continued until disease progression. For patients with hormone receptor–positive disease, endocrine therapy may be added during the maintenance phase. In 2025, trastuzumab deruxtecan, in combination with pertuzumab, was FDA-approved as a first-line HER2-directed therapy based on the DESTINY-Breast09 trial, in which T-DXd/pertuzumab significantly improved progression-free survival compared with THP (40.7 versus 26.9 months; hazard ratio, 0.56). An overall survival benefit has not yet been reached, and unlike THP, the chemotherapy component of this regimen is continued until disease progression, which may have important quality-of-life implications. Thus, selection of first-line therapy requires careful, individualized consideration of efficacy, toxicity profile, hormone receptor status, treatment duration, patient preferences, and long-term quality of life.

Hurvitz SA et al. Trastuzumab deruxtecan versus trastuzumab emtansine in patients with HER2-positive metastatic breast cancer: updated results from DESTINY-Breast03, a randomised, open-label, phase 3 trial. Lancet. 2023;401:105. [PMID: 36495879]

Tolaney SM et al; DESTINY-Breast09 Trial Investigators. Trastuzumab deruxtecan plus pertuzumab for HER2-positive metastatic breast cancer. N Engl J Med. 2026;394:551. [PMID: 41160818]

3. Targeting triple-negative breast cancer with immune checkpoint inhibition—PD-L1 is a protein on cancer cell surfaces (as well as other cells) that couples with T cells. This coupling, or immune checkpoint, protects the cancer cells from being destroyed by T cells. Checkpoint inhibitor drugs prevent the PD-1/PD-L1 coupling from taking place, thus allowing the T cells to attack the tumor. A PD-1-targeted immune checkpoint inhibitor, pembrolizumab, is FDA-approved for patients with PD-L1-positive disease in combination with chemotherapy (taxane or gemcitabine/carboplatin) based on results from the KEYNOTE 355 trial.

Cortes J et al; KEYNOTE-355 Investigators. Pembrolizumab plus chemotherapy in advanced triple-negative breast cancer. N Engl J Med. 2022;387:217. [PMID: 35857659]

4. Targeting Trop-2 in triple-negative and hormone receptor–positive breast cancer—Sacituzumab govitecan is an FDA-approved antibody-drug conjugate that delivers SN-38 (active metabolite of the chemotherapy irinotecan) to cells expressing Trop-2, which is ubiquitously expressed in breast cancer. The phase 3 ASCENT trial demonstrated that sacituzumab govitecan (TRODELVY) is associated with a statistically significant improvement in progression-free and overall survival when compared to single-agent chemotherapy in patients with triple-negative breast cancer who had received at least two prior lines of standard chemotherapy for metastatic disease, making this the first antibody-drug conjugate approved for triple-negative breast cancer. The ASCENT-03 study showed that sacituzumab govitecan is beneficial as first-line treatment. Sacituzumab is also approved for hormone receptor–positive disease based on the results of TROPiCS-02 in which it was associated with improved progression-free and overall survival compared with chemotherapy in patients who had received two to four prior lines of chemotherapy for metastatic disease. Another Trop-2 directed antibody-drug conjugate, datopotamab deruxtecan, demonstrated significant benefits compared with chemotherapy in two phase 3 clinical trials for hormone receptor–positive breast cancer (TROPION-Breast01) and triple-negative breast cancer (TROPION Breast02). Datopotamab deruxtecan is FDA-approved for hormone receptor–positive metastatic breast cancer, but approval for triple-negative disease is pending.

Bardia A et al; TROPION-Breast01 Investigators. Datopotamab deruxtecan versus chemotherapy in previously treated inoperable/metastatic hormone receptor-positive human epidermal growth factor receptor 2-negative breast cancer: primary results from the TROPION-Breast01. J Clin Oncol. 2025;43:285. [PMID: 39265124]

Cortés J et al; ASCENT-03 Clinical Trial Investigators. Sacituzumab govitecan in untreated, advanced triple-negative breast cancer. N Engl J Med. 2025;393:1912. [PMID: 41124233]

5. Targeting PARP in BRCA1/2 mutation–associated breast cancer—Poly (adenosine diphosphate-ribose) polymerase (PARP) is an enzyme important in single-strand DNA repair. Patients who carry germline mutations in *BRCA1* or *BRCA2* have tumors with deficient double-strand DNA repair mechanisms; inhibiting PARP might selectively kill *BRCA1/2*-mutated cancers. A phase 3 clinical trial (OlympiAD) that compared olaparib (an oral PARP inhibitor) to treatment of physician's choice (single-agent chemotherapy) demonstrated a significantly improved progression-free survival (7.0 months versus 4.2 months), an improved response rate, and a lower rate of adverse events than standard therapy. Talazoparib, a second PARP inhibitor, has also been shown to improve outcomes similarly in the phase 3 EMBRACA study. Both olaparib and talazoparib are FDA-approved for *BRCA*-mutated metastatic breast cancer as single agents.

6. Targeting HER2 in HER2-low expressing breast cancer— Although the minority of breast cancer (~15–20%) has overexpression or amplification of HER2 ("HER2-positive" disease), the majority of breast cancer (approximately two-thirds of hormone receptor–positive breast cancer and a third of triple-negative disease) expresses low levels of the HER2 protein. Although "HER2-low" breast cancer is not associated with a different disease biology per se, this level of HER2 expression is used to target T-DXd to the cancer cells. A practice-changing phase 3 trial comparing T-DXd to single-agent chemotherapy (DESTINY-Breast04) demonstrated a significantly improved progression-free and overall survival with T-DXd in patients whose metastatic disease had progressed after standard chemotherapy (and endocrine therapy, if hormone receptor–positive).

Bardia A et al; DESTINY-Breast06 Trial Investigators. Trastuzumab deruxtecan after endocrine therapy in metastatic breast cancer. N Engl J Med. 2024;391:2110. [PMID: 39282896]

C. Palliative Chemotherapy

Cytotoxic medications should be considered for the treatment of metastatic breast cancer if (1) hormonally targeted treatment is unsuccessful or the disease has progressed after an initial response to hormonal manipulation (for hormone receptor–positive breast cancer), or (2) the tumor is ER-negative or HER2-positive. For hormone receptor–positive breast cancer, phase 3 studies (RIGHT Choice and PADMA) have indicated that the use of first-line CDK4/6 inhibitor plus endocrine therapy should be administered prior to chemotherapy even in the presence of life- or organ-threatening visceral metastases. Prior adjuvant chemotherapy does not seem to alter response rates in patients who relapse. A number of chemotherapy medications (including vinorelbine, paclitaxel, docetaxel, gemcitabine, ixabepilone, carboplatin, cisplatin, capecitabine, albumin-bound paclitaxel, eribulin, and liposomal doxorubicin) may be used as single agents with first-line objective response rates ranging from 30% to 50%.

Combination chemotherapy yields statistically significantly higher response rates and progression-free survival rates compared with sequential single-agent therapy but has not been conclusively shown to improve overall survival rates. Combinations with proven efficacy compared with single-agent therapy include capecitabine (Table 43–4)/docetaxel (Table 43–5), gemcitabine (Table 43–4)/paclitaxel (Table 43–5), and capecitabine (Table 43–4)/ixabepilone. It is generally appropriate to treat willing patients with multiple sequential lines of therapy as long as they tolerate the treatment and their performance status is good (eg, at least ambulatory and able to care for self, up out of bed > 50% of waking hours).

National Comprehensive Cancer Network. NCCN Guidelines: Breast Cancer. https://www.nccn.org/guidelines/guidelines-detail?category=1&id=1419

Prognosis

Stage of breast cancer is the most reliable indicator of prognosis (Table 19–6). Axillary lymph node status is the best-analyzed prognostic factor and correlates with survival at all tumor sizes. When cancer is localized to the breast with no evidence of regional spread after pathologic examination, the clinical cure rate with most accepted methods of therapy is 75% to > 90%. In fact, patients with small mammographically detected, biologically favorable tumors and no evidence of axillary spread have a 5-year survival rate > 95%. When the axillary lymph nodes are involved with tumor, the survival rate drops to 50–70% at 5 years and probably around 25–40% at 10 years. The use of biologic markers, such as ER, PR, grade, and HER2, helps identify high-risk tumor types as well as direct treatment used (see Biomarkers & Gene Expression Profiling). Gene analysis can predict disease-free survival for some subsets of patients. The eighth edition of the AJCC Staging Manual has incorporated these factors into staging, resulting in incorporation of biologic factors to predict outcome.

Five-year statistics do not accurately reflect the final outcome of therapy. The mortality rate of breast cancer

Table 19–6. Approximate survival of patients with breast cancer by TNM stage.[1]

TNM Stage	5 Years	10 Years
0	95%	90%
I	85%	70%
IIA	70%	50%
IIB	60%	40%
IIIA	55%	30%
IIIB	30%	20%
IV	5–10%	2%
All	65%	30%

TNM, tumor, node, metastasis.
[1]See text for description of TNM stages.

patients exceeds that of age-matched normal controls for nearly 20 years. Thereafter, the mortality rates are equal, though deaths that occur among breast cancer patients are often directly the result of tumor.

In general, breast cancer appears to be somewhat more aggressive and associated with worse outcomes in younger than in older women, and this may be related to the fact that fewer younger women have ER-positive tumors. Disparities in treatment outcome for different racial and ethnic backgrounds have been reported by several studies. These differences appear to be not only due to different socioeconomic factors (and a resulting difference in access to health care) but also due to differences in the subtype of breast cancer diagnosed.

For those patients whose disease progresses despite treatment, some studies suggest supportive group therapy may improve survival. Especially as they approach the end of life, such patients will require meticulous palliative care (see Chapter 5).

Ellington TD et al. Trends in breast cancer mortality by race/ethnicity, age, and US census region, United States—1999-2020. Cancer. 2023;129:32. [PMID: 36309838]

Gao L et al. Searching for the "Holy Grail" of breast cancer recurrence risk: a narrative review of the hunt for a better biomarker and the promise of circulating tumor DNA (ctDNA). Breast Cancer Res Treat. 2024;205:211. [PMID: 38355821]

Venetis K et al. The evolving role of genomic testing in early breast cancer: implications for diagnosis, prognosis, and therapy. Int J Mol Sci. 2024;25:5717. [PMID: 38891906]

Follow-Up Care

After primary therapy, patients with breast cancer should be monitored long term in order to detect recurrences and to observe the opposite breast for a second primary carcinoma. Local and distant recurrences occur most frequently within the first 2–5 years, especially for hormone receptor–negative tumors. During the first 2 years, most patients should be examined every 6 months, then annually thereafter. Special attention is paid to the contralateral breast because a new primary breast malignancy will develop in 20–25% of patients. In some cases, especially in hormone receptor–positive breast cancer, metastases are dormant for long periods and may appear 20 years or longer after removal of the primary tumor. Although studies have failed to show an adverse effect of hormonal replacement in disease-free patients, it is rarely used after breast cancer treatment, particularly if the tumor was hormone receptor–positive. Even pregnancy has not been associated with shortened survival of patients rendered disease free—yet many oncologists are reluctant to advise a young patient with breast cancer that it is safe to become pregnant. The use of estrogen replacement for conditions such as osteoporosis, vaginal dryness, and hot flushes may be considered for a woman with a history of breast cancer after discussion of the benefits and risks; however, it is not routinely recommended, especially given the availability of nonhormonal agents for these conditions (such as bisphosphonates and denosumab for osteoporosis).

A. Local Recurrence

The incidence of local recurrence correlates with tumor size, the presence and number of involved axillary nodes, the histologic type of tumor, the presence of skin edema or skin and fascia fixation with the primary tumor, and the type of definitive surgery and local irradiation. Local recurrence on the chest wall after total mastectomy and axillary dissection develops in as many as 8% of patients. When the axillary nodes are not involved, the local recurrence rate is < 5%, but the rate is as high as 25% when they are heavily involved. A similar difference in local recurrence rate is noted between small and large tumors. Factors such as multifocal cancer, in situ tumors, lymphovascular invasion, positive resection margins, chemotherapy, and radiotherapy impact local recurrence in patients treated with breast-conserving surgery. Systemic therapy greatly decreases the rate of local recurrence.

Chest wall recurrences usually appear within the first several years but may occur as late as 15 or more years after mastectomy. All suspicious nodules and skin lesions should be biopsied. Local excision or localized radiotherapy may be feasible if an isolated nodule is present. If lesions are multiple or accompanied by evidence of regional involvement in the internal mammary or supraclavicular nodes, the disease is best managed by radiation to the entire chest wall including the parasternal, supraclavicular, and axillary areas as well as systemic therapy.

Local recurrence after mastectomy usually signals widespread disease and is an indication for tests to search for metastases. When there is no evidence of metastases beyond the chest wall and regional nodes, irradiation for cure after complete local excision should be attempted. After partial mastectomy, local recurrence does not have as serious a prognostic significance as after mastectomy. However, those patients in whom a recurrence develops have a worse prognosis than those who do not. Completion of the mastectomy should be done for local recurrence after partial mastectomy; some of these patients will survive for prolonged periods, especially if the breast recurrence is DCIS or occurs > 5 years after initial treatment. Systemic treatment should be used for women in whom disseminated disease develops or those in whom local recurrence occurs. In rare cases, re-irradiation with accelerated partial breast techniques may be effective.

Horan J et al. Assessing mode of recurrence in breast cancer to identify an optimised follow-up pathway: 10-year institutional review. Ann Surg Oncol. 2023;30:6117. [PMID: 37479843]

B. Breast Cancer Survivorship Issues

Given that most women with nonmetastatic breast cancer will be cured, a significant number of women face survivorship issues stemming from either the diagnosis or the treatment of the breast cancer, or both. These challenges include psychological struggles, cognitive dysfunction (also called "chemo brain"), upper extremity lymphedema, weight management problems, cardiovascular issues, bone loss, postmenopausal side effects, and fatigue. One randomized study reported that survivors who received psychological intervention from the time of diagnosis had a lower risk of recurrence and breast cancer-related mortality. A randomized study in older, overweight cancer survivors showed that diet and exercise reduced the rate of self-reported functional decline compared with no intervention.

Cardoso F et al. Elinzanetant for vasomotor symptoms from endocrine therapy for breast cancer. N Engl J Med. 2025;393:753. [PMID: 40454634]

1. Edema of the arm—Significant edema of the arm occurs in about 10–30% of patients after axillary dissection with or without mastectomy. It occurs more commonly in obese women, in women who had radiotherapy, and in women who had postoperative infection. Partial mastectomy with radiation to the axillary lymph nodes is followed by chronic edema of the arm in 10–20% of patients. Sentinel lymph node dissection has proved to be an accurate form of axillary staging without the side effects of edema or infection. Judicious use of radiotherapy, with treatment fields carefully planned to spare the axilla as much as possible, can greatly diminish the incidence of edema, which will occur in only 5% of patients if no radiotherapy is given to the axilla after a partial mastectomy and lymph node dissection.

Late or secondary edema of the arm may develop years after treatment as a result of axillary recurrence or infection in the hand or arm, with obliteration of lymphatic channels. When edema develops, a careful examination of the axilla for recurrence or infection is performed. Infection in the arm or hand on the dissected side should be treated with antibiotics, rest, and elevation. If there is no sign of recurrence or infection, the swollen extremity should be treated with rest and elevation. A mild diuretic may be helpful. If there is no improvement, a compressor pump or manual compression decreases the swelling, and the patient is then fitted with an elastic glove or sleeve. Most patients are not bothered enough by mild edema to wear an uncomfortable glove or sleeve and will treat themselves with elevation or manual compression alone. Rarely, edema may be severe enough to interfere with use of the limb. A prospective randomized study has shown that twice weekly progressive weightlifting improves lymphedema symptoms and exacerbations and improves extremity strength. Surgery to reconnect lymphatics in the axilla to correct lymphedema is being assessed, with several studies showing a decrease in lymphedema rates from the traditional 25–30% to 5–10%.

McEvoy MP et al. Prevention and treatment of lymphedema in breast cancer. Adv Surg. 2024;58:65. [PMID: 39089787]
Shen A et al. Risk factors for breast cancer-related lymphedema: an umbrella review. Ann Surg Oncol. 2024;31:284. [PMID: 37725224]

2. Breast reconstruction—Breast reconstruction is usually feasible after total or modified radical mastectomy. Prior to mastectomy, reconstruction should be discussed with patients because it offers an important psychological focal point for recovery. Reconstruction is not an obstacle to the diagnosis of recurrent cancer. The most common breast reconstruction has been implantation of a silicone gel or saline prosthesis in the subpectoral plane between the pectoralis minor and pectoralis major muscles. Alternatively, autologous tissue can be used for reconstruction.

Autologous tissue flaps have the advantage of not feeling like a foreign body to the patient. The most popular autologous technique is reconstruction using abdominal tissue flaps. This includes the deep inferior epigastric perforator (DIEP) flap and the more traditional transrectus abdominis muscle (TRAM) flap. A latissimus dorsi flap can be swung from the back but offers less volume than the TRAM flap and thus often requires supplementation with an implant. Reconstruction may be performed immediately (at the time of initial mastectomy) or may be delayed until later, usually when the patient has completed adjuvant therapy. When considering reconstructive options, concomitant illnesses should be considered, since the ability of an autologous flap to survive depends on medical comorbidities. In addition, the need for radiotherapy may affect the choice of reconstruction as radiation may increase fibrosis around an implant or decrease the volume of a flap. Skin-sparing and nipple-sparing mastectomies with immediate reconstruction, when feasible, may afford superior cosmetic outcomes.

3. Risks of pregnancy—Clinicians are often asked to advise patients regarding the potential risk of future pregnancy after definitive treatment for early-stage breast cancer. *To date, no adverse effect of pregnancy on survival of women who have had breast cancer has been demonstrated.* When counseling patients, oncologists must take into consideration the patients' overall prognosis, age, comorbidities, and life goals.

In patients with inoperable or metastatic cancer (stage IV disease), induced abortion may be advisable because of the possible adverse effects of hormonally targeted treatment, radiotherapy, or chemotherapy upon the fetus in addition to the expectant mother's poor prognosis. Clinicians need to be aware of laws regarding the availability of abortions in the jurisdiction of their practice.

Arecco L et al. Safety of pregnancy after breast cancer in young women with hormone receptor-positive disease: a systematic review and meta-analysis. ESMO Open. 2023;8:102031. [PMID: 37879234]

Azim HA Jr et al. Fertility preservation and assisted reproduction in patients with breast cancer interrupting adjuvant endocrine therapy to attempt pregnancy. J Clin Oncol. 2024;42:2822. [PMID: 38810178]
Hickey M et al. Managing menopause after cancer. Lancet. 2024;403:984. [PMID: 38458217]
Lambertini M et al. Pregnancy after breast cancer in young BRCA carriers: an international hospital-based cohort study. JAMA. 2024;331:49. [PMID: 38059899]
Radhakrishnan A et al. Oncology and primary care involvement in breast cancer survivorship care more than 5 years after initial treatment. JCO Oncol Pract. 2024 Dec 6. [Epub ahead of print] [PMID: 39642316]

CARCINOMA OF THE MALE BREAST

ESSENTIALS OF DIAGNOSIS

- A painless lump beneath the areola in a man usually over 50 years of age.
- Nipple discharge, retraction, or ulceration may be present.
- Generally poorer prognosis than in women.

General Considerations

Breast cancer in men is a rare disease; the incidence is only about 1% of all breast cancer diagnoses. For men in the United States, ~2670 new cases of invasive breast cancer were expected to be diagnosed in 2026, and an estimated 530 men died of breast cancer. The average age at occurrence is about 70 years, and there may be an increased incidence of breast cancer in men with prostate cancer. As in women, hormonal influences are probably related to the development of male breast cancer. There is a high incidence of both breast cancer and gynecomastia in Bantu men, theoretically owing to failure of estrogen inactivation by associated liver disease. It is important to note that first-degree relatives of men with breast cancer are considered to be at high risk. This risk should be taken into account when discussing options with the patient and family. In addition, *BRCA2* mutations are common in men with breast cancer. Men with breast cancer, especially with a history of prostate cancer, should receive genetic counseling to determine whether genetic testing is indicated.

Clinical Findings

A painless lump, occasionally associated with nipple discharge, retraction, erosion, or ulceration, is the primary complaint. Examination usually shows a hard, ill-defined, nontender mass beneath the nipple or areola. Gynecomastia not uncommonly precedes or accompanies breast cancer in men and may itself be a risk factor. Nipple discharge is an uncommon presentation for breast cancer in men but is an ominous finding associated with carcinoma in nearly 75% of cases.

Breast cancer staging is the same in men as in women. Gynecomastia and metastatic cancer from another site (eg, prostate) must be considered in the differential diagnosis. Benign tumors are rare, and biopsy should be performed on all males with a defined breast mass.

Treatment

Treatment usually consists of modified radical mastectomy in operable patients, who should be chosen by the same criteria as women with the disease. Breast-conserving therapy is rarely performed for men. Irradiation is the first step in treating localized metastases in the skin, lymph nodes, or skeleton that are causing symptoms. Examination of the cancer for hormone receptors and *HER2* overexpression is of value in determining adjuvant therapy. Over 95% of men have ER-positive tumors and < 10% have overexpression of *HER2*. Androgen receptor is also commonly overexpressed in male breast cancer, though this does not impact systemic therapy decisions. Adjuvant systemic therapy and radiation are used for the same indications as in breast cancer in women.

Because breast cancer in men is frequently hormone receptor–positive, diagnosed late, and is a disseminated disease, endocrine therapy is of considerable importance in its management. Tamoxifen (20 mg orally daily) is the main medication for management of advanced breast cancer in men and should be the initial treatment. There are few data regarding the use of AIs in men, but they are used frequently. Castration in advanced breast cancer is a successful measure and more beneficial than the same procedure in women but is rarely used. Objective evidence of regression may be seen in 60–70% of men with endocrine therapy for metastatic disease—approximately twice the proportion in women. Bone is the most frequent site of metastases from breast cancer in men (as in women), and endocrine therapy relieves bone pain in most patients so treated. The longer the interval between mastectomy and recurrence, the longer is the remission following treatment.

Chemotherapy should be administered for the same indications and using the same dosage schedules as for women with metastatic disease or for adjuvant treatment.

Prognosis

A large population-based, international breast cancer study reported that after adjustment for prognostic features (age, stage, treatment), men have a similar relative survival stage for stage compared to women. For node-positive disease, 5-year survival is ~69%, and for node-negative disease, it is about 88%.

For those patients whose disease progresses despite treatment, meticulous efforts at palliative care are essential (see Chapter 5).

Bucalo A et al. Male breast cancer risk associated with pathogenic variants in genes other than BRCA1/2: an Italian case-control study. Eur J Cancer. 2023;188:183. [PMID: 37262986]
Hassett MJ et al. Management of male breast cancer: ASCO guideline. J Clin Oncol. 2020;38:1849. [PMID: 32058842]
Khare VS et al. Male breast cancer: an updated review of patient characteristics, genetics, and outcome. Int J Breast Cancer. 2024;2024:9003572. [PMID: 38559438]

Women's Health Issues

Emmanuelle Yecies, MD, MS
Judith Walsh, MD, MPH

20

AMENORRHEA

ESSENTIALS OF DIAGNOSIS

- Amenorrhea is the abnormal absence of menstruation.
- Amenorrhea is classified as "primary" or "secondary."
- Pregnancy is the most common cause of amenorrhea.

1. Primary Amenorrhea

General Considerations

Primary amenorrhea is the absence of the onset of menses by age 13 in those who lack secondary sexual characteristics (such as body hair or breast development) or by age 15 in those who have developed some secondary sexual characteristics. Excluding pregnancy, the etiologies for primary amenorrhea include:

Low or normal FSH levels:

- Hypothalamic-pituitary causes (with low or normal FSH), which occur most commonly from a constitutional delay of growth and puberty.
- Uterine causes (with normal FSH), including Müllerian agenesis, which result in a missing uterus with vaginal hypoplasia while gonadal structures remain intact.
- Hyperandrogenism (with low or normal FSH), which is excessive testosterone secretion that can result from polycystic ovaries, ovarian tumors, adrenal tumors, or adrenal hyperplasia. Androgenic steroid abuse may also cause this syndrome.
- 46,XY disorders of sexual development (pseudohermaphroditism) are often associated with normal FSH levels.
- Severe illness, vigorous exercise (eg, ballet dancing, running), stressful life events, dieting, or anorexia nervosa (with normal or low FSH levels). However, these conditions should not be assumed to account for amenorrhea without a full endocrinologic evaluation.

High FSH levels:

- Ovarian causes, including gonadal dysgenesis (Turner syndrome and others), are the most common cause of permanent primary amenorrhea.

Clinical Findings

The initial endocrine evaluation should include serum FSH, LH, prolactin, total and free testosterone, TSH, free thyroxine, and β-human chorionic gonadotropin (hCG) (pregnancy test). Pelvic duplex/color sonography is useful, as an absent uterus should prompt karyotype analysis. Patients who are virilized or hypertensive require serum electrolyte determinations and further hormonal evaluation to exclude a congenital adrenal disorder. Those who have a normal uterus and high FSH without features of congenital adrenal hyperplasia require a karyotype to diagnose X chromosome mosaicism, even in the absence of classic features of Turner syndrome. MRI of the hypothalamus and pituitary is used to evaluate teens with primary amenorrhea and low or normal FSH and LH—especially those with high prolactin levels.

2. Secondary Amenorrhea

General Considerations

Secondary amenorrhea is an absence of menses for > 3 months in patients with previously regular cycles and > 6 months in those with previously irregular cycles. The most common cause of secondary amenorrhea is physiologic pregnancy. Other causes include medications, anatomic changes, and endocrinologic abnormalities.

An intact hypothalamic-pituitary-ovarian-uterine axis is required for regular menses. A variety of endocrine-mediated disorders that can result in secondary amenorrhea include hypogonadotropic hypogonadism, polycystic ovary syndrome (PCOS), which is also known as polyendocrine metabolic ovarian syndrome, pituitary dysfunction from prolactinomas, Sheehan syndrome, or infiltrative or inflammatory syndromes of the pituitary gland, thyroid dysfunction, hypercortisolemia, hyperandrogenemia, or primary ovarian insufficiency. Medications that block the dopamine D_2 receptor can increase prolactin levels, disrupt the hypothalamic-uterine axis, and cause subsequent amenorrhea. These medications include first- and second-generation antipsychotics and some antiemetics. Other medications that can cause amenorrhea through less clear mechanisms include cyclic antidepressants, selective serotonin reuptake inhibitors, other antidepressants, and opioid analgesics.

Clinical Findings

A. Symptoms and Signs

Questions should focus on a sexual history, timing of the last menstrual period, and medications, including contraceptives, antipsychotics, antiemetics, and antidepressants (Table 20–1). Symptoms of pregnancy should be elicited, such as breast tenderness or enlargement, nausea,

Table 20–1. Etiology and evaluation of common causes of secondary amenorrhea.

Category	Etiology	Possible Clinical Findings	Key Laboratory or Imaging Studies
Pregnancy	Physiologic amenorrhea	Breast tenderness, nausea, vomiting, increased urinary frequency, weight changes	Positive urine hCG
Hypothalamic	Hypothalamic amenorrhea	Weight loss, excessive exercise, decreased caloric intake, significant psychosocial or other stressors, presence of lanugo, excoriations on extensor surfaces of hands	Normal TSH and prolactin Normal or low FSH Low estradiol
	Infiltrative or inflammatory symptoms	Systemic symptoms of associated disorders (eg, tuberculosis, sarcoidosis)	Variable; often will present with decreased anterior pituitary hormone levels
Pituitary	Prolactinoma	Galactorrhea, headaches, vision changes, including field changes	Elevated prolactin, MRI pituitary
	Other pituitary tumors	Headaches, vision changes; other symptoms dependent on tumor type (eg, acromegaly, corticotroph adenoma)	Variable; dependent on type of tumor; MRI pituitary
	Pituitary apoplexy or infarct	History of significant obstetric emergency, difficulty breastfeeding, hypotension, cold intolerance	Low TSH, FSH, estradiol
Ovarian	Primary ovarian insufficiency	Age < 40, hot flashes, night sweats, sleep disturbance, sexual dysfunction, vaginal dryness	High FSH Low estradiol
	Menopause	Age > 40, symptoms as above, absence of menses for 1 year, vaginal dryness or atrophy	High FSH Low estradiol
	Androgen-secreting tumor	Quickly developing hirsutism, acne, hypertension, acne, facial hair, androgenic alopecia	High testosterone High DHEAS
Uterine	Asherman syndrome or cervical stenosis	History of recurrent pregnancy loss, prior dilatation and curettage procedures, prior radiation or chemotherapy	Normal hormone levels, absent withdrawal bleeding after progestin, hysteroscopic diagnosis
Other Common Causes	PCOS	Weight gain, hirsutism, acne (particularly nonfacial acne), acanthosis nigricans, skin tags	Normal TSH, prolactin, FSH, estradiol
	Thyroid dysfunction (either hyper- or hypothyroidism)	Heat/cold intolerance, palpitations, diarrhea/constipation, hair loss, skin dryness, fatigue	May have polycystic ovaries on pelvic ultrasound
	Hypercortisolism	Weight gain, hirsutism, acne, hypertension, striae, central adiposity, muscle atrophy	High cortisol
	Medications	See text	May have high prolactin depending on the medication

DHEAS, dehydroepiandrosterone sulfate; hCG, β-human chorionic gonadotropin; PCOS, polycystic ovarian syndrome.

vomiting, or weight gain. Symptoms of prolactinoma include galactorrhea, particularly bilateral galactorrhea, with visual field symptoms or headache. PCOS can manifest with hirsutism or excessive acne, particularly on the back or trunk; patients should be asked about the previous presence of these findings since they may have taken medications or used other measures to remove them. Rapid onset of hirsutism may suggest an androgen-producing tumor. A dietary history, exercise history, and evaluation of ongoing social stressors or significant medical events will help to identify patients with hypothalamic amenorrhea. Thyroid dysfunction can lead to heat or cold intolerance, palpitations, hair loss, or constipation; disorders leading to abnormal cortisol can result in weight gain, weakness, headache, fatigue, and other nonspecific symptoms. Estrogen deficiency may manifest with hot flashes, vaginal dryness, interrupted sleep, and decreased libido. A history of an obstetrical emergency, dilatation and curettage, infection, or endometritis can help identify patients with Sheehan syndrome, uterine adhesions, or cervical stenosis.

The physical examination should assess for hyper- or hypotension, tachycardia, and weight changes. The presence of exophthalmos, visual field deficits, facial hair or cystic acne, or enlarged parotoid glands should be sought. The breasts should be examined if the patient endorses tenderness or galactorrhea. The presence of acne on the back or trunk, abdominal striae, dry skin, androgenetic hair loss, or the presence of lanugo should be noted.

B. Laboratory Findings

Initial laboratory testing, after urine hCG to exclude pregnancy, typically includes TSH, FSH, prolactin, and estradiol levels. Subsequent evaluation will depend on the results of the initial testing (Table 20–1).

Treatment

The management of secondary amenorrhea is addressed in sections below based on the cause of secondary amenorrhea.

With hypothalamic amenorrhea, engaging patients in lifestyle changes to balance caloric intake with energy expenditure will often support resumption of menses, and cognitive behavioral therapy is recommended to support patients in engaging in these positive behaviors. The weight at which a woman previously menstruated is an appropriate goal weight. If menses do not resume with 6–12 months of lifestyle efforts, supplementation with estrogen and cyclic progesterone, such as transdermal estradiol 100 mcg continuously and micronized progesterone 200 mcg for 12 days of each month, should be considered for bone health until menses resume.

Practice Committee of the American Society for Reproductive Medicine. Current evaluation of amenorrhea: a committee opinion. Fertil Steril. 2024;122:52. [PMID: 38456861]

Saadedine M et al. Functional hypothalamic amenorrhea: recognition and management of a challenging diagnosis. Mayo Clin Proc. 2023;98:1376. [PMID: 37661145]

MENOPAUSE

ESSENTIALS OF DIAGNOSIS

- Menopause is a retrospective diagnosis after 12 months of amenorrhea.
- ~80% of women experience hot flushes and night sweats.
- High FSH and low estradiol can help confirm the diagnosis, if needed.

General Considerations

Natural menopause is defined as the permanent cessation of menstrual periods. A woman is considered to have gone through menopause once she has not had a menstrual period for 12 months. The average age of menopause in the United States is 51.4 years. **Perimenopause** (or the menopausal transition) occurs before menopause and is characterized by irregular menses, endocrine changes, and symptoms such as hot flashes. **Primary ovarian insufficiency** is defined as menopause that occurs in women aged < 40 years; premature menopause is defined as menopause that occurs in women aged 40–45. Both premature menopause and primary ovarian insufficiency are associated with increased cardiovascular risk, bone loss, and cognitive concerns. Predictors of age at menopause include genetic factors, family history, ethnicity, and cigarette smoking status.

Women who undergo bilateral salpingo-oophorectomy experience "surgical menopause," which is associated with an abrupt onset of menopausal symptoms. Women who undergo pelvic radiation can often have similar symptoms.

Clinical Findings

A. Symptoms and Signs

1. Cessation of menstruation—Menstrual cycles generally become irregular during the early menopause transition. Anovulatory cycles occur more often, with irregular cycle length and occasional menorrhagia. The late menopause transition is evidenced by amenorrhea of over 60 days' duration. Perimenopause includes the late menopause transition and the 12 months following the last menstrual period, with missed periods or episodes of spotting only. When no bleeding has occurred for 1 year, menopause has occurred.

2. Vasomotor symptoms—Hot flushes (feelings of intense heat over the trunk and face, with flushing of the skin and sweating) occur in > 80% of women. Vasomotor symptoms last > 7 years in > 50% of women. Hot flushes occur more frequently at night, causing sweating and insomnia that result in fatigue the following day.

3. Genitourinary syndrome of menopause (GSM)—Decreased estrogen secretion results in less vaginal lubrication. Up to 50% of women experience symptoms of dryness, dyspareunia, burning, vaginal spotting, and pruritus. Estrogen deficiency also causes urinary frequency, urgency, dysuria, and an increased risk of UTIs. GSM does not improve over time, in contrast to hot flushes. These symptoms can be associated with physical discomfort, sexual dysfunction, emotional distress, and reduced quality life. Many women indicate having symptoms of GSM when asked, but very few indicate that their provider initiated a conversation about it. Pelvic examination reveals pale, smooth vaginal mucosa and a small cervix and uterus.

4. Other manifestations seen at the time of menopause— "Brain fog" is described as a constellation of cognitive symptoms experienced by women around the time of menopause. The main difficulties are with memory and attention, such as forgetting intentions (such as why they entered a room) or difficulty maintaining a train of thought. These cognitive changes often occur in the context of vasomotor symptoms, sleep disturbance, and mood changes; treatment of these symptoms may help with the cognitive symptoms. These symptoms resolve for some women but not for all and are not a precursor to cognitive decline.

There is an increased incidence of sleep disturbance and mood changes. Major depression is experienced by about 10% of women during the menopausal transition. Decreased libido is experienced by about 10% of menopausal women and is thought to be related to deficiencies in both estrogen and testosterone. Joint pain is common in women at midlife, and there may be an association with menopausal status. Pain tends to increase, and fibromyalgia symptoms can become more intense. Postmenopausal osteoporosis presents with increasing age after menopause with fragility fractures of long bones and vertebrae.

B. Laboratory Findings

No laboratory testing is required to diagnose normal menopause when amenorrhea occurs at the expected age. The expected age of menopause correlates with a woman's mother's age at menopause and varies among different kindreds and ethnic groups. Elevated hCG overwhelmingly indicates pregnancy; false-positive testing may rarely occur with ectopic hCG secretion (eg, choriocarcinoma or bronchogenic carcinoma). An elevated serum FSH (> 40 IU/L) with a low or low-normal serum estradiol helps confirm the diagnosis. For women aged < 40 years, the diagnosis of premature ovarian insufficiency requires at least two increased FSH levels drawn at least a month apart. Further laboratory evaluation for nonpregnant women includes serum prolactin, LH (elevated in menopause), and TSH.

C. Other Diagnostic Studies

An MRI of the pituitary region should be obtained if there is hyperprolactinemia or hypopituitarism without obvious cause. If there is any bleeding after 6 months from the cessation of menses, pelvic ultrasonography should be obtained to assess the thickness of the endometrial lining, and an endometrial curettage or aspiration should be performed to rule out endometrial cancer.

Treatment

A. Nonpharmacologic Treatment of Vasomotor Symptoms

Several nonpharmacologic strategies have long been recommended for women with vasomotor symptoms. These include dressing in layers, sleeping in a cool room, exercise, yoga, and eliminating triggers for hot flushes, such as smoking cigarettes, alcohol, caffeine, and hot spicy foods. Slow, deep breathing can ameliorate hot flushes. Although evidence for these strategies is limited, many are benign or have other potential health benefits. Nonpharmacologic strategies recommended by the North American Menopause Society include cognitive behavioral therapy, hypnosis, and stellate ganglion block. Although many herbal and complementary therapies such as black cohosh are often advocated, they are not recommended by the North American Menopause Society.

B. Hormonal Therapy for Vasomotor Symptoms

The strategy of using estrogen or progestin to treat menopausal symptoms is called hormone therapy (HT). Although previously referred to as hormone replacement therapy (HRT), HRT now refers to HT given when menopause occurs at an early age, suggesting replacement of declining hormone levels. In contrast, HT refers to using hormones to manage menopausal symptoms. Women who have a uterus must use estrogen-progestin therapy (EPT), as unopposed estrogen can cause endometrial proliferation and increase the risk of uterine cancer; whereas women who have had a hysterectomy can use estrogen therapy (ET) alone. Although most treatments have not been directly compared, HT appears to be the most effective treatment for vasomotor symptoms. Because of some of the potential risks associated with HT (noted below), women are generally encouraged to use the lowest dose for the shortest duration of time.

1. Benefits and risks of HT—The Women's Health Initiative's (WHI) randomized trial compared the impact of EPT in women with a uterus versus ET alone in women who had a hysterectomy in the largest trial of its kind. The main outcomes were heart disease and breast cancer. Subsequent WHI publications have evaluated the impact of EPT and ET alone on many other clinical outcomes, including osteoporosis, thromboembolic disease, and all-cause mortality. In 2002, the WHI trial was halted early due to an unfavorable balance of benefits and risks in those taking EPT, mainly due to an increased risk of breast cancer.

Importantly, the WHI study was designed to evaluate the impact of HT on disease prevention outcomes, not symptoms. The average age of enrolled women was 63 years, which is not reflective of the average age of women who are being considered for symptomatic treatment. Long-term follow-up after 20 years showed that there was no impact on all-cause mortality. Women who took EPT had an increased risk of breast cancer at 20 years but no increase in breast cancer mortality. At 20-year follow-up, ET alone was associated with a decreased risk of breast cancer as well as a decrease in breast cancer mortality. Other important benefits of HT are a reduction in the risk of osteoporosis, including a 33% reduction in hip fracture risk, and possible reduction in CVD and all-cause mortality in younger women.

An additional important risk is an increased risk of thromboembolic disease. This risk appears to be higher in women who take oral ET compared with women who use transdermal HT. Unopposed estrogen in women who have a uterus is associated with an increase in endometrial cancer. Therefore, all women with a uterus who take estrogen must also take progestin.

Finally, when taking into account the risks and benefits of HT, it is not recommended for chronic prevention of any disease.

2. EPT formulations—The most used estrogen formulations are oral and transdermal. Since transdermal estrogen has been associated with a lower risk of thromboembolic disease in observational studies, it is the preferred mode of treatment. Conjugated equine estrogen (Premarin) was studied in the WHI trial, and the "standard" oral dose, the dose that stops hot flashes in 80% of women, is 0.625 mg daily. "Standard doses" of other formulations are 1 mg of oral micronized 17-estradiol daily and 50 mcg of transdermal 17-β estradiol twice weekly. Lower doses are also used but may not be as effective in hot flash reduction and may take longer to reach maximal effect.

For women with a uterus, progestin must be taken. Medroxyprogesterone can be added at a dose of either 2.5 mg orally daily or 10 mg orally daily for 10–12 days a month. Micronized progesterone is the same as the hormone secreted by the ovary and is often perceived as more natural. It is used at a dose of either 100 mg orally daily or 200 mg orally for 10–12 days a month. Some women have problems with progestin so it is recommended to give this less often; however, using micronized progesterone quarterly is not recommended. A combined estrogen/progestin patch is also available. These preparations mix estradiol with either norethindrone acetate or levonorgestrel. Available patches include 0.05 mg estradiol with either 0.14 mg or 0.25 mg norethindrone acetate daily dose (CombiPatch) replaced twice weekly and 0.045 mg estradiol with 0.015 mg levonorgestrel daily dose (Climara Pro) replaced once weekly.

Progestins may cause moodiness, particularly in women with a history of premenstrual dysphoric disorder, and cycled progestins may trigger migraines in some. Many other adverse reactions have been reported, including breast tenderness, alopecia, and fluid retention. For women unable to tolerate oral progestin, a levonorgestrel-containing IUD is often used, although it is not approved by the FDA for this use.

A. Oral estrogen plus selective estrogen receptor modulators—A combination of conjugated equine estrogens (0.45 mg) with bazedoxifene (20 mg) is available (Duavee). Bazedoxifene is a selective estrogen receptor modulator (SERM) that reduces the risk of endometrial hypertrophy and dysfunctional uterine bleeding, without adverse breast effects. This formulation is indicated for moderate to severe vasomotor symptoms and the prevention of postmenopausal osteoporosis.

B. Parenteral estrogen—Rarely, parenteral estrogen injections can be used when other methods have failed.

C. Weighing the risks and benefits of hormone therapy—In light of these considerations, estrogen therapy is most commonly prescribed for women who are aged < 60 years and within the first 5–10 years of menopause, when symptoms are the worst and the benefits are greatest. Transdermal estrogen is favored over oral therapy to reduce the risk of thromboembolism. In women with an intact uterus, a progestin must be added because estrogen replacement without a progestin risks endometrial hypertrophy and dysfunctional uterine bleeding. Although not an FDA-approved use, progestin may be delivered directed to the uterus with a progesterone-eluting IUD. The American College of Obstetricians and Gynecologists and North American Menopause Society have recommended that the decision to continue estrogen therapy past age 65 should include an assessment of risks and benefits, particularly including relief from hot flushes and prevention of osteoporosis, balanced with increased risk of breast cancer and thromboembolic disease. In summary, estrogen is not recommended for chronic disease prevention for any disease.

D. How long to treat with hormonal therapy—Although the general recommendation is to treat with the "lowest dose for the shortest duration," knowing when to stop HT can be challenging. Since menopausal symptoms are self-limited, treatment is also for a limited period. However, ~25% of women will have recurrence of symptoms when they stop HT. It is unclear whether it is best to stop abruptly or to taper. Tapering can be done by decreasing the daily dose, decreasing the number of doses per week, or decreasing the strength of the transdermal estrogen. When tapering, a typical practice is to taper until mild symptoms develop and then maintain that dose until symptoms resolve.

C. Nonhormonal Pharmacologic Treatment of Vasomotor Symptoms

SSRIs are FDA-approved as nonhormonal treatment for vasomotor symptoms. The dose of paroxetine is 7.5 mg orally daily; paroxetine must not be used by women taking tamoxifen, as it interacts with the cytochrome P-450 system involved in tamoxifen metabolism. Escitalopram (10–20 mg orally daily) has also shown effectiveness, regardless of coexisting anxiety or depression. SSRIs often provide modest effects within a week.

The serotonin-norepinephrine reuptake inhibitor venlafaxine extended release (37.5 mg or 75 mg orally daily) is effective for reducing vasomotor symptoms. Compared to its typical use for depression, this dose is lower, and the effects are noticed sooner.

Gabapentin is also effective for hot flash reduction. It is particularly helpful when given at bedtime (300–600 mg orally) for hot flashes that awaken the woman from sleep.

Fezolinetant, a neurokinin B receptor antagonist that acts on the thermoregulatory center of the hypothalamus, is a nonhormonal treatment of vasomotor symptoms. Although it has not been directly compared to other treatments of vasomotor symptoms, a network meta-analysis found that an oral dose of fezolinetant 45 mg daily is equivalent to all HT regiments and that it is more efficacious than all non-HT regimens. When prescribing, liver biochemical tests should be measured at baseline and then every 3 months for the first 9 months of treatment.

Clonidine transdermal patch can reduce hot flashes by up to 40%, but side effects such as orthostatic hypotension can be limiting.

Small studies have suggested that oxybutynin in doses of 5–10 mg orally daily can be helpful in hot flash reduction, but side effects such as dry mouth can be limiting.

D. Treatment of Genitourinary Syndrome of Menopause

1. Vaginal moisturizers and lubricants—Vaginal moisturizers are used several times a week, and vaginal lubricants are used for sexual activity. Although both can improve the symptoms of dryness or coital comfort, they do not impact vaginal atrophy. Over-the-counter moisturizer products include Replens and Vagisil, and vaginal lubricants include Astroglide, K-Y Jelly, and Elegance Woman's.

2. Vaginal estrogen—Local vaginal estrogen is the most effective treatment for symptoms related to vaginal atrophy and also can relieve symptoms of UTIs and urge incontinence. It is moderately effective in reducing symptoms of urogenital atrophy, while minimizing systemic estrogen exposure. Vaginal estrogen can be administered in three different ways: creams, tablets, and rings.

A. ESTROGEN VAGINAL CREAMS—These creams are administered intravaginally with a measured-dose applicator daily for 2 weeks for atrophic vaginitis, then administered one to three times weekly. *Conjugated equine estrogens* are available as Premarin Vaginal (0.625 mg/g cream), dosed as 0.25–2 g cream administered vaginally one to three times weekly. *Estradiol* is available as Estrace Vaginal (0.1 mg/g cream), 1 g cream administered vaginally one to two times weekly.

B. ESTRADIOL VAGINAL TABLETS AND SOFTGEL INSERTS—*Vagifem* and *Yuvafem* (generic equivalent) are available as 10 mcg tablets. *Imvexxy* is a softgel vaginal insert (4 mcg or 10 mcg estradiol in a coconut oil base). Either preparation can be administered intravaginally daily for 2 weeks followed by a maintenance regimen of twice weekly. Vaginal preparations are usually inserted at bedtime.

C. ESTRADIOL VAGINAL RINGS—These rings are inserted manually into the upper third of the vagina, worn continuously, and replaced every 3 months. Only a small amount of the released estradiol enters the systemic circulation. Vaginal rings do not usually interfere with sexual intercourse. If a ring is removed or descends into the introitus, it may be washed in warm water and reinserted. Estring (2 mg estradiol/ring) is most effective for local vaginal symptoms. Femring releases estradiol acetate and is available in two strengths: 12.4 mg/ring releases estradiol acetate 0.05 mg/day or 24.8 mg/ring releases estradiol acetate 0.1 mg/day. Both rings are replaced every 90 days. For women with postmenopausal urinary urgency and frequency, even the low-dose Estring can successfully reduce urinary symptoms and vaginal dryness.

D. VAGINAL DEHYDROEPIANDROSTERONE SULFATE (DHEAS)—Prasterone is a 6.5 mg vaginal insert used daily.

E. OSPEMIFENE—Ospemifene is a novel selective estrogen modulator for treating dyspareunia associated with postmenopausal vaginal and vulvar atrophy. In a trial of women with moderate to severe dyspareunia, the severity of vaginal pain was significantly improved. Unfortunately, hot flashes were the most significant side effects, occurring in up to 10% of women. Ospemifene may be useful for women when vaginal estrogen is not indicated or is difficult to use (eg, severe arthritis).

3. Vaginal androgen—Vaginal androgen is an option for postmenopausal women who are experiencing vaginal dryness and reduced sexual satisfaction. It is also an option for women who cannot use systemic or vaginal estrogen due to breast cancer. Testosterone cream 150–300 mcg (formulated) is administered vaginally daily for 2 weeks and then three times weekly. It improves sexual satisfaction while reducing vaginal dryness and dyspareunia without increasing systemic estrogen or testosterone levels.

4. Laser or energy-based therapies—These therapies may be promising but there are safety concerns, and they are not recommended for the treatment of GSM.

5. Special considerations for women with breast cancer—Topical estrogen has minimal, but not absent, systemic absorption. It is generally best, therefore, to start treatment for GSM with nonhormonal options such as moisturizers and lubricants. Women on aromatase inhibitors should avoid topical estrogens. For women with a low risk of recurrence of breast cancer, the use of topical estrogens is probably acceptable. Decision-making should take place in concert with the oncologist and focus on the advantages and disadvantages.

6. Treatment of GSM—Guidelines published by the American Urologic Association, American Urogynecologic Society, and Society of Urodynamics, Female Pelvic Medicine & Urogenital Reconstruction and endorsed by several other organizations, including The Menopause Society, focus on educating perimenopausal and menopausal women about GSM. Moisturizers and lubricants remain first-line treatment. For women with moderate-to-severe GSM for whom moisturizers and lubricants are not adequate, vaginal estrogen, vaginal DHEAS, or ospemifene are recommended. Systemic ET is recommended if vasomotor symptoms are also present. Although systemic risks with topical ET are highly unlikely, women with a history of breast or endometrial cancer should discuss use with their oncologist. There is no need for progestins or routine endometrial monitoring with topical ET. Treatment should continue as long as bothersome symptoms persist.

Cappola AR et al. Hormones and aging: an Endocrine Society scientific statement. J Clin Endocrinol Metab. 2023;108:1835. [PMID: 37326526]

Crandall CJ et al. Management of menopausal symptoms: a review. JAMA. 2023;329:405. [PMID: 36749328]
Johnson KA et al. Efficacy and safety of fezolinetant in moderate to severe vasomotor symptoms associated with menopause: a phase 3 RCT. J Clin Endocrinol Metab. 2023;108:1981. [PMID: 36734148]
Kaufman MR et al. The AUA/SUFU/AUGS guideline on genitourinary syndrome of menopause. J Urol. 2025;214:242. [PMID: 40298120]
Steunkel CA et al. Primary ovarian insufficiency. N Engl J Med. 2023;388:154. [PMID: 36630623]
The 2023 Nonhormone Therapy Position Statement of The North American Menopause Society Advisory Panel. The 2023 nonhormone therapy position statement of The North American Menopause Society. Menopause. 2023;30:573. [PMID: 37252752]

SEXUALITY & SEXUAL HEALTH IN WOMEN

Approximately 40–50% of women will experience concerns pertaining to sexual health during their lifetime. Female sexual dysfunction includes **female sexual interest/arousal disorder** (previously known as hypoactive sexual desire disorder, HSDD), **sexual arousal disorder, female orgasmic disorder,** and **genitopelvic pain** or **penetration disorder**. When diagnosing any sexual health disorder, symptoms must be present for 6 months, be personally distressing to the patient, and meet at least three of six specific criteria related to symptoms and frequency (outlined in *DSM-5*) to ensure an accurate diagnosis. Duration criteria may limit overdiagnosis as transient factors commonly impact sexual function, such as relationship conflict or other life events.

Although female sexual disorders are common, many women will not seek help from clinicians. Thus, it is important for health care providers to invite women to discuss their sexual concerns by routinely initiating dialogue about sexual health during office visits. Patients who express concerns can be asked a more complete history that includes the onset, duration, and severity of symptoms as well as associated distress.

Female sexual dysfunction: ACOG Practice Bulletin Summary, number 213. Obstet Gynecol. 2019;134:203. [PMID: 31241595]

LOW SEXUAL DESIRE IN WOMEN

Among female sexual function disorders, female sexual interest/arousal disorder is the most prevalent sexual disorder in women. Affected women report at least 6 months of low motivation or desire for sexual activity with associated significant personal distress. The Decreased Sexual Desire Screener is a validated self-administered questionnaire that can aid clinicians in diagnosing this disorder.

Pathophysiologically, female sexual interest/arousal disorder is related to an imbalance of central sexual excitatory and inhibitory pathways. Excitatory pathways involve the action of dopamine, melatonin, oxytocin, vasopressin, and norepinephrine, whereas inhibitory pathways utilize opioid, serotonin, and endocannabinoid systems. Psychological comorbidities, stressors, medications, medical comorbidities, cultural and religious factors, or partner and relationship concerns further contribute to sexual dysfunction.

Clinical Findings

Several medical conditions (eg, depression, anxiety, diabetes mellitus, malignancy) and certain medications (eg, antidepressants, antihyperlipidemics, antihypertensives) can contribute to low sexual desire, so a detailed history is essential for eliciting potentially modifiable risk factors. In certain women, it may be appropriate to perform a gynecologic examination to identify areas of tenderness or discomfort that might be associated with painful intercourse and reduced sexual desire. Laboratory evaluation is not necessary for making the diagnosis, although prolactin and thyroid hormone levels can be measured in select patients where other symptoms raise concern for hormonal abnormalities. Notably, testosterone levels do not correlate with female sexual function and should not be routinely measured.

Treatment

Treatment for low sexual desire includes office-based counseling, psychological therapy, and medications. Office-based counseling can be facilitated using an approach based on the PLISSIT model employed in sex therapy: permission [P], limited information [LI], specific suggestions [SS], and intensive therapy [IT].) In addition to sex therapy, intensive psychological therapy may include cognitive-behavioral training and mindfulness-based stress reduction training.

Based on the understanding of sexual excitatory and inhibitory pathways, medications that increase dopamine or decrease serotonin release or binding can be effective in increasing sexual desire. Two medications are FDA-approved for low sexual desire in premenopausal women: flibanserin and bremelanotide. In a systematic review, flibanserin led to a small increase in the number of satisfying sexual events and sexual desire intensity but had high rates of dizziness and somnolence. Flibanserin 100 mg should be taken orally once nightly and should not be combined with alcohol, which can potentiate side effects. Bremelanotide has shown modest improvements in sexual function compared with placebo in two randomized controlled trials (25% vs 17%). Side effects are common, including nausea in 40%, vomiting, and skin darkening. Contraindications include uncontrolled hypertension and use of naltrexone. Bremelanotide is a subcutaneous injection (1.7 mg) dosed as needed prior to sexual activity and can be used up to once daily and eight times per month.

Several studies have investigated the efficacy of testosterone for the management of low sexual desire in women. While a systematic review showed an increase in sexually satisfying encounters, sexual desire, and orgasms, side effects are common, including increased acne and hair growth. There are no FDA-approved testosterone formulations for women with sexual dysfunction, which limits clinicians to use this medication off-label. Bupropion is commonly used as an adjunct when SSRI-associated decreases in desire are present, and it has also been shown to improve desire in premenopausal women. However, bupropion is not FDA-approved for this indication. Systemic DHEAS failed to show efficacy in a trial of postmenopausal women and should not be used for this indication. Finally, sildenafil has shown mixed, contradictory results for the treatment of female sexual dysfunction and should not be used for this indication outside of research settings.

Shared decision-making focused on the individual risk and benefits profiles of each agent should guide medication selection. The high cost of both flibanserin and bremelanotide may limit their use for many patients.

American College of Obstetricians and Gynecologists. Female sexual dysfunction: ACOG practice bulletin clinical management guidelines for obstetrician-gynecologists, number 213. Obstet Gynecol. 2019;134:e1. [PMID: 31241598]

Burton CS et al. Pharmacologic therapeutic options for sexual dysfunction. Curr Opin Obstet Gynecol. 2022;34:402. [PMID: 36036468]

Pettigrew JA et al. Hypoactive sexual desire disorder in women: physiology, assessment, diagnosis, and treatment. J Midwifery Womens Health. 2021;66:740. [PMID: 34510696]

CHRONIC PELVIC PAIN IN WOMEN

ESSENTIALS OF DIAGNOSIS

- Noncyclic pain.
- Duration of 3–6 months or more.
- Localized to anatomic pelvis, anterior abdominal wall at or below the umbilicus, the lumbosacral back, or buttocks.
- Associated with functional disability.

General Considerations

Chronic pelvic pain is defined as noncyclic pain lasting at least 3–6 months that localizes to the pelvic girdle region; it must be of sufficient severity to cause functional disability or necessitate medical care. This disorder is common, accounting for 10–20% of outpatient visits to a gynecologist, and is associated with decreased quality of life, depression, and sexual dysfunction. Patients with chronic pelvic pain may also experience marital stress, altered relationships at home, and decreased work capacity.

Chronic pelvic pain is a symptom that can arise from a diverse group of disorders, including gynecologic, urologic, GI, musculoskeletal, or neurologic abnormalities. Specific gynecologic conditions that can cause chronic pelvic pain include endometriosis, pelvic adhesions, chronic pelvic inflammatory disease, ovarian remnant, pelvic congestion syndrome, and adenomyosis. Interstitial cystitis (also called bladder pain syndrome [BPS]), irritable bowel syndrome, and pelvic floor myalgia have all been associated with chronic pelvic pain. Musculoskeletal and neurologic causes of pelvic discomfort should also be considered, including disk herniation, lumbar spondylosis, and nerve entrapment. Many women may have more than one diagnosis contributing to their pain, with studies showing that multiple pelvic pain syndromes often coexist such as bladder pain syndrome and irritable bowel syndrome. Chronic pelvic pain may also be diagnosed in the absence of clear identifiable underlying pathology.

Given the overlap of symptoms in many chronic pelvic pain disorders, pathophysiologic models highlight the shared afferent and efferent neurologic pathways between visceral and somatic structures in the pelvis, which can help inform a clinician's approach to these disorders where persistent input from visceral sources leads to perceived pain in somatic structures, and vice versa. Thus, a patient with (somatic) pelvic floor muscle dysfunction may exhibit (visceral) symptoms of urinary frequency or urgency. The mechanisms that exacerbate chronic pelvic pain often include contributions from central pain sensitization, adverse childhood experiences (eg, abuse or trauma), and psychological distress or coexisting mental health diagnoses. History, physical examination, and treatment should address each of these along with possible gynecologic or non-gynecologic diagnoses as noted above.

Clinical Findings

A. Symptoms and Signs

Certain features of the history and physical examination can provide clues to the underlying diagnosis. Patients should be asked about the location, quality, and intensity of their pain as well as the relationship with the menstrual cycle, sexual activity, urination, and defecation. Dysmenorrhea and dyspareunia are often experienced by patients with endometriosis, whereas dysuria, urgency, and frequency in association with pelvic pain are characteristic of interstitial cystitis or myofascial pain syndromes. Patients with irritable bowel syndrome often report abdominal pain, distention, and diarrhea or constipation. Clinicians should ask patients about surgery or direct trauma involving the spine or pelvis, which may suggest musculoskeletal sources of pain. In addition, a thorough gynecologic and obstetric history should be obtained in all women.

Guidelines emphasize the importance of evaluating the impact of the patient's chronic pelvic pain on her quality of life, psychological health, and relationships. Patients can complete a detailed questionnaire prior to the office visit (Pelvic Pain Assessment Form is available at https://www.ucsfhealth.org/-/media/project/ucsf/ucsf-health/pdf/ipps_english.pdf). This survey asks patients to rate the effect of their pain on their emotional well-being and daily functioning and can provide the clinician with valuable information. Additional items on the survey assess for occurrences of physical, sexual, or emotional abuse, which may be risk factors for chronic pelvic pain.

The physical examination, including the pelvic examination, can be painful for patients with chronic pelvic pain; therefore, providers should employ trauma-informed principles, such as explaining all steps of the examination and their rationale before proceeding, giving patients the option to stop the examination at any point, and providing patients with opportunities to ask questions or choose which portions of the examination will be done. Guidelines also recommend performing the physical examination in a particular order, progressing sequentially from the musculoskeletal examination to the examination of the cervix to minimize pain and discomfort. The examination should begin with palpation of the thoracic and lumbar spine, pelvic girdle, and abdomen, which may reveal areas of tenderness that are referred to the pelvic area. A positive Carnett test (an increase in pain when the abdominal muscles are tensed) can be helpful for identifying abdominal wall trigger points.

Next, examination of the external genitalia should be performed using a cotton swab to carefully identify areas of vulvar sensitivity. The single-digit internal vaginal examination is helpful for localizing exact areas of pain, palpating specific pelvic structures (cervix, urethra, bladder base), and assessing for trigger points along the pelvic floor muscles. Palpation of the pelvic viscera can help identify localized areas of tenderness in women with endometriosis or chronic pelvic inflammatory disease. The cervical examination may be performed with a small speculum and should assess for cervical lesions, mucosal abnormalities, and evidence of infection; tenderness localized to the cervix or vaginal fornices may be elicited by palpation with a long cotton swab.

When examining a patient where there is high likelihood of myofascial pain, a standardized examination can be performed that includes palpation of the sacroiliac joints while the patient is seated followed by palpation of the medial anterior superior iliac spine and specific pelvic floor muscles while the patient is supine; the degree of pain experienced by the patient with each maneuver is noted and a diagnosis of myofascial pain is likely when patients have pain at four or more sites.

B. Laboratory Findings

Laboratory evaluation should be guided by the history and physical examination findings. Testing may include a UA, testing for STIs, or cervical cytology.

C. Diagnostic Testing and Imaging

Transvaginal ultrasonography is useful to confirm a suspected diagnosis, such as an ovarian endometrioma or adenomyosis. Laparoscopy is considered the gold standard for diagnosis of gynecologic disorders such as endometriosis or pelvic adhesions.

Differential Diagnosis

Chronic pelvic pain may be associated with gynecologic and non-gynecologic conditions; it is not uncommon for more than one causative diagnosis to be present in a woman. GI disorders (irritable bowel syndrome) and functional urinary syndromes (interstitial cystitis/BPS) are common non-gynecologic diagnoses that may contribute to chronic pelvic pain. Clinicians should perform a careful examination of the GI, urologic, musculoskeletal, and neurologic systems to evaluate for these possibilities.

Treatment

Successful treatment of chronic pelvic pain often requires a multidisciplinary approach, recognizing its impact on a patient's quality of life, psychological health, relationships, and work. Health psychologists, psychiatrists, pain specialists, and physical therapists may all play important roles in helping the patient to manage symptoms and maximize daily functioning and well-being.

A. Medical Treatment

Medical therapy may be general (focused on overall management of the pain) or disease-specific (focused on specific underlying etiologies of pain). The choice of medical therapy should be influenced by side-effect profiles as well as the patient's pregnancy intent.

General therapies include medications that are often used for the treatment of chronic pain syndromes. Initial treatment may begin with simple analgesics, such as acetaminophen or NSAIDs. Some women may also benefit from neuromodulators, including tricyclic antidepressants, duloxetine, gabapentin, and pregabalin. Guidelines acknowledge the limited evidence for the effectiveness of these treatments for the management of chronic pelvic pain; the potential for side effects (such as GI and renal side effects with NSAIDs) may limit long-term use of some treatments. A large, randomized controlled trial of women with chronic pelvic pain demonstrated that side effects of gabapentin—dizziness, drowsiness, and visual disturbances—were common while pain control in the gabapentin group was no better than in the placebo group. However, smaller trials have demonstrated benefit in some patients at 24 weeks of gabapentin treatment. Hormonal therapies are used primarily for treating gynecologic sources of chronic pelvic pain. Women with suspected endometriosis can be empirically treated with hormonal therapy before diagnostic laparoscopy is performed. Combined oral contraceptives, progestins (oral, injectable, and intrauterine), gonadotropin-releasing hormone (GnRH) analogs, and danazol are effective for treating the dysmenorrhea associated with endometriosis, although the side effects vary. The effects on BMD associated with GnRH analog therapy can be mitigated by "add-back" low-dose hormonal therapy (norethindrone, low-dose estrogen, or a combination of estrogen and progesterone), which may also provide symptomatic relief for associated hot flashes and vaginal symptoms. Danazol may be associated with severe androgenic side effects, including hirsutism, acne, and weight changes; therefore, it is not used as first-line therapy. For women who have endometriosis and desire pregnancy, NSAIDs may provide symptomatic relief.

A Cochrane systematic review and meta-analysis investigated the effectiveness of noninvasive treatments for the management of chronic pelvic pain unrelated to endometriosis, primary dysmenorrhea, chronic pelvic inflammatory disease, or irritable bowel syndrome. Treatment with daily high-dose oral medroxyprogesterone (50 mg), compared with placebo, was associated with a reduction in pain that was maintained up to 9 months after therapy; side effects included weight gain and bloating.

Musculoskeletal sources of chronic pelvic pain include pelvic floor myalgia, which is related to spasm of the levator ani muscles, and myofascial trigger points. Treatments include referral to pelvic physical therapy and, if needed, trigger point injections with a local anesthetic or botulinum A toxin, although evidence supporting these therapies are mixed.

Treatment of irritable bowel syndrome and interstitial cystitis/bladder pain syndrome are discussed in Chapters 17 and 26.

B. Surgical Treatment

Patients with endometriosis may be offered laparoscopic surgical destruction of implants; adhesiolysis can be considered if severe and dense adhesions are also present. Uterine artery ablation has been shown to be effective for the treatment of adenomyosis, and pelvic vein embolization improves pain in patients with pelvic venous congestion.

Guidelines note that additional surgical techniques for the management of chronic pelvic pain include presacral neurectomy, laparoscopic uterine nerve ablation, hysterectomy, and salpingo-oophorectomy.

When to Refer

Patients with chronic pelvic pain benefit from a multidisciplinary approach to their care. Clinicians should consider referring to health psychologists, pain specialists, and sex therapists early in treatment.

Patients should be referred to a gynecologist for diagnostic or therapeutic surgical procedures if the underlying diagnosis is unclear or if expertise is needed to manage the side effects associated with medical treatments (ie, GnRH agonist therapy).

Chronic pelvic pain: ACOG practice bulletin, number 218. Obstet Gynecol. 2020;135:e98. [PMID: 32080051]

Engeler D et al. EAU guidelines on chronic pelvic pain. 2023. https://uroweb.org/guideline/chronic-pelvic-pain/

Lamvu G et al. Chronic pelvic pain in women: a review. JAMA. 2021;325:2381. [PMID: 34128995]

Vincent K et al. An update on the management of chronic pelvic pain in women. Anaesthesia. 2021;76 Suppl 4:96. [PMID: 33682093]

HIRSUTISM & VIRILIZATION

ESSENTIALS OF DIAGNOSIS

- Hirsutism, acne, menstrual disorders.
- Virilization: muscularity, androgenic alopecia, deepening voice, clitoromegaly.
- Rarely, a palpable pelvic tumor.
- Serum DHEAS and androstenedione elevated in adrenal disorders; variable in others.
- Serum testosterone is often elevated.

General Considerations

Hirsutism is a condition in women that causes excessive growth of dark or coarse hair in a male-like pattern. The excess hair often appears on the face, chest, and back. Significant hirsutism affects about 5–15% of women, although it varies by ethnicity and cultural norms, including the amount of hair growth considered unacceptable. **Virilization** is the development of male physical characteristics in women, such as pronounced muscle development, deep voice, male pattern baldness, and more severe hirsutism.

Etiology

Hirsutism may be idiopathic, familial, or caused by ovarian or adrenal disorders. Rare causes of hirsutism include medications, acromegaly, or ACTH-induced Cushing disease. Hirsutism is often associated with excessive androgen levels.

A. Idiopathic or Familial

Most women with hirsutism or androgenic alopecia have no detectable hyperandrogenism; hirsutism may be considered normal in the context of their genetic background. Such patients may have hair follicles that are more sensitive to androgens, rather than androgen overproduction.

B. Polycystic Ovary Syndrome (PCOS)

PCOS is the most common cause of hirsutism and accounts for at least 50% of all cases (see Chapter 21). A diagnosis of PCOS must meet two of three criteria: (1) androgen excess with clinical hyperandrogenism or elevated serum free or total testosterone; (2) ovarian dysfunction with oligoanovulation or polycystic ovary morphology; and (3) polycystic ovaries as assessed by ultrasonography or high anti-Müllerian hormone levels. PCOS is a diagnosis of exclusion, and other causes of testosterone excess or anovulation, such as pregnancy, thyroid dysfunction, 21-hydroxylase deficiency, neoplastic testosterone secretion, Cushing syndrome, or hyperprolactinemia, must be ruled out.

Affected women usually have signs of hyperandrogenism, including hirsutism, acne, or male pattern thinning of scalp hair; this persists after natural menopause. They also have elevated serum testosterone or free testosterone levels. About 70% of affected women have polycystic ovaries on pelvic ultrasonography, and 50% have oligomenorrhea or amenorrhea with anovulation.

Obesity and high serum insulin levels (due to insulin resistance) contribute to the syndrome in 70% of women. The serum LH:FSH ratio is often > 2.0. Both adrenal and ovarian androgen hypersecretion are commonly present.

C. 46,XX Karyotype: Congenital Adrenal Hyperplasia (see Chapter 29)

D. 46,XY Karyotype: Defects in Androgen Action or Synthesis (see Chapter 29)

E. Neoplastic Disorders

Ovarian tumors are uncommon causes of hirsutism (0.8%) and include arrhenoblastomas, Sertoli-Leydig cell tumors, dysgerminomas, and hilar cell tumors. Adrenal carcinoma, a rare cause of Cushing syndrome and hyperandrogenism, can be virilizing. Pure androgen-secreting adrenal tumors occur very rarely; about 50% are malignant.

F. Rare Causes of Hirsutism and Virilization

Acromegaly and ACTH-induced Cushing disease are rare causes of hirsutism and virilization. Porphyria cutanea tarda can cause periorbital hair growth in addition to dermatitis in sun-exposed areas. Maternal virilization during pregnancy may result from a luteoma of pregnancy, hyperreactio luteinalis, or polycystic ovaries. In postmenopausal women, diffuse stromal Leydig cell hyperplasia is a rare cause of hyperandrogenism. Pharmacologic causes of hirsutism include minoxidil, cyclosporine, phenytoin, anabolic steroids, interferon, cetuximab, diazoxide, and certain progestins.

Clinical Findings

A. Symptoms and Signs

Modest androgen excess from any source increases male pattern hair growth (chin, upper lip, abdomen, and chest) and increases sebaceous gland activity, producing acne. Menstrual irregularities, anovulation, and amenorrhea are common. If androgen excess is pronounced, defeminization (decrease in breast size, loss of feminine adipose tissue) and virilization (androgenic balding, muscularity, clitoromegaly, and deepening of the voice) occur. Virilization suggests an androgen-producing neoplasm.

Hirsutism is quantitated using the Ferriman-Gallwey score; it is graded from 0 (none) to 4 (severe) in nine areas of the body, with a maximum possible score of 36 (https://myendoconsult.com/learn/ferriman-gallwey-score/).

Hypertension may be present in Cushing syndrome, adrenal 11-hydroxylase deficiency, or cortisol resistance syndrome. A pelvic examination may disclose clitoromegaly or ovarian enlargement that may be cystic or neoplastic.

B. Laboratory Testing and Imaging

Laboratory testing is indicated for women with moderate to severe hirsutism, mild hirsutism with menstrual disturbances, and women with worsening hirsutism despite therapy. Laboratory tests to consider include FSH, LH, total and free testosterone, 17-hydroxyprogesterone, androstenedione, and DHEAS.

A serum testosterone level > 200 ng/dL (6.9 nmol/L) or free testosterone > 40 ng/dL (140 pmol/L) is suggestive of an ovarian or adrenal neoplasm. Evaluation should start with pelvic ultrasonography; if that is unrevealing, follow up with an adrenal CT scan. A serum androstenedione level > 1000 ng/dL (34.9 nmol/L) also suggests an ovarian or adrenal neoplasm.

Women with a serum DHEAS > 700 mcg/dL (35 nmol/L) have an adrenal source of androgen, usually due to adrenal hyperplasia and rarely due to adrenal carcinoma. Women with clinical signs of Cushing syndrome should be evaluated with a 1-mg overnight dexamethasone suppression test (see Chapter 29).

Women with a family history of congenital adrenal hyperplasia and women who are members of some ethnic groups (Ashkenazi Jews, Croatians, Iranians, Yupik Inuit) are at increased risk for "late-onset" congenital adrenal hyperplasia due to 21-hydroxylase deficiency. Patients with congenital adrenal hyperplasia usually have a 17-hydroxyprogesterone level > 300 ng/dL (9.1 nmol/L).

An LH:FSH ratio > 2.0 is common in patients with PCOS. Obtaining a transvaginal ultrasound may not be helpful since about 25–30% of normal young women have polycystic ovaries. Transvaginal ultrasonography or MRI usually detects virilizing tumors of the ovary. However, small virilizing ovarian tumors may not be detectable by imaging studies; selective venous sampling for testosterone may be useful for diagnosis in such patients.

Treatment

The treatment of hirsutism is multimodal, including lifestyle modifications, physical hair removal, and androgen suppression or blockade. Weight loss in patients who are obese decreases androgen levels and hirsutism, and local hair removal, especially with laser, is effective. Underlying medical causes of hirsutism (eg, Cushing syndrome, acromegaly) should be treated, and drugs causing hirsutism should be stopped.

A. Topical and Laser Treatments

Topical treatment of facial hirsutism by shaving, depilatories, waxing, electrolysis, or bleaching is effective. Eflornithine (Vaniqa) 13.9% topical cream retards hair growth when applied twice daily to unwanted facial hair; improvement is noted within 4–8 weeks. Eflornithine can also be used with laser therapy for a more dramatic response, but local skin irritation is common. Hirsutism returns with discontinuation of eflornithine when used alone.

Laser treatment (photoepilation) is particularly effective for facial hirsutism for women with dark hair and light skin. For women of color, a longer-wavelength laser such as Nd:YAG or diode laser with skin cooling is used. Repeated laser treatments are usually required. Laser therapy is not recommended for women with facial hirsutism of Middle Eastern and Mediterranean ancestry, since they have an increased risk of paradoxical hypertrichosis with laser therapy.

B. Medications

Oral contraceptives are preferred as initial therapy for women with hirsutism who are not desiring pregnancy. To reduce DVT risk, an oral contraceptive is recommended with a low-dose of estradiol (20 mcg) and a progestin having a relatively low risk of venous thrombosis (norethindrone, norgestimate). Oral contraceptives that contain particularly antiandrogenic progestins such as desogestrel (Azurette, Kariva), drospirenone (Yaz, Gianvi), norgestimate (Ortho Tri-Cyclen Lo), or cyproterone acetate (Diane 35, not available in United States) more effectively reduce hirsutism and acne; however, the antiandrogenic oral contraceptives are associated with an increased DVT risk compared with norethindrone or levonorgestrel.

Cyproterone acetate is a unique progestin that is used to treat women with hirsutism worldwide, but it is not FDA-approved in United States. Cyproterone acetate blocks androgen receptors as well as 5-α-reductase activity while also suppressing testosterone levels. It is typically given as an oral contraceptive in a dose of 2 mg with ethinyl estradiol 35 mcg.

Combined oral contraceptives are relatively contraindicated for women who are at risk for thromboembolic disease, including those who smoke cigarettes. They are also contraindicated in women who have migraines with aura and women who have hypertension.

Generally, a 6-month trial of oral contraceptive is recommended. If the desired effect is not achieved, an antiandrogen such as spironolactone, flutamide or finasteride can be added.

Spironolactone is effective for reducing hirsutism, acne, and androgenic alopecia. Doses of 100–200 mg orally (taken as a single dose or in two divided doses) are taken on days 5–25 of the menstrual cycle or daily in combination with an oral contraceptive. Spironolactone is contraindicated in pregnancy; reproductive-age women must use reliable contraception during this therapy. Serum potassium should be checked 1 month after beginning therapy or after dosage increases, as hyperkalemia is a rare side effect. Spironolactone should be avoided or used cautiously in women with kidney disease or those on an ACE inhibitor or ARB. Side effects of spironolactone include breast tenderness, irregular menses, headaches, nausea, and fatigue, which often improve with continued treatment or dose reduction; paradoxical scalp hair loss has been reported at higher doses.

Flutamide and **bicalutamide** inhibit testosterone binding to androgen receptors and also suppress serum testosterone. Flutamide reduces abdominal adiposity and serum LDL cholesterol in women with PCOS. They should only be used as a last resort for women with severe hirsutism/virilization and only with very close monitoring for hepatic toxicity and strict contraceptive precautions due to risks of fetal malformations.

Finasteride inhibits 5-α-reductase, the enzyme that converts testosterone to active dihydrotestosterone in the skin. Finasteride is used off-label at a dose of 5 mg daily for its anti-androgen effects to treat women with hirsutism and transgender women. Finasteride can induce pseudohermaphroditism in male fetuses if taken during pregnancy, so contraception is critical for reproductive-age women.

Simvastatin and **atorvastatin** have been shown to reduce hirsutism in women with PCOS. When given to women taking an oral contraceptive, they lead to a greater decrease in hirsutism than an oral contraceptive alone. Statins are not recommended as primary therapy for hirsutism.

Crinecerfont, a corticotropin releasing factor pituitary receptor antagonist, is used to treat hyperandrogenism in women with congenital adrenal hyperplasia (21-hydroxylase deficiency). At a dose of 100 mg twice daily, it dramatically decreases androstenedione production, with a secondary benefit of a reduction in hirsutism. Patients may experience fatigue that usually improves with time and optimization of glucocorticoid replacement.

GnRH agonists are not routinely used for treatment of hirsutism but have been successful in treating postmenopausal women with severe ovarian hyperandrogenism when laparoscopic oophorectomy is contraindicated or declined.

C. Surgery

Laparoscopic resection of androgenizing tumors of the adrenal or ovary is recommended. Postmenopausal women with severe hyperandrogenism should undergo laparoscopic bilateral oophorectomy (if CT scan of the adrenals and ovaries is normal), since small hilar cell tumors of the ovary may not be visible on scans. Women with classic salt-wasting congenital adrenal hyperplasia and infertility or treatment-resistant hyperandrogenism may be treated with laparoscopic bilateral adrenalectomy.

Auchus RJ et al. Phase 3 trial of crinecerfont in adult congenital adrenal hyperplasia. N Engl J Med. 2024;391:504. [PMID: 38828955]

Dumesic DA et al. Randomized clinical trial: effect of low-dose flutamide on abdominal adipogenic function in normal-weight women with polycystic ovary syndrome. Fertil Steril. 2023;119:116. [PMID: 36400597]

Hirschberg AL. Approach to investigation of hyperandrogenism in a postmenopausal woman. J Clin Endocrinol Metab. 2023;108:1243. [PMID: 36409990]

Shrivastava S et al. Polycystic ovary syndrome. Med Clin North Am. 2023;107:227. [PMID: 36759093]

Teede HJ et al. Recommendations from the 2023 International Evidence-based Guideline for the assessment and management of polycystic ovary syndrome. J Clin Endocrinol Metab. 2023;108:2447. [PMID: 37580314]

Gynecologic Disorders

21

Jill Brown, MD, MPH, MHS, FACOG[1]
Logan Peterson, MD, FACOG[1]
Katerina Shvartsman, MD, FACOG[1]

ABNORMAL UTERINE BLEEDING IN PERSONS OF REPRODUCTIVE AGE

ESSENTIALS OF DIAGNOSIS

- Accurate diagnosis of abnormal uterine bleeding (AUB) depends on appropriate categorization and diagnostic tests.
- Evaluating AUB depends on the patient's age and risk factors.
- Pregnancy should always be ruled out as a cause of AUB in persons of reproductive age.

General Considerations

Normal menstrual frequency varies from 24 to 38 days with bleeding lasting an average of 5 days (range, 2–8 days) and a mean blood loss of 40 mL per cycle. *AUB refers to menstrual bleeding of abnormal quantity, duration, or schedule in nonpregnant reproductive age patients.* The International Federation of Gynecology and Obstetrics (FIGO) introduced the classification system for AUB in 2011, which was then endorsed by the American College of Obstetricians and Gynecologists. This classification system pairs AUB with descriptive terms denoting the bleeding pattern (ie, **heavy**, **light, menstrual**, **intermenstrual**) and etiology (the acronym **PALM-COEIN** standing for **P**olyp, **A**denomyosis, **L**eiomyoma, **M**alignancy and hyperplasia, **C**oagulopathy, **O**vulatory dysfunction, **E**ndometrial, **I**atrogenic, and **N**ot yet classified). In adolescents, AUB often occurs because of persistent anovulation due to the immaturity of the hypothalamic-pituitary-ovarian axis. AUB in patients aged 19–39 years is often a result of structural lesions, anovulatory cycles, use of hormonal contraception, or endometrial hyperplasia.

[1]Dr. Brown, Dr. Peterson, and Dr. Shvartsman are employees of the Uniformed Services University (USU). The opinions and assertions expressed in this chapter are the authors' and do not reflect the official policy or position of the USU or the Department of Defense.

Clinical Findings

A. History and Physical

The diagnosis depends on the following: (1) confirming a uterine source of the bleeding; (2) excluding pregnancy and confirming the patient is premenopausal; (3) ascertaining whether the bleeding pattern suggests regular ovulatory bleeding or anovulatory bleeding; (4) determining the contribution of structural abnormalities (PALM), including risk for malignancy/hyperplasia; (5) identifying risk of medical conditions that may impact bleeding (eg, inherited bleeding disorders, endocrine disease, risk of infection); and (6) assessing the contribution of medications, including hormonal contraceptives, anticoagulants, and natural product supplements that may affect bleeding.

B. Laboratory Studies

A CBC, pregnancy test (urine or serum), and thyroid tests should be done. For adolescents with heavy menstrual bleeding and adults with a positive screening history for bleeding disorders, coagulation studies should be considered, including a von Willebrand panel for adolescents, since *up to 18% of persons with heavy menstrual bleeding have an underlying coagulopathy*. For patients with irregular bleeding and prolonged time between menses, checking serum prolactin, FSH, and estradiol levels may be useful. Vaginal or urine samples to test for infectious causes of cervicitis should be considered. If indicated, cervical cytology should also be obtained.

C. Imaging

Transvaginal ultrasound is useful to assess for the presence of fibroids and suspicion of adenomyosis, as well as to evaluate endometrial thickness for potential hyperplasia or endometrial cancer. Sonohysterography or hysteroscopy may help to diagnose endometrial polyps or subserous myomas. MRI is not a primary imaging modality for AUB but can more definitively diagnose submucous myomas and adenomyosis.

D. Endometrial Sampling

The purpose of endometrial sampling is to determine if hyperplasia or carcinoma is present. Sampling methods

Table 21–1. Common gynecologic diagnostic procedures (listed in alphabetical order).

Colposcopy
Visualization of cervical, vaginal, or vulvar epithelium under 5–50 × magnification with and without dilute acetic acid to identify abnormal areas requiring biopsy. An office procedure.
Dilation & curettage (D&C)
Dilation of the cervix and curettage of the entire endometrial cavity, using a metal curette or suction cannula and often using forceps for the removal of endometrial polyps. Can usually be done in the office under local anesthesia or in the operating room under sedation or general anesthesia. D&C is often combined with hysteroscopy for improved sensitivity.
Endocervical curettage
Removal of endocervical epithelium with a small curette for diagnosis of cervical dysplasia and cancer. An office procedure performed with or without local anesthesia.
Endometrial biopsy
Blind sampling of the endometrium by means of a curette or small aspiration device without cervical dilation. Diagnostic accuracy similar to D&C. An office procedure performed with or without local anesthesia.
Hysterosalpingography
Injection of radiopaque dye through the cervix to visualize the uterine cavity and oviducts. Mainly used in investigation of infertility or to identify a space-occupying lesion.
Hysteroscopy
Visual examination of the uterine cavity with a small fiberoptic endoscope passed through the cervix. Curettage, endometrial ablation, biopsies of lesions, and excision of myomas or polyps can be performed concurrently. Can be done in the office under local anesthesia or in the operating room under sedation or general anesthesia. Greater sensitivity for diagnosis of uterine pathology than D&C.
Laparoscopy
Visualization of the abdominal and pelvic cavity through a small fiberoptic endoscope passed through a subumbilical incision. Permits diagnosis, tubal sterilization, and treatment of many conditions previously requiring laparotomy. General anesthesia is used.
Saline infusion sonohysterography
Introduction of saline solution into endometrial cavity with a catheter to visualize submucous myomas or endometrial polyps by transvaginal ultrasound. May be performed in the office with oral or local analgesia, or both.

and other gynecologic diagnostic procedures are described in Table 21–1. Polyps, endometrial hyperplasia, and, occasionally, submucous myomas are identified on endometrial biopsy. *Endometrial sampling should be performed in patients with AUB who are aged ≥ 45 years, or in younger patients with a history of unopposed estrogen exposure (including obesity or chronic ovulatory dysfunction), or failed medical management and persistent AUB.*

Treatment

Treatment for patients with AUB depends on the etiology of the bleeding, determined by history, physical examination, laboratory findings, imaging, and endometrial sampling. Patients with AUB due to structural abnormalities (eg, submucosal myomas, endometrial polyps, or pelvic [endometrial] neoplasms) or bleeding diathesis may require targeted therapy.

Treatment for AUB-O should include consideration of potentially contributing medical conditions. *Often, AUB-O can be treated hormonally.* For patients amenable to using hormonal contraceptives, estrogen-progestin contraceptives and the 52-mg levonorgestrel-releasing IUD are both effective treatments. The choice between the two depends on whether any contraindications to these treatments exist and on patient preference. Oral or injectable progestin-only medications are also generally effective, but there is little consensus on optimal regimens, and they appear to be less effective than other medical therapies like the hormonal IUD, estrogen-progestin contraceptives, and tranexamic acid. *Nonhormonal options* include NSAIDs, such as naproxen or mefenamic acid, in the usual anti-inflammatory doses taken during menses, and tranexamic acid 1300 mg orally three times per day for up to 5 days. Both have been shown to decrease menstrual blood loss by about 40%, with tranexamic acid superior to NSAIDs in direct comparative studies.

Patients experiencing heavier bleeding can be given a taper of any of the combination oral contraceptives (with 30–35 mcg of ethinyl estradiol) to control the bleeding. There are several commonly used contraceptive dosing regimens, including one pill three times daily (every 8 hours) for 1 or 2 days followed by one pill twice daily through day 5 and then one pill daily through day 20; after withdrawal bleeding occurs, pills are taken in the usual dosage for three cycles. In cases of heavy bleeding requiring hospitalization, intravenous conjugated estrogens, 25 mg every 4 hours for three or four doses, can stop acute bleeding. This can be followed by oral conjugated estrogens, 2.5 mg daily, or ethinyl estradiol, 20 mcg orally daily, for 3 weeks, with the addition of medroxyprogesterone acetate, 10 mg orally daily for the last 10 days of treatment, or a combination oral contraceptive daily for 3 weeks. This will stabilize the endometrium and control the bleeding.

For patients with AUB and ineffective results from medical management or who do not desire medical management, surgical options can be considered. *Heavy menstrual bleeding due to structural lesions (eg, fibroids, adenomyosis, polyps) is the most common indication for surgery.* Minimally invasive procedural options for fibroids include uterine artery embolization and focused ultrasound ablation. Surgical options include myomectomy or hysterectomy. For adenomyosis, the definitive treatment is hysterectomy. Polyps can often be excised hysteroscopically. For women without structural abnormalities, endometrial ablation has similar results compared to the 52-mg levonorgestrel IUD in reducing menstrual blood loss. Hysteroscopic surgical approaches include endometrial ablation with electrocautery or, less commonly, laser photocoagulation. Several nonhysteroscopic techniques using different energy sources are available in the United States. The latter methods are well-adapted to outpatient therapy under local anesthesia. While hysterectomy was used commonly in the past for bleeding unresponsive to medical therapy, the low risk of complications and the good short-term results of both endometrial ablation and hormonal IUD make them attractive alternatives to hysterectomy.

Management options for **endometrial hyperplasia without atypia** include surveillance, oral contraceptives, or progestin therapy. Surveillance may be used if the risk of occult cancer or progression to cancer is low, and the inciting factor (eg, anovulation) has been eliminated. Therapy may include cyclic or continuous progestin therapy (medroxyprogesterone acetate, 10–20 mg/day orally, or norethindrone acetate, 15 mg/day orally) or using a hormonal IUD. Repeat sampling should be performed if symptoms recur. Hysterectomy is the preferred treatment for endometrial hyperplasia with atypia (also called *endometrial intraepithelial neoplasia*) or carcinoma of the endometrium. In some patients with endometrial hyperplasia with atypia, progestin therapy with scheduled repeat endometrial sampling may be an alternative to hysterectomy. Patients who elect this approach include those who desire future childbearing or those who are not candidates for surgery.

When to Refer

- If bleeding is not controlled with first-line therapy.
- If expertise is needed for a surgical procedure.

When to Admit

If bleeding is uncontrollable with first-line therapy or the patient is not hemodynamically stable.

Jain V et al. Contemporary evaluation of women and girls with abnormal uterine bleeding: FIGO Systems 1 and 2. Int J Gynaecol Obstet. 2023;162 Suppl 2:29. [PMID: 37538019]

Lebduska E et al. Abnormal uterine bleeding. Med Clin North Am. 2023;107:235. [PMID: 36759094]

Munro MG et al; FIGO Committee on Menstrual Disorders and Related Health Impacts, and FIGO Committee on Reproductive Medicine, Endocrinology, and Infertility. The FIGO ovulatory disorders classification system. Fertil Steril. 2022;118:768. [PMID: 35995633]

Papakonstantinou E et al. Management of pre-, peri-, and postmenopausal abnormal uterine bleeding: when to perform endometrial sampling? Int J Gynaecol Obstet. 2022;158:252. [PMID: 34669187]

POSTMENOPAUSAL UTERINE BLEEDING

ESSENTIALS OF DIAGNOSIS

- Any uterine bleeding in a postmenopausal patient (≥ 12 months following cessation of menses) is abnormal and should be evaluated.
- Transvaginal ultrasound measurement of the endometrium is an important tool in evaluating the cause of postmenopausal bleeding.

General Considerations

Menopause is defined as 1 year without menstrual bleeding in the absence of other biologic or physiologic cause. The most common causes of postmenopausal bleeding are endometrial atrophy, endometrial proliferation or hyperplasia, endometrial or cervical cancer, and administration of estrogens without or with added progestin. Other causes include atrophic vaginitis, trauma, endometrial polyps, abrasion of the cervix associated with prolapse of the uterus, and blood dyscrasias.

Diagnosis

The vulva and vagina should be inspected for areas of bleeding, ulcers, or neoplasms. Cervical cytology should be obtained, if indicated. Endometrial biopsy or transvaginal ultrasound can be used initially to evaluate the endometrium, but it may be less reliable for initial screening in Black individuals. Transvaginal ultrasound is used to measure endometrial thickness. *An endometrial stripe measurement of ≤ 4 mm indicates a low likelihood of hyperplasia or endometrial cancer.* If the endometrial thickness is > 4 mm or if there is persistent bleeding, endometrial sampling is indicated. If there is focal thickening of the endometrium on ultrasound or persistent bleeding despite negative results on endometrial biopsy, guided sampling with hysteroscopy is more appropriate than random endometrial sampling.

Treatment

Treatment for postmenopausal bleeding is dictated by the underlying etiology. Patients with endometrial atrophy can be given reassurance. As described above, endometrial hyperplasia without atypia can be treated with progestin therapy. Hyperplasia with atypia or endometrial cancer is most appropriately treated with hysterectomy.

When to Refer

- Expertise in performing ultrasonography is required.
- Endometrial hyperplasia with atypia is present.
- Hysteroscopy is indicated.

Dell KM et al. Endometrial thickness as diagnostic triage for endometrial cancer among black individuals. JAMA Oncol. 2024;10:1068. Erratum in: JAMA Oncol. 2025;11:354. [PMID: 38935372]

Doll KM et al. Estimated performance of transvaginal ultrasonography for evaluation of postmenopausal bleeding in a simulated cohort of Black and White women in the US. JAMA Oncol. 2021;7:1158. [PMID: 34264304]

Slaager FC et al. Diagnostic workup of patients with benign or inconclusive reports on office endometrial biopsy after first episode of postmenopausal blood loss. Eur J Obstet Gynecol Reprod Biol. 2025;310:113991. [PMID: 40294513]

LEIOMYOMA OF THE UTERUS (Fibroid Tumor)

ESSENTIALS OF DIAGNOSIS

- Irregular enlargement of the uterus (may be asymptomatic).
- Heavy or irregular uterine bleeding.
- Pelvic pain, dysmenorrhea, and pressure.

General Considerations

Uterine leiomyomas are the most common benign neoplasm of the female genital tract. They are discrete, round, firm, often multiple, uterine tumors composed of smooth muscle and connective tissue. The most commonly used classification is by anatomic location: (1) intramural, (2) submucous, (3) subserous, and (4) cervical. Submucous myomas may be pedunculated and descend through the cervix into the vagina.

Clinical Findings

A. Symptoms and Signs

In nonpregnant patients, myomas are frequently asymptomatic. The two most common symptoms of uterine leiomyomas for which patients seek treatment are AUB and pelvic pain or pressure. Occasionally, degeneration occurs, causing intense pain. Torsion of subserosal pedunculated fibroids may lead to necrosis and pain.

B. Laboratory Findings

Iron deficiency anemia may result from heavy uterine bleeding.

C. Imaging

Ultrasonography will confirm the presence of uterine myomas and can be used sequentially to monitor growth. MRI can delineate intramural and submucous myomas accurately and is typically used before uterine artery embolization to determine fibroid size and location in relation to uterine blood supply. Hysterography or hysteroscopy can also confirm cervical or submucous myomas.

Differential Diagnosis

Irregular myomatous enlargement of the uterus must be differentiated from the similar, but symmetric enlargement that may occur with pregnancy or adenomyosis. Subserous myomas must be distinguished from ovarian tumors. Leiomyosarcoma is an unusual malignant tumor occurring in 0.5% of patients undergoing surgery for myomas. It is rare under the age of 40 but increases in incidence thereafter.

Treatment

A. Nonsurgical Measures

Patients who have small asymptomatic myomas can be managed expectantly and evaluated annually. In patients wishing to defer surgical management, nonhormonal therapies (such as NSAIDs and tranexamic acid) have been shown to decrease menstrual blood loss. Patients with heavy bleeding related to fibroids may respond to estrogen-progestin oral contraceptives or the hormonal IUD, although an IUD cannot be used with a distorted cavity or cavity length > 10 cm. Hormonal therapies, such as gonadotropin-releasing hormone (GnRH) agonists and GnRH antagonists, have been shown to reduce myoma volume, uterine size, and menstrual blood loss.

The US FDA has approved two combination treatments using GnRH antagonists for the management of heavy menstrual bleeding associated with uterine fibroids in premenopausal women with a treatment duration of up to 24 months: (1) relugolix 40 mg, estradiol 1 mg, and norethindrone acetate 0.5 mg once daily and (2) elagolix 300 mg twice daily in combination with estradiol 1 mg and norethindrone acetate 0.5 mg once daily. Linzagolix, an oral GnRH antagonist (dispensed as a 100-mg or 200-mg once-daily tablet), is available in Europe for the treatment of moderate to severe fibroid symptoms.

B. Surgical Measures

Surgical intervention is based on the patient's symptoms, desire for future fertility or uterine preservation, and long-term treatment goals. A variety of surgical measures are available for the treatment of myomas: myomectomy (hysteroscopic, laparoscopic, abdominal, or robotic) and hysterectomy (vaginal, laparoscopic-assisted vaginal, laparoscopic, abdominal, or robotic). Submucous myomas may be amenable to hysteroscopic resection. *Myomectomy is the surgical treatment of choice for women who wish to preserve fertility.*

Because the risk of surgical complications increases with the increasing size of the myoma, preoperative reduction of myoma size is sometimes desirable before hysterectomy. GnRH analogs, such as depot leuprolide, available in 1- and 3-month intramuscular formulations, can be used preoperatively for 3- to 4-month periods to temporarily reduce the size of myomas and surrounding vascularity. GnRH analogs can also serve as a bridge to surgery in patients who are anemic. By stopping menses, patients may increase their hemoglobin level, potentially decreasing their need for blood transfusion perioperatively.

Uterine artery embolization is a minimally invasive treatment for uterine fibroids in which embolic materials are injected into the uterine artery via femoral artery catheterization to occlude fibroid blood supply, causing them to shrink. Uterine artery embolization is *not* intended for women who desire future childbearing. Magnetic resonance–guided high-intensity focused ultrasound (MRgFUS), laparoscopic myolysis/radiofrequency ablation (RFA), and laparoscopic uterine vessel occlusion are other interventions used to treat fibroids with outcomes not shown to be superior to UAE.

Prognosis

In patients desiring future fertility, myomectomy may be offered. Patients should be counseled that approximately 12% of patients undergo repeat surgery within 8 years. Additionally, postoperative pelvic adhesions may impact fertility, and cesarean delivery may be necessary for future pregnancy secondary to disruption of the myometrium. Approximately 80% of women have long-term improvement in symptoms following uterine artery embolization. However, direct comparison of patients undergoing myomectomy or uterine artery embolization has shown that fibroid-related quality of life at 2 years post-procedure is higher among women undergoing myomectomy. *Definitive surgical therapy (ie, hysterectomy) is curative.*

When to Refer

Refer to a gynecologist for treatment of symptomatic leiomyomata.

When to Admit

For acute abdomen associated with an infarcted leiomyoma or for hemorrhage not controlled by outpatient measures.

Ali M et al. An evaluation of relugolix/estradiol/norethindrone acetate for the treatment of heavy menstrual bleeding associated with uterine fibroids in premenopausal women. Expert Opin Pharmacother. 2022;23:421. [PMID: 35068291]
Keating MK et al. Uterine fibroids: rapid evidence review. Am Fam Physician. 2025;112:393. [PMID: 41118184]
Lazaridis A et al. Surgical management of uterine fibroids. Curr Opin Obstet Gynecol. 2023;35:440. [PMID: 37548229]
Lee S et al. New treatment options for nonsurgical management of uterine fibroids. Curr Opin Obstet Gynecol. 2023;35:288. [PMID: 37144584]
Stewart EA et al. Uterine fibroids. N Engl J Med. 2024;391:1721. [PMID: 39504521]
Vannuccini S et al. The modern management of uterine fibroids-related abnormal uterine bleeding. Fertil Steril. 2024;122:20. [PMID: 38723935]

CERVICAL POLYPS

ESSENTIALS OF DIAGNOSIS

- Irregular or postcoital bleeding.
- Polyps visible in the cervical os on speculum examination.

Clinical Findings

Cervical polyps commonly occur during the reproductive years, particularly after age 40, and are occasionally noted in postmenopausal patients. Cervical polyps are visible in the cervical os on speculum examination. The cause is not known, but inflammation may play an etiologic role. The principal symptoms are discharge and abnormal vaginal bleeding. However, abnormal bleeding should not be ascribed to a cervical polyp without evaluating the patient for AUB as indicated.

Cervical polyps should be differentiated from polypoid neoplastic disease of the endometrium, small submucous pedunculated myomas, large nabothian cysts, and endometrial polyps. Cervical polyps rarely contain foci of dysplasia (0.5%) or of malignancy (0.5%). Small, asymptomatic polyps in women < age 45 may be left untreated.

Treatment

Small cervical polyps can generally be removed in the office by avulsion with uterine packing forceps or ring forceps.

When to Refer

- Polyp with a wide base.
- Inability to differentiate endocervical from endometrial polyp.

Baker E et al. Approach to cervical polyps in primary care. Can Fam Physician. 2025;71:26. [PMID: 39843194]

PELVIC PAIN

ESSENTIALS OF DIAGNOSIS

- Determine if pain is acute or chronic.
- Categorize if pain is cyclic or continuous.
- Consider nongynecologic causes.

1. Primary Dysmenorrhea

Primary dysmenorrhea is pain associated with menstrual cycles in the absence of pathologic findings. Primary dysmenorrhea usually begins within 1–2 years after menarche and may become progressively more severe. Prevalence increases up to age 20 and then decreases with both increasing age and parity. Half to three-quarters of menstruating people are affected by dysmenorrhea at some time; 5–6% have incapacitating pain.

Clinical Findings

Primary dysmenorrhea is low, midline, wave-like, cramping pelvic pain often radiating to the back or inner thighs. Cramps may last for ≥ 1 day and may be associated with nausea, diarrhea, headache, and flushing. The pain is produced by uterine vasoconstriction, anoxia, and sustained contractions mediated by prostaglandins. The pelvic examination is normal between menses; examination during menses may produce discomfort, but there are no pathologic findings.

Treatment

NSAIDs (ibuprofen, ketoprofen, mefenamic acid, naproxen) are generally helpful. The medication should be started 1–2 days before expected menses. Symptoms can be suppressed with use of combined hormonal contraceptives, depo-medroxyprogesterone acetate (DMPA), etonogestrel subdermal implant (Nexplanon), or the hormonal IUD. Other therapies that have shown some benefit include local heat, exercise, and high-frequency transcutaneous electrical nerve stimulation around the time of menses. These options may be offered to patients who desire nonhormonal therapy, although they have less supporting evidence.

2. Endometriosis

General Considerations

Endometriosis is an aberrant growth of endometrium outside of the uterus, particularly in the dependent parts of the pelvis and in the ovaries. Its principal manifestations are chronic pain and infertility. Although **retrograde menstruation** is the most widely accepted cause, its pathogenesis and natural course are not fully understood. The overall prevalence in the United States is 6–10%.

Clinical Findings

The clinical manifestations of endometriosis are variable and unpredictable in both presentation and course. Dysmenorrhea, chronic pelvic pain, and dyspareunia are among the well-recognized symptoms. Many patients with endometriosis, however, remain asymptomatic, and most patients with endometriosis have a normal pelvic examination. However, in some, pelvic examination can reveal tender nodules in the cul-de-sac or rectovaginal septum, uterine retroversion with decreased uterine mobility, uterine tenderness, or adnexal mass or tenderness.

Endometriosis should be distinguished from pelvic inflammatory disease, ovarian neoplasms, and uterine myomas. Bowel invasion by endometrial tissue may produce blood in the stool that must be distinguished from that produced by bowel neoplasm.

Imaging is useful mainly in the presence of a pelvic or adnexal mass. Transvaginal ultrasonography is the imaging modality of choice to detect the presence of deeply penetrating endometriosis of the rectum or rectovaginal septum; MRI should be reserved for equivocal cases of rectovaginal or bladder endometriosis. A presumptive clinical diagnosis may be made based on the combination of symptoms, physical examination, and imaging findings. However, a definitive diagnosis of endometriosis is made only by histology of lesions removed at surgery.

Treatment

A. Medical Treatment

Medical treatment, including use of NSAIDs or a variety of hormonal therapies, is effective in the amelioration of pain associated with endometriosis. *Hormonal regimens are designed to inhibit ovulation and to lower hormone levels,* thus preventing cyclic stimulation of endometriotic implants and inducing atrophy. The American Society of Reproductive Medicine views endometriosis as *a chronic disease for which medical management should be prioritized and surgical intervention limited.* Commonly used hormonal regimens include the following:

1. *Combined hormonal (estrogen-progestin) contraceptives are first-line treatment because they have a favorable side effect profile and provide relief for many patients.* Continuous use of any of the combination oral contraceptives, the contraceptive patch, or the vaginal ring is the preferred for treatment of endometriosis.
2. Progestins, specifically oral norethindrone acetate and subcutaneous DMPA, have been approved by the US FDA for treatment of endometriosis-associated pain. The etonogestrel implant has also been shown to decrease endometriosis-related pain.
3. The hormonal IUD has been shown to be effective in reducing endometriosis-associated pelvic pain and may be considered before surgery.
4. GnRH agonists (such as leuprolide acetate, 3.75 mg intramuscular injection monthly or 11.25 mg intramuscular injection every 3 months) are highly effective in reducing pain associated with endometriosis; however, they are not superior to other methods such as combined hormonal contraceptives. Side effects of vasomotor symptoms and bone demineralization may be relieved by "add-back" therapy, such as conjugated equine estrogen, 0.625 mg orally daily, or norethindrone acetate, 5 mg orally daily.
5. GnRH antagonists, like GnRH agonists, suppress pituitary gonadotropin production and create a hypoestrogenic state; however, they are effective immediately rather than requiring 7–14 days for GnRH suppression. Injectable and oral forms (eg, cetrorelix and elagolix, respectively) are available.
6. Danazol is an androgenic medication used to treat endometriosis-associated pain but is not commonly used due to androgenic side effects. It may be used for 4–6 months and is typically prescribed orally in divided doses from 400 mg daily to 800 mg daily.
7. Aromatase inhibitors (such as anastrozole or letrozole) in combination with conventional therapy (eg, progestin, combined hormonal contraceptive, or GnRH analog) have been evaluated with positive results in premenopausal patients with endometriosis-associated pain and pain recurrence.

B. Surgical Measures

Surgical treatment of endometriosis—particularly extensive disease—is effective both in reducing pain and in promoting fertility. Laparoscopic ablation of endometrial implants significantly reduces pain. Ablation of implants and, if necessary, removal of ovarian endometriomas enhance fertility, although subsequent pregnancy rates are inversely related to the severity of disease. Patients with disabling pain for whom childbearing is not a consideration can be treated definitively with hysterectomy plus bilateral salpingo-oophorectomy. Hormone therapy should be considered to relieve menopausal symptoms, reduce bone loss, improve cardiovascular parameters, and reduce all-cause mortality after oophorectomy.

Prognosis

There is little systematic research regarding either the progression of the disease or the prediction of clinical outcomes. The prognosis for reproductive function in early or moderately advanced endometriosis appears to be good with conservative therapy. Hysterectomy, with bilateral salpingo-oophorectomy, often is regarded as "definitive" treatment of endometriosis in patients with intractable pelvic pain, adnexal masses, or multiple previous ineffective conservative surgical procedures. However, *symptoms may recur even after hysterectomy and oophorectomy.*

When to Refer

Refer to a gynecologist for laparoscopic diagnosis or surgical treatment.

When to Admit

Rarely necessary except for acute abdomen associated with ruptured or bleeding endometrioma.

3. Other Etiologies of Pelvic Pain

Additional causes of pelvic pain may include adenomyosis, fibroids, pelvic inflammatory disease (PID), malpositioned IUD, or other abnormalities of the pelvic organs, including the bowel or bladder.

Clinical Findings

The history may be suggestive of the causes mentioned above. Physical examination may be useful to narrow the differential diagnosis.

Diagnosis

Targeted physical examination may help identify the anatomic source of pelvic pain. Treatment for PID is advised for sexually active patients with pelvic pain and examination findings of cervical motion tenderness, uterine tenderness, or adnexal tenderness without another explanation for the pain. Pelvic imaging is useful for diagnosing uterine fibroids or other anomalies. **Adenomyosis** (the presence of endometrial glands and stroma within the myometrium) may be detected with ultrasound or MRI. Laparoscopy may help diagnose endometriosis or other pelvic abnormalities not visualized by imaging.

Treatment

Treatment should be directed at the underlying cause. For example, PID should be treated with antibiotics as described below. If pain symptoms are marked or prolonged or unresponsive to medical management, diagnostic laparoscopy may be warranted. Definitive surgery depends on the intraoperative findings and the underlying etiology. For example, adenomyosis or endometriosis may respond to hormonal approaches, but if those are unsuccessful, hysterectomy remains the definitive treatment of choice for patients for whom childbearing is not a consideration.

4. Chronic Pelvic Pain

Chronic pelvic pain is generally defined as noncyclic pain in the pelvic area that has persisted for 3 to 6 months or longer and is unrelated to pregnancy. It is a common gynecologic condition accounting for 20% of all gynecologic referrals. There are multiple potential causes and contributing factors. A stepwise approach is needed to identify and treat all possible causes of the pain. A thorough history that includes timing of onset, duration, location, and any alleviating or aggravating factors may assist in diagnosis. The physical exam should include a systematic evaluation of the pelvic structures to identify the source of pain, including the bladder, bowel, pelvic musculature, and gynecologic organs. Imaging may be helpful if a mass is suspected on exam. Management will depend on the underlying etiology of the pain.

When to Refer

- Standard therapy fails to relieve pain.
- Suspicion of pelvic pathology, such as endometriosis, leiomyomas, adenomyosis, or PID.

As-Sanie S et al. Endometriosis: a review. JAMA. 2025;334:64. [PMID: 40323608]

Horne AW et al. Pathophysiology, diagnosis, and management of endometriosis. BMJ. 2022;379:e070750. [PMID: 36375827]

Meisenheimer ES et al. Chronic pelvic pain in women: evaluation and treatment. Am Fam Physician. 2025;111:218. [PMID: 40106288]

Moïse A et al. Endometriosis and infertility: Gynecological examination practical guide. J Clin Med. 2025;14:1904. [PMID: 40142712]

Schroll JB et al. Combined oral contraceptive pill for primary dysmenorrhoea. Cochrane Database Syst Rev. 2023;7:CD002120. [PMID: 37523477]

Starzec-Proserpio M et al. Effectiveness of nonpharmacological conservative therapies for chronic pelvic pain in women: a systematic review and meta-analysis. Am J Obstet Gynecol. 2025;232:42. [PMID: 39142363]

PELVIC ORGAN PROLAPSE

General Considerations

Pelvic organ prolapse, including cystocele, rectocele, and enterocele, are vaginal hernias commonly seen in multiparous patients. **Cystocele** is a hernia of the bladder wall into the vagina, causing a soft anterior fullness. Cystocele may be accompanied by **urethrocele**, which is not a hernia but a prolapse of the urethra into the vagina. **Rectocele** is a herniation of the terminal rectum into the posterior vagina, causing a collapsible pouch-like fullness. **Enterocele** is a vaginal vault hernia containing small intestine, usually in the posterior vagina and resulting from a deepening of the rectouterine pouch. Two or all three types of hernia may occur in combination. The cause of pelvic organ prolapse is multifactorial. Risk factors include vaginal birth, genetic predisposition, advancing age, prior pelvic surgery, connective tissue disorders, and increased intra-abdominal pressure associated with obesity or straining associated with chronic constipation or coughing.

Clinical Findings

Symptoms of pelvic organ prolapse may include a sensation of a bulge or protrusion in the vagina, a sense of incomplete bladder or bowel emptying, and dyspareunia.

Treatment

Treatment depends on the extent of prolapse, associated symptoms, impact on the patient's quality of life, the patient's age, and desire to retain the uterus and preserve ability for coitus.

A. General Measures

Supportive measures include a high-fiber diet and laxatives to improve constipation. Weight reduction in patients with obesity and limitation of straining and heavy lifting are helpful. Pelvic muscle training (**Kegel exercises**) is a simple, noninvasive intervention that may improve pelvic function; it has demonstrated clear benefit for patients with urinary or fecal symptoms. **Pessaries** may reduce a cystocele, rectocele, or enterocele and are helpful in patients who do not wish to undergo surgery or who are poor surgical candidates.

B. Surgical Measures

The most common surgical procedure is vaginal or abdominal hysterectomy with additional attention to restoring apical support with a suspension procedure, such as by vaginal uterosacral suspension, sacrospinous fixation, or by abdominal sacral colpopexy. Since stress urinary incontinence and urinary retention may coexist with apical prolapse, patients should be evaluated for these conditions before surgery. *An anti-incontinence procedure may be done in conjunction with prolapse surgery if indicated.* Some procedures incorporate the use of surgical mesh. *Due to the finding of serious associated complications, in April 2019, the US FDA withdrew its approval of surgical mesh for the indication of transvaginal repair of pelvic organ prolapse.* Patients who previously have received transvaginal mesh for the surgical repair of pelvic organ prolapse and have no associated symptoms or complications should continue with their annual checkups and other routine follow-up care. They should let their clinician know that they have a surgical mesh implant, especially if they plan to have another pelvic surgery or related medical procedure. In addition, they should notify their clinician if they develop symptoms such as persistent vaginal bleeding or discharge, pelvic or groin pain, or dyspareunia.

Generally, surgical repair of pelvic organ prolapse is reserved until after completion of childbearing. If a patient with symptomatic prolapse desires pregnancy, the same procedures for vaginal suspension can be performed without hysterectomy, though limited data on pregnancy outcomes or prolapse outcomes are available. For older patients who do not desire coitus, colpocleisis (the partial obliteration of the vagina) is an effective and straightforward procedure. Uterine suspension with sacrospinous cervicocolpopexy may be an effective approach in older patients who wish to avoid hysterectomy but preserve coital function.

When to Refer

- Refer to urogynecologist or gynecologist for incontinence evaluation.
- Refer if nonsurgical therapy is ineffective.
- Refer for removal of mesh if symptoms develop.

Padoa A et al. Pelvic organ prolapse: current challenges and future perspectives. J Clin Med. 2025;14:7313. [PMID: 41156187]

PREMENSTRUAL SYNDROME

General Considerations

The **premenstrual syndrome (PMS)** *is a recurrent, variable cluster of troublesome physical and emotional symptoms that develop during the 5 days before the onset of menses and subside within 4 days after menstruation begins.* PMS intermittently affects about 40% of all premenopausal patients, primarily those 25–40 years of age. In about 5–8% of those affected, the syndrome may be severe. Although not every patient experiences all the symptoms or signs at one time, many describe bloating, breast pain, headache, swelling, irritability, aggressiveness, depression, inability to concentrate, libido change, lethargy, and food cravings. When emotional or mood symptoms predominate, along with physical symptoms, and there is a clear functional impairment with work or personal relationships, the term **"premenstrual dysphoric disorder" (PMDD)** may be applied. The pathogenesis of PMS/PMDD is still uncertain, and treatment methods are mainly empiric. The clinician should provide support for both the patient's emotional and physical distress, including the following:

1. Careful evaluation of the patient, with understanding, explanation, and reassurance.
2. Advise to keep a daily diary of all symptoms for 2–3 months, such as the **Daily Record of Severity of Problems**, to evaluate the timing and characteristics of symptoms. If symptoms occur throughout the month rather than in the 2 weeks before menses, the patient may have depression or other mental health diagnosis instead of or in addition to PMS or PMDD.

Treatment

For mild to moderate symptoms, a program of aerobic exercise; reduction of caffeine, salt, and alcohol intake; and use of alternative therapies, such as acupuncture and herbal treatments with *Vitex agnus-castus* (chasteberry) have some data to support their use. However, there are no US FDA-approved herbal treatments for premenstrual symptoms.

Medications that prevent ovulation, such as hormonal contraceptives, may lessen physical symptoms. This includes continuous use of combined hormonal contraceptive (CHC) methods (pill, patch, or vaginal ring). The drospirenone and 20 mcg ethinyl estradiol contraceptive pill (commercial name Yaz) is US FDA-approved for PMDD.

When mood disorders predominate, several SSRIs have been shown to be effective in relieving tension, irritability, and dysphoria with few side effects. First-line medication therapy includes serotonergic antidepressants (citalopram, escitalopram, fluoxetine, sertraline, venlafaxine) either daily or only on symptom days. Fluoxetine, paroxetine, and sertraline are US FDA-approved for PMDD.

GnRH agonist with "add-back" therapy (eg, oral estradiol 1 mg daily with oral micronized progesterone 100 mg daily or an equivalent regimen used for menopausal hormone therapy) is an alternative second-line option in patients who do not respond to CHCs or SSRIs. Cognitive behavioral therapy may also provide some benefit.

ACOG. Management of premenstrual disorders: ACOG Clinical Practice Guideline No. 7. Obstetrics & Gynecology. 2023;142:1516. [PMID: 37973069]

Ciccone N et al. The pharmacotherapeutic management of premenstrual dysphoric disorder. Expert Opin Pharmacother. 2023;24:145. [PMID: 35974667]

MENOPAUSE

See Chapter 20, Women's Health Issues.

POLYCYSTIC OVARY SYNDROME

ESSENTIALS OF DIAGNOSIS

- Clinical or biochemical evidence of hyperandrogenism.
- Oligoovulation or anovulation.
- Polycystic ovaries on ultrasonography.

General Considerations

Polycystic ovary syndrome (PCOS), increasingly referred to as "Polyendocrine Metabolic Ovarian Syndrome (PMOS)", is a common endocrine disorder of unknown etiology affecting 5–10% of those of reproductive age. The **Rotterdam Criteria**, endorsed by the National Institutes of Health, identifies *hyperandrogenism, ovulatory dysfunction, and polycystic ovaries as the key diagnostic features of the disorder in adult menstruating persons*; at least two of these features must be present for diagnosis.

Clinical Findings

PCOS often presents as a menstrual disorder (ranging from amenorrhea to heavy menstrual bleeding) and infertility. Skin disorders due to peripheral androgen excess, including hirsutism and acne, are common. Patients may also show signs of insulin resistance and hyperinsulinemia, with increased risk for early-onset type 2 diabetes mellitus and metabolic syndrome. *Unrecognized or untreated PCOS is a risk factor for CVD.* In addition, prolonged anovulation increases long-term risk of endometrial cancer secondary to chronic exposure to unopposed estrogen. Patients who do become pregnant are at increased risk for perinatal complications, such as gestational diabetes and preeclampsia.

Differential Diagnosis

Anovulation in the reproductive years may also be due to (1) primary ovarian insufficiency (high FSH, low estradiol); (2) functional hypothalamic amenorrhea, often associated with rapid weight loss or extreme physical exertion (low to normal FSH for age); (3) discontinuation of hormonal contraceptives (return to ovulation typically occurs within 90 days); (4) pituitary adenoma with elevated prolactin (galactorrhea may or may not be present); and (5) hyperthyroidism or hypothyroidism. To rule out other etiologies in patients with suspected PCOS, serum FSH, estradiol, prolactin, hCG, and TSH should be evaluated. *Because of the high risk of insulin resistance and dyslipidemia, all patients with confirmed PCOS should have diabetes and lipid screening.* Patients with clinical evidence of androgen excess should have total testosterone and a morning, early follicular phase 17-hydroxyprogesterone measured. Patients with stigmata of Cushing syndrome should have a 24-hour urinary free cortisol or a low-dose dexamethasone suppression test. Congenital adrenal hyperplasia and androgen-secreting adrenal tumors also tend to have high circulating androgen levels and anovulation with polycystic ovaries; these disorders must also be ruled out in patients with presumed PCOS and high serum androgens.

Treatment

In patients with PCOS and obesity, weight reduction and exercise are often effective in reversing the metabolic effects and inducing ovulation. For patients who do not respond to weight loss and exercise and do not desire pregnancy, combined hormonal contraceptives are first-line treatment to manage hyperandrogenism and menstrual irregularities. Intermittent or continuous progestin therapy or a hormonal IUD may be used for endometrial protection in patients who cannot or choose not to use combined hormonal contraceptives. Metformin therapy may be used as a second-line therapy to improve menstrual function. Metformin has little or no benefit in the treatment of hirsutism, acne, or infertility, however. Contraceptive counseling should be offered to prevent unplanned pregnancy in case of a return of ovulatory cycles. For patients who are seeking pregnancy and remain anovulatory, letrozole (first line), clomiphene, or other medications can be used for ovarian stimulation (see section on Infertility below). Patients with PCOS have increased risk for multiple gestation with ovarian stimulation.

If hirsutism does not improve after 6 months of treatment with combined hormonal contraceptives, an antiandrogen, such as spironolactone, may be added. Topical eflornithine cream applied to affected facial areas twice daily for 6 months may be helpful in most women. Hirsutism may also be managed with depilatory creams, electrolysis, and laser therapy. The combination of laser therapy and topical eflornithine may be particularly effective.

Weight loss, exercise, and treatment of unresolved metabolic derangements are important in preventing CVD. *Patients with PCOS should be managed aggressively and should have regular monitoring of lipid profiles and glucose.* Patients who are unable to reduce body weight with lifestyle modifications may benefit from use of GLP-1 receptor agonists to lower body weight, improve metabolic parameters, and normalize menstrual cycles.

When to Refer

- If expertise in diagnosis is needed.
- If patient is infertile.

Alesi S et al. Efficacy and safety of anti-androgens in the management of polycystic ovary syndrome: a systematic review and meta-analysis of randomised controlled trials. EClinicalMedicine. 2023;63:102162. Erratum in: EClinicalMedicine. 2024;79:103009. [PMID: 37583655]
Bader S et al. A systematic review of GLP-1 on anthropometrics, metabolic and endocrine parameters in patients with PCOS. Womens Health (Lond). 2024;20:17455057241234530. [PMID: 38444070]
Christ JP et al. Current guidelines for diagnosing PCOS. Diagnostics (Basel). 2023;13:1113. [PMID: 36980421]
Huddleston HG et al. Diagnosis and treatment of polycystic ovary syndrome. JAMA. 2022;327:274. [PMID: 35040896]

INFERTILITY

A couple is said to be infertile if pregnancy does not result after 1 year of penile-vaginal intercourse without contraception. Up to 20% of couples experience infertility in their reproductive lives; the incidence of infertility increases with age, with a decline in fertility beginning in the early 30s and accelerating in the late 30s. Couples in which the woman is younger than 35 years who do not achieve pregnancy within 1 year of trying may be candidates for infertility treatment, and within 6 months for women aged ≥ 35 years. *The male partner contributes to about 40% of cases of infertility,* and a combination of factors is common.

A. Initial Testing

During the initial interview, the clinician can present an overview of infertility and discuss an evaluation and management plan (including information about adoption, when appropriate). Private consultations with each partner separately are then conducted. Pertinent details (eg, sexually transmitted infection history or prior pregnancies) should be obtained. The ill effects of cigarettes, alcohol, and other illicit or non-prescribed drugs (eg, anabolic steroids and opiates) on fertility should be discussed. Prescription medications that impair male potency and factors that may lead to scrotal hyperthermia, such as tight underwear or frequent use of saunas or hot tubs, should be discussed. The gynecologic history should include the menstrual pattern, the use and types of contraceptives, frequency and success of coitus, and correlation of intercourse with time of ovulation.

General physical and genital examinations are performed on the pregnancy capable partner. Basic laboratory studies include assessment of **ovarian reserve** (eg, antimüllerian hormone, day 3 FSH and estradiol) and thyroid function tests. If the patient has regular menses with moliminal (late luteal phase) symptoms, the likelihood of ovulatory cycles is very high. *A luteal phase serum progesterone above 3 ng/mL establishes ovulation.* Couples should be advised that coitus resulting in conception occurs during the 6-day window before the day of ovulation. Ovulation predictor kits have largely replaced basal body temperatures for predicting ovulation, but temperature charting may be used to identify most fertile days. Basal body temperature charts cannot predict ovulation; they can only retrospectively confirm that ovulation occurred.

A semen analysis should be completed to rule out male factor infertility (see Chapter 26).

B. Further Testing

1. Gross deficiencies of sperm (number, motility, or appearance) require a repeat confirmatory analysis.
2. A screening pelvic ultrasound and hysterosalpingography to identify uterine cavity or tubal anomalies should be performed. **Hysterosalpingography** is performed within 3 days following the menstrual period. This radiographic study will demonstrate uterine abnormalities (septa, polyps, submucous myomas) and tubal obstruction. Patients who have had prior PID or abnormal tubes seen on hysterosalpingography or laparoscopy should receive antibiotic prophylaxis with doxycycline, 100 mg orally twice daily for 5 days.
3. Absent or infrequent ovulation requires additional laboratory evaluation. Elevated FSH and low estradiol and antimüllerian hormone levels indicate ovarian insufficiency. Patients with elevated prolactin levels should be evaluated for pituitary adenoma. Patients aged ≥ 35 years may require further assessment of ovarian reserve. *A markedly elevated FSH (> 15–20 IU/L) on day 3 of the menstrual cycle suggests inadequate ovarian reserve.* Although less widely performed, a **clomiphene citrate challenge test**, with measurement of FSH on day 10 after administration of clomiphene from days 5–9, can help confirm a diagnosis of diminished ovarian reserve. The number of antral follicles during the early follicular phase of the cycle can provide useful information about ovarian reserve and can confirm serum testing. An antimüllerian hormone level can be measured at any time during the menstrual cycle.
4. If all the above testing is normal, **unexplained infertility** is diagnosed.

Treatment

A. Medical Measures

Fertility may be restored by treatment of endocrine abnormalities, particularly hypothyroidism or hyperthyroidism. Patients who are anovulatory because of low body weight or exercise may become ovulatory when they gain weight or decrease their exercise levels; conversely, patients with obesity who are anovulatory may become ovulatory with loss of even 5–10% of body weight.

B. Surgical Measures

Excision of ovarian tumors or ovarian foci of endometriosis can improve fertility. Microsurgical relief of tubal obstruction due to salpingitis or tubal ligation will reestablish fertility in many cases, although with severe disease or proximal obstruction, **in vitro fertilization (IVF)** is preferable. Peritubal adhesions or endometriotic implants often can be treated via laparoscopy.

In a male with a varicocele, sperm characteristics may be improved following surgical treatment. For men who have sperm production but obstructive azoospermia, trans-epidermal sperm aspiration or microsurgical epidermal sperm aspiration has been successful.

C. Induction of Ovulation

Induction of ovulation may be performed in combination with **intrauterine insemination**, in which washed ejaculated sperm are injected directly into the upper uterine cavity using a small catheter threaded through the cervix, for patients with oligoovulation/anovulation or unexplained infertility.

1. Clomiphene citrate—Clomiphene citrate stimulates gonadotropin release, especially FSH. It acts as a selective estrogen receptor modulator, similar to tamoxifen and raloxifene, and binds to the estrogen receptor. A low level of estrogen decreases the negative feedback on the hypothalamus, thereby stimulating GnRH, and increasing the release of FSH and LH from the anterior pituitary. When FSH and LH are present in the appropriate amounts and timing, ovulation occurs.

After a normal menstrual period or induction of withdrawal bleeding with progestin, clomiphene 50 mg orally should be given daily for 5 days, typically on days 3–7 of the cycle. If ovulation does not occur, the clomiphene dosage is increased to 100 mg orally daily for 5 days. While doses of 150 mg may be used, doses > 100 mg do not appear to improve clinical pregnancy rates. The rate of ovulation following clomiphene treatment is approximately 80% in the absence of other infertility factors. The pregnancy rate is 30–40%, and twinning occurs in about 7% of these pregnancies. Three or more fetuses are rare (< 0.5% of cases). Pregnancy is most likely to occur within the first three ovulatory cycles and unlikely to occur after cycle 6. In addition, several studies have suggested a twofold to threefold increased *risk of ovarian cancer* with the use of clomiphene for more than 1 year, so treatment with clomiphene is usually limited to a maximum of six cycles.

2. Letrozole—Available data suggest that the *aromatase inhibitor letrozole is more effective than clomiphene for induction of ovulation in women with PCOS.* There is a reduced risk of multiple pregnancy, a lack of antiestrogenic effects, and a reduced need for ultrasound monitoring. The dose of letrozole is 2.5–7.5 mg daily, starting on day 3 of the menstrual cycle. In patients who have a history of estrogen-dependent tumors, such as breast cancer, letrozole is preferred over other agents because the estrogen levels with this medication are much lower.

3. Human menopausal gonadotropins (hMG) or recombinant FSH—hMG or recombinant FSH is indicated in cases of hypogonadotropism and most other types of anovulation resistant to clomiphene treatment. Because of the complexities, laboratory tests, and expense associated with this treatment, these patients should be referred to an infertility specialist.

D. Artificial Insemination in Azoospermia

If azoospermia is present, artificial insemination by a donor usually results in pregnancy, assuming female function is normal. *Using frozen sperm provides the opportunity for screening for sexually transmitted infections, including HIV infection.*

E. Assisted Reproductive Technology (ART)

Couples who have not responded to traditional infertility treatments and those with occlusive tubal disease, severe endometriosis, oligospermia, immunologic, or unexplained infertility, may benefit from ART. All ART procedures involve ovarian stimulation to produce multiple oocytes, oocyte retrieval by transvaginal ultrasound–guided needle aspiration, and handling of the oocytes outside the body. With **IVF**, the eggs are fertilized in vitro and the embryos transferred to the uterus. **Intracytoplasmic sperm injection** allows fertilization with a single sperm. While originally intended for couples with male factor infertility, it is now used in two-thirds of all IVF procedures in the United States.

The chance of a multiple gestation pregnancy (ie, twins, triplets) is increased in all assisted reproductive procedures, increasing the risk of preterm delivery and other pregnancy complications. However, the increasing use of single embryo transfer has resulted in far fewer multiple births from ART.

Prognosis

The prognosis for conception and normal pregnancy depends on the underlying cause. In the absence of identifiable causes of infertility, 60% of couples will achieve a spontaneous pregnancy within 3 years.

When to Refer

Refer to a reproductive endocrinologist if ART is indicated or surgery is required.

Santoro N et al. Infertility evaluation and treatment. N Engl J Med. 2025;392:1111. [PMID: 40073310]

World Health Organization Guideline Development Group for Infertility et al. Recommendations from the WHO guideline for the prevention, diagnosis, and treatment of infertility. Hum Reprod. 2026;41:25. [PMID: 41312724]

CONTRACEPTION & FAMILY PLANNING

Unintended pregnancies are a worldwide problem but disproportionately impact developing countries. There were 121 million unintended pregnancies annually from 2015 to 2019, corresponding to a global rate of 64 per 1000 women aged 15–49; 61% of these cases resulted in an abortion. In middle- and high-income countries, the unintended pregnancy rate fell by 21% from 1990–1994 to 2015–2019, whereas it fell by 18% in low-income countries over this time frame. Annual average unintended pregnancy rates in the United States were estimated at 35 per 1000 during 2015–2019. It is important for clinicians to educate their patients about the benefits of contraception and to provide options that are appropriate and desirable for the patient. The WHO and the CDC provide medical eligibility criteria based on a patient's medical condition. Additionally, patients who are not in mutually monogamous relationships should use condoms for protection from STIs.

1. Oral Contraceptives

A. Combined Oral Contraceptives

1. Efficacy and methods of use—Combined (estrogen and progestin) oral contraceptives have a perfect use failure rate of 0.3% and a typical use failure rate of 8%. *Their primary mode of action is suppression of ovulation.* The pills can be started on the first day of the menstrual cycle, the first Sunday after the onset of the cycle, or on any day of the cycle. If started more than 5 days after the first day of the cycle, a backup method should be used for the first 7 days. If an active pill is missed at any time, and no intercourse occurred in the past 5 days, two pills should be taken immediately, and a backup method should be used for 7 days. If intercourse occurred in the previous 5 days, emergency contraception should be offered. A backup method should be used for 7 days.

2. Benefits of oral contraceptives—Noncontraceptive benefits of oral contraceptives include lighter menses and improvement of dysmenorrhea, decreased risk of ovarian and endometrial cancer, and improvement in acne. Functional ovarian cysts are less likely with oral contraceptive use. There is also a beneficial effect on bone mass.

3. Selection of an oral contraceptive—*Any of the combination oral contraceptives containing ≤ 35 mcg of ethinyl estradiol, 3 mg of estradiol valerate, or 14.2 mg of estetrol are suitable for most women.* There is some variation in potency of the various progestins in the pills, but there are essentially no clinically significant differences for most patients among the progestins in the low-dose pills. There is insufficient evidence that triphasic oral contraceptives provide any benefit compared to monophasic oral contraceptives in terms of effectiveness, bleeding patterns, or discontinuation rates. Therefore, *monophasic pills are recommended as a first choice for patients starting oral contraceptive use.* Patients with acne or hirsutism may benefit from treatment with desogestrel, drospirenone, or norgestimate since they are the least androgenic progestins. Pills are typically packaged in 21- or 28-day cyclic regimens but may be taken continuously to allow the user to decide if and when to have a withdrawal bleed. *Studies have shown no significant risk from long-term amenorrhea in patients taking continuous oral contraceptives.* The low-dose oral contraceptives commonly used in the United States are listed in Table 21–2.

4. Drug interactions—Several medications interact with oral contraceptives potentially decreasing their efficacy, typically by inducing microsomal enzymes in the liver. Some commonly prescribed medications in this category are phenytoin, phenobarbital (and other barbiturates), primidone, topiramate, carbamazepine, rifampin, and St. John's wort. Patients taking these medications should use another means of contraception for maximum efficacy.

Antiretroviral medications, specifically ritonavir-boosted protease inhibitors, may significantly decrease the efficacy of combined oral contraceptives. Other antiretrovirals, such as nonnucleoside reverse transcriptase inhibitors, have smaller effects on oral contraceptive efficacy.

5. Contraindications and adverse effects—Oral contraceptives have been associated with several adverse effects; they are contraindicated with some conditions and should be used with caution in others (Table 21–3).

A. Myocardial infarction—*The risk of MI is higher with use of oral contraceptives in certain populations, but the risk attributable to oral contraceptives is low in reproductive age women.* Cigarette smoking, obesity, hypertension, diabetes mellitus, and hypercholesterolemia increase this risk. *People aged > 35 years who smoke cigarettes and patients with other cardiovascular risk factors should use other non-estrogen–containing methods of birth control.*

B. Thromboembolic disease—A three- to fivefold increased rate of VTE is found in oral contraceptive users, but the absolute risk is low (5–6 per 100,000 woman-years compared to a rate of 50–300 per 100,000 pregnancies). Several studies have reported a twofold increased risk in users of oral contraceptives containing the progestins gestodene (not available in the United States), drospirenone, or desogestrel, compared with women using oral contraceptives with levonorgestrel and norethindrone. *Users in whom thromboembolism develops should stop using oral contraceptives, as should those at increased risk for thromboembolism associated with surgery, fracture, serious injury, hypercoagulable condition, or immobilization.* Those with a known thrombophilia should not use estrogen-containing contraceptives.

C. Cerebrovascular disease—Overall, a small increased risk of hemorrhagic stroke and subarachnoid hemorrhage and a somewhat greater increased risk of thrombotic stroke have been found; smoking, hypertension, and age > 35 years are associated with increased risk. Users should stop using estrogen-containing contraceptives if such warning symptoms as severe headache, blurred or lost vision, or other transient neurologic disorders develop.

D. Carcinoma—*Oral contraceptives appear to be associated with minimal to no increased risk of breast cancer.* Patients with a family history of breast cancer or those who started oral contraceptive use at a young age are *not* at increased risk. Combination oral contraceptives *reduce* the risk of endometrial carcinoma by 40% after 2 years of use and 60% after ≥ 4 years of use. The risk of ovarian cancer is *reduced* by 30% with pill use for < 4 years, by 60% with pill use for 5–11 years, and by 80% with use for ≥ 12 years. Oral contraceptives have been associated with developing benign hepatocellular adenomas and peliosis hepatis (blood-filled cavities) (but not focal nodular hyperplasia or HCC); hepatocellular adenomas may rarely cause rupture of the liver, hemorrhage, and death. The risk of hepatocellular adenoma increases with higher dosage, longer duration of use, and older age.

E. Hypertension—*Oral contraceptives may cause hypertension in some users*; the risk is increased with longer duration of use and older age. Users in whom hypertension develops while using oral contraceptives should use other non-estrogen–containing contraceptive methods. However, *with regular blood pressure monitoring, nonsmokers*

Table 21–2. Commonly used low-dose oral contraceptives (listed within each category in order of increasing estrogen dose, except for Nextstellis and the Progestin-Only Pill category, which is in alphabetical order).

Name	Progestin	Estrogen (Ethinyl Estradiol, except as noted)
Combination		
Alesse[1,2]	0.1 mg levonorgestrel	20 mcg
Loestrin 1/20[1]	1 mg norethindrone acetate	20 mcg
Multiple brands with this combination available[1,2]	0.15 mg desogestrel	20 mcg
Yaz[1]	3 mg drospirenone	20 mcg
Loestrin 21 1.5/30[1]	1.5 mg norethindrone acetate	30 mcg
Low Ogestrel[1,2]	0.3 mg norgestrel	30 mcg
Levora[1,2]	0.15 mg levonorgestrel	30 mcg
Desogen[1,2]	0.15 mg desogestrel	30 mcg
Yasmin[1,2]	3 mg drospirenone	30 mcg
Brevicon[1,2]	0.5 mg norethindrone	35 mcg
Zovia 1/35[1,2]	1 mg ethynodiol diacetate	35 mcg
Multiple brands with this combination available[1,2]	1 mg norethindrone	35 mcg
Sprintec[1,2]	0.25 mg norgestimate	35 mcg
Gildagia[1] (not available in US)	0.4 mg norethindrone	35 mcg
Nextstellis	3 mg drospirenone	14.2 mg estetrol
Combination: Extended-Cycle		
LoSeasonique (91-day cycle)[1]	0.10 mg levonorgestrel (days 1–84)/0 mg levonorgestrel (days 85–91)	20 mcg (84 days)/10 mcg (7 days)
Amethyst (28-day pack)	90 mcg levonorgestrel	20 mcg
Seasonique (91-day cycle)[1]	0.15 mg levonorgestrel (days 1–84)/0 mg levonorgestrel (days 85–91)	30 mcg (84 days)/10 mcg (7 days)
Triphasic		
Estrostep[1]	1 mg norethindrone acetate (days 1–5) 1 mg norethindrone acetate (days 6–12) 1 mg norethindrone acetate (days 13–21)	20 mcg 30 mcg 35 mcg
Cyclessa[1]	0.1 mg desogestrel (days 1–7) 0.125 mg desogestrel (days 8–14) 0.15 mg desogestrel (days 15–21)	25 mcg
Tri-Lo-Estarylla[1,2]	0.18 mg norgestimate (days 1–7) 0.215 mg norgestimate (days 8–14) 0.25 mg norgestimate (days 15–21)	25 mcg
Trivora[1,2]	0.05 mg levonorgestrel (days 1–6) 0.075 mg levonorgestrel (days 7–11) 0.125 mg levonorgestrel (days 12–21)	30 mcg 40 mcg 30 mcg
Ortho-Novum 7/7/7[1,2]	0.5 mg norethindrone (days 1–7) 0.75 mg norethindrone (days 8–14) 1 mg norethindrone (days 15–21)	35 mcg
Tri Estarylla[1,2]	0.18 mg norgestimate (days 1–7) 0.215 mg norgestimate (days 8–14) 0.25 mg norgestimate (days 15–21)	35 mcg
Multiple brands with this combination available[1,2]	0.5 mg norethindrone (days 1–7) 1 mg norethindrone (days 8–16) 0.5 mg norethindrone (days 17–21)	35 mcg
Quadriphasic		
Natazia	2 mg dienogest (days 3–8) 3 mg dienogest (days 9–26)	Estradiol valerate 3/2/2/1 mg

(continued)

Table 21–2. Commonly used low-dose oral contraceptives (listed within each category in order of increasing estrogen dose, except for Nextstellis and the Progestin-Only Pill category, which is in alphabetical order). (continued)

Name	Progestin	Estrogen (Ethinyl Estradiol, except as noted)
Progestin-Only Pill		
Camila[1,2]	0.35 mg norethindrone to be taken continuously	None
Opill[3]	0.075 mg norgestrel to be taken continuously	None
Slynd	4 mg drospirenone (days 1–24)	None
Zelleta[2]	0.075 mg desogestrel to be taken continuously (not available in United States or Canada)	None

[1]Generic equivalent available.
[2]Multiple other brands available.
[3]Non-prescription oral contraceptive (US only).

with well-controlled mild hypertension may use oral contraceptives.

F. HEADACHE—Migraine or other vascular headaches may occur or worsen with pill use. If severe or frequent headaches develop while using this method, it should be discontinued. *Those with migraine headaches with aura should not use estrogen-containing oral contraceptives due to the increased risk of stroke.*

G. LACTATION—Combined oral contraceptives may impair the quantity of breast milk. Any effects on milk supply are small and are not associated with developmental abnormalities in infants. Combination oral contraceptives should not be started earlier than 4 weeks postpartum to allow for establishment of lactation and to avoid compounding the increased risk of postpartum thromboembolic disease. Progestin-only pills, levonorgestrel implants, and DMPA are alternatives with no adverse effects on milk supply.

Table 21–3. Contraindications to use of combined hormonal contraceptives (listed in alphabetical order within categories).

Absolute contraindications
Active hepatitis
Age ≥ 35 years and smoking ≥ 15 cigarettes daily
Cancer of the breast (known or suspected)
Estrogen-dependent cancer (known or suspected)
Hepatocellular adenoma (past or present)
Known thrombophilia
Migraine with aura
Pregnancy or < 21 days postpartum
Stroke or CAD (past or present)
Surgery or orthopedic injury requiring prolonged immobilization
Thrombophlebitis or thromboembolic disorders (past or present)
Uncontrolled hypertension
Undiagnosed abnormal vaginal bleeding
Relative contraindications
21 to < 30 days postpartum
30 to 42 days postpartum with risk factors for VTE Migraine without aura
Diabetes mellitus (with nephropathy/retinopathy, vascular disease, or > 20 years duration)
Heart or kidney disease
Hypertension
Symptomatic gallbladder disease

H. OBESITY—Traditionally, clinical trials evaluating oral contraceptives generally have only included participants of normal weight. Obesity is an independent risk factor for thromboembolic complications. However, *patients with obesity should not be denied effective contraception because of concerns about oral contraceptive complications or efficacy.* Evidence suggests that efficacy for most oral contraceptives is similar for individuals with obesity or overweight compared to individuals of normal weight. The oral contraceptive pill containing drospirenone/estetrol (commercial name Nextstellis) may have slightly decreased efficacy in those with a BMI > 30.

I. OTHER DISORDERS—Cholestatic jaundice may occur in patients taking birth control pills if they previously experienced it during pregnancy.

6. Minor side effects—Nausea and dizziness may occur in the first few months of pill use. Unscheduled spotting or breakthrough bleeding may occur; this may be helped by switching to a pill of slightly higher estrogen dosage. Missed menstrual periods may occur, especially with low-dose pills. A pregnancy test should be performed if pills have been skipped or an expected menstrual period is missed. Fluid retention may occur. Chloasma may occur, as in pregnancy, and is increased by exposure to sunlight.

B. Progestin-Only Pills

1. Efficacy and methods of use—A formulation containing 0.35 mg of norethindrone alone (minipill) is available in the United States. The efficacy is similar to that of combined oral contraceptives but *depends highly on consistent use* (eg, taking the pill within the same 3-hour window every day). The minipill is believed to prevent conception by causing thickening of the cervical mucus (making it hostile to sperm), by altering ovum transport (which may account for the slightly higher rate of ectopic pregnancy with these pills), and by inhibiting implantation. Ovulation is inhibited inconsistently with this method. The minipill is begun on the first day of a menstrual cycle and then taken continuously for as long as contraception is desired; there is no "placebo week." A progestin-only pill containing drospirenone 4 mg was approved by the US FDA in 2019, and a desogestrel-only pill is available in several countries outside the United States. A norgestrel-only pill was approved for over-the-counter use by the US FDA in 2023. Drospirenone, desogestrel, and norgestrel have longer half-lives than norethindrone, which allows for more forgiveness with the timing of administration. Their main mechanism of action is ovulation suppression.

2. Advantages—*The low dose of progestin and absence of estrogen make progestin-only pills safe for women with contraindications to estrogen therapy.* Because estrogen may decrease initial milk production during lactation, *progestin-only pills are an ideal choice for breastfeeding women.* They may be preferred by patients who want minimal doses of hormones and by patients who are over age 35. Progestin-only pills lack the cardiovascular side effects of combination pills.

3. Complications and contraindications—There are few contraindications to the progestin-only pill (ie, current breast cancer). Progestin-only pills typically should be avoided in patients with malabsorptive disease, current or past ischemic heart disease, and history of stroke. Progestin-only pill users often have bleeding irregularities (eg, prolonged flow, spotting, amenorrhea); such patients may need regular pregnancy tests if there is a concern about contraceptive effectiveness. Many of the absolute contraindications and relative contraindications listed in Table 21–3 apply to the progestin-only pills; however, the contraceptive benefit of progestin-only pills may outweigh the risks for patients who smoke, who are over age 35, or who have conditions such as DVT or superficial venous thrombosis or known thromboembolic disorders or diabetes mellitus with vascular disease. Minor side effects of combination oral contraceptives such as mild headache also may occur with progestin-only pills.

Bearak JM et al. Country-specific estimates of unintended pregnancy and abortion incidence: a global comparative analysis of levels in 2015-2019. BMJ Glob Health. 2022;7:e007151. [PMID: 35332057]
Lee A et al. Estetrol/Drospirenone: a review in oral contraception. Drugs. 2022;82:1117. Erratum in: Drugs. 2022;82:1341. [PMID: 35781795]

2. Contraceptive Injections & Implants (Long-Acting Progestins)

The **injectable progestin depot medroxyprogesterone acetate (DMPA)** is approved for contraceptive use in the United States. There has been extensive worldwide experience with this method over the past three decades. The medication is given as a deep intramuscular injection of 150 mg every 3 months and has a typical use failure rate of 4%. A subcutaneous preparation, containing 104 mg of DMPA is also available in the United States. Common side effects include irregular bleeding, amenorrhea, weight gain, and headache. It is associated with bone mineral loss that is reversible after discontinuation of the method. Users commonly have irregular bleeding initially and subsequently develop amenorrhea. Return to ovulation may be delayed after its discontinuation. Contraindications are similar to those for progestin-only pills.

A **single-rod, subdermal progestin implant, etonogestrel (Nexplanon)**, is approved for use in the United States. Nexplanon is a 40-mm by 2-mm rod containing 68 mg of the progestin etonogestrel that is inserted in the inner aspect of the nondominant arm. It is currently approved for use for 3 years, but data suggest it maintains effectiveness through 5 years. Hormone levels drop rapidly after removal, and there is no delay in the return of fertility. In clinical trials, there were no pregnancies reported through 3 years of use. Typical use failure is 0.1%. The side-effect profile is similar to that of progestin-only pills and DMPA. Irregular bleeding has been the most common reason for discontinuation.

Genazzani AR et al. Hormonal and natural contraceptives: a review on efficacy and risks of different methods for an informed choice. Gynecol Endocrinol. 2023;39:2247093. [PMID: 37599373]
Klein DA et al. Provision of quality contraceptive services: Updates from national guidelines. Am Fam Physician. 2025;112:176. [PMID: 40834374]
Nguyen AT et al. U.S. medical eligibility criteria for contraceptive use, 2024. MMWR Recomm Rep. 2024;73:1. [PMID: 39106314]
Ott MA et al; Committee on Adolescence. Contraceptive counseling and methods for adolescents: clinical report. Pediatrics. 2025;156:e2025072218. [PMID: 40518138]
Zuniga C et al. Effectiveness and efficacy rates of progestin-only pills: a comprehensive literature review. Contraception. 2023;119:109925. [PMID: 36535414]

3. Other Combined Hormonal Contraceptives

A **transdermal contraceptive patch** is available in two formulations. One delivers a daily dose of norelgestromin (150 mcg) and ethinyl estradiol (35 mcg) and measures 14 cm^2. The second delivers 120 mcg levonorgestrel and 30 mcg ethinyl estradiol daily and measures 20 cm^2. The patch is applied to the lower abdomen, upper torso, or buttock once a week for 3 consecutive weeks, followed by 1 week without the patch. It appears that the average steady-state concentration of ethinyl estradiol with the patch is approximately 60% higher than with a 35-mcg pill. However, there is no evidence for an increased incidence of estrogen-related side effects. The mechanism of action, side effects, and efficacy are similar to those associated with oral contraceptives, although compliance may be better. However, discontinuation due to side effects is more frequent. Neither patch is approved for individuals with BMI ≥ 30. The ethinyl estradiol/norelgestromin patch is contraindicated because of increased risk of VTE while the ethinyl estradiol/levonorgestrel patch is contraindicated due to lower efficacy for these users.

A **contraceptive vaginal ring** that releases 120 mcg of etonogestrel and 15 mcg of ethinyl estradiol daily (**NuvaRing**) is available. The ring is soft and flexible and is placed in the upper vagina for 3 weeks, removed, and replaced 1 week later, or can be removed and immediately replaced after 3 weeks for continuous use, similar to oral contraceptives. The **1-year reusable segesterone acetate/ethinyl estradiol vaginal ring (Annovera)** is worn for 3 weeks and removed for 1 week, and that pattern is repeated for a total of 13 cycles. The efficacy, mechanism of action, and systemic side effects of combined hormonal vaginal rings are similar to those associated with oral contraceptives. Ring users may experience increased vaginal discharge.

4. Intrauterine Devices

In the United States, the following IUDs are available: the **hormone (levonorgestrel)-releasing Mirena, Liletta, Kyleena**, and **Skyla** IUDs and the **copper-bearing TCu380A (Paragard) and Miudella.** The Miudella IUD was approved by the FDA in early 2025 and contains 175 mm^2 of copper compared to 380 mm^2 in the Paragard IUD. The mechanism of action of the copper IUD is thought to involve either spermicidal or inhibitory effects on sperm capacitation and transport. The hormonal IUDs' contraceptive effect is through thickening of cervical mucus and suppression of the endometrial lining. They may inhibit ovulation, but not reliably.

Skyla and Miudella are US FDA-approved for use for 3 years, Kyleena for 5 years, Liletta and Mirena for 8 years, and the TCu380A for 10 years. The hormonal IUDs have the advantage of reducing cramping and menstrual flow. The levonorgestrel 52-mg IUD is also US FDA-approved for the treatment (for up to 5 years) of heavy menstrual bleeding.

IUDs are highly effective, with failure rates similar to those achieved with permanent contraception. IUDs may be used in nulliparous women and adolescents. Hormonal IUDs may have a protective effect against upper tract infection similar to that of oral contraceptives.

A. Placement

IUD placement can be performed at any time during the menstrual cycle if pregnancy can be reasonably excluded. At the time of placement, screening for gonorrhea and chlamydia can be performed, but placement should not be delayed for results. All patients should be counseled regarding potential pain during placement and the risks, benefits, and alternatives of different options for pain management. Lidocaine (as paracervical block or topical) may help reduce pain during placement. IUDs can be safely placed in the immediate (within 10 minutes) postpartum and postabortal periods. Both types of IUDs (hormonal and copper-bearing) may be placed after vaginal delivery or prior to closure of the uterus at the time of cesarean delivery. Delayed postpartum placement is also acceptable. Placement immediately following abortion is acceptable if there is no sepsis.

B. Contraindications and Complications

Contraindications to use of IUDs are outlined in Table 21–4.

Table 21–4. Contraindications to IUD use (listed in alphabetical order within categories).

Absolute contraindications
Acute or subacute pelvic inflammatory disease or purulent cervicitis
Breast cancer (hormonal IUD)
Cervical, endometrial, or gestational trophoblastic neoplasia
Pregnancy
Significant anatomic abnormality of uterus
Unexplained uterine bleeding
Wilson disease or copper allergy (copper IUD)
Relative contraindications
Active liver disease (hormonal IUD)
Menorrhagia or severe dysmenorrhea (copper IUD)

1. Pregnancy—An IUD should not be placed in a pregnant uterus. If pregnancy occurs due to IUD failure, there is a greater chance of spontaneous pregnancy loss (spontaneous abortion/miscarriage) if the IUD is left in situ (50%) than if it is removed (25%). *People using an IUD who become pregnant should have the IUD removed if the string is visible.* An IUD can be removed at the time of abortion if that is desired. If the string is not visible and the patient wants to continue the pregnancy, the patient should be informed of the increased risk of pregnancy loss, infection, preterm birth, and abruption. They should be informed that any flu-like symptoms such as fever, myalgia, headache, or nausea warrant immediate medical attention for possible septic abortion. Since the risk of ectopic pregnancy is increased in patients who become pregnant with an IUD in situ, clinicians should search for adnexal masses in the setting of early pregnancy with an IUD in place and should always evaluate for adequate products of conception following abortion.

2. Pelvic infection—The risk of pelvic infection attributable to IUD placement is rare. The subsequent risk of pelvic infection appears to be primarily related to the risk of acquiring STIs.

3. Heavy menstrual bleeding or severe dysmenorrhea—The copper IUD can cause heavier menstrual periods, bleeding between periods, and more cramping, so it is generally not suitable for patients who already suffer from these problems. Alternatively, the levonorgestrel 52-mg IUD is approved by the US FDA to treat heavy menstrual bleeding. NSAIDs are also helpful in decreasing bleeding and pain in IUD users.

4. Complete or partial expulsion—Spontaneous expulsion of the IUD occurs in up to 10% of women during the first year of use. Any IUD should be removed if the body of the device can be seen or felt in the cervical os.

5. Missing IUD strings—If the transcervical string cannot be seen, this may signify unnoticed expulsion, perforation of the uterus with abdominal migration of the IUD, or simply retraction of the string into the cervical canal or uterus. Once pregnancy is ruled out, the clinician may probe for the IUD with sterile sound or forceps designed for IUD removal. If the IUD cannot be detected, pelvic ultrasound will demonstrate if the IUD is intrauterine. Alternatively, anteroposterior and lateral radiographs of the pelvis can evaluate for an extrauterine IUD. If the IUD is in the abdominal cavity, it should generally be removed by laparoscopy or laparotomy.

ACOG Committee Statement No. 21: Access to Contraception. Obstet Gynecol. 2025;146:e88. [PMID: 41100881]
Paradise SL et al. Evidence-based contraception: common questions and answers. Am Fam Physician. 2022;106:251. [PMID: 36126006]

5. Diaphragm & Cervical Cap

The **diaphragm (with a spermicidal gel)** is a safe and effective contraceptive method with features that make it acceptable to some users and not others. When positioned properly, it rests in the vagina behind the pubic bone anteriorly and in the posterior fornix posteriorly. Typical use failure is 17%. The advantages of this method are that it has no systemic side effects and gives significant protection against pelvic infection and cervical dysplasia as well as pregnancy. The disadvantages are that it must be inserted near the time of coitus and that pressure from the rim predisposes some users to cystitis after intercourse.

The **cervical cap (with a spermicidal gel)** is similar to the diaphragm but fits snugly over the cervix only. The cervical cap is more difficult to insert and remove than the diaphragm. The main advantages are that it can be used by patients who cannot be fitted for a diaphragm because of a relaxed anterior vaginal wall or because of repeated bladder infections stemming from diaphragm use. However, reported typical use failure rates are 14% in nulliparous women and 29% in parous women.

Because of the small risk of toxic shock syndrome, a cervical cap or diaphragm should not be left in the vagina for over 24 hours. The cervical cap should not be used during menses.

6. Contraceptive Foam, Cream, Film, Sponge, Jelly, & Suppository

These products are available without prescription, are easy to use, and have typical failure rates of 10–22%. All contain the spermicide **nonoxynol-9**, which also has some viricidal and bactericidal activity. The US FDA requires products containing nonoxynol-9 to include a warning that *the products do not protect against HIV or other STIs;* use of these products can irritate the vagina and rectum and may *increase* the risk of HIV acquisition from an infected partner. A different on-demand vaginal contraceptive, a vaginal pH regulator gel containing lactic acid–citric acid–potassium bitartrate (commercial name **Phexxi**), was US FDA-approved for use in the US in 2020; it requires a prescription. The supporting clinical trial estimated 27.5 pregnancies per 100 woman-years.

7. Condoms

The **male condom** of latex, polyurethane or animal membrane affords protection against pregnancy—equivalent to that of a diaphragm and spermicidal jelly; latex and polyurethane (but not animal membrane) condoms also offer protection against many STIs, including HIV. When a spermicide, such as vaginal foam, is used with the condom, perfect use failure rate is approximately 2% and typical use, 13%. The disadvantages of condoms are dulling of sensation and potential spillage of semen due to condom tearing or slipping, or leakage with detumescence of the penis. Latex condoms should not be used with oil-based lubricants since these can degrade the condom and make it less effective.

Two **female condoms**, one made of polyurethane and the other of synthetic nitrile, are available in the United States. The reported failure rates range from 5% to 21%; the efficacy is comparable to that of the diaphragm. *These are the only female-controlled method that offers significant protection against both pregnancy and STIs.*

8. Contraception Based on Awareness of Fertile Periods

These methods are most effective when the couple restricts intercourse to the post-ovulatory phase of the cycle or uses a barrier method at other times. Well-instructed, motivated couples may achieve low pregnancy rates with fertility awareness methods. Examples of some of these include monitoring cervical mucus changes, basal body temperature fluctuations, and menstrual cycle calculations to avoid having intercourse on fertile days. However, comparative efficacy trials of these methods against other contraceptive methods have not been performed.

9. Emergency Contraception

Emergency contraception can decrease the risk of pregnancy after intercourse but before the establishment of pregnancy. These methods should be started as soon as possible and *within 120 hours* after unprotected coitus: (1) Levonorgestrel, 1.5 mg orally as a single dose (available in the United States prepackaged as **Plan B** and available over the counter for persons aged ≥ 17 years), has a 1–3% failure rate when taken within 72 hours. It remains efficacious up to 120 hours after intercourse, though less so compared with earlier use, and is indicated for use within 72 hours. (2) If the levonorgestrel regimen is not available, a combination oral contraceptive containing ethinyl estradiol and levonorgestrel 1.5 mg given twice in 12 hours may be used. Used within 72 hours, the failure rate of these regimens is approximately 3%, but antinausea medication is often necessary. (3) Ulipristal acetate, a selective progesterone receptor modulator, taken orally as a single 30 mg dose, has been shown to be more effective than levonorgestrel, especially when used between 72 and 120 hours, particularly among patients with overweight and obesity. Patients should wait 5 days after taking ulipristal acetate to start or restart a hormonal contraceptive method and use backup contraception for a week or until the next menses. (4) Copper or levonorgestrel 52-mg IUD placement within 5 days after one episode of unprotected midcycle coitus will also prevent pregnancy. Copper IUD use for emergency contraception is the most effective available method, with first cycle pregnancy rates of 0.1%. *All survivors of sexual violence should be offered emergency contraception.*

Li RHW et al. Oral emergency contraception with levonorgestrel plus piroxicam: a randomised double-blind placebo-controlled trial. Lancet. 2023;402:851. Erratum in: Lancet. 2023;402:850. [PMID: 37597523]
Salcedo J et al. Society of Family Planning Clinical Recommendation: emergency contraception. Contraception. 2023;121:109958. [PMID: 36693445]
Teal S et al. Contraception selection, effectiveness, and adverse effects: a review. JAMA. 2021;326:2507. [PMID: 34962522]

10. Permanent Contraception

In the United States, permanent contraception is the most commonly used method of birth control for couples who do not want more children. Although reversible in some instances, reversal surgery for both women and men is costly, complicated, and not always successful. Therefore, *patients should be counseled carefully regarding permanence of the procedure.*

Female permanent contraception procedures include **laparoscopic bipolar electrocoagulation, salpingectomy, plastic ring application on the uterine tubes**, or **minilaparotomy with tubal resection**. Salpingectomy may be preferred for the added benefit of decreasing ovarian cancer risk. The advantages of laparoscopy are minimal postoperative pain, small incisions, and rapid recovery. The advantages of minilaparotomy are that it can be performed with standard surgical instruments under local or general anesthesia. However, there is more postoperative pain and a longer recovery period. The cumulative 10-year failure rate for all methods combined is 1.85%, varying from 0.75% for postpartum partial salpingectomy and laparoscopic unipolar coagulation to 3.65% for spring clips; this fact should be discussed with patients preoperatively. Some studies have found an increased risk of menstrual irregularities as a long-term complication of tubal ligation, but findings in different studies have been inconsistent.

Male permanent contraception by vasectomy is a safe, simple procedure in which the vas deferens is severed and sealed through a scrotal incision under local anesthesia. Failure rate is reported at 1 in 2000. See also Chapter 26.

When to Refer

Refer to experienced clinicians for etonogestrel subdermal (Nexplanon) placement, IUD placement, tubal occlusion or ligation, or vasectomy.

Fang NZ et al. Female permanent contraception trends and updates. Am J Obstet Gynecol. 2022;226:773. [PMID: 34973178]

11. Abortion

When the procedure of abortion was legalized in the United States in 1973 under the *Roe v. Wade* US Supreme Court decision, the related maternal mortality rate fell markedly because illegal and self-induced abortions were replaced by safer procedures. Abortions in the first trimester of pregnancy are performed by vacuum aspiration under local anesthesia or with medical regimens. Dilation and evacuation, a variation of vacuum aspiration, is generally used in the second trimester. Techniques utilizing intra-amniotic instillation of hypertonic saline solution or various prostaglandin regimens, along with medical or osmotic dilators, are occasionally used after 18 weeks. Several medical abortion regimens using mifepristone and multiple doses of misoprostol have been reported as being effective in the second trimester. Overall, legal abortion in the United States has a mortality rate of < 1:100,000. In 2022, the *Dobbs v. Jackson Women's Health Organization* decision overturned the 1973 US Supreme Court decision and held that the Constitution does not confer a right to abortion. This has left the legality of abortion at the state level and has resulted in various states enacting abortion bans and others blocking such bans. Since the *Dobbs* decision, although abortion has been restricted or banned in many states, a small but consistent *increase* in the national monthly number of abortions has been seen, thought to be driven at least in part by the availability of *abortion services remotely via telehealth*. Yet, an analysis of mortality rates by state abortion restriction level following the *Dobbs* decision found that an increasing number of restrictive abortion laws was associated with increasing maternal and infant mortality, and the presence of a trigger law (a law banning abortion after the *Dobbs decision)* was significantly associated with increased all-cause mortality in reproductive-aged women, maternal mortality, and infant mortality. *Clinicians need to be aware of laws regarding availability of abortion in the jurisdiction of their practice.*

Complications resulting from abortion may include retained products of conception (often associated with infection and heavy bleeding), uterine perforation, and unrecognized ectopic pregnancy. Immediate analysis of the removed tissue for products of conception can exclude or corroborate the diagnosis of ectopic pregnancy. Women who have fever, bleeding, or abdominal pain after abortion should be examined; use of broad-spectrum antibiotics and reaspiration of the uterus are frequently necessary. Hospitalization is advisable if postabortal endometritis requires administration of intravenous antibiotics. Patients undergoing self-managed abortion may need emergency care for hemorrhage, septic shock, or uterine perforation.

Prophylactic antibiotics are recommended before surgical abortion; for example, a single dose of doxycycline 200 mg orally can be given 1 hour before the procedure. Rh immune globulin should be given to Rh-negative women following abortion at or beyond 12 weeks' gestation. Contraception should be thoroughly discussed and provided at the time of abortion, including the option of immediate postabortal IUD placement.

Mifepristone (RU 486) is approved by the US FDA as an oral abortifacient at a dose of 200 mg orally on day 1, followed by misoprostol 800 mcg buccally 24–48 hours later. The WHO recommended regimen includes mifepristone orally followed by misoprostol vaginally, sublingually, or buccally. These combinations are 93% successful in terminating pregnancies of up to 70 days' gestation with few complications. There is a 5–10% risk of incomplete abortion requiring curettage and approximately 1% risk of requiring intervention for excessive bleeding. Overall, the risk of uterine infection is lower with medical than with surgical abortion.

ACOG Clinical Practice Update: Rh D immune globulin administration after abortion or pregnancy loss at less than 12 weeks of gestation. Obstet Gynecol. 2024;144:e140. [PMID: 39255498]

Harper LM et al. All-cause mortality in reproductive-aged females by state: an analysis of the effects of abortion legislation. Obstet Gynecol. 2023;141:236. [PMID: 36318777]

Roth LM et al. Undue burdens: state abortion laws in the United States, 1994–2022. J Health Polit Policy Law. 2023;48:511. [PMID: 36693181]

Society of Family Planning #WeCount report. October 22, 2024. https://societyfp.org/research/wecount/. Accessed February 11, 2026.

Stein RA et al. The far-reaching impact of abortion bans: reproductive care and beyond. Eur J Contracept Reprod Health Care. 2023;28:23. [PMID: 36369860]

FEMALE SEXUAL DYSFUNCTION

General Considerations

Female sexual dysfunction is common and is defined as a sexual problem causing *personal distress in one or more of the following domains: desire, arousal, orgasm, or pain.* Depending on the questions asked, surveys have shown that from 35% to 98% of women report sexual concerns. Questions related to sexual functioning should be asked as part of the routine medical history. Three helpful questions to broach the topic are "*Are you currently involved in a sexual relationship?*," "*With men, women, or both?*," and "*Do you have any sexual concerns or any pain with sex?*" If not involved in a sexual relationship, the patient should be asked if there are any concerns that are contributing to a lack of sexual behavior. If a history of sexual dysfunction is elicited, a complete history of factors that may affect sexual function should be taken. These factors include reproductive history (including pregnancies and mode of delivery) as well as history of infertility, STI, rape or sexual violence, gynecologic or urologic disorders, endocrine abnormalities (such as diabetes mellitus or thyroid disease), neurologic problems, CVD, psychiatric disease and pharmacologic treatment, as well as over-the-counter, illicit, and non-prescribed drug use. A detailed history of the specific sexual dysfunction should be elicited, and a gynecologic examination should focus on findings that may contribute to sexual complaints.

Etiology

A. Disorders of Sexual Desire

Sexual desire in women is a complex and poorly understood phenomenon. Relationship conflict, fear or anxiety related to previous sexual encounters, or history of sexual abuse or violence may contribute to a lack of desire. Physical factors such as chronic illness, fatigue, depression, and specific medical disorders (such as diabetes mellitus, thyroid disease, or adrenal insufficiency) may also contribute. Menopause and attitudes toward aging may play a role. In addition, sexual desire may be influenced by other sexual dysfunction, such as arousal disorders, dyspareunia, or anorgasmia.

B. Sexual Arousal Disorders

Sexual arousal disorders may be both subjective and objective. Sexual stimulation normally leads to genital vasocongestion and lubrication. Some patients may have a physiologic response to sexual stimuli but may not subjectively feel aroused because of factors such as distractions, negative expectations, anxiety, fatigue, depression, or medications, such as SSRIs or oral contraceptives. Others with vaginal atrophy may lack both a subjective and physiologic response to sexual stimuli.

C. Orgasmic Disorders

Despite subjective and physiologic arousal, patients may experience a marked delay in orgasm, diminished sensation of an orgasm, or anorgasmia. The etiology of orgasmic disorders is complex and typically multifactorial, but the cause of a particular patient's orgasmic disorder is usually amenable to treatment.

D. Sexual Pain Disorder

Female sexual dysfunction can include persistent or recurrent challenges with pain, including (1) pain with vaginal penetration, (2) vulvovaginal or pelvic pain during genital contact, (3) marked fear or anxiety about vulvovaginal or pelvic pain in anticipation of, during, or as a result of genital contact, or (4) marked hypertonicity or overactivity of pelvic floor muscles with or without genital contact (ie, vaginismus). Other medical causes of sexual pain may include vulvovaginitis; vulvar disease, including lichen planus, lichen sclerosus, and lichen simplex chronicus; pelvic disease, such as endometriosis or chronic PID; or vulvovaginal atrophy (associated with genitourinary syndrome of menopause or lactation).

Treatment

A. Disorders of Sexual Interest/Arousal

Low libido is the most common sexual problem for females. *In the absence of specific medical disorders, the focus of therapy is psychological.* Cognitive behavioral therapy, sexual therapy, and couples therapy may all play a role. Two pharmacologic treatments, bremelanotide and flibanserin, have been approved by the US FDA for treatment of **hypoactive sexual desire** in premenopausal women. Bremelanotide (Vyleesi), a melanocortin receptor agonist, is given as 1.75 mg subcutaneously at least 45 minutes before sexual activity. Flibanserin (Addyi), a centrally acting serotonin receptor agonist/antagonist, is a pill used daily; however, to be effective, it must be used long term and cannot be taken within 2 hours of alcohol consumption or in combination with CYP3A4 inhibitors. While not US FDA-approved, the use of bupropion and testosterone, with or without estrogen, also has shown success. There are no available testosterone preparations for females in the United States; typical prescribing approach includes use of topical testosterone cream or gel applied in approximately one-tenth of the male prescribed dose. The phosphodiesterase inhibitors used in men do *not* appear to benefit most women with sexual arousal disorders. However, there is evidence to suggest a role for sildenafil in women with sexual dysfunction due to multiple sclerosis, type 1 diabetes mellitus, and spinal cord injury.

B. Orgasmic Disorders

For many women, counseling or sex therapy may be adequate treatment. Vibrators and an US FDA-cleared vacuum device (Eros therapy system) increase clitoral blood flow and may improve the likelihood of orgasm.

C. Sexual Pain Disorders

Specific disorders contributing to sexual pain, such as endometriosis, vulvovaginitis, vulvar dermatoses, or vulvovaginal atrophy, should be treated as outlined in other sections of this chapter. Female sexual pain may be treated initially with sexual counseling, education about anatomy and sexual function, and pelvic floor physical therapy by a specialized provider.

Since the cause of **vulvodynia** (defined as persistent vulvar pain for > 3 months without clear etiology) is unknown, management is difficult. Few treatment approaches have been subjected to methodologically rigorous trials. A variety of topical agents have been tried, although only a few have been useful in improving vulvodynia. Topical estradiol 0.01% cream or compounded estradiol with testosterone 0.05% to 0.1% cream applied at bedtime to the vulvar vestibule benefits some patients, especially those with symptoms beginning after starting hormonal contraceptives. Topical lidocaine may be helpful prior to bothersome sexual activity. Useful oral medications include amitriptyline in gradually increasing doses from 10 mg/day to 50–75 mg/day or gabapentin, starting at 100 mg at bedtime, and increasing to 100 mg three times per day after 3–4 days. Patients who tolerate daytime dosing can be increased to three divided doses of ≥ 300 mg per dose (maximum 1200 mg three times per day). Various SSRIs have also been used. Biofeedback and physical therapy, with a therapist experienced with the treatment of vulvar pain, have been shown to be helpful. Surgery—usually consisting of vestibulectomy—has been useful for women with introital dyspareunia.

When to Refer

- When symptoms or concerns persist despite first-line therapy.
- For expertise in surgical procedures.

Brotto LA et al. New management approaches for female sexual dysfunction. Curr Opin Obstet Gynecol. 2024;36:372. [PMID: 39109594]

Dalrymple SN et al. Female sexual dysfunction: common questions and answers. Am Fam Physician. 2025;111:433. [PMID: 40378324]

Davis SR. Sexual dysfunction in women. N Engl J Med. 2024; 391:736. [PMID: 39167808]

Toledo RG et al. Female sexual desire, arousal, and orgasmic dysfunctions: A systematic review and meta-analysis of treatment options. J Minim Invasive Gynecol. 2026;33:16. [PMID: 40543759]

SEXUAL VIOLENCE

ESSENTIALS OF DIAGNOSIS

- The legal definition of **rape** varies by state and geographic location. The term **"sexual violence"** is used by the CDC and will be used in this discussion. It can be committed by a stranger, but more commonly the assailant is known to the survivor, including a current or former partner or spouse (a form of **intimate partner violence [IPV]**).
- All survivors of sexual violence should be offered emergency contraception.
- The many individuals affected, the enormous health care costs, and the need for a multidisciplinary approach make sexual violence and IPV important health care issues.
- Knowledge of state laws and collection of evidence requirements are essential for clinicians evaluating possible survivors of sexual violence, including IPV.

General Considerations

Types of sexual violence, including rape and sexual assault, are legally defined in different ways in various jurisdictions. Clinicians and emergency department personnel who treat survivors of sexual violence should be familiar with the local laws pertaining to sexual assault. From a medical and psychological viewpoint, *it is essential that persons treating survivors of sexual violence recognize the nonconsensual and violent nature of the crime.* About 95% of people who report sexual violence are women. Each year in the United States, > 433,000 cases of sexual assault or rape are reported. Penetration may be vaginal, anal, or oral and may be by the penis, hand, or a foreign object. The assailant may be unknown to the survivor or, more frequently, may be an acquaintance or even the spouse.

Health care providers can have a significant impact in increasing the reporting of sexual violence and in identifying resources for the survivors. The International Rescue Committee has developed a **multimedia training tool** to encourage competent, compassionate, and confidential clinical care for sexual violence survivors in low-resource settings. This training encourages providers to offer care in the areas of pregnancy and STI prevention as well as assistance for psychological trauma.

Because sexual violence is a personal crisis, each patient will react differently, but anxiety disorders and PTSD are common sequelae. The **rape trauma syndrome** comprises two principal phases: (1) Immediate or acute: shaking, sobbing, and restless activity may last from a few days to a few weeks. The patient may experience anger, guilt, or shame or may repress these emotions. Reactions vary depending on the survivor's personality and the circumstances of the attack. (2) Late or chronic: problems related to the attack may develop weeks or months later. Sexual violence survivors are at increased risk for developing several psychological and behavioral adverse effects, including PTSD, sleep disturbances, anxiety, depression, suicide attempts, and medication misuse.

Clinicians and emergency department personnel who deal with survivors of sexual violence should work with community rape crisis centers or other sources of ongoing psychological support and counseling.

Examination

The clinician who first sees the alleged survivor of sexual violence should be empathetic and prepared with appropriate evidence collection and treatment materials. Standardized information and training, such as the program created by the International Rescue Committee, can be a helpful resource to the providers caring for these patients. Many emergency departments have a protocol for sexual violence survivors and personnel who are trained in interviewing and examining survivors of sexual violence.

Treatment

1. Give analgesics or sedatives if indicated. Administer tetanus toxoid if deep lacerations contain soil or dirt particles.
2. Give ceftriaxone, 500 mg intramuscularly, plus doxycycline 100 mg twice daily for 7 days orally, to prevent gonorrhea and chlamydia. In addition, give metronidazole 500 mg twice daily for 7 days to treat trichomoniasis. Incubating syphilis will probably be prevented by these medications, but syphilis testing should be repeated 6 weeks after the assault.
3. Prevent pregnancy by using one of the methods discussed under Emergency Contraception.
4. Vaccinate against hepatitis B.
5. Vaccinate against HPV for survivors aged 9–26 years who have not been vaccinated or are incompletely vaccinated. Follow-up doses should be administered at 1–2 months and 6 months if age ≥ 15 years and only at 6–12 months if < 15 years.
6. Offer HIV prophylaxis (see Chapter 35).
7. Because women who are sexually assaulted are at increased risk for long-term psychological sequelae, such as PTSD and anxiety disorders, it is critical that the patient and her family and friends have a source of *ongoing counseling and psychological support.*

When to Refer

All women who seek care for sexual assault should be referred to a facility that has expertise in the management of survivors of sexual violence and is qualified to perform expert forensic examination, if requested.

Barbara G et al. Sexual violence in adult women and adolescents. Minerva Obstet Gynecol. 2022;74:261. [PMID: 35147019]
Wiener SJ et al. A trauma-informed guide to caring for adolescents following sexual assault. Curr Opin Pediatr. 2021;33:354. [PMID: 34039900]
Yemane REH et al. Sexual assault/domestic violence. Obstet Gynecol Clin North Am. 2022;49:581. [PMID: 36122986]

BARTHOLIN DUCT CYSTS & ABSCESSES

The Bartholin glands (greater vestibular glands) are located bilaterally at 4 and 8 o'clock in the vulvar vestibule. They provide lubrication to the vagina through a duct 2.5 cm long. Obstruction of the Bartholin duct can lead to pain, swelling, and cyst and abscess formation (Figure 21–1).

Purulent drainage or secretions from the gland should be tested for *Neisseria gonorrhoeae*, *Chlamydia trachomatis*, and other pathogens, and treated accordingly (see Chapter 37); frequent warm sitz baths may be helpful. Abscesses or cysts that are symptomatic should undergo incision and drainage with additional efforts to keep the drainage tract open (eg, Word catheter or marsupialization). Marsupialization should be considered to prevent recurrences. Antibiotics are unnecessary unless cellulitis is present. In women under 40, asymptomatic cysts do not require therapy; in women over age 40, biopsy or removal should be considered to rule out vulvar carcinoma.

When to Refer

When surgical therapy (marsupialization) is indicated.

Bakouei F et al. Comparison of word catheter and marsupialization in the management of Bartholin's glands: a systematic review and meta-analysis. J Obstet Gynaecol Can. 2024;46:102357. [PMID: 38215822]
Illingworth B et al. Evaluation of treatments for Bartholin's cyst or abscess: a systematic review. BJOG. 2020;127:671. [PMID: 31876985]

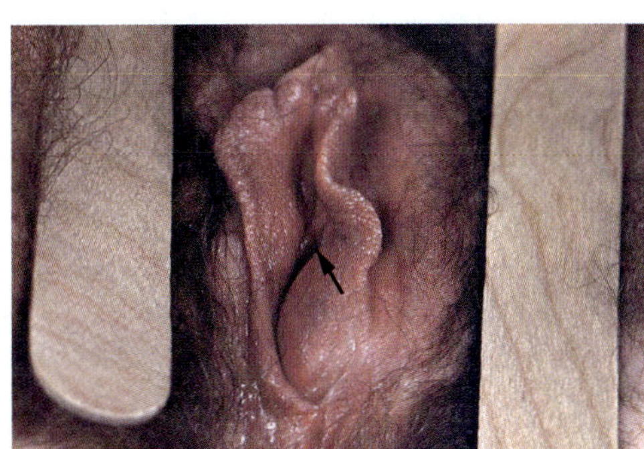

Figure 21–1. Bartholin cyst (abscess). The Bartholin gland is located in the lower two-thirds of the introitus. (From Susan Lindsley, Public Health Image Library, CDC.)

VAGINITIS

ESSENTIALS OF DIAGNOSIS

- Vaginal irritation.
- Pruritus.
- Abnormal or malodorous discharge.

General Considerations

Inflammation and infection of the vagina are common gynecologic complaints, resulting from a variety of pathogens, allergic reactions to vaginal products, vaginal atrophy, or friction during coitus. The normal vaginal pH is 4.5 or less, and *Lactobacillus* is the predominant organism. Normal cervical or vaginal secretions midcycle, or during pregnancy, can be confused with vaginitis.

Clinical Findings

When the patient reports vaginal irritation, pain, pruritus or unusual or malodorous discharge, a history should be taken, noting the onset, location, duration, and characterization of symptoms including triggers and alleviating factors. Additional history should include the last menstrual period; recent sexual activity; use of contraceptives, tampons, or douches; and recent changes in medications or use of antibiotics. The physical examination should include careful inspection of the vulva and speculum examination of the vagina and cervix. A vaginal, cervical, or urine sample can be obtained for detection of gonococcus and chlamydia, if clinically indicated. Evaluation for yeast, bacterial vaginosis, and *Trichomonas* should be performed. The vaginal pH should be tested; it is frequently > 4.5 in infections due to trichomonads and bacterial vaginosis. A bimanual examination to look for evidence of pelvic infection, namely cervical motion, uterine, or adnexal tenderness, should follow. *Point-of-care testing is available for all three main organisms that cause vaginitis and can be used if microscopy is not available or for confirmatory testing of microscopy.*

A. Vulvovaginal Candidiasis

Pregnancy, diabetes mellitus, and use of broad-spectrum antibiotics or corticosteroids may increase risk of *Candida* infections. Heat, moisture, and occlusive clothing also increase risk. Pruritus, vulvovaginal erythema, and a white curd-like discharge that is not malodorous are often found (Figure 21–2). Microscopic examination with 10% potassium hydroxide reveals hyphae and spores. A swab for cultures or for PCR testing may be performed if *Candida* is suspected but not demonstrated.

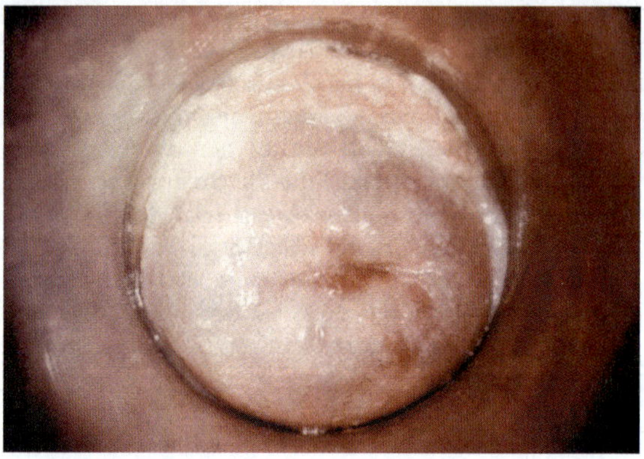

Figure 21–2. Cervical candidiasis. (Public Health Image Library, CDC.)

B. *Trichomonas vaginalis* Vaginitis

This sexually transmitted protozoal flagellate infects the vagina, Skene ducts, and lower urinary tract in women and the lower genitourinary tract in men. Pruritus and a malodorous frothy, yellow-green discharge occur, along with diffuse vaginal erythema and red macular lesions on the cervix in severe cases ("**strawberry cervix**," Figure 21–3). Motile organisms with flagella seen by microscopic examination of a wet mount with saline solution is confirmatory but such organisms are identified in only 60–70% of cases. Nucleic acid amplification tests are highly sensitive and specific to identify *T vaginalis*. Other rapid diagnostic tests with improved sensitivity compared to wet mount (eg, Affirm VP III and OSOM *Trichomonas* Rapid Test) are commercially available.

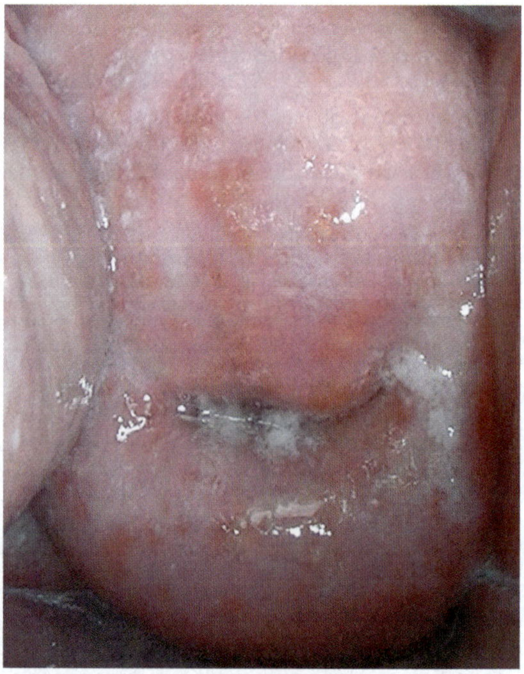

Figure 21–3. **Strawberry cervix in *Trichomonas vaginalis* infection, with inflammation and punctate hemorrhages.** (Reproduced with permission from Richard P. Usatine, MD, in Usatine RP, Smith MA, Mayeaux EJ Jr, Chumley H, Tysinger J. *The Color Atlas of Family Medicine*. McGraw-Hill, 2009.)

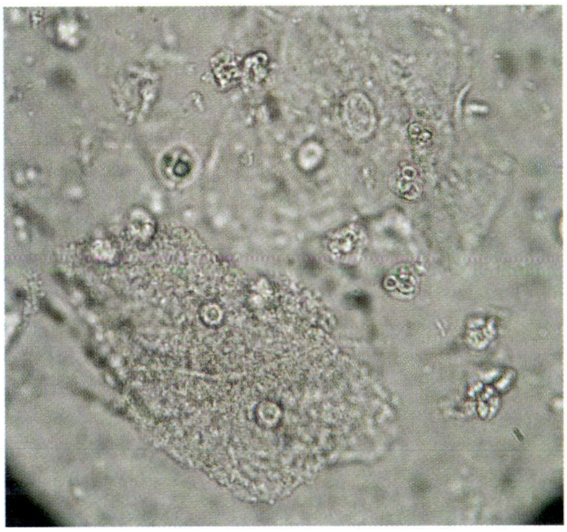

Figure 21–4. Clue cells seen in bacterial vaginosis due to *Gardnerella vaginalis.* (Reproduced with permission from Richard P. Usatine, MD, in Usatine RP, Smith MA, Mayeaux EJ Jr, Chumley H, Tysinger J. *The Color Atlas of Family Medicine.* McGraw-Hill, 2009.)

C. Bacterial Vaginosis

Bacterial vaginosis is a polymicrobial disease that is not considered a STI, although sexual activity is a risk factor. An overgrowth of *Gardnerella* and other anaerobes is often associated with increased malodorous discharge without obvious vulvitis or vaginitis. The discharge is grayish and sometimes frothy, with a pH of 5.0–5.5. An amine-like ("fishy") odor is present if a drop of discharge is alkalinized with 10% potassium hydroxide ("**whiff test**"). On wet mount in saline, epithelial cells are covered with bacteria to such an extent that cell borders are obscured (**clue cells**, Figure 21–4). Vaginal cultures are generally not useful in diagnosis; however, molecular testing is available.

Treatment

A. Vulvovaginal Candidiasis

A variety of topical and oral regimens are available to treat vulvovaginal candidiasis. Women with uncomplicated vulvovaginal candidiasis will usually respond to a 1- to 3-day regimen of a topical azole or a one-time dose of oral fluconazole 150 mg. Vulvovaginal candidiasis in pregnancy is typically treated with a topical imidazole vaginally for 7 days. Women with complicated infection (including three or more episodes in 1 year [**recurrent vulvovaginal candidiasis**], severe symptoms and signs, non-albicans species, uncontrolled diabetes mellitus, HIV infection, or corticosteroid treatment) can be treated with three consecutive doses of oral fluconazole, each 3 days apart. In recurrent non-albicans infections, boric acid 600 mg in a gelatin capsule intravaginally once daily for 2–3 weeks is approximately 70% effective. If recurrence occurs, referral to a gynecologist or an infectious disease specialist is indicated.

1. Single-dose regimens—Effective single-dose regimens include topical miconazole (1200-mg vaginal suppository), tioconazole (6.5% cream, 5 g vaginally), or sustained-release butoconazole (2% cream, 5 g vaginally), or oral fluconazole (150-mg tablet).

2. Three-day regimens—Effective 3-day regimens include clotrimazole (2% cream, 5 g vaginally once daily), terconazole (0.8% cream, 5 g, or 80-mg vaginal suppository once daily), or miconazole (4% cream, 5 g, or 200-mg vaginal suppository once daily).

3. Seven-day regimens—The following regimens are effective when given once daily for 7 days: clotrimazole (1% cream), miconazole (2% cream, 5 g, or 100-mg vaginal suppository), or terconazole (0.4% cream, 5 g).

4. Recurrent vulvovaginal candidiasis (maintenance therapy)—After induction treatment with three doses oral fluconazole every 72 hours, fluconazole 150 mg once weekly for 6 months can be used for maintenance therapy.

5. Alternative therapies—Ibrexafungerp (Brexafemme), US FDA-approved in 2021, is indicated for patients who prefer oral therapy but have an intolerance or allergy to fluconazole or a candidal strain resistant to fluconazole. Two 150 mg pills are taken orally twice a day for one day (4 pills total). Otesconazole (Vivjoa), US FDA-approved in 2022, is indicated for recurrent vulvovaginal candidiasis. It has a 12-week dosing regimen with four 150-mg pills taken orally on day 1, three pills taken on day 2, and then one pill taken weekly for 11 weeks starting on day 14. These medications are not approved to be taken during pregnancy.

B. *Trichomonas vaginalis* Vaginitis

Treatment of both partners simultaneously is recommended; metronidazole, 500 mg orally twice a day for 7 days for women, and metronidazole, 2 g orally as a single dose for men. Metronidazole vaginal gel is not adequate for treatment as the gel does not reliably penetrate vaginal ducts and glands.

In the case of treatment failure with metronidazole, in the absence of reexposure, the patient should be re-treated with metronidazole, as described above, or tinidazole, 2 g orally once daily for 7 days. If this is not effective in eradicating the organisms, a kit for drug-resistance testing can be requested from the CDC via https://www.cdc.gov/laboratory/specimen-submission/detail.html?CDCTestCode=CDC-10239. Women with *T vaginalis* infection have an increased risk for concurrent infection with other STIs and should be offered comprehensive STI testing.

C. Bacterial Vaginosis

The recommended regimens are metronidazole (500 mg orally, twice daily for 7 days), clindamycin vaginal cream (2%, 5 g, once daily for 7 days), or metronidazole gel (0.75%, 5 g, once daily for 5 days). A recent study demonstrated that treatment of male partners with metronidazole 400 mg tablets and 2% clindamycin cream applied to the penile skin, both twice daily for 7 days, along with the recommended treatment regimens for the female patient, resulted in a lower rate of bacterial vaginosis recurrence within 12 weeks compared to standard care. Based on this study, the American College of Obstetricians & Gynecologists updated its clinical recommendations to advise concurrent partner therapy with a combined oral and topical antimicrobial for male sexual partners of adult patients with recurrent, symptomatic bacterial vaginosis. The National STD Curriculum offers a helpful training module to clinicians to review current recommendations for treatment of vaginitis.

Concurrent sexual partner therapy to prevent bacterial vaginosis recurrence. Obstet Gynecol. 2025;146:e111. [PMID: 41100865]

Powell AM et al. Microbiome and vulvovaginitis. Obstet Gynecol Clin North Am. 2023;50:311. [PMID: 37149312]

Vodstrcil LA et al; StepUp Team. Male-partner treatment to prevent recurrence of bacterial vaginosis. N Engl J Med. 2025;392:947. [PMID: 40043236]

PELVIC INFLAMMATORY DISEASE (Salpingitis, Endometritis)

ESSENTIALS OF DIAGNOSIS

- Lower abdominal or pelvic pain.
- Uterine, adnexal, or cervical motion tenderness.
- Absence of a competing diagnosis.

General Considerations

PID is a polymicrobial infection of the upper genital tract associated with the sexually transmitted organisms *N gonorrhoeae* and *C trachomatis* as well as endogenous organisms, including anaerobes, *Haemophilus influenzae*, enteric gram-negative rods, and streptococci. Young age and multiple partners are risk factors for development of PID, a leading cause of infertility and ectopic pregnancy. The use of barrier methods of contraception may provide significant protection.

Clinical Findings

A. Symptoms and Signs

Patients with PID most commonly present with lower abdominal pain. Additional complaints may include AUB and abnormal vaginal discharge. Systemic features such as fever typically indicate more severe disease, including pelvic abscess. Right upper quadrant pain may indicate an associated perihepatitis **(Fitz-Hugh-Curtis syndrome).** *Diagnosis of PID is complicated by the fact that patients may have subtle or mild symptoms that are not readily recognized as PID, such as postcoital bleeding, urinary frequency, or low back pain.*

B. Minimum Diagnostic Criteria

PID is diagnosed clinically. *Patients with cervical motion, uterine, or adnexal tenderness meet diagnostic criteria for PID and should be treated with antibiotics unless there is a competing diagnosis, such as ectopic pregnancy or appendicitis.*

C. Additional Criteria

No single historical, physical, or laboratory finding is definitive for acute PID. The following criteria may be used to enhance the specificity of the diagnosis: (1) oral temperature higher than 38.3°C, (2) abnormal cervical or vaginal discharge with white cells on saline microscopy (> 1 leukocyte per epithelial cell), (3) elevated ESR, (4) elevated CRP, and (5) laboratory documentation of cervical infection with *N gonorrhoeae* or *C trachomatis*. Testing for gonorrhea and chlamydia should be performed. Treatment should not be delayed while awaiting results.

Differential Diagnosis

Appendicitis, ectopic pregnancy, septic abortion, hemorrhagic or ruptured ovarian cysts or tumors, ovarian torsion, degeneration of a myoma, and acute enteritis should be considered in the differential diagnosis. PID is more likely to occur when there is a prior history of PID, recent sexual contact, recent onset of menses, recent placement of an IUD, or recent intercourse with a partner who has a STI. *Acute PID is highly unlikely when recent (within 60 days) intercourse has not taken place.* A sensitive serum pregnancy test should be obtained to rule out pregnancy. Pelvic ultrasonography is helpful to rule out tubo-ovarian abscess (TOA). Laparoscopy should be considered when imaging is not informative, and the patient has not improved after 72 hours of inpatient treatment; it should also be considered when an acutely ill patient has a high suspicion of a competing diagnosis requiring surgical intervention (eg, appendicitis). The appendix should be visualized at laparoscopy to rule out appendicitis. Cultures should be obtained at laparoscopy.

Treatment

A. Antibiotics

Early treatment with appropriate antibiotics effective against *N gonorrhoeae*, *C trachomatis*, and the endogenous organisms listed above is essential to prevent long-term sequelae. *The sexual partner should be treated appropriately.* Most women with mild to moderate disease can be treated successfully as an outpatient. The recommended outpatient regimen is a single dose of ceftriaxone (500 mg intramuscularly; 1 g for persons who weigh ≥ 150 kg) plus doxycycline (100 mg orally twice a day for 14 days) with metronidazole 500 mg orally twice a day **or** a single dose of cefoxitin (2 g intramuscularly) with probenecid (1 g orally) plus doxycycline (100 mg orally twice daily for 14 days) with metronidazole 500 mg orally twice daily for 14 days. For patients with severe disease or those who meet criteria for hospitalization, there are three recommended regimens: cefotetan, 2 g intravenously every 12 hours, or cefoxitin, 2 g intravenously every 6 hours, or ceftriaxone, 1 g intravenously every 24 hours, each given with doxycycline, 100 mg orally or intravenously every 12 hours. If ceftriaxone is used, metronidazole 500 mg orally or intravenously every 12 hours should be added. These regimens should be continued for at least 24 hours after the patient shows significant clinical improvement. Then, an oral regimen should be given for a total course of antibiotics of 14 days with doxycycline, 100 mg orally twice a day and metronidazole, 500 mg orally twice a day.

B. Procedural Interventions

Procedural intervention is reserved for cases of large TOA (> 8 cm), suspected TOA rupture, or cases with a poor response to antibiotics. Interventional radiology drainage may be considered after TOA antibiotic failure or for large TOA. If surgical intervention is pursued, unilateral adnexectomy is acceptable for unilateral abscess. Hysterectomy and bilateral salpingo-oophorectomy may be necessary for overwhelming infection or in cases of chronic disease with intractable pelvic pain.

Prognosis

Despite treatment, long-term sequelae, including repeated episodes of infection, chronic pelvic pain, dyspareunia, ectopic pregnancy, or infertility, develop in one-fourth of women with acute disease. *The risk of infertility increases with repeated episodes of salpingitis*: it is estimated at 10% after the first episode, 25% after a second episode, and 50% after a third episode.

When to Admit

The following patients with acute PID should be admitted for intravenous antibiotic therapy:

- The patient has a TOA (direct inpatient observation for at least 24 hours before switching to outpatient therapy).
- The patient is pregnant.
- The patient cannot follow or tolerate an outpatient regimen.
- The patient has not responded clinically to outpatient therapy within 72 hours.
- The patient has severe illness, nausea and vomiting, or high fever.
- Another surgical emergency, such as appendicitis, cannot be ruled out.

Frock-Welnak DN et al. Identification and treatment of acute pelvic inflammatory disease and associated sequelae. Obstet Gynecol Clin North Am. 2022;49:551. [PMID: 36122985]

CONDYLOMA ACUMINATA

Warty growths on the vulva, perianal area, vaginal walls, or cervix are caused by various types of HPV. Pregnancy and immunosuppression favor growth. Ninety percent of genital warts are caused by HPV 6 and 11. Vulvar lesions may be obviously wart-like or may be diagnosed only after biopsy of suspicious lesions. Vaginal lesions may show diffuse hypertrophy or a cobblestone appearance.

Recommended treatments for vulvar warts include freezing with liquid nitrogen or a cryoprobe, surgical removal, or application of 80–90% trichloroacetic or bichloroacetic acid (with care to avoid the surrounding skin). The pain of bichloroacetic or trichloroacetic acid application can be lessened by a sodium bicarbonate paste applied immediately after treatment. Patient-applied regimens, useful when the entire lesion is accessible to the patient, include imiquimod 5% cream or sinecatechins 15% ointment. Vaginal warts may be treated with cryotherapy with liquid nitrogen or trichloroacetic acid. Extensive warts may require treatment with CO_2 laser, electrocautery, or excision under local or general anesthesia.

CERVICAL INTRAEPITHELIAL NEOPLASIA (CIN) (Dysplasia of the Cervix)

ESSENTIALS OF DIAGNOSIS

- The presumptive diagnosis is made by an abnormal Papanicolaou test.
- Diagnose by colposcopically directed biopsy.

General Considerations

The squamocolumnar junction of the cervix is an area of active squamous cell proliferation. In childhood, this junction is located on the exposed vaginal portion of the cervix. At puberty, because of hormonal influence and possibly because of changes in the vaginal pH, the squamous margin begins to encroach on the single-layered, mucus-secreting epithelium, creating an area of metaplasia (**transformation zone**). Infection with HPV (see Prevention, below) may lead to cellular abnormalities, which over time may develop into squamous cell dysplasia or cancer. There are varying degrees of dysplasia (Table 21–5), defined by the degree of cellular atypia; *all atypia must be observed closely and treatment considered for persistence or progression to high-grade lesions.*

Clinical Findings

There are no specific symptoms or signs of CIN. The presumptive diagnosis is made by cytologic screening of an asymptomatic population with no grossly visible cervical changes. *All visible abnormal cervical lesions should be biopsied* (Figure 21–5).

Screening & Diagnosis

A. Cytologic Examination (Papanicolaou Test) and HPV Testing

For immunocompetent patients, the USPSTF recommends cervical cancer screening beginning at age 21, while the American Cancer Society recommends primary HPV testing every 5 years beginning at age 25. The USPSTF recommendation to start screening at age 21 years regardless of the age of onset of sexual intercourse is based on the very low incidence of cancer in younger patients and the potential for adverse effects associated with treatment of young patients with abnormal cytology screening results.

Table 21–5. Bethesda classification for Papanicolaou tests.

Category	Specifics
Specimen adequacy	Satisfactory for evaluation
	Unsatisfactory for evaluation
General categorization	Negative for intraepithelial lesion or malignancy
	Epithelial cell abnormality
	Other
Epithelial cell abnormalities	
Squamous cell abnormalities	Atypical squamous cells of undetermined significance (ASC-US)
	Atypical squamous cells cannot exclude HSIL (ASC-H)
	Low-grade squamous intraepithelial lesion (LSIL)
	High-grade squamous intraepithelial lesion (HSIL)
	Squamous cell carcinoma
Glandular cell abnormalities	Atypical glandular cells (specify endocervical, endometrial, or not otherwise specified)
	Atypical glandular cells, favor neoplastic
	Endocervical adenocarcinoma in situ
	Adenocarcinoma

In contrast to the high rate of infection with HPV in sexually active adolescents, invasive cervical cancer is very rare in patients younger than age 21 years. The USPSTF 2018 statement recommends screening for cervical cancer in women aged 21–65 years as follows: for women aged 21–29 years, screening with cytology (conventional [Papanicolaou test] or liquid-based) alone every 3 years; and for women aged 30–65 years, screening with cytology alone every 3 years, with high-risk HPV testing alone every 5 years, or with a combination of cytology and high-risk HPV testing (**co-testing**) every 5 years. Self-collected vaginal specimens for primary HPV testing were added as a screening option in 2025. The American Cancer Society recommends screening with self-collection be repeated every 3 years. These recommendations apply to patients who have a cervix, regardless of their sexual history or HPV vaccination status. They do not apply to patients who have a previous diagnosis of cervical cancer or a high-grade precancerous cervical lesion (ie, CIN grade II or III), patients with immune compromise (eg, living with HIV), or those with in utero exposure to diethylstilbestrol; these patients are classified as high risk and may require more frequent screening.

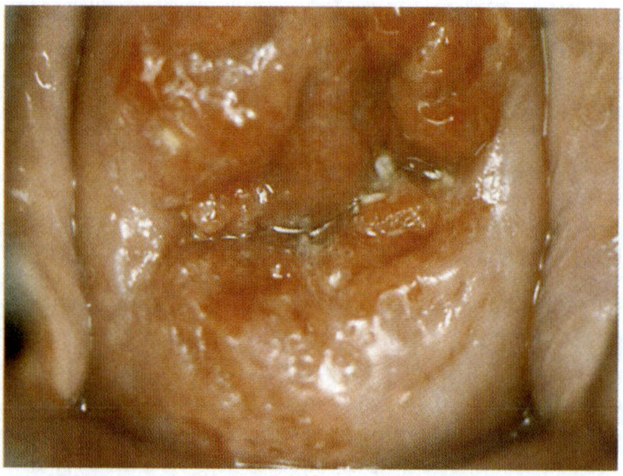

▲ **Figure 21–5.** Erosion of the cervix due to cervical intraepithelial neoplasia (CIN), a precursor lesion to cervical cancer. (Public Health Image Library, CDC.)

The USPSTF recommends *against* cervical cancer screening for women younger than age 21 years, for patients aged ≥ 65 years who have had adequate prior screening and are not otherwise at high risk for cervical cancer, and for those who have had a hysterectomy with removal of the cervix and who have no history of cervical cancer or a high-grade precancerous lesion. The goal of screening is to identify high-grade precancerous cervical lesions and prevent their progression to cervical cancer. These high-grade cervical lesions may be treated with excisional and ablative therapies. Screening and management guidelines are continually undergoing evaluation and change frequently. For the most current guidelines, please consult these sources: https://www.uspreventiveservicestaskforce.org/uspstf/recommendation/cervical-cancer-screening#fullrecommendationstart, https://www.cancer.org/health-care-professionals/american-cancer-society-prevention-early-detection-guidelines/cervical-cancer-screening-guidelines.html, and https://www.asccp.org/guidelines.

Cytologic reports from the laboratory may describe findings in one of several ways. The **Bethesda System** is a commonly used system that classifies epithelial cell abnormalities. The terms to classify squamous cell abnormalities include "atypical squamous cells of unknown significance" (**ASC-US**), "atypical squamous cells cannot exclude high-grade squamous intraepithelial lesion" (**ACS-H**), and "squamous intraepithelial lesions," including low-grade (**LSIL**) or high-grade (**HSIL**) (see Table 21–5). ***HPV DNA testing*** *can be used adjunctively as a triage test to stratify risk in patients aged ≥ 21 years with a cytologic diagnosis of ASC-US or LSIL.*

In 2019, the American Society for Colposcopy and Cervical Pathology (ASCCP) published guidelines for surveillance and management of abnormal screening based on a patient's risk of developing high-grade cervical intraepithelial neoplasia (CIN 3) or higher (adenocarcinoma in situ and cancer). A patient's "risk estimate" is determined by their current cytology and HPV status as well as past results.

Perkins RB et al. Self-collected vaginal specimens for human papillomavirus testing and guidance on screening exit: an update to the American Cancer Society cervical cancer screening guideline. CA Cancer J Clin. 2026;76:e70041. [PMID: 41342729]

B. Colposcopy

Colposcopy is performed by viewing the cervix with 10–20× magnification; this allows for assessment of the size and margins of an abnormal transformation zone and determination of extension into the endocervical canal. The application of 3–5% acetic acid (vinegar) dissolves mucus, and the acid's desiccating action sharpens the contrast between normal and actively proliferating squamous epithelium. Abnormal changes include white patches and vascular atypia, which indicate areas of greatest cellular activity.

C. Biopsy

Colposcopically directed biopsy and endocervical curettage are office procedures used to identify precancerous and cancerous lesions. Data from both cervical biopsy and endocervical curettage are important in deciding on treatment.

Prevention

Virtually all cervical dysplasias and cancers are associated with HPV infection of the cervix. There are over 100 recognized HPV subtypes. Types 6 and 11 tend to cause genital warts and mild dysplasia and rarely progress to cervical cancer; types 16, 18, 31, and others cause higher-grade dysplasia. The **HPV 9-valent recombinant vaccine (9vHPV)** is indicated for the prevention of cervical, vaginal, and vulvar cancers (in women) and anal cancers (in women and men) caused by HPV types 16, 18, 31, 33, 45, 52, and 58; genital warts (in women and men) caused by HPV types 6 and 11; and precancerous/dysplastic lesions of cervix, vagina, vulva (in women), and anus (in women and men) caused by HPV types 6, 11, 16, 18, 31, 33, 45, 52, and 58. *The 9vHPV is recommended for vaccination of females and males aged 9–26 and some adults aged 27 to 45 years old based on risk factors.* The older HPV 4-valent vaccine indicated for prevention of diseases related to HPV types 6, 11, 16, and 18 has been discontinued in the United States. The use of HPV vaccination in the United States continues to increase; however, *the HPV vaccination continues to lag far behind other vaccines recommended for adolescents.* In 2024, 62.9% of adolescents were current with the HPV vaccine series, and 78.2% had received at least one dose of the vaccine.

Because complete coverage of all carcinogenic HPV types is not provided by the 9vHPV vaccine, all women need to have regular cervical cancer screening as outlined above. In addition to vaccination, preventive measures include limiting the number of sexual partners and thus exposure to HPV, correct and consistent condom use, smoking cessation, and avoiding exposure to secondhand smoke.

Treatment

Treatment varies depending on the degree and extent of CIN. Biopsies should precede treatment, except in cases of high-grade cytology and colposcopic impression with concerns for inability to return for follow-up.

A. Ablative Procedures

Ablative procedures using cryosurgery or CO2 laser may be considered for lesions in which the entire squamocolumnar junction has been visualized on colposcopy (ie, adequate colposcopy) and the entire lesion is visualized.

B. Excisional Procedures

An excisional procedure (ie, LEEP [loop electrosurgical excisional procedure], cold knife cone or laser cone biopsy) is the preferred modality when treatment is planned. Excision includes removal of the entire transformation zone of the cervix.

Follow-Up

Because recurrence is possible—especially in the first 2 years after treatment—and because the false-negative rate of a single cervical cytologic test is approximately 20%, *close follow-up after colposcopy and biopsy is imperative.* Following an excisional or an ablative procedure, HPV-based testing should be performed at 6 months and then annually for 2 years followed by HPV-based testing every 3 years for at least 25 years. Colposcopy and endocervical sampling should be performed for any abnormality.

The ASCCP Guidelines for cervical cancer screening and management of abnormal Papanicolaou tests are available online (https://www.asccp.org/guidelines).

When to Refer

- Patients with CIN II/III should be referred to an experienced colposcopist.
- Patients requiring conization biopsy should be referred to a gynecologist.

Perkins RB et al. Cervical cancer screening: a review. JAMA. 2023;330:547. [PMID: 37552298]
Perkins RB et al. Self-collected vaginal specimens for human papillomavirus testing and guidance on screening exit: an update to the American Cancer Society cervical cancer screening guideline. CA Cancer J Clin. 2026;76:e70041. [PMID: 41342729]

CARCINOMA OF THE CERVIX

ESSENTIALS OF DIAGNOSIS

- Increased risk in women who smoke and those with HIV or high-risk HPV types.
- Gross lesions should be evaluated by colposcopically directed biopsies and not cytology alone.

General Considerations

Cervical cancer is the fourth most common cancer in women worldwide and the leading cause of gynecologic cancer death among women in developing countries. It is considered an STI as both squamous cell and adenocarcinoma of the cervix are secondary to infection with HPV, primarily types 16 and 18. Patients infected with HIV and with other forms of immunosuppression are at an increased risk for high-risk HPV infection and CIN. *Smoking appears to be a cofactor for squamous cell carcinoma (SCC).* SCC accounts for approximately 75–80% of cervical cancers, while adenocarcinoma accounts for 15%, and adenosquamous carcinoma for 3–5%; neuroendocrine or small cell carcinomas are rare.

SCC appears first in the intraepithelial layers (the preinvasive stage, or carcinoma in situ). Preinvasive cancer (CIN III) is most commonly diagnosed in women 25–35 years of age. Two to 10 years are required for carcinoma to penetrate the basement membrane and become invasive.

Clinical Findings

A. Symptoms and Signs

Early cervical cancer is often asymptomatic. The most common signs are irregular or heavy bleeding and postcoital spotting. Bladder and rectal dysfunction or fistulas and pain are late sequelae.

B. Cervical Biopsy and Endocervical Curettage or Conization

These procedures are necessary steps after a positive Papanicolaou test to determine the extent and depth of invasion of the cancer. Even if the pap test is positive, definitive diagnosis must be established through biopsy before additional treatment is given.

C. "Staging" or Estimate of Gross Spread of Cancer of the Cervix

Staging of invasive cervical cancer is achieved by clinical evaluation, usually conducted under anesthesia. Further examinations, such as ultrasonography, CT, MRI, lymphangiography, laparoscopy, and fine-needle aspiration, are valuable for treatment planning.

Complications

Metastasis to regional lymph nodes occurs with later-stage disease. Paracervical extension can occur in all directions from the cervix. The ureters may become obstructed lateral to the cervix, causing hydroureter and hydronephrosis and consequently impaired kidney function. Almost two-thirds of patients with untreated carcinoma of the cervix die of uremia when ureteral obstruction is bilateral. Pain in the back, in the distribution of the lumbosacral plexus, is often indicative of neurologic involvement. Gross edema of the legs may be indicative of vascular and lymphatic stasis due to tumor. Vaginal fistulas to the rectum and urinary tract are severe late complications. Hemorrhage causes death in 10–20% of patients with extensive invasive carcinoma.

Prevention

Routine cervical cancer screening and vaccination with the recombinant 9-valent HPV vaccine can prevent cervical cancer. The 9-valent HPV vaccine targets the HPV types that pose the greatest risk and protects against low-grade and precancerous lesions caused by other HPV types (see Cervical Intraepithelial Neoplasia).

Treatment

A. Emergency Measures

Vaginal hemorrhage originates from gross ulceration and cavitation in later-stage cervical carcinoma. Ligation and suturing of the cervix are usually not feasible, but emergent vaginal packing, cautery, tranexamic acid, and irradiation are helpful to stop bleeding temporarily. Ligation, resection, or embolization of the uterine or hypogastric arteries may be lifesaving when other measures fail.

B. Specific Measures

Microinvasive carcinoma (**stage IA1**) is treated with conization (if margins are negative on the diagnostic specimen) or simple, extrafascial hysterectomy. **Stages IA2 and IB1** cancers with limited stromal involvement can be treated with simple hysterectomy and pelvic lymphadenectomy. Patients with early-stage disease at low risk for recurrence may be candidates for fertility-sparing surgery. Women with **IB2** cancers typically undergo radical hysterectomy and pelvic lymphadenectomy. Adjuvant chemotherapy or radiation may be used for women with risk factors for recurrence. Women with locally advanced disease (**stage IB3 to IVA**) usually are treated with primary chemoradiation. Metastatic disease (**stage IVB**) typically is treated with chemotherapy.

Prognosis

The overall 5-year relative survival rate for carcinoma of the cervix is 67% in the United States. Survival rates decrease with more advanced disease, with 5-year survival rates for localized, regional, and distant disease reported at 91, 60, and 19%, respectively.

When to Refer

All patients with invasive cervical carcinoma (stage IA or higher) should be referred to a gynecologic oncologist.

Bhatla N et al. Cancer of the cervix uteri: 2025 update. Int J Gynaecol Obstet. 2025;171 Suppl 1:87. [PMID: 40908766]
Podwika SE et al. Top advances of the year: cervical cancer. Cancer. 2023;129:657. [PMID: 36609769]
Tewari KS. Cervical cancer. N Engl J Med. 2025;392:56. [PMID: 39752299]

CARCINOMA OF THE ENDOMETRIUM

ESSENTIALS OF DIAGNOSIS

- Abnormal uterine bleeding is the presenting sign in 90% of cases.
- After a negative pregnancy test, endometrial sampling is required to confirm the diagnosis.

General Considerations

Adenocarcinoma of the endometrium is the most common cancer of the female genital tract in developed countries. It occurs most often in patients 50–70 years of age. Obesity, nulliparity, diabetes mellitus, polycystic ovaries with prolonged anovulation, unopposed estrogen therapy, early menarche, late menopause, and the extended use of tamoxifen for the treatment of breast cancer are risk factors. Women with a family history of colon cancer (hereditary nonpolyposis colorectal cancer, Lynch syndrome) are at significantly increased risk, with a lifetime incidence as high as 30%.

Abnormal bleeding is the presenting sign in 90% of cases. Prompt endometrial sampling should be performed for patients with prolonged anovulation, those aged > 45 years who report abnormal menstrual bleeding, and those with postmenopausal uterine bleeding.

Papanicolaou test of the cervix occasionally shows atypical endometrial cells but is an insensitive diagnostic tool. *Endocervical and endometrial sampling is the only reliable means of diagnosis and is important to differentiate endometrial cancer from hyperplasia, which often can be treated hormonally.* Endometrial biopsy is approximately 90% sensitive for detecting endometrial cancer and can be accomplished in the office setting. Hysteroscopy can be valuable in identifying polyps or other lesions within the uterine cavity. Pelvic ultrasonography may be used to evaluate the uterine cavity and the thickness of the endometrial lining. *The finding of a thin endometrial lining on ultrasound (4 mm or less) in a postmenopausal patient is clinically reassuring in cases where very little tissue is obtainable through endometrial biopsy.* A thickened or irregular endometrial lining should prompt further evaluation for possible hypertrophy, polyps, or neoplasia.

Prevention

Younger patients with chronic anovulation are at risk for endometrial hyperplasia and subsequent endometrial cancer; they can significantly reduce the risk of hyperplasia with the use of hormonal contraceptive methods or cyclic progestins.

Staging

Staging and prognosis are based on surgical and pathologic evaluation only. Examination under anesthesia, endometrial and endocervical sampling, CXR, intravenous urography, cystoscopy, sigmoidoscopy, transvaginal ultrasound, and MRI will help determine the extent of the disease and its appropriate treatment.

Treatment

Treatment consists of total hysterectomy and bilateral salpingo-oophorectomy. Peritoneal washings for cytologic examination are routinely taken and lymph node sampling may be done. Women with high-risk endometrial cancer (serous adenocarcinoma, clear cell carcinoma, grade 3 deeply invasive endometrioid carcinoma, and stages III/IV disease) are generally treated with surgery followed by chemotherapy, radiation therapy, or both. Molecular subtyping may inform treatment decisions.

Prognosis

With early diagnosis and treatment, the overall 5-year survival for localized disease is approximately 95%. With localized disease, the depth of myometrial invasion is the strongest predictor of survival. Survival rates decrease with increasing stage of disease, with 5-year survival rates reported at 69.8% for regional disease and 18.4% for distant disease.

When to Refer

All patients with endometrial carcinoma should be referred to a gynecologic oncologist.

Bryce C et al. Endometrial cancer: rapid evidence review. Am Fam Physician. 2025;111:526. [PMID: 40531151]
Crosbie EJ et al. Endometrial cancer. Lancet. 2022;399:1412. [PMID: 35397864]
Karpel HC et al. Treatment options for molecular subtypes of endometrial cancer in 2023. Curr Opin Obstet Gynecol. 2023;35:270. [PMID: 36943683]

CARCINOMA OF THE VULVA

ESSENTIALS OF DIAGNOSIS

- Two independent pathways for development: HPV or chronic inflammation.
- History of prolonged vulvar irritation, with pruritus, local discomfort, or slight bloody discharge.
- Early lesions may suggest or include non-neoplastic epithelial disorders.
- Late lesions appear as a mass, an exophytic growth, or a firm, ulcerated area in the vulva.
- Biopsy is necessary for diagnosis.

General Considerations

Most cancers of the vulva are squamous lesions that classically occur in patients over 50. **Vulvar low-grade squamous intraepithelial lesions (LSIL)** are benign and do not require intervention. **Vulvar HSIL** and **differentiated vulvar intraepithelial neoplasia (dVIN)** are premalignant conditions. Vulvar HSIL (VIN usual type) is associated with HPV, while dVIN is associated with vulvar dermatoses, eg, lichen sclerosus. About 70–90% of premalignant lesions are vulvar HSIL, but HSIL is the precursor for only 20% of vulvar cancers, while dVIN is the precursor for approximately 80% of vulvar cancers. Given that high percentages of HSIL and vulvar cancers are HPV-related, immunization with the HPV vaccine is beneficial to reduce the risk of HPV-related vulvar disease.

Differential Diagnosis

Other vulvar lesions must be considered. VIN may resemble vulvar cancer and must be distinguished by histology. Benign vulvar disorders that should be considered in the diagnosis of carcinoma of the vulva include inflammatory vulvar dermatoses (psoriasis, lichen sclerosus, lichen planus), chronic granulomatous lesions (eg, lymphogranuloma venereum, syphilis), condylomas, epidermal inclusion cysts, hidradenomas, or neurofibromas. Lichen sclerosus and other associated leukoplakic changes in the skin should be biopsied. The likelihood that a superimposed vulvar cancer will develop in a patient with a non-neoplastic epithelial disorder is low (1–5%).

Diagnosis

Biopsy is essential for the diagnosis of VIN and vulvar cancer and should be performed for any localized atypical vulvar lesion, including white patches and hyperpigmented lesions. Multiple skin-punch specimens can be taken in the office under local anesthesia. Colposcopy of vulva, vagina, and cervix can help in identifying areas for biopsy and in planning further treatment.

Staging

Vulvar cancer generally spreads by direct extension into the vagina, urethra, perineum, and anus, with discontinuous spread into the inguinal and femoral lymph nodes. Staging is based on a combined clinical and surgical/pathologic system.

Treatment

Invasive carcinoma confined to the vulva without evidence of spread to adjacent organs or to the regional lymph nodes is treated with radical local excision and inguinal lymphadenectomy or radical local excision alone if invasion is < 1 mm. To avoid the morbidity of inguinal lymphadenectomy, some guidelines recommend sentinel lymph node sampling for women with early-stage vulvar cancer. Patients with more advanced disease may receive preoperative radiation, chemotherapy, or both.

Prognosis

Vulvar SCCs seldom metastasize. With adequate excision, the prognosis is excellent. Patients with invasive vulvar SCC 2 cm in diameter or less, without inguinal lymph node metastases, have an 85–90% 5-year survival rate. If the lesion is larger than 2 cm and lymph node involvement is present, the likelihood of 5-year survival is approximately 40%.

When to Refer

All patients with invasive vulvar carcinoma should be referred to a gynecologic oncologist.

Lukovic J et al. Postoperative management of vulvar cancer. Int J Gynecol Cancer. 2022;32:338. [PMID: 35256421]

Olawaiye AB et al. Cancer of the vulva: 2025 update: FIGO Cancer Report 2025. Int J Gynaecol Obstet. 2025;171 Suppl 1(Suppl 1):36. [PMID: 40735881]

Sheern C et al. Vulval squamous cell carcinoma: a review. Clin Exp Dermatol. 2025:l. [PMID: 40834239]

OVARIAN TUMORS & OVARIAN CANCER

ESSENTIALS OF DIAGNOSIS

- Symptoms include vague GI discomfort, pelvic pressure, or pain.
- Many cases of early-stage cancer are asymptomatic.
- Pelvic examination and ultrasound are mainstays of diagnosis.

General Considerations

Ovarian tumors are common. Most are benign, but *malignant ovarian tumors are the leading cause of death from gynecologic cancer.* The wide range of types and patterns of ovarian tumors is due to the complexity of ovarian embryology and differences in tissues of origin.

In patients with no family history of ovarian cancer, the lifetime risk in the United States is 1.3%, whereas a woman with one affected first-degree relative has a 5% lifetime risk. Worldwide, the risk of ovarian cancer is 2.7%. Ultrasound or tumor marker screening for patients with one or no affected first-degree relatives has *not* been shown to reduce mortality from ovarian cancer, and the risks associated with prophylactic surgical procedures outweigh the benefits in low-risk women. For patients with two or more affected first-degree relatives, the lifetime risk is 7%. Approximately 3% of women with two or more affected first-degree relatives will have a **hereditary ovarian cancer syndrome** with a lifetime ovarian cancer risk of 40%. Women with a *BRCA1* gene pathogenic variant have a 45% lifetime risk of ovarian cancer and those with a *BRCA2* pathogenic variant, a 20% risk. *Typically, risk-reducing salpingo-oophorectomy is recommended for patients who have completed childbearing and by age 35–40 years for*

BRCA1 *carriers, while women with* BRCA2 *may consider delaying until age 40–45 years because of later onset of ovarian cancer.*

Clinical Findings

A. Symptoms and Signs

Most patients with both benign and malignant ovarian neoplasms are either asymptomatic or experience only mild nonspecific GI symptoms or pelvic pressure. Patients with advanced malignant disease may experience abdominal pain and bloating, and a palpable abdominal mass with ascites is often present.

B. Laboratory Findings

Serum CA 125 is elevated in 80% of patients with epithelial ovarian cancer overall but in only 50% with early disease. However, CA 125 may be elevated in premenopausal patients with benign disease (such as endometriosis), minimizing its usefulness in ovarian cancer screening. In premenopausal women with ovarian masses, other tumor markers (such as human chorionic gonadotropin [hCG], LD, or α-fetoprotein) may be indicators of the tumor type.

C. Imaging

Transvaginal ultrasound is useful for screening high-risk patients but has inadequate sensitivity for screening low-risk patients. Ultrasound is helpful in differentiating ovarian masses that are benign and likely to resolve spontaneously from those with malignant potential. Color Doppler imaging may further enhance the specificity of ultrasound diagnosis.

Differential Diagnosis

Once an ovarian mass has been detected, it must be categorized as functional, benign neoplastic, or potentially malignant. Predictive factors include age, size of the mass, ultrasound features, serum CA 125 level, the presence of symptoms, and whether the mass is unilateral or bilateral. Simple cysts up to 10 cm in diameter are almost universally benign in both premenopausal and postmenopausal patients. Most will resolve spontaneously and may be monitored without intervention. If the mass is larger or unchanged on repeat transvaginal ultrasound, or if symptomatic, surgical evaluation is warranted.

Treatment

If a malignant ovarian mass is suspected, surgical evaluation should be performed by a gynecologic oncologist. For benign neoplasms, tumor excision or unilateral oophorectomy may be performed if symptomatic. For early-stage ovarian cancer, the standard therapy is complete surgical staging including hysterectomy and bilateral salpingo-oophorectomy with omentectomy and selective lymphadenectomy. With more advanced disease, aggressive removal of all visible tumor improves survival. Except for patients with low-grade ovarian cancer in an early stage, postoperative chemotherapy is indicated (see Table 43–2). Several chemotherapy regimens are effective in halting progression of disease, such as the combination of cisplatin or carboplatin with paclitaxel; however, overall likelihood of recurrence for all stages of disease is 62% and 80–85% for those with stage III or IV disease.

Prognosis

Regional or distant disease is diagnosed in approximately 75% of women with ovarian cancer. The overall 5-year survival is approximately 31.5% with distant disease, but 72.9% with regional and 92.4% with localized disease.

When to Refer

If a malignant mass is suspected, surgical evaluation should be performed by a gynecologic oncologist.

Avesani G et al. ESR Essentials: characterisation and staging of adnexal masses with MRI and CT-practice recommendations by ESUR. Eur Radiol. 2024;34:7673. [PMID: 38849662]

Centers for Disease Control and Prevention (CDC). Ovarian cancer screening. https://www.cdc.gov/ovarian-cancer/screening/?CDC_AAref_Val=https://www.cdc.gov/cancer/ovarian/basic_info/screening.htm. Accessed September 16, 2025.

NCCN Clinical Practice Guidelines in Oncology (NCCN Guidelines®) for Genetic/Familial High-Risk Assessment: Breast, ovarian, pancreatic, and prostate V.2.20226 © National Comprehensive Cancer Network, Inc. 2025. https://www.nccn.org/guidelines/guidelines-detail?category=2&id=1545. Accessed November 4, 2025.

Patel-Lippman KK et al; Expert Panel on GYN and OB Imaging. ACR Appropriateness Criteria® clinically suspected adnexal mass, no acute symptoms: 2023 update. J Am Coll Radiol. 2024;21:S79. [PMID: 38823957]

Wheeler V et al. Adnexal masses: diagnosis and management. Am Fam Physician. 2023;108:580. [PMID: 38215419]

22 Obstetrics & Obstetric Disorders

Vanessa L. Rogers, MD
Scott W. Roberts, MD

DIAGNOSIS OF PREGNANCY

Pregnancy should be diagnosed as promptly as possible. Prenatal care can begin early for a desired pregnancy to eliminate potential risks, such as harmful medications, drug and alcohol use, smoking, and occupational chemical exposure. If an unwanted pregnancy occurs, counseling about options can be provided at an early stage. Clinicians must be aware of laws in their jurisdiction of practice regarding termination.

Pregnancy Tests

All urine or blood pregnancy tests rely on the detection of human chorionic gonadotropin (hCG) produced by the placenta. Levels increase shortly after implantation, approximately double every 48 hours (this rise can range from 30–100% in normal pregnancies), reach a peak at 50–75 days, and fall to lower levels in the second and third trimesters. Pregnancy tests are performed on serum or urine and are accurate at the time of the missed period or shortly after it.

1. In ectopic pregnancies—Compared with intrauterine pregnancies, ectopic pregnancies may show lower levels of hCG that plateau or fall in serial determinations. Quantitative assays of hCG repeated at 48-hour intervals are used in the diagnosis of ectopic pregnancy as well as in cases of molar pregnancy and early pregnancy loss. Comparison of hCG levels between laboratories may be misleading in a given patient because different international standards may produce results that vary by as much as twofold. Consistent follow-up is necessary.

2. In pregnancy of unknown location—Despite a positive pregnancy test, the location and viability of the pregnancy are unknown because it is not seen on transvaginal ultrasound.

Lin Y et al. Management of pregnancy of unknown location. Eur J Obstet Gynecol Reprod Biol. 2025;312:114047. [PMID: 40435713]

Manifestations of Pregnancy

The following symptoms and signs are usually due to pregnancy, but none are diagnostic. A record of the time of coitus or insemination is helpful for diagnosing and dating a pregnancy.

A. Symptoms

Amenorrhea, nausea and vomiting, breast tenderness and tingling, urinary frequency and urgency, "quickening" (perception of first movement noted at about the 18th week), and weight gain are symptoms of pregnancy.

B. Signs (in Weeks From Last Menstrual Period)

Breast changes (enlargement, vascular engorgement, colostrum) begin early in pregnancy and continue until the postpartum period. Cyanosis of the vagina and cervical portio and softening of the cervix occur in about the 7th week. Softening of the cervico-uterine junction takes place in the 8th week, and generalized enlargement and diffuse softening of the corpus occurs after the 8th week. The abdomen typically starts to enlarge in the 16th week but depends on body habitus.

The uterine fundus is palpable above the pubic symphysis by 12–15 weeks from the last menstrual period and reaches the umbilicus by 20–22 weeks. Fetal heart tones can be heard by Doppler at 10–12 weeks' gestation.

Differential Diagnosis

The nonpregnant uterus enlarged by myomas can be confused with the gravid uterus, but it is usually firm and irregular. An ovarian tumor may be found midline, displacing the nonpregnant uterus to the side or posteriorly. Ultrasonography and a pregnancy test will provide a diagnosis in these circumstances.

ESSENTIALS OF PRENATAL CARE

Prenatal visits should begin as early as possible after the diagnosis of pregnancy. The initial visit should include a history, physical examination, advice to the patient, and

Table 22–1. Common drugs that are teratogenic or fetotoxic.[1]

ACE inhibitors	Lithium
Alcohol	Methotrexate
Androgens	Misoprostol
Angiotensin-II receptor blockers	NSAIDs (third trimester)
Antiepileptics (phenytoin, valproic acid, carbamazepine)	Opioids (prolonged use)
	Radioiodine (antithyroid)
Benzodiazepines	Reserpine
Cyclophosphamide	Ribavirin
Diazoxide	Sulfonamides (second and third trimesters)
Diethylstilbestrol	
Disulfiram	Tetracycline (third trimester)
Ergotamine	Thalidomide
Estrogens	Tobacco smoking
Griseofulvin	Warfarin and other coumarin anticoagulants
Isotretinoin	

[1]Many other drugs are also contraindicated during pregnancy. Evaluate any drug for its need versus its potential adverse effects. Further information can be obtained from the manufacturer or from any of several teratogenic registries around the country. Go to https://www.fda.gov/consumers/womens-health-topics/pregnancy-exposure-registries for more information.

appropriate tests and procedures (see *Current Medical Diagnosis & Treatment* on AccessMedicine.com for a discussion of routine prenatal care).

A. Medications

Only medications prescribed or authorized by the obstetric provider should be taken since certain medications are contraindicated during pregnancy (Table 22–1).

B. Alcohol and Other Drugs

Pregnant persons should be encouraged to abstain from alcohol, tobacco, and all recreational ("street") drugs.

1. Fetal alcohol syndrome—No safe level of alcohol intake has been established for pregnancy. Fetal effects of fetal alcohol syndrome include growth restriction; facial, skeletal, and cardiac abnormalities; and serious CNS dysfunction.

2. Cigarette smoking—There is fetal exposure to carbon monoxide and nicotine from cigarette smoking, which may lead to adverse pregnancy outcomes. An increased risk of placental abruption (abruptio placentae), placenta previa, and premature rupture of the membranes is documented among pregnant persons who smoke. Preterm delivery, low birth weight, and ectopic pregnancy are also more likely among persons who smoke cigarettes. Persons who smoke should quit smoking or at least reduce the number of cigarettes smoked per day to as few as possible. Complete cessation is preferred over reduction with the best outcomes seen in persons who stop smoking before 15 weeks' gestation. Clinicians should ask all pregnant persons about their smoking history and offer smoking cessation counseling, since there is more motivation to change at this time. Pregnant persons should also avoid exposure to environmental smoke ("passive smoking"), smokeless tobacco, and e-cigarettes. Pharmacotherapy for smoking cessation has been used with mixed results. Studies of bupropion and nicotine replacement systems are inadequate to properly weigh risks and benefits.

3. Illicit drug use—Cocaine use in pregnancy is associated with an increased risk of premature rupture of membranes, preterm delivery, placental abruption, intrauterine growth restriction, and sudden infant death syndrome. Similar adverse effects on pregnancy are associated with amphetamine use, perhaps reflecting the vasoconstrictive properties of both amphetamines and cocaine. Adverse effects associated with opioid use include intrauterine growth restriction, prematurity, and fetal death. For pregnant persons with opioid use disorder, opioid agonist therapy is the standard of care (see Chapter 47).

C. Radiographs and Noxious Exposures

Radiographs should be avoided unless essential and approved by a clinician. Abdominal shielding should be used whenever possible. The patient should be told to inform her other health care providers that she is pregnant. Chemical or radiation hazards should be avoided as should excessive heat in hot tubs or saunas. Patients should be told to avoid handling cat feces or cat litter and to wear gloves when gardening to avoid infection with toxoplasmosis.

LACTATION

Drugs taken by a nursing mother may accumulate in milk and be transmitted to the infant. LactMed® is an online drug and lactation database for breastfeeding mothers (https://www.ncbi.nlm.nih.gov/books/NBK501922/).

Meek JY et al. Technical report: breastfeeding and the use of human milk. Pediatrics. 2022;150:e2022057989. [PMID: 35921641]

TRAVEL & IMMUNIZATIONS DURING PREGNANCY

During an otherwise normal low-risk pregnancy, travel can be planned most safely up to the 32nd week. Commercial flying in pressurized cabins does not pose a threat to the fetus. An aisle seat will allow frequent walks. Adequate fluids should be taken during the flight.

Travel can increase one's chances of exposure to communicable diseases. Pregnant persons with SARS-CoV-2 infection are at increased risk for preterm birth and for serious illness compared with nonpregnant persons. Pregnant persons should consider risk reduction strategies as appropriate. Vaccination against COVID-19 is recommended for persons who are pregnant, trying to get pregnant, or may become pregnant, and who are breastfeeding. The CDC has determined that the benefits of vaccination outweigh any risks. There is no evidence that vaccination causes problems with fertility in men or women. Pregnant persons who have been vaccinated against COVID-19 may receive a dose of the updated vaccine. The CDC also recommends that persons who are 32–36 weeks pregnant during the RSV season receive the maternal RSV vaccine to help protect their infant from RSV after birth.

Traveling to endemic areas of yellow fever (Africa or Latin America) or of Zika virus (Latin America) is not advisable; since Zika virus can be sexually transmitted, partner travel should also be discussed (see Chapter 36). Similarly, it is inadvisable to travel to areas of Africa or Asia where chloroquine-resistant falciparum malaria is a hazard since complications of malaria are more common in pregnancy.

Ideally, all immunizations should precede pregnancy. *Live virus products are contraindicated during pregnancy (measles, rubella, yellow fever, and smallpox).* Inactivated polio vaccine should be given subcutaneously instead of the oral live-attenuated vaccine. The varicella vaccine should be given 3 months before becoming pregnant. It is not recommended in pregnancy. Vaccines against pneumococcal pneumonia, meningococcal meningitis, and hepatitis A can be used as indicated. Pregnant persons who have not been previously vaccinated against hepatitis B receive the vaccine during pregnancy. The HPV vaccine is not recommended during pregnancy; however, no adverse outcomes have been reported when used during pregnancy. If pregnancy occurs after initiation of the HPV vaccine series, the remaining doses should be deferred until after pregnancy.

The CDC lists pregnancy as a high risk for influenza. Annual influenza vaccination at the appropriate time is indicated in all women who are pregnant or will be pregnant during the "flu season." It can be given in the first trimester. The CDC also recommends that every pregnant woman receive a dose of Tdap during each pregnancy irrespective of her prior vaccination history. The optimal timing for such Tdap administration is between 27–36 weeks' gestation, to maximize the antibody response of the pregnant woman against pertussis and the passive antibody transfer to the infant. For any woman who was not previously vaccinated with Tdap and for whom the vaccine was not given during her pregnancy, Tdap should be administered immediately postpartum. Further, any teenagers or adults not previously vaccinated who will have close contact with the infant should also receive it, ideally 2 weeks before exposure to the infant. This vaccination strategy is called "cocooning," and its purpose is to protect the infant aged < 12 months who is at particularly high risk for lethal pertussis.

Hepatitis A vaccine contains formalin-inactivated virus and can be given in pregnancy when needed. Pooled immune globulin to prevent hepatitis A is safe and does not carry risk of HIV transmission. Chloroquine and proguanil can be used for malaria prophylaxis in pregnancy.

Water should be purified by boiling when there is potential for microbial contamination, since iodine purification may provide more iodine than is safe during pregnancy.

Prophylactic antibiotics or bismuth subsalicylate should not be used during pregnancy to prevent diarrhea. Oral rehydration and treatment of bacterial diarrhea with erythromycin or ampicillin if necessary are preferred.

Centers for Disease Control and Prevention. Guidelines for Vaccinating Pregnant Persons | Pregnancy & Vaccines https://www.cdc.gov/vaccines-pregnancy/hcp/vaccination-guidelines/index.html

OBSTETRIC COMPLICATIONS OF THE FIRST & SECOND TRIMESTERS

VOMITING OF PREGNANCY & HYPEREMESIS GRAVIDARUM

ESSENTIALS OF DIAGNOSIS

- **Vomiting of pregnancy**
  - "Morning sickness" lasts throughout the day.
  - Exerts no adverse effects on the pregnancy and does not presage complications.
- **Hyperemesis gravidarum**
  - Persistent, severe vomiting.
  - Weight loss, dehydration, hypochloremic alkalosis, hypokalemia.
  - May have transient elevation of liver enzymes.
  - Appears related to high or rising serum hCG.
  - Vomiting of pregnancy and hyperemesis gravidarum more common with multifetal pregnancies or hydatidiform mole.

General Considerations

Nausea and vomiting begin soon after the first missed period and cease by the fifth month of gestation. Up to three-fourths of women experience nausea and vomiting during early pregnancy, with the vast majority noting nausea throughout the day.

Persistent, severe vomiting during pregnancy—hyperemesis gravidarum—can be disabling and require hospitalization. Hyperthyroidism can be associated with hyperemesis gravidarum, so it is advisable to determine TSH and free thyroxine (FT_4) values in these patients if they have symptoms of hyperthyroidism.

Treatment

A. Mild Nausea and Vomiting of Pregnancy

In most instances, only reassurance and dietary advice are required. Because of possible teratogenicity, drugs used during the first half of pregnancy should be restricted to those of major importance to life and health.

Pyridoxine (vitamin B_6), 50–100 mg/day orally, is nontoxic and may be helpful in some patients. Pyridoxine alone or in combination with doxylamine (10 mg doxylamine succinate and 10 mg pyridoxine hydrochloride, two tablets at bedtime) is first-line pharmacotherapy. Antiemetics, antihistamines, and antispasmodics are generally unnecessary.

B. Hyperemesis Gravidarum

With more severe nausea and vomiting, it may become necessary to hospitalize the patient. In this case, a private room with limited activity is preferred. It is recommended to give nothing by mouth until the patient is improving and maintain hydration and electrolyte balance by giving appropriate parenteral fluids and vitamin supplements as indicated. Antiemetics such as promethazine (12.5–25 mg orally, rectally, or intravenously every 4–6 hours), metoclopramide (5–10 mg orally or intravenously every 6 hours), or ondansetron (4–8 mg orally or intravenously every 8 hours) should be started. Ondansetron has been associated in some studies with congenital anomalies. Data are limited, but the risks and benefits of treatment should be addressed with the patient. If there is an increased risk, it is probably low. Antiemetics will likely need to be given intravenously initially. Rarely, total parenteral nutrition may become necessary but only if enteral feedings cannot be done. As soon as possible, the patient should be placed on a dry diet consisting of six small meals daily. Antiemetics may be continued orally as needed. After inpatient stabilization, the patient can be maintained at home even if she requires intravenous fluids in addition to her oral intake. There are conflicting studies regarding the use of corticosteroids for the control of hyperemesis gravidarum, and it has also been associated with fetal anomalies, specifically oral clefts. The increase in risk is likely small. However, this treatment should be withheld before 10 weeks' gestation and until more accepted treatments have been exhausted.

When to Refer

- Patient does not respond to first-line outpatient management.
- There is concern for other pathology (ie, hydatidiform mole).

When to Admit

- Patient cannot tolerate any food or water.
- Patient cannot ingest necessary medications.
- Weight loss.
- Presence of a hydatidiform mole.

American College of Obstetricians and Gynecologists. ACOG Practice Bulletin No. 189: nausea and vomiting of pregnancy. Obstet Gynecol. 2018;131:e15. [Reaffirmed 2024] [PMID: 29266076]

SPONTANEOUS PREGNANCY LOSS

ESSENTIALS OF DIAGNOSIS

- Intrauterine pregnancy <20 weeks' gestation.
- Low or falling levels of hCG.
- Bleeding, midline cramping pain.
- Open cervical os.
- Complete or partial expulsion of products of conception.

General Considerations

About three-fourths of spontaneous pregnancy losses (spontaneous abortions/miscarriage) occur before the 16th week; of these, three-fourths occur before the 8th week. Almost 20% of all clinically recognized pregnancies result in a spontaneous loss.

More than 60% of spontaneous losses result from chromosomal defects due to maternal or paternal factors; about 15% appear to be associated with maternal trauma, infections, dietary deficiencies, diabetes mellitus, hypothyroidism, antiphospholipid antibody syndrome, or anatomic malformations. There is no reliable evidence that spontaneous pregnancy loss may be induced by psychic stimuli, such as severe fright, grief, anger, or anxiety. In about one-fourth of cases, the cause cannot be determined. There is no evidence that video display terminals or associated electromagnetic fields are related to an increased risk of spontaneous pregnancy loss.

It is important to distinguish women with a history of incompetent cervix (a problem during the second trimester) from those with early pregnancy loss in the first trimester. Factors that predispose to incompetent cervix are a history of incompetent cervix with a previous pregnancy, cervical conization or surgery, cervical injury, diethylstilbestrol (DES) exposure, and anatomic abnormalities of the cervix. Before pregnancy or during the first trimester, there are no methods for determining whether the cervix will eventually be incompetent. After 14–16 weeks, ultrasound may be used to evaluate the internal anatomy of the lower uterine segment and cervix for the funneling and shortening abnormalities consistent with cervical incompetence.

Clinical Findings

A. Symptoms and Signs

1. Incompetent cervix—Characteristically, incompetent cervix presents as "silent" cervical dilation (ie, with minimal uterine contractions) in the second trimester. Incompetent cervix is a significant (but not inevitable) risk factor for pregnancy loss. When the cervix dilates to ≥ 4 cm, active uterine contractions or rupture of the membranes may occur secondary to the degree of cervical dilation.

2. Threatened spontaneous pregnancy loss—Bleeding or cramping occurs, but the pregnancy continues. The cervix is not dilated.

3. Inevitable spontaneous pregnancy loss—The cervix is dilated, and the membranes may be ruptured, but passage of the products of conception has not yet occurred. Bleeding and cramping persist, and passage of the products of conception is inevitable.

4. Incomplete pregnancy loss—The cervix is dilated. Some portion of the products of conception remains in the uterus. Pregnancy loss is inevitable. Only mild cramps are reported, but bleeding is persistent and often excessive.

5. Early pregnancy loss—The pregnancy has ceased to develop, but the conceptus has not been expelled. Symptoms of pregnancy disappear. There may be a brownish vaginal discharge but no active bleeding. Pain does not develop. The cervix is semifirm and slightly patulous; the uterus becomes smaller and irregularly softened; the adnexa are normal.

B. Laboratory Findings

Pregnancy tests show low or falling levels of hCG. A CBC should be obtained if bleeding is heavy. Determine Rh type and give Rh_0(D) immune globulin if Rh-negative. All tissue recovered should be assessed by a pathologist and may be sent for genetic analysis in selected cases.

C. Ultrasonographic Findings

Transvaginal ultrasound can detect the gestational sac 5–6 weeks from the last menstruation, a fetal pole at 6 weeks, and fetal cardiac activity at 6–7 weeks. Serial observations are often required to evaluate changes in size of the embryo. Diagnostic criteria of early pregnancy loss are a crown-rump length of ≥ 7 mm and no heartbeat or a mean sac diameter of ≥ 25 mm and no embryo.

Differential Diagnosis

The bleeding that occurs in abortion of a uterine pregnancy must be differentiated from the abnormal bleeding of an ectopic pregnancy and anovulatory bleeding in a nonpregnant person. The passage of hydropic villi in the bloody discharge is diagnostic of hydatidiform mole.

Treatment

A. General Measures

1. Threatened spontaneous pregnancy loss—Studies have failed to demonstrate benefit of bedrest for 1–2 days followed by gradual resumption of usual activities. Abstinence from sexual activity has also been suggested without proven benefit. Data are lacking to support the administration of progestins to all women with a threatened pregnancy loss. If an infection is diagnosed (ie, UTI) during the patient's evaluation, it should be treated.

2. Early pregnancy loss—This calls for counseling regarding the fate of the pregnancy and planning for its elective termination at a time chosen by the patient and clinician. Management can be medical or surgical. Each has risks and benefits. Medically induced first-trimester termination with prostaglandins (ie, misoprostol given vaginally in a dose of 800 mcg, followed by one repeat dose if needed 3 hours to 7 days after the first dose) is safe, effective, less invasive, and more private than surgical intervention. If available, a dose of mifepristone, 200 mg orally, should be given 24 hours before administration of misoprostol. If medical management is unsuccessful or if there is excessive bleeding, a surgical procedure (dilation and curettage) may still be needed. Patients must be counseled about the different therapeutic options.

B. Surgical Measures

1. Incomplete pregnancy loss—Prompt removal of any products of conception remaining within the uterus is required to stop bleeding and prevent infection. Analgesia and a paracervical block are useful, followed by uterine exploration with ovum forceps or uterine aspiration. Regional anesthesia may be required.

2. Incompetent cervix—A cerclage is the treatment of choice for incompetent cervix, but a viable intrauterine pregnancy should be confirmed before placement of the cerclage.

Cerclage should be undertaken with caution when there is advanced cervical dilation or when the membranes are prolapsed into the vagina. *Rupture of the membranes and infection are specific contraindications to cerclage.* Testing for *N gonorrhoeae*, *C trachomatis*, and group B streptococci should be obtained before elective placement of a cerclage. *N gonorrhoeae* and *C trachomatis* should be treated before cerclage placement. Testing for group B streptococci is used to guide the need for antibiotics should the patient labor. Patients should consider abstaining from sexual intercourse.

When to Refer

- Patient with history of a second-trimester pregnancy loss.
- Vaginal bleeding that resembles menstruation in a pregnant patient.
- Patient with an open cervical os.
- No signs of uterine growth in serial examinations of a pregnant patient.
- Leakage of amniotic fluid.

When to Admit

- Open cervical os.
- Heavy vaginal bleeding.
- Leakage of amniotic fluid.

American College of Obstetricians and Gynecologists. ACOG Practice Bulletin No. 200: early pregnancy loss. Obstet Gynecol. 2018;132:e197. [Reaffirmed 2025] [PMID: 30157093]

RECURRENT PREGNANCY LOSS

According to the American Society of Reproductive Medicine, recurrent pregnancy loss is defined as the loss of two or more previable (< 24 weeks' gestation or 500 g) pregnancies in succession. Recurrent pregnancy loss affects about 1–5% of pregnancies. Abnormalities related to recurrent pregnancy loss can be identified in approximately 50% of both partners. If a woman has lost three previous pregnancies without identifiable cause, she still has at least a 55% chance of carrying a fetus to viability.

Recurrent pregnancy loss is a clinical rather than pathologic diagnosis. The clinical findings are similar to those observed in other types of pregnancy loss. It is appropriate to begin a medical evaluation in a woman who has had two first-trimester losses.

Treatment

A. Preconception Therapy

Preconception therapy is aimed at detection of maternal or paternal defects that may contribute to pregnancy loss. A thorough history and examination is essential. Maternal testing of a random blood glucose and thyroid function studies (including thyroid antibodies) can be done if the history indicates a possible predisposition to diabetes mellitus or thyroid disease; detection of lupus anticoagulant and other hemostatic abnormalities (proteins S and C and antithrombin deficiency, hyperhomocysteinemia, anticardiolipin antibody, factor V Leiden mutations) and an antinuclear antibody test may be indicated, but in most cases these tests will not be helpful. Hysteroscopy, saline infusion sonogram, or hysterography can be used to exclude submucosal myomas and congenital anomalies of the uterus. In women with recurrent pregnancy losses, resection of a uterine septum, if present, has been recommended. Chromosomal (karyotype) analysis of both partners can be done to rule out balanced translocations (found in 3–4% of infertile partners), but karyotyping is expensive and may not be helpful.

Many therapies have been tried to prevent recurrent loss from immunologic causes. Low-molecular-weight heparin, aspirin, intravenous immunoglobulin, and corticosteroids have been used but the definitive treatment has not been determined (see Antiphospholipid Syndrome, below). Prophylactic low-dose heparin and low-dose aspirin have been recommended for women with antiphospholipid antibodies and recurrent pregnancy loss.

B. Postconception Therapy

The patient should be provided early prenatal care and scheduled frequent office visits. Empiric sex steroid hormone therapy is complicated and should be done by an expert if undertaken.

Prognosis

The prognosis is excellent if the cause of pregnancy losses can be corrected or treated.

Turesheva A et al. Recurrent pregnancy loss etiology, risk factors, diagnosis, and management. Fresh look into a full box. J Clin Med. 2023;12:4074. [PMID: 37373766]

ECTOPIC PREGNANCY

ESSENTIALS OF DIAGNOSIS

- Amenorrhea or irregular bleeding and spotting.
- Pelvic pain, usually adnexal.
- Adnexal mass by clinical examination or ultrasound.
- Failure of serum β-hCG to double every 48 hours.
- No intrauterine pregnancy on transvaginal ultrasound with serum β-hCG > 3500 mIU/mL.

General Considerations

Ectopic implantation occurs in approximately 2% of first trimester pregnancies. About 98% of ectopic pregnancies are tubal. Other sites of ectopic implantation are the peritoneum or abdominal viscera, the ovary, and the cervix. Any condition that prevents or inhibits migration of the fertilized ovum to the uterus can predispose to an ectopic pregnancy, including a history of infertility, pelvic inflammatory disease, ruptured appendix, and prior tubal surgery. Combined intrauterine and extrauterine pregnancy of two embryos (heterotopic) may occur rarely. In the United States, undiagnosed or undetected ectopic pregnancy is one of the most common causes of maternal death during the first trimester.

Clinical Findings

A. Symptoms and Signs

Severe lower quadrant pain occurs in many cases. It is sudden in onset, stabbing, intermittent, and does not radiate. Backache may be present during attacks. Shock occurs in about 10%, often after pelvic examination. At least two-thirds of patients give a history of abnormal menstruation; many have been infertile.

Blood may leak from the tubal ampulla over a period of days, and considerable blood may accumulate in the peritoneum. Slight but persistent vaginal spotting is usually reported, and a pelvic mass may be palpated. Abdominal distention and mild paralytic ileus are often present.

B. Laboratory Findings

The CBC may show anemia and slight leukocytosis. Quantitative serum pregnancy tests will show levels generally lower than expected for normal pregnancies of the same duration. If β-hCG levels are followed over a few days, there may be a slow rise or a plateau rather than the near doubling every 2 days associated with normal early intrauterine pregnancy or the falling levels that occur with spontaneous pregnancy loss.

C. Imaging

Ultrasonography can reliably demonstrate a gestational sac 5–6 weeks from the last menstruation and a fetal pole at 6 weeks if located in the uterus. An empty uterine cavity raises a strong suspicion of extrauterine pregnancy, which can occasionally be revealed by transvaginal ultrasound. A discriminatory zone of serum β-hCG (also known as a threshold level) has been correlated with ultrasound findings of an intrauterine pregnancy; a β-hCG level of ≥ 6500 mIU/mL with an empty uterine cavity by transabdominal ultrasound is highly suspicious for an ectopic pregnancy. Similarly, a β-hCG value ≥ 3500 mIU/mL can be indicative of an ectopic pregnancy if no products of conception are detected within the uterine cavity by transvaginal ultrasound. A discriminatory zone, however, should be used with caution and clinical decisions should not be made solely on β-hCG levels; there have been cases where it is not a reliable indicator of intrauterine or ectopic pregnancy.

D. Special Examinations

Laparoscopy is the surgical procedure of choice both to confirm an ectopic pregnancy and in most cases to permit removal of the ectopic pregnancy without the need for exploratory laparotomy.

Ectopic pregnancy should be suspected when postabortal tissue examination fails to reveal chorionic villi. Steps must be taken for immediate diagnosis, including prompt microscopic tissue examination, ultrasonography, and serial β-hCG titers every 48 hours.

Differential Diagnosis

Clinical and laboratory findings suggestive or diagnostic of pregnancy will distinguish ectopic pregnancy from many acute abdominal illnesses such as acute appendicitis, acute pelvic inflammatory disease, ruptured corpus luteum cyst or ovarian follicle, and urinary calculi. Uterine enlargement with clinical findings similar to those found in ectopic pregnancy is also characteristic of an aborting uterine pregnancy or hydatidiform mole.

Treatment

Patients must be warned about the complications of an ectopic pregnancy and monitored closely. In a stable patient with normal liver and kidney function tests, methotrexate (50 mg/m^2) intramuscularly—given as single or multiple doses—is acceptable medical therapy for early ectopic pregnancy. Criteria favoring a therapeutic response to methotrexate are that the pregnancy is <4 cm in largest dimension and unruptured, with no active bleeding and no fetal heart tones. Several small studies have not found an increased risk of fetal malformations or pregnancy losses in women who conceive within 6 months of methotrexate therapy.

When a patient with an ectopic pregnancy is unstable or when surgical therapy is planned, the patient is hospitalized. Blood is typed and cross-matched. The goal is to diagnose and operate before there is frank rupture of the tube and intra-abdominal hemorrhage. *The use of methotrexate in an unstable patient is absolutely contraindicated.*

Surgical treatment is definitive. In most patients, diagnostic laparoscopy is the initial surgical procedure performed. Depending on the size of the ectopic pregnancy and whether it has ruptured, salpingostomy with removal of the ectopic pregnancy or a partial or complete salpingectomy can usually be performed. Clinical conditions permitting, patency of the contralateral tube can be established by injection of indigo carmine into the uterine cavity and flow through the contralateral tube confirmed visually by the surgeon; iron therapy for anemia may be necessary during convalescence. Rh_0(D) immune globulin (300 mcg) should be given to Rh-negative patients.

Prognosis

Repeat tubal pregnancy occurs in about 10% of cases. This should not be regarded as a contraindication to future pregnancy, but the patient requires careful observation and early ultrasound confirmation of an intrauterine pregnancy.

When to Refer

- Severe abdominal pain.
- Palpation of an adnexal mass on pelvic examination.
- Abdominal pain and vaginal bleeding in a pregnant patient.

When to Admit

Presence of symptoms or signs of a ruptured ectopic pregnancy.

Chong KY et al. Ectopic pregnancy. Nat Rev Dis Primers. 2024;10:94. [PMID: 39668167]

GESTATIONAL TROPHOBLASTIC DISEASE (Hydatidiform Mole & Choriocarcinoma)

ESSENTIALS OF DIAGNOSIS

Hydatidiform mole

- Amenorrhea.
- Irregular uterine bleeding.
- Serum β-hCG > 40,000 mIU/mL.
- Passage of grapelike clusters of enlarged edematous villi per vagina.
- Uterine ultrasound shows characteristic heterogeneous echogenic image and no fetus or placenta.
- Cytogenetic composition is 46,XX (85%), of paternal origin.

Choriocarcinoma

- Persistence of detectable β-hCG after mole evacuation.

General Considerations

Gestational trophoblastic disease is a spectrum of disorders that includes hydatidiform mole (partial and complete), invasive mole (local extension into the uterus or vagina), choriocarcinoma (malignancy often complicated by distant metastases), and placental site trophoblastic tumor. Complete moles show no evidence of a fetus on ultrasonography. The majority are 46,XX, with all chromosomes of paternal origin. Partial moles generally show evidence of an embryo or gestational sac; are triploid, slower-growing, and less symptomatic; and often present clinically as spontaneous pregnancy loss. Partial moles tend to follow a benign course, while complete moles have a greater tendency to become choriocarcinoma.

In North America, the frequency of gestational trophoblastic disease is 1:1500 pregnancies. The highest rates occur in Asian patients. Risk factors include prior spontaneous pregnancy loss, a history of mole, and age younger than 21 or older than 35. Approximately 10% of women require further treatment after evacuation of the mole; choriocarcinoma develops in 2–3% of women.

Clinical Findings

A. Symptoms and Signs

1. Hydatidiform mole—Uterine bleeding, beginning at 6–16 weeks, is observed in most instances. In some cases, the uterus is larger than would be expected in a normal pregnancy of the same duration. Excessive nausea and vomiting may occur. Bilaterally enlarged cystic ovaries are sometimes palpable. They result from ovarian hyperstimulation due to excess β-hCG. Preeclampsia-eclampsia may develop during the second trimester of an untreated molar pregnancy, but this is unusual because most are diagnosed early.

2. Choriocarcinoma—Manifestations may be continued or recurrent uterine bleeding after evacuation of a mole or following delivery, spontaneous pregnancy loss, or ectopic pregnancy. An ulcerative vaginal tumor, pelvic mass, or distant metastases may be the presenting manifestation.

B. Laboratory Findings

Hydatidiform moles are generally characterized by high serum β-hCG values, which can range from high normal to the millions. Levels are higher with complete moles than with partial moles. Serum β-hCG values, if extremely high, can assist in making the diagnosis, but they are more helpful in managing response to treatment. Hemoglobin/hematocrit, creatinine, blood type, liver biochemical tests, and thyroid function tests should also be measured. High β-hCG levels can cause the release of thyroid hormone, and rarely, symptoms of hyperthyroidism.

C. Imaging

The preoperative diagnosis of hydatidiform mole is confirmed by ultrasound. Placental vesicles can be easily seen on transvaginal ultrasound. A preoperative CXR is indicated to rule out pulmonary metastases of the trophoblast.

Treatment

Patients with hyperthyroidism may require β-blocker therapy until the mole has been evacuated.

A. Specific (Surgical) Measures

The uterus should be emptied as soon as the diagnosis of hydatidiform mole is established, preferably by suction curettage. The products of conception should be sent to a pathologist for review. Ovarian cysts should not be resected nor ovaries removed; spontaneous regression of theca lutein cysts will occur with elimination of the mole. Rh_0(D) immune globulin should be given if Rh-negative. In patients who have completed their childbearing, hysterectomy is an acceptable alternative. Hysterectomy does not preclude the need for follow-up of β-hCG levels.

B. Follow-Up Measures

Weekly quantitative β-hCG level measurements are initially required. Following successful surgical evacuation, moles show a progressive decline in β-hCG. After a negative weekly test (< 5 mIU/mL) is achieved, the interval may be increased to every 1 month for an additional 6 months. The purpose of this follow-up is to identify persistent nonmetastatic and metastatic disease, including choriocarcinoma, which is more likely to occur if the initial β-hCG is high and the uterus is large. If levels plateau or begin to rise, the patient should be evaluated by repeat laboratory tests, CXR, and dilation and curettage (D&C) before the initiation of chemotherapy. Effective contraception (preferably birth control pills) should be prescribed to avoid the confusion of elevated β-hCG from a new pregnancy. The β-hCG levels should be negative for 6 months before pregnancy is attempted again. Because the risk of recurrence of a molar pregnancy is 1–2%, an ultrasound should be performed in the first trimester of the pregnancy following a mole to ensure that the pregnancy is normal. In addition, a β-hCG level should then be checked 6 weeks postpartum (after the subsequent normal pregnancy) to ensure there is no persistent trophoblastic tissue, and the placenta should be examined by a pathologist.

C. Antitumor Chemotherapy

If malignant tissue is discovered at surgery or during the follow-up examination, chemotherapy is indicated. For low-risk patients with a good prognosis, methotrexate is considered first-line therapy followed by dactinomycin. Patients with high-risk disease should be referred to a cancer center, where multiple-agent chemotherapy probably will be given.

Prognosis

Five-year survival after courses of chemotherapy, even when metastases have been demonstrated, can be expected in at least 85% of cases of choriocarcinoma.

When to Refer

- Uterine size exceeds that anticipated for gestational age.
- Vaginal bleeding similar to menstruation.
- Pregnant patient with a history of a molar pregnancy.

When to Admit

- Confirmed molar pregnancy by ultrasound and laboratory studies.
- Heavy vaginal bleeding in a pregnant patient under evaluation.

Ngan HYS et al. Diagnosis and management of gestational trophoblastic disease: 2025 update. Int J Gynaecol Obstet. 2025;171 Suppl 1(Suppl 1):78. [PMID: 40631439]

OBSTETRICAL COMPLICATIONS OF THE SECOND & THIRD TRIMESTERS

GESTATIONAL HYPERTENSION, PREECLAMPSIA, & ECLAMPSIA

ESSENTIALS OF DIAGNOSIS

Gestational hypertension

- Blood pressure ≥ 140 mm Hg systolic or > 90 mm Hg diastolic after 20 weeks' gestation.
- Blood pressure was normal before pregnancy and returns to normal postpartum.
- Absence of proteinuria.

Preeclampsia without severe features

- Blood pressure ≥ 140 mm Hg systolic or ≥ 90 mm Hg diastolic after 20 weeks' gestation.
- Proteinuria ≥ 0.3 g in 24 hours.

Preeclampsia with severe features

- Blood pressure ≥ 160 mm Hg systolic or ≥ 110 mm Hg diastolic.
- Progressive kidney injury.
- Proteinuria is not always present.
- If proteinuria is absent, diagnosis should still be considered if hypertension is present along with any of the following:
  - Thrombocytopenia.
  - Hemolysis, elevated liver enzymes, low platelets (HELLP).
  - Pulmonary edema.
  - Vision changes or headache.
- When hypertension is present with severe features of preeclampsia, seizure prophylaxis is beneficial.

Eclampsia

- Seizures with findings of preeclampsia.

General Considerations

Chronic hypertension is defined as hypertension that developed before pregnancy or is evident before 20 weeks' gestation. Gestational hypertension is hypertension (in the absence of proteinuria) that develops 20 weeks or later during pregnancy in a previously normotensive patient whose blood pressure returns to normal postpartum. Chronic hypertension is discussed below. Preeclampsia is defined as the presence of newly elevated blood pressure and proteinuria during pregnancy. Eclampsia is diagnosed when seizures develop in a patient with evidence of preeclampsia. Historically, three elements were required for the diagnosis of preeclampsia: hypertension, proteinuria, and edema. Edema was difficult to objectively quantify and is no longer a required element. In addition, proteinuria may not always be present in preeclampsia with severe features.

Preeclampsia-eclampsia most commonly occurs in the third trimester but can occur any time after 20 weeks' gestation and up to 6 weeks postpartum.

Risk factors for early preeclampsia-eclampsia are maternal comorbid conditions, such as hypertension, kidney disease, and SLE.

Preeclampsia-eclampsia is a disease unique to pregnancy, with the only cure being delivery of the fetus and placenta. Preeclampsia develops in approximately 7% of pregnant persons in the United States; of those, eclampsia will develop in 5% (0.04% of pregnant persons). Primiparas are most frequently affected; however, the incidence of preeclampsia-eclampsia is increased with multifetal gestations, preeclampsia in a previous pregnancy, and comorbid diseases such as chronic hypertension, pregestational diabetes, gestational diabetes, thrombophilia, kidney disease, SLE, prepregnancy BMI > 30, antiphospholipid antibody syndrome, maternal age ≥ 35 years old, assisted reproductive technology, and obstructive sleep apnea. Eclampsia is a significant cause of maternal death.

Clinical Findings

The severity of preeclampsia-eclampsia is based on its effect on six major target areas: the CNS, the kidneys, the liver, the hematologic system, the vascular system, and the fetal-placental unit. By evaluating each of these areas for the presence of mild to severe preeclampsia, the degree of involvement can be assessed, and an appropriate management plan can be formulated that balances the severity of disease and gestational age (Table 22–2).

A. Gestational Hypertension

Preeclampsia and gestational hypertension are defined based on similar blood pressure elevations > 140/90 mm Hg on two occasions at least 4 hours apart but proteinuria is absent with gestational hypertension.

B. Preeclampsia

1. Without severe features—Patients usually have few complaints, and the diastolic blood pressure is < 110 mm Hg. Edema may be present. The platelet count is > 100,000/mcL (100 × 10^9/L), antepartum fetal testing is

Table 22–2. Indicators of mild and severe preeclampsia-eclampsia and gestational hypertension with severe features.

Site	Indicator	Mild	Severe
CNS	Symptoms and signs	Hyperreflexia	Seizures, blurred vision, scotomas, headache, clonus, irritability
Kidney	Proteinuria Urinary output	> 0.3 g/24 hours[1] > 30 mL/hour	> 0.3 g/24 hours[1] < 30 mL/hour
Liver	AST, ALT, LD	Normal liver enzymes	Elevated liver enzymes, epigastric pain, ruptured liver
Hematologic	Platelets Hemoglobin	Normal Normal	< 100,000/mcL (100×10^9/L) Low, normal, or elevated
Vascular	Blood pressure Retina	<160/110 mm Hg Arteriolar spasm	> 160/110 mm Hg Retinal hemorrhages
Fetal-placental unit	Growth restriction Oligohydramnios Fetal distress	Absent Absent Absent	Present Present Present

[1]Proteinuria may not always be present.

reassuring, CNS irritability is minimal, epigastric pain is not present, and liver enzymes are not elevated. Proteinuria is present with urine protein ≥ 0.3 g/24 hours or a protein/creatinine ratio of > 0.3.

2. With severe features—Symptoms are more dramatic and persistent. Patients may complain of headache and changes in vision. The blood pressure is often above 160/110 mm Hg. Thrombocytopenia (platelet count < 100,000/mcL [100×10^9/L]) may be present and progress to disseminated intravascular coagulation. Proteinuria usually exceeds 0.3 g/24 hours. Severe epigastric pain may be present from hepatic subcapsular hemorrhage with significant stretch or rupture of the liver capsule. HELLP syndrome is an advanced form of severe preeclampsia.

C. Eclampsia

The occurrence of seizures defines eclampsia. It is a manifestation of severe CNS involvement. Other findings of preeclampsia are observed.

Differential Diagnosis

Other diseases that can mimic preeclampsia-eclampsia include chronic hypertension, CKD, primary seizure disorders, gallbladder and pancreatic disease, immune thrombocytopenia, thrombotic thrombocytopenic purpura, and hemolytic-uremic syndrome.

Treatment

The American College of Obstetricians and Gynecologists (ACOG) supports considering the use of low-dose aspirin (81 mg orally daily) initiated between 12–28 weeks' gestation (optimally before 16 weeks) and continued daily until delivery for women at increased risk for preeclampsia; risk factors include a history of preeclampsia, multifetal gestation, chronic hypertension, diabetes mellitus, kidney disease, or autoimmune diseases (such as SLE or antiphospholipid syndrome). Clinicians may also consider low-dose aspirin (81 mg orally daily) if more than one of the following moderate risk factors are present: nulliparity, obesity, family history of preeclampsia, Black race, age > 35 years, low socioeconomic status, personal history factors (eg, mother having a previous baby with low birth weight), and in vitro fertilization. Diuretics, dietary restriction or enhancement, sodium restriction, and vitamin-mineral supplements (eg, calcium or vitamins C and E) have not been confirmed to be useful. The only cure is delivery of the fetus at a time as favorable as possible for its survival.

A. Gestational Hypertension

The oral agents that are recommended for treatment of hypertension during pregnancy are labetalol (Table 13–9), nifedipine (Table 13–7) and methyldopa (Table 13–10). The goal of treatment for gestational hypertension is a blood pressure of 140/90 mm Hg. *ACE inhibitors, ARBs, and mineralocorticoid receptor antagonists are teratogenic and contraindicated in pregnancy.* Delivery should take place at term in the absence of severe hypertension.

B. Preeclampsia

Early recognition is the key to treatment. This requires careful attention to the details of prenatal care—especially subtle changes in blood pressure and weight. The objectives are to prolong pregnancy, if possible, to allow fetal lung maturity while preventing progression to severe disease and eclampsia. The critical factors are the gestational age of the fetus, fetal pulmonary maturity, and the severity of maternal disease.

1. Preeclampsia without severe features—Home management may be attempted for these patients if they have a stable home situation. Patients must be reliable and have assistance at home, rapid access to the hospital, and ability to obtain frequent blood pressure readings. Treatment of hypertension is the same as for Gestational Hypertension, above. A home health nurse can often provide frequent home visits and assessments. For preeclampsia without severe features at ≥ 37 weeks' gestation, delivery rather than expectant management (eg watchful waiting or close monitoring) upon diagnosis is recommended. It also is reasonable to deliver patients with gestational hypertension at this time.

2. Preeclampsia-eclampsia with severe features—Hospitalization is required for patients with preeclampsia with severe features or those with unpredictable home situations. Regular assessments of blood pressure, urine protein, and fetal heart tones and activity are required. A CBC with platelet count, electrolyte panel, and liver enzymes should be checked regularly, with frequency dependent on severity. A 24-hour urine collection for total protein and creatinine clearance should be obtained on admission and repeated as indicated. Magnesium sulfate should be given for seizure prophylaxis once the diagnosis of severe preeclampsia is made and delivery is planned (see Eclampsia, below); magnesium sulfate is given intravenously, 4- to 6-g load over 15–20 minutes followed by 2–3 g/hour maintenance. A urinary catheter is inserted to monitor urinary output. If hypertension is present with systolic values ≥ 160 mm Hg or diastolic values ≥ 110 mm Hg, antihypertensive medications should be administered to reduce the blood pressure to 140–150/90–100 mm Hg. Lower blood pressures than this may induce placental insufficiency through reduced perfusion. Hydralazine, given in 5- to 10-mg increments intravenously every 20 minutes, is frequently used to lower blood pressure. Labetalol, 10–20 mg intravenously, every 20 minutes as needed, can also be used. Immediate-release oral nifedipine 10–20 mg may be administered and then repeated in 20 minutes, followed by 10–20 mg every 4–6 hours for a maximum daily dosage of 180 mg. This medication is helpful if the patient does not have intravenous access. Before term, severe preeclampsia-eclampsia requires delivery with few exceptions. Epigastric pain, seizures, severe range blood pressures, thrombocytopenia, and visual disturbances are strong indications for delivery of the fetus. Marked proteinuria alone can be managed more conservatively.

If the fetus is <34 weeks' gestation, corticosteroids (betamethasone 12 mg intramuscularly every 24 hours for two doses, or dexamethasone 6 mg intramuscularly every 12 hours for four doses) should be administered to the mother (preeclampsia-eclampsia with or without severe features). *However, when a patient clearly has unstable severe preeclampsia, delivery should not be delayed.* The impetus for delivery should not necessarily preclude the initiation of corticosteroids.

The method of delivery is determined by the maternal and fetal status. A vaginal delivery is preferred because it has less blood loss than a cesarean section and requires less coagulation factors. Cesarean section is reserved for the usual fetal indications.

C. Eclampsia

1. General care—Eclampsia necessitates delivery once the patient is stabilized. It is important, however, that assessment of the status of the patient and fetus take place first. Continuous fetal monitoring must be performed and maternal blood typed and cross-matched quickly. The ACOG recommends that systolic blood pressures > 160 mm Hg be treated within 60 minutes using an intravenous agent. (See Preeclampsia-eclampsia with severe features, above). The use of a semi-autonomous algorithm to treat these severe blood pressures within 60 minutes has demonstrated improved expeditious treatment.

If the patient is eclamptic, she is turned on her side to prevent aspiration and to improve blood flow to the placenta. The seizure may be stopped by giving an intravenous bolus of magnesium sulfate (the preferred agent), 4–6 g over 4 minutes or until the seizure stops. A continuous intravenous infusion of magnesium sulfate is then started at a rate of 2–3 g/hour unless the patient has reduced kidney function (serum creatinine > 1.0 mg/dL). Reducing maintenance dosing to 1 g/hour or temporarily stopping infusion may be necessary to address instances of kidney dysfunction and magnesium toxicity. Serum magnesium levels may be checked every 4–6 hours and ideally the infusion rate adjusted to maintain a therapeutic blood level (4–7 mEq/L). Urinary output is checked hourly, and the patient assessed for signs of possible magnesium toxicity such as loss of deep tendon reflexes or decrease in respiratory rate and depth, which can be reversed with calcium gluconate, 1 g intravenously over 2 minutes. If seizures continue, an additional dose of magnesium sulfate, 2 g intravenously, may be infused. Alternative agents (eg, benzodiazepines and phenytoin) should be used only if magnesium sulfate is unavailable.

2. Delivery—Delivery is mandated once eclampsia has occurred. Vaginal delivery is preferred. Subsequent prolonged fetal heart rate decelerations are frequent after an eclamptic seizure. However, delivery should proceed only after there is maternal hemodynamic stabilization. Furthermore, maternal resuscitation is usually followed by normalization of the fetal tracing. The rapidity with which delivery must be achieved depends on the fetal and maternal status following the seizure and the availability of laboratory data on the patient. Oxytocin, given intravenously and titrated to a dose that results in adequate contractions, can induce or augment labor. Oxytocin should only be administered by a clinician specifically trained in its use. Regional analgesia or general anesthesia is acceptable. Cesarean section is used for the usual obstetric indications.

3. Postpartum—Magnesium sulfate infusion (2–3 g/hour with noted exceptions, see above) should be continued for 24 hours postpartum. Late-onset preeclampsia-eclampsia can occur during the postpartum period. It is usually manifested by either hypertension or seizures. Treatment is the same as before delivery—ie, with hydralazine and magnesium sulfate.

When to Refer

- New onset of hypertension and proteinuria in a pregnant patient > 20 weeks' gestation.
- New onset of seizure activity in a pregnant patient.

When to Admit

- Symptoms of preeclampsia with severe features in a pregnant patient with elevated blood pressure above baseline.
- Evaluation for preeclampsia when severe features of the disease are suspected.
- Evaluation for preeclampsia in a patient with an unstable home environment.
- Evidence of eclampsia.

American College of Obstetricians and Gynecologists. Practice Bulletin No. 222: gestational hypertension and preeclampsia. Obstet Gynecol. 2020;135:e237. [Reaffirmed 2023] [PMID: 32443079]

ACOG Committee Opinion No. 743: Low-dose aspirin use during pregnancy. Obstet Gynecol. 2018;132:e44. [Reaffirmed 2023] [PMID: 29939940]

Magee LA et al. Preeclampsia. N Engl J Med. 2022;386:1817. [PMID: 35544388]

Tita AT et al; Chronic Hypertension and Pregnancy (CHAP) Trial Consortium. Treatment for mild chronic hypertension during pregnancy. N Engl J Med. 2022;386:1781. [PMID: 35363951]

PRETERM LABOR

ESSENTIALS OF DIAGNOSIS

- Preterm regular uterine contractions approximately 5 minutes apart.
- Cervical dilatation, effacement, or both.

General Considerations

Preterm birth is defined as birth between 20 0/7 and 36 6/7 weeks' gestation. Spontaneous preterm labor with or without premature rupture of the fetal membranes causes at least two-thirds of all preterm births. Prematurity is the largest single contributor to infant mortality, and survivors are at risk for a myriad of short- and long-term complications. It is also the most common reason for antepartum hospitalization. Rates of infant death and long-term neurologic impairment are inversely related to gestational age at birth. The cusp of viability in contemporary practice is 23–25 weeks' gestation, and infants born before 23 weeks rarely survive. About two-thirds of the preterm births occur between 34 weeks and 36 weeks and 6 days (termed "late preterm birth"), and good outcomes are expected at these gestational ages. Importantly, however, even these late preterm infants are at significantly increased risk for both morbidity and mortality when compared to those infants born at term.

Major risk factors for spontaneous preterm labor include a past history of preterm birth and a short cervical length as measured by transvaginal ultrasound. Other known risk associations include Black race, multifetal pregnancies, intrauterine infection, substance use, cigarette smoking, periodontal disease, and socioeconomic deprivation. Numerous preterm births are preceded by ruptured membranes.

Clinical Findings

In women with regular uterine contractions and cervical change, the diagnosis of preterm labor is straightforward. However, symptoms such as pelvic pressure, cramping, or vaginal discharge may be the first complaints in high-risk patients who later develop preterm labor. Because these complaints may be vague and irregular uterine contractions are common, distinguishing which patients merit further evaluation can be problematic. In some cases, this distinction can be facilitated by the use of fetal fibronectin measurement in cervicovaginal specimens. This test is most useful when it is negative (<50 ng/mL) since the negative predictive value for delivery within 7–14 days is 93–97%. A negative test, therefore, usually means the patient can be reassured and discharged home. Because of its low sensitivity, however, fetal fibronectin is not recommended as a screening test in asymptomatic women.

Treatment

A. General Measures

Patients must be educated to identify symptoms associated with preterm labor to avoid unnecessary delay in their evaluation. In patients who are believed to be at increased risk for preterm delivery, randomized trials have failed to demonstrate improved outcomes in women placed on activity restriction. Paradoxically, such recommendations may place a patient at an *increased* risk to deliver preterm. Women with preterm labor at the threshold of viability present unique ethical and obstetric challenges and are best managed in consultation with maternal-fetal medicine and neonatology specialists. The patients in such situations should be actively and continually engaged about decisions regarding the aggressiveness of resuscitative efforts.

B. Corticosteroids

In pregnancies between 24–34 weeks' gestation where preterm birth is anticipated, a single short course of corticosteroids should be administered to promote fetal lung maturity. Between 22–24 weeks' gestation the administration of corticosteroids should be considered. Such therapy has been demonstrated to reduce the frequency of respiratory distress syndrome, intracranial hemorrhage, and even death in preterm infants. Betamethasone, 12 mg intramuscularly repeated once 24 hours later, and dexamethasone, 6 mg intramuscularly repeated every 12 hours for four doses, both cross the placenta and either is the preferred treatment. A single repeat course of antenatal corticosteroids should be considered in women who are at risk for preterm delivery within the next 7 days, and whose prior dose of antenatal corticosteroids was administered > 14 days previously. Rescue course corticosteroids could be provided as early as 7 days from the prior dose, if indicated by the clinical scenario. The Society for Maternal-Fetal Medicine (SMFM) Consult Series recommends offering a single course of antenatal corticosteroids (two doses of 12 mg of intramuscular betamethasone, 24 hours apart) to patients who meet the inclusion criteria of the Antenatal Late Preterm Steroids trial (those with a singleton pregnancy between 34 0/7 and 36 6/7 weeks' gestation who are at high risk for preterm birth within the next 7 days and before 37 weeks' gestation).

C. Antibiotics

Despite the finding that preterm labor is associated with intrauterine infection in certain cases, there is no evidence that antibiotics forestall delivery in women with preterm labor and intact membranes. However, women in preterm labor should receive antimicrobial prophylaxis against group B *Streptococcus* unless a single standard culture of the distal vagina and anorectum has been negative for the organism in the preceding 5 weeks. Notably, there is usually not enough time in this clinical setting to culture and test isolates. The recommended regimen for antimicrobial prophylaxis against group B *Streptococcus* is penicillin G, 5 million units intravenously as a loading dose and then 2.5–3 million units intravenously every 4 hours until delivery. In penicillin-allergic patients not at high risk for anaphylaxis, 2 g of cefazolin can be given intravenously as an initial dose and then 1 g intravenously every 8 hours until delivery. In patients at high risk for anaphylaxis, vancomycin, 20 mg/kg intravenously every 8 hours until delivery, can be used. Clindamycin, 900 mg intravenously every 8 hours until delivery, can also be used after a group B streptococcal isolate has been confirmed to be susceptible.

D. Tocolytic Agents

First-line tocolytic treatment to forestall delivery is with β-adrenergic receptor agonists, calcium channel blockers, or indomethacin. This treatment can prolong pregnancy in the short-term (up to 48 hours) to allow for the administration of antenatal corticosteroids, and (if appropriate), transport the patient to a facility better equipped to care for premature infants. Maintenance therapy (continuation of treatment beyond 48 hours) is not effective at preventing preterm birth and is not recommended.

Before attempts are made to prevent preterm delivery with tocolytic agents, the patient should be assessed for conditions in which delivery would be indicated. Severe preeclampsia, lethal fetal anomalies, placental abruption, and intrauterine infection are all examples of indications for preterm delivery. In such cases, attempts to forestall delivery are inappropriate.

1. β-Adrenergic receptor agonist—Terbutaline can be given every 30 minutes as an intravenous infusion starting at 2.5 mcg/min or as a subcutaneous injection starting at 250 mcg. Oral terbutaline is not recommended because of the lack of proven efficacy and concerns about maternal safety. Serious maternal side effects from terbutaline include tachycardia, pulmonary edema, arrhythmias, metabolic derangements (eg, hyperglycemia and hypokalemia), and even death. Pulmonary edema occurs with increased frequency with concomitant administration of corticosteroids, large-volume intravenous fluid infusion, maternal sepsis, or prolonged tocolysis. Because of these safety concerns, the US FDA warns that terbutaline be administered exclusively in a hospital setting and discontinued after 48–72 hours of treatment.

2. Nifedipine and indomethacin—Nifedipine, 20 mg orally every 6 hours, and indomethacin, 50 mg orally once then 25 mg orally every 6 hours up to 48 hours, have been used with limited success.

3. Magnesium sulfate—This commonly used medication (but no longer recommended as a first-line agent) for tocolysis may also be protective against cerebral palsy in infants born from 24–32 weeks' gestation when given at time of birth. Magnesium sulfate is given intravenously as a 4- to 6-g bolus followed by a continuous infusion of 2 g/hour. Magnesium levels are not typically checked but should be monitored if there is any concern for toxicity. Magnesium sulfate is entirely cleared by the kidney and must, therefore, be used with caution in women with any degree of kidney disease.

Preterm Birth Prevention

In 2003, the US FDA withdrew approval of 17-α hydroxyprogesterone caproate to reduce the risk of recurrent spontaneous preterm birth due to lack of evidence of efficacy. Although the issue has not been settled, there is evidence that progesterone therapy may decrease rates of preterm birth in nulliparous women who have a shortened cervix as measured by transvaginal ultrasound. The ACOG does not recommend universal transvaginal cervical length screening but acknowledges that this strategy may be considered.

There is also evidence that women with a previous spontaneous preterm birth (before 24 weeks' gestation) and a shortened cervix (< 25 mm) may benefit from placement of a cervical cerclage. Incidentally detected short cervical length in the second trimester in the absence of a prior singleton preterm birth is not diagnostic of cervical insufficiency, and cerclage is not indicated in this setting. In twin and triplet gestations, progesterone administration has not been effective at prolonging pregnancy, and this therapy is not recommended. Cervical cerclage is not recommended for prevention of preterm birth if the sole indication is multiple gestations.

When to Refer

- Symptoms of increased pelvic pressure or cramping in high-risk patients.
- Regular uterine contractions.
- Rupture of membranes.
- Vaginal bleeding.

When to Admit

- Cervical dilation of ≥ 2 cm before 34 weeks' gestation.
- Contractions that cause cervical change.
- Rupture of membranes.

American College of Obstetricians and Gynecologists. Practice Advisory: use of antenatal corticosteroids at 22 weeks of gestation. 2022 Oct. https://www.acog.org/clinical/clinical-guidance/practice-advisory/articles/2021/09/use-of-antenatal-corticosteroids-at-22-weeks-of-gestation
American College of Obstetricians and Gynecologists. ACOG Practice Bulletin No. 217: prelabor rupture of membranes. Obstet Gynecol. 2020;135:e80. [Reaffirmed 2023] [PMID: 32080050]
Hoffman MK. ACOG Practice Bulletin, No 234: prediction and prevention of spontaneous preterm birth. Obstet Gynecol. 2021;138:945. [Reaffirmed 2025] [PMID: 34794160]
Reddy UM et al; Society for Maternal-Fetal Medicine. Society for Maternal-Fetal Medicine Consult Series #58: Use of antenatal corticosteroids for individuals at risk for late preterm delivery: replaces SMFM Statement #4. Am J Obstet Gynecol. 2021;225:B36. [PMID: 34363784]

THIRD-TRIMESTER BLEEDING

Five to 10 percent of women have vaginal bleeding in late pregnancy. The clinician must distinguish between placental causes (eg, placenta previa, placental abruption, vasa previa) and nonplacental causes (eg, labor, infection, disorders of the lower genital tract, systemic disease). The approach to bleeding in late pregnancy depends on the underlying cause, the gestational age at presentation, the degree of blood loss, and the overall status of the mother and her fetus. The cause of antepartum bleeding after mid-pregnancy is unknown in one-third of cases.

Treatment

A. General Measures

The patient should initially be observed closely with continuous fetal monitoring to assess for fetal distress. A CBC with platelets and an INR should be obtained and repeated serially if the bleeding continues. If hemorrhage is significant or if there is evidence of acute hypovolemia, the need for transfusion should be anticipated and an appropriate volume of red cells prepared with cross-matching. Ultrasound examination should be performed to determine placental location. Digital pelvic examinations are done only after ultrasound examination has ruled out placenta previa. Administration of anti-D immune globulin may be required for women who are Rh negative.

B. Placenta Previa

Placenta previa occurs when the placenta implants over the internal cervical os. Risk factors for this condition include previous cesarean delivery, increasing maternal age, multiparity, and cigarette smoking. If the diagnosis is initially made in the first or second trimester, the ultrasound should be repeated in the third trimester. Persistence of placenta previa is an indication for cesarean as the route of delivery. Painless vaginal bleeding is the characteristic symptom in placenta previa and can range from light spotting to profuse hemorrhage. Hospitalization for extended evaluation is the appropriate initial management approach. For pregnancies that have reached 37 weeks' gestation or beyond with continued bleeding, cesarean delivery is generally indicated. Pregnancies at 36 weeks or earlier are candidates for expectant management (eg, watchful waiting or close monitoring) provided the bleeding is not prodigious, and a subset of these women can be discharged if the bleeding and contractions completely subside.

C. Morbidly Adherent Placenta

Morbidly adherent placenta is a general term describing an abnormally adherent placenta that has invaded into the uterus. The condition can be further classified depending on whether the depth of invasion is limited to the endometrium (*accreta*), extends into the myometrium (*increta*), or invades beyond the uterine serosa (*percreta*). The most important risk factor for a morbidly adherent placenta is a prior uterine scar—typically from one or more prior cesarean deliveries. The focus of invasion usually involves the scar itself, and *placenta previa* is commonly associated with morbid adherence. The incidence of these syndromes has increased dramatically over the last 50 years commensurate with the increasing cesarean delivery rate.

After delivery of the infant, almost always in a repeat cesarean section, the morbidly adherent placenta does not separate normally, and the bleeding that results can be torrential. Emergency hysterectomy is usually required to stop the hemorrhage, and transfusion requirements are often massive. Because of the considerable increase in both maternal morbidity and mortality associated with this condition, careful preoperative planning is imperative when the diagnosis is suspected antenatally. Ultrasound findings such as intraplacental lacunae, bridging vessels into the bladder, and loss of the retroplacental clear space suggest placental invasion in women who have placenta previa. The 2021 SMFM Placenta Accreta Task Force consensus document contains standardized ultrasound markers for the identification of placenta accreta spectrum. *Importantly, however, even if ultrasound findings are subtle, an abnormally adherent placenta should be suspected in any patient with one or more prior cesarean deliveries and an anterior placenta previa.* Ideally, delivery planning should involve a multidisciplinary team, and the surgery should take place at an institution with appropriate personnel and a blood bank equipped to handle patients requiring massive transfusions. A systematic approach to management with a multidisciplinary team improves patient outcomes. Evidence-based recommendations regarding delivery timing are lacking, but the goal is to have a planned, late-preterm cesarean delivery. As such, delivery at 34–36 weeks in a stable patient seems a reasonable approach.

D. Placental Abruption

Placental abruption is the premature separation of the placenta from its implantation site before delivery. Risk factors for abruption include hypertension, multiparity, cocaine use, cigarette smoking, previous abruption, and thrombophilias. Classic symptoms are vaginal bleeding, uterine tenderness, and frequent contractions, but the clinical presentation is highly variable. There is often concealed hemorrhage when the placenta abrupts, which causes increased pressure in the intervillous space. Excess amounts of thromboplastin escape into the maternal circulation and defibrination occurs. Profound coagulopathy and acute hypovolemia from blood loss can occur in the mother, especially when the abruption is severe enough to kill the fetus. Ultrasound may be helpful to exclude placenta previa, but failure to identify a retroplacental clot does not exclude abruption. In most cases, abruption is an indication for immediate cesarean delivery because of the high risk of fetal death. Quantification of maternal blood loss, as described in statewide quality improvement bundles, has been advocated to reduce maternal hemorrhage associated morbidity.

American College of Obstetricians and Gynecologists. Practice Bulletin No. 183: postpartum hemorrhage. Obstet Gynecol. 2017;130:e168. [Reaffirmed 2024] [PMID: 28937571]

Brandt JS et al. Placental abruption at near-term and term gestations: pathophysiology, epidemiology, diagnosis, and management. Am J Obstet Gynecol. 2023;228:S1313. [PMID: 37164498]

Oyelese Y et al. Placenta previa. Clin Obstet Gynecol. 2025;68:86. [PMID: 39654466]

OBSTETRIC COMPLICATIONS OF THE PERIPARTUM PERIOD

PUERPERAL MASTITIS

Postpartum mastitis occurs sporadically in nursing mothers, usually with symptom onset after discharge from the hospital. *Staphylococcus aureus* is usually the causative agent. Women nursing for the first time and those with difficulty breastfeeding appear to be at greatest risk. Rarely, inflammatory carcinoma of the breast can be mistaken for puerperal mastitis (see also Chapter 19). Unfortunately, strategies aimed at preventing mastitis in breastfeeding women have been unsuccessful.

Mastitis frequently begins within 3 months after delivery and may start with an engorged breast and a sore or fissured nipple. Cellulitis is typically unilateral with the affected area of breast being red, tender, and warm. Fever and chills are common complaints as well. Treatment consists of antibiotics effective against penicillin-resistant staphylococci (dicloxacillin 500 mg orally every 6 hours or a cephalosporin for 10–14 days) and regular emptying of the breast by nursing or by using a mechanical suction device. Although nursing from the infected breast is safe for the infant, local inflammation of the nipple may complicate latching. Failure to respond to usual antibiotics within 2 days may represent an organizing abscess or infection with a resistant organism. The risk for abscess formation is increased when the causative organism is methicillin-resistant *S aureus* (MRSA), compared with infection from nonresistant staphylococcal species. If an abscess is suspected, ultrasound of the breast can help confirm the diagnosis. In these cases, aspiration or surgical evacuation is usually required. Changing antibiotics based on culture sensitivity (to vancomycin or trimethoprim-sulfamethoxazole, for example) is helpful, especially if the clinical course is not improving appropriately.

CHORIOAMNIONITIS & METRITIS

ESSENTIALS OF DIAGNOSIS

- Fever not attributable to another source.
- Uterine tenderness.
- Tachycardia in the mother, fetus, or both.

General Considerations

Pelvic infections are relatively common problems encountered during the peripartum period. Chorioamnionitis is an infection of the amnion and chorion (fetal parts), usually occurring during labor. Uterine infection after delivery is often called endometritis or endomyometritis, but the term "metritis" is probably most accurate to emphasize that the infection extends throughout the uterine tissue. These infections are polymicrobial and are most commonly attributed to urogenital pathogens. The single most important risk factor for puerperal infection is cesarean delivery, which increases the risk 5- to 20-fold. Other recognized risk factors include prolonged labor, use of internal monitors, nulliparity, multiple pelvic examinations, prolonged rupture of membranes, and lower genital tract infections. Although maternal complications such as dysfunctional labor and postpartum hemorrhage are increased with clinical chorioamnionitis, the principal reason to initiate treatment is to prevent morbidity in the offspring. Neonatal complications such as sepsis, pneumonia, intraventricular hemorrhage, and cerebral palsy are increased in the setting of chorioamnionitis. Intrapartum initiation of antibiotics, however, significantly reduces neonatal morbidity.

Clinical Findings

Puerperal infections are diagnosed principally by the presence of fever (≥ 38°C) in the absence of any other source and one or more of the following signs: maternal or fetal tachycardia (or both), and uterine tenderness. Foul-smelling lochia may be present but is an insensitive marker of infection as many women without infection may experience an unpleasant odor. Likewise, some life-threatening infections such as necrotizing fasciitis are typically odorless. Isolated fever of 38–38.9°C can occur, and many clinicians elect to treat given the increased morbidity associated with these infections. Cultures are typically not done because of the polymicrobial nature of the infection.

Treatment

Treatment is empiric with broad-spectrum antibiotics that will cover gram-positive and gram-negative organisms if still pregnant and gram-negative organisms and anaerobes if postpartum. A common regimen for chorioamnionitis is ampicillin, 2 g intravenously every 6 hours, and gentamicin, 2 mg/kg intravenous load then 1.5 mg/kg intravenously every 8 hours. A common regimen for metritis is gentamicin, 2 mg/kg intravenous load then 1.5 mg/kg intravenously every 8 hours, and clindamycin, 900 mg intravenously every 8 hours. Continuation of antibiotics in the postpartum period varies depending on mode of delivery and clinical scenario. No oral antibiotics are subsequently needed after completion of intravenous treatment. Patients with metritis who do not respond in the first 24–48 hours may have an enterococcal component of metritis and require additional gram-positive coverage (such as ampicillin) to the regimen.

MEDICAL CONDITIONS COMPLICATING PREGNANCY

ANEMIA

Normal pregnancy is characterized by an increase in maternal plasma volume of about 50% and an increase in red cell volume of about 25%. Because of these changes, the mean hemoglobin and hematocrit values are lower than in the nonpregnant state. Anemia in pregnancy is considered when the hemoglobin measurement is < 11 g/dL in the first trimester, 10.5 g/dL in the second trimester, and 11 g/dL in the third trimester. By far, the most common causes are iron deficiency and acute blood loss anemia, the latter usually occurring in the peripartum period. Symptoms such as fatigue and dyspnea that would otherwise suggest the presence of anemia in nonpregnant women are common in pregnant women; therefore, periodic measurement of hematocrits in pregnancy is essential so that anemia can be identified and treated. In addition to its impact on maternal health, untoward pregnancy outcomes such as low birthweight and preterm delivery have been associated with second- and third-trimester anemia.

A. Iron Deficiency Anemia

The increased requirement for iron over the course of pregnancy is appreciable to support fetal growth and expansion of maternal blood volume. Dietary intake of iron generally cannot meet this demand, and all pregnant women should receive about 30 mg of elemental iron per day in the second and third trimesters. Oral iron therapy is commonly associated with GI side effects, such as nausea and constipation, and these symptoms often contribute to noncompliance. If supplementation is inadequate, anemia often becomes evident by the third trimester of pregnancy. Because iron deficiency is by far the most common cause of anemia in pregnancy, treatment is usually empiric and consists of 60–100 mg of elemental iron per day and a diet containing iron-rich foods. Iron studies can confirm the diagnosis, if necessary (see Chapter 15), and further evaluation should be considered in patients who do not respond to oral iron. Intermittent iron supplementation (eg, every other day) has been associated with fewer side effects and may be reasonable for women who cannot tolerate daily therapy.

During the third trimester of pregnancy for women with severe and demonstrated iron deficiency anemia, some experts recommend the administration of intravenous ferric carboxymaltose (Injectafer), 1000 mg, over 15 minutes and then repeated in 7 days. Intravenous iron administration has been shown to be more effective than oral iron, which some patients cannot tolerate due to side effects or do not take as prescribed. With severe anemia (hematocrit <25%), intravenous infusion of iron can reduce the need for blood transfusions.

B. Folic Acid Deficiency Anemia

Megaloblastic anemia in pregnancy is almost always caused by folic acid deficiency, since vitamin B_{12} deficiency is uncommon in the childbearing years. Folate deficiency is usually caused by inadequate dietary intake of fresh leafy vegetables, legumes, and animal proteins.

The diagnosis is made by finding macrocytic red cells and hypersegmented neutrophils on a blood smear (see Chapter 15). However, blood smears in pregnancy may be difficult to interpret since they frequently show iron deficiency changes as well. With established folate deficiency, a supplemental dose of 1 mg/day and a diet with increased folic acid will generally correct the anemia.

C. Sickle Cell Anemia

Women with sickle cell anemia are subject to serious complications in pregnancy. The anemia becomes more severe, and acute pain crises often occur more frequently. When compared with women who do not have hemoglobinopathies, women with hemoglobin SS are at increased risk for infections (especially pulmonary and urinary tract), thromboembolic events, pregnancy-related hypertension, transfusion, cesarean delivery, preterm birth, and fetal growth restriction. There also continues to be an increased rate of maternal mortality, despite an increased recognition of the high-risk nature of these pregnancies. Intensive medical treatment may improve the outcomes for both mother and fetus. Prophylactically transfusing packed red cells to lower the level of hemoglobin S and elevate the level of hemoglobin A is a controversial practice without clear benefit. Most women with sickle cell disease will not require iron supplementation, but folate requirements can be appreciable due to red cell turnover from hemolysis.

D. Other Anemias

Although many of the inherited or acquired causes of anemia are relatively rare in women of childbearing age, they can be encountered in pregnancy. The implications for the mother and her offspring vary widely depending on the etiology of anemia. For example, mild microcytic anemia may be caused by iron deficiency, but it could also represent anemia of chronic disease because of previously undiagnosed malignancy. As such, women who have anemia caused by a disorder besides a nutritional deficiency are best managed in conjunction with a maternal-fetal medicine specialist and a hematologist. Additionally, women who have an inherited form of anemia (hemoglobinopathies and thalassemia syndromes, for example) should be offered genetic counseling; prenatal diagnosis, if available, should be discussed if the mother wishes to know whether the fetus is affected.

American College of Obstetricians and Gynecologists. ACOG Practice Bulletin No. 233: anemia in pregnancy. Obstet Gynecol. 2021;138:e55. [Reaffirmed 2024][PMID: 34293770]
Derman RJ et al. Single-dose intravenous iron vs oral iron for treatment of maternal iron deficiency anemia: a randomized clinical trial. RAPIDIRON Trial Group (Appendix). Am J Obstet Gynecol. 2025;233:120.e1. [PMID: 39909327]
Kirthan JPA et al. Pathophysiology and management of iron deficiency anaemia in pregnancy: a review. Ann Hematol. 2024;103:2637. [PMID: 37787837]
Sinkey RG et al. Society for Maternal-Fetal Medicine Consult Series #68; Sickle cell disease in pregnancy. Am J Obstet Gynecol. 2024;230:B17. [PMID: 37866731]

ANTIPHOSPHOLIPID SYNDROME

The antiphospholipid syndrome is characterized by autoantibodies, notably in association with arterial and venous thrombosis and adverse pregnancy outcomes (see Chapter 23).

THYROID DISEASE

Thyroid disease is relatively common in pregnancy, and in their overt states, both hypothyroidism and hyperthyroidism have been consistently associated with adverse pregnancy outcomes. There are gestational age-specific effects that pregnancy has on thyroid function tests; failure to recognize these physiologic alterations can cause misclassification or misdiagnosis. Women who have a history of a thyroid disorder or symptoms that suggest thyroid dysfunction should be screened with thyroid function tests. Screening asymptomatic pregnant women, however, is of unproven benefit and is not recommended.

The most common etiology of hypothyroidism during pregnancy is autoimmune (Hashimoto) thyroiditis. Many of the symptoms of hypothyroidism mimic those of normal pregnancy, making its clinical identification difficult. Maternal hypothyroidism has consistently been associated with an increase in complications such as spontaneous pregnancy loss, preterm birth, preeclampsia, placental abruption, and impaired neuropsychological development in the offspring; the fetus is at least partially dependent on maternal T_4 for its CNS development—particularly in the second trimester. For women who are already taking levothyroxine, one should anticipate a 25% dose increase at pregnancy confirmation.

1. Overt hypothyroidism—An elevated serum TSH level with a depressed FT_4 level define overt hypothyroidism. During pregnancy, several factors occur that affect maternal thyroid hormones: (1) Rising estrogen levels increase thyroxine binding globulin serum concentrations, reducing FT_4 levels. (2) Placental deiodinase promotes the turnover of T_4. (3) Supplemental iron and prenatal multivitamins containing iron can bind to oral T_4 and reduce its intestinal absorption. Pregnant women with overt hypothyroidism or myxedema should be treated immediately with levothyroxine at full replacement doses of 1.6 mcg/kg/day (about 100–150 mcg daily). For titration, the levothyroxine dosage may be increased according to clinical response and serum TSH, which should be measured every 4–6 weeks to keep the TSH level in a trimester-specific gestational reference range. An increase in the dose of levothyroxine may be required in the second and third trimesters, as well. By mid-pregnancy, women require an average of 47% increase in their levothyroxine dosage.

2. Subclinical hypothyroidism—This is defined as an increased serum TSH with a normal FT_4 level. Although some studies have found associations with untoward pregnancy outcomes such as miscarriage, preterm birth, and preeclampsia, others have failed to confirm these findings. There is no evidence that treatment of subclinical hypothyroidism will prevent any of these outcomes. The ACOG and the American Association of Clinical Endocrinologists recommend against universal screening for thyroid disease in pregnancy.

3. Overt hyperthyroidism—There is excessive production of thyroxine with a depressed (usually undetectable) serum TSH level in overt hyperthyroidism, which is also associated with increased risks in pregnancy. Spontaneous pregnancy loss, preterm birth, preeclampsia, and maternal HF occur with increased frequency with untreated thyrotoxicosis. Thyroid storm, although rare, can be a life-threatening complication. Medical treatment of thyrotoxicosis is usually accomplished with the antithyroid drugs propylthiouracil or methimazole. Although teratogenicity has not been clearly established, in utero exposure to methimazole has been associated with aplasia cutis and choanal and esophageal atresia in the offspring. Propylthiouracil is not believed to be teratogenic, but it has been associated with the rare complications of hepatotoxicity and agranulocytosis. Recommendations by the American Thyroid Association are to treat with propylthiouracil in the first trimester and convert to methimazole for the remainder of the pregnancy. The therapeutic target for the FT_4 level is the upper limit of the normal reference range. The TSH levels generally stay suppressed even with adequate treatment. A β-blocker can be used for such symptoms as palpitations or tremors. Fetal hypothyroidism or hyperthyroidism is uncommon but can occur with maternal Graves disease, which is the most common cause of hyperthyroidism in pregnancy. *Radioiodine ablation is absolutely contraindicated in pregnancy because it may destroy the fetal thyroid.*

4. Postpartum thyroiditis—This is discussed in Chapter 29; see Thyroiditis.

American College of Obstetricians and Gynecologists. Practice Bulletin No. 223: thyroid disease in pregnancy. Obstet Gynecol. 2020;135:e261 [Reaffirmed 2023] [PMID: 32443080]

DIABETES MELLITUS

Normal pregnancy can be characterized as a state of increased insulin resistance that helps ensure a steady stream of glucose delivery to the developing fetus. Thus, both mild fasting hypoglycemia and postprandial hyperglycemia are physiologic.

A. Gestational Diabetes Mellitus

Gestational diabetes mellitus is abnormal glucose tolerance in pregnancy and is generally believed to exaggerate the pregnancy-induced physiologic changes in carbohydrate metabolism. Alternatively, pregnancy may unmask an underlying propensity for glucose intolerance, which will be evident in the nonpregnant state at some future time if not in the immediate postpartum period. Indeed, at least 50% of women with gestational diabetes will have an overt diabetes diagnosis in their lifetime. During pregnancy, the principal concern in women with gestational diabetes is excessive fetal growth, which can cause increased maternal and perinatal morbidity. Shoulder dystocia occurs more frequently in infants born to mothers with diabetes because of fetal overgrowth and increased fat deposition on the shoulders. Cesarean delivery and preeclampsia are also significantly increased in women with diabetes, both gestational and overt.

All asymptomatic pregnant women should undergo laboratory screening for gestational diabetes after 24 weeks' gestation. The diagnostic thresholds for glucose tolerance tests in pregnancy are not universally agreed upon, and importantly, adverse pregnancy outcomes appear to occur along a continuum of glucose intolerance even if the diagnosis of gestational diabetes is not formally assigned. A two-stage testing strategy is recommended by the ACOG, starting with a 50-g screening test offered to all pregnant women at 24–28 weeks' gestation. If this test is abnormal, the diagnostic test is a 100-g oral glucose tolerance test (Table 22–3).

Women in whom gestational diabetes is diagnosed should undergo nutrition counseling, and medications are typically initiated for those with persistent fasting hyperglycemia. Insulin remains the standard of care to achieve glycemic control. Oral hypoglycemic agents, principally glyburide and metformin, have been evaluated in short-term clinical trials and appear to achieve similar degrees of glycemic control to insulin without increasing maternal or neonatal morbidity. These medications, however, have not been approved by the US FDA for this indication; the long-term safety of oral agents has not been adequately studied in the women or in their offspring, thus insulin is first-line therapy unless circumstances preclude its use. In those cases, metformin is a reasonable choice. Insulin regimens commonly include multiple daily injections of a split-dose mix of intermediate acting and short acting agents that do not cross the placenta (eg, regular and NPH insulins, insulin lispro and aspart) (see Chapter 31 for a discussion of self-monitoring glucose systems). Once therapy is initiated, blood glucose surveillance is important to assess for adequacy of glycemic control. Capillary blood glucose levels should be checked four times per day, once fasting and three times after meals. Euglycemia is considered to be 60–95 mg/dL (3.3–5.3 mmol/L) while fasting and premeal, and < 120 mg/dL (6.7 mmol/L) 2 hours postprandially. Intensive therapy with dietary modifications or insulin, or both, has been demonstrated to decrease rates of macrosomia, shoulder dystocia, and preeclampsia. Because of the increased prevalence of overt diabetes in women identified to have gestational diabetes, they should be screened at 6–12 weeks' postpartum with a fasting plasma glucose test or a 2-hour oral glucose tolerance test (75-g glucose load).

Table 22–3. Screening and diagnostic criteria for gestational diabetes mellitus.

Screening for gestational diabetes mellitus

1. 50-g oral glucose load, administered between 24 and 28 weeks, without regard to time of day or time of last meal.
2. Venous plasma glucose measured 1 hour later.
3. Value ≥ 140 mg/dL (7.8 mmol/L) in venous plasma indicates the need for a diagnostic glucose tolerance test.

Diagnostic testing for gestational diabetes mellitus

1. 100-g oral glucose load, administered in the morning after overnight fast lasting at least 8 hours but not more than 14 hours, and following at least 3 days of unrestricted diet (> 150 g carbohydrate) and physical activity.
2. Venous plasma glucose is measured fasting and at 1, 2, and 3 hours. Patient should remain seated and should not smoke throughout the test.
3. The diagnosis of gestational diabetes is made when ≥ 2 of the following venous plasma concentrations are met or exceeded: fasting, 95 mg/dL (5.3 mmol/L); 1 hour, 180 mg/dL (10 mmol/L); 2 hours, 155 mg/dL (8.6 mmol/L); 3 hours, 140 mg/dL (7.8 mmol/L).

B. Overt Diabetes Mellitus

Overt diabetes is diabetes mellitus that antedates the pregnancy. There is an inverse relationship between glycemic control and fetal malformations, and women whose periconceptional glycosylated hemoglobin levels are at or near normal levels have rates of malformations that approach baseline. In gestational diabetes, fetal overgrowth from inadequately controlled hyperglycemia remains a significant concern because of the increased maternal and perinatal morbidity that accompany macrosomia. In overt diabetes, additional complications are increased frequency of spontaneous pregnancy losses and third-trimester stillbirths. There is also at least a two- to threefold increased risk for fetal malformations (risk in in normal pregnancies is 2–3%), as hyperglycemia during organogenesis is teratogenic. The most common malformations in offspring of women with diabetes are cardiac, skeletal, and neural tube defects. For the mother, the likelihood of infections and pregnancy-related hypertension is increased.

Preconception counseling and evaluation in a patient with diabetes is ideal to maximize the pregnancy outcomes. This provides an opportunity to optimize glycemic control and evaluate for evidence of end-organ damage. The initial evaluation of women with diabetes should include a complete chemistry panel, HbA_{1c} determination, 24-hour urine collection for total protein and creatinine clearance, funduscopic examination, and an ECG. Hypertension is common and may require treatment. *Optimally, euglycemia should be established before conception and maintained during pregnancy with daily home glucose monitoring by the patient.* A well-planned dietary program is a key component, with an intake of 1800–2200 kcal/day divided into three meals and three snacks. Insulin is given subcutaneously in a split-dose regimen as described above for women with gestational diabetes. The use of continuous insulin pump therapy may be helpful for some patients (see Chapter 31).

Throughout the pregnancy, women with diabetes should be assessed every 2–3 weeks and more frequently depending on the clinical condition. Adjustments in the insulin regimen may be necessary as the pregnancy progresses to maintain optimal glycemic control. A specialized ultrasound is often performed around 20 weeks to screen for fetal malformations. Symptoms and signs of infections should be evaluated and promptly treated. In the third trimester, fetal surveillance is indicated, and women with diabetes should receive serial antenatal testing (usually in the form of a nonstress test or biophysical profile to assess the health of the fetus). The timing of delivery is dictated by the quality of diabetic control, the presence or absence of medical complications, and fetal status. The goal is to reach 39 weeks' gestation (38 completed weeks) and then proceed with delivery. Confirmation of lung maturity may be appropriate if preterm delivery is contemplated.

American College of Obstetricians and Gynecologists. Practice Bulletin No. 201: pregestational diabetes mellitus. Obstet Gynecol. 2018;132:e228. [Reaffirmed 2023] [PMID: 30461693]

American College of Obstetricians and Gynecologists. Practice Bulletin No. 190: gestational diabetes mellitus. Obstet Gynecol. 2018;131:e49. [Reaffirmed 2024] [PMID: 29370047]

American Diabetes Association Professional Practice Committee. 15. Management of Diabetes in Pregnancy: Standards of Care in Diabetes-2024. Diabetes Care. 2024;47(Suppl 1):S282. [PMID: 38078583]

CHRONIC HYPERTENSION

Chronic hypertension is estimated to complicate up to 5% of pregnancies. To establish this diagnosis, hypertension should antedate the pregnancy or be evident before 20 weeks' gestation to differentiate it from pregnancy-related hypertension. This distinction can be problematic when the initial presentation is after 20 weeks, but chronic hypertension is confirmed if the blood pressure remains elevated beyond 12 weeks postpartum. Risk factors for chronic hypertension include older maternal age, Black race, and obesity.

Women with chronic hypertension are at increased risk for adverse maternal and perinatal outcomes. Superimposed preeclampsia develops in up to 20% of women with mild hypertension, but the risk increases up to 50% when there is severe baseline hypertension (≥ 160/110 mm Hg) and may be even higher when there is evidence of end-organ damage. When preeclampsia is superimposed on chronic hypertension, there is a tendency for it to occur at an earlier gestational age, be more severe, and impair fetal growth. Women with chronic hypertension are also at increased risk for placental abruption, cesarean delivery, preterm birth, and perinatal mortality.

Ideally, women with chronic hypertension should undergo a preconceptional evaluation to detect end-organ damage, assess the need for antihypertensive therapy, and discontinue teratogenic medications. The specific tests ordered may vary depending on the severity of the hypertension, but an evaluation of liver, kidney, and cardiac function (eg, 24-hour urine protein and maternal echocardiogram if mother has underlying renal or cardiac disease may be appropriate).

Based on findings from the 2022 Chronic Hypertension and Pregnancy study, the ACOG recommends utilizing 140/90 mm Hg as the threshold for initiation or titration of medical therapy for chronic hypertension in pregnancy, rather than the previously recommended threshold of 160/110 mm Hg. Although methyldopa has the longest record of safety in pregnancy, nifedipine (see Tables 13–7 and 13–16) and labetalol (see Table 13–9) are also acceptable, and these three agents are recommended above all others when initiating therapy in pregnancy. Care must be taken not to excessively reduce the blood pressure, as this may decrease uteroplacental perfusion. The goal is a modest reduction in blood pressure and avoidance of severe hypertension.

If a patient with mild chronic hypertension is stable on a medical regimen when she becomes pregnant, it is usually appropriate to continue this therapy, although the benefits of doing so are not well established. *ACE inhibitors and ARBs, however, are contraindicated in all trimesters of pregnancy.* These medications are teratogenic in the first trimester and cause fetal hypocalvaria and AKI in the second and third trimesters. These medications should be discontinued when pregnancy is diagnosed, and the patient should be counseled about potential teratogenicity.

When there is sustained *severe* hypertension despite multiple medications or significant end-organ damage from hypertensive disease, pregnancy is not likely to be tolerated well. In these situations, therapeutic abortion may be appropriate. Clinicians need to be aware of laws regarding availability of abortion in the jurisdiction of their practice. If the pregnancy is continued, the patient must be counseled that the maternal and perinatal risks are appreciable, and complications such as superimposed preeclampsia and fetal growth restriction should be anticipated.

American College of Obstetricians and Gynecologists. ACOG Practice Bulletin No. 203: chronic hypertension in pregnancy. Obstet Gynecol. 2019;133:e26. [Reaffirmed 2024] [PMID: 30575676]

HEART DISEASE

Normal pregnancy physiology is characterized by cardiovascular adaptations in the mother. Cardiac output increases markedly because of both augmented stroke volume and an increase in the resting heart rate, and the maternal blood volume expands by up to 50%. These changes may not be tolerated well in women with functional or structural abnormalities of the heart. Thus, although only a small number of pregnancies are complicated by cardiac disease, these contribute disproportionately to overall rates of maternal morbidity and mortality. Most cardiac disease in women of childbearing age in the United States is caused by congenital heart disease and not rheumatic heart disease. Ischemic heart disease, however, is seen increasingly in pregnant women due to rising rates of comorbid conditions, such as diabetes mellitus, hypertension, and obesity.

For practical purposes, the best single measurement of cardiopulmonary status is defined by the New York Heart Association Functional Classification. Most pregnant women with cardiac disease have class I or II functional disability, and although good outcomes are generally anticipated in this group, complications such as preeclampsia, preterm birth, and low birth weight appear to occur with increased frequency. Women with more severe disability (class III or IV) are rare in contemporary obstetrics; however, the maternal mortality is markedly increased in this setting and is usually the result of HF. Because of these risks, therapeutic abortion for maternal health should be considered in women who are severely disabled from cardiac disease. Clinicians need to be aware of laws regarding availability of abortion in the jurisdiction of their practice. Specific conditions that have been associated with a high risk for maternal death include Eisenmenger syndrome, primary pulmonary hypertension, Marfan syndrome with aortic root dilatation, and severe aortic or mitral stenosis. In general, these conditions should be considered contraindications to pregnancy.

The importance of preconceptional counseling for women with heart disease cannot be overstated. A thorough evaluation before pregnancy provides an opportunity for comprehensive risk assessment and detailed planning. Once pregnant, women with cardiac disease are best treated by a team of clinicians experienced in caring for such patients. HF and arrhythmias are the most common cardiovascular complications associated with heart disease in pregnancy, and adverse maternal and fetal outcomes are increased when they occur. Volume overload should therefore be evaluated and treated promptly. Labor management depends on the underlying cardiac lesion and the degree of disability. Women with a history of arrhythmia should have continuous cardiac monitoring throughout labor, delivery, and the immediate postpartum period. Cesarean delivery is generally reserved for obstetric indications but may be appropriate for women in whom Valsalva maneuvers are contraindicated. The early postpartum period is a critical time for fluid management. Patients who are predisposed to HF should be monitored closely during the puerperium.

Infective endocarditis prophylaxis is not recommended for most vaginal or cesarean deliveries in the absence of infection, except in the small subset of women at highest risk for adverse outcomes from endocarditis (eg, those with cyanotic heart disease, prosthetic valves, or both). Prophylactic antibiotics for endocarditis, if required, should be given intravenously. If infection is present, such as chorioamnionitis, the underlying infection should be treated with the usual regimen and additional agents are not needed specifically for endocarditis prophylaxis.

American College of Obstetricians and Gynecologists. ACOG Practice Bulletin No. 199: use of prophylactic antibiotics in labor and delivery. Obstet Gynecol. 2018;132:e103. [Reaffirmed 2021] [PMID: 30134425]

Shapiro H et al. Valvular heart disease in pregnancy. Methodist Debakey Cardiovasc J. 2024;20:13. eCollection 2024. [PMID: 38495658]

ASTHMA

(See also Chapter 9.)

Asthma is one of the most common medical conditions encountered in pregnancy. Women with mild to moderate asthma can generally expect excellent pregnancy outcomes, but severe or poorly controlled asthma has been associated with several pregnancy complications, including preterm birth, small-for-gestational-age infants, and preeclampsia. The effects of pregnancy on asthma are likely minimal as asthma severity in the pregnancy is generally similar to its severity during the year preceding the pregnancy. Strategies for treatment are similar to those in nonpregnant women. Patients should be educated about symptom management and avoidance of asthma triggers. Baseline PFTs can objectively assess lung function and may help the patient with self-monitoring of her asthma severity using a peak flow meter. As in nonpregnant women, treatment algorithms generally follow a stepwise approach, and commonly used medications, particularly those for mild to moderate asthma symptoms, are generally considered safe in pregnancy. Concerns about teratogenicity and medication effects on the fetus should be thoroughly discussed with the patient to decrease noncompliance rates. Inhaled β_2-agonists are indicated for all pregnant patients with asthma, and low to moderate dose inhaled corticosteroids are added for persistent symptoms when a rescue inhaler alone is inadequate. Systemic corticosteroid administration is reserved for severe exacerbations but should not be withheld, if indicated, irrespective of gestational age. Cromolyn, leukotriene receptor antagonists, and theophylline are appropriate alternative therapies if first-line management is ineffective. The primary goals of management in pregnancy include minimizing symptoms and avoiding hypoxic episodes to the fetus. Prostaglandin F2a and ergonovine—medications frequently used to treat postpartum uterine atony—should be avoided because they can precipitate bronchospasm in women with asthma.

Dombrowski MP et al; ACOG Committee on Practice Bulletins-Obstetrics. ACOG Practice Bulletin No. 90: asthma in pregnancy. Obstet Gynecol. 2008;111:457. [Reaffirmed 2024] [PMID: 18238988]

Huang J et al. Asthma in pregnancy. JAMA. 2023;329:1981. [PMID: 37234011]

SEIZURE DISORDERS

Epilepsy is one of the most frequent serious neurologic disorders in pregnant women. Many of the commonly used antiepileptic drugs are known human teratogens. Therefore, the principal objectives in managing pregnancy in women with epilepsy are achieving adequate control of seizures while minimizing exposure to medications that can cause congenital malformations. Certain women who are contemplating pregnancy and have been seizure-free for 2–5 years may be considered candidates for discontinuation of antiseizure medication before pregnancy. For those who continue to require treatment, however, therapy with one medication is preferred.

Selecting a regimen should be based on the type of seizure disorder and the risks associated with each medication. Valproic acid should not be considered first-line therapy because it has consistently been associated with higher rates of fetal malformations than most other commonly used antiepileptic drugs, and it may be associated with impaired neurocognitive development in the offspring. Phenytoin and carbamazepine both have established patterns of associated fetal malformations. Concerns about teratogenicity have prompted increasing use of the newer antiepileptic drugs such as lamotrigine, topiramate, oxcarbazepine, and levetiracetam. Experiences from ongoing registries and large, population-based studies suggest that in utero exposure to the newer antiepileptic drugs in the first trimester of pregnancy carries a lower risk of major malformations than older medications. Lamotrigine and levetiracetam are considered the least teratogenic. One birth registry, however, found an increase in oral clefts among women taking lamotrigine. Several small studies have found an association between levetiracetam and low birth weight. Some studies suggest that topiramate is associated with a slightly increased risk of oral clefts. Although it is recommended that pregnant women with epilepsy be given supplemental folic acid, it is unclear if supplemental folate decreases rates of fetal malformations in women taking antiepileptic medications. Serum levels of antiepileptic medications should be followed, when appropriate, because they may be affected by volume of distribution changes in pregnancy.

Darmawan KF et al. Contemporary management of epilepsy in pregnancy. Curr Opin Obstet Gynecol. 2023;35:87. [PMID: 36912246]

Li Y et al. Epilepsy and pregnancy. Continuum (Minneap Minn). 2022;28:34. [PMID: 35133310]

Moise AC et al. Antiseizure medications in pregnancy. Obstet Gynecol Clin North Am. 2023;50:251. [PMID: 36822708]

Wesley SR et al. Neurologic emergencies in pregnancy. Obstet Gynecol 2024;144:25. [PMID: 38626451]

BREAST CANCER OCCURRING DURING PREGNANCY OR LACTATION

(See Chapter 19.)

INFECTIOUS CONDITIONS COMPLICATING PREGNANCY

URINARY TRACT INFECTION

The urinary tract is especially vulnerable to infections during pregnancy because the altered secretions of steroid sex hormones and the pressure exerted by the gravid uterus on the ureters and bladder cause hypotonia and congestion and predispose to urinary stasis. Labor and delivery and urinary retention postpartum also may initiate or aggravate infection. *Escherichia coli* is the offending organism in over two-thirds of cases.

From 2% to 10% of pregnant women have asymptomatic bacteriuria, which some believe to be associated with an increased risk of preterm birth. It is estimated that pyelonephritis will develop in 20–40% of these women if untreated.

An evaluation for asymptomatic bacteriuria at the first prenatal visit is recommended for all pregnant women. If a urine culture is positive, treatment should be initiated. Nitrofurantoin (100 mg orally twice daily), amoxicillin (500 mg orally three times daily), and cephalexin (250 mg orally four times daily) are acceptable medications for 5–7 days. Sulfonamides should be avoided in the third trimester because they may interfere with bilirubin binding and thus impose a risk of neonatal hyperbilirubinemia and kernicterus. Fluoroquinolones are also contraindicated because of their potential teratogenic effects on fetal cartilage and bone. Patients with recurrent bacteriuria should receive suppressive medication (once daily dosing of an appropriate antibiotic) for the remainder of the pregnancy. Acute pyelonephritis requires hospitalization for intravenous antibiotics and crystalloids until the patient is afebrile; this is followed by a full course of oral antibiotics.

ACOG Clinical Consensus No. 4. American College of Obstetricians and Gynecologists. Urinary tract infections in pregnant individuals. Obstet Gynecol. 2023;142:435. [PMID: 39601712]

GROUP B STREPTOCOCCAL INFECTION

Group B streptococci frequently colonize the lower female genital tract, with an asymptomatic carriage rate in pregnancy of 10–30%. This rate depends on maternal age, gravidity, and geographic variation. Vaginal carriage is asymptomatic and intermittent, with spontaneous clearing in approximately 30% and recolonization in about 10% of women. Adverse perinatal outcomes associated with group B streptococcal colonization include UTI, intrauterine infection, premature rupture of membranes, preterm delivery, and postpartum metritis.

Women with postpartum metritis due to infection with group B streptococci, especially after cesarean section, develop fever, tachycardia, and abdominal pain, usually within 24 hours after delivery. Approximately 35% of these women are bacteremic.

Group B streptococcal infection is a common cause of neonatal sepsis. Transmission rates are high, yet the rate of neonatal sepsis is surprisingly low at < 1:1000 live births. Unfortunately, the mortality rate associated with early-onset disease can be as high as 20–30% in premature infants. In contrast, it is approximately 2–3% in those at term. Moreover, these infections can contribute markedly to chronic morbidity, including developmental delays and neurologic disabilities. Late-onset disease develops through contact with hospital nursery personnel. Up to 45% of these health care workers can carry the bacteria on their skin and transmit the infection to newborns.

The 2022 ACOG recommendations for screening and prophylaxis for group B streptococcal colonization, reaffirmed in 2025, are available at https://www.acog.org/clinical/clinical-guidance/committee-opinion/articles/2020/02/prevention-of-group-b-streptococcal-early-onset-disease-in-newborns.

VARICELLA

Commonly known as chickenpox, primary varicella-zoster virus (VZV) infection during pregnancy may cause serious illness to the mother and to the fetus. Approximately 95% of women born in the United States have VZV antibodies by the time they reach reproductive age. Infection results in lifelong immunity. The incidence of primary VZV infection during pregnancy has been reported as up to 7:10,000. *The vaccine is contraindicated in pregnancy because the effects of the vaccine on the fetus are unknown.* Nonpregnant women who are vaccinated should avoid pregnancy for 3 months after injection. Inadvertent vaccination in early pregnancy or within a month of pregnancy is not an indication for termination, although women should be counseled about theoretical risks.

Clinical Findings

A. Symptoms and Signs

The incubation period for this infection is 10–20 days. A primary infection follows and is characterized by a flu-like syndrome with malaise, fever, and development of a pruritic maculopapular rash on the trunk, which becomes vesicular and then crusts. Pregnant women are prone to the development of VZV pneumonia, often a fulminant infection sometimes requiring respiratory support. After a primary infection, the virus becomes latent, ascending to dorsal root ganglia. Subsequent reactivation can occur as zoster, often under circumstances of immunocompromise, although this is rare during pregnancy.

Two types of fetal infection have been documented. The first is congenital VZV syndrome, which typically occurs in 0.4–2% of fetuses exposed to primary VZV infection during the first trimester. Anomalies include limb and digit abnormalities, microphthalmos, and microcephaly. The second type occurs during the second and third trimesters and is less threatening. Maternal IgG crosses the placenta, protecting the fetus. The only infants at risk for severe infection are those born after maternal viremia but before development of maternal protective antibody. Maternal infection manifesting 5 days before or up to 2 days after delivery is the time period believed to be most hazardous for transmission to the fetus.

B. Laboratory Findings

Diagnosis is commonly made on clinical grounds. Laboratory verification is made by ELISA, fluorescent antibody, and hemagglutination inhibition antibody techniques. Vesicular fluid can be sent for qualitative varicella PCR assay.

Treatment

Varicella-zoster immune globulin (VZIG) has been shown to prevent or modify the symptoms of infection in exposed persons. Treatment success depends on identification of susceptible women at or just following exposure. Exposed women with a questionable or negative history of chickenpox should be checked for antibody, since the overwhelming majority will have been previously exposed. If the antibody is negative, VZIG (625 units intramuscularly) should ideally be given within 96 hours of exposure for greatest efficacy, but the CDC reports it can be given for up to 10 days. There are no known adverse effects of VZIG administration during pregnancy, although the incubation period for disease can be lengthened. Infants born to women in whom symptoms develop in the period from 5 days before delivery to 2 days after delivery should also receive VZIG (125 units).

Pregnant women with varicella may benefit from treatment with oral acyclovir, 800 mg orally four times daily for 5 days, if started within 24 hours of rash onset. Treatment has been shown to improve maternal symptoms but does not prevent congenital varicella. Infected pregnant women should be closely observed and hospitalized at the earliest signs of pulmonary involvement. Intravenous acyclovir (10 mg/kg intravenously every 8 hours) is recommended in the treatment of VZV pneumonia.

American College of Obstetricians and Gynecologists. ACOG Practice Bulletin No. 151: cytomegalovirus, parvovirus B19, varicella zoster, and toxoplasmosis in pregnancy. Obstet Gynecol. 2015;125:1510. [Reaffirmed 2024] [PMID: 26000539]

TUBERCULOSIS

Women at high risk for tuberculosis include those from endemic areas, those infected with HIV, those with substance use disorder, health care workers, and close contacts of people with tuberculosis. Both tuberculin skin testing and interferon gamma release assays are acceptable tests in pregnancy. Screening CXRs should only be obtained in pregnant patients who have a positive test or with suggestive findings in the history and physical examination. Abdominal shielding must be used if a CXR is obtained.

Decisions on treatment depend on whether the patient has active disease or is at high risk for progression to active disease. Pregnant women with active disease or who are high risk for progression should be treated during pregnancy as the risks of complications from tuberculosis outweigh the risks of treatment. Pregnant women with latent disease not at high risk for disease progression can receive treatment postpartum, which does not preclude breastfeeding. The concentration of medication in breast milk is neither toxic nor adequate for treatment of the newborn. Isoniazid, ethambutol, and rifampin are used to treat tuberculosis (see Chapters 9 and 37). Because isoniazid therapy may cause vitamin B_6 deficiency, supplemental vitamin B_6, 50 mg orally daily, should be given simultaneously. There is concern that isoniazid, particularly in pregnant women, can cause hepatitis. Liver biochemical tests should be performed monthly in pregnant women who receive treatment. Streptomycin, ethionamide, and most other antituberculosis drugs should be avoided in pregnancy. If adequately treated, tuberculosis in pregnancy has an excellent prognosis.

Hui SYA et al. Tuberculosis in pregnancy. Best Pract Res Clin Obstet Gynaecol. 2022;85:34. [PMID: 36002371]

HIV/AIDS DURING PREGNANCY

Asymptomatic HIV infection is associated with a normal pregnancy rate and no increased risk of adverse pregnancy outcomes. There is no evidence that pregnancy causes AIDS progression.

Previously, two-thirds of neonates positive for HIV acquired their infection close to, or during, the time of delivery. Routine HIV screening in pregnancy, including the use of rapid HIV tests in labor and delivery units, and using antiretroviral drugs have markedly reduced this transmission risk to approximately 1%. In a pregnant person who is HIV-positive, a CD4 count, plasma RNA level, creatinine, liver function tests, and resistance testing (if virus is detectable, and the patient has not already had this) should be obtained at the first prenatal visit. Treatment should not be delayed while waiting for the results of resistance testing. Prior or current antiretroviral use should be reviewed. The patient should be tested for HLA-B*5701 if abacavir may be prescribed; HLA-B*5701 positivity puts the patient at risk for a serious hypersensitivity reaction and its use is contraindicated.

A person already taking and tolerating an acceptable antiretroviral regimen need not discontinue it in the first trimester. Patients should also be tested for hepatitis A, hepatitis C, tuberculosis, and toxoplasmosis.

Women not taking medication should be offered combination antiretroviral therapy (commonly a dual nucleoside reverse transcriptase inhibitor combination and either a ritonavir-boosted protease inhibitor or an integrase strand transfer inhibitor) after counseling regarding the potential impact of therapy on both mother and fetus (see Chapter 35). The preferred regimen in pregnancy is bictegravir (BIC) plus tenofovir alafenamide (TAF) and emtricitabine (FTC) (available as a fixed-dose combination). Antiretroviral therapy should be offered regardless of viral load and CD4 count. Whether to start in the first or second trimester should be determined on a case-by-case basis, but it should be started as early as reasonably possible. It can be started in the first trimester after explanation of risks and benefits, provided the mother is not experiencing nausea and vomiting. Most medications used to treat HIV/AIDS have thus far proven to be safe in pregnancy with an acceptable risk/benefit ratio. The physiologic changes that occur during pregnancy may alter the effect of some medications. Before starting any regimen, the safety and efficacy of the medications selected should be reviewed. Standard of care includes zidovudine (2 mg/kg intravenously over 1 hour followed by 1 mg/kg/hour intravenously) begun 3 hours before cesarean delivery and continued through the surgery until cord clamping in women whose viral load near delivery (after 34–36 weeks' gestation or within 4–6 weeks of delivery) is > 1000 copies/mL or unknown. Antiretroviral therapy on the patient's usual schedule should be continued in labor. Intravenous zidovudine is not required for women who have been compliant with their antiretroviral therapy and whose viral load is ≤ 50 copies/mL near delivery; data are limited in cases where the viral load is between 50–1000 copies/mL.

The use of prophylactic elective cesarean section at 38 weeks' gestation (before the onset of labor or rupture of the membranes) to prevent vertical transmission of HIV infection from mother to fetus has been shown to further reduce the transmission rate. In patients with a viral load of < 1000 copies/mL near delivery, there may be no additional benefit of cesarean delivery, and those women can be offered a vaginal delivery. Amniotomy should not be performed in the setting of viremia unless there is a clear obstetric indication. Amniotomy, however, has not been associated with an increased risk of perinatal transmission when the mother is receiving antiretroviral therapy and virologically suppressed. Internal monitors, particularly the fetal scalp electrode, should be avoided as should operative deliveries (forceps-assisted and vacuum-assisted vaginal deliveries). Methylergonovine (Methergine) (used for postpartum hemorrhage) should be avoided, if possible, in patients receiving regimens that include cytochrome P450 (CYP) 3A4 inhibitors and CYP3A4 enzyme inducers. Women with HIV should be advised not to breastfeed their infants.

The Public Health Task Force provides guidelines for the management of HIV/AIDS in pregnancy (https://clinicalinfo.hiv.gov). In addition, there is the National Perinatal HIV Hotline, which provides free consultation regarding perinatal HIV care (1-888-448-8765).

Panel on Treatment of HIV During Pregnancy and Prevention of Perinatal Transmission. Recommendations for the Use of Antiretroviral Drugs During Pregnancy and Interventions to Reduce Perinatal HIV Transmission in the United States. Department of Health and Human Services. https://clinicalinfo.hiv.gov/en/guidelines/perinatal. Accessed December 8, 2025.

MATERNAL HEPATITIS B & C CARRIER STATE

A. Hepatitis B Virus

There are an estimated 300 million chronic carriers of hepatitis B virus worldwide. In the United States, up to 1.8 million people are infected, with the highest rate among Asian American people. All pregnant women should be screened for HBsAg during every pregnancy. If not previously done, the patient should have a triple-panel screen (HBsAg, anti-HBs, and total antibody to hepatitis B core antigen [total anti-HBc]). Transmission of the virus to the baby is likely if both surface antigen and e antigen are positive. Vertical transmission can be blocked by the immediate postdelivery administration to the newborn of hepatitis B immunoglobulin and hepatitis B vaccine intramuscularly. The vaccine dose is repeated at 1 and 6 months of age. Third trimester administration of tenofovir disoproxil fumarate, 300 mg orally once daily starting at 28–32 weeks and continuing through delivery (first-line), lamivudine, or telbivudine to women with a viral load of > 10^6–10^8 copies/mL has been shown to reduce vertical transmission, particularly if the viral load is <10^6 copies/mL at delivery. This therapy appears safe in pregnancy, although long-term follow-up data are lacking. Pregnant women with chronic hepatitis B should have liver biochemical tests and viral load testing during the pregnancy. Hepatitis B infection is not a contraindication to breastfeeding if the baby has received immunoprophylaxis. Maternal antiviral therapy, if given, need not be continued postpartum.

B. Hepatitis C Virus

This infection is the most common chronic blood-borne infection in the United States. Because risk-based screening misses approximately 50% of cases and postpartum treatment is highly effective, universal screening in pregnancy is recommended. The average rate of hepatitis C virus (HCV) infection among infants born to women positive for HCV and negative for HIV is 5–6%. However, the average infection rate increases to 10–11% when mothers are coinfected with HCV and HIV. The principal factor associated with transmission is HCV RNA in the mother at the time of birth. Treatment is not recommended in pregnancy. Interferon and ribavirin have been considered contraindicated. Ledipasvir/sofosbuvir (Harvoni) has been shown to be safe in animal studies. Direct-acting antiviral regimens should only be initiated during pregnancy if in the setting of a clinical trial. Cesarean section is not recommended solely for a maternal history of hepatitis C. During labor, early rupture of membranes and placement of a fetal scalp electrode should be avoided if safe to do so because of the unknown risk of increased vertical transmission. Breastfeeding is not contraindicated.

Society for Maternal-Fetal Medicine (SMFM); Badell ML et al; SMFM Publications Committee. Society for Maternal-Fetal Medicine Consult Series #69: Hepatitis B in pregnancy: updated guidelines. Am J Obstet Gynecol. 2024;230:B2. [PMID: 38141870]

Viral Hepatitis in Pregnancy: ACOG Clinical Practice Guideline No. 6. Obstet Gynecol. 2023;142:745. [PMID: 37590986]

HERPES GENITALIS

Infection of the lower genital tract by herpes simplex virus type 2 (HSV-2) (see also Chapter 6) is a common STI with potentially serious consequences to pregnant women and their newborn infants. Although up to 25% of pregnant women may have antibodies to HSV-2, a history of the infection is unreliable, and the incidence of neonatal infection is not known. There are estimated to be 1200–1500 cases of neonatal infection annually in the United States. Many infected neonates are born to women with no history, symptoms, or signs of infection.

Women who have had *primary* herpes infection late in pregnancy are at high risk for shedding virus at delivery; however, it can be difficult to differentiate primary from nonprimary infection. Women with a primary infection or nonprimary first outbreak and women with a clinical history of genital herpes should be offered prophylactic acyclovir, 400 mg orally three times daily, starting at 36 weeks' gestation, to decrease the likelihood of active lesions at the time of labor and delivery. For treatment, see Chapter 36.

Women with a history of *recurrent* genital herpes have a lower neonatal attack rate than women infected during the pregnancy, but they should still be monitored with clinical observation and culture of any suspicious lesions. Since asymptomatic viral shedding is unpredictable by antepartum cultures, recommendations do not include routine cultures in individuals with a history of herpes without active disease. However, when labor begins, vulvar and cervical inspection should be performed. Cesarean delivery is indicated at the time of labor if there are prodromal symptoms or active genital lesions.

American College of Obstetricians and Gynecologists. ACOG Practice Bulletin No. 220: management of genital herpes in pregnancy. Obstet Gynecol. 2020;135:e193. [Reaffirmed 2023] [PMID: 32332414]

SYPHILIS, GONORRHEA, & *CHLAMYDIA TRACHOMATIS* INFECTION

These STIs have significant consequences for mother and child (see also Chapters 37 and 38). Untreated syphilis in pregnancy can cause late pregnancy loss, stillbirth, transplacental infection, and congenital syphilis. Gonorrhea can produce large-joint arthritis by hematogenous spread as well as ophthalmia neonatorum. Maternal chlamydial infections are largely asymptomatic but are manifested in the newborn by inclusion conjunctivitis and, at age 2–4 months, by pneumonia. Because of increasing rates of congenital syphilis, all women should be tested for syphilis as part of their routine prenatal care at their initial visit, in the third trimester, and at delivery. Pregnant women aged < 25 years and those at increased risk for *C trachomatis* should be screened for chlamydia at their first prenatal visit. Repeat testing depends on risk factors, prevalence, and state laws. A pregnant person treated for *C trachomatis* should be tested for cure 4 weeks later and then retested 3 months later because of high reinfection rates. Women who remain at high risk should be tested in the third trimester. Women aged < 25 years and those at increased risk should be tested for gonorrhea at their first prenatal appointment. Women with positive tests for gonorrhea should be treated and then retested 3 months later. Women who remain at high risk should be tested in the third trimester. The sexual partners of women with STIs should be identified and treated if possible; the local health department can assist with this process.

ACOG. Screening for Syphilis in Pregnancy. Practice Advisory. April 2024, Reaffirmed October 2025. https://www.acog.org/clinical/clinical-guidance/practice-advisory/articles/2024/04/screening-for-syphilis-in-pregnancy. Accessed December 9, 2025.

Workowski KA et al. Sexually transmitted infections treatment guidelines, 2021. MMWR Recomm Rep. 2021;70:1. [PMID: 34292926]

GASTROINTESTINAL, HEPATIC, & BILIARY DISORDERS OF PREGNANCY

Complications involving the GI tract, liver, and gallbladder are common in pregnancy. Nausea and vomiting in the first trimester affect most pregnant women to some degree (see Obstetric Complications of the First & Second Trimesters).

Nausea and vomiting in the last half of pregnancy, however, are never normal; a thorough evaluation of such complaints is mandatory. Some of these conditions are incidental to pregnancy (eg, appendicitis), while others are related to the gravid state and tend to resolve with delivery (eg, acute fatty liver of pregnancy). Importantly, the myriad anatomic and physiologic changes associated with normal pregnancy must be considered when assessing for a disease state. Likewise, interpretation of laboratory studies must consider the pregnancy-associated changes in hepatic protein production.

For conditions in which surgery is clinically indicated, operative intervention should never be withheld based solely on a person being pregnant. While purely elective surgery is avoided during pregnancy, women who undergo surgical procedures for an urgent or emergent indication during pregnancy do not appear to be at increased risk for adverse outcomes. Obstetric complications, when they occur, are more likely to be associated with the underlying maternal illness. Recommendations are that the optimal time for semi-elective surgery is the second trimester to avoid exposure to anesthesia in the first trimester and the enlarged uterus in the third. Importantly, however, there is no convincing evidence that general anesthesia induces malformations or increases the risk for spontaneous pregnancy loss.

CHOLELITHIASIS & CHOLECYSTITIS

Cholelithiasis is common in pregnancy as physiologic changes such as increased cholesterol production and incomplete gallbladder emptying predispose to gallstone formation. The diagnosis is usually suspected based on classic symptoms of nausea, vomiting, and right upper quadrant pain, usually after meals, and is confirmed with right upper quadrant ultrasound. Symptomatic cholelithiasis without cholecystitis is usually managed conservatively, but recurrent symptoms are common. Cholecystitis results from obstruction of the cystic duct and often is accompanied by bacterial infection. Medical management with antibiotics is reasonable in selected cases, but definitive treatment with cholecystectomy will help prevent complications such as gallbladder perforation and pancreatitis. Cholecystectomy has successfully been performed in all trimesters of pregnancy and should not be withheld based on the stage of pregnancy if clinically indicated. Laparoscopy is preferred in the first half of pregnancy after the first trimester but becomes more technically challenging in the last trimester due to the enlarged uterus and cephalad displacement of abdominal contents.

Obstruction of the common bile duct, which can lead to cholangitis, is an indication for surgical removal of gallstones and establishment of biliary drainage. Endoscopic retrograde cholangiopancreatography (ERCP) with or without sphincterotomy is a nonsurgical alternative. ERCP should only be undertaken when there is therapeutic intent. Pregnant women can safely undergo ERCP provided that precautions are taken to minimize fetal exposure to radiation. There does, however, appear to be a slightly higher rate of post-procedure pancreatitis in pregnant women who undergo ERCP. Magnetic resonance cholangiopancreatography (MRCP) can also be of use in patients with suspected common bile duct obstruction. This study is useful for those women in whom the etiology of common duct dilatation is unclear on ultrasound. MRCP can provide detailed evaluation of the entire biliary system and the pancreas while avoiding ionizing radiation.

The most common cause of acute pancreatitis in pregnancy is gallstone disease. The diagnosis can be confirmed with an appropriate history and an elevated serum amylase or lipase. Although pregnancy is associated with a rise in serum amylase, a value of at least two times the upper limit of normal suggests pancreatitis with the appropriate clinical scenario. Management is conservative, including bowel rest, intravenous fluids, supplemental nutrition if necessary, and analgesics. CT imaging should be avoided unless severe complications such as necrosis, abscess, or hemorrhage are suspected.

Olafson SN et al. The management of gallstones in pregnancy. Adv Surg. 2025;59:109. [PMID: 40769689]

Oldenkamp CL et al. Nonobstetric surgical emergencies in pregnancy. Emerg Med Clin North Am. 2023; 41:259.[PMID: 37024162]

Ray J et al. Lower gastrointestinal tract disorders: clinical updates in women's health care primary and preventive care review. Obstet Gynecol. 2022;139:1201. [PMID: 35675626]

Zhou D et al. Clinical characteristics and pregnancy outcome analysis of 20 cases of acute pancreatitis during pregnancy. Int J Gynaecol Obstet. 2024;166:435. [PMID: 38391228]

ACUTE FATTY LIVER OF PREGNANCY

Acute fatty liver of pregnancy, a disorder limited to the gravid state, occurs in the third trimester of pregnancy and causes acute hepatic failure. With improved recognition and immediate delivery, the maternal mortality rate in contemporary reports is about 4%. The disorder is usually seen after the 35th week of gestation and is more common in primigravidas and those with twins. The incidence is about 1:10,000 deliveries.

The etiology of acute fatty liver of pregnancy is likely poor placental mitochondrial function. Many cases may be due to a homozygous fetal deficiency of long-chain acyl coenzyme A dehydrogenase.

Clinical Findings

Clinical onset is gradual, with nausea and vomiting being the most common presenting symptoms. Varying degrees of flu-like symptoms are also typical. Eventually, symptoms progress to those of fulminant hepatic failure: jaundice, encephalopathy, disseminated intravascular coagulation, and death.

Laboratory findings include marked elevation of alkaline phosphatase but only moderate elevations of ALT and AST. Hypocholesterolemia and hypofibrinogenemia are typical, and hypoglycemia can be extreme. Coagulopathy is also frequently seen with depressed procoagulant protein production. Kidney function should be assessed for hepatorenal syndrome. The WBC count is elevated, and the platelet count is depressed. Liver biopsy is usually not needed for diagnosis.

Differential Diagnosis

The differential diagnosis is that of fulminant hepatitis. Liver aminotransferases for fulminant hepatitis are higher (> 1000 U/mL) than those for acute fatty liver of pregnancy (usually 500–1000 U/mL). Preeclampsia may involve the liver but rarely causes jaundice; the elevations in liver biochemical tests in patients with preeclampsia rarely reach the levels seen in patients with acute fatty liver of pregnancy.

Treatment

Diagnosis of acute fatty liver of pregnancy mandates immediate delivery. Intensive supportive care with ICU-level observation is essential and typically includes administration of blood products and glucose and correction of acidemia. Vaginal delivery is preferred. Resolution of encephalopathy and laboratory derangements occurs over days with supportive care, and recovery is usually complete. Some have found plasma exchange therapy to be helpful. Rare cases of liver transplantation have been reported.

Erez O et al. Preeclampsia and eclampsia: the conceptual evolution of a syndrome. Am J Obstet Gynecol. 2022;226:S786. [PMID: 35177220]
Lan J et al. Risk factors for acute fatty liver of pregnancy complicated by acute liver failure: a retrospective study of 133 cases. BMC Pregnancy Childbirth. 2025;25:960. [PMID: 41029226]
Li L et al. The assessment in patients with acute fatty liver of pregnancy (AFLP) treated with plasma exchange: a cohort study of 298 patients. BMC Pregnancy Childbirth. 2023;23:171. [PMID: 36915067]

INTRAHEPATIC CHOLESTASIS OF PREGNANCY

Intrahepatic cholestasis of pregnancy is characterized by incomplete clearance of bile acids in genetically susceptible women. The principal symptom is pruritus, which can be generalized but tends to have a predilection for the palms and soles. Presentation is typically in the third trimester, and women with multifetal pregnancies are at increased risk. The finding of an elevated serum bile acid level, ideally performed in the fasting state, confirms the diagnosis. Associated laboratory derangements include modest elevations in hepatic transaminase levels and mild hyperbilirubinemia. Although rare, the bilirubin level may be sufficiently elevated to result in clinical jaundice. The symptoms and laboratory abnormalities resolve quickly after delivery but can recur in subsequent pregnancies or with exposure to combination oral contraceptives.

Adverse fetal outcomes, particularly preterm birth, nonreassuring fetal status, meconium-stained amniotic fluid, and stillbirth, have consistently been reported in women with cholestasis of pregnancy. The risk for adverse perinatal outcomes appears to correlate with disease severity as measured by the degree of bile acid elevation, and women with fasting bile acids > 40 mcmol/L have been reported to be at greatest risk. Because of the risks associated with cholestasis of pregnancy, many clinicians recommend antenatal testing in the third trimester, and if cholestasis is present, elective early delivery to reduce the risk of stillbirth. The diagnosis of cholestasis of pregnancy is made when the level of bile salts is ≥ 10 mcmol/L (not necessarily fasting) with maternal symptoms. The 2021 SMFM recommendations are for early delivery (36 weeks' gestation) when the patient's bile acid level is > 100 mcmol/L and other fetal tests are normal; in the symptomatic patient whose bile acid level is < 100 mcmol/L, the SMFM suggests delivery between 36–39 weeks' gestation. The ACOG endorses ursodeoxycholic acid as the first-line agent for the treatment of maternal symptoms of intrahepatic cholestasis of pregnancy.

Girling J et al. Intrahepatic cholestasis of pregnancy: Green-top guideline No. 43 June 2022. Royal College of Obstetricians and Gynaecologists. BJOG. 2022;129:e95. [PMID: 35942656]
Hobson SR et al. Guideline No. 452: Diagnosis and management of intrahepatic cholestasis of pregnancy. J Obstet Gynaecol Can. 2024;46:102618. [PMID: 39089469]
Horgan R et al. Intrahepatic cholestasis of pregnancy: a comparison of Society for Maternal-Fetal Medicine and the Royal College of Obstetricians and Gynaecologists' guidelines. Am J Obstet Gynecol MFM. 2023;5:100838. [PMID: 36503152]

APPENDICITIS

Appendicitis occurs in about 1 of 1500 pregnancies. The diagnosis is more difficult to make clinically in pregnant women where the appendix is displaced cephalad from McBurney point. Furthermore, nausea, vomiting, and mild leukocytosis occur in normal pregnancy, so with or without these findings, any complaint of right-sided pain should raise suspicion. Imaging can help confirm the diagnosis if clinical findings are equivocal. Abdominal sonography is a reasonable initial imaging choice, but nonvisualization of the appendix is common in pregnancy. CT scanning is more sensitive than ultrasound, and with proper shielding, the radiation exposure to the fetus is minimized. MRI in pregnant women is a reasonable alternative to CT scanning.

An operative approach to appendicitis, rather than a conservative nonoperative approach, is indicated for pregnant patients. Conservative management is associated with increases in maternal morbidity, including septic shock, peritonitis, and VTE. Some experts, however, find conservative management acceptable for uncomplicated appendicitis.

Unfortunately, the diagnosis of appendicitis is not made until the appendix has ruptured in at least 20% of obstetric patients. Peritonitis in these cases can lead to preterm labor or spontaneous pregnancy loss. With early diagnosis and appendectomy, the prognosis is good for mother and baby.

Ashbrook M et al. Management of complicated appendicitis during pregnancy. JAMA Netw Open. 2022;5:e227555. [PMID: 35426921]
Ceresoli M et al. Operative and non-operative management of acute appendicitis during pregnancy: a population-based study. Arch Gynecol Obstet. 2025;311:33. [PMID: 39704819]

23 Rheumatologic, Immunologic, & Allergic Disorders

Rebecca L. Manno, MD, MHS
Jinoos Yazdany, MD, MPH
Teresa K. Tarrant, MD
Mildred Kwan, MD, PhD

RHEUMATOLOGIC DISORDERS

Diagnosis & Evaluation

A. Examination of the Patient

Two helpful clinical clues for diagnosing arthritis are the joint pattern and the presence or absence of extra-articular manifestations. The joint pattern is defined by the answers to three questions: (1) Is inflammation present? (2) How many joints are involved? and (3) What joints are affected? Joint inflammation manifests as warmth, swelling, and morning stiffness of at least 30 minutes' duration. Overlying erythema occurs with the intense inflammation of crystal-induced and septic arthritis. Both the number of affected joints and the specific sites of involvement affect the differential diagnosis (Table 23–1). Some diseases—gout, for example—are characteristically monoarticular, whereas other diseases, such as rheumatoid arthritis (RA), are usually polyarticular. The location of joint involvement can also be distinctive. Only two diseases frequently cause prominent involvement of the distal interphalangeal (DIP) joint: osteoarthritis and psoriatic arthritis. Extra-articular manifestations such as fever (eg, gout, Still disease, endocarditis, vasculitis, SLE), rash (eg, SLE, psoriatic arthritis, inflammatory myositis), nodules (eg, RA, gout), or neuropathy (eg, vasculitis) narrow the differential diagnosis further.

B. Arthrocentesis and Examination of Joint Fluid

If the diagnosis is uncertain, synovial fluid should be examined whenever possible (Table 23–2). Most large joints are easily aspirated, and contraindications to arthrocentesis are few. The aspirating needle should never be passed through an overlying cellulitis or psoriatic plaque because of the risk of introducing infection. For patients who are receiving DOACs or warfarin, joints can be aspirated with a small-gauge needle (eg, 22G); the INR should be < 3.0 for patients taking warfarin.

1. Types of studies—

A. GROSS EXAMINATION—Clarity is an approximate guide to the degree of inflammation. Noninflammatory fluid is transparent, mild inflammation produces translucent fluid, and purulent effusions are opaque. Traumatic taps, trauma, and bleeding disorders are the most common causes of bloody effusions.

B. CELL COUNT—Normal synovial fluid contains < 200 WBC/mcL (0.2×10^9/L). Higher synovial fluid white cell counts can discriminate between noninflammatory (< 2000 WBC/mcL [2.0×10^9/L]), inflammatory (2000–75,000 WBC/mcL [$2.0–75 \times 10^9$/L]), and purulent (> 100,000 WBC/mcL [100×10^9/L]) joint effusions (Table 23–2). Synovial fluid glucose and protein levels add little information and should not be ordered.

C. MICROSCOPIC EXAMINATION—Compensated polarized light microscopy distinguishes monosodium urate (gout, negatively birefringent) and calcium pyrophosphate (pseudogout, positive birefringent) crystals. Gram stain has specificity but limited sensitivity (50%) for septic arthritis.

D. CULTURE—Bacterial cultures and special studies for gonococci, tubercle bacilli, or fungi are ordered as appropriate.

2. Interpretation—Synovial fluid analysis is diagnostic in infectious or crystalline arthritis. Although the severity of inflammation in synovial fluid can overlap among various conditions, the synovial fluid white cell count is a helpful guide to diagnosis (Table 23–3).

OSTEOARTHRITIS & CRYSTAL-INDUCED ARTHRITIS

OSTEOARTHRITIS

ESSENTIALS OF DIAGNOSIS

- A progressive joint disorder with minimal articular inflammation.
- No systemic symptoms.
- Pain relieved by rest; morning stiffness brief.
- Radiographic findings: narrowed joint space, osteophytes, increased subchondral bone density, bony cysts.

Table 23–1. Diagnostic value of the joint pattern.

Characteristic	Status	Representative Disease
Inflammatory[1] synovial fluid	Present	Rheumatoid arthritis, SLE, gout, CPPD
	Absent	Osteoarthritis
Number of involved joints	Monoarticular	Gout, CPPD, trauma, septic arthritis, Lyme disease, osteoarthritis
	Oligoarticular (2–4 joints)	Reactive arthritis, psoriatic arthritis, IBD
	Polyarticular (≥ 5 joints)	Rheumatoid arthritis, SLE
Site of joint involvement	Carpometacarpal of the thumb DIP	Osteoarthritis, psoriatic arthritis (not rheumatoid arthritis)
	PIP, MCP, wrists	Rheumatoid arthritis, SLE, calcium pyrophosphate deposition disease (not osteoarthritis)
	First MTP	Gout, osteoarthritis

CPPD, calcium pyrophosphate deposition (pseudogout); DIP, distal interphalangeal; MCP, metacarpophalangeal; MTP, metatarsal phalangeal; PIP, proximal interphalangeal.
[1]See text.

General Considerations

Osteoarthritis, the most common form of joint disease, is chiefly a disease of aging. Ninety percent of all people have radiographic features of osteoarthritis in weight-bearing joints by age 40. Symptomatic disease increases with age. Sex is a risk factor; osteoarthritis develops in women more frequently than in men.

This arthropathy is characterized by degeneration of cartilage and by hypertrophy of bone at the articular margins. Inflammation is usually minimal. Hereditary and mechanical factors may be involved in the pathogenesis.

Obesity is a risk factor for osteoarthritis of the knee, hand, and hip, although the association is strongest for the knee. Recreational running does not increase the incidence of osteoarthritis, but participation in competitive contact sports (eg, football) does. Jobs requiring frequent bending and carrying increase the risk of knee osteoarthritis; arthroscopic meniscal procedures and prior joint injuries are also linked to osteoarthritis (see Chapter 45).

Clinical Findings

A. Symptoms and Signs

Osteoarthritis is categorized into two types: (1) primary, which most commonly affects some or all of the following: the DIP and the proximal interphalangeal (PIP) joints of the fingers, the carpometacarpal joint of the thumb, the hip, the knee, the metatarsophalangeal (MTP) joint of the big toe, and the cervical and lumbar spine; and (2) secondary, which may occur in any joint as a sequela to articular injury. The injury may have been acute, as in a fracture; or chronic, as from occupational overuse of a joint or metabolic disease (eg, hyperparathyroidism, hemochromatosis, ochronosis) or joint inflammation (eg, RA).

The onset is insidious. Initially, there is articular stiffness, seldom lasting > 15 minutes; this develops later into pain on motion of the affected joint and is made worse by activity or weight bearing and relieved by rest. Flexion contracture or varus deformity of the knee is not unusual, and bony enlargements of the DIP (Heberden nodes) and PIP (Bouchard nodes) are occasionally prominent (Figure 23–1). There is no ankylosis, but limitation of motion of the affected joint or joints is common. Crepitus may often be felt over the knee. Joint effusion and other articular signs of inflammation are mild. However, in some cases a one-way valve effect between the knee joint and gastrocnemius-semimembranosus bursa can lead to accumulation of synovial fluid, called a popliteal (Baker) cyst. There are no systemic manifestations.

B. Laboratory Findings

Osteoarthritis does not cause elevation of the ESR or other laboratory signs of inflammation. Synovial fluid is noninflammatory (Table 23–2).

Table 23–2. Examination of joint fluid.

Measure	Normal	Group I (Noninflammatory)	Group II (Inflammatory)	Group III (Purulent)
Volume (mL) (knee)	< 3.5	Often > 3.5	Often > 3.5	Often > 3.5
Clarity	Transparent	Transparent	Translucent to opaque	Opaque
Color	Clear	Yellow	Yellow to opalescent	Yellow to green
WBC per mcL	< 200 (0.2×10^9/L)	< 2000 (2.0×10^9/L)	2000–75,000[1] ($2.0–75.0 \times 10^9$/L)	> 100,000[2] (100×10^9/L)
Polymorphonuclear leukocytes	< 25%	< 25%	≥ 50%	≥ 75%
Culture	Negative	Negative	Negative	Usually positive[2]

[1]Gout, rheumatoid arthritis, and other inflammatory conditions occasionally have synovial fluid WBC counts > 75,000/mcL (75×10^9/L) but rarely > 100,000/mcL (100×10^9/L).
[2]Most purulent effusions are due to septic arthritis. Septic arthritis, however, can present with group II synovial fluid, particularly if infection is caused by organisms of low virulence (eg, *Neisseria gonorrhoeae*) or if antibiotic therapy has been started.

Table 23–3. Differential diagnosis by synovial fluid WBC count.

Noninflammatory (< 2000 WBC/mcL [< 2 × 10^9/L])	Inflammatory (2000–50,000 WBC/mcL [2.0–50.0 × 10^9/L])	Purulent (> 50,000 WBC/mcL [> 50 × 10^9/L])	Hemorrhagic
Osteoarthritis Osteonecrosis Charcot arthropathy Normal joint	Rheumatoid arthritis/JIA SLE/MCTD Idiopathic inflammatory myositis Systemic sclerosis Systemic vasculitides Crystalline arthritis (gout, CPPD)[1] Psoriatic arthritis Reactive arthritis IBD arthritis Sarcoidosis Rheumatic fever Septic arthritis in an immunosuppressed host[2] Nonbacterial infections[3]	Septic arthritis (bacterial)[4]	Trauma Pigmented villonodular synovitis Tuberculosis Neoplasia Coagulopathy

CPPD, calcium pyrophosphate deposition; JIA, juvenile idiopathic arthritis; MCTD, mixed connective tissue disease.
[1]Crystalline arthritis cell count may be > 50,000 WBC/mcL and mimic infection.
[2]Such as a patient receiving a biologic agent for rheumatoid arthritis.
[3]Lyme, viral, mycobacterial, fungal.
[4]Lower synovial fluid WBC counts do not exclude the diagnosis.
Adapted, with permission, from Klippel JH et al (eds). *Primer on the Rheumatic Diseases*, 13th ed. Springer, 2008.

C. Imaging

Radiographs can support the clinical diagnosis of osteoarthritis but are not routinely required. Findings include narrowing of the joint space; osteophyte formation and lipping of marginal bone; and thickened, dense subchondral bone. Bone cysts may also be present.

Differential Diagnosis

Because articular inflammation is minimal and systemic manifestations are absent, osteoarthritis should seldom be confused with other arthritides. The distribution of joint involvement in the hands also helps distinguish osteoarthritis from RA. Osteoarthritis chiefly affects the DIP and PIP joints and spares the wrist and metacarpophalangeal (MCP) joints; RA involves the wrists and MCP joints and spares the DIP joints. Furthermore, the joint enlargement is bony-hard and cool in osteoarthritis but spongy and warm in RA. Degenerative changes in joints—especially in the spine—may cause coexistent metastatic neoplasia, osteoporosis, plasma cell myeloma, or other bone disease to be overlooked.

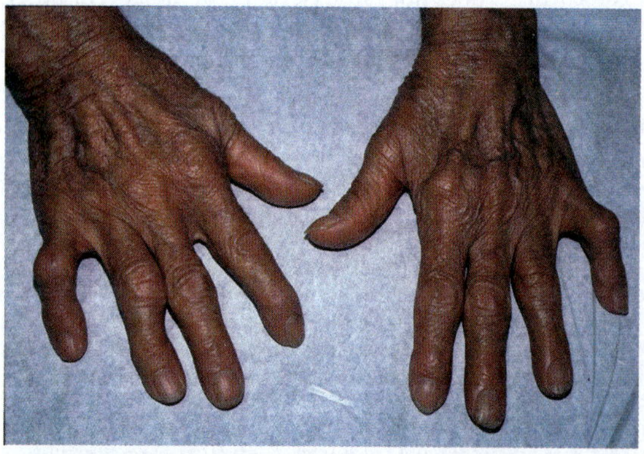

▲ **Figure 23–1.** **Bony enlargement of some distal interphalangeal (DIP) and proximal interphalangeal (PIP) joints consistent with Heberden (DIP) and Bouchard (PIP) nodes.** (Reproduced with permission from Richard P. Usatine, MD, in Usatine RP, Smith MA, Mayeaux EJ Jr, Chumley H. *The Color Atlas of Family Medicine*, 3rd ed. McGraw-Hill, 2019.)

Prevention

Weight reduction and regular physical activity reduce the risk of developing symptomatic knee, hip, and hand osteoarthritis. Correcting leg length discrepancy of > 1 cm with shoe modification may prevent knee osteoarthritis from developing in the shorter leg.

Treatment

A. General Measures

Patients with osteoarthritis of the hand may benefit from assistive devices and instruction on techniques for joint protection; splinting is beneficial for those with symptomatic osteoarthritis of the first carpometacarpal joint. Patients with mild to moderate osteoarthritis of the knee or hip should participate in a regular exercise program (eg, a supervised walking program, hydrotherapy classes) and, if overweight, should lose weight. An RCT of individuals with knee osteoarthritis found that physical therapy was more effective at reducing pain and disability at 1 year than intra-articular glucocorticoid injections. Reduction in pain with weight loss can be significant; one study showed that loss of ≥ 10% of body weight resulted in a 50% reduction in pain scores of knee osteoarthritis. Using assistive devices (eg, a cane on the contralateral side) can improve functional status.

B. Medical Management

1. Topical therapies—Topical NSAIDs (eg, 4 g of diclofenac gel 1% applied to the affected joint four times daily) are effective for knee and hand osteoarthritis. Because they have lower rates of systemic side effects than oral NSAIDs, topical NSAIDs are preferable for patients with one or a few painful joints, particularly knee or hand osteoarthritis, and for those with risk factors for NSAID-induced GI toxicity. Topical NSAIDs are preferred for patients 75 years of age or older. Topical capsaicin may be of benefit for osteoarthritis of the hand or the knee.

2. Oral NSAIDs—Oral NSAIDs (see Table 5–4) can be considered for patients with involvement of multiple joints, those with hip osteoarthritis, or those with inadequate pain relief from topical agents. Oral NSAIDs are more effective than acetaminophen for osteoarthritis but have greater toxicity. NSAIDs inhibit cyclooxygenase (COX), the enzyme that converts arachidonic acid to prostaglandins. COX exists in two isomers—COX-1, which is expressed continuously in many cells and is responsible for the homeostatic effects of prostaglandins, and COX-2, which is induced by cytokines and expressed in inflammatory tissues. Most NSAIDs are nonselective since they inhibit both COX-1 and COX-2 isomers. COX-2 inhibitors have fewer adverse GI effects than COX-1 inhibitors. Celecoxib is the only selective COX-2 inhibitor available in the United States. Whenever possible, limiting the duration of oral NSAIDs to control osteoarthritis pain is preferred to minimize the risk of adverse events.

GI toxicity, such as gastric ulceration, perforation, and GI hemorrhage, are the most common serious side effects of NSAIDs. The overall rate of bleeding with NSAID use in the general population is low (≤ 1:6000 users) but is increased by the risk factors of long-term use; higher NSAID dose; concomitant corticosteroids, anticoagulants, or SSRIs; presence of RA; history of peptic ulcer disease; alcohol use disorder; and age over 70. *PPIs (eg, esomeprazole 20–40 mg orally daily) reduce the incidence of serious GI toxicity and should be used in combination with oral NSAIDs for patients with risk factors for NSAID-induced GI toxicity.* Patients who have recently recovered from an NSAID-induced bleeding gastric ulcer appear to be at high risk for rebleeding (about 5% in 6 months) when an NSAID is reintroduced, even if prophylactic measures (such as PPIs) are used. Compared with nonselective NSAIDs, celecoxib is less likely to cause upper GI tract adverse events, including bleeding.

All NSAIDs, including aspirin and celecoxib, can produce renal toxicity, including interstitial nephritis, nephrotic syndrome, prerenal azotemia, and aggravation of hypertension. Hyperkalemia due to hyporeninemic hypoaldosteronism is seen rarely. Renal toxicity is uncommon but is increased by the following risk factors: CKD, volume depletion from diuretic use or GI loss, HF, cirrhosis, or use of ACE inhibitors or ARBs.

All NSAIDs, except celecoxib and the nonacetylated salicylates (eg, salsalate, sodium salicylate), interfere with platelet function and prolong bleeding time. Aspirin irreversibly inhibits platelet function, so the bleeding time effect resolves only as new platelets are made. In contrast, the effect of nonselective NSAIDs on platelet function is reversible and resolves as the drug is cleared. Concomitant administration of a nonselective NSAID can interfere with the ability of aspirin to acetylate platelets and thus may interfere with the cardioprotective effects of low-dose aspirin. *All NSAIDs are associated with a small increase in the absolute risk of MI and stroke in patients with or without risk factors for heart disease or known heart disease.* While the cardiovascular risk is related to the dose and duration of treatment, stroke and MI can occur within the first week of treatment. Cardiovascular risks associated with naproxen, ibuprofen, and moderate dose celecoxib (200 mg orally daily) are comparable.

3. Acetaminophen, opioids, and supplements—Acetaminophen is not recommended because its impact on pain is frequently negligible and hepatotoxicity can occur from high doses. Opioids are not appropriate for the long-term management of pain from osteoarthritis; tramadol may be considered as a last-line option in selected patients when other therapies have failed, but benefits are modest and adverse effects are common. Chondroitin sulfate and glucosamine, alone or in combination, fish oil, and vitamin D are no better than placebo in reducing the pain of knee or hip osteoarthritis. Boswellia serrata extracts provide modest short-term improvements in pain and function in osteoarthritis trials compared with placebo.

4. Intra-articular injections—Intra-articular corticosteroid injections for knee osteoarthritis provide short-term pain relief lasting weeks, with no sustained structural benefit and potential risks with repeated use. Intra-articular hyaluronic acid shows inconsistent symptomatic benefit over placebo. Evidence about platelet-rich plasma in knee osteoarthritis is conflicting; some placebo-controlled trials show no benefit, but meta-analyses suggest modest pain and function improvements, mainly in early to moderate disease with specific formulations.

5. Semaglutide—In a randomized, double-blind trial of individuals with obesity and pain from knee osteoarthritis, semaglutide 2.4 mg subcutaneously weekly (or 1.7 mg if unacceptable side effects with 2.4 mg) significantly reduced weight and knee pain and improved physical function in patients with obesity and moderate to severe knee osteoarthritis compared with placebo. Beyond weight reduction, GLP-1 receptor agonists may have anti-inflammatory and antidegradative effects.

6. Duloxetine—For patients with osteoarthritis in multiple joints who either have not responded to or cannot use NSAIDs, duloxetine, 30–60 mg orally daily, can reduce pain. Nausea occurs in 6–15% of patients.

7. Physical therapy—Physical therapy is modestly beneficial for knee osteoarthritis. An RCT of patients with knee osteoarthritis compared intra-articular glucocorticoid injections to physical therapy; those receiving physical therapy had less pain and functional disability after 1 year compared to those receiving injections. High-intensity strength training offers no benefits over low-intensity training.

8. Neuromodulation and Denervation Therapies—Transcutaneous electrical nerve stimulation delivers surface electrical currents to modulate pain but provides inconsistent and short-term benefit in knee osteoarthritis. Genicular radiofrequency ablation uses thermal energy to denervate genicular nerves and may reduce pain for up to 6 months, but benefits are not durable and techniques vary, so routine use is not recommended.

C. Surgical Measures

Total hip and knee replacements provide excellent symptomatic and functional improvement when involvement of that joint severely restricts walking or causes pain at rest, particularly at night. Patients should not be excluded from referral for joint replacement based on age, sex, smoking status, comorbidities, or obesity since positive outcomes are achievable in most groups. Arthroscopic surgery for knee osteoarthritis is ineffective. Severe first carpometacarpal osteoarthritis can be treated surgically when other treatments are inadequate.

Prognosis

Symptoms may be severe and limit activity (especially with involvement of the hips, knees, and cervical spine).

When to Refer

Refer patients to an orthopedic surgeon when recalcitrant symptoms or functional impairment, or both, warrant consideration of joint replacement of the hip, knee, or thumb.

Bliddal H et al. Once-weekly semaglutide in persons with obesity and knee osteoarthritis. N Engl J Med. 2024;391:1573. [PMID: 39476339]
Kloppenburg M et al. Osteoarthritis. Lancet. 2025;405:71. [PMID: 39755397]

CRYSTAL DEPOSITION ARTHRITIS

1. Gouty Arthritis

ESSENTIALS OF DIAGNOSIS

- Acute, monoarticular arthritis, often of the first MTP joint; recurrence is common.
- Polyarticular involvement more common with long-standing disease.
- Identification of urate crystals in joint fluid or tophi is diagnostic.
- Dramatic response to NSAIDs.
- With chronicity, urate deposits in subcutaneous tissue, bone, cartilage, joints, and other tissues.

General Considerations

Gout is a heterogeneous metabolic disease, often familial, associated with abnormal deposits of urate in tissues and characterized initially by a recurring acute arthritis, usually monoarticular, and later by chronic deforming arthritis. Urate deposition occurs when serum uric acid is supersaturated (ie, at levels > 6.8 mg/dL [404.5 mcmol/L]). Hyperuricemia is due to overproduction or underexcretion of uric acid—sometimes both. The disease is more common in Asian-Pacific populations (eg, a prevalence > 10% has been reported in the Māori people). Primary gout has a heritable component, and genome-wide surveys have linked the risk of gout to genes whose products regulate urate handling by the kidney. Gout due to secondary hyperuricemia, which also may have a heritable component, is related to acquired causes of hyperuricemia, such as medication use (especially diuretics, low-dose aspirin, cyclosporine, and niacin), myeloproliferative disorders, CKD, and lead poisoning. Alcohol ingestion promotes hyperuricemia by increasing urate production and decreasing the renal excretion of uric acid. Uric acid is created from the metabolism of organic compounds (purines) contained in purine-rich foods or beverages. Beer and spirits are particularly high in purines and ingestion is a common precipitant of gout. Finally, hospitalized patients frequently suffer attacks of gout because of changes in diet (including fasting before procedures), fluid intake, or medications that lead either to rapid reductions or increases in the serum urate level.

Gout is three times more common in men than women, and the incidence increases with each decade of life. In women, the onset is typically postmenopausal. The characteristic lesion is the tophus, a nodular deposit of monosodium urate monohydrate crystals with an associated foreign body reaction. Tophi are found in cartilage, subcutaneous and periarticular tissues, tendon, bone, the kidneys, and elsewhere. The precise relationship of hyperuricemia to gouty arthritis is still obscure, since chronic hyperuricemia is found in people who never develop gout or uric acid stones. Rapid fluctuations in serum urate levels, either increasing or decreasing, are important factors in precipitating acute gout. The mechanism of the late, chronic stage of gouty arthritis is better understood. This is characterized pathologically by tophaceous invasion of the articular and periarticular tissues, with structural derangement and secondary osteoarthritis.

Uric acid kidney stones are present in 14% of patients with gouty arthritis. Hyperuricemia correlates highly with the development of stones, with the risk of stone formation increasing with higher uric acid levels. Chronic urate nephropathy is caused by the deposition of monosodium urate crystals in the renal medulla and pyramids. Although progressive CKD occurs in a substantial percentage of patients with chronic gout, the role of hyperuricemia in causing this outcome is controversial because many patients with gout have numerous confounding risk factors for CKD (eg, hypertension, NSAID use, alcohol use, diabetes). In a randomized trial in patients with CKD and a high risk of its progression, urate-lowering treatment with allopurinol did not slow the decline in eGFR.

Clinical Findings

A. Symptoms and Signs

Acute gouty arthritis is sudden in onset and frequently nocturnal. It may develop without apparent precipitating cause or may follow rapid increases or decreases in serum urate levels. The MTP joint of the great toe is the most susceptible joint ("podagra"), although others, especially those of the feet, ankles, and knees, are commonly affected (Figure 23–2). Gouty attacks may develop in periarticular soft tissues such as the olecranon or prepatellar bursae. Hips and shoulders are rarely affected. More than one joint may occasionally be affected during the same attack; in such cases, the distribution of the arthritis is usually asymmetric. As the attack progresses, the pain becomes intense. The involved joints are swollen and exquisitely tender and the overlying skin tense, warm, and dusky red. Fever is common and may reach 39°C. Tophi may be found in the pinna of the ears, around the joints and extensor tendons of the hands and feet, in the olecranon and prepatellar bursae, and along the Achilles tendon. Tophi usually develop years after the initial attack of gout.

Asymptomatic periods of months or years commonly follow the initial acute attack. After years of untreated hyperuricemia and recurrent severe monoarthritis attacks of the lower extremities, gout can evolve into a chronic, deforming polyarthritis of upper and lower extremities that mimics RA.

Chronic lead intoxication may cause attacks of gouty arthritis (saturnine gout).

B. Laboratory Findings

Although serial measurements of the serum uric acid detect hyperuricemia in 95% of patients, a single uric acid determination during an acute flare of gout is normal in ≥ 25% of cases. A normal serum uric acid level, therefore, does not exclude gout, especially in patients taking urate-lowering drugs. During an acute attack, the peripheral WBC count (neutrophilia) is frequently elevated. The joint fluid is inflammatory (Table 23–2). Identification of sodium urate crystals in joint fluid or material aspirated from a tophus establishes the diagnosis. The crystals, which may be extracellular or found within neutrophils, are needle-like and negatively birefringent when examined by polarized light microscopy.

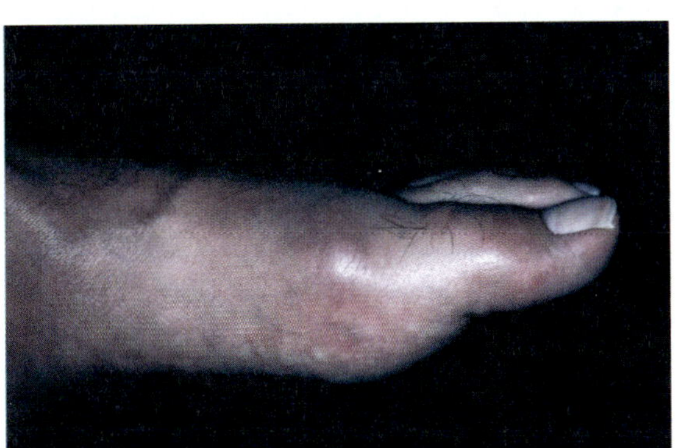

▲ **Figure 23–2.** Typical inflammatory changes of gout at first metatarsophalangeal joint (podagra). (Used, with permission, from Richard P. Usatine, MD in Usatine RP, Smith MA, Mayeaux EJ Jr, Chumley H. *The Color Atlas of Family Medicine,* 3rd ed. McGraw-Hill, 2019.)

C. Imaging

Early in the disease, radiographs show no changes. Later, punched-out erosions with an overhanging rim of cortical bone ("rat bite") develop. When these are adjacent to a soft tissue tophus, they are diagnostic of gout. Ultrasonography and dual-energy CT can be used to confirm the diagnosis of gout; tophi that are too small to appreciate on physical examination and smaller deposits of urate crystals can frequently be detected by these imaging modalities.

Differential Diagnosis

Acute gout is often confused with cellulitis. Bacteriologic studies usually exclude acute pyogenic arthritis, but rarely, acute gout and pyogenic arthritis can coexist. Pseudogout is distinguished by the identification of calcium pyrophosphate crystals (positive birefringence) in the joint fluid, usually normal serum uric acid, and the radiographic appearance of chondrocalcinosis.

Tophaceous arthritis may resemble chronic RA; gout is suggested by an earlier history of monoarthritis and is established by the demonstration of urate crystals in a suspected tophus. Likewise, hips and shoulders are generally spared in tophaceous gout. Biopsy may be necessary to distinguish tophi from rheumatoid nodules.

Treatment

A. Asymptomatic Hyperuricemia

As a general rule, uric acid–lowering drugs should not be instituted until gout, renal calculi, or tophi have become apparent.

B. Acute Attack

Treatment of the acute attack focuses on reducing inflammation, not lowering serum uric acid. If a patient is taking long-term urate-lowering therapies like allopurinol or febuxostat, these drugs should be continued. There is no contraindication to starting urate-lowering therapy during an acute gout attack; however, one of the following therapies is needed to treat the acute attack:

1. NSAIDs—Oral NSAIDs in full dose (eg, naproxen 500 mg twice daily or indomethacin 25–50 mg every 8 hours; see Table 5–4) are effective treatment for acute gout and should be continued until the symptoms have resolved (usually 7–10 days). Contraindications include active peptic ulcer disease, impaired kidney function, cirrhosis, and a history of adverse reaction to NSAIDs.

2. Colchicine—Oral colchicine is an appropriate treatment option for acute gout, and most effective < 36 hours after symptom onset. For acute gout, colchicine should be administered orally as follows: a loading dose of 1.2 mg followed by a dose of 0.6 mg 1 hour later for a total dose of 1.8 mg the first day; thereafter 0.6 mg twice per day is used until resolution. Patients who are already taking prophylactic doses of colchicine and have an acute flare of gout may receive the full loading dose (1.2 mg) followed by 0.6 mg 1 hour later (before resuming the usual 0.6 mg once or twice daily) provided they have not received this regimen within the preceding 14 days (in which case, NSAIDs or corticosteroids should be used). Higher doses of colchicine should be avoided, given a high prevalence of adverse events such as diarrhea. Colchicine dose should be reduced or avoided if there is significant kidney or liver impairment and in patients who are taking a drug that strongly reduces CYP3A4 or that is a P-glycoprotein (P-gp) inhibitor, such as verapamil, clarithromycin, or any protease inhibitor, except fosamprenavir. Using oral colchicine during the intercritical period to prevent gout attacks is discussed below.

3. Corticosteroids—Corticosteroids often give dramatic symptomatic relief in acute episodes of gout and will control most attacks. They are especially useful in patients with contraindications to NSAIDs. Corticosteroids may be given intravenously (eg, methylprednisolone, 0.5 mg/kg/day) or orally (eg, prednisone, 40–60 mg/day). Corticosteroids can be given at the suggested dose for 5–10 days and then simply discontinued or given at the suggested initial dose for 2–5 days and then tapered over 7–10 days. If the patient's gout is monoarticular or oligoarticular, intra-articular administration of the corticosteroid (eg, triamcinolone, 10–40 mg depending on the size of the joint) is very effective. Because gouty and septic arthritis can coexist, albeit rarely, joint aspiration and Gram stain with culture of synovial fluid should be performed when intra-articular corticosteroids are given.

4. Interleukin-1 inhibitors—Anakinra (an interleukin-1 receptor antagonist) and canakinumab (a monoclonal antibody against interleukin-1-β) can be used to treat acute gout in patients in whom comorbidities prevent the use of NSAIDs, colchicine, or glucocorticoids (Table 23–4). Anakinra has a short half-life (6 hours) and may be preferred in patients in whom infection is a concern; canakinumab is FDA-approved to treat gout flares in patients unable to use other therapies.

C. Management Between Attacks

Treatment during symptom-free periods is intended to minimize urate deposition in tissues and to reduce the frequency and severity of recurrences. Potentially reversible causes of hyperuricemia are a high-purine diet, obesity, alcohol consumption, and use of certain medications, such as diuretics. Patients with a single episode of gout who have normal kidney function, can lose weight, and stop drinking alcohol are at low risk for another attack and may not require long-term medical therapy. In contrast, patients with mild CKD or a history of multiple gout attacks will likely benefit from pharmacologic treatment. In general, the higher the uric acid level and the more frequent the attacks, the more likely that long-term medical therapy will be beneficial. All patients with tophaceous gout should receive urate-lowering therapy.

1. Diet and alcohol—Excessive consumption of alcohol, particularly beer, can precipitate attacks and should be avoided. Although dietary purines usually contribute only 1 mg/dL to the serum uric acid level, moderation in eating foods with high purine content is advisable. Sugar-sweetened beverages and foods sweetened with high fructose corn syrup increase serum urate and the risk of gout. A high liquid intake and, more importantly, a daily urinary output of ≥ 2 L will aid urate excretion and minimize urate precipitation in the kidney.

2. Avoidance of hyperuricemic medications—Thiazide and loop diuretics inhibit renal excretion of uric acid and, if possible, should be avoided in patients with gout. Similarly, calcineurin inhibitors (eg, cyclosporine) and some antibiotics (eg, pyrazinamide and ethambutol) can raise uric acid level. Low-dose aspirin (≤ 325 mg/day) also aggravates hyperuricemia.

3. Colchicine prophylaxis—Colchicine can be used when urate-lowering therapy is started to suppress attacks precipitated by abrupt changes in the serum uric acid level. The usual dose is 0.6 mg orally either once or twice a day. Colchicine is renally cleared. Patients with severe CKD (eGFR < 30 mL/min/1.73 m^2) should either avoid colchicine or take a reduced dose (0.3 mg/day); monitoring for peripheral neuromyopathy and other complications of colchicine toxicity is mandatory. In patients with concomitant CAD, chronic colchicine use can reduce major cardiovascular events.

4. Canakinumab prophylaxis—In exceptional situations where alternative preventive treatments are not possible, canakinumab can be used for prophylaxis.

5. Reduction of serum uric acid—Indications for urate-lowering therapy in a person with gout include frequent acute arthritis (two or more episodes per year), tophaceous deposits, or CKD (stage 2 or worse). The American College of Rheumatology (ACR) guidelines recommend treating to a target uric acid of 6 mg/dL (357 mcmol/L) so that urate crystals can begin to solubilize. In some cases, particularly in patients with tophi or frequent attacks, control of gout may require lowering serum uric acid to < 5 mg/dL or 297.4 mcmol/L. Lowering serum uric acid levels does not benefit an acute gout flare. Patients with a high serum uric acid who have *not* had gout, renal calculi or tophi generally do not need urate-lowering medications. Exceptions include patients undergoing treatment for myeloproliferative disorders. Three classes of agents may lower the serum uric acid—xanthine oxidase inhibitors (allopurinol or febuxostat), uricosuric agents, and uricase (pegloticase).

A. Xanthine oxidase inhibitors—Allopurinol and febuxostat are the preferred first-line agents for lowering urate and have similar efficacy. They reduce plasma uric acid levels by blocking the final enzymatic steps in the production of uric acid. Allopurinol and febuxostat should not be used together, but they can be tried sequentially if the initial agent fails to lower serum uric acid to the target level or if it is not tolerated. A frequent adverse effect with either medication is the precipitation of an acute gouty attack; thus, patients generally should be receiving prophylactic doses of colchicine.

Table 23–4. Biologic and targeted synthetic agents (selected list).[1]

Agent	Recommended Regimen[2]	Indication
B-cell–depleting agents		
Inebilizumab	Induction: 300 mg intravenously days 1 and 15 Maintenance: 300 mg intravenously every 6 months	Neuromyelitis optica spectrum disorder, IgG_4-related disease
Rituximab	Induction: 375 mg/m² intravenously once weekly for 4 weeks or 1000 mg days 1 and 15 Maintenance: varies but typically 500 mg–1000 mg intravenously every 4–6 months	ANCA-associated vasculitis (granulomatosis with polyangiitis, microscopic polyangiitis, eosinophilic granulomatosis with polyangitis)
	Induction: 1000 mg intravenously once every 2 weeks for 2 doses Maintenance: 1000 mg intravenously every 2 weeks for 2 doses every 16–24 weeks	RA Doses vary for other diseases (eg, Sjögren disease, hepatitis C–associated cryoglobulinemic vasculitis, SLE, APS, systemic sclerosis, inflammatory myositis, IgG4-RD)
Obinutuzumab	Induction: 1000 mg intravenously days 1 and 15 Maintenance: doses vary	SLE
Calcineurin inhibitors		
Tacrolimus	Doses vary but typically 2 mg orally twice daily	Lupus nephritis
Voclosporin	23.7 mg orally twice daily	Lupus nephritis
Complement pathway–targeted therapies		
Eculizumab	Induction: 900 mg intravenously weekly for 4 weeks Maintenance: 1200 mg intravenously every 4 weeks	APS, complement-mediated TMA
Avacopan	30 mg oral twice daily (in combination with corticosteroids and rituximab or cyclophosphamide induction therapy)	Granulomatosis with polyangiitis, microscopic polyangiitis
IL-1 inhibitors		
Anakinra	100 mg subcutaneously daily	RA, gout, adult-onset Still disease
Canakinumab	150 mg subcutaneously as a single dose at gout flare	Gout, adult-onset Still disease
IL-5 inhibitors		
Mepolizumab	300 mg subcutaneously every 4 weeks	Eosinophilic granulomatosis with polyangitis
Benralizumab	Induction: 30 mg subcutaneously every 4 weeks for the first three doses Maintenance: 30 mg subcutaneously every 8 weeks thereafter	Eosinophilic granulomatosis with polyangitis
IL-6 inhibitors		
Sarilumab	200 mg subcutaneously once every 2 weeks	RA, adult-onset Still disease, PMR
Tocilizumab	162 mg subcutaneously once weekly or 4 mg/kg intravenously every 4 weeks followed by an increase to 8 mg/kg intravenously every 4 weeks based on clinical response	RA, GCA, systemic sclerosis Doses vary by disease
IL-12/23 inhibitors		
Ustekinumab	45 mg subcutaneously at weeks 0, 4, then every 12 weeks Doses vary based on indication	Psoriatic arthritis, Crohn disease
IL-17 inhibitors		
Bimekizumab	160 mg subcutaneously every 4 weeks	Psoriatic arthritis, axial spondyloarthritis
Brodalumab	Induction: 210 mg subcutaneously at weeks 0, 1, and 2 Maintenance: 210 mg subcutaneously every 2 weeks	Psoriatic arthritis
Ixekizumab	Induction: 160 mg subcutaneously at week 0 Maintenance: 80 mg subcutaneously every 4 weeks	Psoriatic arthritis, axial spondyloarthritis
Secukinumab	Induction: 6 mg/kg intravenously at week 0 Maintenance: 1.75 mg/kg (max 300 mg) intravenously every 4 weeks *or* Induction: 150 mg subcutaneously at weeks 0, 1, 2, 3, and 4 Maintenance: 150 mg subcutaneously every 4 weeks (can be increased to 300 mg if lower dose ineffective)	Psoriatic arthritis, axial spondyloarthritis

(*continued*)

Table 23–4. Biologic and targeted synthetic agents (selected list).[1] (continued)

Agent	Recommended Regimen[2]	Indication
IL-23 inhibitors		
Guselkumab	100 mg subcutaneously at weeks 0, 4, then every 8 weeks	Psoriatic arthritis, ulcerative colitis
Risankizumab	150 mg subcutaneously at weeks 0, 4, then every 12 weeks	Psoriatic arthritis, Crohn disease, ulcerative colitis
Janus kinase (JAK) inhibitors		
Baricitinib	2 mg orally daily	RA
Tofacitinib	Immediate-release Tablet: 5 mg orally twice daily Extended-release Tablet: 11 mg orally once daily	RA, axial spondyloarthritis, IBD-associated spondyloarthritis, psoriatic arthritis
Upadacitinib	15 mg orally daily	RA, axial spondyloarthritis, IBD-associated spondyloarthritis, psoriatic arthritis, atopic dermatitis, GCA
Monoclonal antibody type I interferon receptor		
Anifrolumab	300 mg intravenously every 4 weeks	SLE
Monoclonal antibody BAFF inhibitors		
Belimumab	Induction: 10 mg/kg intravenously every 2 weeks for 3 doses Maintenance: 10 mg/kg intravenously every 4 weeks *or* 200 mg subcutaneously once weekly	SLE and lupus nephritis
Multiple tyrosine kinases inhibitor		
Nintedanib	150 mg orally twice daily	Systemic sclerosis
T-cell costimulation modulator		
Abatacept	125 mg weekly subcutaneously *or* Weight-based intravenous dosing: < 60 kg: 500 mg, 60–100 kg: 750 mg, > 100 kg: 1000 mg at weeks 0, 2, 4, then every 4 weeks	RA, psoriatic arthritis
TNF inhibitors		
Adalimumab	40 mg subcutaneously every other week	RA, Behçet disease, psoriatic arthritis, axial spondyloarthritis
Certolizumab pegol	400 mg subcutaneously at week 0, 2, and 4 followed by 200 mg subcutaneously every other week	RA, psoriatic arthritis, axial spondyloarthritis
Etanercept	50 mg subcutaneously once weekly *or* 25 mg subcutaneously twice weekly	RA, psoriatic arthritis, axial spondyloarthritis
Golimumab	50 mg subcutaneously once monthly *or* 2 mg/kg intravenously at weeks 0, 4 and then every 8 weeks thereafter	RA, psoriatic arthritis, axial spondyloarthritis
Infliximab	3–5 mg/kg intravenous infusion; repeat infusions after 2 and 6 weeks, then every 8 weeks	RA, Behçet disease, psoriatic arthritis
	5 mg/kg intravenously at 0, 2, and 6 weeks followed by 5 mg/kg intravenously every 6 weeks thereafter	Axial spondyloarthritis

ANCA, anti-neutrophil cytoplasmic antibodies; APS, antiphospholipid syndrome; GCA, giant cell arteritis; IgG4-RD, IgG4-related disease; PMR, polymyalgia rheumatica; RA, rheumatoid arthritis; TMA, thrombotic microangiopathy.
[1]To be used with active participation of a rheumatologist.
[2]Consult for dose modification for weight and for disorders that require dose adjustment (eg, kidney injury, liver disease).

Hypersensitivity to allopurinol occurs in 0.05% of cases, usually within the first few months of therapy, and it can be life-threatening. The most common initial sign of hypersensitivity is a pruritic rash that may progress to toxic epidermal necrolysis, Stevens-Johnson syndrome (SJS), and drug reaction with eosinophilia and systemic symptoms (DRESS), particularly if allopurinol is continued. *Patients should be instructed to stop allopurinol immediately if a rash develops.* CKD and concomitant thiazide therapy are risk factors. There is a strong association between allopurinol hypersensitivity and HLA-B*58:01, which is a prevalent allele in certain populations. *Screening for HLA-B*58:01 before initiating allopurinol should be considered in persons of Chinese, Thai, and Korean descent, and in Black persons.*

The initial daily dose of allopurinol is 100 mg/day orally (50 mg/day for those with stage 4 or worse CKD), titrating upward every 2–5 weeks to achieve the target serum uric acid level. A typical dose of allopurinol is 300 mg, but many patients require > 300 mg daily to achieve the target uric acid level. The maximum daily dose is 800 mg. Allopurinol interacts with other drugs including azathioprine and 6-MP and can cause life-threatening pancytopenia.

Febuxostat can also rarely cause hypersensitivity reactions, and those with previous hypersensitivity to allopurinol appear to have slightly higher risk. It can be given without dose adjustment to patients with mild to moderate kidney disease. However, abnormal liver tests may develop in 2–3% of patients taking febuxostat. Despite initial concern that febuxostat was associated with more cardiovascular events than allopurinol, a large RCT showed that the two drugs have similar cardiovascular safety. The initial dose of febuxostat is 40 mg/day orally. If the target serum uric acid is not reached in 4 weeks, the dose of febuxostat can be increased to 80 mg/day and then to the maximum dose of 120 mg/day.

B. Uricosuric drugs—Uricosuric drugs lower serum uric acid levels by blocking the tubular reabsorption of filtered urate, thereby increasing uric acid excretion by the kidney. Probenecid is started at 250 mg orally twice daily and titrated up to 2000 mg/day to reach target urate levels. It is generally reserved for patients who do not achieve a serum urate ≤ 6.0 mg/dL with allopurinol or febuxostat alone. Probenecid is ineffective when creatinine clearance is < 50 mL/min and is contraindicated in patients with nephrolithiasis or high urinary uric acid excretion (ie, > 800 mg/24 hour). To reduce the risk of developing uric acid stones, patients should increase fluid intake and may require urinary alkalinization (eg, potassium citrate, 30–80 mEq/day orally) to maintain a urine pH > 6.0.

C. Pegloticase—Pegloticase, a recombinant uricase that must be administered intravenously (8 mg every 2 weeks), is indicated for the rare patient with refractory chronic tophaceous gout. Pegloticase carries an FDA black box warning, which advises administering the drug only in health care settings and by health care professionals prepared to manage anaphylaxis. Methotrexate 15 mg orally per week and folic acid 1 mg orally daily should be started 4 weeks before pegloticase initiation and continued through the end of treatment; use of methotrexate increases response rates and reduces the risk of anaphylaxis. If methotrexate cannot be used, alternative immunosuppressants include mycophenolate mofetil or azathioprine. Pegloticase should be stopped if serum urate levels remain > 6 mg/dL, indicating insufficient uric acid reduction and the development of antidrug antibodies. Pegloticase should be followed by urate-lowering therapy, usually with xanthine oxidase inhibitors.

D. Chronic Tophaceous Arthritis

With rigorous drug adherence, allopurinol, febuxostat, and pegloticase shrink tophi and in time can lead to their disappearance. Resorption of extensive tophi requires maintaining a serum uric acid < 6 mg/dL.

E. Gout in Patients Post Transplant

Hyperuricemia and gout commonly develop in many patients post transplant because they have decreased kidney function and require drugs that inhibit uric acid excretion (especially cyclosporine and diuretics). Often the best approach for monoarticular gout—after excluding infection—is injecting corticosteroids into the joint. In polyarticular gout, because drug–drug interactions can limit colchicine use and reduced kidney function increases NSAID toxicity; systemic corticosteroids may be the safest option for some patients. Since patients who have received a transplant often have multiple attacks of gout, long-term relief requires lowering the serum uric acid with allopurinol or febuxostat. However, both agents inhibit azathioprine and mercaptopurine metabolism and should be avoided in patients receiving these medications.

Prognosis

Without treatment, an acute attack may last from a few days to several weeks. The intervals between acute attacks vary up to years, but the asymptomatic periods often become shorter as the disease progresses. Chronic gouty arthritis occurs after repeated attacks of acute gout, but only after inadequate treatment. The younger the patient at the onset of disease, the greater the tendency to a progressive course. Destructive arthropathy is rarely seen in patients whose first attack is after age 50.

Barry A et al. Comparison of gout flares with the initiation of treat-to-target allopurinol and febuxostat: a post-hoc analysis of a randomized multicenter trial. Arthritis Rheumatol. 2024;76:1552. [PMID: 38925627]

FitzGerald JD. Gout. Ann Intern Med. 2025;178:ITC33. [PMID: 40063960]

Wang Y et al. Target serum urate achievement and chronic kidney disease progression in patients with gout and kidney disease. JAMA Intern Med. 2025;185:74. [PMID: 39585678]

2. Calcium Pyrophosphate Deposition

ESSENTIALS OF DIAGNOSIS

- An acute crystal-induced arthritis ("pseudogout").
- A degenerative arthropathy.
- A chronic inflammatory polyarthritis ("pseudo-rheumatoid arthritis").
- Asymptomatic chondrocalcinosis detected incidentally on radiographs.

General Considerations

Aging is the most significant risk factor for calcium pyrophosphate deposition (CPPD) disease. Rarely, CPPD results from hyperparathyroidism, familial hypocalciuric hypercalcemia, hemochromatosis, or hypomagnesemia.

CPPD has multiple phenotypes, including acute arthritis (pseudogout), chronic CPPD inflammatory arthritis and CPPD with osteoarthritis.

Clinical Findings

Pseudogout is most often seen in persons aged ≥ 60 years, and usually affects joints that are spared in osteoarthritis, such as the radiocarpal, metacarpophalangeal or glenohumeral joints. It is almost always accompanied by radiographic chondrocalcinosis of the affected joints. Pseudogout, like gout, frequently develops 24–48 hours after major surgery. Identification of weakly positively birefringent calcium pyrophosphate crystals in joint aspirates is diagnostic.

The crowned dens syndrome, also diagnostic, is caused by pseudogout of the atlantoaxial junction associated with "crown-like" calcifications around the dens, and manifests with severe neck pain, rigidity, and high fever that can mimic meningitis or giant cell arteritis.

Chronic CPPD inflammatory arthritis is also termed "pseudorheumatoid arthritis". It typically involves the metacarpophalangeal joints and wrists and may resemble RA.

CPPD associated with osteoarthritis preferentially affects joints uncommonly involved in primary osteoarthritis, such as the glenohumeral joint, wrist, and patellofemoral compartment of the knee. Radiographs often show chondrocalcinosis with degenerative changes, including asymmetric joint space narrowing, osteophyte formation, and a squared-off appearance of the second and third metacarpophalangeal joints. CPPD is associated with a 30% increased risk of fracture compared to those with osteoarthritis alone.

Treatment

NSAIDs are helpful in the treatment of acute episodes of pseudogout. Colchicine, up to 1.8 mg orally during the first 24 hours of treatment, followed by 0.6 mg once or twice daily until symptoms resolve can be effective. Aspiration of the inflamed joint and intra-articular injection of triamcinolone, 10–40 mg, depending on the size of the joint, can be effective as can oral prednisone started at a dose of 30–50 mg and tapered over 7–10 days.

For chronic CPPD inflammatory arthritis refractory to standard therapies, early evidence suggests that anakinra or canakinumab (IL-1 inhibition) and, more limitedly, tocilizumab (IL-6 inhibition) may reduce symptoms; however, these therapies are not FDA-approved to treat CPPD. For three or more attacks per year, prophylaxis with colchicine 0.6 mg orally once or twice daily can reduce flares.

Abhishek A et al. The 2023 ACR/EULAR classification criteria for calcium pyrophosphate deposition disease. Arthritis Rheumatol. 2023;75:1703. [PMID: 37494275]

Zhao SS et al. Calcium pyrophosphate deposition disease is associated with increased risk of fractures: a retrospective cohort study using electronic health record data. Osteoarthritis Cartilage. 2025;33:1041. [PMID: 40484271]

RHEUMATOID ARTHRITIS

ESSENTIALS OF DIAGNOSIS

- Usually insidious onset with morning stiffness and joint pain.
- Symmetric polyarthritis with predilection for small joints of the hands and feet; deformities common with progressive disease.
- Radiographic findings: juxta-articular osteoporosis, joint erosions, and joint space narrowing.
- Rheumatoid factor and antibodies to cyclic citrullinated peptides (anti-CCP) are present in 70–80%.
- Extra-articular disease such as subcutaneous nodules and interstitial lung disease.

General Considerations

RA is a chronic systemic inflammatory disease whose major manifestation is synovitis of multiple joints. It has a prevalence of 1% and is more common in women than men (female:male ratio of 3:1). RA can begin at any age, but the peak onset is in the fourth or fifth decade for women and the sixth to eighth decades for men. Susceptibility to RA is genetically determined with multiple genes contributing. Inheritance of HLA-DRB1 alleles encoding a distinctive five-amino-acid sequence known as the "shared epitope" is the best characterized genetic risk factor. Untreated, RA causes joint destruction with consequent disability and shortens life expectancy.

The pathologic findings in the joint include chronic synovitis with formation of a pannus, which erodes cartilage, bone, ligaments, and tendons. Effusion and other manifestations of inflammation are common.

The diagnosis of RA is made using the 2010 ACR/European League Against Rheumatism (EULAR) classification criteria (Table 23–5).

Children with juvenile idiopathic arthritis can have arthritis that persists into adulthood. Although this entity is distinct from RA, the polyarticular form of the disease is often associated with a positive rheumatoid factor and has a similar joint distribution to RA.

Clinical Findings

A. Symptoms and Signs

1. Joint symptoms—The clinical manifestations of RA are highly variable, but joint symptoms usually predominate. Although acute presentations may occur, the onset of articular signs of inflammation is usually insidious, with prodromal symptoms of vague periarticular pain or stiffness. Symmetric swelling of multiple joints with tenderness and pain is characteristic, but monoarticular disease occasionally occurs initially. Stiffness persisting for longer than 30 minutes (and usually many hours) is prominent in the morning. Stiffness may recur after daytime inactivity and be much

Table 23–5. Classification criteria for rheumatoid arthritis.

Patients who have at least one swollen joint that is not better explained by another disease							
Joint Involvement (swollen or tender joints)	**Score**	**Serology**	**Score**	**Acute-Phase Reactants**	**Score**	**Duration of Symptoms**	**Score**
1 large joint	0	Negative RF; negative anti-CCP Ab	0	Normal CRP and ESR	0	< 6 weeks	0
2–10 large joints	1	Low + RF or anti-CCP Ab	2	Abnormal CRP or ESR	1	≥ 6 weeks	1
1–3 small joints (± large joints)	2	High + RF or anti-CCP Ab	3				
4–10 small joints (± large joints)	3			≥ 6/10 points is definite rheumatoid arthritis			
>10 joints (≥ 1 small joint)	5						

CCP, cyclic citrullinated peptides; RF, rheumatoid factor.

Reproduced with permission from Aletaha D, Neogi T, Silman AJ, et al. 2010 Rheumatoid arthritis classification criteria: an American College of Rheumatology/European League Against Rheumatism collaborative initiative. Arthritis Rheum. 2010;62(9):2569–2581.

more severe after strenuous activity. Although any diarthrodial joint may be affected, PIP joints, MCP joints (Figure 23–3), wrists, knees, ankles, and MTP joints are most often involved. Synovial cysts and rupture of tendons may occur. Entrapment syndromes are common—particularly of the median nerve at the carpal tunnel of the wrist. RA can affect the neck but spares the other components of the spine and does not involve the sacroiliac joints. In advanced disease, atlantoaxial (C1–C2) subluxation can lead to myelopathy.

2. Rheumatoid nodules—Twenty percent of patients have subcutaneous rheumatoid nodules, most commonly situated over bony prominences but also observed in the bursae and tendon sheaths (Figure 23–4). Nodules are occasionally seen in the lungs, the sclerae, and other tissues. Nodules correlate with the presence of rheumatoid factor in serum ("seropositivity"), as do most other extra-articular manifestations.

3. Ocular symptoms—Ocular manifestations include episcleritis, scleritis (Figure 23–5), scleromalacia due to scleral nodules, and peripheral ulcerative keratitis. Dryness of the eyes, mouth, and other mucous membranes is found especially in advanced disease (see Sjögren disease).

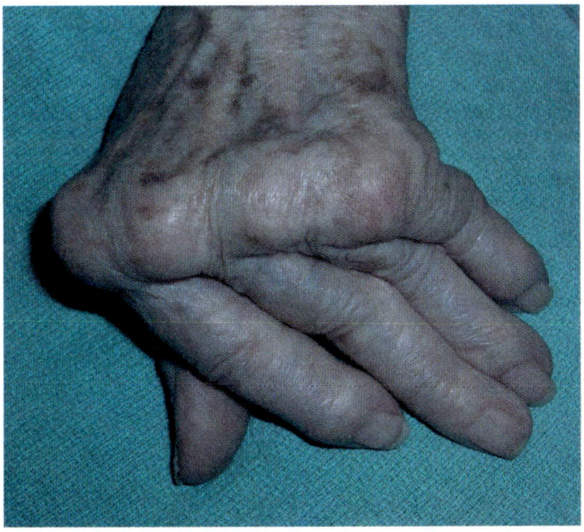

▲ **Figure 23–3.** Ulnar deviation at metacarpophalangeal joints in advanced rheumatoid arthritis. Also note the swelling at the distal interphalangeal joints, seen best on the first finger. (Reproduced with permission from Richard P. Usatine, MD, in Usatine RP, Smith MA, Mayeaux EJ Jr, Chumley H. *The Color Atlas of Family Medicine,* 3rd ed. McGraw-Hill, 2019.)

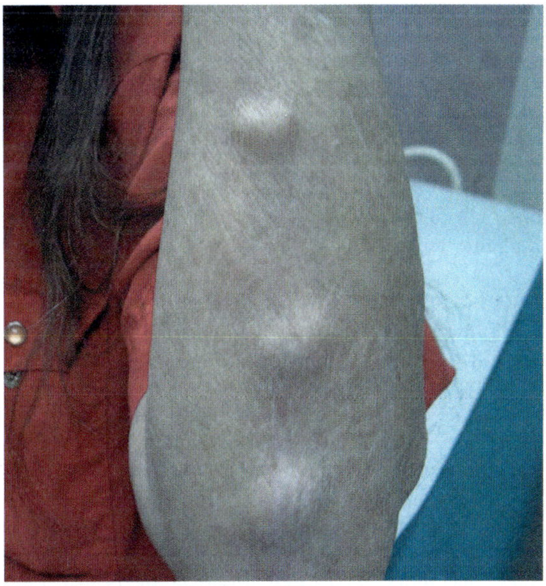

▲ **Figure 23–4.** Rheumatoid nodules over the extensor surface of the forearm. (Used, with permission, from Richard P. Usatine, MD in Usatine RP, Smith MA, Mayeaux EJ Jr, Chumley H. *The Color Atlas of Family Medicine,* 3rd ed. McGraw-Hill, 2019.)

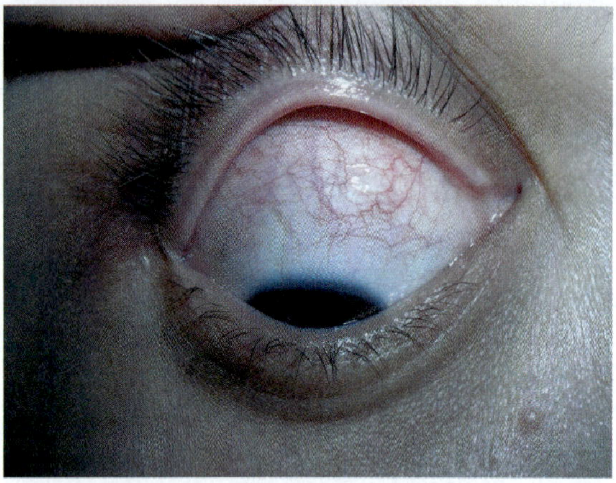

▲ **Figure 23–5.** Scleritis in a young woman with rheumatoid arthritis. Note the violaceous deep vessel engorgement. (Reproduced with permission from Richard P. Usatine, MD, in Usatine RP, Smith MA, Mayeaux EJ Jr, Chumley H. *The Color Atlas of Family Medicine*, 3rd ed. McGraw-Hill, 2019.)

4. Other symptoms—Interstitial lung disease, often asymptomatic and detected by chest imaging, can be clinically significant in about 15% of patients. Pericarditis and pleural disease are usually silent clinically, but symptomatic exudative effusions can develop. Osteoporosis is common in RA. Patients are at significantly increased risk of cardiovascular disease given a higher prevalence of risk factors such as diabetes, hypertension and obesity, as well as the effects of systemic inflammation. Occasionally, a small-vessel vasculitis develops and manifests as tiny hemorrhagic infarcts in the nail folds or finger pulps. Necrotizing arteritis is rare. A small subset of patients with RA have splenomegaly and neutropenia (Felty syndrome), usually in the setting of untreated severe, destructive arthritis. Felty syndrome must be distinguished from large granular lymphoproliferative disorder, with which it shares many features.

B. Laboratory Findings

Anti-CCP antibodies and rheumatoid factor, an IgM antibody directed against the Fc region of IgG, are present in 70–80% of patients with established RA. Rheumatoid factor has a sensitivity of only 50% in early disease. Anti-CCP antibodies are the most specific blood test for RA (specificity ~95%). Rheumatoid factor can occur in other autoimmune diseases and in chronic infections, including hepatitis C, syphilis, subacute bacterial endocarditis, and tuberculosis. The prevalence of rheumatoid factor positivity also rises with age in healthy individuals. Approximately 30% of patients with RA have antinuclear antibodies.

The ESR and levels of CRP are typically elevated in proportion to disease activity. Anemia of chronic disease is common. Initial joint fluid examination confirms the inflammatory nature of the arthritis (see Table 23–2).

Arthrocentesis is needed to diagnose superimposed septic arthritis, which is a common complication of RA and should be considered whenever a patient with RA has one joint inflamed out of proportion to the rest.

C. Imaging

Characteristic radiographic changes greatly aid in the diagnosis of RA. Radiographs obtained during the first 6 months of symptoms, however, are usually normal. The earliest changes occur in the hands or feet and consist of soft tissue swelling and juxta-articular demineralization. Later, uniform joint space narrowing and erosions develop. The erosions are often first evident at the fifth MTP joint and the ulnar styloid and occur at the juxta-articular margin, where the bony surface is not protected by cartilage. Characteristic changes also occur in the cervical spine, with C1–2 subluxation, but these changes usually take many years to develop. MRI and ultrasonography are more sensitive than radiographs in detecting bony and soft tissue changes in RA and can be considered if synovitis is suspected but difficult to confirm by physical examination.

Differential Diagnosis

In contrast to RA, osteoarthritis spares the wrists and the MCP joints. Osteoarthritis is not associated with constitutional manifestations, and the joint pain is characteristically relieved by rest, unlike the morning stiffness of RA. Signs of articular inflammation, prominent in RA, are usually minimal in osteoarthritis. CPPD disease can cause a degenerative arthropathy of the MCPs and wrists; radiographs are usually diagnostic. Although gouty arthritis is almost always intermittent and monoarticular in the early years, it may evolve with time into a chronic polyarticular process that mimics RA. Gouty tophi can resemble rheumatoid nodules but are not associated with rheumatoid factor, whose sensitivity for rheumatoid nodules approaches 100%.

Spondyloarthropathies, particularly earlier in their course, can be a source of diagnostic uncertainty; predilection for lower extremities and involvement of the spine and sacroiliac joints point to the correct diagnosis. Chronic Lyme arthritis typically involves only one joint, most commonly the knee, and is associated with positive serologic tests (see Chapter 38). Acute viral infections, particularly parvovirus B19 and Chikungunya virus, can cause a polyarthritis that mimics early RA. Fever is common and serologic testing confirms recent infection; symptoms usually resolve within weeks, but Chikungunya infection may lead to persistent or chronic CPPD inflammatory arthritis. Chronic infection with hepatitis C can cause a chronic, nonerosive polyarthritis associated with rheumatoid factor; tests for anti-CCP antibodies are negative.

Malar rash, photosensitivity, discoid skin lesions, alopecia, antibodies to double-stranded DNA or Smith, glomerulonephritis, and CNS abnormalities point to SLE. Polymyalgia rheumatica can cause polyarthralgias in patients over age 50, but these patients remain rheumatoid factor–negative and have chiefly proximal muscle pain and stiffness, centered on the shoulder and hip girdles. Joint pain that can be confused with RA presents in some patients with granulomatosis with polyangiitis. Although large joints are commonly affected and the arthritis is typically nonerosive and intermittent, small joints can be involved; recognition of other systemic vasculitic features helps distinguish this condition. A variety of cancers produce paraneoplastic syndromes, including polyarthritis. One form is hypertrophic pulmonary osteoarthropathy most often produced by lung and GI carcinomas, characterized by a rheumatoid-like arthritis associated with clubbing, periosteal new bone formation, and a negative rheumatoid factor.

Treatment

The primary objectives in treating RA are reduction of inflammation and pain, preservation of function, and prevention of deformity. Early, aggressive treatment is the standard of care. Disease-modifying antirheumatic drugs (DMARDs) should be started as soon as the diagnosis of RA is certain and then adjusted to suppress disease activity. NSAIDs provide some symptomatic relief but do not prevent erosions or alter disease progression. They are not appropriate as monotherapy and should only be used in conjunction with DMARDs, if at all. The ACR recommends using standardized assessments, such as the Disease Activity Score 28 Joints or the Clinical Disease Activity Index, to gauge therapeutic responses, with the target of low disease activity or remission by these measures.

A. DMARDs

1. Synthetic DMARDs—

A. METHOTREXATE—Methotrexate is the initial synthetic DMARD of choice for patients with RA. It is generally well tolerated and often produces a beneficial effect in 3–6 weeks; about one-third of patients achieve low disease activity on methotrexate monotherapy. The usual initial dose is 7.5 or 10 mg orally once weekly in older patients or those with comorbidities (eg, mild kidney disease); a starting dose of 15 mg can be used in younger, otherwise healthy individuals. If the patient tolerates methotrexate but has not responded in 1 month, the dose can be increased by 2.5–5 mg orally weekly to reach the maximal oral dose of 20 mg weekly.

The most frequent side effects are gastric irritation and stomatitis. Cytopenia, most commonly leukopenia or thrombocytopenia but rarely pancytopenia from bone marrow suppression, is an important potential problem of methotrexate therapy. The risk of developing pancytopenia is much higher in patients with GFR < 60 mL/min/1.73 m^2. Hepatotoxicity with fibrosis and cirrhosis is a serious toxic effect that correlates with cumulative dose and is uncommon with appropriate monitoring of liver biochemical tests. Methotrexate is contraindicated with any form of chronic hepatitis, in pregnant patients, and in any patient with significant kidney dysfunction (estimated GFR < 30 mL/min/1.73 m^2). Heavy alcohol use increases hepatotoxicity, so patients should be advised to drink alcohol in extreme moderation, if at all. Metabolic dysfunction-associated fatty liver disease, diabetes mellitus, obesity, and kidney disease also increase the risk of hepatotoxicity. Liver biochemical tests should be monitored at least every 12 weeks, along with a CBC. The dose of methotrexate should be reduced if aminotransferase levels are elevated, and the drug should be discontinued if abnormalities persist despite dosage reduction. All patients should be prescribed either daily folate (1 mg orally) or weekly leucovorin calcium (2.5–5 mg taken orally 24 hours after the dose of methotrexate) to reduce gastric irritation, stomatitis, cytopenias, and hepatotoxicity. Hypersensitivity to methotrexate can cause an acute or subacute interstitial pneumonitis that can be life-threatening but usually responds to cessation of the drug and corticosteroids. Methotrexate is teratogenic; women of childbearing age must use effective contraception while taking the medication. A rare adverse event is methotrexate associated lymphoproliferative disorder, which may regress after withdrawal. Methotrexate is also linked to a modestly increased risk of all types of skin cancer, but primarily non-melanoma skin cancers, and a slightly increased risk of B-cell lymphomas, some of which resolve following the discontinuation of the medication. The combination of methotrexate and other folate antagonists, such as trimethoprim-sulfamethoxazole, should be used cautiously since pancytopenia can result. Amoxicillin can decrease renal clearance of methotrexate, leading to toxicity.

B. SULFASALAZINE—This drug is usually combined with methotrexate when methotrexate alone does not adequately control disease activity. The usual starting dose of sulfasalazine is 500 mg orally twice daily and increased weekly to a maximum of 3000 mg daily. Side effects, particularly neutropenia and thrombocytopenia, occur in 10–25% and are serious in 2–5%; nausea is also common. *Sulfasalazine causes hemolysis in patients with glucose-6-phosphate dehydrogenase (G6PD) deficiency, and screening should be considered in those with high-risk backgrounds (Mediterranean, Asian, or African descent, or a family history of G6PD deficiency).* Patients with aspirin sensitivity should not be given sulfasalazine. Patients taking sulfasalazine should have CBC monitored every 2–4 weeks for the first 3 months, then every 3 months.

C. LEFLUNOMIDE—Leflunomide, a pyrimidine synthesis inhibitor, is an alternative for those who cannot take methotrexate. The dose is 20 mg orally once daily. The most frequent side effects are diarrhea, rash, reversible alopecia, and hepatotoxicity. Some patients experience dramatic unexplained weight loss. Leflunomide is teratogenic, and its active metabolite has extensive enterohepatic recirculation, allowing drug levels to persist for up to 2 years without a washout procedure. Thus, it is contraindicated in premenopausal women who wish to bear children.

D. ANTIMALARIALS—Hydroxychloroquine monotherapy should be reserved for patients with very mild disease, as response rates are limited and clinical benefit often requires 3–6 months of treatment. Hydroxychloroquine is often used in combination with other conventional DMARDs, particularly methotrexate and sulfasalazine (so-called "triple therapy"). The advantages of hydroxychloroquine are that it is not immunosuppressive and has comparatively low toxicity, especially at a dosage of 200–400 mg/day orally (not to exceed 5 mg/kg/day). The prevalence of the most important adverse effect, retinal toxicity that can lead to visual loss, is a function of duration of therapy, occurring in < 2% of patients (dosed properly) during the first 10 years of use but rises with prolonged use. Ophthalmologic examinations at baseline and then every 12 months after 5 years of use are required. Rare reactions include neuropathies and myopathies of both skeletal and cardiac muscle, which usually improve when the drug is withdrawn.

E. Janus kinase inhibitors—Tofacitinib, baricitinib, and upadacitinib, inhibitors of Janus kinase (JAK), are oral agents used to manage severe RA that is refractory to methotrexate or other agents (Table 23–4). JAK inhibitors can be used either as monotherapy or in combination with methotrexate. JAK inhibitors increase the risk of infections. Patients should be screened and treated for latent tuberculosis and vaccinated against varicella prior to receiving these drugs. There is an FDA black box warning for JAK inhibitors related to slightly higher risks of serious heart-related events, cancer, blood clots, and death based on data from a large RCT comparing tofacitinib with TNF inhibitors in patients taking methotrexate.

2. Biologic DMARDs (Table 23–4)—

A. Tumor necrosis factor inhibitors—Inhibitors of TNF—a proinflammatory cytokine—are frequently added to the treatment of patients who have not responded adequately to methotrexate and can be used as initial therapy in combination with methotrexate for patients with poor prognostic factors.

Five TNF inhibitors are in use: etanercept, infliximab, adalimumab, golimumab, and certolizumab pegol. Infliximab, etanercept, and adalimumab have biosimilar formulations with demonstrated similar efficacy. Each drug produces substantial improvement in > 60% of patients and is usually well tolerated. Minor irritation at injection sites is the most common side effect of the injectable anti-TNF drugs. TNF inhibitors have been associated with a several-fold increased risk of serious bacterial infections and a striking increase in granulomatous infections, particularly reactivation of tuberculosis. Screening for latent tuberculosis (see Chapter 9) is mandatory before initiating TNF inhibitors. It is prudent to suspend TNF inhibitors when a fever or other manifestations of a clinically significant infection develops. Demyelinating neurologic complications that resemble multiple sclerosis have been reported rarely in patients taking TNF inhibitors, but the true magnitude of this risk—likely small—has not been determined with precision. TNF inhibitors do not appear to increase the overall risk of malignancy compared with conventional DMARDs, though TNF inhibitors are associated with a modestly increased risk of non-melanoma skin cancer. Infliximab was associated with increased morbidity in an HF trial. Therefore, TNF inhibitors should be used with extreme caution in patients with moderate or severe HF (New York Heart Association class III/IV). Infliximab can rarely cause anaphylaxis and induce anti-DNA antibodies (and rarely clinically evident drug-induced SLE).

B. Abatacept—Abatacept, a recombinant protein made by fusing human IgG with a T-cell inhibitory receptor (CTLA4), blocks T-cell costimulation and produces clinically meaningful responses in approximately 50% of individuals whose disease does not respond to the combination of methotrexate and a TNF inhibitor. Abatacept has a relatively lower risk of serious infection and is often preferred in patients with recurrent infections or interstitial lung disease, although its onset of action may be slower than that of TNF inhibitors.

C. Rituximab—Rituximab, a B-cell–depleting monoclonal antibody, is typically used in combination with methotrexate (or leflunomide) for RA that is refractory to TNF inhibitor therapy, although it may be used as monotherapy when other drugs cannot be given. Because rituximab reduces the humoral immune response, it increases susceptibility to infections. Testing for viral hepatitis is mandatory prior to drug initiation since rituximab can lead to reactivation of hepatitis B in patients who are surface antigen or core antibody positive.

D. Tocilizumab and sarilumab—These monoclonal antibodies block the receptor for IL-6, an inflammatory cytokine involved in the pathogenesis of RA. They can be used alone or in combination with methotrexate in patients with disease refractory to TNF inhibitor therapy. Adverse effects include elevated liver enzymes, neutropenia, hyperlipidemia, rare gastrointestinal perforation (especially with diverticular disease), CYP450 drug interactions, and blunted CRP and fever responses that may mask serious infection.

3. Combination DMARDs—DMARDs often have greater efficacy when administered in combination than when used individually. The most used combination is methotrexate with a TNF inhibitor. Still, most patients who require DMARD therapy are given methotrexate monotherapy initially because this regimen is effective in up to one-third of patients and is less expensive and less toxic than combination therapy. The combination of methotrexate, sulfasalazine, and hydroxychloroquine ("triple therapy") is economical, effective, and not inferior to the combination of methotrexate plus etanercept for those who have not responded to methotrexate monotherapy. The choice of a second-line biologic agent for patients who have not responded to TNF inhibitors is often based on comorbidities, patient and provider preference, and insurance coverage. *Biologic DMARDs should not be combined.*

B. Corticosteroids

ACR guidelines recommend avoiding corticosteroids to treat early RA whenever possible because of their well-established toxicity. In some cases, low-dose corticosteroids (eg, oral prednisone 5–10 mg daily) are necessary to produce a prompt anti-inflammatory effect while waiting for disease control with DMARDs. Corticosteroids should be used for the shortest duration possible and generally for < 3 months. Higher doses are used to manage serious extra-articular manifestations (eg, pericarditis, necrotizing scleritis). When corticosteroids are discontinued, they should be tapered gradually according to a planned schedule based on the duration of therapy. In the rare patient in whom long-term corticosteroid therapy is needed, measures should be taken to prevent osteoporosis (Table 30–5).

Intra-articular corticosteroids may be helpful for symptom control if one or two joints are causing symptoms.

Intra-articular triamcinolone, 10–40 mg depending on the size of the joint, may be given but not more than four times a year to prevent cartilage loss.

Course & Prognosis

After months or years, deformities may occur; the most common are ulnar deviation of the fingers (Figure 23–3), boutonnière deformity (hyperextension of the DIP joint with flexion of the PIP joint), "swan-neck" deformity (flexion of the DIP joint with extension of the PIP joint), valgus deformity of the knee, and volar subluxation of the MTP joints. Screening and management of osteoporosis is important. The excess mortality associated with RA is largely due to CVD. Aggressive management of hypertension, diabetes, obesity, avoidance of cigarette smoking, and control of RA-related inflammation can improve outcomes.

When to Refer

Early referral to a rheumatologist is essential for diagnosis and the timely introduction of effective therapy.

Gudu T et al. Contemporary approaches to the management of rheumatoid arthritis: precision and progress. Best Pract Res Clin Rheumatol. 2025;39:102106. [PMID: 41038768]

Liu T et al. Tocilizumab monotherapy or combined with methotrexate for rheumatoid arthritis: a randomized clinical trial. JAMA Netw Open. 2025;8:e2511095 [PMID: 40388166]

ADULT STILL DISEASE

Still disease refers to a systemic inflammatory disorder that occurs in both children (systemic juvenile idiopathic arthritis) and adults (adult-onset Still disease) in which high spiking fevers are often more prominent than arthritis at disease onset. The disease is rare; most affected adults are in their 20s or 30s, and onset after age 60 is uncommon. The fever is dramatic, often with daily spikes to 40°C, associated with sweats and chills, and then plunging to normal or several degrees below normal in the absence of antipyretics. Many patients initially complain of sore throat. An evanescent salmon-colored nonpruritic rash, chiefly on the chest and abdomen, is a characteristic feature. The rash can easily be missed since it often appears only with the fever spike. Many patients have lymphadenopathy and pericardial effusions. Joint symptoms are mild or absent initially, but a destructive arthritis, especially of the wrists, may develop months later. Liver enzyme elevations occur in most patients. Anemia and leukocytosis (predominantly neutrophilia), with peripheral WBC counts often > 15,000/mcL (15×10^9/L), are the rule. Serum ferritin levels are often strikingly elevated (> 3000 ng/mL or 6741 pmol/L). (Other conditions, including viral infections, malignancy, and multiple blood transfusions, can also cause extreme elevations in ferritin levels.) Significant elevations of serum IL-18 or S100 proteins (eg, calprotectin) strongly support the diagnosis, and should be measured if available. The diagnosis of adult Still disease is suggested by the quotidian fever pattern, sore throat, and the classic rash, but it requires exclusion of other causes of fever. About 20% of patients with mild disease respond to NSAIDs. Early use of biologic therapies targeting IL-1 (anakinra or canakinumab) or IL-6 (tocilizumab or sarilumab) improves outcomes and reduces the need for long-term corticosteroids (Table 23–4). The course of adult Still disease can be monophasic, intermittent, or chronic.

Macrophage activation syndrome is a serious, potentially life-threatening complication of Still disease. It manifests as fever; splenomegaly; cytopenia; liver dysfunction; hypertriglyceridemia; hypofibrinogenemia; marked ferritin elevation; elevated soluble CD25; depressed natural cell activity; and hemophagocytosis in bone marrow, spleen, and lymph nodes. Treatment includes high-dose corticosteroids, IL-1 inhibitors, cyclosporine, and interferon-γ inhibitors.

Fautrel B et al. EULAR/PReS recommendations for the diagnosis and management of Still's disease, comprising systemic juvenile idiopathic arthritis and adult-onset Still's disease. Ann Rheum Dis. 2024;83:1614. [PMID: 39317417]

SYSTEMIC LUPUS ERYTHEMATOSUS

ESSENTIALS OF DIAGNOSIS

- Occurs mainly in young women.
- Rash over areas exposed to sunlight.
- Joint symptoms in 90% of patients.
- Anemia, leukopenia, thrombocytopenia.
- Glomerulonephritis and CNS disease are major sources of disease morbidity.
- Serologic findings: antinuclear antibodies (100%), anti–double-stranded DNA antibodies (approximately two-thirds), and low serum complement levels (particularly during disease flares).

General Considerations

SLE is an inflammatory autoimmune disorder of autoantibodies to nuclear antigens. It can affect multiple organ systems. Many of its clinical manifestations are secondary to inflammation resulting from the trapping of antigen-antibody complexes in capillaries of visceral structures or to autoantibody-mediated destruction of host cells (eg, thrombocytopenia). The clinical course is marked by spontaneous remission and relapses. The severity may vary from mild and episodic to a rapidly fulminant, life-threatening illness.

The incidence of SLE is influenced by many factors, including sex, environmental exposures, and genetics. About 90% of patients are women and most cases develop after menarche and before menopause. Among older individuals, the sex distribution is more equal. SLE occurs in 1 in 400 Black women, 1 in 800 Hispanic women, and 1 in 1100 White women; social determinants of health likely contribute to these disparities. There are familial occurrences of SLE, and the disorder is concordant in 25–70% of identical twins. Positive antinuclear antibody serologies are seen in asymptomatic family members, and the prevalence of other rheumatic diseases is increased among close relatives.

The diagnosis of SLE should be suspected in patients having a multisystem disease with a positive test for antinuclear antibodies. It is essential to confirm that the condition is not drug-induced (see Drug-Induced Lupus below).

The 2019 European and American criteria for SLE require an ANA titer of ≥ 80 (Table 23–6), underscoring that SLE is generally not diagnosed in the absence of a positive ANA. Criteria are developed as guidelines for the inclusion of patients in research studies and do not supplant clinical judgment in the diagnosis of SLE.

Clinical Findings

A. Symptoms and Signs

Systemic features of SLE include fever, anorexia, fatigue, and weight loss. Many patients have skin lesions at some

Table 23–6. 2019 European League Against Rheumatism/American College of Rheumatology classification criteria for SLE.

Entry criterion Antinuclear antibodies (ANA) at a titer of ≥ 1:80 on HEp-2 cells or an equivalent positive test (ever)			
↓			
If absent, do not classify as SLE If present, apply additive criteria			
↓			
Additive criteria **Do not count a criterion if there is a more likely explanation than SLE.** **Occurrence of a criterion on at least one occasion is sufficient.** SLE classification requires at least one clinical criterion and ≥ 10 points. **Criteria need not occur simultaneously.** **Within each domain, only the highest weighted criterion is counted toward the total score.**[§]			
Clinical domains and criteria	**Weight**	**Immunology domains and criteria**	**Weight**
Constitutional		***Antiphospholipid antibodies***	
Fever	2	Anticardiolipin antibodies *or*	
Hematologic		Anti-β_2-GP1 antibodies *or*	
Leukopenia	3	Lupus anticoagulant	2
Thrombocytopenia	4	***Complement proteins***	
Autoimmune hemolysis	4	Low C3 OR low C4	3
Neuropsychiatric		Low C3 AND low C4	4
Delirium	2	***SLE-specific antibodies***	
Psychosis	3	Anti-dsDNA antibody* *or*	6
Seizure	5	Anti-Smith antibody	
Mucocutaneous			
Non-scarring alopecia	2		
Oral ulcers	2		
Subacute cutaneous *or* discoid lupus	4		
Acute cutaneous lupus	6		
Serosal			
Pleural or pericardial effusion	5		
Acute pericarditis	6		
Musculoskeletal			
Joint involvement	6		
Renal			
Proteinuria > 0.5 g/24 h	4		
Renal biopsy Class II or V lupus nephritis	8		
Renal biopsy Class III or IV lupus nephritis	10		
Total score:			
↓			
Classify as SLE with a score of ≥ 10 if entry criterion fulfilled.			

Anti-β_2GPI, anti–β_2-glycoprotein I; anti-dsDNA, anti–double-stranded DNA.
§ = additional criteria within the same domain will not be counted; * = in an assay with 90% specificity against relevant disease controls.
Reproduced with permission from Aringer M, Costenbader K, Daikh D, et al. 2019 European League Against Rheumatism/American College of Rheumatology Classification Criteria for Systemic Lupus Erythematosus. *Arthritis Rheumatol.* 2019;71(9):1400–1412.

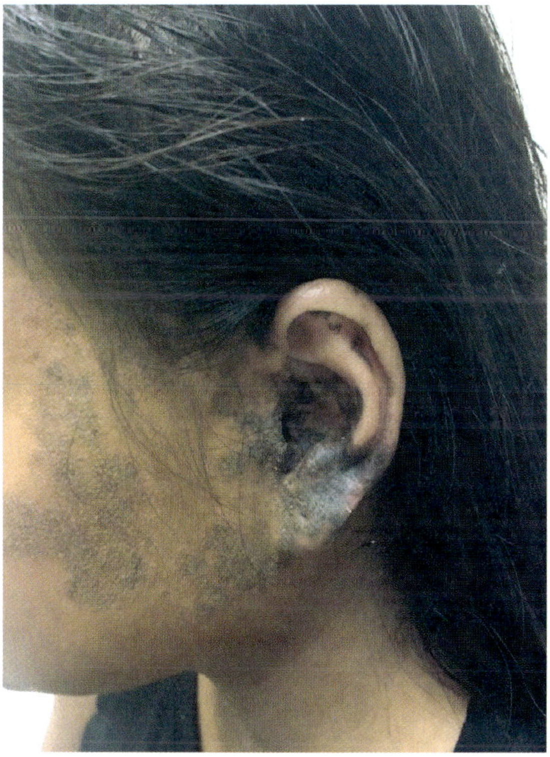

▲ **Figure 23–6.** Discoid lupus in the ear of a patient. (Used, with permission, from Sarah Goglin, MD.)

time; the characteristic "butterfly" (malar) rash affects less than half of patients. Photosensitivity is common and may precipitate or exacerbate cutaneous and systemic disease activity. Other cutaneous manifestations are panniculitis (lupus profundus), discoid lupus (Figure 23–6), and typical fingertip lesions (periungual erythema, nail fold infarcts, and splinter hemorrhages). Alopecia is common. Painless oral or nasal ulcers are a common mucocutaneous manifestation, particularly during disease flares. Raynaud phenomenon is present in about 20% of patients.

Joint symptoms, with or without active synovitis, occur in over 90% of patients and are often the earliest manifestation. The arthritis can lead to reducible swan-neck deformities, but only 10% of patients develop radiographic erosions that are more typical of RA.

Glomerulonephritis may occur, including mesangial, focal proliferative, diffuse proliferative, and membranous forms (see Chapter 25). Some patients may also have interstitial nephritis. With appropriate therapy, survival is favorable even in patients with proliferative lupus nephritis, although a substantial proportion of those with severe disease ultimately progress to ESKD.

Ocular manifestations include keratoconjunctivitis sicca, retinal vasculitis, episcleritis, scleritis, and optic neuropathy.

Pleurisy and pleural effusion are common. Pneumonitis, interstitial lung disease, and pulmonary hypertension can rarely occur. Alveolar hemorrhage is uncommon but life-threatening.

The pericardium is affected in most patients. HF may result from myocarditis and hypertension. Cardiac arrhythmias can occur. Atypical verrucous endocarditis of Libman-Sacks is usually clinically silent but occasionally can produce acute or chronic valvular regurgitation—most commonly mitral regurgitation, which can be a source of systemic emboli.

GI manifestations can include inflammation of the small intestine (lupus enteritis), which can lead to diarrhea and abdominal pain, as well as peritonitis and lupus hepatitis.

Neurologic complications of SLE include psychosis, cognitive impairment, seizures, peripheral and cranial neuropathies, and strokes. Transverse myelitis is a medical emergency and can present with weakness, bowel and bladder dysfunction, and a sensory level deficit. Severe depression and psychosis are sometimes exacerbated by the administration of high doses of corticosteroids.

Hematologic manifestations include leukopenia, autoimmune hemolytic anemia, immune thrombocytopenia, and thrombotic thrombocytopenic purpura. Antiphospholipid syndrome (APS) can occur in association with SLE (see Antiphospholipid Syndrome, below).

B. Laboratory Findings

SLE is characterized by the production of many different autoantibodies (Table 23–7). ANA tests using HEp-2 cells (a human cell line) as a source of nuclei are nearly 100% sensitive for SLE but not specific—ie, they are positive in low titer in up to 20% of healthy adults and also in many patients with other immune-mediated conditions such as RA, thyroid disease, systemic sclerosis, and Sjögren disease, as well as in some infections and malignancies. False-negative ANA results can occur with tests based on multiplex assays that use specific nuclear antigens rather than cell lines. Antibodies to double-stranded DNA and to Sm are specific for SLE but not sensitive, since they are present in only 60% and 30% of patients, respectively. Depressed serum complement—a finding suggestive of disease activity—often returns toward normal in remission. Anti–double-stranded DNA antibody levels also correlate with disease activity in some patients; anti-Sm levels do not. Other autoantibodies commonly seen in SLE include antibodies to SS-A/Ro, SS-B/La, ribonucleoprotein (RNP), and phospholipid. Antibodies to SS-A/Ro are associated with subacute cutaneous lupus; during pregnancy these autoantibodies can cross the placenta and damage the developing fetal conduction system, producing congenital heart block.

During disease flares, ESR elevations are common, but the serum CRP is usually normal unless there is serositis or arthritis. *An elevated CRP in the absence of these manifestations should increase clinical suspicion for infection.* Abnormal urinary sediment (hematuria with or without casts) and persistent proteinuria (eg, urine protein to creatinine ratio ≥ 0.5 g/g) are suggestive of active lupus nephritis and warrant renal biopsy to classify disease and guide therapy.

▶ Differential Diagnosis

The differential diagnosis is broad, including drug-induced lupus, RA, systemic vasculitis, systemic sclerosis, primary APS, inflammatory myopathies, viral hepatitis, sarcoidosis, acute drug reactions, and infections or malignancies with multisystem involvement.

Table 23–7. Major autoantibody associations in the ANA-positive rheumatic diseases.[1]

Condition	Autoantibodies	Prevalence	Notes
SLE	Anti-dsDNA	50–75%	Correlates with disease activity and lupus nephritis
	Anti-Smith	15–30%	Highly specific for SLE
	Anti-U1 RNP	30–40%	Also seen in MCTD
	Anti-SSA (Ro)	25–50%	Associated with Sjögren disease, neonatal lupus, and SCLE. Both Ro52 and Ro60 are seen in SLE; Ro60 has strong association with skin disease
	Anti-SSB (La)	10–30%	Associated with Sjögren disease and neonatal lupus
	Anti-histone	50–70%	Also seen in drug-induced SLE
Sjögren disease	Anti-SSA (Ro)	40–70%	Associated with sicca symptoms and neonatal lupus. Both Ro52 and Ro60 are seen in Sjögren disease, but Ro52 can be associated with interstitial lung disease
	Anti-SSB (La)	30–60%	Associated with sicca symptoms and neonatal lupus
Mixed connective tissue disease	Anti-U1 RNP	100%	Required to diagnose MCTD
Systemic sclerosis	Anticentromere	30–35%	Associated with limited systemic sclerosis (CREST syndrome)
	Anti-Scl-70	20–40%	Associated with diffuse systemic sclerosis and interstitial lung disease
	Anti-RNA polymerase III	5–15%	Associated with diffuse disease, renal crisis, and malignancy
Drug-induced lupus	Anti-histone	75%	Also seen in SLE

MCTD, mixed connective tissue disease.

Reproduced with permission from Aggarwal A. Role of antibody testing. *Best Pract Res Clin Rheumatol.* 2014;28(6):907–920.

Treatment

Since the various manifestations of SLE affect prognosis differently and since SLE activity often waxes and wanes, drug therapy—both the choice of agents and the intensity of their use—must be tailored to match disease severity. Patients should be cautioned against sun exposure and should apply broad-spectrum UVA/UVB sunscreen while outdoors. Mild rashes often respond to topical corticosteroids. Minor joint symptoms can usually be alleviated by NSAIDs.

Hydroxychloroquine reduces the incidence of disease flares and prolongs survival in SLE and therefore is recommended for all patients. Hydroxychloroquine is initial therapy for lupus rashes or joint symptoms. The dose of hydroxychloroquine is 200 or 400 mg/day orally and should generally not exceed 5 mg/kg/day; annual monitoring for retinal toxicity is recommended after 5 years of use. Neuropathy and myopathy are rare adverse effects of hydroxychloroquine and may be erroneously ascribed to the underlying disease.

Corticosteroids should be used judiciously in SLE given significant long-term toxicity; they are generally not necessary for minor skin rashes, leukopenia, or the anemia associated with chronic inflammation. Short courses of prednisone 5–15 mg orally daily can be used to treat flares that are not life-threatening, such as rashes, serositis, or arthritis. Severe manifestations such as proliferative glomerulonephritis, myocarditis, alveolar hemorrhage, CNS involvement, and severe thrombocytopenia or hemolytic anemia all require high-dose corticosteroid treatment combined with other interventions. Methylprednisolone 250–1000 mg given intravenously over 30 minutes daily for 3 days or prednisone 40–60 mg orally is given initially. Corticosteroids should be tapered to the lowest possible dose and eventually stopped if possible (Table 30–5).

Immunosuppressive agents such as mycophenolate mofetil, azathioprine, or methotrexate are used for long-term control of disease; intravenous cyclophosphamide is usually reserved for refractory disease. Belimumab, a monoclonal antibody that inhibits the activity of a B-cell growth factor, is used for active nonrenal and renal lupus that has not responded to standard therapies (eg, antimalarials or immunosuppressive therapies) and is used to permit tapering of prednisone. Voclosporin, a novel calcineurin inhibitor, and obinutuzumab, a B-cell–depleting agent, are approved to treat active lupus nephritis and when either is used in combination with mycophenolate mofetil. Anifrolumab, a type 1 interferon receptor antagonist, is approved to treat nonrenal lupus that has not responded to standard therapies and is especially effective for severe lupus skin rashes (Table 23–4).

1. Induction therapy for lupus nephritis—A renal biopsy is recommended to confirm active disease, and urgent immunosuppression is recommended for those with active proliferative or membranous lupus nephritis on pathology. Mycophenolate mofetil (titrated up to 1000 mg or 1500 mg orally twice daily) is usually the first-line treatment for lupus nephritis and is generally given with corticosteroids to achieve disease control. Cyclophosphamide has equivalent efficacy for lupus nephritis and is usually administered using the Euro-Lupus regimen (500 mg intravenously every 2 weeks for six doses) but can also be administered according to the NIH regimen (3–6 monthly intravenous pulses [0.5–1 g/m^2]). When higher doses of cyclophosphamide are required, gonadotropin-releasing hormone analogs can be given to protect against premature ovarian failure in women. Guidelines recommend combination therapy to further improve renal response either by (1) adding a calcineurin inhibitor (voclosporin or tacrolimus) to mycophenolate mofetil in patients with significant proteinuria (≥ 3 g/day) for rapid reduction of proteinuria; (2) adding belimumab to mycophenolate mofetil or cyclophosphamide in those with lower proteinuria levels; or (3) adding obinituzumab to mycophenolate mofetil. Rituximab can also be considered in refractory disease, including treatment-resistant lupus nephritis (especially if obinutuzumab is not available) and severe extra-renal manifestations such as autoimmune hemolytic anemia or transverse myelitis (Table 23–4).

2. Maintenance therapy for lupus nephritis—Either mycophenolate mofetil or azathioprine is typically used as maintenance therapy for lupus nephritis. Patients whose disease was induced with combination therapy, including belimumab or voclosporin, should generally continue these agents for at least 1 year and often longer, depending on response and tolerability. B-cell–depleting therapies are used initially but are not routinely continued indefinitely. Prednisone should be tapered to ≤ 5 mg by 6 months to reduce toxicity. Close follow-up is needed to watch for potential drug side effects; these agents should be administered by clinicians experienced in their use.

Course & Prognosis

Ten-year survival rates exceeding 85% are routine. In most patients, the illness has a relapsing and remitting course. However, there are some in whom the disease pursues a virulent course, leading to serious impairment of vital structures such as lungs, heart, brain, or kidneys, and the disease may lead to death. Mortality in SLE shows a bimodal pattern. In the early years after diagnosis, infections—especially with opportunistic organisms—are the leading cause of death, followed by active SLE, chiefly due to kidney or CNS disease. In later years, accelerated atherosclerosis, linked to chronic inflammation, becomes a major cause of death. Indeed, the incidence of MI is five times higher in persons with SLE than in the general population. Therefore, patients with SLE should avoid cigarette smoking and minimize other conventional risk factors for atherosclerosis.

Fertility is normal in SLE. Women are advised to pursue pregnancy under close supervision and when SLE is well-controlled and no teratogenic medications are used. Osteoporosis is common; routine screening is recommended for those with corticosteroid exposure. Avascular necrosis of bone, affecting most commonly the hips and knees, is responsible for substantial morbidity.

When to Refer

- Appropriate diagnosis and management of SLE requires the active participation of a rheumatologist.
- The severity of organ involvement dictates referral to other subspecialists, such as nephrologists and pulmonologists.

When to Admit

- Rapidly progressive glomerulonephritis, pulmonary hemorrhage, transverse myelitis, and other severe organ-threatening manifestations of lupus usually require in-patient assessment and management.
- Severe infections, particularly in the setting of immunosuppressant therapy, should prompt admission.

Fanouriakis A et al. EULAR recommendations for the management of systemic lupus erythematosus with kidney involvement: 2025 update. Ann Rheum Dis. 2026;85:75. [PMID: 41107121].

Sammaritano LR et al. 2024 American College of Rheumatology (ACR) guideline for the screening, treatment, and management of lupus nephritis. Arthritis Rheumatol. 2025;77:1115. [PMID: 40331662].

DRUG-INDUCED LUPUS

ESSENTIALS OF DIAGNOSIS

- Symptomatic during exposure to offending drug; symptoms resolve after drug is stopped.
- Unlike in SLE, kidney involvement is unlikely.
- Elevated ANA but unlikely to have anti-DNA antibodies unless secondary to TNF inhibitors.

Drug-induced lupus shares several clinical and serologic features with SLE but is due to ongoing exposure to a drug and resolves when the offending drug is discontinued. In contrast to SLE, the sex ratio is nearly equal. Generally, drug-induced lupus presents with the abrupt onset of fever, arthralgia, myalgia, and serositis but not kidney involvement, neurologic symptoms, or other features of SLE. Serologic testing reveals elevated titers of antinuclear antibodies in all patients, but antibodies to DNA, Sm, RNP, SS-A, and SS-B are rare. Antibodies to histones occur in up to 95% of patients but are also seen in SLE and thus do not distinguish drug-induced lupus from SLE. Complement levels are usually normal. The list of drugs implicated as possible causes of drug-induced lupus is extensive. There are definite associations between the development of drug-induced lupus and the use of hydralazine, isoniazid, and minocycline as well as several less commonly prescribed drugs (procainamide, methyldopa, chlorpromazine). The incidence of drug-induced lupus in patients taking hydralazine for a year or longer is as high as 5–8%; for most other medications, the risk is considerably lower (< 1%). TNF inhibitors can induce antibodies to double-stranded DNA, typically without anti-histone antibodies, and may cause a lupus-like syndrome that is mechanistically distinct from classic drug-induced lupus; however, the incidence is low (0.5–1%). Drug-induced lupus generally resolves within weeks to months after discontinuing the offending agent.

Subacute cutaneous lupus (SCLE) is a distinct entity and drug-induced in more than one-third of patients. Hydrochlorothiazide is a common cause of SCLE;

antifungals (terbinafine), PPIs, antihypertensives (calcium channel blockers, ACE inhibitors), TNF inhibitors, and immune checkpoint inhibitors also have been implicated.

Safaei S et al. Clinical characteristics and management of drug-induced lupus caused by tumor necrosis factor inhibitors: a comprehensive review. Cureus. 2024;16:e72522. [PMID: 39606520]

ANTIPHOSPHOLIPID SYNDROME

ESSENTIALS OF DIAGNOSIS

- Hypercoagulability; recurrent arterial or VTE.
- Thrombocytopenia is common.
- Recurrent or late fetal loss.
- Anticoagulation with warfarin is recommended over DOACs.

General Considerations

APS can occur alone or in association with other autoimmune diseases such as SLE. The clinical features of APS are venous or arterial thrombosis or certain pregnancy complications. Patients have at least one of the following three antiphospholipid antibodies: anticardiolipin antibodies, antibodies to β_2-glycoprotein 1, and lupus anticoagulant.

Catastrophic APS occurs in < 1% of patients with antiphospholipid antibodies. This potentially devastating syndrome leads to diffuse thromboses, thrombotic microangiopathy, and multiorgan system failure. Catastrophic APS has a mortality rate approaching 50%. Triggers of catastrophic APS include infections, surgery, use of estrogen-containing medications, autoimmune disease flares, and discontinuation of anticoagulation.

Clinical Findings

A. Symptoms and Signs

APS can cause thrombotic, microvascular, hematologic, and obstetric complications. Thrombosis may involve either the venous or arterial circulation. Common manifestations include deep vein thrombosis, pulmonary embolism, and ischemic stroke. Less common but well-recognized events include Budd–Chiari syndrome, cerebral venous sinus thrombosis, myocardial or digital infarction, and adrenal hemorrhage secondary to adrenal vein thrombosis. Thromboses can also involve the microvascular circulation, leading to livedo racemosa or vasculopathy, microangiopathic nephropathy, and pulmonary hemorrhage. Cardiac valvular thickening or vegetations can also occur. Obstetric manifestations include ≥ 3 consecutive pregnancy losses < 10 weeks' gestation, one or more unexplained fetal deaths of a morphologically normal fetus ≥ 10 weeks' gestation, or severe preeclampsia, eclampsia or placental insufficiency occurring < 34 weeks with or without fetal death.

The ACR and the EULAR classification of APS assigns scores to assay test results and clinical findings; these criteria highlight the far-ranging manifestations of the syndrome and the need to consider APS in the broad spectrum of differential diagnoses (Table 23–8).

B. Laboratory Findings

Thrombocytopenia occurs in 22–42% of patients and is usually moderate (platelet counts > 50,000/mcL [50×10^9/L]). The presence of thrombocytopenia does not reduce the risk of thrombosis.

Three types of antiphospholipid antibodies are associated with this syndrome: (1) IgG or IgM anticardiolipin antibodies; (2) IgG or IgM antibodies to β_2-glycoprotein; and (3) "lupus anticoagulant" that prolongs certain phospholipid-dependent coagulation tests (see below). APS testing is generally done shortly after an event, followed by confirmatory testing after 12 weeks to ensure the antibody was not transient. Those with all three antibodies ("triple positivity") have the highest risk of thrombosis and pregnancy loss, higher recurrence rates, and usually require lifelong anticoagulation.

Anticardiolipin antibodies can produce a biologic false-positive test for syphilis (ie, a positive rapid plasma reagin but negative specific anti-treponemal assay). In general, IgG anticardiolipin antibodies are believed to be more pathologic than IgM. Presence of the lupus anticoagulant is a stronger risk factor for thrombosis or pregnancy loss than is the presence of antibodies to either β_2-glycoprotein 1 or anticardiolipin. A clue to the presence of a lupus anticoagulant, which may occur in individuals who do not have SLE, is prolongation of the partial thromboplastin time (which, paradoxically, is associated with a thrombotic tendency rather than a bleeding risk). Tests for the lupus anticoagulant use phospholipid-dependent functional assays of coagulation, such as the Russell viper venom time (RVVT). Heparin, warfarin, and DOACs can cause false-positive lupus anticoagulant assays.

Differential Diagnosis

Other genetic or acquired conditions associated with hypercoagulability such as protein C, protein S, or antithrombin deficiency and factor V Leiden should be excluded. Myeloproliferative cancers, heparin-induced thrombocytopenia, and paroxysmal nocturnal hemoglobinuria are additional considerations. Catastrophic APS has a broad differential, including sepsis, pulmonary-renal syndromes, systemic vasculitis, disseminated intravascular coagulation, and thrombotic thrombocytopenic purpura.

Treatment

Patients who have positive anti-phospholipid antibodies but no history of the clinical events described above should not be treated with anticoagulation.

1. Thrombotic APS—Most individuals with either macro- or microvascular thrombosis require lifelong anticoagulation with warfarin to maintain an INR of 2.0–3.0. DOACs are not recommended because they are less effective than

Table 23–8. Criteria for the diagnosis of APS.[1]

Clinical Criteria	Score[2]
Macrovascular	
VTE with high risks for VTE (eg, active malignancy, hospital admission/immobilization, major trauma, obesity, surgery, severe infection, hormonal therapy)	1
VTE without high risks	3
Arterial thrombosis with high risks for CVD (hypertension, CKD, diabetes mellitus, hyperlipidemia, smoking, obesity)	2
Arterial thrombosis without high risks for CVD	4
Microvascular (suspected)	
Livedo racemosa Livedoid vasculopathy lesions Acute or chronic aPL-nephropathy Pulmonary hemorrhage	2
Microvascular (established)	
Livedoid vasculopathy Acute or chronic aPL-nephropathy Pulmonary hemorrhage Myocardial disease Adrenal hemorrhage	5
Obstetric	
≥ 3 consecutive spontaneous pregnancy losses (< 10 weeks' gestation) or early fetal deaths (10–15 weeks' gestation)	1
Fetal death (age 16–33 weeks' gestation) No preeclampsia with severe features or placental insufficiency with severe features	1
Preeclampsia with severe features (< 34 weeks' gestation) ***or*** placental insufficiency with severe features (< 34 weeks' gestation) ± fetal death	3
Preeclampsia with severe features (< 34 weeks' gestation) ***and*** placental insufficiency with severe features (< 34 weeks' gestation) ± fetal death	4
Cardiac valve	
Thickening present	2
Vegetations present	4
Hematology	
Thrombocytopenia (lowest 20–130 × 10^9/L)	2
Laboratory criteria for aPL tests[3]	
Lupus anticoagulant test	
Positive (once)	1
Positive (persistent)	5
Anticardiolipin antibody ELISA and/or anti-β_2-glycoprotein-1 antibodies	
Moderate or high positive (IgM) anticardiolipin ***and/or*** anti-β_2-glycoprotein-1 antibodies	1
Moderate positive (IgG) anticardiolipin ***and/or*** anti-β_2-glycoprotein-1 antibodies	4
High positive (IgG) anticardiolipin ***or*** anti-β_2-glycoprotein-1 antibody	5
High positive (IgG) anticardiolipin ***and*** anti-β_2-glycoprotein-1 antibodies	7

aPL, antiphospholipid antibody; APS, antiphospholipid syndrome.

[1]When considering the diagnosis of APS, an aPL test needs to be positive within 3 years of the appearance of at least one clinical criterion.

[2]**Scoring:** A diagnosis of APS requires a total of 6 points: 3 points from laboratory criteria for the aPL tests **and** 3 points from clinical criteria. Use only the highest point value in category if more than one criteria applies.

[3]aPL tests are the lupus anticoagulant test, or moderate to high titers of anticardiolipin or anti-β 2-glycoprotein-I antibodies (IgG or IgM).

warfarin in APS, especially for arterial thromboses. Patients who have recurrent thrombotic events while taking warfarin may require higher INRs (≥ 3.0), but the bleeding risk increases substantially with this degree of anticoagulation; low-molecular weight heparin is used in patients who have thrombotic events while taking warfarin despite INRs being in the therapeutic range. Patients with thrombotic APS should avoid estrogen-containing contraceptives.

2. Pregnancy-associated APS—The combination of prophylactic doses of low-molecular-weight heparin (Table 16–14) and low-dose aspirin (81 or 162 mg) is the usual approach to prevent pregnancy complications. In pregnant patients with a history of thrombotic events outside of pregnancy, full-dose low-molecular-weight heparin is administered (Table 16–16). Anticoagulation for thromboprophylaxis is typically continued through pregnancy and the early postpartum period; the use of corticosteroids and intravenous immunoglobulin in these patients is not recommended.

3. Catastrophic APS—Either intravenous immunoglobulin or plasmapheresis *plus* intravenous heparin and high doses of corticosteroids are administered for this disorder. Resistant disease may require B-cell depletion (rituximab) or complement component C5 inhibitors (eculizumab), although data to support these therapies are limited to case series (Table 23–4).

Devreese KMJ et al. An update on laboratory detection and interpretation of antiphospholipid antibodies for diagnosis of antiphospholipid syndrome: guidance from the ISTH-SSC Subcommittee on Lupus Anticoagulant/Antiphospholipid Antibodies. J Thromb Haemost. 2025;23:731. [PMID: 39510414]

Knight JS et al. Rethinking antiphospholipid syndrome to guide future management and research. Nat Rev Rheumatol. 2024;20:377. [PMID: 38702511]

RAYNAUD PHENOMENON

ESSENTIALS OF DIAGNOSIS

- Paroxysmal bilateral digital pallor and cyanosis followed by rubor.
- Precipitated by cold or emotional stress; relieved by warmth.
- **Primary form:** benign course; usually affects young women.
- **Secondary form:** more severe, sometimes causing digital ulceration or gangrene.

General Considerations

Raynaud phenomenon (RP) is a syndrome of paroxysmal digital ischemia, most commonly caused by an exaggerated response of digital arterioles to cold or emotional stress. The initial phase of RP, mediated by excessive vasoconstriction, consists of well-demarcated digital pallor or cyanosis; the subsequent (recovery) phase of RP, caused by vasodilation, leads to intense hyperemia and rubor. Although RP chiefly affects fingers, it can also affect toes and other acral areas such as the nose and ears. RP is classified as primary (idiopathic or Raynaud disease) or secondary. Nearly one-third of the population reports being "sensitive to the cold" but does not experience the paroxysms of digital pallor, cyanosis, and erythema characteristic of RP. Primary RP occurs in 3–5% of adults, is especially common in young women, and poses more of a nuisance than a threat to good health. In contrast, secondary RP is less common, is chiefly associated with rheumatic diseases (especially systemic sclerosis) and can be severe enough to cause digital ulceration or gangrene.

Clinical Findings

Early in the course of RP, only one or two fingertips may be affected; as it progresses, all fingers down to the distal palm may be involved. The thumbs are rarely affected. Sensory changes that often accompany vasomotor manifestations include numbness, tingling, diminished sensation, and aching pain. During recovery there may be intense rubor, paresthesia, pain, and slight swelling. Symptom triggers include cold exposure, vibration, smoking/nicotine, sympathomimetic medications (eg, decongestants), β-blockers, amphetamines, and cocaine. Attacks usually terminate spontaneously or upon returning to a warm room or putting the extremity in warm water. The patient is usually asymptomatic between attacks. Primary RP is more common in women aged 15–30 years, symmetrically involving the fingers of both hands, unlike secondary RP (which may be unilateral and may involve only one or two fingers). It tends to be mildly progressive with spasms becoming more frequent and prolonged. Unlike secondary RP, primary RP does not cause digital pitting, ulceration, or gangrene.

Primary RP must be differentiated from the numerous causes of secondary RP (Table 23–9). The history and examination may suggest the diagnosis of systemic sclerosis, SLE, RA, or mixed connective tissue disease; RP is often the first manifestation of limited systemic sclerosis (CREST syndrome). The diagnosis of many of these rheumatic diseases is supported with specific serologic tests.

Secondary RP may occur with thoracic outlet syndromes; involvement is generally unilateral, and symptoms referable to brachial plexus compression tend to dominate the clinical picture. Carpal tunnel syndrome should also be considered, and nerve conduction tests are appropriate in selected cases. Occupations that involve chronic vibration exposure of digits (eg, construction) can result in RP.

Nailfold capillary abnormalities are among the earliest clues of secondary rather than primary RP. Dropout of capillaries and dilation of the remaining capillary loops indicate a secondary form of RP, most commonly systemic sclerosis. While highly specific for secondary RP, nailfold capillary changes have a low sensitivity. Digital pitting or ulceration or other abnormal physical findings (eg, skin tightening, loss of extremity pulse, rash, swollen joints) provides evidence of secondary RP.

Table 23–9. Causes of secondary Raynaud phenomenon.[1]

Rheumatic diseases
Systemic sclerosis
SLE
Mixed connective tissue disease
Idiopathic inflammatory myopathies
Sjögren disease
Vasculitis (polyarteritis nodosa, Takayasu arteritis, thromboangiitis obliterans)
Neurovascular compression and occupational trauma
Carpal tunnel syndrome
Thoracic outlet obstruction
Vibration injury
Drugs and substances
β-Blockers
Serotonin agonists (sumatriptan)
Sympathomimetic drugs (decongestants)
Chemotherapy (bleomycin, vinblastine)
Ergotamine
Interferon therapy
Amphetamines
Caffeine
Nicotine
Cocaine
Epoxy resins
Hematologic disorders
Cryoglobulinemia
Polycythemia vera
Paraproteinemia
Cold agglutinins
Endocrine disorders
Hypothyroidism
Pheochromocytoma
Miscellaneous
Atherosclerosis
Embolic disease
Migraine
Sequela of frostbite

[1]Listed in descending order of frequency.

Differential Diagnosis

The differentiation from Buerger disease (thromboangiitis obliterans) is usually not difficult, since thromboangiitis obliterans is generally a disease of men, particularly those who smoke cigarettes; peripheral pulses are often diminished or absent; and, when RP occurs in association with thromboangiitis obliterans, it is usually in only one or two digits.

In acrocyanosis, cyanosis of the hands is painless, symmetric and not episodic; the sharp and paroxysmal line of demarcation with pallor does not occur with acrocyanosis. Frostbite may lead to chronic RP. Patients with peripheral neuropathy or complex regional pain syndrome can have vasomotor symptoms but also have neuropathic pain, allodynia, and trophic skin changes.

RP may be mimicked by type I cryoglobulinemia, usually associated with plasma cell myeloma or with lymphoproliferative disorders, in which a monoclonal antibody cryoprecipitates in the cooler distal circulation.

Treatment

A. General Measures

Keeping the body warm is a cornerstone of initial therapy. Patients should wear gloves or mittens whenever in temperatures that precipitate attacks. Warm shirts, coats, and hats will help prevent the exaggerated vasospasm that causes RP and that is not prevented by warming only the hands. The hands should be protected from injury; wounds heal slowly, and infections are consequently hard to control. Softening and lubricating lotion to control fissured dry skin should be applied to the hands frequently. Environmental and drug triggers should be avoided. For most patients with primary RP, general measures alone are sufficient to control symptoms. Medical or surgical therapy should be considered in patients who have severe symptoms or are experiencing tissue injury from digital ischemia.

B. Medications

Calcium channel blockers are first-line therapy for RP. They produce a modest benefit and are more effective in primary RP than secondary RP. Slow-release nifedipine (30–120 mg/day orally), amlodipine (5–20 mg/day orally), felodipine, isradipine, and nisoldipine are more effective than verapamil, nicardipine, and diltiazem. In patients with severe, secondary RP refractory to calcium channel blockers, phosphodiesterase inhibitors (eg, sildenafil, tadalafil, and vardenafil) can be added or substituted. Additional therapies include angiotensin II receptor blockers, topical nitrates, or SSRIs (fluoxetine). Bosentan, an endothelin receptor antagonist, can be effective for those with digital ulcerations. Severe or refractory episodes of RP in which there is a threat of digital loss may require treatment with intravenous prostacyclin or prostacyclin analogs (eg, epoprostenol, iloprost, treprostinil).

C. Procedures

Digital sympathectomy may be indicated when ischemia is progressive and other medical measures have failed. RCTs of botulinum toxin injection have not demonstrated efficacy.

Prognosis

Primary RP is benign but bothersome for individuals who are exposed to cold climates or excessive air conditioning. The prognosis of secondary RP depends on the underlying disease; unfortunately, severe pain from ulceration and gangrene is not rare with systemic sclerosis.

When to Refer

Appropriate management of patients with secondary RP often requires consultation with a rheumatologist.

When to Admit

Patients with critical digital ischemia as evidenced by severe pain and demarcation should be admitted for intensive therapy.

Curtiss P et al. Part II: The treatment of primary and secondary Raynaud's phenomenon. J Am Acad Dermatol. 2024;90:237. [PMID: 35809802]

Frech TM et al. Rethinking strategies for a pharmaceutical approach to pain related to connective tissue-related Raynaud phenomenon in the United States. Arthritis Care Res (Hoboken). 2025;78:106 [PMID: 40999744]

SYSTEMIC SCLEROSIS (Scleroderma)

ESSENTIALS OF DIAGNOSIS

- **Limited disease** (CREST syndrome) (80%): skin thickening confined to face, neck, and distal extremities.
- **Diffuse disease** (20%): widespread thickening of skin, with areas of increased pigmentation and depigmentation.
- Raynaud phenomenon (RP) and antinuclear antibodies are present in virtually all patients.
- **Systemic features:** gastroesophageal reflux, GI hypomotility, pulmonary fibrosis, pulmonary hypertension, renal involvement.

General Considerations

Systemic sclerosis is a rare chronic disorder characterized by diffuse fibrosis of the skin and internal organs. Symptoms usually appear in the third to fifth decades, and women are affected two to three times as frequently as men.

Two forms of systemic sclerosis are generally recognized: limited (80% of patients) and diffuse (20%). Limited or diffuse systemic sclerosis refers specifically to the amount of skin involvement. Both can have multisystem internal organ involvement. In general, patients with limited systemic sclerosis have better outcomes than those with diffuse disease, largely because life-threatening lung or kidney disease is less common. Pulmonary hypertension is more characteristic of limited systemic sclerosis.

Clinical Findings

A. Symptoms and Signs

1. Limited systemic sclerosis—RP is usually the initial manifestation and can precede other symptoms by years. Often there is one or more features of the CREST syndrome (calcinosis cutis, RP, esophageal motility disorder, sclerodactyly, and telangiectasia). Hardening of the skin (scleroderma) is limited to the face, neck, and skin distal to the elbows and knees. A small group of patients do not have skin hardening (scleroderma-sine scleroderma). Patients with limited disease are more susceptible to digital ischemia, leading to finger loss, and to life-threatening pulmonary hypertension than are patients with diffuse disease. Renal crisis is rare in limited disease. Small and large bowel hypomotility can cause constipation alternating with diarrhea, malabsorption due to bacterial overgrowth, pseudo-obstruction, and severe bowel distention with rupture. Dysphagia and symptoms of reflux due to esophageal dysfunction are common and result from abnormalities in motility and later from fibrosis. Fibrosis and atrophy of the GI tract cause hypomotility. Large-mouthed diverticula occur in the jejunum, ileum, and colon. GI bleeding from gastric antral vascular ectasia (GAVE, "watermelon stomach") can also occur.

2. Diffuse systemic sclerosis—Polyarthralgia, weight loss, and malaise are common early features of diffuse systemic sclerosis but are infrequent in limited disease. The skin changes of diffuse disease can involve the trunk and proximal extremities, in contrast to limited disease. Cutaneous disease usually, but not always, precedes visceral involvement and can manifest initially as nonpitting subcutaneous edema associated with pruritus. With time the skin becomes thickened and hidebound, with loss of normal folds. Rapid skin progression in the first 3 years is associated with internal organ involvement and mortality. Telangiectasia, pigmentation, and depigmentation are characteristic. The fingertips can ulcerate. Tendon friction rubs over the forearms and shins develop uniquely (but not universally) in diffuse systemic sclerosis. Interstitial lung disease presents early in diffuse systemic sclerosis and affects over half of patients. Pulmonary hypertension may also develop and is frequently secondary to lung disease, although pulmonary arterial hypertension can occur independently. Cardiac abnormalities include pericardial effusions, heart block, myocardial fibrosis, and right HF secondary to pulmonary hypertension. GI manifestations, such as those seen in limited disease, are common. Scleroderma renal crisis, resulting from intimal proliferation of smaller renal arteries and usually associated with acute-onset hypertension and kidney injury, is a life-threatening emergency. Renal crisis is seen most frequently in patients with early, rapidly progressive diffuse disease.

B. Laboratory Findings

Mild anemia is often present. Antinuclear antibody tests are nearly always positive, frequently in high titers. The scleroderma antibody (anti-SCL-70), directed against DNA topoisomerase I, is found in one-third of patients with diffuse systemic sclerosis and in 20% of those with limited disease. Anti-SCL-70 antibodies portend a poor prognosis, with a high likelihood of serious internal organ involvement (eg, interstitial lung disease). Anticentromere antibodies are seen in 50% of those with limited systemic sclerosis. Anticentromere antibodies are highly specific for limited systemic sclerosis, but they also occur occasionally in overlap syndromes. Anti-RNA polymerase III antibodies develop in 10–20% of systemic sclerosis patients overall and are associated with rapidly progressive skin disease, renal crisis, and a higher risk of concomitant solid cancers, especially lung and breast cancers (Table 23–7); cancer risk in this patient group is highest within 2–5 years of disease onset.

In renal crisis, the peripheral blood smear shows findings of microangiopathic hemolytic anemia (from mechanical damage to red blood cells from diseased small vessels). Mild proteinuria, usually < 2 g/24 hours, with few cells or casts, may be present.

C. Special Examinations

Patients should receive pulmonary function testing, HRCT of the chest, and echocardiography at regular intervals to assess cardiopulmonary involvement.

Differential Diagnosis

Early in its course, systemic sclerosis can cause diagnostic confusion with other causes of RP, particularly SLE, mixed connective tissue disease, and the inflammatory myopathies. Scleredema, often associated with diabetes or following infection, is characterized by skin thickening of the posterior neck, shoulders, and upper back; however, this condition spares the fingers and RP is absent. Eosinophilic fasciitis is a rare disorder presenting with skin hardening that resembles diffuse systemic sclerosis, but inflammation is limited to the fascia rather than the dermis and epidermis. Moreover, patients have peripheral blood eosinophilia, the absence of RP, a good response to prednisone, and an association (in some cases) with paraproteinemias. Diffuse skin thickening and visceral involvement are features of scleromyxedema; the presence of a paraprotein, the absence of RP, and distinct skin histology point to scleromyxedema. Diabetic cheiroarthropathy typically develops in long-standing, poorly controlled diabetes mellitus and can mimic sclerodactyly. Morphea and linear scleroderma cause sclerodermatous changes limited to circumscribed areas of the skin and usually have excellent outcomes.

Treatment

Treatment of diffuse and limited systemic sclerosis focuses on the organ systems involved. Although there is no effective therapy for the underlying disease process, interventions for management of specific organ manifestations have improved substantially. There is little or no role for prednisone in the treatment of systemic sclerosis except in patients with debilitating symptoms that cannot be controlled with other therapies, such as severe myositis or inflammatory arthritis. Doses higher than 15 mg daily have been associated with scleroderma renal crisis. Treatment for RP is discussed above.

1. Skin disease—For significant skin involvement, methotrexate (titrated up to 15 or 20 mg orally once weekly) or mycophenolate mofetil (titrated up to 2000 or 3000 mg orally daily), started as early as possible in the disease course, can be modestly effective. Intravenous immunoglobulin, rituximab, and tocilizumab are additional options for refractory disease. The choice of therapy is often driven by other disease manifestations. For example, in patients with arthritis, methotrexate is preferred, while in those with interstitial lung disease, mycophenolate mofetil, rituximab, or tocilizumab is preferred (Table 23–4).

2. Renal crisis—Hypertensive crises in scleroderma renal crisis must be treated urgently and aggressively (in the hospital) with ACE inhibitors, eg, captopril, initiated at 12.5–25 mg orally every 6 hours and titrated up as tolerated to a maximum of 100 mg every 6 hours. A rise in serum creatinine is common; however, the drug should be continued unless severe hypotension or hyperkalemia develops.

3. GI disease—Esophageal reflux can be reduced and the risk of scarring diminished by avoiding late-night meals and using PPIs (eg, omeprazole, 20–40 mg orally once or twice daily), which inhibit gastric acid production and are effective for refractory esophagitis. Patients with delayed gastric emptying maintain their weight better if they eat small, frequent meals and remain upright for at least 2 hours after eating. Oral prokinetic agents such as metoclopramide (10 mg four times daily) can improve dysphagia caused by esophageal hypomotility. Erythromycin (250 mg three times daily) can be used if prokinetic agents fail. Malabsorption due to bacterial overgrowth responds to antibiotics (eg, rifaximin, 550 mg three times orally daily, often prescribed cyclically).

4. Lung disease—For patients who require treatment for interstitial lung disease, mycophenolate mofetil (1000–1500 mg orally twice daily) can improve dyspnea and pulmonary function tests modestly. Cyclophosphamide has some efficacy but greater toxicity; this drug should be administered only by physicians familiar with its use. The IL-6 inhibitor tocilizumab slows the rate of decline in pulmonary function and may be used as an alternative for patients who cannot tolerate mycophenolate mofetil. In patients who do not respond to or cannot take mycophenolate or cyclophosphamide, rituximab is increasingly preferred based on emerging evidence supporting its efficacy and tolerability. Nintedanib, a multitarget tyrosine kinase inhibitor, can further slow disease progression and is FDA-approved for this indication, although the optimal timing and duration of therapy remain under investigation. Azathioprine is also used to treat systemic sclerosis–associated lung disease (Table 23–4). Lung transplantation has favorable outcomes in eligible patients.

5. Pulmonary hypertension—Treatment of pulmonary hypertension in systemic sclerosis is largely extrapolated from general trials of pulmonary hypertension. Therapies include phosphodiesterase type 5 inhibitors (sildenafil, tadalafil), a guanylate cyclase stimulant (riociguat), TGF-β signaling modulator (sotatercept), and endothelin receptor antagonists (bosentan, ambrisentan, macitentan). Calcium channel blockers (eg, amlodipine, nifedipine, extended-release diltiazem) are reserved for rare patients with documented acute vasoreactivity. Combination therapy using two or more agents from different classes is common, although riociguat should not be combined with PDE-5 inhibitors. Refractory pulmonary hypertension may require prostacyclin pathway agonists (epoprostenol, treprostinil, iloprost, selexipag) or lung transplantation.

6. Joint and muscle disease—Arthralgias and myalgias commonly occur, and patients can initially try NSAIDs or acetaminophen. Hydroxychloroquine or methotrexate can be used for inflammatory arthritis, while biologic drugs typically used for RA can be used for refractory disease. Significant inflammatory myositis may initially respond to low-dose prednisone or methotrexate; severe cases require therapies for immune-mediated inflammatory myositides.

Prognosis

The 10-year survival rate in systemic sclerosis averages approximately 70%. Lung disease—pulmonary fibrosis or pulmonary arterial hypertension—is the leading cause of mortality. Persons in whom severe internal organ involvement does not develop in the first 3 years have a substantially better prognosis. Small studies conducted in patients with simultaneous onset of cancer and systemic sclerosis have demonstrated that the disease developed due to an immune response directed at the cancer.

When to Refer

- Appropriate management of systemic sclerosis requires frequent consultations with a rheumatologist.
- Severity of organ involvement dictates referral to cardiologists, pulmonologists, gastroenterologists, or nephrologists.

When to Admit

- Critical digital ischemia, severe pulmonary hypertension or interstitial lung disease with cardiopulmonary compromise, renal crisis.
- Serious GI manifestations such as bowel obstruction, GI bleeding, or severe malabsorption.

Del Galdo F et al. EULAR recommendations for the treatment of systemic sclerosis: 2023 update. Ann Rheum Dis. 2025;84:29. [PMID: 39874231]

Johnson SR et al. Treatment of interstitial lung disease in systemic sclerosis: guidelines and new clinical trial results. Curr Opin Rheumatol. 2024;36:420. [PMID: 39193880]

IMMUNE-MEDIATED INFLAMMATORY MYOPATHIES

ESSENTIALS OF DIAGNOSIS

- Progressive muscle weakness.
- **Dermatomyositis:** characteristic cutaneous manifestations (Gottron papules, heliotrope rash); increased risk of malignancy.
- Elevated creatine kinase, myositis-specific antibodies, diagnostic muscle biopsy.
- Mimics include infectious, metabolic, or drug-induced myopathies.

General Considerations

Immune-mediated inflammatory myopathies are categorized by muscle symptoms and associated autoantibodies. They include antisynthetase syndromes, dermatomyositis, polymyositis, myositis resulting from a rheumatic disease or overlap syndrome, inclusion body myositis (IBM), and immune-mediated necrotizing myopathy. These disorders are characterized by progressive muscle weakness, and most demonstrate an inflammatory infiltrate in muscle tissue.

Antisynthetase syndromes, dermatomyositis, and polymyositis are systemic disorders of unknown cause whose principal manifestation is muscle weakness. Although their clinical presentations (aside from the presence of certain skin findings in dermatomyositis, some of which are pathognomonic) and treatments are similar, the diseases are distinct. They affect persons of any age group, but the peak incidence is in the fifth and sixth decades of life and women are affected twice as commonly as men. There is an increased risk of malignancy in dermatomyositis but not in antisynthetase syndromes. Up to one patient in four with dermatomyositis has an occult malignancy. Malignancies may be evident at the time of presentation with muscle disease or may not be detected until months after diagnosis. The malignancies most commonly associated with dermatomyositis are lung, ovarian, breast, colorectal, cervical, bladder, nasopharyngeal, esophageal, pancreatic, and renal. Patients may have skin disease without overt muscle involvement, a condition termed dermatomyositis sine myositis (or amyopathic dermatomyositis); these patients can have aggressive interstitial lung disease. Polymyositis has become a rarer diagnosis as many cases previously attributed to it are now identified as conditions such as immune-mediated necrotizing myopathy and overlap syndromes. Myositis may be a feature of other connective tissue diseases, especially systemic sclerosis, SLE, mixed connective tissue disease, and Sjögren disease.

IBM affects older men and is characterized by distal weakness in the upper extremities and is generally less symmetric. Immune-mediated necrotizing myopathies include those associated with the signal recognition particle (anti-SRP) or with anti-3-hydroxy-3-methylglutaryl coenzyme A reductase (anti-HMGCR) autoantibodies. Anti-HMGCR myopathy is distinct from the more common statin-induced myopathy, which occurs in about 1% of statin users. Unlike anti-HMGCR necrotizing myopathy, statin-induced myopathy is generally mild and resolves within 6 months of drug discontinuation.

Clinical Findings

A. Symptoms and Signs

1. Antisynthetase syndrome—Presenting symptoms are muscle weakness, particularly of the proximal muscles. Weakness can range from mild to severe. Constitutional symptoms are common. Other clinical findings include inflammatory nonerosive arthritis, fever, Raynaud phenomenon, "mechanic's hands" (hyperkeratosis along the radial and palmar aspects of the fingers), interstitial lung disease, and specific autoantibodies (eg, antibodies to Jo-1, PL-7, PL-12, EJ, OJ, Zo, Ks, Ha, or Ly).

2. Dermatomyositis—Most patients experience symmetric, proximal muscle weakness. There is a characteristic dusky red rash which may appear in a malar distribution, mimicking the classic rash of SLE. Facial erythema beyond the malar distribution (crossing the nasolabial fold) is characteristic of dermatomyositis. Erythema also occurs over other areas of the face, neck, shoulders, and upper

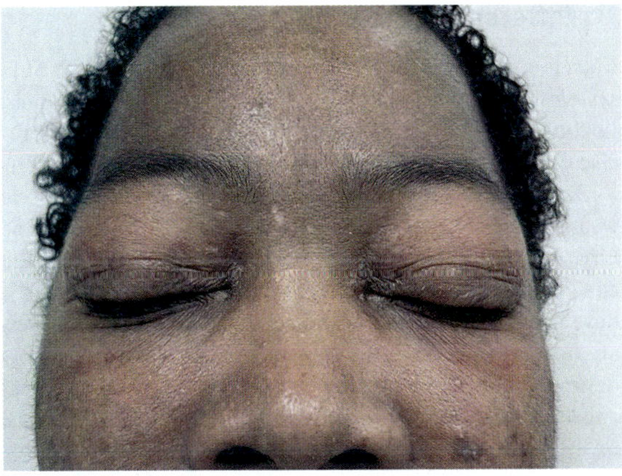

▲ **Figure 23–7.** Heliotrope rash in a patient who has anti-NXP2 dermatomyositis. (Used, with permission, from Rebecca L. Manno, MD.)

chest and back ("shawl sign"). Periorbital edema and a purplish (heliotrope) suffusion over the eyelids are typical signs. Coloration of the heliotrope and other rashes of dermatomyositis can be affected by skin tone. In Black persons, the rashes may appear more hyperpigmented than erythematous or violaceous (Figure 23–7). Periungual erythema, dilations of nailfold capillaries, Gottron papules (raised violaceous lesions overlying the dorsa of DIP, PIP, and MCP joints), and Gottron sign (erythematous rash on the extensors surfaces of the fingers, elbows, and knees) are highly suggestive of dermatomyositis. Scalp involvement by dermatomyositis may mimic psoriasis and intense scalp pruritus is common. Infrequently, the cutaneous findings of this disease precede the muscle inflammation by weeks or months. Autoantibodies include anti-Mi2, anti-TIF-1-γ, anti-NXP2, and anti-MDA5. Each of these autoantibodies is associated with specific clinical features. For example, anti-TIF1-γ and anti-NXP2 are strongly associated with malignancy, whereas anti-MDA5 is associated with punched-out skin ulcerations and rapidly progressive interstitial lung disease (Table 23–10).

3. Polymyositis—There is progressive, symmetrical, proximal muscle weakness without significant skin involvement and negative antibody testing. With current testing, many cases previously labeled as polymyositis are now attributed to more precisely defined myositis subtypes. Therefore, other diagnoses, including IBM, immune-mediated necrotizing myopathy, and overlap syndromes, should be considered in patients with these symptoms.

4. Inclusion body myositis—IBM is a common cause of misdiagnosed "treatment-resistant polymyositis." The typical patient is a man over the age of 50 years. The onset of IBM is more insidious than that of dermatomyositis (ie, occurring over years rather than months) and is characterized by asymmetric distal motor weakness (especially the wrists and hands). Dysphagia occurs in up to half of patients. Foot drop from anterior leg muscle weakness can occur. Creatine kinase levels are often minimally elevated and are normal in 25%. Electromyography may show a mixed picture of myopathic and neurogenic abnormalities. The disease is associated with antibodies to cytoplasmic 5′-nucleotidase 1A (cN1A). IBM is unlikely to respond to immunosuppressive therapy.

5. Immune-mediated necrotizing myopathy—This myopathy is characterized by the presence of muscle necrosis. Autoantibodies aid in diagnosis; anti-SRP

Table 23–10. Myositis-specific autoantibodies.

Antibody	Antigen	Clinical
Jo-1	His-tRNA synthetase	**Synthetase syndrome**: Myositis, mechanic's hands, high-frequency ILD, Gottron papules, arthritis, Raynaud phenomenon
PL-7, PL-12, EJ, OJ, KS, Zo, Ha	Various RNA synthetases	
Mi-2	Nucleosome deacetylase ATPase	**Skin disease (classic dermatomyositis)** Myositis with good response to treatment
p155/140, TIF1γ	Transcription intermediary factor 1-γ	**Cancer-associated dermatomyositis in adults**, severe skin disease Juvenile dermatomyositis
NXP-2 (MJ)	Nuclear matrix protein-2	**Calcinosis** in dermatomyositis Associated with malignancy. Juvenile dermatomyositis
MDA-5 (CADM-140)	Melanoma differentiation factor 5, an RNA helicase	**Skin disease (dermatomyositis) and rapidly progressive lung disease** Often without overt muscle disease = **"Amyopathic dermatomyositis"**
SAE	Small ubiquitin-like modifier-activating enzyme	**Skin disease, dysphagia** Possible cancer association
SRP	Signal recognition peptide	**Necrotizing myopathy, often poor treatment response**, cardiac myositis
HMG CoA reductase	3-hydroxy-3-methyl-glutaryl-CoA reductase (target of statin therapy)	**Necrotizing myopathy. Often associated with statin use** Responds to immunosuppressives

Modified with permission from Wener MH. Laboratory Testing. In: Stone JH. eds. *Current Diagnosis & Treatment: Rheumatology*, 4e. McGraw Hill; 2021.

antibodies are associated with severe muscle weakness, pain, and cardiac involvement. Anti-HMGCR antibodies usually, but not always, occur in the setting of statin use and are associated with profound proximal muscle weakness and marked creatine kinase elevations. Many patients have a severe and unrelenting disease course with persistent weakness, unlike other statin-induced myopathies.

B. Laboratory Findings

Measurement of serum levels of muscle enzymes, especially creatine kinase and aldolase, is useful in diagnosis and in assessment of disease activity. Inflammatory myositis can be misdiagnosed as hepatitis because of elevations in serum levels of muscle-derived ALT and AST levels. ESR and CRP are often normal and are not reliable indicators of disease activity. Antinuclear antibodies may be present, especially when there is an associated connective tissue disease. A number of autoantibodies are seen exclusively in patients with myositis and are associated with distinctive clinical features (Table 23–10). CXRs may show interstitial lung disease, which is common in some IIM phenotypes. Electromyographic abnormalities can point toward a myopathic, rather than a neurogenic, cause of weakness. MRI can detect early and patchy muscle involvement, can guide biopsies, and often is more useful than electromyography for diagnosis. MRI can also determine the extent of fatty replacement in the muscle, a consequence of long-standing severe disease. The search for an occult malignancy should begin with a history and physical examination, a CBC, comprehensive biochemical panel, UA, and age- and risk-appropriate cancer screening tests. Given the especially strong association of ovarian carcinoma and dermatomyositis, transvaginal ultrasonography, CT scanning, and CA-125 levels may be useful in women. No matter how extensive the initial screening, some malignancies will not become evident for months after the initial presentation of the myopathy.

C. Biopsy

Biopsy of clinically involved muscle is often required if patients do not have characteristic dermatomyositis rashes or myositis-specific antibodies. In dermatomyositis, the cellular infiltrate is mostly perifascicular and perivascular, while in polymyositis, the inflammatory infiltrate involves the fascicle itself. Myofiber HLA-DR expression can be diagnostic of antisynthetase myopathy. Necrosis with a paucity of inflammatory cells suggests an immune-mediated necrotizing myopathy. Muscle biopsy in IBM shows characteristic intracellular rimmed vacuoles by light microscopy and either tubular or filamentous inclusions in the nucleus or cytoplasm by electron microscopy. False-negative muscle biopsies sometimes occur in these disorders because of the patchy distribution of pathologic abnormalities and the absence of the primary inflammatory infiltrate from immunosuppression. Skin biopsy in dermatomyositis will show interface dermatitis and is indistinguishable pathologically from lupus.

Differential Diagnosis

Muscle inflammation may occur as a component of SLE, systemic sclerosis, Sjögren disease, and overlap syndromes. In those cases, associated findings usually permit the precise diagnosis of the primary condition.

Hypothyroidism is a common cause of proximal muscle weakness associated with elevations of serum creatine kinase. Patients with polymyalgia rheumatica are over the age of 50 and—in contrast to patients with polymyositis—have pain but no objective weakness; creatine kinase levels are normal with ESR and CRP universally elevated. Disorders of the peripheral nervous system and CNS (eg, chronic inflammatory polyneuropathy, multiple sclerosis, myasthenia gravis, Lambert-Eaton disease, and amyotrophic lateral sclerosis) can produce weakness but are distinguished by characteristic symptoms and neurologic signs and often by distinctive electromyographic abnormalities. Muscle weakness associated with some systemic vasculitides (polyarteritis nodosa, microscopic polyangiitis, eosinophilic granulomatosis with polyangiitis, granulomatosis with polyangiitis, and mixed cryoglobulinemia) is typically distal and asymmetric (such as mononeuritis multiplex), at least in the early stages.

Limb-girdle muscular dystrophy can present in early adulthood with a clinical picture that mimics polymyositis: proximal muscle weakness, elevations in serum creatine kinase, and inflammatory cells on muscle biopsy.

Many drugs, including corticosteroids, alcohol, clofibrate, penicillamine, tryptophan, and hydroxychloroquine, can produce proximal muscle weakness. Long-term use of colchicine, even as low as 0.6 mg per day in patients with moderate CKD, can produce a mixed neuropathy-myopathy that mimics polymyositis. Weakness and muscle enzyme elevation reverse with cessation of the drug. HIV-associated myopathy can cause proximal weakness, elevated muscle enzymes, and an inflammatory muscle infiltrate; antiretroviral therapy can result in mitochondrial myopathy presenting as weakness, myalgias, and fatigue.

Statins can cause myalgias, myopathy, and rhabdomyolysis, in addition to the anti-HMGCR myopathy described above. Although only about 0.1% of patients taking a statin drug alone develop myopathy, concomitant administration of other drugs (especially nirmatrelvir with ritonavir [Paxlovid], gemfibrozil, cyclosporine, niacin, macrolide antibiotics, azole antifungals, and protease inhibitors) increases the risk.

The use of immune checkpoint inhibitors to treat cancer can cause rheumatic and musculoskeletal symptoms, including myalgia and myositis.

Treatment

Most patients with immune-mediated inflammatory myopathy respond to corticosteroids. Initially, prednisone, 40–60 mg or more orally daily is often required. The dose is then adjusted downward while monitoring muscle strength and serum levels of muscle enzymes. Long-term use of corticosteroids is often needed, and the disease may recur when they are withdrawn. Patients with an associated neoplasm have a poor prognosis, although remission may follow treatment of the tumor; corticosteroids may or may not be effective in these patients. Immunosuppressive drugs like methotrexate (15–25 mg orally or subcutaneous weekly), azathioprine (1.5–2 mg/kg orally once daily), or mycophenolate mofetil (1–1.5 g orally twice daily) are often started to reduce cumulative corticosteroid exposure. Intravenous immunoglobulin, an FDA-approved therapy for dermatomyositis, is highly effective for skin, muscle and interstitial lung disease associated with immune-mediated inflammatory myopathies. Along with corticosteroids, IVIG is first-line therapy for anti-HMGCR myopathy. Rituximab or JAK inhibitors may be effective for some inflammatory myositis or skin involvement unresponsive to corticosteroids and other immunosuppressants. Since the rash of dermatomyositis is often photosensitive, patients should limit sun exposure. Immunosuppressive therapy has limited efficacy for IBM. Cricopharyngeal myotomy is a consideration for advanced IBM with dysphagia. All patients with immune-mediated inflammatory myopathies should be encouraged to participate in an exercise program, which is a foundational treatment and a key component of therapeutic interventions.

When to Refer

- All patients with myositis should be referred to a rheumatologist or neurologist.
- All patients with immune-mediated inflammatory myopathies should be referred for physical therapy.
- For patients with IBM and dysphagia, early referral to a speech-language pathologist is important to minimize aspiration risk
- Severe lung disease may require consultation with a pulmonologist.

When to Admit

- Signs of rhabdomyolysis.
- New onset of dysphagia.
- Respiratory insufficiency with hypoxia or carbon dioxide retention.

Fattorini F et al. Idiopathic inflammatory myopathies: one year in review 2024. Clin Exp Rheumatol. 2025;43:167. [PMID: 40018744]

Jensen KY et al. High-intensity resistance training improves quality of life, muscle endurance and strength in patients with myositis: a randomised controlled trial. Rheumatol Int. 2024;44:1909. [PMID: 39192022]

MIXED CONNECTIVE TISSUE DISEASE, OVERLAP, & UNDIFFERENTIATED SYNDROMES

Special attention has been drawn to a subset of patients with positive antinuclear antibodies who have high titers of RNP autoantibodies and overlapping features of SLE, systemic sclerosis, RA, and inflammatory myositis. Swollen or puffy hands are a common early feature of this disease, referred to as mixed connective tissue disease. Raynaud phenomenon, arthralgias, and myalgias are common. Unlike patients with SLE, renal or CNS disease is uncommon. A key reason to identify this subset of patients is that pulmonary hypertension and interstitial lung disease are major causes of mortality, and regular screening for these manifestations is required.

Some patients have features of more than one connective tissue disease (eg, RA and SLE, SLE and systemic sclerosis) without high-titer anti-RNP antibodies. This is called "overlap syndrome." Others have only a few features of autoimmunity and cannot yet be classified ("undifferentiated connective tissue disease"). Treatments are guided by the distribution and severity of patients' organ system involvement.

SJÖGREN DISEASE

ESSENTIALS OF DIAGNOSIS

- Women (average age 50 years) comprise 90% of patients.
- Dryness of eyes and mouth (sicca) are the most common features, but can be a multisystem disease with neurologic, pulmonary, and renal involvement.
- Rheumatoid factor, SSA (anti-Ro60 and Ro52), SSB (anti-La), and antinuclear antibodies are common.
- Increased incidence of lymphoma.

General Considerations

Sjögren disease is a systemic autoimmune disorder whose clinical presentation is usually dominated by dryness of the eyes and mouth due to immune-mediated dysfunction of the lacrimal and salivary glands. The disorder is predominantly seen in women, with a ratio of 9:1; most cases develop between the ages of 40 and 60 years. In general, it is slowly progressive with symptoms and glandular damage occurring over years. A high incidence of lymphoma is observed. Sjögren disease can occur in isolation ("primary" Sjögren disease) or in association with another rheumatic disease ("secondary" Sjögren disease), most frequently RA, but also with SLE, primary biliary cholangitis, systemic sclerosis, and Hashimoto thyroiditis.

Clinical Findings

A. Symptoms and Signs

Keratoconjunctivitis sicca results from inadequate tear production caused by lymphocyte and plasma cell infiltration of the lacrimal glands. For most patients, symptoms of dryness of the mouth (xerostomia) are the most disabling. Patients frequently complain of a "cotton mouth" and difficulty swallowing foods, especially dry foods, like crackers, unless they are washed down with liquids. Persistent xerostomia results in rampant dental caries; caries at the gum line strongly suggest Sjögren disease. Ocular symptoms are directly related to decreased tear production. Burning, itching, and the sensation of having a foreign body or a grain of sand in the eye are common. The initial manifestation in some patients may be the inability to tolerate wearing contact lenses. Photophobia may signal corneal ulceration, a painful complication of severe ocular dryness. Dryness may involve the nose, throat, larynx, bronchi, vagina, and skin. Parotid enlargement, which may be chronic or relapsing, develops in one-third of patients.

Additional systemic autoimmune manifestations of Sjögren disease are rarer than sicca and include inflammatory arthritis (generally small joints), small-vessel vasculitis (often associated with cryoglobulinemia), and lung involvement (interstitial lung disease and pneumonitis). The spectrum of neurologic involvement is broad and can be devastating, including peripheral neuropathy, dysautonomia, and neuromyelitis optica. Renal tubular acidosis (type I, distal) occurs in 20% of patients, and chronic interstitial nephritis may cause impaired kidney function.

B. Laboratory Findings

Laboratory findings include anemia, leukopenia, and mild eosinophilia. Polyclonal hypergammaglobulinemia, rheumatoid factor positivity (70%), and antinuclear antibodies (95%) are common. Antibodies against SS-A (anti-Ro 60 and Ro52) and SS-B (anti-La) are often present in primary Sjögren disease and tend to correlate with the presence of extraglandular manifestations (Table 23–7). Cryoglobulins are associated with a higher risk of vasculitis and subsequent lymphoma.

Useful ocular diagnostic tests include the Schirmer test, which measures the quantity of tears secreted. Lip biopsy, a simple procedure, reveals characteristic lymphoid foci in accessory salivary glands. Sialometry is an easy bedside test to quantify saliva production with a value ≤ 0.1 mL/min for unstimulated whole salivary flow being common, but not alone diagnostic, in Sjögren disease.

Ultrasound of salivary glands show hyperechoic bands and hypoechoic areas and may be a helpful tool for diagnosis and prognosis.

Differential Diagnosis

Isolated complaints of dry mouth are commonly due to medication side effects. Chronic hepatitis C can cause sicca symptoms and rheumatoid factor positivity; minor salivary gland biopsies reveal lymphocytic infiltrates but not to the extent of Sjögren disease, and tests for anti-SS-A and anti-SS-B are negative. Diffuse infiltration of CD8 T cells producing parotid gland enlargement can develop in patients with HIV. Involvement of the lacrimal or salivary glands, or both, in sarcoidosis can mimic Sjögren disease; biopsies reveal noncaseating granulomas. Rarely, amyloid deposits in the lacrimal and salivary glands produce sicca symptoms. IgG_4-related systemic disease can cause lacrimal and salivary gland enlargement.

Treatment & Prognosis

Treatment of mild to moderate sicca symptoms is symptomatic and supportive. Artificial tears applied frequently will relieve ocular symptoms and avert further desiccation. Topical ocular cyclosporine 0.05% or lifitegrast 5% also improve ocular symptoms. The mouth should be kept well lubricated. Sipping water frequently or using sugar-free gums and hard candies usually relieves dry mouth symptoms. Pilocarpine (5 mg orally four times daily) and the acetylcholine derivative, cevimeline (30 mg orally three times daily), may improve xerostomia symptoms. Atropinic (anticholinergic) drugs and decongestants decrease salivary secretions and should be avoided. A program of oral hygiene, including fluoride treatment, is essential to preserve dentition.

Drugs targeting B cells (rituximab) and B-cell activating factor (BAFF) (belimumab, ianalumab, telitacicept) have shown promise in improving composite outcomes in Sjögren disease (Table 23–4). Nipocalimab, a monoclonal antibody with high affinity to block FcRn and reduce levels of circulating immunoglobulin G, has an FDA Breakthrough Therapy designation for patients with moderate to severe Sjögren disease.

Although Sjögren disease may compromise patients' quality of life significantly, the disease is usually associated with a normal life span. Poor prognosis is influenced by the presence and severity of organ involvement (pulmonary, renal, neurologic), vasculitis, and the complication of lymphoma. The patients at greatest risk for developing lymphoma are those with severe exocrine dysfunction, marked parotid gland enlargement, splenomegaly, vasculitis, peripheral neuropathy, anemia, and mixed monoclonal cryoglobulinemia (3–10% of the total Sjögren population).

When to Refer

- Presence of systemic symptoms or signs.
- Ocular dryness not responsive to artificial tears.

When to Admit

Presence of severe systemic signs, such as vasculitis or neurologic, unresponsive to outpatient management.

Gandolfo S et al. Precision medicine in Sjogren's disease. Lancet Rheumatol. 2024;6:e636. [PMID: 38723653]

IgG_4-RELATED DISEASE

ESSENTIALS OF DIAGNOSIS

- Mainly affects men aged > 50 years.
- Lymphoplasmacytic infiltrates causing tumors or fibrosis in any organ or tissue.
- Subacute onset; constitutional symptoms rare.
- Diagnostic histopathology.

General Considerations

IgG_4-related disease is a systemic disorder of unknown cause marked by highly characteristic fibroinflammation that contains IgG_4 plasma cells and can infiltrate virtually any organ. Elevations of serum IgG_4 levels occur often but are not diagnostic. The disorder chiefly affects men (75% of patients) aged > 50 years.

Clinical Findings

A. Symptoms and Signs

IgG_4-related disease can affect any organ of the body, can be localized or generalized, demonstrates the same distinctive histopathology at all sites of involvement, produces protean manifestations depending on location and extent of involvement, and causes disease ranging in severity from asymptomatic to organ- or life-threatening. The inflammatory infiltration in IgG_4-related disease frequently produces tumefactive masses that can be found during physical examination or on imaging. Some of the common presenting manifestations include enlargement of salivary or submandibular glands, lymphadenopathy, proptosis from periorbital infiltration, retroperitoneal fibrosis, mediastinal fibrosis, inflammatory aortic aneurysm, and pancreatic mass with autoimmune pancreatitis. IgG_4-related disease can also affect the thyroid (formerly Riedel thyroiditis), kidney, meninges, pituitary, sinuses, lung, prostate, breast, and coronary arteries. Most symptomatic patients with IgG_4-related disease present subacutely.

B. Laboratory Findings

Serum IgG_4 levels are usually, but not invariably, elevated so this finding cannot be used as the sole diagnostic criterion. Hypocomplementemia may be seen in 40% of patients. The infiltrating lesions in IgG_4-related disease often produce tumors or fibrotic changes that are evident on CT or MRI. However, the cornerstone of diagnosis is histopathology. The key pathological findings are a dense lymphoplasmacytic infiltrate rich in IgG_4 plasma cells, storiform (matted and irregularly whorled) fibrosis, and obliterative phlebitis.

Differential Diagnosis

IgG_4-related disease can mimic many disorders including sarcoidosis, Sjögren disease (lacrimal gland enlargement), pancreatic cancer (pancreatic mass), chronic infections (eg, HIV, hepatitis C, tuberculosis), and granulomatosis with polyangiitis

Treatment & Prognosis

Patients who are asymptomatic and have no organ-threatening disease can be monitored carefully. Spontaneous resolution can occur. Initial therapy is usually oral prednisone 0.6 mg/kg/day, tapered over weeks or months. Corticosteroid monotherapy often fails to control the disease and can cause significant long-term toxicity. Therefore B-cell–depleting therapy with inebilizumab (FDA-approved to treat IgG_4-related disease) or rituximab, should also be used. Azathioprine and mycophenolate mofetil are alternative therapies.

When to Refer

- All patients should be referred to a rheumatologist.
- Presence of organ involvement.
- For initiation of steroid-sparing therapy after prednisone induction.

When to Admit

Presence of severe systemic signs unresponsive to outpatient management.

Stone J. IgG_4-related disease: lessons from the first 20 years. Rheumatology (Oxford). 2025;64(Suppl 1):i24. [PMID: 40071397]

VASCULITIS SYNDROMES

Vasculitis is a heterogeneous group of disorders characterized by inflammation within the walls of affected blood vessels. The first consideration in classifying cases of vasculitis is the size of the major vessels involved: large, medium, or small. The major forms of primary systemic vasculitis are listed in Table 23–11. The presence of the clinical signs and symptoms shown in Table 23–12 helps distinguish among these three groups. After determining the size of the major vessels involved, other issues that contribute to the classification include the following:

- Which organs are involved?
- What are the patient's demographic characteristics (age, sex, ethnicity, cigarette smoking status, comorbidities)?
- Is there hypocomplementemia or other evidence of immune complex deposition?
- Is there granulomatous inflammation on tissue biopsy?
- Are antineutrophil cytoplasmic antibodies (ANCA) present?

Table 23–11. Classification scheme of primary vasculitides according to size of predominant blood vessels involved.

Predominantly large-vessel vasculitides
Takayasu arteritis
Giant cell arteritis (temporal arteritis)
Behçet disease[1]
Predominantly medium-vessel vasculitides
Polyarteritis nodosa
Thromboangiitis obliterans
Primary angiitis of the CNS
Kawasaki disease
Predominantly small-vessel vasculitides
Cutaneous leukocytoclastic angiitis ("hypersensitivity vasculitis")
Immune-complex–mediated
IgA vasculitis (Henoch-Schönlein purpura)
Hypocomplementemic urticarial vasculitis (anti-C1q vasculitis)
Cryoglobulinemic vasculitis[2]
"ANCA-associated" vasculitis[3]
Granulomatosis with polyangiitis[2]
Microscopic polyangiitis[2]
Eosinophilic granulomatosis with polyangiitis[2]

ANCA, antineutrophil cytoplasmic antibodies.
[1]May involve small-, medium-, and large-sized blood vessels (variable vessel vasculitis).
[2]Frequent overlap of small- and medium-sized blood vessel involvement.
[3]Not all forms of these disorders are associated with ANCA positivity.

Table 23–12. Typical clinical manifestations of large-, medium-, and small-vessel vasculitis.

Large Vessel	Medium Vessel	Small Vessel
Fever, weight loss, malaise, arthralgias/arthritis Limb claudication Asymmetric blood pressures Absence of pulses Bruits Aortic dilation	Fever, weight loss, malaise, arthralgias/arthritis Cutaneous nodules Ulcers Livedo reticularis Digital gangrene Mononeuritis multiplex Microaneurysms	Fever, weight loss, malaise, arthralgias/arthritis Purpura Vesiculobullous lesions Urticaria Glomerulonephritis, hematuria Alveolar hemorrhage Cutaneous extravascular necrotizing granulomas Splinter hemorrhages Uveitis Episcleritis Scleritis

In addition to primary vasculitides, "secondary" forms of vasculitis occur in the setting of chronic infections (eg, hepatitis B or C, subacute bacterial endocarditis), connective tissue disorders (SLE, Sjögren disease), IBD, malignancies, and reactions to medications. Only the major primary forms of vasculitis are discussed here.

POLYMYALGIA RHEUMATICA & GIANT CELL ARTERITIS

ESSENTIALS OF DIAGNOSIS

- Age over 50 years.
- Markedly elevated ESR and CRP.
- **Polymyalgia rheumatica:** pain and stiffness in shoulders and hips lasting for several weeks without other explanation.
- **Giant cell arteritis:** headache, jaw claudication, polymyalgia rheumatica; without treatment, permanent blindness may occur.

General Considerations

Polymyalgia rheumatica and giant cell arteritis probably represent a spectrum of one disease. Both affect the same population (patients over the age of 50), and the incidence of the disease increases with each decade of life. Both show preference for the same HLA haplotypes and show similar patterns of cytokines in blood and arteries. Giant cell arteritis is a systemic panarteritis affecting medium-sized and large vessels. Giant cell arteritis was previously called temporal arteritis because the temporal artery is frequently involved, as are other extracranial branches of the carotid artery. However, the aorta and its major branches also may be involved in giant cell arteritis. Polymyalgia rheumatica and giant cell arteritis frequently coexist. Polymyalgia rheumatica alone is not a systemic vasculitis, does not cause blindness, and responds to low-dose (10–20 mg/day orally) prednisone; giant cell arteritis can cause blindness, aortitis, and large artery complications that require high-dose (40–60 mg/day) prednisone.

Clinical Findings

A. Polymyalgia Rheumatica

Polymyalgia rheumatica is a clinical diagnosis based on pain and stiffness of the shoulder and pelvic girdle areas, frequently in association with malaise and weight loss. In approximately two-thirds of cases, polymyalgia occurs in the absence of giant cell arteritis. Because of profound stiffness and pain in the shoulders, hips, and lower back, patients have trouble combing their hair, putting on a coat, or rising from a chair. In contrast to polymyositis and polyarteritis nodosa, polymyalgia rheumatica does not cause muscular weakness either through primary muscle inflammation or secondary to nerve infarction.

B. Giant Cell Arteritis

The 2022 American and European classification criteria for giant cell arteritis highlight the multiple domains important to making the diagnosis of giant cell arteritis: clinical, laboratory, pathologic (temporal artery biopsy), and imaging.

The mean age at onset of giant cell arteritis is 79 years. The classic cranial symptoms are headache, scalp tenderness, visual symptoms (particularly amaurosis fugax or diplopia), and jaw claudication. Of these symptoms, jaw claudication has the highest positive predictive value. The temporal artery can be normal on physical examination but may be nodular, enlarged, tender, or pulseless. Blindness usually results from anterior ischemic optic neuropathy, caused by occlusive arteritis of the posterior ciliary branch of the ophthalmic artery; there may be no funduscopic findings for the first 24–48 hours after the onset of blindness. About 50% of patients with giant cell arteritis have polymyalgia rheumatica.

Asymmetry of pulses in the arms, a murmur of aortic regurgitation, or bruits near the clavicle resulting from subclavian artery stenoses identify patients in whom giant cell arteritis has affected the aorta or its major branches. Clinically evident large artery involvement—characterized chiefly by aneurysm of the thoracic aorta or stenosis of the subclavian, vertebral, carotid, and basilar arteries—occurs in at least 25% of patients with giant cell arteritis, sometimes years after the diagnosis. Subclinical large artery disease is the rule: PET scans reveal inflammation in the aorta and its major branches in nearly 85% of untreated patients. Forty percent of patients with giant cell arteritis have non-cranial symptoms at presentation, including large artery involvement causing aortic regurgitation or arm claudication, respiratory tract problems (most frequently dry cough), mononeuritis multiplex (most frequently with painful paralysis of a shoulder), or fever of unknown origin. Giant cell arteritis accounts for 15% of all cases of fever of unknown origin in patients over the age of 65.In contrast to patients with infection, patients with giant cell arteritis and fever usually have normal WBC counts (before prednisone is started). Thus, in an older patient with fever of unknown origin, elevated acute-phase reactants, and negative infectious workup, giant cell arteritis must be considered even in the absence of cranial giant cell arteritis features.

C. Laboratory Findings

1. Polymyalgia rheumatica—Acute-phase reactants (generally ESR > 30 mm/hour and CRP > 0.5 mg/dL) are universally present.

2. Giant cell arteritis—Nearly 90% of patients with giant cell arteritis have ESRs > 50 mm/hour. The ESR in this disorder is often > 100 mm/hour, but cases in which the ESR is lower or even normal do occur. In one series, 5% of patients with biopsy-proven giant cell arteritis had ESRs < 40 mm/hour. Although the CRP is slightly more sensitive, patients with biopsy-proven giant cell arteritis with normal CRP have also been described. Most patients also have a mild normochromic, normocytic anemia and thrombocytosis. The alkaline phosphatase (liver source) is elevated in 20% of patients with giant cell arteritis.

D. Imaging

Ultrasonography of the temporal artery can demonstrate the "halo sign" with a sensitivity (50–80%) and specificity (80–90%) that is highly operator dependent. For large artery giant cell arteritis (eg, aortitis), magnetic resonance angiography or CT angiography (sensitivity 73–85%, specificity 85–100%) can establish the diagnosis by demonstrating long stretches of narrowing, thickening, or aneurysmal dilation of the aorta and the subclavian and axillary arteries, or both. PET-CT has a sensitivity 85% and specificity 83% to differentiate between clinically active large-vessel vasculitis and noninflammatory conditions.

Thoracic aortic aneurysms occur 17 times more frequently in patients with giant cell arteritis than in normal individuals and can cause aortic regurgitation, dissection, or rupture. The aneurysms can develop at any time but typically occur 7 years after the diagnosis of giant cell arteritis is made; hence, routine screening for this complication with magnetic resonance angiography or CT angiography is recommended for all patients with giant cell arteritis. Ultrasonography may be used to screen for thoracic aortic aneurysms if other modalities are not available and if there is appropriate expertise.

E. Biopsy

Biopsy remains the gold standard for diagnosis in the United States. An adequate biopsy specimen is essential (at least 2 cm in length), because the disease may be segmental. The 2021 guidelines recommend obtaining a unilateral biopsy (positive in approximately 80–85% of patients) since bilateral biopsies increase the yield by < 15%. Although it is prudent to obtain a temporal artery biopsy as soon as possible after instituting treatment, diagnostic findings of giant cell arteritis may still be present 2 weeks (or longer) after starting corticosteroids. Temporal artery biopsy is abnormal in only 50% of patients with large artery giant cell arteritis (eg, aortitis); magnetic resonance angiography or CT angiography will establish the diagnosis.

Differential Diagnosis

The differential diagnosis of malaise, anemia, and striking acute-phase reactant elevations includes rheumatic diseases (such as RA or other systemic vasculitides), occult malignancies, and chronic infections (such as subacute bacterial endocarditis and osteomyelitis).

Treatment

A. Polymyalgia Rheumatica

Patients with isolated polymyalgia rheumatica (ie, those without giant cell arteritis) are treated with prednisone, 10–20 mg/day orally. If the patient does not experience a dramatic improvement within 72 hours, the diagnosis should be revisited. Usually after 2–4 weeks of treatment, slow tapering of prednisone can be attempted. Most patients require some dose of prednisone for a minimum of approximately 1 year; 6 months is too short in most cases. Disease flares are common (≥ 50%) as prednisone is tapered, which may necessitate increasing prednisone. Tapering of prednisone should be based on symptoms and not solely on laboratory values because ESR can fluctuate and is not specific for polymyalgia rheumatica disease activity. However, failure of the ESR and CRP to respond to treatment with corticosteroids should bring alternative diagnoses into consideration. Sarilumab, a human anti-IL-6Rα antibody, is FDA-approved to treat refractory polymyalgia rheumatica and for patients who fail corticosteroid tapering (Table 23–4). Methotrexate (15–25 mg orally weekly) may also have a steroid-sparing role in refractory polymyalgia rheumatica.

B. Giant Cell Arteritis

The urgency of early diagnosis and treatment in giant cell arteritis relates to the prevention of blindness. Once blindness develops, it is usually permanent. Therefore, when a patient has symptoms and findings suggestive of cranial involvement from giant cell arteritis, therapy with prednisone (1 mg/kg/daily or max 80 mg/day orally) should be initiated immediately, and a temporal artery biopsy or temporal artery ultrasound performed promptly thereafter. For patients who seek medical attention for visual loss, intravenous pulse methylprednisolone (eg, 1 g daily for 3 days) should be started; unfortunately, few patients recover vision no matter what the initial treatment.

Prednisone should be continued at a high dose orally for about 1 month before tapering. When tapering and adjusting the dosage of prednisone, the ESR (or CRP) is a useful, but not absolute, guide to disease activity. A common error is treating the ESR rather than the patient. Because older individuals often have baseline ESRs that are above the normal range, mild ESR elevations should not be an occasion for renewed treatment with prednisone in patients who are asymptomatic. Tocilizumab, an inhibitor of the IL-6 receptor, is FDA-approved for giant cell arteritis and can reduce the prolonged use of prednisone and decrease the risk of disease flare. Upadacitanib, a selective JAK1 inhibitor, is also FDA-approved to treat giant-cell arteritis. Upadacitinib 15 mg orally daily with a 26-week corticosteroid taper showed superior efficacy (sustained remission of giant cell arteritis) compared with placebo and a 52-week corticosteroid taper. Giant cell arteritis treatment guidelines are to initiate a steroid-sparing therapy along with corticosteroids for all patients with new or relapsing giant cell arteritis (Table 23–4).

Blockmans D et al. A phase 3 trial of upadacitinib for giant-cell arteritis. N Engl J Med. 2025;392:2013. [PMID: 40174237]
Bolhuis TE et al. Results of a 1-year randomised double-blind placebo-controlled trial with methotrexate 25 mg/week in recently diagnosed polymyalgia rheumatica. Ann Rheum Dis. 2025:S0003-4967(25)04592. [PMID: 41423373]

TAKAYASU ARTERITIS

Takayasu arteritis is a granulomatous vasculitis of the aorta and its major branches. It primarily affects women, and age of onset is < 60 years. Takayasu arteritis can present with nonspecific constitutional symptoms of malaise, fever, and weight loss with or without manifestations of vascular inflammation and damage: diminished pulses, unequal blood pressures in the arms, carotidynia (tenderness over the carotid arteries), bruits over carotid and subclavian arteries, retinopathy, limb claudication, hypertension, or major ischemic events. There are no specific laboratory abnormalities or autoantibodies, although ESR and CRP are elevated in most cases. The diagnosis is established by imaging and clinical presentation. It is important to visualize the entire aorta given the wide distribution of vascular lesions in Takayasu. MRI can detect inflammatory thickening of affected arteries. CT angiography provides images of the stenoses, occlusions, and dilations characteristic of arteritis. High-dose corticosteroids (eg, oral prednisone, 1 mg/kg) are recommended for newly diagnosed or severely relapsing Takayasu arteritis. The addition of methotrexate, azathioprine, mycophenolate mofetil, or TNF inhibitors is recommended for refractory disease and as corticosteroid-sparing agents; TNF inhibitors are first line. There are limited data for other biologic therapies, such as anti-IL-6 therapy (tocilizumab) and JAK inhibitors. Antiplatelets therapy is recommended for patients with active Takayasu arteritis or critical cranial or vertebrobasilar involvement. Takayasu arteritis has a chronic relapsing and remitting course that requires ongoing monitoring and adjustment of therapy.

POLYARTERITIS NODOSA

ESSENTIALS OF DIAGNOSIS

- Medium-sized arteries are affected.
- Clinical findings depend on the arteries involved; lungs are spared.
- Common features include fever, abdominal pain, extremity pain, livedo reticularis, mononeuritis multiplex.
- Kidney involvement causes renin-mediated hypertension.
- Associated with hepatitis B (10% of cases).

General Considerations

Polyarteritis nodosa is a necrotizing arteritis of medium-sized vessels that has a predilection for involving the skin, peripheral nerves, mesenteric vessels (including renal arteries), heart, and brain but spares the lungs. Polyarteritis nodosa is rare with a prevalence of 30 per 1 million people. Approximately 10% of cases of polyarteritis nodosa are caused by hepatitis B and most occur within 6 months of hepatitis B infection. Mutations in the gene for adenosine deaminase 2 have been identified in early-onset familial polyarteritis.

Clinical Findings

A. Symptoms and Signs

The clinical onset is usually insidious, with fever, malaise, weight loss, and other symptoms developing over weeks to months. Pain in the extremities is often a prominent early feature caused by arthralgia, myalgia (particularly affecting the calves), or neuropathy. Polyarteritis nodosa is one of the vasculitides most commonly associated with vasculitic neuropathy. The combination of mononeuritis multiplex (most commonly presenting with foot drop) and features of a systemic illness is one of the earliest clues to the presence of an underlying vasculitis.

In polyarteritis nodosa, the typical skin findings—livedo reticularis (Figure 23–8), subcutaneous nodules, and skin ulcers—reflect the involvement of deeper, medium-sized blood vessels. Digital gangrene is common. The most common cutaneous presentation is lower extremity ulcerations, usually occurring near the malleoli. Involvement of the renal arteries leads to a renin-mediated hypertension (much less characteristic of vasculitides involving smaller blood vessels). For unclear reasons, classic polyarteritis nodosa seldom (if ever) involves the lung, with the occasional exception of the bronchial arteries.

Abdominal pain—particularly diffuse periumbilical pain precipitated by eating—is common but often difficult to attribute to mesenteric vasculitis in the early stages.

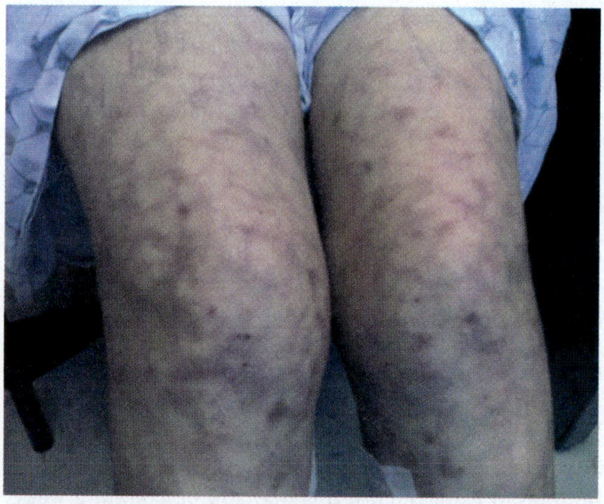

▲ **Figure 23–8.** Livedo reticularis as a manifestation of antiphospholipid antibody syndrome. (Used, with permission, from Imboden JB et al. *Current Diagnosis & Treatment: Rheumatology,* 3rd ed. McGraw-Hill, 2013.)

Nausea and vomiting are frequent symptoms. Some patients present dramatically with an acute abdomen caused by mesenteric vasculitis and gut perforation or with hypotension resulting from rupture of a microaneurysm in the liver, kidney, or bowel.

Subclinical cardiac involvement is common, and overt cardiac dysfunction may occur (eg, MI secondary to coronary vasculitis, or myocarditis).

B. Laboratory Findings

Most patients with polyarteritis nodosa have anemia and leukocytosis. Acute-phase reactants are often (but not always) strikingly elevated. There is no specific autoantibody for polyarteritis nodosa. Patients with classic polyarteritis nodosa are ANCA-negative but may have low titers of rheumatoid factor or antinuclear antibodies, both of which are nonspecific. Tests for active hepatitis B infection (HBsAg, HBeAg, hepatitis B viral load) should be performed. Patients with childhood onset of polyarteritis nodosa should undergo genetic evaluation for mutations in the genes for adenosine deaminase 2.

C. Biopsy and Angiography

The diagnosis of polyarteritis nodosa requires confirmation with either a tissue biopsy or vascular imaging. Biopsies of symptomatic sites such as skin and nerve and muscle (or both) are essential for diagnosis. A deep biopsy, not a punch biopsy, of skin ulcers or nodules should be made to ensure a medium-size artery is included in the sample. Guidelines recommend a biopsy of the nerve and muscle (instead of the nerve alone) in patients with neuropathic symptoms. Patients in whom polyarteritis nodosa is suspected—eg, based on mesenteric ischemia or new-onset hypertension occurring in the setting of a systemic illness—may be diagnosed by the angiographic finding of aneurysmal dilations in the renal, mesenteric, or hepatic arteries.

Differential Diagnosis

Genetic collagen vascular disorders (such as Ehlers-Danlos and Loeys-Dietz syndromes), fibromuscular dysplasia, and segmental arterial mediolysis should be considered when imaging findings suggest polyarteritis nodosa in the absence of other clinical features of the disorder.

Treatment

High-dose pulse methylprednisolone (eg, 1 g intravenously daily for 3 days) is recommended as the initial treatment for severe polyarteritis nodosa. Adding cyclophosphamide lowers the risk of death and morbidity in severe disease. Methotrexate or azathioprine are used to maintain remissions induced by cyclophosphamide. For patients with polyarteritis nodosa associated with hepatitis B, the preferred treatment regimen is a short course of prednisone accompanied by anti-HBV therapy and plasmapheresis (three times a week for up to 6 weeks). TNF-α inhibitors are first-line therapy for the polyarteritis associated with deficiency of adenosine deaminase 2.

Prognosis

Without treatment, the 5-year survival rate in this disorder is about 10%. With appropriate therapy, remissions are often possible and the 5-year survival rate has improved to 60–90%. Poor prognostic factors are CKD with serum creatinine > 1.6 mg/dL (141 mcmol/L), proteinuria > 1 g/day, GI ischemia, CNS disease, and cardiac involvement. In the absence of any of these five factors, 5-year survival is nearly 90%. Survival at 5 years drops to 75% with one poor prognostic factor and to about 50% with two or more factors. In contrast to many other forms of systemic vasculitis, disease relapses in polyarteritis following the successful induction of remission occur in only about 20% of cases.

GRANULOMATOSIS WITH POLYANGIITIS

ESSENTIALS OF DIAGNOSIS

- Classic triad of upper and lower respiratory tract disease and glomerulonephritis.
- Suspect if upper respiratory tract symptoms (eg, nasal congestion, sinusitis) are refractory to usual treatment.
- Kidney disease is often rapidly progressive.
- VTE commonly occurs.
- ANCAs (90% of patients), usually directed against proteinase-3 (but may be directed against myeloperoxidase).
- Tissue biopsy usually necessary for diagnosis.

General Considerations

Granulomatosis with polyangiitis (formerly Wegener granulomatosis), which has an estimated incidence of approximately 12 cases per million individuals per year, is one of three vasculitides associated with ANCA. The other "ANCA-associated vasculitides" are microscopic polyangiitis and eosinophilic granulomatosis with polyangiitis (Table 23–11). Granulomatosis with polyangiitis is characterized by vasculitis of small arteries, arterioles, and capillaries, necrotizing granulomatous lesions of both upper and lower respiratory tract, glomerulonephritis, and other vasculitic organ manifestations. Without treatment, generalized disease is invariably fatal, with most patients surviving < 1 year after diagnosis. It occurs most commonly in the fourth and fifth decades of life and affects men and women with equal frequency.

Clinical Findings

A. Symptoms and Signs

The disorder usually develops over 4–12 months. Upper respiratory tract symptoms develop in 90% of patients and lower respiratory tract symptoms develop in 60%; some patients may have both upper and lower respiratory tract symptoms. Upper respiratory tract symptoms include nasal congestion, sinusitis, otitis media, mastoiditis, inflammation of the gums, or stridor due to subglottic stenosis. Since many of these symptoms are common, the underlying disease is not often suspected until the patient develops systemic symptoms, or the original problem is refractory to treatment. The lungs are affected initially in 40% and eventually in 80%, with symptoms including cough, dyspnea, and hemoptysis. Other early symptoms can include a migratory oligoarthritis with a predilection for large joints; a variety of symptoms related to ocular disease (unilateral proptosis from orbital pseudotumor [Figure 23–9], red eye from scleritis, episcleritis, anterior uveitis, or peripheral ulcerative keratitis); purpura or other skin lesions; and dysesthesia due to peripheral neuropathy. Renal involvement, which develops in three-fourths of the cases, may be subclinical until kidney disease is advanced. Fever, malaise, and weight loss are common.

Physical examination can be remarkable for congestion, crusting, ulceration, bleeding, and even perforation of the nasal septum. Destruction of the nasal cartilage with "saddle nose" deformity occurs late. Otitis media, proptosis, scleritis, episcleritis, and conjunctivitis are other common findings. VTE events (eg, DVT and PE) are a common occurrence in granulomatosis with polyangiitis. Although limited forms of granulomatosis with polyangiitis have been described in which the kidney is spared initially, kidney disease will develop in most untreated patients.

B. Laboratory Findings

1. Serum tests and UA—Most patients have anemia, mild leukocytosis, and elevated acute-phase reactants. If there is kidney involvement, proteinuria occurs and the urinary sediment contains red cells, often with red cell casts.

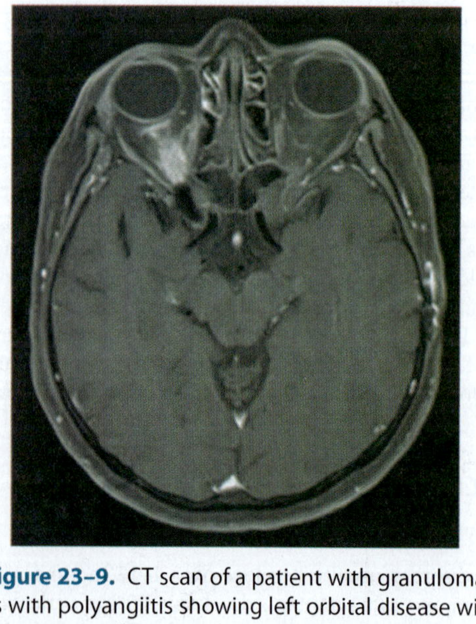

▲ **Figure 23–9.** CT scan of a patient with granulomatosis with polyangiitis showing left orbital disease with optic nerve involvement. (Used, with permission, from Vaughan DG, Asbury T, Riordan-Eva P [editors]. *General Ophthalmology,* 19th ed. McGraw-Hill, 2018.)

Serum tests for ANCA help in the diagnosis of granulomatosis with polyangiitis. ANCA levels, however, correlate erratically with disease activity, and changes in titer should not dictate changes in therapy in the absence of supporting clinical data. The two key ANCA subtypes relevant to systemic vasculitis are those directed against proteinase-3 (PR3) and myeloperoxidase (MPO). Antibodies to these two antigens are termed "PR3-ANCA" and "MPO-ANCA," respectively. The cytoplasmic pattern of immunofluorescence (c-ANCA) caused by PR3-ANCA has a high specificity (> 90%) for granulomatosis with polyangiitis but may less commonly be seen in the other forms of ANCA-associated vasculitis. A substantial percentage of patients with "limited" granulomatosis with polyangiitis, disease that does not pose an immediate threat to life and is often confined to the sinus and upper respiratory tract, are ANCA-negative. The perinuclear (p-ANCA) pattern, caused by MPO-ANCA, is more likely to occur in microscopic polyangiitis or eosinophilic granulomatosis with polyangiitis but may be found in granulomatosis with polyangiitis. Approximately 10–25% of patients with classic granulomatosis with polyangiitis have MPO-ANCA. All positive immunofluorescence assays for ANCA should be confirmed by enzyme immunoassays for the specific autoantibodies directed against PR3 or MPO.

2. Histologic findings—Although ANCA testing is helpful, most cases require diagnostic confirmation by tissue biopsy. Histologic features of granulomatosis with polyangiitis include vasculitis, granulomatous inflammation, geographic necrosis, and acute and chronic inflammation. The full range of pathologic changes is usually evident only on thoracoscopic lung biopsy; granulomas, observed only rarely in kidney biopsy specimens, are found much more commonly on lung biopsy specimens. Nasal biopsies often do not show vasculitis but may show chronic inflammation and other changes that rule out nasopharyngeal cancer or infection. Kidney biopsy discloses a segmental necrotizing glomerulonephritis with multiple crescents; this is characteristic but not diagnostic. The kidney lesion of granulomatosis with polyangiitis (and other forms of "ANCA-associated vasculitis") is characterized as a pauci-immune glomerulonephritis because of the relative absence (compared with immune complex–mediated disorders) of IgG, IgM, IgA, and complement proteins within glomeruli.

C. Imaging

Chest CT is more sensitive than CXR; lesions include infiltrates, nodules, masses, and cavities. Pleural effusions are uncommon. Often the radiographs prompt concern about lung cancer. Other common radiographic abnormalities include extensive sinusitis and even bony sinus erosions.

▶ Differential Diagnosis

Due to refractory and severe sinusitis, granulomatosis with polyangiitis may be misdiagnosed as chronic infectious sinonasal disease and treated with antibiotics alone. Initial complaints of joint pain can lead to a misdiagnosis of RA. Lung cancer may be the first diagnostic consideration for middle-aged patients with cough, hemoptysis, and lung masses. Granulomatosis with polyangiitis shares with SLE, anti–glomerular basement membrane disease, and microscopic polyangiitis the ability to cause an acute pulmonary-renal syndrome. Although both granulomatosis with polyangiitis and microscopic polyangiitis may have MPO-ANCA positivity, microscopic polyangiitis does not involve the sinuses or upper respiratory tract and does not have granulomatous inflammation on histopathology. Cocaine use can destroy midline tissues—the nose and palate—that mimics granulomatosis with polyangiitis. Patients using cocaine may have a drug-induced positive result for PR-3-ANCA, and lesional biopsies may demonstrate vasculitis from exposure to the toxin. COPA syndrome, a rare genetic autoinflammatory interferonopathy condition caused by mutations in the coatomer subunit-α gene, has many features of systemic vasculitis such as diffuse alveolar hemorrhage, glomerulonephritis, and inflammatory arthritis.

Treatment

Early treatment is crucial to prevent the devastating end-organ and catastrophic complications of this disease. Treatment is divided into two phases: induction of remission and maintenance of remission. Plasma exchange is not routinely recommended to treat ANCA-associated vasculitisPlasma exchange should not be used to treat alveolar hemorrhage in ANCA-associated vasculitis.

A. Induction of Remission

Choice of induction therapy is dictated by whether the patient has mild disease (ie, no significant kidney dysfunction) or severe disease (ie, life- or organ-threatening disease such as rapidly progressive glomerulonephritis or pulmonary hemorrhage). American College of Rheumatology/Vasculitis Foundation recommendations to treat granulomatosis with polyangiitis favor rituximab (plus corticosteroids) as first-line induction therapy, particularly for patients who are anti-PR3 positive. Cyclophosphamide also may be used for induction therapy in severe disease. Avacopan, an oral C5a receptor inhibitor, has a considerable steroid-sparing effect and is FDA-approved as add-on treatment for severe ANCA-associated vasculitis induction therapy in combination with rituximab or cyclophosphamide plus corticosteroids. Pulse corticosteroids (1 g intravenously daily for three doses) followed by an oral prednisone taper is standard for induction of remission in ANCA-vasculitis. A reduced-dose corticosteroid regimen (0.5 mg/kg/day prednisone tapered to 5 mg by week 15), has been shown to be as effective as a standard-dose corticosteroid regimen (1 mg/kg/day prednisone tapered to 5 mg by week 23) for induction in ANCA-vasculitis with fewer infections.

1. Rituximab plus prednisone (plus avacopan)—The B-cell–depleting antibody rituximab is FDA-approved in combination with corticosteroids (prednisone 1 mg/kg orally daily) to treat granulomatosis with polyangiitis and microscopic polyangiitis (Table 23–4). Studies demonstrate that rituximab is as effective as cyclophosphamide for remission induction in these conditions. Rituximab is the preferred agent (over cyclophosphamide) for induction therapy in cases of granulomatosis with polyangiitis and microscopic polyangiitis with relapsing disease.

2. Cyclophosphamide plus prednisone (plus avacopan)—Remission can be induced in > 90% of patients treated with prednisone (1 mg/kg daily) plus cyclophosphamide (2 mg/kg/day orally or 15 mg/kg intravenously every 2 weeks for three doses, then every 3 weeks for at least three doses with adjustments required for acute or CKD and patients over age 70). To minimize toxicity, patients are treated with cyclophosphamide for only 3–6 months; once remission is achieved, the patient is switched to a non-cyclophosphamide maintenance regimen.

Both rituximab and cyclophosphamide increase the risk of developing life-threatening opportunistic infections (including progressive multifocal leukoencephalopathy [PML]). *Whenever cyclophosphamide or rituximab is used,* Pneumocystis jirovecii *prophylaxis with one single-strength oral trimethoprim-sulfamethoxazole daily is essential.*

3. Methotrexate plus prednisone—For nonsevere disease without life- or organ-threatening manifestations, methotrexate up to 25 mg orally or subcutaneously weekly, plus prednisone up to 1 mg/kg orally daily may be effective induction therapy. If there is an intolerance or contraindication to methotrexate, mycophenolate mofetil can be used as a second-line induction therapy for nonsevere disease.

B. Maintenance of Remission

Options for maintaining remission in patients with normal or near normal kidney function after rituximab or cyclophosphamide induction include rituximab (500 mg intravenously every 6 months for at least 2 years), azathioprine (up to 2 mg/kg/day orally), methotrexate (20–25 mg/week either orally or subcutaneously), or mycophenolate mofetil (Table 23–4). Per treatment guidelines, intravenous rituximab is favored as first-line maintenance treatment.

When to Refer

All patients should be referred to a rheumatologist; other subspecialty consultations may also be appropriate.

When to Admit

Admit for organ- or life-threatening disease, including alveolar hemorrhage or rapidly progressive glomerulonephritis.

Hellmich B et al. EULAR recommendations for the management of ANCA-associated vasculitis: 2022 update. Ann Rheum Dis. 2024;83:30. [PMID: 36927642]

MICROSCOPIC POLYANGIITIS

ESSENTIALS OF DIAGNOSIS

- Necrotizing vasculitis of small- and medium-sized arteries and veins.
- Most common cause of pulmonary-renal syndrome (diffuse alveolar hemorrhage and glomerulonephritis).
- +p-ANCA (anti-MPO) in 75% of cases.

General Considerations

Microscopic polyangiitis is a pauci-immune nongranulomatous necrotizing vasculitis that (1) affects small blood vessels (capillaries, venules, or arterioles), (2) often causes glomerulonephritis and pulmonary capillaritis, and (3) is often associated with ANCA. Because microscopic polyangiitis may involve medium-sized as well as small blood vessels and because it tends to affect capillaries within the lungs and kidneys, its spectrum overlaps those of both polyarteritis nodosa and granulomatosis with polyangiitis.

In rare instances, medications, particularly propylthiouracil, hydralazine, allopurinol, penicillamine, minocycline, and sulfasalazine, induce a systemic vasculitis associated with high titers of p-ANCA (may be an atypical ANCA) and features of microscopic polyangiitis.

Clinical Findings

A. Symptoms and Signs

A wide variety of findings suggesting vasculitis of small blood vessels may develop in microscopic polyangiitis. These include "palpable" (or "raised") purpura and other signs of cutaneous vasculitis (ulcers, splinter hemorrhages, vesiculobullous lesions).

Microscopic polyangiitis is the most common cause of pulmonary-renal syndromes, being several times more common than anti–glomerular basement membrane disease. Pulmonary hemorrhage may occur with pathologic findings typically of capillaritis. Interstitial lung fibrosis that mimics usual interstitial pneumonitis may be part of the presenting condition and conveys a poor prognosis.

Vasculitic neuropathy (mononeuritis multiplex) is also common in microscopic polyangiitis.

B. Laboratory Findings

Three-fourths of patients with microscopic polyangiitis are ANCA-positive, usually with anti-myeloperoxidase antibodies (anti-MPO-ANCA) that cause a p-ANCA pattern on immunofluorescence testing. ANCA directed against proteinase-3 (PR3-ANCA) can also be observed.

Elevated acute-phase reactants are typical of active disease. Microscopic hematuria, proteinuria, and RBC casts in the urine may occur. The kidney lesion is a segmental, necrotizing glomerulonephritis, often with localized intravascular coagulation and the observation of intraglomerular thrombi upon renal biopsy.

Differential Diagnosis

Distinguishing this disease from granulomatosis with polyangiitis may be challenging. In microscopic polyangiitis, there is no granulomatous inflammation and it is not associated with the chronic destructive upper respiratory tract disease often found in granulomatosis with polyangiitis. Because their treatments may differ, microscopic polyangiitis must also be differentiated from polyarteritis nodosa. COPA syndrome is a rare, genetic, multisystem, autoinflammatory disorder with recurrent pulmonary hemorrhage that mimics microscopic polyangiitis. There may be autoantibodies. COPA often presents in childhood, usually with a striking family history.

Treatment

Microscopic polyangiitis is usually treated in the same way as granulomatosis with polyangiitis: patients with severe disease, typically involving pulmonary hemorrhage and glomerulonephritis, require urgent induction treatment with corticosteroids, avacopan, and either rituximab or cyclophosphamide. Following successful induction of remission, maintenance treatment should be continued with rituximab, as first line, or azathioprine, methotrexate, or mycophenolate (all second-line maintenance therapy). In cases of drug-induced MPO-ANCA–associated vasculitis, the offending medication should be discontinued; significant organ involvement (eg, pulmonary hemorrhage, glomerulonephritis) requires immunosuppressive therapy.

Prognosis

The key to effecting good outcomes is early diagnosis. Compared with patients who have granulomatosis with polyangiitis, those who have microscopic polyangiitis are more likely to have significant fibrosis on renal biopsy because of later diagnosis.

Kronbichler A et al. Diagnosis and management of ANCA-associated vasculitis. Lancet. 2024;403:683. [PMID: 38368016]
Merkel PA et al. Safety of avacopan for the treatment of antineutrophil cytoplasmic antibody-associated vasculitis: combined data from three clinical trials. ACR Open Rheumatol. 2025;7:e70001. [PMID: 40192160]

EOSINOPHILIC GRANULOMATOSIS WITH POLYANGIITIS

ESSENTIALS OF DIAGNOSIS

- **Nonvasculitic manifestations:** sinusitis with polyposis, asthma, transient pulmonary infiltrates
- **Vasculitic manifestations:** necrotizing, granulomatous inflammation, mononeuritis multiplex, rash, glomerulonephritis
- Peripheral eosinophilia is often present
- Eosinophilic infiltration of tissue may be seen on biopsy
- Cardiac involvement (myocarditis, coronary arteritis) is associated with high mortality
- 30-40% ANCA-positive, most commonly anti-MPO

General Considerations

Eosinophilic granulomatosis with polyangiitis (previously called Churg-Strauss syndrome) is an ANCA-associated vasculitis (along with granulomatosis with polyangiitis and microscopic polyangiitis), although the presence of ANCA occurs in < 50% of patients (usually anti-MPO).

Clinical Findings

Eosinophilic granulomatosis with polyangiitis is characterized by peripheral eosinophilia, sinusitis with polyposis, asthma, lung infiltrates, vasculitic skin involvement, glomerulonephritis, and vasculitic neuropathy. Myocarditis can lead to arrhythmias and HF if untreated. Coronary artery vasculitis can lead to myocardial ischemia. Eosinophilic granulomatosis with polyangiitis should be considered in patients with an unexplained peripheral eosinophilia (> 1000 cells/mcL [1.0×10^9/L]) and vasculitis. Laboratory workup for unexplained eosinophilia should include ANCA testing, serum tryptase levels, peripheral flow cytometry for platelet-derived growth factor (PDGF) receptor abnormalities (which can be seen in eosinophilic leukemia), and testing for helminthic infections. Eosinophilic infiltrates on tissue samples (skin, nerve, muscle, nasal polyps) strongly suggest the diagnosis of eosinophilic granulomatosis with polyangiitis, especially if accompanied by vasculitis (purpura, glomerulonephritis, vasculitic ulcers, mononeuritis multiplex).

Treatment

Prednisone (0.5–1mg/kg orally daily) remains first-line treatment with azathioprine and methotrexate demonstrating efficacy for mild to moderate disease. Mepolizumab and benralizumab are IL-5 inhibitors FDA-approved to treat eosinophilic granulomatosis with polyangiitis; guidelines recommend their use for relapsed or nonsevere disease. For severe life- or organ-threatening vasculitic manifestations (cardiac, renal, mononeuritis) or for patients with poor prognostic features (age > 65 years, gastrointestinal manifestations, lack of ear, nose, throat manifestations), induction therapy should be initiated with pulse solumedrol (1g intravenously daily for 3 days) and cyclophosphamide followed by maintenance therapy with azathioprine, methotrexate or mycophenolate mofetil. Rituximab may be considered for induction therapy, maintenance therapy, or both.

Wechsler ME et al. Benralizumab versus mepolizumab for eosinophilic granulomatosis with polyangiitis. N Engl J Med. 2024;390:911. [PMID: 38393328]

CRYOGLOBULINEMIA

Cryoglobulinemia can be associated with an immune-complex–mediated, small and medium vessel vasculitis. The cryoglobulins associated with vasculitis are cold-precipitable immune complexes consisting of rheumatoid factor and IgG (rheumatoid factor is an autoantibody to the constant region of IgG). The rheumatoid factor component can be monoclonal (type II cryoglobulins) or polyclonal (type III cryoglobulins). Type I cryoglobulins are cryoprecipitable monoclonal proteins that lack rheumatoid factor activity; these cause cold-induced hyperviscosity syndromes, not vasculitis, and are associated with B-cell lymphoproliferative diseases. Type II and Type III cryoglobulinemias are associated with chronic infections (hepatitis C, subacute bacterial endocarditis, osteomyelitis, HIV, and hepatitis B) or connective tissue diseases (especially Sjögren disease).

Clinical Findings

Cryoglobulinemic vasculitis typically manifests as recurrent palpable purpura (predominantly on the lower extremities) and peripheral neuropathy. A proliferative glomerulonephritis may develop and can manifest as rapidly progressive glomerulonephritis. Abnormal liver biochemical tests, abdominal pain, digital gangrene, and pulmonary disease may also occur. The diagnosis is based on a compatible clinical picture and a positive serum test for cryoglobulins. The presence of a disproportionately low C4 level or rheumatoid factor or both can be diagnostic clues to the presence of cryoglobulinemia.

Treatment

Antiviral regimens are first-line therapy for hepatitis C–associated cryoglobulinemic vasculitis that is neither life- nor organ-threatening. Interferon-free direct-acting antiviral agents are preferred because of the excellent long-term response in clinical trials. Patients with severe cryoglobulinemic vasculitis (eg, extensive digital gangrene, extensive neuropathy, and rapidly progressive glomerulonephritis) and hepatitis C should receive immunosuppressive therapy with corticosteroids and either rituximab or cyclophosphamide plus antiviral treatment. Plasma exchange may provide additional benefit in selected cases.

Cacoub P et al. Cryoglobulinemia - one name for two diseases. N Engl J Med. 2024;391:1426. [PMID: 39413378]

IgA VASCULITIS (Henoch-Schönlein Purpura)

IgA vasculitis (Henoch-Schönlein purpura), the most common systemic vasculitis in children, occurs in adults as well. Typical clinical features are palpable purpura, arthritis, and hematuria. Abdominal pain occurs less frequently in adults than in children. Pathologic features on skin biopsy include leukocytoclastic vasculitis with IgA deposition. Biopsy of the kidney reveals segmental glomerulonephritis with crescents and mesangial deposition of IgA. The cause is not known.

The purpuric skin lesions are typically located on the lower extremities but may also be seen on the hands, arms, trunk, and buttocks. Joint symptoms are present in most patients, with the knees and ankles being most commonly involved. Abdominal pain secondary to vasculitis of the intestinal tract is often associated with GI bleeding. Children tend to have more frequent and more serious GI vasculitis, whereas adults (especially if aged ≥ 65 years) more often have glomerulonephritis and severe renal disease. Chronic courses with persistent or intermittent skin disease are more likely to occur in adults than in children.

The value of corticosteroids has been controversial. Severe disease in adults is often treated with immunosuppressive agents, such as rituximab or mycophenolate mofetil, but there is no consensus regarding the efficacy of this approach or optimal therapeutic regimen.

Stanway J et al. IgA vasculitis nephritis-outcomes in adult-onset disease. Rheumatology (Oxford). 2025;64:690. [PMID: 38273659]

RELAPSING POLYCHONDRITIS

This disease is characterized by inflammatory destructive lesions of cartilaginous structures, principally the ears, nose, trachea, and larynx (Figure 23–10). Nearly 40% of cases are associated with another disease, especially other immunologic disorders (ANCA-vasculitis, SLE, RA, or Hashimoto thyroiditis), cancers (plasma cell myeloma), or hematologic disorders (myelodysplastic syndrome). Relapsing polychondritis is episodic and affects men and women equally. The cartilage is painful, swollen, and tender during an attack and subsequently becomes atrophic, resulting in permanent deformity. Biopsy of the involved cartilage shows inflammation and chondrolysis. Laryngotracheal and bronchial chondritis can lead to life-threatening airway narrowing and collapse. Noncartilaginous manifestations of the disease include fever, episcleritis, uveitis, deafness, aortic regurgitation, inflammatory arthritis, and rarely, glomerulonephritis. Large-vessel vasculitis is a frequently overlooked but potentially catastrophic complication. Diagnosing this uncommon disease is especially difficult since the signs of cartilage inflammation (such as red ears or nasal pain) may be more subtle than the fever, arthritis, rash, or other systemic manifestations, and there are no serologic markers.

Prednisone, 0.5–1 mg/kg/day orally, is often effective. Dapsone (100–200 mg/day orally) or methotrexate (7.5–20 mg orally per week) may also have efficacy, sparing the need for long-term high-dose corticosteroid treatment. Involvement of the tracheobronchial tree may respond to inhibitors of TNF.

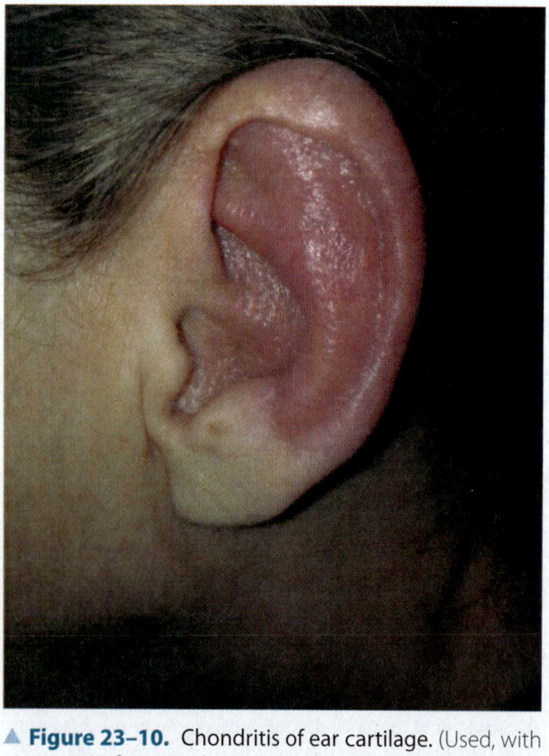

▲ **Figure 23–10.** Chondritis of ear cartilage. (Used, with permission, from Sarah Goglin, MD.)

The genetic syndrome VEXAS (vacuoles, E1 enzyme, X-linked, autoinflammatory, somatic) is caused by somatic mutations in *UBA1* in hematopoietic progenitor cells. Clinical features include hematologic manifestations (cytopenias, macrocytosis, bone marrow failure) and a spectrum of inflammatory findings such as chondritis, vasculitis, fever, and arthritis. This rare syndrome (predominately in males because it is X-linked) should be considered in the differential diagnosis of chondritis, especially in the presence of an unexplained macrocytosis and evidence of systemic inflammation (ie, high ESR/CRP).

Yang R et al. Clinical manifestations and treatment in patients with relapsing polychondritis: a multicenter observational cohort study. ACR Open Rheumatol. 2025;7:e70027. [PMID: 40391876]

BEHÇET DISEASE

ESSENTIALS OF DIAGNOSIS

- Recurrent, painful oral and genital aphthous ulcers.
- Erythema nodosum–like lesions; follicular rash; pathergy phenomenon.
- Anterior or posterior uveitis. Posterior uveitis may be asymptomatic until significant damage to the retina has occurred.
- Neurologic lesions can mimic multiple sclerosis.

General Considerations

Named after the Turkish dermatologist who first described it, Behçet disease is of unknown cause and most commonly occurs in persons of Asian, Turkish, or Middle Eastern background. The protean manifestations result from vasculitis that may involve all types of blood vessels: small, medium, and large, on both the arterial and venous side of the circulation. The hypercoagulability that can occur with Behçet disease is associated with systemic inflammation and disease activity.

Clinical Findings

A. Symptoms and Signs

The hallmark of Behçet disease is painful aphthous ulcerations in the mouth. These lesions, which usually are multiple, may be found on the tongue, gums, and inner surfaces of the oral cavity. Genital lesions, similar in appearance, are common but do not occur in all patients. Other key cutaneous lesions of Behçet disease include tender, erythematous, papular lesions that resemble erythema nodosum, and papulopustular lesions. On biopsy, however, many of these lesions are shown to be secondary to vasculitis rather than septal panniculitis. These erythema nodosum–like lesions tend to ulcerate, which is a major difference between the lesions of Behçet disease and the erythema nodosum seen in sarcoidosis and IBD. An erythematous follicular rash that occurs frequently on the upper extremities may be a subtle feature of the disease. The **pathergy phenomenon** is highly specific for Behçet, although not pathognomonic. In this phenomenon, sterile pustules develop at sites where needles have been inserted into the skin (eg, for phlebotomy).

Nonerosive inflammatory arthritis occurs in about two-thirds of patients most commonly affecting the knees and ankles. Eye involvement is one of the most devastating complications of Behçet disease. Anterior uveitis, associated with the triad of photophobia, blurred vision, and a red eye, is intensely symptomatic. This complication may lead to a hypopyon, the accumulation of pus in the anterior chamber. Posterior uveitis, as a retinal venulitis, may lead to the insidious destruction of large areas of the retina before the patient becomes aware of visual problems.

CNS involvement can cause major morbidity. Findings include sterile meningitis (recurrent meningeal headaches associated with a lymphocytic pleocytosis), cranial nerve palsies, seizures, encephalitis, sinus vein thrombosis, and spinal cord lesions. The CNS lesions may mimic multiple sclerosis radiologically. Aphthous ulcerations of the ileum and cecum and other forms of GI involvement develop in approximately a quarter of patients. Large-vessel vasculitis can lead to pulmonary artery aneurysms and life-threatening pulmonary hemorrhage. Finally, patients have a hypercoagulable tendency that may lead to complicated VTE events, particularly DVT, PE, or cerebral sinus thrombosis.

The clinical course may be chronic but is often characterized by remissions and exacerbations.

B. Laboratory Findings

There are no pathognomonic laboratory features of Behçet disease. Acute-phase reactants are often elevated, and there is no disease specific autoantibody. Behçet disease has a genetic risk factor (HLA B51), but this gene is neither necessary nor sufficient to cause the disease.

Differential Diagnosis

The differential diagnosis for oral ulcerations is broad and includes other forms of vasculitis (ANCA-associated), IBD, celiac disease, IgA deficiency, infections (HIV, histoplasmosis), complex aphthosis, and mucosal skin conditions (pemphigus vulgaris, lichen planus, mucous membrane pemphigoid).

Treatment

Both colchicine (0.6 mg once to three times daily orally) and topical corticosteroids (oral dexamethasone suspension 1 mg twice daily swish and spit of 0.5 mg/5 mL) may ameliorate mucocutaneous ulcerative symptoms. Apremilast, a selective phosphodiesterase-4 inhibitor, is FDA-approved to treat oral ulcers in Behçet disease. Corticosteroids (1 mg/kg/day of oral prednisone) are a mainstay of initial therapy for severe disease manifestations. Azathioprine (2 mg/kg/day orally) may be an effective steroid-sparing agent. TNF-α inhibitors (infliximab, adalimumab) (Table 23–4) or cyclophosphamide are indicated for severe ocular and CNS complications of Behçet disease.

Hatemi G et al. Behçet's syndrome: one year in review 2025. Clin Exp Rheumatol. 2025;43:1699. [PMID: 41133359]

PRIMARY ANGIITIS OF THE CENTRAL NERVOUS SYSTEM

Primary angiitis of the CNS is a rare syndrome that produces small- and medium-sized vasculitis limited to the brain and spinal cord. Biopsy-proved cases have predominated in men who have a history of weeks to months of headaches, encephalopathy, and multifocal strokes. Systemic symptoms and signs are absent, and routine laboratory tests, including ESR, CRP and autoantibodies, are normal. MRI of the brain is almost always abnormal (multiterritorial, bilateral, distal acute stroke lesions) and may also show mass-like lesions. The spinal fluid often reveals a mild lymphocytosis and a modest increase in protein level. Cerebral angiograms classically reveal a "string of beads" pattern produced by alternating segments of arterial narrowing and dilation. However, neither the MRI nor the angiogram appearance is specific for vasculitis. Several conditions, including vasospasm, can produce the same angiographic pattern as vasculitis. Definitive diagnosis requires a compatible clinical picture with exclusion of infection (subacute bacterial endocarditis, syphilis, aspergillosis), neoplasm (especially intravascular lymphoma), genetic conditions (retinal vasculopathy with cerebral leukoencephalopathy and systemic manifestations) or drug exposure (cocaine) that can mimic primary angiitis of the CNS *and* a positive brain biopsy. In contrast to biopsy-proved cases, patients with angiographically defined CNS vasculopathy are chiefly women who have had an abrupt onset of headaches and stroke (often in the absence of encephalopathy) with normal spinal fluid findings. Many patients who fit this clinical profile may have reversible cerebral vasoconstriction rather than true vasculitis. Such cases are best treated with calcium channel blockers (such as nimodipine or verapamil). Biopsy-proven cases of primary angiitis of the CNS usually improve with corticosteroids, but often cyclophosphamide or mycophenolate mofetil is required to induce and maintain remission. Treatment response correlates with the size of arteries involved: vasculitis of small cortical and leptomeningeal vessels is associated with a better response and outcome than vasculitis of larger arteries.

Salvarani C et al. Primary central nervous system vasculitis. N Engl J Med. 2024;391:1028. [PMID: 39292929]

LIVEDO RETICULARIS & LIVEDO RACEMOSA

Livedo reticularis produces a mottled, purplish discoloration of the skin with reticulated cyanotic areas surrounding paler central cores (Figure 23–8). This distinctive "fishnet" pattern is caused by spasm or obstruction of perpendicular arterioles, combined with pooling of blood in surrounding venous plexuses. Idiopathic primary livedo reticularis is a benign condition that worsens with cold exposure, improves with warming, and primarily affects the extremities. Apart from cosmetic concerns, it is usually asymptomatic. The presence of systemic symptoms or the development of cutaneous ulcerations suggests an underlying disease. Livedo reticularis must be distinguished from erythema ab igne, a benign cutaneous disorder caused by exposure to infrared heat source, such as that generated from a heating pad or laptop computer.

Secondary livedo reticularis, called livedo racemosa, occurs with diseases that cause vascular obstruction or inflammation. Livedo racemosa resembles idiopathic livedo reticularis but has a wider skin distribution, including trunk, buttocks, and extremities. Of particular importance is the link with antiphospholipid antibody syndrome. Livedo racemosa is the presenting manifestation in 25% of patients with antiphospholipid antibody syndrome and is strongly associated with the subgroup that has arterial thromboses. Other underlying causes of livedo racemosa include the vasculitides (particularly polyarteritis nodosa), cholesterol emboli syndrome, thrombocythemia, cryoglobulinemia, cold agglutinin disease, primary hyperoxaluria (due to vascular deposits of calcium oxalate), and disseminated intravascular coagulation.

SERONEGATIVE SPONDYLOARTHROPATHIES

The seronegative spondyloarthropathies include axial spondyloarthropathy (radiographic ankylosing spondylitis and nonradiographic), psoriatic arthritis, reactive arthritis, the arthritis associated with IBD, and undifferentiated spondyloarthropathy. In addition to axial inflammation, these disorders share features of asymmetric oligoarthritis of large peripheral joints, enthesopathy (inflammation at the point where ligaments, tendons, and joint capsule insert into bone), ocular inflammation, the absence of autoantibodies, and a striking association with HLA-B27. HLA-B27 is positive in up to 90% of patients with ankylosing spondylitis and 75% with reactive arthritis. HLA-B27 also occurs in 50% of patients with psoriatic arthritis and IBD who have sacroiliitis. Patients with only peripheral arthritis in these latter two syndromes do not show an increase in HLA-B27.

AXIAL SPONDYLOARTHRITIS

ESSENTIALS OF DIAGNOSIS

- Inflammatory back pain: chronic low backache and stiffness in young adults (onset age < 45 years), worst in the morning.
- Progressive limitation of back motion and chest expansion.
- Transient (50%) or persistent (25%) peripheral arthritis of large joints.
- Anterior uveitis in 20–25%.
- Negative serologic tests for rheumatoid factor and anti-CCP antibodies.
- HLA-B27 testing is most helpful when there is an intermediate probability of disease.

General Considerations

Axial spondyloarthritis (axSpA) is a chronic inflammatory disease of the joints of the axial skeleton, manifested clinically by pain and progressive fusion of the spine. axSpA can be radiographic (diagnostic changes of sacroiliac joints or spine visible on plain radiograph) or nonradiographic (axial inflammation [sacroiliitis] is only visualized by MRI). This classification more likely represents a spectrum of disease rather than distinct conditions. Radiographic axSpA has historically been named ankylosing spondylitis, although this nomenclature does not distinguish between the radiographic and nonradiographic forms of the disease. The age at onset is usually in the late teens or early 20s. The incidence is greater in males than in females.

Clinical Findings

A. Symptoms and Signs

The onset of axSpA is usually gradual, with intermittent bouts of back pain that may radiate into the buttocks. The back pain has an "inflammatory quality." It is worse in the morning and associated with profound stiffness that lasts hours. Pain and stiffness improve with activity, in contrast to back pain due to mechanical causes, which improves with rest and worsens with activity. As the disease advances, symptoms progress in a cephalad direction and back motion becomes limited, with the normal lumbar curve flattened and the thoracic curvature exaggerated. Chest expansion is often limited due to costovertebral joint involvement. In advanced cases, the entire spine becomes fused, allowing no motion in any direction. Acute arthritis of large peripheral joints occurs in about 50% of cases, and permanent changes in the peripheral joints—most commonly the hips, shoulders, and knees—are seen in about 25%. Enthesopathy, a hallmark of the spondyloarthropathies, can manifest as swelling of the Achilles tendon at its insertion, plantar fasciitis (producing heel pain), or dactylitis, which is fusiform "sausage" swelling of a finger or toe.

Anterior uveitis occurs in up to 25% of cases and may be a presenting feature of axSpA. Cardiac involvement, characterized by atrioventricular conduction defects, aortic regurgitation, or aortic root widening, occurs in 3–5% of patients with long-standing severe disease. Pulmonary fibrosis of the upper lobes, with progression to cavitation and bronchiectasis, mimicking tuberculosis, may rarely occur long after the onset of skeletal symptoms.

B. Laboratory Findings

ESR is elevated in 85% of cases, and autoantibodies are negative. Anemia of chronic inflammation may be present but is often mild. HLA-B27 is found in 90% of White and 50% of Black patients with axSpA. Because this antigen occurs in 8% of healthy White persons and 2% of healthy Black persons, it is not a specific diagnostic test and is most useful when there is intermediate probability of disease.

C. Imaging

The earliest radiographic changes are usually in the sacroiliac joints. Between 10% and 25% of patients with nonradiographic axial spondyloarthropathy will progress to radiographic spondyloarthropathy (erosion and sclerosis of sacroiliac joints on radiograph) within 10 years. The sacroiliitis of ankylosing spondylitis is bilateral and symmetric. Inflammation where the annulus fibrosus attaches to the vertebral bodies initially causes sclerosis ("the shiny corner sign") and then characteristic squaring of the vertebral bodies. "Bamboo spine" describes the late radiographic appearance of the spinal column in which the vertebral bodies are fused by vertically oriented, bridging syndesmophytes formed by ossification of the annulus fibrosus and calcification of the anterior and lateral spinal ligaments.

Differential Diagnosis

Low back pain due to mechanical causes, disk disease, and osteoarthritis are very common. RA predominantly affects multiple, small, peripheral joints of the hands and feet. RA spares the sacroiliac joints and only affects the cervical component of the spine. Bilateral sacroiliitis indistinguishable from ankylosing spondylitis is seen with spondyloarthropathy associated with IBD. Sacroiliitis associated with reactive arthritis and psoriasis is often asymmetric or even unilateral. Osteitis condensans ilii (sclerosis on the iliac side of the sacroiliac joint) is an asymptomatic, postpartum radiographic finding that is occasionally mistaken for sacroiliitis. Diffuse idiopathic skeletal hyperostosis (DISH) causes exuberant osteophytes ("enthesophytes") of the spine that may be difficult to distinguish from the syndesmophytes of ankylosing spondylitis.

Treatment

NSAIDs remain first-line treatment of axSpA (Table 5–4). TNF inhibitors have well-established efficacy for NSAID-resistant axial disease; responses are often substantial and durable. TNF inhibitors have disease-modifying effects and slow radiographic progression (Table 23–4). Secukinumab and ixekizumab (monoclonal antibodies against soluble IL-17A), bimekizumab (anti-IL17A/F) and tofacitinib and upadacitinib (small-molecule JAK inhibitors) are highly effective and FDA-approved to treat radiographic and nonradiographic axSpA. Sulfasalazine (1000 mg orally twice daily) may be useful for peripheral arthritis but lacks effectiveness for spinal and sacroiliac joint disease. Corticosteroids have minimal impact in ankylosing spondylitis and can worsen osteopenia.

Prognosis

Most patients have persistent symptoms over decades; rare individuals experience long-term remissions. The severity of disease varies greatly, with about 10% of patients having work disability after 10 years. Biologic agents provide symptomatic relief, improve quality of life, and slow disease progression for many patients with axial spondyloarthritis.

When to Refer

- Early referral to a rheumatologist is essential for diagnosis and initiation of effective therapy to prevent damage.
- Refer to an ophthalmologist for symptoms of uveitis.
- All patients should be referred to a physical therapist for instruction in postural exercises and a safe exercise program.

Maksymowych WP et al. Features of axial spondyloarthritis in two multicenter cohorts of patients with psoriasis, uveitis, and colitis presenting with undiagnosed back pain. Arthritis Rheumatol. 2025;77:17. [PMID: 39107875]

PSORIATIC ARTHRITIS

ESSENTIALS OF DIAGNOSIS

- Psoriasis precedes arthritis in 80% of cases.
- **Arthritis:** usually asymmetric, with "sausage" appearance of fingers and toes (dactylitis); polyarthritis that may resemble RA.
- Sacroiliac joint involvement common.
- **Radiographic findings:** osteolysis; pencil-in-cup deformity; relative lack of osteoporosis; bony ankylosis; asymmetric sacroiliitis and atypical syndesmophytes.

General Considerations

Although psoriasis usually precedes the onset of arthritis, arthritis may precede skin disease by up to 2 years or occur simultaneously in approximately 20% of cases.

Clinical Findings

A. Symptoms and Signs

The multiple patterns or subsets of joint involvement in psoriatic arthritis include the following:

1. A symmetric polyarthritis that resembles RA but, usually, fewer joints are involved.
2. An oligoarthritis that may lead to considerable destruction of the affected joints.
3. The DIP joints are primarily affected. Early, this may be monoarticular, and often the joint involvement is asymmetric. Nail pitting and onycholysis frequently accompany DIP involvement.
4. A severe deforming arthritis (arthritis mutilans) with osteolysis.
5. A spondylitic form in which sacroiliitis and spinal involvement predominate; 50% of these patients are HLA-B27 positive.

Arthritis is at least five times more common in patients with severe psoriatic skin disease than in those with only mild skin findings. Occasionally, however, patients may have a single patch of psoriasis (typically hidden in the scalp, gluteal cleft, or umbilicus) and are unaware of its presence. Thus, a detailed search for cutaneous lesions is essential in patients with arthritis of new onset. Also, the psoriatic lesions may have cleared when arthritis appears—in such cases, the history is most useful in diagnosing previously unexplained cases of monoarthritis or oligoarthritis. Nail pitting is sometimes a clue. "Sausage" swelling, or dactylitis, of one or more digits is a common manifestation of enthesopathy in psoriatic arthritis. Uveitis or IBD (or both) may occur in psoriatic arthritis and will influence treatment options.

B. Laboratory Findings

The ESR is elevated in approximately 50% of patients with psoriatic arthritis; normal values do not rule out the diagnosis. Rheumatoid factor and anti-CCP antibodies are not present. Uric acid levels may be high, reflecting the active turnover of skin affected by psoriasis.

C. Imaging

Radiographic findings are most helpful in distinguishing the disease from other forms of arthritis. There are marginal erosions of bone and irregular destruction of joint and bone, which, in the phalanx, gives the appearance of a sharpened pencil. Fluffy periosteal new bone may be marked, especially at the insertion of muscles and ligaments into bone. Such changes will also be seen along the shafts of metacarpals, metatarsals, and phalanges. Psoriatic spondylitis causes asymmetric sacroiliitis.

Treatment

Guidelines for the treatment of psoriatic arthritis recommend a "domain-based" approach (peripheral arthritis, axial disease, enthesitis, dactylitis, skin psoriasis, nail disease, IBD, uveitis) and outline therapeutic options specific to each "domain." A patient may have activity in some, but not all, domains and treatment should be tailored as such. For musculoskeletal and cutaneous domains of psoriatic arthritis, TNF inhibitors, IL-12/23 inhibitors (ustekinumab), IL-17 inhibitors (secukinumab, ixekizumab, brodalumab, bimekizumab), IL-23 inhibitors (guselkumab, risankizumab), phosphodiesterase 4 inhibitors (apremilast), and JAK inhibitors (tofacitinib, upadacitinib) are recommended (Table 23–4). For axial disease, TNF inhibitors, anti-IL-17, and JAK inhibitors are specifically recommended. For nonaxial domains of psoriatic arthritis and skin, conventional DMARDs, specifically methotrexate, may be considered.

Corticosteroids are less effective in psoriatic arthritis than in other forms of inflammatory arthritis and may precipitate pustular psoriasis during tapers.

REACTIVE ARTHRITIS

ESSENTIALS OF DIAGNOSIS

- Oligoarthritis, conjunctivitis, urethritis, keratoderma blennorrhagicum, and mouth ulcers.
- Usually follows dysentery or a sexually transmitted infection.
- HLA-B27–positive in 50–80% of patients.

General Considerations

Reactive arthritis is precipitated by antecedent GI or genitourinary infections and manifests as an asymmetric sterile oligoarthritis, typically of the lower extremities. It is frequently associated with enthesitis. Extra-articular manifestations are common and include urethritis, conjunctivitis, uveitis, keratoderma blennorrhagicum, and mucocutaneous lesions. Reactive arthritis occurs most commonly in young men and is associated with HLA-B27 in 80% of White patients and 50–60% of Black patients.

Clinical Findings

Most cases of reactive arthritis develop within 1–4 weeks after either a GI infection (usually with *Shigella, Salmonella, Yersinia,* or *Campylobacter*) or a sexually transmitted infection (with *Chlamydia trachomatis* or perhaps *Ureaplasma urealyticum*). Whether the inciting infection is sexually transmitted or dysenteric does not affect the subsequent manifestations. Other pathogens known to cause reactive arthritis include *Mycobacterium*, *Streptococcus*, *Staphylococcus*, and SARS-CoV-2. Synovial fluid from affected joints is culture negative. A clinically indistinguishable syndrome can occur without an apparent antecedent infection, suggesting that subclinical infection can precipitate reactive arthritis or that there are other, as yet unrecognized, triggers.

The arthritis is most commonly asymmetric and frequently involves the large weight-bearing joints (knee and ankle); sacroiliitis or ankylosing spondylitis is observed in at least 20% of patients, especially after frequent recurrences. Systemic symptoms including fever and weight loss are common at the onset of disease. The mucocutaneous lesions may include balanitis (Figure 23–11), stomatitis, and keratoderma blennorrhagicum, indistinguishable from pustular psoriasis. Involvement of the fingernails in reactive arthritis mimics psoriatic changes. When present, conjunctivitis is mild and occurs early in the disease course. Anterior uveitis, which can develop at any time in

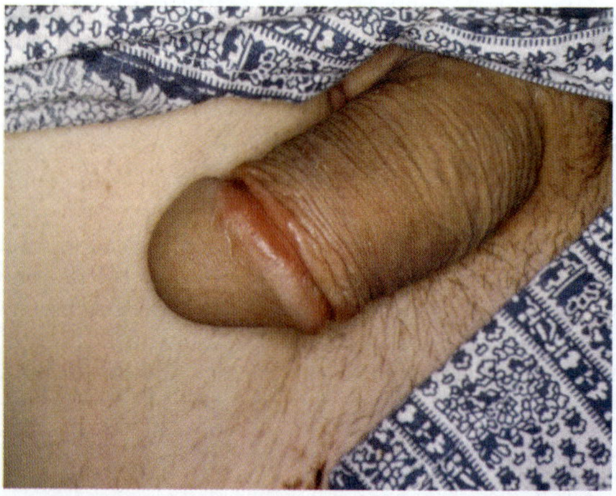

Figure 23–11. Circinate balanitis due to reactive arthritis. (From Susan Lindsley, Dr. M. F. Rein, Public Health Image Library, CDC.)

HLA-B27–positive patients, is a more clinically significant ocular complication. Carditis and aortic regurgitation may occur. While most signs of the disease disappear within days or weeks, the arthritis may persist for several months or become chronic. Recurrences involving any combination of clinical manifestations are common and are sometimes followed by permanent sequelae, especially in the joints (eg, articular destruction).

Differential Diagnosis

Gonococcal arthritis can initially mimic reactive arthritis, but the marked improvement after 24–48 hours of antibiotic administration in gonococcal arthritis and the culture results distinguish the two disorders. New-onset RA, axial spondyloarthritis, and psoriatic arthritis must be considered. By causing similar oral, ocular, and joint lesions, Behçet disease may mimic reactive arthritis. The oral lesions of reactive arthritis, however, are typically painless, in contrast to those of Behçet disease.

Treatment

NSAIDs are the mainstay of therapy (Table 5–4). Antibiotics given at the time of a nongonococcal sexually transmitted infection reduce the chance that reactive arthritis will develop. For chronic reactive arthritis associated with chlamydial infection, a randomized trial demonstrated that 6 months of rifampin (300 mg orally twice daily) in combination with either doxycycline (100 mg orally twice daily) or azithromycin (500 mg orally daily for 5 days then twice weekly) was more effective than placebo. Patients who do not respond to NSAIDs may respond to the DMARDs sulfasalazine (1 g orally twice daily) or methotrexate (up to 25 mg oral or subcutaneous once weekly). Duration of treatment is highly variable and dependent on severity of manifestations and clinical course. For patients with recent-onset disease that is refractory to NSAIDs and traditional DMARDs, anti-TNF agents or other biologics (eg, IL-17 inhibitors), which are effective in the other spondyloarthropathies, may be effective (Table 23–4).

Agarwal A et al. Treatment of reactive arthritis with biological agents. Curr Rheumatol Rep. 2024;26:450. [PMID: 39312088]

INFLAMMATORY BOWEL DISEASE–ASSOCIATED SPONDYLOARTHRITIS

One-fifth of patients with IBD have arthritis. IBD-associated arthritis can have a peripheral arthritis pattern with or without axial involvement. The peripheral arthritis is usually a nondeforming, asymmetric, oligoarthritis of large joints. Peripheral arthritis may pre-date the onset of the IBD and the activity may be independent of intestinal symptoms. Axial involvement with IBD-associated spondyloarthritis is indistinguishable by symptoms or radiographs from axSpA and follows a course independent of the bowel disease. About 50% of these patients are HLA-B27 positive.

Controlling the intestinal inflammation usually eliminates the arthritis. NSAIDs can be effective for mild arthritis but may exacerbate IBD. TNF inhibitors, JAK inhibitors (tofacitinib, upadacitinib), and IL-12/23 inhibitors (ustekinumab) can treat both the bowel and joint/axial inflammation (Table 23–4). Despite their efficacy in spondyloarthritis, anti-IL17A/F agents (secukinumab, ixikizumab, bimikizumab) should be avoided in patients with inflammatory bowel disease due to the risk of colitis specific to this class of biologic agents.

INFECTIOUS ARTHRITIS

NONGONOCOCCAL ACUTE BACTERIAL (Septic) ARTHRITIS

ESSENTIALS OF DIAGNOSIS

- Acute onset of inflammatory monoarticular arthritis, most often in large weight-bearing joints and wrists.
- Common risk factors include previous joint damage and injection drug use.
- Infection with causative organism commonly found elsewhere in body.
- Joint effusions are usually large; synovial fluid WBC counts > 50,000/mcL (50×10^9/L) are common.

General Considerations

Nongonococcal acute bacterial arthritis is most often due to hematogenous seeding of the joint; direct inoculation from penetrating trauma is rare. The key risk factors are bacteremia (eg, injection drug use, endocarditis, infection at other sites), damaged joints (eg, RA), prosthetic joints, compromised immunity (eg, advanced age, diabetes mellitus, advanced CKD, alcohol use disorder, cirrhosis, or immunosuppressive therapy), and loss of skin integrity (eg, cutaneous ulcer or psoriasis). *Staphylococcus aureus* is the most common cause of nongonococcal septic arthritis, accounting for about 50% of all cases. Methicillin-resistant *S aureus* (MRSA) and group B *Streptococcus* are frequent and important causes of septic arthritis. Gram-negative septic arthritis causes about 10% of cases and is especially common with injection drug use and in immunocompromised persons; *Escherichia coli* and *Pseudomonas aeruginosa* are the most common pathogens. Pathologic changes include varying degrees of acute inflammation, with synovitis, effusion, abscess formation in synovial or subchondral tissues, and, if treatment is not adequate, articular destruction.

The arthritis of Lyme disease is discussed in Chapter 38.

Clinical Findings

A. Symptoms and Signs

The onset is acute, with pain, swelling, and heat of the affected joint worsening over hours. The knee is most frequently involved; other commonly affected joints are the hip, wrist, shoulder, and ankle. Unusual sites, such as the sternoclavicular or sacroiliac joint, can be involved in those who use injection drugs. Chills and fever are common but are absent in up to 20% of patients. Infection of the hip usually does not produce apparent swelling but results in groin pain aggravated by walking. More than one joint is involved in 15% of cases of septic arthritis; risk factors for multiple joint involvement include RA, associated endocarditis, and infection with group B streptococci.

B. Laboratory Findings

Synovial fluid analysis is critical for diagnosis. The leukocyte count of the synovial fluid is always inflammatory (> 2000/mcL [2×10^9/L]), usually exceeds 50,000/mcL (50×10^9/L), and often is > 100,000/mcL (100×10^9/L), with ≥ 90% polymorphonuclear cells (Table 23–2). Synovial fluid cell count in septic arthritis may be lower in patients who are immunocompromised, especially those on biologic therapies. Gram stain of the synovial fluid is positive in 75% of staphylococcal infections and 50% of gram-negative infections. Synovial fluid cultures are positive in 70–90% of cases; administration of antibiotics prior to arthrocentesis reduces the likelihood of a positive culture result. Blood cultures are positive in approximately 50% of patients.

C. Imaging

Imaging tests generally add little to the diagnosis of septic arthritis. Other than demonstrating joint effusion, radiographs are usually normal early in the disease; however, evidence of demineralization may develop quickly within just days of onset. Bony erosions and narrowing of the joint space followed by osteomyelitis and periostitis may be seen within 2 weeks.

D. Prosthetic Joint Infection

The clinical and laboratory manifestations of prosthetic joint infection are influenced by whether the infection is early (< 3 months after surgery), delayed (3–12 months after surgery), or late (> 12 months after surgery). Early infections present with acute redness and swelling and are usually caused by *S aureus* and gram-negative organisms. Delayed infections often present with subtle manifestations: pain is common but only 50% of patients will have fever. Less virulent organisms, such as coagulase-negative *Staphylococcus*, *Propionibacterium acnes*, and enterococci, are common causes of delayed infections. Late infections present with acute pain, swelling, and fever and are often caused by hematogenous seeding of *S aureus*, gram-negative bacilli, and hemolytic streptococci. Elevated synovial biomarkers—namely calprotectin, CRP (synovial), α-defensin, and leukocyte esterase—may be useful in identifying infection.

Differential Diagnosis

Gout and pseudogout can cause acute, very inflammatory monoarticular arthritis and fever; failure to find crystals on synovial fluid analysis excludes these diagnoses. The most common articular manifestation of chronic Lyme disease is inflammatory monoarthritis of the knee, which yields synovial fluid that is Gram stain and culture negative. Acute rheumatic fever commonly involves an inflammatory migratory oligoarthritis. Pyogenic arthritis may be superimposed on other types of joint disease, notably RA. Septic arthritis must be excluded by joint fluid examination in any patient with RA who has a joint strikingly more inflamed than the other joints, especially if the patient is receiving biologic DMARD therapy.

Prevention

The American Academy of Orthopedic Surgeons advocates prescribing antibiotic prophylaxis for any patient with a prosthetic joint replacement who undergoes a procedure that can cause bacteremia. However, the topic remains controversial.

Treatment

Treatment of septic arthritis requires appropriate antibiotic therapy together with drainage of the infected joint. If the likely causative organism cannot be determined clinically or from the synovial fluid Gram stain, treatment should be started with broad-spectrum antibiotic coverage against staphylococci, streptococci, and gram-negative organisms. The recommended initial treatment is vancomycin (1 g intravenously every 12 hours, adjusted for age, weight, and renal function) plus a third-generation cephalosporin: ceftriaxone, 1–2 g intravenously daily (or every 12 hours if concomitant meningitis or endocarditis is suspected); or cefotaxime, 1–2 g intravenously every 8 hours. Antibiotic therapy should be adjusted when culture results become available; the duration of antibiotic therapy is usually 4–6 weeks.

Effective drainage is usually achieved through early arthroscopic lavage and debridement. Options for treating prosthetic joint infections depend, in part, on the timing of the infection and include chronic suppression, debridement without removal of the prosthesis, or one- or two-stage exchange of the prosthesis.

Prognosis

The outcome of septic arthritis depends largely on the antecedent health of the patient, the causative organism (eg, *S aureus* bacterial arthritis is associated with a poor functional outcome in about 40% of cases), and the promptness of treatment. The mortality rate is 30% for patients with polyarticular sepsis. Bony ankylosis and articular destruction commonly occur if treatment is delayed or inadequate.

When to Refer

Early orthopedic consultation is essential.

When to Admit

Hospitalization is necessary for intravenous antibiotic therapy and drainage of the joint.

GONOCOCCAL ARTHRITIS

ESSENTIALS OF DIAGNOSIS

- Prodromal migratory polyarthralgias.
- Tenosynovitis is the most common sign.
- Purulent monoarthritis in 50%.
- Characteristic skin lesions, especially of the palms and soles.
- Most common in young women during menses or pregnancy.
- Symptoms of urethritis frequently absent.
- Dramatic response to antibiotics.

General Considerations

In contrast to nongonococcal bacterial arthritis, gonococcal arthritis usually occurs in otherwise healthy individuals. Host factors, however, influence the expression of the disease: gonococcal arthritis is two to three times more common in women than in men, is especially common during menses and pregnancy, and is rare after age 40. Gonococcal arthritis is also common in men who have sex with men, whose high incidence of asymptomatic gonococcal pharyngitis and proctitis predisposes them to disseminated gonococcal infection. Recurrent disseminated gonococcal infection should prompt testing of the patient's CH50 level to evaluate for a congenital deficiency of a terminal complement component (C5, C6, C7, or C8).

Clinical Findings

A. Symptoms and Signs

One to 4 days of migratory polyarthralgias involving the wrist, knee, ankle, or elbow are common at the outset. Thereafter, two patterns emerge. The first pattern is characterized by tenosynovitis that most often affects the wrists, fingers, ankles, or toes and is seen in 60% of patients. The second pattern is purulent monoarthritis that most frequently involves the knee, wrist, ankle, or elbow and is seen in 40% of patients. Less than half of patients have fever, and less than one-fourth have any genitourinary symptoms. Most patients will have asymptomatic, but highly characteristic, skin lesions that usually consist of 2 to 10 small necrotic pustules distributed over the extremities, especially the palms and soles.

B. Laboratory Findings

The peripheral WBC averages about 10,000 cells/mcL (10×10^9/L) and is elevated in less than one-third of patients. The synovial fluid WBC count usually ranges from 30,000 to 60,000 cells/mcL ($30–60 \times 10^9$/L). Positive synovial fluid Gram stain occurs in one-fourth of cases and culture in less than half. Positive blood cultures are uncommon. Urethral, throat, cervical, and rectal cultures should be done in all patients, and are often positive in the absence of local symptoms. Urinary nucleic acid amplification tests have excellent sensitivity and specificity for the detection of *Neisseria gonorrhoeae* in genitourinary sites.

C. Imaging

Radiographs are usually normal or show only soft tissue swelling.

Differential Diagnosis

Reactive arthritis can produce acute monoarthritis, urethritis, and fever in a young person but is distinguished by negative cultures and failure to respond to antibiotics. Lyme disease involving the knee is less acute, does not show positive cultures, and may be preceded by known tick exposure and characteristic rash. The synovial fluid analysis will exclude gout, pseudogout, and nongonococcal bacterial arthritis. Rheumatic fever and sarcoidosis can produce migratory tenosynovitis. Infective endocarditis with septic arthritis can mimic disseminated gonococcal infection. Meningococcemia occasionally presents with a clinical picture that resembles disseminated gonococcal infection; blood cultures establish the correct diagnosis. Rocky mountain spotted fever and dengue can produce arthritis and skin findings. Early hepatitis B infection is associated with circulating immune complexes that can cause an urticarial rash and polyarthralgias.

Treatment

The treatment of disseminated gonorrhea (arthritis-dermatitis syndrome) per CDC guidelines is ceftriaxone (1 g daily intravenously or intramuscularly). Once susceptibility testing has been obtained and it is 24–48 hours after clinical improvement, the antibiotic regimen can be changed to an oral agent to complete a 7-day course.

Prognosis

Generally, gonococcal arthritis responds dramatically after 24–48 hours of antibiotics, and drainage of the infected joint(s) is rarely needed. Complete recovery is the rule.

When to Refer

Consult an infectious disease specialist for questions about antibiotic resistant gonococcal strains. Report to the public health department for tracing contacts.

When to Admit

Hospitalization is indicated to establish the diagnosis and administer intravenous antibiotics until there is clinical improvement.

Vitiello A et al. Antimicrobial resistance in gonorrhea. Microb Drug Resist. 2024;30:297. [PMID: 38579162]

RHEUMATIC MANIFESTATIONS OF HIV INFECTION

Infection with HIV has been associated with various rheumatic symptoms and may coexist with autoimmune rheumatic diseases, such as RA, psoriatic arthritis, or spondyloarthritis. Acute new HIV infection (viremia) causes severe arthralgias in an oligoarticular, asymmetric pattern that resolve within 24 hours; the joint examination is normal. HIV-associated arthritis is an asymmetric oligoarticular process with objective findings of arthritis and a self-limited course that ranges from weeks to months. Along with antiretroviral therapies, immunosuppressive medications, including biologic agents, can be used if necessary in patients with HIV (see Chapter 35, HIV Infection & AIDS). Muscle weakness associated with an elevated creatine kinase can be due to nucleoside reverse transcriptase inhibitor–associated myopathy or HIV-associated myopathy; the clinical presentations of each resemble idiopathic inflammatory myopathies but muscle biopsies show minimal inflammation. Other rheumatic manifestations of HIV include diffuse infiltrative lymphocytosis syndrome (with parotid gland enlargement) and various forms of vasculitis.

VIRAL ARTHRITIS

Arthralgias occur frequently in the course of acute infections with many viruses, but frank arthritis is uncommon with the notable exceptions of acute parvovirus B19 infection and Chikungunya fever. Parvovirus B19 causes an acute polyarthritis in 50–60% of adult cases (infected children develop the febrile exanthem known as "slapped cheek fever"). The arthritis can mimic RA but is almost always self-limited and resolves within several weeks. The diagnosis is established by the presence of IgM antibodies specific for parvovirus B19. Chikungunya fever is an arthropod-borne viral infection that is endemic to West Africa but has spread to multiple locations including the Indian Ocean islands, the Caribbean and Central and Latin America. Clinical manifestations include high fever, rash, and incapacitating bone pain. Acute polyarthralgia and polyarthritis are common and can persist for months or years. For Chikungunya-associated chronic arthritis, treatment with methotrexate or other DMARD agents may be an option. There is an FDA-approved vaccine for individuals 18 and older at risk for Chikungunya infection.

Self-limited polyarthritis is common in acute hepatitis B infection and typically occurs before the onset of jaundice. Urticaria or other types of skin rash may be present. The clinical picture resembles that of serum sickness. Serum transaminase levels are elevated, and tests for hepatitis B surface antigen are positive. Serum complement levels are often low during active arthritis and become normal after remission of arthritis. The incidence of hepatitis B–associated polyarthritis has fallen substantially with the introduction of hepatitis B vaccination.

Chronic infection with hepatitis C is associated with chronic polyarthralgia (up to 20% of cases) and with chronic polyarthritis (3–5%). This can mimic RA; the presence of rheumatoid factor in most hepatitis C infections leads to further diagnostic confusion. RA always causes objective arthritis (not just arthralgias) and can be erosive (hepatitis C–associated arthritis is nonerosive). The presence of anti-CCP antibodies helps to diagnose RA.

SPINAL TUBERCULOSIS (Pott Disease)

ESSENTIALS OF DIAGNOSIS

- Seen primarily in individuals from developing countries or immunocompromised patients.
- Back pain and gibbus deformity with radiographic evidence of vertebral involvement.
- < 20% have active pulmonary tuberculosis.
- Evidence of *Mycobacterium tuberculosis* in aspirate or biopsies of spinal lesions.

General Considerations

In the developing world, children primarily bear the burden of musculoskeletal tuberculosis. In the United States, however, musculoskeletal infection is more often seen in adults who have immigrated from countries where tuberculosis is prevalent, or it develops in the setting of immunosuppression (eg, HIV infection, therapy with biologic agent). Spinal tuberculosis (Pott disease) accounts for about 50% of musculoskeletal infection due to *M tuberculosis* (see Chapter 9). Seeding of the vertebrae may occur through hematogenous spread from the respiratory tract at the time of primary infection, with clinical disease developing years later due to reactivation, or through lymphatics from infected foci in the pleura or kidneys. The thoracic and lumbar vertebrae are the most common sites of spinal involvement; vertebral infection is associated with paravertebral cold abscesses in 75% of cases.

Clinical Findings

A. Symptoms and Signs

Patients have back pain, often present for months and sometimes associated with radicular pain and lower extremity weakness. Constitutional symptoms are usually absent, and < 20% have active pulmonary disease. Destruction of the vertebral body anteriorly can produce the characteristic wedge-shaped gibbus deformity.

B. Laboratory Findings

Most patients have a positive reaction to purified protein derivative or a positive blood interferon-γ release assay. Cultures of paravertebral abscesses and biopsies of vertebral lesions are positive in up to 70–90%. Biopsies reveal characteristic caseating granulomas in most cases. Isolation of *M tuberculosis* from an extraspinal site is sufficient to establish the diagnosis in the proper clinical setting.

C. Imaging

Radiographs can reveal lytic and sclerotic lesions and bony destruction of vertebrae but are normal early in the disease.

CT scanning can demonstrate paraspinal soft tissue extensions of the infection; MRI is the image of choice to detect compression of the spinal cord or cauda equina.

Differential Diagnosis

Spinal tuberculosis must be differentiated from subacute and chronic spinal infections due to pyogenic organisms, *Brucella*, fungi, and malignancy.

Complications

Paraplegia due to compression of the spinal cord or cauda equina is the most serious complication of spinal tuberculosis.

Treatment

Antimicrobial therapy should be administered for 6–9 months, usually in the form of isoniazid, rifampin, pyrazinamide, and ethambutol for 2 months followed by isoniazid and rifampin for an additional 4–7 months (see also Chapter 9). Medical management alone is often sufficient. Surgical intervention, however, may be indicated when there is neurologic compromise or severe spinal instability.

MISCELLANEOUS RHEUMATOLOGIC DISORDERS

FIBROMYALGIA

ESSENTIALS OF DIAGNOSIS

- Most frequent in women aged 20–50.
- Chronic widespread musculoskeletal pain syndrome with multiple tender points.
- Fatigue, headaches, memory problems, dysregulated sleep, mood disorders, and increased sensitivity to sensory input frequently co-occur.
- Objective signs of inflammation absent; laboratory studies normal.

General Considerations

Fibromyalgia is a common nociplastic pain syndrome, affecting 3–10% of the general population. It shares many features with myalgic encephalomyelitis/chronic fatigue syndrome, namely, an increased frequency among women aged 20–50, absence of objective findings, and absence of diagnostic laboratory test results. While many of the clinical features of the two conditions overlap, musculoskeletal pain predominates in fibromyalgia, whereas lassitude dominates myalgic encephalomyelitis/chronic fatigue syndrome.

Although the cause of fibromyalgia is unknown, the pathophysiology is aberrant CNS processing of pain and sensory stimuli. Fibromyalgia may coexist with rheumatic and other medical conditions, such as SLE, hypothyroidism, RA, or sleep apnea.

Clinical Findings

Chronic aching pain and stiffness are the hallmarks of fibromyalgia. The pain frequently involves the entire body but with prominence around the neck, shoulders, low back, and hips. Fatigue, sleep disorders, numbness with paresthesias, chronic headaches, and irritable bowel and bladder symptoms are common. Even minor exertion aggravates pain and increases fatigue. Physical examination is normal. There are no specific biomarkers for fibromyalgia, and laboratory studies are generally normal.

Differential Diagnosis

Fibromyalgia is a diagnosis of exclusion. A detailed history and repeated physical examination can obviate the need for extensive laboratory testing. RA and SLE present with objective physical findings and laboratory abnormalities. Thyroid function tests are useful because hypothyroidism can produce a fibromyalgia-like syndrome. The idiopathic inflammatory myopathies produce demonstrable weakness. Polymyalgia rheumatica produces shoulder and pelvic girdle pain, is associated with an elevated ESR and occurs after age 50. The diagnosis of fibromyalgia should be made hesitantly in a patient over age 50 and should never be invoked to explain fever, weight loss, or any other objective signs or lab abnormalities.

Treatment

A multidisciplinary approach is most effective. Patient education is essential. Patients can be comforted that they have a diagnosable syndrome treatable by specific therapies and that the course is not progressive. Cognitive behavioral therapy, including programs that emphasize mindfulness meditation, is often helpful. Exercise programs are beneficial and should be universally recommended, particularly tai chi, yoga, and resistance exercise. The FDA-approved pharmacotherapies for fibromyalgia are pregabalin (begin with 75 mg orally twice daily and increase to 150 mg twice daily as tolerated), duloxetine (begin with 30 mg orally daily and increase to 60 mg daily as tolerated), milnacipran (begin with 12.5 mg orally daily and increase to 50 mg twice daily as tolerated) and sublingual cyclobenzaprine (TNX-102 SL) begin with 2.8 mg sublingually in the evening and increase to 5.6 mg as tolerated). Other pharmacotherapies that have shown modest efficacy are amitriptyline (begin with 10 mg orally nightly and increase as tolerated or needed to 75 mg nightly), tramadol, fluoxetine, gabapentin, and low-dose naltrexone. NSAIDs are generally ineffective. Cannabinoids may have a role in the treatment of fibromyalgia; however, dose, formulation, and frequency are unknown. Opioids and corticosteroids are ineffective and should not be used. Depression and anxiety are extremely common among patients with fibromyalgia; concurrent treatment of these comorbid conditions is highly recommended.

Prognosis

All patients have chronic symptoms. Progressive or objective findings do not develop.

THORACIC OUTLET SYNDROMES

Thoracic outlet syndromes result from compression of the neurovascular structures supplying the upper extremity. Symptoms and signs arise from intermittent or continuous pressure on elements of the brachial plexus (> 90% of cases) or the subclavian or axillary vessels (veins or arteries) by a variety of anatomic structures of the shoulder girdle region. Most commonly thoracic outlet syndromes are caused by scarred scalene neck muscles secondary to neck trauma or sagging of the shoulder girdle resulting from aging, obesity, or pendulous breasts. Faulty posture, occupation, or thoracic muscle hypertrophy from physical activity (eg, weightlifting, baseball pitching) are other predisposing factors.

CXR will identify patients with cervical ribs (although most patients with cervical ribs are asymptomatic). MRI with the arms held in different positions is useful in identifying sites of impaired blood flow. Intra-arterial or venous obstruction is confirmed by angiography. Determination of conduction velocities of the ulnar and other peripheral nerves of the upper extremity may help localize the site of their compression.

More than 95% of patients can be treated successfully with conservative therapy consisting of physical therapy and avoiding postures or activities that compress the neurovascular bundle. Operative treatment, required by < 5% of patients, is more likely to relieve the neurologic rather than the vascular component that causes symptoms.

COMPLEX REGIONAL PAIN SYNDROME

Complex regional pain syndrome (formerly called reflex sympathetic dystrophy) is a rare disorder of the extremities characterized by autonomic and vasomotor instability. The cardinal symptoms and signs are pain localized to an arm or leg, swelling of the involved extremity, disturbances of color and temperature in the affected limb, dystrophic changes in the overlying skin and nails, and limited range of motion. Strikingly, the findings are not limited to the distribution of a single peripheral nerve. Most cases are preceded by surgery or direct physical trauma, often of a relatively minor nature, to the soft tissues, bone, or nerve. Early mobilization after injury or surgery reduces the likelihood of developing the syndrome. Any extremity can be involved, but the syndrome most commonly occurs in the hand and is associated with ipsilateral restriction of shoulder motion ("shoulder-hand" syndrome). This syndrome proceeds through phases: pain, swelling, and skin color and temperature changes develop early and, if untreated, lead to atrophy and dystrophy. The swelling in complex regional pain syndrome is diffuse ("catcher's mitt hand") and not restricted to joints. Pain is often burning in quality, intense, and greatly worsened by minimal stimuli such as light touch. Complex regional pain syndrome may occur after a knee injury or after knee surgery. There are no systemic symptoms. In the early phases of the syndrome, bone scans are sensitive, showing diffuse increased uptake in the affected extremity; radiographs eventually reveal severe generalized osteopenia. This syndrome should be differentiated from RA, thoracic outlet obstruction, and mononeuritis multiplex, among others.

Early treatment offers the best prognosis for recovery. For mild cases, NSAIDs (eg, naproxen 250–500 mg twice daily orally) can be effective. For more severe cases associated with edema, prednisone, 30–60 mg/day orally for 2 weeks and then tapered over 2 weeks, can be effective. Pain management is important and allows for effective physical therapy, which is critical to restore function. Some patients may benefit from antidepressant agents (eg, nortriptyline initiated at a dosage of 10 mg orally at bedtime and gradually increased to 40–75 mg at bedtime) or anticonvulsants (eg, gabapentin 300 mg three times daily orally). Regional nerve blocks, and dorsal-column stimulation have also been reported to be helpful. The role of bisphosphonates and calcitonin to treat complex regional pain syndrome is controversial. Vitamin C supplementation (1 g orally daily) may have a role in preventing the development of complex regional pain syndrome following surgical procedures known to be a risk factor (eg, total knee replacement, foot or ankle surgery). The prognosis depends on the stage in which the lesions are encountered and the extent and severity of the condition.

RHEUMATOLOGIC MANIFESTATIONS OF CANCER

Rheumatologic syndromes may be the presenting manifestations for a variety of cancers. Dermatomyositis is often associated with cancer. Hypertrophic pulmonary osteoarthropathy, which is characterized by the triad of polyarthritis, clubbing, and periosteal new bone formation, is associated with both malignant diseases (most commonly lung cancer) and nonmalignant ones (eg, cyanotic heart disease, cirrhosis, and lung abscess). Cancer-associated polyarthritis is rare, has both oligoarticular and polyarticular forms, and should be considered when "seronegative RA" develops abruptly in an older patient. Palmar fasciitis manifests as bilateral palmar swelling with finger contractures and may be the first indication of cancer, particularly ovarian. Remitting seronegative synovitis with non-pitting edema ("RS3PE") presents with a symmetric small-joint polyarthritis associated with non-pitting edema of the hands; it can be idiopathic or associated with malignancy. Palpable purpura due to leukocytoclastic vasculitis may be the presenting complaint in myeloproliferative disorders. Hairy cell leukemia can be associated with medium-sized vessel vasculitis such as polyarteritis nodosa. Acute leukemia can produce severe joint and bone pain without florid synovitis. Rheumatic manifestations of myelodysplastic syndromes include cutaneous vasculitis, lupus-like syndromes, neuropathy, and episodic intense arthritis. Erythromelalgia, a painful warmth and redness of the extremities that (unlike Raynaud) improves with cold exposure or with elevation of the extremity, is often associated with myeloproliferative diseases, particularly essential thrombocythemia.

Immune-related adverse events from immune checkpoint inhibitors used to treat a variety of malignancies include pneumonitis, colitis, myositis, vasculitis, myocarditis, and inflammatory arthritis. These events are common and often can be managed with corticosteroids alone and adjustment of immunotherapy. However, the persistence of some autoimmune conditions despite cessation of cancer treatment, namely inflammatory arthritis, may require long-term immunosuppression with methotrexate or biologic agents.

OSTEONECROSIS (Avascular Necrosis of Bone)

Osteonecrosis is a complication of corticosteroid use, alcohol use, trauma, SLE, pancreatitis, gout, sickle cell disease, dysbaric syndromes (eg, "the bends"), factor deficiencies (eg, protein S and antithrombin III) and infiltrative diseases (eg, Gaucher disease). The most commonly affected sites are the proximal and distal femoral heads, leading to hip or knee pain.

Osteonecrosis of the jaw can be a complication of bisphosphonates, usually when high-dose intravenous bisphosphonate therapy is used for treating metastatic cancer or plasma cell myeloma rather than osteoporosis. Initially, radiographs are normal; MRI and CT scan are more sensitive techniques. Treatment involves avoidance of weight bearing on the affected joint for at least several weeks. For osteonecrosis of the hip, a variety of procedures designed to preserve the femoral head have been developed for early disease, including vascularized and nonvascularized bone grafting procedures, platelet-rich plasma and stem cell injections. The value of surgical core decompression is controversial and can be used in combination with structural or biologic interventions. These procedures are most effective in avoiding or forestalling the need for total hip arthroplasty in young patients who do not have advanced disease. Without intervention, the natural history of avascular necrosis is progression of the bony infarction to cortical collapse, resulting in significant joint dysfunction. Total hip replacement is the usual outcome for all patients who are candidates.

ALLERGIC & IMMUNOLOGIC DISORDERS

IMMEDIATE HYPERSENSITIVITY

1. Food Allergy

Immediate hypersensitivity IgE-mediated allergic reactions to foods commonly occur within 2 hours of ingestion and are much less common in adults as a de novo food allergy than in children. Typical systemic reactions include a combination of emesis, diarrhea, urticaria with or without angioedema, bronchial hypersensitivity, and hypotension. A serum tryptase may be elevated during anaphylactic reactions within a few hours after the exposure. The most common systemic food allergies are caused by milk, egg, wheat, soy, fish, shellfish, peanuts, and tree nut allergens. Shellfish, peanuts, and tree nuts are the most common causes of food anaphylaxis in adults; milk and egg allergies are more common in children but often resolve by adulthood. Diagnosis of food allergy is based on a correlative history, skin tests, and serum specific IgE tests. Because of frequent false-positive IgE tests, the use of indiscriminate screening of IgE panels to foods is not recommended; oral food challenge with a reproducible immediate hypersensitivity reaction remains the gold standard for diagnosis. Food challenge, however, should only be conducted by an experienced provider in a setting equipped to treat anaphylaxis. There is no role for specific IgG or IgA testing for evaluating food immediate hypersensitivity. Management of food allergy involves strict avoidance of the food and guaranteed access to epinephrine autoinjectors. The use of oral immunotherapy to treat food allergy in children and adolescents should only be performed by an experienced allergist immunologist.

Other IgE-mediated food reactions include oral allergy syndrome and hypersensitivity to α-gal (galactose-α-1,3-galactose). Oral allergy syndrome and pollen-associated food allergy syndrome result from cross-reactivity between certain food and pollen proteins. Affected individuals have known seasonal pollen allergies (most commonly tree pollens) and experience itching of the oral mucosa upon ingestion of cross-reactive raw fruits and vegetables. In contrast to systemic food allergy, symptoms are mostly limited to the oropharynx.

The enzyme α-gal glycosylates proteins in mammals and is found in mammal-derived meats (ie, beef, pork, lamb, and mutton). Sensitization to this carbohydrate is epidemiologically linked to Lone Star (Amblyomma americanum) tick bites, but the pathogenesis is not entirely clear. In contrast to conventional immediate hypersensitivity IgE-mediated food allergy to proteins, the α-gal IgE-mediated reaction typically occurs 2–12 hours after ingestion, with most reactions occurring within 3–6 hours. Heavily influenced by cofactors (eg, consumption with alcohol, exercise before or after ingestion), α-gal IgE-mediated food reactions do not occur with every exposure. Diagnosis is made by clinical history with confirmatory α-gal IgE testing by an allergist. Surrogate markers beef, pork, and mutton IgE levels may be used if α-gal IgE is not available.

Mollah F et al. What is alpha-gal syndrome? JAMA 2024;331:86. [PMID: 38064235]
Wilson JM et al. Tick bites, IgE to galactose-alpha-1.3-alpha-galactose and urticarial reactions to mammalian meat: the alpha gal syndrome. Allergy. 2024;79:1440. [PMID: 38193233]

2. Venom Allergy

Most systemic allergic reactions to insect stings are caused by honeybees, vespids (yellow jackets, hornets, wasps, honeybee), and fire ants. Systemic anaphylactic reactions can occur at any age after stinging events. Patients at highest risk for anaphylaxis from subsequent stings are those who have had a history of recent or severe reactions, or both; thus, the risk of a systemic reaction declines over elapsed time since the last sting. If a systemic allergy is suspected because symptoms include generalized urticaria, anaphylaxis, angioedema, wheezing, or diarrhea, refer the patient to an allergist for confirmative venom allergy testing; initiation of venom immunotherapy is commonly recommended. In the interim, patients should be given self-administrated epinephrine for those with continuing exposure.

3. Anaphylaxis

General Considerations

Anaphylaxis is the most serious and potentially life-threatening manifestation of mast cell and basophil mediator release. The National Institute of Allergy and Infectious

Table 23–13. NIAID/FAAN consensus criteria for anaphylaxis. Anaphylaxis is likely when any one of the three criteria is fulfilled.

Presentation	Time to Onset of Symptoms	Clinical Manifestations
Criterion 1: Acute onset of illness	Minutes to 2–3 hours	One of the following combinations of symptoms: Skin or mucosal symptoms, or both[1] *with* Respiratory compromise[2] *or* ↓ blood pressure or end-organ dysfunction[3]
Criterion 2: After exposure to *likely* allergens	Minutes to 2–3 hours	Involvement of ≥ 2 of the following systems: Skin or mucosa, or both[1] Respiratory compromise[2] ↓ blood pressure or end-organ dysfunction[3] Persistent GI symptoms[4]
Criterion 3: After exposure to *known* allergens	Minutes to 2–3 hours	Involvement of the cardiovascular system: ↓ blood pressure

FAAN, Food Allergy and Anaphylaxis Network; NIAID, National Institute of Allergy and Infectious Disease.
[1]Indicates presence of pruritus, flushing, hives, or angioedema.
[2]Indicates presence of dyspnea, wheeze-bronchospasm, decreased peak expiratory flow, stridor, or hypoxemia.
[3]Indicates decreased blood pressure; end-organ dysfunction includes collapse, syncope, or incontinence.
[4]Indicates presence of vomiting, crampy abdominal pain, or diarrhea.
Reproduced with permission from Renae Boerneke and Mildred Kwan, University of North Carolina and Sampson HA, Muñoz-Furlong A, Campbell RL, et al. Second symposium on the definition and management of anaphylaxis: summary report–Second National Institute of Allergy and Infectious Disease/Food Allergy and Anaphylaxis Network symposium. *J Allergy Clin Immunol*. 2006;117(2):391–397.

Diseases/Food Allergy and Anaphylaxis Network definition of anaphylaxis and criteria for diagnosis are shown in Table 23–13. Anaphylaxis is likely under these circumstances: (1) an allergen exposure followed by the acute onset of illness involving skin or mucosal tissue and either respiratory compromise or hypotension (systolic blood pressure < 90 mm Hg or 30% less than known baseline); (2) a *likely* allergen exposure followed by the acute onset of two or more of these conditions: skin or mucosal tissue involvement, respiratory compromise, hypotension, and persistent GI symptoms; or (3) a known allergen exposure followed by hypotension.

IgE-dependent anaphylaxis is an acute syndrome initiated by a repeat allergen exposure after a prior exposure has sensitized the patient with anti-allergen IgE antibodies; IgE-mediated anaphylaxis cannot occur on first-time exposure to allergens like medications, insect venoms, latex, and foods. Conversely, other anaphylactic reactions (sometimes called "anaphylactoid"), such as radiocontrast media, certain medications (most NSAIDs, opioids, and vancomycin), and COVID mRNA vaccine reactions, are due to different immunologic mechanisms and can occur with first-time exposure.

Clinical Findings

A. Symptoms and Signs

Symptoms and signs typically start within 30 minutes of initial exposure but may rarely appear up to several hours later. These include: (1) skin manifestations (typically urticaria, flushing, blotchy rashes, and pruritus); (2) respiratory distress (wheezing, stridor, bronchospasm, and airway angioedema); (3) GI symptoms (cramping, emesis, and diarrhea [especially in food allergy]); and (4) hypotension. Anaphylaxis is potentially fatal, especially if untreated.

B. Laboratory Findings

Laboratory evaluation obtained shortly after onset of symptoms can support a diagnosis of anaphylaxis but should not take the place of expedient treatment. Elevated serum tryptase within 4–6 hours following onset of anaphylaxis is most useful because it is a specific biomarker of mast cell degranulation. Plasma histamine generally peaks 30 minutes after onset of symptoms, making it difficult to obtain during peak levels. Referral to an allergist is necessary because of concern for future reactions and need for appropriate education and intervention. Specific serum IgE or skin testing to suspected allergens may be performed optimally 4–6 weeks after a severe reaction; this delayed testing is to avoid falsely negative testing during a post-reaction "refractory" period where IgE consumed during anaphylaxis has not yet been regenerated. The positive predictive value of these tests depends highly on a suggestive temporal relationship to a suspected allergen exposure.

Treatment

Administration of intramuscular epinephrine (0.01 mg/kg of a 1:1000 [1 mg/mL] solution, maximum 0.5 mg in adults) at the onset of suspected anaphylaxis is the cornerstone of therapy and should not be delayed. There is no absolute contraindication to administering intramuscular epinephrine in the setting of anaphylaxis. Supportive measures, such as oxygen, intravenous fluids and, if required, airway management are also appropriate. Adjunctive therapies may include antihistamines, bronchodilators, and corticosteroids. Self-administered epinephrine at the earliest signs of recurrence can be life-sparing, whereas antihistamines and corticosteroids have limited value in reversing anaphylaxis.

When to Refer

Patients with new or unexplained onset of anaphylaxis should be evaluated by an allergist.

Alvarez-Arango S et al. Non-IgE-mediated immediate drug-induced hypersensitivity reactions. J Allergy Clin Immunol Pract. 2024;12:1109. [PMID: 38423288]

Wang J et al. Anaphylaxis in practice: a guide to the 2023 practice parameter update. J Allergy Clin Immunol Pract. 2024;12:2325. [PMID: 38944199]

ALLERGY TESTING

Cutaneous or skin prick allergen testing produces a localized pruritic wheal (induration) and flare (erythema) that is maximal at 15–20 minutes. Such testing is used most commonly to diagnose allergic respiratory disease (rhinitis and asthma) and IgE-mediated allergy to food, drugs (penicillins), and *Hymenoptera* venom. Allergen extracts are available for pollens, fungi, animal danders, and dust mites and are appropriately selected for the patient's geographic area.

ADVERSE DRUG REACTIONS

1. Drug Allergy (IgE-mediated Immediate Hypersensitivity Reactions)

Prick skin testing for most low-molecular-weight drugs is not validated and is interpretable only if the test is positive at a nonirritating concentration. Testing for IgE-mediated allergy to penicillin (PCN) is validated; skin testing with the metabolic determinants of PCN has a high (> 98%) negative predictive value. Referral of individuals with a listed PCN allergy to an allergist for evaluation is worthwhile because > 90% have either lost sensitization or do not have a true PCN allergy. Such patients may then safely receive β-lactam antibiotics, including penicillins and cephalosporins. Allergy testing to non-PCN drugs is more limited; an allergist may provide guidance about whether re-challenging with the drug would be advisable.

Banerji A et al. Drug allergy practice parameter updates to incorporate into your clinical practice. J Allergy Clin Immunol Pract. 2023;11:356. [PMID: 36563781]

2. Non-IgE–Mediated Anaphylactic Drug Reactions

Non-IgE–mediated anaphylaxis induced by drugs resembles immediate hypersensitivity reactions but is not mediated by allergen-IgE cross-linking on mast cells or basophils. Contrary to IgE-mediated reactions, these reactions can often be prevented by prophylactic medical regimens.

A. Radiocontrast Media Reactions

Reactions to radiocontrast media are not usually IgE antibody–mediated, yet they are clinically similar to anaphylaxis and can be life-threatening. If a patient has had an anaphylactoid reaction to conventional radiocontrast media, the risk for a second reaction upon re-exposure may be as high as 30%. Patients with a history of atopy are at increased risk.

Management includes use of low-osmolality contrast preparations and prophylactic administration of prednisone (50 mg orally every 6 hours beginning 13 hours before the procedure) and diphenhydramine (25–50 mg orally, intramuscularly, or intravenously 60 minutes before the procedure). Using lower-osmolality radiocontrast media in combination with the pretreatment regimen decreases the incidence of recurrent reactions to < 1%.

B. Vancomycin Infusion Reaction

Vancomycin infusion reaction causes non-IgE–mediated anaphylaxis with flushing, pruritus, and erythema of the upper body. Initially described as a vancomycin infusion reaction, it can also occur after intravenous infusion of opioids. The reaction is related to the rate of drug administration resulting in direct activation of mast cells. Management includes administration of an antihistamine such as diphenhydramine, 25–50 mg intravenously or intramuscularly, and re-initiation of the vancomycin infusion at no more than half the former rate. In patients who have previously experienced a vancomycin infusion reaction, premedication with an H_1-antagonist (eg, diphenhydramine 50 mg orally or intravenously) and H_2-antagonist (eg, cimetidine 200 mg orally) is recommended 1 hour before the infusion. Although rare, anaphylaxis with vancomycin use can occur. Vancomycin skin testing has not been validated as a diagnostic tool. Induction of tolerance to vancomycin is possible for patients with anaphylaxis without an acceptable alternative antibiotic.

DELAYED DRUG HYPERSENSITIVITY

Type IV delayed hypersensitivity typically occurs 48–72 hours after contact with the antigen.

1. Drug Exanthems

The clinical manifestation of drug exanthems is vast (see Chapter 6), ranging from common morbilliform rashes to severe cutaneous adverse reactions (SCARs) (eg, Stevens-Johnson syndrome [SJS]/toxic epidermal necrolysis [TEN], drug reaction with eosinophilia and systemic symptoms [DRESS], acute generalized exanthematous pustulosis [AGEP]). Given the broad range of cutaneous findings, the differential diagnosis includes miliaria, lichen planus, folliculitis, pityriasis rosea, tinea corporis, and mycosis fungoides. While many drugs can cause exanthems, there are no commercially available laboratory or other diagnostic tests to reliably confirm these adverse reactions.

Management consists of immediate cessation of suspected medications and monitoring for symptom resolution. Systemic corticosteroids may be indicated for extensive dermatitis or other organ involvement.

Wang C et al. Management and Prevention of Hypersensitivity Reactions to Radiocontrast Media: A Consensus Statement from the American College of Radiology and the American Academy of Allergy, Asthma & Immunology. J Allergy Clin Immunol Pract. 2025:S2213-2198(25)00191-6. [PMID: 40332064]

2. Severe Cutaneous Adverse Reactions (SCARs)

A. Stevens-Johnson Syndrome/Toxic Epidermal Necrolysis (SJS/TEN)

SJS and TEN comprise a spectrum of disease that are differentiated by the severity of skin detachment, ranging from < 10% in SJS to > 30% in TEN. Drugs and infections are the main etiologies and include anticonvulsants, sulfonamide antibiotics, NSAIDs, allopurinol, *Mycoplasma pneumoniae,* and herpes simplex virus. Allopurinol hypersensitivity is increased with the HLA-B*58:01 allele, the prevalence of which is highest in Han Chinese, Korean, and Thai persons, as well as in Black individuals. Testing for the HLA-B*58:01 allele before starting allopurinol is conditionally recommended for these patients. Universal testing for HLA-B*58:01 is not recommended. See Chapter 6.

B. Drug Reaction with Eosinophilia & Systemic Symptoms (DRESS)/Drug-Induced Hypersensitivity Syndrome (DIHS)

DRESS typically includes eosinophilia, lymphocytosis, and systemic symptoms such as fever and lymph node enlargement, along with rash. DRESS and DIHS likely are part of a continuum of disease with DIHS representing a more severe form of DRESS with HHV-6 (see Chapter 6). A limited number of drugs are implicated in induction of DRESS including anticonvulsants, sulfonamide antibiotics (eg, sulfasalazine), allopurinol, minocycline, dapsone, and vancomycin. The diagnosis may be aided with the use of the RegiSCAR score for DRESS (https://www.researchgate.net/figure/The-RegiSCAR-scoring-system-for-diagnosing-DRESS-syndrome_tbl1_317485615).

C. Acute Generalized Exanthematous Pustulosis (AGEP)

AGEP is characterized by hundreds of small, pruritic, sterile pustules on an erythematous base distributed mainly on the trunk and intertriginous areas. Onset of AGEP occurs within hours to days following the initiation of the culprit drug. In addition to pustules, mucosal involvement is minimal to none and, if present, is only found in a single site such as the lips or buccal mucosa. Many patients will have fever and neutrophilia (> 7.5×10^6/mL).

Treatment of AGEP includes cessation of the suspected drug with resolution of symptoms within a few days. The area of skin involved desquamates as the patient recovers. Mortality occurs in < 5% of patients. Wet dressings and antiseptic solutions applied while the patient has active pustules is recommended; antibiotics should be used only if there is pustular superinfection. The utility of other treatments such as systemic corticosteroids is unclear.

3. Aspirin- & NSAID-Exacerbated Respiratory Disease

Aspirin- and NSAID-exacerbated respiratory disease is caused by aberrant arachidonic acid metabolism. Patients typically have increased airway responsiveness, bronchospasm, rhinorrhea, and nasal congestion. Chronic rhinosinusitis with nasal polyps and asthma is called aspirin-exacerbated respiratory disease (formally known as Samter's triad). Ocular, cutaneous, and gastric symptoms may also occur. Diagnosis is largely based on history and clinical findings. A positive aspirin challenge can demonstrate NSAID hypersensitivity and may suggest benefit from nasal polypectomy and aspirin desensitization. Long-term aspirin therapy following desensitization has been shown to reduce the need for nasal polypectomy and asthma therapy. Referral to an allergist is appropriate for aspirin desensitization. Treatment may also include montelukast or inhibition of 5-LOX with zileuton.

Haque R et al. Clinical evaluation and diagnosis of aspirin exacerbated respiratory disease. J Allergy Clin Immunol. 2021;148:283. [PMID: 34364538]

PRIMARY IMMUNODEFICIENCY IN ADULTS

Several important immunodeficiency disorders present in adulthood, most notably the antibody deficiency syndromes: selective IgA deficiency, common variable immunodeficiency (CVID), and specific (functional) antibody deficiency. Antibody deficiency predisposes patients to recurrent serious bacterial infections, particularly of the respiratory tract, including refractory chronic rhinosinusitis, bronchitis, pneumonia, and bronchiectasis. Patients are most susceptible to infections with encapsulated bacteria (eg, *Haemophilus influenzae* type b, *Streptococcus pneumoniae, Neisseria meningitides*). However, the innate or cellular immune system also can be defective to varying degrees, which results in infections with different spectra of organisms depending on the severity of the immune defect.

1. Selective IgA Deficiency

Selective IgA deficiency is the most common primary immunoglobulin deficiency and is characterized by undetectable serum IgA levels (< 7 mg/dL) with normal levels of IgG and IgM; its prevalence is about 1 in 500 individuals, with a higher prevalence in White persons. Most individuals are healthy, and the IgA deficiency is found incidentally. A minority of patients have recurrent bacterial infections such as sinusitis, otitis, bronchitis, and GI infections. Selective IgA deficiency is associated with an increase in atopic and autoimmune disorders, including Graves disease, SLE, juvenile RA, type 1 diabetes mellitus, and celiac disease.

Table 23–14. Selected primary immunodeficiency diseases that can present in adulthood.

Disease	Clinical Presentation	Diagnosis[1]	Treatment
Complement disorders	"Early" complement component (C1–C4) deficiencies: autoimmune diseases "Late" complement component (C5–C8) deficiencies: recurrent meningococcal or gonococcal infections	Screen with CH50 and AH50. Obtain individual serum complement levels if abnormal. **Genetic testing if complement level absent to confirm diagnosis.**	Prompt administration of antibiotics and *Neisseria* vaccination if C5–C8 deficient. Immune suppression if C1–4 deficient to treat organ specific autoimmunity.
Good syndrome	Current or past thymoma, recurrent severe sinopulmonary infections, may also have opportunistic infections.	**Hypogammaglobulinemia (IgG, IgM, IgA), absent B cells on flow cytometry**, may present with pure red cell aplasia or cytopenias. **Chest film consistent with thymoma.**	IgG-RT (subcutaneously or intravenously) 300 mg–600 mg/kg/month
Hereditary angioedema	Unpredictable swelling of face, lips, tongue, hands, feet; no urticaria; GI tract swelling causing severe abdominal pain	**Decreased C1 esterase inhibitor serum level and/or function,** decreased serum C4 level. **Genetic testing if C4 or C1 esterase level is absent to confirm diagnosis.**	Prophylactic treatment: Danazol, tranexamic acid Acute treatment: C1 esterase inhibitor product, kallikrein inhibitor, bradykinin receptor antagonist
Granulocyte disorders	Recurrent invasive skin and soft tissue infections, abscesses requiring incision and drainage Common organisms are *Staphylococcus aureus*, gram-negative bacilli, *Nocardia, Aspergillus*	CBC with differential to evaluate neutrophil count. **Dihydrorhodamine assay to confirm defective oxidative burst. Genetic testing to confirm diagnosis.**	Antimicrobial prophylaxis; interferon for chronic granulomatous disease
CXCR4 immunodeficiency (WHIM syndrome)	Neutropenia and lymphopenia. Warts variable and may include genital warts refractory to treatment. Recurrent sinopulmonary and viral infections. Hypogammaglobulinemia variable.	Bone marrow biopsy may reveal myelokathexis. **Genetic testing to confirm diagnosis with a single CXCR4 mutation.**	CXCR4 antagonist mavorixafor, IgG-RT, GCSF, antibiotics, HPV and PCV21 vaccinations

CXCR4, C-X-C motif chemokine receptor 4; GCSF, granulocyte colony stimulating factor; HPV, human papillomavirus; IgG-RT, immune globulin replacement therapy. PCV21, 21-valent pneumococcal conjugate vaccine; WHIM, warts, hypogammaglobulinemia, infections, myelokathexis

[1]**Key diagnostic findings in bold.**

Reproduced with permission from Ashar B, Miller R, Sisson S (editors): *Johns Hopkins Internal Medicine Board Review Certification and Recertification*, 5th ed. Elsevier LTD, 2015 and modified.

Some individuals with undetectable levels of serum IgA have high titers of IgG or IgE anti-IgA antibodies and are at risk for anaphylactic reactions to IgA after infusions of plasma (or other blood transfusions). Immune globulin replacement therapy (IgG-RT) is not indicated for selective IgA deficiency and may result in anaphylaxis from preparations that contain detectable amounts of IgA. Notably, IgG-RT does not treat IgA deficiency since there is little IgA present in IgG-RT products.

When to Refer

- Refer patients with undetectable serum IgA and recurrent sinopulmonary infections, celiac disease, giardiasis, or a family history of immunodeficiency to an immunologist.
- Healthy, asymptomatic individuals with IgA deficiency do not need a referral.

2. Common Variable Immunodeficiency (CVID)

ESSENTIALS OF DIAGNOSIS

- Recurrent, severe sinopulmonary infections secondary to humoral immune deficiency.
- Two or more low (< 2 standard deviations) serum immunoglobulin levels (IgG, IgA, IgM) and deficient functional antibody responses to vaccination. Importantly, other causes for hypogammaglobulinemia and recurrent sinopulmonary infections have been ruled out.

General Considerations

CVID is a heterogeneous immunodeficiency characterized by recurrent, severe sinopulmonary infections with

hypogammaglobulinemia and inadequate vaccination responses. Approximately half of patients with CVID will also have autoimmune disease with or without neoplastic disease. CVID onset is generally in adolescence or early adulthood, but it can occur at any age, mostly due to delay in diagnosis. Most cases are sporadic; about 10–20% are familial. Thus, routine immunoglobulin screening of family members without severe symptoms is not advised, albeit patients with CVID may have family members with a higher incidence of autoimmune disease or IgA deficiency. Since the genetic defect is not known, patients with CVID and their offspring are not recommended to undergo genetic testing unless advised by an immunologist or geneticist.

Clinical Findings

A. Symptoms and Signs

Increased susceptibility to serious infections, especially with encapsulated organisms leading to pneumonia and pyogenic infections, is the hallmark of CVID. Virtually all patients have recurrent bacterial sinusitis, bronchitis, and otitis, but it is the recurrent pneumonia that sets these individuals apart from patients with severe atopy. Infections may be prolonged or associated with unusual complications such as meningitis, empyema, or sepsis. Bronchiectasis occurs in > 25% of patients who are not treated with IgG-RT and is a leading cause of morbidity. Recurrent viral infections are not prototypic of the disease, albeit varicella-zoster reactivation, CMV reactivation, and increased symptomatic disease from other herpes viruses and *Candida* can occur in some patients.

GI infections and autoimmunity are commonly associated with CVID. Many patients will develop an inflammatory sprue-like syndrome or collagenous colitis, with diarrhea, steatorrhea, malabsorption, protein-losing enteropathy, and hepatosplenomegaly. Norovirus and *Giardia* infections can be chronic and refractory to treatment. Paradoxically, there is an increased incidence of autoimmune disease (20%) in patients with CVID, although they rarely display prototypic serologic markers as they are hypogammaglobulinemic. Autoimmune cytopenias are most common, but autoimmune endocrinopathies, seronegative rheumatic disease, and the aforementioned GI disorders are also commonly seen. Lymph nodes may be enlarged in patients with CVID, yet biopsies show marked reduction in plasma cells. Noncaseating granulomas mimicking sarcoidosis can be found in the spleen, liver, lungs, or skin. There is an increased propensity for the development of B-cell neoplasms (50- to 400-fold increased risk of lymphoma) and gastric carcinomas.

B. Laboratory Findings

The serum IgG level is reduced at least two standard deviations below normal in most patients. IgA, IgM, or both, also are reduced two standard deviations below normal; it is common that IgA is undetectable. Demonstration of impaired antibody production in response to vaccination is essential and is performed by checking antibody response to polysaccharide (pneumococcal 23 serotypes, *H influenzae* type b) and protein (tetanus, diphtheria) antigens at baseline and 4–6 weeks after vaccination. The diagnosis is made in patients who have two or more reduced serum immunoglobulin classes and poor antibody response to vaccines after exclusion of secondary causes (eg, proteinuria, protein-losing enteropathy, drug effects from immunosuppressants, antiepileptics, hematologic malignancies).

The absolute B-cell count in the peripheral blood, however, can be normal. A subset of patients with CVID have concomitant T-cell immunodeficiency with increased numbers of activated CD8 cells, splenomegaly, and decreased delayed-type hypersensitivity.

Differential Diagnosis

Secondary causes of hypogammaglobulinemia must be excluded (Table 23–15). Secondary causes of recurrent sinopulmonary infections to also exclude are severe atopic disease, COPD, current or past prolonged cigarette smoking, chronic sinusitis, cystic fibrosis, Kartagener syndrome, and colonization with multi-drug–resistant bacteria.

Treatment

In addition to IgG-RT, patients should be treated aggressively with antibiotics at the first sign of infection. Since antibody deficiency predisposes patients to high-risk pyogenic infections, antibiotic coverage should cover encapsulated bacteria. Infections with other microorganisms can develop including viruses, parasites, and extracellular gram-positive or gram-negative bacteria (such as *S aureus* or *P aeruginosa*). The standard of care for preventive therapy is IgG-RT. The preferred method of administration of IgG-RT is by subcutaneous injections, 300–600 mg/kg monthly in divided weekly doses, which offers the convenience of self-administration and lower incidence of adverse effects. Adjustment of the dosage or injection interval is made primarily based on clinical responses in addition to serum IgG levels. Such therapy is essential for decreasing the incidence of potentially life-threatening infections, increasing quality of life, and reducing the progression of lung disease. IgG-RT can be administered intravenously, but this is less common due to the improved cost, ease of administration, fewer systemic side effects, and more stable IgG levels achieved with subcutaneous administration.

When to Refer

- Refer patients with ≥ 2 low serum immunoglobulins and recurrent serious or unusual infections to a clinical immunologist with expertise in immunodeficiency.
- The presence of bronchiectasis without a known underlying cause such as cystic fibrosis or Kartagener syndrome should raise the suspicion of a primary immunodeficiency and warrants further evaluation by a clinical immunologist.
- Patients with granulomatous disease (resembling sarcoidosis) who have had recurrent, severe infections should be evaluated by a clinical immunologist.

3. Specific (Functional) Antibody Deficiency

Specific antibody deficiency is characterized by decreased or absent IgG antibody response to vaccines in the setting

Table 23–15. Secondary causes of hypogammaglobulinemia.

Medications	Infections	Malignancy and Transplantation	Protein-Losing Enteropathy
Anti-CD20 therapy (rituximab, ocrelizumab, ofatumumab, ublituximab, or biosimilars)	*Clostridioides difficile* with colitis	Chronic lymphocytic leukemia	Amyloidosis
Antiepileptics (carbamazepine, phenytoin, valproate)	Cytomegalovirus	GI malignancy	Celiac disease with diarrhea
Bortezomib	HIV	Good syndrome	Congenital disorders of glycosylation
BTK inhibitors	Small intestinal bacterial overgrowth	Graft-versus-host disease	Congenital heart disease
CD19 CAR-T-cell therapy	Whipple disease	Multiple myeloma	Eosinophilic gastroenteritis
Clozapine		Non-Hodgkin lymphoma	Erosive gastritis
Corticosteroids		Solid organ transplantation	IBD
Cyclophosphamide			Lymphocytic gastritis
Mycophenolate mofetil			NSAID enteropathy
Methotrexate			Peritonitis
Purine analogs (azathioprine, cladribine, fludarabine)			Primary and secondary lymphangiectasia

BTK, Bruton tyrosine kinase inhibitor; CAR-T, chimeric antigen receptor T-cell.

of normal or mildly decreased serum immunoglobulin levels. The clinical spectrum can range from mild symptoms that can be managed with antibiotics and vaccination to, more rarely, recurrent infections with features very similar to CVID. Since this can be a nuanced diagnosis, recommendations are to refer to a clinical immunologist for diagnosis and treatment recommendations.

4. Immunoglobulin Subclass Deficiency

There are four subclasses of IgG: IgG_1, IgG_2, IgG_3, and IgG_4. A low level of at least one IgG subclass has been found incidentally in 2% of the population. Thus, low or absent IgG subclass levels alone are not sufficient for a diagnosis of immunodeficiency, and IgG-RT is not clinically indicated unless other functional impairments (as discussed in the diagnosis of CVID) in the immune system are identified.

5. Secondary Hypogammaglobulinemia

Secondary causes of hypogammaglobulinemia, rather than from a primary genetic defect, are more likely to occur in the older population due to an increase in comorbid conditions and medications. Some malignancies, immunosuppressants, anti-psychotic medications, chronic diarrhea, sepsis, nephrosis, and HIV have known associations with hypogammaglobulinemia (Table 23–15). The principal therapy of secondary hypogammaglobulinemia is treatment of the underlying condition or removal of the offending medication.

6. Less Common Immunodeficiencies in Adulthood

Less common immunodeficiency diseases that present in adulthood can be attributed to an inborn error of immunity or malignancy (Table 23–14). Inborn errors of immunity are being increasingly diagnosed in adulthood; approximately 50% of cases are diagnosed in patients aged > 25 years with an estimated prevalence as high as 1:1200. More than 480 inborn errors of immunity are recognized, due, in part, to scientific advancements and increased accessibility of genetic testing. The cost of genetic testing, including focused gene panels, whole exome sequencing, and whole genome sequencing, may be covered by insurance carriers or research programs. Consider obtaining genetic tests for abnormalities in immune function and for undiagnosed etiologies of severe, recurrent infections.

When to Refer

- Isolated immunoglobulin subclass deficiency does not need to be referred if other immune studies are normal.
- Secondary hypogammaglobulinemia should be referred to an immunologist if hypogammaglobulinemia or recurrent infections are persistent or severe and if vaccination boosters and antibiotics do not result in clinical improvement.
- Consider referral to an immunologist or medical geneticist for any abnormality in immunologic diagnostic workup (Table 23–14).

Otani IM et al. Practical guidance for the diagnosis and management of secondary hypogammaglobulinemia: a work group report of the AAAAI Primary Immunodeficiency and Altered Immune Response Committees. J Allergy Clin Immunol. 2022;149:1525. [PMID: 35176351]

Wang JJF et al. Inborn errors of immunity in adulthood. Allergy Asthma Clin Immunol. 2024;20:6. [PMID: 38233962]

24 Electrolyte & Acid-Base Disorders

Nayan Arora, MD, FASN
J. Ashley Jefferson, MD, FRCP

ASSESSMENT OF THE PATIENT

The pathophysiology of all electrolyte disorders is rooted in basic principles of total body water and its distribution across fluid compartments. The optimal evaluation and treatment of fluid and electrolyte disorders require careful interpretation of serum and urine chemistries, along with a thorough history and physical examination. While classic teaching has focused on physical examination to determine a patient's volume status, such an approach can be challenging because of limitations in accurate bedside analysis of volume status.

A. Body Water and Fluid Distribution

Total body water depends on the relative proportions of muscle and fat in the body. Total body water is typically estimated as 50% of body weight in women and 60% in men, as women, on average, have a higher proportion of fat to body weight (Table 24–1). Total body water tends to decrease with age due to declining muscle mass. Approximately two-thirds of total body water is located in the intracellular compartment and one-third in the extracellular compartment. The volume in the extracellular compartment is further divided into two components: the interstitial fluid (15% of body weight) and the plasma fluid (5% of body weight).

Changes in total body water content are best evaluated by documenting changes in body weight. Extracellular volume (ECV) may be assessed by physical examination (eg, blood pressure, pulse, jugular venous distention, peripheral or central edema). Quantitative assessments of ECV and intravascular volume may be invasive (ie, CVP assessed via a catheter or pulmonary wedge pressure from right heart catheterization) or noninvasive (ie, inferior vena cava diameter and right atrial pressure assessed by surface echocardiography). Intracellular volume (ICV) is assessed using the serum sodium concentration.

Table 24–1. Total body water (as percentage of body weight) in relation to age and sex.

Age	Male	Female
18–40	60%	50%
41–60	60–50%	50–40%
Over 60	50%	40%

B. Serum Electrolytes

Under healthy conditions, serum electrolytes are maintained within a narrow range by the kidneys (homeostasis). The serum level of an electrolyte may be normal, elevated, or decreased, but may not correlate with the total body levels of that electrolyte due to the shift of water or electrolytes into and out of cells.

C. Evaluation of Urine

The urine concentration of an electrolyte can help determine whether the kidney is excreting or retaining the electrolyte in response to high or low serum levels. A 24-hour urine collection for daily electrolyte excretion remains the gold standard for assessing kidney electrolyte handling; however, the collection process can be cumbersome and technically challenging in certain patients. A more convenient method to determine renal electrolyte handling is the use of fractional excretion (FE) of an electrolyte X (FE_x), which is calculated from a spot urine sample and concomitant serum sample, using creatinine (Cr):

$$FE_x(\%) = \frac{Urine_x \times Serum_{Cr}}{Serum_x \times Urine_{Cr}} \times 100$$

A low fractional excretion indicates renal reabsorption (electrolyte retention), while a high fractional excretion indicates renal wasting (electrolyte excretion). Thus, fractional excretion helps determine whether the kidney's response to a specific electrolyte disorder is appropriate.

D. Serum Osmolality

Total solute concentration is measured by osmolality in millimoles per kilogram. Osmolarity is measured in millimoles of solute per liter of solution. These terms are often used interchangeably in clinical medicine. Plasma osmolality is the total concentration of all the solutes contained in plasma, both electrolytes and non-electrolytes, and normally ranges between 285 and 295 mOsm/kg. Differences in osmole concentration across cell membranes lead to the movement of water toward the region of higher osmolality. Substances that easily permeate cell membranes (eg, urea, ethanol) are ineffective osmoles and do not cause fluid shifts across fluid compartments. High serum osmolality stimulates thirst and increases the secretion of antidiuretic hormone (ADH).

Serum osmolality (Osm) can be estimated using the following formula:

$$Osm = 2(Na^{+}\,mEq/L) + \frac{Glucose\ mg/dL}{18} + \frac{BUN\ mg/dL}{2.8}$$

(*Note:* dividing urea by 2.8 converts mg/dL to mmol/L; dividing glucose by 18 converts mg/dL to mmol/L)

Sodium is the major extracellular cation; in the body, doubling the serum sodium in the formula for estimated osmolality accounts for corresponding anions. A discrepancy between measured and calculated osmolality of > 10 mmol/kg suggests an osmolar gap, due to unmeasured osmoles such as ethanol, methanol, isopropanol, and ethylene glycol (see Table 42–5).

DISORDERS OF SODIUM CONCENTRATION

HYPONATREMIA

ESSENTIALS OF DIAGNOSIS

- Must know volume status as well as serum and urine osmolality to determine etiology.
- Hyponatremia usually reflects excess water retention rather than sodium deficiency. The serum sodium concentration is not a measure of total body sodium.
- Hyponatremia in hospitalized patients is commonly caused by the administration of hypotonic fluids.

General Considerations

Hyponatremia is defined as a serum sodium concentration < 135 mEq/L (135 mmol/L) and is the most common electrolyte abnormality encountered in clinical practice. Hyponatremia represents an excess of water relative to sodium in the plasma, leading to a reduction in plasma osmolality and subsequent movement of water from the extracellular fluid into the intracellular fluid compartment. The cellular swelling particularly impacts the brain due to limited space for expansion within the skull. If this movement of water happens acutely, intracranial pressure rises as a consequence of cerebral edema, increasing the risk of seizures and even brain herniation.

Chronic hyponatremia is often asymptomatic or presents with mild confusion, nausea, or falls; cerebral adaptation occurs as the brain cells excrete intracellular osmoles to limit cellular swelling. In this chronic setting, hyponatremia is traditionally corrected slowly due to concern for instigating profound neurologic abnormalities (osmotic demyelination syndrome). However, this concern has been challenged by retrospective, observational studies; in practice, osmotic demyelination is rare, suggesting factors other than correction rates are likely implicated. Regardless, caution is still recommended when correcting chronic hyponatremia in terms of the rate of hypertonic fluid administration.

A common misconception is that hyponatremia is secondary to a deficiency in total body sodium; however, it usually reflects an excess of total body water. The basic pathophysiologic principle is that more water (oral or intravenous) is ingested than the kidney can excrete (commonly due to the action of ADH). A diagnostic algorithm (Figure 24–1) separates the causes of hyponatremia using serum osmolality, urine osmolality, and urine sodium.

Etiology

A. Isotonic and Hypertonic Hyponatremia

Hyponatremia is typically associated with hypoosmolality with two exceptions: pseudohyponatremia and hypertonic hyponatremia.

1. Pseudohyponatremia—This represents a rare laboratory artifact in patients with marked hypertriglyceridemia or hypergammaglobulinemia. In these settings, an increase in the solid components of plasma, relative to plasma water, results in a lower sodium level per given volume. Analyzers that measure serum sodium concentration using indirect ion selective electrodes are particularly vulnerable to this phenomenon as they use diluted specimens. Direct ion-selective electrodes, which are found in point of care devices and blood gas analyzers, do not require dilution and can be used to confirm a suspicion of pseudohyponatremia. There is no need to treat the hyponatremia in these cases.

2. Hypertonic hyponatremia—The best clinical examples of this situation occur in the setting of hyperglycemia. Glucose is an active osmole that increases the tonicity of the extracellular fluid, pulling water from inside cells into the extracellular space, diluting the sodium content. Note, this leads to a reduction in intracellular volume, and therefore, hyponatremia does not cause cerebral edema in this setting. However, cerebral edema may occur in the treatment phase of this condition due to over-rapid correction of hyperglycemia and injudicious use of intravenous fluids. The increased tonicity also stimulates thirst and vasopressin release, further contributing to water retention. To determine whether the hyponatremia can be entirely attributed to hyperglycemia, a sodium correction factor is often used. Most guidelines recommend using a decrease in the serum sodium concentration of 1.6 mEq/L (1.6 mmol/L) for every 100 mg/dL (5.5 mmol/L) rise in plasma glucose above normal for this correction, although more recent work suggests a correction factor of 2.4 for every 100mg/dL rise.

B. Hypotonic Hyponatremia

Most cases of hyponatremia are hypotonic, highlighting sodium's role as the predominant extracellular osmole.

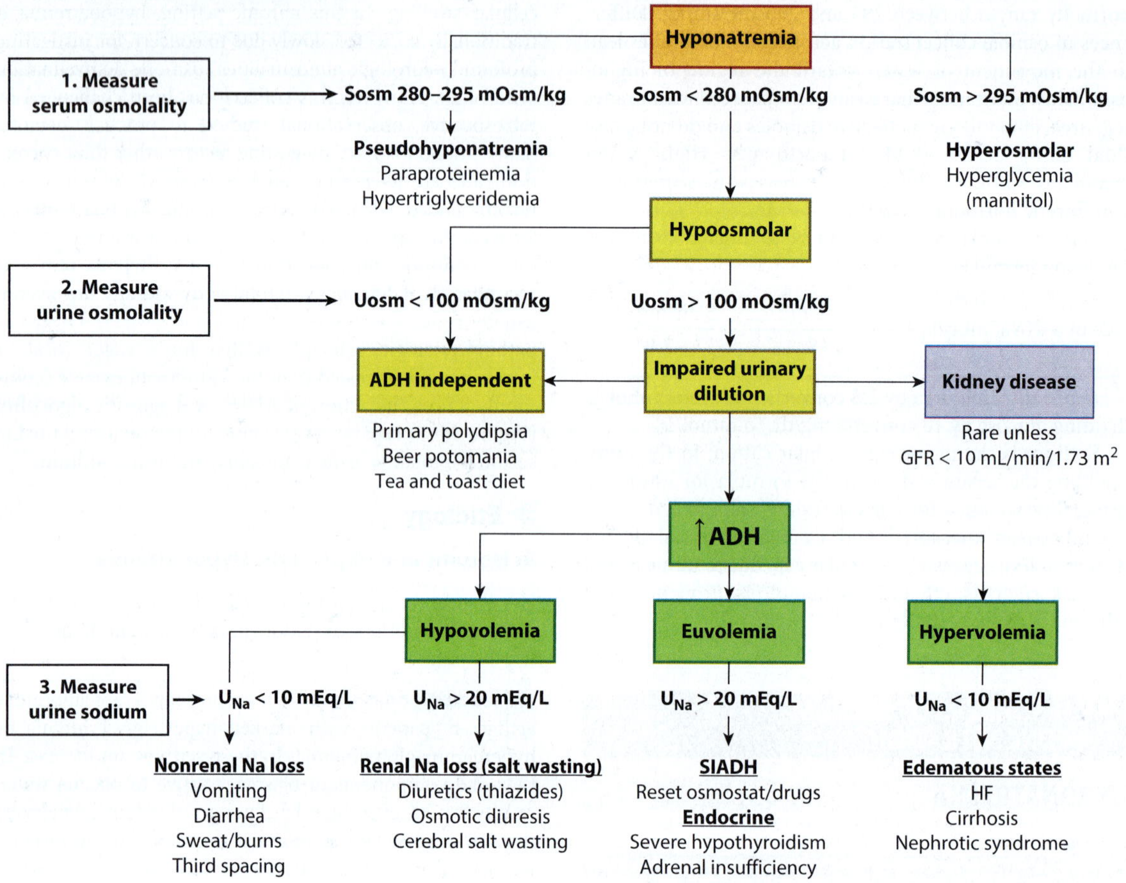

Figure 24–1. A diagnostic algorithm for the causes of hyponatremia using serum osmolality, urine osmolality, and urine sodium.

The presence of hypotonic hyponatremia indicates that water intake exceeds the kidney's excretory capacity. The next step is to classify hypotonic cases as ADH dependent or independent based on the kidney's ability to excrete dilute urine.

1. ADH-independent causes—In rare circumstances, hypotonic hyponatremia can occur when the kidney's ability to excrete free water is intact (urine osmolality < 100 mOsm/kg).

A. Primary polydipsia—This condition develops when excess water intake overwhelms the kidney's capacity to excrete adequately dilute urine. ADH is appropriately suppressed, reflected by a urine osmolality < 100 mOsm/kg. Polydipsia without physiologic thirst occurs primarily in patients with psychiatric disorders. Psychiatric medications may also interfere with water excretion or increase thirst through anticholinergic side effects, further increasing water intake.

B. Low dietary solute intake—Patients who consume large quantities of beer, which is generally very low in sodium (beer drinker's potomania), or those who consume a low-protein, high-carbohydrate ("tea and toast") diet may have a marked reduction in free water excretion due to insufficient dietary solute intake. The kidney's ability to excrete free water depends not only on ADH suppression but also on solute delivery to the distal nephron. Atypical Western diet generates 1000 mOsm of solute, and with a dilute urine of 50 mOsm/kg, will generate 20 L of urine (1000mOsm ÷ 50mosm/L). However, in patients with a low solute content, (eg, 200 mOsm per day), urinary output would be limited to a maximum of 4 L per day; water intake that exceeds this limit may result in hyponatremia.

C. Renal impairment—Patients with advanced renal impairment (GFR < 15 mL/min/1.73 m^2), whether due to severe CKD or AKI, may be unable to dilute their urine. Patients with advanced renal impairment can often achieve a minimum urine osmolality of only 200–250 mOsm/kg even with maximal ADH suppression and therefore are prone to develop water retention and hyponatremia. This can occur in the setting of normal or high plasma osmolality due to the accumulation of urea. Water retention and hyponatremia from the kidney's impaired ability to dilute urine differ from hypertonic hyponatremia because urea is an ineffective osmole and is freely permeable across cell membranes, only minimally pulling water into the plasma space. Therefore, patients with renal impairment and hyponatremia should be treated as a typical hyponatremic patient.

2. ADH-dependent causes—The most common cause of hypotonic hyponatremia involves a failure to suppress

ADH action. This can either be **appropriate** in the setting of hypovolemia, or a reduced effective arterial volume secondary to cirrhosis or HF (hypervolemia), or **inappropriate,** in the absence of hypovolemia or edematous states, which is known as the syndrome of inappropriate antidiuresis (SIAD).

A. Hypovolemic hyponatremia—Hypovolemic hyponatremia occurs with renal or extrarenal volume loss (sodium and water) and subsequent hypotonic fluid replacement (Figure 24–1). Reduced blood pressure increases ADH secretion by the pituitary gland, limiting free water excretion. In this setting, the body sacrifices serum osmolality to preserve intravascular volume.

Cerebral salt wasting is an inadequately understood, rare subset of hyponatremia that occurs with intracranial disease (eg, infections, cerebrovascular accidents, tumors, and neurosurgery). Clinical features include refractory hypotension, often in the setting of large volumes of isotonic crystalloid solutions. The pathophysiology is unclear but has been attributed to renal sodium wasting, although there is uncertainty as to whether cerebral salt wasting represents a distinct entity or SIAD with desalination of the administered saline.

B. Hypervolemic hyponatremia—Hypervolemic hyponatremia commonly occurs in the edematous states of cirrhosis and HF, and rarely in nephrotic syndrome (Figure 24–1). In these settings, a decreased effective arterial blood volume occurs despite an overall increase in extracellular volume (edema), resulting in ADH secretion. In cirrhosis and HF, effective circulating volume is decreased due to systemic vasodilation and reduced cardiac output, respectively.

C. SIAD—In this condition, ADH is secreted in the absence of an appropriate physiologic stimuli such as a decreased effective circulating volume or hyperosmolality. The major causes of SIAD (Table 24–2) are CNS or lung disorders (eg, cancer or infections) and medications. SIAD is a diagnosis of exclusion, which involves ruling out other causes of hyponatremia (eg, low effective circulating volume, decreased solute intake, cortisol deficiency, and severe hypothyroidism).

D. Reset osmostat—This is a rare cause of hyponatremia in which patients regulate vasopressin release around a lower, or hypotonic, set point. Diagnosis involves documentation of dilute urine when the administration of free water lowers serum sodium; however, this is rarely done in clinical practice. The mild hypo-osmolality of pregnancy is a form of reset osmostat.

E. Adrenal insufficiency and hypothyroidism—Cortisol normally provides negative feedback on ADH release, and therefore, cortisol deficiency can lead to uninhibited ADH activity and hyponatremia. Concomitant mineralocorticoid deficiency may result in hyperkalemia and metabolic acidosis. Hyponatremia due to hypothyroidism has been described in the context of myxedema coma; the hyponatremia may be due to appropriate ADH release from reduced cardiac output and concurrent adrenal insufficiency, rather than from the absence of thyroid hormone.

Table 24–2. Common causes of syndrome of inappropriate antidiuresis.

CNS disorders
Stroke
Hemorrhage
Infection
Trauma
Inflammatory and demyelinating diseases
Pulmonary lesions
Infections (viral, bacterial, fungal)
Malignancies
Many but particularly small cell carcinoma of the lung
Drugs (this is only a partial list as many have been implicated)
Antidepressants: SSRIs, tricyclics, MAO inhibitors
Antineoplastics: cyclophosphamide, ifosfamide, methotrexate
Anticonvulsants: carbamazepine, sodium valproate, lamotrigine
Neuroleptics: haloperidol, fluphenazine, trifluoperazine thioridazine, thiothixene
NSAIDs
Amiodarone
Ciprofloxacin
Opioids
Methylenedioxymethamphetamine (MDMA; ecstasy)
Others
HIV
Pain, postoperative, stress
Nausea
Hereditary
Idiopathic

Despite the lack of evidence associating thyroid hormone deficiency with hyponatremia, ruling out hypothyroidism remains a criterion for diagnosing SIAD (Bartter and Schwartz criteria).

F. Nausea, pain, and surgery—Nausea and pain are potent stimulators of ADH release. Severe hyponatremia can develop after elective surgery in healthy patients due to excessive use of hypotonic fluids.

G. Exercise-associated hyponatremia—Hyponatremia during or after exercise, especially endurance events, may be caused by a combination of excessive hypotonic fluid intake and ADH secretion (due to hypovolemia, pain, or nausea). Guidelines that endurance athletes drink water according to thirst rather than according to specified hourly rates of fluid intake are sound and should be followed. Contrary to impressions in the general population, electrolyte-containing sport drinks do not protect against hyponatremia since they are markedly hypotonic relative to serum.

H. Thiazide diuretics and other medication—Thiazides may induce hyponatremia, typically in older patients, within a few weeks of initiating therapy, and may be exacerbated by increased thirst and low solute intake. The conventional suggested mechanism has been that the induction of volume loss leads to ADH release; however, studies have demonstrated thiazide-induced hyponatremia in the absence of volume depletion. Genome-wide association studies have demonstrated a genetic basis for this disorder. Regardless, therapy involves thiazide discontinuation and fluid restriction. Saline infusion should be used with caution due to the propensity for rapid sodium correction.

NSAIDs increase ADH by inhibiting prostaglandin formation. SSRIs (eg, fluoxetine, paroxetine, and citalopram) can also cause hyponatremia, especially in older adults. Enhanced secretion or action of ADH may result from increased serotonergic tone.

Use of 3,4-methylenedioxymethamphetamine (MDMA, also known as ecstasy) can lead to hyponatremia and severe neurologic symptoms, including seizures, cerebral edema, and brainstem herniation. MDMA and its metabolites increase ADH release from the hypothalamus. Polydipsia may contribute to hyponatremia since MDMA users typically increase fluid intake to prevent hyperthermia.

Clinical Findings

A. Symptoms and Signs

Whether hyponatremia is symptomatic depends on both its severity and acuity. **Acute hyponatremia** (defined as lasting < 48 hours) can result in marked neurologic symptoms, even with relatively modest hyponatremia, due to acute brain cell swelling and subsequent rise in intracranial pressure. Early symptoms include headache and decreased attentiveness, which can progress to lethargy, disorientation, and nausea. The most serious symptoms include marked confusion and reduced levels of consciousness, vomiting, seizures, coma, brainstem herniation, and death. **Chronic hyponatremia,** defined as lasting longer than 48 hours, is often diagnosed on routine electrolyte measurements; patients are often asymptomatic as the brain has adapted to the surrounding hypotonicity. Subtle abnormalities, such as mild concentration and cognitive deficits, as well as gait disturbances that can lead to falls, may be present.

Clinical evaluation starts with eliciting a history of medications and noting any changes to drugs and medications, fluid intake (polydipsia, anorexia, intravenous fluid rates and composition), and fluid output (nausea and vomiting, diarrhea, ostomy output, polyuria, oliguria, insensible losses). The physical examination should attempt to categorize volume status (see Body Water and Fluid Distribution, above). The next determination is why ADH is being released and conditions in which release may be halted abruptly, which can impact the approach to therapy.

B. Laboratory Findings

The initial laboratory assessment should include serum and urine electrolytes and osmolality. The severity of hyponatremia can be classified as mild (130–134 mEq/L), moderate (125–129 mEq/L), or severe (< 125 mEq/L), with complications of untreated hyponatremia and rapid/overcorrection most commonly occurring in patients with severe hyponatremia. In clinical practice, ADH levels are not measured; urine osmolality is used as a surrogate for ADH activity. Urine osmolality should be checked not only at the time of diagnosis but serially during therapy. Bedside assessment of volume status is often insensitive; therefore, a urine sodium may help differentiate between hypovolemia and euvolemia, particularly in nonedematous patients (Figure 24–1). The etiology of most cases of hyponatremia will be apparent by appropriate interpretation of the above laboratory values, in addition to patient history and assessment of volume status. Additional testing, such as thyroid and adrenal function tests, may be warranted in the appropriate context.

SIAD is a clinical diagnosis characterized by (1) hyponatremia; (2) decreased plasma osmolality (< 280 mOsm/kg); (3) absence of heart, kidney, or liver disease; (4) normal thyroid and adrenal function (see Chapter 29); and (5) urine sodium usually over 20 mEq/L. Patients with SIAD may have low BUN (< 10 mg/dL [3.6 mmol/L]) and hypouricemia (< 4 mg/dL [238 mcmol/L]), which are not only dilutional but result from increased urea and uric acid clearances in response to the volume-expanded state. Differentiating among these disorders can be challenging. Interpretation of a urine sodium level post saline administration has been shown to improve diagnostic yield.

Treatment

The initial treatment of hyponatremia is contingent on two primary factors, the acuity of onset and the severity of symptoms. **In patients with documented acute hyponatremia (ie, onset within 48 hours), sodium can be corrected at the rate at which it fell. In general, most cases are chronic and therefore typically corrected more slowly to minimize risk of osmotic demyelination.**

A. Symptomatic Hyponatremia

If a patient has hyponatremia and severe symptoms (eg, seizures, confusion), regardless of etiology, then emergent treatment with hypertonic saline should commence. A relatively small increase in serum sodium of 4–5 mEq/L is generally sufficient to promptly reverse severe neurologic symptoms and decrease intracranial pressure. This can be accomplished most effectively by using boluses of 100 mL of 3% NaCl over 10 minutes, which can be repeated twice if needed. Each bolus might be predicted to raise the serum sodium by 1–2 mEq/L. In patients with less severe symptoms, 3% NaCl may be infused intravenously at a rate of 0.5–2 mL/kg/hour.

The importance of frequent laboratory monitoring—every 1–2 hours—during treatment of hyponatremia cannot be overemphasized.

B. Chronic Hyponatremia

The cornerstone of therapy in most patients with chronic hyponatremia, regardless of etiology, is restricting fluid intake below the level of urinary output. However, this strategy is only minimally effective in most patients. The electrolyte free water equation (see Chronic Hypernatremia below) is used to determine what proportion of a patient's urine volume is electrolyte free water. Because urine volume is not always available, the Furst ratio—a calculated ratio of $(U_{Na} + U_K)/P_{Na}$—is sufficient. A ratio > 1 is highly predictive of failure with fluid restriction alone, and other measures to increase free water excretion should be considered. Loop diuretics (with or without salt tablets) are frequently used since they impair the medullary concentration gradient, thereby limiting renal concentration; despite this physiologic principle, this therapy has not been shown to be superior to fluid restriction alone.

Other options include vasopressin receptor antagonists (vaptans), SGLT-2 inhibitors, and oral urea.

Vaptans impair ADH action by inhibiting the vasopressin type 2 (V_2) receptors in the collecting duct, thereby inducing a water diuresis. While a logical target for therapy in refractory hyponatremia, these agents have not been shown to improve outcomes and are associated with risks of liver toxicity and sodium overcorrection. If these agents are used, they should generally be avoided in patients with cirrhosis, duration should be limited to 30 days, and fluid restriction should concurrently be lifted to reduce the risk of excessive serum sodium correction. An alternative option is the use of oral urea to induce an osmotic diuresis, which enhances free water clearance. The disadvantage of the palatability of oral urea alone has been addressed by combining urea with sodium bicarbonate, citric acid, and sucrose in commercially available formulations. SGLT-2 inhibitors may be an option via their ability to induce an osmotic diuresis through glycosuria and have demonstrated greater improvements in serum sodium levels in patients with SIAD, compared with placebo, when combined with standard fluid restriction.

Osmotic demyelination and correction rate—Iatrogenic osmotic demyelination syndrome is thought to be the result of overly rapid correction of serum sodium in patients with chronic hyponatremia, though, as stated above, this paradigm has been challenged. Previously called central pontine myelinolysis, osmotic demyelination syndrome may also occur outside the brainstem. Demyelination generally occurs 2–6 days after inappropriate sodium correction and presents with profound neurologic deficits that are often irreversible. Risk factors for osmotic demyelination syndrome include serum sodium < 110 mmol/L, alcohol use disorder, liver disease, malnutrition, and concurrent hypokalemia. Of note, large cohort studies have associated an inappropriately slow correction of serum sodium with increased mortality.

Despite studies suggesting sodium correction alone is not the sole risk factor for osmotic demyelination, guidelines continue to recommend caution with correction rates. The optimal correction rate for hyponatremia is debated, though typical targets are < 8 mEq/L in a 24-hour period for patients at high risk for ODS and < 10–12 mEq/L in patients at low risk for ODS. It should be emphasized that this represents a limit and not a goal. In fact, in patients who are deemed at high risk for osmotic demyelination syndrome based on the criteria detailed above, a lower goal of 4–6 mEq/L/day may be appropriate. If rapid discontinuation of the effects of vasopressin is anticipated, particularly in patients who are at high risk for osmotic demyelination syndrome, prophylactic use of intravenous desmopressin acetate (DDAVP) clamp to prevent a water diuresis should be considered.

C. Isotonic and Hypertonic Hyponatremia

Pseudohyponatremia from hypertriglyceridemia or hyperproteinemia requires no therapy except confirmation with the clinical laboratory. Hypertonic hyponatremia from translocational hyponatremia due to hyperglycemia can be managed with glucose correction.

D. Hypotonic Hyponatremia

In addition to the considerations discussed above, patients with **hypovolemic hyponatremia** require fluid resuscitation. There is no clear consensus regarding the optimal fluid for resuscitation, due to conflicting data, between normal saline and balanced solutions such as Ringer lactate or Plasma-lyte. Correction of volume depletion removes the stimulus for ADH and permits the renal excretion of dilute urine. The fluid resuscitation should be undertaken carefully because rapid renal excretion of the excess water may correct the serum sodium level too quickly.

When to Refer

- Nephrology consultation should be considered in patients with hyponatremia of uncertain cause or in refractory or complicated cases.
- Aggressive therapies with hypertonic saline, V_2-antagonists, or dialysis mandate specialist consultation.
- Consultation may be necessary with severe liver or heart disease.

When to Admit

Hospital admission is necessary for severe or symptomatic patients or those requiring aggressive therapies (such as hypertonic saline) for close monitoring and frequent laboratory testing.

Chienwichai K et al. Urine sodium levels post-saline infusion in differentiating non-edematous hyponatremia. Sci Rep. 2025;15:28883. [PMID: 40775013]

Krisanapan P et al. Efficacy of furosemide, oral sodium chloride, and fluid restriction for treatment of syndrome of inappropriate antidiuresis (SIAD): an open label randomized controlled study (The EFFUSE-FLUID trial). Am J Kidney Dis. 2020;76:203. [PMID: 32199708]

MacMillan TE et al. Osmotic demyelination syndrome in patients hospitalized with hyponatremia. NEJM Evid. 2023;2:EVIDoa2200215. [PMID: 38320046]

Sterns RH et al. Treatment guidelines for hyponatremia. Stay the course. Clin J Am Soc Nephrol. 2024;19:129. [PMID: 37379081]

HYPERNATREMIA

ESSENTIALS OF DIAGNOSIS

- Increased thirst and water intake are the main defense against hypernatremia.
- Urine osmolality helps differentiate renal from nonrenal water loss.

General Considerations

Hypernatremia is defined as a sodium concentration > 145 mEq/L. All patients with hypernatremia have hyperosmolality (unlike hyponatremic patients, who can have a low, normal, or high serum osmolality). Hypernatremia develops when there is a relative loss of water with inadequate compensation by water ingestion. Rarely, administration of excess sodium in relation to water ingestion or administration contributes to hypernatremia. This is most often encountered in critically ill patients when large amounts of hypertonic fluid are administered.

The primary responses to hypernatremia are stimulation of thirst (to increase water intake) and increased secretion of ADH (to minimize water loss in the urine). Cells in the hypothalamus can sense minimal changes in serum osmolarity, triggering the thirst mechanism and subsequent intake of water. It is nearly impossible to develop hypernatremia in the context of an intact thirst mechanism with appropriate access to water.

Clinical Findings

A. Symptoms and Signs

Acute, severe hypernatremia (serum sodium > 160 mEq/L) can manifest as lethargy, irritability, and weakness sometimes progressing to hyperthermia, delirium, seizures, and coma. Irreversible neurologic damage may occur if the hypernatremia is left untreated. Because water shifts from the cells to the intravascular space to protect volume status, symptoms may be delayed. Symptoms in older adults may not be specific.

B. Laboratory Findings

The first steps in evaluating patients with hypernatremia are assessing the urine volume, osmolality, and the osmole excretion rate. The latter can be calculated by multiplying the urine osmolality and urine volume. The copeptin test is discussed below.

C. Etiology

The initial step for the diagnosis of hypernatremia is to determine whether the patient is oliguric (ie, urine flow < 0.5 mL/min) or nonoliguric. Patients who are nonoliguric can be categorized by measuring urine osmolality.

1. The oliguric patient (urine flow < 0.5 mL/min)—This is found in several scenarios.

A. Reduced water intake—Hypernatremia develops in patients with reduced water intake secondary to the inability to communicate or limited access to water, or both.

B. Nonrenal water losses—Nonrenal sites of water loss include sweat, GI tract, and the respiratory tract. This is most commonly seen in patients with diarrhea or in febrile patients on a ventilator.

C. Shift of water into cells—Rarely, hypernatremia may manifest from a shift of water into cells due to the intracellular gain of an effective osmole. This may be seen with seizures or rhabdomyolysis.

2. The nonoliguric patient (urine flow > 0.5 mL/min)—

A. Urine osmolality < 250 mOsm/kg—Hypernatremia in the setting of dilute urine is characteristic of arginine vasopressin deficiency or resistance formerly known as central and nephrogenic diabetes insipidus, respectively. Arginine vasopressin deficiency (AVP-D) results from inadequate ADH (arginine vasopressin) release from the pituitary because of stroke, tumor, or infiltration. In arginine vasopressin resistance (AVP-R), ADH levels are normal or even elevated, but the kidneys are less sensitive to its effects. Common causes include lithium therapy, post-relief of urinary obstruction, chronic interstitial nephritis, hypercalcemia, and hypokalemia. Arginine vasopressin deficiency and resistance can be distinguished by the response to exogenous DDAVP administration while polyuric. Measuring copeptin (a C-terminal peptide synthesized with vasopressin, which mirrors its concentration over a wide range of plasma osmolalities) assists in the differential diagnosis of AVP. Elevated levels of copeptin in the setting of hypernatremia suggest the presence of vasopressin and therefore exclude a diagnosis of AVP-D. Vasopressin is unstable in isolated plasma, and obtaining levels is not helpful.

B. Urine osmolality > 300 mOsm/kg—Patients with an elevated urine osmolality and a high urine volume have an osmotic diuresis. Both glucose and urea in the urine can promote polyuria by increasing free water excretion.

Treatment

Treatment of hypernatremia includes both correcting the cause of the fluid loss and replacing the water deficit.

A. Choice of Fluid for Replacement

In general, hypernatremia treatment requires induction of a positive water balance by administering hypotonic fluids, either intravenously or enterally, or both. Because correcting large water deficits via the GI tract alone can be difficult, the most common strategy is to infuse 5% dextrose in water (distilled water is contraindicated due to the risk of hemolysis). Although there appears to be little risk in the rapid correction of hypernatremia in adults, caution is advised when infusing large amounts of 5% dextrose in water due to the risk of hyperglycemia. In patients who are concurrently volume-depleted, priority should be to restore euvolemia using isotonic fluids (eg, 0.9% normal saline), followed by hypotonic fluids to correct any remaining free water deficit. In the rare situation when hypernatremia is due to excess sodium balance (sodium ingestion or intravenous hypertonic saline), diuretics may be administered to enhance sodium excretion.

B. Calculation of Water Deficit

Fluid replacement should include correcting the free water deficit and adding maintenance fluid to replace ongoing and anticipated fluid losses.

1. Acute hypernatremia—This is relatively rare and generally encountered in patients with DI who do not have access to water, or even less commonly, in patients with salt poisoning; rapid restoration of water balance is indicated. Infusion of 0.5% dextrose in water is initiated at a rate of 3–6 mL/kg/hour until the serum sodium is below 145 mEq/L, then the infusion is slowed until the serum sodium normalizes (140 mEq/L). DDAVP is needed to reduce urine water losses in patients with central DI. Rarely, renal replacement therapy may be needed in patients with acute hypernatremia and severe kidney injury.

2. Chronic hypernatremia—Restoration of water balance with either intravenous 5% dextrose in water or oral rehydration in clinically stable patients with an adequate ability to tolerate oral intake should be initiated based on water deficit. The water deficit is the amount of water calculated to restore the sodium concentration to normal (140 mEq/L). Total body water (TBW) (see Table 24–1) correlates with muscle mass and therefore decreases with advancing age and cachexia. On average, TBW is lower in women than in men. Current TBW equals 40–60% of body weight. This equation provides a guide for initial therapy and does not negate the need for repeated measurements to assess response to treatment.

$$\text{Water deficit (L)} = \text{Current TBW} \times \frac{S_{Na} - 140}{140}$$

It should be emphasized that the water deficit represents a static period in time. When considering the volume of water needed to restore sodium balance, a critical mistake that is often made is failure to incorporate ongoing water loss via urinary output and insensible losses. Insensible losses can be estimated as 500–1000 mL daily; however, they can vary significantly. The proportion of urine volume that is free water can be estimated by calculating the electrolyte free water (EFW) clearance via the equation below.

$$C_{EFW}\,(L) = \text{Urine volume} \times \left(1 - \frac{U_{Na} + U_K}{S_{Na}}\right)$$

3. Rate of sodium correction—Although it would be appealing to apply similar principles for patients with hyponatremia to patients with hypernatremia, this practice is not supported by the literature. Adverse neurologic symptoms from overly rapid correction of hypernatremia have only been described in children. Furthermore, a large retrospective study found no evidence of morbidity or mortality with rapid correction of hypernatremia in critically ill patients with admission or hospital-acquired hypernatremia; however, a slow rate of correction is usually recommended on the basis of osmotic brain adaptation that occurs with chronic hypernatremia and corresponding theoretical risk of cerebral edema if hypernatremia is corrected too quickly. Common clinical practice is to limit correction of chronic hypernatremia to below 12 mEq/L in 24 hours; however, if this rate is inadvertently exceeded, the serum sodium should not be raised. In patients with acute hypernatremia, the serum sodium should be corrected to normal (ie, 140 mEq/L) within 24 hours.

4. Treatment of the underlying cause—The underlying cause of the hypernatremia should be identified and addressed. For patients who have AVP-D, vasopressin should be replaced by administration of DDAVP.

When to Refer

Patients with refractory or unexplained hypernatremia should always be referred for nephrology consultation.

When to Admit

- Patients with symptomatic hypernatremia require hospitalization for evaluation and treatment.
- Significant comorbidities or concomitant acute illnesses, especially if contributing to hypernatremia, may necessitate hospitalization.

Flynn K et al. Central and nephrogenic diabetes insipidus: updates on diagnosis and management. Front Endocrinol (Lausanne). 2025;15:1479764. [PMID: 39845881]
Tomkins M et al. Diagnosis and treatment of hypernatremia. Best Pract Res Clin Endocrinol Metab. 2026;40:102065. [PMID: 41203493]

DISORDERS OF POTASSIUM CONCENTRATION

HYPOKALEMIA

ESSENTIALS OF DIAGNOSIS

- Serum potassium < 3.5 mEq/L (3.5 mmol/L).
- Severe hypokalemia may induce arrhythmias and rhabdomyolysis.
- Assessment of urine potassium excretion (urine potassium to creatinine ratio) can distinguish renal from nonrenal loss of potassium.

General Considerations

Hypokalemia can result from intracellular shifting of potassium from the extracellular space, potassium loss (renal or extrarenal) (Table 24–3) or, rarely, insufficient dietary potassium intake. Low dietary potassium intake alone is usually insufficient to cause hypokalemia, as the kidneys can lower urine potassium excretion to very low levels (< 15 mEq/L). The shift of potassium into cells is increased by both insulin and β-adrenergic stimulation. Excess potassium excretion by the kidneys is usually due to increased aldosterone action in the setting of preserved delivery of sodium to the distal nephron. Magnesium is an important regulator of potassium handling, and low levels lead to persistent renal potassium excretion; hypokalemia is often refractory to treatment until the magnesium deficiency is corrected. Several classes of diuretics, carbonic anhydrase inhibitors, loop diuretics, and thiazide diuretics cause substantial renal potassium and magnesium losses.

Clinical Findings

A. Symptoms and Signs

Hypokalemia is often asymptomatic but can lead to muscle weakness and cardiac arrhythmias when severe. Hypokalemia can also lead to dysfunction of the smooth muscle of the GI tract, which can result in constipation or ileus. Rhabdomyolysis with associated AKI can be seen with serum potassium levels < 2.5 mEq/L. Hypokalemia may

Table 24–3. Causes of hypokalemia.

Decreased potassium intake
Potassium shift into the cell
Alkalosis
β-Adrenergic agonists
Insulin release (postprandial, exogenous, insulinoma)
Hypokalemic periodic paralysis
Renal potassium loss with metabolic acidosis
Proximal and distal RTAs
Toluene inhalation (glue sniffing)
Renal potassium loss with metabolic alkalosis
Normal/low blood pressure
Vomiting
Magnesium deficiency
Loop/thiazide diuretics
Bartter syndrome
Gitelman syndrome
High blood pressure
Elevated renin and aldosterone
Malignant hypertension
Renin-producing tumor
Renal artery stenosis
Primary aldosteronism (hyperaldosteronism)
Adrenal adenoma
Glucocorticoid-remediable aldosteronism
Adrenal hyperplasia
Depressed renin and aldosterone
Cushing syndrome
Black licorice
Apparent mineralocorticoid excess
Liddle syndrome
Increased GI losses
Diarrhea
Laxative abuse

RTA, renal tubular acidosis.

additionally present as polyuria and polydipsia due to diminished concentrating ability of the kidney (AVP-R) and eventual kidney disease (tubulointerstitial nephritis).

B. Laboratory Findings

Assessment of renal potassium excretion can help distinguish renal from nonrenal causes of hypokalemia. A 24-hour urine collection is the most accurate method for assessing renal potassium handling. A urine potassium level < 25 mEq/day indicates appropriate renal potassium retention, whereas higher values indicate renal potassium wasting. A more immediate assessment can be made by measuring a urine potassium to creatinine ratio (U_K/U_{Cr}) from a spot urine sample (Figure 24–2). In the setting of hypokalemia, a U_K/U_{Cr} ratio < 13 mEq/g (or 1.5 mEq/mmol) is suggestive of a nonrenal etiology, most commonly GI losses, intracellular potassium shifts, or inadequate dietary intake, whereas higher values imply renal potassium wasting.

C. ECG

Hypokalemia leads to a characteristic progression of ECG changes, initially T wave flattening, subsequently ST depressions and T wave inversions, ultimately leading to U waves as the hypokalemia becomes more severe. Such changes can trigger arrhythmias and be life-threatening. There is significant interpatient variability in the degree of hypokalemia and corresponding ECG findings; therefore, typical ECG patterns may not be observed in all patients.

Etiology

1. Inadequate dietary intake—While the kidney can excrete urine that is virtually free of sodium, a small amount of potassium excretion occurs even in the setting of diets devoid of potassium. With extreme potassium-free diets, which can occur with anorexia nervosa and alcohol use disorder, the hypokalemia is worsened by concurrent magnesium depletion.

2. Intracellular shift—The most critical determinants of intracellular potassium shifts are postprandial insulin and catecholamine release. These physiologic conditions can be exacerbated by β-adrenergic agonist administration and high adrenergic states, which can be seen in situations such as alcohol withdrawal and MI. Rare causes include insulinomas and hypokalemic periodic paralysis.

3. GI losses—The most common cause of nonrenal potassium wasting is GI loss, either diarrhea or vomiting. Diarrhea may have a high potassium and bicarbonate content, resulting in hypokalemia with a concurrent normal anion gap (hyperchloremic) metabolic acidosis. Vomiting leads to hypokalemia with a metabolic alkalosis and potassium loss due to renal wasting (secondary to hypovolemia-induced hyperaldosteronism coupled with distal sodium delivery in the form of sodium bicarbonate).

4. Renal wasting—Renal potassium wasting occurs in states where increased distal sodium delivery is coupled to increased aldosterone activity. This most commonly occurs with diuretic use. Renal tubulopathies, such as Bartter syndrome or Gitelman syndrome, or renal tubular acidosis (RTA) may present with hypokalemia.

Primary hyperaldosteronism is due to excess aldosterone production by the adrenal glands, which causes extracellular volume expansion resulting in hypertension associated with hypokalemia and a metabolic alkalosis. Other rare forms of increased mineralocorticoid activity may be identified by measuring plasma renin activity and serum aldosterone levels.

Treatment

Any underlying conditions should be treated and causative drugs discontinued. Magnesium deficiency should be corrected, particularly in refractory hypokalemia. Oral potassium supplementation is the safest treatment for mild to moderate deficiency, although potassium supplements may cause GI upset. With mild to moderate diuretic doses, 20 mEq/day of oral potassium is generally sufficient to prevent hypokalemia, whereas with established hypokalemia, 40–100 mEq/day over days to weeks may be needed to treat hypokalemia and fully replete potassium stores.

Intravenous potassium is generally reserved for severe hypokalemia (< 3.0 mEq/L) and requires careful monitoring due to the risk of transient hyperkalemia. Potassium chloride may be given through a peripheral intravenous line at rates up to 10–15 mEq/hour diluted in 0.45% or 0.9% normal saline, but higher rates (up to 20 mEq/hour) require

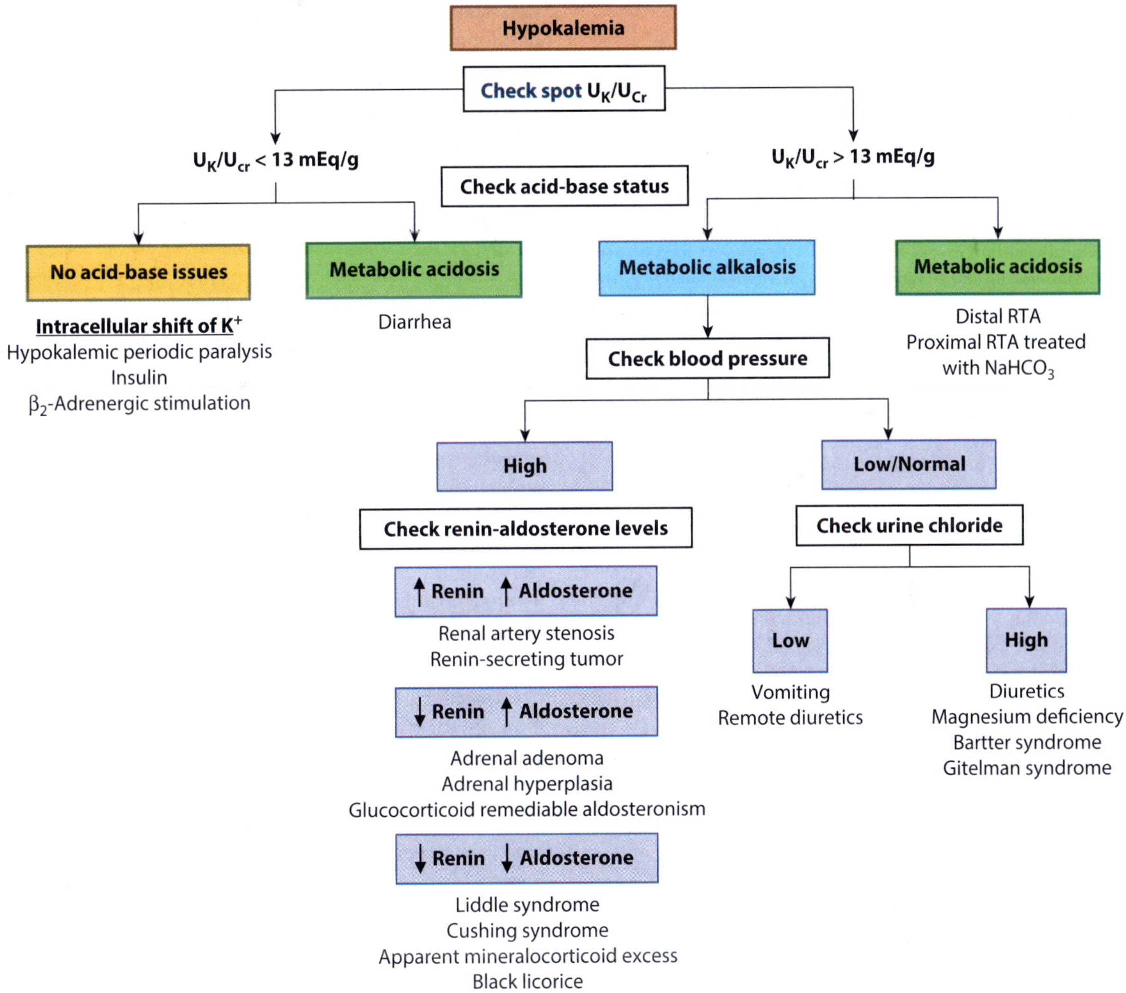

Figure 24–2. Differentiating renal from nonrenal causes of hypokalemia using a spot urine potassium and a spot urine creatinine. $NaHCO_3$, sodium bicarbonate; RTA, renal tubular acidosis; U_K/U_{Cr}, urine potassium to creatinine ratio.

central access due to the risk of peripheral vein irritation. In the event of concurrent metabolic acidosis, potassium repletion should take precedence over alkali administration as correction of the acidosis results in intracellular shift of potassium, further decreasing extracellular potassium concentration. Potassium should be given in a saline rather than dextrose solution, because dextrose will stimulate insulin release resulting in an intracellular potassium shift.

When to Refer

Patients with unexplained hypokalemia, refractory or persistent hypokalemia, or suggestive alternative diagnoses (eg, aldosteronism or RTA) should be referred for nephrology consultation.

When to Admit

Patients with symptomatic or severe hypokalemia (< 2.5 mEq/L), especially with cardiac manifestations, require admission for cardiac monitoring, potassium supplementation, and frequent laboratory testing.

Kim MJ et al. Potassium disorders: hypokalemia and hyperkalemia. Am Fam Physician. 2023;107:59. [PMID: 36689973]
Piner A et al. Disorders of potassium. Emerg Med Clin North Am. 2023;41:711. [PMID: 37758419]

HYPERKALEMIA

ESSENTIALS OF DIAGNOSIS

- Serum potassium > 5.2 mEq/L (5.2 mmol/L).
- Check medications carefully. Hyperkalemia may develop from ACE inhibitors, ARBs, and potassium-sparing diuretics, most commonly in patients with kidney dysfunction.
- The ECG may be normal despite life-threatening hyperkalemia.
- Rule out extracellular potassium shift from cells, especially hyperglycemia.

General Considerations

Hyperkalemia is rare in normal persons due to adaptive mechanisms that prevent extracellular potassium accumulation primarily through enhanced urinary excretion. **Persistent hyperkalemia** generally requires an impairment in renal potassium excretion due to diminished secretion of or hyporesponsiveness to aldosterone, decreased delivery of sodium and water to the distal nephron, or kidney disease (acute or chronic) (Table 24–4). **Transient hyperkalemia** suggests shift of potassium from inside cells into the extracellular fluid, which can occur in the context of tissue damage (rhabdomyolysis, tumor lysis, massive hemolysis, and trauma) or metabolic acidosis.

Clinical Findings

A. Symptoms and Signs

The symptoms of hyperkalemia are due to impaired neuromuscular transmission. The most serious manifestations are cardiac conduction abnormalities and neuromuscular manifestations, such as muscle weakness, which may be profound. This generally occurs with potassium concentrations above 7 mEq/L but can vary depending on the acuity of development of hyperkalemia. Hyperkalemia impairs urinary ammonium excretion and may lead to metabolic acidosis.

B. ECG

ECG is an unreliable method for detecting hyperkalemia; clinical studies show poor correlation between serum potassium and cardiac manifestations. The rapidity in development of hyperkalemia may correlate with the development of ECG changes. Typical sequential changes on the ECG are peaking of the T waves, ST-segment depression, and widening of the PR and QRS intervals. As the QRS continues to widen, sine waves may develop, which are concerning for imminent ventricular fibrillation and ultimately asystole.

Table 24–4. Causes of hyperkalemia.

Pseudohyperkalemia
Repeated fist clenching during phlebotomy, tourniquet application, use of small-bore needles during lab draw
Marked thrombocytosis or leukocytosis with release of intracellular K^+
Extracellular shift of K^+
Metabolic acidosis
Insulin deficiency
Hyperglycemia
α-Adrenergic stimulation
Tissue injury (rhabdomyolysis, hemolysis, tumor lysis)
Hyperkalemic periodic paralysis
Drugs (digoxin overdose, succinylcholine)
Kidney disease, acute and chronic
Renal secretory defects (may or may not have reduced kidney function): interstitial nephritis, SLE, sickle cell disease, amyloidosis, obstructive nephropathy, kidney transplant
Hypoaldosteronism
Addison disease
Type IV renal tubular acidosis
Heparin
Ketoconazole
Drugs that inhibit potassium excretion
Spironolactone, eplerenone, finerenone, drospirenone, NSAIDs, ACE inhibitors, angiotensin II receptor blockers, triamterene, amiloride, trimethoprim, pentamidine, cyclosporine, tacrolimus
Excessive intake of K^+
Especially in patients with diminished kidney excretion

Etiology

1. Increased potassium release from cells—

A. Pseudohyperkalemia—This condition arises during specimen collection due to fist clenching, application of tourniquets, or using small-bore needles during phlebotomy. The presence of hemolysis in the processed sample suggests these etiologies. A more striking example occurs with marked thrombocytosis (> 500,000/mcL [500×10^9/L]) or leukocytosis (> 100,000/mcL [100×10^9/L]), particularly leukemic cells. Centrifugation or pneumatic tube transport causes significant cell damage. If this condition is suspected, a non-centrifuged whole blood sample that is walked to the laboratory is required for confirmation.

B. Tissue breakdown—Tissue damage results in release of intracellular potassium to the extracellular space. Common clinical examples include tumor lysis syndrome, crush injuries, and severe hemolysis. Hyperkalemia is more common when concurrent renal impairment is present.

C. Hyperglycemia—Patients with uncontrolled diabetes may have hyperkalemia, even in the setting of a low total body potassium, due to a combination of insulin deficiency and hyperosmolarity from hyperglycemia.

D. Metabolic acidosis—Acidosis results in potassium shifting out of the intracellular fluid due to buffering of hydrogen ions into cells. Serum potassium concentration rises approximately 0.7 mEq/L for every decrease of 0.1 pH unit. This effect is not seen with organic acidosis, such as lactic acidosis or ketoacidosis.

2. Impaired kidney excretion—

A. AKI—A rapid reduction in kidney function leads to poor renal excretion of potassium and does not allow sufficient time for nonrenal adaptive mechanisms to take effect. Hyperkalemia occurs more commonly in oliguric patients.

B. CKD—The ability to maintain normal serum potassium is generally preserved until GFR declines to < 20–30 mL/min/1.73 m^2. This is primarily due to adaptive mechanisms, particularly increases in potassium excretion by remaining functioning nephrons and by increased GI tract potassium excretion. Hyperkalemia with more modest decreases in GFR is often due to medications that disrupt the renin-angiotensin-aldosterone system, which are commonly used in these patients.

C. Low effective circulating volume—Volume depletion and the edematous states of cirrhosis and HF can cause hyperkalemia due to a decrease in delivery of sodium and water to the distal nephron, which impairs potassium excretion.

D. Reduced aldosterone action—Mineralocorticoid deficiency from Addison disease may cause hyperkalemia due to decreased renal excretion of potassium. Mineralocorticoid resistance due to genetic disorders, interstitial kidney disease, or urinary tract obstruction also leads to hyperkalemia.

3. Medications—Several medications may be implicated in the development of hyperkalemia, and a careful review of a patient's medication list is imperative. Common medications implicated in hyperkalemia include ACE inhibitors, ARBs, and NSAIDs, which reduce aldosterone release. Concomitant use of aldosterone antagonists (spironolactone, eplerenone, or finerenone) or medications that directly block the sodium channels of the principal cells (amiloride, triamterene, or trimethoprim) further increase the risk of hyperkalemia. β-Blockers can cause mild hyperkalemia by interfering with potassium uptake by cells, a phenomenon more commonly observed with nonselective β-blockers. Heparin inhibits aldosterone production in the adrenal glands. Calcineurin inhibitors, such as cyclosporine and tacrolimus, can induce hyperkalemia, partly stimulating the sodium chloride cotransporter in the distal nephron, impairing distal sodium delivery. These medications should be used cautiously in patients with renal impairment, and laboratory monitoring is indicated within 1–2 weeks of drug initiation or dosage increase.

Treatment

The diagnosis of hyperkalemia should be confirmed by repeat laboratory testing to rule out spurious elevation, particularly in the absence of medications that cause hyperkalemia or in patients without kidney disease. The initial treatment is determined by the presence of signs and symptoms and the severity of plasma potassium elevation. In all patients, exogenous sources of potassium should be eliminated, medications that can impair potassium excretion discontinued, volume depletion corrected, and metabolic acidosis treated.

In emergency situations (cardiac toxicity, muscle weakness, or potassium > 6.5 mEq/L), initial therapy should be intravenous calcium gluconate to stabilize the myocardium to protect against arrhythmias, followed by therapies to shift potassium into cells. Insulin and β-agonists shift potassium intracellularly within 10–15 minutes of administration but have a short duration of action (1–2 hours) (Table 24–5). Sodium bicarbonate may help shift potassium into cells in patients with a concurrent metabolic acidosis. Once the patient is stabilized, therapies are focused on potassium excretion.

Renal potassium excretion may be enhanced by three modalities: diuretics, oral potassium-binding agents, and dialysis. Loop diuretics can increase renal potassium excretion, particularly when combined with a saline infusion to maintain distal sodium delivery; however, their acute impact is limited and additional therapies generally required. Patiromer and sodium zirconium cyclosilicate are oral potassium-binding drugs that increase gut potassium excretion. In patients with hyperkalemic emergencies, these have been shown to improve serum potassium levels; sodium zirconium cyclosilicate is preferred due to its more rapid onset of action. Although sodium polystyrene (Kayexalate) has been used for decades, its efficacy and safety have been questioned. It may not increase potassium excretion more than laxatives alone, is associated with colonic necrosis, and is contraindicated in patients with bowel obstruction or postoperative ileus. Hemodialysis may be necessary to remove potassium in patients with acute or chronic kidney injury, particularly in patients who are oliguric. SGLT-2 inhibitors have emerged as an option for decreasing the risk of chronic hyperkalemia with angiotensin and mineralocorticoid antagonists in outpatient settings.

When to Refer

- Nephrology consultation should be obtained for patients with hyperkalemia from kidney disease.
- Transplant patients may need adjustment of their immunosuppression regimen by transplant specialists.

When to Admit

Patients with severe hyperkalemia (> 6 mEq/L), any degree of hyperkalemia associated with ECG changes, or concomitant illness that may worsen hyperkalemia (eg, tumor lysis, rhabdomyolysis, metabolic acidosis) should be sent to the emergency department for immediate treatment.

Lewis H et al. Serum potassium response to single-dose sodium zirconium cyclosilicate for the treatment of asymptomatic hyperkalemia in hospitalized patients. Pharmacotherapy. 2024;44:13. [PMID: 37475499]

Neuen BL et al. Sodium-glucose cotransporter 2 inhibitors and risk of hyperkalemia in people with type 2 diabetes: a meta-analysis of individual participant data from randomized, controlled trials. Circulation. 2022;145:1460. [PMID: 35394821]

DISORDERS OF CALCIUM CONCENTRATION

The normal total plasma (or serum) calcium concentration is 8.5–10.5 mg/dL (2.1–2.6 mmol/L). Ionized calcium (normal: 4.6–5.3 mg/dL [1.16–1.31 mmol/L]) is the physiologically active portion of calcium and is necessary for muscle contraction and nerve function. In most situations, measuring total calcium concentration is sufficient since changes mirror those seen in ionized calcium concentration; the primary exception are those patients with hypoalbuminema.

HYPOCALCEMIA

ESSENTIALS OF DIAGNOSIS

- Usually asymptomatic but can cause cramps or tetany if severe.
- Check for decreased serum parathyroid hormone (PTH), vitamin D, or magnesium levels.
- Total serum calcium may be low with hypoalbuminemia; the diagnosis should be confirmed with an ionized calcium in these patients

Table 24–5. Treatment of hyperkalemia.

Treatment of Hyperkalemia					
Emergent/Stabilizing Therapy					
Modality	**Mechanism of Action**	**Onset**	**Duration**	**Prescription**	**K^+ Removed From Body**
Calcium	Antagonizes cardiac conduction abnormalities	0–5 minutes	1 hour	Intravenous: calcium gluconate 10%, 5–30 mL, or calcium chloride 5%, 5–30 mL	None
Bicarbonate	Distributes K^+ into cells	15–30 minutes	1–2 hours	Intravenous: $NaHCO_3$, 50–100 mEq **Note:** Sodium bicarbonate may not be effective in ESKD patients; dialysis is more expedient and effective. Some patients may not tolerate the additional sodium load of bicarbonate therapy.	None
Insulin	Distributes K^+ into cells	15–60 minutes	4–6 hours	Intravenous: regular insulin, 5–10 units, plus glucose 50%, 25 g	None
Albuterol	Distributes K^+ into cells	15–30 minutes	2–4 hours	Nebulized albuterol, 10–20 mg in 4 mL normal saline, inhaled over 10 minutes **Note:** Much higher doses are necessary for hyperkalemia treatment (10–20 mg) than for airway disease (2.5 mg).	None
Nonemergent/Excretory Therapy					
Modality	**Mechanism of Action**	**Onset of Action**		**Prescription**	**K^+ Removed From Body**
Loop diuretic	Renal K^+ excretion	0.5–2 hours		Intravenous: furosemide, 40–160 mg	Variable
Patiromer	Ca^{2+}-K^+ cation exchange resin	~7 hours		Oral: 4.2–16.8 g once or twice daily	Mean 0.75 mEq/L
Sodium zirconium cyclosilicate	Selective potassium cation trapping agent	1 hour		Oral: 10 g up to three times daily	0.7 mEq/L per 10 g dose
Sodium polystyrene sulfonate (eg, Kayexalate)	Ion-exchange resin binds K^+	1–3 hours		Oral: 15–60 g in 20% sorbitol (60–240 mL) Rectal: 30–60 g in 20% sorbitol **Note:** Resins with sorbitol may cause bowel necrosis and intestinal perforation, especially in patients with abnormal bowel function.	0.5–1 mEq/g resin
Hemodialysis[1]	Extracorporeal K^+ removal	1–8 hours		**Note:** A fast and effective therapy for hyperkalemia, hemodialysis can be delayed by vascular access placement and equipment or staff availability, or both. Serum K can be rapidly corrected within minutes, but post-dialysis rebound can occur.	25–50 mEq/hour
Peritoneal dialysis	Peritoneal K^+ removal	1–4 hours		Frequent exchanges	50–70 mEq/24 hour

[1]Can be both acute immediate and urgent treatment of hyperkalemia.

Reproduced, with permission, from Cogan MG. *Fluid and Electrolytes: Physiology and Pathophysiology.* New York: McGraw-Hill, 1991.

General Considerations

The most common cause of low total serum calcium is hypoalbuminemia, which decreases the amount of bound calcium. Correction factors that adjust total serum calcium for low serum albumin have been shown to be inaccurate; therefore, an ionized calcium level should be obtained.

True hypocalcemia (decreased ionized calcium) implies insufficient action of PTH or active vitamin D. Important causes of hypocalcemia can be differentiated by the presence of high or low PTH levels and are listed in Table 24–6. The most common cause is advanced CKD, in which decreased calcitriol production and hyperphosphatemia both play a role (see Chapter 25). Magnesium depletion reduces both PTH release and tissue responsiveness to PTH, causing hypocalcemia. Hypocalcemia is common in critical illness, likely due to the combination of reductions in calcitriol production and PTH synthesis, as well as end-organ PTH resistance.

Clinical Findings

A. Symptoms and Signs

The hallmark of severe hypocalcemia (ionized calcium below 1 mmol/L) is tetany from increased neuromuscular irritability. Laryngospasm with stridor can obstruct the airway. Convulsions, perioral and peripheral paresthesias, and abdominal pain can develop with hypocalcemia. Less pronounced symptoms include fatigue, anxiety, and depression. Classic physical findings include Chvostek sign (contraction of the facial muscle in response to tapping the facial nerve) and Trousseau sign (carpal spasm occurring with occlusion of the brachial artery by a blood pressure cuff). QT prolongation predisposes to ventricular arrhythmias, though serious dysrhythmias are rare.

Table 24–6. Causes of hypocalcemia.

Decreased intake or absorption
Vitamin D deficit (decreased absorption, decreased production of 25-hydroxyvitamin D or 1,25-dihydroxyvitamin D)
Malabsorption
Small bowel bypass, short bowel
Increased loss
Diuretic therapy
Alcohol use disorder
CKD
Endocrine disease
Hypoparathyroidism, genetic or acquired (including hypo- and hypermagnesemia)
Post-parathyroidectomy (hungry bone syndrome)
Pseudohypoparathyroidism
Calcitonin secretion with medullary carcinoma of the thyroid
Familial hypocalcemia
Associated diseases
Pancreatitis
Rhabdomyolysis
Septic shock
Physiologic causes
Decreased serum albumin[1]
Decreased end-organ response to vitamin D
Hyperphosphatemia
Aminoglycoside antibiotics, plicamycin, loop diuretics, foscarnet

[1]Ionized calcium concentration is normal.

B. Laboratory Findings

A serum total calcium < 8.5 mg/dL (2.1 mmol/L) is low. In true hypocalcemia, the ionized serum calcium concentration is also low (< 4.6 mg/dL [1.15 mmol/L]). Serum phosphate is usually elevated in hypoparathyroidism or in advanced CKD, whereas it is suppressed in vitamin D deficiency. Serum magnesium concentration is often low in hypocalcemia. The ECG shows a prolonged QT interval.

Treatment

A. Severe, Symptomatic Hypocalcemia

In the presence of tetany, arrhythmias, or seizures, intravenous calcium gluconate is indicated. Because of the short duration of action, continuous calcium infusion is usually required. Ten to 15 milligrams of calcium per kilogram body weight, or six to eight 10-mL vials of 10% calcium gluconate (558–744 mg of calcium), are added to 1 L of D_5W and infused over 4–6 hours. By monitoring the serum calcium frequently (every 4–6 hours), the infusion rate is adjusted to maintain the serum calcium at 7–8.5 mg/dL. See Chapter 30 for further discussion of hypoparathyroidism treatment.

B. Asymptomatic Hypocalcemia

Oral calcium (1–2 g of elemental calcium) and vitamin D preparations, including active vitamin D sterols, are used for hypocalcemia without accompanying symptoms. Calcium carbonate is well-tolerated and less expensive than many other calcium tablets, but calcium citrate may have better oral absorption. The low serum calcium associated with hypoalbuminemia does not require replacement therapy. If serum magnesium is low, therapy must include magnesium replacement, which by itself often corrects hypocalcemia.

When to Refer

Patients with complicated hypocalcemia from hypoparathyroidism, familial hypocalcemia, or CKD require referral to an endocrinologist or nephrologist.

When to Admit

Patients with tetany, arrhythmias, seizures, or other symptoms of hypocalcemia require immediate therapy.

Cetani F et al. Unveiling the complexities of hypoparathyroidism: a comprehensive review of clinical manifestations, diagnosis, and novel therapies. J Endocrinol Invest. 2026;49:725. [PMID: 41335198]

Melchers M et al. Management of hypocalcaemia in the critically ill. Curr Opin Crit Care. 2023;29:330. [PMID: 37395330]

HYPERCALCEMIA

ESSENTIALS OF DIAGNOSIS

- Most common causes: primary hyperparathyroidism and malignancy-associated hypercalcemia.
- Asymptomatic, mild hypercalcemia (< 10.5 mg/dL [2.6 mmol/L]) is usually due to primary hyperparathyroidism.
- Symptomatic, severe hypercalcemia (> 14 mg/dL [3.2 mmol/L]) is usually due to malignancy-associated hypercalcemia.

General Considerations

Important causes of hypercalcemia are listed in Table 24–7. Primary hyperparathyroidism and malignancy account for 90% of cases. Primary hyperparathyroidism is the most common cause of hypercalcemia (usually mild) in ambulatory patients. Hypercalcemia above 14 mg/dL is most often associated with malignancy and is rare with primary hyperparathyroidism. Tumor production of PTH-related proteins (PTHrP) is the most common paraneoplastic endocrine syndrome. The neoplasm is clinically apparent in nearly all cases when the hypercalcemia is detected, and the prognosis is poor. Granulomatous diseases, such as sarcoidosis and tuberculosis, cause hypercalcemia via overproduction of active vitamin D (1,25-dihydroxyvitamin D_3).

The entity of "milk-alkali" syndrome (previously attributable largely to excess intake of milk and antacid use for dyspepsia) decreased markedly following the introduction of proton pump inhibitors and histamine H_2-antagonists, but a recent emphasis on calcium supplementation (often with calcium carbonate) for prevention of osteoporosis and dyspepsia has contributed to a resurgence.

Table 24–7. Causes of hypercalcemia.

Increased intake or absorption
Milk-alkali syndrome
Vitamin D or vitamin A excess
Endocrine disorders
Primary hyperparathyroidism
Tertiary hyperparathyroidism
Acromegaly
Adrenal insufficiency
Pheochromocytoma
Thyrotoxicosis
Neoplastic diseases
Tumors producing PTH-related proteins (ovary, kidney, lung)
Plasma cell myeloma (elaboration of osteoclast-activating factor)
Lymphoma (occasionally from production of calcitriol)
Miscellaneous causes
Thiazide diuretics
Granulomatous diseases (production of calcitriol)
Paget disease of bone
Hypophosphatasia
Immobilization
Familial hypocalciuric hypercalcemia
Complications of kidney transplantation
Lithium intake

PTH, parathyroid hormone.

Clinical Findings

A. Symptoms and Signs

The history and physical examination should focus on the duration of hypercalcemia and evidence for a neoplasm. Hypercalcemia may affect GI, kidney, and neurologic function. Mild hypercalcemia (below 12 mg/dL) is often asymptomatic. Moderate hypercalcemia (12–14 mg/dL) may be tolerated if it is longstanding, yet tends to be symptomatic if acute. Severe hypercalcemia (above 14 mg/dL) is frequently symptomatic. Common symptoms include anxiety, lethargy, constipation, anorexia, and cognitive changes, which can progress to lethargy and stupor in severe cases. Pancreatitis from calcium deposition in the pancreatic ducts is a rare complication. Polyuria and dehydration may occur from impaired renal concentrating ability. Other symptoms include renal colic and hematuria from nephrolithiasis. Acute hypercalcemia can shorten the QT interval, though clinically relevant arrhythmias are rare.

B. Laboratory Findings

The serum ionized calcium exceeds 1.32 mmol/L (correct for serum albumin if ionized calcium is unavailable [see Hypocalcemia, above]). Check serum PTH to determine if hypercalcemia is PTH-mediated or non–PTH-mediated.

PTH should be completely suppressed in the presence of hypercalcemia if kidney function is normal. Therefore, "normal" levels of PTH with hypercalcemia do not rule out hyperparathyroidism. Asymptomatic patients with mild hypercalcemia and PTH in the normal or slightly elevated range should have a 24-hour urine calcium or a spot urine calcium-to-creatinine ratio checked for familial hypocalciuric hypercalcemia. If PTH is appropriately suppressed (typically below 20 pg/mL), PTHrP, as well as vitamin D and its metabolites, should be measured. Causes of a suppressed PTH and PTHrP with low or normal 25-OH and 1,25-OH vitamin D_3 levels include plasma cell myeloma, vitamin A intoxication, thyrotoxicosis, and immobilization. Hypocalciuria (below 100 mg/day) occurs in familial hypocalciuric hypercalcemia, thiazide diuretic use, and milk-alkali syndrome. Hypophosphatemia is more common with primary hyperparathyroidism and humoral hypercalcemia of malignancy (elevated PTHrP). In patients with an elevated 1,25-OH vitamin D_3, a CXR may demonstrate the presence of granulomatous disease.

Treatment

Until the primary cause can be identified and treated, therapy is initiated to promote immediate reduction in serum calcium. Asymptomatic patients with mild hypercalcemia (below 12 mg/dL) do not require immediate therapy; patients should be cautioned to avoid measures that exacerbate hypercalcemia, such as volume depletion and thiazide diuretics. Patients with symptomatic hypercalcemia, a sudden rise in serum calcium above 12 mg/dL, and severe hypercalcemia (above 14 mg/dL) should receive immediate therapy. Begin treatment with volume resuscitation, 200–300 mL/hour, or targeting a urinary output of 100–150 mL/hour, until euvolemia is achieved. Traditionally, normal saline is the recommended fluid of choice, although evidence for this is lacking. Loop diuretics to enhance calcium excretion were used more commonly before the availability of more effective calcium-lowering medications, such as bisphosphonates and calcitonin, and should be avoided due to possible complications, such as nephrolithiasis. They may be carefully used in the context of preventing or managing volume overload, particularly in patients with HF or kidney dysfunction.

Calcitonin, 4–8 IU/kg intramuscularly or subcutaneously every 6–12 hours, enhances renal excretion of calcium and decreases bone resorption by interfering with osteoclast activity. The efficacy of calcitonin is limited to 48 hours because of tachyphylaxis. Bisphosphonates are the treatment of choice for hypercalcemia secondary to excessive bone resorption. Denosumab, a monoclonal antibody against RANKL, inhibits osteoclasts, reduces bone resorption and serum calcium levels; this medication is an option when hypercalcemia is refractory to bisphosphonate therapy or when bisphosphonates are contraindicated (ie, severe renal impairment). The calcimimetic agent cinacalcet suppresses PTH secretion and decreases serum calcium concentration; it has been recommended for use in patients with symptomatic or severe primary hyperparathyroidism who are unable to undergo parathyroidectomy and patients with inoperable parathyroid carcinoma. (See Chapters 30 and 43.) Hemodialysis using a low calcium dialysate is an effective therapy for hypercalcemia refractory to the above therapies. Hypercalcemia in granulomatous disease is from overproduction of calcitriol; prednisone inhibits calcitriol synthesis and reduces serum calcium levels within 2–5 days.

Typically, if dialysis patients do not receive proper supplementation of active vitamin D, hypocalcemia and hyperphosphatemia develop. Conversely, hypercalcemia can develop in severe tertiary hyperparathyroidism with high PTH levels or from excess vitamin D supplementation. Metastatic calcification may occur when patients undergoing dialysis have hyperphosphatemia and hypercalcemia.

When to Refer

- Patients may require referral to an oncologist or endocrinologist depending on the cause of hypercalcemia.
- Patients with granulomatous diseases (eg, tuberculosis and other chronic infections, granulomatosis with polyangiitis, and sarcoidosis) may require assistance from infectious disease specialists, rheumatologists, or pulmonologists.

When to Admit

- Patients with symptomatic or severe hypercalcemia require immediate treatment.
- Unexplained hypercalcemia with associated conditions, such as AKI or suspected malignancy, may require urgent treatment and expedited evaluation.

Murray SL et al. Calcium and phosphate disorders: Core Curriculum 2024. Am J Kidney Dis. 2024;83:241. [PMID: 38099870]

Walker MD et al. Hypercalcemia: a review. JAMA. 2022;328:1624. [PMID: 36282253]

DISORDERS OF PHOSPHORUS CONCENTRATION

Plasma phosphorus is mainly inorganic phosphate and represents a small fraction (< 0.2%) of total body phosphate. Important determinants of plasma inorganic phosphate are renal excretion, intestinal absorption, and shift between the intracellular and extracellular spaces. The kidney is the most important regulator of the serum phosphate level. PTH decreases reabsorption of phosphate in the proximal tubule while 1,25-dihydroxyvitamin D increases reabsorption. Renal proximal tubular reabsorption of phosphate is decreased by hypertension, corticosteroids, metabolic acidosis, and proximal tubular dysfunction (as in Fanconi syndrome). Fibroblast growth factor 23 (FGF23) is a potent phosphaturic hormone. Intestinal absorption of phosphate is facilitated by active vitamin D. Cellular phosphate uptake is stimulated by various factors and conditions, including alkalemia, insulin, epinephrine, refeeding syndrome, hungry bone syndrome, and accelerated cell proliferation.

Phosphorus metabolism and homeostasis are intimately related to calcium metabolism.

HYPOPHOSPHATEMIA

ESSENTIALS OF DIAGNOSIS

- Severe hypophosphatemia may cause tissue hypoxia and rhabdomyolysis.
- Renal loss of phosphate can be diagnosed by calculating the fractional excretion of phosphate ($FEPO_4$).
- PTH and FGF23 are the major factors that increase urinary phosphate excretion.

General Considerations

The etiology of hypophosphatemia is due to decreased intestinal absorption, increased urinary excretion, or transcellular shift (Table 24–8). Hypophosphatemia may occur in the presence of normal phosphate stores. Serum phosphate levels decrease transiently after food intake, which stimulates endogenous insulin release. In patients with depleted phosphate stores, such as those who are malnourished or have alcohol use disorder, carbohydrate intake can induce severe hypophosphatemia (refeeding syndrome). Acute respiratory alkalosis can lower serum phosphate concentrations by stimulating glycolysis. Several drugs can impair intestinal

Table 24–8. Causes of hypophosphatemia.

Decreased intestinal absorption
Starvation
Absorption blocked by oral antacids or phosphate binders
Parenteral alimentation with inadequate phosphate content
Malabsorption syndrome, small bowel bypass
Vitamin D–deficient and vitamin D–resistant osteomalacia
Increased urinary excretion
Hyperparathyroidism (primary or secondary)
Hyperthyroidism
Inadequately controlled diabetes mellitus
Renal tubular defects with excessive phosphaturia (congenital, Fanconi syndrome induced by monoclonal gammopathy, heavy metal poisoning), alcohol use disorder
Hypokalemic nephropathy
FGF23 excess (hypophosphatemic rickets, oncogenic osteomalacia)
Phosphaturic medications: intravenous iron, acetazolamide, tenofovir
Transcellular shift of phosphorus (acute)
Acute respiratory alkalosis
Increased insulin secretion (ie, during refeeding)
Anabolic steroids, estrogen, oral contraceptives, β-adrenergic agonists, xanthine derivatives
Hungry bone syndrome
Salicylate poisoning
Other
Electrolyte abnormalities
Hypercalcemia
Hypomagnesemia
Metabolic alkalosis
Abnormal losses followed by inadequate repletion
Diabetes mellitus with acidosis, particularly during aggressive therapy
Recovery from starvation or prolonged catabolic state
Alcohol use disorder, particularly during restoration of nutrition; associated with hypomagnesemia
Recovery from severe burns

FGF23, fibroblast growth factor 23.

absorption of phosphate, particularly calcium-, magnesium-, and aluminum-containing antacids. Elevated PTH causes hypophosphatemia by inhibiting reabsorption in the kidney. Vitamin D deficiency decreases intestinal phosphate and calcium absorption with the resultant hypocalcemia stimulating PTH release, increasing urinary phosphate excretion. Generalized dysfunction in the proximal tubule (Fanconi syndrome) is characterized by hypophosphatemia, metabolic acidosis, glucosuria, and aminoaciduria. Genetic mutations increasing FGF23 levels are associated with urinary phosphorous wasting with rickets or osteomalacia.

Clinical Findings

A. Symptoms and Signs

Phosphorous is a key ingredient component of adenosine triphosphate (ATP), and clinical manifestations are related to ATP deficiency. Symptoms are rare until blood phosphate levels fall below 1.0 mg/dL and are more prominent with acute declines. Symptoms include weakness, paresthesias, and encephalopathy (irritability, confusion, dysarthria, seizures, and coma). Respiratory failure or failure to wean from mechanical ventilation may occur because of diaphragmatic weakness. Decreased myocardial contractility is uncommon but a serious manifestation. Chronic severe depletion may cause anorexia, pain in muscles and bones, and fractures.

B. Laboratory Findings

While the etiology of hypophosphatemia is often revealed from the patient's history and review of medications, urinary phosphate excretion can distinguish between renal and nonrenal causes. Phosphate excretion can be determined by a 24-hour urine collection or by calculation of the $FEPO_4$. The normal renal response to hypophosphatemia is to decrease urinary phosphate excretion to < 100 mg/day and $FEPO_4$ < 5%. Renal wasting of phosphate (or increased $FEPO_4$) occurs most commonly with hyperparathyroidism and Fanconi syndrome (Table 24–8). The clinical usefulness of serum FGF23 levels is undetermined except in uncommon diseases.

Other clinical features may be suggestive of hypophosphatemia, such as hemolytic anemia and rhabdomyolysis. Fanconi syndrome may present with any combination of uricosuria, aminoaciduria, normoglycemic glucosuria, normal anion gap metabolic acidosis, and phosphaturia. In chronic hypophosphatemia, radiographs and bone biopsies show changes resembling osteomalacia.

Treatment

Hypophosphatemia can be prevented by including phosphate in repletion and maintenance fluids. Moderate hypophosphatemia (> 1 mg/dL) and asymptomatic patients should be treated with oral phosphate, typically 40–80 mmol divided into three or four doses over 24 hours. Patients with severe hypophosphatemia (below 1 mg/dL), symptomatic patients, and those who cannot tolerate oral therapy should be treated with intravenous replacement. Hypocalcemia, hypotension, hyperphosphatemia, and ECG abnormalities can be seen with intravenous therapy, which can be avoided by providing moderate doses. A typical dose is 15 mmol over 2 hours; the rate should be decreased if hypotension occurs and monitoring of plasma phosphate and calcium every 6 hours is necessary. Magnesium deficiency often occurs concomitantly and should be treated.

Contraindications to phosphate replacement include hypoparathyroidism, advanced CKD, tissue damage and necrosis, and hypercalcemia. When associated hyperglycemia is treated, phosphate accompanies glucose into cells, and hypophosphatemia may ensue.

When to Refer

- Patients with refractory hypophosphatemia with increased urinary phosphate excretion may require evaluation by an endocrinologist (eg, for hyperparathyroidism and vitamin D disorders) or a nephrologist (eg, for renal tubular defects).
- Patients with decreased GI absorption may require referral to a gastroenterologist.

When to Admit

Patients with severe or refractory hypophosphatemia will require intravenous phosphate.

Murray SL et al. Calcium and phosphate disorders: Core Curriculum 2024. Am J Kidney Dis. 2024;83:241. [PMID: 38099870]

HYPERPHOSPHATEMIA

ESSENTIALS OF DIAGNOSIS

- Advanced CKD is the most common cause.
- Hyperphosphatemia in the presence of hypercalcemia imposes a high risk of metastatic calcification.

General Considerations

The two most common etiologies of hyperphosphatemia are decreased renal phosphate clearance from CKD and transcellular shift. Increased dietary intake of phosphates in the setting of advanced CKD can cause hyperphosphatemia. Phosphate-containing laxatives taken as preparation for a GI procedure can cause hyperphosphatemia in patients with impaired kidney function and are therefore less commonly used. Rapid cell breakdown from tumor lysis syndrome, rhabdomyolysis, and massive hemolysis releases intracellular phosphate. Hyperphosphatemia from insulin deficiency can occur in diabetic ketoacidosis (DKA). These patients, however, are typically phosphate depleted and are at risk for developing hypophosphatemia with insulin therapy. Other causes are listed in Table 24–9.

Table 24–9. Causes of hyperphosphatemia.

Massive load of phosphate into the extracellular fluid
Exogenous sources
Hypervitaminosis D
Laxatives or enemas containing phosphate
Intravenous phosphate supplement
Endogenous sources
Rhabdomyolysis (especially if CKD coexists)
Tumor lysis by chemotherapy, particularly lymphoproliferative diseases
Metabolic acidosis (lactic acidosis, ketoacidosis)
Respiratory acidosis (phosphate incorporation into cells is disturbed)
Decreased excretion into urine
Kidney disease (CKD or AKI)
Hypoparathyroidism
Pseudohypoparathyroidism
Acromegaly
Pseudohyperphosphatemia
Plasma cell myeloma
Hyperbilirubinemia
Hypertriglyceridemia
Hemolysis in vitro

Clinical Findings

A. Symptoms and Signs

Acute hyperphosphatemia is generally asymptomatic, and symptoms are generally associated with concurrent hypocalcemia.

B. Laboratory Findings

In addition to elevated phosphate, blood chemistry abnormalities are those of the underlying disease.

Treatment

Treatment is directed at the underlying cause. Acute hyperphosphatemia with *symptomatic* hypocalcemia and ECG changes (QTc prolongation) can be life-threatening. Intravenous calcium (1–2 g of calcium gluconate over 10–20 minutes) can be given in this situation, though it should be avoided in asymptomatic patients due to the risk of vascular calcification. Hemodialysis may be necessary in patients with impaired kidney function. In chronic hyperphosphatemia, dietary phosphate intake should be decreased and absorption reduced with oral phosphate binders, such as calcium acetate, calcium carbonate, sevelamer, or ferric citrate.

When to Admit

Patients with acute severe hyperphosphatemia require hospitalization for emergent therapy, possibly including dialysis. Concomitant illnesses, such as AKI or cell lysis, may necessitate admission.

Scialla JJ et al. State-of-the-art management of hyperphosphatemia in patients with CKD: an NKF-KDOQI controversies perspective. Am J Kidney Dis. 2021;77:132. [PMID: 32771650]

DISORDERS OF MAGNESIUM CONCENTRATION

Normal plasma magnesium concentration is 1.7–2.1 mg/dL (0.7–0.85 mmol/L). Similar to calcium, only the ionized form is metabolically active. The primary source of magnesium excretion is via the kidney. The physiologic effects of magnesium on the nervous system resemble those of calcium.

Altered magnesium concentration usually provokes an associated alteration of Ca^{2+}. Both hypomagnesemia and hypermagnesemia can decrease PTH secretion or action. Severe hypermagnesemia (> 5 mg/dL [2.1 mmol/L]) suppresses PTH secretion with consequent hypocalcemia; this disorder is typically seen only in patients receiving magnesium therapy for preeclampsia. Severe hypomagnesemia causes PTH resistance in end organs and eventually decreased PTH secretion in severe cases.

HYPOMAGNESEMIA

ESSENTIALS OF DIAGNOSIS

- Serum concentration of magnesium may be normal even in the presence of magnesium depletion. Check urinary magnesium excretion if renal magnesium wasting is suspected.
- Causes neurologic symptoms and arrhythmias.
- Associated with hypocalcemia.

General Considerations

Causes of hypomagnesemia are listed in Table 24–10. Hypomagnesemia and hypokalemia share many etiologies, including diarrhea, alcohol use disorder, and diuretic use. Hypomagnesemia causes renal potassium wasting that is refractory to potassium replacement until magnesium is repleted. Hypomagnesemia also suppresses PTH release and causes end-organ resistance to PTH and low 1,25-dihydroxyvitamin D levels. The resultant hypocalcemia is refractory to calcium replacement until the magnesium is normalized. Normomagnesemia does not exclude magnesium depletion because only 1% of total body magnesium is in the extracellular fluid; magnesium repletion should be considered in patients with risk factors for hypomagnesemia and refractory hypokalemia or hypocalcemia. Finally, there is an FDA warning about hypomagnesemia for patients taking PPIs. The presumed mechanism is decreased intestinal magnesium absorption, but it is not clear why this complication develops in only a small fraction of patients taking these medications. The potassium binder patiromer can additionally cause hypomagnesemia by binding magnesium in the colon.

Table 24–10. Causes of hypomagnesemia.

Diminished absorption or intake
Malabsorption, chronic diarrhea, laxative abuse
Malnutrition
Alcohol use disorder
PPIs
Prolonged GI suction
Small bowel bypass
Total parenteral alimentation with inadequate Mg^{2+} content
Increased renal loss
Volume expansion
Diuretic therapy (loop diuretics, thiazide diuretics, acetazolamide)
Hyperaldosteronism, Gitelman syndrome
Hyperparathyroidism, hyperthyroidism
Hypercalcemia
Tubulointerstitial diseases
Drugs (aminoglycoside, cetuximab, cisplatin, amphotericin B, pentamidine)
Transplant kidney
Others
Diabetes mellitus
Post-parathyroidectomy (hungry bone syndrome)
Respiratory alkalosis
Pregnancy

Clinical Findings

A. Symptoms and Signs

Because hypomagnesemia causes hypokalemia and hypocalcemia, it is difficult to determine whether symptoms are from hypomagnesemia or from potassium and calcium depletion. Marked neuromuscular and CNS hyperirritability may produce tremors, cramps, Trousseau and Chvostek signs, confusion, disorientation, and coma. Weakness is common. Cardiovascular manifestations include hypertension, tachycardia, and ventricular arrhythmias, including torsades de pointes.

B. Laboratory Findings

Urinary excretion of magnesium exceeding 10–30 mg/day or a fractional excretion > 3% indicates renal magnesium wasting. Hypocalcemia and hypokalemia are often present. The ECG may show widening of the QRS complex, peaked T waves with ultimate diminution, and a prolonged PR interval. PTH secretion is often suppressed (see Hypocalcemia).

Treatment

Magnesium oxide, 250–500 mg orally once or twice daily, is useful for treating chronic hypomagnesemia. Slow-release formulations such as magnesium chloride or magnesium lactate may be better tolerated. In patients with refractory hypomagnesemia, potassium-sparing diuretics, such as amiloride, may be effective. SGLT-2 inhibitors have emerged as a novel treatment option for refractory hypomagnesemia. Symptomatic hypomagnesemia requires intravenous magnesium sulfate 1–2 g over 5–60 minutes mixed in either dextrose 5% or 0.9% normal saline. Torsades de pointes in the setting of hypomagnesemia can be treated with 1–2 g of magnesium sulfate in 10 mL of dextrose 5% solution pushed intravenously over 15 minutes. Severe, non–life-threatening deficiency can be treated at a rate to 1–2 g/hour over 3–6 hours. Intravenous magnesium inhibits renal reabsorption and patients will demonstrate increased renal wasting during therapy. Serum levels must be monitored daily and dosage adjusted to keep the concentration from rising above 3 mg/dL (1.23 mmol/L). Tendon reflexes may be checked for the hyporeflexia of hypermagnesemia. K^+ and Ca^{2+} replacement may be required, but patients with hypokalemia and hypocalcemia associated with hypomagnesemia do not recover without magnesium supplementation.

Patients with normal kidney function can excrete excess magnesium; hypermagnesemia should not develop with replacement dosages. In patients with CKD, magnesium replacement should be done cautiously to avoid hypermagnesemia. Reduced doses (50–75% dose reduction) and more frequent monitoring of laboratory values are indicated.

Gommers LMM et al. Mechanisms of proton pump inhibitor-induced hypomagnesemia. Acta Physiol (Oxf). 2022;23:e13846. [PMID: 35652564]

Shah CV et al. Sodium/glucose cotransporter 2 inhibitors and magnesium homeostasis. Am J Kidney Dis. 2024;83:648. [PMID: 38372686]

HYPERMAGNESEMIA

ESSENTIALS OF DIAGNOSIS

- Often associated with advanced CKD and chronic intake of magnesium-containing drugs.

General Considerations

Hypermagnesemia is almost always the result of advanced CKD and impaired magnesium excretion. Antacids and laxatives are underrecognized sources of magnesium. Severe hypermagnesemia can develop in pregnant patients who receive intravenous magnesium for preeclampsia and eclampsia. Magnesium replacement should be done cautiously in patients with CKD; dose reductions up to 75% may be necessary to avoid hypermagnesemia.

Clinical Findings

A. Symptoms and Signs

Muscle weakness, decreased deep tendon reflexes, mental obtundation, and confusion are characteristic manifestations of hypermagnesemia. Weakness, flaccid paralysis, ileus, and hypotension can also occur. Severe findings of this condition include respiratory muscle paralysis, complete heart block, and cardiac arrest.

B. Laboratory Findings and ECG

An elevated serum magnesium level is diagnostic. Since CKD is a common risk factor for hypermagnesemia, BUN, creatinine, potassium, phosphate, and uric acid levels may all be elevated. Moreover, the serum calcium level is often low. The ECG may show an increased PR interval, broadened QRS complexes, and QT prolongation.

Treatment

Exogenous sources of magnesium should be discontinued. Calcium antagonizes Mg^{2+} and may be given intravenously as calcium chloride, 500 mg or more at a rate of 100 mg (4.1 mmol) per minute. Hemodialysis may be necessary to remove magnesium, particularly in the context of severe kidney disease. Finally, the long-term use of magnesium hydroxide and magnesium sulfate should be avoided in patients with advanced stages of CKD.

Adomako EA et al. Magnesium disorders: Core Curriculum 2024. Am J Kidney Dis. 2024;83:803. [PMID: 38372687]
Ribeiro HS et al. Association of magnesium abnormalities at intensive care unit admission with kidney outcomes and mortality: a prospective cohort study. Clin Exp Nephrol. 2022;26:997. [PMID: 35760979]

ACID-BASE DISORDERS

To best evaluate acid-base status, a blood gas and chemistry panel are required. Venous blood pH is typically 0.03–0.04 units lower than arterial blood pH, but still closely approximates arterial blood pH. An ABG should be obtained if a more accurate assessment of blood pH and P_{CO_2} is required. Bicarbonate (HCO_3^-) is calculated from the Henderson-Hasselbalch equation below; therefore, the bicarbonate value measured in the electrolyte panel is typically used.

$$pH = 6.1 + \log \frac{HCO_3^-}{0.03 \times P_{CO_2}}$$

Primary acid-base disorders are secondary to changes in either serum bicarbonate or P_{CO_2}. The first step is to look at the pH of a blood gas (venous or arterial). If changes in pH are secondary to changes in HCO_3^-, a metabolic disorder is present. If changes in pH are secondary to changes in P_{CO_2}, a respiratory disorder is present. If the pH is < 7.40, the primary process is acidosis, either respiratory (P_{CO_2} > 40 mm Hg) or metabolic (HCO_3^- < 24 mEq/L). If the pH is > 7.40, the primary process is alkalosis, either respiratory (P_{CO_2} < 40 mm Hg) or metabolic (HCO_3^- > 24 mEq/L). Normally, the kidneys compensate for respiratory acid-base disorders and the lungs compensate for metabolic disorders to maintain pH in a narrow physiologic range. For example, with metabolic acidosis (low pH, low HCO_3^-), alveolar ventilation increases (P_{CO_2} decreases), returning pH close to the normal range. Similarly, with respiratory acidosis (low pH, high P_{CO_2}), the kidneys excrete H^+ (HCO_3^- increase) to return pH close to the normal range. Such compensation can only bring the pH toward normal, though it can never completely correct it. To normalize pH, the primary disorder must be corrected.

A single respiratory or metabolic disorder with its appropriate compensatory response is a simple acid-base disorder. A mixed acid-base disorder occurs when multiple simple disorders are present simultaneously. Diagnosing an acid-base disorder requires a systematic approach (see box Step-by-Step Analysis of Acid-Base Status). Once the primary disorder has been identified, the clinician should assess whether the compensatory response is appropriate (Table 24–11). An inadequate or exaggerated response indicates the presence of another primary acid-base disturbance.

The serum anion gap should subsequently be calculated (see below) for two reasons. First, it helps identify the cause of a metabolic acidosis, and second, it identifies the presence of a gap metabolic acidosis, which may be present even without a decreased serum bicarbonate concentration. In patients with metabolic acidosis disorders, clinicians should calculate the **Δgap**, which is the difference between the change in anion gap and the change in bicarbonate, to determine if there is a mixed anion gap or normal anion gap metabolic acidosis. In high anion gap acidosis disorders, there should be roughly a millimole for millimole decrease in HCO_3^- as the anion gap increases. The corrected serum HCO_3^- should be calculated by adding the change in serum anion gap to the serum HCO_3^-. A value higher or lower than normal (24 mEq/L) indicates the concomitant presence of metabolic alkalosis or normal anion gap metabolic acidosis, respectively.

Table 24–11. Primary acid-base disorders and expected compensation.

Disorder	Primary Defect	Compensatory Response	Magnitude of Compensation
Respiratory acidosis			
Acute	↑ P_{CO_2}	↑ HCO_3^-	↑ HCO_3^- 1 mEq/L per 10 mm Hg ↑ P_{CO_2}
Chronic	↑ P_{CO_2}	↑ HCO_3^-	↑ HCO_3^- 3.5 mEq/L per 10 mm Hg ↑ P_{CO_2}
Respiratory alkalosis			
Acute	↓ P_{CO_2}	↓ HCO_3^-	↓ HCO_3^- 2 mEq/L per 10 mm Hg ↓ P_{CO_2}
Chronic	↓ P_{CO_2}	↓ HCO_3^-	↓ HCO_3^- 5 mEq/L per 10 mm Hg ↓ P_{CO_2}
Metabolic acidosis	↓ HCO_3^-	↓ P_{CO_2}	↓ P_{CO_2} 1.3 mm Hg per 1 mEq/L ↓ HCO_3^-
Metabolic alkalosis	↑ HCO_3^-	↑ P_{CO_2}	↑ P_{CO_2} 0.7 mm Hg per 1 mEq/L ↑ HCO_3^-

METABOLIC ACIDOSIS

ESSENTIALS OF DIAGNOSIS

- Decreased HCO_3^- with acidemia (low blood pH).
- Classified into increased anion gap acidosis and normal anion gap acidosis.
- Lactic acidosis, ketoacidosis, and toxins produce metabolic acidosis disorders with the largest anion gaps.
- Normal anion gap acidosis is mainly caused by loss of bicarbonate in the GI tract or RTA.

General Considerations

The hallmark of metabolic acidosis is low serum bicarbonate concentration from loss of bicarbonate or gain of acid (Table 24–12); the anion gap detects an increase in plasma anions other than from measured bicarbonate and chloride.

Many clinicians use 12 mEq/L as the normal serum anion gap (range 4–12 mEq/L) due to differences in analyzer methods).

$$\text{Anion Gap} = Na^+ - (HCO_3^- + Cl^-)$$

STEP-BY-STEP ANALYSIS OF ACID-BASE STATUS

Step 1: Look at the pH on a blood gas to determine the primary disorder, either acidemia or alkalemia.

Step 2: Look at the serum HCO_3^- value to determine if the primary disorder is metabolic.

Step 3: Calculate the anion gap (see Table 24–12).

Step 4: Calculate the Δgap.

Step 5: Evaluate magnitude of compensation (see Table 24–11).

Step 6: Examine the patient to determine whether the clinical signs are compatible with the acid-base analysis.

The principal unmeasured anion usually responsible for the anion gap is albumin. The expected anion gap typically is adjusted for hypoalbuminemia; the gap decreases by approximately 2.5 mEq/L for every 1 g/dL reduction in the serum albumin concentration. This common practice however is not supported by clinical evidence.

$$\text{Corrected serum anion gap} = (\text{measured serum anion gap}) + (2.5 \times [4.0 - \text{serum albumin}])$$

In metabolic acidosis from a gain of acid, the anion gap will increase because the addition of acid includes the addition of anions. In normal anion gap or hyperchloremic metabolic acidosis, the anion gap is normal because the rise in chloride parallels the fall in bicarbonate.

Table 24–12. Anion gap in metabolic acidosis.[1]

Increased (> 12 mEq/L)
Metabolic anion
Diabetic ketoacidosis
Alcoholic ketoacidosis
Lactic acidosis
CKD (advanced stages) (PO_4^{3-}, SO_4^{2-})
Starvation ketoacidosis
Drug or chemical anion
Salicylate intoxication
Methanol (formic acid)
Ethylene glycol (oxalic acid)
5-Oxoproline acidosis from acetaminophen toxicity
Normal (4–12 mEq/L)
Loss of HCO_3^-
Diarrhea
Recovery from diabetic ketoacidosis
Pancreatic fluid loss, ileostomy (unadapted)
Carbonic anhydrase inhibitors
Chloride retention
Renal tubular acidosis
Ileal loop bladder
Administration of HCl equivalent or NH_4Cl
Arginine and lysine in parenteral nutrition
Decreased (< 6 mEq/L)
Hypoalbuminemia (decreased unmeasured anion)
Plasma cell dyscrasias
Monoclonal protein (cationic paraprotein accompanied by chloride and bicarbonate)

[1]Reference ranges for anion gap may vary based on laboratory methods.

INCREASED ANION GAP METABOLIC ACIDOSIS

A gap metabolic acidosis is secondary to the addition of acid, either exogenous or endogenous. The major causes are lactic acidosis, ketoacidosis, kidney disease, and ingestions (Table 24–12). A useful mnemonic for the differential diagnosis of increased anion gap metabolic acidosis is GOLDMARK (glycols [ethylene glycol and propylene glycol], oxoproline, L-lactate, D-lactate, methanol, aspirin, renal failure, and ketoacidosis) (Table 24–13).

A. Lactic Acidosis

Lactic acidosis is a common cause of metabolic acidosis, producing an elevated anion gap and decreased serum pH when present without other acid-base disturbances. Lactate is formed from pyruvate in anaerobic glycolysis, primarily in the erythrocytes (which lack enzymes for aerobic oxidation), skeletal muscle, brain, and skin. Normally, lactate levels remain low (1 mEq/L) because of the metabolism of lactate principally by the liver (but also by the kidneys) through gluconeogenesis or oxidation via the Krebs cycle. In lactic acidosis, lactate levels are at least 4–5 mEq/L but commonly significantly higher. There are three types of lactic acidosis summarized below:

Type A (hypoxic) lactic acidosis is the most common, resulting from tissue hypoxia, usually from septic, cardiogenic, or hemorrhagic shock; mesenteric ischemia; respiratory failure; and carbon monoxide poisoning. These conditions increase peripheral lactic acid production and decrease hepatic metabolism of lactate as liver perfusion declines. Aggressive treatment of the precipitating cause to ensure adequate oxygenation and vascular perfusion is the main component of therapy. Alkalinization with intravenous sodium bicarbonate for patients with a pH < 7.1–7.2 and AKI is recommended by some experts; however, this practice remains controversial and has not been demonstrated to improve mortality. Studies suggest that alkali therapy in this situation may delay or mitigate the need for dialysis.

Type B lactic acidosis is secondary to impaired mitochondrial oxygen utilization and may be due to metabolic causes (eg, diabetes mellitus, liver disease, kidney disease, thiamine deficiency, D-lactic acidosis, leukemia, or lymphoma) or toxins (eg, ethanol, methanol, ethylene glycol, cyanide, isoniazid, or metformin). Propylene glycol, which is used as a vehicle for intravenous medications (eg, nitroglycerin, etomidate, and diazepam), can cause lactic acidosis by decreasing liver metabolism. Parenteral nutrition without thiamine causes severe refractory lactic acidosis from deranged pyruvate metabolism.

D-Lactic acidosis may develop in patients with short bowel syndrome due to carbohydrate malabsorption and subsequent fermentation by colonic bacteria. Metabolic acidosis occurs after meals and is associated with neurologic changes (confusion, slurred speech, and ataxia). A specific D-lactic acid assay is required as the standard lactic acid assay only detects the L-isomer.

B. Ketoacidosis

All forms of ketoacidosis share the physiologic state of insulin deficiency and glucagon excess, which shifts the body's primary fuel source from glucose to fatty acid metabolism. There are three types of ketones: acetone, acetoacetate, and β-hydroxybutyrate.

Table 24–13. Common causes and therapy for increased anion gap metabolic acidosis.

Cause	Treatment
Lactic acidosis	Therapy aimed at correcting the underlying cause. Treatment of type A requires improving perfusion and matching oxygen consumption with fluids, packed red cells, vasopressors, and inotropes as needed. Treatment of type B generally requires removal of the offending agent or supplementing key cofactors of anaerobic metabolism.
D-Lactic acidosis	Sodium bicarbonate may be administered in the setting of severe acidemia. Specific antimicrobial agents (metronidazole, neomycin) can be utilized in patients with short gut syndrome. A low-carbohydrate diet can be effective by decreasing substrate delivery to the distal colon. Fecal transplant has been utilized successfully in patients unresponsive to conventional therapies.
Ketoacidosis Diabetes mellitus Starvation Alcoholic	Therapy involves correction of the state of insulin deficiency and glucagon excess. In diabetic ketoacidosis, this requires administration of exogenous insulin, generally with a continuous infusion. In starvation and alcoholic ketoacidosis, dextrose-containing fluids will stimulate endogenous insulin release. In all groups, correction of volume depletion with isotonic fluids as well as judicious repletion of electrolytes (particularly potassium and phosphorous) are imperative.
Kidney failure	Supplemental alkali therapy (sodium bicarbonate or sodium citrate). Hemodialysis when necessary.
Ingestions	
Ethylene glycol Methanol	See Chapter 42.
Salicylic acid	See Chapter 42.
Pyroglutamic acid (5-Oxoproline)	Therapy is directed at the underlying cause. Generally requires withdrawal of the offending agent (acetaminophen) and sodium bicarbonate therapy for severe acidemia. *N*-Acetylcysteine may be effective in restoring glutathione stores.

1. Diabetic ketoacidosis (DKA)—DKA is characterized by hyperglycemia and metabolic acidosis with an increased anion gap from absolute or relative insulin deficiency

$$H^+ + B^- + NaHCO_3 \leftrightarrow CO_2 + NaB + H_2O$$

where B^- is β-hydroxybutyrate or acetoacetate, the ketones responsible for the increased anion gap. DKA may be accompanied by an additional lactic acidosis from tissue hypoperfusion and increased anaerobic metabolism. The anion gap in DKA is often large (> 20 mEq/L) but is variable. The elevated serum glucose leads to a marked osmotic diuresis with sizeable losses of sodium, water, and potassium.

The correction of ketoacidosis via therapeutic maneuvers can be monitored by the measurement of serum β-hydroxybutyrate, measuring the pH, or by normalization of the anion gap. Urine ketones are detected by nitroprusside testing, results of which are rapidly available. However, urinary nitroprusside tests detect both acetoacetate and acetone (albeit to a lesser extent) but do not detect β-hydroxybutyrate. Direct measurement of serum β-hydroxybutyrate is preferred and can be used to monitor response to therapy.

2. Fasting ketoacidosis—Hepatic generation of ketones may occur as a normal response to fasting from relative hypoinsulinemia. Mild ketosis often occurs after 12–14 hours of fasting, peaking after 20–30 hours. The level of acidosis is generally small with fasting, albeit overt ketoacidosis can occur in patients who consume very low carbohydrate diets.

3. Alcoholic ketoacidosis—Chronically malnourished patients who consume large quantities of alcohol may develop alcoholic ketoacidosis. Alcohol metabolism decreases gluconeogenesis, resulting in hepatic production of β-hydroxybutyrate and, to a lesser degree, acetoacetate. Mixed acid-base disorders, such as a combination of metabolic alkalosis from vomiting and respiratory alkalosis from alcohol withdrawal, aspiration, or cirrhosis, are common.

With either fasting or alcohol ketoacidosis, insulin release is suppressed by hypoglycemia or stimulation of the sympathetic nervous system, allowing ketosis to occur. Patients with these disorders can sufficiently produce endogenous insulin and therefore do not require exogenous insulin administration. Treatment should commence with glucose administration to stimulate insulin release and suppress ketogenesis. Potassium should be repleted prior to glucose administration as insulin release will cause intracellular potassium shift, risking hypokalemia.

4. Euglycemic ketoacidosis—A unique form of diabetic ketoacidosis has been increasingly recognized in patients with type 2 diabetes who are treated with SGLT-2 inhibitors. Patients typically have blood glucose levels within the normal range, hence the term "euglycemic" ketoacidosis, which can delay diagnosis. Serum ketones should be checked in any patient taking an SGLT-2 inhibitor who has malaise, nausea, or vomiting. Patients are treated with discontinuation of the SGLT-2 inhibitor, fluid resuscitation, an insulin drip, and dextrose supplementation (to avoid hypoglycemia).

C. Toxins

(See also Chapter 42.) Multiple toxins and drugs increase the anion gap by increasing endogenous acid production. Common examples include methanol (metabolized to formic acid), ethylene glycol (glycolic and oxalic acid), and salicylates (salicylic acid and lactic acid). The latter can cause a mixed disorder of metabolic acidosis with respiratory alkalosis. In toluene poisoning, the metabolite hippurate is rapidly excreted by the kidney, resulting in a normal anion gap acidosis. Isopropanol, which is metabolized to acetone, increases the osmolar gap, but not the anion gap. Long-term acetaminophen use, even at therapeutic doses, can result in an elevated anion gap acidosis from accumulation of 5-oxoproline.

D. Uremic Acidosis

As the GFR drops below 15–30 mL/min/1.73 m², the kidneys are increasingly unable to synthesize ammonium (NH_4). The reduced excretion of H^+ (as NH_4Cl) and accumulation of organic anions from decreased excretion (eg, phosphate and sulfate) result in an increased anion gap metabolic acidosis.

NORMAL ANION GAP METABOLIC ACIDOSIS

The two major causes of a normal anion gap metabolic acidosis are bicarbonate loss from the GI tract or defects in renal acidification (RTA) (Table 24–12 and Table 24–14). The compensatory increase in serum chloride (hyperchloremia) maintains electroneutrality and a normal anion gap. Because urine ammonium is not commonly measured, the urinary anion gap is used as a surrogate to differentiate between these causes; however, studies have shown that the urinary anion gap is not a reliable indicator of urine ammonium.

A. GI HCO_3^- Loss

The GI tract secretes bicarbonate at multiple sites. The most common cause of a normal anion gap metabolic acidosis from the GI tract is diarrhea (loss of bicarbonate rich stool fluid). An infrequent cause is a ureterosigmoidostomy, where ureters are implanted into the sigmoid colon for urinary diversion. Unlike the bladder, colonic mucosa secretes bicarbonate in exchange for chloride, resulting in metabolic acidosis. More commonly, a neobladder is created using a loop of bowel (generally ileum or colon), which has significantly decreased the incidence of metabolic acidosis from diversion, though it can still occur when contact time between urine and mucosa is increased, typically because of an anastomotic stricture.

B. Renal Tubular Acidosis

Hyperchloremic acidosis with a normal anion gap and a normal (or near normal) GFR, in the absence of diarrhea, defines RTA. The defect is either an inability to excrete H^+ as ammonium (inadequate generation of new HCO_3^-) or inadequate reabsorption of filtered HCO_3^-. Three major types can be differentiated by clinical setting, urinary pH, urinary anion gap (or urinary ammonium if available), and serum potassium levels.

1. Distal RTA (type I)—This disorder is characterized by inability to excrete H^+ by the distal nephron. The urine cannot be fully acidified (urine pH remains > 5.5), despite systemic acidosis. Urinary ammonium excretion is therefore decreased, and the urinary anion gap is positive.

Table 24–14. Hyperchloremic, normal anion gap metabolic acidoses.

	Renal Defect	Serum [K^+]	Distal H^+ Secretion		Urinary Anion Gap	Treatment
			Urine pH	Titratable Acid		
GI HCO_3^- loss	None	↓	< 5.5	↑↑	Negative	Na^+, K^+, and HCO_3^- as required
Renal tubular acidosis						
I. Distal	Distal H^+ secretion	↓	> 5.3	↓	Positive	$NaHCO_3$ (1–3 mEq/kg/day)
II. Proximal	Proximal HCO_3^- reabsorption	↓	Variable	Normal	Variable	$NaHCO_3$ or $KHCO_3$ (10–15 mEq/kg/day), thiazide
III. Hyporeninemic hypoaldosteronism	Distal Na^+ reabsorption, K^+ secretion, and H^+ secretion	↑	Variable	↓	Positive	Fludrocortisone (0.1–0.5 mg/day), dietary K^+ restriction, furosemide (40–160 mg/day), $NaHCO_3$ (1–3 mEq/kg/day)

Reproduced, with permission, from Cogan MG. *Fluid and Electrolytes: Physiology and Pathophysiology*. New York: McGraw-Hill, 1991.

Distal RTA (dRTA) is usually secondary to a congenital or acquired decrease in the number of functional H^+ pumps, which reduces H^+ secretion. This is associated with hypokalemia due to enhanced K^+ excretion from a lack of competition from H^+ in the tubular fluid. This form of dRTA is commonly due to Sjögren syndrome, SLE, plasma cell myeloma, toluene inhalation (glue sniffing), Wilson disease, and lithium. dRTA can also be caused by destruction of tubular integrity (eg, by the antifungal amphotericin B). In all types of dRTA, buffering of acid by release of bicarbonate and calcium from bone results in hypercalciuria, which in addition to low urinary citrate from increased reabsorption, can result in nephrolithiasis.

2. Proximal RTA (type II)—Proximal RTA (pRTA) is due to a defect in the ability of the proximal tubule to reabsorb filtered HCO_3. The maximal rate of bicarbonate reabsorption is set by the tubular maximum (Tm), which is normally 26–28 mEq/L. The hallmark of pRTA is a decrease in the Tm for bicarbonate, typically to 14–20 mEq/L. Therefore, this is a self-limited disease with serum bicarbonate levels predicated on the severity of the proximal defect and the ability of the distal nephron to reabsorb bicarbonate. This essentially creates a new steady state, in which the Tm is equivalent to the serum HCO_3^- level, the urine is acidic (because there is no impairment of distal H^+ secretion), and the urine anion gap is negative (because there is no impairment of ammonium excretion). Bicarbonaturia, resulting in alkaline urine (> 5.5), only occurs when the bicarbonate level exceeds the Tm, which has implications in treatment. Fanconi syndrome is a pRTA with other proximal reabsorption defects resulting in glucosuria, aminoaciduria, phosphaturia, and uricosuria. The most common cause of pRTA is proximal tubular toxicity from the monoclonal immunoglobulin light chains in plasma cell myeloma. Other causes include heavy metals; Sjögren syndrome; cystinosis; Wilson disease; and various medications, such as acetazolamide, topiramate, tenofovir, and ifosfamide. The increased delivery of HCO_3^- to the distal nephron enhances K^+ secretion, and hypokalemia results when a patient is treated with HCO_3^- without adequate K^+ supplementation. Similar to dRTA, bone loss from persistent acidosis is common. Rickets can develop in untreated children, while osteomalacia can develop in untreated adults. Unlike dRTA, nephrolithiasis is uncommon in pRTA because of the increased citrate in the urine, which increases calcium solubility.

3. Hyporeninemic hypoaldosteronemic RTA (type IV)— Type IV is the most common RTA in clinical practice. This is primarily a disorder of hyperkalemia secondary to a decrease in aldosterone, which inhibits ammonium production. The clinical presentation is hyperkalemic normal anion gap metabolic acidosis. Common causes include diabetic nephropathy and tubulointerstitial renal diseases. In patients with these disorders, some medications, such as ACE inhibitors, ARBs, spironolactone, and NSAIDs, can worsen the hyperkalemia and acidosis.

C. Other Causes of Normal Anion Gap Acidosis

A dilutional acidosis may occur when the extracellular volume is rapidly expanded with normal saline since it contains neither bicarbonate nor sodium salts that can be metabolized to bicarbonate. Concerns have been raised regarding potential harm from volume expansion with normal saline. In clinical practice, balanced crystalloid solutions, such as lactated Ringer solution, are often preferred; however, data regarding optimal fluid choice are conflicting.

1. Urine anion gap—The normal kidney response to a metabolic acidosis is to increase NH_4Cl excretion to enhance H^+ removal. The daily urinary excretion of NH_4Cl can be increased from 30 mEq at baseline to 200–300 mEq in response to acidosis. Urine ammonium excretion can be estimated using the following urine anion gap equation:

$$\text{Urine anion gap} = U_{Na} + U_K - U_{Cl}$$

The urinary anion gap may help differentiate between GI and renal causes of hyperchloremic acidosis, although concerns have been raised regarding the utility of a urinary anion gap as a surrogate for urinary ammonium. If the cause is GI bicarbonate loss (diarrhea), renal acidification remains intact and NH_4Cl excretion increases appropriately (urinary anion gap will be negative). In a dRTA, ammonium excretion is impaired and the urinary anion gap is positive. In pRTA (type II), the primary problem is impaired HCO_3^- reabsorption, leading to increased HCO_3^- excretion rather than decreased NH_4Cl excretion and the urinary anion gap is often negative until treatment is initiated with exogenous bicarbonate therapy.

2. Urine osmolal gap—When large amounts of other anions (eg, hippurate in toluene poisoning, β-hydroxybutyrate, acetoacetate) are present in the urine, the urinary anion gap may not be reliable. In this situation, the urine osmolal gap may be a better indicator of NH_4^+ excretion, which can be estimated as 50% of the urinary osmolal gap where urine concentrations and osmolality are in mmol/L. A urine osmolal gap below 150 mOsmol/kg suggests impaired ammonium excretion, whereas a urine osmolal gap above 400 mOsmol/kg suggests an intact renal response to acidosis.

$$\text{Urine osmolal gap} = U_{osm} - 2(U_{Na} + U_K) + U_{urea} + U_{glucose}$$

Clinical Findings

A. Symptoms and Signs

Symptoms of metabolic acidosis are mainly those of the underlying disorder. Compensatory hyperventilation is an important clinical sign and may be misinterpreted as a primary respiratory disorder; Kussmaul breathing (deep, regular, sighing respirations) may be seen with severe metabolic acidosis.

B. Laboratory Findings

Blood pH, serum HCO_3^-, and PCO_2 are decreased. Anion gap may be normal (hyperchloremic metabolic acidosis) or increased. Hyperkalemia may be present.

Treatment

A. Increased Anion Gap Acidosis

Treatment is aimed at the underlying disorder, such as insulin and fluid therapy for diabetes and appropriate volume resuscitation to restore tissue perfusion (see Table 24–13). $NaHCO_3$ therapy is controversial in the treatment of increased anion gap metabolic acidosis disorders and is usually reserved for severe cases (arterial pH < 7.1–7.2). Large amounts of $NaHCO_3$ may have deleterious effects, including hypernatremia, hyperosmolality, volume overload, and worsening of intracellular acidosis.

B. Normal Anion Gap Acidosis

Treatment of RTA is mainly achieved by administration of alkali (bicarbonate or citrate) to correct metabolic abnormalities and prevent nephrocalcinosis and CKD.

Large amounts of oral alkali ($NaHCO_3$ or $KHCO_3$ 10–15 mEq/kg/day) (Table 24–14) may be required to treat pRTA because much of the administered alkali is excreted into the urine. This can exacerbate hypokalemia and a mixture of sodium and potassium salts is often required. Treatment of type I dRTA requires less alkali (1–2 mEq/kg/day) than pRTA, and potassium supplementation is typically required.

For type IV RTA, dietary potassium restriction may be necessary and potassium-retaining drugs should be withdrawn. Loop diuretics may be beneficial. Fludrocortisone may be effective in some cases without significant volume expansion. In some cases, oral alkali supplementation (1–2 mEq/kg/day) may be required.

When to Refer

Most clinicians will refer patients with RTA disorders to a nephrologist for evaluation and possible alkali therapy.

When to Admit

Patients require emergency department evaluation or hospital admission depending on the severity of the acidosis and underlying conditions.

Bonner R et al. Renal tubular acidosis: Core Curriculum 2025. Am J Kidney Dis. 2025;85:501. [PMID: 39864011]

Giglio S et al. Distal renal tubular acidosis: a systematic approach from diagnosis to treatment. J Nephrol. 2021;34:2073. [PMID: 33770395]

Uribarri J et al. Beyond the urine anion gap: in support of the direct measurement of urinary ammonium. Am J Kidney Dis. 2022;80:667. [PMID: 35810828]

METABOLIC ALKALOSIS

ESSENTIALS OF DIAGNOSIS

- High HCO_3^- with alkalemia (high pH).
- Evaluate effective circulating volume by physical examination.
- Urinary chloride concentration differentiates saline-responsive alkalosis from saline-unresponsive alkalosis.

General Considerations

Metabolic alkalosis is characterized by high serum HCO_3^- levels. The development of metabolic alkalosis requires its "generation" from loss of acid or gain of alkali, and its "maintenance" from the kidney's inability to excrete excess bicarbonate.

The causes of metabolic alkalosis are classified into two groups based on chloride responsiveness and are generally distinguished using urine chloride values (Figure 24–3). The compensatory increase in PCO_2 rarely exceeds 55 mm Hg; higher PCO_2 values imply a superimposed primary respiratory acidosis. However, the disorders of ion transport do not strictly fit in either category.

Bartter and **Gitelman syndromes** are genetic disorders affecting ion transport. Features of both syndromes include metabolic alkalosis, hypokalemia, and normotension. Bartter syndrome is characterized by abnormalities affecting the NKCC channel in the loop of Henle and mimics a persistent loop diuretic effect. Gitelman syndrome is characterized by abnormalities affecting the NCC channel in the distal tubule, which mimics a persistent thiazide diuretic effect.

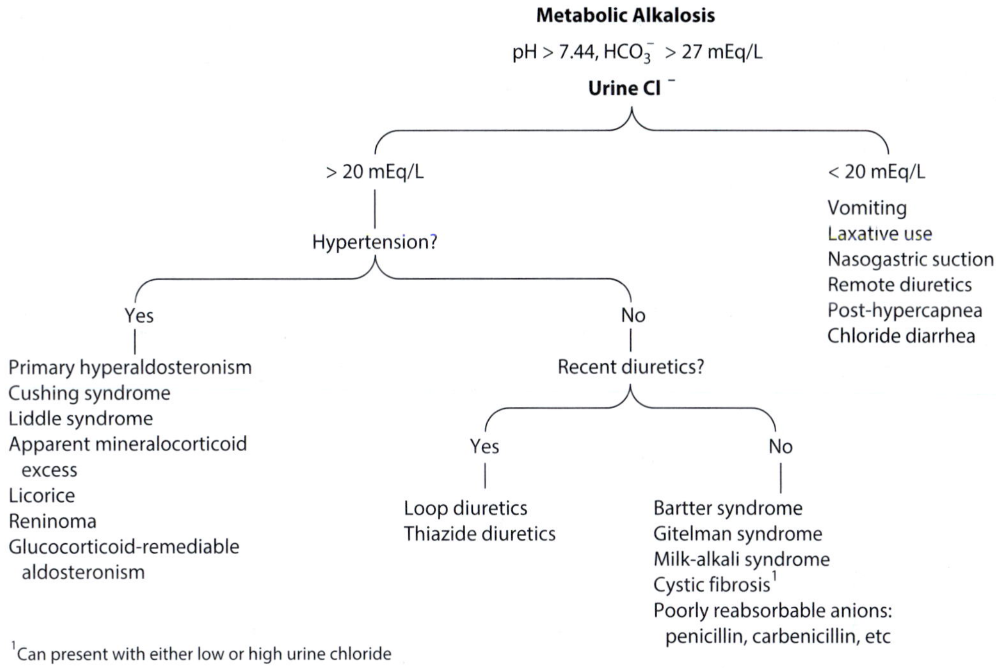

Figure 24–3. Algorithm for metabolic alkalosis on the basis of urine chloride.

A. Chloride-Sensitive Metabolic Alkalosis (U_{Cl}^- < 20 mEq/L)

Chloride-sensitive metabolic alkalosis involves the loss of chloride and extracellular volume. In vomiting and nasogastric suction, loss of acid (HCl) generates alkalosis and volume contraction from chloride loss maintains the alkalosis. Distally acting diuretics that cause chloride loss, eg, loop and thiazide diuretics, are a common cause of metabolic alkalosis. U_{Cl}^- levels can be unreliable in these settings since these diuretics increase U_{Cl}^-. These disorders cause concurrent hypokalemia, which can exacerbate metabolic alkalosis by stimulating H^+ secretion and ammoniagenesis.

In alkalosis, bicarbonaturia causes obligatory sodium excretion as the accompanying cation and U_{Na} levels are unreliable markers of extracellular volume.

B. Chloride-Resistant Metabolic Alkalosis (U_{Cl}^- > 20 mEq/L)

1. Excess mineralocorticoid activity—Mineralocorticoids act directly in the collecting duct to stimulate sodium reabsorption and hydrogen and potassium excretion. The effects on hydrogen excretion are important in the generation of metabolic alkalosis. Important causes of excess mineralocorticoid activity include primary hyperaldosteronism, Cushing disease, congenital adrenal hyperplasia (11-β-hydroxylase and 17-α hydroxylase deficiency), reninoma, excess licorice ingestion, apparent mineralocorticoid excess syndrome, and congenital adrenal hyperplasia (11-β-hydroxylase and 17-α hydroxylase) (Figure 24–3). These disorders are typically associated with hypertension, hypokalemia, metabolic alkalosis, and mild hypernatremia.

2. Alkali administration with decreased GFR—The normal kidney has a substantial capacity for bicarbonate excretion; therefore, metabolic alkalosis usually only develops with HCO_3^- intake (eg, intensive antacid therapy) when there is CKD. In milk-alkali syndrome, sustained heavy ingestion of absorbable antacids and milk causes hypercalcemic kidney injury and metabolic alkalosis. Volume contraction from renal hypercalcemic effects exacerbates the alkalosis.

Clinical Findings

A. Symptoms and Signs

There are no characteristic symptoms or signs. However, hypopnea can be present in severe cases. Concomitant hypokalemia may cause weakness and hyporeflexia. Severe alkalosis with a pH > 7.48 is associated with an increased risk of mortality.

B. Laboratory Findings

The arterial blood pH and bicarbonate are elevated. With respiratory compensation, the arterial P_{CO_2} is increased. Serum potassium and chloride are decreased. The urine Cl^- can differentiate between chloride-responsive (< 20 mEq/L) and unresponsive (> 20 mEq/L) causes.

Treatment

Mild alkalosis is generally well tolerated. Severe or symptomatic alkalosis (pH > 7.60) requires urgent treatment.

A. Chloride-Sensitive Metabolic Alkalosis

Therapy for chloride-sensitive alkalosis involves volume expansion with chloride salts, generally in the form of intravenous normal saline, until a euvolemic state has been achieved. This reduces proximal tubular bicarbonate reabsorption and increases distal tubular delivery of chloride, where it is exchanged for bicarbonate by the luminal Cl^-/HCO_3^- pendrin. In edematous patients with a contraindication to volume expansion (eg, HF), options include Cl^- administration in the form of KCl, which has the added benefit of correcting concurrent hypokalemia if present, and the carbonic anhydrase inhibitor acetazolamide to increase renal bicarbonate excretion.

B. Chloride-Resistant Metabolic Alkalosis

Therapy for chloride-resistant metabolic alkalosis requires therapy targeted to the underlying cause (see Chapter 29).

Emmett M. Metabolic alkalosis: a brief pathophysiologic review. Clin J Am Soc Nephrol. 2020;15:1848. [PMID: 32586924]

RESPIRATORY ACIDOSIS (Hypercapnia)

General Considerations

Respiratory acidosis results from hypoventilation and subsequent hypercapnia. Both pulmonary and extrapulmonary disorders can cause hypoventilation (see Chapter 9, Pulmonary Disorders).

Acute respiratory acidosis is associated with only a modest increase in serum bicarbonate, which is an ineffective buffer due to the impaired carbon dioxide elimination. After 6–12 hours, the primary increase in P_{CO_2} evokes a renal compensation to excrete more acid and to generate more HCO_3^-. Complete metabolic compensation by the kidney takes several days. In acute respiratory acidosis, HCO_3^- increases by 1 mEq/L for every 10 mm Hg increase in P_{CO_2}.

Chronic respiratory acidosis is generally seen in patients with underlying lung disease, such as COPD. Renal excretion of acid as NH_4Cl results in compensatory metabolic alkalosis. In this situation, HCO_3^- increases by 3 mEq/L for every 10 mm Hg increase in P_{CO_2}.

Clinical Findings

A. Symptoms and Signs

With acute-onset respiratory acidosis, somnolence, confusion, mental status changes, asterixis, and myoclonus may develop. Severe hypercapnia increases cerebral blood flow, CSF pressure, and intracranial pressure; papilledema and seizures may be seen.

B. Laboratory Findings

Arterial pH is low and P_{CO_2} is increased. Serum HCO_3^- is elevated but does not fully correct the pH. Respiratory etiologies of respiratory acidosis usually have a wide A-a gradient; a relatively normal A-a gradient in the presence of respiratory acidosis is highly suggestive of global hypoventilation.

Treatment

If opioid overdose is a possible diagnosis or there is no other obvious cause for hypoventilation, the clinician should consider a diagnostic and therapeutic trial of intravenous naloxone (see Chapter 42). Noninvasive or mechanical ventilation may be necessary.

Adrogué HJ et al. Alkali therapy for respiratory acidosis: a medical controversy. Am J Kidney Dis. 2020;75:265. [PMID: 31473018]

RESPIRATORY ALKALOSIS

General Considerations

Respiratory alkalosis is always a disorder of hyperventilation, reducing the P_{CO_2} and increasing serum pH (Table 24–15). In pregnancy, progesterone stimulates the respiratory center, producing an average P_{CO_2} of 30 mm Hg and respiratory alkalosis. Salicylates directly stimulate respiration and aspirin toxicity should be suspected when both respiratory alkalosis and an anion gap metabolic acidosis are present, particularly with alkalemia. Symptoms of acute respiratory alkalosis are related to decreased cerebral blood flow induced by the disorder.

Determination of appropriate metabolic compensation may reveal an associated metabolic disorder.

As in respiratory acidosis, the metabolic compensation is greater if the respiratory alkalosis is chronic (see Table 24–11). In acute respiratory alkalosis, HCO_3^- decreases by 2 mEq/L for every 10 mm Hg decrease in P_{CO_2}, whereas in chronic respiratory alkalosis, HCO_3^- decreases by 4 mEq/L for every 10 mm Hg decrease in P_{CO_2}.

Table 24–15. Causes of respiratory alkalosis.

Hypoxia
Decreased inspired oxygen tension
High altitude
Ventilation/perfusion inequality
Hypotension
Severe anemia
CNS-mediated disorders
Voluntary hyperventilation
Anxiety-hyperventilation syndrome
Neurologic disease
Cerebrovascular accident (infarction, hemorrhage)
Infection
Trauma
Tumor
Pharmacologic and hormonal stimulation
Salicylates
Nicotine
Xanthines
Pregnancy (progesterone)
Liver failure
Gram-negative septicemia
Recovery from metabolic acidosis
Heat exposure
Pulmonary disease
Interstitial lung disease
Pneumonia
PE
Pulmonary edema
Mechanical overventilation

Reproduced with permission from Gennari FJ. *Respiratory acidosis and alkalosis. In: Maxwell and Kleeman's Clinical Disorders of Fluid and Electrolyte Metabolism*, 5th ed. New York: McGraw-Hill,1994.

Clinical Findings

A. Symptoms and Signs

In acute cases (hyperventilation), there is light-headedness, anxiety, perioral numbness, and paresthesias. Tetany occurs from a low ionized calcium, since severe alkalosis increases calcium binding to albumin.

B. Laboratory Findings

Arterial blood pH is elevated, and P_{CO_2} is low. Serum bicarbonate is decreased in chronic respiratory alkalosis.

Treatment

Treatment is directed toward the underlying cause. In acute hyperventilation syndrome from anxiety, the traditional treatment of breathing into a paper bag should be discouraged because it does not correct P_{CO_2} and may decrease P_{O_2}. Reassurance may be sufficient for the anxious patient, but sedation may be necessary if the process persists. Hyperventilation is usually self-limited since muscle weakness caused by respiratory alkalemia will suppress ventilation. Rapid correction of chronic respiratory alkalosis may result in metabolic acidosis as P_{CO_2} is increased with a previous compensatory decrease in HCO_3^-. The severity of hypocapnia in critically ill patients has been associated with adverse outcomes.

Arena A et al. Respiratory acid-base disorders. Emerg Med Clin North Am. 2023;41:863. [PMID: 37758429]
Xu EJ et al. Acid base disorders in cirrhosis. Adv Kidney Dis Health. 2023;30:336. [PMID: 37657880]

FLUID MANAGEMENT

Daily parenteral maintenance fluids and electrolytes for an average adult of 70 kg would include at least 2 L of water in the form of 0.45% saline with 20 mEq/L of potassium chloride. Patients with hypoglycemia, starvation ketosis, or ketoacidosis being treated with insulin may require 5% dextrose-containing solutions. Guidelines for GI fluid losses are shown in Table 24–16.

Weight loss or gain is the best indication of water balance. Insensible water loss should be considered in febrile patients. Water loss increases by 100–150 mL/day for each degree of body temperature over 37°C.

In patients requiring maintenance and possibly replacement of fluid and electrolytes by parenteral infusion, the total daily ration should be administered continuously over 24 hours to ensure optimal utilization.

If intravenous fluids are the only source of water, electrolytes, and calories for longer than a week, parenteral nutrition containing amino acids, lipids, trace metals, and vitamins may be indicated (see Chapter 33).

Balanced crystalloid solutions, such as Ringer lactate, have become the resuscitation fluid of choice, due to concern for metabolic acidosis and reduced GFR associated with normal saline (see Chapter 14). However, studies are conflicting and have not established the superiority of one fluid over another, which may reflect an overall paradigm shift favoring conservative fluid administration and earlier use of vasopressors. Excessive fluid resuscitation and maintenance are complications in hospitalized patients, especially those with critical illness or AKI. These complications have been associated with worsened outcomes, such as prolonged mechanical ventilation, dependence on dialysis, and longer hospitalization with increased mortality.

Ruste M et al. Association of cumulative fluid balance trajectories with haemodynamics, inflammation, and long-term mortality in critically ill patients with circulatory failure. Br J Anaesth. 2026;136:542. [PMID: 41330798]
Zampieri FG et al. Balanced crystalloids versus saline for critically ill patients (BEST-Living): a systematic review and individual patient data meta-analysis. Lancet Respir Med. 2024;12:237. [PMID: 38043564]
Zampieri FG et al. Effect of intravenous fluid treatment with a balanced solution vs 0.9% saline solution on mortality in critically ill patients: the BaSICS randomized clinical trial. JAMA. 2021;326:818. [PMID: 34375394]

Table 24–16. Replacement guidelines for sweat and GI fluid losses.

	Average Electrolyte Composition				Replacement Guidelines per Liter Lost				
	Na^+ (mEq/L)	K^+ (mEq/L)	Cl^- (mEq/L)	HCO_3^- (mEq/L)	0.9% Saline (mL)	0.45% Saline (mL)	D_5W (mL)	KCl (mEq/L)	7.5% $NaHCO_3$ (45 mEq HCO_3^-/amp)
Sweat	30–50	5	30–50			500	500	5	
Gastric secretions	20	10	10			300	700	20	
Pancreatic juice	130	5	35	115		400	600	5	2 amps
Bile	145	5	100	25	600		400	5	0.5 amp
Diarrhea[1]	140	15	110–115	40–45					

[1]In the absence of diarrhea, colonic fluid Na^+ levels are low (40 mEq/L).

25 Kidney Disease

Tonja C. Dirkx, MD
Tyler B. Woodell, MD, MCR

ASSESSMENT OF KIDNEY DISEASE

Kidneys may incur a variety of injuries (Figure 25–1). Although some patients with kidney disease exhibit signs or symptoms such as hypertension, edema, gross hematuria, or uremia that may lead to its discovery, kidney disease is usually discovered incidentally or when screening individuals at high risk for kidney disease. The initial approach is to assess the cause and severity of kidney disease. In addition to a careful history and physical examination, evaluation includes (1) eGFR to characterize disease severity and, when previous eGFR values are available, discern kidney disease duration and rate of progression, (2) urine studies including UA and urinary albumin:creatinine to estimate daily albumin excretion, and (3) renal imaging (usually ultrasonography). Select cases may warrant renal biopsy, particularly when glomerular disease is suspected. Genetic testing is increasingly utilized to elucidate the etiology of kidney disease.

Glomerular Filtration Rate

The primary function of the kidneys is removal of waste products and excess solutes from plasma.

The GFR reflects the amount of plasma ultrafiltered across the glomerular filtration barrier per unit time and serves as the primary metric of kidney function. Daily GFR in normal individuals is variable, ranging from 150–250 L/24 hours or 100–120 mL/min/1.73 m^2 of body surface area. Patients with kidney disease usually have decreased GFR; however, a normal or increased GFR (suggesting glomerular hyperfiltration) may also be seen.

GFR can be measured directly or estimated using validated formulae. Direct measurement is performed by determination of the renal clearance of a plasma substance that is not bound to plasma proteins, is freely filterable across the glomerulus, and is neither secreted nor reabsorbed along the renal tubules; it is defined as:

$$C = \frac{U \times \dot{V}}{P}$$

where C is the clearance, U and P are the respective urine and plasma concentrations of the substance, and V. is volume of urine per unit time (typically mL/min).

The gold standard for GFR measurement is by assessment of clearance of exogenously administered inulin; however, in clinical practice, the clearance of endogenous creatinine (termed **creatinine clearance**) is primarily used. The normal creatinine clearance (C_{cr}) is approximately 100 mL/min in healthy young women and 120 mL/min in healthy young men. The creatinine clearance declines by an average of 0.8 mL/min/year after age 40 years as part of the aging process. Creatinine is a useful biomarker because it is produced at a relatively constant rate as a byproduct of muscle metabolism, is freely filtered by the glomerulus, and is not reabsorbed by the renal tubules. (A small amount also is actively secreted by the tubules into the urine.) However, creatinine clearance is an imperfect measurement for several reasons: (1) the small amount eliminated by tubular secretion progressively increases as GFR declines (thus *over* estimating GFR); (2) in more advanced kidney disease, gut microorganisms degrade creatinine; (3) dietary meat intake and muscle mass affect plasma creatinine levels; (4) several medications impair tubular secretion of creatinine, thereby increasing the plasma creatinine concentration and falsely *under* estimating GFR; and (5) GFR measurement assumes a stable plasma creatinine concentration over a 24-hour period; therefore, it is inaccurate when creatinine concentration is changing, as occurs during the development of and recovery from AKI.

Creatinine clearance is measured with a timed urine collection and a simultaneous plasma creatinine level. An incomplete or prolonged urine collection is a common source of error. The completeness of the collection can be estimated by comparing the amount of creatinine excreted in the collection to that expected over a 24-hour period, which should be constant.

$$U_{cr} \times \dot{V} = 15 - 20 \text{ mg/kg for healthy young women}$$
$$U_{cr} \times \dot{V} = 20 - 25 \text{ mg/kg for healthy young men}$$

Because timed urine collections are cumbersome and often inaccurately collected, GFR is more commonly estimated (denoted **eGFR**) using equations that have been validated using patient characteristics (such as age, sex, and weight) and creatinine levels. The Kidney Disease Improving Global Outcomes workgroup recommends eGFR equations as the primary method for determining GFR; the

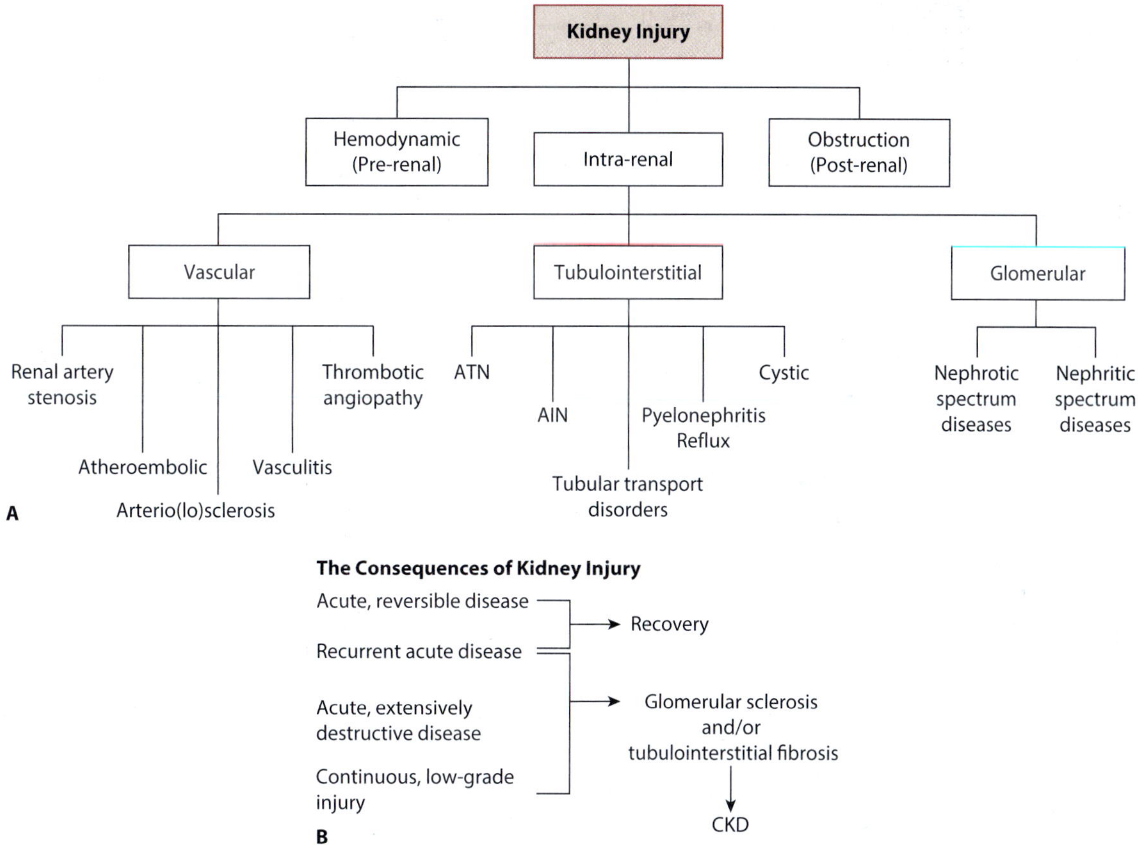

Figure 25–1. A: Kidneys may be damaged by a variety of insults/disease states. **B:** Narrowing the differential diagnosis of kidney disease to a structural compartment can be helpful. AIN, acute interstitial nephritis. (Reproduced, with permission, from Megan Troxell, MD.)

2021 CKD-Epidemiology (EPI) Collaboration creatinine equation is the preferred formula. Most laboratories report the eGFR alongside the plasma or serum creatinine and should specify which equation is in use. eGFR can be estimated by the 2021 CKD-EPI equation using a web-based calculator (eg, https://www.kidney.org/professionals/kdoqi/gfr_calculator).

Cystatin C is another endogenous marker of GFR that is filtered freely at the glomerulus; it is produced at a relatively constant rate by all nucleated cells, so more accurately estimates GFR in conditions with abnormally low muscle mass. Equations which use combined and simultaneous creatinine and cystatin C measurements for eGFR calculation are recommended to improve accuracy in individuals with muscle mass differing from typical body phenotypes (eg, bodybuilders or those with cachexia) and in those with recent African ancestry (see web-based calculator). However, because cystatin C testing is not available in all labs or included in a typical laboratory test sets or bundles, it remains a complementary rather than primary biomarker for estimating GFR.

BUN is another index used to assess kidney function. It is synthesized primarily in the liver as a byproduct of protein catabolism. It is freely filtered by the glomerulus, but 30–70% is reabsorbed in the renal tubules. As such, it *under*estimates GFR and varies widely depending on the clinical situation. For example, renal urea reabsorption increases in hypovolemic patients; a normal BUN:creatinine ratio is approximately 10:1 but can increase to 20:1 or higher with volume depletion. Other causes of increased BUN include increased catabolism (GI bleeding, cell lysis, and corticosteroid use), increased dietary protein, and states leading to decreased renal perfusion with resultant increased BUN reabsorption (eg, HF). Reduced BUN levels are seen in advanced liver disease and SIADH.

Disease Duration

Kidney disease can be acute or chronic. AKI is the worsening of kidney function over hours to days, resulting in retention of waste products (termed "azotemia"). If the etiology of kidney injury is mitigated quickly, AKI may be reversible and without lasting damage. Acute kidney disease (AKD) is the persistence of kidney dysfunction for 7–90 days following injury onset and denotes less reversibility to baseline kidney function. CKD is the persistence of kidney dysfunction beyond 3 months (Figure 25–2). Review of previous creatinine values helps to differentiate between AKI, AKD, and CKD. Additional findings may also be helpful; for example, oliguria is only observed in AKI/AKD, and small kidney size is more consistent with CKD.

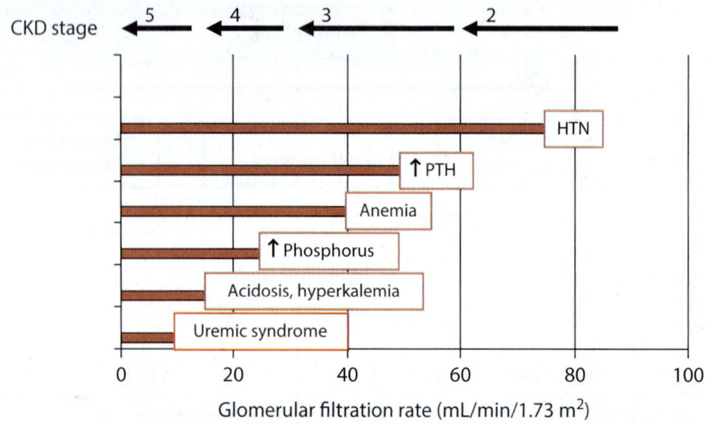

Figure 25–2. Complications of CKD by stage and GFR. Complications arising from CKD tend to occur at the stages depicted, although there is considerable variability noted in clinical practice. HTN, hypertension; PTH, parathyroid hormone. (Reproduced, with permission, from William Bennett, MD.)

Urinalysis

Examination of the urine can provide important clues when evaluating kidney disease. A urine specimen should be collected midstream or by bladder catheterization and examined within 1 hour of collection to avoid destruction of formed elements. UA includes dipstick examination followed by microscopy if the dipstick has positive findings. The dipstick examination measures urinary pH, specific gravity, protein (albumin), hemoglobin (blood or myoglobin), glucose, ketones, bilirubin, nitrites, and leukocyte esterase. Microscopy of centrifuged urinary sediment permits examination of formed elements—crystals, cells, casts, and infectious organisms. When urine flow is low, precipitation of Tamm-Horsfall mucoprotein in the renal tubule causes acellular (also called hyaline) cast formation (Table 25–1), which does not necessarily indicate disease. In contrast, casts containing formed elements do signal underlying damage. Granular casts (also called "muddy brown casts") and renal tubular epithelial cells alone or in casts are hallmarks of ATN. Urinary WBCs (including neutrophils and eosinophils) and WBC casts can be seen with pyelonephritis and interstitial nephritis; however, pyuria alone can also be seen in lower tract infections. The presence of protein on dipstick examination suggests underlying glomerular disease. If the glomerular basement membrane (GBM) is damaged (eg, by inflammation), RBCs may leak into the urinary space and appear dysmorphic. Thus, proteinuria, dysmorphic RBCs, and RBCs casts are highly suggestive of glomerulonephritis. Heavy proteinuria (see next section) accompanied by lipiduria may indicate nephrotic syndrome.

Table 25–1. Significance of specific urinary casts.

Type	Significance
Hyaline casts	Not indicative of kidney disease Concentrated urine, febrile disease, diuretic therapy, after strenuous exercise
RBC casts	Glomerulonephritis
WBC casts	Infection or inflammation Pyelonephritis, interstitial nephritis
Renal tubular cell casts	Can be seen in ATN or interstitial nephritis
Granular (muddy brown) casts	ATN
Broad waxy casts	Indicative of stasis in enlarged collecting tubules, CKD

A. Proteinuria

Albumin is the most abundant protein species in the blood and therefore the most abundant urinary protein species. The terms "proteinuria" and "albuminuria" are often used interchangeably, though there are cases for which this is not accurate. Urinary albumin/protein quantification should be performed in all those at risk for or with kidney disease; this may be done with a spot urine specimen for creatine and either albumin or protein. If both species are reported in the same units (eg, mg/dL), then the resulting dimensionless ratio of ($[U_{albumin}]/[U_{creatinine}]$) or ($[U_{protein}]/[U_{creatinine}]$) estimates the daily urinary albumin (or protein) excretion in g/day (Table 25–2); for example, $[U_{protein}]$ of 400 mg/dL and $[U_{creatinine}]$) of 200 mg/dL estimates a daily urinary protein excretion of 2 g. Twenty-four hour urine collections for protein are rarely necessary. Proteinuria/albuminuria may be the sole sign of kidney damage or may accompany an abnormal eGFR. The degree of albuminuria/proteinuria may help distinguish suspected glomerular disease from non-glomerular disease; is an important prognostic feature; and is used as a target of medical therapy.

There are several reasons proteinuria may develop: (1) **Functional proteinuria** is a benign process due to transient stressors such as acute illness or exercise, and "orthostatic proteinuria." The latter is generally found in people under 30 years of age and usually causes protein excretion < 1 g/day. The orthostatic nature of the proteinuria is confirmed by measuring an 8-hour overnight supine urinary protein excretion, which should be < 50 mg. (2) **Overload proteinuria** occurs when the resorptive capacity of tubules

Table 25–2. Definitions of albuminuria/proteinuria.

	Clinical Results Defining Condition
Normal (with respect to albuminuria)	Albumin < 30 mg/day
Microalbuminuria	Albumin 30–300 mg/day Not detected by urinary dipstick Must evaluate via urinary (micro) ACR
Albuminuria	Albumin > 300 mg/day Detected by urinary dipstick Should be quantified with ACR or UPC
Normal (total) proteinuria	Protein < 150 mg/day
Proteinuria	Protein > 150 mg/day Should be quantified with ACR or UPC Protein > 1 g/day is significant; > 3 g/day is nephrotic-range

ACR, albumin:creatinine ratio; UPC, urine protein:creatinine ratio.

is overwhelmed, which can result from excess production of low-molecular-weight plasma proteins. The most common cause is overproduction of immunoglobulin light chains/Bence-Jones proteins by a plasma cell dyscrasia; in these cases, there may be discordance between the urine dipstick, which detects only negatively charged albumin, and urine protein quantification, which includes both albumin and positively charged light chains. Qualitative urine protein electrophoresis will exhibit a discrete, monoclonal protein spike. Other examples of overload proteinuria include myoglobinuria in rhabdomyolysis and hemoglobinuria in hemolysis. (3) **Glomerular proteinuria** results from damage-induced increased glomerular permeability with increased filtration of albumin, as classically occurs in diabetic nephropathy. Urine protein electrophoresis will exhibit a large albumin spike. (4) **Tubular proteinuria** occurs due to faulty reabsorption of normally filtered proteins in the proximal tubule, such as β-2-microglobulin. Causes may include ATN, toxic injury (lead, aminoglycosides, and certain antiretrovirals), drug-induced interstitial nephritis, and hereditary metabolic disorders (eg, Wilson disease and Fanconi syndrome).

A kidney biopsy may be indicated to determine the cause of proteinuria, particularly if accompanied by abnormal GFR or hematuria. The clinical sequelae of proteinuria are discussed in the section on Nephrotic Spectrum Glomerular Diseases.

B. Hematuria

Hematuria is usually detected incidentally on urine dipstick or following an episode of macroscopic ("gross") hematuria. The diagnosis must be confirmed via microscopic examination, as false-positive dipstick tests can be caused by myoglobin, oxidizing agents, beets and rhubarb, hydrochloric acid, and bacteria. It is considered clinically significant if urine microscopy reveals more than three RBCs per high-power field on at least two occasions.

Hematuria may be due to renal or extrarenal causes. Extrarenal causes are addressed in Chapter 26. Renal causes account for approximately 10% of cases and are classified as either glomerular or extraglomerular. Glomerular causes include glomerulonephritis and heritable abnormalities of the glomerular basement membrane (GBM), thin basement membrane disease, and Alport syndrome. Extraglomerular sources include cysts; calculi; interstitial nephritis; and neoplasms of the kidney, prostate, or bladder (see Chapter 43).

KIDNEY BIOPSY

The kidney is a highly vascular structure; the primary risk of a percutaneous needle biopsy is bleeding. Thus, while pathologic information is helpful in many cases of kidney disease, biopsy is favored for cases in which the potential benefit outweighs the risk—especially those for whom a precise diagnosis will change management. These include (1) suspected nondiabetic glomerular disease, (2) atypical presentations of AKI, and (3) kidney transplant dysfunction. Relative contraindications include a solitary or ectopic kidney (except for transplant allografts), horseshoe kidney, ESKD, congenital anomalies, and multiple cysts. Absolute contraindications include an uncorrected bleeding disorder; severe uncontrolled hypertension; renal infection or neoplasm; hydronephrosis; or uncooperative patients, including those who are unable to lie prone for the procedure.

Anticoagulation should be held for 5–7 days post biopsy if possible. Post-biopsy bleeding most commonly occurs within 72 hours post biopsy but may occur later. More than half of patients will develop a small perinephric hematoma; approximately 1–5% of patients will experience significant bleeding requiring a blood transfusion. Anticoagulation should be held for 5–7 days post biopsy if possible. The risks of nephrectomy or death are about 0.06–0.08%.

GENETIC TESTING

Hundreds of genes are now known to contribute to kidney disease risk. Genetic factors are estimated to contribute to 50% of pediatric and 10% of adult kidney disease. Commercially available gene testing panels increasingly are utilized by nephrologists to help elucidate the etiology of kidney disease; the information provided may be used alongside or in lieu of a kidney biopsy.

Besouna I et al. Nephrogenomics, precision medicine and the role of genetic testing in adult kidney disease management. Nat Rev Nephrol. 2025;21:597. [PMID: 40524009]

Fogazzi GB et al. An updated approach to the evaluation of the urinary sediment. Pediatr Nephrol. 2025;40:933. [PMID: 39377940]

Levey AS et al. Uses of GFR and albuminuria level in acute and chronic kidney disease. N Engl J Med. 2022;386:2120. [PMID: 35648704]

Najafian B et al. Approach to kidney biopsy: core curriculum 2022. Am J Kidney Dis. 2022;80:119. [PMID: 35125261]

Navaneethan SD et al. KDOQI US commentary on the KDIGO 2024 Clinical Practice Guideline for the Evaluation and Management of CKD. Am J Kidney Dis. 2025;85:135. [PMID: 39556063]

ACUTE KIDNEY INJURY

ESSENTIALS OF DIAGNOSIS

- Rapid increase in serum creatinine.
- Oliguria may be present.
- Symptoms and signs depend on cause and severity.

General Considerations

AKI is defined as an acute increase in creatinine occurring over < 7 days, an acute decrease in urine output, or both. It is characterized as oliguric if urine production is < 500 mL/day. In the complete absence of renal function, creatinine will typically increase by 1–1.5 mg/dL daily, although in certain conditions such as rhabdomyolysis it may increase more rapidly. AKI is estimated to occur in approximately 20% of all hospitalized patients and 65% of patients in the ICU. AKI may pose a risk for the development and more rapid progression of CKD, and AKI from any cause is associated with a higher risk for all-cause mortality (likely due to injurious organ cross talk), even if there is substantial renal recovery.

Clinical Findings

A. Symptoms and Signs

Most AKI is subclinical; however, in severe cases, profound accumulation of waste products can cause nonspecific symptoms and signs collectively termed **uremia**: nausea, vomiting, malaise, and altered sensorium. Elevated blood pressure can occur due to impaired sodium homeostasis; however, if hypovolemia has caused the AKI (sometimes termed **prerenal azotemia**), the blood pressure may be low. Hyperkalemia may occur, with attendant risk of heart block and ventricular tachycardia. Uremia may cause prolonged bleeding time due to platelet dysfunction may be seen with uremia. Progressive uremia may also cause neurologic signs such as asterixis, encephalopathy, and seizures. Rarely, it may cause hemorrhagic pericarditis with a friction rub on auscultation and possible tamponade if the effusion is large.

B. Laboratory Findings

Creatinine levels are elevated. Decreased clearance of organic and inorganic acids may lead to metabolic acidosis. Hyperkalemia can occur from impaired renal potassium excretion or from shifting of potassium from cells into the blood as a result of inorganic metabolic acidosis. With hyperkalemia, ECG can reveal peaked T waves, PR prolongation, and QRS widening. A long QT segment can occur with hypocalcemia. Hyperphosphatemia is common. Anemia can occur as a result of decreased erythropoietin production over weeks, and bleeding time may be prolonged.

Classification & Etiology

AKI is diagnostically organized into three anatomic categories: prerenal causes (kidney hypoperfusion), intrinsic kidney disease, and postrenal causes (obstruction to urinary outflow) (Figure 25–1A) (Table 25–3).

A. Prerenal Causes

Prerenal causes are the most common etiology of outpatient AKI, accounting for 40–80% of cases. Prerenal azotemia is a physiologic response to renal hypoperfusion; if reversed quickly (eg, fluid resuscitation), renal parenchymal damage often does not occur. If hypoperfusion persists, prerenal azotemia can develop into intrinsic kidney injury/ATN.

Table 25–3. Classification and differential diagnosis of AKI.

			Intrinsic Renal Disease		
	Prerenal Azotemia	Postrenal Azotemia	ATN	Acute Glomerulonephritis	Acute Interstitial Nephritis
Etiology	Poor renal perfusion	Obstruction of the urinary tract	Ischemia, nephrotoxins, sepsis	Immune complex–mediated, pauci-immune, anti-GBM–related, monoclonal immunoglobulin–mediated, C3 glomerulopathy	Allergic reaction; drug reaction; infection; autoimmune disease
Serum BUN:Cr ratio	> 20:1	> 20:1	< 20:1	> 20:1	< 20:1
U_{Na} (mEq/L)	< 20	Variable	> 20	< 20	Variable
FE_{Na} (%)	< 1	Variable	> 1 (when oliguric)	< 1	Variable
Urine osmolality (mOsm/kg)	> 500	< 400	250–300	Variable	Variable
Urinary sediment	Benign or hyaline casts	Normal or red cells, white cells, or crystals	Granular (muddy brown) casts, renal tubular cell casts	Red cells, dysmorphic red cells, and red cell casts	White cells, white cell casts, with or without eosinophils

BUN:Cr, blood urea nitrogen:creatinine ratio; FE_{Na}, fractional excretion of sodium; GBM, glomerular basement membrane; U_{Na}, urinary concentration of sodium.

Decreased renal perfusion can occur due to a decrease in intravascular volume, a change in vascular resistance, or low cardiac output. Causes of volume depletion include hemorrhage, GI losses, excessive diuresis, burns, and extravascular fluid sequestration (eg, pancreatitis). In states of hypovolemia or decreased effective circulating volume (including poor cardiac output, cirrhosis, and reduced systemic vascular resistance due to sepsis, anaphylaxis, and anesthesia), autoregulation of renal blood flow and maintenance of GFR becomes dependent on prostaglandin-mediated afferent arteriolar vasodilation and angiotensin II-mediated efferent arteriolar vasoconstriction. Blockade of the renin-angiotensin system, as with ACE inhibitors or ARBs, and blockade of prostaglandin production, as with NSAIDs, impair this autoregulation and increase risk for more profound AKI in susceptible states. Renal blood flow may also be impaired due to vasoconstricting agents such as epinephrine, norepinephrine, high-dose dopamine, anesthetic agents, hypercalcemia, and calcineurin inhibitors. Renal artery stenosis causes increased resistance and decreased renal perfusion. Hepatorenal syndrome, a serious complication of decompensated cirrhosis, is another prerenal cause of AKI that results from low effective circulating volume (see Chapter 18).

History, physical examination, and laboratory data are important in the initial evaluation. In prerenal AKI, the BUN:creatinine ratio often exceeds 20:1 due to increased urea reabsorption by functioning tubules. In oliguric patients, a useful index is the fractional excretion of sodium (FE_{Na}). With decreased GFR, the kidney reabsorbs salt and water avidly if there is no intrinsic tubular dysfunction. Thus, oliguric patients with prerenal AKI should have a low fractional excretion of sodium (< 1%). In contrast, oliguric patients with intrinsic kidney dysfunction typically have a high FE_{Na} (> 1–2%), indicating loss of tubular cells' ability to reabsorb sodium. The FE_{Na} is calculated as follows: FE_{Na} = clearance of Na+/GFR = clearance of Na+/C_{cr}:

$$FE_{Na} = \frac{Urine_{Na} / Serum_{Na}}{Urine_{cr} / Serum_{cr}} \times 100\%$$

The equation was created and validated to differentiate *oliguric* ATN and prerenal AKI; its utility in nonoliguric patients is limited. Because diuretics act by increasing sodium excretion, a high FE_{Na} within 12–24 hours after diuretic administration cannot be meaningfully interpreted. In contrast, a low FE_{Na} *despite* receiving diuretics offers strong evidence of prerenal states in oliguric patients.

Urine microscopy is a valuable tool in the evaluation of AKI. Prerenal azotemia results in a bland urine sediment; hyaline casts may be present. In contrast, renal tubular epithelial cells or muddy brown casts are indicative of ATN.

Treatment of prerenal AKI depends on the underlying cause, but achievement of euvolemia, attention to serum electrolytes, and avoidance of nephrotoxic drugs are fundamentals of therapy.

B. Postrenal Causes

Postrenal causes of AKI are the least common, accounting for approximately 5–10% of cases; these occur when urinary flow from both kidneys, or a single functioning kidney, is obstructed. Obstruction leads to elevated intraluminal pressure and resultant kidney parenchymal damage, with marked effects on renal blood flow and tubular function.

Postrenal AKI can occur from obstruction at the level of the urethra, bladder, ureters, or renal pelvises. In men, benign prostatic hyperplasia is the most common cause. Patients taking anticholinergic drugs are at risk for urinary retention. Obstruction can also be caused by bladder, prostate, and cervical cancers; retroperitoneal fibrosis; and neurogenic bladder (eg, from diabetes mellitus). Less common causes include blood clots, bilateral ureteral stones, urethral stones or strictures, and bilateral papillary necrosis.

Obstruction can be constant or intermittent, and partial or complete. Obstruction may cause anuria but can also cause polyuria in the setting of partial obstruction with resultant tubular dysfunction and inability to reabsorb salt and water. Patients may have lower abdominal or back pain, and on examination may have an enlarged prostate, distended bladder, or palpable abdominal mass.

Laboratory examination may initially reveal high urine osmolality, low urine sodium, high BUN:creatinine ratio, and low FE_{Na} (ie, tubular function may not be compromised). These indices are similar to prerenal AKI because extensive intrinsic renal damage has not yet occurred. After several days, however, the urine sodium increases as the kidneys fail and are unable to concentrate urine (isosthenuria). Urine sediment is generally bland, though hematuria may be seen if the obstruction is due to stones, blood clots, or papillary necrosis.

Patients with AKI due to suspected postrenal causes should undergo bedside or formal ultrasonography to assess for hydroureter, hydronephrosis, or large bladder volume (despite recent attempted voiding). Prompt treatment of obstruction within days by catheters, stents, or surgical procedures can result in partial or complete reversal of AKI. After treatment of the obstruction, some patients experience significant increased urinary output (called postobstructive diuresis). In such settings, care should be taken to avoid volume depletion and electrolyte derangements.

C. Intrinsic Acute Kidney Injury

Intrinsic renal disorders account for up to 50% of all cases of AKI. Intrinsic dysfunction is considered after prerenal and postrenal causes have been excluded. The potential sites of injury are the tubules, interstitium, vasculature, and glomeruli. Intrinsic AKI is discussed in greater detail in the following sections.

When to Refer

- AKI that has not reversed over 1–2 weeks, or when the degree of AKI is concerning (eg, doubling of creatinine) and without an immediately reversible cause such as obstruction (see Table 25–7).
- Patients with signs of urinary tract obstruction should be referred to a urologist.

When to Admit

Patients should be admitted if there is sudden loss of kidney function resulting in abnormalities that cannot be appropriately addressed in an outpatient setting (eg, hyperkalemia, volume overload, uremia) or if an acute intervention is needed, such as emergent urologic procedures or dialysis.

Abdelhafez MO et al. Utility of fractional excretion of urea in acute kidney injury with comparison to fractional excretion of sodium: a systematic review and meta-analysis. Am J Med Sci. 2024;368:224. [PMID: 38768779]
Molitoris BA. Low-flow acute kidney injury: the pathophysiology of prerenal azotemia, abdominal compartment syndrome, and obstructive uropathy. Clin J Am Soc Nephrol. 2022;17:1039. [PMID: 35584927]
Patschan D et al. Recovery of kidney function in acute kidney injury. J Nephrol. 2025;38:445. [PMID: 40025396]
Turgut F et al. Acute kidney injury: medical causes and pathogenesis. J Clin Med. 2023;12:375. [PMID: 36615175]
Zarbock A et al. Sepsis-associated acute kidney injury: consensus report of the 28th Acute Disease Quality Initiative workgroup. Nat Rev Nephrol. 2023;19:401. [PMID: 36823168]

ACUTE TUBULAR NECROSIS

ESSENTIALS OF DIAGNOSIS

- AKI.
- Ischemic or toxic insult, or underlying sepsis.
- Urine sediment may reveal granular (muddy brown) casts, renal tubular epithelial cells, or both.

General Considerations

AKI due to tubular damage is called **acute tubular necrosis (ATN)**; it accounts for 85% of intrinsic AKI and the majority of hospitalized cases. ATN may be caused by prolonged renal ischemia, nephrotoxin exposure, or sepsis (even in patients who are normotensive).

A. Exogenous Nephrotoxins

Aminoglycosides are a common cause of ATN, even at therapeutic levels. Nonoliguric AKI typically occurs after 5–10 days of exposure. Predisposing factors include underlying kidney disease, volume depletion, and advanced age. Monitoring drug levels is important, and troughs are helpful in predicting renal toxicity.

Amphotericin B is typically nephrotoxic after a total dose of 2–3 g. This causes a type 1 (distal) renal tubular acidosis with severe vasoconstriction and tubular damage, which can lead to hypokalemia and nephrogenic diabetes insipidus. **Vancomycin**, intravenous **acyclovir**, and **cephalosporins** are also known to cause or be associated with ATN.

Radiographic contrast media may be nephrotoxic; contrast nephropathy refers to a rise in creatinine that occurs 24–48 hours after contrast administration. AKI in association with contrast exposure results from the synergistic combination of direct renal tubular epithelial cell toxicity and renal medullary ischemia in susceptible individuals. The combination of preexisting diabetes mellitus and CKD is associated with the greatest risk; other risk factors include advanced age, volume depletion, HFrEF, multiple myeloma, repeated doses of contrast, and recent exposure to agents which impair renal autoregulation, including NSAIDs, ACE inhibitors/ARBs, and SGLT-2 inhibitors. Prevention of contrast nephropathy in patients who have high risk for injury includes using minimizing contrast volume and the use of non-ionic, low osmolar agents. Other prophylactic measures include infusion of intravenous fluids—usually normal saline given at 3 mL/kg/hour for 1 hour before and 1 mL/kg/hour for 4–6 hours after contrast administration in patients who can tolerate this volume; increasing oral intake of fluids is an alternative, though is likely less protective.

Calcineurin inhibitor (tacrolimus or cyclosporine) toxicity is usually dose-dependent. It causes distal tubular dysfunction (a type 4 renal tubular acidosis) and severe vasoconstriction. Regular blood level monitoring is important to prevent both acute and chronic nephrotoxicity. Acute kidney dysfunction usually improves after reducing the dose or stopping the drug.

Other exogenous agents that can cause ATN include chemotherapeutic agents such as cisplatin; phosphate-based enemas; organic solvents; and heavy metals such as mercury, cadmium, and arsenic. ACE inhibitors, ARBs, and SGLT-2 inhibitors have many long-term benefits for patients with CKD but may cause or contribute to ischemic ATN at times of prolonged hypotension or volume depletion or when administered in combination with NSAIDs. Some traditional medicines and herbal or nutritional supplements may also be nephrotoxic.

B. Endogenous Nephrotoxins

Endogenous nephrotoxins include pigments (myoglobin, hemoglobin, and bilirubin), uric acid, and paraproteins. These products can cause direct tubular toxicity, resulting in ATN. The most common type of pigment nephropathy is rhabdomyolysis, caused by release of myoglobin from muscle. Massive intravascular hemolysis with release of hemoglobin is seen in transfusion reactions and in certain hemolytic anemias. Bile cast nephropathy occurs in severe cholestatic states with resultant bilirubin-induced renal tubular toxicity. Remission of the underlying disorder and volume resuscitation, when clinically appropriate, are mainstays of treatment.

Hyperuricemia can occur in the setting of rapid cell turnover and lysis. Chemotherapy for germ cell and hematologic malignancies (leukemia and lymphoma) is the primary cause; spontaneous tumor lysis syndrome can also occur, though is less common. When serum uric acid levels exceed 15–20 mg/dL, ATN can result from intratubular precipitation of uric acid crystals. Allopurinol or rasburicase can be used prophylactically, and rasburicase with or without dialysis is often used for treatment in established cases.

Paraproteins due to plasma cell myeloma can cause direct tubular toxicity and tubular obstruction. Other renal complications from plasma cell myeloma include hypercalcemia and renal tubular dysfunction, including type 2 (proximal) renal tubular acidosis (see Plasma Cell Myeloma below).

C. Sepsis

The most common etiology of ATN in hospitalized patients is sepsis/severe infection in which circulating inflammatory cytokines act as endogenous nephrotoxins. AKI in these cases is often multifactorial in etiology, including a possible preceding shock state with renal hypoperfusion; renal venous congestion and possible abdominal compartment physiology from volume over-resuscitation; and exposure to potential nephrotoxic antibiotics.

Clinical Findings

A. Symptoms and Signs

See Acute Kidney Injury.

B. Laboratory Findings

Hyperkalemia and hyperphosphatemia are commonly present. The BUN:creatinine ratio is usually < 20:1 due to tubular dysfunction, as described in the general section on AKI (see Table 25–3). Urine sodium concentration and FE_{Na} are usually elevated, also indicative of tubular dysfunction. Granular casts or renal tubular epithelial cells on urine microscopy are strongly predictive of ATN, but their negative predictive value is low (see Table 25–1). Kidney biopsy is not performed in cases of suspected ATN but is sometimes helpful in cases of diagnostic uncertainty.

Treatment

Treatment of ATN is aimed at hastening recovery and avoiding complications. Preventive measures should be taken to avoid volume overload and hyperkalemia. There is no benefit of loop diuretics on either recovery from AKI or death; thus, in critically ill patients with AKI, diuretics should be used only when otherwise clinically indicated (eg, in states of volume overload). Nonresponsiveness to a trial of high-dose diuretics (called "furosemide stress test") has been shown to predict future need for acute dialysis in this population. Ultrafiltration is generally reserved for patients with AKI in need of volume removal who are unresponsive to diuretics; however, this has not been shown to improve survival. Hyperkalemia and hyperphosphatemia can be treated with dietary restriction, potassium-binding agents, or phosphate-binding agents (taken with meals) (see section on CKD. Magnesium-containing antacids and laxatives should be avoided. Dosages of all medications eliminated by the kidney must be adjusted.

Indications for dialysis in AKI from ATN or other intrinsic diseases include life-threatening "AEIOUs" (Acid-base or Electrolyte disturbances [eg, hyperkalemia] refractory to medical management; Intoxications from certain drugs; volume; Overload unresponsive to diuretics; and Uremic complications [eg, encephalopathy, pericarditis, and/or seizures]). In critically ill patients, less severe but worsening abnormalities may also be indications for dialytic support. There is no evidence that more intensive or earlier initiation of renal replacement therapy for patients with AKI confers a benefit of earlier renal recovery or improved survival.

Course & Prognosis

The clinical course of ATN is often divided into three phases: initial injury, maintenance, and recovery. The maintenance phase is expressed as either oliguric (urinary output < 500 mL/day) or nonoliguric. Nonoliguric ATN is associated with better outcomes than oliguric ATN; however, only intrinsic renal recovery/tubular repair can convert an oliguric to a nonoliguric state. Average duration of the maintenance phase is 1–3 weeks, but some cases last several months, during which time cellular repair and clearance of tubular debris begin to occur. The recovery phase can be heralded by diuresis, due both to the inability of recovering renal tubules to reabsorb salt and water appropriately and to solute- and urea-induced diuresis.

The mortality rate associated with AKI is 20–50% in hospitalized patients and up to 70% in ICU patients requiring dialysis. Increased mortality is associated with advanced age, severe underlying disease, and multisystem organ failure due to injurious organ cross talk. Leading causes of death are infections, fluid and electrolyte disturbances, and worsening of underlying disease.

When to Refer

- When uncertainty exists as to the cause of or treatment for AKI.
- For fluid, electrolyte, and acid-base abnormalities that are recalcitrant to interventions.
- Nephrology referral improves outcomes in AKI.

When to Admit

A patient with symptoms or signs of AKI that require immediate intervention, such as administration of intravenous fluids or dialytic therapy, or that require a team approach that cannot be coordinated as an outpatient.

Krishnan N et al. Toxic nephropathies of the tubulointerstitium: core curriculum 2024. Am J Kidney Dis. 2024;83:659. [PMID: 38243994]

Ostermann M et al. Indications for and timing of initiation of KRT. Clin J Am Soc Nephrol. 2023;18:113. [PMID: 36100262]

Yanyan L et al. Contrast-induced acute kidney injury: a review of definition, pathogenesis, risk factors, prevention and treatment. BMC Nephrol. 2024;25:140. [PMID: 38649939]

Zarbock A et al. Sepsis-associated acute kidney injury: consensus report of the 28th Acute Disease Quality Initiative workgroup. Nat Rev Nephrol. 2023;19:401. [PMID: 36823168]

RHABDOMYOLYSIS

ESSENTIALS OF DIAGNOSIS

- Associated with crush injuries to muscle, immobility, drug toxicities, and hypothermia.
- Characterized by serum elevations in muscle enzymes, including creatine kinase, and marked electrolyte abnormalities.
- Release of myoglobin leads to direct renal toxicity.

General Considerations

Rhabdomyolysis is a syndrome of acute skeletal muscle necrosis resulting in markedly elevated plasma creatine kinase levels and myoglobinuria. Excessive urinary myoglobin can cause intrarenal vasoconstriction and pigmented tubular cast formation, leading to intrarenal obstruction and ATN. Rhabdomyolysis can result from crush injuries, prolonged immobility, seizures, substance use (eg, cocaine), vigorous exercise, viral infection (eg, COVID-19), and medications. Concomitant volume depletion in these settings increases risk of rhabdomyolysis and associated ATN. Risk of statin-induced rhabdomyolysis is increased with concomitant kidney or liver disease, diabetes, hypothyroidism, and concurrent use of niacin and fibrate-containing therapy. With the exception of rosuvastatin and pravastatin, risk with statins is also increased with concomitant therapy with drugs that inhibit cytochrome P450 (including protease inhibitors, erythromycin or clarithromycin, itraconazole, diltiazem, and verapamil). Commercially available genetic testing may help identify those at particularly high risk of non–trauma-related rhabdomyolysis.

Clinical Findings

A. Symptoms and Signs

Patients with rhabdomyolysis may be asymptomatic, or have myalgias, weakness, or both. Urine may appear dark due to the presence of myoglobin.

B. Laboratory Findings

Rhabdomyolysis of clinical importance commonly occurs when serum creatine kinase > 16,000–50,000 IU/L. Often, there are elevated serum levels of other skeletal muscle enzymes including AST, ALT, and LDH. The acute muscle enzyme elevations peak quickly and usually resolve within days once the inciting injury has resolved.

The classic laboratory finding in rhabdomyolysis is a urine dipstick test that is positive for "blood" but without RBCs on microscopy; the false-positive result is due to detection of myoglobin rather than hemoglobin. Additionally, rhabdomyolysis causes injured muscle cells to release intracellular components, leading to electrolyte derangements (including hyperkalemia, hyperphosphatemia, hyperuricemia, and hypocalcemia).

Treatment

The mainstay of treatment is aggressive volume repletion with 0.9% normal saline (ie, > 4 L/day) and removal of offending medications thought to have caused or contributed to the disorder. Adjunctive treatments with mannitol and alkalization of the urine have not been proven to change outcomes. As patients recover, calcium can translocate from tissues to plasma, so early exogenous calcium administration for hypocalcemia is not recommended unless the patient is symptomatic or the level becomes exceedingly low in an unconscious patient; calcium repletion can cause precipitation of calcium phosphate given the frequently concurrent hyperphosphatemia.

Myopathic complications of statins usually resolve within several weeks of discontinuing the drug.

When to Refer

Clinically concerning rhabdomyolysis requires immediate attention and inpatient management. Referral for nephrologist management may be appropriate following hospital discharge.

When to Admit

Patients whose serum creatine kinase levels are > 15,000–20,000 IU/L or patients with AKI or electrolyte derangements should be admitted for fluid repletion and serial monitoring of creatine kinase and electrolytes.

Akrivos VS et al. Crush injury and crush syndrome: a comprehensive review. EFORT Open Rev. 2025;10:424. [PMID: 40459168]

Kruijt N et al. 276th ENMC International Workshop: recommendations on optimal diagnostic pathway and management strategy for patients with acute rhabdomyolysis worldwide. 15th-17th March 2024, Hoofddorp, The Netherlands. Neuromuscul Disord. 2025;50:105344. [PMID: 40220353]

INTERSTITIAL NEPHRITIS

ESSENTIALS OF DIAGNOSIS

- Acute or chronic in nature.
- Pyuria, WBC casts, and proteinuria.
- Fever, transient maculopapular rash, or eosinophilia may occur in acute disease.

General Considerations

Acute interstitial nephritis accounts for 10–15% of cases of intrinsic AKI. An interstitial inflammatory response with edema is the typical pathologic finding; tubular damage may be present as well.

Although drugs account for the majority of cases, acute interstitial nephritis may also be caused by infectious diseases and autoimmune disorders. The most commonly implicated drugs are penicillins and cephalosporins, immune checkpoint inhibitors (ICIs), sulfonamides and sulfonamide-containing diuretics, NSAIDs, PPIs, rifampin, and allopurinol. Infectious causes include streptococcal infections, leptospirosis, cytomegalovirus, histoplasmosis, and Rocky Mountain spotted fever. Sjögren syndrome and sarcoidosis can cause interstitial nephritis, as can SLE and cryoglobulinemia, though these latter entities are more commonly associated with glomerulonephritis (Table 25–4).

Clinical Findings

Features of drug-induced acute interstitial nephritis may include fever, rash, arthralgias, and peripheral blood eosinophilia; however, the classic triad of fever, rash, and arthralgias is present in only 10–15% of cases and many have no signs or symptoms. If inflammatory cell infiltration increases renal volume sufficiently, the resultant renal capsular stretch may cause flank pain. Urine microscopy often reveals white cells and white cell casts; red cells may also be present. Proteinuria is often present, particularly in NSAID-induced interstitial

Table 25–4. Causes of acute tubulointerstitial nephritis (abbreviated list).

Drug Reactions
Antibiotics
β-Lactam antibiotics: methicillin, penicillin, ampicillin, cephalosporins
Ciprofloxacin
Erythromycin
Sulfonamides (trimethoprim-sulfamethoxazole, loop and thiazide diuretics)
Tetracycline
Vancomycin
Ethambutol
Rifampin
NSAIDs
Diuretics
Thiazides
Furosemide
Other
Allopurinol
Cimetidine
Phenytoin
PPIs
Systemic Infections
Bacteria
Streptococcus
Corynebacterium diphtheriae
Legionella
Viruses
Epstein-Barr
Other
Mycoplasma
Rickettsia rickettsii
Leptospira icterohaemorrhagiae
Toxoplasma
Idiopathic
Tubulointerstitial nephritis-uveitis

nephritis, but is usually modest (< 2 g/day). Eosinophiluria is neither sensitive nor specific for interstitial nephritis. Although the clinical history and laboratory data often suggest the diagnosis, kidney biopsy is sometimes needed.

Treatment & Prognosis

Acute interstitial nephritis often carries a good prognosis, with recovery occurring over weeks to months. Urgent dialytic support may be necessary in up to one-third of patients before resolution, but patients rarely progress to ESKD in the short-term. Those with prolonged oliguria and advanced age have a worse prognosis. Treatment consists of supportive measures and prompt removal of the inciting agent. If kidney injury persists despite removal of the culprit drug, corticosteroids should be considered, although data to support their use are limited, and their efficacy is diminished if started more than 1–2 weeks after onset of AKI. Short-term, high-dose methylprednisolone (0.25–0.5 g/day intravenously for 1–4 days) or prednisone (60 mg/day orally for 4–6 weeks) followed by a prednisone taper can be used in severe cases of drug-induced interstitial nephritis, including disease due to ICIs.

ICI-associated AKI is becoming increasingly common. General recommendations include holding therapy and treating with a course of corticosteroids. Based on consideration of treatment benefit, re-introduction of ICI therapy after AKI resolution may be considered with careful monitoring. Avoidance of concomitant potentially allergenic medications (eg, PPIs, sulfonamides, and ciprofloxacin) may help prevent AIN due to ICIs.

Herrmann SM et al. Diagnosis and management of immune checkpoint inhibitor-associated nephrotoxicity: a position statement from the American Society of Onconephrology. Kidney Int. 2025;107:21. [PMID: 39455026]

Sahutoglu T et al. Update on acute tubulointerstitial nephritis: clinical features, immunologic insights, and diagnostic and treatment approaches. Kidney Int Rep. 2025;10:1643. [PMID: 40630288]

GLOMERULONEPHRITIS

ESSENTIALS OF DIAGNOSIS

- Hematuria and proteinuria.
- Red cell casts may be seen.
- Dependent edema and hypertension.
- AKI.

General Considerations

Acute glomerulonephritis is an uncommon cause of AKI, accounting for about 5% of cases. In these cases, glomerular inflammation often incites a proliferative response by mesangial cells, glomerular capillary endothelial cells, or both. Glomerular crescents may be seen when severe damage causes breaks in the glomerular walls with exudation of inflammatory cells into the urinary space. Generally, the development of crescents portends a poorer prognosis and increases the urgency for treatment.

Glomerulonephritides (detailed later in this chapter) are classified into five pathophysiologic processes:

Immune-complex glomerulonephritis occurs when autoantibodies combine with antigens to form immune complexes that deposit within glomeruli. There are several distinct immune-complex glomerulonephritides, including IgA nephropathy, infection-related glomerulonephritis, lupus nephritis, and cryoglobulinemic glomerulonephritis (often associated with hepatitis C virus [HCV]).

Anti-GBM–associated acute glomerulonephritis is either confined to the kidney or associated with pulmonary hemorrhage. The latter is called "Goodpasture syndrome." Injury is related to autoantibodies against type IV collagen in the GBM.

Pauci-immune acute glomerulonephritis is a form of small-vessel ANCA-associated vasculitis in which there is kidney damage without direct immune-complex deposition or antibody binding. Tissue injury is believed to be due to neutrophil-mediated immune processes. The two most common ANCA vasculitides are granulomatosis with polyangiitis (GPA) and microscopic polyangiitis. GPA is a systemic necrotizing vasculitis of small arteries and veins associated with intravascular and extravascular granuloma formation; in addition to glomerulonephritis, these patients can have upper airway, pulmonary, and skin manifestations. ANCA subtype testing for proteinase 3 (which is more common in GPA) and myeloperoxidase (which is more common in microscopic polyangiitis) may be helpful in distinguishing these two vasculitides.

ANCA- and anti-GBM–associated acute glomerulonephritis have poor outcomes unless treatment is started early.

Monoclonal immunoglobulin–mediated glomerulonephritis is characterized by the deposition of a monoclonal immunoglobulin in glomeruli, the tubular basement membrane, or both. Immunofluorescent or immunohistochemical staining of kidney biopsies detects monotypic immunoglobulin deposits. Many cases occur in the setting of an identifiable monoclonal gammopathy, but this is not always the case. Serum protein electrophoresis, immunofixation, and free light chain analysis are important diagnostic tests to perform when monoclonal immunoglobulin–mediated glomerulonephritis is suspected or confirmed.

C3 glomerulopathy results from predominant C3 deposition in the glomeruli with or without minimal deposition of immunoglobulins. It is also identified by immunofluorescence or immunohistochemistry. The pathogenesis of C3 glomerulonephropathy stems from abnormalities in regulation of the alternative pathway of complement. Measurement of serum C3 levels may be helpful, but normal levels do not rule out C3 glomerulopathy.

Other vascular causes of glomerulonephritis include hypertensive emergencies and the thrombotic microangiopathies such as hemolytic-uremic syndrome and thrombotic thrombocytopenic purpura (see Chapter 16).

Clinical Findings

A. Symptoms and Signs

Patients with acute glomerulonephritis may be hypertensive and edematous. Extrarenal signs that reflect systemic manifestations of their disease (eg, rash in patients with lupus; cough or sinus congestion in patients with ANCA glomerulonephritis, or subacute fatigue and weight loss in patients with infection or vasculitis) may be present. Macroscopic hematuria is uncommon but may occur in select cases (eg, IgA nephropathy).

B. Laboratory Findings

Creatinine can rise over days to months, reflecting the severity of the underlying process. Urine dipstick shows blood and protein, with urine microscopy demonstrating dysmorphic RBCs (acanthocytes). Urinary sediment may reveal RBC casts—a sign of heavy glomerular bleeding. Red cell casts and acanthocytes are highly specific for glomerulonephritis.

Serum complement levels (C3, C4) may be low in immune complex glomerulonephritis (except for IgA nephropathy) and in C3 glomerulopathy, but normal in pauci-immune, anti-GBM–related, and most monoclonal immunoglobulin–mediated glomerulonephritides. Other serologic evaluations include ASO titers, anti-GBM antibody levels, ANCAs, ANA titers, cryoglobulins, HIV, hepatitis B and C serologies, serum protein electrophoresis, immunofixation, serum free light chains, and blood cultures. Renal ultrasound should be done to ensure there are no anatomic contraindications for renal biopsy. A kidney biopsy is usually necessary to confirm the diagnosis prior to treatment.

Treatment

Treatment is tailored to the specific type and severity of glomerulonephritis. It may include high-dose corticosteroids, rituximab, cytotoxic agents (such as cyclophosphamide), antiproliferative agents (eg, mycophenolate), and calcineurin inhibitors (eg, tacrolimus). Plasma exchange can be used in Goodpasture syndrome as a temporizing measure until chemotherapy can take effect. Treatment and prognosis for specific diseases are discussed below.

Anders HJ et al. Glomerulonephritis: immunopathogenesis and immunotherapy. Nat Rev Immunol. 2023;23:453. [PMID: 36635359]

Qasim H et al. Patterns of glomerular injury: histopathological classification and clinical correlation. Cureus. 2025;6:e91728. [PMID: 41058842]

COVID-19 & THE KIDNEY

ESSENTIALS OF DIAGNOSIS

- Broad array of clinical presentations and kidney pathology.

Clinical Findings & Treatment

Over time, the incidence and severity of AKI in the setting of COVID-19 infection has decreased. ATN is the most common cause of AKI, which is secondary to a high inflammatory state (termed "cytokine storm"). Individuals with high-risk *APOL1* alleles (see section on Nephrotic Spectrum Glomerular Diseases below) may develop COVID-19–associated collapsing glomerulopathy—a type of focal segmental glomerulosclerosis that presents with nephrotic syndrome. Treatment of COVID-19–related AKI is largely supportive, including dialytic support when appropriate. Corticosteroids have been used in COVID-19–associated collapsing glomerulopathy with reported success, but there is a lack of trial data or long-term follow-up to date to confirm efficacy. Although the rates of severe AKI associated with COVID-19 infections have decreased since early stages of the pandemic, there is growing awareness that individuals with milder AKI and those with long COVID are at increased risk for the development and progression of CKD.

Ivkovic V et al. Long COVID and the kidney. Nat Rev Nephrol. 2025;21:833. [PMID: 40908304]
Medina E et al. FSGS and COVID-19 in non-African American patients. Kidney360. 2023;4:687. [PMID: 37229730]

HEPATORENAL SYNDROME

See Chapter 18.

CARDIORENAL SYNDROME (Cardiovascular-Kidney-Metabolic Syndrome)

ESSENTIALS OF DIAGNOSIS

- **Cardiac dysfunction:** acute or chronic HF, ischemic injury, or arrhythmias.
- **Kidney disease:** acute or chronic, depending on the type of cardiorenal syndrome.

General Considerations

Cardiorenal syndrome is a pathophysiologic disorder of the heart and kidneys wherein acute or chronic deterioration of one organ results in the acute or chronic deterioration of the other. Recently, the focus has turned to the common metabolic dysfunction affecting both organ systems, which is more aptly termed "cardiovascular-kidney-metabolic syndrome." Achieving euvolemia, addressing cardiovascular and metabolic risk factors, and implementing guideline-directed medical therapy as tolerated are the overarching therapeutic goals (see Heart Failure section in Chapter 11).

Increasing recognition of the central importance of venous congestion in the development and progression of cardiorenal syndrome has led to an increased emphasis on assessment of right atrial pressure (which may include point-of-care ultrasonography) and strategies to overcome diuretic resistance (if present), including sequential nephron blockade (ie, adding a thiazide to a loop diuretic). If such approaches fail to achieve adequate decongestion, extracorporeal ultrafiltration therapy may be considered. While guideline-directed medical therapy is crucial, caution is required in those with advanced CKD due to increased risk with some agents (alone or in combination) for hyperkalemia or excessive blood-pressure lowering (alone or in combination).

Guaricci AI et al. Assessment and management of heart failure in patients with chronic kidney disease. Heart Fail Rev. 2024;29:379. [PMID: 37728751]
Lo KB et al. Kidney dysfunction in heart failure: core curriculum 2025. Am J Kidney Dis. 2025;86:109. [PMID: 40380970]
Tran P et al. A pragmatic approach to acute cardiorenal syndrome: diagnostic strategies and targeted therapies to overcome diuretic resistance. J Clin Med. 2025;26:2996. [PMID: 40364029]
Zoccali C et al. From cardiorenal syndrome to chronic cardiovascular and kidney disorder: a conceptual transition. Clin J Am Soc Nephrol. 2024;19:813. [PMID: 37902772]

CHRONIC KIDNEY DISEASE

ESSENTIALS OF DIAGNOSIS

- Reduced GFR, urinary abnormalities (eg, proteinuria), or both present for at least 3 months.
- Hypertension is commonly present.
- Bilateral small or echogenic kidneys on ultrasound in advanced disease.
- Symptoms and signs of uremia when nearing end-stage disease.

General Considerations

CKD affects about 14% of Americans and 850 million people worldwide. Many are unaware of their CKD as it is asymptomatic until it becomes advanced. The National Kidney Foundation's staging system helps clinicians formulate practice plans according to stage or severity of CKD (Table 25–5). Over 70% of cases of ESKD in the United States are due to diabetes mellitus or hypertension/vascular disease. Glomerulonephritis, cystic diseases, chronic tubulointerstitial diseases, and other urologic diseases account for the remainder (Table 25–6). Genetic polymorphisms of the *APOL-1* gene are associated with an increased risk of developing CKD in people of sub-Saharan African ancestry.

CKD is typically characterized by progressive decline in kidney function, even if the inciting cause can be identified and treated. Destruction of nephrons leads to compensatory hypertrophy and supranormal GFR of the remaining nephrons in order to maintain overall homeostasis. As a result, serum creatinine may appear normal even in the face of significant loss of renal mass, making it an insensitive marker for early renal damage and scarring. In addition, compensatory hyperfiltration leads to overwork injury in the remaining nephrons, which over time leads to glomerular sclerosis and interstitial fibrosis. ARBs, ACE inhibitors, SGLT-2 inhibitors, and mineralocorticoid receptor antagonists (MRA) help reduce hyperfiltration, which can slow progression of CKD.

CKD is an independent risk factor for CVD, particularly if proteinuria is present. Many patients at earlier stages of CKD will die of underlying CVD prior to progression to ESKD.

Clinical Findings

A. Symptoms and Signs

Stages 1–4 CKD usually are asymptomatic. As GFR declines, symptoms develop slowly, are nonspecific, and often do not manifest until GFR is < ~10 mL/min/1.73 m^2, at which time the accumulation of metabolic waste products (uremic toxins) may cause **uremia**. Uremia is a syndrome characterized by fatigue, anorexia, nausea, and a metallic taste in the mouth. Neurologic features such as memory impairment, insomnia, restless legs, and twitching may develop. Generalized pruritus (without rash) may

Table 25–5. Stages of CKD: a clinical action plan.[1,2]

Stage[3]	Description	GFR (mL/min/1.73 m^2)	Action
1	Kidney damage with normal or ↑↑ GFR	≥ 90	Diagnosis and treatment of underlying etiology if possible. Treatment of comorbid conditions. Estimate progression, work to slow progression. CVD risk reduction.
2	Kidney damage with mildly ↓ GFR	60–89	
3a	Mildly-moderately ↓ GFR	45–59	As above, and evaluating and treating complications.
3b	Moderately-severely ↓ GFR	30–44	
4	Severely ↓ GFR	15–29	Preparation for ESKD.
5	ESKD	< 15 (or dialysis)	Dialysis, transplant, or palliative care.

[1]Based on National Kidney Foundation, KDOQI, and KDIGO Chronic Kidney Disease Guidelines.
[2]CKD is defined as either kidney damage or GFR < 60 mL/min/1.73 m^2 for 3 or more months. Kidney damage is defined as pathologic abnormalities or markers of damage, including abnormalities in blood or urine tests or imaging studies.
[3]At all stages, persistent albuminuria confers added risk for CKD progression and CVD in the following gradations: < 30 mg/day = lowest added risk, 30–300 mg/day = mildly increased risk, > 300–1000 mg/day = moderately increased risk, > 1000 mg/day = severely increased risk.
Reproduced with permission from Kidney Disease: Improving Global Outcomes (KDIGO) CKD Work Group. KDIGO 2012 Clinical Practice Guideline for the Evaluation and Management of Chronic Kidney Disease. *Kidney Int.* 2013;3(1)(Suppl):1–150.

occur, as may decreased libido and menstrual irregularities. Pericarditis, a rare complication of ESKD, may present with pleuritic chest pain. Medications cleared by the kidneys will accumulate as kidney function worsens and toxicity may ensue; an important example is insulin, which carries risk of precipitating hypoglycemia if its dose is not appropriately reduced.

Table 25–6. Causes of CKD.

Glomerular Diseases[1]
Diabetic nephropathy
Focal segmental glomerulosclerosis
IgA nephropathy
Lupus nephritis
Membranous nephropathy
Infection-related glomerulonephritis
Tubulointerstitial Nephritis
Medication hypersensitivity
Heavy metals
NSAIDs/analgesic nephropathy
Reflux/chronic pyelonephritis
Sickle cell nephropathy
Idiopathic
Cystic Diseases
Polycystic kidney disease
Medullary cystic disease
Obstructive Nephropathies
Bladder outlet obstruction
Nephrolithiasis
Retroperitoneal fibrosis
Congenital/reflux
Vascular Diseases
Hypertensive nephrosclerosis
Renal artery stenosis

[1]Most common glomerular diseases worldwide.

The most common physical exam finding in CKD is hypertension, due in part to impaired sodium excretion, which often presents in early stages of CKD and worsens as disease progresses. In later stages of CKD, sodium retention may lead to clinically apparent volume overload. When GFR falls below 10 mL/min/1.73 m^2, signs of mild uremia such as slowed cognition and halitosis (uremic fetor) may be seen. More severe uremic presentations may include a generally sallow and ill appearance, decreased mental status, asterixis, myoclonus, and, rarely, seizures.

The presence of uremia warrants immediate consultation with a nephrologist; those with severe signs and symptoms should be hospitalized for urgent dialysis initiation. Because AKI can often be superimposed on CKD, it is important to identify and correct potentially reversible insults or exacerbating factors (Table 25–7). Urinary obstruction, hypovolemia, hypotension, nephrotoxins (such as NSAIDs, aminoglycosides, or PPIs), hypertensive emergency, and decompensated HF should be excluded.

Table 25–7. Reversible causes of kidney injury.

Reversible Factors	Diagnostic Clues
Obstruction	Post-void residual, bladder catheterization, renal ultrasound
Significant hypotension relative to baseline	Blood pressure and pulse
Extracellular fluid volume depletion	Orthostatic vitals, weight, volume status exam
Hypercalcemia	Serum electrolytes, calcium, phosphate
Nephrotoxic agents	Medication/supplement history
Severe/urgent hypertension	Blood pressure, CXR
HF exacerbation	Physical examination, CXR

B. Laboratory Findings

CKD is defined by the presence of at least one of the following for a minimum of 3 months: reduced eGFR; urinary abnormalities such as proteinuria or hematuria; electrolyte abnormalities (eg, renal tubular acidosis); or imaging abnormalities (eg, polycystic kidneys or a single kidney). Multiple estimates of GFR over time are used to determine the rate and pattern of progression. Although progression rates can vary (eg, a smooth linear slope, or stair-stepping pattern), any acute decline in eGFR should prompt evaluation for potentially reversible causes (see Acute Kidney Injury above). Anemia, hyperphosphatemia, hypocalcemia, hyperkalemia, and metabolic acidosis are common complications of advanced CKD. The urinary sediment may show broad waxy casts as a result of dilated, hypertrophic nephrons. If proteinuria is present, it should be quantified as described above. This can help elucidate the etiology of CKD (Table 25–6). For example, glomerular diseases typically present with protein excretion of > 0.5 g/day. Quantifying proteinuria also informs prognosis (ie, higher rates are associated with more rapid progression of CKD and increased risk of cardiovascular mortality) and guides management (eg, antiproteinuric therapy to slow disease progression).

C. Imaging

Findings of small, echogenic kidneys bilaterally (< 9–10 cm) by ultrasonography suggest chronic scarring of advanced CKD. Large kidneys can be seen with polycystic kidney disease, diabetic nephropathy, HIV-associated nephropathy, plasma cell myeloma, amyloidosis, and obstructive uropathy.

Francis A et al. Chronic kidney disease and the global public health agenda: an international consensus. Nat Rev Nephrol. 2024;20:473. [PMID: 38570631]

Grams M. et al. Chronic kidney disease. Ann Intern Med. 2025;178:ITC129. [PMID: 40921075]

Stevens P et al. KDIGO 2024 Clinical practice guideline for the evaluation and management of chronic kidney disease. Kidney Int. 2024;105:S117. [PMID: 38490803]

Complications

Complications of CKD tend to occur at relatively predictable stages of disease as noted in Figure 25–2.

A. Cardiovascular Complications

CKD confers increased morbidity and mortality risk compared to the general population. Roughly 80% of patients with CKD die before reaching ESKD, primarily of CVD. In patients undergoing dialysis, over 50% will die of a cardiovascular cause. The mechanisms for increased cardiovascular mortality in CKD are complex and include abnormal phosphorus and calcium homeostasis, increased burden of oxidative stress and inflammation, increased vascular reactivity, LVH, and coexistent conditions such as hypertension and diabetes mellitus. The presence of proteinuria is a marker for increased CVD risk.

1. Hypertension—Hypertension is the most common complication of CKD; it tends to be progressive and salt-sensitive. As with other patient populations, control of hypertension is achieved through both pharmacologic and nonpharmacologic therapy (eg, low-salt diet, exercise, weight loss, treatment of obstructive sleep apnea). CKD results in disturbed sodium homeostasis such that the ability of the kidney to adjust to variations in sodium and water intake diminishes as GFR declines. A low-salt diet (2 g/day) is often essential to control blood pressure and prevent volume overload. Diuretics are commonly needed to help control hypertension as disease progresses (see Table 13–9). Thiazides work well through stage 4 CKD. Loop diuretics are often used in those with more overt signs of volume overload and are more effective at blood pressure control when administered twice daily. Recommendations for initial drug therapy in nonproteinuric patients are no different than for the general population. For proteinuric patients, first-line therapy includes ACE inhibitors or ARBs (see Table 13–6), then MRAs if proteinuria persists. Serum creatinine and potassium should be checked 7–14 days after starting these drugs or increasing their dose due to a risk of hyperkalemia. A rise in serum creatinine > 30% from baseline warrants consideration of dose reduction or drug cessation and continued following of the creatinine trajectory. Strategies to mitigate hyperkalemia include addition of a diuretic (loop inhibitor or thiazide), a low-potassium diet, potassium-binding resins, or a combination of these. Patients in whom hyperkalemia develops and who are not able to adhere to recommended mitigation strategies with close follow-up should not be treated with ACE inhibitors, ARBs, or MRAs. An ACE inhibitor and ARB should not be used in combination. CKD is a common cause of resistant hypertension for which agents from multiple classes are often needed. Guidelines differ with respect to blood pressure goals in CKD; the American Heart Association recommends < 130/80 mm Hg, whereas the Kidney Diseases Improving Global Outcomes (KDIGO) committee recommends < 120/80 mm Hg. Patients with CKD are at risk for renal hypoperfusion and AKI with overtreatment of hypertension; it is prudent to individualize the approach to blood pressure control based on patient characteristics and risk factors.

2. Cardiovascular disease—Patients with CKD are at higher risk for death from CVD than the general population. Uremic vascular calcification involving disordered phosphorus homeostasis and other mediators may contribute. Traditional modifiable risk factors for CVD, such as hypertension, diabetes mellitus, tobacco use, and dyslipidemia, should be aggressively treated.

3. Heart failure—CKD complications result in increased cardiac workload due to hypertension, volume overload, and anemia. Patients may also have accelerated rates of atherosclerosis and vascular calcification resulting in vessel stiffness. These factors contribute to LVH and HF with preserved EF, which is common in CKD. Over time, HF with decreased EF may develop. Loop diuretic therapy, in addition to fluid and salt restriction, is often necessary; diuretic dose escalation may be needed as kidney function declines. ACE inhibitors and ARBs can be used for patients with advanced CKD with close monitoring of blood pressure and potassium; MRAs may be used with similar precautions as long as eGFR is > 25 mL/min/1.73 m^2. SGLT-2 inhibitors improve outcomes for both HF and CKD and, therefore, are recommended by both nephrology and cardiology society guidelines.

4. Atrial fibrillation—Patients with advanced CKD and ESKD have increased rates of atrial fibrillation, which approach 20% in patients receiving dialysis. Those with pre-ESKD should be treated as the general population. For patients with ESKD, anticoagulation for prevention of thromboembolic events is challenging due to increased risks of bleeding, although limited data suggest a benefit of anticoagulation for stroke reduction. For nonvalvular atrial fibrillation, DOACs may be safer and more effective than vitamin K antagonists for thromboembolic prophylaxis.

5. Aortic valvular calcification and stenosis—CKD may lead to aortic valvular calcification with valvular stenosis, which may progress rapidly in those with advanced CKD and ESKD.

6. Pericarditis—Pericarditis rarely develops in uremic patients; typical findings include pleuritic chest pain and a friction rub. Because cardiac tamponade can occur with uremic pericarditis, hospitalization and initiation of hemodialysis are essential when consistent with goals of care.

Kramer H. Chronic kidney disease-part 2: management and its complications. Adv Kidney Dis Health. 2025;32:79. [PMID: 40175033]
Marx-Schütt K et al. Cardiovascular disease in chronic kidney disease. Eur Heart J. 2025;46:2148. [PMID: 40196891]
Stambolliu et al. Managing hypertension in chronic kidney disease: the role of diet and guideline recommendations. J Clin Med. 2025;14:3755. [PMID: 40507517]
The EMPA-KIDNEY Collaborative Group; Herrington WG et al. Empagliflozin in patients with chronic kidney disease. N Engl J Med. 2023;388:117. [PMID: 36331190]

B. Mineral Bone Disorders

Mineral bone disorders of CKD refer to the complex disturbances of calcium and phosphorus metabolism, parathyroid hormone (PTH), active vitamin D (calcitriol), and fibroblast growth factor-23 (FGF-23) homeostasis (see Chapter 30 and Figure 25–3). A typical pattern seen in advanced CKD is relative hyperphosphatemia and hypocalcemia with low active vitamin D, resulting in secondary hyperparathyroidism and elevated FGF-23 levels. These abnormalities contribute to bone disease and excess fracture risk, as well to vascular calcification that is partly responsible for the accelerated CVD and excess mortality seen in CKD. Epidemiologic studies associate elevated phosphorus levels with increased risk of cardiovascular mortality in early CKD through ESKD. Data regarding how best to manage mineral bone disorders in these patients are limited; control of mineral and PTH levels per guidelines is discussed below.

Bone disease, or renal osteodystrophy, in advanced CKD is common and manifests in a variety of lesions. The gold standard for diagnosing renal osteodystrophy is bone biopsy, but this is not widely available. The most common

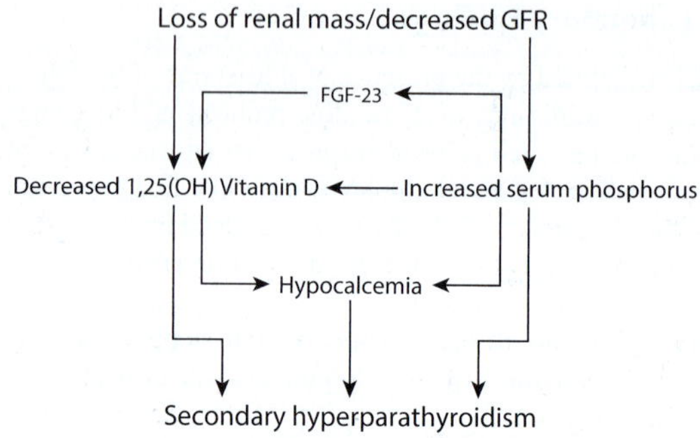

▲ **Figure 25–3.** Mineral abnormalities of CKD. Decline in GFR and loss of renal mass lead directly to increased serum phosphorus and hypovitaminosis D. Both of these abnormalities result in hypocalcemia and hyperparathyroidism. Many CKD patients also have nutritional 25(OH) vitamin D deficiency. PTH, parathyroid hormone. (From Tonja Dirkx, MD.)

bone disease, osteitis fibrosa cystica, is a result of secondary hyperparathyroidism and the osteoclast-stimulating effects of PTH. This is a high-turnover disease with bone resorption and subperiosteal lesions, which can cause bone pain and proximal muscle weakness. Adynamic bone disease, or low bone turnover, is becoming more common and may occur iatrogenically from suppression of PTH or via spontaneously low PTH production. Osteomalacia is characterized by lack of bone mineralization. Although historically associated with aluminum toxicity, osteomalacia is now most commonly due to vitamin D deficiency. Bisphosphonate administration in advanced CKD also may result in osteomalacia.

Management involves correction of calcium, phosphorus, and 25-OH vitamin D levels toward normal values, and mitigation of hyperparathyroidism. Understanding the interplay between these abnormalities can help target therapy (Figure 25–3). Declining GFR leads to phosphorus retention. Loss of renal mass and low 25-OH vitamin D levels often seen in CKD patients result in low 1,25(OH) vitamin D production by the kidney. Hypocalcemia can result from poor gut calcium absorption due to hypovitaminosis D as well as excess phosphate, which complexes with calcium and leads to vascular, valvular and soft tissue calcification. Hyperphosphatemia, hypocalcemia, and hypovitaminosis D are all stimuli for PTH production, and, over time, parathyroid gland hyperplasia.

The foundational step in treating mineral bone disorders is management of serum phosphorus levels. Patients should be instructed to avoid intake of highly bioavailable phosphorus—usually in the form of cola beverages, highly-processed foods, or both. If phosphorus targets are not achieved, further dietary phosphorus restriction may be necessary (see section on dietary management), followed by oral phosphate binders. Oral phosphate binders block absorption of dietary phosphorus and thus are taken with meals. Although target phosphorus levels are not strongly evidenced-based, standard treatment goals in ESKD are levels < 5.5 mg/dL. Calcium-containing binders are relatively inexpensive but may contribute to positive calcium balance and vascular calcification; overt hypercalcemia may also occur. Because of this, guidelines suggest limiting their use in favor of non–calcium-containing binders (sevelamer carbonate; or lanthanum carbonate) and iron-based binders (ferric citrate and sucroferric oxyhydroxide). Ferric citrate should be avoided in patients with iron overload. Aluminum hydroxide is a highly effective phosphorus binder. It can be used in the acute setting for severe hyperphosphatemia or for short periods (eg, 3 weeks) in patients with ESKD, but generally should not be used long-term because it can cause osteomalacia and neurologic complications.

Once serum phosphorus levels are controlled and 25-OH vitamin D stores are repleted, active vitamin D (1,25[OH] vitamin D, or calcitriol) or other vitamin D analogs may be used to treat secondary hyperparathyroidism in advanced CKD and ESKD. Monitoring for calcitriol-induced hypercalcemia and hyperphosphatemia is important; therapy should be dose-reduced or discontinued if either occurs. Calcimimetics such as cinacalcet or etelcalcetide target the calcium-sensing receptors of the parathyroid gland and suppress PTH production. Cinacalcet can be used if elevated serum phosphorus or calcium levels prohibit the use of vitamin D analogs; etelcalcetide is only available intravenously and is administered at hemodialysis units. Because calcimimetics can cause severe hypocalcemia, close monitoring is required. Optimal PTH levels in CKD are not known, but because skeletal resistance to PTH develops with uremia, relatively high levels are targeted in advanced CKD to avoid adynamic bone disease. Expert guidelines suggest goal PTH levels near or just above the upper limit of normal for moderate CKD, and 2- to 9-fold the upper limit of normal for ESKD.

Cupisti A et al. Dietary phosphorus and metabolic health in CKD and ESKD. Clin J Am Soc Nephrol. 2025;20:1289. [PMID: 40111420]
Natale P et al. Phosphate binders for preventing and treating chronic kidney disease-mineral and bone disorder (CKD-MBD). Cochrane Database Syst Rev. 2025;6:CD006023. [PMID: 40576086]
Zaimi M et al. Current therapeutic approach of chronic kidney disease-mineral bone disorder. Ther Apher Dial. 2024;28:671. [PMID: 38898685]

C. Hematologic Complications

1. Anemia—Anemia of CKD is primarily due to decreased erythropoietin production. It often becomes clinically significant at stage 3b–4 disease. The approach to a patient with CKD and anemia begins with ensuring that the bone marrow can respond to erythropoietin. Thus, thyroid function tests, serum vitamin B_{12} levels, reticulocyte count, and iron stores (ferritin and iron saturation) should be checked in the initial evaluation. CKD is also associated with high levels of hepcidin, which blocks GI iron absorption and mobilization of iron from body stores; this results in a functional iron deficiency or "anemia of chronic disease." In patients with CKD and anemia, KDIGO guidelines recommend offering iron supplementation if serum ferritin is < 500 ng/mL and iron saturation is < 30%. Iron therapy usually is withheld if the serum ferritin is > 700 ng/mL, even if iron saturation is low. Oral therapy with ferrous sulfate, gluconate, or fumarate, 325 mg once every other day, is typically prescribed in pre-dialysis CKD; higher doses may result in increasing hepcidin levels. For those who do not respond due to poor GI absorption or intolerance, intravenous iron (eg, iron sucrose or iron gluconate) can be considered.

Erythropoiesis-stimulating agents (ESAs, eg, recombinant erythropoietin and darbepoetin) are used to treat anemia of CKD if other treatable causes are excluded. Initiation of an ESA is usually considered when hemoglobin (Hgb) values are 9–10 g/dL. Typical ESA starting doses are epoetin-α 50–100 U/kg once or twice weekly; darbepoetin 0.45 mcg/kg every 2–4 weeks; or epoetin-β 60–100 mcg every 2–4 weeks. These agents can be given intravenously (eg, during hemodialysis) or subcutaneously; subcutaneous dosing of epoetin-α is roughly 30% more effective than intravenous dosing. ESAs should be titrated to an Hgb of 10–11 g/dL for optimal safety; studies show that targeting a higher Hgb increases the risk of stroke and possibly other cardiovascular events. When titrating doses, Hgb levels should rise no more than 1 g/dL every 3–4 weeks. Other concerns regarding ESA use include possible exacerbation of HTN and acceleration of underlying malignancy growth. For this reason, daprodustat, a hypoxia-inducible factor prolyl hydroxylase inhibitor, has emerged as an alternative to ESAs in treating anemia; however, it is not widely used.

2. Coagulopathy—Bleeding diathesis may occur in stage 4–5 CKD due to platelet dysfunction or severe anemia.

Treatment of bleeding diathesis is required only in patients who are symptomatic. Raising the Hgb to 9–10 g/dL can reduce risk of bleeding via improved clot formation. Desmopressin is a short-lived but effective treatment for platelet dysfunction and can be used in preparation for surgery or kidney biopsy; hyponatremia is a potential adverse effect of this treatment. Dialysis improves platelet function in uremic patients.

Aoun M et al. Erythrocytosis and CKD: a review. Am J Kidney Dis. 2024;84:495. [PMID: 38621632]
Babitt JL et al. Controversies in optimal anemia management: conclusions from a Kidney Disease: Improving Global Outcomes (KDIGO) conference. Kidney Int. 2021;99:1280. [PMID: 33839163]
Johnson H et al. Daprodustat: a hypoxia-inducible factor-prolyl hydroxylase inhibitor for anemia of chronic kidney disease. Ann Pharmacother. 2025;59:71. [PMID: 38616529]
Ku E et al. Novel anemia therapies in chronic kidney disease: conclusions from a Kidney Disease: Improving Global Outcomes (KDIGO) controversies conference. Kidney Int. 2023;104:655. [PMID: 37236424]

D. Hyperkalemia

Potassium balance typically remains intact in CKD until stages 4–5. However, hyperkalemia may occur at earlier stages when certain conditions are present, such as type 4 renal tubular acidosis (seen in patients with diabetes mellitus), high-potassium diets, or medications that decrease renal potassium secretion (amiloride, triamterene, spironolactone, eplerenone, finerenone, NSAIDs, ACE inhibitors, ARBs) or block cellular potassium uptake (β-blockers). Other causes include acidemic states and any process causing release of intracellular contents, such as hemolysis and rhabdomyolysis.

Treatment of acute hyperkalemia is discussed in Chapter 24 (see Table 24–5). Cardiac monitoring is indicated for any ECG changes seen with hyperkalemia or a serum potassium level > 6.0–6.5 mEq/L. Chronic hyperkalemia is best treated with dietary potassium restriction (2 g/day) and minimization or elimination of any medications that may impair renal potassium excretion, as noted above. Diuretics may help control potassium levels; SGLT-2 inhibitors and thiazides are less potent kaliuretics than loop diuretics. Oral potassium-binding resins (patiromer and sodium zirconium cyclosilicate) may permit the continued use of cardio- and reno-protective medications contributing to hyperkalemia, but this strategy should only be utilized in highly adherent patients with routine lab monitoring.

Fujimaru T et al Management of hyperkalemia: strategic clinical actions in real-world practice. Clin Exp Nephrol. 2025;29:1699. [PMID: 40705102]
Kreitzer N et al. EMCREG-International multidisciplinary consensus panel on management of hyperkalemia in chronic kidney disease and heart failure. Cardiorenal Med. 2025;15:133. [PMID: 39809248]
Palmer BF et al. Hyperkalemia treatment standard. Nephrol Dial Transplant. 2024;39:1097. [PMID: 38425037]

E. Acid-Base Disorders

Damaged kidneys are unable to excrete the ~1 mEq/kg/day of acid generated by metabolism of dietary animal protein intake. The resultant non-anion gap metabolic acidosis is primarily due to impaired ammonia genesis; proximal or distal tubular defects also may contribute to or worsen the acidosis. Excess hydrogen ions are buffered by bone; the consequent leaching of calcium and phosphorus from the bone contributes to the mineral bone disorders described above. Chronic acidosis can increase muscle protein catabolism and accelerate CKD progression. Reduction of dietary animal protein, increase in fruit and vegetable intake, and the administration of oral sodium bicarbonate (in titrated doses of 0.5–1.0 mEq/kg/day divided twice daily) may bring serum bicarbonate levels toward normal and is recommended when levels are consistently < 18 mmol/L. Citrate salts increase the absorption of dietary aluminum and should be avoided in CKD.

Mahboobi S et al. Effects of dietary interventions for metabolic acidosis in chronic kidney disease: a systematic review and meta-analysis. Nephrol Dial Transplant. 2025;40:751. [PMID: 39277780]
Poyourow CN et al. The role of dietary acid load on progression of estimated glomerular filtration rate among individuals diagnosed with chronic kidney disease. J Ren Nutr. 2024;34:273. [PMID: 38490515]
Raphael K. Metabolic acidosis in CKD: pathogenesis, adverse effects, and treatment effects. Int J Mol Sci. 2024;25:5187. [PMID: 38791238]

F. Neurologic Complications

Uremic encephalopathy, resulting from the accumulation of uremic toxins, typically does not occur until GFR falls < 5–10 mL/min/1.73 m^2. Symptoms begin with difficulty in concentrating and can progress to lethargy, confusion, seizure, and coma. Physical findings may include altered mental status, weakness, and asterixis. These findings improve with dialysis.

Other neurologic complications of advanced CKD may include peripheral neuropathies (stocking-glove or isolated mononeuropathies), erectile dysfunction, autonomic dysfunction, sleep disorders, restless leg syndrome, and pruritus. These may not improve with dialysis therapy.

Andrews T et al. Uremic toxins, CKD, and cognitive dysfunction. J Am Soc Nephrol. 2025;36:1208. [PMID: 40009460]
Glennon C et al. Skin disorders in kidney disease: core curriculum 2026. Am J Kidney Dis. 2026;87:102. [PMID: 41251635]
Vendeville N et al. Sleep-related disorders in patients with CKD and kidney transplant recipients. Clin J Am Soc Nephrol. 2025;20:1446. [PMID: 40202805]

G. Endocrine Disorders

Hypothyroidism is common in CKD. Men with advanced CKD may experience decreased libido and erectile dysfunction; women may have menstrual disturbances and anovulatory cycles. During pregnancy, a serum creatinine > 1.4 mg/dL is associated with more rapid CKD progression. However, risk in pregnancy is not increased in women with creatinine < 1.4 mg/dL and fetal survival is not compromised unless CKD is advanced.

Brenta G. Kidney diseases and the thyroid: interactions and consequences. Nat Rev Endocrinol. 2026;22:228. [PMID: 41249474]
Griffin TP et al. Thyroid dysfunction and chronic kidney disease: unravelling the connection. Mayo Clin Proc. 2024;99:7. [PMID: 38176835]
Piscitani L et al. Kidney and pregnancy: a comprehensive review. Clin Pract. 2025;15:189. [PMID: 41148787]

Treatment

A. Slowing Progression

Slowing CKD progression is a multipronged task that includes (1) treatment of the underlying cause, (2) blood pressure control, (3) therapy with antiproteinuric agents (ACE inhibitor or ARB, MRA, SGLT-2-inhibitor, or a combination of these) if appropriate, (4) weight loss if a patient has obesity, (5) avoidance of possible nephrotoxins (iodinated contrast agents, NSAIDs, PPIs), and (6) management of cardiovascular risk factors. Treatment of metabolic acidosis is recommended. In patients with diabetes, GLP-1 receptor agonists are effective at slowing disease progression. Laboratory results should be monitored after starting or titrating antiproteinuric agents. An initial fall in eGFR within the first several weeks may be seen, but as long as further testing demonstrates stabilization of kidney function and there is no concerning hyperkalemia, the agent should be continued.

Blum M et al. Risk-directed management of chronic kidney disease. Nat Rev Nephrol. 2025;21:287. [PMID: 39885336]
Perkovic V et al. Effects of semaglutide on chronic kidney disease in patients with type 2 diabetes. N Engl J Med. 2024;391:109. [PMID: 38785209]

Stevens P et al. KDIGO 2024 Clinical Practice Guidelines for the evaluation and management of chronic kidney disease. Kidney Int. 2024;105:S117. [PMID: 38490803]

The EMPA-KIDNEY Collaborative Group; Herrington WG et al. Empagliflozin in patients with chronic kidney disease. N Engl J Med. 2023;388:117. [PMID: 36331190]

B. Dietary Management

Patients with CKD should consult with a renal dietitian. Patient-specific recommendations should be made concerning protein, salt, potassium, and phosphorus intake to help mitigate CKD progression and complications.

1. Protein restriction—Limiting protein intake to 0.6–0.8 g/kg/day in patients with diabetes, and 0.55–0.6 g/kg/day in patients without diabetes, may slow CKD progression; plant-based sources of protein are thought to be better than animal sources for long-term kidney health. Restricting beyond these amounts is not advisable and should be avoided in those with cachexia or low serum albumin.

2. Salt restriction—Efforts should prioritize sodium restriction over water restriction; patients should be encouraged to drink water to thirst so long as they are following guidance on sodium intake appropriately. In advanced CKD, the kidney is unable to adapt to large changes in sodium intake. Intake of > 3–4 g/day can lead to hypertension and hypervolemia, whereas intake of < 1 g day can lead to volume depletion and hypotension. A goal of 2 g/day of sodium is reasonable for most patients.

3. Potassium restriction—Restriction is often needed once the GFR falls < 10–20 mL/min/1.73 m^2, or earlier if the patient is hyperkalemic. Patients should receive detailed lists describing potassium content of foods and should limit their intake to < 50–60 mEq/day (2 g/day). Constipation can contribute to hyperkalemia in CKD, since a higher percentage of potassium is excreted through the GI tract as GFR declines.

4. Phosphorus restriction—Guidelines suggest lowering elevated serum phosphorus levels toward normal in advanced CKD and to a level of < 5.5 mg/dL in ESKD. Initial dietary phosphate restriction should include avoidance of highly bioavailable phosphorus (fast foods and highly processed foods, and cola beverages), and subsequently moderation of intake of other phosphorus-rich foods such as eggs, dairy products, nuts, beans, and meat. Care must be taken to avoid protein malnutrition. When ESKD is reached, dietary restriction alone rarely is sufficient to reach target levels, and phosphorus binders are often required (see section on Mineral Bone Disorders).

Afsar RE et al. Sodium management in kidney disease: old stories, new tricks. Semin Nephrol. 2023;43:15104. [PMID: 37639931]

Carballo-Casla A et al. Protein intake and mortality in older adults with chronic kidney disease. JAMA Netw Open. 2024;7:e2426577. [PMID: 39110456]

Dang Z et al. Plant-based diet and chronic kidney disease: a systematic review and meta-analysis. J Ren Nutr. 2025;35:517. [PMID: 40081608]

Mafra D et al. Low-protein diet for chronic kidney disease: evidence, controversies, and practical guidelines. J Intern Med. 2025;298:319. [PMID: 40739997]

C. Medication Management

Many drugs are excreted by the kidney; dosages should be adjusted for GFR. As CKD advances, patients with diabetes using insulin or sulfonylureas may face increased risk of hypoglycemia due to decreased renal elimination of insulin; patient education and dose appropriate reductions are vital to avoid harm. The risk of lactic acidosis with metformin is due to both dose and eGFR; its dose should be reduced when eGFR is < 45 mL/min/1.73 m^2, and it should be discontinued when eGFR is < 30 mL/min/1.73 m^2.

Magnesium-containing medications, such as laxatives or antacids, and phosphorus-containing medicines (eg, enemas) should be avoided. Active morphine metabolites can accumulate in advanced CKD and should be avoided; this problem is not encountered with other opioid agents. Drugs with potential nephrotoxicity (NSAIDs, intravenous contrast, as well as others noted in the Acute Kidney Injury section) should be avoided. PPIs should be used only when medically necessary and for short courses.

Ammar A et al. Updates in chronic kidney disease management: a systematic review. Pharmacotherapy. 2025;45:291. [PMID: 40152479]

Hall RK et al. Drug stewardship in chronic kidney disease to achieve safe and effective medication use. Nat Rev Nephrol. 2024;20:386. [PMID: 38491222]

Pogson C et al. Medication review interventions for adults living with advanced chronic kidney disease: a scoping review. Br J Clin Pharmacol. 2025;91:1132. [PMID: 39739541]

D. Treatment of ESKD

When GFR declines to 5–10 mL/min/1.73 m^2, kidney replacement therapy (hemodialysis, peritoneal dialysis, or kidney transplantation) may extend life. Patient evaluation and education are crucial for timely preparation for the chosen therapy. Referral to a nephrologist has been shown to improve clinical outcomes. Practice guidelines recommend referral to a nephrologist when the GFR falls < 30 mL/min/1.73m^2, declines rapidly (> 5 mL/min/1.73 m^2 per year), or when > 300 mg/day of albuminuria is present. Preparation for ESKD treatment requires a team approach with the involvement of dietitians, social workers, pharmacists, primary care clinicians, and nephrologists. For older adults (over 80 years), or those with multiple debilitating or life-limiting comorbidities, dialysis may not meaningfully prolong life, and the option of medical management without dialysis should be discussed with the patient and family. Conversely, for patients who are otherwise relatively healthy, evaluation for preemptive kidney transplantation should be considered.

1. Dialysis—Dialysis initiation should be considered when GFR is near 10 mL/min/1.73 m^2 and uremic symptoms are present. Other indications for dialysis, which may occur when GFR is 10–15 mL/min/1.73 m^2, are fluid overload unresponsive to diuresis and refractory hyperkalemia.

A. Hemodialysis—Vascular access for hemodialysis can be an arteriovenous fistula (the preferred method) or prosthetic graft; creation of dialysis access should be considered well before dialysis initiation, and patients and providers should be educated to "save" the nondominant arm for future access creation by avoiding peripherally inserted central catheter (PICC) placement. A tunneled dialysis catheter is used when there is no usable vascular access. Because catheters confer a high risk of bloodstream infection, they should be considered a temporary measure. Fistulae typically last longer than prosthetic grafts but require a longer time after surgical construction for maturation (at least 6–8 weeks for a fistula, versus 2 weeks for a graft). Infection, thrombosis, and aneurysm formation are complications seen more often in grafts than fistulae. *Staphylococcus* species are the most common cause of soft tissue infections and bacteremia.

Treatment at a hemodialysis center typically occurs three times a week. Sessions last 3–4.5 hours, depending on body habitus and patient habits. Home hemodialysis is performed more frequently (4–6 days per week for shorter sessions) and often requires a trained helper. Clinical trials comparing quotidian modalities (nocturnal and frequent home hemodialysis) to conventional in-center dialysis have not shown significant mortality differences, but there may be improvements in blood pressure control, mineral metabolism, and quality of life.

B. Peritoneal dialysis—With peritoneal dialysis, the peritoneal membrane is the "dialyzer."

There are two primary approaches to peritoneal dialysis: continuous ambulatory peritoneal dialysis (CAPD), in which the patient manually exchanges the dialysate four to six times daily; and continuous cyclic peritoneal dialysis (CCPD), which utilizes a cycler machine that automatically perform exchanges at night during sleep.

The most common complication of peritoneal dialysis is peritonitis. Peritonitis may present with nausea and vomiting, abdominal pain, diarrhea or constipation, and fever. The normally clear dialysate becomes cloudy; and a diagnostic peritoneal fluid cell count > 100 WBC/mcL (0.1×10^9/L) with a differential of > 50% polymorphonuclear neutrophils is present. *Staphylococcus aureus* is the most common infecting organism, but streptococci and gram-negative species may also be causative. Empiric intraperitoneal administration of either vancomycin or a first-generation cephalosporin (cefazolin) plus a third-generation cephalosporin (ceftazidime) should be instituted with the first signs of peritonitis and subsequently tailored based on culture results.

2. Kidney transplantation—Many patients with ESKD are otherwise healthy enough to undergo transplantation, although standard criteria for recipient selection are lacking between transplant centers. Two-thirds of kidney allografts come from deceased donors, with the remainder from living related or unrelated donors. Over 100,000 patients are on the waiting list for a deceased donor transplant in the United States; the average wait is 3–7 years, depending on geographic location and recipient blood type.

The 1- and 5-year kidney graft survival rates continue to improve over time and are > 85–90% for both living- and deceased-donor allografts at 5 years posttransplant.

Immunosuppressive regimens to prevent allograft rejection generally include a combination of corticosteroids, an antimetabolite (azathioprine or mycophenolate mofetil), and a calcineurin inhibitor (tacrolimus or cyclosporine) or mTor inhibitor (sirolimus). Any changes in the transplant recipient's medical regimen should occur only after consultation with a trained pharmacist or transplant nephrologist.

3. Medical management of ESKD—As noted above, some patients are not candidates for kidney transplantation and may not benefit from dialysis, and others may elect not to pursue transplantation or dialysis. Frail older adults may die soon after dialysis initiation; those who do not may rapidly lose functional status in the first year of treatment. The decision to initiate dialysis in those with limited life expectancy should be weighed against probable deterioration in quality of life. For patients with ESKD who elect not to undergo dialysis or who withdraw from dialysis, progressive uremia with gradual suppression of sensorium results in a typically painless death within days to months. Hyperkalemia may intervene with a fatal cardiac dysrhythmia. Diuretics, volume restriction, and opioids, as described in Chapter 5, may help decrease the symptoms of volume overload. Involvement of a palliative care team is essential.

Flythe JE et al. Dialysis for chronic kidney failure. JAMA. 2024;332:1559. [PMID: 39356511]

Lok C et al. Hemodialysis vascular access: core curriculum 2025. Am J Kidney Dis. 2025;85:236. [PMID: 39625430]

Montez-Rath ME et al. Effect of starting dialysis versus continuing medical management on survival and home time in older adults with kidney failure: a target trial emulation study. Ann Intern Med. 2024;177:1233. [PMID: 39159459]

Shapiro J et al. Peritoneal dialysis and kidney transplantation: your questions answered. Perit Dial Int. 2025;45:142. [PMID: 39871717]

Prognosis in ESKD

Compared with kidney transplant recipients and age-matched controls, mortality is higher for patients undergoing dialysis. There is likely little difference in survival for well-matched peritoneal versus hemodialysis patients.

Patients undergoing dialysis have an average life expectancy of 3–5 years, but survival for as long as 25 years may be achieved depending on comorbidities, age at which dialysis is initiated, and underlying cause of kidney disease. Overall 5-year survival is estimated at 40%. Five-year Kaplan-Meier survival rates vary from 37% for patients with diabetes to 54% for patients with glomerulonephritis. The most common cause of death is cardiac disease (> 50%). Other causes include infection, cerebrovascular disease, and malignancy.

When to Refer

- A patient should be referred to a nephrologist for management in conjunction with the primary care provider when GFR falls < 30 mL/min/1.73m^2 or declines rapidly (> 5 mL/min/1.73 m^2 per year).
- A patient with other forms of CKD such as those with proteinuria > 300 mg/day or polycystic kidney disease should be referred to a nephrologist at earlier stages.

When to Admit

- Admission should be considered for decompensation of problems related to CKD, such as worsening of acid-base status, electrolyte abnormalities, and volume overload, that cannot be appropriately treated in the outpatient setting.

- Admission is appropriate when a patient needs to start dialysis and is not stable for outpatient initiation.

RENAL ARTERY STENOSIS

ESSENTIALS OF DIAGNOSIS

- Secondary to atherosclerotic occlusive disease (80–90% of patients) or fibromuscular dysplasia (10–15%).
- Hypertension, may be resistant or refractory.
- AKI may occur in patients with bilateral stenosis when ACE inhibitor or ARB therapy is initiated.

General Considerations

Renal artery stenosis is a relatively common cause of secondary hypertension and can lead to CKD and ESKD. Atherosclerotic disease is the usual cause, hence renal artery stenosis typically occurs in older individuals with other cardiovascular risk factors such as diabetes mellitus, hyperlipidemia, tobacco use, or disease in other vessels. Fibromuscular dysplasia, a less common cause of renal artery stenosis, usually occurs in young women.

Clinical Findings

A. Symptoms and Signs

Patients with atherosclerotic renovascular disease may have refractory hypertension, new-onset hypertension, acute pulmonary edema with poorly controlled blood pressure, and/or AKI upon starting an ACE inhibitor or ARB. Physical examination may reveal an audible abdominal bruit on the affected side. Unexplained hypertension in a woman younger than 40 years should raise suspicion for fibromuscular dysplasia.

B. Laboratory Findings

Serum creatinine may be elevated if there is significant renal ischemia. Patients with bilateral renal artery stenosis may have hypokalemia, a finding that reflects activation of the renin-angiotensin-aldosterone system in response to reduced blood flow (a "prerenal" state). Plasma renin concentration/activity is elevated.

C. Imaging

Abdominal ultrasound may reveal asymmetric kidney size (> 1.5 cm difference) if one renal artery is primarily affected, or small hyperechoic kidneys if both are affected.

Screening with Doppler ultrasonography, CT angiography, or magnetic resonance angiography (MRA) is recommended if a corrective procedure would be performed when a positive test result is found. **Doppler ultrasonography** of the renal arteries can be both sensitive and specific but is extremely operator- and patient habitus–dependent.

CT angiography consists of intravenous contrast injection with digital subtraction arteriography and offers good sensitivity and specificity.

MRA is an excellent but expensive way to screen for renal artery stenosis, particularly in those with atherosclerotic disease. The newer-generation gadolinium contrast agents seem to carry little to no risk for nephrogenic systemic fibrosis in those with advanced CKD or ESRD.

Renal angiography is the gold standard for diagnosis but is invasive, requiring femoral artery catheterization. Thus, it is usually performed after a positive screening test in order to confirm the anatomy and to provide interventions when high grade, hemodynamically significant stenotic lesions are identified. There is risk of atheroembolic phenomena after angiography. Fibromuscular dysplasia has a characteristic "beads-on-a-string" appearance on angiography.

Treatment

Treatment of atherosclerotic renovascular disease is controversial. Options include medical management and angioplasty with stenting. Two large randomized trials showed that mechanical intervention is no better than optimal medical management (including ACE inhibitor or ARB and lipid control) in most patients. Risks of stenting include atheroemboli to the ipsilateral kidney and renal artery dissection. Stenting often is not the hoped-for 'panacea' due to its inability to address underlying small vessel disease and renal scarring, which are often present at the time of diagnosis. Angioplasty and stenting nonetheless should be considered for those with high-grade stenosis (> 70%) and any of the following: acute ("flash") pulmonary edema or recurrent episodes of volume overload, refractory HTN, ACE or ARB intolerance, increased rate of eGFR decline, or stenosis in a transplanted kidney artery.

Treatment of fibromuscular dysplasia with percutaneous transluminal angioplasty is often curative.

Matam MB et al. A literature review of renal artery stenosis: presentation, diagnosis, and management options in secondary hypertension. Cureus. 2025;17:e92945. [PMID: 41133069]

Shao C et al. Impact of renal artery stenosis on renovascular hypertension and the therapeutic role of renal artery stenting: a comprehensive review. Kidney Blood Press Res. 2025 Mar 10. [Epub ahead of print] [PMID: 40064159]

GLOMERULAR DISEASES

The glomerulus is a histologically complex structure consisting of the epithelial cells (podocytes), basement membrane, capillary endothelium, and mesangium. A variety of different insults can occur within these structures causing different patterns of injury. Examples of injuries that can affect any or all of the constituents of the glomerulus are (1) overwork injury, as in CKD or obesity; (2) an inflammatory process, such as SLE; (3) a podocyte protein mutation, as in hereditary focal segmental glomerulosclerosis (FSGS); or (4) a deposition disease, as in diabetes or amyloidosis. Different glomerular patterns of injury tend to cause different clinical syndromes or findings, which may help narrow the differential diagnosis, but a kidney biopsy is often needed to confirm the diagnosis.

Classification

Glomerular diseases are clinically classified as either nephritic or nephrotic (Figure 25–4). These are distinguished by the amount of proteinuria, as well as the presence (nephritic) or absence (nephrotic) of significant glomerular hematuria. Differentiation is important because it helps narrow the differential diagnosis of the underlying glomerular disease and guide further serologic evaluation prior to possible kidney biopsy (Tables 25–8 and 25–9).

Nephritic diseases are characterized by proteinuria < 3.5 g/day and glomerular hematuria. At the "least severe" end of the nephritic spectrum, asymptomatic glomerular hematuria (ie, dysmorphic RBCs) with or without subnephrotic proteinuria is characteristic. The mid-portion of the spectrum is the nephritic *syndrome*, where additional features accompany hematuria and proteinuria, such as edema, hypertension, and impaired kidney function (decreased GFR). The "most severe" and clinically urgent end of the spectrum are the rapidly progressive glomerulonephritides (RPGNs).

Nephrotic spectrum diseases demonstrate greater proteinuria with a typically bland urine sediment (no cells or cellular casts). The relatively rare nephrotic *syndrome* is the most severe end of the spectrum, encompassing heavy proteinuria (> 3.5 g/day) in addition to hypoalbuminemia, edema, and hyperlipidemia.

Glomerular diseases can also be classified according to whether they cause renal abnormalities alone (primary renal disease) or represent manifestations of a systemic disease (secondary renal disease), such as diabetes.

Anders HJ et al. Glomerulonephritis: immunopathogenesis and immunotherapy. Nat Rev Immunol. 2023;23:453. [PMID: 36635359]

NEPHRITIC SPECTRUM GLOMERULAR DISEASES

ESSENTIALS OF DIAGNOSIS

- **Mild cases: asymptomatic glomerular hematuria**
  - Hematuria with dysmorphic RBCs
  - Proteinuria typically < 1 g/day
- **More severe cases: nephritic syndrome**
  - Glomerular hematuria (and RBC casts if glomerular bleeding is heavy)
  - Proteinuria typically 1–3.5 g/day
  - Hypertension
  - Edema
  - Worsening kidney function (rising creatinine) over days to months
- **Most severe cases: rapidly progressive glomerulonephritis (RPGN)**
  - AKI with rising creatinine over days to months
  - Glomerular hematuria and RBC casts
  - Proteinuria typically 1–3.5 g/day

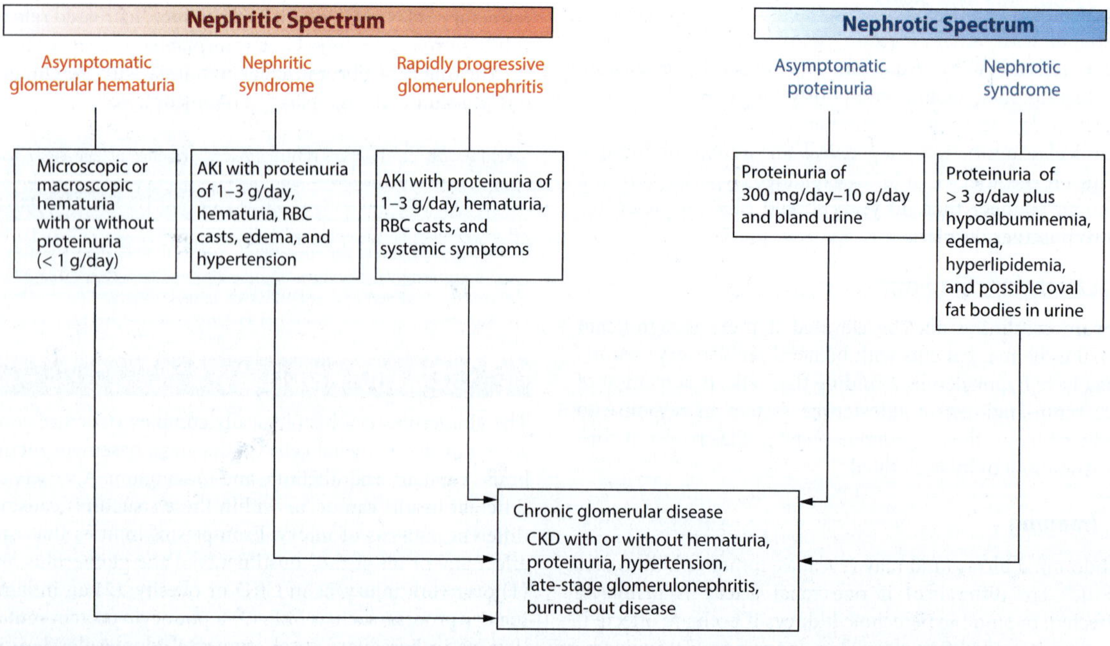

Figure 25–4. Glomerular diseases present within one of the clinical spectra shown; the exact presentation is determined by the severity of the underlying disease and the pattern of injury. Nephritic diseases are characterized by the presence of an active urine sediment with glomerular hematuria and often with proteinuria. Nephrotic spectrum diseases are proteinuric with bland urine sediments (no cells or cellular casts). All glomerular diseases may progress to a chronic, scarred state. (Reproduced, with permission, from Megan Troxell, MD, PhD.)

Table 25–8. Nephritic spectrum glomerular diseases.

	Typical Presentation	Association/Notes	Serology
Postinfectious or infection-related glomerulonephritis	Children: abrupt onset of nephritic syndrome and AKI but can present anywhere in nephritic spectrum	Streptococci, other bacterial infections (eg, staphylococci, endocarditis, shunt infections)	Rising ASO titers, low complement levels, blood cultures
IgA nephropathy (Berger disease) and Henoch-Schönlein purpura, systemic IgA vasculitis	Classically: gross hematuria with respiratory tract infection, but can present anywhere in nephritic spectrum; Henoch-Schönlein purpura with vasculitic rash and GI hemorrhage	Abnormal IgA glycosylation in both primary (familial predisposition) and secondary disease (associated with cirrhosis, HIV, celiac disease) Henoch-Schönlein purpura in children after an inciting infection	No serologic tests helpful; complement levels are normal
Cryoglobulin-associated glomerulonephritis	Often acute nephritic syndrome; often with systemic vasculitis including rash and arthritis	Most commonly associated with chronic hepatitis C; may occur with other chronic infections or some connective tissue diseases	Cryoglobulins positive; rheumatoid factor may be elevated; complement levels low
Lupus nephritis	Anywhere in nephritic spectrum, depending on pattern/severity of injury	Treatment depends on clinical course and International Society of Nephrology and Renal Pathology Society classification on biopsy	High ANA and anti-double-stranded DNA titers; low complement levels
Pauci-immune (granulomatosis with polyangiitis, eosinophilic granulomatosis with polyangiitis, polyarteritis)	Classically: crescentic or RPGN, but can present anywhere in nephritic spectrum; may have respiratory tract/sinus symptoms in granulomatosis with polyangiitis	May be related to environmental exposures including infection	ANCAs: MPO or PR3 titers high; complement levels normal
Anti-GBM glomerulonephritis; Goodpasture syndrome	Classically: crescentic or RPGN, but can present anywhere in nephritic spectrum; pulmonary hemorrhage in Goodpasture syndrome	May develop as a result of respiratory irritant exposure (chemicals or tobacco use)	Anti-GBM antibody titers high; complement levels normal
C3 glomerulopathies (and idiopathic immune-complex MPGN)	Classically: acute nephritic syndrome, but can also have nephrotic syndrome	Most patients are < 30 years old; dysregulation of alternative complement pathway resulting in overactivation	Low complement levels, may have findings of underlying infection or paraproteinemia
Monoclonal immunoglobulin glomerulonephritis (monoclonal gammopathy of renal significance)	Anywhere in nephritic spectrum	Can cause different patterns of renal injury	SPEP with monoclonal protein; serum light chain ratio > 3

ANCAs, antineutrophil cytoplasmic antibodies; ASO, antistreptolysin O; GBM, glomerular basement membrane; MPGN, membranoproliferative glomerulonephritis; MPO, myeloperoxidase; PR3, proteinase 3; RPGN, rapidly progressive glomerulonephritis.

General Considerations

"Glomerulonephritis" is a term given to nephritic diseases and usually signifies an inflammatory process causing kidney dysfunction. Glomerulonephritis is further classified according to one of five pathogenic subtypes: immune-complex (eg, lupus nephritis), pauci-immune, anti-GBM, C3 glomerulopathy, or monoclonal immunoglobulin–mediated. Presentation may be acute (developing over days to weeks), with or without resolution, or may be chronic and indolent with progressive scarring. As noted above, nephritic diseases may present with glomerular hematuria and proteinuria, with nephritic syndrome, or with RPGN.

Clinical Findings

A. Symptoms and Signs

Nephritic syndrome usually presents with an acute decrease in GFR. The resultant sodium retention can lead to hypertension and edema, which is first seen in regions of low tissue pressure such as the periorbital and scrotal areas. Rarely, heavy bleeding from glomerular inflammation may result in gross hematuria ("cola-colored urine").

B. Laboratory Findings

1. Serologic testing—Serologic tests (selected based on the history and physical examination) help narrow the

Table 25–9. Classification and findings in glomerulonephritis: nephrotic spectrum presentations.

Disease	Typical Presentation	Association/Notes
Minimal change disease	Child with sudden onset of nephrotic syndrome	Children: associated with allergy or viral infection Adults: associated with Hodgkin disease, NSAIDs, bee stings
Focal and segmental glomerulosclerosis	Anywhere in nephrotic spectrum; children with congenital disease have nephrotic syndrome	Children: congenital disease with podocyte gene mutation, or in spectrum of disease with minimal change disease Adults: associated with heroin use, HIV infection, reflux nephropathy, obesity, pamidronate, podocyte protein mutations, *APOL1* mutations
Membranous nephropathy	Anywhere in nephrotic spectrum, but nephrotic syndrome not uncommon; particular predisposition to hypercoagulable state	Serologic PLA_2R Ab positivity strongly suggestive of primary MN (may eliminate need for renal biopsy) Secondary may be associated with non-Hodgkin lymphoma, carcinoma (GI, renal, bronchogenic, thyroid), gold therapy, penicillamine, SLE, chronic hepatitis B or C infection
Diabetic kidney disease	High GFR (hyperfiltration) → microalbuminuria → frank proteinuria → decline in GFR	Diabetes diagnosis precedes diagnosis of nephropathy by years
HIV-associated nephropathy	Heavy proteinuria, often nephrotic syndrome, progresses to ESKD relatively quickly	Usually seen in antiviral treatment-naïve patients (rare in antiretroviral therapy era), and in those with 2 *APOL1* risk alleles
Amyloidosis	Usually nephrotic syndrome; may have signs of amyloid deposition in other organs	AL: plasma cell dyscrasia with Ig light chain overproduction and deposition; check SPEP/UPEP, serum light chains AA: serum amyloid protein A overproduction and deposition in response to chronic inflammatory disease (rheumatoid arthritis, IBD, chronic infection)

PLA_2R, phospholipase A_2 receptor; SPEP/UPEP, serum and urine protein electrophoresis.

differential diagnosis. These include C3 and C4 complement levels, ANA, cryoglobulins, hepatitis serologies, serum/urine protein electrophoreses and immunofixation, serum free light chains, ANCAs, anti-GBM antibodies, and anti-pathogen antibodies (eg, antistreptolysin O titers) (Table 25–8).

2. UA—The urine dipstick is positive for protein and blood. Urinary microscopy reveals RBCs that are dysmorphic from traversing a damaged glomerular basement membrane. RBC casts are seen with heavy glomerular bleeding and tubular stasis. When quantified, proteinuria is usually subnephrotic range (< 3.5 g/day).

3. Biopsy—Definitive diagnosis of the underlying glomerular disease cannot be made without a kidney biopsy. Candidates for biopsy are patients for whom test results would influence management or inform prognosis; exceptions include those with advanced underlying CKD, those who cannot adhere to medical therapy, those for whom immunosuppressive therapy is not appropriate, or those for whom the clinical presentation is "classic" for a particular disease (eg, poststreptococcal glomerulonephritis). The major risk of biopsy is bleeding. Contraindications include a bleeding diathesis, thrombocytopenia, and uncontrolled hypertension.

Treatment

General measures include treatment of hypertension and fluid overload, if present. Antiproteinuric therapy with an ACE inhibitor or ARB should be considered for those without AKI. For those with profound AKI, dialysis may be needed. The inflammatory glomerular injury may require immunosuppressive agents (see specific diseases discussed below).

When to Refer

Any patient in whom glomerulonephritis is suspected should be immediately referred to a nephrologist.

When to Admit

Any suspicion for acute nephritic syndrome or RPGN warrants consideration of immediate hospitalization.

Romagnani P et al. The five types of glomerulonephritis classified by pathogenesis, activity and chronicity (GN-AC). Nephrol Dial Transplant. 2023;38:ii3. [PMID: 37218714]

Rovin BH et al. Executive summary of the KDIGO 2021 guideline for the management of glomerular diseases. Kidney Int. 2021;100:753. [PMID: 34556300]

1. Immune Complex Glomerulonephritis: Infection-Related & Postinfectious Glomerulonephritis

ESSENTIALS OF DIAGNOSIS

- Proteinuria.
- Glomerular hematuria.
- Symptoms occur during course of some infections (eg, pneumonia, endocarditis) or 1–3 weeks after some infections (often pharyngitis or impetigo).

General Considerations

Infection-related glomerulonephritis (IRGN) is characterized by glomerular injury during active or recent infection. Although more common in the setting of staphylococcal infections (eg, bloodstream infections, abscesses, endocarditis), IRGN can occur in a variety of infections including viral, fungal, and parasitic causes of glomerulonephritis; these include hepatitis B or C, HIV, cytomegalovirus infection, infectious mononucleosis, coccidioidomycosis, malaria, mycobacteria, syphilis, and toxoplasmosis. Post-infectious glomerulonephritis specifically refers to those cases that arise due to infection with nephritogenic group A β-hemolytic streptococcal infections (pharyngitis or impetigo), and 1–3 weeks after infection (average 7–10 days).

Clinical Findings

A. Symptoms and Signs

Disease presentation varies across the nephritic spectrum from asymptomatic glomerular hematuria with preserved kidney function, to nephritic syndrome with hypertension, edema, and gross glomerular hematuria ("cola-colored urine"); the most severe cases may result in oliguric AKI requiring dialysis.

B. Laboratory Findings

Serum C3 and C4 are low, with C3 levels classically being "disproportionately" lower than C4. In postinfectious glomerulonephritis due to group A streptococcal infection, anti-streptolysin O (ASO) titers may be high. Glomerular hematuria and proteinuria are present. In children with recent streptococcal infection and nephritic features, a diagnosis may be made empirically without a biopsy. When performed, kidney biopsy shows a diffuse proliferative pattern of injury on light microscopy with neutrophils present. Immunofluorescence demonstrates granular deposition of IgG and C3 in the mesangium and along the capillary basement membrane. Electron microscopy shows large, dense subepithelial deposits or "humps". Kidney biopsy findings in IRGN are similar, though some may demonstrate IgA deposition rather than IgG, and others may appear similar to C3 glomerulopathy.

Treatment

Any active infection should be identified and treated appropriately; otherwise, treatment for IRGN is supportive. Although steroids are sometimes considered, evidence does not support their use. Antihypertensives, salt restriction, and diuretics should be used if needed. Prognosis depends on the severity of the glomerular injury and age of the patient. Children are more likely to fully recover; adults are more prone to the development of severe disease (RPGN with crescent formation) and CKD.

Bonner RW et al. Infection-associated glomerulonephritis. Adv Kidney Dis Health. 2024;31:246. [PMID: 39004464]
Dhakal A et al. Acute post-streptococcal glomerulonephritis in children-treatment standard. Nephrol Dial Transplant. 2025;40:1843. [PMID: 40650562]
Sayad R et al. Immunosuppressant use in infective endocarditis-associated glomerulonephritis: a systematic review. Clin Drug Investig. 2025;45:443. [PMID: 40682760]
Wada Y et al. Clinico-pathogenic similarities and differences between infection-related glomerulonephritis and C3 glomerulopathy. Int J Mol Sci. 2023;24:8432. [PMID: 37176142]

2. Immune-Complex Glomerulonephritis: IgA Nephropathy

ESSENTIALS OF DIAGNOSIS

- Proteinuria: minimal to nephrotic-range.
- Glomerular hematuria: microscopic is common; macroscopic (gross) can occur after infection.
- Positive IgA staining on kidney biopsy.

General Considerations

IgA nephropathy results from glomerular mesangial deposition of immune complexes made up of aberrantly glycosylated IgA (a heritable condition) and IgG autoantibodies against these abnormal molecules. IgA nephropathy can be a primary (renal-limited) disease or secondary to cirrhosis, celiac disease, and infections such as HIV and cytomegalovirus. IgA nephropathy is the most common primary glomerular disease worldwide, particularly in Asia. It is most often seen in children and young adults and affects males two to three times more commonly than females.

Clinical Findings

The classic presentation of IgA nephropathy is an episode of gross hematuria associated with a mucosal viral infection, often of the upper respiratory tract 1–2 days after illness onset (in contrast to the longer latent period seen in post-infectious glomerulonephritis). IgA nephropathy can present anywhere along the nephritic spectrum from asymptomatic microscopic hematuria with minimal proteinuria and preserved eGFR to RPGN (see Figure 25–4). Rarely, nephrotic syndrome can also develop.

There are no serologic tests that aid in this diagnosis; serum complements are normal. The typical pattern of injury seen on kidney biopsy is a focal glomerulonephritis with mesangial proliferation; immunofluorescence demonstrates diffuse mesangial IgA and C3 deposits.

Treatment

Treatment recommendations for IgA nephropathy are changing rapidly, and many new therapies have emerged. In general, patients at lowest risk for progression (no hypertension, normal GFR, minimal proteinuria) can be monitored expectantly. Patients at higher risk (proteinuria > 1.0 g/day, decreased GFR, hypertension, or any combination of these three conditions) should be treated with an ACE inhibitor or ARB. Therapy should be titrated to reduce proteinuria to < 0.5 g/day and to control blood pressure to 120/80 mm Hg. SGLT-2 inhibitors are standard care in proteinuric patients. Sparsentan, a dual-acting endothelin and angiotensin II antagonist, is superior to ACE inhibitors or ARBs for proteinuria reduction, but its use may be limited by high cost.

Immunosuppressive therapy is considered for patients at the highest risk, defined as persistent proteinuria > 1.0 g/day despite 90 days of optimized antiproteinuric therapy. Guidelines recommend consideration of systemic corticosteroids to reduce proteinuria reduction and slow progression, but their use must be weighed against risk of adverse effects, including infection. By targeting intestinal mucosal immunogenicity, enteric-coated budesonide therapy reduces proteinuria with fewer adverse effects compared with systemic corticosteroids and can be considered. Additionally, iptacopan, which inhibits factor B in the alternative pathway of complement, has been shown to reduce proteinuria without increasing risk of infection. Small studies support the consideration of mycophenolate mofetil. For the rare patient with IgA nephropathy and a rapidly progressive clinical course with diffuse crescent formation on biopsy, cyclophosphamide and corticosteroid therapy should be considered (see section on ANCA-associated vasculitis below). Kidney transplantation is an excellent option for patients with ESKD, but recurrent disease develops in 30% of patients 5–10 years posttransplant.

Prognosis

Patients with IgA nephropathy are at risk for progression to ESKD, particularly when presenting with proteinuria of > 0.5 g/day, lower GFR, and/or biopsy finding of tubulointerstitial fibrosis and glomerulosclerosis.

Cheung CK et al. The pathogenesis of IgA nephropathy and implications for treatment. Nat Rev Nephrol. 2025;21:9. [PMID: 39232245]

Floege J et al. Executive summary of the KDIGO 2025 Clinical Practice Guideline for the management of immunoglobulin A nephropathy (IgAN) and immunoglobulin A vasculitis (IgAV). Kidney Int. 2025;108:548. [PMID: 40975525]

Lafayette R et al. Efficacy and safety of a targeted-release formulation of budesonide in patients with primary IgA nephropathy (NefIgArd): 2-year results from a randomised phase 3 trial. Lancet. 2023;402:859. [PMID: 37591292]

Perkovic V et al. Alternative complement pathway inhibition with iptacopan in IgA nephropathy. N Engl J Med. 2025;392:531. [PMID: 39453772]

Rovin BH et al. Efficacy and safety of sparsentan versus irbesartan in patients with IgA nephropathy (PROTECT): 2-year results from a randomised, active-controlled, phase 3 trial. Lancet. 2023;402:2077. [PMID: 37931634]

3. Immune-Complex Glomerulonephritis: IgA Vasculitis (Henoch-Schönlein Purpura)

IgA vasculitis, or Henoch-Schönlein purpura, is a systemic small-vessel leukocytoclastic vasculitis associated with IgA subclass 1 deposition in vessel walls. It is most common in children and is often associated with an inciting infection or medication exposure. It classically presents with palpable purpura in the lower extremities and buttocks, arthralgias, abdominal symptoms (nausea, colic, and melena), and AKI with nephritic urine sediment. The renal pattern of injury is the same as IgA nephropathy. Most patients with microscopic hematuria and minimal proteinuria recover fully over several weeks. Progressive CKD is more likely to develop in adults and in those with both nephritic and nephrotic syndromes. Although several treatment regimens of various immunosuppressive agents have been clinically tested, none is proven to alter the course of severe nephritis. Rituximab treatment and plasma exchange have been successful for severe disease according to several case reports, but clinical trials are lacking. Rapidly progressive disease with crescent formation on biopsy should be treated as in ANCA-associated vasculitis (see section below). Further details about IgA vasculitis are provided in Chapter 23.

Hahn D et al. Interventions for preventing and treating kidney disease in IgA vasculitis. Cochrane Database Syst Rev. 2023;2:CD005128. [PMID: 36853224]

Vivarelli M et al. IPNA clinical practice recommendations for the diagnosis and management of children with IgA nephropathy and IgA vasculitis nephritis. Pediatr Nephrol. 2025;40:533. [PMID: 39331079]

Zhang Y et al. IgA vasculitis with nephritis: an overview of the pathogenesis and clinical characteristics. Clin Exp Rheumatol. 2025;43:728. [PMID: 39436720]

4. Immune-Complex Glomerulonephritis: Cryoglobulin-Associated Glomerulonephritis

Systemic vasculitis due to cryoglobulinemia (cold-precipitable immunoglobulins) can cause glomerular disease. The majority of cases are caused by HCV infection. Immune complexes of rheumatoid factor, HCV antigen, and polyclonal anti-HCV IgG deposit in vessels and incite inflammation. Additional causes of polyclonal cryoglobulinemic vasculitis include other overt or occult infections (eg, viral, bacterial, and fungal) and autoimmune diseases (eg, Sjögren syndrome). Disease without an identifiable cause is termed "essential" cryoglobulin-associated glomerulonephritis.

Patients exhibit purpuric and necrotizing skin lesions in dependent areas, arthralgias, fever, and hepatosplenomegaly. Serum complement levels (particularly C4) are low, and rheumatoid factor is often elevated. Kidney biopsy may show different patterns of injury: crescent formation, glomerular capillary thrombi, or a membranoproliferative pattern of injury ("MPGN"). Treatment consists of aggressively targeting the cause, if known. Viral eradication with direct-acting antiviral agents is the cornerstone of treatment of HCV-associated cryoglobulinemic glomerulonephritis (see Chapter 18). Therapy with rituximab and possibly corticosteroids and plasmapheresis should be initiated in patients with severe vasculitis prior to the initiation of antiviral therapy.

Moretti M et al. Cryoglobulinemic vasculitis: a 2023 update. Curr Opin Rheumatol. 2024;36:27. [PMID: 37916482]
Quartuccio L et al. Management of mixed cryoglobulinemia with rituximab: evidence and consensus-based recommendations from the Italian Study Group of Cryoglobulinemia (GISC). Clin Rheumatol. 2023;42:359. [PMID: 36169798]
Sohal A et al. Renal manifestations of chronic hepatitis C: a review. J Clin Med. 2024;13:5536. [PMID: 39337023]
Villa A et al. Renal involvement in mixed cryoglobulinemic vasculitis: current perspectives. J Clin Med. 2025;14:4369. [PMID: 40566113]

5. Immune-Complex Glomerulonephritis: Lupus Nephritis

Lupus nephritis occurs in 35–90% of patients who have SLE, with higher estimates encompassing subclinical disease. Rates of lupus nephritis are highest in non-White patients. The pathogenesis is complex and in part due to autoantibody response to exposed nuclear antigens, ultimately resulting in immune-complex glomerulonephritis. See Chapter 23 for further discussion of SLE.

The term "lupus nephritis" encompasses many patterns of injury; however, most present within the nephritic spectrum (eg, class IV). Non-glomerular syndromes include tubulointerstitial nephritis and vasculitis. All patients with SLE should have routine UAs to monitor for hematuria or proteinuria. If urinary abnormalities are detected, kidney biopsy is often recommended. The International Society of Nephrology and Renal Pathology Society classification of renal glomerular lesions is class I, minimal mesangial nephritis; class II, mesangial proliferative nephritis; class III, focal (< 50% of glomeruli affected with capillary involvement) proliferative nephritis; class IV, diffuse (> 50% of glomeruli affected with capillary involvement) proliferative nephritis; class V, membranous nephropathy (discussed below); and class VI, advanced sclerosis without residual disease activity. Classes III and IV, the most severe forms of lupus nephritis, are further classified as active or chronic, and global or segmental, which confers additional prognostic value.

Treatment

Individuals with **class I** and **class II lesions** generally require antiproteinuric therapy with ACE inhibitors or ARBs. Hydroxychloroquine is recommended in all patients with lupus nephritis, regardless of histological class. Transformation into a more active lesion may occur and is usually accompanied by an increase in lupus serologic activity (eg, rising titers of anti–double-stranded DNA antibodies, and falling C3 and C4 levels) and increasing proteinuria or falling GFR. Repeat biopsy in such patients is recommended.

Patients with active **class III** and **IV lesions** should receive prompt, aggressive immunosuppression. Poor prognostic indicators include elevated serum creatinine, lower complement levels, male sex, presence of antiphospholipid antibodies, nephrotic-range proteinuria, sub-Saharan African descent (unclear association with *APOL1* risk alleles), and poor response to therapy. Immunosuppression for class V lupus nephritis is indicated if superimposed proliferative lesions exist, or if nephrotic syndrome is present. Class VI lesions represent irreversible patterns of injury and do not respond to treatment.

Treatment of class III or IV lupus nephritis consists of approximately 6 months of induction therapy, followed by maintenance therapy. For induction therapy, revised 2024 practice guidelines call for a combination of corticosteroids in combination with one of the following: (1) mycophenolate mofetil; (2) intravenous cyclophosphamide; (3) belimumab (anti-B cell therapy) with either mycophenolate or cyclophosphamide; or (4) mycophenolate mofetil with a calcineurin inhibitor. The decision on which approach to take is based on severity of clinical presentation and patient factors; three-drug regimens are typically considered for more severe presentations. Induction is followed by maintenance therapy with daily oral mycophenolate mofetil (preferred) or azathioprine for at least 3 years. With standard therapy, remission rates with induction vary from 80% for partial remission to 50–60% for full remission. Relapse is common and higher in those who do not experience complete remission. Progression to ESKD is more common in those who relapse more frequently or fail to achieve remission. Some patients may respond to newer steroid-sparing regimens of obinutuzumab in combination with mycophenolate mofetil. Pure class V disease can be treated similarly to classes III/IV, though calcineurin inhibitors appear especially effective.

The levels of various disease activity markers (double-stranded DNA antibodies, serum C3, C4 levels), proteinuria, and sediment activity can be useful in monitoring response to treatment, though repeat renal biopsy yields more reliable information regarding disease activity and may be used to guide maintenance therapy withdrawal. Patients with SLE who undergo dialysis have a favorable prospect for long-term survival; SLE symptoms often become quiescent with the development of ESKD. Patients with SLE undergoing kidney transplants can have recurrent renal disease, although relapse rates are relatively low.

Furie R et al. Efficacy and safety of obinutuzumab in active lupus nephritis. N Engl J Med. 2025;392:1471. [PMID: 39927615]
Hoi A et al. System lupus erythematosus. Lancet. 2024;403:2326. [PMID: 38642569]
Kidney Disease: Improving Global Outcomes (KDIGO) Lupus Nephritis Work Group. KDIGO 2024 Clinical Practice Guideline for the management of lupus nephritis. Kidney Int. 2024;105:S1. [PMID: 38182286]
Parodis I et al. Lupus nephritis. Nat Rev Dis Primers. 2025;11:69. [PMID: 40998820]

6. Pauci-Immune Glomerulonephritis (ANCA-Associated)

Pauci-immune necrotizing glomerulonephritis is caused by the following ANCA-associated vasculitides (AAVs): granulomatosis with polyangiitis, microscopic polyangiitis, and eosinophilic granulomatosis with polyangiitis (see Chapter 23). ANCA-associated glomerulonephritis can also present as a kidney-limited disease without systemic vasculitis. The pathogenesis of these entities appears to involve cytokine-primed neutrophils that present cytoplasmic antigens—proteinase-3 or myeloperoxidase—on their surfaces. Circulating ANCAs bind to these antigens and activate neutrophils with consequent vascular damage; primed neutrophils also appear to activate the alternative complement pathway. Immunofluorescence of kidney biopsy specimens demonstrates lack of or scant immunoglobulin/complement deposition, hence the term "pauci-immune." Renal involvement classically presents as RPGN, but more indolent presentations can be seen. Most cases of AAV are idiopathic, but others may be linked to an infection (including COVID-19), environmental exposure (eg, silica), or drug exposure (eg, levamisole).

Clinical Findings

A. Symptoms and Signs

Symptoms of a systemic inflammatory disease, including fever, malaise, and weight loss, may be present, sometimes for months prior to diagnosis. In addition to the glomerular inflammatory signs of hematuria and proteinuria, vasculitic involvement of dermal capillaries and nerve arterioles may result in purpura and mononeuritis multiplex, respectively. Ninety percent of patients with granulomatosis with polyangiitis have upper (especially sinus) or lower respiratory tract symptoms with nodular lesions that can cavitate and bleed. Hemoptysis is suggestive of alveolar hemorrhage and usually warrants hospitalization and aggressive immunosuppression.

B. Laboratory Findings

Serologically, ANCA subtype analysis is done to determine whether antiproteinase-3 antibodies (PR3-ANCA) or anti-myeloperoxidase antibodies (MPO-ANCA) are present. Most patients with granulomatosis with polyangiitis are PR3 positive, whereas microscopic polyangiitis is generally associated with MPO-ANCA. Renal biopsy reveals necrotizing lesions and crescents on light microscopy; immunofluorescence is negative for immune-complex deposition.

Treatment

Prompt initiation of treatment is essential. A 3–6-month induction therapy course with corticosteroids and cyclophosphamide or rituximab is followed by long-term rituximab (preferred) or azathioprine. The oral complement inhibitor avacopan can be considered in place of corticosteroids during induction. The role of plasma exchange in ANCA vasculitis is controversial; it may be considered in cases of diffuse alveolar hemorrhage with hypoxemia or severe kidney disease (creatinine > 3.4 mg/dL [> 300 mcmol/L]), and it is standard of care if anti-GBM antibodies are also present (see below).

Prognosis

Without treatment, prognosis is extremely poor. With aggressive treatment, complete remission can be achieved in the majority of patients. Prognosis depends on the extent of renal involvement before treatment is started. ANCA titers may be monitored to follow treatment efficacy, though they are only modestly predictive of future disease relapse and should be interpreted in the context of additional clinical data including the urine sediment.

Chevet B et al. Diagnosing and treating ANCA-associated vasculitis: an updated review for clinical practice. Rheumatology. 2023;62:1787. [PMID: 26315063]

Floege J et al. Executive summary of the KDIGO 2024 Clinical Practice Guideline for the Management of ANCA-Associated Vasculitis. Kidney Int. 2024;105:447. [PMID: 38388147]

Odler B et al. The effects of plasma exchange and glucocorticoids on early kidney function among patients with ANCA-associated vasculitis in the PEXIVAS trial. Kidney Int. 2025;107:558. [PMID: 39708998]

7. Anti-Glomerular Basement Membrane Glomerulonephritis & Goodpasture Syndrome

Autoantibodies to epitopes of the GBM cause glomerulonephritis (anti-GBM disease); concomitant immune attack on alveolar basement membranes results in pulmonary hemorrhage as well (Goodpasture syndrome). Anti-GBM–associated glomerulonephritis accounts for 10–20% of patients with acute RPGN. The incidence has a bimodal distribution, peaking in the third decade of life during which time men are predominantly affected and lung involvement is more common, and again in the sixth and seventh decades with less gender specificity and pulmonary involvement. Goodpasture syndrome is associated with pulmonary infection, tobacco use, and exposure to hydrocarbon solvents or alemtuzumab; HLA-DR2 and -B7 antigens may predispose as well.

Clinical Findings

A. Symptoms and Signs

The onset of disease may be preceded by an upper respiratory tract infection; hemoptysis, dyspnea, and respiratory failure may ensue. Kidney laboratory findings are almost always consistent with RPGN, although cases may rarely present more mildly (eg, glomerular hematuria and proteinuria with minimal kidney dysfunction).

B. Diagnostic Findings

Imaging may demonstrate pulmonary infiltrates if pulmonary hemorrhage is present. Serum complement levels are normal. Circulating anti-GBM antibodies are present in over 90% of patients. A small percentage of patients have elevated ANCA titers. Kidney biopsy typically shows crescent formation with light microscopy, with linear IgG staining along the GBM on immunofluorescence.

Treatment

Patients with pulmonary hemorrhage and strong clinical suspicion of Goodpasture syndrome should be treated emergently—often prior to confirming the diagnosis with serology and kidney biopsy. Treatment is a combination of therapeutic plasma exchange daily for up to 2 weeks to remove circulating antibodies, and administration of corticosteroids and cyclophosphamide to prevent formation of new antibodies and control the inflammatory response. Rituximab has been used in a small number of patients with refractory disease. Patients with oliguric AKI or who require dialysis upon presentation have a poor prognosis. Anti-GBM antibody titers should decrease as the clinical course improves.

Bharati J et al. Anti-glomerular basement membrane disease: recent updates. Adv Kidney Dis Health. 2024;31:206. [PMID: 39004460]
Kuang H et al. Epidemiology, clinical features, risk factors, and outcomes in anti-glomerular basement membrane disease: a systematic review and meta-analysis. Autoimmun Rev. 2024;23:103531. [PMID: 38493958]
McAdoo S et al. Anti-glomerular basement membrane disease–treatment standard. Nephrol Dial Transplant. 2025;41:42. [PMID: 40973182]
Ponticelli C et al. Anti-glomerular basement membrane vasculitis. Autoimmun Rev. 2023;22:103212. [PMID: 36252931]

8. C3 Glomerulopathies

C3 glomerulopathy is caused by several inherited or acquired abnormalities in the alternative complement pathway; this diagnosis encompasses two disease expressions/patterns of injury—C3 glomerulonephritis and dense deposit disease. Both frequently result in low circulating C3 levels. Renal biopsy of C3 glomerulonephritis shows varying degrees of mesangial hypercellularity, endocapillary proliferation and capillary wall remodeling resulting in double contours of the GBM ("tram track" appearance) that are characterized as a membranoproliferative pattern of injury (MPGN). While other glomerulonephritides can also display an MPGN pattern of injury on light microscopy, the defining histopathologic characteristic in C3 glomerulonephritis is a lack or paucity of immunoglobulin staining on immunofluorescence. The rare variant of dense deposit disease is characterized by thick ribbon-like deposits on electron microscopy. Evaluation for viral infection, cancer screening, and genetic testing are standard diagnostic tests for C3 glomerulopathy.

Treatment of C3 glomerulopathies is evolving as novel therapies targeting the dysregulated alternative complement cascade are explored. Iptacopan leads to a clinically meaningful reduction in proteinuria. Small, uncontrolled series suggest a benefit of eculizumab in some patients; others may respond to mycophenolate mofetil. Risk of ESKD is relatively high. Less favorable prognostic findings include dense deposit disease, early decline in GFR, hypertension, and persistent disease. C3 glomerulopathy recurs with high frequency after kidney transplantation.

Dixit S et al. C3 glomerulopathy: advancements in diagnostics and therapeutics. Curr Opin Nephrol Hypertens. 2026;35:52. [PMID: 41208293]
Kavanagh D et al. Oral iptacopan therapy in patients with C3 glomerulopathy: a randomized, double-blind, parallel group, multicentre, placebo-controlled phase 3 study. Lancet. 2025;406:1587. [PMID: 41016405]
Vivarelli M et al. The role of complement in kidney disease: conclusions from a Kidney Disease: Improving Global Outcomes (KDIGO) Controversies Conference. Kidney Int. 2024;106:369. [PMID: 38844295]
Wooden B et al. Update on C3 glomerulopathy. Adv Kidney Dis Health. 2024;31:223. [PMID: 39004462]

9. Monoclonal Immunoglobulin Glomerulonephritis

Monoclonal gammopathies which do not otherwise meet criteria for hematologic therapy may nonetheless result in glomerular injury, termed MIg glomerulonephritis or monoclonal gammopathy of renal significance (MGRS). Clinical presentation is varied, ranging from asymptomatic glomerular hematuria and proteinuria to RPGN. Laboratory studies typically reveal some combination of abnormal serum free light chain ratios, signifying accumulation of either kappa or lambda light chains; abnormal serum or urine protein electrophoresis, which determines the concentration of an abnormal monoclonal protein; or abnormal serum or urine immunofixation, which determines the type of monoclonal protein present (eg, IgG kappa). If MIg glomerulonephritis is suspected and the patient is not already on therapy for systemic disease (eg, myeloma), a kidney biopsy is warranted to define the disease process and guide treatment. Although light microscopic findings are variable, all MIg glomerulonephritis have the monotypic presence of immunoglobulins on immunofluorescence.

Treatment of MIg glomerulonephritis is aimed at identifying and targeting the underlying clone of monoclonal immunoglobulin. If the clone derives from plasma cells, daratumumab or bortezomib is recommended (see section on Plasma Cell Myeloma). B-cell clones are responsive to rituximab. Prognosis in MIg glomerulonephritis is dependent upon the eradication of the clone and is favorable if remission is achieved.

Du J et al. Systematic review and meta-analysis of the clinical features of MGRS. BMC Nephrol. 2024;25:22. [PMID: 38229028]
Nasr S et al. Renal Pathology Society/International Kidney and Monoclonal Gammopathy Research Group consensus on pathologic definitions and terminology of monoclonal gammopathy-associated kidney lesions. Kidney Int. 2025;108:184. [PMID: 40280412]
Pinney J et al. Diagnosis and management of monoclonal gammopathy of renal significance: A British Society for Haematology good practice paper. Br J Haematol. 2025;206:447. [PMID: 39777620]
Shankar M et al. Unraveling monoclonal gammopathy of renal significance: a mini review on kidney complications and clinical insights. Front Nephrol. 2024;4:1439288. [PMID: 39328783]

NEPHROTIC SPECTRUM GLOMERULAR DISEASES

ESSENTIALS OF DIAGNOSIS

- Persistent proteinuria with bland urine sediment (few if any cells).
- Nephrotic *syndrome* (if present):
  - Hypoalbuminemia.
  - Peripheral edema.
  - Hyperlipidemia.
- Oval fat bodies may be seen in the urine.

General Considerations

In developed countries, the most common cause of nephrotic disease is diabetes mellitus. Other causes include minimal change disease, FSGS, membranous nephropathy, and amyloidosis. Clinical presentations along the nephrotic spectrum vary based on etiology, with diabetic nephropathy and secondary FSGS typically on the less severe end (bland UA and proteinuria); minimal change disease, membranous nephropathy, and amyloidosis usually present with overt nephrotic *syndrome*. Serum creatinine may be abnormal at the time of presentation, depending on the severity and chronicity of the disease.

Clinical Findings

A. Symptoms and Signs

Patients with isolated proteinuria do not manifest symptoms of kidney disease. In those with nephrotic *syndrome*, peripheral edema is present, likely due to sodium retention and hypoalbuminemia-induced low plasma oncotic pressure. Edema may develop solely in dependent regions, such as the lower extremities, or it may become generalized and include periorbital edema. Dyspnea due to pulmonary edema, pleural effusions, and ascites can occur.

B. Laboratory Findings

1. UA—Proteinuria occurs due to podocyte injury and variable damage to the glomerular filtration barrier. The urine dipstick is a good screening test for albuminuria; if positive, urinary protein excretion should be quantified (see earlier Proteinuria section, Table 25–2). A spot urine protein to urine creatinine ratio gives a reasonable approximation of grams of protein excreted per day; a 24-hour urine sample for protein excretion is more precise but not routinely needed.

The urinary sediment has few cellular elements. However, if marked hyperlipidemia is present, urinary oval fat bodies may be seen. They appear as "grape clusters" under light microscopy and "Maltese crosses" under polarized light.

2. Blood chemistries—Nephrotic *syndrome* results in hypoalbuminemia. Hyperlipidemia occurs in over 50% of patients with nephrotic syndrome, due to falling oncotic pressure that triggers increased hepatic lipid production and decreased clearance of VLDLs with resultant hypertriglyceridemia. An elevated ESR may be seen as a result of increased levels of fibrinogen. Heavy urinary excretion of binding proteins may result in deficiencies of vitamin D, zinc, and copper.

Laboratory testing to help elucidate the underlying cause of the glomerular disease includes complement levels (C3 and C4), serum/urine protein electrophoresis and immunofixation, serum free light chains, ANA, PLA_2R antibody titers, HbA_{1c}, and serologic testing for hepatitis B and C, HIV, and syphilis (Table 25–9).

3. Kidney biopsy—Kidney biopsy is often performed in adults with new onset nephrotic syndrome if a primary renal disease that may require immunosuppressive therapy is suspected. Chronically and significantly decreased GFR suggests irreversible kidney disease which may decrease the utility of kidney biopsy. In the setting of long-standing (> 12 years) diabetes mellitus type 1 or 2, proteinuric kidney disease is not commonly biopsied unless atypical features (eg, significant glomerular hematuria or cellular casts) are also present, or if there is reason to suspect an additional or alternative kidney lesion.

Treatment

A. Proteinuria

In those with isolated proteinuria, dietary protein restriction may be helpful in slowing progression of kidney disease (see CKD section). Anti-proteinuric medications, including ACE inhibitors, ARBs, mineralocorticoid receptor antagonists, and SGLT-2 inhibitors, can help slow progression. They can be used in patients with reduced GFR as long as significant hyperkalemia (potassium > 5.5 mEq/L) does not occur and serum creatinine rises < 30% after drug initiation or dose titration; patients should be counseled on preventive practices to reduce risk of AKI and hyperkalemia. Combination therapy of an ARB and an ACE inhibitor is not recommended. MRA is not recommended when eGFR is < 25 mL/min.

B. Edema

Dietary sodium restriction is essential for managing edema; most patients also require diuretic therapy. Refractory fluid retention can occur due to hypoalbuminemia or decreased delivery of diuretics to the kidney tubule. Higher doses or combination diuretic therapy (multiple classes) may be required.

C. Hyperlipidemia

Hypercholesterolemia and hypertriglyceridemia can occur as noted above. Dietary modification and exercise should be encouraged, but pharmacologic treatment is usually required (see Chapter 32).

D. Hypercoagulable State

Patients with nephrotic *syndrome* have urinary losses of antithrombin, protein C and protein S, and increased platelet activation. Patients with serum albumin < 2.5 g/dL (25 g/L) are at particularly high risk for thrombosis and may develop DVT, renal vein thrombosis, or PE, especially in cases of membranous nephropathy. Anticoagulation therapy is warranted for at least 3–6 months in patients with evidence of thrombosis in any location and may be required indefinitely for renal vein thrombosis, PE, recurrent thromboemboli, or when ongoing nephrotic syndrome poses a risk of thrombosis recurrence.

When to Refer

Any patient with nephrotic *syndrome* should be referred immediately to a nephrologist for volume and blood pressure management, assessment for kidney biopsy, and treatment of the underlying disease. Nephrotic range proteinuria without the nephrotic syndrome also merits nephrology referral, though with less urgency.

When to Admit

Patients with edema refractory to outpatient therapy or rapidly worsening kidney function that requires inpatient interventions should be admitted.

Floege J et al. KDIGO 2025 Clinical Practice Guideline for the management of nephrotic syndrome in children. Kidney Int. 2025;107:S241. [PMID: 40254391]

Jhaveri KD et al. Nephrotic syndrome: have we entered a new era? Adv Kidney Dis Health. 2024;31:265. [PMID: 38935003]

Ponticelli C et al. Nephrotic syndrome: pathophysiology and consequences. J Nephrol. 2023;36:2179. [PMID: 37466816]

NEPHROTIC SPECTRUM DISEASE IN PRIMARY KIDNEY DISORDERS

MINIMAL CHANGE DISEASE

ESSENTIALS OF DIAGNOSIS

- Usually presents with nephrotic syndrome.
- Kidney biopsy shows no changes on light microscopy.
- Diffuse foot-process effacement on electron microscopy.

General Considerations

Minimal change disease is the most common cause of proteinuric kidney disease in children, accounting for approximately 80% of cases. It often remits upon treatment with corticosteroids. Children with nephrotic syndrome are often treated for minimal change disease empirically without a biopsy diagnosis. Minimal change disease is less common in adults, accounting for 20–25% of cases of primary nephrotic syndrome in those over age 40 years. This entity can be idiopathic but also occurs following viral upper respiratory infections (especially in children), in association with neoplasms such as Hodgkin disease, with drugs (lithium), and with hypersensitivity reactions (especially to NSAIDs and bee stings).

Clinical Findings

A. Symptoms and Signs

Patients usually present with sudden onset of nephrotic syndrome, which confers susceptibility to infection, thrombotic events, hyperlipidemia, and protein malnutrition. Minimal change disease can also present with AKI due to renal tubular damage and interstitial edema.

B. Laboratory and Histologic Findings

There is no helpful serologic testing. When kidney biopsy is performed, glomeruli appear normal on light microscopy and immunofluorescence. On electron microscopy, there is a characteristic diffuse effacement of podocyte foot processes. Mesangial cell proliferation may be seen in a subgroup of patients; this finding is associated with more hematuria and hypertension and poor response to standard corticosteroid treatment.

Treatment

First-line treatment is with prednisone, 1 mg/kg/day; remission in steroid-responsive minimal change disease often occurs within 4–8 weeks, though treatment up to 16 weeks is sometimes needed. Treatment should be continued for at least 2 weeks after complete remission, and dosing tapers should be individualized. Roughly half of patients with minimal change disease relapse and require repeated corticosteroid treatment. Patients with frequent relapses or corticosteroid resistance respond well to rituximab, although cyclophosphamide or a calcineurin inhibitor (tacrolimus, cyclosporine) are sometimes utilized to induce and maintain remissions. Progression to ESKD is rare. Complications most often arise from prolonged corticosteroid use.

Barr B et al. New insights into the biology and treatment of minimal change disease and focal segmental glomerulosclerosis. Curr Opin Nephrol Hypertens. 2025;34:450. [PMID: 40726375]

Gomez AC et al. Minimal change disease. Adv Kidney Dis Health. 2024;31:267. [PMID: 39084752]

Isaka Y et al. Rituximab for relapsing nephrotic syndrome in adults: a randomized clinical trial. JAMA. 2025;334:2011. [PMID: 41191364]

Vivarelli M et al. Childhood nephrotic syndrome. Lancet. 2023;402:809. [PMID: 37659779]

FOCAL SEGMENTAL GLOMERULOSCLEROSIS (FSGS)

General Considerations

FSGS is a relatively common pattern of injury resulting from damage to podocytes. It can be a primary/kidney-limited disorder or may be secondary to another underlying disease. Etiologies of primary FSGS fall into three categories: (1) heritable abnormalities in any one of several podocyte proteins or underlying type 4 collagen mutations; (2) polymorphisms in the *APOL1* gene in those of sub-Saharan African ancestry; or (3) increased levels of a circulating permeability factor that has yet to be identified. Secondary causes include kidney overwork injury (eg, history of nephrectomy), obesity, hypertension, chronic urinary reflux, HIV or SARS-CoV-2 infection, or analgesic or bisphosphonate exposure. Genetic testing in primary cases is increasingly available, especially in the pediatric population.

Clinical Findings

Decreased GFR is present in 25–50% of those with FSGS at time of diagnosis. Nephrotic syndrome is commonly seen in those with FSGS caused by a genetic disorder or putative circulating permeability factor; nephrotic syndrome is uncommon in secondary and *APOL1*-associated FSGS.

Diagnosis requires kidney biopsy, and genetic testing may be helpful. Light microscopy shows sclerosis of segments of some, but not all, glomeruli. On immunofluorescence, IgM and C3 are seen in sclerotic lesions, although it is hypothesized that these immune components are simply trapped in the sclerotic glomeruli and not pathologic. As in minimal change disease, electron microscopy shows foot process effacement.

Treatment

Treatment for all forms of FSGS includes ACE inhibitors, ARBs, or MRAs to control proteinuria and hypertension, and statins for hyperlipidemia; SGLT-2 inhibitors may be considered for those not receiving immunosuppression. Immunosuppression (oral prednisone, 1 mg/kg/day for 4–16 weeks followed by a slow taper) is recommended if nephrotic syndrome is present, as this suggests primary FSGS. In those with steroid-resistance or intolerance, calcineurin inhibitors, rituximab, and mycophenolate mofetil can be considered. Kidney transplantation in this subgroup of FSGS patients is complicated by a relatively high relapse rate and risk of graft loss. Those with *APOL1*-associated and hereditary primary FSGS do not appear to benefit from immunosuppression. Patients with secondary FSGS do not benefit from immunosuppressive therapy; treatment should be directed at the underlying cause.

Altintas M et al. Pathogenesis of focal segmental glomerulosclerosis and related disorders. Annu Rev Pathol. 2025;20:329. [PMID: 39854184]

Gembillo G et al. Advances in the pathophysiology and treatment of focal segmental glomerulosclerosis: The importance of a timely and tailored approach. World J Nephrol. 2025;14:103039. [PMID: 40568339]

Sim J et al. Treatment response rates and kidney outcomes among adults with primary FSGS. Clin J Am Soc Nephrol. 2026;21:296. [PMID: 41055958]

Torra R et al. When should the nephrologist think about genetics in patients with glomerular diseases? Clin Kidney J. 2025;18:sfaf044. [PMID: 40115110]

MEMBRANOUS NEPHROPATHY

ESSENTIALS OF DIAGNOSIS

- Varying degrees of proteinuria.
- Most common cause of primary adult nephrotic syndrome.
- Significant risk for thrombosis if nephrotic syndrome present.
- "Spike and dome" pattern on kidney biopsy from subepithelial deposits.
- Secondary causes include hepatitis B virus and cancer.

General Considerations

Membranous nephropathy is the most common cause of nephrotic syndrome in adults, typically presenting in the fifth and sixth decades. Primary membranous nephropathy is an autoimmune disease with reactivity against several possible podocyte antigens. Secondary disease is associated with infections, (such as hepatitis B and C, endocarditis, and syphilis); underlying cancer; SLE (class V); and certain drugs (such as NSAIDs, captopril, and possibly traditional indigenous medicines). The course of primary disease is highly variable, with spontaneous remission in approximately 30% of patients and progression to ESKD over 3–10 years in 50%. Poorer outcome is associated with concomitant tubulointerstitial fibrosis, male sex, elevated serum creatinine on presentation, hypertension, and proteinuria > 10 g/day.

Compared to other causes of nephrotic syndrome, patients with membranous nephropathy have a higher risk of hypercoagulability, including a predisposition to renal vein thrombosis.

Clinical Findings

A. Symptoms and Signs

Patients may be asymptomatic or may have edema. Symptomatic venous thrombosis may be an initial sign. There may be symptoms or signs of an underlying infection or neoplasm (especially lung, stomach, breast, and colon cancers) in secondary membranous nephropathy.

B. Laboratory Findings

Hypoalbuminemia and hyperlipidemia are characteristic laboratory findings in nephrotic syndrome. Evaluation for secondary causes including serologic testing for SLE, syphilis, and viral hepatitides, and age- and risk-appropriate cancer screening should be performed. The presence of circulating PLA_2R antibodies is considered diagnostic for primary membranous nephropathy and often eliminates the need for kidney biopsy. PLA_2R antibody titers can be followed during treatment.

Kidney biopsy findings in membranous nephropathy include increased capillary wall thickness without inflammatory changes or cellular proliferation; on silver stain, a classic "spike and dome" pattern results from projections of excess GBM between the subepithelial immune complex deposits. Immunofluorescence shows IgG, C3, and possibly PLA_2R Ab staining along capillary loops. Electron microscopy reveals deposits along the subepithelial surface of the basement membrane.

Treatment

Secondary causes must be considered prior to consideration of treatment. Primary disease treatment depends on the risk of disease progression. Roughly 30% of patients present with subnephrotic proteinuria (< 3.5 g/day), which portends a favorable prognosis with conservative management, including antiproteinuric therapy with ACE inhibitor or ARB. Spontaneous remission may develop even in those with heavy proteinuria (about 30% of cases). Thus, immunosuppression should be reserved for those at highest risk for progression, including nephrotic syndrome, and with salvageable kidney function and serum creatinine < 3 g/dL. Rituximab or corticosteroids and cyclophosphamide are given for 6 months. Calcineurin inhibitors with or without corticosteroids may be considered as well, though risk of relapse is higher with this drug regimen. Achievement of remission may take 6 months or longer, especially with rituximab-based regimens. Patients with primary membranous nephropathy who progress to ESKD are excellent candidates for transplant.

Avasare R et al. Drug-induced membranous nephropathy: piecing together clues to understand disease mechanisms. J Am Soc Nephrol. 2025;36:1629. [PMID: 40198910]
Caravaca-Fontan F et al. Updated diagnostic and therapeutic management for membranous nephropathy. Curr Opin Nephrol Hypertens. 2025;34:23. [PMID: 39513350]
Sethi S et al. Antigens in membranous nephropathy: discovery and clinical implications. Nat Rev Nephrol. 2025;21:653. [PMID: 40691733]
Zand L et al. What's new in membranous nephropathy and how to incorporate new antigen discoveries into clinical practice: a review. Am J Kidney Dis. 2026;87:93. [PMID: 41110629]

NEPHROTIC SPECTRUM DISEASE FROM SYSTEMIC DISORDERS

DIABETIC KIDNEY DISEASE

ESSENTIALS OF DIAGNOSIS

- Evidence of diabetes mellitus, typically over 10 years.
- Albuminuria usually precedes decline in GFR.
- Other end organ damage, such as retinopathy, is common.

General Considerations

Diabetic kidney disease is the most common cause of ESKD in the United States. The incidence of CKD is approximately 30–40% in both type 1 and type 2 diabetes mellitus. ESKD is much more likely to develop in persons with type 1 diabetes mellitus, in part due to fewer comorbidities and deaths before ESKD ensues. With the current epidemic of obesity and type 2 diabetes mellitus, rates of diabetic nephropathy continue to increase. Those with a family history of kidney disease are at higher risk. Mortality rates are higher for patients with diabetes who have comorbid kidney disease compared to those without CKD.

Clinical Findings

Kidney disease develops about 10 years after the onset of diabetes mellitus but may be present at the time type 2 diabetes mellitus is diagnosed. The first stage is hyperfiltration with an increase in GFR, followed by the development of moderate albuminuria (30–300 mg/day). Over time, albuminuria becomes severe (> 300 mg/day) and can be detected on urine dipstick as overt proteinuria. GFR subsequently declines over time. Yearly screening for moderate albuminuria is recommended for all patients with diabetes to detect disease at its earliest stage, though diabetic kidney disease less commonly can present as nonproteinuric CKD.

The most common lesion in diabetic kidney disease is diffuse glomerulosclerosis, but nodular glomerulosclerosis (Kimmelstiel-Wilson nodules) is pathognomonic. The kidneys are usually enlarged until disease becomes advanced. Kidney biopsy is not required in most patients unless atypical findings are present, such as sudden onset of proteinuria, nephritic features (see above), massive proteinuria (> 10 g/day), urinary cellular casts, or rapid decline in GFR.

Patients with diabetes are prone to other kidney diseases. These include type 4 (hyporeninemic hypoaldosteronemic) renal tubular acidosis and increased susceptibility to AKI from many insults, including intravenous contrast material and concomitant use of an ACE inhibitor or ARB with NSAID.

Treatment

At the onset of moderate albuminuria, treatment is necessary. Strict glycemic control should be emphasized early in diabetic nephropathy, while acknowledging risk of hypoglycemia as CKD becomes advanced (see CKD section). Recommended blood pressure goals should be tailored to the individual patient. In the BPROAD trial, targeting blood pressure below 120/80 mm Hg conferred a composite benefit of reduced risk of death from cardiovascular cause or nonfatal stroke, MI, or hospitalization for HF in patients with diabetes with increased risk of CVD. The 2021 Kidney Disease Improving Global Outcomes (KDIGO) practice guideline on blood pressure management recommends targeting blood pressure below 120/80 mm Hg in patients with diabetes who have CKD, regardless of degree of albuminuria. ACE inhibitors and ARBs in those with moderate albuminuria decrease rate of progression to overt proteinuria and slow progression to ESKD by reducing intraglomerular pressure and via antifibrotic effects; these agents are not absolutely indicated in patients without albuminuria who have diabetes. Patients with diabetes, especially with advanced CKD, are at relatively high risk for AKI and hyperkalemia with inhibition of the renin-angiotensin system, so monitoring for hyperkalemia or a decline in GFR > 30% within ~2 weeks of the initiation or uptitration of this therapy is prudent, with dose reduction or discontinuation of therapy if these complications are encountered. Combination ARB and ACE inhibitor therapy is not recommended due to lack of efficacy and increased adverse events of hyperkalemia and AKI. In addition to their cardioprotective effects, SGLT-2 inhibitors, including canagliflozin, empagliflozin, and dapagliflozin, slow progression of diabetic nephropathy in patients with type 2 diabetes mellitus. Although their use is FDA-authorized only when eGFR is > 30 mL/min/1.73 m^2, dapagliflozin and empagliflozin are safe and effective at eGFRs as low as 25 and 20 mL/min/1.73 m^2, respectively. The combination of mineralocorticoid receptor antagonists and SGLT-2 inhibitors leads to greater reduction in proteinuria than either treatment alone; non-steroidal MRAs (eg, finerenone) are less likely to cause hyperkalemia. GLP-1 agonists, such as semaglutide, are effective treatment options as additional therapy, for those who are intolerant of SGLT-2 inhibitors, or for those with more advanced CKD. Metformin may have kidney-specific benefits but should be discontinued when eGFR is < 30 mL/min/1.73 m^2. Treatment of obesity and other cardiovascular risk factors is vital. Many with diabetes have multiple comorbid conditions, and mortality is high among those who progress to ESKD. Patients who are relatively healthy, however, benefit from kidney transplantation.

Agarwal R et al. Finerenone with empagliflozin in chronic kidney disease and type 2 diabetes. N Engl J Med. 2025;393:533. [PMID: 40470996]

Bi Y et al. Intensive blood-pressure control in patients with type 2 diabetes. N Engl J Med. 2025;392:1155. [PMID: 39555827]

Perkovic V et al. Effects of semaglutide on chronic kidney disease in patients with type 2 diabetes. N Engl J Med. 2024;391:109. [PMID: 38785209]

The EMPA-KIDNEY Collaborative Group; Herrington WG et al. Empagliflozin in patients with chronic kidney disease. N Engl J Med. 2023;388:117. [PMID: 36331190]

HIV-ASSOCIATED NEPHROPATHY

HIV-associated nephropathy usually presents with nephrotic syndrome and declining GFR in patients with active, untreated HIV infection. Most who present with HIV-associated nephropathy are of sub-Saharan African descent with *APOL1* risk alleles (see section on Focal Segmental Glomerulosclerosis). HIV-associated nephropathy is usually associated with low CD4 counts and AIDS, but it can also be the initial presentation of HIV disease. Persons living with HIV are at risk for other kidney diseases, such as toxicity from antiretroviral medications (eg, tenofovir disoproxil fumarate), vascular disease, and diabetes, or immune complex–mediated glomerular disease (HIV-immune complex disease).

Classic HIV-associated nephropathy is characterized by an FSGS pattern of injury with glomerular collapse; severe tubulointerstitial damage may also be present.

HIV-associated nephropathy is less common in the era of HIV screening and more effective antiretroviral therapy. Small, uncontrolled studies have shown that antiretroviral therapy slows progression of disease. ACE inhibitors or ARBs can be used to control blood pressure and proteinuria. Kidney biopsy is necessary for diagnosis and to rule out other causes of kidney dysfunction. Patients who progress to ESKD and are otherwise healthy are good candidates for kidney transplantation.

Diana NE et al. The changing landscape of HIV-associated kidney disease. Nat Rev Nephrol. 2024;20:330. [PMID: 38273026]

Fisher M et al. HIV-associated kidney diseases: progress, gaps, and future directions. Clin Microbiol Rev. 2026;39:e0020725. [PMID: 41294345]

Mejia S et al. Kidney disease in patients with HIV. Curr Opin HIV AIDS. 2025;20:359. [PMID: 40184511]

Wearne N et al. HIV-associated kidney disease: the changing spectrum and treatment priorities. Curr Opin Nephrol Hypertens. 2024;33:603. [PMID: 39155827]

RENAL AMYLOIDOSIS

Amyloidosis is a relatively rare cause of nephrotic syndrome. It is caused by tissue deposition of an overproduced and misfolded protein (amyloid). Different proteins can form amyloid fibrils with renal deposition. Primary amyloidosis, or AL amyloidosis, is the most common form and is due to a plasma cell dyscrasia causing overproduction and deposition of monoclonal Ig light chains (see Chapter 15). Secondary amyloidosis, or AA amyloidosis, rarely occurs in chronic inflammatory disease such as rheumatoid arthritis, IBD, or chronic infection due to deposition of an acute phase reactant, serum amyloid A protein.

Renal involvement in amyloidosis is characterized by proteinuria, decreased GFR, and nephrotic syndrome. Evidence of other organ involvement, such as the heart, is common. Serum and 24-hour urine protein electrophoresis and immunofixation, and serum free light chains (kappa and lambda) should be quantified. Amyloid-infiltrated kidneys are often larger than 10 cm. Pathologically, glomeruli display nodular sclerosis and are filled with amorphous deposits that show green birefringence with Congo red staining; EM reveals fibril deposition.

The prognosis of renal AL amyloidosis depends on the GFR and degree of proteinuria at the time of diagnosis; patients with decreased GFR and high grade (> 5 g/24 hours) proteinuria progress to ESKD in an average of 2–3 years. Five-year overall survival ranges from 15% to 50% and is worse in those with advanced cardiac involvement. Standard treatment is a combination of cyclophosphamide, bortezomib, dexamethasone ('CyBorD'), and daratumumab. Melphalan and autologous stem cell transplantation are associated with a high (45%) mortality rate but can induce remission in 80% of survivors; however, few patients are eligible for this treatment. In AA amyloidosis, remission can occur if the underlying disease is successfully treated. Renal transplantation can be considered, but guidelines suggest it be performed only in patients with minimal extrarenal disease who have achieved a durable remission.

Allinovi M et al. The evolving spectrum of kidney amyloidosis: advances in diagnosis, typing, and treatment. Nephrol Dial Transplant. 2025;40:1826. [PMID: 40036358]
Karam S et al. Renal AA amyloidosis: presentation, diagnosis, and current therapeutic options: a review. Kidney Int. 2023;103:473. [PMID: 36502873]
Murakami N et al. Management recommendations for kidney transplantation in patients with plasma cell dyscrasia. Kidney Int. 2025;108:780. [PMID: 40738478]
Rauf M et al. Revised renal stratification and progression models for predicting long-term renal outcomes in immunoglobulin light chain amyloidosis. Haematologica. 2025;110:3032. [PMID: 40568719]

TUBULOINTERSTITIAL DISEASES

Tubulointerstitial disease may be acute or chronic. Acute disease is most commonly associated with medications, infectious agents, and systemic rheumatologic disorders. Interstitial edema, infiltration with polymorphonuclear neutrophils, and accompanying ATN can be seen. (See Acute Kidney Injury, above, and Table 25–4.) Chronic disease may result from clinically apparent acute disease that was not fully reversible or, more commonly, may develop insidiously over time without a known inciting factor. Interstitial fibrosis and tubular atrophy are present, with a mononuclear cell predominance. The chronic disorders are described below.

CHRONIC TUBULOINTERSTITIAL DISEASES

ESSENTIALS OF DIAGNOSIS

- Kidney size is small.
- Decreased urinary concentrating ability.
- CKD.

General Considerations

There are many identifiable causes of chronic tubulointerstitial disease (also called chronic interstitial nephritis [CIN]), including chronic obstruction, toxic exposures, systemic autoimmune disorders (eg, Sjögren syndrome), granulomatous disease (eg, sarcoidosis) and hereditary forms; however, many cases are of unknown etiology.

Obstructive uropathy is a common cause of CIN. It is the result prolonged or recurrent obstruction, most commonly from prostate disease; bilateral ureteral calculi, or calculus in a single functioning kidney; carcinoma of the cervix, colon, or bladder; and retroperitoneal tumors or fibrosis.

Vesicoureteral reflux, generally a childhood disorder, occurs when an incompetent vesicoureteral sphincter allows urine from the bladder to reflux to the kidney during voiding. Urine can extravasate into the interstitium, triggering an inflammatory response that leads to fibrosis over time.

Analgesic nephropathy can occur in patients who ingest large quantities of anti-inflammatory pain medications such as paracetamol, aspirin, and other NSAIDs; acetaminophen is a possible but less certain culprit. Ingestion of these analgesics of ≥ 1 g/day for several years is considered necessary for kidney dysfunction to develop; however, many patients underestimate their analgesic use. Female sex, older age, and malnutrition are risk factors for analgesic nephropathy. Aspirin and other NSAIDs can cause damage through intermediate metabolites, which can lead to cell necrosis. These drugs also decrease medullary blood flow (via inhibition of prostaglandin synthesis) and decrease glutathione levels, which are necessary for detoxification. Renal papillary tip and inner medullary concentrations of some analgesics are 10-fold higher than in the renal cortex; all of which may result in papillary necrosis in addition to chronic interstitial inflammation and scarring.

Long-term **lithium** use, usually > 10 years, can result in CIN with slowly progressive CKD and renal parenchymal microcysts.

Environmental exposure to **heavy metals**—such as lead, cadmium, mercury, and bismuth—can cause CIN. Individuals at risk for lead-induced tubulointerstitial disease are those with occupational exposure (eg, those who weld, or work with lead-based paint or leaded-gasoline) or who drink alcohol distilled in automobile radiators ("moonshine" whiskey).

CIN in agricultural communities is a form of chronic tubulointerstitial disease seen in workers in tropical and subtropical agricultural communities that can lead to ESKD.

Autosomal dominant tubulointerstitial disease is a rare, but increasingly recognized cause of heritable kidney disease. It may be caused by defects in one of several genes, and the clinical presentation varies with the pathogenic variant.

Clinical Findings

A. General Findings

Polyuria may occur if tubular damage leads to nephrogenic diabetes insipidus, possibly from vasopressin insensitivity. This is especially common in those with lithium exposure. Volume depletion can rarely occur due to salt-wasting defects in some individuals.

Renal tubular acidosis is common and can develop through three mechanisms: (1) reduced ammoniagenesis in the proximal tubules, (2) inability to reabsorb bicarbonate in the proximal tubules, and (3) inability to secrete protons in the distal tubules, which is needed for urinary acidification. Type 1 (hypokalemic) or type 4 (hyperkalemic) renal tubular acidoses may be seen in tubulointerstitial disease; heavy metal exposures tend to damage the proximal tubule and may result in proximal (type 2) renal tubular acidosis. In contrast to *acute* interstitial nephritis, the UA in CIN disease is often bland, either with no findings or a few cells or broad waxy casts. Proteinuria may be present, owing to inability of the proximal tubule to reabsorb freely filtered proteins, but is typically < 2 g/day.

B. Specific Findings

1. Obstructive uropathy—In partial obstruction, patients can exhibit polyuria (from tubular damage) or oliguria (due to decreased GFR). Renin-mediated hypertension may be present. Abdominal, rectal, and genitourinary examinations may be helpful in detecting a distended bladder or large prostate. UA is often bland, but may show hematuria, pyuria, or bacteriuria. Bedside ultrasound for elevated post-void residual bladder volume can be helpful in cases of bladder outlet obstruction. Abdominal ultrasound usually detects hydroureter, and hydronephrosis but may miss obstruction due to retroperitoneal fibrosis. CT scanning or MRI can be considered if suspicion remains despite a normal ultrasound.

2. Vesicoureteral reflux—Vesicoureteral reflux is typically diagnosed in young children with a history of recurrent UTIs but can also develop after kidney transplantation. Renal ultrasound can show renal scarring and hydronephrosis. Most damage occurs before age 5, and progressive deterioration to ESKD is common.

3. Analgesics—Patients may exhibit hematuria, mild proteinuria, polyuria (from tubular damage), anemia (from GI bleeding or erythropoietin deficiency), and sterile pyuria. Sloughed papillae can be found in the urine when papillary necrosis occurs and can lead to obstruction. Although classically diagnosed by IVP, papillary necrosis is more commonly detected by CT imaging or cystoureteroscopy.

4. Heavy metals—Proximal tubular damage from lead exposure can cause decreased secretion of uric acid, resulting in hyperuricemia and saturnine gout. Hypertension is common. Diagnosis of lead nephropathy is established with a calcium disodium edetate (EDTA) chelation test—24-hour urine excretion of > 600 mg of lead following 1 g of EDTA indicates excessive lead exposure. The proximal tubular dysfunction from cadmium can cause hypercalciuria and nephrolithiasis.

5. Chronic interstitial nephritis in agricultural communities—In addition to low-grade proteinuria, hyperuricemia and hypokalemia are often identified among affected individuals. Although not pathognomonic, areas of glomerular ischemia (despite mild vascular disease) that accompany chronic tubulointerstitial injury on kidney biopsy are highly suggestive of CINAC.

Treatment

Treatment depends first on identifying the disorder responsible for kidney dysfunction. Interstitial fibrosis on biopsy reflects irreversible damage, the degree of which is directly associated with the likelihood of progression to ESKD. Treatment of hypertension may slow progression. Tubular dysfunction may require bicarbonate supplementation to treat metabolic acidosis or potassium restriction to mitigate hyperkalemia.

If hydronephrosis is present, the obstruction should be promptly relieved. Prolonged obstruction leads to further tubular damage—particularly in the distal nephron—which may become irreversible. Although surgical correction of reflux may be indicated in select instances, this will unlikely prevent deterioration toward ESKD if fibrosis is extensive.

Patients in whom lead nephropathy is suspected should continue chelation therapy with EDTA if there is minimal evidence of irreversible renal damage; continued exposure to lead should be avoided.

Treatment of analgesic nephropathy requires cessation of all analgesics. Stabilization of or improvement in kidney function may occur if significant interstitial fibrosis is not present. Ensuring volume repletion during exposure to analgesics may also have some beneficial effects.

Patients with chronic interstitial nephritis in agricultural communities should be counseled to remain adequately hydrated and, if possible, minimize heat exposure. NSAIDs should be avoided due to their hemodynamic effects (reduced renal blood flow and glomerular filtration), which may exacerbate renal injury in states of volume depletion and hot climates.

When to Refer

- Patients with stage 3–5 CKD should be referred to a nephrologist. Earlier referral may be appropriate if management of tubular dysfunction, such as renal tubular acidosis, is necessary.
- Patients with urologic abnormalities should be referred to a urologist.

Madero M et al. Chronic kidney disease of unknown etiology: a tubulointerstitial disease. Adv Kidney Dis Health. 2025;32:350. [PMID: 40947150]

Weber N et al. Prognosis and outcomes of acute and chronic tubulointerstitial nephritis. Adv Kidney Dis Health. 2025;32:382. [PMID: 40947154]

Yadav R et al. Environmental toxicants and nephrotoxicity: implications on mechanisms and therapeutic strategies. Toxicology. 2024;504:153784. [PMID: 38518838]

SIMPLE OR SOLITARY CYSTS

Renal cysts are tubular epithelium-lined cavities filled with fluid or semisolid material. Cysts are described as "simple" or "complex" based on scanning characteristics. Simple cysts account for 65–70% of all renal masses and may be noted incidentally on abdominal imaging in 50% of persons over 50 years of age. They are typically asymptomatic but rarely can become infected or cause hematuria. On ultrasonography simple cysts are (1) echo-free, (2) sharply demarcated with smooth walls, and (3) have an enhanced back wall (indicating good transmission through the cyst). On contrast CT scan, simple cysts do not enhance. Simple cysts do not require any specific follow-up, though changes in clinical presentation should prompt repeat imaging. Renal parenchymal scarring and remodeling can lead to simple cyst formation (known as "acquired" cysts) in CKD and ESKD; these cysts carry a small risk of malignant transformation to renal cell carcinoma. Simple cysts must be differentiated from malignancy, abscess, or heritable cystic diseases.

Complex cysts can have thick walls, calcifications, solid components, and mixed echogenicity. Renal cell carcinoma usually demonstrates vascular enhancement, although a small number are avascular. If a cyst has questionable imaging characteristics or is of uncertain significance, periodic reevaluation is recommended, and urologic consultation should be considered. Heritable cystic diseases are

Table 25–10. Clinical features of renal cystic disease.

	Simple Renal Cysts	Acquired Renal Cysts	Autosomal Dominant Polycystic Kidney Disease	Medullary Sponge Kidney	Medullary Cystic Kidney
Prevalence	Common	Dialysis patients	1:1000	1:5000	Rare
Inheritance	None	None	Autosomal dominant	None	Autosomal dominant
Age at onset	...	...	20–40 years	40–60 years	Adulthood
Kidney size	Normal	Small	Large	Normal	Small
Cyst location	Cortex and medulla	Cortex and medulla	Cortex and medulla	Collecting ducts	Corticomedullary junction
Hematuria	Occasional	Occasional	Common	Rare	Rare
Hypertension	None	Variable	Common	None	None
Associated complications	None	Adenocarcinoma in cysts	Hepatic cysts, UTIs, renal calculi, cerebral aneurysms	Renal calculi, UTIs	Polyuria, salt-wasting
Kidney failure	Never	Always	Frequently	Never	Always

associated with many cysts in both kidneys and, depending on type, can progress to ESKD (Table 25–10).

Alrumayyan M et al. Cystic renal masses: old and new paradigms. Urol Clin North Am. 2023;59:227. [PMID: 36948669]
Hanna C et al. Cystic kidney diseases in children and adults: differences and gaps in clinical management. Semin Nephrol. 2023;43:151434. [PMID: 37996359]

AUTOSOMAL DOMINANT POLYCYSTIC KIDNEY DISEASE

ESSENTIALS OF DIAGNOSIS

- Multiple cysts in both kidneys; number of cysts depends on patient age.
- Hypertension and (over time) large palpable kidneys.
- Autosomal dominant pattern of inheritance, although sporadic cases may occur.

General Considerations

Autosomal dominant polycystic kidney disease (ADPKD) is the most common monogenic kidney disease. It has a prevalence of 1:1000 and accounts for 5–10% of all ESKD cases globally. ADPKD is primarily caused by mutations in genes encoding polycystins (*PKD1* for polycystin 1, or *PKD2* for polycystin 2). Affected individuals with the more common *PKD1* mutations tend to develop ESKD by age 50, although disease penetration is variable. Those with the less common *PKD2* mutations (15–20% of patients) have slower progression of disease, with median age at ESKD of 75 years. Sporadic cases without identifiable polycystin gene mutations may occur; these cases tend to have milder, less progressive disease.

Clinical Findings

Hematuria (either microscopic or gross) is present in most patients. A family history of ADPKD is present in 75% of cases. Cyst development and growth over time eventually results in large kidneys that may be palpable on abdominal examination; massively enlarged kidneys can cause early satiety, shortness of breath, or pain. Spontaneous cyst rupture can cause severe intermittent flank pain; gross hematuria episodes may result from bleeding into cysts. Cysts may become infected, causing pain and fever. Roughly half of patients have concurrent hepatic cysts; pancreatic and splenic cysts may occur. UA often shows hematuria and subnephrotic proteinuria. In patients with an established family history of ADPKD, ultrasonography confirms the diagnosis—two or more cysts in patients under age 30 years, two or more cysts in each kidney in patients aged 30–59 years, and four or more cysts in each kidney in patients aged 60 years or older are diagnostic for ADPKD. Importantly, these criteria do *not* apply to individuals without a known family history; these individuals should be evaluated with CT, which is more sensitive. If found, the presence of multiple hepatic cysts helps support the diagnosis. In some cases, genetic testing for *PKD1* and *PKD2* mutations may be required.

Complications & Treatment

A. Pain

Abdominal or flank pain may be caused by cyst infection, rupture or hemorrhage, or nephrolithiasis. Cyst decompression may ameliorate chronic pain.

B. Hematuria

Gross hematuria is most commonly due to cystic rupture into the renal pelvis, but it can also be caused by a kidney stone or UTI. If due to cyst rupture, hematuria typically resolves within several days.

C. Renal Infection

An infected renal cyst should be suspected in patients who have flank pain, fever, and leukocytosis. UA may be normal if the cyst does not communicate directly with the urinary tract. CT evaluation demonstrating increased wall thickness is suggestive of infection, but PET CT provides greater sensitivity. Adequate antibiotic treatment is limited by poor cyst penetration; fluoroquinolones (ciprofloxacin or levofloxacin) or trimethoprim-sulfamethoxazole are agents of choice.

D. Nephrolithiasis

Up to 20% of patients have kidney stones, primarily calcium oxalate. The usual lifestyle modification recommendations for stone prevention should be prescribed.

E. Hypertension

Hypertension is common, likely due to cyst-induced ischemia with activation of the renin-angiotensin system. ACE inhibitors or ARBs are first-line therapy. Intensive blood pressure control (goal ≤ 110/75 mm Hg) is recommended in adults < age 50 with eGFR > 60 mL/min/1.73 m^2; for all other affected individuals, the blood pressure goal is ≤ 130/85 mm Hg.

F. Cerebral Aneurysms

About 10–15% of patients have arterial aneurysms in the circle of Willis. Screening arteriography is controversial; some experts recommend screening for all (with CT or MR angiography) while others reserve screening for those who have a family history of aneurysms or sudden death, are employed in a high-risk profession (eg, airline pilot), or are undergoing elective surgery with a high risk of moderate to severe perioperative hypertension.

G. Other Complications

Individuals with ADPKD are more likely to have mitral valve prolapse (up to 25%), aortic aneurysms, aortic valve abnormalities, and colonic diverticulae. Rates of renal cell carcinoma are 2-fold higher.

Prognosis

Kidney size, reported as total kidney volume, is the best predictor of kidney function decline in patients with autosomal dominant polycystic kidney disease, and can be measured via CT or MRI using the Mayo Classification system (www.mayo.edu/research/documents/pkd-center-adkpkd-classification/doc-20094754). Those at high risk according to this classification system may benefit from treatments that delay cyst growth. Vasopressin receptor antagonists decrease the rate of change in total kidney volume and eGFR decline; tolvaptan is used to slow progression in carefully selected individuals. Liberal ingestion of water will have the same physiologic effect on vasopressin, and patients should be encouraged to drink at least 2 L of water daily. Avoidance of caffeine may prevent cyst formation due to effects on G-coupled proteins.

Borghol AH et al. Intracranial aneurysms in autosomal dominant polycystic kidney disease: a practical approach to screening and management. Mayo Clin Proc. 2025;100:1030. [PMID: 40319406]

Borghol AH et al. Kidney stones and autosomal dominant polycystic kidney disease: a state-of-the-art review. Ren Fail. 2025;47:2570071. [PMID: 41208250]

Gordon CE et al. Autosomal dominant polycystic kidney disease: core curriculum 2025. Am J Kidney Dis. 2025;86:525. [PMID: 40844441]

Torres VE et al. KDIGO 2025 clinical practice guidelines for the evaluation, management, and treatment of autosomal dominant polycystic kidney disease (ADPKD): executive summary. Kidney Int. 2025;107:234. [PMID: 39848746]

MEDULLARY SPONGE KIDNEY

Medullary sponge kidney is a disease involving the distal nephron that affects < 1% of the general population. Although present at birth, it is not usually diagnosed until the third or fourth decade. It is thought to occur due to disruption of the ureteric bud-metanephric mesenchyme interface, often resulting from autosomal dominant mutations in genes responsible for urogenital development. Kidneys have marked, irregular enlargement of the medullary and papillary collecting ducts. This is associated with diffuse medullary cysts, giving a "Swiss cheese" appearance in these regions.

Clinical Findings

Nephrolithiasis is the most common clinical presentation and complication of medullary sponge kidney, affecting up to 70% of patients. Hematuria (either gross or microscopic), recurrent UTIs, or both may also occur. Other findings may include decreased urinary concentrating ability, nephrocalcinosis, and, less commonly, type 1 (distal) renal tubular acidosis. The diagnosis is established clinically through laboratory data and imaging characteristics. CT imaging shows cystic dilatation of the distal collecting tubules with a striated appearance, and calcifications in the renal collecting system. Similar findings on ultrasound may also support the diagnosis.

Treatment

Treatment for medullary sponge kidney is supportive and primarily centered on mitigating risk for stone formation and nephrocalcinosis. Oral alkali therapy (preferably citrate salts); a low salt/low animal protein diet; and ≥ 3 L of fluid intake daily are recommended. Thiazides may help lower urinary calcium excretion.

Prognosis

Medullary sponge kidney is generally considered a benign condition unless there are complications from recurrent UTIs, nephrolithiasis, or uncontrolled acidosis.

Camolese BA et al. Porous perspectives: a comprehensive review of medullary sponge kidney. Int Urol Nephrol. 2025;57:3251. [PMID: 40287601]

MULTISYSTEM DISEASES WITH VARIABLE KIDNEY INVOLVEMENT

PLASMA CELL MYELOMA

Plasma cell myeloma is a malignancy of plasma cells (see Chapter 15); collateral kidney damage due to toxic effects of monoclonal immunoglobulins or light chains may manifest in a variety of renal injury patterns. Cast nephropathy (also called "myeloma kidney") is the most common kidney disease and occurs when immunoglobulin light chains (Bence Jones protein) overwhelm the resorptive capacity of the tubules, leading to precipitation in the distal nephron and tubular obstruction. Proteinuria in cast nephropathy is exclusively due to tubular overflow of light chains which will not be detected by urine dipstick (see section on Proteinuria). Plasma cell myeloma may also cause generalized dysfunction of the proximal tubule (Fanconi syndrome), manifesting as type 2 renal tubular acidosis and euglycemic glycosuria. Another manifestation of plasma cell myeloma is renal amyloidosis with nephrotic syndrome; in these patients, urine dipstick will reveal heavy albuminuria due to glomerular damage. Less common myeloma-related kidney disorders include plasma cell infiltration of the renal parenchyma, hyperviscosity syndrome compromising renal blood flow, and renal effects of hypercalcemia (vasoconstriction, nephrogenic diabetes insipidus). Therapy for AKI (see Acute Kidney Injury, above) attributable to plasma cell myeloma includes correction of hypercalcemia; volume repletion; and chemotherapy for the underlying malignancy, typically with bortezomib-based regimens. Plasmapheresis and hemodialysis are sometimes considered to reduce the burden of circulating free light chains, but results have been equivocal and their use is controversial.

Dimopoulos MA et al. Management of multiple myeloma-related renal impairment: recommendations from the International Myeloma Working Group. Lancet Oncol. 2023;24:e293. [PMID: 37414019]

Wang L et al. Update on kidney injury caused by multiple myeloma. Ann Hematol. 2024;103:5007. [PMID: 38942949]

SICKLE CELL DISEASE

Kidney damage is common with sickle cell disease. Sickling of RBCs in the relatively hypoxic renal medulla results in congestion and stasis, which leads to hemorrhage, interstitial inflammation, papillary infarcts, and necrosis. Hematuria is common; proteinuria can occur and portends a poorer prognosis. Isosthenuria (urine osmolality equal to that of serum) signals damage to renal capillaries with impaired urinary concentrating ability and excess renal water losses; patients can easily become dehydrated. Sickle cell glomerulopathy is less common but inexorably progresses to ESKD. Treatment of the kidney disease centers on control of sickle cell disease and ensuring adequate fluid intake; ACE inhibitors or ARBs should be considered for albuminuric patients; hydroxyurea may also be reno-protective. Sickle cell trait can also result in kidney disease, though at lower rates than are seen in sickle cell disease. For those who progress to ESKD, renal transplantation should be considered.

Abbasi M et al. Management of kidney disease with sickle cell disease. J Am Soc Nephrol. 2025;36:2041. [PMID: 40569673]

Banda K et al. Clinical and genetic predictors of sickle cell nephropathy: a global systematic review. OMICS. 2025;29:353. [PMID: 40719369]

Castro-Sesquen YE et al. Chronic kidney disease in adults with sickle cell trait: a systematic review and meta-analysis. Blood Adv. 2025;9:3644. [PMID: 40300155]

TUBERCULOSIS

Renal tuberculosis usually results from hematogenous spread. Up to 20% of patients with tuberculosis have extra-pulmonary disease, of whom 5% have genitourinary involvement, which often is underdiagnosed. Its classic manifestation is the presence of microscopic pyuria without bacterial growth on urine culture—or "sterile pyuria"; microscopic hematuria may be present. Characteristic findings on imaging include papillary necrosis and cavitation of the renal parenchyma; ureteral strictures resulting in hydronephrosis may also be present. Kidney biopsy demonstrates granulomatous inflammation and tubulointerstitial nephritis; however, a presumptive diagnosis is often made without biopsy confirmation based on positive urine PCR testing. Prompt initiation of antituberculosis treatment is indicated, without which chronic inflammation and obstruction will lead to ESKD. Nephrectomy may be indicated in refractory cases.

Bausch K et al. Genitourinary tuberculosis: a brief manual for urologists on diagnosis and treatment from the European Association of Urology Urological Infections Panel. Eur Urol Focus. 2024;10:77. [PMID: 37541917]

Figueiredo AA et al. Current insights into urogenital tuberculosis in the clinical settings. Expert Rev Anti Infect Ther. 2025;23:1059. [PMID: 41213826]

GOUT & THE KIDNEY

The kidney is the primary organ for uric acid excretion. Patients with CKD have decreased excretion of uric acid and are prone to gouty arthritis attacks. Depending on the pH and uric acid concentration, deposition can occur in the tubules, the interstitium, or the urinary tract. The more alkaline pH of the interstitium causes urate salt deposition, whereas the acidic environment of the tubules and urinary tract causes uric acid crystallization deposition.

Three disorders of renal uric acid overload can develop: (1) uric acid nephrolithiasis, which may result in ureteral obstructive uropathy; (2) acute uric acid nephropathy due to uric acid crystal precipitation in the distal tubule, which results in tubular obstruction and tubulointerstitial toxicity (usually seen in tumor lysis syndrome), and (3) chronic urate nephropathy with deposition of urate crystals of the interstitium, which leads to fibrosis and atrophy.

Those with hyperuricemia should avoid food and drugs causing hyperuricemia (see Chapter 23), ensure adequate fluid intake, and be considered for urate-lowering therapy (eg, allopurinol or febuxostat); SGLT-2 inhibition also may reduce gout flares. Treatment of uric acid nephrolithiasis also includes fluid intake that should exceed 3 L/day, and consideration of a urinary alkalinizing agent. Patients with hyperuricemia but no history of gout or uric acid nephrolithiasis have not been shown to benefit from urate-lowering therapy.

Helget LN et al. Efficacy and safety of allopurinol and febuxostat in patients with gout and CKD: subgroup analysis of the STOP Gout Trial. Am J Kidney Dis. 2024;84:538. [PMID: 38906504]
Ostrowski RA. Gout management in patients with CKD: a review. Am J Kidney Dis. 2025:86:516. [PMID: 40609855]

SARCOIDOSIS

The prevalence of renal damage in the setting of sarcoidosis is unclear, with estimates ranging from 3 to 30%. The most common cause of kidney dysfunction is nephrocalcinosis (parenchymal calcium salts deposition leading to fibrosis) due to chronic hypercalcemia and hypercalciuria; these individuals may also present with calcium-oxalate or -phosphate nephrolithiasis. Sarcoidosis can also cause a granulomatous acute or, more commonly, chronic interstitial nephritis. Individuals with sarcoidosis should be screened at diagnosis and periodically thereafter for kidney involvement with evaluation of plasma calcium level, eGFR, and UA to screen for hematuria and albuminuria. Assessment for nephrocalcinosis and nephrolithiasis burden via ultrasongraphy or non-contrasted CT is also warranted. Early recognition of renal involvement allows for institution of therapy to mitigate the risk of further kidney damage and progression to ESKD. Glucocorticoids are first-line agents to treat granulomatous disease and hypercalcemia; other agents such as azathioprine, hydroxychloroquine, or other biologics may need to be considered in refractory or relapsing cases.

Miao J et al. Clinicopathological characteristics and long-term kidney outcomes in biopsy-proven renal sarcoidosis. Kidney360. 2025;6:1780. [PMID: 40155578]

Urologic Disorders

Mathew Sorensen, MD, MS, FACS
Marah C. Hehemann, MD
Chloe E. Peters, MD

26

HEMATURIA

ESSENTIALS OF DIAGNOSIS

- Gross hematuria requires evaluation: the upper urinary tract should be imaged, and the lower tract evaluated by cystoscopy.
- In microscopic hematuria, the workup should be risk stratified.

General Considerations

An *upper tract source* (kidneys and ureters) can be identified in 10% of patients with gross or microscopic hematuria. For upper tract sources, stone disease accounts for 40%, medical kidney disease (medullary sponge kidney, glomerulonephritis, papillary necrosis) for 20%, renal cell carcinoma for 10%, and urothelial cell carcinoma of the ureter or renal pelvis for 5%. Medication ingestion and associated medical problems may provide diagnostic clues. Analgesic use (**papillary necrosis**), cyclophosphamide (**chemical cystitis**), antibiotics (**interstitial nephritis**), diabetes mellitus, sickle cell trait or disease (**papillary necrosis**), a history of stone disease, or malignancy should all be investigated. The *lower tract source* of gross hematuria (in the absence of infection) is most commonly from bleeding prostatic varices or urothelial carcinoma of the bladder. Microscopic hematuria in the male is most commonly from BPH (13%), kidney stones (6%), or urethral stricture (1.4%). *The presence of hematuria in patients receiving antiplatelet or anticoagulation therapy cannot be presumed to be due to the medication; a complete evaluation consisting of upper tract imaging, cystoscopy, and urine cytology is warranted.* (See Chapter 43 for Bladder Cancer, Cancers of the Ureter & Renal Pelvis, Renal Cell Carcinoma, and Other Primary Tumors of the Kidney.)

Clinical Findings

A. Symptoms and Signs

If gross hematuria occurs, a description of the timing (initial, terminal, total) may provide a clue to the localization of disease. Associated symptoms (ie, renal colic, irritative voiding symptoms, or constitutional symptoms) should be investigated. *The history should be focused on risk factors for urothelial cancer* (age, male sex, smoking history, history of gross hematuria, irritative lower urinary tract voiding symptoms, history of cyclophosphamide or ifosfamide chemotherapy, family history of urothelial carcinoma or Lynch syndrome, occupational exposure to benzene chemicals or aromatic amines, history of chronic indwelling foreign body in the urinary tract such as a Foley or suprapubic catheter) and on nonmalignant causes. The physical examination should look for signs of systemic disease (fever, rash, lymphadenopathy, abdominal or pelvic masses) as well as signs of medical kidney disease (hypertension, volume overload). The urologic evaluation may demonstrate an enlarged prostate, flank mass, or urethral disease. The evaluation of patients with hematuria and their risk stratification should *not* be influenced by whether they are taking any antiplatelet or anticoagulant agents.

B. Laboratory Findings

Initial laboratory investigations include a UA and urine culture. **Microhematuria** is defined as three or more RBCs per high-power field on a microscopic evaluation of the urine. The degree of microscopic hematuria is important in risk stratification according to the 2020 American Urological Association hematuria guidelines (Figure 26–1). A positive dipstick reading for heme merits microscopic examination to confirm or refute the diagnosis of hematuria but is not enough to warrant workup on its own. If UA and culture are suggestive of a UTI, follow-up UA after treatment of the infection is important to ensure resolution of the hematuria. An estimate of kidney function should be obtained, since renal insufficiency may influence the methods of upper tract imaging (eg, ability to obtain a contrast CT or MRI imaging) of patients with hematuria. *Urine cytology and other urinary-based markers are* not *routinely recommended in the evaluation of asymptomatic microscopic hematuria.*

C. Risk Stratification

Following initial evaluation, clinicians should categorize patients with microscopic hematuria as low, intermediate, or high risk for a urothelial malignancy (Figure 26–1).

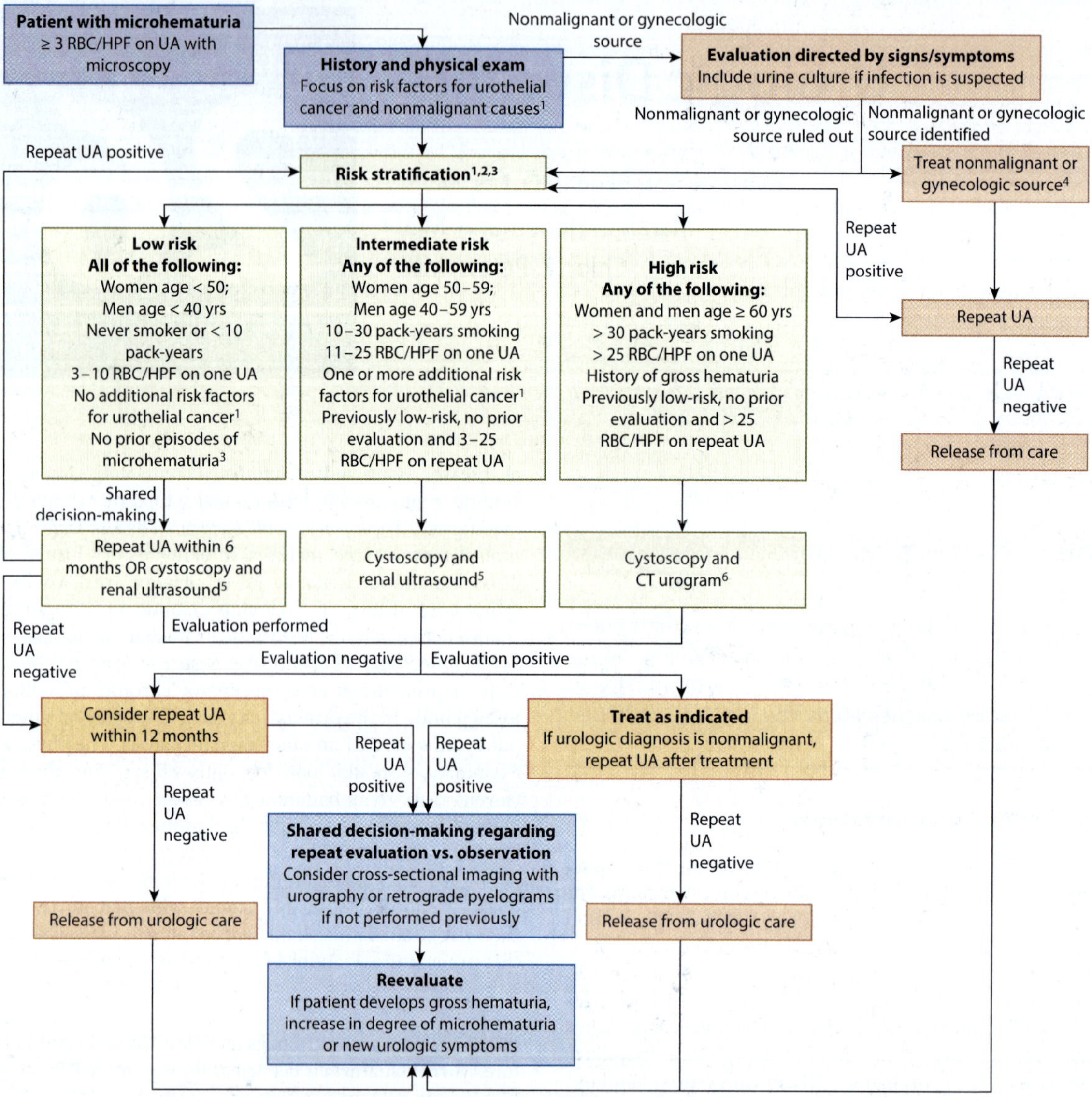

[1]Main risk factors for urothelial cancer are those in the AUA risk stratification system (age, male sex, smoking, degree of microhematuria and history of gross hematuria). Additional risk factors for urothelial carcinoma include but are not limited to irritative lower urinary tract voiding symptoms, history of cyclophosphamide or ifosfamide chemotherapy, family history of urothelial carcinoma or Lynch syndrome, occupational exposures to benzene chemicals or aromatic amines, history of chronic indwelling foreign body in the urinary tract.

[2]If medical kidney disease is suspected, consider nephrologic evaluation, but pursue concurrent risk-based urological evaluation.

[3]Patients may be low-risk at first presentation with microhematuria, but may be considered intermediate- or high-risk if found to have persistent microhematuria.

[4]There are nonmalignant and gynecologic sources of hematuria that do not require treatment and/or may confound the diagnosis of microhematuria. Clinicians can consider catheterized urine specimen in women with vaginal atrophy or pelvic organ prolapse. Clinicians must use careful judgment and patient engagement to decide whether to pursue microhematuria evaluation in the setting of chronic conditions that do not require treatment, such as the aforementioned gynecologic conditions, nonobstructing stones or BPH.

[5]Clinician may perform cross-sectional imaging with urography or retrograde pyelograms if hematuria persists after negative renal ultrasound.

[6]If contraindications to CT urogram, MR urogram or noncontrast imaging plus retrograde pyelograms.

▲ **Figure 26–1.** Microscopic hematuria: algorithmic approach to risk stratification of patients as low risk, intermediate risk, and high risk for urothelial malignancy. HPF, high-powered field. (Reproduced with permission from Barocas DA, Boorjian SA, Alvarez RD, et al. Microhematuria: AUA/SUFU Guideline. J Urol. 2020;204(4):778-786.)

D. Evaluation

Patients with **gross hematuria** should have both complete evaluation of the upper tract by a **CT-intravenous pyelogram (CT-IVP)** or a **magnetic resonance urogram (MR-urogram)** with and without contrast with delayed phases. *No imaging study adequately evaluates the bladder, and visual inspection of the bladder by cystoscopy is required.*

Low-risk patients with microscopic hematuria should undertake a shared decision-making approach with their clinician to decide between repeat urinalyses over the next 6 months or proceeding immediately with cystoscopy and **renal ultrasound**. If microscopic hematuria persists on a repeat UA, then patients who did not initially undergo cystoscopy should be reclassified as intermediate- or high-risk and undergo both upper tract imaging according to their risk group, and lower tract evaluation by cystoscopy.

Intermediate-risk patients should undergo both upper tract imaging with renal ultrasound and lower tract evaluation by cystoscopy.

High-risk patients should undergo upper tract evaluation with CT-IVP (preferred), MR-urogram (if CT-IVP contraindicated), and cystoscopic evaluation of the bladder. If there are contraindications to CT-IVP and MR-urogram, clinicians may perform noncontrast axial imaging along with retrograde pyelography at the time of cystoscopy.

Follow-Up

In patients with negative hematuria evaluations, it is typically recommended that a UA with microscopy be repeated at 6–12 months. Patients with a negative follow-up UA require no further evaluation. If microscopic hematuria persists or recurs on follow-up urinalyses, then providers should engage patients with shared decision-making regarding repeat evaluation. However, patients who develop gross hematuria or increased severity of microscopic hematuria should be referred for repeat upper and lower tract evaluation.

When to Refer

In the absence of a clear benign etiology (such as an infection, menstruation, vigorous exercise, acute stone event, medical renal disease, viral illness, trauma, or recent urologic procedure), hematuria (either gross or microscopic) requires evaluation.

Ballon-Landa E et al. Diagnostic yield of upper tract imaging performed for hematuria screening: results from a national, privately-insured cohort. Urol Oncol. 2024;42:21.e1. [PMID: 39492009]

Barocas DA et al. Updates to microhematuria: AUA/SUFU guideline (2025). J Urol. 2025;213:547. [PMID: 40013563]

Hayden JP et al. Risk of hematuria-related complications associated with anticoagulant and antiplatelet medications: a single-institution retrospective cohort study. Urology. 2025:197:12. [PMID: 39547280]

Messing EM. Urologist and advanced practice providers evaluating hematuria. Bladder Cancer. 2024;10:161. [PMID: 39131871]

GENITOURINARY TRACT INFECTIONS

Urinary tract infections are among the most common entities encountered in medical practice. In acute infections, a single pathogen is usually found, whereas two or more pathogens are often seen in chronic infections. Coliform bacteria are responsible for most non-nosocomial, uncomplicated UTIs, with *Escherichia coli* being the most common. Such infections typically are sensitive to a wide variety of orally administered antibiotics and respond quickly. Nosocomial infections often are due to more resistant pathogens and may require parenteral antibiotics. Renal infections are of particular concern because if they are inadequately treated, loss of kidney function may result. A urine culture is recommended for patients with suspected UTI and ideally should be obtained prior to the initiation of antibiotic therapy. Previously, a colony count > 10^5/mL was considered the criterion for UTI, though up to 50% of women with symptomatic infections may have lower counts. In addition, *the presence of pyuria correlates poorly with the diagnosis of UTI, and thus UA alone is not adequate for diagnosis*. With respect to treatment, *tissue infections* (pyelonephritis, prostatitis) require therapy for 1–2 weeks, while *mucosal infections* (cystitis) require only 1–3 days of therapy.

1. Acute Cystitis

ESSENTIALS OF DIAGNOSIS

- Irritative voiding symptoms.
- Patient usually afebrile.
- Positive urine culture; blood cultures may also be positive.

General Considerations

Acute cystitis is an infection of the bladder, most commonly due to the coliform bacteria (especially *E coli*) and occasionally gram-positive bacteria (enterococci). The route of infection is typically ascending from the urethra. Viral cystitis due to adenovirus is sometimes seen in children but is rare in immunocompetent adults. *Uncomplicated cystitis in men is rare and implies a pathologic process such as infected stones, prostatitis, or chronic urinary retention requiring further investigation.*

Clinical Findings

A. Symptoms and Signs

Irritative voiding symptoms (frequency, urgency, dysuria) and suprapubic discomfort are common. Women may experience gross hematuria, and symptoms may often appear following sexual intercourse. Physical examination may elicit suprapubic tenderness, but examination is often unremarkable. Systemic toxicity is absent.

B. Laboratory Findings

UA should be without squamous cells, indicating a clean collection, and typically shows pyuria, bacteriuria, and varying degrees of hematuria. The degree of pyuria and bacteriuria does not necessarily correlate with the severity of symptoms. Urine culture is positive for the offending organism, but *colony counts exceeding 10^5/mL are not required for the diagnosis. Patients with asymptomatic bacteriuria or colonization are expected to have positive urine cultures but do not require treatment except in pregnant women.* Patients with long-term urinary catheters (indwelling urinary [Foley] or suprapubic catheter) or urostomy urinary diversions are expected to be colonized with bacteria, and thus, UA and urine culture are most helpful in directing therapy rather than determining whether symptomatic infection exists. Symptoms in these patients include worsening urgency, bladder spasms, leakage around a catheter, and fevers. Malodorous or cloudy urine alone is not necessarily indicative of a UTI.

C. Imaging

Because uncomplicated cystitis is rare in men, appropriate investigation is necessary to elucidate the underlying problem and may include abdominal ultrasonography, postvoid residual testing, and cystoscopy. Follow-up imaging using CT scanning is warranted if pyelonephritis, recurrent infections, or anatomic abnormalities are suspected.

Differential Diagnosis

In women, infectious processes such as vulvovaginitis and pelvic inflammatory disease can usually be distinguished by pelvic examination and UA. In men, urethritis and prostatitis may be distinguished by physical examination (urethral discharge or prostatic tenderness). Bacteriuria on urine culture, in the absence of symptoms, generally should not be treated.

Noninfectious causes of cystitis-like symptoms include pelvic irradiation, chemotherapy (cyclophosphamide), bladder carcinoma, interstitial cystitis, voiding dysfunction disorders, bladder irritants, distal ureteral stone, and psychosomatic disorders.

Prevention

The risk of developing a UTI can be reduced by drinking plenty of fluid and completely emptying the bladder frequently. Women in whom UTIs tend to develop after intercourse may benefit from a single dose of postcoital antibiotic. Voiding before and after sex has *not* been shown to reduce risk of UTI. Postmenopausal women with *recurrent UTIs* (three or more episodes per year) treated with vaginal estrogen either as a cream or ring have a significant reduction in infections. Daily cranberry tablets may reduce the risk of cystitis, though the data are conflicting. Methenamine may be used in some patients. Prophylactic antibiotics are generally discouraged. Prior to institution of antibiotic prophylaxis, a thorough urologic evaluation is warranted to exclude any anatomic abnormality (eg, stones, reflux, fistula, prolapse, urethral diverticula). An initial course of 6–12 months of prophylactic antibiotics can be offered, though the benefits of prophylactic antibiotics should be weighed against the risks associated with expected bacterial resistance.

The risk of acquiring a catheter-associated UTI in hospitalized patients can be minimized by using indwelling catheters only when necessary, implementing systems to ensure removal of catheters when no longer needed, using antimicrobial catheters in high-risk patients, maintaining proper insertion techniques, identifying significant elevated postvoid residuals, and utilizing alternatives such as intermittent catheterization and external collection devices (condom catheters) in appropriately selected men.

Treatment

Uncomplicated cystitis is defined as infection confined to the bladder in women or men. A *complicated UTI* is when infection is not confined to the bladder (pyelonephritis, bacteremia) or in populations with neurogenic bladder, urinary obstruction, or catheter-associated UTIs. This is indicated by symptoms such as fever, chills, rigors, flank pain, and costovertebral angle tenderness.

Uncomplicated UTI in women can be treated with short-term antimicrobial therapy, which consists of a single dose or 1–5 days of therapy. Fosfomycin, nitrofurantoin, and trimethoprim-sulfamethoxazole are the medications of choice for uncomplicated cystitis (Table 26–1). The US Food and Drug Administration (FDA) advises restricting fluoroquinolone use for uncomplicated infections. Gepotidacin is a novel antibiotic that received FDA approval for use in uncomplicated UTIs in 2025. Due to emergence of resistant organisms, local patterns of bacterial resistance should be consulted to identify best treatment options. Literature review has proposed that *acute uncomplicated cystitis in women can be diagnosed without office evaluation or urine culture,* and that appropriate first-line therapies include trimethoprim-sulfamethoxazole (160/800 mg twice daily for 3 days), nitrofurantoin (100 mg twice daily for 5 days), or fosfomycin trometamol (3 g single dose). In men, uncomplicated UTI is less common and is more likely associated with urinary retention; thus, the duration of antibiotic therapy depends on the underlying etiology. Hot sitz baths or urinary analgesics (phenazopyridine, 200 mg orally three times daily) may provide additional symptomatic relief. Postmenopausal women with recurrent cystitis can be treated with vaginal estrogen cream 0.5 g nightly for 2 weeks and then twice weekly thereafter.

Prognosis

Infections typically respond rapidly to therapy, and failure to respond suggests resistance to the selected medication or anatomic abnormalities requiring further investigation.

When to Refer

- Suspicion or radiographic evidence of anatomic abnormality.
- Evidence of urolithiasis.
- Recurrent cystitis due to bacterial persistence.

Table 26–1. Empiric therapy for UTIs.

Diagnosis	Antibiotic	Route	Duration
Acute cystitis[a]			
	First-line:		
	Trimethoprim-sulfamethoxazole, 160/800 mg (one DS tablet) every 12 hours[1]	Oral	3 days
	Nitrofurantoin (macrocrystals), 100 mg every 12 hours	Oral	5 days
	Fosfomycin, 3 g packet once	Oral	1 day
	Second-line:		
	Ciprofloxacin, 250 mg every 12 hours[2]	Oral	3 days
	Levofloxacin, 250–500 mg daily[2]	Oral	3 days
	Alternative agents:		
	Cephalexin, 500 mg every 6–12 hours	Oral	7 days
	Amoxicillin/clavulanate, 500/125 mg every 12 hours	Oral	3 days
	Cefpodoxime, 100 mg every 12 hours	Oral	3 days
Acute pyelonephritis[b]			
	Sepsis:		
	Third- or fourth-generation cephalosporins, carbapenems, piperacillin-tazobactam, fluoroquinolones	Intravenous	7 days
	Without sepsis, IV route:		
	Third- or fourth-generation cephalosporins, piperacillin-tazobactam, or fluoroquinolones	Intravenous	7 days
	Without sepsis, oral route:		
	Ciprofloxacin, 500 mg every 12 hours[2]	Oral	7 days
	Levofloxacin, 750 mg daily[2]	Oral	5 days
	Trimethoprim-sulfamethoxazole, 160/800 mg (one DS tablet) every 12 hours[1]	Oral	7 days
Acute bacterial prostatitis[c]			
	Hospitalized:		
	Piperacillin-tazobactam; third-generation cephalosporin	Intravenous	Until afebrile
	Ampicillin, 2 g every 6 hours, plus gentamicin, 1.5 mg/kg every 8 hours	Intravenous	Until afebrile
	Followed by one of these outpatient oral regimens:		
	Trimethoprim-sulfamethoxazole, 160/800 mg (one DS tablet) every 12 hours[1]	Oral	3 weeks
	Ciprofloxacin, 250–500 mg every 12 hours[2]	Oral	3 weeks
	After prostate biopsy:		
	Carbapenems, amikacin, or second-generation cephalosporins	Intravenous	Until afebrile
Chronic bacterial prostatitis[c]			
	First-line:		
	Ciprofloxacin, 500 mg every 12 hours[2]	Oral	1–3 months
	Levofloxacin, 750 mg daily[2]	Oral	28 days
	Second-line:		
	Doxycycline, 100 mg twice daily	Oral	4–12 weeks
	Azithromycin, 500 mg daily	Oral	4–12 weeks
	Clarithromycin, 500 mg daily	Oral	4–12 weeks

(*continued*)

Table 26–1. Empiric therapy for UTIs. (continued)

Diagnosis	Antibiotic	Route	Duration
Acute epididymitis[d]			
Sexually transmitted (under age 35)	Ceftriaxone, 500 mg as single dose, **plus** Doxycycline, 100 mg every 12 hours	Intramuscular Oral	Once 10 days
Sexually transmitted in men who practice insertive anal sex	Ceftriaxone, 500 mg as single dose, **plus** Levofloxacin, 500 mg daily[2]	Intramuscular Oral	Once 10 days
Non–sexually transmitted, usually enteric organisms (age > 35)	Levofloxacin, 500 mg daily[2]	Oral	10 days

[1]Increasing resistance noted (up to 20%).
[2]FDA advises restricting fluoroquinolone use for some uncomplicated infections, including uncomplicated UTIs, because of mental health side effects including disturbances in attention, disorientation, agitation, nervousness, memory impairment, and delirium; musculoskeletal side effect risks of tendinitis and tendon rupture; neuromuscular side effect of peripheral neuropathy and worsening of myasthenia gravis; and endocrine side effect of coma from hypoglycemia.
[3]Indications: adults with complicated UTI, including pyelonephritis, especially those due to extended-spectrum β-lactamase (ESBL) infections caused by *Escherichia coli, Klebsiella, Pseudomonas, Proteus,* and *Enterobacter.*
[4]Infectious Diseases Society of America (IDSA) recommends an initial 24-hour intravenous dose of antibiotic when local resistance of the selected oral regimen exceeds 10%. Please refer to local antibiograms.
Sources:
[a]Treatment regimens based upon Gupta K et al. Treatment of acute uncomplicated cystitis and pyelonephritis in women: a 2010 update by the Infectious Diseases Society of America and European Society for Microbiology and Infectious Diseases. Clin Infect Dis. 2011;52:e103; and Lee RA et al; Scientific Medical Policy Committee of the American College of Physicians. Appropriate use of short-course antibiotics in common infections: Best Practice Advice From the American College of Physicians. Ann Intern Med. 2021;174:822.
[b]Treatment regimens based on IDSA recommendations for complicated urinary tract infections. Trautner BW et al. Clinical practice guideline by Infectious Diseases Society of America (IDSA): 2025 guideline on management and treatment of complicated urinary tract infections: Selection of antibiotic therapy for complicated UTI. Clin Infect Dis. 2025 Dec 19. [Epub ahead of print]
[c]Treatment regimens based upon Coker TJ et al. Acute bacterial prostatitis: diagnosis and management. Am Fam Physician. 2016;93:114; and Su ZT et al. Management of chronic bacterial prostatitis. Curr Urol Rep. 2020;21:29.
[d]Treatment regimens based upon Workowski KA et al; Centers for Disease Control and Prevention. Sexually transmitted diseases treatment guidelines, 2021. MMWR Recomm Rep. 2021;70:1.

Grant A et al. Management of asymptomatic bacteriuria in noncatheterized adults. Urol Clin North Am. 2024;51:561. [PMID: 39349023]
Kaufman MR et al. The AUA/SUFU/AUGS guideline on genitourinary syndrome of menopause. J Urol. 2025;214:242. [PMID: 40298120]
Kwok M et al. Guidelines of guidelines: management of recurrent urinary tract infections in women. BJU Int. 2022;130:11. [PMID: 35579121]
Nelson Z et al. Guidelines for the prevention, diagnosis, and management of urinary tract infections in pediatrics and adults: a WikiGuidelines Group consensus statement. JAMA Netw Open. 2024;7:e2444495. Erratum in: JAMA Netw Open. 2024;7:e2453497. [PMID: 39495518]
Trautner BW et al. Clinical practice guideline by Infectious Diseases Society of America (IDSA): 2025 guideline on management and treatment of complicated urinary tract infections: selection of antibiotic therapy for complicated UTI. Clin Infect Dis. 2025 Dec 19. [Epub ahead of print] [PMID: 41419213]
Wagenlehner F et al. Oral gepotidacin versus nitrofurantoin in patients with uncomplicated urinary tract infection (EAGLE-2 and EAGLE-3): two randomised, controlled, double-blind, double-dummy, phase 3, non-inferiority trials. Lancet. 2024;403:741. [PMID: 38342126]

2. Acute Pyelonephritis

ESSENTIALS OF DIAGNOSIS

- Fever.
- Flank pain.
- Irritative voiding symptoms.
- Positive urine culture.

General Considerations

Acute pyelonephritis is an infectious inflammatory disease involving the kidney parenchyma and renal pelvis. Gram-negative bacteria are the most common causative agents including *E coli, Proteus, Klebsiella, Enterobacter,* and *Pseudomonas.* Gram-positive bacteria are less commonly seen but include *Enterococcus faecalis* and *Staphylococcus aureus.* The infection usually ascends from the lower urinary tract—with the exception of *S aureus,* which usually is spread by a hematogenous route.

Clinical Findings

A. Symptoms and Signs

Symptoms include rigors, flank pain, shaking chills, and irritative voiding symptoms (urgency, frequency, dysuria). Associated nausea and vomiting and diarrhea are common. Signs include fever and tachycardia. *Costovertebral angle tenderness is usually pronounced.*

B. Laboratory Findings

Complete blood cell count shows leukocytosis and a left shift. UA shows pyuria, bacteriuria, and varying degrees of hematuria. White cell casts may be seen. Urine culture demonstrates growth of the offending organism, and blood culture may also be positive.

C. Imaging

In complicated pyelonephritis, renal ultrasound may show hydronephrosis from a stone or other source of obstruction. CT scan may demonstrate decreased perfusion of the kidney or focal areas within the kidney and nonspecific perinephric fat stranding. Renal abscesses can be seen on CT.

Differential Diagnosis

The differential diagnosis includes acute cystitis or a lower urinary source. Acute intra-abdominal disease such as appendicitis, cholecystitis, pancreatitis, or diverticulitis must be distinguished from pyelonephritis. A normal UA is usually seen in gastrointestinal disorders; however, on occasion, inflammation from adjacent bowel (appendicitis or diverticulitis) may result in hematuria or sterile pyuria. Abnormal liver biochemical tests or elevated amylase levels may assist in the differentiation. Lower-lobe pneumonia is distinguishable by abnormal CXR.

In males, the main differential diagnosis for acute pyelonephritis also includes acute epididymitis and acute prostatitis. Physical examination and the location of the pain should permit this distinction.

Complications

Sepsis with shock can occur with acute pyelonephritis. In diabetic patients, emphysematous pyelonephritis resulting from gas-producing organisms may be life-threatening if not adequately treated. **Obstructive pyelonephritis, for example due to a stone, is a surgical emergency and requires urgent attention.** Healthy adults usually recover complete kidney function, yet if coexistent kidney disease is present, scarring or chronic pyelonephritis may result. Inadequate therapy could result in abscess formation.

Treatment

Urine and blood cultures are obtained to identify the causative agent and to determine antimicrobial sensitivity. In the inpatient setting, broad-spectrum intravenous antibiotics should be initiated until organism sensitivities are available (Table 26–1), with antibiotics adjusted according to sensitivities. Third- or fourth-generation cephalosporins, carbapenems, piperacillin-tazobactam, or fluoroquinolones are the first-line choice for patients with sepsis. For patients without sepsis, third- or fourth-generation cephalosporins, piperacillin-tazobactam, or fluoroquinolones should be the initial selection. Intravenous antibiotics can be transitioned to oral antibiotics in patients who are clinically improving and who are able to tolerate oral medications. Shorter antibiotic courses are now recommended; duration should be 5–7 days for a fluoroquinolone and 7 days for a non-fluoroquinolone. Patients with bacteremia who are improving clinically should be treated for 7 days. In the outpatient setting, empiric therapy may be initiated (Table 26–1). *If local antibiograms demonstrate local resistance rates for the oral regimen exceed 10%, an initial 24-hour intravenous dose of antibiotic is required.* Fevers may persist for up to 72 hours even with appropriate antibiotics; failure to respond within 48 hours warrants imaging (CT or ultrasound) to exclude complicating factors that may require intervention (such as a perinephric abscess or an obstructing stone). Catheter drainage may be necessary in the face of urinary retention and ureteral stent or nephrostomy drainage if there is ureteral obstruction.

Prognosis

With prompt diagnosis and appropriate treatment, acute pyelonephritis carries a good prognosis. Complicating factors, underlying kidney disease, and increasing patient age may lead to a less favorable outcome.

When to Refer

- Evidence of complicating factors (urolithiasis, obstruction).
- Failure of clinical improvement in 48 hours.

When to Admit

- Severe infections or complicating factors, evidence of sepsis, or need for parenteral antibiotics.
- Need for radiographic imaging or drainage of urinary tract obstruction.

Al Lawati H et al. Urinary tract infections: core curriculum 2024. Am J Kidney Dis. 2024;83:90. [PMID: 37906240]

Geyer AC et al. Outcomes of high-dose oral beta-lactam definitive therapy compared to fluoroquinolone or trimethoprim-sulfamethoxazole oral therapy for bacteremia secondary to a urinary tract infection. Antimicrob Steward Healthc Epidemiol. 2023;3:e148. [PMID: 37771747]

Veillette JJ et al. Real-world effectiveness of intravenous and oral antibiotic stepdown strategies for gram-negative complicated urinary tract infection with bacteremia. Open Forum Infect Dis. 2024;11:ofae193. [PMID: 38665174]

3. Acute Bacterial Prostatitis

ESSENTIALS OF DIAGNOSIS

- Fever.
- Irritative voiding symptoms.
- Perineal or suprapubic pain; exquisite tenderness common on rectal examination.
- Positive urine culture.

General Considerations

Acute bacterial prostatitis is usually caused by gram-negative rods, especially *E coli* and *Pseudomonas* species, and less commonly by gram-positive organisms (eg, enterococci). The most likely routes of infection include ascent up the urethra and reflux of infected urine into the prostatic ducts. Lymphatic and hematogenous routes are probably rare.

Clinical Findings

A. Symptoms and Signs

Symptoms may follow chronic dysfunctional voiding, urinary retention, and pushing to urinate. Perineal, sacral, or suprapubic pain, fever, and irritative voiding complaints are common. Varying degrees of obstructive symptoms may occur as the acutely inflamed prostate swells, which may lead to urinary retention. High fevers and a warm and often exquisitely tender prostate are detected on examination. Care should be taken to perform a gentle rectal examination, since vigorous manipulations may result in septicemia. *Prostatic massage is contraindicated.*

B. Laboratory Findings

Complete blood count shows leukocytosis and a left shift. UA shows pyuria, bacteriuria, and varying degrees of hematuria. Urine or expressed prostatic secretions cultures will demonstrate the offending pathogen (Table 26–2).

C. Imaging

Acute prostatitis can progress to prostatic abscess, and a pelvic CT or transrectal ultrasound is indicated in patients who do not respond to antibiotics in 24–48 hours.

Differential Diagnosis

Acute pyelonephritis or acute epididymitis should be distinguishable by the location of pain and physical examination. Acute diverticulitis is occasionally confused with acute prostatitis; however, the history and UA should permit clear distinction. Urinary retention from prostatic enlargement is distinguishable by initial or follow-up rectal examination and postvoid residual bladder scan.

Treatment

Hospitalization may be required, and intravenous antibiotics (piperacillin-tazobactam, ceftriaxone, or oral ciprofloxacin) should be initiated until organism sensitivities are available (Table 26–1). After the patient is afebrile for 24–48 hours, oral antibiotics (ciprofloxacin, levofloxacin, or trimethoprim-sulfamethoxazole) are used to complete 2–4 weeks of therapy. If urinary retention develops, an in-and-out catheterization to relieve the initial obstruction or short-term indwelling urinary catheter is appropriate.

Prognosis

Acute bacterial prostatitis is relatively simple to treat, since bacteria are eradicated with appropriate antibiotic therapy. Progression to chronic bacterial prostatitis is rare.

When to Refer

- Evidence of urinary retention.
- Evidence of chronic prostatitis.

When to Admit

- Signs of sepsis.
- Need for surgical drainage of bladder or prostatic abscess.

Borgert BJ et al. Prostatitis: a review. JAMA. 2025;334:1003. [PMID: 40788632]

Lam JC et al. Acute and chronic prostatitis. Am Fam Physician. 2024;110:45. [PMID: 39028781]

Table 26–2. Clinical characteristics of prostatitis and chronic pelvic pain syndrome (listed in alphabetical order).

Findings	Acute Bacterial Prostatitis	Chronic Bacterial Prostatitis	Chronic Nonbacterial Prostatitis	Chronic Pelvic Pain Syndrome
Expressed prostate secretions	Contraindicated	+ WBC + Culture	+ WBC – Culture	– WBC – Culture
Fever	+	–	–	–
Post–prostatic massage urine specimen	Contraindicated	+ Culture	– Culture	– Culture
Urinalysis	+	–	–	–

4. Chronic Bacterial Prostatitis

ESSENTIALS OF DIAGNOSIS

- Irritative voiding symptoms.
- Perineal or suprapubic discomfort, often dull and poorly localized.
- Abnormal expressed prostatic secretions and positive culture.

General Considerations

Although chronic bacterial prostatitis may evolve from acute bacterial prostatitis or recurrent UTI, *over half of affected men have no history of acute infection*. Gram-negative rods are the most common etiologic agents, but only one gram-positive organism (*Enterococcus*) is associated with chronic infection. Routes of infection are the same as discussed for acute infection.

Clinical Findings

A. Symptoms and Signs

Clinical manifestations are variable. Most patients have varying degrees of irritative voiding symptoms, urethral pain, and obstructive urinary symptoms. Low back and perineal pain are common. Many patients (25–43%) report a history of UTIs. Physical examination is often unremarkable, although the prostate may feel normal, boggy, or indurated. *A postvoid residual urine volume should be measured to evaluate for urinary retention.*

B. Laboratory Findings

UA is normal unless a secondary cystitis is present. *Expressed prostatic secretions* or a *post-prostatic massage voided urine* or both demonstrate increased numbers of leukocytes (> 5–10 per high-power field) and bacterial growth when cultured (Table 26–2). *Culture of the secretions and the post-prostatic massage urine specimen is necessary to make the diagnosis.* Leukocyte and bacterial counts from expressed prostatic secretions do not correlate with severity of symptoms. If no organisms are identified on culture, then nonbacterial prostatitis, chronic pelvic pain, or interstitial cystitis should be suspected.

C. Imaging

Imaging tests are typically not necessary.

Differential Diagnosis

Chronic urethritis may mimic chronic prostatitis, though cultures of the fractionated urine may localize the source of infection to the initial specimen, which comes from the urethra. Cystitis may be secondary to prostatitis, but urine samples after prostatic massage may localize the infection to the prostate. Other chronic prostatic conditions, such as nonbacterial prostatitis, chronic pelvic pain, or interstitial cystitis, are distinguished from chronic bacterial prostatitis by examination and culture of prostatic secretions and post-prostatic massage urine sample. Anal disease may share some of the symptoms of prostatitis, but physical examination should distinguish between the two.

Treatment

As in acute prostatitis, if patients are febrile or systemically ill, they may require admission and initial intravenous therapy with broad-spectrum antibiotics, such as ampicillin plus gentamicin, a third-generation cephalosporin, or a fluoroquinolone (Table 26–1). Therapy would then continue with oral trimethoprim-sulfamethoxazole, fluoroquinolone, or extended-spectrum β-lactamase antibiotic based on culture and sensitivities of expressed prostatic secretion or post-prostatic massage urine. The optimal duration of therapy remains controversial, ranging from 4 to 6 weeks. Symptomatic relief may be provided by anti-inflammatory agents (indomethacin, ibuprofen), hot sitz baths, and α-blockers (tamsulosin, alfuzosin, silodosin).

Prognosis

Chronic bacterial prostatitis may be recurrent, can be difficult to cure, and often requires repeated courses of therapeutic antibiotics.

When to Refer

- Persistent symptoms.
- Consideration of enrollment in clinical trials.

Lam JC et al. Acute and chronic prostatitis. Am Fam Physician. 2024;110:45. [PMID: 39028781]

5. Nonbacterial Chronic Prostatitis/Chronic Pelvic Pain Syndrome

ESSENTIALS OF DIAGNOSIS

- Irritative voiding symptoms.
- Perineal or suprapubic discomfort, similar to that of chronic bacterial prostatitis.
- Presence of WBCs in expressed prostatic secretions but negative culture.

General Considerations

Nonbacterial chronic prostatitis and chronic pelvic pain syndromes are incompletely understood with symptoms due to interrelated cascade of inflammatory, immunologic, endocrine, muscular, neuropathic, and psychological mechanisms. There are a variety of subtypes based on the most pronounced symptoms. Chronic perineal, suprapubic, or pelvic pain is the most common presenting symptom, though men may complain of pain in the testes, groin, and low back. *Pain during or after ejaculation is one of the most prominent and bothersome symptoms in many patients.*

Psychosocial factors (depression, anxiety, catastrophizing, poor social support, stress) also likely play an important role in the exacerbation of chronic pelvic pain symptoms. Because the cause of nonbacterial prostatitis remains unknown, the diagnosis is usually one of exclusion, and treatment may require multimodal therapy. Quality of life is greatly decreased for many patients with chronic nonbacterial prostatitis and chronic pelvic pain syndrome.

Clinical Findings

A. Symptoms and Signs

The clinical presentation is identical to that of chronic bacterial prostatitis; however, no history of UTIs is typically present. The National Institutes of Health Chronic Prostatitis Symptom Index (NIH-CPSI) (https://www.med.unc.edu/menshealth/calculator-international-prostatism-symptom-score-ipss) has been validated to quantify symptoms of chronic nonbacterial prostatitis or chronic pelvic pain syndrome.

B. Laboratory Findings

Increased numbers of leukocytes are typically seen in expressed prostatic secretions, but cultures of both expressed prostatic secretions and post–prostatic urine specimens are negative.

Differential Diagnosis

The major distinction is from chronic bacterial prostatitis. *The absence of positive cultures makes the distinction* (Table 26–2). In older men with irritative voiding symptoms and negative cultures, bladder cancer must be excluded with urinary cytologic examination and cystoscopy.

Treatment

Multimodal therapy is recommended according to the various modes of patient presentation. Patients with voiding symptoms are treated with α-blockers (tamsulosin, alfuzosin, silodosin). Antibiotics are used to treat newly diagnosed, antimicrobial-naive patients. Psychosocial disorders are treated with cognitive behavioral therapy, antidepressants, anxiolytics, and, if necessary, referral to mental health specialists. Neuropathic pain is treated with gabapentinoids, amitriptyline, neuromodulation, acupuncture, and if necessary, referral to a pain management specialist (see Chapter 5). Pelvic floor muscle dysfunction may respond to diazepam, biofeedback, physical therapy (Kegel exercises), pelvic shock wave lithotripsy, and heat therapy. Sexual dysfunction with pain is treated with sexual therapy and phosphodiesterase-5 inhibitors (avanafil, sildenafil, tadalafil, vardenafil). Surgery is not recommended for chronic prostatitis.

Prognosis

Annoying, recurrent symptoms are common, but serious sequelae have not been identified.

Lackner JM et al. Cognitive behavioral therapy for chronic pelvic pain: what is it and does it work? J Urol. 2024;211:539. [PMID: 38228093]

Lai HH et al. Male chronic pelvic pain: AUA guideline: Part II treatment of chronic prostatitis/chronic pelvic pain syndrome. J Urol. 2025;214:127. [PMID: 40243102]

Maeda K et al. A review of current treatments for chronic prostatitis/chronic pelvic pain syndrome under the UPOINTS system. Int J Urol. 2023;30:431. [PMID: 36788717]

Qin Z et al. Comparative efficacy of non-pharmacological management for chronic prostatitis/chronic pelvic pain syndrome: a systematic review and network meta-analysis protocol. BMJ Open. 2024;14:e088848. [PMID: 39627138]

6. Acute Epididymitis

ESSENTIALS OF DIAGNOSIS

- Fever.
- Irritative voiding symptoms.
- Painful enlargement of epididymis.

General Considerations

Most cases of acute epididymitis are infectious and can be divided into one of two categories that have different age distributions and etiologic agents. *Sexually transmitted forms* typically occur in men under age 35 years, are associated with urethritis, and result from *Chlamydia trachomatis* or *Neisseria gonorrhoeae*. Men who practice insertive anal intercourse may have acute epididymitis from sexually transmitted and enteric organisms. *Non–sexually transmitted forms* typically occur in men age 35 years and older, are associated with UTIs and prostatitis, and are caused by enteric gram-negative rods. The route of infection is typically via the urethra to the ejaculatory duct and then down the vas deferens to the epididymis. Amiodarone has been associated with self-limited epididymitis in a dose-dependent phenomenon.

Clinical Findings

A. Symptoms and Signs

Symptoms may follow chronic dysfunctional voiding, urinary retention, urethral catheter placement, sexual activity, or trauma. Associated symptoms of urethritis (pain at the tip of the penis and urethral discharge) or cystitis (irritative voiding symptoms) may occur. Pain develops in the scrotum and may radiate along the spermatic cord or to the flank. Scrotal swelling and tenderness are usually apparent. Severe cases may develop systemic symptoms such as fever. Early in the course, the epididymis may be distinguishable from the testis; however, later the two may appear as one enlarged, tender mass. A reactive hydrocele may develop. The prostate may be tender on rectal examination.

B. Laboratory Findings

A CBC shows leukocytosis and a left shift. In the sexually transmitted variety, Gram staining of a smear of urethral discharge may be diagnostic of gram-negative intracellular diplococci (*N gonorrhoeae*). White cells without visible organisms on urethral smear signify nongonococcal urethritis, and *C trachomatis* is the most likely responsible pathogen. In the non–sexually transmitted variety, UA shows pyuria, bacteriuria, and varying degrees of hematuria. Urine cultures will demonstrate the offending pathogen.

C. Imaging

Scrotal ultrasound may aid in the diagnosis if examination is difficult or if there is uncertainty in the diagnosis.

Differential Diagnosis

Scrotal ultrasound is helpful to define the pathology. Tumors generally cause painless enlargement of the testis. UA is negative, and examination reveals a normal epididymis with a palpable testis mass. Testicular torsion usually occurs in prepubertal males but is occasionally seen in young adults. Acute onset of symptoms and a negative UA favor testicular torsion or torsion of one of the testicular or epididymal appendages. **Prehn sign** (elevation of the scrotum improves pain from epididymitis) may be suggestive but is not reliable in its diagnosis. A distal ureteral stone often presents with referred pain into the ipsilateral groin and scrotum, but the scrotum is not tender to palpation and a scrotal ultrasound is normal.

Treatment

Bed rest, ice, and scrotal elevation are important in the acute phase. Treatment is directed toward the identified pathogen (Table 26–3). The sexually transmitted variety in patients under age 35 is treated with a single intramuscular injection of ceftriaxone 500 mg plus 10 days of oral doxycycline 100 mg twice daily; in addition, *any sexual partners from the preceding 60 days must be evaluated and treated as indicated*. Men who practice insertive anal intercourse receive a single intramuscular injection of ceftriaxone 500 mg and 10 days of oral levofloxacin 500 mg daily to cover sexually transmitted and enteric organisms. Non–sexually transmitted forms are treated for 10 days with oral levofloxacin 500 mg daily. Symptoms and signs of epididymitis that do not improve within 3 days require reevaluation of the diagnosis and therapy.

Prognosis

Prompt treatment usually results in a favorable outcome. If a reactive hydrocele or significant scrotal swelling occurs, it may take > 4 weeks to resolve. Delayed or inadequate treatment may result in epididymoorchitis, decreased fertility, or abscess formation.

When to Refer

- Persistent symptoms and infection despite antibiotic therapy.
- Signs of sepsis or abscess formation.

Centers for Disease Control and Prevention (CDC). 2021 Sexually Transmitted Disease Treatment Guidelines: Epididymitis. 2021. Accessed September 17, 2025. https://www.cdc.gov/std/treatment-guidelines/epididymitis.htm

Khastgir J. Advances in the antibiotic management of epididymitis. Expert Opin Pharmacother. 2022;23:1103. [PMID: 35380486]

INTERSTITIAL CYSTITIS

ESSENTIALS OF DIAGNOSIS

- Pain with bladder filling; urinary urgency and frequency.
- Submucosal petechiae or ulcers on cystoscopic examination.
- Diagnosis of exclusion.

General Considerations

Interstitial cystitis (painful bladder syndrome) is characterized by pain with bladder filling that is relieved by emptying and is often associated with urgency and frequency with a dramatic exaggeration of normal sensations. This is a diagnosis of exclusion, and patients must have a negative urine culture and cytology and no other obvious cause such as radiation cystitis, chemical cystitis (cyclophosphamide), vaginitis, urethral diverticulum, or genital herpes. Up to 40% of patients referred to urologists for interstitial cystitis

Table 26–3. Recommended treatment regimens for epididymitis.

Condition	Treatment Regimen
For acute epididymitis most likely caused by chlamydia or gonorrhea	Ceftriaxone 500 mg[1] intramuscularly in single dose **plus** Doxycycline 100 mg orally twice daily for 10 days
For acute epididymitis most likely caused by chlamydia, gonorrhea, or enteric organisms (seen in men who practice insertive anal sex)	Ceftriaxone 500 mg[1] intramuscularly in single dose **plus** Levofloxacin 500 mg orally once daily for 10 days
For acute epididymitis most likely caused by enteric organisms only	Levofloxacin 500 mg orally once daily for 10 days

[1]For persons weighing ≥ 150 kg, 1 g of ceftriaxone should be administered.

Modified from "Recommended Regimens for Epididymitis," in the section on "Epididymitis" from the Division of STD Prevention, National Center for HIV, Viral Hepatitis, STD, and TB Prevention, Centers for Disease Control and Prevention, https://www.cdc.gov/std/treatment-guidelines/epididymitis.htm.

may actually be found to have a different diagnosis after careful evaluation. *What was once considered a bladder disorder is now considered a chronic pain syndrome.*

Population-based studies have demonstrated a prevalence between 18 and 40 per 100,000 people. Both sexes are involved, but most patients are women, with a mean age of 40 years at onset. Patients with interstitial cystitis are more likely to report bladder problems in childhood, especially women. Up to 50% of patients may experience spontaneous remission of symptoms, with a mean duration of 8 months without treatment.

The etiology of interstitial cystitis is unknown, and it is most likely not a single disease but rather several diseases with similar symptoms. Associated diagnoses include severe allergies, irritable bowel syndrome, and inflammatory bowel disease. Theories regarding the cause of interstitial cystitis include increased epithelial permeability, neurogenic causes (sensory nervous system abnormalities), and autoimmunity.

Clinical Findings

A. Symptoms and Signs

Pain, pressure, or discomfort with bladder filling that is relieved with urination, and urgency, frequency, and nocturia are the most common symptoms. Patients should be asked about exposure to pelvic radiation or treatment with cyclophosphamide. Examination should exclude genital herpes, vaginitis, or a urethral diverticulum. Baseline voiding symptoms and pain levels should be obtained to measure subsequent treatment effects.

B. Laboratory Findings

UA, urine culture, and urinary cytology are obtained to examine for infectious causes and bladder malignancy; in interstitial cystitis, they are all normal. Urodynamic testing can be done to assess bladder sensation and compliance and to exclude detrusor instability.

C. Cystoscopy

Cystoscopy should be considered with the diagnosis is in doubt and may reveal glomerulations (submucosal hemorrhage) with hydrodistention of the bladder. Total bladder capacity should be determined. Biopsy of any suspicious lesions should be performed to exclude other causes such as carcinoma, eosinophilic cystitis, and tuberculous cystitis. The presence of submucosal mast cells is *not* needed to make the diagnosis of interstitial cystitis.

Differential Diagnosis

Exposures to radiation or cyclophosphamide are discovered by the history. Bacterial cystitis, genital herpes, or vaginitis can be excluded by UA, culture, and physical examination. A urethral diverticulum may be suspected if palpation of the urethra demonstrates an indurated mass that results in the expression of pus from the urethral meatus. Urethral carcinoma presents as a firm mass on palpation.

Treatment

There is no cure for interstitial cystitis, but most patients achieve symptomatic relief from one of several approaches. Initial treatment should be nonsurgical. Multimodal pain management approaches (pharmacology, stress management, physical therapy) should be initiated. Behavioral/nonpharmacologic treatments include patient education and cognitive behavioral therapy, self-care practices and behavioral modifications, stress management, and manual physical therapy techniques (focused on trigger points, relaxing spastic muscles, scar stretching). Oral pharmacology for pain management should be similar to that for other chronic pain conditions and may include acetaminophen, NSAIDs, opioids (rarely), and urinary analgesics. Amitriptyline, cimetidine, hydroxyzine, pentosan polysulfate sodium (though with the risk of macular damage and vision-related injuries), and silodosin have each demonstrated efficacy in patients with interstitial cystitis. Oral cyclosporine A may be offered for patients with Hunner lesions identified on cystoscopy refractory to fulguration. Intravesical instillations of dimethyl sulfoxide (DMSO), heparin, lidocaine, or a combination of those may also be beneficial.

Hydrodistention is a procedure in which the bladder is filled with short-duration, low-pressure fluid and allowed to stretch under anesthesia; approximately 20–30% of patients will notice symptomatic improvement that lasts 3–6 months. If Hunner lesions are present they can be fulgurated or injected with triamcinolone. Patients with very small bladder capacities (< 200 mL) are unlikely to respond to medical therapy.

Therapies that should *not* be offered include long-term antibiotics, systemic long-term glucocorticoid administration, intravesical instillation of bacillus Calmette-Guérin (BCG), or high-pressure long-duration hydrodistention.

If other treatments have not provided adequate improvement in symptoms and quality of life, further treatment modalities include intradetrusor onabotulinumtoxin A injections (though with the risk of temporary urinary retention requiring self-catheterization) or trial of neuromodulation. Major surgery for interstitial cystitis should be considered only as a last resort and may require cystourethrectomy with urinary diversion.

When to Refer

Persistent and bothersome symptoms in the absence of identifiable cause.

Buford K et al. Global consensus on interstitial cystitis/bladder pain syndrome: an update on therapeutic treatments. Obstet Gynecol Surv. 2025;80:694. [PMID: 41194362]

Chermansky CJ et al. Pharmacologic management of interstitial cystitis/bladder pain syndrome. Urol Clin North Am. 2022; 49:273. [PMID: 35428433]

Homma Y et al. Definition change and update of clinical guidelines for interstitial cystitis and bladder pain symptoms. Low Urin Tract Symptoms. 2024:16:e12532 [PMID: 39267358]

Masterson JM et al. Pathophysiology and clinical biomarkers in interstitial cystitis. Urol Clin North Am. 2023;50:39. [PMID: 36424082]

Park JJ et al. Current updates relating to treatment for interstitial cystitis/bladder pain syndrome: systematic review and network meta-analysis. BMC Urol. 2024;24:95. [PMID: 38658949]

Yu WR et al. The pathomechanism and current treatments for chronic interstitial cystitis and bladder pain syndrome. Biomedicines. 2024;12:2051. [PMID: 39335564]

URINARY STONE DISEASE

ESSENTIALS OF DIAGNOSIS

- Severe flank pain, nausea, and vomiting.
- Fever, infection with obstruction, renal failure.
- Identification on noncontrast CT or ultrasonography.

General Considerations

Urinary stone disease is exceeded in frequency as a urinary tract disorder only by infections and prostatic disease. It affects approximately 1 in 10 Americans per year, representing an approximately threefold relative increase over the prior three decades. Historically men have been much more frequently affected by urolithiasis than women; however, more recently, the prevalence in women has increased 45% (from 6.5% up to 9.4%) while the prevalence in men has remained slightly higher but stable (11.9%). *This persistent increase in prevalence in women has been attributed to increasing obesity and metabolic syndrome rates.* Initial presentation usually occurs in the third through fifth decades, and > 50% of patients will become recurrent stone formers.

There are five major types of urinary stones: **calcium oxalate**, **calcium phosphate**, **struvite (magnesium ammonium phosphate)**, **uric acid**, and **cystine.** The most common types are those composed of calcium oxalate or phosphate (85%), and for that reason most urinary stones are radiopaque on plain abdominal radiographs. Uric acid stones may be radiolucent if pure or partially radiopaque if mixed with calcium. Cystine and struvite stones are faintly visible on radiographs.

Geographic factors contribute to the development of stones. *High humidity and elevated temperatures are contributing factors*, and the incidence of symptomatic ureteral stones is greatest in such areas during hot summer months. Climate change is projected to further increase the burden of disease for individuals and society. Higher incidence of stones has also been associated with sedentary lifestyle, obesity, hypertension, insulin resistance and poor glycemic control, carotid calcification, and cardiovascular disease.

Many commonly prescribed medications increase the risk of formation of kidney stones, including carbonic anhydrase inhibitors (topiramate, zonisamide, acetazolamide), systemic corticosteroids (prednisone), antiretroviral protease inhibitors (indinavir and others), gout medications (probenecid), diuretics (furosemide, bumetanide, torsemide, triamterene), decongestants (guaifenesin, ephedrine), and laxatives (if abused for weight loss). The risk of stones from calcium supplementation is controversial. Thus, if calcium supplementation is medically necessary, it is recommended that the calcium supplement be taken with meals, and that total calcium intake (diet plus supplementation) not exceed 2000 mg daily. Dietary calcium intake should not be restricted unless excessive (> 2000 mg daily). Several large studies of the novel antidiabetic SGLT-2 inhibitors and GLP-1 agonists have demonstrated their safety in patients with kidney stones, with convincing evidence SGLT-2 inhibitors reduce the risk of stones by nearly 40%.

Inadequate hydration is a very important dietary factor in the development of urinary stones for essentially all stone formers. Stone formation requires saturation of the urine with minerals, and increasing fluid intake dilutes the urine, decreasing the risk of new stone formation and stone growth. Excess animal protein and salt intake (> 3500 mg daily) and restricted dietary calcium intake also increase the risk of stones.

Genetic factors may contribute to urinary stone formation. While approximately 50% of calcium-based stones are thought to have a heritable component, other stone types are better characterized genetically. **Cystinuria** is an autosomal recessive disorder where homozygous individuals have markedly increased excretion of cystine and frequently have numerous recurrent episodes of urinary stones. Distal renal tubular acidosis may be transmitted as a hereditary trait, and urolithiasis occurs in up to 75% of affected patients.

Clinical Findings

A. Symptoms and Signs

Obstructing urinary stones usually present with acute, unremitting, and severe colic. Pain most often occurs suddenly, is typically localized to the flank, and may be associated with nausea and vomiting. In sharp contrast to patients with an acute abdomen, *patients with kidney stones are constantly moving*, trying to find a comfortable position. The pain may occur episodically and may radiate anteriorly over the abdomen. As the stone progresses down the ureter, the pain may be referred into the ipsilateral groin, and when the stone reaches the distal ureter near the bladder, patients may complain of marked urinary urgency, frequency, and dysuria. In men, pain may radiate to the tip of the penis; this can be confused as a symptom of a UTI. After the stone passes into the bladder, there is immediate relief of symptoms, then *the stone passes harmlessly through the urethra.* Stone size does not correlate with the severity of the symptoms but does impact the duration and likelihood of successfully passing. If the stone fails to pass and obstruction persists, patients may note a deceptive improvement in symptoms. As many as 25% of patients with resolution of pain will have a persistent stone, and thus, it is recommended patients strain their urine and *follow-up imaging is recommended in all patients if the stone has not been witnessed to pass.*

B. Laboratory Findings

Regardless of symptom severity, UA usually reveals microscopic or gross hematuria (~ 90%). However, the absence of microhematuria does not exclude urinary stones. A single spot urine pH should be interpreted cautiously due to significant fluctuations throughout the day, although a persistent urinary pH < 5.5 may suggest a uric acid stone, while a persistent urinary pH > 7.2 may suggest a struvite (infection-related) or calcium phosphate stone. Patients with an obstructing stone should be evaluated with serum white blood count, electrolytes, renal function, and UA to assess for obstruction with infection, renal insufficiency, or renal failure with electrolyte abnormalities. *Fever or other signs of infection are an indication for urgent intervention with a drainage procedure (ureteral stent or nephrostomy tube) to relieve the obstruction.*

C. Metabolic Evaluation

Stone analysis can facilitate counseling for prevention of recurrence. Patients with uncomplicated first-time stones should undergo dietary counseling as outlined below and can be offered an optional complete metabolic evaluation.

General dietary counseling includes encouraging patients to augment their fluid intake to increase their urine volume (goal urinary output of > 2500 mL/day). This typically requires a fluid intake of 3000 mL/day or more. Stone formers should reduce their sodium intake (goal < 3500 mg/day) and animal protein intake (eggs, fish, chicken, pork, and beef). Stone formers should be encouraged to increase their fruit and vegetable intake but *not* to restrict dietary calcium. Detailed medical and dietary history, serum chemistries, and UA should be obtained for all patients with newly diagnosed nephrolithiasis. A serum parathyroid hormone level should be checked when hyperparathyroidism is suspected as the cause of calcium oxalate or calcium phosphate stones, and a serum uric acid should be obtained to exclude severe hyperuricemia, which can lead to uric acid stones as well as crystal deposition in the kidneys or heart.

A 24-hour urine collection to determine urinary volume, creatinine, pH, calcium, uric acid, oxalate, phosphate, sodium, and citrate excretion is recommended for interested patients with their first stone, for all patients who have recurrent stones, and for patients at high risk for recurrence. Results are used to personalize medical management to individual patient risk factors.

D. Imaging

Noncontrast CT is the most accurate imaging modality for evaluating flank pain given its superior sensitivity and specificity over other tests; however, ultrasonography (which does not use ionizing radiation) is a safe and effective alternative for initial evaluation of renal colic and one that can be used in the emergency department with good accuracy. CT scans should be obtained in the prone position to help differentiate distal ureterovesicular stones from those that have already passed into the urinary bladder. A "low-dose" imaging protocol should be used when available, and repeated CT scans should be minimized due to the substantial cumulative radiation exposure faced by people who form stones recurrently. Stone density can be estimated with Hounsfield units (HU) on CT scans to help determine stone type. All stones, whether radiopaque or radiolucent on plain abdominal radiographs, will be visible on noncontrast CT except the rare calculus caused by a protease inhibitor, or crystalized medication (guaifenesin, triamterene, ciprofloxacin). A plain abdominal radiograph (kidney, ureter, and bladder [KUB]) and renal ultrasound examination will diagnose up to 80% of stones. *Since > 60% of patients with acute renal colic will have a stone in the distal 4 cm of the ureter, attention should be directed to that region when examining radiographs and ultrasonographic studies.* Pain from a kidney stone is due to the dilatation of the ureter and kidney from the obstruction, and thus small nonobstructing kidney stones are typically not associated with pain.

Medical Treatment & Prevention

To reduce the recurrence rate of urinary stones, dietary modification is key. Metabolic evaluation often identifies a modifiable risk factor that can further reduce stone recurrence rates. If no medical treatment is provided, stones will generally recur in 50% of patients within 5 years. Some stone types (eg, uric acid, cystine, brushite, struvite) are prone to rapid recurrence. *Consistent increased fluid intake to dilute the urine and prevent dehydration is the most important dietary risk factor to reduce stone recurrence and may diminish the risk by 50%.* Increasing fluid intake to ensure a voided volume of 2.5 L/day is recommended (normal average voided volume is 1.6 L/day). Urine should be clear or light yellow at each void. Medical therapy should be tailored to the patient's metabolic workup and the activity of their stone disease. Routine follow-up every 6–8 months and annual imaging (ultrasonography with or without kidney, ureters, bladder x-ray) will help encourage medical compliance, assess for interval stone formation or growth, and permit adjustments in medical therapy based on repeat metabolic studies.

A. General Dietary Recommendations

A 24-hour urinary sodium level of > 150 mmol/day indicates excessive sodium intake. Sodium intake should be limited to < 3500 mg daily. Excessive sodium intake will increase renal sodium and calcium excretion, increase urinary monosodium urates (a nidus for stone growth), increase the relative saturation of calcium phosphate, and decrease urinary citrate excretion. All of these factors encourage stone growth.

A urinary sulfate level of > 20 mEq/day indicates excessive animal protein intake. Animal protein intake is best limited to 1 g/kg/day. Excess intake leads to acidic urine, increases urinary calcium, oxalate, and uric acid excretion, and decreases urinary citrate excretion. *Patients should be reminded that animal protein includes animal flesh such as eggs and fish in addition to traditional "red meat."*

Dietary calcium intake should not be restricted because it may paradoxically lead to increased stone formation due to increased oxalate absorption, consequent hyperoxaluria, and increased risk of stones.

Patients should be encouraged to increase dietary fruit, vegetable, and fiber intake as this may increase urinary citrate, provides dietary alkali, and likely replaces consumption of higher-risk foods like animal protein.

B. Calcium Nephrolithiasis

1. Hypercalciuria—Elevated urinary calcium levels (> 4 mg/kg/day or > 250 mg/day for males and > 200 mg/day for females) lead to hypercalciuric calcium nephrolithiasis. After primary hyperparathyroidism has been excluded based on serum calcium and PTH testing, thiazide diuretics should be prescribed since they decrease renal calcium excretion in patients with high urinary calcium and recurrent calcium stones. Chlorthalidone and indapamide are first-line agents since they can be administered once a day, while hydrochlorothiazide for hypercalciuria must be administered twice a day. Despite some evidence questioning the efficacy of thiazides in stone prevention, they remain a mainstay of kidney stone prevention. All patients respond to thiazide diuretics with decreases in urinary calcium unless they have primary hyperparathyroidism or are nonadherent with taking the medication. Clinicians should periodically test patients taking thiazide diuretics for hypokalemia. Patients should be encouraged to increase their dietary potassium intake by focusing on greater fruit and vegetable intake, and if insufficient, some patients may require potassium supplementation. Patients with hypercalciuria are at risk of bone mineral density problems due to the excessive calcium losses in the urine, though treatment with thiazide diuretics can halt and increase bone density 1% per year while receiving therapy.

2. Hypocitraturia—Urinary citrate is the most important inhibitor of stone formation. Urinary citrate binds to calcium, decreasing available calcium for precipitation and subsequent stone formation. Low urine citrate levels (< 450 mg/day) increase the risk of stones. **Hypocitraturic calcium nephrolithiasis** is usually idiopathic. Hypocitraturia can occur secondary to any systemic metabolic acidemia (chronic diarrhea, bowel disease, distal renal tubular acidosis) or with low serum potassium levels (thiazide or loop diuretics, diarrhea, vomiting). Usually, effective treatment in these situations is potassium citrate supplementation: a typical dose is 40–60 mEq total daily intake, divided into two or three daily doses. Alternatively, there are over-the-counter drinks such as lemonade and orange juice that have been shown to modestly increase urinary citrate. However, they must be consumed in fairly large quantities and can contain tremendous calories if not consumed as part of a varied diet. Several supplements have been rigorously tested and are available as an alternative to prescription potassium citrate (Moonstone powder, LithoLyte powder, Kidney COP, KSP tabs, LithoBalance, NOW potassium citrate capsules, TheraLith XR) with varying levels of citrate, alkali, and cost.

3. Hyperoxaluria—**Hyperoxaluric calcium nephrolithiasis** (> 40 mg/day of urinary oxalate) is usually due to either an intestinal malabsorption disorder or a mismatch in dietary calcium and oxalate intake. Patients with a history of chronic diarrhea, inflammatory bowel disease, malabsorption, or gastric bypass surgery are at risk for hyperoxaluria. In these disorders, dietary calcium is bound forming a soap-like product due to increased intestinal fat or bile (or both) preventing calcium from binding with dietary oxalate, leading to free oxalate absorption. Even a small increase in free oxalate absorption significantly increases risk of stone formation. If the process cannot be effectively curtailed, oral calcium should be increased with meals, either by diet or by taking low-dose calcium carbonate supplements (250 mg). When dietary calcium and oxalate are consumed concurrently they bind together in the intestinal tract and are unable to be absorbed systemically. But if dietary calcium is restricted, or if dietary oxalate is excessive, free oxalate is rapidly absorbed and excreted in the urine, leading to hyperoxaluric calcium nephrolithiasis. Treatment includes adhering to a diet containing moderate calcium intake (1000–1200 mg daily). Treatment also involves avoiding high-oxalate-containing foods including potatoes, cocoa powder and chocolate, beets, spinach, rhubarb, Swiss chard, nuts of all types, and soy products. Patients with excess urinary oxalate levels should be reminded to avoid soy milk and nut-based products (peanut butter, almond milk). Patients with lactose intolerance may select rice milk, oat milk, and hemp milk. NOTE: High-dose ascorbic acid (> 2000 mg/day) will substantially increase urinary oxalate levels.

4. Hyperuricosuria—**Hyperuricosuric calcium nephrolithiasis** is defined by elevated urinary uric acid levels (> 800 mg/day for males and > 750 mg/day for females). It is usually secondary to dietary purine excess or endogenous uric acid metabolic defects. Excess uric acid in the urine can lead to uric acid stones if the urine pH is low, or to calcium stones if a crystal forms and then calcifies. Dietary purine restriction can reduce hyperuricosuria in 85% of cases. Patients with hyperuricosuria, normocalciuria, and recurrent calcium oxalate stones can be successfully treated with allopurinol. *However, allopurinol is* not *first-line treatment of uric acid stones; urinary alkalinization is first-line therapy (see below).*

C. Uric Acid Calculi

Urinary pH is the most important contributor to uric acid stone formation, and thus first-line efforts to prevent uric acid stones should focus on alkalinizing the urine with oral potassium citrate or sodium bicarbonate. Efforts to decrease urinary uric acid (with allopurinol 300 mg/day orally) should be reserved for patients continuing to form stones *despite* adequate urinary alkalinization and hydration. In patients who form pure uric acid stones, urine pH is consistently < 5.5. Increasing the urinary pH dramatically increases uric acid solubility, leading to prevention of stone formation (with urine pH > 6.0) and to stone dissolution (with urine pH > 6.5). *Nitrazine pH test strips* (which turn blue with alkaline urine pH > 6.0) are often useful to some patients in reinforcing adherence to urinary alkalinization efforts. Less common contributors to uric acid stone formation include hyperuricemia, myeloproliferative disorders, chemotherapy for malignancies with rapid cell turnover or cell death, abrupt and dramatic weight loss, and uricosuric medications (probenecid).

D. Struvite Calculi

Struvite stones are composed of magnesium-ammonium-phosphate and are faintly visible on plain radiographs. They are most common in women with recurrent UTIs and patients with chronic bladder catheters and are due to urease-producing organisms, including *Proteus*, *Pseudomonas*, *Providencia*, and, less commonly, *Klebsiella*, *Staphylococcus*, and *Mycoplasma* (but not *E coli*). Clinically, they rarely present with colic from a ureteral stone. Instead, a struvite stone is discovered as a large staghorn calculus forming a cast of the renal collecting system and is often associated with recurrent UTIs with the same organism. Urinary pH is high, routinely above 7.2. Appropriate perioperative antibiotics are required prior to removal. They can recur rapidly, and efforts should be taken to remove all of the stone and then to prevent further UTIs and reduce bacterial colonization levels. Some patients who develop recurrent struvite stones benefit from methenamine 1 g twice daily plus vitamin C 500 mg twice daily to suppress bacterial growth. Cases that recur despite methenamine and vitamin C may require a daily prophylactic antibiotic or acetohydroxamic acid, which is typically reserved for refractory cases that have not responded to other treatments as the medication is often poorly tolerated and has a significant side-effect profile.

E. Cystine Calculi

Cystine stones are caused by a genetic metabolic defect resulting in abnormal excretion of cystine. These stones are exceptionally challenging to manage medically. Prevention involves markedly increasing fluid intake during the day and night to achieve a urinary volume of 3–4 L/day, decreasing sodium and dietary cystine intake, and increasing urinary alkalinization (typically with high-dose potassium citrate) with a goal urinary pH > 7.0. Refractory stone formers may be treated with disulfide inhibitors such as tiopronin (α-mercaptoproprionylglycine) or penicillamine. There are no known inhibitors of cystine calculi.

Medical Expulsion & Surgical Treatment

Signs of infection, including associated fever, tachycardia, hypotension, and elevated WBC count, may indicate a UTI behind the obstructing stone. **Any obstructing stone with associated infection is a medical emergency requiring urology consultation and prompt drainage of the kidney with a ureteral stent or a percutaneous nephrostomy tube.** Antibiotics alone are inadequate and only used as an adjunct to drainage of the infected urine behind the obstruction.

In the acute setting, forcing intravenous fluids will not push stones down the ureter. Forced diuresis is counterproductive, as it exacerbates pain and can lead to fluid overload; instead, a euvolemic state should be achieved with many patients requiring some resuscitation due to dehydration from nausea and vomiting.

A. Ureteral Stones

Ureteral stones are usually discovered at three sites: the ureteropelvic junction, the crossing of the ureter over the iliac artery, or the ureterovesicular junction. Stones smaller than 5–6 mm in diameter usually pass spontaneously. **Medical expulsive therapy** with α-blockers (eg, tamsulosin 0.4 mg orally once daily) in combination with an anti-inflammatory agent (eg, ibuprofen 600 mg orally three times per day), with or without a short course of a low-dose oral corticosteroid (eg, prednisone 10 mg orally daily for 5–10 days), may increase the rate of spontaneous stone passage and appears to be most effective for distal stones > 5 mm. Patients should be advised that this use of α-blockers is common but off-label. *Attempted medical expulsive therapy with effective pain medications and imaging follow-up are appropriate for a few weeks. If the stone fails to pass within 4 weeks, the patient has fever, intolerable pain, or persistent nausea or vomiting, or the patient must return to work or anticipates travel, then surgical intervention is indicated.*

Stones in the mid and distal ureter that require surgical removal are best managed with ureteroscopy. Ureteroscopic stone treatment is an outpatient procedure typically performed under general anesthesia involving placement of a small endoscope through the urethra and bladder and into the ureter. Under direct vision, basket extraction or laser fragmentation is performed. Recent evidence supports concurrent treatment of additional kidney stones at the time of ureteral stone treatment, as it dramatically reduces the risk of relapse. A ureteral stent is often placed temporarily to allow drainage of the kidney while the swelling and inflammation from the stone and procedure resolve.

Extracorporeal shock wave lithotripsy (SWL) can be offered as second-line therapy. SWL utilizes an external energy source focused on the stone with the aid of fluoroscopy or ultrasonography. SWL is typically performed under anesthesia or sedation as an outpatient procedure with the goal of stone fragmentation. Stone fragments then pass within a few weeks. Occasionally, the stone fails to fragment adequately and residual fragments obstruct the ureter. Conservative management usually results in spontaneous resolution of the obstruction with eventual passage of the stone fragments. Fragments that have not passed within 6 weeks are unlikely to do so without intervention. SWL is strictly contraindicated in patients who are pregnant, have untreated UTI, have uncorrected coagulopathy, or must continue receiving anticoagulant or antiplatelet therapy. A ureteral stent is typically not necessary with SWL.

Proximal ureteral stones can be treated with SWL or ureteroscopy. SWL is less successful with stones that are larger, dense, or deep. In cases of SWL failure, ureteroscopic treatment is required.

B. Renal Calculi

Patients with small, asymptomatic, nonobstructing renal calculi, without UTI or obstruction, may not warrant surgical treatment. *If surveillance is undertaken, the patient should be monitored with serial abdominal radiographs or renal ultrasonographic examinations every 3–12 months.* If the calculi grow or become symptomatic, intervention is indicated. SWL is most effective for stones < 1 cm in the lower pole of the kidney or < 2 cm elsewhere in the kidney. SWL is less effective for stones that are very hard (cystine, brushite, calcium oxalate stones > 1000–1200 Hounsfield units on CT scan) and for obese patients (skin-to-stone distance > 10–12 cm). SWL is discouraged in staghorn and infectious stones. Ureteroscopy and **laser lithotripsy** are effective for multiple stones and larger stones, although very large stones may require multiple treatment sessions. New vacuum aspiration sheaths and scopes have expanded the limits of ureteroscopic treatment of stones, allowing fragments and dust to be removed. This has resulted in improved visualization and clearance of infectious stone material, reducing residual fragment retention and allowing larger stones to be treated in a single setting. As laser lithotripsy is performed with direct vision, stones tend to be more completely fragmented. Stones > 20 mm and staghorn calculi (large, branched stones occupying at least two renal calices) are best treated via **percutaneous nephrolithotomy**. Percutaneous nephrolithotomy is performed by inserting a needle into the appropriate renal calyx and dilating a tract large enough to allow a nephroscope to pass directly into the kidney. Larger and more complex renal stones can be identified, fragmented, and removed. In unusual cases, laparoscopic, robotic-assisted, or open stone removal may be considered.

When to Refer

- Evidence of urinary obstruction.
- Urinary stone with associated flank pain.
- Anatomic abnormalities, solitary kidney, or CKD.
- Larger stones (approximately 6 mm or larger) including staghorn stones.
- Concomitant pyelonephritis or recurrent UTI.

When to Admit

- Intractable nausea and vomiting or pain.
- Obstructing stone with fever or other signs of infection.

Bargagli M et al. Kidney stone disease: risk factors, pathophysiology and management. Nat Rev Nephrol. 2025;21:794. [PMID: 40790363]

Hsi RS et al. Thiazide dose, urine calcium, and symptomatic kidney stone events. JAMA Netw Open. 2024;7:e2428953. [PMID: 39172453]

Kaufman J et al. The impact of heat on kidney stone presentations in South Carolina under two climate change scenarios. Sci Rep. 2022;12:369. [PMID: 35013464]

Paik JM et al. Sodium-glucose cotransporter 2 inhibitors and nephrolithiasis risk in patients with type 2 diabetes. JAMA Intern Med. 2024;184:265. [PMID: 38285598]

Pearle MS et al. Surgical management of kidney and ureteral stones: AUA guideline (2026) Part I: Evaluation and treatment of patients with kidney and/or ureteral stones. J Urol. 2026;215:113. [PMID: 41263323]

Shastri S et al. Kidney stone pathophysiology, evaluation and management: core curriculum 2023. Am J Kidney Dis 2023;82:617. [PMID: 37565942]

Sorensen MD et al. Removal of small, asymptomatic kidney stones and incidence of relapse. N Engl J Med. 2022;387:506. [PMID: 35947709]

Spiardi R et al. Role of climate change in urologic health: kidney stone disease. Eur Urol Focus. 2023;9:866. [PMID: 37839975]

MALE SEXUAL DYSFUNCTION & ERECTILE DYSFUNCTION

ESSENTIALS OF DIAGNOSIS

- Erectile dysfunction is a common condition that negatively impacts quality of life when left untreated.
- Most erectile dysfunction is related to underlying medical issues, *may be an early sign of cardiovascular disease*, and requires evaluation.
- Peyronie disease is a common disorder caused by scar formation within the erectile bodies of the penis resulting in pain, penile deformity, and sexual dysfunction.
- Peyronie disease is treatable by intralesional medication, surgery, or a combination of both, but is not responsive to oral medications.

General Considerations

Male sexual dysfunction manifests in a variety of ways, and patient history is critical to proper classification and treatment. **Erectile dysfunction** is the consistent inability to attain or maintain a sufficiently rigid penile erection for sexual intercourse. *More than half of men aged 40–70 years have erectile dysfunction, and its incidence increases with age.* Normal male erection relies on intact autonomic and somatic nerves to the penis, arterial blood flow supplied by the cavernosal arteries, and smooth and striated musculature of the corpora cavernosa and pelvic floor. Erection is initiated by nerve impulses in the parasympathetic fibers to the pelvic plexus, which lead to an increase in arterial flow, active relaxation of the smooth muscle within the sinusoids of the corpora cavernosa, and an increase in venous resistance. Contraction of the ischiocavernosus muscle causes further rigidity of the penis with intracavernosal pressures exceeding systolic blood pressure. Nitric oxide is the key neurotransmitter that initiates and sustains erections. Loss of erections may result from neurogenic, arterial, venous, hormonal, or psychological causes. Concurrent medical problems may damage one or more of the mechanisms.

The most common cause of erectile dysfunction is a decrease in arterial flow resultant from progressive vascular disease. Endothelial dysfunction results from the decreased bioavailability of nitric oxide with subsequent impairment of arterial vasodilation. *Erectile dysfunction may be an early manifestation of systemic endothelial dysfunction, which precedes more severe atherosclerotic CVD and should be considered a risk-enhancing factor for CVD.* Many medications, especially antihypertensive, antidepressant, and opioid agents, are associated with erectile dysfunction.

Anejaculation is the absence of seminal emission, which may result from androgen deficiency by decreasing prostate and seminal vesicle secretions, or by sympathetic denervation due to spinal cord injury, diabetes mellitus, or iatrogenic injury secondary to pelvic or retroperitoneal surgery or radiation. **Retrograde ejaculation** may occur as a result of mechanical disruption of the bladder neck due to congenital abnormalities, transurethral prostate surgery, pelvic radiation, sympathetic denervation, or treatment with α-blockers. **Premature ejaculation** refers to ejaculation with minimal stimulation and before a person desires, which may cause significant distress. Primary premature ejaculation may be treated with behavioral modification, sexual health counseling, topical desensitizing agents, and systemic medications used alone or in combination. Secondary premature ejaculation is due to erectile dysfunction and responds to treatment of the underlying disorder. **Peyronie disease** is a fibrotic disorder of the tunica albuginea of the penis resulting in varying degrees of penile pain, curvature, or deformity. Peyronie disease affects up to 10% of men and, like erectile dysfunction, is more common with increased age. The majority of men do not recall a major traumatic event preceding the onset of curvature. While 10% of men improve spontaneously, 50% will stabilize and the remainder will progress if left untreated. Penile deformity can impair normal sexual function and impact self-esteem.

Priapism is prolonged painful penile erection in the absence of sexual stimulation that results in ischemic injury of the corpora cavernosa from venous congestion, blood coagulation within the cavernous sinuses, and complete cessation of arterial inflow (low flow or "ischemic" priapism). **Ischemic priapism is a medical emergency requiring immediate medical or surgical intervention to avoid irreversible penile damage.** Ischemic priapism may be caused by RBC dyscrasias, drug use, and any of the treatments for erectile dysfunction.

Clinical Findings

A. Symptoms and Signs

Erectile dysfunction should be distinguished from problems with libido, orgasm, ejaculation, and penile deformity. The severity, intermittency, timing, and associated symptoms of erectile dysfunction should be noted. The history should include inquiries about dyslipidemia, hypertension, depression, neurologic disease, diabetes mellitus, kidney disease, endocrine disorders, and cardiac or peripheral vascular disease. Pelvic trauma, surgery, or irradiation increases a man's likelihood of erectile dysfunction. Histories of prostate cancer treatment or Peyronie disease should be queried. In the absence of other medical history, the onset of erectile dysfunction may be the first sign of endothelial dysfunction and further cardiovascular risk stratification should be considered. Medication use should be reviewed, with special attention given to the use of nitrate-containing medications. Alcohol, tobacco, marijuana, and other recreational drug use are associated with an increased risk of sexual dysfunction. Validated instruments, such as the Sexual Health Inventory for Men (SHIM) or Erectile Hardness Score (EHS), can be used for screening and diagnosing erectile dysfunction as well as monitoring therapeutic response.

During the physical examination, vital signs, body habitus (obesity), and secondary sexual characteristics should be assessed. Basic cardiovascular and neurologic examinations should be performed. The genitalia should be examined, noting the stretched length of the penis, fibrosis of the penile shaft, and any abnormalities in size or consistency of either testicle.

B. Laboratory Findings

Laboratory evaluation should be performed in select cases based on patient history and physical examination findings. Possible testing includes serum lipid profile, glucose, and testosterone. Patients with an abnormal testosterone should have measurement of free testosterone and LH to distinguish hypothalamic-pituitary dysfunction from primary testicular failure.

Treatment

Treatment of men suffering from sexual dysfunction should be patient-centered and goal-oriented. Lifestyle modification and reduction of cardiovascular risk factors are important components of treatment and should include smoking cessation; reduction of alcohol intake; diet; exercise; and treatment of diabetes, dyslipidemia, and hypertension. Men who have a psychogenic component to their erectile dysfunction or who are experiencing emotional distress will benefit from sexual health therapy or psychological counseling.

A. Hormonal Replacement

In men with hypogonadism who have undergone complete endocrinologic evaluation, restoration of normal testosterone levels may improve sexual function (see Treatment, Male Hypogonadism, Chapter 29).

B. Vasoactive Therapy

1. Oral agents—Sildenafil, vardenafil, tadalafil, and avanafil inhibit phosphodiesterase type 5 (PDE-5), preventing the degradation of cGMP and increasing blood flow into the penis. These medications are similar but have variable effectiveness in different patients. The medications have variable durations of onset, activity, and side effects. Each medication should be initiated at the lowest dose and titrated to achieve the desired effect. These medications are *contraindicated in patients taking nitroglycerin or nitrates,* since there may be exaggerated cardiac preload reduction causing hypotension, syncope, or stroke.

The combination of PDE-5 inhibitors and α-receptor blockers (prescribed for lower urinary tract symptoms) may cause a larger reduction in systemic blood pressure than when PDE-5 inhibitors are used alone. However, these two classes of medication may be safely used in combination if they are initiated and titrated in a stepwise fashion.

2. Injectable or suppository medications—Injection of prostaglandin E_1 into the corpora cavernosa is an acceptable form of treatment for erectile dysfunction in patients with poor response or contraindication to oral therapy.

Injections are performed using a tuberculin-type syringe or a metered-dose injection device. The base and lateral aspect of the penis is used as the injection site to avoid injury to the superficial blood and nerve supply located dorsally. Complications include priapism, penile pain, bruising, fibrosis, and infection. Prostaglandin E_1 is often compounded with papaverine, phentolamine, or atropine to increase effectiveness and reduce side effects, most notably penile discomfort. Patients using such compounded agents should be cautioned about the risk of priapism and variability of drug effect due to differences in compounding. These agents can also be delivered via intraurethral gel obtained through national compounding pharmacies, though effectiveness may be more limited than injectable treatments. Prostaglandin E1 intraurethral suppositories are no longer in production.

C. Vacuum Erection Device

The vacuum erection device creates negative pressure around the penis, drawing blood into the corpora cavernosa and corpus spongiosum. Once tumescence is achieved, an elastic constriction band is placed around the penile base to prevent loss of erection. Serious complications are rare, but such devices can be cumbersome to use and may cause penile discomfort and numbness leading to a high rate of disuse.

D. Penile Prosthetic Surgery

Penile prostheses are surgically implanted into the paired corpora cavernosa and may be semi-rigid (malleable) or inflatable. Inflatable prostheses are self-contained hydraulic devices that result in relatively natural appearance and function. Inflatable prosthetics are used most commonly because they emulate the tumescence and detumescence of the normal erection. Penile prosthesis implantation represents a definitive treatment option and is appropriate for patients who do not achieve a satisfactory response to oral or other less invasive therapies.

E. Medical and Surgical Therapy for Peyronie Disease

Oral medications have been found to have little benefit for reduction of penile curvature associated with Peyronie disease and should not be recommended. Injectable collagenase *Clostridium histolyticum* is approved by the FDA for the treatment of Peyronie disease. Collagenase enzymatically severs disordered collagen fibers after injection into the penile plaque, causing improvement in penile curvature. Penile traction therapy may be used as an adjunctive, nonsurgical treatment in Peyronie disease, with evidence supporting modest improvements in curvature and penile length. Surgical treatment is an alternative for men with compromised sexual function due to severe curvature, with lesions causing penile instability, or with inadequate results from collagenase. The choice of corrective procedure should be tailored to each patient after a detailed evaluation of disease severity and sexual function.

When to Refer

- Patients with erectile dysfunction who have an unsatisfactory response to oral medications.
- Patients with Peyronie disease or other penile deformity.
- Patients with sexual dysfunction and a history of pelvic or perineal trauma, surgery, or radiation.
- Patients with priapism to the emergency department for immediate intervention to allow restoration of penile perfusion.

Kloner RA et al. Princeton IV consensus guidelines: PDE5 inhibitors and cardiac health. J Sex Med 2024;21:90. [PMID: 38148297]

MALE INFERTILITY

ESSENTIALS OF DIAGNOSIS

- Infertility affects approximately one in six couples, and male factors contribute to up to 50% of cases.
- Causes include decreased or absent sperm production or function, or obstruction of the male genital tract.
- Abnormal semen quality and male factor infertility may indicate poor health or increased risk of certain health conditions.

General Considerations

Infertility is the inability of a couple to conceive a child after 1 year of sexual intercourse without contraceptive use. It affects 15–20% of couples in the United States, and *male factors contribute to up to half of cases*. The evaluation of both partners is critical for optimizing treatment. Following a detailed history and physical examination, a semen analysis should be performed at least twice, on two separate occasions (Figure 26–2). Because spermatogenesis takes approximately 75 days, exposures and health events in the prior 3 months should be reviewed. Male infertility is associated with a higher risk of testicular germ cell cancer, medical comorbidities including cardiovascular disease, diabetes, malignancy, and a higher risk of mortality. These men should be counseled, screened appropriately, and taught testicular self-examination.

Clinical Findings

A. Symptoms and Signs

The history should include an assessment of prior testicular insults (torsion, cryptorchidism, trauma), infections (mumps orchitis, epididymitis, sexually transmitted infections, COVID-19), environmental factors (excessive heat,

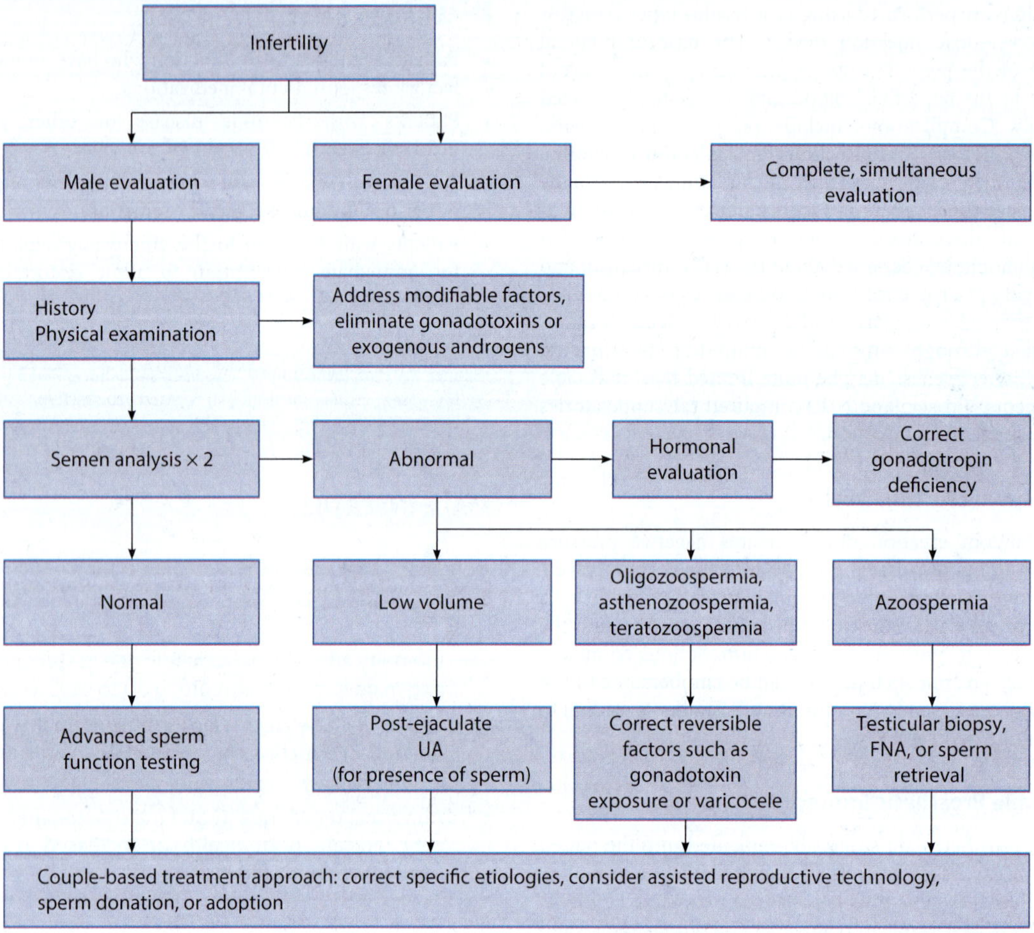

▲ **Figure 26–2.** Couple-based approach to evaluation and treatment of male factor infertility. FNA, fine-needle aspiration.

radiation, chemotherapy, prolonged pesticide exposure), medications (testosterone, finasteride, cimetidine, selective serotonin reuptake inhibitors, and spironolactone may affect spermatogenesis; phenytoin may lower FSH; sulfasalazine and nitrofurantoin affect sperm motility; tamsulosin causes retrograde ejaculation), and other drugs (alcohol, tobacco, marijuana). Sexual function, frequency and timing of intercourse, use of lubricants, and each partner's previous fertility are important. Past medical and surgical history should be surveyed for chronic disease, including obesity, cardiovascular, thyroid, or liver disease (decreased spermatogenesis); diabetes mellitus (decreased spermatogenesis, retrograde or anejaculation); or radical pelvic or retroperitoneal surgery (absent seminal emission secondary to sympathetic nerve injury).

Physical examination should assess features of hypogonadism: underdeveloped sexual characteristics, diminished male pattern hair distribution (axillary, body, facial, pubic), body habitus, gynecomastia, and obesity. Testicular size should be noted (normal size approximately 4.5 × 2.5 cm, volume 18 mL). **Varicoceles** are abnormally dilated, refluxing veins of the pampiniform plexus that can be identified in the standing position by gentle palpation of the spermatic cord and, on occasion, may only be appreciated with the Valsalva maneuver. The vasa deferentia and epididymides should be palpated (absence of all or part of one or both of the vasa deferentia may indicate the presence of a cystic fibrosis variant, congenital bilateral or unilateral absence of the vasa deferentia).

B. Laboratory Findings

Semen analysis should be performed after 2–5 days of ejaculatory abstinence. The specimen should be analyzed within 1 hour after collection. Abnormal sperm concentrations are < 15 million/mL (**oligozoospermia** is the presence of < 15 million sperm/mL in the ejaculate; **azoospermia** is the complete absence of sperm). Normal semen volume should be equal to or > 1.5 mL (lesser volumes may be due to retrograde ejaculation, ejaculatory duct obstruction, congenital bilateral absence of the vasa deferentia, or hypogonadism). Normal sperm motility and morphology demonstrate > 39% motile cells and > 3% normal morphology. Abnormal motility (asthenozoospermia) may result from varicocele, antisperm antibodies, infection, abnormalities of the sperm flagella, or ejaculatory duct obstruction. Abnormal morphology may result from a varicocele, infection, or exposure to gonadotoxins (eg, tobacco, marijuana).

Endocrine evaluation is warranted if sperm concentration is below 10 million sperm/mL or if the history and physical examination suggest an endocrinologic origin. Initial testing should include serum total testosterone and FSH. Specific abnormalities in these hormones should prompt additional testing, including serum LH, free testosterone, prolactin, and estradiol. Elevated FSH and LH levels and low testosterone levels (**hypergonadotropic** or **primary hypogonadism**) are associated with primary testicular failure (see Chapter 29 for primary hypogonadism). Low FSH and LH associated with low testosterone (**hypogonadotropic** or **secondary hypogonadism**) may be of hypothalamic or pituitary origin (see below for secondary hypogonadism). Elevated testosterone and low FSH and LH levels indicate supplemental testosterone use. Elevation of serum prolactin may indicate the presence of prolactinoma. Elevation of estradiol may indicate abnormal peripheral conversion of testosterone to estrogen by aromatase stored in adipocytes.

C. Genetic Testing

Men with sperm concentrations < 1 million/mL should consider testing for Y chromosome microdeletions, and men with sperm concentrations < 5 million/mL should consider testing for karyotypic abnormalities. Gene deletions from the long arm of the Y chromosome may cause azoospermia or oligozoospermia with age-related decline in spermatogenesis that is transmissible to male offspring. When small (5 mL), firm testes are identified, karyotyping should be performed to identify Klinefelter syndrome (see Chapter 44 Genetic & Genomic Disorders). Partial or complete absence of the vasa deferentia should prompt testing for gene pathogenic variants associated with cystic fibrosis.

D. Imaging

Scrotal ultrasound aids in characterizing the testes and may detect a testicular mass or varicocele. Men with low ejaculate volume and no evidence of retrograde ejaculation on postejaculate urinalysis may undergo transrectal ultrasound to evaluate the prostate and seminal vesicles for obstruction. MRI of the sella turcica should be performed in men with elevated prolactin or hypogonadotropic hypogonadism to evaluate the anterior pituitary gland. MRI of the pelvis and scrotum should be considered for men in whom the testes cannot be identified in the scrotum by physical examination or ultrasound. Men with unilateral absence of the vas deferens should have abdominal ultrasound or CT to exclude absence of the ipsilateral kidney.

Treatment

A. General Measures

Education about intercourse timing in relation to the woman's ovulatory cycle as well as the avoidance of spermicidal lubricants should be discussed. In cases of gonadotoxic exposure or medication-related factors, the offending agent should be removed whenever feasible. Patients with active genitourinary tract infections should be treated with appropriate antibiotics. Healthy lifestyle habits, including diet, exercise, and avoidance of gonadotoxins (tobacco, excessive alcohol, and marijuana), should be reinforced.

B. Varicocele

Varicocelectomy is performed to prevent retrograde blood flow in abnormal spermatic cord veins. Surgical ligation, which is accomplished via a subinguinal incision with the aid of a surgical microscope and Doppler ultrasound, is the gold standard approach given its high efficacy and low complication rates. Percutaneous venographic embolization of varicoceles is another approach but incurs both radiation and intravenous contrast exposure. Embolization may be the best approach for recurrence of varicocele after surgery.

C. Endocrine Therapy

Hypogonadotropic hypogonadism may be treated with human chorionic gonadotropin (2000 IU intramuscularly three times a week) once primary pituitary disease has been excluded or treated. If sperm concentration fails to rise after 12 months, recombinant FSH therapy should be initiated (150 IU subcutaneously three times a week). Clomiphene citrate is a selective estrogen receptor modulator (SERM) that stimulates a functioning pituitary gland to increase gonadotropin production. Anastrozole inhibits aromatization of testosterone to estradiol, thereby enhancing gonadotropin production. While studied extensively in men, neither clomiphene nor anastrozole is approved by the US FDA for treatment of male infertility. Therefore, men should be counseled appropriately before using either medication.

D. Ejaculatory Dysfunction Therapy

Patients with retrograde ejaculation may benefit from α-adrenergic agonists (pseudoephedrine, 60 mg orally three times a day) or imipramine (25 mg orally three times a day). Medical failures may require the collection of postejaculation urine for intrauterine insemination. Anejaculation can be treated with vibratory stimulation or electroejaculation in select cases, or may warrant surgical sperm retrieval for use with in vitro fertilization (IVF).

E. Ductal Obstruction

Obstruction of the vas deferens after vasectomy may be treated by microsurgical vasectomy reversal or by surgical sperm retrieval in combination with IVF. Although success depends on the duration of vasectomy, microsurgical vasectomy reversal is highly effective at restoring sperm to the ejaculate.

F. Assisted Reproductive Techniques

Intrauterine insemination and in vitro fertilization (with or without intracytoplasmic sperm injection) are alternatives for patients in whom other means of treating reduced sperm concentration, motility, or functionality have failed.

Intrauterine insemination should be performed only when adequate numbers of motile sperm are noted in an ejaculate sample. With the use of intracytoplasmic sperm injection, some men with azoospermia may still initiate a pregnancy by surgical retrieval of sperm from the testicle, epididymis, or vas deferens.

When to Refer

- Couples with infertility or who are concerned about their fertility potential.
- Men with known genital insults, genetic diagnoses, or syndromes that preclude natural fertility.
- Reproductive-aged men with newly diagnosed cancer or other disease that may require cytotoxic therapies with interest in fertility preservation.

Brannigan RE et al. Updates to male infertility: AUA/ASRM guideline (2024). J Urol. 2024;212:789. [PMID: 39145501]
Caroppo E et al. Are infertile men at a higher risk of morbidity and early mortality? Hum Reprod. 2026;41:148. [PMID: 41237188]
Daniels D et al. Climate change, microplastics, and male infertility. Curr Opin Urol. 2024;34:366. [PMID: 38932480.]
Lo JO et al. Influence of substance use on male reproductive health and offspring outcomes. Nat Rev Urol. 2024;21:534. [PMID: 38664544]

BENIGN PROSTATIC HYPERPLASIA

ESSENTIALS OF DIAGNOSIS

- History and physical examination including digital rectal examination.
- International prostate symptom score and UA.
- In-office testing to assess prostate size and shape, assessment of postvoid residual and urinary flow rate.
- Characterize obstructive or irritative voiding symptoms.
- Absence of UTI, neurologic disorder, stricture disease, prostatic or bladder malignancy.

General Considerations

Benign prostatic hyperplasia is extremely common, and its incidence rises with increasing age. Autopsy studies have shown histologically proven *BPH in 60% of men aged 60 and 80% of men aged 80. Bothersome urinary symptoms related to BPH also increase with age, although it is important to note that these symptoms can occur without significant enlargement on exam.* Obstructive voiding symptoms are reported by approximately 25% of men aged 55 and 50% of men aged 75. *It is critical for the clinician to discriminate between "obstructive" and "irritative" symptoms to target the root cause of that patient's bother.* This may be related to prostatic enlargement, high smooth muscle tone at the bladder neck or prostatic urethra, or underlying detrusor overactivity, which all require specific treatments.

Risk factors for the development of BPH are poorly understood. Some studies have suggested a genetic predisposition and some have noted racial differences. Approximately 50% of men under age 60 years who undergo surgery for BPH may have a heritable form of the disease. This form is most likely an autosomal dominant trait, and first-degree male relatives of such patients carry an increased relative risk of approximately fourfold.

Lower urinary tract symptoms result from the complex interplay of a dynamic system and are often multifactorial.

Clinical Findings

A. Symptoms

The symptoms of BPH can be divided into obstructive and irritative complaints. *Obstructive symptoms* include hesitancy, decreased force and caliber of the stream, sensation of incomplete bladder emptying, double voiding (urinating a second time within minutes), straining to urinate, and postvoid dribbling. *Irritative symptoms* include urgency, dysuria, frequency, and nocturia.

The American Urological Association (AUA) symptom index (Table 26–4) is an important tool used in the evaluation of patients with this disorder and should be calculated for all patients before starting therapy. The answers to seven questions quantitate the severity of obstructive or irritative complaints on a scale of 0–5. Thus, the score can range from 0 to 35 with increasing severity of symptoms. An estimation of **postvoid residual** can provide important information on bladder emptying and the need for more urgent intervention.

A detailed history focusing on the urinary tract should be obtained to exclude other possible causes of symptoms such as prostate cancer, UTI, neurogenic bladder, or urethral stricture. A focused medical history may also reveal other comorbidities that can directly affect urinary symptoms such as metabolic syndrome, HF, Parkinson disease, and obstructive sleep apnea.

B. Signs

A physical examination, digital rectal examination (DRE), and a focused neurologic examination should be performed on all patients. The size and consistency of the prostate should be noted. While prostate size does not correlate perfectly with the severity of symptoms or the degree of obstruction, it can inform treatment decisions. BPH usually results in a smooth, firm, elastic enlargement of the prostate. Induration or a nodule, if detected, must alert the clinician to the possibility of cancer, and further evaluation is needed (ie, PSA testing, transrectal ultrasound, and biopsy). Examination of the lower abdomen may reveal a distended bladder.

C. Laboratory Findings

UA should be performed to exclude infection or hematuria. Clinicians should consider obtaining a serum PSA test in patients within the screening age range.

Table 26–4. American Urological Association symptom index for benign prostatic hyperplasia.[1]

Questions to Be Answered	Not at All	Less Than One Time in Five	Less Than Half the Time	About Half the Time	More Than Half the Time	Almost Always
1. Over the past month, how often have you had a sensation of not emptying your bladder completely after you finish urinating?	0	1	2	3	4	5
2. Over the past month, how often have you had to urinate again less than 2 hours after you finished urinating?	0	1	2	3	4	5
3. Over the past month, how often have you found you stopped and started again several times when you urinated?	0	1	2	3	4	5
4. Over the past month, how often have you found it difficult to postpone urination?	0	1	2	3	4	5
5. Over the past month, how often have you had a weak urinary stream?	0	1	2	3	4	5
6. Over the past month, how often have you had to push or strain to begin urination?	0	1	2	3	4	5
7. Over the past month, how many times did you most typically get up to urinate from the time you went to bed at night until the time you got up in the morning?	0	1	2	3	4	5

[1]Sum of seven circled numbers equals the symptom score. See text for explanation.

Reproduced, with permission, from Barry MJ et al; Measurement Committee of the American Urological Association. The American Urological Association symptom index for benign prostatic hyperplasia. J Urol. 2017;197(2S):S189-97.

D. Imaging

Urologists are advised to consider prostate volume assessment prior to surgical intervention to determine the most appropriate approach (eg, water vapor therapy for smaller glands vs simple prostatectomy for a very large gland). This assessment can be done with cystoscopy; transrectal ultrasound; or cross-sectional imaging of the pelvis.

E. Cystoscopy

Cystoscopy is not required to determine the need for treatment but may assist in determining the best approach in patients opting for surgical therapy.

F. Additional Tests

Uroflowmetry and postvoid residual should be assessed prior to surgical treatment of the prostate and can be useful in tracking response to treatments. Cystometrograms and urodynamic profiles should be reserved for patients with unclear etiology of symptoms, suspected neurologic disease, or those who have not responded to previous prostate surgery.

Differential Diagnosis

A history of prior urethral instrumentation, urethritis, sexually transmitted infections, or trauma should be elucidated to exclude urethral stricture or bladder neck contracture. Hematuria and pain are commonly associated with bladder stones. Carcinoma of the prostate may be detected by abnormalities on DRE or an elevated PSA (see Chapter 43). A UTI can mimic the irritative symptoms of BPH and can be readily identified by UA and culture; however, a UTI can also be a complication of BPH. Carcinoma of the bladder, especially carcinoma in situ, may also present with irritative voiding complaints; however, UA usually shows evidence of hematuria (see Chapter 43). Patients with a neurogenic bladder may also have many of the same symptoms and signs as those with BPH; however, a history of neurologic disease, stroke, diabetes mellitus, or back injury may be obtained, and diminished perineal or lower extremity sensation or alterations in rectal sphincter tone or in the bulbocavernosus reflex might be observed on examination. Simultaneous alterations in bowel function (constipation) might also suggest the possibility of a neurologic disorder. Urodynamics studies can distinguish between neurogenic etiologies and obstructive etiologies for poor bladder emptying.

Treatment

Clinical practice guidelines exist for the evaluation and treatment of patients with BPH. Following the evaluation as outlined above, patients may be offered various forms of therapy for BPH. Patients are advised to consult with their primary care clinicians or urologists to make an educated decision on the basis of the relative efficacy and side effects of the treatment options.

Patients with mild symptoms (AUA scores 0–7) and relatively low bother scores may be managed by watchful waiting only. *Medical therapy is appropriate for those with significant bother attributed to their symptoms. Surgery should be considered for those who have moderate to severe symptoms and have failed medical therapy.* This is defined as a lack of efficacy, progressive symptoms despite medical treatment, or medication side effects or adverse reactions. More serious sequelae of BPH—recurrent UTI, recurrent gross hematuria attributed to the prostate, bladder stones, refractory urinary retention (failing at least one attempt at catheter removal), or obstructive nephropathy—are classic indications for surgery, but patients should generally be trialed on medical management prior to proceeding to surgery.

A. Watchful Waiting

The risk of progression or complications is uncertain. Not all symptoms require treatment, and intervention should be tailored to the degree of bother and impact on quality of life for most men. While men with progressive symptoms and large prostates do have a higher chance of developing urinary retention or requiring surgical intervention in the future, this risk is thought to be relatively low overall.

A large randomized study from 1998 compared finasteride with placebo in men with moderate to severely symptomatic disease and enlarged prostates on DRE. Patients in the placebo arm demonstrated a 7% risk of developing urinary retention over 4 years. Behavioral and lifestyle modifications may be offered prior to medical or surgical therapy.

B. Medical Therapy

1. α-Blockers—α-adrenergic receptors are ubiquitous, but the prostate and bladder neck have high levels of α_{1A}-receptors. Activation of these receptors results in increased prostatic smooth muscle tone, urethral constriction, and impaired urine flow. Blocking these receptors leads to smooth muscle relaxation and reduced resistance at the bladder outlet. α-blockade has been shown to result in both objective and subjective degrees of improvement in the symptoms and signs of BPH. α-blockers can be classified according to their receptor selectivity (Table 26–5) as well as their half-life.

Table 26–5. α-blockade agent treatment for benign prostatic hyperplasia (listed in alphabetical order).

Agent	Action	Oral Dose
Alfuzosin	α_{1A}-blockade	10 mg daily
Doxazosin	α_1-blockade	1–8 mg daily
Silodosin	α_{1A}-blockade	4 or 8 mg daily
Tadalafil	Phosphodiesterase type 5 inhibitor	5 mg daily
Tamsulosin	α_{1A}-blockade	0.4 or 0.8 mg daily
Terazosin	α_1-blockade	1–10 mg daily

Several nonselective α-blockers previously utilized in the treatment of BPH have fallen out of favor for more selective medications. Terazosin and doxazosin can still be offered but require dose titration and have higher rates of orthostatic hypotension and dizziness; prazosin and phenoxybenzamine are not used in BPH treatment.

Long-acting, nonselective α-blockers allow for once-a-day dosing, but dose titration is necessary. Terazosin improves symptoms, and in numerous studies, it is superior to placebo or finasteride. Terazosin is started at a dosage of 1 mg orally daily for 3 days, increased to 2 mg orally daily for 11 days, then 5 mg orally daily. Additional dose escalation to 10 mg orally daily can be performed if necessary. Doxazosin is started at a dosage of 1 mg orally daily for 7 days, increased to 2 mg orally daily for 7 days, then 4 mg orally daily. Additional dose escalation to 8 mg orally daily can be performed if necessary.

α_{1A}-receptors are localized to the prostate and bladder neck. Selective blockade of these receptors results in fewer systemic side effects than nonselective α-blocker therapy thus obviating the need for dose titration. The typical dose of tamsulosin is 0.4 mg orally daily taken 30 minutes after a meal. Alfuzosin is a long-acting α_{1A}-blocker; its dose is 10 mg orally once daily with food, and it does not require titration. Several randomized, double-blind, placebo-controlled trials have been performed comparing terazosin, doxazosin, tamsulosin, and alfuzosin with placebo. All agents have demonstrated safety and efficacy. **Floppy iris syndrome**, a complication of cataract surgery, can occur in patients taking both nonselective α-blockers and α_{1A}-blockers well after cessation of therapy.

2. 5-α-Reductase inhibitors—Finasteride and dutasteride block the conversion of testosterone to dihydrotestosterone, resulting in reduction in size of the gland and improvement in symptoms. *Six months of therapy are required for maximum effects on prostate size* (20–30% reduction) and symptomatic improvement.

Several randomized, double-blind, placebo-controlled trials have been performed comparing finasteride with placebo. Efficacy, safety, and durability are well established. However, symptomatic improvement is seen only in men with enlarged prostates (> 40 mL by ultrasonographic examination). Side effects include decreased libido, decrease in volume of ejaculate, and erectile dysfunction. *Serum PSA is reduced by approximately 50% in patients receiving finasteride therapy, but the % free PSA is unchanged.* Therefore, in order to compare with pre-finasteride PSA levels, the serum PSA of a patient taking finasteride should be doubled.

Studies have shown that finasteride therapy decreases the incidence of urinary retention and the need for operative treatment in men with enlarged prostates and moderate to severe symptoms. The larger the prostate over 40 mL, the greater the relative-risk reduction. Dutasteride is a nonselective 5-α-reductase inhibitor (5ARI) that appears to be similar to finasteride in its effectiveness; it is dosed at 0.5 mg orally daily.

Both 5ARIs have been shown to be effective chemopreventive agents for prostate cancer in large RCTs. A 25% risk reduction was observed in men with both low and high risk for prostate cancer. However, despite the strength of the evidence for 5ARIs in reducing the risk of prostate cancer, an FDA advisory committee recommended against labeling these agents for prostate cancer chemoprevention, citing the *potential increased risk of high-grade cancers* in these studies (1.8% vs 1.0% for finasteride and 1% vs 0.5% for dutasteride), isolated risk reduction in low-grade cancers, and inability to apply the findings to the general population. Moreover, the FDA has included the increased risk of being diagnosed with high-grade prostate cancer in the labels of all 5ARIs.

3. Phosphodiesterase-5 inhibitor—Tadalafil is approved by the FDA to treat the symptoms and signs of BPH (Table 26–5); it is also approved for first-line use in men with both urinary symptoms and erectile dysfunction. The data from two randomized, double-blind, placebo-controlled trials demonstrated significant improvements in standardized measurements of urinary function between 2 and 4 weeks after initiating treatment at 5 mg once daily, with minimal adverse effects.

4. Combination therapy—The Medical Therapy of Prostatic Symptoms (MTOPS) trial (2003) was a large, randomized, placebo-controlled trial comparing finasteride, doxazosin, the combination of the two, and placebo in 3047 men observed for a mean of 4.5 years. Long-term combination therapy with doxazosin and finasteride was safe and reduced the risk of overall clinical progression of BPH significantly more than did treatment with either medication alone. Combination therapy and finasteride alone reduced the long-term risk of acute urinary retention and the need for invasive therapy.

C. Surgical Therapy

Most cases of BPH requiring surgery can be managed with transurethral or minimally invasive techniques. This remains an area of active research and innovation with several new technologies available. An overview of all the surgical options and decision making was published by the American Urological Association (Figure 26–3).

1. Transurethral resection of the prostate (TURP)—Over 95% of prostate surgeries can be performed endoscopically (through the urethra). TURP is the gold standard treatment for surgical treatment of BPH, and it often requires a 1- to 2-day hospital stay. Most head-to-head surgical studies comparing TURP to minimally invasive therapies show that *symptom scores and flow rate improvements are superior following TURP compared with other minimally invasive therapies.* It is one of the most durable treatments available, with patients remaining symptom-free for an average of 5–10 years. The risks of TURP include retrograde ejaculation (75%), erectile dysfunction (5–10%), and urinary incontinence (< 1%). Potential complications include (1) bleeding; (2) urethral stricture or bladder neck contracture; (3) perforation of the prostate capsule with extravasation; and (4) **transurethral resection syndrome**, a hypervolemic, hyponatremic state resulting from absorption of the hypotonic irrigating solution. This is rarely seen currently, as bipolar electrocautery and isotonic saline irrigation have largely replaced monopolar electrocautery for TURP.

2. Transurethral incision of the prostate (TUIP)—Men with moderate to severe symptoms and small prostates (< 30 g) often have posterior commissure hyperplasia or an "elevated bladder neck." These patients will often benefit from incision of the prostate. The procedure is more rapid and less morbid than TURP. Outcomes in well-selected patients are comparable, though a lower rate of retrograde ejaculation has been reported (25%).

3. Photoselective vaporization of the prostate (PVP)—Various laser technologies exist and vary by wavelength and energy produced. The original KTP greenlight laser uses a 532-nm wavelength that is selectively absorbed by hemoglobin, leading to improved hemostasis. Advantages include combined vaporization and coagulation with significant reduction in tissue volume, making this an *ideal choice for anticoagulated patients.* Outcomes are similar to those seen with TURP. Disadvantages include limitations on prostate volume that can be efficiently treated (< 80 mL) and difficulty controlling bleeding from larger venous channels, the lack of tissue for pathologic examination, variable effectiveness, and more frequent irritative voiding during recovery.

4. Aquablation—This ultrasound-guided, robot-executed waterjet ablation of the prostate is designed to relieve prostatic obstruction with limited bleeding, shorter operative time, and preservation of sexual function. It is one of the few size-agnostic transurethral surgical options for BPH and has been shown to effectively treat glands ranging in size from 30 mL to 150 mL. Urinary outcomes have been shown to be comparable to the gold standard TURP with lower risk of stricture, incontinence, and sexual dysfunction. Pretreatment transrectal ultrasound is used to map out the obstructive adenoma to be ablated, while excluding the ejaculatory ducts. Real-time transrectal ultrasound is then used to monitor tissue resection during the procedure. The resection is performed under general or spinal anesthesia using a heat-free water jet from a transurethrally placed robotic handpiece with simultaneous suction of ablation tissue through the device. Following the resection, electrocautery or traction from a three-way catheter is used to obtain hemostasis. A 5-year multicenter clinical trial (2022) showed significant and sustained improvements in urinary flow rate, postvoid residual volume, and quality of life.

5. Laser enucleation—Holmium laser enucleation of the prostate (**HoLEP**) is a technique of enucleating the adenomatous lobes intact and morcellating the tissue within the bladder. Advantages of HoLEP compared with other methods include ability to treat all prostate sizes, low re-treatment rates, few complications, and shorter duration of bladder catheterization. There is a higher rate of transient stress incontinence, but this typically resolves within 3 months. This technique is an attractive alternative to the simple prostatectomy for very large glands (> 100 cc) with comparable outcomes. However, due to the steep learning curve for operators, it is not as widely available as other techniques. It may also be performed via **thulium laser enucleation of the prostate (ThuLEP)** depending upon surgeon experience and preference.

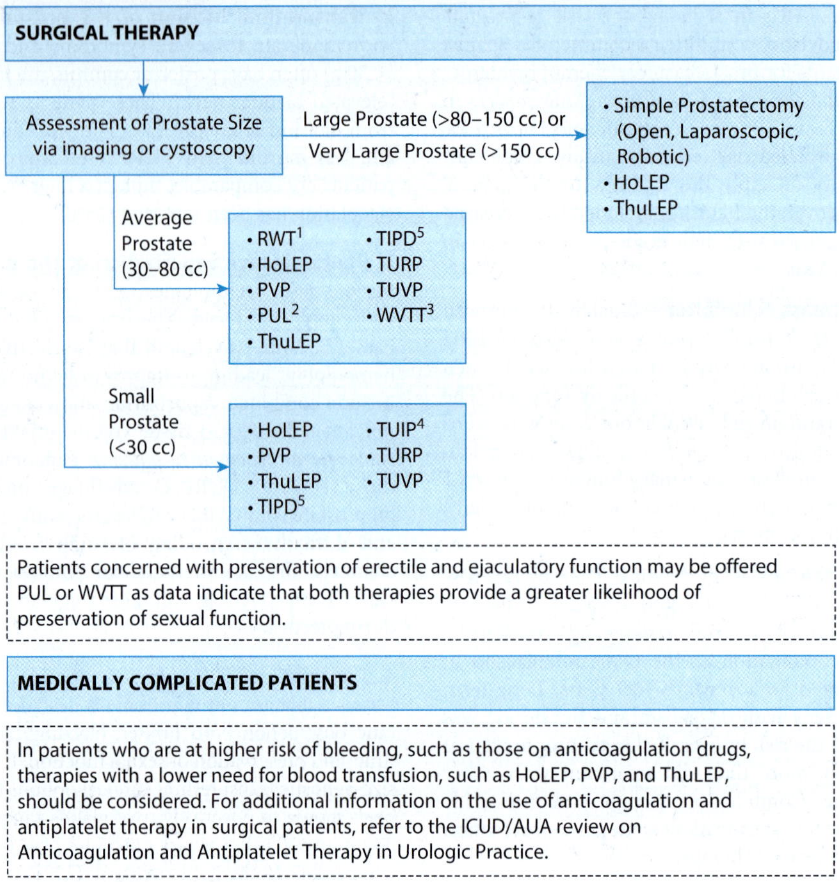

Based on the evidence reports of the current guidelines, the following criteria are recommended when utilizing these approaches:

[1] RWT: prostate volume 30–80 cc.

[2] PUL: absence of obstructing midline prostate tissue and prostate volume 30–80 cc.

[3] WVTT: prostate volume 30–80 cc.

[4] TUIP: prostate volume ≤30 cc.

[5] TIPD: prostate volume 25–75 cc and absence of obstructive middle lobe.

▲ **Figure 26–3.** Surgical management of lower urinary tract symptoms attributed to BPH. HoLEP, holmium laser enucleation of the prostate; PUL, prostatic urethral lift; PVP, photoselective vaporization of the prostate; ThuLEP, thulium laser enucleation of the prostate; TUIP, transurethral incision of the prostate; TUMT, transurethral microwave therapy; TURP, transurethral resection of the prostate; TUVP, transurethral vaporization of the prostate. (Reproduced with permission from Sandu JS et al. Management of lower urinary tract symptoms attributed to benign prostatic hyperplasia (BPH): AUA guideline amendment J Urol. 2023;10;1097.)

D. Minimally Invasive Therapies

1. Prostatic urethral lift (UroLift)—The UroLift system uses permanent nitinol and stainless steel implants placed under cystoscopic guidance to retract the lateral lobes of the prostate and mechanically open the prostatic urethra. The procedure can be performed under local anesthesia in the outpatient setting, and holding anticoagulation medication is not necessary. The ideal candidate has primarily lateral lobe hyperplasia and a prostate volume under 80 cc. Short-term data show improved symptoms and voiding flow rates with no de novo erectile dysfunction or incontinence. Re-treatment rates within 5 years have been reported to be as high as 13.6%.

2. Water vapor thermal therapy (Rezūm)—This minimally invasive technique uses a modified cystoscope to deliver water vapor into the prostatic tissue. As the steam condenses back into water, it releases large amounts of stored thermal energy leading to tissue necrosis and resorption of tissue within about 3 months. This procedure is done in the clinic or ambulatory surgery setting; it requires 3–7 days of bladder catheterization. In contrast to the UroLift procedure, there is a significant reduction in prostate volume over time, about 30% by 6 months, which relieves lower urinary tract symptoms as a result. A 5-year RCT reported significant objective improvement in lower urinary tract symptoms as early as 2 weeks post-procedure, improvement that remained durable throughout the 5-year period. Recommended prostate volume for Rezūm treatment is 30–80 cc. Advantages include the minimally invasive, outpatient nature of the procedure with no significant bleeding risk even for anticoagulated patients, ability to treat the median lobe, and no reports of de novo erectile dysfunction or urinary incontinence. Disadvantages include slower recovery, significant postoperative irritative symptoms, and longer bladder catheterization times compared with TURP and laser procedures. Surgical re-treatment rate at 5 years was reported to be 4.4%, a rate far lower than other minimally invasive options.

3. Optilume balloon dilation—The Optilume BPH catheter system is the first minimally invasive device with a dual mechanical and pharmacological mechanism of action that builds on the device's original use in treating recurrent urethral strictures. The BPH balloon creates an anterior commissurotomy with simultaneous paclitaxel delivery to prevent regrowth or refusion of the anterior prostatic lateral lobes. A double-blind, randomized, sham-controlled study showed improvement in flow rate, post-void residual (PVR), and patient satisfaction scores that were sustained at 1 year. Treatment was limited to prostates ranging in size from 20 to 80 mL, and long-term benefit has yet to be proven.

4. Temporary implantable nitinol device (iTIND)—This procedure involves placing a device with three expanding nitinol struts into the prostatic urethra and bladder neck. It is left in place for 5–7 days and then removed. The resulting ischemic necrosis from the struts leaves grooves or channels, similar to a TUIP. Early data shows benefit in smaller prostates, but more study is needed to determine optimal patient selection and durability.

E. Simple Prostatectomy

When the prostate is very large, a simple prostatectomy by an open or robotic enucleation approach may be considered. Glands > 100 cc are usually considered for enucleation. In addition to size, other relative indications for simple prostatectomy include when there is a concomitant bladder diverticulum or stone, and when dorsal lithotomy positioning of the patient is not possible. The robotic approach has improved recovery, lower blood loss, and shortened hospital stays.

F. Prostate Artery Embolization

Initially described in the 1970s to control bleeding, angioembolization of the bilateral prostatic arteries has been shown to reduce prostate volume, and recent data show some relief of urinary symptoms. Selective embolization using 100- to 500-mcm microspheres results in a low risk of nontarget ischemia. Due to its minimally invasive nature it can be considered in select patients, particularly those with larger glands who are not candidates for other available treatments.

When to Refer

- Obstructive uropathy.
- Patient dissatisfaction with medical therapy.
- Patient interest in surgical treatments.
- Need for further evaluation (cystoscopy) or surgical intervention.

Arnold MJ et al. Benign prostatic hyperplasia: rapid evidence review. Am Fam Physician. 2023;107:613. [PMID: 37327163]
Bhojani N et al. Aquablation therapy in large prostates (80-150 mL) for lower urinary tract symptoms due to benign prostatic hyperplasia: final WATER II 5-year clinical trial results. J Urol. 2023;210:143. [PMID: 37115632]
Kaplan SA et al. The PINNACLE Study: a double-blind, randomized, sham-controlled study evaluating the Optilume BPH Catheter System for the treatment of lower urinary tract symptoms secondary to benign prostatic hyperplasia. J Urol. 2023;210:500. [PMID: 37555604]
Sandu JS et al. Management of lower urinary tract symptoms attributed to benign prostatic hyperplasia (BPH): AUA guideline amendment 2023. J Urol. 2024;211:11. [PMID: 37706750]
Wei JT et al. Lower urinary tract symptoms in men: a review. JAMA. 2025;334:809. [PMID: 40658396]

CANCERS OF THE GENITOURINARY TRACT

(See Chapter 43 for Cancers of the Genitourinary Tract: Prostate Cancer, Bladder Cancer, Cancers of the Ureter & Renal Pelvis, Renal Cell Carcinoma, & Testicular Cancers.)

27 Nervous System Disorders

Vanja C. Douglas, MD
Michael J. Aminoff, MD, DSc, FRCP

HEADACHE

Headache is such a common complaint and can occur for so many different reasons that its proper evaluation may be difficult. New, severe, or acute headaches are more likely than chronic headaches to relate to an intracranial disorder; the approach to such headaches is discussed in Chapter 2. **Chronic headaches** may be primary or secondary to another disorder. Common **primary** headache syndromes include migraine, tension-type headache, and cluster headache. Important **secondary** causes to consider include intracranial lesions, head injury, cervical spondylosis, dental or ocular disease, temporomandibular joint dysfunction, sinusitis, hypertension, depression, and a wide variety of general medical disorders. Although underlying structural lesions are *not* present in most patients presenting with headache, it is nevertheless important to bear this possibility in mind. About one-third of patients with brain tumors, for example, present with a primary complaint of headache.

1. Migraine

ESSENTIALS OF DIAGNOSIS

- Headache, usually pulsatile, lasting 4–72 hours.
- Pain is typically, but not always, unilateral.
- Nausea, vomiting, photophobia, and phonophobia are common accompaniments.
- Pain is aggravated with routine physical activity.
- An aura of transient neurologic symptoms (commonly visual) may precede head pain in one quarter of patients.

General Considerations

The pathophysiology of migraine probably relates to neuronal dysfunction in the trigeminal system resulting in release of vasoactive neuropeptides such as calcitonin gene–related peptide leading to neurogenic inflammation, sensitization, and headache. Migraine aura is hypothesized to result from cortical spreading depression, a wave of neuronal and glial depolarization that moves slowly across the cerebral cortex corresponding to the clinical symptoms (ie, occipital cortex and visual aura). Migraine often exhibits a complex, polygenic pattern of inheritance. Sometimes, an autosomal dominant inheritance pattern is apparent, as in **familial hemiplegic migraine**, in which attacks of lateralized weakness represent the aura.

Clinical Findings

Typical migrainous headache is a lateralized throbbing headache that occurs episodically following its onset in adolescence or early adult life. In many cases, the headaches do not conform to this pattern, although their associated features and response to antimigrainous medications nevertheless suggest a similar basis. In this broader sense, migrainous headaches may be lateralized or generalized, may be dull or throbbing, and are sometimes associated with anorexia, nausea, vomiting, photophobia, phonophobia, osmophobia, cognitive impairment, and blurring of vision. They usually build up gradually and last several hours or longer. Headaches are often preceded by a 24–48 hour prodrome of mood or autonomic symptoms. Focal disturbances of neurologic function (**migraine aura**) may precede or accompany the headaches. Visual disturbances occur commonly and may consist of field defects (**scotoma**); of luminous visual hallucinations such as stars, sparks, unformed light flashes (**photopsia**), geometric patterns, or zigzags of light; or of some combination of field defects and luminous hallucinations (**scintillating scotomas**). Other focal disturbances such as aphasia or numbness, paresthesias, clumsiness, dysarthria, dysequilibrium, or weakness in a circumscribed distribution may also occur.

In rare instances, the neurologic or somatic disturbance accompanying typical migrainous headaches becomes the sole manifestation of an attack ("**migraine aura without headache**"). Rarely, the patient may be left with a permanent neurologic deficit following a migrainous attack, and migraine with aura is a risk factor for stroke.

Patients often give a family history of migraine. Attacks may be triggered by emotional or physical stress, lack or excess of sleep, missed meals, odors, alcoholic beverages, bright lights, loud noise, menstruation, or use of oral contraceptives.

An uncommon variant is **migraine with brainstem aura**, in which blindness or visual disturbances throughout both visual fields are accompanied or followed by dysarthria, dysequilibrium, tinnitus, and perioral and distal paresthesias and are sometimes followed by transient loss or impairment of consciousness or by a confusional state. This, in turn, is followed by a throbbing (usually occipital) headache, often with nausea and vomiting.

In **recurrent painful ophthalmoplegic neuropathy** (previously termed "ophthalmoplegic migraine"), lateralized pain—often about the eye—is accompanied by nausea, vomiting, and diplopia due to transient external ophthalmoplegia. The ophthalmoplegia is due to third nerve palsy, sometimes with accompanying sixth nerve involvement, and may outlast the orbital pain by several days or even weeks. The ophthalmic division of the fifth nerve has also been affected in some patients. The condition is rare and a diagnosis of exclusion; more common causes of a painful ophthalmoplegia are internal carotid artery aneurysms and diabetes.

Treatment

Management of migraine consists of avoidance of any precipitating factors, together with prophylactic or symptomatic pharmacologic treatment if necessary.

A. Symptomatic Therapy

During acute attacks, rest in a quiet, darkened room may be helpful until symptoms subside. A simple analgesic (eg, aspirin, acetaminophen, ibuprofen, or naproxen) taken immediately often provides relief, but prescription medication is sometimes necessary. *To prevent medication overuse, use of simple analgesics should be limited to 15 days or less per month, and, in general, other medications should be limited to no more than 10 days per month.*

1. Ergotamines—Cafergot, a combination of ergotamine tartrate (1 mg) and caffeine (100 mg), is often helpful; one or two tablets are taken at the onset of headache or warning symptoms, followed by one tablet every 30 minutes, if necessary, up to six tablets per attack and no more than 10 days per month. Cafergot given rectally (one-half to one suppository containing 2 mg of ergotamine) or dihydroergotamine mesylate intravenously (0.5–1 mg) or subcutaneously or intramuscularly (1–2 mg), or intranasally (0.5 mg in each nostril) may be useful when vomiting precludes use of oral medications. Ergotamine-containing preparations should be *avoided* during pregnancy, in patients with CVD or its risk factors, and in patients taking potent CYP 3A4 inhibitors.

2. Serotonin agonists—Triptans are 5-$HT_{1b/1d}$ receptor agonists that inhibit release of vasoactive neuropeptides. Sumatriptan is a rapidly effective agent for aborting attacks when given subcutaneously by an autoinjection device (4–6 mg once subcutaneously, may repeat once after 2 hours if needed; maximum dose 12 mg/24 hours). Nasal and oral preparations are available but may be less effective due to slower absorption. Zolmitriptan is available in oral and nasal formulations. The dose is 5 mg orally or in one nostril once; this may be repeated once after 2 hours. The maximum dose for both formulations is 10 mg/24 hours. Other triptans are available, including rizatriptan (5–10 mg orally at onset, may repeat every 2 hours twice [maximum dose 30 mg/24 hours]); naratriptan (1–2.5 mg orally at onset, may repeat once after 4 hours [maximum dose 5 mg/24 hours]); almotriptan (6.25–12.5 mg orally at onset, may repeat once after 2 hours [maximum dose 25 mg/24 hours]); frovatriptan (2.5 mg orally at onset, may repeat once after 2 hours [maximum dose 7.5 mg/24 hours]); and eletriptan (20–40 mg orally at onset; may repeat once after 2 hours [maximum dose 80 mg/24 hours]). Eletriptan is useful for immediate therapy, and frovatriptan, which has a longer half-life, may be worthwhile for patients with prolonged attacks or attacks provoked by menstrual periods. Patients often experience greater benefit when the triptan is combined with naproxen (500 mg orally).

Triptans may cause nausea and vomiting. They are best avoided in persons who are pregnant, and in patients with hemiplegic or basilar migraine, a history of stroke or transient ischemic attack, or uncontrolled hypertension. In patients whose hypertension is controlled, triptans are commonly used safely, although caution is advised. *Triptans are contraindicated in patients with coronary or peripheral vascular disease and Prinzmetal angina.*

Lasmiditan (50–200 mg taken once at headache onset; no more than one dose in 24 hours) is a 5-HT_{1F} receptor agonist that lacks the vasoconstrictive properties of triptans and can be given safely to patients with cardiovascular risk factors. Dizziness and somnolence are common side effects, and patients should not drive within 8 hours of administration.

3. Calcitonin gene-related peptide antagonists—Rimegepant sulfate (75 mg orally dissolved tablet taken once at headache onset; maximum dose 75 mg/24 hours), ubrogepant (50 or 100 mg orally at headache onset, may repeat once after 2 hours; maximum dose 200 mg/24 hours), and zavegepant (10 mg intranasally once in one nostril at headache onset, 10 mg/spray; maximum dose 10 mg/24 hours) achieve pain freedom in 20% and pain relief in 60% of patients within 2 hours. Hypersensitivity reactions may occur immediately or several days after administration with rimegepant.

4. Other agents—Prochlorperazine is effective and may be administered rectally (25 mg suppository), intravenously or intramuscularly (5–10 mg), or orally (5–10 mg). Intravenous metoclopramide (10–20 mg) is also useful in the emergency department setting. Various butalbital-containing combination oral analgesics risk overuse and dependence and should only be used as a last resort. Opioid analgesics should be *avoided* because of high rates of rebound headache and the tendency to develop **medication overuse headache**.

5. Neuromodulation—Sham-controlled trials show that single-pulse transcranial magnetic stimulation aborts migraine with aura, and noninvasive vagus nerve stimulation, transcutaneous trigeminal nerve stimulation, and remote electrical stimulation applied to the upper arm abort migraine with or without aura. Transcranial magnetic stimulation is contraindicated in patients with epilepsy.

B. Preventive Therapy

Preventive treatment may be necessary if migraine headaches occur more frequently than two or three times a month or significant disability is associated with attacks. Avoidance of triggers and maintenance of homeostasis with regular sleep, meals, and hydration should not be neglected; a headache diary may be useful to identify triggers. Some more common agents used for prophylaxis are listed in Table 27–1. The medication chosen first will vary with the individual patient, depending on factors such as comorbid obesity, depression, anxiety, hypertension, and patient preference. Several medications may have to be tried in turn before headaches are brought under control. Once a medication has been found to help, it should be continued for several months. If the patient remains headache-free, the dose may be tapered and the medication eventually withdrawn. Acupuncture reduces headache frequency and intensity in migraine, with and without aura, and is as effective and safer than prophylactic pharmacologic treatment in migraine without aura and **chronic migraine** (at least 15 days per month with headaches lasting 4 hours per day or longer). Botulinum toxin type A injected into selected head and neck muscles reduces headache frequency in chronic migraine. Transcutaneous supraorbital neurostimulation, single-pulse transcranial magnetic stimulation, and non-invasive vagus nerve stimulation reduced headache frequency as reflected in a meta-analysis of RCTs and are approved in the United States. A meta-analysis of placebo-controlled trials showed biofeedback therapy to be highly effective for prevention of migraine.

Chen Y et al. Non-invasive brain stimulation treatments for migraine prophylaxis: a network meta-analysis of randomized controlled trials. Acta Neurol Belg. 2023;123:1481. [PMID: 37184609]

Whealy M et al. The 5-HT1B and 5-HT1D agonists in acute migraine therapy: ergotamine, dihydroergotamine, and the triptans. Handb Clin Neurol. 2024;199:17. [PMID: 38307644]

2. Tension-Type Headache

This is the most common type of primary headache disorder. Patients frequently report pericranial tenderness, poor concentration, and other nonspecific symptoms, in addition to headaches that are often vise-like or tight in quality but not pulsatile. Headaches may be exacerbated by emotional stress, fatigue, noise, or glare. The headaches are usually generalized, may be most intense about the neck or back of the head, and are not associated with focal neurologic symptoms. There is diagnostic overlap with migraine.

Abortive therapy with simple analgesics is usually effective. Anti-migraine preparations are *not* recommended unless the patient has comorbid migraine headaches. Tricyclic antidepressants, such as amitriptyline, are supported for headache prophylaxis by randomized trial evidence and often are tried first. Treatment of comorbid anxiety or depression is important. Behavioral therapies that may be effective include physical therapy, biofeedback therapy, and relaxation training.

Florczyk S et al. Headache treatment options. J Am Board Fam Med. 2024;37:737. [PMID: 39455276]

3. Cluster Headache

Cluster headache affects predominantly middle-aged men. The pathophysiology is unclear but may relate to activation of cells in the ipsilateral hypothalamus, triggering the trigeminal autonomic vascular system. There is often no family history of headache or migraine. Episodes of severe unilateral periorbital pain occur daily for several weeks and are often accompanied by one or more of the following: ipsilateral nasal congestion, rhinorrhea, lacrimation, redness of the eye, and Horner syndrome (ptosis, pupillary meiosis, and facial anhidrosis or hypohidrosis). During attacks, patients are often restless and agitated. Episodes typically occur at night, awaken the patient, and last between 15 minutes and 3 hours. Spontaneous remission then occurs, and the patient remains well for weeks or months before another bout of closely spaced attacks. *Bouts may last for 4 to 8 weeks and may occur up to several times per year.* During a bout, many patients report alcohol triggers an attack; others report that stress, glare, or ingestion of specific foods occasionally precipitates attacks. In occasional patients, remission does not occur. This variant has been referred to as **chronic cluster headache**. In longstanding cases, Horner syndrome may persist between attacks.

Cluster headache is one of the **trigeminal autonomic cephalalgias**, which include hemicrania continua, paroxysmal hemicrania, and short-lasting neuralgiform headache attacks. Similar to cluster headache, the other trigeminal autonomic cephalalgias consist of unilateral periorbital pain associated with ipsilateral autonomic symptoms such as conjunctival injection and tearing; they are distinguished from cluster headache by different attack duration and frequency and, in some cases, their exquisite responsiveness to indomethacin.

Treatment of an individual attack with oral medications is generally unsatisfactory, but subcutaneous (6–12 mg) or intranasal (20 mg/spray) sumatriptan or inhalation of 100% oxygen (12–15 L/min for 15 minutes via a nonrebreather mask) are effective. Zolmitriptan (5–10 mg nasal spray) is also effective. Dihydroergotamine (0.5–1 mg intramuscularly or intravenously), octreotide (100 mcg subcutaneously) or viscous lidocaine (1 mg of 4–6% solution intranasally) is sometimes effective.

Various prophylactic agents include oral medications such as verapamil (start at 240 mg daily, increase by 80 mg every 2 weeks to 960 mg daily, with routine ECG to monitor the PR interval), lithium carbonate (start at 300 mg daily, titrating according to serum levels and treatment response up to a typical total daily dose of 900–1200 mg, divided three or four times), topiramate (100–400 mg daily), and galcanezumab (300 mg subcutaneously monthly until end of cluster period). As there is often a delay before these medications are effective, transitional therapy is often used. Prednisone (60–100 mg daily for 5 days followed by gradual withdrawal over 7–10 days) is effective in 70–80% of patients, and suboccipital corticosteroid injection about the greater occipital nerve is effective in 75%. Ergotamine tartrate can be given as rectal suppositories (0.5–1 mg at

Table 27–1. Pharmacologic prophylaxis of migraine (listed in alphabetical order within classes).

Medication	Usual Adult Oral Daily Dose	Selected Side Effects and Comments
Antiepileptic[1]		
Topiramate[2]	100 mg (divided twice daily)	Somnolence, nausea, dyspepsia, irritability, dizziness, ataxia, nystagmus, diplopia, glaucoma, renal calculi, weight loss, hypohidrosis, hyperthermia.
Valproic acid[2]	500–1000 mg (divided twice daily)	Nausea, vomiting, diarrhea, drowsiness, alopecia, weight gain, hepatotoxicity, thrombocytopenia, tremor, pancreatitis.
Cardiovascular		
Candesartan[2,3]	8–32 mg once daily	Dizziness, cough, diarrhea, fatigue.
Guanfacine[3]	1 mg once daily	Dry mouth, somnolence, dizziness, constipation, erectile dysfunction.
Propranolol[2,4]	80–240 mg (divided twice to four times daily)	Fatigue, dizziness, hypotension, bradycardia, depression, insomnia, nausea, vomiting, constipation.
Verapamil[3,5]	120–240 mg (divided three times daily)	Headache, hypotension, flushing, edema, constipation. May aggravate atrioventricular nodal heart block and HF.
Antidepressant[6]		
Amitriptyline[3,7]	10–150 mg at bedtime	Sedation, dry mouth, constipation, weight gain, blurred vision, edema, hypotension, urinary retention.
Venlafaxine[3]	37.5–150 mg extended-release once daily	Nausea, somnolence, dry mouth, dizziness, diaphoresis, sexual dysfunction, anxiety, weight loss.
Monoclonal Antibodies Against Calcitonin Gene–Related Peptide		
Eptinezumab	100 mg intravenously every 3 months	Hypersensitivity reaction during infusion, nasopharyngitis.
Erenumab	70–140 mg subcutaneously once monthly	Injection site reactions, constipation, muscle cramps, antibody development.
Fremanezumab	225 mg subcutaneously once monthly	Injection site reactions, antibody development.
Galcanezumab	120 mg subcutaneously daily × 2 doses, followed by 120 mg monthly	Injection site reactions, antibody development.
Calcitonin Gene–Related Peptide Receptor Antagonists		
Atogepant	10–30 mg once daily	Nausea, constipation, fatigue.
Rimegepant	75 mg once every other day	Hypersensitivity, nausea.
Other		
Acupuncture		More rapid pain relief and fewer side effects than pharmacologic treatment.
Botulinum toxin	Intramuscular injection	Injection site reaction, hypersensitivity, muscle weakness.
Coenzyme Q10	300 mg once daily	
Magnesium citrate	200–300 mg twice daily	Diarrhea, nausea.
Memantine[3]	5 mg once daily to 10 mg twice daily	Somnolence, sedation, nausea.
Riboflavin	400 mg once daily	Yellow-orange discoloration of urine.
Transcutaneous supraorbital neurostimulation	20 minutes daily	Transient paresthesia at site of stimulation.
Transcranial magnetic stimulation	Up to 4 pulses twice daily	Transient lightheadedness, paresthesias, tinnitus. Contraindicated in patients with implanted medical devices in head or neck, excluding dental work.
Noninvasive vagus nerve stimulation	Two 2-minute treatments twice daily	Contraindicated in patients with implanted medical devices.

[1]Gabapentin and possibly other antiepileptics have also been used successfully.
[2]Caution or avoid during pregnancy.
[3]Not FDA-approved for this indication.
[4]Other β-adrenergic antagonists such as atenolol, metoprolol, nadolol, and timolol are similarly effective.
[5]Other calcium channel antagonists (eg, nimodipine, nicardipine, and diltiazem) may also help.
[6]Depression is commonly comorbid with migraine disorder and may warrant separate treatment.
[7]Other tricyclic antidepressants (eg, nortriptyline and imipramine) may help similarly.

night or twice daily), by mouth (2 mg daily), or by subcutaneous injection (0.25 mg three times daily for 5 days per week). Noninvasive electrical stimulation of the vagus nerve at headache onset successfully aborts pain in 30–50% of attacks; this treatment is approved in the United States.

May A et al. European Academy of Neurology guidelines on the treatment of cluster headache. Eur J Neurol. 2023;30:2955. [PMID: 37515405]

4. Posttraumatic Headache

A variety of nonspecific symptoms may follow closed head injury, regardless of whether consciousness is lost (see Head Injury). Headache is often a conspicuous feature. It usually appears within a day or so following injury, may worsen over the ensuing weeks, and then gradually subsides. It is usually a constant dull ache, with superimposed throbbing that may be localized, lateralized, or generalized. Headaches are sometimes accompanied by nausea, vomiting, or scintillating scotomas and often respond to simple analgesics; severe headaches may necessitate preventive treatment as outlined for migraine.

Teli P et al. Headache management in traumatic brain injury. J Neurol Sci. 2024;463:123002. [PMID: 39047510]

5. Primary Cough Headache

Severe head pain may be produced by coughing (and by straining, sneezing, and laughing) but, fortunately, usually lasts for a few minutes or less. Intracranial lesions, usually in the posterior fossa (eg, Arnold-Chiari malformation), are present in about 10% of cases, and brain tumors or other space-occupying lesions may present in this way. Accordingly, *CT scanning or MRI should be undertaken in all patients.*

The disorder is usually self-limited, although it may persist for several years. For unknown reasons, symptoms sometimes clear completely after lumbar puncture. Indomethacin (75–150 mg daily orally) may provide relief. Similar activity-triggered headache syndromes include primary exertional headache and primary headache associated with sexual activity.

Nandyala A et al. Primary cough headache. Curr Pain Headache Rep. 2023;27:679. [PMID: 377477622]

6. Headache Due to Giant Cell (Temporal or Cranial) Arteritis

This topic is discussed in Chapter 23.

7. Headache Due to Intracranial Mass Lesion

Intracranial mass lesions of all types may cause headache owing to displacement of vascular structures and other pain-sensitive tissues. While pain and location are nonspecific, headache may be worse upon lying down, awaken the patient at night, or peak in the morning after overnight recumbency. *The key feature prompting brain imaging is a new or worsening headache in middle or later life.* Other features suggesting an intracranial lesion include signs or symptoms of infection or malignancy such as fever, night sweats, and weight loss; immunocompromise; or history of malignancy. Signs of focal or diffuse cerebral dysfunction or of increased intracranial pressure (eg, papilledema) also necessitate investigation.

Friedman DI. Approach to the patient with headache. Continuum (Minneap Minn). 2024;30:296. [PMID: 38568485]

8. Medication Overuse (Analgesic Rebound) Headache

In many patients with **chronic daily headaches**, medication overuse is responsible. Patients have chronic pain or severe headache unresponsive to medication (typically defined as no effect after having been used regularly for more than 3 months). Ergotamines, triptans, medications containing butalbital, and opioids cause medication overuse headache when taken on more than 10 days per month; acetaminophen, acetylsalicylic acid, and NSAIDs may also be offenders if taken on more than 15 days per month. Medications such as lasmiditan and the calcitonin gene–related peptide antagonists have not been associated with overuse headaches; nevertheless, their use is also generally restricted to 10 days per month. Dopamine antagonists are unlikely to cause overuse headache, but their use should also be limited to prevent drug-induced parkinsonism or dyskinesia. Early initiation of a migraine preventive therapy, especially with antibodies to calcitonin gene related peptide, permits withdrawal of analgesics and eventual relief of headache.

Koonalintip P et al. Medication-overuse headache: update on management. Life (Basel). 2024;14:1146. [PMID: 39337929]

9. Headache Due to Other Neurologic Causes

Cerebrovascular disease may be associated with headache, but the mechanism is unclear. Headache may occur with internal carotid artery occlusion or carotid dissection and after carotid endarterectomy. Acute severe headache (**"thunderclap"**) accompanies subarachnoid hemorrhage, carotid or vertebral artery dissection, cerebral venous thrombosis, ischemic or hemorrhagic stroke, reversible cerebral vasoconstriction syndrome, hypertensive crisis, posterior reversible leukoencephalopathy syndrome, pituitary apoplexy, spontaneous intracranial hypotension, vasculitis, and meningeal infections; accompanying focal neurologic signs, impairment of consciousness, and signs of meningeal irritation indicate the need for further investigations. Headaches are also a feature of idiopathic intracranial hypertension (pseudotumor cerebri).

Headache is a frequent sequela of lumbar puncture and may last for several days. It is aggravated by the erect posture and alleviated by recumbency. The mechanism is unclear, but the headache is commonly attributed to leakage of CSF through the dural puncture site. Its incidence may be reduced if an atraumatic needle (instead of a beveled, cutting needle) is used for the lumbar puncture. Treatment is with bed rest, hydration, and caffeine. An epidural blood patch may helpful for headaches that are unresponsive to these measures.

Friedman DI. Approach to the patient with headache. Continuum (Minneap Minn). 2024;30:296. [PMID: 38568485]

When to Refer

- Thunderclap onset.
- Increasing headache unresponsive to simple measures.
- History of trauma, hypertension, fever, visual changes.
- Presence of neurologic signs or of scalp tenderness.

When to Admit

Suspected subarachnoid hemorrhage or other structural intracranial lesion.

FACIAL PAIN

1. Trigeminal Neuralgia

ESSENTIALS OF DIAGNOSIS

- Brief episodes of stabbing facial pain.
- Pain is in the territory of the second and third division of the trigeminal nerve.
- Pain exacerbated by touch.

General Considerations

Trigeminal neuralgia ("tic douloureux") is most common in middle and later life. It affects women more frequently than men. Pain may be due to an anomalous artery or vein impinging on the trigeminal nerve.

Clinical Findings

Momentary episodes of sudden lancinating facial pain commonly arise near one side of the mouth and shoot toward the ipsilateral ear, eye, or nostril. The pain may be triggered by such factors as touch, movement, drafts, and eating. To lessen the likelihood of triggering further attacks, many patients try to hold their face still while talking. Spontaneous remissions for several months or longer may occur. As the disorder progresses, the episodes of pain become more frequent, remissions become shorter and less common, and a dull ache may persist between the episodes of stabbing pain. Symptoms remain confined to the distribution of the trigeminal nerve (usually the second or third division) on one side only.

Differential Diagnosis

The characteristic features of the pain in trigeminal neuralgia usually distinguish it from other causes of facial pain. Neurologic examination shows no abnormality except in a few patients in whom trigeminal neuralgia is symptomatic of some underlying lesion, such as multiple sclerosis or a brainstem neoplasm, in which case the finding will depend on the nature and site of the lesion. High-resolution contrast-enhanced brain MRI should be obtained to rule out secondary causes and evaluate for neurovascular compression. Secondary causes are more likely in patients younger than 40 years and those with bilateral symptoms.

Treatment

The medications most helpful for treatment are oxcarbazepine (although not approved by the FDA for this indication) or carbamazepine, with monitoring by serial blood counts and liver biochemical tests. If these medications are ineffective or cannot be tolerated, phenytoin should be tried. Doses and side effects of these medications are shown in Table 27–3. Topiramate (50 mg orally twice daily), lamotrigine (400 mg orally daily), or baclofen (10–20 mg orally three or four times daily) may also be helpful, either alone or in combination with one of these other agents. Gabapentin (up to 3600 mg orally daily) may also relieve pain, especially in patients with multiple sclerosis.

For neuralgia refractory to medical treatment, several surgical treatment options are available that provide initial pain relief in at least 80% of patients. Microvascular surgical decompression with separation of the anomalous vessel (usually not visible on CT scans, MRI, or arteriograms) from the nerve root produces long-term relief of symptoms in roughly 75% of patients. Three less invasive techniques are based on destruction of nociceptive trigeminal nerve fibers, which causes sensory loss in addition to symptom relief in half of patients: (1) radiofrequency rhizotomy produces long-term pain relief in 60% of patients, (2) percutaneous balloon compression of the trigeminal ganglion in 67%, and (3) stereotactic radiosurgery to the trigeminal nerve root in 45%. In older patients, radiofrequency rhizotomy and stereotactic radiosurgery are sometimes preferred because both can be performed without general anesthesia and have few complications. Surgical exploration is inappropriate in patients with trigeminal neuralgia due to multiple sclerosis, but the less invasive techniques are sometimes helpful.

Pergolizzi JV et al. An update on pharmacotherapy for trigeminal neuralgia. Expert Rev Neurother. 2024;24:773. [PMID: 38870050]

2. Atypical Facial Pain

Facial pain without the typical features of trigeminal neuralgia is generally a constant, burning pain that may have a restricted distribution at its onset but soon spreads to the rest of the face on the affected side and sometimes involves the other side, the neck, or the back of the head as well. The disorder is especially common in middle-aged women, many with depression, but it is not clear whether depression is the cause of or a reaction to the pain. Simple analgesics, tricyclic antidepressants, carbamazepine, oxcarbazepine, and phenytoin should be given a trial; however, the response is often disappointing. Opioid analgesics pose a danger of substance use disorder. Attempts at surgical treatment are *not* indicated.

Alshammari AF et al. Systematic review of pharmacotherapy for atypical facial pain: evaluation of pain reduction, depression, anxiety and quality of life. Ann Med. 2025;57:2476050. [PMID: 40084597]

3. Glossopharyngeal Neuralgia

Glossopharyngeal neuralgia is an uncommon disorder in which pain similar in quality to that in trigeminal neuralgia occurs in the throat, about the tonsillar fossa, and sometimes deep in the ear and at the back of the tongue. The pain may be precipitated by swallowing, chewing, talking, or yawning and is sometimes accompanied by syncope. In most instances, no underlying structural abnormality is present; multiple sclerosis is sometimes responsible. Oxcarbazepine and carbamazepine are the treatments of choice and should be tried before surgical procedures are considered. Microvascular decompression is often effective and is generally preferred over destructive surgical procedures such as partial rhizotomy in medically refractory cases.

Nahas SJ. Cranial neuralgias. Continuum (Minneap Minn). 2024;30:473. [PMID: 38568494]

4. Postherpetic Neuralgia

Postherpetic neuralgia develops in about 15% of patients who have herpes zoster (shingles). This complication is especially likely to occur in older or immunocompromised persons, when the rash is severe, and when the first division of the trigeminal nerve is affected. It also relates to the duration of the rash before treatment is instituted. A history of shingles and the presence of cutaneous scarring resulting from shingles aid in the diagnosis. Severe pain with shingles correlates with the intensity of postherpetic symptoms.

Acyclovir (800 mg five times daily) or valacyclovir (1000 mg three times daily), when *given within 72 hours* of rash onset, reduces the incidence of postherpetic neuralgia by almost half; systemic corticosteroids do *not* help prevent postherpetic neuralgia (see Chapter 6). Management of the established complication is with simple analgesics. If they fail to help, a trial of a tricyclic antidepressant (eg, amitriptyline or nortriptyline, up to 100–150 mg daily orally) is often effective. Other patients respond to gabapentin (up to 3600 mg daily orally) or pregabalin (up to 600 mg/daily orally). Subcutaneous injection of botulinum toxin into the affected region produced sustained pain relief in 87% of patients in a small placebo-controlled trial. Topical application of capsaicin cream may be helpful, as may topical lidocaine (5%). *The administration of* ***recombinant zoster vaccine*** *to patients over the age of 50 years is important in reducing the likelihood of herpes zoster or reducing the severity of postherpetic neuralgia.*

Valero EG et al. Analgesic treatment approach for postherpetic neuralgia: a narrative review. J Pain Palliat Care Pharmacother. 2023;37:184. [PMID: 36731106]

5. Facial Pain Due to Other Causes

Facial pain may be caused by temporomandibular joint dysfunction in patients with malocclusion, abnormal bite, or faulty dentures. There may be tenderness of the masticatory muscles, and sometimes pain begins at the onset of chewing. This pattern differs from that of jaw (masticatory) claudication, a symptom of giant cell arteritis, in which pain develops progressively with mastication. Treatment of the underlying joint dysfunction relieves symptoms.

A relationship of facial pain to chewing or temperature changes may suggest a dental disturbance. The cause is sometimes not obvious, and diagnosis requires careful dental examination and radiographs. Sinusitis and ear infections causing facial pain are usually recognized by a history of respiratory tract infection, fever, and, in some instances, nasal or aural discharge. There may be localized tenderness. Radiologic evidence of sinus infection or mastoiditis is confirmatory.

Glaucoma is an important ocular cause of facial pain, usually localized to the periorbital region.

On occasion, pain in the jaw may be the principal manifestation of angina pectoris. Precipitation by exertion and radiation to more typical areas suggest a cardiac origin.

Barad M et al. Orofacial pain. Continuum (Minneap Minn). 2024;30:1397. [PMID: 39445947]

When to Refer

- Worsening pain unresponsive to simple measures.
- Continuing pain of uncertain cause.
- For consideration of surgical treatment (trigeminal or glossopharyngeal neuralgia).

EPILEPSY

ESSENTIALS OF DIAGNOSIS

- Recurrent unprovoked seizures.
- Characteristic electroencephalographic changes accompany seizures.
- Mental status abnormalities or focal neurologic symptoms may persist for hours postictally.

General Considerations

The term "epilepsy" denotes any disorder characterized by *recurrent unprovoked seizures.* A seizure is a transient disturbance of cerebral function due to an abnormal paroxysmal neuronal discharge in the brain. Epilepsy is relatively common, affecting approximately 0.5% of the population in the United States.

Patients with recurrent seizures provoked by a readily reversible cause, such as withdrawal from alcohol or drugs, hypo- or hyperglycemia, or uremia, are not considered to have epilepsy.

Classification of Epilepsy

According to the International League Against Epilepsy classification system, recurrent seizures should be classified first by seizure type, second by epilepsy type, and third, if possible, by epilepsy syndrome. The etiology of recurrent seizures should be sought at each stage of classification (see Etiology of Epilepsy).

A. Seizure Types

The International League Against Epilepsy distinguishes seizures affecting only part of the brain (focal seizures) from those that are generalized.

1. Focal-onset seizures—The initial clinical and electroencephalographic manifestations of focal (partial) seizures indicate that only a restricted part of one cerebral hemisphere has been activated. The ictal manifestations depend on the area of the brain involved. Focal seizures are classified by motor or nonmotor onset as well as by whether awareness is impaired.

A. MOTOR VERSUS NONMOTOR ONSET—Seizures with motor onset may be **clonic**, **tonic**, **atonic**, **myoclonic**, or **hyperkinetic**, or may manifest as **automatisms** or **epileptic spasms**. The most commonly observed focal motor seizures consist of clonic jerking or automatisms. Nonmotor seizures may be manifested by sensory symptoms (eg, paresthesias or tingling, gustatory, olfactory, visual or auditory sensations), behavior arrest, cognitive symptoms (eg, speech arrest, déjà vu, jamais vu), emotional symptoms (eg, fear), or autonomic symptoms or signs (eg, abnormal epigastric sensations, sweating, flushing, pupillary dilation). Focal sensory and motor seizures may spread (or "march") to different parts of the limb or body depending on their cortical representation and were previously called "simple partial" seizures.

B. AWARE VERSUS IMPAIRED AWARENESS—Awareness is defined as knowledge of self and environment and of events occurring during a seizure. Impaired awareness may be preceded, accompanied, or followed by the various motor and nonmotor symptoms mentioned above. Such seizures were previously called "complex partial" seizures.

C. FOCAL TO BILATERAL TONIC-CLONIC—Focal seizures sometimes involve loss of awareness and evolve to bilateral tonic-clonic seizures, in a process previously called "secondary generalization."

2. Generalized onset seizures—Generalized seizures are thought to originate in or rapidly spread to involve *bilateral cortical networks*. In some cases, the distinction between focal and generalized onset can only be made by electroencephalogram (EEG). Generalized seizures are classified into those with motor or nonmotor features. Awareness is typically lost with generalized seizures but may be retained partially in the briefest absence attacks and some myoclonic seizures.

A. NONMOTOR (ABSENCE) SEIZURES—These are characterized by impairment of consciousness, sometimes with mild clonic, tonic, myoclonic, or atonic components (ie, reduction or loss of postural tone), autonomic components (eg, enuresis), or accompanying automatisms. Onset and termination of attacks are abrupt. During conversation, the patient may miss a few words or break off in midsentence for a few seconds. The impairment of external awareness is so brief that the patient is unaware of it. **Absence ("petit mal") seizures** almost always begin in childhood and frequently cease by the age of 20 years or are then replaced by other forms of generalized seizure. Electroencephalographically, such attacks are associated with bursts of bilaterally synchronous and symmetric 3-Hz spike-wave activity. A normal background in the electroencephalogram and normal or above-normal intelligence imply a good prognosis for the ultimate cessation of these seizures. **Atypical absence seizures** may demonstrate more marked changes in tone, or attacks may have a more gradual onset and termination than in typical absence seizures. They commonly occur in patients with multiple seizure types, may be accompanied by developmental delay, and are associated with slower spike-wave discharges than those in typical absence attacks.

B. MOTOR SEIZURES—Types of generalized motor seizures include **tonic-clonic**, **clonic**, **tonic**, **myoclonic**, **myoclonic-tonic-clonic**, **myoclonic-atonic**, **atonic**, and **epileptic spasms**. During tonic-clonic seizures there is sudden loss of consciousness, the patient becomes rigid and falls to the ground, and respiration is arrested. This tonic phase, which usually lasts for under 1 minute, is followed by a clonic phase in which there is jerking of the body musculature that may last for 2 or 3 minutes and is then followed by a stage of flaccid coma. During the seizure, the tongue or lips may be bitten, urinary or fecal incontinence may occur, and the patient may be injured. Immediately after the seizure, the patient may recover consciousness, drift into sleep, have a further convulsion without recovery of consciousness between the attacks **(status epilepticus)**, or after recovering consciousness have a further convulsion **(serial seizures)**. In other cases, patients may behave in an abnormal fashion in the immediate postictal period, without subsequent awareness or memory of events **(postepileptic automatism)**. Headache, disorientation, confusion, drowsiness, nausea, soreness of the muscles, or some combination of these symptoms commonly occurs postictally. Myoclonic seizures consist of single or multiple myoclonic jerks. Atonic seizures consist of brief (< 2 seconds) loss of muscle tone and often result in falls **(epileptic drop attacks)**. **Epileptic spasms** are sudden flexion or extension of truncal muscles; these seizures usually manifest during infancy.

3. Unknown onset seizures—In some circumstances, seizures cannot be classified because of incomplete information or because they do not fit into any category. Generally, with additional information from the history or from video-EEG telemetry, the seizure onset can be correctly classified.

B. Epilepsy Types

The International League Against Epilepsy classifies epilepsy by the seizure type. Thus, epilepsy may be **focal**, **generalized**, or **combined generalized and focal**. The EEG may be helpful in facilitating classification.

C. Epilepsy Syndromes

Epilepsy syndromes are defined by constellations of seizure types, EEG findings, and imaging features, and often also depend on age at onset and comorbidities. Not every patient with epilepsy can be given a syndromic diagnosis. Several well-known epilepsy syndromes exist but are beyond the scope of this chapter.

Etiology of Epilepsy

In parallel to classifying the seizure type, epilepsy type, and epilepsy syndrome (if applicable), the cause of the patient's seizures should be sought. The International League Against Epilepsy lists six broad etiologic categories; sometimes a patient's seizures have more than one etiology.

A. Structural Etiology

1. Pediatric age groups—Congenital abnormalities and perinatal injuries may result in seizures presenting in infancy or childhood.

2. Mesial temporal sclerosis—Hippocampal sclerosis is a recognized cause of focal and secondarily generalized seizures of uncertain etiology.

3. Trauma—Trauma is an important cause of seizures at any age, but especially in young adults. Posttraumatic epilepsy is more likely to develop if the dura mater was penetrated and generally becomes manifest within 2 years following the injury. Seizures developing in the first week after head injury do not necessarily imply that future attacks will occur. Prophylactic anticonvulsant medication treatment does *not* reduce the incidence of posttraumatic epilepsy.

4. Tumors and other space-occupying lesions—Neoplasms may lead to seizures at any age, but they are an especially important cause of seizures in middle and later life, when the incidence of neoplastic disease increases. Seizures are commonly the initial symptoms of the tumor and often are focal in character. They are most likely to occur with structural lesions involving the frontal, parietal, or temporal regions. *Tumors must be excluded by imaging studies (MRI preferred over CT) in all patients with onset of seizures after 20 years of age, focal seizures or signs, or a progressive seizure disorder.*

5. Vascular diseases—Stroke and other vascular diseases become increasingly frequent causes of seizures with advancing age and are the most common cause of seizures with onset at age 60 years or older.

6. Degenerative disorders—Alzheimer disease and other degenerative disorders are a cause of seizures in later life.

B. Genetic Etiology

This category encompasses a broad range of disorders, for which the age at onset ranges from the neonatal period to adolescence or even later in life. Monogenic disorders tend to exhibit an autosomal dominant pattern of inheritance, and where the mutation is known, the responsible gene often encodes a neuronal ion channel. A genetic etiology may also underpin certain epilepsies with a metabolic or structural basis.

C. Infectious Etiology

Infectious diseases must be considered in all age groups as potentially reversible causes of seizures. Seizures may occur with an acute infective or inflammatory illness, such as bacterial meningitis or herpes encephalitis, or in patients with longstanding infections, such as neurosyphilis or cerebral cysticercosis. In patients with AIDS, seizures may result from CNS toxoplasmosis, cryptococcal meningitis, secondary viral encephalitis, or other infective complications. Seizures are a common sequela of supratentorial brain abscess, developing most frequently in the first year after treatment.

D. Metabolic Etiology

Inborn errors of metabolism and other inherited conditions may cause epilepsy as one of their manifestations (eg, pyridoxine deficiency, mitochondrial disease); these disorders typically present during childhood.

E. Immune Etiology

Autoimmune diseases such as SLE and autoimmune limbic encephalitis may cause epilepsy; often the epilepsy can be cured with immunotherapy and lifelong antiepileptic medication treatment is not necessary.

F. Unknown Etiology

In many cases, the cause of epilepsy cannot be determined.

Clinical Findings

A. Symptoms and Signs

Nonspecific changes such as headache, mood alterations, lethargy, and myoclonic jerking alert some patients to an impending seizure hours before it occurs. *These prodromal symptoms are distinct from the aura*; the aura that may precede a generalized seizure by a few seconds or minutes is itself a part of the seizure indicating focal onset from a restricted part of the brain.

Seizures usually occur unpredictably at any time and without any relationship to posture or ongoing activities. Occasionally, they occur at a particular time (eg, during sleep) or in relation to external precipitants such as lack of sleep, missed meals, emotional stress, menstruation, alcohol ingestion (or alcohol withdrawal), or use of certain recreational drugs. Fever and nonspecific infections may also precipitate seizures in patients with epilepsy. In a few patients, seizures are provoked by specific stimuli such as flashing lights or a flickering television set (**photosensitive epilepsy**), music, or reading.

Clinical examination between seizures shows no abnormality in patients with idiopathic epilepsy, but in the immediate postictal period, extensor plantar responses may be seen. The presence of lateralized or focal signs postictally suggests that seizures may have a focal origin. In patients with symptomatic epilepsy, the findings on examination will reflect the underlying cause.

B. Imaging

Imaging should be performed in patients with clinical evidence of a progressive disorder and in those with new onset of seizures after the age of 20 years because of the possibility of an underlying neoplasm. It is also indicated for patients with focal neurologic symptoms or signs, focal seizures, or electroencephalographic findings of a focal disturbance. MRI is the preferred imaging modality in most patients. CT is less sensitive than MRI in detecting small structural brain abnormalities but may be used when MRI is contraindicated or unavailable.

C. Laboratory Studies

Initial investigations after a first seizure should include CBC, serum glucose, electrolytes, creatinine, calcium, magnesium, and liver biochemical tests to exclude various causes of provoked seizures and to provide a baseline for subsequent monitoring of long-term effects of treatment. Routine laboratory investigations usually are unnecessary after recurrent seizures in patients with known epilepsy. A lumbar puncture may be necessary when any sign of infection is present or in the evaluation of new-onset seizures in the acute setting. Elevation of serum lactate above 2.4 mmol/L for up to 3 hours is common after a generalized convulsive epileptic seizure but rare after a psychogenic nonepileptic seizure or transient loss of consciousness from other causes.

D. Electroencephalography

Electroencephalography may support the clinical diagnosis of epilepsy (by demonstrating paroxysmal abnormalities containing spikes or sharp waves), provide a guide to prognosis, and help classify the seizure disorder. Classification of the disorder is important for determining the most appropriate anticonvulsant medication with which to start treatment. For example, absence and focal seizures with impaired awareness may be difficult to distinguish clinically, but their electroencephalographic findings and treatment of choice are different. Finally, by localizing the epileptogenic source, the electroencephalographic findings are important in evaluating candidates for surgical treatment. Inpatient or ambulatory continuous video EEG monitoring is often required to discriminate epileptic from nonepileptic seizures, to determine seizure type, localize for presurgical planning, and detect nonconvulsive seizures as a cause of unexplained encephalopathy.

Differential Diagnosis

The distinction between the various disorders likely to be confused with generalized seizures is usually based on the history. *The importance of obtaining an eyewitness account of the attacks cannot be overemphasized.*

A. Differential Diagnosis of Focal Seizures

1. TIAs—These are distinguished from seizures by their longer duration, lack of spread, and negative (eg, weakness or numbness) rather than positive (eg, convulsive jerking or paresthesias) symptoms. Level of consciousness, which is unaltered, does not distinguish them.

2. Migraine aura—Migraine aura may produce positive or negative symptoms, tends to spread slowly from one part of the body to another (over minutes rather than seconds), and is usually longer in duration (minutes to hours). It is usually, but not always, followed by a typical migraine headache.

3. Transient focal neurologic episodes—Most commonly observed in patients with cerebral amyloid angiopathy, these events resemble migraine aura and are theorized to have a similar pathophysiologic basis in cortical spreading depression triggered by areas of superficial siderosis or convexity subarachnoid hemorrhage.

4. Panic attacks—These may be hard to distinguish from focal seizures unless there is evidence of an anxiety disorder between attacks and the attacks have a clear relationship to external circumstances.

5. Rage attacks—These are situational and lead to goal-directed aggressive behavior.

B. Differential Diagnosis of Generalized Seizures

1. Syncope—Syncopal episodes usually occur in relation to postural change, emotional stress, instrumentation, pain, or straining. They are typically preceded by pallor, sweating, nausea, and malaise and lead to loss of consciousness accompanied by flaccidity; recovery occurs rapidly with recumbency, and there is no postictal headache or confusion. In some instances, however, motor accompaniments and urinary incontinence may simulate a seizure.

2. Cardiac disease—Cerebral hypoperfusion due to a disturbance of cardiac rhythm should be suspected in patients with known cardiac or vascular disease or in older patients who present with episodic loss of consciousness. Prodromal symptoms are typically absent. Cardiac rhythm monitoring may be necessary to establish the diagnosis. A relationship of attacks to physical activity and the finding of a systolic murmur are suggestive of aortic stenosis.

3. Brainstem ischemia—Loss of consciousness is preceded or accompanied by other brainstem signs. Basilar artery migraine and vertebrobasilar vascular disease are discussed elsewhere in this chapter.

4. Psychogenic nonepileptic seizure (PNES)—Simulating an epileptic seizure, a PNES may occur due to a conversion disorder or malingering. Many patients also have epileptic seizures or a family history of epilepsy. A history of childhood physical or sexual abuse is common. Although a PNES tends to occur at times of emotional stress, this may also be the case with epileptic seizures.

Clinically, the attacks superficially resemble tonic-clonic seizures, but there may be obvious preparation before a PNES. Moreover, there is usually no tonic phase; instead, there may be an asynchronous thrashing of the limbs and the attack rarely leads to injury. Eyes are often forcibly closed during PNES, unlike epileptic seizures, in which they are typically open. Consciousness may be normal or "lost," but in the latter context, the occurrence of goal-directed behavior or of shouting or swearing, indicates that it is feigned. Postictally, there are no changes in behavior or neurologic findings. Video EEG is almost always necessary to distinguish PNES from epilepsy.

Treatment

A. General Measures

For patients with epilepsy, medication is prescribed with the goal of preventing further attacks and *usually continued until there have been no seizures for at least 2 years*. Patients should be advised to avoid situations that could be dangerous or life-threatening if further seizures should occur. Legislation may require clinicians to report to the state authorities any patients with seizures or other episodic disturbances of consciousness; *driving cessation for 6 months* or as legislated is appropriate following an unprovoked seizure.

1. Choice of medication—Medication selection depends on seizure type, side effect profile, coexisting medical conditions, route of metabolism, drug interactions, and cost (Tables 27–2 and 27–3). In women of childbearing age, special consideration must be given to potential teratogenicity and interactions with oral contraceptives. *All antiepileptics are potentially teratogenic*, although the teratogenicity of the newer antiseizure medications is less clear. Nevertheless, antiepileptic medication must be given to pregnant persons with epilepsy to prevent seizures, which can pose serious risk to the fetus from trauma, hypoxia, or other factors.

The dose of the selected anticonvulsant is gradually increased until seizures are controlled or until side effects prevent further increases. If seizures continue despite treatment at the maximal tolerated dose, a second medication is added and the dose increased depending on tolerance; the first medication is then gradually withdrawn. In most patients with seizures of a single type, satisfactory control can be achieved with a single anticonvulsant. Treatment with two medications may further reduce seizure frequency or severity but usually at the cost of greater toxicity. Treatment with more than two medications is almost always unhelpful unless the patient is having seizures of different types.

2. Monitoring—Individual differences in drug metabolism cause a given dose of a medication to produce different blood concentrations in different patients, and this will affect the therapeutic response. In general, *the dose of an antiepileptic agent is increased, depending on tolerance, to achieve the desired clinical response regardless of the serum drug level.* When a dose is reached that either controls seizures or is the maximum tolerated, a steady-state trough drug level may be obtained for future reference; rechecking the trough level may be appropriate during pregnancy, if a breakthrough seizure occurs, a dose change occurs, or another (potentially interacting) medication is added to the regimen. A laboratory's therapeutic range for a medication is only a guide; many patients achieve good seizure control with no adverse effect at serum levels that exceed the stipulated range, and in these cases no dose adjustment is needed. The most common cause of a lower concentration

Table 27–2. Approved indications for antiseizure medications (listed in alphabetical order within seizure type or epilepsy syndrome).

Seizure Type or Epilepsy Syndrome	Approved as Monotherapy or Adjunctive Therapy	Approved Only as Adjunctive Therapy
Absence seizures	Clonazepam[2], ethosuximide, valproic acid	
Akinetic (atonic) seizures	Clonazepam	
Cyclin-dependent kinase-like 5 deficiency	Ganaxolone[3]	
Dravet syndrome	Cannabidiol	
Focal onset seizures	Brivaracetam, carbamazepine, cenobamate, eslicarbazepine felbamate[1], lacosamide, lamotrigine, levetiracetam, oxcarbazepine, perampanel, phenobarbital, primidone, topiramate, valproic acid	Clorazepate, gabapentin, pregabalin, tiagabine, vigabatrin, zonisamide
Generalized onset seizures	Carbamazepine, phenobarbital, primidone, topiramate	Lacosamide, lamotrigine, levetiracetam, perampanel
Infantile spasms	Vigabatrin	
Lennox-Gastaut syndrome	Cannabidiol, clonazepam	Clobazam, felbamate[1], lamotrigine, rufinamide, topiramate
Multiple seizure types including absence seizures		Valproic acid
Myoclonic seizures	Clonazepam	Levetiracetam
Tuberous sclerosis complex	Cannabidiol	

[1]Not to be used as a first-line medication; when used, blood counts should be performed regularly (every 2–4 weeks). Should be used only in selected patients because of risk of aplastic anemia and hepatic failure. It is advisable to obtain written informed consent before use.
[2]Approved in patients who have failed to respond to succinimides (ethosuximide).
[3]Approved in patients 2 years or older.

Table 27–3. Medication treatment for seizures in adults (listed in alphabetical order).

Medication[1]	Usual Adult Daily Oral Dose	Minimum No. of Daily Doses	Time to Steady-State Medication Levels	Optimal Medication Level and Laboratory Monitoring[1]	Selected Side Effects and Idiosyncratic Reactions
Brivaracetam	50–100 mg	2	1–2 days	CBC, liver biochemical tests	Somnolence, fatigue, ataxia, vertigo, psychosis, leukopenia, hypersensitivity (bronchospasm and angioedema).
Cannabidiol	5–20 mg/kg	2	11–13 days	Liver biochemical tests at baseline, 1, 3, and 6 months	Somnolence, fatigue, anorexia, weight loss, anemia, diarrhea, rash, sleep disorder, infections. Elevation in liver enzymes may occur; reduce dose in hepatic impairment.
Carbamazepine	400–1600 mg (immediate- or extended-release)	2	3–4 days	4–8 mcg/mL CBC, liver biochemical tests, BUN/Cr	Nystagmus, dysarthria, diplopia, ataxia, drowsiness, nausea, blood dyscrasias, hepatotoxicity, hyponatremia, Stevens-Johnson syndrome.[2] May exacerbate myoclonic seizures.
Cenobamate	200–400 mg	1	14 days	Liver biochemical tests, potassium	Multiorgan hypersensitivity, QT shortening, somnolence, dizziness, cognitive dysfunction, blurred vision.
Clobazam	10–40 mg	2	7–10 days		Lethargy and somnolence, ataxia, insomnia, dysarthria, aggression, constipation, fever, Stevens-Johnson syndrome.
Clonazepam	0.04–0.2 mg/kg	2	7–10 days	20–80 ng/mL CBC, liver biochemical tests	Drowsiness, ataxia, irritability, behavioral changes, exacerbation of tonic-clonic seizures.
Clorazepate	22.5–90 mg	2	10 days		Sedation, dizziness, confusion, ataxia, depression, dependency/abuse.
Ethosuximide	500–1500 mg	2	5–10 days	40–100 mcg/mL CBC, liver biochemical tests, UA	Nausea, vomiting, anorexia, headache, lethargy, unsteadiness, blood dyscrasias, SLE, urticaria, pruritus.
Eslicarbazepine	400–1200 mg	1	4 days	Serum sodium and chloride; liver biochemical tests	As for carbamazepine.
Felbamate[4]	1200–3600 mg	3	4–5 days	CBC and reticulocytes, liver biochemical tests	Anorexia, nausea, vomiting, headache, insomnia, weight loss, dizziness, hepatotoxicity, fatal aplastic anemia. Reserved for refractory epilepsy.
Gabapentin	900–3600 mg	3	1 day		Sedation, fatigue, ataxia, nystagmus, weight loss.
Ganaxolone	450–1800 mg	3	7 days		Sedation, fever, excessive salivation, seasonal allergy.
Lacosamide	100–400 mg	2	3 days	ECG if known cardiac conduction problems or severe cardiac disease	Vertigo, diplopia, nausea, headache, fatigue, ataxia, tremor, anaphylactoid reactions, PR prolongation, cardiac dysrhythmia, suicidality.
Lamotrigine	100–500 mg	2	4–5 days		Sedation, skin rash, visual disturbances, dyspepsia, ataxia.
Levetiracetam	1000–3000 mg	2	2 days		Somnolence, ataxia, headache, behavioral changes.
Oxcarbazepine	900–1800 mg	2	2–3 days	Serum sodium	As for carbamazepine.
Perampanel	4–12 mg	1	3 weeks		Dizziness, somnolence, irritability, weight gain, falls, ataxia, dysarthria, blurred vision.

(*continued*)

Table 27–3. Medication treatment for seizures in adults (listed in alphabetical order). (continued)

Medication[1]	Usual Adult Daily Oral Dose	Minimum No. of Daily Doses	Time to Steady-State Medication Levels	Optimal Medication Level and Laboratory Monitoring[1]	Selected Side Effects and Idiosyncratic Reactions
Phenobarbital	100–200 mg	1	14–21 days	10–40 mcg/mL CBC, liver biochemical tests, BUN/Cr	Drowsiness, nystagmus, ataxia, skin rashes, learning difficulties, hyperactivity.
Phenytoin	200–400 mg	1	5–10 days	10–20 mcg/mL CBC, liver biochemical tests, folate	Nystagmus, ataxia, dysarthria, sedation, confusion, gingival hyperplasia, hirsutism, megaloblastic anemia, blood dyscrasias, skin rashes, fever, SLE, lymphadenopathy, peripheral neuropathy, dyskinesias. May exacerbate myoclonic seizures.
Pregabalin	150–300 mg	2	2–4 days		Somnolence, dizziness, poor concentration, weight gain, thrombocytopenia, skin rashes, anaphylactoid reactions.
Primidone	750–1500 mg	3	4–7 days	5–12 mcg/mL CBC	Sedation, nystagmus, ataxia, vertigo, nausea, skin rashes, megaloblastic anemia, irritability.
Rufinamide	800–3200 mg	2	2 days		Somnolence, headache, dizziness, suicidality, Stevens-Johnson syndrome, leukopenia, shortened QT interval, nausea, vomiting.
Tiagabine	32–56 mg	2	2 days		Somnolence, anxiety, dizziness, poor concentration, tremor, diarrhea.
Topiramate	200–400 mg	2	4 days	Serum bicarbonate, BUN/Cr in older patients	Somnolence, nausea, dyspepsia, irritability, dizziness, ataxia, nystagmus, diplopia, glaucoma, renal calculi, weight loss, hypohidrosis, hyperthermia.
Valproic acid	1500–2000 mg	2–3	2–4 days	50–100 mcg/mL CBC, liver biochemical tests	Nausea, vomiting, diarrhea, drowsiness, alopecia, weight gain, hepatotoxicity, thrombocytopenia, tremor, pancreatitis. Teratogenic; avoid in women of childbearing age.
Vigabatrin	3000 mg	2	2 days		Somnolence, anorexia, nausea, vomiting, agitation, hostility, confusion, suicidality, neutropenia, Stevens-Johnson syndrome, permanent visual field loss.[3]
Zonisamide	200–600 mg	1	14 days	BUN/Cr, serum bicarbonate	Somnolence, ataxia, anorexia, nausea, vomiting, rash, confusion, renal calculi. Do not use in patients with sulfonamide allergy.

Cr, creatinine. Note that many factors influence optimal dose of these drugs including age, tolerance, and concomitant medication.

[1]Patients starting treatment with any antiepileptic drug should be monitored for new or worsening depression or suicidal thoughts, especially during the first weeks of therapy. Baseline measurement of creatinine clearance is advisable in renally metabolized drugs.

[2]Carriers of the HLA-B*1502 allele are at higher risk for Stevens-Johnson syndrome. Patients of Asian ancestry should be tested for this allele prior to initiation of therapy.

[3]Regular ophthalmologic examination is recommended.

[4]Not to be used as a first-line drug; when used, blood counts should be performed regularly (every 2–4 weeks). Should be used only in selected patients because of risk of aplastic anemia and hepatic failure. It is advisable to obtain written informed consent before use.

of medication than expected for the prescribed dose is suboptimal patient adherence. Adherence can be improved by limiting to a minimum the number of daily doses. Recurrent seizures or status epilepticus may result if medications are taken erratically, and in some circumstances nonadherent patients may be better off without any medication. All anticonvulsants have side effects, and many require baseline and regular laboratory monitoring (Table 27–3).

3. Discontinuance of medication—*Only when adult patients have been seizure-free for 2 years should withdrawal of medication be considered.* Unfortunately, there is no way of predicting which patients can be managed successfully without treatment, although seizure recurrence is more likely in (1) patients with a longer duration of epilepsy prior to remission, (2) those with a shorter duration of remission, (3) those who initially did not respond to therapy, (4) those with seizures having focal features or of multiple types, (5) those with onset during adulthood, and (6) those with continuing electroencephalographic abnormalities. Dose reduction should be gradual (over weeks or months), and medications should be withdrawn one at a time. If seizures recur, treatment is reinstituted with the previously effective regimen.

4. Surgical treatment—Patients with seizures refractory to two or more medications may be candidates for operative treatment. Surgical resection is most efficacious when there is a single well-defined seizure focus, particularly in the temporal lobe. Among well-chosen patients, up to 70% remain seizure-free after extended follow-up. Additional surgical techniques for medically refractory epilepsy approved in the United States include laser interstitial thermal therapy, deep brain stimulation, responsive cortical stimulation, and vagus nerve stimulation.

B. Special Circumstances

1. Solitary seizures—In patients who have had only one seizure or a flurry of seizures over a brief period of several hours, investigation as outlined earlier should exclude an underlying cause requiring specific treatment. An electroencephalogram should be obtained, preferably within 24 hours after the seizure. Prophylactic anticonvulsant treatment is generally *not* required unless further attacks occur or investigations reveal underlying pathology. The risk of seizure recurrence varies in different series between about 30% and 70%, with higher risk of recurrence in patients with structural brain lesions or abnormalities on electroencephalogram. Epilepsy should *not* be diagnosed based on a solitary seizure. If seizures occur in the context of transient, nonrecurrent systemic disorders such as hyponatremia or hypoglycemia, the diagnosis of epilepsy is inaccurate, and long-term prophylactic anticonvulsant treatment is unnecessary.

2. Alcohol withdrawal seizures—The characteristic alcohol withdrawal seizure pattern is one or more generalized tonic-clonic seizures that may occur within 48 hours or so of withdrawal from alcohol after a period of high or prolonged intake. If the seizures have consistently focal features, the possibility of an associated structural abnormality, often traumatic in origin, must be considered. Treatment with anticonvulsants is generally not required for alcohol withdrawal seizures, since they are self-limited. Benzodiazepines are effective and safe for preventing further seizures. Status epilepticus may complicate alcohol withdrawal and is managed along conventional lines. Further attacks will not occur if the patient abstains from alcohol.

3. Tonic-clonic status epilepticus—Poor adherence to the anticonvulsant regimen is the most common cause; however, any disorder that can cause a single seizure may be responsible. The mortality rate may be as high as 20%, and among survivors the incidence of neurologic and cognitive sequelae is high. The prognosis relates to the underlying cause as well as the length of time between onset of status epilepticus and the start of effective treatment.

Status epilepticus is a medical emergency. Initial management includes maintenance of the airway and 50% dextrose (25–50 mL) intravenously in case hypoglycemia is responsible. If seizures continue, an intravenous bolus of lorazepam, 4 mg, is given at a rate of 2 mg/min and repeated once after 10 minutes if necessary; alternatively, 10 mg of midazolam is given intramuscularly, and again after 10 minutes if necessary. Diazepam can also be given rectally as a gel (0.2 mg/kg). These measures are usually effective in halting seizures for a brief period. Respiratory depression and hypotension may complicate the treatment and are treated as in other circumstances, including intubation and mechanical ventilation and admission to an ICU.

Regardless of the response to lorazepam or midazolam, fosphenytoin or phenytoin should be administered intravenously. Fosphenytoin (18–20 mg phenytoin equivalents [PE]/kg) is rapidly and completely converted to phenytoin following intravenous administration. It is preferred because it is less likely to cause reactions at the infusion site, can be given with all common intravenous solutions, and may be administered at a faster rate (150 mg PE/min). When fosphenytoin is not available, phenytoin (18–20 mg/kg) is given intravenously at a rate of 50 mg/min. Because arrhythmias may develop during rapid administration of fosphenytoin or phenytoin, ECG monitoring is advised. Hypotension may occur, especially if diazepam has also been given. Alternatively or additionally, intravenous valproate (loading dose 20–40 mg/kg over 15 minutes, maximum dose 3000 mg) or levetiracetam (loading dose 60 mg/kg over 15 minutes, maximum dose 4500 mg) is used for status epilepticus. Although neither is approved by the FDA for this indication, both were equivalent to fosphenytoin in a randomized trial. Due to the teratogenicity of valproate, it should be avoided in persons who may be pregnant.

If seizures continue, phenobarbital is then given in a loading dose of 10–20 mg/kg intravenously by slow or intermittent injection (50 mg/min). Respiratory depression and hypotension are especially common with this therapy.

If these measures fail, general anesthesia with ventilatory assistance may be required; some experts recommend proceeding directly to general anesthesia if convulsions do not cease after the initial 18–20 PE/kg fosphenytoin load. Intravenous midazolam may provide control of refractory status epilepticus; the suggested loading dose is 0.2 mg/kg, followed by 0.05–0.2 mg/kg/hour. Propofol (1–2 mg/kg as an intravenous bolus, followed by infusion at 2–15 mg/kg/hour depending on response) may also be used, as may pentobarbital (5–15 mg/kg intravenously, followed by 0.5–4 mg/kg/hour).

After status epilepticus is controlled, an oral medication program for the long-term management of seizures is started, and investigations into the cause of the disorder are pursued.

4. Nonconvulsive status epilepticus—In some cases, status epilepticus presents not with convulsions, but with a fluctuating abnormal mental status, confusion, impaired responsiveness, and automatism. Electroencephalography establishes the diagnosis. The treatment approach outlined above applies to any type of status epilepticus, although intravenous anesthesia is usually not necessary. The prognosis is a reflection of the underlying cause rather than of continuing seizures.

When to Refer

- Behavioral episodes of uncertain nature.
- Seizures are difficult to control with monotherapy.
- There is a progressive neurologic disorder.

When to Admit

- Status epilepticus.
- Frequent seizures requiring rapid medication titration and electroencephalographic monitoring.
- For inpatient monitoring when PNES is suspected.

Pack AM et al. Teratogenesis, perinatal, and neurodevelopmental outcomes after in utero exposure to antiseizure medication: practice guideline from the AAN, AES, and SMFM. Neurology. 2024;102:e209279. [PMID: 38748979]

Vossler DG. First seizures, acute repetitive seizures, and status epilepticus. Continuum (Minneap Minn). 2025;31:95. [PMID: 39899098]

DYSAUTONOMIA

ESSENTIALS OF DIAGNOSIS

- Postural hypotension or abnormal heart rate regulation.
- Abnormalities of sweating, intestinal motility, sexual function, or sphincter control.
- Syncope may occur.
- Symptoms occur in isolation or any combination.

General Considerations

Dysautonomia may be caused by pathological processes in the central or peripheral nervous system. It is manifested by a variety of symptoms related to abnormalities of blood pressure regulation, thermoregulatory sweating, GI function, sphincter control, sexual function, respiration, and ocular function. The differential diagnosis of autonomic dysfunction depends on the time course and whether it is an isolated symptom or associated with central or peripheral neurologic symptoms and signs.

A. Causes in the Central Nervous System

Disease at certain sites, regardless of its nature, may lead to dysautonomic symptoms. Postural hypotension, which is usually the most troublesome and disabling symptom, may result from spinal cord transection and other myelopathies (eg, due to tumor or syringomyelia) above the T6 level or from brainstem lesions such as syringobulbia and posterior fossa tumors. Sphincter or sexual disturbances may result from cord lesions at any level. Certain primary degenerative disorders are responsible for dysautonomia occurring in isolation (**pure autonomic failure**) or in association with more widespread abnormalities (**multisystem atrophy**) that may include parkinsonism, pyramidal symptoms, and cerebellar deficits. Postural hypotension is a prominent symptom of idiopathic Parkinson disease and dementia with Lewy bodies.

B. Causes in the Peripheral Nervous System

A pure autonomic neuropathy may occur acutely or subacutely after a viral infection or as a paraneoplastic disorder, usually related to small cell lung cancer, in association with certain antibodies, such as anti-Hu or those directed at neuronal nicotinic ganglionic acetylcholine receptors. Dysautonomia often occurs in patients with Guillain-Barré syndrome, manifesting with hypotension, hypertension, or cardiac arrhythmias that may have a fatal outcome. It may also occur with diabetic, uremic, amyloidotic, and other metabolic or toxic neuropathies; in association with leprosy or Chagas disease; and as a feature of certain hereditary neuropathies. Autonomic symptoms are prominent in the crises of hepatic porphyria. Small fiber neuropathies may underlie some cases of postural orthostatic tachycardia syndrome (POTS) due to impaired contractility in denervated venules and resulting preload failure (see below). Patients with botulism or the Lambert-Eaton myasthenic syndrome may have constipation, urinary retention, and a sicca syndrome due to impaired cholinergic function.

Clinical Findings

A. Symptoms and Signs

Dysautonomic symptoms include syncope, postural hypotension, paroxysmal hypertension, persistent tachycardia without other cause, facial flushing, hypo- or hyperhidrosis, vomiting, constipation, diarrhea, dysphagia, abdominal distention, disturbances of micturition or defecation, erectile dysfunction, apneic episodes, and declining night vision. In syncope, prodromal malaise, nausea, headache, diaphoresis, pallor, visual disturbance, loss of postural tone, and a sense of weakness and impending loss of consciousness are followed by actual loss of consciousness. It is usually accompanied by hypotension and bradycardia and may occur in response to emotional stress, postural hypotension, vigorous exercise in a hot environment, obstructed venous return to the heart, acute pain or its anticipation, fluid loss, and a variety of other circumstances. Although the patient is usually flaccid, some motor activity is not uncommon. Urinary (and rarely fecal) incontinence may occur, simulating a seizure. Recovery is rapid once the patient becomes recumbent, but headache, nausea, and fatigue commonly persist.

B. Evaluation of the Patient

The extent and severity of autonomic dysfunction should be determined, and the presence of associated neurologic symptoms and signs ascertained. Bedside testing of autonomic function includes examination of pupillary reactivity, of the skin for areas of excessive or reduced sweating, and of the hands and feet for color or temperature changes. Blood pressure and heart rate should be assessed in the supine position and 3 minutes after standing. With dysautonomia, *postural hypotension is not accompanied by a compensatory rise in heart rate.* Specialized tests include the cardiovascular response to the Valsalva maneuver and deep respiration, the tilt-table test, the thermoregulatory sweat test, the quantitative sudomotor axon reflex test, and the quantitative direct and indirect axon reflex tests. Tests of GI motility and urodynamics may be helpful when symptoms of dysmotility, incontinence, or urinary retention are present.

The neurologic examination should focus on detection of signs of parkinsonism, cerebellar dysfunction, neuromuscular transmission disorders, and peripheral neuropathy. All patients should be tested for vitamin B_{12} deficiency and diabetes. Patients with acute or subacute isolated dysautonomia should undergo testing for ganglionic acetylcholine receptor, anti-Hu, voltage-gated potassium channel complex, and voltage-gated calcium channel antibodies. For those with evidence of peripheral neuropathy, nerve conduction studies; electromyography; and testing for HIV, amyloidosis, Sjögren syndrome, and Fabry disease are indicated. If there is evidence of central pathology, imaging studies will exclude a treatable structural cause. If the neurologic examination is normal, reversible, non-neurologic causes of symptoms must be considered. Isolated postural hypotension and syncope may relate to a reduced cardiac output, paroxysmal cardiac dysrhythmias, volume depletion, various medications, and endocrine and metabolic disorders such as Addison disease, hypo- or hyperthyroidism, pheochromocytoma, and carcinoid syndrome.

Treatment

The most disabling symptoms are usually postural hypotension and syncope. Abrupt postural change, prolonged recumbency, heavy meals, and other precipitants should be avoided. Medications associated with postural hypotension should be discontinued or reduced in dose. Treatment may include wearing waist-high elastic hosiery, salt supplementation, sleeping in a semierect position (which minimizes the natriuresis and diuresis that occur during recumbency), ingestion of 500 mL water 30 minutes before arising, and fludrocortisone (0.1–0.5 mg orally daily). Vasoconstrictor agents may be helpful and include midodrine (2.5–10 mg orally three times daily), droxidopa (100–600 mg orally three times daily), and ephedrine (15–30 mg orally three times daily). Other agents used occasionally are dihydroergotamine, yohimbine, pyridostigmine, atomoxetine, and clonidine; refractory cases may respond to erythropoietin (epoetin-α) or desmopressin. Patients must be monitored for recumbent hypertension. Postprandial hypotension is helped by caffeine. There is no satisfactory treatment for disturbances of sweating, but an air-conditioned environment is helpful in avoiding extreme swings in body temperature.

When to Refer

- When the diagnosis is uncertain.
- When symptoms persist despite conventional treatment.

Hovaguimian A. Dysautonomia: diagnosis and management. Neurol Clin. 2023;41:193. [PMID: 36400555]

POSTURAL ORTHOSTATIC TACHYCARDIA SYNDROME (POTS)

Clinical Findings

In POTS, orthostatic symptoms (tremulousness, lightheadedness, palpitations, visual disturbances, weakness, fatigue, anxiety, hyperventilation, nausea) and significant tachycardia (an increase of 30 beats/min or more or a heart rate of 120 beats/min or more) develop within 10 minutes of standing in the absence of postural hypotension or an autonomic neuropathy. POTS is more common in women than men and in patients between 20 and 50 years of age. Other medical problems causing a tachycardia must be excluded.

Its pathophysiology is uncertain but may involve cardiac deconditioning; impaired peripheral vasoconstriction due to peripheral sympathetic denervation, leading to venous pooling in the legs on standing and a compensatory tachycardia (**"neuropathic POTS"**); or an exaggerated sympathetic response to standing, with tachycardia caused by markedly elevated levels of plasma norepinephrine (**"hyperadrenergic POTS"**). Other possible mechanisms include hypovolemia, possibly from impaired function of the renin-angiotensin system (**"volume dysregulation POTS"**) and excessive mast cell activation leading to inappropriate release of histamine during physical activity. Psychological mechanisms have also been invoked. POTS may be associated with joint hypermobility syndrome and mitral valve prolapse. It may follow pregnancy, surgery, trauma, chemotherapy, vaccinations, or viral infections, including SARS-CoV-2.

Treatment

Regardless of the underlying cause, initial management should include volume repletion (high salt diet and copious fluids), postural and psychophysiologic training, and a graduated exercise program. Treatment for patients with hyperadrenergic POTS may include a β-blocking agent (eg, propranolol 10–40 mg three times daily or metoprolol 12.5–50 mg twice daily), phenobarbital (15 mg in the morning, 60 mg at night), or clonidine (0.2 mg twice daily). If a neuropathic cause is suspected, treatment with midodrine, droxidopa, pyridostigmine, or fludrocortisone at the doses described for postural hypotension may be considered. The long-term prognosis is unclear but approximately 50% of patients recover within 3 years.

Boris JR et al. Long-term POTS outcomes survey: diagnosis, therapy, and clinical outcomes. J Am Heart Assoc. 2024;13:e033485. [PMID: 38958137]

TRANSIENT ISCHEMIC ATTACKS

ESSENTIALS OF DIAGNOSIS

- Focal neurologic deficit of acute onset.
- Clinical deficit resolves completely within 24 hours.
- Risk factors for vascular disease often present.

General Considerations

Transient ischemic attacks (TIAs) are characterized by *focal ischemic cerebral neurologic deficits that last for < 24 hours* (usually < 1–2 hours). About 30% of patients with stroke have a history of TIAs and 5–10% of patients with TIAs will have a stroke within 90 days. The natural history of attacks is variable. Some patients will have a major stroke after only a few attacks, whereas others may have frequent attacks for weeks or months without having a stroke. *The risk of stroke is high in the first 3 months after an attack, particularly in the first month and especially within the first 48 hours.* The stroke risk is greater in patients older than 60 years, in patients with diabetes, or after TIAs that last longer than 10 minutes and with symptoms or signs of weakness, speech impairment, or gait disturbance. Carotid ischemic attacks are more likely than vertebrobasilar ischemic attacks to be followed by stroke.

Urgent intervention in TIA patients reduces rates of subsequent stroke, and *the condition should be treated with a similar sense of urgency as unstable angina.*

Etiology

An important (and most common) cause of transient cerebral ischemia is embolization. In many patients with these attacks, a source is readily apparent in the heart or a major extracranial artery to the head, and emboli sometimes are visible in the retinal arteries. An embolic phenomenon explains why separate attacks may affect different parts of the territory supplied by the same major vessel. Cardiac causes of embolic ischemic attacks include atrial fibrillation, HF, infective and nonbacterial thrombotic endocarditis, atrial myxoma, and mural thrombi complicating MI. Atrial septal defects and patent foramen ovale may permit venous thromboemboli to reach the brain (**paradoxical emboli**). An ulcerated plaque on a major artery to the brain may serve as a source of emboli. In the anterior circulation, atherosclerotic changes occur most commonly in the region of the carotid bifurcation extracranially; these changes may cause a bruit. Atherosclerosis also affects the vertebrobasilar system and the major intracranial vessels including the middle and anterior cerebral arteries.

Less common abnormalities of blood vessels that may cause TIAs include fibromuscular dysplasia, which affects the cervical internal carotid artery; atherosclerosis of the aortic arch; inflammatory arterial disorders such as giant cell arteritis, polyarteritis, and granulomatous angiitis; Fabry disease; and meningovascular syphilis. Critical stenosis of a major extracranial or intracranial artery may cause TIA, especially in the setting of hypotension.

Hematologic causes of TIA include polycythemia, sickle cell disease, hyperviscosity syndromes, and the antiphospholipid antibody syndrome. Severe anemia may also lead to transient focal neurologic deficits in patients with preexisting cerebral arterial disease.

The **subclavian steal syndrome** may lead to transient vertebrobasilar ischemia. Symptoms develop when there is localized stenosis or occlusion of one subclavian artery proximal to the source of the vertebral artery, so that blood is "stolen" from the vertebral artery to supply the arm. A bruit in the supraclavicular fossa, unequal radial pulses, and a difference of 20 mm Hg or more between the systolic blood pressures in the arms should suggest the diagnosis in patients with vertebrobasilar TIAs.

Clinical Findings

A. Symptoms and Signs

The symptoms of TIAs vary markedly among patients; however, the symptoms in a given individual tend to be constant in type. Onset is abrupt and without warning, and recovery usually occurs rapidly, often within a few minutes. The specific symptoms depend on the arterial distribution affected, as outlined in the subsequent section on stroke. Of note, *TIA rarely causes loss of consciousness or acute confusion but is often erroneously blamed for such symptoms.*

B. Imaging

CT or MRI scan is indicated within 24 hours of symptom onset, in part to exclude the possibility of a small cerebral hemorrhage or a cerebral tumor masquerading as a TIA. MRI with diffusion-weighted sequences is sensitive for revealing acute or subacute infarction, which is seen in up to one-third of cases despite resolution of clinical symptoms and indicates a high risk of subsequent stroke. Noninvasive imaging of the cervical vasculature should also be performed; carotid duplex ultrasonography is useful for detecting significant stenosis of the internal carotid artery, and MR or CT angiography permits broader visualization of cervical and intracranial vasculature.

C. Laboratory and Other Studies

Clinical and laboratory evaluation must include assessment for hypertension, heart disease, hematologic disorders, diabetes mellitus, hyperlipidemia, and peripheral vascular disease. It should include CBC, fasting blood glucose, and serum cholesterol determinations, and may include serologic tests for syphilis and HIV infection. An ECG should be obtained. Echocardiography with agitated saline contrast is performed if a cardioembolic source is likely, and blood cultures are obtained if endocarditis is suspected. If the cause of the TIA remains elusive, extended ambulatory ECG monitoring (eg, Zio patch, Holter) is indicated to detect paroxysmal atrial fibrillation, *which may be found in up to 20% of patients.*

Differential Diagnosis

Focal seizures usually cause abnormal motor or sensory phenomena such as clonic limb movements, paresthesias, or tingling, rather than weakness or loss of feeling. Symptoms generally spread ("march") up the limb and may lead to a generalized tonic-clonic seizure.

Classic migraine is easily recognized by the visual premonitory symptoms, followed by nausea, headache, and photophobia, but less typical cases may be hard to distinguish. Patients with migraine are typically younger, commonly have a history of episodes since adolescence, and report that other family members have a similar disorder.

Focal neurologic deficits may occur during periods of hypoglycemia in patients with diabetes receiving insulin or oral hypoglycemic agent therapy.

Treatment

A. Medical Measures

Medical treatment is aimed at preventing further attacks and stroke. Treat diabetes mellitus, hematologic disorders, and hypertension, preferably with an ACE inhibitor or ARB. Among patients with atherosclerosis and LDL > 100 mg/dL, atorvastatin 80 mg orally once daily should be started. The LDL should be measured every 3 to 12 months, and ezetimibe (10 mg once orally once daily) added if necessary to lower the LDL to < 70 mg/dL. In patients with at least two major atherosclerotic cardiovascular events (ischemic stroke, ACS or MI, peripheral arterial disease) or one major such event and multiple risk factors (age over 64 years, cardiac bypass surgery or percutaneous coronary intervention, heterozygous familial hypercholesterolemia, diabetes, hypertension, CKD, or active tobacco smoking), a proprotein convertase subtilisin/kexin type 9 inhibitor (eg, evolocumab or alirocumab) can be added. Cigarette smoking should be stopped, and cardiac sources of embolization should be treated appropriately. Weight reduction and regular physical activity should be encouraged when appropriate. An antiplatelet or anticoagulant should be started as soon as imaging has established the absence of hemorrhage (see Anticoagulation and Antiplatelet therapy below).

1. Hospitalization—Hospitalization should be considered within a week of the attack when patients are at increased risk for early recurrence. A common method for estimating recurrence risk is the **ABCD² score**: age 60 years or older (1 point), blood pressure 140/90 mm Hg or higher (1 point), clinical symptoms of focal weakness (2 points) or speech impairment without weakness (1 point), duration of 60 minutes or longer (2 points) or 10–59 minutes (1 point), or diabetes mellitus (1 point). *An ABCD² score of 4 or more points has been suggested as a threshold for hospital admission.* The **ABCD²I** (with an additional 3 points for any abnormal diffusion-weighted MRI finding or any infarct [new or old] on noncontrast CT) has been proposed as a better predictor of subsequent stroke risk. Admission is also advisable for patients with crescendo attacks, symptomatic carotid stenosis, or a known cardiac source of emboli or hypercoagulable state. Hospitalization facilitates early intervention for stroke recurrence and rapid institution of secondary prevention measures.

2. Anticoagulation—*The chief indication for anticoagulation after TIA is atrial fibrillation.* Patients with mechanical heart valves, left atrial or ventricular thrombus, LV assist devices, and the antiphospholipid antibody syndrome should also receive anticoagulation therapy. In the setting of atrial fibrillation in patients without moderate to severe mitral stenosis (Chapter 12) or a mechanical heart valve, apixaban (2.5–5 mg orally twice daily), dabigatran (150 mg orally twice daily), edoxaban (60 mg orally daily), and rivaroxaban (20 mg orally daily) are *preferred over warfarin for long-term anticoagulation.* Warfarin (target INR 2.0–3.0) is indicated in patients with valvular atrial fibrillation (ie, moderate to severe mitral stenosis), mechanical heart valves, LV assist devices, and the antiphospholipid antibody syndrome. Combination antiplatelet-anticoagulation therapy is only indicated in select patients with mechanical heart valves or those with a separate indication for antiplatelet therapy such as a cardiac stent. In patients with cardiomyopathy and an EF under 35% without atrial fibrillation, warfarin (target INR 2.0–3.0) reduces ischemic stroke risk compared to aspirin but results in a roughly equivalent increase in the risk of major hemorrhage; treatment in this population should therefore be individualized.

3. Antiplatelet therapy—All patients with TIA or ischemic stroke in whom anticoagulation is not indicated should be treated with antiplatelet therapy to reduce the frequency of TIAs and the incidence of stroke. Short-term administration of dual antiplatelet therapy (DAPT) is recommended in two situations. The first is within 12 hours after a high-risk TIA (ABCD² score ≥ 4) or minor stroke (defined by a NIH Stroke Scale of 3 or less); an oral loading dose of clopidogrel (300–600 mg) is followed by 75 mg/day orally plus aspirin (50–325 mg daily orally) for 21 days. Due to an increased risk of hemorrhagic complications, DAPT is *not* recommended beyond 21 days. The second is after a TIA or stroke due to 70–99% stenosis of an intracranial artery; aspirin and clopidogrel (without a loading dose) are given for 90 days. Again, DAPT is *not* recommended beyond 90 days. Dual therapy is sometimes given in other, less common circumstances, but precise indications are evolving. Antiplatelet monotherapy is with aspirin (81 mg daily orally), clopidogrel (75 mg daily orally), or aspirin combined with extended-release dipyridamole (200 mg twice daily orally). Cilostazol (100 mg twice daily) had similar efficacy as aspirin at long-term stroke prevention in an Asian population with less risk of hemorrhage.

B. Surgical or Endovascular Measures

1. Carotid revascularization—When arteriography reveals a surgically accessible high-grade stenosis (70–99% in luminal diameter) on the side appropriate to carotid ischemic attacks, operative treatment (**carotid endarterectomy**) or endovascular intervention reduces the risk of ipsilateral carotid stroke, especially when TIAs are of recent onset (< 1 month) and when the perioperative morbidity and mortality risk is estimated to be < 6%. Endovascular therapy carries a slightly higher procedural stroke risk than endarterectomy in patients older than 70 years and is generally reserved for younger patients whose neck anatomy is unfavorable for surgery. Patients with symptomatic carotid stenosis of 50–69% derive moderate benefit from intervention, but surgery is *not* indicated for mild stenosis (< 50%).

2. Closure of patent foramen ovale—Carefully selected patients with patent foramen ovale (PFO) and right-to-left shunt benefit from PFO closure and antiplatelet therapy. Patients should be considered for PFO closure if they are between 18 and 60 years old; have had a cryptogenic stroke or TIA; and do not have uncontrolled diabetes, hypertension, or a specific indication for long-term anticoagulation. A cryptogenic stroke does not have an identified mechanism, such as large artery atherosclerosis (≥ 30–50% stenosis of the intracranial or cervical arteries or a plaque ≥ 4 mm thick in the aortic arch), known cardioembolic source (eg, atrial fibrillation), small vessel arteriolosclerosis (eg, lacunar stroke smaller than 1.5 cm in diameter), hypercoagulable state, or dissection. Patients with moderate to large interatrial shunts or associated atrial septal aneurysms appear to benefit most from PFO closure. See also Chapter 10.

3. Left atrial appendage closure—The left atrial appendage is the source of embolism in most patients with atrial fibrillation. A meta-analysis of randomized trials showed percutaneous left atrial appendage closure was equivalent to anticoagulation in preventing stroke and systemic embolization, and several devices are approved for this indication in the United States and Europe. The procedure should be considered in patients with a contraindication to long-term anticoagulation, although short-term anticoagulation (45 days) followed by dual antiplatelet therapy (4.5 months) and then indefinite aspirin monotherapy is usually necessary after device placement.

When to Refer

All patients should be referred for urgent investigation and treatment to prevent stroke.

When to Admit

If seen within a week of a TIA, patients should be considered for admission when they have an $ABCD^2$ score of 4 points or more, when outpatient evaluation is impractical, or when there are multiple attacks, carotid stenosis of > 70%, or other concern for early recurrence or stroke.

Joglar JA et al. 2023 ACC/AHA/ACCP/HRS Guideline for the diagnosis and management of atrial fibrillation: a report of the American College of Cardiology/American Heart Association joint committee on clinical practice guidelines. Circulation. 2024;149:e1. [PMID: 38033089]

National Institute of Neurological Disorders and Stroke NIH Stroke Scale. U.S. Department of Health and Human Services, National Institutes of Health. Last reviewed December 8, 2025. https://www.ninds.nih.gov/health-information/stroke/assess-and-treat/nih-stroke-scale.

STROKE

ESSENTIALS OF DIAGNOSIS

- Sudden onset of neurologic deficit of cerebrovascular origin.
- Patient often has hypertension, diabetes mellitus, tobacco use, atrial fibrillation, or atherosclerosis.
- Distinctive neurologic signs reflect the region of the brain involved.

General Considerations

In the United States, stroke is the fourth leading cause of death and a leading cause of disability. Risk factors for stroke include hypertension, diabetes mellitus, hyperlipidemia, cigarette smoking, cardiac disease, HIV infection, trigeminal herpes zoster, recreational drug abuse, heavy alcohol consumption, and a family history of stroke.

Strokes are subdivided pathologically into **infarcts** and **hemorrhages**. The distinction may be difficult clinically; CT scanning is essential to clarify the pathologic basis (Table 27–4).

1. Lacunar Infarction

Lacunar infarcts are small lesions (usually < 1.5 cm in diameter) that occur in the distribution of short penetrating arterioles in the basal ganglia, pons, cerebellum, internal capsule, thalamus, and, less commonly, the deep cerebral white matter (Table 27–4). Lacunar infarcts are associated with poorly controlled hypertension or diabetes and have been found in several clinical syndromes, including contralateral pure motor hemiparesis or pure hemisensory deficit, ipsilateral ataxia with hemiparesis, and dysarthria with clumsiness of the hand. The neurologic deficit may progress over 24–36 hours before stabilizing.

Early mortality and risk of stroke recurrence is higher for patients with nonlacunar than lacunar infarcts. The prognosis for recovery from the deficit produced by a lacunar infarct is usually good, with partial or complete resolution occurring over the following 4–6 weeks in many instances. Treatment is as described for TIA (discussed in the section on TIA) and cerebral infarction.

2. Cerebral Infarction

Thrombotic or embolic occlusion of a major vessel leads to cerebral infarction. Causes are identical to the disorders predisposing to TIAs. The resulting deficit depends on the particular vessel involved and the extent of any collateral circulation. Cerebral ischemia leads to release of excitatory and other neuropeptides that may augment calcium flux into neurons, thereby leading to cell death and increasing the neurologic deficit.

Table 27–4. Features of the major stroke subtypes.

Stroke Type and Subtype	Clinical Features	Diagnosis	Treatment
Ischemic Stroke			
Lacunar infarct	Small (< 1.5 cm) lesions in the basal ganglia, pons, cerebellum, or internal capsule; less often in deep cerebral white matter; prognosis generally good; clinical features depend on location but may worsen over first 24–36 hours.	MRI with diffusion-weighted sequences usually defines the area of infarction; CT is insensitive acutely but can be used to exclude hemorrhage.	Antiplatelet; control risk factors (hypertension, tobacco use, hypercholesterolemia, and diabetes mellitus).
Carotid circulation obstruction	See text—signs vary depending on occluded vessel.	Noncontrast CT to exclude hemorrhage but findings may be normal during first 6–24 hours of an ischemic stroke; diffusion-weighted MRI is gold standard for identifying acute stroke; ECG, carotid duplex studies, echocardiography, blood glucose, CBC, and tests for hyperlipidemia are indicated; ambulatory ECG monitoring, including extended monitoring in selected instances; CTA, MRA, or conventional angiography in selected cases; tests for hypercoagulable states in selected cases.	0–4.5 hours: intravenous thrombolytics (approved in United States up to 3 hours and in Europe up to 4.5 hours). 0–6 hours: endovascular mechanical embolectomy. 6–24 hours: endovascular mechanical embolectomy in select cases. Secondary prevention: antiplatelet agent is first-line therapy; anticoagulation without heparin bridge for cardioembolic strokes due to atrial fibrillation and other select cases when no contraindications exist; control risk factors as above.
Vertebrobasilar occlusion	See text—signs vary based on location of occluded vessel.	As for carotid circulation obstruction.	As for carotid circulation obstruction.
Hemorrhagic Stroke			
Spontaneous intracerebral hemorrhage	Commonly associated with hypertension; also with bleeding disorders, amyloid angiopathy. Hypertensive hemorrhage is located commonly in the basal ganglia, pons, thalamus, cerebellum, and less commonly the cerebral white matter.	Noncontrast CT is superior to MRI for detecting bleeds of < 48 hours duration; laboratory tests to identify bleeding disorder: angiography may be indicated to exclude aneurysm or AVM in younger patients without hypertension. Do *not* perform lumbar puncture.	Lower systolic blood pressure to 130–150 mm Hg; cerebellar bleeds or hematomas with gross mass effect may require urgent surgical evacuation. AVM: surgical resection indicated to prevent further bleeding; other modalities to treat nonoperable AVMs available at specialized centers.
Subarachnoid hemorrhage	Present with sudden onset of worst headache of life, may lead rapidly to loss of consciousness; signs of meningeal irritation often present; etiology usually aneurysm or AVM, but 20% have no source identified.	CT to confirm diagnosis but may be normal in rare instances; if CT negative and suspicion high, perform lumbar puncture to look for RBCs or xanthochromia; angiography to determine source of bleed in candidates for treatment.	Lower systolic blood pressure to < 140 mm Hg immediately. Aneurysm: prevent further bleeding by clipping aneurysm or coil embolization; nimodipine helps prevent vasospasm; once aneurysm has been obliterated intravenous fluids and induced hypertension to prevent vasospasm; angioplasty may also reverse symptomatic vasospasm. AVM: as above.

AVMs, arteriovenous malformations; CTA, computed tomography angiography; MRA, magnetic resonance angiography.

Clinical Findings

A. Symptoms and Signs

Onset is usually abrupt, and there may then be little progression except that due to brain swelling. Clinical evaluation should always include examination of the heart for murmurs and rhythm irregularities. Auscultating over the carotid or subclavian vessels may reveal a bruit but is not sensitive enough to substitute for vascular imaging.

1. Obstruction of carotid circulation—Occlusion of the **anterior cerebral artery** distal to its junction with the anterior communicating artery causes weakness and cortical sensory loss in the contralateral leg and sometimes mild weakness of the arm, especially proximally. There may be a contralateral grasp reflex, paratonic rigidity, abulia (lack of initiative), or frank confusion. Urinary incontinence is not uncommon, particularly if behavioral disturbances are conspicuous. Bilateral anterior cerebral infarction is especially likely to cause marked behavioral changes and memory disturbances. Unilateral anterior cerebral artery occlusion proximal to the junction with the anterior communicating artery is generally well tolerated because of the collateral supply from the other side.

Middle cerebral artery occlusion leads to contralateral hemiplegia, hemisensory loss, and homonymous hemianopia (ie, bilaterally symmetric loss of vision in half of the visual fields), with the eyes deviated to the side of the lesion. If the dominant hemisphere is involved, global aphasia is also present. It may be impossible to distinguish this clinically from occlusion of the internal carotid artery. With occlusion of either of these arteries, there may also be considerable swelling of the hemisphere during the first 72 hours. For example, an infarct involving one cerebral hemisphere may lead to swelling that disturbs the function of the other hemisphere or the rostral brainstem and coma results. Occlusions of different branches of the middle cerebral artery cause more limited findings. For example, involvement of the superior division in the dominant hemisphere leads to a predominantly expressive (**Broca**) aphasia and to contralateral paralysis and loss of sensations in the arm, the face and, to a lesser extent, the leg. Inferior branch occlusion in the dominant hemisphere produces a receptive (**Wernicke**) aphasia and a homonymous visual field defect. With involvement of the nondominant hemisphere, speech and comprehension are preserved, but there may be a left hemispatial neglect syndrome or constructional and visuospatial deficits.

Occlusion of the **ophthalmic or central retinal artery** leads to sudden painless visual loss with retinal pallor and a macular cherry red spot on fundoscopic examination. Sudden, transient vision loss in one eye (**amaurosis fugax**) is a TIA in this arterial territory.

2. Obstruction of vertebrobasilar circulation—Occlusion of the **posterior cerebral artery** may lead to a thalamic syndrome in which contralateral hemisensory disturbance occurs, followed by the development of spontaneous pain and hyperpathia. There is often a macular-sparing homonymous hemianopia and sometimes a mild, usually temporary, hemiparesis. Involuntary movements may occur if the subthalamic nucleus is involved and alexia if the infarct involves the left occipital lobe and the splenium of the corpus callosum. Occlusion of the main artery beyond the origin of its penetrating branches may lead solely to a macular-sparing hemianopia.

Vertebral artery occlusion below the origin of the anterior spinal and posterior inferior cerebellar arteries may be clinically silent because the circulation is maintained by the other vertebral artery. If the remaining vertebral artery is congenitally small or severely atherosclerotic, however, a deficit similar to that of basilar artery occlusion is seen unless there is good collateral circulation from the anterior circulation through the circle of Willis. An obstruction of the **posterior inferior cerebellar artery** or an obstruction of the vertebral artery just before it branches to this vessel leads to the **lateral medullary syndrome**, characterized by vertigo and nystagmus (vestibular nucleus), ipsilateral spinothalamic sensory loss involving the face (trigeminal nucleus and tract), dysphagia (nucleus ambiguus), limb ataxia (inferior cerebellar peduncle), and Horner syndrome (descending sympathetic fibers), combined with contralateral spinothalamic sensory loss involving the limbs.

Occlusion of **both vertebral arteries** or the **basilar artery** leads to coma with pinpoint pupils, flaccid quadriplegia and sensory loss, and variable cranial nerve abnormalities. With partial basilar artery occlusion, there may be diplopia, visual loss, vertigo, dysarthria, ataxia, weakness, or sensory disturbances in some or all of the limbs, and discrete cranial nerve palsies. In patients with hemiplegia of pontine origin, the eyes are often deviated to the paralyzed side, whereas in patients with a hemispheric lesion, the eyes commonly deviate from the hemiplegic side. When the small paramedian arteries arising from the basilar artery are occluded, contralateral hemiplegia and sensory deficit occur in association with an ipsilateral cranial nerve palsy at the level of the lesion.

Occlusion of any of the major **cerebellar arteries** produces vertigo, nausea, vomiting, nystagmus, and ipsilateral limb ataxia. Contralateral spinothalamic sensory loss in the limbs may also be present. Deafness due to cochlear infarction may follow occlusion of the anterior inferior cerebellar artery, which may also cause ipsilateral facial spinothalamic sensory loss and weakness. Massive cerebellar infarction may lead to obstructive hydrocephalus, coma, tonsillar herniation, and death.

B. Imaging

A CT scan of the head (without contrast) should be performed immediately, before the administration of aspirin or other antithrombotic agents, to exclude cerebral hemorrhage (Table 27–4). CT is relatively insensitive to acute ischemic stroke within the first 6–12 hours, and subsequent MRI with diffusion-weighted sequences helps define the distribution and extent of infarction as well as exclude tumor or other differential considerations. **CT angiography of the head and neck** should be performed to identify large vessel occlusions amenable to endovascular therapy in patients presenting within 6 hours of stroke onset and should be considered in those presenting between 6 and 24 hours, together with CT perfusion studies. Regardless of timing of presentation, imaging of the cervical vasculature is indicated as part of a search to identify the source of the stroke. In patients with a PFO and otherwise cryptogenic stroke, the intracranial vasculature must be imaged to rule out large vessel atherosclerosis before PFO closure can be considered.

C. Laboratory and Other Studies

Investigations should include a CBC, blood glucose determination, and fasting lipid panel. Serologic tests for syphilis and HIV infection may be included depending on the circumstances. Screening for antiphospholipid antibodies (lupus anticoagulants, anticardiolipin, and anti-β_2-glycoprotein antibodies); the factor V Leiden mutation; abnormalities of protein C, protein S, or antithrombin; or a prothrombin gene mutation is indicated if a hypercoagulable disorder is suspected (eg, a young patient without apparent risk factors for stroke) or needs to be ruled out prior to PFO closure. While elevated serum homocysteine is a risk factor for stroke, lowering homocysteine levels with vitamin supplementation has not been shown to decrease risk; hence, routine homocysteine testing is *not* recommended. ECG or continuous cardiac monitoring for at least 24 hours will help exclude a recent MI or a cardiac arrhythmia that might be a source of embolization. While atrial fibrillation will be discovered in approximately 10% of patients with ischemic stroke during their hospitalization, an arrhythmia will be found in an additional 10% with prolonged ambulatory ECG monitoring after discharge; this testing is indicated in cases where atrial fibrillation is suspected (eg, nonlacunar stroke and left atrial enlargement on echocardiography or lack of intracranial or carotid atherosclerosis) but has not been demonstrated. Echocardiography (with agitated saline contrast) should be performed in cases of nonlacunar stroke to exclude valvular disease, right-to-left shunting (including PFO), and cardiac thrombus. Blood cultures should be performed if endocarditis is suspected. Examination of the CSF may be helpful if cerebral vasculitis or another inflammatory or infectious cause of stroke is suspected but should be delayed until after CT or MRI to exclude risk of herniation due to mass effect.

Treatment

Management is divided into acute and chronic phases: the first is aimed at minimizing disability and the second at preventing recurrent stroke. A combination of thrombolysis and endovascular therapies is available to patients who present within 24 hours of stroke onset, determined by when the patient was last normal.

Intravenous thrombolytic therapy with recombinant tissue plasminogen activator (rtPA) improves the chance of recovery without significant disability at 90 days from 26% to 39% if given within 3 hours from stroke onset but is still effective up to 4.5 hours from stroke onset. Treatment should be initiated as soon as possible; *outcome is directly related to the time from stroke onset to treatment.* Alteplase (0.9 mg/kg to a maximum of 90 mg, with 10% given as a bolus over 1 minute and the remainder over 1 hour) and tenecteplase (0.25 mg/kg intravenously once, maximum dose 25 mg) are approved in Europe for use up to 4.5 hours from stroke onset but up to 3 hours in the United States, although off-label use during the 3- to 4.5-hour window is standard. Outcomes with these medications are similar; some centers prefer tenecteplase because it can be given as a single bolus. In patients with systolic pressure > 185 mm Hg or diastolic pressure > 110 mm Hg, the blood pressure should be lowered to < 185/110 mm Hg with intravenous labetalol or nicardipine to enable rtPA administration. Due to the risk of hemorrhage, rtPA should not be used beyond 4.5 hours, although some evidence suggests patients with ischemic but not infarcted tissue identified by automated perfusion imaging or MRI may be treated up to 9 hours after onset or upon awakening with stroke symptoms. Physicians who treat patients with acute ischemic stroke should be familiar with the comprehensive list of indications and contraindications for thrombolysis available in published guidelines.

Several randomized trials have demonstrated an increased likelihood of achieving functional independence after **endovascular mechanical embolectomy** by stent retrievers as an adjunct to intravenous rtPA or as a standalone treatment in patients ineligible for rtPA. Patients with large vessel occlusion (about 20% of patients with acute ischemic stroke) in whom treatment can be initiated within 6 hours of stroke onset are eligible for embolectomy, as are patients who present between 6 and 24 hours and have a large ischemic penumbra identified by perfusion CT, perfusion MRI, or diffusion-weighted MRI.

Early management of a completed stroke otherwise requires general supportive measures. Management in a **stroke care unit** has been shown to improve outcomes, likely due to early rehabilitation and prevention of medical complications. During the acute stage, there may be marked brain swelling and edema, with symptoms and signs of increasing intracranial pressure, an increasing neurologic deficit, or herniation syndrome. Elevated intracranial pressure is managed by head elevation and osmotic agents such as mannitol. Maintenance of an adequate cerebral perfusion pressure helps prevent further ischemia. Early decompressive hemicraniectomy (within 48 hours of stroke onset) for malignant middle cerebral artery infarctions reduces mortality and improves functional outcome. Attempts to lower the blood pressure of hypertensive patients during the acute phase (ie, within 72 hours) of a stroke should generally be *avoided* unless the purpose is to enable the safe administration of rtPA, as there is loss of cerebral autoregulation, and lowering the blood pressure may further compromise ischemic areas. However, in patients not treated with rtPA and in those treated with rtPA > 24 hours previously, a systolic pressure > 220 mm Hg can be lowered using intravenous labetalol, nicardipine, or clevidipine with continuous monitoring to 170–200 mm Hg; after 72 hours, it can be reduced to < 140/90 mm Hg. Blood pressure augmentation is usually not necessary in patients with relative hypotension but maintenance of hydration with intravenous fluids if necessary is important.

Prophylactic and medical measures are discussed in the section on TIAs and should guide management. Once hemorrhage has been excluded by CT, **aspirin** (325 mg orally daily) is started immediately unless the patient received thrombolysis, in which case aspirin is initiated at 24 hours after a follow-up CT has ruled out thrombolytic-associated hemorrhage. **Dual antiplatelet therapy** should be used for 21 days in patients with minor stroke (NIH Stroke Scale of 3 or less). **Anticoagulant** medications are started when indicated, as discussed in the section on TIAs. There is generally no advantage in delay, and the common fear of causing hemorrhage into a previously infarcted area is misplaced, since there is a far greater risk of further embolism to the cerebral circulation if treatment is withheld.

Physical therapy has an important role in the management of patients with impaired motor function. Passive movements at an early stage will help prevent contractures. As cooperation increases and recovery begins, active movements will improve strength and coordination. In all cases, early mobilization and active rehabilitation are important. **Occupational therapy** may improve morale and motor skills, while **speech therapy** may help expressive aphasia or dysarthria. Because of the risk for dysphagia following stroke, access to food and drink is typically restricted until an appropriate swallowing evaluation; the head of the bed should be kept elevated to prevent aspiration. Urinary catheters should *not* be placed and, if placed, removed within 24–48 hours.

Prognosis

The prognosis for survival after cerebral infarction is better than after cerebral or subarachnoid hemorrhage. Patients receiving treatment with rtPA are at least 30% more likely to have minimal or no disability at 3 months than those not treated by this means. Those treated with mechanical embolectomy are also at least 30% more likely to achieve functional independence. Loss of consciousness after a cerebral infarct implies a poorer prognosis. The extent of the infarct governs the potential for rehabilitation. Patients who have had a cerebral infarct are at risk for additional strokes and for MIs. The prophylactic treatment measures discussed reduce this risk. Antiplatelet therapy reduces the recurrence rate by 30% among patients with stroke without a cardiac cause who are not candidates for carotid endarterectomy. Nevertheless, the cumulative risk of recurrence of noncardioembolic stroke is 3–7% annually. Management is focused on palliative care when meaningful recovery from massive strokes is unlikely (see Chapter 5).

Grotta JC. Intravenous thrombolysis for acute ischemic stroke. Continuum (Minneap Minn). 2023;29:425. [PMID: 37039403]

3. Intracerebral Hemorrhage

Spontaneous, nontraumatic intracerebral hemorrhage (ICH) in patients with no angiographic evidence of an associated vascular anomaly (eg, aneurysm or angioma) is usually due to hypertension. Hypertensive ICH occurs most frequently in the basal ganglia, pons, thalamus, and cerebellum, and less commonly in the cerebral white matter. Hemorrhage may extend into the ventricular system or subarachnoid space, and signs of meningeal irritation are then found. In older adults, cerebral amyloid angiopathy is another important and frequent cause of hemorrhage, which is usually lobar in distribution, sometimes recurrent, and associated with a better immediate prognosis than hypertensive hemorrhage. Arteriovenous malformations are an important cause of ICH in younger patients.

Other causes of nontraumatic ICH include hematologic and bleeding disorders (eg, leukemia, thrombocytopenia, hemophilia, or disseminated intravascular coagulation), anticoagulant therapy, liver disease, high alcohol intake, cocaine and methamphetamine abuse, herpes simplex encephalitis, vasculitis, Moyamoya disease, reversible cerebral vasoconstriction syndrome, and primary or secondary brain tumors. There is also an association with advancing age and male sex. Bleeding is primarily into the subarachnoid space when it occurs from an intracranial aneurysm, but it may be intraparenchymal as well. Hemorrhage can also occur into arterial and venous cerebral infarcts.

Clinical Findings

A. Symptoms and Signs

With hemorrhage into the cerebral hemisphere, consciousness is initially lost or impaired in one-half of patients. Vomiting occurs frequently at the onset of bleeding, and headache is sometimes present. Focal symptoms and signs then develop, depending on the site of the hemorrhage. With hypertensive hemorrhage, there is generally a rapidly evolving neurologic deficit with hemiplegia or hemiparesis. A hemisensory disturbance is also present with more deeply placed lesions. With lesions of the putamen, loss of conjugate lateral gaze may be conspicuous. With thalamic hemorrhage, there may be a loss of upward gaze, downward or skew deviation of the eyes, lateral gaze palsies, and pupillary inequalities.

Cerebellar hemorrhage may present with sudden onset of nausea and vomiting, dysequilibrium, ataxia of gait, limbs, or trunk; headache; and loss of consciousness that may terminate fatally within 48 hours. Pontine hemorrhage causes some combination of lateral conjugate gaze palsies to the side of the lesion; small reactive pupils; contralateral hemiplegia; peripheral facial weakness; and periodic respiration. These signs may be bilateral with larger pontine hemorrhage, and the patient may become locked in, with quadriplegia and preserved consciousness.

B. Imaging

CT scanning (without contrast) or MRI with magnetic susceptibility weighted sequences (eg, gradient echo) is important in confirming that hemorrhage has occurred and in determining the size and site of the hematoma. Additional vascular imaging is usually unnecessary, but CT or MR angiography to look for an underlying source of hemorrhage is recommended for the following patients: those < age 70 with lobar ICH, those < age 45 with deep or posterior fossa ICH, and those aged 45–70 years with deep or posterior fossa ICH and no history of hypertension. Conventional digital subtraction angiography should be considered when CT or MR angiography is normal, when a vascular lesion is detected on CT or MR angiography, or for cases of isolated intraventricular hemorrhage. CT or MR venography should be considered if the ICH location (eg, parasagittal or temporoparietal regions) suggests cerebral venous thrombosis. In patients with normal vascular imaging and no history of hypertension, a contrast-enhanced MRI may indicate a nonhypertensive cause, such as an underlying neoplasm or cerebral amyloid angiopathy.

C. Laboratory and Other Studies

A CBC, platelet count, prothrombin and partial thromboplastin times, liver biochemical tests, and kidney function tests may reveal a predisposing cause for the hemorrhage. *Lumbar puncture is contraindicated* because it may precipitate a herniation syndrome in patients with a large hematoma, and CT scanning is superior in detecting intracerebral hemorrhage.

Treatment

Patients should be admitted to an ICU for observation and supportive care. Unlike ischemic stroke, in patients with ICH and a presenting systolic pressure > 150 mm Hg, the systolic pressure should be lowered and maintained between 130–150 mm Hg with intravenous labetalol, nicardipine, or clevidipine. Lowering systolic pressure under 130 mm Hg may be harmful in the acute phase. *Long-term treatment of hypertension is imperative to prevent recurrence.* Thrombocytopenia should be treated with platelet transfusion; the specific threshold for treatment and the goal platelet count after transfusion vary with patient characteristics and provider experience. Platelet transfusion should *not* be used to treat antiplatelet-associated ICH unless emergency surgery is necessary. Anticoagulation should be discontinued immediately, and coagulopathies should be reversed using fresh frozen plasma, prothrombin complex concentrates, vitamin K, or specific reversal agents (eg, protamine for heparin; idarucizumab for dabigatran; and andexanet-α or 4-factor prothrombin complex concentrates for apixaban, edoxaban, and rivaroxaban). Activated charcoal can be administered if a direct oral anticoagulant was taken within 2 hours. Hemostatic therapy with recombinant activated factor VII in patients without underlying coagulopathy has not improved survival or functional outcome. Intracranial pressure may require monitoring and osmotic therapy. Ventricular drainage with or without intraventricular thrombolysis may be required in patients with intraventricular hemorrhage and acute hydrocephalus. Decompression or minimally invasive hematoma evacuation may be helpful when a superficial hematoma in cerebral white matter is exerting a mass effect and causing incipient herniation. In patients with cerebellar hemorrhage who are deteriorating neurologically or who have brainstem compression or hydrocephalus, prompt surgical evacuation of the hematoma is appropriate because spontaneous unpredictable deterioration may otherwise lead to a fatal outcome and because operative treatment may lead to complete resolution of the clinical deficit. The treatment of underlying structural lesions or bleeding disorders depends on their nature. There is no specific treatment for cerebral amyloid angiopathy.

Pradilla G et al. Trial of early minimally invasive removal of intracerebral hemorrhage. N Engl J Med. 2024;390:1277. [PMID: 38598795]

4. Spontaneous Subarachnoid Hemorrhage

ESSENTIALS OF DIAGNOSIS

- Sudden ("thunderclap") severe headache.
- Signs of meningeal irritation usually present.
- Obtundation is common.
- Focal deficits frequently absent.

General Considerations

Between 5% and 10% of strokes are due to subarachnoid hemorrhage. Trauma is the most common cause of subarachnoid hemorrhage, the prognosis of which depends on the severity of the head injury. Spontaneous (nontraumatic) subarachnoid hemorrhage frequently results from the rupture of an **arterial saccular ("berry") aneurysm** or from an **arteriovenous malformation**.

Clinical Findings

A. Symptoms and Signs

Subarachnoid hemorrhage has a characteristic clinical picture. Its onset is with sudden ("**thunderclap**") headache of a severity never experienced previously by the patient. This may be followed by nausea and vomiting and by a loss or impairment of consciousness that can either be transient or progress inexorably to deepening coma and death. If consciousness is regained, the patient is often confused and irritable and may show other symptoms of an altered mental status. Neurologic examination generally reveals nuchal rigidity and other signs of meningeal irritation, except in deeply comatose patients.

Most aneurysms are asymptomatic until they rupture, but they may cause a focal neurologic deficit by compressing adjacent structures. Occasional patients with aneurysms have headaches, sometimes accompanied by nausea and neck stiffness, a few hours or days before massive subarachnoid hemorrhage occurs. This has been attributed to "warning leaks" of a small amount of blood from the aneurysm.

A higher risk of subarachnoid hemorrhage is associated with older age, female sex, non-White ethnicity, hypertension, tobacco smoking, high alcohol consumption (exceeding 150 g per week), previous symptoms, posterior circulation aneurysms, and larger aneurysms. Focal neurologic signs are usually absent but, when present, may relate either to a focal intracerebral hematoma (from arteriovenous malformations) or to ischemia in the territory of the vessel with a ruptured aneurysm.

B. Imaging

A CT scan (preferably with CT angiography) should be performed immediately to confirm that hemorrhage has occurred and to search for clues regarding its source. CT is preferable to MRI because it is faster and more sensitive in detecting hemorrhage in the first 24 hours. In patients with suspected hemorrhage but normal CT findings, the CSF must then be examined for the presence of blood or xanthochromia before the possibility of subarachnoid hemorrhage is discounted.

Cerebral arteriography is undertaken to determine the source of bleeding. In general, bilateral carotid and vertebral arteriography are necessary because aneurysms are often multiple, while arteriovenous malformations may be supplied from several sources. The procedure allows an interventional radiologist to treat an underlying aneurysm or arteriovenous malformation by various techniques.

If arteriograms show no abnormality, the examination should be repeated after 2 weeks because vasospasm or thrombus may have prevented detection of an aneurysm or other vascular anomaly during the initial study. CT or MR angiography may also be revealing but is less sensitive than conventional arteriography.

C. Laboratory and Other Studies

The CSF demonstrates an elevated RBC count. Subarachnoid hemorrhage can be differentiated from a traumatic lumbar puncture by the lack of clearing of RBCs from the first and fourth tube of CSF or by the presence of xanthochromia, which occurs due to lysis of RBCs and takes at least 2 hours to develop. The absolute RBC count is also helpful: in the absence of xanthochromia, an RBC count of < 2000/mcL (2.0×10^9/L) is unlikely to be due to subarachnoid hemorrhage. ECG evidence of arrhythmias or myocardial ischemia has been well described and probably relates to excessive sympathetic activity. Peripheral leukocytosis and transient glycosuria are also common findings.

Treatment

All patients should be hospitalized and evaluated by a neurologist. The measures outlined below in the section on stupor and coma are applied to comatose patients. Conscious patients are confined to bed, advised against any exertion or straining, treated symptomatically for headache and anxiety, and given laxatives or stool softeners. The systolic blood pressure should be lowered to 140 mm Hg until the aneurysm is treated definitively. Seizure prophylaxis is *not* necessary unless a convulsion has occurred (see Table 27–3). Patients are generally hospitalized for at least 14 days to monitor, prevent, and treat vasospasm.

The major aim of treatment is to prevent further hemorrhage. The risk of further hemorrhage from a ruptured aneurysm is greatest within a few days of the first hemorrhage; approximately 20% of patients will have further bleeding within 2 weeks and 40% within 6 months. Definitive treatment of an aneurysm, ideally within 2 days of the hemorrhage, requires surgical clipping or endovascular coil embolization by an interventional radiologist; the latter is sometimes feasible even for inoperable aneurysms and has a lower morbidity than surgery.

Complications

Spontaneous subarachnoid hemorrhage may result in severe complications, so monitoring is necessary, usually in an ICU. **Vasospasm** may follow aneurysmal bleeding after a delay of 2–14 days. It sometimes leads to significant cerebral ischemia or infarction (with focal deficits or hemiplegia) and may further aggravate any existing increase in intracranial pressure. Noninvasive transcranial Doppler ultrasound may be used to screen for vasospasm, but conventional arteriography is required to document and treat vasospasm when the clinical suspicion is high. Nimodipine reduces the incidence of ischemic deficits; a dose of 60 mg every 4 hours orally for 21 days is given prophylactically to all patients. After surgical obliteration of aneurysms, symptomatic vasospasm may also be treated by intravascular volume expansion and induced hypertension; transluminal balloon angioplasty of involved intracranial vessels is also helpful.

Acute hydrocephalus sometimes occurs due to CSF outflow disruption by the subarachnoid blood and should be suspected if the patient deteriorates clinically; a repeat CT scan should be obtained. It frequently causes severe intracranial hypertension that may require temporary, and less commonly prolonged or permanent, intraventricular CSF shunting. **Cerebral salt-wasting** is another complication of subarachnoid hemorrhage that may develop abruptly during the first several days of hospitalization. The resulting hyponatremia and cerebral edema may exacerbate intracranial hypertension and may require carefully titrated treatment with oral sodium chloride or intravenous hyperosmotic sodium solution. Daily measurement of the serum sodium level allows for the early detection of this complication. **Hypopituitarism** may occur as a late complication of subarachnoid hemorrhage.

Hoh BL et al. Guideline for the management of patients with aneurysmal subarachnoid hemorrhage: a guideline from the American Heart Association/American Stroke Association. Stroke. 2023;54:e314. [PMID: 37212182]

5. Intracranial Venous Thrombosis

Intracranial venous thrombosis may occur in association with intracranial or maxillofacial infections, hypercoagulable states, polycythemia, sickle cell disease, cyanotic congenital heart disease, and in pregnancy or during the puerperium. Genetic factors are also important. Cases of intracranial venous thrombosis with thrombocytopenia and antiplatelet factor 4 antibodies have rarely been observed after administration of SARS-CoV-2 adenoviral vector vaccines. The disorder is characterized by headache, focal or generalized convulsions, drowsiness, confusion, increased intracranial pressure, and focal neurologic deficits—and sometimes by evidence of meningeal irritation. The diagnosis is confirmed by CT or MR venography or angiography.

Treatment includes anticonvulsants if seizures have occurred (see Table 27–3) and—if necessary—measures to reduce intracranial pressure. Anticoagulation with dose-adjusted intravenous heparin or weight-adjusted subcutaneous low-molecular-weight heparin, followed by oral warfarin anticoagulation for 6 months reduces morbidity and mortality of venous sinus thrombosis. Direct oral anticoagulants are likely acceptable alternatives to warfarin based on one randomized trial comparing dabigatran to warfarin and many observational studies comparing rivaroxaban, apixaban, and dabigatran to warfarin showing similar efficacy. Measurement of antiplatelet factor 4 antibodies and treatment with a non-heparin anticoagulant and intravenous immunoglobulin (1 g/kg daily for 2 days) or therapeutic plasma exchange for 5 to 7 days is recommended in cases following SARS-CoV-2 vaccination. *Concomitant intracranial hemorrhage related to the venous thrombosis does not contraindicate anticoagulant therapy.* In cases refractory to anticoagulation, endovascular techniques including catheter-directed thrombolytic therapy (urokinase) and thrombectomy are sometimes helpful but may increase the risk for major hemorrhage.

Saposnik G et al. Diagnosis and management of cerebral venous thrombosis: a scientific statement from the American Heart Association. Stroke. 2024;55:e77. [PMID: 38284265]

6. Infarction of the Spinal Cord

ESSENTIALS OF DIAGNOSIS

- Sudden onset of back or limb pain and neurologic deficit in limbs.
- Motor, sensory, or reflex changes in limbs depending on level of lesion.
- Imaging studies distinguish between infarct and hematoma.

Infarction of the spinal cord is rare and typically occurs in the territory of the anterior spinal artery; this vessel, which supplies the anterior two-thirds of the cord, is itself supplied by only a limited number of feeders. Infarction usually results from interrupted flow in one or more of these feeders (eg, with aortic dissection, aortic aneurysm, aortography, polyarteritis, severe hypotension, or after surgical repair of the thoracic or abdominal aorta). The paired posterior spinal arteries, by contrast, are supplied by numerous arteries at different levels of the cord. Spinal cord hypoperfusion may lead to a central cord syndrome with distal weakness of lower motor neuron type and loss of pain and temperature appreciation, with preserved posterior column function.

Since the anterior spinal artery receives numerous feeders in the cervical region, infarcts almost always occur caudally. Clinical presentation is characterized by acute onset of flaccid, areflexive paraplegia that evolves after a few days or weeks into a spastic paraplegia with extensor plantar responses. There is an accompanying dissociated sensory loss, with impairment of appreciation of pain and temperature but preservation of sensations of vibration and joint position.

The risk of spinal cord infarction in the setting of abdominal aortic surgery and thoracic endovascular repair may be reduced by intraoperative CSF drainage through a catheter placed in the lumbar subarachnoid space to reduce intraspinal pressure. If signs of infarction are noted after surgery, blood pressure augmentation for 24–48 hours in addition to lumbar drainage has been noted anecdotally to improve outcomes. CSF drainage and blood pressure augmentation are also sometimes attempted in patients with spinal cord infarction due to other causes. Treatment is otherwise symptomatic.

Jadhav AP. Vascular myelopathies. Continuum (Minneap Minn). 2024;30:160. [PMID: 38330477]

7. Spinal Epidural or Subdural Hemorrhage

Epidural or subdural hemorrhage may lead to sudden severe back pain followed by an acute compressive myelopathy necessitating urgent spinal MRI or myelography and surgical evacuation. It may occur in patients with bleeding disorders or those who are taking anticoagulants, sometimes following trauma or lumbar puncture. Epidural hemorrhage may also be related to a vascular malformation or tumor deposit.

Benzon HT et al. Literature review of spinal hematoma case reports: causes and outcomes in pediatric, obstetric, neuraxial and pain medicine cases. Reg Anesth Pain Med. 2024;49:900. [PMID: 38267076]

When to Refer

All patients with stroke should be referred.

When to Admit

All patients should be hospitalized, preferably in a stroke care unit.

ANEURYSMS & VASCULAR MALFORMATIONS

1. Intracranial Aneurysm

ESSENTIALS OF DIAGNOSIS

- Subarachnoid hemorrhage or focal deficit.
- Abnormal imaging studies.

General Considerations

Saccular aneurysms (**"berry" aneurysms**) tend to occur at arterial bifurcations, are frequently multiple (20% of cases), and are usually asymptomatic. They are associated with polycystic kidney disease, Moyamoya disease, familial aldosteronism type 1, and coarctation of the aorta. Risk factors for aneurysm formation include cigarette smoking, hypertension, and female sex. Most aneurysms are located on the anterior part of the circle of Willis—particularly on the anterior or posterior communicating arteries, at the bifurcation of the middle cerebral artery, and at the bifurcation of the internal carotid artery. Mycotic aneurysms resulting from septic embolism occur in more distal vessels and often at the cortical surface. *The most significant complication of intracranial aneurysms is a subarachnoid hemorrhage*, which is discussed in the preceding section.

Clinical Findings

A. Symptoms and Signs

Aneurysms may cause a focal neurologic deficit by compressing adjacent structures. However, most are asymptomatic or produce only nonspecific symptoms until they rupture, at which time subarachnoid hemorrhage results. Its manifestations, complications, and management were outlined in the preceding section.

B. Imaging

Definitive evaluation is by **digital subtraction angiography** (bilateral carotid and vertebral studies), which generally indicates the size and site of the lesion, sometimes reveals multiple aneurysms, and may show arterial spasm if rupture has occurred. Visualization by CT or MR angiography is not usually adequate if operative treatment is under consideration because lesions may be multiple and small lesions are sometimes missed, but these modalities can be used to screen patients who have two or more first-degree relatives with intracranial aneurysms.

Treatment

The major aim of treatment is to prevent hemorrhage. Management of ruptured aneurysms was described in the section on subarachnoid hemorrhage. Symptomatic but unruptured aneurysms merit prompt treatment, either surgically or by endovascular techniques. The decision to treat or monitor asymptomatic aneurysms discovered incidentally is complicated and depends on aneurysm size, location, risk factors for rupture, and treatment-related morbidity; risk scores to guide decision-making are available.

Reddy A et al. Endovascular and medical management of unruptured intracranial aneurysms. Semin Neurol. 2023; 43:480. [PMID: 37517406]

2. Cerebral Arteriovenous Malformations

ESSENTIALS OF DIAGNOSIS

- Sudden onset of subarachnoid and intracerebral hemorrhage.
- Distinctive neurologic signs reflect the region of the brain involved.
- Signs of meningeal irritation in patients presenting with subarachnoid hemorrhage.
- Seizures or focal deficits may occur.

General Considerations

Arteriovenous malformations are congenital vascular malformations that result from a localized maldevelopment of part of the primitive vascular plexus and consist of abnormal arteriovenous communications without intervening capillaries. They vary in size, ranging from massive lesions that are fed by multiple vessels and involve a large part of the brain to lesions so small that they are hard to identify at arteriography, surgery, or autopsy. In approximately 10% of cases, there is an associated arterial aneurysm, while 1–2% of patients presenting with aneurysms have associated arteriovenous malformations. Clinical presentation may relate to hemorrhage from the malformation or an associated aneurysm or may relate to cerebral ischemia due to diversion of blood by the anomalous arteriovenous shunt or due to venous stagnation. Regional maldevelopment of the brain, compression or distortion of adjacent cerebral tissue by enlarged anomalous vessels, and progressive gliosis due to mechanical and ischemic factors may also be contributory.

Clinical Findings

Most cerebral arteriovenous malformations are supratentorial, usually lying in the territory of the middle cerebral artery. *Up to 70% bleed at some point in their natural history*, most commonly before the patient reaches the age of 40 years. Arteriovenous malformations that have bled once are more likely to bleed again, at an approximate rate of 4.5% annually. A higher risk of bleeding is also observed if there is an associated aneurysm, deep venous drainage, or deep brain location; size of the malformation is not associated with risk of hemorrhage.

A. Symptoms and Signs

Initial symptoms consist of hemorrhage in 30–60% of cases, recurrent seizures in 20–40%, headache in 5–25%, and miscellaneous complaints (including focal deficits) in 10–15%. Hemorrhage is commonly intracerebral as well as into the subarachnoid space and is fatal in about 10% of cases. Seizures are more likely with frontal or parietal arteriovenous malformations. Headaches are especially likely when the external carotid arteries are involved in the malformation. These sometimes simulate migraine, but more commonly are nonspecific in character, with nothing about them to suggest an underlying structural lesion. Brainstem and cerebellar arteriovenous malformations may cause obstructive hydrocephalus.

In patients presenting with subarachnoid hemorrhage, examination may reveal an abnormal mental status and signs of meningeal irritation. Additional findings may help localize the lesion and sometimes indicate that intracranial pressure is increased. *A cranial bruit always suggests the possibility of a cerebral arteriovenous malformation*, but bruits may also be found with aneurysms, meningiomas, acquired arteriovenous fistulas, and arteriovenous malformations involving the scalp, calvarium, or orbit. Bruits are best heard over the ipsilateral eye or mastoid region and are of some help in lateralization but of no help in localization. Absence of a bruit *does not exclude* the possibility of arteriovenous malformation.

B. Imaging

In patients with suspected hemorrhage, CT scanning indicates whether subarachnoid or intracerebral bleeding has recently occurred, helps localize its source, and CT angiography may reveal the arteriovenous malformation. Even if the findings on CT angiography suggest arteriovenous malformation, arteriography is required to establish the nature of the lesion with certainty and to determine its anatomic features so that treatment can be planned. The examination must generally include bilateral opacification of the internal and external carotid arteries and the vertebral arteries. Arteriovenous malformations typically appear as a tangled vascular mass with distended tortuous afferent and efferent vessels, a rapid circulation time, and arteriovenous shunting.

In patients presenting without hemorrhage, CT scan or MRI usually reveals the underlying abnormality, and MRI frequently also shows evidence of old or recent hemorrhage that may have been asymptomatic. The nature and detailed anatomy of any focal lesion identified by these means are delineated by angiography, especially if operative treatment is under consideration.

C. Laboratory and Other Studies

Electroencephalography is usually indicated in patients presenting with seizures and may show consistently focal or lateralized abnormalities resulting from the underlying cerebral arteriovenous malformation. This should be followed by CT scanning.

Treatment

Surgical treatment to prevent further hemorrhage is justified in patients with arteriovenous malformations that have bled, provided that the lesion is accessible and the patient has a reasonable life expectancy. Surgical treatment is also appropriate if intracranial pressure is increased and to prevent further progression of a focal neurologic deficit. In patients presenting solely with seizures, anticonvulsant treatment is usually sufficient (see Table 27–3), and operative treatment is unnecessary unless seizures cannot be controlled medically.

Definitive operative treatment consists of excision of the arteriovenous malformation if it is surgically accessible. Stereotactic radiosurgery is used to treat inoperable cerebral arteriovenous malformations. Arteriovenous malformations that are inoperable because of their location are sometimes treated solely by embolization; although the risk of hemorrhage is not reduced, neurologic deficits may be stabilized or even reversed by this procedure. Embolization is more commonly performed as an adjunct to surgery or radiosurgery; it is also used to treat aneurysms associated with the arteriovenous malformations.

Nguyen TN. Management of unruptured intracranial aneurysms and brain arteriovenous malformations. Continuum (Minneap Minn). 2023;29:584. [PMID: 37039411]

3. Spinal Dural Arteriovenous Fistulae

Spinal dural arteriovenous fistulae present with spinal subarachnoid hemorrhage or myeloradiculopathy. Since most of these malformations are located in the thoracolumbar region, they lead to motor and sensory disturbances in the legs and to sphincter disorders. Pain in the legs or back is often severe. Examination reveals an upper, lower, or mixed motor deficit in the legs; sensory deficits are also present and are usually extensive, although occasionally they are confined to a radicular distribution. Cervical spinal dural arteriovenous fistulae lead also to symptoms and signs in the arms. Spinal MRI may not detect the spinal dural arteriovenous fistula, although most cases show either T2 hyperintensity in the cord or perimedullary flow voids. Myelography (performed with the patient prone and supine) may detect serpiginous filling defects due to enlarged vessels. **Selective spinal arteriography** is required to confirm the diagnosis and plan treatment. Most lesions are extramedullary, are posterior to the cord (lying either intradurally or extradurally), and can be treated easily by ligation of feeding vessels and excision of the fistulous anomaly or by embolization procedures. Delay in treatment may lead to increased and irreversible disability or to death from recurrent subarachnoid hemorrhage.

Mamaril-Davis J et al. Recurrence rates following treatment of spinal vascular malformations: a systematic review and meta-analysis. World Neurosurg. 2023;173:e250. [PMID: 36787855]

When to Refer

All patients should be referred.

When to Admit

- All patients with a subarachnoid or cerebral hemorrhage.
- All patients undergoing surgical or endovascular treatment.

INTRACRANIAL & SPINAL MASS LESIONS

1. Primary Intracranial Tumors

ESSENTIALS OF DIAGNOSIS

- Generalized or focal disturbance of cerebral function, or both.
- Increased intracranial pressure in some patients.
- Neuroradiologic evidence of space-occupying lesion.

General Considerations

One-third of primary intracranial neoplasms (Table 27–5) are meningiomas, one-quarter are gliomas, and the remainder are pituitary adenomas (see Chapter 29), neurofibromas, and other tumors. Certain tumors, especially neurofibromas, hemangioblastomas, and retinoblastomas, may have a familial basis, and congenital factors bear on the development of craniopharyngiomas. Tumors may occur at any age, but certain gliomas show particular age predilections.

Clinical Findings

A. Symptoms and Signs

Intracranial tumors typically present with headache, seizures, or focal neurologic deficits. New headaches or symptoms of elevated intracranial pressure, such as headaches awaking a patient from sleep or worsening with Valsalva maneuver, cough, or recumbency, are suggestive of brain tumor. Intracranial tumors may also lead to a generalized disturbance of cerebral function with personality changes, intellectual decline, emotional lability, nausea, and malaise.

Table 27–5. Primary intracranial tumors (listed by major histology grouping and by incidence within each group).

Tumor	Clinical Features	Treatment and Prognosis
Tumors of Meninges		
Meningioma	Originates from the dura mater or arachnoid; compresses rather than invades adjacent neural structures. Increasingly common with advancing age. Tumor size varies greatly. Symptoms vary with tumor site—eg, unilateral proptosis (sphenoidal ridge); anosmia and optic nerve compression (olfactory groove). Tumor is usually benign and readily detected by CT scanning; may lead to calcification and bone erosion visible on plain radiographs of skull.	Treatment is surgical. Tumor may recur if removal is incomplete.
Tumors of Neuroepithelial Origin		
Glioblastoma, IDH-wildtype	Presents commonly with nonspecific complaints and increased intracranial pressure. As it grows, focal deficits develop. O^6-methylguanine-DNA methyltransferase promoter methylation positivity (seen in 40% of cases) carry better prognosis.	Course is rapidly progressive, with poor prognosis (< 20% survival at 2 years). Total surgical removal is usually not possible. Radiation therapy and temozolamide may prolong survival. Tumor treatment fields added to temozolamide after completion of radiation therapy prolong survival.
Astrocytoma, IDH-mutant	Presentation similar to glioblastoma but course more protracted, often over several years. Cerebellar astrocytoma may have a more benign course.	Prognosis is variable. By the time of diagnosis, total excision is usually impossible; tumor may be radiosensitive and temozolamide; procarbazine, lomustine, plus vincristine; or vorasidenib may be used. In cerebellar astrocytoma, total surgical removal is often possible.
Ependymoma	Glioma arising from the ependyma of a ventricle, especially the fourth ventricle; leads to early signs of increased intracranial pressure. Arises also from central canal of cord.	Tumor is best treated surgically if possible. Radiation therapy may be used for residual tumor.
Oligodendroglioma, IDH-mutant, and 1p/19q-codeleted	Slow-growing. Usually arises in cerebral hemisphere in adults. Calcification may be visible on skull radiograph. Co-deletion of 1p/19q and isocitrate dehydrogenase 1/2 mutation required for diagnosis.	Treatment is surgical and usually successful. Radiation and chemotherapy (temozolamide; procarbazine, lomustine, plus vincristine; or vorasidenib) may be used.
Brainstem glioma	Frequently presents during childhood with cranial nerve palsies and then with long tract signs in the limbs. Signs of increased intracranial pressure occur late.	Tumor is inoperable; treatment is by irradiation and shunt for increased intracranial pressure. Diffuse midline glioma with H3K27M mutations can be treated with dordaviprone.
Neuronal and mixed neuronal-glial tumors	Slow-growing; usually arise in cerebral hemispheres; often associated with seizures. Some are benign (eg, dysembryoblastic neuroepithelial tumors) and some have malignant potential (eg, ganglioglioma).	Resection is not always necessary for benign tumors unless seizures are medically refractory but is indicated for those with malignant potential.
Medulloblastoma	Seen most frequently in children. Generally arises from roof of fourth ventricle and leads to increased intracranial pressure accompanied by brainstem and cerebellar signs. May seed subarachnoid space. Wingless activated tumors carry best prognosis (> 90% 5-year survival).	Treatment consists of surgery combined with radiation therapy and chemotherapy; 5-year survival exceeds 70%. Wingless activated tumors may require less aggressive treatment.
Pineal tumor	Presents with increased intracranial pressure, sometimes associated with impaired upward gaze (Parinaud syndrome) and other deficits indicative of midbrain lesion.	Ventricular decompression by shunting is followed by surgical approach to tumor; irradiation is indicated if tumor is malignant. Prognosis depends on histopathologic findings and extent of tumor.
Tumors of the Sellar Region		
Pituitary adenoma	Functioning adenomas present with symptoms of hormone secretion; nonfunctioning adenomas present with symptoms of local mass effect (eg, bitemporal hemianopsia, hypopituitarism) or are found incidentally.	Prolactin-secreting adenomas are treated with bromocriptine or cabergoline. Others are surgically resected. Pituitary hormone replacement may be required.
Craniopharyngioma	Originates from remnants of Rathke pouch above the sella, depressing the optic chiasm. May present at any age but usually in childhood, with endocrine dysfunction and bitemporal visual field defects.	Treatment is surgical, but total removal may not be possible. Radiation may be used for residual tumor.

(*continued*)

Table 27–5. Primary intracranial tumors (listed by major histology grouping and by incidence within each group). (continued)

Tumor	Clinical Features	Treatment and Prognosis
Germ cell tumors (germinomas and nongerminomatous germ cell tumors)	Two most common locations are pineal and suprasellar regions. The pineal region presentation is as described in pineal tumors, above. Suprasellar tumors present with hypothalamic and pituitary dysfunction such as diabetes insipidus, delayed or precocious puberty, or growth hormone deficiency.	Germinomas are treated with radiation; prognosis is good for localized tumors. Chemotherapy is added for nongerminomatous germ cell tumors.
Tumors of Cranial and Spinal Nerves		
Acoustic neurinoma (also referred to as acoustic neuroma)	Ipsilateral hearing loss is most common initial symptom. Subsequent symptoms may include tinnitus, headache, vertigo, facial weakness or numbness, and long tract signs. (May be familial and bilateral when related to neurofibromatosis.) Most sensitive screening tests are MRI and brainstem auditory evoked potential.	Treatment is excision by translabyrinthine surgery, craniectomy, or a combined approach. Outcome is usually good.
Lymphomas		
Primary cerebral lymphoma	Associated with AIDS and other immunodeficient states. Presentation may be with focal deficits or with disturbances of cognition and consciousness. May be indistinguishable from cerebral toxoplasmosis.	Various chemotherapy regimens containing high-dose methotrexate and corticosteroids followed by radiation therapy or stem cell transplant. When associated with AIDS, prognosis depends on CD4 count at diagnosis.
Unclassified		
Cerebellar hemangioblastoma	Presents with dysequilibrium, ataxia of trunk or limbs, and signs of increased intracranial pressure. Sometimes familial. May be associated with retinal and spinal vascular lesions, polycythemia, and renal cell carcinoma.	Treatment is surgical. Radiation is used for residual tumor. Belzutifan can be used for hemangioblastoma in patients with Von Hippel-Lindau disease.

1. Frontal lobe lesions—Tumors of the frontal lobe often lead to progressive intellectual decline, slowing of mental activity, personality changes, and contralateral grasp reflexes. They may lead to expressive aphasia if the posterior part of the left inferior frontal gyrus is involved. Anosmia may also occur as a consequence of pressure on the olfactory nerve. Precentral lesions may cause focal motor seizures or contralateral pyramidal deficits.

2. Temporal lobe lesions—Tumors of the uncinate region may be manifested by seizures with olfactory or gustatory hallucinations, motor phenomena such as licking or smacking of the lips, and some impairment of external awareness without actual loss of consciousness. Temporal lobe lesions also lead to depersonalization, emotional changes, behavioral disturbances, sensations of déjà vu or jamais vu, micropsia or macropsia (objects appear smaller or larger than they are), visual field defects (crossed upper quadrantanopia), and auditory illusions or hallucinations. Left-sided lesions may lead to dysnomia and receptive aphasia, while right-sided involvement sometimes disturbs the perception of musical notes and melodies.

3. Parietal lobe lesions—Tumors in this location characteristically cause contralateral disturbances of sensation and may cause sensory seizures, sensory loss or inattention, or some combination of these symptoms. The sensory loss is cortical in type and involves postural sensibility and tactile discrimination, so that the appreciation of shape, size, weight, and texture is impaired. Objects placed in the hand may not be recognized (astereognosis). Extensive parietal lobe lesions may produce contralateral hyperpathia and spontaneous pain. Involvement of the optic radiation leads to a contralateral homonymous field defect that sometimes consists solely of lower quadrantanopia. Lesions of the left angular gyrus cause **Gerstmann syndrome** (a combination of agraphia, acalculia, right-left confusion, and finger agnosia), whereas involvement of the left submarginal gyrus causes ideational apraxia. Anosognosia (the denial, neglect, or rejection of a paralyzed limb) is seen in patients with lesions of the nondominant (right) hemisphere. Constructional apraxia and dressing apraxia may also occur with right-sided lesions.

4. Occipital lobe lesions—Tumors of the occipital lobe characteristically produce contralateral homonymous hemianopia or a partial field defect. With left-sided or bilateral lesions, there may be visual agnosia both for objects and for colors, while irritative lesions on either side can cause unformed visual hallucinations. Bilateral occipital lobe involvement causes cortical blindness in which there is preservation of pupillary responses to light and lack of awareness of the defect by the patient. There may also be loss of color perception, prosopagnosia (inability to identify a familiar face), simultagnosia (inability to integrate and interpret a composite scene as opposed to its individual elements), and Balint syndrome (failure to turn the eyes to a particular point in space, despite preservation of spontaneous and reflex eye movements). The denial of blindness or a field defect constitutes **Anton syndrome**.

5. Brainstem and cerebellar lesions—Brainstem lesions lead to cranial nerve palsies, ataxia, incoordination, nystagmus, and pyramidal and sensory deficits in the limbs on one or both sides. Intrinsic brainstem tumors, such as gliomas, tend to produce an increase in intracranial pressure only late in their course. Cerebellar tumors produce marked ataxia of the trunk if the vermis cerebelli is involved and ipsilateral appendicular deficits (ataxia, incoordination, and hypotonia of the limbs) if the cerebellar hemispheres are affected.

6. Herniation syndromes—If the pressure is increased in a particular cranial compartment, brain tissue may herniate into a compartment with lower pressure. The most familiar syndrome is herniation of the temporal lobe uncus through the tentorial hiatus, which causes compression of the third cranial nerve, midbrain, and posterior cerebral artery. The earliest sign of this is ipsilateral pupillary dilation, followed by stupor, coma, decerebrate posturing, and respiratory arrest. Another important herniation syndrome consists of displacement of the cerebellar tonsils through the foramen magnum, which causes medullary compression leading to apnea, circulatory collapse, and death.

7. False localizing signs—Tumors may lead to neurologic signs other than by direct compression or infiltration, thereby leading to errors of clinical localization. These false localizing signs include third or sixth nerve palsy and bilateral extensor plantar responses produced by herniation syndromes, and an extensor plantar response occurring ipsilateral to a hemispheric tumor as a result of compression of the opposite cerebral peduncle against the tentorium.

B. Imaging

MRI with gadolinium enhancement is the preferred method to detect the lesion and to define its location, shape, and size; the extent to which normal anatomy is distorted; and the degree of any associated cerebral edema or mass effect. CT scanning with radiocontrast enhancement may be performed, but it is less helpful than MRI for small lesions or tumors in the posterior fossa. The characteristic appearance of meningiomas on MRI or CT scanning is virtually diagnostic, ie, a lesion in a typical site (parasagittal and sylvian regions, olfactory groove, sphenoidal ridge, tuberculum sellae) that appears as a homogeneous area of increased density in noncontrast scans and enhances uniformly with contrast. Additional MRI sequences may be helpful in differentiating gliomas from other intracranial pathology, including perfusion imaging, magnetic resonance spectroscopy, and diffusion-weighted imaging, although none are specific enough to obviate the need for tissue sampling. Arteriography is reserved for presurgical embolization of highly vascular tumors. In patients with an intrasellar mass and normal hormone levels, angiography sometimes is necessary to distinguish between a pituitary adenoma and an arterial aneurysm.

C. Laboratory and Other Studies

When glial neoplasms are suspected, biopsy is necessary for definitive histologic diagnosis and molecular analysis. The WHO classifies glial tumors by both histology and genetic characteristics. Lumbar puncture is rarely necessary; the findings are seldom diagnostic, and the procedure carries the risk of causing a herniation syndrome. Suspected intracranial germ cell tumors are an exception. If lumbar puncture can be performed safely, CSF cytology and determination of α-fetoprotein and β-human chorionic gonadotropin should be performed and serum tumor markers measured.

Treatment

Treatment depends on the type, grade, genetics, and site of the tumor (Table 27–5) and the condition of the patient. Some benign tumors, especially meningiomas discovered incidentally during brain imaging for another purpose, may be monitored with serial annual imaging.

For symptomatic tumors, complete surgical removal may be possible if the tumor is extra-axial (eg, meningioma, acoustic neuroma) or is not in a critical or inaccessible region of the brain (eg, cerebellar hemangioblastoma). Surgery also permits the diagnosis to be verified and tumor genetics to be determined. Even if the neoplasm cannot be removed, surgery may be beneficial in reducing intracranial pressure and relieving symptoms. Clinical deficits are sometimes partly due to obstructive hydrocephalus, for which simple surgical shunting often produces dramatic benefit.

In patients with malignant gliomas, survival correlates to the extent of initial resection. Radiation therapy increases median survival rates regardless of any preceding surgery and its combination with chemotherapy provides additional benefit. Indications for irradiation in the treatment of patients with other primary intracranial neoplasms depend on tumor type and accessibility and the feasibility of complete surgical removal. Long-term neurocognitive deficits may complicate radiation therapy. Temozolomide is a commonly used oral and intravenous chemotherapeutic agent for gliomas. The addition of low-intensity, 200 kHz frequency alternating electric fields (tumor treatment fields) delivered extracranially at least 18 hours daily improves progression-free survival by 2.7 months and median survival by 4.9 months compared to temozolomide alone in glioblastoma. Bevacizumab is approved in the United States but not in Europe for use in recurrent high-grade glioma.

Tumor genetics guide medical treatment. In patients with glioblastoma with methylated methylguanine-DNA methyltransferase (MGMT) promoter, combination therapy with lomustine and temozolomide improved median survival from 31 to 48 months in an RCT. In patients with isocitrate dehydrogenase (IDH)–mutant astrocytoma and IDH–mutant, p1/19q co-deleted oligodendroglioma, combination therapy with radiation, procarbazine, lomustine, and vincristine improves survival. Grade 2 IDH-mutant astrocytomas and oligodendrogliomas may be treated with the IDH inhibitor vorasidenib (40 mg once daily orally), which prolongs progression-free survival.

Corticosteroids help reduce cerebral edema and are usually started before surgery. Herniation is treated with intravenous dexamethasone (10–20 mg as a bolus, followed by 4 mg every 6 hours) and intravenous mannitol (20% solution given in a dose of 1.5 g/kg over about 30 minutes).

Anticonvulsants are commonly administered in standard doses when necessary (see Table 27–3) but are not indicated for prophylaxis in patients who have no history of seizures. For those patients with difficult to treat symptoms or those needing help with advance care planning, specialty palliative care consultation is appropriate (see Chapter 5).

Mellinghoff IK et al. Vorasidenib in IDH1- or IDH2-mutant low-grade glioma. N Engl J Med. 2023;389:589. [PMID: 37272516]
Swensen SN et al. Treatment options for IDH-mutant malignant gliomas. Curr Treat Options Oncol. 2024;25:1594. [PMID: 39612163]

2. Metastatic Intracranial Tumors

A. Cerebral Metastases

Metastatic brain tumors present in the same way as other cerebral neoplasms, ie, with increased intracranial pressure, with focal or diffuse disturbance of cerebral function, or both. In patients with a single cerebral lesion, the metastatic nature of the lesion may become evident only on histopathologic examination. In other patients, there is initial evidence of widespread metastatic disease, or an isolated cerebral metastasis develops during treatment of the primary neoplasm.

The most common source of intracranial metastasis is carcinoma of the lung; other primary sites are the breast, kidney, skin (melanoma), and GI tract. Most cerebral metastases are located supratentorially. Laboratory and radiologic studies used to evaluate patients with metastases are those described for primary neoplasms. They include MRI and CT scanning performed with and without contrast. Lumbar puncture is necessary only in patients with suspected carcinomatous meningitis. In patients with verified cerebral metastasis from an unknown primary, investigation is guided by symptoms and signs. In women, mammography is indicated; in men under 50, germ cell origin is sought.

Treatment of brain metastases is rapidly evolving and a multidisciplinary approach between neurosurgery, radiation oncology, oncology, and palliative care is necessary. In patients with a single, surgically accessible cerebral metastasis who are otherwise well (ie, a high level of functioning and little or no evidence of extracranial disease), surgical resection followed by irradiation may be possible; the latter may also be selected as the sole treatment. Systemic immunotherapy may be an acceptable initial option in select cases. In patients with multiple metastases or widespread systemic disease, stereotactic radiosurgery, whole-brain radiotherapy, or both may help in some instances; systemic chemotherapy or immunotherapy may be options in others, but in many, treatment is palliative only. *Memantine (5 mg once daily orally titrated by 5 mg weekly to 10 mg twice daily) reduces cognitive toxicity associated with whole-brain radiotherapy and is recommended;* this effect can be augmented through intensity modulated radiation therapy with hippocampal avoidance.

B. Leptomeningeal Metastases (Carcinomatous Meningitis)

The neoplasms metastasizing most commonly to the leptomeninges are carcinoma of the breast and lung, lymphomas, and leukemia (see Chapter 43*).* Leptomeningeal metastases lead to multifocal neurologic deficits, which may be associated with infiltration of cranial and spinal nerve roots, direct invasion of the brain or spinal cord, obstructive or communicating hydrocephalus, or some combination of these factors.

The diagnosis is confirmed by examination of the CSF. Findings may include elevated CSF pressure, pleocytosis, increased protein concentration, and decreased glucose concentration. Cytologic studies may indicate that malignant cells are present; if not, lumbar puncture should be repeated at least twice to obtain further samples for analysis.

CT scans may show contrast enhancement in the basal cisterns or showing hydrocephalus without any evidence of a mass lesion. Gadolinium-enhanced MRI is more sensitive and frequently shows enhancing foci in the leptomeninges. Myelography may show deposits on multiple nerve roots.

Treatment is by irradiation to symptomatic areas, combined with intrathecal chemotherapy in select patients. The long-term prognosis is poor—only about 10% of patients survive for 1 year—and palliative care is therefore important (see Chapter 5).

Kumthekar P et al. Brain metastases and leptomeningeal disease. Continuum (Minneap Minn). 2023;29:1727. [PMID: 38085896]

3. Intracranial Mass Lesions in Patients with AIDS

Primary cerebral lymphoma is a common complication in patients with AIDS. This leads to disturbances in cognition or consciousness, focal motor or sensory deficits, aphasia, seizures, and cranial neuropathies. Similar clinical disturbances may result from **cerebral toxoplasmosis**, which is also a common complication in patients with AIDS (see Chapters 35 and 38). **Cryptococcal meningitis** is a common opportunistic infection in patients with AIDS. Clinically, it may resemble cerebral toxoplasmosis or lymphoma, but cranial CT scans are usually normal (see Chapter 40).

4. Primary & Metastatic Spinal Tumors

ESSENTIALS OF DIAGNOSIS

- Paraparesis or quadriparesis or a spinal sensory level, or both.
- New bowel or bladder dysfunction.

General Considerations

Approximately 10% of spinal tumors are intramedullary. Ependymoma is the most common type of intramedullary tumor; the remainder are other types of glioma. Extramedullary tumors may be extradural or intradural in location. Among the primary extramedullary tumors, neurofibromas and meningiomas are relatively common, benign, and may be intradural or extradural. Carcinomatous metastases, lymphomatous or leukemic deposits, and myeloma are usually extradural; in the case of metastases, the prostate, breast, lung, and kidney are common primary sites.

Tumors may lead to spinal cord dysfunction by direct compression, by ischemia secondary to arterial or venous obstruction and, in the case of intramedullary lesions, by invasive infiltration.

Clinical Findings

A. Symptoms and Signs

Symptoms usually develop insidiously. Pain is often conspicuous with extradural lesions; is characteristically aggravated by coughing or straining; may be radicular, localized to the back, or felt diffusely in an extremity; and may be accompanied by motor deficits, paresthesias, or numbness, especially in the legs. Bladder, bowel, and sexual dysfunction may occur. Pain, however, often precedes specific neurologic symptoms from epidural metastases.

Examination may reveal localized spinal tenderness. A segmental lower motor neuron deficit or dermatomal sensory changes (or both) are sometimes found at the level of the lesion, while an upper motor neuron deficit and sensory disturbance are found below it.

B. Imaging

MRI with contrast or CT myelography is used to identify and localize the lesion. *The combination of known tumor elsewhere in the body, back pain, and either abnormal plain films of the spine or neurologic signs of cord compression is an urgent indication to perform imaging.* In patients with a known primary tumor, the diagnosis can often be made radiologically; in others, a biopsy may be necessary but should not delay treatment.

Treatment

Intramedullary tumors are treated by decompression and surgical excision (when feasible) and by irradiation. The prognosis depends on the cause and severity of cord compression before it is relieved.

Treatment of epidural spinal metastases consists of surgical decompression, radiation, or both. Dexamethasone is also given in a high dosage (eg, 10–96 mg once intravenously, followed by 4–25 mg four times daily for 3 days orally or intravenously, followed by rapid tapering of the dosage, depending on initial dose and response) to reduce cord swelling and relieve pain. Radiation alone is often all that is required in patients with radiosensitive tumors. Surgical decompression is reserved for patients with tumors that are unresponsive to irradiation or who have previously been irradiated, for those with spinal instability, and for patients in whom there is some uncertainty about the diagnosis. The long-term outlook is poor, but treatment may at least delay the onset of major disability.

Haro-Perez P et al. Surgery with or without radiotherapy versus radiotherapy alone for malignant spinal cord compression: an updated meta-analysis. Spine (Phila). 2025;50:277. [PMID: 39477818]

5. Brain Abscess

ESSENTIALS OF DIAGNOSIS

- Signs of expanding intracranial mass.
- Signs of primary infection or congenital heart disease are sometimes present.
- Fever may be absent.

General Considerations

Brain abscess presents as an intracranial space-occupying lesion and arises as a sequela of dental, ear, or nose infection, may be a complication of infection elsewhere in the body, or may result from infection introduced intracranially by trauma or surgical procedures. The most common infective organisms are streptococci, staphylococci, and anaerobes; mixed infections also occur.

Clinical Findings

A. Symptoms and Signs

Headache, drowsiness, inattention, confusion, and seizures are early symptoms, followed by signs of increasing intracranial pressure and then a focal neurologic deficit. There may be little or no systemic evidence of infection.

B. Imaging and Other Investigations

A CT scan of the head characteristically shows an area of contrast enhancement surrounding a low-density core. Similar abnormalities may be found in patients with metastatic neoplasms. MRI findings often permit earlier recognition of focal cerebritis or an abscess. Stereotactic needle aspiration may enable a specific etiologic organism to be identified. Examination of the CSF does not help in diagnosis and may precipitate a herniation syndrome. Peripheral leukocytosis is sometimes present.

Treatment

Treatment consists of intravenous antibiotics combined with surgical drainage (aspiration or excision), if necessary, to reduce the mass effect or sometimes to establish the diagnosis. *Abscesses smaller than 2 cm can often be cured medically.* Broad-spectrum antibiotics, selected based on risk factors and likely organisms, are used if the infecting organism is unknown (see Chapter 37). An initial empiric multi-antibiotic regimen typically includes ceftriaxone (2 g intravenously every 12 hours), metronidazole (15 mg/kg intravenous loading dose, followed by 7.5 mg/kg intravenously every 6 hours), and vancomycin (1 g intravenously every 12 hours). The regimen is altered once culture and sensitivity data are available. Antimicrobial treatment is usually continued parenterally for 6–8 weeks and is followed by oral treatment for certain infections, such as nocardiosis, actinomycosis, fungal infections, and tuberculosis. The patient should be monitored by serial CT scans or MRI every 2 weeks and at deterioration. Dexamethasone (4–25 mg four times daily intravenously or orally, depending on severity, followed by tapering of dose, depending on response) may reduce any associated edema, but intravenous mannitol is sometimes required.

When to Refer

All patients should be referred.

When to Admit

- All patients with increased intracranial pressure.
- All patients requiring biopsy, surgical treatment, or shunting procedures.

Omland LH et al. Update and approach to patients with brain abscess. Curr Opin Infect Dis. 2024;37:211. [PMID: 38547383]

NONMETASTATIC NEUROLOGIC COMPLICATIONS OF MALIGNANT DISEASE

A variety of nonmetastatic neurologic complications of malignant disease can occur. **Metabolic encephalopathy** due to electrolyte abnormalities, infections, drug overdose, or the failure of some vital organ may be reflected by drowsiness, lethargy, restlessness, insomnia, agitation, confusion, stupor, or coma. The mental changes are usually associated with tremor, asterixis, and multifocal myoclonus. The electroencephalogram is generally diffusely slowed. Laboratory studies are necessary to detect the cause of the encephalopathy, which must then be treated appropriately.

Immune suppression resulting from either the malignant disease or its treatment (eg, by chemotherapy) predisposes patients to brain abscess, progressive multifocal leukoencephalopathy, meningitis, herpes zoster infection, and other opportunistic infectious diseases. Moreover, an overt or occult CSF fistula, as occurs with some tumors, may also increase the risk of infection. MRI or CT scanning aids in the early recognition of a brain abscess, but metastatic brain tumors may have a similar appearance. Examination of the CSF is essential in the evaluation of patients with meningitis and encephalitis but is of no help in the diagnosis of brain abscess.

Cerebrovascular disorders that cause neurologic complications in patients with systemic cancer include nonbacterial thrombotic endocarditis, septic embolization, and cerebral infarcts due to malignancy-induced hypercoagulability. Cerebral, subarachnoid, or subdural hemorrhages may occur in patients with myelogenous leukemia and may be found in association with metastatic tumors, especially melanoma. Spinal subdural hemorrhage sometimes occurs after lumbar puncture in patients with marked thrombocytopenia.

Disseminated intravascular coagulation occurs most commonly in patients with acute promyelocytic leukemia or with some adenocarcinomas and is characterized by a fluctuating encephalopathy, often with associated seizures, that frequently progresses to coma or death. There may be few accompanying neurologic signs. **Venous sinus thrombosis**, which usually presents with convulsions and headaches, may also occur in patients with leukemia or lymphoma. Examination commonly reveals papilledema and focal or diffuse neurologic signs.

Autoimmune paraneoplastic disorders occur when the immune system reacts against neuronal antigens expressed by tumor cells. The clinical manifestations depend on the autoantibody. Symptoms may precede those due to the neoplasm itself. Several distinct syndromes are common, each associated with specific antibodies and tumors (Table 27–6). Identification of an antibody is not always possible in a suspected autoimmune paraneoplastic condition, and a search for an underlying neoplasm should be undertaken. Treatment of the neoplasm offers the best hope for stabilization or improvement of the neurologic symptoms, which often are not completely reversible. Specific treatment of the antibody-mediated symptoms by intravenous immunoglobulin (IVIG) administration, plasmapheresis, corticosteroids, or other immunosuppressive regimens is frequently attempted despite limited evidence of efficacy. Many of the disorders listed in Table 27–6 can occur either as paraneoplastic phenomena or in isolation; when they occur in the absence of a tumor, the response to immunotherapy is typically more favorable.

Autoimmune disorders may also be triggered as a result of cancer immunotherapy. Encephalitis, hypophysitis, meningitis, transverse myelitis, acute and chronic inflammatory demyelinating polyneuropathy, autonomic neuropathy, myasthenia gravis, and myositis have all been described.

McCombe JA et al. Neurologic manifestations of autoimmunity with immune checkpoint inhibitors. Handb Clin Neurol. 2024;200:449. [PMID: 38494296]

IDIOPATHIC INTRACRANIAL HYPERTENSION (Pseudotumor Cerebri)

ESSENTIALS OF DIAGNOSIS

- Headache, worse on straining.
- Visual obscurations or diplopia may occur.
- Examination reveals papilledema.
- Abducens palsy is commonly present.

General Considerations

There are many causes of this disorder. Thrombosis of the transverse venous sinus (as a complication of otitis media or chronic mastoiditis) and sagittal sinus thrombosis may lead to a clinically similar picture. Other causes include chronic pulmonary disease, SLE, uremia, endocrine disturbances such as hypoparathyroidism, hypothyroidism, or Addison disease, vitamin A toxicity, the use of tetracycline, and withdrawal of corticosteroids following long-term use. In most instances, however, no specific cause can be found, and the disorder remits spontaneously after several months. This idiopathic variety occurs most commonly among overweight women aged 20–44. *In all cases, screening for a space-occupying lesion of the brain is important.*

Table 27–6. Autoimmune paraneoplastic disorders and their associated antibodies and tumors (listed in alphabetical order).

Syndrome	Clinical Features	Associated Antibodies	Typical Associated Tumors
Anti-NMDA receptor–associated encephalitis	Paranoia, delusions, behavioral disturbance, seizure, orofacial dyskinesias, athetosis, dysautonomia, hypoventilation	NMDA receptor[1]	Ovarian teratoma, lung, breast, ovary, testicle
Autoimmune necrotizing myopathy	Weakness	SRP,[1] HMGCR[1]	Lung, breast, GI, bladder
Autonomic neuropathy	Postural hypotension, gastroparesis	Hu, ganglionic AChR[1]	
Cerebellar degeneration	Ataxia, dysarthria, nystagmus	GAD65,[1] KLHL11, mGluR1,[1] NIF,[1] Ri, SOX-1, Tr, VGCC,[1] Yo	Lung, breast, thymus, ovary, testicle, Hodgkin lymphoma
Dermatomyositis	Weakness, heliotrope skin rash	TIF-1 γ	Lung, breast, ovary, GI, lymphoma
Lambert-Eaton myasthenic syndrome	Fatigable weakness, ptosis, diplopia, dry mouth, constipation	VGCC,[1] SOX-1	Lung
Limbic encephalitis/encephalomyelitis	Short-term memory loss, hallucinations, seizures, behavioral disturbance, encephalopathy	AMPA receptor,[1] Caspr2,[1] CRMP5, DPPX,[1] $GABA_A$ receptor,[1] $GABA_B$ receptor,[1] GAD65,[1] GFAP,[1] Hu, LGI1,[1] Ma2, mGluR5,[1] MOG,[1] NIF,[1] thyroglobulin[1]/thyroperoxidase[1]	Lung, breast, thymus, ovary, testicle, Hodgkin lymphoma
Myasthenia gravis	Fatigable weakness, ptosis, diplopia	AChR,[1] LRP4,[1] MuSK[1]	Thymus
Myelitis	Paraparesis, bowel and bladder dysfunction; sensory level	Amphiphysin,[1] aquaporin 4,[1] CRMP5, GFAP,[1] Hu, MOG,[1] NIF,[1] Yo	Lung, breast, lymphoma, leukemia, thyroid, renal
Neuromyotonia	Cramps, stiffness, myokymia, fasciculations	Caspr2,[1] LGI1[1]	Lung, Hodgkin lymphoma, thymoma
Opsoclonus/myoclonus	Erratic, conjugate saccadic eye movements and limb myoclonus	Ri	Lung, breast, ovary, testicle, neuroblastoma (children)
Retinopathy	Vision loss	Anti-recoverin, anti-retinal bipolar cell	Small cell lung, melanoma
Sensorimotor neuropathy	Numbness with or without weakness; may be mild and chronic or acute and severe	Amphiphysin, CRMP5, Hu, MAG[1], Ri	Small cell lung, monoclonal gammopathy, thymoma
Sensory neuronopathy	Pain, numbness, sensory ataxia, hearing loss	Hu	Lung
Stiff person syndrome	Co-contraction of antagonist and agonist muscles	Amphiphysin,[1] GAD65,[1] GlyR[1]	Small cell lung, breast, thymus, lymphoma

AChR, acetylcholine receptor; AMPA, α-amino-3-hydroxy-5-methylisoxazole-4-propionic acid; Caspr2, contactin associated protein-like 2; CRMP, collapsin response-mediator protein; DPPX, dipeptidyl-peptidase-like protein-6; GABA, γ-aminobutyric acid; GAD, glutamic acid decarboxylase; GFAP, glial fibrillary acidic protein; GlyR, glycine receptor; HMGCR, 3-hydroxy-3-methylglutaryl-coenzyme A reductase; KLHL11, kelch-like protein 11; LGI1, leucine rich glioma inactivated; LRP4, LDL receptor-related protein 4; mGluR, metabotropic glutamate receptor; MAG, myelin-associated glycoprotein; MOG, myelin oligodendrocyte glycoprotein; MuSK, muscle-specific tyrosine kinase; NIF, neuronal intermediate filament; NMDA, *N*-methyl-D-aspartate; REM, rapid eye movement; SOX-1, Sry-like high mobility group box transcription factor 1; SRP, signal recognition particle; TIF-1, human transcription intermediary factor-1; VGCC, voltage-gated calcium channel.

[1]Can occur in absence of tumor.

Clinical Findings

A. Symptoms and Signs

Symptoms consist of headache, diplopia, and other visual disturbances due to papilledema and abducens nerve dysfunction. Pulse-synchronous tinnitus may also occur. Examination reveals papilledema and some enlargement of the blind spots, but patients otherwise look well.

B. Imaging

Investigations reveal no evidence of a space-occupying lesion. CT or MRI may show small or normal ventricles, an empty sella turcica, tortuous optic nerves, distension of the optic nerve sheath, and posterior globe flattening. MR venography is important in screening for thrombosis of the intracranial venous sinuses. In some cases, stenosis of one or more of the venous sinuses will be observed.

C. Laboratory Findings

Lumbar puncture is necessary to confirm the presence of intracranial hypertension, but the CSF is normal. Laboratory studies help exclude some of the other causes mentioned earlier.

Treatment

Untreated intracranial hypertension sometimes leads to secondary optic atrophy and permanent visual loss. Acetazolamide (250–500 mg orally three times daily, increasing slowly to a maintenance dose of up to 4000 mg daily, divided two to four times daily) reduces formation of CSF. Like acetazolamide, the antiepileptic medication topiramate (see Table 27–3) is a carbonic anhydrase inhibitor and was shown to be similarly effective in an open-label study; topiramate has the added benefit of causing weight loss. Furosemide (20–40 mg daily) may be helpful as adjunct therapy. Corticosteroids are discouraged. Weight loss is important: bariatric surgery led to a decrease in both intracranial pressure and weight at 2 years compared with a community weight management program in a randomized trial and may be considered in patients with a BMI of 35 or greater. The role of GLP-1 agonists is being investigated. Repeated lumbar puncture to lower the intracranial pressure by removal of CSF is effective as a temporizing measure, but pharmacologic approaches to treatment provide better long-term relief. Treatment is monitored by checking visual acuity and visual fields, funduscopic appearance, and pressure of the CSF. The disorder may worsen after a period of stability, indicating the need for long-term follow-up.

If medical treatment fails to control the intracranial pressure, surgical placement of a lumboperitoneal or ventriculoperitoneal shunt or optic nerve sheath fenestration should be undertaken to preserve vision. Patients with venous sinus stenosis may benefit from stenting.

In addition to the above measures, any specific cause of intracranial hypertension requires appropriate treatment. Thus, hormone therapy should be initiated if there is an underlying endocrine disturbance. Discontinuing the use of tetracycline or vitamin A will allow for resolution of intracranial hypertension due to these agents. If corticosteroid withdrawal is responsible, the medication should be reintroduced and then tapered more gradually.

When to Refer

All patients should be referred.

When to Admit

All patients with worsening vision requiring surgical treatment should be hospitalized.

Azzam AY et al. Venous sinus stenting for idiopathic intracranial hypertension: an updated meta-analysis. J Neurol Sci. 2024;459:122948. [PMID: 38457956]

Horton JC. Idiopathic intracranial hypertension. N Engl J Med. 2025;393:1409. [PMID: 41061234]

SELECTED NEUROCUTANEOUS DISEASES

Because the nervous system develops from the epithelial layer of the embryo, a number of congenital diseases include both neurologic and cutaneous manifestations. Three disorders are discussed below, and **von Hippel-Lindau** disease is discussed in Chapter 29.

1. Tuberous Sclerosis

Tuberous sclerosis may occur sporadically or on a familial basis with autosomal dominant inheritance. Neurologic presentation is with seizures and progressive psychomotor delay beginning in early childhood. The cutaneous abnormality adenoma sebaceum becomes manifest usually between 5 and 10 years of age and typically consists of reddened nodules on the face (cheeks, nasolabial folds, sides of the nose, and chin) and sometimes on the forehead and neck. Other typical cutaneous lesions include subungual fibromas, shagreen patches (leathery plaques of subepidermal fibrosis, situated usually on the trunk), and leaf-shaped hypopigmented spots. Associated abnormalities include retinal lesions and tumors, benign rhabdomyomas of the heart, lung cysts, benign tumors in the viscera, and bone cysts.

The disease is slowly progressive and leads to increasing mental deterioration. Anticonvulsants are indicated to control seizures. Everolimus, a mammalian target of rapamycin (mTOR) inhibitor, is approved in the United States and Europe for medically refractory epilepsy and inoperable subependymal giant cell astrocytomas due to tuberous sclerosis.

Sasongko TH et al. Rapamycin and rapalogs for tuberous sclerosis complex. Cochrane Database Syst Rev. 2023;7:CD011272. [PMID: 37432030]

2. Neurofibromatosis

Neurofibromatosis may occur sporadically or on a familial basis with autosomal dominant inheritance. Two distinct forms are recognized: **Type 1 (Recklinghausen disease)** is characterized by multiple hyperpigmented macules, Lisch nodules, and neurofibromas; **type 2 (NF2-associated schwannomatosis)** is characterized by bilateral eighth nerve tumors, often accompanied by other intracranial or intraspinal tumors.

Neurologic presentation is usually with symptoms and signs of tumor. Multiple neurofibromas characteristically are present and may involve spinal or cranial nerves, especially the eighth nerve. Examination of the superficial cutaneous nerves usually reveals palpable mobile nodules. In some cases, there is marked overgrowth of subcutaneous tissues (**plexiform neuromas**), sometimes with an underlying bony abnormality. Associated cutaneous lesions include axillary freckling and patches of cutaneous pigmentation (**café au lait spots**). Malignant degeneration of neurofibromas occasionally occurs and may lead to peripheral sarcomas. Meningiomas, gliomas (especially optic nerve gliomas), bone cysts, pheochromocytomas, scoliosis, and obstructive hydrocephalus may also occur. Two mitogen-activated protein kinase inhibitors are approved by the

FDA for treatment of inoperable plexiform neurofibromas: selumetinib in children 2 years of age and older and mirdametinib in adults and children. Bevacizumab has been used for rapidly growing vestibular schwannomas in patients with neurofibromatosis type 2.

Sato AA et al. Targeted therapies in neurofibromatosis type 1. Am J Med Genet C Semin Med Genet. 2025;199:154. [PMID: 40968507]

3. Sturge-Weber Syndrome

Sturge-Weber syndrome consists of a congenital, usually unilateral, cutaneous capillary angioma involving the upper face, leptomeningeal angiomatosis, and, in many patients, choroidal angioma. It has no sex predilection and usually occurs sporadically. The cutaneous angioma sometimes has a more extensive distribution over the head and neck and is often quite disfiguring, especially if there is associated overgrowth of connective tissue. Focal or generalized seizures are the usual neurologic presentation and may commence at any age. There may be contralateral homonymous hemianopia, hemiparesis and hemisensory disturbance, ipsilateral glaucoma, and intellectual disability.

Medical treatment is aimed at controlling seizures (see Table 27–3), but surgical treatment may be necessary. Ophthalmologic evaluation is warranted for management of choroidal angioma and increased intraocular pressure.

Hachem ME et al. Multidisciplinary, multicenter consensus for the care of patients affected with Sturge-Weber syndrome. Orphanet J Rare Dis. 2025;20:28. [PMID: 39819452]

MOVEMENT DISORDERS

1. Essential (Familial) Tremor

ESSENTIALS OF DIAGNOSIS

- Postural tremor of hands, head, or voice.
- Family history common.
- May improve temporarily with alcohol.
- No abnormal findings other than tremor.

General Considerations

The cause of essential tremor is uncertain, but it is sometimes inherited in an autosomal dominant manner. Various responsible genes have been identified.

Clinical Findings

Tremor may begin at any age and is enhanced by emotional stress. The tremor usually involves one or both hands, the head, or the hands and head, while the legs tend to be spared. Except in advanced cases, the tremor typically is *not present at rest* but emerges with action. Examination reveals no other abnormalities. Ingestion of a small quantity of alcohol commonly provides remarkable but short-lived relief by an unknown mechanism.

The tremor typically becomes more conspicuous with time. Occasionally, it interferes with manual skills and leads to impairment of handwriting. Speech may also be affected if the laryngeal muscles are involved.

Treatment

Treatment often is unnecessary. When it is required because of disability, propranolol (60–240 mg daily orally) may be helpful. Long-term therapy is typical; however, intermittent therapy is sometimes useful in patients whose tremor becomes exacerbated in specific predictable situations. Primidone may be helpful when propranolol is ineffective, but patients with essential tremor are often sensitive to it. The starting dose is 50 mg daily orally, and the daily dose is increased by 50 mg every 2 weeks depending on the patient's response; a maintenance dose of 125 mg three times daily orally is commonly effective. Occasional patients do not respond to these measures but are helped by alprazolam (up to 3 mg daily orally in divided doses), topiramate (titrated up to a dose of 400 mg daily orally in divided doses over 8 weeks), or gabapentin (1800 mg daily orally in divided doses). Botulinum toxin may reduce tremor, but adverse effects include dose-dependent weakness of the injected muscles.

Disabling tremor unresponsive to medical treatment may be helped by high-frequency thalamic stimulation ("deep brain stimulation") on one or both sides, according to the laterality of symptoms. Focused transcranial ultrasound thalamotomy using MRI guidance is also effective, as is stereotactic radiosurgery for unilateral upper extremity tremor. Transcutaneous electrical stimulation of the median and radial nerves modestly improves function and is an option for tremors that are not controlled by medications or suitable for surgical treatment.

Kondapavulur S et al. A systematic review comparing focused ultrasound surgery with radiosurgery for essential tremor. Neurosurgery. 2023;93:524. [PMID: 37010324]
Shih LC. Essential tremor. Continuum (Minneap Minn). 2025;31:979. [PMID: 40748121]

2. Parkinson Disease

ESSENTIALS OF DIAGNOSIS

- Any combination of tremor, rigidity, bradykinesia, and progressive postural instability ("parkinsonism").
- Cognitive impairment is sometimes prominent.

General Considerations

Parkinsonism is a relatively common disorder that occurs in all ethnic groups, with an approximately equal sex distribution. The most common variety, idiopathic Parkinson disease, begins most often between 45 and 65 years of age and is a progressive disease.

Etiology

In idiopathic Parkinson disease, dopamine depletion due to degeneration of the dopaminergic nigrostriatal system leads to an imbalance of dopamine and acetylcholine, which are neurotransmitters normally present in the corpus striatum. Treatment of the motor disturbance is directed at redressing this imbalance by blocking the effect of acetylcholine with anticholinergic medications or by the administration of levodopa, the precursor of dopamine. Increased physical activity and prior use of ibuprofen, caffeine, or cigarettes are associated with a *decreased* risk of developing Parkinson disease, Factors associated with increased risk of disease include age, family history, male sex, prior head trauma, and exposure to herbicides, pesticides, or chlorinated solvents.

Parkinsonism may rarely occur on a familial basis, especially with onset before age 50, and the parkinsonian phenotype may result from mutations of several different genes. Postencephalitic parkinsonism is becoming rare. Exposure to certain toxins (eg, manganese dust, carbon disulfide) and severe carbon monoxide poisoning may lead to parkinsonism. Reversible parkinsonism may develop in patients receiving neuroleptic medications (see Chapter 28), reserpine, or metoclopramide. Only rarely is hemiparkinsonism the presenting feature of a progressive space-occupying lesion.

Clinical Findings

A. Symptoms and Signs

Tremor, rigidity, bradykinesia, and postural instability are the cardinal motor features of parkinsonism and may be present in any combination. Nonmotor manifestations include affective disorders (depression, anxiety, and apathy), psychosis, cognitive changes, fatigue, sleep disorders, anosmia, autonomic disturbances, sensory complaints or pain, and seborrheic dermatitis. Dementia or mild cognitive impairment will eventually develop in many patients.

The tremor of about four to six cycles per second is *most conspicuous at rest*; it is enhanced by emotional stress and often less severe during voluntary activity. Although it may ultimately be present in all limbs, it is commonly confined to one limb or to limbs on one side for months or years before it becomes more generalized. In some patients, tremor is absent.

Rigidity (an increase in resistance to passive movement) is responsible for the characteristically flexed posture seen in many patients, but *the most disabling symptoms of parkinsonism are due to bradykinesia*, manifested as a slowness of voluntary movement and a reduction in automatic movements such as swinging of the arms while walking. Curiously, effective voluntary activity may be regained briefly during an emergency (eg, the patient is able to leap aside to avoid an oncoming motor vehicle).

Clinical diagnosis of the well-developed syndrome is usually simple. The patient has a relatively immobile face with widened palpebral fissures, infrequent blinking, and a fixity of facial expression. Seborrhea of the scalp and face is common. There is often mild blepharoclonus, and a tremor may be present about the mouth and lips. Repetitive tapping (about twice per second) over the bridge of the nose produces a sustained blink response (**Myerson sign**). Other findings may include saliva drooling from the mouth, perhaps due to impairment of swallowing; soft and poorly modulated voice; a variable rest tremor and rigidity in some or all of the limbs; slowness of voluntary movements; impairment of fine or rapidly alternating movements; and micrographia. There is typically no muscle weakness (provided that sufficient time is allowed for power to be developed) and no alteration in the tendon reflexes or plantar responses. The patient has difficulty rising from a sitting position and when beginning to walk. The gait itself is characterized by small shuffling steps and a loss of the normal automatic arm swing; there may be unsteadiness on turning, difficulty in stopping, and a tendency to fall.

B. Imaging

There are no routine diagnostic imaging tests for Parkinson disease, although brain MRI scan may exclude an underlying structural lesion. Striatal dopamine transporter imaging (DaT scan) is sometimes helpful when the clinical diagnosis is not clear but is usually unnecessary. In Parkinson disease it shows reduced uptake by striatal dopaminergic neurons of a specific radioactive tracer injected into the blood on single photon emission computerized tomography (SPECT) or PET.

C. Laboratory Findings

Misfolded α-synuclein, the neuropathological hallmark of Parkinson disease, may be detected in other tissues such as skin and CSF; assays using both are commercially available in the United States and helpful if the diagnosis is unclear clinically. These assays may also help differentiate between other disorders of misfolded α-synuclein, namely dementia with Lewy bodies and multisystem atrophy.

Differential Diagnosis

Diagnostic problems may occur in mild cases, especially if tremor is minimal or absent. For example, mild hypokinesia or slight tremor is commonly attributed to old age. Depression, with its associated expressionless face, poorly modulated voice, and reduction in voluntary activity, can be difficult to distinguish from mild parkinsonism, especially since the two disorders may coexist. The family history, the character of the tremor, and lack of other neurologic signs should distinguish essential tremor from parkinsonism. Wilson disease can be distinguished by its early age at onset, the presence of other abnormal movements, Kayser-Fleischer rings, and chronic hepatitis, and by increased concentrations of copper in the tissues. Huntington disease presenting with rigidity and bradykinesia may be mistaken for parkinsonism unless the family history and accompanying dementia are recognized. In multisystem atrophy (previously called the Shy-Drager syndrome), autonomic insufficiency (leading to postural hypotension, anhidrosis, disturbances of sphincter control, erectile dysfunction, etc) may be accompanied by parkinsonism, pyramidal deficits, lower motor neuron signs, or cerebellar dysfunction. In progressive supranuclear palsy, bradykinesia and rigidity are accompanied by a supranuclear disorder of eye movements, pseudobulbar palsy, pseudo-emotional lability (**pseudobulbar affect**), and axial dystonia. Creutzfeldt-Jakob disease may be accompanied by features of parkinsonism, but progression is rapid, dementia is usual, myoclonic jerking is common, ataxia and pyramidal signs may be conspicuous, and the MRI and electroencephalographic findings are usually characteristic. In corticobasal degeneration, asymmetric parkinsonism is accompanied by conspicuous signs of cortical dysfunction (eg, apraxia, sensory inattention, dementia, aphasia). Dementia with Lewy bodies is characterized by prominent visual hallucinations and cognitive impairment that begin before or within 1 year of onset of the motor features of parkinsonism.

Treatment

Treatment is symptomatic. There is great interest in developing disease-modifying therapies and gene therapies, but trials of several putative neuroprotective agents have shown little benefit.

A. Medical Measures

Medication is not required early in the course of Parkinson disease, but the nature of the disorder and the availability of medical treatment for use when necessary should be discussed with the patient.

1. Amantadine—Patients with mild symptoms but no disability may be helped by amantadine (100 mg orally two to three times daily [immediate release] or once daily [extended release]). This medication improves all of the clinical features of parkinsonism, but its mode of action is unclear. Side effects are uncommon but may include restlessness, confusion, depression, skin rashes, edema, nausea, constipation, anorexia, postural hypotension, and disturbances of cardiac rhythm. Amantadine also ameliorates dyskinesias resulting from long-term levodopa therapy.

2. Levodopa—Levodopa, which is converted in the body to dopamine, is the recommended initial therapy for treatment of motor symptoms. It improves all of the major features of parkinsonism, including bradykinesia, but *does not stop progression* of the disorder. The most common early side effects of levodopa are nausea, vomiting, and hypotension, but cardiac arrhythmias may also occur. Dyskinesias, restlessness, confusion, and other behavioral changes tend to occur somewhat later and become more common with time. **Levodopa-induced dyskinesias** may take any conceivable form, including chorea, athetosis, dystonia, tremor, tics, and myoclonus. An even later complication is the **wearing off effect** or the **on-off phenomenon**, in which abrupt but transient fluctuations in the severity of parkinsonism occur unpredictably but frequently during the day. *The "off" period of marked bradykinesia* has been shown to relate in some instances to falling plasma levels of levodopa. During the *"on" phase*, dyskinesias are often conspicuous but mobility is increased. However, such response fluctuations may relate to advancing disease rather than to levodopa therapy itself.

Carbidopa, which inhibits the enzyme responsible for the breakdown of levodopa to dopamine, does not cross the blood-brain barrier. When levodopa is given in combination with carbidopa, the extracerebral breakdown of levodopa is diminished. This reduces the amount of levodopa required daily for beneficial effects and lowers the incidence of nausea, vomiting, hypotension, and cardiac irregularities. Such a combination does not prevent the development of response fluctuations and the incidence of other side effects (dyskinesias or psychiatric complications) may actually be increased.

Sinemet, a commercially available preparation that contains carbidopa and levodopa in a fixed ratio (1:10 or 1:4), is generally used. Treatment is started with a small dose—eg, one tablet of Sinemet 25/100 (containing 25 mg of carbidopa and 100 mg of levodopa) three times daily—and gradually increased depending on the response. Sinemet CR is a controlled-release formulation (containing 25 or 50 mg of carbidopa and 100 or 200 mg of levodopa) and is mainly useful when taken at bedtime to lessen motor disability upon awakening. Formulations of carbidopa/levodopa containing both immediate- and delayed-release beads (Rytary or Crexont) provides a smoother response in patients with fluctuations. The commercially available combination of levodopa with both carbidopa and entacapone (Stalevo) may also be helpful in this context and is discussed in the following section on COMT inhibitors. Response fluctuations are also reduced by keeping the daily intake of *protein* at the recommended minimum and taking the main protein meal as the last meal of the day. A continuous infusion of a carbidopa-levodopa enteral suspension through a percutaneous gastrojejunostomy tube reduces "off" time in patients with advanced Parkinson disease. A continuous subcutaneous infusion of foslevodopa-foscarbidopa also reduces "off" time and improves the amount of "on" time without troublesome dyskinesias. Levodopa can also be taken as a dispersible tablet placed sublingually for a faster response, or by inhalation (Inbrija) as a rescue medication for patients developing severe akinesia (off periods).

The dyskinesias and behavioral side effects of levodopa are dose-related, but reduction in dose may eliminate any therapeutic benefit. Levodopa-induced dyskinesias may also respond to amantadine.

Levodopa therapy is contraindicated in patients with psychotic illness or narrow-angle glaucoma. It should not be given to patients taking MAO inhibitors or within 2 weeks of their withdrawal, because hypertensive crises may result. Sudden discontinuation of levodopa can precipitate neuroleptic malignant syndrome and should be avoided.

3. Dopamine agonists—Dopamine agonists, such as pramipexole and ropinirole, act directly on dopamine receptors, and their use in parkinsonism is associated with a lower incidence of the response fluctuations and dyskinesias that occur with long-term levodopa therapy. They are effective in both early and advanced stages of Parkinson disease, although less effective than levodopa. They are often given before the introduction of levodopa or in combination with a low dose of Sinemet 25/100 (carbidopa 25 mg and levodopa 100 mg, one tablet three times daily) when dopaminergic therapy is first introduced in patients younger than 60; the dose of Sinemet is kept constant, while the dose of the agonist is gradually increased.

Pramipexole is started at a dosage of 0.125 mg three times daily orally, and the dose is built up gradually to between 0.5 and 1.5 mg three times daily. Ropinirole is begun at 0.25 mg three times daily orally and gradually increased; most patients require between 2 and 8 mg three times daily for benefit. Extended-release, once-daily formulations of pramipexole and ropinirole have similar efficacy and tolerability as the immediate release versions. Rotigotine is a dopamine agonist absorbed transdermally from a skin patch; it is started at 2 mg once daily and increased weekly by 2 mg daily until achieving an optimal response, up to a maximum of 8 mg daily. Apomorphine can be administered by continuous subcutaneous infusion, which reduces "off" time in patients with motor fluctuations, and by subcutaneous injection for relief of sudden "off" symptoms (starting with a 1 mg test dose given under medical supervision). It usually is prescribed by experienced providers. Premedication with an anti-emetic for 3 days prior to starting apomorphine is recommended. Adverse effects of these various agonists include fatigue, somnolence, nausea, peripheral edema, dyskinesias, confusion, and postural hypotension. Less commonly, an irresistible urge to sleep may occur, sometimes in inappropriate and hazardous circumstances. Impulse control disorders involving gambling, shopping, or sexual activity also occur. Local skin reactions may occur with the rotigotine patch. The **dopamine agonist withdrawal syndrome** develops occasionally in patients in whom a dopamine agonist is tapered. It consists of a combination of distressing physical and psychological symptoms that are refractory to levodopa and other dopaminergic medications. It may persist for months or longer, and there is no effective treatment. The dopamine agonist should be reintroduced and tapered more gradually.

4. Selective MAO inhibitors—Rasagiline, a selective MAO-B inhibitor, has a symptomatic benefit in some patients at a daily oral dose of 1 mg, taken in the morning; it may also be used for adjunctive therapy in patients with response fluctuations to levodopa. Selegiline (5 mg orally with breakfast and lunch) and safinamide (50 mg orally daily, increased to 100 mg daily after 14 days) are also approved as adjunctive treatments. By inhibiting the metabolic breakdown of dopamine, these medications may improve fluctuations or declining response to levodopa.

Studies have suggested (but not proven) that rasagiline may slow the progression of Parkinson disease, and it appears to delay the need for other symptomatic therapies. For these reasons, rasagiline is often started early, particularly for patients who are young or have mild disease.

5. COMT inhibitors—Catecholamine-*O*-methyltransferase (COMT) inhibitors reduce the metabolism of levodopa to 3-*O*-methyldopa and thereby alter the plasma pharmacokinetics of levodopa, leading to more sustained plasma levels and more constant dopaminergic stimulation of the brain. Treatment with entacapone or tolcapone results in reduced response fluctuations, with a greater period of responsiveness to administered levodopa. Tolcapone is given in a dosage of 100 mg or 200 mg three times daily orally, and entacapone is given as 200 mg with each dose of Sinemet. Opicapone, a long-acting, peripherally selective COMT inhibitor, is taken once daily (50 mg) at bedtime at least 1 hour before or after eating. The dose of Sinemet taken concurrently may have to be reduced by up to one-third to avoid side effects. Diarrhea is sometimes troublesome. Because of rare cases of fulminant hepatic failure, tolcapone should be *avoided* in patients with preexisting liver disease. Serial liver biochemical tests should be performed at 2-week intervals for the first year of treatment and at longer intervals thereafter—as recommended by the manufacturer. Serious hepatotoxicity has not been reported with entacapone or opicapone.

Stalevo, the commercial preparation of levodopa combined with both carbidopa and entacapone, is best used in patients already stabilized on equivalent doses of carbidopa/levodopa and entacapone. Stalevo is available in three strengths, which can be tailored to the patient's needs.

6. Istradefylline—This adenosine A_{2A} receptor antagonist (20–40 mg orally once daily) is given to patients taking levodopa or a dopamine agonist to reduce off time; total off time is typically reduced by < 1 hour per day.

7. Anticholinergic medications—Anticholinergics are more helpful in alleviating tremor and rigidity than bradykinesia. Trihexyphenidyl and benztropine are commonly used formulations. Treatment is started with a small dose and gradually increased until benefit occurs or side effects limit further increments. If treatment is ineffective, the medication is gradually withdrawn and another preparation then tried.

These medications are often poorly tolerated, especially in older adults. Side effects include dryness of the mouth, nausea, constipation, palpitations, cardiac arrhythmias, urinary retention, confusion, agitation, restlessness, drowsiness, mydriasis, increased intraocular pressure, and defective accommodation. Anticholinergic medications are contraindicated in patients with prostatic hyperplasia, narrow-angle glaucoma, or obstructive GI disease. They are best avoided whenever cognitive impairment or a predisposition to delirium exists.

8. Antipsychotics—Confusion and psychotic symptoms may occur as a side effect of dopaminergic therapy or as a part of the underlying illness. Pimavanserin (34 mg once daily), a serotonin(2A) agonist, is approved by the FDA specifically for treating the psychosis of Parkinson disease. This may also respond to the atypical antipsychotic agents clozapine and quetiapine, which have few extrapyramidal side effects and do not block the effects of dopaminergic medication. Clozapine may rarely cause marrow suppression, and weekly blood counts are therefore necessary for patients taking it. The dosage is started at 6.25 mg at bedtime and increased gradually to 25–100 mg/day, as needed. In low doses, clozapine may improve iatrogenic dyskinesias. Typical antipsychotic agents and the second-generation antipsychotic agents risperidone and olanzapine may cause worsening of motor symptoms and should be avoided.

B. General Measures

Physical therapy, occupational therapy, and speech therapy helps many patients. A meta-analysis of 15 RCTs and six nonrandomized controlled trials concluded that there were beneficial effects of **tai chi** in improving motor function, depression, balance, and functional mobility in patients with Parkinson disease. Cognitive impairment and psychiatric symptoms may be helped by a cholinesterase inhibitor, such as rivastigmine (3–12 mg orally daily or 4.6 or 9.5 mg/24 hours transdermally daily). Affective disorders, which may be conspicuous during off periods, should be treated by antidepressants or antianxiety agents as necessary. The quality of life can often be improved by the provision of simple aids to daily living, eg, rails or banisters placed strategically about the home, special table cutlery with large handles, nonslip rubber table mats, and devices to amplify the voice.

C. Stimulation and Ablative Treatments

High-frequency stimulation of the subthalamic nuclei or globus pallidus internus may benefit many of the motor features of the disease but does not affect its natural history. Electrical stimulation of the brain has the advantage over ablative thalamotomy and pallidotomy procedures of being reversible and of causing minimal or no damage to the brain; it is therefore the preferred surgical approach to treatment. It is reserved for patients without cognitive impairment or psychiatric disorder who have a good response to levodopa, but in whom dyskinesias or response fluctuations are problematic. It frequently takes 3–6 months after surgery to adjust stimulator programming and to achieve optimal results. Side effects include depression, apathy, impulsivity, executive dysfunction, and decreased verbal fluency in a subset of patients. Focused ultrasound thalamotomy or stereotactic radiosurgery may help patients with medically refractory tremor-predominant parkinsonism who are reluctant to undergo surgery.

Rawls A et al. Parkinson disease. Continuum (Minneap Minn). 2025;31:930. [PMID: 40748114]
Tanner CM et al. Parkinson's disease. N Engl J Med. 2024;391:442. [PMID: 39083773]

3. Huntington Disease

ESSENTIALS OF DIAGNOSIS

- Gradual onset and progression of chorea and dementia or behavioral change.
- Family history of the disorder.

General Considerations

Huntington disease is characterized by chorea and dementia. It is inherited in an autosomal dominant manner and occurs throughout the world, in all ethnic groups, with a prevalence rate of about 5 per 100,000. There is an expanded and unstable CAG trinucleotide repeat in the huntingtin gene at 4p16.3; longer repeat lengths correspond to an earlier age of onset and faster disease progression.

Clinical Findings

A. Symptoms and Signs

Clinical onset is usually between 30 and 50 years of age. The disease is progressive and usually leads to a fatal outcome within 15–20 years. The initial symptoms may consist of either abnormal movements or intellectual changes, but ultimately both occur. The earliest mental changes are often behavioral, with irritability, moodiness, antisocial behavior, or a psychiatric disturbance, but a more obvious dementia subsequently develops. The dyskinesia may initially be no more than an apparent fidgetiness or restlessness, but eventually choreiform movements and some dystonic posturing occur. A parkinsonian syndrome with progressive rigidity and akinesia (rather than chorea) sometimes occurs in association with dementia, especially in cases with childhood onset. The diagnosis is established with a widely available genetic test, although such testing should be pursued under the guidance of a licensed genetic counselor.

B. Imaging

CT scanning or MRI usually demonstrates cerebral atrophy and atrophy of the caudate nucleus in established cases. PET has shown reduced striatal metabolic rate.

Differential Diagnosis

Chorea developing with no family history of choreoathetosis should not be attributed to Huntington disease until other causes of chorea have been excluded clinically and by appropriate laboratory studies. Nongenetic causes of chorea include stroke, SLE and antiphospholipid antibody syndrome, polycythemia vera, nonketotic hyperglycemia, paraneoplastic syndromes and *N*-methyl-D-aspartate receptor encephalitis, infection with HIV, and various medications. In younger patients, self-limiting Sydenham chorea develops after group A streptococcal infections on rare occasions. If a patient presents solely with progressive intellectual failure, it may not be possible to distinguish Huntington disease from other causes of dementia unless there is a characteristic family history or a dyskinesia develops.

Huntington disease–like (HDL) disorders resemble Huntington disease but are caused by other genetic mutations. A clinically similar autosomal dominant disorder (**dentatorubral-pallidoluysian atrophy**), manifested by chorea, dementia, ataxia, and myoclonic epilepsy, is uncommon except in persons of Japanese ancestry. Chorea may also occur in neuroacanthocytosis, Wilson disease, and neuroferritinopathy. Treatment of the chorea is as for Huntington disease.

Treatment

There is no cure for Huntington disease; progression cannot be halted; and treatment is purely symptomatic. Chorea is treated with vesicular monoamine transporter type 2 (VMAT2) inhibitors, three of which are approved in the United States. Tetrabenazine is initiated at 12.5 mg twice or three times daily orally, increasing by 12.5 mg every 5 days depending on response and tolerance; the usual maintenance dose is 25 mg three times daily. Deutetrabenazine's starting dose is 6 mg once daily orally, increased to 6 mg twice daily after 1 week and by 6-mg increments weekly thereafter, to a maximum of 24 mg twice daily. Valbenazine is started at 40 mg once daily orally, increased by 20 mg every 2 weeks to a maximum of 80 mg daily. Side effects of VMAT2 inhibitors include depression, postural hypotension, drowsiness, and parkinsonian features; they should not be given within 14 days of taking MAO inhibitors and are not indicated for the treatment of levodopa-induced dyskinesias. Treatment with medications blocking dopamine receptors, such as phenothiazines or haloperidol, may control the dyskinesia and any behavioral disturbances. Haloperidol treatment is usually begun with a dose of 1 mg once or twice daily orally, which is then increased every 3 or 4 days depending on the response; alternatively, atypical antipsychotic agents such as quetiapine (increasing from 25 mg daily orally up to 100 mg twice daily orally as tolerated) may be tried. Amantadine in a dose of 200 mg to 400 mg daily orally is sometimes helpful for chorea. Deep brain stimulation has been used successfully to treat chorea in a small number of patients. Behavioral disturbances may respond to clozapine.

Offspring should be offered genetic counseling. Genetic testing permits presymptomatic detection and definitive diagnosis of the disease.

Moore KPL. Huntington disease and chorea. Continuum (Minneap Minn). 2025;31:1066. [PMID: 40748130]

4. Idiopathic Torsion Dystonia

ESSENTIALS OF DIAGNOSIS

- Dystonic movements and postures.
- Normal birth and developmental history. No other neurologic signs.
- Investigations (including CT scan or MRI) reveal no cause of dystonia.

General Considerations

Idiopathic torsion dystonia may occur sporadically or on a hereditary basis, with autosomal dominant, autosomal recessive, and X-linked recessive modes of transmission. Symptoms may begin in childhood or later and persist throughout life.

Clinical Findings

The disorder is characterized by the onset of abnormal movements and postures in a patient with a normal birth and developmental history, no relevant past medical illness, and no other neurologic signs. Investigations (including CT scan) reveal no cause for the abnormal movements. Dystonic movements of the head and neck may take the form of torticollis, blepharospasm, facial grimacing, or forced opening or closing of the mouth. The limbs may also adopt abnormal but characteristic postures. About one-third of patients eventually become so severely disabled that they are confined to chair or bed, while another one-third are affected only mildly.

Differential Diagnosis

Perinatal anoxia, birth trauma, and kernicterus are common causes of dystonia, but abnormal movements usually then develop before the age of 5, the early development of the patient is usually abnormal, and a history of seizures is not unusual. Moreover, examination may reveal signs of intellectual disability or pyramidal deficit in addition to the movement disorder. Dystonic posturing may also occur in Wilson disease, Huntington disease, or parkinsonism; as a sequela of encephalitis lethargica or previous neuroleptic medication therapy; and in certain other disorders. In these cases, diagnosis is based on the history and accompanying clinical manifestations.

Treatment

Idiopathic torsion dystonia usually responds poorly to medications. A distinct variety of dystonia is remarkably responsive to levodopa; therefore, *a levodopa trial is warranted in all dystonic patients* (Sinemet 25/100 mg start 0.5 tablet orally once daily and increased depending on response). Failing this, diazepam, clonazepam, anticholinergic medication such as trihexyphenidyl or benztropine (in high dosage), or baclofen is occasionally helpful; if not, a trial of the VMAT2 inhibitor tetrabenazine may be worthwhile. In each case, the dose has to be individualized, depending on response and tolerance; the doses of the latter medications required for benefit often cause mild parkinsonism. Pallidal deep brain stimulation is helpful for disabling generalized dystonia and has a lower morbidity than stereotactic thalamotomy, which is sometimes helpful in patients with predominantly unilateral limb dystonia. Potential adverse events of deep brain stimulation include cerebral infection or hemorrhage, broken leads, affective changes, and dysarthria.

Richardson SP. Dystonia. Continuum (Mineap Minn). 2025;31:1050. [PMID: 40748115]

5. Focal Torsion Dystonia

A number of the dystonic manifestations that occur in idiopathic torsion dystonia may also occur as isolated phenomena. They are best regarded as focal dystonias that either occur as formes frustes of idiopathic torsion dystonia in patients with a positive family history or represent a focal manifestation of the adult-onset form of that disorder when there is no family history. Medical treatment is generally unsatisfactory. A trial of the medications used in idiopathic torsion dystonia is worthwhile, however, since a few patients do show some response. In addition, with restricted dystonias such as blepharospasm or torticollis, local injection of botulinum toxin into the overactive muscles may produce worthwhile benefit for several weeks or months and can be repeated as needed.

Both **blepharospasm** and **oromandibular dystonia** may occur as an isolated focal dystonia. The former is characterized by spontaneous involuntary forced closure of the eyelids for a variable interval. Oromandibular dystonia is manifested by involuntary contraction of the muscles about the mouth causing, for example, involuntary opening or closing of the mouth, roving or protruding tongue movements, and retraction of the platysma. **Cervical dystonia** (spasmodic torticollis), usually with onset between 25 and 50 years of age, is characterized by a tendency for the neck to twist to one side. This initially occurs episodically, but eventually the neck is held to the side. Some patients have a sensory trick ("geste antagoniste") that lessens the dystonic posture, eg, touching the side of the face. Spontaneous resolution may occur in the first year or so. The disorder is otherwise usually lifelong. Local injection of botulinum toxin provides benefit in most cases. Deep brain stimulation of the globus pallidus interna is an option if medical treatment and botulinum toxin injection are unsuccessful.

Writer's cramp is characterized by dystonic posturing of the hand and forearm when the hand is used for writing and sometimes when it is used for other tasks, eg, playing the piano or using a screwdriver or eating utensils. Medication treatment is usually unrewarding, but injections of botulinum toxin are often helpful. Specialized physiotherapy may also be beneficial, especially in reducing pain associated with dystonia.

Kassaye SG. The effectiveness of physiotherapy for patients with isolated cervical dystonia: an updated systematic review and meta-analysis. BMC Neurol. 2024;24:53. [PMID: 38302911]

6. Myoclonus

Occasional myoclonic jerks may occur in anyone, especially when drifting into sleep. **General or multifocal myoclonus** is common in patients with idiopathic epilepsy and is especially prominent in certain hereditary disorders characterized by seizures and progressive intellectual decline, such as the lipid storage diseases. It is also a feature of subacute sclerosing panencephalitis and Creutzfeldt-Jakob disease. Generalized myoclonic jerking may accompany uremic and other metabolic encephalopathies, result from therapy with levodopa or tricyclic antidepressants, occur in alcohol or drug withdrawal states, or follow anoxic brain damage. It also occurs on a hereditary or sporadic basis as an isolated phenomenon in otherwise healthy subjects.

Segmental myoclonus is a rare manifestation of a focal spinal cord lesion. It may also be the clinical expression of **epilepsia partialis continua**, a disorder in which a repetitive focal epileptic discharge arises in the contralateral sensorimotor cortex, sometimes from an underlying structural lesion. An electroencephalogram is often helpful in clarifying the epileptic nature of the disorder, and CT or MRI scan may reveal the causal lesion.

Myoclonus may respond to certain anticonvulsant medications, especially valproic acid or levetiracetam, or to one of the benzodiazepines, particularly clonazepam (see Table 27–3). It may also respond to piracetam (up to 16.8 g daily; not available in the United States). Myoclonus following anoxic brain damage is often responsive to oxitriptan (5-hydroxytryptophan), the precursor of serotonin, and sometimes to clonazepam. Oxitriptan is given in gradually increasing doses up to 1–1.5 mg daily. In patients with segmental myoclonus, a localized lesion should be searched for and treated appropriately.

Vellieux G et al. Multimodal assessment of the origin of myoclonus in Lance-Adams syndrome. Neurology. 2024;103:e209994. [PMID: 39499871]

7. Wilson Disease

In this metabolic disorder, abnormal movement and posture may occur with or without coexisting signs of liver involvement. Psychiatric and neuropsychological manifestations are common. Wilson disease is discussed in Chapter 18.

8. Drug-Induced Abnormal Movements

Medications may produce a wide variety of abnormal movements, including tremor, parkinsonism, akathisia (ie, motor restlessness), acute dystonia, chorea, myoclonus, and tardive dyskinesias or dystonia. **Medication-induced tremor** is usually postural with a low amplitude and high frequency and may occur with β-2-adrenergic agonists, sympathomimetics, serotonergic agents, glucocorticoids, thyroid hormone, antiseizure medications, antiarrhythmics, antipsychotics, chemotherapeutics, immunosuppressants, hypoglycemic agents, and other medications such as lithium, caffeine, and theophylline.

Drug-induced parkinsonism is usually bilateral at onset, tends to have a lower incidence of tremor, and is poorly responsive to levodopa. It may be caused by antidopaminergic medications (eg, typical and atypical antipsychotics, antiemetics, central monoamine depleting agents), serotonergic agents, calcium channel blockers, and lithium.

Chorea may develop in patients receiving antidopaminergic medications (eg, typical and atypical antipsychotics, antiemetics), levodopa, dopamine agonists, anticholinergic medications, certain antiseizure medications, lithium, amphetamines, or oral contraceptives.

Acute dystonia may be produced by antidopaminergic medications (eg, phenothiazines and their derivatives, butyrophenones, metoclopramide) and dopaminergic medications (eg, levodopa, bromocriptine), serotonergic agents, phenytoin, carbamazepine, and lithium. Dyskinesias related to psychiatric medications are discussed in Chapter 28. *With the exception of tardive dyskinesia and dystonia, the movement disorder usually resolves with withdrawal of the offending substance, but parkinsonism may take many months to do so.* When severe, acute dystonia and akathisia are treated with intravenous or intramuscular benztropine or diphenhydramine, drug-induced parkinsonism is treated with oral benztropine, and tardive dyskinesia is treated with deutetrabenazine or valbenazine.

Conn H et al. Drug-induced parkinsonism: diagnosis and treatment. Expert Opin Drug Saf. 2023;23:1503. [PMID: 39419777]

9. Restless Legs Syndrome

This common disorder, affecting 1–5% of people, may occur as a primary (idiopathic) disorder or in relation to Parkinson disease, pregnancy, iron deficiency anemia, or peripheral neuropathy (especially uremic or diabetic). Restless legs syndrome may have a hereditary basis, and several genetic loci have been associated with the disorder. Restlessness and curious sensory disturbances lead to an irresistible urge to move the limbs, especially during periods of relaxation; movement of the limbs provides relief. The urge occurs exclusively in the evening and at night or is worse at night than during the day. Most patients also have **periodic limb movements of sleep** and one-third have periodic limb movements during relaxed wakefulness; both consist of brief involuntary flexion at the ankle, knee, and hip. Disturbed nocturnal sleep and excessive daytime somnolence may result. *Ferritin levels should always be measured*; treatment with oral iron sulfate in patients with ferritin levels ≤ 75 mcg/L (13.4 mcmol/L) and transferrin saturation < 45% should be attempted prior to initiation of other pharmacotherapies. In patients who do not respond to or are ineligible for iron therapy, gabapentin enacarbil (300–1200 mg orally each evening), gabapentin (starting with 300 mg orally daily, increasing to approximately 1800 mg daily, depending on response and tolerance), or pregabalin (150–300 mg orally divided twice to three times daily) should be tried next. Therapy with nonergot dopamine agonists, such as pramipexole (0.125–0.5 mg orally once daily), ropinirole (0.25–4 mg orally once daily 2–3 hours before bedtime), or rotigotine (1–3 mg/24 hours transdermal patch once daily), is helpful but may lead to an augmentation of symptoms. Levodopa also is helpful but also leads to augmentation, so its use is generally reserved for those who do not respond to other measures. Extended-release oxycodone-naloxone (2.5–5 mg to 5–10 mg orally twice daily) is useful in patients with severe symptoms or those who are refractory to first-line therapies.

Winkelman JW et al. Treatment of restless legs syndrome and periodic limb movement disorder: an American Academy of Sleep Medicine systematic review, meta-analysis, and GRADE assessment. J Clin Sleep Med. 2025;21:153. [PMID: 39324664]

10. Gilles de la Tourette Syndrome

ESSENTIALS OF DIAGNOSIS

- Multiple motor and phonic tics.
- Symptoms begin before age 18 years.
- Tics occur frequently for at least 1 year.
- Tics vary in number, frequency, and nature over time.

Clinical Findings

Simple tics occur transiently in up to 25% of children, remit within weeks to months, and do not require treatment. Tourette syndrome is a more complex disorder. **Motor tics** are the initial manifestation in 80% of cases and most commonly involve the face, whereas in the remaining 20%, the initial symptoms are **phonic tics**; ultimately a combination of different motor and phonic tics develop in all patients. Tics are preceded by an urge that is relieved upon performance of the movement or vocalization; they can be temporarily suppressed but eventually the urge becomes overwhelming. These are noted first in childhood, generally between the ages of 2 and 15. Motor tics occur especially about the face, head, and shoulders (eg, sniffing, blinking, frowning, shoulder shrugging, head thrusting). Phonic tics commonly include grunts, barks, hisses, throat-clearing, and coughs, and sometimes also verbal utterances, including coprolalia (obscene speech). There may also be echolalia (repetition of the speech of others), echopraxia (imitation of others' movements), and palilalia (repetition of words or phrases). Some tics may be self-mutilating in nature, such as nail-biting, hair-pulling, or biting of the lips or tongue. The disorder is chronic, but the course may be punctuated by relapses and remissions. OCD and attention deficit hyperactivity disorder (ADHD) are commonly associated and may be more disabling than the tics themselves. A family history is sometimes obtained.

Examination usually reveals no abnormalities other than the tics. In addition to OCD, psychiatric disturbances may occur because of the associated cosmetic and social embarrassment. The diagnosis of the disorder is often delayed for years, the tics being interpreted as psychiatric illness or some other form of abnormal movement. Patients are thus often subjected to unnecessary treatment before the disorder is recognized. The tic-like character of the abnormal movements and the absence of other neurologic signs should differentiate this disorder from other movement disorders presenting in childhood. Wilson disease, however, can simulate the condition and should be excluded.

Treatment

Treatment is symptomatic and may need to be continued indefinitely. Habit reversal training or other forms of behavioral therapy can be effective alone or in combination with pharmacotherapy. α-Adrenergic agonists, such as clonidine (start 0.05 mg orally at bedtime, titrating to 0.3–0.4 mg orally daily, divided three to four times per day) or guanfacine (start 0.5 mg orally at bedtime, titrating to a maximum of 3–4 mg orally daily, divided twice daily), are first-line therapies because of a favorable side-effect profile compared with typical antipsychotics, and are FDA-approved therapies for the disorder. They also have the advantage of improving the symptoms of concomitant ADHD. When a typical antipsychotic is required in cases of severe tics, haloperidol is generally regarded as the medication of choice. It is started in a low dose (0.25 mg daily orally) that is gradually increased (by 0.25 mg every 4 or 5 days) until there is maximum benefit with a minimum of side effects or until side effects limit further increments. A total daily oral dose of between 2 mg and 8 mg is usually optimal, but higher doses are sometimes necessary. Aripiprazole (2.5–20 mg orally daily), fluphenazine (1–15 mg orally daily), pimozide (1–10 mg orally daily), and risperidone (1–6 mg daily orally) are alternatives; haloperidol, aripiprazole, and pimozide are FDA-approved for Tourette syndrome. Typical antipsychotics can cause significant weight gain and carry a risk of tardive dyskinesias and other long-term, potentially irreversible motor side effects. Therefore, many specialists favor the use of a VMAT2 inhibitor (see dosing in the discussion of Huntington disease); tetrabenazine is approved for Tourette syndrome in Canada but not the United States. Small, randomized trials or observational studies have reported benefit from topiramate, nicotine, tetrahydrocannabinol, baclofen, and clonazepam.

Injection of botulinum toxin at the site of the most distressing tics is sometimes worthwhile and has fewer side effects than systemic antipsychotic therapy. Bilateral high-frequency deep brain stimulation at various sites has been helpful in some, otherwise intractable, cases.

Lenka A et al. An update on the pharmacological management of Tourette syndrome and emerging treatment paradigms. Expert Rev Neurother. 2024;24:1025. [PMID: 39034647]

When to Refer

- Patients with essential tremor, Parkinson disease, and restless legs syndrome unresponsive to first-line therapy.
- All patients with Huntington disease, Wilson disease, Gilles de la Tourette syndrome, and dystonia.

When to Admit

Patients undergoing surgical treatment should be admitted.

DEMENTIA

ESSENTIALS OF DIAGNOSIS

- Progressive intellectual decline.
- Not due to delirium or psychiatric disease.
- Age is the main risk factor, followed by family history and vascular disease risk factors.

General Considerations

Dementia is a progressive decline in intellectual function that is severe enough to compromise social or occupational functioning. **Mild cognitive impairment** describes a decline that has not resulted in a change in the level of function. Although a few patients identify a precipitating event, most experience an insidious onset and gradual progression of symptoms.

Dementia typically begins after age 60, and the prevalence doubles approximately every 5 years thereafter; in persons aged 85 and older, around half have dementia (see Chapter 4). In older patients with gradually progressive cognitive symptoms and no other complaint or sign, a neurodegenerative disease is likely (Table 27–7). These conditions are defined by their underlying neuropathology, and their clinical presentation reflects the locations in the brain where the pathology typically accumulates.

Dementia is distinct from delirium and psychiatric disease. **Delirium** is an acute confusional state that often occurs in response to an identifiable trigger, such as drug or alcohol intoxication or withdrawal (eg, Wernicke encephalopathy, described below), medication side effects (especially medications with anticholinergic properties, antihistamines, benzodiazepines, sleeping aids, opioids, neuroleptics, corticosteroids, and other sedative or psychotropic agents), infection (consider occult UTI or pneumonia in older patients), metabolic disturbance (including an electrolyte abnormality; hypo- or hyperglycemia; or a nutritional, endocrine, renal, or hepatic disorder), sleep deprivation, or other neurologic disease (seizure, including a postictal state, or stroke). Delirium typically involves *fluctuating* levels of arousal, including drowsiness or agitation, and it improves after removal or treatment of the precipitating factor. Patients with dementia are especially susceptible to episodes of delirium, but recognition of dementia is not possible until delirium lifts. For this reason, dementia is typically diagnosed in outpatients who are otherwise medically stable, rather than in acutely ill patients in the hospital.

Clinical Findings

A. Symptoms and Signs

Symptoms and signs of the common causes of dementia are detailed in Table 27–7. Clinicians should be aware that a patient's insight into a cognitive change may be vague or absent, and *collateral history is essential to a proper evaluation*. As patients age, primary care clinicians should inquire periodically about the presence of any cognitive symptoms.

Symptoms depend on the area of the brain affected. **Short-term memory loss**, involving the repeating of questions or stories and a diminished ability to recall the details of recent conversations or events, frequently results from pathologic changes in the hippocampus and is most commonly a sign of Alzheimer disease. **Word-finding difficulty** often involves difficulty recalling the names of people, places, or objects, with low-frequency words affected first, eventually resulting in speech laden with pronouns and circumlocutions. This problem is thought to arise from pathology at the temporoparietal junction of the left hemisphere. When aphasia is an early or prominent symptom of dementia, the most frequent underlying disorders are Alzheimer disease and frontotemporal dementia. Problems with articulation, fluency, comprehension, or word meaning are anatomically distinct and less common. **Visuospatial dysfunction** may result in poor navigation and getting lost in familiar places, impaired recognition of previously familiar faces and buildings, or trouble discerning an object against a background. The occipital and right parietal lobes are two of the brain areas implicated in such symptoms and are commonly affected by Alzheimer disease and dementia with Lewy bodies. **Executive dysfunction** may manifest by easy distractibility, impulsivity, mental inflexibility, concrete thought, slowed processing speed, poor planning and organization, or impaired judgment. Localization may vary and could include the frontal lobes or subcortical areas like the basal ganglia or cerebral white matter, which accounts for

Table 27–7. Common causes of age-related dementia (listed by prevalence).

Disorder	Pathology	Clinical Features
Alzheimer disease	Plaques containing β-amyloid peptide, and neurofibrillary tangles containing tau protein, occur throughout the neocortex.	• Most common age-related neurodegenerative disease; incidence doubles every 5 years after age 60. • Short-term memory impairment is early and prominent in most cases. • Variable deficits of executive function, visuospatial function, and language.
Vascular dementia	Multifocal ischemic change.	• Stepwise or progressive accumulation of cognitive deficits in association with repeated strokes. • Symptoms depend on localization of strokes.
Dementia with Lewy bodies	Histologically indistinguishable from Parkinson disease: α-synuclein-containing Lewy bodies occur in the brainstem, midbrain, olfactory bulb, and neocortex. Alzheimer pathology may coexist.	• Cognitive dysfunction, with prominent visuospatial and executive deficits. • Psychiatric disturbance, with anxiety, visual hallucinations, and fluctuating delirium. • Parkinsonian motor deficits with or after other features. • Cholinesterase inhibitors lessen delirium; poor tolerance of neuroleptics and dopaminergics.
Frontotemporal dementia (FTD)	Neuropathology is variable and defined by the protein found in intraneuronal aggregates. Tau protein, TAR DNA-binding protein 43 (TDP-43), or fused-in-sarcoma (FUS) protein account for most cases.	• Peak incidence in the sixth decade; approximately equal to Alzheimer disease as a cause of dementia in patients under 60 years old. • Familial cases result from mutations in genes for tau, progranulin, or others. **Behavioral variant FTD** • Deficits in empathy, social comportment, insight, abstract thought, and executive function. • Behavior is disinhibited, impulsive, and ritualistic, with prominent apathy and increased interest in sex or sweet/fatty foods. • Relative preservation of memory. • Focal right frontal atrophy. • Association with amyotrophic lateral sclerosis. **Semantic variant primary progressive aphasia** • Deficits in word-finding, single-word comprehension, object and category knowledge, and face recognition. • Behaviors may be similar to behavioral variant FTD. • Focal, asymmetric temporal pole atrophy. **Nonfluent/agrammatic variant primary progressive aphasia** • Speech is effortful with dysarthria, phonemic errors, sound distortions, and poor grammar. • Focal extrapyramidal signs and apraxia of the right arm and leg are common; overlaps with corticobasal degeneration. • Focal left frontal atrophy.

the prevalence of executive dysfunction in vascular dementia. **Apathy** or indifference, separate from depression, is common and may have a similar anatomy as executive dysfunction. **Apraxia**, or the loss of learned motor behaviors, may result from dysfunction of the frontal or parietal lobes, especially the left parietal lobe.

The time of symptom onset must be established, but subtle, early symptoms are often apparent only in retrospect. Another event, such as an illness or hospitalization, may lead to new recognition of existing symptoms. Symptoms often accumulate over time, and *the nature of the earliest symptom is most helpful in forming the differential diagnosis*. The history should establish risk factors for dementia, including family history, other chronic illnesses, and vascular disease risk factors. Finally, it is important to document the patient's current capacity to perform **basic and instrumental activities of daily living** (see Chapter 4) and to note the extent of decline from the premorbid level of function. Indeed, *this functional assessment defines the presence and severity of dementia*.

The physical examination is important to identify any occult medical illness. In addition, eye movement abnormalities, parkinsonism, or other motor abnormalities may help identify an underlying neurologic condition. The workup should prioritize the exclusion of conditions that are reversible or require separate therapy. Screening for depression is necessary, along with imaging and laboratory workup, as indicated below.

B. Neuropsychologic Assessment

Brief quantification of cognitive impairment is indicated in a patient reporting cognitive symptoms or if caregivers raise similar concerns. The **Folstein Mini Mental State Exam (MMSE)**, **Montreal Cognitive Assessment (MoCA)**, **Mini-Cog**, and other similar tests are brief, objective, and widely translated and used, but have important limitations: they are insensitive to mild cognitive impairment, they may be biased negatively by the presence of language or attention problems, and they do not correlate with functional capacity (see Chapter 4 for further details).

Psychiatric disease sometimes leads to complaints of impaired cognition (**pseudodementia**). Impaired attention is usually to blame, and in some patients with depression or anxiety, poor focus and concentration may even be a primary complaint. Screening for depression and anxiety in patients presenting with cognitive complaints is imperative.

A **neuropsychiatric evaluation** by a trained neuropsychologist or psychometrician may be appropriate. The goal of such testing is to enhance localization by defining the cognitive domains that are impaired as well as to quantify the degree of impairment. There is no standard battery of tests, but a variety of metrics is commonly used to assess the symptom types highlighted above. Assessments are most accurate when a patient is well rested, comfortable, and otherwise medically stable.

C. Imaging

Brain imaging with MRI or CT without contrast is indicated in any patient with a new, progressive cognitive complaint. The goal is to exclude occult cerebrovascular disease, tumor, or other identifiable structural abnormality, rather than to provide positive evidence of a neurodegenerative disease. Global or focal brain atrophy may be worse than expected for age and could suggest a particular neurodegenerative process, but such findings are rarely specific.

PET with fluorodeoxyglucose (FDG) does not confirm or exclude any specific cause of dementia but may be useful as an element of the workup in specific clinical circumstances, such as discriminating between Alzheimer disease and frontotemporal dementia in a patient with some symptoms of each. PET imaging with a radiolabeled ligand for β-amyloid, one of the pathologic proteins in Alzheimer disease, is highly sensitive to amyloid pathology and may provide positive evidence for Alzheimer disease in a patient with cognitive decline. However, after age 60 or 70, amyloid plaques can accumulate in the absence of cognitive impairment; thus, the specificity of a positive amyloid scan diminishes with age. PET imaging with radiolabeled ligands for tau, a pathogenic protein in Alzheimer disease, progressive supranuclear palsy, and some forms of frontotemporal dementia, also helps refine the diagnosis. Single-photon emission CT offers similar information as FDG-PET but is less sensitive.

D. Laboratory Findings

Serum levels of vitamin B_{12}, free T_4, and TSH should be measured for any patient with cognitive symptoms. A serum rapid plasma reagin (RPR) and testing for HIV should be considered. Other testing should be driven by clinical suspicion, and often includes a CBC, serum electrolytes, glucose, and lipid profile.

Elevated serum phosphorylated Tau217 is correlated with positive amyloid PET and supports the diagnosis of Alzheimer disease in a patient with characteristic symptoms and signs. Spinal fluid protein measurements (with decreased β-amyloid and increased tau protein) also may support the diagnosis of Alzheimer disease in the appropriate clinical context, but testing shares some of the same concerns as amyloid PET imaging. Dementia with Lewy bodies may be suggested by the presence of misfolded α synuclein in spinal fluid.

Although the presence of one or two ApoE ε-4 alleles indicates an increased risk of Alzheimer disease. ApoE genotyping is clinically available; however, it is of *limited clinical utility.* In a young patient with dementia, finding an ApoE ε-4 allele might raise the index of suspicion for Alzheimer disease, but in an older patient obtaining a genotype is unlikely to be helpful. Until a preventative therapy becomes available, testing of an asymptomatic patient as a marker of risk for Alzheimer disease is inappropriate.

Differential Diagnosis

A. Decline Before Age 60 or Atypical Course

Decline beginning before age 60, rapid progression, fluctuating course, unintended weight loss, systemic complaints, or other unexplained symptoms or signs raise suspicion for a process other than a neurodegenerative disease. In this case, the differential is broad and includes infection or inflammatory disease, neoplasm or a paraneoplastic condition, endocrine or metabolic disease, drugs or toxins, or other conditions including rare genetic disorders such as Niemann-Pick disease type C. A lumbar puncture should be considered to screen for cells or antibodies in the spinal fluid, to measure β-amyloid and tau, and to measure the opening pressure if hydrocephalus is suspected.

Normal pressure hydrocephalus is an important but difficult diagnosis to establish. Symptoms include gait apraxia (sometimes described as a "magnetic" gait, as if the feet are stuck to the floor), urinary incontinence, and dementia. CT scanning or MRI of the brain reveals ventricles that are enlarged in obvious disproportion to sulcal widening and overall brain atrophy. When drainage of a large volume (30–50 mL) of CSF by lumbar puncture results in objective improvement of gait (such as in the time to walk 20 feet), consideration often is given to the placement of a lumboperitoneal or ventriculoperitoneal shunt. Unfortunately, gait disorders, incontinence, and cognitive dysfunction often occur together nonspecifically in older patients, and distinguishing normal pressure hydrocephalus from cerebral atrophy is not straightforward. Because of the surgical risks associated with shunt placement, as well as a strong risk for future shunt malfunction requiring further surgical intervention, the procedure should be avoided except in clear-cut cases. In general, it is the gait apraxia that is most likely to improve after surgery; the cognitive impairment is least likely to respond.

B. Rapidly Progressive Dementia

When dementia develops quickly, with obvious decline over a few weeks to a few months, the syndrome may be classified as a **rapidly progressive dementia**. The differential diagnosis for typical dementias is still relevant, but additional etiologies must be considered, including prion disease; infections; toxins; neoplasms; and autoimmune and inflammatory diseases, including corticosteroid-responsive (Hashimoto) encephalopathy and antibody-mediated paraneoplastic and nonparaneoplastic encephalitis (Table 27–6). Workup should begin with brain MRI with contrast and diffusion-weighted imaging, routine laboratory studies (serum vitamin B_{12}, free T_4, and TSH levels), serum RPR, HIV antibody, Lyme serology, rheumatologic tests (ESR, CRP, and antinuclear antibody), anti-thyroglobulin and anti-thyroperoxidase antibody levels, paraneoplastic and nonparaneoplastic autoimmune antibodies (see Table 27–6), and CSF studies (cell count and differential; protein and glucose levels; protein electrophoresis for oligoclonal bands; IgG index [spinal-fluid-to-serum-γ-globulin level] ratio; and VDRL). Depending on the clinical context, it may be necessary to exclude Wilson disease (24-hour urine copper level); heavy metal intoxication (urine heavy metal panel); and infectious encephalitis due to atypical bacteria, viruses, fungi, and mycobacteria.

Creutzfeldt-Jakob disease is a relatively common cause of rapidly progressive dementia (see Chapter 36). Family history is important since mutations in *PRNP*, the gene for the prion protein, account for around 15% of cases. Diffusion-weighted MRI is the most helpful diagnostic tool, classically revealing cortical ribboning (a gyral pattern of hyperintensity) as well as restricted diffusion in the caudate and anterior putamen. An electroencephalogram often shows periodic complexes. Real-time quaking induced conversion (RT-QuIC), in which patient CSF is mixed with recombinant prion protein and aggregation of prion protein is detected, is a sensitive and specific diagnostic test. Reflecting the high rate of neuronal death, CSF levels of the intraneuronal proteins tau, 14-3-3, and neuron-specific enolase are often elevated, although this finding is neither sensitive nor specific.

Treatment

A. Anti-amyloid Therapy

Two anti-amyloid therapies are approved in the United States. Lecanemab (10 mg/kg intravenously every 2 weeks) and donanemab (700 mg intravenously every 4 weeks for 3 doses; then 1400 mg intravenously every 4 weeks) modestly slowed cognitive decline in patients with early Alzheimer disease and reduced brain amyloid burden measured by amyloid PET compared with placebo. The use of these therapies is limited to patients with mild cognitive impairment or mild dementia and amyloid pathology proven by amyloid PET or CSF analysis. Patients and prescribers must adhere to a monitoring regime including frequent brain MRI due to a high risk of complications such as cerebral edema and hemorrhage. Caution should be used in patients with a history of cerebral hemorrhage, evidence of microhemorrhages or superficial siderosis on pretreatment brain MRI, anticoagulant or antiplatelet use other than aspirin, any bleeding disorder, or an ApoE ε-4 allele. Cost effectiveness and long-term risk of these therapies remain uncertain.

B. Cholinesterase Inhibitors and Memantine

Cholinesterase inhibitors provide modest, symptomatic treatment for cognitive dysfunction and may prolong the capacity for independence in Alzheimer disease and dementia with Lewy bodies (Table 27–7) but do *not* prevent disease progression. Commonly used medications include donepezil, rivastigmine, and galantamine. Donepezil treatment starts at 5 mg orally daily for 4 weeks, then increases to 10 mg daily; a 23 mg daily dose is approved for moderate to severe Alzheimer disease, although its modest additional efficacy over the 10 mg dose is overshadowed by an increased risk of side effects. Rivastigmine treatment starts at 1.5 mg orally twice daily, then increases every 2 weeks by 1.5 mg twice daily to a goal of 3–6 mg twice daily; a once daily transdermal patch formulation (4.6, 9.5, or 13.3 mg/24 hours) is also available. Galantamine starts at 4 mg orally twice daily, then increases every 4 weeks by 4 mg twice daily to a goal of 8–12 mg twice daily; a once-daily extended-release formulation is also available. Cholinesterase inhibitors are *not* given for frontotemporal dementia because they may worsen behavioral symptoms. Nausea and diarrhea are common side effects; syncope and cardiac dysrhythmia are uncommon but more serious. An ECG is often obtained before and after starting therapy, particularly in a patient with cardiac disease or a history of syncope.

Memantine (start at 5 mg orally daily, then increase by 5 mg per week up to a target of 10 mg twice daily) is approved for the treatment of moderate to severe Alzheimer disease. It is typically used instead of, not in addition to, the cholinesterase inhibitors. In frontotemporal dementia, memantine is ineffective and may worsen cognition. There is some evidence that memantine may improve cognition and behavior among patients with dementia with Lewy bodies.

C. Other Therapies

Treatment for mood and behavioral disturbances is discussed in Chapter 4, where safety issues are also considered.

When to Refer

- All patients with new, unexplained cognitive decline should be referred, especially those with rapid progression.
- Patients with mild cognitive impairment or early dementia who may be candidates for anti-amyloid therapies.

When to Admit

Admission to the hospital should only occur when essential in patients with dementia due to increased risk of developing hospital-acquired delirium.

Atri A et al. Alzheimer's Association clinical practice guideline for the diagnostic evaluation, testing, counseling, and disclosure of suspected Alzheimer's disease and related disorders (DETeCD-ADRD): executive summary of recommendations for primary care. Alzheimers Dement. 2025;21:e14333. [PMID: 39713942]

Heneka MT et al. Passive anti-amyloid β immunotherapy in Alzheimer's disease: opportunities and challenges. Lancet. 2024;404:2198. [PMID: 39549715]

WERNICKE ENCEPHALOPATHY & KORSAKOFF SYNDROME

Wernicke encephalopathy is characterized by confusion, ataxia, and nystagmus leading to ophthalmoplegia (lateral rectus muscle weakness, conjugate gaze palsies); peripheral neuropathy may also be present. It is *due to thiamine deficiency* and in the United States occurs most commonly in patients with alcohol use disorder. It may also occur in patients with AIDS or hyperemesis gravidarum, and after bariatric surgery. In suspected cases, thiamine (100 mg) is given intravenously immediately and on a daily basis until a satisfactory diet can be ensured after which the same dose is given orally. Some guidelines recommend initial doses of 200–500 mg intravenously three times daily for the first 5–7 days of treatment. Intravenous glucose given *before* thiamine may precipitate the syndrome or worsen the symptoms. The diagnosis is confirmed by the response in 1 or 2 days to treatment, which must not be delayed while awaiting laboratory confirmation of thiamine deficiency. Thiamine diphosphate concentration from a whole blood sample should obtained prior to thiamine administration. **Korsakoff syndrome** occurs in more severe cases; it includes anterograde and retrograde amnesia and sometimes confabulation and may not be recognized until after the initial delirium has lifted.

Eva L et al. Neuropsychiatric and neuropsychological aspects of alcohol-related cognitive disorders: an in-depth review of Wernicke's encephalopathy and Korsakoff's syndrome. J Clin Med. 2023;12:6101. [PMID: 37763040]

STUPOR & COMA

ESSENTIALS OF DIAGNOSIS

- Level of consciousness is depressed.
- Stuporous patients respond only to repeated vigorous stimuli.
- Comatose patients are unarousable and unresponsive.

General Considerations

The patient who is **stuporous** is unresponsive except when subjected to repeated vigorous stimuli, while the **comatose** patient is unarousable and unable to respond to external events or inner needs, although reflex movements and posturing may be present.

Coma is a major complication of serious CNS disorders. It can result from seizures, hypothermia, metabolic disturbances, meningoencephalitis, or structural lesions causing bilateral cerebral hemispheric dysfunction or a disturbance of the brainstem reticular activating system. A mass lesion involving one cerebral hemisphere may cause coma by compression of the brainstem.

Assessment & Emergency Measures

The diagnostic workup of the comatose patient must proceed concomitantly with management. Supportive therapy for respiration or blood pressure is initiated; in hypothermia, all such patients should be rewarmed before the prognosis is assessed.

The patient can be positioned on one side with the neck partly extended, dentures removed, and secretions cleared by suction; if necessary, the patency of the airways is maintained with an oropharyngeal airway. Blood is drawn for serum glucose, electrolyte, and calcium levels; ABGs; liver biochemical and kidney function tests; and toxicologic studies as indicated. Thiamine (100 mg), followed by dextrose 50% (25 g), and naloxone (0.4–1.2 mg) are given intravenously without delay.

Further details are then obtained from attendants of the patient's medical history, the circumstances surrounding the onset of coma, and the time course of subsequent events. Abrupt onset of coma suggests subarachnoid hemorrhage, brainstem stroke, or intracerebral hemorrhage, whereas a slower onset and progression occur with other structural or mass lesions. Urgent noncontrast CT scanning of the head should be performed to identify intracranial hemorrhage, brain herniation, or other structural lesions that may require immediate neurosurgical intervention, and CT angiogram is important to rule out basilar artery occlusion. A metabolic cause is likely with a preceding intoxicated state or agitated delirium. On examination, attention is paid to the behavioral response to painful stimuli, the pupils and their response to light, the response to touching the cornea with a wisp of sterile gauze, position of the eyes and their movement in response to passive movement of the head and ice-water caloric stimulation, and the respiratory pattern.

A. Response to Painful Stimuli

Purposeful limb withdrawal from painful stimuli implies that sensory pathways from and motor pathways to the stimulated limb are functionally intact. Unilateral absence of responses despite application of stimuli to both sides of the body in turn implies a corticospinal lesion; bilateral absence of responsiveness suggests brainstem involvement, bilateral pyramidal tract lesions, or psychogenic unresponsiveness. **Decorticate** (flexor) posturing may occur with lesions of the internal capsule and rostral cerebral peduncle and **decerebrate** (extensor) posturing with dysfunction or destruction of the midbrain and rostral pons. Decerebrate posturing occurs in the arms accompanied by flaccidity or slight flexor responses in the legs in patients with extensive brainstem damage extending down to the pons at the trigeminal level.

B. Ocular Findings

1. Pupils—Hypothalamic disease processes may lead to unilateral Horner syndrome, while bilateral diencephalic involvement or destructive pontine lesions may lead to small but reactive pupils. Ipsilateral pupillary dilation with no direct or consensual response to light occurs with compression of the third cranial nerve, eg, with uncal herniation. The pupils are slightly smaller than normal but responsive to light in many metabolic encephalopathies; however, they may be fixed and dilated following overdosage with atropine or scopolamine, and pinpoint (but responsive) with opioids.

2. Corneal reflex—Touching the cornea with a wisp of sterile gauze or cotton should elicit a blink reflex. The afferent limb of the arc is mediated by the fifth cranial nerve; the efferent limb by the seventh nerve. A unilateral absent corneal reflex implies damage to the ipsilateral pons or a trigeminal deficit. Bilateral loss can be seen with large pontine lesions or in deep pharmacologic coma.

3. Eye movements—Conjugate deviation of the eyes to the side suggests the presence of an ipsilateral hemispheric lesion, a contralateral pontine lesion, or ongoing seizures from the contralateral hemisphere. A mesencephalic lesion leads to downward conjugate deviation. Dysconjugate ocular deviation in coma implies a structural brainstem lesion unless there was preexisting strabismus.

The oculomotor responses to passive head turning and to caloric stimulation relate to each other and provide complementary information. In response to brisk rotation of the head from side to side and to flexion and extension of the head, normally conscious patients with open eyes do not exhibit contraversive conjugate eye deviation (**oculocephalic reflex**) unless there is voluntary visual fixation or bilateral frontal pathology. With cortical depression in lightly comatose patients, a brisk oculocephalic reflex is seen. With brainstem lesions, this oculocephalic reflex becomes impaired or lost, depending on the site of the lesion.

The **oculovestibular reflex** is tested by caloric stimulation using irrigation with ice water. In normal patients, jerk nystagmus is elicited for about 2 or 3 minutes, with the slow component toward the irrigated ear. In unconscious patients with an intact brainstem, the fast component of the nystagmus disappears, so that the eyes tonically deviate toward the irrigated side for 2–3 minutes before returning to their original position. With impairment of brainstem function, the response becomes abnormal and finally disappears. In metabolic coma, oculocephalic and oculovestibular reflex responses are preserved, at least initially.

C. Respiratory Patterns

Diseases causing coma may lead to respiratory abnormalities. **Cheyne-Stokes respiration** (in which episodes of deep breathing alternate with periods of apnea) may occur with bihemispheric or diencephalic disease or in metabolic disorders. **Central neurogenic hyperventilation** occurs with lesions of the brainstem tegmentum; **apneustic breathing** (in which there are prominent end-inspiratory pauses) suggests damage at the pontine level (eg, due to basilar artery occlusion); and **ataxic breathing** (a completely irregular pattern of breathing with deep and shallow breaths occurring randomly) is associated with lesions of the lower pontine tegmentum and medulla.

1. Stupor & Coma Due to Structural Lesions

Supratentorial mass lesions tend to affect brain function in a systematic way. There may initially be signs of hemispheric dysfunction, such as hemiparesis. As coma develops and deepens, cerebral function becomes progressively disturbed, producing a predictable progression of neurologic signs that suggest rostrocaudal deterioration.

Thus, as a supratentorial mass lesion begins to impair the diencephalon, the patient becomes drowsy, then stuporous, and finally comatose. There may be Cheyne-Stokes respiration; small but reactive pupils or an ipsilateral third nerve palsy due to uncal herniation; normal oculocephalic responses with side-to-side head movements but sometimes an impairment of reflex upward gaze with brisk flexion of the head; tonic ipsilateral deviation of the eyes in response to vestibular stimulation with cold water; and initially a positive response to pain but subsequently only decorticate posturing. With further progression, midbrain failure occurs. Motor dysfunction progresses from decorticate to bilateral decerebrate posturing in response to painful stimuli; Cheyne-Stokes respiration is gradually replaced by sustained central hyperventilation; the pupils become middle-sized and fixed; and the oculocephalic and oculovestibular reflex responses become impaired, abnormal, or lost. As the pons and then the medulla fail, the pupils remain unresponsive; oculovestibular responses are unobtainable; respiration is rapid and shallow; and painful stimuli may lead only to flexor responses in the legs. Finally, respiration becomes irregular and stops, the pupils often then dilating widely.

In contrast, a **subtentorial (ie, brainstem) lesion** may lead to an early, sometimes abrupt disturbance of consciousness without any orderly rostrocaudal progression of neurologic signs. Compressive lesions of the brainstem, especially cerebellar hemorrhage, may be clinically indistinguishable from intraparenchymal processes.

2. Stupor & Coma Due to Metabolic Disturbances

Patients with a metabolic cause of coma generally have signs of patchy, diffuse, and symmetric neurologic involvement that cannot be explained by loss of function at any single level or in a sequential manner, although focal or lateralized deficits may occur in hypoglycemia. Pupillary reactivity is usually preserved. Comatose patients with meningitis, encephalitis, or subarachnoid hemorrhage may also exhibit little in the way of focal neurologic signs, however, and clinical evidence of meningeal irritation is sometimes subtle in comatose patients. Examination of the CSF in such patients is essential to establish the correct diagnosis, once a CT scan has ruled out a structural lesion posing risk of cerebral herniation.

In patients with coma due to cerebral ischemia and hypoxia, the absence of pupillary light reflexes 24 hours after return of spontaneous circulation indicates that there is little chance of regaining independence; absent corneal reflexes or absent or extensor motor responses at 72 hours also indicate a grim prognosis. Physical findings are less reliable predictors of outcome among those treated with therapeutic hypothermia, although absent corneal or pupillary light reflexes at 72 hours after rewarming likely indicate a poor prognosis, as do bilaterally absent cortical somatosensory evoked potentials in response to median nerve stimulation after the patient has returned to normothermia.

Treatment of metabolic encephalopathy is of the underlying disturbance and is considered in other chapters. If the cause of the encephalopathy is obscure, all medications except essential ones may have to be withdrawn in case they are responsible for the altered mental status.

3. Brain Death (Death by Neurologic Criteria)

Brain death occurs when there is complete and irreversible cessation of all brain function; although the organs can be maintained with mechanical ventilation for the purposes of donation, in most countries *the diagnosis of brain death is equivalent to a declaration of death.* To diagnose brain death, the cause of coma must be established, be compatible with a known cause of brain death, and be irreversible. Reversible coma simulating brain death may be seen with hypothermia (temperature < 32°C) and overdosage with CNS depressant drugs. These conditions must be excluded by warming the patient and allowing enough time for all sedating medications to be metabolized (ie, at least five half-lives) or by measuring serum levels. Severe blood pressure, electrolyte, acid-base, and endocrine derangements cannot be present.

Finally, a neurologic examination must demonstrate that the patient is comatose (ie, no eye opening and no response to central or peripheral pain); has lost all brainstem reflex responses, including the pupillary, corneal, oculovestibular, oculocephalic, oropharyngeal, and cough reflexes; and has no respiratory drive. The response to pain should be absent or only consist of spinal reflex movements; decerebrate or decorticate posturing is not consistent with brain death. Absence of respiratory drive is demonstrated with an **apnea test** (absence of spontaneous respiratory activity at a pH < 7.30, a $PaCO_2$ of at least 60 mm Hg and a rise of at least 20 mm Hg from baseline).

Certain ancillary tests may assist the determination of brain death if the pupillary light reflex cannot be assessed or an apnea test cannot be performed. These include demonstration of an absent cerebral circulation by intravenous radioisotope cerebral angiography or by four-vessel contrast cerebral angiography. An electroencephalogram, even when combined with brainstem auditory and somatosensory evoked potentials, does not fully evaluate brainstem function and should *not* be used to make a formal determination of brain death.

4. Persistent Vegetative State

Patients with severe bilateral hemispheric disease may show some improvement from an initially comatose state, so that, after a variable interval, they appear to be awake but lie motionless and without evidence of awareness or higher mental activity. This is called a **"persistent" vegetative state** once it has lasted over 4 weeks and has also been variously referred to as akinetic mutism, apallic state, or coma vigil. Patients in a vegetative state from a medical cause (eg, anoxic brain injury) for more than 3 months and from a traumatic brain injury for more than 12 months are said to be in a **"chronic" vegetative state**, from which a few patients may regain consciousness but remain severely disabled.

5. Minimally Conscious State

In this state, patients exhibit inconsistent evidence of consciousness. There is some degree of functional recovery of behaviors suggesting self- or environmental-awareness, such as basic verbalization or context-appropriate gestures, emotional responses (eg, smiling) to emotional but not neutral stimuli, or purposive responses to environmental stimuli (eg, a finger movement or eye blink apparently to command). Further improvement is manifest by the restoration of communication with the patient. The minimally conscious state may be temporary or permanent. Little information is available about its natural history or long-term outlook, which reflects the underlying cause. The likelihood of useful functional recovery diminishes with time; after 12 months, patients are likely to remain severely disabled and without a reliable means of communication. Prognostication is difficult. Amantadine (100–200 mg orally daily) may hasten recovery when given to patients in a vegetative or minimally conscious state 4–16 weeks after traumatic brain injury.

6. Locked-In Syndrome (De-efferented State)

Acute destructive lesions (eg, infarction, hemorrhage, demyelination, encephalitis) involving the ventral pons and sparing the tegmentum may lead to a mute, quadriparetic but conscious state in which the patient is capable of blinking and voluntary eye movement in the vertical plane, with preserved pupillary responses to light. Such a patient can mistakenly be regarded as comatose. Clinicians should recognize that "locked-in" individuals are fully aware of their surroundings. The prognosis is usually poor, but recovery has occasionally been reported in some cases, including resumption of independent daily life. A similar condition may occur with severe Guillain-Barré syndrome and has a better prognosis.

Greer DM et al. Pediatric and adult brain death/death by neurologic criteria consensus guideline: report of the AAN guidelines subcommittee, AAP, CNS, and SCCM. Neurology. 2023;101:1112. [PMID: 37821233]

HEAD INJURY

Trauma is the most common cause of death in young people, and head injury accounts for almost half of these trauma-related deaths. Head injury severity ranges from **concussion** to **severe traumatic brain injury (TBI)**. Concussion is broadly defined as an alteration in mental status caused by trauma with or without loss of consciousness. The term concussion is often used synonymously with mild TBI. Grades of TBI are traditionally defined by the Glasgow Coma Scale (GCS) measured 30 minutes after injury (Table 27–8).

Head trauma may cause cerebral injury through a variety of mechanisms (Table 27–9). Central to management is determination of which patients need head imaging and observation. Of particular concern is identification of patients with epidural and subdural hematoma, who may present with normal neurologic findings shortly after injury (**lucid interval**) but rapidly deteriorate thereafter, and in whom surgical intervention is lifesaving.

Table 27–8. Glasgow Coma Scale.[1]

Points	Eye Opening	Verbal Response	Motor Response
1	None	None	None
2	To pain	Vocal but not verbal	Extension
3	To voice	Verbal but not conversational	Flexion
4	Spontaneous	Conversational but disoriented	Withdraws from pain
5	—	Oriented	Localizes pain
6	—	—	Obeys commands

[1]GCS score indicating severity of traumatic brain injury: **mild**, 13–15; **moderate**, 9–12; **severe**, ≤ 8.
Reproduced, with permission, from Aminoff MJ et al. *Clinical Neurology*, 9th ed, McGraw-Hill Education, 2015; data from Teasdale G, Jennett B. Assessment of coma and impaired consciousness. A practical scale. *Lancet*. 1974;304:81–84.

Clinical Findings

A. Symptoms and Signs

Common symptoms of concussion that develop acutely include headache, nausea, vomiting, confusion, disorientation, dizziness, and imbalance. A period of amnesia encompassing the traumatic event and a variable period of time leading up to the trauma is typical. Loss of consciousness may occur. Additional symptoms of photophobia, phonophobia, difficulty concentrating, irritability, and sleep and mood disturbances may develop over the following hours to days. Examination is usually normal, although orientation and attention, short-term memory, and reaction time may be impaired. Persistent or progressive decline in the level of consciousness after the initial injury, or focal neurologic findings, suggests the need for urgent imaging and neurosurgical consultation.

Patients should also be examined for signs of scalp lacerations, facial and skull fracture, and neck injury. The clinical signs of basilar skull fracture include bruising about the orbit (**raccoon sign**), blood in the external auditory meatus (**Battle sign**), and leakage of CSF (which can be identified by its glucose or β-2-transferrin content) from the ear or nose. Cranial nerve palsies (involving especially the first, second, third, fourth, fifth, seventh, and eighth nerves in any combination) may also occur. The head and neck should be immobilized until imaging can be performed.

B. Imaging and Other Investigations

Recommendations are that head CT be performed in patients with concussion and any of the following: GCS score < 15, focal neurologic deficit, seizure, coagulopathy, aged 60 or older, skull fracture, persistent headache or vomiting, retrograde amnesia exceeding 30 minutes, intoxication, soft tissue injury of the head or neck, or a dangerous mechanism of injury such as pedestrian struck by

Table 27–9. Acute cerebral sequelae of head injury (listed in alphabetical order).

Sequelae	Clinical Features	Pathology
Cerebral contusion or laceration	Loss of consciousness longer than with concussion. Focal neurologic deficits are often present. May lead to death or severe residual neurologic deficit.	Bruising on side of impact (coup injury) or contralaterally (contrecoup injury). Vasogenic edema, multiple petechial hemorrhages, and mass effect. May have subarachnoid bleeding. Herniation may occur in severe cases. Cerebral laceration specifically involves tearing of the cerebral tissue and pia-arachnoid overlying a contusion.
Cerebral hemorrhage	Generally develops immediately after injury. Clinically resembles hypertensive hemorrhage. Surgery to relieve mass effect is sometimes necessary.	Hematoma, visible on CT scan.
Concussion	A transient, trauma-induced alteration in mental status that may or may not involve loss of consciousness. Symptoms and signs include headache, nausea, disorientation, irritability, amnesia, clumsiness, visual disturbances, and focal neurologic deficit.	Unknown; likely mild diffuse axonal injury and excitotoxic neuronal injury. Cerebral contusion may occur.
Diffuse axonal injury	Persistent loss of consciousness, coma, or persistent vegetative state resulting from severe rotational shearing forces or deceleration.	Imaging may be normal or may show tiny, scattered white matter hemorrhages. Histology reveals torn axons.
Epidural hemorrhage	Headache, confusion, somnolence, seizures, and focal deficits occur several hours after injury (lucid interval) and lead to coma, respiratory depression, and death unless treated by surgical evacuation.	Tear in meningeal artery, vein, or dural sinus, leading to hematoma visible on CT scan.
Subdural hemorrhage	Similar to epidural hemorrhage, but interval before onset of symptoms is longer. Neurosurgical consultation for consideration of evacuation.	Hematoma from tear in veins from cortex to superior sagittal sinus or from cerebral laceration, visible on CT scan.

motor vehicle. Otherwise, patients can be sent home as long as a responsible caregiver can check the patient at *hourly intervals* for the next 24 hours. Patients requiring imaging should be admitted unless the head CT is normal, the GCS score is 15, there have been no seizures, there is no predisposition to bleeding, and they can be monitored by a caregiver at home.

Because injury to the spine may have accompanied head trauma, cervical spine radiographs (three views) or CT should always be obtained in comatose patients and in patients with severe neck pain or a deficit possibly related to cord compression.

Treatment

Head injury can often be prevented by helmets, seatbelts, and other protective equipment.

After intracranial bleeding has been excluded clinically or by head CT, treatment of mild TBI is aimed at promoting resolution of postconcussive symptoms and preventing recurrent injury, which increases the risk of chronic neurobehavioral impairment and delays recovery. Rarely, a recurrent concussion while a patient is still symptomatic from a first concussion may lead to fatal cerebral edema (**second impact syndrome**). These observations form the basis of the recommendation that patients at risk for recurrent concussion (eg, athletes) be held out of the risky activity until their concussive symptoms have fully resolved.

In patients hospitalized with moderate or severe TBI, management often requires a multidisciplinary approach due to multiple concomitant injuries. Elevated intracranial pressure can result from diffuse axonal injury or a hematoma requiring surgical evacuation, or from a variety of medical causes. Decompressive craniectomy may reduce otherwise refractory intracranial hypertension but does not improve neurologic outcome. Hypothermia is associated with worsened functional outcomes.

Because bridging veins between the brain and venous sinuses become more vulnerable to shear injury as the brain atrophies, a **subdural hematoma** may develop days or weeks following head injury in older patients or even occur spontaneously. Clinical presentation can be subtle, often with mental changes such as slowness, drowsiness, headache, confusion, or memory disturbance. Focal neurologic deficits such as hemiparesis or hemisensory disturbance are less common. Surgical intervention is indicated if the hematoma is 10 mm or more in thickness or there is a midline shift of 5 mm or more; if there is a decline in GCS score of 2 or more from injury to hospital admission; or if one or both pupils are fixed and dilated.

Scalp lacerations and depressed skull fractures should be treated surgically as appropriate. Simple skull fractures require no specific treatment. If there is any leakage of CSF, conservative treatment, with elevation of the head, restriction of fluids, and administration of acetazolamide (250 mg orally four times daily), is often helpful; if the leak continues for more than a few days, lumbar subarachnoid drainage may be necessary. Antibiotics are given if infection occurs, based on culture and sensitivity studies; vaccination against pneumococcus is recommended (see Table 34–7). Only occasional patients require intracranial repair of the dural defect because of persistence of the leak or recurrent meningitis.

Prognosis

Moderate and severe TBI may result in permanent cognitive and motor impairment depending on the severity and location of the initial injury. Initial GCS and head CT findings have prognostic value. Among patients with a GCS score of 8 or less at presentation, mortality approaches 30% and only one-third of survivors regain functional independence. Cognitive impairment tends to affect frontal and temporal lobe function, causing deficits in attention, memory, judgment, and executive function. Behavioral dysregulation, depression, and disinhibition can impair social functioning. Anosmia, presumably due to shearing of fibers from the nasal epithelium, is common.

Epilepsy can develop after TBI, especially with more severe injury. Among patients with severe TBI (typically loss of consciousness for at least 12–24 hours, intracranial hematoma, depressed skull fracture, or cerebral contusion), phenytoin or levetiracetam is typically given for 7 days to reduce the incidence of early posttraumatic seizures; this is done exclusively to minimize acute complications resulting from such seizures and does not prevent the development of posttraumatic epilepsy.

Among patients with mild TBI, symptoms of concussion resolve in most patients by 1 month and in the vast majority by 3 months. **Prolonged postconcussive symptoms** are uncommon, persisting at 1 year in 10–15% of patients. Risk factors for prolonged postconcussive symptoms include active litigation regarding the injury; repeated concussions; and GCS score of 13 or less at presentation. Headaches often have migrainous features and may respond to tricyclic antidepressants or β-blockers (see Table 27–1). Opioids should be avoided to minimize the risk of medication overuse headache. Mood symptoms may respond to antidepressants, anxiolytics, and cognitive behavioral therapy.

There appears to be an association between head trauma and the later development of neurodegenerative disease, such as Alzheimer disease, Parkinson disease, or amyotrophic lateral sclerosis (ALS). Normal pressure hydrocephalus may also occur. Repetitive, mild head injury, such as that which occurs in athletes or military personnel, can lead to **chronic traumatic encephalopathy**, a distinct pathologic entity associated with mood and cognitive changes and characterized by the abnormal aggregation of tau or other proteins either focally or globally in the cerebral cortex. Whether chronic traumatic encephalopathy is a static response to recurrent head injury or a progressive neurodegenerative disease is not known, but the severity of neuropathology appears to correlate to lifetime exposure to repetitive head injury.

When to Refer

- Patients with focal neurologic deficits, altered consciousness, or skull fracture.
- Patients with late complications of head injury, eg, posttraumatic seizure disorder or normal pressure hydrocephalus.

When to Admit

- Patients with concussion and GCS score < 15, predisposition to bleeding, seizure, or no responsible caregiver at home.
- Patients with abnormal head CT.

American College of Surgeons. Best practice guidelines: the management of traumatic brain injury. American College of Surgeons; 2024. https://www.facs.org/media/vgfgjpfk/best-practices-guidelines-traumatic-brain-injury.pdf.

Valente JH et al. Clinical policy: critical issues in the management of adult patients presenting to the emergency department with mild traumatic brain injury. Ann Emerg Med. 2023;81:e63. [PMID: 37085214]

MULTIPLE SCLEROSIS

ESSENTIALS OF DIAGNOSIS

- Episodic neurologic symptoms.
- Patient usually < 55 years of age at onset.
- Single pathologic lesion cannot explain clinical findings.
- Multiple foci best visualized by MRI.

General Considerations

This common neurologic disorder, which probably has an autoimmune basis, has its greatest incidence in young adults. Epidemiologic studies indicate that multiple sclerosis is much more common in persons who live in temperate zones. Environmental factors hypothesized to increase risk for multiple sclerosis include reduced sunlight exposure, low vitamin D level, and infection with Epstein-Barr virus. A genetic susceptibility to the disease is present. Pathologically, focal—often perivenular—areas of demyelination with reactive gliosis (fibrous proliferation of glial cells in injured areas of the CNS) are found scattered in the white matter of the brain and spinal cord and in the optic nerves. Axonal damage also occurs.

Clinical Findings

A. Symptoms and Signs

The common initial presentation is weakness, numbness, tingling, or unsteadiness in a limb; spastic paraparesis; retrobulbar optic neuritis; diplopia; dysequilibrium; or a sphincter disturbance such as urinary urgency or hesitancy. Symptoms may disappear after a few days or weeks, although examination often reveals a residual deficit.

Several forms of the disease are recognized. Least commonly, symptoms are steadily progressive from their onset, and disability develops at a relatively early stage (**primary progressive disease**). In most patients, there is an interval of months or years after the initial episode before new symptoms develop or the original ones recur (**relapsing-remitting disease**). Eventually, relapses and usually incomplete remissions lead to increasing disability, with weakness, spasticity, and ataxia of the limbs, impaired vision, and urinary incontinence. The findings on examination at this stage commonly include optic atrophy; nystagmus; dysarthria; and pyramidal, sensory, or cerebellar deficits in some or all of the limbs. In some of these patients, the clinical course changes so that a steady deterioration occurs, unrelated to acute relapses (**secondary progressive disease**). The diagnosis cannot be made with confidence unless the total clinical picture indicates involvement of different parts of the CNS (dissemination in space) at different times (dissemination in time), although dissemination in time is less emphasized in the most recent diagnostic criteria. Fatigue is common in all forms of the disease.

A number of factors (eg, infection) may precipitate or trigger exacerbations. Relapses are reduced in pregnancy, are more likely during the 2 or 3 months following pregnancy, but are less likely in women who exclusively breastfeed their infants.

B. Imaging

MRI of the brain and cervical cord has a major role in excluding other causes of neurologic dysfunction and in demonstrating the presence of multiple lesions. In T1-weighted images, hypointense "black holes" probably represent areas of permanent axonal damage. Gadolinium-enhanced T1-weighted images may highlight areas of active inflammation with breakdown of the blood-brain barrier, which helps identify newer lesions. T2-weighted images provide information about disease burden or total number of lesions, which typically appear as areas of high signal intensity. Certain MRI findings (seen best on 3T scanners) are specific for multiple sclerosis; these include the central vein sign (CVS) and paramagnetic rim lesions (PRLs). The CVS is considered positive if there is a vein running through the middle of at least six T2 hyperintense white matter lesions, or in the majority of fewer than ten total lesions. PRLs are T2 hyperintense white matter lesions with a rim of hypointensity that are identified using iron sensitive sequences. CT scans are less helpful than MRI.

In patients with myelopathy alone and no clinical or laboratory evidence of more widespread disease, MRI or myelography is necessary to exclude a congenital or acquired surgically treatable lesion. In patients with mixed pyramidal and cerebellar deficits in the limbs, the foramen magnum region must be visualized to exclude the possibility of Arnold-Chiari malformation, in which parts of the cerebellum and lower brainstem are displaced into the cervical canal.

C. Laboratory and Other Studies

A definitive diagnosis can never be based solely on the laboratory findings. If there is clinical evidence of only a single lesion in the CNS, multiple sclerosis cannot properly be diagnosed unless it can be shown that other regions are affected subclinically. Visual, brainstem auditory, and somatosensory evoked potentials are helpful in this regard, and optical coherence tomography can detect subclinical optic nerve demyelination. Other disorders, however, also may be characterized by multifocal electrophysiologic abnormalities reflecting disease of central white matter. Certain infections (eg, HIV, Lyme disease, syphilis), connective tissue diseases (eg, SLE, Sjögren syndrome), sarcoidosis, metabolic disorders (eg, vitamin B_{12} deficiency), and lymphoma may therefore require exclusion.

There may be mild lymphocytosis or a slightly increased protein concentration in the CSF, especially soon after an acute relapse. Elevated IgG in CSF, discrete bands of IgG (oligoclonal bands), and increased intrathecal production of kappa free light chains are present in many patients. The presence of intrathecal immunoglobulin production, however, is not specific; it has been found in a variety of inflammatory neurologic disorders and occasionally in vascular or neoplastic disorders of the nervous system.

Vitamin D deficiency may be associated with an increased risk of developing multiple sclerosis; randomized trials have *not* shown vitamin D supplementation reduces attack rate or progression in relapsing-remitting disease.

D. Diagnosis

The most widely accepted diagnostic algorithm for multiple sclerosis is the 2024 revised McDonald criteria, which reflects a shift toward biomarker-based diagnosis using MRI, CSF, optical coherence tomography, and visual evoked potentials. In a patient with a typical clinical attack and an initial workup that suggests multiple sclerosis and excludes alternative etiologies, the diagnosis of multiple sclerosis depends on whether there also is dissemination in space (DIS). To fulfill the DIS criterion, MRI should demonstrate at least one lesion in at least two of five typical sites (periventricular, cortical or juxtacortical, infratentorial, spinal, or optic nerve); a lesion in the optic nerve can also be identified by abnormal visual evoked potentials or optical coherence tomography.

If the initial workup is suggestive and the DIS criteria are met, multiple sclerosis can be diagnosed if there are one or more of the following: (1) unique oligoclonal bands or an elevated kappa free light chain index in the CSF (CSF positivity); (2) if MRI demonstrates a positive CVS; (3) if there are lesions in at least four of the five typical sites; or (4) if there is dissemination in time (DIT)—defined by the simultaneous presence of gadolinium-enhancing and non-enhancing lesions at any time, a new lesion appearing on follow-up MRI, or a second clinical attack.

If there are lesions present at only one typical site, multiple sclerosis can be diagnosed if there is CSF positivity and a positive CVS; if there is CSF positivity and at least one PRL; if there is DIT and CVS positivity; or if there is DIT and at least one PRL.

Primary progressive multiple sclerosis is diagnosed with the same criteria but requires at least a year of progression, and DIS criteria can be met if there are at least two spinal lesions.

In patients with a single clinical event who do not satisfy criteria for multiple sclerosis, a diagnosis of a **clinically isolated syndrome** is made. Follow-up MRI should be considered 6–12 months later to assess for the presence of any new lesion. Patients without a typical clinical attack may be diagnosed with **radiologically isolated syndrome** if a brain MRI incidentally demonstrates findings consistent with multiple sclerosis. Multiple sclerosis can then be diagnosed if criteria for DIS are met and there is CSF positivity, a positive CVS, or DIT.

Treatment

At least partial recovery from acute exacerbations can reasonably be expected, but further relapses may occur without warning. Some disability is likely to result eventually, but about half of all patients are without significant disability even 10 years after onset of symptoms. Treatments chiefly are aimed at preventing relapses, thereby reducing disability.

Recovery from acute relapses may be hastened by treatment with corticosteroids, but the extent of recovery is unchanged. Intravenous therapy is often given first—typically methylprednisolone 1 g daily for 3 days—followed by oral prednisone at 60–80 mg daily for 1 week with a taper over the ensuing 2–3 weeks, but randomized trials show similar efficacy whether the initial high dose is given orally or intravenously. Long-term treatment with corticosteroids provides no benefit and does not prevent further relapses. Transient exacerbation of symptoms relating to intercurrent infection or heat requires no added treatment.

In patients with relapsing disease, numerous medications have well-established efficacy at *reducing the frequency of attacks* (Table 27–10). The initial agent is chosen after considering medication tolerance and risks, patient preference, and disease severity. In general, the medications most effective at reducing relapses have stronger immunomodulatory effects and more serious, albeit rare, adverse effects. In a study conducted in Denmark and Sweden, early treatment with highly effective medications (rituximab, natalizumab, or fingolimod) reduced disability progression at 24 weeks compared with more moderately effective medications (teriflunomide, glatiramer acetate, or interferon β-1a). This raises the possibility that early more intensive treatment will lead to a more favorable prognosis. Many of these agents, especially those that deplete or interfere with B-cells, render vaccination ineffective. Prescription of these agents should be managed by a specialist.

Ocrelizumab is the only medication effective in slowing disability progression in primary progressive multiple sclerosis and is approved for this indication by the FDA. For patients with active secondary progressive disease, cladribine, ocrelizumab, ofatumumab, ozanimod, ponesimod, and siponimod can be used. Plasmapheresis is sometimes helpful in patients with severe relapses unresponsive to corticosteroids.

Symptomatic therapy for spasticity, neurogenic bladder, or fatigue may be required. Fatigue is especially common in multiple sclerosis, and modafinil (200 mg orally every morning) is an effective and FDA-approved therapy for this indication. Dalfampridine (an extended-release formulation of 4-aminopyridine administered as 10 mg orally twice daily) is efficacious at improving timed gait in multiple sclerosis. Depression and even suicidality can occur in multiple sclerosis and may worsen with interferon β-1a therapy; screening and conventional treatment of such symptoms are appropriate.

Patients with clinically isolated syndrome are at risk for developing multiple sclerosis and are sometimes offered β-interferon or glatiramer acetate therapy, which may delay progression to clinically definite disease. Teriflunomide

Table 27–10. Treatment of multiple sclerosis (in alphabetical order within categories).[1]

Medication	Dose
Acute Episode, Including Relapse[2]	
Dexamethasone	160 mg orally daily for 3–5 days
Methylprednisolone	1 g intravenously or orally daily for 3–5 days
Plasmapheresis	
Disease-Modifying Therapy (FDA-Approved)	
Alemtuzumab (Lemtrada)[3,4]	12 mg intravenously daily for 5 days; 3-day course given 1 year later
Cladribine (Mavenclad)[3,5,6]	1.75 mg/kg orally divided between weeks 1 and 5, repeated once in 1 year
Dimethyl fumarate (Tecfidera)[3,5]	240 mg orally twice daily
Fingolimod (Gilenya)[3,4,5]	0.5 mg orally daily
Glatiramer acetate (Copaxone, Mylan, Glatopa)[5]	20 mg subcutaneously daily or 40 mg subcutaneously three times weekly
Interferon β-1a (Rebif)[5]	44 mcg subcutaneously three times per week
Interferon β-1a (Avonex)[5]	30 mcg intramuscularly once per week
Interferon β-1b (Betaseron, Extavia)[5]	0.25 mg subcutaneously on alternate days
Mitoxantrone[3]	12 mg/m^2 intravenously every 3 months; maximum lifetime dose, 140 mg/m^2
Natalizumab (Tysabri)[3,4]	300 mg intravenously monthly
Ocrelizumab (Ocrevus)[3,4,5,6,7]	300 mg intravenously on day 1 and day 15, followed by 600 mg every 6 months
Ofatumumab (Kesimpta)[3,4,5,6]	20 mg subcutaneously weeks 0, 1, 2, 4, and monthly thereafter
Ozanimod (Zeposia)[3,4,5,6]	0.23 mg orally daily on days 1–4, 0.46 mg daily on days 5–7, and 0.92 mg daily thereafter
Pegylated interferon β-1a (Plegridy)[5]	125 mg subcutaneously once every 2 weeks
Ponesimod (Ponvory)[3,4,5,6]	Titrate from 2 mg orally daily to 5 mg in 1-mg increments every 2 days, then by 1 mg daily to 10 mg by day 12, and then to 20 mg daily on day 15
Siponimod (Mayzent)[3,4,5,6]	0.25 mg orally daily, titrated over 5 or 6 days to 1 or 2 mg orally daily, depending on CYP2C9 genotype
Teriflunomide (Aubagio)[5]	14 mg or 7 mg orally daily
Ublituximab-xiiy (Briumvi)[3,4,5,6]	150 mg intravenously on day 1 and 450 mg on day 15, followed by 450 mg every 24 weeks (starting from the first 150 mg dose)

[1]Several of these agents require special monitoring or pretreatment; some should be avoided during pregnancy. Readers should refer to the manufacturer's guidelines.
[2]For corticosteroid-refractory relapses, plasmapheresis may be used.
[3]Relapse prevention for disease activity despite use of first-line treatment.
[4]High disease activity (typically with multiple gadolinium-enhancing lesions on MRI).
[5]Relapse prevention, first-line treatment.
[6]Active secondary progressive disease.
[7]Primary progressive disease.

and dimethyl fumarate delay time to first clinical attack in patients with radiologically isolated syndrome.

Prognosis

The prognosis for relapsing remitting multiple sclerosis has substantially improved. With disease modifying therapy, relapses occur once every 10 years, whereas before such treatment was available, they occurred yearly. Early in the disease course, substantial to full recovery from acute exacerbations can be expected. Over time, disability may accumulate as a result of incomplete recovery from attacks and, eventually, progression between attacks (secondary progressive multiple sclerosis). However, modern treatment may slow disability accumulation. Observational cohort studies show that after diagnosis only half of patients experience worsening disability in the first 10 years; less than one fifth of patients progress to secondary progressive multiple sclerosis by 15 years; and one in ten patients require an assistive device to walk 15 years after diagnosis.

When to Refer

All patients, but especially those with progressive disease despite standard therapy, should be referred.

When to Admit

- Patients requiring plasma exchange for severe relapses unresponsive to corticosteroids.
- During severe relapses.
- Patients unable to manage at home.

Gonzalez-Lorenzo M et al. Immunomodulators and immunosuppressants for relapsing-remitting multiple sclerosis: a network meta-analysis. Cochrane Database Syst Rev. 2024;1:CD011381. [PMID: 38174776]

Montalban X et al. Diagnosis of multiple sclerosis: 2024 revisions of the McDonald criteria. Lancet Neurol. 2025;24:850. [PMID: 40975101]

NEUROMYELITIS OPTICA SPECTRUM DISORDER

This disorder is characterized by optic neuritis and acute myelitis with MRI changes that extend over at least three segments of the spinal cord. An isolated myelitis, optic neuritis, or area postrema syndrome characterized by nausea, vomiting, and hiccups may also occur. Previously known as **Devic disease** and once regarded as a variant of multiple sclerosis, neuromyelitis optica is associated with a specific antibody marker (AQP4-IgG) targeting the water channel aquaporin-4 in 80% of cases, and with antibodies to myelin oligodendrocyte glycoprotein (MOG-IgG) in approximately 33% of AQP4-IgG seronegative patients. Widespread white matter involvement is not typically seen on brain MRI but does not exclude the diagnosis. Four immunosuppressive medications that reduce time to first relapse or relapse rate are approved for long-term treatment of neuromyelitis optica spectrum disorder. Eculizumab and ravulizumab are complement inhibitors, inebilizumab is a humanized anti-CD19 antibody that depletes B-cells, and satralizumab is an interleukin-6 receptor antagonist. Use of eculizumab or ravulizumab requires prior immunization against meningococcus. Off-label therapies include rituximab, mycophenolate mofetil, or azathioprine. Acute relapses are treated with corticosteroids at doses similar to those outlined for multiple sclerosis and with plasma exchange for severe relapses unresponsive to corticosteroids.

Antibodies to MOG-IgG are associated with a broader spectrum of disease manifestations than myelitis and optic neuritis, including acute disseminated encephalomyelitis, cerebral cortical encephalitis, seizures, and brainstem or cerebellar involvement. Compared to AQP4-IgG neuromyelitis optica, onset is often younger and attacks are more frequently accompanied by fever or preceded by infection. As many as 50% of patients with an attack of MOG-IgG antibody-associated disease will not experience a second relapse and can be treated with a prolonged tapering corticosteroid course alone; those who relapse are usually offered off-label treatment with a long-term immunosuppressant or periodic IVIG infusions.

Sechi E. NMOSD and MOGAD. Continuum (Minneap Minn). 2024;30:1052. [PMID: 39088288]

VITAMIN E DEFICIENCY

Vitamin E deficiency may produce a disorder somewhat similar to Friedreich ataxia. There is spinocerebellar degeneration involving the posterior columns of the spinal cord and leading to limb ataxia, sensory loss, absent tendon reflexes, slurring of speech, and, in some cases, pigmentary retinal degeneration. (See Chapter 33.)

SPASTICITY

The term "spasticity" is commonly used for an upper motor neuron deficit, but it properly refers to a velocity-dependent increase in resistance to passive movement that affects different muscles to a different extent, is not uniform in degree throughout the range of a particular movement, and is commonly associated with other features of pyramidal deficit. It is often a major complication of stroke, cerebral or spinal injury, static perinatal encephalopathy, and multiple sclerosis. Spasticity may be exacerbated by pressure injuries, urinary or other infections, and nociceptive stimuli.

Physical therapy with appropriate stretching programs is important during rehabilitation after the development of an upper motor neuron lesion and in subsequent management. The aim is to prevent joint and muscle contractures and perhaps to modulate spasticity.

Medication management also is important, but treatment may increase functional disability when increased extensor tone is providing additional support for patients with weak legs. Pharmacologic treatment with baclofen (5–10 mg twice daily orally titrated to 80 mg daily), tizanidine (2–8 mg three time daily orally), diazepam (2–10 mg three times daily orally), or dantrolene (25 mg once daily orally, titrated every 3 days as tolerated to a maximum of 100 mg four times daily) is often helpful. Dantrolene is best avoided in patients with poor respiratory function or severe myocardial disease. Cannabinoids (combination of tetrahydrocannabinol and cannabidiol) also are effective in reducing spasticity, but are associated with side effects, including dizziness, drowsiness, and fatigue. Intramuscular injection of botulinum toxin is used to relax targeted muscles.

In patients with severe spasticity that is unresponsive to other therapies and is associated with marked disability, intrathecal injection of phenol or alcohol may be helpful. Surgical options include implantation of an intrathecal baclofen pump, rhizotomy, or neurectomy. Severe contractures may be treated by surgical tendon release.

Marsden J et al. Treatment of spasticity. Handb Clin Neurol. 2023;196:497. [PMID: 37620087]

MYELOPATHIES IN AIDS

A variety of myelopathies may occur in patients with AIDS. These are discussed in Chapter 35.

MYELOPATHY OF HUMAN T-CELL LEUKEMIA VIRUS INFECTION

Human T-cell leukemia virus (HTLV-1), a human retrovirus, is transmitted by breastfeeding, sexual contact, blood transfusion, and contaminated needles. Most patients are asymptomatic, but after a variable latent period (which may be as long as several years), a myelopathy develops in some instances. The MRI, electrophysiologic, and CSF findings are similar to those of multiple sclerosis, but HTLV-1 antibodies are present in serum and spinal fluid. There is no specific treatment, but intravenous or oral corticosteroids may help in the initial inflammatory phase of the disease.

Roman GC. Tropical spastic paraparesis. Handb Clin Neurol. 2023;196:149. [PMID: 37620067]

SUBACUTE COMBINED DEGENERATION OF THE SPINAL CORD

Subacute combined degeneration of the spinal cord is due to **vitamin B_{12} deficiency**, such as occurs in pernicious anemia. It is characterized by myelopathy with spasticity, weakness, proprioceptive loss, and numbness due to degeneration of the corticospinal tracts and posterior columns. Polyneuropathy, mental changes, or optic neuropathy also develops in some patients. Megaloblastic anemia may also occur, but this does *not* parallel the neurologic disorder, and the former may be obscured if folic acid supplements have been taken. Treatment is with vitamin B_{12}. For pernicious anemia, a convenient therapeutic regimen is 1000 mcg cyanocobalamin intramuscularly daily for 1 week, then weekly for 1 month, and then monthly for the remainder of the patient's life. Oral cyanocobalamin replacement is not advised for pernicious anemia when neurologic symptoms are present. A similar syndrome is caused by recreational abuse of inhaled nitrous oxide due to its interference with vitamin B_{12} metabolism. Copper deficiency, caused by malabsorption or excess zinc ingestion, may also be responsible.

Hassing LT et al. Nitrous-oxide-induced polyneuropathy and subacute combined degeneration of the spine: clinical and diagnostic characteristics in 70 patients, with focus on electrodiagnostic studies. Eur J Neurol. 2024;31:e16076. [PMID: 37754673]

SPINAL TRAUMA

ESSENTIALS OF DIAGNOSIS

- History of preceding trauma.
- Development of acute neurologic deficit.
- Signs of myelopathy on examination.

General Considerations

While spinal cord damage may result from whiplash injury, severe injury usually relates to fracture-dislocation causing compression or angular deformity of the cord either cervically or in the lower thoracic and upper lumbar regions. Extreme hypotension following injury may also lead to cord infarction.

Clinical Findings

Total cord transection results in immediate flaccid paralysis and loss of sensation below the level of the lesion. Reflex activity is lost for a variable period, and there is urinary and fecal retention. As reflex function returns over the following days and weeks, spastic paraplegia or quadriplegia develops, with hyperreflexia and extensor plantar responses, but a flaccid atrophic (lower motor neuron) paralysis may be found depending on the segments of the cord that are affected. The bladder and bowels also regain some reflex function, permitting urine and feces to be expelled at intervals. As spasticity increases, flexor or extensor spasms (or both) of the legs become troublesome, especially if the patient develops bed sores or a UTI. Paraplegia with the legs in flexion or extension may eventually result.

With lesser degrees of injury, patients may be left with mild limb weakness, distal sensory disturbance, or both. Sphincter function may also be impaired, urinary urgency and urge incontinence being especially common. More particularly, a unilateral cord lesion leads to an ipsilateral motor disturbance with accompanying impairment of proprioception and contralateral loss of pain and temperature appreciation below the lesion (**Brown-Séquard syndrome**). A central cord syndrome may lead to a lower motor neuron deficit at the level of the lesion and loss of pain and temperature appreciation below it, with sparing of posterior column functions. With more extensive involvement, posterior column sensation may also be impaired and pyramidal weakness develops. A radicular deficit may occur at the level of the injury—or, if the cauda equina is involved, there may be evidence of disturbed function in several lumbosacral roots.

Treatment

Treatment of the injury consists of immobilization and—if there is cord compression—early decompressive laminectomy and fusion (within 24 hours). Early treatment with high doses of corticosteroids (eg, methylprednisolone, 30 mg/kg by intravenous bolus, followed by 5.4 mg/kg/hour for 23 hours) may improve neurologic recovery if commenced within 8 hours after injury, although the evidence is limited and some neurosurgical guidelines do not recommend their use. Anatomic realignment of the spinal cord by traction and other orthopedic procedures is important. Subsequent care of the residual neurologic deficit—paraplegia or quadriplegia—requires treatment of spasticity and care of the skin, bladder, and bowels.

When to Refer

All patients with focal neurologic deficits should be referred.

When to Admit

- Patients with neurologic deficits.
- Patients with spinal cord injury, compression, or acute epidural or subdural hematoma.
- Patients with vertebral fracture-dislocation likely to compress the cord.

Izzy S. Traumatic spinal cord injury. Continuum (Minneap Minn). 2024;30:53. [PMID: 38330472]

SYRINGOMYELIA

Destruction or degeneration of gray and white matter adjacent to the central canal of the cervical spinal cord leads to cavitation and accumulation of fluid within the spinal cord. The precise pathogenesis is unclear, but many cases are associated with **Arnold-Chiari malformation**, in which there is displacement of the cerebellar tonsils, medulla, and fourth ventricle into the spinal canal, sometimes with accompanying meningomyelocele. In such circumstances, the cord cavity connects with and may merely represent a dilated central canal. In other cases, the cause of cavitation is less clear. There is a characteristic clinical picture, with segmental atrophy, areflexia, and loss of pain and temperature appreciation in a "cape" distribution, owing to the destruction of fibers crossing in front of the central canal in the mid-cervical spinal cord. Thoracic kyphoscoliosis is usually present. With progression, involvement of the long motor and sensory tracts occurs as well, so that a pyramidal and sensory deficit develops in the legs. Upward extension of the cavitation (**syringobulbia**) leads to dysfunction of the lower brainstem and thus to bulbar palsy, nystagmus, and sensory impairment over one or both sides of the face.

Syringomyelia, ie, cord cavitation, may also occur in association with an intramedullary tumor or following severe cord injury, and the cavity then does not communicate with the central canal.

In patients with Arnold-Chiari malformation, CT scans reveal a small posterior fossa and enlargement of the foramen magnum, along with other associated skeletal abnormalities at the base of the skull and upper cervical spine. MRI reveals the syrinx as well as the characteristic findings of the Arnold-Chiari malformation, including the caudal displacement of the fourth ventricle and herniation of the cerebellar tonsils through the foramen magnum. Focal cord enlargement is found at myelography or by MRI in patients with cavitation related to past injury or intramedullary neoplasms.

Treatment of Arnold-Chiari malformation with associated syringomyelia is by suboccipital craniectomy and upper cervical laminectomy, with the aim of decompressing the malformation at the foramen magnum. The cord cavity should be drained and, if necessary, an outlet for the fourth ventricle can be made. In cavitation associated with intramedullary tumor, treatment is surgical, but radiation therapy may be necessary if complete removal is not possible. Posttraumatic syringomyelia is also treated surgically if it leads to increasing neurologic deficits or to intolerable pain.

Prasad AS et al. Efficacy of neurosurgical intervention in syrinx resolution in patients presenting with Chiari malformation type I and syringomyelia: a systematic review and radiological meta-analysis. Neurosurg Rev. 2025;48:724. [PMID: 41111088]

DEGENERATIVE MOTOR NEURON DISEASES

ESSENTIALS OF DIAGNOSIS

- Weakness.
- No sensory loss or sphincter disturbance.
- Progressive course.
- No identifiable underlying cause other than genetic basis in familial cases.

General Considerations

This group of degenerative disorders is characterized clinically by weakness and variable wasting of affected muscles, without accompanying sensory changes.

Motor neuron disease in adults generally commences between 30 and 60 years of age. There is degeneration of the anterior horn cells in the spinal cord, the motor nuclei of the lower cranial nerves, and the corticospinal and corticobulbar pathways. The disorder is usually sporadic, but familial cases may occur and several genetic mutations or loci have been identified. Cigarette smoking may be one risk factor.

Classification

Five varieties have been distinguished on clinical grounds.

A. Progressive Bulbar Palsy

Bulbar involvement predominates owing to disease processes affecting primarily the motor nuclei of the cranial nerves.

B. Pseudobulbar Palsy

Bulbar involvement predominates in this variety also, but it is due to bilateral corticobulbar disease and thus reflects upper motor neuron dysfunction. There may be a "**pseudobulbar affect**," with uncontrollable episodes of laughing or crying to stimuli that would not normally have elicited such marked reactions.

C. Progressive Spinal Muscular Atrophy

This is characterized primarily by a lower motor neuron deficit in the limbs due to degeneration of the anterior horn cells in the spinal cord.

D. Primary Lateral Sclerosis

There is a purely upper motor neuron deficit in the limbs.

E. Amyotrophic Lateral Sclerosis (ALS)

A mixed upper and lower motor neuron deficit is found in the limbs. This disorder is sometimes associated with cognitive decline (in a pattern consistent with frontotemporal dementia), a pseudobulbar affect, or parkinsonism. Up to 10% of ALS cases are familial and have been associated with mutations at several different genetic loci, including a hexanucleotide repeat on chromosome 9 that also associates with frontotemporal dementia. Some (15–20% of familial cases and 1–3% of sporadic cases) are due to mutations in the superoxide dismutase gene, for which a targeted gene therapy is available.

Differential Diagnosis

The spinal muscular atrophies (SMAs) are inherited syndromes caused most often by mutations of the survival motor neuron 1 (*SMN1*) gene on chromosome 5 that usually present during infancy or childhood. There are reports of juvenile SMA due to hexosaminidase deficiency. X-linked spinal and bulbar muscular atrophy

(Kennedy syndrome) is associated with an expanded trinucleotide repeat sequence on the androgen receptor gene and carries a more benign prognosis than other forms of motor neuron disease. Hereditary spastic paraplegia is a diverse genetic syndrome that causes a slowly progressive myelopathy that can usually be distinguished from ALS by the presence of sensory signs and sphincter dysfunction.

Pure motor syndromes resembling motor neuron disease may also occur in association with monoclonal gammopathy or multifocal motor neuropathies with conduction block. A motor neuronopathy may also develop in Hodgkin disease and has a relatively benign prognosis. Infective anterior horn cell diseases (polio virus or West Nile virus infection) can generally be distinguished by the acute onset and monophasic course of the illness, as discussed in Chapter 36. Acute flaccid myelitis following infection with enterovirus may occur, especially in children, without sensory involvement and resembles poliomyelitis. There is no specific treatment. Compressive cervical radiculomyelopathy may cause lower motor neuron signs in the cervical myotomes with upper motor neuron signs in the legs. Benign fasciculations can be distinguished from ALS by a normal neurologic exam and electromyography.

Clinical Findings

A. Symptoms and Signs

Difficulty in swallowing, chewing, coughing, breathing, and talking (dysarthria) occurs with bulbar involvement. In progressive bulbar palsy, there is drooping of the palate; a depressed gag reflex; pooling of saliva in the pharynx; a weak cough; and a wasted, fasciculating tongue. In pseudobulbar palsy, the tongue is contracted and spastic and cannot be moved rapidly from side to side. Limb involvement is characterized by motor disturbances (weakness, stiffness, wasting, fasciculations) reflecting lower or upper motor neuron dysfunction; there are no objective changes on sensory examination, although there may be vague sensory complaints. The sphincters are generally spared. Cognitive changes or pseudobulbar affect may be present. The disorder is progressive, and ALS is usually fatal within 3–5 years; death usually results from pulmonary infections. Patients with bulbar involvement generally have the poorest prognosis, while patients with primary lateral sclerosis often have a longer survival despite profound quadriparesis and spasticity.

B. Laboratory and Other Studies

Electromyography may show signs of acute and chronic partial denervation with reinnervation. In patients with suspected ALS, the diagnosis should not be made with confidence unless such changes are found in at least three spinal regions (cervical, thoracic, lumbosacral) or two spinal regions and the bulbar musculature. Motor conduction velocity is usually normal but may be slightly reduced, and sensory conduction studies are also normal. Biopsy of a wasted muscle shows the histologic changes of denervation but is *not* necessary for diagnosis. The serum creatine kinase may be slightly elevated but never reaches the extremely high values seen in some of the muscular dystrophies. Testing for HIV, Lyme disease, and serum paraproteins can be considered. The CSF is normal. Molecular genetic testing is available when familial disorders are suspected. Reduced hexosaminidase activity is found in serum and leukocytes in patients with juvenile SMA due to hexosaminidase deficiency.

Treatment

Two medications are approved by the FDA for ALS. Riluzole, 50 mg orally twice daily, which reduces the presynaptic release of glutamate, increased short-term survival of patients with ALS in randomized trials. Edaravone, a free radical scavenger, slows disease progression in patients with mild disease. It is administered in monthly cycles as a 60 mg intravenous infusion on days 1–14 in the first month and days 1–10 in the subsequent months, or 105 mg orally once daily following the same dosing schedule. Ultra-high-dose methylcobalamin injections (50 mg intramuscularly twice weekly) slowed functional decline in a placebo-controlled randomized trial of patients within 1 year of symptom onset.

Noninvasive ventilation at least 4 hours per day in patients with a maximal inspiratory pressure < 60 cm H_2O may prolong survival in ALS. Symptomatic and supportive measures to treat spasticity (discussed earlier in the section on spasticity), drooling, and dysphagia, prevent contractures, and preserve mobility are important. Drooling is treated with over-the-counter decongestants, anticholinergic medications (such as trihexyphenidyl, amitriptyline, or atropine), botulinum toxin injections into the salivary glands, or use of a portable suction machine. Physical and occupational therapy are helpful throughout the disease course. Combination dextromethorphan/quinidine (20 mg/10 mg, one tablet orally once or twice daily) may relieve symptoms of pseudobulbar affect. A semiliquid diet or gastrostomy tube feeding may be needed if dysphagia is severe; it is advisable to perform the procedure before the FVC falls below 50% of predicted to minimize the risk of complications. Tracheostomy is sometimes performed if respiratory muscles are severely affected; however, in the terminal stages of these disorders, realistic expectations and advance care planning should be discussed. Information on palliative care is provided in Chapter 5.

Gene therapy is approved by the FDA for patients with ALS caused by SOD1 mutations and SMA.

When to Refer

All patients (to exclude other treatable causes of symptoms and signs) should be referred.

When to Admit

Patients may need to be admitted for initiation or titration of noninvasive ventilation, or for periods of increased requirement of noninvasive ventilator support during pulmonary infections.

Izenberg A. Amyotrophic lateral sclerosis and other motor neuron diseases. Continuum (Minneap Minn). 2023;29:1538. [PMID: 37851042]

PERIPHERAL NEUROPATHIES

When evaluating disorders of peripheral nerves, the first determination should be whether a single nerve is involved in isolation (mononeuropathy) or multiple nerves are involved, either symmetrically (polyneuropathy) or asymmetrically (mononeuropathy multiplex). In all cases, the predominant pathologic feature may be **axonal degeneration** (**axonal neuropathies**) or **demyelination** (**demyelinating neuropathies**). This often critical distinction may be possible based on neurophysiologic findings. Motor and sensory conduction velocity can be measured in accessible segments of peripheral nerves. In axonal neuropathies, conduction velocity is normal or reduced only mildly and needle electromyography provides evidence of denervation in affected muscles. In demyelinating neuropathies, conduction may be slowed considerably in affected fibers, and in more severe cases, conduction is blocked completely, without accompanying electromyographic signs of denervation.

POLYNEUROPATHIES & MONONEUROPATHY MULTIPLEX

ESSENTIALS OF DIAGNOSIS

- Weakness, sensory disturbances, or both in the extremities.
- Pain is common.
- Depressed or absent tendon reflexes.
- May be family history of neuropathy.
- May be history of systemic illness or toxic exposure.

General Considerations

Diffuse **polyneuropathies** lead to a symmetric sensory, motor, or mixed deficit, often most marked distally. They include hereditary, metabolic, and toxic disorders; idiopathic inflammatory polyneuropathy (**Guillain-Barré syndrome**); and peripheral neuropathies that may occur as a nonmetastatic complication of malignant diseases. Involvement of motor fibers leads to flaccid weakness that is most marked distally; dysfunction of sensory fibers causes impaired sensory perception. Tendon reflexes are depressed or absent. Paresthesias, pain, and muscle tenderness may also occur. Multiple mononeuropathies (**mononeuropathy multiplex**) suggest a patchy multifocal disease process such as vasculopathy (eg, diabetes, arteritis), an infiltrative process (eg, leprosy, sarcoidosis), radiation damage, or an immunologic disorder (eg, brachial plexopathy).

Clinical Findings

The cause of polyneuropathy or mononeuritis multiplex is suggested by the history, mode of onset, and predominant clinical manifestations. Laboratory workup includes a CBC, serum protein electrophoresis with reflex to immunofixation or immunotyping, determination of plasma urea and electrolytes, liver biochemical tests, thyroid function tests, vitamin B_{12} level, tests for rheumatoid factor and antinuclear antibody, hepatitis B and C determination, a serologic test for syphilis, fasting blood glucose level and hemoglobin A_{1c}, urinary heavy metal levels, CSF examination, and CXR. These tests should be ordered selectively, as guided by symptoms and signs. Measurement of nerve conduction velocity can confirm the peripheral nerve origin of symptoms and provides a means of following clinical changes, as well as indicate the likely disease process (ie, axonal or demyelinating neuropathy). Cutaneous nerve biopsy may help establish a precise diagnosis (eg, polyarteritis, amyloidosis). In about half of cases, no specific cause can be established; of these, slightly less than half are subsequently found to be familial.

Treatment

Treatment is of the underlying cause, when feasible, and is discussed below under the individual disorders. Physical therapy helps prevent contractures, and splints can maintain a weak extremity in a position of useful function. Anesthetic extremities must be protected from injury. To guard against burns, patients should check the temperature of water and hot surfaces with a portion of skin having normal sensation, measure water temperature with a thermometer, and use cold water for washing or lower the temperature setting of their hot-water heaters. Shoes should be examined frequently during the day for grit or foreign objects in order to prevent pressure lesions.

Patients with polyneuropathies or mononeuritis multiplex are subject to additional nerve injury at pressure points and should therefore avoid such behavior as leaning on elbows or sitting with crossed legs for lengthy periods.

Neuropathic, burning pain may respond to simple analgesics, such as aspirin or NSAIDs, and to gabapentin (300 mg orally three times daily, titrated up to a maximum of 1200 mg orally three times daily as necessary) or pregabalin (50–100 mg orally three times daily). Duloxetine (60 mg orally once or twice daily), venlafaxine (start 37.5 mg orally twice daily, and titrate up to 75 mg orally two to three times daily), or tricyclic antidepressants (eg, amitriptyline 10–150 mg orally at bedtime daily) may be helpful to treat pain associated with peripheral neuropathies. Medical cannabis may provide some relief, but long-term safety data are lacking. The use of a frame or cradle to reduce contact with bedclothes may be helpful. Many patients experience episodic stabbing pains, which may respond to gabapentin, pregabalin, carbamazepine (start 100 mg orally twice daily, and titrate up to 400 mg orally twice daily), or tricyclic antidepressants. Opioids may be necessary for severe hyperpathia or pain induced by minimal stimuli, but their use generally should be avoided. An implanted 10 kHz spinal cord stimulator combined with medical management reduced pain by an average of 80% in an RCT in patients with painful diabetic neuropathy, a result that was sustained for 24 months and was also associated with neurologic improvement in most patients. In a meta-analysis of RCT, scrambler therapy, which consists of transcutaneous electrical nerve stimulation at multiple simultaneous sites, appears effective for neuropathic pain. It has a favorable safety profile and is approved in the United States for treatment of chronic, acute, and postoperative pain.

Symptoms of autonomic dysfunction are occasionally troublesome. Treatment of postural hypotension is discussed earlier in this chapter. Erectile dysfunction can be treated with phosphodiesterase inhibitors; a flaccid neuropathic bladder may respond to parasympathomimetic medications such as bethanechol chloride, 10–50 mg three or four times daily.

Soliman N et al. Pharmacotherapy and non-invasive neuromodulation for neuropathic pain: a systematic review and meta-analysis. Lancet Neurol. 2025;24:413. [PMID: 40252663]

1. Inherited Neuropathies

A. Charcot-Marie-Tooth Disease (HMSN Type I, II)

There are several distinct varieties of Charcot-Marie-Tooth disease, usually with an autosomal dominant mode of inheritance, but occasional cases occur on a sporadic, recessive, or X-linked basis. Clinical presentation may be with foot deformities or gait disturbances in childhood or early adult life. Slow progression leads to the typical features of polyneuropathy, with distal weakness and wasting that begin in the legs, a variable amount of distal sensory loss, and depressed or absent tendon reflexes. Tremor is a conspicuous feature in some instances. **Hereditary motor and sensory neuropathy** (HMSN) **type I** is characterized by demyelination on electrodiagnostic studies and is usually caused by mutations in the peripheral myelin protein 22 or myelin protein zero gene. In **HMSN type II**, electrodiagnostic studies show axonal loss rather than demyelination; one-third of cases are due to mutations in the gene mitofusin 2.

A similar disorder may occur in patients with progressive distal SMAs, but there is no sensory loss; electrophysiologic investigation reveals that motor conduction velocity is normal or only slightly reduced, and nerve action potentials are normal.

B. Dejerine-Sottas Disease (HMSN Type III)

The disorder may occur on a sporadic, autosomal dominant or, less commonly, autosomal recessive basis. Onset in infancy or childhood leads to a progressive motor and sensory polyneuropathy with weakness, ataxia, sensory loss, and depressed or absent tendon reflexes.

C. Friedreich Ataxia

This disorder, the only known autosomal recessive trinucleotide repeat disease, is caused most commonly by expansion of a poly-GAA locus in the gene for frataxin on chromosome 9, leading to symptoms in childhood or early adult life. The gait becomes ataxic, the hands become clumsy, and other signs of cerebellar dysfunction develop accompanied by weakness of the legs and extensor plantar responses. Involvement of peripheral sensory fibers leads to sensory disturbances in the limbs and depressed tendon reflexes. There is bilateral pes cavus. Pathologically, there is a marked loss of cells in the posterior root ganglia and degeneration of peripheral sensory fibers. In the CNS, changes are conspicuous in the posterior and lateral columns of the cord. Electrophysiologically, conduction velocity in motor fibers is normal or only mildly reduced, but sensory action potentials are small or absent. Cardiac disease is the most common cause of death. Omaveloxolone led to functional improvement compared with placebo in a randomized trial and is approved for patients 16 years of age or older.

In the differential diagnosis for Friedreich ataxia are other spinocerebellar ataxias, a growing group of inherited disorders, each involving a different identified gene. These heterogeneous disorders, which frequently (but not exclusively) exhibit an autosomal dominant inheritance pattern and poly-CAG expansion of the affected gene, typically cause cerebellar ataxia and varying combinations of other symptoms (such as peripheral neuropathy, ophthalmoparesis, dysarthria, and pyramidal and extrapyramidal signs).

D. Refsum Disease (HMSN Type IV)

This autosomal recessive disorder is due to a disturbance in phytanic acid metabolism. Pigmentary retinal degeneration is accompanied by progressive sensorimotor polyneuropathy and cerebellar signs. Auditory dysfunction, cardiomyopathy, and cutaneous manifestations may also occur. Motor and sensory conduction velocities are reduced, often markedly, and there may be electromyographic evidence of denervation in affected muscles. Dietary restriction of phytanic acid and its precursors may be helpful therapeutically. Plasmapheresis to reduce stored phytanic acid may help at the initiation of treatment.

E. Porphyria

Peripheral nerve involvement may occur during acute attacks in both **variegate porphyria** and **acute intermittent porphyria**. Motor symptoms usually occur first, and weakness is often most marked proximally and in the upper limbs rather than the lower. Sensory symptoms and signs may be proximal or distal in distribution. Autonomic involvement is sometimes pronounced. The electrophysiologic findings are in keeping with the results of neuropathologic studies suggesting that the neuropathy is axonal in type (see Chapter 42).

F. Familial Amyloid Polyneuropathy

Sensory and autonomic symptoms are especially conspicuous, whereas distal wasting and weakness occur later. The polyneuropathy is axonal and likely results from amyloid deposition within the peripheral nerves due to mutations in the genes encoding transthyretin, apolipoprotein A1, or gelsolin. **Transthyretin amyloidosis** is the most common and is associated with cardiomyopathy, nephropathy, leptomeningeal involvement, and vitreous opacity. It is treatable with liver transplantation, the small interfering ribonucleic acids patisiran and vutrisiran, or the antisense oligonucleotides inotersen and eplontersen. Tafamidis helps transthyretin amyloid cardiomyopathy and may slow the progression of the neuropathy.

Coelho T et al. Eplontersen for hereditary transthyretin amyloidosis with polyneuropathy. JAMA. 2023;330:1448. [PMID: 37768671]

2. Neuropathies Associated with Systemic & Metabolic Disorders

A. Diabetes Mellitus

In this disorder, involvement of the peripheral nervous system may lead to symmetric sensory or mixed polyneuropathy, asymmetric motor radiculoneuropathy or plexopathy (diabetic amyotrophy), thoracoabdominal radiculopathy, autonomic neuropathy, or isolated lesions of individual nerves. These may occur singly or in any combination and are discussed in Chapter 31.

B. Uremia

Uremia may lead to a symmetric sensorimotor polyneuropathy that tends to affect the lower limbs more than the upper limbs and is more marked distally than proximally (see Chapter 25). The diagnosis can be confirmed electrophysiologically because motor and sensory conduction velocity is moderately reduced. The neuropathy improves both clinically and electrophysiologically with kidney transplantation and to a lesser extent with chronic dialysis.

C. Alcohol Use Disorder and Nutritional Deficiency

Many patients with alcohol use disorder have an axonal distal sensorimotor polyneuropathy that is frequently accompanied by painful cramps, muscle tenderness, and painful paresthesias and is often more marked in the legs than in the arms. Symptoms of autonomic dysfunction may also be conspicuous. Motor and sensory conduction velocity may be slightly reduced, even in subclinical cases, but gross slowing of conduction is uncommon. Treatment is similar to diabetic polyneuropathy but also includes abstinence from alcohol. A similar distal sensorimotor polyneuropathy is a well-recognized feature of **beriberi** (thiamine deficiency). In vitamin B_{12} deficiency, distal sensory polyneuropathy may develop but is usually overshadowed by CNS manifestations (eg, myelopathy, optic neuropathy, or intellectual changes).

D. Paraproteinemias

A symmetric sensorimotor polyneuropathy that is gradual in onset, progressive in course, and often accompanied by pain and dysesthesias in the limbs may occur in patients (especially men) with **plasma cell myeloma** (formerly multiple myeloma). The neuropathy is of the axonal type in classic lytic myeloma, but segmental demyelination (primary or secondary) and axonal loss may occur in sclerotic myeloma and lead to predominantly motor clinical manifestations. Both demyelinating and axonal neuropathies are also observed in patients with paraproteinemias without myeloma. A small fraction will develop myeloma if serially followed. The demyelinating neuropathy in these patients may be due to the monoclonal proteins reacting to a component of the nerve myelin. The neuropathy of classic plasma cell myeloma is poorly responsive to therapy. The polyneuropathy of **benign monoclonal gammopathy** may respond to immunosuppressant medications and plasmapheresis.

Polyneuropathy may also occur in association with monoclonal gammopathy of unknown significance, macroglobulinemia, and cryoglobulinemia and sometimes responds to plasmapheresis. Many patients with an IgM M-protein will have antibodies to myelin-associated glycoprotein (MAG); these patients may respond to treatment with rituximab. Entrapment neuropathy, such as carpal tunnel syndrome, is more common than polyneuropathy in patients with (nonhereditary) generalized amyloidosis.

Min YG et al. Neuropathy with anti-myelin-associated glycoprotein antibodies: update on diagnosis, pathophysiology and management. J Neurol Neurosurg Psychiatry. 2025;96:340. [PMID: 39658134]

3. Neuropathies Associated with Infectious & Inflammatory Diseases

A. Leprosy

Leprosy is an important cause of peripheral neuropathy in certain parts of the world. Sensory disturbances are mainly due to involvement of intracutaneous nerves. In tuberculoid leprosy, they develop at the same time and in the same distribution as the nerve; trunks lying beneath the lesion are also involved. In lepromatous leprosy, there is more extensive sensory loss, and this develops earlier and to a greater extent in the coolest regions of the body, such as the dorsal surfaces of the hands and feet, where the bacilli proliferate most actively. Motor deficits result from involvement of superficial nerves where their temperature is lowest, eg, the ulnar nerve in the region proximal to the olecranon groove, the median nerve as it emerges from beneath the forearm flexor muscle to run toward the carpal tunnel, the peroneal nerve at the head of the fibula, and the posterior tibial nerve in the lower part of the leg; patchy facial muscular weakness may also occur owing to involvement of the superficial branches of the seventh cranial nerve.

Motor disturbances in leprosy are suggestive of multiple mononeuropathy, whereas sensory changes resemble those of distal polyneuropathy. Examination, however, relates the distribution of sensory deficits to the temperature of the tissues; in the legs, for example, sparing frequently occurs between the toes and in the popliteal fossae, where the temperature is higher. Treatment is with antileprotic agents (see Chapter 37).

B. AIDS

A variety of neuropathies occur in patients with HIV (see Chapter 35).

C. Lyme Borreliosis

The neurologic manifestations of Lyme disease include meningitis, meningoencephalitis, polyradiculoneuropathy, mononeuropathy multiplex, and cranial neuropathy.

Serologic tests establish the underlying disorder. Lyme disease and its treatment are discussed in depth in Chapter 38.

D. Sarcoidosis

Cranial nerve palsies (especially facial palsy), multiple mononeuropathy and, less commonly, symmetric polyneuropathy may all occur, the latter sometimes preferentially affecting either motor or sensory fibers. Treatment of sarcoidosis is discussed in Chapter 9.

E. Polyarteritis

Involvement of the vasa nervorum by the vasculitic process may result in infarction of the nerve. Clinically, one encounters an asymmetric sensorimotor polyneuropathy (mononeuritis multiplex) that pursues a waxing and waning course. Corticosteroids, cyclophosphamide, or rituximab helps, depending on the specific case (see Chapter 23).

F. Rheumatoid Arthritis

Compressive or entrapment neuropathies, ischemic neuropathies, mild distal sensory polyneuropathy, and severe progressive sensorimotor polyneuropathy can occur in rheumatoid arthritis (see Chapter 23).

Pacut P et al. Top 10 clinical pearls in vasculitic neuropathies. Semin Neurol. 2025;45:112. [PMID: 39348853]

4. Neuropathy Associated with Critical Illness

Patients in ICUs with sepsis and multiorgan failure sometimes develop polyneuropathies. This may be manifested initially by unexpected difficulty in weaning patients from a mechanical ventilator and in more advanced cases by wasting and weakness of the extremities and loss of tendon reflexes. Sensory abnormalities are relatively inconspicuous. The neuropathy is axonal in type. Its pathogenesis is obscure, and treatment is supportive. The prognosis is good provided that patients recover from the underlying critical illness. A myopathy may also occur.

Younger DS. Critical illness-associated weakness and related motor disorders. Handb Clin Neurol. 2023;195:707. [PMID: 37562893]

5. Toxic Neuropathies

Axonal polyneuropathy may follow exposure to industrial agents or pesticides such as acrylamide, organophosphorus compounds, hexacarbon solvents, methyl bromide, and carbon disulfide; metals such as arsenic, thallium, mercury, and lead; medications such as phenytoin, amiodarone, perhexiline, isoniazid, nitrofurantoin; and platinum or taxane chemotherapies, vincristine, and pyridoxine in high doses. Detailed occupational, environmental, and medical histories and recognition of clusters of cases are important in suggesting the diagnosis. Treatment is by preventing further exposure to the causal agent. Cryotherapy or covering the hands and feet with cold gloves and stockings before, during, and after neurotoxic chemotherapy infusion prevented neuropathy and improved quality of life in a meta-analysis of randomized trials. Isoniazid neuropathy is prevented by pyridoxine supplementation.

Diphtheritic neuropathy results from a neurotoxin released by the causative organism and is common in many areas. Palatal weakness may develop 2–4 weeks after infection of the throat, and infection of the skin may similarly be followed by focal weakness of neighboring muscles. Disturbances of accommodation may occur about 4–5 weeks after infection and distal sensorimotor demyelinating polyneuropathy after 1–3 months.

Tai HY et al. Efficacy of cryotherapy in the prevention of chemotherapy-induced peripheral neuropathy: a systematic review and meta-analysis. Support Care Cancer. 2024;32:482. [PMID: 38955817]

6. Neuropathies Associated with Malignant Diseases

A variety of neuropathies have been associated with nonmetastatic complications of malignancy. Some were discussed above in the section on paraproteinemia. A sensory neuronopathy may be observed in association with anti-Hu antibodies, especially in patients with small cell lung cancer.

Shelly S et al. Paraneoplastic neuropathies and peripheral nerve hyperexcitability disorders. Handb Clin Neurol. 2024;200:239. [PMID: 38494281]

7. Acute Idiopathic Polyneuropathy (Guillain-Barré Syndrome)

ESSENTIALS OF DIAGNOSIS

- Acute or subacute progressive polyradiculoneuropathy.
- Weakness is more severe than sensory disturbances.
- Acute dysautonomia may be life-threatening.

General Considerations

This acute or subacute polyradiculoneuropathy sometimes follows infective illness, inoculations, or surgical procedures. There is an association with preceding *Campylobacter jejuni* enteritis. Cohort studies suggest an association with adenovirus vector SARS-CoV-2 vaccines but not with mRNA vaccines. The disorder probably has an immunologic basis, but the precise mechanism is unclear.

Clinical Findings

A. Symptoms and Signs

The main complaint is of weakness that varies widely in severity in different patients and often has a proximal emphasis and symmetric distribution. It usually begins in the legs, spreading to a variable extent but frequently involving the arms and often one or both sides of the face.

The muscles of respiration or deglutition may also be affected. Sensory symptoms are usually less conspicuous than motor ones, but distal paresthesias and dysesthesias are common, and neuropathic or radicular pain is present in many patients. Autonomic disturbances are also common, may be severe, and are sometimes life-threatening; they include tachycardia, cardiac irregularities, hypo- or hypertension, facial flushing, abnormalities of sweating, pulmonary dysfunction, and impaired sphincter control. The axonal subtypes of the syndrome (**acute motor axonal neuropathy** [AMAN] and **acute motor and sensory axonal neuropathy** [AMSAN]) are caused by antibodies to gangliosides on the axon membrane. The **Miller Fisher syndrome**, another subtype, is characterized by the clinical triad of ophthalmoplegia, ataxia, and areflexia, and is associated with anti-GQ1b antibodies.

B. Laboratory Findings

The CSF characteristically contains a high protein concentration with a normal cell count, but these changes may take up to 2 weeks to develop; WBC counts > 50 cells/mcL (0.05×10^9/L) should prompt consideration of alternative diagnoses. Electrophysiologic studies may reveal marked abnormalities, which do not necessarily parallel the clinical disorder in their temporal course.

Differential Diagnosis

When the diagnosis is made, the history and appropriate laboratory studies should exclude the possibility of porphyric, diphtheritic, or toxic (heavy metal, hexacarbon, organophosphate) neuropathies, and of HIV infection. The temporal course excludes other peripheral neuropathies. Poliomyelitis, botulism, and tick paralysis must also be considered as they cause weakness of acute onset. The presence of pyramidal signs, a markedly asymmetric motor deficit, a sharp sensory level, or early sphincter involvement should suggest a focal cord lesion.

Treatment

Treatment with prednisone is *ineffective* and may prolong recovery time. Plasmapheresis or IVIG (400 mg/kg/day for 5 days) is of value. Treatment is best initiated within the first few days of illness and is useful for clinically severe or rapidly progressive cases or those with ventilatory impairment. Patients should be admitted to ICU if their FVC is declining, and intubation is considered if the FVC reaches 15 mL/kg, the maximum inspiratory pressure reaches –30 mm Hg, or dyspnea becomes evident. Declining oxygen saturation is a late indicator of neuromuscular respiratory failure. Respiratory toilet and chest physical therapy help prevent atelectasis. Marked hypotension may respond to volume replacement or pressor agents. Thromboprophylaxis is important.

Prognosis

Most patients eventually make a good recovery, but this may take many months, and about 20% of patients are left with persisting disability. Approximately 3% of patients with acute idiopathic polyneuropathy have one or more clinically similar relapses, sometimes several years after the initial illness.

Censi S et al. Guillain-Barré syndrome and COVID-19 vaccination: a systematic review and meta-analysis. J Neurol. 2024;271:1063. [PMID: 38233678]

8. Chronic Inflammatory Polyneuropathy

Chronic inflammatory demyelinating polyneuropathy, an acquired immunologically mediated disorder, is clinically similar to Guillain-Barré syndrome except that it has a relapsing or steadily progressive course over months or years and that autonomic dysfunction is generally less common. It may present as an exclusively motor disorder or with a mixed sensorimotor disturbance. In the relapsing form, partial recovery may occur after some relapses, but in other instances there is no recovery between exacerbations. Although remission may occur spontaneously with time, the disorder frequently follows a progressive downhill course leading to severe functional disability. Occasional acute presentations may mimic Guillain-Barré syndrome, which are frequently associated with IgG_4 antibodies to proteins expressed at the nodes of Ranvier (neurofascin-155, contactin-1, and contactin associated protein 1 [CASPR1]).

The diagnosis is established through clinical examination, electrodiagnostic studies, and the exclusion of alternative etiologies of chronic demyelinating neuropathy. Electrodiagnostic studies show marked slowing of motor and sensory conduction, and focal conduction block. Signs of partial denervation may also be present owing to secondary axonal degeneration. Nerve biopsy may show chronic perivascular inflammatory infiltrates in the endoneurium and epineurium, without accompanying evidence of vasculitis.

Corticosteroids may arrest or reverse the downhill course. Treatment is usually begun with prednisone, 60–80 mg orally daily, continued for 2–3 months or until a definite response has occurred. If no response has occurred despite 3 months of treatment, a higher dose may be tried. In responsive cases, the dose is gradually tapered, but most patients become corticosteroid-dependent, often requiring prednisone, 20 mg daily on alternate days, on a long-term basis. IVIG can be used in place of, or in addition to corticosteroids, and is best used as the initial treatment in pure motor syndromes (2 g/kg over 2–5 days followed by 1 g/kg every 3 weeks). A weekly regimen of 0.2–0.4 g/kg of a 20% subcutaneous immunoglobulin solution is an effective alternative but has not been compared directly to corticosteroids or IVIG. When both IVIG and corticosteroids are ineffective, plasma exchange may be worthwhile. Weekly subcutaneous injection of efgartigimod-α and hyaluronidase-qvfc (1008 mg/11,200 U), a neonatal Fc receptor blocker, reduced the risk of relapse in CIDP in a randomized trial and is approved in the United States and Europe. Immunosuppressant or immunomodulatory medications (such as azathioprine or rituximab) may be added when the response to other measures is unsatisfactory or to enable maintenance doses of corticosteroids to be lowered. Symptomatic treatment is also important.

Allen JA et al. Safety, tolerability, and efficacy of subcutaneous efgartigimod in patients with chronic inflammatory demyelinating polyradiculoneuropathy (ADHERE): a multicentre, randomised-withdrawal, double-blind, placebo-controlled, phase 2 trial. Lancet Neurol. 2024;23:1013. [PMID: 39304241]

Bus SR et al. Intravenous immunoglobulin for chronic inflammatory demyelinating polyradiculoneuropathy. Cochrane Database Syst Rev. 2024;2:CD001797. [PMID: 38353301]

When to Refer

- All patients with a progressive neuropathy should be referred.
- Painful neuropathy unresponsive to first-line treatment.
- Patients with disabling autonomic symptoms.

When to Admit

- Patients with rapidly progressive symptoms or respiratory compromise.

MONONEUROPATHIES

ESSENTIALS OF DIAGNOSIS

- Focal motor or sensory deficit.
- Deficit is in territory of an individual peripheral nerve.

An individual nerve may be injured along its course or may be compressed, angulated, or stretched by neighboring anatomic structures, especially at a point where it passes through a narrow space (**entrapment neuropathy**). The relative contributions of mechanical factors and ischemia to the local damage are not clear. With involvement of a sensory or mixed nerve, pain is commonly felt distal to the lesion. Symptoms never develop with some entrapment neuropathies, resolve rapidly and spontaneously in others, and become progressively more disabling and distressing in yet other cases. The precise neurologic deficit depends on the nerve involved. Percussion of the nerve at the site of the lesion may lead to paresthesias in its distal distribution.

Entrapment neuropathy may be the sole manifestation of subclinical polyneuropathy, and this must be borne in mind and excluded by nerve conduction studies. Such studies are also indispensable for the localization of the focal lesion. Neuromuscular ultrasound is also useful in this context.

In patients with acute compression neuropathy such as may occur in intoxicated individuals (**Saturday night palsy**), no treatment is necessary. Complete recovery generally occurs, usually within 2 months, presumably because the underlying pathology is demyelination. However, axonal degeneration can occur in severe cases, and recovery then takes longer and may never be complete.

In chronic compressive or entrapment neuropathies, avoidance of aggravating factors and correction of any underlying systemic conditions are important. Local infiltration of the region about the nerve with corticosteroids may be of value; in addition, surgical decompression may help if there is a progressively increasing neurologic deficit or if electrodiagnostic studies show evidence of partial denervation in weak muscles.

Peripheral nerve tumors are uncommon, except in neurofibromatosis type 1, but also give rise to mononeuropathy. This may be distinguishable from entrapment neuropathy only by noting the presence of a mass along the course of the nerve and by demonstrating the precise site of the lesion with appropriate electrophysiologic studies and neuromuscular ultrasound. Treatment of symptomatic lesions is by surgical removal if possible.

1. Carpal Tunnel Syndrome

See Chapter 45.

2. Pronator Teres or Anterior Interosseous Syndrome

The median nerve gives off its motor branch, the anterior interosseous nerve, below the elbow as it descends between the two heads of the pronator teres muscle. A lesion of either nerve may occur in this region, sometimes after trauma or owing to compression from, for example, a fibrous band. With anterior interosseous nerve involvement, there is no sensory loss, and weakness is confined to the pronator quadratus, flexor pollicis longus, and the flexor digitorum profundus to the second and third digits. Weakness is more widespread and sensory changes occur in an appropriate distribution when the median nerve itself is affected. The prognosis is variable. If improvement does not occur spontaneously, decompressive surgery may be helpful.

Richards D et al. Other median neuropathies. Handb Clin Neurol. 2024;201:89. [PMID: 38697748]

3. Ulnar Nerve Lesions

Ulnar nerve lesions are likely to occur in the elbow region as the nerve runs in the condylar groove behind the medial epicondyle and descends into the cubital tunnel. In the condylar groove, the ulnar nerve is exposed to pressure or trauma. Moreover, any increase in the carrying angle of the elbow, whether congenital, degenerative, or traumatic, may cause excessive stretching of the nerve when the elbow is flexed. Ulnar nerve lesions may also result from thickening or distortion of the anatomic structures forming the cubital tunnel, and the resulting symptoms may also be aggravated by flexion of the elbow, because the tunnel is then narrowed by tightening of its roof or inward bulging of its floor. A severe lesion at either site causes sensory changes in the fifth and medial half of the fourth digits and along the medial border of the hand. There is weakness of the ulnar-innervated muscles in the forearm and hand. With milder cubital tunnel lesions, however, there may be relative sparing of the flexor carpi ulnaris muscle. Electrophysiologic evaluation using nerve stimulation techniques allows more precise localization of the lesion.

Initial treatment consists of avoiding pressure on the medial elbow (eg, avoid resting the elbows on arm rests; pad the elbow during sleep) and preventing prolonged elbow flexion, especially at night. Splints are available to keep the elbow from flexing beyond 45 to 90 degrees. If conservative measures are unsuccessful in relieving symptoms and preventing further progression, surgical treatment may be necessary. This consists of nerve transposition if the lesion is in the condylar groove, or a release procedure if it is in the cubital tunnel.

Ulnar nerve lesions may also develop at the wrist or in the palm of the hand, usually owing to repetitive trauma (eg, cycling) or to compression from ganglia or benign tumors. They can be subdivided depending on their presumed site. Compressive lesions are treated surgically. If repetitive mechanical trauma is responsible, this is avoided by occupational adjustment or job retraining.

Hannaford A et al. Ulnar neuropathy. Handb Clin Neurol. 2024;201:103. [PMID: 38697734]

4. Radial Nerve Lesions

The radial nerve can be injured anywhere along its length. It is liable to compression in the axilla (eg, by crutches). This leads to weakness or paralysis of all the muscles supplied by the nerve, including the triceps and the wrist and finger extensors. Sensory changes may also occur but are often surprisingly inconspicuous, being marked only in a small area on the back of the hand between the thumb and index finger. Injuries to the radial nerve in the spiral groove of the humerus occur characteristically during deep sleep, as in intoxicated individuals, but there is sparing of the triceps muscle, which is supplied more proximally. Radial nerve injuries at the elbow may affect the purely motor posterior interosseous branch, which supplies some wrist extensors and all finger extensors. There is sparing of the extensor carpi radialis longus, so that the wrist deviates radially when extended. The superficial radial nerve may be compressed by handcuffs or a tight watch strap, resulting in paresthesias and sensory loss over the dorsal lateral aspect of the hand and dorsal first three-and-a-half fingers.

Chalk C. Radial neuropathy. Handb Clin Neurol. 2024;201:127. [PMID: 38697735]

5. Femoral Neuropathy

The clinical features of femoral nerve palsy consist of weakness and wasting of the quadriceps muscle, with sensory impairment over the anteromedian aspect of the thigh and sometimes also of the leg to the medial malleolus, and a depressed or absent knee jerk. Isolated femoral neuropathy may occur in patients with diabetes or from compression by retroperitoneal neoplasms or hematomas (eg, expanding aortic aneurysm). Femoral neuropathy may also result from pressure from the inguinal ligament when the thighs are markedly flexed and abducted, as in the lithotomy position.

Chalk C et al. Femoral and obturator neuropathies. Handb Clin Neurol. 2024;201:183. [PMID: 38697739]

6. Meralgia Paresthetica

The **lateral femoral cutaneous nerve**, a sensory nerve arising from the L2 and L3 roots, may be compressed or stretched in patients with obesity or diabetes and during pregnancy. The nerve usually runs under the outer portion of the inguinal ligament to reach the thigh, but the ligament sometimes splits to enclose it. Hyperextension of the hip or increased lumbar lordosis—such as occurs during pregnancy—leads to nerve compression by the posterior fascicle of the ligament. However, entrapment of the nerve at any point along its course may cause similar symptoms, and several other anatomic variations predispose the nerve to damage when it is stretched. Pain, paresthesia, or numbness occurs about the outer aspect of the thigh, usually unilaterally, and is sometimes relieved by sitting. The pain stops at the knee, unlike the pain from lower lumbar sciatica that radiates to the foot. Examination shows no abnormalities except in severe cases when cutaneous sensation is impaired in the affected area. Symptoms are usually mild and commonly settle spontaneously. Hydrocortisone injections medial to the anterosuperior iliac spine often relieve symptoms temporarily, while ultrasound-guided hydrodissection with 5% dextrose or surgical nerve decompression may provide more lasting relief.

Xu H et al. A randomized double-blind trial of 5% dextrose versus corticosteroid hydrodissection for meralgia paresthetica. Pain Physician. 2024;27:E835. [PMID: 39621981]

7. Sciatic & Fibular (Common Peroneal) Nerve Palsies

Misplaced deep intramuscular injections are likely the most common cause of sciatic nerve palsy. Trauma to the buttock, hip, or thigh may also be responsible. The resulting clinical deficit depends on whether the whole nerve has been affected or only certain fibers. In general, the fibular fibers of the sciatic nerve are more susceptible to damage than those destined for the tibial nerve. A sciatic nerve lesion may therefore be difficult to distinguish from fibular neuropathy unless there is electromyographic evidence of involvement of the short head of the biceps femoris muscle. The fibular nerve itself may be compressed or injured in the region of the head and neck of the fibula, eg, by sitting with crossed legs or wearing high boots. There is weakness of dorsiflexion and eversion of the foot, accompanied by numbness or blunted sensation of the anterolateral aspect of the calf and dorsum of the foot. If there is poor motor recovery, surgical treatments such as tendon transfer may improve function.

Benstead TJ. Fibular (peroneal) neuropathy. Handb Clin Neurol. 2024;201:149. [PMID: 38697737]

8. Tarsal Tunnel Syndrome

The tibial nerve, the other branch of the sciatic, supplies several muscles in the lower extremity, gives origin to the sural nerve, and then continues as the posterior tibial nerve to supply the plantar flexors of the foot and toes. It passes through the tarsal tunnel behind and below the medial malleolus, giving off calcaneal branches and the medial and lateral plantar nerves that supply small muscles of the foot and the skin on the plantar aspect of the foot and toes. Compression of the posterior tibial nerve or its branches between the bony floor and ligamentous roof of the tarsal tunnel leads to pain, paresthesias, and numbness over the bottom of the foot, especially at night, with sparing of the heel. Muscle weakness may be hard to recognize clinically. Compressive lesions of the individual plantar nerves may also occur more distally, with clinical features similar to those of the tarsal tunnel syndrome. Treatment is surgical decompression.

Miller TA et al. Sciatic and tibial neuropathies. Handb Clin Neurol. 2024;201:165. [PMID: 38697738]

When to Refer

- If there is uncertainty about the diagnosis.
- Symptoms or signs are progressing despite treatment.

BELL PALSY

ESSENTIALS OF DIAGNOSIS

- Sudden onset of lower motor neuron facial palsy.
- Hyperacusis or impaired taste may occur.
- No other neurologic abnormalities.

General Considerations

Bell palsy is an *idiopathic facial paresis of lower motor neuron type* that has been attributed to an inflammatory reaction involving the facial nerve near the stylomastoid foramen or in the bony facial canal. In some instances, this may be due to reactivation of herpes simplex or varicella zoster virus infection in the geniculate ganglion. The disorder is more common in pregnant persons and in persons with diabetes mellitus.

Clinical Findings

The facial paresis (Figure 27–1) generally comes on abruptly, but it may worsen over the following day or so. Pain about the ear precedes or accompanies the weakness in many cases but usually lasts for only a few days. The face itself feels stiff and pulled to one side. There may be ipsilateral restriction of eye closure and difficulty with eating and fine facial movements. A disturbance of taste is common, owing to involvement of chorda tympani fibers, and hyperacusis due to involvement of fibers to the stapedius occurs occasionally. In cases due to herpes zoster infection, vesicles may be observed in the external ear canal.

Differential Diagnosis

Lower motor neuron facial palsy can be differentiated from stroke by clinical examination. A stroke or other central lesion will not cause hyperacusis or disturbance of taste, generally spares the forehead, and is accompanied by other focal deficits. An isolated facial palsy may occur in patients with HIV seropositivity, sarcoidosis, Lyme disease (Figure 27–1; also see Chapter 38), or any process causing an inflammatory reaction in the subarachnoid space, such as meningitis. Whenever facial palsies occur bilaterally, or a facial palsy occurs in conjunction with other neurologic deficits, MRI brain imaging should be undertaken and other investigations considered.

Treatment

Approximately 60% of cases of Bell palsy recover completely without treatment, presumably because the lesion is so mild that it leads merely to conduction block. Treatment with corticosteroids (prednisone 60 mg orally daily for 5 days followed by a 5-day taper, or prednisolone 25 mg orally twice daily for 10 days) increases the chance of a complete recovery at 9–12 months by 12–15%. *Treatment with acyclovir or valacyclovir is only indicated when there is evidence of herpetic vesicles in the external ear canal.* It is helpful to protect the eye with lubricating drops (or lubricating ointment at night) and a patch if eye closure is not possible. There is no evidence that surgical procedures to decompress the facial nerve are of benefit. Physical therapy may improve facial function.

Varelas EA et al. Physical therapy for idiopathic facial paralysis: a systematic review. Am J Otolaryngol. 2024;46:104511. [PMID: 39647183]

DISCOGENIC NECK PAIN

ESSENTIALS OF DIAGNOSIS

- Neck pain, sometimes radiating to arms.
- Restricted neck movements.
- Motor, sensory, or reflex changes in arms with root involvement.
- Neurologic deficit in legs, gait disorder, or sphincter disturbance with cord involvement.

General Considerations

A variety of congenital abnormalities may involve the cervical spine and lead to neck pain; these include hemivertebrae, fused vertebrae, basilar impression, and instability of the atlantoaxial joint. Traumatic, degenerative, infective, and neoplastic disorders may also lead to pain in the neck. When rheumatoid arthritis involves the spine, it tends to affect especially the cervical region, leading to pain, stiffness, and reduced mobility; displacement of vertebrae or atlantoaxial subluxation may lead to cord compression that can be life-threatening if not treated by fixation. Further details are given in Chapter 43 and discussion here is restricted to disk disease.

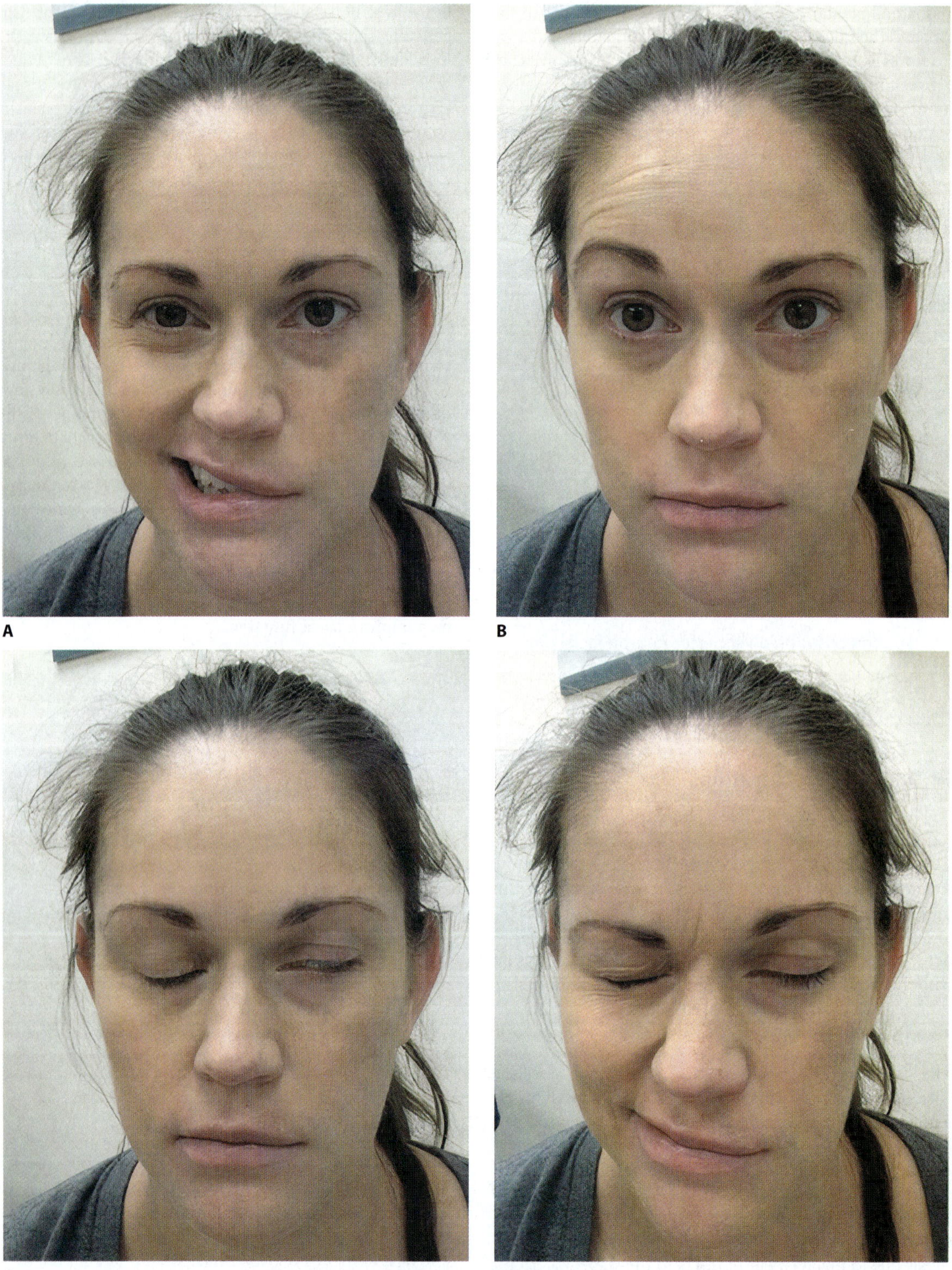

▲ **Figure 27–1.** Left-sided lower motor neuron pattern facial weakness (due to Bell palsy). (Reproduced with permission from Berkowitz AL. *Clinical Neurology & Neuroanatomy: A Localization-Based Approach,* 2nd ed. McGraw-Hill, 2022.)

1. Acute Cervical Disk Protrusion

Acute cervical disk protrusion leads to pain in the neck and radicular pain in the arm, exacerbated by head movement. With lateral herniation of the disk, motor, sensory, or reflex changes may be found in a radicular (usually C6 or C7) distribution on the affected side (Figure 27–2); with more centrally directed herniations, the spinal cord may also be involved, leading to spastic paraparesis and sensory disturbances in the legs, sometimes accompanied by impaired sphincter function. The diagnosis is confirmed by MRI or CT myelography. In mild cases, the prognosis is good and complete recovery occurs in most patients with conservative therapy. Evidence does not support any specific intervention, and some combination of bed rest, activity restriction, immobilization of the neck in a collar for several weeks, and physical therapy is generally prescribed. If these measures are unsuccessful or the patient has a significant neurologic deficit, surgical removal of the protruding disk may be necessary.

2. Cervical Spondylosis

Cervical spondylosis results from chronic cervical disk degeneration, with herniation of disk material, secondary calcification, and associated osteophytic outgrowths. One or more of the cervical nerve roots may be compressed, stretched, or angulated; and myelopathy may also develop as a result of compression, vascular insufficiency, or recurrent minor trauma to the cord. Patients present with neck pain and restricted head movement, occipital headaches, radicular pain and other sensory disturbances in the arms, weakness of the arms or legs, or some combination of these symptoms. Examination generally reveals that lateral flexion and rotation of the neck are limited. A segmental pattern of weakness or dermatomal sensory loss (or both) may be found unilaterally or bilaterally in the upper limbs, and tendon reflexes mediated by the affected root or roots are depressed. The C5 and C6 nerve roots are most commonly involved, and examination frequently then reveals weakness of muscles supplied by these roots (eg, deltoids, supraspinatus and infraspinatus, biceps, brachioradialis), pain or sensory loss about the shoulder and outer border of the arm and forearm, and depressed biceps and brachioradialis reflexes. Spastic paraparesis may also be present if there is an associated myelopathy, sometimes accompanied by urinary urgency, incontinence, or posterior column or spinothalamic sensory deficits in the legs.

Plain radiographs of the cervical spine show osteophyte formation, narrowing of disk spaces, and encroachment on the intervertebral foramina, but such changes are common in middle-aged persons and may be unrelated to the presenting complaint. CT or MRI helps confirm the diagnosis and exclude other structural causes of the myelopathy.

Restriction of neck movements by a cervical collar may relieve pain. Local injection of anesthetics or corticosteroids by a pain management specialist may be of benefit. Operative treatment may be necessary to prevent further progression if there is a significant neurologic deficit; if there are bowel or bladder symptoms; or if root pain is severe, persistent, and unresponsive to conservative measures.

When to Refer

- Pain unresponsive to simple measures.
- Patients with neurologic deficits.
- Patients in whom surgical treatment is under consideration.

When to Admit

- Patients with progressive or significant neurologic deficit.
- Patients with sphincter involvement (from cord compression).
- Patients requiring surgical treatment.

Hejrati N et al. Degenerative cervical myelopathy: where have we been? Where are we now? Where are we going? Acta Neurochir (Wien). 2023;165:1105. [PMID: 37004568]

BRACHIAL & LUMBAR PLEXUS LESIONS

1. Brachial Plexus Neuropathy

Brachial plexus neuropathy may be idiopathic, sometimes occurring in relationship to a number of different nonspecific illnesses or factors. In other instances, brachial plexus lesions follow trauma or result from congenital anomalies, neoplastic involvement, or injury by various physical agents. In rare instances, the disorder occurs on a familial basis.

Idiopathic brachial plexus neuropathy (**neuralgic amyotrophy**) characteristically begins with severe pain about the shoulder, followed within a few days by weakness, reflex changes, and sensory disturbances involving especially the C5 and C6 segments but affecting any nerve in the brachial plexus. Symptoms and signs are usually unilateral but may be bilateral. Wasting of affected muscles is sometimes profound. The disorder relates to disturbed function of cervical roots or part of the brachial plexus, but its precise cause is unknown. Recovery occurs over the ensuing months but may be incomplete. Treatment is purely symptomatic, although emerging evidence suggests that microsurgical neurolysis of hourglass-like constrictions on affected nerves identified by magnetic resonance neurography or high-resolution ultrasound improves outcome in patients who have not recovered after several months of conservative management.

Gabet JM et al. Neuralgic amyotrophy: an update in evaluation, diagnosis, and treatment approaches. Muscle Nerve. 2025;71:846. [PMID: 39402917]

2. Cervical Rib Syndrome

Compression of the C8 and T1 roots or the lower trunk of the brachial plexus by a cervical rib or band arising from the seventh cervical vertebra leads to weakness and wasting of intrinsic hand muscles, especially those in the thenar eminence, accompanied by pain and numbness in the medial two fingers and the ulnar border of the hand and forearm. Electromyography, nerve conduction studies, and somatosensory evoked potential studies may help confirm the diagnosis.

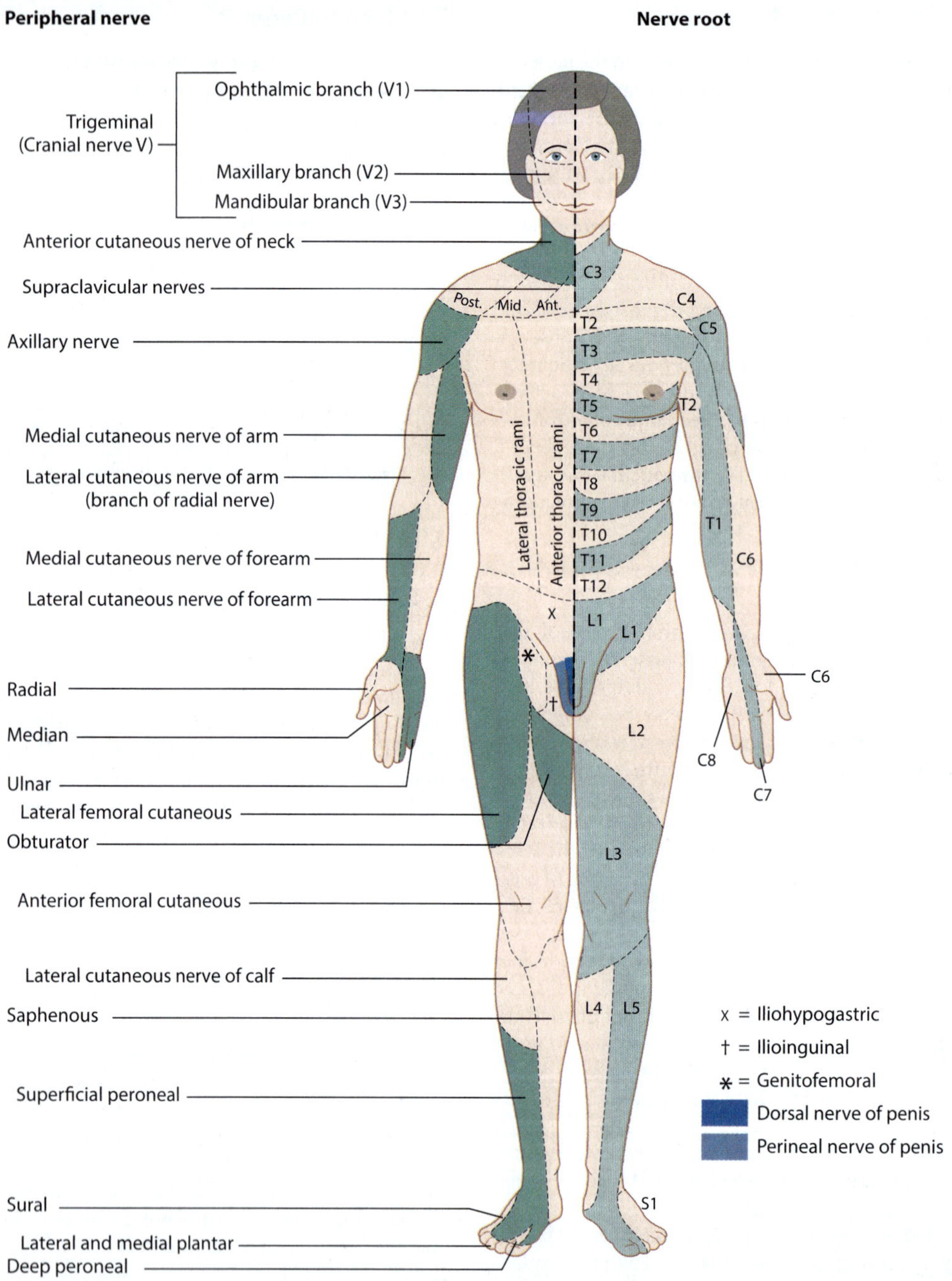

▲ **Figure 27–2.** Cutaneous innervation. The segmental or radicular (root) distribution is shown on the left side of the body and the peripheral nerve distribution on the right side. Segmental maps show differences depending on how they were constructed (single root stimulation or section; local anesthetic injection into single dorsal root ganglia). (Reproduced with permission from Aminoff MJ, Greenberg DA, Simon RP. *Clinical Neurology*, 9th ed. McGraw-Hill Education, 2015.)

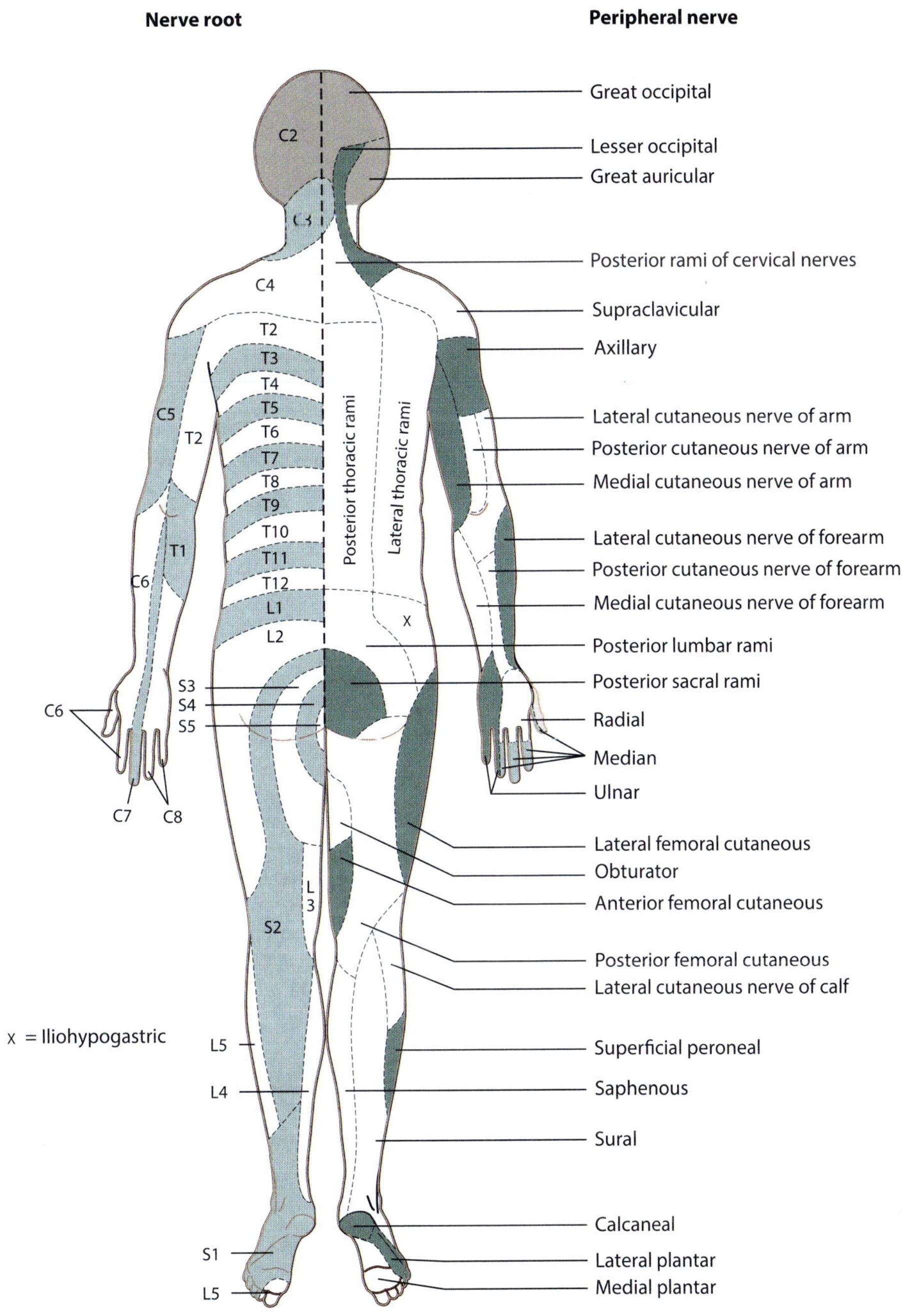

Figure 27–2. *(Continued)*

MRI may be especially helpful in revealing the underlying compressive structure. Plain radiographs or CT scanning sometimes shows the cervical rib or a large transverse process of the seventh cervical vertebra, but normal findings do not exclude the possibility of a cervical band. Treatment of the disorder is by surgical excision of the rib or band.

Khoury MK et al. Systematic review of intermediate and long-term results of thoracic outlet decompression. Semin Vasc Surg. 2024;37:90. [PMID: 38704189]

3. Lumbosacral Plexus Lesions

A lumbosacral plexus lesion may develop in association with diseases such as diabetes, cancer, or bleeding disorders or in relation to injury. It occasionally occurs as an isolated phenomenon similar to idiopathic brachial plexopathy (**nondiabetic lumbosacral radiculoplexus neuropathy**), and pain and weakness then tend to be more conspicuous than sensory symptoms. The distribution of symptoms and signs depends on the level and pattern of neurologic involvement.

McCray BA et al. Atypical diabetic neuropathies. BMJ. 2025;390:e081109. [PMID: 41022466]

DISORDERS OF NEUROMUSCULAR TRANSMISSION

1. Myasthenia Gravis

ESSENTIALS OF DIAGNOSIS

- Fluctuating weakness of commonly used voluntary muscles, producing symptoms such as diplopia, ptosis, and difficulty in swallowing.
- Activity increases weakness of affected muscles.
- Short-acting anticholinesterases transiently improve the weakness.

General Considerations

Myasthenia gravis occurs at all ages, *sometimes in association with a thymic tumor or thyrotoxicosis*, as well as in rheumatoid arthritis and lupus erythematosus. It is most common in young women with HLA-DR3; if thymoma is associated, older men are more commonly affected. Onset is usually insidious, but the disorder is sometimes unmasked by a coincidental infection that leads to exacerbation of symptoms. Exacerbations may also occur before the menstrual period and during or shortly after pregnancy. Symptoms are due to a variable degree of block of neuromuscular transmission caused by autoantibodies binding to acetylcholine receptors; these are found in most patients with the disease and have a primary role in reducing the number of functioning acetylcholine receptors. Additionally, cellular immune activity against the receptor is found.

Clinical Findings

A. Symptoms and Signs

Patients present with ptosis, diplopia, difficulty in chewing or swallowing, respiratory difficulties, limb weakness, or some combination of these problems. Weakness may remain localized to a few muscle groups or may become generalized. The external ocular muscles and certain other cranial muscles, including the masticatory, facial, and pharyngeal muscles, are especially likely to be affected, and the respiratory and limb muscles may also be involved. Symptoms often fluctuate in intensity during the day, and this diurnal variation is superimposed on a tendency to longer-term spontaneous relapses and remissions that may last for weeks. Nevertheless, the disorder follows a slowly progressive course and may have a fatal outcome owing to respiratory complications such as aspiration pneumonia.

Clinical examination confirms the weakness and fatigability of affected muscles. In most cases, the extraocular muscles are involved, and this leads to ocular palsies and ptosis, which are commonly asymmetric. Pupillary responses are normal. The bulbar and limb muscles are often weak, but the pattern of involvement is variable. Sustained activity of affected muscles increases the weakness, which improves after a brief rest. Sensation is normal, and there are usually no reflex changes.

Life-threatening exacerbations of myasthenia (so-called **myasthenic crisis**) may lead to respiratory weakness requiring immediate admission to the ICU, where respiratory function can be monitored and ventilator support is readily available.

B. Laboratory and Other Studies

Assay of serum for elevated levels of circulating **acetylcholine receptor antibodies** is useful because it has a sensitivity of 80–90% for the diagnosis of myasthenia gravis. Certain patients without antibodies to acetylcholine receptors have serum antibodies to muscle-specific tyrosine kinase (MuSK), which should therefore be determined; these patients are more likely to have facial, respiratory, and proximal muscle weakness than those with antibodies to acetylcholine receptors. Rarely, patients with myasthenia gravis may have antibodies to the LDL receptor-related protein 4 (LRP4), which can be tested in those who are double seronegative.

Electrophysiologic demonstration of a decrementing muscle response to repetitive 2- or 3-Hz stimulation of motor nerves indicates a disturbance of neuromuscular transmission. Such an abnormality may even be detected in clinically strong muscles with certain provocative procedures. Needle electromyography of affected muscles shows a marked variation in configuration and size of individual motor unit potentials, and single-fiber electromyography reveals an increased jitter, or variability, in the time interval between two muscle fiber action potentials from the same motor unit. Electrodiagnostic confirmation is helpful in all suspected cases, and especially when serologic testing is negative or when rapid diagnosis is needed.

C. Imaging

A CT scan of the chest with and without contrast should be obtained to demonstrate a coexisting thymoma.

Treatment

Anticholinesterase medications provide symptomatic benefit without influencing the course of the disease. Neostigmine, pyridostigmine, or both can be used, the dose being determined on an individual basis. The usual dose of neostigmine is 7.5–30 mg (average, 15 mg) orally taken four times daily; of pyridostigmine, 30–180 mg (average, 60 mg) orally four times daily. Overmedication may temporarily increase weakness. A wide range of medications (eg, aminoglycosides) may exacerbate myasthenia gravis and should be avoided.

Thymectomy should be performed when a thymoma is present. A multicenter randomized trial demonstrated the benefit of thymectomy even in the absence of a radiologically identifiable thymoma, with improved strength, lower immunosuppression requirements, and fewer hospitalizations in the surgically treated group. Thus, *thymectomy should be considered in all patients younger than age 65 unless weakness is restricted to the extraocular muscles.* If the disease is of recent onset and only slowly progressive, operation is sometimes delayed for a year or so, in the hope that spontaneous remission will occur.

Treatment with corticosteroids is indicated for patients who have responded poorly to anticholinesterase medications. Some patients experience transient exacerbation of weakness and even develop respiratory failure within the first 1–2 weeks if corticosteroids are initiated at high doses (eg, prednisone 1 mg/kg/day). Therefore, in stable patients, corticosteroids are introduced gradually in the outpatient setting. Prednisone can be started at 20 mg orally daily and increased by 10 mg increments weekly to a target of 1 mg/kg/day (maximum daily dose 100 mg). Corticosteroids can be prescribed as alternate-day or daily treatment, with alternate-day therapy potentially mitigating side effects. Once the patient has stabilized at the initial high dose, corticosteroids can gradually be tapered to a relatively low maintenance level (eg, < 7.5 mg prednisone orally daily) as improvement occurs; total withdrawal is difficult, however.

In patients who do not achieve normal clinical function at a low maintenance level of corticosteroids, treatment with a steroid-sparing agent should be initiated. Azathioprine is commonly used; the usual dose is 2–3 mg/kg orally daily after initiation at a lower dose. Other immunosuppressive agents that are used in myasthenia gravis to reduce the corticosteroid dose include mycophenolate mofetil, rituximab, cyclosporine, methotrexate, and tacrolimus. Efgartigimod, rozanolixizumab, and nipocalimab act at the neonatal Fc receptor and reduce circulating IgG, improving motor function within weeks of administration. All are approved by the FDA for acetylcholine antibody–positive myasthenia, and rozanolixizumab and nipocalimab are also approved for patients with MuSK-positive myasthenia. Three complement inhibitors (zilucoplan, ravulizumab, and eculizumab) are approved by the FDA for patients who are acetylcholine receptor antibody positive; a beneficial effect on muscle strength is usually observed within several weeks of starting therapy. Patients must be vaccinated against meningococcus before receiving them. While their role in therapy is still being defined, both neonatal Fc receptor inhibitors and complement inhibitors may be useful while awaiting the effect of thymectomy and long-term immunosuppression with medications such as azathioprine, as rescue therapy in refractory disease, or for patients intolerant of other therapies.

In patients with major disability or weakness requiring ventilatory support (ie, myasthenic crisis), plasmapheresis or IVIG are beneficial, have similar efficacy, and usually yield improved strength within one week. These therapies are also useful for stabilizing patients before thymectomy. Because their beneficial effect only lasts several weeks, patients in crisis should also be treated with corticosteroids with or without a steroid-sparing agent to establish long-term control. Corticosteroids may be started at 1 mg/kg orally in patients recently treated with plasmapheresis or IVIG. Retreatment with plasmapheresis or IVIG every 2 to 4 weeks may be necessary until stabilization with corticosteroids or a steroid-sparing agent is achieved. The neonatal Fc receptor inhibitors and complement inhibitors may also have a role in myasthenic crisis, owing to their rapid onset of action.

Juel VC. Autoimmune myasthenia gravis. Continuum (Minneap Minn). 2025;31:1270. [PMID: 41037173]

2. Myasthenic Syndrome (Lambert-Eaton Myasthenic Syndrome)

ESSENTIALS OF DIAGNOSIS

- Variable weakness, typically improving with activity.
- Dysautonomic symptoms may also be present.
- A history of malignant disease may be obtained.

Clinical Findings

Myasthenic syndrome *may be associated with small cell carcinoma,* sometimes developing before the tumor is diagnosed, and occasionally occurs with certain autoimmune diseases. There is defective release of acetylcholine in response to a nerve impulse, caused by P/Q-type voltage-gated calcium channel antibodies, and this leads to weakness, especially of the proximal muscles of the limbs. Unlike myasthenia gravis, however, power steadily increases with sustained contraction. The diagnosis can be confirmed electrophysiologically, because the muscle response to stimulation of its motor nerve increases remarkably after exercise or if the nerve is stimulated repetitively at high rates (50 Hz), even in muscles that are not clinically weak.

Treatment

Treatment with IVIG, plasmapheresis, and immunosuppressive medication therapy (prednisone and azathioprine) may lead to clinical and electrophysiologic improvement, in addition to therapy aimed at the tumor when present. Prednisone is usually initiated in a daily dose of 60–80 mg orally and azathioprine in a daily dose of 2 mg/kg orally. Symptomatic therapy includes the use of potassium channel antagonists; of these, amifampridine is a 3,4-diaminopyridine (15–80 mg/day orally in three divided doses) and is approved in the United States and Europe. Guanidine hydrochloride (25–50 mg/kg/day orally in divided doses) is an alternative and is occasionally helpful in patients with serious disability, but adverse effects of the medication include marrow suppression. The response to treatment with anticholinesterase medications such as pyridostigmine or neostigmine is usually disappointing.

Lipka AF. Lambert-Eaton myasthenic syndrome. Handb Clin Neurol. 2024;200:307. [PMID: 38494285]

3. Botulism

The toxin of *Clostridium botulinum* prevents the release of acetylcholine at neuromuscular junctions and autonomic synapses. Botulism occurs most commonly following the ingestion of contaminated home-canned food; outbreaks have also occurred among drug abusers due to wound infection after injection of contaminated heroin. The diagnosis should be suggested by the development of sudden, fluctuating, severe weakness with preserved sensation in a previously healthy person. Symptoms begin within 72 hours following ingestion of the toxin and may progress for several days. Typically, there is diplopia, ptosis, facial weakness, dysphagia, and nasal speech, followed by respiratory difficulty and finally by weakness that appears last in the limbs. Blurring of vision (with unreactive dilated pupils) is characteristic, and there may be dryness of the mouth, constipation (paralytic ileus), and postural hypotension. The tendon reflexes are not affected unless the involved muscles are weak. If the diagnosis is suspected, the local health authority should be notified and a sample of serum and contaminated food (if available) sent to be assayed for toxin. Support for the diagnosis may be obtained by electrophysiologic studies; with repetitive stimulation of motor nerves at fast rates, the muscle response increases in size progressively.

Patients should be hospitalized in case respiratory assistance becomes necessary. Treatment is with heptavalent antitoxin, in patients without known allergy to horse serum. Potassium channel antagonists may provide symptomatic relief as they do in Lambert-Eaton myasthenic syndrome. Anticholinesterase medications are of no value. Respiratory assistance and other supportive measures should be provided as necessary. Further details are provided in Chapter 37.

Ramdas S. Botulism, Lambert-Eaton myasthenic syndrome, and congenital myasthenic syndromes. Continuum (Minneap Minn). 2025;31:1303. [PMID: 41037175]

4. Disorders Associated with Use of Aminoglycosides

Aminoglycoside antibiotics (eg, gentamicin) may produce a clinical disturbance similar to botulism by preventing the release of acetylcholine from nerve endings, but symptoms subside rapidly as the responsible medication is eliminated from the body. These antibiotics are dangerous in patients with preexisting disturbances of neuromuscular transmission and are therefore best avoided in patients with myasthenia gravis.

When to Refer

All patients should be referred.

When to Admit

- Patients with suspected botulism, acute exacerbation of myasthenia gravis, or respiratory involvement.
- Patients requiring plasmapheresis.
- For thymectomy.

MYOPATHIC DISORDERS

ESSENTIALS OF DIAGNOSIS

- Muscle weakness without sensory loss, often in a characteristic distribution.
- Serum creatine kinase elevated in most cases.
- Age at onset, time course, and inheritance pattern may suggest underlying disorder.

General Considerations

Myopathies can be inherited or acquired. Acquired myopathies often present acutely or subacutely while inherited myopathies are typically insidious in onset. Patients typically describe *weakness affecting proximal muscles*, such as difficulty climbing stairs, arising from a chair, or reaching overhead, or of head drop. Sensory symptoms are absent. A detailed family history is required.

Examination shows weakness of proximal muscles. In some cases, there is a more specific pattern of weakness (eg, quadriceps and finger flexor weakness in inclusion body myositis). Extraocular muscle involvement is rarely seen, except in certain mitochondrial disorders, oculopharyngeal muscular dystrophy, and hyperthyroidism; when present, it should suggest the possibility of a neuromuscular junction disorder. Reflexes are normal or diminished in proportion to the degree of weakness. Sensation is normal.

Initial testing should include serum creatine kinase determination. Consider testing TSH, cortisol, vitamin D, and calcium. Antibodies specific to certain inflammatory myopathies and connective tissue disease can be checked when these conditions are suspected and may obviate the need for muscle biopsy (see Chapter 23). Electromyography will reveal small motor units and early recruitment; it is helpful in confirming the localization of weakness to the muscle and suggesting a suitable site for biopsy, as does MRI. The electromyographic findings may be normal in corticosteroid and mitochondrial myopathies. Muscle biopsy establishes the diagnosis when inflammatory, mitochondrial, metabolic, or certain inherited myopathies are suspected. In cases where the family history or pattern of weakness suggests a specific genetic disorder, genetic testing can be pursued directly and biopsy may not be needed. Selected common and treatable myopathies are discussed below.

1. Muscular Dystrophies

These inherited myopathic disorders are subdivided by mode of inheritance, age at onset, and clinical features, as shown in Table 27–11. In the **Duchenne type**, pseudohypertrophy of muscles frequently occurs at some stage; intellectual disability is common; and there may be skeletal deformities, muscle contractures, and cardiac involvement. A genetic defect on the short arm of the X chromosome has been identified in Duchenne dystrophy. The affected gene codes for the protein dystrophin, which is markedly reduced or absent from the muscle of patients with the disease.

Table 27–11. Selected muscular dystrophies.[1]

Disorder	Inheritance	Age at Onset (years)	Distribution	Prognosis	Genetic Association
Duchenne type	X-linked recessive	1–5	Pelvic, then shoulder girdle; later, limb and respiratory muscles.	Rapid progression. Death within about 15 years after onset.	Xp21; Dystrophin (loss of functional expression).
Becker	X-linked recessive	5–25	Pelvic, then shoulder girdle.	Slow progression. May have normal life span.	Xp21; Dystrophin (reduced functional expression).
Limb-girdle (Erb)	Autosomal recessive, dominant, or sporadic	10–30	Pelvic or shoulder girdle initially, with later spread to the other.	Variable severity and rate of progression. Possible severe disability in middle life.	Multiple.
Facioscapulohumeral	Autosomal dominant	Any age	Face and shoulder girdle initially; later, pelvic girdle and legs.	Slow progression. Minor disability. Usually normal life span.	4q35.2; Double homeobox protein 4. 18p11.32; Structural maintenance of chromosome's flexible hinge domain-containing protein 1.
Emery-Dreifuss	X-linked recessive or autosomal dominant	5–10	Humeroperoneal or scapuloperoneal.	Variable.	Multiple.
Distal	Autosomal dominant or recessive	40–60	Onset distally in extremities; proximal involvement later.	Slow progression.	Multiple.
Oculopharyngeal	Autosomal dominant	Any age	Ptosis, external ophthalmoplegia, and dysphagia.	Slow progression.	14q11.2–q13; Poly (A)-binding protein-2.
Myotonic dystrophy	Autosomal dominant	Any age (usually 20–40)	Face, neck, distal limbs.	Slow progression.	19q13.32; Myotonin-protein kinase. 3q21.3; Cellular nucleic acid-binding protein.

[1]Not all possible genetic loci are shown.

Dystrophin levels are generally normal in the **Becker** variety, but the protein is qualitatively altered. The diagnosis is usually made with genetic testing; muscle biopsy is needed occasionally. Duchenne muscular dystrophy can be recognized early in pregnancy in about 95% of women by genetic studies; in late pregnancy, DNA probes can be used on fetal tissue obtained for this purpose by amniocentesis.

Four antisense oligonucleotides are approved by the FDA for treatment of Duchenne muscular dystrophy. Patients treated with these antisense oligonucleotides had more functional dystrophin on muscle biopsy than controls and a slower rate of disease progression than matched historical controls. A viral vector transgene encoding a microdystrophin protein, delandistrogene moxeparvovec, increases microdystrophin production and may improve functional outcomes; it is approved by the FDA for ambulatory boys but severe complications may occur. Prednisone (0.75 mg/kg orally daily or 10 mg/kg orally given weekly over 2 days) or deflazacort (0.9 mg/kg orally daily) improves muscle strength and function in boys with Duchenne dystrophy, but side effects need to be monitored. Although both corticosteroid preparations cause similar side effects, weight gain at 1 year is less with deflazacort. Vamorolone (6 mg/kg once daily; maximum daily dose 300 mg) is a novel oral corticosteroid approved for patients ≥ 2 years of age. It is as effective as prednisone but with fewer adverse effects. Givinostat (22.2–53.2 mg twice daily based on body weight) is an oral histone deacetylase inhibitor approved for patients > 6 years of age. In an RCT, it slowed decline over 72 weeks compared with placebo. Prolonged bed rest must be avoided, as inactivity often leads to worsening of the underlying muscle disease. Physical therapy and orthopedic procedures may help counteract deformities or contractures.

Dang UJ et al. Efficacy and safety of vamorolone over 48 weeks in boys with Duchenne muscular dystrophy: a randomized controlled trial. Neurology. 2024;102:e208112. [PMID: 38335499]

Mercuri E et al. Safety and efficacy of givinostat in boys with Duchenne muscular dystrophy (EPIDYS): a multicentre, randomised, double-blind, placebo-controlled, phase 3 trial. Lancet Neurol. 2024;23:393. [PMID: 38508835]

2. Myotonic Dystrophy

Myotonic dystrophy, a slowly progressive, dominantly inherited disorder, usually manifests itself in the third or fourth decade but occasionally appears early in childhood. Two types, with a different genetic basis, have been recognized. Myotonia leads to complaints of muscle stiffness and is evidenced by the marked delay that occurs before affected muscles can relax after a contraction. This can often be demonstrated clinically by delayed relaxation of the hand after sustained grip or by percussion of the belly of a muscle. In addition, there is weakness and wasting of the facial, sternocleidomastoid, and distal limb muscles. Associated clinical features include cataracts, frontal baldness, testicular atrophy, diabetes mellitus, cardiac abnormalities, and intellectual changes. Electromyographic sampling of affected muscles reveals myotonic discharges in addition to changes suggestive of myopathy.

It is difficult to determine whether medication therapy for myotonia is safe or effective. When myotonia is disabling, treatment with a sodium channel blocker—such as phenytoin (100 mg orally three times daily), lamotrigine (slowly titrated to 150 mg orally twice daily), procainamide (0.5–1 g orally four times daily), or mexiletine (150–200 mg orally three times daily)—may be helpful, but the associated side effects, particularly for antiarrhythmic medications, are often limiting. Neither the weakness nor the course of the disorder is influenced by treatment. Cardiac function should be monitored, and pacemaker placement may be considered if there is evidence of heart block.

Perez PG. Myotonic dystrophy. Continuum (Minneap Minn). 2025;31:1437. [PMID:41037177]

3. Myotonia Congenita

Myotonia congenita is commonly inherited as a dominant trait. Generalized myotonia without weakness is usually present from birth, but symptoms may not appear until early childhood. Patients report muscle stiffness that is enhanced by cold and inactivity and relieved by exercise. Muscle hypertrophy, at times pronounced, is also a feature. A recessive form with later onset is associated with slight weakness and atrophy of distal muscles. Mexiletine, procainamide, lamotrigine, phenytoin, and carbamazepine may help the myotonia, as in myotonic dystrophy.

Spillane J et al. Drug treatment for myotonia. Cochrane Database Syst Rev. 2025;4:CD004762. [PMID: 40197813]

4. Mitochondrial Myopathies

The mitochondrial myopathies are a clinically diverse group of disorders that on pathologic examination of skeletal muscle with the modified Gomori stain show characteristic "ragged red fibers" containing accumulations of abnormal mitochondria. Patients may present with progressive external ophthalmoplegia or with limb weakness that is exacerbated or induced by activity. Other patients present with central neurologic dysfunction, eg, myoclonic epilepsy (**myoclonic epilepsy, ragged red fiber syndrome**, or **MERRF**), or the combination of myopathy, encephalopathy, lactic acidosis, and stroke-like episodes (**MELAS**). Migraine is a common symptom. Systemic features include but are not limited to diabetes mellitus, hearing loss, retinopathy, cardiomyopathy, gastric dysmotility, and short stature. The serum creatine kinase is usually normal. Mitochondrial myopathies result from variants in mitochondrial or nuclear DNA. There are no approved treatments for these disorders, but coenzyme Q10, creatine, and levocarnitine are often prescribed; arginine is also given to patients with MELAS because it reduced frequency and severity of stroke-like episodes in an open-label trial.

Bangeas A et al. Advances in management of mitochondrial myopathies. Int J of Mol Sci. 2025;26:5411. [PMID: 40508218]

5. Acid Maltase Deficiency (Pompe Disease)

This is a glycogen storage disease due to mutations in the gene encoding acid α-1,4-glucosidase. Age at presentation ranges from infancy to the late fifties and depends on the degree of residual enzyme activity. The juvenile and adult-onset forms present with slowly progressive proximal weakness that includes respiratory failure. Cardiomyopathy is less common in the adult form. Serum creatine kinase is mildly elevated. Muscle biopsy shows glycogen containing lysosomal vacuoles, but the diagnosis is suggested by detecting reduced acid-1,4-α-glucosidase activity on a dried blood spot and then confirmed by genetic testing. Enzyme replacement with recombinant α-glucosidase stabilizes disease progression and results in improvement in respiratory function. Patients who weigh ≥ 40 kg and are not improving on initial enzyme replacement therapy are eligible for treatment with the combination of cipaglucosidase α-atga and miglustat, which demonstrated similar efficacy to alglucosidase-α in a randomized trial.

Schoser B et al. 104-week efficacy and safety of cipaglucosidase alfa plus miglustat in adults with late-onset Pompe disease: a phase III open-label extension study (ATB200-07). J Neurol. 2024;271:2810. [PMID: 38418563]

6. Dermatomyositis, Anti-Synthetase Syndromes, Immune-Mediated Necrotizing Myopathies, & Polymyositis

See Chapter 23.

7. Inclusion Body Myositis

This disorder, of unknown cause, begins insidiously, usually after middle age, with progressive proximal weakness of first the lower and then the upper extremities, and affecting facial and pharyngeal muscles. Weakness often begins in the quadriceps femoris in the lower limbs and the forearm flexors in the upper limbs. Distal weakness is usually mild. Serum creatine kinase levels may be normal or increased. The diagnosis is confirmed by muscle biopsy. Anticytosolic 5'-nucleotidase 1A antibodies are detected in up to one-half of cases and may be associated with a more severe phenotype. Corticosteroid and immunosuppressive therapies are sometimes offered but are usually ineffective, and IVIG therapy is not recommended.

Naddaf E. Inclusion body myositis. Continuum (Minneap Minn). 2025;31:1372. [PMID: 41037166]

8. Endocrine Myopathies

Myopathy is observed with hypo- and hyperthyroidism, Cushing syndrome and disease, Addison disease, vitamin D deficiency, and both hyper- and hypoparathyroidism (the latter mediated by calcium derangements). In hypothyroidism, there may be associated entrapment neuropathies, and examination may show delayed relaxation of tendon reflexes, muscle enlargement, or myoedema. Hyperthyroidism can cause both distal and proximal weakness and rarely a bulbar myopathy. Serum creatine kinase is normal except in hypothyroid myopathy, which can also be painful. Treatment is of the underlying endocrinopathy.

Reda H. Neurologic complications of endocrine disorders. Continuum (Minneap Minn). 2023;29:887. [PMID: 37341334]

9. Critical Illness Myopathy

Myopathy may occur in association with critical illness, typically in patients who received neuromuscular blocking agents and corticosteroids. It is frequently discovered when patients unexpectedly require prolonged ventilatory support. There can be an associated sensorimotor polyneuropathy. Serum creatine kinase may be elevated initially but has frequently returned to normal or is below normal by the time the condition is suspected. Treatment is supportive.

Younger DS. Critical illness-associated weakness and related motor disorders. Handb Clin Neurol. 2023;195:707. [PMID: 37562893]

10. Toxic Myopathies

Myopathy can occur in patients taking aminocaproic acid, amiodarone, chloroquine, colchicine, corticosteroids, cyclosporine, daptomycin, emetine, fibrates, gemcitabine, nucleoside reverse transcriptase inhibitors, or statin medications. Myopathy also occurs with chronic alcohol use disorder, whereas acute reversible muscle necrosis may occur shortly after acute alcohol, cocaine, or methamphetamine intoxication, and with propofol infusion. Inflammatory myopathy may occur in patients taking penicillamine, statins, and can be induced by immune checkpoint inhibitors; preexisting myotonia may be exacerbated or unmasked by depolarizing muscle relaxants (eg, suxamethonium), β-blockers (eg, propranolol), fenoterol and, possibly, certain diuretics. Valproic acid can precipitate or worsen myopathy in patients with mitochondrial disorders or carnitine palmitoyltransferase II deficiency.

Le Quang M et al. Clinical and pathological aspects of toxic myopathies. J Neurol. 2024;271:5722. [PMID: 38907023]

When to Refer

All patients should be referred to establish the diagnosis and underlying cause.

When to Admit

- For respiratory assistance.
- For rhabdomyolysis.

PERIODIC PARALYSIS SYNDROMES

Periodic paralysis may have a familial (dominant inheritance) basis. The syndromes to be described are *channelopathies* that manifest as abnormal, often potassium-sensitive, muscle-membrane excitability and lead clinically to episodes of flaccid weakness or paralysis, sometimes in association with abnormalities of the plasma potassium level. Strength is initially normal between attacks, but progressive myopathic weakness may develop in up to one-third of patients as they age. **Hypokalemic periodic paralysis** is characterized by attacks that tend to occur on awakening, after exercise, or after a heavy meal and may last for several days. An ongoing attack may be aborted by potassium chloride given orally or intravenously, provided the ECG can be monitored and kidney function is satisfactory. A low-carbohydrate and low-salt diet may help prevent attacks, as may potassium supplementation, carbonic anhydrase inhibitors, and potassium sparing diuretics. It can occur in the setting of hyperthyroidism (**thyrotoxic periodic paralysis**) with or without an underlying genetic polymorphism; treatment of the endocrine disorder prevents recurrences. A nonselective β-adrenergic blocker may prevent attacks until the endocrine abnormality has been treated. In **hyperkalemic periodic paralysis,** attacks also tend to occur after exercise but usually last for < 1 hour. They may also be triggered by potassium-rich foods and cold. They may be terminated by intravenous calcium gluconate (1–2 g), intravenous diuretics (furosemide, 20–40 mg), glucose, glucose and insulin, or inhaled β agonists (albuterol 1–2 puffs of a 90 mcg/actuation metered dose inhaler). Thiazide diuretics or carbonic anhydrase inhibitors are used to prevent attacks. **Normokalemic periodic paralysis** is similar clinically to the hyperkalemic variety, but the plasma potassium level remains normal during attacks. Several randomized trials support the use of dichlorphenamide (50–100 mg orally twice daily) for prevention of attacks in both hyper- and hypokalemic periodic paralysis; acetazolamide (250–750 mg orally daily) is also effective.

When to Refer

All patients should be referred.

When to Admit

Patients with prolonged attacks or attacks involving respiration or deglutition requiring intravenous therapy.

Cannon SC. Periodic paralysis. Handb Clin Neurol. 2024;203:39. [PMID: 39174253]

28 Psychiatric Disorders

Kristin S. Raj, MD
Mohamad Matout, MD, MSc
Nolan R. Williams, MD
Charles DeBattista, DMH, MD

The American Psychiatric Association's *DSM-5* is the common language that clinicians use for psychiatric conditions. It utilizes specific criteria with which to objectively assess symptoms for use in clinical diagnosis and communication.

COMMON PSYCHIATRIC DISORDERS

ADJUSTMENT DISORDERS

ESSENTIALS OF DIAGNOSIS

- Anxiety or depression in reaction to an identifiable stress, though out of proportion to the stressor severity.
- Symptoms not as severe as a major depressive episode or do not have the chronicity of generalized anxiety disorder (GAD).

General Considerations

An individual experiences stress when adaptive capacity is overwhelmed by events. The event may be an insignificant one and even favorable changes (eg, promotion and transfer) can produce stress. Stress is subjectively defined, and the response to stress is a function of each person's personality and physiologic endowment.

Clinical Findings

An individual may react to stress by becoming anxious or depressed, by developing a physical symptom, by running away, drinking alcohol, overeating, starting an affair, or in limitless other ways. Common subjective responses are anxiety, sadness, fear, rage, guilt, and shame. Acute and reactivated stress may be manifested by restlessness, irritability, fatigue, increased startle reaction, and a feeling of tension. Inability to concentrate, sleep disturbances (insomnia, bad dreams), and somatic preoccupations sometimes lead to self-medication, most commonly with alcohol or other CNS depressants. Emotional and behavioral distressing symptomatology in response to stress is called **adjustment disorder**, with the major symptom specified (eg, adjustment disorder with depressed mood, with anxiety, with mixed anxiety and depressed mood, with disturbance of conduct, with mixed disturbance of emotions and conduct, and unspecified). Even with an identifiable stressor, if the patient meets criteria for another disorder such as major depression, the convention is to diagnose a major depression and not an adjustment disorder with depressed mood. Risk factors for developing an adjustment disorder include female gender, younger age, unemployed status, stress, physical illness and injury, low social support, and a history of mental health disorders.

Differential Diagnosis

Adjustment disorders are distinguished from anxiety disorders, mood disorders, bereavement, other stress disorders such as PTSD, personality disorders exacerbated by stress, and from somatic disorders with psychic overlay. Unlike many other psychiatric disorders, adjustment disorders are *wholly situational* and usually resolve when the stressor resolves or the individual effectively adapts to the situation. Adjustment disorders may have symptoms that overlap with other disorders, such as anxiety symptoms, but they occur in reaction to an identifiable life stressor. An adjustment disorder that persists and worsens can potentially evolve into another psychiatric disorder such as major depression or GAD. However, that is not the case for most patients. By definition, an adjustment disorder occurs within 3 months of the onset of an identifiable stressor and symptoms do not persist for more than an additional 6 months once the stress or its consequences have terminated.

Treatment

A. Behavioral

Stress reduction techniques include immediate symptom reduction (eg, progressive muscle relaxation or slowed exhalations) or early recognition and removal from a stress source before full-blown symptoms appear. It is often helpful to keep a daily log of stress precipitators, responses, and alleviators. Relaxation, mindfulness-based stress reduction, and exercise techniques are helpful in improving the reaction to stressful events.

B. Social

The stress reactions of life problems are a function of psychosocial upheaval. It is important for the clinician to establish the framework of the problem, since the patient's denial system may obscure the issues. Clarifying the problem in the patient's psychosocial context facilitates the difficult decisions the patient eventually must make (eg, change of job).

C. Psychological

Prolonged psychotherapy is seldom necessary in cases of isolated stress response or adjustment disorder. Supportive psychotherapy with an emphasis on strengthening of existing coping mechanisms is helpful as the patient's own resiliency restores the previous level of function. In addition, cognitive behavioral therapy is helpful to treat acute stress and facilitate recovery. Brief problem-solving therapy can further aid in identifying practical strategies to navigate stressors effectively. Computerized interventions, including virtual reality, internet-based cognitive behavioral modules, and self-guided apps, have shown some efficacy in improving symptoms by enhancing accessibility and engagement..

D. Pharmacologic

Judicious use of anxiolytics (eg, lorazepam, 0.5–1 mg two or three times daily orally) for a limited time can provide relief from acute anxiety symptoms. Short-term use of SSRIs targeting dysphoria and anxiety may be useful.

Emerging evidence supports nonbenzodiazepine anxiolytics, such as etifoxine, as alternatives for acute anxiety management, offering comparable efficacy with reduced risk of dependence upon discontinuation.

Prognosis

Return to satisfactory function after a short period is expected with this syndrome, provided the stressor resolves or is effectively managed. Resolution may be delayed if others' responses to the patient's difficulties are harmful, the secondary gains outweigh the advantages of recovery, or maladaptive coping patterns persist. The longer the symptoms persist, the worse the prognosis, potentially signaling vulnerability to chronic mood or anxiety disorders.

Cowansage KP et al. Treatments for adjustment disorder: a systematic review and meta-analysis of randomized controlled trials. Psychiatry Res. 2025;353:116739. [PMID: 41005147]

Peter C et al. Nature of stressors, clinical manifestations and diagnostic concurrence with the new ICD-11 criteria in adjustment disorder: a retrospective data review. Nord J Psychiatry. 2025;79:175. [PMID: 40013376]

Poremski D et al. The longitudinal dispositions of people diagnosed with adjustment or severe stress disorders. BMC Psychiatry. 2024;24:457. [PMID: 38890697]

Ohi K et al. Is adjustment disorder genetically correlated with depression, anxiety, or risk-tolerant personality trait? J Affect Disord. 2023;340:197. [PMID: 37557993]

TRAUMA & STRESSOR-RELATED DISORDERS

ESSENTIALS OF DIAGNOSIS

- Exposure to a traumatic or life-threatening event.
- Flashbacks, intrusive images, and nightmares, often represent reexperiencing the event.
- Avoidance symptoms, including numbing, social withdrawal, and avoidance of stimuli associated with the event.
- Increased vigilance, such as startle reactions and difficulty falling asleep.
- Symptoms impair functioning.

General Considerations

Post-traumatic stress disorder (PTSD) has been reclassified from an anxiety disorder to a trauma and stressor-related disorder in the *DSM-5*. PTSD is a syndrome characterized by "reexperiencing" a traumatic event (eg, sexual assault, severe burns, military combat) and decreased responsiveness and avoidance of current events associated with the trauma. The lifetime prevalence of PTSD among adult Americans has been estimated to be 6.8% with a point prevalence of 3.6% and with women having rates twice as high as men. Many individuals with PTSD (20–40%) have experienced other associated problems, including divorce, parenting problems, difficulties with the law, and substance abuse.

Clinical Findings

The key to establishing the diagnosis of PTSD lies in the history of exposure to a perceived or actual life-threatening event, serious injury, serious medical illness, or sexual violence. The symptoms of PTSD include intrusive thoughts (eg, flashbacks, nightmares), avoidance (eg, withdrawal), negative thoughts and feelings, and increased reactivity. Patients with PTSD can experience physiologic hyperarousal, including startle reactions, illusions, overgeneralized associations, sleep problems, nightmares, dreams about the precipitating event, impulsivity, difficulties in concentration, and hyper-alertness. The symptoms may be precipitated or exacerbated by events that are a reminder of the original traumatic event. Symptoms frequently arise after a long latency period (eg, child abuse can result in later-onset PTSD). *DSM-5* includes the requirement that the symptoms persist for at least 1 month. In some individuals, the symptoms fade over months or years, and in others they may persist for a lifetime. Those with comorbid chronic pain tend to have heightened PTSD symptoms compared with those without chronic pain.

Differential Diagnosis

In 75% of cases, PTSD occurs with comorbid depression or panic disorder, and there is considerable overlap in the symptom complexes of all three conditions. Acute stress disorder has many of the same symptoms as PTSD, but symptoms persist for <1 month after the trauma. Another major comorbidity is alcohol and substance abuse. The **Primary Care-PTSD Screen** (https://www.ptsd.va.gov/professional/assessment/documents/pc-ptsd5-screen.pdf) and the **PTSD Checklist** (https://www.ptsd.va.gov/professional/assessment/adult-sr/ptsd-checklist.asp) are two useful screening instruments in primary care clinics or community settings with populations at risk for trauma exposure.

Treatment

A. Psychotherapy

Cognitive processing therapy, cognitive behavioral therapy, Eye Movement Desensitization and Restructuring (EMDR), and prolonged exposure therapy have demonstrated improvement in symptoms of PTSD. In these approaches, the individual confronts the traumatic situation and over time learns to view and experience it with less hyperarousal. PTSD responds to interventions that help patients integrate the event in an adaptive way with some sense of mastery in having survived the trauma. Because partner relationship problems may be an area of concern, couples counseling may be indicated. Addressing interpersonal difficulties may also involve broader attention to social connectedness, trust-building, and addressing patterns of revictimization or social withdrawal.

Treatment of comorbid substance abuse is an essential part of the recovery process for patients with PTSD. There are better outcomes when substance abuse treatment is delivered alongside trauma-focused psychotherapy. Support groups and 12-step programs such as Alcoholics Anonymous are often helpful.

Integration of psychotherapy with pharmacotherapy, when indicated, may enhance overall outcomes, particularly for patients with severe symptom intensity or prominent comorbid depression or anxiety. Attention to sleep disturbance is increasingly prioritized, as persistent insomnia and nightmares can impede recovery and contribute to ongoing functional impairment.

B. Pharmacotherapy

SSRIs and SNRIs are helpful in ameliorating depression, panic attacks, sleep disruption, and startle responses. Recent guidelines continue to emphasize SSRIs and SNRIs as first-line agents, with sertraline, paroxetine, fluoxetine, and venlafaxine having the strongest evidence base. Treatment response requires adequate dosing and duration, often extending beyond the typical timeframe for other anxiety or mood disorders. Early treatment of anxious arousal with β-blockers (eg, propranolol, 80–160 mg orally daily) may lessen the peripheral symptoms of anxiety (eg, tremors, palpitations) but has not been shown to prevent development of PTSD. Similarly, noradrenergic agents such as clonidine (titrated from 0.1 mg orally at bedtime to 0.2 mg three times a day) may help with the hyperarousal symptoms of PTSD. The α-blocking agent prazosin (2–10 mg orally at bedtime) has been widely used to decrease nightmares and improve quality of sleep in PTSD; however, recent large-scale trials have not consistently demonstrated superiority over placebo for this indication. Trazodone (25–100 mg orally at bedtime) is commonly prescribed as a non–habit-forming hypnotic agent. Benzodiazepines, such as clonazepam, are generally thought to be *contraindicated* in the treatment of PTSD because the risks of addiction and increase in intrusive and dissociative symptoms are thought to outweigh the short-term anxiolytic and sleep benefits. Second-generation antipsychotics have not demonstrated utility in the treatment of PTSD, but agents such as quetiapine 50–300 mg/day may have a limited role in treating irritability and sleep disturbance. Phase 2 and 3 studies of methylenedioxymethamphetamine (MDMA) reported large effect sizes and higher remission rates than prior studies of SSRIs. However, independent US Food and Drug Administration (FDA) reviews of these studies found numerous methodologic problems that may have introduced bias. As a result, in 2024 the FDA declined to approve MDMA for the treatment of PTSD. Whether adjunctive psychedelic-assisted therapies may eventually have a role is contingent on resolution of these methodologic and regulatory issues.

Prognosis

Half of patients with PTSD experience chronic symptoms. Prognosis is best in those with good premorbid psychiatric functioning and early symptom onset recognition. Comorbid depression, substance use disorders, and ongoing stressors can complicate recovery and prolong symptom duration. Social support quality and access to evidence-based care are important modifiable prognostic factors.

Patients who receive their preferred treatment are more likely to be adherent, respond to treatment, and have lower self-reported PTSD, depression, and anxiety symptoms, underscoring the value of shared decision-making in treatment planning.

Lang AJ et al. A clinician's guide to the 2023 VA/DoD Clinical Practice Guideline for Management of Posttraumatic Stress Disorder and Acute Stress Disorder. J Trauma Stress. 2024;37:19. [PMID: 38184799]

Yaw LK et al. Long-term outcomes and determinants of new-onset mental health conditions after trauma. JAMA Netw Open. 2025;8:e250349. [PMID: 40063026]

Zhao YF et al. Psychotherapeutic, pharmacological and other active interventions from the NICE guideline for post-traumatic stress disorder with sleep disorder: systematic review and meta-analysis. BMC Psychiatry. 2025;25:699. [PMID: 40665297]

ANXIETY DISORDERS

ESSENTIALS OF DIAGNOSIS

- Persistent excessive anxiety or chronic fear and associated behavioral disturbances.
- Physical symptoms such as muscle tension, restlessness, and becoming easily fatigued.
- Not limited to an adjustment disorder.
- Not a result of physical disorders, other psychiatric conditions (eg, schizophrenia), or drug abuse (eg, cocaine).

General Considerations

Stress, fear, and anxiety may interact. The principal components of anxiety are **psychological** (tension, fears, difficulty in concentration, apprehension) and **somatic** (tachycardia, hyperventilation, shortness of breath, palpitations, tremor, sweating). Sympathomimetic symptoms of anxiety are both a response to a CNS state and a reinforcement of further anxiety. Anxiety can become self-generating, since the symptoms reinforce the reaction, causing it to spiral. Additionally, avoidance of triggers of anxiety reinforces the anxiety. The person continues to associate the trigger with anxiety and never relearns through experience that the trigger need not always result in fear, or that anxiety will improve with prolonged exposure to an objectively neutral stressor.

Clinical Findings

A. Generalized Anxiety Disorder

Anxiety disorders are the most prevalent psychiatric disorders. About 7% of women and 4% of men will meet criteria for GAD over a lifetime. GAD becomes chronic in many patients and lasts longer than 2 years in over half of patients. Anxiety disorder in older adults is twice as common as dementia and four to six times more common than major depression; it is associated with poorer quality of life and contributes to the onset of disability. The anxiety symptoms of apprehension, worry, and difficulty controlling the worry are present more days than not for at least 6 months. Further manifestations can include restlessness, muscle tension, difficulty concentrating, sleep disturbance, and irritability.

B. Panic Disorder

Panic attacks are recurrent, unpredictable episodes of intense surges of anxiety accompanied by marked physiologic manifestations. Symptoms and signs such as dyspnea, tachycardia, palpitations, dizziness, paresthesia, choking, smothering feelings, and nausea are associated with feelings of impending doom (alarm response). These symptoms overlap with some of the complaints found in the somatic symptom disorders; however, the key to the diagnosis of panic disorder is the psychic pain and suffering the individual expresses. **Panic disorder** is diagnosed when panic attacks are accompanied by a chronic fear of the recurrence of an attack or a maladaptive change in behavior to try to avoid potential triggers of the panic attack. Recurrent **sleep panic attacks** (not nightmares) occur in about 30% of panic disorders. Persistent worry about future panic attacks develops in patients with panic disorder and further constricts their daily lives. Panic disorder tends to be familial, with onset usually under age 25; it affects 3–5% of the population, and the female-to-male ratio is 2:1. The premenstrual period is one of heightened vulnerability. Patients frequently undergo evaluations for emergent medical conditions (eg, heart attack or hypoglycemia), which are then ruled out before the correct diagnosis is made. GI symptoms (eg, stomach pain, heartburn, diarrhea, constipation, nausea, and vomiting) are common, occurring in about one-third of cases. MI, pheochromocytoma, hyperthyroidism, and various recreational drug reactions can mimic panic disorder. Patients who have panic disorder can become demoralized, hypochondriacal, agoraphobic, and depressed. These individuals are at increased risk for major depression and suicide. Alcohol abuse (in about 20%) may result from self-treatment and is frequently combined with dependence on sedatives. About 25% of patients with panic disorders also have obsessive-compulsive disorder (OCD).

C. Phobic Disorders

Simple phobias are fears of a specific object or situation (eg, spiders, height) that are out of proportion to the danger posed, which tend to be chronic. **Social phobias** are global or specific; in the former, all social situations are poorly tolerated, while the latter group includes **performance anxiety** (eg, fear of public speaking). Agoraphobia is frequently associated with panic attacks; it often develops in early adult life, potentially making activities of daily living difficult. Patients with agoraphobia experience intense fear about common situations, such as being in open spaces (eg, marketplaces), being in enclosed spaces (eg, theaters), standing in line, or being alone outside of their homes.

Treatment

In all cases, underlying medical disorders must be ruled out (eg, cardiovascular, endocrine, respiratory, and neurologic disorders and substance-related syndromes). Clinicians are encouraged to apply stepwise, measurement-based care that integrates patient education, regular monitoring, and consideration of comorbidities. Minimizing long-term benzodiazepine exposure remains essential due to mounting evidence of cognitive effects and tolerance. Tailoring medication choice to individual profiles, including sleep, substance use, and medical comorbidities, supports safer and more durable outcomes.

A. Pharmacologic

1. Generalized anxiety disorder—Antidepressants including the SSRIs and SNRIs are the first-line pharmacotherapies in the long-term management of GAD. Because benzodiazepines take effect more quickly, they can be beneficial in brief acute management (Table 28–1).

A. BENZODIAZEPINES—The longer-acting benzodiazepines are used for the treatment of anxiety symptoms and alcohol withdrawal; the intermediate medications are useful as sedatives for insomnia (eg, lorazepam), while short-acting agents (eg, midazolam) are used for medical procedures such as endoscopy. In psychiatric disorders, the benzodiazepines are usually given orally. Because lorazepam does not produce active metabolites and has a half-life of 10–20 hours, it is useful in treating older adult patients or those with liver dysfunction. Ultra-short-acting agents, such as triazolam, have half-lives of 1–3 hours and may lead to rebound withdrawal anxiety. Longer-acting benzodiazepines, such as flurazepam, diazepam, and clonazepam, produce active metabolites, have half-lives of 20–120 hours,

Table 28–1. Commonly used antianxiety and hypnotic agents (listed in alphabetical order within classes).

Medication	Usual Daily Oral Doses	Usual Daily Maximum Doses
Benzodiazepines (used for anxiety)		
Alprazolam (Xanax)[1]	0.5 mg	4 mg
Chlordiazepoxide (Librium)[2]	10–20 mg	100 mg
Clonazepam (Klonopin)[2]	1–2 mg	10 mg
Clorazepate (Tranxene)[2]	15–30 mg	60 mg
Diazepam (Valium)[2]	5–15 mg	30 mg
Lorazepam (Ativan)[1]	2–4 mg	4 mg
Oxazepam (Serax)[1]	10–30 mg	60 mg
Benzodiazepines (used for sleep)		
Estazolam (Prosom)[1]	1 mg	2 mg
Flurazepam (Dalmane)[2]	15 mg	30 mg
Quazepam (Doral)[2]	7.5 mg	15 mg
Temazepam (Restoril)[1]	15 mg	30 mg
Triazolam (Halcion)[4]	0.125 mg	0.25 mg
Miscellaneous (used for anxiety)		
Buspirone (Buspar)[1]	10–30 mg	60 mg
Phenobarbital[2]	15–30 mg	90 mg
Miscellaneous (used for sleep)		
Eszopiclone (Lunesta)[3]	2–3 mg	3 mg
Hydroxyzine (Vistaril)[1]	50 mg	100 mg
Lemborexant (Dayvigo)	5 mg	10 mg
Ramelteon (Rozerem)	8 mg	8 mg
Suvorexant (Belsomra)	5–10 mg	20 mg
Zaleplon (Sonata)[4]	5–10 mg	10 mg
Zolpidem (Ambien)[3]	5–10 mg	10 mg

[1]Intermediate physical half-life (10–20 hours).
[2]Long physical half-life (> 20 hours).
[3]Short physical half-life (1–6 hours).
[4]Short physical half-life (about 1 hour).

and should be avoided in older adults; however, some clinicians prefer clonazepam because of its long half-life and thus ease of dosing to once or twice a day. Medication dosage must be individualized, as patients vary widely in their response and effects can be long-lasting.

The side effects of all the benzodiazepine antianxiety agents are patient- and dose-dependent. As the dosage exceeds the levels necessary for sedation, the side effects include disinhibition, ataxia, dysarthria, nystagmus, and delirium.

Paradoxical agitation, anxiety, psychosis, confusion, mood lability, and anterograde amnesia have been reported, particularly with the shorter-acting benzodiazepines. These agents produce cumulative clinical effects with repeated dosage (especially if the patient has not had time to metabolize the previous dose), additive effects when given with other classes of sedatives or alcohol, and residual effects after termination of treatment (particularly in the case of medications that undergo slow biotransformation).

Overdosage results in respiratory depression, hypotension, shock syndrome, coma, and death. Flumazenil, a benzodiazepine antagonist, is effective in overdosage. Overdosage (see Chapter 42) and withdrawal states are medical emergencies. Serious side effects of chronic excessive dosage are development of tolerance, resulting in increasing dose requirements, and physiologic dependence, resulting in withdrawal symptoms similar in appearance to alcohol and barbiturate withdrawal (withdrawal effects must be distinguished from reemergent anxiety). Abrupt withdrawal of sedative medications may cause serious and even fatal convulsive seizures. Psychosis, delirium, and autonomic dysfunction also have been described. Both duration of action and duration of exposure are major factors related to likelihood of withdrawal.

Common withdrawal symptoms after low to moderate daily use of benzodiazepines are classified as somatic (disturbed sleep, tremor, nausea, muscle aches), psychological (anxiety, poor concentration, irritability, mild depression), or perceptual (poor coordination, mild paranoia, mild confusion). The presentation of symptoms will vary depending on the half-life of the medication. The potential for interactions with benzodiazepines and other medications must be considered.

B. Antidepressants—Antidepressants are as effective as benzodiazepines without the risks of tolerance or dependence and are therefore the preferred first-line therapy. SSRIs and SNRIs are selected based on prior treatment response, tolerability, and comorbid conditions such as depressive or somatic symptoms.

Antidepressants can themselves be anxiogenic when first started; therefore patient education with slow titration of SSRIs and SNRIs is recommended. Concomitant short-term treatment with a benzodiazepine sometimes is indicated. The SNRIs venlafaxine and duloxetine are approved for the treatment of GAD in usual antidepressant doses. Initial daily dosing should start low (37.5–75 mg for venlafaxine and 30 mg for duloxetine) and be titrated upward as needed. Buspirone (30–60 mg daily in divided doses) also is effective for generalized anxiety though usage has declined due to its delayed onset and modest effect size. Higher doses are associated with side effects of GI symptoms and dizziness. It remains useful in patients with substance use risk or benzodiazepine intolerance. Patients should be advised that there is a 2- to 4-week delay before antidepressants and buspirone take full effect. Sleep is sometimes negatively affected. Gabapentin (titrated to doses of 900–1800 mg orally daily, with larger doses at night) and pregabalin appear effective but do not have FDA approval for anxiety. Pregabalin may be considered as a first-line or adjunctive option, but clinicians should remain mindful of its controlled substance status and emerging data on misuse potential. Alcohol is the most frequently self-administered drug and should be strongly discouraged.

2. Panic disorder—Antidepressants are the first-line pharmacotherapy for panic disorder. Several SSRIs, including fluoxetine, paroxetine, and sertraline, are approved for treatment. The SNRI venlafaxine also is FDA-approved for treatment.

While panic disorder often responds to high-potency benzodiazepines such as clonazepam and alprazolam, these agents are best prescribed early in the course of treatment concurrently with an antidepressant and their duration limited to minimize cognitive and dependence risks. Once the antidepressant has begun fully working (after 4 or more weeks), the benzodiazepine may be tapered. Patients should be educated that mild early activation or transient worsening of anxiety can occur when initiating SSRIs or SNRIs and that these effects are dose-related and temporary.

β-Blockers have been used in conjunction with antidepressants in resistant cases, although there are limited data to support their use. They block symptoms mediated by sympathetic stimulation (eg, palpitations, tremulousness) but not nonadrenergic symptoms (eg, diarrhea, muscle tension). Propranolol (40–160 mg/day orally) can mute the peripheral symptoms of anxiety without significantly affecting motor and cognitive performance.

3. Phobic disorders—Social phobias (social anxiety disorder) and agoraphobia may be treated with SSRIs, such as paroxetine, sertraline, and fluvoxamine, and often respond to SNRIs such as venlafaxine. Gabapentin in a dosage of 300–3600 mg/day is an alternative to antidepressants. Performance-only social anxiety may respond to as-needed β-blockers such as propranolol, which target peripheral autonomic arousal. Benzodiazepines have a potential role in specific phobias such as those with flight anxiety.

B. Behavioral

Current guidelines emphasize a combination of pharmacotherapy with behavioral interventions to enhance long-term outcomes and reduce relapse following medication discontinuation. Relaxation techniques can sometimes be helpful in reducing anxiety as well as the physiologic symptoms of panic attacks. Desensitization, by exposing the patient to graded doses of a phobic object or situation, is an effective technique.

Emphasis has shifted toward promoting inhibitory learning rather than simple habituation, encouraging patients to approach rather than suppress anxious experiences.

Emotive imagery, wherein the patient imagines the anxiety-provoking situation while at the same time learning to relax, helps decrease the anxiety when the patient faces the real-life situation. Exercise, both aerobic and resistance training, reduces anxiety symptoms across many anxiety disorders.

C. Psychological

Cognitive behavioral therapy is the first-line psychotherapy in treatment of anxiety disorders. It includes a cognitive component of examining the thoughts associated with the fear and a behavioral technique of exposing the individual to the feared object or situation. The combination of medication and cognitive behavioral therapy is more effective than either alone. **Mindfulness meditation** can be effective in decreasing symptoms of anxiety. **Group therapy** is the treatment of choice when the anxiety is clearly a function of the patient's difficulties in dealing with social settings. **Acceptance and commitment therapy** have been used with some success in anxiety disorders. It encourages individuals to keep focused on life goals while they "accept" the presence of anxiety in their lives. **Virtual reality therapy** has similar efficacy to the other established therapies.

D. Social

Peer support groups for panic disorder and agoraphobia have been helpful. Measures such as family counseling can aid acceptance of the patient's symptoms and avoid counterproductive behavior in behavioral training. Any help in maintaining the social structure is anxiety-alleviating, and work, school, and social activities should be maintained whenever feasible.

Prognosis

Anxiety disorders are usually long-standing and may be difficult to treat. All patients can be relieved to varying degrees with medications and behavioral techniques, and with ongoing, collaborative care many achieve sustained symptom reduction and improved functioning. The prognosis is better when treatment is started early, comorbid conditions (such as substance use and major depression) are addressed, and patients remain engaged in maintenance strategies to prevent relapse. Nonetheless, anxiety disorders typically require long-term monitoring and periodic treatment adjustment.

Archer C et al. Beta-blockers for the treatment of anxiety disorders: a systematic review and meta-analysis. J Affect Disord. 2025;368:90. [PMID: 39271062]

de Ponti N et al. The efficacy of psychotherapy for social anxiety disorder, a systematic review and meta-analysis. J Anxiety Disord. 2024;104:102881. [PMID: 38815481]

Bandelow B et al. World Federation of Societies of Biological Psychiatry (WFSBP) guidelines for treatment of anxiety, obsessive-compulsive and posttraumatic stress disorders - Version 3. Part II: OCD and PTSD. World J Biol Psychiatry. 2023;24:118. [PMID: 35900217]

Johnco CJ et al. A systematic review and meta-analysis of diagnostic remission, treatment response, attrition and relapse following cognitive behavior therapy (CBT), other psychological therapies and pharmacological treatments for anxiety disorders in older adults. Am J Geriatr Psychiatry. 2026;34:500. [PMID: 40581526]

Papola D et al. Psychotherapies for generalized anxiety disorder in adults: a systematic review and network meta-analysis of randomized clinical trials. JAMA Psychiatry. 2024;81:250. [PMID: 37851421]

OBSESSIVE-COMPULSIVE DISORDER & RELATED DISORDERS

ESSENTIALS OF DIAGNOSIS

- Preoccupations or rituals (repetitive psychologically triggered behaviors) that are distressing to the individual.
- Symptoms are excessive or persistent beyond potentially developmentally normal periods.

General Considerations

Obsessive-compulsive disorder (OCD) is part of a separate category of Obsessive-Compulsive Disorder and Related Disorders in *DSM-5*. In OCD, the irrational idea or impulse repeatedly and unwantedly intrudes into awareness. **Obsessions** (recurring distressing thoughts, such as fears of exposure to germs) and **compulsions** (repetitive actions such as washing one's hands many times or cognitions such as counting rituals) are recognized by the individual as unwanted or unwarranted and are resisted, but anxiety often is alleviated only by ritualistic performance of the compulsion or by deliberate contemplation of the intruding idea or emotion. Some patients experience only obsessions, while some experience both obsessions and compulsions. Many patients do not volunteer the symptoms and must be asked about them. There is an overlapping of OCD with some features in other disorders ("**OCD spectrum**"), including tics, trichotillomania (hair pulling), excoriation disorder (skin picking), hoarding, and body dysmorphic disorder. The incidence of OCD in the general population is 2–3% and there is a high comorbidity with major depression: major depression will develop in two-thirds of OCD patients during their lifetime. Male-to-female ratios are similar, with the highest rates occurring in the young, divorced, separated, and unemployed. Neurologic abnormalities of fine motor coordination and involuntary movements are common. Under extreme stress, these patients sometimes exhibit paranoid and delusional thoughts, often associated with depression, that can mimic schizophrenia.

Treatment

A. Pharmacologic

OCD responds to serotonergic antidepressants including SSRIs and clomipramine in 60% of cases but usually has a longer time to response than depression (up to 12 weeks). SSRIs are the preferred first-line treatment due to their favorable tolerability. Fluoxetine has been widely used but in doses higher than those used in depression (up to 60–80 mg orally daily). Other SSRI medications are used with comparable efficacy. In SSRI-resistant OCD, clomipramine may be considered in doses equivalent to those used for depression. Plasma levels of clomipramine and its metabolite should be checked 2–3 weeks after a dosing of 50 mg/day has been achieved, with levels kept under 500 ng/mL to avoid toxicity. Emerging evidence supports vortioxetine as a monotherapy option in SSRI-resistant OCD.

B. Behavioral

OCD may respond to a variety of behavioral techniques. The first-line psychotherapeutic intervention is **exposure and response prevention (ERP)**, which is delivered effectively in individual and group formats. As in the treatment of simple phobias, ERP involves gradually exposing the OCD spectrum patient to situations that the patient fears, such as perceived germs. Patients work through a list of their obsessions and compulsions with their therapist by first exposing themselves to the trigger, then working to prevent the habitual thought or compulsion that accompanies it. By gradually exposing patients to increasingly stressful situations and helping them manage their anxiety without performing the unwanted behavior, OCD spectrum patients are often able to develop some mastery over the behaviors. The primary goal is building distress tolerance rather than simply reducing anxiety, ie, learning that distressing thoughts and feelings are tolerable and that feared outcomes typically do not occur.

C. Psychological

OCD may respond to psychological therapies including cognitive behavioral therapy in which the patient learns to identify maladaptive cognitions associated with obsessive thoughts and challenge those cognitions. These cognitions can be identified and gradually replaced with more rational thoughts. Combined cognitive behavioral therapy, ERP, and medications combined can be more effective than a single intervention alone.

D. Social

OCD can have devastating effects on the ability of a patient to lead a normal life. Educating both the patient and family about the course of illness and treatment options is extremely useful in setting appropriate expectations. Severe OCD is commonly associated with vocational disability, and the clinician may sometimes need to facilitate a leave of absence from work, encourage vocational rehabilitation, or promote social skills training to get the patient back to work.

E. Procedures

Transcranial magnetic stimulation is an effective FDA-approved therapy for treatment-resistant OCD. Psychosurgery has a limited place in selected cases of severe unremitting OCD. Deep brain stimulation in OCD is FDA-approved on a humanitarian device exemption basis for refractory OCD patients.

Prognosis

OCD is usually a chronic disorder with a waxing and waning course. As many as 40% of patients in whom OCD problems develop in childhood will experience remission as adults. However, it is less common for OCD to remit without treatment when it develops during adulthood.

Bandelow B et al. World Federation of Societies of Biological Psychiatry (WFSBP) guidelines for treatment of anxiety, obsessive-compulsive and posttraumatic stress disorders - Version 3. Part II: OCD and PTSD. World J Biol Psychiatry. 2023;24:118. [PMID: 35900217]

Evey KJ et al. A systematic review of the use of acceptance and commitment therapy to treat adult obsessive-compulsive disorder. Behav Ther. 2023;54:1006. [PMID: 37863582]

Ganzevoort CO et al. Intensive treatments for children and adolescents with anxiety or obsessive-compulsive disorders: a systematic review and meta-analysis. J Anxiety Disord. 2024;108:102940. [PMID: 39522354]

Miegel F et al. Exposure therapy in mixed reality for obsessive-compulsive disorder: a randomized clinical trial. JAMA Netw Open. 2025;8:e2511488. [PMID: 40392553]

Tjelle K et al. Patient adherence as a predictor of acute and long-term outcomes in concentrated exposure treatment for difficult-to-treat obsessive-compulsive disorder. BMC Psychiatry. 2024;24:327. [PMID: 38689256]

SOMATIC SYMPTOM & RELATED DISORDERS (Abnormal Illness Behaviors)

ESSENTIALS OF DIAGNOSIS

- Prominent physical symptoms may involve one or more organ systems and are associated with distress, impairment, or both.
- Sometimes able to correlate symptom development with psychosocial stresses.
- Combination of biogenetic and developmental patterns.

General Considerations

Somatic symptom disorders encompass somatic disorders that include conversion disorder (functional neurologic symptom disorder), illness anxiety disorder (previously known as hypochondriasis), somatic symptom disorder, and psychological factors affecting other medical conditions. Any organ system can be affected. Vulnerability in one or more organ systems and exposure to family members with somatization problems plays a major role in the development of particular symptoms, and the "functional" versus "organic" dichotomy is a hindrance to good treatment. Clinicians should suspect psychiatric disorders in a number of somatic conditions. For example, 45% of patients describing palpitations had lifetime psychiatric diagnoses including generalized anxiety, depression, panic, and somatic symptom disorders. Similarly, 33–44% of patients who undergo coronary angiography for chest pain but have negative results have been found to have panic disorder. Somatic symptom disorders frequently co-occur with mood disorders (depression) and anxiety conditions.

Clinical Findings

A. Functional Neurologic Disorder/ Conversion Disorder

Functional neurologic disorder (FND) is understood as a disorder of brain functioning in which symptoms reflect abnormal patterns of attention, expectation, and illness beliefs rather than structural neurologic damage. The two most common types of FND are motor (often, weakness or paralysis) or seizure-type symptoms, although sensory, gait, speech (aphonia), and visual symptoms are also encountered. "Conversion" of psychic conflict into physical neurologic symptoms in parts of the body innervated by the sensorimotor system can occur concomitantly with panic disorder or depression. The somatic manifestation that takes the place of anxiety is often paralysis, and in some instances, the dysfunction may have symbolic meaning (eg, arm paralysis in marked anger so the individual cannot use the arm to strike someone). Psychogenic nonepileptic seizures can be difficult to differentiate from intoxication states or panic attacks and can occur in patients who also have epileptic seizures. Lack of postictal confusion, closed eyes during the seizure, ictal crying, and a fluctuating course can suggest nonepileptic seizures; some symptoms such as asynchronous movements or pelvic thrusting can occur in both nonepileptic seizures and frontal lobe seizures (see also Chapter 27). *La belle indifférence* (an unconcerned affect) is not a significant identifying characteristic, as commonly believed, since individuals even with genuine medical illness may exhibit a high level of denial. It is important to identify physical disorders with unusual presentations (eg, multiple sclerosis, SLE).

B. Illness Anxiety Disorder

Illness anxiety disorder is characterized by a persistent preoccupation with having or acquiring a serious medical illness, despite the absence of somatic symptoms or the presence of only mild, commonplace bodily sensations. The key distinction from somatic symptom disorder is that in illness anxiety disorder the distress centers on the possibility or meaning of serious illness rather than on disruptive or prominent physical symptoms themselves. The clinical picture is dominated by health-focused anxiety; patients are often hypervigilant to normal physiologic fluctuations (eg, benign palpitations, transient gastrointestinal discomfort) and misinterpret these as signs of serious disease. Reassurance from physicians, normal diagnostic tests, and lack of corroborating physical findings typically provide only transient relief. Over time, the feared illness may shift (eg, from cancer to neurologic or cardiac disease), but the underlying pattern of preoccupation and anxiety remains stable.

Concomitant mood anxiety disorders, including panic disorder and generalized anxiety disorder, are common and can heighten the intensity of health-related fears. Insight varies; some patients recognize that their worry is excessive but feel unable to control it, whereas others are firmly convinced they are seriously ill, blurring the boundary with overvalued ideas.

C. Somatic Symptom Disorder

Somatic symptom disorder is characterized by one or more somatic symptoms that are associated with significant distress or disability. The somatic symptoms are associated with disproportionate and persistent thoughts about the seriousness of the symptoms, a high level of anxiety about health, or excessive time and energy devoted to these symptoms. The patient's focus on somatic symptoms is usually chronic. The diagnosis rests on the maladaptive thoughts/feelings/behaviors and functional impact, not on whether symptoms are "medically unexplained"; the disorder can co-occur with general medical conditions. Panic, anxiety, and depression are often present, and major depression is an important consideration in the differential diagnosis. There is a significant relationship (20%) to a lifetime history of panic-agoraphobia-depression. It usually occurs before age 30 and is 10 times more common in women. Preoccupation with medical and surgical therapy becomes a lifestyle that may exclude other activities.

Patients' complaints of symptoms should always be first carefully medically evaluated. Even when evaluation is reassuring, patients may experience reassurance regarding their physical condition as only briefly helpful (or dismissive) and may have difficulty accepting that their fears and health concerns are excessive. Management therefore typically benefits from a collaborative approach (often anchored in primary care) with regular, planned follow-up that validates suffering, sets explicit goals for functioning, and continues symptom monitoring and further workup only as clinically indicated.

D. Factitious Disorders

In these disorders, symptom production is intentional and involves conscious deception (in contrast to the unconscious process of the other somatic symptom disorders). They are characterized by self-induced or described symptoms or falsification of physical and laboratory findings for the purpose of deceiving clinicians or other health care personnel. The deceptions may involve self-mutilation, fever, hemorrhage, hypoglycemia, seizures, and an almost endless variety of manifestations—often presented in an exaggerated and dramatic fashion **(Munchausen syndrome). Factitious disorder imposed on another**, previously termed **Munchausen by proxy**, is diagnosed when someone (often a parent) creates an illness in another person (often a child) for perceived psychological benefit of the first person, such as sympathy or a relationship with clinicians. The duplicity may be either simple or extremely complex and difficult to recognize. The patients are frequently connected in some way with the health professions, or otherwise knowledgeable about medical care, and there is no apparent external motivation other than achieving the patient role. If apparent external motivation such as financial gain or avoidance of responsibility are present, malingering should be considered instead. A poor clinician-patient relationship and "doctor shopping" tend to exacerbate the problem and increase iatrogenic risk through repeated investigations and interventions.

Complications

Sedative and analgesic dependency is the most common iatrogenic complication. Patients may pursue medical or surgical treatments that induce iatrogenic problems. Thus, it is important to identify patients with a potential somatic symptom disorder and attempt to limit tests, procedures, and medications that may lead to harm.

Treatment

A. Medical

Medical support with careful attention to *building a therapeutic clinician–patient relationship is the mainstay of treatment.* It must be accepted that the patient's distress is real. Validation is most effective when paired with a clear explanation that links symptoms to stress physiology, illness beliefs, and behavioral responses, while emphasizing that the symptoms are experienced as bodily and not imagined. *Every problem not found to have an organic basis is not necessarily a mental disease.* Conversely, the diagnosis of a somatic symptom disorder does not require that symptoms be "medically unexplained"—and clinically significant health-focused thoughts, feelings, and behaviors may occur alongside a general medical condition. Regular, frequent, short appointments that are not symptom-contingent may be helpful. Visits are often most useful when they are structured around function, coping, and agreed-upon next steps; they should include explicit limits on repeated diagnostic testing and "doctor shopping," which can inadvertently reinforce illness behavior and expose patients to false-positive findings and iatrogenic harm. Medications should *not* be prescribed to replace appointments. When medication is used, it is generally aimed at treatable comorbid conditions (eg, depressive or anxiety disorders) rather than the somatic symptom itself; clinicians should be cautious with sedatives and habit-forming analgesics that can complicate the clinical picture. One person should be the primary clinician, and consultants should be used mainly for evaluation. A coordinated, collaborative model (often primary care with "behind-the-scenes" behavioral health input) can help maintain consistent messaging across clinicians and reduce fragmented care. Ongoing re-evaluation is necessary since somatization can coexist with a concurrent physical illness.

B. Psychological

The primary clinician can use psychological approaches when the patient is ready to make some changes in lifestyle in order to achieve symptomatic relief. Cognitive behavioral therapy (CBT) has been shown to be an effective treatment for somatoform disorders by reducing physical symptoms, psychological distress, and disability. Acceptance- and mindfulness-based variants are options for persistent bodily distress, particularly when comorbid anxiety/depression or experiential avoidance are prominent. Group therapy with other individuals who have similar problems is sometimes of value. Hypnosis used early can be helpful in resolving conversion disorders. If the primary clinician has been working with the patient on psychological problems related to the physical illness, the groundwork is often laid for successful psychiatric referral.

For patients identified as having a factitious disorder, early psychiatric consultation is indicated. In addition, coordinated team communication and a shared plan are important to reduce iatrogenic harm and to avoid the common pattern of splitting that can destabilize care. There are two main treatment strategies for these patients. One consists of a conjoint confrontation of the patient by both the primary clinician and the psychiatrist. The second approach avoids direct confrontation and attempts to provide a face-saving way to relinquish the symptom without overt disclosure of the disorder's origin. Whichever approach is taken, careful, transparent documentation and ongoing attention to safety (including limiting unnecessary high-risk interventions) are central.

C. Behavioral

Behavioral therapy is best exemplified by **biofeedback** techniques. In biofeedback, the abnormality (eg, increased peristalsis) must be recognized and monitored by the patient and therapist (eg, by an electronic stethoscope to amplify the sounds). This is immediate feedback, and after learning to recognize it, the patient can then learn to identify any change thus produced (eg, a decrease in bowel sounds) and so become a conscious originator of the feedback instead of a passive recipient. Relief of the symptom operantly conditions the patient to utilize the maneuver that relieves symptoms (eg, relaxation causing a decrease in bowel sounds). With emphasis on this type of learning, the patient is able to identify symptoms early and initiate the counter-maneuvers, thus decreasing the symptomatic problem. Migraine and tension headaches have been responsive to biofeedback methods.

Physical-based therapies such as speech/occupational/physical also have strong evidence for improving symptoms in those living with a functional neurologic disorder.

D. Social

Social endeavors include family, work, and other interpersonal activity. Family members should come for some appointments with the patient so they can learn how best to live with the patient and to support a consistent, function-focused plan (including helping the patient rely on a stable, coordinated outpatient care relationship rather than repeated urgent visits or fragmented consultations). When significant family conflict or other ongoing stressors are present, brief family-focused interventions can be used to align expectations and reduce interpersonal amplification of distress and disability. Peer support groups provide a climate for encouraging the patient to accept and live with the problem, particularly when they emphasize self-management and functional improvement. Ongoing communication with the employer may be necessary to encourage long-term continued interest in the employee; with the patient's consent, this communication is often most useful when framed around functional capacity, job demands, pacing, and practical workplace adjustments.

Prognosis

The prognosis is better if the primary clinician intervenes early before the situation has deteriorated. After the problem has crystallized into chronicity, it is more difficult to effect change.

Smakowski A et al. Psychological risk factors of somatic symptom disorder: a systematic review and meta-analysis of cross-sectional and longitudinal studies. J Psychosom Res. 2024;181:111608. [PMID: 38365462]

Town JM et al. Halifax somatic symptom disorder trial: a pilot randomized controlled trial of intensive short-term dynamic psychotherapy in the emergency department. J Psychosom Res. 2024;187:111889. [PMID: 39241562]

Wang Y et al. Integrative group psychotherapy for patients with somatic symptom disorder: a randomized controlled trial. Psychiatry Res. 2024;331:115660. [PMID: 38061179]

PSYCHOSEXUAL DISORDERS

The stages of sexual activity include **excitement** (arousal), **orgasm**, and **resolution**. The precipitating excitement or arousal is psychologically determined.

In a well-adjusted person, arousal stimuli lead to vasocongestive and orgasmic responses. These can be considered as separate stages that can produce different syndromes responding to different treatment procedures.

Clinical Findings

There are three major groups of sexual disorders.

A. Paraphilias

In these conditions, the excitement stage of sexual activity is associated with sexual objects or orientations different from those usually associated with adult sexual stimulation. For example, the stimulus may be a woman's shoe, a child, animals, instruments of torture, or incidents of aggression. The pattern of sexual stimulation is usually one that has early psychological roots. Paraphilias are characterized as *paraphilic disorders* when they are associated with intrinsic distress (ie, not merely from societal disapproval) or the behavior includes situations that involve harm (or risk of harm) to others, including unwilling persons or those unable to consent. Some paraphilias or paraphilic disorders include exhibitionism, transvestism, voyeurism, pedophilia, incest, sexual sadism, and sexual masochism.

B. Gender Dysphoria

Gender dysphoria is distress associated with the incongruence between a person's experienced or expressed gender and a person's biological sex. The diagnosis is defined by clinically significant distress or functional impairment, not by transgender identity or gender nonconformity; individuals may experience gender incongruence without meeting criteria for gender dysphoria. Dysphoric distress may fluctuate with developmental stage (including puberty) and with the degree of affirmation or rejection in the person's social context (family, peers, school/work, community). Screening should be done for conditions related to the oppression and stigmatization that transgender people face, including depression, anxiety, substance use, trauma-related symptoms, disordered eating/body image concerns, and social isolation—alongside routine safety assessment for self-harm and suicidality.

C. Sexual Dysfunctions

This category includes a large group of vasocongestive and orgasmic disorders. Often, they involve problems of sexual adaptation, education, and technique that are often initially discussed with, diagnosed by, and treated by the primary care provider. This group is now more commonly framed as disorders of sexual desire, arousal, orgasm, and sexual pain, with attention to contextual and relational factors. A basic evaluation typically includes a focused sexual history (desire, arousal, orgasm, pain), relationship context, mental health symptoms, substance use, and a review of medications that commonly affect sexual function (eg, SSRIs/SNRIs, antipsychotics, antihypertensives, opioids).

There are two conditions common in men: erectile dysfunction and ejaculation disturbances.

Erectile disorder/dysfunction is inability to achieve or maintain an erection firm enough for satisfactory intercourse; patients sometimes use the term incorrectly to mean premature ejaculation. Clinicians should distinguish erectile difficulty from low desire, arousal problems related to inadequate stimulation, orgasmic disorder, and genito-pelvic pain. Depression, anxiety, and sleep disorders can reduce sexual interest and arousal and can also alter erectile function; antidepressants may further contribute. Psychological erectile dysfunction is caused by interpersonal or intrapsychic factors (eg, partner disharmony, depression). Organic factors are discussed in Chapter 26.

Ejaculation disturbances include premature ejaculation, inability to ejaculate, and retrograde ejaculation. Clinicians should differentiate lifelong vs acquired patterns and assess erectile difficulty, anxiety, and medication effects, because these frequently co-occur and influence treatment choice. Pathogenic factors are those that interfere with learning control, most frequently sexual ignorance. Intrapsychic factors (anxiety, guilt, depression) and interpersonal maladaptation (partner problems, unresponsiveness of mate, power struggles) also are common. Organic causes include interference with sympathetic nerve distribution (often due to surgery or radiation) and the effects of pharmacologic agents (eg, SSRIs, other antidepressants, antipsychotics, α-adrenergic agents).

In women, the most common forms of sexual dysfunction include female sexual interest/arousal difficulties, orgasmic disorder, and sexual pain disorders; presentations are often overlapping and context-dependent.

Orgasmic disorder is a complex condition in which there is a general lack of sexual responsiveness. The woman has difficulty in experiencing erotic sensation and the vasocongestive response. Sexual activity varies from active avoidance of sex to an occasional orgasm. **Orgasmic dysfunction**—in which a woman has a vasocongestive response but varying degrees of difficulty in reaching orgasm—is sometimes differentiated from **anorgasmia.** Causes for the dysfunctions include poor sexual techniques, early traumatic sexual experiences, interpersonal disharmony (partner struggles, use of sex as a means of control), and intrapsychic problems (anxiety, fear, guilt). Organic causes include any conditions that might cause pain in intercourse.

Hypoactive sexual desire disorder consists of diminished or absent libido in either sex and may be a function of organic or psychological difficulties (eg, anxiety, phobic avoidance). Relationship satisfaction, stress, trauma history, and body image concerns commonly contribute and should be assessed alongside medical factors. Systemic illnesses (including CKD), endocrine disorders, and hypogonadism may contribute. Untreated mood/anxiety disorders are frequent, reversible contributors. Alcohol, sedatives, opioids, marijuana, and some medications (including antiandrogens) may affect sexual drive and performance; menopause may lead to diminution of sexual desire in some women due to hormonal changes and sexual pain from vulvovaginal atrophy.

Treatment

A. Paraphilias

1. Psychological—Paraphilias, particularly those of a more superficial nature (eg, voyeurism) and those of recent onset, are responsive to psychotherapy in some cases. The prognosis is much better if the motivation comes from the individual rather than the legal system; unfortunately, judicial intervention is frequently the only stimulus to treatment because the condition persists and is reinforced until conflict with the law occurs. Therapies frequently focus on barriers to normal arousal response; the expectation is that the variant behavior will decrease as normal behavior increases. Cognitive behavioral therapy may reduce behaviors such as compulsive pornography use.

2. Behavioral—In some cases, paraphilic disorders improve with modeling, role-playing, and conditioning procedures. Older "aversion" paradigms are used less often in current practice, having largely given way to CBT-based self-management approaches that emphasize skills acquisition, coping with urges, and reductions in risk.

3. Social—Although they do not produce a change in sexual arousal patterns or gender role, self-help groups may facilitate adjustment to an often hostile society. Attention to the family is important in helping people in such groups to accept their situation and alleviate their guilt about the role they think they had in creating the problem; family is also used to support monitoring and reduce environmental access to potential victims.

4. Pharmacologic—Antilibidinal agents require broader medical monitoring (eg, metabolic/cardiovascular and hepatic risk, thromboembolic risk) and coordination with primary care or endocrinology providers. Medroxyprogesterone acetate, a suppressor of libidinal drive, can be used to mute disruptive sexual behavior in men. Onset of action is usually within 3 weeks, and the effects are generally reversible. Fluoxetine or other SSRIs at depression doses may reduce some of the compulsive sexual behaviors including the paraphilias. Current guidelines describe GnRH analogues/agonists as a key option for severe, high-risk paraphilic disorders, usually as part of combined pharmacologic and psychotherapeutic treatment. GnRH agonists require long-term follow-up for hypogonadism-related adverse effects.

B. Gender Dysphoria

The Standards of Care for the Health of Transsexual, Transgender, and Gender Nonconforming People is a publication of the World Professional Association for Transgender Health (WPATH), with the goal to provide clinical guidance for health professionals to assist transsexual, transgender, and gender nonconforming people with a path to maximize their health, psychological well-being, and self-fulfillment. The standards of care are based on the best available science and expert professional consensus.

WPATH Standards of Care are now in an eighth edition, with increased emphasis on individualized assessment, reduction of unnecessary barriers to care, and clinician competence in transgender and gender diverse health.

1. Psychological—Individuals with gender dysphoria often find benefit from psychotherapy, providing them with a safe place to explore and understand their thoughts and feelings, and to identify their own specific needs and desires and adjust to a changing life.

2. Social—Peer support groups, parent psychoeducation and support, and community empowerment are important social components of treatment.

3. Medical—Medical interventions are best conceptualized within a multidisciplinary, longitudinal care model that includes ongoing primary care, gynecologic and urologic care, sexual health, fertility counseling/preservation options when desired, and monitoring for treatment-related risks and general preventive care. Some individuals with gender dysphoria choose to pursue surgery or hormone therapy or both. Most recommendations prior to surgery include that the individual spends significant time prior living as their desired gender; however, the most recent WPATH Standards of Care removed a requirement for "living in role" as a prerequisite. Current practice emphasizes individualized readiness, informed consent, and assessment focused on goals, supports, and capacity to adhere to perioperative care rather than fixed social-transition timelines. Rates of suicide fall significantly after surgery but still remain much higher than in the general population.

C. Sexual Dysfunction

1. Psychological—The use of psychotherapy by itself is best suited for those cases in which interpersonal difficulties or intrapsychic problems predominate. Anxiety and guilt about parental injunctions against sex may contribute to sexual dysfunction. Even in these cases, however, a combined behavioral-psychological approach usually produces results most quickly. Mindfulness may be beneficial. Brief, structured sex therapy is commonly integrated with couples interventions that address desire discrepancy, avoidance cycles, and performance pressure, alongside psychoeducation about normal variability in sexual response across the life cycle.

2. Behavioral—Syndromes resulting from conditioned responses have been treated by conditioning techniques, with excellent results. Masters and Johnson have used behavioral approaches in all sexual dysfunctions, with concomitant supportive psychotherapy and with improvement of the communication patterns of the couple.

3. Social—Social assessment is often broadened to include contextual stressors (caregiving demands, sleep deprivation, privacy constraints, cultural/religious norms, minority stress, and technology-related factors) that may function as chronic inhibitors even in otherwise stable relationships.

4. Medical—Even if the condition is not reversible, identification of the specific cause helps the patient to accept the condition. Partner disharmony, with its exacerbating effects, may thus be avoided. For women following menopause, treatment may address vulvovaginal pain and arousal (eg, lubricants/moisturizers, local estrogen when appropriate, pelvic floor interventions) and, in carefully selected postmenopausal women with distressing low desire, consideration of testosterone therapy with appropriate monitoring. Sildenafil, tadalafil, and vardenafil are phosphodiesterase type 5 inhibitors and effective oral agents for the treatment of penile erectile dysfunction (eg, sildenafil 25–100 mg orally 1 hour prior to intercourse), including SSRI-induced erectile dysfunction. These agents also are effective in some cases for SSRI-associated sexual dysfunction in women. Use of the medications in conjunction with any nitrates (including recreational "poppers") can have significant hypotensive effects leading to death in rare cases. Because of their common effect in delaying ejaculation, the SSRIs have been effective in premature ejaculation; patients should be counseled about the trade-off of reduced desire/arousal or anorgasmia and about on-demand vs daily regimens.

Flibanserin is a 5-HT_{1A}-agonist/5-HT_2-antagonist that is FDA-approved for the treatment of female hypoactive sexual desire disorder. Women treated with flibanserin have a marginally higher number of sexual events. Bremelanotide is FDA-approved medication for the treatment of hypoactive sexual desire disorder in premenopausal women; however, the mechanism of action is unclear and subjective improvement is low. Both flibanserin and bremelanotide have potentially intolerable side effects, and their usage remains low.

Culos C et al. Pharmacological interventions in paraphilic disorders: systematic review and insights. J Clin Med. 2024;13:1524. [PMID: 38541760

de Aquino ACQ et al. Pharmacological treatment of antidepressant-induced sexual dysfunction in women: a systematic review and meta-analysis of randomized clinical trials. Clinics (Sao Paulo). 2025;80:100602. [PMID: 39985829]

Rowen TS et al. Evaluation and management of hypoactive sexual desire disorder in women: recommendations from the 5th International Consultation on Sexual Medicine (ICSM 2024). Sex Med Rev. 2026;14:qeaf057. [PMID: 41092352]

Toledo RG et al. Female sexual desire, arousal, and orgasmic dysfunctions: a systematic review and meta-analysis of treatment options. J Minim Invasive Gynecol. 2026;33:16. [PMID: 40543759]

PERSONALITY DISORDERS

ESSENTIALS OF DIAGNOSIS

- Long history dating back to childhood.
- Recurrent maladaptive behavior.
- Difficulties with interpersonal relationships or society.
- Depression with anxiety when maladaptive behavior fails.

General Considerations

An individual's personality structure, or character, is an integral part of self-image. It reflects genetics, temperament, neurodevelopmental vulnerabilities, interpersonal influences (including attachment and trauma-related experiences), and broader sociocultural context, as well as recurring patterns of behavior adopted to cope with the environment. These patterns tend to become enduring and rigid over time, shaping both self-functioning (eg, identity and self-direction) and interpersonal functioning (eg, empathy and intimacy).

The classification of subtypes of personality disorders depends on the predominant symptoms and their severity. Distinguishing a personality disorder from a personality style requires attention to pervasiveness, inflexibility, cultural context, and associated distress or impairment.

Classification & Clinical Findings

See Table 28–2.

Differential Diagnosis

Patients with personality disorders tend to experience anxiety and depression when pathologic coping mechanisms fail and may first seek treatment when this occurs. The presenting complaints are often mood/anxiety symptoms, trauma-related distress, or substance-related problems, and evaluation should distinguish state-dependent syndromes from enduring maladaptive traits and interpersonal patterns. Occasionally, the more severe cases may decompensate into psychosis under stress and mimic other psychotic disorders.

Treatment

Hospitalization is indicated in the case of serious suicidal or homicidal danger and when the patient cannot be maintained safely in a less restrictive setting. In most cases, treatment can be accomplished in the day treatment center, intensive outpatient setting, or self-help community.

A. Social

Social and therapeutic environments such as day hospitals, halfway houses, and self-help communities utilize peer feedback, modeling, and contingency-based reinforcement to modify the self-destructive behavior. The patient with a personality disorder often has failed to profit from experience, and difficulties with authority, trust, and interpersonal sensitivity can impair the learning experience. When problems are detected early, both the school and the home can serve as foci of intensified social pressure to change the behavior, particularly with the use of behavioral techniques.

B. Behavioral

Dialectical behavioral therapy is a program of individual and group therapy specifically designed for patients with chronic suicidality and borderline personality disorder and now adapted for other problems characterized by emotion dysregulation and self-harm. It blends mindfulness and a cognitive behavioral model to address self-awareness, interpersonal functioning, affective lability, and reactions to stress.

C. Psychological

Psychological interventions can be conducted in group and individual settings. Group therapy is helpful when specific interpersonal behavior needs to be improved, particularly when the group is structured (clear goals, agreed-upon rules, active facilitation) and attends to boundaries, safety, and rupture repair. The group identifies the patient's types of behavior and helps improve the validity of the patient's self-assessment, so that the antecedents of the unacceptable

Table 28–2. Personality disorders: Classification and clinical findings (listed in alphabetical order).

Personality Disorder	Clinical Findings
Antisocial	Selfish, callous, promiscuous, impulsive, unable to learn from experience, often has legal problems.
Avoidant	Fears rejection, hyperreacts to rejection and failure, with poor social endeavors and low self-esteem.
Borderline	Impulsive; has unstable and intense interpersonal relationships; is suffused with anger, fear, and guilt; lacks self-control and self-fulfillment; has identity problems and affective instability; is suicidal (a serious problem—up to 80% of hospitalized borderline patients make an attempt at some time during treatment, and the incidence of death by suicide is as high as 5%); aggressive behavior, feelings of emptiness, and occasional psychotic decompensation.
Dependent	Passive, overaccepting, unable to make decisions, lacks confidence, with poor self-esteem.
Histrionic (hysterical)	Dependent, immature, seductive, egocentric, vain, emotionally labile.
Narcissistic	Exhibitionist, grandiose, preoccupied with power, lacks interest in others, with excessive demands for attention.
Obsessive-compulsive	Perfectionist, egocentric, indecisive, with rigid thought patterns and need for control.
Paranoid	Defensive, oversensitive, secretive, suspicious, hyperalert, with limited emotional response.
Schizoid	Shy, introverted, withdrawn, avoids close relationships.
Schizotypal	Superstitious, socially isolated, suspicious, with limited interpersonal ability, eccentric behaviors, and odd speech.

behavior can be effectively handled, thus decreasing its frequency. Individual therapy should initially be supportive, ie, helping the patient to restabilize, mobilize coping mechanisms, and strengthen capacity for reflection and self-observation. Psychodynamic psychotherapy also can be an effective treatment, as can other specific forms of therapy, including transference-focused psychotherapy, mentalization-based therapy, and schema-focused therapy. The therapist must be able to handle countertransference feelings (which are frequently negative), maintain appropriate boundaries in the relationship, and refrain from premature confrontations and interpretations.

D. Pharmacologic

Pharmacotherapy can be directed to specific symptom clusters, but there is limited evidence for its efficacy in personality disorders; medications are generally adjunctive to psychotherapy rather than primary treatment for core personality pathology. Antidepressants have improved anxiety, depression, and sensitivity to rejection in some patients with borderline personality disorder. SSRIs also have a role in reducing aggressive behavior in impulsive aggressive patients (eg, fluoxetine 20–60 mg orally daily or sertraline 50–200 mg orally daily). Antipsychotics may be helpful in targeting hostility, agitation, and transient stress-related perceptual disturbances, and as adjuncts to antidepressant therapy (eg, olanzapine [2.5–10 mg/day orally], risperidone [0.5–2 mg/day orally], or haloperidol [0.5–2 mg/day orally, split into two doses]); periodic reassessment, metabolic monitoring, and avoidance of polypharmacy are important. In some cases, medications are required only for several days and can be discontinued after the patient has regained a previously established level of adjustment. Patients with a schizotypal personality often improve with antipsychotics, while those with avoidant personality may benefit from strategies that reduce anxiety, including the use of SSRIs and benzodiazepines.

Prognosis

Antisocial and narcissistic categories generally have a guarded prognosis, as engagement in therapy often is limited. Those patients with a history of parental abuse and a family history of mood disorder tend to have the most challenging treatments; continued assessment of personality disorders is needed for targeting of treatments to symptoms and to guide treatment intensity, focus, and risk management over time.

Aslam HM et al. Clinical practice guidelines for the treatment of borderline personality disorder: a systematic review of best practice in anticipation of MAiD MD-SUMC. Borderline Personal Disord Emot Dysregul. 2025;12:13. [PMID: 40211336]

Crotty K et al. Psychotherapies for the treatment of borderline personality disorder: a systematic review. J Consult Clin Psychol. 2024;92:275. [PMID: 37902689]

Keepers GA et al. The American Psychiatric Association Practice Guideline for the Treatment of Patients With Borderline Personality Disorder. Am J Psychiatry. 2024;181:1024. [PMID: 39482953]

Leichsenring F et al. Borderline personality disorder: a review. JAMA. 2023;329:670. [PMID: 36853245]

SCHIZOPHRENIA SPECTRUM DISORDERS

ESSENTIALS OF DIAGNOSIS

- Social withdrawal, usually slowly progressive, with decrease in emotional expression or motivation or both.
- Deterioration in personal care with disorganized behaviors or decreased reactivity to the environment or both.
- Disorganized thinking, often inferred from speech that switches topics oddly or is incoherent.
- Auditory hallucinations, often of a derogatory nature.
- Delusions, fixed false beliefs despite conflicting evidence, frequently of a persecutory nature.

General Considerations

Schizophrenia is the most common psychotic disorder characterized by a loss of contact with reality. It is manifested by a massive disruption of thinking, mood, and overall behavior as well as poor filtering of stimuli, reflecting widespread dysregulation of information processing and integration across multiple neural networks. One percent of the population suffers from schizophrenia. It is a chronic disorder that is characterized by increasing social and vocational disability that begins in late adolescence or early adulthood and tends to continue through life. The average age of onset for men is 18 years and for women is 25 years. The cause of schizophrenia is believed to be multifactorial, with genetic, environmental, and neurotransmitter pathophysiologic components; dopamine and glutamate system dysregulation are prominent but not exclusive contributors. There is no laboratory method for confirming the diagnosis of schizophrenia; the diagnosis remains clinical, based on standardized criteria and exclusion of other medical and substance-related causes of psychosis. There may or may not be a history of a major disruption in the individual's life (failure, loss, physical illness) before gross psychotic deterioration is evident; such stressors are viewed as potential triggers or exacerbating factors in a biologically vulnerable individual rather than primary causes.

Other psychotic disorders on this spectrum are similar to schizophrenia in their acute symptoms but may have a less pervasive influence over the long term, often with better preserved premorbid functioning and less pronounced structural and cognitive decline. The patient usually attains higher levels of functioning. The acute psychotic episodes tend to be less disruptive of the person's lifestyle, with a quick return to previous levels of functioning.

Classification

A. Schizophrenia

Schizophrenia is characterized by disorganized thinking and behavior. **Positive symptoms** include hallucinations, delusions, paranoia, disorganized speech, and grossly disorganized or catatonic behavior, which are thought to be related to increased dopaminergic (D_2) activity in the mesolimbic region. **Negative symptoms** include diminished sociability, restricted affect, and poverty of speech; these symptoms are related to decreased D_2 activity in the mesocortical system. Negative symptoms may reflect broader frontotemporal dysfunction and are strongly associated with impaired motivation, reduced emotional expressiveness, and poor functional outcome.

Diagnostic criteria require at least two core psychotic symptoms (one of which must be delusions, hallucinations, or disorganized speech) after exclusion of mood, substance-induced, and medical causes of psychosis. A marked decline in the level of functioning must be present for at least 6 months from before the onset of symptoms. Schizophrenia now is classified within a spectrum that also includes related psychotic disorders, with the severity characterized across positive, negative, cognitive, and mood symptom domains. Earlier subtypes of schizophrenia (paranoid, disorganized, catatonic, undifferentiated, residual) are no longer used.

B. Delusional Disorder

Delusional disorders are psychoses in which the predominant symptoms are persistent beliefs that are false (delusions) yet remain fixed despite being shown evidence that they are unfounded. For example, the person may have paranoid delusions, of one's partner being unfaithful, or of being related to or loved by a well-known person. Although there is minimal impairment of daily functioning and intellectual and occupational activities, social and partner functioning tends to be markedly impacted. Hallucinations are not usually present; if they occur, they are typically not prominent and are related to the delusional content; however, other characteristic features of schizophrenia are absent. Diagnostic evaluation should also exclude delusions attributable to a primary mood disorder with psychotic features, a substance/medication effect, or another medical condition.

C. Schizoaffective Disorder

Schizoaffective disorders are characterized by a combination of psychotic and mood symptoms over time that do not clearly fit the schizophrenia or affective categories. These patients usually have affective symptoms (either a major depressive episode, manic episode, or hypomanic episode) that precede or develop concurrently with psychotic manifestations. The psychotic symptoms may linger for some time after resolution of the mood episode but do not remain permanently; in addition, clinically significant mood symptoms are present for a substantial portion of the disorder duration. There must also be at least 2 weeks of delusions or hallucinations in the absence of prominent mood symptoms.

D. Schizophreniform Disorders

Schizophreniform disorders are similar in their symptoms to schizophrenic disorders except that the duration of prodromal, acute, and residual symptoms is > 1 month but < 6 months. If symptoms persist beyond 6 months or resolve fully, diagnostic reevaluation is warranted; many cases evolve or remit.

E. Brief Psychotic Disorders

Brief psychotic disorders are defined by the presence of one or more psychotic symptoms (delusions, hallucinations, disorganized speech, or disorganized or catatonic behavior) lasting < 1 month, with eventual return to premorbid functioning (eg, the short duration correlates with a more acute onset that is the result of psychological stress and has a much better prognosis).

Clinical Findings

A. Symptoms and Signs

The symptoms and signs of schizophrenia vary markedly among individuals as well as in the same person at different times. The patient's appearance may be bizarre, although the usual finding is mildly to moderately unkempt. Motor activity is generally reduced, although extremes ranging from catatonic stupor to frenzied excitement occur. Social behavior is characterized by marked withdrawal coupled with disturbed interpersonal relationships and a reduced ability to experience pleasure, reflecting prominent negative symptoms. Dependency and a poor self-image are common. Verbal utterances are variable, the language being concrete yet symbolic, with unassociated rambling statements (at times interspersed with mutism) during an acute episode. Neologisms (made-up words or phrases), echolalia (repetition of words spoken by others), and verbigeration (repetition of senseless words or phrases) are occasionally present. Affect is usually flattened, with occasional inappropriateness; however, the diminished emotional expression may coexist with an internally intense, distressing psychotic experience. Depression is present in many cases but may be less apparent during the acute psychotic episode and more obvious during recovery; careful assessment is required to distinguish primary depressive symptoms from negative symptoms. Depression is sometimes confused with akinetic side effects of antipsychotic medications. Work is generally unavailable and time unfilled, providing opportunities for counterproductive activities such as drug abuse, withdrawal, and increased psychotic symptoms.

Thought content may vary from a paucity of ideas to a rich complex of delusional fantasy with archaic thinking. One frequently notes after a period of conversation that little if any information has been conveyed. Incoming stimuli produce varied responses. In some cases, a simple question may trigger explosive outbursts, whereas at other times there may be no overt response whatsoever (catatonia). When paranoid ideation is present, the patient is often irritable and less cooperative. Delusions (false beliefs) are characteristic of paranoid thinking and usually take the form of a preoccupation with the supposedly threatening behavior exhibited by other individuals. This ideation may cause the patient to adopt active countermeasures such as locking doors and windows, taking up weapons, covering the ceiling with aluminum foil to counteract radar waves, and other unusual efforts. Somatic delusions can revolve around issues of bodily decay or infestation. Perceptual distortions usually include auditory hallucinations—visual hallucinations are more commonly associated with organic mental states—and may include illusions (distortions of reality) such as figures changing in size or lights varying in intensity. Lack of humor, feelings of dread, depersonalization (a feeling of being apart from the self), and fears of annihilation may be present. Any of the above symptoms generate higher anxiety levels, with heightened arousal and occasional panic and suicidal ideation, as the individual fails to cope.

The development of the acute episode in schizophrenia frequently is the end product of a gradual decompensation. Frustration and anxiety appear early, followed by depression and alienation, along with progressive ineffectiveness in day-to-day coping. This often leads to feelings of panic and increasing disorganization, with loss of the ability to test and evaluate the reality of perceptions. The stage of so-called **psychotic resolution** includes delusions, autistic preoccupations, and psychotic insight, with acceptance of the decompensated state. The process can be complicated by using caffeine, alcohol, and other recreational drugs.

B. Imaging

A full medical evaluation should be considered in first episodes of psychosis to rule out organic brain conditions. A medical workup may include neuroimaging in selective cases such as sudden onset, first episode after 30 years of age, or any patient who presents with concurrent neurologic symptoms.

Differential Diagnosis

The diagnosis of schizophrenia is best made over time because repeated observations increase the reliability of the diagnosis. Cases initially diagnosed as schizophrenia later may be rediagnosed as bipolar disorder, which may respond to mood stabilizers rather than antipsychotics. Some manic episodes can have symptoms that overlap with schizophrenia, including thought disorder, auditory hallucinations, and delusions. Psychotic depressions, brief reactive psychosis, delusional disorder, and any illness with psychotic ideation tend to be confused with schizophrenia, partly because of the incorrect tendency to use the terms interchangeably.

In the early stages of illness, medical disorders such as thyroid dysfunction, adrenal and pituitary disorders, reactions to toxic materials (eg, mercury, PCBs), and other organic mental disorders must be ruled out. Postpartum psychosis is discussed under Mood Disorders. Complex partial seizures, especially when psychosensory phenomena are present, are an important differential consideration. Toxic drug states arising from prescription and over-the-counter medications, street drugs, and herbal products may mimic the psychotic disorders. The chronic use of amphetamines, cocaine, and other stimulants frequently produces a psychosis that is almost identical to the acute paranoid schizophrenic episode. Drug-induced psychoses can have all the positive symptoms of schizophrenia but less commonly the negative symptoms. The presence of formication (sensation of insects crawling on or under the skin) and stereotypy suggests the possibility of stimulant abuse. Phencyclidine, a common street drug, may cause a reaction that is difficult to distinguish from other psychotic disorders. Cerebellar signs, excessive salivation, dilated pupils, and increased deep tendon reflexes should alert the clinician to the possibility of a toxic psychosis. Industrial chemical toxicity (both organic and metallic), degenerative disorders, and metabolic deficiencies must be considered in the differential diagnosis.

Catatonia, a psychomotor disturbance that may involve decreased motor activity, decreased interaction, or excessive and odd motor activity, can be present in a number of other organic illnesses and other psychiatric disorders such as bipolar disorder and major depression. Neoplasms, viral and bacterial encephalopathies, CNS hemorrhage, metabolic derangements such as diabetic ketoacidosis, sedative withdrawal, and liver and kidney malfunction have all been implicated. Drug toxicity (eg, overdoses of antipsychotic medications such as fluphenazine or haloperidol) can cause catatonic syndrome, which may be misdiagnosed as a catatonic schizophrenia and inappropriately treated with more antipsychotic medication.

Treatment

A. Pharmacologic

Antipsychotic medications are the treatment of choice. The relapse rate can be reduced by 50% with proper maintenance therapy. Long-acting, injectable antipsychotics are used in patients who are not adherent to medication recommendations or who do not respond to oral medication, or patients who choose the ease of not taking a daily pill. Side effects are discussed below.

Antipsychotic medications include the **"typical or first-generation"** antipsychotics (haloperidol, chlorpromazine, loxapine, perphenazine, fluphenazine and dopamine [D_2]-receptor antagonists) and the **"atypical or second-generation"** antipsychotics (clozapine, risperidone, olanzapine, quetiapine, aripiprazole, ziprasidone, paliperidone, asenapine, iloperidone, lurasidone, cariprazine, and lumateperone, and xanomeline–trospium chloride) (Tables 28–3 and 28–4). Generally, increasing milligram potency of the typical antipsychotics is associated with decreasing anticholinergic and adrenergic side effects and increasing extrapyramidal symptoms. There appears to be similar antipsychotic efficacy for first- and second-generation antipsychotics but second-generation antipsychotics may be better tolerated with fewer extrapyramidal side effects, leading to enhanced compliance.

Clozapine, the first "atypical" (novel) antipsychotic medication developed, has dopamine (D_4) receptor–blocking activity as well as central serotonergic, histaminergic, and α-blocking activity. It is effective in the treatment of about 30% of psychoses resistant to other antipsychotic medications and may have specific efficacy in decreasing suicidality in patients with schizophrenia. Risperidone is an antipsychotic that blocks some serotonin receptors

Table 28–3. Commonly used antipsychotic medications (listed in alphabetical order).

Medication	Usual Daily Oral Dose	Usual Daily Maximum Dose[1]
Aripiprazole (Abilify)	10–15 mg	30 mg
Asenapine (Saphris)	10–20 mg	20 mg
Cariprazine (Vraylar)	1.5–6 mg	6 mg
Chlorpromazine (Thorazine; others)	100–400 mg	1 g
Clozapine (Clozaril)	300–450 mg	900 mg
Fluphenazine (Permitil, Prolixin)[2]	2–10 mg	60 mg
Haloperidol (Haldol)	2–5 mg	60 mg
Iloperidone (Fanapt)	12–24 mg	24 mg
Loxapine (Loxitane)	20–60 mg	200 mg
Lumateperone (Caplyta)	42 mg	42 mg
Lurasidone (Latuda)	40–80 mg	80 mg
Olanzapine (Zyprexa)	5–10 mg	20 mg
Olanzapine/samidorphan (Lybalvi)	5/10 mg	20/10 mg
Paliperidone (Invega)	6–12 mg	12 mg
Perphenazine (Trilafon)[2]	16–32 mg	64 mg
Pimavanserin (Nuplazid)	34 mg	34 mg
Quetiapine (Seroquel)	200–400 mg	800 mg
Risperidone (Risperdal)[3]	2–6 mg	10 mg
Thiothixene (Navane)[2]	5–10 mg	80 mg
Trifluoperazine (Stelazine)	5–15 mg	60 mg
Xanomeline/trospium (Cobenfy)	100/20 mg twice daily	125/30 mg twice daily
Ziprasidone (Geodon)	40–160 mg	160 mg

[1]Can be higher in some cases.
[2]Indicates piperazine structure.
[3]For risperidone, daily doses above 6 mg increase the risk of extrapyramidal syndrome. Risperidone 6 mg is approximately equivalent to haloperidol 20 mg.

($5\text{-}HT_2$) and D_2 receptors. Risperidone causes somewhat fewer extrapyramidal side effects than the typical antipsychotics at doses <6 mg. It appears to be as effective as haloperidol and possibly as effective as clozapine in treatment-resistant patients without necessitating weekly white cell counts, as required with clozapine therapy. Risperidone-induced hyperprolactinemia, even on low doses, has been reported and more commonly than with other atypical antipsychotics. Risperidone is available in a long-acting injectable preparation.

Olanzapine is a potent blocker of $5\text{-}HT_2$ and dopamine D_1, D_2, and D_4 receptors. Higher doses of olanzapine (10–20 mg daily) appear to be more effective than lower doses. The medication appears somewhat more effective than haloperidol in the treatment of negative symptoms, such as withdrawal, psychomotor retardation, and poor interpersonal relationships. It is available in an orally disintegrating form for patients who are unable to tolerate standard oral dosing and in an injectable form for the management of acute agitation associated with schizophrenia and bipolar disorder.

Quetiapine is an antipsychotic with greater $5\text{-}HT_2$ relative to D_2 receptor blockade as well as a relatively high affinity for α-1 and α-2 receptors. It appears to be as efficacious as haloperidol in treating positive and negative symptoms of schizophrenia, with fewer extrapyramidal side effects even at high doses.

Ziprasidone has both anti-dopamine receptor and anti-serotonin receptor effects, with good efficacy for both positive and negative symptoms of schizophrenia. Aripiprazole is a partial agonist at the dopamine D_2 and serotonin $5\text{-}HT_1$ receptors and an antagonist at $5\text{-}HT_2$ receptors, and it is effective against positive and negative symptoms of schizophrenia. It functions as an antagonist or agonist, depending on the dopaminergic activity at the dopamine receptors, which may decrease side effects. Aripiprazole is available as an acute injectable preparation as well as a long-term injectable preparation that is given once monthly in patients who are unable to adhere to daily oral dosing. Asenapine, approved for the treatment of schizophrenia and bipolar disorder (mixed or manic state), appears to be helpful in treating negative symptoms of schizophrenia. It is available in a transdermal form, which may reduce some side effects associated with the sublingual form. Paliperidone, the active metabolite of risperidone, is available as a capsule and

Table 28–4. Relative potency and side effects of antipsychotic medications (listed in alphabetical order).

Medication	Chlorpromazine:Drug Potency Ratio	Anticholinergic Effects[1]	Extrapyramidal Effect[1]
Aripiprazole	1:20	1	1
Chlorpromazine	1:1	4	1
Clozapine	1:1	4	—
Fluphenazine	1:50	1	4
Haloperidol	1:50	1	4
Iloperidone	1:25	1	1
Loxapine	1:10	2	3
Lurasidone	1:5	1	2
Olanzapine	1:20	1	1
Perphenazine	1:10	2	3
Quetiapine	1:1	1	1
Risperidone	1:50	1	3
Thiothixene	1:20	1	4
Trifluoperazine	1:20	1	4
Ziprasidone	1:1	1	1

[1]1, weak effect; 4, strong effect.

a monthly injection. Lurasidone has been shown to be effective in treating acute decompensation in patients with chronic schizophrenia. Cariprazine is a partial agonist of the D_2 and D_3 receptor and is approved by the FDA for the treatment of schizophrenia and bipolar disorder. Akathisia and insomnia are among its more commonly reported side effects. Because cariprazine is not a potent D_2-antagonist, it is less likely to increase prolactin levels than most antipsychotics. Cariprazine demonstrates greater efficacy in reducing negative symptoms of schizophrenia. Lumateperone, another second-generation antipsychotic, appears to have a favorable metabolic profile and appears to act on glutamate as well as D_2 and 5-HT_2 receptors. Unlike other antipsychotics, it does not require dose titration; the starting dose of 42 mg/day is the therapeutic dose. It does not have appreciable antimuscarinic or antihistaminic properties, which reduces side effects associated with other antipsychotics such as sedation or weight gain.

In 2024, the first-in-class muscarinic M1/M4 agonist, **xanomeline–trospium chloride,** was approved for the treatment of schizophrenia. In contrast to all other antipsychotics, it is the first agent that does not act as a dopamine or 5-HT_2 antagonist. Consequently, xanomeline/trospium does not carry many of the side effects associated with traditional antipsychotics, including extrapyramidal symptoms and metabolic complications. As a muscarinic agonist, it has other possible side effects, including nausea, vomiting, constipation, abdominal pain, diarrhea, and gastroesophageal reflux. For treatment of schizophrenia, xanomeline/trospium is at least comparable with other antipsychotics in terms of both positive and negative symptoms. It has demonstrated statistically significant reductions in Positive and Negative Syndrome Scale total scores versus placebo in phase 3 trials and sustained improvements over 1 year in extension studies; it may prove to be a valuable alternative for patients unable to tolerate previous antipsychotic treatments.

Beyond antipsychotics, there is mixed evidence that cannabidiol (CBD) may improve psychotic symptoms in schizophrenia.

1. Clinical indications—The antipsychotics are used to treat all forms of the schizophrenias as well as drug-induced psychoses, psychotic depression, augmentation of unipolar depression, acute mania, and the prevention of mood cycles in bipolar disorder. They are also effective in Tourette syndrome and behavioral dyscontrol in autistic patients. The improvement rate for treating positive symptoms with antipsychotics is about 80%. Patients whose behavioral symptoms worsen with use of antipsychotic medications may have an undiagnosed organic condition such as anticholinergic toxicity.

Symptoms that are ameliorated by these medications include hyperactivity, hostility, aggression, delusions, hallucinations, irritability, and poor sleep. Individuals with acute psychosis and good premorbid function respond quite well. The most common cause of failure in the treatment of acute psychosis is inadequate dosage, and the most common cause of relapse is noncompliance.

Although first-generation antipsychotics are efficacious in the treatment of positive symptoms of schizophrenia, such as hallucinations and delusions, second-generation antipsychotics are thought to have efficacy in reducing positive symptoms and some efficacy in treating negative symptoms. Antidepressant medications may be used in conjunction with antipsychotics if significant depression is present. Resistant cases may require concomitant use of lithium, carbamazepine, or valproic acid. The addition of a benzodiazepine medication to the antipsychotic regimen may prove helpful in treating the agitated or catatonic psychotic patient who has not responded to antipsychotics alone—lorazepam, 1–2 mg orally, can produce a rapid resolution of catatonic symptoms and may allow maintenance with a lower antipsychotic dose.

2. Dosage forms and patterns—The dosage range is quite broad (Table 28–3). For example, risperidone can be effective for some patients with psychotic features at 0.25–1 mg orally at bedtime, whereas up to 6 mg/day may be used in a young patient with acute schizophrenia. In an acutely distressed, psychotic patient one might use haloperidol, 10 mg intramuscularly, which is absorbed rapidly and achieves an initial tenfold plasma level advantage over equal oral doses. Psychomotor agitation, racing thoughts, and general arousal are quickly reduced. The dose can be repeated every 3–4 hours; when the patient is less symptomatic, oral doses can replace parenteral administration in most cases.

After a maintenance dose has been established, most patients can then be maintained on a single daily dose, usually at bedtime. This is appropriate when the sedative effect of the medication is desired for nighttime sleep and undesirable daytime sedative effects can be avoided. For patients who experienced their first psychotic episode, medications should be tapered off after 6 months of stability and then carefully monitored; the rate of relapse is lower for first-episode patients than that of multiple-episode patients.

Psychiatric patients—particularly patients who have paranoia—often neglect to take their medication. In these patients and those who do not respond to oral medication, long-acting fluphenazine enanthate or decanoate (the latter has fewer extrapyramidal side effects) or haloperidol decanoate may be given by deep subcutaneous injection or intramuscularly in the clinician's office with efficacy lasting 7–28 days. The usual dose of the fluphenazine long-acting preparations is 25 mg every 2 weeks, but dosage varies widely from 0.5 mg monthly to 100 mg weekly. Use the smallest effective amount as infrequently as possible.

Intravenous haloperidol, the antipsychotic most commonly used by this route, is often used in critical care units in the management of agitation and delirium. Intravenous haloperidol should be given no faster than 1 mg/min to reduce cardiovascular side effects, such as torsades de pointes. ECG monitoring should be used whenever haloperidol is administered intravenously.

Several long-acting formulations of atypical antipsychotic medications also are available, including risperidone (25–50 mg intramuscularly every 2–4 weeks), olanzapine (every 2–4 weeks), paliperidone (every 3 or 6 months), and aripiprazole (every 2 months). Concomitant use of a benzodiazepine (eg, lorazepam, 2 mg orally twice daily) may permit reduction of the required dosage of oral or parenteral antipsychotic medication.

3. Side effects—For both typical and atypical antipsychotic agents, a range of side effects are reported. The most common anticholinergic side effects include **dry mouth** (which can lead to ingestion of caloric liquids and weight gain or hyponatremia), **blurred near vision, urinary retention** (particularly in older adult men with enlarged prostates), **delayed gastric emptying, esophageal reflux, ileus, delirium**, and precipitation of **acute glaucoma** in patients with narrow anterior chamber angles. Other autonomic effects include **orthostatic hypotension** and **sexual dysfunction**—problems in achieving erection, ejaculation (including retrograde ejaculation), and orgasm in men (approximately 50% of cases) and women (approximately 30%). Delay in achieving orgasm is often a factor in medication noncompliance. **Electrocardiographic changes** occur frequently, but clinically significant arrhythmias are less common. Older adult patients and those with preexisting cardiac disease are at greater risk. The most frequently seen changes include diminution of the T wave amplitude, appearance of prominent U waves, depression of the ST segment, and prolongation of the QT interval (Table 28–5). Ziprasidone can produce QTc prolongation. A pretreatment ECG is indicated for patients at risk for cardiac sequelae (including patients taking other medications that might prolong the QTc interval). In critical care patients, torsades

Table 28–5. Adverse factors associated with atypical antipsychotic medications (listed in alphabetical order).

Medication	Weight Gain	Hyperlipidemia	New-Onset Diabetes Mellitus	QTc Prolongation[1]
Aripiprazole	+/–	–	–	++
Asenapine	+/–	+/–	+/–	+++
Clozapine	+++	+++	+++	+/–
Lurasidone	–	–	–	–
Olanzapine	+++	+++	+++	+/–
Paliperidone	+	+/–	+/–	+++
Quetiapine	++	++	++	+++
Risperidone	++	++	++	+
Ziprasidone	+/–	–	–	+++

[1]QTc prolongation is a side effect of many medications and suggests a possible risk for arrhythmia. Prescriber's Letter 2011;18(12):271207.

de pointes has been associated with the use of high-dose intravenous haloperidol (usually > 30 mg/24 hours).

Many atypical antipsychotics are associated with new-onset **diabetes, hyperlipidemia**, and **weight gain** (Table 28–5). The risk of diabetes mellitus is increased in patients taking clozapine and olanzapine. FDA-approved olanzapine/samidorphan mitigates olanzapine-associated weight gain while retaining antipsychotic efficacy. Monitoring of weight, fasting blood sugar, and lipids prior to initiation of treatment and at regular intervals thereafter is an important part of medication monitoring. The addition of metformin to olanzapine may improve drug-induced weight gain in patients with drug-naïve, first-episode schizophrenia. Emerging adjunctive use of GLP-1 receptor agonists (eg, semaglutide) shows promise in reducing antipsychotic-associated weight gain and improving metabolic parameters. **Lactation and menstrual irregularities** are common. **Bone marrow depression** and **cholestatic jaundice** occur rarely; these are hypersensitivity reactions, and they usually appear in the first 2 months of treatment. They subside on discontinuance of the medication.

Clozapine is associated with a 1.6% risk of **agranulocytosis** (higher in persons of Ashkenazi Jewish ancestry). Updated 2025 guidelines recommend weekly absolute neutrophil count (ANC) for the first 18 weeks, biweekly through 1 year and monthly thereafter, if stable. Before initiating clozapine, genetic testing may be considered for the *HLADQB1* allele that is associated with a 2.5 times higher risk of agranulocytosis. Clozapine has been associated with fatal myocarditis and is contraindicated in patients with severe heart disease. In addition, it lowers the seizure threshold and has many side effects, including sedation, severe constipation, hypotension, increased liver biochemical levels, hypersalivation, respiratory arrest, weight gain, adynamic ileus, and changes in both the ECG and the electroencephalogram.

Photosensitivity, retinopathy, and **hyperpigmentation** are associated with use of high dosages of chlorpromazine. Patients on long-term medication should have periodic eye examinations.

The **neuroleptic malignant syndrome (NMS)** is a catatonia-like state manifested by extrapyramidal signs, blood pressure changes, altered consciousness, and hyperpyrexia; it is an uncommon but serious complication of antipsychotic treatment. Muscle rigidity, involuntary movements, confusion, dysarthria, and dysphagia are accompanied by pallor, cardiovascular instability, fever, pulmonary congestion, and diaphoresis and may result in stupor, coma, and death. The cause may be related to a number of factors, including poor antipsychotic medication dosage control, affective illness, decreased serum iron, dehydration, and increased sensitivity of dopamine receptor sites. Lithium in combination with an antipsychotic medication may increase vulnerability. In most cases, the symptoms develop within the first 2 weeks of antipsychotic drug treatment. The syndrome may occur with small doses of the medications. Intramuscular administration is a risk factor. Elevated creatine kinase and leukocytosis with a shift to the left are present early in about half of cases. Treatment includes controlling the fever and providing fluid support. For mild cases benzodiazepines such as lorazepam are often first-line treatment; dopamine agonists such as bromocriptine, 2.5–10 mg orally three times a day, and amantadine, 100–200 mg orally twice a day, also have been useful. Dantrolene, 50 mg intravenously as needed, is used to alleviate rigidity (do not exceed 10 mg/kg/day due to hepatotoxicity risk). There is ongoing controversy about the efficacy of these agents. ECT has been used effectively in resistant cases. Clozapine has been used with relative safety and fair success as an antipsychotic medication for patients who have had NMS.

Akathisia is the most common (about 20%) extrapyramidal symptom. It usually occurs early in treatment (but may persist after antipsychotics are discontinued) and is frequently mistaken for anxiety or exacerbation of psychosis. It is characterized by a subjective desire to be in constant motion followed by an inability to sit or stand still and consequent pacing. It may induce suicidality or feelings of fright, rage, terror, or sexual torment. Insomnia is often present. It is crucial to educate patients in advance about these potential side effects so that the patients do not misinterpret them as signs of increased illness. In all cases, reevaluate the dosage requirement or the type of antipsychotic medication; switching to an antipsychotic with lower akathisia risk, such as clozapine, may be considered prior to adjunctive agents. Antiparkinsonism medications (such as trihexyphenidyl, 2–5 mg orally three times daily) may be helpful, but first-line treatment often includes a benzodiazepine (such as clonazepam, 0.5–1 mg orally three times daily). In resistant cases, symptoms may be alleviated by propranolol, 30–80 mg/day orally, diazepam, 5 mg orally three times daily, amantadine, 100 mg orally three times daily, low-dose mirtazapine, or vitamin B6.

Acute dystonias usually occur early, although a late (**tardive**) occurrence is reported in patients (mostly men after several years of therapy) who previously had early severe dystonic reactions and a mood disorder. Younger patients are at higher risk for acute dystonias. The most common signs are bizarre muscle spasms of the head, neck, and tongue. Frequently present are torticollis, oculogyric crises, swallowing or chewing difficulties, and masseter spasms. Laryngospasm is particularly dangerous. Back, arm, or leg muscle spasms are occasionally reported. Diphenhydramine, 50 mg intramuscularly, is effective for the acute crisis; one should then give benztropine mesylate, 2 mg orally twice daily, for several weeks, and then discontinue gradually. Few of the extrapyramidal symptoms require long-term use of antiparkinsonism medications.

Drug-induced parkinsonism is indistinguishable from idiopathic parkinsonism, but it is typically reversible, occurs later in treatment than the preceding extrapyramidal symptoms, and in some cases appears after antipsychotic withdrawal. The condition includes the typical signs of apathy and reduction of facial and arm movements (akinesia, which can mimic depression), festinating gait, rigidity, loss of postural reflexes, and pill-rolling tremor. High-potency antipsychotics often require antiparkinsonism medications, which can provide immediate relief in the same dosages as above. The dosage of the antipsychotic drug should also be reduced. After 4–6 weeks, antiparkinsonism medications can often be discontinued with no recurrent symptoms. For any of the extrapyramidal symptoms, amantadine, 100–400 mg orally daily, may be used instead of the antiparkinsonism medications. Antipsychotic-induced catatonia is similar to catatonic stupor with rigidity, drooling, urinary incontinence, and cogwheeling. It usually responds slowly to withdrawal of the offending medication and use of antiparkinsonism agents.

Tardive dyskinesia is a syndrome of abnormal involuntary stereotyped movements of the face, mouth, tongue, trunk, and limbs that may occur after months or (usually) years of treatment with antipsychotic agents. The syndrome affects 20–35% of patients who have undergone long-term antipsychotic therapy. Predisposing factors include older age, many years of treatment, cigarette smoking, and diabetes mellitus. There are no clear-cut differences among the antipsychotic medications in the development of tardive dyskinesia. However, clozapine is unique in that it has been found to treat antipsychotic-induced tardive dyskinesia. Early manifestations of tardive dyskinesia include fine worm-like movements of the tongue at rest, difficulty in sticking out the tongue, facial tics, increased blink frequency, or jaw movements of recent onset. Later manifestations may include bucco-linguo-masticatory movements, lip smacking, chewing motions, mouth opening and closing, disturbed gag reflex, puffing of the cheeks, disrupted speech, respiratory distress, or choreoathetoid movements of the extremities (the last being more prevalent in younger patients). The symptoms do not necessarily worsen even though antipsychotic medications are continued. The dyskinesias do not occur during sleep and can be voluntarily suppressed for short periods. Stress and movements in other parts of the body will often aggravate the condition.

The emphasis should be on prevention of side effects. Use the least amount of antipsychotic medication necessary to improve the psychotic symptoms. If early manifestations of dyskinesias occur, gradually discontinue antipsychotic medications, if clinically feasible. Keep the patient off the medications until reemergent psychotic symptoms dictate their resumption, at which point restart in low doses and gradually increase until there is clinical improvement. Clozapine and olanzapine appear to offer less risk of recurrence. The use of adjunctive agents such as benzodiazepines or lithium may help directly or indirectly by allowing control of psychotic symptoms with a low dosage of antipsychotics. If the dyskinesia syndrome recurs and it is necessary to continue antipsychotic medications to control psychotic symptoms, informed consent should be obtained. Vesicular monoamine transporter 2 (VMAT2) inhibitors, such as valbenazine and deutetrabenazine, amantadine, vitamin B_6, vitamin E, and propranolol all have had some usefulness in treating the dyskinetic side effects. The VMAT2 inhibitors are considered the treatment of choice for tardive dyskinesia and are the only medications FDA-approved for its treatment but are expensive and not covered by some insurance plans.

B. Social

Some individuals with a chronic psychiatric illness may have a history of repeated hospitalizations, a continued low level of functioning, and symptoms that never completely remit. Family rejection and work failure are common. In these cases, board and care homes staffed by personnel experienced in caring for psychiatric patients are most important. Supported housing models and assertive community treatment teams further enhance stability by providing flexible, recovery-oriented on-site and outreach support. Nonresidential self-help groups such as Recovery, Inc., should be utilized whenever possible. Peer-led support groups offer additional avenues for experiential sharing and empowerment. Employment programs such as Individual Placement and Support and work agencies (eg, Goodwill Industries) provide assessment, training, and job opportunities at a level commensurate with the person's clinical condition.

C. Psychological

CBT is an efficacious adjunctive strategy in the treatment of schizophrenia. It involves helping the individual challenge psychotic thinking, particularly improving negative symptoms and altering the response to hallucinations. A newer, specialized approach, AVATAR therapy, uses a digitally created representation of the patient's distressing voice to facilitate structured, therapist-guided dialogues in which the patient gradually develops a more empowered and less fearful stance toward the voice; this brief intervention has shown promise for persistent, medication-resistant auditory hallucinations and is emerging as a targeted option within CBT-informed treatments. Similarly, a form of psychotherapy called acceptance and commitment therapy has shown value in helping prevent hospitalizations in schizophrenia. Cognitive remediation therapy is another approach to treatment that may help patients with schizophrenia become better able to focus their disorganized thinking and enhance overall cognitive performance. Family therapy may also help alleviate the patient's stress and to assist relatives in coping with the patient. Metacognitive training, social skills training, psychoeducation, family interventions, physical exercise, lifestyle interventions, and supported employment are all additional effective strategies. Overall, it is best to employ both medication and psychosocial services early when symptoms begin.

D. Behavioral

Hospitalization may be necessary, particularly early in the course of illness and in those situations when the patient is unable to care for themselves (gravely disabled), a danger to self, or a danger to others. The presence of competent family members or social support lessens the need for hospitalization, and each case should be judged individually. The major considerations are to prevent self-inflicted harm or harm to others and to provide for the patient's basic needs. Assertive community treatment may serve as an alternative to hospitalization for suitable patients with histories of poor service engagement, emphasizing multidisciplinary outreach and crisis resolution.

Behavioral techniques (see above) are most frequently used in therapeutic settings such as day treatment centers, but they can also be incorporated into family situations or any therapeutic setting.

E. Neuromodulation

Electroconvulsive therapy (ECT) has been effective in treating catatonia and in treating schizophrenia when used in combination with medications. Recent studies confirm ECT's efficacy in treatment-resistant cases. Repetitive transcranial magnetic stimulation (rTMS) shows promise for negative symptoms and cognitive deficits with good safety and tolerability.

Prognosis

The course of schizophrenia is heterogeneous. With early intervention, sustained antipsychotic treatment, and psychosocial rehabilitation, a substantial minority achieve meaningful functional recovery, although residual cognitive and negative symptoms are common. For most patients with any psychosis, the prognosis is good for alleviation of positive symptoms such as hallucinations or delusions treated with medication. Negative symptoms such as diminished affect and sociability are much more difficult to treat but may be mildly responsive to atypical antipsychotics. Cognitive deficits, such as the executive dysfunction that is common to schizophrenia, also do not appear as responsive to antipsychotics as do positive symptoms but show benefit from cognitive remediation therapies integrated with psychosocial rehabilitation. Both negative symptoms and cognitive deficits appear to contribute more to long-term disability than do positive symptoms. Comprehensive psychosocial interventions, including cognitive remediation, family interventions, and supported employment, can enhance functional outcomes and mitigate these risks. Unavailability of structured work situations and lack of family therapy or access to other social support are two other reasons why the prognosis is so guarded in such a large percentage of patients. Patients with schizophrenia have a shorter life expectancy than the general population and often have associated comorbid conditions such as the metabolic syndrome, which may be induced or exacerbated by the atypical antipsychotic agents.

Many patients with schizoaffective disorder have ongoing functional impairment, and the long-term prognosis is generally considered intermediate. It is often better than for schizophrenia but not as favorable as for pure mood disorders, depending heavily on the predominance and course of both psychotic and affective symptoms.

Barlati S et al. Evidence-based psychosocial interventions in schizophrenia: a critical review. Curr Opin Psychiatry. 2024;37:131. [PMID: 38410981]

Berendsen S et al. Cognitive behavioural therapy for the treatment of schizophrenia spectrum disorders: an umbrella review of meta-analyses of randomised controlled trials. EClinicalMedicine. 2024;67:102392. [PMID: 38274116]

McCutcheon RA et al; INTEGRATE Advisory Group. INTEGRATE: International guidelines for the algorithmic treatment of schizophrenia. Lancet Psychiatry. 2025;12:384. [PMID: 40179920]

Yeh TC et al. Pharmacological and nonpharmacological augmentation treatments for clozapine-resistant schizophrenia: a systematic review and network meta-analysis with normalized entropy assessment. Asian J Psychiatr. 2023;79:103375. [PMID: 36470132]

MOOD DISORDERS (Depression & Mania)

ESSENTIALS OF DIAGNOSIS

Present in most depressions

- Mood varies from mild sadness to intense despondency and feelings of guilt, worthlessness, and hopelessness.
- Difficulty in thinking, including inability to concentrate, ruminations, and lack of decisiveness.
- Loss of interest, with diminished involvement in work and recreation.
- Somatic complaints such as disrupted, lessened, or excessive sleep; loss of energy; change in appetite; decreased sexual drive.

Present in some severe depressions

- Psychomotor retardation or agitation.
- Delusions of a somatic or persecutory nature.
- Withdrawal from activities.
- Physical symptoms of major severity, eg, anorexia, insomnia, reduced sexual drive, weight loss, and various somatic complaints.
- Suicidal ideation.

Possible symptoms in mania

- Mood ranging from euphoria to irritability.
- Sleep disruption.
- Hyperactivity.
- Racing thoughts.
- Grandiosity or extreme overconfidence.
- Variable psychotic symptoms.

General Considerations

Depression is extremely common, with up to 30% of primary care patients having depressive symptoms. Depression may be the final expression of (1) genetic factors, (2) developmental problems (negative childhood events), or (3) psychosocial stresses (divorce, unemployment).

Mania and hypomania are hallmarks of bipolar disorder. They may occur alone or together with depression either in a mixed episode or in cyclical fashion.

Clinical Findings

There are four major types of depression, with similar symptoms in each group.

A. Adjustment Disorder with Depressed Mood

Depressed mood may occur in reaction to some identifiable stressor or adverse life situation, usually loss of a person by death (grief reaction), divorce, etc; financial reversal (crisis); or loss of an established role, such as being needed. Although sadness and grief are normal responses to loss, depression is not. The symptoms range from mild sadness, anxiety, irritability, worry, and lack of concentration, discouragement, and somatic complaints to the more severe symptoms of frank depression. When the full criteria for major depressive disorder are present, that diagnosis should be made and treatment instituted, even when there is a known stressor. One should not neglect treatment for major depression simply because it appears to be an understandable reaction to a particular stress or difficulty.

B. Depressive Disorders

The subclassifications include major depressive disorder and dysthymia.

1. Major depressive disorder—A major depressive disorder consists of a syndrome of mood, physical, and cognitive symptoms that occurs at any time of life. Complaints vary widely but frequently include a loss of interest and pleasure (**anhedonia**), withdrawal from activities, and feelings of guilt. Also included are inability to concentrate, some cognitive dysfunction, anxiety, chronic fatigue, feelings of worthlessness, somatic complaints (unexplained somatic complaints frequently indicate depression), loss of sexual drive, and thoughts of death. Unemployment has been associated with increase in depression risk. Diurnal variation with improvement as the day progresses is common. Vegetative signs that frequently occur are insomnia, anorexia with weight loss, and constipation. Occasionally, severe agitation and psychotic ideation are present. **Psychotic major depression** occurs in up to 14% of all patients with major depression and 25% of patients who are hospitalized with depression. Psychotic symptoms (delusions, paranoia) are more common in depressed persons who are older than 50 years. Paranoid symptoms may range from general suspiciousness to ideas of reference with delusions. The somatic delusions frequently revolve around feelings of impending annihilation or somatic concerns (eg, that the body is rotting away with cancer). Hallucinations are less common than unusual beliefs and tend not to occur independent of delusions.

In addition to psychotic major depression, other subcategories include **major depression with atypical features** that is characterized by hypersomnia, overeating, lethargy, and mood reactivity in which the mood brightens in response to positive events or news. **Melancholic major depression** is characterized by a lack of mood reactivity seen in atypical depression, the presence of a prominent anhedonia, and more severe vegetative symptoms. **Major depression with a seasonal onset (seasonal affective disorder)** is a dysfunction of circadian rhythms that occurs more commonly in the fall and winter months and is believed to be due to decreased exposure to full-spectrum light. Common symptoms include carbohydrate craving, lethargy, hyperphagia, and hypersomnia. **Major depression with peripartum onset** occurs during pregnancy or starts up to 4 weeks after delivery.

Half of depressions associated with the peripartum period start during pregnancy. Most women (up to 80%) experience some mild letdown of mood in the postpartum period. For some of these (10–15%), the symptoms are more severe and similar to those usually seen in serious depression, with a potential emphasis on concerns related to the baby (obsessive thoughts about harming it or inability to care for it). When psychotic symptoms occur, there is frequently associated sleep deprivation, volatility of behavior, and manic-like symptoms. Postpartum psychosis is much less common (< 2%), often occurs within the first 2 weeks, and requires early and aggressive management. Biologic vulnerability with hormonal changes and psychosocial stressors all play a role. The chances of a second episode are about 25% and may be reduced with prophylactic treatment.

2. Persistent depressive disorder—Persistent depressive disorder (previously known as dysthymia) is a chronic depressive disturbance characterized by a depressed mood with sadness, loss of interest, fatigue, poor appetite, low self-esteem, feelings of hopelessness, and withdrawal from activities over a period of 2 or more years with a relatively persistent course. Generally, the symptoms are milder but longer-lasting than those in a major depressive episode.

3. Premenstrual dysphoric disorder—Depressive symptoms occur during the late luteal phase (last 2 weeks) of the menstrual cycle. (See also Chapter 21.)

C. Bipolar Disorder

Bipolar spectrum illnesses consist of episodic mood shifts into mania, major depression, hypomania, and mixed mood states. The initial diagnosis of bipolar disorder can be difficult due to its ability to mimic aspects of many other coincident major mental health disorders and a high comorbidity with substance abuse. **Bipolar I** is diagnosed when an individual has manic episodes. For individuals who experience hypomanic episodes without frank mania as well as depressive episodes, the diagnosis is **bipolar II**.

1. Mania—A manic episode is a mood state characterized by elation or intense irritability with increased energy or activity, overinvolvement in life activities, flight of ideas, easy distractibility, and little need for sleep. The overenthusiastic quality of the mood and the expansive behavior initially attract others, but the irritability, mood lability with swings into depression, aggressive behavior, and grandiosity usually lead to marked interpersonal difficulties. Activities may occur that are later regretted, eg, excessive spending, resignation from a job, a hasty marriage, sexual acting-out, and exhibitionistic behavior, with alienation of friends and family. Atypical manic episodes can include gross delusions, paranoid ideation of severe proportions, and auditory hallucinations usually related to some grandiose perception. The episodes begin abruptly (sometimes precipitated by life stresses) and may last from several days to months. Generally, the manic episodes are of shorter duration than the depressive episodes. In almost all cases, the manic episode is part of a broader bipolar disorder. Patients with four or more discrete episodes of a mood disturbance in 1 year have "**rapid cycling**." Substance abuse, particularly cocaine, can mimic rapid cycling.

2. Cyclothymic disorder—This is a chronic mood disturbance with episodes of subsyndromal depression and hypomania. The symptoms must have at least a 2-year duration and are milder than those that occur in depressive or manic episodes. Occasionally, the symptoms will escalate into a full-blown manic or depressive episode, in which case reclassification as bipolar I or II would be warranted.

D. Mood Disorders Secondary to Illness and Medications

Any illness, severe or mild, can cause significant depression. Conditions such as rheumatoid arthritis, multiple sclerosis, stroke, and chronic heart disease are likely to be associated with depression, as are other chronic illnesses. Depression is common in cancer, as well, with a particularly high degree of comorbidity in pancreatic cancer. Hormonal variations clearly play a role in some depressions. Varying degrees of depression occur at various times in schizophrenic disorders, CNS disease, and organic mental states. Alcohol dependency frequently coexists with serious depression.

Drug-induced depression has occurred with a number of medications. Corticosteroids are commonly associated with mood changes such as depression and hypomania or psychosis. Medications associated with development of depressive symptoms include digitalis, antiparkinsonian medications, retinoids, interferon, disulfiram, anticholinesterase agents, and clonidine. Stimulant use results in a depressive syndrome when the drug is withdrawn. Alcohol, sedatives, and opioids are depressants but, paradoxically, are often used by patients in self-treatment of depression.

Differential Diagnosis

Since depression may be a part of any illness—either reactively or as a secondary symptom—careful attention must be given to personal life adjustment problems and the role of medications. Schizophrenia, partial complex seizures, organic brain syndromes, panic disorders, and anxiety disorders must be differentiated. Thyroid dysfunction and other endocrinopathies should be ruled out. Malignancies are sometimes associated with depressive symptoms and may antecede the diagnosis of tumor. Strokes, particularly dominant hemisphere lesions, can occasionally present with a syndrome that looks like major depression. Bipolar disorders, particularly bipolar II, warrant careful consideration due to substantial symptom overlap with unipolar depression, often leading to initial misdiagnosis as major depressive disorder.

Complications

The most serious complication of major depression is **suicide**. Recent guidelines emphasize individualized risk formulation over categoric risk stratification (low, medium, high), recognizing the fluctuating nature of suicidal ideation. Suicide rates in the general population vary from 9 per 100,000 in Spain to 15 per 100,000 in the United States to 31 per 100,000 in Russia. Men over the age of 50 are more likely to die by suicide because of their tendency to use more lethal means, particularly guns. Women make more attempts but are less likely to die by suicide. The suicide rate in the younger population, aged 15–35, continues to rise. Suicide rates are higher in patients with previous suicide attempts, a family history of suicide, psychiatric illness (eg, panic disorder, anxiety, severe depression), and severe medical illness. Acute alcohol use is implicated in approximately 50% of all deaths by suicide. Suicide is 10 times more prevalent in patients with schizophrenia than in the general population. Contemplation of violent methods, a humiliating social stressor, and drug use (including long-term sedative or alcohol use) contribute to impulsiveness or mood swings. Patients with cancer, respiratory illnesses, AIDS, and those being maintained on hemodialysis have higher suicide rates.

Patients confronted with acute situational stress may make suicide attempts. These situations include a recent breakup in a relationship, a major disappointment, or a stressful situation with a component of public humiliation (eg, person who has experienced cyberbullying). A suicide attempt in such cases may be an impulsive or aggressive act not associated with significant depression.

The immediate goal of psychiatric evaluation is to assess the current suicidal risk and determine the need for hospitalization versus outpatient management. A useful question is to ask the person whether they have thoughts that life is not worth living. Assessing the risk further by inquiring about intent, plans, means, and suicide-inhibiting factors (eg, strong ties to children or the church) is essential. Alcohol, hopelessness, delusional thoughts, and complete or nearly complete loss of interest in life or ability to experience pleasure are all correlated with increased risk of suicide attempts. In a patient with depression, an apparent dramatic improvement may be due to the patient's decision to die by suicide. Other high-risk individuals are those with psychotic illness who tend not to verbalize their concerns. An attempt is less likely to be suicidal if very small amounts of poison or medication were ingested or scratching of wrists was superficial, if the act was performed near others or with early notification of others, or if the attempt was arranged so that early detection would be anticipated.

The patient's current mood status is best evaluated by direct evaluation of plans and concerns about the future, personal reactions to the attempt, and thoughts about the reactions of others. The patient's immediate resources should also be assessed—people who can be significantly involved, family support, job situation, financial resources, etc. Measurement of mood is often facilitated by using a standardized instrument such as the **Hamilton** or **Montgomery-Asberg** clinician-administered rating scales or the self-administered **Quick Inventory of Depressive Symptomatology (QIDS-SR 16).** Scales allow for initial assessment as well as ongoing treatment tracking. Suicide risk can be specifically assessed using a validated instrument such as the **Columbia-Suicide Severity Risk Scale** (https://cssrs.columbia.edu/wp-content/uploads/C-SSRS_Pediatric-SLC_11.14.16.pdf).

If hospitalization is not indicated after a suicide attempt, the clinician must formulate and institute a treatment plan or make an adequate referral. (The National Suicide Prevention Lifeline, 1-800-273-8255, may be of assistance.) Medication should be dispensed in small amounts to at-risk patients. Although tricyclic antidepressants (TCAs) and SSRIs are associated with an equal incidence of suicide attempts, the risk of death by suicide is much higher with TCA overdose. Guns and medications should be removed from the patient's household. Driving should be cautioned against until the patient improves.

Treatment of Depression

A. Medical

Milder forms of depression usually do not require medication therapy and can be managed by psychotherapy and the passage of time. Hospitalization is necessary if suicide is a major consideration or if complex treatment modalities are required. In severe cases—particularly when vegetative signs are significant and symptoms have persisted for more than a few weeks—antidepressant medication therapy is often effective. Medication therapy is also suggested by a family history of major depression in first-degree relatives or a past history of prior episodes.

The antidepressant medications may be classified into four groups: (1) the newer antidepressants, including the SSRIs, SNRIs, gepirone (selective 5-HT1A receptor agonist), bupropion, vilazodone, vortioxetine, and mirtazapine, (2) the TCAs and clinically similar medications, (3) the MAO inhibitors (Table 28–6), and (4) stimulants.

Medication selection is influenced by the history of previous response or lack thereof if that information is available. A positive family history of response to a particular medication may suggest that the patient will respond similarly. If no background information is available, a medication such as sertraline, 25 mg orally daily and increasing gradually up to 200 mg, depending on response and side effects, or venlafaxine at 37.5 mg/day and titrated gradually, as necessary, to a maximum dose of 225 mg/day can be selected and a full trial instituted. During the medication trial, patients should be monitored for worsening mood or suicidal ideation every 1–2 weeks until week 6. The STAR*D trial suggests that if there is no response to the first medication, the best alternatives are to switch to a second agent that may be from the same or different class of antidepressant; if there is partial response to the first agent, another approach is to try augmenting it with a second agent, such as bupropion (150–450 mg/day), lithium (eg, 300–900 mg/day orally), thyroid medication (eg, liothyronine, 25–50 mcg/day orally), or a second-generation antipsychotic (eg, aripiprazole [5–15 mg/day]). The Agency for Health Care Policy and Research has produced clinical practice guidelines that outline one algorithm of treatment decisions (Figure 28–1).

Cognitive issues such as concentration and memory problems are common to depression; the evidence shows that these issues sometimes persist even after depression has remitted, with a higher risk in those individuals who have had more depressive episodes.

Psychotic depression should be treated with a combination of an antipsychotic and an antidepressant such as an SSRI at their usual doses. Mifepristone may have specific and early activity against psychotic depression. ECT is generally regarded as the single most effective treatment for psychotic depression, with remission rates between 60% and 90%.

Major depression with atypical features or seasonal onset can be treated with bupropion or an SSRI with good results. MAO inhibitors appear more effective than TCAs, and an MAO inhibitor may be used if more benign antidepressant strategies prove unsuccessful.

Melancholic depression may respond to ECT, TCAs, and SNRIs, which are preferable to SSRIs. However, SSRIs are often used in the treatment of melancholic depression and are effective in many cases.

Depressed patients often have suicidal thoughts, and the amount of medication dispensed should be appropriately controlled particularly if prescribing an MAO inhibitor, TCA, and to a lesser extent, venlafaxine. At the same time, adults with untreated depression are at higher risk for suicide than those who are treated sufficiently to reduce symptoms. It has been thought that in children and adolescent populations, antidepressants may be associated with slightly increased risk of suicidality. One meta-analysis indicates that suicidality persists even after symptoms of depression are treated, suggesting other causes such as increased impulsivity among younger patients. After age 25, antidepressants may have neutral or possibly protective effects until age 65 years or older. The older TCAs have a narrow therapeutic index. One advantage of the newer medications is their wider margin of safety. Nonetheless, even with newer agents, because of the possibility of suicidality early in antidepressant treatment, close follow-up is indicated. In all cases of pharmacologic management of depressed states, caution is indicated until the risk of suicide is considered minimal.

1. SSRIs, SNRIs, and atypical antidepressants—SSRIs include fluoxetine, sertraline, paroxetine, fluvoxamine, and citalopram and its enantiomer escitalopram (Table 28–6). The chief advantages of these agents are that they are generally well tolerated, the starting dose is typically a therapeutic dose for most patients, and they have much lower lethality in overdose compared with TCAs or MAO inhibitors. (Citalopram carries a warning regarding QT prolongation in doses above 40 mg, and 20 mg is considered the maximum dose for patients older than 60 years. There is no similar FDA warning for escitalopram.) The SNRIs include venlafaxine, desvenlafaxine, duloxetine, milnacipran, and levomilnacipran. In addition to possessing the strong serotonin reuptake blocking properties of the SSRIs, the SNRIs are also norepinephrine reuptake blockers. The atypical antidepressants are bupropion, nefazodone, trazodone, vilazodone, vortioxetine, and mirtazapine (Table 28–6). All these antidepressants are effective in the treatment of depression, both typical and atypical. The SSRI medications have been effective in the treatment of panic disorder, bulimia, GAD, OCD, and PTSD.

Many of the medications in this group tend to be activating and are given in the morning so as not to interfere with sleep. Some patients, however, may have sedation, requiring that the medication be given at bedtime. The SSRIs can be given in once-daily dosage. Nefazodone and trazodone are usually given twice daily. Bupropion and venlafaxine are available in extended-release formulations and can be given once daily. Venlafaxine appears to be more effective with doses > 200 mg/day orally, although some individuals respond to doses as low as 75 mg/day. There may be some delay in response with medications in

Table 28–6. Commonly used antidepressant medications (listed in alphabetical order within classes).

Medication	Usual Daily Oral Dose (mg)	Usual Daily Maximum Dose (mg)	Sedative Effects[1]	Anticholinergic Effects[1]
SSRIs				
Citalopram (Celexa)	20	40	<1	1
Escitalopram (Lexapro)	10	20	<1	1
Fluoxetine (Prozac, Sarafem)	5–40	80	<1	<1
Fluvoxamine (Luvox)	100–300	300	1	<1
Paroxetine (Paxil)	20–30	50	1	1
Sertraline (Zoloft)	50–150	200	<1	<1
SNRIs				
Desvenlafaxine (Pristiq)	50	100	1	<1
Duloxetine (Cymbalta)	40	60	2	3
Levomilnacipran (Fetzima)	40	120	1	1
Milnacipran (Savella)	100	200	1	1
Venlafaxine XR (Effexor)	150–225	225	1	<1
Tricyclic and Clinically Similar Compounds				
Amitriptyline (Elavil)	150–250	300	4	4
Amoxapine (Asendin)	150–200	400	2	2
Clomipramine (Anafranil)	100	250	3	3
Desipramine (Norpramin)	100–250	300	1	1
Doxepin (Sinequan)	150–200	300	4	3
Imipramine (Tofranil)	150–200	300	3	3
Maprotiline (Ludiomil)	100–200	300	4	2
Nortriptyline (Aventyl, Pamelor)	100–150	150	2	2
Protriptyline (Vivactil)	15–40	60	1	3
Trimipramine (Surmontil)	75–200	200	4	4
Monoamine Oxidase Inhibitors				
Phenelzine (Nardil)	45–60	90	...	...
Selegiline transdermal (Emsam)	6 (skin patch)	12	...	...
Tranylcypromine (Parnate)	20–30	50	...	...
Other Compounds				
Bupropion SR (Wellbutrin SR)	300	400[2]	<1	<1
Bupropion XL (Wellbutrin XL)	300[4]	450[3]	<1	<1
Mirtazapine (Remeron)	15–45	45	4	2
Nefazodone (Serzone)	150–600	600	3	1
Trazodone (Desyrel)	100–300	400	4	<1
Vilazodone (Viibryd)	10–40	40	1	1
Vortioxetine (Brintellix)	10	20	<1	<1

[1] 1, weak effect; 4, strong effect.

[2] 200 mg twice daily.

[3] Wellbutrin XL is a once-daily form of bupropion. Bupropion is still available as immediate release, and, if used, no single dose should exceed 150 mg.

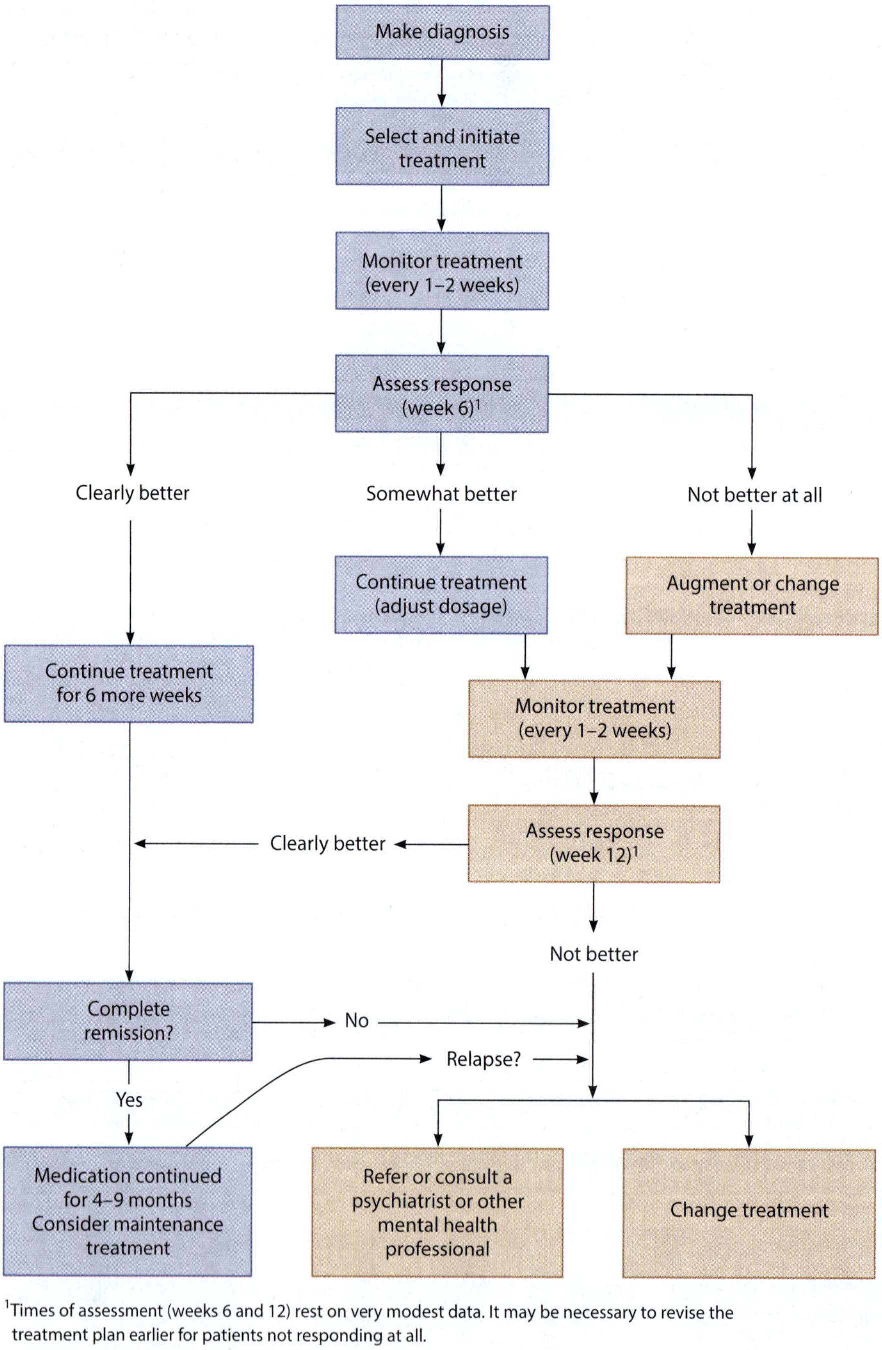

▲ **Figure 28–1.** Overview of treatment for depression. (Reproduced from Agency for Health Care Policy and Research: Depression in Primary Care. Vol. 2: Treatment of Major Depression. United States Department of Health and Human Services, 1993.)

this group; fluoxetine, for example, requires 2–6 weeks to act in depression. The starting dose of fluoxetine (10 mg) is given for 1 week before increasing to the average daily oral dose of 20 mg for depression. Some patients, particularly older adults, may tolerate and benefit from as little as 10 mg/day or every other day. Newer medications such as intranasal esketamine and oral bupropion combined with dextromethorphan work more rapidly. Intravenous brexanolone and oral zuranolone also have more rapid efficacy than traditional antidepressants and specific efficacy for postpartum depression.

The side effects common to these medications are headache, nausea, tinnitus, insomnia, and nervousness. Akathisia has been common with the SSRIs; other extrapyramidal symptoms (eg, dystonias) have occurred infrequently but particularly in withdrawal states. Because SSRIs affect platelet serotonin levels, abnormal bleeding can occur. Sexual side effects of erectile dysfunction, retrograde ejaculation, and anorgasmia are very common with the SSRIs. Oral phosphodiesterase-5 inhibitors (such as sildenafil, 25–50 mg; tadalafil, 5–20 mg; or vardenafil, 10–20 mg taken 1 hour prior to sexual activity) can improve erectile dysfunction in some patients and have been shown to improve other SSRI-induced sexual dysfunction in both men and women. Adjunctive bupropion (75–150 mg orally daily) may also enhance sexual arousal. Taking a "drug holiday," ie, skipping a day of medication periodically when sexual activity is anticipated, can also decrease sexual side effects. The SSRIs are strong serotonin uptake blockers and may in high dosage or in combination with MAO inhibitors cause a **"serotonin syndrome."** This syndrome is manifested by rigidity, hyperthermia, autonomic instability, myoclonus, confusion, delirium, and coma. This syndrome can be troublesome in older adults. SSRIs are safer agents than TCAs in patients with cardiac disease.

Withdrawal symptoms, including dizziness, paresthesias, dysphoric mood, agitation, and a flu-like state, have been reported for the shorter-acting SSRIs and SNRIs but may occur with other classes including the TCAs and MAO inhibitors. These medications should be discontinued gradually over a period of weeks or months to reduce the risk of withdrawal phenomena.

Venlafaxine lacks significant anticholinergic side effects. Nausea, nervousness, and profuse sweating appear to be the major side effects. Venlafaxine appears to have few drug-drug interactions. It does require monitoring of blood pressure because dose-related hypertension may develop in some individuals. Desvenlafaxine, a newer form of the medication, is started at its target dose of 50 mg/day orally and does not require upward titration although higher doses have been well studied and some patients benefit from 100 mg/day. Duloxetine may also result in small increases in blood pressure. Common side effects include dry mouth, dizziness, and fatigue. Milnacipran, approved for the treatment of fibromyalgia, and levomilnacipran, approved for the treatment of major depression, carry many of the side effects common to other SNRIs including a mild tachycardia, hypertension, sexual side effects, mydriasis, urinary constriction, and occasional abnormal bleeding. Levomilnacipran is started at 20 mg/day orally then increased to 40 mg/day after 2–3 days. The target dose is 40–120 mg given once daily. Milnacipran is typically started at 12.5 mg/day orally, titrated to 12.5 mg twice daily after 2 days, and then to 25 mg twice daily after 7 days. The target dose is typically 100–200 mg/day given in in two divided doses. While not approved for the treatment of major depression, the evidence suggests that milnacipran, like levomilnacipran, is an effective antidepressant agent.

Mirtazapine is thought to enhance central noradrenergic and serotonergic activity with minimal sexual side effects compared with the SSRIs. Its action as a potent antagonist of histaminergic receptors may make it a useful agent for patients with depression and insomnia. It is also an effective antiemetic due to its antagonism of the 5-HT_3 receptor. Its most common adverse side effects include somnolence, increased appetite, weight gain, lipid abnormalities, and dizziness. There is a modest association of agranulocytosis (2 of 2796 patients) or a clinically significant neutropenia. It is given in a single oral dose at bedtime starting at 15 mg and titrated up to 45 mg, although 30 mg may be optimal for most people.

Vortioxetine is an antidepressant that blocks serotonin reuptake, is a partial agonist of the 5-HT_{1A} receptor, and affects a variety of other serotonin receptor sites. The side effects attributed to its serotonergic effects include GI upset and sexual dysfunction. It has demonstrated efficacy in improving some cognitive symptoms of depression Vortioxetine is typically dosed at 10 mg/day orally and may be increased to 20 mg/day.

2. Tricyclic antidepressants (TCAs) and clinically similar medications—TCAs were the mainstay of medication therapy for depression for many years. They have also been effective in panic disorder, pain syndromes, and anxiety states. Specific ones have been studied and found to be effective in OCD (clomipramine), enuresis (imipramine), psychotic depression (amoxapine), and reduction of craving in cocaine withdrawal (desipramine).

TCAs are characterized more by their similarities than by their differences. They tend to affect both serotonin and norepinephrine reuptake; some medications act mainly on the former and others principally on the latter neurotransmitter system. Individuals receiving the same dosages vary markedly in therapeutic drug levels achieved (older adult patients require smaller doses), and determination of plasma drug levels is helpful when clinical response has been disappointing. Nortriptyline is usually effective when plasma levels are between 50 and 150 ng/mL; imipramine at plasma levels of 200–250 ng/mL; and desipramine at plasma levels of 100–250 ng/mL. High blood levels are not more effective than moderate levels and may be counterproductive (eg, delirium, seizures). Patients with GI side effects benefit from plasma level monitoring to assess absorption of the drug. Most TCAs can be given in a single dose at bedtime, starting at low doses (eg, nortriptyline 25 mg orally) and increasing by 25 mg every several days as tolerated until the therapeutic response is achieved (eg, nortriptyline, 100–150 mg) or to maximum dose if necessary (eg, nortriptyline, 150 mg). The most common cause of treatment failure is an inadequate trial. A full trial consists of giving a therapeutic daily dosage for at least 6 weeks. Because of marked anticholinergic and sedating side effects, clomipramine is started at a low dose (25 mg/day orally) and increased slowly in divided doses up to 100 mg/day, held at that level for several days, and then gradually increased as necessary up to 250 mg/day. The TCAs have anticholinergic side effects to varying degrees (amitriptyline 100 mg is equivalent to atropine 5 mg). One must be particularly wary of the effect in older adult men with prostatic hyperplasia. The anticholinergic effects also predispose to other medical problems such as constipation, confusion, heat stroke, or dental problems from xerostomia. Orthostatic hypotension is common, is not dose-dependent, and may not remit with time on medication; this may predispose to falls and hip fractures in older adults.

Cardiac effects of the TCAs are functions of the anticholinergic effect, direct myocardial depression, quinidine-like effect, and interference with adrenergic neurons. These factors may produce altered rate, rhythm, and contractility, particularly in patients with preexisting cardiac disease, such as bundle-branch or bifascicular block. Even relatively small overdoses (eg, 1500 mg of imipramine) have resulted in lethal arrhythmias. Electrocardiographic changes range from benign ST segment and T wave changes and sinus tachycardia to a variety of complex and serious arrhythmias requiring a change in medication. Because TCAs have class I antiarrhythmic effects, they should be used with caution in patients with ischemic heart disease, arrhythmias, or conduction disturbances. SSRIs or the atypical antidepressants are better initial choices for this population.

TCAs lower the seizure threshold, which is of particular concern in patients with risk for seizures. Loss of libido and erectile, ejaculatory, and orgasmic dysfunction are common and can compromise compliance. Trazodone rarely causes priapism (1 in 9000), but when it occurs, it requires treatment within 12 hours (epinephrine 1:1000 injected into the corpus cavernosum). Delirium, agitation, and mania are infrequent complications of the TCAs but can occur. Sudden discontinuation of some of these medications can produce "cholinergic rebound," manifested by headaches and nausea with abdominal cramps. Overdoses of TCAs are often serious because of the narrow therapeutic index and quinidine-like effects (see Chapter 42).

3. Monoamine oxidase inhibitors—The MAO inhibitors are generally used as third-line medications for depression (after a failure of SSRIs, SNRIs, TCAs, or the atypical antidepressants) because of the dietary and other restrictions required (Table 28–7). They also should be considered third-line medications for refractory panic disorder. MAO inhibitor skin patches (selegiline) bypass the GI tract, obviating the need for dietary restrictions at the lowest dosage strength (6 mg/24 hours).

The MAO inhibitors commonly cause symptoms of orthostatic hypotension (which may persist) and sympathomimetic effects of tachycardia, sweating, and tremor. Nausea, insomnia (often associated with intense afternoon drowsiness), and sexual dysfunction are common. CNS effects include agitation and toxic psychoses. Dietary limitations (see Table 28–7) and abstinence from medication products containing phenylpropanolamine, phenylephrine, meperidine, dextromethorphan, and pseudoephedrine are mandatory for MAO-A type inhibitors (those marketed for treatment of depression), since the reduction of available MAO leaves the patient vulnerable to exogenous amines (eg, tyramine in foodstuffs).

Table 28–7. Principal dietary restrictions in MAO inhibitor use.

1. Cheese, except cream cheese and cottage cheese and fresh yogurt
2. Fermented or aged meats such as bologna, salami
3. Broad bean pods such as Chinese bean pods
4. Liver of all types
5. Meat and yeast extracts
6. Red wine, sherry, vermouth, cognac, beer, ale
7. Soy sauce, shrimp paste, sauerkraut

4. Other medications—Dextroamphetamine (5–30 mg/day orally) and methylphenidate (10–45 mg/day orally) may be effective for the short-term treatment of some depressive symptoms in medically ill and geriatric patients. The stimulants are notable for rapid onset of action (hours) and a paucity of side effects (tachycardia, agitation) in most patients. These agents may also be useful as adjunctive agents in refractory depression. Intravenous infusion of the dissociative anesthetic ketamine has been shown to lead to a rapid improvement in depressive symptoms in 50–70% of patients with depression. The effects of a single treatment are short-lived (about 3–7 days). Esketamine nasal spray is approved for the treatment of depression for patients who have been inadequately treated by two other antidepressant medications. However, long-term use of esketamine or ketamine may increase the risk of abuse and longer-term impacts on mood and suicidality.

Allopregnanolone, a neurosteroid, is an allosteric modulator of GABA-a receptors and is approved for the treatment of postpartum depression. It is administered intravenously, and the antidepressant effects are rapid. The most common side effects of allopregnanolone are headache, dizziness, and somnolence. There is a rare side effect of loss of consciousness that requires the infusion be monitored in a health care facility An oral analog of brexanolone, zuranolone, was approved in 2023 to treat postpartum depression. It is taken as a once-daily, 50-mg dose over 14 days and appears about as effective as intravenous brexanolone.

5. Switching and combination therapy—If there has been a partial response, evidence supports medication augmentation. If the therapeutic response has been poor after an adequate trial with the chosen medication, the diagnosis should be reassessed. Assuming that the trial has been adequate and the diagnosis is correct, a trial with a second medication is appropriate. In switching from one group to another, an adequate "washout time" must be allowed. This is critical in certain situations—eg, in switching from an MAO inhibitor to a TCA, allow 2–3 weeks between stopping one medication and starting another; in switching from an SSRI to an MAO inhibitor, allow 4–5 weeks for fluoxetine and at least 2 weeks for other SSRIs. In switching within groups—eg, from one TCA to another (amitriptyline to desipramine, etc)—no washout time is needed, and one can rapidly decrease the dosage of one medication while increasing the other. In clinical practice, adjunctive treatment with lithium, buspirone, or thyroid hormone may be helpful in depression. The adjunctive use of low-dose atypical antipsychotics such as aripiprazole, olanzapine, and quetiapine in the treatment of patients with refractory depression may be helpful. The side effect risk is the same as when treating psychosis. Adding an atypical agent requires monitoring BMI, lipids, and glucose. Combining two antidepressants or adding an antipsychotic to an antidepressant requires caution and is usually reserved for clinicians who feel comfortable managing this or after psychiatric consultation.

6. Maintenance and tapering—When clinical relief of symptoms is obtained, medication is continued for 6–12 months in the same dosage required in the acute stage.

Although there is a higher risk of relapse after tapering off medication, there is evidence that cognitive behavioral therapy can prevent symptom relapse and the need for long-term medication. The full dosage should be continued indefinitely when the individual has had three episodes. Major depression generally should be considered a chronic/intermittent disease with most patients having relapses in time and some patients never fully recovering from a depressive episode. If the medication is being tapered, it should be done gradually over several months, monitoring closely for relapse.

7. Drug interactions—There are numerous possible drug interactions that prescribers should consider. Review of potential drug interactions with available online tools or a pharmacist is recommended.

8. Electroconvulsive therapy—ECT is the most effective (about 45–85% remission rate) treatment of severe depression. The mechanism of action is not known, but it is thought to involve major neurotransmitter responses at the cell membrane. In treatment-resistant depression, remission rates from ECT are lower (around 48%). It is particularly effective for the delusions and agitation commonly seen with depression in older adults. It is indicated when medical conditions preclude the use of antidepressants, with nonresponsiveness to these medications, and for extreme suicidality. Comparative controlled studies of ECT in severe depression show that it is more effective than pharmacotherapy. It is also effective in the treatment of mania and catatonia. It has also been shown to be helpful in chronic schizophrenic disorders when clozapine alone is not fully effective.

The most common side effects of ECT are memory disturbance and headache. While some memory deficits may persist, memory loss tends to improve in a few weeks after the last ECT treatment.

Serious complications arising from ECT occur in fewer than 1 in 1000 cases. Most of these problems are cardiovascular or respiratory in nature (eg, aspiration of gastric contents, arrhythmias, MI). Poor patient understanding and lack of acceptance of the technique by the public are some of the biggest obstacles to the use of ECT.

9. Phototherapy—Phototherapy is used in major depression with seasonal onset. It consists of indirect eye exposure to a light source of > 2500 lux for 2 hours daily or 10,000 lux for 20 minutes daily to increase the photoperiod of the day. Light visors are an adaptation that provides greater mobility and an adjustable light intensity but may not be as effective.

10. Repetitive transcranial magnetic stimulation—Repetitive transcranial magnetic stimulation (rTMS) delivers electromagnetic pulses to the prefrontal cortex. It is approved by the FDA for individuals who have not tolerated or responded to at least one or more standard antidepressant medications. Traditionally delivered in a course of 30 sessions over 6 weeks, rTMS does not require general anesthesia and is not associated with cognitive side effects. Several meta-analyses have demonstrated that in nonpsychotic depression, rTMS is noninferior to ECT. The most common side effects are scalp sensitivity under the coil and transient headache. A rapid acting form of rTMS is approved that is delivered over 5 days, termed "SAINT" (Stanford Accelerated Intelligent Neuromodulation Therapy).

11. Other treatments—Vagus nerve stimulation has shown promise in about one-third of extremely refractory cases and is approved by the FDA. Data have demonstrated that the effects plateau around 18 months to 2 years and are durable at 5 years.

B. Psychological

It is often challenging to engage an individual in psychotherapeutic endeavors during the acute stage of a severe depression. While medications may be taking effect, a supportive and behavioral approach to strengthen existing coping mechanisms and appropriate consideration of the patient's continuing need to function at work, to engage in recreational activities, etc, are necessary as the severity of the depression lessens. Behavioral activation, scheduling rewarding activities to counter withdrawal and inactivity, has emerged as a focused, standalone component of supportive approaches during this phase. Therapy during or just after the acute stage may focus on coping techniques, with practice of alternative choices. Depression-specific psychotherapies improve self-esteem, increase assertiveness, and lessen dependency. Interpersonal psychotherapy has shown efficacy in the treatment of acute depression, helping patients master interpersonal stresses and develop new coping strategies. Cognitive behavioral therapy for depression addresses patients' patterns of negative thoughts, called cognitive distortions, which lead to feelings of depression and anxiety. Treatment usually includes homework assignments such as keeping a journal of cognitive distortions and of positive responses to them. The combination of medication therapy plus interpersonal psychotherapy or cognitive behavioral therapy is generally more effective than either modality alone. It is sometimes helpful to involve the spouse or other significant family members early in treatment. Mindfulness-based cognitive therapy is as effective as maintenance medication in preventing relapse. This therapy incorporates meditation and teaches patients to distance themselves from depressive thinking.

C. Social

Flexible use of appropriate social services can be of major importance in the treatment of depression. Since alcohol abuse is often associated with depression, early involvement in alcohol treatment programs such as Alcoholics Anonymous can be important to future success (see Chapter 47). The structuring of daily activities during severe depression is often quite difficult for the patient, and loneliness is often a major factor. Social prescribing, in which link workers connect patients to community activities and resources addressing isolation, has emerged as a valuable approach to enhance engagement and well-being. The help of family, employer, or friends is often necessary to mobilize the patient who experiences no joy in daily activities and tends to remain uninvolved and to deteriorate. Insistence on sharing activities will help involve the patient in simple but important daily functions. In some severe cases, the use of day treatment centers or support groups of a specific type (eg, mastectomy groups, peer-led depression support groups) is indicated. Peer support interventions, often delivered in groups, offer benefits comparable with usual care enhancements in reducing depressive symptoms and improving social functioning. It is not unusual for a patient to have multiple legal, financial, and vocational problems requiring legal and vocational assistance.

D. Behavioral

When depression is a function of self-defeating coping techniques such as passivity, the role-playing approach can be useful. Behavioral techniques, including desensitization, may be used in problems such as phobias where depression is a by-product. When depression is a regularly used interpersonal style, behavioral counseling to family members or others can help in extinguishing the behavior in the patient. Behavioral activation, a technique of motivating depressed patients to begin engaging in pleasurable activities, has been shown to be a useful depression-specific psychotherapy; it is increasingly delivered in digital formats to enhance accessibility. Recent evidence supports exercise, including walking or jogging, yoga, and strength training, in improving depressive symptoms

Treatment of Bipolar Disorder, Manic & Depressive Episodes

Acute manic or hypomanic symptoms will respond to the mood stabilizers lithium or valproic acid after several days of treatment. Antipsychotics may be used as well for mania. High-potency benzodiazepines (eg, clonazepam) may also be useful adjuncts in managing the agitation and sleep disturbance that are features of manic and hypomanic episodes.

A. Antipsychotics

Acute manic symptoms may be treated initially with a second-generation antipsychotic such as olanzapine (eg, 5–20 mg orally), risperidone (2–3 mg orally), or aripiprazole (15–30 mg) in conjunction with a benzodiazepine if indicated. Alternatively, when behavioral control is immediately necessary, olanzapine in an injectable form (2.5–10 mg intramuscularly) or haloperidol, 5–10 mg orally or intramuscularly repeated as needed until symptoms subside, may be used. The dosage of the antipsychotic may be gradually reduced after lithium or another mood stabilizer is started. Olanzapine, quetiapine, ziprasidone, aripiprazole, and the long-acting injectable risperidone are approved as maintenance treatments for bipolar disorder to prevent subsequent cycles of both mania and depression. Antipsychotic medications are FDA-approved medications for treatment of bipolar depression, including quetiapine, lurasidone, fluoxetine/olanzapine combination, cariprazine, and lumateperone. There is also strong evidence for tamoxifen, typically a breast cancer treatment, in treatment of mania. Its mechanism may be inhibition of protein kinase C.

B. Valproic Acid

Valproic acid (divalproex) is a first-line treatment for mania. This issue is particularly important in patients living with AIDS or other medically ill patients prone to dehydration or malabsorption with wide swings in serum lithium levels. Valproic acid has also been used effectively in panic disorder and migraine headache. Treatment is often started at a dose of 750 mg/day orally and titrated to achieve therapeutic serum levels. GI symptoms and weight gain are the main side effects. Liver enzyme biochemical tests, CBCs, glucose levels, and weight should be monitored at 2 weeks, 4 weeks, and 3 months initially and annually or more frequently thereafter based on clinical judgment. Significant teratogenic effects are a concern so pregnancy should be ruled out prior to initiation. Alternatives to valproate should be considered in individuals of childbearing years who might become pregnant.

C. Lithium

Lithium significantly decreases the frequency and severity of both manic and depressive attacks in about 50–70% of patients and is FDA-approved for maintenance and manic episodes.

In addition to its use in bipolar disorder, lithium is sometimes useful in the prophylaxis of recurrent unipolar depressions and in lowering the risk of suicide. Lithium may ameliorate nonspecific aggressive behaviors and dyscontrol syndromes. Many patients with bipolar disease can be managed long-term with lithium alone, although some will require continued or intermittent use of an antipsychotic or lamotrigine to help prevent depressive episodes. An excellent resource for information is the Lithium Information Center (https://www.miminc.org/aboutlithinfoctr.html).

Before treatment, the clinical workup should include a medical history and physical examination; CBC; T_4, TSH, BUN, serum creatinine, and serum electrolyte determinations; UA; and ECG (in patients age > 45 or with a history of cardiac disease).

1. Dosage—The common starting dosage of lithium carbonate is 300–900 mg daily, usually administered in split dosing twice daily, with trough blood levels measured after 4–5 days of treatment and after changes in dose. Blood for lithium levels should be drawn 12 hours after the last dose. A slow-release form or units of different dosage may be used. Lithium citrate is available as a syrup. Dosing for acute manic episodes is adjusted to achieve therapeutic trough ranges from 0.8 mEq/L to 1.2 mEq/L.

For maintenance treatment, lithium levels should be monitored initially every 1–2 months, and then every 6–12 months in stable, long-term patients. For long-term maintenance therapy, many clinicians reduce the medication to achieve trough levels of 0.6–1 mEq/L in order to reduce side effects. Levels should be monitored more closely when there is any condition that causes volume depletion (eg, diarrhea, dehydration, use of diuretics). Once-a-day dosage is acceptable for maintenance therapy.

2. Side effects—Early side effects, which are usually transient, may include mild GI symptoms (take with food and in divided doses), fine tremors (treat with propranolol, 20–60 mg/day orally, only if persistent), slight muscle weakness, and somnolence. Moderate polyuria (reduced renal responsiveness to ADH) and polydipsia (associated with increased plasma renin concentration) are often present. This effect may be blunted by once daily dosing and potassium administration. Weight gain and leukocytosis can occur.

Thyroid side effects include goiter (3%; often euthyroid) and hypothyroidism (10%). Lithium-induced hypothyroidism may be treated with thyroid hormone while continuing lithium therapy. Changes in glucose tolerance, nephrogenic diabetes insipidus, nephrotic syndrome, edema, folate deficiency, and pseudotumor cerebri can occur. Thyroid and kidney function should be checked at 4- to 6-month intervals. Hypercalcemia and elevated parathyroid hormone levels occur in some patients. Electrocardiographic abnormalities (principally T wave flattening or inversion) may occur during lithium administration but are not of major clinical significance. Sinoatrial block may occur, particularly in older adults. Most side effects subside when lithium is discontinued; when residual side effects exist, they are usually not serious.

Side effects from long-term lithium therapy include the development of cogwheel rigidity and, occasionally, other extrapyramidal signs. Lithium-induced delirium with therapeutic lithium levels is an infrequent complication usually occurring in older adults and may persist for several days after serum levels have become negligible. Encephalopathy has occurred in patients receiving combined lithium and antipsychotic therapy and in those who have cerebrovascular disease, thus requiring careful evaluation of patients who develop neurotoxic signs at subtoxic blood levels.

Long-term use of lithium may have adverse effects on kidney function. Persistent polyuria should require an investigation of the kidney's ability to concentrate urine. A rise in serum creatinine levels is an indication for in-depth evaluation of kidney function and consideration of alternative treatments.

Lithium exposure in early pregnancy minimally increases the frequency of rare congenital anomalies. Mothers who take lithium should use formula to feed their newborn, since concentration in breast milk is one-third to half that in serum.

Toxicity usually occurs at blood lithium levels > 2 mEq/L. Because sodium and lithium are reabsorbed at the same loci in the proximal renal tubules, any sodium loss (diarrhea, use of diuretics, or excessive perspiration) increases lithium levels. Symptoms and signs include vomiting and diarrhea. Other symptoms and signs include tremors, muscle weakness, confusion, dysarthria, vertigo, choreoathetosis, ataxia, hyperreflexia, rigidity, lack of coordination, myoclonus, seizures, opisthotonos, and coma. Toxicity is more severe in older adults, who should be maintained on slightly lower serum levels. Significant overdoses of lithium are typically managed with hemodialysis since the medication is excreted completely by the kidneys.

See Chapter 42 for the treatment of patients with massive ingestions of lithium or blood lithium levels > 2.5 mEq/L.

3. Drug interactions—Patients receiving lithium should use diuretics with caution and only under close medical supervision. The thiazide diuretics cause increased lithium reabsorption from the proximal renal tubules, resulting in increased serum lithium levels and adjustment of lithium intake must be made to compensate for this. Potential drug interactions of lithium with other medications should be considered; consultation with a pharmacist or online drug interaction tools is recommended.

D. Carbamazepine

Carbamazepine is used in the treatment of bipolar patients who cannot be satisfactorily treated with lithium (nonresponsive, excessive side effects, or rapid cycling). It is often effective at 800–1600 mg/day orally. Dose-related side effects include sedation and ataxia. Dosages start at 400–600 mg orally daily and are increased slowly to therapeutic levels. Skin rashes and a mild reduction in white count are common. SIAD secretion occurs rarely. Carbamazepine can be effective in conjunction with lithium, although there have been reports of reversible neurotoxicity with the combination. It also lowers T_4, free T_4, and T_3 levels. Cases of fetal malformation (particularly spina bifida) have been reported along with growth deficiency and developmental delay. Liver biochemical tests and CBCs should be monitored in patients taking carbamazepine. Screening for the HLA-B1502 allele in the Han Chinese population and the HLA-A3101 allele in northern Europeans may help target individuals more susceptible to a serious rash.

In current guidelines, carbamazepine is viewed as a second- or third-line option for bipolar disease due to its side-effect profile. Oxcarbazepine appears to carry a and a lower risk of hepatotoxicity than does carbamazepine.

E. Lamotrigine

Lamotrigine is FDA-approved for the maintenance treatment of bipolar disorder. Current guidelines endorse lamotrigine for the prevention of cycles of bipolar depression, but is has limited utility in acute mania. More frequent mild side effects include headache, dizziness, nausea, and diplopia. Any new rash associated with lamotrigine use should be evaluated by a dermatologist. Rashes occur in 10% of patients and may be an indication for immediate cessation of dosing, since lamotrigine has been associated with Stevens-Johnson syndrome (1:1000) and toxic epidermal necrolysis. If the rash is associated with systemic symptoms including fever, lymphadenopathy, and oral mucosa ulcerations, the medication should be stopped and the patient sent to an emergency department. Dosing starts at 25–50 mg/day orally and is titrated upward slowly to decrease the likelihood of rash.

Prognosis

Most depressive episodes are usually time-limited, and the prognosis with treatment is good if a pathologic pattern of adjustment does not intervene. Major affective disorders frequently respond well to a full trial of medication treatment. However, a substantial minority of patients experience persistent symptoms despite optimized pharmacotherapy, often necessitating multimodal interventions. At least 20% of patients will have a more chronic illness lasting two or more years. Many patients do not sustain a complete remission of symptoms and most depressive episodes recur. At least 80% of patients who have a single major depressive episode will have one or more recurrences within 15 years of the index episode. Many patients, therefore, require long-term maintenance therapy with antidepressants.

Mania has a good prognosis with adequate treatment, although patient adherence to treatment is often quite challenging. Many patients with bipolar disorder require treatment with two or more medications such as lithium, antipsychotics, and sleeping agents. Contemporary management increasingly emphasizes personalized combinations of mood stabilizers, atypical antipsychotics, and adjunctive agents to address breakthrough mood instability, particularly in cases with rapid cycling or mixed features. Breakthrough manic or depressive episodes are common, even with adherence to maintenance treatments, although maintenance therapy lessens the risk of recurrent episodes.

Giguère S et al. Effectiveness of psychological therapy for treatment-resistant depression in adults: a systematic review and meta-analysis. J Pers Med. 2025;15:338. [PMID: 40863400]

Huang W et al. Comparative efficacy, safety, and tolerability of pharmacotherapies for acute mania in adults: a systematic review and network meta-analysis of randomized controlled trials. Mol Psychiatry. 2025;30:838. [PMID: 39191865]

Oliva V et al. Switch to mania after acute antidepressant treatment for bipolar depression: a systematic review and network meta-analysis of randomised controlled trials. EClinicalMedicine. 2025;87:103413. [PMID: 40823496]

Voderholzer U et al. Enduring effects of psychotherapy, antidepressants and their combination for depression: a systematic review and meta-analysis. Front Psychiatry. 2024;15:1415905. [PMID: 39664326]

ATTENTION-DEFICIT/HYPERACTIVITY DISORDER

ESSENTIALS OF DIAGNOSIS

- Persistent patterns of inability to sustain attention, excessive motor activity/restlessness/impulsivity, or both.
- Symptoms interfere with daily functioning.
- Symptoms began prior to age 12 and in at least two settings (ie, school/work, home, with friends/family).

Clinical Findings

Attention-deficit/hyperactivity disorder (ADHD) begins in childhood; however, longitudinal studies confirm persistent symptoms in 50–65% of adults, often with evolving symptom profiles necessitating ongoing pharmacotherapy. The prevalence of ADHD in adults is estimated to be 4–5%. In some adult patients, ADHD was not diagnosed during childhood because they were not presented for assessment or were able to compensate for symptoms. The presenting symptoms in adulthood tend to be inattention, restlessness, and impulsivity, whereas hyperactivity has often improved. There are three main subtypes of adult ADHD: predominantly inattentive, predominantly hyperactive-impulsive, and combined. For the predominantly inattentive subtype, at least five inattention symptoms are required to meet diagnostic criteria, such as making careless mistakes, being easily sidetracked, trouble keeping deadlines or with organization, losing belongings, and being forgetful in daily chores/tasks. For the hyperactive-impulsive subtype, at least five hyperactivity/impulsivity symptoms are required, such as feeling restless, leaving a seat though expected to remain, feeling "driven by a motor," interrupting others, inability to wait his or her turn, etc. The diagnosis of combined ADHD is characterized by the presence of both inattentive and hyperactive-impulsive features. Per DSM-5 criteria, these symptoms must have been present before age 12, with current impairment in multiple settings. It is often useful to have patients provide questionnaires to other adult observers, including those who knew them during childhood, such as parents. This collateral data can help prevent diagnosing ADHD in someone who is seeking stimulants but without symptomatology as well as aid in making the diagnosis, since evidence shows that many adults who do have ADHD underreport symptoms. Standardized adult rating scales, such as the Adult ADHD Self-Report Scale or observer versions, enhance diagnostic reliability alongside collateral history.

Treatment

A. Pharmacologic

Stimulants such as methylphenidate and amphetamine are the most effective treatments for ADHD. These come in short-acting and long-acting formulations. Caution should be used prior to prescribing these mediations to assess for potential substance abuse or diversion as well as for comorbid mood disorders that may not respond well to a stimulant. Atomoxetine and viloxazine are nonstimulants that are second-line FDA-approved agents for ADHD. Bupropion is not FDA-approved for ADHD, but meta-analyses suggest benefit in adults; it may be considered in patients in whom a stimulant is contraindicated or in those who also suffer from major depression.

B. Behavioral and Other Treatments

Psychoeducation regarding ADHD should be given to all patients. Many patients are able to implement behavioral changes that either improve their functioning, such as creating calendars and organizational schemes or doing tasks in multiple timed short spurts, or can help them avoid tasks that are challenging for them in favor of complementary tasks they are more suited to (ie, selecting jobs that value more activity rather than sustained focus, or sharing in the chores at home that do not require attention to detail). Cognitive training may help with residual symptoms after medication management has been optimized.

Bellato A et al. Systematic review and meta-analysis: effects of pharmacological treatment for attention-deficit/hyperactivity disorder on quality of life. J Am Acad Child Adolesc Psychiatry. 2025;64:346. [PMID: 38823477]
Ostinelli EG et al. Comparative efficacy and acceptability of pharmacological, psychological, and neurostimulatory interventions for ADHD in adults: a systematic review and component network meta-analysis. Lancet Psychiatry. 2025;12:32. [PMID: 39701638]
Yang X et al. Short-term and long-term effect of non-pharmacotherapy for adults with ADHD: a systematic review and network meta-analysis. Front Psychiatry. 2025;16:1516878. [PMID: 39958157]

AUTISM SPECTRUM DISORDERS

ESSENTIALS OF DIAGNOSIS

- Persistent issues with social communication and interactions.
- Repetitive behaviors, interests, or activities.
- Symptoms interfere with functioning.
- May or may not have accompanying language or intellectual impairment.

Clinical Findings

Autism spectrum disorder is a neurodevelopmental disorder in which patients suffer from pervasive difficulties with social communication and have repetitive, restricted interests and behaviors. It affects about 1% of the adult population with an estimated heritability of about 90%. Observed increases in incidence largely reflect broadened diagnostic criteria, improved awareness and screening, reduced stigma, and diagnostic substitution from other developmental disorders, rather than a true rise in occurrence. Approximately 20–30% of individuals also have a substance use problem, and there is higher risk of ADHD and mood or obsessive-compulsive disorders. Sensory processing differences and motor coordination challenges, including dyspraxia, are increasingly recognized as core clinical features. The National Institute of Health and Care Excellence (NICE) guidelines recommend that assessment of autism spectrum disorder should be a comprehensive and multidisciplinary approach that includes asking about core autism spectrum disorder difficulties, early development, medical and family history, behavior, education, employment, needs assessment, and risks, as well as physical examination, potential laboratory testing, and feedback to the individual. Recent updates emphasize incorporating evaluation of sensory sensitivities and co-occurring neurodevelopmental features during assessment.

Treatment

Risperidone and aripiprazole are FDA-approved antipsychotics for treating irritability in patients with autism spectrum disorders. These antipsychotics can help with some of the behavioral symptoms of autism but carry a risk of metabolic side effects and extrapyramidal symptoms. There is some evidence for use of applied behavioral analysis to address social cognitions and behaviors.

Choi H et al. Pharmacological and non-pharmacological interventions for irritability in autism spectrum disorder: a systematic review and meta-analysis with the GRADE assessment. Mol Autism. 2024;15:7. [PMID: 38263251]
Hirota T et al. Autism spectrum disorder: a review. JAMA. 2023;329:157. [PMID: 36625807]
Manter MA et al. Pharmacological treatment in autism: a proposal for guidelines on common co-occurring psychiatric symptoms. BMC Med. 2025;23:11. [PMID: 39773705]
Yuan LX et al. A systematic review of transcranial magnetic stimulation treatment for autism spectrum disorder. Heliyon. 2024;10:e32251. [PMID: 38933955]

SLEEP-WAKE DISORDERS

Sleep consists of two distinct states as shown by electroencephalographic studies: (1) **REM** (rapid eye movement) sleep, also called dream sleep, D state sleep, or paradoxical sleep, and (2) **NREM** (non-REM) sleep, also called S stage sleep, which is divided into stages 1, 2, 3, and 4 and is recognizable by different electroencephalographic patterns. Stages 3 and 4 are "delta" sleep. Current terminology designates NREM substages as N1, N2, and N3 (formerly stages 1, 2, and 3–4), with N3 encompassing slow-wave "delta" sleep. Dreaming occurs mostly in REM and to a lesser extent in NREM sleep.

Sleep is a cyclic phenomenon, with four or five REM periods during the night accounting for about one-fourth of the total night's sleep (1.5–2 hours). The first REM period occurs about 80–120 minutes after onset of sleep and lasts about 10 minutes. Later REM periods are longer (15–40 minutes) and occur mostly in the last several hours of sleep. Most stage 4 (deepest) sleep occurs in the first several hours.

Age-related changes in normal sleep include an unchanging percentage of REM sleep and a marked decrease in stage 3 and stage 4 sleep, with an increase in wakeful periods during the night. These shifts reflect consolidated N3 reduction and greater N1 fragmentation. These normal changes, early bedtimes, and daytime naps play a role in the increased complaints of insomnia in older people. Variations in sleep patterns may be due to circumstances (eg, "jet lag") or to idiosyncratic patterns ("night owls") in persons who perhaps because of different "biologic rhythms" habitually go to bed late and sleep late in the morning. Creativity and rapidity of response to unfamiliar situations are impaired by loss of sleep. There are also rare individuals who have chronic difficulty in adapting to a 24-hour sleep-wake cycle (**desynchronization sleep disorder**), which can be resynchronized by altering exposure to light. It is particularly prevalent among those who are totally blind.

The three major sleep disorders are discussed below. Additional entities include hypersomnolence disorder, circadian rhythm sleep-wake disorders, and parasomnias. Any persistent sleep disorder that is not attributable to another condition should be evaluated by a sleep specialist.

1. Insomnia

Classification & Clinical Findings

Patients may report difficulty getting to sleep or staying asleep, intermittent wakefulness during the night, early morning awakening, or combinations of any of these. Transient episodes are usually of little significance. Stress, caffeine, physical discomfort, daytime napping, and early bedtimes are common factors. Circadian rhythm disruption, irregular sleep-wake schedules, and excessive use of digital devices before bedtime are increasingly recognized contributors.

Psychiatric disorders are often associated with persistent insomnia. Hyperarousal and altered sleep–wake regulation are central features of insomnia associated with depression and anxiety disorders. In manic disorders, a reduced total sleep time and a decreased need for sleep are cardinal features and important early sign of impending mania. Sleep-related panic attacks occur in the transition from stage 2 to stage 3 sleep in some patients with a longer REM latency in the sleep pattern preceding the attacks.

Abuse of alcohol may cause or be secondary to the sleep disturbance. There is a tendency to use alcohol as a means of getting to sleep without realizing that it disrupts the normal sleep cycle. Acute alcohol intake produces a decreased sleep latency with reduced REM sleep during the first half of the night. REM sleep is increased in the second half of the night, with an increase in total amount of slow wave sleep (stages 3 and 4). Vivid dreams and frequent awakenings are common. Chronic alcohol abuse increases stage 1 and decreases REM sleep, with symptoms persisting for many months after the individual has stopped drinking. Acute alcohol or other sedative withdrawal causes delayed onset of sleep and REM rebound with intermittent awakening during the night. Even moderate alcohol use impairs sleep continuity and architecture, contributing to next-day cognitive and mood disturbances.

Heavy smoking (more than a pack a day) causes difficulty falling asleep—often independently associated with an increase in coffee drinking. Excess intake of caffeine, cocaine, and other stimulants near bedtime causes decreased total sleep time—mostly NREM sleep—with some increased sleep latency.

Sedative-hypnotics—specifically, the benzodiazepines, which are the most commonly prescribed medications to promote sleep—tend to increase total sleep time, decrease sleep latency, and decrease nocturnal awakening, with variable effects on NREM sleep. Nonbenzodiazepine hypnotics have similar effects on sleep as do the benzodiazepines, though some evidence shows improved slow wave sleep and less residual next-morning somnolence with nonbenzodiazepines, such as zolpidem. Withdrawal causes just the opposite effects and results in continued use of the medication for the purpose of preventing withdrawal symptoms. Antidepressants decrease REM sleep (with marked rebound on withdrawal in the form of nightmares) and have varying effects on NREM sleep. The effect on REM sleep correlates with reports that REM sleep deprivation produces improvement in some depressions. Other agents, including dual orexin receptor antagonists and melatonin receptor agonists, now play a growing role in the management of chronic insomnia due to their more physiologic modulation of sleep-wake pathways and reduced risk for dependence.

Persistent insomnias are also related to a wide variety of medical conditions, particularly delirium, pain, respiratory syndromes, uremia, thyroid disorders, and nocturia due to benign prostatic hyperplasia. Sleep apnea and restless leg movement are described below. Adequate analgesia and proper treatment of medical disorders will reduce symptoms and decrease the need for sedatives. There is an increased risk of insomnia among older adults, because sleep is lighter and more easily disrupted with aging, and medical disorders are more common. Comorbid insomnia and sleep apnea are now recognized as common in older adults, often requiring combined behavioral and respiratory treatment approaches.

Treatment

In general, there are two broad classes of treatment for insomnia that may be combined: psychological (cognitive behavioral) and pharmacologic. Contemporary guidelines reinforce cognitive behavioral therapy for insomnia (CBT-I) as the first-line intervention for chronic insomnia, with pharmacotherapy reserved for adjunctive use or when CBT-I is inaccessible or insufficient. In situations of acute distress, such as a grief reaction, short-term pharmacologic measures may be most appropriate. With primary insomnia, however, initial efforts should be psychologically based. This is true in older adults to avoid the potential adverse reactions of medications. A stepped-care approach prioritizes behavioral therapies, progressing to targeted pharmacotherapy based on symptom persistence, comorbidities, and risk profile.

A. Psychological

Psychological strategies include educating the patient regarding good **sleep hygiene:** (1) Go to bed only when sleepy. (2) Use the bed and bedroom only for sleeping and sex. (3) If still awake after 20 minutes, leave the bedroom, pursue a restful activity (such as a bath or meditation), and only return when sleepy. (4) Get up at the same time every morning regardless of the amount of sleep during the night. (5) Discontinue caffeine and nicotine, at least in the evening if not completely. (6) Establish a daily exercise regimen; moderate aerobic exercise and mind–body exercises haves demonstrated efficacy in improving sleep. (7) Avoid alcohol as it may disrupt continuity of sleep. (8) Limit fluids in the evening. (9) Learn and practice relaxation techniques. (10) Establish a bedtime ritual and a routine time for going to sleep. Cognitive behavioral therapy for insomnia is as effective as zolpidem with benefits sustained 1 year after treatment.

B. Pharmacologic

When the above measures are insufficient, the following medications may be used: lorazepam (0.5 mg orally nightly); temazepam (7.5–15 mg orally nightly); zolpidem (5 mg orally in women, 5–10 mg orally in men, nightly); and zaleplon (5–10 mg orally nightly). Zaleplon is often used to treat insomnia characterized by middle-of-the-night awakening with difficulty falling back to sleep. Eszopiclone (2–3 mg orally) is similar in action to zolpidem and zaleplon and has a longer duration of action. A lower dose of 1 mg is indicated in older adults or those with hepatic impairment. In general, it is appropriate to use medications for short courses of 1–2 weeks. Intermittent or as-needed dosing minimizes tolerance and dependency risks across all agents. It is important to note that short-acting agents like triazolam or zolpidem may lead to amnestic episodes if used on a daily ongoing basis.

Longer-acting agents such as flurazepam (half-life of > 48 hours) may accumulate in older adults and lead to cognitive slowing, ataxia, falls, and somnolence.

Antihistamines such as diphenhydramine (25 mg orally nightly) or hydroxyzine (25 mg orally nightly) may also be useful for sleep, as they produce no pharmacologic dependency; their anticholinergic effects may, however, produce confusion or urinary symptoms in older adults. In addition, they are associated with a habituations of response, and long term use has been implicated in cognitive decline in older patients. Trazodone, an atypical antidepressant, is a non–habit-forming, effective sleep medication in lower than antidepressant doses (25–150 mg orally at bedtime). Priapism is a rare side effect requiring emergent treatment. Doxepin, 3–6 mg per night, is a TCA that is also effective for insomnia. It appears to be safe for ongoing use without the development of tolerance.

Melatonin, which is available without a prescription, may improve the time to onset of sleep but is not effective in maintaining sleep. Melatonin (often administered at 0.5–5 mg orally) is most effective when used short term and in combination with behavioral strategies. Ramelteon, 8 mg orally at bedtime, is a melatonin receptor agonist that helps with sleep onset and does not appear to have abuse potential. Tasimelteon (20 mg orally, 1 hour before bedtime) offers similar circadian-modulating effects, primarily for sleep-onset difficulties.

The dual orexin receptor antagonist (DORA) class of hypnotics is approved to help initiate and maintain sleep. DORAs such as suvorexant (10–20 mg orally), lemborexant (5–10 mg orally), and daridorexant (25-50 mg orally) given 30 minutes before bedtime may be more effective than other hypnotics for some patients with potentially fewer next-day residual effects. Their role relative to other hypnotics has not been established, but they may be viable treatment options for patients with chronic insomnia refractory to first-line therapies. DORAs have shown a significant increase in depressive symptoms in a subset of patients, so other hypnotics may be a better choice in depressed patients.

2. Hypersomnias (Disorders of Excessive Sleepiness)

Classification & Clinical Findings

A. Breathing-Related Sleep Disorders

Obstructive sleep apnea is by far the most common of the breathing-related sleep disorders that include **central sleep apnea** and **sleep-related hypoventilation**. Obstructive sleep apnea hypopnea is characterized by snoring, gasping, or breathing pauses during sleep and five or more apneas or hypopneas per hour or evidence by polysomnography. (See Chapter 9.)

B. Narcolepsy Syndrome

Narcolepsy syndrome develops from a selective loss or dysfunction of orexin (also known as hypocretin) neurons of the lateral hypothalamus. Approximately 85–95% of individuals with narcolepsy with cataplexy or hypocretin deficiency are positive for the HLA DQB1*06:02 haplotype. Symptoms often begin between the ages of 15 and 25 years. Narcolepsy consists of recurrent daytime naps or lapses into sleep, at least three times a week, that are accompanied by at least one of the following: (1) hypocretin deficiency; (2) cataplexy—sudden loss of muscle tone involving specific small muscle groups or generalized muscle weakness, often associated with emotional reactions and sometimes confused with seizure disorder; (3) characteristic abnormalities on nocturnal polysomnogram or multiple sleep latency test. The sleep attacks often are characterized by an abrupt transition into REM sleep.

REM sleep behavior disorder, characterized by motor dyscontrol and often violent dreams during REM sleep, may be related to narcolepsy.

C. Kleine-Levin Syndrome

This syndrome, which occurs mostly in young men, is characterized by hypersomnic attacks three or four times a year lasting up to 2 days, with hyperphagia, hypersexuality, irritability, and confusion on awakening. It has often been associated with antecedent neurologic insults and usually remits after age 40.

D. Periodic Limb Movement Disorder

Periodic lower leg movements occur only during sleep with subsequent daytime sleepiness, anxiety, depression, and cognitive impairment. Clinical evaluation includes assessment for iron deficiency and medication adverse effects as potentially modifiable contributors. **Restless leg syndrome** includes movements while awake as well.

E. Shift Work Sleep Disorder

Shift work sleep disorder occurs when there is excessive fatigue as a consequence of work shifts occurring during the normal sleep period.

Treatment

Narcolepsy can be managed by daily administration of a stimulant such as dextroamphetamine sulfate, 10 mg orally in the morning, with increased dosage as necessary. Modafinil and its enantiomer armodafinil are schedule IV medications approved by the FDA for treating the excessive daytime fatigue of narcolepsy, sleepiness associated with obstructive sleep apnea, and shift work sleep disorder. Usual dosing is 200–400 mg orally each morning for modafinil and 150–250 mg orally in the morning for armodafinil. The exact mechanism of action of modafinil and armodafinil is unknown, yet they are thought to be less of an abuse risk than stimulants such as dextroamphetamine that are primarily dopaminergic. Newer agents include the wake-promoting stimulants (eg, solriamfetol, pitolisant, the night-time formulation oxybate). Selection is guided by the symptom profile (excessive sleepiness vs cataplexy), comorbidities (eg, cardiovascular disease, anxiety, substance use risk), and patient preferences.

Cataplexy is often treated with agents that more directly target this symptom burden, including oxybate formulations and pitolisant. Imipramine, 75–100 mg orally daily, has been effective in treatment of cataplexy but not narcolepsy.

Periodic limb movement disorder and REM sleep behavior disorder can be treated with clonazepam with variable results. For REM sleep behavior disorder, attention should be given to fall risk, cognitive vulnerability, and comorbid sleep-disordered breathing; systematic environmental safety measures (eg, removing bedside hazards) should be included as part of treatment planning. There is no treatment for Kleine-Levin syndrome, but lithium is a commonly considered preventive option that nay prevent recurrences in some patients.

Treatment of sleep apnea is discussed in more detail in Chapter 9.

3. Parasomnias (Abnormal Behaviors during Sleep)

These disorders (sleep terror, nightmares, sleepwalking, and enuresis) are common in children but less so in adults.

Hwang JW et al. Systematic review and meta-analysis on fully automated digital cognitive behavioral therapy for insomnia. NPJ Digit Med. 2025;8:157. [PMID: 40075149]

Kishi T et al. Comparative efficacy and safety of daridorexant, lemborexant, and suvorexant for insomnia: a systematic review and network meta-analysis. Transl Psychiatry. 2025;15:211. [PMID: 40555730]

Winkelman JW et al. Treatment of restless legs syndrome and periodic limb movement disorder: an American Academy of Sleep Medicine systematic review, meta-analysis, and GRADE assessment. J Clin Sleep Med. 2025;21:137. [PMID: 39324694]

Xu M et al. Comparative efficacy of exercise modalities on sleep quality in populations with sleep disorders: a systematic review and network meta-analysis. Sleep Med Rev. 2024;73:101877. [PMID: 38006755]

DISORDERS OF AGGRESSION

Aggression and violence are symptoms rather than diseases and are not necessarily associated with an underlying medical condition. Clinicians are unable to predict dangerous behavior with greater than chance accuracy; however, structured professional judgment tools such as the HCR-20 enhance violence risk assessment by systematically evaluating historic, clinical, and risk management factors. Depression, schizophrenia, personality disorders, mania, paranoia, temporal lobe dysfunction, and organic mental states may be associated with acts of aggression. Impulse control disorders are characterized by physical abuse (usually of the aggressor's domestic partner or children), by pathologic intoxication, by impulsive sexual activities, and by reckless driving. Anabolic steroid usage by athletes has been associated with increased tendencies toward violent behavior.

In the United States, a significant proportion of all violent deaths are alcohol related. The ingestion of even small amounts of alcohol can result in pathologic intoxication that resembles an acute organic mental condition. Amphetamines, crack cocaine, and other stimulants are frequently associated with aggressive behavior. Phencyclidine is a drug commonly associated with violent behavior that is occasionally of a bizarre nature, partly due to lowering of the pain threshold.

Treatment

A. Psychological

Management of any acutely potentially violent individual includes appropriate psychological maneuvers. These may be useful in the management of patients who are hospitalized or being held involuntarily for psychiatric evaluation. Move slowly, talk slowly with clarity and reassurance, and evaluate the situation. Strive to create a setting that is minimally disturbing and eliminate people or things threatening to the violent individual. Do not threaten and do not touch or crowd the person. Allow no weapons in the area. Proximity to a door is comforting to both the patient and the examiner. Use a negotiator who the violent person can relate to comfortably. Food and drink can be helpful in defusing the situation. Honesty is important. Make no false promises, bolster the patient's self-esteem, and continue to engage the subject verbally until the situation is under control. This type of individual does better with strong external controls to replace the lack of inner controls over the long term. Close probationary supervision and judicially mandated restrictions can be most helpful. Mentalization-based treatment (MBT), particularly adapted for antisocial personality disorder (MBT-ASPD), has shown promise in reducing aggression when combined with probationary oversight. There should be a major effort to help the individual avoid drug use (eg, Alcoholics Anonymous).

For less acute treatment, community-based programs as well as cognitive bias modification interventions can be useful in decreasing aggressive behaviors. CBT approaches targeting maladaptive thought patterns also demonstrate benefit in managing intermittent explosive outbursts.

B. Pharmacologic

Pharmacologic means are often necessary whether or not psychological approaches have been successful. This is true in the agitated or psychotic patient. The medications of choice in seriously violent or psychotic aggressive states are antipsychotics, given intramuscularly if necessary, every 1–2 hours until symptoms are alleviated. A number of second-generation intramuscular antipsychotics are FDA-approved in the management of acute agitation and include aripiprazole (9.75 mg/1.3 mL), ziprasidone (10 mg/0.5 mL), and olanzapine (10 mg/2 mL). The second-generation antipsychotics appear no more effective than first-generation medications like haloperidol (2.5–5 mg) but are less likely to cause acute extrapyramidal symptoms. Clozapine, particularly at lower doses, is effective in reducing aggression across psychotic and impulsive subtypes, including in treatment-resistant cases. Dexmedetomidine (120–180 mcg) is a sublingual medication that is an alternative to oral and IM antipsychotics for the treatment of acute agitation in patients with bipolar disorder and schizophrenia. Benzodiazepine sedatives (eg, diazepam, 5 mg orally or intravenously every several hours) can be used for mild to moderate agitation but are sometimes associated with a disinhibition of aggressive impulses similar to alcohol. Chronic aggressive states, particularly in patients with intellectual disabilities and brain damage (rule out causative organic conditions and medications such as anticholinergic medications in amounts sufficient to cause confusion), have been ameliorated with risperidone, 0.5–2 mg/day orally, propranolol, 40–240 mg/day orally, or pindolol, 5 mg twice daily orally (pindolol causes less bradycardia and hypotension than propranolol). Carbamazepine and valproic acid are effective in the treatment of aggression and explosive disorders, particularly when associated with known or suspected brain lesions. Lithium and SSRIs are also effective for some intermittent explosive outbursts. Buspirone (10–45 mg/day orally) is helpful for aggression, particularly in patients with intellectual disabilities. Omega-3 fatty acid supplementation has demonstrated efficacy in reducing aggressive behavior.

C. Physical

Physical management is necessary if psychological and pharmacologic means are not sufficient. It requires the active and visible presence of an adequate number of personnel (five or six) to reinforce the idea that the situation is under control despite the patient's lack of inner controls. Such an approach often precludes the need for actual physical restraint. Seclusion rooms and restraints should be used only when necessary (ambulatory restraints are an alternative), and the patient must then be observed at frequent intervals. Narrow corridors, small spaces, and crowded areas exacerbate the potential for violence in an anxious patient.

D. Other Interventions

The treatment of impacted persons (eg, battered women) is challenging and can be complicated by a reluctance to leave the situation. Reasons for staying vary, but common themes include the fear of more violence because of leaving, the hope that the situation may ameliorate (in spite of steady worsening), and the financial aspects of the situation. Concerns for the children may finally compel the person to seek help. An early step is to get the impacted person into a therapeutic situation that provides the support of others in similar straits. Al-Anon is frequently a valuable asset when alcohol is a factor. The group can support the individual while they gather strength to consider alternatives without being paralyzed by fear. Many cities offer temporary emergency centers and counseling. Use the available resources, attend to any medical or psychiatric problems, and maintain a compassionate interest. Some states require clinicians to report injuries caused by abuse or suspected abuse to police authorities.

Jiang S et al. Effectiveness of community-based programs on aggressive behavior among children and adolescents: a systematic review and meta-analysis. Trauma Violence Abuse. 2024;25:2845. [PMID: 38293961]

Kayaoğlu K et al. Effect of cognitive-behavioral therapy–based anger management training on anger and aggression levels of individuals convicted of violent crimes. J Psychosoc Nurs Ment Health Serv. 2024;62:51. [PMID: 38768383]

Raine A et al. Omega-3 supplementation reduces aggressive behavior: a meta-analytic review of randomized controlled trials. Aggress Violent Behav. 2024;78:101956. [PMID: 38911617]

NEUROCOGNITIVE DISORDERS

ESSENTIALS OF DIAGNOSIS

- Transient or permanent brain dysfunction with alterations in awareness or attention.
- Cognitive impairment to varying degrees.
- Impaired recall and recent memory, inability to focus attention and problems in perceptual processing, often with psychotic ideation.
- Random psychomotor activity such as stereotypy.
- Emotional disorders frequently present: depression, anxiety, irritability.
- Behavioral disturbances: impulse control, sexual acting-out, attention deficits, aggression, and exhibitionism.

General Considerations

The term *neurocognitive disorders* refers to cognitive decline that may be a primary brain disorder or a secondary manifestation of some general disorder, rather than psychiatric illness. All of the cognitive disorders show *some degree of impaired thinking* depending on the site of involvement, the rate of onset and progression, and the duration of the underlying brain lesion. ***Delirium*** presents with fluctuating attention and altered consciousness, typically has an acute onset, and is often reversible when the underlying medical cause is addressed. Neuropsychiatric symptoms (including apathy, agitation, disinhibition, and psychosis) are common across neurocognitive disorders and often prompt clinical attention even when cognitive deficits are mild. Depression may coexist with, mimic, or exacerbate cognitive symptoms; careful assessment is needed to determine whether a mood disturbance is primary, reactive, or part of the neurocognitive syndrome itself. Behavioral disturbances tend to be more common with chronicity, tend to be more directly related to the underlying personality or CNS vulnerability to drug side effects, and are not necessarily correlated with cognitive dysfunction. These symptoms may respond to environmental modification, caregiver education, and cautious pharmacologic intervention, though sensitivity to medication side effects is heightened in this population.

The causes of cognitive disorders are listed in Table 28–8.

Table 28–8. Etiology of delirium and other cognitive disorders (listed in alphabetical order).

Disorder	Possible Causes
Cardiovascular disorders	MIs, cardiac arrhythmias, cerebrovascular spasms, hypertensive encephalopathy, hemorrhages, embolisms, and occlusions indirectly cause decreased cognitive function.
Collagen-vascular and immunologic disorders	Autoimmune disorders, including SLE, Sjögren syndrome, and AIDS.
Degenerative diseases	Alzheimer disease, Pick disease, multiple sclerosis, parkinsonism, Huntington chorea, normal pressure hydrocephalus.
Endocrine disorders	Thyrotoxicosis, hypothyroidism, adrenocortical dysfunction (including Addison disease and Cushing syndrome), pheochromocytoma, insulinoma, hypoglycemia, hyperparathyroidism, hypoparathyroidism, panhypopituitarism, diabetic ketoacidosis.
Infections	Septicemia; meningitis and encephalitis due to bacterial, viral, fungal, parasitic, or tuberculous organisms or to CNS syphilis; acute and chronic infections due to the entire range of microbiologic pathogens.
Intoxication	Alcohol, sedatives, bromides, analgesics (eg, pentazocine), psychedelic drugs, stimulants, and household solvents.
Long-term effects of alcohol	Wernicke-Korsakoff syndrome.
Medication withdrawal	Withdrawal from alcohol, sedative-hypnotics, corticosteroids.
Medications	Anticholinergic medications, antidepressants, H_2-blocking agents, digoxin, salicylates (long-term use), and a wide variety of other over-the-counter and prescribed medications.
Metabolic disturbances	Fluid and electrolyte disturbances (especially hyponatremia, hypomagnesemia, and hypercalcemia), acid-base disorders, hepatic disease (hepatic encephalopathy), kidney failure, porphyria.
Neoplasms	Primary or metastatic lesions of the CNS, cancer-induced hypercalcemia.
Nutritional deficiencies	Deficiency of vitamin B_1 (beriberi), vitamin B_{12} (pernicious anemia), folic acid, nicotinic acid (pellagra); protein-calorie malnutrition.
Respiratory disorders	Hypoxia, hypercapnia.
Seizure disorders	Ictal, interictal, and postictal dysfunction.
Trauma	Subdural hematoma, subarachnoid hemorrhage, intracerebral bleeding, concussion syndrome.

Clinical Findings

The many manifestations include problems with orientation, short or fluctuating attention span, loss of recent memory and recall, impaired judgment, emotional lability, lack of initiative, impaired impulse control, inability to reason through problems, depression (worse in mild to moderate types), confabulation (not limited to alcohol organic brain syndrome), constriction of intellectual functions, visual and auditory hallucinations, and delusions. Physical findings will vary according to the cause. Contemporary assessment often integrates structured cognitive testing with observation for fluctuation over time, in order to help distinguish delirium, dementia, and primary psychiatric illness. The electroencephalogram usually shows generalized slowing in delirium.

A. Delirium

Delirium (**acute confusional state**) is a transient global disorder of attention, with clouding of consciousness, usually a result of systemic problems (eg, medications, hypoxemia). See Chapters 4 and 27. Onset is usually rapid. The mental status fluctuates (impairment is usually least in the morning), with varying inability to concentrate, maintain attention, and sustain purposeful behavior. There is a marked deficit of short-term memory and recall. Anxiety and irritability are common. Orientation problems follow the inability to retain information. Perceptual disturbances (often visual hallucinations) and psychomotor restlessness with insomnia are common. "**Sundowning**"—mild to moderate delirium at night—is more common in patients with preexisting dementia and may be precipitated by hospitalization, medications, and sensory deprivation.

Initial management includes early identification of precipitating factors, minimization of deliriogenic medications, and structured reorientation; cautious use of pharmacologic agents should be used when these nonpharmacologic approaches are insufficient.

B. Dementia

Dementia is characterized by chronicity and deterioration of selective mental functions (see Chapters 4 and 27). The term *major neurocognitive disorder* encompasses the various types of dementia, including Alzheimer, Lewy body dementia, vascular dementia, and frontotemporal dementia.

In all types of dementia, loss of impulse control (sexual and language) is common. Early behavioral disinhibition and apathy are particularly characteristic of frontotemporal forms. ***Pseudodementia*** is a term previously applied to depressed patients who appear to be demented. These patients are often identifiable by their tendency to report memory problems vociferously rather than try to cover them up. They usually say they cannot complete cognitive tasks but with encouragement can often do so. They can be considered to have depression-induced reversible dementia that improves when the depression resolves. In many geriatric patients, however, the depression appears to be an insult that often unmasks a progressive dementia. In light of the recognized overlap between depressive cognitive impairment and early neurodegenerative change, longitudinal cognitive monitoring and neuroimaging may be utilized.

In 2025, the first blood test (Lumipulse) to assist in the diagnosis of Alzheimer disease was approved by the FDA. The test measures the ratio of Tau p217 to β-amyloid 1-42. The test is approximately 90% effective in predicting the brain changes consistent with Alzheimer disease up to 3–4 years before the onset of symptoms. However, the test may be inconclusive in up 20% of cases and false positives do occur. Thus, the test is used a part of a comprehensive evaluation of a possible Alzheimer case.

C. Amnestic Syndrome

This is a memory disturbance without delirium or dementia. It is usually associated with thiamine deficiency and chronic alcohol use (eg, Korsakoff syndrome). There is an impairment in the ability to learn new information or recall previously learned information.

D. Substance-Induced Hallucinosis

This condition is characterized by persistent or recurrent hallucinations (usually auditory) without the other symptoms usually found in delirium or dementia. Alcohol or hallucinogens are often the cause. Stimulants, cannabinoids, and certain prescribed medications may provoke similar syndromes. There does not have to be any other mental disorder, and there may be complete spontaneous resolution. Chronic cases can resemble primary psychotic disorders but are distinguished by the clear temporal association with substance exposure and the lack of pervasive disorganization of thinking.

Treatment

See Chapters 4 and 27 for detailed discussion.

Dickerson B et al. Alzheimer's Association clinical practice guideline for the diagnostic evaluation, testing, counseling, and disclosure of suspected Alzheimer's disease and related disorders (DETeCD-ADRD): executive summary of recommendations for primary care. Alzheimers Dement. 2025;21:e14333. [PMID: 39713957]

Livingston G et al. Dementia prevention, intervention, and care: 2024 report of the Lancet Commission. Lancet. 2024;404:572. [PMID: 39096926]

Veronese N et al. Interventions to prevent and treat delirium: an umbrella review of randomized controlled trials. Ageing Res Rev. 2024;97:102313. [PMID: 38677599]

PSYCHIATRIC PROBLEMS ASSOCIATED WITH HOSPITALIZATION & ILLNESS

Diagnostic Categories

A. Acute Problems

1. Delirium with psychotic features secondary to the medical or surgical problem or compounded by effect of treatment.
2. Acute anxiety, often related to ignorance and fear of the immediate problem as well as uncertainty about the future.
3. Anxiety as an intrinsic aspect of the medical problem (eg, hyperthyroidism).
4. Denial of illness, which may present during acute or intermediate phases of illness.

B. Intermediate Problems

1. Depression as a function of the illness or acceptance of the illness, often associated with realistic or fantasied hopelessness about the future.
2. Behavioral problems, often related to denial of illness and, in extreme cases, causing the patient to leave the hospital against medical advice.

C. Recuperative Problems

1. Decreasing cooperation as the patient sees that improvement and compliance are not compelled.
2. Readjustment problems with family, job, and society.

General Considerations

A. Acute Problems

1. "Intensive care unit psychosis"—The ICU environment may contribute to delirium. Critical care unit factors include sleep deprivation, increased arousal, mechanical ventilation, and social isolation. Other causes include those common to delirium and require vigorous investigation (see Delirium, above).

2. Presurgical and postsurgical anxiety states—Anxiety before or after surgery is common. **Presurgical anxiety** is common and is principally a fear of death (many surgical patients make out their wills). Patients may be fearful of anesthesia, the operating room, and the disease processes that might be uncovered by the surgeon. Such fears frequently cause people to delay examinations that might result in a greater chance of cure.

The opposite of this is **surgery proneness**, the quest for surgery to escape from overwhelming life stresses. Some polysurgery patients may be classified as having factitious disorders. Motivations include the need to get dependency needs met, the desire to outwit authority figures, unconscious guilt, or a masochistic need to suffer. Frequent surgery may also be related to a somatic symptom disorder, particularly body dysmorphic disorder (an obsession that a body part is disfigured). Patients with somatic symptom and related disorders often undergo excessive diagnostic procedures and interventions due to heightened illness anxiety. Other reasons include an attempt to get relief from pain and a lifestyle that has become almost exclusively medically oriented.

Postsurgical anxiety states are usually related to pain, procedures, and loss of body image. Acute pain problems are quite different from chronic pain disorders the former are readily handled with adequate analgesic medication (see Chapter 5). Preoperative anxiety has been linked to prolonged recovery times and increased postoperative delirium risk. Alterations in body image (eg, amputations, ostomies, and mastectomies) often raise concerns about relationships with others.

3. Iatrogenic problems—These include medications, complications of diagnostic and treatment procedures, and impersonal and unsympathetic staff behavior. Polypharmacy heightens risks of adverse interactions, reduced adherence, and iatrogenic harm, particularly in vulnerable populations. Patients with unsolved diagnostic problems are at higher risk due to the quest for answers that engenders further diagnostic procedures and risk of complications. The upset patient and family may be anxious and excessively demanding. Such behavior is best handled with calm and measured responses.

B. Intermediate Problems

1. Prolonged hospitalization—Prolonged hospitalization presents unique problems. There often are behavioral difficulties related to length of hospitalization and necessary procedures. Disputes with staff are common and often concern pain medication or ward privileges. Some patients regress to infantile behavior and dependency. Staff members must agree about their approach to the patient in order to ensure the smooth functioning of the unit.

2. Depression—Mood disorders, ranging from mild adjustment disorder to major depressive disorder, frequently occur during prolonged hospitalizations. Depression may be due to the individual's loss of self-esteem; they often think of themselves as worthless and are guilt ridden. Therapeutic medications (eg, corticosteroids) may be a factor. Depression can contribute to irritability and overt anger. Severe depression can lead to anorexia, which further complicates healing and metabolic balance. It is during this period that the issue of disfigurement arises—relief at survival gives way to concern about future function and appearance.

C. Recuperative Problems

1. Anxiety—Anxiety about return to the posthospital environment can cause regression to a dependent position. Complications increase, and staff forbearance again is tested.

2. Posthospital adjustment—Adjustment difficulties after discharge are related to the severity of the deficits and the use of outpatient facilities (eg, physical therapy, rehabilitation programs, psychiatric outpatient treatment). Posttraumatic stress symptoms from medical trauma or injury can persist and impair reintegration. Some patients may experience posttraumatic stress symptoms (eg, from traumatic injuries or from necessary medical treatments). Lack of appropriate follow-up can contribute to depression in the patient, who may feel that he or she is making poor progress and may have thoughts of "giving up." Reintegration into work, educational, and social endeavors may be slow.

Clinical Findings

The symptoms that occur in these patients are similar to those discussed in previous sections of this chapter, eg, delirium, stress and adjustment disorders, anxiety, and depression. Post-hospitalization, delirium is associated with persistent cognitive impairment and heightened risk of PTSD-like symptoms. Behavior problems may include lack of cooperation, increased complaints, demands for medication, sexual approaches to nurses, threats to leave the hospital, and actual signing out against medical recommendations. Such behaviors, often called "difficult patient behaviors," encompass splitting, acting out, avoidance, boundary crossing, false compliance, and dependence, particularly under acute medical stress even without underlying personality pathology. The stress of hospitalization often brings out more primitive defense mechanisms than the patient displays in daily life. Hospitalization may also precipitate clinical instability, exacerbating symptom fluctuations and increasing rehospitalization risk across psychiatric diagnoses.

Complications

Prolongation of hospitalization causes increased expense, deterioration of patient-staff relationships, and increased probabilities of iatrogenic and legal problems. Prolonged stays may also precipitate hospital-associated deconditioning, characterized by physical, cognitive, and psychological vulnerabilities, including delirium, depressive symptoms, and apathy. The possibility of increasing post-hospital treatment problems is enhanced. This vulnerability, often termed *post-hospital syndrome*, elevates risks of readmission, functional decline, and adverse outcomes due to sleep disruption, immobility, medication effects, and psychological stress.

Treatment

A. Medical

It is important to have one clinician in charge, whom the patient trusts and who is able to oversee multiple treatment approaches (see Somatic Symptom & Related Disorders (Abnormal Illness Behaviors), above). In acute problems, attention must be paid to metabolic imbalance, alcohol withdrawal, and previous drug use—prescribed, recreational, or over the counter. Adequate sleep and analgesia are important in enhancing a patient's coping abilities.

Many clinicians are attuned to the early detection of the surgery-prone patient. Plastic and orthopedic surgeons are at particular risk. Appropriate consultations may help detect some problems and mitigate future ones.

Standardized preoperative screening for depression, anxiety, and substance use can support early intervention and reduce postoperative complications.

Postsurgical anxiety states can be alleviated by personal attention from the surgeon. Anxiety is not as effectively lessened by ancillary personnel, whom the patient perceives as lesser authorities, until after the clinician has reassured the patient. "Patient-controlled analgesia" can improve pain control, decrease anxiety, and minimize side effects.

Depression should be recognized early. If moderate to severe, antidepressant medications (see Treatment of Depression, above) may be prescribed. Collaborative care models that embed mental health professionals within general-hospital teams can improve detection and treatment of depression in medically ill inpatients. High levels of anxiety can be lowered with judicious use of anxiolytic agents. Unnecessary medications tend to reinforce the patient's impression that there must be a serious illness or medication would not be required.

B. Psychological

Prepare the patient and family for what is to come. This includes the types of units where the patient will be quartered, the procedures that will be performed, and any disfigurements that will result from surgery. Repetition improves understanding. The nursing staff can be helpful, since patients frequently confide a lack of understanding to a nurse but are reluctant to do so to the physician. Shared-decision-making dialogues and the use of visual aids or decision tools can enhance realistic expectations and reduce later distress.

Denial of illness is frequently a block to acceptance of treatment. This too should be handled with family members present (to help the patient face the reality of the situation) in a series of short interviews (for reinforcement). In illness-anxiety disorder and related presentations, structured psychoeducation and brief cognitive-behavioral strategies can help contain relentless reassurance-seeking and reduce iatrogenic burden. Dependency problems resulting from long hospitalization are best handled by focusing on the changes to come as the patient makes the transition to the outside world. Key figures are teachers, vocational counselors, and physical therapists. Challenges should be realistic and practical and handled in small steps.

Depression is usually related to the loss of familiar hospital supports, and the outpatient therapists and counselors help to lessen the impact of the loss. Early activation-based interventions (behavioral activation) can be particularly useful in post-hospitalization depression, emphasizing graded re-engagement with valued activities rather than passive "restoration" of a prior role. The impact can be alleviated by anticipating, with the patient and family, the signal features of the common depression to help prevent the patient from assuming a permanent sick role.

Suicide is a concern when a patient is faced with despair. An honest, compassionate, and supportive approach will help sustain the patient during this trying period. Systematic suicide-risk assessment and structured safety planning should be integrated into routine care for patients confronting major life-role changes or perceived loss of autonomy.

C. Behavioral

Prior desensitization can significantly allay anxiety about medical procedures. A "dry run" can be done to reinforce the oral description. Modern applications of systematic or graded exposure, often combined with relaxation training, can be tailored to procedures such as imaging, dialysis, or respiratory support and can reduce avoidance and procedural distress. Cooperation during acute problem periods can be enhanced by the use of appropriate reinforcers such as a favorite nurse or helpful family member. People who are positive reinforcers are even more helpful during the intermediate phases when the patient becomes resistant to the seemingly endless procedures (eg, debridement of burned areas).

Specific situations (eg, psychological dependency on the respirator) can be corrected by weaning with appropriate reinforcers (eg, watching a favorite movie on a media player or laptop when disconnected from the ventilator). Behavioral approaches should be used in a positive and optimistic way for maximal reinforcement. Technology-facilitated reinforcement (eg, tablet-based rewards or virtual-reality distraction) can extend the reach of behavioral strategies in hospitalized patients, especially in settings with limited staffing.

Relaxation techniques, hypnosis, and attentional distraction can be used to block side effects of a necessary treatment (eg, nausea in cancer chemotherapy). These techniques are increasingly embedded in integrative oncology and critical-care settings, where brief, protocol-driven interventions can reduce symptom burden and improve treatment adherence.

D. Social

A change in environment requires adaptation. Because of the illness, admission and hospitalization may be more easily handled than discharge. A predischarge evaluation must be made to determine whether the family will be able to cope with the physical or mental changes in the patient. Assessment of "social prescribing" needs (transportation, housing, caregiving) and perceived social support can strongly influence readmission risk and functional outcomes. Working with the family while the patient is in the acute stage may presage a successful transition later on.

Development of a new social life can be facilitated by various self-help organizations (eg, the stoma club). Digital and hybrid support-group options (virtual meetings, moderated forums) can expand access for patients who face mobility, geographic, or stigma-related barriers. Sharing problems with others in similar circumstances eases the return to a social life, which may be quite different from that prior to the illness. Emphasis on peer support and identity-reframing (eg, beyond "patient" status) can strengthen resilience and reduce long-term social isolation.

Prognosis

The prognosis is good in all patients who have reversible medical and surgical conditions. However, even with resolution of the underlying medical illness, associated psychiatric complications such as delirium may confer persistent risks of functional decline, cognitive impairment, and institutionalization. It is guarded when there is serious functional loss that impairs vocational, educational, or societal possibilities—especially in the case of progressive and ultimately life-threatening illness. In such cases, comprehensive postdischarge rehabilitation targeting functional recovery and monitoring for ongoing neuropsychiatric sequelae are essential.

Crone C et al. The American Psychiatric Association Practice Guideline for the Prevention and Treatment of Delirium. Am J Psychiatry. 2025;182:880. [PMID: 40887950]

Lewis K et al. A focused update to the clinical practice guidelines for the prevention and management of pain, anxiety, agitation/sedation, delirium, immobility, and sleep disruption in adult patients in the ICU. Crit Care Med. 2025;53:e711. [PMID: 39982143]

Disorders of the Pituitary, Thyroid, & Adrenal Glands

29

Paul A. Fitzgerald, MD

DISEASES OF THE HYPOTHALAMUS & PITUITARY GLAND

ANTERIOR HYPOPITUITARISM

ESSENTIALS OF DIAGNOSIS

- ACTH deficiency: low adrenal secretion of cortisol and epinephrine; normal aldosterone secretion.
- Growth hormone (GH) deficiency: short stature in children; asthenia, obesity, and increased cardiovascular risk in adults.
- Prolactin (PRL) deficiency: postpartum lactation failure.
- TSH deficiency: secondary hypothyroidism.
- LH and FSH deficiency: hypogonadism and infertility in men and women.

General Considerations

The anterior pituitary hormones are GH, PRL, ACTH, TSH, LH, and FSH. The hypothalamus synthesizes hormones that regulate anterior pituitary secretion, including corticotropin-releasing hormone (CRH), growth hormone–releasing hormone (GHRH), gonadotrophin-releasing hormone (GnRH), thyrotropin-releasing hormone, and somatostatin. The hypothalamus also secretes dopamine that inhibits PRL secretion. These hypothalamic regulatory hormones are transported by a portal venous system down the pituitary stalk to the anterior pituitary. The hypothalamus also synthesizes oxytocin and arginine vasopressin (AVP), also known as ADH. Nerves from the hypothalamus carry oxytocin and AVP to the posterior pituitary, where they are stored and released. Hypopituitarism can be caused by either hypothalamic or pituitary dysfunction. Patients with hypopituitarism may have single or multiple hormonal deficiencies.

1. Hypopituitarism with mass lesions—Lesion in the sellar or perisellar area may cause hypopituitarism by impingement on the hypothalamus, pituitary stalk, or pituitary.

a. Pituitary neuroendocrine tumors—These tumors, also known as pituitary adenomas, can cause anterior hypopituitarism, particularly when they are large macroadenomas (1 cm or larger). Nonfunctioning pituitary neuroendocrine tumors are more likely than functioning pituitary adenomas to grow large enough to cause anterior hypopituitarism; they rarely cause diabetes insipidus. Pituitary adenomas are usually sporadic but 5% arise in kindreds with multiple endocrine neoplasia type 1 (MEN1). Pituitary adenomas most frequently secrete PRL or (less commonly) GH or ACTH.

b. Pituitary metastases—These lesions are usually from breast cancer (45%); 50% present over 10 years after the primary tumor. Lung cancer accounts for about 21% of pituitary metastases that typically present within 1 year of the primary cancer. Pituitary metastases often present with visual loss or ophthalmoplegia, ACTH deficiency (71%), TSH deficiency (65%), diabetes insipidus (26%), or gonadotropin deficiency (88%).

c. Other mass lesions—These lesions include craniopharyngioma, plasmacytoma, germ cell tumors, glioma, lymphomas, cysts (Rathke cleft, dermoid, epidermoid, arachnoid), meningioma, and hemangiopericytoma.

d. Vascular lesions—These lesions include pituitary tumor apoplexy, cavernous sinus aneurysm, and subarachnoid hemorrhage.

e. Inflammatory/infiltrative lesions—These include granulomatosis with polyangiitis, xanthomatosis, giant cell granuloma, Langerhans cell histiocytosis, sarcoidosis, syphilis, hypophysitis, and tuberculosis. Infectious lesions can be bacterial, fungal, or parasitic. Lymphocytic hypophysitis is an autoimmune disorder that is characterized by infiltration of the infundibulum and pituitary by lymphocytes, macrophages, and plasma cells. Spontaneous lymphocytic hypophysitis is more common in women (71%) and most frequently presents during pregnancy or postpartum. Immune checkpoint inhibitor hypophysitis can be caused by several immunity-enhancing drugs.

F. PITUITARY STALK THICKENING—This disorder is caused most frequently by lymphocytic hypophysitis, metastases, neurosarcoidosis, or a congenital ectopic posterior pituitary, but often the cause is never determined. Pituitary stalk damage frequently causes central diabetes insipidus and one or more anterior pituitary hormone deficiencies, including ACTH deficiency with secondary adrenal insufficiency.

2. Hypopituitarism without mass lesions—

A. CONGENITAL HYPOPITUITARISM—This disorder occurs in syndromes such as septo-optic dysplasia and in patients with various gene mutations that cause a progressive loss of anterior pituitary function in childhood. Prader-Willi syndrome is a genetic disorder where genes on the paternal chromosome 15 are deleted or unexpressed. Kallmann syndrome is caused by various gene mutations that impair the development or migration of GnRH-synthesizing neurons from the olfactory bulb to the hypothalamus, causing hypogonadism with hyposmia or anosmia. Congenital GH deficiency occurs as an isolated pituitary hormone deficiency in one-third of cases.

B. ACQUIRED HYPOPITUITARISM—This disorder can result from cranial radiation therapy, pituitary surgery, encephalitis, cerebral malaria, COVID-19 infection, parasitic infection, viper bites, hemochromatosis, autoimmunity, or coronary artery bypass grafting. GH deficiency can also occur following peptide receptor radionuclide therapy for neuroendocrine tumors. *Hypopituitarism can occur acutely, usually with severe secondary adrenal insufficiency that may be fatal unless recognized and treated.* Acute hypopituitarism may also be associated with diabetes insipidus.

At least one pituitary hormone deficiency develops in 25–30% of survivors of moderate to severe **traumatic brain injury** and in about 55% of survivors of **aneurysmal subarachnoid hemorrhage**. Some degree of hypopituitarism, most commonly GH deficiency and hypogonadotropic hypogonadism, occurs in one-third of **ischemic stroke** patients. Other cases of acquired hypopituitarism can be idiopathic or associated with an empty sella on MRI.

Sheehan syndrome refers to hypopituitarism caused by postpartum pituitary necrosis, usually following severe postpartum uterine hemorrhage. It is usually characterized by postpartum amenorrhea and inability to lactate. Hypopituitarism in Sheehan syndrome usually occurs gradually over 10–20 years; the diagnosis is typically delayed an average of 9 years. Manifestations in affected women are typically hyponatremia, hypoglycemia, or anemia. In acute Sheehan syndrome, MRI shows an enlarged pituitary with only a thin rim of enhancement with gadolinium.

C. FUNCTIONAL HYPOPITUITARISM—Functional hypogonadotropic hypogonadism can occur in both women and men secondary to excessive exercise or weight loss. Partial hypogonadotropic hypogonadism commonly develops in men with normal aging or obesity, with serum free testosterone levels that are low or near the lower end of normal reference ranges but normal serum FSH and LH levels. Women may develop hypothalamic amenorrhea during periods of severe emotional or physical stress. LH and FSH deficiency with hypogonadotropic hypogonadism occur in serious illness, malnutrition, anorexia nervosa, alcohol use disorder, Cushing syndrome (spontaneous or iatrogenic), and hyperprolactinemia (drug-induced or spontaneous). Opioid use causes partial hypogonadotropic hypogonadism in about 60% of long-term (including methadone) users and secondary adrenal insufficiency in about 15% of patients; it is less likely to cause GH or TSH deficiency. Therapy with GnRH agonists (eg, leuprolide) also causes hypogonadotropic hypogonadism that can persist after therapy is stopped.

Functional GH deficiency can occur with normal aging, malnutrition, and CKD. ACTH suppression with functional isolated secondary adrenal insufficiency occurs in patients receiving megesterol acetate, high-dose opioid therapy (15%), and endogenous or exogenous corticosteroids. Chemotherapy with **bexarotene** may cause secondary hypothyroidism and hypopituitarism. **Mitotane** therapy for adrenocortical carcinoma causes central hypothyroidism.

Clinical Findings

When hypopituitarism is caused by a mass lesion or hypophysitis, patients may have headaches or visual field defects. Nonspecific symptoms, such as fatigue, dizziness and hypotension, confusion, cognitive dysfunction, sexual dysfunction, polydipsia, or cold intolerance, can develop. Other symptoms and signs attributed to specific pituitary hormone deficiencies are described below.

A. Symptoms and Signs

1. GH (somatropin) deficiency—GH deficiency in adults is often undiagnosed because maximum height has already been reached and other manifestations are nonspecific. Nonspecific symptoms, varying from mild to severe, include mild to moderate central obesity, reduced physical and mental energy, impaired concentration and memory, and depression. Patients may also have reduced muscle mass, increased LDL cholesterol, and reduced cardiac output with exercise. Chronic GH deficiency leads to osteopenia and an increased risk of fractures. When other more recognizable pituitary hormone deficits are present, there is a high likelihood of concurrent GH deficiency.

2. Gonadotropin deficiency (hypogonadotropic hypogonadism)—In gonadotropin deficiency, insufficiencies of LH and FSH cause hypogonadism and infertility.

Congenital gonadotropin deficiency is characterized by partial or complete lack of pubertal development. Isolated hypogonadal hypogonadism occurs in as many as 1 in 4000 males but is less common in females. About 30% of cases have been linked to genetic variants with variable phenotypic expressions. Patients may have normal or abnormal olfaction (Kallmann syndrome), abnormal genitalia, kidney abnormalities, midline craniofacial defects, neurologic deficits, or musculoskeletal malformations. Some affected women have menarche followed by secondary amenorrhea. Affected boys who survive childhood may present with failure to enter puberty.

Prader-Willi syndrome presents with cryptorchidism, mental retardation, short stature, hyperflexibility, autonomic dysregulation, cognitive impairment, obesity, hypogonadotropic hypogonadism, or primary hypogonadism.

Acquired gonadotropin deficiency is characterized by the gradual loss of facial, axillary, pubic, and body hair. Men may note diminished libido, erectile dysfunction, muscle atrophy, infertility, and osteopenia (see Male Hypogonadism). Women have amenorrhea, infertility, and osteoporosis.

3. TSH deficiency—TSH deficiency causes hypothyroidism (see Hypothyroidism, below).

4. ACTH deficiency—Central adrenal insufficiency is caused by ACTH deficiency. There is functional atrophy of the adrenal cortex within 2 weeks of pituitary damage, which results in diminished cortisol. Adrenal mineralocorticoid secretion continues, so manifestations of adrenal insufficiency in hypopituitarism may be less striking than in bilateral adrenal gland destruction (see Primary Adrenal Insufficiency [Addison disease]). Central adrenal insufficiency from pituitary metastases typically presents with nausea, weight loss, and fatigue; these symptoms are often incorrectly attributed to chemotherapy or to the malignancy itself. Patients with partial ACTH deficiency have some cortisol secretion and may not have symptoms until stressed by illness or surgery.

5. PRL deficiency—This presents in women with failure to lactate in the puerperium.

6. Panhypopituitarism—This refers to a deficiency of several or all pituitary hormones. There may be hypogonadotropic hypogonadism (62%), diabetes insipidus (54%), headache (50%), hypothyroidism (48%), ACTH deficiency (47%), GH deficiency (37%), and hyperprolactinemia (36%), which clinicians may mistake for a prolactinoma. Hypopituitarism typically presents in women with amenorrhea.

7. Hypothalamic damage—This can cause obesity and cognitive impairment. Hypopituitarism occurs but usually along with *increased* serum levels of PRL. Local tumor effects can cause headache or optic nerve compression with visual field impairment.

B. Laboratory Findings

Initially, there may be hyponatremia and hypoglycemia, with secondary hypoadrenalism, hypothyroidism, or GH deficiency. Hyponatremia can be caused by hypothyroidism or hypoadrenalism. Hyperkalemia usually does not occur, since aldosterone production is not affected. Patients with lymphocytic hypophysitis frequently have elevated serum antinuclear or anticytoplasmic antibodies. Patients with hypopituitarism without an established etiology should be screened for hemochromatosis with a serum ferritin or iron and transferrin saturation.

Male hypogonadotropic hypogonadism is diagnosed by drawing blood before 10 AM after an overnight fast in men without an acute or subacute illness. Affected men have a low fasting serum total or free serum testosterone with a low or normal serum LH. A serum PRL is also obtained, since hyperprolactinemia of any cause can result in hypogonadism.

Female hypogonadotropic hypogonadism is suspected in nonpregnant women with amenorrhea or oligomenorrhea, who do not have acute illness, hyperthyroidism, or hyperandrogenism. The serum estradiol is low and the serum FSH is low or normal. In nonpregnant women, a serum PRL is obtained, since hyperprolactinemia of any cause can result in hypogonadism. In postmenopausal women, the absence of an elevated serum FSH (in a woman not taking estrogen replacement) indicates gonadotropin deficiency (see Chapter 20).

Central hypothyroidism is diagnosed with a low serum free thyroxine (FT_4) in the setting of pituitary disease. The serum TSH can be low or normal. Central hypothyroidism can emerge when patients begin GH replacement, so thyroid levels must be monitored in that setting. Patients undergoing pituitary surgery should be assessed for central hypothyroidism preoperatively and again 6 weeks postoperatively.

Central adrenal insufficiency is diagnosed after withholding corticosteroid replacement for at least 18–24 hours. Blood is drawn at 8–9 AM for baseline plasma ACTH and serum cortisol. A serum cortisol < 3 mcg/dL (80 nmol/L) usually indicates adrenal insufficiency, whereas AM serum cortisol > 15 mcg/dL (400 nmol/L) usually excludes adrenal insufficiency. For AM cortisol levels between 3 and 15 mcg/dL, a cosyntropin test is often required. For the cosyntropin test, patients should hold any corticosteroid replacement for at least 18–24 hours. At 8–9 AM, blood is drawn for serum cortisol, ACTH, and dehydroepiandrosterone (DHEA); then cosyntropin (synthetic $ACTH_{1-24}$) 0.25 mg is administered intramuscularly or intravenously. Another serum cortisol is obtained 45 minutes after the cosyntropin injection; a stimulated serum cortisol of < 20 mcg/dL (550 nmol/L) indicates probable adrenal insufficiency. With gradual pituitary damage and early in the course of ACTH deficiency, patients can have a stimulated serum cortisol of ≥ 20 mcg/dL (550 nmol/L) but a baseline 8 AM serum cortisol of ≤ 5 mcg/dL (138 nmol/L), which is suspicious for adrenal insufficiency. The baseline serum ACTH level is low or normal in secondary hypoadrenalism, distinguishing it from primary adrenal disease. Serum DHEA is a proxy for ACTH; levels are usually low in patients with secondary adrenal deficiency, helping confirm the diagnosis. Hyponatremia may occur, especially when ACTH and TSH deficiencies are both present.

For patients with signs of secondary adrenal insufficiency (hyponatremia, hypotension, pituitary tumor) but borderline cosyntropin test results, treatment can be instituted empirically and the test repeated at a later date.

GH deficiency in adults is difficult to diagnose, since GH secretion is normally pulsatile and serum GH levels are normally undetectable for much of the day. Also, adults (particularly men) physiologically tend to produce less GH when they are over age 50 or have abdominal obesity. Therefore, pathologic GH deficiency is often inferred by symptoms of GH deficiency in the presence of pituitary destruction or other pituitary hormone deficiencies. GH deficiency is present in 96% of patients with three or more other pituitary hormone deficiencies and a low serum IGF-1. GH stimulates the production of IGF-1, but the serum IGF-1 level is neither a sensitive (about 50%) nor specific test for GH deficiency in adults. Very low serum IGF-1 levels (< 84 mcg/L) are usually indicative of GH deficiency but also occur in malnutrition, prolonged fasting, hypothyroidism, uncontrolled diabetes mellitus, and liver failure, as well as with estrogen therapy. A therapeutic trial of GH therapy should be considered for symptomatic patients who have either a serum IGF-1 < 84 mcg/L or three other pituitary hormone deficiencies.

Provocative GH stimulation testing to help diagnose adult GH deficiency has a sensitivity of only 66%; however, tests are sometimes indicated or required for insurance coverage of GH therapy. In the absence of a serum IGF-1 level < 84 mcg/L or multiple other pituitary hormone deficiencies, provocative GH-stimulation testing may be indicated for the following patients: (1) young adult patients who have completed GH therapy for childhood GH deficiency and have achieved maximal linear growth; (2) patients who have a hypothalamic or pituitary tumor or who have received surgery or radiation therapy to these areas; and (3) patients who have had prior head trauma, cerebrovascular accident, or encephalitis. Testing usually entails measuring serum GH following provocative stimuli, including macimorelin or glucagon.

C. Imaging

MRI of the hypothalamus and pituitary is indicated when a mass lesion is suspected. MRI can detect lesions of the pituitary, hypothalamus or pituitary stalk, including pituitary adenoma, lymphocytic hypophysitis, neurosarcoidosis, Langerhans cell histiocytosis, craniopharyngioma, germinoma, astrocytoma, and metastatic malignancy. MRI shows pituitary enlargement in 75% of cases of ipilimumab-associated hypophysitis but only 25% of cases of anti-PD-1 agent–induced hypophysitis. MRI is not warranted in cases of functional hypopituitarism associated with severe obesity, drugs, or nutritional disorders.

Differential Diagnosis

The failure to enter puberty may simply reflect a constitutional delay in growth and puberty.

Reversible, second hypothyroidism with suppression of TSH and T_4 can be caused by severe illness, hyperthyroxinemia, and administration of triiodothyronine, mitotane, or bexarotene, resulting in temporary central hypothyroidism. Corticosteroids and megestrol reversibly suppress endogenous ACTH and cortisol secretion. High-dose corticosteroid therapy can cause secondary adrenal insufficiency that may persist for many months.

GH deficiency occurs normally with aging and physiologically with obesity (reversible with sufficient weight loss). Very low serum IGF-1 levels can be seen with prolonged fasting, malnutrition, liver failure, hypothyroidism, and uncontrolled diabetes mellitus.

Complications

During a stressful illness, patients with untreated hypoadrenalism may become febrile and comatose and die of hyponatremia and shock.

Rarely, acute hemorrhage may occur in large pituitary tumors, manifested by rapid loss of vision, headache, and evidence of acute pituitary failure (pituitary apoplexy) requiring emergency decompression of the sella. Among patients with craniopharyngiomas, diabetes insipidus is found in 16% preoperatively and in 60% postoperatively. Hyponatremia often presents abruptly during the first 2 weeks following any pituitary surgery. Conventional radiation therapy for intracranial disorders can result in an increased incidence of small vessel ischemic strokes, second tumors and damaged hypothalamic-pituitary function.

Treatment

A. Corticosteroid Replacement

Long-term therapy is initiated with hydrocortisone 10–25 mg orally in the morning and 5–15 mg in the late afternoon. Prednisone or methylprednisolone may also be used; the dosing and timing must be individually tailored. No mineralocorticoid replacement is required. See Corticosteroid Replacement Therapy-Primary Adrenal Insufficiency (Addison Disease) below.

B. Thyroid Hormone Replacement

Levothyroxine is given to correct hypothyroidism only after the patient is assessed for cortisol deficiency or is already receiving corticosteroids (see Hypothyroidism). The typical maintenance dose is about 1.6 mcg/kg body weight, averaging 125 mcg daily with a wide range of 25–300 mcg daily. Because assessment of serum TSH is useless for monitoring patients with hypopituitarism, the optimal replacement dose of levothyroxine is determined clinically by raising or lowering the dose, according to the patient's symptoms and clinical examination. With clinically optimized levothyroxine replacement, serum FT_4 levels are usually in the mid to high-normal range. Some patients do not feel clinically euthyroid until they receive levothyroxine in doses at which the serum FT_4 levels are mildly elevated; however, serum T_3 or FT_3 levels should be in the low-normal range. During pregnancy, clinical status and serum FT_4 or total T_4 levels need to be monitored frequently, since higher doses of levothyroxine are usually required.

C. Sex Hormone and Gonadotropin Hormone Replacement

Hyperprolactinemia-related hypogonadotropic hypogonadism improves or resolves with treatment. Sex hormone replacement may be required. See Male Hypogonadism (later in this chapter) and Female Hypogonadism (Chapter 20).

Women with panhypopituitarism have profound androgen deficiency caused by the combination of both secondary hypogonadism and adrenal insufficiency. When serum DHEA levels are < 400 ng/mL, women may also be treated with compounded USP-grade DHEA 25–50 mg/day orally. DHEA therapy tends to increase pubic and axillary hair and may improve libido, alertness, stamina, and overall psychological well-being.

For men with oligospermia, human chorionic gonadotropin (hCG) (equivalent to LH) may be given at a dosage of 1500–3000 units intramuscularly three times weekly and testosterone replacement discontinued. The dose of hCG is adjusted to normalize serum testosterone levels. After 6–12 months of hCG treatment, if the sperm count remains low, hCG injections are continued along with injections of follitropin β (synthetic recombinant FSH) or urofollitropins (urine-derived FSH). An alternative for patients with an intact pituitary is the use of leuprolide (GnRH analog) by intermittent subcutaneous infusion. With treatment, testicular volumes increase within 5–12 months, and some spermatogenesis occurs in most cases.

For men with secondary hypogonadism, treatment with hCG achieves serum testosterone levels that are typically higher than with transdermal testosterone therapy and more consistent than intramuscular testosterone therapy. Many men prefer hCG over testosterone replacement, even when fertility is not at issue.

Clomiphene, 25–50 mg/day orally, can sometimes stimulate men's own pituitary gonadotropins (when their pituitary is intact), thereby increasing testosterone and sperm production. For fertility induction in females, ovulation may be induced with clomiphene, 50–100 mg/day orally for 5 days every 2 months. Ovulation induction with FSH and hCG can induce multiple births and should be used only by those experienced with their administration (see Hypogonadism).

D. Human Growth Hormone (hGH) Replacement

Symptomatic adults with GH deficiency may be treated with subcutaneous recombinant human growth hormone (rhGH, somatropin) injections, at a starting dose of 0.2 mg/day (0.6 IU/day), administered three times weekly. The dosage of rhGH is increased every 2–4 weeks by increments of 0.1 mg (0.3 IU) until side effects occur or a sufficient salutary response and a normal serum IGF-1 level are achieved. If the desired effects (eg, improved energy and mentation, reduction in visceral adiposity) are not seen within 3–6 months at maximum tolerated dosage, rhGH therapy is discontinued. Serum FT_4 levels require monitoring when beginning hGH therapy.

RhGH may be safely administered to pregnant women with hypopituitarism at their usual pregestational dose during the first trimester, tapering the dose during the second trimester, and discontinuing rhGH during the third trimester.

Treatment of adult GH deficiency usually improves the patient's overall quality of life, with better emotional sense of well-being, increased muscle mass, and decreased visceral fat and waist circumference. Long-term treatment with rhGH does not appear to affect mortality.

Side effects of rhGH therapy may include peripheral edema, hand stiffness, arthralgias and myalgias, paresthesias, carpal tunnel syndrome, tarsal tunnel syndrome, headache, pseudotumor cerebri, gynecomastia, hypertension, and proliferative retinopathy. Treatment with rhGH can also cause sleep apnea, insomnia, dyspnea, sweating, and fatigue. Side effects usually remit promptly after a sufficient reduction in dosage. Replacement therapy with rhGH does not increase the risk of any malignancy or the regrowth of pituitary or brain neoplasms; serum IGF-1 levels should be kept in the normal range.

GH should not be administered during critical illness, since administration of very high doses of rhGH increased mortality in patients receiving intensive care. There is no proven role for GH replacement for the physiologic GH deficiency that is seen with abdominal obesity or normal aging.

E. Other Treatment

Selective transsphenoidal surgery is usually performed to resect non-prolactinoma pituitary masses and Rathke cleft cysts that cause local symptoms or hypopituitarism. Such surgery reverses hypopituitarism in a minority of cases. Patients with lymphocytic hypophysitis have been treated with corticosteroid therapy and other immunosuppressants without much response and without reversing hypopituitarism.

Prognosis

Functionally, most patients with hypopituitarism do well with hormone replacement. Men with infertility who are treated with hCG/FSH or GnRH are likely to resume spermatogenesis if they have had sexual maturation and have descended testicles with a baseline serum inhibin B level over 60 pg/mL. Women under age 40 years with infertility from hypogonadotropic hypogonadism can usually have successful ovulation induction.

Hypopituitarism resulting from a pituitary tumor may be reversible with dopamine agonists for prolactinomas (see Prolactinoma, below) or with careful selective resection of the tumor. Spontaneous recovery from hypopituitarism associated with pituitary stalk thickening has been reported. Patients can also recover from functional hypopituitarism due to excessive exercise or weight loss if they greatly reduce exercise and gain weight; about half of men regain normal serum testosterone levels. Spontaneous reversal of idiopathic isolated hypogonadotropic hypogonadism occurs in about 10% of patients after several years of hormone replacement therapy (HRT). However, hypopituitarism is usually permanent, and long-term HRT is ordinarily required.

Patients with hypopituitarism have an increased mortality risk, particularly women and those in whom diagnosis was made at a younger age, who have a craniopharyngioma, or who required transcranial surgery or radiation therapy. There is also an increased risk of death from infections with adrenal crisis in patients with untreated secondary insufficiency. Some pituitary tumors are locally invasive. Asymptomatic Rathke cleft cysts may not require surgery but do require endocrine, ophthalmic, and scan surveillance.

Aljbor GS et al. Acute and chronic hypopituitarism following traumatic brain injury: a systematic review and meta-analysis. Neurosurg Rev. 2024;47:841. [PMID: 39527353]

Arlien-Søborg MC et al. Consensus and controversies about diagnosing GH deficiency: a Delphi survey by the GH Research Society. 2025;28:57. [PMID: 40335774]

Bando H et al. Hypopituitarism: genetic, developmental, and acquired etiologies with a focus on the emerging concept of autoimmune hypophysitis. Endocrine Journal. 2025;72:649. [PMID: 40139845]
Muir CA et al. Efficacy of gonadotropin treatment for induction of spermatogenesis in men with pathologic gonadotropin deficiency: a meta-analysis. Clin Endocrinol (Oxf). 2025; 102:167. [PMID: 39445789]

ANTIDIURETIC HORMONE DEFICIENCY (Central Diabetes Insipidus)

ESSENTIALS OF DIAGNOSIS

- ADH deficiency with polyuria (2.5–20 L/day) and polydipsia.
- Hypernatremia occurs if fluid intake is inadequate.

General Considerations

Antidiuretic hormone (ADH), also called arginine vasopressin, is secreted by the posterior pituitary. Deficiency of pituitary secretion, also called central diabetes insipidus, is uncommon.

Primary ADH deficiency (ADH-D) without an identifiable lesion noted on MRI of the pituitary and hypothalamus accounts for one-third of cases of diabetes insipidus. It may be idiopathic, caused by autoimmunity against hypothalamic ADH-secreting cells, or due to rare genetic disorders. Reversible central diabetes insipidus can occur with administration of propofol anesthesia, ketamine, temozolomide, or the anti-PD-L1 monoclonal antibody avelumab, and in the myelodysplastic preleukemic phase of acute myelogenous leukemia.

Secondary ADH-D frequently occurs after traumatic brain injury. It usually presents within 2 weeks after injury, although delayed presentations are reported. Other causes of damage to the hypothalamus or pituitary stalk include tumor, hypophysitis, infarction, hemorrhage, anoxic encephalopathy, or surgery involving the pituitary or hypothalamus. Less commonly, it is caused by infection (eg, encephalitis, tuberculosis, syphilis), craniopharyngioma, germinoma, or granulomas (sarcoidosis or Langerhans cell granulomatosis). Metastases to the pituitary or infundibulum are more likely to cause ADH-D (33%) than are pituitary adenomas (1%).

Clinical Findings

A. Symptoms and Signs

The symptoms of ADH-D are intense thirst, especially a craving for ice water, with the volume of ingested fluid varying from 2.5 L to 20 L daily, and polyuria, with large urine volumes and low urine specific gravity (usually < 1.006 with ad libitum fluid intake). The urine is otherwise normal. Partial ADH-D presents with less intense symptoms and should be suspected in patients with enuresis. Most patients with ADH-D are able to maintain fluid balance by continuing to ingest large volumes of water.

Patients with ADH-D who do not have free access to water become dehydrated and develop hypernatremia. Similarly, patients with damage to the anterior hypothalamic thirst center have adipsic central diabetes insipidus (ADI) and develop dehydration and hypernatremia with reduced urine output. ADI commonly occurs following neurosurgical clipping of an anterior communicating artery aneurysm. ADI is usually permanent when associated with hypothalamic damage but may be temporary in patients with critical illness.

B. Laboratory Findings

Diagnosis of ADH-D is a clinical one; there is no single diagnostic laboratory test. Evaluation should include a 24-hour urine collection for volume and creatinine. The urine is collected during ad libitum fluid intake. A urine volume of < 2.5 L/24 hours (in the absence of hypernatremia) rules out diabetes insipidus. Blood testing includes plasma vasopressin and serum glucose, urea nitrogen, calcium, potassium, sodium, and uric acid.

Plasma ADH levels are usually low (< 1 pg/mL) with both central diabetes insipidus and primary polyuria. By contrast, plasma ADH levels are normal or elevated (> 2.5 pg/mL) with nephrogenic diabetes insipidus. Plasma osmolality of 300 mOsm/kg or more implies either central or nephrogenic diabetes insipidus, whereas plasma osmolality of 280 mOsm/kg or less implies primary polydipsia as the diagnosis. Urine osmolality is low (300 mOsm/L or lower) in all three polyuric conditions and is not a helpful test. Hyperuricemia occurs frequently with both central and nephrogenic diabetes insipidus, whereas it is uncommon with primary polydipsia.

The most sensitive test for ADH-D involves the intravenous administration of hypertonic 3% saline (250 mL bolus, followed by a continuous infusion of 0.15 mL/kg/min) with plasma sodium measurements every 30 minutes. When the sodium level reaches 150 mmol/L, a plasma copeptin level of ≤ 4.9 pmol/L helps confirm the diagnosis.

The arginine-stimulation test for ADH-D involves intravenous administration over 30 minutes of l-arginine hydrochloride 0.5 g/kg (maximum of 40 g in 500 mL of 0.9 normal saline). Serum copeptin is measured at 60 and 90 minutes after the start of the infusion. Copeptin levels < 2.4 pmol/L indicate severe ADH-D; levels of 2.4–3.8 pmol/L indicate partial deficiency; and levels of > 3.8 pmol/L indicate primary polydipsia.

A less cumbersome "vasopressin challenge test" may be done. Desmopressin acetate 0.05–0.1 mL (5–10 mcg) intranasally (or 1 mcg subcutaneously or intravenously) is given, with measurement of urine volume for 12 hours before and 12 hours after administration. A serum sodium is obtained at baseline, 12 hours after the desmopressin, and immediately if symptoms of hyponatremia develop. Patients with ADH-D usually notice a distinct reduction in thirst and polyuria; serum sodium usually remains normal. The dosage of desmopressin is doubled if the response is marginal. In patients with primary polydipsia and nephrogenic diabetes insipidus, a desmopressin challenge causes no significant reduction in thirst or urine volume.

C. Imaging

Distinguishing central diabetes insipidus from primary polydipsia may require an MRI of the pituitary and hypothalamus. A posterior pituitary "bright spot" on noncontrast MRI T1-weighted imaging indicates the functional integrity of the posterior pituitary. The bright spot is undetectable or small with central diabetes insipidus whereas it is usually present in primary polydipsia and nephrogenic diabetes insipidus. MRI can also detect pathology responsible for central diabetes insipidus.

Differential Diagnosis

Central diabetes insipidus must be distinguished from polyuria caused by psychogenic polydipsia, diabetes mellitus, Cushing syndrome, hypercalcemia, hypokalemia, and nocturnal polyuria of Parkinson disease.

Vasopressinase-induced diabetes insipidus may be seen in the last trimester of pregnancy, associated with oligohydramnios, preeclampsia, or liver dysfunction, and in the puerperium. Maternal circulating vasopressin is destroyed by placental vasopressinase; however, synthetic desmopressin is unaffected.

Nephrogenic diabetes insipidus is caused by unresponsiveness of the kidney tubules to the normal secretion of vasopressin (see Chapter 24). A congenital form is familial and transmitted as an X-linked trait. Acquired forms are usually less severe and occur in pyelonephritis, recovery following ATN, renal amyloidosis, myeloma, potassium depletion, Sjögren syndrome, sickle cell anemia, chronic hypercalcemia, or caused by medications (eg, certain antimicrobials, lithium) may induce nephrogenic diabetes insipidus.

Complications

If water is not readily available, the excessive output of urine will lead to severe dehydration and worsening hypernatremia (see Chapter 24). Patients with an impaired thirst mechanism are very prone to hypernatremia, as are those with impaired mentation who forget to take their desmopressin. Excessive desmopressin acetate can induce water intoxication and hyponatremia.

Treatment

Mild cases of diabetes insipidus require no treatment other than adequate fluid intake. Reduction of aggravating factors (eg, corticosteroids) will improve polyuria.

Desmopressin acetate is the treatment of choice for central diabetes insipidus and for vasopressinase-induced diabetes insipidus associated with pregnancy or the puerperium. Desmopressin acetate (100 mcg/mL solution) is given intranasally every 8–24 hours as needed for thirst and polyuria. It may be administered via metered-dose nasal inhaler containing 0.1 mL (10 mcg/spray) or via a calibrated rhinal tube. The starting dose is one metered-dose spray or 0.05–0.1 mL every 12–24 hours; the dose is then individualized according to response. Patients with adipsic diabetes insipidus require daily administration of desmopressin on a schedule determined by daily weights and frequent testing of serum sodium concentrations.

Oral desmopressin is useful for patients in whom rhinitis or conjunctivitis develops from the nasal preparation. It is initiated at 0.05 mg twice daily and increased to a maximum of 0.4 mg every 8 hours, if required. Sublingual desmopressin is not available in the United States

Desmopressin can be given intravenously, intramuscularly, or subcutaneously in doses of 1–4 mcg every 12–24 hours as needed.

Desmopressin may cause hyponatremia, but this is uncommon if minimum effective doses are used and the patient allows thirst to occur every 1–2 days. Desmopressin can sometimes cause agitation, emotional changes, and depression with an increased risk of suicide. Patients should be monitored by family, friends, and medical staff when desmopressin therapy is started.

Prognosis

Central diabetes insipidus after pituitary surgery or head trauma usually remits after days to weeks but may be permanent if the hypothalamus or upper pituitary stalk is damaged.

Chronic central diabetes insipidus is ordinarily more an inconvenience than a dire medical condition. Hypernatremia can occur, especially when the hypothalamic thirst center is damaged, but diabetes insipidus does not otherwise reduce life expectancy, and the prognosis is that of the underlying disorder. Treatment with desmopressin allows normal sleep and activity.

Atila C et al. A novel diagnostic score for diagnosing arginine vasopressin deficiency (central diabetes insipidus) or primary polydipsia with basal laboratory and clinical parameters. Lancet Diabetes & Endocrinol. 2025;13:505. [PMID: 40294614]

Newell-Price J et al. Approach to the patient with suspected hypotonic polyuria. J Clin Endocrinol Metab. 2025;110:e506. [PMID: 39148427]

Tomulescu SA et al. Delayed onset arginine vasopressin deficiency after traumatic brain injury. Endocrinol Diabetes Metab Case Rep. 2024;2024:24-0039. [PMID: 39475774]

Varaldo E et al. Desmopressin dose requirements in patients with permanent arginine vasopressin deficiency: a tertiary center experience. Pituitary. 2024;27:714. [PMID: 39266909]

ACROMEGALY & GIGANTISM

ESSENTIALS OF DIAGNOSIS

- Pituitary neuroendocrine tumor with over secretion of GH.
- **Gigantism:** begins before puberty before closure of epiphyses.
- **Acromegaly:** occurs after puberty with excessive growth of hands, feet, jaw, internal organs.
- Amenorrhea, hypertension, headaches, visual field loss, weakness.
- Soft, doughy, sweaty handshake.
- Elevated serum IGF-1.
- Serum GH not suppressed following oral glucose.

General Considerations

GH exerts much of its growth-promoting effects by stimulating the release of IGF-1 from the liver and other tissues.

Acromegaly is a rare condition, with a yearly incidence of about 10 cases per million. It is nearly always caused by a pituitary adenoma. About 70% are macroadenomas (1 cm or larger) when diagnosed. These tumors may be locally invasive, particularly into the cavernous sinus. Less than 1% are malignant. Acromegaly is usually sporadic but may rarely be familial, with < 3% being due to multiple endocrine neoplasia (MEN) types 1 or 4. Acromegaly may also be seen rarely in McCune-Albright syndrome and Carney complex. Acromegaly is rarely caused by ectopic secretion of growth hormone–releasing hormone or GH secreted by a neuroendocrine tumor or lymphoma.

Clinical Findings

A. Symptoms and Signs

Excessive GH causes tall stature and gigantism if it occurs in youth, before closure of epiphyses. Afterward, acromegaly develops. The manifestations of acromegaly usually present insidiously; median time to diagnosis after symptom onset is 10 years. The hands enlarge and a doughy, moist handshake is characteristic. The fingers widen, causing patients to enlarge their rings. Carpal tunnel syndrome is common. The feet also grow, particularly in shoe width. Facial features coarsen since the bones and sinuses of the skull enlarge, commonly causing facial dysmorphia (22%). The mandible becomes more prominent, causing prognathism and malocclusion. Tooth spacing widens. Older photographs of the patient can be a useful comparison.

Macroglossia occurs, as does hypertrophy of pharyngeal and laryngeal tissue, which causes a deep, coarse voice. Snoring and obstructive sleep apnea are common. A goiter may be noted. Hypertension (30%), cardiomegaly (16%), and a dilated LV and HF with reduced EF (10%) may be present. Weight gain is typical, particularly of muscle and bone. Insulin resistance is usually present and frequently causes diabetes mellitus (30%). Polyarticular arthralgias and degenerative arthritis are present in about 70% of patients. Overgrowth of vertebral bone can cause spinal stenosis. Colon polyps are found in about 30%, especially in patients with skin papillomas. The skin may also manifest hyperhidrosis, thickening, cystic acne, skin tags, and acanthosis nigricans.

GH-secreting pituitary tumors usually cause some hypogonadism, either by cosecretion of PRL or by direct pressure upon normal pituitary tissue. Decreased libido and erectile dysfunction are common in men and irregular menses or amenorrhea occur in women. Women who become pregnant have an increased risk of gestational diabetes and hypertension. Secondary hypothyroidism sometimes occurs; hypoadrenalism is unusual. Headaches are frequent. Temporal hemianopia may occur as a result of the optic chiasm being impinged by suprasellar extension of the tumor.

B. Laboratory Findings

For screening purposes, a random serum IGF-1 can be obtained. If it is normal for age, acromegaly is ruled out.

For further evaluation, the patient should be fasting for at least 8 hours (except for water), not be acutely ill, and not have exercised on the day of testing. Assay for the following: serum GH, IGF-1 (increased and usually over five times normal in acromegaly), PRL (cosecreted by many GH-secreting tumors), serum free T_4, and TSH (secondary hypothyroidism is common in acromegaly; primary hypothyroidism may increase PRL). Additional labs should include glucose, serum creatinine, liver enzymes, and serum calcium and phosphorus. Acromegaly is excluded if any serum GH is < 1 mcg/L; however, many normal individuals can have a serum GH above this level. Therefore, the glucose suppression test is usually performed. Glucose syrup (100 g) is administered orally, and serum GH is measured 60 minutes afterward; acromegaly is excluded if the serum GH is suppressed to below 0.4 mcg/L with an ultrasensitive GH assay. The serum IGF-1 and glucose-suppressed GH are usually complementary tests; however, disparities between the two occur in up to 30% of patients.

C. Imaging

MRI shows a pituitary tumor in over 96% of acromegalic patients. When MRI fails to demonstrate a tumor in the pituitary or surrounding bone, CT imaging of the chest and abdomen may demonstrate an ectopic source of GH or GHRH. Radiographs may show an enlarged sella and thickened skull and tufting of the terminal phalanges of the fingers and toes.

Differential Diagnosis

Active acromegaly must be distinguished from familial coarse features, large hands and feet, and isolated prognathism and from inactive ("burned-out") acromegaly in which there has been a spontaneous remission due to infarction of the pituitary adenoma. GH-induced gigantism must be differentiated from familial tall stature and from aromatase deficiency.

High serum GH levels can be caused by exercise or eating just prior to the test; acute illness or agitation; liver failure or kidney disease; malnourishment; diabetes mellitus; or concurrent treatment with oral estrogens, β-blockers, or clonidine. Acromegaly can be difficult to diagnose during pregnancy, since the placenta produces GH and commercial GH assays may not be able to distinguish between pituitary and placental GH. During normal adolescence, serum IGF-1 levels are usually elevated and GH may fail to be suppressed.

Complications

Complications include hypopituitarism, hypertension, hyperglycemia, cardiac enlargement, HF, and colon polyps. Arthritis of hips, knees, and spine can be troublesome as can carpal tunnel syndrome. Cord compression may occur. Visual field defects may be severe and progressive. Acute loss of vision or cranial nerve palsy may occur if the tumor undergoes spontaneous hemorrhage and necrosis (pituitary apoplexy).

Treatment

A. Pituitary Microsurgery

Transsphenoidal pituitary surgery achieves a remission in about 70% of patients. With tumors < 2 cm and GH levels < 50 ng/mL, transsphenoidal pituitary surgery is successful in 80% of patients. Extrasellar extension of the pituitary tumor, particularly cavernous sinus invasion, reduces the likelihood of surgical cure. Complications of transsphenoidal surgery occur in about 12% of patients, including infection, CSF leak, and hypopituitarism.

B. Medications

Acromegalic patients with an incomplete biochemical remission after pituitary surgery may benefit from medical therapy with dopamine agonists, somatostatin analogs, tamoxifen, or pegvisomant.

Cabergoline is the oral dopamine agonist of choice. Cabergoline will shrink one-third of acromegaly-associated pituitary tumors by more than 50%. It appears to be safe during pregnancy.

Somatostatin receptor ligands (SRLs) include: paltusotine, octreotide LAR, and **lanreotide depot.** SRLs inhibit GH secretion and tumor growth by activating tumor somatostatin receptors. **Paltusotine** is a nonpeptide SRL that selectively targets somatostatin receptor type 2 (SST2). It is a first-line oral therapy for patients with acromegaly who are not eligible for surgery or who have failed surgery. In a placebo-controlled trial, 83% of patients taking paltusotine achieved a normal serum IGF-1 level compared to 4% of the placebo group.

Injectable SRLs achieve a normal serum IGF-1 levels in 53% of patients. First generation SRLs include octreotide LAR and lanreotide depot. Mycapssa is an oral form of octreotide; it is less effective than oral paltusotine. Whichever preparation is used, the dosage can be adjusted to achieve serum GH levels under 2 ng/mL. Headaches often improve, and tumor shrinkage of about 30% may be expected.

Pegvisomant, a GH receptor antagonist, can be helpful for patients resistant to other treatments, especially when there is associated diabetes mellitus. It blocks hepatic IGF-1 production but does not shrink GH-secreting tumors. Pegvisomant therapy produces symptomatic relief and normalizes serum IGF-1 levels in 63% of patients.

C. Stereotactic Radiosurgery

Acromegalic patients who do not achieve a complete remission with transsphenoidal surgery or medical therapy may be treated with stereotactic radiosurgery: linear accelerator (eg, CyberKnife), gamma knife radiosurgery, and proton beam radiosurgery. Following any pituitary radiation therapy, patients are advised to take lifelong daily low-dose aspirin because of the increased risk of small-vessel stroke. Stereotactic radiosurgery to pituitary tumors causes anterior hypopituitarism in 35–60% of patients within 5 years, so patients must have regular monitoring of their pituitary function.

Prognosis

Acromegaly is usually chronic and progressive unless treated. Patients with acromegaly experience increased mortality from cardiovascular disorders and progressive acromegalic symptoms. Those who are treated and have a random serum GH < 1.0 ng/mL or a glucose-suppressed serum GH < 0.4 ng/mL with normal age-adjusted serum IGF-1 levels have reduced morbidity and mortality.

Postoperatively, normal pituitary function is usually preserved. Soft tissue swelling regresses but bone enlargement is permanent. Adjuvant medical therapy is successful in treating patients who are not cured by pituitary surgery. Gamma knife or CyberKnife radiosurgery reduces GH levels an average of 77%, with 20% of patients having a full remission after 12 months. Proton beam radiosurgery produces a remission in 80% of patients by 5 years. Radiation therapy eventually produces some degree of hypopituitarism in most patients. Patients must receive lifelong follow-up, with regular monitoring of serum GH and IGF-1 levels. Serum GH levels over 5 ng/mL and rising IGF-1 levels usually indicate a recurrent tumor.

Araujo-Castro M et al. Biomarker-guided therapy increases remission rates and reduces time to control vs standard therapy. Expert Rev Endocrinol Metab. 2025;20:539. [PMID: 41020777]

Biller BMK et al. Rapid and sustained response of biochemically uncontrolled acromegaly to once-daily oral paltusotine treatment. J Clin Endocrinol Metab. 2026;111:e1050. [PMID: 41128642]

Ferone D et al. Octreotide subcutaneous depot for acromegaly: a randomized, double-blind, placebo-controlled phase 3 trial, ACROINNOVA 1. J Clin Endocrinol Metab. 2025;110:1729. [PMID: 39378125]

Giustina A et al. Acromegaly. N Engl J Med. 2025;393:1926. [PMID: 41223366]

Kaparounaki C et al. Medical treatment in acromegaly: a network meta-analysis. Eur J Endocrinol. 2025;193:S83. [PMID: 41140134]

HYPERPROLACTINEMIA

ESSENTIALS OF DIAGNOSIS

- Most common secretory pituitary tumor.
- Women: Oligomenorrhea, amenorrhea; galactorrhea; infertility.
- Men: Hypogonadism; decreased libido and erectile dysfunction; infertility.
- Elevated serum PRL.
- CT or MRI may show a pituitary adenoma.

General Considerations

Some causes of hyperprolactinemia are shown in Table 29–1. PRL-secreting pituitary tumors (prolactinomas) are the most common secretory pituitary tumor; they are usually sporadic but may rarely be familial as part of MEN type 1 or 4. Most are microadenomas (< 1 cm),

Table 29–1. Causes of hyperprolactinemia.

Physiologic Causes	Pharmacologic Causes	Pathologic Causes
Assay interference Breastfeeding Exercise Familial (mutant prolactin receptor) Idiopathic Macroprolactin ("big prolactin") Nipple stimulation Neonatal Pregnancy Sleep (REM phase) Stress (trauma, surgery)	Amoxapine Amphetamines Androgens Anesthetic agents Antipsychotics (conventional and atypical) Butyrophenones Cimetidine (not famotidine or nizatidine) Cocaine use or withdrawal Domperidone Estrogens Hydroxyzine Licorice (real) Lorcaserin MAO inhibitors Methyldopa Metoclopramide Opioids Nicotine Phenothiazines Progestins Protease inhibitors Reserpine SSRIs Tricyclic antidepressants Verapamil	Acromegaly Adrenal insufficiency Chronic chest wall stimulation (thoracotomy, augmentation or reduction mammoplasty, mastectomy, herpes zoster, chest acupuncture, nipple rings, etc) Hypophysitis Hypothalamic or pituitary stalk damage Hypothyroidism Liver disease Multiple sclerosis Optic neuromyelitis Prolactin-secreting tumors Pseudocyesis (false pregnancy) Renal insufficiency (especially with zinc deficiency) Spinal cord lesions SLE

REM, rapid eye movement.

which are more common in women and typically do not grow even with pregnancy or oral contraceptives. Aggressive macroprolactinomas (> 1 cm) are more common in men and can spread into the cavernous sinuses and suprasellar areas; rarely, they may erode the floor of the sella to invade the paranasal sinuses. Hyperprolactinemia (without a pituitary adenoma) may also be familial.

Clinical Findings

A. Symptoms and Signs

Hyperprolactinemia may cause hypogonadotropic hypogonadism and reduced fertility. Men usually have diminished libido and erectile dysfunction that may not respond to testosterone replacement; gynecomastia sometimes occurs.

About 90% of premenopausal women with prolactinomas experience amenorrhea, oligomenorrhea, or infertility. Estrogen deficiency can cause decreased vaginal lubrication, irritability, anxiety, and depression. Galactorrhea (lactation in the absence of nursing) is common. During pregnancy, clinically significant enlargement of a microprolactinoma (< 10 mm) occurs in < 3%; clinically significant enlargement of a macroprolactinoma occurs in about 30%.

Pituitary prolactinomas may cosecrete GH and cause acromegaly. Large tumors may cause headaches, visual symptoms, and pituitary insufficiency.

B. Laboratory Findings

An elevated serum prolactin level should be verified with a repeat determination, ideally in a different laboratory. Evaluate for conditions known to cause hyperprolactinemia, particularly pregnancy (serum hCG), hypothyroidism (serum FT_4 and TSH), kidney disease (BUN and serum creatinine), cirrhosis (liver tests), and hyperparathyroidism (serum calcium). Screen for acromegaly with a random serum IGF-1 level. Men are evaluated for hypogonadism with serum total and free testosterone, LH, and FSH. Women who have amenorrhea are assessed for hypogonadism with serum estradiol, LH, and FSH. Patients with macroprolactinomas or manifestations of possible hypopituitarism should be evaluated for hypopituitarism. Patients with hyperprolactinemia who are relatively asymptomatic and have no apparent cause for hyperprolactinemia should have an assay for macroprolactinemia, which is an increased circulating level of a high molecular weight PRL that is biologically inactive but is detected on assays.

C. Imaging

Patients with hyperprolactinemia not induced by drugs, hypothyroidism, or pregnancy should be examined by pituitary MRI. Small prolactinomas may be demonstrated, but clear differentiation from normal variants is not always possible. The normal pituitary grows during pregnancy. MRI is therefore generally not performed during pregnancy unless there are visual-field defects or other neurologic symptoms, in which case a limited MRI study without gadolinium should be done.

Differential Diagnosis

The differential diagnosis for galactorrhea includes the small amount of breast milk that can normally be expressed from the nipple in many parous women. Nipple stimulation from nipple rings, chest surgery, or acupuncture can cause galactorrhea; serum PRL levels may be normal or minimally elevated. Some women can have idiopathic galactorrhea with normal serum PRL levels. Normal breast milk may be various colors besides white. However, bloody galactorrhea requires evaluation for breast cancer.

About 40% of nonfunctional pituitary macroadenomas produce some degree of hyperprolactinemia. These and other lesions and malignancies can be misdiagnosed as prolactinomas. One distinguishing characteristic is that the serum PRL is usually only marginally elevated in the latter tumors, whereas with pituitary macroprolactinomas the serum PRL typically exceeds 100 mcg/L.

Pregnant women have high serum PRL levels, with physiological hyperplastic enlargement of the pituitary on MRI. Increased pituitary size is a normal variant in young women. Primary hypothyroidism can cause hyperprolactinemia and hyperplasia of the pituitary that can be mistaken for a pituitary adenoma. Macroprolactinemia occurs in 3.7% of the general population and accounts for 10–25% of all cases of hyperprolactinemia.

Treatment

Medications known to increase PRL should be stopped if possible (Table 29–1). Hyperprolactinemia due to hypothyroidism is corrected by levothyroxine.

Women with microprolactinomas who have amenorrhea or who desire contraception may safely take estrogen replacement or oral contraceptives; there is minimal risk of stimulating enlargement of the microadenoma. Patients with infertility and hyperprolactinemia may be treated with a dopamine agonist to improve fertility.

Pituitary macroprolactinomas have a higher risk of progressive growth, particularly during estrogen or testosterone HRT or during pregnancy. Therefore, patients with macroprolactinomas should not be treated with HRT or oral contraceptives unless they are in remission with dopamine agonist medication or surgery.

Pregnant women with macroprolactinomas should continue to receive treatment with dopamine agonists throughout the pregnancy to prevent tumor growth. If dopamine agonists are not used during pregnancy in a woman with a macroprolactinoma, visual field testing is required in each trimester. Measurement of PRL is not useful surveillance for tumor growth due to the fact that PRL increases greatly during normal pregnancy.

A. Dopamine Agonists

Dopamine agonists are the initial treatment of choice for patients with giant prolactinomas and those with hyperprolactinemia desiring restoration of normal sexual function and fertility. Cabergoline is the most effective and usually best-tolerated ergot-derived dopamine agonist. Begin with 0.25 mg orally once weekly for 1 week, then 0.25 mg twice weekly for the next week, then 0.5 mg twice weekly. Further dosage increases may be required monthly, based on serum PRL levels, up to a maximum of 1.5 mg twice weekly. Bromocriptine is an alternative. Aripiprazole may be added to conventional dopamine agonist therapy to optimally reduce high PRL levels caused by antipsychotics or antidepressants. Patients whose tumor is resistant to one dopamine agonist may be switched to another in an effort to induce a remission.

Dopamine agonists are given at bedtime to minimize side effects of fatigue, nausea, dizziness, and orthostatic hypotension, which occur in up to 50% of patients. These symptoms usually improve with dosage reduction and continued use. Dopamine agonists can cause a variety of psychiatric side effects (particularly depression, impulse control disorder, and hypersexuality) that are not dose related and may take weeks to resolve once the drug is discontinued.

Dopamine agonists do not increase the risk of miscarriage or teratogenicity. Pregnant women with microprolactinomas may safely stop treatment during pregnancy and breastfeeding. However, over 20% of macroadenomas enlarge significantly during pregnancy; if therapy is withdrawn, patients must be monitored with serum PRL determinations and computer-assisted visual fields.

B. Surgical Treatment

Transsphenoidal pituitary surgery may be urgently required for large tumors undergoing apoplexy or those severely compromising visual fields. It is also used electively for patients who do not tolerate or respond to dopamine agonists. Surgery is generally well tolerated, with a mortality rate of < 0.5%. For pituitary microprolactinomas, skilled neurosurgeons are successful in normalizing PRL in 87% of patients and some patients prefer surgery to long-term therapy with dopamine agonists.

C. Stereotactic Radiosurgery

Stereotactic radiosurgery is seldom required for prolactinomas since they usually respond to cabergoline or surgery. It is reserved for patients with macroadenomas that are growing despite treatment with dopamine agonists or patients who are intolerant to dopamine agonists.

D. Chemotherapy

Some patients with aggressive pituitary macroadenomas or carcinomas are not surgical candidates and do not respond to dopamine agonists or radiation therapy. A small percentage of patients with aggressive tumors respond to cabergoline with the addition of either temozolomide or everolimus.

Prognosis

Pituitary microprolactinomas are typically indolent, and only 15% grow after diagnosis. However, macroprolactinomas tend to be more aggressive. Prolactinomas generally respond well to dopamine agonist therapy. Ninety percent of patients with prolactinomas experience a fall in serum PRL to 10% or less of pretreatment levels and 80% achieve a normal serum PRL level. Shrinkage of a pituitary adenoma occurs early, but the maximum effect may take up to 1 year. Nearly half of prolactinomas—even massive tumors—shrink > 50%. During pregnancy, growth of a pituitary prolactinoma occurs in 3% of women with a microprolactinoma and in 23% of those with a macroprolactinoma. If cabergoline is stopped after 2 years of therapy, hyperprolactinemia recurs in 68% of patients with idiopathic hyperprolactinemia, 79% with microprolactinomas, and 84% with macroprolactinomas.

The 10-year recurrence rate is 13% for pituitary microadenomas after transsphenoidal surgery; pituitary function can be preserved in > 95% of cases. However, the surgical success rate for macroprolactinomas is much lower, and the complication rates are higher.

Chen Z et al. Presurgical medical treatment in prolactinomas: surgical implications and pathological characteristics from 290 cases. J Clin Endocrinol Metab. 2024;109:1433. [PMID: 38163969]

Fleseriu M et al. Prolactin-secreting adenomas: pathogenesis, diagnosis, and management. Lancet Diabetes Endocrinol. 2025;13:874. [PMID: 40876473]

Fountas A et al. Conservatively managed non-functioning pituitary macroadenomas—cohort study. Eur J Endocinol. 2025;192:680. [PMID: 40305776]

Glezer A et al. Approach to the patient with dopamine-resistant microprolactinoma. J Clin Endocrinol Metab. 2026;111:879. [PMID: 41234156]

NONFUNCTIONING PITUITARY NEUROENDOCRINE TUMORS

ESSENTIALS OF DIAGNOSIS

- Clinical and biochemical evaluation for pituitary hormone hypersecretion is negative.
- MRI shows a pituitary microadenoma (< 1 cm) or macroadenoma (≥ 1 cm).
- Headache, visual field compromise, and anterior hypopituitarism are common with macroadenomas.
- Elevated serum PRL with macroadenomas may be due to stalk compression.

General Considerations

Although pituitary neuroendocrine tumors (PitNETs) may secrete PRL, GH, or ACTH, most are nonfunctional and do not produce symptoms of hormone oversecretion. Pituitary nonfunctioning adenomas occur more frequently in men than women and are more common with age. Pituitary adenomas are found on about 16% of brain MRIs; most are microadenomas < 1 cm diameter.

Clinical Findings

A. Symptoms and Signs

Nonfunctioning pituitary macroadenomas (≥ 1 cm) tend to be more aggressive than functioning pituitary adenomas. Those with nonfunctioning macroadenomas are much more likely to be symptomatic from mass effect with visual field compromise, headache, cranial nerve palsies affecting extraocular muscles, and pituitary apoplexy. Larger macroadenomas frequently cause some hypopituitarism, particularly hypogonadotropic hypogonadism. Nonfunctioning pituitary microadenomas are asymptomatic.

B. Laboratory Findings

1. Pituitary hormone hypersecretion—All patients with a pituitary adenoma require testing for pituitary hormone hypersecretion. Obtain a serum PRL to screen for prolactin hypersecretion; women with hyperprolactinemia are tested for pregnancy with a serum hCG. Testing for Cushing disease or acromegaly should be obtained, if clinically indicated.

2. Anterior hypopituitarism—Patients should have the following tests: serum free T_4, TSH, morning serum testosterone and free testosterone. Serum LH and FSH should be obtained in men with low serum testosterone, women who are postmenopausal, and younger women with amenorrhea. Serum sodium and glucose should be obtained in all patients. A cosyntropin stimulation test is performed for patients with hyponatremia or symptoms of possible hypoadrenalism. A serum IGF-1 is drawn to screen for GH deficiency. Younger patients with short stature who have not fused their epiphyses should have a full evaluation for growth hormone deficiency.

3. Pituitary macroadenomas—Patients with a macroadenoma that impinges upon the optic chiasm require formal visual field testing.

C. Imaging

Pituitary dynamic contrast-enhanced MRI (3T) is the imaging modality of choice for the evaluation and follow-up of pituitary adenomas. Nonfunctioning pituitary microadenomas that are < 0.5 cm require no further MRI follow-up. For nonfunctioning pituitary adenomas ≥ 0.5 cm, repeat MRI is recommended at 6 months, then yearly for 3 years. If no enlargement is noted, MRI surveillance can then be done less frequently.

Differential Diagnosis

Mass lesions that can mimic pituitary adenoma include pituitary craniopharyngiomas, gliomas, meningiomas, skull base osteosarcomas, Rathke cysts, lymphocytic hypophysitis, infection, or metastases. Large normal pituitary glands and physiologic pituitary enlargement during primary hypothyroidism or pregnancy should also be considered; serum prolactin levels are elevated in primary hypothyroidism and pregnancy. Hyperprolactinemia also occurs when there is pituitary stalk compression from pituitary macroadenomas and other mass lesions; with pituitary stalk compression, serum prolactin is typically lower than expected for the size of the pituitary mass.

Treatment

Patients with asymptomatic pituitary nonfunctioning microadenomas ordinarily require no treatment. Surgery is the preferred treatment option for patients whose adenoma is causing mass effect symptoms, premature development of puberty, hormonal deficiencies, or the emergence of symptomatic hormonal hypersecretion. A trial of oral cabergoline may be considered for patients with macroadenomas who have progressive disease. Radiation therapy can be used for select individuals with pituitary macroadenomas.

Prognosis

The prognosis is excellent for patients with nonfunctioning microadenomas < 0.5 cm. Patients with larger nonfunctioning microadenomas also have a very good prognosis but require follow-up. Transsphenoidal surgery is 65% successful in completely resecting pituitary macroadenomas, improves hypopituitarism in 50%, and reverses visual field compromise in 80% of patients. Following surgery, deficiencies of anterior pituitary hormones occur in 10% of patients. The 6-year postoperative recurrence rate has been reported to be 36% following surgery alone and 13% after surgery plus adjuvant radiation therapy. Temozolomide has documented effectiveness against aggressive PitNETs, but most patients have progressive disease.

Costachescu M et al. A study in pituitary neuroendocrine tumors (PitNETs): real-life data amid baseline and serial CT scans. Cancers (Basel). 2024;16:3477. [PMID: 39456571]

Deng C et al. Temozolomide treatment in refractory pituitary adenomas and pituitary carcinomas. Neuroendocrinology. 2025;115:335. [PMID: 39778549]
Fountas A et al. Conservatively managed non-functioning pituitary macroadenomas—cohort study. Eur J Endocinol. 2025;192:680. [PMID: 40305776]
Hefner NA et al. Management of recurrent and aggressive non-functioning pituitary adenomas. J Clin Med. 2025;14:5203. [PMID: 40806825]

DISEASES OF THE THYROID GLAND

THYROIDITIS

ESSENTIALS OF DIAGNOSIS

Autoimmune thyroiditis

- Chronic lymphocytic (Hashimoto) thyroiditis is the most common thyroiditis and often progresses to hypothyroidism.
- Postpartum thyroiditis and subacute lymphocytic thyroiditis (silent thyroiditis) can cause transient hyperthyroidism due to passive release of stored thyroid hormone.
- Thyroid peroxidase antibodies (TPO Ab) or thyroglobulin antibodies (Tg Ab) are usually high.

Painful subacute thyroiditis (de Quervain thyroiditis)

- Tender thyroid gland with painful dysphagia.
- Viral etiology.
- Antithyroid antibodies are absent or low.

Infectious (suppurative) thyroiditis

- Severe, painful thyroid gland.
- Febrile with leukocytosis and elevated ESR.

IgG_4-related thyroiditis (Riedel thyroiditis)

- Most often in middle age or older women.
- Usually part of a systemic fibrosing syndrome.

General Considerations

A. Autoimmune Thyroiditis

Several clinical entities are classified as autoimmune thyroiditis, including chronic lymphocytic thyroiditis, postpartum thyroiditis, and painless (silent) sporadic subacute thyroiditis. Dietary iodine supplementation (especially when excessive) and certain medications can cause autoimmune thyroiditis. The incidence of autoimmune thyroiditis varies by kindred, race, and sex. It is commonly familial. Elevated serum levels of antithyroid antibodies are detectable in the general population in 3% of men and 13% of women. Among United States adults, elevated levels of antithyroid antibodies are found in 14.3% of those who self-identify as White, 10.9% as Latina/Latino, and 5.3% as Black. Subclinical thyroiditis is extremely common; autopsy series have found focal thyroiditis in 40% of women and 20% of men.

1. Chronic lymphocytic thyroiditis—Also known as "Hashimoto thyroiditis," chronic lymphocytic thyroiditis is the most common thyroid disorder in the United States. Cell-mediated T-lymphocyte invasion gives the microscopic appearance of "lymphocytic thyroiditis." Humoral autoimmunity, with detectable serum antithyroid antibodies (TPO Ab or Tg Ab, or both), is present in most but not all affected patients. It is frequently associated with dry eye disease.

2. Postpartum thyroiditis—Postpartum thyroiditis occurs soon after delivery in about 7% of women. The affected thyroid releases stored thyroid hormone, resulting in transient hyperthyroidism (often mild and undiagnosed) followed by hypothyroidism. The thyroid gland is not acutely tender, but some women report mild thyroid discomfort. Most women recover normal thyroid function. Women in whom postpartum thyroiditis develops have a 70% chance of recurrence after subsequent pregnancies. It occurs most commonly in women who have high levels of TPO Ab in the first trimester of pregnancy or immediately after delivery.

3. Painless (silent) sporadic subacute thyroiditis—This form of autoimmune thyroiditis is similar to postpartum thyroiditis, except that it is not related to pregnancy. Causes include amiodarone and immunotherapy. Hyperthyroidism results from the release of stored thyroid hormone. This accounts for about 1% of cases of thyrotoxicosis and is followed by hypothyroidism that may or may not resolve spontaneously.

4. Other causes—Dietary iodine supplementation (especially when excessive) and certain medications, including tyrosine kinase inhibitors, alemtuzumab, interferon-α, interleukin-2, thalidomide, lenalidomide, lithium, amiodarone, and immune checkpoint inhibitors, are other causes of autoimmune thyroiditis. Chronic hepatitis C increases the risk for autoimmune thyroiditis: 21% of affected patients have antithyroid antibodies and 13% have hypothyroidism. COVID-19 infection increases the risk for autoimmune thyroiditis and subacute thyroiditis. Vaccination against SARS-CoV-2 can trigger subacute thyroiditis as well as Graves disease.

Autoimmune thyroiditis often progresses to hypothyroidism, which may be linked to thyrotropin receptor–blocking antibodies, detected in 10% of patients with autoimmune thyroiditis. High serum levels of TPO Ab also predict progression from subclinical to symptomatic hypothyroidism. Although the hypothyroidism is usually permanent, up to 11% of patients experience a remission after several years. Hyperthyroidism can be caused by the destructive release of thyroid hormones (followed by hypothyroidism) or by increased synthesis of thyroid hormones (Graves disease).

Autoimmune thyroiditis is sometimes associated with other endocrine deficiencies as part of autoimmune polyendocrine syndrome type 2 (APS-II). Adults with APS-II are prone to autoimmune thyroiditis, type 1 diabetes mellitus, autoimmune gonadal failure, hypoparathyroidism, and adrenal insufficiency. Thyroiditis is frequently associated with other autoimmune conditions: pernicious anemia, Sjögren syndrome, vitiligo, IBD, celiac disease, and gluten sensitivity.

B. Painful Subacute Thyroiditis

Also called de Quervain thyroiditis, granulomatous thyroiditis, and giant cell thyroiditis, painful subacute thyroiditis is relatively common. Like painless subacute thyroiditis, most affected patients have transient hyperthyroidism, followed by hypothyroidism. Painful subacute thyroiditis is typically associated with viral upper respiratory infection (including COVID-19) and may follow vaccinations, including SARS-CoV-2. Some patients also have antithyroid antibodies. Its incidence peaks in the summer to early autumn. It affects both sexes, but over 75% are middle-aged women. Subacute thyroiditis can also be a sequela of a drug-induced hypersensitivity syndrome.

C. Infectious (Suppurative) Thyroiditis

Infectious thyroiditis is rare among immunocompetent patients. It is usually bacterial but mycobacterial, fungal, and parasitic infections can occur, particularly in immunosuppressed individuals.

D. IgG_4-Related (Riedel) Thyroiditis

IgG_4-related thyroiditis, also called Riedel thyroiditis, invasive fibrous thyroiditis, Riedel struma, woody thyroiditis, ligneous thyroiditis, and invasive thyroiditis, is the rarest form of thyroiditis. It is found most frequently in middle-aged or older women and is usually part of a multifocal systemic fibrosis syndrome. It may occur as a thyroid manifestation of IgG_4-related systemic disease.

Clinical Findings

A. Symptoms and Signs

In **autoimmune thyroiditis**, the thyroid gland may be diffusely enlarged, firm, and finely nodular but is frequently not palpable. One thyroid lobe may be asymmetrically enlarged, raising concerns about neoplasm. Although patients may report neck tightness, pain and tenderness are not usually present. Other patients have no palpable goiter and no neck symptoms. The thyroid is fibrotic and atrophic in about 10% of cases, particularly in older women.

Symptoms and signs are mostly related to levels of thyroid hormone. Affected patients may have combinations of hyperthyroidism and hypothyroidism. For example, a patient with hypothyroidism might later develop hyperthyroidism that can wax and wane. Depression and chronic fatigue are more common, even after correction of hypothyroidism.

About one-third of patients have mild dry mouth (xerostomia) or dry eyes (keratoconjunctivitis sicca) related to Sjögren syndrome. Associated myasthenia gravis is usually of mild severity, mainly affecting the extraocular muscles and having a relatively low incidence of detectable AChR Ab or thymic disease. Associated celiac disease or gluten intolerance can produce fatigue or depression, sometimes in the absence of GI symptoms.

Postpartum thyroiditis is typically manifested by hyperthyroidism that begins 1–6 months after delivery and persists for only 1–2 months. Then, hypothyroidism tends to develop beginning 4–8 months after delivery.

In painless sporadic thyroiditis, thyrotoxic symptoms are usually mild; a small, nontender goiter may be palpated in about 50% of patients. The course is similar to postpartum thyroiditis.

Painful subacute thyroiditis presents with an acute, usually painful enlargement of the one or both lobes of the thyroid gland, often with dysphagia. Those with bilateral involvement are likely to be more hyperthyroid. The majority of patients experience pain that may radiate to the ears, jaw, or upper chest. Patients usually have a low-grade fever and fatigue. The manifestations may persist for weeks or months. Thyrotoxicosis develops in 50% of affected patients and tends to last for several weeks. Subsequently, hypothyroidism develops that lasts 4–6 months. Normal thyroid function typically returns within 12 months, but persistent hypothyroidism develops in 5% of patients.

Infectious suppurative thyroiditis patients usually are febrile and have severe pain, tenderness, redness, and fluctuation in the region of the thyroid gland.

In **IgG_4-related thyroiditis**, thyroid enlargement is often asymmetric; the gland is stony hard and adherent to the neck structures, causing signs of compression and invasion, including dysphagia, dyspnea, pain, and hoarseness. Related conditions include retroperitoneal fibrosis, fibrosing mediastinitis, sclerosing cervicitis, subretinal fibrosis, and sclerosing cholangitis.

B. Laboratory Findings

In **autoimmune thyroiditis** (including postpartum thyroiditis), there are usually increased circulating levels of the antithyroid antibodies TPO Ab (90%) or Tg Ab (40%). However, 5% of patients have no detectable antithyroid antibodies. Most patients with thyroiditis caused by immune checkpoint inhibitors have no detectable antithyroid antibodies. Antithyroid antibodies decline during pregnancy and are often undetectable in the third trimester. Once autoimmune thyroiditis has been diagnosed, monitoring of antibody levels is not helpful. If autoimmune thyroiditis leads to inadequate thyroid hormone release, the serum TSH level is elevated and thyroid hormone levels may be normal or decreased (hypothyroidism). Autoimmune thyroiditis may also lead to passive release of stored thyroid hormones, resulting in hyperthyroidism with increased serum FT_4 levels that are proportionally higher than T_3 levels and suppressed TSH levels. Because T_4 is less active than T_3, the hyperthyroidism seen in autoimmune thyroiditis is usually less severe than with Graves disease.

Patients with autoimmune thyroiditis have a 15% incidence of having serum IgA tissue transglutaminase (tTG) antibody and at least 5% have clinically significant celiac disease.

In **painful subacute thyroiditis**, the ESR is markedly elevated while antithyroid antibody titers are low, distinguishing it from autoimmune thyroiditis. Subacute thyroiditis may result in passive release of stored thyroid hormones, resulting in hyperthyroidism. In **infectious thyroiditis**, both the leukocyte count and ESR are usually elevated.

C. Imaging

Ultrasound typically shows diffuse heterogeneous thyroid density and reduced echogenicity. It is useful to distinguish autoimmune thyroiditis from multinodular goiter, thyroid nodules that are suspicious for malignancy, and Graves disease. In thyroiditis, vascularity is reduced or normal, whereas in Graves disease, the thyroid gland is hypervascular.

Radioiodine (RAI) uptake and scan can help distinguish thyroiditis from Graves disease; painful subacute thyroiditis exhibits very low RAI uptake. RAI uptake may be normal or high with uneven uptake in chronic autoimmune thyroiditis (euthyroid or hypothyroid); CT or MRI is not useful in diagnosis.

[^{18}F] Fluorodeoxyglucose positron emission tomography (^{18}FDG-PET) scanning frequently shows diffuse thyroid uptake of isotope in cases of thyroiditis. Discrete nodular areas of ^{18}FDG-PET uptake within the thyroid have a 50% chance of being malignant.

D. Fine-Needle Aspiration Cytology

Patients with autoimmune thyroiditis who have a thyroid nodule should have an ultrasound-guided FNA biopsy, since the risk of papillary thyroid cancer is about 8% in such nodules. When infectious (suppurative) thyroiditis is suspected, an FNA biopsy with Gram stain and culture is required. FNA biopsy is usually not required for painful subacute thyroiditis but shows characteristic giant multinucleated cells.

Complications

Over 20% of patients with autoimmune thyroiditis eventually develop overt hypothyroidism. Hyperthyroidism may develop, either due to the emergence of Graves disease or due to the release of stored thyroid hormone, a condition variably termed "hashitoxicosis" or "painless sporadic thyroiditis." Euthyroid women with high serum TPO Ab may have an increased risk of miscarriage and preterm birth; unfortunately, treatment with levothyroxine fails to improve these risks. Perimenopausal women with high serum levels of TPO Ab have a higher relative risk of depression, independent of ambient thyroid hormone levels.

Subacute and chronic thyroiditis are complicated by the effects of pressure on the neck structures: dyspnea and, in Riedel struma, vocal cord palsy. Papillary thyroid carcinoma or thyroid lymphoma may rarely be associated with chronic thyroiditis and must be considered in the diagnosis of uneven painless enlargements that continue despite treatment; such patients require FNA biopsy.

Differential Diagnosis

All types of goiters must be considered in the differential diagnosis of thyroiditis, especially if enlargement is rapid. Unlike in goiters, in subacute thyroiditis there is very low RAI uptake and the T_4 and T_3 are elevated. Thyroid autoantibody tests have been helpful in the diagnosis of autoimmune thyroiditis, but the tests are not specific (positive in patients with multinodular goiters, malignancy [eg, thyroid carcinoma, lymphoma], and concurrent Graves disease). The subacute and suppurative forms of thyroiditis may resemble any infectious process in or near the neck structures. Chronic thyroiditis may resemble thyroid carcinoma, especially if the enlargement is uneven and if there is pressure on surrounding structures; both disorders may be present in the same gland.

Treatment

A. Autoimmune Thyroiditis

If hypothyroidism is present, levothyroxine should be given in usual replacement doses (0.05–0.2 mg orally daily) (see Hypothyroidism & Myxedema, below). If hyperthyroidism is present, see Hyperthyroidism (Thyrotoxicosis), below.

In patients with a large goiter and normal or elevated serum TSH, an attempt is made to shrink the goiter with levothyroxine in doses sufficient to drive the serum TSH below the reference range while maintaining clinical euthyroidism. Suppressive doses of T_4 tend to shrink the goiter an average of 30% over 6 months. If the goiter does not regress, lower replacement doses of levothyroxine may be given. If the thyroid gland is only minimally enlarged and the patient is euthyroid, regular observation is indicated, since hypothyroidism may develop, often years later.

Dietary supplementation with selenium 200 mcg/day reduces serum levels of TPO Ab but does not prevent hypothyroidism. The favored formulation is selenomethionine.

B. Painful Subacute Thyroiditis

All treatment is empiric and must be continued for several weeks. Recurrence is common. The drug of choice is aspirin (325–650 mg orally every 4–6 hours, which relieves pain and inflammation) or NSAIDs. For patients with severe pain, prednisone, 20 mg orally daily for about 2 weeks, can be effective. Thyrotoxic symptoms are treated with propranolol, 10–40 mg orally every 6 hours, or propranolol ER, 60–160 mg orally daily. Iodinated contrast agents cause a prompt fall in serum T_3 levels and a dramatic improvement in thyrotoxic symptoms. Ipodate sodium (Bilivist, Oragrafin) or iopanoic acid (Telepaque) is given orally in doses of 500 mg orally daily until serum FT_4 levels return to normal. Transient hypothyroidism is treated with T_4 (0.05–0.1 mg orally daily) if symptomatic.

C. Infectious (Suppurative) Thyroiditis

Treatment is with antibiotics and with surgical drainage when fluctuation is marked. Surgical thyroidectomy may be required.

D. IgG_4-Related (Riedel) Thyroiditis

The treatment of choice is tamoxifen, 20 mg orally twice daily, which must be continued for years. Tamoxifen can induce partial to complete remissions in most patients within 3–6 months. Its mode of action appears to be unrelated to its antiestrogen activity. Short-term corticosteroid treatment may be added for partial alleviation of pain and compression symptoms. Rituximab may be useful for

Riedel thyroiditis that is refractory to tamoxifen and corticosteroids. Surgical decompression usually fails to permanently alleviate compression symptoms; surgery is difficult due to dense fibrous adhesions, making surgical complications more likely.

Prognosis

Patients with Hashimoto autoimmune thyroiditis generally have an excellent prognosis, since the condition either remains stable for years or progresses slowly to hypothyroidism, which is easily treated. Although 80% of women with postpartum thyroiditis subsequently recover normal thyroid function, permanent hypothyroidism eventually develops in about 50% within 7 years. In subacute painful thyroiditis, spontaneous remissions and exacerbations are common; the disease process may smolder for months.

Khachaturov M et al. Hashimoto thyroiditis—what's in a name? Hormones (Athens). 2025;24:389. [PMID: 40172784]
Orth HM et al. Subacute thyroiditis—is it really linked to viral infection? J Clin Endocrinol Metab. 2025;110:2938. [PMID: 39812071]
Randelović K et al. Hashimoto's thyroiditis and dry eye disease. J Clin Med. 2025;14:1710. [PMID: 40095800]
Zhang H et al. Clinical efficacy of selenium supplementation in patients with Hashimoto thyroiditis: a systematic review and meta-analysis. Medicine (Baltimore). 2025;104:e44043. [PMID: 40898469]

HYPOTHYROIDISM & MYXEDEMA

ESSENTIALS OF DIAGNOSIS

- Hashimoto autoimmune thyroiditis is the most common cause.
- Fatigue, cold intolerance, constipation, weight change, depression, menorrhagia, hoarseness.
- Dry skin, bradycardia, delayed return of deep tendon reflexes.
- FT_4 is usually low.
- TSH elevated in primary hypothyroidism.

General Considerations

Hypothyroidism is common, with 0.3% of the population having overt disease. About 85% of affected individuals are women. Thyroid hormone deficiency affects almost all body functions. The degree of severity ranges from mild and unrecognized hypothyroid states to striking myxedema. Maternal hypothyroidism during pregnancy results in offspring with IQ scores that are an average 7 points lower than those of euthyroid mothers.

Hypothyroidism may be due to failure or resection of the thyroid gland itself (primary hypothyroidism) or deficiency of pituitary TSH (secondary hypothyroidism; see Hypopituitarism). Autoimmune thyroiditis is the most common cause of hypothyroidism (see Thyroiditis). A hypothyroid phase also occurs in subacute (de Quervain) viral thyroiditis following initial hyperthyroidism.

Goiter (thyroid enlargement) may be present with thyroiditis, iodide deficiency, genetic thyroid enzyme defects, food goitrogens in iodide-deficient areas (eg, turnips, cassavas), or infiltrating diseases (eg, cancer, sarcoidosis). Goitrogenic medications include iodide, propylthiouracil (PTU) or methimazole, sulfonamides, amiodarone, interferon-α, interferon-β, interleukin-2, and lithium. About 50% of patients taking lithium long term have an ultrasound-detectable goiter. Goiter is often absent in patients with autoimmune thyroiditis or hypothyroidism due to destruction of the gland by head-neck or chest-shoulder radiation therapy or ^{131}I therapy. Total thyroidectomy causes hypothyroidism; after hemithyroidectomy, hypothyroidism develops in 22% of patients.

Amiodarone, because of its high iodine content, causes clinically significant hypothyroidism in 15–20% of patients as well as thyrotoxicosis (see Amiodarone-induced thyrotoxicosis, below). Hypothyroidism occurs most often in patients with preexisting autoimmune thyroiditis. The T_4 level is low or low-normal, and the TSH is elevated, usually > 20 mIU/L. Another 17% of patients taking amiodarone are asymptomatic with normal serum T_4 levels despite elevations in serum TSH; they can be closely monitored without levothyroxine therapy.

Hypothyroidism may also develop in patients with a high iodine intake, especially if they have underlying lymphocytic thyroiditis. Some malignancies overexpress thyroid hormone inactivating enzyme (type 3 deiodinase) and cause "consumptive hypothyroidism." This has occurred with large hemangiomas or a heavy tumor burden of colon cancer, basal cell cancer, fibrous tumors, or gastrointestinal stromal tumors (GISTs).

Chemotherapeutic agents that can cause silent thyroiditis include tyrosine kinase inhibitors, denileukin diftitox, alemtuzumab, interferon-α, interleukin-2, thalidomide, lenalidomide, and immune checkpoint inhibitors. Thyroiditis usually starts with hyperthyroidism (often unrecognized) and then progresses to hypothyroidism. RAI-based targeted radioisotope therapy can also cause hypothyroidism. Mifepristone causes primary hypothyroidism and an increased dose requirement for thyroid hormone replacement. Mitotane causes secondary hypothyroidism.

Clinical Findings

A. Symptoms and Signs

1. Common manifestations—Mild hypothyroidism often escapes detection. Patients typically have nonspecific symptoms that include weight gain, fatigue, lethargy, depression, weakness, dyspnea on exertion, arthralgias or myalgias, muscle cramps, menorrhagia, constipation, dry skin, headache, paresthesias, cold intolerance, carpal tunnel syndrome, and Raynaud syndrome. Physical findings can include bradycardia; diastolic hypertension; thin, brittle nails; thinning of hair; peripheral edema; puffy face and eyelids; and skin pallor or yellowing (carotenemia). Delayed relaxation of deep tendon reflexes may be present. Patients often have a goiter that arises due to elevated serum TSH levels or the underlying thyroid pathology.

2. Less common manifestations—Less common symptoms of hypothyroidism include diminished appetite and weight loss, hoarseness, decreased sense of taste and smell, and diminished auditory acuity. Some patients with goiter may report dysphagia or neck discomfort. Although most menstruating women have menorrhagia, some women have scant menses or amenorrhea. Physical findings may include loss of eyelash and eyebrow hairs; thickening of the tongue; hard pitting edema; and effusions into the pleural and peritoneal cavities as well as into joints. Galactorrhea may also be present. Cardiac enlargement ("myxedema heart") and pericardial effusions may develop. Psychosis "myxedema madness" can occur from severe hypothyroidism or from toxicity of other drugs whose metabolism is slowed in hypothyroidism.

Some hypothyroid patients with autoimmune thyroiditis have symptoms that are not due to hypothyroidism but rather to conditions associated with autoimmune thyroiditis; these include Addison disease, hypoparathyroidism, diabetes mellitus, pernicious anemia, Sjögren syndrome, vitiligo, biliary cirrhosis, gluten sensitivity, and celiac disease.

B. Laboratory Findings

The single best screening test for hypothyroidism is the serum TSH (Table 29–2). In primary hypothyroidism, the serum TSH is increased in a reflex effort to stimulate the failing gland, while the serum FT_4 is low or low-normal. The normal reference range for ultrasensitive TSH levels is generally 0.4–4.0 mIU/L.

Other laboratory abnormalities can include hypoglycemia or anemia (with normal or increased mean corpuscular volume). Hyponatremia due to SIAD (formerly SIADH) or decreased GFR is common. Additional frequent findings include increased serum levels of LDL cholesterol, triglycerides, lipoprotein(a), liver enzymes, creatine kinase, or PRL. In patients with autoimmune thyroiditis, titers of antibodies against TPO and TG are high; serum ANA may be present but are rarely indicative of lupus.

Subclinical hypothyroidism is defined as the state of having a normal serum FT_4 with a serum TSH that is above the reference range. It occurs most often in persons aged 65 years or older, in whom the prevalence is 13%. Subclinical hypothyroidism is often transient, and serum TSH levels normalize spontaneously in about 60% of cases within 5 years. The likelihood of TSH normalization is higher in patients without antithyroid antibodies and those with a marginally elevated serum TSH. The term "subclinical" is somewhat misleading, since it refers to the serum hormone levels and not the patient's symptoms.

C. Imaging

Radiologic imaging is usually not necessary for patients with hypothyroidism. On CT or MRI, a goiter may be noted in the neck or in the mediastinum (retrosternal goiter).

Differential Diagnosis

The differential diagnosis for subclinical hypothyroidism (low serum T_4 or high serum TSH in the absence of hypothyroidism) includes antibody interference with the serum TSH assay, macro-TSH, sleep deprivation, exercise, recovery from nonthyroidal illness, acute psychiatric emergencies, and other conditions and medications (Table 29–3).

Euthyroid sick syndrome should be considered in patients without known thyroid disease who are found to have a low serum FT_4 with a serum TSH that is not elevated. This syndrome can be seen in patients with severe illness, caloric deprivation, or major surgery. Treatment with levothyroxine is not indicated for patients with euthyroid sick syndrome.

Serum TSH tends to be suppressed in severe nonthyroidal illness, making the diagnosis of concurrent primary hypothyroidism difficult, although the presence of a goiter suggests the diagnosis. The clinician must decide whether such severely ill patients (with a low serum T_4 and low TSH) might have hypothyroidism due to hypopituitarism. Patients without symptoms of prior brain lesion or

Table 29–2. Appropriate use of thyroid tests.

	Test	Comment
For screening	Serum TSH Free thyroxine (FT_4)	Most sensitive test for primary hypo- and hyperthyroidism Excellent test
For hypothyroidism	Serum TSH Thyroid peroxidase and thyroglobulin antibodies	High in primary and low in secondary hypothyroidism Elevated in autoimmune (Hashimoto) thyroiditis
For hyperthyroidism	Serum TSH Triiodothyronine (T_3) or free triiodothyronine (FT_3) ^{123}I uptake and scan Thyroid peroxidase and thyroglobulin antibodies Thyroid-stimulating immunoglobulin (TSI)	Suppressed except in TSH-secreting pituitary tumor or pituitary hyperplasia (rare) Elevated Increased uptake; diffuse versus "hot" foci on scan Elevated in Graves disease Usually (65%) positive in Graves disease
For thyroid nodules	Fine-needle aspiration (FNA) biopsy ^{123}I uptake and scan ^{99m}Tc scan Ultrasonography	Best diagnostic method for thyroid cancer Cancer is usually "cold"; less reliable than FNA biopsy Vascular versus less vascular Useful to assist FNA biopsy. Useful in assessing the risk of malignancy (multinodular goiter or pure cysts are less likely to be malignant). Useful to monitor nodules and patients after thyroid surgery for carcinoma.

Table 29–3. Factors that may cause aberrations in laboratory tests that may be mistaken for primary hypothyroidism.[1]

Low Serum T_4 or T_3	High Serum TSH
Acute psychiatric illness	Acute psychiatric illness (transient) (14%)
Cirrhosis	Amiodarone
Familial thyroid-binding globulin deficiency	Anti-mouse antibodies
Laboratory error	Antithyrotropin antibodies
Nephrotic syndrome	Anti-TSH receptor antibodies
Severe illness	Autoimmune disease (assay interference)
Drugs	Drugs
Androgens	Allopurinol
Antiseizure drugs	Amphetamines
Carbamazepine	Atypical antipsychotics
Phenobarbital	Dopamine agonists
Phenytoin	Heroin
Asparaginase	Phenothiazines
Carbamazepine (T_4)	Exercise before testing
Chloral hydrate	Following prolonged primary hypothyroidism
Corticosteroids	Heterophile antibodies
Diclofenac (T_3), naproxen (T_3)	Laboratory error
Didanosine	Macro-thyrotropin
Fenclofenac	Nonadherence to thyroid replacement therapy
5-Fluorouracil	Older adults (especially women)
Halofenate	Pituitary TSH hypersecretion
Imatinib	Recovery from acute nonthyroidal illness (transient)
Mitotane	Strenuous exercise (acute)
Nicotinic acid	Sleep deprivation (acute)
Oxcarbazepine	TSH resistance
Phenobarbital	
Phenytoin	
Salicylates in large doses (T_3 and T_4)	
Sertraline	
Stavudine	
T_3 therapy (T_4)	

[1]True primary hypothyroidism may coexist.
T_4, levothyroxine; T_3, triiodothyronine.

hypopituitarism are very unlikely to suddenly develop hypopituitarism during an unrelated illness. Patients with diabetes insipidus, hypopituitarism, or other signs of a CNS lesion may be given T_4 empirically.

Complications

Severe or long-standing hypothyroidism may increase susceptibility to bacterial pneumonia or rarely cause megacolon or infertility. Organic psychoses with paranoid delusions may occur ("myxedema madness"). Rhabdomyolysis may occur and cause kidney dysfunction. Untreated hypothyroidism during pregnancy often results in miscarriage. Thyroid therapy may exacerbate preexistent CAD or HF and rarely may precipitate adrenal crisis.

Myxedema crisis refers to severe symptoms of hypothyroidism that become a threat to life. Of patients with myxedema crisis, 94% have primary hypothyroidism, 50% have previously undiagnosed hypothyroidism, and 80% are women. Myxedema crisis can also result from failure to take prescription levothyroxine. It can occur spontaneously in severely hypothyroid patients with prolonged exposure to the cold, with resultant hypothermia. It also can also be induced by a stroke, HF, infection (particularly pneumonia), or trauma. Myxedema crisis is often precipitated by the administration of sedatives, antidepressants, hypnotics, anesthetics, or opioids, the metabolism of which is slowed in hypothyroidism. These drugs further impair cognition and respiratory drive and can precipitate respiratory arrest. All patients with myxedema crisis have some degree of obtundation, ranging from somnolence to coma. The term "myxedema coma" is a misnomer, since the alertness of affected patients varies from simple lethargy to coma. Convulsions and abnormal CNS signs may occur. Patients may also present with hyponatremia (65%), hypothermia (50%), hypotension (40%), bradycardia (20%), hypoglycemia (15%), rhabdomyolysis, and AKI. The mortality rate is high.

Treatment

Before beginning therapy with thyroid hormone, the hypothyroid patient requires a clinical assessment for adrenal insufficiency and angina. The presence of either condition requires further evaluation and management.

For patients with subclinical hypothyroidism, levothyroxine therapy is sometimes given to women attempting pregnancy, young adult patients aged 30 years or younger, patients with serum TSH levels 20 mIU/L or higher, and those with significant symptoms attributable to hypothyroidism. Other patients with subclinical hypothyroidism do not require levothyroxine therapy but must be monitored regularly for the emergence of symptoms.

A. Treatment of Hypothyroidism

Synthetic levothyroxine is the preferred preparation for treating most patients with hypothyroidism. Generic levothyroxine preparations have met FDA criteria for bioequivalence. Patients who have difficulty swallowing tablets may prefer Tirosint (capsules or liquid). Lyophilized preparations of levothyroxine are available for reconstitution and intravenous administration, when indicated.

Desiccated natural porcine thyroid preparations containing both T_4 and T_3 (eg, Armour Thyroid, NP Thyroid) are prescribed by some clinicians. Several professional societies discourage the use of desiccated thyroid preparations but many patients prefer them.

Otherwise healthy young and middle-aged adults with hypothyroidism may be treated initially with levothyroxine in average doses of about 1.6 mcg/kg/day. Lower doses can be used for very mild hypothyroidism. The initial hormonal goal of levothyroxine replacement therapy should be to normalize serum TSH levels. Bedtime levothyroxine administration results in somewhat higher serum T_4 and lower TSH levels than morning administration, therefore, administration timing should be kept constant. Significant increases in serum T_4 levels are seen within 1–2 weeks of drug initiation and near-peak levels within 3–4 weeks.

Pregnant women with overt hypothyroidism or myxedema should be treated immediately with levothyroxine at full replacement doses.

Patients with stable CAD or those who are over age 60 years are treated with smaller initial doses of levothyroxine,

25–50 mcg orally daily; higher initial doses may be used if such patients are severely hypothyroid. Likewise, lower initial doses are used for following total thyroidectomy for patients with coronary insufficiency or cardiac dysrhythmias. The dose can be increased by 25 mcg every 1–3 weeks until the patient is euthyroid. Ideally, patients with hypothyroidism and unstable CAD or uncontrolled atrial fibrillation should begin levothyroxine replacement following medical or interventional therapy.

Myxedema crisis can be treated with full replacement doses of oral levothyroxine. Intravenous levothyroxine may be required in some situations, including for obtunded patients with hypercapnia requiring mechanical ventilation. Levothyroxine sodium 500 mcg is given intravenously as a loading dose, followed by 50–100 mcg intravenously daily; the lower dose is given to patients with suspected CAD. In patients with severe myxedema crisis, liothyronine (T_3, Triostat) can be given intravenously with a loading bolus of 10–20 mcg, followed by 10 mcg intravenous boluses every 8–12 hours for the first 48 hours. Patients with hypothermia are warmed only with blankets, since faster warming can precipitate cardiovascular collapse. Patients with hypoglycemia are given 5% dextrose intravenously.

Hyponatremia in any hypothyroid patient requires evaluation for adrenal insufficiency. Medications and hypotonic intravenous solutions that can cause or aggravate hyponatremia are discontinued. Patients who are mildly symptomatic with a serum sodium 120–129 mEq/mL are treated with fluid restriction, unless they are dehydrated. Symptomatic patients with a serum sodium 120–129 mEq/mL must be managed as an inpatient (see Chapter 24, Hyponatremia).

When giving intravenous saline to myxedematous patients, care must be taken to avoid fluid overload.

Patients with hypercapnia require mechanical assistance with ventilation. Opioid medications must be stopped or used in very low doses. Infections must be treated aggressively. Patients in whom concomitant adrenal insufficiency is suspected are treated with hydrocortisone at initial doses of 100 mg intravenously, followed by 25–50 mg every 6–8 hours.

B. Monitoring and Optimizing Treatment of Hypothyroidism

Regular clinical and laboratory monitoring is critical to determine the optimal levothyroxine dose. After initiating levothyroxine replacement, serum TSH levels are monitored monthly and the dose adjusted with an aim to normalize the serum TSH levels (0.4–2.0 mIU/L). The patient should be prescribed sufficient levothyroxine to restore a clinically euthyroid state; this can usually be attained by maintaining the serum TSH levels in the lower half of the reference range (0.4–2.0 mIU/L). Serum levels of both FT_4 and FT_3 are also measured.

Pregnancy usually increases the levothyroxine dosage requirement. Postpartum, levothyroxine replacement requirements ordinarily return to prepregnancy level.

1. Elevated serum TSH level—For most patients, a high serum TSH indicates under-replacement with levothyroxine. However, patient nonadherence to prescribed levothyroxine is surprisingly common; before increasing the levothyroxine dosage, it is important to confirm patient compliance. For patients with CAD or recurrent atrial fibrillation, it may be prudent to administer lower doses of levothyroxine to keep serum TSH in the high-normal or even slightly elevated range.

Increased levothyroxine dosage requirements (low serum T_4 levels) can occur with drugs that increase the hepatic metabolism of levothyroxine and with oral estrogen (Table 29–3). Amiodarone can increase or decrease levothyroxine dose requirements. Malabsorption of levothyroxine can be caused by GI disorders (malabsorption, atrophic gastritis); by coadministration of binding substances, such as iron, fiber; raloxifene; sucralfate; aluminum hydroxide antacids; sevelamer; orlistat; bile acid–binding resins (cholestyramine and colesevelam); PPIs, calcium, magnesium, milk, coffee, and soy milk.

Serum TSH may be elevated transiently in acute psychiatric illness, with antipsychotics and phenothiazines, and during recovery from nonthyroidal illness.

2. Normal serum TSH level—For most patients, the goal of levothyroxine replacement is to maintain the serum TSH in the low normal range (0.4–2.0 mIU/L). Patients taking levothyroxine replacement with normalized serum TSH levels frequently have serum FT_4 levels above the reference range (28%) or serum FT_3 levels below the reference range (7%), which may explain why some patients taking levothyroxine continue to have subjective symptoms of mild hypothyroidism and higher serum LDL cholesterol compared with matched euthyroid controls. Such patients must be assessed for concurrent conditions, such as an adverse drug reaction, Addison disease, depression, hypogonadism, anemia, celiac disease, or gluten sensitivity. If such conditions are not present or are treated and hypothyroid-type symptoms persist, a serum T_3 or free T_3 level may be helpful. Low serum T_3 levels may reflect inadequate peripheral deiodinase activity to convert inactive T_4 to active T_3. Unless contraindicated by unstable angina, such patients with continued hypothyroid-type symptoms may be carefully administered a slightly higher dose of levothyroxine to suppress the serum TSH slightly while achieving clinical euthyroidism and a serum FT_3 in the lower half of the reference range. For most patients with hypothyroidism, an ideal stable maintenance dose of levothyroxine can usually be found.

3. Low or suppressed serum TSH level—A serum TSH level below the reference range (adults 0.4–4.0 mIU/L) is either "low" (0.1–0.39 mIU/L) or "suppressed" (< 0.1 mIU/L). Clinically euthyroid patients receiving levothyroxine who have "low" TSH levels do not have increased morbidity. However, a "suppressed" serum TSH often indicates over-replacement with levothyroxine; such patients may have symptoms of hyperthyroidism with an increased risk for atrial fibrillation, osteoporosis, and clinical hyperthyroidism. The differential diagnosis for a suppressed serum TSH includes hypopituitarism, severe nonthyroidal illness, and some medications. Aside from the latter circumstances, when the serum TSH is suppressed, the dosage of levothyroxine is reduced. However, some patients feel unmistakably hypothyroid while taking the reduced dose of levothyroxine and have low serum T_3 or free T_3 levels. For such patients, a higher levothyroxine dose may be resumed or substituted with desiccated thyroid, with close surveillance for atrial fibrillation, osteoporosis, and subtle manifestations of hyperthyroidism.

Prognosis

Patients with mild hypothyroidism caused by autoimmune thyroiditis have a remission rate of 11%. With levothyroxine treatment of hypothyroidism, return to a normal state is usually the rule, but relapses will occur if treatment is interrupted. Patients with myxedema crisis have a mortality rate of 30–100%, with higher rates in patients with severe symptoms.

When to Refer

- Difficulty titrating levothyroxine replacement to normal TSH or clinically euthyroid state.
- Any patient with significant CAD needing levothyroxine therapy.

When to Admit

- Suspected myxedema crisis.
- Hypercapnia.

Biondi B et al. Critical approach to hypothyroid patients with persistent symptoms. J Clin Endocrinol Metab. 2023;108:2708. [PMID: 37071856]

Chaker L et al. Hypothyroidism. A review. JAMA. 2025;334:1750. [PMID: 40900603]

El Hage L et al. How can I select the right thyroid hormone formulation for my patient with hypothyroidism? Cleve Clin J Med. 2025;92:745. [PMID: 41326191]

Kruitoff ML et al. Thyroid emergencies: a narrative review. Endocr Pract. 2025;31:1310. [PMID: 40553957]

Sankoda A et al. Effects of levothyroxine treatment on fertility and pregnancy outcomes in subclinical hypothyroidism: a systematic review and meta-analysis of randomized controlled trials. Thyroid. 2024;34:519. [PMID: 38368537]

Zhang Y et al. Myxedema coma: challenges and future directions, a systemic survey and review. Thyroid Res. 2025;18:48. [PMID: 41053871]

HYPERTHYROIDISM (Thyrotoxicosis)

ESSENTIALS OF DIAGNOSIS

- Sweating, weight loss or gain, anxiety, palpitations, loose stools, heat intolerance, menstrual irregularity.
- Tachycardia; warm, moist skin; stare; tremor.
- Graves disease: most common cause of hyperthyroidism; palpable goiter in most; ophthalmopathy common.
- Amiodarone: most common cause of thyrotoxic crisis ("thyroid storm").
- Suppressed TSH in primary hyperthyroidism; usually increased T_4, FT_4, T_3, FT_3.

General Considerations

The term "thyrotoxicosis" refers to the clinical manifestations associated with elevated serum levels of T_4 or T_3 that are excessive for the individual (hyperthyroidism).

A. Graves Disease

Graves disease is the most common cause of thyrotoxicosis. It is an autoimmune disorder, characterized by an increase in synthesis and release of thyroid hormones. Autoantibodies, known as thyroid-stimulating immunoglobulins (TSI) or thyrotropin receptor antibodies (TRAb), bind to the TSH receptors in the thyroid cell membranes and stimulate the gland to overproduce thyroid hormones. The presence of these antibodies distinguishes Graves disease from autoimmune chronic lymphocytic (Hashimoto) thyroiditis. Both conditions usually have present serum antithyroid antibodies (TPO Ab or Tg Ab or both).

Graves disease is more common in women than in men (8:1). Its usual onset is between the ages of 20 and 40 years. It may be accompanied by infiltrative ophthalmopathy (Graves exophthalmos) and, less commonly, by infiltrative dermopathy (pretibial myxedema). The thymus gland is typically enlarged and serum ANA levels are usually elevated. Many patients with Graves disease have a family history of either Graves disease or Hashimoto autoimmune thyroiditis.

Viral infections, including infections with SARS-CoV-2, have been reported to precipitate Graves disease. Vaccinations against SARS-CoV-2 also have triggered de novo Graves disease as well as relapses 4–30 days after infection or vaccination.

Patients with Graves disease have an increased risk of other systemic autoimmune disorders, including Sjögren syndrome, celiac disease, pernicious anemia, Addison disease, alopecia areata, vitiligo, type 1 diabetes mellitus, hypoparathyroidism, myasthenia gravis, and cardiomyopathy.

B. Toxic Multinodular Goiter and Thyroid Nodules

Autonomous hyperfunctioning thyroid nodules that produce hyperthyroidism are known as toxic multinodular goiter (Plummer disease). They are more prevalent among older adults and in iodine-deficient regions. A single hyperfunctioning nodule can also produce hyperthyroidism. Thyroid cancer is found in 5% of patients with toxic multinodular goiter (see Thyroid Nodules and Multinodular Goiter, below).

C. Autoimmune (Postpartum or Silent) Thyroiditis and Subacute Thyroiditis

These conditions cause thyroid inflammation with release of stored hormone. They all produce a variable triphasic course: variable hyperthyroidism is followed by transient euthyroidism and progression to hypothyroidism (see Thyroiditis, above).

D. Medication-Induced Hyperthyroidism

1. Amiodarone-induced thyrotoxicosis (AIT)—Amiodarone causes thyrotoxicosis in about 5% of patients in the United States, with a higher incidence in iodine-deficient geographic areas. Amiodarone is 37% iodine by weight and its metabolites have a half-life of about 100 days. In the short term, amiodarone normally increases serum TSH though usually not over 20 mIU/L. Serum T_4 and FT_4 rise about 40% and may become elevated in clinically euthyroid patients, while serum T_3 levels typically decline. After 3 months, the serum TSH usually normalizes. Thyroid function tests (TSH, FT_4, T_3) should be checked before starting amiodarone, after 3–6 months of therapy, and thereafter at least every 6 months (sooner if clinically warranted). Due to early short-term changes, it is best to not check thyroid function tests during the first 3 months of therapy.

Amiodarone-induced thyrotoxicosis (AIT) can occur at any time during treatment and may develop several months after treatment discontinuation. It is diagnosed when serum TSH levels are suppressed and serum T_3 or FT_3 levels are high or high-normal. Amiodarone is the leading cause for thyrotoxic crisis ("thyroid storm"); however, the manifestations can be missed since amiodarone tends to cause bradycardia. Type 1 AIT is caused by the *active* production of excessive thyroid hormone and typically occurs within 2–6 months after starting amiodarone. Type 2 AIT is caused by the *passive* release of stored thyroid hormone and occurs an average of 30 months after starting amiodarone.

2. Iodine-induced hyperthyroidism (Basedow disease)— The recommended iodine intake for nonpregnant adults is 150 mcg/day. Higher iodine intake can precipitate hyperthyroidism in patients with nodular goiters, autonomous thyroid nodules, or asymptomatic Graves disease, and less commonly in patients with no detectable underlying thyroid disorder. Common sources of excess iodine include intravenous oral potassium iodine supplements, certain foods (eg, kelp, nori), topical iodinated antiseptics (eg, povidone iodine), and medications (eg, amiodarone or potassium iodide).

3. Tyrosine kinase inhibitors—Silent autoimmune thyroiditis that releases stored thyroid hormone, resulting in hyperthyroidism, develops in about 3% of patients receiving chemotherapy with tyrosine kinase inhibitors (eg, axitinib, sorafenib, sunitinib). Hypothyroidism usually follows hyperthyroidism and occurs in 19% of patients taking these drugs.

4. Immune checkpoint inhibitor cancer therapy— Immune checkpoint inhibitor therapy directed against either PD-1/PD-L1 or CTLA-4/B7-1/B7-2 frequently precipitates autoimmune adverse reactions. Thyroid autoimmunity commonly causes thyroiditis, hypothyroidism (primary or secondary), or hyperthyroidism from either passive release of thyroid hormone or active production of thyroid hormone (Graves disease).

E. Pregnancy, hCG-Secreting Trophoblastic Tumors, and Testicular Choriocarcinoma

Human chorionic gonadotropin (hCG) can bind to the thyroid's TSH receptors. Very high levels of serum hCG, particularly during the first 4 months of pregnancy may cause sufficient receptor activation to cause gestational thyrotoxicosis. About 20% of pregnant women have a low serum TSH during pregnancy, but only 1% of such women have clinical hyperthyroidism that requires treatment. This condition must be distinguished from true Graves disease in pregnancy, which usually predates conception and may be associated with high serum levels of TSI and antithyroid antibodies or with exophthalmos.

F. Rare Causes of Hyperthyroidism

Thyrotoxicosis factitia is due to intentional or accidental ingestion of excessive amounts of exogenous thyroid hormone. Struma ovarii is thyroid tissue contained in about 3% of ovarian dermoid tumors and teratomas. Pituitary TSH hypersecretion by a pituitary thyrotroph tumor or hyperplasia can rarely cause hyperthyroidism; serum TSH is elevated or inappropriately normal in the presence of true thyrotoxicosis. Metastatic functioning thyroid carcinoma can cause hyperthyroidism in patients with a heavy tumor burden.

High levels of hCG can also cause thyrotoxicosis in some cases of pregnancies with gestational trophoblastic disease (molar pregnancy, choriocarcinoma). Some such pregnancies have produced thyrotoxic crisis. Men have developed hyperthyroidism from high levels of serum hCG secreted by a testicular choriocarcinoma.

Clinical Findings

A. Symptoms and Signs

Thyrotoxicosis can produce nervousness, restlessness, heat intolerance, increased sweating, palpitations, pruritus, fatigue, muscle weakness, muscle cramps, tetany (rarely), frequent bowel movements, weight change (usually loss), or menstrual irregularities (usually lighter flow). There may be fine resting finger tremors, moist warm skin, fever, hyperreflexia, fine hair, hair loss (scalp and lateral eyebrows), and onycholysis. Angina or atrial fibrillation may also be present, sometimes in the absence of other thyrotoxic symptoms (apathetic hyperthyroidism). Chronic thyrotoxicosis may cause osteoporosis.

Patients with Graves disease usually have a diffusely enlarged thyroid that is frequently asymmetric and often accompanied by a bruit. However, there may be no palpable thyroid enlargement. The thyroid gland in painful subacute thyroiditis is usually moderately enlarged and tender. There is often dysphagia and pain that can radiate to the jaw or ear. With toxic multinodular goiter, there are usually palpable nodules. Patients with silent thyroiditis or postpartum thyroiditis have either no palpable goiter or a small, nontender goiter.

Cardiopulmonary manifestations of thyrotoxicosis commonly include a forceful heartbeat, premature atrial contractions, and sinus tachycardia. Patients often have exertional dyspnea. Atrial fibrillation or atrial tachycardia occurs in about 8% of patients with thyrotoxicosis. The ventricular response from the atrial fibrillation may be difficult to control. Thyrotoxicosis can cause a thyrotoxic cardiomyopathy, and the onset of atrial fibrillation can precipitate HF. Echocardiogram reveals pulmonary artery hypertension in about 40% of patients. Even "subclinical hyperthyroidism" increases the risk for atrial fibrillation and overall mortality. Hemodynamic abnormalities and pulmonary hypertension are reversible with restoration of euthyroidism.

Thyrotoxic crisis or "thyroid storm" is an extreme form of severe thyrotoxicosis and an immediate threat to life. The most common manifestations are cardiac (HF, severe sinus tachycardia [60%], ventricular fibrillation [13%], MI, and cardiogenic shock), agitation or delirium (63%), high fever, vomiting, diarrhea, dehydration, and hepatic impairment (52%).

Eye manifestations that occur with hyperthyroidism are discussed in Thyroid Eye Disease, below.

Graves dermopathy (pretibial myxedema) occurs in about 3% of patients with Graves disease. It usually affects the pretibial region but can also affect the dorsal forearms and wrists and dorsum of the feet. It is more common in patients with high levels of serum TSI and severe Graves ophthalmopathy.

Thyroid acropachy is a rare skeletal manifestation of Graves disease. It presents with digital clubbing, swelling of fingers and toes, and radiographic findings of periostitis involving phalangeal and metacarpal bones.

Clinical hyperthyroidism during pregnancy has a prevalence of about 0.2%. It may commence before conception or emerge during pregnancy, particularly the first trimester. Pregnancy can have a beneficial effect on the thyrotoxicosis of Graves disease, with decreasing antibody titers and decreasing serum T_4 levels as the pregnancy advances; about 30% of affected women experience a remission by late in the second trimester. Undiagnosed or undertreated hyperthyroidism carries an increased risk of miscarriage, preeclampsia-eclampsia, preterm delivery, abruptio placenta, maternal HF, and thyrotoxic crisis (thyroid storm). Such thyrotoxic crisis can be precipitated by trauma, infection, surgery, or delivery and confers a fetal/maternal mortality rate of about 25%.

Hypokalemic periodic paralysis occurs in about 15% of Asian or American Indian men with thyrotoxicosis and is 30 times more common in men than women. It is marked by sudden symmetric flaccid paralysis, along with hypokalemia and hypophosphatemia, that occurs during hyperthyroidism (often after intravenous dextrose, oral carbohydrates, or vigorous exercise) despite few, if any, of the classic signs of thyrotoxicosis. Attacks last 7–72 hours.

B. Laboratory Findings

Serum FT_4, T_3, FT_3, and T_4, thyroid resin uptake, and FT_4 index are all usually increased. Sometimes the FT_4 level may be normal but with an elevated serum T_3 (T_3 toxicosis). The severity of the elevation of serum FT_4 and FT_3 levels does not always correlate with the severity of thyrotoxic manifestations; patients with thyrotoxic crisis tend to have serum thyroid levels that are not significantly higher than those with less pronounced symptoms. Serum T_4 or T_3 can be elevated in other nonthyroidal conditions (Table 29–4).

Serum TSH is suppressed in hyperthyroidism. Serum TSH may be misleadingly low in other nonthyroidal conditions (Table 29–4). The term **"subclinical hyperthyroidism"** is used to describe individuals with a low serum TSH but normal serum levels of FT_4 and T_3; in such patients, the overall prevalence of symptomatic hyperthyroidism is 0.7–1.8% in iodine-sufficient patients and 2–15% in patients with iodine deficiency. About two-thirds of patients with subclinical hyperthyroidism have serum TSH levels of 0.1–0.4 mIU/L (mild subclinical hyperthyroidism), while the remainder have serum TSH levels below 0.1 mIU/L (severe subclinical hyperthyroidism).

Hyperthyroidism can cause anemia (usually normochromic normocytic), neutropenia, hypercalcemia, and increased hepatic aminotransferases and alkaline phosphatase. Hyperthyroidism also increases urinary magnesium excretion, which can lead to hypomagnesemia and functional hypoparathyroidism with hypocalcemia. Hypokalemia and hypophosphatemia occur in thyrotoxic periodic paralysis.

About 30% of patients with acute psychiatric disorders have elevated serum T_4 levels without clinical thyrotoxicosis. The TSH is not usually suppressed, distinguishing psychiatric disorder from true hyperthyroidism. T_4 levels return to normal gradually.

In **Graves disease**, serum TSI and serum TRAb levels are usually detectable (90%). Very high serum TSI levels predispose to Graves ophthalmopathy. TPO Ab or Tg Ab are usually elevated, reflecting concurrent autoimmune

Table 29–4. Factors that can cause misleading laboratory tests for hyperthyroidism.

High Serum T_4 or T_3	Low Serum TSH
Laboratory error	Laboratory error
Collection vial contains gel barrier for T_3	African descent (3–4%)
Acute psychiatric problems (30%)	Autonomous thyroid or thyroid nodule
Acute or chronic active hepatitis, primary biliary cirrhosis	Corticosteroids (short-term use)
AIDS (increased TBG)	Drugs
Autoimmunity	Amphetamines
Euthyroid sick	Biotin supplements (certain assays)
Familial thyroid-binding abnormalities	Calcium channel blockers (nifedipine, verapamil)
Familial resistance to thyroid (Refetoff syndrome)	Dobutamine
Pregnancy: morning sickness, hyperemesis gravidarum	Dopamine
Drugs	Dopamine agonists
Amiodarone	Glucocorticoids
Amphetamines	Metformin
Biotin supplements (certain assays)	Somatostatin analogs
Capecitabine	Thyroid hormone
Clofibrate	Elderly euthyroid
Estrogens (oral)	hCG-secreting trophoblastic tumors
Heparin	Hypopituitarism
Heroin, methadone	Nonthyroidal illness (severe)
Perphenazine	Pregnancy (especially with morning sickness)
Tamoxifen	Suppression after recent therapy for hyperthyroidism
Thyroid hormone therapy (excessive or factitious)	TSH variants not detected by commercial assays

hCG, human chorionic gonadotropin; T_4, levothyroxine; T_3, triiodothyronine; TBG, thyroid-binding globulin.

thyroiditis. Serum ANA levels are also usually elevated without evidence of rheumatologic disease.

With painful **subacute thyroiditis**, patients often have an increased WBC, ESR, and CRP. About 25% have antithyroid antibodies (usually in low titer); serum TSI and TRAb levels are normal. Patients with iodine-induced hyperthyroidism have undetectable serum TSI, TRAb, and serum TPO Ab, and an elevated urinary iodine concentration.

With **hyperthyroidism during pregnancy**, women have an elevated serum total T_4 and FT_4 while the TSH is suppressed. The serum T_4 is elevated in most pregnant women; however, values > 20 mcg/dL (257 nmol/L) are encountered only in hyperthyroidism. The T_3 resin uptake is low in normal pregnancy because of high thyroxine-binding globulin (TBG) concentration but is normal or high in thyrotoxic persons.

Since high levels of T_4 and FT_4 are normally seen in patients taking **amiodarone**, a suppressed TSH must be present along with a greatly elevated T_4 (> 20 mcg/dL [257 nmol/L]) or T_3 (> 200 ng/dL [3.1 nmol/L]) in order to diagnose hyperthyroidism. In type 1 amiodarone-induced thyrotoxicosis, the presence of proptosis and serum TSI (TSHrAb) is diagnostic. In type 2 amiodarone-induced thyrotoxicosis, serum levels of interleukin-6 (IL-6) are usually quite elevated.

C. Radioisotope Uptake and Imaging

Note: *All radioisotope testing is contraindicated during pregnancy or breastfeeding.*

Radioiodine (^{123}I) scanning can be helpful in some situations to determine the cause of hyperthyroidism but is unnecessary for diagnosis in patients with obvious Graves disease who have elevated serum TSI or associated Graves ophthalmopathy. A high thyroid RAI uptake is seen in Graves disease and toxic nodular goiter. A low ^{123}I RAI uptake is characteristic of iodine-induced hyperthyroidism and thyroiditis (subacute, silent, or postpartum), distinguishing them from Graves disease.

Technetium (Tc-99m) pertechnetate thyroid uptake is increased or normal with Graves disease, whereas those with thyrotoxicosis from thyroiditis (silent, subacute, postpartum) have reduced uptake.

99mTc-sestamibi (MIBI) scanning usually shows increased uptake with type 1 amiodarone-induced thyrotoxicosis (AIT), decreased uptake in type 2 AIT, and intermediate uptake in mixed AIT.

D. Other Imaging

Thyroid ultrasound can be helpful in hyperthyroid patients with palpable thyroid nodules. Thyroid ultrasound shows a variably heterogeneous, hypoechoic gland in thyroiditis. Color flow Doppler sonography is helpful to distinguish type 1 amiodarone-induced thyrotoxicosis (enlarged gland with normal to increased blood flow velocity and vascularity) from type 2 amiodarone-induced thyrotoxicosis (distorted gland without increased vascularity).

Differential Diagnosis

True thyrotoxicosis must be distinguished from those conditions that elevate serum T_4 and T_3 or suppress serum TSH without affecting clinical status (see Table 29–4). Serum TSH is commonly suppressed in early pregnancy and only about 10% of pregnant women with a low TSH have clinical hyperthyroidism.

States of hypermetabolism without thyrotoxicosis—notably severe anemia, leukemia, polycythemia, cancer, and pheochromocytoma—rarely cause confusion. Acromegaly may also produce tachycardia, sweating, and thyroid enlargement.

The differential diagnosis for thyroid-associated ophthalmopathy includes an orbital tumor (eg, lymphoma) or pseudotumor. Ocular myasthenia gravis is another autoimmune condition that occurs more commonly in Graves disease.

Diabetes mellitus and Addison disease may coexist with thyrotoxicosis and can aggravate the weight loss, fatigue, and muscle weakness seen with hyperthyroidism.

Complications

Hypercalcemia, osteoporosis, and nephrocalcinosis may occur in hyperthyroidism. Decreased libido, erectile dysfunction, diminished sperm motility, and gynecomastia may be noted in men. Other complications include cardiac arrhythmias and HF, thyroid crisis, ophthalmopathy, dermopathy, and thyrotoxic hypokalemic periodic paralysis.

Treatment

A. Treatment of Graves Disease

Table 29–5 outlines the treatment options for hyperthyroidism.

1. Propranolol—Propranolol is used for symptomatic relief of tachycardia, tremor, diaphoresis, and anxiety until the hyperthyroidism is resolved. It is the initial treatment of choice for thyrotoxic crisis and effectively treats thyrotoxic hypokalemic periodic paralysis. Treatment usually starts with propranolol ER, which is given every 12 hours for severe hyperthyroidism due to accelerated metabolism of the propranolol; it may be given once daily as hyperthyroidism improves (Table 29–5).

2. Thiourea drugs—Methimazole or PTU is used for most patients with Graves disease or toxic nodular goiter. Methimazole is preferred, but PTU is used for women planning pregnancy or during pregnancy. See Treatment of Hyperthyroidism During Pregnancy-Planning, Pregnancy, and Lactation, below. There is a 50% chance of remission of hyperthyroidism with long-term thiourea therapy. A better likelihood of long-term remission occurs in patients with small goiters, mild hyperthyroidism, those requiring small doses of thiourea, and those with serum TSI (TSHrAb) < 2 mU/L. Remission is marked by decreasing thiourea dosage requirement, until none is required. Patients whose TPO Ab and Tg Ab remain low after 2 years of therapy have only a 10% rate of relapse. There should be no rush to discontinue thiourea therapy in favor of RAI or surgery, even after years of treatment. Thioureas may be continued long term for patients who are tolerating them well. The exception is women with thyrotoxic Graves disease who are planning pregnancy in the near future; thyroid surgery or RAI

Table 29–5. Medications for the treatment of hyperthyroidism.[1]

Medication	Dose and Frequency	Indications
Propranolol ER	Dose: 60–80 mg orally once daily, increasing every 3 days until heart rate < 90 beats per minute. Maximum dose: 320 mg daily	Symptomatic relief of tachycardia, tremor, diaphoresis, anxiety Thyrotoxic crisis Hypokalemic periodic paralysis
Thiourea: Methimazole	Initial dose: usually 30–60 mg orally once daily Dose may be divided and given twice daily to avoid GI upset Lower dose of 10–20 mg for very mild symptoms During pregnancy or breastfeeding, dose should not exceed 20 mg daily	Young adults Older adult patients Mild thyrotoxicosis Small goiter Fear of isotopes Precautions during pregnancy[2]
Propylthiouracil (PTU)	Dose: 300–600 mg orally daily in four divided doses During pregnancy or breastfeeding, dose should not exceed 200 mg daily	Precautions during pregnancy[2]
Iodinated contrast agents Iopanoic acid or ipodate sodium	Initial dose: 500 mg orally twice daily for 3 days Maintenance dose: 500 mg once daily	Effective temporary treatment of thyrotoxicosis, especially for patients who are very symptomatic Alternative treatment for patients intolerant of thioureas
Radioactive iodine (RAI, ^{131}I)		Destroys overactive thyroid tissue See text for Precautions Avoid with thyroid eye disease (Graves ophthalmopathy)
Prednisone	Initial dose: 0.5–0.7 mg/kg orally daily After 2 weeks: begin to slowly taper and stop after about 3 months	Type 2 amiodarone-induced thyrotoxicosis

[1]See text for expanded discussion of these agents.
[2]See Treatment of Hyperthyroidism During Pregnancy-Planning, Pregnancy, and Lactation in text.

should be considered at least 4 months in advance of conception. Thiourea drugs are also useful for preparing nonpregnant hyperthyroid patients for surgery and older patients for RAI treatment.

Agranulocytosis (absolute neutrophil count < 500/mcL [0.5×10^9/L]) or pancytopenia may occur abruptly in 0.4% of patients taking either methimazole or PTU. All patients receiving thiourea therapy must be informed of the danger of agranulocytosis or pancytopenia and the need to stop the drug and seek medical attention immediately with the onset of any infection or unusual bleeding. Nearly 85% of agranulocytosis cases occur within 90 days of commencing therapy; however, continued long-term blood test monitoring is required. Agranulocytosis generally remits spontaneously with discontinuation of the thiourea.

Other common side effects include pruritus, allergic dermatitis, nausea, and dyspepsia. Since the two thiourea drugs are similar, patients who have a major allergic reaction to one should not be given the other.

The patient's thyroid status is best monitored clinically and with serum FT_4 levels. The patient may become clinically hypothyroid for 2 weeks or more before TSH levels rise.

A. **Methimazole**—Except during the first trimester of pregnancy, methimazole is generally preferred over PTU since it is more convenient to use and is less likely to cause fulminant hepatic necrosis. Methimazole therapy is also less likely to cause ^{131}I treatment failure. Rare complications peculiar to methimazole include serum sickness, cholestatic jaundice, alopecia, nephrotic syndrome, hypoglycemia, and loss of taste.

B. **Propylthiouracil**—Acute liver failure occurs in about 1 in 1000 patients, making PTU a second-line medication for treating patients with Graves hyperthyroidism. The onset of severe liver toxicity varies from 3 days to 12 months after starting PTU. Therefore, PTU is ordinarily reserved for treating women actively seeking fertility and during the first trimester of pregnancy, when it is preferred over methimazole. See Treatment of Hyperthyroidism During Pregnancy-Planning, Pregnancy, and Lactation, below.

3. Iodinated contrast agents—Iopanoic acid (Telepaque) and ipodate sodium (Bilivist, Oragrafin) are iodinated contrast agents that inhibit peripheral 5′-monodeiodination of T_4, thereby blocking its conversion to active T_3. They provide effective temporary treatment for thyrotoxicosis of any cause and are particularly useful for patients who are symptomatically very thyrotoxic. Within 24 hours, serum T_3 levels fall an average of 62%. For patients with **Graves disease**, methimazole is begun first to block iodine organification; the next day, ipodate sodium or iopanoic acid may be added. They offer a therapeutic option for patients with subacute thyroiditis, amiodarone-induced thyrotoxicosis, T_4 overdosage, and for those intolerant to thioureas.

4. Radioactive iodine (RAI, ^{131}I)—^{131}I therapy destroys overactive thyroid tissue (either diffuse or toxic nodular goiter). Patients who have been treated with ^{131}I in adulthood do not have an increased risk of subsequent thyroid cancer, leukemia, or offspring with congenital abnormalities. Conflicting evidence has shown either no increased risk or a slightly increased risk of subsequent solid tumor malignancies following ^{131}I treatment for hyperthyroidism.

Precautions: Because radiation is harmful to the fetus and children, *RAI should not be given to pregnant or lactating women or to mothers who lack childcare. Women are advised to avoid pregnancy for at least 4 months following ^{131}I therapy. A pregnancy test should be obtained within 48 hours before therapy for any woman with childbearing potential. Men have been found to have abnormal spermatozoa for up to 6 months following ^{131}I therapy and are advised to use contraceptive methods during that time.*

Patients may receive ^{131}I while being symptomatically treated with propranolol ER, which is then reduced in dosage as hyperthyroidism resolves. Radioiodine therapy fails to fully correct hyperthyroidism in about 20% of patients, particularly those with larger glands, very high free T_4 levels, and prior thiourea therapy. However, therapy with ^{131}I will usually be effective if methimazole is discontinued at least 3–4 days before RAI therapy.

The presence of Graves ophthalmopathy is a relative contraindication to ^{131}I therapy. Following ^{131}I treatment for hyperthyroidism, Graves ophthalmopathy appears or worsens in 15% of patients. Therefore, patients with Graves ophthalmopathy who are to be treated with ^{131}I should be considered for prophylactic prednisone (20–40 mg orally daily) for 2 months following administration of ^{131}I; among patients receiving prednisone following ^{131}I treatment, preexistent ophthalmopathy improves in 67% and worsens in none.

Cigarette use increases the risk of having a flare in ophthalmopathy following ^{131}I treatment and also reduces the effectiveness of prednisone treatment.

There is a high incidence of hypothyroidism in the months to years after ^{131}I. Patients with Graves disease treated with ^{131}I also have an increased lifetime risk of developing hyperparathyroidism, particularly when ^{131}I therapy was administered in childhood or adolescence. Lifelong clinical follow-up is mandatory, with measurements of serum TSH, FT_4, and calcium when indicated.

5. Thyroid surgery—Surgery may be indicated for patients with Graves disease who are intolerant to thioureas, women planning pregnancy in the near future, patients who choose not to have RAI therapy, and patients with Graves ophthalmopathy. The surgical procedure of choice is a total resection of one lobe and a subtotal resection of the other lobe, leaving about 4 g of thyroid tissue (Hartley–Dunhill operation).

Patients are ordinarily rendered euthyroid preoperatively with a thiourea drug (Table 29–5). Propranolol ER is given until the heart rate is < 90 beats per minute and continued until the serum T_3 (or free T_3) is normal preoperatively. The patient should be euthyroid by the time of surgery.

The risks of subtotal or total thyroidectomy include damage to a recurrent laryngeal nerve, with resultant vocal fold paralysis. Hypoparathyroidism also occurs; serum calcium levels must be checked postoperatively.

B. Treatment of Toxic Solitary Thyroid Nodules

Toxic solitary thyroid nodules are usually benign but may rarely be malignant. If a nonsurgical therapy is elected, the nodule should be evaluated with a fine-needle aspiration (FNA) biopsy. **Medical therapy** for hyperthyroidism caused by a single hyperfunctioning thyroid nodule may be treated symptomatically with propranolol ER and methimazole or PTU, as in Graves disease (Table 29–5). The dose of methimazole should be adjusted to keep the TSH slightly suppressed, so the risk of TSH-stimulated growth of the nodule is reduced. **Surgical treatment** is usually recommended for patients under age 40 years, for healthy older patients with toxic solitary thyroid nodules, and for nodules that are suspicious for malignancy. Postoperative hypothyroidism usually resolves spontaneously, but permanent hypothyroidism occurs in about 14% of patients by 6 years after surgery. **^{131}I therapy** may be offered to patients with a toxic solitary nodule who are over age 40 or in poor health (see **Precautions** for RAI use, above).

Permanent hypothyroidism occurs in about one-third of patients by 8 years after ^{131}I therapy. The nodule remains palpable in 50% and may grow in 10% of patients after ^{131}I.

C. Treatment of Toxic Nodular Goiter

Medical therapy for patients with toxic nodular goiter consists of propranolol ER (while hyperthyroid) and a thiourea, as in Graves disease (Table 29–5). Thioureas (methimazole or PTU) reverse hyperthyroidism but do not shrink the goiter. There is a 95% recurrence rate if the drug is stopped.

Surgical therapy is the definitive treatment for a large toxic nodular goiter, following therapy with a thiourea to render them euthyroid. Surgery is particularly indicated to relieve pressure symptoms or for cosmetic indications. Patients with toxic nodular goiter are not treated preoperatively with potassium iodide. Total or near-total thyroidectomy is recommended, since surgical pathology reveals unsuspected differentiated thyroid cancer in 18.3% of cases.

^{131}I therapy may be used to treat patients with toxic nodular goiter. See **Precautions** for RAI use, above. Any suspicious nodules should be evaluated beforehand for malignancy with FNA cytology.

The patient follows a low-iodine diet in order to enhance the thyroid gland's uptake of ^{131}I, which may be relatively low in this condition (compared to Graves disease). Relatively high doses of ^{131}I are usually required. Hypothyroidism can occur but less commonly than seen with RAI therapy for Graves disease. Recurrent thyrotoxicosis can occur, so patients must be monitored closely. Peculiarly, in about 1–5% of patients with diffusely nodular toxic goiter, the administration of ^{131}I therapy may induce Graves disease.

D. Treatment of Hyperthyroidism from Thyroiditis

Patients with thyroiditis (subacute, postpartum, or silent) are treated with propranolol during the hyperthyroid phase, which usually subsides spontaneously within weeks to months. For symptomatic relief, begin propranolol ER until the heart rate is < 90 beats per minute (Table 29–5). Ipodate sodium or iopanoic acid, 500 mg orally daily, promptly corrects elevated T_3 levels and is continued for

15–60 days until the serum FT_4 level normalizes. Thioureas are ineffective since thyroid hormone production is actually low in this condition. Patients are monitored carefully for the development of hypothyroidism and treated with levothyroxine as needed. With subacute thyroiditis, pain can usually be managed with NSAIDs and corticosteroids, but opioid analgesics are sometimes required.

E. Treatment of Hyperthyroidism During Pregnancy-Planning, Pregnancy, and Lactation

Due to the increased risk of congenital anomalies with every thiourea, all women who are planning to become pregnant are encouraged to consider definitive therapy with ^{131}I or surgery well before conception. Both men and women who are planning pregnancy should not have ^{131}I treatment within about 4 months of conception. See **Precautions** for RAI use, above. Dietary iodine must not be restricted for such women to protect the fetus from iodine deficiency.

First-trimester fetal exposure to thioureas (methimazole or PTU) increases the risk of birth defects by about 2%. The fetal anomalies associated with PTU are typically less severe than those associated with methimazole; therefore, PTU is the preferred thiourea for women actively seeking fertility and during the first trimester of pregnancy, despite the very low risk for hepatic necrosis. Women should be treated with PTU immediately prepregnancy and through the first trimester; during pregnancy, the dose of PTU is kept < 200 mg daily to avoid goitrous hypothyroidism in the infant. PTU can be switched to methimazole in the second trimester (see Thiourea drugs, above). Thiourea should be given in the smallest dose possible, permitting mild subclinical hyperthyroidism to occur, since it is usually well tolerated. About 30% of women with Graves disease experience a remission by the late second trimester.

Both PTU and methimazole cross the placenta and can induce hypothyroidism, with fetal TSH hypersecretion and goiter. Fetal hypothyroidism is rare if the mother's hyperthyroidism is controlled with small daily doses of PTU (50–150 mg/day orally) or methimazole (5–15 mg/day orally). Serum total T_4 levels during pregnancy should be kept at about 1.5 × the prepregnancy level.

Subtotal thyroidectomy is indicated for pregnant women with Graves disease or for fertile women of reproductive age who are sexually active and decline contraceptives, under the following circumstances: (1) severe adverse reaction to thioureas; (2) high dosage requirement for thioureas (methimazole ≥ 30 mg/day or PTU ≥ 450 mg/day); or (3) uncontrolled hyperthyroidism due to nonadherence to thiourea therapy. Surgery is best performed during the second trimester.

Both methimazole and PTU are secreted in breast milk but not in amounts that affect the infant's thyroid hormone levels. No adverse reactions to these drugs have been reported in breastfed infants. Methimazole is generally preferred, due to a lower general risk of hepatotoxicity. See Table 29–5 for recommended doses. It is recommended that the medication be taken just after breastfeeding.

F. Treatment of Amiodarone-Induced Thyrotoxicosis (AIT)

Patients with either type 1 or type 2 AIT require treatment with propranolol ER for symptomatic relief and methimazole (Table 29–5). After two doses of methimazole, iopanoic acid or sodium ipodate may be added to the regimen to further block conversion of T_4 to T_3 until the thyrotoxicosis is resolved. Amiodarone may be withdrawn but this does not have a significant therapeutic impact for several months because of its long half-life. For patients with type 1 AIT, therapy with ^{131}I may be successful, but only for those with sufficient RAI uptake. Patients with type 2 AIT are usually also treated with prednisone for about 2 weeks, which is slowly tapered and withdrawn after about 3 months. Subtotal thyroidectomy should be considered for patients with AIT that is resistant to treatment.

G. Treatment of Complications

1. Thyroid eye disease—See Thyroid Eye Disease (Graves Ophthalmopathy below).

2. Cardiac complications—

A. SINUS TACHYCARDIA—Treatment consists of treating the thyrotoxicosis. A β-blocker such as propranolol is used in the interim unless there is an associated cardiomyopathy.

B. ATRIAL FIBRILLATION—Hyperthyroidism must be treated immediately. Other drugs, including digoxin, β-blockers, and anticoagulants, may be required. Electrical cardioversion is unlikely to convert atrial fibrillation to normal sinus rhythm while the patient is thyrotoxic. Spontaneous conversion to normal sinus rhythm occurs in 62% of patients with return of euthyroidism, but that likelihood decreases with age. Following conversion to euthyroidism, there is a 60% chance that atrial fibrillation will recur, despite normal thyroid function tests. Those with persistent atrial fibrillation may have elective cardioversion following anticoagulation 4 months after resolution of hyperthyroidism.

(1) β-Blockers—β-Blockers will reduce the ventricular rate, but they must be used with caution in patients with HF with reduced EF. Propranolol is generally preferred over metoprolol and other β-blockers for thyrotoxicosis-induced atrial fibrillation. Sotalol is sometimes preferred in patients with HF and reduced LVEF.

(2) Non-dihydropyridine calcium channel blockers (NDCC)—Diltiazem or verapamil slows the ventricular response during atrial fibrillation. However, these drugs have negative inotropic effects and must be used with caution in patients with HF and reduced EF.

(3) Anticoagulants—Thyrotoxicosis induces a prothrombotic state and increases the risk of embolic stroke in atrial fibrillation. Anticoagulation is usually required. DOACs are preferred over warfarin in thyrotoxicosis-induced atrial fibrillation, since DOACs are associated with a lower all-cause mortality and lower risk for hemorrhagic complications.

(4) Digoxin—Digoxin is now a second-line agent for ventricular rate control in thyrotoxicosis-induced atrial fibrillation; larger than normal doses are usually required in thyrotoxicosis. Digoxin doses are reduced as hyperthyroidism

is corrected. Serum digoxin levels should be kept < 1.2 ng/mL, since higher levels are associated with increased mortality.

C. Heart failure—Thyrotoxicosis can cause high-output HF due to extreme tachycardia, cardiomyopathy, or both. Aggressive treatment of the hyperthyroidism is required in either case.

HF may also occur as a result of low-output dilated cardiomyopathy. It is uncommon and may be caused by an idiosyncratic severe toxic effect of hyperthyroidism upon certain hearts. Cardiomyopathy may occur at any age and without preexisting cardiac disease. See Chapter 11 for treatment of HF and dilated cardiomyopathy. The patient should be rendered euthyroid. However, the HF usually persists despite correction of the hyperthyroidism.

D. Apathetic hyperthyroidism—Apathetic hyperthyroidism may present with angina pectoris. Treatment is directed at reversing the hyperthyroidism as well as providing standard antianginal therapy. PCI or coronary artery bypass grafting can often be avoided by prompt diagnosis and treatment.

3. Thyrotoxic crisis or "thyroid storm"—ICU admission is required. A thiourea drug is given (eg, methimazole, 15–25 mg orally every 6 hours, or PTU, 150–250 mg orally every 6 hours). Ipodate sodium (500 mg/day orally) can be helpful if begun 1 hour *after* the first dose of thiourea. Iodide is given 1 hour later as potassium iodide (10 drops three times daily orally). Propranolol is given in a dosage of 0.5–2 mg intravenously every 4 hours or 20–120 mg orally every 6 hours. Hydrocortisone is usually given in doses of 50 mg orally every 6 hours, with rapid dosage reduction as the clinical situation improves. Plasmapheresis has been successfully used in refractory cases to directly remove thyroid hormone. For refractory cases, emergency surgical thyroidectomy is an option.

Supportive care is usually required, including vasopressors, mechanical ventilation, dialysis, and extracorporeal membrane oxygenation (ECMO) for cardiogenic shock.

4. Hyperthyroidism from postpartum thyroiditis—Propranolol ER is given during the hyperthyroid phase followed by levothyroxine during the hypothyroidism phase.

5. Graves dermopathy—Treatment involves application of a topical corticosteroid (eg, fluocinolone) with nocturnal plastic occlusive dressings. Compression stockings may improve any associated edema.

6. Thyrotoxic hypokalemic periodic paralysis—Therapy with oral propranolol, 3 mg/kg in divided doses, normalizes the serum potassium and phosphate levels and reverses the paralysis within 2–3 hours. No intravenous potassium or phosphate is usually required. Intravenous dextrose and oral carbohydrate aggravate the condition and are to be avoided. Therapy is continued with propranolol, 60–80 mg orally every 8 hours (or propranolol ER daily at equivalent daily dosage), along with a thiourea drug (eg, methimazole) to treat the hyperthyroidism.

Prognosis

Mild **Graves disease** may sometimes subside spontaneously. Graves disease that presents in early pregnancy has a 30% chance of spontaneous remission before the third trimester. The ocular, cardiac, and psychological complications can become serious and persistent even after treatment. Permanent hypoparathyroidism and vocal cord palsy are risks of surgical thyroidectomy. If thiourea therapy is stopped, recurrence of hyperthyroidism occurs in about 55% of patients with persistently positive TSI and in about 35% of those with undetectable TSI. Recurrence of hyperthyroidism can also occur after low-dose ^{131}I therapy or subtotal thyroidectomy. With adequate treatment and long-term follow-up, the results are usually good. However, despite treatment for hyperthyroidism, women experience an increased long-term risk of death from thyroid disease, CVD, stroke, and fracture of the femur. Posttreatment hypothyroidism is common. It may occur within a few months or up to several years after RAI therapy or subtotal thyroidectomy. Patients with thyrotoxic crisis have a high mortality rate despite treatment.

Subclinical hyperthyroidism generally subsides spontaneously. Progression to symptomatic thyrotoxicosis occurs at a rate of 1–2% per year in patients without a goiter and at a rate of 5% per year in patients with a multinodular goiter. Most patients do well without treatment and the serum TSH usually reverts to normal within 2 years. In persons over age 60 years, serum TSH is suppressed (below 0.1 mIU/L) in 3% and mildly low (0.1–0.4 mIU/L) in 9%. The chance of developing atrial fibrillation is 2.8% yearly in older patients with a suppressed TSH and 1.1% yearly in those with mildly low TSH. Asymptomatic persons with very low serum TSH are monitored closely but are not treated unless atrial fibrillation or other manifestations of hyperthyroidism develop.

When to Admit

- Thyroid crisis.
- Hyperthyroidism-induced atrial fibrillation with severe tachycardia.
- Thyroidectomy.

Bartalena L et al. Treatment of hyperthyroidism in Graves' disease complicated by thyroid eye disease. J Clin Endocrinol Metab. 2025;110:922. [PMID: 39787151]

Bodnar TW. How do I manage my patients with thyrotoxicosis until they see the endocrinologist? Cleve Clin J Med. 2024;91:727. [PMID: 39622593]

Mounsey A et al. Hyperthyroidism: diagnosis and treatment. Am Fam Physician. 2025;112:146. [PMID: 40834371]

Octaviono YH et al. Exploring current diagnosis and management of amiodarone-induced thyrotoxicosis. Am J Cardiol. 2025;242:75. [PMID: 39924094]

Shah R et al. Management aspects of medical therapy in Graves disease. Endocr Pract. 2025;31:536. [PMID: 39701285]

THYROID EYE DISEASE

General Considerations

In patients with Graves disease, 27% have clinically apparent eye disease and 6% experience moderate to severe orbitopathy. The severity of eye disease is not correlated with the severity of thyrotoxicosis. In fact, about 10% of patients with thyroid eye disease have no clinical or laboratory evidence of Graves disease at presentation or on long-term follow-up; the absence of laboratory evidence requires consideration of other diagnoses.

Thyroid eye disease (TED) has an early inflammatory stage, typically lasting 18–36 months, where there is active lymphocytic infiltration into retrobulbar tissues. The active inflammatory stage then tends to evolve to a chronic, fibrotic, "burned out" stage in which treatment of the exophthalmos is medically resistant to glucocorticoid treatment. Aggravation of TED has occurred with active smoking, thiazolidinediones, and after vaccination against COVID-19. Radioiodine therapy for Graves disease can also aggravate TED.

Clinical Findings

The primary clinical features of TED of any etiology include upper eyelid retraction, lid lag with downward gaze, and a staring appearance. With Graves orbitopathy, there can be exophthalmos, conjunctival chemosis, episcleral inflammation, and weakness of upward gaze. Corneal drying may occur with inadequate lid closure. Eye changes may be asymmetric or unilateral. Patients with severe exophthalmos can experience diplopia from extraocular muscle entrapment and optic nerve compression, causing progressive loss of color vision, visual acuity, and visual fields (inferior especially).

Symptoms of active retrobulbar inflammation include (1) retrobulbar aching, (2) orbital inflammation and edema worse after recumbent sleep, (3) edematous or erythematous eyelids, (4) conjunctival redness or chemosis (edema), (5) recent progression in exophthalmos, (6) recent diplopia or strabismus, and (7) recent loss of visual acuity.

Exophthalmometry is performed on all patients with Graves disease to document their degree of exophthalmos and detect progression of orbitopathy. The protrusion of the eye beyond the orbital rim is measured with a prism instrument (Hertel exophthalmometer).

MRI and CT scanning of the orbits are the imaging methods of choice to visualize Graves ophthalmopathy. The primary imaging features are enlargement of the extraocular muscles, usually affecting both orbits. Imaging is required only in severe or unilateral cases or in euthyroid exophthalmos that must be distinguished from orbital pseudotumor, tumors, and other lesions.

Differential Diagnosis

The clinical and imaging abnormalities of thyroid eye disease may be mimicked by congenital proptosis, asymmetry in orbital protrusion, or dural carotid-cavernous sinus fistula. Ocular myasthenia and TED are associated and may coexist, with the presence of ptosis rather than lid retraction being more characteristic of the former. Other conditions mimicking TED include orbital cellulitis or myositis, immunoglobulin G4-related orbital disease, sarcoidosis, lymphoma, and orbital pseudotumor.

Treatment

General eye protective measures include wearing glasses to protect the protruding eye, use of methylcellulose drops or gels ("artificial tears"), and taping the lids shut during sleep if corneal drying is a problem. Most patients with TED are treated with selenium 100 mcg orally twice daily, which appears to slow its progression. Statins are often prescribed, which are associated with improved outcomes and responses to treatment.

The Mourits clinical activity score helps grade the severity of thyroid eye disease. Therapy in addition to selenium is warranted for active TED with a clinical activity point score ≥ 3.

Medical therapy is begun promptly with intravenous pulse methylprednisolone, 500 mg weekly for 6 weeks, then 250 mg weekly for 6 weeks. Oral prednisone, 40–60 mg daily with dosage reduction over several weeks, can be used but may be less effective. Higher initial daily prednisone doses of 80–120 mg are used when there is optic nerve compression.

Corticosteroid-resistant acute TED may be treated with other medications, such as teprotumumab and tocilizumab. Teprotumumab (Tepezza) is a monoclonal antibody inhibitor of the IFG-1 receptor that is FDA-approved for TED and is effective in reducing proptosis in the majority of affected patients. Tocilizumab (TCZ) is a monoclonal antibody that blocks the interleukin 6 receptor. Although not FDA-approved for TED, it is used off-label for patients with moderate-to-severe TED. It may be preferred over teprotumumab for patients with hearing loss or uncontrolled diabetes mellitus.

Retrobulbar radiation therapy may be used to treat patients with progressive active exophthalmos. Radiation is given over 2 weeks to deliver 20 Gy to extraocular muscles, while avoiding the cornea and lens, with concurrent high-dose prednisone. Patients who respond well to orbital radiation include those with signs of acute inflammation, recent exophthalmos (< 6 months), or optic nerve compression. Patients with chronic proptosis and orbital muscle restriction respond less well.

Diplopia should be treated conservatively (eg, with prisms) in the active stages of the disease and only by surgery when the disease has been static for at least 6 months. For severe cases, orbital decompression surgery may save vision, though diplopia often persists postoperatively.

When to Refer

All patients with TED should be referred to an ophthalmologist, urgently if there is reduced vision.

Hsu GC-Y et al. An appraisal of the preventive effect of statins on the development of Graves' ophthalmopathy: a hospital-based cohort study. Ophthalmol Ther. 2024;13:1499. [PMID: 38581604]

Huang J et al. Postmarketing safety concerns of teprotumumab: a real-world pharmacovigilance assessment. J Clin Endocrinol Metab. 2025;110:159. [PMID: 38878281]

Jay M et al. Treatment of subclinical hyperthyroidism and incident atrial fibrillation. Clin Endocrinol. 2025;102:315. [PMID: 39400387]

Vincent AB et al. Thyroid eye disease: what's the latest? Cleve Clin J Med. 2025;92:693. [PMID: 41184071]

Wiersinga WM et al. Thyroid eye disease (Graves' orbitopathy): clinical presentation, epidemiology, pathogenesis, and management. Lancet Diabetes Endocrinol. 2025;13:600. [PMID: 40324443]

THYROID NODULES & MULTINODULAR GOITER

ESSENTIALS OF DIAGNOSIS

- Single or multiple thyroid nodules are commonly palpated by the patient or clinician or discovered incidentally on imaging studies.
- Thyroid function tests recommended.
- FNA cytology for thyroid nodules ≥ 1 cm or for smaller nodules when prior head-neck or chest-shoulder radiation.
- Ultrasound guidance improves FNA diagnosis for palpable and nonpalpable nodules.
- Clinical follow-up required.

General Considerations

Thyroid nodules are common. Palpable nodules occur in about 5% of adults; however, neck ultrasound reveals a thyroid nodule in 50% of adults. They are more common in women than men and become more prevalent with age. Most patients with a thyroid nodule are euthyroid; however, there is a high incidence of hypo- or hyperthyroidism. Patients with palpable nodules require thyroid function testing and evaluation for thyroid malignancy.

Thyroid nodules may be detected incidentally on neck imaging done for another purpose. When such scans detect a nodule, a thyroid ultrasound is performed to help determine the risk for malignancy and to establish a baseline for follow-up examinations. Most nodules that are 1 cm or more in diameter require fine needle aspiration cytology (FNAc). Smaller nodules may be selected for FNAc if their ultrasound appearance is suspicious for malignancy or if they arise in a patient who has an increased risk for thyroid malignancy.

The overall risk of malignancy (ROM) for thyroid nodules 1 cm or larger in diameter is 1.2% overall and 2.8% in patients under age 30 (excluding papillary microfollicular carcinoma). The risk of a thyroid nodule being malignant is higher in (1) men; (2) patients with a history of head-neck radiation or exposure to radioactive fallout as a child; (3) patients with a personal history of malignancy; (4) patients with a family history of thyroid cancer or a thyroid cancer syndrome, such as multiple endocrine neoplasia type 2, familial polyposis, Carney syndrome, or Cowden syndrome; (5) patients with large solitary nodules; and (6) patients with hoarseness, vocal fold paralysis, adherence to the trachea or strap muscles, or cervical lymphadenopathy.

Clinical Findings

Table 29–6 illustrates how to evaluate thyroid nodules based on the index of suspicion for malignancy.

A. Symptoms and Signs

Most small thyroid nodules cause no symptoms. They may sometimes be detected only by having the patient swallow during inspection and palpation of the thyroid.

A thyroid nodule or multinodular goiter can grow to become visible and of concern to the patient. Large nodular goiters can become a cosmetic embarrassment. Nodules can grow large enough to cause discomfort, hoarseness, or dysphagia. Nodules that cause ipsilateral recurrent laryngeal nerve palsy are more likely to be malignant. Retrosternal large multinodular goiters can cause dyspnea due to tracheal compression. Large substernal goiters may cause superior vena cava syndrome, manifested by facial erythema and jugular vein distention that progress to cyanosis and facial edema when both arms are kept raised over the head.

Goiters and thyroid nodules may be associated with hypothyroidism (autoimmune thyroiditis, endemic goiter) or hyperthyroidism (Graves disease, toxic nodular goiter, subacute thyroiditis, and thyroid cancer with metastases).

Table 29–6. Clinical evaluation of thyroid nodules.[1]

Clinical Evidence	Low Index of Suspicion	High Index of Suspicion
History	Family history of goiter; residence in area of endemic goiter	Previous therapeutic radiation of head, neck, or chest; hoarseness
Physical characteristics	Older women; soft nodule; multinodular goiter	Young adults, men; solitary, firm nodule; vocal fold paralysis; enlarged lymph nodes; distant metastatic lesions
Serum factors	High titer of thyroid peroxidase antibody; hypothyroidism; hyperthyroidism	Elevated serum calcitonin
Fine-needle aspiration cytology	Colloid nodule or adenoma	Papillary carcinoma, follicular lesion, medullary or anaplastic carcinoma
Scanning techniques		
Uptake of ^{123}I	Hot nodule	Cold nodule
Ultrasonogram	Cystic lesion	Solid lesion
Radiograph	Shell-like calcification	Punctate calcification

[1]Clinically suspicious nodules should be evaluated with fine-needle aspiration cytology and molecular testing, when indicated.

B. Laboratory Findings

A serum TSH and FT_4 determine if the thyroid is hyperfunctioning. Patients with a subnormal serum TSH must have a radionuclide (^{123}I or ^{99m}Tc pertechnetate) thyroid scan to examine whether the nodule is hyperfunctioning; hyperfunctioning nodules are usually, but not always, benign. Serum calcitonin is obtained if a medullary thyroid carcinoma is suspected in a patient with a family history of medullary thyroid carcinoma or MEN types 2 or 3.

C. Imaging

Neck ultrasonography should be performed and is generally preferred over CT, MRI, or radioiodine scans. The ACR Thyroid Imaging Reporting and Data System (TI-RADS) classifies thyroid nodules into five categories based on risk of malignancy (in parentheses) with recommended management and follow up:

1. TR1: Benign (0%). No FNA required.
2. TR2: Not suspicious (< 2%). No FNA required.
3. TR3: Mildly suspicious (3%). Nodules ≥ 1.5 cm require follow-up at 1, 3, and 5 years; nodules ≥ 2.5 cm require FNA.
4. TR4: Moderately suspicious (19%). Nodules ≥ 1.0 cm require follow-up at 1, 2, 3, and 5 years; nodules ≥ 1.5 cm require FNA.
5. TR5: Highly suspicious (80%). Nodules ≥ 0.5 cm follow-up annually for 5 years; nodules ≥ 1.0 cm require FNA.

D. Fine-Needle Aspiration & Molecular Testing of Thyroid Nodules

FNA is the best method to assess a thyroid nodule for malignancy. For multinodular goiters, the four largest nodules (≥ 1 cm) usually are biopsied to minimize the risk of missing a malignancy. FNA cytology is reported using The Bethesda System for Reporting Thyroid Cytopathology (TBSRTC):

I. **Nondiagnostic or unsatisfactory:** The malignancy risk is about 12%. The usual management is a repeat FNA under ultrasound guidance.

II. **Benign:** The malignancy risk is about 2%. The usual management is clinical and ultrasound follow-up.

III. **Atypia of undetermined significance (AUS):** The malignancy risk is about 16%, higher with sonographic features of malignancy. The usual management is a repeat FNA, molecular testing, diagnostic thyroid lobectomy, or surveillance.

IV. **Follicular neoplasm (FN):** The malignancy risk is about 23%, higher when Hürthle cells are present and in patients over age 50. The usual management is molecular testing or thyroid lobectomy.

V. **Suspicious for malignancy (SFM):** The malignancy risk is about 65%. The usual management is molecular testing, thyroid lobectomy, or near-total thyroidectomy.

VI. **Malignant:** The malignancy risk is about 94%. The usual management is thyroid lobectomy or near-total thyroidectomy.

Molecular testing of the biopsy is useful when cytopathology is indeterminate for malignancy (Bethesda categories III, IV, or V). The detection of a *BRAF* mutation indicates the presence of a papillary thyroid carcinoma with a 98% probability. Molecular testing reduces the need for surgery by about 50%.

Surveillance & Treatment

All thyroid nodules, including those that are benign, need to be monitored by regular periodic palpation and ultrasound every 6 months initially. After several years of stability, yearly examinations are sufficient. Thyroid nodules should be re-biopsied if growth occurs. Excessive iodine intake should be minimized; a toxic multinodular goiter and hyperthyroidism may develop in patients who have had exposure to large amounts of iodine, either orally (eg, amiodarone) or intravenously (eg, radiographic contrast).

Patients with hyperthyroidism caused by thyroid nodules or multinodular goiter may be treated with propranolol, thioureas, surgery, or radioiodine.

A. Levothyroxine Suppression Therapy

Patients with nodules larger than 2 cm and elevated or normal TSH levels may be considered for TSH suppression with levothyroxine, starting at doses of 50 mcg orally daily. Levothyroxine suppression therapy is not recommended if the serum TSH is low or for small benign thyroid nodules if the serum TSH level is normal. Levothyroxine suppression therapy is more successful in iodine-deficient areas. Long-term levothyroxine suppression of TSH tends to keep nodules from enlarging but only 20% shrink > 50%. Thyroid nodule size increased in 29% of patients treated with levothyroxine versus 56% of patients not receiving levothyroxine. Levothyroxine suppression also reduces the emergence of new nodules: 8% with levothyroxine and 29% without levothyroxine. Levothyroxine suppression therapy is not given to patients with ischemic heart disease since it increases the risk for angina and atrial fibrillation.

Levothyroxine suppression needs to be carefully monitored, since it carries a 17% risk of inducing hyperthyroidism. All patients receiving levothyroxine suppression therapy should have serum TSH levels monitored at least annually, with the levothyroxine dose adjusted to keep the serum TSH mildly suppressed (between 0.1 mIU/L and 0.8 mIU/L).

B. Surgery

Total thyroidectomy is required for thyroid nodules that are malignant on FNA biopsy. More limited thyroid surgery is indicated for benign nodules with indeterminate or suspicious cytologic test results, compression symptoms, discomfort, or cosmetic embarrassment. Surgery may also be used to remove hyperfunctioning "hot" thyroid adenomas or toxic multinodular goiter causing hyperthyroidism.

C. Radiofrequency Ablation

Ultrasound-guided radiofrequency ablation (RFA) is a therapeutic option for cytology-proven benign thyroid nodules that are 3 cm or larger and predominantly solid. Autonomously functioning thyroid nodules can cause subclinical or overt hyperthyroidism that can be reversed by RFA. Radiofrequency ablation shrinks benign thyroid nodules by about 67% after 6 months, improving pressure symptoms and dysphagia in most patients and reducing the size of cosmetically embarrassing thyroid nodules. Side effects include mild neck discomfort, swelling, bruising, and dysphagia that generally resolves within 5 days. Transient hyperthyroidism occurs in 9% and responds to therapy with β blockade. Mild hypothyroidism may also occur. Radiofrequency ablation–induced damage to the recurrent laryngeal nerve can cause hoarseness.

D. Radioiodine (^{131}I) Therapy

^{131}I is a treatment option for hyperthyroid patients with toxic thyroid adenomas, multinodular goiter, or Graves disease. See **Precautions** for RAI use, above. RAI is not recommended for benign, nontoxic thyroid nodules. ^{131}I therapy may be used to shrink large multinodular goiters; it may rarely induce Graves disease or cause hypothyroidism that may develop years after therapy.

Prognosis

Benign thyroid nodules may involute but usually persist or grow slowly. Most thyroid nodules will increase their volume by 15% or more over 5 years. Significant nodule growth (> 2 mm in two dimensions) is more common in younger patients (< 45 years) and in patients with multiple nodules. Cytologically benign nodules that grow are unlikely to be malignant. Very small (< 1 cm), incidentally discovered, nonpalpable thyroid nodules that have a benign ultrasound appearance require no FNA cytology and only yearly palpation and clinical follow-up. Larger nodules (> 1 cm) and small nodules with a suspicious ultrasound appearance may require FNA cytology or thyroid ultrasound every 1–2 years. Thyroid nodules that are benign-appearing on ultrasound and or have benign FNA cytology require yearly follow-up with neck palpation. Ultrasound follow-up can be performed every 3–5 years.

Erdiğan MF et al. Changes in the volume and diameter of benign thyroid nodules: a 10-year follow-up study. Thyroid. 2025;35:31. [PMID: 39692610]
Kostek M et al. Molecular testing in thyroid nodules: how much does it change clinical practice? Biomedicines. 2025;13:1947. [PMID:40868201]
Ryu YJ et al. Radiofrequency ablation of Bethesda category III thyroid nodules with benign molecular testing: preliminary findings from a single institution. Am J Surg. 2025;241:115929. [PMID: 39217057]
Swaminathan N et al. Diagnostic value of molecular testing for evaluating thyroid nodules greater than 4 centimeters. Am J Surg. 2025;252:116755. [PMID: 41352294]

THYROID CANCER

ESSENTIALS OF DIAGNOSIS

- Painless swelling in region of thyroid.
- Thyroid function tests are usually normal.
- Possible history of childhood irradiation to head and neck region.
- Positive thyroid FNA cytology.

General Considerations

Thyroid cancers historically were discovered by detection of a thyroid mass by the patient or provider. Over the last 40 years, small nonpalpable thyroid malignancies have been detected with increasing frequency as a result of the widespread use of ultrasound, CT, MRI, and PET imaging. The yearly incidence of diagnosed thyroid malignancy in the United States has therefore tripled during this period to about 44,000 cases annually, but the mortality has remained relatively stable at 2400 deaths annually. Thyroid cancers are diagnosed three times more frequently in women than men. However, the mortality rate from thyroid cancer is nearly as high in men compared to women. Larger differentiated thyroid cancers (palpable or > 1 cm) are more likely to behave in a malignant fashion and usually require treatment.

Of thyroid cancers that are detected incidentally on imaging, most are nonpalpable, small (< 1 cm) papillary microcarcinomas. Although these microcarcinoma fulfill pathologic criteria for malignancy, they are almost all indolent; as such, a new terminology has been proposed for them: "indolent lesion of epithelial origin (IDLE)." In routine autopsy series, thyroid papillary microcarcinoma (< 1 cm) is found in 11.5% in both women and men.

Four histologic types account for 97% of thyroid cancer: papillary, follicular, medullary, and anaplastic (Table 29–7).

Pure papillary (and mixed papillary-follicular) carcinoma represents over 85% of all diagnosed thyroid cancers. It usually presents as a single thyroid nodule but can arise out of a multinodular goiter. Papillary thyroid carcinoma is commonly multifocal and involves both lobes in 30% of patients.

Papillary thyroid carcinoma is the least aggressive thyroid malignancy. It tends to grow slowly and often remains confined to the thyroid and regional lymph nodes for years. In about 80% of patients, there are microscopic (smaller than 2 mm) metastases to cervical lymph nodes, which does not appear to affect survival. The malignancy may become more aggressive in patients over age 45 years, especially in older adults. The cancer may invade the trachea and local muscles and spread to the lungs.

Childhood exposure to head and neck radiation therapy poses a particular threat because of an increased lifetime risk of developing thyroid cancer, including papillary carcinoma. These cancers may emerge 10–40 years after exposure, with a peak occurrence 20–25 years later.

Papillary thyroid carcinoma can occur in familial syndromes as an autosomal dominant trait, caused by loss of various tumor suppressor genes.

Microscopic "micropapillary" carcinomas (< 2 mm) are found in 24% of thyroidectomies performed for benign thyroid disease. These are invisible on thyroid ultrasound, seldom become clinically significant, and may be considered a variant of normal. Surgical pathology may report such tiny micropapillary carcinomas, but treatment and surveillance are not warranted.

Follicular thyroid carcinoma and its variants (eg, Hürthle cell carcinoma) account for 11% of thyroid malignancies; follicular carcinomas are generally more aggressive than papillary carcinomas. Most absorb iodine, making diagnostic scanning and treatment with ^{131}I after total

Table 29–7. Some characteristics of thyroid cancer.

	Papillary	Follicular	Medullary	Anaplastic
Incidence	Most common	Common	Uncommon	Uncommon
Average age (years)	42	50	50	57
Females	77%	72%	56%	56%
Invasion				
Lymph nodes	+++++	+	++++++	+++
Blood vessels	+	+++	+++	+++++
Distant sites	+	+++	++	++++
^{123}I uptake	+	++++	0	0
10-year disease-specific survival	98%	92%	78%	7.3%

thyroidectomy possible. Poorly differentiated and Hürthle cell (oncocytic) variants of follicular thyroid carcinoma are associated with a higher risk of metastasis and recurrence.

Medullary thyroid carcinoma (MTC) represents 2% of thyroid cancers. They arise from thyroid parafollicular cells that can secrete calcitonin, prostaglandins, serotonin, ACTH, CRH, and other peptides that may cause symptoms and can be used as tumor markers. About one-third are sporadic, one-third are familial, and one-third are associated with MEN type 2A or 2B. Discovery of an MTC makes genetic analysis mandatory. MTC is often caused by an activating mutation of the *ret* protooncogene on chromosome 10.

Anaplastic thyroid carcinoma represents 1% of thyroid cancers. It is the most aggressive thyroid carcinoma and metastasizes early to surrounding nodes and distant sites. It usually presents in an older patient as a rapidly enlarging mass in a multinodular goiter. This tumor does not concentrate iodine, which precludes the therapeutic use of RAI.

Other thyroid malignancies represent about 3% of thyroid cancers. Primary thyroid lymphomas are most commonly diffuse large B-cell lymphomas (50%), mucosa-associated lymphoid tissue lymphoma (23%), or mixed type; other types include follicular, small lymphocytic, and Burkitt lymphoma and Hodgkin disease. Cancers may sometimes metastasize to the thyroid, particularly bronchogenic, breast, renal carcinoma, and melanoma.

Clinical Findings

A. Symptoms and Signs

Thyroid carcinoma usually presents as a palpable, firm, nontender thyroid nodule. Most thyroid carcinomas are asymptomatic, but large thyroid cancers can cause neck discomfort, dysphagia, or hoarseness (due to pressure on the recurrent laryngeal nerve). **Papillary thyroid cancer** presents with palpable lymph node involvement in 10%; it may invade the trachea and local muscles. Occult metastases to the lung occur in 10–15%. **Follicular thyroid carcinoma** commonly metastasizes to neck nodes, bones, and lung, but nearly every organ can be involved (Table 29–7).

Medullary thyroid carcinoma typically metastases to local nodes and adjacent muscle and trachea as well as mediastinal lymph nodes. Metastases may appear in the bones, lungs, adrenals, or liver. It frequently causes flushing and diarrhea (30%), which may be the initial clinical features. Cushing syndrome develops in 5% of patients from tumor secretion of ACTH or CRH.

Anaplastic thyroid carcinoma is more apt to be advanced at the time of diagnosis, presenting with signs of pressure or invasion of surrounding tissue, resulting in dysphagia, hoarseness, or recurrent laryngeal nerve palsy or dyspnea due to lung metastases.

B. Laboratory Findings

FNA cytology is discussed in Thyroid Nodules, above. Thyroid function tests are generally normal unless there is concomitant thyroiditis. However, with a heavy tumor burden, functioning follicular or papillary thyroid carcinomas can sometimes secrete enough thyroid hormone to produce thyrotoxicosis and suppress the serum TSH.

Serum thyroglobulin is high in most metastatic papillary and follicular tumors, making this a useful marker for recurrent or metastatic disease. Caution must be exercised for the following reasons: (1) Circulating Tg Ab can cause erroneous thyroglobulin determinations. However, declining levels of Tg Ab are a good prognostic sign after treatment. (2) Thyroglobulin levels may be misleadingly elevated in thyroiditis, which often coexists with carcinoma. (3) Certain thyroglobulin assays falsely report the continued presence of thyroglobulin after total thyroidectomy and tumor resection, causing undue concern about possible metastases.

Serum calcitonin is usually elevated in MTC, making this a marker for metastatic disease. Serum calcitonin may be elevated in thyroiditis; pregnancy; kidney disease; hypergastrinemia; hypercalcemia; and other malignancies, particularly neuroendocrine tumors (including pheochromocytomas, carcinoid tumors) and carcinomas of the lung, pancreas, breast, and colon. Serum calcitonin and carcinoembryonic antigen (CEA) determinations should be obtained before surgery, then regularly in postoperative follow-up: every 4 months for 5 years, then every 6 months for life. Serum calcitonin levels > 250 ng/L (73 pmol/L) or rising levels of calcitonin are the best indication of recurrence or metastatic disease. Serum pro-calcitonin levels also appear to be a reasonable tumor marker for medullary cancer. Serum CEA levels are elevated but are not specific for MTC.

C. Imaging

1. Ultrasound of the neck—Ultrasound of the neck should be performed on all patients with thyroid cancer for the initial diagnosis and for follow-up. Ultrasound is useful in determining the size and location of the malignancy as well as the location of any neck metastases.

2. Radioactive iodine scanning—RAI (^{131}I or ^{123}I) thyroid and whole-body scanning is used after thyroidectomy for differentiated thyroid cancer utilizing the protocol described later. (See Radioactive Iodine (^{131}I) Therapy for Differentiated Thyroid Cancer, below.) Medullary thyroid cancer does not take up RAI.

3. CT and MRI scanning—CT scanning may demonstrate metastases and is particularly useful for localizing and monitoring lung metastases but is less sensitive than ultrasound for detecting metastases within the neck. Medullary carcinoma in the thyroid, nodes, and liver may calcify, but lung metastases rarely do so. MRI is particularly useful for imaging bone metastases.

4. PET scanning—PET scanning is especially helpful for detecting thyroid cancer metastases that do not have sufficient iodine uptake to be visible on RAI scans. Thyroid cancer metastases may be detected with ^{18}FDG-PET whole-body scanning. Patients with medullary thyroid cancer are monitored with MRI and ^{18}FDG PET/CT scanning. ^{68}Ga-DOTATATE-PET imaging is superior for detecting medullary thyroid cancer metastases in certain patients, particularly those with very high serum calcitonin levels (above 500 pg/mL).

Differential Diagnosis

Head-neck RAI uptake is seen in normal thyroid, salivary glands, nasal mucosa, thyroglossal duct remnants, and sinusitis.

Negative RAI scans are common in early metastatic differentiated thyroid carcinoma. Negative RAI scans also occur frequently with advanced metastatic thyroid carcinoma, making it difficult to detect and to distinguish from nonthyroidal neoplasms. An elevated serum thyroglobulin in patients with a negative RAI scan should arouse suspicion for metastases that are not avid for RAI. MTC does not concentrate iodine.

Complications

Hyperthyroidism can develop in patients with a heavy tumor burden of differentiated thyroid cancer. One-third of MTCs secrete serotonin and prostaglandins, producing flushing and diarrhea. The management of patients with medullary carcinomas may be complicated by the coexistence of pheochromocytomas or hyperparathyroidism.

Treatment of Differentiated Thyroid Carcinoma

A. Surgical Treatment

For low-risk papillary or papillary/follicular thyroid microcarcinoma (smaller than or equal to 1 cm), both active surveillance and unilateral thyroid lobectomy (hemithyroidectomy) are acceptable treatment options; since the 5-year disease-specific survival is over 98%, active surveillance is becoming more common. **For low-risk differentiated thyroid cancers (papillary or follicular) between 1 and 4 cm**, either hemithyroidectomy or total thyroidectomy can be used. Both provide the same overall 5-year survival, although recurrence is more common after hemithyroidectomy. Hemithyroidectomy is increasingly preferred, as it has no risk of hypoparathyroidism, decreased risk for recurrent laryngeal nerve palsy, and a 30% chance that postoperative thyroid replacement will not be required.

For medium and high-risk papillary and follicular thyroid carcinoma, total or near-total thyroidectomy is usually performed, particularly for patients with tumors > 4 cm and those with evidence for local or distant metastases. The advantages of total thyroidectomy for differentiated thyroid carcinoma include the resection of carcinoma foci in the contralateral lobe. Furthermore, it removes all remaining normal thyroid tissue that would otherwise compete with uptake of radioiodine administered for diagnostic scans or treatment of residual cancer. Levothyroxine, 0.05–0.1 mg orally daily, is begun immediately postoperatively. About 2–4 months after surgery, patients require reevaluation and often ^{131}I therapy.

Patients with nodal metastases can have a central neck lymph node dissection at the time of thyroidectomy.

Following surgical resection, permanent injury to one recurrent laryngeal nerve (rarely both) occurs in 1–7% of patients, temporary laryngeal nerve palsies in 5%, and hypoparathyroidism (usually temporary) in 20%. Thyroidectomy requires at least an overnight hospital admission, since late bleeding, airway problems, and tetany can occur. *Ambulatory thyroidectomy is potentially dangerous and should not be done.* Following surgery, staging (Table 29–8) should be done to help determine prognosis and to plan therapy and follow-up. Metastases to the brain are treated surgically or with gamma-knife radiosurgery, since treatment with RAI is ineffective.

In pregnant women with thyroid cancer, surgery is usually delayed until after delivery, except for fast-growing tumors that may be resected after 24 weeks' gestation; there has been no difference in survival or tumor recurrence rates in women who underwent surgery during or after their pregnancy.

Table 29–8. Staging and prognosis for patients with papillary thyroid carcinoma using MACIS scoring.

Total Score[1] - Stage	Percentage of Patients with Papillary Thyroid Carcinoma	20-Year Survival
< 6.0 = Stage I	74.2%	96–99%
6.0–6.99 = Stage II	8.5%	68–89%
7.0–7.99 = Stage III	9.2%	55–56%
≥ 8.0 = Stage IV	8.1%	17–24%

[1]Total score = 3.1 (if aged ≤ 39 years) *or* 0.08 × age (if aged ≥ 40 years) + 0.3 × tumor size (cm), + 1 (if incompletely resected), + 1 (if locally invasive), + 3 (if distant metastases).

MACIS, metastases, age, complete resection, invasion, size.

B. Active Surveillance for Papillary Thyroid Carcinoma

Most papillary thyroid carcinomas (PTCs) that are < 1 cm (microcarcinomas) are indolent with an excellent prognosis. Conservative management is usually warranted for patients with these low-risk tumors. The active surveillance protocol typically consists of clinical examination and neck ultrasound every 6 months. Larger PTCs (1–4 cm) that are intrathyroidal and nonmetastatic are typically treated with hemithyroidectomy; however, active surveillance is increasingly employed for larger PTCs with low-risk characteristics.

C. Levothyroxine Suppression of TSH

Levothyroxine is no longer prescribed for euthyroid patients with low-risk differentiated thyroid cancer (DTC) who have had a unilateral thyroid lobectomy. Levothyroxine is prescribed for other patients with DTC in doses to achieve certain target levels of serum TSH as follows: (1) For high-risk DTC, the target TSH range is 0.1 mIU/L (while maintaining clinical euthyroidism). (2) For intermediate-risk DTC, the serum TSH target is 0.1 to 0.4 mIU/L. (3) For low-risk DTC, the TSH target range is 0.4 to 2 mIU/L. (4) For all patients with DTC who have atrial fibrillation, the serum TSH should be kept at or above 0.1 mIU/L.

D. Radioactive Iodine (^{131}I) Therapy for Differentiated Thyroid Cancer (DTC)

Following total or near-total thyroidectomy for DTC, ^{131}I therapy may improve survival in (1) high-risk patients with gross extrathyroidal extension or distant metastases; (2) intermediate-risk patients with over 5 microscopic lymph node metastases, mediastinal lymph node metastases, primary tumor size above 4 cm diameter with extrathyroidal extension or in patients over age 50, or tumor above 1 cm diameter with aggressive histology or vascular invasion. ^{131}I is usually administered 2–4 months after surgery.

1. RAI thyroid remnant ablation—For patients with low-risk DTC, radioiodine is no longer recommended either for thyroid remnant ablation or for adjuvant therapy following total or near-total thyroidectomy. Low-risk DTC includes a single papillary or follicular thyroid cancer < 2 cm diameter or multiple tumors < 1 cm diameter with no significant nodal disease, no extrathyroidal extension, and no unfavorable histopathology.

2. RAI treatment of metastases—Therapy with ^{131}I improves survival and reduces recurrence rates of differentiated thyroid cancer for patients with stage III–IV cancer and those with stage II cancer having gross extrathyroidal extension. RAI therapy is also given to patients with stage II cancer who have distant metastases, a primary tumor larger than 4 cm, or primary tumors 1–4 cm with lymph node metastases or other high-risk features. Brain metastases do not usually respond to ^{131}I and are best resected or treated with gamma knife radiosurgery.

Staging with RAI scanning or ^{18}FDG-PET/CT scanning assists with determining the activity of ^{131}I to be administered. Patients with differentiated thyroid carcinoma who have little or no uptake of RAI into metastases (about 35% of cases) should not be treated with ^{131}I. Patients with asymptomatic, stable, RAI-resistant metastases should receive levothyroxine to suppress serum TSH and should be carefully monitored for tumor progression.

3. Recombinant human TSH (rhTSH)-stimulated ^{131}I therapy—Recombinant human thyroid-stimulating hormone (rhTSH, Thyrogen) can be given to increase the sensitivity of serum thyroglobulin for residual cancer and to increase the uptake of ^{131}I into residual thyroid tissue (thyroid remnant "ablation") or cancer.

Thyrogen should not be administered to patients with an intact thyroid gland because it can cause severe thyroid swelling and hyperthyroidism. Hyperthyroidism can also occur in patients with significant metastases or residual normal thyroid. Other side effects include nausea (11%) and headache (7%). Thyrotropin has caused neurologic deterioration in 7% of patients with CNS metastases.

4. Thyroid-withdrawal stimulated ^{131}I therapy—Thyroid withdrawal is sometimes used because of its lower cost than rhTSH, despite the discomforts of becoming hypothyroid. Levothyroxine is withdrawn for 14 days and the patient is allowed to become hypothyroid; high levels of endogenous TSH stimulate the uptake of RAI and production of thyroglobulin by thyroid cancer or residual thyroid. Three days after ^{131}I therapy, levothyroxine therapy may be resumed at full replacement dose.

5. Side effects from ^{131}I therapy—Patients treated with ^{131}I have a slightly higher risk of developing secondary malignancies than patients treated with surgery alone.

^{131}I therapy can cause gastritis, temporary oligospermia, sialadenitis, tearing, and xerostomia. It can cause neurologic decompensation in patients with thyroid brain metastases. Cumulative doses of ^{131}I over 500 mCi (18.5 GBq) can cause infertility, pancytopenia (4%), leukemia (0.3%), and pulmonary fibrosis.

E. Other Therapies for Differentiated Thyroid Cancer

Patients with osteolytic metastases to bone from differentiated thyroid cancer may be treated with zoledronic acid or denosumab.

Targeted therapies are available for patients with radioiodine-refractory differentiated thyroid cancer. Recurrence in the neck may be treated with surgical debulking and external beam radiation therapy. Patients with RAI-refractory differentiated thyroid cancer metastases that are advanced and rapidly progressive may be treated with chemotherapy tailored to the genetic defect exhibited by the tumor.

Treatment of Other Thyroid Malignancies

MTC is best treated with surgery for the primary tumor and metastases. MTC does not respond to ^{131}I therapy. Patients should be monitored closely, with serum calcitonin levels checked about every 3 months. Since MTC can be indolent, patients should receive treatment only if they have rapidly progressive metastases, as evidenced by a doubling time of serum calcitonin or CEA of < 2 years.

^{177}Lu-DOTATATE peptide receptor radionuclide therapy (PRRT, Lutathera) is an option for patients with progressive MTC metastases that are very avid for ^{64}Cu-DOTATATE on diagnostic imaging or demonstrate high SSTR2a receptor expression on immunohistochemical staining. Patients with progressing MTCs (with germline or sporadic *RET* proto-oncogene mutations or fusions) are treated with selpercatinib or pralsetinib, selective *RET* inhibitors. *Patients with MTC should not receive diabetic or weight-loss therapy with GLP-1 agonists, because they may stimulate the growth of MTC.*

Anaplastic thyroid carcinoma is treated with local resection and radiation. It does not respond to ^{131}I therapy. Anaplastic thyroid cancers with mTOR mutations may be inhibited by everolimus. In patients with *BRAF*^{V600E} mutant anaplastic thyroid cancer, combined treatment with dabrafenib and trametinib has induced durable responses.

Thyroid lymphoma: Thyroid mucosa-associated lymphoid tissue lymphomas have a low risk of recurrence after simple thyroidectomy. Patients with other thyroid lymphomas are best treated with external radiation therapy; chemotherapy is added for extensive lymphoma (see Table 43–2).

External beam radiation therapy may be delivered to bone metastases, especially those that are without radioiodine uptake or are RAI-refractory. Local neck radiation therapy may also be given to patients with anaplastic thyroid carcinoma. Brain metastases can be treated with gamma knife radiosurgery.

Follow-Up

Most recurrences of differentiated thyroid carcinoma become manifest within 5–10 years after thyroidectomy. All patients require at least a yearly thyroid ultrasound and serum thyroglobulin level (while taking levothyroxine). Patients at higher risk usually require at least two annual consecutively negative stimulated serum thyroglobulin determinations < 1 ng/mL and normal RAI scans (if done) and neck ultrasound scans before they are considered to be in remission. The first surveillance occurs with stimulated postoperative serum thyroglobulin, ^{131}I therapy, and post-therapy scanning about 2–4 and 9–12 months after surgery. Serum thyroglobulin and RAI scanning are stimulated by either rhTSH or thyroid hormone withdrawal according to the protocols described above for ^{131}I treatment. Patients need not have repeated ^{131}I therapies if persistent RAI uptake is confined to the thyroid bed, neck ultrasounds appear normal, and stimulated serum thyroglobulin levels remain < 2 ng/mL. Patients with differentiated thyroid carcinoma must be monitored long term for recurrent or metastatic disease. Further RAI or other scans may be required for patients with more aggressive differentiated thyroid cancer, prior metastases, rising serum thyroglobulin levels, or other evidence of metastases.

1. Levothyroxine suppression for differentiated thyroid cancer—Patients who have had a total or near-total thyroidectomy for differentiated thyroid cancer must take levothyroxine replacement for life. (See Levothyroxine Suppression of TSH, above.) Thyrotoxicosis can be caused by over-replacement with levothyroxine or by the growth of functioning metastases. Patients receiving levothyroxine suppression therapy should have periodic bone densitometry.

2. Serum thyroglobulin—Thyroglobulin is produced by normal thyroid tissue and by most differentiated thyroid carcinomas. After a total or near-total thyroidectomy and ^{131}I remnant ablation, thyroglobulin becomes a useful marker for residual or metastatic tumor in for patients with differentiated papillary or follicular thyroid cancer, particularly for patients who do not have serum Tg Ab. In patients receiving levothyroxine following thyroidectomy (with TSH suppression), baseline thyroglobulin levels are insensitive for detection of residual or recurrent disease. Therefore, *stimulated* serum thyroglobulin measurements should be used. Following stimulation by either rhTSH or levothyroxine withdrawal, serum thyroglobulin levels 2 ng/mL or higher indicate the need for a repeat neck ultrasound and further scanning with RAI or ^{18}FDG-PET (see ^{131}I Treatment).

3. Neck ultrasound—Neck ultrasound should be used in all patients with thyroid carcinoma at 3 months postoperatively and regularly thereafter. Ultrasound is more sensitive for lymph node metastases than either CT or MRI scanning. Ultrasound-guided FNA biopsy should be performed on suspicious lesions.

4. Radioactive iodine (RAI: ^{131}I or ^{123}I) neck and whole-body scanning—Despite its limitations, RAI scanning has traditionally been used to detect metastatic differentiated thyroid cancer and to determine whether it is amenable to treatment with ^{131}I. RAI scanning is particularly useful for high-risk patients and those with persistent Tg Ab that make serum thyroglobulin determinations unreliable.

Following total or near-total thyroidectomy, about 65% of metastases are detectable by RAI scanning. The combination of rhTSH-stimulated scanning and thyroglobulin levels detects a thyroid remnant or cancer with a sensitivity of 84%. It is reasonable to perform a rhTSH-stimulated scan and thyroglobulin level 2–3 months after the initial neck surgery. If the scan is negative and the serum thyroglobulin is < 2 ng/mL, low-risk patients may not require further scanning but should continue to be monitored with neck ultrasound and serum thyroglobulin levels every 6–12 months. In about 21% of low-risk patients, rhTSH stimulates serum thyroglobulin to > 2 ng/mL; such patients have a 23% risk of local neck metastases and a 13% risk of distant metastases. The rhTSH-stimulated RAI neck and whole-body scan detects only about half of these metastases because they are small or not avid for iodine. For higher-risk patients, the rhTSH-stimulated thyroglobulin and RAI scan may be repeated about 1 year after surgery and then again if warranted.

5. Positron emission tomography scanning—^{18}FDG-PET scanning is particularly useful for detecting differentiated thyroid cancer metastases in patients with a detectable serum thyroglobulin (especially serum thyroglobulin levels > 10 ng/mL and rising) who have a normal whole-body RAI scan and an unrevealing neck ultrasound. It is also sensitive for detecting metastases from MTC. ^{18}FDG-PET scanning can be combined with a CT scan; the resultant ^{18}FDG-PET/CT fusion scan is 60% sensitive for detecting metastases that are not visible by other methods. This scan is less sensitive for small brain metastases.

^{68}Ga-DOTATATE-PET scanning is useful for staging patients with MTC. It is also useful to determine whether a patient can be treated with PRRT.

6. Other scanning—Thallium-201 (^{201}Tl) scans may be useful for detecting metastatic differentiated thyroid carcinoma when the ^{131}I scan is normal but serum thyroglobulin is elevated. MRI scanning is useful for imaging metastases in the brain, mediastinum, or bones. CT scanning is useful for imaging and monitoring pulmonary metastases.

Prognosis

1. Papillary thyroid carcinoma—This cancer has an overall mortality rate of 2%. It is best staged using the MACIS (metastasis, age, completeness of resection, invasion, size) scoring system (see Table 29–8). ^{18}FDG-PET scanning showing pulmonary, brain, or bone metastases independently predicts lower overall survival. Unlike other forms of cancer, patients with papillary thyroid carcinoma who have palpable lymph node metastases do not have a particularly increased mortality rate; however, their risk of local recurrence is increased. The best prognosis has been with the follicular variant of papillary thyroid cancer.

2. Follicular thyroid carcinoma—The mortality rate of follicular thyroid carcinoma is 3.4 times higher than that of papillary carcinoma. Patients with primary tumors larger than 1 cm who undergo limited thyroid surgery (subtotal thyroidectomy or lobectomy) have a 2.2-fold increased mortality over those having total or near-total thyroidectomies. Patients who have not received ^{131}I ablation have mortality rates that are increased twofold by 10 years and threefold by 25 years (over those who have received ablation). The risk of cancer recurrence is twofold higher in men than in women and 1.7-fold higher in multifocal than in unifocal tumors.

Patients with a normal ^{18}FDG-PET scan have a 98% 5-year survival. Five-year survival is 95% with local metastases, 70% with regional (supraclavicular, mediastinal) metastases, and 35% with distant metastases.

3. Medullary thyroid carcinoma—This cancer is more aggressive than differentiated thyroid cancer but is typically indolent. MTC with a somatic *RET* codon *M918T* mutation has a poorer prognosis, whereas the gene polymorphism CDKN1B V109G has a more favorable prognosis. Familial cases and those associated with MEN 2A tend to be less aggressive.; cases seen in MEN2B (MEN3) are more aggressive and carry a worse overall prognosis. Patients with sporadic disease usually have lymph node involvement noted at the time of diagnosis, whereas distal metastases may not be noted for years. When postoperative serum calcitonin levels are > 500 pg/mL (146 pmol/L), distant metastases are likely. Patients with metastatic MTC whose serum calcitonin doubling time is over 2 years also have a relatively good prognosis.

4. Other thyroid carcinomas—Lymphoma has a 5-year survival of nearly 100% if localized and 63% if there is extension beyond the thyroid. **Anaplastic thyroid carcinoma** carries a 1-year survival rate of 10% and a 5-year survival rate of 5%; immunotherapy may be used as an adjunct therapy.

Cho YY et al. TSH cutoffs and recurrence risk in differentiated thyroid carcinomas: a systematic review and meta-analysis. J Clin Endocrinol Metab. 2025;110:3588. [PMID: 40811629]

Kiyota N et al. Anticancer drug therapy for anaplastic thyroid cancer. Eur Thyroid J. 2025;14:e240287. [PMID: 40163699]

Kuenstner W et al. Update in papillary thyroid cancer. Endocrinol Metab Clin N Am. 2025;54:329. [PMID: 40716890]

Ringel MD et al. 2025 American Thyroid Association management guidelines for adult patients with differentiated thyroid cancer. Thyroid. 2025;35:841. [PMID: 40844370]

Shariq OA et al. Approach to the patient: hereditary medullary thyroid carcinoma. J Clin Endocrinol Metab. 2025;110:2685. [PMID: 40105880]

Zhang Y et al. Efficacy and safety of targeted therapy for radioiodine-refractory differentiated thyroid cancer. J Clin Endocrinol Metab. 2025;110:873. [PMID: 39292866]

IODINE DEFICIENCY DISORDER & ENDEMIC GOITER

ESSENTIALS OF DIAGNOSIS

- Common in regions with low-iodine diets.
- High rate of congenital hypothyroidism and cretinism.
- Goiters may become multinodular and enlarge.
- Most adults with endemic goiter are euthyroid; however, some are hypo- or hyperthyroid.

General Considerations

Although global rates of iodine deficiency have declined in recent decades, mild to severe iodine deficiency exists in 30 countries; an estimated 1.9 billion people have insufficient iodine intake. Iodine deficiency is reemerging in certain developed countries, such the United Kingdom, Norway, and other parts of Europe. Although the United States is considered "iodine sufficient," iodine supplementation is voluntary and the average iodine consumption has decreased by about 50% over the last 50 years.

Moderate iodine deficiency during gestation and infancy can cause manifestations of hypothyroidism, deafness, and short stature and lower a child's intelligence quotient by 10–15 points. Severe iodine deficiency increases the risk of miscarriage and stillbirth. Cretinism occurs in about 0.5% of live births in iodine-deficient areas.

Although iodine deficiency is the most common cause of endemic goiter, there are other natural goitrogens, including certain foods (eg, sorghum, millet, maize, cassava), mineral deficiencies (selenium, iron, zinc), and water pollutants, which can themselves cause goiter or aggravate a goiter proclivity caused by iodine deficiency.

Clinical Findings

A. Symptoms and Signs

Endemic goiters may become multinodular and very large. Growth often occurs during pregnancy, increasing the size of thyroid nodules and causing new nodules; compressive symptoms may occur.

Substernal goiters are usually asymptomatic but can cause tracheal compression, respiratory distress, dysphagia, superior vena cava syndrome, palsies of the phrenic or recurrent laryngeal nerves, or Horner syndrome. The incidence of significant malignancy is < 1%.

Some patients with endemic goiter may become hypothyroid. Others may become thyrotoxic as the goiter grows and becomes more autonomous, especially if iodine is added to the diet.

B. Laboratory Findings

The serum T_4 and TSH are generally normal. TSH is low in hyperthyroidism if a multinodular goiter has become autonomous and there is sufficient iodine for thyroid hormone synthesis. TSH increases with hypothyroidism. Thyroid RAI uptake is usually elevated, but it may be normal if iodine intake has improved. Serum antithyroid antibodies are usually either undetectable or in low titers. Serum thyroglobulin is often elevated above 13 mcg/L.

Differential Diagnosis

Endemic goiter must be distinguished from other forms of nodular goiter that may coexist in an endemic region.

Prevention

The daily minimum dietary requirement for iodine is 150 mcg daily in nonpregnant adults and 250 mcg daily for pregnant or lactating women. Iodized salt contains iodine at about 20 mg per kg salt. Other sources of iodine include commercial bread, milk, and seafood. Initiating iodine supplementation in an iodine-deficient area greatly reduces the emergence of new goiters but causes an increased frequency of hyperthyroidism during the first year.

Treatment

Most patients with iodine-deficient goiter are euthyroid. Dietary iodine supplementation is recommended to avoid hypothyroidism but has proven ineffective in shrinking such goiters. Thyroidectomy may be required for cosmesis, compressive symptoms, or thyrotoxicosis. There is a high goiter recurrence rate in iodine-deficient geographic areas, so near-total thyroidectomy is preferred when surgery is indicated.

Complications

Dietary iodine supplementation increases the risk of autoimmune thyroid dysfunction, which may cause hypo- or hyperthyroidism. Excessive iodine intake can actually cause endemic goiter. High-dose iodine supplementation may precipitate thyrotoxicosis. Suppression of TSH by administering levothyroxine carries the risk of inducing hyperthyroidism, particularly in patients with autonomous multinodular goiters. Levothyroxine suppression should not be started in patients with a low TSH level. Treating patients with ^{131}I for large multinodular goiter may shrink the gland; however, Graves disease develops in some patients 3–10 months following therapy.

Liang D et al. Perspective: global burden of iodine deficiency: insights and projections to 2050 using XGBoost and SHAP. Adv Nutr. 2025;16:100384. [PMID: 39914495]

Wu Z et al. The burden of iodine deficiency. Arch Med Sci. 2024;20:1484. [PMID: 39649274]

DISEASES OF THE ADRENAL CORTEX

PRIMARY ADRENAL INSUFFICIENCY (Addison Disease)

ESSENTIALS OF DIAGNOSIS

- Deficiency of cortisol secretion from the adrenal cortex.
- Weakness, vomiting, diarrhea; abdominal pain, arthralgias; amenorrhea.
- Increased skin pigmentation, especially of creases, pressure areas, and nipples.
- Hypovolemic hypotension.
- Hyponatremia; hyperkalemia; hypoglycemia; eosinophilia.
- Elevated plasma ACTH level; cosyntropin unable to stimulate serum cortisol to ≥ 20 mcg/dL (550 nmol/L).
- **Acute adrenal crisis:** above manifestations become critical, with fever, shock, confusion, coma, death.

General Considerations

Primary adrenal insufficiency (Addison disease) is caused by dysfunction or absence of the adrenal cortices. Secondary adrenal insufficiency is caused by deficient secretion of ACTH. Addison disease refers to a chronic deficiency of cortisol caused by adrenocortical insufficiency; plasma ACTH and α-MSH levels are consequently elevated, causing pigmentation that ranges from none to strikingly dark.

Addison disease is an uncommon disorder. In the United States, the prevalence is about 90–140 cases per million and the annual incidence is about 5–6 cases per million. Patients with destruction of the adrenal cortices or with classic 21-hydroxylase deficiency also have mineralocorticoid deficiency, typically with hyponatremia, volume depletion, and hyperkalemia. In contrast, mineralocorticoid deficiency is not present in patients with familial corticosteroid deficiency, Allgrove syndrome, or secondary adrenal insufficiency.

Acute adrenal (Addisonian) crisis is an emergency caused by insufficient cortisol. Crisis may occur in the course of treatment of chronic adrenal insufficiency, or it may be the presenting manifestation of adrenal insufficiency. Acute adrenal crisis is more commonly seen in primary adrenal insufficiency (7 cases/100 patient-years) than in secondary adrenal insufficiency (3 cases/100 patient-years). It is usually precipitated by one of the following: (1) severe stress (eg, infection, trauma, surgery, hyperthyroidism, or prolonged fasting), or minor stress (vaccinations) in patients with latent or treated adrenal insufficiency; (2) hyperthyroidism or prescription of thyroid hormone to patients with untreated adrenal insufficiency; (3) nonadherence to glucocorticoid replacement or sudden withdrawal of glucocorticoids (oral, parenteral, or transdermal) in patients with chronic primary or secondary adrenal insufficiency; (4) bilateral adrenalectomy or removal of a functioning adrenal tumor that had suppressed the other adrenal gland; (5) selective resection of an ACTH-producing pituitary tumor; (6) sudden destruction of the pituitary gland (pituitary necrosis) or damage to both adrenals (by trauma, hemorrhage, anticoagulant therapy, thrombosis, infection or, rarely, metastatic carcinoma); or (7) administration of intravenous etomidate (used for rapid anesthesia induction or intubation).

Etiology

Autoimmunity is the most common cause of Addison disease in industrialized countries, accounting for about 90% of spontaneous cases; adrenal function decreases over several years as it progresses to overt adrenal insufficiency. Over half the cases of autoimmune Addison disease occur as part of an autoimmune polyendocrine syndrome (APS-1, APS-2). Addison disease can also occur following treatment for malignancies with a PD-1 immune checkpoint inhibitor (ICI). Symptoms of adrenal insufficiency may emerge at any time after ICI therapy, with a median of 10 weeks.

Bilateral adrenal infiltrative diseases cause primary adrenal insufficiency. Causative neoplasms include lymphomas, breast cancer, and lung cancer. Causative infections include tuberculosis, coccidiomycosis, histoplasmosis, cytomegalovirus, cryptococcus, and syphilis.

Infections of the adrenal glands, particularly with cytomegalovirus, are found in nearly half of patients with untreated HIV at autopsy. However, a much lower percentage have clinical Addison disease. The diagnosis of adrenal insufficiency in patients with HIV is often problematic. A cortisol resistance syndrome has been described in patients with HIV, and a revision of normal range for the cosyntropin test for these patients has been advocated (normal peak cortisol over 22 mcg/dL).

Bilateral adrenal hemorrhage may occur with sepsis, heparin-associated thrombocytopenia, anticoagulation, or the antiphospholipid antibody syndrome. It may occur in association with major surgery or trauma, presenting about 1 week later with pain, fever, and shock. It may also occur spontaneously and present with flank pain. Meningococcemia may be associated with purpura and adrenal insufficiency secondary to adrenal infarction (Waterhouse-Friderichsen syndrome).

Adrenoleukodystrophy is an X-linked peroxisomal disorder causing accumulation of very long-chain fatty acids in the adrenal cortex, testes, brain, and spinal cord. Adrenal insufficiency ultimately occurs in 80% of affected patients. It presents most commonly in childhood or adolescence but can manifest at any age.

Congenital adrenal insufficiency occurs in several conditions. Familial corticosteroid deficiency is an autosomal recessive disease that is caused by germline mutations in the adrenal ACTH receptor (melanocortin 2 receptor, MC2R). It is characterized by isolated cortisol deficiency and ACTH resistance and may present with neonatal hypoglycemia, frequent infections, and dark skin pigmentation. Triple A (Allgrove) syndrome is caused by a mutation in the AAAS gene that encodes a protein known as ALADIN (***al***acrima, ***a***chalasia, a***d***renal ***i***nsufficiency, ***n***eurologic disorder). Cortisol deficiency usually presents in infancy but may not occur until the third decade of life.

Congenital adrenal hyperplasia is caused by various genetic defects in the enzymes responsible for adrenal steroid synthesis. Due to defective cortisol synthesis, patients have variable degrees of adrenal insufficiency and increased levels of ACTH that causes hyperplasia of the adrenal cortex. The most common enzyme defect is *P450c21 (21-hydroxylase deficiency)*, with a prevalence of about 1:18,000. Women with 21-hydroxylase deficiency have a block in adrenal steroid biosynthesis that causes an accumulation of 17-hydroxyprogesterone (17-OHP) and other steroid precursors that are shunted to another biosynthetic pathway to produce excessive androstenedione and testosterone. At birth, affected women may have variable ambiguous genitalia, with fusion of labia and clitoromegaly. Less serious enzymatic blocks may present with hirsutism and virilization, particularly after puberty, which has been called "late onset" congenital adrenal hyperplasia. Males are more prone to escape detection at birth, since they have normal genitalia but then present later in the newborn period with shock and hyponatremia.

Drugs that cause primary adrenal insufficiency include mitotane, abiraterone acetate, and the tyrosine kinase inhibitors lenvatinib and vandetanib. **Rare causes** of adrenal insufficiency include lymphoma, metastatic carcinoma, scleroderma, amyloidosis, and hemochromatosis.

Clinical Findings

A. Symptoms and Signs

The onset of symptoms can occur suddenly but usually develops gradually over months or years. The diagnosis is often delayed, since many early symptoms are nonspecific. Over 90% of patients describe fatigue, reduced stamina, weakness, anorexia, and weight loss. Over 80% of affected patients present with symptoms of orthostatic hypotension (aggravated by dehydration caused by nausea or vomiting), lightheadedness with standing, salt craving, and eventually hyperpigmentation of skin and gums. Abdominal pain, nausea, and vomiting eventually develop in most patients; diarrhea can occur, aggravating dehydration and hypotension. Fevers and lymphoid tissue hyperplasia may also occur. Patients often have significant pain: arthralgias, myalgias, chest pain, abdominal pain, back pain, leg pain, or headache. Psychiatric symptoms include anxiety, irritability, and depression; by the time of diagnosis, over 40% of patients have been told that their symptoms were psychological. Cerebral edema can cause headache, vomiting, gait disturbance, and intellectual dysfunction that may progress to coma. Hypoglycemia can occur and worsen the patient's weakness and mental functioning. Patients treated long-term for adrenal insufficiency appear to be more prone to pneumonia and GI and UTIs.

Skin hyperpigmentation due to increased pituitary secretion of α-MSH varies among affected patients (eg, from none to increased freckling to diffuse darkening that resembles a suntan or a bronze appearance). Sun-exposed areas darken the most, but nonexposed areas darken as well. Hyperpigmentation is often especially prominent over the knuckles, elbows, knees, posterior neck, palmar creases, gingival mucosa, and vermilion border of the lips. Nail beds may develop longitudinal pigmented bands. Nipples and areolas tend to darken. The skin also darkens in pressure areas, such as the belt or brassiere lines and the buttocks. Skin folds and new scars may also become pigmented. Conversely, patches of autoimmune vitiligo can be found in about 10% of patients. Scant axillary and pubic hair typically develops in women.

In pregnancy, undiagnosed adrenal insufficiency is rare, since the condition tends to cause anovulation and reduced fertility. Undiagnosed adrenal insufficiency can cause intrauterine growth retardation and fetal loss. Pregnant women with undiagnosed adrenal insufficiency can experience shock from adrenal crisis, particularly during the first trimester, concurrent illness, labor, or postpartum.

Patients with preexistent type 1 diabetes experience more frequent hypoglycemia with the onset of adrenal insufficiency, such that their insulin dosage must be reduced.

Acute adrenal crisis is an immediate threat to life. Affected patients have magnified symptoms of chronic adrenal insufficiency and experience an acute deterioration in their health, typically with acute GI symptoms and fever that can mimic an abdominal emergency. Infections (lower respiratory, urinary, or GI) are common triggers for acute adrenal crisis. Patients also frequently experience back pain, arthralgias, and profound fatigue. They may have delirium or coma, sometimes aggravated by hypoglycemia. Adrenal crisis is marked by orthostatic dizziness and hypotension (blood pressure below 100 mm Hg systolic or 20 mm Hg lower than their baseline). Most patients have hyponatremia, hyperkalemia, and some degree of lactic acidosis. Severe hypocalcemia has been reported. **Stress (Takotsubo) cardiomyopathy** and HF can also occur. Serum troponins can be extremely high without any coronary insufficiency or permanent myocardial damage. Without glucocorticoid replacement, hypotension can progress to life-threatening shock that is unresponsive to intravenous fluids and vasopressors (see Treatment).

B. Laboratory Findings

Typically, there is mild anemia, moderate neutropenia, lymphocytosis, and eosinophilia (total eosinophil count > 300/mcL). Among patients with chronic adrenal insufficiency, the serum sodium is usually low (88%) and the potassium elevated (64%). However, patients with vomiting or diarrhea may not be hyperkalemic. Fasting hypoglycemia is common. Hypercalcemia may be present.

A plasma cortisol < 3 mcg/dL (83 nmol/L) at 8 AM is diagnostic, especially if accompanied by simultaneous elevation of the plasma ACTH level > 200 pg/mL (44 pmol/L). The diagnosis is confirmed by a simplified cosyntropin stimulation test: (1) Synthetic $ACTH_{1-24}$ (cosyntropin), 0.25 mg, is given intramuscularly. (2) Serum cortisol is obtained 45 minutes after cosyntropin is administered. Normally, serum cortisol rises to at least 20 mcg/dL (550 pmol/L), whereas patients with adrenal insufficiency have stimulated serum cortisol levels < 20 mcg/dL (550 pmol/L). For patients receiving corticosteroid treatment, hydrocortisone must not be given for at least 8 hours before the test. Other corticosteroids (eg, prednisone, dexamethasone) do not interfere with specific assays for cortisol. Cosyntropin is usually well tolerated, but infrequent (< 5%) side effects have included hypersensitivity reactions with nausea, headache, dizziness, dyspnea, palpitations, flushing, edema, and local injection site reactions.

One or more serum anti-adrenal antibodies are found in about 50% of cases of autoimmune Addison disease. The sensitivity of four serum anti-adrenal antibodies is as follows: cytoplasmic antibodies (26%), 21-hydroxylase antibodies (21%), 17-hydroxylase antibodies (21%), and side-chain cleavage antibodies (16%). Antibodies to thyroid (45%) and other tissues may also be present.

Elevated plasma renin activity (PRA) indicates the presence of depleted intravascular volume and the need for fludrocortisone administration. Serum epinephrine levels are low in untreated patients with adrenal insufficiency.

Congenital adrenal hyperplasia due to 21-hydroxylase deficiency is usually diagnosed at birth by "heel prick" screening for high levels of 17-OH progesterone in females due to ambiguous genitalia. Males and patients with milder enzyme defects may present later. In adults, 8 AM serum 17-OHP levels 200–800 ng/dL (6–24 nmol/L) are considered borderline high. For borderline high 17-OHP levels, a cosyntropin stimulation test is performed (0.25 mg subcutaneously) followed 60 minutes later by measurement of serum cortisol and serum 17-OHP. Stimulated levels > 1000 ng/dL (30.3 nmol/L) confirm the diagnosis.

Young men with idiopathic Addison disease are screened for X-linked adrenoleukodystrophy by determining plasma very long-chain fatty acid levels; affected patients have high levels.

C. Imaging

When adrenal insufficiency is not clearly autoimmune, a CT scan of the adrenal glands should be obtained. The adrenals are enlarged in about 85% of cases related to metastatic or granulomatous disease. Adrenal calcifications occur in 50% of tuberculous Addison cases but are also seen with hemorrhage, fungal infection, pheochromocytoma, and melanoma. Small, noncalcified adrenals are seen in autoimmune Addison disease.

Differential Diagnosis

Patients with secondary adrenal insufficiency due to ACTH deficiency have normal mineralocorticoid production and do not develop hyperkalemia (see Hypopituitarism). In contrast to Addison disease, patients with secondary adrenal insufficiency have normal to decreased skin pigmentation that has been described as "alabaster skin." Hemochromatosis also causes bronze skin hyperpigmentation, and hemochromatosis may in fact be the cause of Addison disease. Acute adrenal crisis must be distinguished from other causes of shock (eg, septic, hemorrhagic, cardiogenic).

The constitutional symptoms may be mistaken for cancer, anorexia nervosa, or emotional stress. Acute adrenal insufficiency must be distinguished from an acute abdomen in which neutrophilia is the rule, whereas in adrenal insufficiency there is lymphocytosis and eosinophilia. The neurologic manifestations of Allgrove syndrome and adrenoleukodystrophy (especially in women) may mimic multiple sclerosis. Hyperkalemia can be caused by hyporeninemic hypoaldosteronism from type IV renal tubular acidosis. Hyperkalemia is also seen with rhabdomyolysis, hyperkalemic paralysis, and some drugs (eg, ACE inhibitors, spironolactone, and drospirenone) (see Chapter 24).

Hyponatremia is seen in many other conditions (eg, hypothyroidism, diuretic use, HF, cirrhosis, vomiting, diarrhea, severe illness, or major surgery) (see Figure 24–1). Nearly 40% of critically ill patients have low serum cortisol levels due to low serum albumin levels; their total serum cortisol levels may be low but their serum free cortisol levels are normal.

Complications

Any of the complications of the underlying disease (eg, tuberculosis) are more likely to occur in adrenal insufficiency, and intercurrent infections may precipitate an acute adrenal crisis. Associated autoimmune diseases are common (see above).

Treatment

A. General Measures

Patients and family members must be thoroughly educated about adrenal insufficiency. *Patients are advised to wear a medical alert bracelet or neck medallion reading, "Adrenal insufficiency—takes cortisone."* Patients should also carry a wallet medical card and smartphone medical ID that guides hospital staff on the specific protocol for an adrenal crisis. It is also advisable for patients to carry an emergency kit that includes a supply of oral hydrocortisone or other glucocorticoid for oral stress dosing as well as ondansetron ODT and Solu-Cortef 100 mg injectable hydrocortisone. Patients need to be provided with a dose escalation schedule for increased corticosteroids for illness, accidents, or prior to minor surgical procedures and for increased fludrocortisone for hot weather or prolonged strenuous exercise. Patients must receive advance instructions to seek medical attention at an emergency facility immediately in the event of vomiting or severe illness.

B. Specific Therapy

Replacement therapy should include corticosteroids with mineralocorticoids for primary adrenal insufficiency. In mild cases, corticosteroids alone may be adequate.

1. Corticosteroid replacement therapy—Maintenance therapy for most patients with Addison disease is 15–30 mg of hydrocortisone orally daily in two divided doses (10–20 mg in the morning; 5–10 mg in the evening) or three divided doses (eg, 10 mg at 7 AM, 10 mg at 1 PM, and 5 mg at 7 PM). Adjustments in dosage are made according to the clinical response. The corticosteroid dose should be kept at the lowest level at which the patient feels clinically well.

Patients with partial ACTH deficiency (basal morning serum cortisol above 8 mg/dL [220 mmol/L]) require hydrocortisone replacement in lower doses of about 5 mg orally twice daily or even 10 mg every morning. Some patients feel better with the substitution of prednisone (2–7.5 mg/day orally) or methylprednisolone (2–6 mg/day orally), given in divided doses. Fludrocortisone is not required. For mild illness or mild-moderate surgical stress, corticosteroid doses are doubled or tripled.

Plenadren MR (5- or 20-mg modified-release tablets) is a once-daily dual-release oral preparation of hydrocortisone that may be administered in the morning (usual dose range is 20–30 mg daily). It is not available in the United States but is available in the United Kingdom and European Union.

Patients must be monitored carefully for clinical signs of over- or under-replacement of corticosteroid replacement therapy. A proper corticosteroid dose usually results in clinical improvement. Fatigue may be an indication of suboptimal dosing of medication, electrolyte imbalance, or concurrent hypothyroidism or diabetes mellitus. A WBC count with a differential can be useful, since a relative neutrophilia and lymphopenia can indicate corticosteroid over replacement, and vice versa. Serum ACTH levels vary substantially and should not be used to determine dosing.

Caution: Increased corticosteroid dosing is required in circumstances of infection, trauma, surgery, stressful diagnostic procedures, or other forms of stress. For mild illness or mild-moderate surgical stress, corticosteroid doses are doubled or tripled. For severe illness, trauma, or major surgical stress, hydrocortisone 100 mg is given intravenously, followed by 200 mg daily, given as either a continuous intravenous infusion or as 50 mg boluses given every 6 hours intravenously or intramuscularly and then reduced to usual doses as the stress subsides. Following major trauma, increased doses of replacement hydrocortisone may be required for up to several weeks. Lower doses, oral or parenteral, are used for less severe stress. For immunizations that are given with an adjuvant, such as varicella zoster (Shingrix), there is sufficient local inflammation that increased doses of hydrocortisone are recommended for 5 days following the immunization. The dose is reduced back to normal as the stress subsides. Decreased corticosteroid dosing is required when medications are prescribed that inhibit corticosteroid metabolism by blocking the isoenzyme CYP34A, particularly the antifungals ketoconazole or itraconazole, the antidepressant nefazodone, anti-HIV protease inhibitors, and cobicistat. Rifampin increases hydrocortisone clearance, necessitating increased corticosteroid dosing. During the third trimester of pregnancy, corticosteroid requirements are higher, so usual corticosteroid doses are increased by 50%.

2. Mineralocorticoid replacement therapy—Fludrocortisone acetate has a potent sodium-retaining effect. The dosage is 0.05–0.3 mg orally daily or every other day. In the presence of postural hypotension, hyponatremia, or hyperkalemia, the dosage is increased. Similarly, in patients with fatigue, an elevated PRA indicates the need for a higher replacement dose of fludrocortisone. If edema, hypokalemia, or hypertension ensues, the dose is decreased. The dose of fludrocortisone replacement can also be adjusted based upon serum electrolytes and plasma renin activity. During treatment with hydrocortisone with maximum doses appropriate for stress, fludrocortisone replacement is not required. Some patients cannot tolerate fludrocortisone and must substitute NaCl tablets to replace renal sodium loss.

3. DHEA replacement therapy—In a double-blind clinical trials, women with Addison disease taking DHEA 50 mg orally each morning experienced an improved sense of well-being, decreased depression and anxiety, increased sexuality, increased muscle mass, and a reversal in bone loss at the femoral neck. It requires about 4 months for symptomatic improvements to be fully noted. Women may note unwanted androgenic side effects (acne, increased body hair), which may improve with a dose reduction. Because over-the-counter preparations have variable potencies, it is best to have the pharmacy formulate this with pharmaceutical-grade micronized DHEA.

4. Treatment of hyperandrogenism in women with congenital adrenal hyperplasia (CAH)—Treatment of women with hirsutism and virilism from CAH require glucocorticoid replacement to reduce ACTH levels that drive the adrenal steroidogenic pathways. Typical replacement doses of hydrocortisone, prednisone, or methylprednisolone are usually insufficient; however, supraphysiological glucocorticoid replacement doses are dangerous, resulting in Cushing syndrome and childhood short stature. Therefore, glucocorticoids are usually administered jointly with **crinecerfont** (Crenessity) (100 mg twice daily), an oral medication that blocks corticotrophin releasing factor 1 (CRF_1) receptors on pituitary corticotroph cells, blocking excess pituitary ACTH secretion. Serum androstenedione levels are followed to make glucocorticoid dose adjustments. Crinecerfont is generally well-tolerated, but patients can experience symptoms of adrenal insufficiency if glucocorticoid replacement is inadequate. (See Chapter 20.)

5. Treatment of acute adrenal crisis—If acute adrenal crisis is suspected but the diagnosis of adrenal insufficiency is not yet established, intravenous access must be established. Blood is drawn for cultures, plasma ACTH, serum cortisol, serum glucose, BUN, creatinine, and electrolyte levels. A UA is obtained to screen for a UTI. Without waiting for the results, treatment is initiated *immediately* with hydrocortisone, 100 mg by intravenous bolus followed by 50 mg intravenously every 6 hours as either intravenous boluses or a continuous intravenous infusion. The hydrocortisone dosage may then be reduced according to the clinical picture and laboratory test results.

Intravenous fluids are administered as either 0.9% normal saline or 0.9% normal saline/5% dextrose solutions. A volume of 2–3 L is given quickly and then the intravenous rate is reduced according to clinical parameters and frequent serum electrolytes and glucose determinations. When intravenous saline is stopped, mineralocorticoid replacement is commenced with fludrocortisone, starting with 0.1 mg orally daily and adjusted according to serum electrolyte determinations.

Since bacterial infection frequently precipitates acute adrenal crisis, broad-spectrum antibiotics should be administered empirically while waiting for the results of initial cultures (see Table 34–5). The patient must also be treated for electrolyte abnormalities, hypoglycemia, and dehydration, as indicated.

When the patient can take food by mouth, hydrocortisone is administered orally in doses of 10–20 mg every 6 hours, and the dosage is reduced to maintenance levels as needed. Most patients ultimately require hydrocortisone twice daily (10–20 mg in the morning; 5–10 mg in the evening). Mineralocorticoid replacement is not needed when large amounts of hydrocortisone are given, but as its dose is reduced, it is usually necessary to add fludrocortisone acetate, 0.05–0.2 mg orally daily. Some patients never require fludrocortisone or become edematous at doses of more than 0.05 mg once or twice weekly. Once the crisis has passed, the patient must be evaluated to assess the degree of permanent adrenal insufficiency and to establish the cause, if possible.

Prognosis

The life expectancy of patients with Addison disease is reasonably normal, as long as they are compliant with their medications and knowledgeable about their condition. Cushing syndrome can develop, imposing its own risks, in patients who take excessive doses of corticosteroid replacement.

Adrenal crisis can occur in patients who stop their medication or who experience stress such as infection, trauma, or surgery without appropriately higher doses of corticosteroids. If adrenal crisis is unrecognized and untreated, shock that is unresponsive to fluid replacement and vasopressors can result in death. Acute adrenal crisis usually responds to rapid treatment with stress doses of glucocorticoids. Stress doses usually reverse the cardiomyopathy, however patients may require an intra-aortic balloon pump (IABP) as a critical temporary support. Patients who survive stress cardiomyopathy may develop a dilated cardiomyopathy or pericarditis with pericardial effusion and tamponade.

Auchus RJ et al. Phase 3 trial of crinecerfont in adult congenital adrenal hyperplasia. N Engl J Med. 2024;391:504. [PMID: 38828955]

Heidarpour M et al. Adrenal crisis-induced cardiogenic shock (ACCS): a comprehensive review. Heart Failure Reviews. 2025;30:227. [PMID: 39503801]

Magklis MSK et al. Adrenal insufficiency. Endotext. 2025. [PMID: 25905309]

Vaidya A et al. Adrenal insufficiency in adults. JAMA. 2025;334:714. [PMID: 40522647]

CUSHING SYNDROME (Hypercortisolism)

ESSENTIALS OF DIAGNOSIS

- Central obesity, muscle wasting, hirsutism, purple striae.
- Psychological changes and cognitive impairment.
- Osteoporosis, hypertension, poor wound healing.
- Hyperglycemia, leukocytosis, lymphocytopenia, hypokalemia.
- Elevated serum cortisol and urinary free cortisol. Lack of normal suppression by dexamethasone.

General Considerations

The term Cushing "syndrome" refers to the manifestations of excessive corticosteroids. Endogenous Cushing syndrome refers to increased cortisol production by the adrenal cortex. It is a rare disease with an estimated incidence of about 2.4 cases per million per year in the United States. About 75% of such cases are due to excessive ACTH secretion, while 25% are due to autonomous cortisol production by the adrenal cortex. Exogenous Cushing syndrome is most commonly due to supraphysiologic doses of oral corticosteroid drugs or chronic treatment with potent topical corticosteroids.

A. Cushing Disease with Elevated or Normal ACTH Levels (75%)

About 90% of cases of ACTH-dependent hypercortisolism are due to Cushing "disease," caused by a benign ACTH-secreting pituitary adenoma. The adenoma is typically smaller than 5 mm and located in the anterior pituitary (94%); however, about 6% are ectopic in locations such as the cavernous sinus, sphenoid sinus, ethmoid sinus, or posterior pituitary. Cushing disease is at least three times more frequent in women than men, and the median age is 41 years at diagnosis.

About 10% of cases of ACTH-dependent hypercortisolism are due to nonpituitary neuroendocrine neoplasms that produce ectopic ACTH. Ectopic locations include the lungs (55%), pancreas (9%), mediastinum-thymus (8%), adrenal (6%), GI tract (5%), thyroid (4%), and other sites (13%). About 15% of cases are due to ACTH from a source that cannot be initially located.

B. Cushing Syndrome with Low or Low-Normal ACTH (25%)

About 25% of cases of spontaneous Cushing syndrome are due to excessive *autonomous* secretion of cortisol by the adrenals. Cortisol secretion is independent of ACTH, and plasma ACTH levels are usually low or low-normal. Most cases are due to a unilateral adrenal tumor. Benign adrenal adenomas are generally small and produce mostly cortisol. Adrenocortical carcinomas are usually large when discovered and can produce excessive cortisol as well as androgens but may be nonsecretory. ACTH-independent macronodular adrenal hyperplasia can also produce hypercortisolism due to the adrenal cortex cells' abnormal stimulation by hormones such as catecholamines, arginine vasopressin, serotonin, hCG/LH, or gastric inhibitory polypeptide; in the latter case, hypercortisolism may be intermittent and food-dependent, and plasma ACTH levels may not be completely suppressed. Bilateral primary pigmented adrenal macronodular adrenocortical disease may be an isolated condition or part of the Carney complex, an autosomal dominant condition with additional features consisting of myxomas of the heart and skin with spotty skin pigmentation and facial freckles.

Clinical Findings

A. Symptoms and Signs

The manifestations of Cushing syndrome vary considerably. Early in the course of the disease, patients frequently describe nonspecific symptoms, such as fatigue or reduced endurance but may have few, if any, of the physical stigmata described below. Most patients eventually develop weight gain with central obesity and a plethoric "moon face," "buffalo hump," supraclavicular fat pads, protuberant abdomen, and thin extremities. Muscle atrophy causes weakness, with difficulty standing up from a seated position or climbing stairs. Patients may also experience backache, headache, hypertension, osteoporosis, avascular necrosis of bone, acne, hirsutism, superficial skin infections, and oligomenorrhea or amenorrhea in women or erectile dysfunction and diminished libido in men. Patients may have thirst and polyuria (with or without glycosuria), renal calculi, glaucoma, purple striae (especially around the thighs, breasts, and abdomen, and easy bruising. Unusual bacterial or fungal infections are common. Wound healing is impaired. Cushing syndrome adversely affects the brain, resulting in cognitive impairment and emotional disorders. Patients frequently have diminished ability to concentrate, impaired memory, reduced executive function, increased depression, and increased lability of mood. Anxiety may sometimes be accompanied by psychosis. Hyperglycemia with diabetes mellitus is common. Patients are susceptible to opportunistic infections. Hyperpigmentation is common with ectopic ACTH-secreting neoplasms that tend to produce very high plasma ACTH levels; hyperpigmentation is uncommon with pituitary Cushing disease.

Adrenal carcinomas are functional in 60% of cases. Cushing syndrome occurs in 45%, virilization in 15%, and a mixture of Cushing syndrome and virilization in 20%. At least 40% develop hypokalemia. Symptoms of Cushing syndrome due to adrenal carcinomas typically develop over weeks or months, whereas patients with Cushing disease or benign adrenal secretory tumors typically develop manifestations over months to years. Most patients are symptomatic and have gross metastases by the time of diagnosis. Microscopic metastases can be inferred from the presence of detectable cortisol levels following removal of the primary adrenal tumor in patients with a cortisol-secreting carcinoma and Cushing syndrome. More than 30% patients with adrenal carcinomas are now diagnosed incidentally, which tend to be less symptomatic and have a better prognosis.

B. Laboratory Findings

Glucose tolerance is impaired as a result of insulin resistance. Polyuria is present as a result of increased free water clearance; diabetes mellitus with glycosuria may worsen it. Patients with Cushing syndrome often have leukocytosis with granulocytosis (AGC > 8000 cells/mcL) and relative lymphocytopenia (RLC < 24%). Hypokalemia may be present, particularly in cases of ectopic ACTH secretion.

1. Diagnostic tests for hypercortisolism—Testing for hypercortisolism involves determining whether the following characteristics of Cushing syndrome are present: (1) lack of cortisol diurnal variation, (2) reduced suppressibility of cortisol by dexamethasone, (3) increased 24-hour urine free cortisol. At least two of these three tests must be positive to make a diagnosis of Cushing syndrome. In patients with a known adrenal mass, suppression of plasma ACTH also indicates hypercortisolism. Conflicting results are common.

Late-night (10–11 PM) salivary cortisol determinations are particularly useful, especially for ACTH-dependent hypercortisolism. Normal late-night salivary cortisol levels are < 150 ng/dL (4.0 nmol/L). Late-night salivary cortisol levels that are consistently > 250 ng/dL (7.0 nmol/L) are considered abnormal. The late-night salivary cortisol test has a relatively high sensitivity and specificity for Cushing syndrome.

The **overnight dexamethasone suppression test** is an easy screening test for hypercortisolism and is particularly sensitive for mild ACTH-independent hypercortisolism from an adrenal nodule. Dexamethasone 1 mg is given orally at 11 PM and serum collected for cortisol determination at 8 AM the next morning; a cortisol level < 1.8 mcg/dL (50 nmol/L) excludes Cushing syndrome with some certainty. However, 8% of established patients with pituitary Cushing disease have dexamethasone-suppressed cortisol levels < 2 mcg/dL (55 nmol/L). Several antiseizure drugs and rifampin accelerate the metabolism of dexamethasone, causing a lack of cortisol suppression by dexamethasone. Estrogens—during pregnancy or as oral contraceptives or HRT—may also cause lack of dexamethasone suppressibility.

A 24-hour urinary free cortisol and creatinine is usually used to confirm hypercortisolism in patients with a high late-night salivary cortisol or an abnormal dexamethasone suppression test. A high 24-hour urine free cortisol (> 50 mcg/day or 140 nmol/day in adults), or free cortisol to creatinine ratio of > 95 mcg cortisol/g creatinine, helps confirm hypercortisolism. However, many patients with mild hypercortisolism have a urinary free cortisol that is within the reference range. In pregnancy, urine free cortisol is increased, while 17-hydroxycorticosteroids remain normal and diurnal variability of serum cortisol is normal.

2. Diagnostic tests for the source of hypercortisolism—Once hypercortisolism is confirmed, a plasma ACTH and dehydroepiandrosterone sulfate (DHEAS) are obtained. A plasma ACTH < 6 pg/mL (1.3 pmol/L) indicates a probable adrenal tumor, whereas higher levels are produced by pituitary or ectopic ACTH-secreting tumors. Serum DHEAS levels can be used as a proxy for ACTH, since DHEAS secretion is ACTH-dependent; levels below the reference range and particularly < 40 mcg/dL (1.1 mcmol/L) imply ACTH-independent hypercortisolism from an adrenal tumor.

C. Imaging

In ACTH-independent Cushing syndrome, CT of the adrenals usually detects a mass lesion, which is most often an adrenal adenoma. Adrenocortical carcinomas can usually be distinguished from benign adrenal adenomas since they are generally larger (average 11 cm) and many have metastases that are visible on preoperative scans.

In ACTH-dependent Cushing syndrome, > 90% of pituitary lesions are microadenomas (< 10 mm). MRI of the pituitary gland demonstrates a pituitary lesion in about 70% of cases; however, the remaining 30% are invisible or difficult to discern. Very small lesions (< 5 mm) are not diagnostic. When the pituitary MRI is normal or shows a tiny (< 5 mm) irregularity that may be incidental, selective catheterization of the inferior petrosal sinus veins draining the pituitary is performed. ACTH levels in the inferior petrosal sinus that are more than twice the simultaneous peripheral venous ACTH levels are indicative of pituitary Cushing disease.

When inferior petrosal sinus ACTH concentrations are not above the requisite levels, a search for an ectopic source of ACTH is undertaken. Ectopic sources can be very small (2–5 mm). Location of an ectopic source begins with a whole-body DOTATATE PET/CT with special attention to the lungs (for carcinoid or small cell carcinoma), the thymus, pancreas, thyroid, and adrenals, for which the sensitivity is 80%. For suspected pulmonary sources, CT is used to better discern the tumor. For suspected abdominal sources, MRI is used.

Differential Diagnosis

Cushing syndrome without hypercortisolism is often due to iatrogenic glucocorticoid exposure (oral, topical, or inhaled).

Alcoholic patients can have hypercortisolism and many clinical manifestations of Cushing syndrome. Pregnant women have elevated serum ACTH levels, increased urine free cortisol, and high serum cortisol levels due to high serum levels of cortisol-binding globulin. Critically ill patients frequently have hypercortisolism, usually with suppression of serum ACTH. Depressed patients also have hypercortisolism that can be nearly impossible to distinguish biochemically from Cushing syndrome but are without clinical signs of Cushing syndrome. Anorexia nervosa and bulimia can be mistaken for Cushing syndrome, owing to the muscle wasting and extraordinarily high urine free cortisol levels found in anorexia. Patients with severe obesity frequently have an abnormal dexamethasone suppression test, but the urine free cortisol is usually normal, as is diurnal variation of serum cortisol. Patients with familial cortisol resistance have hyperandrogenism, hypertension, and hypercortisolism without actual Cushing syndrome. Excessive ingestion of γ-hydroxybutyric acid (GHB, sodium oxybate) can also induce ACTH-dependent Cushing syndrome that resolves after the drug is stopped.

Some adolescents develop violaceous striae on the abdomen, back, and breasts; these are known as "striae distensae" and are not indicative of Cushing syndrome. Patients receiving antiretroviral therapy for HIV-1 infection frequently develop partial lipodystrophy with thin extremities and central obesity with a dorsocervical fat pad ("buffalo hump") causing pseudo-Cushing syndrome.

Treatment

Patients must receive treatment for cortisol-dependent comorbidities, including osteoporosis, psychiatric disorders, diabetes mellitus, hypertension, hypokalemia, muscle weakness, and infections. Bone densitometry is recommended for all patients and treatment is commenced for patients with osteoporosis.

A. Surgical Therapy

Pituitary Cushing disease is best treated with transsphenoidal selective resection of the pituitary adenoma, even when the pituitary MRI is normal or inconclusive. With an experienced pituitary neurosurgeon, remission rates range from 80% to 90%. Postoperative hyponatremia occurs frequently; serum sodium should be monitored often for the first 2 weeks postoperatively. The patient should be screened for secondary hypothyroidism with a serum free T_4 within 1–2 weeks after surgery. After successful pituitary surgery, the rest of the pituitary usually returns to normal function; however, the pituitary corticotrophs remain suppressed and require 6–36 months to recover normal function. Therefore, patients receive empiric replacement-dose hydrocortisone postoperatively. The cosyntropin test becomes abnormal by 2 weeks following successful pituitary surgery. Patients with secondary adrenal insufficiency and their families require patient education about the condition and must continue corticosteroid replacement until a cosyntropin stimulation test is normal.

Cushing disease may persist or recur after pituitary surgery, particularly when there has been cavernous sinus involvement. A pituitary MRI is obtained about 3 months postoperatively and repeated as indicated for clinical evidence of recurrent Cushing disease. For patients with persistent or recurrent Cushing disease, repeat transsphenoidal pituitary surgery may be warranted if the recurrent tumor is visible and deemed resectable. Otherwise, bilateral laparoscopic adrenalectomy is usually the best treatment option. Residual or recurrent ACTH-secreting pituitary tumors may also be treated with stereotactic radiosurgery.

Ectopic ACTH-secreting tumors should be surgically resected. If the tumor cannot be localized or is metastatic, laparoscopic bilateral adrenalectomy is usually recommended. Metastatic ACTH-secreting neuroendocrine tumors that are avid for DOTATATE on PET imaging may be treated with peptide receptor radionuclide therapy (PRRT) with a radioisotope-tagged octreotide analogue. Medical treatment with an oral combination of mitotane (3–5 g/24 hours), ketoconazole (0.4–1.2 g/24 hours), and metyrapone (3–4.5 g/24 hours) often suppresses the hypercortisolism.

Cortisol-secreting benign adrenal adenomas may be resected laparoscopically if they are smaller than 6 cm; cure is achieved in most patients. However, most patients experience prolonged secondary adrenal insufficiency. Patients with bilateral adrenal macronodular hyperplasia usually require bilateral adrenalectomies and an evaluation for Carney complex.

Adrenocortical carcinomas are resected surgically. If the adrenocortical carcinoma was functional, postoperative secondary adrenal insufficiency is a good prognostic sign, with an increased chance that the tumor was completely resected without metastases; however, detectable postoperative cortisol levels predict metastases, even if no metastases are detectable on scans.

B. Medical Therapy

For patients with Cushing syndrome who decline surgery or for whom surgery has been unsuccessful, medical therapy may be considered: **Osilodrostat** 2 mg orally twice daily can normalize urine free cortisol and improve the manifestations of hypercortisolism. It reduces cortisol synthesis by blocking the adrenal enzyme 11b-hydroxylase and can be used in patients with florid Cushing syndrome to control cortisol secretion; replacement hydrocortisone is usually required. Adverse effects include adrenal insufficiency, a prolonged cardiac QT interval, hypertension, hirsutism, and acne. **Metyrapone** also may be used for patients with secretory adrenocortical carcinoma whose hypercortisolism is not fully controlled with mitotane. **Etomidate** is an intravenous anesthetic agent that blocks adrenal steroidogenesis. It can be given in sub-anesthetic doses to control severe hypercortisolism in severely ill patients with Cushing syndrome.

Mineralocorticoid hypertension can be treated with spironolactone, eplerenone, finerenone, or dihydropyridine calcium channel blockers. Women with hyperandrogenism may be treated with flutamide. Cabergoline, 0.5–3.5 mg orally twice weekly, reduced hypercortisolemia in 40% of patients with Cushing disease in one small study. Pasireotide, a multireceptor-targeting somatostatin analog, is a treatment option for refractory ACTH-secreting pituitary tumors causing Cushing disease or Nelson syndrome.

Metastatic ACTH-producing tumors visible with ^{64}Cu-DOTATATE-PET imaging respond to therapy with somatostatin analogs; pasireotide LAR (60 mg intramuscularly every 28 days) or octreotide LAR (30–40 mg intramuscularly every 28 days) slows progression of the malignancy and reduces ACTH secretion in up to half such patients. Radionuclide therapy with several cycles of ^{177}Lu-DOTATATE has produced remissions in some patients.

Patients who are successfully surgically treated for Cushing syndrome typically develop "cortisol withdrawal syndrome," even when given replacement corticosteroids for adrenal insufficiency. Manifestations can include hypotension, nausea, fatigue, arthralgias, myalgias, pruritus, and flaking skin. Increasing the hydrocortisone replacement to 30 mg orally twice daily can improve these symptoms; the dosage is then reduced slowly as tolerated.

Mitotane is approved for use with adrenocortical carcinoma and reduces cortisol secretion over several weeks.

Patients with secretory adrenocortical carcinomas are usually treated with mitotane postoperatively, particularly if metastases are visible or cortisol is detectable postoperatively. Patients with non-secretory metastatic adrenocortical carcinomas have also responded to mitotane. It is typically given for 2–5 years postoperatively. Mitotane can cause hypogonadism and primary adrenal insufficiency. Replacement hydrocortisone or prednisone should be started when mitotane doses reach 2 g daily. The replacement dose of oral hydrocortisone starts at 15 mg in the morning and 10 mg in the afternoon but must often be doubled or tripled because mitotane increases cortisol metabolism and cortisol-binding globulin levels; the latter can artifactually raise serum cortisol levels. Mitotane also causes central hypothyroidism in 95% of patients within the first year of treatment.

Combined chemotherapy with etoposide, doxorubicin, cisplatin, and mitotane (EDP-M) is the most effective regimen for recurrent or metastatic adrenocortical carcinoma.

Prognosis

The manifestations of Cushing syndrome regress with time, but patients may have residual cognitive or psychiatric impairment, muscle weakness, osteoporosis, and sequelae from vertebral fractures. Continued impaired quality of life is more common in women compared to men. Younger patients have a better chance for full recovery.

Patients with Cushing syndrome from a benign adrenal adenoma experience a 5-year survival of 95% and a 10-year survival of 90%, following a successful adrenalectomy. Patients with Cushing disease from a pituitary adenoma experience a similar survival if their pituitary surgery is successful, which can be predicted if the postoperative nonsuppressed serum cortisol is < 2 mcg/dL (55 nmol/L). Following successful treatment, overall mortality remains particularly higher for patients with older age at diagnosis, higher preoperative ACTH concentrations, and longer duration of hypercortisolism. Patients in remission from Cushing disease continue to experience a higher mortality rate than expected, particularly from ischemic heart disease and from cerebral infarction, bacterial infections, and suicide.

Patients who have a complete remission after transsphenoidal surgery have a 15–20% chance of recurrence over the next 10 years. Recurrence of hypercortisolism may occur as a result of growth of an adrenal remnant stimulated by high levels of ACTH. The prognosis for patients with ectopic ACTH-producing tumors depends on the aggressiveness and stage of the particular tumor. Patients with ACTH of unknown source have a 5-year survival rate of 65% and a 10-year survival rate of 55%.

In patients with adrenocortical carcinoma, 5-year survival rates of treated patients have correlated with the ENSAT stage. For stage 1, the 5-year survival was 81%; for stage 2, 61%; for stage 3, 50%; and for stage 4, 13%.

Complications

Following bilateral adrenalectomy for Cushing disease, a pituitary adenoma may enlarge progressively (Nelson syndrome), causing local destruction (eg, visual field impairment, cranial nerve palsy) and hyperpigmentation. Following successful therapy for Cushing syndrome, secondary adrenal insufficiency occurs and requires long-term corticosteroid replacement. Five years after successful surgery, secondary hypoadrenalism resolves in about 58% of patients with pituitary Cushing disease, 82% of those with ectopic ACTH, and only 38% of those who had an adrenal tumor.

When to Refer

Dexamethasone suppression test is abnormal.

When to Admit

- Transsphenoidal hypophysectomy.
- Adrenalectomy.
- Resection of ectopic ACTH-secreting tumor.

Fleseriu M et al. Osilodrostat treatment of Cushing syndrome in real-world clinical practice: findings from the ILLUSTRATE study. J Endocr Soc. 2025;9:bvaf046. [PMID: 40226519]
Khalid S et al. Evaluation of hypercortisolism in mild autonomous cortisol secretion. JAMA Intern Med. 2025;185:1387. [PMID: 40892430]
Pfeffer A et al. Efficacy and safety of radiotherapy and systemic treatment in adrenocortical carcinoma: systematic review and meta-analysis. J Clin Endocrinol Metab. 2025;110:3599. [PMID: 40796146]
Rowell NP. Oncological management of adrenocortical carcinoma: an update and critical review. Oncol Ther. 2025;13:307. [PMID: 40979823]
Saini J et al. Dehydroepiandrosterone sulfate in diagnosing mild autonomous cortisol secretion and adrenal insufficiency. J Endocr Soc. 2025;9:braf136. [PMID: 40909019]

PRIMARY ALDOSTERONISM

ESSENTIALS OF DIAGNOSIS

- Hypertension may be severe or drug-resistant.
- Hypokalemia (in minority of patients) may cause polyuria, polydipsia, muscle weakness.
- Low plasma renin; elevated plasma and urine aldosterone levels.

General Considerations

Primary aldosteronism (hyperaldosteronism) refers to excessive adrenal aldosterone excretion associated with low plasma renin activity and serum aldosterone levels that are inappropriately high and nonsuppressible. Hypertension from primary aldosteronism causes more cardiovascular morbidity than does essential hypertension. Although most affected patients have hypertension, some may be normotensive. The prevalence of primary aldosteronism is 5–10% in hypertensive patients and at least 20% in patients with resistant hypertension. Primary aldosteronism should be suspected when the patient has early-onset hypertension or stroke (before age 50 years).

Low-renin hypertension accounts for about 30% of all hypertension cases. Primary aldosteronism and cases of low renin essential hypertension may overlap, making distinguishing between them difficult. Patients of all ages may be affected, but the peak incidence is between 30 years and 60 years. Excessive aldosterone production increases sodium retention; increases renal potassium excretion, which can lead to hypokalemia; and suppresses plasma renin.

Primary aldosteronism is most frequently caused by bilateral adrenal cortical hyperplasia (75%), which is more common in men with a 4:1 ratio, peaking between ages 50 and 60. Primary aldosteronism may be also caused by a unilateral aldosterone-producing adrenal cortical adenoma (Conn syndrome, 25%), which is more common in women with a 2:1 ratio, peaking between ages 30 and 50. It is important to distinguish the two, since a unilateral aldosteronoma (Conn syndrome) may be cured by surgical resection, whereas bilateral adrenal hyperplasia is treated medically.

Clinical Findings

A. Symptoms and Signs

Primary aldosteronism is the most common cause of refractory hypertension in youths and middle-aged adults. Patients have hypertension that is typically moderate but may be severe. Some patients have only diastolic hypertension, without other symptoms and signs. Edema is rarely seen in primary aldosteronism. Hypokalemia can produce muscle weakness, paresthesias with tetany, headache, polyuria, and polydipsia.

B. Laboratory Findings

Plasma potassium should be determined in hypertensive individuals. However, hypokalemia, once thought to be the hallmark of hyperaldosteronism, is present in only 37% of affected patients: 50% of those with an aldosterone-producing adenoma and 17% of those with adrenal hyperplasia. An elevated serum bicarbonate (HCO_3) concentration indicates metabolic alkalosis and is commonly present.

Endocrine society guidelines suggest that all hypertensive patients be screened for primary aldosteronism (PA). A useful single screening blood test should include plasma potassium, plasma renin activity, and serum aldosterone. If an unprepared screening test for PA is suspicious or the test was negative but the patient was taking potentially interfering medications, another prepared test should be ordered: (1) Medications that can *raise* PRA should be held prior to testing; mineralocorticoid receptor antagonists (spironolactone, eplerenone, finerenone) should be held for at least 4 weeks, and ACE inhibitors ARBs, thiazide, and loop diuretics ideally should be held for at least 2 weeks. (2) β-Blockers and clonidine can *suppress* PRA and should be held for at least 2 weeks to prevent a false-positive test. (3) Hypokalemia suppresses serum aldosterone and should be corrected with an oral potassium supplement. (4) The patient should consume a high-salt diet (NaCl > 6 g/day) for 3 days. Following appropriate patient preparation, a plasma potassium, plasma renin activity, and serum aldosterone should be repeated; it is prudent to also obtain a 24-hour urine collection for aldosterone and creatinine.

Table 29–9. Laboratory criteria for primary aldosteronism (PA).

(1) PRA ≤ 1.0 ng/mL/hour *or* DRC ≤ 8.2 mU/L
AND
(2) Serum aldosterone (immunoassay) ≥ 10 ng/dL (≥ 277 pmol/L) *or* (LC-MS/MS) ≥ 7.5 ng/dL (≥ 208 pmol/L)
AND
(3) Increased ARR Aldosterone (immunoassay ng/dL)/PRA (ng/mL/hour) > 20 *or* Aldosterone (LC-MS/MS ng/dL)/PRA (ng/mL/hour) > 15 Aldosterone (immunoassay pmol/L)/DRC (mU/L) > 70 *or* Aldosterone (LC-MS/MS pmol/L/)/DRC 9 mU/L) > 52
(4) Borderline testing for PA can be confirmed with a 24-hour urine aldosterone > 12 mcg/24 hours (> 33 nmol/24 hours) in the presence of a low PRA or DRC.

Modified from Adler GK et al. Primary Aldosteronism: An Endocrine Society Clinical Practice Guideline. J Clin Endocrinol Metab. 2025;110:2453. [PMID: 40658480]

ARR, aldosterone to renin ratio; DRC, direct renin concentration; LC-MS/MS, liquid chromatography—tandem mass spectrometry; PRA, plasma renin activity.

For blood testing, the patient should be out of bed for at least 2 hours and seated for 15–60 minutes before the blood draw, which should preferably be obtained between 8 AM and 10 AM.

Patients with primary aldosteronism have a suppressed PRA below < 1.0 ng/mL/hour, in conjunction with an increased serum aldosterone concentration (Table 29–9). To help confirm the diagnosis of primary aldosteronism, especially for patients with a suppressed PRA but lower serum aldosterone levels, a 24-hour urine aldosterone > 12 mcg/24 hours (> 33 nmol/24 hours) confirms PA.

Genetic testing for familial corticosteroid-remediable aldosteronisms is recommended for patients with confirmed primary aldosteronism by age 20 years and those with a family history of primary aldosteronism or stroke at young age (under age 40).

C. Imaging

All patients with biochemically confirmed primary aldosteronism require a thin-section CT scan of the adrenals to screen for a large adrenal adenoma or rare adrenal carcinoma. In the absence of a large adrenal adenoma, adrenal CT scanning cannot reliably distinguish unilateral from bilateral aldosterone excess (both having 78% sensitivity and specificity). Therefore, adrenal vein sampling is often required. Imaging with ^{11}C-MTO PET-CT can help determine laterality of aldosterone secretion and is an alternative to adrenal vein sampling to detect a small unilateral adenoma.

D. Adrenal Vein Sampling

Bilateral selective adrenal vein sampling is invasive, expensive, and not widely available. Adrenal vein sampling has a sensitivity of 95% and a specificity of 100% but only when performed by an experienced radiologist. This procedure entails a 0.6% risk of major complications.

Adrenal vein sampling therefore is indicated only if surgery is contemplated in order to direct the surgeon to the correct adrenal gland. It may not be required for patients contemplating surgery who are found to have an adrenal nodule and meet all three of the following criteria: (1) patient < aged 35 years; (2) a unilateral adrenal mass > 1 cm is evident on CT; (3) the patient has a very high aldosterone and low potassium. It also may not be required for patients whose blood pressure is already well controlled with spironolactone, eplerenone, or finerenone and for those with familial hyperaldosteronism. Adrenal vein sampling can be useful to identify the adrenal gland to be removed when there is no visible adrenal adenoma on CT imaging. It can also help avoid mistaken removal of an incidental nonsecreting adrenal adenoma. Lateralization is present when the aldosterone:cortisol ratio from one adrenal vein is at least four times that from the opposite adrenal vein. Aldosterone hypersecretion that is lateralized to one adrenal usually indicates that adrenal has a unilateral adenoma or unilateral hyperplasia, particularly when aldosterone secretion from the contralateral adrenal is suppressed. Patients with a unilateral adrenal mass should also be screened for hypercortisolism.

Differential Diagnosis

The differential diagnosis of primary aldosteronism includes other causes of hypokalemia in patients with essential hypertension, especially diuretic therapy; chronic depletion of intravascular volume stimulates renin secretion and secondary hyperaldosteronism (see Table 24–3).

Apparent mineralocorticoid excess syndrome may be caused by real (black) licorice ("natural licorice" or "licorice root") or anise-flavored drinks (sambuca, pastis), which contain glycyrrhizinic acid. Abiraterone, a drug therapy for prostate cancer, causes hypertension and hypokalemia. Similarly, the oral antifungal drugs itraconazole and posaconazolecan cause pseudohyperaldosteronism with hypertension and hypokalemia.

Oral contraceptives may increase aldosterone secretion in some patients. Renal vascular disease can cause severe hypertension with hypokalemia but PRA is high. Excessive adrenal secretion of other corticosteroids (besides aldosterone), certain congenital adrenal enzyme disorders, and primary cortisol resistance may also cause hypertension with hypokalemia. The differential diagnosis also includes Liddle syndrome, an autosomal dominant cause of hypertension and hypokalemia resulting from excessive sodium absorption from the renal tubule; renin and aldosterone levels are low.

Complications

Cardiovascular complications occur more frequently in primary aldosteronism than in idiopathic hypertension. Following unilateral adrenalectomy for Conn syndrome, suppression of the contralateral adrenal may result in temporary postoperative hypoaldosteronism, characterized by hyperkalemia and hypotension.

Treatment

The **unilateral adrenal adenoma** is usually treated by laparoscopic adrenalectomy. During pregnancy, such surgery is best performed during the second trimester. Long-term medical therapy is an option for unilateral hyperaldosteronism, if adequate blood pressure control can be maintained.

Primary aldosteronism from bilateral adrenal hyperplasia is best treated with medical therapy. Direct mineralocorticoid inhibitors are preferred over potassium sparing diuretics such as amiloride or triamterene. **Spironolactone** is the most effective drug. It is initiated at a dose of 25 mg orally once daily and titrated to a maximum of 200 mg daily. Spironolactone has antiandrogen activity and men usually experience breast tenderness, gynecomastia, or reduced libido. Spironolactone might lead to undervirilization of male infants and is contraindicated in pregnancy; reproductive-age women are cautioned to use contraception during therapy. **Canrenone** is an active metabolite of spironolactone that has less antiandrogenic effects; it is available in Europe. **Eplerenone**, 25–50 mg orally twice daily, is favored during pregnancy (FDA pregnancy category B) and for men, since it does not have antiandrogen effects. **Finerenone** is a nonsteroidal mineralocorticoid receptor antagonist with no antiandrogenic effects that has been used successfully for patients with primary aldosteronism. The starting dose is 20 mg/day if eGFR is > 60 mL/min/1.73 m^2, and 10 mg/day if eGFR is 25–60 mL/min/1.73 m^2. If tolerated, the dose may be titrated up to 40 mg/day. **Baxdrostat** is a highly selective aldosterone synthase inhibitor. Treatment with baxdrostat is started at 2 mg per day orally for the first 4 weeks, then increased to 4 mg or 6 mg daily. When beginning these anti-mineralocorticoid medications, blood pressure must be measured daily. Other antihypertensive drugs may be required, particularly amlodipine, ARBs, or ACE inhibitors; however, significant drops in blood pressure may occur when anti-mineralocorticoid and other antihypertensives are used together.

Prognosis

The hypertension from unilateral adrenal adenoma is reversible in about two-thirds of cases but persists or returns despite surgery in the remainder. The prognosis is much improved by early diagnosis and treatment. Only 2% of aldosterone-secreting adrenal tumors are malignant.

Adler GK et al. Primary aldosteronism: an Endocrine Society clinical practice guideline. J Clin Endocrinol Metab. 2025;110:2453. [PMID: 40658480]

Flack JM et al. Efficacy and safety of baxdrostat in uncontrolled and resistant hypertension. N Engl J Med. 2025;393:1363. [PMID: 40888730]

Hu J et al. Efficacy and safety of finerenone in patients with primary aldosteronism: a pilot randomized controlled trial. Circulation. 2025;151:196. [PMID: 39804908]

Teo AED et al. Approach to the patient with primary aldosteronism: role of molecular imaging. J Clin Endocrinol Metab. 2025;110:3559. [PMID: 40690719]

Yang J et al. Outcomes after medical treatment for primary aldosteronism: an international consensus and analysis of treatment response in an international cohort. Lancet Diabetes Endocrinol. 2025;13:119. [PMID: 39824204]

PHEOCHROMOCYTOMA & PARAGANGLIOMA

ESSENTIALS OF DIAGNOSIS

- "Attacks" of headache, perspiration, palpitations, anxiety. Multisystem crisis.
- Hypertension: sustained but often paroxysmal, especially during surgery or delivery; may be orthostatic.
- Elevated plasma free fractionated metanephrines.

General Considerations

Pheochromocytomas and sympathetic paragangliomas (collectively called PPGLs) are a type of neuroendocrine tumor with distinct genetics, secretions, and clinical presentations. They are rare, with a yearly incidence of 2–6 cases/million; however, many cases are undiagnosed during life. These tumors may be located in either or both adrenals; anywhere along the sympathetic nervous chain; and sometimes in the mediastinum, heart, or bladder. Pheochromocytomas arise from the adrenal medulla and are considered "intra-adrenal sympathetic paragangliomas"; they secrete epinephrine and norepinephrine. Paragangliomas arise from sympathetic paraganglia; about 50% of paragangliomas secrete norepinephrine, while the rest are nonfunctional or secrete only dopamine, normetanephrine, or chromogranin A (CgA). Nonsecretory paragangliomas arise in the head or neck, particularly in the carotid body, jugular-tympanic region, or vagal body. All PPGLs are potentially malignant, with metastases occurring in about 10–15% of adrenal pheochromocytomas and 35–40% of paragangliomas.

PPGLs are dangerous and deceptive, causing death in up to one-third of patients prior to diagnosis. They account for < 0.4% of hypertension cases. The incidence is higher in hypertensive children and patients with moderate to severe hypertension, particularly in the presence of suspicious symptoms of headache, significant palpitations, or diaphoretic episodes. Nearly 50% of PPGLs are discovered incidentally on imaging studies. They account for about 4% of adrenal incidentalomas.

PPGLs are more heritable than any other tumor. About 40% of patients harbor a germline mutation in 1 of at least 30 known susceptibility genes, usually in an autosomal dominant manner with incomplete phenotypic penetrance. Genetic testing is recommended for all patients with these tumors.

von Hippel–Lindau (VHL) disease type 2 is associated with a 30% lifetime incidence of pheochromocytoma that can present as early as age 5 years or later in adulthood. The pheochromocytomas in VHL are less likely to be malignant (3.5%) compared to pheochromocytomas without VHL (about 10%). About 25% of these patients are asymptomatic and normotensive at diagnosis. The condition is also associated with hemangiomas of the retina, cerebellum, brainstem, and spinal cord; hyperparathyroidism; pancreatic cysts; endolymphatic sac tumors; cystadenomas of the adnexa or epididymis; pancreatic neuroendocrine tumors; and renal cysts, adenomas, and carcinomas; inheritance is autosomal dominant.

MEN 2 (MEN 2A) is associated with pheochromocytomas, MTC, hyperparathyroidism, and cutaneous lichen amyloidosis. Pheochromocytomas are often silent in MEN 2; at diagnosis, only about 50% have symptoms and fewer are hypertensive. The lack of symptoms may be due to earlier diagnosis through yearly screening of mutation carriers. **MEN 3 (MEN 2B)** may be familial, but usually arises from a de novo *ret* mutation; MEN 3 is associated with pheochromocytoma (50%), aggressive MTC, mucosal neuromas, and Marfan-like habitus.

von Recklinghausen neurofibromatosis type 1 (NF-1) is associated with an increased risk of pheochromocytomas/paragangliomas as well as cutaneous neurofibromas, optic and brainstem gliomas, astrocytomas, vascular anomalies, hamartomas, malignant nerve sheath tumors, and smooth-bordered café au lait spots.

Clinical Findings

A. Symptoms and Signs

Clinical manifestations of PPGLs vary according to the manner in which the tumor is discovered. Among PPGLs that are discovered incidentally on imaging study (64% of PPGLs), hypertension is present in 68% and a triad of headaches, palpitations, and sweats in 14%. Among PPGLs discovered through workup of patients with symptoms (32% of PPGLs), hypertension is present in 93% and the symptom triad in 28%. Approximately 4% of PPGLs are discovered during family surveillance for carriers of pathologic germline mutations, among whom hypertension and other symptoms usually are absent. PPGLs can be lethal unless they are diagnosed and treated appropriately.

PPGLs are "great mimics," presenting with a variety of symptoms that also are seen in more common conditions. Among patients with symptoms suspicious of a PPGLs who undergo diagnostic evaluations, < 1% have a confirmed diagnosis of PPGL. Hypertension may be sustained, paroxysmal, or sustained with paroxysmal spikes. A PPGL should be suspected if hypertension is severe or associated with palpitations or sweats. About 60% of patients have episodic nonspecific "spells." Other symptoms include anxiety, weakness/fatigue, dyspnea, nausea/vomiting, tremor, dizziness, chest pain, abdominal pain, paresthesias, or constipation. Vasospasm during an attack can cause Raynaud syndrome, mottled cyanosis, or facial pallor. As the attack subsides, facial flushing and drenching sweats can occur. Epinephrine secretion by a pheochromocytoma can cause episodic tachyarrhythmias, orthostatic hypotension, or syncope. Cardiac manifestations include acute coronary syndrome, cardiomyopathy, HF, and potentially fatal dysrhythmias. Catecholamine-induced cardiomyopathy can present with shock. Confusion, psychosis, paresthesias, seizures, transient ischemic attacks, or stroke may occur with cerebrovascular vasoconstriction or hemorrhagic stroke. Abdominal pain, nausea, vomiting, and even ischemic bowel can occur. Patients may experience increased appetite, loss of weight, numbness, or fevers. During pregnancy, pheochromocytomas can produce hypertension and proteinuria, mimicking eclampsia; vaginal delivery can produce hypertensive crisis followed by postpartum shock. Painful bony metastases may be a presenting symptom of metastatic pheochromocytoma.

Catastrophic hypertensive crisis and fatal cardiac arrhythmias can occur spontaneously or may be triggered by needle biopsy or manipulation of the mass, glucagon injection, vaginal delivery, trauma, anesthesia, or surgery (both unrelated to the tumor or for its removal). Exercise, bending, lifting, or emotional stress can trigger paroxysms. Bladder paragangliomas may present with paroxysms during micturition. Certain drugs can precipitate attacks: decongestants, amphetamines, cocaine, epinephrine, corticosteroids, fluoxetine and other SSRIs, metoclopramide, MAO inhibitors, caffeine, nicotine, and ionic intravenous contrast.

PPGLs can also produce other "ectopic" peptide hormones that rarely cause Cushing syndrome (ACTH), Verner-Morrison syndrome (VIP), or hypercalcemia (PTHrP). PPGLs can also release cytokines that can cause proteinuria, nephrotic syndrome, and acute respiratory distress syndrome (ARDS) that can occur alone or as part of a **multisystem crisis** (kidney dysfunction, liver failure, cardiomyopathy, cardiovascular collapse, and death).

B. Laboratory Findings

Plasma fractionated free metanephrines is the most sensitive test for secretory PPGLs. Free metanephrines are lower when the patient is supine than when ambulatory. The test is 97% sensitive for secretory tumors, so normal levels rule out secretory pheochromocytoma and paraganglioma with some certainty. Among patients with severe hypertension or "spells" caused by PPGLs, plasma fractionated free metanephrines are ordinarily at least three times the upper limit of normal. Misleading results arise in patients with relatively minor elevations in tumor markers (< 3 times the upper normal limit), in whom a secretory PPGL is rarely confirmed. (The exceptions are patients who are being monitored because they harbor a germline mutation for familial pheochromocytoma.) False-positive test results should be suspected when the ratio of normetanephrine to norepinephrine is < 0.52 or the ratio of metanephrine to epinephrine is < 4.2. In such cases, it is best to repeat biochemical testing under optimal conditions, including discontinuation of drugs and foods associated with false-positive testing for at least 2 weeks and having the patient lying supine in a quiet room for 30–90 minutes before the blood is drawn. Patients with persistent mild elevations in tumor markers may be followed clinically or undergo additional abdominal imaging (especially if they harbor a germline mutation for familial PPGL).

Urinary fractionated metanephrines and creatinine effectively confirm most pheochromocytomas that were detected by elevated plasma fractionated free metanephrines, including patients with marginal elevations. A 24-hour urine specimen is obtained, although an overnight or shorter collection may be used. Patients with pheochromocytomas generally have > 2.2 mcg of total metanephrine per milligram of creatinine, and > 135 mcg total catecholamines per gram creatinine. Urinary assay for total metanephrines is 97% sensitive for detecting functioning pheochromocytomas.

Plasma fractionated catecholamines may be helpful to confirm whether an adrenal tumor is a secretory pheochromocytoma. The test may also be useful for normotensive patients with a paraganglioma; the tumor may secrete only dopamine, which can be followed as a tumor marker.

Serum CgA is elevated in about 85% of patients with pheochromocytoma or paraganglioma and the levels correlate with tumor size, being higher in patients with metastatic disease. Serum CgA must be assayed in the fasting state, since levels rise after meals. Serum CgA is not specific for pheochromocytoma, so its measurement is not very useful for the initial diagnosis.

Clonidine suppression testing can help distinguish whether elevated plasma free normetanephrine levels are physiologic or indicative of pheochromocytoma. Plasma fractionated free metanephrines are measured before the administration of clonidine (0.3 mg orally) and 3 hours afterward. A fall of plasma normetanephrine into the normal range or a fall of > 40% from baseline helps rule out the presence of a tumor.

Hyperglycemia is present in about 35% of patients but is usually mild. Proteinuria is present in about 10–20% of patients. Leukocytosis is common.

C. Imaging

About 95% of pheochromocytomas and sympathetic paragangliomas arise in the abdomen or pelvis. Of these, about 90% are pheochromocytomas located in one or both adrenals. Extra-adrenal paragangliomas can be located anywhere sympathetic ganglia are present, particularly in the periaortic and perinephric region (75%), bladder and pelvis (15%), and thorax (10%). Imaging may also detect distant metastases to bones, lungs, or liver.

1. CT and MRI scanning—When an adrenal pheochromocytoma is suspected, a *noncontrast* CT scan of the abdomen is performed, with thin sections through the adrenals. *Glucagon should not be used during scanning, since it can provoke hypertensive crisis in patients with a pheochromocytoma.*

MRI scanning has the advantage of not requiring intravenous contrast dye; its lack of radiation makes it the imaging of choice during pregnancy and for serial imaging. Both CT and MRI scanning have a sensitivity of 90% for adrenal pheochromocytoma and 95% for adrenal tumors > 0.5 cm. However, both CT and MRI are less sensitive for detecting recurrent tumors, metastases, and paragangliomas. If no adrenal tumor is found, the scan is extended to include the entire abdomen, pelvis, and chest.

2. Nuclear imaging—^{64}**Gu-DOTATATE-PET** scanning is the most sensitive scan, detecting about 90% of pheochromocytomas, paragangliomas, and metastases. However, it is not entirely specific for these tumors. PET imaging gives crisper imaging than scintigraphy. Nuclear imaging is usually combined with volumetric imaging (CT or MRI) to determine the precise size and location of tumors.

^{18}**FDG-PET** scanning detects about 54% of metastases but is more sensitive for patients with *SDHB* germline mutations. However, ^{18}FDG-PET scanning is not specific for pheochromocytoma or paraganglioma.

^{123}**I-MIBG** whole-body scintigraphy can lateralize and confirm adrenal pheochromocytomas with a sensitivity of over 90%, but it is only 67% sensitive for extra-adrenal (paraganglioma) tumors and metastases and is also less sensitive for MEN 2– or MEN 3–related pheochromocytomas. ^{123}I-MIBG scintigraphy is also less sensitive for particularly aggressive tumors. Prior to the scan, the patient is given KI to competitively inhibit the uptake of free ^{123}I into the thyroid. Also, drugs that reduce ^{123}I-MIBG uptake should be avoided. Drug interference is suspected in negative ^{123}I-MIBG scans that do not show normal uptake in salivary glands.

Differential Diagnosis

Conditions that mimic pheochromocytoma include thyrotoxicosis, labile essential hypertension, myocarditis, glomerulonephritis or other renal lesions, eclampsia, acute intermittent porphyria, hypogonadal vascular instability (hot flushes), anxiety attacks, cocaine or amphetamine use, and clonidine withdrawal. Patients taking nonselective MAO inhibitor antidepressants can have hypertensive crisis after eating foods that contain tyramine. Patients with erythromelalgia can have hypertensive crises. Renal artery stenosis can cause severe hypertension. Plasma fractionated free metanephrines can be elevated in sleep apnea or with stressful illness. On CT scan, adrenal pheochromocytomas must be distinguished from adrenal adenomas and other masses.

Complications

All the complications of severe hypertension may be encountered. In addition, a catecholamine-induced cardiomyopathy may develop. Severe HF and cardiovascular collapse may develop in patients during a paroxysm. Sudden death may occur due to cardiac arrhythmia. ARDS and multisystem crisis can occur acutely and thus the initial manifestation of pheochromocytoma may be hypotension or even shock. Hypertensive crises with sudden blindness or cerebrovascular accidents are not uncommon.

After removal of the tumor, a state of severe hypotension and shock (resistant to epinephrine and norepinephrine) may ensue with precipitation of AKI or MI. Hypotension and shock may occur from spontaneous infarction or hemorrhage of the tumor.

Pheochromocytomas and paragangliomas may metastasize. Cells can also be seeded within the peritoneum, either spontaneously or as a complication during surgical resection. Such seeding of the abdomen can lead to multifocal recurrent intra-abdominal tumors, a condition known as pheochromocytomatosis.

Medical Treatment

Patients must receive adequate treatment for hypertension and tachyarrhythmias prior to surgery for pheochromocytoma/paraganglioma. Patients are advised to measure their blood pressures daily and immediately during paroxysms. Some patients with pheochromocytoma or paraganglioma are not hypertensive and do not require preoperative antihypertensive management. α-Blockers or calcium channel blockers can be used, either alone or in combination. Blood pressure should be controlled before cardioselective β-blockers are added for control of tachyarrhythmias.

α-Blockers are usually administered in preparation for surgery. Phenoxybenzamine is a long-acting nonselective α-blocker with a half-life of 24 hours; it is given initially in a dosage of 10 mg orally every 12 hours, increasing gradually by about 10 mg/day about every 3 days until hypertension is controlled. Maintenance doses range from 10 mg/day to 120 mg/day. Doxazosin (half-life 22 hours), a selective α_1-blocker, may also be used in doses of 2–32 mg daily. Optimal α-blockade is achieved when supine arterial pressure is below 140/90 mm Hg or as low as possible for the patient to have a standing arterial systolic pressure above 90 mm Hg.

Dihydropyridine calcium channel blockers (nifedipine ER, nicardipine ER, amlodipine) are very effective and are usually added to α-blockers but may be used alone. Nifedipine ER is initially given orally at a dose of 30 mg/day, increasing the dose gradually to a maximum of 60 mg twice daily. Calcium channel blockers are superior to phenoxybenzamine for long-term use, since they cause less fatigue, nasal congestion, and orthostatic hypotension. However, they should not be used for patients with severe HF. For acute hypertensive crisis (systolic blood pressure higher than 170 mm Hg), a nifedipine 10-mg capsule may be chewed and swallowed. Nifedipine is quite effective for treating acute hypertension in patients with PPGLs; it is reasonably safe as long as the blood pressure is carefully monitored.

β-Blockers (eg, metoprolol XL) are often required after institution of α-blockade or calcium channel blockade. *The use of a β-blocker as initial antihypertensive therapy has resulted in an "unopposed α" status that causes paradoxical worsening of hypertension.* Labetalol has combined α- and β-blocking activity and is an effective agent but can also cause paradoxical hypertension if used as the initial antihypertensive agent.

Surgical Treatment

Surgical removal of pheochromocytomas or abdominal paragangliomas is the treatment of choice. For surgery, a team approach—endocrinologist, anesthesiologist, and surgeon—is critically important. Laparoscopic surgery is preferred, but large and invasive tumors require open laparotomy. Patients with small familial or bilateral pheochromocytomas may undergo selective resection of the tumors, sparing the adrenal cortex; however, there is a recurrence rate of 10% over 10 years.

Prior to surgery, blood pressure control should be maintained for a minimum of 4–7 days or until optimal cardiac status is established. It may take a week or even months to correct ECG changes in patients with catecholamine myocarditis, and it may be prudent to defer surgery until then in such cases. Patients must be very closely monitored during surgery to promptly detect sudden changes in blood pressure or cardiac arrhythmias.

Pheochromocytoma & Paraganglioma in Pregnancy

Although rare, PPGLs must be considered in women with hypertension or tachycardia who are planning pregnancy. Susceptible members of known kindreds with familial pheochromocytoma syndromes should be screened for pheochromocytoma *while planning* pregnancy, even if totally asymptomatic. The diagnosis is typically delayed, since hypertension, tachycardia, abdominal pain, and chest pains are often attributed to preeclampsia and pregnancy itself. PPGL (versus preeclampsia) should be considered when hypertension presents before 20 weeks' gestation, is paroxysmal or severe, or if ankle edema and hyperuricemia are absent. Untreated pheochromocytoma results in mortality rates of 25% for the mother and 50% in the fetus. MRI (without gadolinium contrast) is preferred to detect an adrenal mass. Affected women with hypertension are treated with α blockade with doxazosin or phenoxybenzamine, calcium channel blockade (nifedipine or nicardipine), or both. β-Blockers should be used judiciously, since they can cause intrauterine growth retardation. The optimal time for laparoscopic surgical removal of a pheochromocytoma is during the second trimester and before 24 weeks' gestation. Women with a pheochromocytoma diagnosed after 28 weeks' gestation are best treated medically and usually have an elective cesarean section at 38 weeks' gestation.

Metastatic Pheochromocytoma & Paraganglioma

All PPGLs must be approached as possibly malignant. Surgical histopathology for PPGLs cannot reliably determine whether a tumor is malignant. About 15% of pheochromocytomas and up to 50% of abdominal paragangliomas eventually metastasize. Of patients with metastases, about 35% are detected when the primary tumor is discovered. Other metastases become clinically apparent 5.5 years (range 0.3–53 years) after initial diagnosis. Following initial surgery for PPGLs, it is essential to recheck blood pressure and plasma fractionated free metanephrine levels 6 weeks postoperatively, every 6 months for 5 years, and then yearly for life. Metanephrine levels also should be checked if hypertension, suspicious symptoms, or metastases become evident.

Since some metastases are indolent, it is important to tailor treatment according to the tumor's aggressiveness. Most surgeons resect the main tumor and larger metastases (debulking). Some asymptomatic, indolent metastases may be kept under close surveillance without treatment.

A. Somatostatin Analogs

Nearly 90% of metastatic pheochromocytomas and paragangliomas express somatostatin receptors and are visible on ^{64}Cu-DOTATATE-PET imaging. Patients with such tumors may receive a treatment trial of a somatostatin analog.

B. Chemotherapy

The most common chemotherapy regimen combines intravenous cyclophosphamide, vincristine, and dacarbazine (see Table 43–3). About one-third of patients experience some degree of temporary remission. Another chemotherapy regimen uses temozolomide, which is usually the best-tolerated chemotherapy and is particularly effective for metastatic pheochromocytoma or paraganglioma in patients with *SDHB* germline mutations. Tyrosine kinase inhibitor (TKI) therapy can also produce remissions. Metyrosine reduces catecholamine synthesis but does not slow the growth of metastases. **Belzutifan** targets PPGLs that are associated with germline or somatic mutations associated with a pseudohypoxic signature (eg, SDHx, Von Hippel Lindau, and FH mutations).

C. Targeted Radioisotope Therapy

1. Peptide receptor radionuclide treatment (PRRT)—This therapy uses a radioisotope-tagged somatostatin analog against neuroendocrine tumors that express somatostatin receptors. ^{177}Lu-DOTATATE (Lutathera) is FDA-approved for treating patients with metastatic gastroenteropancreatic neuroendocrine tumors (GEP-NETs); it is being used off-label to treat patients with metastatic PPGLs, 90% of which are avid for DOTATATE. The objective response rate is 25%, and the short-term disease control rate is 84%.

2. ^{131}I-iobenguane—About 60% of metastatic PPGLs have tumors with sufficient uptake of ^{123}I-MIBG scanning to allow for therapy with high-specific-activity ^{131}I-MIBG.

D. Treatment for Bone Metastases

Osteolytic bone metastases may be treated with external beam radiation therapy. Vertebral metastases and spinal cord compression require surgical decompression and kyphoplasty. Intravenous zoledronic acid or subcutaneous denosumab may also be administered to patients with osteolytic bone metastases.

Prognosis

The prognosis is good for patients with PPGLs that are resected before metastases or cardiovascular damage. Hypertension usually resolves after successful surgery but may persist or return in 25% of patients despite successful surgery. In such cases, biochemical reevaluation is required to detect a possible second or metastatic pheochromocytoma.

The surgical mortality is under 3% with the use of laparoscopic surgical techniques, intraoperative monitoring, and preoperative blood pressure control with α-blockers or calcium channel blockers.

Even if no metastases are evident at the time of surgery, lifetime surveillance is indicated for detection of later metastases. Patients with metastatic PPGLs have an extremely variable prognosis. Some metastases are indolent for several decades after the primary tumor diagnosis. Overall survival is better for patients with tumors that are nonfunctional, avid for MIBG, or have a Ki67 below 10%. Metastases from head-neck paragangliomas are particularly slow-growing.

Alkaissi H et al. Approach to the patient with metastatic pheochromocytoma and paraganglioma. J Clin Endocrinol Metab. 2025;110:2946. [PMID: 40317194]

Davidoff DF et al. Outcomes of SDHB pathologic variant carriers. J Clin Endocrinol Metab. 2024;109:2400. [PMID: 38605204]

Fischer A et al. Systemic therapy for patients with metastatic pheochromocytoma and paraganglioma. Best Pract Res Endocrinol Metab. 2025;39:10977. [PMID: 39880697]

Hashmi HZ et al. What is the rationale for the laboratory workup for suspected pheochromocytomas and paragangliomas? Cleve Clin J Med. 2023;90:150. [PMID: 36958610]

Jimenez C et al. Belzutifan for advanced pheochromocytoma or paraganglioma. N Engl J Med. 2025;393:2012. [PMID: 41124218]

Li M et al. Recurrent disease in patients with sporadic pheochromocytoma and paraganglioma. J Clin Endocrinol Metab. 2023;108:397. [PMID: 36190922]

Pacak K et al. Approach to the patient: concept and application of targeted radiotherapy in the paraganglioma patient. J Clin Endocrinol Metab. 2024;109:2366. [PMID: 38652045]

Zawadzka K et al. The role of cortisol secretion in pheochromocytomas and paragangliomas: clinical and perioperative implications. J Clin Endocrinol Metab. 2026;111:e541. [PMID: 40578302]

INCIDENTALLY DISCOVERED ADRENAL MASSES

Incidental adrenal masses (IAMs) are defined as adrenal nodules that are discovered incidentally on abdominal imaging obtained for other reasons. Their incidence is 4%, of which 20% are bilateral. They are uncommon in patients younger than 30 years (0.2%) and more common in patients older than 70 years (7%). About 85% are nonfunctioning adrenal adenomas; however, 14% secrete cortisol or aldosterone, which can cause Cushing syndrome or aldosteronism, respectively, and 7% are pheochromocytomas. Another 4% of IAMs represent metastases or adrenal adenocarcinomas. Other causes may include adrenal infection, hemorrhage, and cysts.

Autonomous cortisol secretion typically results in Cushing syndrome with low or low-normal plasma ACTH and serum DHEAS. Patients should be further assessed with a 1 mg dexamethasone suppression test (DST). (See Cushing Syndrome for details.) On the DST, an 8 AM serum cortisol ≥ 1.8 mcg/dL (50 nmol/L) indicates either Cushing syndrome or mild autonomous cortisol excess and a level ≥ 3 mcg/dL (83 nmol/L) portends an increased mortality risk, even without clinical manifestations of Cushing syndrome.

Patients with hypertension are screened for primary aldosteronism with a PRA and serum aldosterone (see Primary Aldosteronism).

All patients with an adrenal incidentaloma should be screened for pheochromocytoma with plasma fractionated free metanephrines, except those whose nodules meet all the following criteria: (1) normotensive, (2) nodule density on unenhanced CT density 10 HU or less, (3) size 3 cm diameter or less, and (4) morphology not suspicious. (See Pheochromocytoma.)

Surgical resection is recommended in adrenal incidentalomas larger than 4 cm, unless it is an unmistakably benign myelolipoma, hemorrhage, or adrenal cyst. The most important caveat is to not miss an adrenal adenocarcinoma or pheochromocytoma. Carcinomas account for 25% of adrenal masses larger than 6 cm diameter, 6% of masses 4–6 cm diameter, and 2% of masses smaller than 4 cm diameter. Smaller adrenal incidentalomas are usually observed after endocrine testing. Suspicion for malignancy in smaller adrenal incidentalomas is increased in patients under age 40 or and lesions that have suspicious features (heterogeneity or irregularity). A *noncontrast* CT should be performed to determine the density of the mass. Over 99% of adrenal pheochromocytomas and adrenocarcinomas have a density of 10 HU or more; patients with adrenal incidentalomas with densities of 10 HU or more that are not resected require both clinical follow-up and CT follow-up in 6–12 months.

Fassnacht M et al. European Society of Endocrinology clinical practice guidelines on the management of adrenal incidentalomas, in collaboration with the European Network for the Study of Adrenal Tumors. Eur J Endocrinol. 2023;189:G1. [PMID: 37318239]

Grazzini G et al. Adrenal mass evaluation: suspicious radiological signs of malignancy. Cancers (Basel). 2025;17:849. [PMID: 40075696]

Mirica A et al. Adrenal incidentaloma: from silent diagnosis to clinical challenge. Biomedicines. 2025;13:2298. [PMID: 41007858]

Park SS et al. Recent updates on the management of adrenal incidentalomas. Endocrinol Metab (Seoul). 2023;38:373. [PMID: 37583083]

Vassiliadi DA et al. Approach to the patient with bilateral adrenal masses. J Clin Endocrinol Metab. 2024;109:2136. [PMID: 38478374]

MALE HYPOGONADISM

ESSENTIALS OF DIAGNOSIS

- Diminished libido and erections.
- Fatigue, depression, reduced exercise endurance.
- Testes small or normal in size.
- Low serum total testosterone or free testosterone.
- Hypogonadotropic hypogonadism: low or normal serum LH and FSH.
- Hypergonadotropic hypogonadism: testicular failure, high serum LH and FSH.

General Considerations

Male hypogonadism is caused by deficient testosterone secretion by the testes. It may be due to (1) insufficient gonadotropin secretion by the pituitary (hypogonadotropic);

Table 29–10. Causes of male hypogonadism.

Hypogonadotropic (Low or Normal LH)	Hypergonadotropic (High LH)

Aging
Alcohol
Chronic illness
Constitutional delay of growth and puberty
Cushing syndrome
Drugs
  Estrogen
  GnRH agonist (leuprolide)
  Ketoconazole
  Marijuana
  Opioids (oral, injected, or intrathecal)
  Prior androgens
  Spironolactone
Genetic conditions[1]
Granulomatous diseases
Hemochromatosis
Hypopituitarism
Hypothalamic or pituitary tumors
Hypo-, hyperthyroidism
Idiopathic
Kidney disease
Lymphocytic hypophysitis
Major medical or surgical illnesses
Malnourishment
Obesity (BMI > 30)
	Aging
	Anorchia (bilateral)
	Autoimmunity
	Chemotherapy
	Idiopathic
	Klinefelter syndrome
	Leprosy
	Lymphoma
	Male climacteric
	Myotonic dystrophy
	Noonan syndrome
	Orchiectomy (bilateral or unilateral)
	Orchitis
	Radiation or radioisotope therapy
	Sertoli cell-only syndrome
	Testicular trauma
	Tuberculosis
	Uremia
	Viral infections (mumps)
	XY gonadal dysgenesis

[1]See text for discussion.
GnRH, gonadotropin-releasing hormone.

(2) pathology in the testes (hypergonadotropic); or (3) both (Table 29–10). Partial male hypogonadism may be difficult to distinguish from the physiologic reduction in serum testosterone seen in normal aging, obesity, and illness.

Etiology

A. Hypogonadotropic Hypogonadism (Low Testosterone with Normal or Low LH)

A deficiency in FSH and LH may be isolated or associated with other pituitary hormonal abnormalities. Hypogonadotropic hypogonadism can be primary, defined as failure to enter puberty by age 14, or it can be acquired. Causes of primary hypogonadotropic hypogonadism include congenital hypopituitarism, isolated hypogonadotropic hypogonadism, or simple constitutional delay of growth and puberty. Causes of acquired hypogonadotropic hypogonadism include genetic conditions, which account for about 40% of cases of isolated and idiopathic disease with a serum testosterone level < 150 ng/dL (5.2 nmol/L) (Table 29–10).

Partial male hypogonadotropic hypogonadism is defined as a serum testosterone in the range of 150–300 ng/dL (5.2–10.4 nmol/L). The main causes of acquired partial male hypogonadotropic hypogonadism include obesity, poor health, or normal aging, such that it is termed **age-related hypogonadism**. Hypogonadism also occurs commonly in patients with **opioid use disorder**. Other etiologies include pituitary or hypothalamic damage from factors such as tumors or traumatic brain injury. Spermatogenesis is usually preserved.

B. Hypergonadotropic Hypogonadism (Testicular Failure with High LH)

A failure of the testicular Leydig cells to secrete adequate testosterone causes a rise in LH and FSH. Acquired conditions that can cause testicular failure are listed in Table 29–9. Male hypergonadotropic hypogonadism can be caused by XY gonadal dysgenesis, partial 17-ketosteroid reductase deficiency, and a congenital partial deficiency in the steroidogenic enzyme CYP17 (17-hydroxylase). In men who have had a unilateral orchiectomy for cancer, the remaining testicle frequently fails, even in the absence of radiation or chemotherapy.

Klinefelter syndrome (47,XXY and its variants) is the most common chromosomal abnormality among males, with an incidence of about 1:500 (see Chapter 44). Although puberty occurs at the normal time, the degree of virilization is variable. Serum testosterone is usually low and gonadotropins are elevated. Adult men usually have somewhat reduced facial and pubic hair. Over 95% have azoospermia or severe oligospermia, although some sperm production is often present in their early teens. Other common findings include tall stature and abnormal body proportions that are unusual for hypogonadal men (eg, height > 3 cm greater than arm span).

XY gonadal dysgenesis describes several conditions that result in the failure of the testes to develop normally. *SRY* is a gene on the Y chromosome that initiates male sexual development. Mutations in *SRY* result in testicular dysgenesis. Affected individuals lack testosterone, which results in sex reversal: female external genitalia with a blind vaginal pouch, no uterus, and intra-abdominal dysgenetic gonads. Affected individuals appear as normal girls until their lack of pubertal development and amenorrhea leads to the diagnosis. Intra-abdominal rudimentary testes have an increased risk of developing a malignancy and are usually resected.

C. Androgen Insensitivity

Partial resistance to testosterone is a rare condition in which phenotypic males have variable degrees of apparent hypogonadism, hypospadias, cryptorchism, and gynecomastia. Serum testosterone levels are normal.

Clinical Findings

A. Symptoms and Signs

Hypogonadism that is congenital or acquired during childhood presents as delayed puberty. Men with acquired hypogonadism have variable manifestations, known as "testosterone deficiency syndrome." Most men experience decreased libido. Others report erectile dysfunction, poor morning erection, or hot sweats. Men often have depression, fatigue, or decreased ability to perform vigorous physical activity. The presenting complaint may also be infertility, gynecomastia, headache, fracture, or other symptoms related to the cause or result of the hypogonadism. The patient's history often gives a clue to the cause (Table 29–10).

Physical signs associated with hypogonadism may include decreased body, axillary, beard, or pubic hair, but only after years of severe hypogonadism. Men with hypogonadism lose muscle mass and gain weight due to an increase in subcutaneous fat. Examination should include measurements of arm span and height. Testicular size should be assessed with an orchidometer (normal volume is about 10–25 mL; normal length is 3–5 cm). Testicular size may decrease but usually remains within the normal range in men with postpubertal hypogonadotropic hypogonadism, but it may be diminished with testicular injury or Klinefelter syndrome. The testes must be palpated for masses and examined for evidence of trauma, infiltrative lesions (eg, lymphoma), or infection (eg, leprosy, tuberculosis).

B. Laboratory Findings

Serum testosterone circulates as "free" hormone and hormone bound to sex hormone–binding globulin. Serum total and free testosterone levels in men are highest at age 20–30 years. Thereafter, serum testosterone levels decline variably by an average of 1–2% annually; serum free testosterone levels decline even faster since sex hormone–binding globulin increases with age. In evaluating laboratory values for total and free testosterone, it is important to compare with age-adjusted reference ranges. Normal ranges for serum testosterone have been derived from non-fasting morning blood specimens, which tend to be the highest of the day.

The evaluation for hypogonadism begins with a morning (before 10 AM) blood draw for serum "ultrasensitive" total testosterone and free testosterone measurement. Serum total testosterone normal reference ranges vary with the lab and assay. **Serum *total* testosterone levels** are considered low if they are < 300 ng/dL (8.3 nmol/L); levels between 300 ng/dL and 350 ng/dL (12 nmol/L) are considered borderline low. **Serum *free* testosterone levels** are considered low if they are < 35 pg/mL (120 pmol/L); levels between 35 pg/mL and 40 pg/mL (140 pmol/L) are considered borderline low. A low serum testosterone or free testosterone should be verified with a repeat morning non-fasting assay, along with serum LH and PRL levels.

The main comorbid conditions that contribute to a decline in serum testosterone with aging include type 2 diabetes, obesity, metabolic syndrome, CVD, COPD, renal insufficiency, cancer, and opioids. After age 70, LH levels tend to rise, indicating a contribution of primary gonadal dysfunction. Testing for serum free testosterone is especially important for detecting hypogonadism in older men, who generally have high levels of sex hormone binding globulin. Serum LH levels are high in patients with hypergonadotropic hypogonadism but low or inappropriately normal in men with hypogonadotropic hypogonadism or normal aging. High serum estradiol levels are seen in men with obesity-related hypogonadotropic hypogonadism.

Mild anemia is common in men with hypogonadism. For men with long-standing severe male hypogonadism, osteoporosis is common, so bone densitometry is recommended.

1. Hypogonadotropic hypogonadism—A serum PRL determination is obtained to screen for a pituitary prolactinoma (see Table 29–1). Men with no discernible cause for hypogonadotropic hypogonadism should be screened for hemochromatosis. Adult men with hypogonadotropic hypogonadism should have an MRI of the pituitary/hypothalamus to search for a mass lesion in presence of one or more of the following: (1) severe hypogonadism (total testosterone < 150 ng/mL [5.2 nmol/L]), (2) elevated serum PRL, (3) other pituitary hormone deficiencies, or (4) symptoms of a mass lesion (headaches or visual field deficits).

2. Hypergonadotropic hypogonadism—Men with hypergonadotropic hypogonadism have low serum testosterone levels with a compensatory increase in FSH and LH. Klinefelter syndrome can be confirmed by karyotyping or by measurement of leukocyte XIST. Testicular biopsy is usually reserved for younger patients in whom the reason for primary hypogonadism is unclear.

Treatment

Testosterone replacement is reasonable for boys who have not entered puberty by age 14 years. It is also beneficial for most men with primary testicular failure (hypergonadotropic hypogonadism). Testosterone replacement or gonadal stimulation therapy is also warranted for men with severe hypogonadotropic hypogonadism of any etiology with serum testosterone levels < 150 ng/mL (5.2 nmol/L). Testosterone therapy should also be considered for men with low or low-normal serum testosterone or free testosterone, along with elevated serum LH levels. For other men without elevated serum LH levels and an average of at least two morning serum total testosterone levels < 275 ng/dL (9.5 nmol/L, "physiologic hypogonadism"), a trial of testosterone therapy may be considered, particularly if they have at least three of the following six symptoms: erectile dysfunction, poor morning erection, low libido, depression, fatigue, and inability to perform vigorous activity. Prior to treatment, it is prudent to screen for prostate cancer with a serum PSA in men over age 40.

Testosterone replacement should be continued only if a patient clearly derives clinical benefits from therapy. Therapy can be adjusted with an aim to improve clinical symptoms while maintaining normal serum levels of testosterone or free testosterone. Men with physiologic low-normal serum testosterone levels > 325 ng/dL (11.3 nmol/L) are unlikely to benefit from testosterone therapy.

Drug interactions can occur. Testosterone should be administered cautiously to men receiving coumadin, since the combination can increase the INR and risk of bleeding. Testosterone can predispose to hypoglycemia in men with diabetes receiving insulin or oral hypoglycemic agents, so close monitoring of blood sugars is advisable during initiation of testosterone therapy.

A. Therapies for Male Hypogonadism

1. Testosterone topical gels—Topical testosterone is usually applied once daily in the morning after showering. One or two fingers are used to apply the gel evenly to skin, followed by hand washing. Topical testosterone should not be

Table 29–11. Topical testosterone formulations and recommended daily doses.

Medication	Available Formulations	Recommended Daily Dose and Suggestion Application Site
Testosterone 1% gel	*Packets:* 12.5 mg/1.25 g, 25 mg/2.5 g, or 50 mg/5 g *Tubes:* 50 mg/5 g	50–100 mg
Testosterone 2% gel	*Pump:* 10 mg/0.5 g actuation	40–70 mg
Androgel 1% gel	*Packets:* 25 mg/2.5 g, 50 mg/5 g *Pump:* 12.5 mg per actuation	50–100 mg Apply to the shoulders
Androgel 1.6% gel	*Pump:* 20.25 mg per actuation	40.5–81 mg
Testim 1% gel	*Tubes:* 50 mg/5 g	50–100 mg Apply to shoulders, upper arms, or abdomen
Fortesta 2% gel (not available in the United States)	*Pump:* 10 mg per actuation	40–70 mg Apply to shoulders, upper arms, thighs, or abdomen
Testogel (not available in the United States)	*Sachet:* 50 mg/5 g	Apply to shoulders, upper arms, or abdomen
Vogelxo 1% gel	*Packets or tubes:* 50 mg/5 g *Pump:* 12.5 mg/1.25 g per actuation	50–100 mg Apply to the shoulders

applied to the breast or genitals. The gel should be allowed to air-dry (about 10 minutes) before dressing. Before close contact with people, a shirt must be worn or the areas of application washed with soap and water to prevent transfer of testosterone to them. The patient should avoid swimming, showering, or washing the application area for at least 2 hours following application. Table 29–11 lists topical testosterone formulations and dosages.

The serum testosterone level should be determined about 14 days after starting therapy; if the level remains below normal or the clinical response is inadequate, the daily dose may be increased to 1.5–2 times the initial dose. Serum testosterone levels vary considerably during the day after topical testosterone gel application, such that a single serum testosterone level may not accurately reflect the average serum testosterone for that individual.

2. Parenteral testosterone—The dose and injection intervals are adjusted according to the patient's clinical response and serum testosterone levels drawn just before the next injection is due. A target serum testosterone level of 500 ng/dL (17.3 nmol/L) is suggested. **Testosterone cypionate** is an intramuscular testosterone formulation that is available in solutions containing 200 mg/mL. Its main advantage is low cost. The usual dose is 200 mg every 2 weeks or 300 mg every 3 weeks. It is usually injected into the gluteus medius muscle in the upper lateral buttock, alternating sides. The injection technique must include sterile precautions and draw-back prior to injection to ensure against intravenous injection, which can result in pulmonary oil embolism.

Testosterone pellets (Testopel) are a long-lasting depot testosterone formulation that is available as individual vials containing a single 75-mg implantable pellet in each vial. With sterile technique, the skin of the upper-outer buttock is anesthetized with lidocaine; using a trocar, the pellets are injected subcutaneously in doses of 150–450 mg every 3–6 months as an in-office procedure.

Testosterone undecanoate (Aveed in United States and Nebido in Europe) is a long-lasting depot testosterone formulation that is restricted to qualified health care facilities, due to the risk of anaphylaxis and pulmonary oil embolism. Aveed is administered as a 750 mg IM injection every 10 weeks.

3. Testosterone nasal gel—Intranasal gel testosterone (Natesto) is self-administered by a metered-dose nasal pump: one pump actuation (5.5 mg) into each nostril three times daily. The nasal pump needs to be primed by inverting it and pressing the pump 10 times before it is used the first time. It should not be used concurrently with intranasal sympathomimetic decongestants. Adverse effects include nasopharyngitis, sinusitis, bronchitis, epistaxis, nasal discomfort, and headache.

4. Oral testosterone undecanoate—Three oral capsule preparations of testosterone undecanoate include: (1) **Jatenzo** (158 mg, 198 mg, 237 mg, 316 mg, or 396 mg taken twice daily); (2) **Kyzatrex** (100 mg, 150 mg, or 200 mg taken twice daily); (3) **Tlando** (112.5 mg taken as 2 capsules twice daily). The recommended starting doses are Jatenzo, 237 mg twice daily; Kyzatrex, 200 mg twice daily; and Tlando, 225 mg twice daily, each taken with food. Dose adjustments are made after 7 days according to clinical response and serum testosterone levels obtained 3–9 hours (varies with each formulation) after oral dose. Side effects are those of nonoral testosterone with additional side effects including an increase in systolic blood pressure (average 4 mm Hg) with risk of adverse cardiovascular events, polycythemia, and GI intolerance.

5. Clomiphene citrate—Men with functional hypogonadotropic hypogonadism usually respond well to clomiphene citrate that is administered orally in doses that are titrated to achieve the desired clinical response with a serum testosterone level of about 500 ng/dL (17.3 nmol/L). Begin with clomiphene 25 mg on alternate days and increased to 50 mg on alternate days if necessary, with a maximum dose of 50 mg daily. Serum testosterone levels usually normalize while spermatogenesis usually improves.

6. Gonadotropins—Patients with hypogonadotropic hypogonadism may require therapy with gonadotropins, particularly to induce fertility. Men may receive hCG 2000 units subcutaneously three times weekly for 6 months; if the semen analysis shows inadequate sperm, FSH 75 units subcutaneously three times weekly is added. Men often prefer long-term therapy with hCG over transdermal testosterone therapy, since hCG therapy maintains higher serum testosterone levels in the upper-half of the reference range, thereby improving masculinization and muscle strength. The dose of hCG for chronic administration is 1500–2000 units subcutaneously three times weekly, with adjustments according to serum testosterone determinations.

7. Weight loss—When hypogonadotropic hypogonadism is due to morbid obesity, significant weight loss often improves serum testosterone levels. The rise in serum testosterone is proportionate to the weight loss.

B. Benefits of Testosterone Replacement or Stimulation Therapy

Testosterone therapy given for the indications listed under Treatment usually benefits men with low serum testosterone and at least three manifestations of hypogonadism. Replacement testosterone therapy can improve overall mood, sense of well-being, sexual desire, and erectile function. It also improves anemia, bone density, physical vigor, and muscle strength. Testosterone replacement improves exercise endurance and stair climbing ability. Long-term testosterone replacement causes significant weight loss and a reduction in waist circumference. After 2 years of testosterone replacement, muscle mass increases about 4.5%, while fat mass decreases by about 9.1%. Appropriate testosterone replacement therapy also appears to improve longevity.

C. Risks of Testosterone Replacement or Stimulation Therapy

Testosterone therapy does not appear to increase the risk of prostate cancer or BPH above that of normal men, provided serum testosterone levels are maintained in the normal reference range. However, testosterone therapy is contraindicated in the presence of active prostate cancer. Hypogonadal men who have had a prostatectomy for low-grade prostate cancer, and who have remained in complete remission for several years, may have testosterone therapy given cautiously while monitoring serum PSA levels.

In the large double-blind placebo-controlled TRAVERSE study of transdermal testosterone replacement in hypogonadal men at high cardiac risk, there was no increased risk of death, major cardiovascular events, BPH, or prostate cancer. However, there was a small increased risk for PE (0.9% versus 0.5%), atrial fibrillation (3.5% versus 2.4%), and kidney injury (2.3% versus 1.5%). Another study showed a small increased fracture risk (3.5% versus 2.5%).

Erythrocytosis is more common with intramuscular injections of testosterone enanthate than with transcutaneous testosterone. Testosterone therapy tends to aggravate sleep apnea in older men, likely through CNS effects. A formal evaluation for sleep apnea is recommended for all high-risk patients with snoring, obesity, partner's report of apneic episodes, nocturnal awakening, unrefreshing sleep with daytime fatigue, or hypertension.

Testosterone therapy frequently increases acne that is usually mild and tolerated; topical antiacne therapy or a reduction in testosterone replacement dosage may be required. Increases in intraocular pressure have occurred during testosterone therapy. During the initiation of testosterone replacement therapy, gynecomastia develops in some men, which usually is mild and tends to resolve spontaneously; switching from testosterone injections to testosterone transdermal gel may help this condition.

D. Risks of Performance-Enhancing Anabolic Steroids

Performance-enhancing agents, particularly androgenic anabolic steroids, are used by up to 2% of young athletes and by 20–65% of power sport athletes. They are often used as part of a "stacking" polypharmacy that may include nandrolone decanoate, dimethandrolone, testosterone propionate, or testosterone enanthate. These androgens are usually illegal, often contaminated by toxic substances (such as arsenic), and can produce toxic hepatitis, dependence, aggression, depression, dyslipidemias, gynecomastia, acne, male pattern baldness, hepatitis, thromboembolism, and cardiomyopathy.

Prognosis of Male Hypogonadism

If hypogonadism is due to a pituitary lesion, the prognosis is that of the primary disease (eg, tumor, necrosis). The prognosis for restoration of virility is good if testosterone is given. In one large study, cardiovascular risk was reduced in hypogonadal men over age 40 who were receiving testosterone replacement therapy to maintain serum testosterone levels within the normal reference range.

Applewhite J et al. Testosterone replacement therapy in men on active surveillance for prostate cancer. J Sex Med. 2025;22:432. [PMID: 39895152]

Bhasin S et al. Testosterone treatment in middle-aged and older men with hypogonadism. N Engl J Med. 2025;393:581. [PMID: 40768717]

Braga MA et al. Long-term cardiovascular safety of testosterone-replacement therapy in middle-aged and older men: a meta-analysis of randomized controlled trials. Am J Cardiovasc Drugs. 2025;25:767. [PMID: 40694252]

McMahon A, Fantus RJ. Testosterone replacement therapy for testosterone deficiency in older men. Clin Geriatr Med. 2025;41:163. [PMID: 40345771]

Muir CA et al. Efficacy of gonadotropin treatment for induction of spermatogenesis in men with pathologic gonadotropin deficiency: a meta-analysis. Clin Endocrinol (Oxf). 2025;102:167. [PMID: 39445789]

MALE GYNECOMASTIA

ESSENTIALS OF DIAGNOSIS

- Palpable enlargement of the male breast, often asymmetric or unilateral.
- Glandular gynecomastia: typically tender.
- Fatty gynecomastia: typically nontender.
- Must be distinguished from carcinoma or mastitis.

General Considerations

Gynecomastia is defined as the presence of palpable glandular breast tissue in males. Gynecomastia is a common condition, and its incidence is increasing in all age groups. The causes are multiple and diverse. Pubertal gynecomastia develops in 60% of boys, more commonly teenagers who are overweight; the swelling usually subsides spontaneously within a year.

In adult men with gynecomastia, 45% of cases are idiopathic and attributed to obesity or physiologic gynecomastia of older men. Other causes include hypogonadism (11%) and medications (20%), particularly anabolic steroids and spironolactone, and in men with chronic liver or kidney disease. Men with HIV may develop gynecomastia from retroviral therapy with nonnucleoside reverse transcriptase inhibitors, especially efavirenz.

Gynecomastia also commonly develops in men receiving hormonal therapy for prostate cancer. Monotherapy with the androgen receptor pathway inhibitor (ARPI) **bacalutamide** causes gynecomastia in 70%; hence cotreatment with androgen deprivation therapy (ADT) or prophylactic treatment with low-dose tamoxifen or radiation therapy to the breasts commonly is given. Monotherapy with second generation ARPIs (**enzalutamide**, **darolutamide**, **apalutamide**) cause breast pain in about 50% of men. Conversely, treatment with the androgen synthesis inhibitor **abiraterone** rarely causes gynecomastia, since it is usually given with a gonadotropin inhibitor.

Gynecomastia is uncommon in men treated with traditional ADT that blocks GnRH release, such as **leuprolide** (GnRH agonist) injections or oral **relugolix** (GnRH antagonist). The addition of ADT to ARPI therapy reduces the risk of gynecomastia to about 1–4%.

Clinical Findings

A. Symptoms and Signs

The male breasts must be palpated to distinguish firm true glandular gynecomastia from softer fatty pseudogynecomastia in which only adipose tissue is felt. The breasts are best examined both seated and supine. Using the thumb and forefinger as pincers, the subareolar tissue is compared to nearby adipose tissue. Fatty tissue is usually diffuse and nontender. True glandular enlargement beneath the areola may be tender. Pubertal gynecomastia is characterized by tender discoid enlargement of breast tissue 2–3 cm in diameter beneath the areola. The following characteristics are worrisome for malignancy: asymmetry; location not immediately below the areola; unusual firmness; or nipple retraction, bleeding, or discharge. The examination must also include an assessment of masculinization, examination of the testes for size and masses, and examination of the penis for hypospadias.

B. Laboratory Findings

In the presence of true glandular gynecomastia, laboratory studies should be drawn between 7–10 AM due to the circadian rhythm of testosterone. Standard testing should include hepatic transaminases, serum creatinine, serum testosterone, free testosterone, LH, FSH, PRL, TSH, FT_4, β-hCG, and estradiol. These tests help determine whether primary hypogonadism (low serum testosterone, high LH), secondary hypogonadism (low serum testosterone, low or normal LH), or androgen resistance may be present. High serum testosterone levels plus high LH levels characterize partial androgen insensitivity syndrome. A serum PRL is obtained to screen for hyperprolactinemia and pituitary/hypothalamic lesions. Serum β-hCG and estradiol levels are obtained to screen for malignancy-associated gynecomastia. Detectable levels of β-hCG implicate a testicular tumor (germ cell or Sertoli cell) or other malignancy (usually lung or liver). Increased serum estradiol levels may result from testicular tumors, increased β-hCG, liver disease, obesity, adrenal tumors (rare), true hermaphroditism (rare), or aromatase gene gain-of-function mutations (rare). A karyotype for Klinefelter syndrome is obtained in men with persistent gynecomastia without obvious cause.

C. Imaging and Biopsy

Investigation of unclear cases should include bilateral mammography and a chest CT to search for bronchogenic or metastatic carcinoma. Benign mammographic findings make malignancy very unlikely. Suspicious mammographic findings require ultrasound-guided FNA and cytologic examination to distinguish gynecomastia from benign lesions (pseudogynecomastia, lipoma, posttraumatic hematoma/fat necrosis, epidermal inclusion cyst), lymphoma, and male breast cancer. Male breast cancer and gynecomastia may coexist.

Men with a high serum hCG or estradiol levels should have the test confirmed with repeat testing. Confirmed increased levels warrant a testicular ultrasound. If the testicular ultrasound is normal, high serum estradiol levels may warrant a CT of the adrenal glands; high serum hCG levels may warrant additional CT scanning to detect rare hCG-secreting carcinomas of the lung, mediastinum, liver, stomach, or kidney.

Treatment

Pubertal gynecomastia often resolves spontaneously within 1–3 years. Drug-induced gynecomastia resolves within months in most patients after the offending drug is removed. Patients with painful or persistent gynecomastia may be treated with medical therapy, usually for 9–12 months.

Selective estrogen receptor modulator (SERM) therapy is effective for true glandular gynecomastia. Raloxifene, 60 mg orally daily for 3–4 months, reduces breast volume by > 50% in about 90% of patients. Tamoxifen reduces breast volume by > 50% in about 60% of patients.

Aromatase inhibitor (AI) therapy is also reasonably effective. A starting dose of anastrozole for male gynecomastia is 0.5 mg orally three times weekly. Serum estradiol is monitored and the dose adjusted to keep the serum estradiol in the middle of the male reference range. Anastrozole reduces breast volume significantly in about 50% of adolescents over 6 months; significant size reduction can be seen within 1 month. Serum estradiol levels fall while serum testosterone levels rise. Long-term AI therapy in adolescents is not recommended because of the possibility of inducing osteoporosis and of delaying epiphyseal fusion, which could cause an increase in adult height.

Gynecomastia caused by ARPIs for prostate cancer can be prevented or treated with the addition of a GnRH antagonist (relugolix).

Testosterone therapy for men with hypogonadism may improve or worsen preexistent gynecomastia.

Surgical correction is reserved for patients with persistent or severe gynecomastia.

Blackburn J et al. Klinefelter syndrome: a review. Clin Endocrinol (Ocf). 2025;102:565. [PMID: 39806878]

Celik AI, Bezgin T. Spironolactone-induced gynecomastia. N Engl J Med. 2025;393:2151. [PMID: 41297008]

Swerdloff RS et al. Gynecomastia: etiology, diagnosis, and treatment. Endotext (Internet). 2023. [PMID: 25905330]

Tsuboi I et al. Incidence, management, and prevention of gynecomastia and breast pain in patients with prostate cancer undergoing antiandrogen therapy: a systematic review and meta-analysis of randomized controlled trials. Eur Urol Open Sci. 2025;73:31. [PMID: 39935942]

Disorders of Parathyroid Glands & Bone Metabolism

Anne Schafer, MD

30

DISEASES OF THE PARATHYROIDS

The concentration of calcium in the blood is tightly regulated and maintained within a narrow physiologic range. That homeostasis is orchestrated by parathyroid hormone (PTH), which is secreted by the parathyroid glands in response to decreased serum calcium concentration. PTH increases osteoclastic activity in bone, increases the renal tubular reabsorption of calcium, and stimulates the synthesis of 1,25-dihydroxycholecalciferol by the kidney. Meanwhile, PTH inhibits the reabsorption of phosphate and bicarbonate by the renal tubule. All of these effects cause a net increase in serum calcium.

HYPOPARATHYROIDISM & PSEUDOHYPOPARATHYROIDISM

ESSENTIALS OF DIAGNOSIS

- Tetany, carpopedal spasms, tingling of lips and hands, muscle cramps, irritability.
- Chvostek sign and Trousseau phenomenon.
- Hypocalcemia with low serum PTH; serum phosphate high; alkaline phosphatase normal; urine calcium excretion reduced.
- Serum magnesium may be low.

General Considerations

Hypoparathyroidism occurs when there is parathyroid gland destruction or abnormal development, or when there is altered regulation or impaired action of PTH. Pseudohypoparathyroidism results from unresponsiveness of target organs to PTH.

Surgical hypoparathyroidism, caused by the accidental removal or devascularization of one or more parathyroid glands, accounts for 75–80% of cases of hypoparathyroidism. After total thyroidectomy, it is estimated to affect 20–30% of patients transiently and up to 3–4% of patients permanently. The risk of hypoparathyroidism after total thyroidectomy is higher in patients with obesity; vitamin D deficiency; larger thyroid glands; substernal goiter or Graves disease; undergoing a reoperation; and when the surgeon does not perform a large volume of thyroidectomy operations. Hypoparathyroidism is defined as permanent if PTH level is still subnormal or undetectable a year after surgery.

Transient hypocalcemia may occur after surgical removal of one more parathyroid adenomas for primary hyperparathyroidism, due to suppression of the remaining normal parathyroids with low PTH levels. Another form of postoperative hypocalcemia, termed "hungry bone syndrome," may occur in patients with hyperparathyroidism who undergo parathyroidectomy due to accelerated calcium and phosphorus uptake by the skeleton. This is distinguishable from hypoparathyroidism because the PTH level is elevated and the phosphorus level is low. Vitamin D deficiency can make this process more likely and more severe.

With these risks in mind, *all patients undergoing thyroidectomy or parathyroidectomy must be observed closely for 12–24 hours with serum calcium and PTH.*

Autoimmune hypoparathyroidism may be isolated or combined with other endocrine deficiencies, such as in autoimmune polyendocrine syndrome type 1 (APS-1), also known as autoimmune polyendocrinopathy-candidiasis-ectodermal dystrophy (APECED).

PTH deficiency may result from **parathyroid damage** from heavy metals, granulomas, tumors, infection, and neck irradiation.

Magnesium deficiency causes functional hypoparathyroidism, blunting the actions of PTH on target organs. More profound hypomagnesemia (< 1.2 mg/dL) also inhibits PTH secretion. Correction of hypomagnesemia results in rapid disappearance of the condition.

Genetic hypoparathyroidism may be syndromic, such as in DiGeorge syndrome. Genetic hypoparathyroidism also may be nonsyndromic, such as in autosomal dominant hypocalcemia with hypercalciuria type 1, which is due to an activating mutation in the gene encoding the calcium-sensing receptor (CaSR).

Clinical Findings

A. Symptoms and Signs

Symptoms of hypocalcemia depend on its severity as well as its rate of development. Patients with acute hypocalcemia after parathyroidectomy may manifest symptoms despite having mildly low or low-normal serum calcium levels, while patients with chronic severe hypocalcemia may have few symptoms. **Neuromuscular irritability** presents with perioral numbness, paresthesias of the feet or hands, myalgias, muscle cramping, generalized muscle spasms with tetany, hyperactive reflexes, and laryngospasm that can cause respiratory stridor. Chvostek sign (facial muscle contraction on tapping the facial nerve in front of the tragus) is present in 70% of patients with hypocalcemia and 15% of individuals who are normocalcemic. Trousseau sign (flexion of the wrist and metacarpal-phalangeal joints with adduction of the fingers after application of a sphygmomanometer cuff inflated to over systolic blood pressure for 3 minutes) is present in over 90% of patients with hypocalcemia but in only about 1% of normocalcemic individuals. **Cardiovascular** manifestations of acute hypocalcemia include arrhythmias (7%), such as bradycardia, ventricular arrhythmias, and reduced EF. **CNS** manifestations include seizures (11%) as well as depression (12%), psychiatric changes, irritability, fatigue, cognitive impairment, and extrapyramidal symptoms. **Ophthalmic** manifestations include cataracts (17%); severe hypocalcemia may cause papilledema. **Renal** manifestations of chronic hypoparathyroidism occur due to hypercalciuria and include nephrolithiasis or nephrocalcinosis (15%), and renal insufficiency (12%). **Dermatologic** manifestations include dry, rough skin; dry hair; scalp and eyebrow hair loss; and brittle fingernails with transverse grooves. Chronic hypocalcemia with hyperphosphatemia can cause calcifications in soft tissues, such as joints, skin, and arteries.

B. Laboratory Findings

Serum calcium is low. Because serum calcium is largely bound to albumin, the serum *ionized* calcium should be determined in patients with hypoalbuminemia. Alternatively, the serum calcium level can be corrected for serum albumin level as follows:

$$\text{"Corrected" serum } Ca^{2+} = \text{Serum } Ca^{2+} \text{ mg/dL} + (0.8 \times [4.0 - \text{Albumin g/dL}])$$

Serum PTH levels are low, either overtly low or inappropriately low-normal, for the hypocalcemia. To confirm the diagnosis in a stable outpatient, serum PTH and calcium levels should be confirmed on a second test at least 2 weeks apart. Serum magnesium levels should always be measured.

Other lab abnormalities caused by hypoparathyroidism include an elevated serum phosphorus (due to the loss of PTH's phosphaturic effect), low 1,25-dihydroxyvitamin D, and high fractional urinary excretion of calcium.

C. Imaging

The kidneys should be imaged by noncontrast CT to determine the presence of nephrolithiasis or nephrocalcinosis. CT scanning of the brain may reveal calcifications of the basal ganglia and other areas in over 50% of patients with chronic hypocalcemia. The bones may appear denser than normal and bone mineral density (BMD) is usually increased, particularly in the lumbar spine. Cutaneous calcification may occur.

D. Other Examinations

Slit-lamp examination may show early posterior lenticular cataract formation. The ECG may show heart block, a prolonged QTc interval, and ST-T changes suggestive of an MI.

Complications

Acute tetany with stridor, especially if associated with vocal cord palsy, may lead to respiratory obstruction requiring tracheostomy. Seizures are common in untreated patients. Hypocalcemia can also cause HF and dysrhythmias. Ossification of the paravertebral ligaments may occur with nerve root compression; surgical decompression may be required. Overtreatment with vitamin D and calcium may produce nephrocalcinosis and impairment of kidney function. There may be associated autoimmunity causing celiac disease, pernicious anemia, or Addison disease.

Differential Diagnosis

Respiratory alkalosis from hyperventilation causes increased binding of calcium to albumin and thus can cause an acute drop in free ionized calcium.

Hypocalcemia may result from conditions other than hypoparathyroidism. Certain medications can cause hypocalcemia, including loop diuretics, plicamycin, phenytoin, and foscarnet. Denosumab and bisphosphonates, also can cause hypocalcemia, particularly in the setting of chronic kidney disease, or vitamin D deficiency. Hypocalcemia may also be due to malabsorption of calcium, magnesium, or vitamin D. It may develop in patients with osteoblastic metastatic carcinomas (especially breast, prostate) instead of the expected hypercalcemia. Hypocalcemia with hyperphosphatemia (simulating hypoparathyroidism) is seen in azotemia but may also be caused by large doses of intravenous, oral, or rectal phosphate preparations and by chemotherapy of responsive lymphomas or leukemias.

Pseudohypoparathyroidism is a genetic disorder characterized by hypocalcemia due to resistance to PTH. Subtypes are caused by different mutations involving the renal PTH receptor, the receptor's G protein, or adenylyl cyclase. Serum PTH levels are high. Hypocalcemia results from hypercalciuria due to renal tubular resistance to PTH.

Treatment

A. Prophylaxis Against Severe Postoperative Hypocalcemia

Post-thyroidectomy hypocalcemia can be detected early by closely monitoring serum PTH and calcium. If the serum calcium falls below 8.0 mg/dL (2.0 mmol/L) with a serum PTH below 10–15 pg/mL (1.0–1.5 pmol/L) after thyroid or parathyroid surgery, the patient is at high risk for hypocalcemia and can be prophylactically treated with calcitriol and calcium. An oral prophylactic regimen is calcitriol, 0.25–1 mcg twice daily, and calcium carbonate (with meals), 500–1000 mg twice daily.

B. Emergency Treatment for Acute Hypocalcemia

1. Airway—Be sure an adequate airway is present.

2. Intravenous calcium gluconate—For urgent treatment, the preferred intravenous salt is calcium gluconate (10 mL [10% solution] = 1 g calcium gluconate = 90 mg elemental calcium = 4.65 mEq). The first 10 mL is infused slowly over 10 minutes with ECG monitoring; this can be followed by a second 10 mL infused over 10 minutes with the same close monitoring until tetany ceases. Generally, an infusion is then begun. One method is to prepare 11 g calcium gluconate in D5W to provide a final volume of 1000 mL (~1 mg elemental calcium/mL), and to infuse it at a rate of 0.5–2.0 mg elemental calcium/kg/hour, adjusted to restore calcium concentration to the lower end of normal range.

3. Oral calcium—Oral calcium salts that supply 1–2 g of elemental calcium daily should be given as soon as possible.

4. Vitamin D preparations—Vitamin D therapy should be started as soon as oral calcium is begun (Table 30–1). 1,25-dihydroxycholecalciferol (calcitriol) has a very rapid onset of action but is not as long-lasting as vitamin D_3 if hypercalcemia occurs. Begin calcitriol at a dose of 0.25 mcg (1000 IU) orally each morning and titrate upward to near normocalcemia. Ultimately, doses of 0.5–4 mcg/day may be required.

5. Magnesium—If hypomagnesemia (serum magnesium < 1.8 mg/dL or < 0.8 mmol/L) is present, it must be corrected to treat the resulting hypocalcemia. For critical hypomagnesemia (serum magnesium < 1.0 mg/dL or < 0.45 mmol/L), 50% magnesium sulfate solution (5 g/10 mL) is diluted in 250 mL 0.9% saline or 5% dextrose in water and given by an intravenous infusion of 5 g over 3 hours, with further dosing based on serum magnesium levels. Long-term oral magnesium replacement may be given as magnesium oxide 500 mg (60% elemental magnesium) tablets, one to three times daily.

C. Maintenance Treatment of Hypoparathyroidism

Patients with mild hypoparathyroidism may require no therapy but need close monitoring for manifestations of hypocalcemia. Therapy is ordinarily required for symptomatic hypocalcemia or serum calcium below 8.0 mg/dL (2 mmol/L).

Vitamin D, calcium, and magnesium therapy: Patients with hypoparathyroidism have a reduced renal tubular reabsorption of calcium and are thus prone to hypercalciuria and kidney stones if the serum calcium is normalized with calcium and vitamin D therapy. Therefore, the goal is to maintain the serum calcium at the low end of normal or in a slightly low but asymptomatic range, approximately 8–8.6 mg/dL (2–2.15 mmol/L). It is prudent to monitor urine calcium with "spot" urine determinations and keep the level below 30 mg/dL (7.5 mmol/L), if possible. Hypercalciuria may respond to oral hydrochlorothiazide, 25 mg daily. Serum magnesium should be monitored and kept in the normal range with supplemental magnesium, if required. Serum phosphate should also be monitored and the serum calcium × phosphate product kept below 55 mg^2/dL^2 (4.4 $mmol^2/L^2$).

Calcium supplements include calcium carbonate (40% elemental calcium) that is best absorbed at the low gastric pH that occurs with meals. Calcium citrate (21% elemental calcium) is absorbed with or without meals and is a better choice for patients taking PPIs or H_2-blockers; it causes less GI intolerance than calcium carbonate. Calcium supplements are given orally in divided doses, and high doses may be required in hypoparathyroidism.

Vitamin D analogs are generally required for patients with chronic hypoparathyroidism (Table 30–1). The dosage of vitamin D preparations required to maintain target serum calcium levels can vary over time. In hypoparathyroidism, there is a deficiency in renal 1-hydroxylation of vitamin D; therefore, vitamin D analogs that are already 1-hydroxylated (activated) (such as calcitriol and alfacalcidol) are usually used. These active preparations have biologic half-lives of about 8 hours. Monitoring serum calcium, serum phosphate, and serum 25-(OH) vitamin D levels is recommended at least every 3–4 months.

For patients with recurrent hypocalcemia despite treatment with active vitamin D analogs, the use of cholecalciferol (vitamin D_3) or ergocalciferol (vitamin D_2) is a treatment option (Table 30–1). High doses may be needed because patients with hypoparathyroidism have reduced conversion of 1,25-OH_2D to 25-OHD. Because of their prolonged duration of action, if hypercalcemia or

Table 30–1. Vitamin D preparations used in the treatment of hypoparathyroidism.

	Available Preparations	Daily Dose	Duration of Action
Calcitriol	0.25 mcg (1000 IU) and 0.5 mcg (2000 IU) capsules; 1 mcg/mL oral solution; 1 mcg/mL for injection	0.25–2 mcg daily in the morning or divided into 2 doses; initial dose 0.25–0.5 mcg in the morning	3–5 days
Alfacalcidol	0.25 mcg, 0.5 mcg, and 1 mcg capsules	0.25 mcg with calcitriol, 0.5–3.0 mcg without calcitriol	3–5 days
Cholecalciferol (vitamin D_3)	400 IU/mL liquid, 1000–50,000 IU capsules (not available commercially in United States; may be compounded)	400–4000 IU with calcitriol, 10,000–100,000 IU without calcitriol	4–8 weeks
Ergocalciferol, ergosterol (vitamin D_2, calciferol)	8000 IU/mL liquid, 50,000 IU capsules	400–4000 IU with calcitriol, 50,000–200,000 IU without calcitriol	1–2 weeks

hypercalciuria develops, it may persist for weeks after the preparation is discontinued.

PTH-based therapies include **palopegteriparatide** and **teriparatide**. FDA-approved in 2024 for the treatment of adults with hypoparathyroidism, palopegteriparatide is a long-acting prodrug of PTH (1-34) that patients self-administer subcutaneously daily. It is an option for patients with difficulty maintaining stable serum and urinary calcium levels with calcium and vitamin D preparations. Teriparatide does not have regulatory approval for the treatment of hypoparathyroidism but has been used off-label. Due to its shorter half-life, it may be administered subcutaneously twice daily.

Transplantation of cryopreserved parathyroid tissue, removed during prior surgery, restores normocalcemia in about 23% of cases.

Hypoparathyroidism in pregnancy presents special challenges. Maternal hypocalcemia can adversely affect the skeletal development of the fetus and cause compensatory hyperparathyroidism in the newborn. Serum calcium levels should ideally be maintained in the lower half of normal reference range, since maternal hypercalcemia can suppress fetal parathyroid development, resulting in neonatal hypocalcemia. Serum calcium levels should be determined every 4 weeks during pregnancy and breast feeding and more frequently for the 3 months prepartum and postpartum. PTH and PTH analogues as well as thiazide diuretics are generally avoided during pregnancy.

Prognosis

Patients with mild hypoparathyroidism generally do well. Periodic serum calcium levels are required, since changes may call for modification of the treatment schedule. Hypercalcemia that develops in patients with seemingly stable, treated hypoparathyroidism may be a presenting sign of Addison disease.

Despite optimal therapy, patients with moderate-to-severe hypoparathyroidism have an overall reduced quality of life. Chronically affected patients frequently develop calcifications in their kidneys and basal ganglia. They have an increased risk of calcium kidney stones and kidney dysfunction as well as seizures, mood and psychiatric disorders, and a reduced overall sense of well-being. Therapy with rhPTH may prevent or improve these manifestations.

Bollerslev J et al. European Society of Endocrinology clinical practice guideline: treatment of chronic hypoparathyroidism in adults. Eur J Endocrinol. 2025;193:G49. [PMID: 41231236]

Khan AA et al. Efficacy and safety of parathyroid hormone replacement with TransCon PTH in hypoparathyroidism: 26-week results from the phase 3 PaTHway trial. J Bone Miner Res. 2023;38:14. [PMID: 39376010]

Khan S et al. Hypoparathyroidism: diagnosis, management and emerging therapies. Nat Rev Endocrinol. 2025;21:360. [PMID: 39905273]

PRIMARY HYPERPARATHYROIDISM

ESSENTIALS OF DIAGNOSIS

- Often found incidentally by routine blood testing.
- Renal calculi, polyuria, hypertension, constipation, fatigue, mental changes.
- Bone pain; rarely, cystic lesions and pathologic fractures.
- Elevated serum PTH, serum and urine calcium, and urine phosphate; serum phosphate low to normal; alkaline phosphatase normal to elevated.

General Considerations

Hyperparathyroidism is a condition of increased production of the hormone PTH. **Primary hyperparathyroidism** occurs when a parathyroid gland disorder is the cause of increased production. **Secondary hyperparathyroidism** occurs, in contrast, when another condition causes low calcium levels in the blood, which causes the parathyroid glands to respond with increased PTH secretion. Causes of secondary hyperparathyroidism include vitamin D deficiency (see Rickets & Osteomalacia) and CKD (see Chapter 25). **Tertiary hyperparathyroidism** occurs when long-standing secondary hyperparathyroidism (most commonly due to CKD) progresses and results in some degree of parathyroid autonomy. **Primary hyperparathyroidism** is the most common cause of hypercalcemia, with an estimated prevalence of 0.89% of the US population, but it is underdiagnosed and undertreated. It occurs at all ages but most commonly in the seventh decade and in women (74%).

There are typically four parathyroid glands, with two on each side nestled behind the thyroid; however, their number and location may vary. Ectopic parathyroid glands have been found within the thyroid gland, high in the neck or carotid sheath, the retroesophageal space, and the thymus or mediastinum. Hyperparathyroidism is usually caused by a single parathyroid adenoma (80%) and less commonly by hyperplasia or adenomas of two or more parathyroid glands (20%), or carcinoma (< 1%). When hyperparathyroidism presents before age 30 years, there is a higher incidence of multiglandular disease (36%) and parathyroid carcinoma (5%). The size of the parathyroid adenoma correlates with the serum PTH level.

About 5–10% of cases are caused by a hereditary (familial) disorder; a presentation before age 45 has a higher chance of being familial. Primary hyperparathyroidism commonly arises in MEN types 1, 2A, and 4 (see Table 30–4).

Primary hyperparathyroidism usually results in excessive excretion of calcium and phosphate by the kidneys. Although PTH stimulates renal tubular reabsorption of calcium, the increase in calcium in the glomerular filtrate overwhelms tubular reabsorption capacity, resulting in hypercalciuria. At least 5% of renal calculi are associated with this disease. Diffuse parenchymal calcification (nephrocalcinosis) is seen less commonly.

Patients may have **normocalcemic primary hyperparathyroidism**, characterized by elevated PTH level in the setting of persistently normal (generally high-normal) serum calcium level. Diagnosis is challenging, however, because it requires the ruling out of secondary hyperparathyroidism (which is generally associated with low-normal serum calcium levels). The natural history of normocalcemic primary hyperparathyroidism is incompletely understood, and the optimal treatment approach not fully appreciated.

Parathyroid carcinoma is a rare cause of hyperparathyroidism, accounting for < 1% of hyperparathyroidism. Distant metastases arise most commonly in the lungs but also in bones, liver, brain, and mediastinum.

Clinical Findings

A. Symptoms and Signs

Hypercalcemia is often discovered incidentally by routine chemistry panels. Many patients are asymptomatic or have only mild symptoms, such as mild fatigue. Parathyroid adenomas are usually small, located deeply in the neck, and almost never palpable.

Symptomatic patients are said to have problems with "bones, stones, abdominal groans, psychic moans, with fatigue overtones."

1. Skeletal manifestations—Low bone density is typically most prominent at the distal one-third of the radius, a site of mostly cortical bone. Lumbar (trabecular) spine bone density is often spared and is higher compared to the distal radius. Hip bones are a mixture of trabecular and cortical bone, and the risk for hip fractures is increased by 50%. Postmenopausal women are prone to asymptomatic vertebral fractures, but severe vertebral demineralization is uncommon in mild hyperparathyroidism. More commonly, patients experience arthralgias and bone pain, particularly involving the legs. Severe chronic hyperparathyroidism can cause **osteitis fibrosa cystica**, which is the replacement of calcified bone matrix with fibrous tissue forming cystic brown tumors of bone that can be palpable in the jaw.

2. Hypercalcemic manifestations—Mild hypercalcemia may be asymptomatic or cause significant symptoms, particularly depression, constipation, and bone and joint pain. **Neuromuscular** manifestations include paresthesias, muscle cramps and weakness, and diminished deep tendon reflexes. **Neuropsychiatric** manifestations include malaise, headache, fatigue, insomnia, irritability, and depression. Patients may have cognitive impairment that can vary from intellectual weariness to severe disorientation, psychosis, or stupor. **Cardiovascular** manifestations include hypertension, palpitations, prolonged P-R interval, shortened Q-T interval, bradyarrhythmias, heart block, asystole, and sensitivity to digitalis. Overall cardiovascular mortality is increased in patients with chronic moderate to severe hypercalcemia. **Renal** manifestations include polyuria and polydipsia from hypercalcemia-induced nephrogenic diabetes insipidus. Among patients with newly discovered hyperparathyroidism, calcium-containing renal calculi have occurred or are detectable in about 18%. **GI** symptoms of hypercalcemia include anorexia, nausea, heartburn, vomiting, abdominal pain, weight loss, constipation, and obstipation. Pancreatitis occurs in 3%. **Dermatologic** symptoms may include pruritus. Calcium may precipitate in the corneas ("band keratopathy"), in extravascular tissues (calcinosis), and in small arteries, causing small vessel thrombosis and skin necrosis (calciphylaxis).

3. Hyperparathyroidism during pregnancy—Pregnant women having mild hyperparathyroidism with a serum calcium below 11.0 mg/dL (< 2.75 mmol/L) generally tolerate pregnancy well with normal outcomes. However, pregnant women with more severe hypercalcemia may experience complications such as nephrolithiasis, hyperemesis, pancreatitis, muscle weakness, and cognitive changes. About 30% of affected women experience preeclampsia and two-thirds of eclamptic women have preterm delivery. Hypercalcemic crisis may occur, especially postpartum. About 80% of fetuses experience complications of maternal hyperparathyroidism, including fetal demise, preterm delivery, and low birth weight. Newborns have hypoparathyroidism that can be permanent.

4. Parathyroid carcinoma—Hyperparathyroidism with a large palpable neck mass, or vocal fold paralysis from recurrent laryngeal nerve palsy, raises concern for parathyroid carcinoma. Some cases present with smaller tumors, less severe hypercalcemia, and benign-appearing histologic features. *FNA biopsy is not recommended because it may seed the biopsy tract with tumor and cytologic distinction between benign and malignant tumors is problematic.* Parathyroid carcinoma is more frequent in patients with hyperparathyroidism–jaw tumor syndrome as well as patients with MEN1 and MEN2A. Therefore, patients should have genetic testing.

B. Laboratory Findings

The hallmark of primary hyperparathyroidism is hypercalcemia with elevated or inappropriately normal PTH level. Hypercalcemia is defined as serum adjusted total calcium above the upper limit of normal (10.5 mg/dL or 2.6 mmol/L). The adjusted total calcium = measured serum calcium in mg/dL + [0.8 × (4.0 – patient's serum albumin in g/dL)]. Serum ionized calcium levels are elevated (> 1.36 mmol/L). Parathyroid carcinoma must always be suspected in patients with a serum calcium of ≥ 14.0 mg/dL (3.5 mmol/L) or more and a serum PTH ≥ 5 times the upper level of normal.

To confirm the diagnosis of hyperparathyroidism, a 24-hour urinary collection for calcium excretion should be obtained. In primary hyperparathyroidism, urine calcium excretion is normal (100–300 mg/day [25–75 mmol/day]) or high. In the absence of thiazide diuretic usage, a low urine calcium excretion (< 100 mg/day [25 mmol/day]) occurs in only 4% of primary hyperthyroidism. Therefore, PTH-mediated hypercalcemia with a low urine calcium excretion suggests familial hypocalciuric hypercalcemia, for which surgery is not indicated.

In primary hyperparathyroidism, serum phosphate may be < 2.5 mg/dL (0.8 mmol/L) due to an excessive loss of phosphate in the urine (25% of cases). A serum calcium:phosphate (Ca/P) ratio > 2.5 (mg/dL) or 2.17 (mmol/L) helps confirm the diagnosis of primary hyperparathyroidism. The alkaline phosphatase is elevated only if bone disease is present. Plasma chloride and uric acid levels may be elevated. Serum 25-OH vitamin D levels should be measured, since vitamin D deficiency is common in patients with hyperparathyroidism. Serum 25-OH vitamin D levels < 20 mcg/L (50 nmol/L) can aggravate hyperparathyroidism and its bone manifestations.

Patients with normal serum calcium and elevated serum PTH must be evaluated for causes of secondary hyperparathyroidism (eg, vitamin D or calcium deficiency, hyperphosphatemia, CKD). In the absence of secondary hyperparathyroidism, these patients have normocalcemic hyperparathyroidism for which monitoring is required. Although specific guidelines are lacking, a reasonable recommendation is to measure calcium, albumin, creatinine, 25-OHD, and PTH every 1–2 years with periodic monitoring of 24-hour urine calcium.

Genetic testing is recommended for patients with primary hyperparathyroidism who are younger (< aged 40–50 years), have recurrent disease, have a family history of primary hyperparathyroidism or endocrine tumors, have multiglandular disease, or have features of relevant syndromes like MEN1.

C. Imaging

Parathyroid imaging is not necessary for the diagnosis of hyperparathyroidism but is performed for most patients prior to parathyroid surgery.

Ultrasound should scan the neck from the mandible to the superior mediastinum in an effort to locate ectopic parathyroid adenomas. Ultrasound has a sensitivity of 79% for single adenomas but only 35% for multiglandular disease. Ultrasound is useful for the surgeon to localize parathyroid adenomas while also assessing the vocal folds.

Sestamibi scintigraphy with ^{99m}Tc-sestamibi is most useful for localizing parathyroid adenomas. However, false-positive scans are common, caused by thyroid nodules, thyroiditis, or cervical lymphadenopathy. Sestamibi-SPECT imaging improves sensitivity for single parathyroid adenomas. Small benign thyroid nodules are discovered incidentally in nearly 50% of patients with hyperparathyroidism who have imaging with ultrasound or MRI.

^{18}F-flurocholine PET/MRI is a useful scan for patients with primary hyperparathyroidism and negative or discordant localization imaging on neck ultrasound and sestamibi scanning. This scan correctly localizes a parathyroid adenoma in about 75% of cases.

Conventional CT and MRI imaging are not usually required prior to a first neck surgery for hyperparathyroidism. However, a four-dimensional CT (4D-CT) is useful for preoperative imaging when ultrasonography and sestamibi scans are negative. It can also be helpful for patients who have had prior neck surgery and for those with ectopic parathyroid glands. MRI may also be useful for repeat neck operations and when ectopic parathyroid glands are suspected. MRI shows better soft tissue contrast than CT.

Noncontrast CT scanning or ultrasonography of the kidneys in patients with hyperparathyroidism can visualize calcium-containing stones.

Bone density measurements by dual-energy x-ray absorptiometry (DXA) should be obtained in all patients with primary hyperparathyroidism. They are helpful in determining the amount of cortical bone loss and whether there is an indication for parathyroid surgery. In primary hyperparathyroidism, DXA may be performed at the lumber spine and hip, as well as at the forearm where the cortical-bone may be especially sensitive to disease-related bone loss. Vertebral spine assessment by radiography, CT, or DXA can evaluate for spinal compression fractures.

Complications

Primary hyperparathyroidism may cause bone loss (with risk of fracture), nephrolithiasis, and associated hypercalcemic manifestations (see Clinical Findings, above). Ureteral stones may cause obstruction and UTI that may lead to kidney disease and uremia. If the serum calcium level rises rapidly, clouding of sensorium, kidney disease, and rapid precipitation of calcium throughout the soft tissues may occur (calciphylaxis). Peptic ulcer and pancreatitis may be intractable before surgery. In patients with MEN type 1, insulinomas, gastrinomas or pituitary tumors may be associated (see Multiple Endocrine Neoplasia). Pseudogout may complicate hyperparathyroidism both before and after surgical removal of tumors. Hypercalcemia during gestation produces neonatal hypocalcemia.

In tertiary hyperparathyroidism due to CKD, high serum calcium and phosphate levels may cause calciphylaxis; calcification of arteries can result in painful ischemic necrosis of skin and gangrene, cardiac arrhythmias, and respiratory failure.

Differential Diagnosis

Artifactual hypercalcemia is common, so a confirmatory serum calcium level should be drawn after an overnight fast along with a serum protein, albumin, and triglyceride while ensuring that the patient is well-hydrated. Hypercalcemia may be due to high serum protein concentrations; in the presence of very high or low serum albumin concentrations, an adjusted serum calcium or an ionized calcium is necessary to confirm the hypercalcemia. Hypercalcemia may also be seen with dehydration.

When PTH-mediated hypercalcemia is confirmed, familial hypocalciuric hypercalcemia (FHH) must be ruled out before a diagnosis of primary hyperparathyroidism may be made. FHH is an uncommon autosomal dominant inherited disorder. Reduced function of the calcium-sensing receptor (CaSR) causes the parathyroid glands to falsely "sense" hypocalcemia and inappropriately release excessive amounts of PTH. The renal tubule CaSRs are also affected, causing hypocalciuria.

Adults with hypercalcemia due to FHH are either asymptomatic or have nonspecific complaints such as fatigue, weakness, or cognitive issues.

FHH is characterized by a mildly elevated serum calcium that is usually < 11.0 mg/dL (2.75 mmol/L) and a low urine calcium excretion that is usually < 50 mg/24 hours (13 mmol/24 hours). FHH is confirmed with genetic testing for associated genetic mutations. These patients should not be subjected to surgery.

Hypercalcemia may be non–PTH-mediated. If PTH level is low, it indicates that another process is causing the hypercalcemia to which the parathyroid glands are responding appropriately with decreased secretion of PTH. There are many causes of non-PTH-mediated hypercalcemia. **Hypercalcemia of malignancy** occurs most frequently with breast, lung, pancreatic, uterine, and renal cell carcinoma, and paraganglioma. In many cases, the malignancy secretes PTH-related protein (PTHrP), which has structural homologies to PTH, that causes bone resorption and hypercalcemia similar to those caused by PTH. In the presence of elevated serum PTHrP levels, the serum PTH levels are low or low-normal; phosphate is often low. In other cases of malignancy-related hypercalcemia, osteolytic bone metastasis are the underlying cause. Some tumors can secrete excessive 1,25 $(OH)_2$ vitamin D_3, particularly lymphoproliferative and ovarian malignancies. Plasma cell myeloma causes hypercalcemia in older individuals. Other hematologic cancers associated with hypercalcemia include monocytic leukemia, T-cell leukemia and lymphoma, and Burkitt lymphoma. The clinical features of malignant hypercalcemia can closely simulate hyperparathyroidism.

Pseudohyperparathyroidism of pregnancy presents with hypercalcemia during pregnancy. It is caused by hypersensitivity of the breasts to PRL. The breasts become abnormally enlarged and secrete excessive amounts of PTHrP which causes hypercalcemia. Treatment with dopamine agonists reverses the hypercalcemia.

Sarcoidosis and other granulomatous disorders, such as tuberculosis, berylliosis, histoplasmosis, coccidioidomycosis, leprosy, and foreign-body granuloma, can cause non–PTH-mediated hypercalcemia. Sarcoid granulomas can secrete PTHrP, but granulomas secrete $1,25(OH)_2D_3$ and serum levels of $1,25(OH)_2D_3$ are usually elevated in the presence of hypercalcemia.

Dietary factors can cause non–PTH-mediated hypercalcemia. Excessive calcium, vitamin D, or vitamin A ingestion can cause hypercalcemia, especially in patients who concurrently take thiazide diuretics, which reduce urinary calcium loss. Hypercalcemia is reversible following withdrawal of calcium and vitamin D supplements. In vitamin D intoxication, hypercalcemia may persist for several weeks. Serum levels of 25-hydroxycholecalciferol $(25[OH]D_3)$ are helpful to confirm the diagnosis. A brief course of corticosteroid therapy may be necessary if hypercalcemia is severe.

Prolonged immobilization at bed rest commonly causes non–PTH-mediated hypercalcemia, particularly in adolescents, critically ill patients, and patients with extensive Paget disease of bone. Hypercalcemia develops in about one-third of acutely ill patients being treated in ICUs, particularly patients with AKI. Serum calcium elevations are typically mild but may reach 15 mg/dL (3.75 mmol/L). Serum PTH levels are usually slightly elevated, consistent with mild hyperparathyroidism but may be suppressed or normal.

Rare causes of non–PTH-mediated hypercalcemia include untreated adrenal insufficiency. Modest hypercalcemia is occasionally seen in patients taking thiazide diuretics or lithium; the PTH level may be inappropriately nonsuppressed with hypercalcemia. Hyperthyroidism causes increased turnover of bone and occasional hypercalcemia. Bisphosphonates can increase serum calcium in 20% and serum PTH becomes high in 10%, mimicking hyperparathyroidism. Other causes of hypercalcemia are shown in Table 24–7.

Treatment

A. Asymptomatic and Mild Primary Hyperparathyroidism

Truly asymptomatic patients who do not meet criteria for surgical treatment for surgery (parathyroidectomy) may be closely monitored and advised to keep active, avoid immobilization, and drink adequate fluids. For patients with hypercalciuria, hydrochlorothiazide may be used to reduce calciuria; however, serum calcium must be monitored carefully. Patients with primary hyperparathyroidism should avoid large doses of thiazide diuretics, vitamin A, and calcium-containing antacids or supplements. However, if they are not hypercalciuric, they need not avoid ingesting calcium altogether.

Serum calcium and albumin are checked at least twice yearly; kidney function, PTH level, and urine calcium once yearly; and bone density by DXA every 2 years.

B. Medical Measures for Symptomatic Hyperparathyroidism

1. Fluids—Hypercalcemia is treated with a large fluid intake unless contraindicated. Severe hypercalcemia requires hospitalization and intensive hydration with intravenous saline.

2. CaSR activators—Cinacalcet is a calcimimetic agent that binds to sites of the parathyroid glands' extracellular CaSRs to increase the glands' affinity for extracellular calcium, thereby decreasing PTH secretion. Cinacalcet may be used as the initial therapy for patients with hyperparathyroidism or for failed surgical parathyroidectomy. For primary hyperparathyroidism with mild hypercalcemia, begin cinacalcet (15 mg orally) and monitor the serum calcium closely; increase the dose every 2 weeks if hypercalcemia persists until the patient becomes normocalcemic. Patients with parathyroid carcinoma and severe hypercalcemia are treated with cinacalcet in addition to the bisphosphonate zoledronic acid. Cinacalcet is usually well tolerated but may cause nausea and vomiting (11%), myalgia, or malaise. Cinacalcet does not usually correct hypercalciuria. Cinacalcet may cause hypocalcemia.

About 50% of azotemic patients with tertiary hyperparathyroidism have hypercalcemia that presents a contraindication for vitamin D analog therapy. In such cases, surgical parathyroidectomy may be considered. Alternatively, or as an interim therapy, cinacalcet may be given in doses of 30 mg orally daily to a maximum of 250 mg daily, with dosage adjustments based on calcium and PTH levels. Etelcalcetide also activates the parathyroid glands' CaSR and reduces hypercalcemia in dialysis patients; it is given intravenously at the end of hemodialysis sessions, thereby avoiding the GI side effects of cinacalcet.

3. Bisphosphonates—Intravenous bisphosphonates are potent inhibitors of bone resorption and can temporarily treat the hypercalcemia of hyperparathyroidism. Zoledronic acid causes a gradual decline in serum calcium over several days that may last for weeks to months. Oral bisphosphonates, such as alendronate, are not effective for treating the hypercalcemia or hypercalciuria of hyperparathyroidism. However, oral alendronate has been shown to improve BMD in the trabecular bone of the lumbar spine and hip (not distal radius) and may be used for asymptomatic patients with hyperparathyroidism who have a low BMD.

4. Denosumab—For patients with severe hypercalcemia, denosumab 120 mcg subcutaneously may be effective.

5. Vitamin D and vitamin D analogs—For patients with primary hyperparathyroidism and vitamin D deficiency, vitamin D replacement may reduce PTH levels. Aggravation of hypercalcemia or hypercalciuria does not ordinarily occur if replacement is cautious.

6. Other measures—Estrogen replacement reduces hypercalcemia slightly in postmenopausal women with hyperparathyroidism. β-Blockers, such as propranolol, may also be useful for preventing the adverse cardiac effects of hypercalcemia. Parathyroid carcinoma metastases may be treated with radiofrequency ablation or arterial embolization.

C. Surgical Parathyroidectomy

Definitive treatment with parathyroidectomy is recommended for patients with primary hyperparathyroidism who have nephrolithiasis, osteoporotic fracture, or other symptoms of disease, unless there is a contraindication to surgery. Surgery may be appropriate for patients with asymptomatic primary hyperparathyroidism who have at least one of the following: (1) age < 50 years; (2) albumin-adjusted serum calcium > 1 mg/dL (0.25 mmol/L) above the upper limit of normal; (3) reduced BMD by DXA to a T-score of < -2.5 at lumbar spine, hip, or distal 1/3 radius); (4) history of low-energy fracture; or (5) GFR of < 60 ml/min. Further, surgery is recommended if urinary calcium excretion is > 400 mg/day and a urinary stone risk profile shows high stone risk. Surgery may still be considered for patients who do not have one of these indications if there are no medical contraindications. During pregnancy, parathyroidectomy is performed in the second trimester for women who are symptomatic or have an albumin-corrected serum calcium > 11.4 mg/dL (2.85 mmol/L).

Successful parathyroidectomy results in normalization of biochemical indices, higher BMD, reduced fracture risk, and reduced risk of kidney stones. Further, surgery may confer modest benefits in social and emotional well-being and overall quality of life in comparison to similar patients being monitored without surgery. Cognitive function may benefit with improvements in nonverbal abstraction and memory.

Without preoperative localization studies, bilateral neck exploration is usually advisable for the following: (1) patients with a family history of hyperparathyroidism, (2) patients with a personal or family history of MEN, and (3) patients wanting an optimal chance of success with a single surgery. Parathyroid glands are often supernumerary (five or more) or ectopic (eg, intrathyroidal, carotid sheath, mediastinum).

Parathyroid hyperplasia is commonly seen with secondary or tertiary hyperparathyroidism associated with uremia that is resistant to vitamin D analogues. Parathyroidectomy offers lower mortality rates, compared with cinacalcet. When surgery is performed, a subtotal parathyroidectomy is optimal; three and one-half glands are usually removed.

Parathyroid carcinoma surgery consists of either parathyroidectomy or en bloc resection of the tumor and ipsilateral thyroid lobe with care to avoid rupturing the tumor capsule. If the surgical margins are not clear of tumor, postoperative neck radiation therapy may be given. Local and distant metastases may be debulked or irradiated. Chemotherapy has been ineffective for patients with distant metastases. Immunotherapy with anti-hPTH monoclonal antibodies is a treatment option.

Complications—Serum PTH levels fall below normal in 70% of patients within hours after successful surgery, commonly causing hypocalcemic paresthesias or even tetany. Hypocalcemia tends to occur the evening after surgery or on the next day. Frequent postoperative monitoring of serum calcium (or serum calcium plus albumin) is advisable beginning the evening after surgery. Once hypercalcemia has resolved, liquid or chewable calcium carbonate is given orally to reduce the likelihood of hypocalcemia. Symptomatic hypocalcemia is treated with larger doses of calcium; calcitriol (0.25–1 mcg daily orally) may be added, with the dosage depending on symptom severity. Magnesium salts are sometimes required postoperatively, since adequate magnesium is required for functional recovery of the remaining suppressed parathyroid glands.

In about 12% of patients having successful parathyroid surgery, PTH levels rise above normal (while serum calcium is normal or low) by 1 week postoperatively. This secondary hyperparathyroidism is probably due to "hungry bones" and is treated with calcium and vitamin D preparations. Such therapy is usually needed only for 3–6 months but is required long term by some patients.

Hyperthyroidism commonly occurs immediately following parathyroid surgery. It is caused by release of stored thyroid hormone during surgical manipulation of the thyroid. In symptomatic patients, short-term treatment with propranolol may be required for several days.

Prognosis

Patients with symptomatic hyperparathyroidism usually experience worsening disease (eg, nephrolithiasis) unless they have treatment. Conversely, the majority of completely asymptomatic patients with a serum calcium below 11.0 mg/dL (2.75 mmol/L) remain stable with follow-up. However, worsening hypercalcemia, hypercalciuria, and reductions in cortical BMD develop in about one-third of asymptomatic patients. Therefore, asymptomatic patients must be monitored carefully and treated with oral hydration and mobilization.

Surgical removal of apparently single sporadic parathyroid adenomas is successful in 94%.

The bones, in spite of severe cyst formation, deformity, and fracture, will heal if hyperparathyroidism is successfully treated. Kidney damage may progress even after removal of a parathyroid adenoma.

Parathyroid carcinoma is associated with 5- and 10-year survival rates of 78% and 49%, respectively. A positive surgical margins or metastases predict a very poor 5-year survival.

When to Refer

Refer to parathyroid surgeon for parathyroidectomy.

When to Admit

Patients with severe hypercalcemia for intravenous hydration.

El-Hajj Fuleihan G et al. Treatment of hypercalcemia of malignancy in adults: an Endocrine Society Clinical Practice Guideline. J Clin Endocrinol Metab. 2023;108:507. [PMID: 36545746]

Kongsaree N et al. Skeletal effect of parathyroidectomy in patients with primary hyperparathyroidism: a systematic review and meta-analysis. J Clin Endocrinol Metab. 2024;109:31922. [PMID: 38739762]

Liu Y et al. Approach to the patient: normocalcemic primary hyperparathyroidism. J Clin Endocrinol Metab. 2025;110:e868. [PMID: 39319404]

Silva BC et al. Primary hyperparathyroidism. Best Pract Res Clin Endocrinol Metab. 2024;38:101247. [PMID: 30477754]

METABOLIC BONE DISEASE

The term "metabolic bone disease" refers to conditions producing diffuse reductions or increases in bone density that affect bone integrity. **Conditions causing reduced bone density** include osteopenia/osteoporosis and osteomalacia. Osteoporosis is characterized by reduction in both bone matrix and mineral, whereas in osteomalacia the bone matrix is intact but bone mineral is decreased. **Conditions causing increased bone density** are less common and include osteopetrosis and fluorosis. Disorders such as fibrous dysplasia and Paget disease of bone also involve disorganized bone and abnormal bone quality. Some metabolic bone disease includes disruption in calcium or phosphate homeostasis. Metabolic bone diseases may cause bone pain and fractures.

OSTEOPOROSIS & OSTEOPENIA

ESSENTIALS OF DIAGNOSIS

- Asymptomatic until a fracture has occurred.
- Fracture risk may be estimated by FRAX tool.
- Diagnosed by DXA bone density scanning.
- Serum calcium, phosphorus, PTH, and 25-OHD levels may be normal process.

General Considerations

Osteoporosis is a disorder of low bone mass and bone microstructural deterioration, resulting in reduced bone strength and predisposition to fracture. In the United States, osteoporosis causes over 1.6 million fractures annually, which have a tremendous medical and economic impact. Common sites of fragility fractures (those due to a fall or lesser trauma) are the vertebrae, forearm, and hip, but any anatomic site may be affected. Vertebral fractures are the most common osteoporotic fracture. Hip fracture in older adults can be particularly devastating with a 25% mortality by 1-year post-fracture; of those patients who survive, only half recover their pre-fracture functional status.

The risk for fragility fracture varies with age, sex, and race and ethnicity. Age is a strong risk factor. In women, there is an accelerated decline in bone mass at menopause due to the drop in estrogen, followed by a continued lower rate of decline. Because women are at higher risk for fracture than men, osteoporosis often goes unsuspected, undiagnosed, and untreated in men because widespread assumptions by providers and patients that osteoporosis is solely associated with postmenopausal women. Fracture risk is lower in Latino/Latina and Black adults than White adults.

Osteoporosis in postmenopausal women and older men is often due to the effects of aging and the decline in the protective effects of sex steroids. However, a variety of other factors can contribute to loss of bone mass or integrity (Table 30–2). Secondary osteoporosis refers to bone loss due to specific clinical conditions or medications.

DXA is a low-radiation, inexpensive imaging test which measures BMD. DXA is the basis for the diagnosis of osteoporosis and a strong risk predictor of osteoporotic fracture. DXA screening should be performed on all women ≥ 65 years of age, and in younger postmenopausal women with an estimated fracture risk that approximates that of a 65-year-old White woman without other risk factors. DXA is also appropriate for some older men with risk factors. Although routine DXA screening is not routinely performed in premenopausal women and young men, it is warranted in patients with fragility fractures.

DXA is used to measure BMD at the lumbar spine, the proximal femur, and, in some clinical situations, at the distal forearm. In postmenopausal women and men 50 years and older, osteoporosis is defined if BMD at the total lumbar spine, femoral neck, or total hip is ≥ 2.5 standard

Table 30–2. Causes of osteoporosis.[1]

Aging	**Medications**
Alcohol use disorder	Androgen deprivation therapy
Cigarette smoking	Aromatase inhibitors
Female sex	Glucocorticoids
Genetic disorders	Pioglitazone
Aromatase deficiency	PPIs
Collagen disorders	SSRIs (older adults)
Ehlers-Danlos syndrome	SGLT-2 inhibitors
Homocystinuria	Vitamin A excess, vitamin D excess
Hypophosphatasia	**Underweight (BMI < 18.5)**
Idiopathic juvenile and adult osteoporosis	**White race**
Marfan syndrome	**Miscellaneous conditions**
Osteogenesis imperfecta	Anorexia nervosa
Hormone deficiency	Celiac disease
Estradiol (women)	COPD
Testosterone (men)	Cystic fibrosis
Hormone excess	Diabetes mellitus
Cushing syndrome	HIV infection
Hyperparathyroidism	IBD
Thyrotoxicosis	Liver disease
Low physical activity and immobilization	Mastocytosis (systemic)
Malignancy, especially multiple myeloma	Primary biliary cholangitis
	Protein-calorie malnutrition
	Rheumatoid arthritis
	Thalassemia major

[1]See Table 30–3 for causes of osteomalacia.

deviations below the mean for a young adult reference population (T-score of -2.5 or lower). Low bone mass or "osteopenia" is defined as a T-score between -1.0 and -2.49. In premenopausal women or men younger than 50, T-scores are not used to diagnose osteoporosis because the relationships between BMD and fracture risk are less well defined. Instead, Z-scores are used, in which the BMD is expressed the as standard deviations from an age- and sex-matched reference population, with a Z-score 2.0 or lower referred to as "low bone mass for age." The diagnosis of osteoporosis in a premenopausal woman or man younger than 50 generally requires both a low bone mass for age (Z-score) and demonstrated skeletal fragility (ie, a fragility fracture).

Use of T-scores to diagnose osteoporosis and osteopenia (low bone mass) is limited in their failure to account for factors beyond BMD that contribute to skeletal fragility, including age, personal history of fracture, and parental history of hip fracture. Fracture risk estimators such as the Fracture Risk Assessment Tool (FRAX) account for these other risk factors. For a postmenopausal woman or man 50 years or over, FRAX predicts 10-year risks of major osteoporotic fracture and hip fracture. The Bone Health and Osteoporosis Foundation recommends that pharmacologic therapy for osteoporosis be considered for postmenopausal women and men 50 and over who have: osteoporosis by T-score; or osteopenia with a personal history of hip or vertebral fracture; or a 10-year risk of major osteoporotic fracture of at least 20% or hip fracture of at least 3%.

Clinical Findings

A. Symptoms and Signs

Osteoporosis is asymptomatic until a fracture occurs. Fractures can be painful and reduce independence and quality of life. Vertebral fractures may be painful or asymptomatic, presenting as loss of height or kyphosis, or diagnosed incidentally on radiograph. Even when asymptomatic, vertebral fractures are associated with a substantially higher risk of future fracture (vertebral or nonvertebral).

B. Laboratory Findings

Laboratory testing is required to evaluate for secondary causes of osteoporosis or and to rule out osteomalacia. Basic testing should include serum determinations for calcium, albumin, phosphate, creatinine, PTH, 25-OHD, TSH, and alkaline phosphatase. In men, a morning total testosterone level evaluates for hypogonadism.

The extent of further laboratory work-up depends on the clinical suspicion for a secondary cause of low bone mass or osteoporosis. A serum protein electrophoresis to evaluate for myeloma, may be appropriate in the setting of vertebral fracture or when kidney disease or hypercalcemia are present. Determination of 24-hour urinary calcium level may provide valuable additional information in the setting of primary or secondary hyperparathyroidism. When there is suggestive history, signs, or symptoms, additional laboratory testing may be warranted to rule out Cushing syndrome or celiac disease. In patients with severe osteoporosis (severely low BMD, multiple fractures, or both) or in premenopausal women and younger men with demonstrated skeletal fragility, a more extensive search for an underlying process may be appropriate.

Biochemical markers of bone turnover are available at commercial laboratories, including CTX (serum C-telopeptide of type 1 collagen), a marker for bone resorption; and P1NP (serum N-propeptide of type 1 procollagen), a marker for bone formation. They are not generally helpful in diagnosis but can be useful measures of medication adherence and efficacy. A clinical response to treatment is expected if the CTX and P1NP drop by at least 50% after commencing therapy. Specimens should be obtained in the morning, fasting, using the same laboratory for sequential testing.

C. Imaging

DXA, as **described above, is used to measure BMD for screening, diagnosis, or monitoring** treatment response. Quantitative CT (QCT) of the spine and hips measures volumetric bone density and can be useful in patients for whom degenerative disk disease interferes with the accurate measurement of spinal areal BMD by DXA. Vertebral radiographs may be helpful for detection of asymptomatic compression fractures.

Differential Diagnosis

Osteoporosis and osteomalacia are indistinguishable by bone densitometry. (See Rickets & Osteomalacia.) They must be differentiated based on clinical history and other laboratory testing, or tetracycline-labeled iliac crest bone biopsy, which is infrequently performed. Other disorders of bone matrix are discussed below.

Prevention & Treatment

A. Nonpharmacologic Measures

For prevention and treatment of osteoporosis, the diet should be adequate in protein, total calories, calcium, and vitamin D. Recommended dietary allowance for calcium is 1300 mg daily during adolescence, 1000 mg for adult women through age 50 years and men through age 70, and 1200 mg for women age 51 and older and men 70 and older. This intake can be achieved from dietary sources, including fortified foods, or from a combination of diet and supplements. Measurement of calcium concentration in the blood is not useful in determining whether calcium intake is adequate, as homeostatic mechanisms usually ensure that calcium concentration stays within normal range. At elevated PTH due to secondary hyperparathyroidism or low 24-hour urinary calcium may indicate that calcium intake or intestinal absorption is inadequate.

Recommended daily allowance for vitamin D in adults is 600 IU per day up to age 70 years and 800 IU per day for those 71 and older. As with calcium, this intake can be achieved from dietary sources, including fortified foods, or from a combination of diet and supplements. Adequacy of vitamin D intake can be assessed by measurement of serum 25-OHD level. For the general population, a 25-OHD level of ≥ 20 ng/mL is considered adequate. For patients with osteoporosis or osteopenia, a goal of ≥ 30 ng/mL is recommended. Levels > 60 ng/mL should be avoided as they do not provide additional benefits for fracture reduction and may cause hypercalciuria (with risk for nephrolithiasis) or hypercalcemia.

Pharmacologic corticosteroids should be avoided or reduced in dose and duration if possible. Cigarette smoking cessation is essential. Excessive alcohol intake must be avoided. Exercise is strongly recommended both for its direct effects on bone strength and its reduction of fall risk through improved balance and body strength. Other fall prevention measures include adequate home lighting, handrails on stairs, handholds in bathrooms, and appropriate walking aids (canes or walkers) for patients with weakness or balance problems. Medications that cause orthostasis, dizziness, or confusion should be avoided.

B. Pharmacologic Measures

Pharmacologic treatment should be considered for: patients with osteoporosis on DXA. It also should be considered in postmenopausal women and men ≥ 50 years with osteopenia and a high risk for fracture demonstrated either by a fragility fracture of the hip or spine, or by a FRAX-determined 10-year risk of hip fracture > 3%, or risk of major osteoporotic fracture > 20%. Select premenopausal women or men younger than 50 with low bone mass for age and demonstrated skeletal fragility may also benefit from treatment.

For patients at high risk of fracture, first-line therapy generally is with a bisphosphonate. Patients at very high risk of fracture are candidates for anabolic therapy with teriparatide or abaloparatide, or for therapy with the mixed antiresorptive/anabolic agent romosozumab.

1. Bisphosphonates—Bisphosphonates are antiresorptive medications that inhibit osteoclast-induced bone resorption. They are the first-line therapy for patients with high enough risk for fracture to warrant pharmacologic therapy. Available in oral and intravenous formulations, bisphosphonates increase bone density significantly and all reduce the incidence of vertebral fractures; all but ibandronate have been demonstrated to also reduce the risk of nonvertebral fractures. Bisphosphonates are also effective in preventing corticosteroid-induced osteoporosis.

Oral bisphosphonates include alendronate, risedronate, and ibandronate. Alendronate is administered orally once weekly; risedronate may be given weekly or monthly; and ibandronate is taken once monthly. To ensure intestinal absorption, oral bisphosphonates must be taken in the morning with at least 8 oz of plain water and at least 40 minutes before consumption of food or other medications or supplements (particularly those containing calcium). The patient must remain upright after taking bisphosphonates to reduce the risk of esophagitis. Oral bisphosphonates are relatively contraindicated in patients with CrCl < 30 mL/min.

Intravenous bisphosphonates are available for patients who cannot take oral bisphosphonates. Zoledronic acid is most commonly used and is a potent osteoclast inhibitor. It is administered once yearly in a dose of 5 mg intravenously over at least 15–30 minutes. In a study of postmenopausal women with osteoporosis, once yearly intravenous zoledronic acid reduced the 3-year incidence of hip fractures by 41% (from 2.5% to 1.4%) and clinical vertebral fractures by 77% (from 2.6% to 0.5%). Intravenous bisphosphonates are relatively contraindicated in patients with CrCl < 35 mL/min.

Because of the very rare but serious potential side effects of cumulative doses of antiresorptive therapy described below (including atypical fractures of the femur, osteonecrosis of the jaw), the benefit and risk of bisphosphonate treatment is reassessed after approximately 3 years of intravenous bisphosphonate or 4–5 years of oral bisphosphonate therapy. If the patient is deemed to be at continued high risk of fracture as assessed by repeat DXA bone densitometry and evaluation or the current clinical history, continued bisphosphonate therapy for a total of 8–10 years may be appropriate. Alternatively, if risk is more moderate, a bisphosphonate "drug holiday" may be pursued.

Side effects of bisphosphonates—Oral bisphosphonates can cause nausea, chest pain, and hoarseness. Erosive esophagus can occur, particularly in patients with hiatal hernia and gastroesophageal reflux.

After the first intravenous infusion of zoledronic acid, symptoms of an acute-phase response occurs in 42% of patients, usually within the first day or two including fever, chills, or flushing (20%); musculoskeletal pain (20%); nausea, vomiting, or diarrhea (8%); and nonspecific symptoms such as fatigue, dyspnea, edema, headache, or dizziness (22%). Although they may last up to several days, the symptoms are transient and resolve spontaneously. They may recur with subsequent doses but diminish in intensity with time. Symptoms may be treated with acetaminophen or

NSAIDs. Patients who experience an especially severe acute-phase response can be given prophylactic corticosteroids (eg, intravenous hydrocortisone) immediately prior to subsequent bisphosphonate infusions.

Osteonecrosis of the jaw is a rare complication of antiresorptive therapy. After tooth extraction or implantation, a painful, necrotic, nonhealing lesion of the mandible or maxilla occurs. The risk is increased with older age, in women, and in patients concomitantly receiving chemotherapy or corticosteroid therapy. About 95% of medication-related osteonecrosis of the jaw has occurred with high-dose bisphosphonate therapy for treatment of malignancy. Only 5% of cases have occurred in patients receiving bisphosphonates for osteoporosis. The incidence of osteonecrosis is about 1:100,000 patients treated for osteoporosis with oral bisphosphonates versus 1:100 in patients being treated for cancer with intravenous bisphosphonates. With this risk in mind, patients should be queried about dental health prior to initiation of antiresorptive therapy and examined by a dentist if appropriate. If dental extractions are needed or implants are planned, those procedures should be completed before initiation of the antiresorptive medication.

Atypical fractures of the femur are another rare complication of antiresorptive therapy. Atypical fractures are often subtrochanteric, occur with little or no trauma, and are usually transverse as opposed to the more typical comminuted or spiral femoral shaft fractures. Patients may have prodromal thigh pain prior to the fracture. The risk for atypical femoral fractures is higher among Asian women, patients taking chronic glucocorticoid therapy, and those receiving bisphosphonate treatment for > 5 years. Although atypical femoral fractures are a serious consideration, the risk is outweighed by the benefits of bisphosphonates. In a large cohort analysis, for every 10,000 women taking bisphosphonates for 3 years, 149 hip fractures were prevented and 2 atypical femur fractures occurred in White women, while 91 hip fractures were prevented and 8 atypical femur fractures occurred in Asian women.

Bisphosphonate (and other antiresorptive) therapy can induce hypocalcemia, particularly in the setting of vitamin D deficiency and if calcium intake or absorption is low. Therefore, vitamin D deficiency should be corrected before starting therapy, and adequate calcium and vitamin D intake are crucial (from supplements, if needed), especially with intravenous bisphosphonate therapy.

2. Denosumab—Denosumab is a monoclonal antibody that inhibits the proliferation and maturation of preosteoclasts into mature osteoclast bone-resorbing cells. It is indicated for treatment of osteoporosis and considered an alternative to bisphosphonates for treatment of patients at high risk of fracture. It also is FDA-approved for patients with high fracture risk who are receiving sex hormone suppression therapy for breast cancer or prostate cancer. Treatment reduces vertebral fractures by 68% and hip fractures by 40%. Denosumab is administered in doses of 60 mg subcutaneously every 6 months.

Denosumab is relatively well tolerated. There is a small incidence of flu-like symptoms (8%), eczema, and cellulitis. Like bisphosphonates, rare cases of osteonecrosis of the jaw and atypical femoral fractures have been reported. Hypocalcemia may occur, particularly in the setting of vitamin D deficiency and if calcium intake or absorption is low. Therefore, vitamin D deficiency should be corrected before starting the medication, and adequate calcium and vitamin D intake (from supplements if needed) are crucial.

Unlike bisphosphonates, denosumab can be given to patients with stage 4 and 5 CKD; however, the risk of hypocalcemia in this population is heightened. A large retrospective cohort study of women on dialysis reported severe hypocalcemia (serum calcium level < 7.5 mg/dL [1.88 mmol/L]) in 41% receiving denosumab (some resulting in life-threatening events, hospitalizations, and death) versus 2% receiving oral bisphosphonates. In 2024, the FDA issued a black box warning about the risk of severe hypocalcemia in patients with advanced CKD, especially those with related mineral bone disorder.

Importantly, following a missed dose or discontinuation of denosumab, there is accelerated bone loss with an increased risk of multiple vertebral fractures. Therefore, denosumab must be given on-schedule without the "drug holidays" applied to bisphosphonate therapy. Once started, denosumab should either be continued indefinitely, or transitioned to another antiresorptive agent (eg, a bisphosphonate), with the intensity and duration of the other therapy dependent on the duration of the denosumab treatment.

3. Other antiresorptive agents—Estrogen has antiresorptive effects, and menopausal hormone therapy with conjugated equine estrogens increases BMD and reduces risk of hip and vertebral fractures. Because alternate therapies for osteoporosis exist without the potential risks of estrogen, estrogen is no longer prescribed for the purpose of treating osteoporosis.

Selective estrogen receptor modulators (SERMS) act as estrogens in some tissues but block estrogens in other tissues. Raloxifene, taken orally daily, is FDA approved for the treatment of postmenopausal osteoporosis. It reduces the risk of vertebral fractures by about 40% but does not reduce the risk of nonvertebral fractures. Unlike estrogen, raloxifene does not reduce hot flushes or relieve vaginal dryness, but it does not cause endometrial hyperplasia, and risk of breast cancer is reduced 76% in women taking raloxifene for 3 years. Raloxifene increases the risk for thromboembolism. Bazedoxifene is available in a fixed-dose combination with conjugated estrogens and is FDA approved for the prevention of osteoporosis in postmenopausal women with an intact uterus.

Intranasal and injectable **calcitonin** are approved for osteoporosis treatment, although they are used infrequently because they have not been shown to reduce nonvertebral or hip fractures, and they have various side effects. Calcitonin may provide some analgesia in patients with pain from vertebral compression fractures. The intranasal spray may cause rhinitis and epistaxis, and the injectable form may cause flu-like symptoms and local injection reactions. Calcitonin increases overall risk of malignancy by about 1.1% and has been withdrawn from the market in Canada and Europe.

4. PTH and PTHrP analogs—Teriparatide and abaloparatide are analogs of PTH and PTHrP, respectively. These analogs are anabolic agents that stimulate bone formation, particularly in the spine. They are options for patients with osteoporosis who are at very high fracture risk, particularly those who have severely low BMD of the spine or have suffered vertebral fracture. Patients self-administer subcutaneous teriparatide or abaloparatide daily for up to 2 years, using a prefilled pen. Following this anabolic agent treatment course, treatment with an antiresorptive agent (usually a bisphosphonate or denosumab) is provided. Teriparatide is also FDA approved for the treatment of glucocorticoid-induced osteoporosis.

Side effects of teriparatide and abaloparatide include hypercalcemia and hypercalciuria. In patients with a history of nephrolithiasis, caution is advised and investigation warranted before prescribing these agents. Patients are excluded from receiving teriparatide or abaloparatide if they have an increased risk of osteosarcoma due to the following: Paget disease of bone, prior radiation therapy to bones, open epiphyses, or a past history of skeletal malignancies.

5. Romosozumab—Romosozumab is an injectable monoclonal antibody that inhibits sclerostin, increasing new bone formation and decreasing bone resorption (ie, it is a mixed anabolic/antiresorptive agent). It is administered once monthly for 12 months in a clinical setting, following which antiresorptive therapy is provided either with a bisphosphonate or denosumab. In one large cohort of women with osteoporosis and fragility fractures, romosozumab treatment for 12 months followed by alendronate for 12 months resulted in a 48% lower risk of vertebral fractures and a 38% lower risk of hip fracture compared to women receiving alendronate alone. Romosozumab is reserved for patients with severe osteoporosis, such as those with osteoporosis on DXA plus a history of fragility fracture. Because of a potential increased risk of major adverse cardiovascular events, a black box warning cautions that it should not be used in patients who have had an MI or stroke within the previous year.

Prognosis

DXA monitoring in an untreated patient can determine whether there is a clinically meaningful decrease in bone density over time. Although DXS can measure improvements in bone density among patients undergoing pharmacologic treatment for osteoporosis, the reduction in fracture risk afforded by treatment is only partially explained by an increase in BMD; randomized trial data demonstrate that patients with little or no significant increase in BMD in response to bisphosphonate therapy still have reduced fracture risk compared to placebo. Osteoporosis should ideally be prevented since it can be only partially reversed.

Cosman et al. Goal-directed osteoporosis treatment: ASBMR/BHOF task force position statement 2024. J Bone Miner Res. 2024;39:1393. [PMID: 39073912]
Ensrud KE et al. Osteoporosis. Ann Int Med. 2024;177:ITC1. [PMID: 38190715]
Fuggle NR et al. Evidence-based guideline for the management of osteoporosis in men. Nat Rev Rheumatol. 2024;20:241. [PMID: 38485753]
McClung MR. Sequential and long-term therapy for osteoporosis. Curr Osteoporos Rep. 2025;23:15. [PMID: 40119973]
Solling AS et al. Denosumab discontinuation. Curr Osteoporos Rep. 2023;21:95. [PMID: 36564572]
Walker MD et al. Postmenopausal osteoporosis. N Engl J Med. 2023;389:1979. [PMID: 37991856]

RICKETS & OSTEOMALACIA

ESSENTIALS OF DIAGNOSIS

- Low bone density from defective mineralization.
- Caused by deficiency in calcium, phosphorus, or low alkaline phosphatase.
- **Rickets:** defective bone mineralization in childhood or adolescence before epiphyseal fusion.
- **Osteomalacia:** defective bone mineralization in adults with fused epiphyses.
- Bone pain; painful proximal muscle weakness (especially pelvic girdle).
- Low serum 25-hydroxy-vitamin D (25-OHD), hypocalcemia, hypocalciuria, hypophosphatemia, secondary hyperparathyroidism.
- Classic radiologic features may be present.

General Considerations

Defective mineralization of the growing skeleton in childhood causes permanent bone deformities (rickets). Defective skeletal mineralization in adults (acquired) is known as osteomalacia. Both are caused by inadequate calcium or phosphate mineralization of bone osteoid.

Etiology

Causes of osteomalacia are listed in Table 30–3.

A. Vitamin D Deficiency & Disorders

Vitamin D deficiency is the most common cause of osteomalacia. In some cases, its cause is low exposure to sunlight caused by urbanization, living at high latitudes, winter season, institutionalization, sunscreen use, or very modest dressing. Other risk factors for vitamin D deficiency include older age, obesity, dark skin, inadequate dietary intake (malnutrition, vegan diets), and intestinal malabsorption. Anticonvulsants may inhibit the hepatic production of 25-OHD. About 36% of adults in the United States are deficient in vitamin D.

Vitamin D–dependent rickets type 1 is a rare autosomal recessive disorder caused by a mutation in the 1-α-hydroxylase gene *CYP27B*. Vitamin D–dependent rickets type 2 (also called vitamin D–resistant rickets) is caused by a germline mutation in the vitamin D receptor.

Table 30–3. Causes of osteomalacia.[1]

Vitamin D disorders
Insufficient sunlight exposure
Nutritional vitamin D deficiency: vegan diet, starvation
Intestinal malabsorption: aging, bariatric surgery, celiac disease, pancreatic enzyme deficiency
Kidney: CKD, nephrotic syndrome
Drugs: Phenytoin, carbamazepine, valproate, or barbiturate therapy (chronic)
Vitamin D–dependent rickets types 1 and 2
Dietary calcium deficiency
Phosphate homeostasis disorders
Intestinal malabsorption
Nutritional deficiency of phosphorus
Adefovir therapy for hepatitis B
Alcohol use disorder
Diuretics
FGF23-related: tumoral hypophosphatemic osteomalacia, X-linked hypophosphatemic rickets
Hyperparathyroidism
Phosphate-binding antacid therapy
Renal tubular loss: Fanconi syndrome, oral contraceptives (idiosyncratic), parenteral iron, renal tubular acidosis
Other disorders: glycogen storage diseases, neurofibromatosis, paraproteinemias, Wilson disease
Inhibitors of mineralization
Aluminum toxicity
Bisphosphonates
Disorders of bone matrix
Hypophosphatasia
Osteogenesis imperfecta
Axial osteomalacia
Fibrogenesis imperfecta ossium

[1]See Table 30–2 for causes of osteoporosis.

B. Calcium Deficiency

Recommended dietary allowances for calcium are 1300 mg daily during adolescence, 1000 mg for adult women up through age 50 years and men up through age 70, and 1200 mg for women age 51 and older and men 70 and older. Patients who have deficient calcium intake may develop rickets (childhood) or osteomalacia (adulthood) even in the presence of sufficient vitamin D. A nutritional deficiency of calcium can occur in vegans and in any severely malnourished patient. Some degree of calcium deficiency is common in older adults, since intestinal calcium absorption declines with age.

C. Phosphate Homeostasis Disorders

Osteomalacia develops in patients with hypophosphatemia due to lack of sufficient phosphate to mineralize bone osteoid. Such patients typically have musculoskeletal pain and muscle weakness and are prone to fractures.

1. Genetic disorders—Fibroblast growth factor-23 (FGF23) is a phosphaturic factor (phosphatonin) that is secreted by bone osteoblasts in response to elevated serum phosphate levels. Various germline mutations can result in high serum FGF23 levels, causing hypophosphatemia and bone mineral depletion. The most common of these genetic conditions is X-linked hypophosphatemic rickets (XLH).

2. Tumor-induced osteomalacia—This rare paraneoplastic syndrome usually involves overproduction of FGF23, with marked hypophosphatemia and hyperphosphaturia due to renal phosphate wasting. Such tumors are usually nonmalignant phosphaturic mesenchymal tumors. The tumors are often small and difficult to find, frequently lying in the sinuses or extremities.

3. Secondary hypophosphatemia—With calcium or vitamin D deficiency, calciopenia stimulates counterregulatory PTH secretion, resulting in hypophosphatemia due to renal phosphate wasting. Hypophosphatemia causes impaired bone mineralization and hypertrophy of chondrocytes at active growth plates, resulting in the bulbous enlargement at costochondral junctions that is seen with rickets.

4. Other causes of hypophosphatemia—Hypophosphatemia can be caused by alcohol use disorder, poor nutrition, and prolonged parenteral nutrition. Tenofovir therapy (tenofovir disoproxil fumarate more so than tenofovir alafenamide) can cause renal phosphate wasting and hypophosphatemia. Hypophosphatemia can also be caused by chelation of phosphate in the gut by aluminum hydroxide antacids, calcium acetate, or sevelamer hydrochloride. Excessive renal phosphate losses are also seen in proximal renal tubular acidosis, Fanconi syndrome, intravenous iron, and in some women using oral contraceptives.

D. Inhibition of Mineralization

Bone mineralization is inhibited by aluminum, so osteomalacia may occur in patients receiving long-term renal hemodialysis with tap water dialysate, or aluminum-containing antacids. Fluoride administered at very high doses with inadequate calcium supplementation may also cause bone formation that is poorly mineralized.

E. Disorders of Bone Matrix

Hypophosphatasia is a heritable rickets or osteomalacia characterized by low activity of the tissue-nonspecific isoenzyme of alkaline phosphatase. There is a range of severity, with perinatal, infantile, childhood, and adult presentations. Adult hypophosphatasia can present in adulthood with premature loss of teeth, metatarsal stress fractures, thigh pain due to femoral pseudofractures, or arthritis due to chondrocalcinosis. Bone density is low, and the osteomalacia is commonly misdiagnosed as osteoporosis. Serum alkaline phosphatase is usually low (< 40 U/L in adults and may be < 20 U/L in severe cases). The differential diagnosis includes other causes of low serum alkaline phosphatase, such as early pregnancy, hypothyroidism, myeloma, severe anemia, or vitamin D intoxication; alkaline phosphatase may also be low in a patient who has been treated with an antiresorptive medication like a bisphosphonate.

Clinical Findings

Older children and adolescents can have bone pain and muscle weakness and may develop the skeletal deformities of classic rickets, such as delayed longitudinal growth.

Hypertrophy of chondrocytes at growth plates causes bulbous enlargements of joints with bowed legs or knock-knees. Thickening at the costochondral joints can cause widening of the chest and deformities known as a "rachitic rosary." Kyphoscoliosis or lumbar lordosis is common.

In adults, osteomalacia is initially asymptomatic. Non-specific complaints include fatigue, reduced endurance and muscle strength, and pain in the bones involving their shoulders ribs, low back, and thighs develop. Pathologic fractures can occur with little or no trauma.

Hypocalcemia causes a reduced quality of life, with fatigue, irritability, depression, anxiety, cognitive impairment, lethargy, and paresthesias in the circumoral area, hands, and feet. More severe manifestations of hypocalcemia include muscle weakness or cramps, carpopedal spasm, convulsions, tetany, laryngospasm, and stridor. Primary or secondary hypophosphatemia can cause severe major muscle weakness, reduced endurance, dysphagia, diplopia, cardiomyopathy, and respiratory muscle weakness. Patients may also have impaired cognition.

Diagnostic Tests

DXA is used to determine the presence of low bone density that can be due to osteoporosis, osteomalacia, or both.

Serum is obtained for calcium, albumin, phosphate, alkaline phosphatase, PTH, and 25-OHD determinations. Vitamin D *deficiency* is defined as a serum 25-OHD < 20 ng/mL (50 nmol/L). Patients with severe osteomalacia may have chronic severe vitamin D deficiency (eg, serum 25-OHD < 12 ng/mL [25 nmol/L]).

Patients with otherwise unexplained hypophosphatemia should have a measurement of serum or plasma FGF23. Patients with high FGF23 levels can have genetic testing for skeletal disorders that includes XLH (*PHEX*), ADHR (*FGF23*), and ARHR (*DMP1, ENPP1*). In patients with hypophosphatemia without an identified mutations, searching for a tumor causing tumor-induced osteomalacia is reasonable, particularly in patients with bone pain or fractures.

Patients with hypophosphatasia have low serum levels of alkaline phosphatase (below 40 U/L in adults and below 20 U/L in severe cases). However, immediately following a fracture, serum alkaline phosphatase rises and may obscure the diagnosis. Provided vitamin B_6 is not being supplemented, an elevated pyridoxal 5'-phosphate is a good marker for the disease. Serum calcium is usually normal. Genetic testing can evaluate for mutations in the *TNSALP* gene, and clinical diagnostic criteria now exist to further guide clinicians.

Differential Diagnosis

Osteomalacia often coexists with osteoporosis. The relative contribution of the two entities to diminished bone density may not be apparent until treatment (eg, repleting vitamin D deficiency) since a dramatic rise in bone density is often seen with therapy for osteomalacia. Phosphate deficiency must be distinguished from hypophosphatemia seen in hyperparathyroidism.

Prevention & Treatment

In children and adolescents, empiric vitamin D supplementation is suggested to prevent nutritional rickets. This may include intake of vitamin D-fortified foods or daily intake of a vitamin D supplement. In adults, recommended daily allowance for vitamin D is 600 IU per day up to age 70 years, then 800 IU per day for those 71 and older. Humans naturally receive about 90% of their vitamin D from sunlight; vitamin D supplementation may be appropriate in patients who are sunlight-deprived or using sunscreen. Patients at risk for vitamin D deficiency or who have metabolic bone disease should have 25-OHD levels monitored.

The main natural food source of vitamin D is fish, particularly salmon, mackerel, cod liver oil, and sardines or tuna canned in oil. Most commercial cow's milk is fortified with vitamin D.

Most vitamin D supplements contain cholecalciferol (vitamin D_3), which is the preferred form for supplementation and treatment. Common supplement doses are 1000 IU or 2000 IU daily, but due to variable absorption and metabolism, a person with low 25-OHD levels may need more. Severe vitamin D deficiency can be treated with high-dose capsules of 50,000 IU each, which are more commonly ergocalciferol (D_2) than cholecalciferol. A common repletion course is 50,000 IU orally once or twice weekly for 8–12 doses. It is ideal to provide a daily supplement (eg, 1000–2000 IU daily) concurrently and extending after the short-term high-dose repletion course, so that 25-OHD levels do not fall again as soon as the repletion course ends. Serum levels of 25-OHD should be monitored, and the dosage of vitamin D adjusted to achieve and maintain a goal level of at least 20 ng/mL in the general population and 30–60 ng/mL in those with metabolic bone disease.

Patients with malabsorption or poor nutrition may need supplemental calcium in addition to vitamin D, which may be in the form of calcium carbonate or citrate.

For patients with tumoral hypophosphatemia, resection of the tumor normalizes serum phosphate levels; about 20% experience recurrence, usually in the same location. With both tumoral and genetic FGF23-related hypophosphatemia, therapy with burosumab improves osteomalacia.

Patients with hypophosphatasia may be treated with asfotase alfa, which replaces the deficient enzyme. Teriparatide can improve bone pain and fracture healing. Bisphosphonates are contraindicated.

Demay MB et al. Vitamin D for the prevention of disease: an Endocrine Society Clinical Practice Guideline. J Clin Endocrinol Metab. 2024;109:1907. [PMID: 38828931]

Korkmaz HA et al. Approach to nutritional rickets. J Pediatr Endocrinol Metab. 2023;36:335. [PMID: 36843296]

Minisola S et al. Tumor-induced osteomalacia: a comprehensive review. Endocr Rev. 2023;44:323. [PMID: 36327295]

Seefried L et al. Diagnosis and treatment of hypophosphatasia. Calcif Tissue Int. 2025;116:46. [PMID: 40047955]

PAGET DISEASE OF BONE (Osteitis Deformans)

ESSENTIALS OF DIAGNOSIS

- Often asymptomatic.
- Bone pain may be the first symptom.
- Kyphosis, bowed tibias, large head, deafness, and fractures.
- Serum calcium and phosphate normal; elevated alkaline phosphatase and biochemical markers of bone turnover.
- Osteolytic or sclerotic lesions, expanded bones on radiographs.

General Considerations

Paget disease of bone is manifested by one or more localized bony lesions having high bone turnover and disorganized osteoid formation. The involved bone first has increased osteoclast activity, causing lytic lesions that may progress at about 1 cm/year. Increased osteoblastic activity follows, producing a high rate of disorganized bone formation. Involved bones become vascular, weak, and deformed. Eventually, there is a final burned-out phase with markedly reduced bone cell activity and abnormal bones that may be enlarged with skeletal deformity.

The prevalence of Paget disease has declined over the recent decades. It is most common in the United Kingdom and in areas of European migration, and it is rare in Africa, Asia, and Scandinavia. In the United States, Paget disease affects about 1% of White persons over age 55 years, with it increasing prevalence over age 40 years. Most cases are discovered incidentally during radiology imaging or because of incidentally discovered elevations in serum alkaline phosphatase.

Clinical Findings

A. Symptoms and Signs

Paget disease is mild and asymptomatic in about 75% of cases. It involves multiple bones (polyostotic) in 72% and only a single bone (monostotic) in 28%. It occurs most commonly in the sacrum, vertebrae, femur, skull, pelvis, and humerus. The disease typically involves affected bones simultaneously and tends not to involve additional bones during its course. When symptomatic, pain, often described as aching, deep, and worse at night, is the usual initial symptom. Increased vascularity over the involved bones may cause increased warmth. Joint surfaces can be involved and cause arthritic pain. The poor bone quality can lead to bowing deformities of the femurs or tibias, kyphosis, and fractures, particularly of weight-bearing bones. If the skull is involved, the patient may report headaches and an increased head size. Involvement of the temporal bone can damage the cochlea, causing hearing loss.

B. Laboratory Findings

Serum total alkaline phosphatase and bone alkaline phosphatase levels are usually elevated, often markedly so. Other biochemical markers of bone turnover such as the C-terminal telopeptide of type 1 collagen (CTx) are also usually elevated. Serum calcium and phosphate are typically normal in untreated disease, although hypercalcemia may result if a patient sustains a fracture and is on bedrest.

C. Imaging

Plain x-rays or CT scans demonstrate osteolytic lesions in Paget disease, with focal radiolucencies. These may include advancing flame-shaped lytic lesions in long bones or "osteoporosis circumscripta" in the skull. In vertebrae, the lesions may display a "clover" or "heart" appearance ("Mickey Mouse sign"), helping distinguish them from bone metastases. Bone lesions can have a lytic phase, mixed phase, or sclerotic phase. The affected bones eventually become thickened and deformed. Radionuclide bone scans (eg, Technetium-99m pyrophosphate) are helpful in delineating activity of bone lesions and finding additional lesions in other locations.

Differential Diagnosis

Paget disease must be differentiated from primary bone lesions (eg, osteogenic sarcoma, plasma cell myeloma, and fibrous dysplasia) and from secondary bone lesions (eg, osteitis fibrosa cystica and metastatic carcinoma to bone). Rare familial types of sclerosing bone dysplasias share phenotypic homologies with Paget disease of bone.

Complications

If immobilization occurs, hypercalcemia and hypercalciuria (with risk of renal calculi) may develop. Arthritis frequently develops in joints adjacent to involved bone. Pathologic fractures may occur in weakened bones, and surgery for fractured long bones may be complicated by excessive blood loss from vascular lytic lesions.

Skull involvement may cause hearing loss or cranial nerve palsies.

Sarcoma or giant cell tumor develops in <1% of longstanding lesions.

Treatment

Treatment is with a bisphosphonate, which suppresses osteoclast activity. Indications for treatment are to relieve symptoms or to prevent future complications. Some asymptomatic patients may require only clinical surveillance, but those who have involvement of the skull, weight-bearing long bones, or vertebrae may benefit from medical therapy.

Zoledronic acid is the treatment of choice for Paget disease and is superior to other bisphosphonates. Administered intravenously as a single 5-mg dose, it normalizes the serum alkaline phosphatase in 89% of patients by 6 months and in 98% by 2 years. In some patients, biochemical remission will be achieved with a single dose of zoledronic acid. If the serum alkaline phosphatase level rises above normal or increases > 25% above the nadir level, the infusion may be repeated.

Following intravenous zoledronic acid, patients frequently experience a flu-like reaction of fever, headache, myalgia, bone pain, or a combination of these, which may be treated with acetaminophen or NSAIDs. Bisphosphonate-induced hypocalcemia may be severe, especially if the patient has vitamin D deficiency or is taking a loop diuretic. Therefore, vitamin D deficiency should be corrected before administering the bisphosphonate, and adequate supplementation of calcium and vitamin D is crucial, especially in the initial days and weeks following treatment.

Prognosis

The prognosis is good, with many patients experiencing sustained response to bisphosphonate therapy, although relapse can occur. By 6.5 years after initial therapy, the recurrence rate is 12.5% after treatment with zoledronic acid and 62% after risedronate. Patients must be monitored long term, measuring serum alkaline phosphatase every 6–12 months. In the most severe forms, marked deformity, intractable pain, and additional complications may occur if not treated with bisphosphonates.

Ayalon-Dangur I et al. Long-term effectiveness of zoledronic acid in patients with Paget's disease of bone – a retrospective cohort study. Endocrine. 2024;85:873. [PMID: 38555314]

Phillips J et al. Randomised trial of genetic testing and targeted intervention to prevent the development and progression of Paget's disease of bone. Ann Rheum Dis. 2024;83:529. [PMID: 38123339]

Ralston SH. Latest developments in Paget's disease of bone. Eur J Endocrinol. 2025;193:R43. [PMID: 41037515]

MULTIPLE ENDOCRINE NEOPLASIA (MEN)

ESSENTIALS OF DIAGNOSIS

- **MEN1:** principal manifestations are tumors of the parathyroid glands, anterior pituitary, and endocrine pancreas and duodenum; may also include tumors of the adrenals and thymus, carcinoid tumors, lipomas, and facial angiofibromas.
- **MEN2A:** medullary thyroid cancer, primary hyperparathyroidism, pheochromocytoma.
- **MEN2B:** medullary thyroid cancer, pheochromocytoma, mucosal neuromas, marfanoid habitus, intestinal ganglioneuroma.
- **MEN4:** a rare mimic of MEN1, usually presenting with tumors of the parathyroid glands and anterior pituitary.

Syndromes of MEN are inherited as autosomal dominant traits that cause a predisposition to the development of tumors of two or more different endocrine glands (Table 30–4). MEN syndromes are caused by germline mutations with tumors arising when additional somatic mutations occur in predisposed organs. Patients with MEN should have genetic testing so that their first-degree relatives may then be tested for the specific mutation.

MEN1

Multiple endocrine neoplasia type 1 (MEN1, Wermer syndrome) is a tumor syndrome with a prevalence of 2–10 per 100,000 persons in the United States. A clinical diagnosis of MEN1 is made when an individual has at least two of the three MEN1-associated tumors: primary hyperparathyroidism, duodenopancreatic neuroendocrine tumor, and

Table 30–4. Multiple endocrine neoplasia (MEN) syndromes: incidence of tumor types.

Tumor Type	MEN1	MEN2A	MEN2B	MEN4
Parathyroid	95%	20–30%	Rare	Common
Enteropancreatic	30–80%			Common
Pituitary	35–65%			Common
Medullary thyroid carcinoma		80–100%	> 95%	
Pheochromocytoma	Rare	50%	50%	
Mucosal and GI ganglioneuromas		Rare	> 90%	
Subcutaneous lipoma	30%			
Adrenocortical adenoma	40%			Observed
Thoracic carcinoid	15%			
Thymic neuroendocrine tumor	< 10%			
Facial angiofibromas and collagenomas	85%			
Breast cancer	27%			

anterior pituitary adenoma (Table 30–4). Patients with MEN1 are also predisposed to develop many other endocrine tumors. A genetic diagnosis is made by identifying a germline pathogenic variant in the *MEN1* gene, regardless of clinical manifestations. Timely diagnosis is very important so that an individual can undergo appropriate screening for MEN1-associated tumors.

Tumor penetrance increases with age, but the timing and nature of the presentation of MEN1 is variable, even in the same kindred. Increased genetic testing and guideline-driven screening has resulted in earlier diagnoses and earlier identification of clinical manifestations. Many patients with MEN1 will develop at least one MEN1-associated tumor in their teens, most commonly with primary hyperparathyroidism identified first. By the time they are in their 40s, almost all patients with MEN1 will have evidence of primary hyperparathyroidism, typically from multiglandular parathyroid tumors.

Enteropancreatic tumors, including gastrinoma, insulinoma, nonfunctioning and pancreatic polypeptide-secreting tumors, glucagonoma, and vasoactive intestinal peptide-overproducing tumor, occur in up to 80% of patients with MEN1. Gastrinomas occur in about 40% of patients.

Insulinomas occur in about 10% of patients. Extrapancreatic neuroendocrine tumors are common in MEN1; they are frequently malignant and include carcinoid tumors (usually in foregut locations [69%]) that may arise in the lung, thymus, duodenum, or stomach and can metastasize, especially to the liver. (See GEP-NETs and Chapter 43.)

Pituitary adenomas are the presenting tumor in 29% of patients with MEN1 and eventually are found in 35–65%. About 42% of the pituitary adenomas secrete PRL, while others secrete GH (6%), ACTH (3%), gonadotrophins (2%), or multiple hormones (5%). About 42% of pituitary adenomas are nonsecretory. Nonsecretory pituitary microadenomas (< 1 cm and detected on routine MRI screening) are usually indolent; 25% of nonsecretory pituitary adenomas are macroadenomas (≥ 1 cm) and more aggressive.

Adrenal adenomas or hyperplasia occur in about 40% of patients with MEN1; 50% are bilateral. They are generally benign and nonfunctional. These adrenal lesions are ACTH-independent.

Thymic neuroendocrine tumors occur in 3.4% of affected patients, with a 10-year survival of 25%. Lung neuroendocrine tumors occur in 13%, with a 10-year survival of 71%.

Nonendocrine tumors occur commonly in MEN1, particularly small head-neck angiofibromas (85%) and lipomas (30%). Collagenomas are common (70%), presenting as firm dermal nodules. Affected patients may also be more prone to meningiomas, breast cancer, colorectal cancers, prostate cancer, and malignant melanomas.

MEN2A

Multiple endocrine neoplasia type 2A (MEN2A, Sipple syndrome) is a rare autosomal-dominant tumor syndrome that arises in patients with a germline gain-of-function *ret* protooncogene mutation. Genetic testing identifies about 95% of affected individuals.

Manifestations include medullary thyroid carcinoma (80–100%); hyperparathyroidism (20–30%) (with hyperplasia or multiple parathyroid gland adenoma developing in most cases); and pheochromocytomas (50%) (which are often bilateral and frequently asymptomatic). Hirschsprung disease or cutaneous lichen amyloidosis may develop. Prophylactic thyroidectomy and annual screening for manifestations are recommended; the underlying RET mutation determines the optimal age for preventive surgery and the age for initiation of screening of each manifestation. Patients with MEN2A should not receive therapy for diabetes with GLP-1 agonists, which may increase the risk for medullary thyroid carcinoma. Before any surgical procedure, MEN2A carriers should be screened for pheochromocytoma and for medullary thyroid carcinoma.

MEN2B

Multiple endocrine neoplasia type 2B (MEN2B), formerly MEN3, is a familial, autosomal dominant multiglandular syndrome that is also caused by a germline gain-of-function mutation of the *ret* protooncogene. Like MEN2A, MEN2B is characterized by medullary thyroid carcinoma and pheochromocytomas, but primary hyperparathyroidism is rare. MEN2B involves a number of somatic manifestations including mucosal neuromas (> 90%) with bumpy and enlarged lips and tongue, marfanoid habitus (75% with skeletal abnormalities [pes cavus and pectus excavatum]), and intestinal ganglioneuromas. Medullary thyroid carcinoma presents early in life, has a penetrance of nearly 100%, and is aggressive.

MEN4

Multiple endocrine neoplasia type 4 (MEN4) is a rare autosomal-dominant familial tumor syndrome caused by germline mutations in the gene *CDKN1B*. It may mimic MEN1, so screening should be considered in patients with an MEN1-like phenotype who do not have an MEN1 gene mutation. Affected patients are particularly prone to parathyroid adenomas, pituitary adenomas, and gastroenteropancreatic neuroendocrine tumors.

Brandi ML et al. Multiple endocrine neoplasia type 1 (MEN1): recommendations and guidelines for best practice. Lancet Diabetes Endocrinol. 2025;13:699. [PMID: 40523372]

Chevalier B et al. Beyond MEN1, when to think about MEN4? Retrospective study on 5600 patients in the French population and literature review. J Clin Endocrinol Metab. 2024;109:e1482. [PMID: 38288531]

English KA et al. Treatments for MEN1-associated endocrine tumours: three systematic reviews and a meta-analysis. Lancet Diabetes Endocrinol. 2025;13:685. [PMID: 40523371]

Frye CC et al. Evaluation and surgical management of multiple endocrine neoplasias. Surg Clin North Am. 2024;104:909. [PMID: 38944508]

ADVERSE EFFECTS OF SYSTEMIC GLUCOCORTICOIDS

Prolonged treatment with high-dose corticosteroids causes toxic effects that can be life threatening. Besides oral and parenteral administration, transdermal and inhaled

Table 30–5. Management of patients receiving systemic glucocorticoids to decrease risk of adverse effects.

Recommendations for prescribing
- Do not administer systemic corticosteroids unless absolutely indicated or more conservative measures have failed.
- Keep dosage and duration of administration to the minimum required for adequate treatment.
- When glucocorticoids are no longer needed, if duration has been > 3–4 weeks, taper therapy rather than abruptly stopping.

Monitoring recommendations
- Screen patients on high-dose therapy for latent infections such as tuberculosis.
- Screen for pregnancy in reproductive age women; recommend contraceptive measures.
- Screen for type 2 diabetes before and during treatment.
- Screen for hypertension before and during treatment.
- Screen for glaucoma and cataracts before moderate- to high-dose treatment and during treatment.
- Monitor weight; use comprehensive lifestyle interventions to avoid or treat obesity and optimize nutrition.
- Assess bone densitometry by DXA at baseline and monitor during treatment at a frequency determined by risk group; measure and monitor height.
- Watch for fungal or yeast infections of skin, nails, mouth, vagina, and rectum, and treat appropriately.

Patient information
- Prepare the patient and family for possible adverse effects on mood, memory, and cognitive function.
- Inform the patient about other possible side effects, such as weight gain, diabetes, osteoporosis, and skin changes.
- Counsel about adrenal insufficiency and the importance of stress-dose glucocorticoids in times of illness or trauma.
- Encourage the wearing of a medical alert bracelet documenting risk of adrenal insufficiency.

Prophylactic measures and treatment of complications
- Institute a vigorous physical exercise and isometric regimen tailored to each patient's abilities or disabilities.
- Recommend calcium and vitamin D intakes according to published recommended dietary allowances: total daily calcium intakes (from diet plus supplements) of 1000 mg/day for adult women to age 50 and men to age 70, and 1200 mg/day for women > 50 and men > 70; vitamin D 600 IU/day for adults to age 70 and 800 IU/day for adults > 70.
- Treat with antiosteoporosis pharmacotherapy if fracture risk is high or very high, with a bisphosphonate (first-line) or anabolic agent (if very high risk for fracture).
- Avoid prolonged bed rest that will accelerate muscle weakness and bone mineral loss.
- Institute fall prevention strategies.
- Treat diabetes as one would treat type 2 diabetes in the general population.
- For ulcer prophylaxis, if administering glucocorticoids with NSAIDs, prescribe a PPI (not required for glucocorticoids alone).
- Immunize patients according to guidelines, and avoid live virus vaccines to specific groups on high-dose therapy.

corticosteroids have some systemic absorption and can cause similar adverse effects. Patients should be thoroughly informed of the major possible side effects of treatment: insomnia, cognitive and personality changes, weight gain with central obesity, skin thinning and bruising, striae, muscle weakness, polyuria, renal calculi, diabetes mellitus, glaucoma, cataracts, sex hormone suppression, candidiasis, and opportunistic infections (Table 30–5). Prolonged high-dose corticosteroids also increase the risk of hypertension, dyslipidemia, MI, stroke, atrial fibrillation or flutter, and HF. Gastric ulceration is more common with high-dose corticosteroids, particularly when patients take NSAIDs concurrently. High-dose inhaled corticosteroids predispose to oral thrush and pulmonary nontuberculous mycobacterial infection. To reduce risks, the dosage and duration of corticosteroid administration must be minimized. Immediately following inhaled corticosteroids, proper mouth-washing and gargling can reduce systemic absorption.

Prolonged oral, inhaled, intravenous, or high-dose topical corticosteroid therapy commonly suppresses pituitary ACTH secretion, causing secondary adrenal insufficiency. Symptoms of glucocorticoid-induced adrenal insufficiency, including hypotension, fatigue, nausea, hyponatremia, and hypoglycemia, may manifest when glucocorticoids are abruptly discontinued or decreased below physiologic doses. Thus, patients no longer requiring chronic glucocorticoids should undergo a taper prior to stopping therapy (Table 30–5). Adrenal insufficiency also may manifest during times of physiologic stress such as infection or trauma, due to an inability of endogenous cortisol production to increase in response to heightened glucocorticoid requirements (see Chapter 29).

Most corticosteroids (dexamethasone, prednisone, hydrocortisone, budesonide) are metabolized by the enzyme CYP34A. When drugs that inhibit CYP34A are administered along with even modest doses of corticosteroids (oral, inhaled, intravenous), the blood levels of the corticosteroids rise and can cause iatrogenic Cushing syndrome and secondary adrenal insufficiency. Medications that strongly inhibit CYP34A include itraconazole, ketoconazole, nefazodone, protease inhibitors, and cobicistat.

In pregnancy, corticosteroids taken by the mother are transmitted across the placenta to the fetus, causing adverse effects on fetal growth and development as well as childhood cognition and behavior. Therefore, women who are to receive high-dose corticosteroids should be screened for pregnancy and counseled to use contraception.

Chronic glucocorticoids negatively affect bone by increasing bone resorption and decreasing bone formation. Osteoporotic fractures (especially vertebral) ultimately occur in about 40% of patients receiving long-term glucocorticoid therapy. Osteoporotic fractures can occur even in patients receiving long-term therapy at relatively low doses (eg, 5–7.5 mg prednisone daily). Pharmacologic therapy is recommended for patients with high fracture risk, which can be determined accounting for age, sex, menopausal status, BMD, fracture history, and glucocorticoid exposure (dose and duration). Guidelines from professional societies including the American College of Rheumatology recommend specific glucocorticoid-corrected thresholds for FRAX risk scores. When fracture risk is high enough to warrant pharmacologic therapy, bisphosphonates (eg, oral alendronate or intravenous zoledronic acid) are first-line (Table 30–5). The anabolic agent teriparatide is FDA approved for treatment of glucocorticoid-induced osteoporosis and an option for those at very high risk of fracture.

Another bone complications of chronic glucocorticoid therapy are avascular necrosis of bone (especially hips), which develops in about 15% of patients who receive glucocorticoids at high doses for > 1 month with cumulative prednisone doses of ≥ 10 g.

Beuschlein F et al. European Society of Endocrinology and Endocrine Society joint clinical guideline: diagnosis and therapy of glucocorticoid-induced adrenal insufficiency. J Clin Endocrinol Metab. 2024;109:1657. [PMID: 38724043]

Hofbauer LC et al. Glucocorticoid-induced osteoporosis: novel concepts and clinical indications. Lancet Diabetes Endocrinol. 2025;13:964. [PMID: 41022095]

Humphrey MB et al. 2022 American College of Rheumatology guideline for the prevention and treatment of glucocorticoid-induced osteoporosis. Arthritis Care Res (Hoboken). 2023;75:2405. [PMID: 37884467]

Vaidya A et al. Adrenal insufficiency in adults: a review. JAMA. 2025;334:714. [PMID: 40522647]

Diabetes Mellitus & Hypoglycemia

31

Savitha Subramanian, MD
Amy Eby, MD

DIABETES MELLITUS

ESSENTIALS OF DIAGNOSIS

Type 1 diabetes

- Polyuria, polydipsia, and weight loss with random plasma glucose ≥ 200 mg/dL (11.1 mmol/L).
- Plasma glucose ≥ 126 mg/dL (7.0 mmol/L) after an overnight fast, documented on more than one occasion.
- Ketonemia, ketonuria, or both.
- Islet autoantibodies frequently present.
- Generally progresses from stage 1 (autoantibodies but normal glucose tolerance) to stage 2 (autoantibodies with glucose intolerance) to stage 3 (symptomatic disease).

Prediabetes

- An intermediate stage of glucose dysregulation between normal blood glucose and type 2 diabetes.
- Fasting plasma glucose 100–125 mg/dL (6.1–6.9 mmol/L), plasma glucose 2 hours after 75 g oral glucose 140–199 mg/dL (7.8–11 mmol/L), and/or HbA_{1c} 5.7–6.4%.
- More than one in three US adults have prediabetes.

Type 2 diabetes

- Most patients are > 40 years of age and have obesity, but onset at any age is possible.
- Polyuria and polydipsia, ketonuria, and weight loss are less common at time of diagnosis.
- Candidal vaginitis may be an initial manifestation, or asymptomatic.
- Plasma glucose ≥ 126 mg/dL (7.0 mmol/L) after an overnight fast on more than one occasion, and/or plasma glucose ≥ 200 mg/dL (11.1 mmol) 2 hours after 75 g oral glucose.
- HbA_{1c} ≥ 6.5%.

Epidemiologic Considerations

As of 2021, an estimated 38.4 million persons (11.6%) in the United States have diabetes mellitus, of whom approximately 5–10% have type 1 diabetes and most others (90–95%) have type 2 diabetes. There is a global epidemic of type 2 diabetes, and the economic burden is significant. A third group designated as "other specific types" by the American Diabetes Association (ADA) numbers in the thousands (https://www.cdc.gov/diabetes/php/data-research/).

Classification & Pathogenesis

A. Type 1 Diabetes Mellitus

Type 1 diabetes is an autoimmune disorder with progressive destruction of pancreatic islet β cells resulting in endogenous insulin deficiency and hyperglycemia. In this catabolic disorder, circulating insulin is virtually absent, plasma glucagon is elevated (since not suppressed by insulin), and pancreatic β cells fail to respond to all insulinogenic stimuli. Exogenous insulin is required to reverse the catabolic state, prevent ketosis, reduce hyperglucagonemia, and decrease blood glucose.

The rate of β cell destruction is variable, being rapid in some individuals and slow in others. There are three distinct stages in the development of type 1 diabetes. Stage 1 occurs when there is β cell autoimmunity (presence of islet autoantibodies) but there is normoglycemia. Stage 2 occurs with there is abnormal glucose tolerance but patients remain asymptomatic. Stage 3 is the development of symptomatic type 1 diabetes.

Although type 1 diabetes commonly occurs in children and young adults, it can occur at any age and 50% of new cases are diagnosed in adults. Misclassification of type 1 diabetes in adults is common, and > 40% of those developing type 1 diabetes after age 30 years are initially treated for type 2 diabetes. The term *latent autoimmune diabetes of adults* (LADA) has been used to identify adults who develop immune-mediated type 1 diabetes. The rate of β cell destruction in patients with LADA is slower than in those who have a "classic" presentation of type 1 diabetes (diabetic ketoacidosis [DKA]). While there is a debate as to whether the term LADA should be used as a diagnosis, the ADA Standards of Care suggests that for the purpose of classification, any form of diabetes mediated by autoimmune β cell destruction should be classified as type 1 diabetes. Therefore, the use of the term LADA in adults who may have progressive autoimmune β cell destruction is acceptable since it can increase clinicians' diagnostic awareness and accelerate appropriate insulin initiation to prevent diabetic ketoacidosis. Some individuals may retain enough β cell function to avoid ketosis, but as their β cell mass diminishes, the need for insulin therapy develops. Surveys for islet cell antibodies among persons of northern European descent indicate that up to 15% of patients with "type 2" diabetes may have LADA.

Many patients with type 1 diabetes mellitus have circulating antibodies to islet cells (ICA), glutamic acid decarboxylase 65 (GAD65), insulin (IAA), tyrosine phosphatase IA2 (ICA-512), and zinc transporter 8 (ZnT8) at the time of diagnosis; screening with these autoimmune markers may identify 98% of patients who have an autoimmune basis for their β cell loss. These antibodies also facilitate screening of siblings of affected children and adults with atypical features of type 2 diabetes mellitus. Up to 10% of patients with new-onset type 1 diabetes have no detectable islet autoantibodies; therefore, the absence of autoantibodies does not exclude type 1 diabetes. Antibody levels also decline with increasing duration of disease.

Patients with type 1 diabetes who do not have evidence of pancreatic β cell autoimmunity do have insulinopenia and can develop ketoacidosis. This subgroup of patients is classified as having "idiopathic type 1 diabetes." Although only a minority of patients with type 1 diabetes fall into this group, most of these individuals are of Asian or sub-Saharan African origin. About 4% of West Africans with ketosis-prone diabetes are homozygous for a sub-Saharan African ancestry-specific allele in *PAX-4* (*Arg133Trp*)—a transcription factor that is essential for the development of pancreatic islets.

Multiple genetic and unidentified factors likely play a role in the etiology of pancreatic autoimmune β cell destruction. Although the risk for developing type 1 diabetes is much higher for relatives of patients with the disease, > 85% of persons who develop type 1 diabetes do not have a first-degree relative with the disease. Most sporadic cases occur because ~ 40% of persons in the general population carry the high-risk human leukocyte antigen (HLA) alleles for diabetes. Family members of probands with diabetes are at increased lifetime risk for developing type 1 diabetes. A child whose mother has type 1 diabetes has a 2% risk of developing the disease and a 6% risk if the child's father has it. The risk in siblings is related to the number of HLA haplotypes that the sibling shares with the proband having diabetes. If one haplotype is shared, the risk is 6% and if two haplotypes are shared, the risk increases to 12–25%. The highest risk is for monozygotic twins, where the concordance rate is 25–50%. Evidence for environmental factors playing a role in the development of type 1 diabetes includes the observation that the disease is more common in Scandinavian countries and becomes progressively less frequent in countries nearer to the equator. Which environmental factor is responsible for the increased risk of type 1 diabetes is not known. Improvements in public health and reduced infections (especially parasitic) may lead to immune system dysregulation and development of autoimmune disorders such as asthma and type 1 diabetes (the hygiene hypothesis).

The use of checkpoint inhibitor immunotherapies, such as nivolumab, pembrolizumab, and ipilimumab, can precipitate autoimmune disorders, including type 1 diabetes; the onset of diabetes can be rapid and is permanent, with diabetic ketoacidosis at presentation. Autoantibodies against islet antigens are present in < 50% of patients; therefore individuals receiving these drugs should be carefully monitored for the development of autoimmune diabetes.

B. Prediabetes for Type 2 Diabetes

A fasting plasma glucose level of 70–99 mg/dL (3.9–5.9 mmol/L) and a glucose level <140 mg/dL (<7.8 mmol/L) 2 hours after a meal are considered normal. The ADA definition of prediabetes is impaired fasting glucose (fasting plasma glucose 100–125 mg/dL [6.1–6.9 mmol/L]), impaired glucose tolerance 2 hours after an oral glucose tolerance test (plasma glucose 140–199 mg/dL [7.8–11mmol/L]), and/or an elevated HbA_{1c} (5.7–6.4%). The ADA calls prediabetes a high-risk state for developing diabetes. The WHO uses the term *intermediate hyperglycemia*, and the WHO criteria for intermediate hyperglycemia include impaired fasting glucose (fasting plasma glucose 110–125 mg/dL [6.1–6.9 mmol/L]) and impaired glucose tolerance (plasma glucose 140–200 mg/dL [7.8–11.0 mmol/L]) 2 hours after ingestion of 75 g of oral glucose, or a combination of the two.

Risk factors for prediabetes include overweight or obesity, older age, lifestyle factors, and genetic predisposition. Microvascular complications, including retinopathy, neuropathy, and nephropathy, can occur with prediabetes and it is established as a risk factor for the development of atherosclerotic CVD. It is estimated that in 2024, 100 million adults in the United States or 37.7% of the population age 18 and older had prediabetes. Annually, 5–15% of US adults progress from prediabetes to diabetes and a similar number each year revert to normoglycemia (https://www.cdc.gov/diabetes/php/data-research/).

C. Type 2 Diabetes Mellitus

Type 2 diabetes is defined by several characteristic abnormalities including resistance to the action of insulin in peripheral tissues (muscle, liver, and fat), defective β cell insulin secretion, decreased skeletal muscle glucose uptake, and increased production of glucose by the liver. β Cell function is not completely lost and is usually sufficient to prevent ketoacidosis but is inadequate to prevent hyperglycemia. This form of diabetes used to occur predominantly in adults, but it is now more frequently encountered in children and adolescents. The clinical presentation of type 2 diabetes is heterogeneous, with widely variable age at onset, severity of the condition, and degree of obesity.

Genetic and environmental factors combine to cause both β cell loss and insulin resistance. Most epidemiologic data indicate strong genetic influences since in monozygotic twins > 40 years of age, concordance develops in > 70% of cases within a year whenever type 2 diabetes develops in one twin. Genome-wide association studies have identified > 700 risk variants and putative regulator mechanisms for type 2 diabetes. Several environmental factors may play a crucial role in the development of the type 2 diabetes. These include excessive caloric intake leading to obesity, a sedentary lifestyle, medications that cause metabolic abnormalities, and disruption of the gut microbiome and circadian rhythm.

Obesity is the most important environmental factor causing insulin resistance. The degree and prevalence of obesity with type 2 diabetes vary among different racial groups. In patients with type 2 diabetes, obesity or overweight is apparent in 50% of Chinese and Japanese patients, 80% of North American or European patients, 50–80% of African patients, and nearly 100% of patients who are Pima Indians or Pacific Islanders from Nauru or Samoa.

Central or visceral obesity, due to accumulation of fat in the omental and mesenteric regions, is strongly linked to insulin resistance; subcutaneous abdominal fat is less associated with insulin insensitivity and may be protective against insulin resistance. *Metabolic obesity* is a term used to describe increased visceral fat in patients with type 2 diabetes without overt obesity.

D. Other Specific Types of Diabetes Mellitus

1. Pancreatic diabetes—A single episode of severe acute pancreatitis, chronic pancreatitis, or subtotal pancreatectomy (resected volume > 40%) reduces the number of functioning β cells and results in insulin deficiency similar to type 1 diabetes, sometimes labeled type 3c diabetes; concomitant reduction in pancreatic α cells may reduce glucagon secretion so that relatively lower doses of insulin replacement are needed. Screening for diabetes is recommended within 3–6 months after an episode of pancreatitis and annually thereafter.

2. Cystic fibrosis–related diabetes (CFRD)—Nineteen percent of adolescents and 40–50% of adults with cystic fibrosis develop CFRD, primarily due to insulin deficiency. CFRD presents initially as impaired glucose tolerance with fasting hyperglycemia occurring late in the disease, so the HbA_{1c} alone can miss postprandial hyperglycemia. Screening with a 2-hour oral glucose tolerance test is recommended annually starting at age 10; insulin is the treatment of choice. Carbohydrate-restricted diet is not recommended for these patients who often have low body weight and malnutrition risk. CFRD is associated with higher pulmonary morbidity and mortality and should be aggressively managed, which can improve pulmonary outcomes.

3. Diabetes related to malnutrition—Malnutrition-related diabetes has been reclassified as type 5 diabetes by the International Diabetes Federation. Type 5 diabetes occurs because of undernutrition, particularly in early childhood and adolescence. Poor maternal nutrition, frequent infections, and food scarcity can result in pancreatic atrophy and insulin deficiency without autoimmunity. Patients have low BMI (< 19) and presenting symptoms of weight loss, fatigue, polyuria and polydipsia, usually without DKA. They are insulin sensitive.

4. Maturity-onset diabetes of the young (MODY)—This subgroup of monogenic disorders is characterized by non–insulin-requiring diabetes with autosomal dominant inheritance and an age at onset of 25 years or younger. MODY is characterized by impaired glucose-induced secretion of insulin and the absence of obesity. Six types of MODY account for > 80% of cases, but at least 14 have been described. Patients age < 30 with a negative autoantibody screen and endogenous insulin production (urinary C-peptide/creatinine ratio of ≥ 0.2 nmol/mmol) are candidates for genetic screening for MODY.

5. Diabetes mellitus associated with a variant of mitochondrial DNA—Diabetes due to variants in mitochondrial DNA occurs in < 2% of patients with diabetes. Diabetes is usually diagnosed when these patients, who may also have hearing loss (maternally inherited diabetes and deafness [MIDD]), are in their late 30s. In some patients, the β cell failure can be rapidly progressive and patients require insulin soon after diagnosis. Other patients can be managed by diet or oral agents for a while but most eventually require insulin. Patients with MIDD are not usually overweight; they resemble patients with type 1 diabetes mellitus but without evidence for autoimmunity.

6. Wolfram syndrome—Wolfram syndrome is an autosomal recessive neurodegenerative disorder first evident in childhood. It consists of diabetes insipidus, diabetes mellitus, optic atrophy, and deafness, hence the acronym DIDMOAD. Cranial diabetes insipidus and sensorineural deafness develop during the second decade in 60–75% of patients. Ureterohydronephrosis, neurogenic bladder, cerebellar ataxia, peripheral neuropathy, and psychiatric illness develop later in many patients.

7. Autosomal recessive syndromes—Homozygous variants in a number of pancreatic transcription factors, such as *NEUROG3, PTF1A, RFX6,* and *GLI-similar 3 (GLIS3),* cause neonatal or childhood diabetes. Patients with variant in the *EIF2AK3* gene have neonatal diabetes, epiphyseal dysplasia, developmental delay, and liver and kidney dysfunction (Wolcott-Rallison syndrome).

8. Diabetes mellitus secondary to other causes—Endocrine tumors secreting growth hormone, glucocorticoids, catecholamines, glucagon, or somatostatin can cause glucose intolerance (Table 31–1). In the first four of these situations, peripheral responsiveness to insulin is impaired. With excess of glucocorticoids, catecholamines, or glucagon, increased hepatic output of glucose is a contributory factor; in the case of catecholamines, decreased insulin release is an additional factor in producing carbohydrate intolerance, and with somatostatin, inhibition of insulin secretion is the major factor. Diabetes mainly occurs in individuals with underlying defects in insulin secretion, and hyperglycemia typically resolves when the hormone excess is resolved.

High-titer anti-insulin receptor antibodies that inhibit insulin binding cause a clinical syndrome characterized by severe insulin resistance, glucose intolerance or diabetes mellitus, and acanthosis nigricans. These patients usually have other autoimmune disorders.

Table 31–1. Secondary causes of hyperglycemia.

Hyperglycemia due to tissue insensitivity to insulin
Medications (corticosteroids, sympathomimetic drugs, niacin, alpelisib, sirolimus)
Hormonal tumors (acromegaly, Cushing syndrome, glucagonoma, pheochromocytoma)
Liver disease (cirrhosis, hemochromatosis)
Muscle disorders (myotonic dystrophy)
Adipose tissue disorders (lipodystrophy, truncal obesity)
Hyperglycemia due to reduced insulin secretion
Medications (thiazide diuretics, β-blockers, phenytoin, pentamidine, calcineurin inhibitors, atypical antipsychotics)
Hormonal tumors (somatostatinoma, pheochromocytoma)
Pancreatic disorders (pancreatitis, hemosiderosis, hemochromatosis)

Many medications are associated with the development of carbohydrate intolerance or diabetes by decreasing insulin secretion, increasing insulin resistance, or both (Table 31–1). The calcineurin inhibitors cyclosporine and tacrolimus impair insulin secretion; sirolimus increases insulin resistance. These agents contribute to the development of new-onset diabetes after solid-organ transplantation. Corticosteroids increase insulin resistance but may also impair β cell function. Screening with an oral glucose tolerance test is recommended; HbA_{1c} and a fasting morning glucose test may miss the hyperglycemia, which is primarily daytime and postprandial. Thiazide diuretics and β-blockers modestly increase the risk of diabetes. Treating hypokalemia due to thiazides may reverse the hyperglycemia. Atypical antipsychotics, particularly olanzapine and clozapine, are associated with increased risk of glucose intolerance; risperidone and quetiapine are associated with an intermediate risk. These drugs cause weight gain and insulin resistance but may also impair β cell function; an increased rate of DKA has been reported.

Diabetes Prevention

A. Prevention of Type 1 Diabetes

At the time of diagnosis of type 1 diabetes, residual β cell pancreatic function remains. This explains why soon after diagnosis and following the initiation of insulin therapy, the diabetes goes into partial clinical remission and little or no insulin is required ("honeymoon effect"). The honeymoon period may reflect temporary slowing or recovery of β cell loss. The incidence and duration of clinical remission varies, and eventually most patients lose all β cell function and develop worsening glucose control. Immune therapies targeting the disease mechanism to prolong this partial clinical remission are used to prevent or delay the loss of functional β cell mass. The CD3 complex present on the T cell modifies CD8-positive T cells that mediate β cell death and preserve regulatory T cells. Teplizumab is a humanized monoclonal antibody against the CD3 molecule on T cells. When teplizumab was administered to patients with new-onset type 1 diabetes, it did not restore glycemic control despite C peptide preservation. However, in a phase 2 study of early intervention in nondiabetic relatives of patients with type 1 diabetes (note that these relatives were at high risk for the development of diabetes since they had two or more diabetes-related autoantibodies and glucose intolerance), a single course of teplizumab delayed progression to clinical type 1 diabetes by about 2 years. Teplizumab is thus approved by the US Food and Drug Administration (FDA) for use in individuals 8 years and older at high risk for type 1 diabetes (two positive β cell autoantibodies and impaired glucose tolerance) to delay its onset. Adverse reactions are common, including transient lymphopenia and generalized leukopenia; serious infections such as gastroenteritis, cellulitis, pneumonia, and sepsis; hypersensitivity reactions; rash; and headache.

Greenbaum C et al. Evolving concepts in pathophysiology, screening, and prevention of type 1 diabetes: report of diabetes mellitus interagency coordinating committee workshop. Diabetes. 2024;73:1780. [PMID: 39167668]

Wadivkar P et al. Classifying a distinct form of diabetes in lean individuals with a history of undernutrition: an international consensus statement. Lancet Glob Health. 2025;13:e1771. [PMID: 40975084]

B. Prevention of Type 2 Diabetes

Several large RCTs have demonstrated that lifestyle intervention with a decreased-calorie meal plan is highly effective in preventing or delaying the onset of type 2 diabetes and decreasing cardiometabolic risk. The Diabetes Prevention Program offers the strongest evidence for diabetes prevention; it studied whether lifestyle intervention or metformin could prevent the onset of type 2 diabetes in overweight men and women with impaired glucose tolerance. Intervention with a low-fat diet and 150 minutes of moderate exercise (such as a brisk walk) per week reduced the risk of incident diabetes by 58% over 3 years. Participants who took metformin 850 mg twice daily reduced their risk of developing type 2 diabetes by 31%, but this intervention was ineffective in those with a lesser degree of obesity or who were older. Of the persons in the Diabetes Prevention Program, 88% continued follow-up in the Diabetes Prevention Program Outcome Study. At 15 years of follow-up, the cumulative incidence of diabetes was 55% in the lifestyle group and 62% in the control group. The SURMOUNT-1 trial has demonstrated that a 3-year treatment with tirzepatide at 5-mg, 10-mg, and 15-mg doses reduced the risk of developing type 2 diabetes by 94% in individuals with prediabetes and obesity or overweight. Participants who took tirzepatide had weight reduction of up to 20% that was sustained over 3 years, and the risk of progression to type 2 diabetes was markedly lower compared with placebo. No medication is yet approved by the FDA to prevent the development of type 2 diabetes.

American Diabetes Association Professional Practice Committee for Diabetes. 3. Prevention or Delay of Diabetes and Associated Comorbidities: Standards of Care in Diabetes—2026. Diabetes Care. 2026;49:S50. [PMID: 41358891]

Ghannam N et al. Addressing the continuum of dysglycaemia and vascular complications in prediabetes and type 2 diabetes: need for early and intensive treatment. Diabetes Metab Syndr Obes. 2023;16:105. [PMID: 36760588]

Jastreboff AM et al. Tirzepatide for obesity treatment and diabetes prevention. N Engl J Med. 2025;392:958. [PMID: 39536238]

Clinical Findings

A. Distinguishing the Different Types of Diabetes

Type 2 diabetes accounts for 90–95% of all diagnosed diabetes. At the time of diagnosis, though, it is important to differentiate between type 1 and type 2 diabetes or other specific types such as MODY to personalize therapy. Features that suggest end-organ insulin insensitivity, such as visceral obesity, acanthosis nigricans, or both, may help diagnose type 2 diabetes but the presence of obesity no longer characterizes only type 2 diabetes. An increase in the rate and severity of obesity has resulted in a major change in the type 1 diabetes phenotype in recent years. In the general population, including persons with type 1 diabetes, sedentary lifestyles and increased consumption of processed foods, refined sugars, and saturated fat have resulted in increased obesity. It is important to assess for a family history of diabetes, including the age at onset, association with obesity, the need for insulin, and whether there were complications. Measurement of GAD65, IAA, ICA 512, and zinc transporter 8 antibodies can help distinguish between type 1 and type 2 diabetes. Many patients with newly diagnosed type 1 diabetes still have significant endogenous insulin production, and therefore measuring C-peptide levels does not reliably distinguish between type 1 and type 2 diabetes.

B. Symptoms and Signs

1. Type 1 diabetes—The hallmark symptom complex of type 1 diabetes is polyuria and polydipsia from hyperosmolality and hyperketonemia from the accumulation of circulating glucose and fatty acids. When absolute insulin deficiency is of acute onset, there is abrupt increase in urination, thirst, blurred vision, weight loss, paresthesias, and altered level of consciousness. Ketoacidosis exacerbates the dehydration and hyperosmolality by producing anorexia and nausea and vomiting, interfering with oral fluid replacement. Symptoms occur a few weeks before diagnosis. Type 1 diabetes can develop in any decade of life; up to 50% of all new cases occur in adults. Adults may present more variably and without the classic symptom complex that occurs in children and young persons,

A. INCREASED URINATION AND THIRST—These symptoms are consequences of osmotic diuresis secondary to sustained hyperglycemia. The diuresis results in a loss of glucose as well as free water and electrolytes in the urine.

B. BLURRED VISION—As the lenses are exposed to hyperosmolar fluids, blurred vision often develops.

C. WEIGHT LOSS—Despite usual or increased appetite, weight loss is a common feature of type 1 diabetes when it develops subacutely. The weight loss is initially due to depletion of water, glycogen, and triglycerides; thereafter, reduced muscle mass occurs as amino acids are diverted to form glucose and ketone bodies. Loss of subcutaneous fat and muscle wasting are features of more slowly developing insulin deficiency. Lowered plasma volume produces symptoms of postural hypotension, which is a serious prognostic sign. Total body potassium loss and the general catabolism of muscle protein contribute to the weakness.

D. LEVEL OF CONSCIOUSNESS—The patient's level of consciousness can vary depending on the degree of hyperosmolality. When insulin deficiency develops relatively slowly and sufficient water intake is maintained, patients remain relatively alert and physical findings may be minimal. When vomiting occurs from worsening ketoacidosis, dehydration progresses and compensatory mechanisms become inadequate to keep serum osmolality < 320–330 mOsm/L. Stupor or even coma may occur when the serum osmolality is > 320–330 mOsm/L. The fruity breath odor of acetone further suggests the diagnosis of DKA.

2. Type 2 diabetes—While increased urination and thirst may be presenting symptoms in some patients with type 2 diabetes, many patients have an insidious onset and are asymptomatic, with hyperglycemia noted during routine laboratory studies. Occasionally, when the disease has been occult for some time, patients may have evidence of neuropathic or cardiovascular complications at the time of presentation. Hyperglycemic hyperosmolar coma can also be present when the serum osmolality exceeds 320–330 mOsm/L; in these cases, patients are profoundly dehydrated, hypotensive, lethargic, or comatose but without the Kussmaul respirations of ketoacidosis. When relative insulin deficiency is profound, ketoacidosis can develop.

A. SKIN MANIFESTATIONS—Diabetes should be suspected in women with chronic candidal vulvovaginitis and in men with balanoposthitis (inflammation of the foreskin and glans in uncircumcised men). Other common skin infections include hordeola, furuncles, folliculitis, carbuncles, and paronychia.

Acanthosis nigricans is associated with significant insulin resistance. The skin in the axilla, groin, and back of neck is hyperpigmented and hyperkeratotic (Figure 31–1). Some patients with chronic hyperglycemia develop multifactorial chylomicronemia (plasma triglycerides > 2000 mg/dL) with eruptive xanthomas on the flexor surface of the limbs and on the buttocks, lipemia retinalis, and a significantly increased risk of developing acute pancreatitis.

B. BODY HABITUS—Patients who develop type 2 diabetes are often overweight or obese. Even those who are not

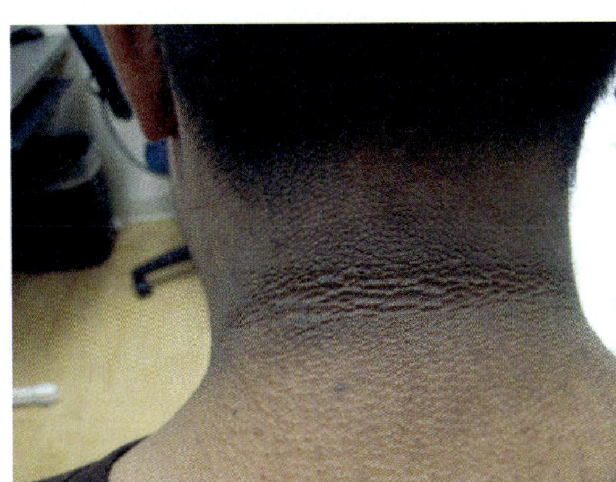

▲ **Figure 31–1.** Acanthosis nigricans of the nape of the neck, with typical dark and velvety appearance. (Used, with permission, from Umesh Masharani, MB, BS, MRCP [UK].)

significantly obese often have characteristic localization of fat deposits on the upper segment of the body (especially the abdomen, chest, neck, and face) and relatively little to no fat on the limbs, which can appear lean and muscular. This centripetal fat distribution is characterized by a high waist circumference; a waist circumference > 40 inches (102 cm) in men and > 35 inches (88 cm) in women is associated with an increased risk of insulin resistance, diabetes and dyslipidemia. Hypertension is often present in patients with diabetes and obesity.

c. Obstetrical complications—Type 2 diabetes should be considered in patients who have delivered babies larger than 9 lb (4.1 kg) or have had polyhydramnios, preeclampsia, or unexplained fetal losses. Gestational diabetes is discussed in Chapter 22.

C. Laboratory Findings and Diagnostic Tests

Diagnostic criteria are the same for all types of diabetes. Abnormal tests of glycemia must be present on two different occasions in the absence of symptoms. HbA_{1c} should be obtained initially and then every 3–6 months. Laboratory evaluation at initial and subsequent annual evaluations includes measurement of lipid panel, liver function tests, urine albumin/creatinine ratio, serum potassium, serum creatinine and estimated GFR (eGFR), CBC, and vitamin B_{12} (when on metformin). TSH should be measured annually in individuals with type 1 diabetes.

1. Plasma or serum glucose—A plasma glucose level ≥ 126 mg/dL (7 mmol/L) on more than one occasion after at least 8 hours of fasting is diagnostic of diabetes mellitus (Table 31–2).

2. Glycated hemoglobin (hemoglobin A_{1C})—Hemoglobin becomes spontaneously glycated when glucose enters the erythrocyte through the glucose transporter 1 (GLUT1). HbA_{1c} reflects glucose bound to hemoglobin within RBCs. Since the average RBC life span is about 120 days, the HbA_{1c} is a weighted average of recent blood glucose exposure during the preceding 8–12 weeks, providing an indirect method of assessing mean glucose. HbA_{1c} is a primary technique to diagnose diabetes and assess management. However, there is substantial inter- and intra-individual variability in HbA_{1c}, and caution should be exercised in estimating average glucose levels from measured HbA_{1c}. For example, for HbA_{1c} values between 6.9% and 7.1%, the glucose levels can range from 125 mg/dL to 205 mg/dL (6.9–11.4 mmol/L); therefore the use of glucose measurements in addition to HbA_{1c} is important for making treatment decisions.

The ADA established diagnostic criterion for diabetes is HbA_{1c} ≥ 6.5% (Table 31–2). The cutoff value of 6.5% (48 mmol/mol) was chosen because the risk for retinopathy increases substantially above this value. The advantages of using the HbA_{1c} over fasting plasma glucose and the oral glucose tolerance test to diagnose and treat diabetes include stability of the assay and convenience (fasting is not needed) with fewer day-to-day changes due to stress, illness, or nutritional status.

Several factors can interfere with assays and affect the accuracy of HbA_{1c}. In patients with hemoglobin variants such as high levels of hemoglobin F, immunoassays give falsely low values of HbA_{1c}. The National Glycohemoglobin Standardization Program website (https://ngsp.org) provides information on how hemoglobin variants and traits impact results of commonly used HbA_{1c} assays.

HbA_{1c} may not be a suitable diagnostic test when factors affecting hemoglobin concentration or RBC turnover are present. Any condition that decreases erythrocyte survival or mean erythrocyte age (eg, recovery from acute blood loss, hemolytic anemia) will falsely lower HbA_{1c}, irrespective of the assay method used. Intravenous iron and erythropoietin therapy for treatment of anemia in CKD falsely lower HbA_{1c} levels. Alternative methods of assessing glycemia such as fructosamine (see below) should be considered in these situations. Vitamins C and E may falsely lower test results, possibly by inhibiting glycation of hemoglobin. Conditions that increase erythrocyte survival such as splenectomy for hereditary spherocytosis will falsely raise HbA_{1c} levels. Iron-deficiency anemia also is associated with higher HbA_{1c} levels.

3. Oral glucose tolerance test—In an asymptomatic nonpregnant adult in whom diabetes is suspected, a standardized oral glucose tolerance test can diagnose diabetes. This test can identify individuals with diabetes whose diagnoses might otherwise be missed, such as those with posttransplant diabetes or cystic fibrosis–related diabetes. In order to optimize insulin secretion and effectiveness, a minimum of 150–200 g of carbohydrate daily should be included in the diet for 3 days before the test. The patient should eat nothing after midnight before the test day. The test is performed in the morning because of diurnal variation in oral glucose tolerance; patients should not smoke or be active during the test. On the morning of the test, patients consume 75 g of glucose in 300 mL of water within 5 minutes. Blood samples for plasma glucose are obtained at 0 and 120 minutes after ingestion of glucose. A fasting value ≥ 126 mg/dL (7 mmol/L) or a 2-hour value > 200 mg/dL (11.1 mmol/L) is diagnostic of diabetes mellitus (Table 31–2). Patients with a

Table 31–2. Criteria for the diagnosis of diabetes.

	Normal Glucose Tolerance[1]	Prediabetes or Impaired Glucose Tolerance[1]	Diabetes Mellitus[2]
Fasting plasma glucose mg/dL (mmol/L)	< 100 (5.6)	100–125 (5.6–6.9)	≥ 126 (7.0)
Plasma glucose mg/dL (mmol/L) 2 hours after glucose load	< 140 (7.8)	≥ 140–199 (7.8–11.0)	≥ 200 (11.1)
HbA_{1c} (%)	< 5.7	5.7–6.4	≥ 6.5

[1]See text for the oral glucose tolerance test protocol.
[2]A fasting plasma glucose ≥ 126 mg/dL (7.0 mmol) is diagnostic of diabetes if confirmed by *repeat testing.* A fasting plasma glucose ≥ 126 mg/dL (7.0 mmol) and HbA_{1c} ≥ 6.5% on the *same sample* also is diagnostic of diabetes.

2-hour value of 140–199 mg/dL (7.8–11.1 mmol/L) have impaired glucose tolerance. False-positive results may occur in patients who are malnourished, are bedridden, or have an infection or severe emotional stress.

4. Urine and blood ketones—Qualitative detection of ketone bodies can be accomplished by nitroprusside tests (Acetest or Ketostix). Although these tests do not detect β-hydroxybutyric acid, which lacks a ketone group, the semiquantitative estimation of ketonuria is nonetheless usually adequate for clinical purposes. Many laboratories measure β-hydroxybutyric acid, and there are meters available (Precision Xtra; Nova Max Plus) for patient use that measure β-hydroxybutyric acid in capillary glucose samples. β-Hydroxybutyrate levels > 0.6 mmol/L require evaluation. Patients with levels > 3.0 mmol/L, equivalent to very large urinary ketones, require hospitalization.

5. Glycated proteins—**Serum fructosamine** is formed by nonenzymatic glycosylation of several serum proteins (90% albumin) when exposed to glucose and turned into ketamines. Since serum albumin has a much shorter half-life than hemoglobin (14–20 days), serum fructosamine generally reflects the average glucose for the preceding 2–3 weeks. The glycation rate of proteins is not affected by RBC lifespan or hemoglobin variants; therefore fructosamine can be used in conditions when HbA_{1c} may not be a reliable marker, such as in the presence of abnormal hemoglobins or hemolytic states or when an earlier response to treatment is required, or in pregnancy. Conditions that reduce serum albumin (eg, nephrotic state, protein-losing enteropathy, or severe liver disease) will lower the serum fructosamine. Normal values vary in relation to the serum albumin concentration and are 200–285 mcmol/L when the serum albumin level is 5 g/dL. HbA_{1c} values and serum fructosamine are highly correlated. Serum fructosamine levels of 300, 367, and 430 mcmol/L approximate to HbA_{1c} values of 7%, 8%, and 9%, respectively. Limitations to the use of fructosamine include uncertainty about the frequency of measurements, lack of standardization, and established clinical cut points. Similarly, **glycated albumin** measures only the glycosylated form of albumin with the same advantages and disadvantages as serum fructosamine measurements. The reference range for glycated albumin is 11.9–15.8%.

6. Lipids—Lipid abnormalities are often present in patients with diabetes. When type 1 diabetes is suboptimally managed, hypertriglyceridemia develops from the absolute insulin deficiency. Once type 1 diabetes is optimally managed or hyperglycemia is corrected, often there is no underlying lipid abnormality. In type 2 diabetes, a distinct "diabetic dyslipidemia" is present and is characteristic of underlying insulin resistance. Dyslipidemia of type 2 diabetes is typified by high serum triglycerides (300–400 mg/dL [3.4–4.5 mmol/L]), low HDL cholesterol (<30 mg/dL [0.8 mmol/L]), and a qualitative change in LDL particles, resulting in smaller dense particles that carry higher amounts of free cholesterol. These small dense LDL particles are more susceptible to oxidation, rendering them atherogenic. These lipid abnormalities can exist even with good glycemic management. Lifestyle adjustments including healthy eating patterns with decreased consumption of sugar-sweetened beverages, refined carbohydrates and alcohol, and regular physical activity all have a beneficial impact on diabetic dyslipidemia. Primary disorders of lipid metabolism may coexist with diabetes; therefore persistence of lipid abnormalities after weight reduction and improvement in blood glucose should prompt a diagnostic workup and possible pharmacotherapy of the lipid disorder (see Chapter 32).

7. Glucose monitoring systems—**Diabetes technology** is a term that encompasses all devices, hardware, and software that individuals with diabetes use to aid self-management. Diabetes technology includes insulin administration devices, blood glucose monitoring (BGM) systems, and continuous glucose monitoring (CGM) systems. Diabetes devices should be offered to all individuals with diabetes based on individual needs and preferences; appropriate training and education should be provided for effective use on an ongoing basis.

A. Self-monitoring glucose systems—Capillary BGM using a glucose meter is an important aspect of diabetes management, especially for individuals on insulin. BGM is a tool for monitoring responses to nutrition, physical activity, and response to therapy and to avoid hypoglycemia. Glucose meters use an enzymatic reaction with either glucose oxidase or glucose dehydrogenase. Many blood glucose meters are available, and accuracy rates are mostly equivalent, but they vary with regard to speed, convenience, size of blood samples required, reporting capability, and cost. Several brands are available, including LifeScan (OneTouch), Bayer Corporation (Contour), Roche Diagnostics (Accu-Chek), and Abbott Laboratories (Precision, FreeStyle). Blood glucose meters range from $15 to $60 each. Test strips remain a major expense, costing up to about $1.50 apiece. The meters also come with a lancet device and disposable 26- to 33-gauge lancets. Most meters can store from 100 to 1000 glucose values, and stored data can be downloaded onto a computer or smartphone. Some glucose meters have integrated speech that can read glucose values aloud to benefit individuals with visual impairment.

BGM systems have limitations to their use. Testing strips have limited lifespans, and improper storage (high temperature, open vial) can affect their accuracy. Patients with diabetes should be advised against using expired strips and purchasing second-hand test strips. All meters have a temperature range for accurate function, as the glucose reaction is temperature sensitive. Increases or decreases in hematocrit can affect measured glucose values. Meters and test strips are calibrated over the glucose concentrations ranging from 60 mg/dL (3.3 mmol/L) to 160 mg/dL (8.9 mmol/L), and the accuracy is not as good for higher and lower glucose levels. When the glucose is <60 mg/dL (3.3 mmol/L), the difference between the meter and the laboratory value may be as much as 20%. Glucose oxidase–based meters underestimate glucose levels in the presence of high oxygen tension (for example, in the critically ill receiving supplemental oxygen); under these circumstances, a glucose dehydrogenase–based system may be preferable as it is not affected by oxygen tension.

Glucose dehydrogenase–based systems may report falsely high glucose levels in patients who are receiving parenteral products containing nonglucose sugars such as maltose, galactose, or xylose or their metabolites. Impaired circulation to the fingers (for example, in patients with Raynaud disease) will artificially lower fingerstick glucose measurements (pseudohypoglycemia).

Despite improved accuracy and precision of BGM, it remains a static measure of glucose without information on patterns unless there are many readings per day.

B. Continuous glucose monitoring systems—CGM systems measure glucose concentrations in the interstitial fluid, which correlate with plasma glucose levels. CGM is the standard for monitoring glucose in adults with type 1 diabetes and for all patients with diabetes who use agents that increase risk of hypoglycemia. These systems require the user to insert a sensor (small filament) into the subcutaneous space to continuously measure glucose concentrations. CGM devices are either owned by the user (personal CGM device) or owned by clinical practices (professional CGM devices). Two types of personal CGM devices are available. "Real-time CGM" systems send a continuous stream of glucose data that is displayed on a receiver, mobile application on a smartphone, a smartwatch, or an insulin pump (eg, Dexcom G7, Dexcom G7 15 Day, Abbott Freestyle Libre 3 plus, Libre 2 plus used with smartphone, Eversense implantable CGM, Medtronic Simplera). The second type, "intermittently scanned CGM" (Abbott Freestyle Libre 2 plus when used with a reader), requires the user to scan the sensor using a reader device. These CGM systems require a prescription. Most prescription CGM devices have similar characteristics; they provide a continuous stream of data, do not require swiping to obtain readings, and have adjustable alarms and alerts to inform the user of rapidly rising or falling glucose values. Non-implantable sensors (placed on the skin) can be worn up to 15 days, and implantable sensors (placed under the skin) can be worn for 365 days. Family members can remotely monitor glucose values and be alerted. Direct-to-consumer CGM systems without alarm features (Abbott Lingo and Dexcom Stelo) can be purchased by anyone, including those with prediabetes or those without diabetes who wish to assess their glycemic responses to food choices and exercise. Personalized glucose management using CGM has resulted in improved glycemic control and diabetes-related outcomes in patients with both type 1 and type 2 diabetes. Several RCTs using real-time CGM have demonstrated improvement in HbA_{1c} and reduction in hypoglycemia when worn consistently. Review of CGM reports (Ambulatory Glucose Profile report) provides key metrics that can guide therapeutic decision-making for the provider and the patient; glucose data offers the user insight on food choices, insulin dosing, and changes in physical activity (Table 31–3). The percentage of "time in range" or glucose levels 70–180 mg/day (3.9–10 mmol/L), glucose levels that are "above range" or "below range," glucose average and variability can be assessed. In general, glucose levels that are ≥ 70% "time in range" are acceptable and correlate with an HbA_{1c} of ~ 7%. Sensor measurement errors can occur from interfering substances (high doses of vitamin C, hydroxyurea, mannitol), faulty placement, defective sensors, or pressure on the sensor location. Contact dermatitis (both irritant and allergic) from the adhesive can develop with all CGM devices that are attached to the skin.

Table 31–3. Standardized continuous glucose monitoring metrics for adults with diabetes.

Metric	Most Adults	Older Individuals
Number of days sensor is worn	≥ 14 days	≥ 14 days
Average glucose	Goal < 154 mg/dL	Individualized
Glucose management indicator	< 7%	Individualized, 7–8% based on comorbid conditions
Coefficient of variation	< 36%	< 36%
Time in range	> 70%	> 50%
Time below range < 70 mg/dL	< 4%	< 1%
Time below range < 54mg/dL	< 1%	< 1%
Time above range > 180mg/dL	< 25%	—
Time above range > 250 mg/dL	< 5%	< 10%

Ajjan RA et al. Continuous glucose monitoring for the routine care of type 2 diabetes mellitus. Nat Rev Endocrinol. 2024;20:426. [PMID: 38589493]

American Diabetes Association Professional Practice Committee for Diabetes. 7. Diabetes Technology: Standards of Care in Diabetes—2026. Diabetes Care. 2026;49:S150. [PMID: 41358889]

Treatment

Foundational aspects of the management of individuals with diabetes include building positive health behaviors and maintaining psychosocial wellbeing. To achieve this, diabetes self-management education and support (DSMES), medical nutrition therapy (MNT), routine physical activity, adequate-quality sleep, support for cessation of tobacco products and vaping, counseling on health behaviors, and psychosocial care are vital. Individuals living with diabetes should receive person-centered collaborative care that involves shared decision-making in the treatment plan and facilitated access to medical, technological, psychosocial, and behavioral health resources and support.

A. Diabetes Self-Management Education and Support

The main goal of DSMES is to empower individuals with diabetes by providing them with tools to make informed self-management decisions. It is recommended that all persons with diabetes participate in DSMES to facilitate informed decision-making, self-care behaviors, problem-solving, and active collaboration with the health care team.

These services should be culturally appropriate and responsive to individual preferences, needs, and values and are commonly offered in group or individual settings.

B. Medical Nutrition Therapy (MNT)

Nutrition therapy plays an integral role in diabetes management, and each person with diabetes should actively engage in education, self-management, and treatment planning with the health care team. There has been a vast change in how individuals with diabetes are counselled on nutrition, moving away from emphasizing macronutrients (carbohydrates, proteins, and fats), and micronutrients (vitamins and minerals) and instead focusing on foods. Patients are encouraged to think about eating patterns, also known as dietary patterns or food patterns, or the totality of the foods and beverages they consume. Promoting consumption of nutrient-dense food cho_ces, such as foods high in micronutrients while being relatively low in calories (eg, vegetables, fruits, and legumes), is useful because people eat food, not nutrients, and nutrition recommendations need to be applicable to what patients actually eat. MNT, when delivered by a registered dietitian, is highly beneficial to persons living with diabetes. MNT is associated with HbA_{1c} reduction of 1.0–1.9% for persons with type 1 diabetes and 0.3–2.0% for those with type 2 diabetes. There is no one-size-fits-all eating pattern for persons with diabetes, and participation in collaboratively developing an individualized meal plan should be highly encouraged. Eating patterns should emphasize inclusion of nonstarchy vegetables, whole fruits, legumes, lean proteins, whole grains, nuts and seeds, and low-fat dairy or nondairy alternatives while minimizing consumption of red meat, sugar-sweetened beverages, sweets, refined grains, and processed and ultra-processed foods for individuals with prediabetes and diabetes. A Mediterranean-style eating pattern (a diet supplemented with walnuts, almonds, hazelnuts, and olive oil) improves glycemic control and lowers combined endpoints for cardiovascular events and stroke. Use of supplements or herbs is not recommended. Alcohol consumption can result in hypoglycemia and/or delayed hypoglycemia (particularly for those using insulin or insulin secretagogue therapies), weight gain, and hyperglycemia (when consumed in excessive amounts). Persons with diabetes should be educated about the risks of alcohol consumption and encouraged to monitor glucose frequently before and after drinking alcohol.

C. Weight Management

One of the primary modes of therapy for patients with obesity and type 2 diabetes is weight reduction. Normalization of glycemia can be achieved by weight loss resulting in improved tissue sensitivity to insulin. A combination of caloric restriction, increased exercise, and behavioral modification can constitute a weight reduction program.

Subcutaneous liraglutide (Victoza) and tirzepatide (Mounjaro), and subcutaneous (Ozempic) and oral semaglutide (Rybelsus), are approved for treatment of persons with diabetes who also require weight loss in addition to glycemic management along with diet and exercise (see GLP-1 receptor agonists, below); these same medications but with different doses and trade names (eg, Saxenda instead of Victoza, Wegovy instead of Ozempic or Rybelsus, and Zepbound instead of Mounjaro) also are approved for weight loss in persons without diabetes (see Obesity in Chapter 33 for discussion of weight loss in patients without diabetes). In a 68-week study in adults without diabetes, patients taking subcutaneous semaglutide lost 14.9% of their initial body weight compared with 2.4% body weight loss in patients taking placebo. In a 72-week study, patients taking tirzepatide 15 mg lost about 21% of their initial body weight compared to 3.1 % with placebo. Common adverse reactions include nausea, vomiting, and diarrhea. Serious side effects include pancreatitis. The medication should not be used in patients with MEN 2 or personal or family history of medullary thyroid cancer.

Other medical options for weight loss include orlistat, phentermine/topiramate, and naltrexone/extended-release bupropion (see Chapter 33).

Bariatric surgery (Roux-en-Y, gastric banding, gastric sleeve, biliopancreatic diversion/duodenal switch) results in substantial weight loss and improvement in glucose levels. A meta-analysis examining the impact of bariatric surgery on patients with diabetes and BMI ≥ 40 noted that 82% of patients had resolution of clinical and laboratory manifestations of diabetes in the first 2 years after surgery and 62% remained free of diabetes > 2 years after surgery. The improvement was most marked in the procedure that caused the greatest weight loss (biliopancreatic diversion/duodenal switch). There was, however, a high attrition of patients available for follow-up, and there was little information about how results vary by ethnicity. Weight regain does occur after bariatric surgery, and it can be expected that 20–25% of the lost weight may be regained over 10 years. The impact of this weight gain on diabetes recurrence depends principally on the degree of β cell dysfunction. In a 2024 pooled analysis of patients from four randomized controlled trials, compared with medical management, bariatric surgery was associated with better long-term improvement of glycemic control, use of fewer medications, and greater weight loss at 7 to 12 years of follow-up. Increased rates of diabetes remission and reductions in medication use (including insulin) were observed in participants who underwent bariatric surgery.

Courcoulas AP et al. Long-term outcomes of medical management vs bariatric surgery in type 2 diabetes. JAMA. 2024;331:654. [PMID: 38411644]

Jastreboff AM et al. Tirzepatide once weekly for the treatment of obesity. N Engl J Med. 2022;387:205. [PMID: 35658024]

Wilding JPH et al. Once-weekly semaglutide in adults with overweight or obesity N Engl J Med. 2021;384:989. [PMID: 33567185]

D. Medications for Treating Hyperglycemia

The medications for treating type 2 diabetes are listed in Table 31–4.

1. Incretin-based therapies—Incretins, principally GLP-1 and glucose-dependent insulinotropic polypeptide (GIP), are hormones released from the gut that increase glucose clearance after nutrient ingestion. After an oral glucose

Table 31–4. Medications for treatment of type 2 diabetes mellitus (oral doses unless otherwise noted).

Drug	Tablet Size	Daily Dose	Duration of Action
GLP-1 Receptor Agonists			
Dulaglutide (Trulicity)	0.75-, 1.5-, 3.0-, 4.5-mg single-dose pens or prefilled syringe	*Usual dose:* 1.5–3.0 mg subcutaneously once weekly *Maximal dose:* 4.5 mg subcutaneously once weekly	1 week
Liraglutide (Victoza)	Prefilled, multidose pens delivering 0.6, 1.2, or 1.8 mg	*Initial dose:* 0.6 mg subcutaneously once daily. Increase to 1.2 mg after a week if tolerated. *Maximal dose:* 1.8 mg subcutaneously once daily.	24 hours
Semaglutide (Ozempic, Rybelsus)	Prefilled multidose pens delivering 0.25, 0.5, 1, or 2 mg	*Initial dose:* 0.25 mg weekly for 1 month and increase to 0.5 mg weekly. Increase dose to 1 mg weekly or 2 mg weekly for additional glucose lowering and/or weight loss as needed (a 2.4-mg weekly dose is approved for weight loss).	1 week
	1-, 3-, 7-, and 14-mg tablets	*Initial dose:* 3 mg for 1 month and then increase to 7 mg. Take fasting daily with water and wait 30 minutes to eat. *Maximal dose:* 14 mg daily.	Daily
Dual GIP/GLP-1 Receptor Agonists			
Tirzepatide (Mounjaro)	Single-dose vial or pen: 2.5, 5, 7.5, 10, 12.5, and 15 mg	*Initial dose*: 2.5 mg weekly for 1 month and increase to 5 mg weekly. Increase dose by 2.5 mg weekly at 1-month intervals for additional glucose lowering and/or weight loss as needed. *Maximal dose*: 15 mg weekly.	1 week
DPP-4 Inhibitors			
Alogliptin (Nesina)	6.25, 12.5, and 25 mg	25 mg once daily if eGFR ≥ 60 mL/min/1.73 m^2 12.5 mg daily if eGFR 30–59 mL/min/1.73 m^2 6.25 mg daily if eGFR < 30 mL/min/1.73 m^2	24 hours
Linagliptin (Tradjenta)	5 mg	5 mg daily	24 hours
Sitagliptin (Januvia)	25, 50, and 100 mg	100 mg once daily if eGFR > 45 mL/min/1.73 m^2 50 mg once daily if eGFR 30–45 mL/min/1.73 m^2 25 mg once daily if eGFR < 30 mL/min/1.73 m^2	24 hours
Vildagliptin (Galvus) (not available in United States)	50 mg	50 mg once or twice daily ***Avoid*** if eGFR ≤ 60 mL/min/1.73 m^2 or AST/ALT three times upper limit of normal	24 hours
SGLT-2 Inhibitors			
Bexagliflozin (Brenzavvy)	20 mg	20 mg once daily ***Avoid*** if eGFR < 30 mL/min/1.73 m^2 for glycemic control	24 hours
Canagliflozin (Invokana)	100 and 300 mg	100–300 mg daily if eGFR > 60 mL/min/1.73 m^2 100 mg daily if eGFR is 30–60 mL/min/1.73 m^2 ***Avoid*** if eGFR < 30 mL/min/1.73 m^2.	24 hours
Dapagliflozin (Farxiga)	5 and 10 mg	5–10 mg daily ***Avoid*** if eGFR < 45 mL/min/1.73 m^2 for glycemic control	24 hours
Empagliflozin (Jardiance)	10 and 25 mg	*Usual dose*: 10 mg daily *Maximal dose*: 25 mg ***Avoid*** if eGFR < 30 mL/min/1.73 m^2 for glycemic control	24 hours
Ertugliflozin (Steglatro)	5 and 15 mg	*Usual dose*: 5 mg daily *Maximal dose*: 15 mg ***Avoid*** if eGFR < 45 mL/min/1.73 m^2 for glycemic control	24 hours
Biguanides			
Metformin (Glucophage)	500, 625, 750, 850, and 1000 mg	500–1000 mg twice daily If eGFR is 30–45 mL/min/1.73 m^2, do not start metformin; if already taking metformin, dose is < 1000 mg daily ***Avoid*** if eGFR < 30 mL/min/1.73 m^2	4 hours

(*continued*)

Table 31–4. Medications for treatment of type 2 diabetes mellitus (oral doses unless otherwise noted). (continued)

Drug	Tablet Size	Daily Dose	Duration of Action
Metformin extended release, 24 hour (Glucophage XL)	500, 750, and 1000 mg	500–2000 mg once daily ***Avoid*** if eGFR < 30 mL/min/1.73 m^2	Up to 24 hours
Thiazolidinediones			
Pioglitazone (Actos)	15, 30, and 45 mg	15–45 mg daily	Up to 24 hours
Rosiglitazone	2, 4, and 8 mg	4–8 mg daily (can be divided)	Up to 24 hours
Sulfonylureas			
Acetohexamide (Dymelor) (not available in United States)	250 and 500 mg	250–1000 mg as single dose; 1500 mg in two divided doses *Maximal dose*: 1500 mg/day	12–24 hours
Chlorpropamide (Diabinese) (not available in United States)	100 and 250 mg	100–500 mg as single dose *Maximal dose*: 750 mg/day	24–72 hours
Gliclazide (not available in United States)	80 mg	40–80 mg as single dose; 160–320 mg divided dose *Maximal dose*: 320 mg/day	12 hours
Glimepiride (Amaryl)	1, 2, 3, and 4 mg	*Usual dose:* 1–4 mg once daily *Maximal dose:* 8 mg once daily ***Avoid*** if eGFR < 15 mL/min/1.73 m^2	Up to 24 hours
Glipizide, immediate release (Glucotrol, immediate release)	5 and 10 mg	*Usual dose:* 2.5–10 mg once daily 30 minutes before meals *Maximal dose:* 10 mg twice daily 2.5 mg once daily if eGFR < 30 mL/min/1.73 m^2 ***Avoid*** if eGFR < 10 mL/min/1.73 m^2	6–12 hours
Glipizide, extended release (Glucotrol XL)	2.5, 5, and 10 mg	*Usual dose:* 2.5–10 mg once daily *Maximal dose:* 20 mg once daily 2.5 mg once daily if eGFR < 30 mL/min/1.73 m^2 ***Avoid*** if eGFR < 10 mL/min/1.73 m^2	Up to 24 hours
Glyburide (glibenclamide)			
(Micronase, DiaBeta, conventional tablets) (not available in United States)	1.25, 2.5, and 5 mg	1.25–20 mg as single dose or in two divided doses *Maximal dose:* 20 mg/day ***Avoid*** if eGFR < 60 mL/min/1.73 m^2	Up to 24 hours
(Glynase PresTab, micronized tablets)	1.25, 1.5, 2.5, 3, 5, and 6 mg	1.5–12 mg as single dose or in two divided doses *Maximal dose:* 12 mg/day ***Avoid*** if eGFR < 60 mL/min/1.73 m^2	Up to 24 hours
Tolazamide (Tolinase)	100, 250, and 500 mg	100–500 mg as single dose; > 500 mg in two divided doses *Maximal dose:* 1000 mg/day	Up to 24 hours
Tolbutamide (Orinase) (not available in United States)	250 and 500 mg	250–3000 mg in two or three divided doses *Maximal dose:* 3000 mg/day	6–24 hours
Meglitinide Analogs			
Mitiglinide (available in Japan)	5 and 10 mg	5 or 10 mg three times daily before meals	2 hours
Repaglinide (Prandin)	0.5, 1, and 2 mg	*Usual dose:* 0.5 to 4 mg three times daily 15 minutes before meals *Maximal dose:* 16 mg daily	3 hours
D-Phenylalanine Derivative			
Nateglinide (Starlix)	60 and 120 mg	60 or 120 mg three times daily before meals *Maximal dose:* 360 mg/day 60 mg three times daily if eGFR < 30 mL/min/1.73 m^2	4 hours
α-Glucosidase Inhibitors			
Acarbose (Precose)	25, 50, and 100 mg	25–100 mg three times daily just before meals *Maximal dose:* ≤ 60 kg: 50 mg three times daily; > 60 kg: 100 mg three times daily	4 hours

(*continued*)

Table 31–4. Medications for treatment of type 2 diabetes mellitus (oral doses unless otherwise noted). (continued)

Drug	Tablet Size	Daily Dose	Duration of Action
Miglitol (Glyset)	25, 50, and 100 mg	25–100 mg three times daily just before meals	4 hours
Voglibose (not available in United States)	0.2 and 0.3 mg	0.2–0.3 mg three times daily just before meals	4 hours
Other			
Pramlintide (Symlin)	SymlinPen 60 or SymlinPen 120	For insulin-treated type 2 diabetes, start at 60 mcg subcutaneously three times daily. Increase to 120 mcg three times daily if no nausea for 3–7 days. Give immediately before meal. For type 1 diabetes, start at 15 mcg three times daily and increase by increments of 15 mcg to a maximum of 60 mcg three times daily, as tolerated. To avoid hypoglycemia, lower insulin dose by 50% on initiation of therapy.	2 hours

load, the release of gut incretin hormones provokes a three- to fourfold higher insulin secretory response than an equivalent intravenous glucose load. This higher insulin response to oral glucose compared to intravenous glucose is called the "incretin effect."

GLP-1 also inhibits glucagon secretion, thereby delaying gastric emptying, increasing satiety, and reducing the drive for food intake. GLP-1 also mediates nonglycemic effects such as reducing inflammation and oxidative stress, improving endothelial function, and preserving pancreatic β cell function. In patients with type 2 diabetes, GLP-1 action is impaired and its secretion is decreased.

A. GLP-1 RECEPTOR AGONISTS—The GLP-1 receptor agonists semaglutide, liraglutide, dulaglutide, and lixisenatide are available for treatment of diabetes. Liraglutide, semaglutide, and dulaglutide are metabolized by proteolysis and are preferred choices in patients with kidney failure.

Semaglutide (Ozempic) is a synthetic analog of GLP-1 with a half-life of about 1 week and is the only GLP-1 receptor agonist that is available in oral and injectable forms. The three multiuse pens available for subcutaneous injection are 0.25-mg or 0.5-mg dose in a starter pen, and 1-mg and 2-mg pens. Dose is escalated every 4 weeks as needed for glucose control, as tolerated. Semaglutide lowers HbA_{1c} by 1.5–2.1%. Weight loss of up to 4.5 kg at the 1-mg dose and 6.4 kg at the 2-mg dose was noted in a trial.

Oral semaglutide (Rybelsus) is formulated with an absorption enhancer to avoid degradation by gastric acid and therefore is taken fasting with a small amount of water (up to 4 oz/120 mL). Intake of food and other medicines should be delayed by 30 minutes thereafter. The starting dose is 3 mg daily for the first month; then the dose is increased to 7–14 mg daily as needed for glucose control, if tolerated. Oral semaglutide decreases A_{1c} by 1–1.3% and results in weight loss of 2.4–3.7 kg.

Liraglutide (Victoza) is a long-acting GLP-1 analog with a half-life of about 12 hours, allowing once-daily injection from a multidose pen. It decreases A_{1c} levels by 1.0–1.5% and results in weight loss of ~4 kg. Dosing is initiated at 0.6 mg daily; it is increased after 1 week to 1.2 mg daily, and then to 1.8 mg daily after 4 weeks if needed for glucose control and if tolerated. Liraglutide can be added to oral agents or basal insulin.

Dulaglutide (Trulicity) has a half-life of about 5 days. It is available in four fixed-dose, single-use pens (0.75 mg, 1.5 mg, 3.0 mg, and 4.5 mg). Dose is increased after at least 4 weeks if needed for glucose control and if tolerated. Dulaglutide monotherapy and combination therapy (eg, with metformin, sulfonylureas, thiazolidinediones, or insulin) lowers HbA_{1c} by about 1.5–1.8%. Weight loss is 2–3 kg on higher doses.

Lixisenatide has a half-life of 3 hours and is administered as a daily injection. It is available in the United States only as a combined medication with insulin glargine. Outside the United States, it is dispensed as two daily-injection fixed-dose pens (10 mcg and 20 mcg). HbA_{1c} lowering ranges from 0.4% to 0.6%, with very modest weight loss. Antibodies to lixisenatide can develop in up to 70% of individuals and impair glycemic efficacy.

(1) Nonglycemic effects of GLP-1 receptor agonists—Many large studies have demonstrated that GLP-1 receptor–based therapies reduce the risk of atherosclerotic cardiovascular events. Both subcutaneous and oral semaglutide significantly reduce the risk of major adverse cardiovascular events in patients with type 2 diabetes at high cardiovascular risk. Studies of liraglutide, semaglutide, and dulaglutide have demonstrated beneficial kidney outcomes with decrease in albuminuria or its progression and a reduction in decline in eGFR. Studies on metabolic associated steatotic liver disease have demonstrated improvement of liver enzymes, decrease in liver fat content, and improved systemic and hepatic inflammation without effect on fibrosis.

(2) Safety concerns—The most frequent adverse reactions of the GLP-1 receptor agonists are gastrointestinal, including nausea (40–50%), vomiting (4–13%), and diarrhea (9–17%). These side effects are transient, are

dose-dependent, and can be lessened by starting at a low dose with gradual stepwise dose escalation. Occasionally, severe and persistent gastrointestinal effects may limit fluid intake and result in dehydration and AKI. Cholecystitis, cholelithiasis, and biliary obstruction, sometimes requiring cholecystectomy, can develop following treatment with GLP-1 receptor agonists due to rapid weight loss, a known risk factor for gallbladder disease. Hair loss due to telogen effluvium and androgenic alopecia is common. It may be related to rapid weight loss and nutritional deficiencies, and can improve once weight stabilizes. Consistent reduction in lean body mass, ranging from 30% to 45%, has been noted and patients should be advised to pursue combining resistance training with adequate protein intake (>1.2 g/kg/day) to help preserve fat-free mass.

Links between GLP-1 receptor agonist use and pancreatitis, pancreatic cancer, and metabolic bone disease have not been supported by several large-scale trials, meta-analyses, or real-world data.

GLP-1 receptor agonists stimulate C-cell neoplasia and cause medullary thyroid carcinoma in rodent studies, which led to a warning of possible thyroid risks in humans; these drugs are contraindicated in individuals with a personal or family history of medullary thyroid carcinoma or multiple endocrine neoplasia type 2. No increased thyroid cancer has been noted with these agents.

An increase in diabetic retinopathy was observed in the semaglutide-treated group in one clinical trial, perhaps from rapid glucose lowering with the drug. Semaglutide may be associated with non-arteritic anterior ischemic optic neuropathy, which may be due to rapid lowering of glucose and relative hypoglycemia, particularly in patients with crowded optic discs. Encouraging full eye examinations is recommended in patients with longstanding severe hyperglycemia.

Prescribing information for GLP-1 receptor agonists contains caution about possible suicidal thoughts. Health care professionals are advised to monitor for and advise patients using GLP-1 receptor agonists to report new or worsening depression, suicidal thoughts, or any unusual changes in mood or behavior.

B. Dual GIP/GLP-1 receptor agonists—Tirzepatide is a dual receptor co-agonist that activates GIP and GLP-1 receptors. Acylation results in enhanced albumin binding, allowing for prolonged action and once-weekly dosing. Treatment with tirzepatide has resulted in dose-dependent HbA_{1c} reductions of 1.7–2.6% from the starting HbA_{1c}. The average weight loss ranges from 6.2 to 12.9 kg. The recommended starting dose is 2.5 mg injected subcutaneously weekly. The dosing regimen ranges from 2.5 to 15 mg; if further glucose lowering and/or weight loss is needed, the dose can be incrementally increased every 4 weeks to a maximum dose of 15 mg.

Beyond its glycemic effects, tirzepatide improves lipid profile, lowers blood pressure, and decreases fatty liver. In patients with type 2 diabetes and major atherosclerotic cardiovascular events, tirzepatide was noninferior to dulaglutide for the composite endpoint of death from cardiovascular causes, myocardial infarction, and stroke. The safety profile is similar to that of the GLP-1 receptor agonists. GI side effects (nausea, vomiting, diarrhea) occur more frequently at higher doses. However, tirzepatide may have fewer gastrointestinal side effects compared with dulaglutide and semaglutide. Tirzepatide use may decrease absorption of oral contraceptives and result in decreased effectiveness.

C. DPP-4 inhibitors—Inhibition of the enzyme DPP-4 prolongs the action of endogenously released, intact, biologically active GLP-1 and GIP. DPP-4 inhibitors are therefore incretin enhancers since they modestly increase the levels of GLP-1 and GIP, which then increase β cell insulin secretion in the pancreas, thereby reducing postprandial and fasting hyperglycemia. Four oral DPP-4 inhibitors, alogliptin, linagliptin, saxagliptin and sitagliptin, are available in the United States for the treatment of type 2 diabetes. Vildagliptin is available in Europe. Other DPP-4 inhibitors—gemigliptin, anagliptin, teneligliptin, trelagliptin, omarigliptin, evogliptin, and gosogliptin—are approved outside of the United States and European Union. DPP4 inhibitors as a class decrease HbA_{1c} by 0.6–0.8% and are generally well-tolerated oral agents. They do not cause weight gain, weight loss, or hypoglycemia. These agents should not be used in combination with the GLP-1 receptor agonists. All DPP-4 inhibitors are noninferior to placebo in cardiovascular outcomes trials and are safe to use in patients with known atherosclerotic cardiovascular disease (ASCVD), but they do not have any demonstrable benefits on cardiovascular outcomes. There is no impact on liver fat accumulation.

Sitagliptin is dosed at 100 mg orally once daily. Since it is cleared by the kidneys, the dose is reduced to 50 mg daily if eGFR is 30–50 mL/min/1.73 m^2 and to 25 mg for eGFR < 30 mL/min/1.73 m^2. Alogliptin is dosed at 25 mg orally daily; a 12.5-mg dose is used in patients with eGFR of 30–60 mL/min/1.73 m^2, and 6.25 mg for clearance < 30 mL/min/1.73 m^2. Linagliptin dose is 5 mg orally daily, and since it is primarily excreted unmetabolized via the bile, no dose adjustment is needed in patients with kidney disease. Saxagliptin is dosed at 2.5 mg and 5 mg. The dose of vildagliptin (available outside of the United States) is 50 mg once or twice daily.

(1) Safety concerns—A predisposition to nasopharyngitis or upper respiratory tract infection is observed in clinical trials. Rare hypersensitivity reactions, including anaphylaxis, angioedema, and exfoliative skin conditions (such as Stevens-Johnson syndrome and bullous pemphigoid), have been reported. There does not appear to be a clear association of immune effects, pancreatitis, or pancreatic cancer with these agents. Rare cases of hepatic dysfunction, including hepatitis, have been reported with the use of vildagliptin; liver biochemical testing is recommended quarterly during the first year of use and periodically thereafter. Vildagliptin is also associated with increased left ventricular volume but no increase in HF. Saxagliptin has been associated with a slightly increased rate of HF, but this is not believed to be a class effect. DPP-4 inhibitors can occasionally cause severe joint pains that resolve after stopping the drug. Overall, DPP-4 inhibitors are safe to use, especially in older individuals and in those with comorbid conditions or kidney impairment.

Nauck MA et al. Glucagon-like receptor agonists and next-generation incretin-based medications: metabolic, cardiovascular, and renal benefits. Lancet. 2026:S0140-6736(25)02105-1. [PMID: 41547366]

2. Sodium-glucose co-transporter (SGLT) 2 inhibitors— Glucose is freely filtered by the kidney glomeruli and is reabsorbed in the proximal tubules by the action of SGLTs. SGLT-2 accounts for ~ 90% of glucose reabsorption, and its inhibition causes glycosuria in persons with diabetes, lowering plasma glucose levels. The FDA-approved oral SGLT-2 inhibitors for treatment of diabetes are canagliflozin, dapagliflozin, empagliflozin, ertugliflozin, and bexagliflozin. SGLT-2 inhibitors reduce the threshold for glycosuria by 30–50% and lower HbA_{1c} by 0.5–1% when used alone or in combination with other oral agents or insulin. The loss of calories results in modest weight loss of 2–5 kg. Dapagliflozin and empagliflozin reduce risk of major cardiovascular endpoints; canagliflozin, dapagliflozin, empagliflozin, and ertugliflozin reduce risk of hospitalization for HF; canagliflozin, dapagliflozin, and empagliflozin are indicated for reducing the risk of decline in GFR and progression to ESKD.

Canagliflozin is dosed at 100 mg daily, but up to 300 mg daily can be used in patients with normal kidney function. The dose of dapagliflozin is 10 mg daily but 5 mg daily is the recommended initial dose in patients with liver failure. The usual dosage of empagliflozin is 10 mg daily, but a higher dose of 25 mg daily can be used. The recommended starting dose of ertugliflozin is 5 mg, but the dose can be increased to 15 mg daily if additional glucose lowering is needed. Bexagliflozin is dosed at 20 mg daily, and for mild to moderate kidney impairment (eGFR 30–89 mL/min/1.73 m^2) no dosage adjustment is required. Bexagliflozin is not recommended for severe kidney impairment (eGFR < 30 mL/min/1.73 m^2).

(1) Cardiovascular benefits—Landmark clinical trials have demonstrated that several SGLT2 inhibitors have cardiovascular benefits that extend beyond their glucose-lowering effects, including reduced cardiovascular mortality and hospitalization for heart failure. Empagliflozin reduces the risk of major adverse cardiovascular events (cardiovascular death, nonfatal MI, or nonfatal stroke) by 14%, and decreases the risk of cardiovascular death by 38%. Subsequent data has shown reductions in cardiovascular death and hospitalizations in patients with heart failure, irrespective of diabetes status. Empagliflozin lowers the risk of progression of kidney disease or death from cardiovascular causes in individuals with CKD. Dapagliflozin decreases cardiovascular events and death in patients with heart failure with and without diabetes. Canagliflozin has been shown to reduce the risk of major adverse cardiovascular events, cardiovascular death, and progression of CKD.

(2) Kidney benefits—SGLT-2 inhibitors are recommended for kidney protection in patients with eGFR as low as 20 mL/min/1.73 m^2 and can be continued until dialysis initiation. The kidney benefit is independent of the glucose-lowering effect. In the DAPA-CKD trial, dapagliflozin reduced the risk of a composite kidney outcome (worsening renal function, end-stage kidney disease, or death from renal or cardiovascular causes) in patients with CKD, regardless of diabetes status. Similarly, empagliflozin resulted in a reduced risk of kidney disease progression or death from cardiovascular causes in a diverse group of patients with CKD, with or without diabetes. SGLT2 inhibitors also decrease proteinuria in diabetes, an independent risk factor for CVD and CKD. These results have reinforced the crucial role of SGLT2 inhibitors in preventing CKD progression. The mechanisms involved in these beneficial effects remain unclear but may be through increased urinary glucose excretion and reduced glomerular hyperfiltration.

(3) Safety concerns—SGLT-2 inhibitors are less effective at glucose lowering with advancing CKD (eGFR < 45 mL/min/1.73 m^2), as their ability to lower glucose through glucosuria is proportional to eGFR. They can cause a transient increase in creatinine after initiation, especially in patients with kidney impairment. The main side effects of this class are increased incidence of genital mycotic infections and UTIs, affecting ~ 8–9% of patients. Cases of necrotizing fasciitis of the perineum (Fournier gangrene) have been reported. There also have been reports of pyelonephritis and septicemia requiring hospitalization. The glycosuria can cause intravascular volume contraction and hypotension. When SGLT-2 inhibitors are used in individuals also taking diuretics, dose adjustment to minimize the risk of hypotension may be required. SGLT-2 inhibitors do not cause hypoglycemia on their own; however, the risk increases when they are combined with insulin or insulin secretagogues. In such cases, a reduction in insulin dose may be necessary. In the CANVAS trial, canagliflozin was associated with increased risk of toe amputations. However, subsequent trials with canagliflozin or other agents in this class have not demonstrated this risk. Nevertheless, it is prudent to avoid SGLT2 inhibitor use in those at increased risk of amputation. In addition, guidelines recommend that all people with diabetes have their feet examined at SGLT2 inhibitor initiation and at least annually.

Canagliflozin causes a decrease in bone mineral density at the lumbar spine and the hip. In a pooled analysis of eight clinical trials (mean duration 68 weeks), a 30% increase in fractures was observed in patients taking canagliflozin. All SGLT-2 inhibitors cause a modest increase in LDL cholesterol levels (3–8%).

Euglycemic DKA is a rare but serious side effect in patients with type 2 diabetes and insulin deficiency, in ketosis-prone diabetes, and with off-label use of SGLT-2 inhibitors with type 1 diabetes. Patients with diabetes who are prescribed SGLT-2 inhibitors should be educated to hold the medication when oral intake is severely decreased, to increase fluid intake during this time, to monitor for ketones, and to seek medical attention for severe symptoms and/or elevated ketones. Patients are instructed to discontinue SGLT-2 inhibitors 3 days before any planned major surgery that will require prolonged periods with nothing by mouth.

O'Hara DV et al. Applications of SGLT2 inhibitors beyond glycaemic control. Nat Rev Nephrol. 2024;20:513. [PMID: 38671190]

3. Medications for type 2 diabetes that primarily lower glucose by their actions on the liver, muscle, and adipose tissue—

A. METFORMIN—Metformin is a first-line therapy for patients with type 2 diabetes—especially in patients without established cardiovascular or kidney disease, in which case other agents may be preferred. It can be used alone or in conjunction with other oral agents or insulin in the treatment of patients with type 2 diabetes. It is ineffective in patients with type 1 diabetes. The major site of action of metformin is the liver, where it decreases hepatic gluconeogenesis and hepatic insulin resistance, resulting in decreased hyperglycemia. Metformin has a half-life of 1.5–3 hours and is not bound to plasma proteins or metabolized. It is excreted unchanged by the kidneys. Hypoglycemia does not occur with therapeutic doses of metformin.

The maximum dosage of metformin is 2550 mg, although little benefit is seen above a total dose of 2000 mg. Metformin is available in immediate release (IR) and extended release (ER) formulations. When initiating metformin, it is important to start with a low dose and increase the dosage gradually; it should be taken with food to reduce gastrointestinal side effects. Nausea, vomiting, abdominal cramps, and diarrhea occur in up to 20% of patients. Up to 48% of patients initiated on metformin may discontinue treatment. The ER formulation has fewer gastrointestinal side effects and may result in better adherence. A common schedule is one 500-mg tablet three times a day (IR formulation) with meals or one 850- or 1000-mg tablet twice daily at breakfast and dinner. Up to 2000 mg of the ER preparation can be taken once a day.

(1) Safety concerns—GI side effects are dose-related, tend to occur at onset of therapy, and often are transient. However, discontinuation of metformin may be required in some individuals due to persistent gastrointestinal discomfort. An eGFR should be obtained in all individuals before initiating metformin. The dose of metformin should be reduced to 50% of maximal dose (1000 mg daily) in patients with eGFRs between 30 and 45 mL/min/1.73 m^2 and in older adults who are at higher risk for AKI from reduced renal functional reserve. Metformin is contraindicated and should be discontinued if the eGFR drops below 30 mL/min/1.73 m^2. Patients with liver failure, excessive alcohol intake, or hypotension should not receive this medication because of the risk of lactic acidosis.

Metformin-induced liver injury with cholestasis is rare but has been described. Metformin interferes with the calcium-dependent absorption of vitamin B_{12}–intrinsic complex in the terminal ileum; thus vitamin B_{12} deficiency can occur. *Measurements of vitamin B_{12} levels is advisable every few years during therapy*, especially in patients with peripheral neuropathy (which may be erroneously attributed to diabetic neuropathy) or if macrocytosis develops. Increased intake of dietary calcium may prevent metformin-induced B_{12} malabsorption.

Lactic acidosis has been reported as a side effect of metformin but is rare (incidence of <10/10,000 patient-years). Almost all reported cases have involved patients with associated risk factors (sepsis, hypoxia, dehydration, heart failure, liver or kidney dysfunction, and alcohol use disorder). AKI can occur rarely in patients taking metformin who receive radiocontrast agents. Metformin therapy should be temporarily halted on the day of radiocontrast administration in patients with eGFR 30–60 mL/min/1.73 m^2 and restarted 48 hours later, after confirmation that kidney function has not deteriorated.

B. THIAZOLIDINEDIONES (TZDS)—The thiazolidinediones (rosiglitazone and pioglitazone) improve insulin sensitivity and lower glucose levels by causing a favorable expansion of the subcutaneous adipose depot. Rosiglitazone, however, is no longer widely used worldwide.

TZDs are effective as monotherapy and in combination with sulfonylureas or metformin or insulin, lowering HbA_{1c} by 1–2%. When used in combination with insulin, they can result in a 30–50% reduction in insulin dosage, and some patients can come off of insulin completely. Pioglitazone is available as a generic agent and is inexpensive; the oral dosage is 15–45 mg daily and can be taken with or without food. These agents do not cause hypoglycemia when used as monotherapy or in combination with other agents.

Pioglitazone potently enhances insulin sensitivity by its action on adipose tissue, liver, and skeletal muscle, and it effectively decreases plasma glucose and HbA_{1c} levels. Pioglitazone also preserves β cell function. Beyond glucose-lowering, pioglitazone can lower blood pressure and has favorable effects on plasma lipids. There is reduction in triglycerides (9%) and increase in HDL-C (15%) without significant changes in total and LDL-cholesterol. Multiple studies have demonstrated that pioglitazone reduces hepatic fat content and reverses hepatic fibrosis. Pioglitazone can decrease urinary albumin and protein excretion in type 2 diabetes; there are no studies in patients with low eGFR. Pioglitazone is metabolized by CYP 2C8 and CYP 3A4.

(1) Safety concerns—Weight gain is common with pioglitazone therapy (1–4 kg over a year [2–5% body weight]). Interestingly, the greater the weight gain, the greater the decline in HbA_{1c} and improvement in insulin sensitivity. Weight gain can be minimized by not exceeding a dose of 30 mg/day (a dose that accounts for 80% of maximal glucose lowering). Pioglitazone used in combination with metformin can limit weight gain. Combination therapy with an SGLT-2 inhibitor or with a GLP-1 receptor agonist reduces weight gain and fluid retention (see below).

(2) Cardiovascular benefit—A large body of evidence from observational RCTs and mechanistic studies suggests that pioglitazone decreases recurrent cardiovascular events in individuals with and without diabetes.

(3) Fluid retention and heart failure—Edema occurs in about 5–10% of patients treated with pioglitazone and is dose related. Edema results from peripheral vasodilation and renal sodium retention. The edema occurs more frequently (10–15%) in patients receiving concomitant sulfonylurea or insulin therapy and may result in heart failure. Pioglitazone is contraindicated in patients with type 2 diabetes with New York Heart Association Class III and IV heart failure. It should also not be started if edema is present on clinical examination. Patients should be instructed to report new-onset edema or shortness of breath. Salt and

water retention from pioglitazone respond best to diuretics that act in the distal tubule such as spironolactone, triamterene, and amiloride. If more than trace edema is present, dietary sodium restriction should be advised, the dose of pioglitazone should be decreased, and treatment should be initiated with a distally acting diuretic.

(4) Bone fractures—An increase in bone fractures has been reported in individuals with type 2 diabetes treated with TZDs. The fractures appear to occur more commonly in postmenopausal women in the distal long bones of the hands and feet and are secondary to trauma. Decrease in lumbar spine bone density also can occur. Fractures are uncommon in premenopausal women and men. Pioglitazone should be used cautiously or avoided in individuals at high risk for fracture, including postmenopausal women with osteoporosis or those with prior fractures.

(5) Bladder cancer—Clinical studies have reported conflicting results regarding an association of bladder cancer with pioglitazone use. A 10-year observational cohort study of patients taking pioglitazone failed to find an association with bladder cancer. A large multipopulation pooled analysis (1.01 million persons over 5.9 million person-years) also failed to find an association between cumulative TZD exposure and incidence of bladder cancer. Another population-based study, however, generating 689,616 person-years of follow-up, did find that pioglitazone was associated with an increased risk of bladder cancer (hazard ratio 1.63). Thus, the FDA still cautions about bladder cancer risk and recommends avoiding use of pioglitazone in patients with type 2 diabetes and active bladder cancer or history of bladder cancer.

Bailey CJ. Metformin: therapeutic profile in the treatment of type 2 diabetes. Diabetes Obes Metab. 2024;26 Suppl 3:3. [PMID: 38784991]

4. Medications for type 2 diabetes that primarily stimulate insulin secretion by binding to the sulfonylurea receptor on the β cell—

A. SULFONYLUREAS—The primary mechanism of action of the sulfonylureas is to stimulate insulin release from pancreatic β cells; thus, they are used in type 2 diabetes. Sulfonylureas are metabolized by the liver, and apart from acetohexamide, whose metabolite is more active than the parent compound, the metabolites of all the other sulfonylureas are weakly active or inactive. The metabolites are excreted by the kidney and, in the case of the second-generation sulfonylureas, partly excreted in the bile.

Safety Concerns: Hypoglycemia is a common adverse reaction with the sulfonylureas. Weight gain also is common, especially in the first year of use. The mechanisms of the weight gain include improved glucose control and increased food intake in response to hypoglycemia. Idiosyncratic reactions are rare, with skin rashes or hematologic toxicity (leukopenia, thrombocytopenia) occurring in <0.1% of users.

(1) First-generation oral sulfonylureas (tolazamide, acetohexamide, chlorpropamide)—The use of these first-generation agents has been generally supplanted by newer generation oral sulfonylureas. Chlorpropamide has a prolonged biologic effect, and severe hypoglycemia can occur especially in older adults as their renal clearance declines with aging. Its other side effects include alcohol-induced flushing and hyponatremia due to increased vasopressin secretion and action.

(2) Second-generation sulfonylureas (glipizide, gliclazide, glimepiride, glyburide)—These medications should be used with caution and at lower doses in the elderly and in those with liver and kidney disease, due to higher risk of hypoglycemia. Evidence also suggests that sulfonylurea use is associated with increased risk of ventricular arrhythmias. In some studies, glyburide has been associated with increased risk of myocardial infarction, and there is some evidence of increased major adverse cardiovascular outcomes with glipizide.

Glipizide is the most commonly prescribed sulfonylurea in the United States. The starting dose is 5 mg/day, titrated up to 15 mg/day as a single daily oral dose before breakfast. When higher daily doses are required, they should be divided and given before meals. The maximum recommended dose is 40 mg/day, although doses above 10–15 mg probably provide little additional benefit. For maximum effect in reducing postprandial hyperglycemia, glipizide should be ingested 30 minutes before meals, since rapid absorption is delayed when the medication is taken with food. Glipizide therapy should not be used in patients with liver failure. Because of its lower potency and shorter duration of action, it is preferable to glyburide in older patients and for those patients with kidney disease. The extended release formulation of glipizide offers greater effectiveness in lowering prebreakfast hyperglycemia than the shorter-duration immediate-release standard glipizide.

Gliclazide (not available in the United States) is an intermediate-duration sulfonylurea with a duration of action of about 12 hours. See Table 31–4 for dosing options. The medication is metabolized by the liver; the metabolites and conjugates have no hypoglycemic effect. An extended-release preparation is available.

Glimepiride has a long duration of effect with a half-life of 5 hours allowing once- or twice-daily dosing. Glimepiride achieves blood glucose lowering with the lowest dose of any sulfonylurea compound. A single daily dose of 1 mg/day has been shown to be effective, and the maximal recommended dose is 8 mg. It is completely metabolized by the liver to relatively inactive metabolic products.

Glyburide is usually started at an oral dose of 2.5 mg/day. The average maintenance dose is 5–10 mg/day given as a single morning dose; maintenance doses higher than 20 mg/day are not recommended. Glyburide is metabolized in the liver, and the metabolic products have hypoglycemic activity. This can cause prolonged hypoglycemia, and glyburide should not be used in older patients or in patients with liver failure or CKD. Flushing has rarely been reported after ethanol ingestion.

B. MEGLITINIDE ANALOGS—Repaglinide is an insulin secretagogue structurally similar to glyburide but lacks the sulfonic acid–urea moiety. It acts by binding to the sulfonylurea receptor and closing the ATP-sensitive potassium channel. It is rapidly absorbed from the intestine and then undergoes complete metabolism in the liver to inactive biliary products, giving it a very short plasma half-life of < 1 hour. The medication therefore causes a brief but rapid pulse of insulin. The starting dose is 0.5 mg three times a day 15 minutes before each meal. The maximum dose is 4 mg with each meal. Metabolism is by cytochrome P450 3A4 isoenzyme, and other medications that induce or inhibit this isoenzyme may increase or inhibit the metabolism of repaglinide. Like the sulfonylureas, repaglinide can be used in combination with metformin. Hypoglycemia is the main side effect. Like the sulfonylureas, repaglinide can cause weight gain. Repaglinide may be useful in patients for whom nocturnal hypoglycemia needs to be avoided, in kidney impairment, or in older adults.

5. Medications that affect absorption of glucose— α-Glucosidase inhibitors competitively inhibit the α-glucosidase enzymes in the gut that digest dietary starch and sucrose. Two of these medications—acarbose and miglitol—are available in the United States. Voglibose, another α-glucosidase inhibitor, is available in Japan, Korea, and India. Both acarbose and miglitol delay the absorption of carbohydrate and lower postprandial glycemic excursion. To maximize tolerance, the starting dose of these medications should be low (eg, one-fourth of the maximum dose), taken just once daily, with dose and frequency slowly increased over a period of weeks or months.

A. Acarbose—Acarbose reduces postprandial hyperglycemia by 30–50%, and its overall effect is to lower the HbA_{1c} by 0.5–1%. It can be used as adjunctive therapy in type 2 diabetes. The recommended starting dose of acarbose is 50 mg orally twice daily, gradually increasing to 100 mg three times daily. For maximal benefit on postprandial hyperglycemia, acarbose should be given with the first mouthful of food.

(1) Safety Concerns—The principal adverse effect that limits its use is flatulence, which occurs in 20–30% of individuals. In 3% of cases, troublesome diarrhea occurs. The GI discomfort tends to discourage excessive carbohydrate consumption and promotes improved adherence to diet prescriptions in patients with type 2 diabetes. When acarbose is given alone, hypoglycemia does not occur. However, if acarbose is combined with insulin or sulfonylureas, it might increase the risk of hypoglycemia from the latter two agents. A slight rise in hepatic aminotransferases has been noted in clinical trials with acarbose (5% vs 2% in placebo controls, and particularly with doses > 300 mg/day). The levels generally return to normal on stopping the medication.

B. Miglitol—Miglitol is similar to acarbose in terms of its clinical effects. It is indicated for use in diet- or sulfonylurea-treated patients with type 2 diabetes. GI side effects occur as with acarbose. The medication is not metabolized and is excreted unchanged by the kidney. Miglitol should not be used in ESKD, when its clearance is affected.

6. Others—Pramlintide is a synthetic analog of islet amyloid polypeptide (IAPP or amylin). Given subcutaneously before a meal, it delays gastric emptying, suppresses glucagon secretion, and decreases appetite. It is approved for use both in type 1 diabetes and in insulin-treated type 2 diabetes. In 6-month clinical studies of patients with type 1 and insulin-treated type 2 diabetes, those taking the medication had ~ 0.4% reduction in HbA_{1c} and ~ 1.7-kg weight loss compared with placebo. The HbA_{1c} reduction was sustained for 2 years, but some of the weight was regained. Hypoglycemia can occur, and it is recommended that the short-acting or premixed insulin doses be reduced by 50% when pramlintide is started. Since pramlintide slows gastric emptying, recovery from hypoglycemia can be a problem because of delay in absorption of fast-acting carbohydrates. Nausea affects 30–50% of persons but tends to improve with time. In patients with type 1 diabetes, the initial dose of pramlintide is 15 mcg before each meal and titrated up by 15-mcg increments to a maintenance dose of 30 mcg or 60 mcg before each meal. In patients with type 2 diabetes, the starting dose is 60 mcg before meals, increased to 120 mcg in 3–7 days if no significant nausea occurs.

7. Medication combinations—Various medication combinations are available in different dose sizes to allow for decrease in number of pills taken. Metformin is available in combination with glyburide, glipizide, repaglinide, pioglitazone, sitagliptin, linagliptin, alogliptin, dapagliflozin, canagliflozin, and empagliflozin. Pioglitazone is available in combination with glimepiride and alogliptin. Combinations of SGLT-2 inhibitors and DPP4 inhibitors also exist. Combinations of insulin degludec and liraglutide (Xultophy), as well as insulin glargine and lixisenatide (Soliqua), are available in the United States. These medication combinations limit the clinician's ability to optimally adjust dosage of the individual medications.

E. Insulin

Insulin is the primary treatment for individuals with type 1 diabetes. Insulin is also indicated for patients with progressive type 2 diabetes with insulin deficiency when hyperglycemia does not respond to other antihyperglycemic agents.

1. Characteristics of insulin preparations—Available insulins include human insulins—regular (R) or NPH (N) formulations—or insulin analogs. Human insulins are bioengineered and structurally similar to endogenous human insulin. Insulin analogs are insulin molecules that are modified by genetic engineering and recombinant DNA technology. The amino acid structure of insulin is altered, and this changes certain properties of insulin—time of onset, peak, and duration of action—compared with human regular insulin (Table 31–5). Importantly, the biologic properties and stability of the insulin molecule remain intact. Six analogs of human insulin—three rapidly acting (insulin lispro, insulin aspart, insulin glulisine) and three long-acting (insulin glargine, insulin detemir, insulin degludec)—are available for clinical use. All currently available insulins are "purified" to preserve their potency so that refrigeration is recommended but not crucial. During travel, reserve supplies of insulin can be readily transported for weeks without losing potency if protected from extremes of heat or cold. All the insulins for human use are available in a concentration of 100 U/mL (U-100) and dispensed in 10-mL vials or 0.3-mL cartridges or prefilled

Table 31–5. Summary of bioavailability characteristics of the insulins.

Insulin Preparations[1]	Onset of Action	Peak Action	Effective Duration
Insulins lispro,[2] aspart,[3] glulisine	5–15 minutes	1–1.5 hours	4–6 hours
Human regular	30–60 minutes	2 hours	6–8 hours
Human NPH	2–4 hours	6–10 hours	10–16 hours
Insulin glargine	0.5–1 hour	Flat	~ 23 hours
Insulin degludec	0.5–1.5 hours	Flat	> 42 hours
Inhaled insulin	Seconds	12–17 min	2–3 hours

[1]Insulin administered subcutaneously unless otherwise noted.
[2]Insulin lispro formulated with treprostinil and citrate (Lyumjev, lispro-aabc) has an 11-minute faster onset of action.
[3]Insulin aspart formulated with niacinamide (Fiasp) has a ~ 10-minute faster onset of action.
NPH, neutral protamine Hagedorn.

disposable pens. Insulins available at higher concentrations are insulin glargine, 300 U/mL (U-300); insulin degludec, 200 U/mL (U-200); insulin lispro, 200 U/mL (U-200); and regular insulin, 500 U/mL (U-500).

2. Insulin preparations—See Table 31–6. *All rapidly acting insulin analogs and long-acting insulins are designed for subcutaneous administration; only regular insulin and insulin aspart can be given intravenously.* Based on their action profiles, insulin products are categorized as follows:

A. Rapid-acting: insulin analogs
B. Short-acting: regular insulin
C. Intermediate-acting: NPH
D. Long-acting insulin analogs, including ultra-long-acting and weekly insulins
E. Premixed insulin
F. Concentrated insulin
G. Inhaled insulin

Table 31–6. Insulin preparations available in the United States.[1]

Rapid-acting insulin analogs
Insulin lispro (Humalog, Lyumjev, Lilly; Admelog, Sanofi)
Insulin aspart (Novolog, Fiasp, Novo Nordisk; Merilog[2]; Kirsty, Biocon)
Insulin glulisine (Apidra, Sanofi)
Inhaled regular insulin (Afrezza)
Short-acting regular insulin
Regular insulin (Lilly, Novo Nordisk)
Short and intermediate-acting regular insulin
Regular insulin, concentrated (Humulin R U-500)
Intermediate-acting insulin
NPH insulin (Lilly, Novo Nordisk)
Premixed insulins
70% NPH/30% regular (70/30 insulin—Lilly, Novo Nordisk)
75% NPL/25% insulin lispro (Humalog Mix 75/25—Lilly)
50% NPL/50% insulin lispro (Humalog Mix 50/50—Lilly)
70% insulin aspart protamine/30% insulin aspart (Novolog Mix 70/30—Novo Nordisk)
70% insulin degludec/30% insulin aspart (Ryzodeg, Novo Nordisk)
Long-acting human insulin analogs
Insulin glargine (Lantus [U-100], Toujeo [U-300], Sanofi Aventis; Basaglar [U-100], Lilly; Semglee, Mylan; Rezvoglar, Lilly)
Insulin degludec (Tresiba, Novo Nordisk)

[1]All insulins available in the United States are recombinant human or human insulin analog origin. All the above insulins are dispensed at U-100 concentration. There is an additional U-500 preparation of regular insulin; U-300 preparation of insulin glargine; U-200 preparation of insulin lispro; and U-200 preparation of insulin degludec.
[2]First rapid-acting biosimilar to insulin aspart (insulin-aspart-szji) to be FDA approved.
NPH, neutral protamine Hagedorn.

A. Rapid-acting insulin analogs—This category includes insulin lispro, aspart, and glulisine. When injected subcutaneously, these insulins have a rapid onset of action in 15–30 minutes, peak in 30–90 minutes, and have an effective duration of 4–5 hours. They have a shorter duration of action compared with human regular insulin because they do not self-aggregate in solution. Clinical trials have demonstrated that the optimal time for premeal injection is 20 minutes for rapid-acting insulin. Another desirable feature of rapid-acting insulin analogs is that their duration of action remains at about 4 hours for most commonly used dosages.

Ultra-rapid-acting insulin aspart (Fiasp) contains aspart with niacinamide (vitamin B_3) to allow for rapid absorption from the injection site and onset of action 10 minutes faster than the standard insulin aspart formulation. It can therefore be injected right before the start of a meal or within 20 minutes after the start of a meal, allowing for some flexibility of dosing. The ultra-rapid-acting formulation of insulin lispro (Lyumjev) contains treprostinil to induce local vasodilation and citrate to increase vascular permeability. Its onset of action is 11 minutes faster than the standard insulin lispro formulation and has lower 1- and 2-hour postprandial glucose excursions.

Insulin aspart is approved for intravenous use (eg, in hyperglycemic emergencies) but does not have any advantage over intravenous regular insulin.

B. Short-acting insulin—Recombinant regular insulin is structurally similar to endogenous human insulin. It consists of dissolved zinc–insulin crystals that, when injected subcutaneously, self-aggregate and result in its effect in 30 minutes. It peaks at 2–3 hours and lasts 6–8 hours. For effective use, it needs to be injected at least 20–30 minutes before meals. Regular insulin increases the risk for hypoglycemia due to its prolonged duration of action. Intravenous infusions of regular insulin are particularly useful in the treatment of DKA and during the perioperative management of patients with diabetes who require insulin.

C. Intermediate-acting insulins—

(1) NPH (neutral protamine Hagedorn or isophane) insulin—NPH insulin is an intermediate-acting insulin that combines recombinant human insulin with protamine, which results in crystal formation. After subcutaneous injection, slow release of precipitated crystals of NPH insulin result in a longer duration of action compared with regular insulin. Its onset of action is 2–4 hours, with peak response in about 6–10 hours. Duration of action often ranges from 12 to 20 hours; therefore most patients require twice-daily dosing for adequate basal coverage. The action of NPH can vary within the same patient and between individuals. NPH insulin is dispensed as a turbid suspension at neutral pH with protamine in phosphate buffer. Occasional vials of NPH insulin show unusual clumping of their contents or "frosting" of the container, with considerable loss of bioactivity. This instability is rare and occurs less frequently if NPH human insulin is refrigerated when not in use and if bottles are discarded after 1 month of use.

(2) Insulin glargine—Insulin glargine is a clear insulin that, when injected into the neutral pH environment of the subcutaneous tissue, forms microprecipitates that slowly release the insulin into the circulation. It has no pronounced peak and a duration of action of 20–24 hours in most patients, allowing for once-daily basal dosing. Occasionally, twice-daily dosing may be needed. Insulin glargine should not be mixed with any other insulin, as it is solubilized in acidic pH.

A more concentrated form of insulin glargine (U-300) also is available (see below). Although limited clinical data suggest that insulin glargine is safe in pregnancy, it is not approved for this use.

(3) Insulin degludec—Insulin degludec is an ultra-long-acting insulin analog with a half-life of 25 hours. Its onset of action is 30–90 minutes and its duration of action is at least 42 hours. Due to this long duration of action, the daily injection time of insulin degludec can be varied without compromising glycemic control or safety. This long duration of action should be considered when a patient is fasting for a procedure or when switching to a different basal insulin, since residual insulin degludec action can last for up to 42 hours. Insulin degludec is available in two concentrations, U-100 and U-200, and dispensed in prefilled disposable pens.

(4) Insulin icodec—This basal insulin analog is given once weekly. It is dispensed in a disposable pen form, 700U/mL, and approved for use in Europe, Canada, Australia, China, and Japan. A loading dose is given on week 1, and a lower weekly maintenance dose conversion chart is provided by the manufacturer.

D. Mixed insulin preparations—Patients sometimes mix a mealtime insulin and intermediate-acting NPH insulin, "free mixing," to provide both basal and bolus coverage while limiting the number of daily injections. Regular insulin or rapid-acting insulin analog is drawn first from the vial followed by NPH insulin and injected immediately. Although free mixing is still practiced, premixed insulin formulations are popular in many parts of the world. These premixed insulins add to the convenience and prevent mixing errors while also achieving reasonable glucose control. Stable premixed insulins (70% NPH and 30% regular) are also beneficial to individuals with vision issues or impaired manual dexterity (Table 31–6). Premixed preparations of insulin lispro and NPH insulins are unstable; stability is achieved by replacing the NPH insulin with NPL (neutral protamine lispro). This insulin has the same duration of action as NPH insulin. Premixed combinations of NPL and insulin lispro (75% NPL/25% insulin lispro mixture [Humalog Mix 75/25] and 50% NPL/50% insulin lispro mixture [Humalog Mix 50/50]) are available for clinical use. Similarly, a 70% insulin aspart protamine/30% insulin aspart (NovoLog Mix 70/30) is available. Advantages of using insulin mixtures are that they can be given within 15 minutes of starting a meal and they are superior in controlling the postprandial glucose rise after a carbohydrate-rich meal. These benefits have not translated into improvements in HbA_{1c} levels when compared with the usual 70% NPH/30% regular mixture. Insulin glargine cannot be mixed with either regular insulin or the rapidly acting insulin analogs. Insulin degludec, however, can be mixed and is available as 70% insulin degludec/30% insulin aspart and is injected once or twice a day.

E. Concentrated insulins—Concentrated insulins are able to deliver more insulin in a lesser volume with fewer injections and less pain at the injection site compared with U-100 insulin, potentially improving adherence. When total daily dose requirements exceed 200 units, concentrated insulins are indicated. It is important to understand that switching from U-100 insulin to U-500 insulin should be done carefully, as they are not bioequivalent.

(1) Concentrated insulin analogs—When U-100 glargine is concentrated threefold, its duration of action is prolonged. U-300 glargine is delivered in one-third of the volume of U-100 glargine, with longer and flatter (more consistent) effects. Since a smaller volume is injected into less surface area in the subcutaneous space, there is slower release of insulin monomers. U-300 glargine results in less hypoglycemia compared with U-100 glargine. U-200 degludec, a twofold concentrated U-100 degludec, also is available. A U-200 concentration of insulin lispro is available in a disposable prefilled pen.

(2) U-500 insulin—This fivefold concentrated regular insulin is administered two to three times a day without basal insulin. Due to its concentration, the action is prolonged and variable; it is recommended only for patients who require ≥ 200 units per day of insulin. This form of regular insulin both provides mealtime coverage and has basal insulin properties. Its onset of action is 30–60 minutes, peak action is 2–4 hours, and duration is at least 8–13 hours. It is available only in a disposable 3-mL pen that contains 1500 units of insulin; the pen doses insulin in 5-unit increments up to a maximum of 300 units at a time. Caution should be used while prescribing U-500 insulin, as there may be confusion among clinicians, pharmacists, nurses, and patients about the risk of hypoglycemia that may develop hours after meals.

F. INHALED INSULIN—Technosphere insulin (Afrezza) is a dry-powder formulation of recombinant human regular insulin that can be inhaled. This insulin is rapidly absorbed, with peak insulin levels reached in 12–15 minutes and declining to baseline in 3 hours; the median time to maximum effect with inhaled insulin is approximately 1 hour. In contrast, the median time to maximum effect with subcutaneous insulin lispro is about 2 hours, declining to baseline in 4 hours. In clinical trials, Technosphere insulin combined with basal insulin was as effective in glucose lowering as rapid-acting insulin analogs combined with basal insulin. It is formulated as a single-use, color-coded cartridge delivering 4, 8, or 12 units immediately before the meal. The manufacturer provides a dose conversion table; patients injecting up to 4 units of rapid-acting insulin analog should use the 4-unit cartridge. Those injecting 5–8 units should use the 8-unit cartridge. If the dose is 9–12 units of rapid-acting insulin premeal, then one 4-unit cartridge and one 8-unit cartridge or one 12-unit cartridge should be used. The most common adverse reaction of inhaled insulin is cough, affecting about 27% of patients. A small decrease in pulmonary function (FEV_1) is seen in the first 3 months of use persisting over 2 years of follow-up. Inhaled insulin is contraindicated in patients who smoke cigarettes or have recently quit, and in those with chronic lung disease, such as asthma and COPD. Spirometry should be performed to identify potential lung disease prior to initiating therapy. During clinical trials, there were two cases of lung cancer in patients who were taking inhaled insulin and none in the comparator-treated patients. All the patients in whom lung cancer developed had a history of prior cigarette smoking. Cases of lung cancer were also reported in persons who smoked cigarettes using a previously available inhaled insulin preparation (Exubera). A follow-up study in 2019 was not able to exclude an increased risk of lung cancer–related mortality associated with Exubera use. The absolute increased risk of lung cancer–related mortality was 0.48 cases per 1000 person-years.

3. Sites of insulin injection—Any part of the body covered by loose skin can be used, such as the abdomen, thighs, upper arms, flanks, and upper buttocks. Preparation with alcohol is not required prior to injection as long as the skin is clean. Rotation of sites is recommended to prevent development of lipohypertrophy or scarred adipose tissue that results from repeated use of a single site. Exercise can increase absorption when the injection site is adjacent to the exercised muscle. For most patients, the abdomen is the recommended region for injection because it provides adequate area in which to rotate sites. The effect of anatomic regions appears to be much less pronounced with the analog insulins.

4. Methods of insulin delivery—

A. INSULIN VIALS, SYRINGES, AND NEEDLES—Plastic disposable syringes are available in 1-mL, 0.5-mL, and 0.3-mL sizes, and the needle gauges (G) are 28, 30, and 31 G. The three lengths of needles are 6 mm, 8 mm, and 12.7 mm. Long needles are preferable in patients with obesity to reduce variability of insulin absorption.

B. INSULIN PENS—Insulin delivery by disposable or reusable insulin pens has replaced vials and syringes in many parts of the world. Insulin pens are simple, convenient, and portable. They contain a cartridge carrying insulin that is injected into the subcutaneous tissue through a fine, replaceable needle. Insulin pens are available as disposable pens with prefilled cartridges or reusable pens with replaceable insulin cartridges. Most insulins are available in pen form. Pen needles are available in 29, 31, and 32 gauges and 4-, 5-, 6-, 8-, and 12.7-mm lengths.

Bluetooth-connected insulin pens and pen caps are smart pens that are integrated into a dedicated mobile application on a smartphone. The pens contain reusable insulin cartridges and have a battery duration of 1 year. Their features include the ability to record the timing and amount of each administered insulin dose, display the last dose, make dosing recommendations based on prespecified information, and provide reminders to administer insulin. Pen caps attach to disposable, prefilled pens of long-acting or rapid-acting insulin. Both smartpens and pen caps integrate with traditional BGM or selected CGM systems. These devices also connect with software, and data can be reviewed retrospectively with the clinician.

C. INSULIN PUMPS—Continuous subcutaneous insulin infusion (CSII) is the most precise way to mimic physiologic insulin secretion. An insulin pump is a computerized mechanical device that can automatically deliver insulin in a physiologic manner throughout the day. Individuals can accommodate changes related to eating, exercise, illness, or varying work and travel schedules by modifying insulin availability. Pumps are small battery-operated devices and house a reservoir or cartridge for insulin. Pumps can be tubed or tubeless. Pumps with tubing have an infusion set that is required for insulin delivery. A catheter or tubing connects the insulin reservoir to a needle or cannula that is inserted subcutaneously to deliver the insulin. The catheter connecting the insulin reservoir to the subcutaneous cannula can be disconnected, allowing the patient to remove the pump temporarily (eg, for bathing). The abdomen is the preferred site for such pumps because of convenience and consistent insulin absorption. The upper outer quadrant of the buttocks, upper thighs, and triceps fat pad of the arms also may be used. Patients may also choose the convenience of a tubeless pump. This pump consists of disposable "pods" that are discarded every 3 days. The pods are small, self-contained, all-in-one units with an internal insulin cartridge, insertion needle, and cannula. Insulin is infused directly from the pod through a catheter without the use of tubing based on wirelessly transmitted instructions from a smartphone or personal digital assistant. All pumps have software that can assist the patient to calculate boluses based on glucose reading and carbohydrates to be consumed. The pumps keep track of the time elapsed since the last insulin bolus, reminding patients of the elapsed time when they attempt to give additional correction bolus before the effect of the previous bolus has worn off.

This reminder feature reduces the risk of overcorrecting and subsequent hypoglycemia. Sensor-augmented pumps communicate with a CGM system and can suspend insulin when glucose levels are low or are predicted to fall low. These systems are effective in reducing nocturnal hypoglycemia. Rapid-acting insulin analogs are almost always used in insulin pumps. Pump therapy can be successfully started at the time of diagnosis of type 1 diabetes, as well as in older individuals with long-standing disease, and it is recommended for patients with type 2 diabetes who require multiple daily insulin injections.

Automated insulin delivery (AID) systems reflect exponential improvements in CGM technologies and refined insulin dosing pump algorithms that minimize insulin delivery burden. The AID system consists of three components: an insulin pump that continuously delivers rapid-acting insulin, a CGM that measures interstitial fluid glucose at frequent intervals, and a control algorithm that resides in the insulin pump, smartphone application, or handheld device and adjusts the insulin delivery. All AID systems are referred to as "hybrid" closed loop systems that adjust basal insulin delivery in real time. Users are required to manually enter insulin boluses pre-meal and when they exercise, but insulin delivery is automated at nighttime and between meals. AID systems are preferred over non-automated pumps and multiple daily injection regimens in persons with type 1 diabetes. AID systems, regardless of the type used, improve glycemic control and quality of life, are cost effective, and decrease anxiety in persons with type 1 diabetes.

Successful use of AID systems requires proficiency at using both the insulin pump and a continuous glucose monitor. Patients should be trained on what to do if there are unexpected high and low glucose levels. Known complications of insulin pump therapy include problems with infusion sets (occlusion, kinking), skin complications such as lipohypertrophy, and pump-site infection. When insulin delivery is interrupted, ketoacidosis can occur; it must be recognized immediately.

Do-it-yourself (DIY) closed loop systems have been developed by persons with type 1 diabetes to self-adjust insulin by modifying their individually owned pumps. These systems are built using widely available open-source code with compatible medical devices by persons who can build their own system. DIY systems are patient-driven and employ "off-label" use of technology; the patient assumes full responsibility for use of the DIY system, and those systems are not approved by regulatory bodies. It is important for clinicians caring for these patients to ensure the user has basic diabetes skills, including pump-site maintenance and knowledge about how to troubleshoot.

D. Mechanical patch pumps—Mechanical insulin delivery devices can enhance adherence to mealtime insulin dosing. V-Go (MannKind Corporation) is a wearable 24-hour patch pump designed for patients with type 2 diabetes who use a basal/bolus insulin regimen. The device delivers rapid-acting insulin continuously and is preset to deliver one of three fixed and flat basal rates (0.83 units/hour, 1.25 units/hour, or 1.67 units/hour) for 24 hours, after which it must be replaced. The V-Go also has an on-demand bolus button that delivers insulin in 2-unit increments to cover meals and lower high glucose excursions. CeQur Simplicity (CeQur Corporation) is a wearable 3-day mechanical patch device that holds 200 units of rapid-acting insulin and delivers 2 units per press of a button to cover meals and to lower high glucose excursions.

E. Complications of insulin therapy—

(1) Hypoglycemia—Hypoglycemia is the most common complication that occurs in patients with diabetes treated with insulin. Hypoglycemia in insulin-treated patients is a consequence of three factors: dosing issues, impaired counterregulatory systems, and complications of diabetes. The signs and symptoms of hypoglycemia may be divided into those resulting from stimulation of the autonomic nervous system and those from neuroglycopenia (insufficient glucose for normal CNS function). When the blood glucose falls to around 54 mg/dL (3 mmol/L), the patient starts to experience both sympathetic (tachycardia, palpitations, sweating, tremulousness) and parasympathetic (nausea, hunger) autonomic nervous system symptoms. If these autonomic symptoms are ignored and the glucose levels fall further (to around 50 mg/dL [2.8 mmol/L]), then neuroglycopenic symptoms appear, including irritability, confusion, blurred vision, tiredness, headache, and difficulty speaking. If untreated, worsening hypoglycemia can lead to loss of consciousness, seizures, or sometimes death.

Common dosing reasons for hypoglycemia include injecting too much insulin for the amount of ingested carbohydrates, exercise, and excessive consumption of alcoholic beverages. In patients with type 1 diabetes, hypoglycemia can occur during or several hours after exercise; therefore, glucose levels need to be monitored and food and insulin adjusted. Aggressive self-management of diabetes with repeated insulin boluses in close intervals ("insulin stacking") can result in hypoglycemia.

Impaired counterregulation resulting in hypoglycemia includes reduced glucagon and sympathoadrenal responses and cortisol deficiency. Patients with diabetes for > 5 years lose their glucagon response to hypoglycemia and lack adequate counterregulation against falling glucose levels. Once the glucagon response is lost, the sympathoadrenal responses take on added importance. Aging, autonomic neuropathy, or hypoglycemia unawareness from repeated low glucose levels further blunts the sympathoadrenal responses. In persons with type 1 diabetes mellitus who develop primary adrenal insufficiency, insulin requirements drop significantly and the insulin dose must be reduced to prevent recurrent hypoglycemia.

Complications of diabetes that increase the risk for hypoglycemia include autonomic neuropathy, gastroparesis, and ESKD. Tachycardia, palpitations, sweating, and tremulousness are important symptoms of the sympathetic nervous system to alert the individual of a falling glucose level. Failure of the sympathoadrenal responses increases the risk of hypoglycemia. If insulin is given before a meal to patients with gastroparesis, hypoglycemia may develop because the insulin action may peak before the food is absorbed. Hypoglycemia can occur with ESKD, presumably because of decreased insulin clearance and loss of renal gluconeogenesis.

Hypoglycemia can develop in patients taking sulfonylureas, repaglinide, and nateglinide, particularly if the patient is older, has kidney or liver disease, or is taking other medications that alter the metabolism of the sulfonylureas (eg, sulfonamides or warfarin). Hypoglycemia occurs even more frequently with the use of long-acting sulfonylureas than with shorter-acting agents. Though not absolutely contraindicated, β-blockers must be used with caution in patients who use insulin. β-Blockers can blunt most sympathetic symptoms of hypoglycemia except sweating; therefore, β-1-selective blocking agents are preferred.

(2) Hypoglycemic unawareness—Repeated episodes of hypoglycemia lead to adaptation; autonomic symptoms do not occur until the blood glucose levels are much lower and the first symptoms are often due to neuroglycopenia. This "hypoglycemia unawareness" can be reversed by keeping glucose levels at a higher range for several weeks.

To prevent and treat insulin-induced hypoglycemia, a patient with diabetes should carry glucose tablets or juice at all times. For most episodes, ingestion of 15 g of carbohydrate is sufficient to reverse the hypoglycemia. The patient should be instructed to check the blood glucose in 15 minutes and treat again if the glucose level is still low. *A parenteral (1 mg) or nasal inhalation (3 mg) glucagon emergency kit should be provided to every patient with diabetes who is receiving insulin therapy.* Family or friends should be instructed how to inject glucagon subcutaneously or intramuscularly into the buttock, arm, or thigh or administer a nasal dose in the event that the patient is unconscious or will not ingest food. Glucagon can occasionally cause vomiting, and the unconscious patient should be turned on his or her side to protect the airway. Glucagon mobilizes glycogen from the liver, raising the blood glucose by about 36 mg/dL (2 mmol/L) in about 15 minutes. After the patient recovers consciousness, additional oral carbohydrate should be given. *Patients with diabetes receiving medications that can cause hypoglycemia should wear an identification MedicAlert bracelet or necklace or carry a card in their wallet (800-ID-ALERT, www.medicalert.org).*

Medical personnel treating severe hypoglycemia can give 50 mL of 50% glucose solution by rapid intravenous infusion. If intravenous access is not available, 1 mg of glucagon can be injected intramuscularly or 3 mg given by nasal spray.

5. Immunopathology of insulin therapy—With the switch to human and purified pork insulin, the various immunopathologic syndromes such as insulin allergy, immune insulin resistance, and lipoatrophy have become quite rare since the titers and avidity of these induced antibodies are generally quite low.

A. INSULIN ALLERGY—Insulin allergy, or immediate-type hypersensitivity, is a rare condition in which local or systemic urticaria is due to histamine release from tissue mast cells sensitized by adherence of anti-insulin IgE antibodies. Immediate insulin allergic reactions can be from the insulin itself or from commonly used additives within the insulin preparation such as protamine, cresol, or, rarely, latex. In severe cases, anaphylaxis results. When only human insulin has been used from the onset of insulin therapy, insulin allergy is exceedingly rare. Antihistamines, corticosteroids, and desensitization may be required, especially for systemic hypersensitivity.

B. IMMUNE INSULIN RESISTANCE—A low titer of circulating IgG anti-insulin antibodies that neutralize the action of insulin to a small extent develops in most insulin-treated patients. This is rarely of clinical importance with the switch to human or highly purified pork insulins from the old animal insulins and has not been reported with the analogs.

C. LIPODYSTROPHY—Atrophy of subcutaneous fatty tissue leading to disfiguring excavations and depressed areas may rarely occur at the site of insulin injection. This complication results from an immune reaction, and it has become rarer with the use of human and highly purified insulin preparations. Lipohypertrophy, on the other hand, is a consequence of the pharmacologic effects of insulin being injected in the same location repeatedly. Rotation of injection sites and avoiding needle reuse will prevent lipohypertrophy.

Home PD. An overview of insulin therapy for the non-specialist. Diabetes Obes Metab. 2025;27 Suppl 5:3. [PMID: 40035222]

G. Transplantation

1. Pancreas transplantation—Whole pancreas transplantation involves complex abdominal surgery and lifelong immunosuppressive therapy and is limited by organ donor availability. Today, pancreas transplants are usually performed simultaneously using two organs from the same donor (simultaneous pancreas-kidney transplant) or as pancreas transplant alone. Patients undergoing simultaneous pancreas and kidney transplantation have an 83% chance of pancreatic graft survival at 1 year and 69% at 5 years. Solitary pancreatic transplantation in the absence of a need for kidney transplantation is considered only in those rare patients who do not respond to all other insulin therapeutic approaches and who have frequent severe hypoglycemia, or who have life-threatening complications related to their lack of metabolic control. Solitary pancreas transplant graft survival is 78% at 1 year and 54% at 5 years. All patients with ESKD and type 1 diabetes who are candidates for a kidney transplant are potential candidates for a pancreas transplant. Eligible candidates include those younger than 55 and those with minimal cardiovascular risk. Extensive CAD and peripheral vascular disease, as well as significant obesity (weight > 100 kg), are contraindications to transplantation.

2. Islet transplantation—Islet transplantation can be pursued in select patients with type 1 diabetes who experience severe hypoglycemia and hypoglycemia unawareness to help restore the α cell response critical for responding to hypoglycemia. Islet transplantation involves donor pancreas procurement followed by steps to isolate, purify, culture, and infuse the islets. Multiple donors are needed to provide enough islet cells. Survival of the islet grafts, limited donor supply, and need for lifelong immunosuppression are major challenges. Islet transplantation is offered in a few specialized centers around the world.

Clinical Trials About Optimum Diabetic Glucose Control

Findings of the Diabetes Control and Complications Trial (DCCT) in type 1 diabetes and of the United Kingdom Prospective Diabetes Study (UKPDS) in type 2 diabetes have confirmed the beneficial effects of improved glycemic control in both type 1 and type 2 diabetes.

A. Type 1 Diabetes

The DCCT, a long-term therapeutic study involving 1441 patients with type 1 diabetes mellitus, reported that "near" normalization of blood glucose resulted in a delay in the onset and a major slowing of the progression of established microvascular and neuropathic complications of diabetes.

The intensive treatment group had a mean HbA_{1c} of 7.2% while in the conventionally treated group, the HbA_{1c} averaged 8.9%. Over the study period, which averaged 7 years, the intensive treatment group had a ~ 60% reduction in risk for diabetic retinopathy, nephropathy, and neuropathy compared with the other group. The intensively treated group also had a nonsignificant reduction in the risk of macrovascular disease of 41% (95% CI, –10% to 68%). Intensively treated patients had a threefold greater risk of serious hypoglycemia as well as a greater tendency toward weight gain; however, there were no deaths definitely attributable to hypoglycemia in any persons in the DCCT study, and no evidence of posthypoglycemic cognitive damage was detected.

The general consensus of the ADA is that intensive insulin therapy associated with comprehensive self-management training should be standard therapy in patients with type 1 diabetes after the age of puberty. Exceptions include those with advanced CKD and older adults since the detrimental risks of hypoglycemia outweigh the benefits of tight glycemic control in these groups.

B. Type 2 Diabetes

The UKPDS, a multicenter study, was designed to establish whether the risk of macrovascular or microvascular complications could be reduced by intensive blood glucose control with oral hypoglycemic agents or insulin and whether any particular therapy was more beneficial than the other for patients with type 2 diabetes.

Findings from the UKPDS support that glycemic control to HbA_{1c} levels of 7% show benefit in reducing total diabetes endpoints, including a 25% reduction in microvascular disease compared with HbA_{1c} levels of 7.9%. This reassures those who have questioned whether the value of intensive therapy, so convincingly shown by the DCCT in type 1 diabetes, can safely be extrapolated to older patients with type 2 diabetes. It also argues against the concept of a "threshold" of glycemic control since in this group there was a benefit from this modest reduction of HbA_{1c} below 7.9%, whereas in the DCCT a threshold was suggested in that further benefit was less apparent at HbA_{1c} levels below 8%. In addition, tight control of blood pressure (median value 144/82 mm Hg vs 154/87 mm Hg) substantially reduced the risk of microvascular disease and stroke but not MI. Reducing blood pressure had substantially greater impact on microvascular outcomes than that achieved by lowering HbA_{1c} from 7.9% to 7%. The UKPDS data showed that every 10–mm Hg decrease in mean systolic blood pressure was associated with 11% reduction in risk for MI. More than half of the patients needed two or more medications for adequate antihypertensive therapy, and there was no demonstrable advantage of ACE inhibitors over β-blockers regarding diabetes endpoints. Use of a calcium channel blocker as combination therapy in either treatment group appeared safe over the long term despite some controversy in the literature about its safety in this population of patients with diabetes.

Steps in the Management of Diabetes

A. Patient Education (Self-Management Training)

Since diabetes is a lifelong disorder, education of the patient and the family is a most important obligation of the clinician who provides care. The best persons to manage a disease that is affected so markedly by daily fluctuations in environmental stress, exercise, diet, and infections are the patients themselves and their families. The "teaching curriculum" should include explanations by the clinician or nurse of the nature of diabetes and its potential acute and chronic hazards and how they can be recognized early and prevented or treated. Self-monitoring of blood glucose should be emphasized, especially in patients with diabetes who require insulin, and instructions must be given on proper testing and recording of data.

Patients taking insulin should understand the actions of basal and bolus insulins. They should be taught to determine whether the basal dose is appropriate and how to adjust the rapidly acting insulin dose for the carbohydrate content of a meal. Patients and their families and friends should be taught to recognize signs and symptoms of hypoglycemia and how to treat low glucose reactions. Strenuous exercise can precipitate hypoglycemia, and patients must be taught to reduce their insulin dosage in anticipation of strenuous activity or to take supplemental carbohydrate. Injection of insulin into a site farthest away from the muscles most involved in the exercise may help ameliorate exercise-induced hypoglycemia, since insulin injected in the proximity of exercising muscle may be more rapidly mobilized. Exercise training also increases the effectiveness of insulin, and insulin doses should be adjusted accordingly. Infections can cause insulin resistance, and patients should be instructed on how to manage the hyperglycemia with supplemental rapidly acting insulin.

Advice on personal hygiene, including detailed instructions on foot and dental care, should be provided. All infections (especially pyogenic ones) provoke the release of high levels of insulin antagonists, such as catecholamines or glucagon, and thus bring about a marked increase in insulin requirements. Patients who are taking oral glucose-lowering agents may decompensate and temporarily require insulin. Patients should be told about community agencies, such as ADA chapters, that can serve as a continuing source of instruction.

Finally, vigorous efforts should be made to persuade patients with newly diagnosed or established diabetes who smoke cigarettes to stop, since large vessel peripheral vascular disease and debilitating retinopathy are less common in nonsmoking patients with diabetes.

B. Medications

Treatment must be individualized on the basis of the type of diabetes and specific needs of each patient. However, certain general principles of management can be outlined for hyperglycemic states of different types.

1. Type 1 diabetes—A combination of rapidly acting insulin analogs and long-acting insulin analogs allows for more physiologic insulin replacement. Table 31–7 illustrates a regimen with a rapidly acting insulin analog and long-acting basal insulin that might be appropriate for a 70-kg person with type 1 diabetes eating meals providing standard carbohydrate intake and moderate to low fat content.

Insulin glargine or insulin degludec is usually given once in the evening to provide 24-hour coverage. There are occasional patients in whom insulin glargine does not last for 24 hours, and in such cases, it needs to be given twice a day.

The 24-hour basal dosage is usually based on age and body weight. An adolescent might need as much as 0.4 unit/kg/day; a young adult (<25 years), 0.35 unit/kg/day; and an older adult, 0.25 unit/kg/day. Insulin pumps allow the setting of different basal rates throughout the 24 hours and permit bolus dose adjustments by as little as 0.05-unit increments. For example, a 70-kg, 30-year-old person may require a basal rate of 0.7 unit per hour throughout the 24 hours with the exception of 3 AM to 8 AM, when 0.8 unit per hour might be appropriate (given the "**dawn phenomenon**"—reduced tissue sensitivity to insulin between 5 AM and 8 AM). The meal bolus varies based on the time of day and the person's age. Adolescents and young adults usually require 1 unit for about 10 g of carbohydrate. Older adults usually require about 1 unit for 15 g of carbohydrate. The correction factor—how much insulin is needed to lower glucose levels by 50 mg/dL—can be calculated from the insulin-to-carbohydrate ratios. For example, if 1 unit is required for 15 g of carbohydrate, then 1 unit will lower glucose levels by 50 mg/dL. If 1.5 units of insulin are required for 15 g of carbohydrate (that is, 1 unit for 10 g carbohydrate), then 1.5 units of insulin will lower glucose levels by 50 mg/dL (that is, 1 unit will lower glucose level by 33 mg/dL). For a 70-kg, 30-year-old person, bolus ratios of 1 unit for 12–15 g of carbohydrate plus 1 unit for 50 mg/dL of blood glucose over a target value of 120 mg/dL would be reasonable starting point. Further adjustments to basal and bolus dosages would depend on the results of blood glucose monitoring. One of the more difficult therapeutic problems in managing patients with type 1 diabetes is determining the proper adjustment of insulin dose when the prebreakfast blood glucose level is high. Occasionally, the prebreakfast hyperglycemia is due to the **Somogyi effect**, in which nocturnal hypoglycemia leads to a surge of counterregulatory hormones to produce high blood glucose levels by 7 AM. However, a more common cause for prebreakfast hyperglycemia is the waning of circulating insulin levels by the morning.

The diagnosis of the cause of prebreakfast hyperglycemia can be facilitated by self-monitoring of blood glucose at 3 AM in addition to the usual bedtime and 7 AM measurements or by analyzing data from the continuous glucose monitor. This is required for only a few nights, and when a particular pattern emerges from monitoring blood glucose levels overnight, appropriate therapeutic measures can be taken. The Somogyi effect can be treated by lowering the basal insulin dose at bedtime or by eating a snack at bedtime. When a waning insulin level is the cause, then either increasing the evening basal insulin dose or shifting it from dinnertime to bedtime (or both) can be effective.

The currently available closed-loop systems enable patients to achieve close to normal glucose levels in the morning with a low risk of nocturnal hypoglycemia and to improve overall glucose control. ***All patients with type 1 diabetes who have good self-management skills should be using these systems.***

Table 31–7. Examples of intensive insulin regimens using rapidly acting insulin analogs (insulin lispro, aspart, or glulisine) and long-acting insulin analogs (insulin glargine or degludec, NPH insulin) in a 70-kg man with type 1 diabetes.[1-3]

	Pre-breakfast	Pre-lunch	Pre-dinner	At Bedtime
Rapid-acting insulin analog	5 units	4 units	6 units	—
Insulin glargine or degludec[3]		—		15–16 units
or				
Rapid-acting insulin analog	5 units	4 units	6 units	
NPH[3]	6–7 units			8–9 units

[1]Assumes that patient is consuming approximately 75 g carbohydrate at breakfast, 60 g at lunch, and 90 g at dinner.
[2]The dose of rapid-acting insulin can be raised by 1 or 2 units if extra carbohydrate (15–30 g) is ingested or if premeal blood glucose is > 170 mg/dL (9.4 mmol/L).
[3]Insulin glargine or NPH must be given as a separate injection.
NPH, neutral protamine Hagedorn.

2. Type 2 diabetes—Therapeutic recommendations are based on the relative contributions of β cell insufficiency and insulin insensitivity in individual patients. The possibility that the individual patient has a specific etiologic cause for diabetes always should be considered, especially when the patient does not have a family history of type 2 diabetes or does not have any evidence of central obesity or insulin resistance. Such patients should be evaluated for other types of diabetes such as **autoimmune (type 1)**, prior pancreatic injury, or MODY. Patients with **autoimmune diabetes** should be prescribed insulin when the disease is diagnosed. Importantly, many patients with type 2 diabetes mellitus have a progressive loss of β cell function and will require additional therapeutic interventions with time.

Glucose-lowering agents—Figure 31–2 outlines the treatment approach based on a consensus algorithm by the ADA and the European Association for the Study of Diabetes.

For all patients with type 2 diabetes:
- Diabetes self-management education, exercise, nutrition management, weight loss counseling with prescribed agents for desired benefit.
- Offer diabetes technology.

↓

Choose GLP1-RA or SGLT-2i agent with desired benefit to maximally tolerated dose to meet goals. If high risk for CVD, known CVD, HF, or CKD:
- Start GLP1-RA or SGLT-2i with proven CVD and/or kidney benefit regardless of glycemic control.
- Even if at glycemic goal, these agents should be prioritized over other agents.

↓

If glycemic goals are not met:
- Add additional agent (GLP1-RA or SGLT-2i)
- SGLT-2i + GLP1-RA combination therapy is necessary only for beginning treatment of severely uncontrolled diabetes with glucose toxicity; step-wise therapy is indicated for routine treatment.*

↓

If glycemic goals still are not met:
- Add metformin, pioglitazone, DPP4i (if not taking GLP1-RA), sulfonylurea, or insulin.
- Insulin is preferred agent for severe hyperglycemia (HbA_{1C} > 10%, glucose > 300 mg/dL); start concurrent GLP1-RA (if no contraindications).
- DPP4i has only intermediate glucose lowering.

Cardiovascular and kidney effects:
- Semaglutide, liraglutide, dulaglutide have proven decreases in the major CV endpoints of nonfatal MI and stroke.
- SGLT-2is decrease risk of ESKD and death in patients with CKD and decrease hospitalizations for HF.
- Metformin decreased all-cause mortality and CV mortality in older studies of type 2 diabetes, especially if patients were overweight; await results of ongoing studies that have dedicated CV outcomes.

Weight management:
- If weight management is a priority, provide weight management counseling, choose diabetes agents with most weight loss potential, offer pharmacologic agents for obesity not related to diabetes (eg, topiramate); consider bariatric surgery.
- GLP1-RA/GIP RA, GLP1-RA, and SGLT-2i promote weight loss.
- Sulfonylureas, insulins, pioglitazone promote weight gain.
- DPP4i and metformin are weight neutral.

Potential benefit for MASLD or MASH benefit:
- GLP1-RA or GLP-RA/GIP RA (outcome pending), pioglitazone
- Insulin if decompensated cirrhosis

Major side effects:
- GLP1-RA or GLP1-RA/GIP RA: nausea, vomiting, constipation, diarrhea, pancreatitis
- SGLT2is: mycotic genital infections, dehydration, UTI
- Metformin: diarrhea, rarely lactic acidosis
- Pioglitazone: fluid retention, fracture risk, macular edema, possible bladder cancer
- DPP4is: diarrhea, nasopharyngeal infections, angioedema, pancreatitis risk (conflicting evidence, small risk)
- Sulfonylureas: hypoglycemia, weight gain
- Insulin: hypoglycemia

Cost:
- All agents except metformin, sulfonylureas, and pioglitazone are expensive.
- Insulins are expensive if additional cost of monitoring is considered; bioequivalent options are improving cost.

*Step-wise therapy is indicated because abrupt normalization of glucose can worsen retinopathy, for example.

CV, cardiovascular; DPP4i, dipeptidyl peptidase-4 inhibitor; GIP RA, glucose-dependent insulinotropic polypeptide receptor agonist; GLP1-RA, glucagon-like peptide-1 receptor agonist; MASH, metabolic dysfunction-associated steatohepatitis; MASLD, metabolic dysfunction-associated steatotic liver disease; SGLT-2i, sodium-glucose cotransporter 2 inhibitor.

▲ **Figure 31–2.** Algorithm for the treatment of type 2 diabetes based on the 2022 recommendations of the consensus panel of the American Diabetes Association/European Association for the Study of Diabetes.

The recommendation is to start pharmacologic therapy at diagnosis and not wait to see whether the patient can achieve target glycemic control with weight management and exercise. See discussion of the individual medications, above.

(1) Initial pharmacologic therapy—The presence of cardiovascular and/or kidney disease is an indication for prescribing a GLP-1 receptor agonist or an SGLT-2 inhibitor as initial therapy for type 2 diabetes. Dulaglutide, liraglutide, and semaglutide are considered first line for patients with established atherosclerotic CVD and have proved beneficial for CKD, particularly albuminuria. The SGLT-2 inhibitors canagliflozin, dapagliflozin, and empagliflozin improve cardiovascular outcomes; these are especially beneficial in patients with HF, diabetes-associated nephropathy, or both. GLP-1 or dual GIP/GLP-1 receptor agonists should be used in patients with or without CAD in need of weight loss. Metformin remains an effective agent if there is not underlying cardiovascular or kidney disease, and if weight loss is not desirable; it is lower in cost.

(2) When initial pharmacologic therapy does not control glucose adequately—A second agent, usually a GLP-1 or GIP/GLP-1 receptor agonist or an SGLT-2 inhibitor, or metformin is added. Combined GLP-1 or GIP/GLP-1 receptor agonist and SGLT-2 inhibitor therapies should be considered for patients with CVD and/or kidney disease. Sulfonylureas have the propensity to cause hypoglycemia and weight gain. In patients who experience hyperglycemia after a carbohydrate-rich meal (such as dinner), a short-acting secretagogue (repaglinide or nateglinide) before meals may suffice to get glucose levels into the target range. Patients with severe insulin resistance may be candidates for pioglitazone. Pioglitazone may also reduce the risk for recurrent stroke in patients who have a history of stroke or transient ischemic attack. If two agents are inadequate, then a third agent is added. The combination of metformin, a GLP-1 receptor agonist, and an SGLT-2 inhibitor should be considered in patients with obesity, heart disease, and kidney disease.

When the combination of non-insulin agents fails to achieve euglycemia in patients with type 2 diabetes, insulin treatment should be instituted. Various insulin regimens may be effective. One proposed regimen is to continue the oral agents (and injectable GLP-1 or dual GIP/GLP-1 receptor agonists) and then simply add a bedtime dose of long-acting insulin analog (insulin glargine, or degludec) to reduce excessive nocturnal hepatic glucose output and improve fasting glucose levels. If the patient does not achieve target glucose levels during the day, then daytime insulin treatment can be initiated. If this regimen fails to achieve satisfactory glycemic goals or is associated with unacceptable frequency of hypoglycemic episodes, then a more intensive regimen of multiple insulin injections can be instituted as in patients with type 1 diabetes (see Methods of Insulin Delivery). Metformin principally reduces hepatic glucose output, and it is reasonable to continue with this medication when insulin therapy is instituted. Pioglitazone, which improves peripheral insulin sensitivity, can be used together with insulin but this combination is associated with more weight gain and peripheral edema. Sulfonylureas, GLP-1 receptor agonists, DPP-4 inhibitors, and SGLT-2 inhibitors also have been shown to be of continued benefit and may be continued with close monitoring for hypoglycemia. Weight-reducing interventions should continue even after initiation of insulin therapy and may allow for simplification of the therapeutic regimen in the future.

American Diabetes Association Professional Practice Committee for Diabetes. 9. Pharmacologic Approaches to Glycemic Treatment: Standards of Care in Diabetes—2026. Diabetes Care. 2026;49:S183. [PMID: 41358900]

C. Acceptable Levels of Glycemic Control

A reasonable aim of therapy is to approach normal glycemic excursions without provoking severe or frequent hypoglycemia. Table 31–8 summarizes blood glucose and HbA_{1c} goals for different patient groups. *The UKPDS study demonstrated that blood pressure control was as significant or more significant than glycemic control in patients with type 2 diabetes regarding the prevention of microvascular as well as macrovascular complications.*

Chronic Complications of Diabetes

Late manifestations of diabetes include pathologic changes that involve small and large blood vessels (microvascular and macrovascular complications), the skin, and the lens of the eye. This damage leads to hypertension, kidney disease, vision loss, autonomic and peripheral neuropathy, amputations of the lower extremities, MI, and stroke. These late manifestations correlate with the duration of diabetes. CVD is the major cause of mortality in patients with type 1 and type 2 diabetes, followed by complications of kidney disease. Cigarette use adds significantly to the risk of both microvascular and macrovascular complications in diabetes.

A. Ocular Complications

Diabetic retinopathy is the most common microvascular complication of diabetes and the leading cause of blindness in adults worldwide (see Chapter 7). Risk factors include duration of diabetes, chronic hyperglycemia, rapid improvement in glycemic control, hypertension, dyslipidemia, cigarette smoking, genetics, and the presence of nephropathy. Large prospective randomized studies have demonstrated that intensive diabetes management with early and/or subsequent near-normoglycemia prevents and/or delays the onset and progression of diabetic retinopathy, reduces the need for future ocular procedures, and potentially improves vision. The ADA recommends an annual dilated and comprehensive eye examination at the time when type 2 diabetes is diagnosed, and 5 years after type 1 diabetes is diagnosed. A retinal examination is important before pregnancy attempts in patients with diabetes and also in each trimester of pregnancy. Annual dilated eye examinations help detect retinopathy; with its early treatment the risk of blindness can be reduced by 95%. In-office retinal photography can improve access to eye screening, but regular comprehensive eye examinations by an eye specialist are still encouraged.

Table 31–8. Glycemic targets for different groups of adults with either type 1 or type 2 diabetes.

	Blood Glucose mg/dL (mmol/L) Targets	HbA_{1c} % (mmol/mol) Targets
Nonpregnant healthy adults	Premeal glucose 90–130 (5–7.2) 1-hour peak < 180 (10) 2-hour peak < 150 (8.3)	< 7 (53). Aim for < 6.5 (48) if it can be achieved without significant hypoglycemia or polypharmacy.
Pregnant women	Premeal glucose < 95 (5.3) 1-hour peak ≤ 140 (7.8) 2-hour peak ≤ 120 (6.7)	6–6.5 (42–48). Aim for < 6 (42) if possible without significant hypoglycemia.
Older adults		
Healthy	Premeal 90–130 (5–7.2) Bedtime 90–150 (5–8.3)	< 7.5 (58)
Frail with limited life expectancy	Premeal 100–180 (5.6–10) Bedtime 110–200 (6.1–11.1)	< 8.5 (69)
Patients with history of severe hypoglycemia	Premeal 90–150 (5–8.3) Bedtime 100–180 (5.6–10)	< 8 (64)
Hospitalized patients	140–180 (7.8–10)	—
Patients with CKD	Glycemic targets in CKD are the same as those without CKD. HbA_{1c} and fructosamine values may not be accurate in ESKD, and greater reliance should be placed on the home glucose measurements	

Studies on the effect of GLP-1 receptor agonists on eye health have been conflicting. In randomized trials, liraglutide, semaglutide, and dulaglutide are associated with a risk of mildly worsening diabetic retinopathy perhaps due to rapid glucose improvement. Thus, retinopathy status should be assessed before intensifying diabetes therapy using GLP-1 receptor agonists. Some GLP-1 receptor agonists are linked to an increased risk of non-arteritic anterior ischemic optic neuropathy and age-related macular degeneration, but further studies are needed. Diabetes also increases the risk for cataracts, age-related macular degeneration, and glaucoma; maintaining glucose control early in the diagnosis of diabetes decreases these long-term risks. See Chapter 7 for assessment and treatment of diabetes-related proliferative and nonproliferative retinopathy and macular edema.

B. Diabetes and Chronic Kidney Disease (see Chapter 25)

CKD attributed to diabetes occurs in 20–40% of adults with diabetes. CKD may develop 10 or more years after a diagnosis of type 1 diabetes but can be present at the time of diagnosis of type 2 diabetes. CKD can progress to kidney failure requiring dialysis or kidney transplantation; diabetes is the leading cause of kidney failure in the United States. Major risk factors for development of CKD in diabetes include duration of diabetes, uncontrolled hyperglycemia, and uncontrolled hypertension. Other risk factors include obesity, cigarette smoking, dyslipidemia, and family history of kidney disease. Screening is recommended annually after 5 years of type 1 diabetes and starting at diagnosis of type 2 diabetes; screening is with a spot urine albumin creatinine ratio and serum creatinine measurement for GFR calculation. Two separate measurements at least 3 months apart are needed to confirm the finding of albuminuria. Severe hyperglycemia, recent exercise, fever, infection, and HF can cause a rise in urine albumin independent of kidney damage. From an early morning spot urine, a ratio of albumin (mg/dL) to creatinine (g/dL) < 30 mg/g is normal, a ratio of 30–300 mg/g suggests moderately increased albuminuria, and a ratio > 300 mg/g suggests severe albuminuria, and *there can be declining GFR without albuminuria*. Rapidly increasing albuminuria, active urinary sediment (WBC and RBC), or rapidly decreasing GFR suggest an etiology different than diabetes; a nephrology consult should be obtained and a kidney biopsy may be necessary. Nephrology should be consulted for advanced kidney disease such as eGFR < 30 mL/min/1.73 m^2 or for an urine albumin–creatinine ratio > 300 mg/g.

Glycemic control (HbA_{1c} ≤ 7%) is the only proven primary prevention for CKD. The ADA and Kidney Disease: Improving Global Outcomes Consensus statement for diabetes-related kidney disease recommends healthy diet, regular physical activity, smoking cessation, and weight management. Treatment of hypertension with ACE inhibitors or ARBs to maximally tolerated doses is beneficial when the urine albumin–creatinine ratio is > 300 mg/g. The goal of treatment should be to lower albuminuria by 30%. For type 2 diabetes, the addition of SGLT-2 inhibitors (for eGFR ≥ 20 mL/min/1.73 m^2) and metformin (half dose for eGFR 30–45 mL/min/1.73 m^2 and stopped for eGFR < 30 mL/min/1.73 m^2) are recommended for kidney protection and glycemic management. The GLP-1 receptor agonists are recommended for those with type 2 diabetes and kidney disease who have not met glycemic goals to lower albuminuria and reduces decline in eGFR. There is some evidence that the GLP-1 receptor agonist class is beneficial for weight and glucose control in persons with type 1 diabetes, but these agents are not FDA approved for these indications. SGLT-2 inhibitors may be beneficial for patients with type 1 diabetes and kidney disease, but these agents are not approved for use in type 1 diabetes due to the excessive risk of diabetic ketoacidosis. The nonsteroidal mineralocorticoid finerenone has been shown to delay decline in kidney function, kidney failure, cardiovascular death, nonfatal heart attack, and hospitalization for heart failure and is recommended for persons with type 2 diabetes and CKD with eGFR > 25 mL/min/1.73 m^2; potassium levels should be monitored 1 month after initiation.

C. Diabetes-Related Neuropathy

Diabetes-related neuropathies, the most common complications of diabetes with a lifetime prevalence of 50%, negatively impact quality of life and ability to work. Peripheral neuropathy may be present at the time of diagnosis of type 2 diabetes and after a longer duration of type 1 diabetes. It affects 10–30% of adults with prediabetes and 8–17% of youth with type 2 diabetes. Diagnosis is one of exclusion; other causes of neuropathy should be considered and treated such as hypothyroidism, vitamin B_{12} deficiency, toxins such as alcohol and chemotherapy, and structural cardiac or gastrointestinal abnormalities.

1. Peripheral neuropathy—

A. Distal symmetric polyneuropathy—

The most common form of diabetes-related peripheral neuropathy presents with symmetrical symptoms in the feet before progressing proximally in a stocking-glove pattern with toes and feet, and then fingertips, affected. This length-dependent axonal neuropathy manifests as pain, altered sensation, or complete loss of sensation, increasing risk for wounds and amputation. Screening with physical examination is recommended at least annually in all patients with type 2 diabetes and after 5 years in patients with type 1 diabetes. Patients with loss of sensation should have their feet examined at every visit to assess for wounds, calluses, and erythema.

Early-stage neuropathy presents with pain and dysesthesia from small fiber damage and altered temperature or pain sensation. Later, large fiber damage can present as balance difficulty and diminished or absent light touch sensation. Patients who have a sensory neuropathy should be examined using a 5.07/10g Semmes-Weinstein filament on the plantar surfaces of the feet. Loss of protective sensation is diagnosed by the absence of the monofilament sensation and signifies a much higher risk of ulcer, delayed healing, and amputation. Patients should be counseled to perform daily foot inspection (with help from a partner or a mirror) to look for mild injury or wounds. Patients should wear supportive shoes that are sufficiently wide and cover the feet and toes at all times. Concurrent autonomic neuropathy leads to altered sweat glands; dry skin is at risk for cracking, and hydrating lotions are recommended. The combination of neuropathy with a foot deformity, such as bunion, hammertoe, pes planus, or callus, warrants podiatric referral and custom-molded shoes and inserts to offload pressure points. The presence of peripheral arterial disease and/or nicotine use increases the risk of chronic wounds, 15% of which may require amputation. Assessment of pulses, presence of rubor or pallor on examination, and history of claudication or rest pain can help identify peripheral arterial disease. Vascular testing should be considered for all patients with nonhealing wounds, since up to 50% may have arterial disease.

Neuropathy can cause denervation of the small muscles of the foot. These changes alter the biomechanics and increase plantar pressures, causing callus and ulcer (Figure 31–3). The combination of peripheral neuropathy, autonomic neuropathy, and repeated trauma predisposes to the development of **Charcot arthropathy**. Acutely presenting with pain and swelling, if left untreated, Charcot arthropathy leads to a "rocker bottom" deformity and ulceration.

Hypersensitivity and "burning" pain, which is most bothersome at night, can become physically and emotionally disabling. Glucose lowering is vital to slow the rate of progression of neuropathy. Weight management and exercise may help improve balance. Smoking cessation counseling is important. *Treatment of concurrent sleep disorders and mood disorders is important.* The ACCORD trial showed that treatment of hypertension can decrease the relative risk for neuropathy by 25%. Although dyslipidemia is an independent risk factor, lipid-lowering therapy has not been shown to slow disease progression.

FDA-approved treatments for painful peripheral neuropathy include pregabalin, duloxetine, topical capsaicin 8% patch (applied in a physician office only), and high-frequency spinal cord stimulation (though its benefit is not supported by data). These agents can be used alone or in combination (with the agents from differing class and mechanisms of action) using stepwise increases in dosing and agents to ensure tolerability and avoid excessive sedation. Pregabalin, a congener of gabapentin, is a schedule V controlled substance. The starting dose of pregabalin is

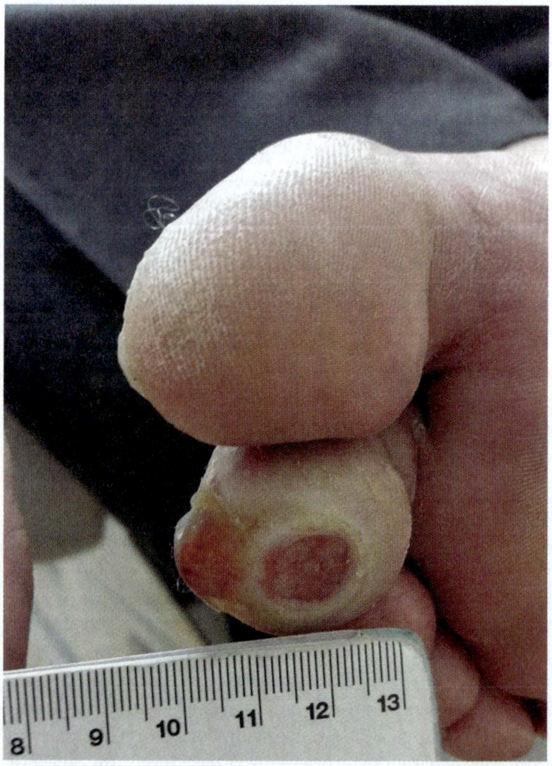

▲ **Figure 31–3.** Neuropathic foot ulcer in a patient with diabetes.

50 mg orally once daily, then increased to three times daily, with an optimal dose for most patients of 100 mg three times daily; decreased renal dosing is required for eGFR < 45 mL/min/1.73 m^2. Pregabalin can cause dizziness and sedation and must be tapered off slowly. Duloxetine is a serotonin and norepinephrine reuptake inhibitor with antidepressant properties; the dose is 60–120 mg once daily. In clinical trials, this medication reduced the pain sensitivity score by 40–50%. Other treatments for painful peripheral neuropathy that lack FDA approval for this indication are gabapentin, venlafaxine, and tricyclic antidepressants. Gabapentin has similar efficacy and side effects as pregabalin; the starting dose is 100 mg orally three times daily or 300 mg at night, then increased to 300 mg three times daily or higher. Gabapentin requires decreased dosing for eGFR < 45 mL/min/1.73 m^2. Venlafaxine, a serotonin and norepinephrine reuptake inhibitor, has a benefit similar to that of duloxetine. The tricyclic antidepressants nortriptyline, desipramine, or amitriptyline may provide dramatic relief, often within 48–72 hours. Tricyclic antidepressants should be discontinued if improvement has not occurred after 5 days; they are to be avoided in patients age > 65 and in patients with ischemic heart disease. Thus, utility is limited in this population as safer options are available. Capsaicin is an over-the-counter cream (Zostrix 0.025%, Zostrix HP 0.075%) rubbed into the skin over the painful region two to four times daily. Capsaicin 8% is approved only for in-office application, usually by a pain specialist.

Patients should be advised to seek immediate medical care if a diabetic foot ulcer develops. Treatment of neuropathic ulcers includes mechanical offloading with a special shoe or boot, management of infection with debridement and antibiotics, physiologic dressings, and ensuring adequate vascular supply and revascularization as appropriate. Deep-wound culture-guided oral antibiotic agents are typically amoxicillin-clavulanate, cephalosporin, dicloxacillin, or clindamycin; if osteomyelitis is present, intravenous agents include piperacillin-tazobactam, vancomycin, and other broad spectrum antibiotics. Local antibiotic resistance patterns and coverage for methicillin-resistant *Staphylococcus aureus* should be considered. The incidence of gangrene of the feet in patients with diabetes is 30 times that of age-matched controls. The factors responsible for its development are peripheral neuropathy with loss of pain sensation and peripheral vascular disease, while concurrent cigarette smoking increases the risk. The GLP-1 receptor agonists, when compared with the SGLT-2 inhibitors, have a decreased risk of adverse lower extremity events, including amputation.

B. Isolated peripheral neuropathy—A less common neuropathy of diabetes is involvement of only one nerve ("mononeuropathy") or of several nerves ("mononeuropathy multiplex"), characterized by sudden onset with subsequent recovery of all or most of the function. This neuropathy has been attributed to vascular ischemia or traumatic damage. Cranial and femoral nerves may be involved. The patient with cranial nerve involvement usually has diplopia and single third, fourth, or sixth nerve weakness but the pupil is spared from the microvascular ischemia. A full recovery of function occurs in 6–12 weeks.

C. Diabetic amyotrophy—The presenting symptom is onset of severe pain in the front of the thigh. Within a few days or weeks of the onset of pain, weakness, and wasting of the quadriceps develops. As the weakness appears, the pain tends to improve. Management includes analgesia and improved diabetes control. The symptoms improve over 6–18 months.

2. Autonomic neuropathy—This neuropathy occurs principally in diabetes of long duration. The cardiovascular, gastrointestinal, and genitourinary systems can be affected, and it is a diagnosis of exclusion. Symptoms may include dizziness, tachycardia, early satiety, nausea, urinary urgency, and sexual dysfunction.

A. Cardiovascular autonomic neuropathy—The prevalence of this neuropathy is 20–60% in patients with long-standing diabetes. Decreased heart rate variability with deep breathing is seen in the early stages, with resting tachycardia and orthostatic hypotension occurring in late stages. This neuropathy can negatively impact underlying CVD, increasing mortality and sudden death risk. After other causes are excluded (anemia, thyroid disease, adrenal insufficiency, substance abuse, structural heart disease, and cardiomyopathy), this diagnosis is supported by positive results on tilt table testing and orthostatic blood pressure measurements. Use of compression stockings, tilting the head of the bed upward, and arising slowly from the supine position can help treat symptoms of orthostatic hypotension. When such measures are inadequate, fludrocortisone 0.1–0.2 mg orally daily can be given but can result in supine hypertension and hypokalemia. The α-agonist midodrine (10 mg orally three times a day) also can be used. Supine hypertension is common, and short-acting antihypertensives such as enalapril or clonidine may be used for overnight blood pressure control. Diuretics should be avoided.

B. GI neuropathy—This neuropathy, which can manifest as nausea, vomiting, postprandial fullness, reflux or dysphagia, constipation or diarrhea (or both), and fecal incontinence, is a diagnosis of exclusion. Gastroparesis should be considered in patients with diabetes in whom unexpected fluctuations and variability in blood glucose levels develop after meals. A gastric emptying study with scintigraphy may show marked delay in gastric emptying; the glucose must be < 250 mg/dL at the time of the test. Normal testing does not exclude a diagnosis of gastroparesis, however. Glucose control is important to lower the risk of progression of gastrointestinal neuropathy and improve symptoms.

Metoclopramide has weak evidence of benefit and is FDA-approved for treatment but only for < 12 weeks. The dose is 10 mg orally three or four times a day, 30 minutes before meals and at bedtime. Drowsiness, restlessness, fatigue, and lassitude are common adverse effects. Tardive dyskinesia and extrapyramidal effects can occur, especially when used for longer than 3 months. Erythromycin, 250 mg orally three times daily, appears to bind to gastric motilin receptors and may improve gastric emptying in the short term, but its effectiveness likely diminishes over time. In selected patients, injections of botulinum toxin into the pylorus can reduce pylorus sphincter resistance and enhance gastric emptying.

Refractory diabetes-related diarrhea is often associated with impaired sphincter control and fecal incontinence. Loperamide, 4–8 mg orally daily, or diphenoxylate with atropine, two tablets (5 mg of diphenoxylate) up to four times a day, may provide relief after other causes of diarrhea have been excluded and offending medications removed. Constipation usually responds to bulking agents or stimulant laxatives.

c. Genitourinary system—Diabetic autonomic neuropathy can result in genitourinary disturbances, including sexual dysfunction and bladder dysfunction. Symptoms include urinary urgency, recurrent UTI, decreased libido, painful intercourse, inadequate lubrication, and erectile dysfunction. Glucose control is important. Recurrent UTIs warrant urologic evaluation of bladder function. Women should be offered vaginal lubricants and low-dose hormone therapy when appropriate. Male erectile dysfunction can result from neurologic, psychological, or vascular causes, or a combination of these causes (see Chapter 26, Male Sexual Dysfunction & Erectile Dysfunction).

D. Cardiovascular Complications

1. Hypertension—Hypertension is common in persons with diabetes and is a major risk for ASCVD, HF, and microvascular complications. Hypertension is defined as a systolic blood pressure ≥ 130 mm Hg or a diastolic blood pressure ≥ 80 mm Hg based on an average of at least two measurements obtained on at least two occasions. The ADA recommends a treatment target blood pressure of < 130/80 mm Hg in persons with diabetes. The Systolic Blood Pressure Intervention Trial (SPRINT) reported that treating to a systolic blood pressure of < 120 mm Hg reduced cardiovascular events by 25% and death from cardiovascular causes by 43%, but individuals with diabetes were excluded from this study. The Strategy of Blood Pressure Intervention in the Elderly Hypertensive Patients (STEP) trial included nearly 20% of persons with diabetes; cardiovascular events were decreased when blood pressure was treated to a systolic goal of < 130 mm Hg. Meta-analyses of hypertension trials suggest that lowering systolic blood pressure to < 130 mm Hg reduces the risk of stroke, retinopathy, and albuminuria, but effects on other ASCVD outcomes and heart failure have not been evident. Patients with type 2 diabetes who have CAD or albuminuria should be treated with an ACE inhibitor or ARB as first-line therapy. Multidrug therapy is often required. If blood pressure is ≥ 150/90 mm Hg, two agents should be initiated (ACE inhibitor/ARB, calcium channel blocker or diuretic). A mineralocorticoid receptor antagonist should be considered in resistant hypertension if the patient is on three classes of antihypertensives and blood pressure is not at goal (see Chapter 13). There are no data to guide blood pressure targets in persons with type 1 diabetes, but a similar target of < 130/80 mm Hg is recommended. Blood pressure goals should be individualized, taking into consideration the risk of potential adverse effects of antihypertensive therapy such as hypotension, syncope, falls, acute kidney injury, and electrolyte abnormalities.

2. Cardiovascular disease—ASCVD—which includes CAD, stroke, and peripheral arterial disease—is the leading cause of morbidity and mortality in diabetes. Individuals with type 2 diabetes often have cardiovascular risk factors including lipid abnormalities, central adiposity, hypertension, and hepatic steatosis, many of which predate the development of diabetes. In the past two decades, ASCVD mortality has decreased in patients with diabetes, likely due to improved care delivery, more stringent risk factor targets, and better risk factor control through lifestyle intervention and newer pharmacologic therapies. The risk of ASCVD in those with diabetes, however, remains two- to fourfold higher than in age- and sex-matched persons without diabetes. ASCVD risk is high in individuals with well-managed type 1 diabetes even in the absence of lipid abnormalities. Mechanisms involved in the atherosclerotic process in diabetes are complex with contributions from hyperglycemia, insulin resistance, dyslipidemia, chronic inflammation, and oxidative stress.

Lowering LDL cholesterol reduces first events of coronary disease in patients without known CAD (primary prevention) and secondary events in patients with known CAD (secondary prevention). Multiple randomized controlled trials have demonstrated the benefits of LDL lowering for primary and secondary ASCVD prevention in individuals with and without diabetes. Statins remain the mainstay of LDL lowering in those with diabetes. For individuals with diabetes and known ASCVD, high-intensity statin therapy is recommended to lower LDL ≥ 50% of baseline with the target goal of < 55 mg/dL due to the very high-risk status of these individuals. If the LDL goal is not attained, addition of ezetimibe, bempedoic acid, and/or PCSK9 inhibitor therapy is indicated. For primary ASCVD risk reduction in adults age 40–75 years, an LDL goal of < 70 mg/dL is recommended. For patients with type 2 diabetes age 20–39 years, statin therapy should be considered if there are additional ASCVD risk factors such as hypertension, obesity, CKD, or family history of ASCVD. Moderate-intensity statin therapy is recommended for those with diabetes age > 75 after assessment of the risk-benefit profile and statin dose reduction, as needed. In persons with hypertriglyceridemia (fasting triglycerides > 150 mg/dL), lifestyle interventions and identifying and treating secondary factors such as medications that raise triglycerides, kidney disease, or hypothyroidism are recommended. For individuals with established ASCVD or with risk factors for CVD and elevated triglycerides (150–499 mg/dL) after maximizing statin therapy, icosapent ethyl may be added. Although data on ASCVD risk reduction in adults with type 1 diabetes are limited, an approach similar to that used in type 2 diabetes should be employed and statin therapy should be initiated, especially with risk factors such as hypertension, obesity, dyslipidemia, or CKD. Routine screening for CAD is not recommended in asymptomatic individuals with diabetes, especially since ASCVD risk factors already should be aggressively managed in these individuals.

Aspirin 81–325 mg orally daily is recommended for reducing cardiovascular morbidity and mortality in patients who have a history of MI or stroke (secondary prevention). For primary prevention, the use of aspirin should be considered only for patients with diabetes who have at least one major risk factor (eg, cigarette smoking, hypertension, obesity, dyslipidemia) and do not have an increased bleeding risk such as age > 70 years, anemia, or kidney disease. If there is an allergy to aspirin, clopidogrel should be used for patients with ASCVD. Dual antiplatelet therapy with aspirin and a P2Y12 receptor antagonist is indicated after acute coronary syndromes, coronary revascularization with stenting, acute ischemic stroke, and transient ischemic attack with duration of therapy determined in conjunction with specialists.

A. Heart failure—Several longitudinal and observational studies have demonstrated that patients with diabetes are at increased risk for developing HF, which may be the first presenting cardiovascular complication. Risk factors for HF include diabetes duration, suboptimal glycemic control, uncontrolled hypertension, hyperlipidemia, higher BMI, microalbuminuria, CKD, CAD, and peripheral artery disease. Individuals with diabetes may develop "diabetic cardiomyopathy," a left ventricular systolic or diastolic dysfunction in the absence of other causes such as hypertension or CAD; women appear to be at higher risk. HF with preserved EF as well as reduced EF can be seen in diabetes, and the diagnosis of both types is often overlooked. Early identification and treatment of risk factors and asymptomatic stages of HF reduce the risk for progression to symptomatic HF in patients with diabetes. The ADA suggests screening asymptomatic adults with diabetes for the development of cardiac structural or functional abnormalities (stage B HF) by measuring BNP or NT-proBNP. Elevated BNP levels ≥ 50 pg/mL and NT-proBNP levels ≥ 125 pg/mL warrant echocardiography and implementation of guideline-directed medical therapy. Treatment includes use of ACE inhibitors or ARBs, β-blockers, an SGLT-2 inhibitor with proven HF prevention benefit, or a dual GIP/GLP-1 receptor agonist or GLP-1 receptor agonist with demonstrated benefit for reducing HF symptoms. Medical therapy for symptomatic HF in patients with and without diabetes is similar and should be in collaboration with a cardiovascular specialist.

B. Peripheral arterial disease (PAD)—Patients with diabetes are at increased risk for developing peripheral arterial disease; risk factors include age, longer duration of diabetes, cigarette smoking, hypertension, dyslipidemia, suboptimal glycemic management, presence of microvascular complications, and a history of CVD. The presence of microvascular disease is associated with an increased risk for future limb amputation. Patients with PAD are often asymptomatic; claudication pain is often not reported due to limited physical activity or to the presence of other comorbid conditions. Screening is recommended with a history and physical examination for asymptomatic PAD; finding an abnormal ankle-brachial index may lead to intensifying pharmacologic therapies such as LDL lowering and initiating GLP-1 receptor agonists, which offer benefit in those with diabetes and PAD (age ≥ 65 years, diabetes duration ≥ 10 years, microvascular disease, presence of foot complications, or end-organ damage from diabetes). If a foot ulcer is present with abnormal noninvasive testing, immediate referral for vascular evaluation is warranted.

E. Skin and Mucous Membrane Complications

Skin infections are highly prevalent in patients with diabetes. Uncontrolled hyperglycemia can lead to chronic or recurrent pyogenic skin infections. *Candida* infections are common and can involve the mucosa (thrush, vulvovaginitis), intertriginous areas (breasts, groin), or nails (paronychia). Intertriginous *Candida* infections may be pruritic or painful and present with erythematous areas. Glycosuria due to SGLT-2 administration can increase the risk for candidal vulvovaginitis and balanoposthitis. Candidiasis is treated with topical or oral antifungal agents containing miconazole or clotrimazole. Improved glycemic control and keeping the affected areas dry are beneficial.

Necrobiosis lipoidica diabeticorum is a rare chronic granulomatous dermatologic disease that occurs most frequently in patients with diabetes and is more common in women than men. It begins as one or a group of well-demarcated rounded erythematous papules that expand and aggregate into plaques with red-brown borders and a yellow atrophic center containing telangiectasias. Lesions are usually located over the anterior surfaces of the legs or the dorsal surfaces of the ankles. Necrobiosis lipoidica diabeticorum is a chronic, debilitating condition for patients and difficult for clinicians to manage. First-line therapy includes topical and subcutaneous corticosteroids. Therapies such as cyclosporine, infliximab, and hydroxychloroquine have been used. Appropriate wound care should be implemented at the earliest for ulcerated lesions, including topical antibiotics, emollients, and compression bandaging.

"Shin spots" (diabetes-related dermopathy) may appear in adults with diabetes. They are brownish, rounded, painless atrophic lesions of the skin in the pretibial area.

F. Bone and Joint Complications

Long-standing diabetes can cause progressive stiffness of the hand secondary to contracture and tightening of skin over the joints (diabetes-related cheiroarthropathy), frozen shoulder (adhesive capsulitis), carpal tunnel syndrome, and Dupuytren contractures. These complications may be due to glycosylation of collagen and perhaps other proteins in connective tissue, and there may be an inflammatory component. Bursitis, particularly of the shoulders and hips, occurs more frequently than expected in patients with diabetes.

Data on bone mineral density and fracture risk in patients with diabetes are contradictory. Patients with type 2 diabetes appear to be at increased risk for nonvertebral fractures. Women with type 1 diabetes have an increased risk of fracture compared with women without diabetes. Other factors, such as duration of diabetes, and diabetes complications, such as neuropathy and kidney disease, likely affect both the bone mineral density and fracture risk.

Diffuse idiopathic skeletal hyperostosis is characterized by ossification of the anterior longitudinal ligaments of the spine and various extraspinal ligaments. It causes stiffness and decreased range of spinal motion. The peripheral joints most commonly affected are the metacarpophalangeal joints, elbows, and shoulders. Diabetes, obesity, hypertension, and dyslipidemia are risk factors.

Hyperuricemia, acute and tophaceous gout, and osteoarthritis are more common in type 2 diabetes.

American Diabetes Association Professional Practice Committee for Diabetes. 10. Cardiovascular Disease and Risk Management: Standards of Care in Diabetes—2026. Diabetes Care. 2026;49:S216. [PMID: 41358899]

American Diabetes Association Professional Practice Committee for Diabetes. 11. Chronic Kidney Disease and Risk Management: Standards of Care in Diabetes—2026. Diabetes Care. 2026;49:S246. [PMID: 41358881]

American Diabetes Association Professional Practice Committee for Diabetes. 12. Retinopathy, Neuropathy, and Foot Care: Standards of Care in Diabetes—2026. Diabetes Care. 2026;49:S261. [PMID: 41358886]

Amini A et al. Semaglutide and non-arteritic anterior ischaemic optic neuropathy: review and interpretation of reported association. Acta Ophthalmol. 2025;103:615. [PMID: 40055951]

Dillon BR et al. Spectrum of diabetic neuropathy: new insights in diagnosis and treatment. Annu Rev Med. 2024;75:293. [PMID: 38285516]

Pop-Busui R et al. Heart failure: an underappreciated complication of diabetes. A consensus report of the American Diabetes Association. Diabetes Care. 2022;45:1670. [PMID: 35796765]

Special Situations

A. Diabetes Management in the Hospital

Initial evaluation should include identification of the type of diabetes (type 1, type 2, gestational, pancreatic, stress hyperglycemia, or drug induced such as from corticosteroids). For all patients with diabetes or those with any glucose abnormality identified at the time of admission, HbA_{1c} C should be measured if no such test result is available from the previous 3 months. A HbA_{1c} value ≥ 6.5% on admission suggests that the onset of diabetes preceded hospitalization. In hospitalized individuals, hyperglycemia is defined as any blood glucose level > 140 mg/dL. Hypoglycemia is defined as blood glucose < 70 mg/dL.

1. Glycemic goals in hospitalized patients—Based on several large randomized clinical trials, insulin and/or other therapies should be initiated for the treatment of persistent hyperglycemia ≥ 180 mg/dL with a glucose goal of 140–180 mg/dL recommended for most critically ill individuals. Tighter glucose goals, such as 110–140 mg/dL, may be considered for select individuals (e.g., critically ill individuals undergoing cardiac surgery) if these goals can be achieved without hypoglycemia. In non–critically ill patients, glucose goals of 100–180 mg/dL are appropriate, whether hyperglycemia is from pre-existing diabetes, stress induced, or from newly diagnosed diabetes.

2. Glucose monitoring in the hospital—In hospitalized patients with diabetes who are eating, point-of-care (POC) blood glucose monitoring should be performed before meals with an FDA-approved hospital-calibrated system; if the patient is not eating, glucose monitoring can be performed every 4–6 hours. If intravenous insulin is used, frequent (typically every 1 hour) POC blood glucose monitoring is recommended for safety. Patients using CGM systems can continue using their devices if clinically appropriate. However, no CGM systems are approved for use in the hospital setting. When insulin dosing decisions need to be made, POC glucose should be used.

3. Insulin pump use in the hospital—Data on inpatient use of automated insulin delivery devices are limited. Best practices on safe use of these devices for hospitalized patients are evolving and limited by access to specialty diabetes care and trained staff. Continued use of an insulin pump or automated insulin delivery system should be supported during hospitalization for patients who are willing and able to self-manage their devices with staff supervision. Patients should be transitioned to a basal bolus subcutaneous insulin regimen if they are unable to manage their pump and/or CGM because of their illness. Pumps should be removed if radiologic studies or hospital procedures are performed based on hospital policies.

4. Treatment of hyperglycemia in hospitalized patients—In the critically ill, continuous intravenous insulin infusion achieves specific glycemic goals and avoids hypoglycemia. There are many validated written or computerized protocols that allow for predefined adjustments in the insulin infusion rate based on glucose values and insulin infusion rates. For individuals who are eating but are receiving an intravenous insulin infusion, prandial insulin coverage using extra subcutaneous rapid-acting insulin can avoid large fluctuations in intravenous insulin dosing and hypoglycemia risk.

5. Transitioning from intravenous to subcutaneous insulin—When transitioning from intravenous insulin to subcutaneous insulin, basal insulin should be given 2 hours before the intravenous infusion is discontinued to minimize rebound hyperglycemia while the subcutaneous insulin becomes effective.

On acute care inpatient services, subcutaneous insulin regimens are often preferred. Basal insulin, or a basal plus bolus correction rapid-acting insulin schedule, is the preferred treatment for non–critically ill hospitalized patients with inadequate or restricted oral intake. An insulin schedule with basal, prandial, and correction components is the preferred treatment for most non–critically ill hospitalized patients with diabetes with adequate nutritional intake. Correctional insulin dosing typically starts at ~ 150 mg/dL. Correctional scales should be based on the total daily dose of insulin—a low-dose scale for insulin doses < 40 units/day, a medium dose scale for insulin 40–80 units/day, and a high-dose scale for insulin > 80 units/day. Standardized order sets reduce errors and include algorithms for recognition and treatment of hypoglycemia. For all hospitalized patients with type 1 diabetes, an insulin schedule with basal and correction scale insulin is critical, even for those not eating, and prandial insulin should be added when patients are eating.

6. Noninsulin therapies—SGLT-2 inhibitors are not recommended for glycemic management in the hospital setting, but they may be initiated or continued in patients with type 2 diabetes hospitalized with HF if there are no contraindications. SGLT-2 inhibitors should be stopped 3 days before scheduled surgeries and held in severe illness, in patients with ketonemia or ketonuria, and during prolonged fasting. GLP-1 receptor agonists should be held in hospitalized, acutely ill patients.

Preoperative and perioperative diabetes management strategies are discussed in Chapter 3.

B. Diabetes in Pregnancy

See Chapter 22.

HYPERGLYCEMIC CRISES

Hyperglycemic crises result in 1% of all hospital admissions in patients with diabetes. Coma may be due to causes directly or not directly related to diabetes and requires differentiation (Table 31–9). Causes of coma directly related to diabetes are (1) hypoglycemic coma from excessive insulin or oral hypoglycemic agents; (2) hyperglycemic coma with either severe insulin deficiency (DKA) or mild to moderate insulin deficiency (hyperglycemic hyperosmolar state); and (3) lactic acidosis, particularly when patients with diabetes have severe infections or cardiovascular collapse.

1. Diabetic Ketoacidosis

ESSENTIALS OF DIAGNOSIS

- Hyperglycemia ≥ 200 mg/dL (13.9 mmol/L) or history of diabetes regardless of glucose value.
- Ketosis with serum β-hydroxybutyrate concentration > 3.0 mmol/L or urine ketone test strip ≥ 2+.
- Metabolic acidosis with blood pH < 7.3 and/or serum bicarbonate < 15 mEq/L.

General Considerations

DKA is a life-threatening hyperglycemic emergency that primarily occurs in patients with type 1 diabetes but can occasionally occur in patients with type 2 diabetes who have severe illness, such as sepsis or trauma. DKA may be the initial manifestation of type 1 diabetes or may be precipitated by an acute stressor or omission of insulin therapy in individuals with diagnosed type 1 diabetes. The classic triad of DKA is hyperglycemia, increased ketone levels in the blood and/or urine, and metabolic acidosis.

DKA results from severe insulin deficiency and increased levels of counterregulatory hormones (glucagon, cortisol, epinephrine, and growth hormone). Insulin deficiency and increased counterregulatory hormones lead to release of free fatty acids from adipose tissue, leading to hepatic fatty acid oxidation, excess ketone body production, ketonemia, and metabolic acidosis.

Precipitating Factors

DKA is most commonly precipitated by acute infections, eg, UTI or pneumonia. DKA may be the initial presentation of newly diagnosed type 1 diabetes. Presence of medical or surgical intercurrent illnesses such as stroke or myocardial infarction, alcohol and substance use, acute pancreatitis, and trauma can precipitate DKA, as can use of drugs such as corticosteroids, SGLT-2 inhibitors, atypical antipsychotics, and immune checkpoint inhibitors. Poor adherence or rationing of insulin therapy, often in the setting of psychosocial stressors, is an important cause of DKA. In patients with type 1 diabetes who use insulin pumps, DKA can occur from error in self-management and intercurrent illness; pump malfunction also can be a cause.

While DKA can occur at any age, many cases of DKA occur in adults < 45 years of age who have type 1 diabetes. However, in the United States, more than half of Black/African American and Hispanic/Latino adults with DKA

Table 31–9. Laboratory diagnosis of diabetic coma.

	Urine Glucose	Urine Ketones	Plasma Glucose	Serum Bicarbonate	Serum Ketones
Related to Diabetes					
Hypoglycemia	0[1]	0 or +	Low	Normal	0
Diabetic ketoacidosis	++++	++++	High	Low	++++
Hyperglycemic hyperosmolar state coma	++++	0 or +	High	Normal or slightly low	0
Lactic acidosis	0 or +	0 or +	Normal or low or high	Low	0 or +
Unrelated to Diabetes					
Alcohol or other toxic drugs	0 or +	0 or +	May be low	Normal or low[2]	0 or +
Cerebrovascular accident or head trauma	+ or 0	0	Often high	Normal	0
Uremia	0 or +	0	High or normal	Low	0 or +

[1]Leftover urine in bladder might still contain glucose from earlier hyperglycemia.
[2]Alcohol can elevate plasma lactate as well as keto acids to reduce pH.

and newly diagnosed diabetes have type 2 diabetes. DKA rates have increased in the past decade. Recurrent episodes of DKA are common in the same individual; therefore, it is important to identify triggers to prevent frequent episodes. Reported mortality during hospital admission for DKA ranges from 0.20% in type 1 diabetes to 1.04% in type 2 diabetes. After an episode of DKA, there is a 1-year age-corrected 13-fold increase in mortality rate compared with the general population.

Clinical Findings

A. Symptoms and Signs

In DKA, the time between initial symptoms and acute presentation may range from hours to a few days. Common presenting symptoms include nausea, vomiting, and abdominal pain. Marked fatigue and malaise may be reported, and osmotic symptoms such as polyuria and polydipsia and unintentional weight loss leading up to presentation can often be elicited. Mental status varies. With mild DKA, the patient's mental status is alert, with moderate DKA, the mental status is alert or drowsy, and with severe DKA, the patient may have a headache or be stuporous, confused, or comatose. On physical examination, volume status should be assessed with vital signs. Hypotension with tachycardia, dry mucous membranes, and decreased skin turgor are indicative of profound fluid and electrolyte depletion, and mild hypothermia can be present. Kussmaul breathing (deep, labored breathing) may be present, and a "fruity" breath odor due to the presence of acetone (a breakdown product of a ketone) is a distinct sign and strongly suggests the diagnosis. Generalized abdominal pain and tenderness may be present, mimicking an acute abdomen. Abdominal pain often occurs in severe metabolic acidosis. Conversely, cholecystitis or pancreatitis may occur with minimal symptoms and signs. Abdominal pain typically resolves in the first 24 hours of initiating treatment, and a lack of improvement of abdominal pain should prompt a search for other causes. Patients should be examined for signs of infection, ischemia, and other potential precipitating factors. An ECG should be performed to assess the presence of repolarization abnormalities from hyperkalemia and to rule out myocardial ischemia.

B. Laboratory Findings

All three of the following criteria must be present to establish the diagnosis of DKA.

1. Hyperglycemia ≥ 200 mg/dL (11.1 mmol/L) or a prior history of diabetes irrespective of the glucose value on presentation.
2. Ketosis: elevated ketone body concentration as detected by venous or capillary β-hydroxybutyrate ≥ 3.0 mmol/L or urine ketone ≥ 2+.
3. Metabolic acidosis: pH < 7.3 and/or bicarbonate concentration < 18 mmol/L.

The severity of DKA can be classified as mild, moderate, or severe based on the degree of metabolic acidosis (blood pH, serum bicarbonate, and ketone levels) and the presence of altered mental status (see above).

1. Mild DKA—Glucose is ≥ 200 mg/dL; pH is 7.25–7.30 or serum bicarbonate 15–18 mmol/L; β-hydroxybutyrate is 3–6 mmol/L.

2. Moderate DKA—Glucose is ≥ 200 mg/d; pH is 7.0–7.25; serum bicarbonate is 10 to < 15 mmol/L; β-hydroxybutyrate is 3–6 mmol/L.

3. Severe DKA—Glucose is ≥ 200 mg/dL; pH is < 7.0; serum bicarbonate is < 10 mmol/L; β-hydroxybutyrate is > 6 mmol/L.

4. Hyperglycemia—Although hyperglycemia is a key diagnostic criterion of DKA, a wide range of plasma glucose concentrations can be observed on presentation. About 10% of patients with DKA present with euglycemic DKA, with plasma glucose levels < 200 mg/dL (see below). In recognition of this wide range of glucose levels, the updated criteria for diagnosis include a lower glucose value of > 200 mg/dL and a prior history of diabetes (irrespective of the glucose levels at diagnosis).

5. Ketonemia—The key diagnostic test in DKA is the detection of elevated circulating ketone body concentrations. Assessment of ketones is performed quantitatively by direct measurement of β-hydroxybutyrate in blood from capillary point-of-care testing or in the laboratory. Semi-quantitative measurements using the nitroprusside reaction in urine or serum measures acetoacetic acid (but not β-hydroxybutyrate, the main ketone in DKA). Both types of ketones have similar diagnostic sensitivity, but measuring β-hydroxybutyrate in blood is more specific for DKA than measuring acetoacetate in urine. Using acetoacetate urine ketone measurements alone can underestimate the severity of ketonemia and should be avoided.

6. Anion gap—Most patients with DKA have a high-anion-gap metabolic acidosis. The anion gap is calculated by subtracting the major measured anions (chloride and bicarbonate) from the major measured cation (sodium). An anion gap > 12 mmol/L indicates the presence of a high-anion-gap metabolic acidosis consistent with DKA. However, in at least a third of patients presenting with DKA, mixed acid–base disorders are present; there is metabolic acidosis from DKA, metabolic alkalosis from volume contraction (due to nausea and vomiting) and osmotic diuresis and natriuresis (due to hyperglycemia), and compensatory respiratory alkalosis from hyperventilation (Kussmaul breathing). Also, a hyperchloremic normal-anion-gap acidosis often follows successful treatment of DKA, which can be mistaken for persistent DKA resulting in delayed transition to subcutaneous insulin. Therefore, the anion gap is not recommended as a first-line diagnostic or resolution criterion, but it may still have clinical utility when blood ketone measurement is unavailable.

7. Euglycemic ketoacidosis—Patients with DKA may have only modestly elevated plasma glucose (< 200 mg/dL (11.1 mmol/L)) with ketonemia and metabolic acidosis (euglycemic DKA). It is commonly caused by SGLT-2 inhibitor use but can also occur from decreased food intake, pregnancy, or impaired gluconeogenesis (eg, alcohol use, liver failure).

8. Other laboratory findings—Hyperkalemia occurs despite total body potassium depletion because of the shift of potassium from the intracellular to extracellular spaces that occurs in systemic acidosis. The average total body potassium deficit resulting from osmotic diuresis, acidosis, and GI losses is ~ 3–5 mEq/kg. Similarly, despite the elevated serum phosphate, total body phosphate is generally depleted. Serum sodium is generally reduced due to loss of sodium ions (7–10 mEq/kg) by polyuria and vomiting and because severe hyperglycemia shifts intracellular water into the interstitial compartment. For every 100 mg/dL of plasma glucose, serum sodium decreases by 1.6 mEq/L (5.56 mmol/L). The decrease in serum sodium may be greater when patients have more severe hyperglycemia (> 400 mg/dL, 22.2 mmol/L), and a correction factor of 2.4 mEq/L may be used. Hypertriglyceridemia should be considered if the corrected sodium is very low.

Leukocytosis is common with DKA and may be due to an acute stress response. However, a WBC count > 25,000/mcL (25 × 109/L) indicates underlying infection and needs investigation. Nonspecific elevations of serum amylase and lipase occur in about 16–25% of cases of DKA, but an imaging study to rule out acute pancreatitis should be considered, as indicated.

Treatment

A. Patient Triage

The severity of DKA is classified as mild, moderate, or severe based on the degree of metabolic acidosis and the presence of altered mental status (see above). This categorization can help triage where a patient should receive care and whether patients with mild DKA can receive subcutaneous insulin dosing rather than intravenous insulin infusion. In general, if close nursing supervision and monitoring are available, patients with mild DKA can be treated in a regular or observation unit and patients with moderate DKA can be treated in a step-down or intermediate care unit. Patients with severe DKA or with critical illness as a precipitating cause require treatment in the ICU. All criteria need not be fulfilled for classification as mild, moderate, or severe, and the decision for where a patient receives care in the hospital should be a clinical one.

B. General Measures

The basics of managing DKA include administration of intravenous fluids, insulin, and electrolytes, with identification and treatment of the precipitating cause. A comprehensive flow sheet that includes vital signs, serial laboratory data, and therapeutic interventions (eg, fluids, insulin) should be meticulously maintained by clinicians responsible for the patient's care. Capillary blood glucose testing should be performed every 1–2 hours using a hospital-calibrated glucose meter, and blood should be drawn every 4 hours for determination of electrolytes, phosphate, creatinine, β-hydroxybutyrate, and venous pH, until resolution of DKA. Neurologic status should be monitored where appropriate. The patient should not receive sedatives or opioids to avoid masking signs and symptoms of impeding cerebral edema (see Complications & Prognosis).

C. Fluid Replacement

Initial intravenous fluid resuscitation restores circulating intravascular volume, improves renal perfusion (which promotes renal excretion of glucose and ketone bodies), corrects electrolyte deficits, and decreases plasma osmolarity. Correction of a fluid deficit also improves insulin sensitivity by reducing counterregulatory hormone concentrations. Plasma glucose levels can decrease by approximately 50–70 mg/dL/hour (2.8–3.9 mmol/L/hour) with intravenous fluid administration only in the absence of insulin. The fluid deficit can be 4–5 L, but in severe DKA the fluid depletion can be as high as 100 mL/kg. The initial resuscitation fluid in adults is 0.9% saline or lactated Ringer, infused at an initial rate of 500–1000 mL/hour over the first 2–4 hours. If the serum sodium is > 150 mEq/L, 0.45% ("half normal") saline solution should be used. After the initial fluid resuscitation, the state of hydration and the serum sodium concentration should guide subsequent management. If intravascular volume is restored (hydration assessed by measuring blood pressure, heart rate, and fluid balance) and the patient is not hyponatremic, the saline infusion rate can be reduced to 250 mL/hour or the infusion changed to 0.45% sodium chloride (250–500 mL/hour). Failure to give enough volume replacement (at least 3–4 L in 8 hours) to restore normal perfusion is one of the most serious therapeutic shortcomings adversely influencing satisfactory recovery. Excessive fluid replacement (> 5 L in 8 hours) may contribute to acute respiratory distress syndrome or cerebral edema. Plasma glucose concentrations decrease to < 250 mg/dL (13.9 mmol/L) within 4–8 hours before ketoacidosis resolves. Therefore, when blood glucose falls to ~ 250 mg/dL (13.9 mmol/L), the fluids should be changed to a 5–10% dextrose-containing solution with 0.9% sodium chloride to prevent hypoglycemia and allow for continued insulin administration until ketonemia resolves.

D. Insulin Replacement

Insulin therapy is the mainstay of treatment of DKA; therefore immediately after initiation of fluid replacement, regular insulin should be administered intravenously in a loading dose of 0.1 unit/kg as a bolus to prime the tissue insulin receptors. Following the initial bolus, intravenous doses of insulin as low as 0.1 unit/kg/hour are continuously infused or given hourly as an intramuscular injection; this is sufficient to replace the insulin deficit in most patients. A prospective randomized study showed that a bolus dose is not required if patients are given a continuous insulin infusion of 0.14 unit/kg hourly. Replacement of insulin deficiency helps correct the acidosis by reducing the flux of fatty acids to the liver, reducing ketone production by the liver, and also improving removal of ketones from the blood.

The insulin infusion should be "piggy-backed" into the fluid line so the rate of fluid replacement can be changed without altering the insulin delivery rate. If the plasma glucose level fails to fall at least 10% in the first hour, a repeat loading dose of intravenous insulin (0.1 or 0.14 unit/kg) is recommended. The insulin dose should be adjusted to lower the glucose concentration by about 50–70 mg/dL/hour (2.8–3.9 mmol/L). Once the blood glucose falls below 250 mg/dL (13.9 mmol/L), 5–10% dextrose should be added to the fluids infusion and the insulin infusion rate should be reduced to 0.05 units/kg/hour. Thereafter, intravenous insulin infusion should be adjusted to maintain glucose levels at about 200 mg/dL (11.1 mmol/L) and continued until the ketoacidosis resolves. If clinical circumstances prevent use of an insulin infusion, then the insulin can be given intramuscularly. An initial 0.15 unit/kg of regular insulin is given intravenously, and at the same time, the same size dose is given intramuscularly. Subsequently, regular insulin is given intramuscularly hourly at a dose of 0.1 unit/kg until the blood glucose falls to around 250 mg/dL, when the insulin can be given subcutaneously. Patients who take insulin glargine or degludec can be given their usual maintenance doses subcutaneously during the initial treatment of the DKA, as this results in lesser insulin requirements and also allows for a smoother transition from intravenous insulin infusion to the subcutaneous regimen.

E. Potassium

Total-body potassium deficit from osmotic diuresis and vomiting may be as high as 3–6 mmol/kg. However, due to potassium shifts from the intracellular to the extracellular space as a consequence of acidosis, serum potassium is usually normal to slightly elevated at initial presentation. As the acidosis is corrected, potassium flows back into the cells, and hypokalemia can develop if potassium replacement is not instituted. To avoid hypokalemia, serum potassium should be measured 2 hours after starting intravenous insulin and every 4 hours thereafter until DKA resolves. Volume expansion, insulin therapy, correction of acidosis, and increased urinary potassium losses all decrease serum potassium. If urinary output is adequate, potassium chloride in doses of 10–30 mEq/hour should be infused during the second and third hours after beginning therapy as soon as the acidosis starts to resolve. Replacement should be started sooner if the initial serum potassium is inappropriately normal or low and should be delayed if serum potassium fails to respond to initial therapy and remains > 5 mEq/L, as in cases of CKD. Occasionally, when the serum potassium level is < 3.5 mEq/L, initiating insulin therapy should be delayed until the potassium level is corrected to > 3.5 mEq/L to prevent life-threatening arrythmias. Severe hypokalemia ≤ 2.5 mEq/L during treatment of DKA is associated with a threefold increase in mortality.

F. Bicarbonate

Routine bicarbonate administration for treatment of DKA is not recommended, as intravenous fluid replacement and insulin administration are usually sufficient to resolve the metabolic acidosis. Data from several studies have demonstrated that bicarbonate administration in DKA does not improve the rate of recovery of hyperglycemia and ketoacidosis or the cardiac or neurologic outcomes. Harmful consequences of bicarbonate therapy include hypokalemia, tissue anoxia, and cerebral edema and acidosis. However, if very severe acidosis is present (arterial blood pH ≤ 7.0), administration of bicarbonate is recommended with careful monitoring to prevent overcorrection. If needed, an isotonic solution of 100 mmol of sodium bicarbonate (8.4% solution) in 400 mL of sterile water can be given intravenously every 2 hours to achieve a pH of 7.1. (Note: Addition of sodium bicarbonate to 0.9% saline would produce a markedly hypertonic solution that could aggravate the hyperosmolar state already present.) *Bicarbonate should not be given if the pH is ≥ 7.1* since additional bicarbonate would increase the risk of rebound metabolic alkalosis as ketones are metabolized. Alkalosis shifts potassium from serum into cells, which could precipitate a fatal cardiac arrhythmia.

G. Phosphate

Hypophosphatemia can occur due to phosphate shifts from the intracellular to the extracellular space and from urinary losses. Phosphate replacement is seldom required in treating DKA; several randomized studies have shown no clinical benefit from phosphate administration, and aggressive replacement can precipitate severe hypocalcemia with tetany. Phosphate replacement should be strongly considered in patients with cardiac dysfunction, anemia, or respiratory depression. If severe hypophosphatemia of < 1.0–1.5 mg/dL (0.3–0.5 mmol/L) develops during insulin therapy, replacement with 20–30 mmol of potassium phosphate added to the replacement fluids is recommended; the average deficit of 20–30 mmol of phosphate should be replaced intravenously at a rate *no greater than 3–4 mmol/hour* in a 60- to 70-kg person. (Additional potassium should be administered as potassium chloride to provide a total of 10–30 mEq of potassium/hour, as noted above.) If the serum phosphate remains < 2.5 mg/dL (0.8 mmol/L) after this infusion, a repeat 5-hour infusion can be given. Phosphate levels should be monitored at least every 4–6 hours during treatment, and more frequently (every 2–3 hours) if not receiving phosphate replacement.

H. Hyperchloremic Acidosis During Therapy

During the initial phase of DKA treatment, ketoacids are lost in the urine. These ketoacids are substrate for regeneration of bicarbonate, and therefore correction of the total bicarbonate deficit is hampered. A portion of the bicarbonate deficit is replaced with chloride ions infused in large amounts of 0.9% saline to correct the dehydration. Thus, as the ketoacidosis clears with insulin replacement, a hyperchloremic, low-bicarbonate pattern may emerge with a normal anion gap. This hyperchloremic non-anion-gap metabolic acidosis that occurs during the recovery phase of DKA is a benign condition that reverses itself over the subsequent 12–24 hours once intravenous saline is discontinued. Using a balanced electrolyte solution with a pH of 7.4 and 98 mEq/L chloride such as lactated Ringer instead of normal saline (pH ~ 5.5; chloride 154 mEq/L) can prevent hyperchloremic acidosis.

I. Treatment of Associated Infection

The most common precipitant of DKA in adults is infection (gastrointestinal, lung, or urinary tract). Antibiotics are prescribed as indicated (Table 34–5). Cholecystitis and pyelonephritis may be particularly severe in these patients. The conditions should be treated in parallel with DKA management.

J. Resolution of DKA

DKA is resolved when plasma ketone levels are < 0.6 mmol/L, venous pH is ≥ 7.3 or bicarbonate is ≥ 18 mmol/L, and blood glucose is < 200 mg/dL (11.1 mmol/L). The anion gap is no longer used as a criterion to assess DKA resolution, as it may be misleading due to the presence of hyperchloremic metabolic acidosis (see above) from the large volumes of administered 0.9% sodium chloride. Similarly, urinary ketone measurement is not used to assess DKA resolution.

K. Transition to Subcutaneous Insulin Regimen

Once the DKA is controlled and the patient is awake and able to eat, subcutaneous insulin can be initiated. To transition from intravenous to subcutaneous insulin, the total daily dose of insulin should be estimated. This estimated total daily dose of insulin may be calculated using weight, preadmission insulin regimen, or intravenous insulin requirements during current admission. A weight-based formula may be considered for total daily dose calculation using 0.5–0.6 units/kg/day in insulin-naïve patients with newly diagnosed type 1 diabetes. If risk factors for hypoglycemia are present, such as kidney failure or frailty, a lower insulin dose (0.3 units/kg/day) may be more appropriate. The total daily dose can also be calculated using the amount of intravenous insulin required in the previous 12–24 hours; half the total daily dose can be given as a long-acting basal insulin and the other half as premeal rapid-acting insulin (Table 31–5). Basal insulin should be initiated at least 1–2 hours before stopping the intravenous insulin infusion. In patients with preexisting diabetes, giving their basal insulin by subcutaneous injection at initiation of treatment simplifies the transition from intravenous to subcutaneous regimen. Patients with type 2 diabetes and DKA due to severe illness may initially require insulin but can often transition back to oral agents during outpatient follow-up.

▶ Complications & Prognosis

Low-dose insulin infusion and fluid and electrolyte replacement combined with careful monitoring of patients' clinical and laboratory responses to therapy have dramatically reduced the mortality rates of DKA to < 5% in individuals < 40 years of age. However, DKA remains a significant risk in older individuals who have mortality rates > 20% and in patients in profound coma in whom treatment has been delayed. Acute MI and infarction of the bowel following prolonged hypotension worsen the outlook. A serious prognostic sign is ESKD, and prior kidney dysfunction worsens the prognosis considerably because the kidney plays a key role in compensating for massive pH and electrolyte abnormalities. Symptomatic cerebral edema occurs primarily in the pediatric population. Risk factors for its development include severe baseline acidosis, rapid correction of hyperglycemia, and excess volume administration in the first 4 hours. A declining level of consciousness, lethargy, and headache should raise suspicion for cerebral edema. If untreated, it can progress to bradycardia, seizures, and respiratory arrest, with a high risk of permanent neurologic damage and mortality. The exact cause of neurologic damage remains unclear, but it may involve osmotic shifts, hypoperfusion, and inflammatory processes. Intravenous mannitol at a dosage of 1–2 g/kg given over 15 minutes is the mainstay of treatment. Excess crystalloid infusion can precipitate pulmonary edema. Acute respiratory distress syndrome is a rare complication of treatment of DKA.

After recovery and stabilization, patients should be instructed on how to recognize the early symptoms and signs of ketoacidosis. Urine ketones or capillary blood β-hydroxybutyrate should be measured in patients with signs of infection or in insulin pump-treated patients when capillary blood glucose remains unexpectedly and persistently high. When heavy ketonuria and glycosuria persist on several successive examinations, supplemental rapid-acting insulin should be administered and liquid foods such as lightly salted tomato juice and broth should be ingested to replenish fluids and electrolytes. The patient should be instructed to contact the clinician if ketonuria persists, especially if there is vomiting and inability to keep down fluids. Recurrent episodes of severe ketoacidosis often indicate poor adherence with the insulin regimen, and these patients will require intensive counseling.

▶ When to Refer

Consultation with a diabetes specialist is advisable, which may reduce length of stay and improve outcomes.

▶ When to Admit

See Patient Triage. Umpierrez GE et al. Hyperglycemic crises in adults with diabetes: a consensus report. Diabetes Care 2024;47:1257. [PMID: 39052901]

2. Hyperglycemic Hyperosmolar State

ESSENTIALS OF DIAGNOSIS

- Hyperglycemia: glucose ≥ 600 mg/dL (33.3 mmol/L).
- Hyperosmolarity: calculated serum osmolality ≥ 300 mOsm/kg or measured total serum osmolality ≥ 320 mOsm/kg.
- Absence of significant ketonemia: β-hydroxybutyrate ≤ 3.0mmol/L or urine ketone strip ≤ 2+.
- Absence of acidosis: blood pH ≥ 7.3 and serum bicarbonate ≥ 15 mEq/L.
- All four criteria are required for diagnosis.

General Considerations

Hyperglycemic hyperosmolar state is the second most common form of hyperglycemic coma. It is characterized by severe hyperglycemia in the absence of significant ketosis, with hyperosmolality and dehydration. It usually occurs in older patients but may occur in young adults as the first presentation of newly diagnosed diabetes. The true incidence is not known, but according to data on hospital discharges it is less common than DKA even in older age groups. Common precipitating factors include infections, ASCVD events, initiation of certain medications such as phenytoin, diazoxide, corticosteroids, and diuretics, and procedures associated with glucose loading such as peritoneal dialysis. Underlying CKD or HF is common, and the presence of either worsens the prognosis.

Pathogenesis

In a hyperglycemic hyperosmolar state, insulin is present but there is not enough being produced. There is sufficient insulin to prevent ketogenesis, but there is insufficient insulin to prevent hyperglycemia from increased hepatic glucose production and decreased glucose utilization by peripheral tissues. Severe hyperglycemia eventually results, leading to osmotic diuresis, volume depletion, and hemoconcentration. Inadequate fluid intake can lead to marked dehydration and a hyperosmolar state with renal impairment and a decline in cognitive function.

Clinical Findings

A. Symptoms and Signs

Onset may be insidious over a period of days or weeks, with weakness, polyuria, and polydipsia. The lack of features of DKA (eg, vomiting, rapid deep breathing, acetone odor) may delay recognition and therapy until dehydration becomes more profound than in ketoacidosis. Reduced intake of fluid is a common historic feature due to inappropriate lack of thirst, nausea, or inaccessibility of fluids to patients who are bedridden and frail. A history of ingestion of large quantities of glucose-containing fluids, such as soft drinks or orange juice in attempts to quench polydipsia, may contribute to severe hyperglycemia. Tachycardia and hypotension correlate with severity of hypovolemia. Assessment for signs of infection, ischemia, and other potential precipitants of a hyperglycemic crisis is important. Lethargy and confusion develop as serum osmolality exceeds 310 mOsm/kg, and convulsions and coma can occur if osmolality exceeds 320–330 mOsm/kg.

B. Laboratory Findings

Severe hyperglycemia is present, with blood glucose values ranging from 600 mg/dL to 2400 mg/dL (44.4 mmol/L to 133.2 mmol/L) (Table 31–9). In mild cases, where dehydration is less severe, dilutional hyponatremia as well as urinary sodium losses may reduce serum sodium to 120–125 mEq/L, which protects to some extent against extreme hyperosmolality. However, as dehydration progresses, serum sodium can exceed 140 mEq/L, producing serum osmolality readings of 330–440 mOsm/kg. Ketosis and acidosis are usually absent or mild. Prerenal azotemia is the rule, with serum urea nitrogen elevations > 100 mg/dL (35.7 mmol/L) being typical.

Treatment

A. Fluid Replacement

Fluid replacement is of paramount importance in treating the nonketotic hyperglycemic state. Fluid deficit may be as much as 6–10 L. The primary goal of treatment is to replace ~ 50% of the fluid deficit within the first 12 hours and the remainder in the following 12 hours. More caution is needed in fluid replacement rates when there is underlying heart failure, pregnancy, or severe kidney disease. The initial administration of fluids during the first 2–4 hours should be with isotonic (0.9%) saline at a rate of 500–1000 mL/hour. Fluid replacement alone can effectively decrease hyperglycemia by restoring intravascular volume, which then increases glomerular filtration and renal excretion of glucose. Serum osmolality also decreases with fluid replacement, and water shifts into the intracellular space. This water shifting results in increasing sodium levels, but this is not an indication for hypotonic solution unless the serum osmolality does not adequately decrease. A rise in serum sodium > 2.4 mmol/L for every 90- to 120-mg/dL fall in blood glucose suggests inadequate fluid replacement and requires a higher infusion rate. If fluid replacement is adequate but glucose and osmolality are not falling at the desired rate, then switching to 0.45% sodium chloride solution should be considered. The goals of treatment are to decrease osmolality by 3–8 mOsmol/kg/hour, reduce serum sodium by no more than 10 mmol/L in 24 hours, and decrease serum glucose by 90–120 mg/dL/hour to avoid the risk of neurologic complications and cerebral edema.

Once blood glucose reaches 250 mg/dL (13.9 mmol/L), fluid replacement should include 5% dextrose. The rate of dextrose infusion should be adjusted to maintain glycemic levels of 250–300 mg/dL (13.9–16.7 mmol/L) in order to reduce the risk of cerebral edema.

B. Insulin

Less insulin may be required to reduce the hyperglycemia in nonketotic patients compared to those with diabetic ketoacidotic coma. Fluid replacement alone can effectively decrease glucose levels (see Fluid Replacement, above). If a hyperglycemic hyperosmolar state is present without ketosis or with only mild to moderate ketonemia without acidosis (β-hydroxybutyrate ≥ 1.0 to < 3.0 mmol/L or urine ketones < 2+), a fixed-rate intravenous insulin infusion should be started at 0.05 units/kg/hour (no bolus needed) and titrated to lower blood glucose levels by 50–70 mg/dL/hour (2.8–3.9 mmol/L/hour). Once the patient has stabilized and the blood glucose falls to around 250 mg/dL (13.9 mmol/L), insulin can be given subcutaneously.

C. Potassium

With the absence of acidosis, there may be no initial hyperkalemia unless associated ESKD is present. This results in less severe total potassium depletion than in DKA, and less potassium replacement is needed. However, because initial serum potassium is usually not elevated and because it declines rapidly as insulin drives potassium intracellularly, it is recommended that potassium replacement be initiated earlier than in patients who are ketotic, assuming that no CKD or oliguria is present. Potassium chloride (10 mEq/L) can be added to the initial bag of fluids if the patient's serum potassium is not elevated.

D. Phosphate

If severe hypophosphatemia (serum phosphate < 1 mg/dL [0.32 mmol/L]) develops during insulin therapy, phosphate replacement can be given as described for ketoacidotic patients (at 3 mmol/hour).

Complications & Prognosis

The severe dehydration and low output state may predispose the patient to complications such as MI, stroke, PE, mesenteric vein thrombosis, and disseminated intravascular coagulation. Fluid replacement is the primary approach to the prevention of these complications. Low-dose heparin prophylaxis is reasonable (Table 16–14), but benefits of routine anticoagulation remain doubtful. Rhabdomyolysis is a recognized complication and should be looked for and treated.

The mortality rate of hyperglycemic hyperosmolar state coma is > 10 times that of DKA, chiefly because of its higher incidence in older patients, who may have compromised cardiovascular systems or associated major illnesses and whose dehydration is often excessive because of delays in recognition and treatment. (When patients are matched for age, the prognoses of these two hyperglycemic emergencies are reasonably comparable.) When prompt therapy is instituted, the mortality rate can be reduced from nearly 50% to that related to the severity of coexistent disorders.

After the patient is stabilized, the appropriate form of long-term management of diabetes must be determined. Insulin treatment should be continued for a few weeks, but patients usually recover sufficient endogenous insulin secretion to make a trial of diet or diet plus oral agents worthwhile. When the episode occurs in a patient who has known diabetes, then education of the patient and caregivers should be instituted. They should be taught how to recognize situations (nausea and vomiting, infection) that predispose to recurrence of the hyperglycemic, hyperosmolar state, as well as detailed information on how to prevent the escalating dehydration that culminates in hyperosmolar coma (small sips of sugar-free liquids, increase in usual hypoglycemic therapy, or early contact with the clinician).

When to Refer

Consultation with a diabetes specialist is advisable and may reduce length of stay and improve outcomes.

When to Admit

Most patients require ICU admission for careful fluid therapy to treat severe volume depletion and hyperglycemia.

American Diabetes Association Professional Practice Committee for Diabetes. Diabetes Care in the Hospital: Standards of Care in Diabetes—2026. Diabetes Care. 2026;49:S339. [PMID: 41358892]

Mustafa OG et al; Joint British Diabetes Societies (JBDS) for Inpatient Care Group. Management of hyperosmolar hyperglycaemic state (HHS) in adults: an updated guideline from the Joint British Diabetes Societies (JBDS) for Inpatient Care Group. Diabet Med. 2023;40:e15005. [PMID: 36370077]

Umpierrez GE et al. Hyperglycemic crises in adults with diabetes: a consensus report. Diabetes Care. 2024;47:1257. [PMID: 39052901]

THE HYPOGLYCEMIC STATES

Spontaneous hypoglycemia in adults is of two principal types: fasting and postprandial. Symptoms begin at plasma glucose levels in the range of 60 mg/dL (3.3 mmol/L) and impairment of brain function begins at approximately 50 mg/dL (2.8 mmol/L). Fasting hypoglycemia is often subacute or chronic and usually presents with neuroglycopenia as its principal manifestation; postprandial hypoglycemia is relatively acute and is often heralded by symptoms of neurogenic autonomic discharge (sweating, palpitations, anxiety, tremulousness).

Differential Diagnosis

Fasting hypoglycemia may occur in certain endocrine disorders, such as hypopituitarism, Addison disease, or myxedema; in disorders related to liver malfunction, such as acute alcohol use disorder, or liver failure; and in instances of ESKD, particularly in patients requiring dialysis (Table 31–10). These conditions are usually obvious, with hypoglycemia being only a secondary feature. When fasting hypoglycemia is a primary manifestation developing in adults without apparent endocrine disorders or inborn metabolic diseases from childhood, the principal diagnostic possibilities include (1) hyperinsulinism, due to either pancreatic β cell tumors or iatrogenic or surreptitious administration of insulin or sulfonylurea; and (2) hypoglycemia due to extrapancreatic tumors.

Table 31–10. Common causes of hypoglycemia in adults.[1]

Fasting hypoglycemia
Pancreatic β cell tumor
Surreptitious administration of insulin or sulfonylureas
Extrapancreatic tumors
Postprandial hypoglycemia
Gastric surgery
Occult diabetes mellitus
Alcohol-related hypoglycemia
Immunopathologic hypoglycemia
Idiopathic anti-insulin antibodies (which release their bound insulin)
Antibodies to insulin receptors (which act as agonists)
Drug-induced hypoglycemia

[1]In the absence of clinically obvious endocrine, kidney, or liver disorders and exclusive of diabetes mellitus treated with hypoglycemic agents.

Postprandial (reactive) hypoglycemia may occur after GI surgery and is particularly associated with the dumping syndrome after gastrectomy and Roux-en-Y gastric bypass surgery. Occult diabetes very occasionally presents with postprandial hypoglycemia.

Alcohol-related hypoglycemia is due to hepatic glycogen depletion combined with alcohol-mediated inhibition of gluconeogenesis. It is most common in malnourished individuals with excessive alcohol intake but can occur in anyone who is unable to ingest food after acute alcohol use followed by gastritis and vomiting.

Immunopathologic hypoglycemia is an extremely rare condition in which anti-insulin antibodies or antibodies to insulin receptors develop spontaneously.

HYPOGLYCEMIA DUE TO PANCREATIC β CELL TUMORS

ESSENTIALS OF DIAGNOSIS

- Hypoglycemic symptoms—often neuroglycopenic (confusion, blurred vision, anxiety, convulsions).
- Immediate recovery upon administration of glucose.
- Blood glucose 40–50 mg/dL (2.2–2.8 mmol/L) with serum insulin ≥ 6 microunits/mL.

General Considerations

Fasting hypoglycemia in an otherwise healthy, well-nourished adult is rare and is most commonly due to an adenoma of the islets of Langerhans. Ninety percent of such tumors are single and benign, but multiple adenomas can occur as well as malignant tumors with functional metastases. Adenomas may be familial, and multiple adenomas have been found in conjunction with tumors of the parathyroids and pituitary (MEN type 1 [MEN 1]). More than 99% of insulinomas are located within the pancreas and < 1% in ectopic pancreatic tissue.

Clinical Findings

A. Symptoms and Signs

The most important prerequisite to diagnosing an insulinoma is simply to consider it, particularly in relatively healthy-appearing persons who have fasting hypoglycemia with some degree of CNS dysfunction such as confusion or atypical behavior. A delay in diagnosis can result in unnecessary treatment for epilepsy or psychiatric disorders and may cause irreversible brain damage. In long-standing cases, obesity can result from overeating to relieve symptoms.

The so-called Whipple triad is characteristic of hypoglycemia regardless of the cause. It consists of (1) a history of hypoglycemic symptoms, (2) an associated low plasma glucose level (40–50 mg/dL), and (3) relief of symptoms upon ingesting fast-acting carbohydrates in approximately 15 minutes. The hypoglycemic symptoms in insulinoma often develop in the early morning or after missing a meal. Occasionally, they occur after exercise.

Patients typically have neuroglycopenic symptoms such as blurred vision or diplopia, headache, feelings of detachment, slurred speech, and weakness. Personality and mental changes vary from anxiety to psychotic behavior, and neurologic deterioration can result in convulsions or coma. Hypoglycemic unawareness is very common, and adrenergic symptoms of palpitations and sweating may be blunted. Patients can sometimes document blood glucose levels in the 40s and 50s with a home blood glucose monitor at the time of symptoms. Access to sulfonylureas or insulin should be explored—does a family member have diabetes, or does the patient or family member work in the medical field? Medication-dispensing errors should be excluded—has the patient's prescription medication changed in shape or color? Patients with insulinoma or factitious hypoglycemia usually have an unremarkable physical examination.

B. Laboratory Findings

β Cell adenomas do not reduce secretion of insulin in the presence of hypoglycemia, and the critical diagnostic test is to demonstrate inappropriately elevated serum insulin, proinsulin, and C-peptide levels at a time when the plasma glucose level is < 45 mg/dL or when the patient has neuroglycopenic symptoms.

The diagnostic criteria for insulinoma after a 72-hour fast are listed in Table 31–11. Other causes of hyperinsulinemic hypoglycemia include factitious administration of insulin or sulfonylureas. Factitious use of insulin will result in suppression of endogenous insulin secretion and low C-peptide levels. In patients who have injected insulin, the insulin/C-peptide ratio (pmol/L) will be > 1. An elevated circulating proinsulin level in the presence of fasting hypoglycemia is characteristic of most β cell adenomas and does not occur in factitious hyperinsulinism. Thus, C-peptide levels (by immunochemiluminometric assays [ICMA]) of > 200 pmol/L and proinsulin levels (by radioimmunoassay [RIA]) of > 5 pmol/L are characteristic of insulinomas. In patients with insulinoma, plasma β-hydroxybutyrate levels are suppressed to ≤ 2.7 mmol/L. No single hormone

Table 31–11. Diagnostic criteria for insulinoma after a 72-hour fast.

Laboratory Test	Result
Plasma glucose	< 45 mg/dL (2.5 mmol/L)
Plasma insulin (RIA)	≥ 6 microunits/mL (36 pmol/L)
Plasma insulin (ICMA)	≥ 3 microunits/mL (18 pmol/L)
Plasma C-peptide	≥ 200 pmol/L (0.2 nmol/L, 0.6 ng/mL)
Plasma proinsulin	≥ 5 pmol/L
β-Hydroxybutyrate	≤ 2.7 mmol/L
Sulfonylurea screen (including repaglinide and nateglinide)	Negative

ICMA, immunochemiluminometric assays; RIA, radioimmunoassay.

measurement (insulin, proinsulin, C-peptide) is 100% sensitive and specific for the diagnosis of insulinoma, and persons diagnosed with insulinoma can have insulin levels <3 microunits/mL (ICMA assay) or proinsulin level < 5 pmol/L. These hormonal assays are also not standardized, and there can be significant variation in the test results. Therefore, the diagnosis should be based on multiple biochemical parameters.

In patients with epigastric distress, a history of renal calculi, or menstrual or erectile dysfunction, a serum calcium, gastrin, or prolactin level may be useful in screening for MEN 1 associated with insulinoma.

C. Diagnostic Tests

If the history is consistent with episodic spontaneous hypoglycemia, patients should be given a home blood glucose monitor and advised to monitor blood glucose levels at the time of symptoms and before consumption of carbohydrates, if this can be done safely. Patients with insulinomas frequently report fingerstick blood glucose levels between 40 mg/dL (2.2 mmol/L) and 50 mg/dL (2.8 mmol/L) at the time of symptoms. The diagnosis, however, cannot be made based on a fingerstick blood glucose. It is necessary to have a low laboratory glucose concomitantly with elevated plasma insulin, proinsulin, and C-peptide levels and a negative sulfonylurea screen. When patients give a history of symptoms after only a short period of food withdrawal or with exercise, then an outpatient assessment can be attempted. The patient should be brought by a family member to the office after an overnight fast and observed in the office. Activity such as walking should be encouraged and fingerstick blood glucose measured repeatedly during observation. If symptoms occur or fingerstick blood glucose is <50 mg/dL (2.8 mmol/L), then samples for plasma glucose, insulin, C-peptide, proinsulin, sulfonylurea screen, serum ketones, and antibodies to insulin should be sent. If outpatient observation does not result in symptoms or hypoglycemia and if the clinical suspicion remains high, then the patient should undergo an inpatient supervised 72-hour fast. A suggested protocol for the supervised fast is shown in Table 31–12.

In 30% of patients with insulinoma, the blood glucose levels often drop below 45 mg/dL (2.5 mmol/L) after an overnight fast, but some patients require up to 72 hours to develop symptomatic hypoglycemia. However, the term "72-hour fast" is actually a misnomer in most cases since the fast should be immediately terminated as soon as symptoms appear and laboratory confirmation of hypoglycemia is available. Typically, in men, the blood glucose does not fall below 55–60 mg/dL (3.1–3.3 mmol/L) during a 3-day fast. In contrast, for normal premenopausal women, the plasma glucose can reach values as low as 35 mg/dL (1.9 mmol/L). In these cases, however, the women are not symptomatic, presumably owing to the development of sufficient ketonemia to supply energy needs to the brain. Insulinoma patients, on the other hand, become symptomatic when plasma glucose drops to subnormal levels, since inappropriate insulin secretion restricts ketone formation. Moreover, the demonstration of a nonsuppressed insulin level of 3 microunits/mL or more using an ICMA assay

Table 31–12. Suggested hospital protocol for supervised fast in diagnosis of insulinoma.

(1) Place intravenous cannula and obtain baseline plasma glucose, insulin, proinsulin, β-hydroxybutyrate, and C-peptide measurements at onset of fast.
(2) Permit only calorie-free and caffeine-free fluids and encourage supervised activity (such as walking).
(3) Obtain fingerstick glucose measurements every 4 hours until values < 60 mg/dL are obtained. Then increase the frequency of fingersticks to 1–2 hours, and when capillary glucose value is < 45 mg/dL send a venous blood sample to the laboratory for plasma glucose.[1] Check frequently for manifestations of neuroglycopenia.
(4) At 48 hours into the fast, send a venous blood sample for plasma glucose, insulin, proinsulin, C-peptide, β-hydroxybutyrate, and sulfonylurea measurement.
(5) If symptoms of hypoglycemia occur ***or*** if a laboratory value of serum glucose is < 45 mg/dL, ***or*** if 72 hours have elapsed, conclude the fast with a final blood sample for plasma glucose,[1] insulin, proinsulin, C-peptide, β-hydroxybutyrate, and sulfonylurea measurements. Then give oral fast-acting carbohydrate followed by a meal. If the patient is confused or unable to take oral agents, administer 50 mL of 50% dextrose intravenously over 3–5 minutes. Do not conclude a fast based simply on a capillary blood glucose measurement—wait for the laboratory glucose value—unless the patient is very symptomatic and it would be dangerous to wait.

[1]Glucose sample should be collected in sodium fluoride containing tube on ice to prevent glycolysis and the plasma separated immediately upon receipt at the laboratory. Arrange for the laboratory to run the glucose samples "stat."

(> 6 microunits/mL using an RIA assay) in the presence of hypoglycemia suggests the diagnosis of insulinoma. If hypoglycemia does not develop in a male patient after fasting for up to 72 hours—and particularly when this prolonged fast is terminated with a period of moderate exercise—insulinoma must be considered an unlikely diagnosis.

An oral glucose tolerance test is of no value in the diagnosis of insulin-secreting tumors. HbA_{1c} levels may be low, but there is considerable overlap with patients who do not have insulinomas and no particular value is diagnostic.

D. Preoperative Localization of β Cell Tumors

After the diagnosis of insulinoma has been unequivocally made by clinical and laboratory findings, studies to localize the tumor should be initiated. Most tumors are in the pancreas, and ectopic cases are rare.

Because of the small size of these tumors (averaging 1.5 cm in diameter in one large series), imaging studies do not necessarily identify all of them. A pancreatic dual phase helical CT scan with thin section can identify 82–94% of the lesions. MRI scans with gadolinium can be helpful in detecting a tumor in 85% of cases. One case report suggests that diffusion-weighted MRI can be useful for detecting and localizing small insulinomas, especially for those with no hypervascular pattern. PET/CT scans using gallium-labeled somatostatin analogs such as DOTA-1-NaI3-octreotide (DOTA-NOC) have been reported to be useful in localizing the tumors. Insulinomas express

GLP-1 receptors, and radiolabeled GLP-1 receptor agonists such as Lys(40)(Ahx-hydrazinonicotinamide [HYNIC]-[(99m)Tc)NH(2)]-exendin-4 for SPECT/CT have also been reported to visualize the tumors. If the imaging study is normal, then an endoscopic ultrasound should be performed. In experienced hands, about 80–90% of tumors can be detected with this procedure. Fine-needle aspiration of the identified lesion can be attempted to confirm the presence of a neuroendocrine tumor. If the tumor is not identified or the imaging result is equivocal, then the patient should undergo selective calcium-stimulated angiography, which has been reported to localize the tumor to a particular region of the pancreas approximately 90% of the time. In this test, angiography is combined with injections of calcium gluconate into the gastroduodenal, splenic, and superior mesenteric arteries, and insulin levels are measured in the hepatic vein effluent. The procedure is performed after an overnight fast. Calcium stimulates insulin release from insulinomas but not normal islets, and so a step-up from baseline in insulin levels (twofold or greater) regionalizes the source of the hyperinsulinism to the head of the pancreas for the gastroduodenal artery, the uncinate process for the superior mesenteric artery, and the body and tail of the pancreas for the splenic artery calcium infusions. These studies combined with careful intraoperative ultrasonography and palpation by a surgeon experienced in insulinoma surgery identifies up to 98% of tumors.

Treatment

The treatment of choice for insulin-secreting tumors is surgical resection. While waiting for surgery, patients should be given oral diazoxide. Divided doses of 300–400 mg/day usually suffice, although an occasional patient may require up to 800 mg/day. Side effects include edema due to sodium retention, gastric irritation, and mild hirsutism. Hydrochlorothiazide, 25–50 mg daily, can be used to counteract the sodium retention and edema as well potentiate diazoxide's hyperglycemic effect.

Of patients with a single benign pancreatic β cell adenoma, 90–95% are cured at the first surgical attempt when intraoperative ultrasound is used by a skilled surgeon.

In patients with inoperable functioning islet cell carcinoma with and without hepatic metastasis and in approximately 5–10% of MEN 1 cases when subtotal removal of the pancreas has failed to produce cure, the treatment approach is the same as for other types of pancreatic neuroendocrine tumors (pNETs). Diazoxide is the treatment of choice in preventing hypoglycemia. Frequent carbohydrate feedings (every 2–3 hours) also can be helpful, although weight gain can become a problem. The somatostatin analogs octreotide or lanreotide should be considered if diazoxide is ineffective or if there is tumor progression. Surgery or embolization (bland, chemo-, and radio-) or thermal ablation (radiofrequency, microwave, and cryoablation) can be used to reduce tumor burden and also provide symptomatic relief. Chemotherapy regimens that can be considered include combination of streptozocin, 5-fluorouracil, and doxorubicin; capecitabine and oxaliplatin; and capecitabine and temozolomide. Everolimus, an inhibitor of mTOR, is approved for treatment of advanced pNETs. Sunitinib has been shown to slow growth of pNETs. Treatment with radioisotopes (indium-111, yttrium-90, or lutetium-177) linked to a somatostatin analog has been reported to show benefit in a proportion of patients.

NONISLET CELL TUMOR HYPOGLYCEMIA

These rare causes of hypoglycemia include mesenchymal tumors such as retroperitoneal sarcomas, hepatocellular carcinomas, adrenocortical carcinomas, and miscellaneous epithelial-type tumors. The tumors are frequently large and readily palpated or visualized on CT scans or MRI.

In many cases the hypoglycemia is due to the expression and release of an incompletely processed insulin-like growth factor 2 (IGF-2) by the tumor.

The diagnosis is supported by serum insulin levels <5 microunit/mL with plasma glucose levels of ≤ 45 mg/dL (2.5 mmol/L). Values for growth hormone and IGF-1 are also decreased. Levels of IGF-2 may be increased but often are "normal" in quantity, despite the presence of the immature, higher-molecular-weight form of IGF-2, which can be detected only by special laboratory techniques.

Not all patients with non–islet cell tumor hypoglycemia have elevated pro-IGF-2. Ectopic insulin production has been described in bronchial carcinoma, ovarian carcinoma, and small cell carcinoma of the cervix. Hypoglycemia due to IgF-1 released from a metastatic large cell carcinoma of the lung has also been reported. GLP-1–secreting tumors (ovarian and pNETs) can also cause hypoglycemia by stimulating insulin release from normal pancreatic islets.

The prognosis for these tumors is generally poor, and surgical removal should be attempted when feasible. Dietary management of the hypoglycemia is the mainstay of medical treatment.

POSTPRANDIAL HYPOGLYCEMIA

1. Hypoglycemia Following Gastric Surgery

Hypoglycemia sometimes develops in patients who have undergone gastric surgery (eg, gastrectomy, vagotomy, pyloroplasty, gastrojejunostomy, Nissan fundoplication, Billroth II procedure, and Roux-en-Y), especially when they consume foods containing high levels of readily absorbable carbohydrates. This late dumping syndrome occurs about 1–3 hours after a meal and is a result of rapid delivery of high concentration of carbohydrates in the proximal small bowel and rapid absorption of glucose. The hyperinsulinemic response to the high carbohydrate load causes hypoglycemia. Excessive release of GI hormones such as GLP-1 likely play a role in the hyperinsulinemic response. The symptoms include lightheadedness, sweating, confusion and even loss of consciousness after eating a high carbohydrate meal. To document hypoglycemia, the patient should consume a meal that leads to symptoms during everyday life. An oral glucose tolerance test is not recommended because many persons without diabetes have false-positive test results. There have been case reports of insulinoma in patients with hypoglycemia following Roux-en-Y surgery. It is unclear how often this occurs. A careful history may identify patients who have a history of hypoglycemia with exercise or missed meals, and these individuals may require a formal 72-hour fast to rule out an insulinoma.

Treatment for secondary dumping includes dietary modification, but this may be difficult to sustain. Patients can try more frequent meals with smaller portions of less rapidly digested carbohydrates. α-Glucosidase therapy may be a useful adjunct to a low-carbohydrate diet. Octreotide 50 mcg subcutaneously two or three times a day 30 minutes prior to each meal has been reported to improve symptoms due to late dumping syndrome. Treatment with exendin 9-39 (avexitide), a GLP-1 receptor agonist, may prevent post gastric bypass hypoglycemia. SGLT-2 inhibitors may ameliorate the postprandial glucose rise, the subsequent insulin response, and hypoglycemia. There is a report of a patient with Roux-en-Y surgery who had complete resolution of both hyperglycemia and hypoglycemia when given canagliflozin. Various surgical procedures to delay gastric emptying have been reported to improve symptoms but long-term efficacy studies are lacking.

2. Functional Alimentary Hypoglycemia

Patients have symptoms suggestive of increased sympathetic activity, including anxiety, weakness, tremor, sweating, or palpitations, after meals. Physical examination and laboratory tests are normal. It is not recommended that patients with symptoms suggestive of increased sympathetic activity undergo either a prolonged oral glucose tolerance test or a mixed meal test. Instead, the patients should be given home blood glucose monitors (with memories) and instructed to monitor fingerstick glucose levels at the time of symptoms. Only patients who have symptoms when their fingerstick blood glucose is low (<50 mg/dL) and who have resolution of symptoms when the glucose is raised by eating rapidly released carbohydrate need additional evaluation. Patients who do not have evidence for low glucose levels at time of symptoms are generally reassured by their findings. Counseling and support should be the mainstays in therapy, with dietary manipulation only an adjunct.

3. Occult Diabetes

This condition is characterized by a delay in early insulin release from pancreatic β cells, resulting in initial exaggeration of hyperglycemia during a glucose tolerance test. In response to this hyperglycemia, an exaggerated insulin release produces a late hypoglycemia 4–5 hours after ingestion of glucose. These patients frequently have obesity and a family history of diabetes mellitus.

Patients with this type of postprandial hypoglycemia often respond to reduced intake of refined sugars with multiple, spaced, small feedings high in dietary fiber. In patients with obesity, treatment is directed at weight reduction to achieve ideal weight. These patients should be considered to have prediabetes or early diabetes (type 1 or 2) and advised to have periodic medical evaluations.

4. Autoimmune Hypoglycemia

Patients with autoimmune hypoglycemia have early postprandial hyperglycemia followed by hypoglycemia 3–4 hours later. The hypoglycemia is attributed to a dissociation of insulin-antibody immune complexes, releasing free insulin.

The disorder is associated with methimazole treatment for Graves disease, although it can also occur in patients treated with various other sulfhydryl-containing medications (captopril, penicillamine) as well as other drugs such as hydralazine, isoniazid, and procainamide. In addition, it has been reported in patients with autoimmune disorders such as rheumatoid arthritis, SLE, and polymyositis as well as in plasma cell myeloma and other plasma cell dyscrasias where paraproteins or antibodies cross-react with insulin. There is also an association with the HLA class II alleles (DRB1*0406, DQA1*0301, and DQB1*0302). These alleles are 10 to 20 times more common in Japanese and Korean populations, which explains why the disorder has been reported mostly in Japanese patients.

High titers of insulin autoantibodies, usually IgG class, can be detected. Insulin, proinsulin, and C-peptide levels may be elevated, but the results may be erroneous because of the interference of the insulin antibodies with the immunoassays for these peptides.

In most cases, the hypoglycemia is transient and usually resolves spontaneously within 3–6 months of diagnosis, particularly when the offending medications are stopped. The most consistent therapeutic benefit in management of this syndrome has been achieved by dietary treatment with small, frequent low-carbohydrate meals. Prednisone (30–60 mg orally daily) has been used to lower the titer of insulin antibodies.

FACTITIOUS HYPOGLYCEMIA

Factitious hypoglycemia may be difficult to document. A suspicion of self-induced hypoglycemia is supported when the patient is associated with the health professions or has access to diabetic medications taken by a member of the family who has diabetes. Insulin and C-peptide are secreted in a 1:1 molar ratio. The triad of hypoglycemia, high immunoreactive insulin, and suppressed plasma C-peptide immunoreactivity is pathognomonic of exogenous insulin administration. A large fraction of the endogenous insulin is cleared by the liver, whereas C-peptide, which is cleared by the kidney, has a lower metabolic clearance rate. For this reason, the molar ratio of insulin and C-peptide in a hypoglycemic patient should be < 1.0 in cases of insulinoma and is > 1.0 in cases of exogenous insulin administration (see Hypoglycemia Due to Pancreatic β Cell Tumors, above). When sulfonylureas, repaglinide, and nateglinide are suspected as a cause of factitious hypoglycemia, a plasma level of these medications to detect their presence may be required to distinguish laboratory findings from those of insulinoma.

HYPOGLYCEMIA DUE TO INSULIN RECEPTOR ANTIBODIES

Hypoglycemia due to insulin receptor autoantibodies is an extremely rare syndrome; most cases have occurred in women often with a history of autoimmune disease. Almost all of these patients have also had episodes of insulin-resistant diabetes and acanthosis nigricans. Their hypoglycemia may be either fasting or postprandial and is often severe and is attributed to an agonistic action of the antibody on the insulin receptor. Balance between the antagonistic and agonistic effects of the antibodies determines whether insulin-resistant diabetes or hypoglycemia occurs. Hypoglycemia was found to respond to corticosteroid therapy but not to plasmapheresis or immunosuppression.

MEDICATION- & ETHANOL-INDUCED HYPOGLYCEMIA

A number of medications apart from diabetic medications can occasionally cause hypoglycemia. Common offenders include the fluoroquinolones such as gatifloxacin and levofloxacin, pentamidine, quinine, ACE inhibitors, salicylates, and β-adrenergic blocking agents. The fluoroquinolones, particularly gatifloxacin, have been associated with both hypoglycemia and hyperglycemia. It is thought that the drug acts on the ATP-sensitive potassium channels in the β cell. Hypoglycemia is an early event, and hyperglycemia occurs several days into therapy. Intravenous pentamidine is cytotoxic to β cells and causes acute hyperinsulinemia and hypoglycemia followed by insulinopenia and hyperglycemia. Fasting patients taking noncardioselective β-blockers can have an exaggerated hypoglycemic response to starvation. The β-blockade inhibits fatty acids and gluconeogenesis substrate release and reduces plasma glucagon response. Therapy with ACE inhibitors increases the risk of hypoglycemia in patients who are taking insulin or sulfonylureas presumably because these drugs increase sensitivity to circulating insulin by increasing blood flow to the muscle. Some opioids cause hypoglycemia. Tramadol has been associated with increased risk of hospitalization for hypoglycemia. Methadone overdose has also been reported to cause hypoglycemia, and a rapid dose escalation of methadone in patients with cancer can lower glucose levels.

Ethanol-associated hypoglycemia may be due to hepatic alcohol dehydrogenase activity depleting nicotinamide adenine dinucleotide (NAD). The resultant change in the redox state—increase in nicotinamide adenine dinucleotide + hydrogen (NADH) to NAD+ ratio—causes a partial block at several points in the gluconeogenic pathway. With prolonged starvation, glycogen reserves become depleted within 18–24 hours and hepatic glucose output becomes totally dependent on gluconeogenesis. Under these circumstances, a blood concentration of ethanol as low as 45 mg/dL (9.8 mmol/L) can induce profound hypoglycemia by blocking gluconeogenesis. Neuroglycopenia in a patient whose breath smells of alcohol may be mistaken for alcoholic stupor. Prevention consists of adequate food intake during ethanol ingestion. Therapy consists of glucose administration to replenish glycogen stores until gluconeogenesis resumes.

When sugar-containing soft drinks are used as mixers to dilute alcohol in beverages (gin and tonic, rum and cola), there seems to be a greater insulin release than when the soft drink alone is ingested and a tendency for more of a late hypoglycemic overswing to occur 3–4 hours later. Prevention would consist of avoiding sugar mixers while ingesting alcohol and ensuring supplementary food intake to provide sustained absorption.

Lipid Disorders

Michael J. Blaha, MD, MPH

32

The "Lipid Hypothesis" of CVD—stating that cholesterol is causal in the development of atherosclerotic CVD (ASCVD) and that lowering cholesterol produces lower cardiovascular event rates—is nearly universally accepted throughout the medical community. For patients with known ASCVD (secondary prevention), studies have shown that cholesterol lowering leads to a consistent reduction in total mortality and in recurrent cardiovascular events in men and women; other studies have documented lowered mortality and events in middle-aged and older patients. Among patients without ASCVD (primary prevention), the data are generally consistent, with rates of cardiovascular events, heart disease mortality, and all-cause mortality differing among studies. Treatment guidelines have been designed to assist clinicians in selecting patients for cholesterol-lowering therapy based predominantly on their overall risk of developing CVD as well as their baseline cholesterol levels.

There are several genetic disorders that provide insight into the pathogenesis of lipid-related diseases. **Familial hypercholesterolemia**, rare in the homozygous state (about one per million), causes markedly high LDL-C levels and early ASCVD. The most common genetic defects involve absent or defective LDL receptors, resulting in unregulated LDL metabolism, genetic pathogenic variants of apolipoprotein B, or gain of function in proprotein convertase subtilisin/kexin type 9 (PCSK9), a protein that regulates breakdown of LDL receptors. Patients with two abnormal genes (homozygotes) have extremely high levels—up to eight times normal—and present with atherosclerotic disease in childhood. Patients with two abnormal genes (homozygotes) may require liver transplantation or plasmapheresis to correct their severe lipid abnormalities; early treatment with statins appears to confer lifetime benefits in such patients. Those with one defective gene (heterozygotes) have LDL concentrations up to two or three times normal; persons with this condition have variable risk, but CVD may develop as early as in their 30s or 40s. With current treatment options, nearly all patients with heterozygous familial hypercholesterolemia can achieve normal cholesterol values with combinations of therapies.

Another rare condition is caused by an abnormality of lipoprotein lipase, the enzyme that enables peripheral tissues to take up triglyceride from chylomicrons and very-low-density lipoprotein (VLDL) particles. Patients with this condition, one cause of **familial chylomicronemia syndrome (FCS)**, have marked hypertriglyceridemia with recurrent pancreatitis and hepatosplenomegaly in childhood. The first medication therapy for FCS, an apoC-III inhibitor called olezarsen, was approved in 2024. Plozasiran was approved for FCS in 2025.

Numerous other genetic abnormalities of lipid metabolism are named for the abnormality noted when serum is electrophoresed (eg, dysbetalipoproteinemia, characterized by elevated levels of remnant lipoproteins) or from polygenic combinations of lipid abnormalities in families (eg, familial combined hyperlipidemia). **Sitosterolemia** is an autosomal recessive condition causing abnormalities in the ability to pump plant sterols from the body, resulting in mild to moderate elevations in total cholesterol, atherosclerosis, and very high blood levels of sitosterol identified on specialized blood tests.

When to Refer

Refer to a lipidologist or preventive cardiologist for:

- Known genetic lipid disorders.
- Striking family history of hyperlipidemia or premature atherosclerosis.
- Extremely high serum LDL cholesterol (LDL-C), triglycerides, and/or lipoprotein(a), as well as extremely low or extremely high serum HDL-C.
- Intolerance to several routine lipid-lowering therapies.

Huang J et al. Low-density lipoprotein cholesterol time in target range and clinical outcomes in the general population. JACC Adv. 2025;4:102184. [PMID: 40972357]

LIPID FRACTIONS & THE RISK OF CORONARY HEART DISEASE

In serum, cholesterol is carried primarily on three different lipoproteins—VLDL, LDL, and HDL. Total cholesterol equals the sum of these three components:

$$\text{Total cholesterol} = \text{HDL cholesterol} + \text{VLDL cholesterol} + \text{LDL cholesterol}$$

Traditionally, the **Friedewald equation** has been used to estimate LDL-C.

Modern research has questioned several of the assumptions underlying the Friedewald equation, particularly the assumption that VLDL is always best estimated as triglycerides/5, which is inaccurate when triglycerides are > 150 mg/dL and when LDL-C is < 70 mg/dL. Therefore, many commercial laboratories have switched to the **Martin-Hopkins equation**, which uses a flexible factor for deriving VLDL from triglycerides (as opposed to always using 5). The Martin-Hopkins equation reduces the systematic underestimation of LDL-C when triglycerides are > 150 mg/dL and LDL is < 70 mg/dL and is more accurate in estimating LDL from nonfasting blood specimens.

Non–HDL-C is increasingly recognized as an important measure of the total quantity of apolipoprotein B–containing atherogenic lipid particles. Non–HDL-C is calculated as: total cholesterol – HDL-C. Advantages of calculating non–HDL-C are that it is directly measured, requires no additional cost, is less sensitive to fasting status, and is a better predictor of cardiovascular risk compared to LDL-C. The serum concentration of apolipoprotein B (ApoB) can also be directly measured, and ApoB treatment targets can be considered alongside or in place of non–HDL-C targets.

Lipoprotein(a), a subfraction of LDL that is largely genetically determined, has also been recognized as a causal factor in atherosclerosis.One-time measurement of lipoprotein(a) in patients with a strong family history, with manifestations of early ASCVD, or with familial hypercholesterolemia is useful. As of 2024, the National Lipid Association recommends one-time screening of the entire adult population and recommends cascade screening in family members of those with severe hypercholesterolemia, including elevated lipoprotein(a). Values > 50 mg/dL or > 100 nmol/L are considered elevated. A novel antisense oligonucleotide therapy (pelacarsen) associated with a nearly 80% reduction in lipoprotein(a) is being tested in a pivotal phase 3 cardiovascular outcomes trial of patients with prior MI, stroke, or peripheral artery disease and high lipoprotein(a). The results from this Lp(a) HORIZON trial are due in 2026. Lipoprotein(a) should be much more commonly measured and used as a risk-enhancing factor favoring early and more aggressive statin treatment.

It becomes difficult to assign a "normal" range for serum lipids. This is because our cholesterol values are vastly higher than our evolutionary ancestors (whose LDL-C may have been 30–50 mg/dL). Mean LDL-C levels are currently declining in the United States, including in youths. There is *no* evidence available that adult cholesterol levels can be "too low"; that is, there is *no* evidence that very low LDL-C is linked with any major side effects (eg, cognitive dysfunction).

Aggarwal R et al. Trends in lipid concentrations and lipid control among US adults, 2007-2018. JAMA. 2022;328:737. [PMID: 35997731]

Koschinsky ML et al. A focused update to the 2019 NLA scientific statement on use of lipoprotein(a) in clinical practice. J Clin Lipidol. 2024;18:e308. [PMID: 38565461]

Reyes-Soffer G et al. Lipoprotein(a): a genetically determined, causal, and prevalent risk factor for atherosclerotic cardiovascular disease: a Scientific Statement from the American Heart Association. Arterioscler Thromb Vasc Biol. 2022;42:e48. [PMID: 34647487]

Soffer DE et al. Role of apolipoprotein B in the clinical management of cardiovascular risk in adults: an expert clinical consensus from the National Lipid Association. J Clin Lipidol. 2024;18:e647. [PMID: 39256087]

THERAPEUTIC EFFECTS OF LOWERING CHOLESTEROL

Reducing cholesterol levels in healthy middle-aged men without CHD (primary prevention) reduces risk in direct proportion to the reduction in LDL-C. Treated adults have clinically important reductions in the rates of MIs, new cases of angina, need for coronary artery bypass or other revascularization procedures, peripheral artery disease, and stroke. The West of Scotland Study showed a 31% decrease in MIs in middle-aged men treated with pravastatin compared with placebo. The Air Force/Texas Coronary Atherosclerosis Prevention Study (AFCAPS/TexCAPS) study showed similar results with lovastatin. As with any primary prevention interventions, large numbers of healthy patients need to be treated to prevent a single event. The numbers of patients needed to treat (NNT) to prevent one nonfatal MI or one CAD death in these two studies were 46 and 50, respectively. The Anglo-Scandinavian Cardiac Outcomes Trial (ASCOT) study of atorvastatin in persons with hypertension and other risk factors but without CHD demonstrated a 36% reduction in CHD events. The Justification for the Use of Statins in Prevention: An Intervention Trial Evaluating Rosuvastatin (JUPITER) study showed a 44% reduction in a combined end point of MI, stroke, revascularization, hospitalization for unstable angina, or death from cardiovascular causes in both men and women. The estimated 5-year NNT to prevent one event was 20. The Heart Outcomes Prevention Evaluation (HOPE-3) trial of rosuvastatin showed a 24% reduction in cardiovascular events. The NNT over 5.6 years was 91. The Randomized Trial to Prevent Vascular Events in HIV (REPRIEVE) showed a 35% reduction in cardiovascular death, MI, hospitalization for unstable angina, stroke, transient ischemic attack, peripheral arterial ischemia, revascularization, or death from an undetermined cause using pitavastatin in 7769 persons with HIV at low to moderate risk of CVD. The 5-year number needed to treat was 106. However, primary prevention studies have found a less consistent effect on total mortality.

In secondary prevention studies among patients with established ASCVD, the mortality benefits of cholesterol lowering are clearer. *Major trials with statins have shown significant reductions in cardiovascular events, cardiovascular deaths, and all-cause mortality in men and women with CAD.* The NNT to prevent a nonfatal MI or a CAD death in these studies was between 12 and 34. Aggressive cholesterol lowering with these agents causes regression of atherosclerotic plaques in some patients, reduces the progression of atherosclerosis in saphenous vein grafts, and can slow or reverse carotid artery atherosclerosis. Results with other classes of medications, particularly those with little effect on LDL or the LDL receptor, have been less consistent. The benefits and adverse effects of cholesterol lowering may be specific to each type or mechanism of medication.

The disparities in absolute event lowering between primary and secondary prevention studies highlight a critical aspect of clinical cholesterol lowering. *The net benefits from cholesterol lowering depend on the underlying risk of ASCVD as well as the competing risks of other diseases.* In middle-aged patients with atherosclerosis and high cholesterol, morbidity and mortality rates are high, and measures that reduce cholesterol-related risk are more likely to provide a robust net benefit to the patient. In older patients with little atherosclerosis and lower cholesterol levels, there may be no meaningful net clinical benefit to cholesterol lowering.

Grinspoon SK et al; REPRIEVE Investigators. Pitavastatin to prevent cardiovascular disease in HIV infection. N Engl J Med. 2023;389:687. [PMID: 37486775]
Mhaimeed O et al. The importance of LDL-C lowering in atherosclerotic cardiovascular disease prevention: lower for longer is better. Am J Prev Cardiol. 2024;18:100649. [PMID: 38576462]
US Preventive Services Task Force; Mangione CM et al. Statin use for the primary prevention of cardiovascular disease in adults: US Preventive Services Task Force recommendation statement. JAMA. 2022;328:746. [PMID: 35997723]

SECONDARY CONDITIONS THAT AFFECT LIPID METABOLISM

Several factors, including medications, can influence serum lipids. These are important for two reasons: abnormal lipid levels (or changes in lipid levels) may be the presenting sign of some of these conditions, and correction of the underlying condition may obviate the need to treat an apparent lipid disorder. Thyroid disease, particularly hypothyroidism, is associated with a high LDL-C. Poorly controlled diabetes mellitus and alcohol use are commonly associated with high triglyceride levels that decline with improvements in glycemic control or reduction in alcohol use, respectively. Thus, secondary causes of high blood lipids should be considered in each patient with a lipid disorder before lipid-lowering therapy is started.

CLINICAL PRESENTATIONS

Most patients with high cholesterol levels have no specific symptoms or signs. The vast majority of patients with lipid abnormalities are detected by the laboratory, either as part of the workup of a patient with CVD or as part of a preventive screening strategy. Extremely high levels of chylomicrons or VLDL particles (triglyceride level above 1000 mg/dL or 10 mmol/L) result in the formation of **eruptive xanthomas** (Figure 32–1) (red-yellow papules, especially on the buttocks). High LDL-C concentrations result in **tendinous xanthomas** on certain tendons (Achilles, patella, back of the hand). Such xanthomas usually indicate one of the underlying genetic hyperlipidemias.

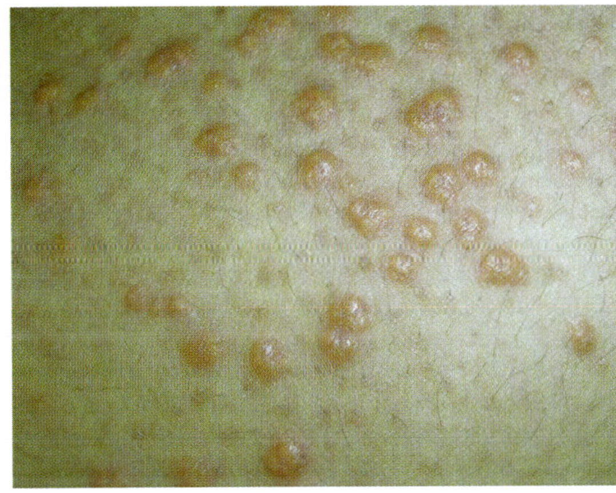

Figure 32–1. Eruptive xanthomas on the arm of a man with untreated hyperlipidemia and diabetes mellitus. (Reproduced with permission from Richard P. Usatine, MD, in Usatine RP, Smith MA, Mayeaux EJ Jr, Chumley H. *The Color Atlas of Family Medicine,* 2nd ed. McGraw-Hill, 2013.)

SCREENING & TREATMENT OF HIGH BLOOD CHOLESTEROL

While screening of all children for cholesterol disorders remains controversial, *all adults should have their lipids checked before middle age (age 35 in men and 45 in women).* In addition, lipids should always be checked within the age range 20–35 years in men and 20–45 years in women when other cardiovascular risk factors are present. Patients with documented atherosclerosis and diabetes mellitus deserve the most scrutiny of their lipids since these patients are at the highest risk for suffering additional manifestations in the near term and thus have the most to gain from lipid lowering. Additional risk reduction measures for atherosclerosis are discussed in Chapter 10; lipid lowering should be just one aspect of a program to reduce the progression and effects of atherosclerosis.

Several algorithms have been developed to guide the clinician in treatment decisions, but management decisions must always be individualized based on the patient's ASCVD risk to maximize net benefit.

The 2018 American Heart Association/American College of Cardiology (AHA/ACC)/Multi-society guidelines recommend screening of all adults aged 20 years or older for high blood cholesterol. The 2016 USPSTF guidelines recommend beginning at age 20 years only if there are other cardiovascular risk factors such as tobacco use, diabetes, hypertension, obesity, or a family history of premature CVD. For men without other risk factors, screening is recommended beginning at age 35 years.

Individuals without CVD should have their 10-year risk of CVD calculated, with lifetime risk also considered. *Although those with LDL-C > 190 mg/dL (4.91 mmol/L) are recommended for treatment independent of their 10-year risk of CVD, all other patients are recommended for treatment based on their overall cardiovascular risk.* While other calculators (such as *SCORE2* or *QRISK*) may be more appropriate for other parts of the world, *the best method for estimating 10-year ASCVD risk in the United States is the* ***Pooled Cohort Equations***. First introduced in the 2013 ACC/AHA guidelines, the Pooled Cohort Equations include separate equations for White and Black patients and estimate the 10-year risk of heart attack, stroke, and cardiovascular death. The ACC/AHA risk estimator can be found at https://tools.acc.org/ASCVD-Risk-Estimator-Plus/#!/calculate/estimate, and mobile apps are available. While it has been shown to overestimate risk in some modern populations, the ACC/AHA risk estimator remains an excellent starting point for a risk discussion. The **LIFE-CVD model** is the best for illustrating lifetime risk and benefit of therapy (https://www.u-prevent.com/calculators/lifeCvd). The **PREVENT equations** were released in 2023 to model the combined risk of ASCVD and HF over both 10- and 30-year time horizons in addition to adding other cardiometabolic risk factors and social determinants, while eliminating race from the equations.

Shared decision-making is a central part of cholesterol management in primary prevention. Therefore, the 2018 AHA/ACC/Multi-society guidelines and the 2019 ACC/AHA primary prevention guidelines identify a set of "*risk-enhancing factors*" that might influence a clinician and patient to favor cholesterol-lowering treatment. Table 32–1 lists these risk-enhancing factors that may be considered, particularly for patients at borderline to intermediate risk (5–20% 10-year cardiovascular risk).

Importantly, the 2018 AHA/ACC/Multi-society guidelines and the 2019 ACC/AHA primary prevention guidelines also identify the **coronary artery calcium score** as the single best test for additional risk stratification. The coronary calcium score is a simple noncontrast cardiac-gated CT scan that takes about 10–15 minutes to perform, is associated with approximately 1 mSv of radiation, and costs between \$50 and \$300. As opposed to the risk-enhancing factors, which may incline a clinician and patient toward treatment, *the coronary artery calcium score may also help identify patients who are unlikely to benefit from cholesterol-lowering therapy*. For example, when the coronary artery calcium score is zero in the absence of smoking or diabetes, the patient is low risk and less likely to receive net benefit from therapy; instead, the coronary artery calcium score can be repeated in approximately 3 years for higher-risk patients and 7 years for lower-risk patients. High coronary artery calcium scores (> 300–1000) are considered generally equivalent to secondary prevention-level risk.

Statins are nearly always the first-line therapy (Tables 32–2 and 32–3). Treatment decisions are based on the presence of clinical CVD or diabetes, LDL-C > 190 mg/dL (4.91 mmol/L), patient age, and the estimated 10-year risk of developing CVD. The 2018 AHA/ACC/Multi-society guidelines define four groups of patients who benefit from statin medications: (1) individuals with clinical ASCVD; (2) individuals with primary elevation of LDL-C > 190 mg/dL (4.91 mmol/L); (3) individuals aged 40–75 with diabetes and LDL ≥ 70 mg/dL (1.81 mmol/L); and (4) individuals aged 40–75 without clinical ASCVD or diabetes, with LDL 70–189 mg/dL (1.81–4.91 mmol/L), and estimated 10-year ASCVD risk of 7.5% or higher.

Ezetimibe, PCSK9 inhibitors, and bempedoic acid (Table 32–2) have the strongest recommendations as second-line therapy for patients with (1) CVD whose LDL on statin therapy remains above the relevant treatment threshold of 55 mg/dL or 70 mg/dL; (2) possible familial hypercholesterolemia with baseline LDL > 190 mg/dL (4.91 mmol/L) whose LDL remains above the 100 mg/dL treatment threshold; or (3) documented statin intolerance. *Statin intolerance is commonly defined as inability or perceived inability to tolerate at least two different statin therapies, including at least one attempt at the lowest approved dose or a trial of an alternate-day dosing strategy.* Table 32–4 outlines modified versions of the 2022 ACC therapeutic recommendations for adults with hypercholesterolemia who are intolerant of statins. In high-risk patients, ezetimibe therapy is favored in part due to reduced cost, while in very high-risk patients, PCSK9 inhibitor therapy should be considered. As shown in the CLEAR OUTCOMES trial, bempedoic acid is an excellent alternative when documented statin intolerance is present.

Table 32–1. Risk-enhancing factors that help identify patients who may benefit most from lipid-lowering therapy: 2018 AHA/ACC/Multi-society guidelines.

Family history of premature disease (males, age < 55 years; females, age < 65 years)
Primary hypercholesterolemia (LDL-C, 160–189 mg/dL [4.1–4.8 mmol/L]; non–HDL-C, 190–219 mg/dL [4.9–5.6 mmol/L])
Metabolic syndrome
CKD (not ESKD)
Chronic inflammatory conditions, such as psoriasis, rheumatoid arthritis, or HIV/AIDS
History of preeclampsia or of premature menopause before age 40 years
High-risk race/ethnicities (eg, South Asian ancestry)
Persistently high triglycerides ≥ 175 mg/dL
Elevated high-sensitivity CRP (≥ 2.0 mg/L)
Elevated lipoprotein(a) (≥ 50 mg/dL or ≥ 125 nmol/L)
Elevated apolipoprotein B (≥ 130 mg/dL)
Ankle brachial index < 0.9

AHA/ACC, American Heart Association/American College of Cardiology; HDL-C, high-density lipoprotein cholesterol; LDL-C, low-density lipoprotein cholesterol.

Screening & Treatment in Older Patients

Meta-analysis of evidence relating cholesterol to CVD in older adults suggests that cholesterol is a somewhat weaker risk factor for CVD for persons over age 75 years. The 2018 AHA/ACC/Multi-society guidelines suggest continuing statin treatment in patients over age 75 who have CVD. The guidelines, however, suggest selectively treating patients over the age of 75 who do not have evidence of CVD. Individual patient decisions to discontinue statin therapy should be based on overall functional status and life expectancy, comorbidities, and patient preference and should be made in context with overall therapeutic goals and end-of-life decisions.

Table 32–2. Effects of selected lipid-modifying medications (listed in alphabetical order).

Medication	Lipid-Modifying Effects			Regimens	Approximate Cost[1]
	LDL-C	HDL-C	Triglyceride		
Alirocumab (Praluent)[2]	−45 to −60%	±	±	*Initial:* 75 mg once subcutaneously every 2 weeks *Maximum:* 150 mg once subcutaneously every 2 weeks	$$$
Atorvastatin (Lipitor)	−25 to −40%	+5 to 10%	↓↓	*Initial:* 10 mg orally once daily *Maximum:* 80 mg orally once daily	$
Bempedoic acid (Nexletol)	−17 to −20%	−6%	±	*Initial:* 180 mg orally once daily *Maximum:* 180 mg orally once daily	$$$
Cholestyramine (Questran, others)	−15 to −25%	+5%	±	*Initial:* 4 g orally twice a day *Maximum:* 24 g orally, divided	$$
Colesevelam (WelChol)	−10 to −20%	+10%	±	*Initial:* 625 mg, 6–7 tablets orally once daily *Maximum:* 625 mg, 6–7 tablets orally once daily	$$
Colestipol (Colestid)	−15 to −60%	+5%	±	*Initial:* 5 g orally twice a day *Maximum:* 30 g orally, divided	$$
Evinacumab (Evkeeza)[3]	−47%	−52%	↓↓	*Initial:* 15 mg/kg intravenously every 4 weeks *Maximum:* 15 mg/kg intravenously every 4 weeks	$$$$
Evolocumab (Repatha)[2]	−50 to −60%	±	±	*Initial:* 140 mg subcutaneously once every 2 weeks *Maximum:* 420 mg subcutaneously once monthly	$$$
Ezetimibe (Zetia)	−15 to −20%	+5%	±	*Initial:* 10 mg orally once daily *Maximum:* 10 mg orally once daily	$
Fenofibrate (Tricor, others)	−10 to −15%	+15 to 25%	↓↓	*Initial:* 48 mg orally once daily *Maximum:* 145 mg orally once daily	$$
Fenofibric acid (Trilipix)	−10 to −15%	+15 to 25%	↓↓	*Initial:* 45 mg orally once daily *Maximum:* 135 mg orally once daily	$$
Fluvastatin (Lescol)	−20 to −30%	+5 to 10%	↓	*Initial:* 20 mg orally once daily *Maximum:* 40 mg orally once daily	$
Gemfibrozil (Lopid, others)	−10 to −15%	+15 to 20%	↓↓	*Initial:* 600 mg orally once daily *Maximum:* 1200 mg orally, divided	$
Inclisiran (Leqvio)[2]	−50 to −52%	+5 to 6%	↓	*Initial:* 284 mg subcutaneously at baseline and 3 months *Maintenance:* 284 mg subcutaneously every 6 months	$$$
Lerodalcibep-liga (Lerochol)	−55 to −60%	±	±	*Initial:* 300 mg subcutaneously once monthly *Maximum:* 300 mg subcutaneously once monthly	$$$
Lomitapide (Juxtapid)[3,4]	−40 to −50%	−7%	↓↓	*Initial:* 5 mg orally once daily *Maximum:* 60 mg orally once daily	$$$$
Lovastatin (Mevacor, others)	−25 to −40%	+5 to 10%	↓	*Initial:* 10 mg orally once daily *Maximum:* 80 mg orally, divided	$
Niacin (OTC, Niaspan)[2]	−15 to −25%	+25 to 35%	↓↓	*Initial:* 100 mg orally once daily *Maximum:* 3–4.5 g orally, divided	$
Olezarsen (Tryngolza)[5]	−8%	+40%	↓↓↓	*Initial:* 80 mg subcutaneous once monthly *Maximum:* 80 mg subcutaneous once monthly	$$$$
Omega-3 fatty acid ethyl esters (Lovaza)	±	±	↓↓	*Initial:* 4 g orally once daily *Maximum:* 4 g orally once daily	$$
Omega-3 fatty acid icosapent ethyl (Vascepa)	±	±	↓↓	*Initial:* 2 g orally twice a day *Maximum:* 2 g orally twice a day	$$
Pitavastatin (Livalo, Zypitamag)	−30 to −40%	+10 to 25%	↓↓	*Initial:* 2 mg orally once daily *Maximum:* 4 mg orally once daily	$$

(*continued*)

Table 32–2. Effects of selected lipid-modifying medications (listed in alphabetical order). (continued)

Medication	Lipid-Modifying Effects			Regimens	Approximate Cost[1]
	LDL-C	HDL-C	Triglyceride		
Plozasiran (Redemplo)[2,5]	+1 to 10%	+45 to 50%	↓↓↓	*Initial:* 25 mg subcutaneously once every 3 months *Maximum:* 25 mg subcutaneously once every 3 months	$$$$
Pravastatin (Pravachol)	−25 to −40%	+5 to 10%	↓	*Initial:* 20 mg orally once daily *Maximum:* 80 mg orally once daily	$
Rosuvastatin (Crestor)	−40 to −50%	+10 to 15%	↓↓	*Initial:* 10 mg orally once daily *Maximum:* 40 mg orally once daily	$
Simvastatin (Zocor, others)	−25 to −40%	+5 to 10%	↓↓	*Initial:* 5 mg orally once daily *Maximum:* 40 mg orally once daily	$

[1]Cost ranging from $ = least expensive to $$$$= most expensive. Cost estimates based on average wholesale price (AWP, for AB-rated generic when available).
[2]Also associated with reduction in lipoprotein(a).
[3]Restricted to patients with homozygous familial hypercholesterolemia.
[4]FDA Black Box warning regarding hepatotoxicity. Can only be prescribed in the context of a Food and Drug Administration Risk Evaluation and Mitigation Strategies plan.
[5]Restricted to patients with familial chylomicronemia syndrome.
± variable, if any; HDL-C, high-density lipoprotein cholesterol; LDL-C, low-density lipoprotein cholesterol; OTC, over the counter.

Screening & Treatment in Patients with HIV

Patients with HIV have higher CVD risk than matched patients without HIV, independent of traditional cardiovascular risk factors. The mechanisms for this include immune activation, inflammation, and the impact of HIV therapies on risk factors including cholesterol. The striking results of the REPRIEVE cardiovascular outcomes trial, in which baseline LDL was just 108 mg/dL, argues for routine statin therapy for nearly all patients with HIV who have no contraindications. Treatments with pitavastatin may have fewer drug-drug interactions than certain other statins (ie, simvastatin).

Dennison Himmelfarb CR et al. Shared decision-making and cardiovascular health: a scientific statement from the American Heart Association. Circulation. 2023;148:912. [PMID: 37577791]

Table 32–3. Indications for high-intensity and moderate-intensity statins: recommendations of the 2018 AHA/ACC/Multi-society guidelines.

Indications	Treatment Recommendation
Presence of clinical ASCVD	High-intensity statin[1] or moderate-intensity statin[2] if over age 75 years
Primary elevation of LDL-C ≥ 190 mg/dL (4.91 mmol/L)	High-intensity statin
Age 40–75 years Presence of diabetes LDL-C ≥ 70 mg/dL (1.81 mmol/L)	Moderate-intensity statin or high-intensity statin if diabetes and 10-year CVD risk ≥ 7.5% or other risk-enhancing criteria[3]
Age 40–75 years No clinical ASCVD or diabetes LDL-C 70–189 mg/dL (1.81–4.91 mmol/L) Estimated 10-year CVD risk ≥ 7.5% or coronary artery calcium score ≥ 100 or ≥ 75th percentile	Moderate- to high-intensity statin

[1]High-intensity statins include atorvastatin 40–80 mg orally daily or rosuvastatin 20–40 mg orally daily.
[2]Moderate-intensity statin includes following oral agents: atorvastatin, 10–20 mg daily; fluvastatin, 40 mg twice daily; lovastatin, 40–80 mg daily; pitavastatin, 1–4 mg daily; pravastatin, 40–80 mg daily; rosuvastatin, 5–10 mg daily; or simvastatin, 20–40 mg daily.
[3]Diabetes duration > 10 years, microalbuminuria, CKD, and ankle brachial index < 0.9 favor aggressive treatment even for patients aged 20–39 years.
AHA/ACC, American Heart Association/American College of Cardiology; ASCVD, atherosclerotic CVD; LDL-C, low-density lipoprotein cholesterol.

Table 32–4. Modified 2022 ACC therapeutic recommendations for adult hypercholesterolemic patients with statin intolerance.[1]

Indications	Treatment Recommendations		
	First-Line Therapy	Second-Line Therapy	Third-Line Therapy
No clinical ASCVD but at increased risk[2]	Ezetimibe	Bempedoic acid (ie, ezetimibe/bempedoic acid combination)	BAS (eg, colesevelam)
No clinical ASCVD but with LDL-C ≥ 190 mg/dL (≥ 5.1 mmol/L)	Ezetimibe and/or PCSK9 inhibitor (monoclonal antibody)	Bempedoic acid or inclisiran	Evinacumab for HoFH
Clinical ASCVD but not at very high risk[3]	Ezetimibe and/or PCSK9 inhibitor (monoclonal antibody)	Bempedoic acid or inclisiran	
Clinical ASCVD at very high risk[3] or with LDL-C ≥ 190 mg/dL (≥ 5.1 mmol/L)	Ezetimibe and/or PCSK9 inhibitor (monoclonal antibody)	Bempedoic acid or inclisiran	Evinacumab for HoFH

[1]Statin intolerance is defined as development of statin-associated side effects (myopathy or rhabdomyolysis, hepatic inflammation, hyperglycemia, memory loss or confusion) on at least two statins with one attempt on the lowest FDA-approved daily dose (or a trial of an alternative dosing regimen).
[2]For example, diabetes or with coronary artery calcium score ≥ 100 or ≥ 75th percentile.
[3]Very high risk ASCVD includes patients with an ACS within the past 12 months, or history of MI or ischemic stroke, or peripheral vascular disease.
ACC, American College of Cardiology; ASCVD, atherosclerotic cardiovascular disease; BAS, bile acid sequestrant such as colesevelam; HoFH, homozygous familial hypercholesterolemia; LDL-C, low-density lipoprotein cholesterol; PCSK9, proprotein convertase subtilisin/kexin type 9.
Data from the 2022 ACC Expert Consensus Decision Pathway on the Role of Nonstatin Therapies for LDL-Cholesterol Lowering in the Management of Atherosclerotic Cardiovascular Disease Risk. J Am Coll Cardiol. 2022;80:1366. [PMID: 36031461]

Kalra DK et al. Dyslipidemia in human immunodeficiency virus disease: JACC Review Topic of the Week. J Am Coll Cardiol. 2023;82:171. [PMID: 37407116]
Khan SS et al; American Heart Association. Novel prediction equations for absolute risk assessment of total cardiovascular disease incorporating cardiovascular-kidney-metabolic health: a scientific statement from the American Heart Association. Circulation. 2023;148:1982. [PMID: 37947094]

TREATMENT OF HIGH LDL CHOLESTEROL

Reduction of LDL-C with statins is just one part of a program to reduce the risk of CVD. Other measures—including diet, exercise, smoking cessation, hypertension control, weight management, diabetes control, and antithrombotic therapy—are also of central importance. For example, exercise (and weight loss) may reduce the LDL-C, increase the HDL, and markedly decrease triglycerides.

*The use of medications to raise the HDL-C has **not** been demonstrated to provide additional benefit.* The addition of niacin to statins has been carefully studied in the AIM-HIGH trial and the HPS2-THRIVE trial in patients at high risk for CVD; no cardiovascular outcome benefit has been shown.

Banach M et al; International Lipid Expert Panel (ILEP). 2024 recommendations on the optimal use of lipid-lowering therapy in established atherosclerotic cardiovascular disease and following acute coronary syndromes: a position paper of the International Lipid Expert Panel (ILEP). Drugs. 2024;84:1541. [PMID: 39497020]

Diet Therapy

Studies of nonhospitalized adults have reported only modest cholesterol-lowering benefits of individual dietary therapies, typically in the range of a 5–10% decrease in LDL-C, and even less over the long term. The effect of diet therapies, however, may be additive; some patients will have striking reductions in LDL-C—up to a 25–30% decrease—whereas others will have clinically important increases. Thus, the results of diet therapy should be assessed about 4–12 weeks after initiation.

Several nutritional approaches to diet therapy are available. Most Americans eat over 35% of calories as fat, of which 15% is saturated fat. A traditional cholesterol-lowering diet recommends reducing total fat to 25–30% and saturated fat to < 7% of calories, with complete elimination of trans fats. These diets replace fat, particularly saturated fat, with carbohydrate. Other diet plans, including the Dean Ornish Diet and most vegetarian diets, restrict fat even further. Low-fat, high-carbohydrate diets may, however, result in insulin resistance, elevated triglycerides, and reductions in HDL-C. This is particularly true when "real" foods are replaced with ultra-processed foods, particularly ultra-processed carbohydrates. *Emphasis has therefore shifted to healthier fats.*

A strategy with strong supporting evidence is the **Mediterranean diet**, which maintains total fat at approximately 35–40% of total calories but replaces saturated fat with monounsaturated fat such as that found in canola oil and in olives, peanuts, avocados, and their oils. This diet, which like others calls for elimination of highly processed or prepackaged food, is equally effective at lowering LDL-C and is less likely to lead to reductions in HDL-C. Several studies have suggested that this diet may also be associated with reductions in endothelial dysfunction, insulin resistance, and markers of vascular inflammation. A clinical trial demonstrated reduced cardiovascular events in persons on a Mediterranean diet supplemented with additional nuts or extra-virgin olive oil compared to persons on a less intensive standard Mediterranean diet.

Other dietary changes may also result in beneficial changes in blood lipids. **Soluble fiber**, such as that found in oat bran or psyllium, may reduce LDL-C by 5–10%. **Plant stanols and sterols** can reduce LDL-C by 10%. *Studies have suggested that when all of these elements are combined into a single dietary prescription, the impact of diet on LDL-C may approach that of statin medications, lowering LDL-C by close to 30%.* In contrast, over-the-counter supplements (ie, garlic, cinnamon, turmeric, etc) have been tested and are generally *ineffective* at lowering LDL-C, especially when directly compared to rosuvastatin in a head-to-head trial.

2025 Focused Update of the 2019 ESC/EAS Guidelines for the management of dyslipidaemias: Developed by the task force for the management of dyslipidaemias of the European Society of Cardiology (ESC) and the European Atherosclerosis Society (EAS). Eur Heart J. 2025;46:4359. [PMID: 41417047]

Laffin LJ et al. Comparative effects of low-dose rosuvastatin, placebo and dietary supplements on lipids and inflammatory biomarkers. J Am Coll Cardiol. 2023;81:1. [PMID: 36351465]

Volpp KG et al; American Heart Association. Food is medicine: a presidential advisory from the American Heart Association. Circulation. 2023;148:1417. [PMID: 37767686]

Pharmacologic Therapy

There are eight classes of medications available for consideration in patients who require pharmacologic treatment of an elevated cholesterol (statins, ezetimibe, PCSK9 inhibitors, omega-3 fatty acids, bempedoic acid, bile-acid–binding resins, fibrates, and niacin). As discussed above, statins are the cornerstone of nearly all medical regimens, and guidelines define four groups of patients who benefit from statin medications (*adults with diabetes mellitus, those with existing ASCVD, LDL-C > 190 mg/dL, or 10-year risk of ASCVD > 7.5%*). Among non-statin medications that are considered for managing LDL-C, the evidence is strongest for ezetimibe, PCSK9 inhibitors, and bempedoic acid; for triglycerides, the evidence is strongest for adding prescription-grade omega-3 fatty acid preparations. There is far less evidence for cholesterol absorption inhibitors, fibrates, and niacin; these medications should generally be used sparingly.

A. Statins (Hydroxymethylglutaryl-Coenzyme A [HMG-CoA] Reductase Inhibitors)

The statins (HMG-CoA reductase inhibitors) work by inhibiting the rate-limiting enzyme in the formation of cholesterol. Cholesterol synthesis in the liver is reduced, with a compensatory increase in hepatic LDL receptors (so that the liver can take more of the cholesterol that it needs from the blood) and a reduction in the circulating LDL-C level by 50% or more at the highest doses. There are also modest increases in HDL levels, substantial decreases in triglyceride levels, and marked reductions in high-sensitivity CRP levels.

The 2018 AHA/ACC/Multi-society guidelines divide statins into two categories: "*high-intensity*" and "*moderate-intensity*" statins (Table 32–3). High-intensity statins lower LDL-C by approximately 50%. Examples include high-dose atorvastatin 40–80 mg/day and rosuvastatin 20–40 mg/day (Table 32–2). Moderate-intensity statins lower LDL-C by approximately 30–50%. Examples include pitavastatin 2–4 mg/day, simvastatin 20–40 mg/day, and pravastatin 40–80 mg/day, as well as low-dose atorvastatin 10–20 mg/day and rosuvastatin 5–10 mg/day. All statins are given once daily in the morning or evening.

Statin-associated muscle aches, with normal serum creatine kinase levels, occur in up to 10% of patients, and often such patients can tolerate the statin upon rechallenge. The SAMSON trial demonstrated the importance of the nocebo effect with perceived statin intolerance (reported side effects being due to patient expectations); in this trial, 90% of the symptoms associated with statin rechallenge were also noted with placebo. The **Statin-Associated Muscle Symptom Clinical Index (SAMS-CI)** is a useful tool to help differentiate statin-related symptoms from symptoms unrelated to statins. More serious, but very uncommon, muscle disease includes myositis and rhabdomyolysis, with moderate and marked elevations of serum creatine kinase levels, respectively. Such muscle disease occurs more often in older patients and when the statin is taken with niacin or a fibrate, as well as with erythromycin, antifungal medications, nefazodone, or cyclosporine. Liver disease, with elevations of serum transaminases, is another uncommon side effect of statin therapy. Manufacturers of statins recommend monitoring liver enzymes before initiating therapy and only as clinically indicated thereafter; current guidelines do *not* recommend routine monitoring. Finally, *statin therapy is associated with a 10% dose-dependent increase in risk of developing diabetes mellitus in at-risk individuals* (eg, those with the metabolic syndrome).

B. Ezetimibe

Ezetimibe inhibits the intestinal absorption of dietary and biliary cholesterol across the intestinal wall by inhibiting a cholesterol transporter. The fixed dose of ezetimibe is 10 mg/day orally and it is a generic medication. Ezetimibe reduces LDL-C between 15% and 20% when used as monotherapy, reduces high-sensitivity CRP, and can further reduce LDL-C in patients taking statins in whom the therapeutic goal has not been reached (Table 32–2). GI side effects are uncommon. While beneficial effects of ezetimibe monotherapy on cardiovascular outcomes are available only from a large open-label trial, the double-blind IMPROVE-IT trial showed that adding ezetimibe to a statin resulted in a small incremental 5–10% relative risk reduction in detrimental cardiovascular outcomes. At the end of 7 years of study, patients taking ezetimibe-simvastatin had a 2% absolute reduction in cardiovascular events compared to patients taking simvastatin alone. *Current guidelines recommend adding ezetimibe therapy to maximally tolerated statin therapy in patients at high risk for CVD whose LDL-C remains above the treatment threshold of 70 mg/dL.*

C. Proprotein Convertase Subtilisin/Kexin Type 9 (PCSK9) Inhibitors

The most commonly used PCSK9 inhibitors are fully human monoclonal antibodies that inhibit PCSK9-mediated

LDL-receptor degradation and lower LDL-C levels by 50–60% and lipoprotein(a) by up to 20–30%. Two agents, alirocumab and evolocumab, are FDA-approved for use in patients with familial hypercholesterolemia or in patients with CVD or high risk of CVD who require further lowering of LDL-C. These medications are injected subcutaneously every 2–4 weeks. No significant increase in adverse events has been observed compared to placebo. The FOURIER trial compared evolocumab with placebo in 27,564 patients with established atherosclerotic disease already taking statin therapy; participants were monitored for a median of 2.2 years. LDL-C was reduced by 59% to a mean value of ~30 mg/dL. Patients receiving the evolocumab plus statin had a 15% reduction in the primary composite endpoint of cardiovascular death, MI, stroke, hospital admission for unstable angina, or coronary revascularization and a 20% reduction in the secondary outcome of cardiovascular death, MI, or stroke. The ODYSSEY-OUTCOMES study randomized 18,924 patients with recent ACS to alirocumab or placebo, demonstrating a 15% reduction in the primary composite cardiovascular endpoint and a 15% reduction in all-cause mortality in secondary statistical testing after median 2.8-year follow-up. The VESALIUS trial extended the benefits of PCSK9 inhibitors to patients without prior MI or stroke; in VESALIUS, among 12,257 patients with no prior ASCVD but established advanced atherosclerosis, evolocumab decreased the primary cardiovascular endpoint by 25%.

However, despite these remarkable results from multiple clinical trials, their high cost meant that initial cost-effectiveness models found that these PCSK9 inhibitors were not cost-effective. Over time, PCSK9 inhibitors have moved closer to being cost-effective and experts now believe that they remain underused; however, *most guidelines still indicate that their relatively high cost must remain part of any consideration regarding their use.* Current guidelines recommend addition of PCSK9 inhibitors to statins at maximally tolerated doses in patients with coronary artery calcium scores > 1000 or at very high risk for recurrent CVD when on-treatment LDL-C remains well above 55 or 70 mg/dL (or above 100 mg/dL in patients with familial hypercholesterolemia without known CVD). Patients considered to be at very high-risk for CVD include those with recent ACS within 12 months; multiple prior MIs or strokes; significant unrevascularized CAD; and polyvascular disease (CAD plus cerebrovascular or peripheral vascular disease). The 2025 ESC cholesterol guidelines also recommend consideration of targeting to an LDL < 40 mg/dL for patients experiencing a second CVD event while already on maximally tolerated statin therapy ("extreme risk").

The PCSK9 inhibitor inclisiran reduces overproduction of PCSK9 protein by approximately 80%. After an initial subcutaneous dose and another at 3 months, inclisiran can be administered subcutaneously every 6 months (two doses annually). This regimen produces sustained LDL-C reductions of approximately 51%. Twice-yearly dosing is novel for lipid-lowering therapy; inclisiran enables new delivery strategies, including in-clinic administration. The results of the large cardiovascular outcomes trial testing inclisiran, called ORION-4, will likely be available in 2026.

The newest PCSK9 inhibitor lerodalcibep-liga is a recombinant fusion protein that blocks the PCSK9 protein and can be given as a monthly subcutaneous injection. In 2026, there is expected approval of the first oral PCSK9 inhibitor called enlicitide (60% LDL-C lowering).

D. Bempedoic Acid

Like statins, bempedoic acid targets cholesterol synthesis in the liver, ultimately resulting in upregulation of expression of the LDL receptor. Bempedoic acid is a small-molecule prodrug that inhibits adenosine triphosphate citrate lyase, an enzyme that is two steps upstream of the mechanism of statins (inhibition of HMG-CoA reductase, the rate-limiting step). Because bempedoic acid is not activated in skeletal muscle, muscle-specific side effects are more limited than they are with statins. Bempedoic acid lowers LDL-C approximately 17–20% on top of the lowering produced by moderate- to high-intensity statins. Bempedoic acid is also marketed in combination with ezetimibe; this combination provides approximately 38% LDL-C reduction on top of background lipid-lowering therapy. Treatment with bempedoic acid may mildly decrease both high-sensitivity CRP and risk of diabetes mellitus. Patients treated with bempedoic acid should be monitored for hyperuricemia and potential onset or worsening of gout as well as cholelithiasis. Bempedoic acid also appears to modestly increase the risk of tendon rupture. Bempedoic acid should not be used with > 20 mg of simvastatin daily or 40 mg of pravastatin daily. The CLEAR OUTCOMES study reported that bempedoic acid reduces cardiovascular events by approximately 13% in patients with established CVD (or in primary prevention and at high risk for CVD), documented statin intolerance, and LDL-C ≥ 100 mg/dL.

E. Omega-3 Fatty Acid Preparations

Omega-3 fatty acids are essential fatty acids that must be consumed in the diet and are a prominent feature of Mediterranean-style diets. In pharmacologic doses, omega-3 fatty acid preparations can lower triglycerides by up to 30%. Pharmacologic therapy should be differentiated from dietary omega-3 fatty acid supplements. The former is an FDA-approved product usually given at a much higher dose; dietary supplements are variable, the supporting evidence is much weaker, and they are not currently regulated.

There is modest evidence from meta-analyses that omega-3 fatty acid supplementation reduces MIs, although with no reduction in total or cardiovascular mortality. Omega-3 ethyl esters have not been associated with cardiovascular event reduction when added to statin therapy.

In contrast, icosapent ethyl, which is a highly purified eicosapentaenoic acid (EPA) only preparation, was shown to reduce cardiovascular deaths, nonfatal MIs, nonfatal strokes, coronary revascularizations, and unstable angina by 25% in statin-treated patients with triglycerides > 135 mg/dL in the 8179 person REDUCE-IT randomized clinical trial compared to a mineral oil placebo. The mechanism of action of icosapent ethyl is not yet clear but likely involves multiple mechanisms beyond lipid lowering, including antiplatelet activity, anti-inflammatory activity, and ventricular arrhythmia prevention. Icosapent ethyl is FDA approved for the broad indication of CVD event–lowering in patients with triglycerides over 150 mg/dL and either established CVD or diabetes mellitus plus two or more additional risk factors for CVD. However, there remains controversy about the efficacy of omega-3 therapies, since the 2020 STRENGTH trial showed no CVD benefit of omega-3 carboxylic acids; it remains unclear if this result was due to a different omega-3 fatty acid preparation, to a much smaller benefit of omega-3 fatty acids preparations than originally demonstrated, to use of a different placebo (corn oil versus mineral oil), or to chance.

F. Bile Acid–Binding Resins

The bile acid–binding resins include cholestyramine, colesevelam, and colestipol. In the pre-statin era, treatment with these agents reduced the incidence of coronary events in middle-aged men by about 20%, with no significant effect on total mortality. The resins work by binding bile acids in the intestine. The resultant reduction in the enterohepatic circulation causes the liver to increase its production of bile acids, using hepatic cholesterol. Thus, hepatic LDL-receptor activity increases, with a decline in plasma LDL-C levels. The triglyceride level tends to increase in some patients treated with bile acid–binding resins; these resins should be used with caution in patients with elevated triglycerides and not at all in patients who have triglyceride levels > 500 mg/dL. The clinician can anticipate a reduction of 15–25% in the LDL-C level, with insignificant effects on the HDL level. Resins are the only lipid-modifying medication considered safe in pregnancy.

These agents may interfere with the absorption of fat-soluble vitamins (thereby complicating the management of patients receiving warfarin) and may bind other drugs in the intestine. They often cause GI symptoms, such as constipation and gas.

G. Fibric Acid Derivatives

The fibrates are peroxisome proliferative-activated receptor-α (PPAR-α) agonists that result in significant reductions of plasma triglycerides and increases in HDL-C. They reduce LDL-C levels by about 10–15% (although the result is variable) and triglyceride levels by about 40% and raise HDL levels by about 15–20%. The fibric acid derivatives or fibrates approved for use in the United States are gemfibrozil and fenofibrate.

Gemfibrozil monotherapy reduced CHD rates in hypercholesterolemic middle-aged men free of coronary disease in the Helsinki Heart Study. The effect was observed only among those who also had lower HDL-C levels and high triglyceride levels. In a Veterans Affairs study, gemfibrozil monotherapy was also shown to reduce cardiovascular events in men with existing CHD whose primary lipid abnormality was a low HDL-C.

However, fibrates have *not* been shown to reduce cardiovascular events in all statin-treated patients with CVD or diabetes. For example, in the ACCORD study, addition of fenofibrate to statin in patients with diabetes and mild triglyceride elevations resulted in no benefit. Clinical interest in using fibrates has declined after publication of the PROMINENT trial of a newer fibrate, pemafibrate, which is a selective PPAR-α receptor modulator. The results of this large trial showed that pemafibrate did not impact the incidence of cardiovascular events. Fenofibrate has fewer side effects than gemfibrozil.

H. Niacin (Nicotinic Acid)

Niacin reduces the production of VLDL particles, with secondary reduction in LDL-C and increases in HDL-C levels; niacin also lowers lipoprotein(a) levels by 15–25%. The average effect of full-dose niacin therapy is a 15–25% reduction in LDL-C and a 25–35% increase in HDL-C.

There is very little evidence to support the use of niacin. In two large pivotal clinical trials, AIM-HIGH and HPS2-THRIVE, extended-release niacin did not reduce cardiovascular events when added to statin therapy in high-risk patients. Therefore, niacin should be rarely used.

Treatment Algorithms

For patients who require a lipid-modifying medication, an HMG-CoA reductase inhibitor (statin) is recommended. In patients with ASCVD, this generally should be at its maximally tolerated dose.

Combination therapy has become commonplace in clinical practice; changing to combination therapy reduces LDL-C and improves clinical outcomes more than increasing the dose of monotherapy. Combination therapy is indicated for (1) patients with familial hypercholesterolemia in whom LDL-C remains above 100 mg/dL with treatment; (2) patients with advanced subclinical atherosclerosis (coronary artery calcium scores > 100 particularly those > 1000), or high-risk patients with existing CVD in whom LDL-C remains above 70 mg/dL with treatment; (3) very high-risk patients with existing CVD in whom LDL-C remains above 55 mg/dL with treatment; and (4) many high-risk patients with triglycerides > 150 mg/dL or non–HDL-C > 100 mg/dL. Based on the 2025 ESC cholesterol guidelines, it is becoming increasingly common to *begin treatment* with combination therapy in (1) very high-risk patients or (2) at the time of an ACS.

Patients with heterozygous familial hypercholesterolemia, premature atherosclerosis, or CVD may need two or more additive medications to get below the treatment threshold, while those without CVD or without advanced subclinical atherosclerosis (primary prevention) will less commonly require multiple medications. The 2018 AHA/ACC/Multi-society guidelines prioritize addition of ezetimibe in high-risk patients, while reserving PCSK9 inhibitor therapy for very high-risk patients or those taking maximally tolerated statin therapy and ezetimibe with LDL-C still not below 70 mg/dL (Table 32–5). Notably, the 2019 ESC guidelines were the first to endorse an LDL-C treatment goal of < 55 mg/dL in very high-risk patients, which uniquely include patients with at least two 50% coronary artery stenoses identified by coronary CT angiography, or in the carotid arteries by ultrasound. These guidelines and the 2025 ESC cholesterol guidelines further endorse an LDL-C goal of < 40 mg/dL in extreme risk patients with multiple recent CVD events. In 2022, the ACC Expert Consensus Decision Pathway likewise endorsed an LDL-C of < 55 mg/dL in very high-risk patients (Table 32–5).

Patients with homozygous familial hypercholesterolemia may need plasmapheresis, special lipid-lowering therapies, or both (see Table 32–2).

Table 32–5. Therapeutic recommendations for adult hypercholesterolemic patients with clinical ASCVD.

Indications	Therapeutic Recommendations		
	First-Line	Second-Line	Third-Line
Very high-risk ASCVD[1]	High-intensity statin[2]/maximal-dose statin	If LDL-C remains > 55 mg/dL [1.8 mmol/L] on maximal-dose statin, add ezetimibe[3]	If LDL-C still > 55 mg/dL [1.8 mmol/L], add PCSK9 inhibitor[4]
Not very high-risk ASCVD[1]			
Age ≤ 75 years	High-intensity statin[2]; if high-intensity not tolerated, use moderate-intensity statin[5]	If on maximal-dose statin and LDL-C remains > 70 mg/dL [1.8 mmol/L], add ezetimibe[3]	
Age > 75 years	Moderate-intensity statin[5]	High-intensity statin[2]	

[1]Very high-risk ASCVD includes those patients with an ACS in the past 12 months, those with significant unrevascularized CAD, and those with history of multiple prior MIs or ischemic strokes.
[2]High-intensity statin includes atorvastatin, 40–80 mg orally daily; or rosuvastatin, 20–40 mg orally daily.
[3]Ezetimibe, 10 mg orally daily.
[4]PCSK9 inhibitors include evolocumab, 140 mg subcutaneously every 2 weeks; alirocumab, 75 mg subcutaneously every 2 weeks; or optionally inclisiran, 284 mg at baseline, 3 months, then every 6 months.
[5]Moderate-intensity statin includes atorvastatin, 10–20 mg orally daily; fluvastatin, 40 mg orally twice daily; lovastatin, 40–80 mg orally daily; pitavastatin, 1–4 mg orally daily; pravastatin, 40–80 mg orally daily; rosuvastatin, 5–10 mg orally daily; or simvastatin, 20–40 mg orally daily.
ASCVD, atherosclerotic cardiovascular disease; LDL-C, low-density lipoprotein cholesterol; PCSK9, proprotein convertase subtilisin/kexin type 9 inhibitor.
Data from the 2022 ACC Expert Consensus Decision Pathway on the Role of Nonstatin Therapies for LDL-Cholesterol Lowering in the Management of Atherosclerotic Cardiovascular Disease Risk. J Am Coll Cardiol. 2022;80:1366. [PMID: 36031461]

Banach M et al; International Lipid Expert Panel (ILEP). 2024 recommendations on the optimal use of lipid-lowering therapy in established atherosclerotic cardiovascular disease and following acute coronary syndromes: a position paper of the International Lipid Expert Panel (ILEP). Drugs. 2024;84:1541. [PMID: 39497020]

Bohula EA et al; VESALIUS-CV Investigators. Evolocumab in patients without a previous myocardial infarction or stroke. N Engl J Med. 2026;394:117. [PMID: 41211925]

Cholesterol Treatment Trialists' Collaboration. Effect of statin therapy on muscle symptoms: an individual participant data meta-analysis of large-scale, randomised, double-blind trials. Lancet. 2022;400:832. [PMID: 36049498]

Lloyd-Jones DM et al. 2022 ACC Expert Consensus decision pathway on the role of nonstatin therapies for LDL-cholesterol lowering in the management of atherosclerotic cardiovascular disease risk: a report of the American College of Cardiology Solution Set Oversight Committee. J Am Coll Cardiol. 2022;80:1366. [PMID: 36031461]

Nissen SE et al; CLEAR Outcomes Investigators. Bempedoic acid and cardiovascular outcomes in statin-intolerant patients. N Engl J Med. 2023;388:1353. [PMID: 36876740]

HIGH BLOOD TRIGLYCERIDES

Patients with very high levels of serum triglycerides (> 1000 mg/dL) are at risk for pancreatitis. The pathophysiology is not certain since pancreatitis never develops in many patients with very high triglyceride levels. Most patients with congenital abnormalities in triglyceride metabolism present in childhood; hypertriglyceridemia-induced pancreatitis first presenting in adults is more commonly due to an acquired problem in lipid metabolism.

Although there are no clear triglyceride levels that predict pancreatitis, most clinicians consider treating fasting levels above 500 mg/dL (5 mmol/L). The risk of pancreatitis may be more related to the triglyceride level following consumption of a fatty meal. Because postprandial increases in triglyceride are inevitable if fat-containing foods are eaten, fasting triglyceride levels in persons prone to pancreatitis should be kept well below that level.

The primary therapy for high triglyceride levels is dietary, avoiding alcohol, simple sugars, refined starches, and saturated and trans fatty acids, and restricting total calories. Control of secondary causes of high triglyceride levels may also be helpful. In patients with fasting triglycerides ≥ 500 mg/dL (5 mmol/L) despite adequate dietary adherence—and certainly in those with a previous episode of pancreatitis—therapy with a triglyceride-lowering medication (eg, statins, omega-3 preparations, or fibric acid derivatives) is indicated. Olezarsen and plozasiran can be used for patients with FCS and may soon be approved for severe hypertriglyceridemia.

Pharmacologic treatment for patients with triglycerides > 150 mg/dL (1.5 mmol/L) but < 500 mg/dL is reserved for those with established CVD with well-controlled LDL-C on maximally tolerated therapy with statins or other agents. Data are strongest for icosapent ethyl, while GLP1-RAs are also highly effective in the setting of being overweight or having obesity.

Stroes ESG et al; Balance Investigators. Olezarsen, acute pancreatitis, and familial chylomicronemia syndrome. N Engl J Med. 2024;390:1781. [PMID: 38587247]

Watts GF et al; PALISADE Study Group. Plozasiran for managing persistent chylomicronemia and pancreatitis risk. N Engl J Med. 2025;392:127. [PMID: 39225259]

33 Nutrition, Nutritional Disorders, & Obesity

Katherine H. Saunders, MD, FTOS, DABOM
Leon I. Igel, MD, FACP, FTOS, DABOM
Sarah Fink, RD, CDN, CNSC

NUTRITIONAL DISORDERS

PROTEIN–ENERGY MALNUTRITION

ESSENTIALS OF DIAGNOSIS

- Inadequate intake of energy and/or protein, increased nutrient losses, or increased nutrient requirements.
- **Kwashiorkor:** caused by protein deficiency.
- **Marasmus:** caused by combined protein and energy deficiency.
- Protein–calorie malnutrition may be mild, moderate, or severe.
- Protein loss correlates with weight loss.
- 35–40% total body weight loss due to malnutrition can be fatal.

General Considerations

Protein–energy malnutrition occurs because of a relative or absolute deficiency of energy and protein. It may be primary, due to inadequate food intake; secondary, as a result of other illness and associated inflammation; or a combination of both. For many developing nations, primary protein–energy malnutrition remains a significant health problem. There are two distinct syndromes: **kwashiorkor**, which is caused by a deficiency of protein in the presence of adequate energy, and **marasmus**, which is caused by combined protein and energy deficiency.

In industrialized societies, malnutrition is more often a sequela of other diseases than starvation. Although there is no universally accepted definition of malnutrition, there are several internationally recognized malnutrition assessment tools that have been developed to standardize malnutrition identification and promote nutrition interventions. Examples include the Subjective Global Assessment (SGA), the American Society for Parenteral and Enteral Nutrition (ASPEN) and Academy of Nutrition and Dietetics (AND) Criteria, the European Society for Parenteral and Enteral Nutrition (ESPEN) Criteria, and the Global Leadership Initiative on Malnutrition (GLIM) Criteria. The widely used ASPEN/AND criteria have an etiology-based approach that recognizes the role of inflammation in the development of malnutrition.

Clinical Findings

Clinical manifestations of protein–energy malnutrition include mild growth restriction in children, weight loss in adults, and several distinct clinical syndromes. Clinical manifestations of protein–energy malnutrition are determined by the patient's nutritional status prior to illness, the disease process itself, associated treatments, and severity of the malnutrition.

Performing a nutrition-focused physical assessment is essential to determine clinical manifestations of protein–energy malnutrition. Wasting begins with weight loss and can be seen in adipose tissue, muscle mass, or both. Cachexia is defined as loss of lean body mass only, irrespective of adipose tissues changes, and it is associated with inflammation and protein catabolism. Muscle mass depletion is seen in the temples, clavicles, shoulders, scapulae, hands, thighs, and calves. Subcutaneous body fat loss may be evident in orbital areas, triceps, and around the rib cage. Dependent edema, ascites, or anasarca may develop and can be assessed on physical examination. Laboratory studies may be unremarkable—serum albumin, for example, tends to be normal in patients with malnutrition related to social, behavioral, or environmental etiologies; however, levels decline in the presence of inflammation and tend to be low in patients who have malnutrition related to acute and chronic diseases. Overall, albumin is not considered a good marker of malnutrition and should not be used as part of diagnosis. Similarly, laboratory assessment of micronutrient deficiencies may not be reliable in the presence of inflammation.

Treatment

The treatment of protein–energy malnutrition should be a slow process and requires great care, especially in chronic and severe cases. In early treatment, the focus is to prevent refeeding syndrome, which is defined as a range of electrolyte alterations following the provision of calories (glucose) after a period of decreased or absent caloric intake. Patients who are refed too quickly are at risk for developing HF due to fluid and electrolyte shifts.

The initial phase of treatment corrects fluid and electrolyte abnormalities, particularly phosphorus, potassium, and magnesium. The second phase of treatment cautiously repletes calories, protein, and micronutrients. Although patients can receive adequate amounts of protein, this may be difficult to achieve with the conservative initiation and advancement of total calories. Depending on the severity of malnutrition, patients may benefit from as little as 10–20 kcal/kg/day for the first few days with advancement of calories as tolerated over the next 7 days. Once out of the initial refeeding window, most patients should receive at least 30–35 kcal/kg/day and 1.5 g protein/kg/day, although some may require significantly more depending on their BMI and severity of malnutrition. All patients should receive thiamine 100 mg daily for at least 5–7 days.

Refeeding edema is benign but must be differentiated from HF. Changes in renal sodium reabsorption and poor skin and blood vessel integrity may result in dependent edema. Treatment includes elevation of the edematous area and sodium restriction, if appropriate. Diuretics should not be used.

Nutrition screening is essential to identify malnourished patients and those at risk of malnutrition. These patients require a formal nutrition assessment with targeted interventions and close monitoring.

Cristancho C et al. Malnutrition in patients with obesity: an overview perspective. Nutr Clin Pract. 2024;39:1300. [PMID: 39439423]

Tomasiewicz A et al. Advancing the understanding of malnutrition in the elderly population: current insights and future directions. Nutrients. 2024;16:2502. [PMID: 39125381]

OBESITY

ESSENTIALS OF DIAGNOSIS

- Disorder of energy homeostasis; BMI ≥ 30; however, definitions are evolving.
- Central obesity (abdomen and flank) is a greater cardiometabolic health risk than excess weight in the lower body (buttocks and thighs).
- Associated with numerous comorbid conditions including type 2 diabetes mellitus, hypertension, hyperlipidemia, heart disease, stroke, and obstructive sleep apnea.

Definition & Measurement

Obesity is a multifactorial, chronic disease characterized by an accumulation of fat, which promotes adipocyte dysfunction. Obesity predisposes to a wide variety of comorbid conditions. **BMI** typically correlates with excess adipose tissue but does not reflect body composition. BMI is calculated by dividing body weight in kilograms by height in meters squared (kg/m^2). The NIH defines healthy BMI as 18.5–24.9. Overweight is defined as BMI 25–29.9. BMI for class I obesity is 30–34.9, class II is 35–39.9, and class III is 40 and above. Central obesity (excess adipose tissue around the waist and flank) is a greater cardiometabolic health risk than lower body obesity (adipose tissue in the thighs and buttocks). Patients with obesity and increased abdominal circumference (> 102 cm or 40 inches in men and 88 cm or 35 inches in women) or high waist–hip ratios (> 1.0 in men and 0.85 in women) have a greater risk of weight-related comorbid conditions and early death than patients with the same BMI and lower ratios. There are different BMI and abdominal circumference thresholds for different populations. Visceral fat is more hazardous to health than subcutaneous fat. Over 40% of American adults and over 16% of adults globally have obesity.

Health Consequences of Obesity

Obesity is associated with significant increases in both morbidity and mortality, and many disorders occur with greater frequency in patients with obesity. Obesity-related comorbidities include leading causes of preventable death such as heart disease, stroke, type 2 diabetes, and a variety of cancers. Over 200 health conditions ranging from hypertension and CAD to thromboembolic and skin disorders are more prevalent in patients with obesity. Patients with obesity have increased surgical and obstetric risks, and most patients with excess weight have experienced weight bias, stigma, and discrimination.

Etiology

Most obesity develops from interactions among multiple contributors, including genes, certain medical conditions, obesogenic medications, environmental influences, behavioral factors, and social determinants of health. Twin studies demonstrate that genetics account for 40–90% of variation in body weight, although only a small percentage is due to single gene mutations.

Medical Evaluation of the Patient with Obesity

A comprehensive medical evaluation is necessary to determine contributors to obesity, complications of obesity, and barriers to obesity treatment. In addition to a thorough medical history, a weight-specific history should include age at onset of weight gain; lifetime weight fluctuations; previous obesity interventions; family history of obesity; physical activity; dietary recall; eating behaviors; and psychosocial factors, including assessment for sleep, mood, and eating disorders.

Physical examination should assess BMI, body composition when possible, and nutritional status. There is an ongoing debate about the best approach to diagnose and risk stratify obesity. While BMI has been widely used, growing evidence suggests that the body roundness index (BRI) may be more accurate in measuring weight distribution and the medical risks associated with obesity. The BRI estimates visceral adipose tissue from a formula that includes waist circumference, hip circumference, and height. The higher the BRI, the greater the risk is for developing CVD, diabetes, and hypertension.

Signs of secondary causes of obesity should be pursued; however, < 1% of patients have an identifiable cause. Cushing syndrome is an example that can be diagnosed by physical examination and laboratory testing (see Chapter 29). All patients should be screened for weight-related comorbid conditions, including obstructive sleep apnea. Blood pressure, waist circumference, fasting glucose, comprehensive metabolic profile, lipid panel, TSH, and hemoglobin A_{1c} should be measured as well as other clinically indicated laboratory tests.

Treatment

Weight loss of 5–10% total body weight is sufficient for many patients with obesity to achieve clinically relevant health benefits, and the magnitude of these benefits is "dose-related." Magnitude of weight loss at 1 year is strongly associated with improvements in many parameters including blood glucose, blood pressure, triglycerides, HDL cholesterol, and various inflammatory markers.

Successful treatment of obesity requires a multidisciplinary approach to counteract the body's resistance to weight loss, a personalized plan to address the heterogeneity of the disease, and ongoing support to prevent weight regain. While diet, physical activity, and behavioral modifications are the cornerstone of obesity care, most individuals with obesity require medical obesity treatment for long-term disease management. Lifestyle interventions alone lead to an average weight loss of only 3–5%, and weight regain is common. As a result, the conversation surrounding **dietary strategies** should focus on health improvements instead of weight loss. Recommendations for specific diets should be tailored to a patient's dietary preferences, as adherence is associated with better outcomes. Dietary instructions should emphasize intake of predominantly "unprocessed" whole foods while limiting foods that provide large amounts of calories without other nutrients, such as ultra-processed foods, sugary drinks, fast food, junk food, and sweets. A Mediterranean diet can be a good option for patients at high cardiovascular risk, since it has been shown to reduce the incidence of major cardiovascular events. A low-glycemic-index diet can curb hunger and decrease cravings by reducing blood glucose fluctuations. Registered dietitians can provide dietary education and customize dietary plans.

Long-term changes in eating behavior as well as **behavior modification** strategies are necessary to support ongoing obesity management. It is important to emphasize meal planning and self-monitoring, including weighing at regular intervals. Some patients maintain a food log to track caloric intake. Self-monitoring aids in behavioral change and provides the clinician with data to guide recommendations. Weight maintenance is often more challenging than initial weight loss, so it is important to continue regular follow-up to reinforce ongoing adherence to a treatment plan and to address challenges as they arise.

Physical activity is an important component of obesity treatment. Aerobic exercise increases daily energy expenditure and partially prevents the decrease in basal energy expenditure (BEE) resulting from weight loss. It supports long-term weight maintenance and helps preserve lean body mass. The combination of exercise and diet results in greater weight loss than diet or exercise alone. Up to 1 hour of moderate exercise per day is associated with long-term weight maintenance.

The American College of Sports Medicine recommends 150 minutes of moderate-intensity aerobic physical activity (such as tennis or brisk walking) per week, 75 minutes of vigorous-intensity aerobic exercise (such as jogging or swimming laps) per week, or an equivalent combination of moderate- and vigorous-intensity aerobic activity. Exercise should be spread throughout the week. Resistance training is also recommended at least twice per week. Exercise physiologists and physical therapists can provide support for patients.

Prescription and over-the-counter medications can have unpredictable and variable effects on weight, so it is important to review patients' medication regimens and balance benefits against the probability of weight gain. **Obesogenic medications** are associated with weight gain and include corticosteroids; contraceptives (and other hormonal agents); and certain antidiabetic, antihypertensive, antidepressant, antipsychotic, antiepileptic, and antihistamine agents. Table 33–1 provides an overview of weight-gaining medications as well as potential alternatives. When possible, clinicians should prescribe weight-neutral– or weight-loss–promoting medications. If there are no alternatives, weight gain can be prevented or mitigated by selecting the lowest effective medication dose for the shortest duration. Lifestyle interventions, self-monitoring, and concomitant obesity medications can also counteract weight gain associated with obesogenic medications.

Weight loss achieved by lifestyle modification alone is generally limited and difficult to maintain because reduced calorie intake and increased energy expenditure are counteracted by adaptive physiologic responses. Appetite increases and resting metabolic rate (RMR) decreases disproportionately to what would be expected based on changes in body composition. This phenomenon is called metabolic adaptation or adaptive thermogenesis. It inhibits weight loss and leads to weight regain. As a result, most patients with obesity require medical intervention with obesity medications, bariatric surgery, devices, endoscopic bariatric therapies, or a combination of treatments to treat their obesity effectively and sustainably.

Obesity medications (OMs) (Table 33–2) should be considered in patients with a BMI 30 or higher, or a BMI 27 or higher with weight-related comorbidities. Most agents affect mechanisms regulating appetite through nutrient-stimulated hormone, serotonergic, dopaminergic, or noradrenergic pathways. They target the arcuate nucleus

Table 33–1. Medications and their effects on weight.

Drug Class	Result: Weight Gain	Result: Weight Neutral (or Minor Weight Gain)	Result: Weight Loss
Antidiabetics	Insulin Meglitinides Sulfonylureas Thiazolidinediones	α-Glucosidase inhibitors Bromocriptine Colesevelam DPP-4 inhibitors	GLP-1 agonists GLP-1/GIP dual agonist Metformin SGLT-2 inhibitors
Antihypertensives	α-Blockers β-Blockers (atenolol, metoprolol, nadolol, propranolol)	ACE inhibitors ARBs β-Blockers (carvedilol, nebivolol) Calcium channel blockers Thiazides	
Antidepressants	Lithium MAO inhibitors Mirtazapine SNRIs (duloxetine, venlafaxine) SSRIs (citalopram, paroxetine) Tricyclic antidepressants (amitriptyline, desipramine, doxepin, imipramine, nortriptyline)	SSRIs (fluoxetine, sertraline)	Bupropion
Antipsychotics	Clozapine Haloperidol Olanzapine Quetiapine Risperidone	Lurasidone Ziprasidone	
Antiepileptics	Carbamazepine Gabapentin Pregabalin Valproic acid	Lamotrigine Levetiracetam Phenytoin	Topiramate Zonisamide
Contraceptives	Medroxyprogesterone acetate	Barrier methods IUDs Surgical sterilization	
Antihistamines	First-generation antihistamines	Second- and third-generation antihistamines	
Steroids	Glucocorticoids	Inhaled steroids Topical steroids	

DPP-4, dipeptidyl peptidase-4; GIP, glucose-dependent insulinotropic polypeptide.
Reproduced with permission from Igel LI et.al. Practical use of pharmacotherapy for obesity. Gastroenterology. 2017;152(7):1765–1779.

of the hypothalamus to stimulate the anorexigenic pro-opiomelanocortin (POMC) neurons, which promote satiety. OMs should be prescribed as part of a comprehensive, personalized, and long-term treatment plan including lifestyle intervention (dietary counseling, physical activity, and behavioral modification), education, and close monitoring. The seven most widely prescribed FDA-approved OMs are phentermine, orlistat, phentermine/topiramate extended-release (ER), naltrexone sustained-release (SR)/bupropion SR, liraglutide 3.0 mg, semaglutide 2.4 mg, and tirzepatide. In addition to producing weight loss, each OM improves biomarkers including blood glucose, blood pressure, and lipids. Because obesity is a heterogeneous disease and there is tremendous variability in response to any treatment, medication dosing and titration should be personalized based on efficacy and tolerability. Three OMs have stopping rules, which provide weight loss thresholds after 12–16 weeks of treatment under which medication discontinuation is suggested. When a patient reaches weight and health goals, they should transition to weight maintenance phase of management to prevent weight gain.

Liraglutide 3.0 mg daily and **semaglutide 2.4 mg weekly** are subcutaneous injectable GLP-1 receptor agonists. GLP-1 is a hormone released by GI L-cells during a meal that delays gastric emptying, stimulates glucose-dependent insulin secretion, and reduces food intake. Liraglutide 1.8 mg and semaglutide 2.0 mg are FDA-approved for the treatment of type 2 diabetes, and **liraglutide 3.0 mg** is approved for weight management. It is initiated at a dose of 0.6 mg subcutaneously daily and can be increased by 0.6 mg each week to a maximum of 3.0 mg daily. In a meta-analysis of 8 RCTs, liraglutide 3.0 mg is associated with 4.81% greater total body weight loss than placebo. **Semaglutide 2.4 mg** also is FDA-approved for the treatment of obesity and is the first FDA-approved OM to lower the risk of cardiovascular death, non-fatal heart attack, or non-fatal stroke in adults with established CVD who are overweight or have obesity; it is initiated at a dose

Table 33–2. Medications tested in clinical trials for treatment of obesity.

Medication	Mechanism, Dosage, and Available Formulations	Trial and Duration	Trial Arms	Weight Loss (%)	Most Common Adverse Events	Good Candidates	Poor Candidates
Phentermine (Adipex,[1] Lomaira[2]) Schedule IV controlled substance NOTE: approved for short-term use (up to 3 months)	Adrenergic agonist 8–37.5 mg daily (8 mg dose can be prescribed up to three times daily) Capsule, tablet	Aronne LJ et al[3] 28 weeks	15 mg daily 7.5 mg daily Placebo (topiramate extended-release and phentermine/topiramate extended-release arms excluded)	6.06* 5.45* 1.71	Dry mouth, insomnia, dizziness, irritability	Younger patients who need assistance with appetite suppression	Patients with uncontrolled hypertension, active or unstable coronary disease, hyperthyroidism, glaucoma, anxiety, insomnia, or general sensitivity to stimulants Patients with a history of drug abuse or recent MAO inhibitor use Patients who are pregnant
Orlistat (Alli,[4] Xenical[5])	Lipase inhibitor 60–120 mg three times daily with meals Capsule	XENDOS[6] 208 weeks	120 mg three times daily Placebo	9.6 (week 52)* 5.25 (week 208)* 5.61 (week 52) 2.71 (week 208)	Fecal urgency, oily stool, flatus with discharge, fecal incontinence	Patients with hypercholesterolemia and/or constipation who can limit their intake of dietary fat	Patients with malabsorption syndromes or other GI conditions that predispose to GI upset/diarrhea Patients who cannot modify the fat content of their diets Patients who are pregnant
Phentermine/Topiramate Extended-release (Qsymia)[7] Schedule IV controlled substance	Adrenergic agonist/neurostabilizer 3.75/23–15/92 mg daily Capsule	EQUIP[8] 56 weeks	15/92 mg daily 3.75/23 mg daily Placebo	10.9* 5.1* 1.6	Paresthesias, dizziness, dysgeusia, insomnia, constipation, dry mouth	Younger patients who need assistance with appetite suppression	Patients with uncontrolled hypertension, active or unstable coronary disease, hyperthyroidism, glaucoma, anxiety, insomnia, or general sensitivity to stimulants Patients with a history of drug abuse or recent MAO inhibitor use Patients with a history of nephrolithiasis Patients who are pregnant or trying to conceive

Naltrexone/Bupropion sustained-release (Contrave)[9]	Opioid receptor antagonist/ dopamine and norepinephrine reuptake inhibitor 8/90 mg daily to 16/180 mg twice daily Tablet	COR-I[10] 56 weeks	16/180 mg twice daily 8/180 mg twice daily Placebo	6.1* 5.0* 1.3	Nausea, vomiting, constipation, headache, dizziness, insomnia, dry mouth	Patients who describe cravings for food and/or addictive behaviors related to food; patients who are trying to quit smoking, reduce alcohol intake, and/or who have concomitant depression	Patients with uncontrolled hypertension, uncontrolled pain, recent MAO inhibitor use, history of seizures, or any condition that predisposes to seizure, such as anorexia/ bulimia nervosa, abrupt discontinuation of alcohol, benzodiazepines, barbiturates, or antiepileptic medications Patients who are pregnant
Liraglutide 3.0 mg (Saxenda)[11]	GLP-1 receptor agonist 0.6–3.0 mg daily Prefilled pen for subcutaneous injection	SCALE Obesity and Prediabetes[12] 56 weeks	3.0 mg daily Placebo	8.0* 2.6	Nausea, vomiting, diarrhea, constipation, dyspepsia, abdominal pain	Patients who experience inadequate meal satiety, and/or have type 2 diabetes, prediabetes, or impaired glucose tolerance Patients requiring use of concomitant psychiatric medications	Patients with a history of pancreatitis, personal/family history of MTC or MEN 2 Patients with an aversion to needles Patients who are pregnant
Subcutaneous Semaglutide 2.4 mg (Wegovy)	GLP-1 receptor agonist 0.25–2.4 mg weekly Prefilled pen for subcutaneous injection	STEP 1[13] 68 weeks	Placebo 2.4 mg weekly	2.4 14.9*	Nausea, vomiting, diarrhea, constipation, dyspepsia, abdominal pain	Patients who experience inadequate meal satiety, and/or have type 2 diabetes, prediabetes, or impaired glucose tolerance Patients requiring use of concomitant psychiatric medications Patients with established cardiovascular disease	Patients with a history of pancreatitis, personal/family history of MTC or MEN 2 Patients with an aversion to needles Patients who are pregnant
Oral Semaglutide	GLP-1 receptor agonist 25 mg once daily (gradual escalation every 30 d: 1.5 mg, 4 mg, 9 mg, 25 mg)	OASIS 64 weeks	Placebo 25 mg daily	2.2% 13.6%	Nausea, vomiting, constipation, dyspepsia, diarrhea, headache, eructation	Same as injectable semaglutide	Same as injectable semaglutide

(continued)

Table 33–2. Medications tested in clinical trials for treatment of obesity. (continued)

Medication	Mechanism, Dosage, and Available Formulations	Trial and Duration	Trial Arms	Weight Loss (%)	Most Common Adverse Events	Good Candidates	Poor Candidates
Tirzepatide (Zepbound)	GLP-1/GIP dual agonist 2.5–15 mg weekly Prefilled pen for subcutaneous injection	SURMOUNT 1[15] 72 weeks	Placebo 5 mg weekly 10 mg weekly 15 mg weekly	3.1% 15%* 19.5%* 20.9%*	Nausea, diarrhea, vomiting, constipation, abdominal pain, dyspepsia	Patients who experience inadequate meal satiety, and/or have type 2 diabetes, prediabetes, or impaired glucose tolerance Patients requiring use of concomitant psychiatric medications Patients with obstructive sleep apnea	Patients with a history of pancreatitis, personal/family history of MTC or MEN 2 Patients with an aversion to needles Patients who are pregnant

*$P < 0.001$ versus placebo.

GIP, glucose-dependent insulinotropic polypeptide; MEN 2, multiple endocrine neoplasia type 2; MTC, medullary thyroid cancer.

[1]Adipex [package insert]. Tulsa, OK: Physicians Total Care, Inc; 2012.
[2]Lomaira [package insert]. Newtown, PA: KVK-TECH, INC; 2016.
[3]Aronne LJ et al. Evaluation of phentermine and topiramate versus phentermine/topiramate extended-release in obese adults. Obesity (Silver Spring). 2013;21:2163.
[4]Alli [package insert]. Moon Township, PA: GlaxoSmithKline Consumer Healthcare, LP; 2015.
[5]Xenical [package insert]. South San Francisco, CA: Genentech USA, Inc; 2015.
[6]Torgerson JS et al. XENical in the prevention of diabetes in obese subjects (XENDOS) study: a randomized study of orlistat as an adjunct to lifestyle changes for the prevention of type 2 diabetes in obese patients. Diabetes Care. 2004;27:155.
[7]Qsymia [package insert]. Mountain View, CA: VIVUS, Inc; 2012.
[8]Allison DB et al. Controlled-release phentermine/topiramate in severely obese adults: a randomized controlled trial (EQUIP). Obesity (Silver Spring). 2012;20:330.
[9]Contrave [package insert]. Deerfield, IL: Takeda Pharmaceuticals America, Inc; 2014.
[10]Greenway FL et al. Effect of naltrexone plus bupropion on weight loss in overweight and obese adults (COR-I): a multicentre, randomised, double-blind, placebo-controlled, phase 3 trial. Lancet. 2010;376:595.
[11]Saxenda [package insert]. Plainsboro, NJ: Novo Nordisk; 2014.
[12]Pi-Sunyer X et al. A randomized, controlled trial of 3.0 mg of liraglutide in weight management. N Engl J Med. 2015;373:11.
[13]Wilding JPH et al. Once-weekly semaglutide in adults with overweight or obesity. N Engl J Med. 2021;384:989.
[14]Wharton S et al. Oral Semaglutide at a Dose of 25 mg in Adults with Overweight or Obesity. N Engl J Med. 2025;393(11):1077-1087. [PMID: 40934115]
[15]Jastreboff AM et al; SURMOUNT-1 Investigators. Tirzepatide once weekly for the treatment of obesity. N Engl J Med. 2022;387:205.

of 0.25 mg subcutaneously weekly and can be titrated to a maximum dose of 2.4 mg weekly. In a meta-analysis of eight RCTs, semaglutide was associated with a 10.8% greater mean total body weight loss than placebo. In the 2023 SELECT cardiovascular outcomes trial, semaglutide 2.4 mg reduced the risk of major adverse cardiovascular events (MACE) by 20% in adults aged 45 and older with BMI > 27 and preexisting CVD without type 2 diabetes. In 2025, semaglutide 2.4 mg also was approved for the treatment of noncirrhotic metabolic dysfunction-associated steatohepatitis (MASH) in adults with moderate to advanced liver fibrosis. Both liraglutide and semaglutide may cause nausea, vomiting, constipation, or diarrhea, and a small increase in pancreatitis and cholecystitis. There is a boxed warning that both liraglutide and semaglutide may cause thyroid C-cell tumors (including medullary thyroid carcinoma) in rodents; however, there is no evidence that GLP-1 receptor agonists cause C-cell tumors in humans.

Tirzepatide is a subcutaneous injectable agonist targeting receptors of both GLP-1 as well as glucose-dependent insulinotropic polypeptide (GIP), another nutrient-stimulated hormone that regulates energy balance through signaling in the brain and adipose tissue. Tirzepatide is FDA-approved for the treatment of type 2 diabetes and obesity management, and in 2024 received an expanded indication for the treatment of moderate to severe obstructive sleep apnea in adults with obesity. It is initiated at a dose of 2.5 mg subcutaneously weekly and can be increased by 2.5 mg each month to a maximum of 15 mg subcutaneously weekly. In the SURMOUNT-1 trial, tirzepatide 15 mg weekly produced a 20.9% total body weight loss compared to 3.1% with placebo. Tirzepatide is associated with the same contraindications, adverse events, and boxed warnings as liraglutide and semaglutide, but is typically better tolerated. Tirzepatide delays gastric emptying and has the potential to decrease absorption of oral medications including contraceptives.

In 2025, **oral semaglutide** was the first oral GLP-1 receptor agonist to receive FDA approval to reduce excess body weight and maintain long-term weight reduction in adults with obesity or who are overweight with at least one weight-related comorbid condition; it was also approved to reduce the risk of MACE in adults with obesity or who are overweight who have established CVD. Oral semaglutide is initiated at a dose of 1.5 mg daily and can be increased every 30 days to 4 mg, 9 mg, and then 25 mg daily. The tablets are administered once daily on an empty stomach in the morning with water (up to 4 ounces) at least 30 minutes before eating food, drinking beverages, or taking other oral medications. In the OASIS 4 trial, oral semaglutide was associated with 13.6% total body weight loss at 64 weeks compared to 2.2% with placebo in adults without diabetes who had obesity or who were overweight with one or more weight-related comorbidities. As incretin-based medications rapidly gain popularity, prescription practices for OM are shifting away from adrenergic agonists, including phentermine (which has been the most prescribed OM agent) and other agents (including diethylpropion, benzphetamine, and phendimetrazine). In a meta-analysis of seven short-term RCTs, phentermine was associated with 3.63% greater total body weight loss than placebo. The maximum recommended dosage of phentermine is 37.5 mg daily, but the dosage should be individualized to the lowest effective dose. Phentermine is indicated for short-term use (3 months), as there are no longer-term trials of phentermine monotherapy. However, many clinicians may prescribe it for long-term OM as obesity is a chronic disease, depending on state restrictions.

Phentermine is approved for long-term OM in combination with **topiramate ER**. The combination of phentermine and topiramate ER (3.75 mg/23 mg orally daily for 14 days, then 7.5 mg/46 mg orally daily, to a maximum dosage of 15 mg/92 mg orally daily) targets two different weight-regulation mechanisms simultaneously. In a 56-week clinical trial, participants taking 15/92 mg lost significantly more weight (9.8%) than those assigned to 7.5/46 mg (7.8%) or placebo (1.2%). A meta-analysis of three RCTs with 52–56 weeks of follow-up found that phentermine/topiramate ER resulted in 8.45% greater total body weight loss than placebo. There is a potential increased risk of orofacial clefts in infants exposed to topiramate during the first trimester of pregnancy.

The combination of **naltrexone SR** and **bupropion SR** (8 mg/90 mg, increasing from 1 tablet orally daily by 1 additional daily tablet each week to a maximum of 2 tablets twice daily) reduces both appetite and food cravings by targeting two areas of the brain: the arcuate nucleus of the hypothalamus and the mesolimbic dopamine reward circuit. Naltrexone 32 mg/bupropion 360 mg is associated with a 6.1% reduction in body weight compared to 1.3% with placebo after 56 weeks. As with all antidepressants, bupropion carries a black box warning related to a potential increase in suicidality among patients under age 24 years during the early phase of treatment.

Orlistat works in the GI tract to inhibit intestinal lipase, thus reducing dietary fat absorption. Orlistat may thereby cause steatorrhea, fecal urgency, abdominal discomfort, and reduced absorption of fat-soluble vitamins. A meta-analysis of RCTs found that individuals taking orlistat lost 2.8% more total body weight compared with placebo. Orlistat is used infrequently in current clinical practice given newer OMs with greater efficacy and tolerability.

Metabolic and bariatric surgery is associated with significant and sustained weight loss, reduction or resolution of obesity-related comorbidities, and improved quality of life. Metabolic and bariatric surgery is also associated with lower incidence of cardiovascular events, decreased number of cardiovascular deaths, and reduced overall mortality compared to usual care. The two most common metabolic and bariatric procedures in the United States are the sleeve gastrectomy and the Roux-en-Y gastric bypass. The laparoscopic adjustable gastric band and other surgical procedures are performed less frequently. In general, metabolic and bariatric surgery should be considered in patients with a BMI ≥ 40 or with a BMI ≥ 35 with at least one obesity-related complication who failed to achieve sufficient or sustained disease management following lifestyle modification, with or without OM. Long-term medical follow-up, lifestyle changes, and adherence to a vitamin regimen are crucial to the success of metabolic and bariatric surgery.

Many patients experience some degree of weight regain. Despite the known benefits of metabolic and bariatric surgery, < 1% of eligible patients undergo surgery to treat their obesity. This is likely due to limited patient knowledge of the health benefits of surgery, limited provider comfort in recommending surgery, inadequate insurance coverage, and the growing list of effective OMs.

The **sleeve gastrectomy** removes approximately 70% of the stomach body and antrum along the greater curvature. Sleeve gastrectomy is associated with approximately 25% total body weight loss after 1 year. Because this procedure is mainly restrictive (versus the Roux-en-Y gastric bypass, which is also malabsorptive), there is a lower risk of nutritional deficiencies. In general, sleeve gastrectomy is associated with fewer complications than the Roux-en-Y gastric bypass. Late complications include gastroesophageal reflux, nutritional deficiencies, and stomach expansion, leading to decreased restriction.

The **Roux-en-Y gastric bypass** involves a staple partition across the proximal stomach with attachment of the small proximal stomach to a jejunal limb, thus bypassing the remainder of the stomach, duodenum, and the proximal jejunum. Roux-en-Y gastric bypass is associated with approximately 30% total body weight loss at 1 year and greater improvements in comorbid disease markers compared to the sleeve gastrectomy. It is associated with a lower rate of gastroesophageal reflux than the sleeve gastrectomy and can even alleviate gastroesophageal reflux in patients who have it. It is often recommended over sleeve gastrectomy for patients with type 2 diabetes because it leads to greater long-term remission. Late adverse events include nutritional deficiencies (eg, vitamins B_1, B_{12}, D, and iron) and anastomosis ulceration. Dumping syndrome can develop at any time. Roux-en-Y gastric bypass is technically a reversible procedure; however, it is generally only reversed in extreme circumstances.

Patients who cannot achieve clinically meaningful weight loss with OMs and who are not candidates or choose not to undergo bariatric surgery fall into a "treatment gap." Several **devices and endoscopic procedures** are available that are reversible and minimally invasive. In addition, they may be less expensive and safer than metabolic and bariatric surgery for poor surgical candidates.

When to Refer

- Patients with obesity (BMI ≥ 30) and patients who are overweight (BMI ≥ 27) with at least one weight-related comorbid condition may be referred to an obesity medicine specialist.
- Patients with a BMI ≥ 40 or ≥ 35 with at least one obesity-related comorbid condition who have not achieved sufficient weight loss to address health goals following behavioral treatment, with or without obesity medication, may be referred to a bariatric surgeon.

Aronne LJ et al. Continued treatment with tirzepatide for maintenance of weight reduction in adults with obesity: the SURMOUNT-4 randomized clinical trial. JAMA. 2024;331:38. [PMID: 38078870]

Jordan G et al. Weight loss pharmacotherapy: current and future therapies. Gastrointest Endosc Clin N Am. 2024;34:591. [PMID: 39277293]

McGowan B et al. Framework for the pharmacological treatment of obesity and its complications from the European Association for the Study of Obesity (EASO). Nat Med. 2025;31:3229. [PMID: 41039115]

Rubino F et al. Definition and diagnostic criteria of clinical obesity. Lancet Diabetes Endocrinol. 2025;13:221. [PMID: 39824205]

Thomsen RW et al. Real-world evidence on the utilization, clinical and comparative effectiveness, and advance effects of newer GLP-1RA-based weight-loss therapies. Diabetes Obes Metab. 2025;27:66. [PMID:40196933]

EATING DISORDERS

ANOREXIA NERVOSA

ESSENTIALS OF DIAGNOSIS

- Restriction of energy intake leading to a significantly low body weight in the context of age, sex, developmental trajectory, and physical health.
- Intense fear of gaining weight or behavior that prevents weight gain.
- Distorted perception of body image, with exaggerated influence of weight on self-worth.
- Denial of the medical seriousness of underweight status.

General Considerations

Anorexia nervosa is characterized by low body weight, intense fear of gaining weight, and distorted perception of body image. Anorexia nervosa typically begins in the years between adolescence and young adulthood but often persists into older adulthood.

The prevalence of anorexia nervosa is greater than previously suggested. The American Psychiatric Association's *DSM-5* classifies the severity of anorexia according to BMI: mild, BMI 17–18.49; moderate, BMI 16–16.99; severe, BMI 15–15.99; extreme, BMI < 15.

There are two subtypes of anorexia nervosa: binge-eating/purging type and restricting type. The binge-eating/purging subtype is characterized by recurrent episodes of binge-eating or purging (ie, self-induced vomiting and/or abuse of diuretics, laxatives, enemas, cathartics). The restricting subtype is characterized by dieting, fasting, or excessive exercising without associated binge-eating or purging.

The cause of anorexia nervosa is not known. Although multiple endocrinologic abnormalities exist in patients with anorexia nervosa, most authorities believe they are secondary to malnutrition and not the primary disorder. Most experts favor a primary psychiatric origin, but no hypothesis explains all cases. The patient characteristically comes from a family whose members are highly goal oriented.

Patients are often perfectionistic in behavior, exhibit obsessional personality characteristics, or have preoccupation with food.

Clinical Findings

A. Symptoms and Signs

Patients with anorexia nervosa may exhibit severe emaciation and frequently report cold intolerance or constipation. Bradycardia, hypotension, and hypothermia may be present in severe cases. Physical examination demonstrates loss of body fat, dry and scaly skin, and increased lanugo body hair. Parotid enlargement and edema may also occur. In women of reproductive age, cessation of menstruation (functional hypothalamic amenorrhea) is common.

B. Laboratory Findings

Laboratory findings are variable but may include anemia, leukopenia, electrolyte abnormalities, and elevations of BUN and serum creatinine. Serum cholesterol levels are often increased. Endocrine abnormalities include depressed levels of LH and FSH and impaired response of LH to gonadotropin-releasing hormone.

Diagnosis & Differential Diagnosis

The diagnosis is based on energy restriction, significantly low body weight, distorted body image, intense fear of weight gain or of loss of control over food intake, and refusal to exceed a minimal healthy weight. Other medical or psychiatric illnesses that can account for anorexia and weight loss must be excluded.

The differential diagnosis includes bulimia nervosa, binge-eating disorder, endocrine and metabolic disorders (eg, panhypopituitarism, Addison disease, hyperthyroidism, and diabetes mellitus), GI disorders (eg, Crohn disease and gluten enteropathy), chronic infections (eg, tuberculosis), cancers (eg, lymphoma), and rare CNS disorders (eg, hypothalamic tumor).

Treatment

The goal of treatment is restoration of healthy body weight and improvement in psychological comorbidities. Hospitalization may be necessary, especially when refeeding syndrome and severe electrolyte abnormalities are anticipated. Treatment programs delivered by experienced teams successfully restore healthy weight in approximately two-thirds of cases. The remainder continue to experience difficulties with underweight, disordered eating behaviors, and associated psychiatric conditions. Up to 6% of patients die of complications of the disorder or by suicide.

Various treatment methods have been used without clear evidence of superiority of one over another. Supportive care by clinicians and family is the most important feature of any therapy. Cognitive-behavioral therapy, intensive psychotherapy, and family therapy may be tried. A variety of medications including tricyclic antidepressants, SSRIs, and lithium are effective in some cases. Patients with severe malnutrition must be hemodynamically stabilized and may require enteral or parenteral feeding. Forced feedings should be reserved for life-threatening situations, since the goal of treatment is to reestablish healthy eating behavior.

When to Refer

- Adolescents and young adults with otherwise unexplained profound weight loss should be evaluated by a psychiatrist or eating disorders specialist.
- All patients with diagnosed anorexia nervosa should be treated by a multidisciplinary team, including physicians, psychiatrists, social workers, and dietitians.

When to Admit

- Signs of hypovolemia, major electrolyte disorders, and severe protein–energy malnutrition.
- Failure to improve with outpatient management.

Attia E et al. Eating disorders: a review. JAMA. 2025;333:1242. [PMID: 40048192]

Baenas I et al. Medical complications in anorexia and bulimia nervosa. Med Clin (Barc). 2024;162:67. [PMID: 37598049]

Himmerich H et al. Anorexia nervosa: diagnostic, therapeutic, and risk biomarkers in clinical practice. Trend Mol Med. 2024;30:350. [PMID: 38331700]

Voderholzer U et al. Anorexia nervosa–an update. Nervenarzt. 2025;96:220. [PMID: 40434418]

BULIMIA NERVOSA

ESSENTIALS OF DIAGNOSIS

- Uncontrolled episodes of binge-eating at least weekly for 3 months.
- Recurrent inappropriate compensatory behavior to prevent weight gain such as self-induced vomiting, laxatives, diuretics, fasting, or excessive exercise.
- Excessive concern with body weight and body shape, with exaggerated influence of weight on self-worth.

General Considerations

Bulimia nervosa is the episodic uncontrolled ingestion of large quantities of food followed by recurrent compensatory behavior to prevent weight gain, such as self-induced vomiting, diuretic or cathartic use, strict dieting, or vigorous exercise. Bulimia nervosa is harder to diagnose than anorexia as patients often maintain a normal or elevated BMI.

Clinical Findings

Patients with bulimia nervosa typically consume large quantities of easily ingested high-calorie foods, usually in secrecy. Some patients may have several such episodes per day over multiple days; others report regular and persistent patterns of binge-eating. Binging is usually followed by vomiting, cathartics, or diuretics and accompanied by feelings of guilt or depression. Periods of binging may be followed by intervals of self-imposed starvation. Body weight may fluctuate but generally remains within 20% of normal BMI.

Family and psychological conditions are generally similar to those of patients with anorexia nervosa. Patients with bulimia, however, have a higher incidence of obesity, greater use of cathartics and diuretics, and more impulsive or antisocial behavior. Menstruation is typically preserved.

Medical complications are numerous. Gastric dilatation and pancreatitis have been reported after binges. Vomiting can result in poor dentition, pharyngitis, esophagitis, aspiration, and electrolyte abnormalities. Cathartic and diuretic abuse can also cause electrolyte abnormalities or dehydration. Constipation is common.

Treatment

Treatment of bulimia nervosa includes supportive care and psychotherapy. Individual, group, family, and behavioral therapy are all options. Antidepressant medications may be helpful, especially fluoxetine and other SSRIs. Although death from bulimia is rare, the long-term psychiatric prognosis is worse for severe bulimia than anorexia nervosa.

When to Refer

All patients with diagnosed bulimia should be treated by a multidisciplinary team, including physicians, psychiatrists, social workers, and dietitians.

Attia E et al. Eating disorders: a review. JAMA. 2025;333:1242. [PMID: 40048192]

Baenas I et al. Medical complications in anorexia and bulimia nervosa. Med Clin (Barc). 2024;162:67. [PMID: 37598049]

Matheson BE. Bulimia nervosa and binge-eating disorder across the lifespan. Focus (Am Psychiatr Publ). 2024;22:278. [PMID: 38988471]

Wilson K et al. Bulimia nervosa and treatment-related disparities: a review. Front Psychol. 2024;15:1386347. [PMID: 39205982]

DISORDERS OF VITAMIN METABOLISM

THIAMINE (B_1) DEFICIENCY

Most thiamine deficiency in the United States is due to alcohol use disorder, with poor dietary intake of thiamine and impaired thiamine absorption, metabolism, and storage. It is also associated with malabsorption (eg, following metabolic and bariatric surgery), dialysis, and other causes of chronic protein–calorie undernutrition. Thiamine depletion can be precipitated when patients with low thiamine are given a large carbohydrate load, such as enteral or parenteral nutrition.

Clinical Findings

Early manifestations of thiamine deficiency include anorexia, muscle cramps, paresthesia, and irritability. Advanced deficiency primarily affects the cardiovascular system ("wet beriberi") or the nervous system ("dry beriberi"). Wet beriberi occurs in thiamine deficiency accompanied by severe physical exertion and high carbohydrate intake. Dry beriberi occurs in thiamine deficiency accompanied by inactivity and low-calorie intake.

Wet beriberi is characterized by marked peripheral vasodilation resulting in high-output HF with dyspnea, tachycardia, cardiomegaly, pulmonary edema, and peripheral edema with warm extremities mimicking cellulitis.

Dry beriberi involves both the peripheral and central nervous system. Peripheral nerve involvement is typically a symmetric motor and sensory neuropathy with pain, paresthesia, and loss of reflexes. Legs are affected more than arms. CNS involvement results in Wernicke-Korsakoff syndrome. Wernicke encephalopathy consists of nystagmus progressing to ophthalmoplegia, truncal ataxia, and confusion. Korsakoff syndrome includes amnesia, confabulation, and impaired learning.

Diagnosis

In most instances, the clinical response to empiric thiamine therapy is used to support a diagnosis of thiamine deficiency. The most common biochemical tests measure thiamine concentration directly, while other assays measure erythrocyte transketolase activity and urinary thiamine excretion. Normal thiamine values typically range from 70 nmol/L to 180 nmol/L.

Treatment

Thiamine deficiency is treated with large parenteral doses of thiamine. Fifty to 100 mg/day is initially administered intravenously, followed by daily oral doses of 5–100 mg/day. It is important to note that thiamine supplementation is only effective if magnesium is replete. All patients should simultaneously receive therapeutic doses of other water-soluble vitamins. Treatment results in complete resolution in one-fourth of patients immediately and another one-fourth over days, but half achieve only partial or no benefit.

When to Refer

Patients with signs of dry beriberi or Wernicke-Korsakoff syndrome should be referred to a neurologist. Patients with signs of wet beriberi should be referred to a cardiologist.

THIAMINE TOXICITY

There is no known toxicity of thiamine.

Panda A et al. Thiamine deficiency in diabetes, obesity and bariatric surgery: recipes for diabetes ketoacidosis. J Family Med Prim Care. 2024;13:1620. [PMID: 38948636]

RIBOFLAVIN (B_2) DEFICIENCY

Clinical Findings

Riboflavin deficiency usually occurs in combination with other vitamin deficiencies. Dietary inadequacy, interactions with medications, alcohol use disorder, and other causes of protein–calorie undernutrition are the most common causes.

Manifestations of riboflavin deficiency include cheilosis, angular stomatitis, glossitis, seborrheic dermatitis, weakness, corneal vascularization, and anemia.

Diagnosis

Riboflavin deficiency can be confirmed by measuring the riboflavin-dependent enzyme erythrocyte glutathione reductase.

Treatment

When suspected, riboflavin deficiency is usually treated empirically with foods such as meat, fish, and dairy products or with oral preparations of the vitamin. Administration of 10–20 mg/day until clinical findings resolve is usually adequate. Riboflavin can also be given parenterally.

RIBOFLAVIN TOXICITY

There is no known toxicity of riboflavin.

Zhang B et al. Riboflavin deficiency and apoptosis: a review. J Nutr. 2025;155:27. [PMID: 39510506]

NIACIN DEFICIENCY

"Niacin" is a generic term for nicotinic acid and other derivatives with similar nutritional activity. Unlike most other vitamins, niacin can be synthesized from the amino acid tryptophan. Niacin is an essential component of the co-enzymes nicotinamide adenine dinucleotide (NAD) and nicotinamide adenine dinucleotide phosphate (NADP), which are involved in many oxidation-reduction reactions. The main dietary sources of niacin are proteins containing tryptophan (meat, fish, poultry) and enriched cereals and grains.

Niacin in the form of nicotinic acid is used therapeutically for the treatment of hypercholesterolemia and hypertriglyceridemia. Niacinamide (the form of niacin generally used to treat niacin deficiency) does not exhibit the lipid-lowering effects of nicotinic acid.

Clinical Findings

As with other B vitamins, early manifestations of niacin deficiency are nonspecific—anorexia, weakness, irritability, mouth soreness, glossitis, stomatitis, and weight loss. More advanced deficiency results in the classic triad of pellagra: dermatitis, diarrhea, and dementia. Dermatitis is symmetric, involving sun-exposed areas. Skin lesions are dark, dry, and scaly. Dementia begins with insomnia, irritability, and apathy and progresses to confusion, memory loss, hallucinations, and psychosis. Diarrhea can be severe and may result in malabsorption due to atrophy of the intestinal villi. Advanced pellagra can result in death.

Diagnosis

In early deficiency, diagnosis requires a high index of suspicion. Low levels may be found in patients with generalized undernutrition. In advanced cases, the diagnosis of pellagra can be made clinically. Niacin can be measured in urine, serum, or plasma.

Treatment

Niacin deficiency can be treated effectively with oral niacin, usually given as nicotinamide (10–150 mg/day). Advanced stages of pellagra are treated via intramuscular injections of nicotinic acid (50–100 ng/day) three times daily for 3 to 4 days, followed by oral therapy of nicotinic acid.

NIACIN TOXICITY

At the high doses of niacin used to treat hyperlipidemia, side effects are common. These include gastric irritation and cutaneous flushing. Flushing can be partially prevented by pretreatment with aspirin, 81–325 mg/day, and use of extended-release nicotinic acid preparations. Elevation of liver enzymes, hyperglycemia, and gout are less common side effects.

Pan J et al. Dietary niacin intake and mortality among individuals with nonalcoholic fatty liver disease. JAMA. 2024;7:e2354277. [PMID: 38300619]

VITAMIN B_6 DEFICIENCY

Vitamin B_6 deficiency most commonly occurs because of alcohol use disorder or interactions with medications, especially isoniazid, and oral contraceptives. Several inborn errors of metabolism and other pyridoxine-responsive syndromes, particularly pyridoxine-responsive anemia, are not clearly due to vitamin deficiency but commonly respond to high doses of the vitamin. Patients with common variable immunodeficiency may have concomitant vitamin B_6 deficiency.

Clinical Findings

Vitamin B_6 deficiency results in clinical symptoms similar to those of other B vitamin deficiencies, including mouth soreness, glossitis, cheilosis, weakness, and irritability. Severe deficiency can result in peripheral neuropathy, anemia, and seizures.

Diagnosis

The diagnosis of vitamin B_6 deficiency can be confirmed by measurement of pyridoxal phosphate in blood, urinary excretion of 4-pyridoxic acid, and erythrocyte AST or ALT.

Treatment

Vitamin B_6 deficiency can be treated effectively with vitamin B_6 supplements (100 mg/day orally). Some patients taking medications that interfere with pyridoxine metabolism (such as isoniazid) may require prophylactic vitamin B_6 (50–100 mg/day orally) to prevent deficiency. This is true for patients who are more likely to have diets low in vitamin B_6, such as older adults and patients with alcohol use disorder.

VITAMIN B_6 TOXICITY

A sensory neuropathy, at times irreversible, can occur in patients receiving large doses of vitamin B_6 (200–2000 mg/day).

Kato N et al. Relationship of low vitamin B6 status with sarcopenia, frailty, and mortality: a narrative review. Nutrients. 2024;16:177. [PMID: 38202006]

VITAMIN B_{12} & FOLATE

Vitamin B_{12} (cobalamin) and folate are reviewed in Chapter 15.

VITAMIN C (ASCORBIC ACID) DEFICIENCY

Most cases of vitamin C deficiency in the United States are due to dietary inadequacy in older adults, malabsorptive disorders, and alcohol use disorder. Patients with chronic illnesses such as cancer and individuals who smoke cigarettes are also at risk.

Clinical Findings

Early manifestations of vitamin C deficiency are nonspecific and include malaise and weakness. In more advanced stages, the typical features of scurvy develop. Manifestations include perifollicular hemorrhages, perifollicular hyperkeratotic papules, petechiae, purpura, splinter hemorrhages, bleeding gums, hemarthroses, and subperiosteal hemorrhages. Anemia is common, and wound healing is impaired. The late stages of scurvy are characterized by edema, oliguria, neuropathy, intracerebral hemorrhage, and death.

Diagnosis

The diagnosis of advanced scurvy can be made clinically based on skin lesions in the proper clinical setting. Atraumatic hemarthrosis is also highly suggestive. The diagnosis can be confirmed with decreased plasma ascorbic acid levels, typically < 0.2 mg/dL.

Treatment

Adult scurvy can be treated with ascorbic acid 300–1000 mg/day orally. Improvement generally occurs within days.

Golder JE et al. Exploring the relationship between vitamin C deficiency and protein-energy malnutrition in adult hospitalised patients: a cross-sectional study. Nutr Diet. 2025;82:152. [PMID: 39648345]

VITAMIN C TOXICITY

Excessive doses of vitamin C can cause gastric irritation, flatulence, or diarrhea. With adequate renal function, toxicity is rare. Patients with renal failure, kidney stones, iron overload, or those receiving heparin or warfarin should avoid large doses. Vitamin C can confound common diagnostic tests by causing false-negative results for some fecal occult blood tests and both false-negative and false-positive results for urine glucose.

VITAMIN A DEFICIENCY

Clinical Findings

Vitamin A deficiency is one of the most common vitamin deficiency syndromes, particularly in developing countries. In certain regions, it is the most common cause of blindness. In the United States, it is usually due to fat malabsorption syndromes or mineral oil laxative abuse, and it occurs most commonly in older adults and patients with malabsorptive conditions.

Night blindness is the earliest symptom. Dryness of the conjunctiva (xerosis) and the development of small white patches on the conjunctiva (Bitot spots) are early signs. Ulceration and necrosis of the cornea (keratomalacia), perforation, endophthalmitis, and blindness are late manifestations. Xerosis and hyperkeratinization of the skin and loss of taste may also occur.

Diagnosis

Abnormalities of dark adaptation are strongly suggestive of vitamin A deficiency. Serum levels below the normal range of 30–65 mg/dL are commonly seen in advanced deficiency.

Treatment

Night blindness, poor wound healing, and other signs of severe deficiency can be effectively treated with vitamin A 30,000 IU orally daily for 1 week. Oral administration of vitamin A 10,000–15,000 IU daily is recommended to enhance wound healing in patients who are concurrently receiving steroid therapy. In patients with malabsorptive conditions and vitamin A insufficiency, longer term supplementation with 2500–3500 IU daily can be considered.

VITAMIN A TOXICITY

Excess intake of β-carotene (hypercarotenosis) results in staining of the skin a yellow-orange color but is otherwise benign. Skin changes are most marked on the palms and soles, while sclerae remain white, clearly distinguishing hypercarotenosis from jaundice.

Excessive vitamin A (hypervitaminosis A), on the other hand, can be toxic. Chronic toxicity usually occurs after ingestion of daily doses of over 50,000 IU/day for > 3 months. Early manifestations include dry, scaly skin, hair loss, mouth sores, painful hyperostosis, anorexia, and vomiting. More serious findings include hypercalcemia, increased intracranial pressure with papilledema, headaches, decreased cognition, and hepatomegaly, which can progress to cirrhosis. Acute toxicity can result from ingestion of excessive doses of vitamin A via medications or supplements. Manifestations include nausea, vomiting, abdominal pain, headache, papilledema, and lethargy.

The diagnosis can be confirmed by elevations of serum retinol levels. The only treatment is withdrawal of vitamin A from the diet. Most signs and symptoms improve rapidly.

Andres E et al. Fat-soluble vitamins A, D, E, and K: review of the literature and points of interest for the clinician. J Clin Med. 2024;13:3641. [PMID: 38999209]

Rao S et al. Vitamin A and its related diseases. Food Sci Nutr. 2025;13:e70630. [PMID: 40672537]

VITAMIN D

Vitamin D is reviewed in Chapter 30.

VITAMIN E DEFICIENCY

Clinical Findings

Clinical deficiency of vitamin E is most common in patients with fat-malabsorptive disorders, such as Crohn disease, cystic fibrosis, compromised biliary function, or resection of the ileum or small intestine. Deficiency may produce spinocerebellar degeneration of the posterior columns of the spinal cord. Manifestations include slurring of speech, sensory loss, areflexia, disturbances of gait, decreased vibration and proprioception, and ophthalmoplegia. (See Chapter 27.)

Diagnosis

Normal plasma vitamin E levels are 0.5–0.7 mg/dL or higher. Since vitamin E is normally transported in lipoproteins, the serum level should be interpreted in relation to plasma cholesterol levels.

Treatment

The optimal therapeutic dose of vitamin E has not been defined; however, the suggested range is 200–2000 mg/day. Large doses, often administered parenterally, can improve the neurologic complications seen in abetalipoproteinemia and cholestatic liver disease. Vitamin E supplementation may also provide benefit in patients with nonalcoholic fatty liver disease.

VITAMIN E TOXICITY

Clinical trials have suggested an increase in all-cause mortality with high-dose (> 400 IU/day) vitamin E supplements. Large doses of vitamin E can also increase the vitamin K requirement and result in bleeding in patients taking oral anticoagulants.

Kaye AD et al. Vitamin E (a-tocopherol): emerging clinical role and adverse risks of supplementation in adults. Cureus. 2025;17:e78679. [PMID: 40065887]

VITAMIN K

Vitamin K is reviewed in Chapter 16.

DIET THERAPY

Specific therapeutic diets can complement the medical management of most common illnesses. Dietary modifications can be difficult to sustain, and patients may benefit from the support of a registered dietitian. Eliciting a dietary recall is a helpful strategy to provide insight into a patient's dietary preferences and restrictions, and it provides information about nutrient content. Ongoing food tracking can improve dietary adherence for certain patients.

Therapeutic diets can be divided into three groups: (1) diets that alter food consistency, (2) diets that restrict or modify dietary components, and (3) diets that supplement dietary components.

DIETS THAT ALTER CONSISTENCY

Clear Liquid Diet

This diet provides adequate water, 500–1000 kcal as simple sugar, and some electrolytes. It is fiber-free and requires minimal digestion or intestinal motility.

A clear liquid diet is useful for patients with resolving postoperative ileus, acute gastroenteritis, partial intestinal obstruction, and in preparation for diagnostic GI procedures. It is commonly used as the first diet for patients who have been taking nothing by mouth for a long period due to impaired GI function. Because of the low calorie and minimal protein content of the clear liquid diet, it is used only for short durations unless it is in addition to other means of nutrition support.

Full Liquid Diet

The full liquid diet provides adequate water and can be designed to provide sufficient calories and protein. Vitamins and minerals may be inadequate and should be provided in the form of supplements. Dairy products, protein shakes, and pureed soups are used to supplement clear liquids.

This diet is low in residue and can be useful for patients with difficulty chewing or swallowing due to orofacial trauma or surgery, with GI partial obstructions, postoperative (eg, bariatric surgery), or in preparation for certain diagnostic procedures. The full liquid diet should be used temporarily during recovery until it is deemed safe to eat regular foods.

Modified Consistency Diets

Modified consistency diets are designed for patients unable to chew or swallow hard food. Textures range from pureed to easy-to-chew foods. Texture modified diets are commonly used in patients with dysphagia or poor dentition, patients who have undergone head and neck surgery, patients with esophageal strictures, and in postoperative patients to assist in progression from liquid diets to regular diets. Modified consistency diets can be designed to meet all nutritional requirements.

DIETS THAT RESTRICT NUTRIENTS

Diets can be designed to restrict (or eliminate) virtually any nutrient or food component. The most common restricted diets are those that limit sodium, fat, carbohydrate, or protein. Other restrictive diets include gluten restriction for patients with gluten enteropathy, potassium and phosphate reduction in patients with CKD, and elimination of certain allergens for patients with food allergies.

Sodium-Restricted Diets

Low-sodium diets can be useful in the treatment of patients with hypertension and conditions in which sodium retention and edema are prominent features, particularly HF, liver disease, and CKD. For patients taking diuretics, sodium restriction may allow lower dosages of diuretic medications and may prevent side effects. For example, sodium restriction decreases diuretic-related potassium losses by reducing distal tubule sodium delivery.

Typical American diets contain 4–6 g (175–260 mEq) of sodium per day. A no-added-salt diet contains approximately 3 g (132 mEq) of sodium per day. Further restriction can be achieved with diets of 2 or 1 g of sodium per day. Diets with more severe restriction are difficult to adhere to and rarely used. National Academies of Sciences, Engineering, and Medicine guidelines recommend 2.3 g of sodium (approximately 1 teaspoon of salt) per day.

Dietary sodium includes sodium naturally occurring in foods, sodium added during food processing, and sodium added during cooking and at the table. Approximately 80% of dietary intake in American diets is from processed and pre-prepared foods. Diets designed for 2.3 g of sodium per day require elimination of most processed foods, added salt, and foods with high sodium content. Patients with mild hypertension may achieve significant reductions in blood pressure (approximately 5 mm Hg diastolic) with this degree of sodium restriction.

Fat-Restricted Diets & Low–Saturated Fat Diets

Traditional fat-restricted diets are useful in the treatment of patients with fat malabsorption syndromes and following surgical procedures such as cholecystectomy and pancreatic resection. Such diets may improve the symptoms of diarrhea with steatorrhea independent of the primary physiologic abnormality by limiting the quantity of fatty acids that reach the colon. The degree of fat restriction necessary to control symptoms must be individualized. Patients with severe malabsorption may limit fat to 40–60 g per day. Diets containing 60–80 g of fat per day can be designed for patients with less severe abnormalities.

Fat-restricted diets that specifically restrict saturated fats are the mainstay of dietary treatment of hyperlipidemia with elevated LDL cholesterol (see Chapter 32). Similar diets are often recommended for the prevention of CAD (see Chapter 10). The Women's Health Initiative Dietary Modification Trial, however, did not show significant benefit of a low-fat diet for weight control or prevention of CVD or cancer. In contrast, a study of Mediterranean diets, supplemented by nuts or extra-virgin olive oil, demonstrated a reduction in cardiovascular events. Plant-based diets, defined by low consumption of animal products, have been increasingly recommended for their health benefits. Numerous studies have found diets enriched with high-quality plant foods, such as whole grains, fruits, vegetables, and nuts, to be associated with lower cardiovascular risk.

The aim of low-fat diets is to restrict total fat to < 30% of calories and saturated fat to < 7% of calories. More extreme restriction offers little additional advantage in modification of serum lipids. Low-fat diets can be augmented with plant stanols and sterols and with soluble dietary fiber to further reduce serum lipids.

Carbohydrate-Restricted Diets

Low-carbohydrate diets typically restrict carbohydrate intake to 50–180 g/day. Consumption of foods that contain higher protein and fat with lower carbohydrate content has been shown to promote satiety. Carbohydrate-restricted diets, including low-glycemic-index diets (see Chapter 31), can be helpful for patients with type 2 diabetes and other forms of insulin resistance to reduce blood sugar and weight. Several studies investigating the efficacy of low-fat versus low-carbohydrate diets for weight loss show no clear benefit of one versus the other.

Protein-Restricted Diets

Protein-restricted diets are recommended for patients with advanced CKD to slow the progression of early disease and to decrease symptoms of uremia in more severe disease.

Protein restriction is intended to limit the production of nitrogenous waste products. Energy intake must be adequate to facilitate the efficient use of dietary protein. Enough protein (at least 0.6 g/kg/day in most patients) must be provided to meet minimal requirements.

DIETS THAT SUPPLEMENT NUTRIENTS

High-Fiber Diets

Dietary fiber is a diverse group of plant constituents that is resistant to digestion by the human digestive tract. Guidelines suggest that adult men should eat 30–38 g of fiber per day and adult women 21–25 g/day. Typical US diets, however, contain about half of that amount. Epidemiologic evidence suggests that populations consuming greater quantities of fiber may have a lower incidence of certain GI disorders, including diverticulitis, colon cancer, and CVD. A meta-analysis of 22 studies suggested that each 7 g of dietary fiber was associated with a 9% decrease in first cardiovascular event.

Diets high in dietary fiber (21–38 g/day) are commonly recommended to patients with a variety of GI disorders such as irritable bowel syndrome and recurrent diverticulitis. Diets high in fiber, particularly soluble fiber, may also be useful to reduce blood glucose in patients with diabetes and to reduce cholesterol in patients with hypercholesterolemia. Good sources of soluble fiber are oats, nuts, seeds, legumes, and most fruits. Foods with insoluble fiber include whole wheat, brown rice, other whole grains, and most vegetables. For some patients, the addition of psyllium or methylcellulose may be a useful adjunct to increase dietary fiber.

Feng S et al. Carbohydrate-restricted diet types and macronutrient replacements for metabolic health in adults: a meta-analysis of randomized trials. Clin Nutr. 2025;54:27. [PMID: 41004974]

Li L et al. Effects of healthy low-carbohydrate diet and time-restricted eating on weight and gut microbiome in adults with overweight or obesity: feeding RCT. Cell Rep Med. 2024;5:101801. [PMID: 39454570]

NUTRITIONAL SUPPORT

Nutritional support is the provision of nutrients to patients who cannot meet their nutritional requirements through standard diets. Nutrients may be delivered enterally via oral nutrition supplements and feeding tubes, or parenterally using lines or catheters inserted directly into veins. Nutritional support techniques permit adequate nutrition delivery; however, their use should be considered only when likely to improve a patient's outcome.

INDICATIONS FOR NUTRITIONAL SUPPORT

Nutritional support is indicated in patients who are malnourished or at risk of malnutrition. Common indications for enteral nutrition include inability to meet nutritional needs orally, GI dysfunction (eg, proximal GI obstruction/mass, gastroparesis, etc.), neurologic conditions including dysphagia, mechanical ventilation, and head and neck cancer. Parenteral nutrition is required when enteral nutrition is contraindicated, or when the GI tract has diminished function due to underlying conditions, including small bowel obstructions, paralytic ileus, short bowel syndrome, and fistulae.

The ASPEN recommendations for the rational use of nutritional support emphasize the need to individualize the decision to begin nutritional support, weighing the risks, benefits, costs, and goals of care. The guidelines also highlight the need to perform comprehensive nutrition assessments to identify patients who may benefit from aggressive nutrition interventions.

Nutritional Support Methods

Selection of the most appropriate nutritional support method involves consideration of GI function, anticipated duration of nutritional support, and ability of each method to meet the patient's nutritional requirements. The chosen method should meet the patient's nutritional needs with the lowest risk and cost. For most patients, enteral feeding is safer and less expensive, and it offers significant physiologic advantages. An algorithm for selection of the most appropriate nutritional support method is presented in Figure 33–1.

Prior to initiating specialized enteral nutritional support, efforts should be made to supplement food intake. Attention to patient food preferences, liberalizing diet orders, timing of meals in relation to diagnostic procedures and required medications, and the use of foods brought to the hospital by family and friends can often increase oral intake. Patients unable to eat enough at regular mealtimes to meet nutritional requirements can be given **oral supplements** as snacks or to replace low-calorie beverages. Oral supplements with different nutritional compositions are available to meet the specific needs of patients with various clinical conditions. Formulations vary in fiber and lactose content, caloric density, protein level, and electrolyte concentrations.

Patients with functioning GI tracts who are unable to take adequate oral nutrition or swallow safely are appropriate candidates for enteral nutritional support (tube feeding). Short-term enteral access devices that terminate in the stomach or small bowel can be placed into the nose or mouth. Examples are orogastric, nasogastric, nasoduodenal, and nasojejunal tubes. Bedside placement of short-term enteral access devices is typically successful; however, it may be difficult to achieve post-pyloric placement. Some patients require fluoroscopic or endoscopic guidance to insert the feeding tube distal to the gastric pylorus. Correct feeding tube placement should always be confirmed radiographically prior to initiation of feeding. Long-term enteral access devices that are placed directly into the stomach or small bowel are called tube enterostomies. Percutaneous gastrostomies, jejunostomies, and gastrojejunostomies can be placed by an endoscopist, interventional radiologist, or surgeon.

When selecting the appropriate enteral access device, it is important to consider anticipated duration of use, patient anatomy, aspiration risk, and quality of life. Patients who are at increased risk of aspiration may benefit from small bowel feeding; however, this may not prevent aspiration,

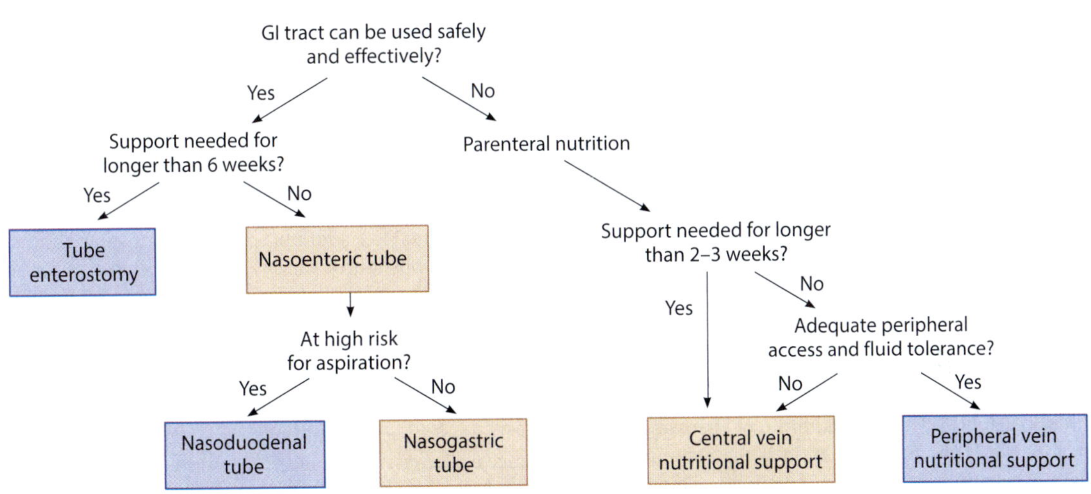

Figure 33–1. Nutritional support method decision tree.

particularly if the pylorus is patulous. Patients fed via the stomach can receive bolus, intermittent, or continuous tube feeding. Patients fed via the small bowel require pump-assisted continuous or cycled tube feeding; bolus feeds are generally not well tolerated in the small intestine.

Patients with impaired GI tracts who require nutritional support are candidates for **parenteral nutritional support**. The choice to use parenteral nutrition via central line or peripheral line is based on nutrition status, duration of use, and whether the patient can tolerate large volumes.

Central parenteral nutrition is reserved for patients who are malnourished and anticipated to require nutritional support for > 7–14 days. It is delivered via intravenous catheters placed percutaneously using sterile technique. Proper placement in the superior vena cava must be documented radiographically before the solution is infused, and catheters must be carefully maintained by experienced nursing staff to prevent infection and other catheter-related complications.

Peripheral parenteral nutrition is most often considered in patients who are not malnourished or who require short-term parenteral nutritional support (< 2 weeks). Peripheral vein nutritional support is administered via standard intravenous lines. Serious adverse events are infrequent, but there is a high incidence of phlebitis, infiltration of intravenous lines, and volume overload.

NUTRITIONAL REQUIREMENTS

Prior to initiation of nutritional support, the patient's estimated nutritional requirements must be determined. In general, solutions of equal nutrient value can be designed for delivery via enteral and parenteral routes, but differences in absorption should be considered. A complete nutritional support solution contains water, carbohydrates, amino acids, fat, electrolytes, vitamins, and minerals.

Water

One method for calculating fluid requirements in adults is to allot 1500 mL for the first 20 kg of body weight with the addition of 20 mL for every kilogram above 20 kg. Another way to calculate fluid requirements is 25–35 mL/kg or approximately 1 mL/kcal energy required. It is important to note that patients with certain medical conditions benefit from fluid restriction.

Energy

Indirect calorimetry is considered the gold standard for estimating energy requirements, but it is not available in most clinical settings. In its absence, predictive energy expenditure equations and simple weight-based calculations can be utilized.

The most widely used and validated predictive energy expenditure equations for healthy individuals include the Harris-Benedict Equation and Mifflin-St. Jeor Equation, which calculate RMR with the addition of stress and activity factors. The Penn State Equation is the recommended predictive equation for critically ill patients. This formula calculates RMR combined with dynamic physiological variables such as maximum temperature in a 24-hour period and minute ventilation. Different versions of the equation exist for patients over 60 years of age or with obesity. Actual body weight should be used for all predictive equations.

Energy requirements can also be estimated by multiplying actual body weight in kilograms by 25–35 kcal/kg/day. Although this method is simple and easy to use, its accuracy is under 50%.

The above methods provide imprecise estimates of actual energy expenditure, especially for markedly underweight, overweight, and critically ill patients who are ideal candidates for indirect calorimetry. Studies using indirect calorimetry have demonstrated that as many as 30–40% of patients have measured expenditures 10% above or below estimated values.

In standard diets and balanced nutritional support solutions, carbohydrates provide the greatest amount of energy compared to the other macronutrients; however, protein and fat are required in optimal amounts to provide the body energy and support other functions.

Protein

Protein and energy requirements are closely related. If adequate calories are provided, stable and non-stressed patients should receive 0.8–1.2 g/kg/day of protein. Patients under moderate to severe stress require at least 1.5 g/kg/day, although patients with trauma and burns may need closer to 2.5 g/kg/day. Actual weight should be used for patients with a healthy weight or underweight while adjusted body weight should be used for patients with obesity.

Patients who receive protein without adequate calories catabolize protein for energy rather than utilize it for protein synthesis. As a result, when energy intake is low, excess protein is needed for nitrogen balance.

Fat

Patients receiving nutritional support should be given 2–4% of their total calories as linoleic acid and 0.25–0.5% as α-linolenic acid to prevent essential fatty acid deficiency (EFAD). Most enteral formulas contain adequate essential fatty acids. Patients receiving parenteral nutrition should be given 250 mL of a 20% soy-based lipid emulsion at least twice weekly to prevent EFAD.

Electrolytes, Minerals, Vitamins, & Trace Elements

Requirements for sodium, potassium, magnesium, calcium, and phosphorus vary widely depending on a patient's cardiovascular, renal, endocrine, and GI status as well as measurements of serum concentration.

Patients receiving enteral nutritional support should receive adequate vitamins and minerals according to recommended daily allowances. Most enteral formulations provide sufficient vitamins, minerals, electrolytes, and trace elements if adequate volumes are administered. Certain formulas, like those intended for patients with renal disease, have a lower electrolyte profile.

Patients receiving parenteral nutritional support typically require 1–2 mEq/kg/day of sodium and potassium, 10–15 mEq/day of calcium, 8–20 mEq/day of magnesium, and 20–40 mmol/day of phosphorus.

Parenteral formulations also contain the trace elements zinc, copper, manganese, selenium, and chromium. Patients with diarrhea may require additional zinc to replace fecal losses. Copper and manganese may be excluded from a parenteral formulation in patients with liver disease due to impaired excretion and risk for toxicity. It is important to note that trace element products do not contain iron, so patients on long-term parenteral nutrition may require external iron supplementation.

Vitamins are provided daily in the parenteral nutrition solution. Injectable multivitamin products for adults contain vitamins A, D, E, K, B_1, B_2, B_6, B_{12}, niacinamide, dexpanthenol, biotin, folic acid, and ascorbic acid.

ENTERAL NUTRITIONAL SUPPORT SOLUTIONS

Patients who require enteral nutritional support in an acute care setting receive commercially prepared enteral formulas (Table 33–3). Most enteral formulations have been designed to provide adequate proportions of water, energy, protein, and micronutrients. Some formulas contain less free water for patients who require fluid restriction. Modular products are also available to provide specific macronutrients (eg, protein, carbohydrate, and fat) to supplement commercially available formulas for patients with unique nutrition requirements.

Table 33–3. Enteral formulations.

Standard products
Blenderized commercially prepared (eg, Compleat, Liquid Hope, Real Food Blends)
Intact protein, lactose-free, low-residue:
1 kcal/mL (eg, Isosource 1.0, Kate Farms Standard 1.0)
1.5 kcal/mL (eg, Isosource 1.5, Osmolite 1.5, Nutren 1.5, Kate Farms 1.4)
2 kcal/mL (eg, TwoCal HN, Nutren 2.0, Resource 2.0)
Intact protein, lactose-free, high-residue:
1 kcal/mL (eg, Jevity,[1] Nutren with fiber,[1] Fibersource HN)
"Disease-specific" products
Advanced CKD: with adjusted protein content, fluid concentration, and electrolytes (eg, Nepro, Nepro with Carb Steady, Suplena with Carb Steady, Novosource Renal, Renalcal, Kate Farms Renal Support)
Type 2 diabetes: with lower carbohydrate content (eg, Glucerna 1.0, 1.2, or 1.5, Nutren Glytrol, Diabetisource AC, Kate Farms Glucose Support 1.2)
Malabsorption: with partially or fully hydrolyzed nutrients (eg, Peptamen, Peptamen 1.5, Peptamen AF, Peptamen with Prebio, Peptamen Intense VHP, Tolerex, Vital 1.0 and 1.5, Vital AF 1.2, Vital High Protein, Kate Farms Peptide, Vivonex T.E.N., Vivonex RTF, Vivonex Plus)
Respiratory failure: with > 50% calories from fat (eg, Pulmocare, Nutren Pulmonary, Oxepa)
Hepatic encephalopathy: with high amounts of branched-chain amino acids (eg, Nutri-Hep)
Wound healing: with high protein content (eg, Promote, Replete, Perative)
Modular products
Protein (eg, ProMod, ProStat Sugar Free, Beneprotein, Unjury)
Carbohydrate (eg, Polycose, SolCarb)
Fat (eg, MCT Oil, Microlipid)

[1]Isotonic.

Enteral formulas can be classified as standard (polymeric), peptide-based (elemental or semi-elemental) or disease specific. The classification is based on the overall composition of the formula and its contained macronutrients. Most enteral formulas are lactose-free.

Standard polymeric formulas are typically isotonic with moderate amounts of intact macronutrients, and they may contain fiber. Normal digestive and absorptive capacity are needed for the use of polymeric formulas. Isotonic formulas contain 1 kcal/mL, whereas concentrated formulas contain 1.2–2 kcal/mL. Standard polymeric formulas are well tolerated in most patients.

Semi-elemental and elemental formulas are designed for patients with impaired GI function who have demonstrated malabsorption and maldigestion with standard polymeric formulas. Elemental formulas contain free amino acids, whereas semi-elemental formulas contain partially hydrolyzed oligopeptides. Elemental formulas contain minimal amounts of fat, typically in the form of medium chain triglycerides, which can increase the risk of EFAD when used long-term.

Disease-specific enteral formulas have been designed for immune-nutrition, wound healing, and patients with diabetes, kidney disease, hepatic encephalopathy, and respiratory failure. However, the majority have not been shown to be superior to standard polymeric formulas for most patients.

When initiating enteral nutrition, a continuous pump-infusion is generally preferred. In critically ill patients, enteral nutrition is commonly started at 10–40 mL/hour and advanced to goal rate by 10–20 mL/hour every 8–12 hours. Stable non-critically ill patients can tolerate initiation of enteral nutrition at goal rate; however, this is not appropriate for patients at risk for refeeding syndrome who benefit from more conservative initiation and advancement. In patients with long-term enteral access devices, transitioning to bolus feeds (in patients with gastric feeding tubes only) or cycled/nocturnal feeds (in patients with either gastric or small bowel feeding tubes) can improve quality of life.

COMPLICATIONS OF ENTERAL NUTRITIONAL SUPPORT

Enteral nutrition is the preferred feeding method in patients with functional GI tracts; however, complications occur in 10–15%. Minor mechanical complications are common and include tube occlusion and dislodgment. Common GI complications include diarrhea, nausea, vomiting, and constipation. GI bleeding from feeding tube placement may occur but is less common. The most common complication is diarrhea, which may be caused by the formula itself (ie, intolerance to a hyperosmotic load or to a specific component in the formula), medications, infections, or a primary disease of the intestine. All possibilities should be considered before attributing diarrhea to the enteral nutrition.

One of the most serious complications of enteral nutritional support is aspiration. Aspiration can be prevented by identifying patients at risk and utilizing protocols to reduce risks, as appropriate, including elevating the head of bed to 30 degrees, utilizing promotility agents, placing post-pyloric feeding tubes, and checking gastric volumes every 4 hours (if deemed appropriate). In ICUs that choose to check, feeds should not be held for gastric residual volume < 500 mL in the absence of other signs of EN intolerance.

Metabolic complications during enteral nutritional support are less likely caused by the enteral nutrition itself and more likely related to underlying conditions that predispose patients to metabolic alterations. The most common complications include refeeding syndrome, electrolyte derangements, hyperglycemia, and dehydration.

PARENTERAL NUTRITIONAL SUPPORT SOLUTIONS

The parenteral nutrition formulation is a complex solution containing up to 40 different nutrients. The basic parenteral solution is composed of dextrose, amino acids, lipids, electrolytes, minerals, trace elements, vitamins, and water. Medications can also be added.

Parenteral nutrition administered via a central vein allows for administration of hyperosmolar solution (> 1800 mOsm/L) and adequate nutrition delivery. The dextrose, amino acids, and electrolytes contribute to the osmotic load and can be administered in higher concentrations as compared to peripheral parenteral nutrition. Lipid emulsions are isotonic and can be administered via a central or peripheral vein.

Solutions with lower osmolarities (< 900 mOsm/L) must be administrated via peripheral veins. Solutions for peripheral infusion usually contain 5–10% dextrose and 3% amino acids. These lower osmolarity solutions result in a high incidence of thrombophlebitis and line infiltration. These solutions may provide adequate protein for some patients, but inadequate total energy from dextrose, depending on volume limitations. Additional energy can be provided with lipid emulsions since these solutions are isotonic and well tolerated by peripheral veins.

Lipid emulsions can prevent EFAD and provide energy to patients on parenteral nutrition. There are four lipid emulsion products available for use in the United States. For all lipid emulsions, providers should follow manufacturer dosing recommendations to prevent complications associated with EFAD.

Parenteral nutrition solutions should be initiated at half of the estimated energy requirement, or approximately 100–150 g dextrose for the first 24 hours. They are increased daily as tolerated to prevent hyperglycemia and electrolyte abnormalities in patients at risk for refeeding syndrome. Amino acids and lipid emulsions can be started at target goals.

COMPLICATIONS OF PARENTERAL NUTRITIONAL SUPPORT

Parenteral nutrition is considered a high-risk nutrition therapy, which can result in mechanical, infectious, and metabolic complications. Patients require close monitoring for prevention, detection, and treatment.

Catheter-related complications can occur during insertion or while the catheter is in place. Pneumothorax, arterial laceration, air emboli, and brachial plexus injury can occur during catheter placement. Radiographic imaging must be performed to confirm proper placement of central venous access prior to initiating parenteral nutrition. Additional catheter-related complications include thrombotic occlusions and non-thrombotic occlusions caused by drug-nutrient interactions, precipitates, and residue.

Catheter-related bloodstream infections are the most serious complications. Patients with indwelling central vein catheters who develop a fever without an apparent source should have their lines removed or changed immediately, at which time the catheter tip should be cultured, and empiric antibiotics initiated. Quantitative tip cultures and blood cultures narrow antibiotic therapy. Catheter-related sepsis occurs in 2–3% of patients even if optimal efforts are made to prevent infection. "Central line bundles" are evidence-based practices designed to reduce the incidence of central line–associated infections. The use of peripheral parenteral nutrition over central parenteral nutrition when appropriate is another strategy to prevent catheter-related bloodstream infections.

Metabolic complications of central vein nutritional support include hyperglycemia, hypoglycemia, EFAD, hypertriglyceridemia, fluid and electrolyte abnormalities, hepatobiliary disorders, and metabolic bone disease. A skilled nutritional support clinician is necessary to safely prescribe, monitor, and address potential parenteral nutrition–associated complications. Examples of metabolic complications and suggested solutions are outlined in Table 33–4.

PATIENT MONITORING DURING NUTRITIONAL SUPPORT

Every patient receiving enteral or parenteral nutritional support should be monitored closely. Formal nutritional support teams composed of a physician, a nurse, a dietitian, and a pharmacist have been shown to decrease the rate of complications.

Patients should be monitored both for the adequacy of treatment and to prevent complications or detect them early when they occur. Because estimates of nutritional requirements are imprecise, frequent reassessment is necessary. Daily intakes should be recorded and compared with estimated requirements. Body weight, hydration status, and overall clinical status should be followed. Patients who do not appear to be responding as anticipated should have an indirect calorimetry study performed if possible, and they should be evaluated for nitrogen balance with the following equation:

$$\text{Nitrogen balance} = \frac{\text{24-hour protein intake (g)}}{6.25} - \left(\text{24-hour urinary nitrogen (g)} + 4\right)$$

Patients who receive calorie prescriptions comparable to the results of the indirect calorimetry study and

Table 33–4. Metabolic complications of parenteral nutritional support.

Complication	Common Causes	Possible Solutions
Hyperglycemia	Too rapid infusion of dextrose, "stress," corticosteroids	Decrease glucose infusion; insulin; replacement of dextrose with fat
Hyperosmolar nonketotic dehydration	Severe, undetected hyperglycemia	Insulin, hydration, potassium
Hyperchloremic metabolic acidosis	High chloride administration	Decrease chloride
Azotemia	Excessive protein administration	Decrease amino acid concentration
Hypophosphatemia, hypokalemia, hypomagnesemia	Extracellular to intracellular shifting with refeeding	Increase solution concentration and provide repletion outside of parenteral nutrition bag; do not advance dextrose further
Liver enzyme abnormalities	Lipid trapping in hepatocytes, fatty liver	Decrease dextrose and lipid to a more balanced solution, cycle parenteral nutrition
Acalculous cholecystitis	Biliary stasis	Encourage oral diet or tube feeding as able
Zinc deficiency	Diarrhea, small bowel fistulas	Increase concentration
Copper deficiency	Biliary fistulas	Increase concentration

who have positive nitrogen balances can continue their current regimens, whereas patients not meeting their energy targets or who have negative nitrogen balances should receive moderate increases in calorie and protein before reassessment. Monitoring for metabolic complications includes daily measurements of basic metabolic panels, magnesium, and phosphorus levels. Once the patient is stabilized on the goal nutritional support regimen, labs can be obtained 1–2 times per week. Liver function tests and triglyceride levels should be monitored weekly. Vitamins and trace elements should be assessed every 3–6 months in patients receiving long-term nutritional support.

Baik SM et al. Comparison of early enteral nutrition verses early parenteral nutrition in critically ill patients: a systematic review and meta-analysis. Nutrients. 2024;17:10. [PMID: 39796444]

Bidgood E et al. Peripheral parenteral nutrition: a retrospective observational study to evaluate utility and complications. Nutr Clin Pract. 2025;40:942. [PMID: 39467781]

Lew CCH et al. The association between malnutrition and high protein treatment on outcomes in critically ill patients: a post hoc analysis of the EFFORT protein randomized trial. Chest. 2024;165:1380. [PMID: 38354904]

Patel JJ et al. Contemporary rationale for delivering enteral nutrition in critically ill adults. Crit Care Med. 2025;53:e1481. [PMID: 40396870]

34 Common Problems in Infectious Diseases & Antimicrobial Therapy

Monica Fung, MD, MPH
Katherine Gruenberg, PharmD, MAEd
Peter V. Chin-Hong, MD

COMMON PROBLEMS IN INFECTIOUS DISEASES

FEVER OF UNKNOWN ORIGIN (FUO)

ESSENTIALS OF DIAGNOSIS

- Illness of at least 3 weeks in duration.
- Fever ≥ 38.3°C on at least three occasions.
- Diagnosis has not been made despite a minimum set of diagnostic tests.

General Considerations

The intervals specified in the criteria for the diagnosis of FUO are arbitrary ones intended to exclude patients with protracted but self-limited illnesses and to allow time for the usual radiographic, serologic, and cultural studies to be performed. The criteria for FUO are met when *a diagnosis has not been made despite a minimum standard of diagnostic tests. These include blood tests (CBC with differential, comprehensive metabolic panel including calcium and liver function tests, ESR, CRP, TSH, rheumatoid factor, antineutrophil cytoplasmic antibodies, and ANA), microbiologic tests (three sets of blood cultures, urinalysis, HIV antibody/antigen, and tuberculin skin test or interferon-γ release assay), and imaging (abdominal ultrasound and CXR or CT of the chest/abdomen/pelvis).*

Added categories of FUO include complications of current health care scenarios: (1) **Hospital-associated FUO** refers to the hospitalized patient with fever of 38.3°C or higher on several occasions, due to a process not present or incubating at the time of admission, in whom initial cultures are negative and the diagnosis remains unknown after 1 week of investigation (see Health Care–Associated Infections, below); (2) **Neutropenic FUO** includes patients with fever of 38.3°C or higher on several occasions with < 500 neutrophils per microliter in whom initial cultures are negative and the diagnosis remains uncertain after 3 days (see Chapter 2 and Infections in the Immunocompromised Patient, below); (3) **HIV-associated FUO** pertains to patients with HIV and fever of 38.3°C or higher who have been febrile for 4 weeks or more as an outpatient or 3 days as an inpatient, in whom the diagnosis remains uncertain after 3 days of investigation with at least 2 days for cultures to incubate (see Chapter 35). Although not usually considered separately, **FUO in solid organ transplant recipients** and **FUO in the returning traveler** are common scenarios, each with a unique differential diagnosis, and are also discussed in this chapter.

For a general discussion of fever, see the section on fever and hyperthermia in Chapter 2.

A. Common Causes

Most cases represent unusual manifestations of common diseases and not rare or exotic diseases—eg, tuberculosis, endocarditis, gallbladder disease, and HIV (primary infection or opportunistic infection) are more common causes of FUO than Whipple disease or familial Mediterranean fever.

B. Age of Patient

In adults, infections (25–40% of cases) and cancer (25–40% of cases) account for the majority of FUOs. Autoimmune disorders occur with equal frequency in adults and children (10–20% of cases), but the diseases differ. Juvenile rheumatoid arthritis is common in children, whereas SLE, granulomatosis with polyangiitis, and polyarteritis nodosa are more common in adults. Still disease, giant cell arteritis, and polymyalgia rheumatica occur exclusively in adults. In adults > 65 years of age, multisystem immune-mediated diseases such as temporal arteritis, polymyalgia rheumatica, sarcoidosis, rheumatoid arthritis, and granulomatosis with polyangiitis account for 25–30% of all FUOs.

C. Duration of Fever

The cause of FUO changes dramatically in patients who have been febrile for 6 months or longer. Infection, cancer, and autoimmune disorders combined account for only 20% of FUOs in these patients. Instead, other entities such as granulomatous diseases (granulomatous hepatitis, Crohn disease, ulcerative colitis) and factitious fever become important causes. One-fourth of patients who say they have been febrile for 6 months or longer actually have no true fever or underlying disease. Instead, the usual normal circadian variation in temperature (temperature 0.5–1°C higher in the afternoon than in the morning) is interpreted as abnormal. Patients with **episodic** or **recurrent fever** (ie, those who meet the criteria for FUO but have fever-free periods of 2 weeks or longer) are similar to those with **prolonged fever**. Infection, malignancy, and autoimmune disorders account for only 20–25% of such fevers, whereas various miscellaneous diseases (Crohn disease, familial Mediterranean fever, allergic alveolitis) account for another 25%. *Approximately 50% of cases remain undiagnosed but have a benign course with eventual resolution of symptoms.*

D. Immunologic Status

In the neutropenic patient, fungal infections and occult bacterial infections are important causes of FUO. In the patient taking immunosuppressive medications (particularly organ transplant patients), cytomegalovirus (CMV) infections are a frequent cause of fever, as are fungal infections, nocardiosis, *Pneumocystis jirovecii* pneumonia, and mycobacterial infections.

E. Classification of Causes of FUO

Most patients with FUO will fit into one of five categories.

1. Infection—Both systemic and localized infections can cause FUO. *Tuberculosis and endocarditis are the most common systemic infections associated with FUO*, but mycoses, viral diseases (particularly infection with Epstein-Barr virus and CMV), toxoplasmosis, brucellosis, Q fever, cat-scratch disease, salmonellosis, malaria, and many other less common infections have been implicated. Primary infection with HIV or opportunistic infections associated with AIDS—particularly mycobacterial infections—also can present as FUO. *The most common form of localized infection causing FUO is an occult abscess.* Liver, spleen, kidney, brain, and bone abscesses may be difficult to detect. A collection of pus may form in the peritoneal cavity or in the subdiaphragmatic, subhepatic, paracolic, or other areas. Cholangitis, osteomyelitis, UTI, dental abscess, or paranasal sinusitis may cause prolonged fever.

2. Neoplasms—Many cancers can present as FUO. The most common are lymphoma (both Hodgkin and non-Hodgkin) and leukemia. Posttransplant lymphoproliferative disorders may also present with fever. Other diseases of lymph nodes, such as angioimmunoblastic lymphoma and Castleman disease, can also cause FUO. Primary and metastatic tumors of the liver are frequently associated with fever, as are renal cell carcinomas. Atrial myxoma is an often-forgotten neoplasm that can result in fever. Chronic lymphocytic leukemia and multiple myeloma are rarely associated with fever, and the presence of fever in patients with these diseases should prompt a search for infection.

3. Autoimmune disorders—Still disease, SLE, cryoglobulinemia, and polyarteritis nodosa are the most common causes of autoimmune-associated FUO. Giant cell arteritis and polymyalgia rheumatica are seen almost exclusively in patients > 50 years of age and are nearly always associated with an elevated ESR (> 40 mm/h).

4. Miscellaneous causes—Many other conditions have been associated with FUO but less commonly than the foregoing types of illness. Examples include thyroiditis, sarcoidosis, Whipple disease, familial Mediterranean fever, recurrent pulmonary emboli, alcoholic hepatitis, drug fever, and factitious fever.

5. Undiagnosed FUO—Despite extensive evaluation, the diagnosis remains elusive in about one-half of patients. Of these patients, the fever abates spontaneously in ~75% with no diagnosis; in the remainder, more classic manifestations of the underlying disease appear over time.

Clinical Findings

Because the evaluation of a patient with FUO is costly and time-consuming, it is imperative to first document the presence of fever. This is done by observing the patient while the temperature is being taken to ascertain that fever is not factitious (self-induced). Associated findings that accompany fever include tachycardia, chills, and piloerection. A thorough history—including family, occupational, social (sexual practices, use of injection drugs), dietary (unpasteurized products, raw meat), exposures (animals, chemicals), and travel—may give clues to the diagnosis. Repeated physical examination may reveal subtle, evanescent clinical findings essential to diagnosis.

A. Laboratory Tests

In addition to routine laboratory studies, *three sets of blood cultures should always be obtained*, preferably when the patient has not taken antibiotics for several days, and should be held by the laboratory for 2 weeks to detect slow-growing organisms. Cultures on special media are requested if *Legionella*, *Bartonella*, or nutritionally deficient streptococci are possible pathogens. "Screening tests" with immunologic or microbiologic serologies ("febrile agglutinins") are of low yield and should *not* be done. If the history or physical examination suggests a specific diagnosis, specific serologic tests with an associated fourfold rise or fall in titer may be useful. Because infection is the most common cause of FUO, other body fluids are usually cultured, ie, urine, sputum, stool, CSF, and morning gastric aspirates (if one suspects tuberculosis). Direct examination of blood smears may establish a diagnosis of malaria or relapsing fever (*Borrelia*). Molecular diagnostics, including plasma metagenomic next-generation sequencing, are being applied increasingly in this setting.

B. Imaging

All patients with FUO should have chest and abdominal imaging—this can be a combination of CXR and abdominal ultrasound or CT of the chest, abdomen, and pelvis if readily available. Studies such as sinus CT, upper GI series with small bowel follow-through, barium enema, proctosigmoidoscopy, and evaluation of gallbladder function are reserved for patients who have symptoms, signs, or a history that suggest disease in these body regions. CT scan of the abdomen and pelvis is also frequently performed and is particularly useful for looking at the liver, spleen, and retroperitoneum. When the CT scan is abnormal, the findings often lead to a specific diagnosis. A normal CT scan is not quite as useful; more invasive procedures such as biopsy or exploratory laparotomy may be needed. The role of MRI in the investigation of FUO has not been evaluated. In general, however, MRI is better than CT for detecting lesions of the nervous system and is useful in diagnosing various vasculitides. Ultrasound is sensitive for detecting lesions of the kidney, pancreas, and biliary tree. Echocardiography should be used if one is considering endocarditis or atrial myxoma. *Transesophageal echocardiography is more sensitive than surface echocardiography for detecting valvular lesions, but even a negative transesophageal study does not exclude endocarditis (10% false-negative rate).* Guidelines currently suggest the use of nuclear medicine studies, particularly fludeoxyglucose-PET/CT (FDG-PET/CT), earlier in the course of FUO. Diagnostic yields of FDG-PET/CT for underlying causes are 84–98%, with patients with infection or malignancy benefiting more. Furthermore, FDG-PET/CT may assist with prognostication with patients with negative studies being five times more likely to experience spontaneous remission.

C. Biopsy

Invasive procedures are often required for diagnosis. Any abnormal finding should be aggressively evaluated: headache calls for lumbar puncture to rule out meningitis; skin rash should be biopsied for cutaneous manifestations of collagen vascular disease or infection; and enlarged lymph nodes should be aspirated or biopsied for neoplasm and sent for culture. Bone marrow aspiration with biopsy is a relatively low-yield procedure (15–25%; except in patients with HIV, in whom mycobacterial infection is a common cause of FUO), but the risk is low and the procedure should be done if other less invasive tests have not yielded a diagnosis, particularly in persons with hematologic abnormalities. Liver biopsy will yield a specific diagnosis in 10–15% of patients with FUO and should be considered in any patient with abnormal liver tests even if the liver is normal in size. CT scanning and MRI have decreased the need for exploratory laparotomy; however, surgical visualization and biopsies should be considered when there is continued deterioration or lack of diagnosis.

Treatment

Although an empiric course of antimicrobials is sometimes considered for FUO, it is rarely helpful and may impact infectious diseases diagnoses (eg, by reducing the sensitivity of blood cultures).

When to Refer

- Any patient with FUO and progressive weight loss and other constitutional signs.
- Any immunocompromised patient (eg, transplant recipients and patients with HIV).
- Infectious diseases specialists may also be able to coordinate and interpret specialized testing (eg, Q fever serologies) with outside agencies, such as the US CDC.

When to Treat Empirically

- Any patient who is hemodynamically unstable with high risk of sepsis.
- If FUO is present in immunocompromised patients, such as those who are neutropenic from recent chemotherapy or those who have undergone transplantation (particularly in the previous 6 months).
- High clinical suspicion for tuberculosis (requires Infectious Diseases consultation).
- Patients with suspected giant cell arteritis with visual complaints.

Antoniadou C et al. Fever and inflammation of unknown origin in the 21st century. Eur J Intern Med. 2025;142:106443. [PMID: 40841245]

Betrains A et al. Comparison of diagnostic spectrum between inflammation of unknown origin and fever of unknown origin: a systematic review and meta-analysis. Eur J Intern Med. 2024;124:115. [PMID: 38431500]

Haidar G et al. Fever of unknown origin. N Engl J Med. 2022;386:463. [PMID: 35108471]

Marra AR et al. Metagenomic next-generation sequencing in patients with fever of unknown origin: a comprehensive systematic literature review and meta-analysis. Diagn Microbiol Infect Dis. 2024;110:116465. [PMID: 39059148]

Palestro CJ et al. FDG PET in evaluation of patients with fever of unknown origin: *AJR* Expert Panel narrative review. AJR Am J Roentgenol. 2023;221:151. [PMID: 36722759]

van Rijsewijk ND et al. Molecular imaging of fever of unknown origin: an update. Semin Nucl Med. 2023;53:4. [PMID: 35902280]

Wright WF et al. Fever of unknown origin. BMJ. 2025;388:e080847. [PMID: 39761983]

INFECTIONS IN THE IMMUNOCOMPROMISED PATIENT

ESSENTIALS OF DIAGNOSIS

- Fever and other symptoms may be blunted because of immunosuppression.
- A contaminating organism in an immunocompetent individual may be a pathogen in an immunocompromised one.
- The interval since transplantation and the degree of immunosuppression can narrow the differential diagnosis.
- Empiric broad-spectrum antibiotics may be appropriate in high-risk patients whether or not symptoms are localized.

General Considerations

Immunocompromised patients have acquired or inborn defects in their natural defense mechanisms resulting in an increased risk for infection. In addition, infection is often severe, rapidly progressive, and life-threatening. Organisms that are not usually problematic in the immunocompetent person may be important pathogens in the compromised patient (eg, *Staphylococcus epidermidis*, *Bacillus* species).

Therefore, culture results must be interpreted with caution, and isolates should not be disregarded as solely contaminants. Although the type of immunodeficiency is associated with specific infectious disease syndromes, *nearly any pathogen can cause infection in any immunosuppressed patient*. Thus, a systematic evaluation is required to identify a causative pathogen, and expert consultation is required to interpret identification of microbiologic organisms.

A. Impaired Humoral Immunity

Defects in humoral immunity are often congenital, although hypogammaglobulinemia can occur in multiple myeloma, chronic lymphocytic leukemia, small lymphocyte lymphoma, and in patients who have undergone splenectomy. Patients with ineffective humoral immunity lack opsonizing antibodies and are *at particular risk for infection with encapsulated organisms*, such as *Haemophilus influenzae*, *Neisseria meningitides*, and *Streptococcus pneumoniae*. Although rituximab is normally thought of as being linked to impaired cellular immunity, it has been associated with the development of *Pneumocystis jirovecii* infection and progressive multifocal leukoencephalopathy (PML) as well as with hepatitis B reactivation.

B. Neutropenia

Neutropenia is common following hematopoietic stem cell transplantation and among patients with solid tumors—as a result of myelosuppressive chemotherapy—and in acute leukemias. *The risk of infection begins to increase when the absolute neutrophil count falls below 1000/mcL, with a dramatic increase in frequency and severity when the neutrophil count falls below 200/mcL.* The infection risk is also increased with a rapid rate of decline of neutrophils and with a prolonged period of neutropenia. Patients with granulocytopenia are particularly susceptible to infections with gram-negative enteric organisms, *Pseudomonas*, gram-positive cocci (particularly *Staphylococcus aureus* and viridans streptococci), *Candida, Aspergillus*, and other fungi such as *Scedosporium*, *Fusarium*, and the mucormycoses.

C. Impaired Cellular Immunity

Patients with cellular immune deficiency encompass a large and heterogeneous group, including patients with HIV infection (see Chapter 35); patients with lymphoreticular malignancies, such as Hodgkin disease; and patients receiving immunosuppressive medications, such as corticosteroids, cyclosporine, tacrolimus, and other cytotoxic medications. This latter group—those who are immunosuppressed because of medications—includes patients who have undergone solid organ transplantation, many patients receiving therapy for solid tumors, and patients receiving prolonged high-dose corticosteroid treatment (eg, for asthma, temporal arteritis, SLE). Patients taking TNF inhibitors, such as etanercept and infliximab, also are included in this category. Patients with cellular immune dysfunction are susceptible to infections by a large number of organisms, particularly ones that replicate intracellularly. Examples include bacteria, such as *Listeria*, *Legionella*, *Salmonella*, and mycobacteria; viruses, such as herpes simplex, varicella, and CMV; fungi, such as *Cryptococcus*, *Coccidioides*, *Histoplasma*, and *Pneumocystis;* and protozoa, such as *Toxoplasma*.

D. Hematopoietic Cell Transplant Recipients

The length of time it takes for complications to occur in hematopoietic cell transplant recipients can be helpful in determining the etiologic agent. In the *early (pre-engraftment) posttransplant period (days 1–21)*, patients will become severely neutropenic for 7–21 days. Patients are at risk for gram-positive (particularly catheter-related) and gram-negative bacterial infections, as well as herpes simplex virus, respiratory syncytial virus, and fungal infections. In contrast to solid organ transplant recipients, the source of fever is unknown in 60–70% of hematopoietic cell transplant patients. *Between 3 weeks and 3 months posttransplant*, infections with CMV, adenovirus, *Aspergillus*, and *Candida* are most common. *P jirovecii* pneumonia is possible, particularly in patients who receive additional immunosuppression for treatment of graft-versus-host disease. Patients continue to be at risk for infectious complications *beyond 3 months following transplantation,* particularly those who have received allogeneic transplantation and those who are taking immunosuppressive therapy for chronic graft-versus-host disease. Varicella zoster is common, and *Aspergillus* and CMV infections are increasingly seen in this period as well.

E. Solid Organ Transplant Recipients

The length of time it takes for infection to occur following solid organ transplantation can also be helpful in determining the infectious origin. *Immediate postoperative infections* often involve the transplanted organ. Following lung transplantation, pneumonia and mediastinitis are common; following liver transplantation, intra-abdominal abscess, cholangitis, and peritonitis may be seen; after kidney transplantation, UTIs, perinephric abscesses, and infected lymphoceles can occur.

Most infections that occur in the *first 2–4 weeks posttransplant* are related to the operative procedure and to hospitalization itself (wound infection, intravenous catheter infection, UTI from an indwelling urinary catheter) or are related to the transplanted organ. In rare instances, donor-derived infections (eg, West Nile virus, tuberculosis) may present during this time period. Compensated organ transplants obtained abroad through "medical tourism" can introduce additional risk of infections, which vary by country and by transplant setting. Infections that occur *between the first and sixth months* are often related to immunosuppression. During this period, reactivation of viruses, such as herpes simplex, varicella zoster, and CMV is quite common. Opportunistic infections with fungi (eg, *Candida, Aspergillus, Cryptococcus, Pneumocystis*), *Listeria monocytogenes*, *Nocardia*, and *Toxoplasma* also are common. *After 6 months*, if immunosuppression has been reduced to maintenance levels, infections that would be expected in any population occur. Patients with poorly functioning allografts receiving long-term immunosuppression therapy continue to be at risk for opportunistic infections.

F. Tumor Necrosis Factor Inhibitor Recipients

Patients taking TNF inhibitors (infliximab, etanercept, adalimumab, certolizumab pegol, golimumab) have specific defects that increase risk of bacterial, mycobacterial (particularly tuberculosis), viral (HBV reactivation and HCV progression), and fungal infections (*Pneumocystis*, molds, and endemic mycoses). Infection risk may be highest shortly after therapy is initiated (within the first 3 months) and with a higher dose of medications.

G. Recipients of Other Biologics

In addition to TNF inhibitors, other biologics target a variety of immunologic pathways that are involved in immunologic mediated disease and in cancer replication. Disruption of these pathways include, but are not limited to, impact on B cells, T cells, complement, and leukocytes. *This may result in not only serious infections, but the development of autoimmune disease and malignancies as well.* Some medications have been observed to have specific associations with opportunistic infections (eg, natalizumab and PML, or eculizumab and meningococcal disease). Other biologics such as chimeric antigen receptor T (CAR-T) cells also carry infection risks of up to 40% post-infection or may have adverse effects that mimic infection (eg, cytokine release syndrome). Checkpoint inhibitors (eg, anti–PD-1 and CTLA antibodies) used for the treatment of advanced malignancies also may have *effects that mimic infection via immune enhancement.* Prolonged immunosuppression used to treat immune-associated adverse events in CAR-T and checkpoint inhibitor therapy (eg, TNF inhibitors and corticosteroids) can then result in opportunistic and other infections. As more biologics are developed, such as bispecific antibodies, clinicians must remain vigilant for the possibility of serious infectious disease risk.

H. Other Immunocompromised States

A large group of patients who are not specifically immunodeficient are at increased risk for infection due to debilitating injury (eg, burns or severe trauma), invasive procedures (eg, chronic central intravenous catheters, indwelling urinary catheters, dialysis catheters), CNS dysfunction (which predisposes patients to aspiration pneumonia and pressure injuries), obstructing lesions (eg, pneumonia due to an obstructed bronchus, pyelonephritis due to nephrolithiasis, cholangitis secondary to cholelithiasis), and use of broad-spectrum antibiotics. Patients with diabetes mellitus have alterations in cellular immunity, resulting in mucormycosis, emphysematous pyelonephritis, and foot infections.

Clinical Findings

A. Laboratory Findings

Routine evaluation includes CBC with differential, complete metabolic panel, and blood cultures, with a low threshold for cross-sectional imaging; urine and respiratory cultures should be obtained if indicated clinically or radiographically. Any focal symptoms (eg, localized pain, headache, rash) should prompt imaging and cultures appropriate to the site.

Patients who remain febrile without an obvious source should be evaluated for viral infection (serum CMV PCR), abscesses (which usually occur near previous operative sites), candidiasis involving the liver or spleen, or aspergillosis. Serologic evaluation may be helpful if toxoplasmosis or an endemic fungal infection (coccidioidomycosis, histoplasmosis) is a possible cause. Antigen-based assays may be useful for the diagnosis of aspergillosis (detected by galactomannan level in serum or bronchoalveolar lavage fluid), or other invasive fungal disease, including *Pneumocystis* infection (serum β-D-glucan level).

B. Special Diagnostic Procedures

Special diagnostic procedures should also be considered. The cause of pulmonary infiltrates can be easily determined with simple techniques in some situations—eg, induced sputum yields a diagnosis of *Pneumocystis* pneumonia in 50–80% of patients with AIDS with this infection. In other situations, more invasive procedures may be required (bronchoalveolar lavage, transbronchial biopsy, open lung biopsy). Skin, liver, or bone marrow biopsy may be helpful in establishing a diagnosis. Next-generation DNA-sequencing analysis (eg, of plasma, bronchoalveolar lavage, CSF) is an increasingly used and validated option for diagnosis of infectious diseases in immunocompromised persons.

Differential Diagnosis

Allograft rejection, organ ischemia and necrosis, thrombophlebitis, and malignancy including posttransplant lymphoproliferative disease may all present as fever and must be considered in the differential diagnosis.

Prevention

While prophylactic antimicrobial medications are used commonly, the optimal medications or dosage regimens are debated. *Hand washing is the simplest and most effective means of decreasing hospital-associated infections*, especially in the compromised patient. Invasive devices such as central and peripheral lines and indwelling urinary catheters are potential sources of infection. Some centers use *laminar airflow isolation* or *high-efficiency particulate air (HEPA) filtering* in hematopoietic cell transplant patients. Rates of infection and episodes of febrile neutropenia, but not mortality, are decreased if *colony-stimulating factors* are used (typically in situations where the risk of febrile neutropenia is ≥ 20%) during chemotherapy or during stem cell transplantation.

A. *Pneumocystis* & Herpes Simplex Infections

Trimethoprim-sulfamethoxazole (TMP-SMX), one double-strength tablet orally three times a week, one double-strength tablet twice daily on weekends, or one single-strength tablet daily, can prevent *Pneumocystis* infections. In patients allergic to TMP-SMX, dapsone, 50 mg orally daily or 100 mg three times weekly, is recommended. Glucose-6-phosphate dehydrogenase (G6PD) levels should be assessed before dapsone is instituted. Acyclovir prevents herpes simplex infections in bone marrow and solid organ transplant recipients and is given to seropositive patients who are not receiving ganciclovir or valganciclovir for CMV prophylaxis. The usual dose is 400 mg orally three times daily for 4 weeks (hematopoietic cell transplants) to 12 weeks (solid organ transplants).

B. CMV

The two approaches to CMV prevention are *universal prophylaxis* or *preemptive therapy*. Among solid organ transplant recipients (liver, kidney, heart, lung), the strategy chosen depends on the serologic status of the donor and recipient and the organ transplanted, which determines the level of immunosuppression sought after transplant. The greatest risk of developing CMV disease is in seronegative recipients who receive organs from seropositive donors. These high-risk patients often receive prophylaxis with oral valganciclovir for 3–6 months, potentially longer in lung transplant recipients. Other solid organ transplant recipients (seropositive recipients) are at lower risk for developing CMV disease but still usually receive either prophylaxis with oral valganciclovir for 3 months or preemptive management in which they are monitored for the presence of CMV by PCR. If CMV is detected, then therapy is instituted with treatment-dose oral valganciclovir for a minimum of 2–3 weeks. The newest agent for refractory or resistant CMV is maribavir. The lowest-risk group for the development of CMV disease is in seronegative patients who receive organs from seronegative donors. Typically, no CMV prophylaxis is used in this group. Ganciclovir and valganciclovir also prevent herpes virus reactivation. Because immunosuppression is increased during periods of rejection, patients treated for rejection either receive CMV prophylaxis or are monitored preemptively during rejection therapy.

Recipients of hematopoietic cell transplants are more severely immunosuppressed than recipients of solid organ transplants, are at greater risk for developing serious CMV infection (usually CMV reactivation), and thus usually receive more aggressive prophylaxis. Like in solid organ transplant recipients, all high-risk patients (seropositive patients who receive allogeneic transplants) receive oral prophylaxis to day 100. Because valganciclovir is associated with significant bone marrow toxicity, letermovir is first line for high-risk hematopoietic cell transplant (HCT) recipients. Moderate- and low-risk hematopoietic cell transplant recipients undergo the preemptive approach over prophylaxis. Patients who receive lymphocyte-depleting monoclonal antibodies (eg, alemtuzumab) generally also have weekly CMV surveillance for at least 2 months after completing treatment. Other preventive strategies include use of *CMV-negative* or *leukocyte-depleted blood products* for CMV-seronegative recipients.

C. Other Organisms

Routine decontamination of the GI tract to prevent bacteremia in the neutropenic patient is *not* recommended. The use of prophylactic antibiotics in the afebrile, asymptomatic neutropenic patient is debated, although many centers have adopted this strategy. Rates of bacteremia are decreased, but overall mortality is *not* affected and emergence of resistant organisms takes place. Use of intravenous immunoglobulin is reserved for the small number of patients with severe hypogammaglobulinemia (IgG < 400 mg/dL) following hematopoietic stem cell transplantation and should not be routinely administered to all transplant patients.

Prophylaxis with antifungal agents to prevent invasive mold (primarily *Aspergillus*) and yeast (primarily *Candida*) infections is routinely used, but the optimal agent, dose, and duration are also debated. Lipid-based preparations of amphotericin B, echinocandins, as well as systemic fluconazole, voriconazole, posaconazole, or isavuconazole are all prophylactic options in the neutropenic patient. Voriconazole and posaconazole are superior to amphotericin for documented *Aspergillus* infections, and posaconazole prophylaxis (compared with fluconazole) results in fewer cases of invasive aspergillosis among allogeneic stem cell transplant recipients with graft-versus-host disease; thus, one approach to prophylaxis is to use oral fluconazole (400 mg/day) for patients at low risk for developing fungal infections (autologous stem cell transplants) and oral voriconazole (200 mg twice daily) or oral posaconazole (200 mg suspension three times daily or 300 mg [three 100-mg tablets] sustained-release tablets once daily) for those at high risk (allogeneic transplants, graft-versus-host disease) at least until engraftment (usually 30 days). Echinocandins (eg, micafungin 100 mg intravenously daily) and isavuconazole (372 mg intravenously or orally daily) can be considered as alternative prophylactic agents for patients who are unable to tolerate other azoles due to drug interactions, transaminitis, or QT prolongation. In solid organ transplant recipients, the risk of invasive fungal infection varies considerably (1–2% in liver, pancreas, and kidney transplants and 6–8% in heart and lung transplants). Whether universal prophylaxis or observation with preemptive therapy is the best approach has not been determined. Although fluconazole is effective in preventing yeast infections, emergence of fluconazole-resistant *Candida* and molds (*Fusarium*, *Aspergillus*, *Mucor*) has raised concerns about its routine use as a prophylactic agent in the general solid organ transplant population. However, liver transplant recipients with additional risk factors, such as having undergone a choledochojejunostomy, having had a high transfusion requirement, or having developed kidney disease, may benefit from abbreviated postoperative *Candida* prophylaxis.

Given the high risk of reactivation of tuberculosis in patients taking TNF inhibitors, all patients should be screened for latent tuberculosis infection (LTBI) with a tuberculin skin test or an interferon-γ release assay prior to the start of therapy. If LTBI is diagnosed, treatment with the TNF inhibitors should be delayed until treatment for LTBI has been initiated and consistently tolerated. There is also a marked risk of reactivation of hepatitis B and hepatitis C in patients taking TNF inhibitors; patients should also be screened for these viruses when TNF inhibitor treatment is being considered. Providers should also ensure that patients' vaccinations are up to date before starting TNF inhibitor therapy.

Treatment

A. General Measures

Because infections in the immunocompromised patient can be rapidly progressive and life-threatening, diagnostic procedures must be performed promptly, and empiric therapy is usually instituted.

While reduction or discontinuation of immunosuppressive medication may risk rejection of the transplanted organ or worsening of underlying disease, this measure may be necessary if the infection is life-threatening. Hematopoietic growth factors (granulocyte and granulocyte-macrophage colony-stimulating factors) stimulate proliferation of bone marrow stem cells, resulting in an increase in peripheral leukocytes. These agents shorten the period of neutropenia and have been associated with reduction in infection.

B. Specific Measures

Antimicrobial medication therapy ultimately should be tailored to culture results. While combinations of antimicrobials are used with the intent of providing synergy or preventing resistance, the primary reason for empiric combination therapy is broad-spectrum coverage of all likely pathogens.

Empiric therapy is often instituted at the earliest sign of infection in the immunosuppressed patient because prompt therapy favorably affects outcome, particularly in febrile neutropenia. The antibiotic or combination of antibiotics used depends on the degree of immune compromise and the site of infection. For example, in the *high-risk febrile neutropenic patient, an algorithmic approach to therapy is often used.* Febrile neutropenic patients should be empirically treated with broad-spectrum agents active against selected gram-positive bacteria, *Pseudomonas aeruginosa*, and other aerobic gram-negative bacilli (such as cefepime 2 g every 8 hours intravenously). The addition of vancomycin, 10–15 mg/kg/dose intravenously every 12 hours, should be considered in those patients with suspected infection due to methicillin-resistant *S aureus* (MRSA). Continued neutropenic fever in an unstable patient necessitates broadening of antibacterial coverage from cefepime to agents such as meropenem 1 g every 8 hours intravenously along with an additional gram-negative agent (ciprofloxacin or tobramycin) if the patient is critically ill. Antifungal agents (such as voriconazole, 200 mg intravenously or orally every 12 hours) should be added if fevers continue after 5–7 days of broad-spectrum antibacterial therapy. *While the traditional approach was to continue antibiotics until resolution of neutropenia, practice has shifted to earlier discontinuation of antibiotics in the neutropenic patient who becomes afebrile for 72 hours if no signs or symptoms of infection persist.*

Patients with fever and *low-risk neutropenia* (neutropenia expected to persist for <10 days, no comorbid complications requiring hospitalization, and cancer adequately treated) can be treated with oral antibiotic regimens, such as ciprofloxacin, 750 mg every 12 hours, plus amoxicillin-clavulanic acid, 500 mg every 8 hours for patients not receiving fluoroquinolone prophylaxis. *Antibiotics are usually continued as long as the patient is neutropenic even if a source is not identified.* In the organ transplant patient with interstitial infiltrates, the main concern is infection with *Pneumocystis* or *Legionella* species, so that empiric treatment with a macrolide or fluoroquinolone (*Legionella*) and TMP-SMX, 15 mg/kg/day, dosed on the trimethoprim component, orally or intravenously (*Pneumocystis*), would be reasonable in those patients not receiving TMP-SMX prophylaxis. If the patient does not respond to empiric treatment, a decision must be made to add more antimicrobial agents or perform invasive procedures to make a specific diagnosis. By making a definite diagnosis, therapy can be specific, thereby reducing selection pressure for resistance and superinfection.

When to Refer

- Any immunocompromised patient with an opportunistic infection.
- Patients with potential drug toxicities and drug interactions related to antimicrobials where alternative agents are sought.
- Patients with latent tuberculosis, HBV, and HCV infection in whom therapy with TNF inhibitors is planned.

When to Admit

Immunocompromised patients who are febrile, or those without fevers in whom an infection is suspected, particularly in the following groups: solid organ or hematopoietic stem cell transplant recipient (particularly in the first 6 months), neutropenic patients, patients receiving TNF inhibitors, and transplant recipients who have had recent rejection episodes (including graft-versus-host disease).

Chean D et al. Severe community-acquired pneumonia in immunocompromised patients. Semin Respir Crit Care Med. 2024;45:255. [PMID: 38266998]

Chen Y-H et al. Efficacy and safety of early antibiotic de-escalation in febrile neutropenia for patients with hematologic malignancy: a systematic review and meta-analysis. Antimicrob Agents Chemother. 2025;69:e0159724. [PMID: 40079575]

Giannella M et al; ECCMID study groups on Invasive Fungal Infection and Infection in Immunocompromised Hosts. Invasive fungal disease in the immunocompromised host: changing epidemiology, new antifungal therapies, and management challenges. Clin Microbiol Infect. 2025;31:29. [PMID: 39142631]

Grossi PA et al. Recent advances in cytomegalovirus infection management in solid organ transplant recipients. Curr Opin Organ Transplant. 2024;29:131. [PMID: 38288947]

Kamboj M et al. Vaccination of adults with cancer: ASCO Guideline. J Clin Oncol. 2024;42:1699. [PMID: 38498792]

Ljungman P et al. Recommendations from the 10th European Conference on Infections in Leukaemia for the management of cytomegalovirus in patients after allogeneic haematopoietic cell transplantation and other T-cell-engaging therapies. Lancet Infect Dis. 2025;25:e451. [PMID: 40188837]

Sandherr M et al. 2024 update of the AGIHO guideline on diagnosis and empirical treatment of fever of unknown origin (FUO) in adult neutropenic patients with solid tumours and hematological malignancies. Lancet Reg Health Eur. 2025;51:101214. [PMID: 39973942]

Shahid Z et al. Best practice considerations by the American Society of Transplant and Cellular Therapy: infection prevention and management after chimeric antigen receptor T cell therapy for hematological malignancies. Transplant Cell Ther. 2024;30:955. [PMID: 39084261]

HEALTH CARE–ASSOCIATED INFECTIONS

ESSENTIALS OF DIAGNOSIS

- Acquired during the course of receiving health care treatment for other conditions.
- Most cases are preventable.
- Hospital-associated infections are defined as not being present or incubating at the time of hospital admission and developing ≥ 48 hours after admission.
- Hand washing is the most effective prevention and should be done routinely even when gloves are worn.

General Considerations

Worldwide, approximately 10% of patients acquire a health care–associated infection, resulting in prolongation of the hospital stay, increase in cost of care, and significant morbidity and mortality. The most common infections are UTIs, usually associated with indwelling urinary catheters or urologic procedures; bloodstream infections, most commonly from indwelling catheters but also from secondary sites, such as surgical wounds, abscesses, pneumonia, the genitourinary tract, and the GI tract; pneumonia in intubated patients or those with altered levels of consciousness; surgical wound infections; MRSA infections; and *Clostridioides difficile* infection. There has been hospital-associated transmission of respiratory viruses.

Some general principles are helpful in preventing, diagnosing, and treating health care–associated infections:

1. Many infections are a direct result of the use of *invasive devices* for monitoring or therapy, such as intravenous catheters, indwelling urinary catheters, shunts, surgical drains, catheters placed by interventional radiology for drainage, nasogastric tubes, and orotracheal or nasotracheal tubes for ventilatory support. *Early removal of such devices reduces the possibility of infection.*
2. Patients in whom health care–associated infections develop are often critically ill, have been hospitalized for extended periods, and have received several courses of broad-spectrum antibiotic therapy. As a result, *health care–associated infections are often due to multidrug-resistant pathogens and differ from those encountered in community-acquired infections.* For example, *S aureus* and *S epidermidis* (a frequent cause of prosthetic device infection) are often resistant to methicillin and require vancomycin for therapy; *Enterococcus faecium* is often resistant to ampicillin and vancomycin; gram-negative infections caused by *Pseudomonas, Citrobacter, Enterobacter, Acinetobacter, Stenotrophomonas*, extended-spectrum β-lactamase (ESBL)–producing *E coli, Klebsiella*, and carbapenem-resistant Enterobacterales may be resistant to most antibacterials. When choosing antibiotics to treat the seriously ill patient with a health care–associated infection, the individual patient's prior infection history and local antibiogram (antimicrobial resistance patterns) must be considered. In the most seriously ill patients, broad-spectrum coverage with vancomycin and a carbapenem with or without an aminoglycoside is recommended. Once a pathogen is isolated and susceptibilities are known, the most narrow-spectrum, least toxic, most cost-effective regimen should be used.

Widespread use of antimicrobial medications contributes to the selection of drug-resistant organisms; thus, *every effort should be made to limit the spectrum of coverage and unnecessary duration.* All too often, unreliable or uninterpretable specimens are obtained for culture that result in unnecessary use of antibiotics. The best example of this principle is the diagnosis of line-related or bloodstream infection in the febrile patient. To avoid unnecessary use of antibiotics, thoughtful consideration of culture results is mandatory. A positive wound culture without signs of inflammation or infection, a positive sputum culture without pulmonary infiltrates on CXR, or a positive urine culture in a catheterized patient without symptoms or signs of pyelonephritis are all likely to represent *colonization*, not infection.

Clinical Findings

A. Symptoms and Signs

Catheter-associated infections have a variable presentation, depending on the type of catheter used (peripheral or central venous catheters, nontunneled or tunneled). Local signs of infection may be present at the insertion site, with pain, erythema, and purulence. Fever is often absent in uncomplicated infections and, if present, may indicate more disseminated disease such as bacteremia, cellulitis and septic thrombophlebitis. Often signs of infection at the insertion site are absent.

1. Fever in an ICU patient—*Fever complicates up to 70% of patients in ICUs, and the etiology of the fever may be infectious or noninfectious.* Common infectious causes include catheter-associated infections, hospital-acquired and ventilator-associated pneumonia (see Chapter 9), surgical site infections, UTIs, and sepsis. Clinically relevant sinusitis is relatively uncommon in the patient in the ICU.

An important noninfectious cause is thromboembolic disease. Fever in conjunction with refractory hypotension and shock may suggest sepsis; however, adrenal insufficiency, thyroid storm, and transfusion reaction may have a similar clinical presentation. Drug fever is difficult to diagnose and is usually a diagnosis of exclusion unless there are other signs of hypersensitivity, such as a typical maculopapular rash (most common with β-lactams).

2. Fever in the postoperative patient—Postoperative fever is common and noninfectious fever resolves spontaneously. Timing of the onset of the fever in relation to the surgical procedure may be of diagnostic benefit.

a. Immediate fever (in the first few hours after surgery)—Immediate fever can be due to medications that were given perioperatively, to surgical trauma, or to infections that were present before surgery. Necrotizing fasciitis due to group A streptococci or mixed organisms may present in this period. **Malignant hyperthermia** is rare and presents 30 minutes to several hours following inhalational anesthesia and is characterized by extreme hyperthermia, muscle rigidity, rhabdomyolysis, electrolyte abnormalities, and hypotension. Aggressive cooling and dantrolene are the mainstays of therapy. Aspiration of acidic gastric contents during surgery can result in a chemical pneumonitis (**Mendelson syndrome**) that develops rapidly, is transient, and does not require antibiotics. Fever due to surgical trauma usually resolves in 2–3 days; however, it may be longer in more complicated operative cases and in patients with head trauma.

b. Acute fever (within 1 week of surgery)—Acute fever is usually due to common causes of hospital-associated infections, such as ventilator-associated pneumonia (including aspiration pneumonia in patients with decreased gag reflex) and line infections. Noninfectious causes include alcohol withdrawal, gout, PE, and pancreatitis. *Atelectasis following surgery is commonly invoked as a cause of postoperative fever, but there is no good evidence to support a causal association between the presence or degree of atelectasis and fever.*

c. Subacute fever (at least 1 week after surgery)—Surgical site infections commonly present at least 1 week after surgery. The type of surgery that was performed predicts specific infectious etiologies. Patients undergoing cardiothoracic surgery may be at higher risk for pneumonia and deep and superficial sternal wound infections. Meningitis without typical signs of meningismus may complicate neurosurgical procedures. Postoperative deep abdominal abscesses may require drainage.

B. Laboratory Findings

Blood cultures are universally recommended, and CXRs are frequently obtained. A properly prepared sputum Gram stain and sputum cultures may be useful in selected patients where there is a high pretest probability of pneumonia but multiple exclusion criteria probably limit generalizability in most patients, such as immunocompromised patients and those with drug resistance. Other diagnostic strategies will be dictated by the clinical context (eg, transesophageal echocardiogram in a patient with *S aureus* bacteremia).

Any fever in a patient with a central venous catheter should prompt the collection of blood. The best method to evaluate bacteremia is to gather *at least two peripherally obtained blood cultures.* Blood cultures from unidentified sites, a single blood culture from any site, or a blood culture through an existing line will often be positive for coagulase-positive staphylococci, particularly *S epidermidis*, often resulting in the inappropriate use of vancomycin. *Unless two separate venipuncture cultures are obtained—not through catheters—interpretation of results is impossible,* and unnecessary therapy often results with resulting increase in bacterial resistance pressure, laboratory costs, antibiotic use, and length of stay. Microbiologic evaluation of the removed catheter can sometimes be helpful, but only in addition to (not instead of) blood cultures drawn from peripheral sites. The *differential time to positivity* measures the difference in time that cultures simultaneously drawn through a catheter and a peripheral site become positive. A positive test (central blood culture positive ≥ 120 minutes before peripheral blood culture) supports a catheter-related bloodstream infection, while a negative test suggests catheters may be retained.

Complications

Complications such as septic thrombophlebitis, endocarditis, or metastatic foci of infection (particularly with *S aureus*) may be suspected in patients with persistent bacteremia and fever despite removal of the infected catheter. Additional studies such as venous Doppler studies, transesophageal echocardiogram, and CXRs may be indicated, and 4–6 weeks of antibiotics may be needed. In the case of septic thrombophlebitis, anticoagulation with heparin is also recommended if there are no contraindications.

Differential Diagnosis

Although most fevers are due to infections, about 25% of patients will have fever of noninfectious origin, including drug fever, nonspecific postoperative fevers (tissue damage or necrosis), hematoma, pancreatitis, PE, MI, and ischemic bowel disease.

Prevention

*The concept of **universal precautions** emphasizes that all patients are treated as though they have a potential blood-borne transmissible disease, and thus all body secretions are handled with care to prevent spread of disease.* Body substance isolation requires use of gloves whenever a health care worker anticipates contact with blood or other body secretions. *Even though gloves are worn, health care workers should routinely wash their hands, since it is the easiest and most effective means of preventing hospital-associated infections.* Application of a *rapid drying, alcohol-based antiseptic* is simple, takes less time than traditional hand washing with soap and water, is more effective at reducing hand colonization, and promotes compliance with hand decontamination. *For prevention of transmission of C difficile infection, hand washing is more effective than alcohol-based antiseptics.* Consequently, even after removing gloves, providers should always wash hands in cases of proven or suspected *C difficile* infection.

Peripheral intravenous lines should be replaced no more frequently than every 3–4 days. Some clinicians replace only when clinically indicated or if the line was put in emergently. Arterial lines and lines in the central venous circulation (including those placed peripherally) can be left in place indefinitely and are changed or removed when they are clinically suspected of being infected, when they are nonfunctional, or when they are no longer needed. Using sterile barrier precautions (including cap, mask, gown, gloves, and drape) is recommended while inserting central venous catheters. *Antibiotic-impregnated (minocycline plus rifampin or chlorhexidine plus silver sulfadiazine) venous catheters* reduce line infections. *Silver alloy–impregnated indwelling urinary catheters* reduce the incidence of catheter-associated bacteriuria, but not consistently catheter-associated UTIs. Best practices to prevent ventilator-associated pneumonia include avoiding intubation if possible, minimizing and daily interruption of sedation, pooling/draining of subglottic secretions above the tube cuff, and elevating the head of the bed. Silver-coated endotracheal tubes may reduce the incidence of ventilator-associated pneumonia but have limited impact on hospital stay duration or mortality, so they are not generally recommended. *Catheter-related UTIs and intravenous catheter-associated infections are not Medicare-reimbursable conditions in the United States. Preoperative skin preparation* with chlorhexidine and alcohol (versus povidone-iodine) reduces the incidence of infection following surgery. Another strategy that can prevent surgical site infections is the *identification and treatment of S aureus nasal carriers* with 2% mupirocin nasal ointment and chlorhexidine soap. *Daily bathing of ICU patients* with chlorhexidine-impregnated washcloths versus soap and water results in lower incidence of health care–associated infections and colonization. Selective decontamination of the digestive tract with nonabsorbable or parenteral antibiotics, or both, does not decrease mortality and is in limited use because of the concern of the development of antibiotic resistance. *Prevention bundles* (implementing more than one intervention concomitantly) are commonly used as a practical strategy to enhance care.

Attentive nursing care (positioning to prevent pressure injuries, wound care, elevating the head during tube feedings to prevent aspiration) is critical in preventing hospital-associated infections. In addition, monitoring of high-risk areas by hospital epidemiologists is critical in the prevention of infection. Some guidelines advocate rapid screening (active surveillance cultures) for MRSA on admission to acute care facilities among certain subpopulations of patients (eg, those recently hospitalized, admission to the ICU, patients undergoing hemodialysis). However, outside the setting of an MRSA outbreak, it is not clear whether this strategy decreases the incidence of hospital-associated MRSA infections.

Vaccines, including hepatitis A, hepatitis B, and the varicella, pneumococcal, influenza, and SARS-CoV-2 vaccinations, are important adjuncts. (See Immunization Against Infectious Diseases, below.)

Treatment

A. Fever in an ICU Patient

Unless the patient has a central neurologic injury with elevated intracranial pressure or has a temperature > 41°C, there is less physiologic need to maintain euthermia. *Empiric broad-spectrum antibiotics (see* Table 34–1*) are recommended for neutropenic and other immunocompromised patients and in patients who are clinically unstable.*

B. Catheter-Associated Infections

Factors that inform treatment decisions include the type of catheter, the causative pathogen, the availability of alternate catheter access sites, the need for ongoing intravascular access, and the severity of disease.

In general, catheters should be removed if there is purulence at the exit site; if the organism is *S aureus*, gram-negative rods, or *Candida* species; if there is persistent bacteremia (> 48 hours while receiving antibiotics); or if complications, such as septic thrombophlebitis, endocarditis, or other metastatic disease, exist. Central venous catheters may be exchanged over a guidewire provided there is no erythema or purulence at the exit site and the patient does not appear to be septic. Methicillin-resistant, coagulase-negative staphylococci are the most common pathogens; thus, empiric therapy with vancomycin, 15 mg/kg/dose intravenously twice daily, should be given assuming normal kidney function. Empiric gram-negative coverage should be used in patients who are immunocompromised or who are critically ill (see Table 34–1).

Antibiotic treatment duration depends on the pathogen and the extent of disease. For uncomplicated bacteremia, 5–7 days of therapy is usually sufficient for coagulase-negative staphylococci, even if the original catheter is retained. Fourteen days of therapy are generally recommended for uncomplicated bacteremia caused by gram-negative rods, *Candida* species, and *S aureus*. *Antibiotic lock therapy* involves the instillation of supratherapeutic concentrations of antibiotics with heparin in the lumen of catheters. The purpose is to achieve adequate concentrations of antibiotics to kill microbes in the biofilm. Antibiotic lock therapy can be used for catheter-related bloodstream infections caused by both gram-positive and gram-negative bacterial pathogens and when the catheter is being retained in a salvage situation.

When to Refer

- Any patient with multidrug-resistant infection.
- Any patient with fungemia, *S aureus* bacteremia, or persistent bacteremia of any organism.
- Patients whose catheters cannot be removed.
- Patients with multisite infections.
- Patients with impaired or fluctuating kidney function for assistance with dosing of antimicrobials.
- Patients with refractory or recurrent *C difficile* infection.

Cymbal M et al. Management of *Clostridioides difficile* infection: diagnosis, treatment, and future perspectives. Am J Med. 2024;137:571. [PMID: 38508330]

Huston JM et al; Therapeutics and Guidelines Committee. The Surgical Infection Society Guidelines on the management of intra-abdominal infection: 2024 Update. Surg Infect (Larchmt). 2024;25:419. [PMID: 38990709]

Juul FE et al. Fecal microbiota transplantation versus vancomycin for primary *Clostridioides difficile* infection: a randomized controlled trial. Ann Intern Med. 2025;178:940. [PMID: 40523286]

Metersky ML et al. Management of ventilator-associated pneumonia: guidelines. Infect Dis Clin North Am. 2024;38:87. [PMID: 38280768]

Rosenthal VD et al. Preventing ventilator-associated pneumonia: a position paper of the International Society for Infectious Diseases, 2024 update. Int J Infect Dis. 2025;151:107305. [PMID: 39551087]

Table 34–1. Examples of initial antimicrobial therapy for acutely ill, hospitalized adults pending identification of causative organism (listed in alphabetical order by suspected clinical diagnosis).

Suspected Clinical Diagnosis	Likely Etiologic Diagnosis	Medication of Choice
Brain abscess	*Staphylococcus aureus*, gram-negative bacilli, streptococci, mixed anaerobes	Ceftriaxone, 2 g intravenously every 12 hours **plus** metronidazole, 500 mg orally/intravenous every 8 hours, **plus** vancomycin, 15–20 mg/kg intravenously every 8–12 hours[1]
Endocarditis, acute	*S aureus*, *Enterococcus faecalis*, viridans streptococci	Vancomycin, 15–20 mg/kg/dose intravenously every 8–12 hours[1]
Fever in neutropenic patient receiving cancer chemotherapy	*S aureus*, *Pseudomonas*, *Klebsiella*, *Escherichia coli*	Cefepime, 2 g intravenously every 8 hours. If concerned for MRSA infection, add vancomycin 15–20 mg/kg intravenously every 8–12 hours[1]
Intra-abdominal sepsis (eg, postoperative, peritonitis, cholecystitis)	Gram-negative bacteria, anaerobic bacteria (ie, *Bacteroides*), enterococcus	Piperacillin-tazobactam, 4.5 g intravenously every 6–8 hours, **or** ertapenem, 1 g every 24 hours
Meningitis, bacterial, age 18–50 years, community-acquired	Pneumococcus,[3] meningococcus	Ceftriaxone, 2 g intravenously every 12 hours,[3] **plus** vancomycin, 15–20 mg/kg intravenously every 8–12 hours[1]
Meningitis, bacterial, age > 50 years, community-acquired	*Streptococcus pneumoniae* (pneumococcus), *Neisseria meningitidis* (meningococcus), *Listeria monocytogenes*,[2] gram-negative bacilli, group B streptococcus	Ampicillin, 2 g intravenously every 4 hours, **plus** ceftriaxone, 2 g intravenously every 12 hours, **plus** vancomycin, 15–20 mg/kg intravenously every 8–12 hours[1]
Meningitis, postoperative (or posttraumatic)	*S aureus*, gram-negative bacilli, coagulase-negative staphylococci, diphtheroids (eg, *Cutibacterium acnes*)	Vancomycin, 15–20 mg/kg intravenously every 8–12 hours,[1] **plus** cefepime, 2 g intravenously every 8 hours
Osteomyelitis	*S aureus*, secondarily gram-negative aerobes	Vancomycin 15–20 mg/kg intravenously every 8–12 hours,[1] **plus** ceftriaxone 2 g intravenously every 24 hours
Pneumonia, community-acquired, non-ICU hospital admission	Pneumococci, *Haemophilus influenzae*, *Mycoplasma pneumoniae*, *Legionella*, *Chlamydia pneumoniae*	Ceftriaxone, 1 g intravenously every 24 hours or ampicillin-sulbactam 1.5–3 g intravenously every 6 hours) **plus** azithromycin, 500 mg intravenously every 24 hours; **or** a respiratory fluoroquinolone[4] alone
Pneumonia, postoperative or nosocomial	*S aureus*, gram-negative bacilli	Cefepime, 2 g intravenously every 8 hours; **or** ceftazidime, 2 g intravenously every 8 hours; **or** piperacillin-tazobactam, 4.5 g intravenously every 6–8 hours; **or** imipenem, 500 mg intravenously every 6 hours; **or** meropenem, 1 g intravenously every 8 hours **plus** vancomycin, 15–20 mg/kg/dose intravenously every 8–12 hours[1] Empiric combination therapy for gram-negative bacilli may be considered based on local susceptibility patterns. Secondary agents include ciprofloxacin, 400 mg intravenously every 8 hours **or** tobramycin, 5–7 mg/kg intravenously every 24 hours
Pyelonephritis with flank pain and fever	*E coli*, *Klebsiella*, *Proteus*	Ceftriaxone, 1 g intravenously every 24 hours; **or** if culture results confirm susceptibility, ciprofloxacin, 400 mg intravenously every 12 hours (500 mg orally); **or** levofloxacin, 500 mg once daily (intravenously/orally)
Septic arthritis	*S aureus*, *Neisseria gonorrhoeae*	Ceftriaxone, 1–2 g intravenously every 24 hours **plus** vancomycin 15–20 mg/kg/dose intravenously every 8–12 hours[1]
Septic thrombophlebitis	*S aureus*, gram-negative aerobic bacteria	Vancomycin, 15–20 mg/kg/dose intravenously every 8–12 hours,[1] **plus** ceftriaxone, 1 g intravenously every 24 hours

[1]Vancomycin serum levels should be monitored. Select drug interval based on estimated kidney function and dose rounded to nearest 250 mg.
[2]TMP-SMX can be used to treat *Listeria monocytogenes* in patients allergic to penicillin in a dosage of 15–20 mg/kg/day of TMP in three or four divided doses. Dose reduction is necessary for patients with reduced kidney function.
[3]Including penicillin-resistant isolates.
[4]Levofloxacin 750 mg/day, moxifloxacin 400 mg/day.

Simniceanu A et al. Infection prevention and control of epidemic-prone acute respiratory infections in healthcare setting. Curr Opin Pulm Med. 2025;31:230. [PMID: 40013505]
SuDDICU Investigators for the Australia and New Zealand Intensive Care Society Clinical Trials Group and the Canadian Critical Care Trials Group. Selective decontamination of the digestive tract during ventilation in the ICU. N Engl J Med. 2025 Oct 29. [Epub ahead of print] [PMID: 41159880]
Vaughn BP et al. Diagnosis and management of *Clostridioides difficile* in inflammatory bowel disease. Am J Gastroenterol. 2025;120:313. [PMID: 39230037]
Ye Q et al. Meta-analysis of risk factors for infection by multidrug-resistant organisms in intensive care unit patients. J Hosp Infect. 2025;158:1. [PMID: 39924114]

INFECTIONS OF THE CENTRAL NERVOUS SYSTEM

ESSENTIALS OF DIAGNOSIS

- CNS infection is a medical emergency.
- Symptoms and signs common to all CNS infections include headache, fever, sensorial disturbances, neck and back stiffness, positive Kernig and Brudzinski signs, and CSF abnormalities.

General Considerations

Infections of the CNS can be caused by almost any infectious agent, including bacteria, mycobacteria, fungi, spirochetes, protozoa, helminths, and viruses.

Etiologic Classification

CNS infections can be divided into several categories that usually can be readily distinguished from each other by CSF examination as the first step toward etiologic diagnosis (Table 34–2).

A. Purulent Meningitis

Patients with bacterial meningitis usually seek medical attention within hours or 1–2 days after onset of symptoms. The organisms responsible depend primarily on the age of the patient as summarized in Table 34–3. The diagnosis is usually based on the Gram stain (positive in 60–90%) or culture (positive in > 90%) of the CSF.

B. Chronic Meningitis

The presentation of chronic meningitis is less acute than purulent meningitis. Patients with chronic meningitis usually have a history of symptoms lasting weeks to months. The most common pathogens are *Mycobacterium tuberculosis*, atypical mycobacteria, fungi (*Cryptococcus*, *Coccidioides*, *Histoplasma*), and spirochetes (*Treponema pallidum* and *Borrelia burgdorferi*). The diagnosis is made by culture or in some cases by serologic tests (cryptococcosis, coccidioidomycosis, syphilis, Lyme disease).

C. Aseptic Meningitis

Aseptic meningitis—a more benign and self-limited syndrome than purulent meningitis—is *caused principally by viruses*, especially herpes simplex virus and the enterovirus group (including coxsackieviruses and echoviruses). Infectious mononucleosis may be accompanied by aseptic meningitis. Leptospiral infection is also usually placed in the aseptic group because of the lymphocytic cellular response and its relatively benign course. This type of meningitis also occurs during secondary syphilis and disseminated Lyme disease. Prior to the routine administration of measles-mumps-rubella (MMR) vaccines, mumps was the most common cause of viral meningitis. Drug-induced

Table 34–2. Typical CSF findings in various CNS diseases (listed in alphabetical order after "Normal").

Diagnosis	Cells/mcL	Glucose (mg/dL)	Protein (mg/dL)	Opening Pressure
Normal	0–5 lymphocytes	45–85[1]	15–45	70–180 mm H_2O
Aseptic meningitis, viral meningitis, or meningoencephalitis[2]	25–2000 (0.025–2.0 × 10^9/L), mostly lymphocytes[3]	Normal or low	High (> 50)	Slightly elevated
Granulomatous meningitis (mycobacterial, fungal)[3]	100–1000 (0.1–1.0 × 10^9/L), mostly lymphocytes[3]	Low (< 45)	High (> 50)	Moderately elevated
"Neighborhood reaction"[4]	Variably increased	Normal	Normal or high	Variable
Purulent meningitis (bacterial)[5] community-acquired	200–20,000 (0.2–20 × 10^9/L), polymorphonuclear neutrophils	Low (< 45)	High (> 50)	Markedly elevated
Spirochetal meningitis	100–1000 (0.1–1.0 × 10^9/L), mostly lymphocytes[3]	Normal	High (> 50)	Normal to slightly elevated

[1]CSF glucose must be considered in relation to blood glucose level. Normally, CSF glucose is 20–30 mg/dL lower than blood glucose, or 50–70% of the normal value of blood glucose.
[2]Viral isolation from CSF early; antibody titer rise in paired specimens of serum; PCR for herpesvirus.
[3]Polymorphonuclear neutrophils may predominate early.
[4]May occur in mastoiditis, brain abscess, epidural abscess, sinusitis, septic thrombus, brain tumor. CSF culture results usually negative.
[5]Organisms in smear or culture of CSF; counterimmunoelectrophoresis or latex agglutination may be diagnostic.

Table 34–3. Initial antimicrobial therapy for purulent meningitis of unknown cause.

Population	Usual Microorganisms	Standard Therapy
18–50 years	*Streptococcus pneumoniae, Neisseria meningitidis*	Vancomycin[1] **plus** ceftriaxone[2]
Over 50 years	*S pneumoniae, N meningitidis, Listeria monocytogenes*, enteric gram-negative bacilli, group B streptococcus	Vancomycin[1] **plus** ampicillin,[3] **plus** ceftriaxone[2]
Impaired cellular immunity	*L monocytogenes*, gram-negative bacilli, *S pneumoniae*	Vancomycin[1] **plus** ampicillin,[3] **plus** cefepime[4]
Postsurgical or posttraumatic	*Staphylococcus aureus, S pneumoniae*, aerobic gram-negative bacilli, coagulase-negative staphylococci,[5] diphtheroids (eg, *Cutibacterium acnes*)[5] (uncommon)	Vancomycin[1] **plus** cefepime[4]

[1]Given to cover highly penicillin- or cephalosporin-resistant pneumococci. The dose of vancomycin is 15–20 mg/kg intravenously every 8–12 hours. Doses should be adjusted to achieve a target area under the curve (AUC) between 400 and 600 mg*h/L for confirmed methicillin-resistant *Staphylococcus aureus* (MRSA) or target trough 15–20 mcg/mL for non-MRSA infections. Vancomycin should be stopped if the causative organism is susceptible to ceftriaxone.

[2]Ceftriaxone 2 g intravenously every 12 hours can often be used safely in most patients with a history of low-risk (eg, not IgE-mediated) penicillin allergy. Aztreonam, dosed at 2 g intravenously every 6–8 hours, can be considered for empiric coverage of gram-negative bacilli in patients with type 1 IgE-mediated (anaphylactic) penicillin and cephalosporin allergy. If the organism is susceptible to penicillin, then penicillin 4 million units intravenously every 4 hours is given.

[3]In severely ill patients, ampicillin 2 g intravenously every 4 hours is used when *L monocytogenes* infection is a consideration. For confirmed infection due to *L monocytogenes*, gentamicin is sometimes added to ampicillin. (For patients with type 1 IgE-mediated penicillin allergy, trimethoprim-sulfamethoxazole [TMP-SMX] in a dosage of 15–20 mg/kg/day of TMP in three or four divided doses can be considered.)

[4]Cefepime is given in a dose of 2 g intravenously every 8 hours.

[5]Primarily associated with presence of hardware.

aseptic meningitis has been reported with NSAIDs, sulfonamides, and certain monoclonal antibodies.

D. Encephalitis

Encephalitis (due to herpesviruses, arboviruses, rabies virus, flaviviruses [West Nile encephalitis, Japanese encephalitis], and many others) produces disturbances of the sensorium, seizures, and many other manifestations. Patients are more ill than those with aseptic meningitis. CSF may be entirely normal or may show some lymphocytes and, in some instances (eg, herpes simplex), red cells as well. Influenza has been associated with encephalitis, but the relationship is not clear. An autoimmune form of encephalitis associated with *N*-methyl-D-aspartate receptor antibodies should be suspected in younger patients with encephalitis and associated seizures, movement disorders, and psychosis.

E. Partially Treated Bacterial Meningitis

Previous effective antibiotic therapy given for 12–24 hours will decrease the rate of positive CSF Gram stain results by 20% and culture by 30–40% but will have little effect on cell count, protein, or glucose. Occasionally, previous antibiotic therapy will change a predominantly polymorphonuclear response to a lymphocytic pleocytosis, and some of the CSF findings may be similar to those seen in aseptic meningitis.

F. Neighborhood Reaction

As noted in Table 34–2, this term denotes a purulent infectious process in close proximity to the CNS that spills some of the products of the inflammatory process—WBCs or protein—into the CSF. Such an infection might be a brain abscess, osteomyelitis of the vertebrae, epidural abscess, subdural empyema, or bacterial sinusitis or mastoiditis.

G. Noninfectious Meningeal Irritation

Carcinomatous meningitis, sarcoidosis, SLE, chemical meningitis, and certain medications—NSAIDs, TMP-SMX, IVIG, monoclonal antibodies, and others—can also produce symptoms and signs of meningeal irritation with associated CSF pleocytosis, increased protein, and low or normal glucose. Meningismus with normal CSF findings occurs in the presence of other infections such as pneumonia and shigellosis.

H. Brain Abscess

Brain abscess presents as a space-occupying lesion; symptoms may include vomiting, fever, change of mental status, or focal neurologic manifestations. When brain abscess is suspected, a CT scan should be performed. If positive, lumbar puncture should *not* be performed since results rarely provide clinically useful information and herniation can occur. The bacteriology of brain abscess is usually polymicrobial and includes *S aureus*, gram-negative bacilli, streptococci, and mouth anaerobes (including anaerobic streptococci and *Prevotella* species).

I. Health Care–Associated Meningitis

This infection may arise as a result of invasive neurosurgical procedures (eg, craniotomy, internal or external ventricular catheters, external lumbar catheters), complicated head trauma, or hospital-acquired bloodstream infections. Outbreaks have been associated with contaminated epidural or paraspinal corticosteroid injections. In general, the microbiology is distinct from community-acquired meningitis, with gram-negative organisms (eg, *Pseudomonas*), *S aureus*, and coagulase-negative staphylococci and, in the outbreaks associated with contaminated corticosteroids, mold and fungi (*Exserohilum rostratum* and *Aspergillus fumigatus*) playing a larger role.

Clinical Findings

A. Symptoms and Signs

The classic triad of fever, stiff neck, and altered mental status has a low sensitivity (44%) for bacterial meningitis. However, *nearly all patients with bacterial meningitis have at least two of the following symptoms—fever, headache, stiff neck, or altered mental status.*

B. Laboratory Tests

Evaluation of a patient with suspected meningitis includes a blood count, blood culture, lumbar puncture followed by careful study and culture of the CSF, and a CXR. The fluid must be examined for cell count, glucose, and protein, and a smear stained for bacteria (and acid-fast organisms when appropriate) and cultured for pyogenic organisms and for mycobacteria and fungi when indicated. Latex agglutination tests can detect antigens of encapsulated organisms (*S pneumoniae, H influenzae, N meningitidis*, and *Cryptococcus neoformans*) but are rarely used except for detection of *Cryptococcus* or in partially treated patients. PCR testing of CSF has been used to detect bacteria (*S pneumoniae, H influenzae, N meningitidis, M tuberculosis, B burgdorferi*, and *Tropheryma whipplei*) and viruses (herpes simplex, varicella zoster, CMV, Epstein-Barr virus, and enteroviruses) in patients with meningitis. The greatest experience is with PCR for herpes simplex, varicella zoster, and JC virus. These tests are very sensitive (> 95%) and specific. In addition to its use in meningitis, molecular methods such as PCR and next-generation sequencing are being used increasingly for the diagnosis of encephalitis, transverse myelitis, and brain abscess. In general, molecular diagnostic tests may provide a more sensitive and rapid alternative to traditional culture and serology methods. However, it is difficult to ascertain the true sensitivity of many molecular tests for CNS infections given the absence of a gold standard. In some cases, tests to detect several organisms may not be any more sensitive than culture (or serology), but the *real value is the rapidity* with which results are available, ie, hours compared with days or weeks.

C. Lumbar Puncture and Imaging

Since performing a lumbar puncture in the presence of a space-occupying lesion (brain abscess, subdural hematoma, subdural empyema, necrotic temporal lobe from herpes encephalitis) may result in brainstem herniation, *a CT scan is performed prior to lumbar puncture if a space-occupying lesion is suspected on the basis of papilledema, seizures, or focal neurologic findings.* Other indications for CT scan are an immunocompromised patient or moderately to severely impaired level of consciousness. If delays are encountered in obtaining a CT scan and bacterial meningitis is suspected, blood cultures should be drawn and antibiotics and corticosteroids administered even before CSF is obtained for culture to avoid delay in treatment (Table 34–2). *Antibiotics given within 4 hours before obtaining CSF probably do not affect culture results.* MRI with contrast of the epidural injection site and surrounding areas is recommended (sometimes repeatedly) for those with symptoms following a possibly contaminated corticosteroid injection to exclude epidural abscess, phlegmon, vertebral osteomyelitis, discitis, or arachnoiditis.

Treatment

Although it is difficult to prove with existing clinical data that early antibiotic therapy improves outcome in bacterial meningitis, *prompt therapy is still recommended.* In purulent meningitis, the identity of the causative microorganism may remain unknown or doubtful for a few days and initial antibiotic treatment as set forth in Table 34–3 should be directed against the microorganisms most common for each age group.

The duration of therapy for bacterial meningitis varies depending on the etiologic agent: *H influenzae*, 7 days; *N meningitidis*, 3–7 days; *S pneumoniae*, 10–14 days; *L monocytogenes*, 14–21 days; and gram-negative bacilli, 14–21 days.

For adults with pneumococcal meningitis, dexamethasone 10 mg administered intravenously 15–20 minutes before or simultaneously with the first dose of antibiotics and continued every 6 hours for 4 days decreases morbidity and mortality. Patients most likely to benefit from corticosteroids are those infected with gram-positive organisms (*S pneumoniae* or *S aureus*), and those who are HIV negative. It is unknown whether patients with meningitis due to *N meningitidis* and other bacterial pathogens benefit from the use of adjunctive corticosteroids. Increased intracranial pressure due to brain edema often requires therapeutic attention. Hyperventilation, mannitol (25–50 g intravenously as a bolus), and even drainage of CSF by repeated lumbar punctures or by placement of intraventricular catheters have been used to control cerebral edema and increased intracranial pressure. Dexamethasone (4 mg intravenously every 4–6 hours) also may decrease cerebral edema.

Therapy of brain abscess consists of drainage (excision or aspiration) in addition to 3–4 weeks of systemic antibiotics directed against isolated organisms. An empiric regimen often includes metronidazole, 500 mg intravenously or orally every 8 hours, plus ceftriaxone, 2 g intravenously every 12 hours (CNS dosing), with or without vancomycin, 10–15 mg/kg/dose intravenously every 12 hours. Vancomycin trough serum levels should be > 15 mcg/mL in such patients; however, achievement of an area under the curve/minimal inhibitory concentration (AUC/MIC) ratio of 400–600 is a better predictor of outcome and should be used in confirmed MRSA abscesses. In cases where abscesses are smaller than 2 cm, where there are multiple abscesses that cannot be drained, or if an abscess is located in an area where significant neurologic sequelae would result from drainage, antibiotics for 6–8 weeks can be used without drainage.

In addition to antibiotics, in cases of health care–associated meningitis associated with an external intraventricular catheter, the probability of cure is increased if the catheter is removed. In infections associated with internal ventricular catheters, removal of the internal components and insertion of an external drain is recommended. After collecting CSF, epidural aspirate, or other specimens for culture, routine empiric treatment for other pathogens (as above) is recommended until the specific cause of the patient's CNS or parameningeal infection has been identified. In addition, early consultation with a neurosurgeon is recommended for those found to have an epidural abscess, phlegmon, vertebral osteomyelitis, discitis, or arachnoiditis to discuss possible surgical management (eg, debridement).

Therapy of other types of meningitis is discussed elsewhere in this book (fungal meningitis, Chapter 40; syphilis and Lyme borreliosis, Chapter 38; tuberculous meningitis, Chapter 37; herpes encephalitis, Chapter 36).

When to Refer

- Patients with acute meningitis, particularly if culture negative or atypical (eg, fungi, syphilis, Lyme disease, *M tuberculosis*), or if hospital-acquired, associated with an intraventricular catheter, or if the patient is immunosuppressed.
- Patients with chronic meningitis.
- All patients with brain abscesses and encephalitis.
- Patients with suspected hospital-acquired meningitis (eg, in patients who have undergone recent neurosurgery or epidural or paraspinal corticosteroid injection).
- Patients with recurrent meningitis.

When to Admit

- Patients with suspected acute meningitis, encephalitis, and brain or paraspinous abscess should be admitted for urgent evaluation and treatment.
- There is less urgency to admit patients with chronic meningitis; these patients may be admitted to expedite diagnostic procedures and coordinate care, particularly if no diagnosis has been made in the outpatient setting.

Allos H et al. Aseptic meningitis: a foundation review. Curr Opin Infect Dis. 2025;38:261. [PMID: 40152185]

Beltran-Reyes P et al. Update on diagnosis and treatment of fungal meningitis: lessons from recent outbreaks. Curr Opin Infect Dis. 2024;37:437. [PMID: 39259683]

Chang CC et al. Global guideline for the diagnosis and management of cryptococcosis: an initiative of the ECMM and ISHAM in cooperation with the ASM. Lancet Infect Dis. 2024;24:e495. Erratum in: Lancet Infect Dis. 2024;24:e485. [PMID: 38346436]

Fagre AC et al. West Nile Virus and other nationally notifiable arboviral diseases - United States, 2021. MMWR Morb Mortal Wkly Rep. 2023;72:901. [PMID: 37616182]

Habis R et al. Absence of cerebrospinal fluid pleocytosis in encephalitis. Clin Infect Dis Off Publ Infect Dis Soc Am. 2025;81:179. [PMID: 39096271]

Ivaska L et al. Distinguishing community-acquired bacterial and viral meningitis: microbes and biomarkers. J Infect. 2024;88:106111. [PMID: 38307149]

Smyth M et al. Chronic meningitis: diagnostic and therapeutic challenges. Curr Opin Infect Dis. 2025;38:252. [PMID: 40183580]

Xu Y et al. Advances in the pathogenesis and treatment of pneumococcal meningitis. Virulence. 2024;15:2387180. [PMID: 39192572]

ANIMAL & HUMAN BITE WOUNDS

ESSENTIALS OF DIAGNOSIS

- Cat and human bites have higher rates of infection than dog bites.
- Hand bites are particularly concerning for the possibility of closed-space infection.
- Antibiotic prophylaxis indicated for noninfected bites of the hand and hospitalization required for infected hand bites.
- All infected wounds need to be cultured to direct therapy.

General Considerations

About 1000 dog bite injuries require emergency department attention each day in the United States, most often in urban areas. Dog bites occur most commonly in the summer months. Biting animals are usually known by their victims, and most biting incidents are *provoked* (ie, bites occur while playing with the animal or after surprising the animal while eating or waking it abruptly from sleep). *Failure to elicit a history of provocation is important because an unprovoked attack raises the possibility of rabies.* Human bites are usually inflicted by children while playing or fighting; in adults, bites are associated with alcohol use and closed-fist injuries that occur during fights.

The animal inflicting the bite, the location of the bite, and the type of injury inflicted are all important determinants of whether they become infected. *Cat bites are more likely to become infected than human bites*—between 30% and 50% of all cat bites become infected. Infections following human bites are variable. Bites inflicted by children rarely become infected because they are superficial, and bites by adults become infected in 15–30% of cases, with a high rate of infection in closed-fist injuries. Dog bites, for unclear reasons, become infected only 5% of the time. Bites of the head, face, and neck are less likely to become infected than bites on the extremities. "Through and through" bites (eg, involving the mucosa and the skin) have an infection rate similar to closed-fist injuries. Puncture wounds become infected more frequently than lacerations, probably because the latter are easier to irrigate and debride.

The bacteriology of bite infections is polymicrobial. Following dog and cat bites, > 50% of infections are caused by aerobes and anaerobes and 36% are due to aerobes alone. Pure anaerobic infections are rare. *Pasteurella* species are the single most common isolate (75% of infections caused by cat bites and 50% of infections caused by dog bites). Other common aerobic isolates include streptococci, staphylococci, *Moraxella*, and *Neisseria;* the most common anaerobes are *Fusobacterium*, *Bacteroides*, *Porphyromonas*, and *Prevotella*. The median number of isolates following human bites is four (three aerobes and one anaerobe). Like dog and cat bites, infections caused by most human bites are a mixture of aerobes and anaerobes (54%) or are due to aerobes alone (44%). Streptococci and *S aureus* are the most common aerobes. *Eikenella corrodens* (found in up to 30% of patients), *Prevotella*, and *Fusobacterium* are the most common anaerobes. Although the organisms noted are the most common, innumerable others have been isolated—including *Capnocytophaga* (dog and cat), *Pseudomonas*, and *Haemophilus*—emphasizing the point that *all infected bites should be cultured to define the microbiology.*

HIV can be transmitted from bites (either from biting or receiving a bite from a patient with HIV) but has rarely been reported.

Treatment

A. Local Care

Vigorous cleansing and irrigation of the wound as well as debridement of necrotic material are the most important factors in decreasing the incidence of infections. Radiographs should be obtained to look for fractures and the presence of foreign bodies. Careful examination to assess the extent of the injury (tendon laceration, joint space penetration) is critical to appropriate care.

B. Suturing

If wounds require closure for cosmetic or mechanical reasons, suturing can be done. However, *one should never suture an infected wound, and wounds of the hand should generally not be sutured since a closed-space infection of the hand can result in loss of function.*

C. Prophylactic Antibiotics

Prophylaxis is indicated in high-risk bites and in high-risk patients. *Cat bites in any location and hand bites by any animal, including humans, should receive prophylaxis.* Individuals with certain comorbidities (diabetes, liver disease) are at increased risk for severe complications and should receive prophylaxis even for low-risk bites, as should patients without functional spleens who are at increased risk for overwhelming sepsis (primarily with *Capnocytophaga* species). Amoxicillin-clavulanate (Augmentin) 500 mg /125 mg orally three times daily for 5–7 days is the regimen of choice. For patients with serious allergy to penicillin, a combination of clindamycin 300 mg orally three times daily together with one of the following is recommended for 5–7 days: doxycycline 100 mg orally twice daily, or double-strength TMP-SMX orally twice daily, or a fluoroquinolone (ciprofloxacin 500 mg orally twice daily or levofloxacin 500–750 mg orally once daily). Moxifloxacin, a fluoroquinolone with good aerobic and anaerobic activity, may be suitable as monotherapy at 400 mg orally once daily for 5–7 days. Agents such as dicloxacillin, cephalexin, macrolides, and clindamycin should *not be used alone* because they lack activity against *Pasteurella* species. TMP-SMX has poor activity against anaerobes and should be used only in combination with clindamycin.

Because the risk of HIV transmission is so low following a bite, routine postexposure prophylaxis is not recommended. Each case should be evaluated individually and consideration for prophylaxis should be given to those who present within 72 hours of the incident, the source is known to be HIV infected, and the exposure is high risk.

D. Antibiotics for Documented Infection

For wounds that are infected, antibiotics are clearly indicated. How they are given (orally or intravenously) and the need for hospitalization are individualized clinical decisions. The most commonly encountered pathogens require treatment with ampicillin-sulbactam (Unasyn), 1.5–3.0 g intravenously every 6–8 hours; or amoxicillin-clavulanate (Augmentin), 500 mg /125 mg orally three times daily; or ertapenem, 1 g intravenously daily. For the patient with severe penicillin allergy, a combination of clindamycin, 600–900 mg intravenously every 8 hours, plus a fluoroquinolone (ciprofloxacin, 400 mg intravenously every 12 hours; levofloxacin, 500–750 mg intravenously once daily) is indicated. Duration of therapy is usually 2–3 weeks unless complications such as septic arthritis or osteomyelitis are present; if these complications are present, therapy should be extended to 4 and 6 weeks, respectively.

E. Tetanus and Rabies

All patients must be evaluated for the need for tetanus (see Chapter 37) and rabies (see Chapter 36) prophylaxis.

When to Refer

- If septic arthritis or osteomyelitis is suspected.
- For exposure to bites by dogs, cats, reptiles, amphibians, and rodents.
- When rabies is a possibility.

When to Admit

- Patients with infected hand bites.
- Deep bites, particularly if over joints.

Cottrell DB et al. Animal and human bites: navigating evaluation and care. Nurse Pract. 2024;49:21. [PMID: 38941076]

Lacy M et al. Human rabies treatment-from palliation to promise. Viruses. 2024;16:160. Erratum in: Viruses. 2024;16:26. [PMID: 38275970]

Maurer M et al. Animal bite injuries to the face: a retrospective evaluation of 111 cases. J Clin Med. 2023;12:6942. [PMID: 37959407]

Ortiz DD et al. Dog and cat bites: rapid evidence review. Am Fam Physician. 2023;108:50. [PMID: 37983702]

Schlein S et al. Animal bites and attacks. Emerg Med Clin North Am. 2024;42:639. [PMID: 38925779]

SEXUALLY TRANSMITTED INFECTIONS

ESSENTIALS OF DIAGNOSIS

- All sexually transmitted infections (STIs), also known as sexually transmitted diseases (STDs), have subclinical or latent periods, and patients may be asymptomatic.
- Simultaneous infection with several organisms is common.
- All patients who seek STI testing should be screened for syphilis and HIV.
- Partner notification and treatment are important to prevent further transmission and reinfection of the index case.

General Considerations

The rate of STIs were on the rise prior to and immediately after the COVID-19 pandemic but have been declining since 2023. The most common STIs are gonorrhea,* syphilis,* HPV-associated condyloma acuminatum, chlamydial genital infections,* herpesvirus genital infections, trichomonas vaginitis, chancroid,* granuloma inguinale, scabies, louse infestation, and bacterial vaginosis (among women who have sex with women). However, shigellosis;* hepatitis A, B, and C;* amebiasis; giardiasis;* cryptosporidiosis;* salmonellosis;* campylobacteriosis; dermatophytes (tinea); and mpox may also be transmitted by sexual (oral–anal) contact, especially in men who have sex with men. Ebola virus and Zika virus have both been associated with sexual transmission. Both homosexual and heterosexual contact are risk factors for the transmission of HIV (see Chapter 35). All STIs have *subclinical* or *latent phases* that play an important role in long-term persistence of the infection or in its transmission from infected (but largely asymptomatic) persons to other contacts. *Simultaneous infection by several different agents is common.*

Infections typically present in one of several ways, each of which has a defined differential diagnosis, which should prompt appropriate diagnostic tests.

A. Genital Ulcers

Common etiologies include herpes simplex virus, primary syphilis, and chancroid. Other possibilities include lymphogranuloma venereum (see Chapter 37), granuloma inguinale caused by *Klebsiella granulomatis* (see Chapter 37), mpox, and lesions caused by infection with Epstein-Barr virus and HIV. Noninfectious causes are Behçet disease (see Chapter 23), neoplasm, trauma, drugs, and irritants.

B. Urethritis With or Without Urethral Discharge

The most common infections causing urethral discharge are *Neisseria gonorrhoeae* and *Chlamydia trachomatis*. *N gonorrhoeae* and *C trachomatis* are also frequent causes of prostatitis among sexually active men. Other STIs that can cause urethritis include *Mycoplasma genitalium* and, less commonly, *Ureaplasma urealyticum* and *Trichomonas vaginalis*. Noninfectious causes of urethritis include reactive arthritis with associated urethritis.

C. Vaginal Discharge

Common causes of vaginitis are bacterial vaginosis (caused by overgrowth of anaerobes such as *Gardnerella vaginalis*), candidiasis, and *T vaginalis* (see Chapter 21). Less common infectious causes of vaginitis include HPV-associated condylomata acuminata and group A streptococcus. Noninfectious causes are physiologic changes related to the menstrual cycle, irritants, and lichen planus. Even though *N gonorrhoeae* and *C trachomatis* are frequent causes of cervicitis, they *rarely* produce vaginal discharge.

Screening & Prevention

All persons who seek STI testing should undergo routine screening for HIV infection, using rapid HIV testing (if patients may not follow-up for results obtained by standard methods) or nucleic acid amplification followed by confirmatory serology (if primary HIV infection may be a possibility) as indicated. *Most algorithms now start with an antigen/antibody combination HIV-1/2 immunoassay with a confirmatory HIV-1/HIV-2 antibody differentiation immunoassay.* Patients in whom certain STIs have been diagnosed and treated (chlamydia or gonorrhea, and trichomonas in women) are at a high risk for reinfection and should be encouraged to be *rescreened for STIs at 3 months* following the initial STI diagnosis.

Asymptomatic patients often request STI screening at the time of initiating a new sexual relationship. Routine HIV testing and hepatitis B serology testing should be offered to all such patients. In sexually active women who have not been recently screened, cervical Papanicolaou testing and nucleic acid amplification testing of a urine specimen for gonorrhea and chlamydia are recommended. Among men who have sex with men, additional screening is recommended for syphilis; hepatitis A; urethral, pharyngeal, and rectal gonorrhea; as well as urethral and rectal chlamydia. Nucleic acid amplification testing is recommended for gonorrhea or chlamydia. There are no recommendations to screen heterosexual men for urethral chlamydia, but this could be considered in STI clinics, adolescent clinics, or correctional facilities. The periodicity of screening thereafter depends on sexual risk, but *most screening should be offered at least annually to sexually active adults (particularly to those 25 years old and under).* Clinicians should also evaluate transgender persons for STI screening, based on current anatomy and behaviors practiced. If not immune, *hepatitis B vaccination is recommended for all sexually active adults,* and hepatitis A vaccination in men who have sex with men. Persons between the ages of 9 and 26 should be routinely offered vaccination against HPV (9-valent).

The risk of developing an STI following a sexual assault is difficult to accurately ascertain given high rates of

*Reportable to public health authorities.

baseline infections and poor follow-up. People who have been sexually assaulted have a high baseline rate of infection (*N gonorrhoeae*, 6%; *C trachomatis*, 10%; *T vaginalis*, 15%; and bacterial vaginosis, 34%), and the risk of acquiring infection as a result of the assault is significant but often lower than the preexisting rate (*N gonorrhoeae*, 6–12%; *C trachomatis*, 4–17%; *T vaginalis*, 12%; syphilis, 0.5–3%; and bacterial vaginosis, 19%). Patients should be evaluated within 24 hours of the assault, and nucleic acid amplification tests for *N gonorrhoeae* and *C trachomatis* should be performed. Vaginal secretions are obtained for *Trichomonas* wet mount and culture, or point-of-care testing. If a discharge is present, if there is itching, or if secretions are malodorous, a wet mount should be examined for *Candida* and bacterial vaginosis. In addition, a blood sample should be obtained for immediate serologic testing for syphilis, hepatitis B, and HIV. Follow-up examination for STIs should be repeated within 1–2 weeks, since concentrations of infecting organisms may not have been sufficient to produce a positive test at the time of initial examination. If prophylactic treatment was given (may include postexposure hepatitis B vaccination without hepatitis B immune globulin; treatment for chlamydial, gonorrheal, or trichomonal infection; and emergency contraception), tests should be repeated only if the patient has symptoms. If prophylaxis was not administered, the individual should be seen in 1 week so that any positive tests can be treated. Follow-up serologic testing for syphilis and HIV infection should be performed in 6, 12, and 24 weeks if the initial tests are negative. The usefulness of presumptive therapy is controversial, with some feeling that all patients should receive it and others that it should be limited to those in whom follow-up cannot be ensured or to patients who request it.

Although seroconversion to HIV has been reported following sexual assault when this was the only known risk, this risk is believed to be low. The likelihood of HIV transmission from vaginal or anal receptive intercourse when the source is known to be HIV positive is 1 per 1000 and 5 per 1000, respectively. Although prophylactic antiretroviral therapy has not been studied in this setting, the Department of Health and Human Services recommends the *prompt institution of postexposure prophylaxis with antiretroviral therapy if the person seeks care within 72 hours of the assault, the source is known to be HIV positive, and the exposure presents a substantial risk of transmission.*

In addition to screening asymptomatic patients with STIs, other strategies for preventing further transmission include evaluating sex partners and administering preexposure prophylaxis of preventable STIs to individuals at risk; additional strategies include the consistent use of male and female condoms and male circumcision. Adult male circumcision has been shown to decrease the transmission of HIV by 50%, and of herpes simplex virus and HPV by 30% in heterosexual couples in sub-Saharan Africa. Note that vaginal spermicides and condoms containing nonoxynol-9 provide *no* additional protection against STIs. Among persons with HIV, viral suppression with antiretroviral therapy can prevent HIV acquisition in an uninfected sex partner. Also, preexposure prophylaxis with either a once-daily or on-demand pill containing emtricitabine plus tenofovir or long-acting injectable cabotegravir has been shown to be effective in preventing HIV infection among high-risk men who have sex with men, heterosexual women and men, transgender women, and persons who inject drugs. Postexposure prophylaxis with doxycycline appears to reduce bacterial STIs among individuals disproportionately affected by STIs. Antiviral suppression of HSV can decrease risk of transition to an uninfected sex partner. For each patient with an STI, there are one or more sexual contacts who require diagnosis and treatment. Prompt treatment of contacts by giving antibiotics to the index case to distribute to all sexual contacts (*patient-delivered therapy*) is an important strategy for preventing further transmission and to prevent reinfection of the index case.

When to Refer

- Patients with a new diagnosis of HIV.
- Patients with persistent, refractory, or recurrent STIs, particularly when drug resistance is suspected.

Chua TP et al. Evolving patterns of macrolide and fluoroquinolone resistance in *Mycoplasma genitalium*: an updated systematic review and meta-analysis. Lancet Microbe. 2025;6:101047. [PMID: 40147462]

Hanft W et al. Sexually transmitted human papillomavirus and related sequelae. Clin Microbiol Rev. 2025;38:e0008523. [PMID: 39950806]

Kelley CF et al. Twice-yearly lenacapavir for HIV prevention in men and gender-diverse persons. N Engl J Med. 2025;392:1261. [PMID: 39602624]

Patel R et al. 2024 European guidelines for the management of genital herpes. J Eur Acad Dermatol Venereol. 2025;39:742. [PMID: 39620271]

Raccagni AR et al. When is it a sexually transmitted infection? Intimate contact transmission of pathogens not traditionally defined as STIs. Curr Opin Infect Dis. 2025;38:65. [PMID: 39745336]

Sankaran M et al. Doxycycline postexposure prophylaxis and sexually transmitted infection trends. JAMA Intern Med. 2025;185:266. [PMID: 39761052]

Traeger MW et al. Doxycycline postexposure prophylaxis and bacterial sexually transmitted infections among individuals using HIV preexposure prophylaxis. JAMA Intern Med. 2025;185:273. [PMID: 39761062]

INFECTIONS IN PERSONS WHO INJECT DRUGS

ESSENTIALS OF DIAGNOSIS

- Common infections that occur with greater frequency in persons who inject drugs include:
  - Skin infections, aspiration pneumonia, tuberculosis.
  - Hepatitis A, B, C, D; STIs; HIV/AIDS.
  - Pulmonary septic emboli, infective endocarditis.
  - Osteomyelitis and septic arthritis.

General Considerations

There is a high incidence of infection among persons with opioid use disorder, particularly among people who inject drugs. Increased risk of infection is likely associated with poor hygiene and colonization with potentially pathogenic organisms, contamination of drugs and equipment, increased sexual risk behaviors, and impaired immune defenses. The use of parenterally administered recreational drugs has increased enormously in recent years, fueled in part by an epidemic of prescription opioid misuse and abuse. More than 3 million persons in North America are estimated to have used injection drugs in the past year, with opioid deaths increasing during the COVID-19 pandemic particularly in low-income urban neighborhoods.

Skin infections are associated with poor hygiene and use of nonsterile technique when injecting drugs. *S aureus* (including community-acquired methicillin-resistant strains) and oral flora (streptococci, *Eikenella, Fusobacterium, Peptostreptococcus*) are the most common organisms, with enteric gram-negatives generally more likely seen in those who inject into the groin. Cellulitis and subcutaneous abscesses occur most commonly, particularly in association with subcutaneous ("skin-popping") or intramuscular injections and the use of cocaine and heroin mixtures (probably due to ischemia). Myositis, clostridial myonecrosis, and necrotizing fasciitis occur infrequently but are life-threatening. Wound botulism in association with black tar heroin occurs sporadically but often in clusters.

Aspiration pneumonia and its complications (lung abscess, empyema, brain abscess) result from altered consciousness associated with drug use. Mixed aerobic and anaerobic mouth flora are usually involved.

Tuberculosis also occurs in persons who use drugs, and infection with HIV has fostered the spread of tuberculosis in this population. Morbidity and mortality rates are increased in individuals with HIV and tuberculosis. Classic radiographic findings are often absent; *tuberculosis is suspected in any patient with infiltrates who does not respond to antibiotics.*

Hepatitis is common among persons who inject drugs and is transmissible both by the parenteral (hepatitis B, C, and D) and by the fecal-oral route (hepatitis A). Multiple episodes of hepatitis with different agents can occur. Hepatitis C has also been associated with noninjection heroin use as well as intranasal use of other drugs, likely secondary to blood on shared straws.

Pulmonary septic emboli may originate from venous thrombi or right-sided endocarditis.

STIs are not directly related to drug use, but the practice of exchanging sex for drugs has resulted in an increased frequency of STIs. Syphilis, gonorrhea, and chancroid are the most common.

HIV/AIDS has a high incidence among persons who inject drugs and their sexual contacts and among the offspring of infected women (see Chapter 35).

Infective endocarditis in persons who inject drugs is most commonly caused by *S aureus, Candida* (usually *C albicans* or *C parapsilosis*), *Enterococcus faecalis*, other streptococci, and gram-negative bacteria (especially *Pseudomonas* and *Serratia marcescens*). See Chapter 37.

Other vascular infections include septic thrombophlebitis and mycotic aneurysms. Mycotic aneurysms resulting from direct trauma to a vessel with secondary infection most commonly occur in femoral arteries and less commonly in arteries of the neck. Aneurysms resulting from hematogenous spread of organisms frequently involve intracerebral vessels and thus are seen in association with endocarditis.

Osteomyelitis and *septic arthritis* involving vertebral bodies, sternoclavicular joints, the pubic symphysis, the sacroiliac joints, and other sites usually results from hematogenous distribution of injected organisms or septic venous thrombi. Pain and fever precede radiographic changes, sometimes by several weeks. While *S aureus*—often methicillin-resistant—is most common, *Serratia, Pseudomonas, Candida* (often not *C albicans*), and other pathogens rarely encountered in spontaneous bone or joint disease are found in persons who inject drugs.

Treatment

A common and difficult clinical problem is management of a person known to inject drugs who presents with fever. In general, *after obtaining appropriate cultures (blood, urine, and sputum if the CXR is abnormal), empiric therapy is begun.* If the CXR is suggestive of a community-acquired pneumonia (consolidation), therapy for inpatient pneumonia is begun with ceftriaxone, 1 g intravenously every 24 hours, plus either azithromycin (500 mg orally or intravenously every 24 hours) or doxycycline (100 mg orally or intravenously twice daily). If the CXR is suggestive of septic emboli (nodular infiltrates), therapy for presumed endocarditis is initiated, usually with vancomycin 15 mg/kg/dose every 12 hours intravenously (due to the high prevalence of MRSA and the possibility of enterococcus). If the CXR is normal and no focal site of infection can be found, *endocarditis is presumed.* While awaiting the results of blood cultures, empiric treatment with vancomycin is started. If blood cultures are positive for organisms that frequently cause endocarditis in drug users (see above), endocarditis is presumed to be present and treated accordingly. In the instance of confirmed methicillin-susceptible *S aureus* infection, vancomycin should be discontinued and treatment initiated with cefazolin or an antistaphylococcal penicillin (eg, nafcillin). If blood cultures are positive for an organism that is an unusual cause of endocarditis, evaluation for an occult source of infection should go forward. In this setting, *a transesophageal echocardiogram may be quite helpful since it is 90% sensitive in detecting vegetations and a negative study is strong evidence against endocarditis.* If blood cultures are negative and the patient responds to antibiotics, therapy should be continued for 7–14 days (oral therapy can be given once an initial response has occurred). In every patient, careful examination for an occult source of infection (eg, genitourinary, dental, sinus, gallbladder) should be done. *Clinicians also can have a significant role to play in integrating treatment of opioid use disorder when patients present with infectious disease complications.* This includes screening for opioid use disorder, undergoing specific training for and prescribing opioid use disorder medications, treatment of withdrawal symptoms, and linkage to community-based treatment after hospital discharge.

When to Refer

- Any patient with suspected or proven infective endocarditis.
- Patients with persistent bacteremia.

When to Admit

- Persons who inject drugs with fever.
- Patients with abscesses or progressive skin and soft tissue infections that require debridement.

Akritidou O et al. A review of current insights in fungal endocarditis. J Clin Med. 2025;14:6149. [PMID: 40943909]
Leis BT et al. Management of infective endocarditis secondary to injection drug use: practical recommendations for clinicians from a Canadian working group. Can J Cardiol. 2026;42:575. [PMID: 41276214]
Marks LR et al. Infectious complications of injection drug use. Med Clin North Am. 2022;106:187. [PMID: 34823730]
Swets MC et al. Clinical subphenotypes of *Staphylococcus aureus* bacteremia. Clin Infect Dis. 2024;79:1153. [PMID: 38916975]
Thompson GR 3rd et al. Fungal endocarditis: pathophysiology, epidemiology, clinical presentation, diagnosis, and management. Clin Microbiol Rev. 2023;36:e0001923. [PMID: 37439685]
Tong SYC et al. Management of *Staphylococcus aureus* bacteremia: a review. JAMA. 2025;334:798. [PMID: 40193249]

ACUTE INFECTIOUS DIARRHEA

ESSENTIALS OF DIAGNOSIS

- Acute diarrhea: lasts < 2 weeks.
- Chronic diarrhea: lasts > 2 weeks.
- Mild diarrhea: ≤ 3 stools per day.
- Moderate diarrhea: ≥ 4 stools per day with local symptoms (abdominal cramps, nausea, tenesmus).
- Severe diarrhea: ≥ 4 stools per day with systemic symptoms (fever, chills, dehydration).

General Considerations

Acute diarrhea can be caused by a number of different factors, including emotional stress, food intolerance, inorganic agents (eg, sodium nitrite), organic substances (eg, mushrooms, shellfish), medications, and infectious agents (including viruses, bacteria, and protozoa) (Table 34–4). From a diagnostic and therapeutic standpoint, it is helpful to classify infectious diarrhea into syndromes that produce inflammatory or bloody diarrhea and those that are noninflammatory, nonbloody, or watery. In general, the term **inflammatory diarrhea** suggests colonic involvement by invasive bacteria or parasites or by toxin production. Patients report frequent bloody, small-volume stools, often associated with fever, abdominal cramps, tenesmus, and fecal urgency. Common causes of this syndrome include *Shigella*, *Salmonella*, *Campylobacter*, *Yersinia*, invasive strains of *Escherichia coli*, and other Shiga-toxin–producing strains of *E coli* (STEC), *Entamoeba histolytica*, and *C difficile*. Tests for fecal leukocytes or the neutrophil marker lactoferrin are frequently positive, and definitive etiologic diagnosis requires stool culture. **Noninflammatory diarrhea** is generally milder and is caused by viruses or toxins that affect the small intestine and interfere with salt and water balance, resulting in large-volume watery diarrhea, often with nausea, vomiting, and cramps. Common causes of this syndrome include viruses (eg, rotavirus, norovirus, astrovirus, enteric adenoviruses), vibriones (*Vibrio cholerae*, *Vibrio parahaemolyticus*), enterotoxin-producing *E coli*, *Giardia lamblia*, cryptosporidia, and agents that can cause food-borne gastroenteritis. In developed countries, viruses (particularly norovirus) are an important cause of hospitalizations due to acute gastroenteritis among adults.

The term **food poisoning** denotes diseases caused by toxins present in consumed foods. When the incubation period is short (1–6 hours after consumption), the *toxin is usually preformed*. Vomiting is usually a major symptom, and fever is usually absent. Examples include intoxication from *S aureus* or *Bacillus cereus*, and toxin can be detected in the food. When the incubation period is longer—between 8 hours and 16 hours—the organism is present in the food and *produces toxin after being ingested*. Vomiting is less prominent, abdominal cramping is frequent, and fever is often absent. The best example of this disease is that due to *Clostridium perfringens*. Toxin can be detected in food or stool specimens.

The inflammatory and noninflammatory diarrheas discussed above can also be transmitted by food and water and usually have incubation periods between 12 and 72 hours. *Cyclospora*, cryptosporidia, and *Isospora* are protozoans capable of causing disease in both immunocompetent and immunocompromised patients. Characteristics of disease include profuse watery diarrhea that is prolonged but usually self-limited (1–2 weeks) in the immunocompetent patient but can be chronic in the compromised host. Epidemiologic features may be helpful in determining etiology. Recent hospitalization or antibiotic use suggests *C difficile*; recent foreign travel suggests *Salmonella*, *Shigella*, *Campylobacter*, *E coli*, or *V cholerae;* undercooked hamburger suggests STEC; outbreak in long-term care facility, school, or cruise ship suggests norovirus (including newly identified strains, eg, GII.4 Sydney); and fried rice consumption is associated with *B cereus* toxin. Prominent features of some of these causes of diarrhea are listed in Table 34–4.

Treatment

A. General Measures

In general, *most cases of acute gastroenteritis are self-limited and do not require therapy other than supportive measures.* Treatment usually consists of replacement of fluids and electrolytes and, rarely, management of hypovolemic shock and respiratory compromise. In mild diarrhea, increasing ingestion of juices and clear soups is adequate. In more severe cases of dehydration (postural light-headedness, decreased urination), oral glucose-based rehydration solutions can be used (Ceralyte, Pedialyte).

Table 34–4. Acute bacterial diarrheas and "food poisoning" (listed in alphabetical order by organism).

Organism	Incubation Period	Vomiting	Diarrhea	Fever	Associated Foods	Diagnosis	Clinical Features and Treatment
Bacillus cereus (diarrheal toxin)	10–16 hours	±	+++	–	Toxin in meats, stews, and gravy.	Clinical. Food and stool can be tested for toxin.	Abdominal cramps, watery diarrhea, and nausea lasting 24–48 hours. Treatment: Supportive care.
Bacillus cereus (preformed toxin)	1–8 hours	+++	±	–	Reheated fried rice causes vomiting or diarrhea.	Clinical. Food and stool can be tested for toxin.	Acute onset, severe nausea and vomiting lasting 24 hours. Treatment: Supportive care.
Campylobacter jejuni	2–5 days	±	+++	+	Raw or undercooked poultry, unpasteurized milk, water.	Stool culture on special medium.	Fever, diarrhea that can be bloody, cramps. Usually self-limited in 2–10 days. May be associated with Guillain-Barré syndrome. Treatment: Azithromycin. Fluoroquinolones can be used if susceptibility is confirmed.
Clostridioides difficile	Usually occurs after 7–10 days of antibiotics. Can occur after a single dose or several weeks after completion of antibiotics.	–	+++	++	Associated with antibacterial drugs; clindamycin and β-lactams most commonly implicated. Fluoroquinolones associated with hypervirulent strains.	Stool tested for toxin.	Abrupt onset of diarrhea that may be bloody; fever. Treatment: fidaxomicin or oral vancomycin. IV metronidazole can be added to oral vancomycin for fulminant disease.
Clostridium botulinum	12–72 hours	±	–	–	Clostridia grow in anaerobic acidic environment, eg, canned foods, fermented fish, foods held warm for extended periods.	Stool, serum, and food can be tested for toxin. Stool and food can be cultured.	Diplopia, dysphagia, dysphonia, respiratory embarrassment. Symptoms can last for days to months. Treatment: clear airway, ventilation, and intravenous polyvalent antitoxin.
Clostridium perfringens	8–16 hours	±	+++	–	Clostridia grow in rewarmed meat and poultry dishes and produce an enterotoxin.	Stools can be tested for enterotoxin or cultured.	Abrupt onset of profuse diarrhea, abdominal cramps, nausea; vomiting occasionally. Treatment: Recovery usually without treatment in 24–48 hours. Supportive care; antibiotics not needed.
Enterohemorrhagic *Escherichia coli*, including STEC	1–8 days	+	+++	–	Undercooked beef, especially hamburger; unpasteurized milk and juice; raw fruits and vegetables.	STEC can be cultured on special medium. Other toxins can be detected in stool.	Usually abrupt onset of diarrhea, often bloody; abdominal pain. In adults, it is usually self-limited to 5–10 days. In children, it is associated with HUS. Treatment: Antibiotic therapy may increase risk of HUS. Plasma exchange may help patients with STEC-associated HUS.
Enterotoxigenic *E coli*	1–3 days	±	+++	±	Water, food contaminated with feces.	Stool culture. Special tests required to identify toxin-producing strains.	Watery diarrhea and abdominal cramps, usually lasting 3–7 days. Treatment: In travelers, fluoroquinolones shorten disease.

Noroviruses and other caliciviruses	12–48 hours	++	+++	+	Shellfish and fecally contaminated foods touched by infected food handlers.	Clinical diagnosis with negative stool cultures. PCR available on stool.	Nausea, vomiting (more common in children), diarrhea (more common in adults), fever, myalgias, abdominal cramps. Lasts 12–60 hours. Treatment: Supportive care.
Rotavirus	1–3 days	++	+++	+	Fecally contaminated foods touched by infected food handlers.	Immunoassay on stool.	Acute onset, vomiting, watery diarrhea that lasts 4–8 days. Treatment: Supportive care.
Salmonella species	1–3 days	–	++	+	Eggs, poultry, unpasteurized milk, cheese, juices, raw fruits and vegetables.	Routine stool culture.	Gradual or abrupt onset of diarrhea and low-grade fever. Treatment: No antimicrobials unless high risk (ie, immunosuppressed persons), systemic dissemination is suspected, or isolation of *Salmonella enterica* serotype Typhi or Paratyphi. If susceptibility is confirmed, treatment with ceftriaxone, ciprofloxacin, TMP-SMX, or amoxicillin is recommended. Prolonged carriage can occur.
Shigella species (mild cases)	24–48 hours	±	+	+	Food or water contaminated with human feces. Person to person spread.	Routine stool culture.	Abrupt onset of diarrhea, often with blood and pus in stools, cramps, tenesmus, and lethargy. Stool cultures are positive. Treatment: Azithromycin, ciprofloxacin, and ceftriaxone are drugs of choice. Avoid fluoroquinolones if the ciprofloxacin MIC is 0.12 mcg/mL or greater even if the laboratory report identifies the isolate as susceptible. Do not give opioids. Often mild and self-limited.
Staphylococcus (preformed toxin)	1–8 hours	+++	±	±	Staphylococci grow in meats, dairy, and bakery products and produce enterotoxin.	Clinical. Food and stool can be tested for toxin.	Abrupt onset, intense nausea and vomiting for up to 24 hours, recovery in 24–48 hours. Treatment: Supportive care.
Vibrio cholerae	24–72 hours	+	+++	–	Contaminated water, fish, shellfish, street vendor food.	Stool culture on special medium.	Abrupt onset of liquid diarrhea in endemic area. Treatment: Prompt intravenous or oral replacement of fluids and electrolytes. Doxycycline is drug of choice if antibiotics are indicated. Ciprofloxacin, azithromycin, or ceftriaxone are alternatives.
Vibrio parahaemolyticus	2–48 hours	+	+	±	Undercooked or raw seafood.	Stool culture on special medium.	Abrupt onset of watery diarrhea, abdominal cramps, nausea and vomiting. Treatment: Supportive; recovery is usually complete in 2–5 days.
Yersinia enterocolitica	24–48 hours	±	+	+	Undercooked pork, contaminated water, unpasteurized milk, tofu.	Stool culture on special medium.	Severe abdominal pain (appendicitis-like symptoms), diarrhea, fever. Polyarthritis, erythema nodosum in children. Treatment: If severe, give TMP-SMX. Alternatives are cefotaxime and ciprofloxacin. Without treatment, self-limited in 1–3 weeks.

HUS, hemolytic-uremic syndrome; MIC, minimum inhibitory concentration; STEC, Shiga-toxin–producing *E coli* strains; TMP-SMX, trimethoprim-sulfamethoxazole.

B. Specific Measures

In immunocompetent adults, empiric antimicrobial therapy for bloody diarrhea while waiting for results is recommended only with the following circumstances: (1) documented fever, abdominal pain, bloody diarrhea, and **bacillary dysentery** (frequent scant bloody stools, fever, abdominal cramps, tenesmus) presumptively due to *Shigella*; and (2) returning travelers with a temperature of at least 38.5°C or signs of sepsis.

Either a fluoroquinolone or azithromycin should be used as empiric antimicrobial therapy for bloody diarrhea. Empiric antibacterial treatment should be considered in immunocompromised people with severe illness and bloody diarrhea. Loperamide may be given to immunocompetent adults with acute watery diarrhea but should be avoided with *Shigella* infection or in suspected or proven toxic megacolon.

Bai GH et al. Unraveling the interplay between norovirus infection, gut microbiota, and novel antiviral approaches: a comprehensive review. Front Microbiol. 2023;14:1212582. Erratum in: Front Microbiol. 2023;14:1324539. [PMID: 37485533]

Flynn TG et al. Viral gastroenteritis. Lancet Lond Engl. 2024;403:862. [PMID: 38340741]

Moritz ED et al. Foodborne illness outbreaks at retail food establishments - National Environmental Assessment Reporting System, 25 State and Local Health Departments, 2017-2019. MMWR Surveill Summ. 2023;72:1. [PMID: 37252900]

Ressler AM et al. Current approaches to treat and prevent recurrence of *Clostridioides difficile*. Gastroenterol Clin North Am. 2025;54:259. [PMID: 40348487]

Scallan Walter EJ et al. Foodborne illness acquired in the United States-major pathogens, 2019. Emerg Infect Dis. 2025;31:669. [PMID: 40133035]

INFECTIOUS DISEASES IN THE RETURNING TRAVELER

ESSENTIALS OF DIAGNOSIS

- Most infections are common and self-limited.
- Identify patients with transmissible diseases that require isolation.
- The incubation period may be helpful in diagnosis.
  - Less than 3 weeks following exposure may suggest dengue, leptospirosis, and yellow fever.
  - More than 3 weeks suggests typhoid fever, malaria, and tuberculosis.

General Considerations

The differential diagnosis of fever in the returning traveler is broad, ranging from self-limited viral infections to life-threatening illness. *The evaluation is best done by identifying whether a particular syndrome is present, then refining the differential diagnosis based on an exposure history*. The travel history should include directed questions regarding geography (rural versus urban, specific country and region visited), time of year, animal or arthropod contact, unprotected sexual intercourse, ingestion of untreated water or raw foods, historical or pretravel immunizations, and adherence to malaria prophylaxis.

Etiologies

The most common infectious causes of fever—excluding simple causes such as upper respiratory infections, bacterial pneumonia and UTIs—in returning travelers are malaria (see Chapter 39), diarrhea (see next section), and dengue (see Chapter 36). Others include mononucleosis (associated with Epstein-Barr virus or cytomegalovirus), respiratory infections, including seasonal influenza, influenza A/H1N1 "swine" influenza, and influenza A/H5N1 or A/H7N9 "avian" influenza (see Chapter 36); leptospirosis (see Chapter 38); typhoid fever (see Chapter 37); and rickettsial infections (see Chapter 36). Coronaviruses cause regional and global outbreaks of various sizes (SARS-CoV, MERS-CoV, and the massive global pandemic from SARS-CoV-2). Foreign travel is increasingly recognized as a risk factor for colonization and disease with resistant pathogens, such as ESBL-producing gram-negative organisms. Systemic febrile illnesses without a diagnosis also occur commonly, particularly in travelers returning from sub-Saharan Africa or Southeast Asia.

A. Fever and Rash

Potential etiologies include dengue, Ebola, Chikungunya, and Zika viruses, viral hemorrhagic fever, leptospirosis, meningococcemia, yellow fever, typhus, *Salmonella typhi*, and acute HIV infection.

B. Pulmonary Infiltrates

Tuberculosis, *Ascaris*, *Paragonimus*, and *Strongyloides* can all cause pulmonary infiltrates.

C. Meningoencephalitis

Etiologies include *N meningitidis*, leptospirosis, arboviruses, rabies, and (cerebral) malaria.

D. Jaundice

Consider hepatitis A, yellow fever, hemorrhagic fever, leptospirosis, and malaria.

E. Fever Without Localizing Symptoms or Signs

Malaria, typhoid fever, acute HIV infection, rickettsial illness, visceral leishmaniasis, trypanosomiasis, and dengue are possible etiologies.

F. Traveler's Diarrhea

See next section.

Clinical Findings

Fever and rash in the returning traveler should prompt blood cultures and serologic tests based on the exposure history. The workup of a pulmonary infiltrate should include the placement of a PPD or use of an interferon-γ release assay, examination of sputum for acid-fast bacilli and possibly for ova and parasites. Patients with evidence of meningoencephalitis should receive lumbar puncture, blood cultures, thick/thin smears of peripheral blood, history-guided serologies, and a nape biopsy (if rabies is suspected). Jaundice in a returning traveler should be evaluated for hemolysis (for malaria), and the following tests should be performed: liver biochemical tests, thick/thin smears of peripheral blood, and directed serologic testing. The workup of traveler's diarrhea is presented in the following section. Finally, patients with fever but no localizing signs or symptoms should have blood cultures performed. Routine laboratory studies usually include CBC with differential, electrolytes, liver biochemical tests, UA, and blood cultures. Thick and thin peripheral blood smears should be done (and repeated in 12–24 hours if clinical suspicion remains high) for malaria if there has been travel to endemic areas. Other studies are directed by the results of history, physical examination, and initial laboratory tests. They may include stool for ova and parasites, CXR, HIV test, and specific serologies (eg, dengue, leptospirosis, rickettsial disease, schistosomiasis, *Strongyloides*). Bone marrow biopsy to diagnose typhoid fever could be helpful in the appropriate patient. Increasingly, next-generation sequencing of plasma or body fluids such as CSF is used as an adjunctive modality for diagnosis when traditional methods have not yielded a diagnosis.

When to Refer

Travelers with fever, particularly if immunocompromised.

When to Admit

Any evidence of hemorrhage, respiratory distress, hemodynamic instability, and neurologic deficits.

Avrami S et al. Comparison of clinical and laboratory parameters of primary vs secondary dengue fever in travellers. J Travel Med. 2023;30:taad129. [PMID: 37877966]

Kuehn R et al. Enteric (typhoid and paratyphoid) fever. Lancet. 2025;406:1283. [PMID: 40914181]

Morrison A et al. Oropouche Virus Disease among U.S. travelers - United States, 2024. MMWR Morb Mortal Wkly Rep. 2024;73:769. [PMID: 39236058]

Rolfe RJ et al. Mosquito-borne infections in international travelers. Wilderness Environ Med. 2025;36:572. [PMID: 40686432]

Warner JC et al. Infections in travellers returning to the UK: a retrospective analysis (2015-2020). J Travel Med. 2023;30: taad003. [PMID: 36708032]

TRAVELER'S DIARRHEA

ESSENTIALS OF DIAGNOSIS

- Usually a benign, self-limited disease occurring about 1 week into travel.
- Prophylaxis *not* recommended unless there is a comorbid disease (inflammatory bowel syndrome, HIV, immunosuppressive medication).
- Single-dose therapy of a fluoroquinolone usually effective if significant symptoms develop.

General Considerations

Whenever a person travels from one country to another—particularly if the change involves a marked difference in climate, social conditions, or sanitation standards and facilities—diarrhea may develop within 2–10 days. Bacteria cause 80% of cases of traveler's diarrhea, with enterotoxigenic *E coli*, *Shigella* species, and *Campylobacter jejuni* being the most common pathogens. Less common are *Aeromonas*, *Salmonella*, noncholera vibriones, *E histolytica*, and *G lamblia*. Contributory causes include unusual food and drink, change in living habits, occasional viral infections (adenoviruses or rotaviruses), and change in bowel flora. Chronic watery diarrhea may be due to amebiasis or giardiasis or, rarely, tropical sprue.

Clinical Findings

A. Symptoms and Signs

There may be up to 10 or even more loose stools per day, often accompanied by abdominal cramps and nausea, occasionally by vomiting, and rarely by fever. The stools are usually watery and not associated with fever when caused by enterotoxigenic *E coli*. With invasive bacterial pathogens (*Shigella*, *Campylobacter*, *Salmonella*), stools can be bloody and fever may be present. The illness usually subsides spontaneously within 1–5 days, although 10% remain symptomatic for 1 week or longer, and symptoms persist for longer than 1 month in 2%. Traveler's diarrhea is also a significant risk factor for developing irritable bowel syndrome.

B. Laboratory Findings

In patients with fever and bloody diarrhea, stool culture is indicated, but *in most cases, cultures are reserved for those who do not respond to antibiotics*.

Prevention

A. General Measures

Avoidance of fresh foods and water sources that are likely to be contaminated is recommended for travelers to developing countries, where infectious diarrheal illnesses are endemic.

B. Specific Measures

Because not all travelers will have diarrhea and because most episodes are brief and self-limited, the recommended approach is to *provide the traveler with a supply of antimicrobials. Prophylaxis* is recommended for those with significant underlying disease (IBD, AIDS, diabetes mellitus, heart disease in older adults, conditions requiring immunosuppressive medications) and for those whose full activity status during the trip is so essential that even short periods of diarrhea would be unacceptable.

Prophylaxis is started upon entry into the destination country and is continued for 1 or 2 days after leaving. For stays of > 3 weeks, prophylaxis is not recommended because of the cost and increased toxicity. For prophylaxis, several oral antimicrobial once-daily regimens are effective, such as ciprofloxacin, 500 mg, or rifaximin, 200 mg.

Bismuth subsalicylate is effective but turns the tongue and the stools black and can interfere with doxycycline absorption, which may be needed for malaria prophylaxis; it is rarely used.

Treatment

For most individuals, the affliction is short-lived, and symptomatic therapy with loperamide is all that is required, provided the patient is not systemically ill (fever 39°C or higher) and does not have dysentery (bloody stools), in which case antimotility agents should be avoided. Packages of oral rehydration salts to treat dehydration are available over the counter in the United States (Enfalyte, Pedialyte, others) and in many foreign countries.

When treatment is necessary, in areas where toxin-producing bacteria are the major cause of diarrhea (Latin America and Africa), loperamide (4 mg oral loading dose, then 2 mg after each loose stool to a maximum of 16 mg/day) with a single oral dose of ciprofloxacin (750 mg), levofloxacin (500 mg), or ofloxacin (200 mg) cures most cases of traveler's diarrhea. If diarrhea is associated with bloody stools or persists despite a single dose of a fluoroquinolone, 1000 mg of azithromycin should be taken. In pregnant women and in areas where invasive bacteria more commonly cause diarrhea (Indian subcontinent, Asia, especially Thailand where fluoroquinolone-resistant *Campylobacter* is prevalent), azithromycin is the medication of choice. Rifaximin, a nonabsorbable agent, is also approved for therapy of traveler's diarrhea at a dose of 200 mg orally three times per day or 400 mg twice a day for 3 days. Because luminal concentrations are high, but tissue levels are insufficient, it should not be used in situations where there is a high likelihood of invasive disease (eg, fever, systemic toxicity, or bloody stools).

When to Refer

- Cases refractory to treatment.
- Persistent infection.
- Immunocompromised patient.

When to Admit

Patients who are severely dehydrated or hemodynamically unstable should be admitted to the hospital.

Anderson MS et al. Etiology and epidemiology of travelers' diarrhea among US military and adult travelers, 2018-2023. Emerg Infect Dis. 2024;30:19. [PMID: 39530798]

Carroll SC et al. Incidence and risk factors for travellers' diarrhoea among short-term international adult travellers from high-income countries: a systematic review with meta-analysis of cohort studies. J Travel Med. 2025;32:taae008. [PMID: 38224319]

Gaspar C et al. Landscape of bacterial enteric disease and traveler's diarrhea in South America. J Infect Dis. 2025;231:S10. [PMID: 39928383]

Stürchler D. Infections transmitted via the faecal-oral route: a simple score for a global risk map. J Travel Med. 2023;30: taad069. [PMID: 37158467]

ANTIMICROBIAL THERAPY

SELECTED PRINCIPLES OF ANTIMICROBIAL THERAPY

Specific steps (outlined below) are required when considering antibiotic therapy for patients. Medications within classes, medications of first choice, and alternative medications are presented in Table 34–5.

A. Etiologic Diagnosis

Based on the organ system involved, the organism causing infection can often be predicted. See Table 34–1 and Table 34–6.

B. "Best Guess"

Select an empiric regimen that is likely to be effective against the suspected pathogens.

C. Laboratory Control

Specimens for laboratory examination should be obtained before institution of therapy to determine susceptibility.

D. Clinical Response

Based on clinical response and other data, the laboratory reports are evaluated and then the desirability of changing the regimen is considered. If the specimen was obtained from a normally sterile site (eg, blood, CSF, pleural fluid, joint fluid), the recovery of a microorganism in significant amounts is meaningful even if the organism recovered is different from the clinically suspected agent, and this may force a change in treatment. Isolation of unexpected microorganisms from the respiratory tract, GI tract, or surface lesions (sites that have a complex flora) may represent colonization or contamination, and cultures must be critically evaluated before medications are abandoned that were judiciously selected on a "best guess" basis.

E. Drug Susceptibility Tests

Some microorganisms are predictably inhibited by certain medications; if such organisms are isolated, they need not be tested for drug susceptibility. For example, all group A hemolytic streptococci are inhibited by penicillin. Other organisms (eg, enteric gram-negative rods) are variably susceptible and generally require susceptibility testing whenever they are isolated. Organisms that once had predictable susceptibility patterns are associated with resistance and require testing. Examples include the pneumococci, which may be resistant to multiple medications (including penicillin, macrolides, and tetracyclines); the enterococci, which may be resistant to penicillin, aminoglycosides, and vancomycin; and ESBL-producing *E coli* resistant to third-generation cephalosporins, aminoglycosides, and fluoroquinolones.

When culture and susceptibility results have been finalized, clinicians must use the most narrow-spectrum agent

Table 34–5. Medication of choice for suspected or documented microbial pathogens (listed in alphabetical order, within classes).

Suspected or Proved Etiologic Agent	Medication(s) of First Choice	Alternative Medication(s)
Gram-Negative Cocci		
Moraxella catarrhalis	Cefuroxime axetil, amoxicillin clavulanic acid	Ceftriaxone, a fluoroquinolone,[1] a macrolide,[2] a tetracycline,[3] TMP-SMX[4]
Neisseria gonorrhoeae (gonococcus)	Ceftriaxone ± doxycycline[5]	Gentamicin + azithromycin or cefixime ± doxycycline[5]
Neisseria meningitidis (meningococcus)	Penicillin[6]	Ceftriaxone, ampicillin
Gram-Positive Cocci		
Enterococcus faecalis	Ampicillin ± gentamicin[7] Ampicillin ± ceftriaxone	Vancomycin ± gentamicin
Enterococcus faecium	Vancomycin ± gentamicin[7]	Linezolid,[8] daptomycin,[8] tigecycline,[8] tedizolid,[8] oritavancin[8]
Staphylococcus, methicillin-resistant	Vancomycin	TMP-SMX,[4] doxycycline, minocycline, linezolid,[8] tedizolid,[8] daptomycin,[8] televancin,[8] dalbavancin,[8] oritavancin,[8] ceftaroline, delafloxacin
Staphylococcus, methicillin-susceptible	Cefazolin or Penicillinase-resistant penicillin[9]	Vancomycin, a cephalosporin,[10] clindamycin, amoxicillin-clavulanic acid, ampicillin-sulbactam
Streptococcus, hemolytic, groups A, B, C, G	Penicillin[6]	Macrolide,[2] a cephalosporin,[10] vancomycin, clindamycin
Streptococcus pneumoniae[11] (pneumococcus)	Penicillin[6]	A cephalosporin,[10] vancomycin, clindamycin, a tetracycline,[3] respiratory fluoroquinolones[1]
Viridans streptococci	Penicillin[6]	Cephalosporin,[10] vancomycin
Gram-Negative Rods		
Acinetobacter	Imipenem, meropenem, ampicillin-sulbactam	Tigecycline, minocycline, aminoglycosides,[12] polymyxin B, cefiderocol, sulbactam/durlobactam
Bacteroides, GI strains	Metronidazole	Ampicillin-sulbactam, piperacillin-tazobactam, ertapenem
Brucella	Doxycycline + rifampin	TMP-SMX[4] ± gentamicin; ciprofloxacin + rifampin
Burkholderia pseudomallei (melioidosis) and *Burkholderia mallei* (glanders)	Ceftazidime initially followed by TMP-SMX[4]	Meropenem initially followed by amoxicillin-clavulanic acid
Campylobacter jejuni	Azithromycin	A fluoroquinolone[1]
Enterobacter	Ertapenem, imipenem, meropenem, cefepime	Aminoglycoside, a fluoroquinolone,[1] TMP-SMX[4]
Escherichia coli (complicated, hospitalized)[13]	Ceftriaxone if high local susceptibility rates, otherwise select an alternative	Ertapenem,[13] aminoglycosides,[12] aztreonam, piperacillin-tazobactam, ceftazidime-avibactam,[13,14] ceftolozane-tazobactam,[13] meropenem/vaborbactam,[14] imipenem/cilastatin-relebactam[13,14]
Escherichia coli (uncomplicated outpatient UTI)	Nitrofurantoin	Fluoroquinolones,[1] fosfomycin, TMP-SMX,[4] oral cephalosporin
Haemophilus (respiratory infections, otitis)	Amoxicillin-clavulanate	Doxycycline, azithromycin, ceftriaxone, cefuroxime sodium, cefuroxime axetil, TMP-SMX[4]
Haemophilus (serious infection)	Ceftriaxone	Aztreonam
Helicobacter pylori	PPI, bismuth subsalicylate, tetracycline, and metronidazole if high local susceptibility rates, otherwise select an alternative	PPI, amoxicillin, rifabutin
Klebsiella[13]	Ceftriaxone if high local susceptibility rates, otherwise select an alternative	Cefepime, TMP-SMX,[4] aminoglycoside,[12] ertapenem,[13] fluoroquinolone,[1] aztreonam, piperacillin-tazobactam, ceftazidime-avibactam,[13] ceftolozane-tazobactam,[13] meropenem/vaborbactam,[14] imipenem/cilastatin-relebactam[13,14]

(continued)

Table 34–5. Medication of choice for suspected or documented microbial pathogens (listed in alphabetical order, within classes). (continued)

Suspected or Proved Etiologic Agent	Medication(s) of First Choice	Alternative Medication(s)
Legionella species (pneumonia)	Azithromycin, or fluoroquinolones[1] ± rifampin	Doxycycline ± rifampin
Prevotella, oropharyngeal strains	Clindamycin	Metronidazole
Proteus mirabilis	Ampicillin	TMP-SMX,[4] a fluoroquinolone,[1] a cephalosporin,[10] ertapenem or meropenem[13]
Proteus vulgaris and other species *(Morganella, Providencia)*	Ceftriaxone	Ertapenem or meropenem, TMP-SMX,[4] a fluoroquinolone[1]
Pseudomonas aeruginosa	Piperacillin-tazobactam or ceftazidime or cefepime, or imipenem or meropenem or doripenem or aztreonam	Ceftazidime-avibactam[13,15]; ceftolozane-tazobactam,[13,15] cefiderocol,[15] imipenem/cilastatin-relebactam[15]
Salmonella (bacteremia)	Ceftriaxone	A fluoroquinolone[1]
Serratia	Ceftriaxone, piperacillin-tazobactam	TMP-SMX,[4] a fluoroquinolone,[1] a carbapenem
Shigella	Azithromycin, ciprofloxacin, or ceftriaxone	TMP-SMX[4]
Vibrio (cholera, sepsis)	A tetracycline[3]	Azithromycin, a fluoroquinolone,[1] ceftriaxone
Yersinia pestis (plague)	A fluoroquinolone,[1] or streptomycin, or gentamicin	TMP-SMX,[5] tetracycline[3]
Gram-Positive Rods		
Actinomyces	Penicillin[6]	Tetracycline,[3] clindamycin
Bacillus (including anthrax)	Penicillin[6]	A macrolide,[2] a fluoroquinolone[1]
Clostridium (eg, gas gangrene, tetanus)	Penicillin[6]	Metronidazole, clindamycin, imipenem, or meropenem
Corynebacterium diphtheria	Macrolide[2]	Penicillin[6]
Corynebacterium jeikeium	Vancomycin	Linezolid
Listeria	Ampicillin ± aminoglycoside[12]	TMP-SMX[4]
Acid-Fast Rods		
Mycobacterium avium complex	Clarithromycin or azithromycin + ethambutol, ± rifabutin	Amikacin, ciprofloxacin
Mycobacterium fortuitum-chelonae	Cefoxitin + clarithromycin	Amikacin, rifampin, sulfonamide, doxycycline, linezolid
Mycobacterium kansasii	INH + rifampin ± ethambutol	Clarithromycin, azithromycin, ethionamide, cycloserine
Mycobacterium leprae	Dapsone + rifampin ± clofazimine	Minocycline, ofloxacin, clarithromycin
Mycobacterium tuberculosis[16]	Isoniazid (INH) + rifampin + pyrazinamide ± ethambutol	Other antituberculous drugs (see Chapter 9)
Nocardia	TMP-SMX[4]	Minocycline, imipenem or meropenem, linezolid
Spirochetes		
Borrelia burgdorferi (Lyme disease)	Doxycycline, amoxicillin, cefuroxime axetil	Ceftriaxone, penicillin, azithromycin
Borrelia recurrentis (relapsing fever)	Doxycycline[3]	Penicillin[6]
Leptospira	Penicillin[6]	Doxycycline,[3] ceftriaxone
Treponema pallidum (syphilis)	Penicillin[6]	Doxycycline
Treponema pertenue (yaws)	Penicillin[6]	Doxycycline

(continued)

Table 34–5. Medication of choice for suspected or documented microbial pathogens (listed in alphabetical order, within classes). (continued)

Suspected or Proved Etiologic Agent	Medication(s) of First Choice	Alternative Medication(s)
Mycoplasmas	Azithromycin or doxycycline	A fluoroquinolone[1]
Chlamydiae		
C pneumoniae	Doxycycline[3]	Azithromycin, a fluoroquinolone[1,17]
C psittaci	Doxycycline	Azithromycin, clarithromycin
C trachomatis (urethritis or pelvic inflammatory disease)	Doxycycline	Azithromycin, levofloxacin
Rickettsiae	Doxycycline[3]	A fluoroquinolone[1]

[1]Fluoroquinolones include ciprofloxacin, levofloxacin, moxifloxacin, and others. Levofloxacin, and moxifloxacin, the respiratory fluoroquinolones, demonstrate the most reliable activity against penicillin-resistant *S pneumoniae* and other respiratory infection pathogens. Delafloxacin is predictably active against methicillin-resistant *S aureus* (MRSA).
[2]Azithromycin is the preferred macrolide due to increased safety profile and minimal drug interaction potential.
[3]All tetracyclines have similar activity against most microorganisms. Minocycline (the most active tetracycline) and doxycycline are more active than tetracycline against *S aureus*.
[4]TMP-SMX is a mixture of 1 part trimethoprim and 5 parts sulfamethoxazole.
[5]Add doxycycline if *Chlamydia* has not been ruled out.
[6]Penicillin G is preferred for parenteral injection, penicillin V for oral administration.
[7]Addition of gentamicin indicated only for severe enterococcal infections (eg, endocarditis, meningitis).
[8]Linezolid, tedizolid, tigecycline, daptomycin, telavancin, dalbavancin, and oritavancin should be reserved for the treatment of vancomycin-resistant isolates or in patients intolerant of vancomycin.
[9]Parenteral nafcillin or oxacillin; oral dicloxacillin, cloxacillin, or oxacillin.
[10]Most intravenous cephalosporins (with the exception of ceftazidime) are active against streptococci and methicillin-susceptible staphylococci.
[11]Infections caused by isolates with intermediate resistance may respond to high-dose penicillin or ceftriaxone or the respiratory fluoroquinolones (levofloxacin and moxifloxacin). Infections caused by highly penicillin-resistant isolates should be treated with vancomycin. Penicillin-resistant pneumococci are often resistant to macrolides, tetracyclines, and TMP-SMX.
[12]Aminoglycosides—gentamicin, tobramycin, amikacin, plazomicin—should be chosen on the basis of local patterns of susceptibility.
[13]Extended β-lactamase–producing (ESBL) isolates should be treated with a carbapenem. If a carbapenem cannot be used, ceftazidime-avibactam or possibly ceftolozane-tazobactam or imipenem/cilastatin-relebactam can be considered.
[14]Consider in cases of infection due to carbapenemase-producing *Enterobacterales*.
[15]Ceftolozane-tazobactam, cefiderocol, imipenem/cilastatin-relebactam and occasionally ceftazidime-avibactam may be active against multidrug-resistant *P aeruginosa*.
[16]Resistance is common and susceptibility testing must be performed.
[17]Ciprofloxacin has inferior antichlamydial activity compared with levofloxacin or ofloxacin.
±, alone or combined with.

and the shortest duration possible to decrease the selection pressure for antibacterial resistance.

Antimicrobial drug susceptibility tests may be performed on solid media as disk diffusion tests, in broth, in tubes, in wells of microdilution plates, or as E-tests (strips with increasing concentration of antibiotic). The latter three methods yield results expressed as MIC. In most infections, the MIC is the appropriate in vitro test to guide selection of an antibacterial agent. When there appear to be marked discrepancies between susceptibility testing and clinical response, the following possibilities must be considered:

1. Selection of an inappropriate medication, medication dosage, or route of administration.
2. Failure to drain a collection of pus or to remove a foreign body.
3. Failure of a poorly diffusing drug to reach the site of infection (eg, CNS) or to reach intracellular phagocytosed bacteria.
4. Superinfection in the course of prolonged chemotherapy.
5. Emergence of drug resistance in the original pathogen or superinfection with a new more resistant organism.
6. Participation of two or more microorganisms in the infectious process, of which only one was originally detected and used for medication selection.
7. Inadequate host defenses, including immunodeficiencies and diabetes mellitus.
8. Noninfectious causes, including drug fever, malignancy, and autoimmune disease.

F. Promptness of Response

Response depends on a number of factors, including the patient (immunocompromised patients respond slower than immunocompetent patients), the site of infection (deep-seated infections such as osteomyelitis and endocarditis respond more slowly than superficial infections such as cystitis or cellulitis), the pathogen (virulent organisms such as *S aureus* respond more slowly than viridans streptococci; mycobacterial and fungal infections respond

Table 34–6. Examples of empiric choices of antimicrobials for adult outpatient infections (listed in alphabetical order, except for syphilis).

Suspected Clinical Diagnosis	Likely Etiologic Agents	Medications of Choice	Alternative Medications
Acute sinusitis	*Streptococcus pneumoniae, Haemophilus influenzae, Moraxella catarrhalis*	Amoxicillin-clavulanate,[1] 875/125 mg orally twice daily for 5–7 days	For patients allergic to penicillin, doxycycline, 100 mg twice daily for 5–7 days
Aspiration pneumonia	Mixed oropharyngeal flora	Amoxicillin-clavulanate 875/125 mg orally twice daily for 5–7 days	Levofloxacin 750 mg orally once daily or moxifloxacin 400 mg orally once daily for 5–7 days
Cystitis (uncomplicated)	*Escherichia coli, Staphylococcus saprophyticus, Klebsiella pneumoniae, Proteus* species, other gram-negative rods or enterococci	Nitrofurantoin monohydrate macrocrystals 100 mg twice daily for 5–7 days (unless pregnant); fosfomycin 3 g orally as a single dose	Cephalexin, 500 mg orally four times daily for 7 days, for uncomplicated cystitis. Due to increasing bacterial resistance, TMP-SMX and fluoroquinolones are *not* recommended as first-line therapy for empiric treatment.
Erysipelas, impetigo, nonpurulent cellulitis, ascending lymphangitis	Group A streptococcus	Penicillin V, 250–500 mg orally four times daily for 5–7 days	Cephalexin, 500 mg orally four times daily for 5–7 days
Furuncle with surrounding cellulitis	*Staphylococcus aureus*	Dicloxacillin, 500 mg orally four times daily for 5–7 days for MSSA. For CA-MRSA: TMP-SMX[2] one to two double-strength tablet twice daily for 5–7 days; **or** clindamycin 300 mg orally three to four times daily for 5–7 days	Cephalexin, 500 mg orally four times daily for 5–7 days for MSSA. For CA-MRSA, doxycycline, 100 mg orally twice daily, is a reasonable alternative.
Gastroenteritis	*Salmonella, Shigella, Campylobacter, Entamoeba histolytica*	See footnote 3	
Otitis media	*S pneumoniae, H influenzae, M catarrhalis*	Amoxicillin-clavulanate[1] 875/125 mg orally twice daily for 7–10 days	Cefuroxime, 500 mg orally twice daily; **or** cefpodoxime, 200–400 mg daily; **or** doxycycline, 100 mg twice daily
Pelvic inflammatory disease	*Neisseria gonorrhoeae, Chlamydia trachomatis*, anaerobes, gram-negative rods	Ceftriaxone 500 mg intramuscularly once plus doxycycline 100 mg orally twice daily for 14 days **plus** metronidazole 500 mg orally twice daily for 14 days; **or** cefoxitin 2 g intramuscularly once **plus** probenecid 1 g orally once, **plus** doxycycline 100 mg orally twice daily for 14 days **plus** metronidazole 500 mg orally twice daily for 14 days	Cefotaxime **plus** doxycycline 100 mg orally twice daily for 14 days **plus** metronidazole 500 mg orally twice daily for 14 days
Pharyngitis	Group A streptococcus	Penicillin V, 500 mg orally two times daily, **or** amoxicillin, 500 mg orally two times daily for 10 days	For patients with history of mild penicillin allergy, cephalexin, 500 mg orally four times daily for 10 days; for patients with IgE-mediated reaction, clindamycin, 300 mg orally four times daily for 10 days; **or** azithromycin, 500 mg on day 1 and 250 mg on days 2–5
Pneumonia	*S pneumoniae, Mycoplasma pneumoniae, Legionella pneumophila, Chlamydia pneumoniae*	Amoxicillin, 1 g three times daily **or** Doxycycline, 100 mg orally twice daily	For patients at high risk for infection due to resistant pneumococci: amoxicillin-clavulanate **or** cefpodoxime **or** cefuroxime + macrolide **or** doxycycline **or** monotherapy with a respiratory fluoroquinolone[4]

(continued)

Table 34–6. Examples of empiric choices of antimicrobials for adult outpatient infections (listed in alphabetical order, except for syphilis). (continued)

Suspected Clinical Diagnosis	Likely Etiologic Agents	Medications of Choice	Alternative Medications
Pyelonephritis	*E coli, K pneumoniae, Proteus* species, *S saprophyticus*	Fluoroquinolones[5] for 7 days if prevalence of resistance among uropathogens is <10%	TMP-SMX,[2] one to two double-strength tablets twice daily for 7–14 days for susceptible pathogens. Oral β-lactams are less effective than fluoroquinolones or TMP-SMX
Urethritis, epididymitis	*N gonorrhoeae, C trachomatis*	Ceftriaxone, 500 mg intramuscularly once for *N gonorrhoeae*; doxycycline, 100 mg orally twice daily for 7 days, for *C trachomatis*	Gentamicin 240 mg intramuscularly once **or** cefixime 800 mg orally once for *N gonorrhoeae*[6] Alternatives for *C trachomatis* include azithromycin 1 g orally once **or** levofloxacin 500 mg orally once daily for 7 days
Syphilis			
Early syphilis (primary, secondary, or latent of <1 year's duration)	*Treponema pallidum*	Benzathine penicillin G, 2.4 million units intramuscularly once	Doxycycline, 100 mg orally twice daily for 2 weeks. Ceftriaxone, 1 g intravenously or intramuscularly once daily for 10 days
Latent syphilis of > 1 year's duration or cardiovascular syphilis	*T pallidum*	Benzathine penicillin G, 2.4 million units intramuscularly once a week for 3 weeks (total: 7.2 million units)	Doxycycline, 100 mg orally twice daily for 28 days
Neurosyphilis	*T pallidum*	Aqueous penicillin G, 18–24 million units/day intravenously divided every 4 hours for 10–14 days	Procaine penicillin G 2.4 million units intramuscularly once daily + probenecid 500 mg orally four times daily for 10–14 days

[1]Amoxicillin-clavulante is available as a combination of amoxicillin, 250 mg, 500 mg, or 875 mg, plus 125 mg of clavulanic acid. Augmentin XR is a combination of amoxicillin 1 g and clavulanic acid 62.5 mg.
[2]TMP-SMX is a fixed combination of 1 part trimethoprim and 5 parts sulfamethoxazole. Single-strength tablets: 80 mg TMP, 400 mg SMX; double-strength tablets: 160 mg TMP, 800 mg SMX.
[3]The diagnosis should be confirmed by culture before therapy. *Salmonella* gastroenteritis generally does not require therapy. For susceptible *Shigella* isolates, give ciprofloxacin, 500 mg orally twice daily for 5 days. For *Campylobacter* infection, give azithromycin, 1 g orally for one dose, or ciprofloxacin, 500 mg orally twice daily for 5 days. For *E histolytica* infection, give metronidazole, 750 mg orally three times daily for 5–10 days, followed by an intraluminally active drug such as paromomycin 10 mg/kg orally three times daily for 7 days.
[4]Fluoroquinolones with activity against *S pneumoniae*, including penicillin-resistant isolates, include levofloxacin (500–750 mg orally once daily) or moxifloxacin (400 mg orally once daily). Use fluoroquinolones as medication of choice if recent non-fluoroquinolone antibiotic use within 3 months.
[5]Fluoroquinolones and dosages include ciprofloxacin, 500 mg orally twice daily; ofloxacin, 400 mg orally twice daily; and levofloxacin, 500 mg orally daily.
[6]Test of cure recommended if ceftriaxone is not used.
CA-MRSA, community-acquired methicillin-resistant *Staphylococcus aureus*; MRSA, methicillin-resistant *S aureus*; MSSA, methicillin-susceptible *S aureus;* TMP-SMX, trimethoprim-sulfamethoxazole.

slower than bacterial infections), and the duration of illness (in general, the longer the symptoms are present, the longer it takes to respond). Thus, depending on the clinical situation, persistent fever and leukocytosis several days after initiation of therapy may not indicate improper choice of antibiotics but may be due to the natural history of the disease being treated. In most infections, either a bacteriostatic or a bactericidal agent can be used. *In some infections (eg, infective endocarditis and meningitis), a bactericidal agent should be used.* When potentially toxic medications (eg, aminoglycosides, flucytosine) are used, serum levels of the medication are measured to minimize toxicity and ensure appropriate dosage. In patients with altered renal or hepatic clearance of medications, the dosage or frequency of administration must be adjusted; it is best to measure levels in older adults, in patients with morbid obesity, or in those with altered kidney function when possible and adjust therapy accordingly.

G. Duration of Antimicrobial Therapy

Generally, effective antimicrobial treatment results in reversal of the clinical and laboratory parameters of active infection and marked clinical improvement. However, varying periods of treatment may be required for cure. Key factors include (1) the type of infecting organism (bacterial infections generally can be cured more rapidly than fungal or mycobacterial ones), (2) the location of the process (eg, endocarditis and osteomyelitis require prolonged therapy), and (3) the immunocompetence of the patient.

H. Adverse Reactions and Toxicity

These include hypersensitivity reactions, direct toxicity, superinfection by drug-resistant microorganisms, and drug interactions. If the infection is life-threatening and treatment cannot be stopped, the reactions are managed symptomatically or another medication is chosen that does not cross-react with the offending one (Table 34–5). If the infection is less serious, it may be possible to stop all antimicrobials and monitor the patient closely.

I. Route of Administration

Intravenous therapy is preferred for acutely ill patients with serious infections (eg, endocarditis, meningitis, sepsis, severe pneumonia) when dependable levels of antibiotics are required for successful therapy. Certain medications (eg, doxycycline, fluconazole, voriconazole, rifampin, metronidazole, TMP-SMX, and fluoroquinolones) are so well absorbed that they generally can be administered orally in seriously ill—but not hemodynamically unstable—patients.

Food does not significantly influence the bioavailability of most oral antimicrobial agents. However, the tetracyclines (particularly tetracycline) and the quinolones chelate multivalent cations resulting in decreased oral bioavailability; these effects can be mitigated by separating antibiotic administrations from multivalent cations by several hours.

A major complication of intravenous antibiotic therapy is infection due to the manipulation of the intravenous catheter. Peripheral catheters are changed every 48–72 hours to decrease the likelihood of catheter-associated infection, and antimicrobial-coated central venous catheters (minocycline and rifampin, chlorhexidine and sulfadiazine) have been associated with a decreased incidence of these infections. Most of these infections present with local signs of infection (erythema, tenderness) at the insertion site. *In a patient with fever who is receiving intravenous therapy, the catheter must always be considered a potential source.* Small-gauge (20–23F) peripherally inserted silicone or polyurethane catheters (Per-Q-Cath, A-Cath, Ven-A-Cath, and others) are associated with a low infection rate and can be maintained for 3–6 months without replacement. Such catheters are ideal for long-term outpatient antibiotic therapy.

J. Cost of Antibiotics

The cost of these agents can be substantial. In addition to acquisition costs and monitoring costs (drug levels, liver biochemical tests, electrolytes, etc), the cost of treating adverse reactions, the cost of treatment failure and superinfection, and the costs associated with drug administration must be considered.

K. Antimicrobial Stewardship

Antimicrobial stewardship is a critically important tool intended to optimize clinical outcomes while minimizing unintended consequences of antimicrobial use. These consequences include drug toxicity, superinfection, emergence of bacterial resistance, and impact upon the human microbiome. *The Infectious Diseases Society of America recommends establishment of an antimicrobial stewardship team at all acute care facilities.* The core members of a stewardship team should include an infectious diseases physician and a clinical pharmacist with infectious diseases training. If possible, the addition of a clinical microbiologist, an information system specialist, an infection control professional, and a hospital epidemiologist would be preferable. Key strategies for a stewardship team, as well as the individual prescriber, should include questions associated with the "Four Moments of Antibiotic Decision Making": (1) Does this patient have an infection that requires antibiotics? (2) Have the appropriate cultures been ordered before starting antibiotics? (3) After a few days of empiric antibiotics have passed, can antibiotics be stopped? Can therapy be narrowed? Can therapy be switched from intravenous to oral? (4) What duration of antibiotic therapy is necessary for this patient's diagnosis? Stewardship interventions centered upon one or more of the above questions have been demonstrated to decrease the risk of *C difficile* and *Candida* superinfection as well as attenuate the negative impact of antibiotics on the human microbiome.

Adefisoye MA et al. Antimicrobial resistance expansion in pathogens: a review of current mitigation strategies and advances towards innovative therapy. JAC Antimicrob Resist. 2023;5:dlad127. [PMID: 38089461]

Cantón R et al. Relevance of the consensus principles for appropriate antibiotic prescribing in 2022. J Antimicrob Chemother. 2022;77(Suppl_1):i2. [PMID: 36065724]

MacNair CR et al. Alternative therapeutic strategies to treat antibiotic-resistant pathogens. Nat Rev Microbiol. 2024;22:262. [PMID: 38082064]

HYPERSENSITIVITY

Penicillin Allergy

All penicillins are cross-sensitizing and cross-reacting. Skin tests using penicilloyl-polylysine and undegraded penicillin can identify most individuals with IgE-mediated reactions (eg, hives, bronchospasm). In those patients with positive reaction to skin tests, the incidence of subsequent immediate severe reactions associated with penicillin administration is high. *A history of a remote penicillin reaction is often not reliable.* Only a small proportion (<5%) of patients with a stated history of penicillin allergy experience an adverse reaction when challenged with the medication. The decision to administer penicillin or related medications (other β-lactams) to patients with an allergic history depends on the severity of the reported reaction, the severity of the infection being treated, and the availability of alternative medications. For patients with a history of severe reaction (anaphylaxis), alternative medications should be used. In the rare situations when there is a strong indication for using penicillin (eg, syphilis in pregnancy) in allergic patients, desensitization can be performed. If the reaction is mild (nonurticarial rash), the patient may be rechallenged with penicillin or may be given another β-lactam antibiotic.

Allergic reactions include anaphylaxis, serum sickness (urticaria, fever, joint swelling, angioedema 7–12 days after exposure), skin rashes, fever, interstitial nephritis, eosinophilia, hemolytic anemia, other hematologic disturbances, and vasculitis. The incidence of hypersensitivity to penicillin is estimated to be 1–5% among adults in the United States. *Life-threatening anaphylactic reactions are rare (0.05%).* Ampicillin produces maculopapular skin rashes more frequently than other penicillins, but many ampicillin (and other β-lactam) rashes are not allergic in origin. The nonallergic ampicillin rash usually occurs after 3–4 days of therapy, is maculopapular, is more common in patients with coexisting viral illness (especially Epstein-Barr infection), and resolves with continued therapy. The maculopapular rash may or may not reappear with rechallenge. β-Lactams can induce nephritis with primary tubular lesions associated with anti–basement membrane antibodies.

If an intradermal test is negative, desensitization is not necessary, and a full dose of penicillin may be given. If the test is positive, alternative medications should be strongly considered. If that is not feasible, desensitization is necessary.

Patients with a history of allergy to penicillin are also at an increased risk for having a reaction to cephalosporins or carbapenems. A common approach to these patients is to assess the severity of the reaction. If an IgE-mediated reaction to penicillin can be excluded by history, a cephalosporin can be administered. When the history justifies concern about an immediate-type reaction, penicillin skin testing should be performed. If the test is negative, cephalosporin or carbapenem can be given. If the test is positive, there is a *5–10% chance of cross-reactivity* with cephalosporins, and the decision whether to use cephalosporins depends on the availability of alternative agents, the type of cephalosporin, and the severity of the infection. The exception is cefazolin, which has low cross-reactivity with penicillin due to its distinct side chain. While carbapenems were considered highly cross-reactive with penicillins, the cross-reactivity appears to be minimal (< 1%).

Copaescu AM et al. Efficacy of a clinical decision rule to enable direct oral challenge in patients with low-risk penicillin allergy: the PALACE randomized clinical trial. JAMA Intern Med. 2023;183:944. [PMID: 37459086]

Fu M et al. The burden of β-lactam allergy labels in health care: a systematic review and meta-analysis. Lancet Infect Dis. 2025;25:896. [PMID: 40122092]

Göcebe D et al. Evaluation of the PEN-FAST clinical decision rule in non-beta-lactam antibiotic allergy assessment. Ann Allergy Asthma Immunol. 2025;135:443. [PMID: 40550265]

Nolan TJ et al. Antimicrobial stewardship in critical care. Future Microbiol. 2025;20:1225. [PMID: 41363878]

Reza N et al. Antimicrobial use and resistance. BMJ. 2025;391:e082681. [PMID: 41386779]

Sousa J et al. Algorithms for the classification of patients with a β-lactam allergy label: a systematic review. Curr Opin Allergy Clin Immunol. 2025;25:247. [PMID: 40539896]

IMMUNIZATION AGAINST INFECTIOUS DISEASES

RECOMMENDED IMMUNIZATION FOR ADULTS

Immunization is one of the most important tools (along with sanitation) used to prevent morbidity and mortality from infectious diseases. **Passive immunization** occurs when preformed antibodies are given (eg, immune globulin from pooled serum), resulting in temporary protection. However, the administration of most vaccinations induces a durable antibody response (**active immunity**). The two variants of active immunization are *live attenuated vaccines* (which are believed to result in an immunologic response more like natural infection) and *inactivated or killed vaccines.*

The schedule of vaccinations varies based on the risk of the disease being prevented by vaccination, whether a vaccine has been given previously, the immune status of the patient (probability of responding to vaccine) and safety of the vaccine (live versus killed product, as well as implications for the fetus in pregnant women). Recommendations for healthy adults as well as special populations based on medical conditions are summarized in Table 34–7, which can be accessed online at https://www.cdc.gov/vaccines/. Recommendations for SARS-CoV-2 vaccinations and boosters are being updated regularly.

1. Healthy Adults

Vaccination recommendations are made by the Advisory Committee on Immunization Practices (ACIP) of the US CDC (Table 34–7). Note that for adolescents and children, we recommend following the guidelines from the American Academy of Pediatrics with the endorsement of 12 other medical groups. Characteristics of selected COVID-19 vaccines can be found online and in Chapter 36.

2. Pregnant Women

The following vaccinations are recommended during pregnancy: tetanus (transfer of maternal antibodies across the placenta is important to prevent neonatal tetanus), diphtheria, pertussis, and influenza. Influenza can be a serious infection if acquired in pregnancy, and *all pregnant women should be offered influenza (inactivated) vaccination.* The live attenuated (intranasal) influenza vaccine is *not* recommended during pregnancy. We recommend respiratory syncytial virus vaccination for patients 32–36 weeks pregnant during September through January. We also recommend SARS-CoV-2 vaccination for pregnant persons if they have not received one in the past year. Live vaccines are avoided during pregnancy.

Table 34–7. Recommended adult immunization schedule—United States, 2026.

Vaccine	19–26 years	27–49 years	50–64 years	≥65 years
COVID-19	1 or more doses of 2024–2025 vaccine (See Notes)			2 or more doses of 2024–2025 vaccine (See Notes)
Influenza inactivated (IIV3, ccIIV3) **Influenza recombinant** (RIV3)	1 dose annually			1 dose annually (HD–IIV3, RIV3, or aIIV3 preferred)
Influenza inactivated (aIIV3; HD–IIV3) **Influenza recombinant** (RIV3)	Solid organ transplant (See Notes)			
Influenza live, attenuated (LAIV3)	1 dose annually			
Respiratory syncytial virus (RSV)	Seasonal administration during pregnancy (See Notes)		50 through 74 years (See Notes)	≥75 years
Tetanus, diphtheria, pertussis (Tdap or Td)	1 dose Tdap each pregnancy; 1 dose Td/Tdap for wound management (See Notes) 1 dose Tdap, then Td or Tdap booster every 10 years			
Measles, mumps, rubella (MMR)	1 or 2 doses depending on indication (if born in 1957 or later)			For health care personnel (See Notes)
Varicella (VAR)	2 doses (if born in 1980 or later)		2 doses	
Zoster recombinant (RZV)	2 doses for immunocompromising conditions (See Notes)		2 doses	
Human papillomavirus (HPV)	2 or 3 doses depending on age at initial vaccination or condition	27 through 45 years		
Pneumococcal (PCV15, PCV20, PCV21, PPSV23)			See Notes	See Notes
Hepatitis A (HepA)	2, 3, or 4 doses depending on vaccine			
Hepatitis B (HepB)	2, 3, or 4 doses depending on vaccine or condition			
Meningococcal A, C, W, Y (MenACWY)	1 or 2 doses depending on indication (See Notes for booster recommendations)			
Meningococcal B (MenB)	19 through 23 years 2 or 3 doses depending on vaccine and indication (See Notes for booster recommendations)			
***Haemophilus influenzae* type b** (Hib)	1 or 3 doses depending on indication			
Mpox	2 doses			
Inactivated poliovirus (IPV)	Complete 3-dose series if incompletely vaccinated. Self-report of previous doses acceptable (See Notes)			

Recommended vaccination for adults who meet age requirement, lack documentation of vaccination, or lack evidence of immunity

Recommended vaccination for adults with an additional risk factor or another indication

Recommended vaccination based on shared clinical decision-making

No Guidance/ Not Applicable

Always use this table in conjunction with the schedule by age group and the Notes that follow. Medical conditions or indications are often not mutually exclusive. If multiple medical conditions or indications are present, refer to guidance in all relevant columns. See Notes for medical conditions or indications not listed.

VACCINE	Pregnancy	Immunocompromised (excluding HIV infection)	HIV infection CD4 percentage and count		Men who have sex with men	Asplenia, complement deficiency	Heart or lung disease	Kidney failure, End-stage renal disease or on dialysis	Chronic liver disease; alcoholism[a]	Diabetes	Health care Personnel[b]
			<15% or <200/mm³	≥15% and ≥200/mm³							
COVID-19		See Notes									
Influenza inactivated Influenza recombinant		Solid organ transplant (See Notes)	1 dose annually								
LAIV3					1 dose annually if age 19–49 years		1 dose annually if age 19–49 years				
RSV	Seasonal administration (See Notes)	See Notes					See Notes		Liver disease (See Notes)	See Notes	
Tdap or Td	Tdap: 1 dose each pregnancy	1 dose Tdap, then Td or Tdap booster every 10 years									
MMR	*										
VAR	*			See Notes							
RZV		See Notes									
HPV	*	3-dose series if indicated									
Pneumococcal											
HepA											
HepB	See Notes									Age ≥ 60 years	
MenACWY											
MenB											
Hib		HSCT: 3 doses[c]				Asplenia: 1 dose					
Mpox	See Notes				See Notes						See Notes
IPV		Complete 3-dose series if incompletely vaccinated. Self-report of previous doses acceptable (See Notes)									

Legend:
- Recommended for all adults who lack documentation of vaccination, **OR** lack evidence of immunity
- Not recommended for all adults, but recommended for some adults based on either age **OR** increased risk for or severe outcomes from disease
- Recommended based on shared clinical decision-making
- Recommended for all adults, and additional doses may be necessary based on medical condition or other indications. See Notes.
- Precaution: Might be indicated if benefit of protection outweighs risk of adverse reaction
- Contraindicated or not recommended *Vaccinate after pregnancy, If indicated
- No Guidance/ Not Applicable

a. Precaution for LAIV3 does not apply to alcoholism.

b. See Notes for influenza; hepatitis B; measles, mumps, and rubella; and varicella vaccinations.

c. Hematopoietic stem cell transplant.

(continued)

Table 34–7. Recommended adult immunization schedule—United States, 2026. (continued)

NOTES

For vaccination recommendations for persons ages 18 years or younger, see the Recommended Child and Adolescent Immunization Schedule, 2025: www.cdc.gov/vaccines/hcp/imz-schedules/child-adolescent-age.html

Additional Information

- For calculating intervals between doses, 4 weeks = 28 days. Intervals of ≥4 months are determined by calendar months.
- Within a number range (e.g., 12–18), a dash (–) should be read as "through."
- Vaccine doses administered ≤4 days before the minimum age or interval are considered valid. Doses of any vaccine administered ≥5 days earlier than the minimum age or minimum interval should not be counted as valid and should be repeated. **The repeat dose should be spaced after the invalid dose by the recommended minimum interval.** For further details, see Table 3–2, Recommended and minimum ages and intervals between vaccine doses, in *General Best Practice Guidelines for Immunization* at https://www.cdc.gov/vaccines/hcp/imz-best-practices/timing-spacing-immunobiologics.html.
- Information on travel vaccination requirements and recommendations is available at www.cdc.gov/travel/.
- For vaccination of persons with immunodeficiencies, see Table 8–1, Vaccination of persons with primary and secondary immunodeficiencies, in *General Best Practice Guidelines for Immunization* at https://www.cdc.gov/vaccines/hcp/imz-best-practices/altered-immunocompetence.html?CDC_AAref_Val=https://www.cdc.gov/vaccines/hcp/acip-recs/general-recs/immunocompetence.html
- For information about vaccination in the setting of a vaccine–preventable disease outbreak, contact your state or local health department.
- The National Vaccine Injury Compensation Program (VICP) is a no–fault alternative to the traditional legal system for resolving vaccine injury claims. All vaccines included in the adult immunization schedule except PPSV23, RSV, RZV, Mpox, and COVID–19 vaccines are covered by the National Vaccine Injury Compensation Program (VICP). Mpox and COVID–19 vaccines are covered by the Countermeasures Injury Compensation Program (CICP). For more information, see www.hrsa.gov/vaccinecompensation or www.hrsa.gov/cicp.

COVID–19 vaccination

Routine vaccination

Age 19–64 years

- **Unvaccinated:**
  - 1 dose 2024–25 Moderna or Pfizer-BioNTech
  - 2 doses 2024–25 Novavax at 0, 3–8 weeks
- **Previously vaccinated before 2024–25 vaccine with:**
  - **1 or more doses Moderna or Pfizer-BioNTech:** 1 dose 2024–25 Moderna or Novavax or Pfizer-BioNTech at least 8 weeks after the most recent dose.
  - **1 dose Novavax:** 1 dose 2024–25 Novavax 3–8 weeks after most recent dose. If more than 8 weeks after most recent dose, administer 1 dose 2024–25 Moderna or Novavax or Pfizer-BioNTech.
  - **2 or more doses Novavax:** 1 dose 2024–25 Moderna or Novavax or Pfizer-BioNTech at least 8 weeks after the most recent dose.
  - **1 or more doses Janssen:** 1 dose 2024–25 Moderna or Novavax or Pfizer-BioNTech.

Age 65 years and older

- **Unvaccinated:** follow recommendations above for unvaccinated persons ages 19–64 years **and** administer dose 2 of 2024–25 Moderna or Novavax or Pfizer-BioNTech 5 months later (minimum interval 2 months).
- **Previously vaccinated before 2024–25 vaccine:** follow recommendations above for previously vaccinated persons ages 19–64 years **and** administer dose 2 of 2024–25 Moderna or Novavax or Pfizer-BioNTech 6 months later (minimum interval 2 months).

Special situations

Persons who are moderately or severely immunocompromised. Use vaccine from the same manufacturer for all doses in the initial vaccination series.

- **Unvaccinated:**
  - 4 doses (**3-dose initial series 2024–25 Moderna** at 0, 4 weeks, and at least 4 weeks after dose 2, followed by 1 dose 2024–25 Moderna or Novavax or Pfizer-BioNTech 6 months later [minimum interval 2 months]). May administer additional doses.*
  - 4 doses (**3-dose initial series 2024–25 Pfizer-BioNTech** at 0, 3 weeks, and at least 4 weeks after dose 2, followed by 1 dose 2024–25 Moderna or Novavax or Pfizer-BioNTech 6 months later [minimum interval 2 months]). May administer additional doses.*
  - 3 doses (**2-dose initial series 2024–25 Novavax** at 0, 3 weeks, followed by 1 dose Moderna or Novavax or Pfizer-BioNTech 6 months later [minimum interval 2 months]) May administer additional doses.*
- **Incomplete initial vaccination series before 2024–25 vaccine:**
  - **Previous vaccination with Moderna**

    1 dose Moderna: complete initial series with 2 doses 2024–25 Moderna at least 4 weeks apart (administer dose 1 4 weeks after most recent dose), followed by 1 dose 2024–25 Moderna or Novavax or Pfizer-BioNTech 6 months later (minimum interval 2 months). May administer additional doses.*

    2 doses Moderna: complete initial series with 1 dose 2024–25 Moderna at least 4 weeks after most recent dose, followed by 1 dose 2024–25 Moderna or Novavax or Pfizer-BioNTech 6 months later (minimum interval 2 months). May administer additional doses.*

- **Previous vaccination with Pfizer-BioNTech**
  - **1 dose Pfizer-BioNTech:** complete initial series with 2 doses 2024–25 Pfizer-BioNTech at least 4 weeks apart (administer dose 1 3 weeks after most recent dose), followed by 1 dose 2024–25 Moderna or Novavax or Pfizer-BioNTech 6 months later (minimum interval 2 months). May administer additional doses.*
  - **2 doses Pfizer-BioNTech:** complete initial series with 1 dose 2024–25 Pfizer-BioNTech at least 4 weeks after most recent dose, followed by 1 dose 2024–25 Moderna or Novavax or Pfizer-BioNTech 6 months later (minimum interval 2 months). May administer additional doses.*
- **Previous vaccination with Novavax**
  - **1 dose Novavax:** complete initial series with 1 dose 2024–25 Novavax at least 3 weeks after most recent dose, followed by 1 dose 2024–25 Moderna or Novavax or Pfizer-BioNTech 6 months later (minimum interval 2 months). May administer additional doses.*

- **Completed the initial vaccination series before 2024–25 vaccine with:**
  - **3 or more doses Moderna or 3 or more doses Pfizer-BioNTech:** 2 doses 2024–25 Moderna or Novavax or Pfizer-BioNTech 6 months apart (minimum interval 2 months). Administer dose 1 at least 8 weeks after the most recent dose. May administer additional doses.*
  - **2 or more doses Novavax:** 2 doses 2024–25 Moderna or Novavax or Pfizer-BioNTech 6 months apart (minimum interval 2 months). Administer dose 1 at least 8 weeks after the most recent dose. May administer additional doses.*

***Additional doses of 2024–25 COVID-19 vaccine for moderately or severely immunocompromised:** based on shared clinical decision-making and administered at least 2 months after the most recent dose (see Table 2 at www.cdc.gov/vaccines/covid-19/clinical-considerations/interim-considerations-us.html#table-02.). For description of moderate and severe immunocompromising conditions and treatment, see www.cdc.gov/vaccines/covid-19/clinical-considerations/interim-considerations-us.html#immunocompromising-conditions-treatment.

Unvaccinated persons have never received any COVID-19 vaccine doses. There is no preferential recommendation for the use of one COVID-19 vaccine over another when more than one recommended age-appropriate vaccine is available. Administer an age-appropriate COVID-19 vaccine product for each dose.

For information about interchangeability of COVID-19 vaccines, see wcms-wp.cdc.gov/vaccines/covid-19/clinical-considerations/interim-considerations-us.html#Interchangeability.

Current COVID-19 schedule and dosage formulation available at www.cdc.gov/covidschedule. For more information on Emergency Use Authorization (EUA) indications for COVID-19 vaccines, see https://www.fda.gov/emergency-preparedness-and-response/coronavirus-disease-2019-covid-19/covid-19-vaccines-2024-2025.

***Haemophilus influenzae* type b vaccination**

Special situations

- **Anatomical or functional asplenia (including sickle cell disease):** 1 dose if previously did not receive Hib vaccine
  - **Elective splenectomy:** 1 dose preferably at least 14 days before splenectomy
- **Hematopoietic stem cell transplant (HSCT):** 3-dose series 4 weeks apart starting 6–12 months after successful transplant, regardless of Hib vaccination history

Hepatitis A vaccination

Routine vaccination

- **Any person who is not fully vaccinated and requests vaccination** (identification of risk factor not required): complete 2-dose series HepA (Havrix 6–12 months apart or Vaqta 6–18 months apart [minimum interval: 6 months]) or 3-dose series HepA–HepB (Twinrix at 0, 1, 6 months [minimum intervals: dose 1 to dose 2 = 4 weeks; dose 2 to dose 3 = 5 months])

Special situations

- **Any person who is not fully vaccinated and who is at risk for hepatitis A virus infection or severe disease from hepatitis A virus infection:** complete 2-dose series HepA or 3-dose series HepA–HepB as above. Risk factors include:
  - **Chronic liver disease** including persons with hepatitis B, hepatitis C, cirrhosis, fatty liver disease, alcoholic liver disease, autoimmune hepatitis, alanine aminotransferase (ALT) or aspartate aminotransferase (AST) level greater than twice the upper limit of normal.
  - **HIV infection**
  - **Men who have sex with men**
  - **Injection or noninjection drug use**
  - **Persons experiencing homelessness**
  - **Work with hepatitis A virus** in research laboratory or with nonhuman primates with hepatitis A virus infection
  - **Travel in countries with high or intermediate endemic hepatitis A:** HepA–HepB (Twinrix) may be administered on an accelerated schedule of 3 doses at 0, 7, and 21–30 days, followed by a booster dose at 12 months.
  - **Close, personal contact with international adoptee** (e.g., household or regular babysitting) in first 60 days after arrival from country with high or intermediate endemic hepatitis A: dose 1 as soon as adoption is planned; preferably at least 2 weeks before adoptee's arrival.
  - **Pregnancy** if at risk for infection or severe outcome from infection during pregnancy
  - **Settings for exposure,** including health care setting serving persons who use injection or noninjection drugs, or group homes and nonresidential day care facilities for developmentally disabled persons (individual risk factor screening not required)

(continued)

Table 34–7. Recommended adult immunization schedule—United States, 2026. (continued)

Hepatitis B vaccination
Routine vaccination
- **Age 19 through 59 years:** complete a 2- or 3- or 4-dose series
  - 2-dose series only applies when 2 doses of Heplisav–B are used at least 4 weeks apart
  - 3-dose series Engerix–B, PreHevbrio*, or Recombivax HB at 0, 1, 6 months (minimum intervals: dose 1 to dose 2 = 4 weeks; dose 2 to dose 3 = 8 weeks; dose 1 to dose 3 = 16 weeks)
  - 3-dose series HepA–HepB (Twinrix) at 0, 1, 6 months (minimum intervals: dose 1 to dose 2 = 4 weeks; dose 2 to dose 3 = 5 months)
  - 4-dose series HepA–HepB (Twinrix) accelerated schedule of 3 doses at 0, 7, and 21–30 days, followed by a booster dose at 12 months

***Note:** PreHevbrio is not recommended in pregnancy due to lack of safety data in pregnant women.
- **Age 60 years or older without** known risk factors for hepatitis B virus infection **may** receive a HepB vaccine series.
- **Age 60 years or older with** known risk factors for hepatitis B virus infection **should** receive a HepB vaccine series.
- **Any adult age 60 years of age or older** who requests HepB vaccination **should** receive a HepB vaccine series.
  - **Risk factors for hepatitis B virus infection include:**
    - **Chronic liver disease** including persons with hepatitis C, cirrhosis, fatty liver disease, alcoholic liver disease, autoimmune hepatitis, alanine aminotransferase (ALT) or aspartate aminotransferase (AST) level greater than twice the upper limit of normal.
    - **HIV infection**
    - **Sexual exposure risk** e.g., sex partners of hepatitis B surface antigen (HBsAg)–positive persons, sexually active persons not in mutually monogamous relationships, persons seeking evaluation or treatment for a sexually transmitted infection, men who have sex with men
    - **Current or recent injection drug use**
    - **Percutaneous or mucosal risk for exposure to blood** e.g., household contacts of HBsAg–positive persons, residents and staff of facilities for developmentally disabled persons, health care and public safety personnel with reasonably anticipated risk for exposure to blood or blood–contaminated body fluids, persons on maintenance dialysis (including in–center or home hemodialysis and peritoneal dialysis), persons who are predialysis, and patients with diabetes**
  - **Incarceration**
  - **Travel in countries with high or intermediate endemic hepatitis B**

****Age 60 years or older with diabetes:** Based on shared clinical decision making, 2-, 3-, or 4-dose series as above.

Special situations
- **Patients on dialysis:** complete a 3- or 4-dose series
  - 3-dose series Recombivax HB at 0, 1, 6 months (Note: Use Dialysis Formulation 1 mL = 40 mcg)
  - 4-dose series Engerix–B at 0, 1, 2, and 6 months (Note: Use 2 mL dose instead of the normal adult dose of 1 mL)
- **Age 20 years or older with an immunocompromising condition:** complete a 2- or 3- or 4-dose series.
  - 3-dose series Recombivax HB at 0, 1, 6 months (Note: Use Dialysis Formulation 1 ml = 40 mcg)
  - 4-dose series Engerix–B at 0, 1, 2, and 6 months (Note: Use 2mL dose instead of the normal adult dose of 1mL)
  - 2-dose series Heplisav–B at 0, 1 months
  - 3-dose series PreHevbrio* at 0, 1, 6 months

Human papillomavirus vaccination
Routine vaccination
- **All persons through age 26 years:** complete 2– or 3-dose series depending on age at initial vaccination or condition.
  - **Age 9–14 years at initial vaccination and received 1 dose or 2 doses less than 5 months apart:** 1 additional dose
  - **Age 9–14 years at initial vaccination and received 2 doses at least 5 months apart:** HPV vaccination series complete, no additional dose needed
  - **Age 15 years or older at initial vaccination:** 3-dose series at 0, 1–2 months, 6 months (minimum intervals: dose 1 to dose 2 = 4 weeks; dose 2 to dose 3 = 12 weeks; dose 1 to dose 3 = 5 months; repeat dose if administered too soon)
- No additional dose recommended when any HPV vaccine series of any valency has been completed using the recommended dosing intervals.

Shared clinical decision–making
- **Adults age 27–45 years:** Based on shared clinical decision–making, complete a 2-dose series (if initiated age 9–14 years) or 3-dose series (if initiated ≥15 years).

For additional information on shared clinical decision–making for HPV; see www.cdc.gov/vaccines/hcp/admin/downloads/isd–job–aid–scdm–hpv–shared–clinical–decision–making–hpv.pdf

Special situations
- **Age ranges recommended above for routine and catch–up vaccination or shared clinical decision–making also apply in special situations**
  - **Immunocompromising conditions, including HIV infection:** complete 3-dose series, even for those who initiate vaccination at age 9 through 14 years.
  - **Pregnancy**: Pregnancy testing is not needed before vaccination. HPV vaccination is not recommended until after pregnancy. No intervention needed if inadvertently vaccinated while pregnant.

Influenza vaccination
Routine vaccination
- **Age 19 years or older:** 1 dose any influenza vaccine appropriate for age and health status annually
  - **Solid organ transplant recipients aged 19 through 64 years receiving immunosuppressive medications:** HD–IIV3 and aIIV3 are acceptable options. No preference over other age–appropriate IIV3 or RIV3.
  - **Age 65 years or older:** Any one of HD-IIV3, RIV3, or aIIV3 is preferred. If none of these three vaccines is available, then any other age–appropriate influenza vaccine should be used.
- For the 2024–25 season, see www.cdc.gov/mmwr/volumes/73/rr/rr7305a1.htm
- For the 2025–26 season, see the 2025–26 ACIP influenza vaccine recommendations.

Special situations
- **Close contacts (e.g., caregivers, healthcare workers) of severely immunosuppressed persons who require a protected environment:** should not receive LAIV3. If LAIV3 is given, they should avoid contact with/caring for such immunosuppressed persons for 7 days after vaccination.

Note: Persons with an egg allergy can receive any influenza vaccine (egg-based or non–egg based) appropriate for age and health status.

Measles, mumps, and rubella vaccination
Routine vaccination
- **No evidence of immunity to measles, mumps, or rubella:** 1 dose
  - **Evidence of immunity:** Born before 1957 (except for health care personnel, see below), documentation of receipt of MMR vaccine, laboratory evidence of immunity or disease (diagnosis of disease without laboratory confirmation is not evidence of immunity)

Special situations
- **Pregnancy with no evidence of immunity to rubella:** MMR contraindicated during pregnancy; after pregnancy (before discharge from health care facility): 1 dose
- **Nonpregnant women of childbearing age with no evidence of immunity to rubella:** 1 dose
- **HIV infection with CD4 percentages ≥15% and CD4 count ≥200 cells/mm3 for at least 6 months and no evidence of immunity to measles, mumps, or rubella:** complete 2-dose series at least 4 weeks apart; MMR contraindicated for HIV infection with CD4 percentage <15% or CD4 count <200 cells/mm^3
- **Severe immunocompromising conditions:** MMR contraindicated
- **Students in postsecondary educational institutions, international travelers, and household or close, personal contacts of immunocompromised persons with no evidence of immunity to measles, mumps, or rubella:** complete 2-dose series at least 4 weeks apart if previously did not receive any doses of MMR or 1 dose if previously received 1 dose MMR
- **In mumps outbreak settings,** for information about additional doses of MMR (including 3rd dose of MMR), see www.cdc.gov/mmwr/volumes/67/wr/mm6701a7.htm
- **Health care personnel:**
  - **Born before 1957 with no evidence of immunity to measles, mumps, or rubella:** Consider 2-dose series at least 4 weeks apart for protection against measles or mumps or 1 dose for protection against rubella.
  - **Born in 1957 or later with no evidence of immunity to measles, mumps, or rubella:** complete 2-dose series at least 4 weeks apart for protection against measles or mumps or at least 1 dose for protection against rubella.

Meningococcal vaccination
Special situations for MenACWY
- **Anatomical or functional asplenia (including sickle cell disease), HIV infection, persistent complement component deficiency, complement inhibitor (e.g., eculizumab, ravulizumab) use:** 2-dose primary series Menveo or MenQuadfi at least 8 weeks apart; 1 booster dose 5 years after primary series and every 5 years if risk remains
- **Travel in countries with hyperendemic or epidemic meningococcal disease, or for microbiologists routinely exposed to *Neisseria meningitidis*:** 1 dose Menveo or MenQuadfi; 1 booster dose 5 years after primary series and every 5 years if risk remains
- **First–year college students who live in residential housing (if not previously vaccinated at age 16 years or older) or military recruits:** 1 dose Menveo or MenQuadfi

For MenACWY recommendations **in outbreak setting** (e.g., in community or organizational settings, or among men who have sex with men) and **additional meningococcal vaccination** information, see www.cdc.gov/mmwr/volumes/69/rr/rr6909a1.htm

Shared clinical decision–making for MenB
- **Adolescents and young adults age 16–23 years (age 16–18 years preferred)* not at increased risk for meningococcal disease:** based on shared clinical decision–making
  - **Bexsero or Trumenba (use same brand for all doses):** 2-dose series at least 6 months apart (if dose 2 is administered earlier than 6 months, administer dose 3 at least 4 months after dose 2)

*To optimize rapid protection (e.g., for students starting college in less than 6 months), a 3-dose series (0, 1–2, 6 months) may be administered.

For additional information on shared clinical decision–making for MenB, see https://www.cdc.gov/vaccines/media/pdfs/2025/03/2024-isd-job-aid-scdm-menb-508-remediated.pdf?CDC_AAref_Val=https://www.cdc.gov/vaccines/hcp/admin/downloads/isd-job-aid-scdm-mening-b-shared-clinical-decision-making.pdf

Special situations for MenB
- **Anatomical or functional asplenia (including sickle cell disease), persistent complement component deficiency, complement inhibitor (e.g., eculizumab, ravulizumab) use, or microbiologists routinely exposed to *Neisseria meningitidis*.**
  - **Bexsero or Trumenba (use same brand for all doses including booster doses):** 3-dose primary series at 0, 1–2, 6 months (if dose 2 was administered at least 6 months after dose 1, dose 3 not needed; if dose 3 is administered earlier than 4 months after dose 2, a 4th dose should be administered at least 4 months after dose 3).
  - **Booster doses:** 1 booster dose one year after primary series and every 2–3 years if risk remains

(continued)

Table 34–7. Recommended adult immunization schedule—United States, 2026. (continued)

- **Pregnancy:** Delay MenB until after pregnancy due to lack of safety data in pregnant women. May administer if at increased risk and vaccination benefits outweigh potential risks.

For MenB recommendations **in outbreak setting** (e.g., in community or organizational settings, or among men who have sex with men) and **additional meningococcal vaccination** information, see www.cdc.gov/mmwr/volumes/69/rr/rr6909a1.htm.

Note: MenB vaccines may be administered simultaneously with MenACWY vaccines if indicated, but at a different anatomic site, if feasible.
Adults may receive a single dose of Penbraya (MenACWY–TT/MenB–FHbp) as an alternative to separate administration of MenACWY and MenB when both vaccines would be given on the same clinic day. For adults not at increased risk, if Penbraya is used for dose 1 MenB, then MenB–FHbp (Trumenba) should be administered for dose 2 MenB. For adults at increased risk of meningococcal disease, Penbraya may be used for additional MenACWY and MenB doses (including booster doses) if both would be given on the same clinic day **and** at least 6 months have elapsed since most recent Penbraya dose.

Mpox vaccination
Special situations
- **Any person at risk for mpox infection:** complete 2-dose series, 28 days apart.
- **Risk factors for mpox infection include:**
  - Gay, bisexual, or other MSM, or a person who has sex with gay, bisexual, or other MSM who in the past 6 months have had one of the following:
    - A new diagnosis of at least 1 sexually transmitted disease
    - More than 1 sex partner
    - Sex at a commercial sex venue
    - Sex in association with a large public event in a geographic area where mpox transmission is occurring
  - Persons who are sexual partners of the persons described above
  - Persons who anticipate experiencing any of the situations described above
- **Pregnancy:** There is currently no ACIP recommendation for Jynneos use in pregnancy due to lack of safety data in pregnant women. Pregnant women with any risk factor described above may receive Jynneos.
- **Health care personnel:** Vaccination to protect against occupational risk in healthcare settings is not routinely recommended.

For detailed information, see www.cdc.gov/mpox/hcp/vaccine-considerations/vaccination-overview.html.

Pneumococcal vaccination
Routine vaccination
- **Age 50 years or older who have:**
  - **Not previously received a dose of PCV13, PCV15, PCV20, or PCV21 or whose previous vaccination history is unknown:** 1 dose PCV15 or 1 dose PCV20 or 1 dose PCV21
    - If PCV15 is used, administer 1 dose PPSV23 at least 1 year after the PCV15 dose (may use minimum interval of 8 weeks for adults with an immunocompromising condition,* cochlear implant, or cerebrospinal fluid leak).
  - **Previously received only PCV7:** follow the recommendation above.
  - **Previously received only PCV13:** 1 dose PCV20 or 1 dose PCV21 at least 1 year after the last PCV13 dose
  - **Previously received only PPSV23:** 1 dose PCV15 or 1 dose PCV20 or 1 dose PCV21, at least 1 year after the last PPSV23 dose.
    - If PCV15 is used, no additional PPSV23 doses are recommended.
  - **Previously received both PCV13 and PPSV23 but NO PPSV23 was received at age 65 years or older:** 1 dose PCV20 or 1 dose PCV21 at least 5 years after the last pneumococcal vaccine dose.
  - **Previously received both PCV13 and PPSV23, AND PPSV23 was received at age 65 years or older:** Based on shared clinical decision–making, 1 dose of PCV20 or 1 dose of PCV21 at least 5 years after the last pneumococcal vaccine dose.

Special situations
- **Age 19–49 years with certain underlying medical conditions or other risk factors** who have:**
  - **Not previously received a PCV13, PCV15, PCV20, or PCV21 or whose previous vaccination history is unknown:** 1 dose PCV15 or 1 dose PCV20 or 1 dose PCV21
    - If PCV15 is used, administer 1 dose PPSV23 at least 1 year after the PCV15 dose (may use minimum interval of 8 weeks for adults with an immunocompromising condition,* cochlear implant, or cerebrospinal fluid leak).
  - **Previously received only PCV7:** follow the recommendation above.
  - **Previously received only PCV13:** 1 dose PCV20 or 1 dose PCV21 at least 1 year after the last PCV13 dose
  - **Previously received only PPSV23:** 1 dose PCV15 or 1 dose PCV20 or 1 dose PCV21, at least 1 year after the last PPSV23 dose.
    - If PCV15 is used, no additional PPSV23 doses are recommended.

- **Previously received PCV13 and 1 dose of PPSV23:**
  - Cochlear implant, cerebrospinal fluid leak, or an immunocompromising condition*: 1 dose PCV20 or 1 dose PCV21 at least 5 years after the last pneumococcal vaccine dose.
  - Alcoholism, chronic heart/liver/lung disease, cigarette smoking, or diabetes mellitus: no additional PCV or PPSV23 doses recommended at this time. Review pneumococcal recommendations when age 50 years or older.

Adults aged 19 years and older who have received PCV20 or PCV21: no additional pneumococcal vaccine dose recommended.

Pregnancy: no recommendation for PCV or PPSV23 due to limited data. Summary of existing data on pneumococcal vaccination during pregnancy can be found at www.cdc.gov/mmwr/volumes/72/rr/rr7203a1.htm.

PPSV23 not available: adults aged 19 years or older who received PCV15 but have not yet completed PPSV23 series, can complete the series with either 1 dose of PCV20 or 1 dose of PCV21 if they no longer have access to PPSV23.

For guidance on determining which pneumococcal vaccines a patient needs and when, please refer to the mobile app which can be downloaded here: www.cdc.gov/pneumococcal/hcp/vaccine-recommendations/app.html.

***Note:** Immunocompromising conditions include chronic renal failure, nephrotic syndrome, immunodeficiencies, iatrogenic immunosuppression, generalized malignancy, HIV infection, Hodgkin disease, leukemia, lymphoma, multiple myeloma, solid organ transplant, congenital or acquired asplenia, or sickle cell disease or other hemoglobinopathies.

****Note:** Underlying medical conditions or other risk factors include alcoholism, chronic heart/liver/lung disease, chronic renal failure, cigarette smoking, cochlear implant, congenital or acquired asplenia, CSF leak, diabetes mellitus, generalized malignancy, HIV infection, Hodgkin disease, immunodeficiencies, iatrogenic immunosuppression, leukemia, lymphoma, multiple myeloma, nephrotic syndrome, solid organ transplant, or sickle cell disease or other hemoglobinopathies.

Poliovirus vaccination
Routine vaccination
- **Adults known or suspected to be unvaccinated or incompletely vaccinated:** administer remaining doses (1, 2, or 3 IPV doses) to complete a 3-dose primary series.* Unless there are specific reasons to believe they were not vaccinated, most adults who were born and raised in the United States can assume they were vaccinated against polio as children.

Special situations
- **Adults at increased risk for exposure to poliovirus who completed primary series*:** may administer one lifetime IPV booster.

***Note:** Complete primary series consists of at least 3 doses of IPV or trivalent oral poliovirus vaccine (tOPV) in any combination.
For detailed information, see www.cdc.gov/vaccines/vpd/polio/hcp/recommendations.html

Respiratory syncytial virus vaccination
Routine vaccination
- **Pregnant women of any age:**
  - **Pregnant at 32 weeks 0 days through 36 weeks and 6 days gestation from September through January in most of the continental United States*:** 1 dose **Abrysvo**. Administer RSV vaccine regardless of previous RSV infection.
  - Either maternal RSV vaccination with Abrysvo or infant immunization with nirsevimab (RSV monoclonal antibody) is recommended to prevent severe respiratory syncytial virus disease in infants.
  - **All other pregnant women:** RSV vaccine not recommended
  - **Subsequent pregnancies:** additional doses not recommended. No data are available to inform whether additional doses are needed in subsequent pregnancies. Infants born to pregnant women who received RSV vaccine during a previous pregnancy should receive nirsevimab.

***Note:** Providers in jurisdictions with RSV seasonality that differs from most of the continental United States (e.g., Alaska, jurisdictions with tropical climate) should follow guidance from public health authorities on timing of administration. Refer to the 2025 Child and Adolescent Immunization Schedule for considerations regarding nirsevimab administration to infants.

<u>**Age 75 years or older**</u>
- **Unvaccinated:** 1 dose (Arexvy or Abrysvo or mResvia). Additional doses not recommended
- **Previously vaccinated:** additional doses not recommended. No data are available to inform whether additional doses are needed.

Special situations
- **Age 60–74 years:**
  - **Unvaccinated and at increased risk of severe RSV disease**:** 1 dose (Arexvy or Abrysvo or mResvia). Additional doses not recommended.
  - **Previously vaccinated:** additional doses not recommended. No data are available to inform whether additional doses are needed.

Persons 60 years and older can get RSV vaccine at any time but it is best to administer in late summer and early fall before RSV spreads in communities—ideally August through October in most of continental United States. For further guidance, see www.cdc.gov/mmwr/volumes/73/wr/mm7332e1.htm.

****Note: *People can self–attest to the presence of a risk factor.* The following medical and other conditions increase the risk of severe RSV disease:**
- Chronic cardiovascular disease e.g., heart failure, coronary artery disease, congenital heart disease. Excludes isolated hypertension.
- Chronic lung or respiratory disease e.g., chronic obstructive pulmonary disease, emphysema, asthma, interstitial lung disease, cystic fibrosis
- End stage renal disease or dependence on hemodialysis or other renal replacement therapy
- Diabetes mellitus complicated by chronic kidney disease, neuropathy, retinopathy, or other end–organ damage
- Diabetes mellitus requiring treatment with insulin or sodium–glucose cotransporter 2 (SGLT2) inhibitor

(continued)

Table 34–7. Recommended adult immunization schedule—United States, 2026. (continued)

- Neurologic or neuromuscular conditions causing impaired airway clearance or respiratory muscle weakness e.g., post-stroke dysphagia, amyotrophic lateral sclerosis, muscular dystrophy. Excludes history of stroke without impaired airway clearance.
- Chronic liver disease e.g., cirrhosis
- Chronic hematologic conditions e.g., sickle cell disease, thalassemia
- Severe obesity (body mass index ≥ 40 kg/m^2)
- Moderate or severe immune compromise
- Residence in a nursing home
- Other chronic medical conditions or risk factors that a health care provider determines would increase the risk of severe disease due to viral respiratory infection e.g., frailty, concern for presence of undiagnosed chronic medical conditions, residence in a remote or rural community where escalation of medical care is challenging.

Tetanus, diphtheria, and pertussis vaccination
Routine vaccination
- **Completed primary series and received at least 1 dose Tdap at age 10 years or older:** Td or Tdap every 10 years thereafter
- **Completed primary series and did NOT receive Tdap at age 10 years or older:** 1 dose Tdap, then Td or Tdap every 10 years thereafter
- **Unvaccinated or incomplete primary vaccination series for tetanus, diphtheria, or pertussis:** administer remaining doses (1, 2, or 3 doses) to complete 3-dose primary series. 1 dose Tdap followed by 1 dose Td or Tdap at least 4 weeks later, and a third dose of Td or Tdap 6–12 months later (Tdap is preferred as first dose and can be substituted for any Td dose), then Td or Tdap every 10 years thereafter.

Special situations
- **Pregnancy:** 1 dose Tdap during each pregnancy, preferably in early part of gestational weeks 27–36
- **Wound management:** Persons with 3 or more doses of tetanus–toxoid–containing vaccine: For clean and minor wounds, administer Tdap or Td if more than 10 years since last dose of tetanus–toxoid–containing vaccine; for all other wounds, administer Tdap or Td if more than 5 years since last dose of tetanus–toxoid–containing vaccine. Tdap is preferred for persons who have not previously received Tdap or whose Tdap history is unknown. If a tetanus–toxoid–containing vaccine is indicated for a pregnant woman, use Tdap. For detailed information, see www.cdc.gov/mmwr/volumes/69/wr/mm6903a5.htm

Varicella vaccination
Routine vaccination
- **No evidence of immunity to varicella:** 2-dose series 4–8 weeks apart if previously did not receive varicella–containing vaccine (VAR or MMRV [measles–mumps–rubella–varicella vaccine] for children); if previously received 1 dose varicella–containing vaccine, 1 dose at least 4 weeks after first dose.
  - **Evidence of immunity:** U.S.–born before 1980 (except for pregnant women and health care personnel [see below]), documentation of 2 doses varicella–containing vaccine at least 4 weeks apart, diagnosis or verification of history of varicella or herpes zoster by a health care provider, laboratory evidence of immunity or disease.

Special situations
- **Pregnancy with no evidence of immunity to varicella:** VAR contraindicated during pregnancy; after pregnancy (before discharge from health care facility), 1 dose if previously received 1 dose varicella–containing vaccine or dose 1 of 2-dose series (dose 2: 4–8 weeks later) if previously did not receive any varicella–containing vaccine, regardless of whether U.S.–born before 1980.
- **Health care personnel with no evidence of immunity to varicella:** 1 dose if previously received 1 dose varicella–containing vaccine; 2-dose series 4–8 weeks apart if previously did not receive any varicella–containing vaccine, regardless of whether U.S.–born before 1980.
- **HIV infection with CD4 percentages ≥15% and CD4 count ≥200 cells/mm^3 with no evidence of immunity:** Vaccination may be considered (2 doses 3 months apart); VAR contraindicated for HIV infection with CD4 percentage <15% or CD4 count <200 cells/mm^3.
- **Severe immunocompromising conditions:**
VAR contraindicated

Zoster vaccination
Routine vaccination
- **Age 50 years or older*:** 2-dose series recombinant zoster vaccine (RZV, Shingrix) 2–6 months apart (minimum interval: 4 weeks; repeat dose if administered too soon), regardless of previous herpes zoster or history of zoster vaccine live (ZVL, Zostavax) vaccination.

***Note:** Serologic evidence of prior varicella is not necessary for zoster vaccination. However, if serologic evidence of varicella susceptibility becomes available, providers should follow ACIP guidelines for varicella vaccination first. RZV is not indicated for the prevention of varicella, and there are limited data on the use of RZV in persons without a history of varicella or varicella vaccination.

Special situations
- **Pregnancy:** There is currently no ACIP recommendation for RZV use in pregnancy. Consider delaying RZV until after pregnancy.
- **Immunocompromising conditions (including persons with HIV regardless of CD4 count)**:** 2-dose series recombinant zoster vaccine (RZV, Shingrix) 2–6 months apart (minimum interval: 4 weeks; repeat dose if administered too soon). For detailed information, see www.cdc.gov/shingles/hcp/vaccine–considerations/immunocompromised–adults.html

****Note:** If there is no documented history of varicella, varicella vaccination, or herpes zoster, providers should refer to the clinical considerations for use of RZV in immunocompromised adults aged ≥19 years and the ACIP varicella vaccine recommendations for further guidance: www.cdc.gov/mmwr/volumes/71/wr/mm7103a2.htm

3. Adults with HIV

Patients with HIV have impaired cellular and B-cell responses. Inactivated or killed vaccinations can generally be given without any consequence, but the recipient may not be able to mount an adequate antibody response. Live or attenuated vaccines are generally avoided with some exceptions (ie, in patients with CD4+ T lymphocytes > 200 cells/mcL [0.2×10^9/L]). Guidelines for vaccinating patients with HIV have been issued jointly by the CDC, the US National Institutes of Health, and the HIV Medical Association of the IDSA. Timing of vaccination is important to optimize response. If possible, vaccination should be given early in the course of HIV disease or following immune reconstitution.

4. Hematopoietic Cell Transplant Recipients

HCT recipients have varying rates of immune reconstitution following transplantation, depending on (1) the type of chemotherapy or radiotherapy used pretransplant (in autologous HCT), (2) the preparative regimen used for the transplant, (3) whether graft-versus-host disease is present, and (4) the type of immunosuppression used posttransplantation (in allogeneic HCT). Vaccines may not work immediately in the posttransplant period. B cells may take 3–12 months to return to normal post-transplant, and naïve T cells that can respond to new antigens appear only 6–12 months posttransplant. B cells of posttransplant patients treated with rituximab may take up to 6 months to fully recover after the last dose of the medication. Vaccines are therefore administered 6–12 months following transplantation with a minimum of 1 month between doses to maximize the probability of response.

5. Solid Organ Transplant Recipients

Solid organ transplant recipients demonstrate a broad spectrum of immunosuppression, depending on the reason for and type of organ transplantation and the nature of the immunosuppression (including T cell–depleting agents during treatment of organ rejection). These factors affect the propensity for infection posttransplantation and the ability to develop antibody responses to vaccination. In many cases, the time between placing a patient on a transplant list and undergoing the transplantation takes months or years. Providers should take this opportunity to ensure that indicated *vaccines are given during this pretransplant period to optimize antibody responses.* If this is not possible, most experts give vaccines 3–6 months following transplantation. Live vaccines are contraindicated in the post-transplant period.

RECOMMENDED IMMUNIZATIONS FOR TRAVELERS

Individuals traveling to other countries frequently require immunizations in addition to those routinely recommended and may benefit from chemoprophylaxis against various diseases. Vaccinations against yellow fever and meningococcus are the only ones required by certain countries. These and other travel-specific vaccines are listed at http://wwwnc.cdc.gov/travel/destinations/list.

Various vaccines can be given simultaneously at different sites. Some, such as cholera, plague, and typhoid vaccine, cause significant discomfort and are best given at different times. In general, live attenuated vaccines (measles, mumps, rubella, yellow fever, and oral typhoid vaccine) should *not* be given to immunosuppressed individuals or household members of immunosuppressed people or to pregnant persons. Immunoglobulin should not be given for 3 months before or at least 2 weeks after live virus vaccines, because it may attenuate the antibody response.

Chemoprophylaxis of malaria is discussed in Chapter 39.

VACCINE SAFETY

Most vaccines are safe to administer. *In general, it is recommended that the use of live vaccines be avoided in immunocompromised patients, including pregnant women.* Vaccines are generally not contraindicated in the following situations: mild, acute illness with low-grade fevers (<40.5°C); concurrent antibiotic therapy; soreness or redness at the site; and family history of adverse reactions to vaccinations. *Absolute contraindications to vaccines are rare* (Table 34–8).

Centers for Disease Control and Prevention (CDC). Adult immunization schedules by age. Addendum updated November 21, 2024. Accessed September 22, 2025. https://www.cdc.gov/vaccines/hcp/imz-schedules/adult-age.html

Centers for Disease Control and Prevention (CDC). CDC Yellow Book 2024. Health information for international travel. Accessed September 22, 2025. https://wwwnc.cdc.gov/travel/page/yellowbook-home

Kobayashi M et al. Use of 21-valent pneumococcal conjugate vaccine among U.S. adults: recommendations of the Advisory Committee on Immunization Practices - United States, 2024. MMWR Morb Mortal Wkly Rep. 2024;73:793. [PMID: 39264843]

West Coast Health Alliance. Consensus WCHA 2025-2026 Respiratory Virus Season Immunization Recommendations. Accessed March 11, 2026. https://www.oregon.gov/oha/PH/PREVENTIONWELLNESS/VACCINESIMMUNIZATION/GETTINGIMMUNIZED/Documents/2025-26-Respiratory-Virus-Vaccine-Recommendations.pdf

Wodi AP et al. Advisory Committee on Immunization Practices recommended immunization schedule for adults aged 19 years or older - United States, 2025. MMWR Morb Mortal Wkly Rep. 2025;74:30. [PMID: 39820474]

Table 34–8. Adverse effects and contraindications to commonly used vaccines in adults (listed in alphabetical order).

Vaccine	Adverse Effects	Contraindications[1]
Haemophilus influenzae type b (Hib)	Minimal. Consist mainly of pain at the injection site.	Any severe allergic reaction (eg, anaphylaxis) after a previous dose or to a vaccine component.
Hepatitis A	Minimal. Consist mainly of pain at the injection site.	Any severe allergic reaction (eg, anaphylaxis) after a previous dose or to a vaccine component.
Hepatitis B	Minimal. Consist mainly of pain at the injection site.	Any severe allergic reaction (eg, anaphylaxis) after a previous dose or to a vaccine component.
HPV	Minimal. Consist mainly of mild to moderate localized pain, erythema, swelling. Systemic reactions, mainly fever, seen in 4% of recipients.	Any severe allergic reaction (eg, anaphylaxis) after a previous dose or to a vaccine component.
Influenza (intramuscular inactivated and intranasal live attenuated vaccines)	**Intramuscular, inactivated vaccine:** Local reactions (erythema and tenderness) at the site of injection are common, but fevers, chills, and malaise (which last in any case only 2–3 days) are rare. **Either inactivated or live attenuated vaccine:** A potential association between Guillain-Barré syndrome (3000–6000 cases per year in the United States, usually following respiratory infections) and vaccination with intramuscular, inactivated influenza vaccine has been reported (possibly, 1–2 persons per million persons vaccinated), but this rate is lower than the risk of the syndrome developing after influenza itself (given that approximately 750 persons per million adults are hospitalized annually with influenza, and many more cases remain as outpatients). Influenza vaccination may be associated with multiple false-positive serologic tests to HIV, HTLV-1, and hepatitis C, but it is self-limited, lasting 2–5 months.	Contraindication to both inactivated and live attenuated vaccine: History of Guillain-Barré syndrome, especially within 6 weeks of receiving a previous influenza vaccine. Any severe allergic reaction (eg, anaphylaxis) after a previous dose or to a vaccine component, including egg protein.[2] Intranasal, live attenuated vaccine (FluMist) should not be used in: People 50 years of age and over Immunosuppressed individuals and those on immunosuppressive therapy Household members of immunosuppressed individuals Health care workers, or others with close contact with immunosuppressed persons Presence of reactive airway disease (eg, asthma) or chronic underlying metabolic (eg, kidney), pulmonary, or heart diseases (use intramuscular inactivated vaccine) Pregnancy[3] It is recommended that salicylates should be avoided for 6 weeks following vaccination (to prevent Reye syndrome).
Meningococcal, oligosaccharide conjugate (MCV4 or MenACWY [Menveo, MenQuadfi]); meningococcal group B, recombinant (MenB) [Bexsero, Trumenba]; meningococcal serogroup ABCWY [Penbraya]	Minor reactions (fever, redness, swelling, erythema, pain) occur slightly more commonly with MCV4. Major reactions are rare. A potential association between Guillain-Barré syndrome (3000–6000 cases per year in the United States, usually following respiratory infections) and vaccination with MCV4 has been reported, but recommendations favor continued use of MCV4, since the benefits of preventing the serious consequences of meningococcal infection outweigh the theoretical risk of Guillain-Barré syndrome.	Any severe allergic reaction (eg, anaphylaxis) to a previous dose or to a vaccine component (eg, persons with history of adverse reaction to diphtheria toxoid should not receive meningococcal oligosaccharide conjugate and polysaccharide conjugate vaccines since the protein conjugate used in them is diphtheria toxoid).
MMR[4]	Fever will develop in about 5–15% of unimmunized individuals, and a mild rash will develop in about 5% 5–12 days after vaccination. Fever and rash are self-limited, lasting only 2–3 days. Local swelling and induration are common in individuals previously vaccinated with inactivated vaccine.	Pregnancy[5] Known severe immunodeficiency (eg, from hematologic and solid cancers, receipt of chemotherapy, congenital immunodeficiency, long-term immunosuppressive therapy [eg, > 2 weeks of prednisone 20 mg daily or higher]), other disease- or therapy-related immune suppression, or patients with HIV infection who are severely immunocompromised. May be used in asymptomatic individuals with HIV whose CD4 count is > 200/mcL (0.2×10^9/L). Severe allergic reaction (eg, anaphylaxis) to a previous dose or to a vaccine component (eg, neomycin or to related agents such as streptomycin).

Mpox vaccine (Mpox) [Jynneos]	Mild local reactions (redness, soreness, swelling, and itching) and systemic reactions (fatigue, headache, muscle pain).	Any severe allergic reaction (eg, anaphylaxis) after a previous dose or to a vaccine component.
Pneumococcal conjugate (PCV13) [Prevnar]; pneumococcal polysaccharide (PPSV23) [Pneumovax]	Mild local reactions (erythema and tenderness) occur in up to 50% of recipients, but systemic reactions are uncommon. Similarly, revaccination at least 5 years after initial vaccination is associated with mild self-limited local but not systemic reactions.	Any severe allergic reaction (eg, anaphylaxis) after a previous dose or to a vaccine component (eg, for PCV13 to any vaccine containing diphtheria toxoid).
Respiratory syncytial virus vaccine (RSV) [Arexvy, Abrysvo]	Mild local reactions (pain, redness, swelling) and systemic reactions (fatigue, fever, headache, nausea, diarrhea, muscle or joint pain). Rarely: Guillain-Barré syndrome In pregnancy: preterm birth, high blood pressure, pre-eclampsia.	Any severe allergic reaction (eg, anaphylaxis) to a vaccine component.
Tetanus, diphtheria, and pertussis (DTP, Tdap); tetanus, diphtheria (Td)	Minimal. Consist mainly of pain at the injection site.	Any severe allergic reaction (eg, anaphylaxis) after a previous dose or to a vaccine component. For pertussis-containing vaccines: any history of unexplained encephalopathy (eg, coma, decreased level of consciousness, or prolonged seizures) within 7 days of administration of a previous dose of Tdap or diphtheria and tetanus toxoids and pertussis (DTP) or diphtheria and tetanus toxoids and acellular pertussis (Tdap) vaccine.
Varicella	Can occur as late as 4–6 weeks after vaccination. Tenderness and erythema at the injection site are seen in 25%, fever in 10–15%, and a localized maculopapular or vesicular rash in 5%; a diffuse rash, usually with five or fewer vesicular lesions, develops in a smaller percentage. Spread of virus from vaccinees to susceptible individuals is possible, but the risk of such transmission even to immunocompromised patients is small, and disease, when it develops, is mild and treatable with acyclovir.	Known severe immunodeficiency (eg, from hematologic and solid cancers, receipt of chemotherapy, congenital immunodeficiency, long-term immunosuppressive therapy [eg, > 2 weeks of prednisone 20 mg daily or higher; other immunosuppressive medications], other disease- or therapy-related immune suppression, or patients with HIV infection who are severely immunocompromised). Pregnancy. Severe allergic reaction (eg, anaphylaxis) after a previous dose or to a vaccine component (eg, neomycin). For theoretical reasons, it is recommended that salicylates should be avoided for 6 weeks following vaccination (to prevent potential for Reye syndrome).
Zoster	Mild and limited to local reactions. Although it is theoretically possible to transmit the virus to susceptible contacts, no such cases have been reported.	Known severe immunodeficiency (eg, from hematologic and solid cancers, receipt of chemotherapy, congenital immunodeficiency, long-term immunosuppressive therapy [eg, > 2 weeks of prednisone 20 mg daily or higher; other immunosuppressive medications], other disease- or therapy-related immune suppression, or patients with HIV infection who are severely immunocompromised. May be used in asymptomatic individuals with HIV whose CD4 count is > 200/mcL [0.2×10^9/L]). Pregnancy. Any severe allergic reaction (eg, anaphylaxis) after a previous dose or to a vaccine component (eg, gelatin or neomycin).

[1]Adapted from Centers for Disease Control and Prevention. Contraindications and precautions to commonly used vaccines in adults. General recommendations on immunization: recommendations of the Advisory Committee on Immunization Practices. https://www.cdc.gov/vaccines/hcp/imz-best-practices/contraindications-precautions.html, accessed April 1, 2025; from Hamborsky J et al (editors). Appendix A. Epidemiology and prevention of vaccine preventable diseases. 13th edition. Washington, DC, Public Health Foundation, 2015. Available at https://www.cdc.gov/pinkbook/hcp/table-of-contents/; and from Centers for Disease Control and Prevention. Vaccine Information Statements. Available at: https://www.cdc.gov/vaccines/hcp/current-vis/. Accessed April 1, 2025.

[2]The vaccine has typically been prepared using embryonated chicken eggs. However, a new vaccine using mammalian cell culture is FDA-approved.

[3]The inactivated influenza vaccine can be given during any trimester.

[4]MMR vaccine can be safely given to patients with a history of egg allergy even when severe.

[5]Although vaccination of pregnant women is *not* recommended, with the available RA27/3 vaccine strain, the congenital rubella syndrome does not occur in the offspring of those inadvertently vaccinated during pregnancy or within 3 months before conception.

35 HIV Infection & AIDS

Monica Gandhi, MD, MPH
Matthew A. Spinelli, MD, MAS

ESSENTIALS OF DIAGNOSIS

ESSENTIALS OF DIAGNOSIS

- Criteria for diagnosis of HIV with or without AIDS.
- Laboratory testing for HIV antibody, antigen, and HIV viral RNA.
- Prominent systemic complaints: sweats, diarrhea, weight loss, and wasting.
- Opportunistic infections due to diminished cellular immunity—often life-threatening.
- Increased risk of some cancers.

General Considerations

The CDC AIDS case definition (Table 35–1) includes opportunistic infections and malignancies that rarely occur in the absence of severe immunodeficiency (eg, *Pneumocystis* pneumonia, CNS lymphoma, cytomegalovirus retinitis). It also classifies persons as having AIDS if they have a positive HIV antibody test and certain infections and malignancies that can occur in immunocompetent hosts but that are more common among people with HIV (eg, pulmonary tuberculosis, invasive cervical cancer). Several nonspecific conditions, including dementia and wasting (documented weight loss)—in the presence of a positive HIV test—are also classified as AIDS. The definition includes criteria for both definitive and presumptive diagnoses of certain infections and malignancies. Finally, persons with a positive HIV test whose CD4 lymphocyte count drops below 200 cells/mcL or a CD4 lymphocyte percentage below 14% are considered to have AIDS.

Inclusion of persons with low CD4 counts as AIDS cases reflects the recognition that *immunodeficiency is the defining characteristic of AIDS*. The choice of a cutoff point at 200 cells/mcL is supported by several cohort studies showing that AIDS will develop within 3 years in over 80% of persons with counts below this level in the absence of antiretroviral therapy (ART). Fortunately, the prognosis of people with HIV has dramatically improved due to the development of ART. One consequence is that fewer people with HIV ever develop an infection or malignancy or have a low enough CD4 count to classify them as having AIDS, which means that *the CDC definition has become a less useful measure of the impact of HIV/AIDS in the United States*. Conversely, persons in whom AIDS had been previously diagnosed based on a serious opportunistic infection, malignancy, or immunodeficiency may now be markedly healthier, with high CD4 counts, due to the use of ART. Therefore, the Social Security Administration, as well as most social service agencies, now focus on *functional assessment for determining eligibility for benefits* rather than the simple presence or absence of an AIDS-defining illness, as in the past.

Epidemiology

The modes of transmission of HIV are similar to those of hepatitis B, in particular with respect to sexual, parenteral, and vertical transmission. Although certain sexual behaviors (eg, receptive anal intercourse) confer higher risk than other sexual behaviors (eg, insertive vaginal intercourse), it is difficult to quantify per-contact risks. Nonetheless, the best available estimates indicate that the risk of HIV transmission with receptive anal intercourse is 138 per 10,000 exposures, with insertive anal intercourse being 11 per 10,000 exposures. Receptive vaginal intercourse results in HIV transmission in 8 per 10,000 exposures, with insertive vaginal intercourse being 4 per 10,000 exposures, and a negligible risk with insertive or receptive oral intercourse.

A number of *cofactors* are known to increase the risk of HIV transmission during a given encounter, including the presence of ulcerative or inflammatory sexually transmitted diseases, trauma, active menses, and the absence of male circumcision.

The risk of acquiring HIV infection from a needlestick with blood infected with HIV is estimated to be 23 per 10,000 exposures. Factors known to increase the risk of transmission include depth of penetration, hollow bore needles, visible blood on the needle, and advanced stage of disease in the source. The risk of HIV transmission from a mucosal splash with infected blood is unknown but is assumed to be significantly lower.

The risk of acquiring HIV infection from injection drug use with sharing of needles from a person with HIV is

Table 35–1. CDC AIDS case definition for surveillance of adults and adolescents.

Definitive AIDS Diagnoses (with or without laboratory evidence of HIV infection)
1. Candidiasis of the esophagus, trachea, bronchi, or lungs.
2. Cryptococcosis, extrapulmonary.
3. Cryptosporidiosis with diarrhea persisting > 1 month.
4. Cytomegalovirus disease of an organ other than liver, spleen, or lymph nodes.
5. Herpes simplex virus infection causing a mucocutaneous ulcer that persists > 1 month; or bronchitis, pneumonitis, or esophagitis of any duration.
6. Kaposi sarcoma in a patient < 60 years of age.
7. Lymphoma of the brain (primary) in a patient < 60 years of age.
8. *Mycobacterium avium* complex or *Mycobacterium kansasii* disease, disseminated (at a site other than or in addition to lungs, skin, or cervical or hilar lymph nodes).
9. *Pneumocystis jirovecii* pneumonia.
10. Progressive multifocal leukoencephalopathy.
11. Toxoplasmosis of the brain.
Definitive AIDS Diagnoses (with laboratory evidence of HIV infection)
1. Coccidioidomycosis, disseminated (at a site other than or in addition to lungs or cervical or hilar lymph nodes).
2. HIV encephalopathy.
3. Histoplasmosis, disseminated (at a site other than or in addition to lungs or cervical or hilar lymph nodes).
4. Isosporiasis with diarrhea persisting > 1 month.
5. Kaposi sarcoma at any age.
6. Lymphoma of the brain (primary) at any age.
7. Other non-Hodgkin lymphoma of B cell or unknown immunologic phenotype.
8. Any mycobacterial disease caused by mycobacteria other than *Mycobacterium tuberculosis*, disseminated (at a site other than or in addition to lungs, skin, or cervical or hilar lymph nodes).
9. Disease caused by extrapulmonary *M tuberculosis*.
10. Salmonella (nontyphoid) septicemia, recurrent.
11. HIV wasting syndrome.
12. CD4 lymphocyte count < 200 cells/mcL or a CD4 lymphocyte percentage < 14%.
13. Pulmonary tuberculosis.
14. Recurrent pneumonia.
15. Invasive cervical cancer.
Presumptive AIDS Diagnoses (with laboratory evidence of HIV infection)
1. Candidiasis of esophagus: (a) recent onset of retrosternal pain on swallowing; and (b) oral candidiasis.
2. Cytomegalovirus retinitis. A characteristic appearance on serial ophthalmoscopic examinations.
3. Mycobacteriosis. Specimen from stool or normally sterile body fluids or tissue from a site other than lungs, skin, or cervical or hilar lymph nodes, showing acid-fast bacilli of a species not identified by culture.
4. Kaposi sarcoma. Erythematous or violaceous plaque-like lesion on skin or mucous membrane.
5. *Pneumocystis jirovecii* pneumonia: (a) a history of dyspnea on exertion or nonproductive cough of recent onset (within the past 3 months); and (b) chest film evidence of diffuse bilateral interstitial infiltrates or gallium scan evidence of diffuse bilateral pulmonary disease; and (c) ABG analysis showing an arterial oxygen partial pressure < 70 mm Hg or a low respiratory diffusing capacity < 80% of predicted values or an increase in the alveolar-arterial oxygen tension gradient; and (d) no evidence of a bacterial pneumonia.
6. Toxoplasmosis of the brain: (a) recent onset of a focal neurologic abnormality consistent with intracranial disease or a reduced level of consciousness; and (b) brain imaging evidence of a lesion having a mass effect or the radiographic appearance of which is enhanced by injection of contrast medium; and (c) serum antibody to toxoplasmosis or successful response to therapy for toxoplasmosis.
7. Recurrent pneumonia: (a) more than one episode in a 1-year period; and (b) acute pneumonia (new symptoms, signs, or radiologic evidence not present earlier) diagnosed on clinical or radiologic grounds by the patient's clinician.
8. Pulmonary tuberculosis: (a) apical or miliary infiltrates and (b) radiographic and clinical response to antituberculous therapy.

estimated at 63 per 10,000 exposures. Use of clean needles markedly decreases the chance of HIV transmission but does not eliminate it if other drug paraphernalia are shared (eg, cookers).

When blood transfusion from a donor with HIV occurs, the risk of transmission is 93%. Fortunately, since 1985, blood donor screening for HIV has been universally practiced in the United States. HIV antigen and viral load testing have been added to the screening of blood to further lower the chance of HIV transmission. This essentially eliminates donations from persons who have acquired HIV but have not yet developed a positive antigen/antibody test (ie, persons in the "window" period). With these precautions, the chance of HIV transmission with receipt of blood transfusion in the United States is about 1:2,000,000.

Between 13% and 40% of children born to a mother with HIV contract HIV infection when the mother has not received treatment or when the child has not received perinatal HIV prophylaxis. The risk is higher with vaginal than with cesarean delivery; higher among mothers with high viral loads; and higher among those with detectable viremia who breastfeed their children. The combination of prenatal HIV testing and counseling, ART for mothers with HIV during pregnancy and for the infant immediately after birth, scheduled cesarean delivery if the mother has a viral load that is unknown or not virally suppressed at delivery, and initial avoidance of breastfeeding has reduced the rate of perinatal transmission of HIV to < 1% in the United States and Europe. Importantly, breastfeeding has important nutritional and immunologic benefits for children, so international guidelines *recommend* lactating mothers living with HIV on ART breastfeed their infants (https://clinicalinfo.hiv.gov/en/guidelines/perinatal/introduction; https://www.who.int/news-room/questions-and-answers/item/hiv-aids-infant-feeding-and-nutrition). In the United States, the guidelines changed in 2023 to endorse shared decision-making for women with HIV on ART with undetectable viral loads who wish to breastfeed their infants (https://oar.nih.gov/news-and-updates/oar-updates/update-clinical-guidelines-infant-feeding-supports-shared-decision-making).

HIV has not been shown to be transmitted by respiratory droplet spread, by vectors such as mosquitoes, or by casual nonsexual contact. Saliva, sweat, stool, and tears are not considered infectious fluids.

Approximately 1.2 million adults and adolescents in the United States are estimated to be living with HIV. In 2022 31,800 people received an HIV diagnosis in the United States and 6 dependent areas—a 12% decrease from 2018. In 2022, men who have sex with men (MSM) were the population most affected by HIV in the United States and accounted for 67% of all diagnoses (25,422). People who acquired HIV through heterosexual contact made up 22% of HIV diagnoses (7000) in the United States in 2022, with heterosexual women accounting for 15% of new diagnoses. People who inject recreational drugs (including MSM who use injection drugs) accounted for 7% of new HIV diagnoses in 2022. *Among persons with HIV in the United States, the prevalence of infection in Black, Indigenous, and People of Color is disproportionally higher than among White people.* In 2022, people who self-identify as Black represented 12% of the US population but accounted for 37% of new HIV diagnoses, and people who self-identify as Latino/Latina (who represent 19% of the US population) accounted for 33% of new HIV diagnoses.

In general, the progression of HIV-related illness is similar regardless of sex, although women generally have lower viral loads then men early in infection. There are other important differences. Women are at risk for gynecologic complications of HIV, including recurrent candidal vaginitis, pelvic inflammatory disease, and cervical dysplasia and carcinoma. Violence directed against women, pregnancy, and frequent occurrence of drug use and poverty all complicate the treatment of women with HIV.

Worldwide there are an estimated 40.8 million people with HIV, with heterosexual spread being the most common mode of transmission for men and women. There were 1.3 million new HIV infections worldwide in 2024, with 630,000 deaths from HIV/AIDS. Since the beginning of the HIV pandemic, 44.1 million people have died. The reason for the greater risk for transmission with heterosexual intercourse in Africa and Asia than in the United States may relate to cofactors such as general health status, the presence of genital ulcers, relative lack of male circumcision, the number of sexual partners, and different HIV serotypes. Worldwide, 77% of adults have access to lifesaving ART and the overall rates of virologic suppression is estimated at 73%. In the United States, rates of virologic suppression vary by type of care. The Ryan White Care HIV program provides a comprehensive system of primary medical care, ART, and essential support services to people with HIV, including a specific focus on supporting community needs. In 2024 in the United States, the rate of virologic suppression among people with HIV treated in Ryan White Care–funded clinics is 91%, whereas the overall rate of virologic suppression in the United States remains at 67% according to data released by the Centers of Disease Control and Prevention (CDC) in 2025.

HIV.gov. U.S. Statistics. Accessed February 25, 2026. https://www.hiv.gov/hiv-basics/overview/data-and-trends/statistics

National HIV Prevention and Care Objectives: 2025 Update. Accessed February 25, 2026. https://www.cdc.gov/hiv-data/nhss/national-hiv-prevention-and-care-objectives-2025.html

UNAIDS. 2025 Global AIDS Update—AIDS, crisis and the power to transform. July 10, 2025. Accessed February 25, 2026. https://www.unaids.org/en/resources/documents/2025/2025-global-aids-update

Pathophysiology

Clinically, the syndromes caused by HIV infection are usually explicable by one of three known mechanisms: immunodeficiency, autoimmunity, and allergic and hypersensitivity reactions.

A. Immunodeficiency

Immunodeficiency is a direct result of the effects of HIV upon immune cells as well as the indirect impact of a generalized state of inflammation and immune activation due to chronic viral infection. A spectrum of infections and neoplasms is seen, as in other congenital or acquired immunodeficiency states. Two remarkable features of HIV immunodeficiency are the low incidence of certain infections such as listeriosis and aspergillosis and the frequent occurrence of certain neoplasms such as lymphoma or Kaposi sarcoma. This latter complication has been seen primarily in MSM, and its incidence steadily declined through the first 15 years of the epidemic. A herpesvirus (HHV-8) is the cause of Kaposi sarcoma.

B. Autoimmunity and Allergic & Hypersensitivity Reactions

Autoimmunity can occur as a result of disordered cellular immune function or B lymphocyte dysfunction. Examples of both lymphocytic infiltration of organs (eg, lymphocytic interstitial pneumonitis) and autoantibody production (eg, immunologic thrombocytopenia) occur. These phenomena may be the only clinically apparent disease or may coexist with obvious immunodeficiency. Moreover, people with HIV appear to have higher rates of allergic reactions to unknown allergens as seen with **eosinophilic pustular folliculitis** ("itchy red bump syndrome") as well as increased rates of hypersensitivity reactions to medications (for example, the fever and sunburn-like rash seen with trimethoprim-sulfamethoxazole reactions).

Clinical Findings

The complications of HIV-related infections and neoplasms affect virtually every organ. The general approach to people with HIV with symptoms is to evaluate the organ systems involved, aiming to diagnose treatable conditions rapidly. As shown in Figure 35–1, *the CD4 lymphocyte count level enables the clinician to focus on the diagnoses most likely to be seen at each stage of immunodeficiency.* Certain infections may occur at any CD4 count, while others rarely occur unless the CD4 lymphocyte count has dropped below a certain level. For example, a CD4 count of 600 cells/mcL, cough, and fever may be due to a bacterial pneumonia but would be very unlikely to result from ***Pneumocystis jirovecii*** **pneumonia**, which manifests usually with CD4 cell counts < 200 cells/mcL.

A. Symptoms and Signs

Many people with HIV remain asymptomatic for years even without ART, with a mean time of approximately 10 years between infection and development of AIDS. When symptoms occur, they may be remarkably protean and nonspecific. Since virtually all the findings may be seen with other diseases, a combination of complaints is more suggestive of HIV infection than any one symptom.

Physical examination may be entirely unremarkable. Abnormal findings range from completely nonspecific to highly specific for HIV infection. Some opportunistic infections specific to HIV infection include oral hairy leukoplakia (due to Epstein-Barr virus) of the tongue, disseminated Kaposi sarcoma, and cutaneous bacillary angiomatosis (due to *Bartonella*). Generalized lymphadenopathy, which is nonspecific, is common early in infection.

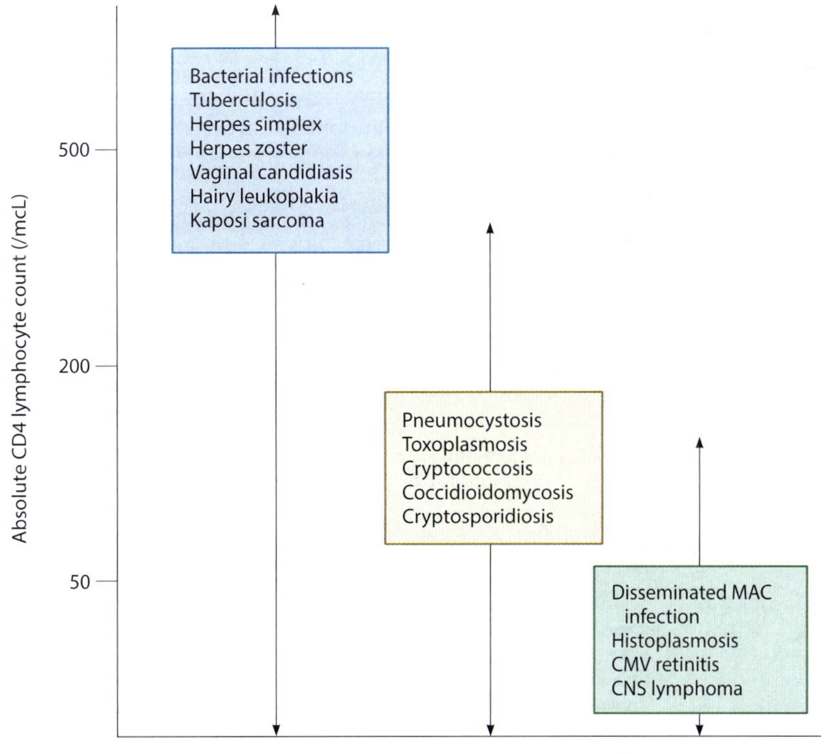

Figure 35–1. Relationship of CD4 count to development of opportunistic infections. MAC, *Mycobacterium avium* complex; CMV, cytomegalovirus.

The specific presentations and management of the various complications of HIV infection are discussed under the Complications section below.

Dillon SM et al. Gut innate immunity and HIV pathogenesis. Curr HIV/AIDS Rep. 2021;18:128. [PMID: 33687703]
Sonti S et al. HIV-1 persistence in the CNS: mechanisms of latency, pathogenesis and an update on eradication strategies. Virus Res. 2021;303:198523. [PMID: 34314771]

B. Laboratory Findings

Specific tests for HIV include antibody, antigen, and HIV viral load detection (Table 35–2). Initial testing for HIV should use a **fourth-generation HIV antigen/antibody immunoassay**. This test detects both HIV-1 and HIV-2 antibodies and HIV-1 p24 antigen. Reactive specimens are then tested with an **HIV-1/HIV-2 differentiation immunoassay** to confirm infection and to distinguish HIV-1 from HIV-2. For patients who are reactive on both tests, the sensitivity and specificity for chronic HIV approach 100%. Patients who have a reactive HIV antigen/antibody immunoassay but a negative HIV-1/HIV-2 differentiation immunoassay should have an **HIV viral load test (nucleic acid test)**; those with positive viral loads despite a negative differentiation assay are likely to have acute HIV infection. Persons who are reactive on the initial test and then negative on the confirmatory test and have nondetectable viral loads are presumed to have a false-positive test, which may occur with recent influenza vaccination, autoantibodies (eg, with collagen vascular or autoimmune diseases), or alloantibodies from pregnancy. With fourth-generation tests, antibodies will be detectable in 99% of persons within 6 weeks after infection, with the median time to detection of about 2 weeks.

Rapid HIV antibody tests of blood or oral fluid provide results within 10–20 minutes and can be performed in clinician offices, including by personnel without laboratory training and without a Clinical Laboratory Improvement Amendment (CLIA)–approved laboratory. Persons who test positive on a rapid test require confirmation with standard testing as above. Rapid testing is particularly helpful in settings where a result is needed immediately (eg, a woman in labor who has not recently been tested for HIV; with use of intramuscular cabotegravir as HIV prevention) or when the patient is unlikely to return for a result. Rapid HIV home tests that allow the testers to learn their status privately by simply swabbing along their gum lines are also available (www.oraquick.com).

Nonspecific laboratory findings with HIV infection may include anemia, leukopenia (particularly lymphopenia), and thrombocytopenia in any combination, elevation of the ESR, polyclonal hypergammaglobulinemia, and hypocholesterolemia. Cutaneous anergy is common with immunosuppression.

The **absolute CD4 lymphocyte count** is the most widely used marker to provide prognostic information and to guide decisions for prophylaxis of opportunistic infections (Table 35–2). As counts decrease, the risk of serious opportunistic infection over the subsequent 3–5 years increases. There are many limitations to using the CD4 count, including diurnal variation, depression with intercurrent illness or vaccination for another pathogen, and intra-laboratory and interlaboratory variability. Therefore, *the trend is more important than a single determination* and the CD4 percentage can circumvent some of the

Table 35–2. Commonly ordered tests for HIV infection (listed in alphabetical order).

Test	Significance
Absolute CD4 lymphocyte count	Best test for determining stage of HIV infection. Risk of progression to an AIDS opportunistic infection or malignancy is high with CD4 count < 200 cells/mcL in the absence of treatment.
CD4 lymphocyte percentage	Percentage may be more reliable than the CD4 count. Risk of progression to an AIDS opportunistic infection or malignancy is high with percentage < 14% in the absence of treatment.
HIV-1/HIV-2 antibody differentiation immunoassay	Serves as confirmatory test and differentiates HIV-1 and HIV-2. Tests that are reactive on HIV-1/2 antigen/antibody immunoassay but negative on this confirmatory test should have an HIV-1 viral load test. Sensitivity and specificity of combination of reactive antigen/antibody immunoassay and positive differentiation assay approach 100% for chronic infection.
HIV-1/2 antigen/antibody immunoassay	Detects antibodies for HIV-1 and HIV-2 along with HIV-1 p24 antigen. Positive specimens require testing with HIV-1/HIV-2 antibody differentiation assay.
HIV rapid antibody test	Screening test for HIV. Produces results in 10–20 minutes. Can be performed by personnel with limited training. Sensitivity and specificity for chronic infection are > 99%, although the sensitivity in acute infection is lower. Positive results must be confirmed with standard HIV testing using the HIV-1/2 antigen/antibody immunoassay and the HIV-1/HIV-2 antibody differentiation assay.
HIV-1 viral load tests	This nucleic acid test measures the amount of actively replicating HIV virus. Patients who have a negative result on the HIV-1/2 antigen/antibody immunoassay or the HIV-1/HIV-2 antibody differentiation assay, or both, but have a positive HIV viral load are likely experiencing acute HIV infection; however, caution is warranted when the test result shows low-level viremia (ie, < 1000 copies/mL) as this may represent a false-positive result. Besides its use in diagnosing acute HIV infection, HIV viral load is the most accurate indicator of viral activity and response to treatment.

limitations of a single absolute CD4 count. The frequency of performance of counts depends on the patient's health status and whether or not they are receiving ART. **All patients regardless of CD4 count should be offered ART and the CD4 count monitored regularly until virologic suppression achieved**; regular CD4 monitoring after the achievement of a CD4 count > 350 cells/mcL and virologic suppression is not necessary. Initiation of *Pneumocystis jirovecii* prophylactic therapy is recommended when the CD4 count drops below 200 cells/mcL, with prophylaxis of *Toxoplasma gondii* recommended in those who are IgG-positive for the pathogen with CD4 count < 100 cells/mcL. Initiation of *Mycobacterium avium complex* prophylaxis is now only recommended in the rare cases of individuals with CD4 counts < 50 cells/mcL who do not initiate ART (eg, per patient preference). The **percentage of CD4 lymphocytes** can be a more reliable indicator of prognosis than the absolute counts (with a percentage < 14% roughly predictive of a CD4 count < 200 cells/mcL), particularly in the setting of acute illness. While the CD4 count measures immune dysfunction, it does not provide a measure of how actively HIV is replicating in the body. HIV viral load tests assess the level of viral replication and provide useful prognostic information that is independent of the information provided by CD4 counts. *The goal of ART is virologic suppression below or at the limits of detection of the assay.*

Differential Diagnosis

HIV infection may mimic a variety of other medical illnesses. Specific differential diagnosis depends on the mode of presentation. In patients presenting with constitutional symptoms such as weight loss and fevers, differential considerations include cancer, chronic infections such as tuberculosis and endocarditis, autoimmune conditions, and endocrinologic diseases such as hyperthyroidism. When pulmonary processes dominate the presentation, acute and chronic lung infections must be considered as well as other causes of diffuse interstitial pulmonary infiltrates, including SARS-CoV-2 infection (COVID-19). When neurologic disease is the mode of presentation, conditions that cause mental status changes or neuropathy—eg, alcohol use disorder, liver disease, kidney dysfunction, thyroid disease, and vitamin deficiency—should be considered. If a patient presents with headache and a CSF pleocytosis, other causes of chronic meningitis enter the differential. When diarrhea is a prominent complaint, infectious enterocolitis, antibiotic-associated colitis, IBD, and malabsorptive syndromes must be considered.

Complications

A. Systemic Complaints

Fever, night sweats, and weight loss are common symptoms in people with HIV and may occur without a complicating opportunistic infection. Patients with persistent fever and no localizing symptoms should nonetheless be carefully examined and evaluated with a CXR (*Pneumocystis* pneumonia can present with subtle respiratory symptoms), bacterial blood cultures if the fever is > 38.0°C, as well as serum cryptococcal antigen and mycobacterial cultures of the blood in those with low CD4 cell counts. Abdominal CT scans can be considered to evaluate occult intrabdominal infections or cancers. If these studies return unremarkable results, patients should be observed closely. Antipyretics are useful to prevent dehydration.

Pahwa S et al. NIH Workshop on HIV-associated comorbidities, coinfections, and complications: summary and recommendation for future research. J Acquir Immune Defic Syndr. 2021;86:11. [PMID: 33306561]

1. Weight changes—Weight loss is a particularly distressing complication of long-standing HIV infection. Patients typically have *disproportionate loss of muscle mass*, with maintenance or less substantial loss of fat stores. The mechanism of HIV-related weight loss is not completely understood but appears to be multifactorial, with some of the older thymidine analog medications implicated. In the setting of the newer medications, weight gain has been seen with some ART regimens, with integrase strand transfer inhibitors associated with greater weight gain than protease inhibitors or nonnucleoside reverse transcriptase inhibitors. Among nucleoside/tide reverse transcriptase inhibitors, tenofovir alafenamide is associated with greater weight gain than tenofovir disoproxil fumarate or abacavir. However, removal of the older ART agents, such as tenofovir disoproxil fumarate or efavirenz, each of which seem to be associated with weight loss, also has been implicated with the weight gain seen with newer regimens.

A. Presentation—Patients with AIDS frequently experience anorexia, nausea, and vomiting, all of which contribute to weight loss by decreasing caloric intake. In some cases, these symptoms are secondary to a specific infection, such as viral hepatitis. In other cases, however, evaluation of the symptoms yields no specific pathogen, and it is assumed to be due to a primary effect of HIV. Malabsorption also plays a role in decreased caloric intake. Patients may suffer diarrhea from infections with bacterial, viral, or parasitic agents.

B. Management—Several strategies have been developed to slow **AIDS wasting**. In the long term, nothing is as effective as ART, since it treats the underlying HIV infection. In the short term, effective fever control decreases the metabolic rate and may slow the pace of weight loss, as does treating any underlying opportunistic infection. Food supplementation with high-calorie drinks and appetite stimulants may enable patients with low appetite to maintain their intake.

Two pharmacologic approaches for increasing appetite and weight gain are the progestational agent megestrol acetate liquid suspension (400–800 mg orally daily in divided doses) and the antiemetic agent dronabinol (2.5–5 mg orally three times a day), but *neither of these agents increases lean body mass.* Side effects from megestrol acetate are rare, but thromboembolic phenomena, edema, nausea, vomiting, and rash have been reported. In 3–10% of patients using dronabinol, euphoria, dizziness, paranoia, and somnolence and even nausea and vomiting have been reported. Dronabinol contains only one of the active ingredients in marijuana, and some patients experience better relief of nausea and improvement of appetite with medical cannabis (THC is thought to be more effective than CBD; administered via smoking, vaporization, essential oils, or cooked in food). In the United States, 38 states and the District of Columbia and 3 US territories have legalized medical marijuana, and 23 states and the District of Columbia and Guam have legalized recreational (nonmedical) use. However, the use and sale of marijuana are still illegal under federal law.

Saeteaw M et al. Efficacy and safety of pharmacological cachexia interventions: systematic review and network meta-analysis. BMJ Support Palliat Care. 2021;11:75. [PMID: 33246937]

2. Nausea—Nausea leading to weight loss is sometimes due to esophageal candidiasis. Patients with oral candidiasis and nausea should be empirically treated with an oral antifungal agent. Patients with weight loss due to nausea of unclear origin may benefit from use of antiemetics or promotility agents prior to meals (ondansetron, 8 mg three times daily; prochlorperazine, 10 mg three times daily; or metoclopramide, 10 mg three times daily). Dronabinol (5 mg three times daily) or medical cannabis can also be used to treat nausea, although in some individuals it can worsen nausea and vomiting. Depression and adrenal insufficiency are two potentially treatable causes of weight loss.

B. Pulmonary Disease

1. *Pneumocystis* pneumonia—(See also Chapter 40.) *P jirovecii* pneumonia is the most common opportunistic infection associated with AIDS. *Pneumocystis* pneumonia may be difficult to diagnose because the symptoms—fever, cough, and shortness of breath—are nonspecific and typically subacute. Furthermore, the severity of symptoms ranges from fever and no respiratory symptoms through mild cough or dyspnea to frank respiratory distress.

Hypoxemia may be severe, with a $PO_2 < 60$ mm Hg. *The cornerstone of diagnosis is the CXR or CT scan* (Figure 35–2). Diffuse or perihilar infiltrates are most characteristic, but only two-thirds of patients with *Pneumocystis* pneumonia have this finding. Normal CXRs are seen in 5–10% of patients with *Pneumocystis* pneumonia, although sensitivity is increased with CT scanning, while the remainder have diffuse ground glass opacities. Severe cases can lead to pneumothoraces. Large pleural effusions are uncommon with *Pneumocystis* pneumonia; their presence suggests bacterial pneumonia, other infections such as tuberculosis, or pleural Kaposi sarcoma.

Definitive diagnosis can be obtained in 70–90% of cases by *Wright-Giemsa stain* or *direct fluorescence antibody (DFA) test* of induced sputum. PCR testing is also available and has high sensitivity and specificity. Sputum induction is performed by having patients inhale an aerosolized solution of 3% saline produced by an ultrasonic nebulizer. Patients should not eat for at least 8 hours and should not use toothpaste or mouthwash prior to the procedure since they can interfere with test interpretation. The next step for patients with negative sputum examinations in whom *Pneumocystis* pneumonia is still suspected should be

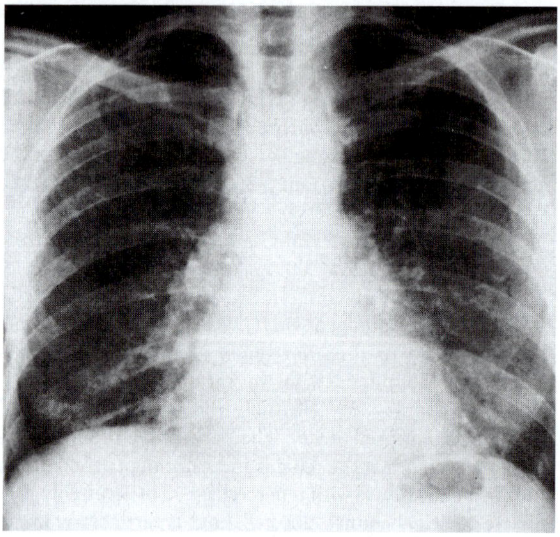

▲ **Figure 35–2.** ***Pneumocystis*** **pneumonia** in a Haitian woman (she/her) in whom underlying HIV/AIDS is suspected. Typical CXR showing bilateral diffuse interstitial infiltrates extending out from the hilar areas. (Reproduced, with permission, from Grippi MA, Elias JA, Fishman JA et al (editors). *Fishman's Pulmonary Diseases and Disorders*, 5th ed. McGraw-Hill, 2015.)

bronchoalveolar lavage. This technique establishes the diagnosis in over 95% of cases.

In patients with symptoms suggestive of *Pneumocystis* pneumonia but with negative or atypical CXRs and negative sputum examinations, other diagnostic tests may provide additional information in deciding whether to proceed to bronchoalveolar lavage. Elevation of *serum LD* occurs in 95% of cases of *Pneumocystis* pneumonia, but the specificity of this finding is at best 75%. A normal *serum β-glucan test* makes *Pneumocystis* pneumonia unlikely, although a variety of factors can cause a false-positive serum β-glucan test. Either a normal *diffusing capacity of carbon monoxide* (DL_{CO}) or a *high-resolution CT scan* of the chest that demonstrates no interstitial lung disease makes the diagnosis of *Pneumocystis* pneumonia very unlikely. In addition, a CD4 count > 250 cells/mcL within 2 months prior to evaluation of respiratory symptoms makes a diagnosis of *Pneumocystis* pneumonia unlikely; only 1–5% of cases occur above this CD4 count level (see Figure 35–1). This is true even if the patient previously had a CD4 count lower than 200 cells/mcL but has had an increase with ART. Pneumothoraces can be seen in people with HIV with a history of *Pneumocystis* pneumonia.

Trimethoprim-sulfamethoxazole is the preferred treatment of *Pneumocystis* pneumonia (Table 35–3). In addition to specific anti-*Pneumocystis* treatment, corticosteroid therapy has been shown to improve the course of patients with moderate to severe *P jirovecii* pneumonia ($PaO_2 < 70$ mm Hg on room air or alveolar-arterial O_2 gradient greater or equal to 35 mm Hg) when administered within 72 hours of the start of anti-*Pneumocystis* treatment. Steroids should be started as early as possible after initiation of treatment, using prednisone 40 mg orally twice daily for days 1–5, 40 mg

Table 35–3. Treatment of AIDS-related opportunistic infections and malignancies[1] (listed in alphabetical order).

Infection or Malignancy	Treatment	Complications[2]
Cryptococcal meningitis	Preferred regimen: Induction: Liposomal amphotericin B, 3–4 mg/kg/day intravenously, with flucytosine, 25 mg/kg/dose orally four times daily for minimum of 2 weeks (adjust flucytosine dose for kidney function), then fluconazole, 400 mg orally daily for a minimum of 8 weeks (consolidation), then 200 mg orally daily to complete a minimum of 1 year of therapy (maintenance)	Liposomal amphotericin: fever, chills, hypokalemia, kidney disease Flucytosine: bone marrow suppression, kidney disease, hepatitis Fluconazole: hepatitis
	Induction: Amphotericin B, 0.7–1.0 mg/kg/day intravenously, with flucytosine, 25 mg/kg/dose orally four times daily for a minimum of 2 weeks (adjust flucytosine dose for kidney function), then fluconazole, 400 mg orally daily for a minimum of 8 weeks (consolidation), then 200 mg orally daily to complete a minimum of 1 year of therapy (maintenance)	Amphotericin: fever, chills, hypokalemia, kidney disease Flucytosine: bone marrow suppression, kidney disease, hepatitis Fluconazole: hepatitis
	Fluconazole, used alone, is inferior to amphotericin B as induction therapy; it is recommended only for patients who cannot tolerate or do not respond to the preferred regimen above. If used for primary induction therapy, give fluconazole, 1200 mg orally daily, with flucytosine, 25 mg/kg/dose orally four times daily for a minimum of 2 weeks (adjust flucytosine dose for kidney function), then 400 mg orally daily for a minimum of 8 weeks (consolidation), then 200 mg orally daily to complete a minimum of 1 year of therapy.	Hepatitis
Cytomegalovirus retinitis (immediate sight-threatening)	Preferred regimen: First-line therapy is oral valganciclovir, 900 mg orally twice a day with food for 21 days followed by 900 mg daily (maintenance). For sight-threatening infections involving the macula or optic nerve, add intravitreal ganciclovir (2 mg/injection) or foscarnet (2.4 mg/injection) for 1–4 doses/day for 7–10 days	For valganciclovir: neutropenia, anemia, thrombocytopenia (avoid in patients with hemoglobin < 8 g/dL, neutrophil count below 500 cells/mcL [0.5×10^9/L] or platelet count below 25,000/mcL [25×10^9/L]). Potentially embryotoxic.
	Ganciclovir, 10 mg/kg/day intravenously in two divided doses for 14–21 days, followed by 5 mg/kg daily (maintenance)	Neutropenia, anemia, thrombocytopenia Adjust ganciclovir dose for kidney function. Potentially embryotoxic.
	Foscarnet, 90 mg/kg intravenously every 12 hours for 14 days, followed by 90–120 mg/kg once daily	Nausea, hypokalemia, hypocalcemia, hyperphosphatemia, azotemia Adjust foscarnet dose for kidney function.
	Cidofovir, 5 mg/kg/week intravenously for 2 weeks, then 5 mg/kg every other week with probenecid, 2 g orally 3 hours before dose, 1 g orally 2 hours after dose, and 1 g orally 8 hours after dose	Nephrotoxicity (to reduce likelihood, pre- and post-saline hydration, along with probenecid), ocular hypotony, anterior uveitis, neutropenia Avoid in patients with sulfa allergy because of cross hypersensitivity with probenecid.
Esophageal candidiasis or recurrent vaginal candidiasis	Fluconazole, 100–200 mg orally daily for 14–21 days for esophageal disease and > 7 days for recurrent vaginal disease	Hepatitis, development of azole resistance. Fluconazole should *not* be given to women who are or may be pregnant because of risk of spontaneous abortion.
Herpes simplex infection	Acyclovir, 400 mg orally three times daily for 5–10 days; or acyclovir, 5 mg/kg intravenously every 8 hours for severe cases	Resistant herpes simplex with long-term therapy
	Valacyclovir, 1 g orally twice daily for 5–10 days	Nausea
	Famciclovir, 500 mg orally twice daily for 5–10 days	Nausea
	Foscarnet, 40 mg/kg intravenously every 8 hours, for acyclovir-resistant cases	Nausea, hypokalemia, hypocalcemia, hyperphosphatemia, azotemia Adjust foscarnet dose for kidney function.

(continued)

Table 35–3. Treatment of AIDS-related opportunistic infections and malignancies[1] (listed in alphabetical order). (continued)

Infection or Malignancy	Treatment	Complications[2]
Herpes zoster	Preferred regimen: Valacyclovir, 1000 mg orally three times daily for 7–10 days	Nausea
	Preferred regimen: Famciclovir, 500 mg orally three times daily for 7–10 days	Nausea
	Acyclovir, 800 mg orally five times daily for 7–10 days. Intravenous therapy at 10 mg/kg every 8 hours for extensive cutaneous or visceral disease until clinical improvement, then switch to oral therapy to complete a 10- to 14-day course. For ocular involvement, consult an ophthalmologist immediately.	Nausea
Kaposi sarcoma		
Mild to moderate	Initiation or optimization of antiretroviral treatment	Side effects of antiretroviral treatment
Advanced disease	Chemotherapy (eg, liposomal doxorubicin or daunorubicin)	Bone marrow suppression, cardiac toxicity
	Pomalidomide, 5 mg/day orally on days 1–21 of every 28-day cycle; alternative to chemotherapy	Fatigue, asthenia, dyspnea, anemia, neutropenia; contraindicated in pregnancy
Mycobacterium avium complex infection	Clarithromycin, 500 mg orally twice daily, or azithromycin, 600 mg once daily with ethambutol, 15 mg/kg/day orally (maximum, 1 g). May also add:	Clarithromycin: hepatitis, nausea, diarrhea Ethambutol: hepatitis, optic neuritis
	Rifabutin, 300 mg orally daily	Rash, hepatitis, uveitis
Non-Hodgkin lymphoma	Combination chemotherapy (eg, R-CHOP and G-CSF). CNS disease: Radiation treatment with dexamethasone for edema	Nausea, vomiting, anemia, neutropenia, thrombocytopenia, cardiac toxicity (with doxorubicin)
Pneumocystis jirovecii infection[3]	Preferred regimen: Trimethoprim-sulfamethoxazole, 15 mg/kg/day (based on trimethoprim component) intravenously or one double-strength tablet orally three times a day for 21 days. Add prednisone when PaO_2 < 70 mm Hg on room air or alveolar-arterial O_2 gradient > 35 mm Hg: 40 mg orally twice a day on days 1–5, 40 mg orally daily on days 6–10, 20 mg orally daily on days 11–21	Nausea, neutropenia, anemia, hepatitis, rash, Stevens-Johnson syndrome
	Pentamidine, 3–4 mg/kg/day intravenously for 21 days plus prednisone when indicated as above	Hypotension, hypoglycemia, anemia, neutropenia, pancreatitis, hepatitis
	Primaquine, 30 mg/day orally, and clindamycin, 600 mg every 8 hours orally, for 21 days plus prednisone when indicated as above	Primaquine: hemolytic anemia in patients with G6PD deficiency,[3] methemoglobinemia, neutropenia, colitis Clindamycin: rash, nausea, abdominal pain, colitis
	Not recommended for severe disease: Trimethoprim, 15 mg/kg/day orally in three divided doses, with dapsone, 100 mg/day orally, for 21 days,[3] plus prednisone when indicated as above	Nausea, rash, hemolytic anemia in patients with G6PD deficiency[3]; methemoglobinemia (weekly levels should be < 10% of total hemoglobin)
	Not recommended for severe disease: Atovaquone, 750 mg orally twice daily with food for 21 days, plus prednisone when indicated as above	Rash, elevated aminotransferases, anemia, neutropenia
Toxoplasmosis	Preferred regimen: Pyrimethamine, 200 mg orally as loading dose, followed by 50 mg daily (weight ≤ 60 kg) or 75 mg daily (weight > 60 kg), combined with sulfadiazine, 1000 mg orally four times daily (weight ≤ 60 kg) or 1500 mg orally four times daily (weight > 60 kg), and leucovorin, 10–25 mg orally daily, for at least 6 weeks. Longer courses are necessary for extensive disease or incomplete clinical or radiographic resolution. Maintenance therapy with pyrimethamine, 25–50 mg orally, plus sulfadiazine, 2000–4000 mg in two to four divided doses, plus leucovorin, 10–25 mg orally daily. Long-term treatment should be maintained until immune reconstitution with antiretroviral treatment occurs.	Pyrimethamine: leukopenia, anorexia, vomiting Sulfadiazine: nausea, vomiting, Stevens-Johnson syndrome

(continued)

Table 35–3. Treatment of AIDS-related opportunistic infections and malignancies[1] (listed in alphabetical order). (continued)

Infection or Malignancy	Treatment	Complications[2]
	For patients who are intolerant of sulfa who cannot be desensitized: Substitute clindamycin, 600 mg intravenously or orally every 6 hours, for the sulfadiazine in the above regimen	Clindamycin: rash, nausea, abdominal pain, colitis
	If pyrimethamine not available: Trimethoprim-sulfamethoxazole, 10 mg/kg/day (based on trimethoprim component)	Nausea, neutropenia, anemia, hepatitis, rash, Stevens-Johnson syndrome

[1]Recommendations drawn from Centers for Disease Control and Prevention. Guidelines for the prevention and treatment of opportunistic infections in HIV-infected adults and adolescents. February 11, 2020. Downloaded from https://aidsinfo.nih.gov/guidelines on February 14, 2020.
[2]List of complications is not exhaustive.
[3]Prior to use of primaquine or dapsone, check glucose-6-phosphate dehydrogenase (G6PD) level in Black patients and those of Mediterranean origin.
G-CSF, granulocyte colony-stimulating factor (filgrastim); R-CHOP, rituximab, cyclophosphamide, doxorubicin, vincristine, prednisolone.

daily for days 6–10, and 20 mg daily for days 11–21 (for patients who cannot take oral medication, intravenous methylprednisolone can be substituted at 75% of the oral dose). The mechanism of action for the steroids to improve outcomes is presumed to be a decrease in alveolar inflammation.

US Department of Health and Human Services. Guidelines for the prevention and treatment of opportunistic infections in adults and adolescents with HIV. Accessed August 30, 2014. https://clinicalinfo.hiv.gov/en/guidelines/adult-and-adolescent-opportunistic-infection/whats-new-guidelines

2. Other infectious pulmonary diseases—Other infectious causes of pulmonary disease in patients with AIDS include bacterial, mycobacterial, and viral etiologies.

A. BACTERIAL—*Community-acquired pneumonia is the most common cause of pulmonary disease in people with HIV*. The incidence of pneumococcal pneumonia with septicemia and *Haemophilus influenzae* pneumonia is higher among people with HIV. *Pseudomonas aeruginosa* is an important respiratory pathogen in advanced disease and, more rarely, pneumonia from *Nocardia* species or *Rhodococcus equi* infection can occur sometimes along with concomitant brain abscesses in advanced AIDS. Since B-cell dysfunction is more common early on in HIV infection, recurrent bacterial infections can be one clue of a new diagnosis.

B. MYCOBACTERIAL—Tuberculosis occurs in an estimated 4.2% of persons in the United States who have HIV. Patients with active tuberculosis and CD4 counts above 350 cells/mcL are likely to present with upper lobe and hilar infiltrates and paratracheal adenopathy, findings similar to persons without HIV (Figure 35–3). With advanced immunodeficiency, lower lobe, middle lobe, interstitial, and miliary infiltrates are more common, along with mediastinal adenopathy and extrapulmonary involvement. Although a *purified protein derivative (PPD)* test or an *interferon* γ *release assay* (IGRA)—including the QuantiFERON and T-SPOT tests—should be performed on all people with HIV in whom a diagnosis of tuberculosis is being considered, the lower the CD4 cell count, the greater the likelihood of falsely negative PPD or IGRA test results or of indeterminate IGRA test results. It is recommended to repeat PPD or IGRA testing following improvement in the CD4 count for those with CD4 count < 200 cells/mcL.

In cases of active tuberculosis, treatment of people with HIV is similar to that of people without HIV. However, *rifampin should* not *be given to patients receiving a boosted protease inhibitor (PI) regimen*. In these cases, rifabutin may be substituted, but it may require dosing modifications

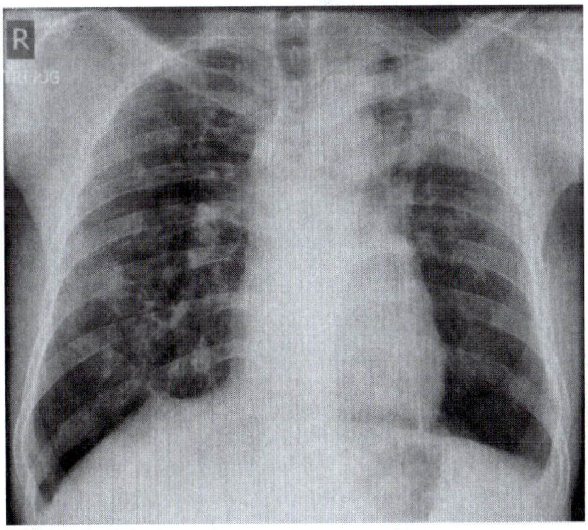

▲ **Figure 35–3.** A 36-year-old man (he/him) with **pulmonary tuberculosis.** There is an opacification of a portion of the left upper lung in association with a cavity, findings consistent with pulmonary tuberculosis. Also, there is an infiltrate in the right lung. The extent of his disease raises the specter that he has underlying HIV/AIDS. (Reproduced, with permission, from Richard P. Usatine, MD, in Usatine RP, Smith MA, Mayeaux EJ Jr, Chumley H. *The Color Atlas of Family Medicine*, 3rd ed. McGraw-Hill, 2019.)

depending on the antiretroviral regimen. Tenofovir alafenamide should not be used with rifampin at its usual dose; tenofovir disoproxil fumarate (TDF) should be used instead. Dolutegravir may be given with rifampin but should be dose adjusted to twice daily. **Multidrug-resistant tuberculosis (MDR)** has been a major problem in several metropolitan areas of the developed world, and cases of **extremely resistant tuberculosis** in patients with HIV are an important global concern. Nonadherence with prescribed antituberculous medications is a major risk factor. Several of the reported outbreaks appear to implicate nosocomial spread. *The emergence of medication resistance makes it essential that antibiotic sensitivities be performed on all positive cultures.* Medication therapy should be individualized. Patients with MDR *M tuberculosis* infection should receive at least three medications to which their organism is sensitive. The rise of MDR TB and extensively resistant TB in Eastern Europe and Russia has prompted increasing use of bedaquiline/pretomanid/linezolid–based regimens.

Atypical mycobacteria can cause pulmonary disease in patients with AIDS with or without preexisting lung disease and responds variably to treatment. Distinguishing between *M tuberculosis* and atypical mycobacteria is typically accomplished using *M tuberculosis* nucleic acid amplification (NAA) if available, which can also identify rifampin resistance rapidly, or via culture. DNA probes allow for presumptive identification usually within days of a positive culture. Definitive species identification for nontuberculous mycobacteria typically requires culture of sputum specimens. While awaiting definitive diagnosis, if clinical suspicion is high, clinicians should err on the side of treating patients as if they have *M tuberculosis* infection. Clinicians may wait for definitive diagnosis if the person is smear-negative for acid-fast bacilli, *M tuberculosis* NAA negative, clinically stable, and not living in a communal setting. It is important to note that isolated *M avium complex* pneumonia is relatively uncommon in AIDS, so diagnostic work-up for unexplained pneumonia should continue if preexisting structural lung disease is not present.

Centers for Disease Control and Prevention (CDC). Provisional CDC guidance for the use of pretomanid as part of a regimen [bedaquiline, pretomanid, and linezolid (BPaL)] to treat drug-resistant tuberculosis disease. Accessed March 15, 2026. https://archive.cdc.gov/#/details?url=https://www.cdc.gov/tb/hcp/treatment/bpal.html

C. Viral (SARS-CoV-2 and Other)—COVID-19, the illness caused by SARS-CoV-2, causes a very wide spectrum of illness, ranging from no symptoms to a mild upper respiratory tract illness with fever and cough, to a clinical triad of fever, cough, and dyspnea, to pneumonia, to acute respiratory distress syndrome (ARDS), and even to fulminant multisystem organ failure and death. CXRs and CT scans may be normal early in the disease course, then may show nonspecific diffuse ground glass opacities, multilobar infiltrates, and consolidations, some progressing to full-blown ARDS (see Chapter 36).

People with HIV prior to COVID-19 vaccines have a greater propensity for severe COVID-19 disease, in part related to higher rates of medical comorbidities (eg, CVD, lung disease, long-term smoking), although low CD4 counts and virologic nonsuppression also portend higher risk. *People with HIV should be considered a priority group for preventive strategies,* including boosting the initial vaccination series, and early treatment approaches with antivirals.

People with HIV should not alter their ART regimens or add medications for the purpose of possibly preventing or treating SARS-CoV-2 infection. With ongoing vaccination and natural infection, population immunity has risen in all groups, including people living with HIV. When COVID-19 is diagnosed in a person with HIV, ART should be continued, even if Paxlovid is initiated, since the course of the latter is only 5 days, despite the potential for drug-drug interactions.

Isolation of cytomegalovirus (CMV) from bronchoalveolar lavage fluid occurs commonly in patients with AIDS but does not establish a definitive diagnosis, with CMV pneumonitis remaining a very rare opportunistic infection among people with AIDS. Diagnosis of CMV pneumonitis typically requires biopsy; response to treatment is poor. Histoplasmosis, coccidioidomycosis, and cryptococcal disease as well as more common respiratory viral infections should also be considered in the differential diagnosis of unexplained pulmonary infiltrates.

US Department of Health and Human Services. Guidance for COVID-19 and persons with HIV. Accessed March 15, 2026. https://clinicalinfo.hiv.gov/sites/default/files/guidelines/archive/guidelines-covid-19-hiv-2022-02-22.pdf

3. Noninfectious pulmonary diseases—

A. Presentation—Noninfectious causes of lung disease in HIV infection include Kaposi sarcoma, non-Hodgkin lymphoma, interstitial pneumonitis, primary effusion lymphoma, and increasingly, in the current ART era, lung cancer. Some of these cancers (eg, lymphoma, Kaposi sarcoma) have an underlying viral etiology. In patients with known Kaposi sarcoma, pulmonary involvement complicates the course in approximately one-third of cases. However, pulmonary involvement is rarely the presenting manifestation of Kaposi sarcoma. Non-Hodgkin lymphoma may involve the lung as the sole site of disease, but more commonly involves other organs as well, especially the brain, liver, and GI tract. Both of these processes may show nodular or diffuse parenchymal involvement, pleural effusions, and mediastinal adenopathy on CXRs.

Nonspecific interstitial pneumonitis may mimic *Pneumocystis* pneumonia. Lymphocytic interstitial pneumonitis seen in lung biopsies has a variable clinical course. Typically, these patients present with several months of mild cough and dyspnea; CXRs show interstitial infiltrates. Performed rarely, transbronchial biopsies demonstrate interstitial inflammation ranging from an intense lymphocytic infiltration (consistent with lymphoid interstitial pneumonitis) to a mild mononuclear inflammation.

4. Sinusitis—Chronic sinusitis can be a frustrating problem for people with HIV. Symptoms include sinus congestion and discharge, headache, and fever. Some patients may have radiographic evidence of sinus disease on sinus CT scan in the absence of significant symptoms.

C. Central Nervous System Disease

CNS disease in people with HIV can be divided into intracerebral space-occupying lesions, encephalopathy, meningitis, and spinal cord processes. Many of these complications have declined markedly in prevalence in the era of effective ART. Cognitive declines, however, may be more common in persons with HIV, especially as they age (older than 50 years), even among those who remain virologically suppressed.

Stephens RJ et al. Central nervous system infections in the immunocompromised adult presenting to the emergency department. Emerg Med Clin North Am. 2021;39:101. [PMID: 33218652]

1. Toxoplasmosis—Toxoplasmosis used to be one of the most common CNS space-occupying lesion in people with HIV. Headache, focal neurologic deficits, seizures, or altered mental status may be presenting symptoms. The diagnosis is usually made presumptively based on the characteristic appearance of cerebral imaging studies in an individual known to be seropositive for *Toxoplasma*. Typically, *toxoplasmosis appears as multiple contrast-enhancing lesions on CT scan that do not reduce on diffusion on MRI scan.* Lesions tend to be peripheral, with a predilection for the basal ganglia.

Single lesions are atypical of toxoplasmosis. When a single lesion has been detected by CT scanning, MRI scanning may reveal multiple lesions because of its greater sensitivity. *If a patient has a single lesion on MRI and is neurologically stable, clinicians may pursue a 2-week empiric trial of toxoplasmosis therapy.* A repeat scan should be performed at 2 weeks. If the lesion has not diminished in size, biopsy of the lesion should be performed. A positive *Toxoplasma* serologic test does *not* confirm the diagnosis because many people with HIV have detectable titers without having active disease. Conversely, < 3% of patients with toxoplasmosis have negative titers. Therefore, negative *Toxoplasma* titers in a patient with HIV infection and a space-occupying lesion should be a cause for aggressively pursuing an alternative diagnosis. The preferred treatment of toxoplasmosis is with pyrimethamine and sulfadiazine (Table 35–3). If pyrimethamine is not available, patients can be treated with oral trimethoprim-sulfamethoxazole.

2. CNS lymphoma—Primary non-Hodgkin lymphoma is the second most common CNS space-occupying lesion in people with HIV. Symptoms are similar to those with toxoplasmosis. While imaging techniques cannot distinguish these two diseases with certainty, lymphoma more often is solitary. Other less common lesions should be suspected if there is preceding bacteremia, tuberculosis risk factors, fungemia, or injection drug use. These include bacterial abscesses, cryptococcomas, tuberculomas, and *Nocardia* lesions.

Stereotactic brain biopsy should be strongly considered if lesions are solitary or do not respond to toxoplasmosis treatment, especially if they are easily accessible. Diagnosis of lymphoma is important because many patients benefit from treatment (radiation therapy). A positive PCR assay of CSF for Epstein-Barr virus (EBV) DNA is consistent with a diagnosis of lymphoma; a *PCR for EBV DNA in CSF is 100% sensitive and 98.5% specific for AIDS-associated primary CNS lymphoma*, making it useful as a diagnostic tumor marker.

3. HIV-associated dementia and neurocognitive disorders—Patients with HIV-associated neurocognitive disorders, including dementia typically have difficulty with cognitive tasks (eg, memory, attention), exhibit diminished motor function, and have emotional or behavioral problems. Patients may first notice a deterioration in their handwriting. The manifestations of cognitive impairment or dementia may wax and wane, with persons exhibiting periods of lucidity and confusion over the course of a day. The diagnosis of HIV-associated dementia most commonly occurs in untreated patients with advanced HIV infection, and is one of exclusion based on a brain imaging study and on spinal fluid analysis that excludes other pathogens. Neuropsychiatric testing is helpful in distinguishing patients with dementia from those with depression. Many patients improve with ART. However, slowly progressive neurocognitive deficits may still develop in patients taking ART as they age.

Metabolic abnormalities may also cause changes in mental status: hypoglycemia, hyponatremia, hypoxia, and drug overdose are important considerations in this population. Other less common infectious causes of encephalopathy include progressive multifocal leukoencephalopathy (discussed below), CMV, syphilis, and herpes simplex encephalitis.

4. Cryptococcal meningitis—Cryptococcal meningitis typically presents with fever and headache. Less than 20% of patients have meningismus. Diagnosis is based on a positive latex agglutination test of serum or CSF that detects cryptococcal antigen (or "CrAg") or positive culture of spinal fluid for *Cryptococcus. Approximately 99% of patients with cryptococcal meningitis have a positive serum CrAg.* Thus, a negative serum CrAg test makes a diagnosis of cryptococcal meningitis unlikely and can be useful in the initial evaluation of a patient with headache, fever, and normal mental status. Treatment has three phases: induction, consolidation, and maintenance. Induction treatment is given for a minimum of 2 weeks plus evidence of clinical improvement and a negative CSF culture on repeat lumbar puncture. The preferred induction treatment is liposomal amphotericin with flucytosine (Table 35–3), followed by an oral fluconazole treatment, and then secondary prophylaxis. Prophylaxis can be stopped if the patient is asymptomatic, has a CD4 cell count of > 100/mcL for at least 3 months, and has suppressed viral load on ART. Of note, a 2022 study showed that an alternative induction regimen of just a single dose of liposomal amphotericin B with 14 days of flucytosine and concomitant fluconazole was noninferior to the longer course of amphotericin B; this can be considered an alternative approach in resource-limited settings or if liposomal amphotericin B is not tolerated.

5. Meningococcal meningitis—People with HIV infection are at increased risk for bacterial meningococcal disease. Treatment is the same as in people without infection. The Advisory Committee on Immunization Practices recommends the *meningococcal conjugate vaccine* routinely (serogroups A, C, W, and Y) for all persons aged 2 months or older with HIV infection. In settings of meningococcal outbreaks, the meningococcal B vaccine may be administered to adolescents and young adults with HIV, not necessarily all patients with HIV, for short-term protection against most strains of serogroup B meningococcal disease. Routine administration of meningococcal B vaccine to patients with HIV, however, is *not* indicated.

National Institutes of Health (NIH). HIVinfo. Guidelines for the Prevention and Treatment of Opportunistic Infections in Adults and Adolescents with HIV. Accessed August 31, 2024. https://clinicalinfo.hiv.gov/en/guidelines/hiv-clinical-guidelines-adult-and-adolescent-opportunistic-infections/immunizations

6. HIV meningitis and HIV myelopathy—HIV meningitis, characterized by lymphocytic pleocytosis of the spinal fluid with negative culture, is common early in HIV infection. Spinal cord function may also be impaired in individuals with HIV infection. HIV myelopathy presents with leg weakness and incontinence. Spastic paraparesis and sensory ataxia are seen on neurologic examination. Myelopathy is usually a late manifestation of HIV disease, and most patients will have concomitant HIV encephalopathy. Pathologic evaluation of the spinal cord reveals vacuolation of white matter. Because HIV myelopathy is a diagnosis of exclusion, symptoms suggestive of myelopathy should be evaluated by lumbar puncture to rule out CMV polyradiculopathy (described below) and an MRI or CT scan to exclude epidural lymphoma.

Leffert J et al. HIV-vacuolar myelopathy: an unusual early presentation in HIV. Int J STD AIDS. 2021;32:205. [PMID: 33323068]

7. Progressive multifocal leukoencephalopathy (PML)— PML is a viral infection (with the JC polyomavirus) of the white matter of the brain seen in patients with very advanced HIV infection. It typically results in focal neurologic deficits such as aphasia, hemiparesis, and cortical blindness. Imaging studies are strongly suggestive of the diagnosis if they show non-enhancing white matter lesions without mass effect; the diagnosis is verified by JC virus positivity via PCR in the CSF. Patients can stabilize or improve after ART initiation; there is no other treatment. In the setting of wide-scale ART and because PML occurs at very low CD4 counts, the prevalence of this condition is rare.

Cortese I et al. Progressive multifocal leukoencephalopathy and the spectrum of JC virus-related disease. Nat Rev Neurol. 2021;17:37. [PMID: 33219338]

D. Peripheral Nervous System

A. PRESENTATION—Peripheral nervous system syndromes include inflammatory polyneuropathies, sensory neuropathies, and mononeuropathies.

An **inflammatory demyelinating polyneuropathy** similar to Guillain-Barré syndrome can occur in people with HIV, usually prior to frank immunodeficiency. The syndrome in many cases improves with plasmapheresis, supporting an autoimmune basis of the disease. CMV can cause an ascending polyradiculopathy characterized by lower extremity weakness and a neutrophilic pleocytosis on spinal fluid analysis with a negative bacterial culture. Transverse myelitis can be seen with herpes zoster or CMV.

Peripheral neuropathy is common among people with HIV. Patients typically complain of numbness, tingling, and pain in the lower extremities. Symptoms are disproportionate to findings on gross sensory and motor evaluation. Beyond HIV infection itself, the most common cause is prior ART with a thymidine analog, such as stavudine or didanosine (although both are no longer available in the United States). Unfortunately, medication-induced neuropathy was not always reversed when the offending agent was discontinued. Patients with advanced disease may also develop peripheral neuropathy; in some cases, it occurs among those with suppressed viral loads. In many patients, the neuropathy improves after persistent virologic suppression is achieved. Evaluation should rule out other causes of sensory neuropathy such as alcohol use disorder, thyroid disease, diabetes, vitamin B_{12} deficiency, and syphilis.

B. MANAGEMENT—Treatment of peripheral neuropathy is aimed at symptomatic relief; those not taking ART consistently should be encouraged to improve their ART adherence and achieve virologic suppression. Those with comorbid diabetes should be encouraged to improve diabetes control. Patients may be treated initially with gabapentin (start at 300 mg at bedtime and increase to 300–900 mg orally three times a day) or other co-analgesics for neuropathic pain (see Chapter 5). Opioid analgesics should be avoided because the condition tends to be chronic and patients are likely to become dependent on these agents without significant improvement in their functional status.

Julian T et al. Human immunodeficiency virus-related peripheral neuropathy: a systematic review and meta-analysis. Eur J Neurol. 2021;28:1420. [PMID: 33226721]

E. Rheumatologic and Bone Manifestations

Arthritis, involving single or multiple joints, with or without effusion, has been commonly noted in people with HIV. Involvement of large joints is most common. Although the cause of HIV-related arthritis is unknown, most patients will respond to NSAIDs. Patients with a sizable effusion, especially if the joint is warm or erythematous, should have the joint aspirated, followed by culture of the fluid to rule out suppurative arthritis as well as fungal and mycobacterial disease.

Several rheumatologic syndromes, including reactive arthritis, psoriatic arthritis, sicca syndrome, and SLE, are reported in people with HIV (see Chapter 23). However, it is unclear if the prevalence is greater than in the general population. Cases of avascular necrosis of the femoral heads have been reported sporadically, generally in the setting of advanced disease with long-standing infection and in patients receiving long-term ART. The etiology is not clear but is probably multifactorial in nature.

Osteoporosis and osteopenia appear to be more common in people with HIV with chronic infection and is associated with long-term use of TDF and PI-based ART. Vitamin D deficiency appears to be quite common among people with HIV and monitoring vitamin D levels and instituting replacement therapy for detected deficiency are recommended. Bone mineral density scans for postmenopausal women with HIV and men 50 years old or older are also recommended.

F. Myopathy

Myopathies are infrequent in the era of effective ART but can be related to either HIV infection or ART, particularly with use of the older agent zidovudine (azidothymidine [AZT]). Proximal muscle weakness is typical, and patients may have varying degrees of muscle tenderness. Given its long-term toxicities, zidovudine is no longer recommended when alternative treatments are available. Integrase strand transferase inhibitors rarely have been associated with creatine phosphokinase elevations and myopathy.

G. Retinitis

In people with HIV, complaints of visual changes must be evaluated immediately by an ophthalmologist familiar with the manifestations of HIV disease. CMV retinitis, characterized by perivascular hemorrhages and white fluffy exudates, is the most common retinal infection in patients with AIDS, usually with CD4 counts < 50 cells/mcL, and can be rapidly progressive (Figure 35–4). In contrast, cotton wool spots, which also are common in people with HIV, are benign, remit spontaneously, and appear as small indistinct white spots without exudation or hemorrhage. Ocular syphilis also should be considered, with the incidence of syphilis rising over time among people with HIV. Other rare retinal processes include other herpesvirus infections or toxoplasmosis. Choice of treatment for CMV retinitis (Table 35–3) depends on severity and location of lesions, as well as the patient's overall condition and circumstances.

Ballard B et al. CMV retinitis. EyeWiki. Accessed August 31, 2024. https://eyewiki.org/CMV_Retinitis

H. Oral Lesions

A. Presentation—Oral candidiasis can be bothersome to patients, many of whom experience an unpleasant taste or mouth dryness. The two most common forms of oral candidiasis seen are *pseudomembranous* (removable white plaques) and *erythematous* (red friable plaques). Angular cheilitis—fissures at the sides of the mouth—is usually due to *Candida* as well.

Oral hairy leukoplakia is caused by the Epstein-Barr virus. The lesion is not usually troubling to patients and sometimes regresses spontaneously. Hairy leukoplakia is commonly seen as a white lesion on the lateral aspect of the tongue. It may be flat or slightly raised, is usually corrugated, and has vertical parallel lines with fine or thick ("hairy") projections (see Figure 8–6). Unlike oral candidiasis, this lesion cannot be scraped off, a distinguishing feature in the physical examination.

The presence of oral candidiasis or hairy leukoplakia is significant for several reasons. First, these lesions are highly suggestive of HIV infection in patients who have no other obvious cause of immunodeficiency. Second, several studies have indicated that patients with candidiasis have a high rate of progression to AIDS even with statistical adjustment for CD4 count.

Gingival disease is common in people with HIV and is thought to be due to an overgrowth of microorganisms. Aphthous ulcers are painful and may interfere with eating.

Other lesions seen in the mouths of people with HIV include Kaposi sarcoma (usually on the hard palate) and oral warts.

B. Management—Treatment of mild oral candidiasis is with topical agents such as clotrimazole 10-mg troches (one troche four or five times a day). Patients with moderate to severe disease or with candidiasis that does not respond to topical antifungals can be treated with fluconazole (100–200 mg orally once a day for 7–14 days). Angular cheilitis can be treated topically with ketoconazole cream (2%) twice a day.

Gingival disease usually responds to professional dental cleaning and chlorhexidine rinses. A particularly

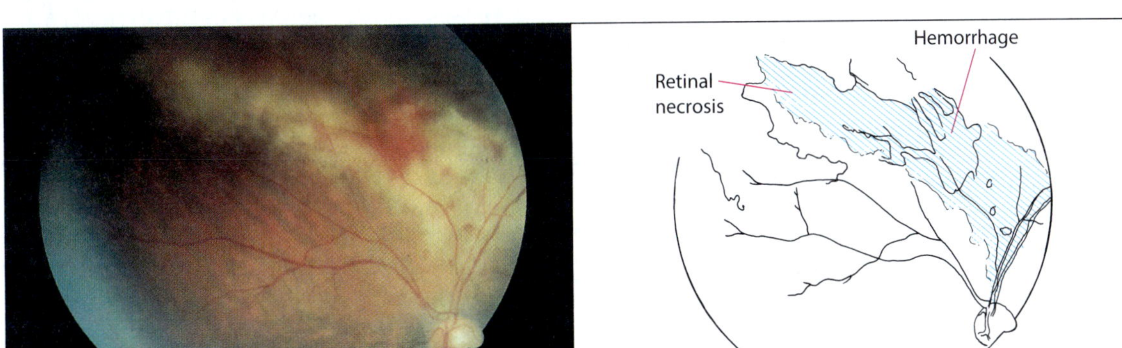

Figure 35–4. CMV retinitis. Retina has classic "pizza pie" or "cheese and ketchup" appearance, with hemorrhages and dirty white, granular appearing retinal necrosis adjacent to major vessels (see diagrammatic map). (Left: Photo contributed by Richard E. Wyszynski, MD. Right: Reproduced with permission from Knoop KJ, Stack LB, Storrow AB, Thurman RJ. *The Atlas of Emergency Medicine*, 5th ed. McGraw Hill, 2021.)

aggressive gingivitis or periodontitis will develop in some people with HIV; these patients should be given antibiotics that cover anaerobic oral flora (eg, metronidazole, 250 mg four times a day for 4 or 5 days) and referred to oral surgeons with experience with these entities.

Aphthous ulcers can be treated with fluocinonide (0.05% ointment mixed 1:1 with plain Orabase and applied six times a day to the ulcer). For lesions that are difficult to reach, patients should use dexamethasone swishes (0.5 mg in 5 mL elixir three times a day). The pain of the ulcers can be relieved with an anesthetic spray (10% lidocaine).

I. Gastrointestinal Manifestations

1. Candidal and other esophagitis—(See also Chapter 17.) Esophageal candidiasis is a common AIDS complication. In a patient with characteristic symptoms, empiric antifungal treatment is begun with fluconazole (200–400 mg orally daily for 14–21 days). Improvement in symptoms should be apparent within 1–2 days of antifungal treatment. If there is no improvement, fungal culture to exclude fluconazole resistance, and further evaluation to identify other causes of esophagitis (herpes simplex, CMV) is recommended.

2. Hepatic disease—

A. PRESENTATION—Autopsy studies have demonstrated that the liver is a frequent site of infections and neoplasms in people with HIV. However, many of these infections are not clinically symptomatic. Mild elevations of alkaline phosphatase and aminotransferases are often noted on routine chemistry panels. Mycobacterial disease, CMV, hepatitis B virus, hepatitis C virus, and lymphoma cause liver disease and can present with varying degrees of nausea, vomiting, right upper quadrant abdominal pain, and jaundice. Sulfonamides, imidazole medications, antituberculous medications, pentamidine, and clarithromycin have also been associated with hepatitis. *The thymidine analog medications in the nucleoside reverse transcriptase inhibitor (NRTI) class (ie, zidovudine) can cause lactic acidosis and hepatic steatosis, which can be fatal.* However, these medications, especially didanosine and stavudine, are rarely used in ART regimens any longer and are not available in the United States. Finally, people with HIV with chronic hepatitis may have more rapid progression of liver disease because of the concomitant immunodeficiency or hepatotoxicity of ART. Percutaneous liver biopsy may be helpful in diagnosing liver disease, but some common causes of liver disease (eg, *M avium* complex, lymphoma) can be determined by less invasive measures (eg, blood culture, biopsy of a more accessible site).

B. MANAGEMENT—With patients living longer as a result of advances in ART, advanced liver disease and hepatic failure due to chronic active hepatitis B or hepatitis C, or both, are increasing causes of morbidity and mortality. *People with HIV who also have hepatitis B infection should be treated with antiretroviral regimens that include two medications with activity against both viruses (TDF or tenofovir alafenamide [TAF], and lamivudine or emtricitabine).* It is important to be extremely cautious about discontinuing these medications in coinfected patients as sudden discontinuation could lead to a fatal flare of hepatitis B infection. Hepatitis D co-infection is underdiagnosed in patients with hepatitis B but may require greater screening in the future since a new antiviral (bulevirtide) has been approved for its treatment in Europe. Nonalcoholic fatty liver disease is a growing concern among people with HIV, particularly given concerns for weight gain and insulin resistance with integrase inhibitors and tenofovir alafenamide. Treatment involves lifestyle modification, avoidance of alcohol, and optimization of diabetes control. If nonalcoholic steatohepatitis (NASH) with fibrosis is identified on biopsy, vitamin E therapy can be considered.

Hepatitis C is more virulent in patients with HIV and should be treated using HCV direct-acting antivirals (DAAs) (see Table 18–6). Prior to treatment, the patient's HCV viral load and HCV genotype should be determined. Pan-genotypic regimens such as glecaprevir/pibrentasvir are increasingly used. Because new DAAs are available and because HCV treatment is a rapidly changing field, clinicians should check the guidelines of the American Association for the Study of Liver Disease (ASLD)/Infectious Diseases Society of America (IDSA) (https://www.hcvguidelines.org/) to see the latest recommended regimens (see also Tables 18–6 and 18–7).

Although the recommended regimens are the same for people with HIV, potential drug interactions with ART may complicate treatment. Clinicians should check the guidelines of the AASLD/IDSA and US Department of Health and Human Services or the guidelines of the University of Liverpool to determine interactions between proposed hepatitis C regimen and HIV regimen. Ritonavir-containing protease inhibitor regimens for HIV are the most likely to cause drug–drug interactions.

Liver transplants have been performed successfully in people with HIV. This strategy is most likely to be successful in persons who have CD4 counts > 100 cells/mcL and nondetectable viral loads.

Buti M. Hepatitis D virus: more attention needed. Nat Rev Gastroenterol Hepatol. 2022;19:556. [PMID: 35883011]

Lake JE et al. Expert panel review on nonalcoholic fatty liver disease in persons with human immunodeficiency virus. Clin Gastroenterol Hepatol. 2022;20:256. [PMID: 33069882]

University of Liverpool. HEP drug interactions. Accessed August 31, 2024. https://www.hep-druginteractions.org

3. Biliary disease—Cholecystitis presents with manifestations similar to those seen in immunocompetent hosts but is more likely to be acalculous. Sclerosing cholangitis and papillary stenosis have also been reported in people with HIV. Typically, the syndrome presents with severe nausea, vomiting, and right upper quadrant pain. Liver enzymes generally show alkaline phosphatase elevations disproportionate to elevation of the aminotransferases. Although dilated ducts can be seen on ultrasound, the diagnosis is made by endoscopic retrograde cholangiopancreatography, which reveals intraluminal irregularities of the proximal intrahepatic ducts with "pruning" of the terminal ductal branches. Stenosis of the distal common bile duct at the papilla is commonly seen. CMV, *Cryptosporidium*, and microsporidia are thought to play inciting roles in this syndrome, but these conditions are rarely seen unless the patient is experiencing very advanced HIV-related immunodeficiency.

4. Enterocolitis—

A. PRESENTATION—Enterocolitis is a common problem in people with HIV. Organisms known to cause enterocolitis include bacteria (*Campylobacter*, *Salmonella*, *Shigella*), viruses (CMV, adenovirus, SARS-CoV-2), and protozoans (*Cryptosporidium*, *Entamoeba histolytica*, *Giardia*, *Isospora*, microsporidia, *Cyclospora*). HIV itself may cause enterocolitis. Several of the organisms causing enterocolitis in people with HIV also cause diarrhea in immunocompetent persons. However, people with HIV tend to have more severe and more chronic symptoms, including high fevers and severe abdominal pain that can mimic acute abdominal catastrophes. Bacteremia and concomitant biliary involvement are also more common with enterocolitis in people with HIV. Relapses of enterocolitis following adequate therapy have been reported with both *Salmonella* and *Shigella* infections.

Because of the wide range of agents known to cause enterocolitis, a stool culture and multiple stool examinations for ova and parasites (including modified acid-fast staining for *Cryptosporidium* and *Giardia* antigen testing) should be performed. Patients who have *Cryptosporidium* in one stool with improvement in symptoms in < 1 month should *not* be considered to have AIDS, as *Cryptosporidium* is a cause of self-limited diarrhea in HIV-negative persons. More commonly, people with HIV with subsequent immunodeficiency with *Cryptosporidium* infection have persistent enterocolitis with profuse watery diarrhea.

B. MANAGEMENT—For individuals who do not improve with ART initiation, nitazoxanide (500–1000 mg twice daily) has been FDA-approved for the treatment of cryptosporidiosis, and paromomycin has been used occasionally in refractory cases based on data from small randomized studies. The diarrhea can be treated symptomatically with loperamide or diphenoxylate with atropine (one or two tablets orally three or four times a day). Durable remission usually requires immune reconstitution with ART.

Patients with a negative stool examination and persistent symptoms should be evaluated with colonoscopy and biopsy. Patients whose symptoms last longer than 1 month with no identified cause of diarrhea are considered to have a presumptive diagnosis of HIV enteropathy. Patients may respond to ART initiation, antimotility agents, or crofelemer (an antidiarrheal agent).

5. Other disorders—Two other important GI abnormalities in people with advanced AIDS are gastropathy and malabsorption. It has been documented that some people with HIV do not produce normal levels of stomach acid and therefore are unable to absorb medications that require an acid medium. This decreased acid production may explain, in part, the susceptibility of people with HIV to *Campylobacter*, *Salmonella*, and *Shigella*, all of which are sensitive to acid concentration. There is no evidence that *Helicobacter pylori* is more common in people with HIV.

A malabsorption syndrome occurs commonly in patients with AIDS. It can be due to infection of the small bowel with *M avium* complex, *Cryptosporidium*, or microsporidia.

J. Endocrinologic Manifestations

Hypogonadism is probably the most common endocrinologic abnormality in men with HIV. The adrenal gland is also a commonly afflicted endocrine gland in patients with AIDS, either from HIV, TB, CMV, histoplasmosis or other mycobacterial organisms. Abnormalities demonstrated on autopsy include infection, especially with CMV and *M avium* complex (ie, those with severe immunocompromise), infiltration with Kaposi sarcoma, and injury from hemorrhage and presumed autoimmunity. The prevalence of clinically significant adrenal insufficiency is low. Patients with suggestive symptoms should undergo a cosyntropin stimulation test.

Although frank deficiency of cortisol is rare, an isolated defect in mineralocorticoid metabolism may lead to salt-wasting and hyperkalemia. Such patients should be treated with fludrocortisone (0.1–0.2 mg orally daily). Trimethoprim-sulfamethoxazole also may cause hyperkalemia through its effects on the distal nephron, so it should be used with caution.

Patients with AIDS appear to have abnormalities of thyroid function tests different from those of patients with other chronic diseases. Patients with AIDS have been shown to have high levels of triiodothyronine (T_3), thyroxine (T_4), and thyroid-binding globulin and low levels of reverse triiodothyronine (rT_3). The causes and clinical significance of these abnormalities are unknown and generally improve with ART initiation.

Pezzaioli LC et al. The importance of SHBG and calculated free testosterone for the diagnosis of symptomatic hypogonadism in HIV-infected men: a single-centre real-life experience. Infection. 2021;49:295. [PMID: 33289905]
Santi D et al. The prevalence of hypogonadism and the effectiveness of androgen administration on body composition in HIV-infected men: a meta-analysis. Cells. 2021;10:2067. [PMID: 34440836]

K. Skin Manifestations

The skin manifestations that commonly develop in people with HIV can be grouped into viral, bacterial, fungal, neoplastic, and nonspecific dermatitides.

1. Viral dermatitides—

A. HERPES SIMPLEX INFECTIONS—These infections (Figure 35–5) occur more frequently, tend to be more severe, and are more likely to disseminate in patients with AIDS than in immunocompetent persons. Because of the risk of progressive local disease, *all herpes simplex attacks should be treated for 5–10 days with valacyclovir (1000 mg orally twice daily), acyclovir (400 mg orally three times a day), or famciclovir (250 mg orally three times a day)* (Table 35–3). To avoid the complications of attacks, many clinicians recommend suppressive therapy for people with HIV with a history of recurrent herpes. Options for suppressive therapy include valacyclovir (1000 mg orally

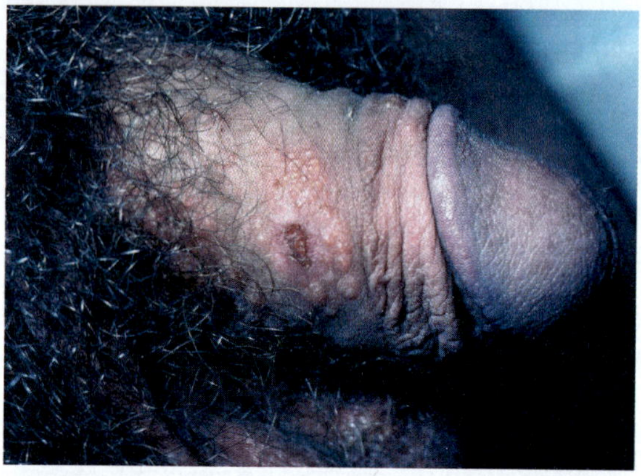

Figure 35–5. Herpes simplex viral skin infection, frequently found in men (he/him) with HIV. Shown are grouped vesicles typical of herpes simplex on the penis, with both intact vesicles of initial eruption and visible crusts of resolving lesions. (Reproduced, with permission, from Eric Kraus, MD, in: Usatine RP, Smith MA, Mayeaux EJ Jr, Chumley H. *The Color Atlas and Synopsis of Family Medicine*, 3rd ed. McGraw-Hill, 2019.)

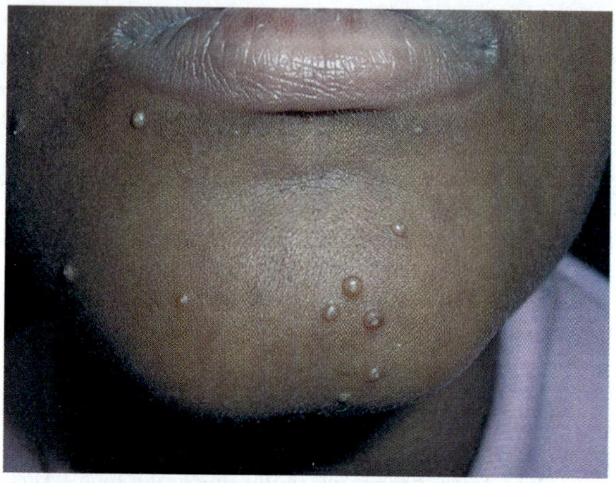

Figure 35–6. Molluscum contagiosum. Extensive molluscum contagiosum lesions on the face of a young person, suggestive of HIV. (Reproduced, with permission, from Richard P. Usatine, MD, in Usatine RP, Smith MA, Mayeaux EJ Jr, Chumley H. *The Color Atlas of Family Medicine*, 3rd ed. McGraw-Hill, 2019.)

daily), acyclovir (400 mg orally twice daily), or famciclovir (250 mg orally twice daily). Long-term suppressive herpes prophylaxis with acyclovir does not reduce HIV transmission between heterosexual men and women from low- and middle-income countries.

B. Varicella zoster—This is a common manifestation of HIV infection. Patients with varicella zoster infections should be treated for 7–10 days with valacyclovir (1000 mg three times a day) or famciclovir (500 mg orally three times a day). Acyclovir can also be used, but it requires more frequent dosing (800 mg orally five times per day for 7 days). Vesicular lesions should be cultured if there is any question about their origin, since herpes simplex requires much lower doses of acyclovir than does varicella zoster. Disseminated zoster and cases with ocular involvement should be treated with intravenous acyclovir (10 mg/kg every 8 hours for 7–10 days). *The recombinant zoster vaccine (Shingrix, two doses administered 2–6 months apart) should be given to people with HIV*, and there is no longer an age requirement in these patients. Because it is not a live virus like the previous zoster vaccine (Zostavax), it is not contraindicated in patients with immune deficiency—but, based on other vaccines, people with HIV are likely to develop more robust immune response to the vaccine when their CD4 count is > 200/mcL.

Harbecke R et al. Herpes zoster vaccines. J Infect Dis. 2021;224:S429. [PMID: 34590136]

C. Molluscum contagiosum—This infection is caused by a pox virus and is seen in people with HIV, as in other immunocompromised patients. The characteristic umbilicated fleshy papular lesions have a propensity for spreading widely over the patient's face and neck (Figure 35–6) and should be treated with topical liquid nitrogen.

D. Mpox (monkeypox)—Mpox (formerly called "monkeypox") is an orthopoxvirus in the same genus as the variola and vaccinia viruses (virus that causes smallpox and virus that is used in the smallpox vaccine, respectively). Cowpox is the fourth orthopoxvirus in the family, and borealpox has recently been added as the fifth member. Although originally isolated in a colony of laboratory monkeys, mpox can be isolated in a variety of rodents, with humans as incidental hosts. Prior to a global outbreak of clade II mpox in 2022, the majority of transmissions were thought to be from rodents to humans in mpox-endemic regions in Western and Central Africa. However, in May 2022, cases of mpox from non-endemic countries were reported, prompting the WHO to declare a global health emergency of international concern in July 2022. The vast majority of the cases (98–99%) were in men and mostly among MSM. With viable virus isolated from anal and urethral swabs and its particular distribution, mpox was reclassified by some organizations as an STI. As of 2024, > 100,000 mpox cases had been reported from 115 countries, although incidence started dropping worldwide in the early fall of 2022 due to a combination of natural infection in the population, mpox vaccination of affected populations, and behavioral change. On May 11, 2023, the global health emergency was declared over by the WHO as the clade II mpox outbreak worldwide was considered to be largely controlled, although cases were ongoing worldwide despite the vaccine being available in high-income countries. However, later in 2023, a clade I outbreak was detected in the Democratic Republic of the Congo, with cases identified throughout Central and East Africa. As the clade I outbreak spread, the WHO declared a new public health emergency of international concern on August 14, 2023. Sporadic travel-related cases of clade I mpox have been identified worldwide, including in the United States linked to travel to Central and/or East Africa.

In the clade II outbreak which began in 2022, a higher rate of mpox cases occurred among people with HIV (~ 40% of all cases), although it is unclear if this due to greater susceptibility to the virus, the disproportionate outbreak among MSM, proclivity toward orthopoxviruses with HIV infection, or other factors. Risk factors for greater severity of mpox disease in HIV include having a CD4+ T-cell count < 200 cells/mcL, although some studies suggest greater rash burden among people with HIV regardless of T-cell count. Patients may first develop fevers, chills, and myalgias, which are then followed by the characteristic rash, which begins as small macules that then evolve into papules, vesicles, and pseudo-pustules filled with cell debris rather than pus. The lesions eventually crust over and fall off approximately 7–14 days after the beginning of the rash. The rash is often painful and, in the most recent outbreak, frequently occurs in the anogenital or perioral areas. Proctitis occurring with the disease may or may not be associated with anorectal lesions. Ocular lesions may occur, and coalescence of lesions may lead to bacterial superinfection. Cases of encephalitis, sepsis, myocarditis, and bowel obstruction have been described, but are rare. Diagnosis is made by orthopoxvirus DNA PCR performed on swab of the lesions. Most patients will recover with supportive care, although tecovirimat therapy can be considered for individuals with or at risk for severe disease, including uncontrolled HIV, those with lesions in the eyes, confluent lesions, severe oral lesions limiting oral intake, or systemic life-threatening disease. In the PALM007 trial, tecovirimat was safe but not effective in reducing the duration of MPOX lesions in children and adults in the clade I outbreak in the Democratic Republic of the Congo. The NIH-sponsored STOMP trial demonstrated the same finding, that tecovirimat was safe but ineffective in reducing the duration or severity of mpox lesions in the United States. With these findings, there is now no effective antiviral for mpox and prevention relies on vaccination. A modified vaccinia vaccine (called Modified Vaccinia Ankara [MVA] or Jynneos) was the mainstay of prevention during the mpox global outbreak and is safe for people with HIV. Anyone with risk factors for mpox or who have had a recent exposure should be vaccinated. See also Chapter 36.

Allan-Blitz LT, Gandhi M et al. A position statement on Mpox as a sexually transmitted disease. Clin Infect Dis. 2023;76:1508. [PMID: 36546646]

Centers for Disease Control and Prevention (CDC). Interim clinical guidance for treatment of monkey pox. Updated 2022 Oct 31. https://www.cdc.gov/poxvirus/monkeypox/clinicians/treatment.html

Centers for Disease Control and Prevention (CDC). Severe manifestations of monkeypox among people who are immunocompromised due to HIV or other conditions. Accessed August 31, 2024. https://archive.cdc.gov/#/details?url=https://www.cdc.gov/han/2022/han00475.html

World Health Organization (WHO). Mpox outbreak 2022. Accessed August 31, 2024. https://www.who.int/emergencies/situations/monkeypox-oubreak-2022

World Health Organization (WHO). 2022 Mpox (monkeypox) outbreak: global trends. Accessed August 31, 2024. https://worldhealthorg.shinyapps.io/mpx_global/

2. Bacterial dermatitides—

A. STAPHYLOCOCCAL INFECTION—*Staphylococcus* is the most common bacterial cause of skin disease in people with HIV; it usually presents as folliculitis, superficial abscesses (furuncles), or bullous impetigo. These lesions should be treated aggressively since sepsis can occur. Folliculitis is initially treated with topical mupirocin or clindamycin, and patients may benefit from regular washing with benzoyl peroxide. Intranasal mupirocin, bleach baths, and cleaning intact skin with chlorhexidine soap have been used successfully for staphylococcal decolonization in other settings. In people with HIV with recurrent staphylococcal infections, weekly intranasal mupirocin should be considered in addition to topical care and systemic antibiotics. Abscesses often require incision and drainage. Patients may need antistaphylococcal antibiotics as well. Due to high frequency of methicillin-resistant *Staphylococcus aureus* (MRSA) skin infections in people with HIV, *coverage of MRSA in empiric regimens is necessary*. Recommendations for empiric treatment of serious infections are either (1) trimethoprim-sulfamethoxazole (one double-strength tablet orally twice daily); (2) doxycycline (100 mg orally twice daily); or (3) linezolid (600 mg orally twice daily) with close follow-up.

Hatlen TJ et al. Staphylococcal skin and soft tissue infections. Infect Dis Clin North Am. 2021;35:81. [PMID: 33303329]

B. BACILLARY ANGIOMATOSIS—It is caused by two closely related organisms: *Bartonella henselae* and *Bartonella quintana*. The epidemiology of these infections suggests zoonotic transmission from fleas of infected domestic cats (*henselae*) or contact with human body louse feces (*quintana*). The most common manifestation is raised, reddish, highly vascular skin lesions that can mimic lesions of Kaposi sarcoma. Fever is a common manifestation of this infection; involvement of bone, lymph nodes, liver (peliosis hepatis due to *B henselae*) and endocarditis have also been reported. The infection is treated with doxycycline, 100 mg orally twice daily and rifampin, 300 mg orally twice daily for a prolonged period depending on the seriousness of the infection. Patients who are seriously ill with visceral involvement or endocarditis may require at least 6 months of therapy.

Ding F et al. Clinical and echocardiographic characteristics of Bartonella infective endocarditis: an 8-year single-centre experience in the United States. Heart Lung Circ. 2022;31:350. [PMID: 34456130]

3. Fungal rashes—

A. RASHES DUE TO DERMATOPHYTES AND *CANDIDA*—Most fungal rashes afflicting patients with AIDS are due to dermatophytes and *Candida*. While particularly common in the inguinal region, they may occur anywhere on the body. Fungal rashes generally respond well to topical clotrimazole (1% cream twice a day) or ketoconazole (2% cream twice a day).

B. EOSINOPHILIC FOLLICULITIS—Eosinophilic folliculitis is a pruritic skin eruption with eosinophilic infiltration of hair follicles leading to papules or pustules, predominantly located on the scalp, face, neck, and torso. Eosinophilic folliculitis in advanced HIV is thought to be noninfectious although the pathophysiology is unknown. The mainstay of treatment is topical corticosteroids with ART and isotretinoin therapy in severe cases.

C. SEBORRHEIC DERMATITIS—This is more common in people with HIV. Scrapings of seborrhea have revealed *Malassezia furfur* (*Pityrosporum ovale*), implying that the seborrhea is caused by this fungus. A consistent finding is that seborrhea responds well to topical clotrimazole (1% cream) as well as hydrocortisone (1% cream).

4. Neoplastic dermatitides—See Chapter 6 and the Kaposi sarcoma section below.

5. Nonspecific dermatitides—

A. XEROSIS—This condition presents in people with HIV with severe pruritus. The patient may have no rash, or nonspecific excoriations from scratching. Treatment is with emollients (eg, absorption base cream) and antipruritic lotions (eg, camphor 9.5% and menthol 0.5%).

B. PSORIASIS—Psoriasis can be very severe in people with HIV. Phototherapy, topical retinoids, and etretinate (0.25–9.75 mg/kg/day orally in divided doses) may be used for recalcitrant cases in consultation with a dermatologist.

L. HIV-Related Malignancies

Four cancers are included in the CDC classification of AIDS: Kaposi sarcoma, non-Hodgkin lymphoma, primary lymphoma of the brain, and invasive cervical carcinoma. Epidemiologic studies have shown that between 1973 and 1987, among single men in San Francisco, the risk of Kaposi sarcoma increased more than 5000-fold and the risk of non-Hodgkin lymphoma more than 10-fold. In the current treatment era, cancers not classified as AIDS-related, such as lung cancer, are being increasingly diagnosed in aging people with HIV despite optimal ART. *Cohort studies suggest that adults with HIV are at increased risk for a variety of cancers compared with age-matched adults who do not have HIV.* Mortality secondary to malignancies represents an increasing cause of death in people with HIV.

Chiao EY et al. The effect of non-AIDS-defining cancers on people living with HIV. Lancet Oncol. 2021;22:e240. [PMID: 34087151]

Pumpalova YS et al. The impact of HIV on non-AIDS defining gastrointestinal malignancies: a review. Semin Oncol. 2021;48:226. [PMID: 34593219]

1. Kaposi sarcoma—

A. PRESENTATION—Kaposi sarcoma is caused by human herpesvirus-8 (HHV-8) and can occur at any CD4 count although the risk increases at lower CD4 cell counts. Lesions may appear anywhere; careful examination of the eyelids, conjunctiva, pinnae, palate, and toe webs is mandatory to locate potentially occult lesions. In light-skinned individuals, Kaposi lesions usually appear as purplish, nonblanching lesions that can be papular or nodular. In dark-skinned individuals, the lesions may appear browner. In the mouth, lesions are most often palatal papules, though exophytic lesions of the tongue and gingivae may also be seen. Kaposi lesions may be confused with other vascular lesions such as angiomas and pyogenic granulomas. Pulmonary Kaposi sarcoma can present with chronic cough, hemoptysis, or both and is associated with peribronchovascular nodules on CT scan. It can be diagnosed via bronchoscopy following visualization of the typical lesions. Gastrointestinal Kaposi sarcoma most often manifests as GI bleeding. Kaposi sarcoma lesions can occur shortly after initiating ART, especially in patients starting ART who have advanced immunodeficiency. In this situation, Kaposi sarcoma is likely to be an immune reconstitution reaction (see Inflammatory Reactions, below).

B. MANAGEMENT—Patients with mild to moderate forms of Kaposi sarcoma do not require specific treatment as the lesions usually resolve with effective ART. However, it should be noted that the lesions may flare when ART is first initiated—probably as a result of an immune reconstitution process. Advanced disease is treated with chemotherapy (Table 35–3).

Alves CGB et al. Clinical and laboratory profile of people living with HIV/AIDS with oral Kaposi sarcoma. AIDS Res Hum Retroviruses. 2021;37:870. [PMID: 34538064]

Gouveia-Moraes F et al. Conjunctival Kaposi's sarcoma. N Engl J Med. 2021;385:e36. [PMID: 34525288]

Ngalamika O et al. Antiretroviral therapy for HIV-associated cutaneous Kaposi's sarcoma: clinical, HIV-related, and sociodemographic predictors of outcome. AIDS Res Hum Retroviruses. 2021;37:368. [PMID: 33386064]

2. Non-Hodgkin lymphoma—

A. PRESENTATION—Non-Hodgkin lymphomas in HIV-infected persons tend to be very aggressive. These malignancies are usually of B-cell origin and characterized as diffuse large-cell tumors. Over 70% of the malignancies are extranodal.

B. MANAGEMENT—The prognosis of patients with systemic non-Hodgkin lymphoma depends primarily on the degree of immunodeficiency at the time of diagnosis. Patients with high CD4 counts do markedly better than those diagnosed with lower CD4 counts. Patients with primary CNS lymphoma typically are treated by oncology with high-dose methotrexate-based chemotherapy with or without rituximab.

3. Hodgkin disease—Although Hodgkin disease is not included as part of the CDC definition of AIDS, studies have found that HIV infection is associated with a fivefold increase in the incidence of Hodgkin disease. HIV-infected persons with Hodgkin disease are more likely to have mixed cellularity and lymphocyte depletion subtypes of Hodgkin disease and to seek medical attention at an advanced stage of disease.

4. Anal dysplasia and squamous cell carcinoma—These lesions are generally a result of HPV infection and noted in people of all genders with HIV. Although many report a history of anal warts or have visible warts, a significant percentage have silent papillomavirus infection. Cytologic (using Papanicolaou smears) and papillomavirus DNA studies can be performed on specimens obtained by anal swab. Because of the risk of progression from dysplasia to cancer in patients with HIV, *regular anal cytologic examinations or high-resolution anoscopy should be performed.* An *anal Papanicolaou smear* is performed by rotating a moistened Dacron swab about 2 cm into the anal canal. The swab is immediately inserted into a cytology bottle. Some experts also recommend high-risk HPV PCR testing be included. In the large ANCHOR study, which involved nearly 4500 individuals with anal high-grade squamous intraepithelial lesions (HGSIL), nine patients who were assigned to aggressive therapy (mostly office-based electrocautery) developed anal cancer compared with 21 of those in an active monitoring group (no treatment), representing a 57% decrease in relative risk of anal cancer over the median 25.8-month follow-up period. This pivotal study has changed care toward more aggressive screening for HGSIL and treatment to prevent progression to anal cancer among people with HIV.

HPV also plays a causative role in cervical dysplasia and carcinoma in women with HIV (discussed below).

Palefsky JM et al; ANCHOR Investigators Group. Treatment of anal high-grade squamous intraepithelial lesions to prevent anal cancer. N Engl J Med. 2022;386:2273. [PMID: 35704479]

M. Gynecologic Manifestations

Vaginal candidiasis, cervical dysplasia and neoplasia, and pelvic inflammatory disease are more common in women with HIV than in women without HIV. These manifestations also tend to be more severe when they occur in association with HIV infection. Therefore, *women with HIV need frequent gynecologic care.* Vaginal candidiasis may be treated with topical agents or a single dose of oral fluconazole (150 mg) (see Chapter 21). Recurrent vaginal candidiasis should be treated with fluconazole (100–200 mg) for at least 7 days. A single dose of fluconazole 150 mg to treat vaginal candidiasis is considered category C, although other uses are considered category D given the risk of rare birth defects.

Women with HIV have a sixfold increased risk of cervical cancer compared with women without HIV. Because of this finding, *recommended screening for women with HIV is more extensive than for women without HIV* (see Chapter 21). For women younger than age 30 years, a Papanicolaou smear should be performed within a year of the onset of sexual activity, but no later than age 21 years. If normal, Papanicolaou smears should be performed yearly. After three negative examinations, screening should be done every 3 years. HPV DNA testing of the cervical specimen is *not* recommended for women younger than age 30 years.

For women aged 30 years or older, screening should continue beyond age 65 years (unlike the general population). There are two accepted screening protocols: cytology alone and cytology with HPV DNA co-testing. A Papanicolaou smear is done when HIV is diagnosed and every 12 months thereafter, and after three negative smears, ongoing screening can be performed every 3 years. Alternatively, a Papanicolaou smear with co-testing for HPV DNA can be performed when HIV is diagnosed or starting when patients are 30 years old. If Papanicolaou smear is normal and HPV test is negative, then the next screening can be in 3 years.

The American Society of Colposcopy and Cervical Pathology recommends colposcopy for all results of HPV-positive ASC-US or higher, or LSIL or higher regardless of HPV status, among women with HIV. If HPV testing is not performed and the result is ASC-US, then cytology should be repeated in 6–12 months, with referral for colposcopy pursued if the repeat result is ASC-US or higher or if HPV positive. Treatment should follow the consensus guidelines in the references below.

While pelvic inflammatory disease appears to be more common in women with HIV, the bacteriology of this condition appears to be the same as among women without HIV. Women with HIV who have pelvic inflammatory disease should be treated with the same regimens as women without HIV (see Chapter 21).

Castle PE et al. Cervical cancer prevention and control in women living with human immunodeficiency virus. CA Cancer J Clin. 2021;71:505. [PMID: 34499351]
Strickler HD et al. Primary HPV and molecular cervical cancer screening in US women living with HIV. Clin Infect Dis. 2021;72:1529. [PMID: 32881999]

N. Coronary Artery Disease

People with HIV are at higher risk for CAD than age- and sex-matched controls. Part of this increase in CAD may be due to residual inflammation that can occur despite ART. Results from the practice-changing 2023 REPRIEVE study indicate that *statin treatment can benefit patients with HIV at low to moderate risk of cardiovascular disease, with the greatest benefit occurring among those with an ASCVD risk score of ≥ 5%.* Some data suggest abacavir may be associated with MI, possibly related to increased platelet aggregation, although this association has not been found in all studies. Some of the risk appears to be due to HIV infection, independent of its therapy. It is important that clinicians pay close attention to this issue because MIs tend to present at a younger age in individuals with HIV than in individuals without HIV. People with HIV with symptoms of CAD such as chest pain or dyspnea should be rapidly evaluated. Clinicians should aggressively treat conditions that result in increased risk of heart disease, especially smoking, hypertension, hyperlipidemia, obesity, diabetes mellitus, and sedentary lifestyle.

Grinspoon SK et al; REPRIEVE Investigators. Pitavastatin to prevent cardiovascular disease in HIV infection. N Engl J Med. 2023;389:687. [PMID: 37486775]
Patel AA et al. Coronary artery disease in patients with HIV infection: an update. Am J Cardiovasc Drugs. 2021;21:411. [PMID: 33184766]

O. Inflammatory Reactions (Immune Reconstitution Inflammatory Syndromes)

With initiation of ART, some patients experience inflammatory reactions that appear to be associated with immune reconstitution as indicated by a rapid increase in CD4 count.

These inflammatory reactions may present with generalized signs of fevers, sweats, and malaise with or without more localized manifestations that usually represent unusual presentations of opportunistic infections. For example, vitreitis has developed in patients with CMV retinitis after they have been treated with ART.

M avium can present as focal even suppurative lymphadenitis or granulomatous masses in patients receiving ART. Tuberculosis may paradoxically worsen with new or evolving pulmonary infiltrates and lymphadenopathy. PML and cryptococcal meningitis may also behave atypically. Clinicians should be alert to these syndromes, which are most often seen in patients who have initiated ART in the setting of advanced disease and who show rapid decreases in HIV viral load and increases in CD4 counts with treatment. The diagnosis of immune reconstitution inflammatory syndrome (IRIS) is one of exclusion and can be made only after recurrence or new opportunistic infection has been ruled out as the cause of the clinical deterioration. Management of IRIS is conservative and supportive with use of corticosteroids only for severe reactions, with ART continued.

Prevention

A. Primary Prevention

Prevention of HIV infection depends on HIV testing and counseling, including initiation of ART among people with HIV as a prevention tool for transmission to others, pre-exposure and postexposure use of antiretrovirals, precautions regarding sexual practices and injection drug use, perinatal management including antiretroviral treatment of the mother, screening of blood products, and infection control practices in the health care setting.

1. HIV testing and counseling—Primary care clinicians should routinely obtain a sexual history and provide risk factor assessment of their patients. *The USPSTF recommends that clinicians screen for HIV infection in adolescents and adults ages 15 to 65 years at least once in a lifetime.* Younger adolescents and older adults who are at increased risk should also be screened, with repeat screening as often as indicated for anyone at ongoing risk. Clinicians should review the risk factors for HIV infection with the patient and discuss HIV prevention strategies and safer needle use as well as the meaning of a positive test. Although the CDC recommends "opt-out" testing in medical settings, some states require specific written consent. For people whose test results are positive, it is critically important that they be connected to medical care. *Public health guidelines and HIV specialists advocate for initiating care and treatment the same day that someone tests positive, including patients in safety-net settings* (see Antiretroviral Therapy below). Referrals for partner-notification services, social services, mental health services, and HIV prevention services should also be provided.

For patients whose test results are negative, clinicians should review HIV prevention strategies, needle use practices, or both. Pre-exposure prophylaxis (PrEP) and post-exposure prophylaxis are highly effective HIV prevention strategies and are reviewed below. To prevent sexual transmission of HIV, only *latex or polyurethane condoms* should be used, along with a water-soluble lubricant. Although nonoxynol-9, a spermicide, kills HIV, it is *contraindicated* because in some patients it may cause genital ulcers that could facilitate HIV transmission. Patients should be counseled that condoms are not 100% effective, and may be ineffective among MSM if not used reliably with all partners. They should be made familiar with the use of condoms, including, specifically, the advice that condoms must be used every time, that space should be left at the tip of the condom as a receptacle for semen, that intercourse with a condom should not be attempted if the penis is only partially erect, that men should hold on to the base of the condom when withdrawing the penis to prevent slippage, and that condoms should not be reused. Several randomized trials in Africa demonstrated that *male circumcision* significantly reduced HIV incidence in men and, eventually, in female partners. This has led to circumcision rollout programs across the African continent.

Persons using injection drugs should be cautioned not to share needles or other drug paraphernalia. When sterile needles are not available, bleach does appear to inactivate HIV and can be used to clean needles. PrEP is an effective prevention option if clean needles are not readily available (see below).

2. ART for decreasing transmission of HIV to others (treatment as prevention)—Besides preventing progression of HIV disease, effective ART decreases the risk of HIV transmission between sexual partners. Among serodiscordant couples (MSM or heterosexual), stably suppressing HIV with ART to an HIV viral load < 200 copies/mL completely eliminated the risk of HIV transmission to the uninfected partner in three large cohort studies. Although HIV-negative persons in stable long-term partnerships with persons with HIV represent only one group of at-risk persons, increasing the use of ART among the population of people with HIV appears to decrease community-wide transmission of HIV. *Despite major improvements in effectiveness and tolerability of ART, only about two-thirds of people with HIV in the United States are virally suppressed. Persons in whom the HIV virus remains consistently suppressed (< 200 copies/mL) do not transmit HIV sexually.* The efficacy of treatment as prevention for transmission via injection drug use is less clear; people with HIV or at risk of HIV should be encouraged to avoid sharing injection equipment to prevent forward transmission.

3. Pre-exposure ART prophylaxis—Several large randomized double-blind placebo-controlled trials demonstrated that administering tenofovir disoproxil fumarate/emtricitabine (TDF/FTC) can reduce the risk of sexual transmission of HIV among uninfected individuals at high risk for infection. Pre-exposure tenofovir has also been shown to reduce HIV infection among people from Thailand who inject recreational drugs. In addition, real-world studies and demonstration projects of MSM and cisgender women, where adherence with emtricitabine/TDF has been adequate (average of at least four doses/week), have found **PrEP** to be highly effective in preventing HIV infection. Subsequent trials and open-label studies have also shown high efficacy with the use of *event-based dosing* (two tablets 2 to 24 hours prior to sex, and then one tablet 24 hours later, and a final tablet 24 hours after that) for TDF/FTC among MSM. And, finally, tenofovir alafenamide (TAF)/FTC was also shown to be noninferior to TDF/FTC among MSM and transgender women so is approved for non-vaginal sex. TAF/FTC is associated with lower bone and renal toxicity than TDF/FTC but increased weight gain and dyslipidemia. TAF/FTC is not approved for prevention with vaginal sex. Moreover, event-based PrEP dosing (ie, 2-1-1 dosing) is not approved for cisgender women. Cabotegravir, a long-acting medication for PrEP, was approved by the FDA in 2021 for use as PrEP as an injectable medication, every 8 weeks. This medication has been shown to be superior to oral TDF/FTC in preventing HIV infection among MSM, transgender women who have sex with men, and cisgender women. The most common adverse reaction to cabotegravir are injection site reactions, although these improve with subsequent injections and most patients do not discontinue therapy as a result of injection site reactions. Given the potential for delayed seroconversion to occur in individuals who develop an HIV breakthrough infection on injectable cabotegravir, HIV RNA testing is recommended at initiation. The use of HIV RNA testing at follow-up visits is being debated, due to the potential for false positives (the positive predictive value of a positive HIV RNA is only 18.5%) and the challenges that frequent RNA testing poses for implementation of injectable cabotegravir in many settings. An isolated positive HIV RNA result at cabotegravir PrEP follow-up, particularly if it is at the limit of detection (ie, < 20 but detected), should be repeated and the patient should be counseled that there is a higher probability of false positives than a true positive.

Approval of a new long-acting PrEP agent, biyearly subdermal lenacapavir (LEN), occurred in June 2025, given the positive results reported from the PURPOSE 1 study, which found 100% efficacy of lenacapavir among cisgender women (0 HIV infections with LEN compared with background HIV incidence of 2.4 per 100 person-years and 39 infections with emtricitabine/tenofovir alafenamide), and PURPOSE-2, finding 96% efficacy among cisgender gay, bisexual, and other men, transgender women, transgender men, and gender-nonbinary individuals compared with background HIV incidence.

CDC guidelines recommend that all sexually active adults and adolescents be informed about PrEP for prevention of HIV acquisition. Risk for HIV is a combination of the likelihood of having a partner who is living with HIV and the likelihood that the behavior (eg, type of intercourse, shared needles) puts them at risk of HIV transmission. MSM and transgender women are the groups with the highest HIV seroprevalence in the United States, and they are likely to have partners who may be living with HIV or of unknown HIV status. Those who have receptive anal intercourse have the highest risk of HIV because the behavior is more efficient at transmitting HIV than other sexual practices. People who use drugs are also at high risk for HIV infection if they do not consistently use clean needles or if they trade drugs for sex. It can be difficult to assess the risk of heterosexual people who are not at risk from drug use because it requires assessing the likelihood that their partners have HIV risks. However, it is important to assess risk as accurately as possible among cisgender women in order to offer PrEP when indicated. Factors known to increase the risk of HIV transmission and potential exposure to HIV are shown in Table 35–4. CDC guidelines also acknowledge that sexual histories taken by medical providers may be inaccurate, or patients may not feel comfortable reporting their sexual practices; hence, *any patient who requests PrEP should be offered PrEP.*

Finally, for PrEP to be effective, patients need to have adequate adherence, particularly around the time of exposure. Following results of the 2-1-1 event-based dosing protocol showing high efficacy among MSM, *taking a double dose on the first day 2–24 hours prior to sex is recommended to shorten the time to maximum protection.* This approach has not been studied among transgender women, heterosexuals, and people who inject drugs. Based on pharmacology modelling, it takes at least 7–10 days for PrEP to reach maximum efficacy for receptive vaginal sex. MSM and transgender women study participants who took at least four daily doses in a week were protected as well as those who took the drug every day, indicating that occasional missed doses do not render the treatment ineffective. PrEP demonstration projects conducted in cisgender women show similar findings. For patients preparing to stop PrEP, dosing should be continued for at least 2 days beyond the last exposure for MSM based on the 2-1-1 protocol. It is not clear how long other groups should continue PrEP following the last exposure, with some clinicians recommending 28 days based on postexposure prophylaxis studies, although this is likely conservative.

Recommendations on initial and follow-up assessments are shown in Table 35–4. TDF/FTC is contraindicated for persons with kidney disease (creatinine clearance < 60 mL/min) because of the small risk of kidney toxicity with TDF. Decreases in bone mineral density have been documented in persons taking TDF/FTC for PrEP at 24 weeks; whether this decrease will have clinical significance is unknown, and declines appear to reverse after stopping PrEP. For MSM who have creatinine clearance < 60 mL/min but > 30 mL/min, or osteoporosis/osteopenia (or at risk for these conditions), clinicians may opt to use TAF/FTC or injectable cabotegravir PrEP. Oral lead-in dosing of cabotegravir prior to injection should be considered optional, as breakthrough seroconversions occurred during the oral lead-in period in one of the cabotegravir studies, and injectable cabotegravir is well tolerated. When using injectable cabotegravir, the most sensitive HIV testing available should be used (ideally HIV RNA testing), given the potential for delayed seroconversion to occur with this therapy. The *cabotegravir tail* (detectable drug levels persistent after last medicine administration) should be covered after discontinuation while at ongoing risk of HIV with TDF/FTC or TAF/FTC, with quarterly HIV RNA testing performed for a year.

High rates of STIs have also been seen in persons taking PrEP, indicating the importance of regular follow-up in patients using PrEP. Regular asymptomatic STI screening and subsequent treatment among PrEP users (including rectal and pharyngeal testing for people exposed at those sites) can make substantial impact on the worsening non-HIV STI epidemic. Some patients are reluctant to use

Table 35–4. Recommendations for preexposure prophylaxis (PrEP) of HIV infection.

Patients for whom PrEP should definitely be considered as a good option for HIV prevention
Sexually active MSM, transgender persons who have sex with men, and heterosexuals and bisexual women who are likely to have partners with HIV risks
Injection drug users
Factors that increase the likelihood that PrEP is a good option
Patient has receptive anal intercourse
Patient has a partner with a known HIV infection without durable virologic suppression, or a partner of unknown HIV status
Patient has a history of STIs
Patient has a high number of sex partners
Patient is a commercial sex worker
Patient with inconsistent or no condom use
Patient who has been incarcerated or who has partners that have been incarcerated
Patient is from or whose partners are from an area where HIV incidence is high
Patient who is sharing needles or related paraphernalia ("works")
Initial assessment before prescribing PrEP
HIV antibody test to confirm HIV-negative (HIV RNA if using injectable cabotegravir)
Symptom review to exclude primary HIV infection (eg, no history of acute illness with fever and rash in prior month)
STI tests: syphilis; gonorrhea (at risk site-specific); and chlamydia (at risk site-specific)
Serum creatinine and eGFR[1]
Confirm immunity to HBV or vaccinate if nonimmune[2]
Pregnancy test
Discuss that PrEP does not protect against other STIs and review common side effects
Counsel patients that they can use latex or polyurethane condoms to prevent STIs and clean needles to prevent bacterial infections and hepatitis C, in addition to PrEP
Assess illicit substance use and offer treatment, if needed
Discuss importance of adherence to daily medication, every 8-week injections, or 2-1-1 PrEP around the time of exposures
PrEP prescription
Emtricitabine/TDF (Truvada) 1 tablet orally daily, 90-day prescription supply recommended. (Double dose is recommended on day 1 for MSM but would shorten the time to therapeutic drug levels in any patient)
Emtricitabine/TAF (Descovy) 1 tablet orally daily, 90-day prescription supply recommended (MSM and transgender women only)
Cabotegravir (Apretude) 600 mg injection given 1 month apart (loading) then every 2 months. Medication may be prescribed with oral cabotegravir 30 mg daily for 4 weeks as a lead-in or without (optional)
Follow-up assessment
HIV test every 3 months (every 8 weeks HIV RNA if using injectable cabotegravir)
Serum creatinine every 6–12 months (optional with cabotegravir)
Pregnancy test every 3 months
STI tests: syphilis, gonorrhea (at risk site-specific); and chlamydia (at risk site-specific)
Assess and support medication adherence
Reinforce benefits of using latex or polyurethane condoms and clean needles with PrEP
Assess substance use and offer treatment, if needed

[1]Emtricitabine/TDF is contraindicated if creatinine clearance < 60 mL/min.
[2]Persons with HBV infection may experience HBV reactivation and liver damage if emtricitabine/TDF is stopped.
HBV, hepatitis B virus; MSM, men who have sex with men; TAF, tenofovir alafenamide fumarate; TDF, tenofovir disoproxil fumarate.
PrEP checklists for providers and patients are available at https://www.cdc.gov/hiv/risk/prep/index.html (Last reviewed August 31, 2024).

insurance to cover the cost of the medication for fear of revealing that they are at risk for HIV; without insurance, the cost is high. Programs are available from the medication manufacturer to cover the cost of treatment for low-income uninsured persons and to cover insurance copays for insured patients. Studies demonstrating the efficacy of doxycycline postexposure prophylaxis among MSM and transgender women with and without HIV (single 200 mg dose after sex up to 72 hours) have shown it effective in preventing chlamydia and syphilis. The study among HIV-negative cisgender women did not show efficacy, although adherence was low in this study. However, one study presented at the 2024 AIDS conference did demonstrate a large reduction in chlamydia and syphilis infections after initiating doxycycline *pre*-exposure prophylaxis with daily doxycycline 100 mg in a pre/post study among 40 female sex workers in Japan. Finally, latex or polyurethane condoms will prevent other STIs and pregnancy.

Abe S et al. Doxycycline PrEP prevents STIs without affecting vaginal bacterial flora in female sex workers in Tokyo. JAC Antimicrob Resist. 2025;7:dlaf054. [PMID: 40390838]
Bekker LG et al. Twice-yearly lenacapavir or daily F/TAF for HIV prevention in cisgender women. N Engl J Med. 2024;391:1179. [PMID: 39046157]
Delany-Moretlwe S et al. Cabotegravir for the prevention of HIV-1 in women: results from HPTN 084, a phase 3, randomised clinical trial. Lancet. 2022;399:1779. [PMID: 35378077]
Kelley CF et al. Twice-yearly lenacapavir for HIV prevention in men and gender-diverse persons. N Engl J Med. 2025;392:1261. [PMID: 39602624]

Landovitz RJ et al; HPTN 083 Study Team. Cabotegravir for HIV prevention in cisgender men and transgender women. N Engl J Med. 2021;385:595. [PMID: 34379922]

Landovitz RJ et al. Site-based HIV testing assay performance for cabotegravir and TDF-FTC PrEP failure in HPTN 083. https://www.croiconference.org/abstract/site-based-hiv-testing-assay-performance-for-cabotegravir-and-tdf-ftc-prep-failure-in-hptn-083/

Luetkemeyer AF et al; DoxyPEP Study Team. Postexposure doxycycline to prevent bacterial sexually transmitted infections. N Engl J Med. 2023;388:1296. [PMID: 37018493]

4. Postexposure prophylaxis for sexual and drug use exposures to HIV—The goal of *postexposure prophylaxis* is to reduce or prevent local viral replication prior to dissemination such that the infection can be aborted. Although there is no prior clinical trial showing that administration of antiretroviral medications following a sexual or parenteral drug use exposure reduces the likelihood of infection, there is suggestive data from animal models, perinatal experience, and a case-control study of health care workers who experienced a needle stick.

Treatment of persons who have been exposed to HIV should be within 72 hours, but sooner is better. All exposed persons should first receive HIV testing to exclude the possibility that they already have infection. If rapid tests are not available, treatment should begin pending the results of a standard HIV test.

The choice of antiretroviral agents and the duration of treatment are the same as those for exposures that occur through the occupational route; the preferred regimen is tenofovir 300 mg with emtricitabine 200 mg daily with dolutegravir 50 mg once daily. In contrast to those with occupational exposures, some individuals may present very late after exposure. Because the likelihood of success declines with length of time from HIV exposure, *treatment is not recommended after > 72 hours after exposure.* In addition, because the psychosocial issues involved with postexposure prophylaxis for sexual and drug use exposures are complex, it should be offered with prevention counseling. Counseling should focus on how to prevent future exposures. Individuals with ongoing risk for HIV infection should be considered candidates for PrEP, sometimes called PEP-to-PrEP. Clinicians needing more information on postexposure prophylaxis for occupational or nonoccupational exposures should contact the *National Clinicians' Post-Exposure Prophylaxis Hotline* (1-888-448-4911; http://nccc.ucsf.edu/clinician-consultation/pep-post-exposure-prophylaxis/).

Centers for Disease Control and Prevention (CDC). Preventing HIV with PEP. Accessed March 15, 2026. https://www.cdc.gov/hiv/prevention/pep.html

O'Connell KA et al. HIV post-exposure prophylaxis in the emergency department: an updated assessment and opportunities for HIV prevention identified. Am J Emerg Med. 2021;46:323. [PMID: 33069548]

5. Prevention of perinatal transmission of HIV—Prevention of perinatal transmission of HIV begins by offering HIV counseling and testing to all women who are pregnant or considering pregnancy. Women with HIV who are pregnant should start ART with at least three medications as quickly as possible. The recommended regimens include a dual-NRTI combination and dolutegravir. Cesarean delivery should be planned if HIV viral load is unsuppressed or unknown near the time of delivery and one or more antiretroviral medications administered to the newborn for 6 weeks to reduce the risk of perinatal acquisition. The infant feeding guidelines in the United States changed in 2023 to allow for shared decision-making with the mother on the decision to breastfeed.

6. Prevention of HIV transmission in health care settings—In health care settings, *universal body fluid precautions* should be used, including use of gloves when handling body fluids and the addition of gown, mask, and goggles for procedures that may result in splash or droplet spread, and use of specially designed needles with sheath devices to decrease the risk of needle sticks.

Epidemiologic studies show that needle sticks occur commonly among health care professionals, especially among surgeons performing invasive procedures, inexperienced hospital house staff, and medical students. Efforts to reduce needle sticks should focus on avoiding recapping needles and use of safety needles whenever doing invasive procedures under controlled circumstances. The risk of HIV transmission from a needle stick with blood from a patient with HIV infection is approximately 1:300, although determinants of risk include deep punctures, large inoculum, and source patients with high viral loads. The risk from mucous membrane contact and contact to non-intact skin is 1:1000 or less.

Health care professionals who sustain needle sticks should be counseled and offered HIV testing as soon as possible. HIV testing is done to establish a negative baseline in case there is a subsequent conversion. Follow-up testing is usually performed at 6 weeks and 3 months. With the patient's permission, their blood can be tested for HIV, with postexposure prophylaxis and further follow-up discontinued for the healthcare worker if the source patient tests negative.

A case-control study by the CDC indicates that administration of zidovudine following a needle stick decreased the rate of HIV seroconversion by 79%. Therefore, *clinicians should be offered ART as soon as possible after exposure and continued for 4 weeks.* Modern antiretrovirals have not been studied, but the efficacy is expected to be higher with more potent and better-tolerated integrase inhibitor–based three-drug regimens. The preferred regimen is TDF 300 mg with emtricitabine 200 mg (Truvada) daily with dolutegravir 50 mg once daily. Clinicians who have exposures to persons who are likely to have antiretroviral medication resistance (eg, persons receiving therapy who have detectable viral loads) should have their therapy individualized, using at least two medications to which the source is unlikely to be resistant.

Centers for Disease Control and Prevention (CDC). HIV occupational transmission. Accessed March 15, 2026. https://www.cdc.gov/hiv/causes/occupational-transmission.html

7. Prevention of transmission of HIV through blood or blood products—Current efforts in the United States to screen blood and blood products have lowered the risk of HIV transmission with transfusion of a unit of blood to 1:2,000,000. Use of blood and blood products should be judicious and only when clinically indicated.

8. HIV vaccine—Primate model data have suggested that development of a protective vaccine may be possible, but clinical trials in humans have been disappointing. Only one vaccine trial has shown any degree of efficacy. In this randomized, double-blind, placebo-controlled trial, a recombinant canarypox vector vaccine plus two booster injections of a recombinant gp120 vaccine reduced the risk of HIV among a primarily heterosexual population in Thailand, but efficacy was too low (31%) for widespread use. A mosaic HIV vaccine resulted in a strong immune response among adult humans and protection against infection with an HIV-like virus in rhesus monkeys. Unfortunately, initial results from a phase 2b trial in cisgender women using this mosaic vaccine (Imbokodo study) did not show efficacy. In January 2023, a phase 3 study (Mosaico) using a different formulation of the mosaic vaccine among 3900 MSM and transgender women conducted in Latin America, North America, and Europe had to be discontinued for lack of efficacy in preventing HIV infection. The latest trial of two vaccine candidates in combination, called the PrEPVacc trial, being tested in 1500 participants in Uganda, Tanzania, and South Africa, also closed early in December 2023 due to lack of efficacy. Although the results from these HIV vaccine trials were disheartening, prior vaccine candidates for HIV have not managed to elicit broadly neutralizing antibodies and T cells against the virus. However, preliminary work with a novel mRNA vaccine developed for HIV shows the development of both. Moreover, protection against simian HIV infection was demonstrated in a small group of macaques using the adapted mRNA HIV vaccine.

National Institute of Allergy and Infectious Diseases (NIAID). News Releases: NIH launches clinical trial of three mRNA HIV vaccines. Accessed August 31, 2024. https://www.niaid.nih.gov/news-events/nih-launches-clinical-trial-three-mrna-hiv-vaccines

National Institutes of Health (NIH). News Releases: Experimental HIV vaccine regimen safe but ineffective, study finds. Accessed August 31, 2024. https://www.nih.gov/news-events/news-releases/experimental-hiv-vaccine-regimen-safe-ineffective-study-finds

National Institutes of Health (NIH). News Releases: HIV vaccine candidate does not sufficiently protect women against HIV infection. Accessed August 31, 2024. https://www.nih.gov/news-events/news-releases/hiv-vaccine-candidate-does-not-sufficiently-protect-women-against-hiv-infection

Zhang P et al. A multiclade env–gag VLP mRNA vaccine elicits tier-2 HIV-1-neutralizing antibodies and reduces the risk of heterologous SHIV infection in macaques. Nat Med. 2021;27:2234. [PMID: 34887575]

B. Secondary Prevention

In the era prior to the development of effective ART, cohort studies of individuals with documented dates of seroconversion demonstrate that AIDS developed within 10 years in approximately 50% of untreated seropositive persons. With currently available treatment, progression of disease has been markedly decreased. In addition to ART, prophylactic regimens can prevent opportunistic infections and improve survival. Prophylaxis and early intervention prevent several infectious diseases, including tuberculosis and syphilis, which are transmissible to others. Recommendations for screening tests, vaccinations, and prophylaxis are listed in Table 35–5.

1. Tuberculosis—Because of the increased occurrence of tuberculosis among people with HIV, these patients should undergo an intradermal PPD test or an IGRA blood test at baseline and yearly thereafter if they remain at risk of exposure (eg, incarcerated, living in congregate settings). Those with a positive PPD (defined for people with HIV as > 5 mm of induration) or a positive IGRA assay (results that are reported as positive and not negative or indeterminate) should be clinically evaluated for active tuberculosis, including by a CXR. Patients with an opacity in any location, especially if accompanied by mediastinal adenopathy, should have sputum sent for acid-fast staining and nucleic acid amplification testing. Patients with active tuberculosis should be treated as outlined in Chapter 9 (see Table 9–15). Patients with a positive PPD or IGRA assay, and a normal CXR or negative sputum evaluation for active tuberculosis are classified as having latent tuberculosis infection. Patients with latent tuberculosis infection who have not been previously treated for (active or latent) tuberculosis should receive once-weekly isoniazid (900 mg orally weekly for patients > 50 kg) and rifapentine (900 mg orally weekly for patients > 50 kg) for 12 weeks. Other preferred regimens are rifampin daily (10 mg/kg; maximum and usual adult dose is 600 mg orally daily) for 4 months, although all people with HIV should be evaluated for drug interactions, including with ART and 3 months of once daily rifampin and isoniazid once daily (300 mg orally daily). The WHO also recommends 1 month of daily isoniazid and daily rifapentine (300 mg daily for a weight of < 35 kg, 450 mg daily for a weight of 35 to 45 kg, and 600 mg for a weight of > 45 kg) as a short-course regimen, although this regimen is not recommend in conjunction with integrase inhibitors due to concern for induction of metabolism by daily rifapentine. An alternative, less preferred regimen given low completion rates, is 9 months of daily isoniazid. In patients with advanced immunodeficiency, both the PPD and IGRA assay are more likely to be falsely negative or (for IGRA assay) indeterminant. Therefore, it may be worth obtaining a CXR, tuberculosis sputum evaluation, or both in people at high risk for tuberculosis, and retesting patients with initially low CD4 counts once they have received ART and have immune reconstitution (CD4 count ≥ 200 cells/mcL).

2. Syphilis—Because of the increased number of cases of syphilis among MSM, including those living with HIV, *all such men should be screened for syphilis by a syphilis enzyme immunoassay, rapid plasma reagin (RPR), or Venereal Disease Research Laboratories (VDRL) test every 3–6 months.* Increases of syphilis cases among people with HIV are of particular concern because these individuals are at increased risk for neurosyphilis and other complications of syphilis.

Table 35–5. Health care maintenance and monitoring of people with HIV.

For all people with HIV:
CD4 counts every 3–6 months (can decrease to every 12 months if viral load suppressed on ART for 2 years and CD4 count > 300 cells/mcL, optional if consistently above 500 cells/mcL)
Viral load tests every 3–6 months and 2–4 weeks following a change in therapy
Genotypic resistance testing at baseline and if viral load not fully suppressed and patient taking ART
CBC, chemistry profile, transaminases and total bilirubin, at baseline and every 3–6 months
UA at baseline and annually during ART (every 6 months if ART regimen includes TDF)
Glucose or hemoglobin A_{1c} at baseline and annually during ART
Lipid panel at baseline, 4–8 weeks after starting or changing an ART regimen that affects lipids, and annually for everyone over 40 years of age
PPD or IGRA at baseline and annually if at high risk for exposure to persons with active TB
Latent TB infection treatment for those with positive PPD or IGRA, normal CXR, and no history of treatment for active or latent TB
RPR or VDRL at entry and periodically based on sexual activity
Toxoplasma IgG serology at baseline
Hepatitis serologies: hepatitis A antibody, hepatitis B surface antigen, hepatitis B surface antibody, hepatitis B core antibody, hepatitis C antibody
Pneumococcal vaccine
Meningococcal vaccine
Herpes zoster vaccine[1]
Inactivated influenza vaccine annually in season
Hepatitis A vaccine for those without immunity to hepatitis A
Hepatitis B vaccine for those who are hepatitis B surface antigen and antibody negative (use 40 mcg formulation at 0, 1, and 6 months; repeat if no immunity 1 month after three-vaccine series)
Combined tetanus, diphtheria, pertussis vaccine
COVID-19 vaccination
HPV vaccine for women aged 26 years or younger with HIV
Haemophilus influenzae type b vaccination
Bone mineral density monitoring for postmenopausal women and men aged 50 years or older
Papanicolaou smears annually; if three smears are negative, can switch to longer intervals (see Complications, Section M. Gynecologic Manifestations)
Consider anal swabs for cytologic evaluation
For people with HIV with CD4 < 200 cells/mcL:
Pneumocystis jirovecii prophylaxis (see Treatment, Section A. Prophylaxis for Complications of HIV Infection and Table 35–6)
For people with HIV with CD4 < 100 cells/mcL and Toxoplasma IgG-positive:
Ensure current prophylaxis covers toxoplasma, and if not, add toxoplasma prophylaxis (see Treatment, Section A. Prophylaxis for Complications of HIV Infection and Table 35–6)

[1]Consider in patients age > 50 years, should not give live vaccine (Zostavax) to individuals with CD4 T-cells < 200 cells/mcL.
ART, antiretroviral therapy; CMV, cytomegalovirus; IgG, immunoglobulin G; IGRA, interferon γ release assay; INH, isoniazid; PPD, purified protein derivative; RPR, rapid plasma reagin; TB, tuberculosis; TDF, tenofovir disoproxil fumarate; VDRL, Venereal Disease Research Laboratories.

People with HIV may lose fluorescent treponemal antibody absorption (FTA-ABS) reactivity after treatment for syphilis, particularly if they have low CD4 counts. Thus, *in this population, a nonreactive treponemal test does not rule out a past history of syphilis*. People with HIV should be evaluated carefully for otic, ophthalmic, or any other neurologic symptoms after a diagnosis of syphilis, with lumbar puncture pursued if there are neurologic symptoms, assuming empiric treatment is not pursued due to the presence of unexplained ophthalmic or otic symptoms. CSF cell count and CSF-VDRL should be examined in these cases. Those without neurologic symptoms or a normal CSF evaluation are treated as having *early latent syphilis* (prior syphilis evaluation within 1 year or symptoms of early syphilis) with one dose of benzathine penicillin G, 2.4 million units intramuscularly. Those with unknown or > 1 year since a prior syphilis evaluation are treated as *late latent syphilis* (benzathine penicillin G, 2.4 million units intramuscularly weekly for 3 weeks). Those with a pleocytosis or a positive CSF-VDRL test are treated as having *neurosyphilis* (aqueous penicillin G, 2–4 million units intravenously every 4 hours for 10–14 days). Given higher rates of clinical failure, people with HIV should be evaluated for treatment response, with nonresponse defined as lack of fourfold decrease in titers in 1 year after early latent syphilis treatment or 2 years after late latent syphilis treatment. These individuals should be evaluated for neurosyphilis, particularly if there is no clinical evidence of reinfection. For a more detailed discussion of this topic, see Chapter 38.

3. Immunizations—Patients with HIV should receive immunizations as outlined in Table 35–5. Patients without evidence of hepatitis B surface antigen or surface antibody should receive hepatitis B vaccination, using the 40-mcg formulation (the higher dose is to increase the chance of developing protective immunity) or using the two-dose CpG-adjuvanted hepatitis B vaccine (Heplisav-B). Although the CpG-adjuvanted vaccine was not initially studied among people with HIV, data presented from an HIV clinical trials network demonstrated that a three-dose regimen led to excellent serologic responses. It is not clear if a three-dose regimen or two-dose regimen should be used among people with HIV. If the patient does not have immunity 1 month after series completion, then the series should be repeated. People with HIV should also receive the standard inactivated vaccines such as tetanus, diphtheria, and pertussis boosters that would be given to uninfected persons. *Most live vaccines, such as yellow fever vaccine, should be avoided in people with CD4+ T-cell counts < 200 cells/mcL.* However, the mpox vaccine (which is a live attenuated vaccine) was found to be safe when administered to people with HIV with a range of CD4 cell counts in the 2022 mpox outbreak. Measles vaccination, while a live virus vaccine, appears relatively safe when administered to patients with HIV and should be given if the patient has never had measles (with the vaccine developed in 1963) or been adequately vaccinated. The recombinant adjuvanted herpes zoster vaccine (Shingrix), two doses 2–6 months apart, is recommended for people all adults with HIV. COVID-19 vaccines are safe and effective for people with HIV. Although most people with HIV will produce a serologic response to vaccination, there is evidence of reduced serologic response among some people with HIV, particularly those with low CD4+ T-cell counts or unsuppressed viral loads. Booster vaccination is therefore recommended for this population.

Spinelli MA et al. Differences in post-mRNA vaccination severe acute respiratory syndrome coronavirus 2 (SARS-CoV-2) immunoglobulin G (IgG) concentrations and surrogate virus neutralization test response by human immunodeficiency virus (HIV) status and type of vaccine: a matched case-control observational study. Clin Infect Dis. 2022;75:e916. [PMID: 34864962]

4. Other measures—STI screening should continue as there are high rates of syphilis, gonorrhea, and chlamydia infection among people with HIV. Postexposure prophylaxis (PEP) with doxycycline has been shown to reduce the incidence of STIs among MSM and transgender women and is recommended for those groups if sexual risk is ongoing. Substance use treatment should be recommended for persons with substance use disorders, as this can improve adherence and treatment engagement. They should be warned to avoid consuming raw meat, eggs, or shellfish to avoid infections with *Toxoplasma, Campylobacter*, and *Salmonella*. Those with CD4+ counts < 200 cells/mcL should wash their hands thoroughly after cleaning cat litter or should forgo this household chore to avoid possible exposure to toxoplasmosis. To reduce the likelihood of infection with *Bartonella* species, patients with low CD4 counts should avoid activities that might result in cat scratches or bites.

Treatment

Treatment for HIV infection can be broadly divided into the following categories: (1) prophylaxis for opportunistic infections, malignancies, and other complications of HIV infection; (2) treatment of opportunistic infections, malignancies, and other complications of HIV infection; and (3) treatment of the HIV infection itself with ART.

A. Prophylaxis for Complications of HIV Infection

In general, decisions about prophylaxis of opportunistic infections are based on the CD4 count, recent HIV viral load, and a history of having had the infection in the past. Studies have shown that *in patients with robust improvements in immune function—as measured by increases in CD4 counts above the levels that are used to initiate treatment—or prolonged virologic suppression in the setting of poor immunologic response, prophylactic regimens can safely be discontinued.*

Because people with advanced HIV infection are susceptible to a number of opportunistic pathogens, the use of agents with activity against more than one pathogen is preferable.

1. Prophylaxis against *Pneumocystis* pneumonia— Patients with CD4 counts below 200 cells/mcL, a CD4 lymphocyte percentage below 14%, or oral candidiasis should be offered primary prophylaxis for *Pneumocystis* pneumonia. Patients with a history of *Pneumocystis* pneumonia should receive secondary prophylaxis until their viral load is undetectable and they have maintained a CD4 count of 200 cells/mcL or more while receiving ART for longer than 3 months. Regimens for *Pneumocystis* prophylaxis are given in Table 35–6.

Table 35–6. *Pneumocystis jirovecii* prophylaxis (listed in order of preference).

Medication	Dose	Side Effects	Limitations
Trimethoprim-sulfamethoxazole	One double-strength tablet three times a week to one tablet daily	Rash, neutropenia, hepatitis, Stevens-Johnson syndrome	Hypersensitivity reaction is common but, if mild, it may be possible to treat through.
Dapsone	50–100 mg orally daily or 100 mg two or three times per week	Anemia, nausea, methemoglobinemia, hemolytic anemia	Less effective than above. Glucose-6-phosphate dehydrogenase (G6PD) level should be checked prior to therapy. Check methemoglobin level after 1 month of treatment.
Atovaquone	1500 mg orally daily with a meal	Rash, diarrhea, nausea	Less effective than suspension trimethoprim-sulfamethoxazole; equal efficacy to dapsone, but more expensive.
Aerosolized pentamidine	300 mg monthly	Bronchospasm (pretreat with bronchodilators); rare reports of pancreatitis	Apical *P jirovecii* pneumonia, extrapulmonary *P jirovecii* infections, pneumothorax.

2. Prophylaxis against *M avium* complex infection— Prophylaxis against *M avium* complex is *no longer recommended* in most individuals who are initiating ART, including in those with CD4+ counts < 50 cells/mcL. The incidence of *M avium* complex infection is very low among those on ART. In rare cases where individuals delay ART (eg, per patient preference) whose CD4 counts fall to below 50 cells/mcL, prophylaxis against *M avium* complex infection should be offered. Clarithromycin (500 mg orally twice daily) and azithromycin (1200 mg orally weekly) are the recommended regimens. The azithromycin regimen is generally preferred based on high adherence and low cost. Prophylaxis against *M avium* complex infection may be discontinued in patients who initiate ART.

3. Prophylaxis against toxoplasmosis—Toxoplasmosis prophylaxis is desirable in patients with a positive IgG toxoplasma serology and CD4 counts below 100 cells/mcL. Trimethoprim-sulfamethoxazole (one double-strength tablet daily) offers good protection against toxoplasmosis, as does a combination of pyrimethamine, 25 mg orally once a week, plus dapsone, 50 mg orally daily, plus leucovorin, 25 mg orally once a week. A glucose-6-phosphate dehydrogenase (G6PD) level should be checked prior to dapsone therapy, and a methemoglobin level should be checked at 1 month. Prophylaxis can be discontinued when the CD4 cells have increased to > 200 cells/mcL for > 3 months.

B. Treatment of Complications of HIV Infection

Treatment of common AIDS-related complications is detailed above and in Table 35–3. In the era prior to the use of ART, patients required lifelong treatment for many infections, including CMV retinitis, toxoplasmosis, and cryptococcal meningitis. However, *among patients who have a good response to ART, maintenance therapy for opportunistic infections can be terminated.* For example, in consultation with an ophthalmologist, maintenance treatment for CMV infection can be discontinued when persons receiving ART have had a sustained increase in CD4 count to > 100 cells/mcL for at least 3–6 months. Similar results have been observed in patients with *M avium* complex bacteremia, who have completed a year or more of therapy for *M avium* complex and have an increase in their CD4 count to 100 cells/mcL for > 6 months while receiving ART. Cessation of secondary prophylaxis for *Pneumocystis* pneumonia is described above.

Treating patients with repeated episodes of the same opportunistic infection can pose difficult therapeutic challenges. For example, patients with second or third episodes of *Pneumocystis* pneumonia may have developed allergic reactions to standard treatments with a prior episode. Fortunately, there are several alternatives available for the treatment of *Pneumocystis* infection. Trimethoprim with dapsone and primaquine with clindamycin are two combinations that often are tolerated in patients with a prior allergic reaction to trimethoprim-sulfamethoxazole and intravenous pentamidine.

C. Antiretroviral Therapy

The availability of agents that in combination suppress HIV replication (Table 35–7) has had a profound impact on the natural history of HIV infection. Indeed, *with the advent of effective ART, the life expectancy of people with HIV approaches that of people without infection when treatment is initiated early in the course of the disease and maintained.*

The recognition that HIV damages the immune system from the beginning of infection, even when the damage is not easily measured by conventional tests, combined with the greater potency, the improved side-effect profile, and the decreased pill burden of modern HIV regimens, have led to the recommendation to **start treatment as soon as possible for all people with HIV, including patients having acute HIV infection, regardless of CD4 count.**

Rapid initiation programs have been created, where treatment can be started on the same day that patients test positive for HIV, so patients can start receiving treatment promptly and avoid being lost to follow-up. The clinician should provide sufficient resources to help patients cope with these major events in a short time, receive sufficient insurance and benefits coverage, and connect to other social services resources (ie, food assistance, housing, etc). If treatment is started before the results of resistance testing are available, a nonnucleoside reverse transcriptase inhibitor (NNRTI) should not be used given the possibility of transmitted drug resistance. Recommended regimens for initiating treatment before resistance testing results are available include (1) dolutegravir plus TAF/emtricitabine or TDF/emtricitabine (or lamivudine), (2) bictegravir/TAF/emtricitabine, or (3) boosted darunavir plus TAF/emtricitabine or TDF/emtricitabine (or lamivudine). The latter regimen is recommended (until resistance testing is known) if a patient developed an HIV seroconversion while on cabotegravir-based PrEP due to the possibility of the development of integrase inhibitor resistance. Also, patients requiring abacavir as part of their regimen should not start treatment prior to the results of HLA-B*5701 allele testing or hepatitis B testing.

The primary goal of therapy should be complete suppression of viral replication as measured by the serum viral load. Partially suppressive combinations should be avoided. Similarly, if toxicity develops, it is preferable to change the offending medication given availability of multiple effective and well-tolerated medications.

Although the HIV treatment protocol has traditionally included three medications from at least two different classes, *several two-drug regimens using medications from at least two different classes have been shown to be effective.* A combination of dolutegravir plus lamivudine (Table 35–8) has been shown to be noninferior to dolutegravir plus TDF and emtricitabine as initial therapy in patients with HIV viral load of < 500,000 copies/mL. A second exception is the coformulation of dolutegravir and rilpivirine (Table 35–8); this combination is FDA-approved as an alternative treatment for patients who have been successfully virally suppressed for at least 6 months, have no history of treatment failure, and are not resistant to either of the two component agents. A third approved two-drug regimen is cabotegravir with rilpivirine provided as intramuscular injections given every 4 or 8 weeks in patients who have first achieved virologic suppression on oral ART. Data from a randomized clinical trial has shown the

Table 35–7. Antiretroviral therapy agents by class (listed in alphabetical order within classes).

Medication	Dose	Common Side Effects	Special Monitoring[1]
Nucleoside Reverse Transcriptase Inhibitors (NRTIs)			
Abacavir (Ziagen)	600 mg orally once daily	Rash, fever—if occur, rechallenge may be fatal	No special monitoring
Emtricitabine (Emtriva)	200 mg orally once daily	Skin discoloration palms/soles (mild)	No special monitoring
Lamivudine (Epivir)	150 mg orally twice daily or 300 mg daily	Rash, peripheral neuropathy	No special monitoring
Zidovudine (AZT) (Retrovir)	600 mg orally daily in two divided doses	Anemia, neutropenia, nausea, malaise, headache, insomnia, myopathy	CBC with differential 4–8 weeks after starting AZT
Nucleotide Reverse Transcriptase Inhibitors (NRTIs)			
Tenofovir alafenamide (TAF)/emtricitabine (Descovy)	25 mg of TAF with 200 mg of emtricitabine once daily	Weight gain; dyslipidemia; lower but still present risk of nephrotoxicity and bone resorption	Creatinine at baseline, at 2–8 weeks, then every 3–6 months; UA and urine glucose and protein at baseline and repeated as clinically indicated; HBsAg, liver enzymes at baseline, at 2–8 weeks, then every 3–6 months, continue for months after discontinuation; consider bone densitometry
Tenofovir (TDF) (Viread)	300 mg orally once daily	Kidney dysfunction, bone resorption, GI distress	Creatinine at baseline, at 2–8 weeks, then every 3–6 months; UA and urine glucose and protein at baseline and repeated as clinically indicated; consider bone densitometry
Nonnucleoside Reverse Transcriptase Inhibitors (NNRTIs)			
Doravirine (Pifeltro)	100 mg daily	Headache, fatigue, abdominal pain	No special monitoring
Efavirenz (Sustiva)	600 mg orally daily	Neurologic disturbances, rash, hepatitis	No special monitoring
Etravirine (Intelence)	200 mg orally twice daily	Rash, peripheral neuropathy	No special monitoring
Nevirapine (Viramune)	200 mg orally daily for 2 weeks, then 200 mg orally twice daily	Rash	No special monitoring
Rilpivirine (Edurant)	25 mg daily	Depression, rash	No special monitoring
Protease Inhibitors (PIs)			
Atazanavir (Reyataz)	400 mg orally once daily or 300 mg atazanavir with 100 mg ritonavir daily	Hyperbilirubinemia	Bilirubin level every 3–4 months
Atazanavir/cobicistat (Evotaz)	300 mg of atazanavir with 150 mg of cobicistat orally once daily	Hyperbilirubinemia	Bilirubin level every 3–4 months
Darunavir/cobicistat (Prezcobix)	800 mg of darunavir and 150 mg of cobicistat orally once daily	Rash	No special monitoring
Darunavir/ritonavir (Prezista/Norvir)	**PI-experienced patients:** 600 mg of darunavir and 100 mg of ritonavir orally twice daily **For PI-naïve patients:** 800 mg of darunavir and 100 mg of ritonavir orally daily	Rash	No special monitoring
Lopinavir/ritonavir (Kaletra)	400 mg/100 mg orally twice daily	Diarrhea	No special monitoring
Ritonavir (Norvir)	600 mg orally twice daily or in lower doses (eg, 100 mg orally once or twice daily) for boosting other PIs	GI distress, peripheral paresthesias	No special monitoring

(continued)

Table 35–7. Antiretroviral therapy agents by class (listed in alphabetical order within classes). (continued)

Medication	Dose	Common Side Effects	Special Monitoring[1]
Entry Inhibitors			
Enfuvirtide (Fuzeon)	90 mg subcutaneously twice daily	Injection site pain and allergic reaction	No special monitoring
Integrase Inhibitors			
Bictegravir	50 mg orally daily. No longer marketed as a single agent; used in antiretroviral combination (Table 35–8)	Diarrhea, nausea, headache	No special monitoring
Cabotegravir	Oral regimen of 30 mg daily with rilpivirine 25 mg daily for 1 month (optional); then intramuscular loading dose of 600 mg with rilpivirine 900 mg intramuscularly in separate buttock injections; followed by (1) this dosage every 8 weeks or (2) monthly intramuscular injections of 400 mg with 600 mg rilpivirine thereafter	Injection site reactions with intramuscular dose	No special monitoring
Dolutegravir (Tivicay)	Treatment-naïve or integrase-naïve patients: 50 mg daily When administered with efavirenz or rifampin: 50 mg twice daily When administered to integrase-experienced patients with suspected integrase resistance: 50 mg twice daily	Hypersensitivity, insomnia, fatigue, headache, rash	No special monitoring
Elvitegravir	No longer marketed as a single agent; used in antiretroviral combinations (Table 35–8)	Diarrhea, headache	No special monitoring
Raltegravir (Isentress)	400 mg orally twice daily	Diarrhea, nausea, headache	No special monitoring
Entry and Fusion Inhibitors			
Enfuvirtide (Fuzeon)	90 mg subcutaneously twice daily	Injection site pain and allergic reaction	No special monitoring
Ibalizumab (Trogarzo)	Loading dose of 2000 mg intravenously over 30 minutes; maintenance dose of 800 mg intravenously every 2 weeks thereafter	Diarrhea, dizziness, nausea, rash, elevated creatinine, lymphopenia	Monthly CBC, creatinine, bilirubin, glucose, lipase
Maraviroc (Selzentry)	150 mg orally twice daily or 300 mg orally twice daily	Cough, fever, rash	No special monitoring
Capsid Inhibitor			
Lenacapavir	At first, 927 mg (2 vials) injected under the skin and 600 mg (2 tablets) once a day on day 1. Followed by 600 mg (2 tablets) once a day on day 2. For maintenance, 927 mg (2 vials) injected under the skin once a day every 6 months.	Subcutaneous nodules and injection site pain	No special monitoring
Attachment Inhibitor			
Fostemsavir	600 mg orally twice a day	Nausea	No special monitoring

[1]Standard monitoring is CBC and differential, basic chemistries, serum aminotransferases, and total bilirubin every 3–6 months, UA at baseline and annually during antiretroviral treatment, fasting glucose or hemoglobin A_{1c} at baseline and annually during antiretroviral treatment, and fasting lipid profile at baseline, 4–8 weeks after starting an antiretroviral treatment regimen that affects lipids, and annually for everyone over 40 years of age.

Table 35–8. Fixed-dose antiretroviral combinations (listed in alphabetical order by brand name).

Brand Name	Components	Dosing and Special Considerations
Atripla	TDF 300 mg Emtricitabine 200 mg Efavirenz 600 mg	One pill daily constitutes a complete ART regimen.
Biktarvy	Emtricitabine 200 mg TAF 25 mg Bictegravir 50 mg	One pill daily constitutes a complete ART regimen. One of the recommended initial treatment regimens.
Complera	TDF 300 mg Emtricitabine 200 mg Rilpivirine 25 mg	One pill daily constitutes a complete ART regimen. Only for patients with HIV viral load < 100,000/mL.
Delstrigo	TDF 300 mg Lamivudine 300 mg Doravirine 100 mg	One pill daily constitutes a complete ART regimen.
Descovy	TAF 25 mg Emtricitabine 200 mg	One pill daily along with an NNRTI, PI, integrase inhibitor, or maraviroc (entry inhibitor). The difference between Descovy and Truvada is that Descovy has a different form of tenofovir (TAF) that has less effect on kidney function and bone mineral density than the form of tenofovir (TDF) in Truvada. Descovy is approved for use as a single agent for PrEP in men (not studied in women).
Dovato	Dolutegravir 50 mg Lamivudine 300 mg	One pill daily constitutes a complete ART regimen in adults with no prior antiviral treatment and no known substitutions associated with resistance to either component.
Epzicom	Abacavir 600 mg Lamivudine 300 mg	One pill daily along with an NNRTI, PI, integrase inhibitor, or maraviroc (entry inhibitor).
Genvoya	TAF 10 mg Emtricitabine 200 mg Elvitegravir 150 mg Cobicistat 150 mg	One pill daily constitutes a complete ART regimen. Although it contains four medications, one component (cobicistat) is a medication booster only. The only difference between Stribild and Genvoya is that Genvoya has a different form of tenofovir (TAF) that appears to be safer than tenofovir TDF with less effect on kidney function and bone mineral density.
Juluca	Dolutegravir 50 mg Rilpivirine 25 mg	One pill daily with a meal for patients who have been virologically suppressed (viral load < 50 copies/mL) on a stable ART regimen for ≥ 6 months and no history of treatment failure or resistance to dolutegravir or rilpivirine.
Odefsey	TAF 25 mg Emtricitabine 200 mg Rilpivirine 25 mg	One pill daily constitutes a complete ART regimen. Only for patients with no history of HIV viral load ≥ 100,000 copies/mL. Or for replacement of stable antiretroviral regimen in patients fully suppressed for > 6 months, with no history of treatment failure, and with no known resistance to components of the drug combination.
Stribild	TDF 300 mg Emtricitabine 200 mg Elvitegravir 150 mg Cobicistat 150 mg	One pill daily constitutes a complete ART regimen. Although it contains four medications, one component (cobicistat) is a medication booster only.
Symtuza	TAF 10 mg Emtricitabine 200 mg Darunavir 800 mg Cobicistat 150 mg	One pill daily constitutes a complete ART regimen. Although it contains four medications, one component (cobicistat) is a medication booster only. One of the recommended initial treatment regimens.
Triumeq	Abacavir 600 mg Lamivudine 300 mg Dolutegravir 50 mg	One pill constitutes a complete ART regimen. One of the recommended initial treatment regimens.
Trizivir	Abacavir 300 mg Lamivudine 150 mg Zidovudine 300 mg	One tablet twice daily with an NNRTI, PI, integrase inhibitor, or maraviroc (entry inhibitor). Although it contains three medications it *does not* constitute a complete ART regimen.
Truvada	TDF 300 mg Emtricitabine 200 mg	One pill daily with an NNRTI, PI, integrase inhibitor, or maraviroc (entry inhibitor). Tenofovir is the most commonly used NRTI backbone. Associated with less weight gain and lipid abnormalities than TAF. Truvada is approved for use as a single agent for PrEP.

ART, antiretroviral therapy; NNRTI, nonnucleoside reverse transcriptase inhibitor (eg, delavirdine, efavirenz, etravirine, nevirapine, rilpivirine); NRTI, nucleoside/nucleotide reverse transcriptase inhibitor (eg, abacavir, didanosine, emtricitabine, lamivudine, stavudine, tenofovir, zidovudine); PI, protease inhibitor; PrEP, pre-exposure prophylaxis; TAF, tenofovir alafenamide; TDF, tenofovir disoproxil fumarate.

benefit of long-acting cabotegravir/rilpivirine among people with HIV with adherence challenges. Finally, data from demonstration projects have demonstrated the benefit of this long-acting combination among people living with HIV with viremia due to adherence challenges taking oral ART. United States–based ART guidelines changed in 2024 to permit the use of long-acting injectables in those without virologic suppression.

The presence of an acute opportunistic infection in most cases does not preclude the initiation of ART. Randomized trials compared early initiation of ART (within 2 weeks of starting treatment for an opportunistic infection or tuberculosis) with ART that was deferred until after treatment of the opportunistic infection was completed (6 weeks after its start); results demonstrated that early initiation reduced death or AIDS progression by 50%. The reduced progression rates were related to more rapid improvements in CD4 counts in patients with advanced immunodeficiency. Furthermore, IRIS and other adverse events were no more frequent in the early ART arm.

Several randomized studies have also demonstrated improved clinical outcomes in HIV/tuberculosis coinfected patients who initiate ART early in the setting of active treatment for tuberculosis and whose CD4 counts are < cells/mcL. *The exception to early ART in the setting of active infections may be in patients with a CNS-associated infection, such as cryptococcal or tuberculosis meningitis.* Several studies from low-income countries have shown high mortality rates with early ART initiation in this setting.

An initial antiretroviral regimen should be chosen to minimize side effects. For hospitalized patients, initiating treatment in patients with opportunistic infections requires close coordination between inpatient and outpatient clinicians to ensure that treatment is continued once patients are discharged.

D. Choosing an Antiretroviral Treatment Regimen

HIV antiretroviral medications can be grouped into six major categories: nucleoside and nucleotide reverse transcriptase inhibitors (NRTIs); NNRTIs; PIs; integrase inhibitors; entry and fusion inhibitors; and attachment inhibitors. A capsid inhibitor administered as a subcutaneous injection (lenacapavir) every 26 weeks is FDA-approved for multidrug-resistant HIV in combination with oral antiretroviral agents with residual activity.

1. Nucleoside and nucleotide reverse transcriptase inhibitors—There are currently six NRTI agents available (counting TDF and TAF as separate agents) for use. The choice of which agent to use depends primarily on the patient's prior treatment experience, results of resistance testing, medication side effects, other underlying conditions, and convenience of formulation. However, most clinicians use fixed-dose combinations (see Table 35–8) of including either emtricitabine/TDF, emtricitabine/TAF, or abacavir/lamivudine (ABC/lamivudine), all of which can be given once a day. Abacavir should be given only to HLA-B*5701-negative persons due to a risk of hypersensitivity in those who are HLA-B*5701-positive. In patients with viral loads > 100,000 copies/mL, ABC/lamivudine was less effective than emtricitabine/TDF when combined with efavirenz or ritonavir-boosted atazanavir. However, ABC/lamivudine appears to be equally efficacious as emtricitabine/TDF in patients with viral loads > 100,000 copies/mL when combined with dolutegravir. In some studies, abacavir increased risks of MI, and therefore should be avoided in patients at high risk for CVD. Zidovudine is now rarely used due to toxicity (eg anemia or neutropenia). Of the available agents, zidovudine is the most likely to cause anemia or neutropenia. Emtricitabine, TDF, TAF, and lamivudine have activity against hepatitis B. TDF, TAF, emtricitabine, abacavir, and lamivudine can be administered once daily. Information specific to each medication is given below and in Table 35–7.

A. **Lamivudine**—Lamivudine is a safe and well-tolerated agent. The dosage is 300 mg orally once a day. The dose should be reduced in patients with CKD, although toxicity is not anticipated. There are no significant side effects with lamivudine; it has activity against hepatitis B, though HBV resistance to it is an increasing problem, and it is always given with tenofovir in the setting of HIV/hepatitis B coinfection.

B. **Emtricitabine**—Emtricitabine is dosed at 200 mg orally once daily. Emtricitabine also has activity against hepatitis B, but should not be used as monotherapy. Its dosage should be reduced in patients with CKD.

C. **Abacavir**—Abacavir is dosed at 600 mg once daily. Prior to initiation of abacavir, patients should undergo testing for HLA typing. *Those with the B*5701 allele should not be treated with abacavir because the likelihood of a hypersensitivity reaction developing is high*; the reaction is characterized by a flu-like syndrome with rash and fever that worsens with successive doses. Unfortunately, the absence of this allele does not guarantee that the patient will avoid the hypersensitivity reaction. Individuals in whom the hypersensitivity reaction develops should *not* be rechallenged with this agent because subsequent hypersensitivity reactions can be fatal. Abacavir, specifically recent use, has also been associated with an increased risk of MI in some cohort studies, generally in patients who have underlying risks for CVD. Abacavir is usually prescribed as a fixed-dose combination pill with lamivudine for use as a once-daily pill (Epzicom; Table 35–8).

D. **Tenofovir**—Tenofovir is the only licensed nucleotide analog. It comes in two forms: TDF and tenofovir alafenamide (TAF). TDF is available for use both in the form of a single pill at an oral dose of 300 mg once daily and as an oral fixed-dose combination pill with emtricitabine 200 mg (Truvada; Table 35–8) once daily. Several other single-tablet once-a-day complete regimens include TDF (Atripla, Complera, Stribild) (Table 35–8). Tenofovir is active against hepatitis B, including isolates that have resistance to lamivudine. TDF is associated with a clinically modest loss of kidney function, a small increased risk of AKI, and increased rate of bone resorption. In patients taking boosted therapy (eg, therapy including cobicistat or ritonavir), TAF appears to cause fewer problems with kidney dysfunction and bone loss and is the preferred choice.

TAF attains higher levels in cells with a much lower plasma level. For this reason, it appears to cause less harm to kidneys and less bone resorption. TAF should not be used with rifamycins. TDF appears to be associated with lower lipid levels, and TAF seems to be associated with greater weight gain when combined with integrase inhibitors.

2. Nonnucleoside reverse transcriptase inhibitors— NNRTIs inhibit reverse transcriptase at a site different from that of the nucleoside and nucleotide agents described above. The major advantage of NNRTIs is that four of them (efavirenz, rilpivirine, doravirine, and nevirapine) have potencies comparable to that of PIs (next section), at least for patients with viral loads under 100,000 copies/mL—with lower pill burden and fewer side effects. However, they have lower barrier to resistance compared with PIs and integrase inhibitors. Unlike PIs, they do *not* cause lipodystrophy and do not seem to cause weight gain; patients with cholesterol and triglyceride elevations who are switched from a PI to an NNRTI may have improvement in their lipids. The resistance patterns of NNRTIs are distinct from those of the PIs. Because these agents may cause alterations in the clearance of PIs, dose modifications may be necessary when these two classes of medications are administered concomitantly. There is a high degree of cross-resistance among the "first-generation" NNRTIs, such that resistance to one medication in this class uniformly predicts resistance to other medications. However, the "second-generation" NNRTIs etravirine, rilpivirine, and doravirine can have consistent antiviral activity in patients with prior exposure and resistance to nevirapine or efavirenz, although genotypic analysis is needed first in these contexts. In particular, the *K103N* pathologic variant does not have an impact on etravirine, doravirine, or rilpivirine. There is no therapeutic reason for using more than one NNRTI at the same time.

A. EFAVIRENZ—Efavirenz can be given once daily in a single dose (600 mg orally) and is available in a once-daily fixed-dose combination with TDF and emtricitabine in a single pill (Atripla; Table 35–8). The major side effects are rash and psychiatric/neurologic complaints, with patients reporting symptoms ranging from lack of concentration and strange dreams to delusions and mania. These side effects tend to wane over time, usually within a month or so; however, there are some patients who cannot tolerate these effects, especially if they persist longer than a month. Participant level data from four randomized trials of efavirenz regimens versus non-efavirenz-containing regimens found *increased suicidality* (hazard ratio of 2.6) among those taking efavirenz. As a result of these neuropsychiatric side effects, efavirenz is no longer a preferred regimen. Administration of efavirenz with food, especially fatty food, may increase its serum levels and consequent neurotoxicity. Therefore, it should be taken on an empty stomach; taking before bedtime may also reduce patients' experience of neuropsychiatric symptoms.

B. DORAVIRINE—Dosed at 100 mg orally daily, this medication can be taken with or without food. Two 48-week phase 3 studies showed that, in previously untreated individuals, doravirine, when used with two NRTIs resulted in similar levels of viral suppression as efavirenz plus two NRTIs or darunavir/ritonavir plus two NRTIs. It is also available as a single-pill combination with TDF and lamivudine (Delstrigo; Table 35–8). It is well tolerated. In cases of virologic failure, NNRTI cross-resistance may develop.

C. RILPIVIRINE—This medication, dosed at 25 mg once daily, is equal in efficacy to efavirenz in patients with HIV viral loads below 100,000 copies/mL. Oral rilpivirine should *not* be used in patients with baseline viral loads of 100,000 copies/mL or greater or those with CD4 counts below 200 cells/mcL because of greater risk of viral failure. As is true of efavirenz, rilpivirine is available in a once-daily fixed-dose combination with TDF and emtricitabine (Complera; Table 35–8) and with TAF and emtricitabine (Odefsey; Table 35–8) to be taken with a meal. It is also available in a two-drug regimen with dolutegravir (Juluca; Table 35–8). PPIs should not be given with rilpivirine. Rilpivirine has fewer neurologic side effects than efavirenz. The FDA has approved a long-acting formulation of rilpivirine for monthly or every 8-week intramuscular injections to be given with the integrase inhibitor cabotegravir (see below).

D. ETRAVIRINE—Etravirine is an NNRTI approved for the treatment of patients with prior NNRTI intolerance or resistance. Etravirine has been shown to be effective in treatment-experienced patients even when some degree of NNRTI resistance is present, making it a true "second-generation" medication in this class. Etravirine dosage is one 200 mg tablet twice daily or 400 mg once daily. The most common side effects are nausea and rash; rarely, the rash can be severe (toxic epidermal necrolysis). *Patients with signs of severe rash or hypersensitivity reactions should immediately discontinue the medication.* Prior rash due to treatment with one of the other NNRTIs does not make rash more likely with etravirine. Etravirine should not be taken by people with severe liver disease or administered with atazanavir/ritonavir, full-dose ritonavir, or PIs without low-dose ritonavir.

3. Protease inhibitors—Four PIs—ritonavir, lopinavir (in combination with ritonavir), atazanavir, and darunavir—are still available (with others used rarely). Darunavir boosted with ritonavir or cobicistat is the most commonly used PI in the United States; a single-pill combination of darunavir/cobicistat with TAF/FTC has been available since 2018. PIs are potent suppressors of HIV replication and are administered as part of a combination regimen.

All of the PIs—to differing degrees—are metabolized by the cytochrome P450 system, and each can inhibit and induce various P450 isoenzymes. Therefore, medication interactions are common and difficult to predict. Clinicians should consult the product inserts before prescribing PIs with other medications. Medications that are known to induce the P450 system, such as rifampin, should be avoided.

The fact that the PIs are dependent on metabolism through the cytochrome P450 system has led to the use of ritonavir to *boost* the medication levels of other PIs, allowing use of lower doses and simpler dosing schedules of these PIs. A second boosting agent, cobicistat, is coformulated with the PI atazanavir (Evotaz) and darunavir (Prezcobix and Symtuza). Similar to ritonavir, cobicistat also inhibits liver enzymes that metabolize other HIV medications.

All PIs have been linked to varying degrees of metabolic side effects, including elevated cholesterol levels, elevated triglyceride levels, insulin resistance, diabetes mellitus, and changes in body fat composition (eg, abdominal obesity). The lipid abnormalities and body habitus changes are referred to as *lipodystrophy*. Although lipodystrophy is commonly associated with PIs, it has been seen also in people with HIV who have never been treated with these agents. In particular, the lipoatrophy effects seen in patients receiving ART appear to be more related to the nucleoside toxicity and in particular to the thymidine analogs (ie, zidovudine).

Of the different manifestations of lipodystrophy, the dyslipidemias that occur are of particular concern because of the likelihood that increased levels of cholesterol and triglycerides will result in increased prevalence of heart disease. *All patients taking PIs should have fasting serum cholesterol, LDL cholesterol, and triglyceride levels assessed.* Clinicians should assess for CHD (see Chapter 32) and consider initiating dietary changes or medication therapy (or both). PIs inhibit statin metabolism. Lovastatin and simvastatin should be avoided. In general, the least interaction is with pravastatin (20 mg daily orally). Atorvastatin (10 mg daily orally) or rosuvastatin (5 mg/day orally initially; maximum 10 mg/day) may also be used cautiously. Patients with persistently elevated fasting serum triglyceride levels of 500 mg/dL or more who do not respond to dietary intervention should be treated with one of the statin medications, followed by gemfibrozil (600 mg twice daily prior to the morning and evening meals). PIs are associated with abnormalities in cardiac conduction, especially prolongation of the PR interval.

A. Ritonavir—Use of this potent PI at full dose (600 mg orally twice daily) has been limited by its inhibition of the cytochrome P450 pathway causing a large number of drug-drug interactions and by its frequent side effects of fatigue, nausea, and paresthesias. However, it is widely used in lower dose (eg, 100 mg daily to 100 mg twice daily) as a booster or pharmacokinetic enhancer of other PIs.

B. Lopinavir/r—Lopinavir/r is lopinavir (200 mg) coformulated with a low dose of ritonavir (50 mg) to maximize the bioavailability of lopinavir. The usual dose is lopinavir 400 mg with ritonavir 100 mg (two tablets) orally twice daily with food. When given along with efavirenz or nevirapine, a higher dose (600 mg/150 mg—three tablets) is usually prescribed. The most common side effect is diarrhea, and lipid abnormalities are frequent. Because of these side effects, lopinavir/r has fallen off the list of medications recommended as part of first-line treatment regimens.

C. Atazanavir—Atazanavir is available alone and coformulated with cobicistat (Evotaz). Atazanavir can be dosed as 400 mg (two 200-mg capsules) daily with food or it can be dosed as 300 mg in combination with 100 mg of ritonavir once daily with food. When coformulated with cobicistat, it is dosed at 300-mg atazanavir and 150-mg cobicistat. The most common side effect is mild hyperbilirubinemia that resolves with discontinuation of the medication. Nephrolithiasis and cholelithiasis have also been reported with this PI. Both tenofovir and efavirenz lower the serum concentration of atazanavir. Therefore, when either of these two medications is used with atazanavir, it should be boosted by administering ritonavir or given coformulated with cobicistat. PPIs are contraindicated in patients taking atazanavir because atazanavir requires an acidic pH to remain in solution.

D. Darunavir—Darunavir has impressive antiviral activity in the setting of significant PI resistance and in treatment-naïve patients. It is formulated by itself and coformulated with cobicistat (Prezcobix). When formulated without cobicistat it requires boosting with ritonavir. For initial treatment of HIV or for treatment-experienced patients without darunavir-related resistance pathologic variants, daily dosing is 800 mg of darunavir with 100 mg of ritonavir or with 150 mg of cobicistat. Darunavir 800 mg is also available in a coformulated tablet with emtricitabine, TAF, and cobicistat (Symtuza, Table 35–8). For patients with PI resistance (with 1–3 pathologic variants known to impact darunavir), darunavir should be dosed at 600 mg orally twice daily, with ritonavir, 100 mg orally twice daily. Darunavir has a safety profile similar to other PIs, such as ritonavir-boosted lopinavir, but is generally better tolerated. Darunavir is a sulfa-containing medication, and its use should be closely monitored in patients with sulfa allergy.

4. Integrase inhibitors—Integrase inhibitors slow HIV replication by blocking the HIV integrase enzyme needed for the virus to multiply. *They are now the preferred regimens for initiating therapy because of the combination of efficacy, ease of administration, and low incidence of side effects.* Five integrase inhibitors are currently available: raltegravir; elvitegravir; dolutegravir; bictegravir; and cabotegravir, which is given via injections along with injections of rilpivirine every 4 or 8 weeks. Clinical trials of available integrase inhibitors reveal a consistent pattern of more rapid decline in viral load compared with more standard PI/r or NNRTI-based regimens. Integrase inhibitors are effective (when combined with other active medications) in the treatment of people with HIV with documented resistance to each of the three main classes of antiretroviral medications (nucleoside analogs, PIs, NNRTIs). Avoid administering oral integrase inhibitors with antacids or other medications with divalent cations (Ca^{2+}, Mg^{2+}, Al^{2+}, Fe^{2+}) because chelation of the integrase inhibitor by the cation reduces absorption. When these medications must be taken with integrase inhibitors, they should either be taken together with food or the integrase inhibitor taken 2 hours before divalent cations. Integrase inhibitors have been associated with weight gain, with or without tenofovir alafenamide.

A. Raltegravir—The dose of raltegravir is 400 mg orally twice daily or 1200 mg orally once daily (two pills of 600 mg). It has been found to be superior to efavirenz and ritonavir-boosted darunavir and ritonavir-boosted atazanavir. Common side effects are diarrhea, nausea, and headache, but overall, it is well tolerated and has the additional advantage over PI-based regimens and efavirenz-based regimens in that it appears to have little impact on lipid profiles or glucose metabolism. Given the higher barrier to resistance with good tolerability of once-daily dosing, second-generation integrase inhibitors (dolutegravir, bictegravir), raltegravir is now rarely used.

B. Elvitegravir—Elvitegravir is not manufactured as a single agent. It can be prescribed in a once-a-day combination pill (Stribild) that contains 125 mg of elvitegravir and 150 mg of cobicistat, a boosting agent, along with standard doses of TDF and emtricitabine (Table 35–8). Stribild has been shown to be noninferior to two preferred first-line regimens: Atripla and boosted atazanavir with emtricitabine/TDF. The main side effect of Stribild is an increase in serum creatinine levels that has been shown to be related to the cobicistat inhibition of tubular secretion of creatinine by the kidney and is thought to be nonpathologic and reversible. However, because of this effect, *Stribild is recommended in patients with estimated creatinine clearance > 70 mL/min.* A UA should be done at baseline and at initial follow-up to look for proteinuria and glycosuria, which are signs of tubulopathy. Diarrhea and rash may also occur, although overall the medication is well tolerated. Elvitegravir is also coformulated with emtricitabine and TAF along with cobicistat boosting in a single once-a-day pill (Genvoya, Table 35–8). Given the higher barrier to resistance and decreased drug interactions of second-generation integrase inhibitors (dolutegravir, bictegravir), elvitegravir is rarely used.

C. Dolutegravir—Dolutegravir shows excellent potency and tolerability and is dosed once a day in most circumstances. It has been shown to be superior to efavirenz and darunavir. Unlike elvitegravir, dolutegravir does not require a boosting agent and has fewer drug-drug interactions. Similar to cobicistat, it inhibits tubular secretion of creatinine by the kidney, resulting in small increases in serum creatinine levels. The standard dosage used in treatment-naïve, integrase-naïve patients is 50 mg/day. It is available combined with abacavir and lamivudine in a single once a day tablet (Triumeq, Table 35–8). In patients receiving efavirenz or rifampin, the dose should be increased to 50 mg twice daily. It should also be dosed at 50 mg twice daily in integrase-experienced patients in whom dolutegravir resistance is documented or suspected. Indeed, when combined with other active medications, it has been shown to provide some activity in patients with integrase resistance who have not responded to prior raltegravir- or elvitegravir-containing regimens. Dolutegravir has demonstrated impressive results in clinical trials of treatment-naïve patients, in terms of effectiveness, tolerability, and high barrier to resistance, when compared with NNRTI, boosted PI, and raltegravir-containing regimens. Dolutegravir is coformulated in combination with rilpivirine (Juluca, Table 35–8) for use as a once-a-day (to be taken with a meal) treatment for patients who are virologically suppressed (viral load < 50 copies/mL) on a stable regimen for at least 6 months, with no history of treatment failures or resistance to either of the two agents. *A combination of dolutegravir-TDF and lamivudine is considered first-line or second-line therapy worldwide.*

D. Bictegravir—Bictegravir is dosed once daily, does not require boosting, and has a high barrier to resistance. It is dosed at 50 mg daily. It has been shown to be noninferior to dolutegravir. It is not available as a single agent but is marketed as a fixed-dose combination of bictegravir with emtricitabine and TAF (Biktarvy, Table 35–8).

E. Cabotegravir—Cabotegravir is an integrase inhibitor that has been approved for use in the United States, Canada, and in the European Union. Cabotegravir comes in two forms: an oral tablet and an injectable formulation. In both forms, it is intended to be given with rilpivirine. When given intramuscularly in combination with rilpivirine, the cabotegravir and rilpivirine are given as separate injections at the same time, one in each buttock. The first intramuscular loading doses are cabotegravir 600 mg and rilpivirine 900 mg. Thereafter, monthly intramuscular dosing is 400 mg of cabotegravir and 600 mg of rilpivirine. The advantage of this combination is that it is complete therapy for patients in whom the viral load is stable and suppressed (< 50 copies) on their current regimen, which is then stopped in favor of cabotegravir/rilpivirine. Additionally, the combination of cabotegravir 600 mg and rilpivirine 900 mg given every 8 weeks via injection has been approved. The most common side effect is injection site reaction.

5. Entry and fusion inhibitors—

A. Enfuvirtide—Enfuvirtide (Fuzeon) is known as a fusion inhibitor; it blocks the entry of HIV into cells by blocking the fusion of the HIV envelope to the cell membrane. The addition of enfuvirtide to an optimized antiretroviral regimen improved CD4 counts and lowered viral loads in heavily pretreated patients with multidrug-resistant HIV. Unfortunately, resistance to enfuvirtide develops rapidly in patients receiving a nonsuppressive treatment regimen. The dose is 90 mg by subcutaneous injection twice daily; unfortunately, painful injection site reactions develop in most patients, which makes long-term use problematic.

B. Maraviroc—Maraviroc is a CCR5 co-receptor antagonist. Medications in this class prevent the virus from entering uninfected cells by blocking the CCR5 co-receptor. Before starting therapy, a viral tropism assay should be performed because this class of entry inhibitors is *active only against "CCR5-tropic virus."* This form of the HIV-1 virus tends to predominate early in infection, while so-called dual/mixed tropic virus (which utilizes either R5 or CXCR4 co-receptors) emerges later as infection progresses. Approximately 50–60% of previously treated people with HIV have circulating CCR5-tropic HIV. The medication has been shown to be effective in people with HIV who have CCR5-tropic virus and ongoing viral replication despite being heavily treated. The dose of maraviroc is 150–300 mg orally twice daily, based on the other medications the patient is taking at the time—in combination with a ritonavir-boosted PI, 150 mg daily of maraviroc has been used successfully. Common side effects are cough, fever, rash, musculoskeletal problems, abdominal pain, and dizziness; however, maraviroc is generally well tolerated with limited impact on serum lipids.

C. Ibalizumab—Ibalizumab is a monoclonal antibody that blocks the entry of HIV into the CD4 cell by blocking the CD4 receptor. Given as an intravenous infusion therapy along with other oral HIV medications, it is used as rescue therapy for patients with multidrug-resistant HIV that is not controlled by other treatments. It is given every 2 weeks and can now be given intravenously over 30 seconds.

Common side effects include diarrhea, dizziness, nausea, rash, elevations in creatinine, and lymphopenia.

6. Attachment inhibitor—

FOSTEMSAVIR—The active metabolite of fostemsavir, temsavir, binds to the viral envelope glycoprotein 120, near to the CD4 binding site, such that the virus does not attach to the CD4 cells and cannot enter them. With its unique mechanism, it has no cross-resistance with other antiretrovirals. Unlike maraviroc, it is effective regardless of HIV-1 tropism. It is FDA-approved for use in heavily treatment-experienced adults with multidrug-resistant HIV-1 infection who are not responding to their current regimen. The dosage of fostemsavir is 600 mg orally twice daily, along with an optimized regimen of other antiretroviral medications. It should not be used in conjunction with medications that are strong P450 (CYP)3A inducers, such as rifampin, phenytoin, and St John's wort.

7. Capsid inhibitor—

LENACAPAVIR—Lenacapavir is a first-in-class capsid inhibitor that is very potent and can be given as a single subcutaneous injection every 26 weeks after two oral loading doses. Lenacapavir has been FDA-approved in combination with oral antiretrovirals with residual activity for those with multidrug-resistant HIV, based on the results of the CAPELLA study.

Segal-Maurer S et al; CAPELLA Study Investigators. Capsid inhibition with lenacapavir in multidrug-resistant HIV-1 infection. N Engl J Med. 2022;386:1793. [PMID: 35544387]

8. Constructing an initial regimen—Guidelines for starting ART are shown in Table 35–9. *The regimens with the strongest evidence all contain integrase inhibitors.* This reflects their high efficacy, high barrier to resistance, tolerability, low pill burden, and safety profile. The two best-tolerated, high barrier to resistance integrase inhibitors are bictegravir and dolutegravir and so they form the backbone of the recommended regimens. Integrase inhibitors are typically given with a backbone of two NRTIs (although see discussion of two-drug therapy below). With respect to NRTIs, the most commonly used combination is TDF or TAF with emtricitabine or lamivudine. *From an efficacy standpoint, there is no difference between TDF or TAF*; for patients on a boosted regimen (ie, one including cobicistat or ritonavir), those with renal dysfunction or osteoporosis or osteopenia (or risk for these conditions) should receive TAF. However, TAF is associated with increased weight gain and dyslipidemia, so TDF may be considered in individuals with obesity or dyslipidemia. Also, choosing between TDF and TAF may depend on convenience: which one is coformulated with other desired partner drugs. Emtricitabine and lamivudine are essentially the same from the point of view of efficacy and side effects. The next most commonly used two-drug NRTI backbone is abacavir and lamivudine (coformulated as part of Epzicom or with dolutegravir in Triumeq). Given the need to perform B*5701 allele and hepatitis B testing, abacavir-containing regimens are not appropriate for rapid ART initiation.

The only two-drug regimen approved for initial ART is dolutegravir plus lamivudine, which is available as a single pill for once-a-day treatment (Dovato, Table 35–8). (All other recommended first-line initial regimens contain three medications, sometimes with a fourth agent as a booster.) This two-drug regimen is not recommended for patients with high HIV viral load (> 500,000 copies/mL), or for patients with HBV coinfection (because of development of resistance by the hepatitis B virus to lamivudine when used as monotherapy with possibility of severe flares of hepatitis), or for patients for whom the results from HIV resistance or HBV testing are not yet available. There is also concern about its use in patients with CD4 cell counts < 200/mL. Dolutegravir/rilpivirine (Juluca) and injectable cabotegravir/rilpivirine (Cabenuva) are approved only in the setting of prior virologic suppression without prior treatment failure or drug resistance, although there are promising observational data regarding its use among patients who are not virologically suppressed but do not have resistance to its components and cannot take oral ART.

Studies have shown dolutegravir/abacavir/lamivudine to be superior to efavirenz/TDF/emtricitabine and have shown dolutegravir to be superior to ritonavir-boosted darunavir (both combined with either abacavir/lamivudine or TDF/emtricitabine). A network meta-analysis adjusting for NRTI backbone found that dolutegravir had superior efficacy in suppressing viral load compared with regimens containing ritonavir-boosted atazanavir, ritonavir-boosted darunavir, efavirenz, or ritonavir-boosted lopinavir. Discontinuation due to adverse events was also statistically lower with the dolutegravir regimens.

The emergence of generic antiretroviral medications can affect prescribing choices when equally effective regimens are available at different costs. For instance, for PrEP, the manufacturer of TDF/FTC and TAF/FTC will no longer allow patients to use their assistance program unless the patient is using branded TAF/FTC. There are generic versions available for abacavir, atazanavir, efavirenz, lamivudine, and TDF.

For patients who cannot take an integrase inhibitor, alternative regimens are recommended (Table 35–9).

Resistance testing should be performed prior to starting ART. Of people with newly diagnosed infections in some urban areas of the United States, 8–10% have transmitted drug resistance (most commonly to NNRTIs followed by NRTIs).

The most important determinant of treatment efficacy is adherence to the regimen. Therefore, it is vitally important that the regimen chosen be one to which the patient can easily adhere (Figure 35–7). In general, patients are more adherent if their medication regimens (Table 35–9) offer complete therapy in one pill that needs to be taken only once a day, do not require special timing with regard to meals, can be taken at the same time as other medications, do not require refrigeration or special preparation, and do not have bothersome side effects. Given the high level of effectiveness of recommended regimens, patients for whom the viral load does not fully suppress are likely to be encountering adherence challenges. Pharmacists and other specially trained clinicians can be very effective in helping patients improve their adherence by taking the time to understand why patients miss their

Table 35–9. Recommended and alternative initial antiretroviral therapy regimens (listed in alphabetical order within categories).

Regimen	Advantages	Disadvantages
Recommended Initial Regimens		
Bictegravir + TAF + emtricitabine (Biktarvy)	Single pill once-a-day regimen Low risk of resistance Noninferior to dolutegravir	Less experience in heavily treated patients than with dolutegravir
Dolutegravir (50 mg daily)[1] + Either: emtricitabine/TDF or emtricitabine/TAF or lamivudine/TDF or lamivudine/TAF	Has activity in some patients with integrase resistance Once-a-day regimen Dolutegravir plus either abacavir/lamivudine or emtricitabine/TDF is superior to darunavir/ritonavir plus either of the NRTI backbones	No single tablet available When used in patients with integrase resistance or combined with certain other medications, requires twice-a-day dosing
Dolutegravir + abacavir + lamivudine (Triumeq)	Single pill once-a-day regimen Low risk of resistance Superior to Atripla Dolutegravir plus either abacavir/lamivudine or emtricitabine/TDF is superior to darunavir/ritonavir plus either of the NRTI backbones	Abacavir should be used only in HLA-B*5701-negative persons Should not be used in patients with hepatitis B coinfection When used in patients with integrase resistance or combined with certain other medications, requires twice-a-day dosing Fixed-dose combination should not be used in patients with creatinine clearance < 50 mL/min
Dolutegravir + lamivudine (Dovato)	Only recommended initial two-drug regimen Single pill once-a-day regimen	Not for use in patients with HIV RNA > 500,000 copies/mL, or patients initiating therapy during an opportunistic infection, or patients with hepatitis B coinfection, or patients in whom antiretroviral therapy is being started prior to results of HIV genotypic resistance testing or hepatitis B testing.
Other Integrase Inhibitor Regimens		
Raltegravir (400 mg twice daily or 1200 mg once daily) + Either: emtricitabine/TDF or emtricitabine/TAF or lamivudine/TDF or lamivudine/TAF	Fewest drug interactions of integrase inhibitors	Lower barrier to resistance than bictegravir and dolutegravir Requires twice-a-day dosing or taking two pills once a day No single tablet available
Alternative Initial Regimens That Are Non–Integrase Inhibitor-Based		
Darunavir (800 mg daily) with cobicistat + Either: emtricitabine/TDF or emtricitabine/TAF or lamivudine/TDF or lamivudine/TAF (boosted PI regimen)	Single tablet once-a-day regimen (with emtricitabine and TAF, Symtuza)	Cobicistat boosting causes similar drug-drug interactions as ritonavir; increases in serum creatinine (nonpathologic)

(*continued*)

Table 35–9. Recommended and alternative initial antiretroviral therapy regimens (listed in alphabetical order within categories). (continued)

Regimen	Advantages	Disadvantages
Darunavir (800 mg daily) with ritonavir (100 mg daily) boosting + Either: emtricitabine/TDF or emtricitabine/TAF or lamivudine/TDF or lamivudine/TAF (boosted PI regimen)	Potent boosted PI Can be given once daily Limited risk of resistance with poor adherence	Not available as a single tablet May cause rash in patients with sulfa allergy Ritonavir boosting required Has metabolic side effects
Doravirine with Either: emtricitabine/TDF or emtricitabine/TAF or lamivudine/TDF or lamivudine/TAF	Avoids the use of both integrase inhibitors and PIs Available as a single pill with lamivudine and TDF (Delstrigo) Does inhibit or induce the cytochrome P450 3A4 enzyme	In cases of viral virologic failure, NNRTI cross-resistance may develop.
Rilpivirine/emtricitabine/TDF (Complera) or with emtricitabine/TAF (Odefsey) Non-integrase, non-PI regimens	Single tablet once-a-day regimens Noninferior to Atripla in patients with baseline viral load < 100,000/mL Limited metabolic side effects	Requires taking with a meal Cannot be used with PPIs Use only in patients with viral loads < 100,000 copies/mL and CD4 counts > 200 cells/mcL Do not use in patients with viral loads > 100,000 copies/mL or CD4 counts < 200 cells/mcL

[1]Usual medication doses are supplied when not part of a fixed-dose preparation.
NNRTI, nonnucleoside reverse transcriptase inhibitor (eg, delavirdine, efavirenz, etravirine, nevirapine, rilpivirine); NRTI, nucleoside/nucleotide reverse transcriptase inhibitor (eg, abacavir, didanosine, emtricitabine, lamivudine, stavudine, tenofovir, zidovudine); PI, protease inhibitor; TAF, tenofovir alafenamide; TDF, tenofovir disoproxil fumarate.

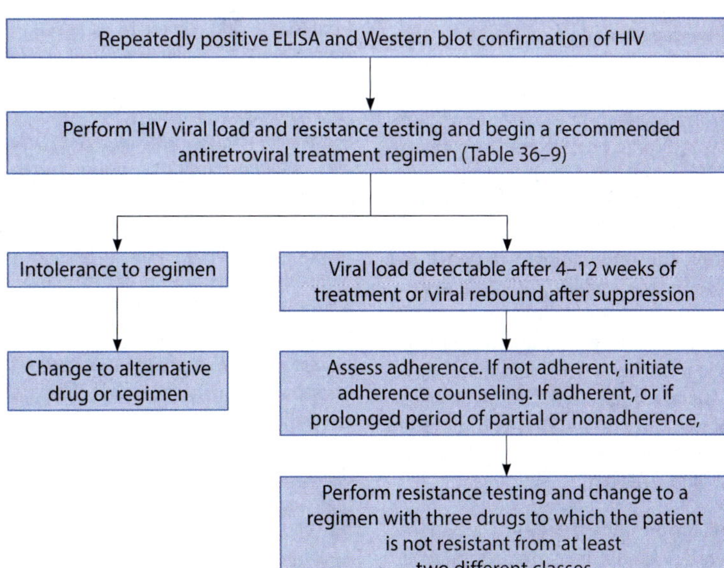

▲ **Figure 35–7.** Approach to monitoring initial and subsequent antiretroviral therapy.

medications and to problem solve (eg, take medicine at same time every day, keep a supply in the car or at work in case they forget). Demonstration projects are examining long-acting cabotegravir and rilpivirine as injectables in people challenged by adherence or viremia, with high virologic suppression achieved in one demonstration project in San Francisco, with 98% of the 129 starting with viremia achieving virologic suppression at 48 weeks compared with 99% in 241 who started with virologic suppression (P = 0.61). In the ACTG5359/LATTITUDE study, participants with adherence challenges were provided financial incentives to achieve viral suppression using oral ART and then were randomized to continue their oral regimen or switch to cabotegravir/rilpivirine. The long-acting ART arm experienced 7.2% cumulative risk of virologic failure compared with 25.4% in the oral ART arm. The International Antiviral Society–USA and DHHS now recommend cabotegravir/rilpivirine among those at high risk of HIV progression who cannot take oral ART, with virus susceptible to both agents. For individuals with HIV resistant to rilpivirine, some clinicians are using cabotegravir and lenacapavir together off label. A case series of 34 individuals using this regimen at 4 academic medical centers achieved high virologic suppression (94%). For certain populations (eg, unstably housed individuals), specially tailored programs may be beneficial.

E. Monitoring Antiretroviral Treatment

1. Goals of monitoring ART—Monitoring of ART (Figure 35–7) has two goals: evaluate for *toxicity* and measure *efficacy* using objective markers to determine whether to maintain or change regimens. Laboratory evaluation for toxicity depends on the specific medications in the combination but generally should be done approximately every 3–6 months once a patient is on a stable regimen. Patients who are intolerant of their initial regimen should be changed to one of the other initial recommended or alternative regimens in Table 35–9. The second aspect of monitoring is to measure HIV viral load, the objective marker of efficacy. The HIV viral load should be repeated 2–4 weeks after the initiation or change of antiretroviral regimen and every 3–6 months thereafter in clinically stable patients. With integrase regimens, a two-$\log_{10}$ reduction is expected within 2 weeks of starting therapy, and approximately 80% of patients will have undetectable HIV viral load at 1 month. *All patients should have undetectable viral loads by 3 months; if not, the usual problem is nonadherence* (see below). CD4+ counts are most useful in determining the immunologic response to ART, although the response can vary significantly, and determining whether opportunistic infection prophylaxis can be discontinued. CD4+ counts should be monitored approximately every 3–6 months in individuals newly initiating ART. For those who have consistently suppressed HIV viral loads over the first 1–2 years of therapy with a CD4+ count > 300 cells/mcL, monitoring can occur yearly, and is optional in those with CD4+ counts > 500 cells/mcL.

2. The challenge of medication adherence—In a patient who is adherent to an integrase inhibitor regimen, viral load should drop by 100-fold within 2 weeks. *For patients in whom viral loads do not decrease adequately, or who have viral rebound after suppression, the major question facing the clinician is whether the patient is nonadherent or has resistance to the regimen, or both.* Patients who are having trouble adhering to their treatment should receive adherence counseling. In patients who are adherent or who have missed enough doses to make resistance possible, resistance testing should be performed. Based on the results of resistance testing, if there is no treatment-emergent resistance, and the patient is tolerating the regimen well, the patient should continue the regimen with assessment of potential barriers to adherence (ie, mental health, substance use, medication coverage, or housing challenges). If resistance has emerged, the patient should be switched to a high-barrier-to-resistance regimen with at least two, but ideally three, active agents (ie, three-drug dolutegravir, bictegravir, or boosted darunavir-based regimen).

Once ART has been initiated, it is not advisable to stop the therapy. So-called drug holidays or structured treatment interruptions are not recommended because they have been shown to increase risk of AIDS-related complications, increase CD4 declines, and increase morbidity from non–AIDS-related complications (eg, MIs and liver failure).

3. The challenge of medication resistance—Resistance to HIV-1 medication has been documented for all currently available antiretrovirals. Although HIV medication resistance was common in the past, high-level resistance has been declining in the past few years, likely related to better tolerated, easier to use, and more efficacious antiretroviral agents. Resistance also occurs in patients who are ART-naïve but who are infected with a medication-resistant strain—called *"primary" or "transmitted" medication resistance.* Cohort studies of ART-naïve patients entering care in North America and Western Europe show that roughly 8–10% of people with a recent infection have a medication-resistant strain of HIV-1.

In addition to being part of a standard baseline evaluation, resistance testing is recommended for patients who are receiving ART and have suboptimal viral suppression (typically a viral load > 500 copies/mL is needed for resistance testing be performed). *Both genotypic and phenotypic resistance tests are commercially available, and in randomized controlled studies, genotypic resistance testing has been shown to result in improved short-term virologic outcomes compared with making treatment choices without resistance testing.* Furthermore, multiple retrospective studies have conclusively demonstrated that resistance tests provide prognostic information about virologic response to newly initiated therapy that cannot be gleaned from standard clinical information (ie, treatment history, examination, CD4 count, and viral load tests).

Because of the complexity of resistance tests, many clinicians require expert interpretation of results. In the case of genotypic assays, results may show that the pathologic variants that are selected for during ART are medication-specific or contribute to broad cross-resistance to multiple medications within a therapeutic class. An example of a medication-specific pathologic variant for the reverse transcriptase inhibitors would be the *M184V* pathologic variant that is selected for by lamivudine or emtricitabine therapy—this pathologic variant causes resistance only to those two medications. Conversely, the thymidine analog pathologic variants ("TAMs") of *M41L,*

D67N, K70R, L210W, T215Y/F, and *T219Q/K/E* are selected for by either prior zidovudine or stavudine therapy, but cause resistance to all the medications in the class and often extend to the nucleotide inhibitor tenofovir when three or more of these TAMs are present. The combination of *M184V* and *K65R* is important to know as it causes resistance to all NRTIs except zidovudine and would typically necessitate change to an NRTI-sparing regimen. The most common pathologic variants associated with medication resistance and cross-resistance patterns for NRTIs, NNRTIs, PIs, and integrase inhibitors can be found at https://hivdb.stanford.edu (see specific references below). Phenotypic resistance testing can provide complementary data and is usually provided with an interpretation about susceptibility to the virus.

Resistance results may be misleading if a patient is not taking antiretroviral medications at the time of testing because the dominant virus is likely the wild-type, even if there are resistant viruses in the body that can become dominant with the selective pressure of antivirals. Thus, resistance results do not replace a careful history of what medications a patient has taken in the past and for how long. Also, the results of resistance testing should be viewed cumulatively—ie, if resistance is reported to an agent on one test, it should be presumed to be present thereafter even if subsequent tests do not give the same result.

The Stanford University HIV Drug Resistance Database (https://hivdb.stanford.edu/) provides a genotypic resistance interpretation algorithm.

F. Constructing Antiretroviral Treatment Regimens for Patients with Resistance

In designing second-line regimens for patients with resistance to initial therapy, the goal is to identify three medications from at least two different classes to which the virus is not resistant. Even without resistance testing, certain forms of cross-resistance between medications within a class can be assumed. For example, the resistance patterns of raltegravir and elvitegravir are overlapping, and patients with treatment-emergent resistance to these regimens potentially harboring resistance to second-generation integrase inhibitors such as bictegravir and dolutegravir. Fostemsavir (an attachment inhibitor), ibalizumab (a monoclonal antibody), and lenacapavir (a subcutaneously administered capsid inhibitor) are specifically FDA approved for heavily treated adults with multidrug-resistant HIV who are not responding to their existing regimen. They are used in combination with other antiretroviral drugs.

In constructing regimens, toxicities should be nonoverlapping and agents that are either virologically antagonistic or incompatible in terms of drug-drug interactions should be avoided. For example, dolutegravir and etravirine should not be coadministered without inclusion of a ritonavir-boosted PI, as etravirine will reduce the plasma concentrations of dolutegravir. The combination of TDF and boosted PIs should ideally be avoided given the potential for increased tenofovir toxicity with this regimen. Coformulated TAF and boosted PI regimens (ie, emtricitabine/TAF/darunavir or Symtuza) are preferred in this setting given these are the only formulations where a lower dose of TAF is available (10 mg versus typical 25 mg dose). Lamivudine and emtricitabine are very similar medications and so are not used together.

Given the availability of new class medications and new generation medications, *a combination of ART can successfully treat virtually all patients—no matter how much resistance is present.*

Course & Prognosis

With improvements in therapy, patients who have access to effective regimens and are adherent to treatment should have life spans that approach the mean. A population-based study conducted in Denmark found that people aged 25 years with HIV without hepatitis C had a life expectancy similar to that of a 25-year-old without HIV. Unfortunately, there are racial and ethnic disparities in the uptake of ART. *Studies consistently show disparities in uptake and maintenance of ART among patients with HIV who self-identify as Black and those with housing insecurity or who inject recreational drugs.* For patients whose disease progresses even though they are receiving appropriate treatment, palliative care must be provided (see Chapter 5), with attention to pain control, spiritual needs, and family (biologic and chosen) dynamics.

When to Refer

- People with HIV in whom viral loads cannot be fully suppressed on one of the initial recommended regimens should be treated in consultation with a specialist.
- Specialty consultation is particularly important for those patients with detectable viral loads on ART; those intolerant of standard medications; those in need of systemic chemotherapy; and those with complicated opportunistic infections, particularly when invasive procedures or experimental therapies are needed.

When to Admit

Admit patients with opportunistic infections who are acutely ill (eg, who are febrile, who have had rapid change of mental status, or who are in respiratory distress) or who require intravenous medications.

Gandhi M et al. Demonstration project of long-acting antiretroviral therapy in a diverse population of people with HIV. Ann Intern Med. 2023;176:969. [PMID: 37399555]

Gandhi M et al. Case series of people with HIV on the long-acting combination of lenacapavir and cabotegravir: call for a trial. Open Forum Infect Dis. 2024;11:ofae125. [PMID: 38628952]

Gistand N et al. Long-term virologic suppression rates in the Ward 86 HIV Clinic's Long-Acting ART Program (SPLASH). Accessed March 15, 2026. https://www.natap.org/2025/CROI/croi_185.htm

Panel on Opportunistic Infections in Adults and Adolescents with HIV. Guidelines for the prevention and treatment of opportunistic infections in adults and adolescents with HIV. Accessed March 15, 2026. https://clinicalinfo.hiv.gov/en/guidelines/hiv-clinical-guidelines-adult-and-adolescent-opportunistic-infections/whats-new

Segal-Maurer S et al; CAPELLA Study Investigators. Capsid inhibition with lenacapavir in multidrug-resistant HIV-1 infection. N Engl J Med. 2022;386:1793. [PMID: 35544387]

36 Viral & Rickettsial Infections

John Szumowski, MD, MPH
James H. Acuff, MD
Wayne X. Shandera, MD

Over the last few decades, the recognition and impact of viral and rickettsial diseases have increased dramatically—especially following COVID-19. Emerging and re-emerging, clinically important viruses and rickettsial/tick-borne pathogens include those that have adapted to new environments because of travel and importation (eg, West Nile virus, chikungunya, mpox), climate change, and expanded vector ranges (eg, dengue, Zika, Japanese encephalitis, tick-borne encephalitis viruses, *Ehrlichia*), and tightening of human-animal interfaces (eg, avian influenza, coronaviruses, Ebola, murine typhus). The most notable new viral pathogen to enter human populations was SARS-CoV-2, the causative agent of COVID-19. The global scientific community has responded to many of these threats by working together to develop new diagnostics, therapeutics, vaccines, and public health interventions, and to improve access to existing ones.

For viral pathogens, novel immunotherapies have been successful against some (eg, CAR T-cell therapy for cytomegalovirus in immunocompromised patients), and novel and repurposed antiviral agents are now widely available for others (remdesivir, molnupiravir, nirmatrelvir/ritonavir for SARS-CoV-2). Novel vaccines and therapeutics have been recently developed for RSV for patients 60 years and older, pregnant women, and neonates. In contrast, older, well-known viruses (eg, rabies, arboviruses, common cold coronaviruses) continue to cause extensive and sometimes severe disease in the absence of new therapeutic and preventive agents. Less attention has been paid to rickettsial diseases, although pathogens such as *Rickettsia rickettsii* and *R typhi* infect increasingly large swaths of the population. Perhaps as important as effective diagnostics, therapeutics, and vaccines, dedicated attention to environmental and climate issues is urgently needed to control and prevent diseases due to new, variant, and re-emerging viral and rickettsial pathogens. Our knowledge of these pathogens is advancing rapidly because of exciting technological leaps in vaccinology, multiomics (proteomics, transcriptomics, genomics, metabolomics), and diagnostics.

VIRAL DISEASES

HUMAN HERPESVIRUSES

1. Herpesviruses 1 & 2

ESSENTIALS OF DIAGNOSIS

- Spectrum of illness: stomatitis, urogenital lesions, Bell palsy, encephalitis.Variable intervals between exposure and clinical disease since herpes simplex virus (HSV) causes both primary and reactivation disease.

General Considerations

HSV-1 and HSV-2 affect primarily the oral and genital areas, respectively (but can cause disease at either site). Most persons with HSV-2 infection in the United States are unaware they are infected. Asymptomatic shedding of either virus is common, but it is more common with HSV-2 and from genital areas. Most infected individuals shed virus at least once a month, which may contribute to transmission. Individuals with asymptomatic HSV-2–infection shed the virus less often than those with symptomatic infection. Total and subclinical shedding of HSV-2 virus decreases after the first year of initial infection, although viral shedding continues for years thereafter.

HSV-2 seropositivity is associated with higher risk of HIV acquisition, and HSV-2 reactivates more often in advanced HIV infection. HIV replication is increased by interaction with HSV proteins. Suppression of HSV-2 decreases HIV plasma levels and genital tract shedding of HIV, which can contribute to a reduction in the sexual transmission of HIV. Pregnancy is also associated with reactivation of HSV-2.

Clinical Findings

A. Symptoms and Signs

1. Mucocutaneous disease—See Chapter 6 for HSV-1 mucocutaneous disease ("**herpes labialis**" or "**gingivostomatitis**"). Digital lesions (herpetic **whitlow**) (Figure 36–1) are an occupational hazard in medicine and dentistry. Contact sports (eg, wrestling) are associated with skin infections ("**herpes gladiatorum**").

Vesicles form moist, painful ulcers after several days and epithelialize over 1–2 weeks if untreated. Primary infection is usually more severe than recurrences but may be asymptomatic. Recurrences often involve fewer lesions, tend to be labial, heal faster, and may be triggered by stress, fever, infection, sunlight, and chemotherapy.

HSV-2 lesions largely involve the genital tract. The virus typically remains latent in the presacral ganglia, and shedding of HSV-2 can occur for years after acquisition (see Chapter 6). Occasionally, lesions arise in the perianal region or on the buttocks and upper thighs. Dysuria, cervicitis, and urinary retention may occur in women. Urethritis may occur in men. Proctitis and extensive, ulcerating, sacral lesions may be presenting symptoms in patients with HIV with low CD4 counts.

Two distinct dermatologic signs are reported in immunosuppressed patients with HSV2 infection: a knife-cut sign and dorsal glossitis.

2. Ocular disease—HSV can cause uveitis, keratitis, blepharitis, and keratoconjunctivitis (see Chapter 7). Lesions limited to the epithelium usually heal without affecting vision, whereas stromal involvement can cause uveitis, scarring, and eventually blindness. HSV is the second most common infectious cause of acute retinal necrosis, after varicella-zoster virus (VZV).

3. Neonatal and congenital infection—HSV-1 or HSV-2 can infect the fetus and induce congenital malformations (organomegaly, bleeding, and CNS abnormalities). Neonatal transmission during delivery is more common than intrauterine infection. The global rate of neonatal herpes is estimated to be about 10 cases per 100,000 live births. Maternal infection during the third trimester is associated with the highest risk of neonatal transmission, but about 70% of these infections are asymptomatic or unrecognized. Invasive fetal monitoring and vacuum or forceps delivery increase the risk of herpesvirus transmission. Neonatal disease can present primarily with cutaneous findings (involving skin, eyes, and mouth) but can also cause disseminated disease, including CNS involvement.

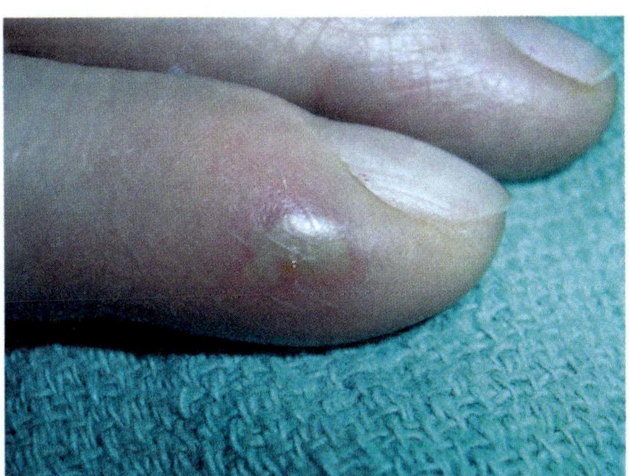

▲ **Figure 36–1.** Herpetic whitlow. (Reproduced with permission from Richard P. Usatine, MD, in Usatine RP, Smith MA, Mayeaux EJ Jr, Chumley H. *The Color Atlas of Family Medicine,* 2nd ed. McGraw-Hill, 2013.)

4. CNS disease—Traditionally, herpes simplex encephalitis is associated with HSV-1 infection and aseptic meningitis with HSV-2 infection. Both viruses, however, can cause encephalitis and may affect both immunocompromised and immunocompetent persons. Encephalitis presents with nonspecific symptoms: a flu-like prodrome followed by headache, fever, behavioral and speech disturbances, and focal or generalized seizures. The temporal lobe is often involved. Untreated disease and presentation with coma are associated with high mortality. Ischemic stroke, although infrequent, can complicate the course of HSV meningitis or encephalitis or can happen in isolation due to HSV-induced cerebral vasculitis. Many survivors suffer neurologic sequelae, which are observed more frequently among patients with HSV-1 infection. While primary HSV infection may present with aseptic meningitis, HSV-2 is also associated with benign recurrent lymphocytic (Mollaret) meningitis.

5. Disseminated infection—Disseminated HSV infection occurs most often in immunosuppression, either primary or iatrogenic, or rarely with pregnancy. In disseminated disease, skin lesions are not always present. Disseminated skin lesions are a particular complication in patients with atopic eczema (**eczema herpeticum**) and burns. Elevated hepatocellular enzymes suggest hepatic involvement, which may cause severe liver disease (see below).

6. Bell palsy—HSV-1 is a cause of Bell palsy (facial nerve paralysis) (see also Chapter 27).

7. Esophagitis and proctitis—HSV-1 can cause esophagitis in immunocompromised patients, particularly those with advanced HIV. The lesions are smaller and deeper than those observed in patients with cytomegalovirus (CMV) esophagitis. Rarely HSV esophagitis is accompanied by significant upper GI hemorrhage. Proctitis occurs mainly in men who have sex with men.

8. Erythema multiforme—HSV infections are a leading cause of erythema multiforme minor ("**herpes-associated erythema multiforme**") and a more severe skin condition, Stevens-Johnson syndrome/toxic epidermal necrolysis (see also Chapter 6).

9. Hepatitis—HSV infection causes approximately 1% of cases of acute liver failure, particularly in pregnant patients and those with immunosuppression. HSV hepatitis may not be associated with a rash. The mortality of fulminant hepatitis is nearly 75%, necessitating a low clinical suspicion for HSV in these cases.

10. Pneumonitis—Pulmonary disease is uncommon and noted primarily in heavily immunocompromised persons (such as persons with hematologic malignancies), where it is associated with high mortality. In addition to causing tracheitis, HSV may manifest as focal pulmonary disease or bilateral interstitial pneumonitis.

11. Alzheimer disease—There are neuropathologic studies and observational evidence supporting an association between HSV-1 infection and Alzheimer's disease. However, the evidence remains insufficient to establish a causal relationship because HSV infection is highly prevalent, there are many interacting cofactors, and randomized clinical trials of antiviral therapy have not yet demonstrated prevention of Alzheimer's disease.

B. Laboratory Findings

1. Mucocutaneous disease—See Chapter 6.

2. Ocular disease—Herpes keratitis is diagnosed by branching (dendritic) ulcers that stain with fluorescein. The extent of epithelial injury in herpes keratitis correlates well with PCR positivity. HSV uveitis is often diagnosed clinically, although PCR assays (including a multiplex assay that includes VZV) on anterior chamber aspirate may assist in making the diagnosis.

3. Encephalitis and meningitis—CSF typically shows a lymphocyte-predominant pleocytosis and elevated protein; RBCs or xanthochromia also may be noted. CSF findings may be atypical in immunosuppressed patients. HSV PCR of the CSF is a rapid, sensitive, and specific tool for early diagnosis and can be included in a multiple rapid array panel. HSV CSF PCR is rarely negative when tested very early in the illness, and it should be repeated after 3–5 days if clinical suspicion persists. Viral culture has limited sensitivity, and assay turnaround times are longer than PCR testing. MRI brain may demonstrate increased signal in the temporal and frontal lobes. Temporal lobe seizure foci may be shown on electroencephalograms (EEGs).

4. Esophagitis, proctitis, and other GI disease—Esophagitis is diagnosed by endoscopic biopsy with PCR and cultures. Proctitis may be diagnosed by rectal swab for PCR or culture. Complicated cases may require biopsy.

5. Pneumonia—Pneumonia is diagnosed by clinical, pathologic, and radiographic findings. The CT findings include diffuse or multifocal areas of ground-glass attenuation or consolidative changes or both and are best confirmed using HRCT techniques. Positive HSV PCR from respiratory specimens usually represents contamination from oral HSV reactivation, especially in immunocompetent patients. Tissue biopsy demonstrating viral inclusions provides stronger evidence for pneumonia but is infrequently done.

6. Disseminated disease—In addition to the organ-specific testing noted above, blood PCR may be positive.

Prevention

Multiple interventions should be considered to reduce the risk of HSV transmission. These include suppressive antiviral therapy for the infected individual (see above and also Chapter 6), patient counseling, and use of barrier protection such as condoms. Disclosure to sexual partners of HSV-seropositive status is associated with about a 50% reduction in HSV-2 acquisition. Male circumcision is also associated with a lower incidence of acquiring HSV-2 infection.

Standard precautions should be used by healthcare personnel caring for persons with active HSV infection. Contact precautions (eg, use of a gown) should be employed in cases with more extensive mucocutaneous disease until herpetic lesions are dry and crusted. Staff with active lesions (eg, whitlows) should not have contact with patients. No herpes vaccine is publicly available, although several vaccine candidates have undergone clinical trials.

Treatment & Prophylaxis

Medications that inhibit replication of HSV-1 and HSV-2 include acyclovir and related compounds (famciclovir, valacyclovir), foscarnet, cidofovir, and trifluridine and vidarabine (both for keratitis) (Table 36–1). Agents under study include the helicase-primase inhibitors pritelivir and amenamevir, which have activity against VZV and HSV. Pritelivir is being further evaluated in a phase 3 trial for treating acyclovir-resistant mucocutaneous HSV in immunocompromised patients. Brincidofovir, a lipid conjugate of cidofovir, showed in vitro activity against HSV/VZV and was effective in one retrospective study in hematopoietic cell transplant recipients as HSV/VZV prophylaxis; however, further clinical trial data are needed.

A. Mucocutaneous Disease

See Chapter 6.

B. Keratitis and Uveitis

For treating acute epithelial keratitis, oral antiviral agents such as valacyclovir or famciclovir are first-line therapies (see Chapter 7). Topical corticosteroids may exacerbate the infection, although systemic corticosteroids may help with selected cases of stromal infection. Long-term treatment (> 1 year) with acyclovir at a dosage of 800 mg/day orally decreases recurrence rates of keratitis, conjunctivitis, or blepharitis due to HSV.

C. Neonatal Disease

Counseling (but not serologic screening) should be offered to pregnant mothers. The use of maternal antenatal suppressive therapy with acyclovir (400 mg orally three times daily) or valacyclovir (500 mg twice daily) beginning at 36 weeks' gestation decreases the presence of detectable HSV, the rates of recurrence at delivery, and the need for cesarean delivery. Cesarean delivery is recommended for pregnant persons with active genital lesions or typical prodromal symptoms. Infants with proven or suspected HSV should receive treatment with intravenous acyclovir (20 mg/kg every 8 hours for 14 days, extended to 21 days with CNS involvement). Management of neonatal herpes is beyond the scope of this chapter, and cases should be managed with assistance of a pediatric infectious diseases specialist.

Table 36–1. Agents for viral infections (listed in alphabetical order).[1]

Drug	Dosing[2]	Spectrum	Toxicities
Acyclovir	**HSV and VZV infections:** 400 mg orally three times daily or 200 mg orally five times daily; 10 mg/kg intravenously every 8 hours (total 30 mg/kg/day) for 7–10 days **Acute herpes encephalitis:** 10 mg/kg intravenously every 8 hours (total 30 mg/kg/day) for 14–21 days	HSV, VZV	Neurotoxic reactions, reversible kidney dysfunction, local reactions
Baloxavir	<80 kg: 40 mg orally as a single dose ≥ 80 kg: 80 mg orally as a single dose	Influenza A and B strains	Diarrhea, vomiting, and bronchitis
Cidofovir	5 mg/kg intravenously weekly for 2 weeks, then every other week	CMV	Neutropenia, kidney disease, ocular hypotonia
Famciclovir	**Acute VZV:** 500 mg orally three times daily for 7 days **Genital or cutaneous HSV-1/HSV-2:** 250 mg three times daily for 7–10 days; 125 mg twice daily for 5 days for recurrences (500 mg twice daily for 5–10 days if HIV-positive)	HSV, VZV	Early angioedema; later rarely, GI symptoms, headaches, rashes
Foscarnet	**Induction:** 90 mg/kg intravenously every 12 hours or 60 mg/kg intravenously every 8 hours for 14–21 days **Maintenance:** 90–120 mg/kg intravenously once daily **HSV:** 40 mg/kg/dose intravenously every 8 to 12 hours for 14–21 days	HSV resistant to acyclovir, CMV, VZV, HIV-1	Nephrotoxicity, genital ulcerations, calcium disturbances
Ganciclovir	**Induction:** 5 mg/kg intravenously every 12 hours for 14–21 days **Maintenance:** 6 mg/kg/day intravenously for 5 days each week	CMV	Neutropenia, thrombocytopenia, CNS side effects
Idoxuridine (not available in the United States)	Topical, 0.1% every 1–2 hours for 3–5 days	HSV keratitis	Local reactions
Interferon alfa-2b	**HBV infection:** 10 million units subcutaneously three times weekly or 5 million units daily[1] **Condylomata:** 1 million units intralesionally in up to five warts three times weekly for 3 weeks	HBV, HCV, HPV	Influenza-like syndrome, myelosuppression, neurotoxicity
Interferon alfa-n3	**Refractory or recurring external condylomata acuminata:** 0.05 mL (250,000 units) per wart intralesionally twice weekly for up to 8 weeks; 0.5 mL (2.5 million units) is the maximum dose per treatment session	HPV, HCV	Local reactions Influenza-like syndrome, myelosuppression, neurotoxicity
Nirmatrelvir/ritonavir	300/100 mg orally twice daily for 5 days	SARS-CoV-2	Adjust for renal dysfunction, multiple drug interactions
Oseltamivir	75 mg orally twice daily for 5 days	Influenza A and B	Adjust for renal dysfunction
Palivizumab	15 mg/kg intramuscularly every month in RSV season	RSV	Upper respiratory infection symptoms
Penciclovir	Topical 1% cream every 2 hours during waking hours for 4 days	HSV	Local reactions
Peramivir	600 mg intravenously as a single dose	Uncomplicated influenza A	Nausea, vomiting, diarrhea, neutropenia
Remdesivir	200 mg intravenously on day 1 followed by 100 mg intravenously once daily for 4 days for non-ICU patients, 9 more days for ICU patients	SARS-CoV-2	Transaminitis, fatigue, headaches, nausea
Ribavirin	**RSV infection:** one vial (6 g) dissolved and delivered through a small particle aerosol generator (SPAG-2) over a continuous 12- to 18-hour period daily for 5 consecutive days	RSV, severe influenza A or B, Lassa fever	Wheezing, hemolytic anemia
Trifluridine	Topical, 1% drops every 2 hours during waking hours (maximum 9 drops per day)	HSV keratitis	Local reactions

(*continued*)

Table 36–1. Agents for viral infections (listed in alphabetical order).[1] (continued)

Drug	Dosing[2]	Spectrum	Toxicities
Valacyclovir	**Acute VZV:** 1 g orally three times daily for 7 days **Primary genital HSV-1/HSV-2:** 1 g orally twice daily for 7–10 days **Recurrent genital HSV-1/HSV-2:** 500 mg orally twice daily for 3 days or 1 g orally once daily for 5 days **Suppressive therapy:** 1 g orally daily; 500 mg orally daily if fewer than 9 recurrences/year (Dose depends on immune status and number of recurrences.)	VZV, HSV	Thrombotic thrombocytopenic purpura or hemolytic-uremic syndrome in AIDS
Valganciclovir	900 mg orally twice daily for 3 weeks; 900 mg daily as maintenance	CMV	See ganciclovir
Zanamivir	Two inhalations (10 mg) twice daily for 5 days	Uncomplicated influenza A and B	Bronchospasm in patients with asthma

Sources: Data from Drugs.com and Lexicomp Online.

[1]Agents used exclusively in the management of HIV infection and AIDS are found in Chapter 36. Agents used in the management of HBV and HCV infections are found in Chapter 16.

[2]Dosing varies considerably by indication and may require adjustment based on patient's clinical state and type of viral infection. Consultation with a pharmacist is recommended.

CMV, cytomegalovirus; HBV, hepatitis B virus; HCV, hepatitis C virus; HSV, herpes simplex virus; VZV, varicella-zoster virus.

D. Encephalitis and Meningitis

Because of the need for rapid treatment to decrease mortality and neurologic sequelae, intravenous acyclovir (10 mg/kg every 8 hours for 10 days or more, adjusting for kidney disease) should be started in those patients with suspected HSV encephalitis, *stopping only if another diagnosis is established.* If the PCR of CSF is negative but clinical suspicion remains high, an LP should be repeated and acyclovir continued. Note that the recommended duration of therapy is longer (14–21 days) for immunosuppressed patients. Acyclovir resistance in herpes simplex encephalitis has been reported but is unusual. Long-term neurologic sequelae of HSV encephalitis are common, and relapse is recognized.

The role for antiviral therapy of aseptic meningitis in immunocompetent persons remains uncertain, as the condition is typically self-limiting; early transition to oral antiviral therapy can be considered in cases where treatment is pursued. Long-term oral valacyclovir prophylaxis, however, does not appear to prevent recurrences of HSV-2 aseptic meningitis.

E. Disseminated Disease

Disseminated disease responds best to parenteral acyclovir when treatment is initiated early.

F. Bell Palsy

While steroids have been demonstrated to improve time to clinical recovery, the role for antiviral therapy in cases of Bell palsy is less clear. Antivirals are not typically recommended but are nevertheless sometimes considered in cases of more severe disease.

G. Esophagitis and Proctitis

Patients with severe disease should receive intravenous acyclovir (5–10 mg/kg every 8 hours) and can be transitioned to oral antiviral therapy (acyclovir, valacyclovir, or famciclovir) once they can swallow and when absorption is felt to be adequate. Duration of therapy depends on resolution of symptoms, typically at least 5 days. Secondary prophylaxis pending immune recovery is typically recommended in immunocompromised persons with following an episode of severe disease or with frequent recurrences.

H. Erythema Multiforme

Suppressive therapy with oral acyclovir (400 mg twice a day for 6 months) decreases the recurrence rate of HSV-associated erythema multiforme. Valacyclovir (500 mg orally twice a day) may be effective in cases unresponsive to acyclovir.

Cohen PR. Clinical features of atypical presentations of mucocutaneous herpes simplex virus infection observed in immunosuppressed individuals. Part I: herpetic geometric glossitis. Dermatol Online J. 2024;30(1). [PMID: 38762852]

Cohen PR. Clinical features of atypical presentations of mucocutaneous herpes simplex virus infection observed in immunosuppressed individuals. Part II: the knife-cut sign. Dermatol Online J. 2024;30(1). [PMID: 38762853]

Cho YE et al. Heterogeneous population of macrophages in the development of non-alcoholic fatty liver disease. Liver Res. 2022;7:16. [PMID: 39959694]

Dovrat S et al. Analysis of HSV1/2 infection reveals an association between HSV-2 reactivation and pregnancy. Viruses. 2024; 16:1370. [PMID: 39339846]

2. Varicella (Chickenpox) & Herpes Zoster (Shingles)

ESSENTIALS OF DIAGNOSIS

- **Varicella rash:** pruritic, centrifugal, papular changing to vesicular ("dew drops on a rose petal"), pustular, and finally crusting.
- **Zoster rash:** tingling, pain, eruption of vesicles in a dermatomal distribution, evolving to pustules and then crusting.

General Considerations

VZV manifests as chickenpox (varicella) following primary infection and as shingles (herpes zoster) following reactivation.

Chickenpox generally presents during childhood and has an incubation period of 10–20 days (average 2 weeks). It is highly contagious, spreading by inhalation of infective droplets or contact with lesions.

The incidence and severity of herpes zoster ("**shingles**"), which *affects up to 30% of persons during their lifetime*, increase with age due to an age-related decline in immunity against VZV. More than half of all patients in whom herpes zoster develops are older than 60 years, and the incidence of herpes zoster reaches 10 cases per 1000 patient-years by age 80 (by which time 50% are infected with VZV), although the global burden of VZV disease in those 70 and over is slightly decreasing because of improved management strategies. The annual incidence of 1 million cases in the United States is increasing as the population ages. Patients who are immunocompromised as a result of advanced HIV, malignancy, transplantation status, or other immunosuppressive therapies are also at increased risk of zoster and zoster-related complications such as disseminated disease.

Clinical Findings

A. Varicella

1. Symptoms and signs—Fever and malaise are mild in children and more marked in adults. The pruritic rash begins prominently on the face, scalp, and trunk and later involves the extremities (Table 36–2). The macular/papular rash evolves within a few hours to vesicles that become pustular and eventually form crusts (Figure 36–2) (Figure 36–3). New lesions may erupt for 1–5 days, so different stages of the eruption are usually present simultaneously. The crusts slough in 7–14 days. The vesicles and pustules are superficial and elliptical, with slightly serrated borders. Although the disease is often mild, complications (such as secondary bacterial infection, pneumonitis, and encephalitis) occur in ~1% of cases and often lead to hospitalization.

Varicella is more severe in older patients and immunocompromised persons (including pregnancy). In the latter, atypical presentations, including widespread dissemination in the absence of skin lesions, are often described. After the primary infection, the virus remains dormant in cranial nerve sensory ganglia and spinal dorsal root ganglia. *Latent VZV will reactivate as herpes zoster in about 30% of persons.*

2. Laboratory findings—Leukopenia and subclinical transaminase elevation are often present, and thrombocytopenia occasionally occurs. Diagnosis is usually made clinically, with confirmation by direct immunofluorescent antibody staining or PCR of scrapings from lesions or CSF, both of which are more sensitive than culture. The exception is VZV vasculopathy, which can be diagnosed via anti-VZV IgG detection in the CSF with a reduced serum/CSF ratio. Note that anti-VZV **IgG** will typically become detectable in the CSF after 2 weeks of illness, while VZV DNA may be detectable only for the first 2 weeks of infection. Although elevation of varicella IgM is occasionally used to diagnose a primary VZV infection, the assay has poor performance and is generally not recommended. A varicella skin test and interferon γ (IFN-γ) enzyme-linked immunospot (ELISPOT) can screen for VZV susceptibility.

B. Herpes Zoster

Herpes zoster ("shingles") usually occurs among adults, but cases are reported among infants and children. Shingles incidence rises markedly with age because of immunosenescence and loss of specific immunity to VZV, with rates of 8 to 12 per 1000 person-years in individuals older than 80 years. Skin lesions typically develop into clusters of vesicles over 3–5 days and can be painful or pruritic. Superficial sensory symptoms such as pain are often severe and commonly *precede* the appearance of rash by several days. Lesions follow a dermatomal distribution, with thoracic and lumbar roots being the most common. In most cases, a single unilateral dermatome is involved, but occasionally, neighboring and distant areas are involved. If lesions cover three or more dermatomes, disease is considered to be *disseminated.* Lesions eventually dry and crust over; in untreated immunocompetent individuals they take 2–4 weeks to heal and can leave hyperpigmented macular scars. Lesions on the tip of the nose, inner corner of the eye, and root and side of the nose **(Hutchinson sign)** indicate involvement of the trigeminal nerve **(herpes zoster ophthalmicus).** Facial palsy and lesions of the external ear with or without tympanic membrane involvement, vertigo, tinnitus, or deafness signify geniculate ganglion involvement **(Ramsay Hunt syndrome** or **herpes zoster oticus).** Shingles is a common and serious complication among immunosuppressed patients.

Complications

A. Varicella

Secondary bacterial skin superinfections, particularly with group A *Streptococcus* and *Staphylococcus aureus*, are the most common complications. Cellulitis, erysipelas, and scarlet fever are described. Bullous impetigo and necrotizing fasciitis are less often seen. Other associations with varicella include epiglottitis, necrotizing pneumonia, osteomyelitis, septic arthritis, epidural abscess, meningitis, endocarditis, pancreatitis, giant cell arteritis, IBD, and purpura fulminans.

Interstitial VZV pneumonia is more common in adults (especially those who smoke cigarettes, patients with HIV, and pregnant persons) and may result in acute respiratory distress syndrome. After healing, numerous densely calcified lesions are seen throughout the lung fields on CXRs.

Historically, neurologic complications developed in about 1 in 2000 children (cerebellar ataxia in 1:4000, specifically). A limited course and complete recovery are the rule. Encephalitis is similarly infrequent, occurs mostly in adults, and is characterized by delirium, seizures, and focal neurologic signs. The rates for both mortality and long-term neurologic sequelae are about 10%. Ischemic strokes in the wake of acute VZV infection present at a mean of

Table 36–2. Diagnostic features of some acute exanthems (listed in alphabetical order).

Disease	Prodromal Signs and Symptoms	Nature of Eruption	Other Diagnostic Features	Laboratory Tests
Chikungunya fever	2–4 (sometimes 1–12) days, fever, headaches, abdominal complaints, myalgias, arthralgias.	Maculopapular, centrally distributed, pruritus, can be bullous with sloughing in children, occasional facial edema and petechiae.	History of mosquito bites, epidemiologic factors.	ELISA-based IgM or IgG (fourfold increase in titers); PCR and cultures are infrequently available.
Eczema herpeticum	None.	Vesiculopustular lesions in area of eczema.		HSV isolated in cell culture. Multinucleated giant cells in smear of lesion.
Ehrlichiosis	Headache, malaise.	Rash in one-third, similar to Rocky Mountain spotted fever.	Pancytopenia, elevated liver biochemical tests.	PCR, immunofluorescent antibody.
Enterovirus infections	1–2 days of fever, malaise.	Maculopapular rash resembling rubella, rarely papulovesicular or petechial.	Aseptic meningitis.	Virus isolation from stool or CSF; complement fixation titer rise.
Erythema infectiosum (Parvovirus B19)	None. Usually in epidemics.	Red, flushed cheeks; circumoral pallor; maculopapules on extremities.	"Slapped face" appearance.	WBC count normal.
Exanthema subitum (HHV-6, 7; roseola)	3–4 days of high fever.	As fever falls, pink maculopapules appear on chest and trunk; fade in 1–3 days.		WBC count low.
Infectious mononucleosis (EBV)	Fever, adenopathy, sore throat.	Maculopapular rash resembling rubella, rarely papulovesicular.	Splenomegaly, tonsillar exudate.	Atypical lymphocytes in blood smears; heterophile agglutination (Monospot test).
Kawasaki disease	Fever, adenopathy, conjunctivitis.	Cracked lips, strawberry tongue, maculopapular polymorphous rash, peeling skin on fingers and toes.	Edema of extremities. Angiitis of coronary arteries.	Thrombocytosis, electrocardiographic changes.
Measles (rubeola)	3–4 days of fever, coryza, conjunctivitis, and cough.	Maculopapular, brick red; begins on head and neck; spreads downward and outward, in 5–7 days rash brownish, desquamating.	Koplik spots on buccal mucosa.	WBC count low. Virus isolation in cell culture. Antibody tests by hemagglutination inhibition or neutralization.
Meningococcemia	Hours of fever, vomiting.	Maculopapules, petechiae, purpura.	Meningeal signs, toxicity, shock.	Cultures of blood, CSF. WBC count high.
Rocky Mountain spotted fever	3–4 days of fever, vomiting.	Maculopapules, petechiae, initial distribution centripetal (extremities to trunk, including palms).	History of tick bite.	Indirect fluorescent antibody; complement fixation.
Rubella	Little or no prodrome.	Maculopapular, pink; begins on head and neck, spreads downward, fades in 3 days. No desquamation.	Lymphadenopathy, postauricular or occipital.	WBC count normal or low. Serologic tests for immunity and definitive diagnosis (hemagglutination inhibition).
Scarlet fever	One-half to 2 days of malaise, sore throat, fever, vomiting.	Generalized, punctate, red; prominent on neck, in axillae, groin, skin folds; circumoral pallor; fine desquamation involves hands and feet.	Strawberry tongue, exudative tonsillitis.	Group A β-hemolytic streptococci in cultures from throat; antistreptolysin O titer rise.

(*continued*)

Table 36–2. Diagnostic features of some acute exanthems (listed in alphabetical order). (continued)

Disease	Prodromal Signs and Symptoms	Nature of Eruption	Other Diagnostic Features	Laboratory Tests
Typhus	3–4 days of fever, chills, severe headaches.	Maculopapules, petechiae, initial distribution centrifugal (trunk to extremities).	Endemic area, lice.	Complement fixation.
Varicella (chickenpox)	0–1 day of fever, anorexia, headache.	Rapid evolution of macules to papules, vesicles, crusts; all stages simultaneously present; lesions superficial, distribution centripetal.	Lesions on scalp and mucous membranes.	Specialized complement fixation and virus neutralization in cell culture. Fluorescent antibody test of smear of lesions.

[1]https://www.cdc.gov/smallpox EBV, Epstein-Barr virus; EM, electron microscopy; HHV, human herpesvirus; HSV, herpes simplex virus; Ig, immunoglobulin.

4 months after rashes (highest relative risk within 1 month after infection) and may be due to an associated vasculitis. Multifocal encephalitis (described without a rash in solid organ transplant recipients), ventriculitis, myeloradiculitis, arterial aneurysm formation, Ramsay Hunt syndrome, optic neuritis (with zoster ophthalmicus), and arteritis are also described in immunosuppressed individuals, especially those with HIV. When seizures develop in immunosuppressed patients, especially those taking corticosteroids, disseminated zoster should be considered.

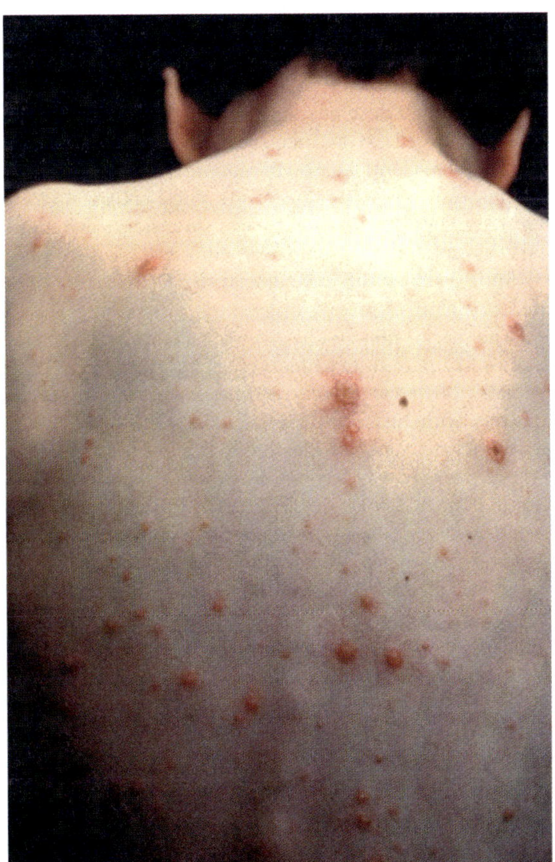

▲ **Figure 36–2.** Primary varicella (chickenpox) skin lesions. (Public Health Image Library, CDC.)

Clinical hepatitis is uncommon and mainly presents in the immunosuppressed patient but can be fulminant and fatal. **Reye syndrome** (fatty liver with encephalopathy) also rarely complicates varicella (and other viral infections, especially influenza B virus), usually in childhood, and is associated with aspirin therapy (see Influenza, below).

When contracted during the first or second trimesters of pregnancy, varicella carries a minuscule risk of congenital malformations, including cicatricial lesions of an extremity, growth retardation, microphthalmia, cataracts, chorioretinitis, deafness, and cerebrocortical atrophy. If varicella develops around the time of delivery, the newborn is at risk for disseminated disease.

B. Herpes Zoster

Postherpetic neuralgia occurs in 10–13% of patients who have herpes zoster and are older than 60 years. The pain

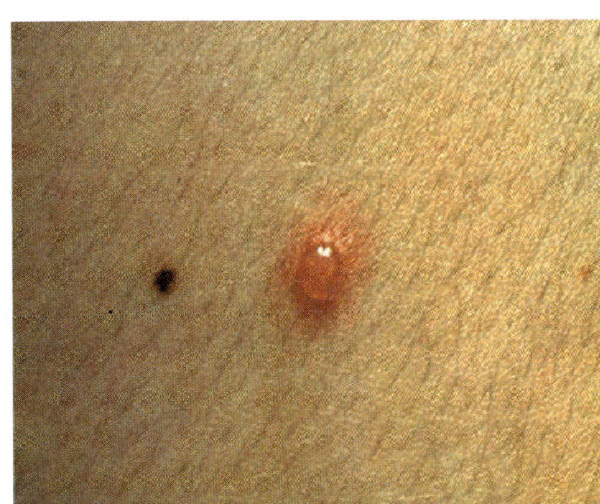

▲ **Figure 36–3.** Chickenpox (varicella) with classic "dew drop on rose petal" appearance. (Reproduced with permission from Richard P. Usatine, MD, in Usatine RP, Smith MA, Mayeaux EJ Jr, Chumley H. *The Color Atlas of Family Medicine,* 2nd ed. McGraw-Hill, 2013.)

can be prolonged and debilitating. Risk factors for postherpetic neuralgia include advanced age, female sex, the presence of a prodrome, obstructive sleep apnea and other comorbidities, and presence/severity of rash or pain. Treatment within 3 days of rash onset appears to prevent the development of postherpetic neuralgia.

Other complications include the following: (1) bacterial skin superinfections; (2) herpes zoster ophthalmicus (HZO), which occurs with involvement of the trigeminal nerve, is a *sight-threatening complication* (especially when it involves the iris), and is a marker for vasculopathic stroke over the ensuing year with the highest risk in the month immediately following the herpes zoster episode—but also evolves into uveitis in about 50% of those with HZO, and this usually appears in the second week of HZO; (3) rarely, unilateral ophthalmoplegia; (4) keratitis; (5) involvement of the geniculate ganglion of cranial nerve VII as well as cranial nerves V, VIII, IX, and X; (6) aseptic meningitis; (7) peripheral motor neuropathy; (8) transverse myelitis, which can become chronic; (9) encephalitis; (10) acute cerebellitis; (11) stroke; (12) vasculopathy; (13) acute retinal necrosis; (14) progressive outer retinal necrosis (largely among patients with HIV); (15) temporal arteritis; and (16) sacral meningoradiculitis (Elsberg syndrome). Visceral dissemination in immunocompromised patients is rare and fatal over half the time. VZV is a major cause of Bell palsy in patients who are HSV seronegative.

Diagnosis of neurologic complications generally requires detection of VZV DNA in CSF or tissue. The exception is VZV vasculopathy, which can be diagnosed via VZV antibodies (see Laboratory findings, above). **Zoster sine herpete** (pain without rash) can also be associated with most of the above complications. A molecular assay can help distinguish HSV from VZV for patients with keratitis.

Varicella-zoster increases maternal and fetal morbidity, and pregnant persons should be advised to avoid exposure to VZV.

Prevention

Healthcare workers should be screened for varicella and vaccinated if seronegative. Patients with active varicella or herpes zoster are promptly separated from seronegative patients. For patients with varicella, airborne and contact isolation is recommended, whereas for those with zoster, contact precautions are sufficient. However, airborne precautions should be added if disease affects three or more dermatomes. For immunosuppressed patients with zoster, precautions should be the same as if the patient had varicella. Exposed serosusceptible patients should be placed in isolation and exposed serosusceptible employees should stay away from work for 8–21 days after exposure. Healthcare workers with zoster should receive antiviral agents during the first 72 hours of disease and withdraw from work until lesions are crusted. The need for postexposure prophylaxis should be assessed.

A. Varicella

1. Vaccination—Universal childhood vaccination against varicella is effective. The varicella vaccine is *live and attenuated*, safe, and > 98.1% effective when given after 13 months of age. A single antigen live attenuated vaccine (VARIVAX, VARILRIX) or a quadrivalent measles, mumps, rubella, and varicella (MMRV) vaccine (ProQuad) is available (the combination is immunogenic). The first dose of the single antigen vaccine should be administered at 12–18 months of age and the second at 4–6 years. Alternatively, the MMRV vaccine can be given as a first dose at 12–15 months of age and the second dose before elementary school entry. *Aspirin should be avoided for at least 6 weeks after vaccination because of the risk of Reye syndrome.* The single-antigen vaccine is safe and well-tolerated, but the quadrivalent MMRV vaccine is associated with a small risk of febrile seizures 5–12 days after vaccination in infants aged 12–23 months. Because of this risk, the CDC recommends using separate varicella and MMR vaccines for the first dose in children younger than 48 months old. Rashes, when secondary to the varicella vaccine, appear 15–42 days after vaccination. Rare cases of keratitis are associated with zoster and varicella vaccines.

For serosusceptible individuals older than 13 years, two doses of varicella vaccine (single antigen) administered 4–8 weeks apart are recommended. For those who previously received a single dose, a *catch-up second dose* is advised, especially in the epidemic setting (where it is effective when given during the first 5 days postexposure). Household contacts of immunocompromised patients should adhere to these recommendations. Susceptible pregnant persons (who should not be vaccinated with live varicella or zoster vaccines during pregnancy) must receive the first dose of single antigen vaccine before discharge after delivery and the second dose 4–8 weeks later. The Advisory Committee on Immunization Practices (ACIP) recommends administration of the single-antigen varicella vaccine as two doses 3 months apart to children living with HIV aged 12 months or older with CD4 cell percentage > 15% and adolescents and adults with CD4 cell counts 200/mcL or higher (regardless of age).

The vaccine may also be given to patients with impaired humoral immunity, to patients receiving corticosteroids, to pediatric oncology patients receiving chemotherapy, and to patients with juvenile rheumatoid arthritis who receive methotrexate. Patients receiving high-dose corticosteroids for > 2 weeks may be vaccinated 1 month after discontinuing therapy. Patients with leukemia, lymphoma, or other malignancies whose disease is in remission and who have not undergone chemotherapy for at least 3 months may be vaccinated. Kidney and liver transplant patients should be vaccinated if they are susceptible to varicella.

The incidence of varicella in the United States is significantly reduced with the varicella vaccine. Although uncommon, the varicella vaccine, like other live varicella-zoster vaccines, can reactivate and cause clinical disease. Vaccination against varicella is thought to provide less protection against future zoster than natural varicella infection. The incidence of varicella-associated group A streptococcal infection and varicella neurologic complications are both diminished with the advent of varicella vaccination.

The FDA no longer maintains a registry for exposed pregnant persons because of the low rate of such incidents and the general safety of varicella vaccines. Incidents can be reported to Merck (877-888-4231) or through the Vaccine Adverse Events Registry System Vaccine (https://vaers.hhs.gov/index).

2. Postexposure—Postexposure vaccination is recommended for unvaccinated persons without other evidence of immunity. **Varicella-zoster immune globulin** available in the United States only as VariZIG should be considered for susceptible exposed patients (for up to 10 days after exposure but as soon as feasible) who should not receive the vaccine, including immunosuppressed patients, neonates from mothers with varicella around the time of delivery, exposed premature infants born from serosusceptible mothers at > 28 weeks' gestation, and neonates born at <28 weeks' gestation regardless of maternal serostatus. Varicella and zoster vaccines are not recommended for pregnant persons.

No controlled studies have evaluated the use of acyclovir in this setting. VariZIG is given by intramuscular injection in a dosage of 125 IU/10 kg, to a maximum of 625 IU with a weight-based (2-kg cutoff) minimum dose of 62.5 or 125 IU), with a repeat identical dose in 3 weeks if a high-risk patient remains exposed. VariZIG has no place in therapy of established disease; however, it reduces severity of varicella in high-risk children or adults (ie, those with impaired immunity and infants exposed peripartum) if given within 4 days of exposure. Varicella vaccination should be delayed at least 5 months after VariZIG administration. If VariZIG is unavailable, standard pooled intravenous immunoglobulin (IVIG) (400 mg/kg given in one dose) can be given. Acyclovir (40–80 mg/kg) for 5 days or the varicella vaccine (if not contraindicated) can also be given as postexposure prophylaxis within 3 days of exposure. Either of these options offers an efficacy of 70–85% compared with 90% efficacy for VariZIG.

Further information may be obtained by calling the CDC's Immunization Information Hotline (1-800-232-4636).

B. Herpes Zoster

Shingrix, HZ/su (GlaxoSmithKline Biologicals), an adjuvanted recombinant subunit vaccine, is approved by the FDA for VZV and is recommended for immunocompetent individuals aged 50 years or older, as well as for adults aged 19 years or older who are or will be immunodeficient or immunosuppressed because of disease or therapy (including people living with HIV). *Shingrix is preferred over the older live attenuated VZV vaccine* (Zostavax, no longer available in the United States). Shingrix is particularly effective in reducing the incidence of herpes zoster infection and postherpetic neuralgia in adults aged 70 years or older; immunosenescence to the vaccine does not appear to occur in older patients; strong, persistent immune responses are seen > 7 years after initial vaccination. Vaccine efficacy has ranged from 70% to 100% in different studies over a follow-up period of 2–7 years, with more rapidly waning efficacy seen in patients who only received one dose (48% by year 3). Shingrix is safe in persons with HIV and with immune restoration (typically CD4 cell counts > 50/mcL), recipients of autologous stem cell transplants, and adults with autoimmune disease taking immunosuppressive therapy. However, it may be less efficacious in immunocompromised hosts, as reported in patients taking corticosteroids at the time of immunization.

Even if the person has had a prior episode of herpes zoster, Shingrix vaccine has efficacy and should be administered. No specific recommendations exist regarding how long to wait between a zoster outbreak and administering the vaccine; the CDC recommends waiting until the outbreak has resolved, and other experts suggest waiting up to a year as herpes zoster itself will boost VZV-specific immunity for several years. Concurrent administration of the adjuvanted recombinant subunit VZV vaccine with pneumococcal vaccine, adjuvanted influenza vaccine (Fluad), and/or COVID-19 vaccines is safe. The CDC recommends that recombinant and adjuvanted vaccines, such as Shingrix, be administered concomitantly with other adult vaccines at different anatomic sites.

If a varicella vaccine is mistakenly administered to an adult instead of the adjuvanted recombinant subunit vaccine zoster vaccine, the dose should be considered invalid, and the patient should be administered a dose of zoster vaccine at the same visit. The zoster vaccine cannot be used in children in place of varicella vaccine; if the vaccine is accidentally given to a child, the event should be reported to the CDC. If Zostavax is administered to an adult when Shingrix is indicated, the Shingrix series can be initiated 8 weeks later.

A new herpes zoster mRNA vaccine (ZOSAL) has shown superior vaccine immunity and safety profile compared with Shingrix in mice and rhesus macaques, but it has yet to be studied in humans.

Treatment

A. General Measures

In general, patients with varicella should be isolated until primary lesions have crusted. Pruritus can be relieved with antihistamines, calamine lotion, and colloidal oatmeal baths. Fever can be treated with acetaminophen (*not* aspirin). Fingernails can be closely cropped to avoid skin excoriation and infection. Hospitalized individuals with open, disseminated herpes zoster skin lesions (ie, lesions that cross three or more dermatomes) should be placed on both contact and airborne isolation until lesions crust over.

B. Antiviral Therapy

1. Varicella—Uncomplicated disease in otherwise healthy children and adolescents does not require antiviral therapy. Acyclovir, 20 mg/kg (max 800 mg per dose) orally four times daily for 5–7 days, should be given within the first 24 hours after the onset of varicella rash and should be considered for patients older than 12 years, secondary household contacts (disease tends to be more severe in secondary cases), patients with chronic cutaneous and cardiopulmonary diseases, and children receiving long-term therapy with salicylates (to decrease the risk of Reye syndrome). Famciclovir is not approved for anyone under 18 years of age. Valacyclovir can be given for patients 2 and older at a dose of 20 mg/kg (max 1000 mg) three times daily for 5 days. Children under 2 should be treated with acyclovir, as the safety of valacyclovir has not been established for this age group. There is no consensus dosing for acyclovir for this age group.

In immunocompromised patients, in pregnant persons during the third trimester, and in patients with extracutaneous disease (encephalitis, pneumonitis), antiviral therapy with high-dose intravenous acyclovir (30 mg/kg/day in three divided doses for at least 7 days, 10 days for encephalitis) *should be started once the diagnosis is suspected.* The oral alternative is 800 mg four times daily for 5–10 days, based on the disease state treated. Corticosteroids may be useful in the presence of pneumonia. Prolonged prophylactic acyclovir is important to prevent VZV reactivation in profoundly immunosuppressed patients. Adjuvant treatment with VSV-specific immunoglobulins for patients with pneumonia is advocated by some experts.

2. Herpes zoster—For uncomplicated herpes zoster, valacyclovir or famciclovir is preferable to acyclovir due to dosing convenience and higher drug levels in the body (Table 36–1). *Therapy should start within the first 72 hours of the onset of the lesions* and be continued until the lesions have all crusted over (typically 7–14 days). Bromovinyl deoxyuridine (brivudine) is another therapy for herpes zoster used primarily in Europe (not available in the United States). *Antiviral therapy reduces the duration of herpetic lesions and associated episodes of acute pain but does not decrease the risk of postherpetic neuralgia.* Corticosteroids (a tapering course, eg, starting at prednisone 60 mg/day, for 2–3 weeks or methylprednisolone 24 mg/day for 1–2 weeks) are safe in immunocompetent patients and may be useful in the acute management of disease to hasten the resolution of zoster-related pain.

Intravenous acyclovir is used for extradermatomal complications of zoster. Adjunctive therapy may be considered in retinal disease (eg, vitreal foscarnet infections) and acute herpes zoster (eg, sorivudine, a topical antiviral). In cases of prolonged or repeated acyclovir use, immunosuppressed patients may require a switch to intravenous foscarnet due to the development of acyclovir-resistant VZV infections.

C. Treatment of Postherpetic Neuralgia

Once established, postherpetic neuralgia is difficult to treat, and less than half of patients achieve adequate pain relief. This condition may respond to neuropathic pain agents such as gabapentin or lidocaine patches. Tricyclic antidepressants and capsaicin cream are also widely used and effective; use of opioids in managing neuropathic pain is controversial and based on limited evidence, and their long-term use should be avoided. The epidural injection of corticosteroids and local anesthetics appears to modestly reduce herpetic pain at 1 month but, as with oral corticosteroids, is not effective for prevention of long-term postherpetic neuralgia. Transcutaneous electrical nerve stimulation or pulsed radiofrequency is reportedly successful. Gabapentin appears to show efficacy as a preventive medication in reducing the risk of postherpetic neuralgia in patients with diabetes and neuropathy. Duloxetine initiated during the initial outbreak may also reduce pain scores at 12 weeks, although randomized, *placebo-controlled* studies on this are lacking. Available evidence suggests that vaccination with the recombinant zoster vaccine (Shingrix; see Herpes Zoster section under Vaccination, below) significantly reduces the duration of herpes zoster–related pain.

Prognosis

The total duration of varicella from onset of symptoms to disappearance of crusts rarely exceeds 2 weeks. Fatalities are rare except in immunosuppressed patients, where in hospitalized patients it was as high as 8% in one French cohort study.

Herpes zoster resolves in 2–6 weeks. Antibodies persist longer and at higher levels than with primary varicella. Eye involvement with herpes zoster necessitates periodic future examinations.

A long-term association under study is the development of Alzheimer disease. Studies from two San Francisco Bay–area medical schools among those vaccinated with the recombinant vaccine (now replaced with Shingrix) show a decrease over several years in the onset of Alzheimer disease. Studies using Shingrix are needed for confirmation, but these and HSV-1/2 studies suggest an important association between herpesviruses and the development of late-term neurodegenerative disorders.

Eyting M et al. A natural experiment on the effect of herpes zoster vaccination on dementia. Nature. 2025;641:438. [PMID: 40175543].

Meyer JJ et al. Herpes zoster ophthalmicus uveitis: onset and complications. Am J Ophthalmol. 2024;268:409. [PMID: 39307262]

Wang Y et al. Effect of antivirals plus low-dose, short-term glucocorticoids on post-herpetic neuralgia. Eur J Dermatol. 2023;33:413. [PMID: 37823492]

Zerbo O et al. Effectiveness of recombinant zoster vaccine against herpes zoster in a real-world setting. Ann Intern Med. 2024;177:189. [PMID: 38190712]

3. Epstein-Barr Virus & Infectious Mononucleosis

ESSENTIALS OF DIAGNOSIS

- Malaise, fever, and sore throat
- Palatal petechiae, lymphadenopathy, splenomegaly; occasionally, a maculopapular rash.
- Positive heterophile agglutination test (Monospot).
- Atypical large lymphocytes in blood smear; lymphocytosis.
- Complications: hepatitis, myocarditis, neuropathy, encephalitis, airway obstruction from adenitis, hemolytic anemia, thrombocytopenia.

General Considerations

Epstein-Barr virus (EBV) is one of the most ubiquitous human viruses, infecting > 95% of adults worldwide.

Infectious mononucleosis is a common manifestation of EBV and may occur at any age following primary infection. In the United States, the incidence of EBV infection is declining, although it remains high for those 12–19 years old. In low- and middle-income countries, infectious mononucleosis occurs at younger ages and tends to be less symptomatic. EBV is largely transmitted by saliva but can also be recovered from genital secretions. Saliva may remain infectious for 6 months or longer after symptom onset. Although infectious mononucleosis is generally a benign condition, EBV has also been linked to malignancies and other chronic conditions, as discussed further below.

Clinical Findings

A. Symptoms and Signs

The early phase of infectious mononucleosis is classically marked by fever, sore throat, fatigue, malaise, anorexia, and myalgia. Physical findings include lymphadenopathy (discrete, nonsuppurative, slightly painful, especially along the posterior cervical chain), transient upper lid edema (**Hoagland sign**), and splenomegaly (in up to 50% of patients and sometimes massive). A maculopapular or petechial rash may occur in 20% of patients; historically rash was associated with ampicillin treatment but appears to be less common in more recent reports. Conjunctival hemorrhage, soft palate petechiae, tonsillar exudates, and uvular edema also may be noted.

Other manifestations include hepatitis, interstitial pneumonitis (sometimes with pleural involvement), cholestasis, gastritis, kidney disease (mostly interstitial nephritis), and epiglottitis. Involvement of the nervous system is uncommon (1–5% of cases) and can manifest in diverse ways such as aseptic meningitis, encephalitis, cerebellitis, peripheral and optic neuritis, transverse myelitis, or Guillain-Barré syndrome. Airway obstruction from lymph node enlargement can occur. Complications of acute disease are more common among older adults.

B. Laboratory Findings

An initial phase of granulocytopenia is followed within 1 week by lymphocytic leukocytosis with atypical lymphocytes (larger than normal mature lymphocytes that may demonstrate irregular shape) constituting > 10% of the leukocyte count. Hemolytic anemia occurs occasionally, as does thrombocytopenia.

Diagnosis is typically made based on characteristic manifestations and serologic evidence of infection. Historically, heterophile antibody tests (eg, Monospot) were used. However, the Monospot test suffers from limited sensitivity—particularly in younger children and early in infection—and has been largely replaced with EBV-specific serologic panels. During acute illness, immunoglobulin M (IgM) antibody to EB virus capsid antigen (VCA) rises and falls, and immunoglobulin G (IgG) antibody to VCA rises and persists for life. Antibodies (IgG) to EBV nuclear antigen (EBNA) appear after 4 weeks of onset and persist thereafter. Absence of IgG and IgM VCA or the presence of IgG EBNA should make one reconsider the diagnosis of acute EBV infection.

EBV PCR testing is available but is usually not used in the routine evaluation of a patient being evaluated for possible infectious mononucleosis.

Differential Diagnosis

CMV infection, toxoplasmosis, acute HIV infection, secondary syphilis, HHV-6 infection, rubella, and drug hypersensitivity reactions (eg, to the anticonvulsants carbamazepine or phenytoin) may mimic infectious mononucleosis due to EBV, but exudative pharyngitis is usually absent and the heterophile antibody tests are negative. With acute HIV infection, rash and mucocutaneous ulceration are common but atypical lymphocytosis is much less common. Heterophile-negative infectious mononucleosis with nonsignificant lymphocytosis (especially if rash or mucocutaneous ulcers are present) should prompt investigation for acute HIV infection. CMV, toxoplasmosis, and, on occasion, EBV can cause heterophile-negative infectious mononucleosis with atypical lymphocytosis. *Mycoplasma* infection may also present as pharyngitis, though lower respiratory symptoms usually predominate.

The differential diagnosis of acute exudative pharyngitis includes gonococcal and streptococcal infections, as well as infections with adenovirus and herpes simplex. Head and neck soft-tissue infections (pharyngeal and tonsillar abscesses) may occasionally be mistaken for the lymphadenopathy of mononucleosis.

Complications

Splenic rupture (0.5–1%) is a rare but dramatic complication, and a history of preceding trauma can be elicited in 50% of cases. Acalculous cholecystitis, fulminant hepatitis with massive necrosis, pericarditis, myocarditis, and hemophagocytic lymphohistiocytosis (HLH) are also infrequent complications of acute EBV infection. Additional EBV-associated conditions are discussed below.

Treatment

A. General Measures

More than 95% of patients with acute EBV-associated infectious mononucleosis recover without specific therapy. Treatment is supportive. Antiviral therapy targeting EBV has not shown clinical benefit, possibly due to absent viral DNA polymerase expression during latent infection. Corticosteroid therapy, although widespread, is *not* recommended in uncomplicated cases; its use is reserved for impending airway obstruction from enlarged lymph nodes, hemolytic anemia, and severe thrombocytopenia. The value of corticosteroid therapy in impending splenic rupture, pericarditis, myocarditis, and nervous system involvement is less well established. Ampicillin and amoxicillin are traditionally avoided with concomitant EBV because of the frequent association with rash (90%); if rash occurs, it does not preclude future challenge with amoxicillin or ampicillin.

B. Treatment of Complications

Hepatitis, myocarditis, and encephalitis are treated symptomatically. Splenic rupture is associated with vigorous physical activity and requires splenectomy. *Patients should avoid contact or collision sports for at least 4 weeks to decrease the risk of splenic rupture (even if splenomegaly is not detected by physical examination, which can be insensitive).*

Prognosis

In uncomplicated cases, fever disappears in 10 days and lymphadenopathy and splenomegaly in 4 weeks. The debility sometimes lingers for 2–3 months.

Death is uncommon and is usually due to splenic rupture, hypersplenic phenomena (severe hemolytic anemia, thrombocytopenic purpura), or encephalitis.

4. Other EBV-Associated Conditions

Persons living with HIV, particularly at lower CD4 counts, may have **oral hairy leukoplakia**. This condition is generally asymptomatic and can be mistaken for oral candidiasis. It classically affects the lateral aspect of the tongue and, unlike candidiasis, does not scrape off with a tongue blade.

EBV is also associated with multiple malignancies, including nasopharyngeal carcinoma, Burkitt lymphoma (particularly endemic and HIV-associated types), a subset of Hodgkin lymphomas, and primary CNS lymphoma among others. Antiviral therapy has not shown benefit in these cases. Immunosuppression should be reduced if possible, and persons with HIV should be started on antiretroviral therapy. Rituximab is shown to be a useful supplement to chemotherapy for patients in Africa with Burkitt lymphoma.

Both solid organ and stem cell transplant recipients are at risk for **posttransplant lymphoproliferative disorder (PTLD)**. EBV-driven B-cell proliferation accounts for up to 50% of PTLD cases. Clinical presentation can vary from asymptomatic disease to acute illness, and PTLD can involve the allograft, lymph nodes, and other extranodal tissues such as the gastrointestinal tract and the central nervous system. In addition to reduction of immunosuppression, B cell–targeted therapies such as rituximab are commonly used in these cases. About 30–40% of PTLD patients are refractory to low-dose therapy and require aggressive chemotherapy.

EBV is also implicated in multiple chronic conditions, though demonstrating causality has been challenging. Associations with gastric conditions including gastric cancer are pathologically approaching causation. Recent work has demonstrated a potential mechanism (molecular mimicry) that suggests a causal link between EBV infection and some cases of multiple sclerosis.

When to Admit

Presence of severe complications of EBV disease including the following:

- Acute meningitis, encephalitis, or Guillain-Barré syndrome.
- Severe thrombocytopenia; significant hemolysis.
- Potential splenic rupture.
- Airway obstruction from severe adenitis.
- Pericarditis.
- Abdominal findings mimicking an acute abdomen.

El-Mallawany NK et al. EBV and post-transplant lymphoproliferative disorder: a complex relationship. Hematology Am Soc Hematol Educ Program. 2024;2024:728. [PMID: 39644052]

Naughton P et al. Infectious mononucleosis: new concepts in clinical presentation, epidemiology, and host response. Curr Opin Infect Dis. 2024;37:157. [PMID: 38529804]

Putukian M et al. American Medical Society of Sports Medicine Position Statement: mononucleosis and athletic participation. Clin J Sport Med. 2023 May 15. [Epub ahead of print] [PMID: 37186809]

5. Cytomegalovirus Disease

ESSENTIALS OF DIAGNOSIS

- Mononucleosis-like syndrome.
- Frequent pathogen seen in populations with compromised cellular immunity, such as transplant recipients.
- Diverse clinical syndromes in HIV (retinitis, esophagitis, colitis, encephalitis).
- Important infectious cause of congenital abnormalities.

General Considerations

CMV infection is common. In high-income countries, the seroprevalence in adults is about 60–80%; it is even higher in low- and middle-income countries.Transmission occurs through sexual contact, receipt of blood products, or transplantation. In pediatric cases, important routes of transmission include close contact (as in day-care centers), breastfeeding, and intrauterine transmission. *Most CMV infections are asymptomatic.* Severe disease occurs primarily in immunocompromised persons, including those post–organ transplant, with advanced HIV, and with IBD.

Three recognizable clinical syndromes exist: (1) perinatal disease and CMV inclusion disease, (2) diseases in immunocompetent persons, and (3) diseases in immunocompromised persons. Congenital CMV infection is the most common congenital infection in high-income countries (about 0.6% of live births, with higher rates in underdeveloped areas and among lower socioeconomic groups). Transmission is much higher from mothers with primary disease than those with reactivation (40% compared with 0.2–1.8%). About 10% of infected newborns will be symptomatic with CMV inclusion disease.

In immunocompetent persons, acute CMV infection is the most common cause of the mononucleosis-like syndrome with negative heterophile antibodies. In critically ill immunocompetent adults, CMV reactivation is associated with prolonged hospitalization and death.

CMV is usually disseminated in persons with compromised cellular immunity, leading to several different clinical manifestations, described below. Solid organ and bone marrow transplant patients are at highest risk for disease from CMV reactivation for a year after allograft transplantation (but especially during the first 100 days post-transplantation) and in particular when graft-versus-host disease is present. For solid organ transplant recipients, the risk is increased when the donor is CMV-seropositive and the recipient is seronegative. On the other hand, for patients undergoing stem cell transplantation, the risk of CMV reactivation and CMV disease is highest in cases of CMV-seronegative donor and seropositive recipient. Depending on the serostatus of the donor and recipient, disease may present as primary infection or reactivation. The risk of CMV disease is proportionate to the degree of immunosuppression and manifestations may differ by the cause. CMV may contribute to transplanted organ dysfunction, which often mimics organ rejection.

Clinical Findings

A. Symptoms and Signs

1. Perinatal disease and CMV inclusion disease—CMV inclusion disease in infected newborns is characterized by hepatitis, thrombocytopenia, microcephaly, periventricular CNS calcifications, mental retardation, and motor disability. Hearing loss develops in > 50% of infants who are symptomatic at birth, making CMV a leading cause of pediatric hearing loss. Most infected neonates are asymptomatic, but neurologic deficits may ensue later in life, including hearing loss in 15% and cognitive impairment in 10–20%. Perinatal infection acquired through breastfeeding or blood products typically has a benign clinical course.

2. Disease in immunocompetent persons—Symptomatic disease in uncommon among immunocompetent adults. Acute CMV infection may present as a mononucleosis-like illness with fever, malaise, myalgias, arthralgias, and splenomegaly. In comparison with EBV-associated mononucleosis, in CMV infection exudative pharyngitis or cervical lymphadenopathies are uncommon whereas cutaneous rashes are common. The mean duration of symptoms is 7–8 weeks. Complications include mucosal GI damage, encephalitis, hepatitis, thrombocytopenia, Guillain-Barré syndrome, pericarditis, and myocarditis. A mononucleosis-like syndrome due to CMV can also occur post-splenectomy, often years later, and is associated with a protracted fever, marked lymphocytosis, and impaired anti-CMV IgM response.

3. Disease in immunocompromised persons—Distinguishing between CMV *infection* (with evidence of CMV replication) and CMV *disease* (evidence for systemic symptoms or organ invasion by pathologic diagnosis) is important. In addition to patients with HIV, transplant recipients (solid organ or hematopoietic stem cell) show a broad spectrum of disease including ocular, GI (eg, colitis, esophagitis, and acute cholecystitis), kidney, and CNS disease.

A. CMV RETINITIS—A funduscopic examination reveals neovascular, proliferative lesions ("pizza-pie" retinopathy). Immune restoration with ART is associated with CMV vitritis and cystoid macular edema.

B. GI AND HEPATOBILIARY CMV—Esophagitis presents with odynophagia. Gastritis can occasionally cause bleeding, and small bowel disease may mimic IBD or may present as ulceration or perforation. Colonic CMV disease causes diarrhea, hematochezia, abdominal pain, fever, and weight loss and may mimic IBD. CMV hepatitis causes a range of liver pathology from asymptomatic transaminase elevation with primary CMV infection to acute liver failure.

C. RESPIRATORY CMV—CMV pneumonitis is characterized by cough, dyspnea, and relatively little sputum production. Co-infection with *Pneumocystis jirovecii* can be seen, and the interaction with CMV may be synergistic.

D. NEUROLOGIC CMV—Neurologic syndromes associated with CMV include polyradiculopathy, transverse myelitis, ventriculoencephalitis, and encephalitis. These manifestations are more prominent in patients with advanced HIV in whom the encephalitis has a subacute onset.

B. Laboratory Findings

1. Mothers and newborns—Congenital CMV disease is confirmed by the presence of the virus in amniotic fluid or an IgM assay from fetal blood. Amniocentesis is less reliable before 21 weeks' gestation (due to inadequate fetal urinary development and release into the amniotic fluid), but amniocentesis is associated with greater risk when performed after 21 weeks' gestation. PCR assays or culture of the newborn's urine, saliva, or blood specimens obtained during the first 3 weeks of life are used to diagnose congenital CMV infection. CMV viral load in blood and urine appears to correlate with clinical disease.

2. Immunocompetent persons—The acute mononucleosis-like syndrome is characterized by initial leukopenia; within 1 week, it is followed by absolute lymphocytosis with atypical lymphocytes. Abnormal liver biochemical tests are common in the first 2 weeks of the disease (often 2 weeks after the fever). Detection of CMV DNA, specific IgM, or a fourfold increase of specific IgG levels supports the diagnosis of acute infection.

3. Immunocompromised persons—Tissue biopsy is the gold standard for diagnosing CMV end-organ disease, though it is not always feasible. In CMV retinitis, however, clinical exam findings in a typical host (eg, patient with advanced AIDS) are sufficient to make a presumptive diagnosis. Fluid cultures may lack specificity, as viral shedding is common in immunocompromised persons. Serologic testing has limited utility given high baseline seropositivity in many populations. However, among patients with HIV, a negative CMV IgG lowers the likelihood of CMV disease.

PCR testing has proved useful for diagnosing CMV in immunocompromised populations. Blood/plasma PCR testing can be challenging to interpret given frequency of herpes virus viremia in association with serious illness and immunocompromise. Nevertheless, quantitative PCR testing is commonly used in transplant recipients to guide treatment and prevention. Serial PCR should be compared using the same specimen type (ie, whole blood or plasma). CSF should be sent for CMV PCR in cases of suspected neurologic involvement. Reactivation of CMV is very common (791.4%) among ICU-treated, CMV IgG–positive patients.

C. Imaging

The CXR findings of CMV pneumonitis are consistent with interstitial pneumonia.

D. Biopsy

Tissue confirmation is especially useful in diagnosing CMV pneumonitis and CMV GI disease; the diagnosis of colonic CMV disease is made by mucosal biopsy showing characteristic CMV histopathologic findings of intranuclear ("owl's eye") and intracytoplasmic inclusions. When biopsy does not yield diagnostic findings but CMV colitis is suspected, CMV DNA PCR might help identify additional cases.

Prevention

Primary prevention is best accomplished by good hand hygiene and use of barrier methods during sexual activity.

A major source of CMV for pregnant persons is their own young children, particularly those in childcare. Measures to decrease their risk of contracting primary CMV include practicing hand hygiene after changing diapers and after contact with respiratory secretions, as well as avoiding sharing utensils, food, and cleansing objects that have been in contact with children's secretions.

Antiretroviral therapy is effective in preventing CMV disease among patients with HIV. While secondary prophylaxis is routine following an episode of CMV retinitis pending CD4 reconstitution, primary prophylaxis is not recommended.

The use of leukocyte-depleted blood products effectively reduces the incidence of CMV disease in transplant recipients. Prophylactic and preemptive strategies (eg, antiviral agents only when antigen detection or PCR assays show evidence of active CMV replication) appear equally effective in preventing invasive disease and mortality after hematopoietic stem cell transplant. The appropriate management of transplant patients is based on the serostatus of the donor and the recipient. All effective anti-CMV therapies can serve as prophylactic agents for CMV-seropositive transplants or for CMV-seronegative recipients of CMV-positive organ transplants. In addition to valganciclovir, letermovir is useful in prophylaxis against CMV infections in adult allogenic hematopoietic stem cell transplant recipients. It is given as 480 mg orally daily using a loading dose with dose adjustments for cyclosporine administration and for advanced kidney dysfunction. Recommended duration of CMV prophylaxis in posttransplant patients and in other immunocompromised patients varies by the type of transplant. In high-risk patients, treatment longer than 100 days may be needed.

CMV immune globulin is used in some centers as part of the prophylaxis in kidney, liver, and lung transplantation patients.

Treatment & Prognosis

In immunocompetent persons, CMV infection is usually self-limited, and no specific antiviral therapy is needed. In contrast, in immunocompromised persons, treatment of CMV disease is necessary. CMV disease in immunocompromised patients is generally treated initially with intravenous ganciclovir (5 mg/kg every 12 hours, adjusted for kidney function). Oral valganciclovir (900 mg every 12 hours, adjusted for kidney function) is an acceptable alternative in patients with non–life-threatening disease.

Foscarnet and cidofovir are reserved for treatment of resistant CMV infections due to their toxicities and requirement for parenteral administration. Maribavir is a recently available oral option for CMV viremia clearance and symptom control in patients with posttransplant refractory CMV infection and recent pharmacologic recommendations suggest that 400 mg twice daily may be insufficient.

CMV infections in immunosuppressed patients require a reduction of immunosuppression when possible. Persons living with HIV should be started on antiretroviral therapy, although a short delay due to concern for immune reconstitution inflammatory syndrome (IRIS) can be considered in cases of retinitis or CNS disease. Therapy for CMV retinitis is maintained until there is sustained CD4 recovery > 100 cells/mcL and retinal lesions appear quiescent; a decision to stop CMV therapy should involve ophthalmology input. The use of secondary prophylaxis following CMV disease without retinal involvement is more individualized and takes into account the extent of disease and immune reconstitution.

In liver transplant patients, CMV infection is more common when cyclosporine is also used, among the younger recipients and those with higher MELD scores, and among those with higher pretransplant CMV status.

Treatment of CMV retinitis is discussed in Chapter 7.

When to Refer

- Patients with advanced HIV with retinitis, esophagitis, colitis, hepatobiliary disease, or encephalitis.
- Transplant recipients

When to Admit

- Concern for severe manifestations such as inability to swallow, severe abdominal pain, or altered mental status.
- Initiation of intravenous anti-CMV agents.

Buchfellner M et al. From diagnosis to management: current perspectives on congenital cytomegalovirus infection. Curr Opin Infect Dis. 2024;37:232. [PMID: 38748563]

Doss KM et al. Updates in cytomegalovirus prevention and treatment in solid organ transplantation. Infect Dis Clin North Am. 2023;37:e1. [PMID: 37989636]

Yong MK et al. CMV prevention strategies in allogeneic hematopoietic cell transplantation; the role of prophylaxis and pre-emptive monitoring in the era of letermovir. Transpl Infect Dis. 2023;25:e14171. [PMID: 37864299]

6. Human Herpesviruses 6, 7, & 8

HHV-6 is a B-cell lymphotropic virus that is the principal cause of **exanthema subitum** (roseola infantum, sixth disease). Infection during pregnancy and congenital transmission is recognized. Primary HHV-6 infection occurs most commonly in children under 2 years of age and is a major cause of infantile febrile seizures. Primary infection in immunocompetent adults is uncommon but can produce a mononucleosis-like illness. Other manifestations in immunocompetent persons such as encephalitis, myocarditis or hepatitis are unusual. HHV-6 is on occasion also associated with drug-induced hypersensitivity syndromes. Some studies link the virus to systemic exertion intolerance disease (SEID).

Most cases of HHV-6 reactivation occur in immunocompromised persons. Reactivation is associated with graft rejection, graft-versus-host disease, and bone marrow suppression in transplant patients and with encephalitis and pneumonitis in patients with advanced HIV. In recipients of hematopoietic stem cell transplants, HHV-6 may cause fever. It is also associated with limbic encephalitis, particularly among recipients of umbilical cord hematopoietic cell transplants. Temporal lobe abnormalities are common on MRI in these cases.

HHV-6 integrates into the telomere of most people in childhood, but in a small percentage the virus is inherited integrated in the genome (with some areas such as Scotland showing nearly 3% integration). The health implications of this are under further study, but an association with angina is established.

Diagnosis in immunocompromised patients is typically made via PCR. This testing can be challenging to interpret, as some patients have chromosomally integrated HHV6 accounting for viremia; infectious diseases consultation is advised. Ganciclovir, cidofovir, and foscarnet have in vitro activity against HHV-6, although optimal therapy remains uncertain.

HHV-7 is a T-cell lymphotropic virus related to HHV-6 that is associated with roseola, febrile seizures, and, rarely, encephalitis. It appears to be a rare cause of disease in adult patients.

HHV-8 (see also Chapter 35) is associated with a spectrum of disease including Kaposi sarcoma, primary effusion lymphoma, and multicentric Castleman disease (MCD), among others. HHV-8 infection is endemic in Africa; transmission seems to be primarily horizontal in childhood from intrafamilial contacts. In the United States, on the other hand, sexual transmission (particularly among men having sex with men) is thought to be most important. Although HHV-8 related malignancies are often associated with HIV infection, Kaposi sarcoma is also well described in solid organ transplant recipients and noted in other patient populations. Antiviral therapy targeting KSHV has not demonstrated efficacy in associated malignancies.

Kampouri E et al. Human herpesvirus-6, HHV-8 and parvovirus B19 after allogeneic hematopoietic cell transplant: the lesser-known viral complications. Curr Opin Infect Dis. 2024;37:245. [PMID: 38726832]

Wood ML et al. Inherited chromosomally integrated human herpesvirus 6: regional variation in prevalence, association with angina, and identification of ancestral viral lineages in two large UK studies. J Virol. 2025;99:e0216024. [PMID: 40470957]

MAJOR VACCINE-PREVENTABLE VIRAL INFECTIONS

1. Measles

ESSENTIALS OF DIAGNOSIS

- Onset of prodrome 7–18 days after exposure in an unvaccinated patient.
- Prodrome: fever, coryza, cough, conjunctivitis, malaise, irritability, photophobia, Koplik spots.
- Rash: brick red, maculopapular; appears 3–4 days after onset of prodrome; begins on the face and proceeds "downward and outward," affecting the palms and soles last.
- Leukopenia.

General Considerations

Measles is a reportable acute systemic paramyxoviral infection transmitted by direct contact with infectious droplets or by airborne spread. It is the most highly contagious febrile rash illness, infecting up to 90% of susceptible close contacts. Missed vaccines and increasing vaccine hesitancy have increased the number of measles cases seen worldwide over recent years. In 2023, the WHO estimates there were 10,341,000 cases of measles worldwide and 136,000 deaths, mostly in children.

The WHO previously considered measles eliminated in most countries worldwide, including the Americas. Though effective vaccination averted an estimated 60.3 million global measles deaths between 2000 and 2023, reduced measles vaccination rates since the COVID-19 pandemic have led to a resurgence of the disease. Measles outbreaks are occurring worldwide; the countries reporting the highest number of measles cases between March 2025 and September 2025, in order, were Yemen (19,420 cases), Pakistan, India, Nigeria, Indonesia, Afghanistan, Kyrgyzstan, Russian Federation, Mexico, and Canada (3815 cases). Measles deaths were reported to decrease by about 8% in 2023 compared with 2022, attributable primarily to an increased number of cases occurring in countries with lower risk for death.

Most measles cases in the United States were formerly imported. However, a number of measles outbreaks have been reported in the United States in recent years due to lower vaccination rates, with a notable increase in parents filing for medical or religious exemptions to childhood vaccines. A total of 800 measles cases and 10 outbreaks were reported in the United States during the first 16 weeks of 2025, which represents a 180% increase over the 285 total cases reported in the United States during all of 2024. In 2024, a total of 285 measles cases were reported by 32 US jurisdictions, with the epicenter in Gaines County, Texas, among a group of unvaccinated Amish individuals. Similar to previous years, almost all (96%) cases occurred in persons who were unvaccinated or whose vaccination status was unknown. During the 2024–2025 school year, coverage for measles vaccines among children continued to decline, now at 92.5%. This level of vaccination coverage and resultant measles outbreaks in the United States is threatening the status of measles elimination in the country (declared in 2000).

Clinical Findings

A. Symptoms and Signs

The incubation period for measles is 10–14 days. The illness starts with a prodromal phase manifested by high-grade fever (often as high as 40–40.6°C), malaise, coryza (nasal obstruction, sneezing, and sore throat resembling upper respiratory infections), persistent cough, and conjunctivitis (redness, swelling, photophobia, and discharge). These symptoms intensify over 2–4 days before onset of the rash and peak on the first day of the rash. The fever persists through the early rash (about 5–7 days) (Table 36–2).

The characteristic measles rash appears on the face and behind the ears. Initial lesions are pinhead-sized papules that coalesce to form a brick-red, irregular, blotchy maculopapular rash. The rash spreads to the trunk and extremities, including the palms and soles. It lasts for 3–7 days and fades in the same manner it appeared. Other findings include pharyngeal erythema, tonsillar exudate, moderate generalized lymphadenopathy, and, at times, splenomegaly.

Koplik spots (small, irregular, and red with whitish center on the mucous membranes) are pathognomonic of measles (Figure 36–4). They appear about 2 days before the rash and last 1–4 days as tiny "table salt crystals" on the palatal or buccal mucosa opposite the molars.

B. Laboratory Findings

Leukopenia is usually present unless secondary bacterial complications exist. A lymphocyte count under 2000/mcL (2.0×10^9/L) is a poor prognostic sign. Thrombocytopenia and proteinuria are common.

Detection of IgM measles antibodies with ELISA or a fourfold rise in serum hemagglutination inhibition antibody supports the diagnosis. IgM assays can be falsely negative the first few days of infection and falsely positive in the presence of rheumatoid factor or with acute rubella, erythrovirus (formerly parvovirus B19), or HHV-6 infection.

Measles virus is technically difficult to culture. Real-time reverse transcriptase–PCR (RT-PCR), available from the CDC and some public health laboratories, can help establish a diagnosis promptly (nasopharyngeal and throat swabs preferred over serum or urine specimens).

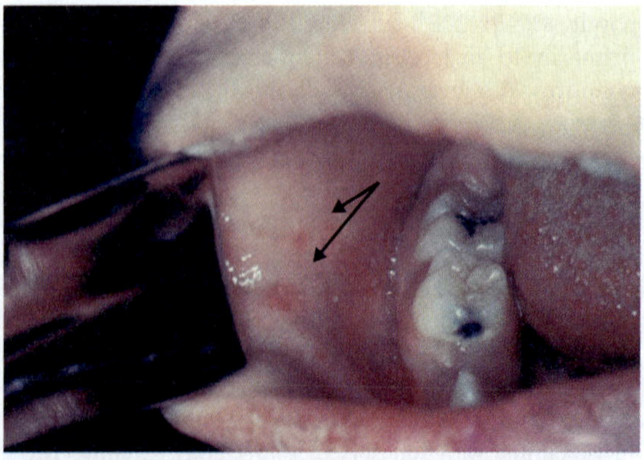

▲ **Figure 36–4.** Very small, bright red spots on the buccal mucosa indicative of Koplik spots. (Public Health Image Library, CDC.)

Differential Diagnosis

Measles is usually diagnosed clinically but may be mistaken for Kawasaki disease and other exanthematous infections (Table 36–2). Frequent difficulty in establishing a diagnosis suggests that measles may be more prevalent than is recognized.

Complications

A. Respiratory Tract Disease

Early in the course of the disease, bronchopneumonia or bronchiolitis due to the measles virus may occur in up to 5% of patients and result in serious respiratory difficulties. Bronchiectasis may occur in up to a quarter of unvaccinated children. The incidence of severe respiratory disease may be increased among immunocompromised children and pregnant persons.

B. Central Nervous System

Postinfectious encephalomyelitis occurs in 0.05–0.1% of cases, with higher rates occurring in adolescents. It is an acute demyelinating disease that usually starts 3–7 days after the rash. Seizures, coma, and other neurologic symptoms and signs may develop. Treatment is symptomatic and supportive. Virus isolation from the CNS is uncommon. Mortality is 10–20%, and morbidity includes 33% of survivors left with neurologic deficits.

Measles inclusion body encephalitis is another form of neurologic complication that results in neurologic deterioration and death within months of the acute illness among patients with impaired cellular immunity. Treatment is supportive, including stopping immunosuppressants when feasible. Interferon and ribavirin are variably successful.

Subacute sclerosing panencephalitis is a very rare, fatal CNS complication that occurs 5–15 years after infection. It is characterized by progressive deterioration of motor and cognitive function leading to death. It is more common in those infected with measles before 2 years of age.

C. Other Complications

Immediately following measles, secondary bacterial infection, particularly otitis media (the most common complication), cervical adenitis, and pneumonia, occurs in about 15% of patients. Keratoconjunctivitis is a serious complication that caused blindness before the widespread use of measles vaccine and vitamin A supplementation. Diarrhea and protein-losing enteropathy (prodromal rectal Koplik spots may occur) are significant complications among malnourished children, although the mortality associated with diarrhea is primarily 1 week before and 4 weeks after the measles rash, with no longer-term mortality shown with measles-associated diarrhea.

Prevention

The measles vaccine is a *live* vaccine available worldwide as part of the trivalent MMR vaccine or the quadrivalent MMRV vaccine. Because measles is highly contagious, the vaccine coverage rates must exceed 95% to prevent outbreaks. Illness confers permanent immunity. One vaccine dose is about 93% effective, two doses 97% protective. The effect of the COVID outbreak was considerable in reducing the vaccination rates, with 83% of the world's children having received one dose of vaccine by their first birthday—the lowest rate since 2008. Geographic disparities and clustering of unvaccinated individuals increases the likelihood of an outbreak.

At 6 months of age, > 99% of infants of vaccinated women and 95% of infants of naturally immune women lose maternal antibodies. There are conflicting studies on the optimal timing of MMR vaccination—one suggested higher measles susceptibility in adults who received the vaccine before 15 months due to the impact of residual maternal antibodies. However, another study showed lower initial seroprotection rates after the first dose of MMR when given at 5–7 months, but no negative impact on the short-term responses to subsequent MMR vaccinations.

In the United States, children receive their first dose of MMR vaccine at 12–15 months of age (https://www.cdc.gov/vaccines/hcp/imz-schedules/child-adolescent-age.html). The second dose is given at age 4–6, before school entry. Studies from Guinea-Bissau, where routine administration occurs at 9 months of age, fail to show a statistically significant benefit from a second dose of measles vaccination at 18 months of age. Older children, teens, and adults without evidence of immunity should receive two MMR doses separated by 28 days. *For individuals born before 1957, herd immunity is assumed.* Persons at high risk for measles exposure (eg, teachers, health care workers, post-high school students, travelers to low- and middle-income countries) should also receive two vaccination doses at least 28 days apart. Immigrants and refugees should be screened and vaccinated if necessary. The MMRV vaccines may be used in place of the traditional MMR vaccine. Data on febrile convulsions after vaccination show a slightly increased risk associated with MMRV over MMR vaccination separate from vaccinia vaccination—but with the statistical weakness of the association, experts recommend that the two be separated only when there is an indication such as a family history of convulsions.

MMR and MMRV vaccine should *not* be administered to pregnant persons, patients with anaphylactic reactions to neomycin, and patients with known primary or acquired immunodeficiency. Asymptomatic patients living with HIV infection with CD4 cell counts higher than 200/mcL should receive the MMR vaccine but not the MMRV vaccine. Recent data also suggest that the MMR vaccine is both safe and effective in children post chemotherapy and hematopoietic stem cell transplant, as well as those post liver and kidney transplant (notably, mean time post-transplant was 6.3 years and 73% were on low-level monotherapy for immunosuppression at time of vaccination).

There are new measles and rubella vaccines in development, utilizing microarray patches rather than injections. In a phase 1 clinical trial and another phase 1/2 clinical trial, this new method has shown promising results with seroconversion rates equivalent to MMR injections in adults, toddlers (age 15–18 months), and infants (age 9–10 months). Safety profile also is encouraging: the most common adverse reaction from the microarray patches are mild localized induration and discoloration at the patch site.

Repeated studies fail to show an association between vaccination and autism. MMR vaccine may cause fever and transient rash, which are generally mild and self-limited. Severe allergic reactions are rare. Quadrivalent MMRV vaccine is associated with an increased risk of febrile seizures that appear to be age-related, with an estimated incidence of 1 per 3000–4000 vaccinated patients; the risk is highest when MMRV is given to infants 12–23 months of age. Postimmunization seizures appear in whole genome studies to be associated with an IFN receptor and a measles receptor. Immune thrombocytopenia is another documented side effect, with an estimated risk of 1 in 40,000 vaccinated individuals. Rare cases of postimmunization encephalitis are reported.

In case of an outbreak, when susceptible individuals are exposed to measles, MMR vaccine can be given as postexposure prophylaxis if administered within 3 days of exposure. Immunoglobulin should be administered within 6 days of exposure in any high-risk person exposed to measles, followed by active immunization 3 months later if no contraindications exist. All infants younger than 1 year of age should receive intramuscular immunoglobulin (0.5 mL/kg, maximum dose 15 mL). For infants aged 6–12 months, MMR vaccination with repeat at 15 months can be given in place of intramuscular immunoglobulin. Pregnant women and severely immunocompromised persons who are exposed to active measles cases should receive IVIG (400 mg/kg).

Patients with measles should be isolated for 4 days after the onset of rash. In the hospital setting, patients with measles should be placed under airborne precautions.

Treatment

Treatment is symptomatic, including antipyretics and fluids as needed. *Vitamin A supplementation for children reduces pediatric morbidity and measles-associated mortality.* Data are less substantial for adult supplementation, although many advocate megadose vitamin A given to the mother at delivery to boost infant vitamin levels.

Measles virus is susceptible to ribavirin and other antivirals in vitro. Ribavirin is used in selected severe cases of pneumonitis, but insufficient data prevent recommending antiviral use. Zinc has a role in maintaining normal immune functions, but routine zinc supplementation to children with measles is *not* recommended, again for lack of data.

Prognosis

In the United States, the case fatality rate is around 2 per 1000 reported cases, with deaths due principally to respiratory and neurologic complications. Deaths in the developing world are mainly related to acute diarrhea and protein-losing enteropathy. Pregnant persons with measles may be at increased risk for death. Historically famines are particularly associated with high measles mortality.

When to Refer

- Any suspect cases should be reported to public health authorities.
- HIV infection.
- Pregnancy.

When to Admit

- Meningitis, encephalitis, or myelitis.
- Severe pneumonia.
- Diarrhea that significantly compromises fluid or electrolyte status.

Adigweme I et al. A measles and rubella vaccine microneedle patch in The Gambia: a phase 1/2, double-blind, double-dummy, randomised, active-controlled, age de-escalation trial. Lancet. 2024;403:1879. [PMID: 38697170]

Do LAH et al. Measles 2025. N Engl J Med. 2025;393:2447. [PMID: 40561553]

Leung J et al. The effects of vaccination status and age on clinical characteristics and severity of measles cases in the United States in the postelimination era, 2001–2022. Clin Infect Dis. 2025;80:663. [PMID: 39271123]

Mathis AD et al. Measles Update — United States, January 1–April 17, 2025. MMWR Morb Mortal Wkly Rep. 2025;74:232. [PMID: 40273019]

Siddiqui E et al. Measles resurgence in Texas: a public health wake-up call. Ann Med Surg (Lond). 2025;87:6893. [PMID: 41180769]

Stoneman EK. Measles. JAMA. 2025 Aug 14. [Epub ahead of print] [PMID: 40811055]

2. Mumps

ESSENTIALS OF DIAGNOSIS

- Exposure 12–25 days before onset.
- Painful, swollen salivary glands, usually parotid.
- Frequent involvement of testes, pancreas, and meninges in unvaccinated individuals.
- Mumps can occur in appropriately vaccinated persons in highly vaccinated communities.

General Considerations

Mumps is a paramyxoviral disease spread by respiratory droplets. Children are most commonly affected; however, in outbreaks, infection can affect patients in their second or third decades of life. Mumps can spread rapidly in congregate settings, such as colleges and schools. The incubation period is 12–25 days (average, 16–18 days). The mumps virus spreads through direct contact with respiratory secretions, saliva, or infected surfaces. Transmission can also be airborne or via droplets. Up to one-third of affected individuals have subclinical infection, which is still transmissible. Since the MMR vaccine was introduced in 1989 in the United States, the mumps case rate has decreased by > 99%, with only a few hundred cases reported most years. The CDC reported 154 cases of mumps in 2021, 399 in 2022, 436 in 2023, and 400 in 2024. A combination of factors contributes to outbreaks, including efficacy of vaccines; waning individual immunity; and crowded conditions, which promote transmission.

The ubiquitous nature of mumps requires that travelers maintain vaccination coverage but not supplement coverage (see below). More than 500,000 cases occur globally per year. Outbreaks are common in countries with low MMR vaccination rates (eg, India). However, as immunity wanes post MMR immunization, endemic transmission is still reported in countries where it is included in the routine vaccination schedule (eg, Canada and the United States).

Clinical Findings

A. Symptoms and Signs

Mumps is more serious in adults than children and appears to occur more commonly in male children, adolescents, and adults. *Parotid tenderness* and *overlying facial edema* (Figure 36–5) are the most common physical findings and typically develop within 48 hours of the prodromal symptoms. Usually, one parotid gland enlarges before the other, but unilateral parotitis occurs in 25% of patients. The parotid duct (orifice of Stensen) may be red and swollen. Trismus may result from parotitis. The parotid glands return to normal within 1 week. Involvement of other salivary glands (submaxillary and sublingual) occurs in 10% of cases. Fever and malaise are variable but often minimal in young children. The entire course of mumps rarely exceeds 2 weeks.

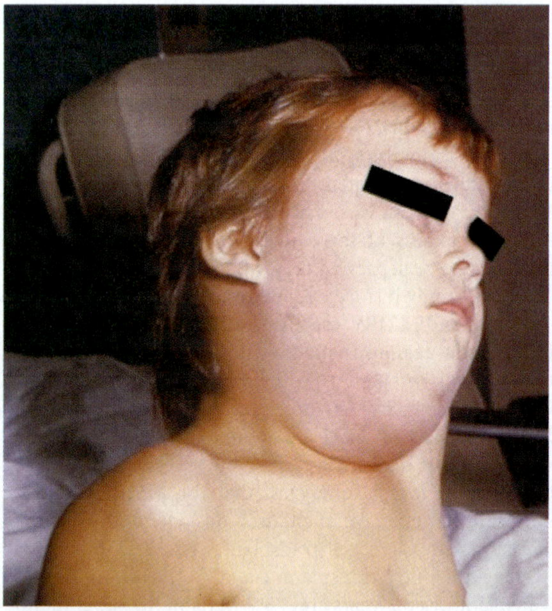

Figure 36–5. Mumps. (Public Health Image Library, CDC.)

The testes are the most common extrasalivary disease site in adults. High fever, testicular swelling, and tenderness (unilateral in 75% of cases) denote *orchitis*, which usually develops 7–10 days after the onset of parotitis. In a review of cases in the United States between 2018 and 2023, approximately 10.7% of infected men developed orchitis, which was twice as prevalent in unvaccinated compared with vaccinated persons. Lower abdominal pain and ovarian enlargement suggest oophoritis, which is usually unilateral and occurs in < 1% of postpubertal women.

Other rare complications, occurring in <1% of cases, are meningitis, encephalitis, Guillain-Barré syndrome, hearing loss, priapism or testicular infarction from orchitis, pancreatitis, thyroiditis, keratitis, neuritis, hepatitis, myocarditis, thrombocytopenia, migratory arthralgias, and nephritis. A rare cause of mumps is iodine exposure in medical procedures ("iodide mumps"). Mumps-related deaths continue to be exceedingly rare in the vaccine era.

B. Laboratory Findings

Mild leukopenia with relative lymphocytosis may be present. Elevated serum amylase usually reflects salivary gland involvement rather than pancreatitis. Mild kidney injury is found in up to 60% of patients.

The characteristic clinical picture usually suffices for diagnosis. An elevated serum IgM is considered diagnostic. Repeat testing 2–3 weeks after the onset of symptoms is recommended if the first assay is negative because the rise in IgM may be delayed, especially in vaccinated persons. A fourfold rise in complement-fixing antibodies to mumps virus in paired serum IgG also confirms infection. Anti-mumps IgM and IgG in the CSF can confirm the diagnosis of mumps-associated meningitis. Nucleic acid amplification techniques, such as RT-PCR (of a buccal swab), are more sensitive than viral cultures and are available from some commercial laboratories, selected state laboratories, and the CDC. Diagnostic yield is highest if collected during the first 3 days of illness. Confirmatory diagnosis of mumps is also made by isolating the virus, preferably from a swab of the parotid duct or another affected salivary gland. The virus can also be isolated from CSF early in aseptic meningitis. Vaccinated persons may shed virus for shorter periods than unvaccinated individuals.

Differential Diagnosis

Swelling of the parotid gland may be due to calculi in the parotid ducts, tumors, or cysts. Other causes include sarcoidosis, cirrhosis, diabetes, bulimia, pilocarpine usage, and Sjögren syndrome. Parotitis may be produced by pyogenic organisms (eg, *S aureus*, gram-negative organisms [particularly in debilitated individuals with poor oral intake]), drug reactions (phenothiazines, propylthiouracil), and other viruses (HIV, influenza A, parainfluenza, EBV infection, coxsackieviruses, adenoviruses, HHV-6). Swelling of the parotid gland must be differentiated from inflammation of the lymph nodes located more posteriorly and inferiorly than the parotid gland.

Prevention

Vaccination is the most effective way to prevent mumps, though factors such as waning immunity and antigenic mismatch between vaccine-strain mumps virus and circulating wild-type virus have led to an increase in mumps incidence observed in fully vaccinated young adults since 2006.

The vaccination schedule, indications, and contraindications are described in the measles section. The mumps vaccine component of the MMR is less effective than the measles and rubella components. One dose is 78% (range: 49–92%) protective. Two vaccine doses are 88% (range: 66–95%) effective. Rare reported complications of mumps vaccination include immune thrombocytopenic purpura and aseptic meningitis. The CDC recommends a third dose of vaccine in case of an outbreak but does not recommend additional doses for travel to areas with a mumps outbreak.

A new live attenuated mumps vaccine is reported from China, and it appears to be safe and effective.

Suspected cases should be isolated. For outbreak control, the most important step is to vaccinate all susceptible individuals. The MMR vaccine is *not* effective in preventing the disease in unvaccinated patients who already have been exposed to the virus. In the health care setting, the following steps should be taken: implement droplet and standard precautions, isolate patients until swelling subsides (about 9 days from onset), and provide vaccination to health care workers with no evidence of immunity.

Treatment

Treatment is symptomatic. Topical compresses may relieve parotid discomfort. Some clinicians advocate IVIG for complicated disease (eg, thrombocytopenia), although its definitive role is unproven. No specific treatment exists for orchitis.

When to Refer

Any suspect cases should be reported to public health authorities.

When to Admit

- Trismus; meningitis; encephalitis; myocarditis; pancreatitis.
- Severe testicular pain; priapism.
- Severe thrombocytopenia.

Hu W et al. Safety analysis of a live attenuated mumps vaccine in healthy adolescents in China: a phase 4, observational, open-label trial. PLoS One. 2023;18:e0291730. [PMID: 37733724]

Liu Y et al. Epidemiological characteristics of breakthrough mumps infection cases from 2019 to 2023 in Chongqing, China. Hum Vaccin Immunother. 2024;20:2426273. [PMID: 39539039]

Shao J et al. Evaluating the impact of different MMR vaccination strategies on mumps incidence in Shapingba, China: an interrupted time series analysis. Vaccine. 2025;67:127885. [PMID: 41166928]

Tappe J et al. Characteristics of reported mumps cases in the United States: 2018–2023. Vaccine. 2024;42:126143. [PMID: 39019661]

3. Rubella

ESSENTIALS OF DIAGNOSIS

- Exposure 14–21 days before onset.
- No prodrome in children, mild prodrome in adults; mild symptoms (fever, malaise, coryza) coincide with, or precede by up to 5 days, the eruption of rash.
- Posterior cervical and postauricular lymphadenopathy 5–10 days before rash.
- Fine maculopapular rash of 3 days' duration; face to trunk to extremities.
- Leukopenia, thrombocytopenia.

General Considerations

Rubella is a systemic disease caused by a togavirus transmitted by inhalation of infective droplets. It is moderately communicable and can be spread by both asymptomatic and symptomatic individuals. Infection usually confers permanent immunity. The incubation period is 14–21 days. The disease is transmissible from 1 week before the rash appears until around 8 days afterward.

The last cases of endemic rubella and **congenital rubella syndrome** were reported in 2009 from the Americas region. Each year in the United States, fewer than 10 cases of rubella are reported, all due to the arrival of infected persons from other countries. In 2015, the WHO declared the Americas the first region free of rubella and congenital rubella syndrome. Some European countries face a challenge with lower immunization coverage among refugees and migrants. Worldwide, cases are decreasing due to widespread implementation of rubella-containing vaccines (81% decline in rubella incidence: 93,816 cases in 2012 to 17,407 in 2022). As of 2024, the vaccine has been added to the national vaccine schedule in 175 of 194 countries (90%), although it is important to note that extensive variation in the rate of national coverage exists. The countries that have not introduced rubella vaccination are mainly in Africa and the Eastern Mediterranean. Of note, the number of reported cases of congenital rubella syndrome is increasing, particularly in Africa and Southeast Asia. The increase in congenital rubella syndrome is likely secondary to increased surveillance and reporting of congenital rubella cases.

Clinical Findings

A. Postnatal Rubella

Rubella is a common childhood disease; most cases are asymptomatic. The clinical picture of rubella is difficult to distinguish from other viral illnesses, such as infectious mononucleosis, measles, echovirus infections, and coxsackievirus infections. Fever and malaise, usually mild, accompanied by tender suboccipital adenitis, may precede the eruption by 1 week. Early posterior cervical and postauricular lymphadenopathy is common. A fine, pink maculopapular rash appears and fades from the face, trunk, and extremities in rapid progression (2–3 days), usually lasting 1 day in each area (Table 36–2).

B. Congenital Rubella

The principal importance of rubella lies in its devastating effects on the fetus in utero causing fetal death, preterm delivery, and teratogenic effects. The severity of symptoms is directly related to the gestational age; fetal infection during the first trimester leads to congenital rubella in at least 80% of fetuses; however, an infection during the fourth month can lead to a 10% risk of a single congenital disability. In the second trimester of pregnancy, deafness is the primary complication.

C. Laboratory Findings

When rubella is suspected, the diagnosis requires serologic confirmation. Diagnosis of acute rubella infection is based on elevated IgM antibody, fourfold or greater rise in IgG antibody titers, or virus isolation. Serosensitivity to rubella is thought to change with subsequent pregnancies, although data from Hong Kong (lower immunity) and the United Kingdom (higher immunity) differed in their findings.

IgM is detectable in 50% of patients on day 1 of the rash but in most on day 5 after rash onset. Antibody testing can be performed on serum or saliva. An isolated IgM-positive test does not necessarily imply acute infection. IgM antibodies can persist after an infection or could be false-positive due to cross-reactivity with other antigens such as EBV, CMV, erythrovirus (Parvovirus B19), and rheumatoid factor. *This distinction is very important to make when infection is suspected in pregnancy.* High-avidity anti-rubella IgG assays can distinguish between recent and remote infection. Low-avidity IgG is observed in acute rubella infections and lasts up to 3 months postinfection. After 3 months, low-avidity antibodies are replaced by high-avidity antibodies indicating remote infection.

The CDC can test for the virus by RT-PCR from throat swabs, oral fluids, or nasopharyngeal secretions. The timing of sample collection is important and is best if collected within the first 3 days of an acute illness and within 3 months in case of congenital rubella syndrome. After 3 months of age, up to 50% of infants with congenital rubella syndrome will not shed the virus.

Complications

Complications of rubella are rare aside from the congenital rubella syndrome. Polyarticular arthritis and arthralgia occur more commonly in adult women; involve the fingers, wrists, and knees; and usually subside within 7 days but may persist for weeks. Hemorrhagic manifestations due to thrombocytopenia and vascular damage occur more commonly in children, unlike other complications. Hepatitis has been reported. Encephalitis, another rare complication, occurs more commonly in adults and has a high mortality rate.

Prevention

Patients with rubella should be isolated for 7 days after rash onset.

In the United States, monovalent rubella vaccine is not produced. *Live attenuated* rubella virus vaccine is included in the MMR or MMRV vaccine. It is recommended that the first dose be given between 12 months and 15 months. The second dose is given between ages 4 and 6, before school entry. More details on scheduling, side effects, and contraindications are explained in the measles section. It is important that girls are immune to rubella before menarche. In the United States, about 80% of 20-year-old women are immune to rubella.

Rubella vaccine is safe and highly efficacious; a single dose of MMR vaccine is about 97% effective at preventing rubella. Vaccination outside the recommended age range (> 7 years) is shown to be effective, and vaccine adherence is not affected by coadministration with yellow fever vaccine (in Argentina) or typhoid vaccine (in India and Malawi). Vaccination of health care workers is effective in augmenting overall rates (Italy), and selective immunization of males has been effective in Japan, where past policies included targeted vaccination of junior high school girls.

The immune status of pregnant persons should be evaluated because antibody titers fall in about 10% of vaccinated individuals within 12 years of vaccination. While no evidence exists for adverse outcomes with MMR immunization of pregnant persons, it is still recommended that women avoid pregnancy for at least 4 weeks after vaccination. *Opportunities should be made available to vaccinate all women of childbearing age.*

The administration of live vaccines to immunocompromised patients is controversial. In patients receiving immunosuppressive therapy and those who have undergone solid organ or bone marrow transplantation, seroconversion is higher in rubella compared with measles, mumps, and varicella. In addition, response to live attenuated vaccines may be lessened due to presence of antibodies from IVIG or other blood products.

Safety is another concern when administering live attenuated vaccines to immunocompromised patients. Because MMR vaccine has historically been considered contraindicated in solid organ transplant recipients, evidence recommends that seronegative patients receive one or two doses of the MMR vaccine at least 4 weeks before solid organ transplantation. Patients who have undergone bone marrow transplant lose antigen-specific antibodies and should be revaccinated regardless of their vaccination history. The guidelines recommend MMR and varicella vaccines be given to seronegative patients without graft-versus-host disease 2 years after hematopoietic stem cell transplantation. See the Prevention section under Measles, above, for more discussion of rubella vaccination in transplant patients.

Treatment

Rubella infection, including complications, is treated symptomatically.

Prognosis

Rubella typically is a mild illness and rarely lasts > 3–4 days. Congenital rubella has a high fetal mortality rate, and the associated congenital disabilities are largely permanent.

When to Refer

- Pregnancy.
- Meningitis/encephalitis.
- Significant vaccination reactions.
- Any suspected cases should be reported to public health authorities.

De Melo LC et al. Congenital rubella syndrome in the post-elimination era: why vigilance remains essential. J Clin Med. 2025;14:3986. [PMID: 40507747]

Ou AC et al. Progress toward rubella and congenital rubella syndrome elimination – worldwide, 2012–2022. MMWR Morb Mortal Wkly Rep. 2024;73:162. [PMID: 38421933]

Vynnycky E et al. Estimates of the global burden of congenital rubella syndrome, 1996–2019. Int J Infect Dis. 2024;137:S25. [PMID: 37690575]

Winter AK et al. Rubella. Lancet. 2022;399:1336. [PMID: 35367004]

4. Poliomyelitis

ESSENTIALS OF DIAGNOSIS

- Incubation period 7–14 days after exposure.
- Headache, stiff neck, fever, vomiting, sore throat.
- Lower motor neuron lesion (flaccid myelitis) with decreased deep tendon reflexes and muscle wasting; sensation intact.

General Considerations

Poliomyelitis virus, an enterovirus, is highly contagious through the fecal-oral route, especially during the first week of infection. Three wild poliovirus serotypes exist; however, only wild poliovirus type 1 (WPV1) has remained endemic since 2012. Pakistan and Afghanistan are the only countries with endemic wild-type poliovirus transmission, with 74 and 25 cases reported in 2024, respectively. Of concern is an increase in circulating vaccine-derived polio (cVDPV) outbreaks. In 2024, a total of 319 cVDPV cases were reported worldwide. The WHO currently classifies 38 countries as currently undergoing outbreaks throughout Europe (Germany, UK, Spain), the Middle East (Yemen, Israel), southeast Asia (Indonesia, Papua New Guinea), and Africa. A complete list and associated cVDPV can be found at https://polioeradication.org. In July 2022 a case of paralytic poliomyelitis due to VDPV2 was identified in the United States (in Rockland County, New York). Wastewater testing detected VDPV2 in Rockland County and neighboring counties from August 2022 to February 2023, but samples have been clear since then. Guatemala, Israel, and the United Kingdom have reported positive environmental samples. Specifically, although declared polio-free since 1999, VDPV2 was detected in the wastewater in Gaza amid a precipitous drop in vaccination rates during the ongoing armed conflict, and the first case in humans was detected in a 10-month-old infant in August, 2024.

Cases of acute flaccid myelitis (formerly acute flaccid paralysis) resembling polio but not due to poliomyelitis virus are being reported (see Acute Flaccid Myelitis, below).

Clinical Findings

A. Symptoms and Signs

At least 95% of infections are asymptomatic. Patients who become symptomatic can present with abortive poliomyelitis, nonparalytic poliomyelitis, or paralytic poliomyelitis. Less than 1% of wild poliovirus infections result in paralysis. Post-poliomyelitis syndrome is the constellation of symptoms that affect polio survivors and is not infectious.

1. Abortive poliomyelitis—Nonspecific symptoms of this minor illness include fever, headache, vomiting, diarrhea, constipation, and sore throat lasting 2–3 days.

2. Nonparalytic poliomyelitis—In addition to the above symptoms, signs of meningeal irritation and muscle spasm occur in the absence of frank paralysis.

3. Paralytic poliomyelitis—Characterized as a flaccid asymmetric paralysis affecting mostly the proximal muscles of the lower extremities; the febrile period is present over 2–3 days. Sensory loss is very rare. Paralytic poliomyelitis is divided into two forms, which may coexist: (1) **spinal poliomyelitis** involving the muscles innervated by the spinal nerves, and (2) **bulbar poliomyelitis** involving the muscles supplied by the cranial nerves (especially nerves IX and X) and of the respiratory and vasomotor centers. The most life-threatening aspect of bulbar poliomyelitis is respiratory paralysis. The incidence of paralytic poliomyelitis is higher when infections are acquired later in life.

4. Post-poliomyelitis syndrome—The syndrome presents with signs of chronic and new denervation. The most frequent symptoms are progressive muscle limb paresis, muscle atrophy, fasciculations, and fibrillation during rest activity. Restless leg syndrome also is reported.

B. Laboratory Findings

The virus may be recovered from throat washings (early) and stools (early and late), and PCR of washings, stool, or CSF can also facilitate diagnosis. CSF findings include the following: (1) normal or slightly increased pressure and protein, (2) glucose is not decreased, and (3) WBC count usually < 500/mcL (0.5×10^9/L) and are principally lymphocytes after the first 24 hours. CSF findings are normal in 5% of patients. Neutralizing and complement-fixing antibodies appear during the first or second week of illness. Serologic testing cannot distinguish between wild-type and vaccine-related virus infections.

Differential Diagnosis

Acute inflammatory polyneuritis (Guillain-Barré syndrome), Japanese encephalitis virus infection, West Nile virus infection, and tick paralysis may resemble poliomyelitis. In Guillain-Barré syndrome (see Chapter 27), the weakness is more symmetric and ascending in most cases, but the Miller Fisher variant of Guillain-Barré is similar to bulbar poliomyelitis. Paresthesia is uncommon in poliomyelitis but common in Guillain-Barré syndrome. The CSF usually has high protein content but normal cell count in Guillain-Barré syndrome. While no evidence of poliomyelitis infection exists in acute flaccid myelitis that resembles polio, enteroviruses are isolated in some cases of acute flaccid myelitis.

Prevention

Given the epidemiologic distribution of poliomyelitis and the continued concern about vaccine-associated disease with the trivalent live OPV, the inactive (Salk) parenteral vaccine (IPV) is used in the United States for all four recommended doses (at ages 2 months, 4 months, 6–18 months, and 4–6 years).

Because most circulating vaccine-derived poliovirus and vaccine-associated poliomyelitis are live OPV type 2, the WHO replaced worldwide the trivalent live OPV (containing types 1, 2, and 3) with the bivalent live OPV (type 1 and 3) in 2016. *The goal is to replace all live OPV with inactive parenteral vaccination to eliminate poliovirus circulation.* The advantages of oral vaccination, however, are the ease of administration, low cost, effective local GI and circulating immunity, and herd immunity. Monovalent OPV type 2 (mOPV2) and trivalent OPV are used for control in countries with vaccine-derived type 2 outbreaks. A novel oral polio vaccine type 2 (nOPV2) has been developed in response to the ongoing circulating vaccine-derived type 2 poliovirus outbreaks and is safe and immunogenic in previously immunized adults. Studies so far have shown that nOPV2 is more genetically stable than the mOPV2 and therefore less prone to reverting to neurovirulence. The nOPV2 was recommended for initial use under the WHO's Emergency Use Listing Procedure in November 2020 and has since been recommended for full licensure and WHO prequalification as of December 2023.

A variety of measures with inactivated vaccines lower costs and increase coverage, including newer adjuvants, new delivery systems with microneedle patches, and developing multimode and combination formats including fractional doses (Bangladesh).

Routine immunization of adults in most parts of the United States is *no longer recommended* because of the low incidence of the disease. Due to the growing concern for polio transmission in New York in 2022, the New York State Health Department recommended that previously unvaccinated adults receive the vaccine, and persons starting the vaccine series after age four should receive three doses. Vaccination should be considered for adults not vaccinated within the prior decade who are exposed to poliomyelitis or who plan to travel to endemic areas and adults engaged in high-risk activities (eg, laboratory workers handling stools).

Treatment

In the acute phase of paralytic poliomyelitis, patients should be hospitalized. In cases of respiratory weakness or paralysis, intensive care is needed. Intensive physiotherapy may help recover some motor function with paralysis. Attention to psychological disorders in longstanding disease is important.

Immunodeficient individuals have prolonged excretion of poliovirus leading to virus circulation and threatening the polio eradication efforts.

Immune modulators, such as prednisone, IFN, and IVIG, do *not* show any clear benefit in the treatment of post-poliomyelitis syndrome.

Prognosis

The death-to-case ratio for paralytic polio ranges between 2% and 30%, depending on age. Bulbar poliomyelitis carries a mortality rate of up to 75%.

When to Refer

Any suspicious cases should be referred to public health authorities.

Fischer TK et al. Poliovirus circulation in the WHO European region, 2015–2022: a review of data from WHO's three core poliovirus surveillance systems. Lancet Reg Health Eur. 2024;47:101104. [PMID: 39498118]

Liang J et al. Advances and challenges in poliomyelitis vaccines: a comprehensive review of development, production, and global deployment. Front Public Health. 2025;13:1611028. [PMID: 40740383]

Mercer LD et al. Safety and immunogenicity of novel live attenuated type 1 and type 3 oral poliomyelitis vaccines in healthy adults in the USA: a first-in-human, observer-masked, multicentre, phase 1 randomised controlled trial. Lancet Infect Dis. 2025;25:1363. [PMID: 40818478]

Sun L et al. A real-world based study for immunogenicity and safety for three immunization schedules of polio vaccine. Sci Rep. 2025;15:6185. [PMID: 39979345]

World Health Organization (WHO). Global Polio Eradication Initiative. Polio today. https://polioeradication.org/polio-today

5. Acute Flaccid Myelitis

ESSENTIALS OF DIAGNOSIS

- Viral illness precedes neurologic signs.
- Flaccid paralysis usually affects upper limbs or all four limbs.
- Enterovirus is commonly isolated; poliomyelitis must be ruled out.

General Considerations

Before widespread polio vaccination in the 1950s, polio was the most common cause of acute flaccid myelitis (also known as acute flaccid paralysis). More recently, nonpolio enteroviruses including enterovirus D68 (EV-D68), enterovirus A71, and human rhinovirus are most often the cause of acute flaccid myelitis. This disease has been reported throughout Africa (20 countries), the Eastern Mediterranean region (5 countries), intermittently in Europe (Germany and France), and the United States (50 states and the District of Colombia). The CDC began surveillance for acute flaccid myelitis in 2014. Since then, there have been three outbreaks in the United States. The largest to date occurred in 2018, with 238 confirmed cases; most had a preceding viral illness in the month before presentation of neurologic signs. Neurologic symptoms most commonly affect the upper limbs or all four limbs. In all instances, poliomyelitis was ruled out, but the exact cause of acute flaccid myelitis was not always determined. Cases in the United States have declined since the 2018 outbreak, with a reported 25 cases in all of 2024. Updated US case counts can be found at https://www.cdc.gov/acute-flaccid-myelitis/cases-in-us.html.

Clinical Findings

Acute flaccid myelitis is usually a childhood disease; the average age of presentation is 5 years. Cases usually present in late summer or early fall. The three clinical stages of acute flaccid myelitis are prodromal illness, acute neurologic injury, and convalescence.

A. Symptoms and Signs

The prodrome typically consists of fever, upper respiratory symptoms, and GI symptoms. One to four weeks later, neurologic symptoms begin and usually manifest as flaccid limb weakness with decreased reflexes. Fever may recur, and the patient experiences myalgia and flaccid weakness in one or more limbs. Upper extremities are affected more often than lower extremities. Once new neurologic symptoms have subsided, the convalescent phase can last months to years. During this time, patients may experience residual muscle weakness and atrophy.

B. Laboratory Findings

CSF analysis shows pleocytosis (WBC count > 5/mcL [0.005×10^9/L]) often paired with elevated protein level (and a normal glucose concentration).

All individuals with suspected acute flaccid myelitis should be tested for enteroviruses (including D68 and A71) and rhinovirus from relevant anatomic sites. Testing for arboviruses, adenovirus, and herpesviruses should also be considered. All suspected cases should be reported to the state health department, the CDC, or both.

C. Imaging

MRIs of the brain and spinal cord should be accompanied by lumbar puncture. MRI typically shows disease of the central gray matter within the spinal cord in the location of the anterior horn cells.

Prevention

Three effective enterovirus-A71 vaccines have been licensed in China for children.

Treatment

No specific treatment exists for acute flaccid myelitis. Management consists of supportive care. Many adjunctive therapies have been used, including IVIG, high-dose corticosteroids, and plasmapheresis, but none have shown efficacy. A monoclonal antibody to EV-D68 is currently in the early stages of investigation via animal models. Neurologists specializing in the management of acute flaccid myelitis can be contacted through the AFM Physician Consult and Support Portal at https://wearesrna.org/srna/.

Long-term therapy during the convalescent phase should include physical therapy and any other necessary forms of physical rehabilitation.

Liu X et al. Immunogenicity and safety of an inactivated enterovirus 71 vaccine co-administered with measles-mumps-rubella vaccine and live attenuated Japanese encephalitis vaccine: a phase 4, single-center, randomized controlled trial. Hum Vaccin Immunother. 2021;17:5348. [PMID: 34905446]

Kalam N et al. Emerging therapeutics in the fight against EV-D68: a review of current strategies. Influenza Other Respir Viruses. 2024;18:e70064. [PMID: 39702696]

Kozlowski J et al. Acute flaccid myelitis: review of clinical features, diagnosis, and management with nerve transfers. Plast Reconstr Surg. 2023;151:85e. [PMID: 36219869]

Rudy MJ et al. EV68-228-N monoclonal antibody treatment halts progression of paralysis in a mouse model of EV-D68 induced acute flaccid myelitis. mBio. 2025;16:e0390624. [PMID: 40126012]

Whitehouse ER et al. Surveillance for acute flaccid myelitis — United States, 2018–2022. MMWR Morb Mortal Wkly Rep. 2024;73:70. [PMID: 38300829]

OTHER NEUROTROPIC VIRUSES

1. Rabies

ESSENTIALS OF DIAGNOSIS

- History of animal bite.
- Paresthesias, hydrophobia, rage alternating with calm.
- Convulsions, paralysis, thick tenacious saliva.

General Considerations

Rabies is a viral (rhabdovirus) encephalitis transmitted by infected saliva that enters the body by an animal bite or an open wound. Worldwide, > 17 million cases of animal bites are reported every year, and it is estimated that about 59,000 deaths annually are attributable to rabies. Rabies is endemic in > 150 countries; it is estimated that > 40% of the world's population lives in areas without rabies surveillance. About 95% of cases of rabies occur in Africa and Asia. In low- and middle-income countries, > 90% of human cases and 99% of human deaths from rabies are secondary to bites from infected dogs. Rabies among travelers to rabies-endemic areas is usually associated with animal injuries (including dogs in North Africa and India, cats in the Middle East, and nonhuman primates in sub-Saharan Africa and Asia), with most travel-associated cases occurring within 10 days of arrival. Rabies-free areas include much of Western Europe, Australia, New Zealand, Japan, and Hawaii in the United States. A map outlining these areas is available on Wikimedia Commons (https://commons.wikimedia.org/wiki/File:Rabies_Free_Countries_and_Territories.svg).

In the United States, domestically acquired rabies cases are rare (approximately 90.4% of cases are associated with wildlife) but probably underreported. Reports largely from the East Coast show an increase in rabies among cats, with about 1% of tested cats showing rabies seropositivity. The annual caseload in the United States is 0–3 cases (https://www.cdc.gov/rabies/php/protecting-public-health/). The most recent case confirmed by the CDC involved a Minnesota resident who was bitten by a bat in 2024. Between 1960 and 2018, 125 human rabies cases were reported in the United States. These included 36 cases (28%) with a history of dog bites during international travel. The remaining 89 cases (72%) were acquired in the United States, most often from bats.

Surveillance for animal rabies in 2022 showed 3579 animal and zero human cases occurring in 54 US jurisdictions. *Wild animals accounted for 90.4% of cases, and among wild animals, bats were the most common animal (35%), followed by raccoons (29%), skunks (17%), and foxes (8%).* Wildlife reservoirs, with each species having its own rabies variant(s), follow a unique geographic distribution in the United States: raccoons on the East Coast; skunks in the Midwest, Southwest, and California; and foxes in the Southwest and in Alaska. However, some areas have all three wildlife reservoirs (eg, the hill country of Texas). Rodents and lagomorphs (eg, rabbits) are unlikely to spread rabies because they cannot survive the disease long enough to transmit it (woodchucks and groundhogs are exceptions). Wildlife epizootics present a constant public health threat in addition to the danger of reintroducing rabies to domestic animals. Vaccination is the key to controlling rabies in small animals and preventing rabies transmission to human beings. Due to successful animal vaccination efforts, animal rabies cases are rarely seen in domestic animals in the United States. Greater than 90% of domestic animal cases are due to cats, dogs, and cattle.

The virus enters dogs' salivary glands 5–7 days before their death from rabies, thus limiting their period of infectivity. Less common transmission routes include contamination of mucous membranes with saliva or brain tissue, aerosol transmission, and corneal transplantation. Recognized mutations in rabies virus proteins can subvert the host immune system. Transmission through solid organ and vascular segment transplantation from donors with unrecognized infection is also reported. Most recently in the United States, a Michigan resident died after receiving a kidney transplant from an infected donor in December 2024. Postexposure prophylaxis can be administered to these patients and may prevent the development of disease.

The incubation period may range from 10 days to many years but is usually 3–7 weeks depending in part on the distance of the wound from the CNS. The virus travels via the nerves to the brain, multiplies there, and then migrates along the efferent nerves to the salivary glands. Rabies virus infection forms cytoplasmic inclusion bodies similar to Negri bodies. These Negri bodies are thought to be the sites of viral transcription and replication.

Clinical Findings

A. Symptoms and Signs

While patients usually report an animal bite, bat bites may not be recognized. Median incubation period ranges from 60 to 71 days with high variability amongst individuals. The prodromal syndrome consists of pain at the site of the bite in association with fever, malaise, headache, nausea, and vomiting. The skin is sensitive to changes of temperature, especially air currents (aerophobia). Percussion myoedema (a mounding of muscles after a light pressure stimulus) can be present and persist throughout the disease. Abnormal sexual behavior is also a recognized presenting symptom of rabies; such behavior includes priapism and frequent ejaculation in men and hypersexuality in women.

The CNS stage begins about 10 days after the prodrome and may be either encephalitic ("furious") or paralytic ("dumb"). The **encephalitic form** (about 80% of the cases) produces the classic rabies manifestations of delirium alternating with periods of calm, extremely painful laryngeal spasms on attempting drinking (hydrophobia), autonomic stimulation (hypersalivation), and seizures. In the less common **paralytic form**, an acute ascending paralysis resembling Guillain-Barré syndrome predominates with relative sparing of higher cortical functions initially. Both forms progress relentlessly to coma, autonomic nervous system dysfunction, and death.

B. Laboratory Findings

Biting animals that appear well should be quarantined and observed for 10 days. Sick or dead animals should be tested for rabies. A wild animal, if captured, should be sacrificed and the head shipped on ice to the nearest laboratory qualified to examine the brain for evidence of rabies virus. *When the animal cannot be examined, raccoons, skunks, bats, and foxes should be presumed to be rabid.*

Direct fluorescent antibody testing of skin biopsy material from the posterior neck of the potentially infected animal (where hair follicles are highly innervated) shows high sensitivity and specificity. The latest guidelines are available from the CDC (https://www.cdc.gov/rabies/hcp/clinical-care/).

Quantitative RT-PCR, nucleic acid sequence-based amplification, direct rapid immunohistochemical test, and viral isolation from the patient's CSF or saliva are advocated as definitive diagnostic assays. Pathologic specimens often demonstrate round or oval eosinophilic inclusion bodies (Negri bodies) in the cytoplasm of neuronal cells, but the finding is neither sensitive nor specific. MRI signs are diffuse and nonspecific.

Prevention

Immunization of household dogs and cats and active immunization of persons with significant animal exposure (eg, veterinarians) are important. The most important decisions, however, concern animal bites. Animals that are frequent sources of infection to travelers are dogs, cats, and nonhuman primates.

In the developing world, education, surveillance, and animal (particularly dog) vaccination programs (at recurrent intervals) are preferred over mass destruction of dogs, which is followed typically by invasion of susceptible feral animals into urban areas. In some Western European countries, oral vaccination campaigns of wild animals led to the elimination of rabies in wildlife.

A. Local Treatment of Animal Bites and Scratches

Thorough cleansing, debridement, and repeated flushing of wounds with soap and water are important. Rabies immune globulin (RIG) or antiserum should be given as stated below. Wounds caused by animal bites should not be sutured.

B. Postexposure Immunization

The decision to treat should be based on the circumstances of the bite, including the extent and location of the wound, the biting animal, the history of prior vaccination, and the local epidemiology of rabies. *Any contact or suspected contact with a bat, skunk, or raccoon is usually deemed a sufficient indication to warrant prophylaxis (eg, observing a bat in your room upon awakening).* Consultation with state and local health departments is recommended. Postexposure treatment including both immune globulin and vaccination should be administered as promptly as possible when indicated.

For patients who had not received rabies vaccination before possible exposure, the optimal form of **passive immunization** is human RIG (HRIG), 20 IU/kg, administered once, although 2020 data from Côte d'Ivoire make its utility unclear. As much as possible of the full dose should be infiltrated around the wound, with any remaining injected intramuscularly at a site distant from the wound. Finger spaces can be safely injected without development of compartment syndrome. Topical 2% lidocaine is shown to reduce the pain of injection. If HRIG is unavailable and appropriate tests for horse serum sensitivity are done, equine rabies antiserum (40 IU/kg) can be used.

Two vaccines containing inactivated rabies viruses are licensed for **active immunization** and available for use in humans in the United States: a human diploid cell vaccine (HDCV, Imovax) and a purified chick embryo cell vaccine (PCECV, RabAvert). Several postexposure prophylaxis strategies are recommended. The most commonly used one is the "abbreviated Essen" strategy, where either of the current vaccines is given as four intramuscular injections of 1 mL in the deltoid or, in small children, into the anterolateral thigh muscles on days 0, 3, 7, and 14 after exposure (the fifth dose at 28 days after exposure is no longer recommended except among immunosuppressed patients). Although not currently routinely recommended, some centers suggest serologic testing for all over age 70, as inadequate titer levels have been seen in up to 6.5% of patients in this age group after the recommended four-dose vaccine schedule, with appropriate levels reached after a fifth booster dose. The vaccine should not be given in the gluteal area due to suboptimal response. An alternative intramuscular vaccination strategy that takes only 1 week, with injections on days 0, 3, and 7 after exposure with a purified Vero cell rabies vaccine (PVRV, Verorab), was reportedly successful in achieving adequate neutralizing titers at days 14 and 28 in a study from Thailand; this vaccine is not available in the United States. Several new rabies vaccines remain in clinical trials, including replication-defective chimpanzee adenovirus vaccines (ChAd155-RG and ChAdOx2 RabG), an mRNA vaccine (CureVac CV7202), and a reformulated serum-free, highly purified rabies vaccine (PRV-NG2).

An alternative to RIG, a monoclonal antibody cocktail called SYN023, developed by a Taiwanese company with Chinese and American support, published results of a phase 3 trial in August 2025. It reduces RIG efficacy if given simultaneously with vaccination, and may moderate long-term immune response to vaccination. Studies from China support using recombinant human rabies antibody (NM57) as equal in efficacy to human rabies immunoglobulin (HRIG). A new monoclonal antibody, also from China, ormutivimab, was shown to be safe with less interference when given with a rabies vaccine and with fewer adverse reactions than RIG. It was recently proven to be noninferior to HRIG in a phase 3 trial.

The WHO supports an intradermal vaccination strategy using Verorab and the inactivated rabies virus vaccine Rabipur (an alternative formulation of the purified chick embryo cell) (0.1 mL per intradermal injection) for regions of the world where vaccine is in short supply. Either vaccine can be given at two sites on days 0, 3, 7, and 28. A 2024 phase 3 trial found comparable immunogenicity and safety of this vaccine compared with other standard-of-care vaccines. A study of three human rabies vaccines used internationally (HDCV, PVRV, and PCECV) showed similar immunogenicity, although HDCV shows fewer side effects.

Rabies vaccines and HRIG should never be given in the same syringe or at the same site. Allergic reactions to the vaccine are rare and include a report of sudden unilateral sensorineural hearing loss and immune thrombocytopenic purpura, although local reactions (pruritus, erythema, tenderness) occur in about 25% and mild systemic reactions (headaches, myalgias, nausea) in about 20% of recipients. Rare cases of postimmunization encephalitis have been reported. Intradermal vaccines appear to be better tolerated than intramuscular vaccines, especially among young children (while titers achieved with intramuscular vaccinations are higher, the titers achieved with intradermal vaccination are deemed sufficient for protection against clinical rabies). The vaccines are commercially available or can be obtained through health departments. Adverse reactions to HRIG seem to be more frequent in women and rare in young children.

In patients with history of past vaccination, the need for HRIG is eliminated (HRIG is in short supply worldwide), but postexposure vaccination is still required. The vaccine should be given 1 mL in the deltoid twice (on days 0 and 3). Neither the passive nor the active form of postexposure prophylaxis is associated with fetal abnormalities and thus pregnancy is not considered a contraindication to vaccination. Peripartum rabies transmission occurs but is rare. Neonates may also receive both forms of postexposure prophylaxis at birth.

The WHO has a program to eliminate dog-transmitted human rabies by 2030.

C. Preexposure Immunization

Preexposure prophylaxis with two doses of rabies vaccine administered intramuscularly has been officially endorsed by the CDC in 2022 based on recommendations from the Advisory Committee on Immunization Practices Rabies Work Group. Before 2022 a three-dose series was recommended for preexposure prophylaxis. Injections of human diploid cell vaccine (Imovax) or purified chick embryo cell vaccine (RabAvert) intramuscularly (1 mL on days 0 and 7) are recommended for preexposure prophylaxis. The Work Group also redefined the risk categories. The highest risk categories (1 and 2) include exposures that might be unrecognized and apply to laboratory personnel working with rabies virus diagnostics, persons who frequently perform necropsies, or those who handle bats. The recommendation to check the rabies antibody titers periodically following vaccination in these categories was upheld. Veterinarians, veterinary technicians, animal control officers, their students or trainees, and long-term travelers to remote areas in endemic countries were classified as risk category 3. Short-term travelers with no expected high-risk travel past 3 years after vaccination constitute risk category 4. Both category 3 and 4 are associated with only recognized exposures; checking serial titers for these persons is unnecessary because recognized exposures should always prompt evaluation for postexposure prophylaxis. For risk category 3, a one-time titer check during years 1–3 after a two-dose primary series and a booster vaccine is recommended if titer is <0.5 IU/mL. Alternatively, preemptive booster vaccine without checking titer levels between day 21 and year 3 after two-dose primary vaccination can be considered.

Immunosuppressive illnesses and agents including corticosteroids and antimalarials—particularly chloroquine—may diminish the antibody response.

Among persons with temporary immunocompromising conditions, it is recommended when possible to delay the vaccination until the immunocompromising condition resolves; if it cannot be resolved or temporarily reserved then rabies vaccination can be administered. The antibody titer should be checked after 2–4 weeks following the completion of the two-dose vaccination. If the titer is <0.5 IU/mL, a booster dose should be administered, followed by a subsequent titer check. Local or state public health authorities should be consulted for guidance if two boosters fail to elicit response.

Treatment & Prognosis

Management requires intensive care with attention to the airway, maintenance of oxygenation, and control of seizures. Universal precautions are essential. Corticosteroids are of no use. Once symptoms appear, survival is rare, and data are insufficient to provide estimate of success.

If postexposure prophylaxis (discussed below) is given expediently, before clinical signs develop, it is nearly 100% successful in disease prevention. There is one documented case of death from rabies in a patient who received appropriate postexposure prophylaxis; they had inadequate neutralizing antibodies on later testing, with attributable risk factors of age, monoclonal gammopathy of unknown significance, and metastatic prostate cancer. Once symptoms have appeared, death almost inevitably occurs after 7 days, usually from respiratory failure. Most deaths occur in persons with unrecognized disease who do not seek medical care or in individuals who do not receive postexposure prophylaxis. The very rare cases in which patients recover without intensive care are referred to as "abortive rabies."

When to Refer

Suspicion of rabies requires contact with public health personnel to initiate appropriate passive and active prophylaxis and observation of suspect cases. A set of guidelines to determine need for treatment based on type of exposure is available at the WHO website: https://www.who.int/newsroom/fact-sheets/detail/rabies.

When to Admit

- Respiratory, neuromuscular, or CNS dysfunction consistent with rabies.
- Patients with suspect rabies require initiation of therapy until the disease is ruled out in suspected animals, and this requires coordination of care based on likelihood of patient compliance, availability of inpatient and outpatient facilities, and response of local public health teams.

Ashwini MA et al. Laboratory diagnosis of rabies in an endemic country: progress and challenges on the path to elimination. Diagn Microbiol Infect Dis. 2026;114:117123. [PMID: 41061569]

Jones NJ et al. Temperature stability of rabies neutralizing antibodies. J Immunol Methods. 2025:113982. [PMID: 41072607]

Liu X et al. The efficacy and safety of SYN023 (zamerovimab and mazorelvimab injection), the recombinant humanized anti-rabies virus monoclonal antibody mixture, combined with rabies vaccine in a WHO category III rabies post-exposure population: a randomized, double-blind, positive control, phase III clinical trial. Vaccine. 2025;61:127289. [PMID: 40479926]

Maiti A et al. Primary local wound management practices and initiation of post-exposure prophylaxis among animal bite victims in a teaching institution hospital of Central India. J Family Med Prim Care. 2025;14:3778. [PMID: 41089986]

Pineda-Peña A et al. Immunogenicity and safety of a purified Vero rabies vaccine-serum free, compared with 2 licensed vaccines, in a simulated rabies post-exposure regimen in healthy adults in France: a randomized, controlled, phase 3 trial. Clin Infect Dis. 2024;78:1748. [PMID: 38478634]

2. Arbovirus Encephalitides

ESSENTIALS OF DIAGNOSIS

- Acute febrile illness; rash may be present; stiff neck progressing to stupor, coma, and convulsions.
- Upper motor neuron lesion signs: exaggerated deep tendon reflexes, absent superficial reflexes, and spastic paralysis.
- CSF opening pressure and protein are often increased with lymphocytic pleocytosis.

General Considerations

The arboviruses are arthropod-borne viral pathogens carried by mosquitoes or ticks that produce clinical manifestations in humans. The **mosquito-borne pathogens** include: togaviruses, most of which are of the genus *Alphavirus,* including Eastern, Venezuelan, and Western equine virus (EEEV, VEEV, WEEV) encephalitis, chikungunya, and Mayaro virus; flaviviruses (West Nile, St. Louis encephalitis [the epidemiology of which shows a westward migration in the United States], Japanese encephalitis, Murray Valley encephalitis, dengue, Zika, yellow fever, and Rocio viruses); and orthobunyaviruses, including the California serogroup viruses (Jamestown Canyon [seen largely in the American Northeast], La Crosse [seen primarily in the upper Midwest and mid-Atlantic], and Keystone viruses). Three cases of EEEV in 2025 were reported from Maine, New York, and South Carolina.

The **tick-borne** causes of encephalitis include the flaviviruses Powassan virus (North American Northeast and Great Lakes) and tick-borne encephalitis virus (Europe and Asia), and the Colorado tick fever reovirus. Only those viruses causing primarily encephalitis in the United States are discussed here. The most commonly encountered arboviruses from data to date in 2025 were West Nile virus (1977 cases, of which 1361 were neuroinvasive), Powassan virus (53 cases), St. Louis encephalitis (2 cases in Arizona), La Crosse virus (100 cases, Ohio and Tennessee accounting for the most cases with 52 in Ohio and 26 in Tennessee), Jamestown Canyon virus (21 cases, 10 in Michigan), and eastern equine encephalitis (3 cases in ME, NY, and SC). Neuroinvasive disease was widely prevalent among all reported arboviruses. **West Nile virus** is the leading cause of domestically acquired arboviral disease in the United States. West Nile virus disease is a nationally notifiable condition. The states reporting the most neuroinvasive disease cases in 2025 were Colorado (284), California (149), and Texas (125). Asymptomatic seroconversion is frequent, perhaps the norm, and is not reported.

Outbreaks with West Nile infection tend to occur between mid-July and early September (85% of cases). Climatic factors, including elevated mean temperatures and rainfall, correlate with increased West Nile infection. In Africa as of December 2022, at least 28 countries report isolating the agent among humans, animals, and vectors.

West Nile virus circulates between mosquitoes (mainly *Culex* species) and birds. In cases of West Nile virus outbreak, infected birds develop high-level viremia that leads to substantial avian mortality and a high incidence of mosquito infection. Infected mosquitoes bite and infect humans and other mammals. However, humans and other mammals are "dead-end" hosts since they do not transmit the virus on to other biting mosquitoes (although new data suggest that white-tailed deer may play a role in West Nile virus and other arboviral circulation); only dengue and VEEV produce viremias high enough to allow continued transmission to other mosquitoes and ticks between humans and vectors. Human-to-human transmission is usually related to blood transfusion and organ transplantation. Since 2003, all blood donations in the United States are screened with nucleic acid amplification assays for West Nile virus. In an international series of 74 transfusion-transmitted arboviruses, West Nile virus was responsible for 57% of such transmissions.

Clinical Findings

A. Symptoms and Signs

West Nile virus infection has an incubation period of 2–14 days. The infection is symptomatic in about 20% of cases and < 1% progress to neuroinvasive disease, including meningitis, encephalitis, and flaccid paralysis. The case fatality rate is 3–15% in symptomatic patients.

Symptoms include acute febrile illness, and a nonpruritic maculopapular rash is variably present. Meningitis is indistinguishable from other viral meningitis. West Nile virus encephalitis presents with fever and altered mental status. Other signs include tremors, seizures, cranial nerve palsies, Bell palsy, and other pathologic reflexes. Acute flaccid (poliomyelitis-like) paralysis, which is asymmetric and can involve facial and respiratory muscles, is a well-known complication and is less commonly seen with other arboviruses infection. West Nile virus can also present as Guillain-Barré syndrome with radiculopathy. The disease manifestations associated with West Nile virus infection are strongly *age-dependent*: the acute febrile syndrome and mild neurologic symptoms are more common in the young, aseptic meningitis and poliomyelitis-like syndromes are seen in middle-aged persons, and frank encephalopathy is seen more often in older adults. All forms of disease tend to be severe in immunocompromised persons in whom neuroinvasive manifestations and associated high mortality are more apt to develop. Other risk factors for development of neuroinvasive disease and increased mortality include Black race, diabetes, CKD, and hepatitis C virus infection.

Host genetic variation in the IFN response pathway is associated with both risk for symptomatic West Nile virus infection and increased likelihood of West Nile virus disease progression. Quasispecies intrahost variation is also documented for eastern equine encephalitis.

B. Laboratory Findings

The peripheral WBC count is typically normal. Usually, CSF lymphocytic pleocytosis is present, and polymorphonuclear cells predominate early. The diagnosis of arboviral encephalitides depends on serologic tests. For West Nile virus, an IgM capture ELISA in serum or CSF is almost always positive by the time the disease is clinically evident, and the presence of IgM in CSF indicates neuroinvasive disease. Documentation of a fourfold increase in acute/convalescent IgG titers is confirmatory for all arboviruses. Antibodies to arboviruses persist for life, and the presence of IgG in the absence of a rising titer of IgM may indicate past exposure rather than acute infection. Serologic tests are available commercially and through local and state health departments. Cross-reactivity exists among the different flaviviruses, so a plaque reduction assay may be needed to definitively distinguish between West Nile fever, St. Louis encephalitis, and others. PCR assays (available through state laboratories and the CDC) can detect viral RNA in serum, CSF, or tissue early after illness onset and may be particularly useful in immunocompromised patients with abnormal antibody responses. Blood products are best screened using nucleic acid assays. Brain MRI may reveal increased T2-weighted sequences with leptomeningeal, basal ganglia, thalamic, periventricular enhancement, or a combination of these.

Differential Diagnosis

Mild forms of encephalitis must be differentiated from aseptic meningitis, lymphocytic choriomeningitis, and nonparalytic poliomyelitis. A concurrent outbreak of West Nile and St. Louis encephalitis in 2015 in Maricopa County, Arizona, showed that distinguishing the two clinically may be difficult.

Severe forms of arbovirus encephalitides are to be differentiated from other causes of viral encephalitis (HSV, mumps virus, poliovirus or other enteroviruses, HIV), encephalitis accompanying exanthematous diseases of childhood (measles, varicella, infectious mononucleosis, rubella), encephalitis following vaccination or infection (a demyelinating type seen after rabies, measles, pertussis vaccination), toxic encephalitis (from drugs, poisons, or bacterial toxins such as *Shigella dysenteriae* type 1), Reye syndrome, and severe forms of stroke, brain tumors, brain abscess, autoimmune processes such as lupus cerebritis, and intoxications. In the California Encephalitis Project, anti-*N*-methyl-D-aspartate receptor (anti-NMDAR) encephalitis is a more common cause of encephalitis than viral diseases, especially in the young, with 65% of cases of encephalitis due to anti-NMDAR occurring among patients 18 or younger.

Complications

Bronchial pneumonia, urinary retention and infection, prolonged weakness, and pressure injuries may occur. Retinopathy occurs in 24% of patients with a history of West Nile virus infection and is associated with increased risk in those with encephalitis. Individuals with chronic symptoms after West Nile virus infection may show persistent kidney infection for up to 6 years with West Nile virus RNA present in urine; kidney infection may lead to progressive renal pathology.

Prevention

Mosquito avoidance (eg, repellents, protective clothing, and insecticide spraying) is effective prevention. Laboratory precautions are indicated for handling all these pathogens. No human vaccine is available for the arboviruses prevalent in North America, although an NIH-sponsored, phase 1, randomized clinical trial of a trivalent virus-like particle vaccine against EEEV, WEEV, and VEEV is underway. A chimeric live attenuated West Nile virus vaccine is tested in phase 2 clinical trials and is shown to be safe and immunogenic in healthy adults. No licensed treatment protects against the other arboviral encephalitis. Transfusion products should be assayed for arboviruses, particularly the West Nile virus.

Treatment

Although specific antiviral therapy is not available for most causative entities, vigorous supportive measures can be helpful. Some studies suggest improved outcomes with the use of IVIG enriched with West Nile virus antibody; however, a randomized, controlled trial of IVIG did *not* show a benefit. A host of agents are under development for the encephalitic arboviruses EEEV, VEEEV, and WEEV, and their conserved mechanisms of pathogenesis offer potential for broadly acting medications, with one leading candidate being CID15997213, a quinazolinone compound effective in vitro against VEEV and WEEV, but not EEEV.

Prognosis

Although most infections are mild or asymptomatic, the prognosis is always guarded, especially at the extremes of age. WEEV can be severely pathogenic in younger patients where mortality in those under 1 year of age is 90%, and EEV shows a case fatality rate of 30%, with up to 70% in some outbreaks. Most fatalities occur with neuroinvasive disease.

Most patients with non-neuroinvasive West Nile virus disease or West Nile virus meningitis recover completely, but a syndrome of fatigue, malaise, and weakness can linger for weeks or months. Patients who recover from West Nile virus encephalitis or poliomyelitis often have residual neurologic deficits. The recovery of persons with severe neurologic compromise may take 6 months or longer. The sequelae of West Nile virus infection include a poliomyelitis-like syndrome, cognitive complaints, movement disorders, epilepsy, and depression; and they may become apparent late in the course of what appears to be a successful recovery.

Another entity (nonprimary infection), characterized by elevated serum IgG, absent serum IgM, and occasional detection of West Nile virus RNA in blood or CSF, is associated with underlying psychiatric disorders, hospitalization during times not associated with peak West Nile transmission, fever, and increased in-hospital mortality.

The long-term prognosis is generally better for Western equine than Eastern equine or St. Louis encephalitis.

Giménez-Richarte A et al. Transfusion-transmitted arboviruses: update and systematic review. PLoS Negl Trop Dis. 2022;16:e0010843. [PMID: 36201547]
Kehn-Hall K et al. Understanding host responses to equine encephalitis virus infection: implications for therapeutic development. Expert Rev Anti Infect Ther. 2022;20:1551. [PMID: 36305549]
Lindsey NP et al. Multistate outbreak of eastern equine encephalitis virus—United States, 2019. MMWR Morb Mortal Wkly Rep. 2020;69:50. [PMID: 31945032]
Vahey GM et al. West Nile virus and other domestic nationally notifiable arboviral diseases—United States, 2019. MMWR Morb Mortal Wkly Rep 2021;70:1069. [PMID: 34383731]

3. Japanese Encephalitis

ESSENTIALS OF DIAGNOSIS

- Most important vaccine-preventable cause of encephalitis in the Asia-Pacific region.
- Transmitted by mosquitoes, especially *Culex* species.
- Wide symptom spectrum; most infections are asymptomatic.

General Considerations

Japanese encephalitis virus (JEV) is a flavivirus akin to those causing West Nile and St. Louis encephalitis. It is the most common cause of encephalitis in East Asia, with > 100,000 estimated annual cases and 25,000 annual deaths. It primarily affects children in endemic countries, but there has been an increase in cases among adults. Climate change, terrain modification, and altered human–animal interfaces are deemed responsible for these changes, as they are for many expanding viral diseases.

Most cases occur in the summer and late fall, although in tropical and subtropical areas transmission occurs throughout the year. Major outbreaks every 2–15 years often correlate with patterns of agricultural development. The virus is transmitted by mosquitoes, especially *Culex* species. Wading birds (such as herons) and pigs more commonly sustain the infection as reservoirs in nature, since the viremia in humans is transient and not usually high enough to sustain transmission. Travelers to major urban areas for <1 month are at minimal risk for Japanese encephalitis. Transmission by blood transfusion is documented.

Clinical Findings

A. Symptoms and Signs

The median incubation period is 5–15 days. Most persons remain asymptomatic. The 1% of patients in whom disease develops report sudden-onset headaches, nausea, and vomiting, followed by mental status changes, parkinsonian movement disorders, and in a smaller percentage, seizures.

Japanese encephalitis most closely resembles St. Louis encephalitis and West Nile encephalitis, although epidemiologic data readily distinguish these infections in most instances. The clinical course is less severe in patients with a history of dengue virus infection. Myelitis with flaccid paralysis has been reported, as have Guillain-Barré syndrome and dystonia.

B. Laboratory Findings and Diagnosis

The disease should be suspected in patients with symptoms of CNS infection who recently visited or reside in an endemic area.

Common laboratory abnormalities include leukocytosis, mild anemia, and hyponatremia. CSF typically has a mild to moderate pleocytosis with a lymphocytic predominance, slightly elevated protein, and normal glucose. MRI findings include T2/FLAIR and diffusion restriction in the thalamus, substantia nigra, and basal ganglia.

Diagnosis is confirmed by finding anti-JEV IgM in CSF or serum using ELISA. Definitive diagnosis requires a fourfold increase in virus-specific IgG confirmed by plaque reduction neutralization assay. Because of low levels of viremia in humans, RT-PCR is not recommended. Serologic cross-reactivity is common with other flaviviruses (the viruses causing dengue, West Nile, and Zika infections).

Prevention

Using mosquito repellents; wearing long sleeves, long pants, and socks; and using air-conditioned facilities and bed nets are essential means of protection.

In the United States, formalin inactivated Vero cell culture-derived Japanese encephalitis vaccine (IXIARO) is licensed to prevent Japanese encephalitis in nonpregnant persons 2 months or older. Travelers who plan to spend > 1 month in endemic areas should receive the vaccine. Vaccine should also be considered for travelers who plan to spend < 1 month in endemic areas but are at increased risk for Japanese encephalitis (based on season, location, activities). Primary vaccination requires two doses administered 28 days apart, to be completed > 1 week before travel. For adults, a booster dose is recommended in case of potential re-exposure or continued risk for infection if the primary series of the vaccine was administered > 1 year earlier. No studies exist detailing the safety of IXIARO in pregnant persons. Therefore, administering this vaccine to pregnant persons should be deferred, unless the risk of infection outweighs the risk of vaccine complications.

Treatment

Treatment is supportive, including antipyretics, analgesics, bed rest, and fluids. Corticosteroids may result in clinical improvement of opsoclonus-myoclonus syndrome.

Prognosis & Complications

The case fatality rates have decreased from 26% in the 1960–1970s to < 20% since 2000. Just under half (46%) of survivors live normally, but 49% (with a wide estimate range, 3–86%) show neurologic sequelae. The sequelae include a variety of cognitive, neurologic, and psychiatric complications, including memory impairment and intellectual impairment. Sequelae can persist at least 1–2 years after the acute infection. Opsoclonus myoclonus syndrome is rarely reported.

Centers for Disease Control and Prevention (CDC). Japanese encephalitis vaccine information for healthcare providers. https://www.cdc.gov/japanese-encephalitis/hcp/vaccine/

Cheng Y et al. Estimates of Japanese encephalitis mortality and morbidity: a systematic review and modeling analysis. PLoS Negl Trop Dis. 2022;16:e0010361. [PMID: 35613183]

Islam N et al. Persistence of antibodies, biostability, and interchangeability of Japanese encephalitis vaccines: a systematic review and dose-response meta-analysis. Vaccine. 2022;40:3546. [PMID: 35568587]

4. Tick-Borne Encephalitis

ESSENTIALS OF DIAGNOSIS

- Flaviviral encephalitis found in Eastern, Central, and occasionally Northern Europe and Asia.
- Transmitted via ticks or rarely ingestion of unpasteurized dairy products.
- Long-term neurologic sequelae in 2–25% of cases.
- Therapy is largely supportive.
- Prevention: vaccinate and avoid tick exposure and unpasteurized milk

General Considerations

Tick-borne encephalitis (TBE) is an infection caused by multiple viruses within the Flavivirus family. TBE virus (TBEV) is one of the most common causes with three antigenic subtypes: **European**, **Siberian**, and **Far Eastern.** The principal reservoirs and vectors for TBEV are ticks with small rodents as the amplifying host; humans are an accidental host. The vectors for most cases are *Ixodes ricinus* (European subtype) and *Ixodes persulcatus* (Siberian and Far Eastern subtype), but *Dermacentor reticularis* also is a vector. Infection results from tick bites during outdoor activities in forested areas (it is known to predominate in a "beech climate"), predominantly in the late spring through fall. Because TBEV is present in saliva of the infected tick, transmission occurs early during feeding. Ingestion of unpasteurized milk from viremic livestock (goats, sheep, and cattle) is also a recognized mode of transmission. Transmission by transplantation of solid organs is reported, leading to fatal outcomes. TBE is endemic in certain parts of Europe (where its prevalence has been expanding in recent years), Asia (principally China but a few cases from Japan as well), and where a variety of subtypes extend beyond the original three (Western, Siberian, and Far Eastern). The WHO reports 10,000–12,000 cases per year, which is considered a gross underestimate, with the actual number of reported cases annually fluctuating significantly depending on surveillance, human activities, socioeconomic factors, ecology, and climate. The incubation period is 7–14 days for tick-borne exposures but only 3–4 days for milk ingestion.

Powassan virus is another flavivirus that is similar to TBEV, and it is the only North American member of the tick-borne encephalitides (discussed under Arboviruses, above). Its vector is several *Ixodes* ticks. Most cases occur in older men (majority over age 60; death occurred in 12%

of cases), primarily from Northeast and North Central states. It is also reported from Canada and Russia. Most reported cases are neuroinvasive with presentations including acute encephalitis and aseptic meningitis. The incubation period can range from 1 to 5 weeks, although pinpointing the date of actual exposure is often difficult. It is reportedly transmitted by renal transplantation.

Clinical Findings

A. Symptoms and Signs

Most cases are subclinical, with an estimated two-thirds of patients experiencing asymptomatic infection. When symptomatic, many resemble an influenza-like syndrome with 7–10 (reported extreme range, 4–28) days of fever (usually with malaise, headache, and myalgias). In some cases, the disease is biphasic where the initial flu-like period is followed by a 1- to 21-day symptom-free interval followed by a second phase with fevers and neurologic symptoms (cases from Asia appear not to show this biphasic pattern). The neurologic manifestations range from febrile headache to aseptic meningitis and encephalitis with or without myelitis (preferentially of the cervical anterior horn) and spinal paralysis (usually flaccid). A myeloradiculitic form can also develop but is less common. Peripheral facial palsies, sometimes bilateral, tend to occur infrequently late in the course of infection, usually after encephalitis and generally are associated with a favorable outcome within 30–90 days. Acute myositis and CNS vasculitis are rare but can be associated with severe disease. The main sequela of disease is paresis. Other causes of long-term morbidity include protracted cognitive dysfunction and persistent spinal nerve paralysis. Alimentary infection occurs within 3–4 days of ingesting unpasteurized milk and dairy products, is reported throughout Central Europe, occurs in family or small outbreaks, is commonly (38.9% incidence) biphasic with frequent nonsevere meningoencephalitis, and has a very high probability of recovery.

The **post-encephalitic syndrome** is characterized by headache, difficulties concentrating, balance disorders, dysphasia, hearing defects, and chronic fatigue. A progressive motor neuron disease and partial continuous epilepsy are complications. Longstanding psychiatric complications are reported and include attention deficits, slowness of thought and learning impairment, depression, lability, and mutism.

Mortality in TBE is usually a consequence of brain edema or bulbar involvement.

B. Laboratory Findings and Diagnosis

Leukopenia alternating with leukocytosis can be seen. Abnormal CSF findings include an inconsistent pleocytosis that may persist for up to 4 months. Hyponatremia is more commonly seen than with other viral encephalitides. Neuroimaging might show cerebral atrophy and hyperintense lesions in the thalamus, brainstem, and basal ganglia. In research studies, viral load correlates with disease severity in cases where the CNS is not involved.

The European Centre for Disease Prevention and Control has a case definition for diagnosis, split into possible, probable (clinical + probable laboratory criteria, *or* clinical criteria + epidemiologic link), and confirmed (clinical + confirmed laboratory criteria). Clinical criteria are any symptoms of CNS inflammation. Laboratory criteria for confirmation are any of the following five:

- Serum TBE IgM AND IgG
- CSF TBE IgM
- Fourfold increase or seroconversion of TBE antibodies in convalescent samples
- Viral nucleic acid detection in a clinical specimen
- Isolation of TBE virus from a clinical specimen

Laboratory criteria for a probable diagnosis is detection of serum TBE IgM antibodies only. Epidemiological criterion is exposure to a common source such as unpasteurized milk or ticks.

Note that when neurologic symptoms develop, the TBE virus is typically no longer detectable in blood and CSF samples. Cross-reactivity with other flaviviruses or a vaccinated state may require confirmation by detecting TBE virus-specific antibodies by plaque reduction neutralization tests.

Differential Diagnosis

The differential diagnosis includes other causes of aseptic meningitis, such as enteroviral infections; poliomyelitis (no longer reported from Eastern Europe); herpes simplex encephalitis; and a variety of tick-borne pathogens, including tularemia, the rickettsial diseases, babesiosis, Lyme disease, and other flaviviral infections. Autoimmune encephalitis also may be considered. Coinfections are documented with *Anaplasma, Babesia,* and *Borrelia* infections.

Prevention

An inactivated, whole-virus vaccine (TicoVac; known as FSME-Immun in Europe) was approved for use in the United States in 2021 for adults and children. The vaccine is safe and effective and should provide cross-protection against all three TBE virus subtypes. The initial vaccination schedule requires three doses given over 6 or more months with booster 3 years after initial vaccination. Five other TBE vaccines licensed internationally are not available in the United States. Breakthrough TBE in vaccinated individuals is reported, especially among recipients > 50 years of age and those who are immunosuppressed, such as those receiving anti-TNF therapy or methotrexate, indicating the need for a modified immunization strategy in such patients. Data, based on an impaired immune response in older adults, support adding an extra booster vaccine dose for individuals age 50 years and older (with a schedule of 0–7–21–360 days). Neuritis and neuropathies of peripheral nerves (plexus neuropathy—paresis of lower limb muscles, polyradiculopathy) are recognized complications of TBE vaccination. The vaccine is indicated for those residing and traveling to endemic areas (and the disease is now extending to higher altitudes with climate change).

The low popularity of the vaccine in endemic countries is responsible for the limited ability to control the disease.

When utilized, it is quite effective: a systematic review of 25 European countries from 2003–2023 (primarily looking at the FSME-IMMUN and Encepur vaccines) reported vaccine efficacy > 92%, with thousands of deaths prevented by vaccination. Other prevention recommendations include avoiding tick exposure and pasteurizing cow and goat milk.

Treatment

No specific antiviral treatment is available, and therapy is largely supportive. Recombinant antibody therapy is under development. Minocycline has reduced TBE viral levels in vitro, but clinical data are lacking.

Prognosis

The three subtypes of TBE have different prognoses. The European subtype is usually milder with up to 2% mortality and 30% neuroinvasive disease. The Siberian subtype is associated with 3% mortality and chronic, progressive disease. The Far Eastern subtype is usually more severe with up to 40% mortality and higher likelihood of neurologic involvement. All three subtypes are more severe among older adults compared with children. Coinfection with *Borrelia burgdorferi* (the agent of Lyme disease; transmitted by the same tick vector) may result in more severe disease. A European cohort showed increased odds of severe disease in patients with autoantibodies to type 1 IFNs, although only present in 10% of severe TBE cases. In cases without CNS involvement, the mean duration of illness is around 7 days.

Angulo FJ et al. Tick-borne encephalitis vaccine effectiveness and public health impact in the Baltic countries of Estonia, Latvia, and Lithuania, 2019–2023. IJID Reg. 2025;16:100727. [PMID: 40989722]

Dziubek D et al. Cerebrovascular manifestation of tick-borne encephalitis virus infection. Neurol Neurochir Pol. 2025 Oct 7. [Epub ahead of print] [PMID: 41055388]

Gervais A et al. Autoantibodies neutralizing type I IFNs underlie severe tick-borne encephalitis in ~10% of patients. J Exp Med. 2024;221:10. [PMID: 39316018]

Johnston A et al. Powassan virus encephalitis in an immunocompromised patient: a diagnostic challenge with case report and literature review. Case Rep Infect Dis. 2025;2025:4453384. [PMID: 40994990]

5. Lymphocytic Choriomeningitis

ESSENTIALS OF DIAGNOSIS

- "Influenza-like" prodrome of fever, chills, and cough, followed by a meningeal phase.
- Aseptic meningitis: stiff neck, headache, vomiting, lethargy.
- CSF: slight increase of protein, lymphocytic pleocytosis (500–3000/mcL [$0.5–3.0 \times 10^9$/L]).
- Complement-fixing antibodies within 2 weeks.

General Considerations

The lymphocytic choriomeningitis virus (LCMV) is an arenavirus (related to the pathogen causing Lassa fever, discussed below) that primarily infects the CNS. Its main reservoir is the house mouse (*Mus musculus*), and the prevalence of LCM correlates with the expansion of rodents. Other rodents (such as rats, guinea pigs, porcupines, and pet hamsters), monkeys, shrews, dogs, and swine also are potential reservoirs. The infected animal sheds lymphocytic choriomeningitis virus in nasal secretions, urine, and feces; transmission to humans probably occurs through aerosolized particles and mucosal exposure, percutaneous inoculation, direct contact, or animal bites.

The disease in humans is underdiagnosed and occurs most often in autumn and early winter. The lymphocytic choriomeningitis virus is typically not spread person to person, although vertical transmission is reported. It is considered to be an *underrecognized teratogen*. Rare cases related to solid organ transplantation also are reported. Most of these cases are donor derived, though two separate cases of non–donor-derived infections in the United States were reported in early 2025. Outbreaks are uncommon and usually occur in laboratory settings among those workers with significant rodent exposure.

The ubiquitous nature of its reservoir and the large distribution of the reported cases suggest a widespread geographic risk of lymphocytic choriomeningitis virus infection. Serologic surveys in the United States show significant variability in prior infection, from < 1% in New York to 3–5% in southern and eastern United States.

Clinical Findings

A. Symptoms and Signs

The incubation period is 8–13 days to the appearance of systemic manifestations and 15–21 days to the appearance of meningeal symptoms. Most infections either are asymptomatic or cause a mild self-limited illness. In more severe presentations, symptoms are biphasic, with a prodromal illness characterized by fever, chills, headache, myalgia, cough, and vomiting, occasionally with lymphadenopathy and maculopapular rash. After 3–5 days, the fever subsides only to return after 2–4 days along with the meningeal phase, characterized by headache, nausea and vomiting, lethargy, and variably present meningeal signs. Arthralgias can develop late in the course. Transverse myelitis, deafness, Guillain-Barré syndrome, and transient and permanent hydrocephalus are reported. Lymphocytic choriomeningitis virus is an increasingly recognized cause of congenital infection frequently complicated with obstructive hydrocephalus, periventricular calcifications, chorioretinitis, ventriculomegaly, and microcephaly. In fetuses and newborns with ventriculomegaly or other abnormal neuroimaging findings, screening for congenital lymphocytic choriomeningitis may be considered; mothers are asymptomatic half the time. In over one-third of cases, rodent exposure is reported retrospectively. Occasionally, a syndrome resembling viral hemorrhagic fevers is described in transplant recipients of infected organs and patients with lymphoma.

B. Laboratory Findings

Leukocytosis or leukopenia and thrombocytopenia may be initially present. During the meningeal phase, CSF analysis frequently shows lymphocytic pleocytosis (total count is often 500–3000/mcL [0.5–3.0 × 10^9/L]) with a slight increase in protein, while a low to normal glucose is seen in at least 25%. The virus may be recovered from the blood and CSF by mouse inoculation. Complement-fixing antibodies appear during or after the second week. Detection of specific IgM by ELISA is widely used. Detection of lymphocytic choriomeningitis virus by PCR is available in research settings.

Differential Diagnosis

The influenza-like prodrome and latent period may distinguish this from other aseptic meningitides as well as and bacterial and granulomatous meningitis. A history of exposure to mice or other potential vectors is an important diagnostic clue.

Prevention

Pregnant persons should be advised of the dangers to their unborn children inherent in exposure to rodents. Infection risk can be reduced by limiting contact with pet rodents and rodent trappings.

Treatment

Treatment is supportive. In several survivors of transplant-associated outbreaks, ribavirin (effective against other arenaviruses) has been used successfully along with decreasing immunosuppression. Ongoing studies are evaluating favipiravir and umifenovir, both anti-influenza agents. Favipiravir has been tried unsuccessfully in early COVID-19 infection, and umifenovir (unavailable in the United States) is used for influenza in Russia and China and has activity against several arenavirus infections. Its use in pregnancy also needs further investigation. Trametinib (a mitogen-activated protein kinase inhibitor) has recently been evaluated as a novel therapeutic option.

Prognosis

Complications and fatalities are rare in the general population. The illness usually lasts 1–2 weeks, though convalescence may be prolonged. Congenital infection is more severe, with a ~ 30% mortality rate among infected infants, and > 90% of survivors suffer long-term neurologic abnormalities. Lymphocytic choriomeningitis in solid organ transplant recipients is associated with a poor prognosis; the mortality rate may exceed 80%.

Bartman CR et al. Systemic metabolic changes in acute and chronic lymphocytic choriomeningitis virus infection. Mol Metab. 2025;99:102194. [PMID: 40581045]

Mao W et al. Antiviral activity of the MEK1/2 inhibitor trametinib against lymphocytic choriomeningitis virus. J Med Virol. 2025;97:e70267. [PMID: 40008425]

Sayyad LE et al. Severe non-donor-derived lymphocytic choriomeningitis virus infection in 2 solid organ transplant recipients. Open Forum Infect Dis. 2025;12(2). [PMID: 39896983]

6. Prion Diseases

ESSENTIALS OF DIAGNOSIS

- Rare in humans.
- Rapidly progressive cognitive decline.
- Myoclonic fasciculations, ataxia, visual disturbances, and pyramidal and extrapyramidal symptoms.
- Variant form presents in younger persons with prominent psychiatric or sensory symptoms.
- Specific EEG patterns.

General Considerations

The **transmissible spongiform encephalopathies** are a group of fatal neurodegenerative diseases affecting humans and animals. They are caused by proteinaceous infectious particles called **prions**. These agents show slow replicative capacity and long latent intervals in the host. They induce the conformational change ("misfolding") of a normal brain protein (prion protein; PrP[C]) into an abnormal isoform (PrP[Sc]) that accumulates and causes neuronal vacuolation (spongiosis), reactive proliferation of astrocytes and microglia, and, in some cases, the deposition of β-amyloid oligomeric plaques.

Prion disease is classified as familial, sporadic, or acquired in humans. **Familial** disorders (10% of all CJD cases) are caused by germline mutations in the PRNP gene and are inherited in an autosomal dominant pattern with variable penetrance. This gene is also associated with Gerstmann-Sträussler-Scheinker syndrome and fatal familial insomnia. Another uncommon hereditary disorder is PrP systemic amyloidosis.

Sporadic Creutzfeldt-Jakob disease (sCJD) is the most common of the human prion diseases, accounting for approximately 85% of cases. Acquired prion disease is described only for kuru and Creutzfeldt-Jakob disease in its **iatrogenic (iCJD)** and **variant (vCJD)** form. Iatrogenic transmission of CJD is associated with prion contaminated human corneas, dura mater grafts, pituitary-derived growth hormone, gonadotropins, stereotactic electroencephalography, electrodes, and neurosurgical instruments. A subset of cases with a history of neurosurgical intervention shows hyperintense thalamic lesions, but no periodic sharp wave complexes on EEG (which may be a presymptomatic sign for most cases of sCJD). Abnormal prion proteins have been detected in the nasal mucosa and urine of patients with Creutzfeldt-Jakob disease, raising health concerns about possible transmission.

Kuru, once prevalent in central New Guinea, is now rare, a decline in prevalence that started after the abandonment of cannibalism in the late 1950s.

More than 200 cases of vCJD (**bovine spongiform encephalopathy** [BSE] or "mad cow disease") were reported in the United Kingdom since the first documented cases there in the mid-1990s. It is far less common in North America, with only four cases reported in the United States (the last one in 2015) and two deaths in Canada from definite or probable vCJD. Of the US-reported cases, none are confirmed to have acquired the disease locally (two of them acquired the infection in the United Kingdom, one in Saudi Arabia, one possibly in a Middle Eastern or Eastern European country). The overall annual incidence of prion disease worldwide is approximately 1–2 persons per million and decreasing. BSE is characterized by its bovine-to-human transmission through ingestion of meat from cattle infected with BSE. BSE does not spread from animal to animal, and milk and its derived products are not considered infectious. Reports of secondary transmission of vCJD due to blood transfusions from asymptomatic donors are reported in the United Kingdom.

A **chronic wasting disease** also due to a transmissible spongiform encephalopathic agent is increasing; occurs among deer, elk, and moose; and is reported from 26 states including most of Wyoming and parts of Colorado but is present in the East and South as well. Although no cases of transmission to humans are documented, transmission in the laboratory to squirrel monkeys has occurred, and the CDC recommends refraining from killing bizarrely acting animals, not handling or eating roadkill, and wearing gloves when dressing wild game. Testing for the virus in game animals may be useful, but its efficacy is not established.

Clinical Findings

A. Symptoms and Signs

Both sCJD and fCJD usually present in the sixth or seventh decade of life, whereas the iCJD form tends to occur in a much younger population. Clinical features of these three forms of disease usually involve mental deterioration (dementia, behavioral changes, loss of cortical function) that is progressive over several months, as well as myoclonus and extrapyramidal (hypokinesia) and cerebellar manifestations (ataxia, dysarthria). Finally, coma ensues, usually associated with an akinetic state and less commonly decerebrate/decorticate posturing. Like iCJD, vCJD usually affects younger patients (averaging ~28 years), but the duration of disease is longer (about 1 year). The degree of organ involvement is often extensive, and the clinical symptoms are unique, mainly characterized by prominent psychiatric and sensory symptoms.

B. Laboratory and Imaging Findings

CJD should be diagnosed in the proper clinical scenario, in the absence of alternative diagnoses after routine investigations. Abnormalities in CSF are subtle and rarely helpful. The detection of 14-3-3 protein in the CSF is helpful for the diagnosis of sCJD but not in vCJD and fCJD. Its sensitivity and specificity are widely variable among different studies and may be increased with use of tau protein assays. CSF detection of total PrP can differentiate CJD from atypical Alzheimer disease with 82% sensitivity and 91% specificity.

A blood-based assay and PCR in CSF may help diagnose vCJD with high specificity but just 71% sensitivity. The assay, as well as 14-3-3 protein assay and a "quaking-induced conversion" assay, are all available through referral laboratories. It is also recognized that the presence of a variant with low titers ("very low peripheral prion colonization") in peripheral tissue, including frequently biopsied tonsillar tissue, may be responsible for the underrecognition of vCJD. A skin biopsy, CSF sample, or nasal brushings using a prion "real-time quaking induced conversion" (RT-QuIC) is commercially available in some countries and may be the most sensitive diagnostic tool for sCJD, showing 89–92.9% sensitivity and 100% specificity.

The currently recommended diagnostic criteria for sporadic CJD include neuropsychiatric symptoms plus (1) RT-QuIC as described above, (2) detecting small amounts of CJVD-specific prion protein, and (3) clinically correlated diffusion-weighted images on MRI. The applicability of these assays beyond CJD is unknown and challenging to ascertain due to low case numbers.

The CDC has guidelines for sCJD diagnosis (https://www.cdc.gov/creutzfeldt-jakob/hcp/clinical-overview/#cdc_clinical_overview_test_dia-diagnosis). Definite sCJD requires neuropathologic diagnosis. A probable diagnosis can be assigned with a neuropsychiatric disorder plus positive RT-QuIC in the CSF or other tissues. A probable diagnosis can also be made in the presence of rapidly progressive dementia *and* two of four clinical features (myoclonus, visual or cerebellar signs, pyramidal/extrapyramidal signs, and akinetic mutism) *and* a positive laboratory assay (typical EEG, positive 14-3-3 CSF assay with duration < 2 years) *and* MRI hyperintensity in the caudate nucleus/putamen and/or at least two cortical regions (occipital, parietal, and temporal) on diffusion-weighted imaging or fluid-attenuated inversion recovery (FLAIR) imaging. In sCJD, the EEG typically shows a pattern of paroxysms with high voltages and slow waves, while the MRI is characteristic for bilateral areas of increased signal intensity, predominantly in the caudate and putamen. MRI findings of cortical and subcortical atrophy occur in both fast and slow progressors; the modality is more sensitive in patients < 80 years old (91.4% vs 67.8%). An MRI can improve early diagnosis of sCJD because clinical findings are often missed. When an experienced neuroradiologist or a prion disease expert reviews the MRI, the MRI's diagnostic sensitivity for sCJD increases to 91%.

Differential Diagnosis

Autoimmune encephalitis can have a similar clinical picture. High-titer autoantibodies (eg, to the NMDA receptor) in the CSF is consistent with autoimmune encephalitis. A presentation suggesting cerebrovascular accident can also be seen with sCJD, complicating the diagnostic profile.

Treatment & Prevention

CJD does not have a specific treatment. Once symptoms appear, the infection invariably leads to death. Flupirtine (an analgesic medication) is sometimes useful in slowing the associated cognitive decline but does not affect survival. Antibodies against PrP are also proposed as a therapeutic strategy. Studies continue to identify epitopes for vaccine development, but no promising candidates currently exist.

Iatrogenic CJD can be prevented by limiting patient exposure to potentially infectious sources as mentioned above. Prevention of vCJD relies on monitoring livestock for possible infection. The American Red Cross does not accept blood donations from persons with a family history of CJD or with a history of dural grafts or pituitary-derived growth hormone injections.

The United States no longer defers blood donors with a history of transfusion in the United Kingdom—and Europe imports US plasma, exposing the inconsistency of some EU guidelines.

Murrieta-Hernández I et al. Incidence of sporadic Creutzfeldt-Jakob disease in the emergency department. Am J Alzheimer Dis Other Demen. 2025;40:15333175251391561. [PMID: 41138234]

Rai B et al. Insights into Creutzfeldt-Jakob disease with a case series from a district general hospital and a literature review. Cureus. 2025;17:e92026. [PMID: 41084699]

Zemlyankina I et al. Genetic variation and strain dynamics in chronic wasting disease. Viruses. 2025;17:1308. [PMID: 41157580]

Zerr I et al. Creutzfeldt-Jakob disease and other prion diseases. Nat Rev Dis Primers. 2024;10:14. [PMID: 38424082]

7. Progressive Multifocal Leukoencephalopathy (PML)

PML is a rare demyelinating CNS disorder caused by the reactivation of two Polyoma viruses, the **JC virus** (John Cunningham virus or JCV) and, less commonly, the **BK virus** (associated with nephropathy). The JC virus usually causes its primary infection during childhood with about 80% of adults typically being seropositive. The virus remains latent in the kidneys, lymphoid tissues, epithelial cells, peripheral blood leukocytes, bone marrow, and possibly brain until *reactivation* occurs and symptoms become evident. This reactivation is usually seen in adults with impaired cell-mediated immunity, especially patients with AIDS (5–10% of whom develop PML), as well as those with idiopathic CD4 lymphopenia syndrome. Although the prevalence of PML is only ~0.56% in people living with HIV (PLWH) in general, they constitute anywhere from 43.7% to 84.8% of PML cases. It is also reported among those with lymphoproliferative and myeloproliferative disorders; in those with granulomatous, inflammatory, and rheumatic diseases (SLE and rheumatoid arthritis in particular); in those who have undergone solid and hematopoietic cell transplantation; and occasionally in those who have other medical comorbidities, including cirrhosis and kidney disease. Diagnostic criteria that use clinical, imaging, pathologic, and virologic manifestations of JCV are available from the American Academy of Neurology.

Medication-associated PML is described with the use of natalizumab, rituximab, infliximab, alemtuzumab, fingolimod, azathioprine with corticosteroids, cyclophosphamide, mycophenolate mofetil, dimethyl fumarate, and sphingosine 1-phosphate receptor modulators—as well as possibly the newer disease-modifying agents siponimod (for multiple sclerosis), ofatumumab (for leukemia), and a few other drugs. Natalizumab, a monoclonal antibody used in the treatment of multiple sclerosis, is associated with the risk of PML developing in 3–4 per 1000 treated patients, with the rate increasing with duration of therapy. The risk of clinical PML appears to increase up to 36 months of therapy and levels off thereafter. The mean interval between the use of a medication and the diagnosis of PML is 5.5 months. JCV is detected in the CSF of up to one-half of all patients treated with natalizumab. An immune reconstitution inflammatory state (IRIS) may follow cessation of natalizumab or other monoclonal antibody therapy, although the JCV presence and the residual neurologic deficits may not clear for years after therapy is stopped. The risk of developing PML associated with rituximab is at least 1 in 10,000 exposed patients with cases reported in various autoimmune conditions treated with rituximab (SLE, rheumatoid arthritis, multiple sclerosis). Although the exact relationship between latent JCV and frank PML remains unclear, higher JC viral loads are detected among immunosuppressed patients and among those who have HIV infection with lower CD4 cell counts.

PML is rarely reported in the immunocompetent population, and the average age for the progressive neurodegeneration in such patients is 57.5, with a male predominance.

Clinical Findings

A. Symptoms and Signs

JCV causes lytic infection of oligodendrocytes in the white matter and symptoms presenting subacutely, reflecting the diverse areas of CNS involvement. Symptoms include altered mental status, aphasia, ataxia, hemiparesis or hemiplegia, and visual field disturbances. Seizures occur in about 18%, and status epilepticus is seen with a particular PnP variant (E200K). Involvement of cranial nerves and the cervical spine is rare.

B. Laboratory Findings

Quantitative PCR for JCV in CSF is used to diagnose patients with compatible clinical and radiologic findings. Serum and urinary JCV PCR are not predictive of PML, and utilization is not recommended in routine clinical practice. An anti-JCV IgG was higher 6 months before diagnosis but was not predictive of PML in a cohort of patients living with HIV infection. Serum neurofilament levels are increased in natalizumab-treated patients with multiple sclerosis who develop PML compared with those who do not and may provide prognostic utility (specificity 67%, specificity 80%).

C. Imaging

MRI of the brain shows multifocal areas of white matter demyelination without mass effect or, usually, contrast enhancement. Lesions are more often bilateral than unilateral and often do not conform to vascular territories. The findings may not be distinguishable from IRIS. Increased methionine uptake with concomitant decreased fluorodeoxyglucose uptake on PET may be helpful for diagnosis. In patients with HIV, a syndrome of cerebellar degeneration is described. Case reports attest to the variability of MRI findings and should not be relied upon solely for diagnosis.

Treatment & Prevention

There are no effective antiviral drugs against the JC virus. *Limiting the immunosuppressed state without inducing IRIS represents the mainstay of therapy for HIV-associated PML.* Treatment of HIV with ART reduces the incidence of PML, improves the clinical symptoms, reverses some of the radiographic abnormalities, and improves the 1-year mortality rate, regardless of baseline CD4 cell count. ART with enhanced CNS penetration has not seemed to have any benefit over other ART regimens in controlling PML. Immune recovery can induce worsening of the clinical picture in a few cases. Immune reconstitution syndromes do not alter mortality but are associated with a form of PML called **non-determined leukoencephalopathy** associated with a chemokine polymorphism. Significant neurologic sequelae to PML infections are common, and deficits may persist for years. In the modern ART era, 1-year mortality has decreased to 22–38.2% and is even lower in those with CD4 > 50 cells/mcL at time of diagnosis (11%) and those with CD4 > 50 cells/mcL *and* no opportunistic infections at the time of diagnosis (4.5%).

Decreasing immunosuppression in patients without HIV but with PML (eg, patients with multiple sclerosis or those who have undergone transplant) is important. Cidofovir may be beneficial in non-HIV-related cases, while corticosteroids may be useful with immune reconstitution. Because the JCV infects cells through serotonin receptors, some clinicians recommend using risperidone and mirtazapine. Anecdotal reports show that premature stopping of natalizumab in multiple sclerosis may itself lead to IRIS states and that the combination of teriflunomide with IFN may hold PML symptoms in abeyance while allowing for control of underlying multiple sclerosis. Plasma exchange, which theoretically reduces the plasma level of agents associated with PML, may be useful in natalizumab-associated PML but is associated with a high risk of IRIS. In post-kidney transplant patients, a preinduction regimen with IVIG and rituximab and transplantation with lymphocyte-depleted cells appears to reduce the risk of PML. Titers of JC antibody are not shown to significantly increase before clinical onset of PML in patients who have undergone solid organ transplantation.

Among patients with PML without any obvious immune impairment, treatment responses are reported with mirtazapine and IV pulse methylprednisolone, but in one series the mortality within months of initiating such therapy was 50%.

Current investigational therapies under evaluation include use of programmed cell death protein (PD-1) inhibitors (also known as "immune checkpoint inhibitors"), virus-specific T cell therapies (VSTs) that utilize allogenic T cells targeting JC virus, and cytokine-based immune augmentation (notably IL-7) for immune reconstitution.

Chen J et al. The boundaries between PML and PML-IRIS: difficult to define, pathology may predict. Front Cell Infect Microbiol. 2025;15:1607428. [PMID: 40654580]

Elbaz M et al. JC polyomavirus infection: a narrative review. Infect Dis Ther. 2025;14:2007. [PMID: 40715945]

Mendoza MA et al. Polyomaviruses after allogeneic hematopoietic stem cell transplantation. Viruses. 2025;17:403. [PMID: 40143330]

Zhou R et al. Diagnosing progressive multifocal leukoencephalopathy: positive predictive value of CSF JC virus quantitative PCR and importance of recognizing suggestive neuroimaging findings. J Neurol Sci. 2025;469:123379. [PMID: 39764914]

8. Human T-Cell Lymphotropic Virus (HTLV)

HTLV-1 and -2 are retroviruses that infect CD4 and CD8 T cells, respectively, where they persist as a lifelong latent infection. HTLV-1 infects an estimated 5–10 million individuals worldwide. The Caribbean basin and southwestern Japan historically show the highest prevalence of infection (4–37%, 13% of Caribbean pregnant women).

In the United States, studies done on blood donors show a seroprevalence of HTLV-1 of 0.005% and HTLV-2 of 0.014%. The virus is transmitted sexually, vertically (intrauterine, peripartum, and prolonged breastfeeding), and parenterally (injection drug use and blood transfusion). Coinfection with HIV-1 occurs (in < 5% in a series from Spain) but is likely underrecognized. Transmission via organ transplant has been reported. Disease may flare when biologic agents are used for rheumatoid conditions. HTLV-1 infection is associated with **HTLV-1 adult T-cell lymphoma/leukemia (ATL)** and **HTLV-1–associated myelopathy/tropical spastic paraparesis (HAM/TSP).** In contrast, HTLV-2 is significantly less pathogenic, with few reported cases of HAM/TSP and or other neurologic manifestations.

Clinical Findings

A. Symptoms and Signs

The lifetime risk of developing ATL among HTLV-1–seropositive persons is estimated to be 3% in women and 7% in men, with an incubation period of at least 15 years.

ATL clinical syndromes may be classified as chronic, acute (leukemic), smoldering, or lymphomatous. A primary cutaneous tumor is also described and shows a worse prognosis compared with the smoldering type. Clinical features of ATL include diffuse lymphadenopathy, maculopapular skin lesions that may evolve into erythroderma, periodontitis, a bronchoalveolar disorder, organomegaly, lytic bone lesions, and hypercalcemia. Opportunistic infections, such as *P jirovecii* pneumonia and cryptococcal meningitis, are common. Chronic infectious eczema is often associated with HTLV infection and in a review of chronic crusted scabies, 8.5% of cases were associated with HTL-1 infections.

HAM/TSP, associated with HTLV-1 and HTLV-2, develops in 0.3–4% of seropositive individuals and is more common in women and older individuals. Chronic inflammation of the CNS and spinal cord leads to intense and progressive motor weakness and symmetric spastic paraparesis, bilateral facial palsies, cognitive impairment, falls, nociceptive low back pain, and paraplegia with hyperreflexia. Bladder and sexual disorders (eg, dyspareunia, erectile dysfunction), sensory disturbances, and constipation are also common. Both viruses can also induce motor abnormalities, such as leg weakness, impaired tandem walk, and vibratory sensory findings, without overt HTLV-associated myelopathy.

HTLV-1 seropositivity is associated with an increased risk of tuberculosis, *Strongyloides stercoralis* hyperinfection, crusted scabies, and infective dermatitis.

HTLV-2 appears to cause a milder, slower-to-progress myelopathy than HAM.

B. Laboratory Findings

In persons with ATL, the peripheral smear can show atypical lymphoid cells with basophilic cytoplasm and convoluted nuclei (flower cells). The diagnostic standard for HTLV-1 is evidence of clonal integration of the proviral DNA genome into tumor cells. The identification of HTLV-1 antibodies supports the diagnosis.

Treatment, Prevention, & Prognosis

No vaccine or antiviral therapy exists to prevent and treat HTLV infections.

Management of ATL is beyond the scope of this section. Prophylaxis against infections is needed in ATL because patients show a profound immunodeficiency.

HAM is treated with a variety of immune-modulating agents (including corticosteroids) without consistent results. A monoclonal antibody targeting CCR4 expressing T cells (the target of HTLV-1), mogamulizumab, showed initial promise but its overall role in therapy remains to be determined. Antiretroviral therapy with agents developed for HIV appears not to be beneficial.

Screening of the blood supply for HTLV-1 is required in many countries including the United States. HTLV-1 and HTLV-2 have significant serologic cross-reactivity, but PCR can distinguish the two. Antenatal screening and avoiding breastfeeding (where the virus can be transmitted) are also important preventive measures.

Altieri A et al. HTLV-1 and ATLL: epidemiology, oncogenesis, and opportunities for community-informed research in the United States. Viruses. 2025;17:1333. [PMID: 41157604]

Bangam CR et al. HTLV-1-associated myelopathy/tropical spastic paraparesis. Nat Rev Dis Primers. 2015:1:15012. [PMID: 27188208]

Sato et al. Multicenter, randomized, double-blind, placebo-controlled phase 3 study of mogamulizumab with open-label extension study in a minimum number of patients with human T-cell leukemia virus type-1-associated myelopathy. J Neurol. 2024;271:3471. [PMID: 38430272]

VIRAL HEMORRHAGIC FEVERS

1. Ebola Viral Disease (EVD)

ESSENTIALS OF DIAGNOSIS

- Early-stage EVD: a nonspecific febrile illness.
- Later-stage EVD: severe GI symptoms, then neurologic symptoms and hypovolemic shock.
- Hemorrhagic manifestations are late-stage manifestations.
- Uveitis is prominent.
- Travel and contact history from an Ebola-affected country raise suspicion.
- Virus is detected via RT-PCR.

General Considerations

Members of the *Ebolavirus* genus are single-stranded RNA viruses in the Filoviridae family; four different species have been recognized to cause human disease. Fruit bats are possible animal reservoirs for *Ebolavirus*, and zoonotic transmission to humans occurs via contact with the reservoir or an infected primate. To acquire EVD, the virus must enter the body via mucous membranes, nonintact skin, sexual intercourse, breastfeeding, or percutaneous exposures (e.g., needlesticks). *Ebolavirus can continue to be transmitted among humans who have direct contact with infected body fluids.* Traditional burial practices in some African communities and unprotected direct care of persons with EVD are associated with highest transmission risk.

EVD has a 2–21-day incubation period. Prior to manifestation of symptoms, *Ebolavirus* is not transmissible. Even at symptom onset, the risk of transmission is low but increases over time. Of note, *Ebolavirus* has been detected in semen up to 9 months after recovery from infection (see Prevention, below).

Since the first simultaneous epidemic outbreak in 1976 in the Democratic Republic of Congo and South Sudan, > 20 outbreaks have occurred across West, Central, and East Africa. The estimated average case fatality rate is 60%. Many cases and deaths in these countries occurred among healthcare workers.

Clinical Findings

A. Symptoms and Signs

At symptom onset, **early-stage EVD** most typically presents as a nonspecific febrile illness. Along with fever, patients experience headaches, weakness, dizziness, malaise, fatigue, myalgia, and arthralgia. After 3–5 days, patients with **later-stage EVD** may develop abdominal pain, severe nausea, vomiting, and diarrhea. This stage of the illness may continue for a week, during which time neurologic symptoms gain prominence. Encephalitis is commonly observed and manifested as confusion, slowed cognition, agitation, and occasional seizures. Hypovolemic shock develops in most patients, but hemorrhagic manifestations (GI bleeding, diffuse mucosal bleeding, conjunctival bleeding) develop in only 1–5% of patients. Respiratory symptoms are uncommon, although interstitial pneumonia and respiratory failure are reported.

B. Laboratory Findings

During the first few days of symptoms, diagnosis may be made via several modalities, including antigen-capture ELISA, IgM ELISA, RT-PCR, or virus isolation. Blood samples obtained within the first 3 days of illness and tested by a molecular method should be repeated if results are negative and clinical symptoms and signs persist. RNA levels peak at a median of 7 days after illness onset. Later in the disease course or after recovery, IgM and IgG serologic tests may be sent. Postmortem diagnosis may be made using immunohistochemistry, RT-PCR, or virus isolation. The WHO recommends blood nucleic acid amplification tests (NAATs) from symptomatic patients, and rapid antigen detection tests if NAATs are unavailable. Oral fluid can be tested when blood collection is not possible. **Importantly, patient samples are extreme biohazard risks and should be handled accordingly using appropriate personal protective equipment.**

Laboratory findings typically include a low platelet count, leukopenia, and transaminitis (AST > ALT). As nonspecific symptoms progress to a severe systemic inflammatory response, coagulopathy with evidence of platelet dysfunction and disseminated intravascular coagulopathy (DIC) develop. Additional observed laboratory abnormalities include hypoalbuminemia, electrolyte imbalance, and increased serum creatinine level. Elevated BUN, AST, and creatinine upon presentation are associated with higher mortality.

Differential Diagnosis

The differential diagnosis varies with the stage of illness. Early-stage EVD is commonly mistaken for malaria, typhoid, or other viral illnesses. As GI symptoms develop, health providers should also consider viral hepatitis, toxins, leptospirosis, and rickettsial diseases. In later stage EVD, bacterial, viral, and parasitic illnesses, including cholera and, in children, rotavirus infection, can present with severe gastroenteritis and shock. Encephalitis must be differentiated from the confusion associated with uremia. Hemorrhagic manifestations raise suspicion for EVD but could be due to leukemia, thrombotic thrombocytopenic purpura, hemolytic-uremic syndrome, or DIC. Travel and contact history are crucial when considering the differential diagnosis in areas where Ebola is not endemic.

Complications

Hypovolemic shock and multiorgan failure are the most common complications of EVD. Hemorrhage can occur in late stages. Rhabdomyolysis is reported frequently and may explain many of the associated laboratory abnormalities. Coinfections with malaria or bacteria (or both) are important considerations. The virus is known to persist in immunologically privileged sites, such as the CNS, eye, and testes; however, viral relapse is uncommon. Post-EVD musculoskeletal pain, headache, auditory symptoms including hearing loss, and ocular complications (such as uveitis) may develop. EVD survivors exhibit high rates of neuropsychological long-term sequelae including depression, anxiety, insomnia, and PTSD.

Prevention

Risk reduction should focus on preventing wildlife-to-human transmission and reducing human-to-human transmission by surveillance, early detection and isolation of cases, contact tracing, containment measures (disinfection, hygiene, and sanitation), strict droplet and contact precautions in health care settings, and reduction of sexual transmission in Ebola survivors. The WHO recommends that *men avoid sexual activity or use barrier protection* during intercourse for 12 months from onset of symptoms or until their semen tests negative twice for Ebola virus.

The recombinant vesicular stomatitis virus (rVSV)-based vaccine expressing Z ebolavirus (ZEBOV) glycoprotein (rVSV-ZEBOV, marketed as Ervebo) is a live attenuated single-dose vaccine, effective in disease prevention as soon as 10 days from vaccine administration, and seems to generate a long-lived immune response. Side effects, such as fever, myalgia, chills, fatigue, headaches, and oligoarthritis, develop in most patients who received the vaccine. rVSV-ZEBOV was approved by the European Medicines Agency (EMA) and the US FDA in 2019. A second vaccine, an adenovirus/vaccinia virus vector vaccine (marketed as Zabdeno and Mvabea), approved by the EMA in 2020, is a two-dose series of two different vaccines but is not currently available.

Risk stratification may help determine when and for whom to administer postexposure prophylaxis. A high-risk exposure is defined as (1) percutaneous injury from a contaminated device or through contaminated gloves or clothing or (2) contact of non-intact skin or mucous membranes with an infected patient or their bodily fluids. The rVSV-ZEBOV vaccine was used for postexposure prophylaxis among healthcare workers and was found to be effective. The vaccine-mediated immunity requires an average of 10 days to develop and might not be fast enough in certain cases to prevent infection.

Treatment

Treatment is primarily supportive. Several studies have shown that *intravenous fluids can reduce the mortality rates to <50%.* Despite the wide availability of oral rehydration salts, mortality is high, ranging from 25% to 90%. Almost all patients treated in the United States or Europe received intravenous fluids, electrolyte supplementation, and empiric antibiotic therapy. Invasive or noninvasive mechanical ventilation and continuous renal replacement therapy are necessary in many cases. This increased level of intervention likely contributed to the decreased mortality (19%) among these patients.

Two monoclonal antibody cocktails (Inmazeb [known as REGN-EB3] and Ebanga [known as mAb114]) were approved for the treatment of infection with the *Zaire ebolavirus* species in adults and children by the United States in 2020. In 2022, the WHO published the first guidelines for treatment of EVD, making a strong recommendation for treatment with mAb114 or REGN-EB3 for patients with PCR confirmed EVD caused by *Zaire ebolavirus* species and neonates 7 days or younger born to mother with confirmed EVD caused by *Zaire ebolavirus*.

Prognosis

Children under 5 years of age and adults older than 40 have a high risk of death from EVD. Pregnancy is a risk factor for severe illness and death. In the 2014–2016 outbreak, the average maternal mortality was 86%. Immunosuppressed patients had shorter incubation time, rapid progression of disease, and poor outcomes. A higher baseline viral load was also a strong predictor of mortality. Among survivors, protective antibodies persist for at least 10 years.

When to Admit

Persons living in or returning from a country with high rates of Ebola transmission should be monitored for 21 days and admitted to a health care facility when symptoms meeting the WHO case definition of a suspected EVD case develop, in accordance with the screening protocol designated by the respective country's governmental health decision-making body. **Careful and early coordination with hospital Infection Control, clinical laboratory, and state/local Public Health are paramount in suspected cases.**

Choi MJ et al. Use of Ebola vaccine: recommendations of the Advisory Committee on Immunization Practices, United States, 2020. MMWR Recomm Rep. 2021;70:1. [PMID: 33417593]

Moso MA et al. Prevention and post-exposure management of occupational exposure to Ebola virus. Lancet Infect Dis. 2024;24:e93. [PMID: 37722397]

Mulangu S et al. A randomized, controlled trial of Ebola virus disease therapeutics. N Engl J Med. 2019;381:2293. [PMID: 31774950]

World Health Organization (WHO). Therapeutics for Ebola virus disease. 2022 Aug 19. https://www.who.int/publications/i/item/9789240055742

2. Other Hemorrhagic Fevers

This diverse group of illnesses results from infection with one of several single-stranded RNA viruses (members of the families Arenaviridae, Bunyaviridae, Filoviridae, Flaviviridae, and Nairoviridae). Flaviviruses, such as the pathogens causing dengue and yellow fever, and Filoviridae, causing EVD, are discussed in separate sections.

Lassa fever is a rodent-associated disease caused by an Old World *arenavirus*. Rodents shed the virus in urine and droppings and transmit the virus to humans either by direct contact with these materials, ingestion, or inhalation of aerosolized particles. Lassa fever is mostly endemic in West Africa, where 100,000 to 300,000 cases and 5000 deaths are seen annually. Case fatality rates in hospitalized patients in West Africa are up to 50%.

The **bunyavirus hemorrhagic fevers** include hantaviruses (discussed separately), Crimean-Congo hemorrhagic fever, Rift Valley fever, and several newly emerging viruses such as one that causes severe fever with thrombocytopenia syndrome.

Crimean-Congo hemorrhagic fever (CCHF) is transmitted from ticks and livestock. Human-to-human transmission can occur in the community or hospital setting by contact with infected body secretions. The geographic distribution is widespread with cases reported from Africa, Asia, the Middle East, Eastern Europe, particularly the East Mediterranean region.

Rift Valley fever is transmitted by infected livestock, mosquitoes, and flies. No human-to-human transmission is reported. Risk factors for acquiring Rift Valley fever include working with abortive animal tissue; slaughtering, skinning, or sheltering animals; and drinking unpasteurized milk. Rift Valley fever causes outbreaks in Africa and the Arabian Peninsula.

A new bunyavirus was identified in 2009 in central and northeastern China and was named for its symptoms: **severe fever with thrombocytopenia syndrome (SFTS)** virus. SFTS is transmitted by tick bite (Ixodidae family, including the tick *Haemaphysalis longicornis,* which is found in Asia and the eastern United States). It may also be transmitted between humans through direct contact with infected blood or secretions. Another virus (**Heartland virus**), identified in the United States, is similar to the SFTS virus. Transmission occurs via the Lone Star tick (*Amblyomma americanum*). The virus appears to be amplified in deer and raccoons. In the United States, most cases are reported from the Midwest and southern states.

Oropouche virus, belonging to *Orthobunyavirus,* was first detected in 1955 in Trinidad and Tobago. It is spread primarily by the bite of infected midges and some mosquitoes. One report describing a traveler from Cuba noted higher levels of Oropouche viral RNA in semen, raising concern for human-to-human transmission via sexual encounters. Most outbreaks have been identified in areas within the Amazon Basin and recently in 2024 have affected new regions in South America including Cuba, the Dominican Republic, and Guyana.

Clinical Findings

A. Symptoms and Signs

Viral hemorrhagic fevers initially present with nonspecific symptoms and are important to consider in persons who have spent time in endemic areas. The incubation period varies between species, ranging from 2 to 21 days. The clinical symptoms in the early phase of a viral hemorrhagic fever are indistinguishable from other viral illnesses. Later phases are characterized by organ failure, altered mental status, and hemorrhage. Exanthems and mucosal lesions can occur.

In patients with Lassa fever, advanced illness can be complicated by edema and pleural effusion, though fewer hemorrhagic manifestations compared with EVD. Hearing loss is the most common complication of Lassa fever infection. Mortality is high among pregnant patients and with fetal infection.

CCHF has more prominent hemorrhagic manifestations. Patients have red eyes, flushed face, red throat, and petechiae that progress to bleeding. Severe headaches are common in CCHF and correlate with the severity of vascular damage, vasodilatation, and cytokine release.

Rift Valley fever disease can present with three distinct syndromes: (1) ocular disease; retinitis is the most common complication and permanent vision loss develops in 1–10% of patients; (2) meningoencephalitis occurs in < 1% of cases; these patients have headache, coma, or seizures 1–4 weeks after initial symptoms and a low mortality but a high morbidity with neurologic deficits that can be severe; and (3) hemorrhagic fever; patients present 2–4 days after illness and show evidence of severe liver impairment and later hemorrhages; the hemorrhagic state occurs in < 1% of patients, but the case fatality reaches about 50%.

Oropouche virus disease typically presents with abrupt onset of fever, severe headaches, chills, myalgia, and arthralgia (similar to Dengue and Chikungunya infections, which are important differential diagnoses) and less commonly has hemorrhagic symptoms with epistaxis, gingival bleeding, melena, menorrhagia, and petechiae. About 4% of patients may develop neurologic symptoms; cases of meningitis or encephalitis have been noted. The Pan American Health Organization (PAHO) has issued an alert about vertical transmission of the Oropouche virus with adverse pregnancy outcomes in Brazil.

B. Laboratory Findings

Laboratory features usually include thrombocytopenia, leukopenia (although leukocytosis can be noted in cases of Lassa fever), anemia, elevated liver biochemical tests, and abnormalities consistent with DIC.

Special care should be taken when handling clinical specimens of suspected cases. Laboratory personnel should be warned about the diagnostic suspicion, and, in the United States, the CDC should be contacted for guidance. The diagnosis may be made by PCR, antigen detection (by ELISA), or demonstration of a fourfold rise in antibody titer. Lassa virus can be cultured from blood, urine, or throat swabs; however, isolation of the virus in culture requires a biosafety level 4 laboratory. CCHF is best diagnosed with RT-PCR, but ELISA or antigen detection test also can be used. Serologic assays may produce early false-negative results, and serial testing may be required.

Differential Diagnosis

The differential diagnosis for hemorrhagic fever includes meningococcemia or other septicemias, rickettsial infection, dengue, typhoid fever, and malaria. SFTS differential diagnosis includes anaplasmosis, hemorrhagic fever with renal syndrome, or leptospirosis. The likelihood of acquiring hemorrhagic fevers among travelers is low.

Treatment & Prevention

Patients should be placed in private rooms with standard contact and droplet precautions. Barrier precautions to prevent contamination of skin or mucous membranes should also be adopted by health care providers. Airborne precautions should be considered in patients with significant pulmonary involvement or undergoing procedures that stimulate cough.

Supportive care is the mainstay of therapy for most agents of hemorrhagic fever. No antiviral medication is approved for use against Lassa virus, but ribavirin may reduce mortality if administered early in the course. An RCT comparing ribavirin and favipiravir for Lassa fever has been completed (NCT04907682), but results have not yet been published. While ribavirin's efficacy as treatment for CCHF remains uncertain, it has also been used for postexposure prophylaxis. Interventions targeting animal reservoirs also have an important role in reducing the burden of human illness with certain hemorrhagic fever infections.

When to Admit

- Persons with symptoms of any hemorrhagic fever and who have been in possible endemic areas should be isolated for diagnosis and symptomatic treatment.
- Isolation is particularly important because diseases due to some of these agents, such as the Lassa virus, are highly transmissible to healthcare workers. As with Ebola, close and careful coordination with hospital infection control, clinical laboratories, and state/local health departments is paramount.

Güllü D et al. Viral hemorrhagic fevers - therapeutic trial advances and challenges. Expert Rev Anti Infect Ther. 2025;23:1235. [PMID: 41243891]

Raabe V et al. Lassa virus infection: a summary for clinicians. Int J Infect Dis. 2022;119:187. [PMID: 35395384]

Wang Z et al. Clinical presentation of Oropouche virus infection: a systematic review and meta-analysis. PLoS Negl Trop Dis. 2025;19:e0012962. [PMID: 40173204]

3. Dengue

ESSENTIALS OF DIAGNOSIS

- Incubation period 7–10 days.
- Sudden onset of high fever, chills, myalgias and arthralgias, headache, and retroorbital pain.
- Severe dengue is defined by the presence of plasma leakage, hemorrhage, or organ involvement.
- Signs of hemorrhage such as ecchymoses, GI bleeding, and epistaxis appear later in the disease.

General Considerations

Dengue virus belongs to the genus *Flavivirus* and has four distinct serotypes that can cause infection. Infection with one serotype does not confer immunity to the other serotypes. Dengue is transmitted primarily from human to human by the bite of the *Aedes* mosquito. Healthcare-associated transmission (needlestick or mucocutaneous exposure) and vertical transmission occur rarely. Transmission via bone marrow and solid organ transplant also is known to occur. Dengue is endemic in more than 100 countries, mostly in tropical and subtropical regions; most cases occur in Asia and Latin America.

An estimated 100–400 million cases of dengue fever occur annually. Case numbers have increased over the last two decades; this surge of cases is associated with climatic factors, travel, and urbanization. Thus, along with malaria, *dengue is one of the two most common vector-borne diseases of humans.* Dengue is also the *second overall cause of a febrile illness (after malaria and excluding common upper respiratory viral infections) in travelers returning from low- and middle-income countries.*

Dengue has been a nationally notifiable condition in the United States since 2010. Even though dengue is endemic in Northern Mexico and the *Aedes* mosquito is common in the southern US states, outbreaks are uncommon in the continental United States. Locally acquired dengue cases have been reported in Florida, California, Texas, and Arizona. Most cases occur in travelers, immigrants, or inhabitants of US territories that are endemic to the dengue virus.

The incubation period is usually 7–10 days. When the virus is introduced into susceptible populations, usually by viremic travelers from endemic countries, epidemic attack rates range from 50% to 70%.

Clinical Findings

A. Symptoms and Signs

A history of travel to a dengue-endemic area within 14 days of symptom onset helps establish a diagnosis. Most infected patients are asymptomatic. Only 20% develop symptoms ranging from mild disease (**dengue fever**) to severe hemorrhagic fever to fatal shock (**dengue shock syndrome**). In 1997 the WHO classified symptomatic dengue into dengue fever, dengue hemorrhagic fever, and dengue shock syndrome. The 2009 WHO classification of dengue is the following: dengue without warning signs; dengue with warning signs; and severe dengue. This updated classification is not universally adopted.

After the incubation period, the febrile phase can begin abruptly with nonspecific symptoms, high fever, chills, facial flushing, malaise, retroorbital eye pain, generalized body pain, and arthralgia. Some patients might have maculopapular rash, sore throat, and conjunctival injection. Not all patients have fever. Mild hemorrhagic manifestations can be seen. Most patients will recover, and fever is usually cleared by day 8.

A subset of patients may progress to severe dengue, which is defined by the presence of plasma leakage, hemorrhage, or organ involvement. The risk of severe dengue is increased among persons with prior dengue infection who are later exposed to a different serotype of the virus. Hematocrit increase may be the earliest sign of plasma leakage. Pleural effusion and ascites may be detected by lateral decubitus chest radiograph or ultrasound before becoming clinically apparent. Increasing liver size, persistent vomiting, and severe abdominal pain also are indicators of plasma leakage. Signs of hemorrhage such as ecchymoses, GI bleeding, and epistaxis may appear. Severe organ involvement may develop, such as hepatitis, encephalitis, and myocarditis.

Shock develops in patients after a critical volume of plasma has been lost through leakage. Decrease in the level of consciousness, hypothermia, metabolic acidosis, progressive organ impairment, and DIC leading to severe hemorrhage should raise concern for shock. AKI in dengue largely occurs with shock syndrome and shows a high mortality.

B. Laboratory Findings

Leukopenia is characteristic, and elevated transaminases are common in dengue fever. Thrombocytopenia, fibrinolysis, and hemoconcentration occur more often in the hemorrhagic form of the disease. In other forms of disease, especially in children, anemia is more common.

The nonspecific nature of the illness mandates laboratory verification for diagnosis. During the first few days of infection, virus can be detected in blood by NAAT or assays for the NS1 protein (ELISA available in US; rapid testing available elsewhere). After 7 days, serologic testing is used; paired acute and convalescent tests can be helpful. Of note, cross-reactivity of IgM with other Orthoflavivirus members can be seen. Thrombocytopenia and blood vessel fragility in remote settings can be assessed with a tourniquet test (see below). General evaluation recommendations include testing dengue serotype and monitoring platelet count, serum albumin, AST, and ALT during the febrile phase of illness to screen for severe disease.

Differential Diagnosis

Distinguishing between dengue and other causes of febrile illness in endemic areas is difficult. Fevers due to dengue are more often associated with neutropenia and thrombocytopenia and with myalgias, arthralgias/arthritis, and lethargy among adults. Rickettsial diseases may have a similar presentation but can often be distinguished by differences in epidemiology and cutaneous manifestations. Chikungunya is more apt to cause chronic arthritis. The arboviral encephalitides require additional epidemiologic information and serologic data to make the diagnosis. Influenza and malaria are easily confused early in disease, although rhinitis and malaise should help distinguish influenza, and the cyclicity of fevers and presence of splenomegaly should suggest malaria.

Complications

Usual complications include pneumonia, bone marrow failure, hepatitis, iritis, retinal hemorrhages, maculopathy, orchitis, and oophoritis. Neurologic complications (such as encephalitis, Guillain-Barré syndrome, phrenic neuropathy, subdural hematoma, cerebral vasculitis, and transverse myelitis) are less common. Acute disseminated encephalomyelitis has been linked with infection and the live dengue vaccine. Bacterial superinfection can occur.

Maternal infection poses a risk of hemorrhage in both the mother and the infant if infection occurs near term. Severe dengue is a risk factor for obstetric complications, cesarean delivery, fetal distress, and maternal morbidity.

Prevention

Measures to reduce mosquito exposure should be encouraged, such as use of screens and insect repellents, particularly during early morning and late afternoon exposures. Interventions to reduce mosquito breeding sites (eg, sites of standing water around households) also are recommended.

Dengvaxia (CYD-TDV), a recombinant, live, attenuated, tetravalent dengue vaccine, received FDA approved for children 9–16 years old with previous history of dengue infection who live in endemic areas, but it has been discontinued. An alternative vaccination (Q-denga, TAK-003) is available outside the United States and is recommended by the WHO for children age 6–16 in areas with high rates of dengue transmission.

Treatment

No specific therapeutic options are available for the clinical management of dengue besides supportive care. Treatment entails the appropriate use of volume replacement, blood products, and vasopressors. Acetaminophen is recommended for analgesic and antipyretic treatment. NSAID usage should be minimized and preferably avoided to decrease the risk of gastritis and bleeding, particularly in patients with a predilection for hemorrhage or with abnormalities in platelets, liver function, or clotting factors.

Platelet counts do not usefully predict clinically significant bleeding. Platelet transfusions may be considered for severe thrombocytopenia (< 10,000/mcL [10.0×10^9/L]) or for patients who are bleeding. Benefit in the absence of bleeding, however, may not be observed, and harm may be caused by delay in count recovery. Monitoring vital signs and blood volume may help anticipate the complications of dengue hemorrhagic fever or shock syndrome.

Prognosis

Although fatalities occur with severe disease, the estimated mortality (2.5% of severe cases) appears to be diminishing, likely due to improved recognition of the disease and wider availability of supportive treatment. Causes of death include hemorrhagic fever (seen with recurrent disease) and occasionally fulminant hepatitis. Thrombocytopenia and acute hepatitis are predictors of severe dengue and higher mortality. AKI in dengue shock syndrome portends poor prognosis. In general, the more severe forms of disease (hemorrhagic fever and shock) occur more often in Asia than in the Americas. Comorbidities of CVD, diabetes, stroke, pulmonary disease, kidney disease, and older age are associated with more severe dengue.

Centers for Disease Control and Prevention. Clinical assessment. Tourniquet test. https://www.cdc.gov/dengue/training/cme/ccm/page73112.html

Sangkaew S et al. Risk predictors of progression to severe disease during the febrile phase of dengue: a systematic review and meta-analysis. Lancet Infect Dis. 2021;21:1014. [PMID: 33640077]

World Health Organization. Vaccines and immunization: dengue. https://www.who.int/news-room/questions-and-answers/item/dengue-vaccines

4. Hantaviruses

ESSENTIALS OF DIAGNOSIS

- Transmitted by rodents and causes two clinical syndromes.
- **Hemorrhagic fever with renal syndrome (HFRS):** mild to severe illness.
- **Hantavirus pulmonary syndrome (HPS):** 40% mortality rate.

General Considerations

Hantaviruses are enveloped RNA bunyaviruses naturally hosted in rodents, moles, and shrews. Globally, hantaviruses infect > 200,000 persons annually, and their collective mortality rate is about 35–40%. Hantavirus infection in humans can cause several disease syndromes. HFRS is primarily caused by Old World hantaviruses, namely Dobrava-Belgrade virus, Puumala virus, Seoul virus, and Hantaan virus in Asia and Europe. HPS is caused mainly by Sin Nombre virus and Andes virus, the New World Hantaviruses in the Americas.

The deer mouse is the primary animal reservoir for the Sin Nombre virus. Aerosols of virus-contaminated rodent urine and feces are thought to be the main vehicle for transmission to humans. Person-to-person transmission was reported only with the Andes virus; however, the data are limited. *Occupation is the main risk factor for transmission of all hantaviruses*: animal trappers, forestry workers, laboratory personnel, farmers, and military personnel are at highest risk. *Climate change* appears to be impacting the incidence of hantavirus infection mainly through effects on reservoir ecology.

Clinical Findings

A. Symptoms and Signs

Vascular leakage is the hallmark of the disease for both syndromes, with kidneys being the main target with variants associated with HFRS and the lungs with variants associated with HPS.

1. HFRS—HFRS manifests as mild, moderate, or severe illness depending on the causative strain. A 2- to 3-week incubation period is followed by a protracted clinical course. Various degrees of kidney involvement are usually seen. Other potential complications include thromboembolic phenomena and secondary hemophagocytic lymphohistiocytosis. Pulmonary edema is not typically seen but when present usually occurs in the final stages of disease (oliguric and diuretic phase). Patients may have persistent hematuria, proteinuria, or hypertension up to 35 months after infection.

2. HPS—The clinical course of HPS is divided into a febrile prodrome, a cardiopulmonary stage, oliguric and diuretic phase, followed by convalescence. A 14- to 17-day incubation period is followed by a prodromal phase, typically lasting 3–6 days, associated with myalgia; malaise; abdominal pain, nausea, vomiting, and diarrhea; headache; chills; and fever of abrupt onset. An ensuing cardiopulmonary phase is characterized by the acute onset of pulmonary edema. In this stage, cough is generally present, abdominal pain and symptoms as above may dominate the clinical presentation, and in severe cases, significant myocardial depression occurs. AKI and myositis may occur. Sequelae include neuropsychological impairments in some HPS survivors.

B. Laboratory Findings

Laboratory features include hemoconcentration and elevation in LD, serum lactate, and hepatocellular enzymes. Early thrombocytopenia and leukocytosis (as high as 90,000 cells/mcL [90.0×10^9/L] in HPS) are seen in both HFRS and HPS. In HPS, immunoblasts (activated lymphocytes with plasmacytoid features) can be seen in blood, lungs, kidneys, bone marrow, liver, and spleen.

An indirect fluorescent assay and enzyme immunoassay are available to detect specific IgM or low-avidity IgG virus-specific antibodies that remain detectable for 6–8 months. A quantitative RT-PCR is available. However, the viremia of human hantavirus infections is brief; therefore viral RNA cannot usually be readily detected in the blood or urine of patients.

A plaque reduction neutralization test remains a gold standard serologic assay and distinguishes between the different hantavirus species, although cross-reaction between Old and New World viruses exists. This test must be performed in a laboratory with appropriate biosafety measures (level 3).

Differential Diagnosis

The differential diagnosis of the acute febrile syndrome seen with HFRS or early HPS includes scrub typhus, leptospirosis, and dengue. HPS requires differentiation from other respiratory infections caused by such pathogens as SARS-CoV-2, *Legionella*, *Chlamydia*, and *Mycoplasma*. Coxsackievirus infection should also be considered in the differential diagnosis.

Prevention

Because infection is thought to occur through inhalation of rodent waste, prevention focuses on eradicating rodents in houses and avoiding exposure to rodent excreta. Inactivated vaccines are used in several Asian countries where patients are at risk for HFRS.

Treatment

Treatment is mainly supportive. Cardiorespiratory support with vasopressors is frequently needed; extracorporeal membrane oxygenation may be required in severe cases of HPS. Intravenous ribavirin is used in HFRS (Hantaan virus) with some success in decreasing the severity of the kidney injury. Its effectiveness in HPS, however, is not established.

Prognosis

The outcome is highly variable depending on severity of disease. HPS is a more severe disease than HFRS, with a mortality rate of about 40%. In Sin Nombre virus infections, the persistence of elevated IgG titers correlates with a favorable outcome.

Afzal S et al. Hantavirus: an overview and advancements in therapeutic approaches for infection. Front Microbiol. 2023:14:1233433. [PMID: 37901807]

5. Yellow Fever

ESSENTIALS OF DIAGNOSIS

- Endemic area exposure: tropical and subtropical South America and Africa.
- Sudden onset of severe headache, aching in legs, and tachycardia.
- Brief (1-day) remission, followed by bradycardia, hypotension, jaundice, hemorrhagic tendency.
- Albuminuria, leukopenia, bilirubinemia.

General Considerations

Yellow fever is a zoonotic flavivirus infection transmitted by *Aedes* mosquitoes. The three types of transmission cycles include **sylvatic** (or jungle; humans working or traveling in the forest are bitten by infected mosquitoes), **intermediate** (most common type of outbreak in Africa; mosquitoes infect both monkeys and humans leading to outbreaks in separate villages), and **urban** (seen in large epidemics; infected mosquitoes transmit the virus from person to person). Elevated temperatures and increased rainfall are major determinants of transmission.

Yellow fever occurs in endemic countries in Africa and in Central and South America. Around 90% of cases reported every year occur in sub-Saharan Africa. The number of persons at risk for infection with yellow fever virus worldwide is estimated to be between 394 million and 473 million. The last decade has seen a resurgence of yellow fever, likely due to suboptimal vaccination coverage and waning population-level immunity.

Clinical Findings

A. Symptoms and Signs

Most patients have no illness or only mild illness. The incubation period is 3–6 days.

1. Mild form—Symptoms include malaise, headache, fever, retroorbital pain, nausea, vomiting, and photophobia. Relative bradycardia (a lower-than-expected heart rate for the degree of body temperature elevation), conjunctival injection, and facial flushing may be present.

2. Severe form—Severe illness develops in about 15%. Initial symptoms are similar to the mild form, but a brief afebrile period (hours to a few days) is followed by a "period of intoxication" manifested by fever and relative bradycardia, hypotension, jaundice, hemorrhage (GI, nasal, oral), and delirium that may progress to coma.

B. Laboratory Findings

Leukopenia along with elevated liver enzymes and bilirubin can occur. Proteinuria is present and usually disappears completely with recovery. Bleeding dyscrasias with elevated prothrombin and partial thromboplastin times, decreased platelet count, and presence of fibrin-split products may be seen.

In the early stages of the disease (up to 10 days), diagnosis is confirmed if yellow fever virus RNA is detected by RT-PCR in blood from a person with no history of recent yellow fever vaccination.

In later stages, serologic diagnosis can be made by using ELISA to measure IgM 3 days after the onset of symptoms; however, yellow fever vaccination and infection with other flaviviruses, including dengue, West Nile, and Zika viruses, may give a false-positive ELISA test result. If ELISA is positive for other flaviviruses, the more specific plaque reduction neutralization assay should be done in reference laboratories.

Differential Diagnosis

It may be difficult to distinguish yellow fever from other viral hepatitides, malaria, leptospirosis, louse-borne relapsing fever, dengue, and other hemorrhagic fevers on clinical grounds alone. *Albuminuria* is a consistent feature in yellow fever patients, and its presence helps differentiate yellow fever from other viral hepatitides. Serologic confirmation is often needed.

Prevention

Four live attenuated yellow fever virus vaccines (all derived from the 17D strain) are prequalified by the WHO. All are given as a single dose and are safe and effective. A single dose of vaccine in the past was considered to provide lifelong immunity. While the 10-year booster dose is no longer recommended for most patients, persistent seropositivity at 8 years postvaccination is only 85% (and below 60% in children vaccinated at 9–12 months of age). Thus, at-risk groups with waning immunity and high probability of exposure may consider receiving a second dose of vaccine after 10 years. (These groups are listed at https://www.cdc.gov/yellow-fever/hcp/vaccine/.)

Yellow fever vaccine is recommended for persons age > 9 months who are traveling to or living in areas at risk for yellow fever virus transmission. *This vaccine should never be given to children under 6 months old* due to their higher risk of developing encephalitis related to the vaccine. *The WHO recommends that all endemic countries include yellow fever vaccine in their national immunization programs and provides a list of countries requiring yellow fever vaccination for entry.* The vaccine is contraindicated in persons with severe egg allergies or who are severely immunocompromised, including patients with primary immunodeficiencies, HIV infection with CD4+ cell count < 200 cells/mm^3, thymus disorder with abnormal immune function, malignant neoplasms, transplantation, or immunosuppressive and immunomodulatory therapies. Persons age > 60 are at higher risk for vaccine-related complications (see below) but might still be offered vaccination in select cases after considering risks and benefits. Pregnant persons and breastfeeding patients should receive the vaccine only if they cannot defer travel to endemic areas (Chapter 34). Clinicians should be aware of rare but frequently fatal vaccine-induced reactions, including anaphylaxis, yellow fever vaccine–associated viscerotropic disease, and yellow fever vaccine–associated neurologic disease.

Mosquito avoidance is an important complement to vaccination. If not in an endemic area, the patient should be isolated from mosquitoes to prevent local transmission.

Treatment

No specific antiviral therapy is available. Treatment is directed toward symptomatic relief and management of complications.

Prognosis

The mortality rate of the severe form is 20–50%, with death occurring most commonly between the sixth and the tenth days. Convalescence is prolonged, including 1–2 weeks of asthenia. Infection confers lifelong immunity to those who recover.

Centers for Disease Control and Prevention. Yellow fever vaccine 2023: information for health care professionals advising travelers. https://www.train.org/cdctrain/course/1111879/compilation

Kling K et al. Duration of protection after vaccination against yellow fever: a systematic review and meta-analysis. Clin Infect Dis. 2022;75:2266. [PMID: 35856638]

Waters TW et al. Updated yellow fever entry requirements and recommendations from WHO as of August 2020. J Travel Med. 2020;27:taaa152. [PMID: 32889538]

OTHER SYSTEMIC VIRAL DISEASES

1. Zika Virus

ESSENTIALS OF DIAGNOSIS

- Most infected persons asymptomatically seroconvert.
- Clinical symptoms resemble those of chikungunya virus infection but with less arthritis.
- Complications include microcephaly and ocular abnormalities in infants born to mothers infected during pregnancy, as well as Guillain-Barré.
- No effective antiviral or vaccine is available.

General Considerations

Zika is a flavivirus, akin to the viruses that cause dengue fever, Japanese encephalitis, and West Nile infection.

The virus was noted in Africa and Asia during the 1950s–1980s but first spread beyond those two continents in 2007. A large outbreak occurred in French Polynesia in 2013. The virus then spread to the Western hemisphere and was first noted in northeastern Brazil in 2015. Zika virus spread rapidly throughout the Americas, including the United States and worldwide. Despite distinct lineages, Zika virus exists as only one serotype.

Aedes species mosquitoes, particularly *Aedes aegypti*, are primarily responsible for Zika virus transmission. The biodistribution of the species largely determines the area of prevalence for Zika virus. Rarely, a few other mosquito species including *Anopheles* and *Culex* may serve as vectors for Zika virus. The virus can also be transmitted via blood transfusion, vertical transmission and sexual transmission.

Since the onset of the first reported cases in the United States in 2015, most transmissions were reported in Puerto Rico, with limited local transmission reported in Florida and Texas. No confirmed Zika cases in US territories have been reported since 2019.

Clinical Findings

A. Symptoms and Signs

The incubation period is 3–14 days. Most (50–80%) of Zika virus infections are asymptomatic. Symptoms include acute-onset fever, maculopapular rash that is usually pruritic, nonpurulent conjunctivitis, and arthralgias. Rash may outlast the fever but is not always present. Symptoms last up to 7 days. Viral infections most often confused with Zika include dengue and chikungunya virus infections.

B. Laboratory Findings and Diagnostic Studies

Diagnosis is made by detecting viral RNA (nucleic acid testing) in patients presenting with onset of symptoms <7 days. Nucleic acid testing can be performed within 14 days of illness onset. People tested 14 days or more after symptom onset should be tested using IgM serology. Commercial RT-PCR assays and IgM ELISAs are available. Matched serum and urine specimens should be tested simultaneously. Although not routinely recommended, RT-PCR can be performed on amniotic fluid, CSF, and placental tissue. A positive RT-PCR test definitively diagnoses Zika virus infection and does not require additional confirmatory testing. A negative test does *not* exclude the presence of the virus in other tissues and does not rule out infection. Persons with negative NAATs and symptoms of Zika infection should undergo further testing for Zika virus IgM antibody and other arboviral infections. Serologic testing for Zika virus should only be conducted by laboratories with experience in performing flavivirus serology.

Recommended serologic assays include enzyme immunoassays and immunofluorescence assays and neutralization assays. The Zika MAC-ELISA can be performed on serum or CSF. Anti-Zika IgM antibodies are observed in CSF of children with congenital infection. Neutralizing antibodies can cross-react with dengue and other flaviviruses, so samples testing positive should be sent to public health laboratories for confirmation.

In the United States, testing for asymptomatic pregnant persons is not recommended by the CDC even after travel to an area with Zika activity. The WHO, however, still recommends testing via IgM antibody for asymptomatic pregnant persons who could have had contact with vector-borne or sexually transmitted Zika virus. In areas with active Zika transmission, asymptomatic pregnant persons should be tested for IgM antibodies as part of routine obstetric care. Persistent Zika virus RNA in serum has been reported in pregnancy. Pregnant persons with confirmed or suspected Zika virus infection may be monitored by serial ultrasounds at 3- to 4-week intervals, assessing fetal anatomy and growth. With a declining prevalence of Zika virus infection, positive antibody tests run the risk of more likely being false-positives.

Complications

Two neurologic complications are of particular concern: (1) **congenital microcephaly**, often associated with brain calcifications and other abnormalities; and (2) **Guillain-Barré syndrome**. The incidence of Guillain-Barré syndrome is estimated at 2–3 cases per 10,000 Zika virus infections. In addition to microcephaly, Zika causes a spectrum of congenital disabilities of the CNS that collectively are termed **congenital Zika syndrome**. These include fetal brain disruption sequence, subcortical calcifications, pyramidal and extrapyramidal signs, and ocular abnormalities. Newborns of women infected with Zika virus during pregnancy have a 5–14% risk of congenital Zika syndrome and a 4–6% risk of Zika virus–associated microcephaly. Spontaneous abortions and rare deaths related to Zika virus infection are reported.

As with Ebola virus, the Zika virus can persist in semen for months; in the male reproductive tract the prostate gland and the testes are the presumed reservoirs. Persistence of the virus in the female reproductive tract is possible.

Prevention

The most effective means of Zika prevention include measures to reduce mosquito contact and limit mosquito breeding grounds. Because of the association between microcephaly and Zika virus infection during pregnancy, *pregnant persons should avoid travel to areas where Zika virus is circulating*. Guidelines for testing pregnant persons potentially exposed are available through the CDC. The CDC recommends that pregnant couples use condoms or abstain from sex for the entire pregnancy if the pregnant person's partner had a possible Zika virus exposure. Infected individuals should refrain from sexual intercourse (https://www.cdc.gov/zika/hcp/sexual-transmission/) and blood donations for months (at least 3 months for men, 2 months for women). No approved vaccine against the Zika virus exists.

Treatment

No antivirals are approved for treatment of Zika virus; thus, management should focus on supportive care. Aspirin and NSAIDs are avoided during illness caused by the flavivirus dengue because of its propensity to cause hemorrhage. Zika virus infections, however, do not appear to be associated with major hemorrhagic complications.

Kovacs A. Zika, the newest TORCH infectious disease in the Americas. Clin Infect Dis. 2020;70:2673. [PMID: 31346608]

Major CG et al. Risk estimation of sexual transmission of Zika virus—United States, 2016-2017. J Infect Dis. 2021;224:1756. [PMID: 33822107]

World Health Organization. Zika epidemiology update – May 2024.https://www.who.int/publications/m/item/zika-epidemiology-update-may-2024

2. Chikungunya Fever

Chikungunya ("that which bends up" in the Kimakonde language) fever is an alphavirus infection transmitted to humans by *A. aegypti* and *A. albopictus* and is considered a classic "arthritogenic" virus. The first documented clinical cases in India were derivative of the E/C/S African strains with later reports of outbreaks in Kenya in 2004. Subsequently, reports emerged from areas adjoining the Indian Ocean, Southeast Asia and its neighboring islands (2005–2007), South India (2005), and the island of La Réunion (2005–2006), with further spread including autochthonous cases in Italy and France (2007). Chikungunya virus is ubiquitous in endemic countries in Africa, the Americas, Asia, and Europe. The CDC reported 0 locally acquired cases and 225 travel-associated US cases in 2025.

Among naïve populations, attack rates are often as high as 50%. On Saint Martin, 39% of infections were asymptomatic. Vertical transmission may occur if the mother is viremic at time of delivery, but transmission does not appear to occur throughout pregnancy as it does with Zika virus. Endemicity of *A. aegypti* in the Americas and the introduction of *A. albopictus* into Europe and the New World raise concern for further extension of the epidemic.

Clinical Findings

A. Symptoms and Signs

After an incubation period of 1–12 days (estimated median 3), the acute presentation is characterized by a viremic phase (5–10 days with abrupt fever; headache; polyarthralgia affecting small, large, and axial joints; myalgia; and cutaneous rash) followed by a postviremic phase (6–21 days) with sustained polyarthralgia/arthritis, fatigue, and myalgia. The simultaneous involvement of > 10 joints and tenosynovitis (especially in the wrist) are characteristic. The *stooped posture* of patients gives the disease its name. Joint symptoms persist for 4 months in 33% and linger for years in about 10%. A centrally distributed pigmented or pruritic maculopapular rash is reported in 10–40% of patients. Mucosal disease occurs in about 15%. Facial edema and localized petechiae are reported. Neurologic complications, including encephalitis, myelopathy, peripheral neuropathy, Guillain-Barré syndrome, myeloneuropathy, and myopathy, are usually found in persons younger than 5 years or older than 49 years. Hemorrhagic fever–like presentations are unusual. Coinfection with other respiratory viruses and with dengue is common. Some of the neuropathology may be immune-mediated, and these cases are usually in those over age 20 and associated with longer latencies and better outcomes. Death is rare and usually related to underlying comorbidities. The differential diagnosis includes other tropical febrile diseases, such as malaria, leishmaniasis, or dengue.

B. Laboratory Findings

Diagnosis is made epidemiologically and clinically. Mild leukopenia occurs as does thrombocytopenia, which is seldom severe. Radiographs of affected joints are normal during the acute phase. Bone lesions are visible in some patients with chronic symptoms.

Serologic confirmation requires elevated IgM titers or a fourfold increase in convalescent IgG levels using an ELISA. RT-PCR and ELISA are commercially available; no ELISA kit is FDA-cleared. Culture techniques require BSL 3 (biosafety level 3) containment. Directions on submitting specimens for testing may be obtained from the CDC Arboviral Diseases Branch, 970-221-6400. Suspected cases in the United States should be promptly reported to public health authorities.

Complications & Prognosis

Common complications of chikungunya fever are long-term weakness, asthenia, myalgia, arthralgia, and arthritis, noted to be present in 25–66.5% of cases at 1 year. Risk factors for long-term arthralgias include the existence of such symptoms at 4 months after onset of disease and age > 35 years. Persons with preexisting arthritis are also at increased risk for prolonged symptoms after chikungunya infection. Comorbid conditions, including hypertension, diabetes, and cardiac diseases, may contribute to severe outcomes; although in some series, patients with significant neurologic complications do not show comorbidities.

Treatment & Prevention

Treatment is supportive with NSAIDs and corticosteroids. Chronic joint disease may require disease-modifying antirheumatic medications such as methotrexate.

A live-attenuated Chikungunya vaccination, Ixchiq (VLA1553), is not available any longer in the United States due to concern for risk of severe Chikungunya-like symptoms including encephalitis. However, Vimkunya, a recombinant chikungunya vaccine, remains available for individuals 12 years and older who are traveling to regions experiencing a Chikungunya outbreak and also for laboratory workers. As for other arboviral illnesses, measures to minimize mosquito exposures are also important for disease prevention.

Centers for Disease Control and Prevention. Chikungunya virus in the United States. https://www.cdc.gov/chikungunya/data-maps/chikungunya-us.html

Ng WH et al. Chronic chikungunya disease (CCD): clinical insights, immunopathogenesis and therapeutic perspectives. QJM. 2024;117:489. [PMID: 38377410]

COMMON VIRAL RESPIRATORY INFECTIONS

1. Severe Acute Respiratory Syndrome—Coronavirus 2019 (SARS-CoV-2)

ESSENTIALS OF DIAGNOSIS

- When symptomatic, adults often have respiratory tract illness with fever and cough; upper tract symptoms are more prominent with more recently circulating variants.
- Advanced pulmonary complications (pneumonia, acute respiratory distress syndrome [ARDS]) occur with fulminant disease.

- High predilection for older adults and patients who are immunocompromised, have chronic diseases, and live in crowded conditions.
- Now in endemic phase, with WHO declaring the end of the pandemic phase on May 5, 2023 (with ongoing management with yearly booster vaccinations recommended for older persons and those with risk factors, and treatment when indicated).

General Considerations

Coronaviruses are a large family of viruses commonly found in humans and other species of animals, including bats, camels, cattle, cats, white-tailed deer, and hamsters. There are four genera of coronaviruses, of which only the alphacoronaviruses (coronavirus NL63 and 229E) and the betacoronaviruses affect humans. Like SARS-CoV-1, MERS-CoV, and the human common cold coronaviruses HC43 and HKU1, the SARS-CoV-2 virus is a betacoronavirus. All coronaviruses likely originated in bats.

A. Transmission

R_0 is the basic reproductive number signifying the number of contacts infected by one individual. Calculations of R_0 for SARS-CoV-2 have varied, but the true R_0 likely lies somewhere between 2 and 3, although transmission rates vary by SARS-CoV-2 strain. While the case fatality rate was far higher with the 2003 SARS-CoV-1 virus and with the MERS virus, the rate of person-to-person spread and the number of infected cases is much higher with SARS-CoV-2 than with either the SARS-CoV-1 or MERS viruses. Transmission is particularly efficient within higher-density living facilities and employment settings and is increased among newer variants such as Omicron (see below). Presymptomatic spread accounts for many cases, and the viral load for SARS-CoV-2 was highest the day before symptoms developed prior to widespread population immunity. After population immunity from vaccines and natural infection, the highest viral load for SARS-CoV-2 was on day four of symptoms, with most of the current spread occurring during active symptoms.

The incubation period for SARS-CoV-2 ranges from 2 to 24 days with an average of about 5 days. The principal mode of transmission is respiratory droplets (such as saliva) rather than by air (aerosolization), though aerosolization can occur during activities such as heavy exercise and singing. Simply talking (or singing) in close quarters may efficiently spread the virus. In a medical setting, the WHO and CDC recommend that healthcare providers use both *droplet* and *contact* precautions for all patients with suspected or confirmed COVID-19. Additionally, these organizations recommend that healthcare providers use *airborne* precautions when performing aerosol-generating medical procedures (such as collecting induced sputum or intubating the patient).

In utero transmission of SARS-CoV-2 is reported but appears to be rare. In general, the virus does *not* seem to be transmitted in breast milk.

Superspreading events (ie, when a person infected with SARS-CoV-2 is at the most infectious stage [usually around day 4 of infection] and infects a disproportionate number of susceptible persons) can play an important role in SARS-CoV-2 transmission. The importance of venues outside the home for spreading infection is evident from a Japanese review in which 61% of all national cases were traceable to clusters outside the home, including restaurants, bars, event venues, and workplaces. In a study from the University of Colorado at Boulder, the role of "supercarriers" also was identified, with just 2% of infected individuals carrying 90% of the virions circulating within the community. These persons may be superspreaders.

B. Risk Factors

Data from the United States early in the COVID-19 epidemic showed that the infection rate was highest among young and middle-aged adults, with nearly 25% of confirmed cases occurring in persons age 20–29 and about 20% in those age 50–64. Data from the southern United States showed increases in incidence among persons age 20–39 precede the increases among those age > 60 by 4–15 days. *COVID-19 mortality rates are distinctly higher over the age of 50* and among persons with comorbid medical conditions *such as diabetes, obesity, hypertension, chronic heart, lung, or kidney disease, and prior stroke.* In one large multiethnic cohort study of adults hospitalized with COVID-19, obesity was associated with a 113% increased risk of hospitalization and a 43% increased risk of death.

Children are just as susceptible to SARS-CoV-2 acquisition as adults, although they are much *less* likely to manifest symptoms. Younger individuals, including children, are more likely to have been previously exposed to benign cold-causing coronaviruses that may provide relative protection from severe SARS-CoV-2 infection. Additionally, children have lower concentrations of ACE-2 receptors—the receptor used by SARS-CoV-2 to infect host cells—in lung tissue, which may explain their lower propensity toward severe infection.

1. COVID-19 in immunosuppressed patients—Immunocompromised persons (ie, persons with malignancy, solid organ and hematopoietic stem cell transplant recipients, persons living with HIV, and individuals receiving biologic treatments for autoimmune or other conditions, among others) are at increased risk of severe illness due to COVID-19, though risks vary by patient population in this heterogeneous category. Patients with cancer, especially those with metastatic tumors or lymphomas, or who have recently received chemotherapy, show higher risks of adverse outcomes when infected with SARS-CoV-2. In one review, the subgroups of cancer patients who had disproportionately high COVID-19 mortality included those with lung cancer (case fatality rate [CFR] 18–55%) and those with hematologic malignancy (CFR 33–41%). Immunocompromised individuals may demonstrate prolonged viral shedding and can show a reduced response to vaccination, particularly persons who have received B cell–depleting agents such as rituximab.

2. COVID-19 in pregnancy—See also Chapter 22. While pregnancy is not clearly associated with an increased risk of *acquisition* of SARS-CoV-2, complications develop in pregnant patients at a higher rate than in nonpregnant patients. In a large multinational cohort study of pregnant patients, COVID-19 is shown to be associated consistently with higher maternal morbidity and mortality including increased rates of preeclampsia and eclampsia, severe maternal infections, and maternal ICU admissions. While miscarriage rates are not increased, SARS-CoV-2 can rarely cause placentitis which may lead to stillbirth. In addition, SARS-CoV-2 infection during pregnancy has been associated with preterm birth in some but not all studies.

C. SARS-CoV-2 Variants

Multiple SARS-CoV-2 genetic variants have been identified to date; detailed information on current variants can be found on the WHO (https://www.who.int/en/activities/tracking-SARS-CoV-2-variants/) and CDC websites (https://covid.cdc.gov/covid-data-tracker/#variants-genomic-surveillance).

Most reported mutations are within the spike ("S") protein and can be associated with reduced neutralization by antispike antibodies. Indeed, the evolution of the S protein in the current-era variants have rendered all former monoclonal antibody treatments ineffective.

Clinical Findings

A. Symptoms and Signs

Most infected individuals are asymptomatic, although the ratio of asymptomatic to symptomatic infection changes as more individuals are tested and has evolved with increasing vaccination and infection-inducted immunity. Adults can manifest a wide range of symptoms from mild to severe illness that typically begin 2–14 days after exposure to SARS-CoV-2. Symptomatic patients may have cough, fever, chills/rigors, myalgias, or pharyngitis. Dyspnea is variable but common in severe infection. No one symptom should be used as a discriminant for disease. Less frequent early symptoms include rhinitis, pharyngitis, abdominal symptoms such as nausea and diarrhea, headaches, anosmia, and ageusia (absence of taste) or dysgeusia (disordered taste). At the pandemic's beginning, 15–20% of adults with SARS-CoV-2 infection required hospitalization and 3–5% required critical care. These rates evolved substantially throughout the pandemic with the development of inpatient treatment (eg, remdesivir, dexamethasone) and, later, administration of the COVID-19 vaccines.

B. Laboratory Findings

Hematologic findings include neutrophilia, absolute lymphopenia, and an increased neutrophil-to-lymphocyte ratio. As disease advances, blood chemistry findings often include elevated liver biochemical tests and total bilirubin. Serum markers of systemic inflammation increase in most patients with severe COVID-19, including LD, ferritin, CRP, procalcitonin, and interleukin 6 (IL-6). A coagulopathy is often seen in severe COVID-19, identified by elevated von Willebrand factor (VWF) antigen, elevated D-dimer, and fibrin/fibrinogen degradation products; the prothrombin time, partial thromboplastin time, and platelet counts are usually unaffected initially (see Chapter 14).

C. Diagnostic Studies

The three commonly used types of diagnostic tests are *molecular* tests (most sensitive and specific) and *rapid antigen detection* tests (inexpensive and fast but not as sensitive). *Antibody (serologic)* tests are infrequently used because they generally cannot distinguish vaccination from infection (depending on the assay). Viral culture can be done in research settings but is not used in clinical practice given slower turnaround and lab biosafety requirements.

1. Molecular tests—Reverse transcriptase polymerase chain reaction (RT-PCR) assays have remained a mainstay of COVID-19 diagnosis. These tests detect genetic material and do not directly assess the presence of replicating virus. Isolation of the virus by nucleic acid assays > 10 days after the onset of symptomatic infection (or 15 days after exposure, on average) is usually not associated with replicative infectious particles. Prolonged viral shedding of viral RNA is common (particularly among immunocompromised persons) and underpins guidelines to avoid retesting for SARS-CoV-2 within 90 days of prior infection in most instances. RT-PCR testing is generally done on upper respiratory swabs such as nasopharyngeal swabs. Patients may have positive tests from lower respiratory samples (eg, bronchoalveolar lavage fluid) despite negative samples from the upper respiratory tract.

2. Rapid antigen detection tests—Rapid antigen detection tests are available both in healthcare settings and as home tests. These tests generally are performed on specimens from the upper respiratory tract. Sensitivity of antigen-based testing is lower than that of nucleic acid–based testing, particularly among asymptomatic persons, but performance improves substantially among symptomatic persons (85% compared with culture-based standard in one CDC study). Antigen-based testing may therefore have a role in triaging a case's potential infectiousness.

3. Antibody (serologic) tests—A number of antibody assays are available; they are not useful in diagnosing SARS-CoV-2 infection but can be used to determine immune status. In setting of widespread population immunity, serologic testing is generally not clinically useful for immunocompetent persons. These tests generally are performed on blood (specifically, serum) specimens.

D. Imaging

Early in the disease course, neither CXRs nor chest CT scans provide diagnostic utility, since both may be normal, and the nonspecific findings overlap with those of many respiratory viral infections. Later in the disease course, nonspecific diffuse ground-glass opacities (which may be peripherally-based) and/or multilobar infiltrates become more common. Chest ultrasonography, MRI, and PET/CT findings tend to confirm the CT findings of an evolving organizing pneumonia.

Differential Diagnosis

The clinical presentation of COVID-19 overlaps considerably with other respiratory viruses (including influenza, RSV, and others), necessitating specific testing. Community COVID-19 rates (based on clinical testing or wastewater surveillance data) inform the likelihood of a positive COVID-19 diagnosis. Seasonal influenza infection can usually be ruled out by a nasal PCR. Concomitant infection with influenza or other respiratory pathogens is reported. A useful table comparing symptoms of an upper respiratory infection, influenza, and COVID-19 is available at https://www.medicalnewstoday.com/articles/coronavirus-vs-flu#symptoms.

Complications

Many extrapulmonary complications are reported, and most of these are likely related to SARS-CoV-2–induced inflammatory reactions.

1. SARS-CoV-2–related immune activation—Individuals with more severe COVID-19 disease show pronounced systemic inflammation at presentation, often called a "cytokine storm" in the later phase of illness. Persistent immune activation in predisposed patients can lead to uncontrolled amplification of cytokine production (including IL-6), leading to multiorgan failure and death. An increased incidence of autoimmune diseases is reported, including Guillain-Barré syndrome, autoimmune hepatitis, autoimmune thyroiditis, and autoimmune encephalitis.

2. Pulmonary complications—The most common system involved with complications of severe COVID-19 is pulmonary. Some patients progress to ARDS akin to the coronavirus infections that cause SARS and MERS. In a large Veterans Affairs database early in the pandemic, the risk for such progression was 19-fold greater among COVID-19 patients than among influenza patients. Determination of need for noninvasive ventilation versus intubation versus extracorporeal membrane oxygenation (ECMO) is based on disease severity and likelihood of progressive ARDS.

3. Coagulation complications—See also Chapter 14. **COVID-19-related coagulopathy** is well described and associated with a predisposition to pulmonary embolism and deep venous thrombosis. In general, *outpatients* with COVID-19 should not receive anticoagulant or antiplatelet therapy to prevent venous or arterial thrombosis unless other strong indications are present. Therapeutic anticoagulation with heparin has been recommended for *hospitalized* patients requiring supplemental oxygen (but **not** high-flow nasal cannula oxygen or noninvasive or mechanical ventilation) with elevated d-dimer and without increased bleeding risk. Prophylactic-dose heparin is recommended for other persons hospitalized with COVID-19 who do not have another indication for therapeutic anticoagulation, including critically ill patients requiring high-flow nasal canula oxygen or noninvasive or mechanical ventilation. The reader is directed to online guidance for the most current recommendations on anticoagulant management.

Vaccine-induced thrombosis and thrombocytopenia are discussed below (see Vaccine-associated reactions and complications, below).

4. Cardiac complications—In a multicenter US cohort study, MI occurred in 14% of patients with COVID-19; survival was infrequent (2.9%) in those with infarction who were older than 80 years. A fulminant myocarditis occurs in about 15% of ICU patients, which can be further complicated by HF, cardiac arrhythmias, ACS, stress cardiomyopathy, cardiac aneurysms, vasculitis, and sudden death. The rates of myocarditis and pericarditis following infection are considerably higher than the rates following vaccination.

5. Renal complications—AKI occurred in approximately 12% of patients hospitalized with COVID-19 early in the pandemic. Of these, > 20% required renal replacement therapy. Overactive bladders and increased incidences of UTIs are seen with long COVID (see below).

6. Rheumatologic complications—Examples include inflammatory arthritis, SLE, and less often rhabdomyolysis and myositis. An IgA vasculitis has been reported in patients with long COVID.

7. GI complications—SARS-CoV-2 is shed in the stool in up to 80% of patients and, in a small subset (3.8%), is shed for up to 7 months. Such patients are more likely to report GI symptoms, particularly abdominal pain, nausea, and vomiting (but not diarrhea, which is infrequent). A particularly strong association existed between acute pancreatitis and SARS-CoV-2 infection. LFT abnormalities occur in 53% of healthy vaccinees.

8. Neurologic complications—Commonly reported neurologic complications are headaches; seizures; strokes; and more often, a loss of taste and smell (ageusia and anosmia). The loss of smell without significant rhinorrhea or nasal congestion suggests a neurotropism by this coronavirus. SARS-CoV-2–related meningitis as well as other neurologic complications, including impairment of consciousness to a comatose state, Guillain-Barré syndrome, paresthesia, and acute hemorrhagic necrotizing encephalopathy, have been reported. Such neurologic manifestations were associated with higher in-hospital mortality.

9. Psychiatric complications—Acute psychiatric diagnoses occurring at increased frequency include anxiety, depression, substance use disorder, and PTSD. Increased social isolation resulting from lockdowns was one of several factors contributing to worsened mental health during the early years of the pandemic. Opioid use disorders increased and were attendant with a decrease in outpatient visits for management and a possible decrease in access to naloxone.

10. Dermatologic complications—Skin manifestations are diverse and, on occasion, the presenting sign. Approximately 5–20% of patients with COVID-19 have dermatologic symptoms. One review of patients with COVID-19 identified acral lesions as the most common rash type, followed by erythematous maculopapular rashes, vesicular rashes, urticarial rashes, and many others. COVID-19 has also been associated with increased risk of herpes zoster virus (VZV) reactivation (shingles) in adults 50 years and older.

11. Infectious complications—One systematic review found that approximately 8% of patients hospitalized with COVID-19 have bacterial coinfection or secondary infection. Invasive pulmonary aspergillosis and mucormycosis have been recognized in some cases.

12. Endocrine complications—A host of endocrine abnormalities are reported including diabetic ketoacidosis, subacute thyroiditis with clinical thyrotoxicosis, new-onset Graves disease, autoimmune (Hashimoto) thyroiditis, and new-onset adrenal insufficiency.

13. Multisystem inflammatory syndrome—A hyperinflammatory syndrome akin to atypical Kawasaki disease (KD) is called **multisystem inflammatory syndrome in children (MIS-C)** and rarely **in adults (MIS-A)** in the United States. The leading systems involved are GI (the nonspecific symptoms have been diagnosed as appendicitis), cardiovascular, hematologic, mucocutaneous, and pulmonary. MIS-A presents with inflammatory complications weeks after mild or asymptomatic SARS-CoV-2 infection.

14. Long COVID—*While it is common for symptoms such as mild fatigue to slowly resolve after COVID-19, some individuals report persistent symptoms and deficits for 3 months or more following infection ("long COVID"). The prevalence of long COVID appeared to be between 4% and 7% of those who had acute COVID-19 infection early in the pandemic. With more population immunity and a less severe variant (ie, Omicron), the rate of postinfectious complications is now much lower at 0.2%.* A compilation of nine studies of **post-acute COVID-19 syndrome** demonstrates that the most common complications are fatigue (32%), smell or taste disorder (22%), dyspnea (16%), headache (12%), memory impairment (11%), hair loss (10%), and sleep disorder (10%). Vaccination is shown to reduce the incidence of long COVID substantially, regardless of variant, vaccine type, number of vaccine doses received, or severity of the acute infection.

Prevention

A. Personal and Public Health Measures

Recommended or required population-level and individual public health precautions have varied over the course of the pandemic and by locale. Precautions remain important in communities where SARS-CoV-2 continues to circulate, or most community members are unvaccinated, or both. COVID-19 rates have been more challenging to estimate in recent years due to reduced testing (among other factors), prompting interest in metrics such as wastewater testing to estimate disease activity.

1. Masks—Well-fitted and filtering masks can reduce transmission of respiratory viruses. For healthcare personnel, correctly sized but expired N95 masks with intact elastic bands and masks subjected to sterilization procedures had unchanged fitted filtration efficiencies (FFEs) of > 95%. Portable high-efficiency particulate air (HEPA) cleaners reduce aerosol exposure up to 90% when combined with universal masking. Data have been mixed regarding the real-world effectiveness of masks at reducing the risk of transmission of respiratory viral infections including COVID-19, but masking remains an important intervention to consider for the most medically vulnerable populations including elderly and immunocompromised.

2. Other nonpharmaceutical interventions—Current CDC guidelines recommend that persons with COVID-19 isolate at home until they have been fever-free for at least 24 hours (without fever-suppressive medications such as acetaminophen or NSAIDs) and show symptomatic improvement. These guidelines differ from those in healthcare settings, where time-based criteria (which can be shortened in some cases by follow-up negative testing) remain in use.

Prior to the availability of vaccines and treatments, the nonpharmaceutical interventions used for COVID-19 were physical distancing, face masks, ventilation, avoidance of indoor gatherings, testing, and contact tracing. Widespread asymptomatic testing did not seem to decrease transmission over other infection-prevention controls in healthcare settings, and the Society of Healthcare Epidemiology of America (SHEA) recommended against preadmission and preprocedure testing in 2022. After the availability and uptake of vaccines in high-income countries, and after the milder Omicron variant emerged, most countries stopped using lockdowns to curb viral transmission, given the negative impacts on overall public health.

3. Vaccines—Current vaccines targeting SARS-CoV-2 stimulate the production of neutralizing antibodies against the viral spike protein. In the United States, these vaccines include mRNA-based vaccines (manufactured by both Pfizer and Moderna) and less commonly a protein-based vaccine (Novavax). An adenovirus vector–based vaccine from Janssen/Johnson & Johnson is no longer available. All persons 6 months and older without contraindications are eligible for COVID vaccination in the United States. As vaccination guidance has been evolving, the reader is directed to online resources for the most current guidance.

While current COVID-19 vaccines provide modest efficacy against viral infection, they remain highly protective against severe illness. The continued evolution of SARS-CoV-2 has led to successive vaccine updates to better match circulating viral variants. Immunocompromised individuals are less likely to develop protective immunity following vaccination, prompting interest in passive immunotherapy with monoclonal antibodies, though providing durable protection in face of new viral variants remains a challenge. Mucosal vaccines are an active area of research and offer the hope of long-lasting immunity. Further research is also needed among solid organ transplant recipients who show very low response rates to COVID vaccines. It is advised that solid organ transplant patients receive a supplementary COVID booster dose.

4. Vaccine-associated reactions and complications—The COVID-19 vaccines are generally safe and well-tolerated. CDC data show that non–COVID-19–associated death rates among those vaccinated show lower mortality than the rates among the nonvaccinated, with appropriate cofactor adjustments (sex, age, race, ethnicity, location), thus confirming the safety profile of COVID-19 vaccines. Commonly reported side effects post–mRNA vaccine administration include nausea, low-grade fevers, injection-site soreness, headaches, and fatigue. Surveillance data show that myocarditis/pericarditis occurs disproportionately in young adults age 12–39 years at an excess rate of 6.3 per million doses during the week following vaccination. Rates are slightly higher after the second dose and for younger males. The ability to reduce the viral load is weaker for the adenovirus vector vaccines. Vaccines against COVID all show good efficacy against variants other than the original target, although nucleic acid vaccines offer the most protection.

Other postvaccination adverse events include autoimmune hepatitis akin to that seen with native disease but at lower frequency, polyarthritis (more common among patients with psoriatic than rheumatoid arthritis, uveitis, a set of neurologic complications of which Bell palsy is the most common followed by headache, cerebrovascular events, Guillain- Barré syndrome, function neurologic disorder, and CNS demyelination, most occurring after the Pfizer or prior AstraZeneca vaccine) and oral disorders (ageusia, xerostomia) akin to those of native disease but again at lower frequency.

5. Vaccination in pregnant and lactating patients—Vaccine registry data indicate that mRNA vaccines are safe in pregnant patients; thus pregnant patients and those planning pregnancy should be targeted for vaccination with the mRNA vaccines. Among vaccinated patients, SARS-CoV-2 vaccine antibodies appear in breastmilk by 2 weeks after vaccination and persist for 7 weeks; thus lactating patients and their breastfeeding children likely benefit from vaccination.

Treatment

The WHO (https://www.who.int/teams/health-care-readiness/covid-19), and the Infectious Diseases Society of America (IDSA) (https://www.idsociety.org/practice-guideline/covid-19-guideline-treatment-and-management/) provide guidance for the management of COVID-19 patients from screening to discharge.

While previously vaccinated and otherwise healthy persons with COVID-19 may require only supportive care, additional treatments (discussed below) should be offered to persons with increased risk for complications including unvaccinated, elderly, and immunocompromised individuals. Because of the biphasic nature of *advanced* cases, antiviral therapies may be most efficacious early on in the illness, with a greater role for anti-inflammatory agents at later stages.

A. Viral Protease Inhibitors

The oral boosted protease inhibitor nirmatrelvir/ritonavir (**Paxlovid**) is FDA-approved for the treatment of mild to moderate COVID-19 in outpatients age 12 years or older weighing ≥ 40 kg who are at high risk for progression to severe COVID-19. Treatment should be initiated within 5 days of symptom onset. Akin to protease inhibitors used in the treatment of HIV, nirmatrelvir is boosted with ritonavir, a potent CYP3A4 inhibitor. In phase 2/3 trials, nirmatrelvir/ritonavir showed a relative risk reduction of about 85% for hospitalization or death for patients at high risk of severe disease. The dose is 300 mg nirmatrelvir/100 mg ritonavir orally every 12 hours for 5 days (nirmatrelvir dose adjusted to 150 mg for GFR 30–60 mL/min/1.73 m^2 and contraindicated with GFR <30 mL/min/1.73 m^2). The benefit of nirmatrelvir/ritonavir among otherwise healthy vaccinated persons is less clear, but treatment is still recommended for persons at increased risk of severe disease based on age or medical comorbidities (particularly settings of immunocompromise).

Recurrent symptomatic viremia ("rebound") has been reported in up to 6.6% of patients after nirmatrelvir/ritonavir is stopped, but this phenomenon has also been noted with molnupiravir therapy and in the absence of antiviral therapy. Recurrent symptoms tend to be mild. The use of nirmatrelvir/ritonavir requires screening for potentially serious drug interactions (see https://www.covid19-druginteractions.org/checker), including with several anticonvulsants and antidepressants. Suspension of certain medications during nirmatrelvir/ritonavir treatment may be considered, but when CYP3A4 enzyme inducers are being used (eg, phenytoin, rifampin), alternative anti-COVID therapy is needed. For patients with a creatinine clearance <30 mL/min, nirmatrelvir/ritonavir should *not* be given.

Ensitrelvir, an oral SARS-CoV-2 3C-like protease inhibitor currently available in Japan, was found to reduce symptom duration by about 1 day compared to placebo among patients treated within <72 hours of disease onset in the SCORPIO-SR trial.

B. RNA Polymerase Inhibitors

Remdesivir (Veklury) is a viral RNA-dependent RNA polymerase (RdRp) inhibitor approved by the FDA for the treatment of hospitalized COVID-19 patients. Although trials have not demonstrated a mortality benefit from remdesivir, existing data suggest it improves time to clinical recovery. Remdesivir is recommended for hospitalized patients requiring supplemental oxygen therapy, but its benefit among patients receiving mechanical ventilation or ECMO is uncertain. Among hospitalized patients, 5 days of remdesivir was found to be noninferior to 10 days of remdesivir. In some cases, treatment beyond 5 days may be considered depending on the patient's clinical trajectory. Remdesivir also has a role in treatment of outpatients with mild to moderate COVID-19 who are at increased risk for severe disease based on age ≥ 60 or comorbidities and are seen within 7 days of symptom onset. Treatment duration is 3 days in these cases, and was associated with an 87% reduction in risk of death or hospitalization in a study done before COVID-19 vaccinations were widely available. Remdesivir is available only for intravenous use. Liver function test monitoring is recommended during treatment.

Molnupiravir is an oral antiviral that targets the SARS-CoV-2 RdRp and induces mutations that prohibit coronaviral propagation. While molnupiravir has been associated with reduced mortality compared to placebo, its overall role at a time when COVID-19 related mortality is low remains to be defined. Concern has also been raised about its mutagenic potential. Thus, molnupiravir should not be used in pregnant or breastfeeding women or those under 18 years of age (in whom it may affect bone and cartilage growth). Persons who are of childbearing potential or who have sexual partners of childbearing potential should use effective contraception while taking molnupiravir and subsequent to completing molnupiravir therapy (4 days for females, 3 months for males). In the United States, an FDA EUA has been granted for molnupiravir (800 mg every 12 hours for 5 days) *for the treatment of mild to moderate COVID-19* in adults with positive SARS-CoV-2 tests provided they are: (1) evaluated within 5 days of symptom onset; (2) at high risk for progression to severe disease, hospitalization, or death; and (3) not able to receive other FDA-approved COVID-19 antiviral therapies (ie, nirmatrelvir/ritonavir [Paxlovid] or remdesivir).

C. Corticosteroids

Dexamethasone has been shown to reduce the risk of death among hospitalized patients with severe respiratory complications of COVID-19. *Dexamethasone is recommended only for the treatment of patients with severe disease* (ie, those who require supplemental oxygen and those who are mechanically ventilated or need ECMO). A 10-day course of therapy is standard but can be abbreviated in cases with quick clinical improvement. Very lengthy steroid courses should be avoided due to the potential for multiple adverse effects, including superinfection, bleeding, hyperglycemia, hypertension, and neuropsychiatric complications, among others. Patients without hypoxia and who do not require mechanical ventilation or ECMO should *not* be given corticosteroids. If dexamethasone is unavailable, the NIH COVID-19 treatment guidelines recommend using alternative glucocorticoids, including prednisone, methylprednisolone, or hydrocortisone.

D. IL-6 Receptor Inhibitors

The IL-6 receptor inhibitors tocilizumab and sarilumab were developed and FDA-approved for treatment of a variety of autoimmune/inflammatory conditions including rheumatoid arthritis and were subsequently evaluated as adjunctive therapeutics for severe COVID-19 based on the recognition that high levels of IL-6 are a key component of the "cytokine storm" associated with severe SARS-CoV-2 infection. Of the two agents, there is greater clinical experience with tocilizumab. IL-6 inhibitors can be considered for patients with rapidly increasing respiratory needs and evidence of systemic inflammation, as well as those within 24 hours of admission to the ICU. They are not recommended in the setting of an underlying immunocompromising condition or concurrent (non–COVID-19) infection. IL-6 inhibitors can be used concurrently with corticosteroids, but JAK inhibitors such as baricitinib or tofacitinib (discussed below) should not be given with tocilizumab or sarilumab.

E. Janus Kinase Inhibitors

The Janus kinase (JAK) inhibitors baricitinib and tofacitinib also have attracted interest as adjunctive anti-inflammatory therapies in COVID-19. Like the IL-6 antagonists, these agents are also FDA-approved for treatment of autoimmune/inflammatory conditions including rheumatoid arthritis. In the context of COVID-19, JAK inhibitors have been associated with reduced disease progression and may be associated with reduced mortality. They may be most beneficial for persons receiving high-flow supplemental oxygen or noninvasive ventilation. Baricitinib has been studied in combination with remdesivir and may be considered as an alternative to corticosteroids among persons unable to tolerate corticosteroids. Due to venous thromboembolism risk, persons receiving JAK inhibitors should receive at least prophylactic-dose anticoagulation.

Prognosis

In the earlier COVID-19 surges, the infection fatality rate was < 1% for persons age < 65 years but increased to 15% for persons age ≥ 85 years. The severity of the infection has evolved as variants have appeared and population immunity has increased from infection, vaccination, or both. In a large CDC analysis conducted from December 2020 to October 2021 among > 1.2 million adults who completed primary vaccination, the rate of COVID-19 severe breakthroughs was 0.015% and the rate of COVID-19 death after a vaccine breakthrough was 0.0033%. A large analysis of severe breakthrough infections after 2 vaccine doses across 30 million individuals in the United Kingdom showed that age ≥ 80 years, chronic kidney disease, being on immunosuppressants, or having ≥ 5 comorbidities were continued risk factors for severe diseases. These kinds of population-level studies allow the public health community to target those at risk of severe breakthroughs (older patients and those on immunosuppressants) for booster vaccination and antiviral treatment.

When to Admit

The principal complications requiring admission for adults with COVID-19 are respiratory. Progression to respiratory failure and ARDS can be rapid, and any patient in a high-risk category for complications (eg, those with advanced age, immunosuppression, or chronic diseases, such as hypertension, obesity, and diabetes) or any patient with evident thrombotic, neurologic, or multiple organ system disease should be admitted for observation and placed under intensive care based on respiratory parameters.

Alonso Castillo R et al. Neurological manifestations associated with COVID-19 vaccine. Neurologia (Engl Ed). 2025;40:66. [PMID: 36288776]

Bhimraj A et al. Infectious Diseases Society of America guidelines on the treatment and management of patients with COVID-19. Clin Infect Dis. 2024;78:e250. [PMID: 36063397]

Hoang TNA et al. How well do different COVID-19 vaccines protect against different viral variants? A systematic review and meta-analysis. Trans R Soc Trop Med Hyg. 2025;119:1. [PMID: 39495246]

Janes H et al. Association between SARS-CoV-2 viral load and COVID-19 vaccination in 4 phase 3 trials. J Infect Dis. 2024;230:1384. [PMID: 39225478]
Rudolph AE et al. Factors affecting the impact of COVID-19 vaccination on post COVID-19 conditions among adults: a systematic literature review. Hum Vaccin Immunother. 2025;212474772. [PMID: 40079963]
Siegal DM et al. American Society of Hematology living guidelines on use of anticoagulation for thromboprophylaxis in patients with COVID-19: executive summary. Blood Adv. 2025;9:1247. [PMID: 39437797]
Watanabe A et al. Protective effect of COVID-19 vaccination against long COVID syndrome: a systematic review and meta-analysis. Vaccine. 2023;41:1783. [PMID: 36774332]
World Health Organization. COVID-19 dashboard. https://data.who.int/dashboards/covid19/cases

2. Respiratory Syncytial Virus (RSV) & Other Paramyxoviruses

ESSENTIALS OF DIAGNOSIS

- RSV is a major cause of morbidity and mortality at the extremes of age (< 5 years and > 65 years).
- Treatment is largely supportive.
- No active vaccination for RSV is available.

General Considerations

RSV is a paramyxovirus that causes annual outbreaks during the wintertime with usual onset of pulmonary symptoms between mid-October and early January in the continental United States, although RSV incidence first decreased then increased at unseasonable times in 2022 after the peak of the COVID-19 pandemic. Outside the United States, RSV usually peaks during wet months in areas with high annual precipitation and during cooler months in hot and dry areas. Infections occur earlier in urban areas. RSV is also shown to be increased among refugees and asylum seekers. Each year RSV causes > 3.6 million hospitalizations and ~100,000 deaths in children <5 years of age. The virus also causes significant disease among older adults.

There are two major subtypes of RSV: A and B. The A subtype may be associated with severe disease. RSV is a frequent cause of hospitalization in US children, with annual hospitalization rates of 6 per 1000 children younger than 5 years. RSV is the most common cause of bronchiolitis and pneumonia in children younger than 1 year in the United States. Prematurity and bronchopulmonary dysplasia are major risk factors for severe disease. Early RSV bronchiolitis in children, along with a family history of asthma, are associated with persistence of airway reactivity later in life.

RSV also causes upper and lower respiratory tract infection in older adults, with the virus entering through contact with mucous membranes. RSV occurs with increasing severity in those with comorbid conditions, older adults (accounting for a rate of 4 per 1000 hospitalizations and 14,000 deaths annually), persons with severe combined immunodeficiency, and patients after lung or bone marrow transplantation (because CD8 T cells are not available for viral clearance). An IL-1 receptor polymorphism is associated with more severe bronchiolitis. Recurrences occur throughout life. In 2023, major advances in combating RSV occurred, with three RSV vaccines being approved for individuals 60 years and older and for pregnant women between 32 and 36 weeks' gestation to protect the neonate. A monoclonal antibody for RSV (nirsevimab) was approved for infants and young children for severe disease. The average incubation period is 5 days. Up to 10% of disease classified as invasive pneumococcal disease is thought to be RSV or influenza.

In immunocompromised patients, such as bone marrow transplant recipients, serious pneumonia can occur, and outbreaks with a high mortality rate (> 70%) are reported.

Other paramyxoviruses important in human disease include human metapneumovirus, parainfluenza virus, and Nipah virus.

Human metapneumovirus is a ubiquitous seasonal virus circulating during late winter to early spring. It is divided into subgroups A and B. Metapneumovirus accounted for 7.3% of childhood (younger than 16 years old) pneumonia in a Norwegian series of 3650 patients in which RSV accounted for 28.7%. Clinical presentations range from mild upper respiratory tract infections to severe lower respiratory tract infections (eg, bronchiolitis, croup, and pneumonia). Lower respiratory tract (sometimes severe) infections are observed among immunocompromised and older adults, especially residents of nursing homes. In lung transplant recipients, human metapneumovirus is a common cause of respiratory illness and may increase the risk of acute and chronic graft rejection. Ribavirin appears to be well tolerated in lung transplant recipients with metapneumovirus infection. The control of RSV infection in modeling studies reduces the incidence of human metapneumovirus infection.

Human parainfluenza viruses (HPIVs) are commonly seen in children and are the most common cause of laryngotracheitis (croup). Four different serotypes are described, and they differ in their clinical presentations as well as epidemiology. HPIV-1 and HPIV-2 are responsible for croup. HPIV-3 is associated with bronchiolitis and pneumonia. HPIV-4 is a less frequently reported pathogen. Reinfections are common throughout life. HPIVs can also cause severe disease in older individuals, immunocompromised persons, and patients with chronic illnesses.

Nipah virus is a highly virulent paramyxovirus first described in 1999. Cases are concentrated mainly in Southeast Asia (Malaysia, Singapore, Bangladesh, and India). Fruit bats are identified as the natural host of the virus. An outbreak of 14 cases, 8 fatal, occurred in Bangladesh associated with drinking date palm sap between 2010 and 2014. Direct pig-human, cow-human, human-human, and nosocomial transmission are reported. Nipah virus causes acute encephalitis with a high fatality rate (67–92%), although respiratory symptoms are also described. Cranial nerve palsies, encephalopathy, and dystonia are among neurologic sequelae (15–32%) seen in infected individuals. Relapses occurring weeks and months after initial infection are described (3.4–7.5%).

Clinical Findings

A. Symptoms and Signs

In RSV bronchiolitis, proliferation and necrosis of bronchiolar epithelium develop, producing obstruction from sloughed epithelium and increased mucus secretion. Signs of infection include low-grade fever, tachypnea, and wheezing. Apnea is a common presenting symptom. Hyperinflated lungs, decreased gas exchange, and increased work of breathing are present. Pulmonary hemorrhage is reported. *In children, RSV is globally a common cause of acute lower respiratory infection and acute and recurrent otitis media.*

B. Laboratory Findings

A rapid diagnosis of RSV infection is made by viral antigen identification of nasal washings using an ELISA or immunofluorescent assay; molecular rapid tests are also used. Multiplex assays in conjunction with other respiratory viruses, most commonly influenza and SARS-CoV-2, are available commercially. RSV viral load assay values at day 3 of infection may correlate with requirement of intensive care and respiratory failure in children.

Human metapneumovirus is best diagnosed by PCR. Tests for rapid detection of viral antigens with immunofluorescence, ELISA, and PCR techniques are widely available for detection of HPIV. Culture also may be used. ELISA (serum and CSF) and PCR (urine and respiratory secretions but not blood) are both used for Nipah virus infection diagnosis.

Treatment & Prevention

Treatment of RSV consists of supportive care, including hydration, humidification of inspired air, monoclonal antibody therapy in neonates, antibiotic therapy (to reduce other respiratory morbidity) if concomitant bacterial pneumonia is suspected, and ventilatory support as needed. Neither bronchodilating agents nor corticosteroids show efficacy in bronchiolitis although individual patients with significant bronchospasm or history of asthma may respond to them.

The use of aerosolized ribavirin or RSV-enriched IVIG, or both, can be considered in high-risk patients, such as those with a history of bone marrow transplantation, and appears to lessen mortality.

The prophylactic monoclonal antibody **palivizumab** was the first monoclonal released for RSV and shows an excellent record as a highly effective preventive agent for RSV in high-risk infants. While recommended for and effective in such high-risk infants (premature infants < 32 weeks' gestation as well as infants 32–25 weeks' gestation with additional risk factors such as congenital heart and lung diseases and Down syndrome), it is not of proven efficacy among adults with RSV.

The monoclonal antibody **nirsevimab** also effectively prevents RSV-associated lower respiratory tract infections in premature and term infants. It is currently available in the United States, Europe, and the United Kingdom to prevent RSV in neonates during their first season at risk (and extended in the United States through their second at-risk season). The antibody targets the F fusion protein on the surface of RSV and is generally tolerated well (8% incidence of adverse effects) and shows an efficacy of 82% at 180 days after treatment.

Another monoclonal antibody with a distinct mechanism of action acting at pre- and postfusion RSV binding sites is clesrovimab-cfor (Enflonsia), which received FDA approval for use in infants during their first season at risk for RSV.

Other small-molecule RSV fusion inhibitors that bind to the surface F protein under study as potentially effective in adults 18–59 with chronic immunosuppressive diseases include ziresovir and sisunatovir.

While at least 24 vaccines are currently in development, 3 vaccines are currently approved and available for use in adults in the United States: Arexvy (GSK), Abrysvo (Pfizer), and mResvia (Moderna). The CDC recommends that one of these agents be given to all adults age 75 and older and adults 50–74 with certain immunosuppressive or chronic disease states such as asthma. The vaccines are well-tolerated and can be given with the influenza vaccines. The need for a second booster dose is not fully established. Vaccination of pregnant women (studied with Abrysvo) between 32 and 36 weeks of pregnancy is recommended to reduce the incidence of neonatal RSV infection. A prefusion F protein vaccine is showing promise as an additional RSV vaccine for adults with high-risk conditions.

Long-term complications of RSV include increases in cardiovascular and functional outcomes for those adults hospitalized with RSV. Infants can develop bronchiolitis and asthma; treatment of mothers with vaccine and passive immunization of infants appears to reduce acute and long-term RSV morbidity.

Prevention in hospitals entails rapid diagnosis, handwashing, contact isolation, and, perhaps, passive immunization. (Passive immunization is costly but is associated with improved antiviral titers in hematologic stem cell transplant recipients.) The use of conjugated pneumococcal vaccination appears to decrease the incidence of concomitant pneumonia associated with viral infections in children in some countries. Viral shedding averages 11 days and correlates inversely with age and directly with severity of infection.

Therapeutic modalities for human metapneumovirus and parainfluenza virus infections under investigation include intravenous ribavirin administration.

Alandijany TA et al. Evaluating the efficacy, safety, and immunogenicity of FDA-approved RSV vaccines: a systematic review of Arexvy, Abrysvo, and mResvia. Front Immunol. 2025;16:1624007. [PMID: 40901480]

Carbonell-Estrany X et al. Twenty-five years of palivizumab: a global historic review of its impact on the burden of respiratory syncytial virus disease in children. Expert Rev Anti Infect Ther. 2025;23:359. [PMID: 40111069].

Davis M et al. Bivalent RSVpreF vaccine in adults 18 to <60 years old with high-risk conditions. Clin Infect Dis. 2025;80:911. [PMID: 39523547]

Doty B et al. Incidence of RSV in adults: a comprehensive review of observational studies and critical gaps in information. J Infect Dis. 2024;230:e1182. [PMID: 38934801]

Faus-Cotino J et al. Nipah virus: a multidimensional update. Viruses. 2024;16:179. [PMID: 38399954]
Lee B et al. Real-world effectiveness and safety of nirsevimab, RSV maternal vaccine and RSV vaccines for older adults: a living systematic review and meta-analysis. Thorax. 2025;80:838. [PMID: 40930981]
Wang L et al. Nipah virus: epidemiology, pathogenesis, treatment, and prevention. Front Med. 2024;18:969. [PMID: 39417975]

3. Seasonal Influenza

ESSENTIALS OF DIAGNOSIS

- *Cases usually in epidemic pattern.*
- Onset with fever, chills, malaise, cough, coryza, and myalgias.
- Aching, fever, and prostration out of proportion to catarrhal symptoms.
- Leukopenia.

General Considerations

Influenza (an orthomyxovirus) is a highly contagious disease transmitted by the respiratory route in humans. Transmission occurs primarily by *droplet nuclei* rather than fomites or direct contact. Three types of influenza viruses infect humans. While type A can infect a variety of mammals (humans, swine, horses, etc) and birds, types B and C almost exclusively infect humans. Type A viruses are further divided into subtypes based on the hemagglutinin (H) and the neuraminidase (N) expressed on their surface. Eighteen subtypes of hemagglutinin and 11 subtypes of neuraminidase are identified. Type B virus has only one subtype but with two distinct lineages. Annual epidemics usually appear in the fall or winter in temperate climates. Up to 5 million cases of severe influenza and 500,000 deaths are estimated by the WHO to occur annually, with approximately 0.5 million annual deaths. Influenza epidemics affect 10–20% of the global population (3–11% with a mean of 8% in the United States) on average each year and are typically the result of minor antigenic variations of the virus, or **antigenic drift**, which occur often in influenza A virus. On the other hand, pandemics—associated with higher mortality—appear at longer and varying intervals (decades) as a consequence of major genetic reassortment of the virus (**antigenic shift**) or adaptation of an avian or swine virus to humans (as with the pandemic H1N1 virus of 1918).

The highly pathogenic avian influenza subtypes are discussed in the next section. The novel swine-origin influenza A (pandemic H1N1) virus emerged in Mexico in 2009 and quickly spread throughout North America and the world causing a pandemic. This virus originated from triple-reassortment of North American swine, human, and avian virus lineages and Eurasian swine virus lineages and replaced the previous H1N1 seasonal virus.

Clinical Findings

A. Symptoms and Signs

Type A and B seasonal influenza viruses produce clinically indistinguishable infections, whereas type C usually causes mild illness. The incubation period is 1–4 days. In unvaccinated persons, uncomplicated influenza often begins abruptly. Symptoms range widely from nearly asymptomatic to a constellation of systemic symptoms (including fever, chills, headache, malaise, and myalgias) and respiratory symptoms (including rhinorrhea, congestion, pharyngitis, hoarseness, nonproductive cough, and substernal soreness). GI symptoms and signs may occur, particularly among young children with influenza B virus infections. Fever lasts 1–7 days (usually 3–5). Older patients especially may present with lassitude and confusion, often without fever or respiratory symptoms. Signs include mild pharyngeal injection, flushed face, and conjunctival redness. Moderate enlargement of the cervical lymph nodes and tracheal tenderness may be observed. The presence of fever (> 38.2°C) and cough during the influenza season is highly predictive of influenza infection in individuals aged > 4 years. Idiopathic thrombocytopenic purpura also is a recognized complication.

Influenza is also a travel-associated illness, and providers need be aware of the differential seasonality of the disease in assessing potential travel-associated illnesses.

B. Laboratory Findings

Rapid influenza diagnostic tests for detecting influenza antigens from nasal or throat swabs are widely available, highly specific, and produce fast results but have low sensitivity leading to high false-negative results. Because of this, *the CDC recommends empirically treating patients in whom influenza is suspected.* Not all commercial rapid influenza diagnostic tests can differentiate between influenza A and influenza B, and none of the available rapid influenza diagnostic tests can provide information on influenza A subtypes. Newer digital immunoassays and rapid nucleic acid amplification tests are more sensitive than traditional rapid influenza diagnostic tests; however, the sensitivity and specificity of newer PCR techniques are compromised early in the season during low-prevalence periods. A nasopharyngeal swab, nasal aspirate, combined nasopharyngeal swab with oropharyngeal swab, or material from a bronchoalveolar lavage can be tested for any influenza strain. When influenza pneumonia is suspected, lower respiratory tract specimens should be collected and tested for influenza viruses by RT-PCR or the above assays.

Differential Diagnosis

The differential diagnoses for influenza-like infections include a variety of viral respiratory infections (SARS-CoV-2, parainfluenza, RSV, atypical dengue, adenovirus, enterovirus, coronavirus) or other viral infections (flavivirus, CMV, EBV, acute HIV infection), as well as bacterial infections such as mycobacterial infection (atypical pneumonia), pertussis, and Legionnaire disease. Epidemiologic factors can suggest Legionnaire (older adults who smoke cigarettes).

Chronicity of cough may suggest adenovirus, mycobacterial, or pertussis infection. Leukocytosis and lymphadenopathy are more often seen with CMV and EBV. Distinguishing influenza from dengue requires attention to rhinitis (influenza) and thrombocytopenia (dengue) and travel history.

Complications

Hospitalization or ICU admission for influenza is often a consequence of diffuse viral pneumonitis with severe hypoxemia and sometimes shock. Patients with asthma, residents of nursing homes and long-term care facilities, adults aged 65 years or older, persons who have morbid obesity, and persons with underlying medical conditions (pulmonary, renal, cardiovascular, hepatic, hematologic, neurologic, and neurodevelopmental conditions; and immune-deficient conditions, such as HIV, diabetes, and cirrhosis) are at high risk for complications. Infection during pregnancy increases the risk for hospitalization and may be associated with severe illness, sepsis, pneumothorax and respiratory failure, spontaneous abortion, preterm labor, and fetal distress.

Influenza causes necrosis of the respiratory epithelium, increased adherence of bacteria to infected cells, and ciliary dysfunction, which predispose to secondary bacterial infections. Pneumococcal pneumonia is the most common secondary infection, and staphylococcal pneumonia is the most serious. *Haemophilus* spp infections also occur. Other frequent complications are acute sinusitis, otitis media, and purulent bronchitis.

CVDs are a complication of influenza infection, in particular among older adults, and influenza is postulated to be a significant trigger for MI, cerebrovascular disease, and sudden death. Several studies suggest that influenza vaccination protects against major adverse cardiovascular events. Neurologic complications, including seizures, Guillain-Barré syndrome, myelitis, and encephalopathy, may occur. Encephalopathic complications of influenza are uncommon, but the role of influenza in the evolution of stroke and dementia is showing increased documentation.

Influenza has been variably associated with autoimmune conditions including Guillain-Barré syndrome, type 1 diabetes mellitus, and antiphospholipid syndrome.

Reye syndrome is a rare and severe complication of influenza (usually B type) and other viral diseases (especially varicella), particularly in young children. It consists of rapidly progressive hepatic failure and encephalopathy, and the mortality rate is 30%. The pathogenesis is unknown, but the syndrome is associated with aspirin use in the management of viral infections.

Prevention

Annual influenza vaccination is the most effective measure for preventing influenza and its complications. Seasonal influenza vaccines can reduce influenza hospitalizations by up to an estimated 60%, although the efficacy varies considerably by year (as low as 19% during the 2014–2015 season, but 60% from the 2010–2011 season). Vaccination of health care workers is associated with decreased mortality among hospitalized patients and those in long-term care facilities. Vaccination prevents influenza illness among pregnant patients and their infants during the first months of life. Electronic nudges are shows to be helpful in increasing influenza vaccination utilization.

Multiple measures of CVD are improved with influenza vaccinations including the incidence of myocardial infarction, TIA, cardiac arrest, stroke, and overall mortality.

The ACIP and the American College of Obstetricians and Gynecologists Committee recommend annual influenza vaccination for all persons > 6 months of age with no contraindications. Vaccination is emphasized for high-risk groups and their contacts and caregivers.

Several Cochrane database analyses have examined the efficacy of the influenza vaccines in select populations. The studied groups include patients with COPD (a documented reduction in exacerbations with inactivated vaccine), older adults (where vaccination shows some efficacy), adults with cancer (weak evidence, some lower mortality and influenza-related outcomes), healthy adults (established efficacy with inactivated vaccine, but only modest effects in pregnant patients and newborns), and healthy children (where both live and inactivated vaccines lower the rate of influenza infections).

Other reviews establish the efficacy and safety of influenza vaccination in patients with rheumatoid arthritis, asthma, or myasthenia gravis, and older nursing home patients. Patients with obesity have an impaired response to the influenza vaccine.

Multiple influenza vaccine products are licensed in the United States and available from different manufacturers (see Table 34–8). As of the 2024–2025 influenza season, quadrivalent vaccines are no longer recommended. Available vaccines include the standard- or high-dose vaccine. The CDC publishes its annual influenza recommendations in the late summer (https://www.cdc.gov/acip-recs/hcp/vaccine-specific/flu.html).

Adults > 18 years, including pregnant patients, can receive any influenza vaccine, with few exceptions. Patients 65 years or older should receive a high-dose trivalent inactivated influenza vaccine containing several times more hemagglutinin than standard-dose influenza vaccines. Some data suggest intradermal vaccination is more effective than intramuscular vaccination in older adults. A European series shows efficacy differences based on age with limited protection against H3N2 infections among older individuals, and a meta-analysis among those age ≥ 65 shows improved efficacy with high-dose, adjuvanted or recombinant influenza vaccines compared with standard-dose unadjuvanted influenza vaccines. The immunosuppressed should receive a high-dose inactivated or adjuvanted inactivated influenza vaccine. *The COVID-19 vaccines can be safely coadministered with the inactivated seasonal influenza vaccines with an acceptable reactogenicity profile and without evidence of immunointerference.* Several combined influenza and SARS-CoV-2 vaccines are under study.

Vaccination is contraindicated for persons with a history of severe allergic reaction to an influenza vaccine. Precautions should be taken if patients report a history of

Guillain-Barré syndrome 6 weeks following an influenza vaccine and if patients have a moderate to severe acute illness with or without fever until clinical improvement. The new recommendation for those with egg allergy is that only those with urticarial reactions should be observed closely but all vaccinated patients should be followed for possible reactions regardless of egg allergy history. Dendritic targeting is a new form of vaccine strategy. Additional vaccine information can be found at https://www.cdc.gov/flu/professionals/.

When antiviral chemoprophylaxis is used, it prevents 70–90% of influenza infections. *Chemoprophylaxis is not routinely recommended and is not recommended prior to exposure to prevent development of resistance.* Chemoprophylaxis may be considered for persons at increased risk for complications from infection who are exposed to an infected patient within 2 weeks of vaccination, for persons unlikely to respond to vaccination because of immunosuppression after exposure to an infected person, for persons for whom vaccination is contraindicated and who are at high risk for complications after exposure to an infected person, and for prevention of infection in residents of institutions during an outbreak. Alternatively, a person can be monitored closely, and antiviral therapy initiated at the first onset of symptoms after exposure. Initiation of chemoprophylaxis is not recommended > 48 hours after exposure. Patients taking chemoprophylaxis should seek urgent medical care if an influenza-like illness develops.

Chemoprophylaxis against influenza A and B is accomplished with daily administration of the neuraminidase inhibitors oseltamivir (75 mg/day, oral) or zanamivir (10 mg/day, inhaled) to continue through 7 days after last known exposure. For outbreak control in long-term care facilities and hospitals, a minimum of 2 weeks is recommended, including in vaccinated persons if the seasonal vaccine is not well matched to the circulating strain, to continue until 1 week after identification of the last known case. Zanamivir should not be given as chemoprophylaxis to asthmatic persons, nursing home residents, or children younger than 5 years.

Breakthrough infections with influenza occur with neuraminidase inhibitors (in a study with zanamivir) and with vaccination. The efficacy of chemoprophylaxis is proven for individuals and households but not community settings.

Hand hygiene and surgical facemasks appear to prevent household transmission of influenza virus isolates when implemented within 36 hours of symptom recognition in an index patient. Such nonpharmaceutical interventions help mitigate the spread of pandemic and interpandemic influenza to unvaccinated persons. In one study, patients with seasonal H1N1 influenza infection were infectious from 1 day before through ~7 days following illness onset. Children and immunosuppressed persons exhibit prolonged viral shedding and may be infectious longer. Winter school breaks during periods of high influenza transmission appear to decrease rates of visits to primary care practitioners for influenza illness among children and adults.

Any hospital patient with suspected infection should be isolated in an individual room with standard and droplet precautions. CDC guidelines recommend the equivalent of N95 masks for aerosol-generating procedures (eg, bronchoscopy, elective intubation, suctioning, administering nebulized medications). For such procedures, an airborne infection isolation room can be used, with air exhausted directly outside or recirculated after filtration by a HEPA filter. Strict adherence to hand hygiene with soap and water or an alcohol-based hand sanitizer and immediate removal of gloves and other equipment after contact with respiratory secretions is essential. Precautions should be maintained until 7 days from symptom onset or until 24 hours after symptom resolution, whichever is longer. Postexposure prophylaxis or close monitoring and early treatment should be considered for close contacts of patients who are at high risk for complications of influenza and may be considered for healthcare personnel, public health workers, or first responders who experienced a recognized, unprotected close contact exposure to a person with influenza virus infection during that person's infectious period.

Treatment

Treatment is supportive. While no one antiviral agent is comprehensively inclusive, antiviral therapy should be considered for all persons with acute illness, in particular those at high risk for developing complications who have a suggestive clinical presentation or with laboratory-confirmed influenza. Clinical trials show a reduction in the duration of symptoms, hospital admissions, and secondary complications such as otitis, sinusitis, or pneumonia, but not mortality when using these agents. Maximum benefit is expected with the earliest initiation of therapy. Although the benefit of antiviral therapy after 48 hours of illness is reduced, it should be initiated if the patient is hospitalized or critically ill. Benefit has been noted up to 4–5 days into illness.

The antiviral treatment of choice should be based on the susceptibility of the circulating virus. Since high levels of resistance to the adamantanes (amantadine and rimantadine) persist among seasonal H1N1 and H3N2 influenza A viruses and these agents are not effective against influenza B viruses, amantadine and rimantadine are not recommended for treatment.

Three neuraminidase inhibitors are FDA-approved for treatment of influenza A and B: oral oseltamivir, inhaled zanamivir, and intravenous peramivir. The CDC recommends treatment with **oral oseltamivir** (75 mg twice daily for 5 days) as the medication of choice for patients of any age, pregnant persons, and patients who are hospitalized or have complicated infection. Absorption of oral oseltamivir is considered reliable, except in patients with impaired gastric motility or GI bleeding. Oseltamivir is, however, not shown to reduce hospitalization when used by otherwise healthy adults. A retrospective review shows no increased incidence of neuropsychiatric problems among oseltamivir users.

Inhaled zanamivir (10 mg, two inhalations twice daily for 5 days) is indicated for uncomplicated acute influenza in patients aged 7 years or older, is relatively contraindicated among persons with asthma because of the risk of bronchospasm and is not formulated for use in mechanically ventilated patients. Inhaled zanamivir lacks efficacy in pneumonia, probably due to poor bioavailability in the peripheral lungs.

Intravenous peramivir (600 mg in single dose) is used for outpatient treatment of uncomplicated infection in patients aged 18 years or older. It is also recommended if concern exists about inadequate oral absorption of oseltamivir. The efficacy of peramivir in patients with severe illness or influenza B is not well established. Some studies showed that repeated doses of intravenous peramivir for up to 5 days are safe and effective and shorten the duration of influenza illness.

Resistance to neuraminidase inhibitors (oseltamivir, zanamivir, and peramivir) can occur during or after prolonged use in immunocompromised patients, particularly in persons who have undergone hematopoietic stem cell transplant. **Intravenous zanamivir** is an investigational drug that could be requested for clinical use if concern exists for an oseltamivir-resistant influenza strain. **Laninamivir** is a long-acting inhaled neuraminidase inhibitor used for the treatment of seasonal influenza, including infection caused by oseltamivir-resistant virus. It is licensed in Japan and South Korea but not in the United States, although advanced development studies are underway with Biota Technology.

Baloxavir (a selective inhibitor of influenza cap-dependent endonuclease given as a single oral dose) is FDA-approved for treating uncomplicated influenza A and B infections and postexposure prophylaxis. It is widely used in Japan. It is given as 40 mg or 80 mg orally as a single dose depending on weight (the higher dose for persons 80 kg or more) and should be given within the first 48 hours of infection. Its side effects include diarrhea, headache, sinusitis, and bronchitis. The unique mechanism of baloxavir may be beneficial as part of multidrug therapy for resistant or severe disease, however, an RCT (FLAGSTONE) of patients hospitalized with severe influenza, comparing baloxavir plus a neuraminidase inhibitor versus placebo plus a neuraminidase inhibitor did not indicate that combining antivirals improved outcomes. For complicated disease, especially in immunosuppressed patients, the combination of oseltamivir, amantadine, and ribavirin appears to produce faster viral clearance but no definite clinical improvement.

Updated advice is available at http://www.cdc.gov/flu/.

Prognosis

The duration of the uncomplicated illness is 1–7 days, and the prognosis is excellent in healthy adults and children. Hospitalization typically occurs in those with underlying medical disease, at the extremes of age, and in pregnant patients. *Most fatalities are due to bacterial pneumonia, although exacerbations of other disease processes, in particular cardiac diseases, occur.* Pneumonia resulting from influenza has a high mortality rate among pregnant patients and persons with a history of rheumatic heart disease. Mortality among adults hospitalized with influenza ranges from 4% to 8%, although higher mortality (> 10–15%) may be seen during pandemics and among immunocompromised individuals. At least 64% of pneumonia and influenza deaths occurred among older persons in the United States, who comprised only 16% of the population.

If the fever recurs or persists for > 4 days with productive cough and white cell count > 10,000/mcL (10.0×10^9/L), secondary bacterial infection should be suspected.

When to Admit

- Limited availability of supporting services.
- Pneumonia or decreased oxygen saturation.
- Changes in mental status.
- Consider with pregnancy.

Antoon JW et al. Influenza with and without oseltamivir treatment and neuropsychiatric events among children and adolescents. JAMA Neurol. 2025;82:1013. [PMID: 40758339]

Do THT et al. Influenza B virus neuraminidase: a potential target for next-generation vaccines? Expert Rev Vaccines. 2024;23:39. [PMID: 38037386]

Drugs and Lactation Database (LactMed®) [Internet]. Bethesda (MD): National Institute of Child Health and Human Development; 2006. Influenza Vaccines. 2024 Aug 15. [PMID: 30000049]

Egorova M et al. Maternal influenza and offspring neurodevelopment. Curr Issues Mol Biol. 2024;46:355. [PMID: 38248325]

Falsey AR. Neurologic complications of influenza and potential protective vaccine effects. Influenza Other Respir Viruses. 2025;19:e70071. [PMID: 40045906]

Ferdinands JM et al. Protection against influenza hospitalizations from enhanced influenza vaccines among older adults: a systematic review and network meta-analysis. J Am Geriatr Soc. 2024;72:3875. [PMID: 39230284]

Grohskopf LA et al. Prevention and control of seasonal Influenza with vaccines: Recommendations of the Advisory Committee on Immunization Practices — United States, 2024–25 Influenza Season. MMWR Recomm Rep. 2024;73(No. RR-5):1. [PMID: 39197095]

Johansen ND et al. Electronic nudges to increase influenza vaccination in patients with chronic diseases: a randomized clinical trial. JAMA. 2024;3321900. [PMID: 39392741]

4. Avian Influenza

ESSENTIALS OF DIAGNOSIS

- Most human cases occur after exposure to infected poultry.
- Clinically indistinguishable from seasonal influenza.
- Epidemiologic factors assist in diagnosis.
- Rapid antigen assays confirm diagnosis but do not distinguish avian from seasonal influenza.

General Considerations

Avian influenza was first reported in humans in 1977. The genetic diversity of these zoonotic viruses is the source of considerable consternation, and avian influenza is felt by many virologists to be a likely basis for the next global pandemic.

Zoonotic influenza viruses are distinct from human seasonal influenza viruses and do not traditionally easily transmit between humans. The WHO reports increasing numbers of H5, H7, and H9 subtypes including HPA (highly pathogenic H5 infections) and in 2024 reported > 28,800 cases and 1000 deaths from at least 28 countries worldwide from H5 and H7 subtypes.. For avian influenza viruses, birds are the natural hosts. Around the world and in North America, avian influenza A outbreaks occur in poultry from time to time and the virus has become endemic in poultry in some countries, mostly China and Egypt. Avian influenza viruses may occasionally infect humans or other mammals, including domestic cats and dogs. In 2024, spread to cattle was first documented and 300 herds were reported infected in the United States. Illness in humans ranges from mild disease to rapid progressive severe disease and death depending on the subtype In the United States in 2024, 72 human cases of avian influenza were reported to the CDC, with the largest number from California and Washington State, and 1 death occurred in Louisiana.

The primary risk factor for human infection is direct or indirect exposure to infected live or dead poultry or contaminated environments, such as live bird markets. Slaughtering and handling carcasses of infected poultry are also risk factors.

A number of viral genetic changes are required for adaptation to humans The emergence of H5, H7, and H9 avian influenza virus subtypes in humans raises concern that the virus may undergo genetic reassortment or mutations in some of the genes. Such new isolates could develop greater human-to-human transmissibility with the potential to produce a global pandemic. Fatal avian influenza virus infections acquire their internal gene segments usually but not exclusively from H9N2 viruses.

Human cases of H5N1 have been reported since 1997, and H1N2 was reported from Mexico in 2024. Advanced H5N1 cases are often fatal, and to date, highly pathogenic H5N1 avian isolates (HPA), which are typically associated with the clade 2.3.4.4b, have been reported in mammals since 2003 with spread from originally birds to terrestrial and marine mammals. H5N1 cases have been reported sporadically in 912 cases with a 51.5% mortality from 24 countries. This unique clade has been reported as of late 2024 from 15 patients, 12 with bird, 3 with cattle, and 1 with unknown exposure. The widespread and increasing prevalence of H5N1 isolates from a variety of birds and mammals necessitates the need for surveillance and additional studies.

Clinical Findings

A. Symptoms and Signs

Distinguishing avian influenza from regular influenza is difficult. History of exposure to dead or ill birds or live poultry markets in the prior 10 days, recent travel to Southeast Asia or Egypt, or contact with known cases should be investigated. Patients infected by H5N1 or H7N9 avian influenza A viruses have an aggressive clinical course, and neurovirulence is especially seen with H5Nx subtypes. The symptoms and signs include fever followed by lower respiratory symptoms (cough, dyspnea). Upper respiratory tract symptoms occur less often. GI symptoms are reported more frequently in H5N1 infections. Conjunctivitis is reported in influenza H7 infections. Other systems can also be involved leading to neurologic manifestations (encephalopathy, seizure) and liver impairment. Prolonged febrile states and generalized malaise are common. Respiratory failure, multiorgan dysfunction, and septic shock are the usual causes of death. Bacterial superinfections are reported. Pregnant women and their fetuses are at high risk with avian influenza infection and show mortality rates of 90% and 86% respectively.

B. Laboratory Findings

Commercial rapid antigen tests are not optimally sensitive or specific for detecting H5N1 influenza and should *not* be the definitive test for influenza. More sensitive RT-PCR assays are available through many hospitals and state health departments. Diagnostic yield can be improved by early sample collection, preferably within 7 days of illness onset. Throat swabs or lower respiratory specimens (such as tracheal aspirate or bronchoalveolar lavage fluid) may provide higher yield of detection than nasal swabs. When highly pathogenic strains, such as H5N1 influenza virus infections, are suspected, extreme care in the handling of these samples must be observed during preliminary testing. Positive samples must then be forwarded to the appropriate public health authorities for further investigation (eg, culture) in laboratories with the adequate level of biosafety (level 3). With the spread of avian influenza isolates to a variety of mammals, it is important that a variety of reliable diagnostic methods be made available.

Prevention

The most effective method of prevention is *avoidance of exposure*. Those who work with poultry should practice good hand hygiene and use appropriate personal protective equipment. These workers should also be vaccinated against seasonal influenza since this can reduce the likelihood of coinfection with avian and seasonal influenza. All persons, especially those with influenza risk factors, should avoid visiting live poultry markets and contact with ill birds. There is no risk of acquiring avian influenza from consuming well-cooked poultry products. The US government bans the importation of poultry from infected areas. Culling of animals has been effective in ending outbreaks of highly pathogenic avian influenza but is difficult with H7-infected poultry because most are asymptomatic. Policies regarding the closure of live poultry markets during avian epidemics are controversial. The H5N1 avian influenza strain that entered dairy cows was found in pasteurized milk in the spring of 2024 but was not live or considered contagious.

Persons with exposure should monitor themselves for 10 days after the last known exposure and seek prompt medical attention if new fever or respiratory symptoms develop. Postexposure prophylaxis is not recommended for persons working with noninfected birds or who have used appropriate personal protective equipment while working with infected birds. For persons with exposure to infected persons, postexposure prophylaxis is recommended for household and family members and may be considered for health care personnel with close unprotected contact. Postexposure prophylaxis regimens include oseltamivir, 75 mg orally, or zanamivir, 10 mg inhaled twice daily for 5 or 10 days from the last known exposure, depending on the length of the exposure. Careful surveillance for human cases and prudent stockpiling of medications with establishment of an infrastructure for dissemination are essential control modalities. Nonpharmacologic means of control include masks, social distancing, quarantine, travel limitations, and infrastructure development, particularly for emergency departments.

Vaccines do not provide cross-protection against strains of the H5, H7, and H9 influenza viruses, although they lower the likelihood of new recombinants emerging. The US government has prepandemic stockpiles of adjuvanted H5N1 and H7N9 vaccines that are not available to the public. The highly diverse genetic nature and the rapid evolution of the avian influenza viruses have resulted in the emergence of viruses that are not covered by stockpiled vaccines. The FDA approved an adjuvanted influenza A (H5N1) monovalent vaccine (Audenz) in January 2020. It is approved for patients 6 months of age and older. An adjuvanted recombinant hemagglutinin H7 vaccine against avian influenza A subtype H7N9 is shown to be safe and immunogenic in healthy adults. The global increase in H5N8 in birds is a particular concern.

Control of infection among the poultry population is key to preventing human disease. Vaccination of poultry as a sole means of control is ineffective. Closing live poultry markets can interrupt outbreaks. Additional adjunctive measures, such as days where live markets are closed temporarily for disinfection (which can decrease viral loads in surrounding groundwater) or separation of land-based poultry from waterfowl, are needed for improved control.

Because the potential for pandemic influenza for many of the new reassortment viruses is not fully known, continued surveillance is essential, and stockpiling of vaccines, adjuvant, and medications (oseltamivir and zanamivir) is warranted at the public health level.

Treatment

Persons with severe illness and confirmed and probable cases with mild disease should receive treatment as soon as possible. The first-line recommendation is to use the neuraminidase inhibitor oseltamivir, 75 mg orally twice daily for 5 days administered within 48 hours from onset of illness. Longer courses of therapy (eg, 10 days) should be considered in hospitalized patients with severe illness and persistent viral shedding. Data are lacking for inhaled zanamivir or peramivir for severe avian influenza. Overall oseltamivir, by modeling, is associated with a 49% reduction in mortality from H5N1 avian influenza virus infections. As with seasonal influenza, enteric oseltamivir is well absorbed in critically ill persons without gastric stasis, known malabsorption, or GI bleeding. Daily intravenous peramivir (600 mg, reduced to 200 mg for kidney dysfunction) for a minimum of 5 days and a maximum of 10 or more days (depending on severity of illness) or zanamivir (10 mg inhaled daily for 10 days) may be considered in such patients. Combination therapy with amantadine or rimantadine (in countries where H5N1 influenza virus A strains are likely susceptible to adamantanes) may be considered in patients with pneumonia or progressive disease. Resistance of avian H5N1 influenza strains to amantadine and rimantadine is widespread. Resistance to neuraminidase inhibitors (oseltamivir, zanamivir, and peramivir) can occur in patients with H5NA and H7N9 avian infection. Successful treatment with administration of convalescent plasma is reported.

Cargnin Faccin F et al. Pandemic preparedness through vaccine development for avian influenza viruses. Hum Vaccin Immunother. 2024;20:2347019. [PMID: 38807261]

Mostafa A et al. Avian influenza A (H5N1) virus in dairy cattle: origin, evolution, and cross-species transmission. mBio. 2024;15:e0254224. [PMID: 39535188]

Plaza PI et al. Recent changes in patterns of mammal infection with highly pathogenic avian influenza A(H5N1) virus worldwide. Emerg Infect Dis. 2024;30:444. [PMID: 38407173]

Purcell R et al. Systematic review of avian influenza virus infection and outcomes during pregnancy. Emerg Infect Dis. 2025;31:50. [PMID: 39668388]

Webby RJ et al. An update on highly pathogenic avian influenza A (H5N1) virus, clade 2.3.4.4b. J Infect Dis. 2024;230:533. [PMID: 39283944]

5. Severe Acute Respiratory Syndrome (SARS-CoV-1)

ESSENTIALS OF DIAGNOSIS

- Mild, moderate, or severe respiratory illness.
- Travel to endemic areas within 10 days before symptom onset, including mainland China, Hong Kong, Singapore, Taiwan, Vietnam, and Toronto.
- Persistent fever; dry cough, dyspnea in most.
- Diagnosis confirmed by antibody testing or isolation of virus.
- There is no specific treatment; mortality is as high as 14% in clinically diagnosed cases.

General Considerations

SARS-CoV-1 (previously referred to as "SARS") is a respiratory syndrome caused by a coronavirus, transmitted through direct or indirect contact of mucous membranes with infectious respiratory droplets. The virus is shed in stools, but the role of fecal-oral transmission is unknown. The natural reservoir appears to be the horseshoe bat (which eats and drops fruits ingested by civets, the earlier presumed reservoir and a likely amplifying host), which can carry a variety of different coronavirus strains.

The earliest cases were traced to a healthcare worker in Guangdong Province in China in late 2002, with rapid spread thereafter throughout Asia and Canada, considered a consequence of spread through travel. The last cases were reported in 2004. The 2003 outbreak involved 8098 probable cases from 29 countries, with 774 fatalities. Nine additional cases associated with a research laboratory were reported in China in 2004 with no further cases reported since then anywhere in the world. A 29-base pair deletion evolved during the course of human-to-human transmission, and it is thought to be responsible in part for the abeyance of the outbreak.

6. Middle East Respiratory Syndrome–Coronavirus (MERS-CoV)

ESSENTIALS OF DIAGNOSIS

- Mild, moderate, or severe respiratory illness.
- Travel to endemic areas, including the Arabian Peninsula and neighboring countries, within 14 days before symptom onset.
- Contact with camels has been reported in many cases.
- Fever, cough, and dyspnea.
- CDC can assist with RT-PCR.
- Supportive treatment; mortality 36–45%.

General Considerations

MERS-CoV is a syndrome associated with a coronavirus similar to the cause of SARS. Patients with MERS have had a history of residence or travel in the Middle East, in particular Saudi Arabia, or contact with such patients. The virus can be transmitted between humans through direct or indirect contact of mucous membranes with infectious respiratory droplets, although there is much less human-to-human transmission compared with other coronaviruses. The virus is shed in stool, but the role of fecal-oral transmission is unknown. The earliest cases were identified in 2012 in the Kingdom of Saudi Arabia, and 75% of all cases have occurred there. Additional cases have occurred throughout the Middle East, Africa, and Europe, with a reported death rate of 37%, though the WHO acknowledges this may be an overestimation as mild or asymptomatic cases may not be diagnosed (https://www.who.int/health-topics/middle-east-respiratory-syndrome-coronavirus-mers). Only two cases have ever been identified in the United States; both were reported in 2014 in health care providers who lived and worked in Saudi Arabia. As of November 2025, 2630 cases of MERS had been reported to the WHO, including 947 deaths; most were reported from Saudi Arabia.

So-called superspreaders are often responsible for propagating the pathogen in the early stages of an outbreak. It is also recognized more often that asymptomatic cases are frequent, especially among children, and they may contribute to disease transmission. Person-to-person transmission can occur within families; hospital-associated cases comprise 10–25% of reported infections. The median incubation period is 5 days (range, 2–14) with the mean age of 50 (range 9 months to 99 years) and 65% occurring among men. Over 90% of patients have an underlying medical condition, including diabetes mellitus (68%), hypertension (34%), or chronic heart or kidney disease. Those with diabetes, kidney disease, chronic lung disease, or other immunocompromising conditions are at highest risk for severe disease.

Camels (especially female camels) appear to be the principal reservoir, and several studies show that contact with dromedary herds of camels is greater among cases than controls. Raw camel milk is considered a potential source. Persons who work with camels are more likely to have antibody evidence of past infection. Camels most commonly infected with MERS are females, dromedary, young, in free herds, and imported.

Clinical Findings

A. Symptoms and Signs

MERS is an acute respiratory syndrome, with the most common symptoms being fever (98%), cough (83%), and dyspnea (72%). Chills and rigors are common (87%). GI symptoms may occur, with diarrhea being most common (26%), followed by nausea and abdominal pain, and may precede respiratory symptoms. Mild and asymptomatic cases are reported.

B. Laboratory Findings and Imaging

Hematologic findings in the largest series to date include thrombocytopenia (36%), lymphopenia (34%), and lymphocytosis (11%). Moderate elevations in LD (49%), AST (15%), and ALT (11%) are recognized. CXR abnormalities are nearly universal and include increased bronchovascular markings, patchy infiltrates or consolidations, interstitial changes, opacities (reticular and nodular) and pleural effusions, and total lung opacification. Ground-glass opacities and consolidation are most commonly seen. The findings mimic those of many other causes of pneumonia.

Serum serologies and RT-PCR are available through the CDC (https://www.cdc.gov/mers/hcp/diagnosis-testing/). Highest viral loads are found in lower respiratory tract specimens, including bronchoalveolar lavage fluid, sputum, and tracheal aspirates. These samples are preferred for diagnosis. The CDC recommends sending lower respiratory tract specimens, nasopharyngeal and oropharyngeal swabs, and serum for testing. In confirmed cases, serial sample collection (perhaps every 2–4 days) from multiple sites is recommended to increase understanding of virus shedding kinetics. In cases where symptom onset occurred > 14 days prior and symptoms are ongoing, serum should be sent to the CDC for serologic testing and the above specimens should be sent for RT-PCR.

C. Case Definition

A patient with severe illness shows the following characteristics: fever (38°C, 100.4°F or higher) and pneumonia or ARDS (based on clinical or radiologic evidence); and either history of travel in or near the Arabian Peninsula within 14 days before symptom onset; or close contact with a symptomatic traveler in whom fever and acute respiratory illness (not necessarily pneumonia) developed within 14 days after traveling in or near the Arabian Peninsula (above); or is a member of a cluster of patients with severe acute respiratory illness (eg, fever and pneumonia requiring hospitalization) of unknown etiology in which MERS-CoV is being evaluated, in consultation with state and local health departments.

In milder illness, patients have fever and symptoms of respiratory illness (not necessarily pneumonia; eg, cough, shortness of breath) and history of having close contact with a confirmed MERS case as well as a history of being in a health care facility (as a patient, worker, or visitor) within 14 days of symptom onset in a country or territory within the Arabian Peninsula in which recent healthcare-associated cases of MERS have been identified.

Of note, fever may *not* be present in certain patients, including very young, older adults, immunosuppressed individuals, or those taking certain medications.

Complications

Respiratory failure is such a common complication that in a series from Saudi Arabia, 89% of patients required intensive care and mechanical ventilation. Patients with MERS-CoV appear to advance faster to respiratory failure than do those with SARS.

Prevention

Isolation and quarantine of cases are authorized by the CDC. Strict infection control measures are essential as well as care and management of household contacts and hospital workers engaged in the care of patients. Travelers to Saudi Arabia (including many pilgrims to the holy sites) should practice frequent handwashing and avoid contact with people with respiratory symptoms. Evaluation of patients with suspect symptoms within 14 days of return from Saudi Arabia is essential. Because healthcare workers engaged in procedures that involve contact with respiratory droplets are at risk, isolation of high-risk patients is essential, as are simple hygienic measures. Limiting the number of hospital contacts and visits is important. Control measures, including quarantining high-risk exposed persons at home and using facemasks to prevent hospital-acquired infections, are important. Assisting public health authorities with case reporting and surveillance is essential. Postexposure prophylaxis with ribavirin and lopinavir/ritonavir for healthcare workers is associated with a 40% decrease in the risk of acquiring infection.

Camel workers, including slaughterhouse and market workers, veterinarians, and racing personnel, should wear facial protection and protective clothing, practice good personal hygiene, including frequent handwashing after touching animals, and receive education about the syndrome. Family members of such personnel should not be exposed to work paraphernalia including clothing and shoes and workers should shower at the site of employment rather than the home. Avoiding direct contact with camels (who may be asymptomatic but can transmit the virus through nasal or ocular discharge, milk, urine, and feces) is important. Infected camels should be segregated from other livestock and kept off the market, including their meat products, and buried or destroyed. Epidemiologic factors addressed above can be used to avoid contact with most likely infected camels.

Treatment

Respiratory support is essential. No vaccine or known antiviral therapy exists to combat MERS, though mRNA vaccinations are currently in development. Current therapies are adapted from SARS treatments, which include IFNs, ribavirin, lopinavir-ritonavir, or mycophenolate mofetil. The use of macrolides is not associated with reduced mortality. A small retrospective study found improved survival at 14 days with ribavirin and IFN-α but not at 28 days.

Prognosis

The overall mortality rate of identified cases is about 37%. Factors associated with mortality include the use of corticosteroids and also the use of continuous renal replacement therapy. A set of radiographic criteria (diffuse involvement, fibrosing sequela) are associated with a worse prognosis and the need for intubation. Advanced age is associated with a poor prognosis. Functional outcomes of survivors are similar to those of other non-MERS severe acute respiratory virus illnesses.

Dandachi I et al. MERS-COV in the Middle East, a one health concept approach. One Health. 2025;21:101282. [PMID: 41403560]

Liu Q et al. MERS-CoV RBD-mRNA presents better immunogenicity and protection than the Spike-mRNA. Cells. 2025;14:1928. [PMID: 41369417]

ADENOVIRUS INFECTIONS

General Considerations

Adenoviruses are non-enveloped, double-stranded DNA viruses with a worldwide distribution and cause illness year-round. These infections are usually self-limited or clinically inapparent and occur most commonly among infants, young children, and military recruits. However, adenovirus infections are important causes of morbidity and mortality in immunocompromised persons. Adenoviruses have also received recognition through their *role as vectors in gene therapy and vaccine development.*

Clinical Findings

A. Symptoms and Signs

Adenovirus infection presents as various overlapping clinical syndromes with an incubation period of 4–9 days. Viral or bacterial coinfections occur with adenovirus in 15–20% of cases. **The common cold** is characterized by rhinitis, pharyngitis, and malaise without fever, often accompanied by conjunctivitis. Non-streptococcal exudative pharyngitis manifests as fever lasting 2–12 days, malaise, and myalgia. Lower respiratory tract infection may occur, including bronchiolitis or pneumonia. Pharyngoconjunctival fever presents with fever and malaise, conjunctivitis (often unilateral), mild pharyngitis, and cervical adenitis. Epidemic keratoconjunctivitis manifests in adults with bilateral conjunctival redness, pain, tearing, and an enlarged preauricular lymph node. Enteric adenovirus causes acute gastroenteritis, mesenteric adenitis, acute appendicitis, rhabdomyolysis, and intussusception. Adenovirus is commonly identified in endomyocardial tissue of patients with myocarditis and dilated cardiomyopathy.

Hepatitis, pneumonia, and hemorrhagic cystitis tend to develop in infected liver, lung, or kidney transplant recipients, respectively. Patients undergoing hematopoietic stem cell transplant and CAR T therapy are at risk of developing hepatitis, pneumonia, diarrhea, hemorrhagic cystitis, tubulointerstitial nephritis, colitis, and encephalitis.

B. Laboratory Findings and Imaging

Antigen detection assays including direct fluorescence assay or enzyme immunoassay are rapid and show sensitivity of 60–77% compared with viral culture, which may be as low as 50%. Samples with negative rapid assays require PCR assays or viral cultures for diagnosis. Quantitative real-time rapid-cycle PCR is useful in distinguishing disease from colonization, especially in hematopoietic stem cell transplant patients. Typing of isolates is useful epidemiologically and in distinguishing transmission from endogenous reactivation.

On chest CT, adenovirus infection may manifest as a multifocal consolidation or ground-glass opacity without airway inflammatory findings.

Treatment & Prognosis

Treatment is symptomatic. Cidofovir is used in immunocompromised individuals with occasional success, although it is attendant with significant renal toxicity. Brincidofovir, the lipid-conjugated prodrug of cidofovir, has superior oral bioavailability and tolerability, and it achieves higher intracellular concentrations. However, brincidofovir is available only through compassionate use mechanisms. Complications of adenovirus pneumonia in children include bronchiolitis obliterans. Deaths are reported on occasion.

The control of epidemic adenoviral conjunctivitis is often difficult and requires meticulous attention to hand hygiene, the use of disposable gloves, equipment sterilization, cohorting of cases, and furloughing employees. Treatment with a combination of povidone-iodine 1.0% eyedrops and dexamethasone 0.1% eyedrops four times a day can reduce symptoms and expedite recovery. Prolonged shedding can be seen.

Vaccines are not available for general use. The use of live oral vaccines containing attenuated type 4 and type 7 was reinstated in military personnel in 2013 and has been associated with a significant decrease in adenoviral disease.

Kajon AE. Adenovirus infections: new insights for the clinical laboratory. J Clin Microbiol. 2024;62:e0083622. [PMID: 39189703]

Narsana N et al. Treating adenovirus infection in transplant populations: therapeutic options beyond cidofovir? Viruses. 2025;17:599. [PMID: 40431613]

POXVIRUSES & OTHER EXANTHEMATOUS VIRAL INFECTIONS

1. Mpox

ESSENTIALS OF DIAGNOSIS

- Characteristic rash and lymphadenopathy in most unvaccinated persons.
- Previous smallpox vaccination provides protection.
- Transmission is mainly by skin-to-skin contact.

General Considerations

Mpox (previously known as the monkeypox virus) is an orthopoxvirus. Two clades, I and II, are recognized, previously known as Congo Basin and West African, respectively. Clade IIb caused a global outbreak in 2022 and is still currently circulating in low levels. A clade I mpox outbreak began in 2023 in the Democratic Republic of the Congo and spread to neighboring countries in 2024. It can be transmitted when humans encounter infected animals (primates, rodents, rabbits) and by direct contact with infected humans including sexual and skin-to-skin contact.

Mpox was first diagnosed in 1970 in the Democratic Republic of the Congo and later in Central Africa (particularly Nigeria) and West Africa. In 2022, outbreaks of clade II mpox were reported in multiple nonendemic regions, including Europe and the United States. Gay, bisexual, and other men who have sex with men make up the majority of cases; deaths have occurred. The WHO's global situation update can be accessed at https://worldhealthorg.shinyapps.io/mpx_global/#2_Global_situation_update.

Clinical Findings

The incubation period averages 13 days with a range of 1–21 days in the current outbreak. The prodromal period includes a host of symptoms from fever and chills (62%) to lethargy (41%), myalgias (31%), and headaches (27%). Lymphadenopathy is prominent (56%) and can be generalized or localized. Skin lesions occur in almost all cases 1–3 days after the fever starts. The lesions are deep seated and well circumscribed at all stages of development and progress centrifugally. Classic lesions appear in four stages, from macules, to papules, to vesicles, to pustules, eventually scabbing over and resolving. Historically, rashes were seen on the face or the palms and soles; in the current outbreak, lesions on the trunk and anogenital regions and mucosal lesions are more common. Lesions vary in number from 1 to 10, although they can be diffuse. Rash may be confined to one location and may not be disseminated in the current outbreak. Anorectal lesions, common in the current outbreak, present with intense pain, tenesmus, and possibly diarrhea. Keratitis is a recognized ocular manifestation, and a congenital syndrome may occur.

Laboratory Findings

Mpox virus DNA can be detected for prolonged periods in upper respiratory isolates. If skin lesions are present, swabs should be collected and sent for PCR (see resources at https://www.sf.gov/cityclinic-providers-mpox). False-positive assays occur among those recently vaccinated and serologies are not routinely used for diagnosis. Clinicians should notify state and local health officials and the CDC for assistance with diagnostic confirmation. **It is important to test persons with suspected mpox for HIV and other STIs such as gonorrhea and chlamydia.**

Differential Diagnosis

The differential includes varicella (which shares all stages of rash development), syphilis, scabies, herpes, and measles. Confusion with smallpox and varicella occurs; however, both lymphadenopathy (seen in up to 90% of unvaccinated persons) and a febrile prodrome are distinct features of mpox infection. The mpox rash is distinguished by its deep-seated and well-circumscribed nature, lesions at various stages of development (like varicella but unlike smallpox), and centrifugal progression (including palms and soles).

Prevention

Two vaccines are currently available in the United States. JYNNEOS (Imvamune or Imvanex), a live, replication-incompetent vaccinia virus (modified Ankara virus) is the currently preferred mpox vaccine. It was first developed as a smallpox vaccine and is effective and FDA-approved to prevent mpox. It is usually given subcutaneously (0.5 mL) as two doses 1 month apart. Postexposure vaccination is advised for documented contacts of infected persons or animals within 3–4 days up to 14 days of exposure.

ACAM2000 (a live, replication-competent vaccinia virus) is an older vaccine that historically was used for smallpox eradication and is available only under the CDC's expanded-access investigational new drug protocol. This vaccine should not be given to those with eczema or severe immune deficiency, including bone marrow transplant patients. The side effects associated with this vaccine include rare instances of myocarditis, encephalitis, and blindness. Thus, it should not be used in patients with cardiac disease, eye disease treated with steroids, congenital or acquired immune deficiency, eczema, infants under 1 year of age, and pregnant persons.

PPE should include gown, gloves, eye protection, and N95 respirator. *Hospitalized patients should be housed in single rooms with dedicated staff and respiratory equipment, PPE for staff, and airflow isolation for respiratory procedures.* Cases are considered infectious until all scabs have fallen off.

Treatment

Most patients with mpox will have mild, self-limited disease. However, **persons with severe illness or those at risk for severe illness** (including immunocompromised persons, persons having conditions associated with a compromised skin barrier such as atopic dermatitis, children, and pregnant persons) should be considered for antiviral therapy (https://www.cdc.gov/mpox/hcp/clinical-care/). No treatments currently have FDA approval for mpox treatment, but therapies developed for smallpox have been used in some cases.

Tecovirimat (TPOXX; 600 mg orally twice daily for 2 weeks) is available in the United States through the CDC's expanded access investigational new drug (IND) protocol. Clinical studies have shown that tecovirimat is generally well tolerated, but it has not been associated with faster resolution of skin lesions or pain among persons with mild to moderate disease severity. Other possible systemic therapies for mpox include vaccinia immunoglobulin, cidofovir, and brincidofovir. Cidofovir use is limited by potential nephrotoxicity. Clinical experience with brincidofovir in the management of mpox is limited. Brincidofovir is available through an FDA-authorized single-patient emergency use IND for persons (1) with severe mpox or at risk for severe disease and (2) who have no durable response to tecovirimat, are ineligible for tecovirimat, or are severely immunocompromised. **Expert consultation should be sought to guide decision-making when considering mpox therapeutics.**

Vaccinia immunoglobulin intravenous (VIGIV) may be considered in severe cases when there is insufficient antibody response and is available upon request to CDC on a case-by-case basis.

Prognosis

Though acute disease may last several weeks, the prognosis is generally excellent. Rare fatalities have been reported in the 2022–2023 outbreak and fatalities have been somewhat higher in the 2023–2024 ongoing outbreak (where the case fatality rate is about 3.6%). The immunosuppressed are more prone to complications, including bronchopneumonia, sepsis, encephalitis, and keratitis with rare visual loss.

When to Refer

Any patient with suspicious lesions should be referred to an infectious diseases consultant or the local health department. Patients with severe disease (particularly those presenting with oral or anogenital disease) should immediately be referred to the emergency department.

When to Admit

Any patient at risk for development of severe complications such as sepsis, pneumonia, encephalitis, or keratitis should be admitted.

Centers for Disease Control and Prevention (CDC). Treatment and vaccine recommendations https://www.cdc.gov/mpox/hcp/clinical-care/

San Francisco City Clinic. Mpox resources. https://www.sf.gov/cityclinic-providers-mpox

Titanji BK et al. Mpox clinical presentation, diagnostic approaches, and treatment strategies: a review. JAMA. 2024;332:1652. [PMID: 39401235]

2. Variola (Smallpox) & Vaccinia

ESSENTIALS OF DIAGNOSIS

- Prodromal high fever.
- Eruption progressing from papules to vesicles to pustules, then crusts.
- All lesions in the *same* stage.
- Face and distal extremities (including palms and soles) favored.

Historically, smallpox caused millions of deaths worldwide before its eradication in 1980. Concern for the use of smallpox virus as a bioterrorist weapon has led to the reintroduction of vaccination in some segments of the population (first responders and the military).

The face is the initial site of involvement, followed by the upper and lower extremities and trunk, with complete evolution over 1 week. Lesions exhibit relative uniformity within each anatomic region.

3. Molluscum Contagiosum

Molluscum contagiosum is caused by a pox virus, *Molluscipoxvirus*, that may be transmitted sexually, by close contact, or by contaminated fomites. The incubation period averages 2–3 months and is self-limited in most people. The disease presents as pearly, raised, umbilicated skin nodules sparing the palms and soles. Keratoconjunctivitis can occur. Most ocular lesions are typical umbilicated dome-shaped lesions, but a variety of atypical ocular lesions are reported often in immunocompetent patients, more often in women and young adults (mean age 19 years). Rare anal and scalp lesions are reported.

There may be an association with atopic dermatitis or eczema. Marked and persistent lesions in patients with AIDS respond readily to combination ART. Treatment options include destructive therapies (curettage, cryotherapy, cantharidin, 10–15% hydrogen peroxide, 10% potassium hydroxide, and keratolytics, among others), immunomodulators (imiquimod, cimetidine, tuberculin-purified protein derivatives [PPDs], and *Candida* antigen), and antiviral agents (topical cidofovir is effective anecdotally in refractory cases; brincidofovir is approved for the treatment of Ebola but is still off-label for molluscum contagiosum, where it shows some efficacy). No treatment is uniformly effective. Multiple courses of therapy are often needed.

Hebert AA et al. Molluscum contagiosum: epidemiology, considerations, treatment options, and therapeutic gaps. J Clin Aesthet Dermatol. 2023;16:S4. [PMID: 37636018]

4. Orf and Paravaccinia

Orf (contagious pustular dermatitis, or ecthyma contagiosa) and paravaccinia (milker's nodules) are occupational diseases acquired by contact with sheep/goats and cattle, respectively. Household meat processing and animal slaughter are identified as risk factors. Orf is a common infection in sheep, goats, and reindeer globally, with farmers, veterinarians, and hunters at heightened risk. The incubation period ranges from 3 to 7 days. Clinically it presents as a solitary 1-cm hand pustule, progressing through six clinically distinct dermatologic stages, and typically heals in 3–6 weeks without scarring. The use of nonporous gloves when handling animals is recommended, especially for immunosuppressed individuals. Molecular tests are used to confirm clinical diagnosis. Although orf has no specific treatment, it anecdotally responds to imiquimod. Cidofovir has been suggested as potential treatment as well. A live vaccine is available for animals.

Incubation period for paravaccinia is 5–15 days. The lesion progresses as papules (reddish blue, firm) to painless vesicular nodules with erythematous ring, then to exudative nodules followed by dry, crusting formation. It then becomes papillomatous nodules and finally involutes without a scar. Management is usually supportive treatment. Treatment of domestic pet animals is recommended to ensure complete management.

Poudel GP et al. Milker's nodule: an under-reported and under-diagnosed occupational infection. Clin Case Rep. 2020;8:1162. [PMID: 32695349]
Thompson HJ et al. Orf virus in humans: case series and clinical review. Cutis. 2022;110:48. [PMID: 36179231]

5. Erythroparvovirus Infections

Primate erythroparvovirus 1, more commonly known as **parvovirus B19,** infects human erythroid precursor cells. It is widespread, and its transmission occurs through respiratory secretions and saliva, through the placenta, and through administration of blood products. The incubation period is 4–14 days. Chronic forms of the infection can occur in immunocompromised persons. Bocavirus, another erythroparvovirus, is a cause of respiratory disease in children and adults.

Clinical Findings

A. Symptoms and Signs

Parvovirus B19 causes several syndromes and manifests differently in various populations as discussed below. Infection may be asymptomatic but can also present with a biphasic course. The first phase (most contagious, lasting for ~ 5 days) is characterized by fever, myalgia, and malaise, and the second phase 7–10 days after the first is associated with rash, joint pain, anemia, thrombocytopenia, or leukopenia.

1. Children—In children, an exanthematous illness ("**fifth disease**" or **erythema infectiosum**) is characterized by a fiery red "slapped cheek" appearance, circumoral pallor, and a subsequent lacy, maculopapular, evanescent rash on the trunk and limbs. Parvovirus B19 infection is also one of the most common causes of myocarditis in childhood.

2. Healthy adults—A limited, nonerosive symmetric polyarthritis resembling SLE and rheumatoid arthritis can develop in middle-aged persons (especially women). Rashes, especially facial, are less common in adults.

3. Persons with underlying red cell disorders—Parvovirus may provoke a transient aplastic crisis requiring transfusion support in persons with conditions such as sickle cell or spherocytosis.

4. Immunocompromised patients—Prolonged viremia and pure RBC aplasia may occur in persons with advanced HIV or malignancy, in transplant recipients, or in those with other immunocompromising conditions. Bone marrow aspirates reveal absence of mature erythroid precursors and characteristic giant pronormoblasts.

5. Pregnant persons—Transplacental transmission occurs in 30% of cases of maternal infection, leading to complications such as premature labor, hydrops fetalis, fetal anemia, and fetal loss necessitating testing and monitoring for symptomatic pregnant individuals.

B. Laboratory Findings

The diagnosis of fifth disease is clinical (Table 36–2). Parvovirus may be diagnosed via elevated serum IgM antibodies or with PCR of serum or bone marrow. In an immunocompetent patient, viremia has often cleared by the time common symptoms such as rash or polyarthropathy present, but IgM antibodies are likely present. In immunocompromised patients, PCR is more useful. Autoimmune antibodies (antiphospholipid and antineutrophil cytoplasmic antibodies) can be present and are thought to result from molecular mimicry.

Treatment

Treatment in otherwise healthy persons is symptomatic. Red cell transfusions are used to support patients through aplastic crises. In immunosuppressed patients including those with HIV, IVIG is effective in the short-term reduction of anemia. Relapses tend to occur about 4 months after administration of IVIG. Reduction of immunosuppressive treatments can be considered. Intrauterine blood transfusion can be considered in severe fetal anemia, especially during 18–35 weeks of gestation.

Prevention & Prognosis

Several nosocomial outbreaks are documented. In these cases, standard and droplet precautions, including hand washing after patient exposure and avoiding contact with pregnant persons, are paramount. Pregnant and immunocompromised patients should be monitored for Parvovirus B19 infection especially during outbreaks. Among infected, pregnant persons, the presence of fetal hydrops is associated with a poor prognosis.

Because transfusion-transmitted parvovirus is very rare, blood banks do *not* routinely screen for parvovirus in the United States or abroad. Most infected donor patients have concomitant antibodies, most recipients have had prior parvovirus infection, and the levels of viremia are considered too low in infected patients to transmit the virus. Transfusion specialists recommend DNA screening of vulnerable patients after transfusion.

The prognosis is generally excellent in immunocompetent individuals. In immunosuppressed patients, persistent anemia may lead to prolonged transfusion dependence. Remission of parvovirus B19 infection in patients with AIDS may occur with antiretroviral therapy.

There is no vaccine available for Parvovirus B19 infection.

Bloise S et al. Parvovirus B19 infection in children: a comprehensive review of clinical manifestations and management. Ital J Pediatr. 2024;50:261. [PMID: 39696462]

Mendes-de-Almeida DP et al. Clinical presentation of parvovirus B19 infection in adults living with HIV/AIDS: a case series. Viruses. 2023;15:1124. [PMID: 37243210]

VIRUSES & GASTROENTERITIS

Viruses are responsible for at least 30–40% of cases of infectious diarrhea in the United States. Rotaviruses and noroviruses are responsible for most nonbacterial cases of gastroenteritis.

Rotaviruses are reoviruses associated with significant morbidity and mortality. In 2021, 108,322 deaths were attributed to rotavirus compared with 316,382 in 2000. Children age 6 months to 2 years are the most affected; by age 5, virtually every child has been infected with this pathogen. Rotavirus infections follow an endemic pattern, especially in the tropics and low-income countries, but they peak during the winter in temperate regions. The virus is transmitted by the fecal–oral route and can be shed in feces for up to 3 weeks. In outbreak settings (eg, day care centers), the virus is ubiquitously found in the environment, and secondary attack rates are between 16% and 30%. Nosocomial outbreaks are reported.

The disease is usually mild and self-limiting. A 2- to 3-day prodrome of fever and vomiting is followed by nonbloody diarrhea lasting for 1–4 days. Patients with gastroenteritis are not routinely tested for rotavirus because the results do not alter treatment. Oral and intravenous rehydration solutions are the primary treatment options. Neurologic complications are rare but include encephalitis, cerebellitis, and encephalocerebellitis, with long-term complications more common with older age at diagnosis or the presence of encephalocerebellitis.

Vaccines have been highly successful in reducing the global burden of rotavirus. In the United States, two rotavirus vaccines have been approved since 2006: RotaTeq (given at 2, 4, and 6 months of age) and a live, oral attenuated monovalent human rotavirus vaccine (HRV, Rotarix or RV1; given at 2 and 4 months of age). One advantage of these vaccines is the evidence of *heterotypic immunity* (prevention against rotavirus strains not included in the vaccine). Accordingly, some data suggest that rotavirus vaccination confers herd immunity to children under 1 year of age. Rotavirus vaccination has been associated with a low risk of intussusception shortly after vaccination, but rotavirus vaccination remains recommended given its efficacy against severe diarrhea.

With the control of rotavirus, **noroviruses** such as Norwalk virus are now *the major cause of diarrhea globally.*

Noroviruses are a leading cause of foodborne disease in the United States and are significantly associated with military deployment as well as travel-associated and nosocomial infections. Globally, each year, norovirus gastroenteritis is responsible for nearly 700 million infections and up to 20% of all cases of diarrhea in children and adults, with an estimated 200,000 deaths. Outbreak environments include long-term care facilities, restaurants, hospitals, schools, day care centers, vacation destinations (including cruise ships), and military bases. Persons at particular risk are younger individuals, older adults, those who are institutionalized, and immunosuppressed individuals. Transmission occurs readily through multiple mechanisms (eg, contaminated food or water, contact with sick person or contaminated surface). A short incubation period (24–48 hours), a short symptomatic illness (12–60 hours, but up to 5 days in hospital-associated cases), a high frequency (> 50%) of vomiting, and absence of bacterial pathogens in stool samples are highly predictive of norovirus gastroenteritis. Rare neurologic complications of norovirus infection occur, including seizures and encephalitis. Prolonged diarrhea can occur in immunocompromised persons. RT-PCR of stool samples is used for diagnostic and epidemiologic purposes. No long-lasting protective immunity develops, and reinfections are common.

Outbreak control for both rotavirus and norovirus infections includes strict adherence to general hygienic measures. Despite the promise of alcohol-based sanitizers to control pathogen transmission, *such cleansers may be relatively ineffective against the noroviruses compared with antibacterial soap and water.* Cohorting of sick patients, contact precautions for symptomatic hospitalized patients, and proper decontamination procedures are crucial. Symptomatic staff should be excluded from work until symptom resolution (or 48–72 hours afterward for norovirus disease).

Vetter V et al. Established and new rotavirus vaccines: a comprehensive review for healthcare professionals. Hum Vaccin Immunother. 2022;18:1870395. [PMID: 33605839]

Wang G et al. Impact of vaccination with different types of rotavirus vaccines on the incidence of intussusception: a randomized controlled meta-analysis. Front Pediatr. 2023;11:1239423. [PMID: 37583623]

ENTEROVIRUSES THAT PRODUCE SEVERAL SYNDROMES

The most famous enterovirus, the poliomyelitis virus, is discussed above under Major Vaccine-Preventable Viral Infections. The best-known nonpolio enteroviruses (enterovirus D68, enterovirus A71, and coxsackie viruses A6 and A16) and other clinically relevant enteroviral infections are discussed in this section.

1. Coxsackievirus Infections

Coxsackievirus infections cause several clinical syndromes. As with other enteroviruses, infections are most common during the summer. Two groups, A and B, are defined either serologically or by mouse bioassay. More than 50 serotypes have been identified.

Clinical Findings

A. Symptoms and Signs

The clinical syndromes associated with coxsackievirus infection are summer grippe; herpangina; epidemic pleurodynia; aseptic meningitis and other neurologic syndromes; acute nonspecific pericarditis; myocarditis; hand, foot, and mouth disease; epidemic conjunctivitis; and other syndromes.

1. Summer grippe (A and B)—A febrile illness, principally of children, summer grippe usually lasts 1–4 days. Minor upper respiratory tract infection symptoms are often present.

2. Herpangina (A2–6, 10; B3)—There is sudden onset of fever, which may be as high as 40.6°C, sometimes with febrile convulsions. Other symptoms are headache, myalgia, and vomiting. The sore throat is characterized early by petechiae or papules on the soft palate that ulcerate in about 3 days and then heal. Treatment is symptomatic.

3. Epidemic pleurodynia (Bornholm disease) (B1–5)—Pleuritic pain is prominent. Tenderness, hyperesthesia, and muscle swelling are present over the area of diaphragmatic attachment. Other findings include headache, sore throat, malaise, nausea, and fever. Orchitis and aseptic meningitis occur in <10% of patients. Most patients are ill for 4–6 days.

4. Aseptic meningitis (A and B) and other neurologic syndromes—Fever, headache, nausea, vomiting, stiff neck, drowsiness, and CSF lymphocytosis without chemical abnormalities may occur, and pediatric clusters of group B (especially B5) meningitis are reported. Focal encephalitis and transverse myelitis are reported with coxsackievirus group A. Disseminated encephalitis occurs after group B infection, and acute flaccid myelitis is reported in both coxsackievirus groups A and B.

5. Acute nonspecific pericarditis (B types)—Sudden onset of anterior chest pain, often worse with inspiration and in the supine position, is typical. Fever, myalgia, headache, and pericardial friction rub appear early and are often transient. Evidence for pericardial effusion on imaging studies is often present, and the occasional patient has a paradoxical pulse. Electrocardiographic evidence of pericarditis is often present. Relapses may occur.

6. Myocarditis (B1–5)—HF in the neonatal period is secondary to in utero myocarditis, and > 20% of adult cases of myocarditis and dilated cardiomyopathy are associated with group B (especially B3) infections.

7. Hand, foot, and mouth disease (A5, 6, 10, 12, and 16, B5)—This disease can be epidemic. It is characterized by stomatitis, vesicular rash on hands and feet (Figure 36–6), nail dystrophies, and onychomadesis (nail shedding), with some cases showing higher fevers, long duration, and more severe skin manifestations. Enteroviruses 71 and 33 also are causative agents, the former of usually more severe disease. A16 disease is usually mild. Coxsackie virus A6 (CVA6) is noted to be an important public health issue, as epidemiologic surveillance has shown its incidence increase in recent years worldwide.

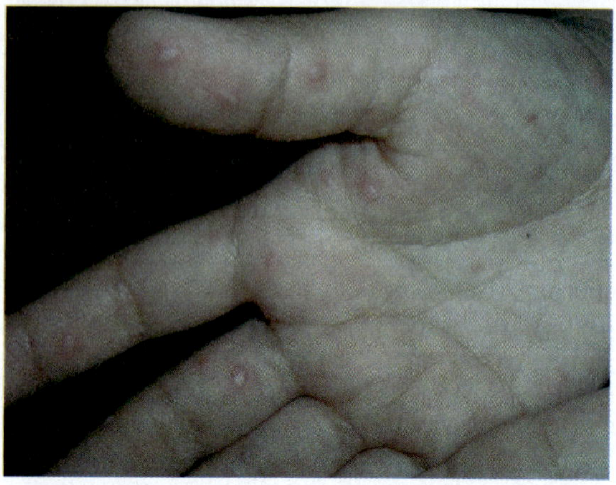

▲ **Figure 36–6.** Rash of hand, foot, and mouth disease. Typical flat, gray, oval vesicular lesions on the ventral hand and fingers. (Reproduced with permission from Richard P. Usatine, MD, in Usatine RP, Smith MA, Mayeaux EJ Jr, Chumley H. *The Color Atlas and Synopsis of Family Medicine,* 3rd ed. McGraw-Hill, 2019.)

8. Epidemic conjunctivitis—As with enterovirus 70, the A24 variant of coxsackievirus is associated with acute epidemic hemorrhagic conjunctivitis in tropical areas with outbreaks reported in southern China, Pakistan, southern Sudan, the Comoros, Uganda, Cuba, and Thailand. It is also reported as a cause of corneal endotheliitis after cataract surgery.

9. Myalgic encephalitis/chronic fatigue syndrome—This is associated in one Korean series with Borna disease virus, while searches for associations with other enteroviruses (as well as herpes and parvoviruses) were unsuccessful.

10. Other syndromes associated with coxsackievirus infections—These include rhabdomyolysis, fulminant neonatal hepatitis (occurs rarely), pancreatitis with concomitant hepatitis and myocarditis (A4), glomerulopathy (group B infections), onychomadesis (B1), neonatal hemophagocytic lymphohistiocytosis (B1), types 1 and 2 diabetes mellitus (mainly group B infections), and thyroid disease (group B4), although definitive causality is not established. A pathogenic role in primary Sjögren syndrome and acute MI has also been proposed for group B coxsackievirus infections. A report of confirmed infective endocarditis due to coxsackievirus B2 in a patient with a prosthetic cardiac patch used in repair of a child with complete atrial ventricular septic defect suggests that viral etiologies of culture-negative infective endocarditis should be considered even in cases of cardiac surgery.

B. Laboratory Findings

Routine laboratory studies show no characteristic abnormalities. Neutralizing antibodies appear during convalescence. The virus may be isolated from throat washings or stools inoculated into suckling mice. Viral culture is expensive and labor-intensive, and it requires several days for results. A PCR test for enterovirus RNA is available and, although it cannot identify the serotype, may be useful, particularly in cases of meningitis.

▶ Treatment & Prognosis

Treatment is symptomatic. Except for meningitis, myocarditis, pericarditis, diabetes, and rare illnesses such as pancreatitis or poliomyelitis-like states, the most common syndromes caused by coxsackieviruses are benign and self-limited. Two controlled trials showed a potential clinical benefit with pleconaril for patients with enteroviral meningitis although the compassionate use of this medication has stopped (clinicians can contact ViroPharma). Anecdotal reports describe success with IVIG in severe disease. Vaccines against the most common etiologic agents in a given country, including three hand foot and mouth vaccines in China in 2016, have been developed, but simultaneous circulation of more than one virus makes coxsackievirus vaccines based on a single agent relatively ineffective. Due to its possible association with type 1 diabetes, a multivalent coxsackie B virus vaccine has been developed with good safety, tolerability, and immunogenicity in a phase 1 clinical trial.

Lee MF et al. Antiviral strategies targeting enteroviruses: current advances and future directions. Viruses. 2025;17:1178. [PMID: 41012605]

Zhang X et al. Clinical characteristics of fatal cases of hand, foot and mouth disease in children. Front Pediatr. 2025;13:1522164. [PMID: 40746350]

Zhou X et al. Recent advances on coxsackievirus A6 vaccine research. Front Immunol. 2025;16:1603028. [PMID: 40547039]

2. Echovirus Infections

Echoviruses (enteric cytopathic human orphan viruses) are enteroviruses that produce several clinical syndromes, particularly in children. Infections are most common during summer. Among reported specimens, death ensues in about 3%. Adolescents and men younger than 20 years are more commonly infected than other persons.

More than 30 serotypes of echoviruses are recognized, and the most common serotypes for disease are E types 6, 9, 11, 19, 29, 30, and 33 as well as C99. Aseptic meningitis is the most common presentation, which may be associated with a rubelliform rash. A highly pathogenic variant of echovirus 11 (E11) was reported in France and other European countries from 2022 to 2023. Transmission is primarily fecal-oral. Handwashing is an effective control measure in outbreaks of aseptic meningitis. Outbreaks related to fecal contamination of water sources, including drinking water and swimming and bathing pools, were reported previously.

Besides meningitis, other conditions associated with echoviruses range from common respiratory diseases (which increased significantly since the SARS-2 pandemic) and epidemic diarrhea to myocarditis, a hemorrhagic obstetric syndrome, keratoconjunctivitis, severe hepatitis with coagulopathy, leukocytoclastic vasculitis, encephalitis with sepsis, interstitial pneumonitis, pleurodynia, rhabdomyolysis, hemophagocytic syndromes (in children with cancer), sudden deafness, encephalitis, acute flaccid myelitis (a leading cause in India), optic neuritis, uveitis, neonatal sepsis, and septic shock. Echoviruses and enteroviruses are also a common cause of nonspecific exanthems.

As with other enterovirus infections, diagnosis is best established by correlation of clinical, epidemiologic, and laboratory evidence. Cytopathic effects are produced in tissue culture after recovery of the virus from throat washings, blood, or CSF. An enterovirus PCR of the CSF can assist in the diagnosis and is associated with a shorter duration of hospitalization in febrile neonates. Fourfold or greater rises in antibody titers signify systemic infection.

Treatment is usually symptomatic, and the prognosis is excellent, although mild paralysis after CNS infection is reported. In vitro data suggest some role for amantadine or ribavirin, but clinical studies supporting these findings are not available.

From a public health standpoint, clustered illnesses, such as among travelers swimming in sewage-infested seawater, suggest point-source exposure. Preventing fecal-oral contamination and maintaining pool hygiene through chlorination and pH control are important public health measures.

Gad B et al. Intensified circulation of echovirus 11 after the COVID-19 pandemic in Poland: detection of a highly pathogenic virus variant. Viruses. 2024;16:1011. [PMID: 39066174]

Weiss SL et al. A novel post-mortem pathogen discovery program detects an outbreak of Echovirus E7: Uganda, 2022–2023. Front Microbiol. 2025;16:1557576. [PMID: 40666800]

3. Enteroviruses 68, 70, 71, & Related Agents

Enteroviruses are nonenveloped, single-stranded viruses in the *Picornaviridae* family. They are divided into 12 species (A to L; human enteroviruses include species A to D). Several distinct clinical syndromes are described in association with enteroviruses.

Enterovirus D68 (EV-D68) is a unique enterovirus that shares epidemiologic characteristics with human rhinovirus and is typically associated with respiratory illness including asthma exacerbations. It is characterized by biennial resurgences since its first recognized global outbreak in 2014. Outbreaks have occurred in Asia, Europe, South America, West Africa, and the United States. Outbreaks associated with acute flaccid myelitis occurred in the United States in 2014, 2016, and 2018. EV-D68 is one of the most commonly implicated viruses resulting in acute flaccid myelitis (see Acute Flaccid Myelitis, above). The virus is also implicated in aseptic meningitis and encephalitis. A US surveillance study between 2017 and 2022 noted a total of 976 children with EV-D68 positive testing, with approximately 55% resulting in hospitalization. Wastewater surveillance is an effective means of monitoring, with levels correlating to confirmed cases.

Enterovirus 70 (EV-A70), a ubiquitous virus responsible for abrupt bilateral eye discharge and subconjunctival hemorrhage with occasional systemic symptoms, is most commonly associated with acute hemorrhagic conjunctivitis (AHC). Its incidence has been decreasing since the 2010s, with Coxsackievirus A24 variant now resulting in the majority of AHC outbreaks.

Enterovirus 71 (EV-A71) almost always occurs in the Asia-Pacific region (but with reports from the United States since the 1980s) and is associated with (1) hand, foot, and mouth disease, which can be severe or even fatal; (2) herpangina; (3) a form of epidemic encephalitis associated on occasion with pulmonary edema; and (4) acute flaccid myelitis mimicking poliomyelitis.

Human enteroviruses are neurotropic. They may have a role in amyotrophic lateral sclerosis. EV-D68 has been reported in a case of fatal meningitis/encephalitis. Several nonpolio type C enteroviruses are associated with polio-like syndromes, and surveillance for these are most active in China. Enterovirus infection of the pancreas can trigger cell-mediated autoimmune destruction of β cells resulting in diabetes. Enterovirus myocarditis can be a serious infection in neonates, complicated by cardiac dysfunction and arrhythmias. An association with hemophagocytosis also is reported.

Mortality is especially high in EV-A71–associated brainstem encephalitis, which is often complicated by pulmonary edema, particularly when it occurs in children younger than 5 years. A complication is autonomic nervous system dysregulation, which may precede pulmonary edema. Because of lower herd immunity, hand, foot, and mouth disease tends to infect children under age 5 in non-endemic areas. Clinical and epidemiologic findings aided by isolating the suspect agent from conjunctival scraping for EV-A70; vesicle swabs, body secretions, or CSF for EV-A71; and respiratory secretions for D68 facilitate diagnosis of these enteroviral entities. Enzyme immunoassays and complement fixation tests show good specificity but poor sensitivity (< 80%). RT-PCR may increase the detection rate in enterovirus infections and is useful in the analysis of CSF samples among patients with meningitis and of blood samples among infants with a sepsis-like illness.

Treatment of these entities remains largely symptomatic. A study in China showed that recombinant human IFN-α 1b in EV-A71–associated hand, foot, and mouth disease was associated with decreased fever duration, healing time of typical skin or oral mucosal lesions, and EV-A71 viral load. Clinicians report anecdotal success in managing myocarditis with immunoglobulins. In vitro studies show reduced viral replication when exposed to doxycycline, but clinical studies are lacking.

The major complication associated with EV-A70 is the rare development of an acute neurologic illness with motor paralysis akin to poliomyelitis. Treatment of acute flaccid myelitis related to EV-A71 with IVIG does not appear to improve neurologic outcomes. Attention-deficit/hyperactivity disorder occurs in about 20% of confirmed cases.

EV-D68 requires supportive care with particular attention to respiratory support. The CDC's National Enterovirus Surveillance System should receive reports of disease at https://www.cdc.gov/ness/contact/.

Household contacts, especially children < 6 months of age, are at particular risk for EV-A71 acquisition. As with other enteroviruses, hand hygiene is essential for preventing transmission. A commercial disinfectant, Virkon S at 1–2% application, appears to reduce infectivity of fomites. A stage-based supportive treatment for EV-A71 infections, recognizing the potential for late-onset CNS disease and cardiopulmonary failure, is important. No EV-A71 vaccine is commercially available in the United States, although three separate inactivated vaccines produced in China appear to be successful against EV-A71–associated hand, foot, and mouth disease and herpangina (efficacy 63.2–90.8%). Decreases in antibody titers suggest booster doses of these vaccines may be needed.

Enterovirus 72 (EV-A72) is another term for hepatitis A virus (see Chapter 18). **Enterovirus EV-A104** is related to rhinoviruses and associated with respiratory illness in reports from Italy and Switzerland.

Bifani AM et al. Enterovirus A71 priorities, challenges, and future opportunities in humoral immunity and vaccine development. NPJ Vaccines. 2025;10:194. [PMID: 40817335]

Clopper BR et al. Enterovirus D68-associated respiratory illness in children. JAMA Netw Open. 2025;8:e259131. [PMID: 40338550]

Fall A et al. Enhanced genomic surveillance of enteroviruses reveals a surge in enterovirus D68 cases, the Johns Hopkins health system, Maryland, 2024. J Clin Microbiol. 2025;63:e0046925. [PMID: 40492725]

Yan X et al. The efficacy and effectiveness of enterovirus A71 vaccines against hand, foot, and mouth disease: a systematic review and meta-analysis. PLoS One. 2025;20:e0323782. [PMID: 40402938]

4. Human Parechovirus Infection

Human parechovirus is classified among 19 genotypes among a distinct genus of picornaviruses and causes a wide variety of diseases in humans, especially in neonates. The pathogen is present worldwide and mainly affects small children during the summer and early fall, although disease can also occur in older adults. Virus type A3 is the most commonly reported isolate in the United States. A parechovirus outbreak occurred in the United States (Tennessee) between April and May 2022 involving 29 infants, including 23 with meningoencephalitis. Clinical presentation is mainly driven by GI and respiratory illness, although otitis, neonatal sepsis, hepatitis, flaccid paralysis, myalgias (which may be epidemic), diffuse maculopapular and palmar-plantar rashes, aseptic meningitis, intracranial hemorrhage, seizures, pericarditis, and an acute disseminated encephalitis are described in the literature. Co-infection with other pathogens is common. Mortality and long-term morbidity are exceedingly rare, although a recent retrospective cohort reports double the baseline prevalence of attention-deficit/hyperactivity disorder by age 8 in children with severe parechovirus infection as infants.

Type A6 typically affects individuals older than 20 years, while type A3 is responsible for meningitis/encephalitis and neonatal sepsis (13% of late-onset neonatal sepsis in one series was due to parechovirus) and was reported in association with necrotizing enterocolitis and hepatitis. It is the most common cause of neonatal meningitis and is the picornavirus most often found in CSF samples of CNS-related infections in very young children. The encephalitis can be severe, and Guillain-Barré syndrome is also reported with parechovirus type A6. CSF parameters include a normal count in > 90% and an abnormal protein in <50%. CNS infection may be seen with virus type A4 as well. Respiratory and GI illnesses are seen with types A4–A6, A10, A13, and A15.

Treatment is largely supportive and rapid identification of the viral antigen by PCR in stools, respiratory samples, and CSF may decrease use of unnecessary antibiotics and shorten hospital stay, although current PCR assays are not always sufficiently sensitive to exclude parechoviruses. Intravenous immunoglobulin was anecdotally successful in one case of parechovirus dilated cardiomyopathy and maternal antibodies to parechovirus type 3 are protective. Reported complications of neonatal cerebral infections include learning disabilities, epilepsy, and cerebral palsy. Because intrafamilial transmission is well documented, diagnosis may help isolate the affected children.

Alam F et al. Parechovirus: neglected for too long? J Virol. 2025;99:e0184624. [PMID: 40130875]

Brisco L et al. Early life parechovirus infection neuropsychological outcomes at 8 years: a cohort study. Child Neuropsychol. 2024;30:1135. [PMID: 38258280]

Freeman MC et al. Enterovirus and parechovirus neurologic infections in children: clinical presentations and neuropathogenesis. J Pediatric Infect Dis Soc. 2025;14:piae069. [PMID: 39776161]

Sasidharan A et al. Diagnosis, management, and outcomes of parechovirus infections in infants: an overview. J Clin Microbiol. 2024;62(6). [PMID: 38647282]

RICKETTSIAL DISEASES

TYPHUS GROUP

1. Epidemic (Louse-Borne) Typhus

ESSENTIALS OF DIAGNOSIS

- Prodrome of headache, then chills and fever.
- Severe, intractable headaches, prostration, persistent high fever.
- Macular rash appearing on days 4–7 on the trunk and in the axillae, spreading to the rest of the body but sparing the face, palms, and soles.
- Diagnosis confirmed by complement fixation, microagglutination, or immunofluorescence.

General Considerations

Epidemic louse-borne typhus is caused by *Rickettsia prowazekii* and transmitted by the body louse *Pediculus humanus* (Table 36–3). It was particularly prevalent during and after WW1 when urban density and social conditions favored transmission. Transmission is favored by crowded, unsanitary living conditions such as those seen during wartime and among persons experiencing homelessness. After biting a person infected with *R prowazekii*, the louse becomes infected by the organism, which persists in the louse's gut and is excreted in its feces. When the infected louse bites an uninfected individual, the feces enter the bloodstream when

Table 36–3. Rickettsial diseases (listed in alphabetical order, within groups).

Disease	Rickettsial Pathogen	Geographic Areas of Prevalence	Insect Vector	Mammalian Reservoir	Travel Association
Typhus Group					
Endemic (murine) typhus	*Rickettsia typhi*	Worldwide; small foci (United States: southeastern Gulf Coast)	Flea	Rodents, opossums	Often
Epidemic (louse-borne) typhus	*Rickettsia prowazekii*	South America, Northeastern and Central Africa	Louse	Humans, flying squirrels	Rare
Scrub Typhus Group					
Scrub typhus	*Orientia tsutsugamushi*	Southeast Asia, Japan, Australia, Western Siberia	Mite[1]	Rodents	Often
Spotted Fever Group					
African tick bite fever	*Rickettsia africae*	Rural sub-Saharan Africa, Eastern Caribbean	Tick[1]	Cattle	Often
California flea rickettsiosis	*Rickettsia felis*	Worldwide	Flea	Cats, opossums	
Lymphangitis-associated rickettsiosis	*R sibirica mongolitimonae*	Europe, Africa, Mongolia	Tick[1]	Unknown	Unknown
Mediterranean spotted fever, Boutonneuse fever, Kenya tick typhus, South African tick fever, Indian tick typhus	*Rickettsia conorii*	Africa, India, Mediterranean regions	Tick[1]	Rodents, dogs	Often
Queensland tick typhus	*Rickettsia australis*	Eastern Australia	Tick[1]	Rodents, marsupials	Rare
Rocky Mountain spotted fever, Brazilian spotted fever	*Rickettsia rickettsii*	Western Hemisphere; United States (especially mid-Atlantic coast region) Southeastern Brazil	Tick[1]	Rodents, dogs, porcupines, capybaras for Brazilian spotted fever	Rare
Siberian Asian tick typhus	*Rickettsia sibirica*	Siberia, Mongolia	Tick[1]	Rodents	Rare
Tick-borne lymphadenopathy/*Dermacentor*-borne necrosis erythema lymphadenopathy/scalp eschar neck lymphadenopathy	*R slovaca, R raoultii, Candidatus R rioja*	Europe	Tick	Unknown	Occasional
Transitional Group					
Rickettsialpox	*Rickettsia akari*	United States, Korea, former USSR	Mite[1]	Mice	Occasional
Ehrlichiosis/Anaplasmosis					
Human granulocytic anaplasmosis	*Anaplasma phagocytophilum, Ehrlichia ewingii, Ehrlichia muris eauclairensis*[2] *Neorickettsia sennetsu*[2]	Northeastern United States and upper Midwest (*E muris eauclairensis*) Southeast Asia (*N sennetsu*)	Tick[1]	Rodents, deer, sheep	Occasional
Human monocytic ehrlichiosis	*Ehrlichia chaffeensis, Ehrlichia canis*	Southeastern United States	Tick[1]	Dogs	Occasional
Q fever	*Coxiella burnetii*	Worldwide	None[3]	Cattle, sheep, goats	Occasional

[1]Also serve as arthropod reservoirs by maintaining rickettsiae through transovarian transmission.
[2]Limited data available on exact cell involved in pathogenesis.
[3]Human infection results from inhalation of dust.

the person scratches the wound. Louse feces may also enter via the respiratory tract; because of aerosol transmissibility, *R prowazekii* is considered a possible bioterrorism agent.

R prowazekii can survive in lymphoid and adipose (in endothelial reservoirs) tissues after primary infection and, years later, produce recrudescence of disease (**Brill-Zinsser disease**) without exposure to infected lice. This phenomenon can serve as a point source for future outbreaks.

Flying squirrels (*Glaucomys volans*) are a zoonotic reservoir of *R prowazekii* in the United States. Transmission to humans, known as sylvatic typhus, usually causes mild disease. Foci of sylvatic typhus are found in the eastern United States and are reported to occur in Brazil, Ethiopia, and Mexico.

Clinical Findings

A. Symptoms and Signs

Prodromal malaise, cough, headache, backache, arthralgia, myalgia, and chest pain begin after an incubation period of 10–14 days, followed by an abrupt onset of chills, high fever, and prostration, with flu-like symptoms progressing to delirium and stupor. Headache is severe, and fever is prolonged (Table 36–2).

Facial flushing and macular rash (that may become confluent) appear; the rash appears first in the axillae and then over the trunk, spreading to the extremities but sparing the palms and soles. Severely ill patients may develop hemorrhagic rash and hypotension. Pneumonia, thromboses, vasculitis, myocarditis, uremia, and seizures may occur. Improvement begins 13–16 days after onset.

B. Laboratory Findings

The WBC count is variable. Thrombocytopenia, elevated liver enzymes, proteinuria, and hematuria commonly occur. Serum obtained 5–12 days after onset of symptoms usually shows specific antibodies for *R prowazekii* antigens as demonstrated by complement fixation, microagglutination, or immunofluorescence. In primary rickettsial infection, early antibodies are IgM; in recrudescence (Brill-Zinsser disease), early antibodies are predominantly IgG. A PCR test exists, but its availability is limited.

C. Imaging

Radiographs of the chest may show patchy consolidation.

Differential Diagnosis

The prodromal symptoms and the early febrile stage lack enough specificity to permit diagnosis in nonepidemic situations. The rash is sufficiently distinctive for diagnosis, but it may be absent in up to 50% of cases or may be difficult to observe in dark-skinned persons. A variety of other acute febrile diseases should be considered, including typhoid fever, meningococcemia, dengue, leptospirosis, and measles.

Prevention

Prevention consists of louse control with insecticides, particularly by applying chemicals to clothing or treating it with heat, and frequent bathing. A deloused and bathed typhus patient is not infectious. The disease is not transmitted from person to person. No vaccine is available to prevent *R prowazekii* infection.

Treatment

Treatment consists of doxycycline, 100 mg orally twice daily, for 7–10 days or for at least 3 days after the fever subsides. A single dose of 200 mg of doxycycline may be effective; however, some patients may relapse. Chloramphenicol is considered less effective than doxycycline, but it is still the drug of choice in pregnancy.

Prognosis

The prognosis depends greatly on the patient's age and immune status. The mortality rate is 10% in the second and third decades of life but has in the past reached 60% in the sixth decade. Brill-Zinsser disease is rarely fatal.

Centers for Disease Control and Prevention (CDC). About epidemic typhus. https://www.cdc.gov/typhus/about/epidemic.html
Deng YP et al. Emerging bacterial infectious diseases/pathogens vectored by human lice. Travel Med Infect Dis. 2023;55:102630. [PMID: 37567429]

2. Endemic (Murine) Typhus

Rickettsia typhi, a ubiquitous pathogen recognized on all continents, is transmitted between rats via fleas (Table 36–3). Serosurveys of animals show high prevalence of antibodies to *R typhi* in opossums, dogs, and cats. Humans usually acquire the infection in an urban or suburban setting when bitten by an infected flea. Rare human cases in the developed world occur in travelers, usually to Southeast Asia, Africa, or the Mediterranean area, although other pockets of infection are also known to occur. Murine typhus is recognized in the United States along the Gulf Coast (in Texas murine typhus accounts for more than one-half of all zoonotic infections), Southern California, and Hawaii. The surge in cases is attributed to climate change, vector expansion, and increased recognition.

Clinical Findings

A. Symptoms and Signs

The presentation is nonspecific, including fever, headache, myalgia, and chills. Relative bradycardia is reported. Maculopapular rash occurs in around 50% of cases; it is concentrated on the trunk, mostly sparing the palms and soles, and fades rapidly. Rare presentations include pain or painful genital (Lipschutz) ulcers, meningitis, and meningoencephalitis. Untreated infections last an average of 12–15 days.

Even if untreated, endemic typhus is usually self-limited, and the prognosis is excellent. Murine typhus in pregnancy is often associated with transaminitis and usually has a favorable prognosis. However, it can be associated with maternal death, miscarriage, preterm birth, and low birth weight if acquired early during pregnancy.

B. Laboratory Findings

A fourfold rise in serum antibody titers between the acute and the convalescent phase is diagnostic. It is important to note that *R. typhi* serologic tests frequently cross-react with *R. prowazekii.* During the first week of illness, PCR is the most sensitive test if samples are taken before doxycycline administration. Anemia, thrombocytopenia, leukopenia, hyponatremia, and elevated levels of liver enzymes commonly occur. PCR or culture are preferred to serologies (being positive two weeks earlier) but are not available at most diagnostic laboratories.

Differential Diagnosis

The most common differential diagnosis is Rocky Mountain spotted fever, usually occurring after rural exposure and with a different rash (centripetal rather than the centrifugal rash seen in epidemic or endemic typhus). Murine typhus has been confused with COVID and is also associated with a multisystem inflammatory syndrome.

Complications

Murine typhus can be associated with pneumonia, pleural effusion, and respiratory failure. Other complications include neurologic seen in one-third of cases (facial nerve paralysis, meningitis with or without encephalitis, stroke, extrapyramidal movement disorders as well as generalized ataxia, and seizures), renal (acute kidney injury and focal segmental glomerulosclerosis), myocarditis, and ocular disease. Less commonly, multiorgan failure, disseminated intravascular coagulation, and hemophagocytic lymphohistiocytosis may occur.

Treatment

Doxycycline, 100 mg orally twice daily, for 3 days (or until the patient is afebrile for 48 hours) is the medication of choice, except during pregnancy. Ciprofloxacin (500–750 mg orally twice daily) and ampicillin (500 mg orally three times a day) are reportedly successful in pregnant patients. Azithromycin is frequently used but is inferior to doxycycline and is not associated with improved fetal outcomes.

Prevention

Preventive measures are directed at control of rats and fleas.

Prognosis

Endemic typhus is usually a self-limited. A large case series from Texas reported a fatality rate of 0.4%. When encephalitis or meningitis occurs the mortality is as high as 27%.

Anstead GM. A One Health perspective on the resurgence of flea-borne typhus in Texas in the 21st century: part 1: the bacteria, the cat flea, urbanization, and climate change. Pathogens. 2025;14:154. [PMID: 40005529]

Blanton LS. Murine typhus: a review of a reemerging flea-borne rickettsiosis with potential for neurologic manifestations and sequalae. Infect Dis Rep. 2023;15:700. [PMID: 37987401]

Roxas PB et al: Typhus group Rickettsia community-acquired bacterial central nervous system infections: we must think outside the box! J Neurol Sci. 2024;466:123281. [PMID: 39447222]

3. Scrub Typhus

ESSENTIALS OF DIAGNOSIS

- Exposure to mites in endemic South and East Asia, the western Pacific (including Korea), and Australia.
- Black eschar at site of the bite, with regional and generalized lymphadenopathy.
- High fever, relative bradycardia, headache, myalgia, and a short-lived macular rash.
- Frequent pneumonitis, encephalitis, and myocarditis.

General Considerations

Scrub typhus is caused by *Orientia tsutsugamushi* and is transmitted by mites (chiggers). The mites live on vegetation but complete their maturation cycle by biting humans. The disease is endemic in Southeast Asia (Table 36–3) in an area known as the "tsutsugamushi triangle." Scrub typhus is a cause of acute febrile illness in India and China and is a recognized cause of fever of unknown origin. The disease is more common in rural areas, but urban cases have also been described. Vertical transmission may occur, and transmission has also been recognized via transfusion and occupational exposures (eg, among laboratory workers). Cases among travelers are increasingly recognized. Climate change (increase temperatures and precipitation) is associated with increasing numbers of cases, as is the increased prevalence of greenhouse gases and air pollution in endemic areas.

Clinical Findings

A. Symptoms and Signs

After a 1- to 3-week incubation period, malaise, chills, headache, and backache develop. At the site of the bite, a papule evolves into a black eschar; this finding is suggestive when it is present but was recognized in only 19% of patients in a South Korean series. Regional (and sometimes generalized) lymphadenopathy occurs. Fever rises during the first week of infection, and the rash is usually macular and primarily on the trunk. The rash can be fleeting or more severe, peaking at 8 days but lasting up to 21 days after onset of infection. Relative bradycardia frequently accompanies scrub typhus infection. GI symptoms, including nausea, vomiting, and diarrhea, occur in nearly two-thirds of patients and correspond to the presence of superficial mucosal hemorrhage, multiple erosions, or ulcers in the GI tract. Acute kidney injury and other renal abnormalities are frequently present.

A wide range of complications can be seen in association with scrub typhus including pneumonitis, myocarditis, encephalitis or aseptic meningitis, pancreatitis, and acute kidney injury among other less common manifestations. ARDS or hemophagocytosis may develop during the second or third week. Congenital cases are reported, and women who acquire infections during pregnancy have a higher rates of fetal loss especially when the woman develops pneumonia. Infection confers prolonged immunity against homologous strains and transient immunity against heterologous strains.

B. Laboratory Findings

Thrombocytopenia and elevation of liver enzymes, bilirubin, and creatinine are common. Indirect immunofluorescent assay and indirect immunoperoxidase assays are the gold standard for scrub typhus diagnosis. These tests are expensive and have limited availability. An ELISA detecting *Orientia*-specific antibodies in serum is available. PCR (from the eschar or blood) is the most sensitive diagnostic test. Culture of the organism from blood obtained in the first few days of illness can be done but requires a specialized BSL 3 laboratory. Use of both ELISA and PCR is recommended.

Differential Diagnosis

Leptospirosis, typhoid, dengue, malaria, Q fever, hemorrhagic fevers, meningitis, and other rickettsial infections should be considered. The headache may mimic trigeminal neuralgia. Scrub typhus is a recognized cause of obscure tropical fevers, especially in children. The presence of an eschar, lymphocytosis, and elevated CRP may help distinguish scrub typhus from dengue. Coinfection with malaria may exist.

Prevention

Insect repellents on clothing and skin and protective clothing are effective preventive measures. Although chemoprophylaxis with doxycycline has been used, the CDC does not recommend antibiotic prophylaxis for asymptomatic travelers. Permethrin-treated uniforms are shown to be associated with fewer cases among troops in Northern Australia. No effective vaccines are available.

Treatment & Prognosis

Without treatment, fever subsides spontaneously after 2 weeks, but the mortality rate may be 10–30%. Poor prognostic factors include hypotension requiring vasopressors, ICU care, age > 60 years, absence of an eschar (making the diagnosis difficult), pregnancy, and laboratory findings such as leukocytosis or hypoalbuminemia. Most patients recover without neurologic sequelae. Late hospitalizations for heart failure and new-onset atrial fibrillation are both increased among scrub typhus survivors. Autoimmune markers also are increased among survivors. Thromboembolic complications are correlated with rifampin treatment, advanced age, history of atrial fibrillation, and a particular genotype (Taguchi).

The treatment of choice is doxycycline (100 mg twice daily) or minocycline (100 mg twice daily). Patients should be treated for at least 3 days after their fever subsides. Shorter duration of therapy is associated with relapse. A clinical trial comparing doxycycline, azithromycin, and both for severe scrub typhus showed no difference between doxycycline and azithromycin monotherapy, but found lower incidence of 28-day mortality, complications at day 7, and persistent fever at day 5 with combination therapy. Alternative therapies for pregnant patients and those with doxycycline allergy include chloramphenicol and azithromycin. Azithromycin appears to have similar efficacy to doxycycline with fewer adverse effects.

Chen C et al. Antibiotics in the treatment of scrub typhus: A network meta-analysis and cost-effectiveness analysis. J Infect Dev Ctries. 2025;19:67. [PMID: 39977469]
Majumdar S et al. Neurological manifestations of scrub typhus: the clinical spectrum, determinants, and outcome. Neurol India. 2025;73:88. [PMID: 40652474]

SPOTTED FEVERS

1. Tick Typhus (Rickettsial Fever)

The term *tick typhus* denotes a variety of spotted rickettsial fevers, often named by their geographic location (including Rocky Mountain spotted fever, Mediterranean spotted fever, and African tick bite fever, among others) or by morphology (eg, boutonneuse fever). More than 30 species of spotted fever group rickettsioses are found worldwide, 21 of which are pathogenic in humans. These illnesses are caused by various rickettsial organisms (eg, *R rickettsii*, *R africae*, *R australis*, *R conorii*, *R japonica*, *R massiliae*, *R parkeri*, *R sibirica*, and *R 364D*) and are transmitted by various tick species. Dogs and wild animals, usually rodents and even reptiles, may serve as reservoirs for rickettsial fevers. Travel is a risk factor for disease, particularly among older adult ecotourists. *R conorii*–associated tick typhus is the most common rickettsial infection in Israel.

The pathogens may produce an eschar or black spot ("tache noire") at the site of the tick bite that may be useful in diagnosis. Common symptoms include fever, headache, myalgias, and rash. **The severity of illness varies by *Rickettsia* species, and infections not caused by *R. rickettsiae* tend to have a better prognosis (detailed further below).** Painful lymphadenopathy or lymphangitis also may occur. Rarely, papulovesicular lesions may be present (as described with Rickettsialpox). Regional adenopathy, kidney disease, splenic rupture, hepatitis, and retinitis have been reported. Neurologic complications, coronary involvement, purpura fulminans, and hemophagocytic syndrome are rare.

The diagnosis is clinical, with serologic methods or PCR of the buffy coat of blood or an eschar used for confirmation. Oral treatment with doxycycline (100 mg twice daily) or chloramphenicol (50–75 mg/kg/day in four divided doses) for 7–10 days is indicated. Fluoroquinolones or macrolides can be considered as alternatives for less severely ill persons when doxycycline cannot be given, though data are more limited.

Prevention entails protective clothing, repellents, and inspection for and removal of ticks.

Cohen R et al. Spotted fever group rickettsioses in Israel, 2010–2019. Emerg Infect Dis. 2021;27:2117. [PMID: 34286684]

2. Rocky Mountain Spotted Fever

ESSENTIALS OF DIAGNOSIS

- Exposure to tick bite in an endemic area.
- Influenza-like prodrome followed by fever, severe headache, and myalgias; occasionally, delirium and coma.
- Red macular rash appears between days 2 and 6 of fever, first on the wrists and ankles and then spreading centrally ("centripetal spread"); it may become petechial.
- Mortality > 70% in untreated patients.
- Serial serologic examinations by indirect fluorescent antibody confirm the diagnosis retrospectively.

General Considerations

Rocky Mountain spotted fever (RMSF) is caused by *R rickettsii* and is endemic in parts of the Americas (Table 36–3). In the United States, the number of RMSF cases has increased over the last two decades. **Despite its name, most cases of RMSF occur *outside* the Rocky Mountain area.** More than half of US cases are from five states: Arkansas, Missouri, North Carolina, Tennessee, and Virginia.

R rickettsii is transmitted to humans by the bite of ticks. Several hours of contact between the tick and the human host are required for transmission. Ticks that can transmit the infection include the Rocky Mountain wood tick, *Dermacentor andersoni*, in the western United States, and the American dog tick, *Dermacentor variabilis*, in the eastern United States. The brown dog tick, *Rhipicephalus sanguineus*, is a vector in eastern Arizona, Southern California, and Mexico, associated with peridomestic habitats. Epidemic RMSF, as described in Arizona and Mexico, is associated with massive local infestations of the brown dog tick in domestic dogs. The tribal communities of Arizona are particularly impacted by RMSF, and since 2003 more than 500 cases and 28 deaths have been reported. The One Health initiative is active in coordinating MRSF public health activities among its other activities.

Clinical Findings

A. Symptoms and Signs

RMSF can cause severe multiorgan dysfunction and fatality rates of up to 73% if left untreated, making it *the most serious rickettsial disease*. Two to 14 days (mean, 7 days) after the bite of an infectious tick, symptoms begin with the abrupt onset of high fever, chills, headache, nausea and vomiting, myalgias, restlessness, insomnia, and irritability. The characteristic rash (faint macules progressing to maculopapules and then petechiae) appears between days 2 and 6 of fever. It initially involves the wrists and ankles, spreading *centrally* to the arms, legs, and trunk over the next 2–3 days. Involvement of the palms and soles is characteristic. Eschars are not usually seen. Facial flushing, conjunctival injection, and hard palate lesions (Figure 36–7) may occur. In about 10% of cases, however, no rash or only a minimal rash is seen. Cough and pneumonitis may develop, and delirium, lethargy, seizures, stupor, and coma may also appear in more severe cases. Splenomegaly, hepatomegaly, jaundice, myocarditis (which may mimic an ACS), adrenal hemorrhage, polyarticular arthritis, or uremia are occasionally present. ARDS and necrotizing vasculitis, when present, are of greatest concern.

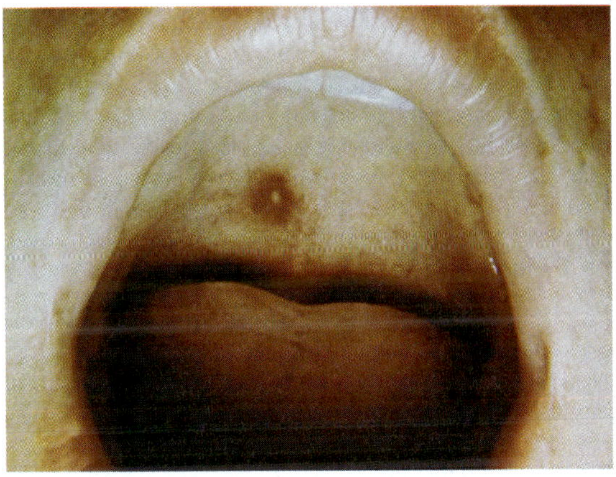

Figure 36–7. Hard palate lesion caused by Rocky Mountain spotted fever. (Public Health Image Library, CDC.)

B. Laboratory and Imaging Findings

Thrombocytopenia, hyponatremia, elevated aminotransferases, and hyperbilirubinemia are common. CSF may show hypoglycorrhachia and mild pleocytosis. DIC is observed in severe cases. Diagnosis during the acute phase of the illness can be made by immunohistologic or PCR demonstration of *R rickettsii* in skin biopsy specimens (or cutaneous swabs of skin lesions). Performing such studies as soon as skin lesions become apparent maximizes sensitivity.

A characteristic MRI appearance has been noted among RMSF patients with meningoencephalitis (a "starry sky" appearance with numerous foci showing increased signal on T2 and diffusion-weighted sequences) but may be less common among adult patients.

Diagnosis is most commonly made serologically. Most patients do not mount an antibody response until the second week of illness. The indirect fluorescent antibody IgG test is most commonly used. It is important to use paired sera (acute and convalescent) whenever possible to establish an acute infection. **Due to the slow turnaround of testing and risk of mortality, it is important to initiate empirical antibiotic therapy when a diagnosis of RMSF is being considered.**

Differential Diagnosis

The diagnosis is challenging because early symptoms resemble those of many other infections. The classic triad of fever, rash, and tick bite is rarely recognized, with up to 40% of patients not recalling a tick bite. Moreover, the rash may be confused with that of measles, typhoid, ehrlichiosis, or—most importantly—meningococcemia. Co-infections may mask the diagnosis. Some spotted fever rickettsioses may also mimic RMSF but will not be detected by routine serologic testing for RMSF.

Prevention

Protective clothing, tick-repellent chemicals, and the removal of ticks at frequent intervals are helpful measures. Aggressive campaigns to decrease ticks exist in many communities with high RMSF attack rates. Prophylactic therapy after a tick bite is not recommended. Control of dog ticks is important, and the San Carlos Apache tribe along with the CDC is masterminding a prevention project entitled RMSF Rodeo including dog and tick control and community education.

Treatment & Prognosis

Treatment with doxycycline (100 mg orally twice daily for 5–7 days or for at least 3 days after the fever subsides) is recommended for all ages, including pregnant patients. Chloramphenicol (50–100 mg/kg/day in four divided doses, orally or intravenously for 4–10 days) is the only alternative medication to treat RMSF; however, patients who are treated with chloramphenicol may be at higher risk for death than patients treated with a tetracycline. Note that oral formulations of chloramphenicol are not available in the United States and that use of chloramphenicol potentially has adverse risks such as aplastic anemia. Patients usually defervesce within 48–72 hours, and therapy should be continued for at least 3 days after defervescence occurs.

The reported mortality rate for treated patients in the United States is about 3–5%, although in northern Mexico the rates are often as high as 50%. Complications include seizures, encephalopathy and encephalitis, peripheral neuropathy, paraparesis, bowel and bladder incontinence, cerebellar and vestibular dysfunction, hearing loss, and motor deficits. Features associated with increased risk of poor outcomes include (1) older age; (2) the presence of atypical clinical features (absence of headache, no history of tick attachment, GI symptoms) and underlying chronic diseases; and (3) a delay in initiation of appropriate antibiotic therapy. The usual cause of death is pneumonitis with respiratory or cardiac failure. A fulminant form of RMSF can be seen in patients with glucose-6-phosphate dehydrogenase deficiency.

Álvarez-Hernández G et al. Rocky Mountain spotted fever in Mexico: a call to action. Am J Trop Med Hyg. 2024;111:1070. [PMID: 39288751]

Chiang L et al. Rocky Mountain spotted fever in children along the US-Mexico border, 2017–2023. Emerg Infect Dis. 2024;30:2288. [PMID: 39387516]

Foley J et al. Focus on brown dog tick-transmitted Rocky Mountain spotted fever in dogs and people: shared threats and solutions. J Am Vet Med Assoc. 2025;263:293. [PMID: 39879657]

OTHER RICKETTSIAL & RICKETTSIAL-LIKE DISEASES

1. Ehrlichiosis & Anaplasmosis

ESSENTIALS OF DIAGNOSIS

- Infection of monocytes or granulocytes by tick-borne gram-negative bacteria.
- Nine-day incubation period; clinical disease ranges from asymptomatic to life-threatening.
- Malaise, nausea, fever, and headaches.
- Excellent response to therapy with tetracyclines.

General Considerations

Human ehrlichiosis and anaplasmosis are endemic in the United States. The three species of ehrlichiosis found in the United States are *E chaffeensis*, *E ewingii*, and *E muris eauclairensis*.

Ehrlichia chaffeensis (Table 36–3) is the most common *Ehrlichia* species infecting humans and is seen primarily in the south-central United States (Arkansas and Missouri lead the US case load). Cases are also reported from Mexico City and Japan, suggesting it is more widely distributed than was formerly recognized.

Human granulocytic anaplasmosis, formerly called human granulocytic ehrlichiosis, is caused by *Anaplasma phagocytophilum*; most cases in the United States are reported from New England, New York, Minnesota, and Wisconsin. Anaplasmosis is increasingly reported in Asia and Europe, with its recognition in 97 vectors and 208 wildlife species.

In North America, the major tick-borne rickettsial disease vectors for these pathogens are (1) the Lone Star tick (*Amblyomma americanus*), which is the vector for *E chaffeensis* and *E ewingii*; (2) the black-legged tick (*Ixodes scapularis),* which is a vector for *B burgdorferi* (Lyme disease), *Babesia microti* (babesiosis), and *A phagocytophilum* (anaplasmosis), and a possible vector for *Ehrlichia muris eauclairensis*; and (3) the western black-legged tick (*Ixodes pacificus*), which is a vector for *A phagocytophilum* along the Pacific coast of the United States. The principal reservoirs for human monocytic ehrlichiosis and human granulocytic anaplasmosis are the white-tail deer and the white-footed mouse, respectively. Other mammals are implicated as well. Transfusion-transmitted anaplasmosis has been reported.

Clinical Findings

A. Symptoms and Signs

Clinical disease of human monocytic ehrlichiosis ranges from mild to life-threatening. Typically, after a 1- to 2-week incubation period and a prodrome consisting of malaise, myalgias, rigors, and nausea, high fever and headache develop. A pleomorphic rash may occur. Presentation in immunosuppressed patients (including transplant patients) and older patients tends to be more severe. Rare serious sequelae include acute respiratory failure and ARDS; neurologic complications, the most common being meningoencephalitis and aseptic meningitis; acute kidney disease; hemophagocytic syndrome; and multiorgan failure.

The clinical manifestations of human granulocytic anaplasmosis are similar to those of human monocytic ehrlichiosis. Asymptomatic infection is recognized. Rash, however, is infrequent. If a rash is present, coinfection with other tick-borne diseases or an alternative diagnosis should be suspected. Persistent fever and malaise are reported to occur for 2 or more years. Reported complications of anaplasmosis include hyponatremia, leukopenia, thrombocytopenia, pulmonary hypertension, and an acute cerebral infarction.

Coinfection with anaplasmosis and Lyme disease or babesiosis has been well described. The clinical manifestations (including fever and cytopenias) are more severe with anaplasmosis than with Lyme disease. A spirochete, *Borrelia miyamotoi*, may mimic anaplasmosis in its clinical manifestations.

B. Laboratory Findings

Diagnosis can be made by the history of tick exposure followed by a characteristic clinical presentation. Leukopenia, absolute lymphopenia, thrombocytopenia, and transaminitis occur often. Thrombocytopenia occurs more often than leukopenia in human granulocytic ehrlichiosis. Hyponatremia from volume depletion is reported. Examination of peripheral blood with Giemsa stain may reveal characteristic intraleukocytic vacuoles (morulae) in up to 20% of patients. An indirect fluorescent antibody assay is available through the CDC and requires acute and convalescent sera. A blood PCR assay can help make the diagnosis early in the disease course. PCR assay is most sensitive in the first week of illness and can be used as a confirmatory test, although public health studies in North Carolina suggest that < 1% of cases have PCR testing performed.

Treatment & Prevention

Treatment for human ehrlichiosis and anaplasmosis is with doxycycline, 100 mg twice daily (orally or intravenously) for 10–14 days or until 3 days of defervescence. Rifampin is an alternative for pregnant patients. Treatment should not be withheld while awaiting confirmatory serology when suspicion is high. Lack of clinical improvement and defervescence 48 hours after doxycycline initiation suggests an alternate diagnosis. Some patients may continue to have headache, weakness, and malaise for weeks despite adequate treatment. The case fatality rate is 1% with *E chaffeensis* infections and 0.3% among cases of human anaplasmosis.

Tick control is the essence of prevention. Given the increasing prevalence and recognition of these diseases, screening for solid organ transplants and blood transfusions should be established to prevent posttransplant infections. Travel history is also important, with data from Texas and North Carolina emphasizing travel as a factor associated with transmission.

Adams SN et al. National surveillance of human ehrlichiosis caused by *Ehrlichia ewingii*, United States, 2013–2021. Emerg Infect Dis. 2025;31:222. [PMID: 39983701]

Siegler AM et al. Contribution of limited molecular testing to low ehrlichiosis diagnosis in high incidence area, North Carolina, USA. Emerg Infect Dis. 2025;31:281. [PMID: 39983688]

2. Q Fever (*Coxiella burnetii* Infection)

ESSENTIALS OF DIAGNOSIS

- Exposure to sheep, goats, cattle, or their products; some infections are laboratory-acquired.
- Acute or chronic febrile illness: headache, cough, prostration, and abdominal pain.
- Pneumonitis, hepatitis, or encephalopathy; less often, endocarditis, vascular infections, osteomyelitis, or chronic fatigue syndrome.
- A common cause of culture-negative endocarditis.

General Considerations

Q fever, a reportable and significantly underestimated disease in the United States, is caused by the gram-negative obligate intracellular coccobacillus *C burnetii*. It is considered a neglected zoonotic disease per the WHO. *Coxiella* infections occur globally (with increasing recognition in several countries, including Brazil and South Korea), mostly in cattle, sheep, and goats, and cause mild or subclinical disease (Table 36–3). In these animals, reactivation of the infection occurs during pregnancy and causes abortions or low birth weight offspring. *Coxiella* is resistant to heat and drying and remains infective in the environment for months. Its incidence appears to be increasing, and modes of transmission in outbreaks are transitioning from occupational to community acquisition. *C burnetii* is isolated from about 25% of cheese samples.

Human infection occurs via inhalation of aerosolized bacteria (in dust or droplets) from feces, urine, milk, or products of conception of infected animals. Ingestion and skin penetration are other recognized routes of transmission. Animal handlers, slaughterhouse workers, veterinarians, laboratory workers, and other workers exposed to animal products are at risk due to their occupations. Nonetheless, in a review of 81 human outbreaks, over half occurred outside traditional occupational at-risk settings. In the United States, > 60% of cases do not report an exposure to potentially infectious animals, but cases are more than twice as likely as non-cases to report drinking raw milk. An Italian group has identified *Coxiella*-like agents in birds and postulate they may also be involved in the pathogenesis of *C burnetii* infection.

Human-to-human transmission does *not* seem to occur, but maternal-fetal infection can occur, and infection after liver transplant is reported. Rare tick-borne transmission is suspected, but ticks may be important in ruminant transmission. In Europe, 4.8% of ticks carry *C burnetii*.

Clinical Findings

A. Symptoms and Signs

Asymptomatic infection is common. For the remaining cases, a febrile illness develops after an incubation period of 2–3 weeks, usually accompanied by headache, relative bradycardia, prostration, and muscle pains. The clinical course may be acute, chronic (6 months or longer), or relapsing. Pneumonia and granulomatous hepatitis are the predominant manifestations in the acute form (and these may vary in incidence geographically), whereas other less common manifestations include skin rashes (maculopapular or purpuric), fever of unknown origin, myocarditis, pericarditis, aortic aneurysms, aseptic meningitis, encephalitis, orchitis, iliopsoas abscess, peripheral neuropathy (from mononeuritis multiplex to plexopathy and Guillain-Barré syndrome), spondylodiscitis, tenosynovitis, granulomatous osteomyelitis (more often seen in children and infrequently associated with full joint recovery), and regional (mediastinal) or diffuse lymphadenopathies.

It has been recommended that the term *chronic Q fever* be abandoned to avoid confusion and be replaced with *persistent localized infections*. The most common presentation in patients with persistent localized infections is culture-negative endocarditis. Risk factors for endocarditis are an immunocompromised state, preexisting valvular conditions, male sex, and age above 40. Valvular prosthesis (mechanical or bioprosthesis) represents the most important risk factor. In a series of post-cardiac surgery patients with culture-negative endocarditis, Q fever is the most common cause (about 40% of cases). In a Dutch series of 107 patients with Q fever endocarditis risk factors and positive serologies, follow-up at a median of 64 months after initial screening showed that 4.7% went on to develop a persistent localized infection (one person despite an intermediate negative serology), while 23.4% became seronegative, and most (72%) showed a pattern of resolved infection.

The clinical manifestations of endocarditis are nonspecific with fever, night sweats, and weight loss. Rarely, urticaria, edema, erythema nodosum, and arthralgias are reported. Sudden cardiac insufficiency, stroke, or other embolic and mycotic aneurysms can also develop. Vascular infections, particularly of the aorta (causing mycotic aneurysms) and of graft prostheses, are the second most common presentation and are associated with a high mortality (25%). Endocarditis due to coinfections occurs rarely. A post–Q fever chronic fatigue syndrome (1 year after acute infection with chronic symptoms) is controversial and of unknown pathophysiology. Cognitive behavioral therapy is effective in reducing fatigue severity in patients with Q fever fatigue syndrome; long-term treatment with doxycycline is not effective. Recurrent osteoarticular infections in children can also be due to long-term Q fever infection.

New infection or reactivation of Q fever can occur in pregnant persons and is associated with spontaneous abortions, intrauterine growth retardation, intrauterine fetal death, and premature delivery. *C burnetii* infection during the first trimester can cause oligohydramnios.

B. Laboratory Findings

Laboratory examination during the acute phase may show elevated liver biochemical tests and occasional leukocytosis. Patients with acute Q fever usually produce antibodies to *C burnetii* phase II antigen. Phase II antigens are formed in vitro from deleted avirulent mutants and are more commonly seen in acute disease, whereas phase I antigens, seen in nature and laboratory infections, are found in the IgG form in chronic disease. A fourfold rise between acute and convalescent sera by indirect immunofluorescence is considered diagnostic. Real-time PCR for *C burnetii* DNA is helpful only in early diagnosis of Q fever. *C burnetii* DNA becomes undetectable in serum as serologic responses develop. The positive predictive value of antibodies to phase II antigens in acute disease is at most 65%, and considerable intertest variability exists with phase 2 antigens. Diagnostic tests combining PCR with ELISA (Immuno-PCR) improve sensitivity and specificity during the first 2 weeks after the onset of symptoms.

While persistent infection can be diagnosed based on serologic tests done at 3- and 6-month intervals (with an IgG titer against phase I antigen of 1:800 or greater), the sensitivity of such serologies is often low, and the diagnosis of Q fever is often made clinically. An automated epifluorescence assay has > 95% sensitivity for detecting phase I antigens in persistent infection. The presence of elevated levels of anticardiolipin antibodies has a high positive predictive value for acute endocarditis.

Diagnosis of Q fever endocarditis is often made during valve replacement with PCR of tissue samples. *C burnetii* may also be isolated from affected valves using the shell-vial technique. Newer methods including metagenomic next-generation sequencing (mNGS) are emerging as another tool that may assist in diagnosis of *C burnetii* along with other causes of culture negative endocarditis.

C. Imaging

Chest radiographs may show patchy pulmonary infiltrates. *All patients with acute Q fever should be screened for underlying valvular disease with echocardiography.* Initial imaging and follow-up with serial 18-FDG PET/CT scan may help identify chronic infection and monitor treatment response.

Differential Diagnosis

Viral, *Mycoplasma*, and bacterial pneumonias; viral hepatitis; brucellosis; Legionnaire disease; murine or scrub typhus; Kawasaki disease; tuberculosis; psittacosis; and other animal-borne diseases can have similar clinical presentations to Q fever. Q fever should be considered in cases of unexplained fevers with negative blood cultures in association with embolic or cardiac disease. Cases of Q fever can mimic autoimmune disease. Coinfection with typhus and leptospirosis is reported.

Treatment & Prognosis

Doxycycline is the most effective medication against *C burnetii*; doxycycline resistance is rare. Isolates remain susceptible to levofloxacin, moxifloxacin, and to a lesser extent ciprofloxacin. No resistance to sulfamethoxazole-trimethoprim is reported to date.

For acute infection, treatment with doxycycline (100 mg orally twice daily) for 14 days or at least 3 full days after defervescence is recommended. The mortality rate is usually low in untreated patients, except when endocarditis develops. For children under age 8 years, ciprofloxacin-based therapy is preferred, combined with rifampin or trimethoprim-sulfamethoxazole.

No consensus guidelines exist for the treatment of persistent *C burnetii* infections. Most experts recommend a combination oral therapy with doxycycline (100 mg twice a day) plus hydroxychloroquine for approximately 18 months for native valve endocarditis and 24 months for prosthetic valve endocarditis. The use of alternative combination regimens with a quinolone or rifampin shows some efficacy.

Serologic responses can be monitored during and after completion of therapy and treatment can be extended in the absence of favorable serologic response. The general variability of serologic data, however, limits their utility, and providers usually rely on clinical criteria. Patients should be monitored for an extended period, generally at least several years per expert opinion, due to the risk of relapse.

For patients with endocarditis, clinical cure is possible without valve replacement. Heart valve replacement is *not* associated with better survival, except in patients with a valvular prosthesis. Given the difficulty in treating endocarditis, *transthoracic echocardiography is recommended to screen for predisposing valvulopathy in all patients with acute Q fever*, and the same therapy for 1 year should be offered if valvulopathy is present. In addition, patients undergoing routine valve surgery in endemic countries should be evaluated via Q fever serology and treated if positive.

All infected pregnant patients should be given long-term trimethoprim-sulfamethoxazole (320/1600 mg orally for the duration of pregnancy, but not beyond 32 weeks' gestation) to prevent obstetric complications.

In retrospective studies, an increased risk of diffuse B-cell lymphoma and follicular lymphoma was found in patients with Q fever compared with the general population. Patients with persistent focalized infections were at higher risk for lymphadenitis and progression to lymphoma.

Prevention

Prevention is based on detecting infection in livestock, reducing contact with infected and parturient animals or contaminated dust; special care when working with animal tissues; and effective pasteurization of milk. A whole-cell Q fever vaccine is available in Australia (Q-VAX) for persons with high-risk exposures (where the overall seroprevalence of antibodies to *Coxiella* is only 19%). Severe reactogenic responses are associated with Q fever vaccines and are a major barrier to use of such vaccines. Clinicians report vaccine failure > 15 days after vaccination, and recipients with a prior exposure to *C burnetii* are at higher risk for adverse reactions that include nodules and abscesses at the injection sites. Because of this the vaccine should never be used as a booster. New vaccines under development target immunogenic, especially cytoplasmic and inner and outer membrane, proteins, and the antigens are formulated as subunit vaccines, multi-epitope DNA vaccines, and synthetic LPS-targeted peptide mimickers.

The organism is highly transmissible to laboratory workers, and culture techniques require a biosafety level 3 setting. *C burnetii* is a category B bioterrorism agent. In the setting of a bioterrorist attack, postexposure prophylaxis with doxycycline 100 mg orally twice a day for 5–7 days should be administered within 8–12 days of exposure. Pregnant patients may take trimethoprim-sulfamethoxazole as an alternative.

Heinzen RA et al. Control of human Q fever by vaccination: the journey to Q-VAX and beyond. Infect Immun. 2025;93:e0028025. [PMID: 41196302]

Latifian M et al. Evidence of *Coxiella burnetii* infection among pregnant and aborted women: a systematic review and meta-analysis. New Microbes New Infect. 2025;67:101619. [PMID: 41050738]

Mohammadi MR et al. *Coxiella burnetii:* Emerging threats, molecular insights, and advances in diagnosis and control measures. J Microbiol Methods. 2025;237:107213. [PMID: 40774611]

Rahal M et al. Global epidemiology and molecular typing of *Coxiella burnetii*: a systematic review of Q fever in humans and animals. Comp Immunol Microbiol Infect Dis. 2025;123:102401. [PMID: 40902447]

KAWASAKI DISEASE

ESSENTIALS OF DIAGNOSIS

- Fever, conjunctivitis, oral mucosal changes, rash, cervical lymphadenopathy, peripheral extremity changes.
- Elevated ESR and CRP levels.
- Risk for coronary arteritis and aneurysms.

General Considerations

Kawasaki disease is a worldwide multisystem disease. It is also known as the "**mucocutaneous lymph node syndrome**." It occurs mainly in children between the ages of 3 months and 5 years (with a case reported also in a neonate) but can occur occasionally in adults. Kawasaki disease occurs most often in persons of Asian or native Pacific Islander descent. Its incidence in Japan is twice that of the United States, and in general, cases are more often reported from the developed world, but cases are also reported from developing countries such as Kenya. It occurs among siblings at twice the incidence of cases and at higher rates among parents of cases. These findings plus the known seasonality (higher incidence in winter and early spring) and occasional epidemic pattern of cases point to the inadequate current understanding of the etiology of this disease.

Kawasaki disease is an acute, self-limiting, mucocutaneous vasculitis characterized by the infiltration of small or medium vessel walls with mononuclear cells and later by IgA-secreting plasma cells that can result in the destruction of the tunica media and subsequent aneurysm formation. The cause remains unknown. Epidemiologic studies show an increased risk with advanced maternal age, mother of foreign birth, maternal group B *Streptococcus* colonization, and early infancy hospitalization for a bacterial illness. Genetic factors are considered to play an important role in the pathogenesis of the disease. Ongoing analyses identify many gene polymorphisms, which significantly correlate with Kawasaki disease susceptibility (at least 23 to disease, and 10 to the presence of coronary aneurysms).

The Kawasaki-like disease called **multisystem inflammatory syndrome in children (MIS-C)** is described in the section above on SARS-CoV-2. In summary, the chief differences are the age and sex distribution. Kawasaki typically occurs among younger children and men of East Asian ethnicity, whereas MIS-C is more common among children of African and Hispanic heritage. IL-17 is elevated in Kawasaki disease; IL-15 and IFN-γ are elevated in MIS-C.

Clinical Findings

A. Symptoms and Signs

Clinical manifestations typically present in three phases: acute, subacute, and convalescent. The acute phase usually lasts for up to 14 days. A clinical diagnosis of classic or "**complete**" **Kawasaki disease** requires the presence of at least 5 days of fever, usually high-grade (> 39°C to 40°C) and four of the following five criteria: (1) bilateral nonexudative conjunctivitis (begins shortly after the onset of fever), (2) oral changes of erythema and cracking of lips, strawberry tongue, and erythema of oral and pharyngeal mucosa (ulcers and pharyngeal exudates are not consistent with Kawasaki disease), (3) peripheral extremity changes (erythema and edema of the hands and feet in the acute phase, or periungual desquamation, or both, within 2 to 3 weeks after the onset of fever), (4) polymorphous rash, and (5) cervical lymphadenopathy (> 1.5 cm, usually unilateral; least common of the clinical features). The revised case definition allows the diagnosis to be made as early as day 4 in the presence of more than four principal clinical criteria, particularly when redness and swelling of the hands and feet are present.

A diagnosis of atypical or "**incomplete**" **Kawasaki disease** can be made in patients with unexplained fever and fewer than four principal criteria if accompanied by compatible laboratory tests or findings of aneurysms detected by echocardiography or angiography.

A wide spectrum of rare diagnostic and recognized presentations includes an erythema multiforme rash, onychomycosis, cervical lymphadenopathy, a retropharyngeal abscess, febrile seizures, cheilitis, torticollis, facial nerve palsy, Beau lines of the nails, scrotal and penile edema, and UTI. In patients who previously received BCG vaccination, development of erythema/crusting/and induration at the site of prior vaccination is considered a strong specific indicator of Kawasaki disease.

Major complications include arteritis and aneurysms of the coronary vessels. Arteritis begins 6–8 days after the onset of disease, occurs in about 15–25% of untreated patients, and occasionally causes MI. Patients appropriately treated with IVIG have rates reduced to around 3–5%. Coronary complications are more common among patients older than 6 years or younger than 1 year of age; males; and those unresponsive to IVIG, who received a smaller dose of IVIG, or did not receive treatment within 10 days of symptom onset. While myocarditis can be found in all patients with Kawasaki disease on histologic specimens and is prominent during the acute stage, only a small percentage of patients are clinically symptomatic.

Cardiac complications include LV dysfunction, which usually normalizes promptly with IVIG therapy, and mitral regurgitation, which occurs early and does not appear to persist. The newer cardiac concept of global longitudinal strain may be of diagnostic utility but is especially useful in MIS-C patients.

The multisystemic findings of Kawasaki disease show it to be a systemic disease that affects medium-sized arteries of multiple organs, causing elevations in serum transaminases, interstitial pneumonitis, abdominal pain, vomiting, diarrhea, gallbladder hydrops, pancreatitis, lymphadenopathy, hypoalbuminemia, arrhythmias, aseptic meningitis, acute encephalopathy with biphasic seizures and late reduced diffusion, retinal and choroidal detachment, pulmonary complications (effusions, empyema, pneumothorax and an ARDS referred to as "Kawasaki disease shock syndrome"), and pyuria. CSF pleocytosis with a mononuclear cell predominance, normal glucose levels, and protein levels is seen in one-third of children who undergo lumbar puncture.

Other diseases with similar presentation that should be considered include measles in unimmunized children as well as other viral infections, such as SARS-CoV-2, adenovirus, scarlet fever, hemophagocytic lymphohistiocytosis syndrome, and toxic shock syndrome; rickettsial infections; or leptospirosis and drug hypersensitivity reactions.

B. Laboratory Findings

Laboratory findings in the acute phase of Kawasaki disease typically include leukocytosis with neutrophilic predominance, anemia, and an elevated ESR and CRP. High platelet counts are characteristic but occur in the second week. N-terminal moiety of BNP (NT-proBNP), likely indicative of myocardial involvement, may be elevated in some patients with Kawasaki disease.

C. Imaging

Noninvasive diagnosis of coronary complications can be made with CT coronary angiography (the most sensitive test), magnetic resonance angiography, or transthoracic echocardiography (advocated for early screening). Kawasaki shock syndrome is a complication, with an estimated incidence of 7%, possibly caused by a decrease in peripheral vascular resistance, myocarditis with or without myocardial ischemia, and capillary leakage.

Treatment & Prevention

All patients meeting the diagnostic criteria for Kawasaki disease (complete and incomplete), including patients with recurrent Kawasaki disease, should be treated as soon as the diagnosis is suspected to reduce inflammation and arterial damage.

A single dose of IVIG should be given in the first 7–10 days of the illness. Patients in whom the diagnosis was made later than the tenth day may still benefit from IVIG treatment if they have elevated inflammatory markers (ESR or CRP), persistent fever, or coronary artery aneurysms. When IVIG treatment is not given, coronary artery aneurysms occur in 20% of children. Even when treated with IVIG within the first 10 days of illness, coronary artery aneurysms may still develop in 5% of patients. In a Cochrane database review, IVIG was most effective in controlling fever and reducing coronary artery aneurysm incidence at 30 days. Rare cases of aseptic meningitis are reported with IVIG. Coombs-positive hemolytic anemia, especially in individuals with AB blood type, and anaphylactic reactions to immunoglobulins with selective IgA deficiency are other complications associated with IVIG administration.

Although aspirin does not lower the frequency of development of coronary abnormalities, it has important anti-inflammatory and antiplatelet activity. Concomitant aspirin with IVIG should be started at 80–100 mg/kg/day orally (divided into four doses and not exceeding 4 g/day) until the patient is afebrile for 48 hours and then reduced to 3–5 mg/kg/day until markers of acute inflammation normalize. A 2019 meta-analysis indicates that low-dose aspirin (3–5 mg/kg/day) may be as effective as high-dose aspirin (30 mg/kg/day or more) for the initial treatment of Kawasaki disease. Since ibuprofen antagonizes the irreversible platelet inhibition induced by aspirin, it should be avoided when aspirin is given.

The use of corticosteroids for children with Kawasaki disease is controversial. According to the 2017 published guidelines by the American Heart Association, single-dose pulse methylprednisolone should not be used routinely for patients with Kawasaki disease. A course of corticosteroid therapy with tapering over 2–3 weeks could be considered in addition to IVIG and aspirin for patients at high risk for not responding to IVIG.

Resistant Kawasaki disease, defined as having recrudescent or persistent fever at least 36 hours after the end of the first IVIG infusion when no other source of fever is found, develops in about 10–20% of patients. Coronary artery abnormalities on the initial echocardiogram and their presence before day 5 of fever predict nonresponse to IVIG in one Israeli study. Prognostic markers for resistance to therapy include most prominently CRP to albumin ratio (CAR) but also neutrophil-to-lymphocyte ratio (indicating markers for inflammation versus immune regulatory response), CRP absolute level, platelet-to-lymphocyte ratio (PLR) (megakaryocytes indicate inflammation), and NLR (neutrophil to lymphocyte ratios)/PLR ratio.

Options for refractory cases include a second dose of IVIG (the full validity of which needs further study), high-dose pulse corticosteroids over 3 days with or without a subsequent oral taper course, longer oral tapering course of corticosteroids over 2–3 weeks together with IVIG and aspirin. The TNF-α blocker **infliximab** is safe, well tolerated, and effective in treating patients with IVIG resistant KD and results in shorter duration of fever, reduced need for additional therapy, less severe anemia, prevents the progression of arterial lesions, and shorter hospitalization compared with a second IVIG infusion. The side effects of infliximab include rash, arthritis, respiratory disease, infusion reactions, and hepatomegaly.

Other options include the anti-inflammatory IL-1 receptor antagonist anakinra, low-dose methotrexate, and calcineurin inhibitors. Immunomodulatory monoclonal antibody therapy and cytotoxic agents or (rarely) plasma exchange should be considered in highly refractory cases only when other therapy has failed. Variation in two types of available IVIG is shown in Taiwan to affect the outcome.

The most common serious complication in the acute phase is thrombotic occlusion of a coronary artery aneurysm leading to MI or sudden death. An echocardiogram is recommended within 1–2 weeks and 4–6 weeks after treatment for uncomplicated patients, and exercise stress echocardiograms are especially sensitive in assessing myocardial dysfunction. More frequent imaging is recommended for patients with significant and evolving coronary artery abnormalities. Coronary artery aneurysms with smaller diameter, especially smaller than 6 mm, tend to regress earlier, typically within 6 months of infection.

Anticoagulation with warfarin or low-molecular-weight heparin is indicated, along with aspirin, in patients with rapidly expanding coronary artery aneurysms. Aspirin, a second antiplatelet agent, and anticoagulation with warfarin, low-molecular-weight heparin, or DOACs (which need further study in this population) may be considered for patients with large or giant aneurysms (at least 8 mm) (which correlate with delay in diagnosis) and a recent history of coronary artery thrombosis. Platelets from patients with Kawasaki disease treated with antiplatelet agents do show decreased platelet aggregation function. Systemic arterial aneurysms are also recognized and always occur concomitantly with coronary aneurysms, and large systemic aneurysms show a high rate of regression.

If MI occurs, therapy with thrombolytics, percutaneous coronary intervention, coronary artery bypass grafts, and even cardiac transplantation should be considered. Manifestations of coronary artery aneurysms can occur as late as in the third or fourth decade of life, with a study showing a prevalence of 5% coronary sequelae from Kawasaki disease among young adults evaluated with angiography. Calcified coronary aneurysms on CT scans are less likely to regress.

Breastfeeding is associated with a reduced risk of Kawasaki disease but not with a reduced risk of coronary artery lesions or with improved resistance to IVIG therapy.

Prognosis

The reported recurrence rate is 3% in a Japanese study. The highest risk of recurrence occurs in the first 2 years after the first episode. The mortality peaks between 15 and 45 days after the onset of fever, at the time of coronary artery vasculitis, thrombocytosis, and a hypercoagulable state.

Over the long-term, the risk for clinical cardiac events in patients with no coronary artery abnormalities is similar to the general population. For patients in whom coronary artery abnormalities developed, the risk for cardiac complications, such as thrombosis, stenosis, MI, and death, ranges between 1% and 48%. Follow-up is especially needed among the subset of patients with neutropenia who have been treated with IVIG. The administration of IVIG is shown to improve LV function. The American Heart Association recommends risk stratification based on the assessment of coronary luminal dimensions by echocardiogram, under cardiologic supervision. The frequency of clinical follow-up, diagnostic testing, reproductive counseling, indications for medical therapy (β-blockers, statins), and thromboprophylaxis (aspirin and anticoagulation) depends on the individual's risk assessment.

When to Refer

All cases of Kawasaki disease merit referral to specialists.

Centers for Disease Control and Prevention (CDC). Multisystem inflammatory syndrome in children. https://www.cdc.gov/mis/

Kang C et al. Global incidence of Kawasaki disease: a systematic review. Cardiol Young. 2025;35:1028. [PMID: 40336299]

Lao F et al. Long-term cardiovascular outcomes and mortality following Kawasaki disease: a systematic review and meta-analysis. Paediatr Child Health. 2025;30:406. [PMID: 40917273]

Noval Rivas M et al. Kawasaki disease vasculitis: from diagnosis to new concepts in pathophysiology and therapeutic approaches. Annu Rev Med. 2026;77:87. [PMID: 41160750]

Safar FM et al. The effectiveness of no or low-dose versus high-dose aspirin in treating acute Kawasaki disease: a systematic review and meta-analysis. Clin Pract. 2024;14:1296. [PMID: 39051299]

Bacterial & Chlamydial Infections

37

Kelly A. Johnson, MD, MPH
Emma D. Bainbridge, MD, MPH

INFECTIONS CAUSED BY GRAM-POSITIVE BACTERIA

STREPTOCOCCAL INFECTIONS

Group A β-hemolytic streptococci (*Streptococcus pyogenes*) are the most common bacterial cause of pharyngitis, a topic that is covered along with tonsillitis in Chapter 8.

1. Pharyngitis & Tonsillitis (see Chapter 8)

2. Acute Rheumatic Fever & Scarlet Fever

General Considerations

Group A streptococci are gram-positive, β-hemolytic bacteria that can cause infections ranging from pharyngitis to skin infections to endocarditis and osteomyelitis. Streptococcal pyrogenic exotoxins, known as erythrogenic toxins, can cause scarlet fever in susceptible patients. Moreover, acute streptococcal infections, such as pharyngitis and skin infections, can be followed by nonsuppurative complications due to the production of autoantibodies. For instance, acute rheumatic fever may follow pharyngitis beginning 1–4 weeks after the onset of symptoms. Effectively controlling rheumatic fever depends on identifying and treating primary streptococcal infection and secondary prevention of recurrences. Glomerulonephritis is another rare nonsuppurative complication following acute streptococcal infection with a nephritogenic strain of *Streptococcus* group A (eg, types 4, 12, 2, 49, and 60), more commonly on the skin than in the throat, which can begin 1–3 weeks after the onset of the infection. Group A streptococcal infections must therefore be monitored closely for both acute and, rarely, postacute complications.

Clinical Findings

S pyogenes (group A *Streptococcus* [GAS]) pharyngitis is usually a self-limited condition, lasting 3–5 days. Please see Chapter 8 for a comprehensive discussion of pharyngitis and tonsillitis.

1. Scarlet fever—Scarlet fever may appear 1–2 days after the onset of GAS pharyngitis. The rash of scarlet fever (also called *scarlatina*) is diffusely erythematous and resembles a sunburn, with superimposed fine red papules giving the skin a sandpaper consistency; it can be most intense in the groin and axillary areas. The rash blanches on pressure, may become petechial, and fades in 2–5 days, leaving a fine desquamation. The face is flushed, with circumoral pallor, and the tongue is coated with enlarged red papillae (labeled strawberry tongue). The diagnosis is clinically made in the setting of streptococcal pharyngitis.

2. Rheumatic fever—The diagnosis of acute rheumatic fever relies on a constellation of signs, symptoms, and laboratory findings, known as the Jones criteria: major criteria include presence of pancarditis, polyarthritis, subcutaneous nodules, erythema marginatum, chorea, and minor criteria include presence of heart block, arthralgia, elevated ESR or CRP, fever, leukocytosis, or history of prior rheumatic fever. At least two major Jones criteria, or one major and two minor criteria, plus evidence of recent GAS infection by bacterial culture data, rapid strep testing, or elevated anti-strep antibody titers are required to establish a diagnosis. These complications are more common in children.

Treatment

Antimicrobial therapy of pharyngitis reduces the risk of complications (see Chapter 8). There is no additional treatment of scarlet fever or acute rheumatic fever beyond that of the underlying streptococcal pharyngitis. Group A streptococcal species are universally susceptible to penicillin.

Prevention of Recurrent Rheumatic Fever

Patients who have had rheumatic fever should be treated with continuous antimicrobial prophylaxis for at least 5 years. Effective oral regimens are penicillin V, 500 mg orally daily or erythromycin, 250 mg orally twice daily in patients allergic to penicillin. Intramuscular penicillin G benzathine given every 28 days may be used but should be avoided in patients with severe, symptomatic valvular disease, New York Heart Association class III or IV HF, or ventricular dysfunction.

Hirani K et al. Acute rheumatic fever. Lancet. 2025;405:2164. [PMID: 40484016]

Sanyahumbi A et al. Penicillin reactions in patients with severe rheumatic heart disease: a presidential advisory from the American Heart Association. J Am Heart Assoc. 2022;11:e024517. [PMID: 35049336]

3. Streptococcal Skin Infections

Group A β-hemolytic streptococci are not normal skin flora. Streptococcal skin infections result from colonization of normal skin by contact with other infected individuals or from a preceding streptococcal upper or lower respiratory tract infection.

Clinical Findings

A. Symptoms and Signs

Erysipelas is a painful superficial cellulitis that is well demarcated from the surrounding normal skin and frequently involves the face (Figure 37–1). This manifestation has a proclivity for skin with impaired lymphatic drainage, such as edematous lower extremities or wounds.

Impetigo is a focal, vesicular, pustular lesion with a thick, amber-colored crust with a "stuck-on" appearance (see Chapter 6).

B. Laboratory Findings

Cultures obtained from a wound or pustule will likely grow group A streptococci. Blood cultures are occasionally positive.

Treatment

Although penicillin is the treatment of choice for streptococcal infections, distinguishing staphylococcal from streptococcal infections can be difficult. In practice, initial therapy for patients with risk factors for *Staphylococcus aureus* (eg, injection drug use, diabetes mellitus, wound infection) should cover this organism and *Streptococcus pyogenes*. Parenteral therapy with either intravenous nafcillin or cefazolin (which can also be given intramuscularly) is a reasonable choice. In patients at risk for methicillin-resistant *S aureus* (MRSA) infection or with a serious and documented penicillin allergy (ie, anaphylaxis), intravenous vancomycin or daptomycin should be used (Table 37–1).

Patients who do not require parenteral therapy and in whom *S aureus* infection is less likely may be treated only with streptococcal coverage, with amoxicillin, 500 mg three times daily or 875 mg twice daily for 7–10 days. A first-generation oral cephalosporin, eg, cephalexin, or clindamycin is an alternative to amoxicillin (Table 37–1). If MRSA is diagnosed, antibiotics like doxycycline, linezolid, or trimethoprim-sulfamethoxazole often cover the infection. In patients with recurrent leg cellulitis, maintenance therapy (for at least 1 year) with penicillin V 250 mg orally twice daily may reduce relapses.

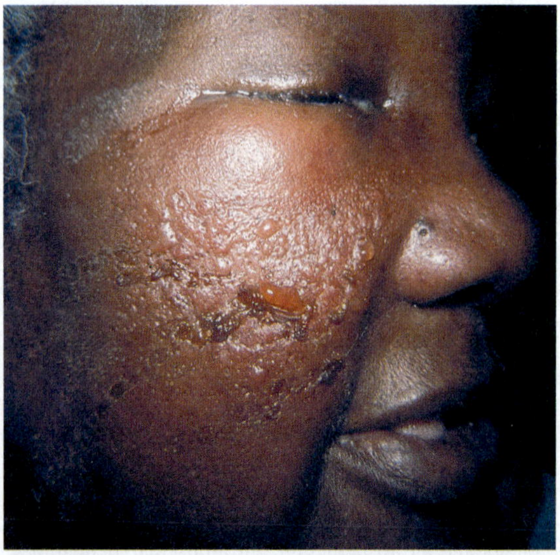

▲ **Figure 37–1.** Erysipelas of the face with edema, bright red erythema, and serosanguineous discharge from the severely swollen cheek. (Public Health Image Library, CDC.)

Bouza E et al. Current international and national guidelines for managing skin and soft tissue infections. Curr Opin Infect Dis. 2022;35:61. [PMID: 35067522]

4. Necrotizing Fasciitis

Necrotizing fasciitis is a rapidly spreading infection involving the fascia of deep muscle often located on an extremity, head and neck, perianal, or genital area (called "Fournier gangrene" in this region). Some patients have a preceding skin or blunt trauma injury. Immunosuppressed patients, have diabetes, are at extremes of age (older adults or neonates), or are affected by liver disease are generally more susceptible.

Necrotizing fasciitis is most often monomicrobial due to *S pyogenes* (group A β-hemolytic streptococci), but it can also be caused by other streptococcal species or *S aureus*. Infections can also be polymicrobial (mixed aerobic and anaerobic bacteria). A history of exposure to brackish water or marine life should raise suspicion for *Vibrio vulnificus, Erysipelothrix rhusiopathiae,* or *Aeromonas* species. Patients with burn injuries are susceptible to *Pseudomonas* species. Necrotizing myositis, which may present similarly and involves both fascia and skeletal muscle, is often caused by *Clostridia* species (clostridial myonecrosis or "gas gangrene"). See Clostridial Diseases, below.

Clinical Findings

A. Symptoms and Signs

The clinical findings at presentation may be those of severe cellulitis, but the presence of systemic toxicity and severe pain, which may be followed by anesthesia of the involved area due to destruction of nerves as infection advances through the fascial planes, is a clue to

Table 37–1. Treatment of common skin and soft tissue infections (SSTIs).

SSTI Type	Common Pathogens	Treatment
Purulent (abscess, furuncle, carbuncle, cellulitis with purulence)	*Staphylococcus aureus*	Incision and drainage is the primary treatment Consider the addition of antibiotics in select situations[1] **Oral antibiotic regimens**[2] Dicloxacillin, 500 mg four times daily, *or* cephalexin, 500 mg four times daily if low suspicion or low prevalence of MRSA Clindamycin, 300 four times daily or 450 mg three times daily *or* trimethoprim-sulfamethoxazole, one double-strength tablet twice daily, *or* doxycycline (or minocycline), 100 mg twice daily if moderate or high suspicion or prevalence of MRSA **Intravenous antibiotic regimens**[2] Nafcillin, 1–2 g four to six times daily, *or* cefazolin, 1 g three times daily for MSSA Vancomycin, 1 g twice daily, *or* daptomycin, 4 mg/kg once daily for MRSA
Nonpurulent (cellulitis, erysipelas)	β-Hemolytic streptococci (*S aureus* less likely)	**Oral antibiotic regimens**[2] Amoxicillin, 500 mg three times daily or 875 mg twice daily Cephalexin, 500 mg four times daily *or* clindamycin, 300 mg four times daily[2] **Intravenous antibiotic regimens**[2] Nafcillin, 1–2 g four to six times daily *or* cefazolin, 1 g three times daily Vancomycin, 1 g twice daily, *or* daptomycin, 4 mg/kg once daily

[1]Antibiotic therapy should be given in addition to incision and drainage for purulent SSTIs if the patient has any of the following: severe or extensive disease, symptoms and signs of systemic illness, purulent cellulitis/wound infection, comorbidities and extremes of age, abscess in area difficult to drain or on face/hand, associated septic phlebitis, or lack of response to incision and drainage alone. Antibiotic doses may vary based on weight and kidney function. Dosages listed assume normal renal and hepatic function, as well as average weight. Reevaluate dosing with renal/hepatic impairment.

[2]Other drugs that are FDA-approved for treating SSTIs include linezolid, 600 mg intravenously or orally twice daily for 10–14 days; daptomycin, 4 mg/kg intravenously once daily for 7–14 days; tedizolid, 200 mg orally once daily for 6 days; tigecycline, 100 mg intravenously once followed by 50 mg intravenously twice a day for 5–14 days; ceftaroline, 600 mg twice a day for 7–14 days; dalbavancin, 1500 mg as a single intravenous dose; oritavancin, 1200 mg as a single intravenous dose; telavancin, 10 mg/kg intravenously once daily for 7–14 days; and delafloxacin, 450 mg orally or 300 mg intravenously twice daily for 5–14 days.

the diagnosis. Pain is often severe. Infection can progress rapidly, debridement is almost always indicated, and multiorgan failure is common.

B. Laboratory Findings

Nonspecific serum markers include elevated WBC, ESR, and CRP. Elevated creatine kinase may indicate muscle involvement. The Laboratory Risk Indicator for Necrotizing Fasciitis (LRINEC) score is a diagnostic tool that uses WBC count, hemoglobin, sodium, glucose, creatinine, and C-reactive protein to predict the likelihood that a soft-tissue infection is due to necrotizing fasciitis. Because the sensitivity of the LRINEC score is poor, it should not be used to rule out necrotizing fasciitis, especially when clinical suspicion is high. Blood cultures and wound cultures should be obtained, as well as tissue cultures from surgical specimens during debridement. Histologic specimens may demonstrate extensive tissue destruction, thrombosis of blood vessels, and bacteria spreading along fascial planes.

C. Imaging

CT or MRI of the affected area may show gas in tissues or fascial plane infection. Imaging may also appear normal, so rely on clinical suspicion and surgical evaluation.

Treatment

Timely surgical exploration is mandatory when the diagnosis is suspected. Early, extensive, and often repeated debridement is essential for survival. **Surgical evaluation should not be delayed while awaiting imaging or other diagnostic tests, especially in the setting of rapid progression of clinical manifestations.**

Broad-spectrum antibiotic therapy should be initiated whenever the diagnosis is suspected and should cover aerobic and anaerobic organisms. Initial therapy for patients with normal kidney function typically consists of intravenous therapy with a carbapenem (meropenem, 2 g every 8 hours or imipenem, 1 g every 6 hours) or piperacillin-tazobactam, 3.375 g every 6 hours (unless *Pseudomonas* is suspected, in which case the dose should be increased to 4.5 g every 6 hours), plus an agent with activity against methicillin-resistant *S aureus* (vancomycin, linezolid, or daptomycin), plus clindamycin for its antitoxin effects against toxin-producing strains of streptococci and staphylococci. Clindamycin should be used at high doses, 600–900 mg every 8 hours, for presumptive toxin-mediated illness. Patients with exposure histories suggesting less common etiologies should also receive therapy targeted to those organisms. Antibiotic therapy should then be tailored to culture results and continued until all infected tissue has been removed and the patient has stabilized; the final duration depends on individual patient factors.

In addition to surgical and antibiotic therapy, the use of intravenous immunoglobulin for streptococcal necrotizing soft tissue infections has been shown to reduce mortality. The dose is 1 g/kg on day 1, followed by 0.5 g/kg on days 2 and 3.

Hua C et al. Necrotising soft-tissue infections. Lancet Infect Dis. 2023;23:e81. [PMID: 36252579]

5. Other Group A Streptococcal Infections

Septic arthritis, pneumonia, empyema, endocarditis, and toxic shock–like syndrome are relatively uncommon infections that may be caused by group A streptococci.

Septic arthritis generally occurs in association with cellulitis. In addition to therapy with penicillin G, 3 million units intravenously every 4 hours (or cefazolin or vancomycin if there is a penicillin allergy or less frequent dosing is required), the infected joint effusions should be drained by percutaneous needle aspiration or open surgical drainage. Treatment duration is not well studied but is generally 2–4 weeks, with final duration dependent upon clinical improvement and normalization of inflammatory markers (ESR, CRP).

Pneumonia and **empyema** often are characterized by extensive tissue destruction and an aggressive, rapidly progressive clinical course associated with significant morbidity and mortality. High-dose penicillin G, 4 million units intravenously every 4 hours and chest tube drainage are indicated for treatment of group A streptococcal empyema. Vancomycin is an acceptable substitute in penicillin-allergic patients. Duration of therapy is guided by clinical improvement, with a minimum of 5 days for pneumonia. Adequate drainage is key for managing empyema, and serial imaging is usually necessary to assess for resolution.

Group A streptococci can cause **endocarditis** in rare instances. Endocarditis should be treated with 24 million units of penicillin G intravenously either continuously or in four to six divided doses for 4–6 weeks. Ceftriaxone 2 g daily is an appropriate alternate regimen. Vancomycin, starting at 1 g intravenously every 12 hours but titrated to keep a trough level of 15–20 mcg/mL, is recommended for patients allergic to penicillin. Daptomycin 6 mg/kg/day is an acceptable alternative for treating endocarditis caused by most gram-positive organisms.

Any streptococcal infection—and necrotizing fasciitis in particular—can be associated with **streptococcal toxic shock syndrome**, typified by invasion of skin or soft tissues, acute respiratory distress syndrome, and kidney failure. Young persons, older adults, and those with underlying medical conditions are at high risk for invasive disease. Accompanying bacteremia occurs in most cases. Skin rash and desquamation may not be present. Mortality rates can be up to 80%. A β-lactam, such as penicillin G, 4 million units intravenously every 4 hours, remains the drug of choice for treatment of serious streptococcal infections, but clindamycin should also be administered at a dose of 900 mg every 8 hours intravenously for invasive disease, especially in the presence of shock. Intravenous immune globulin can be considered for streptococcal toxic shock syndrome for possible therapeutic benefit from specific antibodies to streptococcal exotoxins in immune globulin preparations. Many dosing regimens have been used, including 1 g/kg on day 1, followed by 0.5 g/kg on days 2 and 3.

6. Non–Group A Streptococcal Infections

Non–group A β-hemolytic streptococci (eg, groups B, C, and G) produce a spectrum of disease like group A streptococci. The treatment of infections caused by these strains is generally similar to treatment regimens for group A streptococci. However, some isolates of groups C and G streptococci can exhibit tolerance to penicillin, so antibiotic susceptibility profiles should be assayed for these species.

Group B streptococci are an important cause of sepsis, bacteremia, and meningitis in neonates. Antepartum screening to identify carriers and peripartum antimicrobial prophylaxis are recommended in pregnancy. This organism, part of the normal vaginal flora, may cause septic abortion, endometritis, or peripartum infections and, less commonly, cellulitis, bacteremia, and endocarditis in adults. Treatment of infections caused by group B streptococci is with either penicillin or vancomycin in doses recommended for treatment of group A streptococci skin and soft tissue infections (Table 37–1).

Group D streptococci include *Streptococcus gallolyticus* (formerly known as *S bovis*) and bacteria now classified as enterococci. *S gallolyticus* is a cause of endocarditis in association with bowel neoplasia or cirrhosis and is usually treated with β-lactam antibiotics, although susceptibility to penicillin must first be determined. The species described above are generally β-hemolytic, with a clear zone of hemolysis around the bacterial colonies on a blood agar plate.

Viridans streptococci, which are nonhemolytic or α-hemolytic (ie, producing an incomplete or green zone of hemolysis on blood agar), are part of the normal oral and gut flora. Although these strains may cause focal pyogenic infections, they are most known as the leading cause of native valve endocarditis. Viridans streptococcal species can also be part of mixed bacterial infections at multiple sites or agents of bacteremia with serious GI or genitourinary infections.

PNEUMOCOCCAL (*Streptococcus pneumoniae*) INFECTIONS

1. Pneumococcal Pneumonia

ESSENTIALS OF DIAGNOSIS

- Productive cough, fever, rigors, dyspnea, early pleuritic chest pain.
- Consolidating lobar pneumonia on CXR.
- Gram-positive diplococci on Gram stain of sputum.

General Considerations

Pneumococcus is the most common cause of community-acquired pyogenic bacterial pneumonia. Alcohol use disorder, asthma, HIV infection, sickle cell disease, splenectomy, and hematologic disorders are predisposing factors. Mortality rates remain high in cases of advanced age, multilobar disease, hypoxemia, extrapulmonary complications, and bacteremia.

Clinical Findings

A. Symptoms and Signs

Presenting symptoms and signs include high fever, productive cough, occasional hemoptysis, and pleuritic chest pain. Rigors may occur initially but are uncommon later in the course. Bronchial breath sounds are an early sign.

B. Laboratory Findings

There is often leukocytosis, or occasionally leukopenia, but neither finding should be used to decide whether to admit (see When to Admit, below).

Diagnosis requires isolation of the organism in culture, although the Gram stain of sputum can be suggestive. Sputum and blood cultures, positive in 60% and 25% of cases of pneumococcal pneumonia, respectively, should be obtained before initiating antimicrobial therapy when feasible in patients admitted to the hospital. A good-quality sputum sample (<10 epithelial cells and > 25 polymorphonuclear leukocytes per high-power field) typically shows gram-positive diplococci. A rapid urinary antigen test for *Streptococcus pneumoniae*, with sensitivity of 70–80% and specificity > 95%, can assist with early diagnosis.

C. Imaging

Pneumococcal pneumonia is classically a lobar pneumonia with radiographic findings of consolidation and, occasionally, an effusion. Differentiating it from other pneumonias is not possible radiographically or clinically because of significant overlap in presentations.

Treatment

A. Specific Measures

Initial antimicrobial therapy for pneumonia is empiric (see Table 9–10) pending isolation and identification of the causative agent. Once *S pneumoniae* is identified as the infecting pathogen, any of several antimicrobial agents may be used depending on the clinical setting, community patterns of penicillin resistance, and susceptibility of the particular isolate.

1. Outpatient therapy—Uncomplicated pneumococcal pneumonia (ie, arterial PO_2 > 60 mm Hg, no coexisting medical problems, and single-lobe disease without signs of extrapulmonary infection) caused by penicillin-susceptible strains of pneumococcus may be treated on an outpatient basis with amoxicillin, 1 g orally three times daily until patient is afebrile and for a minimum of 5 days. Cephalosporins including cefpodoxime, 200 mg orally twice daily, also may be used. For penicillin-allergic patients, alternatives include azithromycin, one 500-mg dose orally on the first day and 250 mg for the next 4 days; doxycycline, 100 mg orally twice daily or levofloxacin, 750 mg orally for 5–7 days. Because pneumococcal species have increasing resistance to penicillin, antimicrobial susceptibilities should be examined. Patients should be monitored for clinical response (eg, less cough, defervescence within 2–3 days) on their antibiotic regimen.

Outpatients with high-risk comorbid conditions (such as pulmonary disease, diabetes, cardiac disease, or alcohol use disorder) may benefit from broader combination therapy (eg, amoxicillin/clavulanate or cephalosporin *plus* doxycycline or a macrolide) if anaerobic or other mixed bacteria are suspected in combination with the pneumococcus, unless a fluoroquinolone (eg, levofloxacin or moxifloxacin) is chosen for monotherapy. Fluoroquinolones also cover gram-positive anaerobes and some gram-negative bacteria.

2. Inpatient therapy—Parenteral therapy is generally recommended for the hospitalized patient at least until there has been clinical improvement. Ceftriaxone, 1 g intravenously every 24 hours, is effective for strains that are penicillin-susceptible (ie, strains for which the minimum inhibitory concentration [MIC] of penicillin is 2 mcg/mL or less for non-CNS specimens). For serious penicillin allergy or infection caused by a highly penicillin-resistant strain, vancomycin, 1 g intravenously every 12 hours or a dose to reach a trough level of 15–20 mcg/mL, is effective. Additionally, azithromycin (500 mg orally on the first day and 250 mg for the next 4 days) or doxycycline (100 mg orally twice daily) is typically added to cover atypical organisms (eg, *Mycoplasma pneumoniae*, *Chlamydia pneumoniae*). Alternatively, a respiratory fluoroquinolone (eg, levofloxacin, 750 mg once daily) can be used. The total duration of therapy is not well defined, but 5–7 days is appropriate for patients who have an uncomplicated infection and demonstrate a good clinical response. Corticosteroid use remains controversial in community-acquired bacterial pneumonia and should not be administered routinely.

B. Penicillin-Resistant Pneumococci

In cases of pneumococcal pneumonia where the isolate is not susceptible to penicillin, cephalosporin cross-resistance is common, and a non–β-lactam antimicrobial, such as vancomycin, 1 g intravenously every 12 hours, or a fluoroquinolone with enhanced gram-positive activity (eg, levofloxacin, 750 mg intravenously or orally once daily, or moxifloxacin, 400 mg intravenously or orally once daily), is recommended. Penicillin-resistant strains of pneumococci may be resistant to macrolides and trimethoprim-sulfamethoxazole, and susceptibility testing must be documented prior to their use. All blood and CSF isolates should be tested for penicillin resistance.

Complications

Pleural effusions developing after initiation of antimicrobial therapy usually are sterile, and thoracentesis need not be performed if the patient is otherwise improving. Thoracentesis is indicated for an effusion present before initiation of therapy and in the patient who has not responded to antibiotics after 3–4 days. Empyema occurs in 5% or less of cases and is differentiated from sympathetic effusion clinically and by the presence of organisms on Gram-stained fluid or positive pleural fluid cultures. Empyema most often requires chest tube drainage for resolution. Echocardiography should be done if pericardial effusion is suspected. Patients with pericardial effusion who are responding to antibiotic therapy and have no signs of tamponade may be monitored and treated with indomethacin, 50 mg orally three times daily, for pain. In patients with increasing effusion, unsatisfactory clinical response, or evidence of tamponade, pericardiocentesis will determine whether the pericardial space is infected. Infected fluid must be drained either percutaneously (by tube placement or needle aspiration), by placement of a pericardial window, or by pericardiectomy. Pericardiectomy eventually may be required to prevent or treat constrictive pericarditis.

Pneumococcal endocarditis usually involves the aortic valve and often occurs in association with meningitis and pneumonia (with the three manifestations sometimes referred to as Austrian or Osler triad). Refer to the Infective Endocarditis section of this chapter for appropriate treatment regimens of pneumococcal endocarditis.

Prevention

See Chapter 35 for discussion of pneumococcal vaccines. As of 2025, the CDC recommends pneumococcal conjugate vaccination for all adults aged 50 years or older, and for adults aged 19–50 years with certain underlying medical conditions (including HIV) who have not previously received a pneumococcal conjugate vaccine or whose previous vaccination hist ory is unknown. The 20-valent or 21-valent pneumococcal conjugate vaccines (PCV20 or PCV21, respectively) each represents a complete vaccination course; if the 15-valent vaccine (PCV15) is used, then pneumococcal polysaccharide vaccine (PPSV23) must also be administered 1 year later to complete the vaccination course. All patients should be screened for smoking cessation.

When to Refer

- Seriously ill patient with pneumonia, particularly in the setting of comorbid conditions (eg, liver disease).
- Progression of pneumonia or failure to improve on antibiotics.

When to Admit

- Failure of outpatient pneumonia therapy, including inability to maintain oral intake and medications.
- All patients with pneumococcal pneumonia that is multilobar or is associated with significant hypoxemia.
- Exacerbations of underlying disease (eg, HF) by pneumonia that would benefit from hospitalization.
- Risk scores for illness severity using PSI (Pneumonia Severity Index) and CURB-65 (Confusion, Urea, Respiratory rate, Blood pressure, Age ≥ 65 years) can aid in the decision about whether to admit a patient.
- All patients in whom pneumococcal endocarditis or meningitis is suspected or documented should be admitted for observation, infectious disease specialist consultation, and empiric therapy.

Kobayashi M et al. Use of 21-valent pneumococcal conjugate vaccine among U.S. adults: Recommendations of the Advisory Committee on Immunization Practices — United States, 2024. MMWR Morb Mortal Wkly Rep 2024;73:793. [PMID: 39264843]

Metlay JP et al. Diagnosis and treatment of adults with community-acquired pneumonia. An official clinical practice guideline of the American Thoracic Society and Infectious Diseases Society of America. Am J Respir Crit Care Med. 2019;200:e45. [PMID: 31573350]

Vaughn VM et al. Community-acquired pneumonia: a review. JAMA. 2024;332:1282. [PMID: 39283629]

2. Pneumococcal Meningitis

ESSENTIALS OF DIAGNOSIS

- Fever, headache, altered mental status.
- Meningismus.
- Gram-positive diplococci on Gram stain of CSF.

General Considerations

S pneumoniae is the most common cause of bacterial meningitis in adults. Head trauma with CSF leaks, sinusitis, and pneumonia may precede it.

Clinical Findings

A. Symptoms and Signs

The onset is rapid, with fever, headache, meningismus, and altered mentation. Pneumonia may be present. Compared with meningitis caused by the meningococcus, pneumococcal meningitis lacks a rash. Obtundation, focal neurologic deficits, and cranial nerve palsies are more prominent features and may lead to long-term sequelae.

B. Laboratory Findings

The CSF has a WBC count typically > 1000/mcL (1.0×10^9/L), more than 60% of which are polymorphonuclear leukocytes; the glucose concentration is < 40 mg/dL (2.22 mmol/L), or < 50% of the simultaneous serum concentration; and the protein usually exceeds 150 mg/dL (1500 mg/L). Not all cases of meningitis will have these typical findings, and alterations in CSF analysis may be surprisingly minimal, overlapping with those of aseptic meningitis.

Gram stain of CSF shows gram-positive cocci in 80–90% of cases, and in untreated cases, blood or CSF cultures are almost always positive. Urine antigen tests may be positive but are not sufficiently sensitive to exclude the diagnosis.

Treatment

Antibiotics should be given as soon as the diagnosis is suspected. If lumbar puncture must be delayed (eg, while awaiting results of an imaging study to exclude a mass lesion), the patient should be treated empirically with ceftriaxone, 2 g intravenously every 12 hours, plus vancomycin, 15 mg/kg every 12 hours to maintain trough levels in the 15–20 mcg/mL range, plus dexamethasone, 0.15 mg/kg every 6 hours administered concomitantly after blood cultures (positive in 50% of cases) have been obtained. Once susceptibility to penicillin has been confirmed, vancomycin may be discontinued and penicillin, 24 million units intravenously daily in six divided doses, or ceftriaxone, 2 g every 12 hours intravenously, is continued for 10–14 days in documented cases.

Susceptibility testing is essential for proper management. Penicillin-resistant strains (MIC > 0.06 mcg/mL) are often cross-resistant to the third-generation cephalosporins as well as other antibiotics. If the MIC of ceftriaxone or cefotaxime is 0.5 mcg/mL or less, single-drug therapy with either of these cephalosporins is likely to be effective; when the MIC is 1 mcg/mL or more, treatment with a combination of ceftriaxone, 2 g intravenously every 12 hours, plus vancomycin, 30 mg/kg/day intravenously in two or three divided doses, is recommended. If a patient with a penicillin-resistant organism is slow to respond clinically, repeat lumbar puncture may be indicated to assess bacteriologic response.

Adjunctive dexamethasone given with antibiotics has been associated with a reduction in mortality and neurologic complications such as hearing loss. It is recommended that dexamethasone be given immediately prior to or concomitantly with the first dose of appropriate antibiotic and continued every 6 hours thereafter for a total of 4 days. The effect of dexamethasone on the outcome of meningitis caused by penicillin-resistant organisms is not known.

Hasbun R. Progress and challenges in bacterial meningitis: a review. JAMA. 2022;328:2147. [PMID: 36472590]

ENTEROCOCCAL INFECTIONS

Two species, *Enterococcus faecalis* and *Enterococcus faecium*, are responsible for most human enterococcal infections. Enterococci cause wound infections, UTIs, bacteremia, and endocarditis. Infections caused by penicillin-susceptible strains should be treated with ampicillin, 2 g every 4 hours, or penicillin, 3–4 million units every 4 hours; if the patient is penicillin-allergic, vancomycin, 15–20 mg/kg every 12 hours intravenously, can be given to achieve a trough level of 15–20 mcg/mL. Refer to the Infective Endocarditis section of this chapter for appropriate treatment regimens of enterococcal endocarditis.

Resistance to vancomycin, penicillin, and gentamicin is common among enterococcal isolates, especially *E faecium;* it is essential to determine antimicrobial susceptibility patterns of isolates. Consultation with an infectious disease specialist is strongly advised when treating infections caused by resistant strains of enterococci. Linezolid is active against both *E faecalis* and *E faecium* and approved by the FDA for treatment of infections caused by vancomycin-resistant strains of enterococci. The dose is 600 mg twice daily intravenously or orally. Daptomycin, tigecycline, tedizolid, and oritavancin are not specifically approved for the treatment of vancomycin-resistant strains of enterococci, although they are frequently active in vitro.

Cairns KA et al. Therapeutics for vancomycin-resistant enterococcal bloodstream infections. Clin Microbiol Rev. 2023;36:e0005922. [PMID: 37067406]
Rosselli Del Turco E et al. How do I manage a patient with enterococcal bacteraemia? Clin Microbiol Infect. 2021;27:364. [PMID: 33152537]

STAPHYLOCOCCUS AUREUS INFECTIONS

1. Skin & Soft Tissue Infections

ESSENTIALS OF DIAGNOSIS

- Localized erythema with induration and purulent drainage.
- Abscess formation.
- Gram stain of pus shows gram-positive cocci in clusters; cultures usually positive.

General Considerations

About one-quarter of individuals are asymptomatic nasal carriers of *S aureus*, which is spread by direct contact. Carriage often precedes infection, which occurs as a consequence of disruption of the cutaneous barrier or impairment of host defenses. *S aureus* tends to cause more purulent skin infections than streptococci; abscess formation is common. The prevalence of methicillin-resistant strains in many communities is high and should influence antibiotic choices when antimicrobial therapy is needed.

Clinical Findings

A. Symptoms and Signs

S aureus skin infections may begin around one or more hair follicles, causing folliculitis; may become localized to form boils (or furuncles); or may spread to adjacent skin and deeper subcutaneous tissue (ie, a carbuncle). Deep abscesses involving muscle or fascia may occur, often in association with a deep wound or other inoculation or injection (Figure 37–2). Necrotizing fasciitis (discussed above) has been reported with community strains of methicillin-resistant *S aureus*.

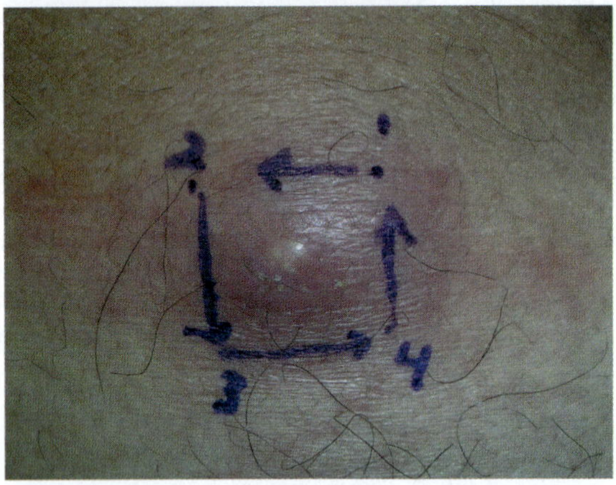

▲ **Figure 37–2.** Methicillin-resistant *Staphylococcus aureus* (MRSA) abscess on the back of the neck. (Reproduced with permission from Richard P. Usatine, MD, in Usatine RP, Smith MA, Mayeaux EJ Jr, Chumley HS. *The Color Atlas and Synopsis of Family Medicine*, 3rd ed. McGraw-Hill, 2019.)

B. Laboratory Findings

Cultures of the wound or abscess material will almost always yield the organism. In patients with systemic signs of infection, blood cultures should be obtained to evaluate for bacteremia, endocarditis, osteomyelitis, or metastatic seeding of other sites. Bacteremic patients should have blood cultures repeated every 24–28 hours during therapy to exclude persistent bacteremia, an indicator of severe or complicated infection.

Treatment

Proper drainage of abscess fluid or other focal infections is the mainstay of therapy. Incision and drainage alone is highly effective for treating most uncomplicated, small cutaneous abscesses. A small benefit can be obtained from adding antimicrobials following incision and drainage (Table 37–1). In areas where methicillin resistance among community *S aureus* isolates is high, recommended oral antimicrobial agents include clindamycin, trimethoprim-sulfamethoxazole, or doxycycline. When the risk of methicillin resistance is low or methicillin susceptibility has been confirmed by testing of the isolate, consider dicloxacillin or cephalexin. Amoxicillin may be used when strains are both methicillin- and penicillin-sensitive. Treatment for 5–7 days is sufficient in most cases.

For complicated infections with extensive cutaneous or deep tissue involvement or systemic symptoms such as fever, initial parenteral therapy is often indicated. When methicillin resistance rates are > 10% in the community, empiric vancomycin is the drug of choice. For infections caused by methicillin-susceptible isolates, cefazolin or a penicillinase-resistant penicillin such as nafcillin or oxacillin administered intravenously is preferred. Total duration of therapy for soft tissue infections depends on clinical response and effectiveness of drainage/debridement. Courses of 7 days with early transition to oral therapy are effective in many cases.

Linezolid is FDA-approved for treating skin and skin-structure infections and hospital-acquired pneumonia caused by methicillin-resistant strains of *S aureus*; it is clinically as effective as vancomycin for these indications. Intravenous daptomycin is increasingly becoming the drug of choice to treat skin and soft tissue infections with methicillin-resistant *S aureus*. Routine creatinine phosphokinase and CBC monitoring should be done in patients taking daptomycin. Other FDA-approved drugs for treating skin and soft tissue infections are listed in Table 37–1.

Tiseo G et al. The future approach for the management of acute bacterial skin and skin structure infections. Curr Opin Infect Dis. 2025;38:128. [PMID: 39831591]

2. Osteomyelitis

ESSENTIALS OF DIAGNOSIS

- Fever associated with pain and tenderness of involved bone.
- Microbiologic diagnosis often made from blood cultures.
- Elevated ESR and CRP.
- Radiographs early in the course are typically negative.

General Considerations

S aureus causes approximately 60% of all cases of osteomyelitis. Osteomyelitis may be caused by (1) hematogenous spread, (2) extension from a contiguous focus of infection or open wound (eg, open fracture or as a result of surgery), and (3) skin breakdown in the setting of vascular insufficiency. Long bones and vertebrae are the usual sites. Epidural abscess is a common complication of vertebral osteomyelitis and should be suspected if fever and severe back or neck pain are accompanied by radicular pain or evidence of spinal cord compression (eg, incontinence, extremity weakness, pathologic extremity reflexes).

Clinical Findings

A. Symptoms and Signs

1. Hematogenous osteomyelitis—Osteomyelitis resulting from bacteremia is a disease associated with sickle cell disease, injection drug use, diabetes mellitus, or older age. Patients with this form of osteomyelitis often present with sudden-onset high fever, chills, and pain and tenderness of the involved bone. The site of osteomyelitis and the causative organism depend on the host. Osteomyelitis in injection drug users develops most commonly in the spine. Although in this setting *S aureus* is most common, gram-negative infections, especially *P aeruginosa* and *Serratia* species, are also frequent pathogens. Among patients with hemoglobinopathies such as sickle cell anemia, osteomyelitis is caused most often by salmonellae; *S aureus* is the second most common cause. Rapid progression to epidural abscess causing fever, pain, and sensory and motor loss is not uncommon. In older patients with hematogenous osteomyelitis, the most common sites are the thoracic and lumbar vertebral bodies. Risk factors for these patients include diabetes, intravenous catheters, and indwelling urinary catheters. These patients often have more subtle presentations, with low-grade fever and gradually increasing bone pain, with neurologic abnormalities a late finding.

2. Osteomyelitis from a contiguous focus of infection— Prosthetic joint replacement or other orthopedic surgery, neurosurgery, and trauma most frequently cause soft tissue infections that can spread to bone. *S aureus* and *Staphylococcus epidermidis* are the most common organisms. Polymicrobial infections, rare in hematogenously spread osteomyelitis, are more common in osteomyelitis due to contiguous spread. Localized signs of inflammation are usually evident, but high fever and other signs of toxicity are usually absent. Septic arthritis and cellulitis can also spread to contiguous bone.

3. Osteomyelitis associated with vascular insufficiency— Patients with diabetes mellitus and vascular insufficiency are susceptible to developing a very challenging form of osteomyelitis. The foot and ankle are commonly affected sites, and the hip and sacrum are also affected due to pressure injury (formerly called pressure ulcer). Infection originates from an ulcer or other break in the skin that is usually still present but may appear disarmingly unimpressive. Polymicrobial infections are common due to contiguous spread, often involving aerobic gram-negative bacilli and anaerobes. Occasionally, *S aureus* may be found as a single pathogen. Bone pain is often absent or muted by the associated neuropathy. Fever is also commonly absent. Two of the best bedside clues to the presence of osteomyelitis are the ability to easily advance a sterile probe to bone through a skin ulcer and an ulcer area > 2 cm × 2 cm.

B. Laboratory Findings

The diagnosis is made by isolating *S aureus* (or another organism) from the blood, bone, or a contiguous focus in a patient with symptoms and signs of focal bone infection. Blood culture will be positive in approximately 60% of untreated cases. The ESR and serum CRP are almost always elevated and can be useful parameters to follow during therapy. Bone biopsy and culture are valuable to guide targeted therapy. Cultures from overlying ulcers, wounds, or fistulas are often contaminated with skin flora and do not correlate with deep tissue or bone culture.

C. Imaging

Plain bone films early in the course of infection are often normal but will become abnormal in most cases even with effective therapy. Spinal infection (unlike malignancy) traverses the disk space to involve the contiguous vertebral body. CT is more sensitive than plain bone radiographs and helps localize associated abscesses. MRI is slightly less sensitive than bone scan but has a specificity of 90%. It is indicated when epidural abscess is suspected in association with vertebral osteomyelitis.

Treatment

Identification of the causative organism and determination of antibiotic susceptibility dictate therapy; consultation with an infectious disease specialist is recommended.

Prolonged therapy (4–6 weeks or longer) is recommended for staphylococcal osteomyelitis. Traditionally, intravenous therapy has been preferred, particularly during the acute phase of the infection for patients with systemic toxicity. Intravenous therapy with cefazolin, 2 g every 8 hours, or alternatively, nafcillin or oxacillin, 9–12 g/day in six divided doses, are the drugs of choice for infection with methicillin-sensitive isolates. Patients with infections due to methicillin-resistant strains of *S aureus* or who have severe penicillin allergies should be treated with vancomycin, 30 mg/kg/day intravenously divided in two or three doses. Doses should be adjusted to achieve a vancomycin trough level of 15–20 mcg/mL. Daptomycin is an alternative agent and should be given in doses of 6–8 mg/kg/dose intravenously every 24 hours.

In terms of shortening the course of intravenous therapy, studies have also demonstrated noninferiority of oral regimens following 2 weeks of intravenous therapy. In patients with *S aureus* isolates susceptible to oral agents, combination oral therapy has been shown to be effective if given for 4–6 weeks following 2 weeks of induction therapy with an intravenous agent as above. Levofloxacin, 750 mg orally daily, or ciprofloxacin, 750 mg orally twice daily, in combination with rifampin, 300 mg twice daily, is an oral regimen with the most data supporting efficacy. Trimethoprim-sulfamethoxazole, doxycycline, or clindamycin may be options for oral therapy depending on the antimicrobial susceptibilities of the organism.

Surgical treatment is often indicated under the following circumstances: (1) staphylococcal osteomyelitis with associated epidural abscess and spinal cord compression (urgent neurosurgical decompression may be required), (2) other abscesses (psoas, paraspinal), (3) extensive disease, or (4) recurrent or persistent infection despite standard medical therapy. Follow-up imaging may not be needed in patients who demonstrate symptom improvement and normalization of inflammatory markers.

Haddad N et al. A review of the clinical utilization of oral antibacterial therapy in the treatment of bone infections in adults. Antibiotics (Basel). 2023;13:4. [PMID: 38275315]

Masters EA et al. Skeletal infections: microbial pathogenesis, immunity and clinical management. Nat Rev Microbiol. 2022;20:385. [PMID: 35169289]

Senneville É et al. IWGDF/IDSA guidelines on the diagnosis and treatment of diabetes-related foot infections (IWGDF/IDSA 2023). Diabetes Metab Res Rev. 2024;40:e3687. [PMID: 37779323]

3. Staphylococcal Bacteremia

S aureus readily invades the bloodstream and infects sites distant from the primary site of infection. Whenever *S aureus* is recovered from blood cultures, the possibility of endocarditis, osteomyelitis, or other metastatic deep infection must be considered. Bacteremia that persists for > 48–96 hours after initiation of therapy is strongly predictive of worse outcome and complicated infection. Given the relatively high risk of infective endocarditis in patients with *S aureus* bacteremia, transesophageal echocardiography is recommended for most patients as a sensitive and cost-effective method for excluding underlying endocarditis. However, transthoracic echocardiography may be sufficient in select patients considered to be at low risk for endocarditis, namely those who meet all the following criteria: (1) no permanent intracardiac device, (2) sterile follow-up blood cultures within 4 days after the initial set, (3) no hemodialysis dependence, (4) nosocomial acquisition of *S aureus* bacteremia, and (5) no clinical signs of infective endocarditis or secondary foci of infection. If these conditions are not met, transesophageal echocardiography is more sensitive to exclude endocarditis, especially left-sided valvular endocarditis.

Empiric therapy of staphylococcal bacteremia should be with vancomycin, 15–20 mg/kg/dose intravenously every 8–12 hours (titrated to achieve a trough level of 15–20 mcg/mL), or daptomycin, 6 mg/kg/day intravenously, until results of susceptibility tests are known. If the *S aureus* isolate is methicillin-susceptible, treatment should be narrowed to cefazolin, 2 g every 8 hours, or nafcillin or oxacillin, 2 g intravenously every 4 hours. Cefazolin is as effective as nafcillin or oxacillin and has been associated with fewer adverse events during treatment. In patients with methicillin-resistant *S aureus*, treatment should be with vancomycin, 15–20 mg/kg/dose intravenously every 8–12 hours; a trough level of 15–20 mcg/mL is recommended. Daptomycin 6–10 mg/kg/day is also an FDA-approved option as long as the patient does not require treatment for concomitant *S aureus* pneumonia, as pulmonary surfactant inactivates daptomycin in the lungs. Adding rifamycins to standard antimicrobial therapy is not beneficial in the absence of indwelling prosthetic material and is associated with more adverse events. Duration of antibiotic therapy for *S aureus* bacteremia is 4–6 weeks, but patients with uncomplicated infection may complete treatment within 14 days. A patient with uncomplicated bacteremia must meet all the following criteria: (1) infective endocarditis has been excluded, (2) no implanted prostheses are present, (3) follow-up blood cultures drawn 2–4 days after the initial set are sterile, (4) the patient defervesces within 72 hours of initiation of effective antibiotic therapy, and (5) no evidence of metastatic infection is present on examination. When present at the time of diagnosis, central venous catheters should be removed. Vancomycin treatment failures are relatively common, particularly for complicated bacteremia and among infections involving foreign bodies. Improved outcomes have been demonstrated when consultation with an infectious disease specialist is obtained and is recommended in all cases of *S aureus* bacteremia.

Minter DJ et al. Contemporary management of *Staphylococcus aureus* bacteremia—controversies in clinical practice. Clin Infect Dis. 2023;77(11):e57. [PMID: 37950887]
Tong SYC et al. Management of *Staphylococcus aureus* bacteremia: a review. JAMA. 2025;334:798. [PMID: 40193249]

4. Toxic Shock Syndrome

S aureus produces toxins that cause three important entities: "scalded skin syndrome" in children, toxic shock syndrome in adults, and enterotoxin food poisoning. Toxic shock syndrome is characterized by abrupt onset of high fever, vomiting, and watery diarrhea. Sore throat, myalgias, and headache are common. Hypotension with kidney injury and HF is associated with a poor outcome. A diffuse macular erythematous rash and nonpurulent conjunctivitis are common, and desquamation, especially of palms and soles, is typical during recovery (Figure 37–3). Fatality rates may be as high as 15%. Although originally associated with tampon use, any focus (eg, nasopharynx, bone, vagina, rectum, abscess, wound) harboring a toxin-producing *S aureus* strain can cause toxic shock syndrome. Classically, blood cultures are negative because symptoms are due to the effects of the toxin and not systemic infection. Other entities associated with toxic shock include invasive group A streptococcal infection and certain *Clostridium* species.

Important aspects of treatment include rapid rehydration, targeted antimicrobials (antistaphylococcal therapy when *S aureus* is implicated) (Table 37–1), management of multiorgan failure, and addressing sources of toxin, eg, removal of tampon or drainage of abscess. Clindamycin, 900 mg every 8 hours intravenously, is often added to inhibit toxin production. Intravenous immune globulin may be considered, although there are limited data compared with *Streptococcus* toxic shock syndrome (see above).

5. Infections Caused by Coagulase-Negative Staphylococci

Coagulase-negative staphylococci are an important cause of infections of intravascular and prosthetic devices and of wound infection following cardiothoracic surgery. These organisms infrequently cause infections such as osteomyelitis

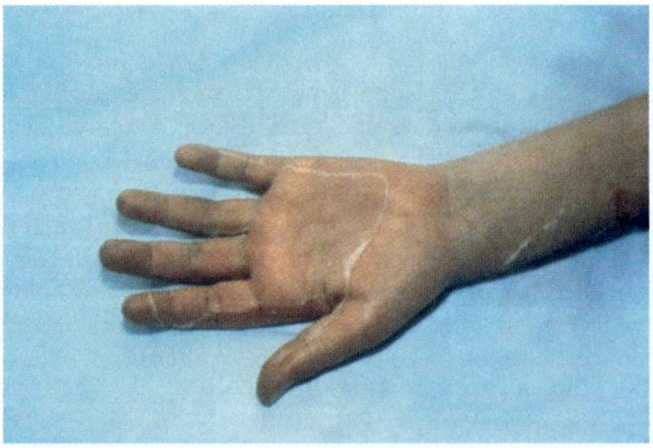

▲ **Figure 37–3.** Marked desquamation due to toxic shock syndrome, which develops late in the disease. (Public Health Image Library, CDC.)

and endocarditis in the absence of a prosthesis. Most human infections are caused by *Staphylococcus epidermidis*, *S haemolyticus*, *S hominis*, *S saprophyticus*, and *S lugdunensis*. With the exception of *S lugdunensis*, these common pathogens are less virulent than *S aureus*, and the infections they cause tend to be more indolent. *S lugdunensis* may cause severe endocarditis with bulky vegetations similar to *S aureus*; this diagnosis is often missed when the coagulase-negative staphylococcal species is dismissed as a contaminant.

Because coagulase-negative staphylococci are normal inhabitants of human skin, it is difficult to distinguish infection from contamination, the latter perhaps accounting for three-fourths of blood culture isolates. Infection is more likely if the patient has a foreign body (eg, sternal wires, prosthetic joint, prosthetic cardiac valve, pacemaker, intracranial pressure monitor, CSF shunt, peritoneal dialysis catheter) or an intravascular device in place. Purulent or serosanguineous drainage, erythema, pain, or tenderness at the site of the foreign body or device suggests infection. Joint instability and pain are signs of prosthetic joint infection. Fever, a new murmur, instability of the prosthesis, and signs of systemic embolization are evidence of prosthetic valve endocarditis.

Infection is also more likely if the same strain is consistently isolated from two or more blood cultures (particularly if samples were obtained at different times and have the same antimicrobial susceptibility patterns) and from the foreign body site.

Whenever possible, the intravascular device or foreign body suspected of being infected should be removed. However, removal and replacement of some devices (eg, prosthetic joint, prosthetic valve, CSF shunt) can be a difficult or risky procedure, and it may sometimes be preferable to treat with antibiotics alone, knowing that the probability of cure is reduced, that suppressive antibiotics may be needed long term, and that surgical management may eventually be necessary.

Coagulase-negative staphylococci are commonly resistant to β-lactams and multiple other antibiotics. For patients with normal kidney function, the treatment of choice until susceptibility to penicillinase-resistant penicillins or other agents has been confirmed is vancomycin, 15–20 mg/kg/dose intravenously every 8–12 hours (titrated to achieve a trough level of 15–20 mcg/mL). Duration of therapy has not been established for relatively uncomplicated infections, such as those from intravenous devices, which may be eliminated by simply removing the device. Infection involving bone or a prosthetic valve should be treated for 6 weeks. A combination regimen of vancomycin plus rifampin, 300 mg orally twice daily, plus gentamicin, 1 mg/kg intravenously every 8 hours, is recommended for treatment of prosthetic valve endocarditis caused by methicillin-resistant strains.

Baddour LM et al. Update on cardiovascular implantable electronic device infections and their prevention, diagnosis, and management: a Scientific Statement From the American Heart Association: Endorsed by the International Society for Cardiovascular Infectious Diseases. Circulation. 2024;149:e201. [PMID: 38047353]

CLOSTRIDIAL DISEASES

1. Clostridial Myonecrosis (Gas Gangrene)

ESSENTIALS OF DIAGNOSIS

- Sudden onset of pain and edema in and around a contaminated wound.
- Brown to blood-tinged watery exudate, with skin discoloration of surrounding area.
- Gas in the tissue by palpation or radiograph.
- Gram-positive rods in culture or smear of exudate.

General Considerations

Gas gangrene or clostridial myonecrosis is a life-threatening muscle infection produced by any one of several clostridia, which are anaerobic organisms, most commonly *Clostridium perfringens*. Trauma and injection drug use are common predisposing conditions. Toxins produced in devitalized tissues under anaerobic conditions result in shock, hemolysis, and myonecrosis.

Clinical Findings

A. Symptoms and Signs

The onset is usually sudden, with rapidly increasing pain in the affected area, hypotension, and tachycardia. Fever is present but is not proportionate to the severity of the infection. In the last stages of the disease, severe prostration, stupor, delirium, and coma occur.

The wound becomes swollen, and the surrounding skin is pale. There is a foul-smelling brown, blood-tinged serous discharge. As the disease advances, the surrounding tissue changes from pale to dusky and finally becomes deeply discolored, with coalescent, red, fluid-filled vesicles. Gas may be palpable in the tissues. Pain is often severe, not concomitant with initial findings, which can be diagnostic.

B. Laboratory Findings

Gas gangrene is a clinical diagnosis, and empiric therapy is indicated if the diagnosis is suspected. Radiographic studies may show gas within the soft tissues, but this finding is not sensitive or specific. Anaerobic culture confirms the diagnosis. It is important to inform the microbiology laboratory that an anaerobic organism is suspected so that the cultures can be appropriately handled and grown.

Differential Diagnosis

Clostridial myonecrosis may present similarly to necrotizing group A streptococcal infections and wound infections due to curved gram-negative organisms, such as *Vibrio vulnificus*. Other bacteria, including enteric gram-negative organisms and anaerobes, can also produce gas in infected tissue.

Treatment

Emergent surgical debridement of infected areas is essential, with radical surgical excision often necessary. Penicillin, 3–4 million units every 4 hours intravenously, is an effective adjunct, and clindamycin, 600–900 mg every 8 hours intravenously, may decrease bacterial toxin production.

Hussain H et al. Clostridial myonecrosis: a comprehensive review of toxin pathophysiology and management strategies. Microorganisms. 2024;12:1464. [PMID: 39065232]

2. Tetanus

ESSENTIALS OF DIAGNOSIS

- History of contaminated or penetrating wound.
- Jaw muscle stiffness ("lock jaw"), then spasms (trismus) with spasms of the facial muscles termed "risus sardonicus" and spasm of the back causing arching or "opisthotonos."
- Neck stiffness, dysphagia, irritability, hyperreflexia.
- Finally, painful convulsions precipitated by minimal stimuli.

General Considerations

Tetanus is caused by the neurotoxin tetanospasmin, elaborated by *C tetani*. Spores of this organism are ubiquitous in soil and may germinate when introduced into a wound. The incubation period is 5 days to 15 weeks, with the average being 8–12 days.

Most cases occur in unvaccinated individuals. Tetanus toxoid vaccine boosters should be provided every 10 years. Older adults, migrant workers, newborns, and persons who inject drugs are at risk. While puncture wounds are prone to causing tetanus, any wound, including bites or decubiti, may become infected by *C tetani*.

Clinical Findings

A. Symptoms and Signs

The first symptom may be pain and tingling at the site of inoculation, followed by spasticity of the muscles nearby. Stiffness of the jaw, neck stiffness, dysphagia, and irritability are other early signs. Hyperreflexia develops later, with spasms of the jaw muscles (trismus) or facial muscles ("risus sardonicus") and rigidity and spasm of the muscles of the abdomen, neck, and back (opisthotonos). Painful tonic convulsions precipitated by minor stimuli are common. Spasms of the glottis and respiratory muscles may cause acute asphyxia and apnea. The patient usually remains conscious and the sensory examination is normal. The temperature is normal or only slightly elevated.

B. Laboratory Findings

The diagnosis of tetanus is made clinically.

Differential Diagnosis

Tetanus must be differentiated from various acute CNS infections such as meningitis. Trismus may occasionally develop with odontogenic infections or the use of phenothiazines. Strychnine poisoning should also be considered.

Complications

Airway obstruction is common. Urinary retention and constipation may result from spasm of the sphincters. Respiratory arrest and cardiac failure are late events.

Prevention

Active immunization prevents tetanus (see Table 34–7). For primary immunization of adults, Td (tetanus and diphtheria toxoids vaccine) is administered as two doses 4–6 weeks apart, with a third dose 6–12 months later. For one of the three doses, Tdap (tetanus toxoid, reduced-dose diphtheria toxoid, acellular pertussis vaccine) should be substituted for Td. Booster Td doses are given every 10 years or at the time of major injury if it occurs > 5 years after a dose; a single dose of Tdap is preferred to Td for wound management if the patient has not been previously vaccinated with Tdap. Women should receive Tdap with each pregnancy, preferably between 27–36 weeks' gestation, with immunization at 27–30 weeks' gestation associated with the highest antibody concentrations.

Passive immunization with tetanus immune globulin, 250 units intramuscularly, should be used in nonimmunized individuals and those whose immunization status is uncertain whenever a wound is contaminated or likely to have devitalized tissue. Active immunization with tetanus toxoid vaccine is started concurrently. Table 37–2 provides a guide to prophylactic management.

Treatment

A. Specific Measures

Human tetanus immune globulin, 500 units, should be administered intramuscularly within the first 24 hours of presentation. Tetanus does not produce natural immunity, so a full course of infection immunization with tetanus toxoid should be administered once the patient has recovered.

B. General Measures

Debridement of wounds should be undertaken if implicated as the source. Metronidazole, 500 mg administered intravenously or orally every 6 hours, is preferred and should be administered to all patients. Penicillin, 3 million units intravenously every 4 hours, is an alternative. Minimal stimuli can provoke spasms, so the patient should be placed on bed rest and excess light and noise should be avoided. Sedation with benzodiazepines, paralysis with curare-like agents, and mechanical ventilation are often necessary. Enteral nutritional support should be given early.

Table 37–2. Guide to tetanus prophylaxis in wound management.

History of Absorbed Tetanus Toxoid	Clean, Minor Wounds		All Other Wounds[1]	
	Tdap or Td[2]	TIG[3]	Tdap or Td[2]	TIG[3]
Unknown or < 3 doses	Yes	No	Yes	Yes
3 or more doses	No[4]	No	No[5]	No

[1]Examples include wounds contaminated with dirt, feces, soil, or saliva; puncture wounds; avulsions; and wounds from missiles, crushing, burns, and frostbite.
[2]Td indicates tetanus toxoid and diphtheria toxoid vaccine, adult form. Tdap indicates tetanus toxoid, reduced diphtheria toxoid, and acellular pertussis vaccine, which may be substituted as a single dose for Td. Unvaccinated individuals should receive a complete series of three doses, one of which is Tdap.
[3]Human tetanus immune globulin, 250 units intramuscularly.
[4]Yes if > 10 years have elapsed since last dose.
[5]Yes if > 5 years have elapsed since last dose. (More frequent boosters are not needed and can enhance side effects.) Tdap has been safely administered within 2 years of Td vaccination, although local reactions to the vaccine may be increased.

Prognosis

High mortality rates are associated with a short incubation period, early onset of convulsions, and delay in treatment. Contaminated lesions about the head and face are more dangerous than wounds elsewhere.

Sudarshan R et al. Tetanus: recognition and management. Lancet Infect Dis. 2025;25:e645. [PMID: 40543524]

3. Botulism

ESSENTIALS OF DIAGNOSIS

- Recent ingestion of home-canned or smoked foods; recovery of toxin in serum or food.
- Injection drug use.
- Diplopia, dry mouth, dysphagia, dysphonia; muscle weakness leading to respiratory paralysis; normal sensory examination.
- Pupils are fixed and dilated in most cases.

General Considerations

Botulism is a paralytic disease caused by the botulinum toxin, produced by *Clostridium botulinum*, a ubiquitous, strictly anaerobic, spore-forming bacillus found in soil. Botulinum toxin is extremely potent and is classified by the CDC as a high-priority agent because of its potential for use as an agent of bioterrorism. Naturally occurring botulism exists in three forms: foodborne botulism, infant botulism, or wound botulism. Foodborne botulism is caused by ingestion of preformed toxin present in canned, smoked, or vacuum-packed foods such as home-canned vegetables, smoked meats, and vacuum-packed fish. Commercial foods have been associated with outbreaks of botulism. Infant botulism (associated with ingestion of honey) and wound botulism (often in association with injection drug use) result from *C tetani* organisms present in the gut or wound that secrete toxin.

Clinical Findings

A. Symptoms and Signs

Twelve to 36 hours after ingestion of the toxin, visual disturbances appear, particularly diplopia and loss of accommodation. Ptosis, cranial nerve palsies with impairment of extraocular muscles, and fixed dilated pupils are characteristic signs. The sensory examination is normal. Other symptoms are dry mouth, dysphagia, and dysphonia. Nausea and vomiting may be present, particularly with type E toxin. The sensorium remains clear and the temperature normal. Symmetric, descending flaccid paralysis progressing to respiratory failure and death may occur unless mechanical assistance is provided.

B. Laboratory Findings

A presumptive diagnosis should be made based on clinical findings. Toxin in foods and patients' serum can be demonstrated by mouse inoculation and identified with specific antiserum, but confirmation of results may take several days.

Differential Diagnosis

Because the clinical presentation of botulism is so distinctive and the differential diagnosis limited, botulism once considered is not easily confused with other diseases. Cranial nerve involvement may be seen with vertebrobasilar insufficiency, the Miller Fisher variant of Guillain-Barré syndrome, myasthenia gravis, or any basilar meningitis (infectious or carcinomatous).

Treatment

If botulism is suspected, the clinician should contact health authorities or the CDC for advice, procurement of equine serum heptavalent botulism antitoxin, and assistance in obtaining assays for toxin in serum, stool, or food. Skin testing is recommended to exclude hypersensitivity to the antitoxin preparation. Antitoxin should be administered as early as possible, ideally within 24 hours of symptom onset;

its administration should not be delayed for laboratory confirmation of the diagnosis. Respiratory failure is managed with intubation and mechanical ventilation. Parenteral fluids or alimentation should be given while swallowing difficulty persists. The removal of unabsorbed toxin from the gut may be attempted. In the case of wound botulism, penicillin, 3 g intravenously every 4 hours, or metronidazole, 500 mg intravenously every 8 hours, may be helpful in arresting the organism.

Kobaidze K et al. Botulism in the 21st century: a scoping review. Brown J Hosp Med. 2023;2:72707. [PMID: 40046154]
Rao AK et al. Clinical guidelines for diagnosis and treatment of botulism, 2021. MMWR Recomm Rep. 2021;70:1. [PMID: 33956777]

LISTERIOSIS

ESSENTIALS OF DIAGNOSIS

- Ingestion of contaminated food product.
- Fever in a pregnant woman in her third trimester.
- Altered mental status and fever in an older or immunocompromised patient.
- Blood and CSF cultures confirm the diagnosis.

General Considerations

Listeria monocytogenes is a facultative, motile, gram-positive rod. Most cases of infection caused by *L monocytogenes* are sporadic, but outbreaks have been traced to eating contaminated food, including unpasteurized dairy products, delicatessen meats, cantaloupes, and soft cheeses. Outbreaks have been associated with significant morbidity and mortality in patients with infection.

Clinical Findings

Five types of severe infection are recognized:

1. **Infection during pregnancy**, usually in the last trimester, is a mild febrile illness without an apparent primary focus and may resolve without specific therapy. However, approximately one in five pregnancies complicated by listeriosis result in spontaneous abortion or stillbirth and surviving infants are at risk for clinical neonatal listeriosis.
2. **Granulomatosis infantisepticum** is a neonatal infection acquired in utero, characterized by disseminated abscesses, granulomas, and a high mortality rate.
3. **Bacteremia** with or without sepsis syndrome is an infection of neonates or immunocompromised adults. Presentation is a febrile illness without a recognized source.
4. **Meningitis** caused by *L monocytogenes* affects infants under 2 months of age and older adults, ranking third after pneumococcus and meningococcus as common causes of bacterial meningitis. CSF often shows *lymphocytic* pleocytosis, with variable protein and glucose findings. Adults with meningitis are often immunocompromised, and cases have been associated with advanced HIV as well as the use of glucocorticoids and TNF inhibitors such as infliximab.
5. **Focal infections**, including adenitis, brain abscess, endocarditis, osteomyelitis, and arthritis, occur rarely.

Prevention

At-risk patients (eg, pregnant women, people living with HIV) should avoid unpasteurized milk products, including raw cheeses. Smoked seafoods, cold cuts, hot dogs, and meat spreads also carry risk. Thoroughly cook animal source food and wash raw vegetables.

Treatment

Ampicillin, 8–12 g/day intravenously in four to six divided doses (the higher dose for meningitis), is the treatment of choice. Gentamicin, 5 mg/kg/day intravenously once or in divided doses, is synergistic with ampicillin against *Listeria*, and the use of combination therapy may be considered during the first few days of treatment to enhance eradication of organisms. In patients with penicillin allergies, trimethoprim-sulfamethoxazole has excellent intracellular and CSF penetration and is an appropriate alternative. The dose is 10–20 mg/kg/day intravenously divided every 6–12 hours of the trimethoprim component. Mortality and morbidity rates still are high. Therapy should be administered for at least 2–3 weeks. Longer durations—between 3 and 6 weeks—have been recommended for treatment of bacteremia, especially in immunocompromised patients.

Khsim IEF et al. Listeriosis in pregnancy: an umbrella review of maternal exposure, treatment and neonatal complications. BJOG. 2022;129:1427. [PMID: 34954888]
Koopmans MM et al. Human listeriosis. Clin Microbiol Rev. 2023;36:e0006019. [PMID: 36475874]

INFECTIVE ENDOCARDITIS

ESSENTIALS OF DIAGNOSIS

- Fever.
- Underlying valvular disease or prosthetic endovascular material.
- Positive blood cultures.
- Evidence of vegetation on echocardiography.
- Evidence of systemic emboli.

General Considerations

Endocarditis is a bacterial or fungal (or rarely aseptic) infection of the valvular or endocardial surface of the heart. The clinical presentation depends on the infecting organism and the infected valve or valves. More virulent organisms—*S aureus* in particular—tend to produce a more rapidly progressive and destructive infection. Endocarditis caused by more virulent organisms often presents as an acute febrile illness and is complicated by early embolization, acute valvular regurgitation, and myocardial abscess formation. Viridans strains of streptococci, enterococci, other bacteria (including intracellular bacteria), yeasts, and fungi tend to cause a more subacute picture.

Predisposing valvular abnormalities include a variety of congenital heart disorders, rheumatic involvement of any valve, bicuspid aortic valves, calcific or sclerotic aortic valves, hypertrophic subaortic stenosis, and mitral valve prolapse. Regurgitation lesions are more susceptible than stenotic ones.

The initiating event in native valve endocarditis is colonization of the valve by bacteria or yeast that gain access to the bloodstream. Transient bacteremia is common during dental, upper respiratory, urologic, and lower GI diagnostic and surgical procedures. Intravascular devices are also a portal of access for microorganisms into the bloodstream. A large proportion of cases of *S aureus* endocarditis are attributable to health care–associated bacteremia.

Native valve endocarditis is usually caused by *S aureus*, viridans streptococci, enterococci, or HACEK organisms (an acronym for *Haemophilus aphrophilus* [now *Aggregatibacter aphrophilus*], *Actinobacillus actinomycetemcomitans* [now *Aggregatibacter actinomycetemcomitans*], *Cardiobacterium hominis*, *Eikenella corrodens*, and *Kingella* species). *S aureus* is the leading cause of native valve endocarditis. Gram-negative organisms and fungi account for a small percentage.

In injection drug users, *S aureus* accounts for > 60% of all endocarditis cases and for 80–90% of cases in which the tricuspid valve is infected. Enterococci and streptococci comprise most of the balance in about equal proportions. Other causative organisms are gram-negative aerobic bacilli, fungi, and unusual organisms, such as *Bartonella* and *Coxiella* species.

The microbiology of **prosthetic valve endocarditis** is distinctive. Early infections (ie, those occurring within 2 months after valve implantation) are commonly caused by staphylococci—both coagulase-positive and coagulase-negative—gram-negative organisms, and fungi. In late prosthetic valve endocarditis, streptococci are commonly identified, although staphylococci still cause many cases.

Clinical Findings

A. Symptoms and Signs

Virtually all patients have fever at some point in the illness, although it may be very low grade (<38°C) in older individuals and in patients with HF or kidney failure. Rarely, there may be no fever at all.

The duration of illness typically is a few days to a few weeks. Nonspecific constitutional symptoms are common. The initial symptoms and signs of endocarditis may be caused by direct arterial, valvular, or cardiac damage. Although a changing regurgitant murmur is significant diagnostically, it is the exception rather than the rule. Symptoms also may occur as a result of embolization, metastatic infection or immunologically mediated phenomena. These include cough; dyspnea; arthralgias or arthritis; diarrhea; and abdominal, back, or flank pain.

The characteristic peripheral lesions—petechiae (on the palate, conjunctiva, or beneath the fingernails), subungual ("splinter") hemorrhages (Figure 37–4), Osler nodes (painful, violaceous raised lesions of the fingers, toes, or feet), Janeway lesions (painless erythematous lesions of the palms or soles), and Roth spots (exudative lesions in the retina)—occur in about 25% of patients. Strokes and major systemic embolic events are present in about 25% of patients and tend to occur before or within the first week of antimicrobial therapy. Hematuria and proteinuria may result from emboli or immunologically mediated glomerulonephritis. Septic emboli to the lungs are common in endocarditis affecting the right-sided valves.

B. Imaging

Echocardiography is useful in identifying vegetations and other characteristic features suspicious for endocarditis and may provide adjunctive information about the specific valve or valves that are infected. The sensitivity of transthoracic echocardiography is around 75%; it cannot reliably rule out endocarditis but may confirm a clinical suspicion. Transesophageal echocardiography is 90% sensitive in detecting vegetations and is useful for identifying valve ring abscesses and prosthetic valve endocarditis. CXR may show evidence for the underlying cardiac

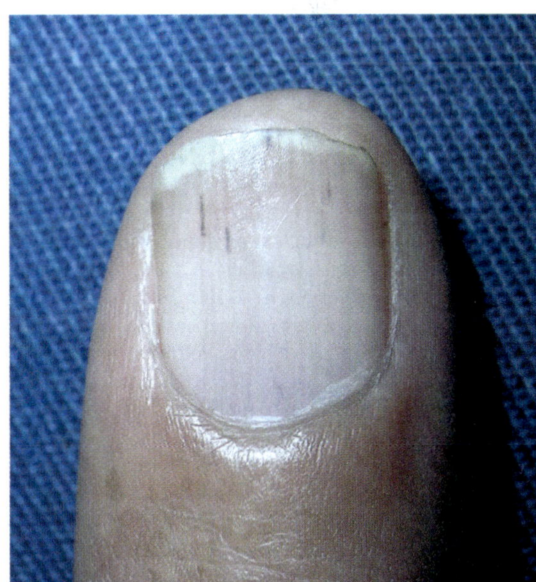

Figure 37–4. Splinter hemorrhages appearing as red linear streaks under the nail plate and within the nail bed, in endocarditis, psoriasis, and trauma. (Reproduced with permission from Richard P. Usatine, MD, in Usatine RP, Smith MA, Mayeaux EJ Jr, Chumley H, Tysinger J. *The Color Atlas of Family Medicine*. McGraw-Hill, 2009.)

abnormality and, in right-sided endocarditis, pulmonary infiltrates. New conduction abnormalities on ECG, such as prolongation of the PR interval, suggest myocardial abscess formation.

C. Diagnostic Studies

1. Blood cultures—Three sets of blood cultures from different venipuncture sites (which may be collected simultaneously or several hours apart) are recommended before starting antibiotics to maximize microbiologic diagnosis. Adequate volume is important; each culture bottle should be filled with 10 mL of blood since half of adults have <1 colony forming unit of bacteria per mL blood.

Less than 10% of cases will be culture-negative, usually attributable to administration of antimicrobials prior to cultures. If antimicrobial therapy has been administered before obtaining cultures and the patient is clinically stable, it is reasonable to withhold antimicrobial therapy for 2–3 days so that appropriate cultures can be obtained. Culture-negative endocarditis may also be due to organisms that require special media for growth (eg, *Bartonella, Abiotrophia* species, formerly referred to as nutritionally deficient streptococci), organisms that do not grow on artificial media and most often require serologic diagnosis (eg, *Tropheryma whipplei*, *Coxiella burnetii*), or those that may require prolonged incubation (eg, *Brucella*, anaerobes, HACEK organisms). *B quintana* and *B henselae* are important causes of culture-negative endocarditis, which is most frequent among those with marginal housing status and are typically diagnosed by serologies.

2. 2023 Duke-International Society for Cardiovascular Infectious Disease (ISCVID) criteria—The 2023 Duke-ISCVID criteria establish a diagnosis of endocarditis by pathologic criteria (ie, microorganisms or histopathologic findings of endocarditis identified on tissue, such as a vegetation, cardiac tissue, or an explanted prosthetic valve or cardiac device) in the context of clinical signs of endocarditis. A definite diagnosis can also be made by meeting two major clinical criteria, one major and three minor clinical criteria, or five minor clinical criteria. **Major criteria** include (1) two positive blood cultures for a microorganism that typically causes infective endocarditis or persistent bacteremia, three or more positive blood cultures for a microorganism that occasionally or rarely causes endocarditis, or blood tests consistent with acute infection with *Coxiella burnetii*, *Bartonella* species, or *Tropheryma whipplei;* (2) evidence of endocardial involvement documented by echocardiography showing definite vegetation, myocardial abscess, new partial dehiscence of a prosthetic valve, or new valvular regurgitation or FDG PET/CT imaging demonstrating abnormal metabolic activity involving cardiac tissue or prosthetic material; and (3) directly observed evidence of endocarditis during cardiac surgery. **Minor criteria** include the presence of a predisposing condition; fever of 38°C or higher; vascular phenomena, such as cutaneous hemorrhages, aneurysm, systemic emboli, or pulmonary infarction; immunologic phenomena, such as glomerulonephritis, Osler nodes, Roth spots, or rheumatoid factor; positive blood cultures not meeting the major criteria or other laboratory evidence of an active infection; abnormal FDG PET/CT metabolic activity within 3 months of implantation of endovascular prosthetic material; and new valvular regurgitation (worsening or changing of a preexisting murmur is insufficient). A possible diagnosis of endocarditis is made if one major and one minor criterion or three minor criteria are met. If fewer criteria are found, or a sound alternative explanation for illness is identified, or the patient's febrile illness has resolved within 4 days, endocarditis is unlikely.

Complications

The course of infective endocarditis is determined by the degree of heart damage, the site of infection (right-sided versus left-sided, aortic versus mitral valve), the presence of metastatic foci of infection, the occurrence of embolization, and immunologically mediated processes. Destruction of infected heart valves is especially common and precipitous with *S aureus* but can occur with any organism and can progress even after bacteriologic cure. The infection can also extend into the myocardium, resulting in abscesses leading to conduction disturbances, and involving the wall of the aorta, creating sinus of Valsalva aneurysms.

Peripheral embolization to the brain and myocardium may result in infarctions. Embolization to the spleen and kidneys is also common. Peripheral emboli may initiate metastatic infections or may become established in vessel walls, leading to mycotic aneurysms. Right-sided endocarditis (usually the tricuspid valve) causes septic pulmonary emboli, occasionally with infarction and lung abscesses.

Prevention

The American Heart Association recommends antibiotic prophylaxis for infective endocarditis in a relatively small group of patients with predisposing congenital or valvular anomalies undergoing invasive dental procedures that involve manipulation of gingival tissue or the periapical region of teeth or perforation of oral mucosa. Prophylaxis is not routinely recommended for other types of procedures.

Treatment

Empiric regimens for endocarditis while culture results are pending should include agents active against staphylococci, streptococci, and enterococci. Vancomycin, 1 g every 12 hours intravenously titrated to achieve a trough level of 15–20 mcg/mL, plus ceftriaxone, 2 g every 24 hours, provides appropriate coverage pending definitive diagnosis; consultation with an infectious disease expert is strongly recommended when initiating treatment. Intravenous therapy has been the mainstay of treatment for infective endocarditis. Some data, however, support the use of oral antibiotic therapy following 2 weeks of intravenous antibiotic regimens for certain organisms.

A. Viridans Streptococci

For penicillin-susceptible viridans streptococcal endocarditis (ie, MIC 0.12 mcg/mL or less), penicillin G, 18 million units intravenously either continuously or in four to six equally divided doses, or ceftriaxone, 2 g intravenously once daily for 4 weeks, is recommended. For patients unable to tolerate penicillin or ceftriaxone, vancomycin, 15 mg/kg intravenously every 12 hours for 4 weeks, is given with a desired trough level of 15–20 mcg/mL. Prosthetic valve endocarditis is treated with a 6-week course of penicillin or ceftriaxone and the clinician can consider adding 2 weeks of gentamicin at the start of therapy.

Viridans streptococci relatively resistant to penicillin (ie, MIC > 0.12 mcg/mL but ≤ 0.5 mcg/mL) should be treated for 4 weeks. Penicillin G, 24 million units intravenously either continuously or in four to six equally divided doses, is combined with gentamicin, 3 mg/kg intravenously every 24 hours for the first 2 weeks. Ceftriaxone may be a reasonable alternative treatment option. In patients with IgE-mediated allergy to penicillin, vancomycin alone, 15 mg/kg intravenously every 12 hours for 4 weeks with achievement of adequate trough levels, should be administered. Prosthetic valve endocarditis is treated with a 6-week course of penicillin or ceftriaxone plus gentamicin as above.

Endocarditis caused by viridans streptococci with an MIC > 0.5 mcg/mL or by *Abiotrophia* species should be treated the same as enterococcal endocarditis.

B. Enterococci (Formerly Group D Streptococci)

For enterococcal endocarditis, penicillin or ampicillin alone is inadequate. One recommended regimen is ampicillin, 2 g intravenously every 4 hours, or penicillin G, 4 million units intravenously every 4 hours plus gentamicin, 1 mg/kg intravenously every 8 hours. The second recommended regimen is ampicillin, 2 g intravenously every 4 hours, plus ceftriaxone, 2 g intravenously every 12 hours. The recommended duration of therapy is 4–6 weeks (the longer duration for patients with symptoms for > 3 months, relapse, or prosthetic valve endocarditis). The combination of ampicillin plus ceftriaxone is recommended for patients with creatinine clearance <50 mL/min or whose enterococcal isolates are resistant to gentamicin. In patients who cannot tolerate penicillin and ampicillin or who have an enterococcal isolate resistant to these agents, vancomycin plus gentamicin can be used. Endocarditis caused by strains resistant to penicillin and vancomycin are difficult to treat and should always be managed with an infectious disease specialist.

C. Staphylococci

For methicillin-susceptible *S aureus* isolates, nafcillin or oxacillin, 12 g intravenously daily given continuously or in four to six divided doses, or cefazolin, 6 g intravenously daily given continuously or in three divided doses for 6 weeks, is the preferred therapy. In cases of brain abscess resulting from methicillin-susceptible *S aureus* endocarditis, nafcillin should be used instead of cefazolin. For patients with history of immediate type hypersensitivity to β-lactams, a desensitization protocol should be undertaken. For patients with a history of non-anaphylactoid reactions to penicillins, cefazolin should be used. Patients who are infected with methicillin-resistant *S aureus* or who are unable to tolerate β-lactam therapy should receive vancomycin, 30 mg/kg/day intravenously divided in two or three doses, to achieve a goal trough level of 15–20 mcg/kg, or daptomycin 8–12 mg/kg intravenously once daily. Aminoglycoside combination regimens are not recommended. The effect of rifampin with antistaphylococcal drugs is variable, and its routine use is not recommended.

Because coagulase-negative staphylococci—a common cause of prosthetic valve endocarditis—are routinely resistant to methicillin, β-lactam antibiotics should not be used unless the isolate is demonstrated to be susceptible. A combination of vancomycin, 30 mg/kg/day intravenously divided into two or three doses for 6 weeks; rifampin, 300 mg every 8 hours for 6 weeks; and gentamicin, 3 mg/kg intravenously every 8 hours for the first 2 weeks, is recommended for prosthetic valve infection. If the organism is sensitive to methicillin, nafcillin, oxacillin, or cefazolin can be combined with rifampin and gentamicin. Combination therapy with nafcillin or oxacillin (vancomycin or daptomycin for methicillin-resistant strains), rifampin, and gentamicin is also recommended for treatment of *S aureus* prosthetic valve infection.

D. HACEK Organisms

HACEK organisms are slow-growing, fastidious, gram-negative coccobacilli or bacilli that are normal oral flora and cause <5% of all cases of endocarditis. They may produce β-lactamase, and thus the treatment of choice is ceftriaxone (or another third-generation cephalosporin), 2 g intravenously once daily for 4 weeks. Prosthetic valve endocarditis should be treated for 6 weeks. In penicillin-allergic patients, experience is limited, but fluoroquinolones have in vitro activity and should be considered. HACEK organisms have previously required extended incubation periods but can now grow within the standard incubation period of 5 days due to automated blood culture systems.

E. Culture-Negative Endocarditis

Failure to culture microorganisms from patients with suspected infective endocarditis may be due to infection from organisms not recovered in routine microbiology testing or previous administration of antimicrobial agents before blood cultures were obtained. These cases must be managed with the assistance of an infectious disease specialist. Pathogens that cannot be cultured by commonly used techniques include *Bartonella* species, *Coxiella* species, *Chlamydia* species, *Brucella* species, and *Tropheryma whipplei*. Serologic testing should be performed in patients who have epidemiologic risk factors for these infections. Increasingly, universal PCR testing is being employed in infectious diseases to make difficult diagnoses. Treatment should be directed at likely pathogens while awaiting serologic results; treatment of patients given prior antimicrobials before cultures were obtained must also consider likely pathogens.

F. Role of Surgery

While many cases can be successfully treated medically, operative management is frequently required. Acute HF unresponsive to medical therapy is an indication for valve replacement even if active infection is present. Infections unresponsive to appropriate antimicrobial therapy after 7–10 days (ie, persistent fevers, positive blood cultures despite therapy) are more likely to be eradicated if the valve is replaced. Surgery is nearly always required for cure of fungal endocarditis and is more often necessary with highly resistant bacteria. It is also indicated when the infection involves the sinus of Valsalva or produces septal abscesses. Recurrent infection with the same organism prompts an operative approach, especially with infected prosthetic valves. Continuing embolization presents a difficult problem when the infection is otherwise responding; surgery may be the proper approach. Particularly challenging is a large and fragile vegetation demonstrated by echocardiography in the absence of embolization. Most clinicians favor an operative approach with vegetectomy and valve repair if the patient is a good candidate. Operation without delay may be considered in patients with endocarditis and an embolic stroke who have an indication for surgery. If not urgent or if intracranial hemorrhage is present, a delay of at least 4 weeks should be considered.

G. Role of Anticoagulation

Anticoagulation is contraindicated in native valve endocarditis because of an increased risk of intracerebral hemorrhage from mycotic aneurysms or embolic phenomena. The role of anticoagulant therapy during prosthetic valve endocarditis is more controversial. Reversal of anticoagulation may result in thrombosis of the mechanical prosthesis, particularly in the mitral position. Conversely, anticoagulation during active prosthetic valve endocarditis caused by *S aureus* has been associated with fatal intracerebral hemorrhage. One approach is to discontinue anticoagulation during the septic phase of *S aureus* prosthetic valve endocarditis. In patients with *S aureus* prosthetic valve endocarditis complicated by a CNS embolic event, anticoagulation should be discontinued for the first 2 weeks of therapy. Indications for anticoagulation following prosthetic valve implantation for endocarditis are the same as for patients with prosthetic valves without endocarditis (eg, nonporcine mechanical valves and valves in the mitral position).

▶ Response to Therapy

If infection is caused by viridans streptococci, enterococci, or coagulase-negative staphylococci, defervescence occurs in 3–4 days on average; with *S aureus* or *Pseudomonas aeruginosa*, fever may persist for longer. Blood cultures should be obtained every 1–2 days to document sterilization. Other causes of persistent fever are myocardial or metastatic abscess, sterile embolization, superimposed hospital-acquired infection, and drug reaction. Most relapses occur within 1–2 months after completion of therapy. Obtaining one or two blood cultures during this period is prudent.

▶ When to Refer

- Consider consulting an infectious diseases specialist in all cases of suspected infective endocarditis.
- Consult a cardiac surgeon as discussed in the Role of Surgery section above to prevent further embolic disease, HF, and other complications, including death.

▶ When to Admit

Patients with infective endocarditis should be hospitalized for expedited evaluation and treatment.

Delgado V et al. 2023 ESC Guidelines for the management of endocarditis. Eur Heart J. 2023;44:3948. [PMID: 37622656] Erratum in: Eur Heart J. 2023;44:4780. [PMID: 37738322]

Fowler VG et al. The 2023 Duke-International Society for Cardiovascular Infectious Diseases Criteria for Infective Endocarditis: Updating the Modified Duke Criteria. Clin Infect Dis. 2023;77:518. [PMID: 37138445]

INFECTIONS CAUSED BY GRAM-NEGATIVE BACTERIA

BORDETELLA PERTUSSIS INFECTION (Whooping Cough)

ESSENTIALS OF DIAGNOSIS

- Predominantly in children under age 2 years; adolescents and adults are reservoirs of infection.
- Two-week prodromal catarrhal stage of malaise, cough, coryza, and anorexia.
- Paroxysmal cough ending in a high-pitched inspiratory "whoop."
- Absolute lymphocytosis, often striking; culture confirms diagnosis.

▶ General Considerations

Pertussis is an acute infection of the respiratory tract caused by *B pertussis* that is transmitted by respiratory droplets. The incubation period is 7–17 days. Half of all cases occur before age 2 years. Neither immunization nor disease confers lasting immunity to pertussis, requiring ongoing booster vaccination. Consequently, adults can be an important reservoir of the disease.

▶ Clinical Findings

The symptoms of classic pertussis last about 6 weeks and are divided into three consecutive stages. The catarrhal stage is characterized by its insidious onset, with lacrimation, sneezing, and coryza, anorexia and malaise, and a hacking night cough that becomes diurnal. The paroxysmal stage is characterized by bursts of rapid, consecutive coughs followed by a deep, high-pitched inspiration (whoop). The convalescent stage begins 4 weeks after onset of the illness with a decrease in the frequency and severity of paroxysms of cough. Atypical presentations are more common in adults and individuals who were previously vaccinated. Cough persisting > 2 weeks is suggestive. Infection may also be asymptomatic, and apnea may be the only manifestation in infants.

The WBC count is usually 15,000–20,000/mcL ($15–20 \times 10^9$/L) with lymphocytosis. The diagnosis is established by isolating the organism from a nasopharyngeal culture on special medium (eg, Bordet-Gengou agar). PCR assays for *B pertussis* may be available in some clinical or health department laboratories.

Prevention

Acellular pertussis vaccine is recommended for all infants, combined with diphtheria and tetanus toxoids (DTaP). Infants and susceptible adults with significant exposure should receive prophylaxis with an oral macrolide. In recognition of their importance as a reservoir of disease, vaccination of adolescents and adults against pertussis is recommended (see Table 34–7). Adolescents aged 11–18 years (preferably between 11 and 12 years of age) who have completed the DTP or DTaP vaccination series should receive a single dose of either Tdap product instead of Td (tetanus and diphtheria toxoids vaccine) for booster immunization against tetanus, diphtheria, and pertussis. Tdap, which immunizes against the same bacteria as DTaP, is a booster immunization; Tdap contains the same amount of tetanus toxoid (T) as DTaP but reduced diphtheria toxoid and acellular pertussis (hence the lower case -dap). Adults of all ages (including those aged 65 years or older) should receive a single dose of Tdap. In addition, pregnant women should receive a dose of Tdap during each pregnancy regardless of prior vaccination history, ideally between 27 and 36 weeks of gestation, to maximize the antibody response of the woman and the passive antibody transfer to the infant. For any woman who was not previously vaccinated with Tdap and for whom the vaccine was not given during her pregnancy, Tdap should be administered immediately postpartum. The CDC has eliminated the recommendation that a 2-year period window is needed between receiving the Td and Tdap vaccines based on data showing no increased risk of adverse events.

Treatment

Antibiotic treatment should be initiated in all suspected cases. Treatment options include azithromycin, 500 mg orally on day 1 and 250 mg for 4 more days, or clarithromycin, 500 mg orally twice daily for 7 days. Trimethoprim-sulfamethoxazole, 160–800 mg orally twice daily for 14 days, is also effective. Treatment shortens the duration of carriage and may diminish the severity of coughing paroxysms. These same regimens are indicated for prophylaxis of contacts to an active case of pertussis who are exposed within 3 weeks of the onset of cough in the index case.

Christie CDC. Resurgence of pertussis: whopping the '100-day cough'. Curr Opin Pediatr. 2025;37:508. [PMID: 40842393].

Kline JM et al. Pertussis: common questions and answers. Am Fam Physician. 2021;104:186. [PMID: 34383446]

MENINGOCOCCAL MENINGITIS

ESSENTIALS OF DIAGNOSIS

- Fever, headache, vomiting, delirium, convulsions.
- Petechial rash on skin and mucous membranes.
- Neck and back stiffness and positive Kernig and Brudzinski signs are characteristic.
- Purulent spinal fluid with gram-negative intracellular and extracellular diplococci.
- Culture of CSF, blood, or petechial aspiration confirms the diagnosis.

General Considerations

Meningococcal meningitis is caused by *Neisseria meningitidis* of groups A, B, C, Y, and W-135, among others. Up to 40% of persons are nasopharyngeal carriers of meningococci, but disease develops in relatively few of these persons. Infection is transmitted by droplets. Clinical illness may take the form of meningococcemia (a fulminant form of septicemia without meningitis), meningococcemia with meningitis, or meningitis. Recurrent meningococcemia with fever, rash, and arthritis is seen rarely in patients with certain terminal complement deficiencies. Asplenic patients are also at risk.

Clinical Findings

A. Symptoms and Signs

High fever, chills, nausea, vomiting, headache, back, abdominal, and extremity pains are typical. Rapidly developing confusion, delirium, seizures, and coma occur in some. In infants and in older adults, fever or stiff neck is often missing, and altered mental status may dominate the picture. On examination, nuchal and back rigidity are typical. Positive Kernig sign (pain in the hamstrings upon extension of the knee with the hip at 90-degree flexion) and Brudzinski sign (flexion of the knee in response to flexion of the neck) are specific but not sensitive findings of meningitis. A petechial rash appearing all over the body, including mucous membranes, the lower extremities, and pressure points, is found in most cases. Petechiae may vary in size from pinpoint lesions to large ecchymoses or even skin gangrene that may later slough.

B. Laboratory Findings

Lumbar puncture typically reveals a cloudy or purulent CSF, with elevated pressure, increased protein, and decreased glucose content. The fluid usually contains a cell count > 1000/mcL (1.0×10^9/L) with polymorphonuclear cells predominating and containing gram-negative intracellular diplococci. The organism is usually demonstrated by smear and culture of the CSF, oropharynx, blood, or aspirated petechiae. The absence of organisms in a Gram-stained smear of the CSF sediment does not rule out the diagnosis. The capsular polysaccharide can be demonstrated in CSF or urine by latex agglutination; this is useful in partially treated patients, although sensitivity is 60–80%.

Disseminated intravascular coagulation is an important complication of meningococcal infection and is typically present in toxic patients with ecchymotic skin lesions.

Differential Diagnosis

Meningococcal meningitis must be differentiated from other meningitides. Rickettsial, echovirus, and, rarely, other bacterial infections (eg, staphylococcal infections, scarlet fever) also cause petechial rash.

Prevention

There are two quadrivalent vaccines with coverage against meningococcal serogroups A, C, W, and Y, and two monovalent vaccines with coverage against meningococcal serogroup B. The quadrivalent vaccines are conjugate vaccines (MenACWY-TT and MenACWY-CRM, collectively termed MCV4) indicated for persons age 2–55 years. The two monovalent vaccines against meningococcal serogroup B are MenB-FHbp and MenB-4C; they are approved for persons aged 10–25 years and are not interchangeable. There are also two pentavalent conjugate vaccines targeting the five major serogroups approved for use in the United States.

The Advisory Committee on Immunization Practices recommends immunization with a dose of MCV4 for preadolescents age 11–12 years with a booster at age 16 years. For ease of program implementation, persons aged 21 years or younger should have documentation of receipt of a dose of MCV4 not more than 5 years before enrollment to college. If the primary dose was administered before the 16th birthday, a booster dose should be administered before enrollment. The vaccine is also recommended as a two-dose primary series administered 2 months apart for persons aged 2–54 years with persistent complement deficiency, persons with functional or anatomic asplenia, and adolescents with HIV infection. All other persons at increased risk for meningococcal disease (eg, military recruits, microbiologists routinely exposed to isolates of *N meningitidis*, or travelers to an epidemic or highly endemic country) should receive a single dose. One of the meningococcal serogroup B vaccines may be administered to persons 10 years or older at increased risk for meningococcal disease. These individuals include those with persistent complement deficiencies, persons with anatomic or functional asplenia, microbiologists, and persons identified to be at increased risk because of a serogroup B meningococcal disease outbreak. Vaccination of persons aged 16–23 years may provide short-term protection against most strains of serogroup B meningococcal disease and is indicated if there is a dormitory or school outbreak. The pentavalent vaccine is recommended when both MCV4 and MenB vaccines are indicated.

Eliminating nasopharyngeal carriage of meningococci is an effective prevention strategy in closed populations and to prevent secondary cases in household or otherwise close contacts. Rifampin, 600 mg orally twice a day for 2 days, ciprofloxacin, 500 mg orally once, or one intramuscular 250-mg dose of ceftriaxone is effective. Ciprofloxacin should not be used as prophylaxis if there have been two or more cases of invasive meningococcal disease due to ciprofloxacin-resistant strains, and ≥ 20% of all reported cases are caused by ciprofloxacin-resistant strains in a local catchment area during a rolling 12-month period. School and work contacts ordinarily need not be treated. Hospital contacts receive therapy only if intense exposure has occurred (eg, mouth-to-mouth resuscitation). Accidentally discovered carriers without known close contact with meningococcal disease do not require prophylactic antimicrobials.

Treatment

Blood cultures must be obtained and intravenous antimicrobial therapy started immediately. This may be done before lumbar puncture in patients whose diagnosis is not straightforward and for those in whom MR or CT imaging is indicated to exclude mass lesions. Ceftriaxone, 2 g intravenously every 12 hours, is the empiric antibiotic of choice pending results of susceptibility testing. The prevalence of intermediate resistance to penicillin in vitro (MICs 0.1–1 mcg/mL) is increasing, particularly in Europe. Penicillin-intermediate strains thus far remain susceptible to ceftriaxone and other third-generation cephalosporins used to treat meningitis. If penicillin susceptibility is confirmed (MIC < 0.1 mcg/mL), either penicillin G, 4 million units intravenously every 4 hours, or ceftriaxone may be used. Treatment should be continued for at least 4 days in adults and 5 days in children and can be extended to 7 days for severe presentations or delayed responses to therapy.

When to Admit

All patients with suspected meningococcal infection should be admitted for evaluation and empiric intravenous antibiotic therapy.

Amin AB et al. Use of the GSK MenACWY-CRM/MenB-4C pentavalent meningococcal vaccine among persons aged ≥10 years: recommendations of the Advisory Committee on Immunization Practices - United States, 2025. MMWR Morb Mortal Wkly Rep. 2026;75:7. [PMID: 41505372]

Berry I et al. Selection of antibiotics as prophylaxis for close contacts of patients with meningococcal disease in areas with ciprofloxacin resistance - United States, 2024. MMWR Morb Mortal Wkly Rep. 2024;73:99. [PMID: 38329923]

INFECTIONS CAUSED BY *HAEMOPHILUS SPECIES*

H influenzae and other *Haemophilus* species may cause sinusitis, otitis, bronchitis, epiglottitis, pneumonia, cellulitis, septic arthritis, meningitis, and endocarditis. Alcohol use disorder, smoking, chronic lung disease like COPD, advanced age, and HIV are risk factors.

For adults with sinusitis, otitis, or respiratory tract infections, appropriate oral antibiotics include amoxicillin (500–1000 mg three times daily, if organism is susceptible) or amoxicillin-clavulanate (875/125 mg twice daily, for β-lactamase producing strains). Other oral antibiotic options may include cefuroxime axetil (500 mg twice daily), cefdinir (600 mg once daily), fluroquinolones (levofloxacin 750 mg daily or moxifloxacin 400 mg daily), doxycycline (100 mg twice daily), or azithromycin (500 mg orally once followed by 250 mg daily). Duration of therapy depends on the clinical syndrome; 5–7 days is often adequate. In more seriously ill patients (eg, those with multilobar pneumonia), ceftriaxone, 1 g/day intravenously, or an intravenous fluoroquinolone (also appropriate for penicillin-allergic patients; dosages as above) can be used.

Epiglottitis is characterized by an abrupt onset of high fever, drooling, and inability to handle secretions. A severe sore throat despite an unimpressive pharyngeal examination can be a diagnostic clue. Stridor and respiratory distress result from laryngeal obstruction. The diagnosis is best made by direct visualization of the cherry-red, swollen epiglottis during laryngoscopy. Because laryngoscopy may provoke laryngospasm and obstruction, especially in children, it should be performed in an intensive care unit or similar setting, and only when intubation can be performed promptly if required. Ceftriaxone, 2 g intravenously every 24 hours is the initial drug of choice, with total duration of therapy typically 7–10 days. Fluoroquinolones (see above for dosage) may be used in patients with severe penicillin allergies.

While rare in adults, *Haemophilus* is a consideration in patients who have **meningitis** associated with sinusitis or otitis. Initial therapy for suspected *H influenzae* meningitis should be with ceftriaxone, 2 g intravenously every 12 hours, unless the strain is proven not to produce β-lactamase. Meningitis due to *H influenzae* is treated for at least 7–10 days. Dexamethasone, 0.15 mg/kg intravenously every 6 hours for the first 4 days of treatment, may reduce the incidence of long-term sequelae, principally hearing loss.

Metlay JP et al. Diagnosis and treatment of adults with community-acquired pneumonia. An official clinical practice guideline of the American Thoracic Society and Infectious Diseases Society of America. Am J Respir Crit Care Med. 2019;200:e45. [PMID: 31573350]

Jones BE et al. Diagnosis and management of community-acquired pneumonia. An Official American Thoracic Society Clinical Practice Guideline. Am J Respir Crit Care Med. 2026;212:24. [PMID: 40679934]

LEGIONNAIRES' DISEASE

ESSENTIALS OF DIAGNOSIS

- Patients are often immunocompromised, smoke cigarettes, or have chronic lung disease.
- Scant sputum production, pleuritic chest pain, toxic appearance.
- CXR: focal patchy infiltrates or consolidation.
- Gram stain of sputum: polymorphonuclear leukocytes and no organisms.

General Considerations

Legionella is an important cause of community or hospital acquired pneumonia and should be considered whenever the etiology of pneumonia is in question. Legionnaires' disease (*Legionella* pneumonia) is more common in persons who smoke cigarettes and in those with chronic lung disease or who are immunocompromised. Outbreaks have been associated with contaminated water sources, such as showerheads and faucets in patient rooms and air conditioning cooling towers.

Clinical Findings

A. Symptoms and Signs

Legionnaires' disease is one of the atypical pneumonias, so called because a Gram-stained smear of sputum does not demonstrate organisms. However, many features of Legionnaires' disease are more like typical pneumonia, with high fevers, toxic appearance, and pleurisy. Associated clinical findings may include nausea, vomiting, diarrhea, and relative bradycardia. Classically, this pneumonia is caused by *Legionella pneumophila*, though other *Legionella* species can cause identical disease.

B. Laboratory Findings

Laboratory findings may include hyponatremia and/or elevated liver enzymes, BUN, creatinine, and creatine kinase. *Legionella* requires special media (charcoal–yeast extract agar or similar enriched media) and is difficult to detect in culture. PCR testing on respiratory samples (ideally sputum or bronchoalveolar lavage) detects all clinically relevant *Legionella* species/serotypes. *Legionella* urinary antigen testing detects only *L pneumophila* serotype 1, which causes 80–90% of *legionella* cases in the United States. *Legionella* serology (acute and convalescent) is a less sensitive diagnostic method.

Treatment

Azithromycin (500 mg orally or intravenously once daily) or a fluoroquinolone (eg, once-daily levofloxacin 750 mg or moxifloxacin 400 mg, administered either orally or intravenously) are drugs of choice for treatment of legionellosis. Duration of therapy is generally 7–10 days, although a 14- to 21-day course of therapy is recommended for immunocompromised patients or those with severe disease.

Rello J. Severe Legionnaires' disease. Ann Intensive Care. 2024;14:51. [PMID: 38565811]

GRAM-NEGATIVE BACTEREMIA & SEPSIS

Gram-negative bacteremia can originate in several sites, the most common being the genitourinary system, hepatobiliary tract, GI tract, and lungs. Less common sources include intravenous lines, infusion fluids, surgical wounds, drains, and pressure injuries. Patients with sepsis secondary to gram-negative bacteremia, particularly those who are immunocompromised, may be severely ill, with mortality rates approaching up to 40% or higher.

Clinical Findings

A. Symptoms and Signs

Most patients have fevers and chills, often with abrupt onset, though some patients may be hypothermic or normothermic. Hyperventilation with respiratory alkalosis and changes in mental status can be early manifestations. Hypotension and shock are unfavorable prognostic signs.

B. Laboratory Findings

Neutropenia or neutrophilia, often with increased numbers of immature forms of polymorphonuclear leukocytes, are the most common laboratory abnormalities in septic patients. Patients may also have thrombocytopenia, laboratory evidence of coagulation abnormalities, or overt disseminated intravascular coagulation. Blood cultures may not always be positive; obtaining two sets of blood cultures from separate sites, ideally before starting antibiotics (if there is no substantial delay in starting antibiotics thereafter), can increase culture yield.

Treatment

Several factors are important in the management of sepsis, including that attributable to gram-negative bacteremia.

A. Removal of Predisposing Factors

When possible, this may mean decreasing or stopping immunosuppressive medications and, in certain circumstances, giving granulocyte colony-stimulating factor (filgrastim; G-CSF) to patients with neutropenia.

B. Identifying the Source of Bacteremia

By finding the source of bacteremia and removing (central venous catheter) or draining it (abscess), a potentially fatal disease becomes treatable.

C. Supportive Measures

The use of fluids, vasopressors, and corticosteroids in septic shock is discussed in Chapter 14. Management of disseminated intravascular coagulation is discussed in Chapter 16.

D. Antibiotics

Antibiotics should be given as soon as sepsis is suspected, since delays in therapy have been associated with increased mortality rates, particularly once hypotension develops. In general, bactericidal antibiotics should be used and given intravenously to ensure therapeutic serum levels up front. Antibiotics that penetrate the primary site of infection are critical for successful treatment—ie, if the infection originates in the CNS, antibiotics that penetrate the blood–brain barrier should be used (such as third- or fourth- but not first-generation cephalosporins, which penetrate poorly). Because sepsis caused by gram-positive organisms cannot be differentiated on clinical grounds from that due to gram-negative bacteria, initial therapy should include antibiotics active against both types of organisms.

The number of antibiotics necessary remains controversial and depends on the source of bacteremia. Table 34–6 provides a guide for empiric therapy. Although a combination of antibiotics may be recommended in patients who are critically ill and/or at risk for multidrug-resistant organisms, a single-drug regimen (such as a third-generation cephalosporin, piperacillin-tazobactam, or carbapenem) is often appropriate. If multiple drugs are used initially, the regimen should be modified and coverage narrowed based on culture and sensitivity testing results. Rapid molecular diagnostic testing on positive blood cultures can decrease time to species identification and detection of resistance mechanisms.

Uncomplicated gram-negative bacteremia (such as a bacteremic urinary tract infection secondary to *E coli*) may be successfully treated with as few as 7 days of antibiotic therapy. In patients with presumed septic shock who respond clinically to antibiotic therapy—but in whom blood cultures remain negative and the source of infection is unclear—consider extending therapy to 10–14 days.

Evans L et al. Surviving sepsis campaign: international guidelines for management of sepsis and septic shock 2021. Intensive Care Med. 2021;47:1181. [PMID: 34599691]

Yahav D et al; Bacteremia Duration Study Group. Seven versus 14 days of antibiotic therapy for uncomplicated gram-negative bacteremia: a noninferiority randomized controlled trial. Clin Infect Dis. 2019;69:1091. [PMID: 30535100]

SALMONELLOSIS

Salmonellosis includes infection by any of > 2000 serotypes of salmonellae. Human infections are caused almost exclusively by *S enterica* subsp *enterica*, of which three serotypes—Typhi, Typhimurium, and Enteritidis—are predominantly isolated. Clinical patterns of infection include enteric fever (eg, typhoid fever due to *Salmonella enterica* subsp *enterica* serovars Typhi or Paratyphi) and acute enterocolitis (typically caused by non-typhoidal *Salmonella* serotypes). All types are typically acquired via ingestion of the organism, usually from contaminated food or drink.

1. Enteric Fever (Typhoid Fever)

ESSENTIALS OF DIAGNOSIS

- Gradual onset of headache, vomiting, abdominal pain.
- Rose spots, relative bradycardia, splenomegaly, and abdominal distention and tenderness.
- Slow (stepladder) rise of fever to maximum and then slow return to normal.
- Leukopenia; blood, stool, and urine cultures positive for *Salmonella*.

General Considerations

Enteric fever is a clinical syndrome characterized by GI and constitutional symptoms such as fever, malaise, and headache. The infection may have a long incubation period (6–30 days), and the GI symptoms may resolve but then recur. Enteric fever is caused by typhoidal serotypes of *Salmonella*, namely Typhi and, to a lesser extent, Paratyphi (subtypes A, B, and C).

Infection begins when organisms breach the mucosal epithelium of the intestines. Having crossed the epithelial barrier, the organisms invade and replicate in macrophages in Peyer's patches, mesenteric lymph nodes, and the spleen. Bacteremia occurs, and the infection then localizes principally in the lymphoid tissue of the small intestine. Peyer's patches become inflamed and may ulcerate, with greatest involvement during the third week of disease. The organism may disseminate to the lungs, gallbladder, kidneys, or CNS.

Clinical Findings

A. Symptoms and Signs

During the prodromal stage, patients experience increasing malaise, headache, cough, and sore throat, often with abdominal pain and constipation, while their fever ascends in a stepwise fashion. After about 7–10 days, the fever plateaus, and the patient is much more ill. Marked constipation, especially early, or "pea soup" diarrhea may develop; abdominal distention also occurs. If there are no complications, the patient's condition will gradually improve over the next 7–10 days, though relapse may occur for up to 2 weeks following defervescence.

There are few physical exam findings during the early prodrome. Later, splenomegaly, abdominal distention and tenderness, relative bradycardia, and occasionally meningismus occur. A rash (known as rose spots) commonly appears during the second week of disease. Rose spots are found principally on the trunk, appear as pink papules 2–3 mm in diameter that fade on pressure, and disappear in 3–4 days.

B. Laboratory Findings

Unlike other causes of gram-negative bacteremia, most patients with enteric fever do not have leukocytosis; leukopenia may be observed instead. Transaminitis is common; anemia and thrombocytopenia may also occur. Typhoid fever is best diagnosed by blood culture, which may be positive in the first week of illness in approximately 80% of patients who have not taken antimicrobials. The rate of positivity declines thereafter, but one-fourth of patients or more may still have positive blood cultures in the third week. Cultures of bone marrow are occasionally positive when blood cultures are not. Stool cultures are often negative by the time systemic symptoms develop.

Differential Diagnosis

Enteric fever must be distinguished from other GI illnesses and from other infections that have few localizing findings. Examples include tuberculosis, infective endocarditis, brucellosis, lymphoma, and Q fever. There is often a history of recent travel to endemic areas (such as Eastern or Southern Asia, Africa, the Caribbean, Central or South America, and the Middle East); consider viral hepatitis, malaria, and amebiasis in the differential.

Complications

Complications occur in about 30% of untreated cases and may result in mortality. Intestinal hemorrhage, manifested by a sudden drop in blood pressure and signs of shock followed by dark or fresh blood in the stool, or intestinal perforation, accompanied by abdominal pain and tenderness, are most likely to occur during the third week. Appearance of leukocytosis and tachycardia should suggest these complications. Urinary retention, pneumonia, thrombophlebitis, myocarditis, neurologic complications, cholecystitis, nephritis, osteomyelitis, and meningitis are less often observed.

Prognosis

The mortality rate of typhoid fever is about 2% in treated cases. Older or debilitated patients are likely to have worse outcomes. With complications, the prognosis is poor. Relapses occur in up to 10% of patients. A residual carrier state may persist despite therapy.

Prevention

Immunization is not always effective but should be considered for household contacts of a typhoid carrier, for travelers to endemic areas, and during epidemic outbreaks. A multiple-dose oral vaccine and a single-dose intramuscular vaccine are available. Their efficacies are similar, but the oral vaccine causes fewer side effects. Boosters, when indicated, should be given every 5 and 2 years for oral and parenteral preparations, respectively.

Adequate waste disposal and protection of food and water supplies from contamination are important public health measures to prevent salmonellosis. Carriers cannot work as food handlers.

Treatment

A. Specific Measures

Globally, most *S enterica* subsp *enterica* serotypes Typhi and Paratyphi isolates remain susceptible to azithromycin and ceftriaxone. When treating empirically, ceftriaxone (2 g intravenous daily for 7–14 days) or azithromycin (1 g orally once, then 500 mg orally for 5–7 days) are reasonable choices for most patients returning from international travel. Due to high rates of antimicrobial resistance, patients who acquire typhoid fever in Pakistan or Iraq (or who did not travel internationally before becoming ill) should be treated with either azithromycin (for uncomplicated disease; dosages as above) or meropenem (for complicated disease; 1–2 g given intravenously every 8 hours). Combination therapy (ceftriaxone or meropenem plus azithromycin) should be considered for all hospitalized patients.

Dexamethasone (3 mg/kg initially, then 1 mg/kg every 6 hours for 48 hours) is indicated in critically ill patients, such as those with shock or encephalopathy. Fluoroquinolones (levofloxacin 750 mg once daily, given orally or intravenously, or twice-daily ciprofloxacin given as 500 mg orally or 400 mg intravenously) can be used when isolates are known to be susceptible. When an infection is caused by a multidrug-resistant strain, select an antibiotic to which the isolate is susceptible in vitro.

B. Treatment of Carriers

Fluoroquinolones (eg, ciprofloxacin, 500–750 mg orally twice a day for 4 weeks) have proved to be effective in eradicating the carrier state. When the isolate is susceptible, treatment of carriage with amoxicillin, ampicillin, or trimethoprim-sulfamethoxazole may be successful. *Salmonella* may sequester in the gallbladder; cholecystectomy may be required if prolonged antimicrobial therapy fails.

Kuehn R et al. Enteric (typhoid and paratyphoid) fever. Lancet. 2025;406:1283. [PMID: 40914181]

2. *Salmonella* Gastroenteritis

By far the most common form of salmonellosis is acute enterocolitis, which is typically caused by non-typhoidal *Salmonella*. The incubation period is 6–72 hours after ingesting contaminated food or liquid.

Symptoms and signs consist of fever (often with chills), nausea and vomiting, cramping abdominal pain, and diarrhea, which may be grossly bloody, lasting 4–7 days; the differential diagnosis also includes viral gastroenteritis, food poisoning, shigellosis, amoebic dysentery, and acute ulcerative colitis. The diagnosis is made by culturing the organism from stool. The disease is usually self-limited, but bacteremia with localization in joints or bones may occur, especially in patients with sickle cell disease.

In most cases, treatment of uncomplicated enterocolitis is symptomatic only, since most illnesses are self-limited and antimicrobial treatment may prolong bacterial shedding. However, certain patients—including those who are malnourished or severely ill, have sickle cell disease, or are immunocompromised (including those with advanced HIV)—should be treated, typically with fluoroquinolones (ciprofloxacin, 500 mg orally twice a day, or once-daily oral levofloxacin 500 mg) if their infection was locally acquired. Patients requiring treatment after international travel should instead be treated with daily azithromycin (500 mg orally) or ceftriaxone (2 g intravenously). Duration of therapy depends on severity of disease and the patient's immune status; patients are generally treated for 7–14 days (14 days for immunocompromised patients).

Patel P et al. Updates and current knowledge on the common forms of gastroenteritis: a review. J Clin Med. 2025;14:3465. [PMID: 40429459]

Shane AL et al. 2017 Infectious Diseases Society of America clinical practice guidelines for the diagnosis and management of infectious diarrhea. Clin Infect Dis. 2017;65:1963. [PMID: 29194529]

3. Complications of *Salmonella* Bacteremia

Salmonella infections may manifest as prolonged or recurrent fevers accompanied by bacteremia and local infection in bone, joints, pleura, pericardium, lungs, or other sites. Mycotic aortic aneurysms may also occur. These complications tend to occur in immunocompromised patients, including those with advanced HIV, or in older adults with preexisting aneurysms or atherosclerotic plaques. Serotypes other than Typhi may be isolated. Treatment requires systemic antimicrobial therapy (duration depends on the site of infection) plus drainage of any abscesses. In patients with HIV infection, relapse is common, and suppressive therapy may be needed until immune reconstitution has been achieved with antiretroviral therapy. If the organism is susceptible, a fluoroquinolone—such as ciprofloxacin, 750 mg orally twice a day—may be effective both for therapy of acute infection and for suppression of recurrence (when needed). Incidence of infections caused by drug-resistant strains may be on the rise.

SHIGELLOSIS

ESSENTIALS OF DIAGNOSIS

- Diarrhea, often with blood and mucus.
- Crampy abdominal pain and systemic toxicity.
- Leukocytes in stool; positive stool culture.

General Considerations

Shigella dysentery is a common disease, often self-limited and mild but occasionally serious. *S sonnei* is the leading cause in the United States, followed by *S flexneri*. *S dysenteriae* causes the most serious form of illness. Shigellae are invasive organisms. Because the infective dose is low (on the order of 10 to 100 organisms), shigellosis is highly transmissible via the fecal-oral route—including ingestion of contaminated food and water as well as oral–anal sexual contact, particularly in men who have sex with men. There has been a rise in strains resistant to multiple antibiotics.

Clinical Findings

A. Symptoms and Signs

The illness usually starts abruptly, with diarrhea, lower abdominal cramps, and tenesmus. The diarrhea is often mixed with blood and/or mucus and associated with abdominal tenderness. Systemic symptoms include fever, chills, anorexia and malaise, and headache. Sigmoidoscopic examination, if done, reveals an inflamed, engorged mucosa with punctate and sometimes large areas of ulceration.

B. Laboratory Findings

The stool contains many leukocytes and red cells. Stool culture is positive for *Shigella* in most cases, but blood cultures rarely grow the organism (0–7% of cases).

Differential Diagnosis

Dysentery due to *Shigella* must be distinguished from *Salmonella* enterocolitis and from infections due to enterotoxigenic *Escherichia coli, Campylobacter*, and *Yersinia enterocolitica*. Amoebic dysentery may have a similar clinical presentation and is diagnosed by finding amoebas in a fresh stool specimen. Ulcerative colitis is another cause of bloody diarrhea.

Complications

Temporary disaccharidase deficiency, resulting in carbohydrate malabsorption and symptoms like irritable bowel syndrome, may follow the diarrhea. Reactive arthritis is an uncommon complication, usually occurring in HLA-B27 positive individuals infected with *Shigella*. Hemolytic-uremic syndrome also occurs rarely. Intestinal complications may include proctitis, intestinal obstruction, and colonic perforation.

Treatment

Antibiotics are not required for uncomplicated, self-resolving gastroenteritis. On the other hand, along with treatment of dehydration and hypotension, antibiotics are recommended in severe cases, and in immunocompromised patients. Antimicrobial therapy should ideally be guided by antibiotic susceptibility testing. Options generally include either a fluoroquinolone (oral or intravenous ciprofloxacin, 750 mg once or twice daily, or levofloxacin, 500 mg once daily for 3–5 days) or ceftriaxone, 1–2 g intravenously once daily for 5 days. If the isolate is susceptible, trimethoprim-sulfamethoxazole, 160/80 mg orally twice daily for 5 days, or azithromycin, 500 mg orally once daily for 3 days, are also effective. Longer durations of therapy (7–10 days) may be indicated for immunocompromised patients. High rates of resistance to amoxicillin and ampicillin make these less effective treatment options. There are also increasing concerns regarding resistance to ceftriaxone, azithromycin, and fluoroquinolones, particularly among men who have sex with men.

Patel P et al. Updates and current knowledge on the common forms of gastroenteritis: a review. J Clin Med. 2025;14:3465. [PMID: 40429459]

Shane AL et al. 2017 Infectious Diseases Society of America clinical practice guidelines for the diagnosis and management of infectious diarrhea. Clin Infect Dis. 2017;65:1963. [PMID: 29194529]

GASTROENTERITIS CAUSED BY *ESCHERICHIA COLI*

E coli causes gastroenteritis by a variety of mechanisms. Enterotoxigenic *E coli* (ETEC) elaborates either a heat-stable or heat-labile toxin that mediates the disease; this pathogen, along with enteroaggregative *E coli* (EAEC), is an important cause of traveler's diarrhea, which is typically watery (see Chapter 34, Traveler's Diarrhea). Enteroinvasive *E coli* (EIEC), which is uncommon in the United States, differs from other *E coli* bowel pathogens in that these strains invade cells, causing bloody diarrhea and dysentery-like infection. Neither ETEC nor EIEC strains are routinely identified from stool cultures, but they can be detected on stool-based PCRs that detect specific virulence genes. Antimicrobial therapy, such as oral azithromycin (either 1000 mg × 1 or 500 mg daily for 3 days) or ciprofloxacin (750 mg daily for 3 days), shortens the clinical course, but the disease is usually self-limited.

Shiga-toxin–producing *E coli* (STEC) infection can result in either asymptomatic carriage, diarrhea that may begin as watery, hemorrhagic colitis, hemolytic-uremic syndrome, or thrombotic thrombocytopenic purpura. Although *E coli* O157:H7 is responsible for most cases of STEC infection in the United States, other STEC strains that cause severe disease have been reported. *E coli* O157:H7 has caused several outbreaks of diarrhea and hemolytic-uremic syndrome related to consumption of products including undercooked hamburger, raw flour, unpasteurized apple juice, and spinach. Older individuals and young children are most affected, with hemolytic-uremic syndrome being more common in the latter group. STEC identification can be difficult. The CDC recommends that all stools submitted for routine testing from patients with acute community-acquired diarrhea be simultaneously cultured for *E coli* O157:H7 and tested for Shiga toxins to detect non-O157 STEC. Antimicrobial therapy does not alter the course of the disease and may increase the risk of hemolytic-uremic syndrome. Treatment is primarily supportive. Hemolytic-uremic syndrome or thrombotic thrombocytopenic purpura occurring in association with a diarrheal illness suggests the diagnosis and should prompt evaluation for STEC. Confirmed STEC infections should be reported to public health officials.

Collins JP et al. Preliminary incidence and trends of infections with pathogens transmitted commonly through food—Foodborne Diseases Active Surveillance Network, 10 U.S. Sites, 2016-2021. MMWR Morb Mortal Wkly Rep. 2022;71:1260. [PMID: 36201372]

Patel P et al. Updates and current knowledge on the common forms of gastroenteritis: a review. J Clin Med. 2025;14:3465. [PMID: 40429459]

CHOLERA

ESSENTIALS OF DIAGNOSIS

- History of travel to endemic area or contact with infected person.
- Voluminous diarrhea (up to 1 L/hour).
- Characteristic "rice water stool."
- Rapid development of marked dehydration.
- Positive stool cultures.

General Considerations

Cholera is an acute diarrheal illness caused by certain serotypes of *Vibrio cholerae*. The disease is toxin-mediated, and fever is unusual. The toxin activates adenylyl cyclase in intestinal epithelial cells of the small intestines, producing hypersecretion of water and chloride ion and resulting in significant diarrhea of up to 1 L/hour. The resulting profound hypovolemia can lead to death. Cholera occurs in epidemics, typically under conditions of crowding, war, and famine (eg, in refugee camps) and where sanitation is inadequate. The infection is acquired via ingestion of contaminated food or water.

Clinical Findings

Cholera is characterized by a sudden onset of severe, frequent watery diarrhea (up to 1 L/hour). The liquid stool is gray and turbid, without fecal odor, blood, or pus ("rice water stool"). Dehydration and hypotension develop rapidly. Definitive diagnosis is based on positive stool culture. Rapid stool antigen and PCR-based stool testing are also available.

Treatment

Treatment is primarily via fluid replacement. In mild or moderate illness, oral rehydration is usually adequate. A simple oral replacement fluid can be made from 1/2 teaspoon of table salt and 6 level teaspoons of sugar added to 1 L of water. Intravenous fluids are indicated for patients with signs of severe hypovolemia and those who cannot take adequate fluids orally. Lactated Ringer infusion is satisfactory.

Antimicrobial therapy shortens the course of illness and is indicated for severely ill patients. Antimicrobials active against *V cholerae* include doxycycline (300 mg orally in a single dose), azithromycin (1 g orally in a single dose), or ciprofloxacin (also 1 g orally in a single dose) as an alternative. Multidrug-resistant strains exist, so susceptibility testing, if available, is advisable.

Prevention

Oral cholera vaccines confer some protection and may be required for entry into or re-entry after travel to some countries. One live attenuated oral vaccine is approved for use in the United States for persons traveling to areas of active cholera transmission. Supplies of the oral vaccine have been limited.

When to Admit

- Severe diarrhea.
- Moderate to severe dehydration in need of parenteral fluid replacement.
- Inability to maintain fluid replacement because there can be rapid development of dehydration.

Collins JP et al. Cholera vaccine: recommendations of the Advisory Committee on Immunization Practices, 2022. MMWR Morb Mortal Wkly Rep. 2022;71:1. [PMID: 36173766]

Kanungo S et al. Cholera. Lancet. 2022;399:1429. [PMID: 35397865]

INFECTIONS CAUSED BY OTHER *VIBRIO* SPECIES

Vibrios other than *V cholerae* that cause human disease are *V parahaemolyticus*, *V vulnificus*, and *V alginolyticus*. All are halophilic marine organisms. Infection is acquired by exposure to organisms in contaminated, undercooked, or raw crustaceans or shellfish and/or warm (> 15–20°C) ocean waters and estuaries. Infections are more common during the summer months, in regions along the Atlantic coast and the Gulf of Mexico in the United States and from tropical waters worldwide. Oysters are implicated in up to 90% of food-related cases.

V parahaemolyticus causes acute watery diarrhea with crampy abdominal pain and fever, typically occurring within 24 hours after ingestion of contaminated shellfish. The disease is self-limited, and antimicrobial therapy is usually not necessary. Patients with chronic liver disease and those who are immunocompromised should be cautioned to avoid eating raw oysters. *V parahaemolyticus* may also cause cellulitis and sepsis, though these findings are more characteristic of *V vulnificus* infection.

V vulnificus and *V alginolyticus* are important causes of cellulitis, wound infections, and primary bacteremia following exposure to sea water or ingestion of contaminated shellfish. Cellulitis with or without sepsis may be accompanied by bulla formation and necrosis with extensive soft tissue destruction, at times requiring debridement or amputation. The infection can be rapidly progressive and is particularly severe in immunocompromised individuals—especially those with cirrhosis or other hepatic disease—with death rates exceeding 50%.

For severe disease caused by non-*cholerae Vibrio* species, primary antibiotic regimens include intravenous ceftazidime (1 g every 8 hours) or ceftriaxone (2 g daily), given with either doxycycline (100 mg orally or intravenously every 12 hours) or ciprofloxacin (750 mg orally twice per day or 400 mg intravenously every 12 hours).

INFECTIONS CAUSED BY *CAMPYLOBACTER* SPECIES

Campylobacter organisms are microaerophilic, motile, gram-negative rods. *Campylobacter* enteritis is typically caused by either *C jejuni* or *C coli*, both of which cause a gastroenteritis associated with fever, abdominal pain, and diarrhea characterized by loose, watery, or bloody stools. Dairy cattle and poultry are an important reservoir for campylobacters. Outbreaks of enteritis have been associated with consumption of raw milk. The differential diagnosis includes shigellosis, *Salmonella* gastroenteritis, and enteritis caused by *Y enterocolitica* or invasive *E coli*. The disease is self-limited, but its duration can be shortened modestly (by about 1 day) with antimicrobial therapy. Azithromycin (1 g orally as a single dose or 500 mg orally daily for 3 days) is effective therapy for uncomplicated gastroenteritis due to *C jejuni or C coli*. Isolates may be resistant to fluoroquinolones and doxycycline, particularly if acquired outside of the United States.

A third species of *Campylobacter*, *C fetus* causes systemic infections that can be fatal, including primary bacteremia, endocarditis, meningitis, and focal abscesses. It infrequently causes gastroenteritis. Patients infected with *C fetus* are often older, debilitated, or immunocompromised. Systemic infections can be treated with intravenous imipenem-cilastatin (500 mg every 6 hours), meropenem (1 g every 8 hours), ertapenem (1 g daily), or ampicillin (100 mg/kg/day, given in divided doses every 6 hours). Meropenem at 2 g intravenously every 8 hours is appropriate for CNS infections due to its ability to penetrate the blood–brain barrier.

Patel P et al. Updates and current knowledge on the common forms of gastroenteritis: a review. J Clin Med. 2025;14:3465. [PMID: 40429459]

Shane AL et al. 2017 Infectious Diseases Society of America clinical practice guidelines for the diagnosis and management of infectious diarrhea. Clin Infect Dis. 2017;65:1963. [PMID: 29194529]

PLAGUE

ESSENTIALS OF DIAGNOSIS

- History of exposure to rodents in endemic area.
- Sudden onset of high fever, muscle pains, and prostration.
- Axillary, cervical, or inguinal lymphadenitis (buboes).
- Pustule or ulcer at inoculation site.
- Pneumonia or meningitis may be fatal.
- Positive smear and culture from bubo and positive blood culture.

General Considerations

Plague is a zoonotic infection carried by wild rodents and caused by *Yersinia pestis*, a small gram-negative rod with bipolar staining on Wright, Giemsa, or Wayson stains. Most human cases in the United States occur in California, Arizona, Nevada, Oregon, Colorado, and New Mexico. Countries with the most cases worldwide include the Democratic Republic of the Congo, Madagascar, and Peru. Plague is transmitted among rodents and to humans by the bites of fleas or from contact with infected animals. Following a fleabite, the organisms spread through the lymphatics to the lymph nodes, which become greatly enlarged (buboes). They may then reach the bloodstream and disseminate to involve all organs. When pneumonia or meningitis develops, the outcome may be fatal. Patients with pneumonia can transmit the infection to others via droplets. The incubation period for bubonic plague is 2–8 days. Because of its extreme virulence and potential for dissemination and person-to-person transmission, plague is considered a high-priority agent for bioterrorism.

Clinical Findings

A. Symptoms and Signs

The onset of plague is sudden, with high fever, malaise, tachycardia, intense headache, delirium, and severe myalgias; patients appear profoundly ill and may have a pustule or ulcer at the site of inoculation. Axillary, inguinal, or cervical lymph nodes become enlarged and tender and may suppurate and drain (bubonic plague). With hematogenous spread (septicemic or bacteremic plague), patients may rapidly become toxic and comatose, with purpuric spots (black plague) appearing on the skin. There may be signs of meningitis.

If pneumonia develops, tachypnea, productive cough, blood-tinged sputum, and cyanosis also occur. Primary pneumonic plague is a fulminant pneumonitis with bloody, frothy sputum and sepsis. It is usually fatal unless treatment is started within a few hours after onset.

B. Laboratory Findings

The plague bacillus may be found in smears from aspirates of buboes examined with Gram staining or other special stains. Cultures from bubo aspirate or pus, blood, CSF, and sputum can be positive, but the organism may grow slowly. Acute and convalescent serum samples can help make the diagnosis serologically (using agglutination tests). In cases where tissue is available—such as from lymph nodes, lung, liver, or bone marrow—direct detection methods using PCR or direct fluorescent antibody testing also may be helpful.

Differential Diagnosis

The lymphadenitis of plague may be mistaken for the lymphadenitis accompanying either staphylococcal or streptococcal infections of the extremities, sexually transmitted infections such as lymphogranuloma venereum or syphilis, or tularemia. Systemic manifestations resemble those of enteric or rickettsial fevers, malaria, or influenza, while pneumonia and meningeal infections attributable to plague resemble those caused by other bacteria.

Prevention

Avoiding exposure to rodents and fleas in endemic areas is the best prevention strategy. Drug prophylaxis may provide temporary protection for those exposed to plague, particularly via the respiratory route. Doxycycline, 100 mg orally twice daily for 7 days, is effective as prophylaxis, as are fluoroquinolones (ciprofloxacin, 500–750 mg orally every 12 hours, levofloxacin, 750 mg orally once daily, or moxifloxacin, 400 mg orally once daily; all are given for 7-day courses). No vaccine is available.

Treatment

Therapy should be started immediately once plague is suspected. Either a fluoroquinolone (ciprofloxacin, 400 mg intravenously every 8 hours, or 750 mg orally every 12 hours; levofloxacin, 750 mg intravenously or orally every 24 hours; or moxifloxacin, 400 mg intravenously or orally every 24 hours) or an aminoglycoside (such as intravenous gentamicin, 5 mg/kg every 24 hours) is effective. The duration of therapy is 10–14 days. Combination therapy with two different classes of antimicrobials is recommended for the initial treatment of patients with severe pneumonic or septicemic plague. Alternative treatment options include doxycycline (200-mg loading dose, then 100 mg every 12 hours intravenously or orally) or trimethoprim-sulfamethoxazole (5 mg/kg of the trimethoprim component, given intravenously or orally every 8 hours). Patients with plague pneumonia are placed in strict respiratory isolation, and prophylactic therapy is given to any person who had contact with the patient.

Nelson CA et al. Antimicrobial treatment and prophylaxis of plague: recommendations for naturally acquired infections and bioterrorism response. MMWR Recomm Rep. 2021;70:1. [PMID: 34264565]

GONOCOCCAL INFECTIONS

ESSENTIALS OF DIAGNOSIS

- Purulent, profuse urethral discharge with dysuria; classically yields positive Gram stain.
- Urethritis, epididymitis, prostatitis, proctitis, pharyngitis.
- Cervicitis with purulent discharge; vaginitis; salpingitis.
- Preferred method of diagnosis at a mucosal site is testing with nucleic acid amplification
- Disseminated disease: fever, rash, tenosynovitis, and arthritis; can also cause bacteremia, septic arthritis, and endocarditis.

General Considerations

Gonorrhea is caused by *Neisseria gonorrhoeae*, a gram-negative diplococcus typically found inside polymorphonuclear cells. It is transmitted during sexual activity and has its greatest incidence in the 15- to 29-year-old age group. The incubation period is usually 2–8 days.

Clinical Findings

A. Urethritis and Cervicitis

1. Penile/urethral infections—Initial symptoms include burning on urination and a serous or milky discharge. One to 3 days later, urethral pain is more pronounced, and the discharge becomes yellow, creamy, and profuse, occasionally blood-tinged. The symptoms may regress and become more chronic or progress to involve the prostate, epididymis, and periurethral glands with painful inflammation. Chronic infection can lead to prostatitis or urethral strictures. Rectal infection (proctitis) is common in men who have sex with men. Extragenital mucosal sites of primary infection (eg, the pharynx or rectum) must always be considered. Asymptomatic infection can occur in all genders.

2. Cervicovaginal infections—Cervicovaginal gonococcal infections may present with dysuria, urinary frequency and urgency, and/or a purulent discharge. Infections may be asymptomatic or present with only slightly increased vaginal discharge and moderate cervicitis on exam. Infections may also persist as chronic cervicitis, serving as an important reservoir for gonococci. Cervicovaginal gonorrhea can progress to involve the uterus and Fallopian tubes with acute and chronic salpingitis, potentially resulting in scarring and infertility. In pelvic inflammatory disease, anaerobes and chlamydia often accompany gonococci. Rectal infection may result from spread of the organism from the genital tract or from receptive anal intercourse.

Nucleic acid amplification tests have excellent sensitivity and specificity; they are the preferred method for diagnosing gonorrhea at all mucosal sites, regardless of gender or sex. In patients with suspected cervicovaginal infections, endocervical or vaginal swabs (preferred; clinician- or self-collected) as well as first-catch morning urine samples are options for testing. In people with suspected penile/urethral infections, first-catch AM urine is recommended. Nucleic acid amplification tests are also recommended for gonorrhea screening and testing at pharyngeal and rectal sites. Urine testing does not detect oropharyngeal or rectal gonorrhea unless there is concurrent genital infection. Gram stain of urethral, cervicovaginal, or rectal discharge may show gram-negative diplococci in polymorphonuclear leukocytes. Cultures and antimicrobial susceptibility testing should be obtained to evaluate for antimicrobial resistance whenever there is concern for gonococcal treatment failure at any mucosal site.

B. Disseminated Disease

Disseminated gonococcal infection (DGI) occurs rarely when gonorrhea invades the bloodstream from a mucosal site and travels to distant sites of the body. DGI can present as an arthritis–dermatitis syndrome, with skin lesions, arthralgias, and tenosynovitis. In this syndrome, arthritis and arthralgias can occur in one or more joints and may be migratory. Skin lesions, when present, can range from maculopapular to petechial, pustular, or hemorrhagic; they tend to be few in number and appear most often on the distal extremities (including the palms and soles). Tenosynovitis is often found in the hands, wrists, feet, and ankles. These unique findings can help distinguish DGI from other infectious syndromes.

DGI can also present as purulent mono- or oligoarticular septic arthritis, or—more rarely—as perihepatitis, bacteremia, meningitis, osteomyelitis, or endocarditis. Antimicrobial susceptibility testing should always be performed whenever the organism grows on culture from a disseminated site (eg, blood, cerebrospinal fluid, synovial fluid). Nucleic acid amplification testing can be performed on synovial fluid (if available) and may be more sensitive for the diagnosis. Host factors that increase the likelihood of DGI include complement deficiencies, systemic lupus erythematosus, and receipt of the monoclonal antibody eculizumab.

C. Conjunctivitis

The most common form of eye involvement is direct inoculation of gonococci into the conjunctival sac. In adults, this occurs by autoinoculation in persons with genital infections. Purulent conjunctivitis may rapidly progress to pan-ophthalmitis and loss of vision unless treated promptly.

Differential Diagnosis

Gonococcal urethritis and cervicovaginal infections must be differentiated from those caused by other pathogens (many of which are also sexually transmitted) such as *Chlamydia trachomatis* and *Trichomonas vaginalis*. Vaginal discharge can also be caused by non-sexually transmitted pathogens, including *Candida* species and *Gardnerella vaginalis*. Patients with mucosal-site gonococcal infections should be evaluated for any symptoms to suggest complications, such as DGI or pelvic inflammatory disease. They should also be screened for other sexually transmitted infections, including chlamydia, syphilis, and HIV, since coinfections are common. Reactive arthritis (urethritis, conjunctivitis, arthritis) may mimic manifestations of gonorrhea or coexist with it.

Prevention

Prevention is based on education and mechanical or biomedical prophylaxis. Condoms, if properly used, can reduce the risk of infection. Partner notification and referral of sexual contacts for gonorrhea testing and empiric treatment is recommended. In cases where partners are unable or unwilling to come into care for testing and treatment, patient-delivered expedited partner therapy with oral cefixime (800 mg in a single dose) is a helpful strategy. In terms of biomedical prevention, doxycycline 200 mg taken orally as postexposure prophylaxis preferably taken within 24 (but up to 72) hours after sex has been shown to significantly reduce the incidence of syphilis, chlamydia, and—in some studies, albeit to a lesser extent—gonorrhea among men who have sex with men and transgender women. This strategy, known as doxy PEP, seems to have contributed to reductions in incidence of chlamydia and syphilis in municipalities (such as San Francisco, CA, United States) that quickly adopted the intervention.

Treatment

Gonorrhea has developed resistance to multiple antibiotics, including penicillin, doxycycline, and ciprofloxacin. These antibiotics should not be used for treatment unless antimicrobial susceptibilities are known. Resistance to azithromycin and ceftriaxone also has been reported, although the latter is rare. Patients and their sexual partners should be treated for gonorrhea and tested for other STIs (such as HIV, chlamydia, and syphilis).

A. Uncomplicated Gonorrhea

For uncomplicated gonococcal infections of the cervix, urethra, rectum, and pharynx, the recommended treatment is ceftriaxone (500 mg intramuscularly for patients who weigh <150 kg and 1 g intramuscularly for patients who weigh 150 kg or more). Cefixime, 800 mg orally as a single dose, can be used for non-pharyngeal infections when an oral cephalosporin is the only option. When chlamydial infection has not been excluded, co-treatment of chlamydia with oral doxycycline, 100 mg twice daily for 7 days, is recommended in nonpregnant patients with gonorrhea. For penicillin-allergic patients, the recommended treatment regimen consists of gentamicin, 240 mg intramuscularly, and azithromycin, 2 g orally. As of late 2025, two new oral medications, gepotidacin and zoliflodacin, have been demonstrated in randomized controlled trials to be noninferior to the combination of ceftriaxone and azithromycin for the treatment of uncomplicated urogenital gonorrhea. These newer oral medications may be incorporated into treatment guidelines in the future.

B. Complicated Gonorrhea

Disseminated gonococcal infection (including arthritis and arthritis-dermatitis syndromes) should be treated with ceftriaxone (1–2 g intravenously or intramuscularly daily). For the arthritis-dermatitis syndrome, therapy may be switched to an oral regimen, guided by antimicrobial susceptibility testing, within 24–48 hours after substantial clinical improvement, for a total treatment course of at least 7 days. Gonococcal endocarditis should be treated with ceftriaxone (2 g every 24 hours intravenously) for at least 4 weeks.

For patients admitted to the hospital, pelvic inflammatory disease (PID) is initially treated with ceftriaxone (1 g intravenously daily) plus doxycycline (100 mg orally or intravenously twice daily) and metronidazole (500 mg orally or intravenously every 12 hours). Admitted patients can also be treated with cefoxitin (2 g intravenously every 6 hours) or cefotetan (2 g intravenously every 12 hours), both given with doxycycline (100 mg orally or intravenously twice daily). Within 24–48 hours after substantial clinical improvement, patients initially treated with intravenous therapy can be transitioned to intramuscular or oral therapy (often with doxycycline and metronidazole at the doses listed above) to complete a total 14-day course. Outpatients with PID can be treated with a one-time dose of either ceftriaxone (500 mg intravenously) or cefoxitin (2 g intramuscularly, given with a single dose of probenecid 1 g orally), both with doxycycline (100 mg orally twice daily) and metronidazole (500 mg orally twice daily) for a total of 14 days.

Luetkemeyer A et al. Postexposure doxycycline to prevent bacterial sexually transmitted infections. N Engl J Med. 2023;388:1296. [PMID: 37018493]

Tang EC et al. Characterizing the rise of disseminated gonococcal infections in California, July 2020-July 2021. Clin Infect Dis. 2023;76:194. [PMID: 36189949]

Workowski KA et al. Sexually transmitted infections treatment guidelines, 2021. MMWR Recomm Rep. 2021;70:1. [PMID: 34292926]

CHANCROID

Chancroid is an STI caused by the short gram-negative bacillus *Haemophilus ducreyi.* The incubation period is 3–7 days. A papule forms at the site of inoculation, subsequently developing into a pustule that then breaks down to form a painful, soft ulcer with a necrotic base, surrounding erythema, and undermined edges. There may be multiple lesions due to autoinoculation. Associated lymphadenitis is usually unilateral and consists of tender, matted nodes of moderate size with overlying erythema. The diagnosis can be made by culturing a swab of the lesion onto a special medium or using a lab-developed nucleic acid amplification test, but neither testing modality is widely available. In the United States, a probable case of chancroid can be diagnosed if a patient has a consistent ulcer (with or without regional lymphadenopathy) and the alternative, more common diagnoses of syphilis and herpes simplex virus have been ruled out.

Chancroid must be differentiated from other causes of genital ulcers. The chancre of syphilis is clean and classically painless, with a hard base and raised border, whereas the ulcer of chancroid is nonindurated, deep, and painful, with serpiginous borders and often a purulent exudate. Coinfections with other sexually transmitted pathogens (including syphilis, herpes simplex virus, and HIV) are very common, as is super-infection of the chancroid ulcer with other bacteria.

A single dose of either azithromycin, 1 g orally, or ceftriaxone, 250 mg intramuscularly, is recommended to treat chancroid. Effective multidose regimens are erythromycin base, 500 mg orally three times a day for 7 days, or ciprofloxacin, 500 mg orally twice a day for 3 days.

Gravett RM et al. An ulcer by any other name: non-herpes and non-syphilis ulcerative sexually transmitted infections. Infect Dis Clin North Am. 2023;37:369. [PMID: 37005160]

Workowski KA et al. Sexually transmitted infections treatment guidelines, 2021. MMWR Recomm Rep. 2021;70:1. [PMID: 34292926]

Gravett RM et al. An ulcer by any other name: non-herpes and non-syphilis ulcerative sexually transmitted infections. Infect Dis Clin North Am. 2023;37:369. [PMID: 37005160]

MYCOPLASMA GENITALIUM

The gram-negative intracellular pathogen *M genitalium* is a newly emerged sexually transmitted infection. Clinical manifestations include symptomatic urethritis and cervicitis. *M genitalium* is implicated in 15–20% of nongonococcal urethritis and 40% of persistent or recurrent urethritis cases, respectively. Cervical *M genitalium* infections have been associated with PID, preterm delivery, spontaneous pregnancy loss, and infertility (although evidence is insufficient to establish a causal relationship between *M genitalium* and pregnancy complications). Asymptomatic genitourinary and rectal carriage is common, although the clinical implications of colonization remain unclear.

Routine screening for *M genitalium* is not recommended, but testing should be performed in symptomatic people, particularly those with persistent or recurrent urethritis/cervicitis. The organism is extremely slow growing (with culture requiring up to 6 months); the diagnosis can be made instead using nucleic amplification testing on urine or urethral, penile meatal, endocervical, or vaginal swabs. Molecular tests for markers of macrolide (azithromycin) or quinolone (moxifloxacin) resistance are not widely available in the United States but may be used in other countries.

Antibiotic resistance is common, and treatment requires two different antibiotics used in sequential order. When *M genitalium* resistance testing is not available or the organism is known to be macrolide-resistant, the recommended treatment consists of doxycycline 100 mg orally twice per day for 7 days (to reduce *M genitalium* bacterial load), followed by moxifloxacin 400 mg daily by mouth for another 7 days. If resistance testing is available and the organism retains macrolide sensitivity, treatment can instead be with doxycycline 100 mg orally twice daily for 7 days followed by azithromycin (1 g orally on day 1, followed by 500 mg orally once per day for 3 more days). Sex partners of patients with confirmed *M genitalium* infections should be tested for *M genitalium* and provided treatment if their test results are positive.

Neither doxycycline nor moxifloxacin are recommended for use in pregnant patients, so *M genitalium* treatment decisions in pregnancy are made on a case-by-case basis, considering symptom severity, patient preferences, and risk/benefit discussions. Clinical consultation for complex cases involving sexually transmitted infections is available online at stdccn.org.

Workowski KA et al. Sexually transmitted infections treatment guidelines, 2021. MMWR Recomm Rep. 2021;70:1. [PMID: 34292926]

BARTONELLA SPECIES

Bartonella species are responsible for a wide variety of clinical syndromes. **Bacillary angiomatosis**, an important manifestation of bartonellosis, is discussed in Chapter 35. A variety of atypical infections, including retinitis, encephalitis, osteomyelitis, persistent bacteremia, and endocarditis (especially consider in culture-negative endocarditis), have been described.

1. *Bartonella quintana*—*B quintana* classically causes **trench fever,** a louse-borne relapsing febrile illness. The disease has occurred epidemically in louse-infested troops and civilians during wars and endemically in residents of scattered geographic areas. An urban equivalent of trench fever has been described among people experiencing homelessness. Humans acquire the infection when infected lice feces enter sites of skin breakdown. Symptom onset is abrupt: fever lasts 2–5 days, with relapses, although isolated febrile episodes or prolonged persistent fevers also can occur. Patients may report weakness and headache, with severe pain behind the eyes and in the back and legs (especially shins). Lymphadenopathy, splenomegaly, and a transient maculopapular rash may appear. The differential diagnosis includes other febrile, self-limited illnesses such as dengue, leptospirosis, malaria, relapsing fever, and typhus. Optimal therapy is uncertain, but experts suggest doxycycline, 100 mg orally twice daily for 4 weeks, given with either gentamicin (3 mg/kg intravenously once daily) or rifampin (300 mg orally twice daily) during the first 2 weeks of treatment.

2. *Bartonella henselae*—*B henselae* classically causes **cat-scratch disease,** an acute infection of children and young adults that is transmitted from cats to humans as the result of a scratch or bite, and most commonly presents as a regional lymphadenitis. Within a few days after exposure, a papule or ulcer may develop at the inoculation site. One to 3 weeks later, fever, headache, and malaise occur. Regional lymph nodes become enlarged, often tender, and may suppurate. Lymphadenopathy from cat scratch disease resembles that due to neoplasm, tuberculosis, lymphogranuloma venereum, or bacterial lymphadenitis. The diagnosis is usually made clinically. Serology can confirm the diagnosis, as can PCR or special stains performed on lymph node aspirates or biopsy. Excisional biopsy is rarely necessary, but—if done—reveals a necrotizing granulomatous lymphadenitis (which itself is not specific for cat-scratch disease). Cat-scratch disease is usually self-limited, but treatment for lymphadenitis (eg, with azithromycin, 500 mg orally once, followed by 250 mg orally daily for 4 days) is recommended to shorten the duration of illness and reduce complications. Disseminated cat-scratch disease occurs rarely but can involve either hepatosplenic or neurologic infection (including encephalitis and/or ocular manifestations).

Disseminated Forms of *Bartonella* Infection

Other disseminated forms of *Bartonella* infection—such as bacillary angiomatosis, peliosis hepatis, endocarditis, and retinitis—occur most commonly in immunocompromised patients such as those with advanced HIV or solid organ transplants. *B quintana* or *B henselae* are most often involved, although other *Bartonella* species also can cause human disease. In bacillary angiomatosis, histopathologically distinct vasculoproliferative lesions due to *Bartonella* infection develop in the skin or internal organs. In *Bartonella*-associated endocarditis, blood cultures will typically be negative. Due to the fastidious nature of the organism and its special growth requirements, serologic testing (eg, demonstration of a high antibody titer in an indirect immunofluorescence assay) or PCR tests performed on tissue or blood are often required to establish a diagnosis.

Disseminated *Bartonella* infections require prolonged courses of antibiotic therapy, with exact regimens and duration depending on the particular manifestation. Endocarditis due to *Bartonella* species can be effectively treated with doxycycline (200 mg orally or intravenously in two divided doses per day) plus either rifampin (300 mg orally or intravenously, given twice daily for the first 6 weeks) or 2 weeks of gentamicin (3 mg/kg/day intravenously, if unable to take rifampin), followed by doxycycline monotherapy for a total duration of at least 3 months. Valve surgery, if performed, may change the duration of antibiotic therapy. Relapses may occur.

DeSimone DC. Blood culture–negative endocarditis: a scientific statement from the American Heart Association. J Am Heart Assoc. 2025;14:e040218. [PMID: 40094211]

Okaro U et al. *Bartonella* species, an emerging cause of blood-culture-negative endocarditis. Clin Microbiol Rev. 2017;30:709. [PMID: 28490579]

ANAEROBIC INFECTIONS

Important types of infections caused by anaerobic organisms are listed below. Treatment of these infections may consist of surgical exploration and excision in conjunction with antimicrobial medications.

1. Head & Neck Infections

Prevotella species and anaerobic spirochetes, among other bacteria, are commonly involved in periodontal infections. These organisms, *Fusobacterium* species, and anaerobic streptococci may be implicated in chronic sinusitis, peritonsillar abscess, deep neck space infections, chronic otitis media, and/or mastoiditis. *F necrophorum* has been recognized as a cause of pharyngitis in adolescents and young adults; infection with this organism has also been associated with septic internal jugular thrombophlebitis (Lemierre syndrome), which can cause septic pulmonary embolization and/or hematogenous dissemination to other sites. Surgical debridement and drainage are as important as antimicrobials in treating many head and neck infections. Penicillin alone is generally inadequate for oral anaerobes because of penicillin resistance, usually due to β-lactamase production. Ampicillin/sulbactam 3 g intravenously every 6 hours (if parenteral therapy is required), or amoxicillin/clavulanic acid 875 mg/125 mg orally twice daily are often reasonable choices instead. Antibiotics are typically continued for a few days after symptoms and signs of infection have resolved. Indolent, established infections (like mastoiditis or osteomyelitis) may require prolonged courses of therapy, eg, 4–6 weeks or longer, using antimicrobials that penetrate bone.

2. Chest Infections

Often in the setting of poor oral hygiene and periodontal disease, aspiration of saliva may lead to necrotizing pneumonia, lung abscesses, or empyema. Polymicrobial infections are common, and anaerobes—such as *Bacteroides* species, oral gram-negative anaerobes, or anaerobic streptococci—are often among the etiologic agents. Most pulmonary infections respond to antimicrobial therapy alone. Percutaneous chest tube or surgical drainage is indicated for empyema.

Depending on the microbiology, preferred regimens may include ampicillin-sulbactam (3 g intravenously every 6 hours, followed by amoxicillin/clavulanic acid 875/125 mg orally twice daily); ceftriaxone (1–2 g intravenously every 24 hours) given with metronidazole (500 mg intravenously or orally every 6–8 hours); piperacillin-tazobactam (4.5 g intravenously every 8 hours); or moxifloxacin (400 mg intravenously or orally once daily). Clindamycin (300–450 mg orally three times daily) may be another option. Because these infections respond slowly, a prolonged course of therapy (eg, 4–6 weeks) may be recommended for complicated infections.

3. Central Nervous System

Anaerobes (especially *Bacteroides* species) are a common cause of brain abscess, subdural empyema, and septic CNS thrombophlebitis. The organisms reach the CNS by direct extension from sinusitis, otitis, or mastoiditis or by hematogenous spread from chronic lung infections. Antimicrobial therapy—eg, ceftriaxone, 2 g intravenously every 12 hours, plus metronidazole, 500 mg intravenously or orally every 8 hours—is an important adjunct to surgical drainage and should be tailored to the microbiology. Duration of therapy is 6–8 weeks but should be based on follow-up imaging. Some small brain abscesses can be treated with antibiotics alone without surgical drainage.

4. Intra-Abdominal Infections

Anaerobes—predominantly *B fragilis*, clostridia, and anaerobic streptococci—constitute > 90% of colonic bacteria. These organisms play a central role in most intra-abdominal abscesses following trauma to the colon, as well as in diverticulitis, appendicitis, perirectal or hepatic abscesses, and cholecystitis. The bacteriology of such infections typically includes anaerobes as well as other organisms, eg, enteric gram-negative rods and occasionally enterococci. Empiric therapy for intra-abdominal infections should thus be directed against both anaerobes and gram-negative aerobes. Agents that are typically active against *B fragilis* include metronidazole, piperacillin-tazobactam, or carbapenems (eg, ertapenem, imipenem-cilastatin, doripenem, or meropenem); amoxicillin-clavulanate may be an option for milder disease. Whenever source control procedures are performed, intra-abdominal fluid cultures should be obtained to further elucidate the microbiology and guide antimicrobial selection.

5. Female Genital Tract & Pelvic Infections

The normal flora of the vagina and cervix includes several species of *Bacteroides*, anaerobic and group B streptococci, lactobacilli, coliform bacteria, and, occasionally, spirochetes and clostridia. These organisms commonly cause genital tract infections and may disseminate from there.

While salpingitis is often caused by gonococci and chlamydiae, tubo-ovarian and pelvic abscesses are also commonly associated with anaerobes. Similarly, while postpartum infections may be caused by aerobic streptococci or staphylococci, anaerobes are also often involved. The most severe cases of postpartum or postabortion sepsis may be associated with clostridia and/or *Bacteroides* species. These infections have a high mortality rate without prompt treatment, generally using antimicrobials directed against both anaerobes and coliforms, combined with abscess drainage or early hysterectomy when appropriate. Potential antibiotic options for chorioamnionitis, septic abortion, or postpartum endometritis include intravenous piperacillin-tazobactam (4.5 g intravenously every 8 hours) or meropenem (1–2 g as loading dose, then 0.5–1 g every 8 hours).

6. Bacteremia & Endocarditis

Complications of anaerobic infections of the GI tract, female genital tract, oropharynx, or pressure injuries can include bacteremia and endocarditis. Cases of endocarditis due to microaerophilic or anaerobic streptococci may be effectively treated with 12–18 million units of intravenous aqueous crystalline penicillin G given daily for 4–6 weeks, although optimal therapy of anaerobic bacterial endocarditis must often rely on laboratory guidance. *Cutibacterium acnes*, clostridia, *Lactobacillus* species, and *Bacteroides* species also occasionally cause endocarditis.

7. Skin & Soft Tissue Infections

Anaerobic infections of the skin and soft tissues usually follow trauma, ischemia, or surgery and are most common in areas contaminated by oral or fecal flora. These infections also occur in persons who inject drugs or have sustained animal bites. There may be progressive tissue necrosis (Figure 37–5) and a putrid odor.

Several terms, such as *bacterial synergistic gangrene*, *synergistic necrotizing cellulitis*, *necrotizing fasciitis*, and *nonclostridial crepitant cellulitis*, have been used to classify these infections. Although there can be some differences in microbiology among them, differentiation on clinical grounds alone is difficult. All are mixed infections caused

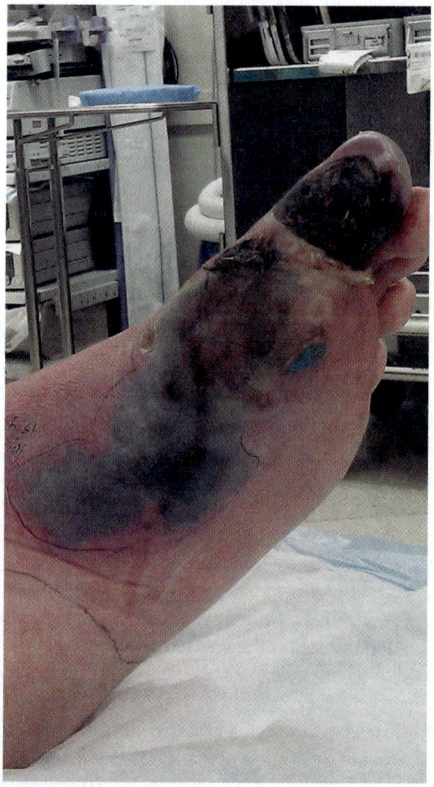

▲ **Figure 37–5.** Left foot gangrene, with plantar extension. (Used, with permission, from Dean SM, Satiani B, Abraham WT. *Color Atlas and Synopsis of Vascular Diseases*. McGraw-Hill, 2014.)

by aerobic and anaerobic organisms; they require aggressive surgical debridement of necrotic tissue for cure.

Broad-spectrum antibiotics active against both anaerobes and gram-positive and gram-negative aerobes should be instituted empirically and modified by culture results. In cases of necrotizing fasciitis, reasonable empiric regimens include either intravenous vancomycin plus piperacillin tazobactam with intravenous clindamycin, or piperacillin-tazobactam plus linezolid. Antibiotics are given for about a week after progressive tissue destruction has been controlled and the wound margins remain free of inflammation.

Bonomo RA et al. 2024 Clinical practice guideline update by the Infectious Diseases Society of America on complicated intra-abdominal infections: risk assessment, diagnostic imaging, and microbiological evaluation in adults, children, and pregnant people. Clin Infect Dis. 2024;79:S81. [PMID: 38965057]

ACTINOMYCOSIS

ESSENTIALS OF DIAGNOSIS

- Recent dental infection, abdominal trauma, or intrauterine contraception device placement.
- Chronic pneumonia or indolent cervicofacial or intra-abdominal abscess.
- Sinus tract formation.

General Considerations

Actinomyces israelii and other species of *Actinomyces* occur in the normal flora of the mouth and tonsillar crypts. When introduced into traumatized tissue and associated with other anaerobic bacteria, these actinomycetes become pathogens.

The most common site of infection is the cervicofacial area (about 60% of cases). Infection typically follows extraction of a tooth or other trauma. Lesions may develop in the GI tract or lungs following ingestion or aspiration of the organism from its endogenous source in the mouth.

Clinical Findings

A. Symptoms and Signs

1. Cervicofacial actinomycosis—Cervicofacial actinomycosis develops slowly, often after dental work or jaw trauma. The affected area becomes markedly indurated, and the overlying skin becomes reddish or cyanotic. Abscesses eventually draining to the surface persist for long periods. "Sulfur granules"—masses of filamentous organisms—may be found in the pus. There is usually little pain unless there is another secondary infection. Trismus indicates that the muscles of mastication are involved. Radiographs may reveal bony involvement. Cervicofacial or thoracic disease may occasionally involve the CNS, most commonly causing brain abscesses or meningitis.

2. Thoracic actinomycosis—Thoracic involvement begins with fever, cough, sputum production, night sweats and weight loss. Pleuritic pain may be present. Multiple sinus tracts may extend through the chest wall, to the heart, or into the abdominal cavity. Ribs may be involved. Radiography shows areas of consolidation and sometimes pleural effusion.

3. Abdominal and pelvic actinomycosis—Abdominal actinomycosis may occur after abdominal surgery and usually causes pain in the ileocecal region, spiking fever and chills, vomiting, and weight loss; it may be confused with Crohn disease. Irregular abdominal masses may be palpated. PID caused by actinomyces may involve tubo-ovarian abscesses and has been associated with prolonged use of intrauterine contraceptive devices. Sinuses draining to the exterior may develop. CT scanning may reveal an inflammatory mass extending to involve bone.

B. Laboratory Findings

The anaerobic, gram-positive organism may be demonstrated as a granule or as scattered branching gram-positive filaments in pus. Anaerobic culture is necessary to distinguish actinomycetes from *Nocardia* species because treatment differs for the two infections. Histopathologic examination of affected tissue and bone is useful in identifying organisms that are fastidious and slow to culture.

Treatment

Initial treatments of choice include intravenous penicillin G (10–20 million units per day, given in divided doses every 4–6 hours for 4–6 weeks) or intravenous ampicillin (200 mg/kg/day divided in 3–4 doses for 2–6 weeks), followed by prolonged oral therapy with penicillin VK (2–4 g per day, divided into four daily doses) or amoxicillin (2 g orally twice per day). Alternatives include intravenous ceftriaxone (2 g daily) for 2–6 weeks, followed by oral penicillin VK, amoxicillin (dosages as above), or doxycycline (100 mg orally twice per day, used for less severe disease). Response to therapy is slow. Therapy should be continued for weeks to months after clinical manifestations have disappeared to ensure cure. Surgical procedures such as drainage and resection may be beneficial. With optimal antimicrobial therapy and surgery, the prognosis is favorable. However, because actinomycosis is difficult to diagnose, extensive tissue destruction may occur before the diagnosis is confirmed and treatment initiated.

Xu Y et al. Disseminated actinomycosis. N Engl J Med. 2018;379:1071. [PMID: 30207906]

NOCARDIOSIS

ESSENTIALS OF DIAGNOSIS

- Indolent pneumonia with dissemination to CNS, skin, and bone or primary cutaneous disease.
- Suspect in setting of chronic lung disease or immunocompromised person.

General Considerations

Nocardia species are aerobic filamentous soil bacteria that can cause primary cutaneous, lymphocutaneous, pulmonary, and/or systemic nocardiosis. Common *Nocardia* species include members of the *Nocardia nova* complex, *Nocardia farcinica*, *Nocardia cyriacigeorgica*, *Nocardia brasiliensis*, and *Nocardia abscessus*. Bronchopulmonary abnormalities (eg, bronchiectasis) may predispose to colonization, while infection is more likely to occur in patients who are receiving systemic corticosteroids or are otherwise immunosuppressed.

Clinical Findings

Primary cutaneous nocardiosis represents ~20% of nocardia infections; the presentation resembles other forms of bacterial cellulitis, typically occurring after a traumatic injury. In the lymphocutaneous form of the disease, cellulitis is accompanied by ascending regional lymphadenopathy. Pulmonary nocardiosis typically presents with a cough productive of purulent sputum, often associated with malaise, weight loss, fever, and night sweats. Pulmonary infiltrates may become cavitary and may be accompanied by pleural effusions or empyema; they may also invade through the ribs and penetrate exteriorly through the chest wall.

Disseminated nocardiosis can involve any organ, with the CNS being one of the more common sites of dissemination. Even in the absence of clinical symptoms and signs of CNS infection, clinicians should pursue MRI brain imaging in patients diagnosed with nocardiosis to rule out occult CNS abscess.

Diagnostically, *Nocardia* species are usually found as delicate, branching, gram-positive filaments. They may be weakly acid-fast, occasionally causing diagnostic confusion with tuberculosis. Identification is typically made by culture with antimicrobial susceptibility testing to guide treatment options.

Treatment

For isolated primary cutaneous infections or lymphadenitis, therapy is initiated with trimethoprim-sulfamethoxazole orally or intravenously (5–10 mg/kg/day based on trimethoprim, given in 2–4 divided doses). Surgical procedures such as drainage and resection may be needed as adjunctive therapy. For pulmonary or disseminated infections, a higher dose of trimethoprim-sulfamethoxazole (15 mg/kg/day based on trimethoprim in 2–4 divided doses) should be used, typically in combination with at least one other antibiotic. Other agents generally active against *Nocardia* species include imipenem-cilastatin (500 mg intravenously every 6 hours); meropenem (2 g intravenously every 8 hours); amikacin (7.5 mg/kg intravenously every 12 hours); linezolid (600 mg intravenously or orally every 12 hours); or (for lymphadenitis and/or skin abscess) minocycline (100–200 mg orally or intravenously twice daily). Consultation with an infectious disease expert is encouraged.

Response to treatment may be slow; therapy should be continued for at least 3, 6, and 12 months for skin, lung, and CNS infections, respectively. The prognosis in systemic nocardiosis is poor when diagnosis and therapy are delayed.

Yetmar ZA et al. State-of-the-art review: modern approach to nocardiosis-diagnosis, management, and uncertainties. Clin Infect Dis. 2025;80:e53. [PMID: 40305688]

INFECTIONS CAUSED BY MYCOBACTERIA

NONTUBERCULOUS MYCOBACTERIAL DISEASES

Nontuberculous mycobacterial infections are among the most common opportunistic infections in advanced HIV but may also cause disease in immunocompetent persons. These organisms occur ubiquitously in the environment, are not communicable from person to person, have distinctive laboratory characteristics, and may be resistant to standard antitubercular drugs.

1. Pulmonary Infections

Mycobacterium avium-intracellulare complex (MAC) causes a chronic, slowly progressive pulmonary infection resembling tuberculosis in immunocompetent patients—classically those with underlying pulmonary disease. Pulmonary disease is often classified as nodular, bronchiectatic, or fibrocavitary. Treatment of pulmonary MAC requires a three-drug regimen, and macrolide susceptibility testing should be performed on all clinical isolates. For nodular or bronchiectatic disease in immunocompetent hosts, treatment may include azithromycin (500 mg), ethambutol (25 mg/kg) and rifampin (600 mg), with all three drugs given orally three times per week. For cavitary disease, treatment may consist of azithromycin (250–500 mg orally per day) plus ethambutol (15 mg/kg/day orally) plus rifampin (10 mg/kg/day up to 600 mg orally per day) and amikacin (15–25 mg/kg intravenously or intramuscularly three times weekly for the first 2–3 months). Therapy is continued for at least 12 months after sterilization of sputum cultures.

M kansasii can produce clinical disease resembling tuberculosis, but the illness progresses more slowly. Most pulmonary infections occur in patients with preexisting lung disease. Microbiologically, *M kansasii* is similar to *M tuberculosis* and is sensitive to the same drugs except pyrazinamide, to which it is resistant. Therapy with daily oral azithromycin (250–500 mg, preferred) or isoniazid 300 mg (given with pyridoxine 50 mg), plus ethambutol (15 mg/kg) and rifampin (600 mg), for at least 12 months has been successful.

Less common causes of pulmonary disease include *M xenopi*, *M szulgai*, and *M malmoense*. These organisms have variable sensitivities, and treatment is based on results of sensitivity tests. The rapidly growing mycobacteria—*M abscessus*, *M chelonae*, and *M fortuitum*—can also occasionally cause pneumonia.

Daley CL et al. Treatment of nontuberculous mycobacterial pulmonary disease: an official ATS/ERS/ESCMID/IDSA clinical practice guideline. Eur Respir J. 2020;56:2000535. [PMID: 32636299]

Nasiri MJ et al. Antibiotic therapy success rate in pulmonary *Mycobacterium avium* complex: a systematic review and meta-analysis. Expert Rev Anti Infect Ther. 2020;18:263. [PMID: 31986933]

2. Lymphadenitis

Most cases of mycobacterial cervical lymphadenitis (scrofula) in adults are caused by *M tuberculosis* and can be a manifestation of disseminated disease. In children, most cases are due to nontuberculous mycobacterial species. Infection with nontuberculous mycobacteria has been successfully treated by surgical excision with or without antituberculous drugs.

3. Skin & Soft Tissue Infections

Skin and soft tissue infections such as abscesses, septic arthritis, and osteomyelitis can result from direct inoculation, from hematogenous dissemination, or as a complication of surgery.

The rapidly growing nontuberculous mycobacteria (*M abscessus*, *M chelonae*, and *M fortuitum*) may cause these types of infections. Most cases occur on the extremities, initially presenting as nodules that may then ulcerate and form abscesses. These organisms are resistant to the usual antituberculosis drugs but (depending on the species) may have susceptibility to azithromycin, clarithromycin, amikacin, imipenem, cefoxitin, linezolid, tetracyclines, fluoroquinolones, sulfonamides, clofazimine, or bedaquiline, among other agents; antibiotic susceptibility testing is recommended. Treatment often includes surgical debridement along with at least two active antibiotics. Treatment is usually continued for at least 3–6 months, although duration must ultimately be determined based on clinical response.

M marinum infection ("swimming pool" or "fish tank" granuloma) presents as a nodular skin lesion following exposure to nonchlorinated water. Surgical excision may be recommended. Therapy is based on susceptibility testing and often involves 2–3 active agents; isolates may be susceptible to rifampin, ethambutol, and clarithromycin, among other agents.

4. Disseminated *Mycobacterium avium-intracellulare* Complex Infection

MAC causes disseminated, multiorgan disease in immunocompromised patients, especially those with HIV who have a CD4 cell count <50/mcL (see Pulmonary Disease Caused by Nontuberculous Mycobacteria, Chapter 9, for a discussion of the infection in immunocompetent patients). Signs and symptoms are nonspecific, including fever, weight loss, fatigue, night sweats, diarrhea, abdominal pain, hepatosplenomegaly, and/or lymphadenopathy. Lab abnormalities can include anemia and alkaline phosphatase elevations. The organism may be cultured from multiple sites, including blood, lymph nodes, bone marrow, or other normally sterile sites. Blood culture is the preferred means of establishing the diagnosis, with a sensitivity of 98%.

Agents with proven activity against MAC are rifabutin, azithromycin, clarithromycin, and ethambutol. A combination of two or more active agents should be used to prevent rapid emergence of secondary resistance. Clarithromycin, 500 mg orally twice daily, plus ethambutol, 15 mg/kg/day orally, with or without rifabutin, 300 mg/day orally, is the treatment of choice. Azithromycin, 500–600 mg orally once daily, may be used instead of clarithromycin in cases of drug–drug interactions or intolerance. In more severe or refractory cases, a fourth drug—such as a fluoroquinolone, injectable aminoglycoside, bedaquiline, linezolid, tedizolid, or omadacycline—may be considered. MAC therapy is usually continued for at least 12 months, although shorter durations may be possible in patients who have a high degree of immune recovery following the initiation of antiretroviral therapy. CD4 counts should exceed 100/mcL (0.1×10^9/L) for ≥ 6 months while receiving antiretroviral therapy before stopping MAC treatment.

Antimicrobial prophylaxis of MAC prevents disseminated disease and prolongs survival in certain patients with HIV. Prophylaxis is recommended for patients with HIV who have CD4 counts of ≤ 50/mcL (0.05×10^9/L) and are not on antiretroviral therapy, remain viremic despite antiretroviral therapy, or do not have options for a fully suppressive HIV regimen. MAC prophylaxis is no longer recommended in patients with HIV who immediately initiate ART or are on a fully suppressive ART regimen. In contrast to active infection, single-drug oral regimens of clarithromycin (500 mg twice daily), azithromycin (either 1200 mg once weekly or 600 mg twice weekly), or rifabutin (300 mg once daily) are appropriate for MAC prevention. Clarithromycin and azithromycin are preferred, as they are more effective and better tolerated. When previously initiated, primary prophylaxis for MAC infection can be stopped in adult and adolescent patients who are continuing fully suppressive ART.

Panel on Opportunistic Infections in Adults and Adolescents with HIV. Guidelines for the prevention and treatment of opportunistic infections in adults and adolescents with HIV: Disseminated mycobacterium avium complex disease. https://clinicalinfo.hiv.gov/en/guidelines/hiv-clinical-guidelines-adult-and-adolescent-opportunistic-infections/disseminated

MYCOBACTERIUM TUBERCULOSIS INFECTIONS

Tuberculosis is discussed in Chapter 9. Further information and expert consultation can be obtained from the Curry International Tuberculosis Center at www.currytbcenter.ucsf.edu or by telephone at (877) 390-6682.

TUBERCULOUS MENINGITIS

ESSENTIALS OF DIAGNOSIS

- Gradual onset of listlessness and anorexia.
- Headache, vomiting, and seizures common.
- Cranial nerve abnormalities typical.
- Tuberculosis focus may be evident elsewhere.
- CSF shows several hundred lymphocytes, low glucose, and high protein.

General Considerations

Tuberculous meningitis is often basilar-predominant. It may result from rupture of a meningeal tuberculoma (itself the result of earlier hematogenous seeding of tubercle bacilli from a primary pulmonary focus), or it may be a consequence of miliary spread.

Clinical Findings

A. Symptoms and Signs

The onset is usually gradual, with listlessness, irritability, anorexia, and fever, followed by headache, vomiting, convulsions, and coma. In older patients, headache and behavioral changes are prominent early symptoms. Nuchal rigidity and cranial nerve palsies occur as the meningitis progresses. Evidence of active tuberculosis elsewhere or a history of prior tuberculosis are often present.

B. Laboratory Findings

The spinal fluid is frequently yellowish, with increased opening pressure, cell count 100–500/mcL ($0.1–0.5 \times 10^9/L$) (predominantly lymphocytes, though neutrophils may be present early during infection), increased protein, and decreased glucose. Acid-fast stains of CSF are often negative, and cultures also may be negative (sensitivity up to 50–60%). Nucleic acid amplification tests are valuable tools that allow for rapid diagnosis when positive. CXRs often reveal abnormalities compatible with tuberculosis but may instead be normal. Tuberculin skin testing and interferon γ release assays do not distinguish between active and latent tuberculosis and may be negative in CNS infection.

Differential Diagnosis

Tuberculous meningitis may be confused with any other type of meningitis, but the gradual onset, predominantly lymphocytic pleocytosis of the spinal fluid, and evidence of tuberculosis elsewhere often point to the diagnosis. Fungal and other granulomatous meningitides, syphilis, and carcinomatous meningitis are in the differential diagnosis.

Complications

Complications of tuberculous meningitis include seizures, cranial nerve palsies, stroke, and obstructive hydrocephalus with impaired cognitive function. These result from inflammatory exudate primarily affecting the basilar meninges and arteries.

Treatment

Presumptive diagnosis followed by early, empiric antituberculous therapy is essential for survival and to minimize sequelae. Even if CSF cultures are negative, a full course of therapy is warranted if the clinical scenario is suggestive of tuberculous meningitis.

Regimens that are effective for pulmonary tuberculosis are effective also for tuberculous meningitis. The current standard of care regimen for drug-susceptible tuberculous meningitis includes isoniazid and rifampin with ethambutol and pyrazinamide (the latter two drugs given only for the first 2 months; total treatment duration 9–12 months). Some experts may opt to treat tuberculous meningitis with higher doses of rifampin (up to 20 mg/kg/day) for better blood–brain barrier penetration, and/or may opt to use other antibiotics (such as levofloxacin and linezolid) in place of ethambutol. Expert consultation is strongly advised when treating tuberculous meningitis.

Many authorities recommend adding corticosteroids as adjunctive therapy, as this has been shown to reduce mortality from tuberculous meningitis. Dexamethasone (0.4 mg/kg/day intravenously for week 1, then 0.3 mg/kg/day for week 2, then 0.2 mg/kg/day for week 3, then 0.1 mg/kg/day for week 4, and then tapered over 3–4 more weeks) may be used for this purpose.

Nahid P et al. Official American Thoracic Society/Centers for Disease Control and Prevention/Infectious Diseases Society of America clinical practice guidelines: treatment of drug-susceptible tuberculosis. Clin Infect Dis. 2016;63:e147. [PMID: 27516382]

LEPROSY (Hansen Disease)

ESSENTIALS OF DIAGNOSIS

- Pale, anesthetic macular—or nodular and erythematous—skin lesions.
- Superficial nerve thickening with resultant anesthesia.
- History of residence in endemic area in childhood.
- Acid-fast bacilli in skin lesions or nasal scrapings, or characteristic histologic nerve changes.

General Considerations

Hansen disease (leprosy) is a chronic infectious disease caused by the acid-fast atypical mycobacteria *M leprae* and *M lepromatosis*. The primary mode of transmission is likely respiratory (versus zoonotic, associated with armadillos) and involves prolonged exposures. The disease is endemic in tropical and subtropical Asia, Africa, South America, and the Pacific regions, and seen sporadically in the United States, particularly in the south and southeast. There have been reports of leprosy occurring in Florida and Georgia without traditional risk factors, raising concerns for endemicity in the soil.

Clinical Findings

A. Symptoms and Signs

The onset is insidious, and the lesions involve cooler body tissues: skin, superficial nerves, nose, pharynx, larynx, eyes, and testicles. Skin lesions may occur as pale, anesthetic macular lesions; discrete erythematous, infiltrated nodules; or diffuse skin infiltration. Neurologic disturbances are caused by nerve infiltration and thickening, with resultant anesthesia and motor abnormalities. Bilateral ulnar neuropathy is highly suggestive. In untreated cases, disfigurement due to skin infiltration and nerve involvement may be extreme, leading to trophic ulcers, bone resorption, and loss of digits.

Hansen disease is divided into two distinct types for treatment purposes The **multibacillary type** typically occurs in patients with defective cellular immunity. The course is progressive, with diffuse skin involvement that may become nodular, slow and symmetric nerve involvement, abundant acid-fast bacilli in the skin lesions, and a negative lepromin skin test. In the **paucibacillary type**, cellular immunity is intact. The course is more benign and less progressive, with macular skin lesions, sudden-onset severe and asymmetric nerve involvement, few bacilli present in the lesions, and a positive lepromin skin test. Eye involvement (keratitis and iridocyclitis), nasal ulcers, epistaxis, anemia, and lymphadenopathy may occur.

B. Laboratory Findings

Laboratory confirmation of leprosy requires the demonstration of acid-fast bacilli in a skin biopsy. Skin or nerve biopsies may also show a typical histologic picture. *M leprae* does not grow in artificial media but does grow in the foot pads of armadillos.

Differential Diagnosis

The skin lesions of leprosy often resemble those of SLE, sarcoidosis, syphilis, erythema nodosum, erythema multiforme, cutaneous tuberculosis, and vitiligo.

Complications

Kidney failure and hepatomegaly from secondary amyloidosis may occur with long-standing disease.

Treatment

Combination therapy is currently recommended for treatment of leprosy. The US National Hansen's Disease Program recommends a triple oral drug regimen of rifampin (600 mg), moxifloxacin (400 mg), and minocycline (100 mg), all administered once monthly for 12 and 24 months in paucibacillary and multibacillary cases, respectively. For resource-constrained settings, the WHO recommends combination oral therapy with monthly rifampin (600 mg), daily dapsone (100 mg), and clofazimine (50 mg daily and 300 mg once monthly), given for 6 months in paucibacillary infections (though the evidence is weaker for use of clofazimine in this scenario) and 12 months in multibacillary infections.

Randhawa A et al. Leprosy: what is new? Int J Dermatol. 2022;61:733. [PMID: 34826151]

INFECTIONS CAUSED BY CHLAMYDIAE

CHLAMYDIA TRACHOMATIS INFECTIONS

1. Lymphogranuloma Venereum

ESSENTIALS OF DIAGNOSIS

- Evanescent primary genital lesion.
- Inguinal buboes with suppuration and draining sinuses.
- Proctitis or proctocolitis, with risk of colorectal strictures and fistulae.
- Diagnosis supported by positive nucleic amplification test for *C trachomatis* in right clinical context.

General Considerations

Lymphogranuloma venereum (LGV) is an acute and chronic sexually transmitted infection caused by *C trachomatis* serovars L1–L3. The disease is acquired during intercourse or through contact with contaminated exudate from active lesions. The incubation period is between 3–30 days. A self-limited ulcer or papule may form at the initial site of inoculation. After the genital lesion disappears, the infection spreads to the lymph nodes of the genital and rectal areas.

Clinical Findings

A. Symptoms and Signs

The initial papule or ulcerative lesion (usually on the external genitalia) is evanescent and often goes unnoticed. Patients may present instead with tender inguinal or femoral lymphadenopathy or buboes, which appear 1–4 weeks after exposure, are typically unilateral, and tend to fuse, soften, and break down to form multiple draining sinuses with extensive scarring. In people engaging in receptive anal sex, LGV most commonly presents with symptoms of proctocolitis. Early anorectal manifestations include proctitis with tenesmus and bloody purulent discharge; late manifestations include chronic cicatrizing inflammation of the rectal and perirectal tissue. These changes can lead to obstipation, rectal stricture and, occasionally, rectovaginal and perianal fistulas.

B. Laboratory Findings

A diagnosis of LGV can be confirmed only with LGV-specific molecular tests (ie, polymerase chain reaction), which can differentiate LGV from non-LGV *C trachomatis* infections. These LGV-specific tests, however, are not widely available, and can have prolonged turnaround times. Instead, the diagnosis of LGV can be made when a patient has a positive nucleic amplification test for chlamydia at a symptomatic site (frequently the rectum) in the appropriate clinical context. Chlamydia serology (complement fixation or microimmunofluorescence) should not be used routinely but may be helpful in cases of isolated inguinal or femoral lymphadenopathy when nucleic amplification testing is unavailable.

Differential Diagnosis

Early LGV lesions must be differentiated from ulcers caused by syphilis, genital herpes, or chancroid; lymph node involvement must be distinguished from that due to tularemia, tuberculosis, plague, neoplasm, or pyogenic infection. Rectal strictures attributable to LGV must be distinguished from those due to malignancy or IBD.

Treatment

If diagnostic testing for LGV is not available, patients with a clinical presentation suggestive of LGV should be treated empirically. The antibiotic of choice (for nonpregnant patients only) is doxycycline, 100 mg orally twice daily for 21 days. Erythromycin, 500 mg orally four times a day for 21 days, is an alternative treatment. Azithromycin, 1 g orally once weekly for 3 weeks, also may be effective.

DeVries et al. Lymphogranuloma venereum, an invasive and destructive sexually transmitted infection with many faces. Clin Dermatol. 2026;44:29. [PMID: 41038545]

Workowski KA et al. Sexually transmitted infections treatment guidelines, 2021. MMWR Recomm Rep. 2021;70:1. [PMID: 34292926]

2. Chlamydial Urethritis & Cervicitis

ESSENTIALS OF DIAGNOSIS

- *C trachomatis*: common cause of nongonococcal urethritis and cervicitis.
- Diagnosis made by nucleic acid amplification testing from a mucosal site (ie, urine sample or swab from the rectum, pharynx, cervix, or vagina).

General Considerations

C trachomatis serotypes D–K are a common cause of nongonococcal urethritis and cervicitis. *Mycoplasma genitalium* is another potential cause of these syndromes. Co-infections with other sexually transmitted pathogens, including gonorrhea, are common. *C trachomatis* infections can occasionally cause epididymitis, prostatitis, or proctitis; sequelae following cervicovaginal infections can include PID, ectopic pregnancy, and infertility.

Clinical Findings

A. Symptoms and Signs

Urethral or cervical discharge due to *C trachomatis* tends to be less painful, less purulent, and more watery than that due to *N gonorrhoeae*. Cervicovaginal chlamydial infections may be asymptomatic or may present with signs and symptoms of cervicitis, salpingitis, or PID. Long-term sequelae may include ectopic pregnancy and infertility.

B. Laboratory Findings

Patients with signs and symptoms of urethritis or cervicitis are assumed to have chlamydial infection until proven otherwise. The diagnosis should be confirmed, whenever possible, by FDA-approved, highly sensitive nucleic acid amplification tests performed on urine, or urethral, cervical or vaginal swabs. A negative urogenital nucleic acid amplification test can reliably exclude the diagnosis of chlamydial urethritis or cervicitis. Urogenital testing does not exclude infection at other sites, such as the rectum or pharynx.

C. Screening

Screening for chlamydial infection is recommended for certain populations: all sexually active women age ≥ 25 years; women age > 25 years with risk factors for sexually transmitted infections; pregnant persons age <25 or at increased vulnerability to sexually transmitted infections; patients with HIV; and men with risk factors for sexually acquired infections, such as men who have sex with men.

Treatment

Doxycycline, 100 mg orally twice daily for 7 days, is the preferred regimen for urogenital, rectal, and pharyngeal chlamydial infections in nonpregnant people. A single oral 1-g dose of azithromycin (alternative regimen, preferred in pregnancy), or 500 mg of levofloxacin once daily for 7 days, can alternatively be used. Empiric chlamydia treatment may be indicated for some patients, such as: (1) people with gonococcal infections in whom no chlamydial testing was performed, or a test other than a nucleic acid amplification test was used to exclude the diagnosis, or (2) people with pending chlamydia test results who are considered unlikely to follow up. Sex partners of patients with confirmed chlamydial infections also should be tested and treated empirically for chlamydia. Screening for HIV, gonorrhea, and syphilis should also be performed in all patients with an STI diagnosis.

Hocking JS et al. Update on the epidemiology, screening, and management of *Chlamydia trachomatis* infection. Infect Dis Clin North Am. 2023;37:267. [PMID: 37005162]

Workowski KA et al. Sexually transmitted infections treatment guidelines, 2021. MMWR Recomm Rep. 2021;70:1. [PMID: 34292926]

CHLAMYDIA PSITTACI & PSITTACOSIS (Ornithosis)

ESSENTIALS OF DIAGNOSIS

- Fever, chills, and cough; headache common.
- Atypical pneumonia with slightly delayed appearance of signs of pneumonitis.
- Contact with infected bird (psittacine, pigeons, many others) 5–14 days previously.
- Isolation of chlamydiae or rising antibody titers.

General Considerations

Psittacosis is acquired from contact with infected birds (parrots, parakeets, pigeons, chickens, ducks, and many others), which may or may not be ill.

Clinical Findings

Most patients with psittacosis experience a mild illness, similar to other respiratory illnesses, with onset 5–14 days after exposure. Symptoms include fever, chills, myalgia, dry cough, and headache. Signs include relative bradycardia (temperature-pulse dissociation), dullness to percussion, and rales. Pulmonary findings may be absent early in the clinical course. Dyspnea and cyanosis may occur later. Culture-negative endocarditis may occasionally occur. Rarely, patients may experience fulminant disease with multiorgan failure. The radiographic findings in psittacosis are usually those of atypical pneumonia—which tends to be interstitial and diffuse in appearance—although consolidation also can occur. Psittacosis is thus indistinguishable from other bacterial or viral pneumonias by radiography.

The organism is rarely isolated from respiratory cultures. Instead, the diagnosis is usually made serologically by either complement fixation or microimmunofluorescence and can be supported by a fourfold or greater rise in antibody titers between acute and convalescent samples (collected 2 weeks apart, to a titer of ≥ 1:32) or a single IgM titer of ≥ 1:16 (by microimmunofluorescence). If available, polymerase chain reaction testing of lower respiratory tract, sputum, nasopharyngeal, or stool samples may provide a more rapid diagnosis.

Differential Diagnosis

The illness is indistinguishable from viral, mycoplasma, or other atypical pneumonias except for the history of contact with birds. Psittacosis is on the differential diagnosis for culture-negative endocarditis.

Treatment

Treatment is with doxycycline 100 mg orally twice daily for 7–10 days. Azithromycin, 500 mg orally on day 1, and then 250 mg once daily for 4 days, may be effective as well.

Li X et al. Clinical, radiological and pathological characteristics of moderate to fulminant psittacosis pneumonia. PLoS One. 2022;17:e0270896. [PMID: 35816485]

CHLAMYDOPHILA PNEUMONIAE INFECTION

C pneumoniae causes pneumonia, pharyngitis, sinusitis, and bronchitis. The organism may be the second most common cause of atypical pneumonia (after mycoplasma) and presents similarly, with fever and nonproductive cough. Nucleic acid amplification testing performed on specimens such as nasopharyngeal swabs, sputum, or bronchial washings is the most sensitive diagnostic method. When a diagnosis of pneumonia due to *C pneumoniae* is confirmed, recommended treatments include levofloxacin (750 mg orally or intravenously for at least 5–7 days) or azithromycin (500 mg on day 1, then 250 mg daily for 4 more days, given orally or intravenously). Doxycycline (100 mg twice daily, given orally or intravenously for at least 5–7 days) is an alternative treatment option.

Metlay JP et al. Diagnosis and treatment of adults with community-acquired pneumonia. An official clinical practice guideline of the American Thoracic Society and Infectious Diseases Society of America. Am J Respir Crit Care Med. 2019;200:e45. [PMID: 31573350]

Tagini F et al. From coughs to complications: the story of *Chlamydia pneumoniae*. J Med Microbiol. 2025;74:002006. [PMID: 40279169]

38 Spirochetal Infections

Ina Park, MD, MS

SYPHILIS

NATURAL HISTORY & PRINCIPLES OF DIAGNOSIS & TREATMENT

Syphilis is a complex infectious disease caused by *Treponema pallidum*, a spirochete capable of infecting almost any organ or tissue in the body and causing protean clinical manifestations. Transmission occurs most frequently during sexual contact (including oral sex) or via the placenta from mother to fetus (congenital syphilis). The risk of acquiring syphilis after unprotected sex with an individual with infectious syphilis is approximately 30–50%. Rarely, it can also be transmitted through nonsexual contact or blood transfusion. The natural history of acquired syphilis is generally divided into two major groups: early syphilis, which is ≤ 1 year in duration and infectious, and late syphilis, which is present for > 1 year and not infectious. Ocular syphilis, otosyphilis, and neurosyphilis can occur at any stage and may occur alone or concurrently with other symptoms.

1. Early syphilis (primary, secondary, and early latent)— *The hallmark of the lesions of primary and secondary syphilis is an abundance of spirochetes*; tissue reaction is usually minimal (Table 38–1).

Primary syphilis lesions include a chancre (usually solitary and painless but multiple lesions can occur and may be painful) and regional lymphadenopathy.

Secondary syphilis lesions commonly involve the skin (rash) and mucous membranes—and occasionally bone, CNS, or liver, when dissemination of *T pallidum* produces systemic signs.

Early latent disease is without signs or symptoms, although relapsing symptoms/lesions may occur.

Congenital syphilis findings (eg, rhinitis, osteitis, skin lesions) are categorized as early disease.

The progression of syphilis without treatment is from the primary stage (chancre at the site of inoculation) to resolution of the lesion(s), and a period of latency. Secondary lesions can arise as the treponemes disseminate; these also can resolve without treatment, and this stage is called early latent syphilis if it has been < 1 year since infection. Thus, there are two distinct periods of early latent syphilis, one after the primary lesion resolves and another after the secondary lesions resolve. During the early latent period after secondary syphilis, there can be a relapse back into secondary signs and symptoms.

Whether an infection occurred within the last year (and therefore is early syphilis) may be determined by the patient recalling primary or secondary lesions—or, more commonly, by confirming the date of the patient's last known negative syphilis serology.

2. Late syphilis (late latent, latent of unknown duration, and tertiary)—Late latent disease is infection acquired > 1 year prior without active lesions, while tertiary disease is characterized by gummatous lesions involving skin, bones, and viscera; CVD (principally aortitis); and CNS and ocular syndromes (Table 38–1). These late forms of syphilis are not contagious. The lesions contain few demonstrable spirochetes, but tissue reactivity (vasculitis, necrosis) is severe and suggestive of hypersensitivity phenomena.

3. Syphilis data and statistics—Public health efforts to control syphilis focus on the diagnosis and treatment of early infectious cases and their sexual partners. In 2024, cases of syphilis declined by 22% over 2023 (190,242 total cases), largely driven by reductions of infections among men, and potentially related to use of doxycycline as post-exposure prophylaxis for STIs (doxy-PEP). However, congenital syphilis increased for the 12th consecutive year. Globally, the WHO estimates 8 million total incident syphilis infections occurred in 2022.

COURSE & PROGNOSIS

The lesions associated with primary and secondary syphilis are self-limiting, even without treatment, and resolve with few or no residua. Ocular and otologic syphilis have been associated with permanent vision and hearing loss. Tertiary and congenital syphilis may be highly destructive and permanently disabling, and may lead to death. While infection is rarely eradicated completely in the absence of treatment, most infections likely remain latent without sequelae, and only a small number of latent infections progress to further disease.

Table 38–1. Stages of syphilis and common clinical manifestations.

Stage	Manifestations
Early (infectious) syphilis	
Primary	Chancre: painless ulcer with clean base and firm indurated borders, can present with multiple or painful lesions Regional lymphadenopathy
Secondary	Skin and mucous membranes Rash: diffuse (may include palms and soles), macular, papular, pustular, and combinations Condylomata lata Mucous patches: painless, silvery ulcerations or elevated plaques of mucous membrane with surrounding erythema Generalized lymphadenopathy Constitutional symptoms Fever, usually low-grade Malaise, anorexia Arthralgias and myalgias CNS Asymptomatic Symptomatic Meningitis Cranial neuropathies (II–VIII) Other Ocular: anterior, posterior or panuveitis (can also affect retina, optic nerve, or cornea) Renal: glomerulonephritis, nephrotic syndrome Hepatitis Musculoskeletal: arthritis, periostitis
Early latent	No signs or symptoms
Late (noninfectious) syphilis	
Late latent	No signs or symptoms
Tertiary	Late benign (gummatous): granulomatous lesion usually involving skin, mucous membranes, and bones but any organ can be involved Cardiovascular Aortic regurgitation Coronary ostial stenosis Aortic aneurysm Neurosyphilis Asymptomatic Meningovascular Tabes dorsalis General paresis

Note: CNS involvement may occur at any stage.

CLINICAL STAGES OF SYPHILIS

1. Primary Syphilis

ESSENTIALS OF DIAGNOSIS

- Typically, painless solitary ulcer on genitalia, perianal area, rectum, pharynx, tongue, lip, or elsewhere.
- Fluid expressed from ulcer contains *T pallidum* by immunofluorescence or darkfield microscopy.
- Nontender enlargement of regional lymph nodes.
- Serologic nontreponemal and treponemal tests may be positive.

Clinical Findings

A. Symptoms and Signs

The typical lesion is the chancre at the site or sites of inoculation, most frequently located on the penis (Figure 38–1), labia, cervix, or anorectal region. Anorectal lesions are especially common among MSM. Chancres also occur occasionally in the oropharynx (lip, tongue, or tonsil) and rarely on the breast or finger or elsewhere. An initial small erosion appears 10–90 days (average, 3–4 weeks) after inoculation and rapidly develops into a single, painless, superficial ulcer with a clean base and firm, indurated margins. Although the "classic" chancre of syphilis has been described as nontender, nonpurulent, and indurated, only 31% of patients have this triad. Bacterial superinfection of the chancre may occur and may be painful. Healing of the chancre occurs without treatment, but a scar may form, especially with secondary bacterial infection. Multiple chancres may be present, particularly in patients with HIV. At the primary stage there is often enlargement of regional lymph nodes, which are rubbery, discrete, and nontender.

B. Laboratory Findings

1. Microscopic examination—In early syphilis, darkfield microscopic examination by a skilled observer of fresh exudate from moist lesions or material aspirated from regional lymph nodes is up to 90% sensitive for diagnosis but is usually only available in select sexual health clinics.

An immunofluorescent staining technique for demonstrating *T pallidum* in dried smears of fluid taken from early syphilitic lesions is performed in only a few laboratories.

2. Serologic tests for syphilis—Serologic tests for antibodies (the mainstay of syphilis diagnosis) fall into two general categories: (1) **Nontreponemal** tests detect antibodies to

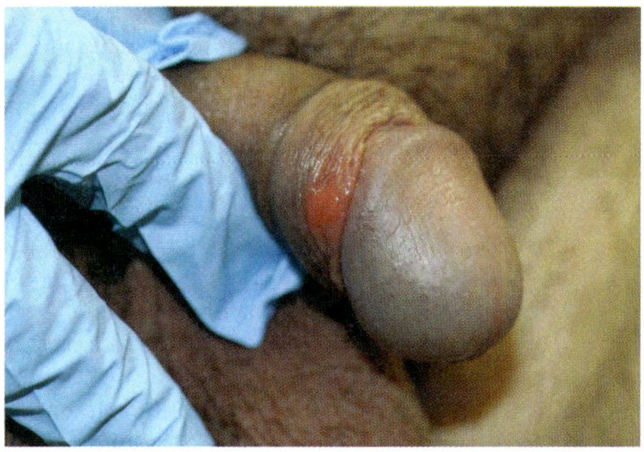

Figure 38–1. Chancre from primary syphilis. Used with permission from Christopher Ried, MD, Orange County Public Health.

Table 38–2. Percentage of patients with positive serologic tests for syphilis.[1]

Test	Stage		
	Primary	Secondary	Tertiary
VDRL or RPR	63–78%	100%	47–64%
FTA-ABS, TPPA	78–100%	100%	94–98%
MHA-TP	46–89%	90–100%	NA
EIA or CIA	54–100%	100%	NA

[1]Based on untreated cases.

CIA, chemiluminescence immunoassay; EIA, enzyme immunoassay; FTA-ABS, fluorescent treponemal antibody absorption assay; MHA-TP, microhemagglutination assay for *T pallidum*; RPR, rapid plasma reagin test; TPPA, *T pallidum* particle agglutination; VDRL, Venereal Disease Research Laboratory test.

lipoidal antigens present in both the host cell membrane as well as *T pallidum*; and (2) **Treponemal** tests use live or killed *T pallidum* as antigen to detect antibodies specific for pathogenic treponemes (Table 38–2).

A. Nontreponemal antibody tests—The most commonly used nontreponemal antibody tests are the Venereal Disease Research Laboratory (VDRL) and rapid plasma reagin (RPR) tests. A patient infected with syphilis produces antibodies that react with lipoidal antigens such as cardiolipin and lecithin; the VDRL and RPR tests detect these antibodies. The traditional term *nontreponemal* is a misnomer because the RPR detects antibodies against antigens in both the host and *T pallidum*.

Nontreponemal tests generally become positive 4–6 weeks after infection or 1–3 weeks after the appearance of a primary lesion; they are almost always positive in the secondary stage.

(1) False-positive nontreponemal tests—False-positive serologic reactions are encountered in many conditions, including infection with non–sexually transmitted treponematoses, autoimmune diseases, infectious mononucleosis, malaria, febrile diseases, leprosy, injection drug use, infective endocarditis, advanced age, and hepatitis C infection, and can occur with the use of COVID-19 mRNA vaccines. False-positive nontreponemal tests are usually of low titer (eg, < 1:8) and may be distinguished from true-positive results by correlating with clinical findings and performing a treponemal-specific antibody test.

(2) False-negative nontreponemal tests—False-negative results can occur in very early infection or paradoxically, when very high antibody titers are present ("prozone phenomenon"). If syphilis is strongly suspected and the nontreponemal test is negative, the laboratory should be instructed to dilute the specimen to detect a positive reaction.

Nontreponemal antibody titers are used to monitor the response to therapy and should decline over time. When these tests are used to follow disease activity, the same testing method should be used, preferably at the same laboratory. The rate of decline depends on various factors. In general, persons with repeat infections, higher initial titers, more advanced stages of disease, or uncontrolled HIV infection at the time of treatment have a slower seroconversion rate and are more likely to remain serofast (ie, titers decline but do not become nonreactive).

B. Treponemal antibody tests—These tests measure antibodies that react with *T pallidum* antigens. The *T pallidum* particle agglutination (TPPA) test and the fluorescent treponemal antibody absorption test (FTA-ABS) are two of the most commonly used treponemal tests. Other treponemal tests include enzyme immunoassays (EIA) and chemiluminescence immunoassays (CIA), which are often used as initial screening tests.

In the traditional screening algorithm, the treponemal tests are used to confirm a positive nontreponemal test (RPR or VDRL). Because of their sensitivity, particularly in the late stages of the disease, treponemal tests are also of value when there is clinical evidence of syphilis, but the nontreponemal serologic test for syphilis is negative. Treponemal tests are reactive in many patients with primary syphilis and in almost all patients with secondary syphilis (Table 38–2). Although a reactive treponemal-specific serologic test remains reactive throughout a patient's life in most cases, it may (like nontreponemal antibody tests) revert to negative with adequate therapy. Final decisions about the significance of the results of serologic tests for syphilis must be based on a clinical appraisal and may require expert consultation. The CDC provides consultation services through the STD Clinical Consultation Network (https://stdccn.org).

C. Enzyme immunoassay (EIA)- or chemiluminescence immunoassay (CIA)-based screening algorithms—Newer screening algorithms reverse the traditional test order and begin with an automated treponemal antibody test (eg, EIA or CIA) followed by a nontreponemal test (RPR or VDRL) if the treponemal EIA or CIA is positive. This is faster and decreases labor costs to laboratories when compared with traditional screening. The EIA and CIA tests generally have high sensitivity and specificity (95–100%), though lower specificity has been reported in some studies.

The reverse algorithms can cause challenges in clinical management. A positive treponemal test with a negative RPR or VDRL (eg, CIA-positive, RPR-negative) may represent prior treated syphilis, untreated latent syphilis, or a false-positive treponemal test. Such results should be evaluated with a second, different treponemal test as a "tiebreaker" such as the *T pallidum* particle agglutination test. Both traditional and reverse algorithms are recognized by the CDC and several international organizations including the International Union Against Sexually Transmitted Infections.

D. Rapid treponemal tests—Both a treponemal and a dual HIV/treponemal rapid point of care test are approved for use in the United States. These tests can be performed outside of clinic settings but must undergo competency testing to ensure that standards are met for accuracy and reliability. Additionally, an FDA-approved over-the-counter treponemal rapid test is available. Numerous other tests are available internationally and are commonly used in limited-resource settings. Sensitivity ranges widely from 60% to 100% in most published studies, with specificity typically ranging from 90% to 100% when using combined RPR and VDRL plus a treponemal test as the reference standard.

3. PCR—In the United States, there are no commercially available, FDA-approved *T pallidum* PCR test kits. However, kits are available as a laboratory-developed test in selected research, referral, and public health laboratories and have the highest yield in primary and secondary lesions. There are no standards for these tests, but PCR has many advantages as a tool for direct detection, including high sensitivity and ability to use a wide range of clinical specimen types, including CSF. PCR testing of blood has low sensitivity and is not recommended.

4. CSF examination—See Neurosyphilis, below.

Differential Diagnosis

The syphilitic chancre may be confused with genital herpes, chancroid (usually painful and uncommon in the United States), lymphogranuloma venereum, or neoplasm. Simultaneous evaluation for herpes simplex virus types 1 and 2 using PCR or culture should be done in these cases.

Prevention & Screening

Avoidance of sexual contact is the only completely reliable method of prevention but is an impractical public health measure. Latex or polyurethane condoms are effective only if all infectious lesions are covered. MSM should be screened at least annually, and as often as every 3 months for those who have multiple partners, those on HIV PrEP, or those who have sex in conjunction with the use of drugs. Because of epidemic increases in congenital syphilis, the CDC recommends universal screening among 15- to 44-year-olds in counties where the syphilis morbidity is high in women of reproductive age (> 4.6 cases per 100,000). The American College of Obstetrics and Gynecology recommends screening three times during pregnancy: at the first prenatal visit, during the third trimester, and at delivery. Additional screening can be considered based on risk factors: new partner(s), history of incarceration, transactional sex work, illicit drug use, or history of STIs. Patients treated for other STIs should also be tested for syphilis, and persons who have known or suspected sexual contact with patients who have syphilis should be evaluated and presumptively treated to abort development of infectious syphilis (see Treating Syphilis Contacts, below).

Treatment

A. Antibiotic Therapy

Penicillin remains the preferred treatment for syphilis, since there have been no documented cases of penicillin-resistant *T pallidum* (Table 38–3). In pregnancy, penicillin is the only option that reliably treats the fetus.

The most commonly used alternatives to penicillin for nonpregnant patients include doxycycline and ceftriaxone; a 2024 meta-analysis found similar serologic cure rates between the three therapies. While azithromycin is effective in some parts of the world, it should not be used in the United States due to resistance and documented treatment failures. All patients treated with a non-penicillin regimen must have close clinical and serologic follow-up.

B. Managing Jarisch–Herxheimer Reaction

The Jarisch–Herxheimer reaction, manifested by fever, headache, myalgia, and tachycardia in the hours following treatment, is a cytokine-mediated immunologic reaction to endotoxins released from the killed bacteria. This reaction is most common in early syphilis, particularly secondary syphilis, where it can occur in 66% of cases.

The Jarisch–Herxheimer reaction may be blunted by simultaneous administration of antipyretics, although no proven method of prevention exists. In cases with increased risk of morbidity due to the reaction (including CNS or cardiac involvement and pregnancy), consultation with an infectious disease expert is recommended. Patients should be reminded that the reaction does not signify an allergy to penicillin.

C. Local Measures (Mucocutaneous Lesions)

Local treatment is usually not necessary. No local antiseptics or topical antibiotics should be applied to a lesion until specimens for microscopy have been obtained.

D. Public Health Measures

Counsel patients with infectious syphilis to abstain from sexual activity for 7 days after treatment. All cases of syphilis must be reported to the appropriate local public health agency to identify and treat sexual contacts of early cases. In addition, all patients with syphilis who are not known to be living with HIV should have an HIV test at the time of diagnosis. Those with a negative HIV test should be offered HIV preexposure prophylaxis (HIV PrEP) because syphilis is associated with an increased risk of future HIV acquisition.

E. Treating Syphilis Contacts

Patients who have been sexually exposed to infectious syphilis within the preceding 3 months may be infected but seronegative and, thus, should be treated for early syphilis even if serologic tests are negative. Persons exposed > 3 months previously should be treated based on serologic results; however, if patient follow-up is unreliable, empiric therapy is indicated. Sexual contacts of the persons with syphilis should be evaluated for HIV PrEP.

Follow-Up Care

Because treatment failures and reinfection may occur, patients treated for syphilis should be monitored clinically and serologically with nontreponemal titers (RPR or VDRL) at 6 and 12 months. In primary and secondary syphilis, titers are expected to decrease fourfold by

Table 38–3. Recommended treatment for syphilis.[1]

Stage of Syphilis	Treatment	Alternative[2]	Comment
Early syphilis			
Primary, secondary, or early latent	Benzathine penicillin G 2.4 million units intramuscularly once	Doxycycline 100 mg orally twice daily for 14 days or Tetracycline 500 mg orally four times daily for 14 days or Ceftriaxone 1 g intramuscularly or intravenously daily for 10 days[3]	HIV testing is recommended at diagnosis or treatment
Late syphilis			
Late latent or uncertain duration	Benzathine penicillin G 2.4 million units intramuscularly weekly for 3 weeks	Doxycycline 100 mg orally twice daily for 28 days or Tetracycline 500 mg orally four times daily for 28 days	No routine CSF evaluation is needed unless there are neurologic symptoms Obtain an HIV test
Tertiary without neurosyphilis	Benzathine penicillin G 2.4 million units intramuscularly weekly for 3 weeks	Consult with an infectious disease specialist	CSF evaluation and an HIV test are recommended in all patients
Neurosyphilis	Aqueous penicillin G 18–24 million units intravenously daily, given every 3–4 hours or as continuous infusion for 10–14 days[4]	Procaine penicillin, 2.4 million units intramuscularly daily with probenecid 500 mg orally four times daily for 10–14 days or Ceftriaxone 2 g intramuscularly or intravenously daily for 10–14 days	Follow treatment with benzathine penicillin G 2.4 million units intramuscularly weekly for 1–3 weeks Obtain an HIV test

[1]Penicillin is the only documented effective treatment in pregnancy; pregnant patients with true allergy should be desensitized and treated with penicillin according to stage of disease as above.
[2]Patients treated with alternative therapies require close clinical and serologic monitoring.
[3]Fewer data for ceftriaxone treatment; optimal dose or duration not known.
[4]Because the 10- to 14-day treatment course for neurosyphilis is less than the 21 days recommended for treatment of late syphilis, CDC guidelines state that clinicians may consider giving an additional 2.4 million units of benzathine penicillin G intramuscularly once weekly for 1–3 weeks at the conclusion of the intravenous treatment.

12 months after treatment. However, titers in up to 20% of patients may not decrease; optimal management of these patients is unclear, but at a minimum, close clinical and serologic follow-up is indicated. In patients without HIV, an HIV test should be repeated; a thorough neurologic history and examination should be performed and lumbar puncture considered because unrecognized neurosyphilis can be a cause of treatment failure. If symptoms or signs persist or recur after initial therapy or there is a fourfold or greater increase in nontreponemal titers, the patient has reinfection (more likely) or the therapy failed (more likely if a non-penicillin regimen was used). In those individuals, an HIV test should be performed, a lumbar puncture done (unless reinfection is a certainty), and re-treatment given as indicated above.

Callado GY et al. Syphilis treatment: systematic review and meta-analysis investigating nonpenicillin therapeutic strategies. Open Forum Infect Dis. 2024;11:ofae142. [PMID: 38595955]

Papp JR, Park IU et al. CDC laboratory recommendations for syphilis testing, United States, 2024. MMWR Recomm Rep. 2024;73:1. [PMID: 38319847]

2. Secondary Syphilis

ESSENTIALS OF DIAGNOSIS

- Generalized maculopapular rash; condylomata lata may appear in moist anogenital skin.
- Mucous membrane lesions (eg, white patches in oral cavity).
- Generalized nontender lymphadenopathy.
- Fever may be present.
- Meningitis, hepatitis, osteitis, arthritis, iritis.
- Many treponemes in moist lesions by immunofluorescence or darkfield microscopy.
- Positive serologic tests for syphilis.

Clinical Findings

The secondary stage of syphilis usually appears a few weeks (or up to 6 months) after development of the chancre, when dissemination of *T pallidum* produces systemic signs

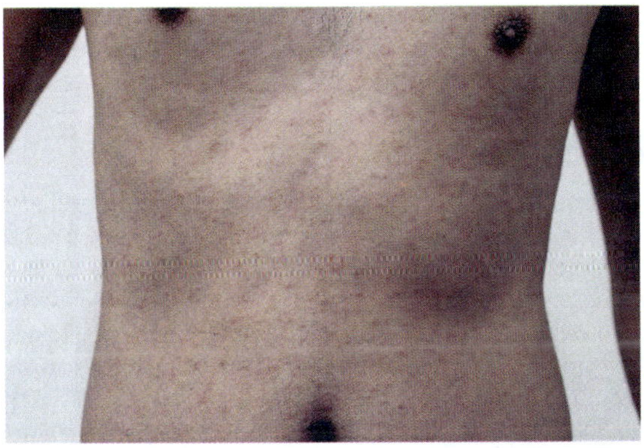

▲ **Figure 38–2.** Maculopapular rash on torso from secondary syphilis. Used with permission from Christopher Ried, MD, Orange County Public Health.

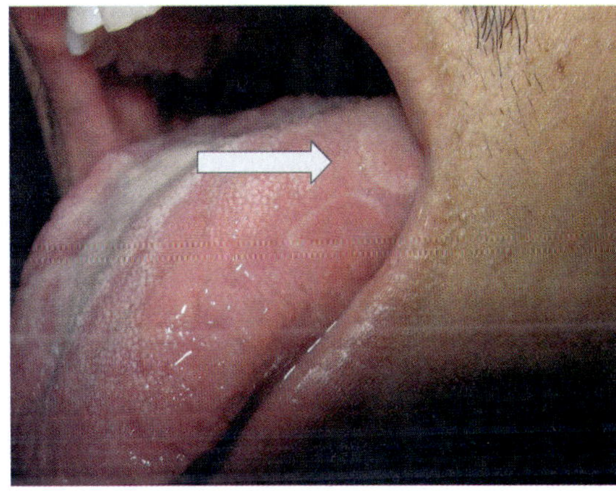

▲ **Figure 38–4.** Mucous patches on the tongue from secondary syphilis. Used with permission from Christopher Ried, MD, Orange County Public Health.

(fever, lymphadenopathy) or infectious lesions at sites distant from the site of inoculation. The most common manifestations are skin and mucosal lesions. The skin lesions are nonpruritic, macular, papular, pustular, or follicular (or combinations of any of these types, but generally *not* vesicular) and generalized (Figure 38–2) (Figure 38–3); involvement of the palms and soles occurs in 80% of cases. Annular lesions simulating ringworm may be observed. Transillumination may help identify faint rashes, or rashes in persons with darker skin color. Mucous membrane lesions may include mucous patches (Figure 38–4), which can be found on the lips, mouth, throat, genitalia, and anus. Condylomata lata, which are weeping papules on the moist skin areas and mucous membranes (and are often fused), are sometimes mistaken for genital warts (Figure 38–5). Unlike the dry rashes, the mucous membrane lesions are highly infectious.

Meningeal (aseptic meningitis or acute basilar meningitis), hepatic, renal, bone, and joint invasion may occur, with resulting cranial nerve palsies, jaundice, nephrotic syndrome, and periostitis. Alopecia (moth-eaten appearance) (Figure 38–6) and uveitis also may occur.

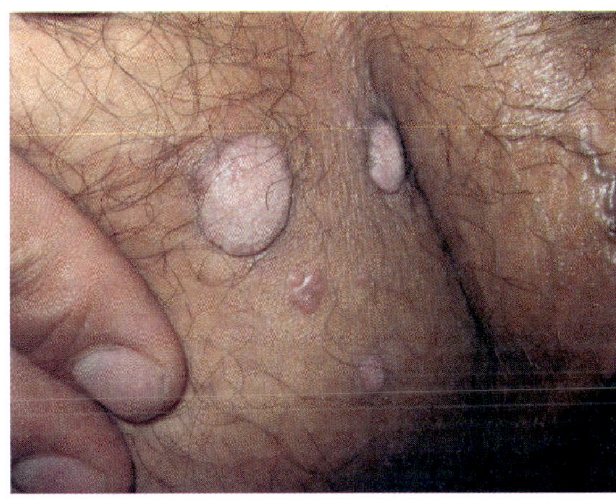

▲ **Figure 38–5.** Condyloma lata from secondary syphilis. Used with permission from Christopher Ried, MD, Orange County Public Health.

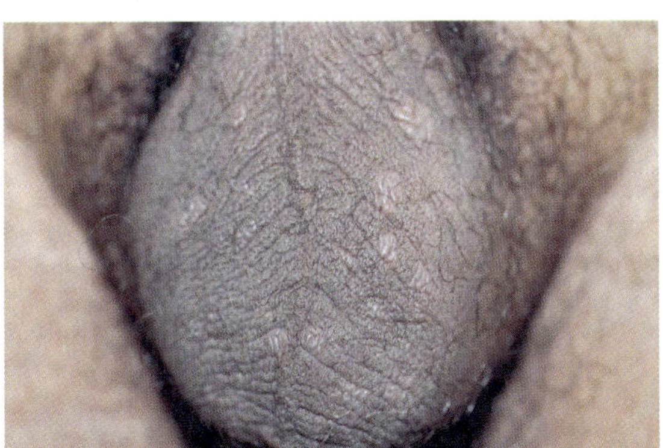

▲ **Figure 38–3.** Scrotal rash from secondary syphilis. Used with permission from Christopher Ried, MD, Orange County Public Health.

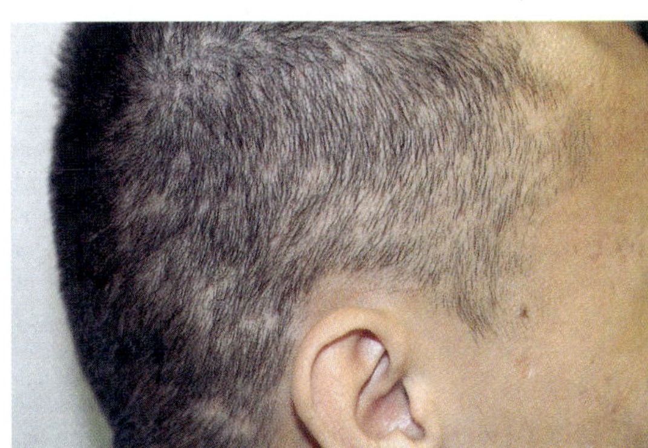

▲ **Figure 38–6. Patchy alopecia from secondary syphilis.** Used with permission from Christopher Ried, MD, Orange County Public Health.

Serologic tests for syphilis are almost always positive (see Primary Syphilis, below, and Table 38–2). The moist cutaneous and mucous membrane lesions often show *T pallidum* on darkfield microscopic examination. A transient CSF lymphocytic pleocytosis (cell count usually < 50–100/mcL [0.05–0.1 × 10^9/L]) is seen in 40% of patients with secondary syphilis. There may be evidence of hepatitis or immune complex nephritis as circulating immune complexes are deposited in blood vessel walls.

Skin lesions may be confused with the infectious exanthems, pityriasis rosea, and drug eruptions. Visceral lesions may suggest nephritis or hepatitis due to other causes.

Treatment

Treatment is as for primary syphilis unless CNS or ocular disease or neurologic signs or symptoms are present, in which case a lumbar puncture should be performed. If examination of the fluid is positive (see Spinal fluid examination, below), treatment for neurosyphilis should be given (see Table 38–3). See Primary Syphilis, above, for follow-up care and treatment of contacts.

3. Latent Syphilis

ESSENTIALS OF DIAGNOSIS

- **Early latent syphilis:** infection ≤ 1 year.
- **Late latent syphilis:** infection > 1 year.
- No physical signs.
- May have history of syphilis with inadequate treatment.
- Positive serologic tests for syphilis.

General Considerations

Latent syphilis is the clinically quiescent phase in the absence of lesions; the diagnosis is made by positive serologic tests.

1. Early latent syphilis—Defined as the first year after primary infection, early latent syphilis may relapse to secondary syphilis if undiagnosed or inadequately treated. Relapse is almost always accompanied by a rising titer in quantitative serologic tests; indeed, a rising titer may be the first or only evidence of relapse. About 90% of relapses occur during the first year after infection. Early latent infection can be diagnosed if there was documented seroconversion or a fourfold increase in nontreponemal titers in the past 12 months; the patient can recall symptoms of primary or secondary syphilis; or the patient had a sex partner with documented primary, secondary, or early latent syphilis.

2. Late latent stage—After the first year of latent syphilis, the patient is said to be in the late latent stage and noninfectious to sex partners. Transplacental transmission to a fetus, however, is possible in any stage. A diagnosis of late latent syphilis is justified only when the history and physical examination show no evidence of tertiary disease or neurosyphilis. The latent stage may last from months to decades.

Treatment

Treatment of early latent syphilis is the same as for primary syphilis unless CNS disease is present (see Table 38–3). Treatment of late latent syphilis is intended to prevent late sequelae (see Table 38–3). If there is evidence of CNS involvement, a lumbar puncture should be performed and, if positive, the patient should receive treatment for neurosyphilis (see Spinal fluid examination, below). Titers may not decline as rapidly following treatment compared to early syphilis. Nontreponemal serologic tests should be repeated at 6, 12, and 24 months. If titers increase fourfold or if initially high titers (≥ 1:32) fail to decrease fourfold by 24 months or if symptoms or signs consistent with syphilis develop, an HIV test should be repeated in patients not known to have HIV, lumbar puncture should be performed, and re-treatment given according to the stage of the disease.

4. Tertiary (Late Symptomatic) Syphilis

ESSENTIALS OF DIAGNOSIS

- Infiltrative tumors of skin, bones, liver (gummas).
- Aortitis, aortic aneurysms, aortic regurgitation.
- CNS disorders: meningovascular and degenerative changes, paresthesias, shooting pains, abnormal reflexes, dementia, or psychosis.

General Considerations

This stage may occur at any time after secondary syphilis, even after years of latency, and is rarely seen in developed countries in the modern antibiotic era. Late lesions are thought to represent an immunologic reaction to the organism and are usually divided into two types: (1) a localized hyperproliferative gummatous reaction with a relatively rapid onset and generally prompt response to therapy and (2) diffuse inflammation of a more insidious onset that characteristically involves the CNS and large arteries, may not improve despite treatment, and is often fatal if untreated. Gummas may involve any area or organ of the body but most often affect the skin or long bones. CVD is usually manifested by aortic aneurysm, aortic regurgitation, or aortitis. Various forms of diffuse or localized CNS involvement may occur.

Late syphilis must be differentiated from neoplasms of the skin, liver, lung, stomach, or brain; other forms of meningitis; and primary neurologic lesions.

Although almost any tissue and organ may be involved in late syphilis, the following are the most common sites of involvement: skin, mucous membranes, skeletal system, eyes, respiratory system, GI system, cardiovascular system, and nervous system.

Clinical Findings

A. Symptoms and Signs

1. Skin—Cutaneous lesions of late syphilis are of two varieties: (1) multiple nodular lesions that eventually ulcerate (lues maligna) or resolve by forming atrophic, pigmented scars; and (2) solitary gummas that start as painless subcutaneous nodules, then enlarge, attach to the overlying skin, and eventually ulcerate.

2. Mucous membranes—Late lesions of the mucous membranes are nodular gummas or leukoplakia, highly destructive to the involved tissue.

3. Skeletal system—Bone lesions are destructive, causing periostitis, osteitis, and arthritis with little or no associated redness or swelling but often marked myalgia and myositis of the neighboring muscles.

4. Eyes—Late ocular lesions are gummatous iritis, chorioretinitis, optic atrophy, and cranial nerve palsies, in addition to the lesions of CNS syphilis.

5. Respiratory system—Respiratory involvement is caused by gummatous infiltrates into the larynx, trachea, and pulmonary parenchyma, producing discrete pulmonary densities. There may be hoarseness, respiratory distress, and wheezing secondary to the gummatous lesion itself or to subsequent stenosis occurring with healing.

6. GI system—Gummas involving the liver may be benign but can cause cirrhosis. Gastric involvement can consist of diffuse infiltration into the stomach wall or focal lesions that endoscopically and microscopically can be confused with lymphoma or carcinoma. Epigastric pain, early satiety, regurgitation, belching, and weight loss are common.

7. Cardiovascular system—Cardiovascular lesions (10–15% of tertiary syphilitic lesions) are often progressive, disabling, and life-threatening. CNS lesions are often present concomitantly. Involvement usually starts as an arteritis in the supracardiac portion of the aorta and progresses to one or more of the following: (1) narrowing of the coronary ostia, with resulting decreased coronary circulation, angina, and acute MI; (2) scarring of the aortic valves, producing aortic regurgitation, and eventually HF; and (3) weakness of the wall of the aorta, with saccular aneurysm formation and associated pressure symptoms of dysphagia, hoarseness, brassy cough, back pain (vertebral erosion), and occasionally rupture of the aneurysm. Recurrent respiratory infections are common as a result of pressure on the trachea and bronchi.

8. Nervous system (neurosyphilis)—See next section.

Treatment

Treatment of tertiary syphilis (excluding neurosyphilis) is the same as late latent syphilis (see Table 38–3); symptoms may not resolve after treatment. Positive serologic tests do not usually become negative.

The pretreatment clinical and laboratory evaluation should include neurologic, ocular, cardiovascular, psychiatric, and CSF examinations. *In the presence of definite CSF or neurologic abnormalities, treat for neurosyphilis.*

5. Neurosyphilis

ESSENTIALS OF DIAGNOSIS

- Can occur at any stage of disease.
- Consider both clinical presentation and laboratory data.
- Perform neurologic examination on all patients; consider CSF evaluation for atypical symptoms or lack of decrease in nontreponemal serology titers.

General Considerations

Neurosyphilis can occur at any stage of disease and can be a progressive, disabling, and life-threatening complication. Asymptomatic CSF abnormalities and meningovascular syphilis occur earlier (months to years after infection, sometimes coexisting with primary and secondary syphilis) than tabes dorsalis and general paresis (2–50 years after infection).

Clinical Findings

A. Classification

1. Asymptomatic neuroinvasion—This form has been reported in up to 40% of patients with early syphilis and is characterized by spinal fluid abnormalities (positive CSF serology [VDRL], lymphocytic pleocytosis, occasionally increased protein) without symptoms or signs of neurologic involvement. There are no clear data to support that these asymptomatic CSF abnormalities have clinical significance.

2. Meningovascular syphilis—This form is characterized by meningeal involvement or changes in the vascular structures of the brain (or both), producing symptoms of acute or chronic meningitis (headache, irritability); cranial nerve palsies (basilar meningitis); unequal reflexes; irregular pupils with poor light and accommodation reflexes; and when large vessels are involved, cerebrovascular accidents. The CSF shows lymphocytic pleocytosis (cell count of 100–1000/mcL [$0.1–1.0 \times 10^9$/L]) and elevated protein and may have a positive serology (CSF VDRL). The symptoms of acute meningitis are rare in late syphilis.

3. Ocular syphilis and otosyphilis—Changes in vision or hearing may occur with or without meningitis. In cases of isolated ocular symptoms or signs (without cranial nerve deficits or other neurologic symptoms), CSF examination is not necessary before treatment. In cases of isolated auditory symptoms, the CDC recommends against performing CSF examination before treatment as CSF is likely to be normal. Patients with ocular or otic syphilis should be treated with the same regimen as for neurosyphilis.

4. Tabes dorsalis—This is a chronic progressive degeneration of the parenchyma of the posterior columns of the spinal cord and of the posterior sensory ganglia and nerve roots. The symptoms and signs are impairment of proprioception and vibration sense, Argyll Robertson pupils (which react poorly to light but accommodate for near focus), and muscular hypotonia and hyporeflexia. Impaired proprioception results in a wide-based gait and inability to walk in the dark. Paresthesias, analgesia, or sharp recurrent pains in the muscles of the leg ("shooting" or "lightning" pains) may occur. Joint damage may occur because of lack of sensory innervation (Charcot joint). The CSF may have a normal or increased lymphocytic cell count, elevated protein, and variable results of serologic tests.

5. General paresis—This is generalized involvement of the cerebral cortex with insidious onset of symptoms. There is usually a decrease in concentrating power, memory loss, dysarthria, tremor of the fingers and lips, irritability, and mild headaches. Most striking is the change of personality; the patient may become slovenly, irresponsible, confused, and psychotic. The CSF findings resemble those of tabes dorsalis. Combinations of the various forms of neurosyphilis (especially tabes and paresis) are not uncommon.

B. Laboratory Findings

See Serologic Tests for Syphilis, above, and Table 38–2; these tests should also be performed in cases of suspected neurosyphilis.

1. Indications for a lumbar puncture—In early syphilis (primary and secondary syphilis and early latent syphilis), invasion of the CNS by *T pallidum* with CSF abnormalities occurs commonly, but clinical neurosyphilis rarely develops in patients who have received standard therapy. Thus, unless clinical symptoms or signs of neurosyphilis or ocular involvement (uveitis, neuroretinitis, optic neuritis, iritis) are present, a lumbar puncture is not routinely recommended. CSF evaluation is recommended, however, if neurologic or ophthalmologic symptoms or signs are present, if there is evidence of treatment failure (see earlier discussion), or if there is evidence of active tertiary syphilis (eg, aortitis, iritis, optic atrophy, the presence of a gumma).

2. Spinal fluid examination—CSF findings in neurosyphilis are variable. In "classic" cases, there is elevated total protein > 46 mg/dL, lymphocytic pleocytosis with a cell count of 5–100/mcL (0.005–0.1 × 10^9/L), and a positive CSF nontreponemal test. VDRL is more sensitive and preferred over RPR. The serum nontreponemal titers will be reactive in most cases. Because the CSF VDRL may be negative in 30–70% of cases of neurosyphilis, *a negative test does not exclude neurosyphilis*, while a positive test confirms the diagnosis. The CSF FTA-ABS is sometimes used; it is a highly sensitive test but lacks specificity. A negative FTA-ABS can help rule out a diagnosis of neurosyphilis.

Treatment

Neurosyphilis is treated with high doses of aqueous penicillin to achieve better penetration and higher drug levels in the CSF than is possible with benzathine penicillin G (see Table 38–3). There are some observational data that support using ceftriaxone (with close follow-up) to treat neurosyphilis, but in some cases, patients with a history of an IgE-mediated reaction to penicillin may require skin testing for allergy to penicillin and, if positive, should be desensitized.

All patients treated for neurosyphilis should have nontreponemal serologic tests done every 3–6 months. CDC guidelines recommend that for patients with HIV who are taking antiretroviral therapy and those without HIV, clinical response and serum nontreponemal titers can be followed in lieu of repeated CSF examinations. If symptoms persist or titers do not normalize, consider repeating the CSF analysis; expert consultation may be helpful in this scenario.

6. Syphilis in Patients with HIV

Syphilis is common among individuals with HIV. Some data suggest that syphilis coinfection is associated with an increase in HIV viral load and a decrease in CD4 count that normalizes with therapy; other studies have not found an association with HIV disease progression. For optimal patient care as well as prevention of transmission to partners, guidelines for the primary care of patients with HIV recommend syphilis screening at least annually.

Interpretation of serologic tests should be the same for persons with or without HIV. If the diagnosis of syphilis is suspected on clinical grounds but nontreponemal antibody tests are negative, consider the prozone effect caused by high titers (see Nontreponemal Antibody Tests, above), or try direct examination of primary or secondary lesions for spirochetes.

Patients with HIV and with primary and secondary syphilis should have careful clinical and serologic follow-up at 3-month intervals. The use of antiretroviral therapy has been associated with reduced serologic failure rates after syphilis treatment.

The diagnosis of neurosyphilis in patients with HIV is complicated because mild CSF abnormalities (eg, pleocytosis) may be found in HIV infection alone. Evaluate patients for visual and hearing changes, since ocular and auditory syphilis may not result in CSF abnormalities. As in patients without HIV, routine lumbar puncture is not recommended in asymptomatic patients; it should be reserved for cases in which neurologic symptoms or signs are present or there is concern for treatment failure. Following treatment, CSF WBC counts should normalize within 12 months regardless of HIV status, while the CSF VDRL may take longer. As discussed above, the same criteria for failure apply to patients with and without HIV, and re-treatment regimens are the same.

For all stages and sites of syphilitic infection, treatment does not differ by HIV infection status.

7. Syphilis in Pregnancy

All pregnant persons should have a nontreponemal serologic test for syphilis at the time of the first prenatal visit (see Chapter 22). The American College of Obstetrics and Gynecology recommends screening three times during pregnancy: at the first prenatal visit, during the third trimester (eg, 28 weeks), and at delivery. The serologic status of mother and infant should be confirmed before discharge from the hospital. Patients who are seropositive should be considered infected and should be treated unless adequate prior treatment and serologic response are documented.

The only recommended treatment for syphilis in pregnancy is penicillin in dosage schedules appropriate for the stage of disease (see Table 38–3). Penicillin prevents congenital syphilis in 90% of cases, even when treatment is given late in pregnancy. Patients with a history of penicillin allergy should be skin tested and desensitized if necessary. *Tetracycline and doxycycline are not recommended in pregnancy.*

The infant should be evaluated immediately at birth, and, depending on the likelihood of infection, monitored for clinical and serologic manifestations in the first year of life.

8. Congenital Syphilis

Prevention of Syphilis

A study of doxycycline postexposure prophylaxis (PEP) for bacterial STIs among MSM in France resulted in a 73% reduction in syphilis and 70% reduction in chlamydia. A subsequent trial among MSM and transgender women in Seattle and San Francisco demonstrated a 77–87% reduction in syphilis, a 74–88% reduction in chlamydia, and a 55–57% reduction in gonorrhea. The CDC provided guidelines for the use of doxycycline as PEP in 2024 (https://www.cdc.gov/mmwr/volumes/73/rr/rr7302a1.htm).

When to Refer

- Consultation with the local public health department may help obtain all prior positive syphilis serologic results and may be helpful in complicated or atypical cases.
- Early (infectious) syphilis cases may be contacted for partner notification and treatment by local public health authorities.

When to Admit

- Pregnant women with syphilis and true penicillin allergy should be admitted for desensitization and treatment.
- Women in late pregnancy treated for early syphilis should have close outpatient monitoring or be admitted because the Jarisch–Herxheimer reaction can induce premature labor.
- Patients with neurosyphilis usually require admission for treatment with aqueous penicillin.

Bachmann LH et al. CDC clinical guidelines on the use of doxycycline postexposure prophylaxis for bacterial sexually transmitted infection prevention, United States, 2024. MMWR Recomm Rep. 2024;73:1. [PMID: 38833414]

Hook EW 3rd et al. One dose versus three doses of benzathine penicillin G in early syphilis. N Engl J Med. 2025;393:869. [PMID: 40902161]

Papp JR, Park IU et al. CDC laboratory recommendations for syphilis testing, United States, 2024. MMWR Recomm Rep. 2024;73:1. [PMID: 38319847]

Workowski KA et al; Centers for Disease Control and Prevention (CDC). Sexually transmitted infections treatment guidelines, 2021. MMWR Recomm Rep. 2021;70:1. [PMID: 34292926]

SELECTED SPIROCHETAL DISEASES

RELAPSING FEVER

Several species of *Borrelia* bacteria cause relapsing fever. The infection has two forms: tick-borne and louse-borne.

A. Tick-Borne Relapsing Fever

Rodents serve as the main reservoir of infection for ticks. Tick-borne relapsing fever may also be transmitted transovarially from one generation of ticks to the next. Humans can be infected by tick bites or by rubbing crushed tick tissues or feces into the bite wound. Tick-borne relapsing fever is endemic but is not transmitted from person to person. In the United States, the two types of infected ticks are *Ixodes pacficus* in the western states and *Ixodes scapularis* in the Northeast and upper Midwest, but clinical cases are uncommon in humans.

B. Louse-Borne Relapsing Fever

The louse-borne form is primarily seen in the developing world, and humans are the only reservoir. Large epidemics may occur in louse-infested populations, and transmission is favored by crowding, malnutrition, and cold climate.

Clinical Findings

A. Symptoms and Signs

For both tick-borne and louse-borne relapsing fever, an abrupt onset of fever, chills, tachycardia, nausea and vomiting, arthralgia, and severe headache may occur as soon as 3 days after infection. A large analysis of US surveillance data found the most common symptoms of tick-borne disease were fever (89%), fatigue (75%), headache (72%), chills (68%), and arthralgia (55%). In both tick-borne and louse-borne relapsing fever, hepatomegaly and splenomegaly may develop, as well as various types of rashes (macular, papular, petechial) that usually occur at the end of a febrile episode. Delirium occurs with high fever, and there may be various neurologic and psychological abnormalities. The attack terminates, usually abruptly, after 3–10 days. After an interval of 1–2 weeks, relapse occurs, but often it is somewhat milder. Before recovery in tick-borne disease, 3–10 relapses may occur; louse-borne disease is associated with only 1 or 2 relapses.

B. Laboratory Findings

During episodes of fever, large spirochetes are seen in thick and thin blood smears stained with Wright or Giemsa stain. The organisms can be cultured in special media but rapidly lose pathogenicity. The spirochetes can multiply in injected rats or mice and can be seen in their blood.

A variety of anti-*Borrelia* antibodies develop during the illness; sometimes the Weil–Felix test for rickettsioses and nontreponemal serologic tests for syphilis may be falsely positive. Infection can cause false-positive indirect fluorescent antibody and Western blot tests for *Borrelia burgdorferi*, causing some cases to be misdiagnosed as Lyme disease. PCR assays can be performed on blood, CSF, and tissue but are not always available in endemic regions. CSF abnormalities occur in patients with meningeal involvement. Mild anemia and thrombocytopenia are common. Leukopenia is less common and reported in 37% of patients with tick-borne relapsing fever.

Differential Diagnosis

The manifestations of relapsing fever may be confused with malaria, leptospirosis, meningococcemia, yellow fever, typhus, or rat-bite fever.

Prevention

Prevention of tick bites (as described for rickettsial diseases) and delousing procedures applicable to large groups can prevent illness. There are no vaccines for relapsing fever.

Postexposure prophylaxis with doxycycline 200 mg orally on day 1 and 100 mg daily for 4 days has been shown to prevent relapsing fever following tick bites in highly endemic areas.

Treatment

A. Tick-Borne Relapsing Fever

Treatment begins with penicillin G, 3 million units intravenously every 4 hours, or ceftriaxone, 1 g intravenously daily; with clinical improvement, a 10-day course can be completed with 0.5 g of tetracycline or erythromycin given orally four times daily. If CNS invasion is suspected, intravenous penicillin G or ceftriaxone should be continued for 10–14 days. Jarisch–Herxheimer reactions occur commonly following treatment and may be life-threatening, so patients should be closely monitored (see Syphilis, above). In louse-borne relapsing fever, administration of anti-TNF antibodies prior to antibiotic therapy can be effective in preventing the reaction. All pregnant women with tick-borne disease should be treated for 14 days, ideally with intravenous penicillin or ceftriaxone.

B. Louse-Borne Relapsing Fevers

A single dose of tetracycline or erythromycin, 0.5 g orally, or a single dose of procaine penicillin G, 600,000–800,000 units intramuscularly likely constitutes adequate treatment for this infection; however, some experts advocate for longer courses of treatment to prevent persistent infection.

Prognosis

The mortality rate without treatment ranges from 5% to as high as 50–70%. Fatalities are most common in older, debilitated, or very young patients. Treatment shortens the initial attack and often prevents relapses. The Jarisch–Herxheimer reaction is more common in louse-borne relapsing fever (55.8%) compared with tick-borne relapsing fever (19.3%).

RAT-BITE FEVER

Rat-bite fever is an uncommon acute infectious disease caused by the treponeme *Spirillum minus* (Asia) or the bacteria *Streptobacillus notomytis* (Asia) or *Streptobacillus moniliformis* (North America). Because this disease is transmitted to humans from rat bites and from ingesting rat feces, inhabitants of rat-infested dwellings, owners of pet rats, and laboratory workers are at greatest risk.

Clinical Findings

A. Symptoms and Signs

In *Spirillum* infections, the original rat bite, unless secondarily infected, heals promptly. However, one to several weeks later, the site becomes swollen, indurated, and painful; it assumes a dusky purplish hue and may ulcerate. Regional lymphangitis and lymphadenitis, fever, chills, malaise, myalgia, arthralgia, and headache are present. Splenomegaly may occur. A sparse, dusky-red maculopapular rash appears on the trunk and extremities in many cases, and there may be frank arthritis.

After a few days, both the local and systemic symptoms subside, only to reappear several days later. This relapsing pattern of fever for 3–4 days alternating with afebrile periods lasting 3–9 days may persist for weeks. The other features, however, usually recur only during the first few relapses.

S moniliformis infections have similar clinical features as *Spirillum* infections but have a shorter incubation period of up to 7 days and a diffuse rash. Endocarditis, osteomyelitis, arthritis, meningitis, and sepsis are rare complications.

B. Laboratory Findings

Leukocytosis is often present, and the nontreponemal test for syphilis (eg, RPR) is often falsely positive. *S minus* may be identified in darkfield examination of the ulcer exudate or aspirated lymph node material. *S minus* has not been cultured in artificial media.

Differential Diagnosis

Clinically, the severe arthritis and myalgias seen in streptobacillary disease are rarely seen in disease caused by *S minus*. Reliable differentiation requires an increasing titer of agglutinins against *S moniliformis* or isolation of the causative organism. Other diseases in the differential include tularemia, rickettsial disease, *Pasteurella multocida* infections, and relapsing fever.

Treatment

In acute illness in adults, intravenous penicillin, 1–2 million units every 4–6 hours, is given initially; ceftriaxone 1 g intravenously daily is another option; higher doses are used for rare severe complications including endocarditis. Once improvement has occurred, therapy may be switched to oral penicillin V 500 mg four times daily, or amoxicillin 500 mg three times daily, to complete 10–14 days of therapy. For the penicillin-allergic patient, tetracycline 500 mg orally four times daily or doxycycline 100 mg twice a day can be used.

Prognosis

The reported mortality rate of about 10% should be markedly reduced by prompt diagnosis and antimicrobial treatment.

LEPTOSPIROSIS

ESSENTIALS OF DIAGNOSIS

- Clinical illness can vary from asymptomatic to fatal liver and kidney failure.
- **Anicteric leptospirosis:** more common and milder form of the disease.
- **Icteric leptospirosis (Weil syndrome):** impaired kidney and liver function, abnormal mental status, hemorrhagic pneumonia; 5–40% mortality rate.

General Considerations

Leptospirosis is an acute and sometimes severe treponemal infection that is caused by several species within the genus *Leptospira*. This worldwide disease is among the most common zoonotic infections. The leptospires enter through minor skin lesions and probably via the conjunctiva. Cases have occurred in international travelers after swimming or rafting in contaminated water, and occupational cases occur among sewer workers, rice planters, abattoir workers, and farmers. Sporadic urban cases have been seen in unhoused persons exposed to rat urine.

Clinical Findings

A. Symptoms and Signs

1. Anicteric leptospirosis—The more common and milder form of the disease, anicteric leptospirosis is often biphasic. After an incubation period of 2–20 days, the initial or acute phase begins with abrupt fever to 39–40°C, chills, abdominal pain, severe headache, and myalgias, especially of the calf muscles. There may be marked conjunctival suffusion. Following a 1- to 3-day period of improvement in symptoms and absence of fever, the second or "immune" phase begins; however, in severe disease the phases may appear indistinct. Aseptic meningitis often occurs; uveitis, rash, nausea, vomiting, diarrhea, and adenopathy also may occur. A rare but severe manifestation is hemorrhagic pneumonia. The illness is usually self-limited, lasting 4–30 days, and complete recovery is the rule.

2. Icteric leptospirosis (Weil syndrome)—The more severe form of the disease, icteric leptospirosis is characterized by fever, impaired kidney and liver function including jaundice, abnormal mental status, hemorrhagic pneumonia, hypotension, and a 5–40% mortality rate. Symptoms and signs often are continuous and not biphasic.

Leptospirosis with jaundice must be distinguished from hepatitis, yellow fever, rickettsial disease, and relapsing fever.

B. Laboratory Findings

1. Anicteric leptospirosis—The leukocyte count may be normal, low, or high with neutrophils predominating. The urine may contain bile, protein, casts, and red cells. Oliguria is common, and in severe cases uremia may occur. In the acute phase, leptospires can be identified by nucleic acid amplification tests (NAATs) or by culture from blood, CSF, urine, and tissue. Blood cultures are most often positive within the first week if obtained before antibiotics are given. In the immune phase, aseptic meningitis is characterized by pleocytosis and elevated protein. Leptospires are absent from blood and CSF but are still present in the kidney (and can be detected in the urine), and specific antibodies appear.

2. Icteric leptospirosis—Features may initially overlap with nonicteric disease. Elevated bilirubin and aminotransferases are seen in 75%, and elevated serum creatinine (> 1.5 mg/dL) (132.6 mcmol/L) is seen in 50% of cases. Serum creatine kinase is usually elevated in persons with leptospirosis and normal in persons with other types of hepatitis. Pulmonary hemorrhage is associated with laboratory findings of disseminated intravascular coagulation; elevated PT, PTT, and D-dimer and low fibrinogen.

3. Both icteric and nonicteric leptospirosis—In both types of disease, diagnosis is usually made by serologic tests, including the microscopic agglutination test and ELISA. PCR molecular diagnostics are sensitive, specific, positive early in disease, and able to detect leptospiral DNA in blood, urine, CSF, and aqueous humor.

Complications

Myocarditis, aseptic meningitis, AKI, and pulmonary infiltrates with hemorrhage are not common but are the usual causes of death. Iridocyclitis may occur.

Prevention

The mainstay of prevention is avoidance of potentially contaminated food and water.

A 2024 meta-analysis did not find that pre- or postexposure prophylaxis reduced infection or all-cause mortality. Prophylaxis with doxycycline (200 mg orally once a week) can be considered if a person is at high risk due to being in an area or season (eg, monsoon flooding) when exposure would be more likely. Human vaccine is used in some limited settings but is not widely available.

Treatment

Many cases are self-limited without specific treatment. Although therapy for mild disease is controversial, most clinicians treat for 7 days with doxycycline (100 mg orally twice daily) or amoxicillin (50 mg/kg, divided into three doses daily); azithromycin (500 mg once daily) for 3 days also may be used. For severe disease, the CDC recommends penicillin (eg, 1.5 million units every 6 hours intravenously) as first-line therapy; other options include ceftriaxone (1 g daily intravenously), cefotaxime (1 g every 6 hours intravenously), or doxycycline (100 mg every 12 hours orally or intravenously for 7 days), without clear mortality benefit between any of these treatments. Jarisch–Herxheimer reactions may occur (see Syphilis, above).

Prognosis

Without jaundice, the disease is almost never fatal. With jaundice, the mortality rate is 5% for those aged < 30 years and 40% for those aged > 60 years.

When to Admit

Patients with jaundice or other evidence of severe disease should be admitted for close monitoring and may require admission to an ICU.

Win TZ et al. Antibiotics for treatment of leptospirosis. Cochrane Database Syst Rev. 2024;3:CD014960. [PMID: 38483092]
Win TZ et al. Antibiotic prophylaxis for leptospirosis. Cochrane Database Syst Rev. 2024;3:CD014959. [PMID: 38483067]

LYME DISEASE (Lyme Borreliosis)

ESSENTIALS OF DIAGNOSIS

- Erythema migrans: a flat or slightly raised red lesion that expands with central clearing.
- Headache or stiff neck.
- Arthralgias, arthritis, and myalgias; arthritis is often chronic and recurrent.

General Considerations

This illness, named after the town of Old Lyme, Connecticut, is the most common tick-borne disease in the United States and Europe. Most US cases are reported from the mid-Atlantic, northeastern, and north central regions of the country. The true incidence of Lyme disease is not known for several reasons: (1) serologic tests are not standardized (see Laboratory Findings, below); (2) clinical manifestations are nonspecific; and (3) even with reliable testing, serology is insensitive in early disease.

The tick vector of Lyme disease varies geographically and is *Ixodes scapularis* in the northeastern, north central, and mid-Atlantic regions of the United States; *Ixodes pacificus* on the West Coast; *Ixodes ricinus* in Europe; and *Ixodes persulcatus* in Asia. The disease also occurs in Australia. Mice and deer make up the major animal reservoir of *B burgdorferi*, but other rodents and birds may also be infected. Domestic animals such as dogs, cattle, and horses can also develop clinical illness, usually arthritis.

Under experimental conditions, ticks must feed for 24–36 hours or longer to transmit infections. Most cases are reported in the spring and summer months. In addition, the percentage of ticks infected varies on a regional and local basis. The description of exposure is important; a history of brushing a tick off the skin (ie, the tick was not feeding) or removing a tick on the same day as exposure (ie, the tick did not feed long enough) decreases the likelihood that infection will develop.

Because the *Ixodes* tick is so small, the bite is usually painless and goes unnoticed. After feeding, the tick drops off in 2–4 days. If a tick is found, it should be removed immediately. The best way to accomplish this is to use fine-tipped tweezers to pull firmly and repeatedly on the tick's mouth part—not the tick's body—until the tick releases its hold. Saving the tick in a bottle of alcohol for future identification may be useful, especially if symptoms develop.

Clinical Findings

The three stages of Lyme disease are classified based on early or late manifestations of the disease and whether it is localized or disseminated.

A. Symptoms and Signs

1. Stage 1, early localized infection—Stage 1 infection is characterized by erythema migrans (see Figure 6–18). About 1 week after the tick bite (range, 3–30 days; median, 7–10 days), a flat or slightly raised red lesion appears at the bite site, which is commonly seen in areas of tight clothing such as the groin, thigh, or axilla. This lesion expands over several days. Although originally described as a lesion that progresses with central clearing ("bulls-eye" lesion), often there is a more homogeneous appearance or even central intensification. About 10–20% of patients either do not have typical skin lesions or the lesions go unnoticed, which may lead to misdiagnosis. Vesicular, urticarial, and evanescent erythema migrans have all been reported. Most patients with erythema migrans will have a concomitant viral-like illness (the "summer flu") characterized by myalgias, arthralgias, headache, and fatigue. Fever may or may not be present. Even without treatment, the symptoms and signs of erythema migrans resolve in 3–4 weeks.

Completely asymptomatic disease, without erythema migrans or flu-like symptoms, can occur but is uncommon in the United States.

2. Stage 2, early disseminated infection—Up to 50–60% of patients with erythema migrans are bacteremic, and within days to weeks of the original infection, secondary skin lesions develop in about 50% of patients. These lesions are similar in appearance to the primary lesion but are usually smaller. Malaise, fatigue, fever, headache (sometimes severe), neck pain, and generalized achiness are common with the skin lesions. Most symptoms are transient. After hematogenous spread, some patients experience cardiac (4–10% of patients) or neurologic (10–15% of patients) manifestations, including myopericarditis, with atrial or ventricular arrhythmias and heart block. Neurologic manifestations include both the central and peripheral nervous systems. The most common CNS manifestation is aseptic meningitis with mild headache and neck stiffness. The most common peripheral manifestation is a cranial nerve VII neuropathy, ie, facial palsy (usually unilateral but can be bilateral, see Figure 27–1). A sensory or motor radiculopathy and mononeuritis multiplex occur less frequently. Conjunctivitis, keratitis, and, rarely, panophthalmitis can also occur. Rarely, a cutaneous hypopigmented skin lesion called a borrelial lymphocytoma develops.

3. Stage 3, late persistent infection—Stage 3 infection occurs months to years after the initial infection and again primarily manifests itself as musculoskeletal, neurologic, and skin disease. In early reports, musculoskeletal complaints developed in up to 60% of patients, but with early recognition and treatment of disease, this has decreased to < 10%. The classic manifestation of late disease is a monoarticular or oligoarticular arthritis most commonly affecting the knee or other large weight bearing joints. While these joints may be quite swollen, these patients generally report less pain compared to patients with bacterial septic arthritis. Even if untreated, the arthritis is self-limited, resolving in a few weeks to months. Multiple recurrences are common but are usually less severe. Joint fluid reflects an inflammatory arthritis with a mean WBC count of 25,000/mcL (25×10^9/L) with a predominance of neutrophils. Chronic arthritis can develop in about 10% of patients; this pathogenesis may be an immunologic phenomenon rather than persistence of infection.

Rarely, the nervous system (both central and peripheral) can be involved in late Lyme disease. In the United States, a subacute encephalopathy, characterized by memory loss, mood changes, and sleep disturbance, is seen. In Europe, a more severe encephalomyelitis caused by *B garinii* occurs and presents with cognitive dysfunction, spastic paraparesis, ataxia, and bladder dysfunction. Peripheral nervous system involvement includes intermittent paresthesias, often in a stocking glove distribution, or radicular pain.

The cutaneous manifestation of late infection, which can occur up to 10 years after infection, is acrodermatitis chronicum atrophicans. It has been described mainly in Europe after infection with *B afzelii*. There is usually bluish-red discoloration of a distal extremity with associated swelling. These lesions become atrophic and sclerotic with time and eventually resemble localized scleroderma. Cases of diffuse fasciitis with eosinophilia, an entity that resembles scleroderma, have been rarely associated with *B burgdorferi* infections.

B. Laboratory Findings

The diagnosis of Lyme disease is based on both clinical manifestations and laboratory findings. The US Surveillance Case Definition specifies a person with exposure to a potential tick habitat (within the 30 days prior to developing erythema migrans) with (1) erythema migrans diagnosed by a clinician or (2) at least one late manifestation of the disease and (3) laboratory confirmation as fulfilling the criteria for Lyme disease.

Nonspecific laboratory abnormalities can occur, particularly in early disease. The most common are an elevated ESR of > 20 mm/hour seen in 50% of cases and mildly abnormal liver biochemical tests in 30% of cases (these are usually transient and return to normal within a few weeks of treatment). The CBC is usually normal. Mild anemia, leukocytosis (11,000–18,000/mcL [$11–18 \times 10^9$/L]), and microscopic hematuria (secondary to IgA nephropathy or minimal change disease) have been reported in ≤ 10% of patients.

Laboratory confirmation requires serologic tests to detect specific antibodies to *B burgdorferi* in serum, preferably by ELISA and not by indirect immunofluorescence assay (IFA), which is less sensitive and specific and can cause misdiagnosis. A two-test approach is recommended for the diagnosis of active Lyme disease, with all specimens positive or equivocal by ELISA then confirmed with either a Western immunoblot assay that can detect both IgM and IgG antibodies or with a different ELISA. A negative Western immunoblot following an initial positive ELISA indicates a false-positive ELISA; the patient does not have evidence of exposure to *B burgdorferi*. A positive immunoblot requires that antibodies are detected against two (for IgM) or five (for IgG) specific protein antigens from *B burgdorferi*.

If a patient with suspected early Lyme disease has negative serologic studies, acute and convalescent titers should be obtained since up to 50% of patients with early disease can be antibody negative in the first several weeks of illness. A fourfold rise in antibody titer would be diagnostic of recent infection. Antibiotic therapy early in disease can abort subsequent seroconversion.

The diagnosis of late nervous system Lyme disease is often difficult since clinical manifestations, such as subtle memory impairment, may be difficult to document. Patients with late disease and peripheral neuropathy almost always have positive serum antibody tests, usually have abnormal neurophysiology tests, and may have abnormal nerve biopsies showing perivascular collections of lymphocytes; however, the CSF is usually normal and does not demonstrate local antibody production.

Caution should be exercised in interpreting serologic tests because they are not subject to national standards, and inter-laboratory variation is a major problem. In addition, some laboratories perform tests that are entirely unreliable and should never be used to support the diagnosis of Lyme disease (including Lyme urinary antigen tests or PCR on inappropriate specimens such as blood or urine). Finally, testing is often done in patients with nonspecific symptoms such as headache, arthralgia, myalgia, fatigue, and palpitations. For these reasons, the CDC and Infectious Diseases Society of America have guidelines for laboratory evaluation of suspected Lyme disease:

1. The diagnosis of early Lyme disease is clinical (ie, exposure in an endemic area, with clinician-documented erythema migrans) and does *not* require laboratory confirmation. (Tests are often negative at this stage.) If lesions are atypical, serology performed on acute and convalescent sera (collected 14–21 days later) can help confirm the diagnosis.
2. Late disease requires objective evidence of clinical manifestations (recurrent brief attacks of monoarticu-

lar or oligoarticular arthritis of the large joints; lymphocytic meningitis, cranial neuritis [facial palsy]; peripheral neuropathy or, rarely, encephalomyelitis—but *not* headache, fatigue, paresthesias, or stiff neck alone; atrioventricular conduction defects with or without myocarditis) and laboratory evidence of disease (two-stage testing with ELISA or IFA followed by Western blot or a second ELISA, as described above).

3. Patients with nonspecific symptoms without objective signs of Lyme disease should *not* have serologic testing done. False-positive tests occur more commonly than true-positive tests in this setting.
4. When assessing for CNS Lyme disease in an appropriate clinical syndrome, serum antibody testing is recommended over CSF serology or PCR.
5. Serum antibody testing is recommended to diagnose Lyme arthritis; PCR can be done on synovial fluid or tissue if needed to confirm the diagnosis and guide treatment.

Erythema migrans is a clinical diagnosis; cultures and PCR of the lesions for *B burgdorferi* are not recommended.

Complications

B burgdorferi infection in pregnant women has *not* been associated with congenital syndromes, unlike other spirochetal illnesses such as syphilis.

Some patients and advocacy groups have claimed either a post–Lyme disease syndrome (in the presence of positive laboratory tests and after appropriate treatment) or "chronic Lyme disease" in which tests may all be negative. Both entities include nonspecific symptoms such as fatigue, myalgias, and cognitive difficulties (see Prognosis, below). Expert groups agree that there are no data to support that ongoing infection is the cause of either syndrome.

Differential Diagnosis

Chemical reactions to tick and spider bites (these usually recede in 24–48 hours, whereas erythema migrans increases in size during this period), drug eruptions, urticaria, and staphylococcal and streptococcal cellulitis have been mistaken for erythema migrans. Southern tick–associated rash illness (STARI) is transmitted by the tick bite of *Amblyomma americanum*. The bite may present with flu-like symptoms and a rash similar to that of erythema migrans or tick-associated rashes, but these bites generally occur in the southern United States only. It is uncertain what borrelial species, if any, is transmitted by the *A americanum*, but STARI is distinct from Lyme disease.

Lyme arthritis may resemble bacterial arthritis, although the former is usually less painful. Lyme carditis presenting as atrioventricular heart block may resemble infectious bacterial endocarditis or noninfectious autoimmune disease. Lyme meningitis must be distinguished from other causes of aseptic meningitis, such as viral meningitis. In early disseminated or late Lyme disease, clinical findings such as erythema migrans and positive serologic tests help confirm the diagnosis.

Prevention

There is no human vaccine available. Measures such as avoiding tick-infested areas, covering exposed skin with long-sleeved shirts, tucking long trousers into socks, wearing light-colored clothing, using repellents, and inspecting for ticks after exposure reduce the risk of tick bites.

Prophylactic antibiotic treatment following tick bites is recommended in certain high-risk situations if all of the following criteria are met: (1) a tick identified as an adult or nymphal *I scapularis* has been attached for at least 36 hours; (2) prophylaxis can be started within 72 hours of the time the tick was removed; (3) more than 20% of ticks in the area are known to be infected with *B burgdorferi*; and (4) there is no contraindication to the use of doxycycline (not pregnant, not allergic). The medication of choice for prophylaxis is a single 200-mg dose of doxycycline. If doxycycline is contraindicated, no prophylaxis should be given since short-course prophylactic therapy with other agents has not been studied. The patient should be closely monitored for early disease, and if early disease does develop, appropriate therapy is effective in preventing long-term sequelae. Individuals who have removed ticks (including those who have had prophylaxis) should be monitored carefully for 30 days for possible coinfections.

Coinfections

Lyme disease, babesiosis (see Chapter 40), and human granulocytic anaplasmosis (see Chapter 37) are endemic in similar regions and are transmitted by the same tick, *I scapularis*. Coinfection with two or all three of these organisms can occur, causing a clinical picture that is not "classic" for any of these diseases. The presence of erythema migrans is highly suggestive of Lyme disease, whereas flu-like symptoms without rash are more suggestive of babesiosis or anaplasmosis. *Coinfection should be considered and excluded in patients who have persistent high fevers 48 hours after starting appropriate therapy for Lyme disease; in patients with persistent symptoms despite resolution of rash; and in those with anemia, leukopenia, or thrombocytopenia.*

Treatment

Recommendations for therapy are outlined in Table 38–4. For erythema migrans, antibiotic therapy shortens the duration of rash and prevents late sequelae. Doxycycline is most commonly used and has the advantage of being active against anaplasmosis, a common coinfection; it has proven effective in shorter courses of 7–10 days compared with other regimens. The Infectious Diseases Society of America guidelines recommend 10 days of doxycycline treatment while a European study demonstrated efficacy with 7 days of treatment. Amoxicillin is also effective and is recommended for pregnant or lactating women and for those who cannot tolerate doxycycline.

Isolated facial palsy (without meningitis or peripheral neuropathy) can be treated with doxycycline, amoxicillin, or cefuroxime axetil for 14–21 days. Therapy does not

Table 38–4. Treatment of Lyme disease.

Manifestations	Medication and Dosage
Tick bite	No treatment in most circumstances (see text); observe
Erythema migrans	Doxycycline, 100 mg orally twice daily for 10 days, or amoxicillin, 500 mg orally three times daily for 14 days, or cefuroxime axetil, 500 mg orally twice daily for 14 days An alternative is azithromycin, 500 mg orally daily for 7 days with monitoring for resolution
Neurologic disease	
Facial palsy (without meningitis)	Doxycycline, 100 mg orally twice daily, or amoxicillin, 500 mg orally three times daily, or cefuroxime axetil, 500 mg orally twice daily—all for 14–21 days
Meningitis (without parenchymal disease of brain or spinal cord)	Ceftriaxone, 2 g intravenously once daily, or cefotaxime, 2 g intravenously every 8 hours, or penicillin G, 18–24 million units daily intravenously in six divided doses—all for 14–21 days or doxycycline, 100 mg orally twice daily for 14–21 days
Parenchymal brain or spinal cord disease	Ceftriaxone, 2 g intravenously once daily, or cefotaxime, 2 g intravenously every 8 hours, or penicillin G, 18–24 million units daily intravenously in six divided doses—all for 14–28 days
Cardiac disease	
Atrioventricular block and myopericarditis[1]	
Outpatient	Doxycycline, 100 mg orally twice daily, or amoxicillin, 500 mg orally three times daily, or cefuroxime axetil, 500 mg orally twice daily—all for 14–21 days
Inpatient	Ceftriaxone, 2 g intravenously once daily; patients can be switched to an oral agent (doxycycline is first-line therapy) to complete 14–21 days of total antibiotic treatment if clinically improving
Arthritis	Doxycycline, 100 mg orally twice daily, or amoxicillin, 500 mg orally three times daily, or cefuroxime axetil, 500 mg orally twice daily—all for 28 days. An oral agent is preferred as initial treatment and can be repeated if needed. If no response to initial treatment or worsening after initial treatment, ceftriaxone, 2 g intravenously once daily, can be given for 14–28 days (see text)
Acrodermatitis chronicum atrophicans	Doxycycline, amoxicillin, or cefuroxime axetil as above for 21–28 days
"Chronic Lyme disease" or "post–Lyme disease syndrome"	Symptomatic therapy; prolonged antibiotics are *not* recommended

[1]Symptomatic patients, those with second- or third-degree block, and those with first-degree block with a PR interval ≥ 300 milliseconds should be hospitalized for observation.

affect the rate of resolution of the cranial neuropathy, but it does prevent development of late disease manifestations.

Some clinicians perform lumbar puncture on all patients with facial palsy and others only if there are symptoms or signs of meningitis. If meningitis is present, either parenteral therapy with ceftriaxone, cefotaxime, or penicillin G or oral doxycycline is recommended. The best initial agent will depend on the clinical scenario; patients who initially receive parenteral therapy can be switched to oral therapy to complete 14–21 total days of treatment. Patients with parenchymal brain or spinal cord disease should be treated with intravenous antibiotics for 14–28 days.

Atrioventricular block or myopericarditis (or both) can be treated with either oral or parenteral agents for 14–21 days. Hospitalization is indicated for symptomatic patients, those with second- or third-degree block, and those with first-degree block with a PR interval of 300 milliseconds or more. Once stabilized, hospitalized patients can be transitioned to one of the oral regimens to complete therapy.

Therapy of arthritis is difficult because some patients do not respond to any therapy, and those who do respond may do so slowly. Oral agents (doxycycline, amoxicillin, or cefuroxime axetil) are as effective as intravenous regimens (ceftriaxone, cefotaxime, or penicillin). A reasonable approach to the patient with Lyme arthritis is to start with oral therapy for 28 days. If there is partial resolution, re-treat with an additional 28 days of the same oral regimen. However, if there has been no response or worsening with initial oral therapy, switch to intravenous ceftriaxone for 14–28 days. If arthritis persists after re-treatment, symptomatic therapy with NSAIDs is recommended. For severe refractory pain, synovectomy may be required.

Acrodermatitis chronicum atrophicans can be treated with oral doxycycline, amoxicillin, or cefuroxime axetil for 21–28 days.

Based on limited data, therapy of Lyme disease in pregnancy should be the same as therapy in other patients, with the exception that doxycycline should not be used.

Clinicians may encounter patients with nonspecific symptoms (such as fatigue and myalgias) and positive serologic tests for Lyme disease who request therapy for their illness. When treating these patients, clinicians must remember (1) that nonspecific symptoms alone are not diagnostic; (2) that serologic tests are fraught with difficulty (as noted above), and in areas where disease prevalence is low, false-positive serologic tests are much more common than true-positive tests; and (3) that parenteral therapy with ceftriaxone for 2–4 weeks can cause significant adverse effects, including cholelithiasis and *Clostridioides difficile* colitis, and is costly. Parenteral therapy should be reserved for those most likely to benefit, ie, those with characteristic cutaneous, neurologic, cardiac, or rheumatic manifestations of Lyme disease.

Prognosis

Most patients respond to appropriate therapy with prompt resolution of symptoms within 4 weeks. True treatment failures are uncommon, and in most cases, re-treatment or prolonged treatment of Lyme disease is instituted because of misdiagnosis or misinterpretation of serologic results (both IgG and IgM antibodies can persist for prolonged periods despite adequate therapy) rather than inadequate therapy or response. Prolonged courses of antibiotic therapy for nonspecific symptoms that persist after completion of appropriate assessment (and treatment, if necessary) for Lyme disease are not recommended.

The long-term outcome of adult patients with Lyme disease is generally favorable, but some patients have chronic complaints. Joint pain, memory impairment, and poor functional status because of pain are common subjective complaints, but physical examination and neurocognitive testing fail to document the presence of these symptoms as objective sequelae.

Immunity is not complete after Lyme disease. Reinfection, although uncommon, is predominantly seen in patients successfully treated for early disease (erythema migrans) in whom antibody titers do not develop. Clinical manifestations and serologic response are similar to an initial infection.

When to Refer

Consultation with an infectious diseases specialist experienced in Lyme disease can be helpful in atypical or prolonged cases.

When to Admit

Admission for parenteral antibiotics is indicated for symptomatic CNS or cardiac disease, second- or third-degree atrioventricular block, or first-degree block with a PR interval of 300 milliseconds or more.

Kobayashi T et al. Diagnostic testing for Lyme disease. Infect Dis Clin North Am. 2022;36:605. [PMID: 36116838]

Lantos PM et al. Clinical Practice Guidelines by the Infectious Diseases Society of America (IDSA), American Academy of Neurology (AAN), and American College of Rheumatology (ACR): 2020 guidelines for the prevention, diagnosis and treatment of Lyme disease. Clin Infect Dis. 2021;72:e1. [PMID: 33417672]

Stupica D et al. Treatment of erythema migrans with doxycycline for 7 days versus 14 days in Slovenia: a randomised open-label non-inferiority trial. Lancet Infect Dis. 2023;23:371. [PMID: 36209759]

Protozoal & Helminthic Infections

39

Philip J. Rosenthal, MD

PROTOZOAL INFECTIONS

AFRICAN TRYPANOSOMIASIS (Sleeping Sickness)

ESSENTIALS OF DIAGNOSIS

- Exposure to tsetse flies; chancre at bite site more common with East African disease.
- **Hemolymphatic disease:** Irregular fever, headache, joint pain, rash, edema, lymphadenopathy.
- **Meningoencephalitic disease:** Somnolence, severe headache, progressing to coma.
- Trypanosomes in blood or lymph node aspirates; positive serologic tests.
- Trypanosomes and increased white cells and protein in CSF.

General Considerations

African trypanosomiasis is caused by the hemoflagellates *Trypanosoma brucei rhodesiense* and *Trypanosoma brucei gambiense*. The organisms are transmitted by bites of tsetse flies (genus *Glossina*), which inhabit shaded areas along streams and rivers. Trypanosomes ingested in a blood meal develop over 18–35 days in the fly; when the fly feeds again on a mammalian host, the infective stage is injected. Human disease occurs in rural areas of sub-Saharan Africa from south of the Sahara to about 30 degrees south latitude. *T b gambiense* causes West African trypanosomiasis and is transmitted in the moist sub-Saharan savannas and forests of west and central Africa. *T b rhodesiense* causes East African trypanosomiasis and is transmitted in the savannas of east and southeast Africa.

T b rhodesiense infection is primarily a zoonosis of game animals and cattle; humans are infected sporadically. Humans are the principal mammalian host for *T b gambiense*, but domestic animals can be infected. After major decreases in incidence, <1000 cases have been reported annually in recent years, mostly due to *T b gambiense*, with the largest number in the Democratic Republic of the Congo. Infections are rare among travelers, including visitors to game parks.

Clinical Findings

A. Symptoms and Signs

1. West African trypanosomiasis (*T b gambiense*)— Chancres at the site of the bite are uncommon. After an asymptomatic period that may last for months, hemolymphatic disease presents with fever, headache, myalgias, arthralgias, weight loss, and lymphadenopathy, with discrete, nontender, rubbery nodes, referred to as Winterbottom sign when in a posterior cervical distribution. Other common signs are mild splenomegaly, transient edema, and a pruritic erythematous rash. Febrile episodes may be broken by afebrile periods of up to several weeks. The hemolymphatic stage progresses over months to meningoencephalitic disease, with somnolence, irritability, personality changes, severe headache, and parkinsonian symptoms progressing to coma and death.

2. East African trypanosomiasis (*T b rhodesiense*)— Chancres at the bite site are more commonly recognized with this infection, with a painful lesion of 3–10 cm and regional lymphadenopathy that appears about 48 hours after the tsetse fly bite and lasts 2–4 weeks. East African disease follows a much more acute course, with the onset of symptoms usually within a few days of the insect bite. The hemolymphatic stage includes intermittent fever and rash, but lymphadenopathy is less common than with West African disease. Myocarditis can cause tachycardia and death due to arrhythmias or heart failure. If untreated, East African trypanosomiasis progresses over weeks to months to meningoencephalitic disease, somnolence, coma, and death.

B. Laboratory Findings

Diagnosis can be difficult, and definitive diagnosis requires identification of trypanosomes. Microscopic examination of fluid expressed from a chancre or lymph node may show motile trypanosomes or, in fixed specimens, parasites stained with Giemsa. During the hemolymphatic stage, detection of parasites in Giemsa-stained blood smears is common in East African disease but difficult in West African disease. Serial specimens should be examined, since parasitemias vary greatly over time. Meningoencephalitic disease is defined by the WHO as CSF showing at least five mononuclear cells per microliter, elevated protein, or presence of trypanosomes. Concentration techniques can aid identification of parasites in blood or CSF. Serologic tests are also available. The card agglutination test for trypanosomes (CATT) has excellent sensitivity and specificity for West African disease and can be performed in the field, but the diagnosis should be confirmed by identification of the parasites. Field-applicable immunochromatographic lateral flow rapid diagnostic tests that cost less than CATT and are simpler to perform are available.

Treatment

Detection of trypanosomes is a prerequisite for treatment of African trypanosomiasis because of the significant toxicity of therapies. Treatment recommendations depend on the type of trypanosomiasis (Table 39–1), which is determined by geography, and stage of disease. Fexinidazole is recommended by the WHO as first-line therapy and is FDA-approved for treatment of early (no CNS disease) and advanced (CNS) West African disease. Acoziborole has demonstrated effective and simpler single-dose oral therapy, but is not yet FDA-approved. Suramin, eflornithine, and melarsoprol are available in the United States from the CDC Drug Service (https://www.cdc.gov/laboratory/drugservice).

A. West African Trypanosomiasis (Table 39–1)

Fexinidazole is effective and safe when administered orally to persons age > 6 years (for weight > 35 kg, give 1800 mg once daily for 4 days, followed by 1200 mg once daily for 6 days). It is recommended for persons with a CSF leukocyte count < 100/mcL (0.1×10^9/L). Evaluation of the CSF can be avoided if there is no suspicion of severe CNS disease. Fexinidazole greatly simplifies therapy compared with parenteral regimens, but relapse and death after treatment may be more common than after treatment with eflornithine plus nifurtimox. Side effects from fexinidazole include headache, nausea, vomiting, insomnia, anxiety, weakness, tremor, and decreased appetite. For children age < 6 years without evidence of CNS disease (CNS leukocytes < 100/mcL [0.1×10^9/L]) pentamidine (4 mg/kg intramuscularly daily for 7 days) is the drug of choice. For advanced CNS disease (CNS leukocytes > 100/mcL [0.1×10^9/L]) at any age, a combination of intravenous eflornithine (400 mg/kg/day in two doses for 7 days) and oral nifurtimox (15 mg/kg/day in three doses for 10 days) is recommended. Eflornithine, although less toxic than older trypanocidal drugs, can cause GI symptoms, bone marrow suppression, seizures, and alopecia. Pentamidine toxicities include hypotension, tachycardia, and dyspnea during infusions and subsequent pancreatic (hypo- or hyperglycemia), renal, and liver toxicity.

B. East African Trypanosomiasis (Table 39–1)

Fexinidazole has replaced suramin and melarsoprol (previously first-line for early and CNS disease, respectively) for individuals age > 6 years with body weight ≥ 20 kg. As the drug is effective for all disease stages, lumbar punctures are no longer routinely required. For younger children, recommendations remain to treat early disease with suramin and CNS disease with melarsoprol. Suramin toxicities include vomiting and, rarely, seizures and shock during infusions as well as subsequent fever, rash, headache, neuropathy, and kidney and bone marrow dysfunction.

Immediate side effects of melarsoprol include fever and GI symptoms. The most important side effect is a reactive encephalopathy that can progress to seizures, coma, and death. To help avoid this side effect, corticosteroids are coadministered (dexamethasone 1 mg/kg/day intravenously for 2–3 days or oral prednisolone 1 mg/kg/day for 5 days, and then 0.5 mg/kg/day until treatment completion). Increasing resistance to melarsoprol is a serious concern.

Table 39–1. Treatment of African trypanosomiasis.

Disease	Stage	Age	Treatment	
			First Line	Alternative
West African	Early[1]	< 6 years[2]	Pentamidine	Pentamidine
		≥ 6 years	Fexinidazole	Suramin Eflornithine
	CNS involvement	< 6 years	Eflornithine + nifurtimox	Melarsoprol
	CNS involvement	≥ 6 years		
	< 100 CSF leukocytes/mcL (0.1×10^9/L)		Fexinidazole	
	> 100 CSF leukocytes/mcL (0.1×10^9/L)		Eflornithine + nifurtimox	
East African	Early[1]	< 6 years[2]	Suramin	Pentamidine
		≥ 6 years	Fexinidazole	
	CNS involvement	< 6 years[2]	Melarsoprol	
		≥ 6 years	Fexinidazole	Melarsoprol

[1]Without CNS involvement.
[2]Also for body weight < 20 kg.

Prevention & Control

Individual prevention in endemic areas should include neutral-colored clothes (eg, long sleeve shirts and pants), insect repellents, and mosquito nets. Control programs focusing on vector elimination and treatment of infected persons and animals have shown good success in many areas but suffer from limited resources.

Álvarez-Rodríguez A et al. Recent progress in diagnosis and treatment of human African trypanosomiasis has made the elimination of this disease a realistic target by 2030. Front Med (Lausanne). 2022;9:1037094. [PMID: 36405602]

Kumeso VKB et al. Effectiveness and safety of fexinidazole for gambiense human African trypanosomiasis and exploration of adherence in outpatients: a phase 3b, prospective, open-label, non-randomised, cohort study. Lancet Glob Health. 2025;13:e900. [PMID: 40288399]

Kumeso VKB et al. Efficacy and safety of acoziborole in patients with human African trypanosomiasis caused by *Trypanosoma brucei gambiense*: a multicentre, open-label, single-arm, phase 2/3 trial. Lancet Infect Dis 2023;23:463. [PMID: 36460027]

Lejon V et al. Human African trypanosomiasis. Lancet. 2025;405:937. [PMID: 40089378]

Lindner AK et al. New WHO guidelines for treating rhodesiense human African trypanosomiasis: expanded indications for fexinidazole and pentamidine. Lancet Infect Dis. 2025;25:e77. [PMID: 39389073]

Matovu E et al. Fexinidazole as a new oral treatment for human African trypanosomiasis due to Trypanosoma brucei rhodesiense: a prospective, open-label, single-arm, phase 2–3, non-randomised study. Lancet Glob Health. 2025;13:e910. [PMID: 40288400]

AMERICAN TRYPANOSOMIASIS (Chagas Disease)

ESSENTIALS OF DIAGNOSIS

Acute stage

- Inflammatory lesion at inoculation site.
- Fever.
- Hepatosplenomegaly; lymphadenopathy.
- Myocarditis.
- Parasites in blood are diagnostic.

Chronic stage

- Heart failure, cardiac arrhythmias.
- Thromboembolism.
- Megaesophagus; megacolon.
- Serologic tests are usually diagnostic.

General Considerations

Chagas disease is caused by *Trypanosoma cruzi*, a protozoan parasite found only in the Americas; it infects wild animals and, to a lesser extent, humans from southern South America to the southern United States. An estimated 6–7 million persons are infected, mostly in rural areas, with the highest national prevalence in Bolivia, Argentina, Paraguay, Ecuador, El Salvador, and Guatemala. An estimated 288,000 infected persons live in the United States. Control efforts in endemic countries have decreased disease incidence to about 30,000 new infections and 12,000 deaths per year. The disease is often acquired in childhood. In many countries in South America, Chagas disease is the most important cause of heart disease. The vector is endemic in the southern United States where animals are infected, and locally transmitted human infections have been reported.

T cruzi is transmitted by reduviid (triatomine) bugs infected by ingesting blood from animals or humans who have circulating trypanosomes. Multiplication occurs in the digestive tract of the bug and infective forms are eliminated in feces. Infection in humans occurs when infected bugs bite humans and the parasite penetrates the skin through the bite wound, mucous membranes, or conjunctiva. Transmission can also occur by blood transfusion, organ or bone marrow transplantation, congenital transfer, or ingestion of food contaminated with vector feces. From the bloodstream, *T cruzi* invades many cell types but has a predilection for myocardium, smooth muscle, and CNS glial cells. Multiplication causes cellular destruction, inflammation, and fibrosis, with progressive disease over decades.

Clinical Findings

A. Symptoms and Signs

As many as 70% of infected persons remain asymptomatic.

1. Acute infection—This stage is seen principally in children and lasts 1–2 months. The earliest findings are at the site of inoculation either in the eye—Romaña sign (unilateral edema, conjunctivitis, and lymphadenopathy)—or in the skin—a chagoma (swelling with local lymphadenopathy). Subsequent findings include fever, malaise, headache, mild hepatosplenomegaly, and generalized lymphadenopathy. Acute myocarditis and meningoencephalitis are rare but can be fatal.

2. Asymptomatic latent period—This indeterminate phase may last for life, but symptomatic disease develops in 10–30% of infected individuals, commonly many years after infection.

3. Chronic Chagas disease—Chronic disease generally manifests as abnormalities in cardiac and smooth muscle. Cardiac disease includes arrhythmias, heart failure, and embolic disease. Smooth muscle abnormalities lead to megaesophagus and megacolon, with dysphagia, regurgitation, aspiration, constipation, and abdominal pain. These findings can be complicated by superinfections. In immunosuppressed persons, including patients with AIDS and transplant recipients, latent Chagas disease may reactivate; findings have included brain abscesses and meningoencephalitis.

B. Diagnostic Testing

1. Acute infection—The diagnosis is made by detecting parasites in persons with suggestive findings who have resided in an endemic area. Evaluation of fresh blood or buffy coats may show motile trypanosomes, and fixed preparations may show Giemsa-stained parasites. Concentration methods increase diagnostic yields. Trypanosomes may be identified in lymph nodes, bone marrow, or pericardial or spinal fluid. Molecular tests are highly sensitive and can be used to detect parasites in organ transplant recipients or after accidental exposure. When initial tests are unrevealing, xenodiagnosis using laboratory vectors, laboratory culture, or animal inoculation may provide a diagnosis, but these methods are expensive and slow.

2. Chronic Chagas disease—This is usually diagnosed serologically. Many serologic assays, including rapid diagnostic tests, are available, but sensitivity and specificity are not ideal; confirmatory assays are advised after an initial positive test, as is standard for blood bank testing in South America. The diagnosis of chronic disease with PCR remains suboptimal.

Treatment

Treatment is inadequate because the two drugs used, benznidazole and nifurtimox, often cause severe side effects, must be used for long periods, and are ineffective against chronic infection. In acute and congenital infections, the drugs can reduce the duration and severity of infection, and apparent cure is achieved in about 70–90% of patients. During the chronic phase of infection, although parasitemia may disappear in up to 70% of patients, treatment does not clearly alter the progression of Chagas disease. Nevertheless, there is general consensus that treatment should be considered in all persons infected with *T cruzi* regardless of clinical status or time since infection. In particular, treatment is recommended for acute, congenital, and reactivated infections and for children and young adults with chronic disease.

Both benznidazole and nifurtimox are FDA-approved for the treatment of Chagas disease. Benznidazole is generally preferred to nifurtimox due to better efficacy and safety profiles. The dose is 5 mg/kg/day orally in two divided doses for 60 days; shorter (2–4 week) regimens offer good efficacy. Its side effects include granulocytopenia, rash, and peripheral neuropathy. The dose of nifurtimox is 8–10 mg/kg orally in four divided doses after meals for 90–120 days. Side effects include GI (anorexia, vomiting) and neurologic (headaches, ataxia, insomnia, seizures) symptoms, which appear to be reversible and to lessen with dosage reduction. For both drugs, some recommendations suggest higher dosing for acute infections. Patients with chronic Chagas disease may benefit from antiarrhythmic therapy, standard therapy for heart failure, and conservative and surgical management of megaesophagus and megacolon.

Prevention & Control

In South America, a major eradication program based on improved housing, use of residual pyrethroid insecticides and pyrethroid-impregnated bed curtains, and screening of blood donors has achieved striking reductions in new infections. In endemic areas and ideally in donors from endemic areas, blood should not be used for transfusion unless at least two serologic tests are negative.

Beatty NL et al. Chagas disease, an endemic disease in the United States. Emerg Infect Dis. 2025;31:1691. [PMID: 40866797]

de Sousa AS et al. Chagas disease. Lancet. 2024;403:203. [PMID: 38071985]

Swett MC et al. Chagas disease: epidemiology, diagnosis, and treatment. Curr Cardiol Rep. 2024;26:1105. [PMID: 39115799]

LEISHMANIASIS

ESSENTIALS OF DIAGNOSIS

- Sand fly bite in an endemic area.
- **Visceral leishmaniasis:** irregular fever, progressive hepatosplenomegaly, pancytopenia, wasting.
- **Cutaneous leishmaniasis:** chronic, painless, moist ulcers or dry nodules.
- **Mucocutaneous leishmaniasis:** destructive nasopharyngeal lesions.
- Amastigotes in macrophages in aspirates, touch preparations, or biopsies.
- Positive culture, serologic tests, PCR, or skin test.

General Considerations

Leishmaniasis is a zoonosis transmitted by bites of sand flies of the genus *Lutzomyia* in the Americas and *Phlebotomus* elsewhere. When sand flies feed on an infected host, the parasitized cells are ingested with the blood meal. Leishmaniasis is caused by about 20 species of *Leishmania;* taxonomy is complex. Clinical syndromes are generally dictated by the infecting species, but some species can cause more than one syndrome.

The estimated annual incidence of disease has been decreasing, with estimates of 600,000 to 1 million annual cases of cutaneous disease and 50,000–90,000 cases of visceral disease. Progress against visceral disease has been greatest on the Indian subcontinent.

1. Visceral leishmaniasis (kala azar)—This is caused mainly by *Leishmania donovani* in the Indian subcontinent and East Africa; *Leishmania infantum* in the Mediterranean, Middle East, China, parts of Asia, and Horn of Africa; and *Leishmania chagasi* in South and Central America. Other species may occasionally cause visceral disease. More than 90% of cases occur in seven countries: Brazil, Ethiopia, India, Kenya, Somalia, South Sudan, and Sudan. In each locale, the disease has particular clinical and epidemiologic features. The incubation period is usually 4–6 months (range: 10 days to 24 months). Without treatment, the fatality rate reaches 90%. Early diagnosis and treatment reduce mortality to 2–5%.

2. Cutaneous leishmaniasis—About 90% of cases occur in Afghanistan, Pakistan, Syria, Saudi Arabia, Algeria, Iran, Brazil, and Peru. Old World cutaneous leishmaniasis is caused mainly by *Leishmania tropica*, *Leishmania major*, and *Leishmania aethiopica* in the Mediterranean, Middle East, Africa, Central Asia, and Indian subcontinent. New World cutaneous leishmaniasis is caused by *Leishmania mexicana*, *Leishmania amazonensis*, and the species listed below for mucocutaneous disease in Central and South America. Mucocutaneous leishmaniasis (espundia) occurs in lowland forest areas of the Americas and is caused by *Leishmania braziliensis*, *Leishmania panamensis*, and *Leishmania peruviana*.

Clinical Findings

A. Symptoms and Signs

1. Visceral leishmaniasis (kala azar)—Most infections are subclinical, but a small number progress to full-blown disease. A local nonulcerating nodule at the site of the sand fly bite may precede systemic manifestations but usually is inapparent. The onset of illness may be acute, within 2 weeks of infection, or insidious. Symptoms and signs include fever, chills, sweats, weakness, anorexia, weight loss, cough, and diarrhea. The spleen progressively becomes greatly enlarged, firm, and nontender. The liver is somewhat enlarged, and generalized lymphadenopathy may occur. Hyperpigmentation of skin can be seen, leading to the name kala azar ("black fever"). Other signs include skin lesions, petechiae, gingival bleeding, jaundice, edema, and ascites. As the disease progresses, severe wasting and malnutrition are seen; death eventually occurs, often due to secondary infections, within months to a few years. Post–kala azar dermal leishmaniasis may appear after apparent cure in the Indian subcontinent and Sudan. It may simulate leprosy, with hypopigmented macules or nodules developing on preexisting lesions. Viscerotropic leishmaniasis entails a relatively mild systemic febrile illness, mostly after *L tropica* infections.

2. Old World and New World cutaneous leishmaniasis—Cutaneous swellings appear 1 week to several months after sand fly bites and can be single or multiple. Characteristics of lesions and courses of disease vary depending on the leishmanial species and host immune response. Lesions begin as small papules and develop into nonulcerated dry plaques or large encrusted ulcers with well-demarcated raised and indurated margins (Figure 39–1). Satellite lesions may be present. The lesions are painless unless secondarily infected. Local lymph nodes may be enlarged. Systemic symptoms are uncommon, but fever, constitutional symptoms, and regional lymphadenopathy may be seen. For most species, healing occurs spontaneously in months to a few years, but scarring is common.

Leishmaniasis recidivans is a relapsing form of *L tropica* infection associated with hypersensitivity, in which the primary lesion heals centrally, but spreads laterally, with extensive scarring. Diffuse cutaneous leishmaniasis involves spread from a primary lesion, with local dissemination of nodules and a protracted course. Disseminated cutaneous leishmaniasis involves multiple nodular or ulcerated lesions, often with mucosal involvement.

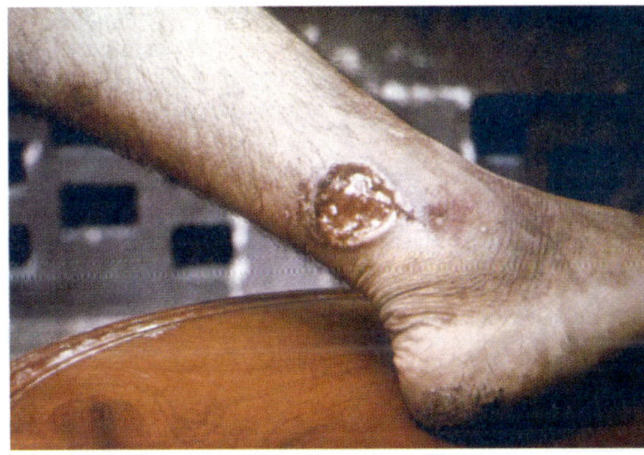

Figure 39–1. Skin ulcer due to cutaneous leishmaniasis. Note the classic morphologic characteristics of this wound with its erythematous, nodular interior, surrounded by a raised border. (From Dr. Mae Melvin, Public Health Image Library, CDC.)

3. Mucocutaneous leishmaniasis (espundia)—In Latin America, mucosal lesions develop in a small percentage of persons infected with *L braziliensis* and some other species, usually months to years after resolution of a cutaneous lesion. Nasal congestion is followed by ulceration of the nasal mucosa and septum, progressing to involvement of the mouth, lips, palate, pharynx, and larynx. Extensive destruction can occur, and secondary bacterial infection is common.

4. Infections in patients with AIDS—Leishmaniasis is an opportunistic infection in persons with AIDS. Visceral leishmaniasis can present late in the course of HIV infection, with fever, hepatosplenomegaly, and pancytopenia. The GI tract, respiratory tract, and skin may also be involved.

B. Laboratory Findings

Identifying amastigotes within macrophages in tissue samples provides a definitive diagnosis.

1. Visceral leishmaniasis—Fine-needle aspiration of the spleen for culture and tissue evaluation is generally safe and yields a diagnosis in > 95% of cases. Bone marrow aspiration is less sensitive but safer and diagnostic in most cases, and Giemsa-stained buffy coat of peripheral blood may occasionally show organisms. Cultures with media available from the CDC will grow promastigotes within a few days to weeks. Molecular assays can be diagnostic. Immunochromatographic strip assays using the rK39 antigen have shown good sensitivity and specificity; one such test is approved by the FDA.

2. Cutaneous leishmaniasis—Biopsies should be taken from the raised border of a skin lesion, with samples for histopathology, touch preparation, and culture. The histopathology shows inflammation with mononuclear cells. Macrophages filled with amastigotes may be present, especially early in infection. An intradermal leishmanin

(Montenegro) skin test is positive in most individuals with cutaneous disease but negative in those with progressive visceral or diffuse cutaneous disease; this test is not approved in the United States.

3. Mucocutaneous leishmaniasis—Diagnosis is established by detecting amastigotes in scrapings, biopsy preparations, or aspirated tissue fluid, but organisms may be rare. Cultures from these samples may grow organisms. Serologic studies are often negative, but the leishmanin skin test is usually positive.

Treatment

A. Visceral Leishmaniasis

1. Amphotericin B—The treatment of choice for visceral leishmaniasis on the Indian subcontinent is liposomal amphotericin B (approved by the FDA), which is generally effective and well tolerated but expensive. Standard dosing is 3 mg/kg/day intravenously on days 1–5, 14, and 21. Simpler regimens that have shown good efficacy in India include four doses of 5 mg/kg over 4–10 days and a single dose of 15 mg/kg, but efficacies of shorter regimens have been lower outside India. A single infusion of an amphotericin B lipid emulsion, which is more affordable than liposomal preparations, showed excellent efficacy, albeit lower than that of the liposomal formulation. Conventional amphotericin B deoxycholate, which is much less expensive, is also highly effective but with more toxicity. It is administered as a slow intravenous infusion of 1 mg/kg/day for 15–20 days or 0.5–1 mg/kg every second day for up to 8 weeks. Infusion-related side effects with conventional or liposomal amphotericin B include GI symptoms, fever, chills, dyspnea, hypotension, and hepatic and renal toxicity.

2. Pentavalent antimonials—These agents remain the most commonly used drugs to treat leishmaniasis in most areas outside India, where resistance is a major problem. Two preparations are available: meglumine antimonate in Latin America and francophone countries and sodium stibogluconate in many other areas. The compounds appear to have comparable activities. Sodium stibogluconate is no longer available in the United States. Standard dosing for either antimonial is 20 mg/kg once daily intravenously (preferred) or intramuscularly for 20 days for cutaneous leishmaniasis and 28 days for visceral or mucocutaneous disease. Toxicity increases over time, with development of GI symptoms, fever, headache, myalgias, arthralgias, pancreatitis, and rash. Intramuscular injections can cause sterile abscesses. Monitoring should include serial ECGs, and changes are indications for discontinuation to avoid progression to serious arrhythmias.

3. Miltefosine—This is the first oral drug for the treatment of leishmaniasis, and it is registered in India for this indication, though efficacy is decreasing due to drug resistance. The daily oral dose is 2.5 mg/kg in two divided doses for 28 days. This same 28-day course of miltefosine is also effective for the treatment of New World cutaneous leishmaniasis. Vomiting, diarrhea, and elevations in transaminases and kidney function studies are common, but generally short-lived, side effects.

4. Paromomycin—Paromomycin (11 mg/kg/day intramuscularly for 21 days) was shown to be similarly efficacious to amphotericin B for the treatment of visceral disease in India, where it is approved for this indication. It is much less expensive than liposomal amphotericin B or miltefosine. The drug is well tolerated; side effects include ototoxicity and reversible elevations in liver enzymes.

5. Combination therapy—The use of drug combinations can improve treatment efficacy, shorten treatment courses, and reduce the selection of resistant parasites.

A. India—In India, compared with a standard 30-day (treatment on alternate days) course of amphotericin, noninferior efficacy and decreased adverse events were seen with a single dose of liposomal amphotericin plus a 14-day course of miltefosine, a single dose of liposomal amphotericin plus a 10-day course of paromomycin (15 mg/kg/day intramuscularly), or a 10-day course of miltefosine plus paromomycin.

B. East Africa—In East Africa, the efficacy of amphotericin B is lower than in Asia, and the standard treatment is a combination of sodium stibogluconate (20 mg/kg/day intravenously) plus paromomycin (15 mg/kg/day intramuscularly) for 17 days, with demonstrated excellent efficacy; paromomycin plus miltefosine, a simpler regimen, has demonstrated equivalent efficacy. Liposomal amphotericin B may be considered in older adults or pregnant persons due to toxicity concerns.

B. Cutaneous Leishmaniasis

In the Old World, cutaneous leishmaniasis is generally self-healing over some months and does not metastasize to the mucosa, so it may be justified to withhold treatment in regions without mucocutaneous disease if lesions are small and cosmetically unimportant. Lesions on the face or hands are generally treated. New World leishmaniasis has a greater risk of progression to mucocutaneous disease, so treatment is more often warranted, but choice of therapy is complex. Standard therapy has been with pentavalent antimonials for 20 days, as described above. Two alternatives are increasingly used: miltefosine, which benefits from oral dosing and relatively little toxicity; and amphotericin B, which is fairly toxic, but highly effective. In studies in South America, a 28-day course of miltefosine was superior to a 20-day course of meglumine antimoniate, and oral fluconazole also showed good efficacy. In the United States, miltefosine and amphotericin B are available; meglumine antimoniate may be obtained via investigator-initiated investigational new drug protocol from the CDC. Topical therapy has included intralesional antimony, intralesional pentamidine, paromomycin ointment, cryotherapy, local heat, and surgical removal. In Brazil, intralesional meglumine antimoniate was as effective and better tolerated than systemic therapy with the drug. Diffuse cutaneous leishmaniasis and related chronic skin processes generally respond poorly to therapy.

C. Mucocutaneous Leishmaniasis

Cutaneous infections from regions where parasites include those that cause mucocutaneous disease (eg, *L braziliensis* in parts of Latin America) should all be treated to help prevent disease progression. Treatment of mucocutaneous disease with antimonials (eg, meglumine antimoniate) is disappointing, with responses in only about 60% in Brazil. Other therapies listed above for visceral leishmaniasis may also be used, although they have not been well studied for this indication.

Prevention & Control

Personal protection measures for avoidance of sand fly bites include use of insect repellants, fine-mesh insect netting, long sleeves and pants, and avoidance of warm shaded areas where flies are common. Disease control measures include destruction of animal reservoir hosts, mass treatment of humans in disease-prevalent areas, residual insecticide spraying in dwellings, limiting contact with dogs and other domesticated animals, and use of permethrin-impregnated collars for dogs.

Lyra MR et al. A randomized, controlled, noninferiority, multicenter trial of systemic vs intralesional treatment with meglumine antimoniate for cutaneous leishmaniasis in Brazil. Clin Infect Dis. 2023;77:574. [PMID: 37100061]

Mathison BA et al. Review of the clinical presentation, pathology, diagnosis, and treatment of leishmaniasis. Lab Med. 2023;54:363. [PMID: 36468667]

Musa AM. Paromomycin and miltefosine combination as an alternative to treat patients with visceral leishmaniasis in eastern Africa: a randomized, controlled, multicountry trial. Clin Infect Dis. 2023;76:e1177. [PMID: 36164254]

MALARIA

ESSENTIALS OF DIAGNOSIS

- Exposure to anopheline mosquitoes in a malaria-endemic area.
- Intermittent attacks of chills, fever, and sweating.
- Headache, myalgia, vomiting, splenomegaly; anemia, thrombocytopenia.
- Intraerythrocytic parasites identified in thick or thin blood smears or positive rapid diagnostic tests.
- **Falciparum malaria complications:** cerebral malaria, severe anemia, hypotension, pulmonary edema, AKI, hypoglycemia, acidosis, and hemolysis.

General Considerations

Malaria is the most important parasitic disease of humans, causing hundreds of millions of illnesses and hundreds of thousands of deaths each year. The disease is endemic in most of the tropics, including much of South and Central America, Africa, the Middle East, the Indian subcontinent, Southeast Asia, and Oceania; transmission, morbidity, and mortality are greatest in Africa, where most deaths are in young children. Malaria is also common in travelers from nonendemic areas to the tropics. Although the disease remains a major problem, impressive advances have been made in many regions. However, after marked gains, progress has stalled, particularly in Africa, where about 95% of cases occur. The WHO estimated that 282 million cases of malaria occurred in 2024 with 610,000 deaths.

Five species of the genus *Plasmodium* classically cause human malaria:

1. *Plasmodium falciparum* is responsible for nearly all severe disease, since it uniquely infects erythrocytes of all ages and mediates the sequestration of infected erythrocytes in small blood vessels, thereby evading clearance by the spleen. *P falciparum* is endemic in most malarious areas and is by far the predominant species in Africa.
2. *Plasmodium vivax* is about as common as *P falciparum* outside of Africa. *P vivax* uncommonly causes severe disease, although this outcome may be more common than previously appreciated.
3. *Plasmodium ovale* (composed of *P ovale curtisi* and *P ovale wallikeri*) is a much less common cause of disease and generally does not cause severe illness.
4. *Plasmodium malariae* is a relatively uncommon cause of disease and usually does not cause severe illness.
5. *Plasmodium knowlesi*, a parasite of macaque monkeys, causes illnesses in humans, including some severe disease, in Southeast Asia.

Malaria is transmitted by the bite of infected female anopheline mosquitoes. During feeding, mosquitoes inject sporozoites, which circulate to the liver, and rapidly infect hepatocytes, causing asymptomatic liver infection.

Merozoites are subsequently released from the liver, and they rapidly infect erythrocytes to begin the asexual erythrocytic stage of infection that is responsible for human disease. Multiple cycles of erythrocytic development, with production of merozoites that invade additional erythrocytes, lead to large numbers of circulating parasites and clinical illness. Some erythrocytic parasites develop into sexual gametocytes, which are infectious to mosquitoes, allowing completion of the life cycle and infection of others.

Malaria may uncommonly be transmitted from mother to infant (congenital malaria), by blood transfusion, and in nonendemic areas by mosquitoes infected after biting infected immigrants or travelers. In *P vivax* and *P ovale*, parasites also form dormant liver hypnozoites, which are not killed by most drugs, allowing subsequent relapses of illness after initial elimination of erythrocytic infections. For all plasmodial species, parasites may recrudesce following initial clinical improvement after suboptimal therapy.

In highly endemic regions, where persons are infected repeatedly, antimalarial immunity prevents severe disease in most older children and adults. However, relatively nonimmune young children are at high risk for severe disease from *P falciparum* infection, and this population is responsible for most deaths from malaria. Pregnant persons are also at increased risk for severe falciparum malaria. In areas with lower endemicity, individuals of all ages commonly present with uncomplicated or severe malaria. Travelers, who are generally nonimmune, are at high risk for severe disease from falciparum malaria at any age.

Clinical Findings

A. Symptoms and Signs

An acute attack of malaria typically begins with a prodrome of headache and fatigue, followed by fever. A classic malarial paroxysm includes chills, high fever, and then sweats. Patients may appear to be remarkably well between febrile episodes. Fevers are usually irregular, especially early in the illness, but without therapy may become regular, with 48-hour (*P vivax* and *P ovale*) or 72-hour (*P malariae*) cycles, especially with non-falciparum disease. Headache, malaise, myalgias, arthralgias, cough, chest pain, abdominal pain, anorexia, nausea, vomiting, and diarrhea are common. Seizures may represent simple febrile convulsions or evidence of severe neurologic disease. Physical findings may be absent or include signs of anemia, jaundice, splenomegaly, and mild hepatomegaly. Rash and lymphadenopathy are not typical in malaria, and thus suggestive of another cause of fever.

In the developed world, it is imperative that all persons with suggestive symptoms, in particular fever, who have traveled in an endemic area be evaluated for malaria. The risk for falciparum malaria is greatest within 2 months of return from travel; other species may cause disease many months—and occasionally > 1 year—after return from an endemic area.

Severe malaria is principally a result of *P falciparum* infection. It is characterized by signs of severe illness, organ dysfunction, or a high parasite load (peripheral parasitemia > 5% or > 200,000 parasites/mcL). Severe falciparum malaria can include dysfunction of any organ system, including neurologic abnormalities progressing to alterations in consciousness, repeated seizures, and coma (cerebral malaria); severe anemia; hypotension and shock; noncardiogenic pulmonary edema and acute respiratory distress syndrome; AKI due to ATN or, less commonly, severe hemolysis; hypoglycemia; acidosis; hemolysis with jaundice; hepatic dysfunction; retinal hemorrhages and other fundoscopic abnormalities; bleeding abnormalities, including disseminated intravascular coagulation; and secondary bacterial infections, including pneumonia and *Salmonella* bacteremia. In the developing world, severe malaria and deaths from the disease are mostly in young children, in particular from cerebral malaria and severe anemia. Cerebral malaria is a consequence of a single severe infection, while severe anemia follows multiple malarial infections, intestinal helminths, and nutritional deficiencies.

Uncommon disorders resulting from immunologic responses to chronic infection are massive splenomegaly and, with *P malariae* infection, immune complex glomerulopathy with nephrotic syndrome. Patients with HIV infection are at increased risk for malaria and for severe disease, in particular with advanced immunodeficiency.

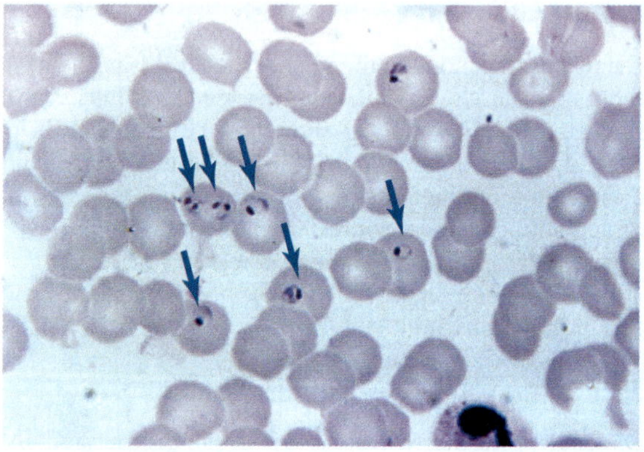

Figure 39–2. Thin film Giemsa-stained micrograph with *Plasmodium falciparum* ring forms. (From Steven Glenn, Laboratory & Consultation Division, Public Health Image Library, CDC.)

B. Laboratory Findings

Giemsa-stained blood smears remain the mainstay of diagnosis. Thick smears provide efficient evaluation of large volumes of blood, but thin smears are simpler for inexperienced personnel and better for discrimination of parasite species (Figure 39–2). Single smears are usually positive in infected individuals, although parasitemias may be low in nonimmune individuals. If illness is suspected, repeating smears at 8- to 24-hour intervals is appropriate. The severity of malaria correlates only loosely with the quantity of infecting parasites, but high parasitemias (especially > 10–20% of erythrocytes infected or > 200,000–500,000 parasites/mcL) or the presence of malarial pigment (a breakdown product of hemoglobin) in > 5% of neutrophils is associated with a particularly poor prognosis.

A second means of diagnosis is rapid diagnostic tests to identify circulating plasmodial antigens. These tests offer sensitivity and specificity near that of high-quality blood smear analysis and are simpler to perform. However, *P falciparum* that is lacking the most common rapid diagnostic test antigen, histidine-rich protein 2 (HRP2), has been identified in some areas (especially parts of South America and the Horn of Africa), so HRP2-based tests may miss some cases of falciparum malaria.

Serologic tests indicate history of disease but are not useful for diagnosis of acute infection. PCR and related molecular tests (eg, loop-mediated isothermal amplification [LAMP]) are highly sensitive but are not available for routine diagnosis. In immune populations, highly sensitive molecular tests, such as PCR, have limited value because subclinical infections, which are not routinely treated, are common.

Other diagnostic findings with uncomplicated malaria include thrombocytopenia, anemia, leukocytosis or leukopenia, liver function abnormalities, and hepatosplenomegaly. Severe malaria can present with the laboratory abnormalities expected for the advanced organ dysfunction discussed above.

Treatment

Malaria is the most common cause of fever in much of the tropics and in travelers seeking medical attention after return from endemic areas. Fevers are often treated presumptively in endemic areas, but treatment should follow definitive diagnosis, especially in nonimmune individuals. Symptomatic malaria is caused only by the erythrocytic stage of infection. Most antimalarial drugs act against this stage, except for primaquine and tafenoquine, which act principally against hepatic parasites.

A. Non-Falciparum Malaria

The first-line drug for non-falciparum malaria from most areas remains chloroquine (Table 39–2).

1. *P vivax*—Due to increasing resistance of *P vivax*, alternative therapies to chloroquine are recommended when resistance is suspected, particularly for infections acquired in Indonesia, Oceania, and South America. These infections can be treated with artemisinin-based combination therapies (ACTs) or other first-line regimens for *P falciparum* infections (as discussed below) plus primaquine.

2. *P vivax* or *P ovale*—For these species, eradication of erythrocytic parasites with chloroquine should be accompanied by treatment with primaquine or tafenoquine (after evaluating for glucose-6-phosphate dehydrogenase [G6PD] deficiency; see below) to eradicate dormant liver stages (hypnozoites), which may lead to relapses with

Table 39–2. Treatment of malaria.

Clinical Setting	Drug Therapy[1]	Alternative Drugs
Chloroquine-sensitive *Plasmodium falciparum* and *Plasmodium malariae* infections	Chloroquine phosphate, 1 g at 0 hours, then 500 mg at 6, 24, and 48 hours or Chloroquine phosphate, 1 g at 0 hours and 24 hours, then 0.5 g at 48 hours	
Plasmodium vivax and *Plasmodium ovale* infections	Chloroquine (as above), then (if G6PD normal) primaquine, 30-mg base daily for 14 days or tafenoquine 300 mg once	For infections from Indonesia, Papua New Guinea, and other areas with suspected resistance: therapies listed for uncomplicated chloroquine-resistant *P falciparum* plus primaquine
Uncomplicated infections with chloroquine-resistant *P falciparum*	Coartem (artemether 20 mg, lumefantrine 120 mg), four tablets twice daily for 3 days or Malarone, four tablets (total of 1 g of atovaquone, 400 mg of proguanil) daily for 3 days or Quinine sulfate, 650 mg three times daily for 3–7 days plus One of the following (when quinine given for <7 days) Doxycycline, 100 mg twice daily for 7 days or Clindamycin, 600 mg twice daily for 7 days	Mefloquine, 15 mg/kg once or 750 mg, then 500 mg in 6–8 hours or Dihydroartemisinin-piperaquine[2] (dihydroartemisinin 40 mg, piperaquine 320 mg), four tablets daily for 3 days or ASAQ[2] (artesunate 100 mg, amodiaquine 270 mg), two tablets daily for 3 days
Severe or complicated infections with *P falciparum*	Artesunate 2.4 mg/kg intravenously every 12 hours for 1 day, then daily[3]	Quinidine gluconate,[4,5] 10 mg/kg intravenously over 1–2 hours, then 0.02 mg/kg intravenously/min or Quinidine gluconate,[4,5] 15 mg/kg intravenously over 4 hours, then 7.5 mg/kg intravenously over 4 hours every 8 hours or Quinine dihydrochloride,[2,4,5] 20 mg/kg intravenously over 4 hours, then 10 mg/kg intravenously every 8 hours or Artemether,[2,3] 3.2 mg/kg intramuscularly, then 1.6 mg/kg/day intramuscularly

[1]All dosages are oral and refer to salts unless otherwise indicated. See text for additional information on all agents, including toxicities and cautions. See CDC guidelines (phone: 877-FYI-TRIP; https://www.cdc.gov/malaria/) for additional information and pediatric dosing.
[2]Not available in the United States.
[3]With all parenteral regimens, change to an oral regimen as soon as the patient can tolerate it.
[4]Cardiac monitoring should be in place during intravenous administration of quinidine or quinine.
[5]Avoid loading doses in persons who have received quinine, quinidine, or mefloquine in the prior 24 hours.
G6PD, glucose-6-phosphate dehydrogenase.

recurrent erythrocytic infection and malaria symptoms after weeks to months if left untreated.

3. *P malariae* and *P knowlesi*—Infections caused by these species need only be treated with chloroquine.

B. Uncomplicated Falciparum Malaria

P falciparum is resistant to chloroquine and sulfadoxine-pyrimethamine in most areas, and falciparum malaria should not be treated with these drugs. ACTs, all including a short-acting artemisinin and longer-acting partner drug, are first-line therapies in nearly all endemic countries. The WHO recommends six ACTs to treat falciparum malaria (Table 39–3). Triple ACTs under development, including an artemisinin plus two partner drugs, have shown excellent treatment efficacy, and their use may delay the spread of resistance. In developed countries, malaria is an uncommon but potentially life-threatening infection of travelers and immigrants. Nonimmune individuals with falciparum malaria should generally be admitted to the hospital due to risks of rapid progression of disease. Several options are available for the treatment of uncomplicated falciparum malaria in the United States (Table 39–2).

C. Severe Falciparum Malaria

Severe malaria is a medical emergency. Parenteral treatment is indicated for severe malaria, as defined above, and with inability to take oral drugs. With appropriate prompt therapy and supportive care, rapid recoveries may be seen even in very ill individuals.

Intravenous artesunate is FDA-approved and the standard of care for severe malaria. It has superior efficacy and better tolerability than quinine (Table 39–2). If artesunate cannot be obtained promptly, severe malaria should be treated with intravenous quinine (available in most countries but not the United States) or an oral agent until intravenous artesunate is available. In endemic regions, if parenteral therapy is not available, intrarectal administration of artemether or artesunate is also effective. Patients receiving intravenous quinine should receive continuous cardiac monitoring; if QTc prolongation exceeds 25% of baseline, the infusion rate should be reduced. Blood glucose should be monitored every 4–6 hours, and 5–10% dextrose may be coadministered to decrease the likelihood of hypoglycemia.

Appropriate care of severe malaria includes maintenance of fluids and electrolytes; respiratory and hemodynamic support; and consideration of blood transfusions, anticonvulsants, antibiotics for bacterial infections, and hemofiltration or hemodialysis. Exchange transfusion is sometimes used for those with high parasitemia (> 5–10%), but beneficial effects have not clearly been demonstrated.

D. Antimalarial Drugs

1. Chloroquine—Chloroquine is the drug of choice for the treatment of non-falciparum and sensitive falciparum malaria (Table 39–2). Chloroquine is active against erythrocytic parasites of all human malaria species. It is the preferred chemoprophylactic agent in malarious regions without resistant falciparum malaria. It does not eradicate hepatic stages. Chloroquine-resistant *P falciparum* is widespread in nearly all areas of the world with falciparum malaria, with the exceptions of Central America west of the Panama Canal and Hispaniola. Chloroquine-resistant *P vivax* has been reported, most notably from Southeast Asia and Oceania.

Chloroquine is usually well tolerated, even with prolonged use. Pruritus is common, primarily in patients from sub-Saharan Africa. Nausea, vomiting, abdominal pain, headache, malaise, blurring of vision, and urticaria are uncommon. Dosing after meals may reduce side effects.

2. Amodiaquine, piperaquine, and pyronaridine—Amodiaquine is a 4-aminoquinoline that is closely related to chloroquine. Amodiaquine has been widely used to treat malaria because of its low cost, limited toxicity, and, in some areas, effectiveness against chloroquine-resistant strains of *P falciparum*. Chemoprophylaxis with amodiaquine should be avoided because of rare but serious side effects, notably agranulocytosis, aplastic anemia, and hepatotoxicity. However, serious side effects appear to be rare with short-term use, and artesunate-amodiaquine is one of the standard ACTs recommended to treat falciparum malaria (Table 39–3).

Piperaquine is another 4-aminoquinoline that has been coformulated with dihydroartemisinin in an ACT. Piperaquine is well tolerated, and in combination with dihydroartemisinin offers a highly efficacious therapy for falciparum and vivax malaria. Due to the long half-life of piperaquine (~3 weeks), dihydroartemisinin-piperaquine offers the

Table 39–3. WHO recommendations for the treatment of uncomplicated falciparum malaria.

Regimen	Notes
Artemether-lumefantrine (Coartem, Riamet)	Coformulated, first-line therapy in many countries. Approved in the United States.
Artesunate-amodiaquine (ASAQ)	Coformulated, first-line therapy in multiple African countries.
Artesunate-mefloquine	First-line therapy in parts of Southeast Asia and South America but efficacy decreasing in parts of Thailand.
Artesunate-pyronaridine	Coformulated. Most recently approved regimen; used in some Southeast Asian countries.
Artesunate-sulfadoxine-pyrimethamine	First-line in some countries, but efficacy lower than other regimens in most areas.
Dihydroartemisinin-piperaquine	Coformulated. First-line in some countries, but efficacy decreasing in parts of Southeast Asia.

From World Health Organization: Guidelines for Malaria. https://www.who.int/publications/i/item/guidelines-for-malaria.

longest period of posttreatment prophylaxis of available ACTs. However, resistance to piperaquine, with consequent treatment failures of dihydroartemisinin-piperaquine, has emerged in Southeast Asia.

Pyronaridine is a benzonaphthyridine active against many drug-resistant strains of *P falciparum*. The combination of artesunate plus pyronaridine has shown excellent efficacy against falciparum and vivax malaria and has been well tolerated, although elevated transaminases can be seen.

3. Mefloquine—Mefloquine is effective against many chloroquine-resistant strains of *P falciparum* and against other malarial species. Although toxicity is a concern, mefloquine is also a recommended chemoprophylactic drug. Resistance to mefloquine has been reported sporadically from many areas, but it appears to be uncommon except in regions of Southeast Asia with high rates of multidrug resistance (especially border areas of Thailand). For uncomplicated malaria, mefloquine can be given as a single dose or in two doses over 1 day (Table 39–2). It is used in combination with artesunate for falciparum malaria, although resistance limits efficacy in Southeast Asia and tolerability limits its use elsewhere. It should be taken with meals and swallowed with a large amount of water. Mefloquine is recommended by the CDC for chemoprophylaxis in all malarious areas except those with no chloroquine resistance (where chloroquine is preferred) and some rural areas of Southeast Asia with a high prevalence of mefloquine resistance.

Side effects with weekly dosing of mefloquine for chemoprophylaxis include nausea, vomiting, dizziness, sleep and behavioral disturbances, epigastric pain, diarrhea, abdominal pain, headache, rash and, uncommonly, seizures and psychosis. There is an FDA black box warning about neuropsychiatric toxicity, possibly including rare, irreversible effects. Mefloquine should be avoided in persons with histories of psychiatric disease or seizures.

Side effects are more common (up to 50% of treatments) with the higher dosages of mefloquine required for treatment. These effects may be lessened by splitting administration into two doses separated by 6–8 hours. Serious neuropsychiatric toxicities (depression, confusion, acute psychosis, or seizures) have been reported in <1 in 1000 treatments, but some authorities believe that these are more common. Mefloquine can also alter cardiac conduction, and so it should not be coadministered with quinine. Mefloquine is generally considered safe in young children and pregnant persons.

4. Quinine—While artesunate is the standard of care for severe falciparum malaria, quinine dihydrochloride also is effective, although it was shown to be inferior to artesunate in large trials, and toxicity concerns complicate therapy (Table 39–2). Resistance of *P falciparum* to quinine is common in some areas of Southeast Asia, where the drug may fail to treat falciparum malaria if used alone. However, quinine still provides at least a partial therapeutic effect in most patients.

Quinine can be administered in divided doses or by continuous intravenous infusion; treatment should begin with a loading dose to rapidly achieve effective plasma concentrations and include cardiac monitoring. Therapy should be changed to an oral agent as soon as the patient has improved and can tolerate oral medications.

Oral quinine sulfate is an alternative first-line therapy for uncomplicated falciparum malaria, although poor tolerance may limit compliance. Quinine is commonly used with a second drug (most often doxycycline) to shorten the duration of use (to 3 days) and limit toxicity. Therapeutic dosages of quinine commonly cause tinnitus, headache, nausea, dizziness, flushing, and visual disturbances. Hematologic abnormalities include hemolysis (especially with G6PD deficiency), leukopenia, agranulocytosis, and thrombocytopenia. Therapeutic doses may cause hypoglycemia through stimulation of insulin release; this is a particular problem in severe infections and in pregnant patients, who have increased sensitivity to insulin. Overly rapid infusions can cause severe hypotension. ECG abnormalities (QT prolongation) are common, but dangerous arrhythmias are uncommon when the drugs are administered appropriately. Quinine should not be given concurrently with mefloquine.

5. Primaquine and tafenoquine—Primaquine phosphate, a synthetic 8-aminoquinoline, is the drug of choice for the eradication of dormant liver forms of *P vivax* and *P ovale* (Table 39–2). Primaquine is active against hepatic stages of all human malaria parasites. This action is optimal soon after therapy with chloroquine or other agents. Primaquine also acts against erythrocytic stage parasites, although this activity is too weak for the treatment of active disease, and against gametocytes. The addition of a single low dose of primaquine to treatment of falciparum malaria with an ACT is a strategy to lower transmission to mosquitoes.

For *P vivax* and *P ovale* infections, chloroquine or other drugs are used to eradicate erythrocytic forms, and if the G6PD level is normal, a 14-day course of primaquine is initiated to eradicate liver hypnozoites and prevent a subsequent relapse; a 7-day course at twice the daily dose was equally effective, but with somewhat higher risk of toxicity. Some strains of *P vivax*, particularly in New Guinea and Southeast Asia, are relatively resistant to primaquine, and the drug may fail to eradicate liver forms.

Standard chemoprophylaxis does not prevent a relapse of *P vivax* or *P ovale* infections, since liver hypnozoites are not eradicated by chloroquine or other standard treatments. To diminish the likelihood of relapse, some authorities advocate the use of a treatment course of primaquine after the completion of travel to an endemic area. Primaquine can also be used for chemoprophylaxis to prevent *P falciparum* and *P vivax* infection in persons with normal levels of G6PD.

Primaquine in recommended doses is generally well tolerated. It infrequently causes nausea, epigastric pain, abdominal cramps, and headache, especially when taken on an empty stomach. Rare side effects include leukopenia, agranulocytosis, leukocytosis, and cardiac arrhythmias. Standard doses of primaquine may cause hemolysis or methemoglobinemia (manifested by cyanosis), especially in persons with G6PD deficiency or other hereditary metabolic defects. Patients should be tested for G6PD deficiency before primaquine is prescribed. Primaquine should be discontinued if there is evidence of hemolysis or anemia and should be avoided in pregnancy.

Tafenoquine, an 8-aminoquinoline, has a much longer half-life than primaquine. These two medications share the risk of hemolysis with G6PD deficiency and probably other toxicities; tafenoquine should not be used during pregnancy or in those with G6PD deficiency. Tafenoquine is FDA-approved for patients at least 16 years of age for two indications, but with different formulations. To eliminate hepatic stages of *P vivax*, a single dose (Krintafel, two 150-mg tablets once daily) is taken with food soon after initiation of primary therapy (with chloroquine or other agents). For malaria chemoprophylaxis, the drug (Arakoda, two 100-mg tablets) is taken once daily for 3 days and then weekly until 1 week after the last exposure.

6. Inhibitors of folate synthesis—Sulfadoxine and pyrimethamine are inhibitors of two parasite enzymes involved in folate metabolism, dihydropteroate synthase (DHPS) and dihydrofolate reductase (DHFR). They are used in combination for the treatment and prevention of malaria.

Fansidar is a fixed combination of sulfadoxine (500 mg) and pyrimethamine (25 mg). It is not advised for long-term chemoprophylaxis due to rare serious side effects with long-term dosing, although it is a component of intermittent chemopreventive regimens. For treatment, advantages of sulfadoxine-pyrimethamine include ease of administration (a single oral dose) and low cost. However, resistance is a major problem.

Sulfadoxine-pyrimethamine is recommended by the WHO for monthly preventive therapy in pregnant women and perennial malaria chemoprevention in children in areas of high endemicity, although its efficacy is limited by resistance. Amodiaquine plus sulfadoxine-pyrimethamine is recommended monthly during the rainy season (known as seasonal malaria chemoprevention [SMC]) for chemoprevention in regions of West Africa with seasonal malaria transmission and limited drug resistance.

7. Artemisinins—Artemisinins act rapidly against all erythrocytic-stage human malaria parasites. Of concern, delayed clearance of parasites after treatment with artemisinins, termed *artemisinin partial resistance*, and failures of ACTs (when there is resistance also to partner drugs) were first seen in southeast Asia, and resistance has emerged in Africa.

Artemisinins play a vital role in the treatment of malaria, including multidrug-resistant *P falciparum* malaria. Due to their short plasma half-lives, recrudescence rates are unacceptably high after short-course therapy, leading to approved use only as initial therapy for severe malaria and in ACTs for uncomplicated malaria. The ACTs that are most advocated in Africa are artemether plus lumefantrine (Coartem) and artesunate plus amodiaquine (ASAQ), each available as a coformulated product. Artesunate plus mefloquine is not as well tolerated and is used mostly outside of Africa; its efficacy has declined in parts of Southeast Asia. Dihydroartemisinin-piperaquine has shown excellent efficacy and is a first-line regimen in some countries, but efficacy has declined in Cambodia due to decreased activity of both components of the regimen. The newest approved ACT, artesunate-pyronaridine, has demonstrated excellent efficacy.

Artemisinins are very well tolerated. The most commonly reported side effects have been nausea, vomiting, and diarrhea, which may often be due to acute malaria, rather than drug toxicity. Neutropenia, anemia, hemolysis, and elevated levels of liver enzymes have been noted rarely. Hemolysis may occur weeks after therapy with intravenous artesunate. Artesunate and artemether also effectively treat severe malaria when administered rectally, offering a valuable treatment modality when parenteral therapy is not available. Artemisinins are teratogenic in animals, but with the good safety profile seen in humans and the importance of effectively treating malaria during pregnancy, the WHO recommends ACTs to treat uncomplicated malaria and intravenous artesunate to treat complicated malaria during all trimesters of pregnancy.

8. Atovaquone plus proguanil (Malarone)—Atovaquone, a hydroxynaphthoquinone, is not effective when used alone, due to rapid development of drug resistance. However, Malarone, a fixed combination of atovaquone (250 mg) and the antifolate proguanil (100 mg), is highly effective for both the treatment and chemoprophylaxis of falciparum malaria, and it is approved for both indications in the United States (Table 39–2). It also appears to be active against other species of malaria parasites. Unlike most other antimalarials, Malarone provides activity against both erythrocytic and hepatic stage parasites.

For treatment, Malarone is given at an adult dose of four tablets daily for 3 days. For chemoprophylaxis, Malarone must be taken daily (Table 39–4). It has an advantage over mefloquine and doxycycline in requiring shorter durations of treatment before and after the period at risk for malaria transmission, due to activity against liver-stage parasites. It should be taken with food.

Malarone is generally well tolerated. Side effects include abdominal pain, nausea, vomiting, diarrhea, headache, and rash, and these are more common with the higher dose required for treatment. Reversible elevations in liver enzymes have been reported. The safety of atovaquone in pregnancy is unknown.

9. Antibiotics—A number of antibacterials in addition to the folate antagonists and sulfonamides are slow-acting antimalarials. None of the antibiotics should be used as single agents for the treatment of malaria due to their slow rate of action.

Doxycycline is commonly used in the treatment of falciparum malaria in conjunction with quinine, allowing a shorter and better-tolerated course of those drugs (Table 39–2). Doxycycline is also a standard chemoprophylactic drug (Table 39–4). Its side effects include GI symptoms, candidal vaginitis, and photosensitivity. The drug should be taken while upright with a large amount of water to avoid esophageal irritation. Clindamycin can be used in conjunction with quinine in those for whom doxycycline is not recommended, such as children and

Table 39–4. Drugs for the prevention of malaria in travelers.[1]

Drug	Use[2]	Adult Dosage (all oral)[3]
Chloroquine	Areas without resistant *Plasmodium falciparum*	500 mg weekly
Malarone	Areas with multidrug-resistant *P falciparum*	1 tablet (250-mg atovaquone/100-mg proguanil) daily
Mefloquine	Areas with chloroquine-resistant *P falciparum*	250 mg weekly
Doxycycline	Areas with multidrug-resistant *P falciparum*	100 mg daily
Primaquine[4]	Terminal prophylaxis of *Plasmodium vivax* and *Plasmodium ovale* infections; alternative for *P falciparum* prophylaxis	30-mg base daily: for terminal prophylaxis take for 14 days after travel For chemoprevention begin 1–2 days before travel, take during travel and for 7 days after travel
Tafenoquine[4]	Alternative for *P falciparum* prophylaxis	200 mg once daily for 3 days and then weekly until 1 week after last exposure

[1]Recommendations may change, as resistance to all available drugs is increasing. See text for additional information on toxicities and cautions. For additional details and pediatric dosing, see CDC guidelines (phone: 800-CDC-INFO; https://wwwnc.cdc.gov/travel/). Travelers to remote areas should consider carrying effective therapy (see text) for use if a febrile illness develops, and they cannot reach medical attention quickly.
[2]Areas without known chloroquine-resistant *P falciparum* are Central America west of the Panama Canal, Haiti, Dominican Republic, Egypt, and most malarious countries of the Middle East. Malarone or mefloquine is currently recommended for other malarious areas except for border areas of Thailand, where doxycycline is recommended.
[3]For drugs other than primaquine, begin 1–2 weeks before departure (except 2 days before for doxycycline and Malarone) and continue for 4 weeks after leaving the endemic area (except 1 week for Malarone). All dosages refer to salts unless otherwise indicated.
[4]Screen for glucose-6-phosphate dehydrogenase deficiency before using primaquine.
Reproduced with permission from Katzung BG. *Basic & Clinical Pharmacology*, 14th edition. McGraw-Hill, 2018.

pregnant persons (Table 39–2). The most common toxicities with clindamycin are GI.

10. Lumefantrine—Lumefantrine, an aryl alcohol, is available only as a fixed-dose combination with artemether (Coartem or Riamet). Oral absorption is highly variable and improved when the drug is taken with food. Use of Coartem with a fatty meal is recommended. Coartem is highly effective for the treatment of falciparum malaria, but it requires twice-daily dosing. Despite this limitation, due to its reliable efficacy against falciparum malaria, Coartem is the first-line therapy for malaria in many malarious countries and is the most widely used antimalarial in the world. Coartem is well tolerated; side effects include headache, dizziness, loss of appetite, GI symptoms, and palpitations. Coartem does not generally cause QT prolongation or serious cardiac toxicity.

Prevention

1. General approach—Malaria is transmitted by night-biting anopheline mosquitoes. Bed nets, in particular nets treated with permethrin insecticides, are heavily promoted as inexpensive means of antimalarial protection, but effectiveness varies in part due to widespread insecticide resistance. Permethrin-treated baby wraps and transfluthrin-based spatial repellents both reduced the incidence of malaria in African studies. Indoor spraying of insecticides is generally highly effective in Africa but limited by resource constraints. When travelers from nonendemic to endemic countries are counseled on the prevention of malaria, it is imperative to emphasize measures to prevent mosquito bites (insect repellents, insecticides, and bed nets), since no chemoprophylactic regimen is fully protective.

2. Malaria vaccine—The RTS,S vaccine, which is based on a sporozoite antigen, has been widely studied; multiple trials showed about 25–50% protection against malaria in children in the year after immunization, but lower levels of protection in very young children, in areas of highest malaria exposure, and over longer periods of time. Seasonal malaria immunization, using the RTS,S vaccine in conjunction with SMC during the high transmission season, has shown excellent preventive efficacy. The R21 vaccine, with the same antigen as RTS,S but a different adjuvant, showed at least equivalent protection. Both the RTS,S and R21 vaccines are being rolled out for young children in Africa. Other approaches under study include vaccines containing erythrocytic, liver-stage, and sexual-stage antigens, and use of radiation-attenuated or molecularly attenuated sporozoites.

3. Chemoprophylaxis—Chemoprophylaxis is recommended for all travelers from nonendemic regions to endemic areas, although risks vary greatly for different locations, and some tropical areas entail no risk; specific recommendations for travel to different locales are available from the CDC (https://www.cdc.gov/). Recommendations from the CDC include the use of chloroquine for chemoprophylaxis in the few areas with only chloroquine-sensitive malaria parasites (principally the Caribbean and Central America west of the Panama Canal), and Malarone, mefloquine, or doxycycline for other areas (Table 39–4). Primaquine and tafenoquine are also effective but not used as often. In some circumstances, it may be appropriate for travelers to not use chemoprophylaxis but to carry supplies of drugs (ACTs or Malarone) with them in case a febrile illness develops and medical attention is unavailable. Most authorities do not recommend routine terminal prophylaxis with primaquine to eradicate dormant hepatic stages of *P vivax* and *P ovale* after travel, but this may be appropriate for travelers with major exposure to these parasites.

Regular chemoprophylaxis is not a standard management practice in developing world populations due to the expense and potential toxicities of long-term therapy. However, intermittent preventive therapy, whereby at-risk populations receive antimalarial therapy at set intervals, may decrease the incidence of malaria while allowing antimalarial immunity to develop. During pregnancy, intermittent preventive therapy with sulfadoxine-pyrimethamine, provided monthly during the second and third trimesters, has improved pregnancy outcomes, probably in part due to non-malarial benefits. With increasing resistance, the preventive efficacy of sulfadoxine-pyrimethamine is likely falling, and the long-acting ACT dihydroartemisinin-piperaquine is a promising replacement. In areas with seasonal malaria transmission and limited drug resistance, principally the Sahel subregion of West Africa, SMC, with monthly amodiaquine plus sulfadoxine-pyrimethamine administered monthly to children during the transmission season, is widely practiced. For children in other regions of Africa, SMC or perennial malaria chemoprevention with monthly sulfadoxine-pyrimethamine in areas with perennial transmission is advocated but not yet widely implemented; efficacy will likely be limited by drug resistance. Injection of long-acting monoclonal antibodies to prevent malaria has shown promise in clinical trials.

Prognosis

When treated appropriately, uncomplicated malaria generally responds well, with resolution of fevers within 1–2 days and a mortality of about 0.1%. Severe malaria can commonly progress to death, but many children respond well to therapy. In the developed world, mortality from malaria is mostly in adults, and often follows extended illnesses and secondary complications long after eradication of the malarial infection. Pregnant persons are at particular risk during their first pregnancy. Malaria in pregnancy also increases the likelihood of poor pregnancy outcomes, with increased prematurity, low birth weight, and mortality.

When to Refer

- Referral to an expert on infectious diseases or travel medicine is important with all cases of malaria in the United States.
- For falciparum malaria, referral should not delay initial diagnosis and therapy, since delays in therapy can lead to severe illness or death.

When to Admit

- Admission for non-falciparum malaria is warranted only if specific problems that require hospital management are present.
- Patients with falciparum malaria are generally admitted because the disease can progress rapidly to severe illness; exceptions may be made with individuals who are from malaria-endemic areas, and thus expected to have a degree of immunity, who are without evidence of severe disease, and who are judged able to return promptly for medical attention if their disease progresses.

Daily JP et al. Malaria. N Engl J Med. 2025;392:1320. [PMID: 40174226]

Duffy PE et al. Malaria vaccines: a new era of prevention and control. Nat Rev Microbiol. 2024;22:756. [PMID: 39025972]

Kamya MR et al. Efficacies of artemether-lumefantrine, artesunate-amodiaquine, dihydroartemisinin-piperaquine, and artesunate-pyronaridine for the treatment of uncomplicated Plasmodium falciparum malaria in children aged 6 months to 10 years in Uganda: a randomised, open-label, phase 4 clinical trial. Lancet Infect Dis. 2026;26:67. [PMID: 40845863]

Poespoprodjo JR et al. Malaria. Lancet. 2023;402:2328. [PMID: 37924827]

Rosenthal PJ et al. Emergence, transmission dynamics and mechanisms of artemisinin partial resistance in malaria parasites in Africa. Nat Rev Microbiol. 2024;22:373. [PMID: 38321292]

World Health Organization. *World Malaria Report 2025.* Geneva, Switzerland: WHO; 2025. https://www.who.int/teams/global-malaria-programme/reports/world-malaria-report-2025ß

BABESIOSIS

ESSENTIALS OF DIAGNOSIS

- History of tick bite or exposure to ticks.
- Fever, flu-like symptoms, anemia.
- Intraerythrocytic parasites on Giemsa-stained blood smears.
- Positive serologic tests.

General Considerations

Babesiosis is an uncommon intraerythrocytic infection caused by *Babesia* species and transmitted by *Ixodes* ticks. In the United States, hundreds of cases of babesiosis have been reported, and infection is caused by *Babesia microti,* which also infects wild mammals. Most babesiosis in the United States occurs in the coastal northeast, with some cases also in the upper Midwest, following the geographic range of the vector *Ixodes scapularis*, and Lyme disease and anaplasmosis, which are spread by the same vector. Babesiosis is caused by *Babesia divergens* and related species in Europe and Asia. Babesiosis due to other *Babesia*-like organisms has been reported uncommonly from the western United States. Babesiosis can also be transmitted by blood transfusion, but blood supplies are not screened. A survey of a large set of blood samples from endemic regions of the United States identified approximately 0.4% as potentially infectious for *B microti*.

Clinical Findings

A. Symptoms and Signs

Serosurveys suggest that asymptomatic infections are common in endemic areas. With *B microti* infections, symptoms appear one to several weeks after a tick bite; parasitemia is evident after 2–4 weeks. Patients usually do not recall the tick bite. The typical flu-like illness develops gradually and is characterized by fever, malaise, fatigue, headache, anorexia, and myalgia. Other findings may include nausea, vomiting, abdominal pain, arthralgia, sore throat, depression, emotional lability, anemia, thrombocytopenia, elevated transaminases, and splenomegaly. Parasitemia may continue for months to years, with or without symptoms, and the disease is usually self-limited. Severe complications are most likely to occur in older persons or in those who have had splenectomy. Serious complications include respiratory failure, hemolytic anemia, disseminated intravascular coagulation, heart failure, and AKI. In a study of hospitalized patients, the mortality rate was 6.5%. Most recognized *B divergens* infections in Europe have been in patients who have had splenectomy. These infections progress rapidly with high fever, severe hemolytic anemia, jaundice, hemoglobinuria, and AKI, with death rates > 40%.

B. Laboratory Findings

Identification of the intraerythrocytic parasite on Giemsa-stained blood smears establishes the diagnosis. Repeated smears are often necessary because well under 1% of erythrocytes may be infected, especially early in infection, although parasitemias can exceed 10%. Diagnosis can also be made by PCR, which is more sensitive than blood smear. An indirect immunofluorescent antibody test for *B microti* is available from the CDC; antibody is detectable within 2–4 weeks after the onset of symptoms and persists for months, and a fourfold increase in antibody titer between acute and convalescent sera confirms acute infection.

Treatment

Most patients have a mild illness and recover without therapy. Standard therapy for mild to moderate disease is a 7-day course of atovaquone (750 mg orally every 12 hours) plus azithromycin (600 mg orally once daily), which is equally effective and better tolerated than the alternative regimen, a 7-day course of quinine (650 mg orally three times daily) plus clindamycin (600 mg orally three times daily). However, there is more experience using quinine plus clindamycin, and this regimen is recommended by some experts for severe disease. Exchange transfusion has been used successfully in severely ill asplenic patients and those with parasitemia > 10%.

Asquith M et al. Human babesiosis: the past, present and future. Expert Rev Mol Med. 2025;27:e30. [PMID: 40908571]

Heller HM. Babesiosis in immunosuppressed hosts: pathogenesis, diagnosis and management. Curr Opin Infect Dis. 2024;37:327. [PMID: 39109671]

TOXOPLASMOSIS

ESSENTIALS OF DIAGNOSIS

- Infection confirmed by isolation of *Toxoplasma gondii* or identification of tachyzoites in tissue or body fluids.

Primary infection

- Fever, malaise, headache, sore throat.
- Lymphadenopathy.
- Positive IgG and IgM serologic tests.

Congenital infection

- After acute infection in seronegative mothers, CNS abnormalities and retinochoroiditis in offspring.

Infection in immunocompromised persons

- Reactivation leads to encephalitis, retinochoroiditis, pneumonitis, myocarditis.
- Positive IgG but negative IgM serologic tests.

General Considerations

T gondii, an obligate intracellular protozoan, is found worldwide in humans and in many species of mammals and birds. The definitive hosts are cats. Humans are infected after ingestion of cysts in raw or undercooked meat, including wild game, ingestion of oocysts in food or water contaminated by cats, transplacental transmission of trophozoites or, rarely, direct inoculation of trophozoites via blood transfusion or organ transplantation. *Toxoplasma* seroprevalence varies widely. It is < 20% in the United States, but higher in other countries in both the developed and developing worlds, where it may exceed 80%. In the United States, *T gondii* is estimated to infect 1.1 million persons each year, with resultant chorioretinitis developing in 21,000 and vision loss in 4800.

Clinical Findings

A. Symptoms and Signs

The clinical manifestations of toxoplasmosis may be grouped into four syndromes.

1. Primary infection in the immunocompetent person—After ingestion, *T gondii* infection progresses from the GI tract to lymphatics, and then dissemination. Most acute infections are asymptomatic. About 10–20% are symptomatic after an incubation period of 1–2 weeks. Acute infections in immunocompetent persons typically present as mild, febrile illnesses that resemble infectious mononucleosis. Nontender cervical or diffuse lymphadenopathy may persist for weeks to months. Systemic findings may include fever, malaise, headache, sore throat, rash, myalgias, hepatosplenomegaly, and atypical lymphocytosis. Rare severe manifestations are pneumonitis, meningoencephalitis, hepatitis, myocarditis, polymyositis, and retinochoroiditis. Symptoms may fluctuate; most patients recover spontaneously within a few months.

2. Congenital infection—Congenital transmission occurs as a result of infection, which may be symptomatic or asymptomatic, in a nonimmune woman during pregnancy. Fetal infection follows maternal infection in 30–50% of cases, but this risk varies by trimester: 10–25% during the first, 30–50% during the second, and 60% or higher during the third trimester. In the United States, an estimated 400 to 4000 congenital infections occur yearly. While the risk of fetal infection increases, the risk of severe fetal disease decreases over the course of pregnancy. Early fetal infections commonly lead to spontaneous abortion, stillbirths, or severe neonatal disease, including neurologic manifestations. Retinochoroiditis and other sight-threatening eye lesions may develop. Infections later in pregnancy less commonly lead to major fetal problems. Most infants appear normal at birth, but they may have subtle abnormalities and progress to symptoms and signs of congenital toxoplasmosis later in life.

3. Retinochoroiditis—The most common late presentation of congenital toxoplasmosis is retinochoroiditis, which presents weeks to years after congenital infection, commonly in teenagers or young adults. Retinochoroiditis also occurs in persons who acquire infection early in life, and these patients more often present with unilateral disease. Uveitis is also seen. Disease presents with pain, photophobia, and visual changes, usually without systemic symptoms. Signs and symptoms eventually improve, but visual defects may persist. Rarely, progression may result in glaucoma and blindness.

4. Disease in the immunocompromised person—Reactivated toxoplasmosis occurs in patients with AIDS, cancer, or those taking immunosuppressive drugs. In advanced AIDS, the most common manifestation is encephalitis, with multiple necrotizing brain lesions. The encephalitis usually presents subacutely, with fever, headache, altered mental status, focal neurologic findings, and other evidence of brain lesions. Less common manifestations of toxoplasmosis in AIDS are chorioretinitis and pneumonitis. Chorioretinitis presents with ocular pain and alterations in vision. Pneumonitis presents with fever, cough, and dyspnea. Toxoplasmosis can develop in recipients of solid organ or bone marrow transplants due to reactivation or, rarely, transmission of infection. Reactivation also can occur in those with hematologic malignancies or treated with immunosuppressive drugs. With primary or reactivated disease in those with immunodeficiency due to malignancy or immunosuppressive drugs, toxoplasmosis is similar to that in individuals with AIDS, but pneumonitis and myocarditis are more common.

B. Diagnostic Testing

1. Identification of parasites—Organisms can be seen in tissue or body fluids, although they may be difficult to identify; special staining techniques can facilitate identification. The demonstration of tachyzoites indicates acute infection; cysts may represent either acute or chronic infection. With lymphadenopathy, examination of lymph nodes usually does not show organisms. Parasite identification can also be made by inoculation of tissue culture or mice. PCR can be used for sensitive identification of organisms in amniotic fluid, blood, CSF, aqueous humor, and bronchoalveolar lavage fluid.

2. Serologic diagnosis—Multiple serologic methods are used, including the Sabin-Feldman dye test, ELISA, indirect fluorescent antibody test, and agglutination tests. IgG antibodies are seen within 1–2 weeks of infection and usually persist for life. IgM antibodies peak earlier than IgG and decline more rapidly, although they may persist for years. In immunocompromised individuals in whom reactivation is suspected, a positive IgG assay indicates distant infection, and thus the potential for reactivated disease; a negative IgG argues strongly against reactivation toxoplasmosis. With reactivation in immunocompromised persons, IgM tests are generally negative.

3. During pregnancy and in newborns—Maternal conversion from a negative to positive serologic test or rising titers are suggestive of acute infection, but tests are not routinely performed during pregnancy. When pregnant persons are screened, negative IgG and IgM assays exclude active infection, but indicate the risk of infection during the pregnancy. Positive IgG with negative IgM is highly suggestive of chronic infection, with no risk of congenital disease unless the mother is severely immunocompromised. A positive IgM test is concerning for new maternal infection because of the risk of congenital disease. Confirmatory testing should be performed before consideration of treatment or possible termination of pregnancy due to the limitations of available tests. Tests of the avidity of antibodies can be helpful, but a battery of tests is needed for confirmation of acute infection during pregnancy. When acute infection during pregnancy is suspected, PCR of amniotic fluid offers a sensitive assessment for congenital disease. In newborns, positive IgM or IgA antibody tests are indicative of congenital infection, although the diagnosis is not ruled out by a negative test. Positive IgG assays may represent transfer of maternal antibodies without infection of the infant, but persistence of positive IgG beyond 12 months of age is diagnostic of congenital infection. PCR of blood, CSF, or urine can also be helpful for early diagnosis of congenital disease.

4. In immunocompetent individuals—Individuals with a suggestive clinical syndrome should be tested for IgG and IgM antibodies. Seroconversion, a 16-fold rise in antibody titer, or an IgM titer > 1:64 is suggestive of acute infection, although false-positive results may occur. Acute infection can also be diagnosed by detection of tachyzoites in tissue, culture of organisms, or PCR of blood or body fluids. Histologic evaluation of lymph nodes can show characteristic morphology, with or without organisms.

5. In immunocompromised individuals—A presentation consistent with toxoplasmic encephalitis warrants imaging of the brain. CT and MRI scans typically show multiple ring-enhancing cerebral lesions, most commonly involving the corticomedullary junction and basal ganglia. MRI is the more sensitive imaging modality. In patients with AIDS who have a positive IgG serologic test and no recent anti-*Toxoplasma* or antiviral therapy, the predictive value of a typical imaging study is about 80%. The other common diagnosis in this setting is CNS lymphoma, which more typically causes a single brain lesion. The differential diagnosis also includes tuberculoma, bacterial brain abscess, fungal abscess, and carcinoma. Diagnosis of CNS toxoplasmosis is most typically made after a therapeutic trial, with clinical and radiologic improvement expected within 2–3 weeks. Definitive diagnosis requires brain biopsy and search for organisms and typical histology. In retinochoroiditis, funduscopic examination shows vitreous inflammatory reaction, white retinal lesions, and pigmented scars. Diagnosis of other clinical entities in immunocompromised individuals is generally based on histology.

Treatment

A. Approach to Treatment

1. For immunocompetent persons—Therapy is generally not necessary in immunocompetent persons, since the primary illness is self-limited. However, for severe, persistent, or visceral disease, treatment for 2–4 weeks may be considered. Treatment is appropriate for primary infection during pregnancy because the risk of fetal transmission or the severity of congenital disease may be reduced. For retinochoroiditis, most episodes are self-limited, and opinions vary on indications for treatment. Treatment is often advocated for episodes with decreases in visual acuity, multiple or large lesions, macular lesions, significant inflammation, or persistence for > 1 month.

2. For immunocompromised persons—Patients with active infection must be treated. For those with transient immunodeficiency, therapy can be continued for 4–6 weeks after cessation of symptoms. For those with persistent immunodeficiency, such as patients with AIDS, full therapy for 4–6 weeks is followed by maintenance therapy with lower doses of drugs. Immunodeficient patients who are asymptomatic but have a positive IgG serologic test should receive long-term chemoprophylaxis.

B. Medications

Drugs for toxoplasmosis are active only against tachyzoites, so they do not eradicate infection. Standard therapy is the combination of pyrimethamine (200-mg orally as a loading dose, then 50–75 mg [1 mg/kg] once daily) plus sulfadiazine (1–1.5 g orally four times daily), with folinic acid (10–20 mg orally once daily) to prevent bone marrow suppression. Patients should be screened for a history of sulfonamide sensitivity (skin rashes, GI symptoms, hepatotoxicity). To prevent sulfonamide crystal-induced nephrotoxicity, good urinary output should be maintained. Pyrimethamine side effects include headache and GI symptoms. Even with folinic acid therapy, bone marrow suppression may occur; platelet and WBC counts should be monitored at least weekly. A first-line alternative is pyrimethamine plus clindamycin (600 mg orally four times daily). Another alternative is TMP-SMZ. Pyrimethamine is not used during the first trimester of pregnancy due to its teratogenicity. Standard therapy for acute toxoplasmosis during pregnancy is spiramycin (1 g orally three times daily until delivery), which reduces the frequency of transmission to the fetus by about 60%. Spiramycin does not cross the placenta, so when fetal infection is documented or for acute infections late in pregnancy (which commonly lead to fetal transmission), treatment with combination regimens as described above is indicated.

Prevention

Prevention of primary infection centers on avoidance of undercooked meat or contact with material contaminated by cat feces, particularly for seronegative pregnant persons and immunocompromised persons. Irradiation, cooking to 66°C, or freezing to –20°C kills tissue cysts. Thorough cleaning of hands and surfaces is needed after contact with raw meat or areas contaminated by cats. Oocysts passed in cat feces can remain infective for a year or more, but fresh oocysts are not infective for 48 hours. For best protection, litter boxes should be changed daily and soaked in boiling water for 5 minutes, gloves should be worn when gardening, fruits and vegetables should be thoroughly washed, and ingestion of dried meat should be avoided.

Universal screening of pregnant persons for *T gondii* antibodies is conducted in some countries but not the United States. Pregnant persons should ideally have their serum examined for IgG and IgM antibody, and those with negative titers should adhere to the prevention measures described above. Seronegative women who continue to have environmental exposure should undergo repeat serologic screening several times during pregnancy.

For immunocompromised individuals, chemoprophylaxis to prevent primary or reactivated infection is warranted. For hematopoietic cell transplant recipients and patients with advanced AIDS, chemoprophylaxis with TMP-SMZ (one double-strength tablet orally daily or two tablets three times weekly), used for protection against *Pneumocystis*, is effective against *T gondii*. Alternatives are pyrimethamine plus either sulfadoxine or dapsone (various regimens). In patients with AIDS, chemoprophylaxis can be discontinued if antiretroviral therapy leads to immune reconstitution.

Beltrame A et al, Human toxoplasmosis: current advances in the field. Curr Opin Infect Dis. 2025;38:392. [PMID: 40747642]
Cerisola A et al. Congenital toxoplasmosis. Semin Pediatr Neurol. 2025;54:101203. [PMID: 40701684]
Miyagaki M et al. Ocular toxoplasmosis: advances in *Toxoplasma gondii* biology, clinical manifestations, diagnostics, and therapy. Pathogens. 2024;13:898. [PMID: 39452769]

AMEBIASIS

ESSENTIALS OF DIAGNOSIS

- Organisms or antigen present in stools or abscess aspirate.
- Positive serologic tests with colitis or hepatic abscess, but these may represent prior infections.
- Mild to moderate colitis with recurrent diarrhea.
- Severe colitis: bloody diarrhea, fever, and abdominal pain, with potential progression to hemorrhage or perforation.
- Hepatic abscess: fever, hepatomegaly, and abdominal pain.

General Considerations

The *Entamoeba* complex contains three morphologically identical species: *Entamoeba dispar* and *Entamoeba moshkovskii*, which are avirulent, and *Entamoeba histolytica*, which may be an avirulent intestinal commensal or lead to serious disease. Disease follows penetration of *E histolytica* into the intestinal wall, resulting in diarrhea, and with severe involvement, dysentery or extraintestinal disease, most commonly liver abscess.

E histolytica infections are present worldwide but are most prevalent in subtropical and tropical areas under conditions of crowding, poor sanitation, and poor nutrition. Of the estimated 500 million persons worldwide infected with *Entamoeba*, most are infected with *E dispar* and an estimated 10% with *E histolytica*. The prevalence of *E moshkovskii* is unknown. Mortality from invasive *E histolytica* infections is estimated at 100,000 per year.

Humans are the only established *E histolytica* host. Transmission occurs through ingestion of cysts from fecally contaminated food or water, facilitated by person-to-person spread, flies and other arthropods as mechanical vectors, and use of human excrement as fertilizer. Urban outbreaks have occurred because of common-source water contamination.

Clinical Findings

A. Symptoms and Signs

1. Intestinal amebiasis—In most infected persons, the organism lives as a commensal, and the carrier is without symptoms. With symptomatic disease, diarrhea usually begins after an incubation period of 2–4 weeks (but may begin within a week of infection), with gradual onset of abdominal pain and diarrhea. Fever is uncommon. Periods of remission and recurrence may last days, weeks, or longer. Abdominal examination may show distention, tenderness, hyperperistalsis, and hepatomegaly. Microscopic hematochezia is common. More severe presentations include colitis and dysentery, with worse diarrhea (10–20 stools per day) and bloody stools. With dysentery, physical findings include high fevers, prostration, vomiting, abdominal pain and tenderness, hepatic enlargement, and hypotension. Severe presentations are more common in young children, pregnant persons, those who are malnourished, and those receiving corticosteroids. Thus, in endemic regions, corticosteroids should not be started for presumed IBD without first ruling out amebiasis. Fulminant amebic colitis can progress to necrotizing colitis, intestinal perforation, mucosal sloughing, and severe hemorrhage, with mortality rates > 40%. More long-term complications include chronic diarrhea with weight loss, which may last for months to years; bowel ulcerations; and amebic appendicitis. Localized granulomatous lesions (amebomas) can present after either dysentery or chronic intestinal infection. Clinical findings include pain, obstructive symptoms, and hemorrhage and may suggest intestinal carcinoma.

2. Extraintestinal amebiasis—The most common extraintestinal manifestation is amebic liver abscess. This can occur with colitis, but more frequently presents without a history of prior intestinal symptoms. Patients have acute or gradual onset of abdominal pain, fever, an enlarged and tender liver, anorexia, and weight loss. Diarrhea is present in a small number of patients. Physical examination may show intercostal tenderness. Abscesses are most commonly single and in the right lobe of the liver, and they are much more common in men. Without prompt treatment, amebic abscesses may rupture into the pleural, peritoneal, or pericardial space, which is often fatal. Amebic infections may rarely occur throughout the body, including the lungs, brain, and genitourinary system.

B. Laboratory Findings

Laboratory studies with intestinal amebiasis show leukocytosis and hematochezia, with fecal leukocytes not present in all cases. With extraintestinal amebiasis, leukocytosis and elevated liver function studies are seen.

C. Diagnostic Testing

1. Intestinal amebiasis—Diagnosis is most commonly made by identifying organisms in the stool. *E histolytica* and *E dispar* cannot be distinguished, but the identification of amebic trophozoites or cysts in a symptomatic patient is highly suggestive of amebiasis. Stool evaluation for organisms is not highly sensitive (~30–50% for amebic colitis), and at least three stool specimens should be evaluated after concentration and staining. Multiple serologic assays are available; these tests are sensitive, although sensitivity is lower (~70% in colitis) early in illness, and they cannot distinguish recent and old disease, as they remain positive for years after infection. Commercially available stool antigen tests (TechLab II, CELISA, QUIK CHEK) can distinguish *E histolytica* from nonpathogenic species and offer improved sensitivity (> 90% for colitis). The QUIK CHEK assay is FDA-approved, offers rapid point-of-care diagnosis, and is available in a combined assay for amebiasis, giardiasis, and cryptosporidiosis. Highly sensitive molecular tests are not used routinely but available in some high-resource settings within commercial panels for identifying gut pathogens. Colonoscopy of uncleansed bowel typically shows no specific findings in mild intestinal disease; in

Table 39–5. Treatment of *E histolytica* amebiasis.[1]

Clinical Setting	Drugs of Choice and Adult Dosage	Alternative Drugs and Adult Dosage
Asymptomatic intestinal infection	**Luminal agent:** Diloxanide furoate,[2] 500 mg orally three times daily for 10 days or Iodoquinol, 650 mg orally three times daily for 21 days or Paromomycin, 10 mg/kg orally three times daily for 7 days	
Mild to moderate intestinal infection	Metronidazole, 750 mg orally three times daily (or 500 mg intravenously every 6 hours) for 10 days or Tinidazole, 2 g orally daily for 3–5 days **plus** Luminal agent (see above)	Luminal agent (see above) **plus** either Tetracycline, 250 mg orally three times daily for 10 days or Erythromycin, 500 mg orally four times daily for 10 days
Severe intestinal infection	Metronidazole, 750 mg orally three times daily (or 500 mg intravenously every 6 hours) for 10 days or Tinidazole, 2 g orally daily for 3–5 days **plus** Luminal agent (see above)	Luminal agent (see above) **plus** either Tetracycline, 250 mg orally three times daily for 10 days or Dehydroemetine[2] or emetine,[2] 1 mg/kg subcutaneously or intramuscularly for 3–5 days
Hepatic abscess, ameboma, and other extraintestinal disease	Metronidazole, 750 mg orally three times daily (or 500 mg intravenously every 6 hours) for 10 days or Tinidazole, 2 g orally daily for 5 days **plus** Luminal agent (see above)	Dehydroemetine[2] or emetine,[2] 1 mg/kg subcutaneously or intramuscularly for 8–10 days, followed by (liver abscess only) chloroquine, 500 mg orally twice daily for 2 days, then 500 mg daily for 21 days **plus** Luminal agent (see above)

[1]See text for additional details and cautions.
[2]Not available in the United States.

severe disease, ulcers may be found with intact intervening friable mucosa, resembling IBD. Examination of fresh ulcer exudate for motile trophozoites and for *E histolytica* antigen may yield a diagnosis.

2. Hepatic abscess—Serologic tests for anti-amebic antibodies are almost always positive, except very early in the infection. Thus, a negative test in a suspicious case should be repeated in about a week. The TechLab II antigen test can be used to test serum with good sensitivity if used before the initiation of therapy. Examination of stools for organisms or antigen is frequently negative; the antigen test is positive in approximately 40% of cases. As imaging studies cannot distinguish amebic and pyogenic abscesses, when a diagnosis is not available from serologic studies, percutaneous aspiration may be indicated, ideally with an image-guided needle. Aspiration typically yields brown or yellow fluid. Detection of organisms in the aspirate is uncommon, but detection of *E histolytica* antigen is very sensitive and diagnostic. The key risk of aspiration is peritoneal spillage leading to peritonitis from amoebas or other (pyogenic or echinococcal) organisms.

D. Imaging

Liver abscesses can be identified by ultrasonography, CT, or MRI, typically with round or oval low-density nonhomogeneous lesions, with abrupt transition from normal liver to the lesion, and hypoechoic centers. Abscesses are most commonly single, but more than one may be present. The right lobe is usually involved.

Treatment

Treatment of amebiasis generally entails the use of metronidazole or tinidazole to eradicate tissue trophozoites and a luminal amebicide to eradicate intestinal cysts (Table 39–5).

1. Asymptomatic infection with *E dispar*—This infection does not require therapy. This organism cannot be differentiated morphologically from *E histolytica*, but serology for *E histolytica* is negative. *E dispar* colonization is likely, and treatment is not indicated.

2. Asymptomatic infection with *E histolytica*—This infection is treated with a luminal agent. Effective luminal agents are diloxanide furoate, iodoquinol (diiodohydroxyquinoline), and paromomycin. Side effects associated with luminal agents are flatulence with diloxanide furoate, mild diarrhea with iodoquinol, and GI symptoms with paromomycin. Relative contraindications are thyroid disease for iodoquinol and kidney disease for iodoquinol or paromomycin.

3. Intestinal amebiasis with *E histolytica*—Treatment of intestinal amebiasis requires metronidazole or tinidazole plus a luminal agent (Table 39–5). Tinidazole offers simpler dosing, a more rapid clinical response, and fewer side effects than metronidazole. Side effects from either agent include transient nausea, vomiting, epigastric discomfort, headache, or a metallic taste. A disulfiram-like reaction may occur if alcohol is co-ingested. Metronidazole and tinidazole should be avoided in pregnant or nursing mothers, if possible. Fluid and electrolyte replacement is also important for patients with significant diarrhea. Surgical management of acute complications of intestinal amebiasis is best avoided whenever possible. Successful therapy of severe amebic colitis may be followed by postdysenteric colitis, with continued diarrhea without persistent infection; this syndrome generally resolves in weeks to months.

4. Amebic hepatic abscess—This is also treated with metronidazole or tinidazole plus a luminal agent (even if intestinal infection is not documented; Table 39–5). Metronidazole can be used intravenously when necessary. With failure of initial response to metronidazole or tinidazole, chloroquine, emetine, or dehydroemetine may be added. Needle aspiration may be helpful for large abscesses (> 5–10 cm), in particular if the diagnosis remains uncertain, if there is an initial lack of response, or if a patient is very ill, suggesting imminent abscess rupture. With successful therapy, abscesses disappear slowly (over months).

Prevention & Control

Prevention requires safe water supplies; sanitary disposal of human feces; adequate cooking of food; protection of food from fly contamination; hand washing; and, in endemic areas, avoidance of fruits and vegetables that cannot be cooked or peeled. Water supplies can be boiled, treated with iodine (0.5-mL tincture of iodine per liter for 20 minutes; cysts are resistant to standard concentrations of chlorine), or filtered.

Kumar R et al. Amebic liver abscess: an update. World J Hepatol. 2024;16:316. [PMID: 38577528]

COCCIDIOSIS (Cryptosporidiosis, Cystoisosporiasis, Cyclosporiasis, Sarcocystosis) & MICROSPORIDIOSIS

ESSENTIALS OF DIAGNOSIS

- Acute diarrhea, especially in children in developing countries.
- Outbreaks of diarrhea secondary to contaminated water or food.
- Prolonged diarrhea in immunocompromised persons.
- Diagnosis mostly by identifying organisms in specially stained stool specimens.

General Considerations

The causes of coccidiosis are *Cryptosporidium* species (*C parvum*, *C hominis*, and others); *Cystoisospora* (formerly *Isospora*) *belli*; *Cyclospora cayetanensis*; and *Sarcocystis* species. Microsporidiosis is caused by at least 14 species, most commonly *Enterocytozoon bieneusi* and *Encephalitozoon intestinalis*. These infections occur worldwide, particularly in the tropics and in regions where hygiene is poor. They cause endemic childhood gastroenteritis (particularly in malnourished children in developing countries); institutional and community outbreaks of diarrhea; traveler's diarrhea; and acute and chronic diarrhea in immunosuppressed patients, in particular those with AIDS. They are all notable for the potential to cause prolonged diarrhea, often lasting for a number of weeks. Clustering occurs in households, day care centers, and among sexual partners.

The infectious agents are oocysts (coccidiosis) or spores (microsporidiosis) transmitted from person to person or by contaminated drinking or swimming water or food. Ingested oocysts release sporozoites that invade and multiply in enterocytes, primarily in the small bowel. Coccidian oocysts and microsporidian cysts can remain viable in the environment for years.

Cryptosporidiosis is a zoonosis (*C parvum* principally infects cattle), but most human infections are acquired from humans, in particular with *C hominis*. Cryptosporidia are highly infectious. They have caused large community outbreaks due to contaminated water supplies and are the leading cause of recreational water–associated outbreaks of gastroenteritis. In the developing world, cryptosporidiosis is a leading cause of childhood diarrhea. In a study of causes of moderate-to-severe diarrhea in Asia and Africa, *Cryptosporidium* was the second most commonly identified pathogen in children under 2 years of age.

C belli and *C cayetanensis* appear to infect only humans. *C cayetanensis* has caused a number of food-borne outbreaks in the United States in recent years, most commonly associated with imported fresh produce. *Sarcocystis* infects many species; humans are intermediate hosts (infected by ingestion of fecal sporocysts) for some species but definitive hosts for *Sarcocystis bovihominis* and *Sarcocystis suihominis* (infected by ingestion of tissue cysts in undercooked beef and pork, respectively).

Clinical Findings

A. Symptoms and Signs

1. Coccidiosis—

A. CRYPTOSPORIDIOSIS—The incubation period appears to be approximately 14 days. In developing countries, disease is primarily in children age < 5, causing 5–10% of childhood diarrhea. Presenting symptoms include acute watery diarrhea, abdominal pain, and cramps, with rapid resolution in most patients; however, symptoms quite commonly persist for 2 weeks or more. In developed countries, most patients are adults. Diarrhea in immunocompetent individuals typically lasts 5–10 days; it is usually watery, with accompanying abdominal pain and cramps, nausea, vomiting, and fever. Relapses may follow initial resolution of symptoms. Mild illness and asymptomatic infection are also common.

Cryptosporidiosis is a well-characterized cause of diarrhea in those with AIDS. It was common before the advent of highly active antiretroviral therapy, particularly with advanced immunosuppression. Clinical manifestations are variable, but patients commonly have chronic diarrhea with frequent foul-smelling stools, malabsorption, and weight loss. Severe, life-threatening watery diarrhea may be seen. Cryptosporidiosis also causes extraintestinal disease with AIDS, including pulmonary infiltrates with dyspnea and biliary tract infection with sclerosing cholangitis and AIDS cholangiopathy.

B. CYSTOISOSPORIASIS—The incubation period for *C belli* is about 1 week. In immunocompetent persons, it usually causes a self-limited watery diarrhea lasting 2–3 weeks, with abdominal cramps, anorexia, malaise, and weight loss. Fever is unusual. Chronic symptoms may persist for months. In immunocompromised patients, cystoisosporiasis more commonly causes severe and chronic diarrhea, with complications including marked dehydration, malnutrition, and hemorrhagic colitis. Extraintestinal disease has been reported rarely.

C. CYCLOSPORIASIS—*C cayetanensis* oocysts must undergo a period of sporulation of ≥ 7 days after shedding before they become infectious. Therefore, person-to-person spread is unlikely, and spread has typically been due to contaminated food (especially fresh produce) and water. The incubation period is 1–11 days. Infections can be asymptomatic. Cyclosporiasis causes an illness similar to that described for the other pathogens included in this section, with watery diarrhea, abdominal cramps, nausea, fatigue, and anorexia. Fever is seen in 25% of cases. Symptoms typically continue for ≥ 2 weeks and may persist for months without therapy. Relapses of diarrhea are common. Diarrhea may be preceded by a flu-like prodrome and followed by persistent fatigue. In immunocompromised patients, cyclosporiasis is typically more severe and prolonged, with chronic fulminant watery diarrhea and weight loss.

D. SARCOCYSTOSIS—*Sarcocystis* infection is common in some developing countries but is usually asymptomatic. Infection most commonly follow the ingestion of undercooked beef or pork, leading to the development of cysts in muscle, with myalgias, fever, bronchospasm, pruritic rash, lymphadenopathy, and subcutaneous nodules. Ingestion of fecal sporocysts may lead to GI symptoms.

2. Microsporidiosis—Microsporidia are obligate intracellular protozoans that cause a wide spectrum of diseases. Many infections are of zoonotic origin, but human-to-human transmission has been documented. Infection is mainly by ingestion of spores, but also by direct inoculation of the eyes. In immunocompetent hosts, microsporidian infections most commonly present as self-limited diarrhea. Ocular infections have also been described. Disease from microsporidia is seen mainly in immunocompromised persons, particularly those with AIDS. Infections in patients with AIDS are most commonly with *E bieneusi* and *E intestinalis*. They cause chronic diarrhea, with anorexia, bloating, weight loss, and wasting, especially in those with advanced immunodeficiency. Fever is usually not seen. Other illnesses in immunocompromised persons associated with microsporidians (including the genera *Enterocytozoon, Encephalitozoon, Brachiola, Vittaforma, Pleistophora, Trachipleistophora,* and *Microsporidium*) include biliary tract disease (AIDS cholangiopathy), genitourinary infection with cystitis, kidney disease, hepatitis, peritonitis, myositis, respiratory infections including sinusitis, CNS infections including granulomatous encephalitis, and disseminated infections. Ocular infections with *Encephalitozoon* species cause conjunctivitis and keratitis, presenting as redness, photophobia, and loss of visual acuity.

B. Laboratory Findings

1. Coccidiosis—

A. CRYPTOSPORIDIOSIS—Typically, stool is without blood or leukocytes. Diagnosis is traditionally made by detecting the organism in stool using a modified acid-fast stain; this technique is relatively insensitive, and multiple specimens should be evaluated before ruling out the diagnosis. Of note, routine evaluation for ova and parasites typically does not include a modified acid-fast stain, so this must be specifically requested in many laboratories. Various detection methods for stool antigens, including immunofluorescence microscopy, ELISA, and immunochromatography, offer improved sensitivity and specificity, both > 90% with available assays, and these methods may be considered the optimal means of diagnosis. Molecular diagnostic panels that recognize *Cryptosporidium* and other enteropathogens in stool are available but expensive.

B. CYSTOISOSPORIASIS —Diagnosis of cystoisosporiasis is by examination of stool wet mounts or after modified acid-fast staining, in which the organism is clearly distinguishable from other parasites. Other stains also show the organism. Shedding of oocysts may be intermittent, so the sensitivity of stool evaluation is not high, and multiple samples should be examined. The organism may also be identified in duodenal aspirates or small bowel biopsies.

C. CYCLOSPORIASIS—Diagnosis is made by examination of stool wet mounts or after modified acid-fast staining. Multiple specimens may need to be examined to make a diagnosis; concentration of specimens improves sensitivity. The organism can also be identified in small bowel aspirates or biopsy specimens. Molecular assays with high sensitivity and specificity, including multi-pathogen panels, are available.

D. SARCOCYSTOSIS—Eosinophilia and elevated creatine kinase may be seen. Diagnosis is by identification of the acid-fast organisms in stool or by identification of trophozoites or bradyzoites in tissue biopsies.

2. Microsporidiosis—Diagnosis can be made by identification of organisms in specially stained stool, fluid, or tissue specimens, for example with Weber chromotrope-based stain. Electron microscopy is helpful for confirmation of the diagnosis and speciation. PCR and culture techniques are available but not used routinely.

Treatment

Most acute infections with these pathogens in immunocompetent persons are self-limited and do not require treatment.

Supportive treatment for severe or chronic diarrhea includes fluid and electrolyte replacement and, in some cases, parenteral nutrition.

1. Coccidiosis—

A. CRYPTOSPORIDIOSIS—Treatment of cryptosporidiosis is challenging. No agent is clearly effective. Modest benefits have been seen in some (but not other) studies, generally in immunocompetent hosts, with nitazoxanide, which is FDA-approved for this indication (500 mg–1 g orally twice daily for 3 days in immunocompetent patients and 2–8 weeks in patients with advanced AIDS), and paromomycin, a nonabsorbed aminoglycoside (25–35 mg/kg orally for 14 days). Other agents that have been used with mixed success in patients with AIDS include azithromycin, spiramycin, bovine hyperimmune colostrum, and octreotide. Reversing immunodeficiency with effective antiretroviral therapy is of greatest importance.

B. CYSTOISOSPORIASIS—Cystoisosporiasis is effectively treated in immunocompetent and immunosuppressed persons with TMP-SMZ (160 mg/800 mg orally two to four times daily for 10 days, with the higher dosage for patients with AIDS). An alternative therapy is pyrimethamine (75 mg orally in four divided doses) with folinic acid (10–25 mg/day orally). Maintenance therapy with low-dose TMP-SMZ (160 mg/800 mg daily or three times per week) or Fansidar (1 tablet weekly) prevents relapse in those with persistent immunosuppression.

C. CYCLOSPORIASIS—Cyclosporiasis is also treated with TMP-SMZ (dosing as for cystoisosporiasis). With AIDS, long-term maintenance therapy (160 mg/800 mg three times weekly) helps prevent relapse. For patients intolerant of TMP-SMZ, ciprofloxacin (500 mg orally twice daily for 7 days) showed efficacy, albeit with less ability to clear the organism than TMP-SMZ.

D. SARCOCYSTOSIS—For sarcocystosis, no specific treatment is established, but patients may respond to therapy with albendazole or TMP-SMZ.

2. Microsporidiosis—Treatment of microsporidiosis is complex. Infections with most species, including those causing GI and other manifestations, should be treated with albendazole (400 mg orally twice daily for 2–4 weeks), which has activity against a number of species, but relatively poor efficacy (about 50%) against *E bieneusi*, the most common microsporidial cause of diarrhea in patients with AIDS. Fumagillin, which is used to treat honeybees and fish with microsporidian infections, has shown benefit in clinical trials at a dose of 20 mg three times per day for 14 days; treatment was accompanied by reversible thrombocytopenia. As with cryptosporidiosis, the best means of controlling microsporidiosis in patients with AIDS is to restore immune function with effective antiretroviral therapy. Ocular microsporidiosis can be treated with topical fumagillin solution (3 mg/mL); this probably should be given with concurrent systemic albendazole. Adjunctive management may include topical corticosteroids to decrease inflammation.

Prevention

Water purification is important for control of these infections. Chlorine disinfection is not effective against cryptosporidial oocysts, so other purification measures are needed. Immunocompromised patients should boil or filter drinking water and should consider avoidance of lakes and swimming pools. Routine precautions (hand washing, gloves, disinfection) should prevent institutional patient-to-patient spread. Optimal means of preventing microsporidial infections are not known, but water purification and body substance precautions for immunocompromised and hospitalized individuals are likely effective.

Diptyanusa A et al. Treatment of human intestinal cryptosporidiosis: a review of published clinical trials. Int J Parasitol Drugs Drug Resist. 2021;17:128. [PMID: 34562754]

Rosenthal BM. Zoonotic Sarcocystis. Res Vet Sci. 2021;136:151. [PMID: 33626441]

GIARDIASIS

ESSENTIALS OF DIAGNOSIS

- Acute diarrhea may be profuse and watery.
- Chronic diarrhea with greasy, malodorous stools.
- Abdominal cramps, distention, flatulence.
- Cysts or trophozoites in stools.

General Considerations

Giardiasis is a protozoal infection of the upper small intestine caused by the flagellate *Giardia lamblia* (also called *Giardia intestinalis* and *Giardia duodenalis*). The parasite occurs worldwide, most abundantly in areas with poor sanitation. In developing countries, young children are very commonly infected. In the United States and Europe, the infection is the most common intestinal protozoal pathogen; the US estimate is 1 million new infections leading to 5000 hospital admissions yearly. Groups at special risk include travelers to *Giardia*-endemic areas, those who swallow contaminated water during recreation or wilderness travel, men who have sex with men, and persons with impaired immunity. Outbreaks are common in households, children's day care centers, and residential facilities, and may occur from contaminated water supplies.

The organism occurs in feces as a flagellated trophozoite and as a cyst. Only the cyst form is infectious by the oral route; trophozoites are destroyed by gastric acidity. Humans are a reservoir for the pathogen; dogs, cats, beavers, and other mammals have been implicated but not confirmed as reservoirs. Under suitable moist, cool conditions, cysts can survive in the environment for weeks to months. Cysts are transmitted as a result of fecal contamination of water or food, by person-to-person contact, or by anal-oral sexual contact. The infectious dose is low, requiring as few as 10 cysts. After the cysts are ingested, trophozoites emerge in the duodenum and jejunum. Epithelial damage and mucosal invasion are uncommon. Hypogammaglobulinemia, low secretory IgA levels in the gut, achlorhydria, and malnutrition favor the development of infection.

Clinical Findings

A. Symptoms and Signs

It is estimated that about 50% of infected persons have no discernable infection, about 10% become asymptomatic cyst passers, and 25–50% develop an acute diarrheal syndrome. Acute diarrhea may clear spontaneously but is commonly followed by chronic diarrhea. The incubation period is usually 1–3 weeks but may be longer. The illness may begin gradually or suddenly. The acute phase may last days or weeks and is usually self-limited. The initial illness may include profuse watery diarrhea, and hospitalization may be required due to dehydration, particularly in young children. Typical symptoms of chronic disease are abdominal cramps, bloating, flatulence, nausea, malaise, and anorexia. Fever and vomiting are uncommon. Diarrhea is usually not severe in the chronic stage of infection; stools are greasy or frothy and foul smelling, without blood, pus, or mucus. The diarrhea may be daily or recurrent; intervening periods may include constipation. Symptoms can persist for weeks to months. Weight loss is frequent. Chronic disease can include malabsorption, including fat and protein-losing enteropathy and vitamin deficiencies.

B. Laboratory Findings

Most patients seek medical attention after having been ill for > 1 week, commonly with weight loss of ≥ 5 kg. Stool is generally without blood or leukocytes. Diagnosis is traditionally made by the identification of trophozoites or cysts in stool. Microscopy with direct fluorescent antibody testing is the diagnostic test of choice. A wet mount of liquid stool may identify motile trophozoites. Stained fixed specimens may show cysts or trophozoites. Sensitivity of stool analysis is not ideal, estimated at 50–80% for a single specimen and > 90% for three specimens. Duodenal biopsy may be helpful in very ill or immunocompromised patients. When giardiasis is suspected, stool antigen assays are simpler and cheaper than repeated stool examinations, but these will not identify other stool pathogens. Multiple tests that identify antigens of trophozoites or cysts in stool, including rapid immunochromatographic cartridge assays and enzyme immunoassays, are available. They are generally quite sensitive (85–98%) and specific (90–100%). Molecular diagnostic panels that recognize *Giardia* and other enteropathogens in stool are available but expensive.

Treatment

The treatments of choice for giardiasis are tinidazole (2 g orally once) or metronidazole (250 mg orally three times daily for 5–7 days). The drugs are not universally effective; cure rates for single courses are typically about 80–95%. Toxicities are as described for treatment of amebiasis, but the lower dosages used for giardiasis limit side effects. Albendazole (400 mg orally once daily for 5 days) and nitazoxanide (500 mg orally twice daily for 3 days) both appear to have similar efficacy and fewer side effects compared with metronidazole, but a meta-analysis suggested that tinidazole is more efficacious than albendazole. Nitazoxanide is generally well tolerated but may cause mild GI side effects. Other drugs with activity against *Giardia* include furazolidone (100 mg orally four times a day for 7 days), which is about as effective as the other named drugs but causes GI side effects, and paromomycin (500 mg orally three times a day for 7 days), which appears to have somewhat lower efficacy but, unlike metronidazole, tinidazole, and furazolidone, is safe in pregnancy. Symptomatic giardiasis should always be treated. Treatment of asymptomatic patients should be considered, since they can transmit the infection. With a suggestive presentation but negative diagnostic studies, an empiric course of treatment may be appropriate. Household or day care contacts with an index case should be tested and treated if infected.

Prevention

Community chlorination (0.4 mg/L) of water is relatively ineffective for inactivating cysts, so filtration is required. For wilderness or international travelers, bringing water to a boil for 1 minute or filtration with a pore size <1 mcm is adequate. In day care centers, appropriate disposal of diapers and frequent hand washing are essential.

Loderstädt U et al. Antimicrobial resistance of the enteric protozoon *Giardia duodenalis*—a narrative review. Eur J Microbiol Immunol (Bp). 2021;11:29. [PMID: 34237023]

TRICHOMONIASIS

Trichomoniasis is caused by the protozoan *Trichomonas vaginalis* and is among the most common STIs, causing vaginitis in women (see Vaginitis in Chapter 21) and nongonococcal urethritis in men. *T vaginalis* is often harbored asymptomatically. For women with symptomatic disease, after an incubation period of 5 days to 4 weeks, a vaginal discharge develops, often with vulvovaginal discomfort, pruritus, dysuria, dyspareunia, or abdominal pain. Examination shows a copious yellow or green discharge, which is usually not foul smelling. Most men infected with *T vaginalis* are asymptomatic, but it can be isolated from about 10% of men with nongonococcal urethritis. The urethral discharge is generally scantier than with other causes of urethritis.

Diagnosis is traditionally made by identifying motile organisms in vaginal or urethral secretions, but point-of-care nucleic acid amplification assays, including multiplex assays that identify multiple pathogens, offer improved sensitivity and excellent specificity.

The treatment of choice is metronidazole, 500 mg orally twice daily for 7 days in women, and as a single 2-g dose in men. An alternative is tinidazole as a 2-g single oral dose for both women and men. Toxicities are discussed in the section on amebiasis. All infected persons should be treated, even if asymptomatic, to prevent subsequent symptomatic disease and limit spread. Treatment failure suggests reinfection, but metronidazole-resistant organisms have been reported. These may be treated with tinidazole, longer courses of metronidazole, intravaginal paromomycin, or other experimental therapies (see Chapter 21).

Ibáñez-Escribano A et al. The past, present, and future in the diagnosis of a neglected sexually transmitted infection: trichomoniasis. Pathogens. 2024;13:126. [PMID: 38392864]
Muzny CA et al. Trichomoniasis and other sexually transmitted parasitic diseases in women. Clin Obstet Gynecol. 2025;68:194. [PMID: 40226933]

HELMINTHIC INFECTIONS

TREMATODE (Fluke) INFECTIONS

SCHISTOSOMIASIS (Bilharziasis)

ESSENTIALS OF DIAGNOSIS

- History of freshwater exposure in an endemic area.
- **Acute schistosomiasis:** fever, headache, myalgias, cough, urticaria, diarrhea, and eosinophilia.
- **Intestinal schistosomiasis:** abdominal pain, diarrhea, and hepatomegaly, then anorexia, weight loss, and portal hypertension.
- **Urinary schistosomiasis:** hematuria and dysuria, then hydronephrosis and urinary infections.
- **Diagnosis:** characteristic eggs in feces or urine; biopsy of rectal or bladder mucosa; positive serology.

General Considerations

Schistosomiasis, which affects > 200 million persons worldwide, leads to severe consequences in 20 million persons and about 100,000 deaths annually (although estimates vary widely). The disease is caused by six species of trematode blood flukes. Five species cause intestinal schistosomiasis, with infection of mesenteric venules: *Schistosoma mansoni*, present in Africa, the Arabian Peninsula, South America, and the Caribbean; *Schistosoma japonicum*, endemic in China and Southeast Asia; *Schistosoma mekongi*, endemic near the Mekong River in Southeast Asia; and *Schistosoma intercalatum* and *Schistosoma guineensis*, which occur in parts of Africa. The sixth species, *Schistosoma haematobium*, causes urinary schistosomiasis, with infection of venules of the urinary tract, and is endemic in Africa and the Middle East. Transmission of schistosomiasis is focal, with greatest prevalence in poor rural areas. Control efforts have diminished transmission in many areas, but high-level transmission remains in sub-Saharan Africa and some other areas. Prevalence of infection and illness typically peaks at about 15–20 years of age.

Humans are infected with schistosomes after contact with freshwater containing cercariae released by infected snails. Infection is initiated by penetration of skin or mucous membranes. After penetration, schistosomulae migrate to the portal circulation, where they rapidly mature. After about 6 weeks, adult worms mate and migrate to terminal mesenteric or bladder venules, where females deposit their eggs. Some eggs reach the lumen of the bowel or bladder and are passed with feces or urine, while others are retained in the bowel or bladder wall or transported in the circulation to other tissues, in particular the liver. Disease in endemic areas is primarily due to a host response to eggs, with granuloma formation and inflammation, eventually leading to fibrosis. Chronic infection can result in scarring of mesenteric or vesicular blood vessels, leading to portal hypertension and alterations in the urinary tract. In previously uninfected individuals, such as travelers with freshwater contact in endemic regions, acute schistosomiasis may occur, with a febrile illness 2–8 weeks after infection.

Clinical Findings

A. Symptoms and Signs

1. Cercarial dermatitis (swimmer's itch)—Following cercarial penetration, localized erythema develops in some individuals, which can progress to a localized pruritic maculopapular rash that persists for some days. Dermatitis can be caused by human schistosomes and, in nontropical areas, by bird schistosomes that cannot complete their life cycle in humans (swimmer's itch).

2. Acute schistosomiasis (Katayama syndrome)—A febrile illness may develop 2–8 weeks after exposure in persons without prior infection, most commonly after heavy infection with *S mansoni* or *S japonicum*. Symptoms and signs include acute onset of fever; headache; myalgias; cough; malaise; urticaria; diarrhea, which may be bloody; hepatosplenomegaly; lymphadenopathy; and pulmonary infiltrates. Localized lesions may occasionally cause severe manifestations, including CNS abnormalities and death. Acute schistosomiasis usually resolves in 2–8 weeks.

3. Chronic schistosomiasis—Many persons have light infections and are asymptomatic, but an estimated 50–60% have symptoms and 5–10% have advanced organ damage. Asymptomatic infected children may suffer from anemia and growth retardation. Symptomatic patients with intestinal schistosomiasis typically experience abdominal pain, fatigue, diarrhea, and hepatomegaly. Over years, anorexia, weight loss, weakness, colonic polyps, and portal hypertension develop. Late manifestations include hematemesis from esophageal varices, hepatic failure, and pulmonary hypertension. Urinary schistosomiasis may present within months of infection with hematuria and dysuria, most commonly in children and young adults. Fibrotic changes in the urinary tract can lead to hydroureter, hydronephrosis, bacterial urinary infections and, ultimately, kidney disease or bladder cancer. Chronic genital schistosomiasis is associated with local lesions and increased risks of incontinence, infertility, and HIV infection.

B. Laboratory Findings

Microscopic examination of stool or urine for eggs, evaluation of tissue, or serologic tests establish the diagnosis. Characteristic eggs can be identified on smears of stool or urine. The most widely used stool test is the Kato-Katz technique. Quantitative tests that yield > 400 eggs per gram of feces or 10 mL of urine are indicative of heavy infections with increased risk of complications. Diagnosis can also be made by biopsy of the rectum, colon, liver, or bladder. Serologic tests include an ELISA available from the CDC that is 99% specific for all species but cannot distinguish acute and past infection. Sensitivity of the test is 99% for *S mansoni*, 95% for *S haematobium*, but <50% for *S japonicum*. Serology is of limited use in endemic settings but can be helpful in travelers from nonendemic regions. The most widely used point-of-care assays detect circulating schistosome antigens in serum and urine. Antigen tests have better sensitivity than stool smears, especially for *S mansoni*; sensitivity is lower for *S haematobium*. Molecular tests for schistosomiasis are not routinely used for diagnosis. In acute schistosomiasis, leukocytosis and marked eosinophilia may occur; serologic tests may become positive before eggs are seen in stool or urine. After therapy, eggs may be shed in stool or urine for months, and so the identification of eggs in fluids or tissue cannot distinguish past or active disease. With a diagnosis of schistosomiasis, evaluation for the extent of disease is warranted, including liver function studies and imaging of the liver for those with intestinal disease and ultrasound or other imaging studies of the urinary system for those with urinary disease.

Treatment

Treatment is indicated for all schistosome infections. In areas where recurrent infection is common, treatment is valuable in reducing worm burdens and limiting clinical complications. The drug of choice is praziquantel. The drug is usually administered for 1 day at an oral dose of 40 mg/kg (in one or two doses) for *S mansoni, S haematobium, S intercalatum*, and *S guineensis* infections and a dose of 60 mg/kg (in two or three doses) for *S japonicum* and *S mekongi*, but a divided dose of 80 mg/kg yielded improved cure rates for *S mansoni* infections. Praziquantel is active against invading cercariae but not developing schistosomulae. Therefore, the drug may not prevent illness when given after exposure and, for recent infections, a repeat course after a few weeks may be appropriate. Praziquantel may be used during pregnancy. Resistance to praziquantel has been reported. Toxicities include abdominal pain, diarrhea, urticaria, headache, nausea, vomiting, and fever, and may be due both to direct effects of the drug and responses to dying worms. Alternative therapies are oxamniquine for *S mansoni* infection and metrifonate for *S haematobium* infection. Both drugs have limited availability (they are not available in the United States), and resistance may be a problem. No second-line drug is available for *S japonicum* infections. The antimalarial drug artemether has activity against schistosomulae and adult worms and may be effective in chemoprophylaxis; however, it is expensive, and long-term use in malarious areas might select for resistant malaria parasites. With severe disease, use of corticosteroids in conjunction with praziquantel may decrease complications. Treatment should be followed by repeat examinations for eggs about every 3 months for 1 year after therapy, with re-treatment if eggs are seen.

Prevention

Travelers to endemic areas should avoid freshwater exposure. Vigorous toweling after exposure may limit cercarial penetration. Chemoprophylaxis with artemether has shown efficacy but is not standard practice. Community control of schistosomiasis includes improved sanitation and water supplies, elimination of snail habitats, and preventive treatment to limit worm burdens.

Buonfrate D et al. Human schistosomiasis. Lancet. 2025;405:658. [PMID: 39986748]
Bustinduy AL et al. Safety and efficacy of praziquantel 40 mg/kg versus 80 mg/kg in preschool-aged children with intestinal schistosomiasis in Uganda: a 2 × 2 factorial, double-blind, placebo-controlled, phase 2 randomised trial. Lancet Glob Health. 2025;13:e1091 [PMID: 40412398]
LoVerde PT. Schistosomiasis. Adv Exp Med Biol. 2024;1454:75. [PMID: 39008264]

LIVER & LUNG FLUKES

FASCIOLIASIS

Human infection by *Fasciola hepatica*, the sheep liver fluke, results from ingestion of encysted metacercariae on watercress or other aquatic vegetables. Infection is prevalent in sheep-raising areas in many countries, especially parts of South America, the Middle East, and southern Europe, and it has increasingly been recognized in travelers to these areas. *Fasciola gigantica* has a more restricted distribution in Asia and Africa and causes similar findings. Eggs are passed from host feces into freshwater, leading to infection of snails, and then deposition of metacercariae on vegetation. In humans, metacercariae excyst, penetrate the peritoneum, migrate through the liver, and mature in the bile ducts, where they cause local necrosis and abscess formation.

Two clinical syndromes are seen, related to acute migration of worms and chronic infection of the biliary tract. Symptoms related to migration of larvae present 6–12 weeks after ingestion. Typical findings are abdominal pain, fever, malaise, weight loss, urticaria, eosinophilia, and leukocytosis. Tender hepatomegaly and elevated liver biochemical tests may be seen. Rarely, migration to other organs may lead to localized disease. The symptoms of worm migration subside after 2–4 months, followed by asymptomatic infection by adult worms or intermittent symptoms of biliary obstruction, with biliary colic and, at times, cholangitis. Early diagnosis is difficult, as eggs are not found in the feces during the acute migratory phase of infection. Clinical suspicion should be based on clinical findings and marked eosinophilia in at risk individuals. CT and other imaging studies show hypodense migratory lesions of the liver. Definitive diagnosis is made by the identification of characteristic eggs in stool. Repeated examinations may be necessary. In chronic infection, imaging studies show masses obstructing the extrahepatic biliary tract. Serologic assays have sensitivity and specificity above 90% but cannot distinguish between past and current infection. Antigen tests with excellent sensitivity and specificity are available in veterinary medicine and show promise for humans.

The treatment of choice is triclabendazole. Standard dosing of 10 mg/kg orally in a single dose or two doses over 12 hours achieves a cure rate of about 80%, but repeat dosing is indicated if abnormal radiologic findings or eosinophilia do not resolve. Of concern, resistance to triclabendazole has been widely reported in animal infections. The second-line drug is bithionol (30–50 mg/kg/day orally in three divided doses on alternate days for 10–15 days); this drug is not available in the United States. Treatment with either drug can be accompanied by abdominal pain and other GI symptoms. Other potential therapies are emetine and dehydroemetine, both widely used in the past but quite toxic, and nitazoxanide. Prevention of fascioliasis involves avoidance of ingestion of raw aquatic plants.

CLONORCHIASIS & OPISTHORCHIASIS

Infection by *Clonorchis sinensis*, the Chinese liver fluke, is endemic in areas of Japan, Korea, China, Taiwan, Southeast Asia, and the far eastern part of Russia. An estimated 15 million persons are infected (13 million in China); in some communities, prevalence can reach 80%. Opisthorchiasis is principally caused by *Opisthorchis felineus* (regions of the former Soviet Union) or *Opisthorchis viverrini* (Thailand, Laos, Vietnam). Clonorchiasis and opisthorchiasis are clinically indistinguishable. Parasite eggs are shed into water in human or animal feces, where they infect snails, which release cercariae, which infect fish. Human infection follows ingestion of raw, undercooked, or pickled freshwater fish containing metacercariae. These parasites excyst in the duodenum and ascend into the biliary tract, where they mature and remain for many years, shedding eggs in the bile.

Most patients harbor few parasites and are asymptomatic. An acute illness can occur 2–3 weeks after initial infection, with fever, malaise, abdominal pain, anorexia, tender hepatomegaly, urticaria, and eosinophilia. The acute syndrome is difficult to diagnose, since ova may not appear in the feces until 3–4 weeks after onset of symptoms. In chronic heavy infections, findings include abdominal pain, anorexia, weight loss, and tender hepatomegaly. Recurrent bacterial cholangitis and sepsis, cholecystitis, liver abscess, and pancreatitis can occur. An increased risk of cholangiocarcinoma has been documented.

Early diagnosis is presumptive, based on clinical findings and epidemiology. Subsequent diagnosis is made by finding characteristic eggs in stool or duodenal or biliary contents. The stool Kato-Katz test is widely used; performing repeated tests improves sensitivity. Imaging studies show characteristic biliary tract dilatations with filling defects due to flukes. Serologic assays for clonorchiasis with excellent sensitivity are available but cannot distinguish between past and current infection. Molecular tests have been developed but are not widely used.

The drug of choice is praziquantel, 25 mg/kg orally three times daily for 2 days, which provides cure rates > 90% and egg reduction rates of nearly 100%. One day of treatment may be sufficient. Re-treatment may be required, especially in areas with known decreased praziquantel efficacy. The second-line drug is albendazole (400 mg orally twice daily for 7 days), which appears to be somewhat less effective. Tribendimidine, which is approved in China, has shown efficacy for clonorchiasis similar to that of praziquantel.

PARAGONIMIASIS

Eight species of *Paragonimus* lung flukes cause human disease. The most important is *Paragonimus westermani*. *Paragonimus* species are endemic in East Asia, Oceania, West Africa, and South America, where millions of persons are infected; rare infections caused by *Paragonimus kellicotti* have occurred in North America. Eggs are released into freshwater, where parasites infect snails, and then cercariae infect crabs and crayfish. Human infection follows consumption of raw, undercooked, or pickled freshwater shellfish. Metacercariae then excyst, penetrate the peritoneum, and pass into the lungs, where they mature into adult worms over about 2 months.

Most infected persons have moderate worm burdens and are asymptomatic. In symptomatic cases, abdominal pain and diarrhea develop 2 days to 2 weeks after infection, followed by fever, cough, chest pain, urticaria, and eosinophilia. Acute symptoms may last for several weeks. Chronic infection can cause cough productive of brown sputum, hemoptysis, dyspnea, and chest pain, with progression to chronic bronchitis, bronchiectasis, bronchopneumonia, lung abscess, and pleural disease. Ectopic infections can cause disease in other organs, most commonly the CNS, where disease can present with seizures, headaches, and focal neurologic findings due to parasite meningitis and to intracerebral lesions.

The diagnosis of paragonimiasis is made by identifying characteristic eggs in sputum or stool or identifying worms in biopsied tissue. Multiple examinations and concentration techniques may be needed. Serologic tests may be helpful; an ELISA available from the CDC has sensitivity and specificity > 95%. CXRs may show varied abnormalities of the lungs or pleura, including infiltrates, nodules, cavities, and fibrosis, and the findings can be confused with those of tuberculosis. With CNS disease, skull radiographs can show clusters of calcified cysts, and CT or MRI can show clusters of ring-enhancing lesions.

Treatment is with praziquantel (25 mg/kg orally three times daily for 2 days), with efficacy of at least 90%. Alternative therapies are bithionol and triclabendazole. As with cysticercosis, for cerebral paragonimiasis, praziquantel should generally be used with corticosteroids. Chronic infection may lead to permanent lung dysfunction and pleural disease requiring drainage procedures.

Blair D. Paragonimiasis. Adv Exp Med Biol. 2024;1454:203. [PMID: 39008267]

Chai JY et al. General overview of the current status of human foodborne trematodiasis. Parasitology. 2022;149:1262. [PMID: 35591777]

Qian M-B et al. Clonorchiasis and opisthorchiasis: epidemiology, transmission, clinical features, morbidity, diagnosis, treatment, and control. Clin Microbiol Rev. 2024;37:e0000923. [PMID: 38169283]

CESTODE INFECTIONS

NONINVASIVE CESTODE INFECTIONS

The four major tapeworms that cause noninvasive infections in humans are the beef tapeworm *Taenia saginata*, the pork tapeworm *Taenia solium*, the fish tapeworm *Diphyllobothrium latum*, each of which can reach many meters in length, and the dwarf tapeworm *Hymenolepis nana*. *Taenia* and *Hymenolepis* species are broadly distributed, especially in the tropics; *D latum* is most prevalent in temperate regions. Other tapeworms that can cause noninvasive human disease include the rodent tapeworm *Hymenolepis diminuta*, the dog tapeworm *Dipylidium caninum*, and other *Taenia* and *Diphyllobothrium* species. Invasive tapeworm infections, including *T solium* (when infective eggs, rather than cysticerci are ingested) and *Echinococcus* species, will be discussed separately.

1. Beef Tapeworm

Infection is most common in cattle breeding areas. Humans are the definitive host. Gravid segments of *T saginata* are passed in human feces to soil, where they are ingested by grazing animals, especially cattle. The eggs then hatch to release embryos that encyst in cattle muscle as cysticerci. Humans are infected by eating raw or undercooked infected beef. Most individuals infected with *T saginata* are asymptomatic, but abdominal pain and other GI symptoms may be present. Eosinophilia is common. The most common presenting finding is the passage of proglottids in the stool, which look like grains of rice and may be motile.

2. Pork Tapeworm

T solium is transmitted to pigs that ingest human feces. Humans can be either the definitive host (after consuming undercooked pork, leading to tapeworm infection) or the intermediate host (after consuming food contaminated with human feces containing *T solium* eggs, leading to cysticercosis, which is discussed under Invasive Cestode Infections). As with the beef tapeworm, infection with *T solium* adult worms is generally asymptomatic, but GI symptoms may occur. Infection is generally recognized after passage of proglottids. Autoinfection with eggs can progress to cysticercosis.

3. Fish Tapeworm

Infection with *D latum* follows ingestion of undercooked freshwater fish, most commonly in temperate regions. Eggs from human feces are taken up by crustaceans, these are eaten by fish, which are then infectious to humans. Infection with multiple worms over many years can occur. Infections are most commonly asymptomatic, but nonspecific GI symptoms, including diarrhea, may occur. Diagnosis usually follows passage of proglottids. Prolonged heavy infection can lead to megaloblastic anemia and neuropathy from vitamin B_{12} deficiency, which is due to infection-induced dissociation of the vitamin from intrinsic factor and to utilization of the vitamin by worms.

4. Dwarf Tapeworm

H nana is the only tapeworm that can be transmitted between humans. Infections are common in warm areas, especially with poor hygiene and institutionalized populations. Infection follows ingestion of food contaminated with human feces. Eggs hatch in the intestines, where oncospheres penetrate the mucosa, encyst as cysticercoid larvae, and then rupture after about 4 days to release adult worms. Autoinfection can lead to amplification of infection. Infection with *H nana*, the related rodent tapeworm *H diminuta*, or the dog tapeworm *D caninum* can also follow accidental ingestion of infected insects. *H nana* are dwarf in size relative to other tapeworms but can reach 5 cm in length. Heavy infection is common, especially in children, and can be accompanied by abdominal discomfort, anorexia, and diarrhea.

Laboratory Findings

Diagnosis is usually made based on the identification of characteristic eggs or proglottids in stool. Egg release may be irregular, so examination of multiple specimens or concentration techniques may be needed.

Treatment

The treatment of choice for noninvasive tapeworm infections is praziquantel. A single dose of praziquantel (5–10 mg/kg orally) is highly effective, except for *H nana*, for which the dosage is 25 mg/kg. Treatment of *H nana* is more difficult, as the drug is not effective against maturing cysts. Therefore, a repeat treatment after 1 week and examination of stool after therapy to document cure are appropriate with heavy infections. Therapy can be accompanied by headache, malaise, dizziness, abdominal pain, and nausea.

The alternative therapy is niclosamide. A single dose of niclosamide (2 g chewed) is effective against *D latum*, *Taenia*, and *D caninum* infections. For *H nana*, therapy is continued daily for 1 week. Niclosamide may cause nausea, malaise, and abdominal pain.

Panti-May JA et al. Worldwide overview of human infections with *Hymenolepis diminuta*. Parasitol Res. 2020;119:1997. [PMID: 32211990]

INVASIVE CESTODE INFECTIONS

1. Cysticercosis

ESSENTIALS OF DIAGNOSIS

- Exposure to *T solium* through fecal contamination of food.
- Focal CNS lesions; seizures, headache.
- Brain imaging shows cysts; positive serologic tests.

General Considerations

Cysticercosis is due to tissue infection with cysts of *T solium* that develop after humans ingest food contaminated with eggs from human feces, thus acting as an intermediate host for the parasite. Prevalence is high where the parasite is endemic, in particular Mexico, Central and South America, the Philippines, and Southeast Asia. An estimated 20 million persons are infected with cysticerci yearly, leading to about 400,000 persons with neurologic symptoms and 50,000 deaths. Antibody prevalence rates up to 10% are recognized in some endemic areas, and the infection is one of the most important causes of seizures in the developing world and in immigrants to the United States from endemic countries. In Latin America, it is estimated that 0.5–1.5 million persons are affected by epilepsy secondary to cysticercosis.

Clinical Findings

A. Symptoms and Signs

Neurocysticercosis can cause intracerebral, subarachnoid, and spinal cord lesions and intraventricular cysts. Single or multiple lesions may be present. Lesions may persist for years before symptoms develop, generally due to local inflammation or ventricular obstruction. Presenting symptoms include seizures, focal neurologic deficits, altered cognition, and psychiatric disease. Symptoms develop more quickly with intraventricular cysts, with findings of hydrocephalus and meningeal irritation, including severe headache, vomiting, papilledema, and visual loss. A particularly aggressive form of the disease, racemose cysticercosis, involves proliferation of cysts at the base of the brain, leading to alterations of consciousness and death. Spinal cord lesions can present with progressive focal findings.

Cysticercosis of organ systems, other than the CNS is usually clinically benign. Involvement of muscles can uncommonly cause discomfort and is identified by radiographs of muscle showing multiple calcified lesions. Subcutaneous involvement presents with multiple painless palpable skin lesions. Involvement of the eyes can present with ptosis due to extraocular muscle involvement or intraocular abnormalities.

B. Laboratory Findings and Imaging

Diagnosis generally requires consideration of both laboratory and imaging findings. The 2017 revised Del Brutto diagnostic criteria have demonstrated good sensitivity and specificity.

CSF examination may show lymphocytic or eosinophilic pleocytosis, decreased glucose, and elevated protein. Serology plays an important role in diagnosis; both antibody and antigen detection assays are available. ELISAs and related immunoblot assays have excellent sensitivity and specificity, but sensitivity is lower with only single or calcified lesions.

With neuroimaging by CT or MRI, multiple parenchymal cysts are most typically seen. Parenchymal calcification is also common. Performing both CT and MRI is ideal because CT is better for identification of calcification and MRI for smaller and ventricular lesions. Typical findings can be highly suggestive of the diagnosis.

Treatment

The medical management of neurocysticercosis has been controversial because the benefits of cyst clearance must be weighed against potential harm of an inflammatory response to dying worms. Antihelminthic therapy hastens radiologic improvement in parenchymal cysticercosis, but some randomized trials have shown that corticosteroids alone are as effective as specific therapy plus corticosteroids for controlling seizures. Overall, most authorities recommend treatment of active lesions, in particular lesions with a high likelihood of progression, such as intraventricular cysts. At the other end of the spectrum, inactive calcified lesions probably do not benefit from therapy. In addition, cysticidal therapy should be avoided if there is a high risk of hydrocephalus, as with subarachnoid involvement. When treatment is deemed appropriate, standard therapy consists of albendazole (10–15 mg/kg/day orally for 8 days) or praziquantel (50 mg/kg/day orally for 15–30 days). Albendazole is probably preferred, since it has shown better efficacy in some comparisons and since corticosteroids appear to lower circulating praziquantel levels but increase albendazole levels. Increasing the dosage of albendazole to 30 mg/kg/day orally may improve outcomes. Combining albendazole with praziquantel improved outcomes compared with albendazole alone in patients with multiple viable intraparenchymal cysts. Corticosteroids are usually administered concurrently, but dosing is not standardized. Patients should be observed for evidence of localized inflammatory responses. Anticonvulsant therapy should be provided if needed, and shunting performed if required for elevated intracranial pressure. Surgical removal of cysts may be helpful for some difficult cases of neurocysticercosis and for symptomatic non-neurologic disease.

Coyle CM et al. Current challenges in neurocysticercosis: recent data and where we are heading. Curr Opin Infect Dis. 2024;37:313. [PMID: 39088697]

de Haes TM et al. Advances and controversies in the diagnosis and management of neurocysticercosis: a clinical perspective. Expert Rev Anti Infect Ther. 2025;23:705. [PMID: 40684313]

Del Brutto OH. Human neurocysticercosis: an overview. Pathogens. 2022;1:1212. [PMID: 36297269]

Pineda-Reyes R et al. Neurocysticercosis: an update on diagnosis, treatment, and prevention. Curr Opin Infect Dis. 2022;35:246. [PMID: 35665719]

Singh G et al. Neurocysticercosis: current diagnostic and treatment paradigms. Curr Opin Neurol. 2025;38:380. [PMID: 40605684]

White AC et al. Diagnosis and treatment of neurocysticercosis: 2017 Clinical Practice Guidelines by the Infectious Diseases Society of America (IDSA) and the American Society of Tropical Medicine and Hygiene (ASTMH). Am J Trop Med Hyg. 2018;98:945. [PMID: 29644966]

2. Echinococcosis

ESSENTIALS OF DIAGNOSIS

- History of exposure to dogs or wild canines in an endemic area.
- *E granulosus* cystic hydatid disease: large cystic lesions, most commonly in the liver or lung.
- *E multilocularis* alveolar hydatid disease: infiltrative disease of the liver
- Positive serologic tests.

General Considerations

Echinococcosis occurs when humans are intermediate hosts for canine tapeworms. Infection is acquired by ingesting food contaminated with canine feces containing parasite eggs. The principal species that infect humans are *Echinococcus granulosus*, which causes cystic hydatid disease, and *Echinococcus multilocularis*, which causes alveolar hydatid disease. *E granulosus* is transmitted by domestic dogs in areas with livestock (sheep, goats, camels, and horses) as intermediate hosts, including Africa, the Middle East, southern Europe, South America, Central Asia, Australia, New Zealand, and the southwestern United States. *E multilocularis*, which much less commonly causes human disease, is transmitted by wild canines and is endemic in northern forest areas of the Northern Hemisphere, including central Europe, Siberia, northern Japan, northwestern Canada, and western Alaska. An increase in the fox population in Europe has been associated with an increase in human cases. The disease range has also extended southward in Central Asia and China. Other species that cause limited disease in humans are endemic in South America and China.

After humans ingest parasite eggs, the eggs hatch in the intestines to form oncospheres, which penetrate the mucosa, enter the circulation, and encyst in specific organs as hydatid cysts. *E granulosus* forms cysts most commonly in the liver (65%) and lungs (25%), but the cysts may develop in any organ, including the brain, bones, skeletal muscles, kidneys, and spleen. Cysts are most commonly single. The cysts can persist and slowly grow for years. Alveolar hydatid disease is tumor-like, infiltrating the liver parenchyma and other organs.

Clinical Findings

A. Symptoms and Signs

Infections are commonly asymptomatic and may be noted incidentally on imaging studies or present with symptoms caused by an enlarging or superinfected mass. Findings may include abdominal or chest pain, biliary obstruction, cholangitis, portal hypertension, cirrhosis, bronchial obstruction leading to segmental lung collapse, and abscesses. Cyst leakage or rupture may be accompanied by a severe allergic reaction, including fever and hypotension. Seeding of cysts after rupture may extend the infection to new areas.

E multilocularis generally causes a more aggressive disease than *E granulosus*, with initial infection of the liver, but then local and distant spread commonly suggesting a malignancy. Symptoms based on the areas of involvement gradually worsen over years, with the development of obstructive findings in the liver and elsewhere.

B. Laboratory Findings

Serologic tests, including ELISA and immunoblot, offer sensitivity and specificity > 80% for *E granulosus* liver infections, but lower sensitivity for involvement of other organs. Serology is somewhat more reliable for *E multilocularis* infections. Serologic tests may also distinguish the two major echinococcal infections.

C. Imaging

Diagnosis is usually based on imaging studies, including ultrasonography, CT, and MRI. In *E granulosus* infection, a large cyst containing multiple daughter cysts that fill the cyst interior is highly suggestive of the diagnosis. In *E multilocularis* infection, imaging shows an irregular mass, often with areas of calcification.

Treatment

The treatment of *cystic* hydatid disease is with albendazole, often with cautious surgical resection of cysts. When used alone, as in cases where surgery is not possible, albendazole (10–15 mg/kg/day orally) has demonstrated efficacy, with courses of ≥ 3 months duration; alternating cycles of treatment and rest may be used. Mebendazole (40–50 mg/kg/day orally) is an alternative drug, and praziquantel may also be effective. In some cases, medical therapy is begun, with surgery performed if disease persists after some months of therapy. Another approach, in particular with inoperable cysts, is percutaneous puncture, aspiration, injection, and re-aspiration (PAIR). In this approach (which should not be used if cysts communicate with the biliary tract), patients receive antihelminthic therapy, and the cyst is partially aspirated. After diagnostic confirmation by examination for parasite protoscolices, a scolicidal agent (95% ethanol, hypertonic saline, or 0.5% cetrimide) is injected, and the cyst is re-aspirated after about 15 minutes. PAIR includes a small risk of anaphylaxis (about 2% of procedures), but death due to anaphylaxis has been rare. Treatment of *alveolar* cyst disease is challenging, generally relying on wide surgical resection of lesions. Therapy with albendazole before or during surgery may be beneficial and may also provide improvement or even cure in inoperable cases.

Chiodini PL. Medical management of cystic echinococcosis. Curr Opin Infect Dis. 2023;36:303. [PMID: 37593991]

Rostami A et al. Human alveolar echinococcosis—a neglected zoonotic disease requiring urgent attention. Int J Mol Sci. 2025;26:2784. [PMID: 40141427]

World Health Organization. WHO guidelines for the treatment of patients with cystic echinococcosis. Geneva, Switzerland: WHO; 2025. https://www.who.int/publications/i/item/9789240110472

INTESTINAL NEMATODE (Roundworm) INFECTIONS

ASCARIASIS

ESSENTIALS OF DIAGNOSIS

- Transient cough, urticaria, pulmonary infiltrates, eosinophilia.
- Nonspecific abdominal symptoms.
- Eggs in stool; adult worms occasionally passed.

General Considerations

Ascaris lumbricoides is the most common of the intestinal helminths, causing about 800 million infections, 12 million acute cases, and 10,000 or more deaths annually worldwide. Prevalence is high wherever there is poor hygiene and sanitation or where human feces are used as fertilizer. Heavy infections are most common in children.

Infection follows ingestion of eggs in contaminated food. Larvae hatch in the small intestine, penetrate into the bloodstream, migrate to the lungs, and then travel via airways back to the GI tract, where they grow to adult worms of up to 40 cm in length, and live for 1–2 years.

Clinical Findings

Most persons with *Ascaris* infection are asymptomatic. In a small proportion of patients, symptoms develop during migration of worms through the lungs, with fever, nonproductive cough, chest pain, dyspnea, and eosinophilia, occasionally with eosinophilic pneumonia. Rarely, larvae lodge ectopically in the brain, kidney, eye, spinal cord, and other sites and may cause local symptoms.

Light intestinal infections usually produce no symptoms. With heavy infection, abdominal discomfort may be seen. Adult worms may also migrate and be coughed up, be vomited, or may emerge through the nose or anus. They may also migrate into the common bile duct, pancreatic duct, appendix, and other sites, which may lead to cholangitis, cholecystitis, pyogenic liver abscess, pancreatitis, obstructive jaundice, or appendicitis. With very heavy infestations, masses of worms may cause intestinal obstruction, volvulus, intussusception, or death. Although severe manifestations of infection are uncommon, the very high prevalence of ascariasis leads to large numbers of individuals, especially children, with important sequelae. Moderate to high worm loads in children are also associated with nutritional abnormalities due to decreased appetite and food intake and also decreased absorption of nutrients.

The diagnosis of ascariasis is made after adult worms emerge from the mouth, nose, or anus, or by identifying characteristic eggs in the feces, usually with the Kato-Katz technique. Imaging studies demonstrate worms, with filling defects in contrast studies and at times evidence of intestinal or biliary obstruction. Eosinophilia is marked during worm migration but may be absent during intestinal infection.

Treatment

All infections should be treated. Treatments of choice are albendazole (single 400-mg oral dose), mebendazole (single 500-mg oral dose or 100 mg twice daily for 3 days), or pyrantel pamoate (single 11-mg/kg oral dose, maximum 1 g). These drugs are well tolerated but may cause mild GI toxicity. They are considered safe for children above 1 year of age and in pregnant persons, although use in the first trimester is best avoided. An alternative (but not in children <35 kg or pregnant persons) is ivermectin (single 200-mcg/kg oral dose). In endemic areas, reinfection after treatment is common. Intestinal obstruction usually responds to conservative management and antihelminthic therapy. Surgery may be required for appendicitis and other GI complications.

TRICHURIASIS

Trichuris trichiura, the whipworm, infects about 500 million persons throughout the world, particularly in humid tropical and subtropical environments. Infection is heaviest and most frequent in children. Infections are acquired by ingestion of eggs. The larvae hatch in the small intestine and mature in the large bowel to adult worms of about 4 cm in length. The worms do not migrate through tissues.

Most persons with infection are asymptomatic. Heavy infections may be accompanied by abdominal cramps, tenesmus, diarrhea, distention, nausea, and vomiting. The *Trichuris* dysentery syndrome may develop, particularly in malnourished young children, with findings resembling IBD including bloody diarrhea and rectal prolapse.

Trichuriasis is diagnosed by identification of characteristic eggs and sometimes adult worms in stools. Eosinophilia is common. Treatment has typically been with albendazole (400 mg/day orally) or mebendazole (200 mg/day orally), for 1–3 days for light infections or 3–7 days for heavy infections, but cure rates are lower than for ascariasis or hookworm infection. Recent studies have shown improved efficacy with a combination of albendazole (400 mg orally) plus ivermectin (200 mcg/kg orally) once daily for 1–3 days. Single-dose albendazole plus moxidectin also was superior to albendazole monotherapy. Oxantel pamoate (one dose of 15–30 mg/kg) has shown good efficacy in clearing infection, but it has low efficacy against *Ascaris* and hookworm infection.

HOOKWORM DISEASE

ESSENTIALS OF DIAGNOSIS

- Transient pruritic skin rash and lung symptoms.
- Anorexia, diarrhea, abdominal discomfort.
- Iron deficiency anemia.
- Characteristic eggs and occult blood in the stool.

General Considerations

Infection with the hookworms *Ancylostoma duodenale* and *Necator americanus* is very common, especially in most tropical and subtropical regions. Both worms are broadly distributed. Prevalence is estimated at about 500 million, causing approximately 65,000 deaths each year worldwide. The eggs hatch when deposited on warm moist soil, releasing larvae that remain infective for up to 1 week. With contact, the larvae penetrate skin and migrate in the bloodstream to the pulmonary capillaries. In the lungs, the larvae penetrate into alveoli and then are carried by ciliary action upward to the bronchi, trachea, and mouth. After being swallowed, they reach and attach to the mucosa of the upper small bowel, where they mature to adult worms. *Ancylostoma* infection can also be acquired by ingestion of the larvae in food or water. Hookworms attach to the intestinal mucosa and suck blood. Blood loss is proportionate to the worm burden.

Clinical Findings

A. Symptoms and Signs

Most persons with infection are asymptomatic. A pruritic maculopapular rash (ground itch) may occur at the site of larval penetration, usually in previously sensitized persons. Pulmonary symptoms may be seen during larval migration through the lungs, with dry cough, wheezing, and low-grade fever, but these symptoms are less common than with ascariasis. About 1 month after infection, as maturing worms attach to the small intestinal mucosa, GI symptoms may develop, with epigastric pain, anorexia, and diarrhea, especially in previously unexposed individuals. Persons chronically infected with large worm burdens may have abdominal pain, anorexia, diarrhea, and findings of marked iron deficiency anemia and protein malnutrition. Anemia can lead to pallor, weakness, dyspnea, and heart failure, and protein loss can lead to hypoalbuminemia, edema, and ascites. These findings may be accompanied by impairment in growth and cognitive development in children. Infection with the dog hookworm *Ancylostoma caninum* can uncommonly lead to abdominal pain, diarrhea, and eosinophilia, with intestinal ulcerations and regional lymphadenitis.

B. Laboratory Findings

Diagnosis is based on the demonstration of characteristic eggs in feces; concentration techniques are usually not needed. Microcytic anemia, occult blood in the stool, and hypoalbuminemia are common. Eosinophilia is common, especially during worm migration.

Treatment

Treatment is usually with albendazole (single 400-mg oral dose) or mebendazole (100 mg orally twice daily for 3 days). Occasional side effects are diarrhea and abdominal pain. A recent trial showed improved efficacy for albendazole plus ivermectin (dosing as for trichuriasis), with three daily doses superior to a single dose. Pyrantel pamoate and levamisole are also effective. Anemia should be managed with iron replacement and, for severe symptomatic anemia, blood transfusion. Mass treatment of children with single doses of albendazole or mebendazole at regular intervals limits worm burdens and the extent of disease and is advocated by WHO.

STRONGYLOIDIASIS

ESSENTIALS OF DIAGNOSIS

- Transient pruritic skin rash and lung symptoms.
- Anorexia, diarrhea, abdominal discomfort.
- Larvae detected in stool.
- Hyperinfection in the immunocompromised; larvae detected in sputum or other fluids.
- Eosinophilia.

General Considerations

Strongyloidiasis is caused by infection with *Strongyloides stercoralis*. Although much less prevalent than ascariasis, trichuriasis, or hookworm infections, strongyloidiasis is nonetheless a significant problem, infecting tens of millions of individuals in tropical and subtropical regions. Infection is also endemic in some temperate regions of North America, Europe, Japan, and Australia. Of particular importance is the predilection of the parasite to cause severe infections in immunocompromised individuals due to its ability to replicate in humans. A related parasite, *Strongyloides fuelleborni*, infects humans in parts of Africa and New Guinea.

Hyperinfection syndrome is the most dangerous manifestation of *S stercoralis* infection, with dissemination of large numbers of filariform larvae to the lungs and other tissues in immunocompromised individuals. Mortality with this syndrome approaches 100% without treatment and has been about 25% with treatment. The hyperinfection syndrome is seen in patients receiving corticosteroids and other immunosuppressive medications; patients with hematologic malignancies, malnutrition, or alcohol use disorder; or persons with AIDS. The risk seems greatest for those receiving corticosteroids.

Clinical Findings

A. Symptoms and Signs

As with other intestinal nematodes, most infected persons are asymptomatic. An acute syndrome can be seen at the time of infection, with a pruritic, erythematous, maculopapular rash, usually of the feet. These symptoms may be followed by pulmonary symptoms (including dry cough, dyspnea, and wheezing) and eosinophilia after several days, followed by GI symptoms after some weeks. Chronic infection may be accompanied by epigastric pain, nausea, diarrhea, and anemia. Maculopapular or urticarial rashes of the buttocks, perineum, and thighs, due to migrating larvae, may be seen. Large worm burdens can lead to malabsorption or intestinal obstruction. Eosinophilia is common but may fluctuate.

With hyperinfection, large numbers of larvae can migrate to many tissues, including the lungs, CNS, kidneys, and liver. GI symptoms can include abdominal pain, nausea, vomiting, diarrhea, and more severe findings related to intestinal obstruction, perforation, or hemorrhage. Bacterial sepsis, probably secondary to intestinal ulcerations, is a common presenting finding. Pulmonary findings include pneumonitis, cough, hemoptysis, and respiratory failure. Sputum may contain adult worms, larvae, and eggs. CNS disease includes meningitis and brain abscesses; the CSF may contain larvae. Various presentations can progress to shock and death.

B. Laboratory Findings

The diagnosis of strongyloidiasis can be difficult, as eggs are seldom found in feces. Diagnosis is usually based on the identification of rhabditiform larvae in the stool or duodenal contents. These larvae must be distinguished from hookworm larvae, which may hatch after stool collection. Repeated examinations of stool or examination of duodenal fluid may be required for diagnosis because the sensitivity of individual tests is only about 30%. Hyperinfection is diagnosed by the identification of large numbers of larvae in stool, sputum, or other body fluids. An ELISA from the CDC offers about 90% sensitivity and specificity, but cross-reactions with other helminths may occur. PCR and related molecular diagnostic methods are useful. Eosinophilia and mild anemia are common, but eosinophilia may be absent with hyperinfection. Hyperinfection may include extensive pulmonary infiltrates, hypoproteinemia, and abnormal liver function studies.

C. Screening

It is important to be aware of the possibility of strongyloidiasis in persons with even a distant history of residence in an endemic area, since the infection can be latent for decades. Screening of at-risk individuals for infection is appropriate before institution of immunosuppressive therapy. Screening can consist of serologic tests, with stool examinations in those with positive serologic tests, but consideration of presumptive treatment is warranted even if the stool evaluations are negative.

▶ Treatment

Full eradication of *S stercoralis* is more important than with other intestinal helminths due to the ability of the parasite to replicate in humans. The treatment of choice for routine infection is ivermectin (200 mcg/kg orally daily for 1–2 days). Less effective alternatives are albendazole (400 mg orally twice daily for 3 days) and thiabendazole (25 mg/kg orally twice daily for 3 days). For hyperinfection, ivermectin should be administered daily until the clinical syndrome has resolved and larvae have not been identified for at least 2 weeks. Follow-up examinations for larvae in stool or sputum are necessary, with repeat dosing if the infection persists. With continued immunosuppression, eradication may be difficult, and regular repeated therapy (eg, monthly ivermectin) may be required.

ENTEROBIASIS

ESSENTIALS OF DIAGNOSIS

- Nocturnal perianal pruritus.
- Identification of eggs or adult worms on perianal skin or in stool.

▶ General Considerations

Enterobius vermicularis, the pinworm, is a common cause of intestinal infections worldwide, with maximal prevalence in school-aged children. Enterobiasis is transmitted person-to-person via ingestion of eggs after contact with the hands or perianal region of an infected individual, food or fomites that have been contaminated by an infected individual, or infected bedding or clothing. Autoinfection also occurs. Eggs hatch in the duodenum and larvae migrate to the cecum. Females mature in about a month and remain viable for about another month. During this time, they migrate through the anus to deposit large numbers of eggs on the perianal skin. Due to the relatively short life span of these helminths, continuous reinfection, as in institutional settings, is required for long-standing infection.

▶ Clinical Findings

A. Symptoms and Signs

Most individuals with pinworm infection are asymptomatic. The most common symptom is perianal pruritus, particularly at night, due to the presence of the female worms or deposited eggs. Insomnia, restlessness, and enuresis are common in children. Perianal scratching may result in excoriation and impetigo. Mild GI symptoms have been attributed to enterobiasis, but associations are not proven. Serious sequelae are uncommon. Rarely, worm migration results in inflammation or granulomatous reactions of the GI or genitourinary tracts. Colonic ulceration and eosinophilic colitis have been reported.

B. Laboratory Findings

Pinworm eggs are usually not found in stool. Diagnosis is made by finding adult worms or eggs on the perianal skin. A common test is to apply clear cellophane tape to the perianal skin, ideally in the early morning, followed by microscopic examination for eggs. The sensitivity of the tape test is about 50% for a single test and 90% for three tests. Nocturnal examination of the perianal area or gross examination of stools may reveal adult worms, which are about 1 cm in length. Eosinophilia is rare.

▶ Treatment

Treatment is with single oral doses of albendazole (400 mg), mebendazole (100 mg), or pyrantel pamoate (11 mg/kg, to a maximum of 1 g). The dose is repeated in 2 weeks due to frequent reinfection. Other family members with infection should be treated concurrently, and treatment of all close contacts may be appropriate when rates of reinfection are high in family, school, or institutional settings. Standard hand washing and hygiene practices help limit spread. Perianal scratching should be discouraged. Washing of clothes and bedding should kill pinworm eggs.

Buonfrate D et al. Human strongyloidiasis: complexities and pathways forward. Clin Microbiol Rev. 2023;36:e0003323. [PMID: 37937980]

Khurana S et al. diagnostic techniques for soil-transmitted helminths—recent advances. Res Rep Trop Med. 2021;12:181. [PMID: 34377048]

Krolewiecki A et al. Albendazole-ivermectin co-formulation for the treatment of Trichuris trichiura and other soil-transmitted helminths: a randomised phase 2/3 trial. Lancet Infect Dis. 2025;25:548. [PMID: 39805305]

Schnoz A et al. Efficacy and safety of moxidectin-albendazole combination therapy for *Trichuris trichiura* infections in school-aged children: a double-blind, randomised, controlled, superiority trial. Lancet Infect Dis. 2025;25:1325. [PMID: 40675166]

INVASIVE NEMATODE (Roundworm) INFECTIONS

ANGIOSTRONGYLIASIS

Nematodes of rats of the genus *Angiostrongylus* cause two distinct syndromes in humans. *Angiostrongylus cantonensis*, the rat lungworm, causes eosinophilic meningoencephalitis, primarily in Southeast Asia and some Pacific islands, Hawaii (82 reported cases in 2007–2017), and Australia, but evidence for disease in other areas, including the southern United States, is growing. In one study, *A cantonensis* was responsible for most cases of eosinophilic meningitis in Vietnam. *Angiostrongylus costaricensis* causes GI inflammation. In both diseases, human infection follows ingestion of larvae within slugs or snails (also crabs, prawns, or centipedes for *A cantonensis*) or on material, such as salads, contaminated by these organisms. Since the parasites are not in their natural hosts, they cannot complete their life cycles, but they can cause disease after migrating to the brain or GI tract. *A cantonensis* can also migrate from the brain to the pulmonary arteries. The disease is caused primarily by worm larvae migrating through the CNS and by the inflammatory response to dying worms.

Clinical Findings

A. *A cantonensis* Infection

After an incubation period of 1 day to 2 weeks, presenting symptoms and signs include headache, stiff neck, nausea, vomiting, cranial nerve abnormalities, and paresthesias. Most cases resolve spontaneously after 2–8 weeks, but serious sequelae and death have been reported. The diagnosis is strongly suggested by the finding of eosinophilic CSF pleocytosis (> 10% eosinophils) in a patient with a history of travel to an endemic area. Peripheral eosinophilia may not be present. The diagnosis can be confirmed with PCR of CSF or blood, but this may be negative early in disease.

B. *A costaricensis* Infection

Parasites penetrate ileocecal vasculature and develop into adults, which lay eggs, but do not complete their life cycle. Disease is due to an inflammatory response to dying worms in the intestinal tract, with an eosinophilic granulomatous response, at times including vasculitis and ischemic necrosis. Common findings are abdominal pain, vomiting, and fever. Pain is most commonly localized to the right lower quadrant, and a mass may be appreciated, all mimicking appendicitis. Symptoms may recur over months. Uncommon findings are intestinal perforation or obstruction, or disease due to migration of worms to other sites. Biopsy of inflamed intestinal tissue may show worms localized to mesenteric arteries and eosinophilic granulomas.

Treatment

Antihelminthic therapy for *A cantonensis* infection may be harmful, since responses to dying worms may worsen with therapy. Some experts, however, recommend prompt therapy for any suspected infection, even for a known accidental snail or slug ingestion in an endemic area, as therapy is likely most beneficial early in the course of disease. Albendazole is probably the best choice, and therapy should be prompt (within 3 weeks of exposure). Corticosteroids are probably appropriate if antihelminthics are provided. Ocular infection is treated surgically. It is not known if antihelminthic therapy is helpful for *A costaricensis* infection. Many cases are managed surgically, usually for suspected appendicitis.

Ansdell V et al. Guidelines for the diagnosis and treatment of neuroangiostrongyliasis: updated recommendations. Parasitology. 2021;148:227. [PMID: 32729438]

Jarvi S et al. *Angiostrongylus cantonensis* and neuroangiostrongyliasis (rat lungworm disease): 2020. Parasitology. 2021;148:129. [PMID: 33315004]

CUTANEOUS LARVA MIGRANS (Creeping Eruption)

Cutaneous larva migrans is caused principally by larvae of the dog and cat hookworms, *Ancylostoma braziliense* and *A caninum*. Other animal hookworms, gnathostomiasis, and strongyloidiasis may also cause this syndrome. Infections are common in warm areas, including the southeastern United States. They are most common in children. The disease is caused by the migration of worms through skin; the nonhuman parasites cannot complete their life cycles, so only cause cutaneous disease.

Clinical Findings

Intensely pruritic erythematous papules develop, usually on the feet or hands, followed within a few days by serpiginous tracks marking the course of the parasite, which may travel several millimeters per day (Figure 39–3). Several tracks may be present. The process may continue for weeks, with lesions becoming vesiculated, encrusted, or secondarily infected. Systemic symptoms and eosinophilia are uncommon.

The diagnosis is based on the characteristic appearance of the lesions. Biopsy is usually not indicated.

Treatment

Without treatment, the larvae eventually die and are absorbed. Mild cases do not require treatment. Systemic therapy is effective, with ivermectin (200 mcg/kg orally as a single dose) being superior to albendazole (400 mg orally once or twice daily for 3–5 days). Thiabendazole (10% aqueous suspension) can be applied topically three times daily for 5 or more days.

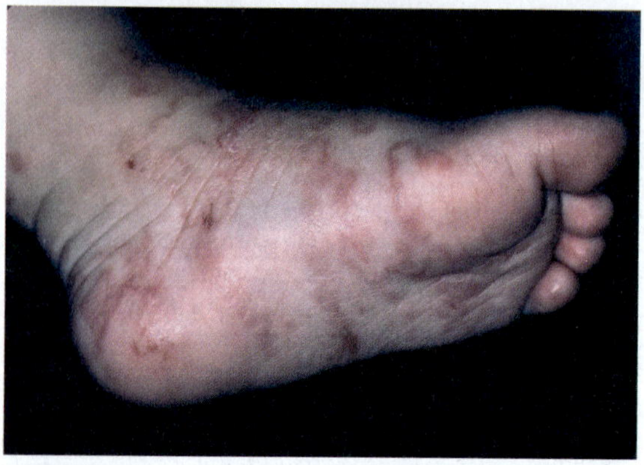

▲ **Figure 39–3.** Serpiginous cutaneous larva migrans. (Reproduced with permission from Richard P. Usatine, MD, in Usatine RP, Smith MA, Mayeaux EJ Jr, Chumley H. *The Color Atlas of Family Medicine*, 3rd ed. McGraw-Hill, 2019.)

Palaniappan V et al. Cutaneous larva migrans. Clin Exp Dermatol. 2025:llaf375. [PMID: 40795202]

FILARIASIS

LYMPHATIC FILARIASIS

ESSENTIALS OF DIAGNOSIS

- Episodic attacks of lymphangitis, lymphadenitis, and fever.
- Chronic progressive swelling of extremities and genitals; hydrocele; chyluria; lymphedema.
- Microfilariae in blood, chyluria, or hydrocele fluid; positive serologic tests.

General Considerations

Lymphatic filariasis is caused by three filarial nematodes: *Wuchereria bancrofti*, *Brugia malayi*, and *Brugia timori*, and is among the most important parasitic diseases of man. Approximately 120 million persons are infected with these organisms in tropical and subtropical countries, about a third of these suffer clinical consequences of the infections, and many are seriously disfigured. *W bancrofti* causes about 90% of episodes of lymphatic filariasis. It is transmitted by *Culex*, *Aedes*, and *Anopheles* mosquitoes and is widely distributed in the tropics and subtropics, including sub-Saharan Africa, Southeast Asia, the western Pacific, India, South America, and the Caribbean. *B malayi* is transmitted by *Mansonia* and *Anopheles* mosquitoes and is endemic in parts of China, India, Southeast Asia, and the Pacific. *B timori* is found only in islands of southeastern Indonesia. *Mansonella* are filarial worms transmitted by midges and other insects in Africa and South America.

Humans are infected by the bites of infected mosquitoes. Larvae then move to the lymphatics and lymph nodes, where they mature over months to thread-like adult worms, and then can persist for many years. The adult worms produce large numbers of microfilariae, which are released into the circulation, and infective to mosquitoes, particularly at night (except for the South Pacific, where microfilaremia peaks during daylight hours).

Clinical Findings

A. Symptoms and Signs

Many infections remain asymptomatic despite circulating microfilariae. Clinical consequences of filarial infection are principally due to inflammatory responses to developing, mature, and dying worms. The initial manifestation of infection is often acute lymphangitis, with fever, painful lymph nodes, edema, and inflammation spreading peripherally from involved lymph nodes (in contrast to bacterial lymphangitis, which spreads centrally). Lymphangitis and lymphadenitis of the upper and lower extremities are common (Figure 39–4); genital involvement, including epididymitis and orchitis, with scrotal pain and tenderness, occurs principally only with *W bancrofti* infection. Acute attacks of lymphangitis last for a few days to a week and may recur a few times per year. Filarial fevers may also occur without lymphatic inflammation.

The most common chronic manifestation of lymphatic filariasis is swelling of the extremities or genitals due to chronic lymphatic inflammation and obstruction. Extremities become increasingly swollen, with a progression over time, including pitting or nonpitting edema or sclerotic changes of the skin that are referred to as elephantiasis. Genital involvement, particularly with *W bancrofti*, occurs more commonly in men, progressing from painful epididymitis to hydroceles that are usually painless but can become very large, with inguinal lymphadenopathy, thickening of the spermatic cord, scrotal lymphedema, thickening and fissuring of the scrotal skin, and occasionally chyluria. Lymphedema of the female genitalia and breasts may also occur.

Tropical pulmonary eosinophilia is a distinct syndrome that principally affects young adult men with either *W bancrofti* or *B malayi* infection, but typically without microfilaremia. This syndrome is characterized by asthma-like symptoms,

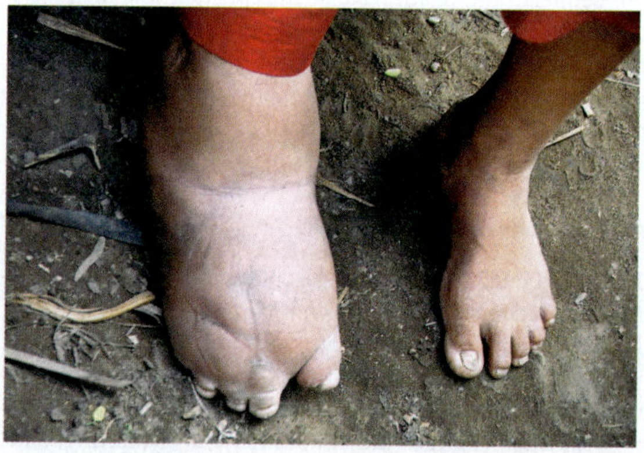

▲ **Figure 39–4.** Elephantiasis of legs due to filariasis. (Used with permission from Rungtip Chatadee/Alamy Stock Photo.)

with cough, wheezing, dyspnea, and low-grade fevers, usually at night. Without treatment, tropical pulmonary eosinophilia can progress to interstitial fibrosis and chronic restrictive lung disease. *Mansonella* can inhabit serous cavities, the retroperitoneum, the eye, or the skin, and cause abnormalities related to inflammation at these sites.

B. Laboratory Findings

The diagnosis of lymphatic filariasis is strongly suggested by characteristic findings of lymphangitis or lymphatic obstruction in persons with risk factors for the disease. The diagnosis is confirmed by finding microfilariae, usually in blood, but microfilariae may be absent, especially early in the disease progression (first 2–3 years) or with chronic obstructive disease. To increase yields, blood samples are obtained at about midnight in most areas, but during daylight hours in the South Pacific. Smears are evaluated by wet mount to identify motile parasites and by Giemsa staining; these examinations can be delayed until the following morning, with storage of samples at room temperature. Of note, the periodicity of microfilaremia is variable, and daytime samples may yield positive results. Microfilariae may also be identified in hydrocele fluid or chylous urine. Eosinophilia is usually absent, except during acute inflammatory syndromes. Serologic tests may be helpful but cannot distinguish past and active infections. Rapid antigen tests with sensitivity and specificity > 90% are available for detection of *W bancrofti*. These are the diagnostic tests of choice and are used to guide control programs. However, cross-reactivity with *Loa* infections has been described. Due to potential severe toxicity, caution is appropriate before ivermectin treatment for positive *W bancrofti* antigen tests in areas also endemic for *L loa* infection. Multiple molecular tests, including field-friendly LAMP assays, are available. Adult worms may also be found in lymph node biopsy specimens (although biopsy is not usually clinically indicated) or by ultrasound of a scrotal hydrocele or lymphedematous breast. When microfilaremia is lacking, especially if sophisticated techniques are not available, diagnoses may need to be made on clinical grounds.

Treatment & Control

A. Drug Treatment

Diethylcarbamazine is the drug of choice, but it cannot cure infections due to its limited action against adult worms. Asymptomatic infection and acute lymphangitis are treated with this drug (2 mg/kg orally three times daily) for 10–14 days, leading to a marked decrease in microfilaremia. Therapy may be accompanied by allergic symptoms, including fever, headache, malaise, hypotension, and bronchospasm, probably due to release of antigens from dying worms. For this reason, treatment courses may begin with a lower dosage, with escalation over the first 4 days of treatment. Single annual doses of diethylcarbamazine (6 mg/kg orally), alone or with ivermectin (400 mcg/kg orally) or albendazole (400 mg orally) may be as effective as longer courses of diethylcarbamazine. Combination therapy with a single dose of each of the three drugs (ivermectin, diethylcarbamazine, and albendazole [IDA]) cleared parasites in > 95% of persons for 3 years and offered superior clearance compared with two drugs; triple-drug therapy was as safe and well tolerated. When onchocerciasis or loiasis is suspected, it may be appropriate to withhold diethylcarbamazine to avoid severe reactions to dying microfilariae; rather, ivermectin plus albendazole may be given, although these drugs are less active than diethylcarbamazine against adult worms. Another promising regimen is moxidectin (approved for onchocerciasis) plus albendazole, with evidence for improved clearance of microfilariae compared to ivermectin plus albendazole. Appropriate management of advanced obstructive disease is uncertain. Drainage of hydroceles provides symptomatic relief, although they will recur. Therapy with diethylcarbamazine cannot reverse chronic lymphatic changes but is typically provided to lower worm burdens. An interesting approach under study is to treat with doxycycline (100–200 mg/day orally for 4–6 weeks), which kills obligate intracellular *Wolbachia* bacteria, leading to death of adult filarial worms. Doxycycline is also effective at controlling *Mansonella perstans* infection, which does not respond well to standard antifilarial drugs. Secondary bacterial infections must be treated. Surgical correction may be helpful in some cases.

B. Disease Control

Avoidance of mosquitoes is a key measure; preventive measures include the use of screens, bed nets (ideally treated with insecticide), and insect repellents. Community-based treatment with single annual doses of effective drugs offers a highly effective means of control. Combination IDA therapy offers improved efficacy and may become the standard of care for the prevention of lymphatic filariasis.

Dubray CL et al. Safety and efficacy of co-administered diethylcarbamazine, albendazole and ivermectin during mass drug administration for lymphatic filariasis in Haiti: results from a two-armed, open-label, cluster-randomized, community study. PLoS Negl Trop Dis. 2020;14:e0008298. [PMID: 32511226]
Koudou GB et al. Moxidectin combination therapies for lymphatic filariasis: an open-label, observer-masked, randomised controlled trial. Lancet Infect Dis. 2025;25:1075. [PMID: 40345209]

ONCHOCERCIASIS

ESSENTIALS OF DIAGNOSIS

- Conjunctivitis progressing to blindness.
- Severe pruritus; skin excoriations, thickening, and depigmentation; and subcutaneous nodules.
- Microfilariae in skin snips and on slit-lamp examination; adult worms in subcutaneous nodules.

General Considerations

Onchocerciasis, or river blindness, is caused by *Onchocerca volvulus*. An estimated 37 million persons are infected worldwide, of whom 3–4 million have skin disease, 500,000 have severe visual impairment, and 300,000 are blinded. More than 99% of infections are in sub-Saharan Africa, especially the West African savanna, with about half of cases in Nigeria and Congo. In some hyperendemic African villages, close to 100% of individuals are infected, and 10% or more of the population is blind. The disease is also prevalent in the southwestern Arabian Peninsula and Latin America, including southern Mexico, Guatemala, Venezuela, Colombia, Ecuador, and northwestern Brazil. Onchocerciasis is transmitted by *Simulium* flies (blackflies). These insects breed in fast-flowing streams and bite during the day.

After the bite of an infected blackfly, larvae are deposited in the skin, where adults develop over 6–12 months. Adult worms live in subcutaneous connective tissue or muscle nodules for a decade or more. Microfilariae are released from the nodules and migrate through subcutaneous and ocular tissues. Disease is due to responses to worms and to intracellular *Wolbachia* bacteria.

Clinical Findings

A. Symptoms and Signs

After an incubation period of up to 1–3 years, the disease typically produces an erythematous, papular, pruritic rash, which may progress to chronic skin thickening and depigmentation. Itching may be severe and unresponsive to medications, such that more disability-adjusted life-years are lost to onchocercal skin problems than to blindness. Numerous firm, nontender, movable subcutaneous nodules of about 0.5–3 cm, which contain adult worms, may be present. Due to differences in vector habits, these nodules are more commonly on the lower body in Africa but on the head and upper body in Latin America. Inguinal and femoral lymphadenopathy is common, at times resulting in a "hanging groin," with lymph nodes hanging within a sling of atrophic skin. Patients may also have systemic symptoms, with weight loss and musculoskeletal pain.

The most serious manifestations of onchocerciasis involve the migration of microfilariae through the eyes. Findings include punctate keratitis and corneal opacities, progressing to sclerosing keratitis and blindness. Iridocyclitis, glaucoma, choroiditis, and optic atrophy may also lead to vision loss. The likelihood of blindness after infection varies greatly based on geography, with the risk greatest in savanna regions of West Africa.

B. Diagnostic Testing

The diagnosis is made by identifying microfilariae in skin snips, by visualizing microfilariae in the cornea or anterior chamber by slit-lamp examination, by identification of adult worms in a biopsy or aspirate of a nodule or, uncommonly, by identification of microfilariae in urine. Skin snips from the iliac crest (Africa) or scapula (Americas) are allowed to stand in saline for 2–4 hours or longer, and then examined microscopically for microfilariae. Deep punch biopsies are not needed, and if suspicion persists after a skin snip is negative, the procedure should be repeated. Ultrasound may identify characteristic findings suggestive of adult worms in skin nodules. When the diagnosis remains difficult, the Mazzotti test can be used; exacerbation of skin rash and pruritus after a topical or 50-mg oral dose of diethylcarbamazine is highly suggestive of the diagnosis, but this test can elicit severe skin and eye reactions in heavily infected individuals. Eosinophilia is a common but inconsistent finding. Antigen and antibody detection tests are under study.

Treatment & Control

The treatment of choice is ivermectin, which kills microfilariae, but not adult worms, so disease control requires repeat administrations. Treatment is with a single oral dose of 150 mcg/mL, but schedules for re-treatment have not been standardized. One regimen is to treat every 3 months for 1 year, followed by treatment every 6–12 months for the suspected life span of adult worms (about 15 years). Treatment results in marked reduction in numbers of microfilariae in the skin and eyes, although its impact on the progression of visual loss remains uncertain. Toxicities of ivermectin are generally mild; fever, pruritus, urticaria, myalgias, edema, hypotension, and tender lymphadenopathy may be seen, presumably due to reactions to dying worms. Ivermectin should be used with caution in patients also at risk for loiasis, since it can elicit severe reactions including encephalopathy. As with lymphatic filariasis, combination drug therapy with ivermectin, diethylcarbamazine, and albendazole offers improved long-term clearance of parasites. Moxidectin is FDA-approved for the treatment of onchocerciasis. Moxidectin is well tolerated and superior to ivermectin in suppressing skin microfilariae and offers another agent for treatment and control. As with other filarial infections, doxycycline acts against *O volvulus* by killing intracellular *Wolbachia* bacteria. A course of 100 mg orally daily for 4–6 weeks kills the bacteria and prevents parasite embryogenesis for at least 18 months. Doxycycline shows promise as a first-line agent to treat onchocerciasis because of its improved activity against adult worms compared with other agents and limited toxicity due to the slow action of the drug.

Protection against onchocerciasis includes avoidance of biting flies. Major efforts are underway to control insect vectors in Africa. In addition, mass distribution of ivermectin for intermittent administration at the community level is ongoing, and the prevalence of severe skin and eye disease is decreasing.

Opoku NO et al. A randomized, open-label study of the tolerability and efficacy of one or three daily doses of ivermectin plus diethylcarbamazine and albendazole (IDA) versus one dose of ivermectin plus albendazole (IA) for treatment of onchocerciasis. PLoS Negl Trop Dis. 2023;17:e0011365. [PMID: 37205721]

40 Mycotic Infections

Stacey R. Rose, MD, FACP, FIDSA
Richard J. Hamill, MD, FIDSA

CANDIDIASIS

ESSENTIALS OF DIAGNOSIS

- Common normal flora but opportunistic pathogen.
- Typically, mucosal disease, particularly vaginitis and oral thrush/esophagitis.
- Persistent, unexplained oral or vaginal candidiasis: check for HIV or diabetes mellitus.
- (1,3)-β-D-glucan results may be positive in candidemia even when blood cultures are negative.

General Considerations

Candida albicans can be cultured from the mouth, vagina, and feces of most people. Cellular immunodeficiency predisposes to mucocutaneous disease. When no other underlying cause is found, persistent oral or vaginal candidiasis should raise suspicion for HIV infection or diabetes. Risk factors for invasive candidiasis include prolonged neutropenia, abdominal surgery, broad-spectrum antibiotics, corticosteroids, kidney disease, and the presence of intravascular catheters. Although *C albicans* remains the most common cause of both mucocutaneous and systemic candidiasis, non-*albicans* strains are of considerable importance in certain contexts and may impact therapy owing to antifungal resistance.

Clinical Findings

A. Mucosal Candidiasis

1. Vulvovaginal candidiasis—This condition occurs in an estimated 75% of women during their lifetime. Risk factors include pregnancy, uncontrolled diabetes mellitus, broad-spectrum antimicrobial treatment, corticosteroid use, and HIV infection. Symptoms include acute vulvar pruritus, burning vaginal discharge, and dyspareunia.

2. Esophageal candidiasis—Substernal odynophagia, gastroesophageal reflux, or nausea without substernal pain can be presenting symptoms. Oral candidiasis, though often associated, is not invariably present. Diagnosis is best confirmed by endoscopy with biopsy and culture.

B. Candidal Funguria

Most cases of candidal funguria are asymptomatic and represent specimen contamination or bladder colonization, and do not warrant antifungal therapy. However, symptoms and signs of true *Candida* UTIs are indistinguishable from bacterial UTIs and can include urgency, hesitancy, fever, chills, or flank pain.

C. Invasive Candidiasis

Invasive candidiasis can be (1) candidemia (bloodstream infection) without deep-seated infection; (2) candidemia with deep-seated infection (typically eyes, kidney, or abdomen); and (3) deep-seated candidiasis in the absence of bloodstream infection (ie, hepatosplenic candidiasis); the ratio of these clinical entities depends on the predominating risk factors for affected patients (ie, neutropenia, indwelling vascular catheters, postsurgical). The clinical presentation of candidemia varies from minimal fever to septic shock that can resemble a severe bacterial infection. The diagnosis of invasive *Candida* infection is challenging since *Candida* species are often isolated from mucosal sites in the absence of invasive disease while blood cultures are positive only 50% of the time in invasive infection. Consecutively positive (1,3)-β-D-glucan results can guide empiric therapy in high-risk patients even in the absence of positive blood cultures.

Hepatosplenic candidiasis can occur following prolonged neutropenia with hematologic cancers, but this entity is less common in the era of widespread antifungal prophylaxis. Typically, fever and abdominal pain present weeks after chemotherapy when neutrophil counts have recovered. Blood cultures are generally negative, though hepatosplenic abscesses may be seen on abdominal imaging.

D. Candidal Endocarditis

Candidal endocarditis is a rare infection affecting patients with prosthetic heart valves or prolonged candidemia, such as with indwelling catheters. The diagnosis is established definitively by isolating *Candida* by culture or molecular testing from vegetations at the time of valve replacement.

Treatment

See Table 40–1.

A. Mucosal Candidiasis

1. Vulvovaginal candidiasis—This condition can be treated with oral or topical azoles. A single 150-mg oral dose of fluconazole is equivalent to topical treatments with better patient acceptance. Topical azole preparations include clotrimazole, 100-mg vaginal tablet for 7 days, or miconazole, 200-mg vaginal suppository for 3 days. Disease recurrence is common but can be decreased with weekly oral fluconazole therapy (150 mg weekly). Vulvovaginal candidiasis caused by non-*albicans* strains—eg, *C glabrata*—may require alternative therapies (such as intravaginal boric acid) in the setting of azole resistance. Oral ibrexafungerp, a highly bioavailable glucan synthase inhibitor, may treat vulvovaginal candidiasis from any disease-causing strains, including azole-resistant pathogens. Oteseconazole is an alternative treatment option for recurrent vulvovaginal candidiasis.

Table 40–1. Agents for systemic mycoses.[1]

Drug	Dosing	Renal Clearance?	CSF Penetration?	Toxicities	Spectrum of Activity
Polyenes					
Amphotericin B	0.3–1.5 mg/kg/day intravenously	No	Poor	Rigors, fever, azotemia, hypokalemia, hypomagnesemia, renal tubular acidosis, anemia	All major pathogens except *Scedosporium*
Amphotericin B lipid complex	5 mg/kg/day intravenously	No	Poor	Fever, rigors, nausea, hypotension, anemia, azotemia, tachypnea	Same as amphotericin B, above
Amphotericin B, liposomal	3–6 mg/kg/day intravenously	No	Poor	Fever, rigors, nausea, hypotension, azotemia, anemia, tachypnea, chest tightness	Same as amphotericin B, above Preferred agent for CNS
Azoles					
Fluconazole	Systemic infection: 400–2000 mg/day intravenously or orally Mucosal infection: 100–200 mg/day orally	Yes	Yes	Nausea, rash, xerosis, alopecia, headache, hepatic enzyme elevations	Mucosal candidiasis (including urinary tract), cryptococcosis, histoplasmosis, coccidioidomycosis
Isavuconazole	200 mg orally or intravenously every 8 hours for six doses (48 hours) as loading dose, followed by 200 mg/day orally or intravenously	No	Low in CSF, high in brain	Nausea, diarrhea, upper abdominal pain, dizziness	Broad range of activity including invasive aspergillosis and mucormycosis (limited data for *Mucorales*)
Itraconazole	Oral solution and capsule formulations both dosed at 200 mg three times daily for 3 days, then 200 mg once or twice daily[2]	No	Variable	Nausea, hypokalemia, edema, hypertension, peripheral neuropathy, exacerbation of HF	Histoplasmosis, coccidioidomycosis, blastomycosis, paracoccidioidomycosis, mucosal candidiasis (except urinary), sporotrichosis, aspergillosis, chromomycosis
SUBA-itraconazole	130 mg orally once daily (two 65-mg capsules)	No	Variable	Nausea, hypokalemia, edema, hypertension, peripheral neuropathy, exacerbation of HF	Histoplasmosis, blastomycosis, aspergillosis

(*continued*)

Table 40–1. Agents for systemic mycoses.[1] (continued)

Drug	Dosing	Renal Clearance?	CSF Penetration?	Toxicities	Spectrum of Activity
Ketoconazole	200–800 mg/day orally in one or two doses with food or acidic beverage	No	Poor	Anorexia, nausea, suppression of testosterone and cortisol, rash, headache, hepatic enzyme elevations, hepatic failure	Nonmeningeal histoplasmosis and coccidioidomycosis, blastomycosis, paracoccidioidomycosis, mucosal candidiasis (except urinary)
Oteseconazole	12-week oteseconazole-only regimen:[3] Day 1: 600 mg orally, then Day 2: 450 mg orally, then Day 14: 150 mg orally weekly for 11 weeks	Yes	Unknown	Headache; nausea; hot flush; dysuria; menorrhagia; metrorrhagia; vulvovaginal irritation; elevated serum CK; contraindicated in women of reproductive potential and in pregnant women due to risk of ocular abnormalities in fetus (based on animal data)	Recurrent vulvovaginal candidiasis
Posaconazole	Delayed-release tablet formulation preferred over oral solution due to more predictable absorption For delayed-release tablet or intravenous formulation: 300 mg twice daily for two doses (1 day) as loading dose followed by 300 mg daily	No	Yes	Nausea, vomiting, abdominal pain, diarrhea, and headache; pseudohyperaldosteronism	Broad range of activity including the *Mucorales*
Voriconazole[4]	Systemic infection: 6 mg/kg intravenously every 12 hours for 24 hours loading dose, followed by 4 mg/kg intravenously every 12 hours or 200–300 mg orally every 12 hours Mucosal infection: 200–300 mg orally[2] every 12 hours (no loading dose required)	Yes	Yes	Transient visual disturbances, rash, photosensitivity, fluoride excess with periostitis, peripheral neuropathy, squamous cell skin cancers, hepatic enzyme elevations	All major pathogens except the *Mucorales* and sporotrichosis
Echinocandins					
Anidulafungin	200 mg intravenous loading dose, followed by 100 mg/day intravenously	<1%	Poor	Diarrhea, hepatic enzyme elevations, histamine-mediated reactions	Mucosal and invasive candidiasis
Caspofungin acetate	70 mg intravenous loading dose, followed by 50 mg/day intravenously	<50%[5]	Poor	Transient neutropenia; hepatic enzyme elevations when used with cyclosporine	Aspergillosis, mucosal and invasive candidiasis, empiric antifungal therapy in febrile neutropenia
Micafungin sodium	100 mg/day intravenously	No	Poor	Rash, rigors, headache, phlebitis	Mucosal and invasive candidiasis, prophylaxis in hematopoietic stem cell transplantation

(*continued*)

Table 40–1. Agents for systemic mycoses.[1] (continued)

Drug	Dosing	Renal Clearance?	CSF Penetration?	Toxicities	Spectrum of Activity
Rezafungin	400 mg intravenous loading dose, followed by 200 mg intravenously weekly (safety beyond 4 weeks not yet established)	No	Unknown but likely poor	Hypokalemia, pyrexia, diarrhea, vomiting, nausea, hypomagnesemia, abdominal pain, constipation, hypophosphatemia	Candidemia and invasive candidiasis in patients ≥ 18 years old who have limited or no alternative treatment options; not studied in endocarditis, osteomyelitis, meningitis
Antimetabolite					
Flucytosine (5-FC)	100–150 mg/kg/day orally in four divided doses	Yes	Yes	Leukopenia,[6] hemorrhagic colitis,[6] rash, diarrhea, hepatitis, nausea, vomiting	Cryptococcosis,[7] candidiasis, chromomycosis
Allylamine					
Terbinafine	250 mg once daily orally	Yes	Poor	Nausea, abdominal pain, taste disturbance, rash, diarrhea, and hepatic enzyme elevations	Dermatophytes, sporotrichosis, chromomycosis, eumycetoma
Triterpenoid (inhibits glucan synthase)					
Ibrexafungerp	300 mg orally every 12 hours for two doses (600 mg total) Dose reduction if concomitant use with CYP3A inhibitors	No	Unknown	Diarrhea, nausea, abdominal pain, dizziness, vomiting; may cause fetal harm (not for use in pregnancy)	Vaginal candidiasis (including azole-resistant strains); under investigation for treatment of invasive mold infections
Gepix					
Fosmanogepix	1000 mg intravenously twice daily (day 1), followed by 600 mg intravenously once daily, with transition to oral therapy (800 mg daily) after day 4 of therapy if clinically stable	Unknown; appears safe in renal insufficiency	Unknown	Headache	Currently available for "expanded access;" under investigation for treatment of invasive candidiasis including resistant isolates (eg, *C auris*) and invasive mold infections
Orotomide (targets dihydroorotate dehydrogenase in pyrimidine synthesis pathway)					
Olorofim	Loading dose of 150 mg twice a day on day 1, followed by 90 mg twice daily	Unknown; metabolized by CYP3A4 thus caution advised for drug–drug interactions	Unknown	Gastrointestinal intolerance Elevated liver function tests	Available through "orphan drug" and "breakthrough therapy" designations for invasive aspergillosis (including azole-resistant species), other molds and dimorphic fungi; lacks activity against yeasts or *Mucorales* species

[1]General information provided, but specific dosing may vary by indication and other patient characteristics; an infectious diseases specialist should be consulted for complex cases.
[2]Oral solution preferred due to less variable absorption; capsule should be taken with food and acidic beverages to enhance absorption. For severe infections, blood levels should be measured to ensure adequate exposure.
[3]An alternative regimen using a combination of fluconazole and oteseconazole is also available.
[4]Some authorities advocate therapeutic drug monitoring in patients who are not responding to therapy. Administration with drugs that are metabolized by the cytochrome P450 system is contraindicated or requires careful monitoring of liver function. Intravenous formulation is contraindicated for patients with CrCl <50 mL/min because of accumulation of cyclodextrin.
[5]No dosage adjustment required for CKD; dosage adjustment necessary with moderate to severe hepatic dysfunction.
[6]To prevent leukopenia or hemorrhagic colitis, drug levels should be monitored or dosing adjusted according to creatinine clearance.
[7]In combination with amphotericin B.
CK, creatine kinase.

2. Esophageal candidiasis—If patients can swallow and take adequate amounts of fluid orally, fluconazole, 200–400 mg orally daily for 14–21 days, is recommended. Patients who are unable to tolerate oral therapy should receive intravenous fluconazole, 400 mg daily, or an echinocandin for 14–21 days. Options for patients with fluconazole-refractory disease include 14–21 days of oral itraconazole solution, 200 mg daily; oral or intravenous voriconazole, 200 mg twice daily; oral posaconazole, 300 mg daily; or an intravenous echinocandin (caspofungin, 70-mg loading dose, then 50 mg/day; anidulafungin, 200 mg/day; or micafungin, 150 mg/day). Relapse is common with all agents in persons with HIV without adequate immune reconstitution.

B. Candidal Funguria

Candidal funguria frequently resolves with discontinuance of antibiotics or removal of bladder catheters. Clinical benefit from treatment of asymptomatic candiduria has not been demonstrated, but persistent funguria should raise the suspicion of invasive infection. When symptomatic funguria persists, oral fluconazole, 200 mg/day for 7–14 days, can be used.

C. Invasive Candidiasis

The 2025 global guidelines for the diagnosis and management of candidiasis recommend an intravenous echinocandin as first-line therapy (ie, caspofungin [70 mg once, then 50 mg daily], micafungin [100 mg daily], or anidulafungin [200 mg once, then 100 mg daily]). Rezafungin (400 mg intravenously once, then 200 mg intravenously weekly) is FDA-approved as a long-acting echinocandin for candidemia and invasive candidiasis when there are limited or no alternative treatment options. Intravenous or oral fluconazole (400 to 800 mg daily) is an acceptable alternative for less critically ill patients without recent azole exposure.

Therapy for candidemia should be continued for 2 weeks after the last positive blood culture and resolution of symptoms and signs of infection. A dilated fundoscopic examination may be advised for patients with candidemia to exclude endophthalmitis and repeat blood cultures should be drawn to demonstrate organism clearance. Susceptibility testing is recommended on all bloodstream *Candida* isolates; after 5 days of parenteral therapy, step down to an oral azole is advised, provided the patient is clinically stable with confirmed drug susceptibility, clearance of *Candida* from the bloodstream, and source control. Removal or exchange of intravascular catheters is recommended for patients with candidemia in whom the catheter is the suspected source of infection.

Non-*albicans* species of *Candida* often have resistance patterns that are different from *C albicans*. An echinocandin is recommended for treatment of *C glabrata* infection with transition to oral fluconazole or voriconazole for patients with susceptible isolates. For isolates with resistance to azoles and echinocandins, lipid formulation amphotericin B (3–5 mg/kg intravenously daily) may be used. *C krusei* is inherently fluconazole-resistant and should be treated with an alternative agent, such as an echinocandin or voriconazole. Health care–associated infections due to multidrug-resistant *Candida auris* may be treated with echinocandins plus environmental source control.

D. Candidal Endocarditis

Best results are achieved with a combination of medical and surgical therapy (valve replacement). Intravenous lipid-formulation amphotericin B (3–5 mg/kg/day) or an intravenous echinocandin—eg, caspofungin (70 mg once, then 50 mg daily), micafungin (150 mg daily with or without fluconazole 400 to 800 mg daily), or anidulafungin (200 mg once, then 100 mg daily)—is recommended as initial therapy with a minimum duration of 12 weeks. Step-down or long-term suppressive therapy for nonsurgical candidates may be done with fluconazole at 6–12 mg/kg orally daily for susceptible organisms.

E. Prevention of Invasive Candidiasis

In high-risk patients undergoing induction chemotherapy or hematopoietic stem cell, liver, small bowel, and pancreas transplantation, prophylaxis with antifungal agents has been shown to prevent invasive fungal infections, although the effect on mortality and the preferred agent(s) remain debated. Critically ill patients are at higher risk for invasive candidiasis, but antifungal prophylaxis has not shown clear clinical benefit.

Aslam S et al. Candida infections in solid organ transplantation: guidelines from the American Society of Transplantation Infectious Diseases Community of Practice.Clin Transplant. 2019;33:e13623. [PMID: 31155770]

Bays DJ et al. Epidemiology of invasive candidiasis. Clin Epidemiol. 2024;16:549. [PMID: 39219747]

Cornely OA et al. Global guideline for the diagnosis and management of candidiasis: an initiative of the ECMM in cooperation with ISHAM and ASM. Lancet Infect Dis. 2025;25:e280. [PMID: 39956121]

Soriano A et al. Clinical and mycological outcomes of candidaemia and/or invasive candidiasis by *Candida* spp. and antifungal susceptibility: pooled analyses of two randomised trials of rezafungin versus caspofungin. Clin Microbiol Infect. 2025;31:250. [PMID: 39581541]

HISTOPLASMOSIS

ESSENTIALS OF DIAGNOSIS

- Exposure to bird and bat droppings; common along river valleys (especially the Ohio River and the Mississippi River valleys).
- Most patients asymptomatic; respiratory illness most frequent clinical problem.
- Disseminated disease common in AIDS or other immunosuppressed states; poor prognosis.
- Blood and bone marrow cultures and urine polysaccharide antigen are useful in diagnosis of disseminated disease.

General Considerations

Histoplasmosis is caused by *Histoplasma capsulatum* and *Histoplasma duboisii*, fungi that have been isolated from soil contaminated with bird or bat droppings in endemic areas (central and eastern United States, eastern Canada, Mexico, Central America, South America, Africa, and Southeast Asia). Infection presumably takes place by inhalation of conidia. These convert into small budding cells that are engulfed by phagocytes in the lungs. The organism proliferates and undergoes lymphohematogenous spread to other organs.

Clinical Findings

A. Symptoms and Signs

Most cases of histoplasmosis are asymptomatic or mild and thus go unrecognized. Past infection is recognized by pulmonary and splenic calcification noted on incidental radiographs. Symptomatic infection may present with mild influenza-like illness, often lasting 1–4 days. Moderately severe infections are frequently diagnosed as atypical pneumonia. These patients have fever, cough, and mild central chest pain lasting 5–15 days.

Clinically evident infections occur in several forms:

1. **Acute pulmonary histoplasmosis** frequently occurs in epidemics, often when soil containing infected bird or bat droppings is disturbed. Clinical manifestations can vary from a mild influenza-like illness to severe pneumonia. The illness may last from 1 week to 6 months but is almost never fatal.
2. **Progressive disseminated histoplasmosis** most frequently occurs in patients with HIV infection (with CD4 cell counts usually <100 cells/mcL) or other conditions of impaired cellular immunity. Disseminated histoplasmosis has also been reported in patients from endemic areas taking TNF-α inhibitors. It is characterized by fever and multiple organ system involvement. CXRs may show a miliary pattern. Presentation may be fulminant, simulating septic shock, with death ensuing rapidly unless treatment is provided. Symptoms usually consist of fever, dyspnea, cough, loss of weight, and prostration. Ulcers of the mucous membranes of the oropharynx may be present. The liver and spleen are nearly always enlarged, and all the organs of the body can be involved, particularly the adrenal glands; *this results in adrenal insufficiency in about 50% of patients.* GI involvement may mimic IBD. CNS invasion occurs in 5–10% of individuals with disseminated disease.
3. **Chronic pulmonary histoplasmosis** is usually seen in older patients who have underlying chronic lung disease. CXRs show various lesions including complex apical cavities, infiltrates, and nodules.
4. **Complications of pulmonary histoplasmosis** include granulomatous mediastinitis characterized by persistently enlarged mediastinal lymph nodes and fibrosing mediastinitis in which an excessive fibrotic response to *Histoplasma* infection results in compromise of pulmonary vascular structures.

B. Laboratory Findings

Sputum culture is rarely positive in acute pulmonary histoplasmosis but often positive in chronic disease. The combination of urine and serum polysaccharide antigen assays has an 83% sensitivity for the diagnosis of acute pulmonary histoplasmosis. Antigen testing of bronchoalveolar lavage fluid may be helpful in acute disease.

Most patients with chronic pulmonary disease show anemia of chronic disease. Bone marrow involvement with pancytopenia may be prominent in disseminated forms. Marked LD and ferritin elevations are also common, as are mild elevations of serum AST.

Blood cultures using lysis centrifugation methods or bone marrow cultures from immunocompromised patients with progressive disseminated disease are positive > 80% of the time but may take several weeks for growth. The urine antigen assay has a sensitivity of > 90% for disseminated disease in immunocompromised patients and a declining titer can be used to follow response to therapy. Both CSF antigen and antibody testing should be performed in patients suspected of having meningitis.

Treatment

Specific therapy can be withheld in immunocompetent individuals with asymptomatic noncalcified pulmonary nodules and mild acute pulmonary disease. For progressive localized disease and for mild to moderately severe nonmeningeal disseminated disease in immunocompetent or immunocompromised patients, itraconazole, 200–400 mg/day orally divided into two doses, is the treatment of choice with an overall response rate of approximately 80% (Table 40–1). Duration of therapy ranges from weeks to several months depending on the severity of illness. The oral solution is better absorbed than the capsule formulation, which requires gastric acid for absorption. Therapeutic drug monitoring of itraconazole levels should be performed to assess adequacy of drug absorption. Intravenous liposomal amphotericin B, 3 mg/kg/day, is used with more severe disseminated disease and meningitis for 1–2 weeks until patients are clinically stable, followed by oral itraconazole. Patients with AIDS-related histoplasmosis require lifelong suppressive therapy with itraconazole, 200 mg/day orally, although secondary prophylaxis may be discontinued if immune reconstitution occurs in response to antiretroviral therapy. Criteria for discontinuing secondary prophylaxis include 1 year of successful antifungal therapy along with a CD4 cell count > 150 cells/mcL and 6 months or more of antiretroviral treatment (ART). There is no clear evidence that antifungal agents are of benefit for patients with fibrosing mediastinitis, although oral itraconazole is often used. Rituximab, in conjunction with corticosteroids, may slow progression of the fibrosing process and provide some clinical benefit. Reported outcomes in patients with fibrosing mediastinitis treated with either surgical procedures or nonsurgical intravascular interventions appear to be relatively good in the short term.

Eichelberger EM et al. Histoplasmosis. Infect Dis Clin North Am. 2025;39:145. [PMID: 39701897]
Pappas P et al. 2025 clinical practice guideline update by the Infectious Diseases Society of America on histoplasmosis: treatment of mild or moderate acute pulmonary histoplasmosis in adults, children, and pregnant people. Clin Infect Dis. 2026;81:i39. [PMID:40637160]

COCCIDIOIDOMYCOSIS

ESSENTIALS OF DIAGNOSIS

- Acute infection: influenza-like illness, fever, backache, headache, fatigue, and cough; erythema nodosum is common.
- Dissemination may result in meningitis, bony lesions, or skin and soft tissue abscesses; common opportunistic infection in patients with AIDS who reside in endemic regions.
- CXR findings vary from pneumonitis to cavitation.
- Serologic tests useful; large spherules containing endospores demonstrable in sputum or tissues.

General Considerations

Coccidioidomycosis should be considered in the diagnosis of any obscure illness in a patient who has lived in or visited an endemic area. Infection results from the inhalation of arthroconidia of *Coccidioides immitis* or *C posadasii*; both organisms are molds that grow in soil in certain arid regions of the southwestern United States, in Mexico, and in Central and South America. Less than 1% of immunocompetent persons show dissemination, but among these patients, the mortality rate is high.

In patients with AIDS who reside in endemic areas, coccidioidomycosis is a common opportunistic infection. In these patients, disease ranges from focal pulmonary infiltrates to widespread miliary disease with multiple organ involvement and meningitis; severity is inversely related to the extent of control of the HIV infection.

Clinical Findings

A. Symptoms and Signs

1. Primary coccidioidomycosis—Symptoms occur in about 40% of primary infections. Symptom onset (after an incubation period of 10–30 days) is usually that of a respiratory tract illness with fever and occasionally chills. Coccidioidomycosis is a common, frequently unrecognized etiology of community-acquired pneumonia in endemic areas. Erythema nodosum may appear 2–20 days after onset of symptoms. Persistent pulmonary lesions, varying from cavities and abscesses to parenchymal nodular densities or bronchiectasis, occur in about 5% of cases.

2. Disseminated disease—This occurs in about 0.1% of White and 1% of non-White patients. Patients who are Filipino or Black are especially susceptible, as are pregnant women of all races.

Any organ may be involved. Pulmonary findings usually become more pronounced, with mediastinal lymph node enlargement, cough, and increased sputum production. Lung abscesses may rupture into the pleural space, producing an empyema. Complicated skin, bone and joint infections may develop. Fungemia is characterized clinically by a diffuse miliary pattern on CXR and by early death. The course may be particularly rapid in immunosuppressed patients. Clinicians caring for immunosuppressed patients in endemic areas need to consider that patients may have latent infection.

Meningitis occurs in 30–50% of cases of dissemination and may result in chronic basilar meningitis. Subcutaneous abscesses and verrucous skin lesions are especially common in fulminating cases. Patients with AIDS and disseminated disease have a higher incidence of miliary infiltrates, lymphadenopathy, and meningitis, but skin lesions are uncommon.

B. Laboratory Findings

In primary coccidioidomycosis, there may be moderate leukocytosis and eosinophilia. Serologic testing is useful for both diagnosis and prognosis. Both the immunodiffusion test (which is highly sensitive and specific) and ELISA detect IgM antibodies within 1–3 weeks of disease onset, are useful for diagnosis early in the disease process, and should be followed by IgG complement fixation testing.

A persistently rising IgG complement fixation titer (1:16 or more) is suggestive of disseminated disease. Complement fixation titers can be used to assess the adequacy of therapy. Serum complement fixation titers may be low when there is meningitis but no other disseminated disease. In patients with HIV-related coccidioidomycosis, the false-negative rate may reach 30%. Blood cultures are rarely positive.

Patients in whom coccidioidomycosis is diagnosed should undergo evaluation for meningeal involvement when CNS symptoms or neurologic signs are present. Spinal fluid findings include increased cell count with lymphocytosis and reduced glucose. Spinal fluid culture is positive in approximately 30% of meningitis cases. Demonstrable complement-fixing antibodies in spinal fluid are diagnostic of coccidioidal meningitis (found in > 90% of cases). CSF *Coccidioides* antigen or (1,3)-β-D-glucan testing may augment (not replace) CSF antibody testing.

C. Imaging

Radiographic findings vary, but patchy, nodular, and lobar upper lobe pulmonary infiltrates are most common. Hilar lymphadenopathy may be seen in localized disease; mediastinal lymphadenopathy suggests dissemination. There may be pleural effusions and lytic lesions in bone with accompanying complicated soft tissue collections.

Treatment

General symptomatic therapy should be provided as needed for disease limited to the chest with no evidence of progression. Itraconazole (400 mg orally daily divided into two doses) or fluconazole (200–400 mg or higher orally once or twice daily) should be given for disease in the chest, bones, and soft tissues; therapy must be continued for 6 months or longer after the disease is inactive to prevent relapse (Table 40–1). Response to therapy should be monitored by following the clinical response and progressive decrease in serum complement fixation titers.

For progressive pulmonary or extrapulmonary disease, liposomal amphotericin B intravenously should be given, although oral azoles may be used for mild cases. Duration of therapy is determined by a declining complement fixation titer and a favorable clinical response. For meningitis, treatment usually is high-dose oral fluconazole (400–1200 mg/day), although lumbar or cisternal intrathecal administration of amphotericin B in increasing doses up to 1–1.5 mg/day is used initially by some experts or in cases refractory to fluconazole. Systemic therapy with liposomal amphotericin B, 3–5 mg/kg/day intravenously, is usually given concurrently with intrathecal therapy, but is not sufficient alone for the treatment of meningeal disease. Once the patient is clinically stable, lifelong oral therapy with an azole, usually fluconazole (400–800 mg orally daily), is the recommended alternative to intrathecal amphotericin B therapy.

Surgical drainage is necessary for management of soft tissue abscesses, necrotic bone, and complicated pulmonary disease (eg, rupture of coccidioidal cavity).

Prognosis

The prognosis for patients with limited disease is good. Serial complement fixation titers should be performed after therapy for coccidioidomycosis; rising titers warrant reinstitution of therapy because relapse is likely. Late CNS complications of adequately treated meningitis include cerebral vasculitis with stroke and communicating hydrocephalus that may require shunting. There may be a benefit from short-term systemic corticosteroids following cerebrovascular events associated with coccidioidal meningitis. Disseminated and meningeal forms have mortality rates exceeding 50% in the absence of therapy.

Donovan FM et al. Coccidioidomycosis. Infect Dis Clin N Am. 2025;39:183. [PMID:39710556]

PNEUMOCYSTOSIS (*Pneumocystis Jirovecii* Pneumonia)

ESSENTIALS OF DIAGNOSIS

- Fever, dyspnea, dry cough, hypoxia with exertion.
- Often only slight lung physical findings.
- CXR: diffuse interstitial disease or normal.
- Detection of *P jirovecii* in sputum, bronchoalveolar lavage fluid, or lung tissue; PCR of bronchoalveolar lavage; (1,3)-β-D-glucan in blood.

General Considerations

Pneumocystis jirovecii, the *Pneumocystis* species that affects humans, is found worldwide.

Overt infection is characterized by a subacute interstitial pneumonia that occurs among older children and adults with abnormal or altered cellular immunity, either due to an underlying condition (eg, AIDS, cancer, malnutrition, hematopoietic stem cell or solid organ transplantation, autoimmune disease) or treatment with immunosuppressive medications (eg, corticosteroids or cytotoxic agents).

Pneumocystis pneumonia occurs in up to 80% of patients with AIDS not receiving prophylaxis and is a major cause of morbidity and mortality. Its incidence increases in direct proportion to the fall in CD4 cells, with most cases occurring at CD4 cell counts <200/mcL. In patients without AIDS receiving immunosuppressive therapy, symptoms frequently begin after corticosteroids have been tapered or discontinued.

Clinical Findings

A. Symptoms and Signs

Findings are usually limited to the pulmonary parenchyma. In patients with AIDS, onset may be subacute, characterized by dyspnea on exertion and nonproductive cough. Physical findings may be slight and disproportionate to the degree of illness and radiologic findings. Evidence of HIV-associated disease, including fever and weight loss, may precede the respiratory illness by several months. In patients without HIV, the disease presentation may be more acute. Without treatment, *Pneumocystis infection* carries a high mortality in patients with and without AIDS.

B. Laboratory Findings

Arterial blood gas determinations usually show hypoxemia with hypocapnia but may be normal; however, rapid desaturation occurs if patients exercise before samples are drawn. Serum (1,3)-β-D-glucan levels have reasonable sensitivity but lack specificity as elevated levels occur in other fungal infections. The organism cannot be cultured, and definitive diagnosis depends on demonstration of the organisms in respiratory specimens using specific stains, such as immunofluorescence. PCR of bronchoalveolar lavage is overly sensitive since the test can be positive in colonized, uninfected persons. A negative PCR from bronchoalveolar lavage rules out disease. Lung biopsy is infrequently required but may aid in diagnosing a granulomatous form of *Pneumocystis*.

C. Imaging

CXRs most often show diffuse "interstitial" infiltration, which may be heterogeneous, miliary, or patchy early in infection. There may also be diffuse or focal consolidation, cystic changes, nodules, or cavitation within nodules. About 5–10% of patients with *Pneumocystis* pneumonia have normal chest films. High-resolution chest CT scans may be quite suggestive of *P jirovecii* pneumonia, helping distinguish it from other causes of pneumonia.

Treatment

It is appropriate to start empiric therapy for *P jirovecii* pneumonia if the disease is suspected clinically; however, in both patients with or without AIDS with mild to moderately severe disease, continued treatment should be based on a proven diagnosis because of the toxicity of therapy and potential for coinfections. Initial antimicrobial therapy (typically with TMP SMZ) should be continued for at least 5–10 days before considering changing agents, as fever, tachypnea, and pulmonary infiltrates persist for 4–6 days after starting treatment. Some patients have a transient worsening of their disease during the first 3–5 days, which may be related to an inflammatory response. Early addition of corticosteroids may attenuate this response and improve clinical outcomes (see below). A longer duration of treatment (21 days) is recommended for AIDS-associated *Pneumocystis* pneumonia; 14 days of treatment is generally appropriate for non-AIDS cases. For patients with AIDS, a diagnosis of *Pneumocystis* should also prompt initiation of antiretroviral therapy.

A. Trimethoprim-Sulfamethoxazole

There are strong data indicating that TMP-SMZ is the optimal first-line therapy for *Pneumocystis* pneumonia. The dosage of TMP-SMZ is 15–20 mg/kg/day (based on trimethoprim component) given orally or intravenously daily in three or four divided doses for 14–21 days. Patients with AIDS have a high frequency of hypersensitivity reactions (approaching 50%).

B. Primaquine/Clindamycin

Primaquine 30 mg orally daily, plus clindamycin 600 mg orally four times daily or 900 mg orally three times daily, is the best second-line therapy with superior results compared with pentamidine. Primaquine may cause hemolytic anemia in patients with glucose-6-phosphate dehydrogenase (G6PD) deficiency.

C. Other Medications

Atovaquone may be used for patients with mild to moderate disease who cannot tolerate TMP-SMZ or other alternative agents, but failure is reported in 15–30% of cases. The dosage is 750 mg orally (taken with a fatty meal) two times daily for 14–21 days. Trimethoprim, 15 mg/kg/day in three divided doses daily, plus dapsone, 100 mg/day, is an another alternative for mild to moderate disease or for continuation of therapy after intravenous therapy is no longer needed.

D. Prednisone

Based on studies done in patients with AIDS, prednisone is given for moderate to severe pneumonia (when PaO_2 on admission is <70 mm Hg or oxygen saturation is <90%) in conjunction with antimicrobials. The addition of corticosteroids in such patients is associated with significant reduction in morbidity and mortality; administration of adjunctive corticosteroids within 72 hours is preferred. The dosage of prednisone is 40 mg twice daily orally for 5 days, then 40 mg daily for 5 days, and then 20 mg daily until therapy is completed (total course, 21 days). Observational studies suggest that adjunctive corticosteroids are associated with reduced mortality in patients without AIDS with *Pneumocystis* pneumonia and severe hypoxia ($PaO_2 \leq 60$ mm Hg).

Prevention

Primary prophylaxis for *Pneumocystis* pneumonia in patients with HIV should be given for CD4 counts < 200 cells/mcL, a CD4 percentage below 14%, or weight loss or oral candidiasis. Persons with HIV who have a history of *Pneumocystis* pneumonia should receive secondary prophylaxis until they have had a durable virologic response to antiretroviral therapy or maintained a CD4 count of > 200 cells/mcL for at least 3–6 months, or both.

Primary prophylaxis is also beneficial for hematologic malignancy, in transplant recipients, and in patients receiving high-dose corticosteroid therapy, although precise recommendations have not been established. Oral TMP-SMZ is the preferred prophylactic agent (dose for at-risk patients with HIV: TMP-SMZ 1 DS or SS tablet orally daily, or alternatively 1 DS tablet orally three times weekly; dose for patients without HIV: TMP-SMZ 1 SS tablet orally daily or 1 DS tablet orally three times weekly).

Prognosis

In the absence of adequate treatment, the fatality rate for *Pneumocystis* pneumonia in patients with AIDS is nearly 100%. Early treatment reduces the mortality to ~ 10–20%, but recurrence is common without prophylaxis. The mortality rate in other immunodeficient disorders is still > 50%, in part due to delays in diagnosis.

Fragoulis GE et al. 2022 EULAR recommendations for screening and prophylaxis of chronic and opportunistic infections in adults with autoimmune inflammatory rheumatic diseases. Ann Rheum Dis. 2023;82:742. [PMID: 36328476]

Hänsel L et al. How to diagnose and treat a patient without human immunodeficiency virus infection having *Pneumocystis jirovecii* pneumonia? Clin Microbiol Infect. 2023;29:1015. [PMID: 37086781]

Lagrou K et al. *Pneumocystis jirovecii* disease: basis for the revised EORTC/MSGERC invasive fungal disease definitions in individuals without human immunodeficiency virus. Clin Infect Dis. 2021;72(Suppl 2):S114. [PMID: 33709126]

Panel on Guidelines for the Prevention and Treatment of Opportunistic Infections in Adults and Adolescents with HIV. Guidelines for the Prevention and Treatment of Opportunistic Infections in HIV-infected Adults and Adolescents: Recommendations from the Centers for Disease Control and Prevention, the National Institutes of Health, and the HIV Medicine Association of the Infectious Diseases Society of America. Accessed Dec 10,2025. https://clinicalinfo.hiv.gov/en/guidelines/hiv-clinical-guidelines-adult-and-adolescent-opportunistic-infections/pneumocystis-0

CRYPTOCOCCOSIS

ESSENTIALS OF DIAGNOSIS

- Most common cause of fungal meningitis.
- Predisposing factors: chemotherapy for hematologic malignancies, Hodgkin lymphoma, corticosteroids, structural lung diseases, transplant recipients, TNF-α inhibitors, and AIDS.
- Headache, abnormal mental status; meningismus occasionally, although rarely in patients with AIDS.
- Demonstration of capsular polysaccharide antigen or positive culture in CSF is diagnostic.

General Considerations

Cryptococcosis is mainly caused by *Cryptococcus neoformans*, an encapsulated budding yeast that is found worldwide in soil and on dried pigeon dung. *Cryptococcus gattii* is a closely related species that also causes disease in humans, although *C gattii* may affect more ostensibly immunocompetent persons. It is a major cause of cryptococcosis in the Pacific northwestern region of the United States and may result in more severe disease than *C neoformans*.

Infections are acquired by inhalation. In the lung, the infection may remain localized, heal, or disseminate. Clinically apparent cryptococcal pneumonia rarely develops in immunocompetent persons. Progressive lung disease and dissemination most often occur in the setting of cellular immunodeficiency, including hematologic malignancies under treatment, Hodgkin lymphoma, long-term corticosteroid therapy, solid organ transplant, TNF-α inhibitor therapy, or uncontrolled HIV infection.

Clinical Findings

A. Symptoms and Signs

Pulmonary disease from either *C neoformans* or *C gattii* ranges from simple nodules to widespread infiltrates leading to respiratory failure. Disseminated disease may involve any organ, but CNS disease predominates. Headache is usually the first symptom of meningitis. Confusion and other mental status changes as well as cranial nerve abnormalities, nausea, and vomiting may be seen as the disease progresses. Nuchal rigidity and meningeal signs occur about 50% of the time but are uncommon in patients with AIDS. Communicating hydrocephalus may complicate the course. *C gattii* infection frequently presents with respiratory symptoms along with neurologic signs caused by space-occupying lesions in the CNS. Primary *C neoformans* infection of the skin may mimic bacterial cellulitis, especially in persons receiving immunosuppressive therapy such as corticosteroids. The immune reconstitution inflammatory syndrome (IRIS), which is paradoxical clinical worsening associated with improved immunologic status and treatment, can occur in patients with HIV and transplant recipients with cryptococcosis, as well as patients without AIDS being treated for *C gattii* infection.

B. Laboratory Findings

Respiratory tract disease is diagnosed by culture of respiratory secretions or pleural fluid. For suspected meningeal disease, lumbar puncture is the preferred diagnostic procedure. Spinal fluid findings include increased opening pressure, variable pleocytosis, increased protein, and decreased glucose, although as many as 50% of patients with AIDS have no pleocytosis. Gram stain of the CSF usually reveals budding, encapsulated fungi. In patients with AIDS, the serum cryptococcal antigen is a sensitive screening test for meningitis, being positive in > 95% of cases. Cryptococcal capsular antigen in CSF and culture together establish the diagnosis > 90% of the time. Antigen testing by lateral flow assay has improved sensitivity and specificity over the conventional latex agglutination test and can provide more rapid diagnostic results. MRI is more sensitive than CT in finding CNS abnormalities, such as cryptococcomas.

Treatment

A. For Patients with AIDS

1. Induction therapy—Because of decreased efficacy, initial therapy with an azole alone is not recommended for treatment of acute cryptococcal meningitis. Initial combination induction therapy is with liposomal amphotericin B, 3–4 mg/kg/day intravenously along with flucytosine 100 mg/kg/day orally (divided into four equal doses and given every 6 hours) for 2 weeks, followed by 8 weeks of fluconazole, 800 mg/day orally for consolidation (Table 40–1). This regimen achieves clinical responses and CSF sterilization in > 70% of patients. The addition of flucytosine has been associated with improved survival, but toxicity is common. Hematologic parameters should be closely monitored during flucytosine therapy, and it is important to adjust the dose for any decreases in kidney function. Fluconazole (800–1200 mg orally daily) may be given with amphotericin B when flucytosine is not available or patients cannot tolerate it. Comparative studies performed in countries with limited resources have demonstrated equivalent efficacy of induction regimens that include a single high dose of intravenous liposomal amphotericin B, 10 mg/kg, along with 14 days of oral flucytosine 100 mg/kg/day (divided into 4 doses) and oral fluconazole 1200 mg daily. Some clinicians in the United States have started using this regimen, although it has not yet been included in US treatment guidelines but is recommended by WHO guidelines. Frequent, repeated lumbar punctures or ventricular shunting should be performed to relieve high CSF pressures or if hydrocephalus is a complication. *Failure to adequately relieve raised intracranial pressure is a major cause of morbidity and mortality.* Corticosteroids should not be used in acute disease.

2. Maintenance therapy—The end points for amphotericin B therapy and for switching to maintenance with oral fluconazole are a favorable clinical response (decrease in temperature; improvement in headache, nausea, vomiting, and Mini-Mental State Examination scores), improvement in CSF biochemical parameters and, most importantly, conversion of CSF culture to negative. Maintenance antifungal therapy is important after treatment of an acute episode in AIDS-related cases, since otherwise the rate of relapse is > 50%. Fluconazole, 200 mg/day orally, is the maintenance therapy of choice, decreasing the relapse rate approximately tenfold compared with placebo and threefold compared with weekly amphotericin B in patients whose CSF has been sterilized by the induction therapy. After successful therapy of cryptococcal meningitis, it is possible to discontinue maintenance therapy with fluconazole in individuals with AIDS who have had a satisfactory response to antiretroviral therapy (eg, CD4 cell count > 100–200 cells/mcL for at least 6 months).

B. For Patients without AIDS

Guidelines recommend similar drug therapy for patients without AIDS, although the mortality rate is somewhat higher.

1. Induction therapy—In patients without AIDS, induction therapy should be extended to 4–6 weeks, followed by consolidation therapy with fluconazole, 400–800 mg/day for an additional 8 weeks.

2. Maintenance therapy—Fluconazole can be used for 6–12 months in patients without AIDS following successful treatment of the acute illness.

Prognosis

Factors that indicate a poor prognosis include the activity of the predisposing disease, older age, organ failure, lack of spinal fluid pleocytosis, high initial antigen titer in either serum or CSF, decreased mental status, increased intracranial pressure, and the presence of disease outside the nervous system.

ASPERGILLOSIS

ESSENTIALS OF DIAGNOSIS

- Most common cause of non-candidal invasive fungal infection in transplant recipients and in patients with hematologic malignancies.
- Risk factors for invasive disease: leukemia, hematopoietic stem cell or solid organ transplantation, corticosteroid use, AIDS, and COVID-19 coinfection.
- Pulmonary, sinus, and CNS are most common disease sites.
- Detection of galactomannan in serum or other body fluids is useful for early diagnosis in at-risk patients.

General Considerations

Aspergillus fumigatus is the usual cause of aspergillosis, though several species of *Aspergillus* cause a wide spectrum of disease. The lungs, sinuses, and brain are the organs most often involved. Clinical illness results either from an aberrant immunologic response or tissue invasion.

Clinical Findings

A. Symptoms and Signs

1. Allergic forms of aspergillosis—Allergic bronchopulmonary aspergillosis (ABPA) occurs in patients with preexisting asthma or cystic fibrosis. Patients develop worsening bronchospasm and fleeting pulmonary infiltrates. Allergic *Aspergillus* sinusitis produces chronic sinus inflammation characterized by eosinophilic mucus and noninvasive hyphal elements.

2. Chronic aspergillosis—Chronic pulmonary aspergillosis usually occurs when there is preexisting lung damage without significant immunocompromise. Disease manifestations range from aspergillomas that develop in a lung cavity to chronic fibrosing pulmonary aspergillosis in which most of the lung tissue is replaced with fibrosis. Long-standing (> 3 months) pulmonary and systemic symptoms such as cough, shortness of breath, weight loss, and malaise are common. Chronic pulmonary aspergillosis is associated with significant morbidity; one systematic review noted a mortality rate of 32% at 5 years.

3. Invasive aspergillosis—Invasive aspergillosis most commonly occurs in patients who are profoundly immunodeficient, such as those with prolonged, severe neutropenia due to acute leukemia or following hematopoietic stem cell transplantation, but it can occur among critically ill immunocompetent patients as well, or in association with COVID-19 infection (termed *COVID-19–associated pulmonary aspergillosis*, or *CAPA*). Pulmonary disease is most common, with patchy infiltration leading to a severe necrotizing pneumonia. Invasive sinus disease also occurs. At any time, there may be hematogenous dissemination to the CNS, skin, and other organs. Early diagnosis and reversal of any correctable immunosuppression are essential.

B. Laboratory Findings

In ABPA, there is eosinophilia with high levels of IgE and IgG *Aspergillus* precipitins in the blood. Diagnosis of chronic pulmonary aspergillosis requires symptoms or signs for at least 3 months with identification of lung cavitation or nodules, plus microbiologic evidence of *Aspergillus* (such as culture or tissue identification from biopsy or serology) and exclusion of alternative diagnoses (eg, mycobacterial infection).

For invasive aspergillosis, definitive diagnosis requires demonstration of *Aspergillus* in tissue or culture from a sterile site; however, given the morbidity of the disease and the low yield of culture, clinicians must maintain a high index of suspicion and use a combination of host, radiologic, and mycologic criteria to yield a probable diagnosis of invasive aspergillosis in at-risk patients. Indirect diagnostic assays include detection of galactomannan (a component of the *Aspergillus* cell wall) in serum or bronchoalveolar lavage, and serum assays for (1,3)-β-D-glucan (a fungal cell wall component that is not specific for *Aspergillus*). To improve the reliability of serum galactomannan testing, serial determinations should be done, though sensitivity is decreased in patients receiving anti-mold prophylaxis. Higher galactomannan levels are correlated with increased mortality, and failure of galactomannan levels to fall in response to therapy portends a worse outcome. *Aspergillus* DNA in serum or bronchoalveolar lavage may aid in diagnosis, particularly when used in combination with other biomarkers. Isolation of *Aspergillus* from pulmonary secretions does not necessarily imply invasive disease, although its positive predictive value increases with more advanced immunosuppression. Clinical suspicion for invasive aspergillosis should prompt CT scanning of the chest, which may aid in early detection and help direct additional diagnostic procedures. Common radiologic findings include nodules, wedge-shaped infarcts, or a characteristic "halo sign".

Prevention

The high mortality rate and difficulty in diagnosis of invasive aspergillosis warrants the use of prophylactic therapy for patients with profound immunosuppression. The best-studied prophylaxis includes mold-active triazole therapy with posaconazole (300 mg orally daily) and voriconazole (200 mg orally twice daily). The National Comprehensive Cancer Network (NCCN) 2024 guidelines recommend posaconazole for patients with myelodysplastic syndrome or acute myeloid leukemia who are neutropenic, and for hematopoietic stem cell transplant recipients on immune suppressive therapy for acute graft-versus-host disease (GVHD). Mold-active triazole therapy is less strongly advised for patients with allogeneic hematopoietic stem cell transplants who are neutropenic. Prophylaxis is recommended until the underlying risk factor has been resolved (ie, neutropenia or GHVD). Anti-mold prophylaxis is not universally recommended for patients with solid organ transplantation; rather, recommendations vary based on the type of transplantation (with lung being highest risk for invasive aspergillosis) and other clinical factors (such as the need for reoperation or renal replacement therapy in liver transplant recipients). Widespread use of broad-spectrum azoles raises concern for development of breakthrough invasive disease by highly resistant fungi.

Treatment

1. Allergic forms of aspergillosis—For allergic *Aspergillus* sinusitis, surgical treatment with polypectomy and sinus washout with intranasal corticosteroids is advised, with antifungal therapy (such as itraconazole 100 to 200 mg twice daily) reserved for refractory cases. For acute exacerbations of ABPA, oral prednisone is begun at a dose of 0.5 mg/kg/day and then tapered slowly over several months. Itraconazole, 200 mg orally twice daily for 16 weeks, appears to improve pulmonary function and decrease corticosteroid requirements in these patients.

2. Chronic aspergillosis—The most effective therapy for symptomatic aspergilloma is surgical resection. Other forms of chronic aspergillosis may be treated with at least 4–6 months of oral azole therapy (itraconazole 200 mg twice daily, voriconazole 200 mg twice daily, posaconazole 300 mg daily, or isavuconazole 200 mg daily) (Table 40–1).

3. Invasive aspergillosis—The 2016 Infectious Diseases Society of America guidelines consider voriconazole (6 mg/kg intravenously twice on day 1 and then 4 mg/kg every 12 hours thereafter) as optimal therapy for invasive aspergillosis. However, the 2017 European Society for Clinical Microbiology and Infectious Diseases, the European Confederation of Medical Mycology, and the European Respiratory Society (ESCMID-ECMM-ERS) joint clinical guidelines indicate either isavuconazole (200 mg intravenously every 8 hours for six doses, then 200 mg daily) or voriconazole as first-line therapy. Other alternatives include a lipid formulation of amphotericin B (3–5 mg/kg/day), caspofungin (70 mg intravenously on day 1, then 50 mg/day thereafter), micafungin (100–150 mg intravenously daily), and posaconazole oral tablets (300 mg twice daily on day 1, then 300 mg daily thereafter).

Treatment duration may vary depending on the clinical response, but 6–12 weeks is generally recommended. Antifungal susceptibility testing of *Aspergillus* isolates is recommended in patients who are unresponsive to therapy or with clinical suspicion for azole resistance. Therapeutic drug monitoring should be considered for both voriconazole and posaconazole given variations in metabolism and absorption.

Surgical debridement is generally done for sinusitis, and can be useful for focal pulmonary lesions. The mortality rate of pulmonary or disseminated disease in the immunocompromised patient remains high, particularly in patients with refractory neutropenia.

Epelbaum O et al. Treatment of invasive pulmonary aspergillosis and preventive and empirical therapy for invasive candidiasis in adult pulmonary and critical care patients. An official American Thoracic Society clinical practice guideline. Am J Respir Crit Care Med. 2024;211:34. [PMID: 39556361]

Kanaujia R et al. Aspergillosis: an update on clinical spectrum, diagnostic schemes, and management. Curr Fungal Infect Rep. 2023:1. [Epub ahead of print] [PMID: 37360858]

Patterson TF et al. Practice guidelines for the diagnosis and management of aspergillosis: 2016 update by the Infectious Diseases Society of America. Clin Infect Dis. 2016;63:e1. [PMID: 27365388]

MUCORMYCOSIS

ESSENTIALS OF DIAGNOSIS

- Most common cause of non-*Aspergillus* invasive mold infection.
- Risk factors: uncontrolled diabetes, hematologic malignancy, hematopoietic stem cell or solid organ transplantation, direct inoculation of wounds (trauma, burns), and COVID-19.
- Pulmonary, rhino-orbital-cerebral, and skin are most common disease sites.
- Rapidly fatal without multidisciplinary interventions.

General Considerations

The term *mucormycosis* describes an opportunistic infection caused by a member of the genera *Rhizopus*, *Mucor*, *Lichtheimia* (formerly *Absidia*), *Saksenaea*, *Apophysomyces*, or *Cunninghamella*. Predisposing conditions include hematologic malignancy; hematopoietic or solid organ transplantation; diabetes; iron overload; or treatment with deferoxamine, corticosteroids, or cytotoxic drugs. COVID-19 is associated with mucormycosis, particularly rhino-orbital-cerebral disease. Immunocompetent patients may develop infection due to direct inoculation of wounds (eg, due to trauma or burns).

Clinical Findings

Invasive disease of the sinuses, orbits, and the lungs may occur. Diabetes is associated with rhino-orbital-cerebral disease, while hematologic malignancy predisposes to pulmonary infection. Necrosis is common due to hyphal tissue invasion that may manifest as ulceration of the palate or hemoptysis. Widely disseminated disease can occur. Biopsy of involved tissue remains the cornerstone of diagnosis; the organisms appear in tissue as broad, branching non-septate hyphae. Molecular identification (eg, PCR) from tissue or blood may aid in the diagnosis; cultures are frequently negative. For pulmonary disease, a reverse "halo sign" (focal area of ground-glass diminution surrounded by a ring of consolidation) may be seen on chest CT.

Treatment

Optimal therapy of mucormycosis involves reversal of predisposing conditions (if possible), surgical debridement, and prompt antifungal therapy. A prolonged course of intravenous liposomal amphotericin B (5–10 mg/kg with higher doses given for CNS disease) should be started early. Oral posaconazole (300 mg/day) or isavuconazole (200 mg every 8 hours for 1–2 days, then 200 mg daily thereafter) can be used for less severe disease, as step-down therapy after disease stabilization, or as salvage therapy due to poor response to or tolerance of amphotericin (Table 40–1). In patients with breakthrough invasive mold infections despite mold-active antifungal prophylaxis, clinicians should initiate treatment with a different class of antifungal agents than was used for prophylaxis. Combination therapy with amphotericin and posaconazole or isavuconazole is not proven but is commonly used because of the poor response to monotherapy. Control of diabetes and other underlying conditions, along with extensive surgical removal of necrotic, nonperfused tissue, is essential. Even with these measures, the prognosis remains guarded.

Cornely OA et al. Global guideline for the diagnosis and management of mucormycosis: an initiative of the European Confederation of Medical Mycology in cooperation with the Mycoses Study Group Education and Research Consortium. Lancet Infect Dis. 2019;19:e405. [PMID: 31699664]

Czech MM. Updates in mucormycosis. Infect Dis Clin N Am. 2025;39:121. [PMID: 39638718]

BLASTOMYCOSIS

Blastomycosis occurs most often in men infected during occupational or recreational activities outdoors and in a geographically limited area of the south, central, and midwestern United States and Canada. Disease usually occurs in immunocompetent individuals.

Pulmonary infection is most common and may be asymptomatic. With dissemination, lesions most frequently occur in the skin, bones, and urogenital system.

Cough, moderate fever, dyspnea, and chest pain are common. These may resolve or progress, with purulent sputum production, pleurisy, fever, chills, loss of weight, and prostration. Radiologic studies, either CXRs or CT scans, usually reveal lobar consolidation or masses.

Raised, verrucous cutaneous lesions are commonly present in disseminated blastomycosis. Bones—often the ribs and vertebrae—are frequently involved. Epididymitis, prostatitis, and other involvement of the male urogenital system may occur. Although they do not appear to be at greater risk for acquisition of disease, infection in persons with HIV may progress rapidly, with dissemination common.

Laboratory findings usually include leukocytosis and anemia. The organism is found in clinical specimens, such as expectorated sputum or tissue biopsies, as a 5- to 20-mcm thick-walled cell with a single broad-based bud. It grows readily on culture. Urine, serum, and CSF antigen assays are available with the urinary antigen being most sensitive; it has considerable cross-reactivity with other dimorphic fungi but may be useful in monitoring disease resolution or progression. A serum enzyme immunoassay based on the surface protein BAD-1 has much better sensitivity and specificity than the urinary antigen test but is not yet commercially available.

Itraconazole, 200–400 mg/day orally for at least 6–12 months, is the therapy of choice for nonmeningeal disease, with a response rate of > 80% (Table 40–1). Liposomal amphotericin B, 3–5 mg/kg/day intravenously, should be given initially for severe disease, treatment failures, or CNS involvement.

Clinical follow-up for relapse should be made regularly for several years so that therapy may be resumed or another drug instituted.

Saravanababu T et al. Diagnosing blastomycosis: a review of laboratory methods and clinical utility. J Fungi. 2025;11:589. [PMID: 40863541]

Zhou S et al. Blastomycosis. Infect Dis Clin N Am. 2025;39:163. [PMID: 39701898]

SPOROTRICHOSIS

Sporotrichosis is a chronic fungal infection caused by organisms of the *Sporothrix schenckii* complex. It is worldwide in distribution; most patients have had contact with soil, sphagnum moss, or decaying wood. Infection takes place when the organism is inoculated into the skin—usually on the hand, arm, or foot, especially during gardening, or puncture from a rose thorn.

The most common form of sporotrichosis begins with a hard, nontender subcutaneous nodule. This later becomes adherent to the overlying skin and ulcerates. Within a few days to weeks, lymphocutaneous spread along the lymphatics draining this area occurs, which may result in ulceration. Cavitary pulmonary disease occurs in individuals with underlying chronic lung disease.

Disseminated sporotrichosis is rare in immunocompetent persons but may present with widespread cutaneous, lung, bone, joint, and CNS involvement in immunocompromised patients, especially those with cellular immunodeficiencies, including AIDS and alcohol use disorder.

Cultures are needed to establish diagnosis. The usefulness of serologic tests is limited, but they may be helpful in diagnosing disseminated disease, especially meningitis.

Itraconazole, 200–400 mg orally daily for 3–6 months, is the treatment of choice for localized disease and some milder cases of disseminated disease (Table 40–1). Terbinafine, 500 mg orally twice daily, also has good efficacy in lymphocutaneous disease. Intravenous amphotericin B, 0.7–1.0 mg/kg/day, or a lipid amphotericin B preparation, 3–5 mg/kg/day, for 6–12 months are used for severe systemic infection. Surgery may be indicated for complicated pulmonary cavitary disease, and joint involvement may require arthrodesis.

The prognosis is good for lymphocutaneous sporotrichosis; pulmonary, joint, and disseminated disease respond less favorably.

Rodrigues AM et al. Current progress on epidemiology, diagnosis, and treatment of sporotrichosis and their future trends. J Fungi (Basel). 2022;8:776. [PMID: 35893145]

OTHER OPPORTUNISTIC MOLD INFECTIONS

Fungi previously considered to be harmless colonizers, including *Pseudallescheria boydii (Scedosporium apiospermum), Lomentospora prolificans, Fusarium, Paecilomyces, Trichoderma longibrachiatum*, and *Trichosporon*, are now significant pathogens in immunocompromised patients. Opportunistic infections with these agents are seen in patients being treated for hematologic malignancies, in hematopoietic stem cell or organ transplant recipients, and in those receiving broad-spectrum antifungal prophylaxis. Infection may be localized in the skin, lungs, or sinuses, or widespread disease may appear with lesions in multiple organs. Fusariosis should be suspected in severely immunosuppressed persons who develop multiple, painful skin lesions; blood cultures are often positive.

Less commonly, opportunistic molds may cause infection in immunocompetent hosts from direct inoculation. In 2023, an outbreak of fungal meningitis due to *Fusarium solani* occurred in patients receiving epidural anesthesia. Fungal keratitis due to *Paecilomyces lilacinus* has been described in association with ocular surgery, environmental trauma, and contact lens usage.

Nonpigmented septate hyphae are seen in tissue and are indistinguishable from those of *Aspergillus* when infections are due to *S apiospermum* or species of *Fusarium, Paecilomyces, Penicillium*, or other hyaline molds. The differentiation of *S apiospermum* and *Aspergillus* is particularly important since the former is uniformly resistant to amphotericin B but may be sensitive to azole antifungals. Fusariosis may be treated with amphotericin, voriconazole, or combination therapy; there are limited data on the use of isavuconazole or posaconazole for this disease. Novel antifungal agents such as fosmanogepix may be of benefit. In addition to antifungal therapy for patients who are immunocompromised, reversal of underlying immunosuppression is essential for treatment of invasive molds.

Infection by melanin-pigmented dematiaceous or "black" molds is designated as phaeohyphomycosis. These black molds (eg, *Exophiala, Bipolaris, Cladophialophora, Curvularia, Alternaria*) are common in the environment, especially on decaying vegetation. In tissues of patients with phaeohyphomycosis, the mold is seen as black or faintly brown hyphae, yeast cells, or both. Culture on appropriate medium is needed to identify the agent. Histologic demonstration of these organisms provides definitive evidence of invasive infection; positive cultures must be interpreted cautiously and not assumed to be contaminants in immunocompromised persons.

Arcobello JT et al. Phaeohyphomycosis. Semin Respir Crit Care Med. 2020;41:131. [PMID: 32000289]

Jacobs SE et al. Non-*Aspergillus* hyaline molds: emerging causes of sino-pulmonary fungal infections and other invasive mycoses. Semin Respir Crit Care Med. 2020;41;115. [PMID: 32000288]

HOUSEHOLD MOLDS

ESSENTIALS OF DIAGNOSIS

- Molds are very common indoors where moisture exists in enclosed spaces.
- Most common indoor molds are *Cladosporium, Penicillium, Aspergillus*, and *Alternaria*.
- People most at risk for health problems include those with allergies, asthma, and underlying immunocompromising conditions.

Molds are commonly present in homes, particularly in the presence of moisture, and patients will commonly seek assessment for whether their illness is due to molds. Well-established health problems due to molds can be considered in three categories: (1) There is the potential for allergy to environmental mold species, which can manifest in the typical manner with allergic symptoms such as rhinitis and eye irritation. Furthermore, in predisposed individuals, exposure to certain molds can trigger asthma or asthmatic attacks. These types of manifestations are reversible with appropriate therapies. More chronic allergic effects can be seen with disorders such as ABPA (see Allergic Forms of Aspergillosis); (2) Susceptible individuals can develop hypersensitivity reactions upon exposure to mold antigens; these include occupational disorders (eg, farmer's lung and pigeon breeder's disease) as well as hypersensitivity pneumonitis in response to a large antigenic exposure. Affected patients have fever, lymph node swelling, and pulmonary infiltrates. These disease manifestations are transient and improve with removal of the offending antigen; (3) Invasive mold disease (see Invasive Aspergillosis).

At the present time, there are no data to support that mold exposure can induce immune dysfunction. Similarly, the concept of toxic-mold syndrome or cognitive impairment due to inhalation of mycotoxins has not been validated despite scrutiny by expert panels. The presence of mold in the household is typically easily discernable with visual inspection or detection by odor; if present, predisposing conditions should be corrected by individuals experienced in mold remediation.

Several laboratories offer testing for the evaluation of patients who suspect they have a mold-induced disorder, such as testing homes for mold spores, measuring urinary "mycotoxins," and performing serum IgG assays to molds. However, these tests should not be obtained as most are not validated and do not provide meaningful results upon which to make therapeutic decisions.

Chang C et al. The myth of mycotoxins and mold injury. Clin Rev Allergy Immunol. 2019;57:449. [PMID: 31608429]

Hurraβ J et al. Indoor molds. Dt Sch Arztebl Int. 2024;121:265. [PMID: 38381662]

41 Disorders Related to Environmental Emergencies

Jacqueline A. Nemer, MD, FACEP
Marianne A. Juarez, MD

COLD & HEAT

The human body maintains a steady temperature through the balance of internal heat production and environmental heat loss. Heat exchange between the body and environment occurs via four common processes: *radiation*, *evaporation*, *conduction*, and *convection*. In extreme temperatures, the body's thermoregulation may fail, resulting in the core body temperature moving toward the temperature of the external environment. Cold and heat exposure may cause a wide spectrum of conditions ranging in severity from mild, to potentially life-threatening, to death. Many of these conditions are preventable with appropriate education and planning.

The likelihood and severity of extreme temperature-related conditions depend on physiologic and environmental factors. Physiologic risk factors include extremes of age; cognitive impairment; pregnancy; poor physical conditioning, sedentary lifestyle, or immobility; poor acclimatization; concurrent injury; prior temperature-related injury; and numerous underlying medical conditions, especially those affecting cognition and thermoregulation. Pharmacologic risk factors include medications, holistic or alternative treatments, illicit drugs, tobacco, and alcohol. Medications impacting sweating and the CNS, or affecting cutaneous blood flow, such as peripheral vasoconstrictors or vasodilators, are more likely to worsen temperature-related conditions. Environmental risk factors include changing weather conditions, inadequate clothing or housing, climate change, and occupational or recreational exposure.

DISORDERS DUE TO HEAT

ESSENTIALS OF DIAGNOSIS

- **Spectrum of preventable heat-related illnesses:** heat cramps, heat exhaustion, heat syncope, and heat stroke.
- **Heat stroke:** hyperthermia with cerebral dysfunction in a patient with heat exposure.
- **Best outcome:** early recognition, removal from hot environment, and initiation of rapid cooling; delays in cooling result in higher morbidity and mortality in patients with heat stroke.
- **Best choice of cooling method:** whichever can be instituted the fastest with the least compromise to the patient.

General Considerations

Heat-related illnesses are among the most commonly seen environmental emergencies presenting to emergency departments. The amount of heat retained in the body is determined by internal metabolic function and environmental conditions, including temperature and humidity, with heat loss occurring primarily through sweating and peripheral vasodilation. **Hyperthermia** results from the body's inability to maintain normal internal temperature through heat loss, from either compromised heat dissipation mechanisms or abnormally high heat production. Increased metabolic rate is the most important factor in elevation of body temperature. The direct transfer of heat from the skin to the surrounding air, by convection or conduction, occurs with diminishing efficiency as ambient temperature rises, *especially above 37.2°C (the point at which heat transfer reverses direction)*. At normal temperatures, evaporation accounts for approximately 20% of the body's heat loss, but at high temperatures, it becomes the primary mechanism for dissipation of heat. This mechanism diminishes as humidity rises.

Heat stress can be caused by a combination of environmental and metabolic heat. *Climate change may significantly contribute to the risk of heat-related conditions and worsen existing inequities faced by structurally marginalized populations.*

There is a spectrum of preventable heat stress conditions, ranging from mild forms, such as heat cramps, to severe forms, such as heat stroke. Risk factors include longer duration of exertion, hot environment, insufficient acclimatization, and dehydration. Additional risk factors include medical conditions that inhibit sweat production or evaporation, pregnancy, obesity, prolonged seizures, hypotension, reduced cutaneous blood flow, reduced cardiac output, the use of medications that increase metabolism or muscle activity or impair sweating, and withdrawal syndromes. Illicit drug use can cause increased muscle activity and thus generate increased body heat.

Classic (nonexertional) heat-related illness may occur in any individual in a hot, relaxing environment despite minimal physical activity, with increased severity in individuals with the risk factors mentioned above.

Heat cramps are exercise-associated painful involuntary muscle contractions during or immediately after exercise. They result from dilutional hyponatremia as sweat losses are replaced with water alone. **Heat exhaustion** is characterized by dehydration, sodium depletion, or isotonic fluid loss with accompanying cardiovascular changes. It results from prolonged strenuous activity in a hot environment without adequate water or salt intake.

Heat syncope is defined as a transient loss of consciousness with spontaneous return to normal mentation. It results from volume depletion and cutaneous vasodilation with subsequent systemic and cerebral hypotension. Exercise-associated postural hypotension is usually the cause of heat syncope and may occur during or immediately following exercise. **Heat stroke** is a severe form of heat-related illness resulting in cerebral dysfunction with core body temperature over 40°C. It may present in one of two forms: classic and exertional. **Classic (nonexertional) heat stroke** occurs in patients with impaired thermoregulatory mechanisms or in extreme environmental conditions. **Exertional heat stroke** occurs in healthy persons undergoing strenuous exertion in a hot or humid environment. Persons at greatest risk are those who are at the extremes of age, chronically debilitated, or taking medications that interfere with heat-dissipating mechanisms.

Clinical Findings

When diagnosing and treating heat-related illnesses, *it is necessary to use an internal (rectal, Foley, or esophageal) thermometer since the skin temperature may not accurately reflect core body temperature.* Heat cramps are painful skeletal muscle contractions and severe muscle spasms with onset during or shortly after exercise. Examination findings typically include stable vital signs; normal or slightly increased core body temperature; moist and cool skin; and tender, hard, lumpy, muscles that may be twitching. The diagnosis is made clinically.

Heat exhaustion is diagnosed based on clinical findings of a core body temperature slightly elevated but < 40°C, tachycardia, and moist skin. Symptoms are like those of heat cramps and heat syncope. Additional symptoms may include nausea, vomiting, malaise, myalgias, hyperventilation, thirst, and weakness. CNS symptoms include headache, dizziness, fatigue, anxiety, paresthesias, impaired judgment, and occasionally psychosis. Heat exhaustion may progress to heat stroke if sweating ceases and mental status declines.

Heat syncope generally occurs in the setting of prolonged vigorous physical activity or prolonged standing in a hot humid environment followed by sudden collapse. Physical examination may reveal cool and moist skin, a weak pulse, and low systolic blood pressure.

Heat stroke is a life-threatening emergency. *The hallmark of heat stroke is cerebral dysfunction when the core body temperature is over 40°C.* Presenting symptoms include all findings seen in heat exhaustion with additional neurologic symptoms such as dizziness, weakness, emotional lability, confusion, delirium, blurred vision, convulsions, collapse, and unconsciousness. Physical examination findings may be variable and therefore unreliable. Exertional heat stroke may present with sudden collapse and loss of consciousness followed by irrational behavior. Sweating may not be present. Clinicians must be vigilant in monitoring for kidney injury, liver failure, metabolic derangements, respiratory compromise, coagulopathy, and ischemia since initial laboratory findings may be nonspecific.

Treatment

A. Heat Cramps

Move the patient to a shaded, cool environment and provide oral isotonic or hypertonic rehydration solution to replace both electrolytes and water. *Oral salt tablets are not recommended.* Advise the patient to rest for at least 2 days with continued dietary supplementation before returning to work or resuming strenuous activity in the heat.

B. Heat Exhaustion

Move the patient to a shaded, cool environment, provide adequate fluid and electrolyte replacement, and initiate active cooling measures if necessary. Physiologic saline or isotonic glucose solution may be administered intravenously when oral administration is not appropriate. At least 48 hours of rest and rehydration are recommended.

C. Heat Syncope

Treatment is essentially the same as for heat exhaustion: rest and recumbency in a shaded, cool place, and fluid and electrolyte replacement by mouth, or intravenously if necessary.

D. Heat Stroke

Initially, the patient's ABCs (airway, breathing, circulation) must be addressed and stabilized, then treatment is aimed at rapidly *reducing the core body temperature within 1 hour* while supporting circulation and perfusion. Patients should be placed on pulse oximetry and cardiac monitors while continuing to measure core body temperature and fluid intake and output. The patient should be observed for complications such as hypovolemic or cardiogenic shock, metabolic abnormalities, cardiac arrhythmias, coagulopathy, acute respiratory distress syndrome (ARDS), hypoglycemia, rhabdomyolysis, seizures, organ dysfunction, infection, and severe edema that can progress to a compartment syndrome. Circulatory failure in heat-related illness is mostly due to shock from relative or absolute hypovolemia. Oral or intravenous fluid administration must be provided to ensure adequate urinary output. Clinicians must also assess for and treat concurrent conditions such as infection, trauma, and medication effects.

Choice of cooling method depends on which can be instituted the fastest with the least compromise to the overall care of the patient. Evaporative cooling is preferred for nonexertional heat stroke and conductive-based cooling for exertional heat stroke. **Evaporative cooling** is a noninvasive, effective, quick, and easy way to reduce temperature. This is accomplished by placing the undressed patient in lateral recumbent position or supported in a hands-and-knees position to expose maximum skin surface to the air while the entire body is sprayed with lukewarm water (20°C) and cooled by large fans circulating room air. Addition of inhaled cool air or oxygen may aid in cooling but must not be used alone. **Conductive-based cooling** involves cool fluid infusion, gastric or bladder lavage, ice packs, and immersion into ice water or cool water. Ice water or cold water immersion is the preferred method of cooling for exertional heat stroke in the field when available. Ice packs are most effective when covering the whole body, as opposed to the traditional method of placing them in the axilla and groin only. Intravascular heat exchange catheter systems as well as hemodialysis using cold dialysate (30–35°C) have also been successful in reducing core body temperature.

Shivering must be avoided because it inhibits the effectiveness of cooling by increasing internal heat production. Medications can be used to suppress shivering including magnesium, quick-acting opioid analgesics, benzodiazepines, and quick-acting anesthetic agents. Skin massage is recommended to prevent cutaneous vasoconstriction. *Antipyretics (aspirin, acetaminophen) have no effect on environmentally induced hyperthermia and are contraindicated.* Treatment must be continued until the core body temperature drops to 39°C.

Prevention

Education is necessary to improve prevention and early recognition of heat-related disorders. Individuals may take steps to reduce personal risk factors and to gradually acclimatize to hot environments. For prevention of occupational heat-related illness, a comprehensive preventive program should assess personal risk factors, estimated time and amount of direct sun exposure, workload, acclimatization status, and early symptom recognition.

Coaches, athletic trainers, athletes, and parents of young athletes must be educated about heat-related illness, specifically about prevention, risks, symptoms and signs, and treatment. Medical evaluation and monitoring should be used to identify at-risk individuals and weather conditions that increase the risk of heat-related disorders.

Those who are physically active in a hot environment must increase fluid consumption before, during, and after physical activities. Fluid consumption should include balanced electrolyte fluids and water. Water consumption alone may lead to electrolyte imbalance, particularly hyponatremia. *It is not recommended to have salt tablets available for use because of the risk of hypertonic hypernatremia.* Close monitoring of fluid and electrolyte intake and early intervention are recommended in situations necessitating exertion or activity in hot environments.

Prognosis

Mortality is high from heat stroke, most frequently secondary to multiorgan dysfunction. The patient is also at risk for rhabdomyolysis, ARDS, and inflammation even after core temperature has normalized. Following heat stroke, immediate re-exposure to ambient heat must be avoided.

When to Refer

Potential consultants include a surgeon for suspicion of compartment syndrome, nephrologist for kidney injury, and transplant surgeon for fulminant liver failure.

When to Admit

All patients with suspected heat stroke must be admitted to a hospital with intensive care capability for close monitoring.

Bauman J et al. Heat-related illnesses. Emerg Med Clin North Am. 2024;42:485. [PMID: 38925769]

Bell ML et al. Climate change, extreme heat, and health. N Engl J Med. 2024;390:1793. [PMID: 38749034]

Green S et al. Approach to heat-related illness. Can Fam Physician. 2024;70:546. [PMID: 39271209]

ACCIDENTAL SYSTEMIC HYPOTHERMIA

ESSENTIALS OF DIAGNOSIS

- Systemic hypothermia is a core body temperature < 35°C.
- Accurate core body temperature measurement must be obtained using a low-reading core temperature probe that measures as low as 25°C.
- Core body temperature must be > 32°C before terminating resuscitation efforts.
- Extracorporeal membrane oxygenation (ECMO) or cardiopulmonary bypass may be considered in hypothermic patients with hemodynamic instability or cardiac arrest.

General Considerations

Systemic **hypothermia** is defined as core body temperature below 35°C. This may be primary, from exposure to prolonged ambient, extremely low temperature, or secondary, due to thermoregulatory dysfunction. Both may be present at the same time.

Hypothermia must be considered in any patient with prolonged exposure to an ambient cold environment, especially in patients with prior cold weather injury as well as the risk factors listed in the Cold & Heat section.

In prolonged or repetitive cold exposure, hypothermia ensues if the body's thermoregulatory responses become impaired.

Clinical Findings

Symptoms and signs of hypothermia are typically nonspecific and markedly variable based on the patient's underlying health and circumstances of cold exposure. All patients must be evaluated for associated conditions including hypoglycemia, trauma, infection, overdose, and peripheral cold injury. Laboratory studies should assess acid-base status; electrolytes, particularly potassium and glucose; kidney, liver, and pancreas function; coagulation; and rhabdomyolysis. Inaccurate laboratory values will occur if the blood sample is warmed to 37°C for testing.

Accurate core body temperature measurements must be obtained using a core temperature probe that measures as low as 25°C. **Stage I hypothermia** is seen when the core body temperature is between 32°C and 35°C and is defined by shivering and possibly poor judgment or coordination but with hemodynamic stability and a normal level of consciousness. **Stage II hypothermia** correlates with core body temperature 28–32°C. *Shivering stops*; bradycardia, dilated pupils, slowed reflexes, cold diuresis, and confusion and lethargy ensue. The ECG may reveal a J wave or Osborn wave (positive deflection in the terminal portion of the QRS complex, most notable in leads II, V_5, and V_6) (Figure 41–1). When the core body temperature is below 28°C, the likelihood of hemodynamic instability and cardiac arrest increases dramatically. **Stage III hypothermia** (core body temperature 24–28°C) is characterized by loss of consciousness but present vital signs. **Stage IV hypothermia** (core body temperature < 24°C) is the loss of vital signs. Coma, loss of reflexes, asystole, or ventricular fibrillation may falsely lead the clinician to assume the patient is dead despite reversible hypothermia.

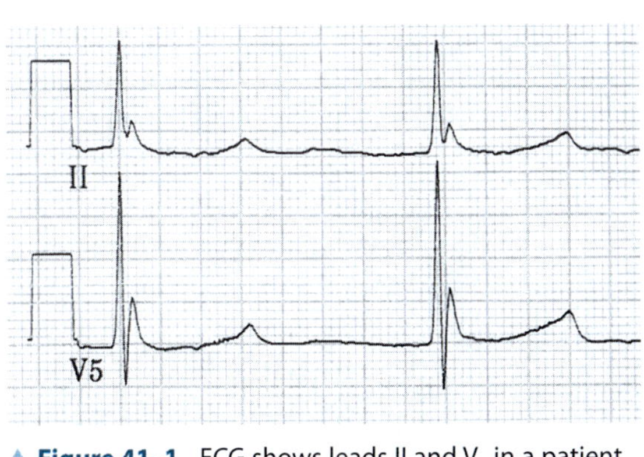

Figure 41–1. ECG shows leads II and V_5 in a patient whose body temperature is 24°C. Note the bradycardia and Osborn waves. These findings become more prominent as the body temperature lowers and gradually resolve with rewarming. Osborn waves have an extra positive deflection in the terminal portion of the QRS complex and are best seen in the inferior and lateral precordial leads (most notably in leads II, V_5, and V_6).

Treatment

Rewarming is the initial, imperative treatment for all hypothermic patients. Resuscitation begins with rapid assessment and support of airway, breathing, and circulation, simultaneously with the initiation of rewarming, and prevention of further heat loss. All cold, wet clothing must be removed and replaced with warm, dry clothing and blankets.

Mild or stage I hypothermia can be treated with **passive external rewarming** (eg, removing and replacing wet clothes with dry ones) or by active external rewarming. In contrast to those with more severe hypothermia, it is safe and recommended for the uninjured patient with mild hypothermia to become physically active to generate heat. **Active external rewarming** is noninvasive, highly effective, and safe for mild hypothermia. It involves applying external heat to the patient's skin. Examples include warm bedding, heated blankets, heat packs, and immersion into a 40°C bath. Patients with mild hypothermia and previous good health usually respond well to passive and active external rewarming.

Stage II and III hypothermia are treated as above with the addition of more aggressive rewarming strategies. This requires close monitoring of vital signs and cardiac rhythm during rewarming. Warm intravenous fluids (38–42°C) are considered minimally invasive and effective.

As hypothermia becomes more severe, there are increased complications of both hypothermia itself and of rewarming. Complications of rewarming occur as colder peripheral blood returns to central circulation. This may result in **core temperature afterdrop**, rewarming lactic acidosis from shunting lactate into the circulation, rewarming shock from peripheral vasodilation and hypovolemia, ventricular fibrillation, and other cardiac arrhythmias. Afterdrop can be lessened by active external rewarming of the trunk but not the extremities and by avoiding any muscle movement by the patient. Extreme caution must be taken when handling the hypothermic patient to avoid triggering potentially fatal arrhythmias in a phenomenon known as rescue collapse.

Patients with hemodynamic instability or cardiac arrest should be transferred to a facility with ECMO or cardiopulmonary bypass capability.

Early recognition and advanced management guidelines are needed for patients with stage IV hypothermia. *For hypothermic patients in cardiac arrest, high-quality CPR must be initiated and continued until the patient's core body temperature is at least 32°C.* Below 30°C, arrhythmias and asystole may be refractory to drug therapy until the patient has been rewarmed; therefore, treatment should focus on excellent CPR technique in conjunction with aggressive rewarming of the patient. Epinephrine may be given in cardiac arrest of the severely hypothermic patient. The International Commission for Mountain Emergency Medicine recommends extracorporeal life support as the treatment of choice for patients at high risk for hypothermic cardiac arrest. Extracorporeal life support has been shown to substantially improve survival of patients with unstable circulation or cardiac arrest.

Hypothermic patients with return of spontaneous circulation are at high risk of subsequent multiorgan system failure.

When to Admit

Hypothermia patients must undergo close monitoring for potential complications. This is typically done during an inpatient admission or prolonged emergency department observation.

Ádám K et al. Accidental hypothermia in emergency care: multifactorial triage-based prediction of early critical outcomes in a temperate-climate cohort. PLoS One. 2025;20:e0334328. [PMID: 41066376]

Hara C et al. Association between rewarming rate and survival and neurologic outcome of accidental hypothermia. Crit Care Med. 2025;53:e1416. [PMID: 40459372]

Mendrala K et al. Extracorporeal life support in accidental hypothermia. JAMA. 2025;334:1846. [PMID: 41060623]

HYPOTHERMIA OF THE EXTREMITIES

ESSENTIALS OF DIAGNOSIS

- *"Keep warm, keep dry, and keep moving"* to prevent cold-induced injury.
- Rewarming of the extremity suffering cold-induced injury must be performed as soon as possible once there is no risk of refreezing; exercise, rubbing, or massage must be avoided during rewarming.

Clinical Findings

Cold exposure of the extremities produces immediate localized and then generalized vasoconstriction, which may result in a wide range of injuries. Tissue damage occurs because of ischemia and intravascular thromboses, endothelial damage, or actual freezing. Freezing (frostbite) may occur when skin temperatures drop or in the presence of wind, water, immobility, malnutrition, or vascular disease.

For all forms of cold-induced injury to an extremity, caution must be taken to avoid rubbing or massaging the injured area and to avoid applying moisture, ice, or heat. The cold-injured extremity must be protected from trauma, secondary infection, and further cold exposure.

Prevention

"Keep warm, keep dry, and keep moving." For optimal prevention of frostbite, individuals must wear warm, dry clothing. Arms, legs, fingers, and toes must be exercised to maintain circulation. Wet clothing, socks, and shoes must be replaced with dry ones. Risk factors include underlying diseases or medications that decrease tissue perfusion and prolonged cold environmental exposure. Caution must be taken to avoid cramped positions; wet or constrictive clothing; prolonged dependency of the feet; use of tobacco, alcohol, and sedative medications; and exposure to wet, muddy ground and windy conditions.

FROSTNIP & CHILBLAINS (Erythema Pernio)

Frostnip is a superficial nonfreezing injury causing local paresthesias of the involved area that completely resolves with passive external rewarming.

Chilblains, or **erythema pernio,** are inflammatory skin changes caused by exposure to cold without actual freezing of the tissues. These skin lesions may be red or purple papular lesions, which are painful or pruritic, with burning or paresthesias. They may be associated with edema or blistering and aggravated by warmth. With continued exposure, ulcerative or hemorrhagic lesions may appear and progress to scarring, fibrosis, and atrophy. Treatment consists of elevating and passively externally rewarming the affected part.

IMMERSION FOOT OR TRENCH FOOT

Immersion foot ("trench foot") or **hand** is caused by prolonged immersion in cold water or mud, usually below 15°C. **Prehyperemic stage** is marked by early symptoms of cold and anesthesia of the affected area. **Hyperemic stage** follows with a hot sensation, intense burning, and shooting pains. **Posthyperemic stage** occurs with ongoing cold exposure; the affected part becomes pale or cyanotic with diminished pulsations due to vasospasm. This may result in blistering, swelling, redness, ecchymoses, hemorrhage, necrosis, peripheral nerve injury, or gangrene.

Treatment consists of air drying and gradual rewarming by exposure to air at room temperature. Affected parts are elevated to aid in removal of edema fluid. Pressure sites are protected with cushions. Bed rest is required until all ulcers have healed.

FROSTBITE

Frostbite is injury from tissue freezing and formation of ice crystals in the tissue. Most tissue destruction follows reperfusion of the frozen tissues resulting in further tissue damage. In mild cases, only the skin and subcutaneous tissues are involved. Symptoms include numbness, prickling, itching, and pallor. With increasing severity, deeper structures become involved; the skin appears white or yellow, loses elasticity, and becomes immobile. Edema, hemorrhagic blisters, necrosis, gangrene, paresthesias, and stiffness may occur.

Treatment

A. Immediate Treatment

Evaluate and treat the patient for associated systemic hypothermia, concurrent conditions, and injury. Early use of systemic analgesics is recommended for nonfrozen injuries. Hydrate the patient to avoid hypovolemia and to improve perfusion.

1. Rewarming—Rapid rewarming at temperatures slightly above normal body temperature may significantly decrease tissue necrosis and reverse the tissue crystallization. *If there* *is any possibility of refreezing, the frostbitten part must not be thawed.* Ideally, the frozen extremity should not be used, but if required for evacuation, the affected frozen extremity must be padded and splinted to avoid additional injury. *Rewarming is best accomplished by warm bath immersion.* The frozen extremity is immersed in a moving water bath heated to 37–39°C for approximately 30 minutes until the area becomes soft and pliable to the touch. Water in this temperature range feels warm but not hot to the normal hand or wrist. If warm water is not available, then passive thawing in a warm environment must be allowed. Dry heat is not recommended because it is more difficult to regulate and increases the likelihood of accidental burns. Thawing may cause tenderness and burning pain. Once the frozen part has thawed and returned to normal temperature, discontinue external heat. *In the early stage, rewarming by exercise, rubbing, or friction is contraindicated.* The patient must be kept on bed rest with the affected parts elevated and uncovered at room temperature. Avoid application of casts, occlusive dressings, or bandages. Blisters should be left intact unless signs of infection develop.

2. Anti-infective measures and wound care—Frostbite increases susceptibility to tetanus and infection. Tetanus prophylaxis status should be verified and updated as needed. Infection risk may be reduced by aseptic wound care. Topical wound care such as aloe vera cream or gel or antibiotic ointment should be applied to the thawed tissue before application of dressings. Nonadherent sterile gauze and fluffy dressing must be loosely applied to wounds and cushions used for all areas of pressure. Systemic antibiotics should not be administered empirically.

B. Medical and Surgical Treatment Options

Telemedicine may be used so that specialists can provide advice on early field treatment of patients in remote areas, thereby improving outcomes. NSAIDs should be administered (in the absence of contraindications) until frostbite wounds are healed or surgical management occurs. Clinicians must watch for evidence of compartment syndrome and need for fasciotomy. Eschar formation without evidence of infection may be conservatively treated. The underlying skin may heal spontaneously with the eschar acting as a biologic dressing. Rates of amputation have been reduced with intravenous infusions of synthetic prostaglandins and tissue plasminogen activators, and with intra-arterial administration of a thrombolytic within 24 hours of exposure. The rate of tissue salvage decreases with every hour of delay from rewarming to thrombolytic therapy.

C. Follow-Up Care

Patient education must include ongoing care of the cold injury and prevention of future hypothermia and cold injury. Gentle, progressive physical therapy to promote circulation should be instituted as tolerated.

Prognosis

Recovery from frostbite depends on the underlying comorbidities, the extent of initial tissue damage, the rewarming reperfusion injury, and the late sequelae. The involved extremity may be at increased susceptibility for discomfort and injury upon re-exposure to cold. Neuropathic sequelae include pain, numbness, tingling, hyperhidrosis, and cold sensitivity of the extremities. Nerve conduction abnormalities may persist for many years after a cold injury.

When to Admit

- Management of tissue damage, comorbidities, associated injuries.
- Need for hospital-based interventions.
- Psychosocial factors that could compromise patient safety or recovery.

Egro FM et al. Update on cold-induced injuries. Clin Plast Surg. 2024;51:303. [PMID: 38429050]
Persitz J et al. Frostbite of the extremities—recognition, evaluation and treatment. Injury. 2022;53:3088. [PMID: 35914986]
Sharifzadeh A et al. An evidence-based review of perniosis (Chilblains): therapeutic strategies and integration with Raynaud's syndrome management. Int J Dermatol. 2025;64:1781. [PMID: 40272049]
Wibbenmeyer L et al. American Burn Association clinical practice guidelines on the treatment of severe frostbite. J Burn Care Res. 2024;45:541. [PMID: 37045447]

DROWNING

ESSENTIALS OF DIAGNOSIS

- The first requirement of rescue is immediate rescue breathing and CPR.
- Clinical manifestations include hypoxemia, pulmonary edema, and hypoventilation.
- Patients must be assessed for hypothermia, hypoglycemia, concurrent injuries, and medical conditions.

General Considerations

According to the WHO, drowning is the third leading cause of unintentional injury death worldwide. Drowning, as defined by the WHO, is any "process of experiencing respiratory impairment from submersion/immersion in liquid." Drowning may result in asphyxiation (from fluid aspiration or laryngospasm), hypoxemia, hypothermia, and acidemia. Outcomes from drowning range from life without morbidity to death. Morbidity may be immediate or delayed. A patient may be deceptively asymptomatic during the initial recovery period only to deteriorate or die from acute respiratory failure within the following 12–24 hours. Disseminated intravascular coagulation may also lead to bleeding after asphyxiation from drowning.

Drowning is a leading cause of death in children worldwide and is highly preventable in all ages with implementation of educational and safety measures. Clinicians must provide patient education and guidance about drowning prevention.

Clinical Findings

A. Symptoms and Signs

The patient's appearance may vary from asymptomatic to marked distress with abnormal vital signs. Symptoms and signs include respiratory difficulty, trismus, chest pain, dysrhythmia, hypotension, cyanosis, and hypothermia (from cold water or prolonged submersion). A pink froth from the mouth and nose indicates pulmonary edema. The patient may experience headache, neurologic deficits, and altered level of consciousness.

B. Laboratory Findings

Metabolic acidosis is common and ABG results may be helpful in determining the degree of injury since initial clinical findings may appear benign. PaO_2 is usually decreased; $PaCO_2$ may be increased or decreased; pH is decreased. Bedside blood glucose must be checked rapidly. Other testing is based on clinical scenario.

Prevention

Education and prevention are critical given the high burden of disease from drowning.

Preventive measures must be taken to reduce morbidity and mortality from drowning. Conditions that increase risk of submersion injury include the use of alcohol, psychotropics, and other drugs, inadequate water safety skills, poor physical health, hyperventilation, sudden acute illness, acute trauma, decompression sickness, dangerous water conditions, and environmental hazards (eg, lack of fencing around pools).

Treatment

A. First Aid

1. The first requirement of rescue is immediate basic life support treatment and CPR. At the scene, immediate airway management and measures to combat hypoxemia are critical to improve outcome.
2. Patient must be assessed for hypothermia, hypoglycemia, concurrent medical conditions, and associated trauma.
3. Rescuer must not attempt to drain water from the person's lungs.
4. Resuscitation and basic life support efforts must be continued until core body temperature reaches 32°C.

B. Subsequent Management

1. Ensure optimal ventilation and oxygenation—The onset of hypoxemia exists even in the alert, conscious patient who appears to be breathing normally. Supplemental oxygen should be administered immediately at the highest available concentration to maintain oxygen saturation at 90% or higher.

Serial physical examinations and CXRs must be performed to detect possible pneumonitis, atelectasis, and pulmonary edema. Bronchodilators may be used to treat wheezing. Nasogastric suctioning may be necessary to decompress the stomach.

2. Cardiovascular support—Intravascular volume status must be monitored and supported by vascular fluid replacement, vasopressors, or diuretics as needed.

3. Correction of blood pH and electrolyte abnormalities—Metabolic acidosis is present in most persons who drown but typically corrects through adequate ventilation and oxygenation. Glycemic control improves outcome.

4. Cerebral and spinal cord injury—CNS damage may progress despite apparently adequate treatment of hypoxia and shock.

5. Hypothermia—Core body temperature must be measured and managed as appropriate (see Accidental Systemic Hypothermia, above).

Course & Prognosis

Favorable prognosis is related to a duration of submersion < 5 minutes, with worsening outcomes correlating with increased submersion times. Respiratory damage is often severe in the minutes to hours following a drowning. With appropriate respiratory supportive treatment, patients may improve rapidly over the first few days following the drowning. Long-term complications of drowning may include neurologic impairment, seizure disorder, and pulmonary or cardiac damage. Prognosis is directly correlated with the patient's age, submersion time, rapidity of prehospital resuscitation and subsequent transport to a medical facility, clinical status at time of arrival to hospital, Glasgow Coma Scale score, pupillary reactivity, and overall health assessment (APACHE II score).

When to Admit

Most patients with significant drowning or concurrent medical or traumatic conditions require inpatient monitoring following the event. This includes continuous monitoring of cardiorespiratory, neurologic, renal, and metabolic function. Pulmonary edema may not appear for 24 hours.

Davis CA et al. Drowning. Emerg Med Clin North Am. 2024;42:541. [PMID: 38925773]
Peden AE et al. Drowning and disasters: climate change priorities. Lancet Planet Health. 2024;8:e345. [PMID: 38849173]

THERMAL BURNS

ESSENTIALS OF DIAGNOSIS

- Estimates of the burn location, size, and depth greatly determine the treatment plan.
- The first 48 hours of burn care offer the greatest impact on morbidity and mortality of a patient with burns.

Worldwide, burns are a common cause of injury and potential morbidity and mortality. Burn prognosis is affected by the type of environment where the burn occurred. Low-resource settings are associated with delays in and suboptimal access to standard burn treatments.

The first 48 hours after thermal burn injury offer the greatest opportunity to impact the survival of the patient. Early surgical intervention, wound care, enteral feeding, glucose control and metabolic management, infection control, and prevention of hypothermia and compartment syndrome have contributed to significantly lower mortality rates and shorter hospitalizations.

General Considerations

A. Classification

Burns are classified by extent, depth, patient age, and associated illness or injury. Accurate estimation of burn size and depth is necessary to quantify the parameters of resuscitation.

1. Extent—In adults, the "*rule of nines*" (Figure 41–2) is useful for rapidly assessing the extent of a burn. It is important to expose the entire patient to make an accurate assessment of skin findings on initial and subsequent examinations. One rule of thumb is that the palm of an open hand in adult patients constitutes 1% of *total body surface area (TBSA)*. TBSA is calculated for partial- and full-thickness burns.

2. Depth—Judgment of depth of injury is difficult. **Superficial burns** may appear red or gray but will demonstrate excellent capillary refill and are not blistered initially. If the wound is blistered and appears pink and wet, this represents a **superficial partial-thickness burn**. **Deep partial-thickness burns** appear white and wet, and bleed if poked; cutaneous sensation is maintained. **Full-thickness burns** result in a loss of adnexal structures and may appear white-yellow or may have a black charred appearance. This stiff, dry skin does not bleed when poked and cutaneous sensation is lost.

Deep partial-thickness and full thickness burns are treated in a similar fashion. Both require early debridement and grafting to heal appropriately, without which the skin becomes thin and scarred.

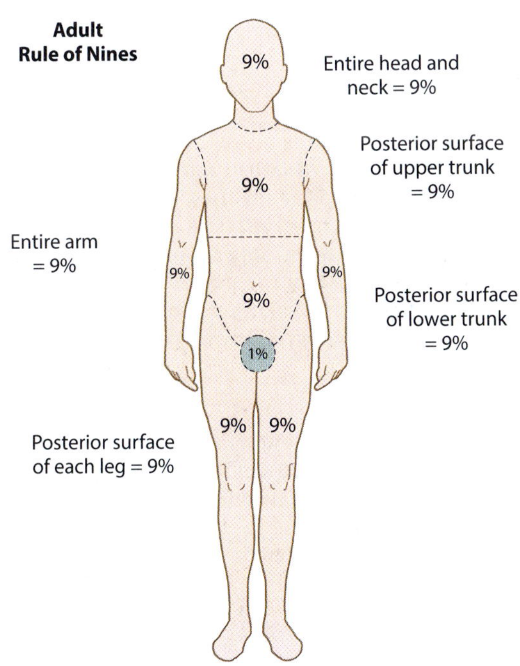

Figure 41–2. Estimation of body surface area in burns.

B. Survival After Burn Injury

Transfer to a burn unit is determined by large burn size, circumferential burn, or burn involving a joint or high-risk body part, and by comorbidities. Mortality rates have been significantly reduced due to treatment advances including improvements in wound care, treatment of infection, early burn excision, skin substitute usage, and early nutritional support.

C. Associated Injuries or Illnesses

Smoke inhalation, trauma, and electrical injuries are commonly associated with burns. Severe burns from any source may result in similar complications (eg, infections, respiratory compromise, multiorgan dysfunction, VTE, and GI complications).

D. Systemic Reactions to Burn Injury

Burns larger than approximately 20% of TBSA may lead to systemic metabolic derangements requiring intensive support. The inflammatory cascade can result in shock and coagulopathy.

Treatment

A. Initial Resuscitation

1. Primary survey—Patients with severe burns require a full trauma assessment, starting with "ABCDE" (airway, breathing, circulation, disability, exposure).

A. AIRWAY CONTROL—Serial assessments of airway and breathing are necessary because airway compromise and ARDS may develop, particularly in those with inhalation injury.

B. VASCULAR ACCESS—Vascular access must be obtained on all patients with severe burns.

C. FLUID RESUSCITATION—Patients with burns > 15% of TBSA require intravascular fluid administration of large volumes of crystalloid. The most widely recognized guideline for fluid resuscitation is the **Parkland formula** (https://www.mdcalc.com/parkland-formula-burns) in which the fluid requirement in the first 24 hours is estimated as 4 mL/kg × body weight per percentage of body surface area burned. Half the calculated fluid is given in the first 8-hour period from the time of injury. The remaining fluid is delivered over the next 16 hours. An extremely large volume of fluid may be required. Crystalloid solutions alone may be insufficient to restore cardiac preload during the period of burn shock and colloid adjuncts may be considered to optimize fluid resuscitation. Clinicians must monitor for clinical signs of volume overload as it may lead to pulmonary complications or compartment syndromes. Electrical burns and inhalation injury may increase the fluid requirement.

B. Management

1. Pain control—Pain control is critical in patients with burn injuries. Treatment is with (oral or intravenous) NSAIDs and opioids (see Chapter 5).

2. Chemoprophylaxis—

A. TETANUS IMMUNIZATION—Verify and update tetanus prophylaxis status *in all patients with burns.* (See Chapter 37.)

B. ANTIBIOTICS—All nonsuperficial wounds need to be covered with topical antibiotics. Prophylaxis with systemic antibiotics is not indicated.

3. Surgical management—

A. ESCHAROTOMY—As tissue swelling occurs, ischemia may develop under any constricting eschar of an extremity, neck, or chest, or in circumferential full-thickness burns of the trunk. Escharotomy incisions can be limb- and life-saving.

B. FASCIOTOMY—Fasciotomy is indicated for any compartment syndrome. Clinicians must frequently monitor patients for development of early signs of a compartment syndrome, particularly in those with circumferential burns.

C. DEBRIDEMENT, DRESSINGS, AND TOPICAL AND SYSTEMIC ANTIBIOTIC THERAPY—Minor burn wounds must be debrided to determine the depth of the burn and then thoroughly cleansed. Thereafter, *daily wound care must consist of debridement as needed, topical antibiotics, and wound dressings.* Patient compliance and adequate pain control is essential for successful outpatient treatment. The wound must be reevaluated by the treating clinician within 24–72 hours to evaluate for signs of infection.

The goal of burn wound management is to protect the wound from desiccation and avoid further injury or infection. Regular and thorough cleansing of burned areas is critical. Topical antibiotics may be applied after wound cleansing. Silver sulfadiazine is *no longer recommended.*

It is imperative to closely monitor for and treat systemic infection, since this remains a leading cause of morbidity among patients with major burn injuries. Health care–associated infections are increasingly common.

D. WOUND MANAGEMENT—*The goal of therapy after fluid resuscitation is rapid and stable closure of the wound.* Wounds that do not heal spontaneously in 7–10 days (eg, deep partial-thickness or full-thickness burns) are best treated by a specialist through excision and autograft to avoid development of granulation and infection. The quality of the skin in regenerated deep partial-thickness burns is marginal because of the very thin dermis that emerges.

Cultured allogeneic keratinocyte grafts can provide rapid early coverage for superficial burn injuries. Skin substitution with cultured grafts may be life-saving for severe burns. Although the replaced dermis has nearly normal histologic dermal elements, there are no adnexal structures present, and very few, if any, elastic fibers.

E. ABDOMINAL COMPARTMENT SYNDROME—Abdominal compartment syndrome is a potentially lethal condition that may develop in severely burned patients, with mortality rates of approximately 60% despite surgical intervention. Diagnosis is confirmed by bladder pressures > 30 mm Hg in at-risk patients. Surgical abdominal decompression may improve ventilation and oxygen delivery but may not impact survival.

C. Patient Support

Patients with severe burns require extensive supportive care, both physiologically and psychologically. It is important to maintain normal core body temperature and avoid hypothermia, by maintaining environmental temperature at or above 30°C, in patients with burns over more than 20% of TBSA. These patients are at risk for many complications such as respiratory injury, ARDS or respiratory failure unresponsive to maximal ventilatory support, sepsis, multiorgan failure, and VTE.

Patients with severe burns have increased metabolic and energy needs for wound healing and require careful assessment and provision of optimal nutrition. Early aggressive nutrition (by parenteral or enteral routes) reduces infections, recovery time, noninfectious complications, length of hospital stay, long-term sequelae, and mortality.

Prevention of long-term scars remains a formidable problem in seriously burned patients.

Prognosis

Prognosis depends on the extent and location of the burn tissue damage, associated injuries, comorbidities, and complications. Hyperglycemia is a predictor of worse outcomes. Common complications include sepsis; gangrene requiring limb amputation; or neurologic, cardiac, cognitive, or psychiatric dysfunction. Psychiatric support may be necessary following burn injury.

When to Refer

Transfer to a **burn unit** is indicated for large burn size (for partial-thickness burns > 10% of TBSA or for full-thickness burns > 5% of TBSA), circumferential burn, inhalation injury, or burn involving a joint or high-risk body part (face, hands, feet, genitalia), and for patients with comorbidities.

When to Admit

- All patients with severe burns require extensive supportive care, both physiologically and psychologically.

- Significant burns (based on location and extent).
- Patients with significant comorbidities and suboptimal home situations.
- *Burn center consultation* can advise which patients require transfer and which can be managed via telemedicine/telephone consultation.
- Monitoring includes vital signs, wound care, and observation for potential complications of electrolyte abnormalities, AKI, hepatic failure, cardiopulmonary compromise, hyperglycemia, and infection.

Cartotto R et al. American Burn Association clinical practice guidelines on burn shock resuscitation. J Burn Care Res. 2024;45:565. [PMID: 38051821]
Davis BN et al. Acute burn care. Plast Reconstr Surg. 2024;153:804e. [PMID: 38546365]
Gwyn-Jones A et al. Major burns in adults: a practice review. Emerg Med J. 2024;41:630. [PMID: 38886061]
Żwierełło W et al. Burns: classification, pathophysiology, and treatment: a review. Int J Mol Sci. 2023;24:3749. [PMID: 36835171]

ELECTRICAL INJURY

ESSENTIALS OF DIAGNOSIS

- After an electrical injury, clinical findings suggestive of death are unreliable; resuscitation must begin immediately.
- Extent of damage from electrical injury is determined by the type, amount, duration, and pathway of current.
- Electrical injury skin findings are not indicative of the depth of tissue injury and may appear misleadingly minor.

General Considerations

Electricity injuries occur by exposure to electrical current of low voltage, high voltage, or lightning. Electrical current type is either alternating current or direct current and is measured in volts (V). Electrical injury is caused by a combination of direct thermal injury and tissue damage, muscle tetany, coagulation necrosis, associated trauma, and delayed sequelae. Treatment is different than for other types of burns. Electricity-induced injuries are common and yet most are preventable.

Alternating current is an electric current thatmay cause muscle tetany, which prolongs the duration and amount of exposure. Alternating current can be low voltage or high voltage. Most households and businesses use electric power of alternating current at low voltages (< 1000 V). Low-voltage electrical injuries range from minor to significant damage and death. High-voltage (> 1000 V) alternating current electrical injuries are often related to occupational exposure and associated with deep tissue damage, and higher morbidity and mortality. *Direct current* is unidirectional electrical flow (eg, lightning, batteries). It is more likely to cause a single intense muscle contraction and asystole. Lightning differs from other high-voltage electrical shock because lightning delivers a direct current of millions of volts in a fraction of a second.

The extent of damage from electrical injury is determined by the current type, amount (voltage), duration of exposure, pathway of current, tissue resistance, moisture, associated trauma, and comorbidities. Current is the most important determinant of tissue damage and causes direct thermal injury. Tissue resistance varies throughout the body with nerve cells being the most vulnerable and bone the most resistant to electrical current.

Clinical Findings

Electrical burns are of three types: *flash (arcing) burns, flame (clothing) burns,* and the *direct heating effect* of tissues by the current.

Skin damage does not correlate with the degree of injury. Symptoms and signs may range from very subtle to death. The presence of entrance and exit burns signifies an increased risk of deep tissue damage and compartment syndrome. Current passing through skeletal muscle can cause muscle necrosis and contractions severe enough to result in bone fracture.

Resuscitation must be initiated on all victims of electrical injury since clinical findings of death are deceptive and unreliable.

Complications

Complications may include cardiac or respiratory arrest; dysrhythmias; neurologic and neuropsychological sequelae; vascular injury from thrombosis and capillary damage; tissue edema and necrosis; compartment syndrome; associated traumatic injuries; pneumothorax; rhabdomyolysis; AKI; hypovolemia from third spacing; infections; otic damage; ocular complications; sepsis; gangrene; and cognitive or psychiatric dysfunction.

Treatment

A. Emergency Measures

The patient must be safely separated from the electrical current prior to CPR initiation and treatment. Resuscitation must be initiated since clinical findings suggesting death are unreliable. The patient must be assessed and treated for acute medical conditions and trauma.

B. Hospital Measures

Electric burn assessment follows the full trauma assessment starting with airway, breathing, circulation, disability, and exposure. Fluid resuscitation is important. Initial evaluation includes ECG, cardiac monitoring, cardiac enzymes, CBC, electrolytes, kidney tests, liver chemistries, creatine phosphokinase or urine myoglobin, and UA. Patients must be evaluated for injuries including burns, blunt trauma, dehydration, hypertension, acid-base disturbances, and neurologic and psychological trauma.

Electrical burn wounds can be devastating with wide-ranging and significant complications. Superficial skin may appear deceivingly benign. *It is important to maintain a high suspicion for extensive deep tissue necrosis, which may lead to profound tissue swelling and high risk of compartment syndrome.*

Pain management is important throughout initial treatment and subsequent rehabilitation.

Prognosis

Prognosis is determined by the degree and location of electrical injury, initial tissue damage, associated injuries, comorbidities, and complications.

When to Refer

- An ophthalmologist for possible ocular complications; an otologist for ear trauma or hearing loss.
- Surgical specialists for fasciotomy for compartment syndrome, debridement, or microvascular reconstruction.
- A psychiatrist may assess any psychological impact.

When to Admit

Indications for hospitalization include high-voltage exposure; arrhythmia or ECG changes; large burn size; neurologic, pulmonary, or cardiac symptoms; suspicion of significant deep tissue or organ damage; transthoracic current pathway; history of cardiac disease or other significant comorbidities or injuries; and need for surgery.

Chen J et al. Characteristics and risk factors for electrical burn injuries: a study based on World Health Organization Global Burn Registry. Burns. 2024;50:1116. [PMID: 38402118]

Goffeng LO et al. Low-voltage electrical accidents, immediate reactions and acute health care associated with self-reported general health 4 years later. Burns. 2023;49:329. [PMID: 35610077]

Khor D et al. Electrical injuries and outcomes: a retrospective review. Burns. 2023;49:1739. [PMID: 37005139]

RADIATION EXPOSURE

ESSENTIALS OF DIAGNOSIS

- Damage from radiation is determined by the radiation type, quantity, duration, accumulated exposures, and the patient's underlying conditions.
- Clinicians and patients must be educated regarding the risks of medical diagnostic radiation weighed against the benefits of the medical imaging needed.

General Considerations

Radiation exposure may occur from environmental, occupational, medical care, accidental, or intentional causes. The extent of damage from radiation exposure depends on the type, quantity, and duration of radiation exposure; the organs exposed; and the patient's age, comorbidities, and accumulated radiation exposures.

Radiation occurs from both nonionizing and ionizing radiation sources. **Nonionizing radiation** is low energy, causing local thermal damage. **Ionizing radiation** is high energy, causing damage in several ways. Exposure may be external, internal, or both. Radiation causes multiple metabolic changes resulting in tissue-specific damage.

The *International Commission on Radiological Protection (ICRP)* website provides the most current recommendations for protection against ionizing radiation (http://www.icrp.org/index.asp). The WHO publishes guidelines on radiation emergencies (https://www.who.int/health-topics/radiation-emergencies#tab=tab_1). These guidelines include recommended interventions during the early, intermediate, and late emergency phases and the management of their psychosocial impact.

Clinical Findings

Radiation exposure results in acute and delayed effects. It is important to obtain the event history, radiation exposure, and coexisting injuries or conditions. Acute effects over hours to days after exposure involve damage to rapidly dividing cells (eg, the mucosa, skin, and bone marrow). *Acute findings* include mucositis, nausea, vomiting, GI edema and ulcers, skin burns, and bone marrow suppression. *Delayed effects* include malignancy, reproduction abnormalities, and liver, kidney, CNS, and immune system dysfunction.

Acute radiation syndrome is a clinical syndrome due to an exposure to high dose(s) of ionizing radiation over a brief time course. Acute radiation syndrome involves multiple organ systems, including hematopoietic, cardiopulmonary, GI, neurovascular, and cutaneous systems. The symptom onset is within hours to days depending on the dose. Symptoms include anorexia, nausea, vomiting, weakness, exhaustion, dehydration, lassitude, prostration, anemia, and infection; these symptoms may occur singly or in combination. The CDC offers information regarding acute radiation syndrome (https://www.cdc.gov/radiation-emergencies/hcp/clinical-guidance/ars.html?CDC_AAref_Val=https://www.cdc.gov/nceh/radiation/emergencies/ars-physicianfactsheet.htm).

Treatment for acute radiation exposure includes close monitoring of the GI, cutaneous, hematologic, cardiopulmonary, and neurovascular systems from initial exposure and over time.

Therapeutic Radiation Exposure

Radiation therapy has been a successful component in the treatment of many malignancies. Unfortunately, these radiation-treated cancer survivors have a higher risk of a second malignancy; obesity; and pulmonary, cardiac, and thyroid dysfunction, as well as an increased overall risk of chronic health conditions and mortality.

Medical Imaging Radiation Exposure

Medical imaging with ionizing radiation exposure has dramatically increased over the past few decades. With the rising use of medical imaging, there is international focus on improving the safety by standardization and regulation of radiation dosing in medical diagnostics and education for clinician and the public. Prevention includes individual risk assessment and medical imaging using dosing "As Low As Reasonably Achievable" (ALARA).

The American College of Radiology (ACR) provides "*ACR Appropriateness Criteria*," which are evidence-based guidelines created by expert panels to serve as a reference for best practices for imaging decisions by health care providers (https://www.acr.org/Clinical-Resources/ACR-Appropriateness-Criteria). Clinicians and patients must carefully weigh the risks and benefits of radiation exposure when deciding on an imaging test.

Occupational & Environmental Radiation Exposure

Useful resources for professionals include the *CDC "Radiation Emergencies" website* (https://www.cdc.gov/nceh/radiation/emergencies/index.htm) and the *National Nuclear Security Administration's Radiation Emergency Assistance Center*, which provides 24-hour access to expert consultation services (telephone: 1-865-576-1005 or website: https://orise.orau.gov/reacts/index.html).

With the rising prominence of 5G systems, cellular, and computer device usage, there is cautious monitoring and research to assess risk of high-frequency and long-term exposure to radiofrequency electromagnetic fields (RF-EMF). The **International Commission on Non-Ionizing Radiation Protection (ICNIRP)** and the **IEEE** establish regulatory guidelines for exposure limits.

Treatment

Treatment is focused on decontamination, on management of coexisting conditions or injuries, and on supportive care. Specific supportive treatments are determined by the dose, route, and effects of exposure and associated conditions present.

Prognosis

Prognosis is determined by the radiation dose, duration, and frequency as well as by the underlying condition of the patient. Death following acute radiation exposure is usually due to hematopoietic failure, mucosal damage, CNS damage, widespread vascular injury, or secondary infection.

Carcinogenesis is related to the radiation type, total dose, duration, and accumulated exposure, and to the susceptibility of the patient. Radiation-related cancer risks persist throughout the exposed person's life span.

With the increased use of ionizing radiation for medical diagnostics and treatments, there is an iatrogenic increase in radiation-induced cancer risks. There are age-related sensitivities to radiation; pregnant women and younger persons are more susceptible to carcinogenesis.

When to Admit

Most patients with significant ionizing radiation exposure require admission for close monitoring and supportive treatment.

Arnautou P et al. Management of acute radiation syndrome. Transfus Clin Biol. 2024;31:253. [PMID: 39025400]

Berrington de Gonzalez A et al. Epidemiological studies of CT scans and cancer risk: the state of the science. Br J Radiol. 2021;94:20210471. [PMID: 34545766]

Chen J et al. Radiation exposure in recurrent medical imaging: identifying drivers and high-risk populations. Front Public Health. 2025;13:1626906. [PMID: 40756407]

Melnick RL et al; International Commission on the Biological Effects of Electromagnetic Fields (ICBE-EMF). The WHO-commissioned systematic reviews on health effects of radiofrequency radiation provide no assurance of safety. Environ Health. 2025;24:70. [PMID: 41034851]

ENVIRONMENTAL DISORDERS RELATED TO ALTITUDE

DYSBARISM & DECOMPRESSION SICKNESS

ESSENTIALS OF DIAGNOSIS

- Early recognition of symptoms temporally related to recent large changes in altitude or pressure and prompt treatment of decompression illness are extremely important for optimal outcome.
- Patients with decompression illness must also be assessed for hypothermia, trauma, hypoglycemia, and other medical conditions.
- Decompression illness must be considered if symptoms are temporally related to recent diving or rapid changes in altitude or pressure within 48 hours after surfacing.
- Consultation with diving medicine or hyperbaric oxygen specialist is indicated.

General Considerations

Dysbarism and decompression illness may result from altitude changes and effects of environmental pressure on the gases in the body. These are more likely to occur when scuba diving is followed closely by rapid ascent, or when the scuba diver is not adherent to the conservative dive guidelines for dive duration, course, depth, and surface times between dives.

As a diver descends, the gases in the body compress and dissolve throughout areas of the body that are both compressible (lungs, GI tract) and noncompressible (sinuses, joints). As the diver descends further, the increased pressure on the body's gases increases the amounts of gases dissolved into the bloodstream and tissues. During the dive ascent, these dissolved gases expand within the body, which can cause dysbarism and decompression illness.

Dysbarism results from barotrauma when gas compression or expansion occurs in parts of the body that are noncompressible or have limited compliance. **Pulmonary overinflation syndrome** is one of the most serious and potentially fatal results of barotrauma. This syndrome is due to an inappropriately rapid ascent causing alveoli rupture and air bubble extravasation into the vital organs or the cerebral circulation.

Decompression illness occurs when the pressure change from higher pressure to lower pressure is too rapid causing gas bubbles to form and cause damage to their location in the body. Decompression illness symptoms depend on the released gas bubbles' size, number, and location. Scuba diving risk of decompression illness depends on multiple factors: the dive details (depth, duration, number of dives, interval surface time between dives, and water conditions). Patient factors include age, weight, overall health, physical condition, physical exertion, the rate of ascent, and the length of time between the low altitude and high altitude. Predisposing factors include obesity, injury, hypoxia, lung, or cardiac disease, right to left cardiac shunt, dehydration, alcohol and medication effects, and stress response. Decompression illness may also occur in those who take hot showers after cold dives.

Preventive measures include pre-dive medical screening and dive planning; diver education and training; strict adherence to dive course, timing, and depths; and a slow and controlled ascent with proper control of buoyancy. Conservative recommendation is to *avoid high altitudes (ground ascent or air travel) for at least 24 hours after surfacing* from the dive, especially following multiple dives. Physiologic monitoring can be useful in prevention and early detection.

Clinical Findings

Clinical manifestations depend on the location of the gas bubble formation or the compressibility of gases in the body. Symptom onset may be immediate or within minutes or hours (up to 48 hours later). Decompression illness symptoms are wide-ranging: pain in the joints; skin pruritus or burning; cardiac; neurologic (symptoms may or may not follow typical neuroanatomic distribution patterns); respiratory compromise; pain in ears or sinuses, or both; coma; and death.

Decompression illness involving the brain and spinal cord may occur due to air bubbles causing arterial occlusion, venous obstruction, or in situ toxicity.

The initial assessment must include assessment of associated conditions of hypothermia, hypoglycemia, hypovolemia, aspiration, near-drowning, trauma, envenomation, and concurrent medical conditions.

Treatment

Early recognition and prompt treatment are extremely important including consultation with diving medicine or hyperbaric oxygen specialists. Decompression illness must be considered if symptoms arise temporally related to recent diving or rapid changes in altitude or pressure within the past 48 hours. Continuous administration of 100% oxygen is indicated and beneficial for all patients. Hyperbaric oxygen treatment is the mainstay of treatment recommended for decompression illness symptoms. Immediate consultation with a diving medicine or hyperbaric oxygen specialist is indicated even if mild decompression illness symptoms resolve. NSAIDs, acetaminophen, or aspirin may be given for pain control if there are no contraindications. Opioids must be used very cautiously since these may obscure the response to recompression.

When to Admit

Rapid transportation to a hyperbaric treatment facility for recompression is imperative since this is the recommended treatment by specialists. The *Divers Alert Network* is an excellent worldwide resource for emergency advice 24 hours daily for the management of diving-related conditions (https://dan.org/).

Beatty P et al. Physiological monitoring to prevent diving disorders. Front Physiol. 2024;15:1517361. [PMID: 39744705]

Tello Montoliu A et al. Cardiovascular considerations on recreational scuba diving. SEC-Clinical Cardiology Association/SEC-Working Group on Sports Cardiology consensus document. Rev Esp Cardiol (Engl Ed). 2024;77:566. [PMID: 38580141]

Vezzoli A et al. Oxy-inflammation in humans during underwater activities. Int J Mol Sci. 2024;25:3060. [PMID: 38474303]

HIGH-ALTITUDE ILLNESS

ESSENTIALS OF DIAGNOSIS

- The severity of high-altitude illness is affected by the rate and height of ascent and the individual's susceptibility.
- Prompt recognition and medical treatment of early findings of high-altitude illness may prevent progression.
- Clinicians must assess for conditions that may coexist or mimic symptoms of high-altitude illness.
- Immediate descent is the definitive treatment for **high-altitude cerebral edema (HACE)** and **high-altitude pulmonary edema (HAPE).**

General Considerations

As altitude increases, there is a decrease in both barometric pressure and oxygen partial pressure resulting in hypobaric hypoxia. High-altitude illnesses are due to hypobaric hypoxia at high altitudes (usually > 2000 meters or 6562 feet). High-altitude illnesses include a spectrum of disorders categorized by end-organ effects (mostly cerebral and pulmonary) and exposure duration. Acute high-altitude illnesses are **acute hypoxia, acute mountain sickness (AMS), high-altitude cerebral edema (HACE),** and **high-altitude pulmonary edema (HAPE).** Diagnosis is based on clinical features with cautious exclusion of other diagnoses.

Acclimatization occurs over time as a physiologic response to the increasing altitude and increasing hypobaric hypoxia. *High-altitude illness results when the hypoxic stress is greater than the individual's ability to acclimatize.* The key determinants of high-altitude illness risk and severity include both individual susceptibility factors and altitudinal factors, such as rate and height of ascent and total change in altitude over time. Risk factors for high altitude illness include inadequate education and preparation, individual susceptibility, previous high-altitude illness, and increased physical activity with insufficient acclimatization.

Individual susceptibility factors include underlying conditions such as genetics, medications, social habits, and preexisting medical conditions. Those with symptomatic neurologic, cardiovascular, or pulmonary disease must avoid high altitudes.

Patient assessment for high-altitude illness must also include evaluation for other conditions, which may coexist or may present in a similar manner.

1. High-Altitude–Associated Neurologic Conditions: AMS & HACE

There is a spectrum of neurologic conditions caused by high altitude, ranging from AMS to HACE, the most serious form.

AMS includes symptoms such as headache (the most severe and persistent symptom), lassitude, drowsiness, dizziness, chilliness, nausea and vomiting, and difficulty sleeping. Later symptoms include irritability, difficulty concentrating, anorexia, insomnia, and increased headaches.

HACE includes the severe symptoms of AMS plus the results of cerebral vasogenic edema and cerebral cellular hypoxia. This usually occurs at elevations above 2500 meters (8202 feet) but may occur at lower elevations. HACE hallmarks are altered mental status, ataxia, severe lassitude, and encephalopathy. Examination findings may include confusion, ataxia, urinary retention or incontinence, focal neurologic deficits, papilledema, and seizures. Symptoms may progress to obtundation, coma, and death.

Treatment

Definitive treatment is immediate descent of at least 610 meters (2001 feet), and then continued descent until symptoms improve. Descent is essential if symptoms are persistent, severe, or worsening, or in the setting of HACE or HAPE. If immediate descent is not possible, portable hyperbaric chambers can provide symptomatic relief but must not delay descent.

Initial treatment involves oxygen administration to keep the pulse oximetry S_pO_2 > 90% and medications. Acetazolamide is an effective medication for both prophylaxis and treatment of mild symptoms of AMS. Dexamethasone is given for moderate to severe AMS. Dexamethasone is also the primary treatment for HACE. Acetazolamide can be added as an adjunct in severe HACE cases. Typically, symptoms resolve within 24–48 hours. HACE treatment must continue for at least 24 hours after resolution of symptoms or until descent is completed. Dexamethasone should not be given for longer than 7 days.

It is imperative for the clinician to assess for HAPE and other conditions which may mimic or coexist with AMS and HACE. If HAPE symptoms and signs are present along with HACE, nifedipine or a selective phosphodiesterase inhibitor may be added with caution for pulmonary vasodilation.

2. Acute HAPE

HAPE is the leading cause of death from high-altitude illness. The hallmark is markedly elevated pulmonary artery pressure followed by pulmonary edema. Early symptoms may appear within a few hours up to 36 hours after ascent to high-altitude. HAPE symptoms include incessant dry cough, headache, dyspnea disproportionate to exertion, decreased exercise performance, fatigue, dyspnea at rest, and chest tightness. Strenuous exertion must be avoided. As pulmonary edema progresses, wheezing, orthopnea, and hemoptysis may develop.

Physical findings may include hypoxia, tachycardia, mild fever, tachypnea, cyanosis, rales, wheezing, and rhonchi. The clinician must assess for other potential medical conditions that may mimic or coexist. Diagnosis is usually clinical; tests are nonspecific. Prompt recognition and medical attention to early symptoms of HAPE may prevent progression.

Treatment

Immediate descent (at least 610 meters [2000 feet]) is essential, although this may not be immediately possible and may not alone improve symptoms.

The patient must be placed at rest, reclined with head elevated, with oxygen administration to keep the pulse oximetry S_pO_2 > 90%. Recompression in portable hyperbaric chambers will reduce symptoms but must not delay rapid or immediate descent.

If descent, oxygen, or portable hyperbaric chambers are not available or successful, nifedipine can be used as an adjunct. Selective phosphodiesterase inhibitors may provide effective symptom relief as an alternative or if nifedipine is not available, and these also may be used for HAPE prevention. Administering both nifedipine plus a phosphodiesterase inhibitor as pulmonary vasodilators is *not* recommended. Treatment for ARDS (see Chapter 9) is required for some patients. If neurologic symptoms are present concurrently with HAPE and do not resolve with improved oxygenation, dexamethasone may be added per HACE treatment guidelines.

There is an international effort to advance the understanding of HAPE through the research and database registry (https://www.altitude.org).

Prevention of High-Altitude Disorders

Pre-trip preventive measures include participant education, medical evaluation, pre-trip planning, optimal physical conditioning before travel, and adequate rest and sleep the day before travel and during the trip. Preventive efforts during ascent include reduced food intake, avoidance of alcohol and tobacco, and limiting any unnecessary physical activity during travel.

Gradual ascent is the most effective way to allow acclimatization. Low-risk ascension rate is 2 or more days to arrive at 2500–3000 meters. *The altitude reached during waking hours is not as important as the altitude at which the hiker sleeps.*

Medication prophylaxis may be prescribed for AMS and HACE if no contraindications exist. Prophylactic low-dose acetazolamide has been shown to reduce the incidence and severity of AMS and HACE when started 3 days prior to ascent and continued for 48–72 hours at high altitude. Dexamethasone is an alternative prophylactic medication for AMS and HACE.

Individuals with a history of HAPE should use medication prophylaxis to reduce the risk of recurrence. Nifedipine started the day before ascent and continued through the fourth day at target elevation, or through the seventh day if the ascent rate was faster, is recommended. As an adjunct to nifedipine, salmeterol can be added beginning 24 hours prior to ascent.

Phosphodiesterase inhibitors may be beneficial in the treatment of HAPE based on their physiologic effects of decreased pulmonary arterial pressures and pulmonary vasodilation.

When to Admit

- All patients with HACE or HAPE must be hospitalized for further observation.
- Hospitalization must also be considered for any patient who remains symptomatic after treatment and descent.
- Pulmonary symptoms and hypoxia may be worsened by complications requiring admission.

Gatterer H et al. Altitude illnesses. Nat Rev Dis Primers. 2024;10:43. [PMID: 38902312]

Luks AM et al. Wilderness Medical Society clinical practice guidelines for the prevention, diagnosis, and treatment of acute altitude illness: 2024 update. Wilderness & Environmental Medicine. 2023;35:2S. [PMID: 37833187]

Richalet JP et al. Cardiovascular physiology and pathophysiology at high altitude. Nat Rev Cardiol. 2024;21:75. [PMID: 37783743]

van Veelen MJ et al. Emergency care for high-altitude trekking and climbing. High Alt Med Biol. 2025;26:70. [PMID: 39073038]

Wang B et al. Recent advances in predicting acute mountain sickness: from multidimensional cohort studies to cutting-edge model applications. Front Physiol. 2024;15:1397280. [PMID: 38978820]

SAFETY OF AIR TRAVEL & SELECTION OF PATIENTS FOR AIR TRAVEL

The medical safety of air travel depends on the nature and severity of the traveler's preflight condition and factors such as travel duration and frequency of travel, in-flight exercise type and frequency, cabin altitude pressure, onboard medical supplies, infectious diseases, and the presence of health care professionals on board. Air travel has been associated with an increased risk of transmission of infectious diseases. A WHO website includes the most updated information on travel health risks and infectious diseases (https://www.who.int/travel-advice). Flight crews and passengers are susceptible to a wide range of flight-related problems: pulmonary, VTE, cardiac, GI, ocular, immunologic, infectious, syncope, neuropsychiatric, metabolic, trauma, radiation, and substance-related conditions. Air travel risks are higher for air travelers with preexisting medical conditions.

Hypobaric hypoxia is the underlying etiology of most serious medical emergencies in-flight due to cabin altitude. Despite commercial aircraft pressurization requirements, there is significant hypoxemia, dyspnea, gas expansion, and stress in travelers, particularly in those with underlying pulmonary disease.

Any form of prolonged travel involving immobilization is associated with increased risk of VTE. Risks for VTE in long-distance travelers include the following: (1) travel time of 4 or more hours, (2) hypercoagulable disorders, and (3) acquired risks. VTE risk is more relevant for those with additional VTE risk factors. VTE prevention measures include wearing graduated compression stockings; frequent exercise and position changes during travel; and in high-risk travelers, the use of thromboprophylaxis.

Air travel is not advised for anyone who is "incapacitated" or has any "unstable conditions." The Air Transport Association of America defines an incapacitated passenger as "one who is suffering from a physical or mental disability and who, because of such disability or the effect of the flight on the disability, is incapable of self-care; would endanger the health or safety of such person or other passengers or airline employees; or would cause discomfort or annoyance of other passengers." Unstable conditions include any condition requiring active treatment immediately.

Pregnancy

Pregnant travelers have unique travel-related and location-specific risks. A clinician's authorization is required if travel is essential during the ninth month of pregnancy or earlier in a complicated or high-risk pregnancy.

Long travel increases risk of VTE for the pregnant traveler. Pregnant travelers are also at higher risk from infection transmission and air travel radiation exposure.

Prevention

Air travel complications may be reduced by the following preventive measures: passenger prescreening, passenger education, and in-flight positioning and activity. Prescreening evaluation is recommended for all high-risk patients including preexisting requirement for oxygen, underlying lung disease, comorbidities worsened by hypoxemia, previous respiratory distress during air travel, recent pneumothorax, and recent (within 6 weeks) acute respiratory illness. Patients at risk for hypoxia must be assessed prior to air travel to determine if there is a need for supplemental in-flight oxygen.

Air travel education must include risk reduction for VTE, infectious diseases, and exacerbations of underlying medical conditions. Long-distance travelers can reduce VTE risk by avoiding constrictive clothing, staying well-hydrated, changing position frequently, avoiding cramped position and leg crossing, engaging in frequent (at least hourly) in-flight leg stretching exercises, and *walking for 5 minutes every hour*. Clinicians must assess those with high risk of VTE prior to air travel to determine whether anticoagulation is indicated (see Table 16–14).

Altundağ İ et al. Presentation, risk assessment, and clinical outcomes of patients with air travel-related emergencies in the emergency department. Am J Emerg Med. 2025;98:130. [PMID: 40865261]

Hodkinson PD et al. Implications of the hypobaric cabin environment during commercial air travel for passenger fitness to fly. Thorax. 2024;79:897. [PMID: 39153861]

Katoch T et al. Hearts in the sky: understanding the cardiovascular implications of air travel. Future Cardiol. 2024;20:651. [PMID: 39301896]

Papadakis E et al. Fright of long-haul flights: focus on travel-associated thrombosis. Semin Thromb Hemost. 2025;51:438. [PMID: 40015328]

Ram S et al. Air travel during pregnancy and the risk of venous thrombosis. Am J Obstet Gynecol MFM. 2023;5:100751. [PMID: 36115570]

42 Poisoning

Craig Smollin, MD

INITIAL EVALUATION: POISONING OR OVERDOSE

Patients with drug overdoses or poisoning may initially have no symptoms or they may have varying degrees of overt intoxication. The asymptomatic patient may have been exposed to or may have ingested a lethal dose, but not yet exhibit any manifestations of toxicity. It is important to *(1) quickly assess the potential danger, (2) consider gut and skin decontamination to prevent absorption, (3) treat complications if they occur, and (4) observe the asymptomatic patient for an appropriate interval.*

Assess the Danger

If the drug or poison is known, its danger can be assessed by consulting a text or computerized information resource or by calling a **regional poison control center.** (In the United States, dialing **1-800-222-1222** will direct the call to the regional poison control center.) Assessment considers the dose ingested; the time since ingestion; the presence of any symptoms or clinical signs; preexisting cardiac, respiratory, kidney, or liver disease; and, occasionally, specific serum drug or toxin levels. Be aware that the history given by the patient or family may be incomplete or unreliable.

IMMEDIATE 24-HOUR TOXICOLOGY CONSULTATION

Call your **regional poison control center**
US toll-free **1-800-222-1222**

Observe the Patient

Asymptomatic or mildly symptomatic patients should be observed for at least 4–6 hours. Longer observation is indicated if the ingested substance is a sustained-release preparation or is known to slow GI motility (eg, opioids, anticholinergics, aspirin) or may cause a delayed onset of symptoms (eg, acetaminophen, colchicine, hepatotoxic mushrooms). After that time, the patient may be discharged if no symptoms have developed. *Before discharge, psychiatric evaluation should be performed to assess suicide risk.* Intentional ingestions in adolescents should raise the possibility of unwanted pregnancy or sexual abuse.

THE SYMPTOMATIC PATIENT

In symptomatic patients, treatment of life-threatening complications takes precedence over in-depth diagnostic evaluation. Patients with mild symptoms may deteriorate rapidly; therefore, *all potentially significant exposures should be observed in an acute care facility.* The following complications may occur, depending on the type of poisoning.

COMA

Assessment & Complications

Coma is commonly associated with ingestion of large doses of antihistamines (eg, diphenhydramine), benzodiazepines and other sedative-hypnotic drugs, ethanol, opioids, antipsychotic drugs, or antidepressants. The most common cause of death in comatose patients is respiratory failure, which may occur abruptly. Pulmonary aspiration of gastric contents may also occur, especially in patients who are deeply obtunded or convulsing. Hypoxia and hypoventilation may cause or aggravate hypotension, arrhythmias, and seizures. Thus, *protection of the airway and assisted ventilation are the most important treatment measures for any poisoned patient.*

Treatment

A. Emergency Management

The initial emergency management of coma can be remembered by the mnemonic ***ABCD***, for **Airway**, ***Breathing***, **Circulation**, and ***Drugs*** (thiamine, then dextrose and naloxone), respectively.

1. Airway—Establish a patent airway by positioning, suction, or insertion of an artificial nasal or oropharyngeal airway. If the patient is deeply comatose or if airway reflexes are depressed, perform endotracheal intubation. These airway interventions may not be necessary if the patient is intoxicated by an opioid and responds to intravenous naloxone.

2. Breathing—Clinically assess the quality and depth of respiration and provide assistance, if necessary, with a bag-valve-mask device or mechanical ventilator. Administer supplemental oxygen, if needed. The arterial or venous blood CO_2 tension, or noninvasive end-tidal CO_2 monitoring, is useful in determining the adequacy of ventilation. The arterial blood PO_2 determination may reveal hypoxemia, which may be caused by respiratory depression, bronchospasm, pulmonary aspiration, or noncardiogenic pulmonary edema. *Pulse oximetry provides an assessment of oxygenation but is unreliable in patients with methemoglobinemia or carbon monoxide poisoning.*

3. Circulation—Measure the pulse and blood pressure and estimate tissue perfusion (eg, by measurement of urinary output, skin signs, arterial blood pH). Place the patient on continuous ECG monitoring. Insert an intravenous line, and draw blood for glucose, electrolytes, serum creatinine and liver tests, and possible quantitative toxicologic testing.

4. Drugs—

A. DEXTROSE AND THIAMINE—Unless promptly treated, severe hypoglycemia can cause irreversible brain damage. Therefore, *in all obtunded, comatose, or convulsing patients, give 50% dextrose, 50–100 mL by intravenous bolus, unless a rapid point-of-care blood glucose test rules out hypoglycemia.* In patients with alcohol use disorder or malnourishment who may have marginal thiamine stores, give thiamine, 100 mg intramuscularly, *before* the dextrose, or in the intravenous fluids.

B. OPIOID ANTAGONISTS—Naloxone, 0.4–2 mg intravenously or 2–4 mg by intranasal spray, may reverse opioid-induced respiratory depression and coma. *It is often given empirically to any comatose patient with depressed respirations.* If opioid overdose is strongly suspected, give additional doses of naloxone (up to 5–10 mg may be required to reverse the effects of potent opioids). **Note:** *Naloxone has a shorter duration of action (2–3 hours) than most common opioids; repeated doses may be required, and continuous observation for at least 3–4 hours after the last dose is mandatory.*

C. FLUMAZENIL—Flumazenil, 0.2–0.5 mg intravenously, repeated as needed up to a maximum of 3 mg, may reverse benzodiazepine-induced coma. **Caution:** *In most circumstances, use of flumazenil is not advised as the potential risks outweigh its benefits.*

HYPOTHERMIA

Assessment & Complications

Hypothermia commonly accompanies coma due to opioids, ethanol, hypoglycemic agents, phenothiazines, barbiturates, benzodiazepines, and other sedative-hypnotics and CNS depressants. Hypothermic patients may have a barely perceptible pulse and blood pressure. Hypothermia may cause or aggravate hypotension, which will not reverse until the temperature is normalized.

Treatment

Treatment of hypothermia is discussed in Chapter 41. Gradual rewarming is preferred unless the patient is in cardiac arrest.

HYPOTENSION

Assessment & Complications

Hypotension may be due to poisoning by many different drugs, including antihypertensives, β-blockers, calcium channel blockers, disulfiram (ethanol interaction), iron, trazodone, quetiapine, and other antipsychotic agents and antidepressants. Poisons causing hypotension include cyanide, carbon monoxide, hydrogen sulfide, aluminum or zinc phosphide, arsenic, and certain mushrooms.

Hypotension in the poisoned or drug-overdosed patient may be caused by venous or arteriolar vasodilation, hypovolemia, depressed cardiac contractility, or a combination of these effects.

Treatment

Most hypotensive poisoned patients respond to empiric treatment with repeated 200 mL intravenous boluses of 0.9% saline or other isotonic crystalloid up to a total of 1–2 L; much larger amounts may be needed if the patient is profoundly volume-depleted (eg, as with massive diarrhea due to *Amanita phalloides* mushroom poisoning). Monitoring the CVP using bedside cardiac ultrasound can help determine whether further fluid therapy is needed. If fluid therapy is not successful after adequate volume replacement, give vasopressors by intravenous infusion.

Hypotension caused by certain toxins may respond to specific treatment. For hypotension caused by overdoses of tricyclic antidepressants or other sodium channel blockers, administer sodium bicarbonate, 50–100 mEq by intravenous bolus injection. Norepinephrine 4–8 mcg/min by intravenous infusion is more effective than dopamine in some patients with overdoses of tricyclic antidepressants or of drugs with predominantly vasodilating effects. For β-blocker overdose, glucagon (5–10 mg intravenously) may be of value. For calcium channel blocker overdose, administer calcium chloride, 1–2 g intravenously (repeated doses may be necessary; doses of 5–10 g and more have been given in some cases). High-dose insulin (0.5–1 U/kg/hour intravenously) euglycemic therapy may also be used (see the sections Beta-Adrenergic Blockers and Calcium Channel Blockers, below). Intralipid 20% lipid emulsion has been reported to improve hemodynamics in some cases of intoxication by highly lipid-soluble drugs such as bupivacaine, bupropion, clomipramine, and verapamil. Intravenous methylene blue and extracorporeal membrane oxygenation (ECMO) have been employed in some refractory cases; ECMO may offer temporary hemodynamic stabilization while the offending drug is eliminated.

Cao D et al. Part 10: Adult and pediatric special circumstances of resuscitation: 2025 American Heart Association guidelines for cardiopulmonary resuscitation and emergency cardiovascular care. Circulation. 2025;152:S578. [PMID: 41122889]

Kaiser SK et al. The roles of antidotes in emergency situations. Emerg Med Clin North Am. 2022;40:381. [PMID: 35461629]
Kim HK et al. Veno-venous extracorporeal membrane oxygenation (VV-ECMO) for acute poisonings in United States: a retrospective analysis of the Extracorporeal Life Support Organization Registry. Clin Toxicol (Phila). 2025;63:204. [PMID: 39868599]
Lee SH et al. Lipid emulsion treatment for drug toxicity caused by nonlocal anesthetic drugs in pediatric patients: a narrative review. Pediatr Emerg Care. 2023;39:53. [PMID: 35981328]

HYPERTENSION

Assessment & Complications

Hypertension may be due to poisoning with amphetamines and synthetic stimulants, anticholinergics, cocaine, performance-enhancing products (eg, containing caffeine, phenylephrine, ephedrine, or yohimbine), MAO inhibitors, and other drugs.

Severe hypertension (eg, diastolic blood pressure > 105–110 mm Hg in a person who does not have chronic hypertension) can result in acute intracranial hemorrhage, MI, or aortic dissection.

Treatment

Treat hypertension if the patient is symptomatic or if the diastolic pressure is higher than 105–110 mm Hg—especially if there is no prior history of hypertension.

Hypertensive patients who are agitated or anxious may benefit from a sedative (such as lorazepam, 2–3 mg intravenously) or an antipsychotic drug (eg, haloperidol or olanzapine). For persistent hypertension, administer phentolamine, 2–5 mg intravenously, or nitroprusside sodium, 0.25–8 mcg/kg/min intravenously. If excessive tachycardia is present, *add* esmolol, 25–100 mcg/kg/min intravenously, or labetalol, 0.2–0.3 mg/kg intravenously. **Caution:** *Do not give β-blockers alone, since doing so may paradoxically worsen hypertension in some cases as a result of unopposed α-adrenergic stimulation.*

ARRHYTHMIAS

Assessment & Complications

Arrhythmias may occur with a variety of drugs or toxins (Table 42–1). They may also occur from hypoxia, metabolic acidosis, or electrolyte imbalance (eg, hyperkalemia, hypokalemia, hypomagnesemia, or hypocalcemia), or following exposure to chlorinated and fluorinated solvents and propellants. Polymorphic ventricular tachycardia (torsades de pointes) is often associated with drugs that prolong the QT interval.

Treatment

Hypoxia or electrolyte imbalance should be sought and treated. If ventricular arrhythmias persist, administer lidocaine or amiodarone at usual antiarrhythmic doses. **Note:** *Wide QRS complex tachycardia in the setting of tricyclic antidepressant overdose (or diphenhydramine or class Ia antiarrhythmic drugs) should be treated with sodium bicarbonate, 50–100 mEq intravenously by bolus infusion.* **Caution:** *In such cases, avoid class Ia antiarrhythmic agents (eg, procainamide, disopyramide) and amiodarone, which may aggravate arrhythmias caused by tricyclic antidepressants.* Torsades de pointes associated with prolonged QT interval may respond to intravenous magnesium (2 g intravenously over 2 minutes) or overdrive pacing. Treat digitalis-induced arrhythmias with digoxin-specific antibodies.

For tachyarrhythmias induced by chlorinated or fluorinated solvents, chloral hydrate, Freons, or sympathomimetic agents, use propranolol or esmolol (see doses in the Hypertension section, above).

Table 42–1. Common toxins or drugs causing arrhythmias (listed in alphabetical order by arrhythmia).[1]

Arrhythmia	Common Causes
Atrioventricular block	β-Blockers, calcium channel blockers, class Ia antiarrhythmics (including quinidine), carbamazepine, clonidine, digitalis glycosides, lithium
QT interval prolongation and torsades de pointes	Arsenic, class Ia and class III antiarrhythmics, citalopram, droperidol, lithium, methadone, pentamidine, sertraline, sotalol, and many other drugs[2]
Sinus bradycardia	β-Blockers, calcium channel blockers, clonidine, digitalis glycosides, organophosphates
Sinus tachycardia	β-Agonists (eg, albuterol), amphetamines, anticholinergics, antihistamines, caffeine, cocaine, pseudoephedrine, tricyclic and other antidepressants
Ventricular premature beats and ventricular tachycardia	Amphetamines, cocaine, ephedrine, caffeine, chlorinated or fluorinated hydrocarbons, digoxin, aconite (found in some Chinese herbal preparations), fluoride, theophylline. QT prolongation can lead to atypical ventricular tachycardia (torsades de pointes)
Wide QRS complex	Class Ia and class Ic antiarrhythmics, phenothiazines (eg, thioridazine), potassium (hyperkalemia), propranolol, tricyclic antidepressants, bupropion, lamotrigine, diphenhydramine (severe overdose)

[1]Arrhythmias may also occur as a result of hypoxia, metabolic acidosis, or electrolyte imbalance (eg, hyperkalemia or hypokalemia, hypocalcemia, hypomagnesemia).
[2]https://crediblemeds.org/

SEIZURES

Assessment & Complications

Seizures may be caused by many poisons and drugs, including amphetamines, antidepressants (especially tricyclic antidepressants, bupropion, and venlafaxine), antihistamines (especially diphenhydramine), antipsychotics, camphor, synthetic cannabinoids and cathinones, cocaine, isoniazid (INH), chlorinated insecticides, piperazines, tramadol, and theophylline. The onset of seizures may be delayed for up to 18–24 hours after extended-released bupropion overdose.

Seizures may also be caused by hypoxia, hypoglycemia, hypocalcemia, hyponatremia, withdrawal from alcohol or sedative-hypnotics, head trauma, CNS infection, or idiopathic epilepsy.

Prolonged or repeated seizures may lead to hypoxia, metabolic acidosis, hyperthermia, and rhabdomyolysis.

Treatment

Administer lorazepam, 2–3 mg, or diazepam, 5–10 mg, intravenously, or—if intravenous access is not immediately available—midazolam, 5–10 mg intramuscularly. If convulsions continue, administer phenobarbital, 15–20 mg/kg slowly intravenously over no less than 30 minutes. (For drug-induced seizures, phenobarbital is the preferred agent.) Levetiracetam and propofol infusion have also been reported effective for some resistant drug-induced seizures.

Seizures due to a few drugs and toxins may require antidotes or other specific therapies (as listed in Table 42–2).

Kishihara Y et al. Efficacy of second-line anticonvulsant agents with adult status epilepticus: a systematic review and network meta-analysis. Am J Emerg Med. 2024;82:183. [PMID: 38941904]

Table 42–2. Seizures related to toxins or drugs requiring special consideration (listed in alphabetical order by toxin or drug).[1]

Toxin or Drug	Comments
Isoniazid	Administer pyridoxine.
Lithium	May indicate need for hemodialysis.
Methylenedioxymethamphetamine (MDMA; "Ecstasy")	Seizures may also be due to hyponatremia or hyperthermia.
Organophosphates	Administer pralidoxime (2-PAM) and atropine in addition to usual anticonvulsants.
Strychnine	"Seizures" are actually spinally mediated muscle spasms and usually require neuromuscular paralysis and mechanical ventilation.
Theophylline	Seizures indicate need for hemodialysis.
Tricyclic antidepressants	Hyperthermia and cardiotoxicity are common complications of repeated seizures; paralyze early with neuromuscular blockers to reduce muscular hyperactivity.

[1]See text for dosages.

HYPERTHERMIA

Assessment & Complications

Hyperthermia may be associated with poisoning by amphetamines and other synthetic stimulants (cathinones, piperazines), atropine and other anticholinergic drugs, cocaine, salicylates, strychnine, 2,4 dinitrophenol, tricyclic antidepressants, and various other medications. Overdoses of serotonin reuptake inhibitors (eg, fluoxetine, paroxetine, sertraline) or their use in a patient taking an MAO inhibitor may cause agitation, hyperactivity, myoclonus, and hyperthermia (**"serotonin syndrome"**). Antipsychotic agents can cause rigidity and hyperthermia (**neuroleptic malignant syndrome**). (See Chapter 28.) **Malignant hyperthermia** is a rare disorder associated with general anesthetic agents.

Hyperthermia is a rapidly life-threatening complication. Severe hyperthermia (temperature > 40–41°C) can rapidly cause brain damage and multiorgan failure, including rhabdomyolysis, AKI, and coagulopathy (see Chapter 41).

Treatment

Treat hyperthermia aggressively. Options for cooling include spraying the skin with tepid water, and high-volume fanning, or alternatively, placing the patient in an ice water bath (not simply applying ice to selected surfaces). If external cooling is not rapidly effective, as shown by a normal rectal temperature within 20–30 minutes, or if there is significant muscle rigidity or hyperactivity, induce neuromuscular paralysis with a nondepolarizing neuromuscular blocker (eg, rocuronium, vecuronium). Once paralyzed, the patient must be intubated and mechanically ventilated and sedated. While the patient is paralyzed, the absence of visible muscular convulsive movements may give the false impression that brain seizure activity has ceased; bedside electroencephalography may be useful in recognizing continued nonconvulsive seizures.

Dantrolene (2–5 mg/kg intravenously) may be effective for hyperthermia associated with muscle rigidity that does not respond to neuromuscular blockade (ie, malignant hyperthermia). Bromocriptine, 2.5–7.5 mg orally daily, has been recommended for neuroleptic malignant syndrome. Cyproheptadine, 4 mg orally every hour for three or four doses, or chlorpromazine, 25 mg intravenously or 50 mg intramuscularly, has been used to treat serotonin syndrome.

Mikkelsen N et al. Serotonin syndrome-a focused review. Basic Clin Pharmacol Toxicol. 2023;133:124. [PMID: 37309284]
Sorensen C et al. Treatment and prevention of heat-related illness. N Engl J Med. 2022;387:1404. [PMID: 36170473]
Wijdicks EFM et al. Neuroleptic malignant syndrome. N Engl J Med. 2024;391:1130. [PMID: 39321364]

ANTIDOTES & OTHER TREATMENT

ANTIDOTES

Give an antidote (if available) when there is reasonable certainty of a specific diagnosis (Table 42–3). Be aware that some antidotes themselves may have serious side effects.

Table 42–3. Some toxic agents for which there are specific antidotes (listed in alphabetical order by toxic agent).[1]

Toxic Agent	Specific Antidote
Acetaminophen	*N*-acetylcysteine
Anticholinergics (eg, atropine)	Physostigmine
Anticholinesterases (eg, organophosphate pesticides)	Atropine and pralidoxime (2-PAM)
Benzodiazepines	Flumazenil (rarely used)[2]
Carbon monoxide	Oxygen (hyperbaric oxygen of uncertain benefit)
Cyanide	Sodium nitrite, sodium thiosulfate; hydroxocobalamin
Digitalis glycosides	Digoxin-specific Fab antibodies
Heavy metals (eg, lead, mercury, iron) and arsenic	Specific chelating agents
Isoniazid	Pyridoxine (vitamin B_6)
Methanol, ethylene glycol	Ethanol (ethyl alcohol) or fomepizole (4-methylpyrazole)
Opioids	Naloxone, nalmefene
Snake venom	Specific antivenin
Sulfonylurea oral hypoglycemic drugs	Glucose, octreotide

[1]See text for indications and dosages.
[2]May induce seizures in patients with preexisting seizure disorder, benzodiazepine addiction, or concomitant tricyclic antidepressant or other convulsant overdose. If seizures occur, diazepam and other benzodiazepine anticonvulsants will not be effective. As with naloxone, the duration of action of flumazenil is short (2–3 hours) and resedation may occur, requiring repeated doses.

The indications and dosages for specific antidotes are discussed in the respective sections for specific toxins.

Kaiser SK et al. The roles of antidotes in emergency situations. Emerg Med Clin North Am. 2022;40:381. [PMID: 35461629]

DECONTAMINATION OF THE SKIN

Corrosive agents rapidly injure the skin and eyes and must be removed immediately. In addition, many toxins are readily absorbed through the skin, and systemic absorption can be prevented only by rapid action.

Wash the affected areas with copious quantities of lukewarm water or saline, taking care to limit exposure to health care providers. Wash carefully behind the ears, under the nails, and in skin folds. For oily substances (eg, pesticides), wash the skin at least twice with plain soap and shampoo the hair. *Specific decontaminating solutions or solvents (eg, alcohol) are rarely indicated and in some cases may paradoxically enhance absorption.* For exposure to chemical warfare poisons such as nerve agents or vesicants, some authorities recommend use of a dilute hypochlorite solution (household bleach diluted 1:10 with water), but not in the eyes.

DECONTAMINATION OF THE EYES

Act quickly to prevent serious damage. Flush the eyes with copious amounts of saline or water. (If available, instill local anesthetic drops in the eye before beginning irrigation.) Remove contact lenses if present. Lift the tarsal conjunctiva to look for undissolved particles and to facilitate irrigation. Continue irrigation for 15 minutes or until each eye has been irrigated with at least 1 L of solution. If the toxin is an acid or a base, check the pH of the tears after irrigation, and continue irrigation until the pH is between 7 and 7.4. An amphoteric decontamination solution (Diphoterine, Prevor) is used in some countries for treatment of alkali injuries to the eye.

After irrigation is complete, perform a careful examination of the eye, using fluorescein and a slit lamp or Wood lamp to identify areas of corneal injury. Patients with serious conjunctival or corneal injury should be immediately referred to an ophthalmologist.

GASTROINTESTINAL DECONTAMINATION

Removal of ingested poisons by induced emesis or gastric lavage was a routine part of emergency treatment for decades. However, *prospective randomized studies have failed to demonstrate improved clinical outcome after gastric emptying.* For small or moderate ingestions of most substances, toxicologists often recommend oral **activated charcoal** alone without prior gastric emptying; in some cases, when the interval after ingestion has been > 1–2 hours and the ingestion is non–life-threatening, even charcoal is withheld (eg, if the estimated benefit is outweighed by the potential risk of pulmonary aspiration of charcoal). *Exceptions are large ingestions of anticholinergic compounds and salicylates, which often delay gastric emptying, and ingestion of sustained-release or enteric-coated tablets, which may remain intact for several hours. In these cases, delayed gut decontamination may be indicated.*

Gastric emptying is not generally used for ingestion of corrosive agents or petroleum distillates, because further esophageal injury or pulmonary aspiration may result. However, in certain cases, removal of the toxin may be more important than concern over possible complications. Consult a medical toxicologist or regional poison control center (1-800-222-1222) for advice.

A. Activated Charcoal

Activated charcoal effectively adsorbs almost all drugs and poisons. Poorly adsorbed substances include iron, lithium, potassium, sodium, mineral acids, and alcohols.

1. Indications—Activated charcoal can be used for prompt adsorption of drugs or toxins in the stomach and intestine. However, evidence of benefit in clinical studies is lacking. Administration of charcoal, especially if mixed with sorbitol, can provoke vomiting, which could lead to pulmonary aspiration in an obtunded patient.

2. Contraindications—Activated charcoal should *not* be used for comatose or convulsing patients unless it can be given by gastric tube and the airway is first protected by a cuffed endotracheal tube. It is also contraindicated for patients with ileus or intestinal obstruction or those who have ingested corrosives for whom endoscopy is planned.

3. Technique—Administer activated charcoal, 50–100 g orally or via gastric tube, mixed in aqueous slurry. Repeated doses may be given to ensure GI adsorption or to enhance elimination of some drugs.

B. Whole Bowel Irrigation

Whole bowel irrigation uses large volumes of a balanced polyethylene glycol-electrolyte solution to mechanically cleanse the entire intestinal tract. Because of the composition of the irrigating solution, there is no significant gain or loss of systemic fluids or electrolytes.

1. Indications—Whole bowel irrigation is particularly effective for massive iron ingestion in which intact tablets are visible on abdominal radiographs. It has also been used for ingestions of lithium, sustained-release and enteric-coated tablets, and swallowed drug-filled packets.

2. Contraindications—Do *not* use in patients with suspected intestinal obstruction. Use with caution in patients who are obtunded or have depressed airway protective reflexes.

3. Technique—Administer a balanced polyethylene glycol-electrolyte solution (CoLyte, GoLYTELY) into the stomach via gastric tube at a rate of 1–2 L/hour until the rectal effluent is clear. This may take several hours. It is most effective when patients can sit on a commode to pass the intestinal contents.

C. Increased Drug Removal

1. Urinary manipulation—*Forced diuresis is hazardous; the risk of complications (fluid overload, electrolyte imbalance) usually outweighs its benefits.* Some drugs (eg, salicylates, phenobarbital) are more rapidly excreted with an alkaline urine. To alkalinize the urine, add 100 mEq (two ampules) of sodium bicarbonate to 1 L of 5% dextrose in 0.225% saline (¼ normal saline), and infuse this solution intravenously at a rate of about 150–200 mL/hour. Acidification (sometimes promoted for amphetamines, phencyclidine) is not effective and should *not* be used.

2. Hemodialysis—The indications for dialysis are as follows: (1) known or suspected potentially lethal amounts of a dialyzable drug (Table 42–4); (2) poisoning with deep coma, apnea, severe hypotension, fluid and electrolyte or acid-base disturbance, or extreme body temperature changes that cannot be corrected by conventional measures; or (3) poisoning in patients with severe kidney, cardiac, pulmonary, or hepatic disease who will not be able to eliminate toxin by the usual mechanisms.

Continuous renal replacement therapy (including continuous venovenous hemodiafiltration and similar techniques) may be of benefit for elimination of some poisons and has the advantage of gradual removal of the toxin and correction of any accompanying acidosis. Its use has been reported in the management of a variety of poisonings, including lithium intoxication. The *Extracorporeal Treatments in Poisoning (EXTRIP) workgroup* publishes valuable summary recommendations for several important dialyzable toxins (see https://www.extrip-workgroup.org/recommendations).

Table 42–4. Recommended use of hemodialysis in selected poisonings (listed in alphabetical order).[1]

Poison	Common Indications[1]
Carbamazepine	Seizures, severe cardiotoxicity; serum level > 60 mg/L
Ethylene glycol	Acidosis, serum level > 50 mg/dL
Lithium	Severe symptoms; level > 4–5 mEq/L, especially if kidney impairment Note: dialysis of uncertain value; consult with medical toxicologist
Methanol	Acidosis, serum level > 50 mg/dL
Phenobarbital	Intractable hypotension, acidosis despite maximal supportive care
Salicylate	Severe acidosis, CNS symptoms, serum level > 100 mg/dL (acute overdose) or > 60 mg/dL (chronic intoxication)
Theophylline	Seizures, severe cardiotoxicity, serum level > 100 mg/L (acute overdose) or > 60 mg/L (chronic intoxication)
Valproic acid	Serum level > 900–1000 mg/L or deep coma, severe acidosis

[1]See text for further discussion of indications.

3. Repeat-dose charcoal—Repeated doses of activated charcoal, 20–30 g orally or via gastric tube every 3–4 hours, may hasten elimination of some drugs (eg, phenytoin, carbamazepine, dapsone) by absorbing drugs excreted into the gut lumen ("gut dialysis"). However, clinical studies have failed to prove better outcome using repeat-dose charcoal. *Sorbitol or other cathartics should not be used with each dose*, or else the resulting large stool volumes may lead to dehydration or hypernatremia.

DIAGNOSIS OF POISONING

The identity of the ingested substance or substances is usually known, but occasionally a comatose patient is found with an unlabeled container or the patient is unable or unwilling to give a coherent history. By performing a directed physical examination and ordering common clinical laboratory tests, the clinician can often make a tentative diagnosis that may allow empiric interventions or may suggest specific toxicologic tests.

Physical Examination

Important diagnostic variables in the physical examination include blood pressure, pulse rate, temperature, pupil size, sweating, muscle tone, level of consciousness, and the presence or absence of peristaltic activity. Poisonings may present with one or more of the following common syndromes.

A. Sympathomimetic Syndrome

The blood pressure and pulse rate are elevated, though with severe hypertension reflex bradycardia may occur. The temperature is often elevated, pupils are dilated, and the skin is sweaty, though mucous membranes are dry. Patients are usually agitated, anxious, or frankly psychotic.

Examples: Amphetamines, cocaine, ephedrine, pseudoephedrine, synthetic cathinones, and cannabinoids.

B. Sympatholytic Syndrome

The blood pressure and pulse rate are decreased, and body temperature is low. The pupils are small or even pinpoint. Patients are usually obtunded or comatose.

Examples: Barbiturates, benzodiazepines and other sedative-hypnotics, γ-hydroxybutyrate (GHB), clonidine and related antihypertensives, ethanol, opioids.

C. Cholinergic Syndrome

Stimulation of *muscarinic receptors* causes bradycardia, miosis (constricted pupils), sweating, and hyperperistalsis as well as bronchorrhea, wheezing, excessive salivation, and urinary incontinence. *Nicotinic receptor* stimulation may produce initial hypertension and tachycardia as well as fasciculations and muscle weakness. Patients are usually agitated and anxious.

Examples: Carbamates, nicotine, organophosphates (including nerve agents), physostigmine.

D. Anticholinergic Syndrome

Tachycardia with mild hypertension is common, and the body temperature is often elevated. Pupils are widely dilated. The skin is flushed, hot, and dry. Peristalsis is decreased, and urinary retention is common. Patients may have myoclonic jerking or choreoathetoid movements. Agitated delirium is frequently seen, and severe hyperthermia may occur.

Examples: Atropine, scopolamine, other naturally occurring and pharmaceutical anticholinergics, antihistamines, tricyclic antidepressants.

Laboratory Tests

The following clinical laboratory tests are recommended for screening of the overdosed patient: measured serum osmolality and calculated osmol gap (if toxic alcohol ingestion is in the differential diagnosis), electrolytes and anion gap, glucose, creatinine, BUN, creatine kinase (CK), UA (eg, oxalate crystals with ethylene glycol poisoning, myoglobinuria with rhabdomyolysis), and ECG. *Quantitative serum acetaminophen and ethanol levels should be determined in all patients with drug overdoses as well as a serum or urine pregnancy test when appropriate.*

A. Osmol Gap

The osmol gap (Table 42–5) is increased in the presence of large quantities of low-molecular-weight substances, most commonly ethanol. Other common poisons associated with increased osmol gap are acetone, ethylene glycol, isopropyl alcohol, methanol, and propylene glycol.

Table 42–5. Use of the osmol gap in toxicology.

The osmol gap (Δ osm) is determined by subtracting the calculated serum osmolality from the measured serum osmolality.

$$\text{Calculated osmolality (osm)} = 2[\text{Na}^+(\text{mEq/L})] + \frac{\text{Glucose (mg/dL)}}{18} + \frac{\text{BUN (mg/dL)}}{2.8}$$

Δ osm = Measured osmolality − Calculated osmolality = 0 ± 10

Serum osmolality may be increased by contributions of exogenous substances such as alcohols and other low-molecular-weight substances. Since these substances are not included in the calculated osmolality, there will be a gap proportionate to their serum concentration. Contact a medical toxicologist or poison control center for assistance in calculating and interpreting the osmol gap.

Reproduced with permission from Stone CK, Humphries RL (editors): *Current Emergency Diagnosis & Treatment*, 5th ed. McGraw-Hill, 2004.

Note: *Severe alcoholic ketoacidosis and diabetic ketoacidosis can also cause an elevated osmol gap resulting from the production of ketones and other low-molecular-weight substances.*

B. Anion Gap

Metabolic acidosis associated with an elevated anion gap is usually due to an accumulation of lactic acid or other acids (see Chapter 24). Common causes of elevated anion gap in poisoning include carbon monoxide, cyanide, ethylene glycol, propylene glycol, iron, INH, methanol, metformin, ibuprofen, and salicylates. Massive acetaminophen overdose can cause early-onset anion gap metabolic acidosis.

The osmol gap should also be checked; combined elevated anion and osmol gaps suggests poisoning by methanol or ethylene glycol, though this may also occur in patients with diabetic ketoacidosis and alcoholic ketoacidosis.

C. Toxicology Laboratory Testing

A comprehensive toxicology screen is of little value in the initial care of the poisoned patient because results usually do not return in time to influence clinical management. *Specific quantitative levels of certain drugs may be extremely helpful (Table 42–6), however, especially if specific antidotes or interventions (eg, dialysis) would be indicated based on the results.*

Many hospitals can perform a quick but limited urine screen for "drugs of abuse" (typically these screens include only opiates, amphetamines, and cocaine, and some add benzodiazepines, barbiturates, methadone, oxycodone, phencyclidine, and tetrahydrocannabinol [marijuana]). There are numerous false-positive and false-negative results. For example, synthetic opioids, such as fentanyl, oxycodone, and methadone, are often not detected by routine opiate immunoassays.

Abdominal Imaging

A plain film (or CT scan) of the abdomen may reveal radiopaque iron tablets, drug-filled condoms, or other toxic material. Studies suggest that few tablets are predictably visible (eg, ferrous sulfate, sodium chloride, calcium

Table 42–6. Specific quantitative levels and potential therapeutic interventions (listed in alphabetical order by drug or toxin).[1]

Drug or Toxin	Treatment
Acetaminophen	Specific antidote (*N*-acetylcysteine) based on serum level
Carbamazepine	High level may indicate need for hemodialysis
Carbon monoxide	High carboxyhemoglobin level indicates need for 100% oxygen, consideration of hyperbaric oxygen
Digoxin	On basis of serum digoxin level and severity of clinical presentation, treatment with Fab antibody fragments (eg, DigiFab) may be indicated
Ethanol	Low serum level may suggest nonalcoholic cause of coma (eg, trauma, other drugs, other alcohols); serum ethanol may also be useful in monitoring ethanol therapy for methanol or ethylene glycol poisoning
Iron	Level may indicate need for chelation with deferoxamine
Lithium	Serum levels can guide decision to institute hemodialysis
Methanol, ethylene glycol	Acidosis, high levels indicate need for hemodialysis, therapy with ethanol or fomepizole
Methemoglobin	Methemoglobinemia can be treated with methylene blue intravenously
Salicylates	High level may indicate need for hemodialysis, alkaline diuresis
Theophylline	Immediate hemodialysis or hemoperfusion may be indicated based on serum level
Valproic acid	Elevated levels may indicate need to consider hemodialysis or L-carnitine therapy, or both

[1]Some drugs or toxins may have profound and irreversible toxicity unless rapid and specific management is provided outside of routine supportive care. For these agents, laboratory testing may provide the serum level or other evidence required for administering a specific antidote or arranging for hemodialysis.

carbonate, and potassium chloride). Thus, the radiograph is useful only if abnormal.

When to Refer

Consultation with a regional poison control center (1-800-222-1222) or a medical toxicologist is recommended when the diagnosis is uncertain; there are questions about what laboratory tests to order; when dialysis is being considered to remove the drug or poison; or when advice is needed regarding the indications, dose, and side effects of antidotes.

When to Admit

- The patient has symptoms and signs of intoxication that are not expected to clear within a 6- to 8-hour observation period.
- Delayed absorption of the drug might be predicted to cause a later onset of serious symptoms (eg, after ingestion of a sustained-release product).
- Continued administration of an antidote is required (eg, *N*-acetylcysteine for acetaminophen overdose).
- Psychiatric or social services evaluation is needed for suicide attempt or suspected drug abuse.

Olson KR, Smollin C (editors). *Poisoning & Drug Overdose*, 8th ed. McGraw-Hill, 2022.

SELECTED POISONINGS

ACETAMINOPHEN

Acetaminophen (paracetamol in the United Kingdom, Europe) is a common analgesic found in many nonprescription and prescription products. After absorption, it is metabolized mainly by glucuronidation and sulfation, with a small fraction metabolized via the P450 mixed-function oxidase system (2E1) to a highly toxic reactive intermediate. This toxic intermediate is normally detoxified by cellular glutathione. With acute acetaminophen overdose (> 150–200 mg/kg, or 8–10 g in an average adult), hepatocellular glutathione is depleted and the reactive intermediate attacks other cell proteins, causing necrosis. *Patients with enhanced P450 2E1 activity, such as patients who have alcohol use disorder and patients taking INH, are at increased risk for developing hepatotoxicity.* Hepatic toxicity may also occur after overuse of acetaminophen—eg, as a result of taking two or three acetaminophen-containing products concurrently or *exceeding the recommended maximum dose of 4 g/day for several days.* The amount of acetaminophen in US oral prescription combination products (eg, hydrocodone/acetaminophen) is limited by the FDA to no more than 325 mg per tablet.

Clinical Findings

Shortly after ingestion, patients may have nausea or vomiting, but there are usually no other signs of toxicity until 24–48 hours after ingestion, when hepatic aminotransferase levels begin to increase. With severe poisoning, fulminant hepatic necrosis may occur, resulting in jaundice, hepatic encephalopathy, AKI, and death. Rarely, massive ingestion (eg, serum levels > 500–1000 mg/L [33–66 mmol/L]) can cause early-onset acute coma, seizures, hypotension, and metabolic acidosis unrelated to hepatic injury.

The risk of hepatotoxicity after acute overdose is based on measurement of the serum acetaminophen level. An acute overdose is defined as an ingestion occurring within a 24-hour period. Plot the serum level versus the time since ingestion on the **acetaminophen nomogram** shown in Figure 42–1. Ingestion of sustained-release products or coingestion of an anticholinergic agent, salicylate, or opioid drug may cause delayed elevation of serum levels, which can make it difficult to interpret the nomogram. The nomogram cannot be used after chronic or staggered overdoses occurring over more than 24 hours.

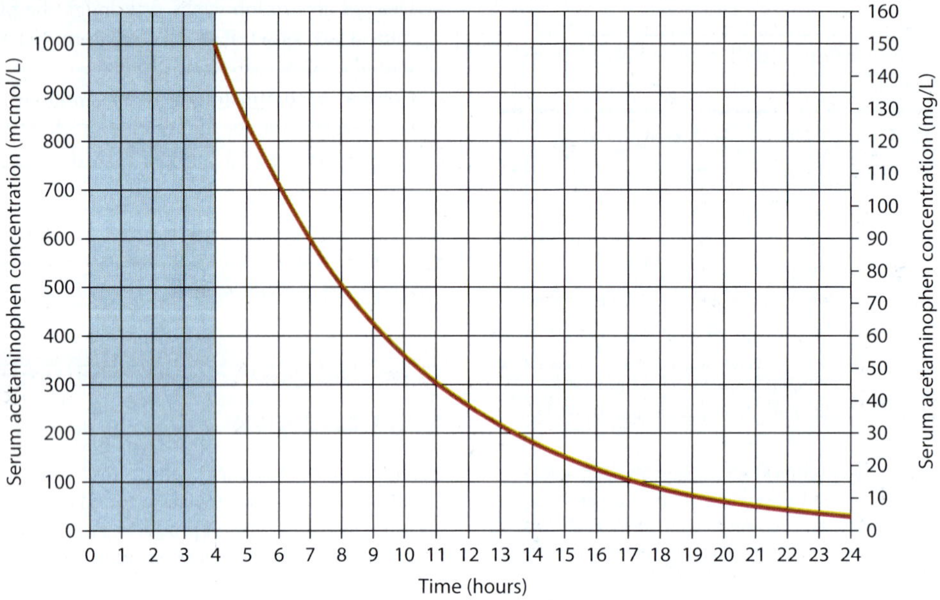

Figure 42–1. Nomogram for prediction of acetaminophen hepatotoxicity following acute overdosage. Patients with serum levels above the line after acute overdose should receive antidotal treatment. (Reproduced with permission from Daly FF, Fountain JS, Murray L, Graudins A, Buckley NA; Panel of Australian and New Zealand clinical toxicologists. Guidelines for the management of paracetamol poisoning in Australia and New Zealand—explanation and elaboration. A consensus statement from clinical toxicologists consulting to the Australasian poisons information centres. Med J Aust. 2008;188(5):296–301.)

Treatment

A. Emergency and Supportive Measures

Administer activated charcoal if it can be given within 1–2 hours of the ingestion. Although charcoal may interfere with absorption of the oral preparation of the antidote acetylcysteine, this is not considered clinically significant.

B. Specific Treatment

If the serum or plasma acetaminophen level falls above the line on the nomogram (Figure 42–1), treatment with *N*-acetylcysteine is indicated; it can be given orally or intravenously. Oral treatment begins with a loading dose of *N*-acetylcysteine, 140 mg/kg, followed by 70 mg/kg every 4 hours. Dilute the solution to about 5% with water, juice, or soda. If vomiting interferes with oral *N*-acetylcysteine administration, consider giving the antidote intravenously. The conventional oral *N*-acetylcysteine protocol in the United States calls for 72 hours of treatment. However, other regimens have demonstrated equivalent success with 20–48 hours of treatment.

The FDA-approved 21-hour intravenous regimen of acetylcysteine (Acetadote) calls for a loading dose of 150 mg/kg given intravenously over 60 minutes, followed by a 4-hour infusion of 50 mg/kg, and a 16-hour infusion of 100 mg/kg. High-risk acetaminophen ingestions (reported ingestions of > 30 g or if the measured serum acetaminophen level is greater than twice the nomogram line) may require a higher dose of *N*-acetylcysteine, and providers should contact a regional poison control center or medical toxicologist for assistance. Novel simplified intravenous regimens are under investigation and may replace the traditional three-bag dosing described above.

Treatment with N-acetylcysteine is most effective if it is started within 8–10 hours after ingestion. Fomepizole, a cytochrome 2E1 inhibitor, has been proposed as an adjunctive therapy, but is not routinely used. Hemodialysis is rarely indicated but might be needed in some patients with massive overdose.

Dart RC et al. Management of acetaminophen poisoning in the US and Canada: a consensus statement. JAMA Netw Open. 2023;6:e2327739. Erratum in: JAMA Netw Open. 2023;6:e2337926. [PMID: 37552484]

Pourbagher-Shahri AM et al. Use of fomepizole (4-methylpyrazole) for acetaminophen poisoning: a scoping review. Toxicol Lett. 2022;355:47. [PMID: 34785186]

Sudanagunta S et al. Comparison of two-bag versus three-bag N-acetylcysteine regimens for pediatric acetaminophen toxicity. Ann Pharmacother. 2023;57:36. [PMID: 35587124]

AMPHETAMINES & COCAINE

See Chapter 47, Substance Use Disorder.

ANTICOAGULANTS

Warfarin and related compounds (including ingredients of many commercial rodenticides, the so-called *superwarfarins* such as brodifacoum, difenacoum, and related compounds) inhibit the normal clotting system by blocking hepatic synthesis of vitamin K–dependent clotting factors. After ingestion of "superwarfarins," inhibition of clotting factor synthesis may persist for several weeks or even months after a single dose. DOACs include the direct thrombin inhibitor dabigatran and the factor Xa inhibitors apixaban, edoxaban, and rivaroxaban. Some of these, especially dabigatran, are largely eliminated by the kidney and may accumulate in patients with kidney dysfunction.

Excessive anticoagulation may cause hemoptysis, gross hematuria, bloody stools, hemorrhages into organs, widespread bruising, and bleeding into joint spaces.

Treatment

A. Emergency and Supportive Measures

Discontinue the drug at the first sign of gross bleeding and determine the prothrombin time (INR). The prothrombin time is increased within 12–24 hours (peak 36–48 hours) after overdose of warfarin or "superwarfarins." **Note:** *DOACs (dabigatran, apixaban, edoxaban, and rivaroxaban) do not predictably alter routine coagulation studies (prothrombin time, partial thromboplastin time, and INR), and these tests are of limited use.* Specialized coagulation studies including the hemaclot and ecarin clotting assay and the anti-factor Xa activity may be helpful but are not widely available.

If the patient has ingested an acute overdose, administer activated charcoal.

B. Specific Treatment

1. Warfarin—*In cases of warfarin and "superwarfarin" overdose, do not treat prophylactically with vitamin K*—wait for evidence of anticoagulation (elevated prothrombin time). See Table 16–21 for the management of INR above therapeutic range. Doses of vitamin K as high as 200 mg/day have been required after ingestion of "superwarfarins." Give prothrombin complex concentrate or activated factor VII as needed to rapidly correct the coagulation factor deficit if there is serious bleeding (fresh-frozen plasma can be administered if PCC is not available). If the patient is chronically anticoagulated and has strong medical indications for being maintained in that status (eg, prosthetic heart valve), give much smaller doses of vitamin K (1 mg orally) and prothrombin complex concentrate (or both) to titrate to the desired prothrombin time. If the patient has ingested brodifacoum or a related superwarfarin, prolonged observation (*over weeks*) and repeated administration of large doses of vitamin K may be required.

2. DOACs—Vitamin K does not reverse the anticoagulant effects of the DOACs. Idarucizumab has been approved by the FDA for reversal of the thrombin inhibitor dabigatran. Evidence supports the use of prothrombin complex concentrates or activated prothrombin complex concentrates for reversal of factor Xa inhibitors.

Rodrigues A et al. Urgent reversal of direct oral anticoagulants in critical and life-threatening bleeding: a multidisciplinary expert consensus. J Clin Med. 2024;13:6842. [PMID: 39597986]

Tran HA et al. 2025 Guidelines for direct oral anticoagulants: a practical guidance on the prescription, laboratory testing, peri-operative and bleeding management. Intern Med J. 2025;55:1174. [PMID: 40448969]

ANTIPSYCHOTIC DRUGS

Drugs in this group include "conventional" antipsychotics (eg, chlorpromazine, haloperidol, droperidol) and "atypical" antipsychotics (eg, risperidone, olanzapine, ziprasidone, quetiapine, aripiprazole). While conventional drugs act mainly on CNS dopamine receptors, atypical drugs also interact with serotonin receptors.

Therapeutic doses of conventional phenothiazines (particularly chlorpromazine) induce drowsiness and mild orthostatic hypotension in as many as 50% of patients. Larger doses can cause obtundation, miosis, severe hypotension, tachycardia, convulsions, and coma. Abnormal cardiac conduction may occur, resulting in prolongation of QRS or QT intervals (or both) and ventricular arrhythmias. Among the atypical agents, quetiapine is more likely to cause coma and hypotension. Hypotension is probably related to blockade of peripheral α-adrenergic receptors, causing vasodilatation.

With therapeutic or toxic doses, an acute extrapyramidal dystonic reaction may develop in some patients, with spasmodic contractions of the face and neck muscles, extensor rigidity of the back muscles, carpopedal spasm, and motor restlessness. This reaction is more common with haloperidol and other butyrophenones and less common with newer atypical antipsychotics. Severe rigidity accompanied by hyperthermia and metabolic acidosis (**neuroleptic malignant syndrome**) may occasionally occur and is life-threatening (see Chapter 28). Atypical antipsychotics have also been associated with weight gain and diabetes mellitus, including diabetic ketoacidosis.

Treatment

A. Emergency and Supportive Measures

Administer activated charcoal for large or recent ingestions. For severe hypotension, treatment with intravenous fluids and vasopressor agents may be necessary. Treat hyperthermia as outlined. Maintain ECG monitoring.

B. Specific Treatment

Hypotension often responds to intravenous saline boluses; cardiac arrhythmias associated with widened QRS intervals on the ECG may respond to intravenous sodium bicarbonate as is given for tricyclic antidepressant overdoses. Prolongation of the QT interval and torsades de pointes are usually treated with intravenous magnesium or overdrive pacing.

For extrapyramidal signs, give diphenhydramine, 0.5–1 mg/kg intravenously, or benztropine mesylate, 0.01–0.02 mg/kg intramuscularly. Treatment with oral doses of these agents should be continued for 24–48 hours.

Bromocriptine (2.5–7.5 mg orally daily) may be effective for mild or moderate neuroleptic malignant syndrome. Dantrolene (2–5 mg/kg intravenously) has also been used for muscle rigidity but is not a true antidote. For severe hyperthermia, perform rapid neuromuscular paralysis.

Berling I et al. QT interval prolongation in acute antipsychotic poisoning: systematic review and recommendations. Clin Toxicol (Phila). 2025;63:810. [PMID: 41255343] Erratum in: Clin Toxicol (Phila). 2026;64:78. [PMID: 41255343]
Wijdicks EFM et al. Neuroleptic malignant syndrome. N Engl J Med. 2024;391:1130. [PMID: 39321364]

ATROPINE & ANTICHOLINERGICS

Atropine, scopolamine, belladonna, *Datura stramonium*, *Hyoscyamus niger*, some mushrooms, tricyclic antidepressants, and antihistamines are antimuscarinic agents with variable CNS effects. Symptoms of toxicity include dryness of the mouth, thirst, difficulty in swallowing, and blurring of vision. Physical signs include dilated pupils, flushed skin, tachycardia, fever, delirium, myoclonus, and ileus. Antidepressants and antihistamines may also induce convulsions.

Antihistamines are commonly available with or without prescription. Diphenhydramine commonly causes delirium, tachycardia, and seizures. Massive diphenhydramine overdose may mimic tricyclic antidepressant cardiotoxic poisoning.

Treatment

A. Emergency and Supportive Measures

Administer activated charcoal. External cooling and sedation, or neuromuscular paralysis in rare cases, are indicated to control high temperatures.

B. Specific Treatment

For severe anticholinergic syndrome (eg, agitated delirium), give physostigmine salicylate, 0.5–1 mg slowly intravenously over 5 minutes, with ECG monitoring; repeat as needed to a total dose of no more than 2 mg. Oral rivastigmine 3–6 mg also can be used as an alternative. **Caution:** *Bradyarrhythmias and convulsions are a hazard with physostigmine administration, and the drug should be avoided in patients with evidence of cardiotoxic effects (eg, QRS interval prolongation) from tricyclic antidepressants or other sodium channel blockers.*

Chiew AL et al. Rivastigmine for the management of anticholinergic delirium. Clin Toxicol (Phila). 2024;62:82. [PMID: 38465631]
Huber S et al. Safety of physostigmine for pediatric antimuscarinic poisoning. J Med Toxicol. 2024;20:263. [PMID: 38265619]

β-ADRENERGIC BLOCKERS

There are a wide variety of β-adrenergic blocking drugs, with varying pharmacologic and pharmacokinetic properties (see Table 13–9). *The most toxic β-blocker is propranolol, which not only blocks β_1- and β_2-adrenoceptors but also has direct membrane-depressant and CNS effects.*

Clinical Findings

The most common findings with mild or moderate intoxication are hypotension and bradycardia. Cardiac depression from more severe poisoning is often unresponsive to conventional therapy with β-adrenergic stimulants such as dopamine and norepinephrine. In addition, with propranolol and other lipid-soluble drugs, seizures and coma may occur. Propranolol, oxprenolol, acebutolol, and alprenolol also have membrane-depressant effects and can cause conduction disturbance (wide QRS interval) similar to tricyclic antidepressant overdose.

The diagnosis is based on typical clinical findings. Routine toxicology screening does not usually include β-blockers.

Treatment

A. Emergency and Supportive Measures

Attempts to treat bradycardia or heart block with atropine (0.5–2 mg intravenously), isoproterenol (2–20 mcg/min by intravenous infusion, titrated to the desired heart rate), or an external transcutaneous cardiac pacemaker are often ineffective, and specific antidotal treatment may be necessary.

For drugs ingested within an hour of presentation (or longer after ingestion of an extended-release formulation), administer activated charcoal.

B. Specific Treatment

For persistent bradycardia and hypotension, give glucagon, 5–10 mg intravenously, followed by an infusion of 1–5 mg/hour. Glucagon is an inotropic agent that acts at a different receptor site and is therefore not affected by β-blockade. High-dose insulin (0.5–1 U/kg/hour intravenously) along with glucose supplementation has also been used to reverse severe cardiotoxicity. Membrane-depressant effects (wide QRS interval) may respond to boluses of sodium bicarbonate (50–100 mEq intravenously) as for tricyclic antidepressant poisoning. Vasopressors (norepinephrine and epinephrine) improve hemodynamics and likely survival in case series and animal studies. Intravenous lipid emulsion (Intralipid 20%, 1.5 mL/kg) has been used successfully in severe propranolol overdose. ECMO should be considered for refractory shock.

Cole JB et al. Cardiotoxic medication poisoning. Emerg Med Clin North Am. 2022;40:395. [PMID: 35461630]
Goldfine CE et al. Beta-blocker and calcium-channel blocker toxicity: current evidence on evaluation and management. Eur Heart J Acute Cardiovasc Care. 2024;13:247. [PMID: 37976176]
Isoardi KZ et al. A prospective study of acute propranolol overdose defining dose thresholds of severe toxicity (ATOM-9). Clin Toxicol (Phila). 2025;63:1. [PMID: 39655516]

CALCIUM CHANNEL BLOCKERS

In therapeutic doses, nifedipine, nicardipine, amlodipine, felodipine, isradipine, nisoldipine, and nimodipine act mainly on blood vessels, while verapamil and diltiazem act mainly on cardiac contractility and conduction. However, these selective effects can be lost after acute overdose. Patients may present with bradycardia, atrioventricular

(AV) nodal block, hypotension, or a combination of these effects. Hyperglycemia is common due to blockade of insulin release. With severe poisoning, cardiac arrest may occur.

Treatment

A. Emergency and Supportive Measures

For ingested drugs, administer activated charcoal. In addition, *whole bowel irrigation should be initiated as soon as possible if the patient has ingested a sustained-release product.*

B. Specific Treatment

Treat symptomatic bradycardia with atropine (0.5–2 mg intravenously), isoproterenol (2–20 mcg/min by intravenous infusion), or a transcutaneous cardiac pacemaker. For hypotension, give calcium chloride 10%, 10 mL, or calcium gluconate 10%, 20 mL. Repeat the dose every 3–5 minutes. The optimum (or maximum) dose has not been established, but many toxicologists recommend raising the ionized serum calcium level to as much as twice the normal level. Calcium is most useful in reversing negative inotropic effects and is less effective for AV nodal blockade and bradycardia. High doses of insulin (0.5–1 U/kg intravenous bolus followed by 0.5–1 U/kg/hour infusion) along with sufficient dextrose to maintain euglycemia have been reported to be beneficial, but there are no controlled studies. Vasopressors (norepinephrine and epinephrine) should also be used for refractory hypotension and shock. Infusion of Intralipid 20% lipid emulsion has been reported to improve hemodynamics in animal models and case reports of calcium channel blocker poisoning. Methylene blue (1–2 mg/kg) was reported to reverse refractory shock due to profound vasodilation in a patient with amlodipine poisoning. Angiotensin II has also been reported to improve vasoplegic shock in case reports of amlodipine poisoning. ECMO has been recommended for refractory shock.

Cao D et al. Part 10: Adult and pediatric special circumstances of resuscitation: 2025 American Heart Association guidelines for cardiopulmonary resuscitation and emergency cardiovascular care. Circulation. 2025;152:S578. [PMID: 41122889]

Goldfine CE et al. Beta-blocker and calcium-channel blocker toxicity: current evidence on evaluation and management. Eur Heart J Acute Cardiovasc Care. 2024;13:247. [PMID: 37976176]

Simpson MD et al. Developments in the epidemiology of calcium channel blocker poisoning and implications for management. Curr Opin Crit Care. 2024;30:603. [PMID: 39503210]

CARBON MONOXIDE

Carbon monoxide is a colorless, odorless gas produced by the combustion of carbon-containing materials. Poisoning may occur as a result of *suicidal or accidental exposure* to automobile exhaust, smoke inhalation in a fire, or accidental exposure to an improperly vented gas heater, generator, or other appliance. Carbon monoxide can be generated during degradation of some anesthetic gases by carbon dioxide adsorbents. Carbon monoxide avidly binds to hemoglobin, with an affinity approximately 250 times that of oxygen. This results in reduced oxygen-carrying capacity and altered delivery of oxygen to cells (see also Smoke Inhalation in Chapter 9).

Clinical Findings

At low carbon monoxide levels (carboxyhemoglobin saturation 10–20%), patients may have headache, dizziness, abdominal pain, and nausea. With higher levels, confusion, dyspnea, and syncope may occur. Hypotension, coma, and seizures are common with levels > 50–60%. Survivors of acute severe poisoning may develop permanent obvious or subtle neurologic and neuropsychiatric deficits. The fetus and newborn may be more susceptible because of high carbon monoxide affinity for fetal hemoglobin.

Carbon monoxide poisoning should be suspected in any person with severe headache or acutely altered mental status, especially during cold weather, when improperly vented heating systems may have been used. Diagnosis depends on specific measurement of the arterial or venous carboxyhemoglobin saturation, although the level may have declined if high-flow oxygen therapy has already been administered, and levels do not always correlate with clinical symptoms. *Routine ABG testing and pulse oximetry are* ***not*** *useful because they give falsely normal* PaO_2 *and oxyhemoglobin saturation determinations, respectively.* (Some specialized pulse oximetry devices are capable of distinguishing oxyhemoglobin from carboxyhemoglobin with variable accuracy.)

Treatment

A. Emergency and Supportive Measures

Maintain a patent airway and assist ventilation, if necessary. Remove the patient from exposure. Treat patients with coma, hypotension, or seizures as described at the beginning of this chapter.

B. Specific Treatment

The half-life of the carboxyhemoglobin (CoHb) complex is about 4–5 hours in room air but is reduced dramatically by high concentrations of oxygen. Administer 100% oxygen by tight-fitting high-flow reservoir face mask or endotracheal tube. *Hyperbaric oxygen (HBO)* can provide 100% oxygen under higher than atmospheric pressures, further shortening the half-life; it may also reduce the incidence of subtle neuropsychiatric sequelae. Randomized controlled studies disagree about the benefit of HBO, but commonly recommended indications for HBO in patients with carbon monoxide poisoning include a history of loss of consciousness, CoHb > 25%, metabolic acidosis, age over 50 years, and cerebellar findings on neurologic examination.

Juurlink DN. Hyperbaric oxygen should not be used routinely for carbon monoxide poisoning. Br J Clin Pharmacol. 2023;89:942. [PMID: 36385706]

Ramponi G et al. The diagnostic accuracy of carbon monoxide pulse oximetry in adults with suspected acute carbon monoxide poisoning: a systematic review and meta-analysis. Front Med (Lausanne). 2023;10:1250845. [PMID: 38223786]

Vural A et al. Early and late adverse clinical outcomes of severe carbon monoxide intoxication: a cross-sectional retrospective study. PLoS One. 2024;19:e0301399. [PMID: 39213322]

COCAINE

See Chapter 47, Substance Use Disorder.

ETHANOL, BENZODIAZEPINES, & OTHER SEDATIVE-HYPNOTIC AGENTS

The group of agents known as sedative-hypnotic drugs includes a variety of products used for the treatment of anxiety, depression, insomnia, and epilepsy. Besides common benzodiazepines, such as lorazepam, alprazolam, clonazepam, diazepam, oxazepam, chlordiazepoxide, and triazolam, this group includes the newer benzodiazepine-like hypnotics zolpidem, zopiclone, and zaleplon, the muscle relaxants baclofen and carisoprodol, and barbiturates such as phenobarbital. Toxicity and fatal overdoses from novel designer benzodiazepines (eg, etizolam, bromazolam), often coingested with fentanyl, are increasingly reported. Phenibut, a $GABA_B$ agonist, is associated with CNS depression and a withdrawal syndrome. Ethanol and other selected agents are also popular recreational drugs. All of these drugs depress the CNS reticular activating system, cerebral cortex, and cerebellum.

Clinical Findings

Mild intoxication produces euphoria, slurred speech, and ataxia. Ethanol intoxication may produce hypoglycemia, even at relatively low concentrations, in children and in fasting adults. With more severe intoxication, stupor, coma, and respiratory arrest may occur. Carisoprodol (Soma) commonly causes muscle jerking or myoclonus. *Death or serious morbidity is usually the result of pulmonary aspiration of gastric contents.* Bradycardia, hypotension, and hypothermia are common. Patients with massive intoxication may appear to be dead, with no reflex responses and even absent electroencephalographic activity. Diagnosis and assessment of severity of intoxication are usually based on clinical findings. Ethanol serum levels > 300 mg/dL (0.3 g/dL; 65 mmol/L) can produce coma in infrequent drinkers, while regular drinkers may remain awake at much higher levels.

Treatment

A. Emergency and Supportive Measures

Administer activated charcoal if the patient has ingested a massive dose and the airway is protected. Repeat-dose charcoal may enhance elimination of phenobarbital, but it has not been proved to improve clinical outcome. Hemodialysis may be necessary for patients with severe phenobarbital intoxication.

B. Specific Treatment

Flumazenil is a benzodiazepine receptor-specific antagonist; it has no effect on ethanol, barbiturates, or other sedative-hypnotic agents. If used, flumazenil is given slowly intravenously, 0.2 mg over 30–60 seconds, and repeated in 0.2–0.5 mg increments as needed up to a total dose of 3–5 mg. **Caution:** *Flumazenil should rarely be used because it may induce seizures in patients with preexisting seizure disorder, benzodiazepine tolerance, or concomitant tricyclic antidepressant or other convulsant overdose.* If seizures occur, diazepam and other benzodiazepine anticonvulsants may not be effective. As with naloxone, the duration of action of flumazenil is short (2–3 hours) and resedation may occur, requiring repeated doses.

Peng L et al. Benzodiazepines and related sedatives. Med Clin North Am. 2022;106:113. [PMID: 34823725]
Rodda LN. The surge of bromazolam-related fatalities replacing other novel designer benzodiazepines-related fatalities in San Francisco. Addiction. 2024;119:1487. [PMID: 38679868]

γ-HYDROXYBUTYRATE (GHB)

GHB is a popular recreational drug. It originated as a short-acting general anesthetic and is occasionally used in the treatment of narcolepsy. It gained popularity among bodybuilders for its alleged growth hormone stimulation and found its way into social settings, where it is consumed as a liquid. It has been used to facilitate sexual assault (the *"date-rape" drug*). Symptoms after ingestion include drowsiness and lethargy followed by coma with respiratory depression. Muscle twitching and seizures are sometimes observed. Recovery is usually rapid, with patients awakening within a few hours. Other related chemicals with similar effects include butanediol and γ-butyrolactone (GBL). A prolonged withdrawal syndrome has been described in some heavy users.

Treatment

Monitor the airway and assist breathing if needed. There is no specific treatment. Most patients recover rapidly with supportive care. GHB withdrawal syndrome may require very large doses of benzodiazepines; baclofen has also been used.

Dufayet L et al. Gamma-hydroxybutyrate (GHB), 1,4-butanediol (1,4BD), and gamma-butyrolactone (GBL) intoxication: a state-of-the-art review. Regul Toxicol Pharmacol. 2023;142:105435. [PMID: 37343712]
Tay E et al. Current insights on the impact of gamma-hydroxybutyrate (GHB) abuse. Subst Abuse Rehabil. 2022;13:13. [PMID: 35173515]

HYPOGLYCEMIC DRUGS

Medications used for diabetes mellitus include insulin, sulfonylureas and other insulin secretagogues, α-glucosidase inhibitors (acarbose, miglitol), biguanides (metformin), thiazolidinediones (pioglitazone, rosiglitazone), SGLT-2 inhibitors, and peptide analogs (pramlintide, exenatide) or enhancers (sitagliptin) (see Chapter 31). Of these, insulin and the insulin secretagogues are the most likely to cause hypoglycemia. Metformin can cause lactic acidosis, especially in patients with impaired kidney function or after intentional drug overdose. Euglycemic diabetic ketoacidosis has been reported with SGLT-2 use. Table 31–4 lists the duration of hypoglycemic effect of oral hypoglycemic agents and Table 31–5 the extent and duration of various types of insulins.

Clinical Findings

Hypoglycemia may occur quickly after injection of short-acting insulins or may be delayed and prolonged, especially if a large amount has been injected into a single area, creating a "depot" effect. Hypoglycemia after sulfonylurea ingestion is usually apparent within a few hours but may be delayed several hours, especially if food or glucose-containing fluids have been given.

Treatment

Give sugar and carbohydrate-containing food or liquids by mouth, or intravenous dextrose if the patient is unable to swallow safely. For severe hypoglycemia, start with D50W, 50 mL intravenously (25 g dextrose); repeat, if needed. Follow up with dextrose-containing intravenous fluids (D5W or D10W) to maintain a blood glucose > 70–80 mg/dL.

For hypoglycemia caused by sulfonylureas and related insulin secretagogues, consider use of octreotide, a synthetic somatostatin analog that blocks pancreatic insulin release. A dose of 50–100 mcg octreotide subcutaneously every 6–12 hours can reduce the need for exogenous dextrose and prevent rebound hypoglycemia from excessive dextrose dosing.

Admit all patients with symptomatic hypoglycemia after sulfonylurea overdose. Observe asymptomatic overdose patients for at least 12 hours.

Consider hemodialysis for patients with metformin overdose accompanied by severe lactic acidosis (lactate > 20 mmol/L or pH < 7.0).

Lee D et al. Clinical features and outcomes of diabetic ketoacidosis in patients using SGLT2 inhibitors: a systematic review and meta-analysis. Diabetes Obes Metab. 2025;27:5805. [PMID: 40692313]

Roberts DM et al. Expanding the evidence for managing metformin poisoning to support decision-making. Clin Toxicol (Phila). 2023;61:203. [PMID: 37129225]

LEAD

Lead is used in a variety of industrial and commercial products, such as firearms ammunition, storage batteries, solders, paints, pottery, plumbing, and gasoline and is found in some traditional Latino/Latina and Ayurvedic ethnic medicines. *Lead toxicity usually results from chronic repeated exposure and is rare after a single ingestion.* Lead produces a variety of adverse effects on cellular function and primarily affects the nervous system, GI tract, and hematopoietic system.

Clinical Findings

Lead poisoning often goes undiagnosed initially because presenting symptoms and signs are nonspecific and exposure is not suspected. Common symptoms include colicky abdominal pain, constipation, headache, and irritability. Severe poisoning may cause coma and convulsions. Chronic intoxication can cause learning disorders (in children) and motor neuropathy (eg, wrist drop). Lead-containing bullet fragments in or near joint spaces can result in chronic lead toxicity.

Diagnosis is based on measurement of the blood lead level. Whole blood lead levels above 3.5 mcg/dL warrant public health investigation. Levels between 1 and 25 mcg/dL have been associated with subclinical impaired neurobehavioral development in children. Levels of 25–60 mcg/dL may be associated with headache, irritability, subclinical neuropathy, slowed reaction time and other neuropsychiatric effects. Levels of 60–80 mcg/dL are associated with moderate toxicity, and levels > 80–100 mcg/dL are often associated with severe poisoning. Other laboratory findings of lead poisoning include microcytic anemia with basophilic stippling and elevated free erythrocyte protoporphyrin.

Treatment

A. Emergency and Supportive Measures

The most critical intervention in the treatment of lead poisoning is identification of and removal from the source of exposure. For patients with encephalopathy, maintain a patent airway and treat coma and convulsions as described at the beginning of this chapter.

For recent acute ingestion, if a large lead-containing object (eg, fishing weight) is still visible in the stomach on abdominal radiograph, whole bowel irrigation, endoscopy, or even surgical removal may be necessary to prevent subacute lead poisoning. (The acidic gastric contents may corrode the metal surface, enhancing lead absorption. Once the object passes into the small intestine, the risk of toxicity declines.)

The US Occupational Safety and Health Administration establishes workplace standards for lead exposure. Contact the regional office for more information. Several states mandate reporting of cases of confirmed lead poisoning.

B. Specific Treatment

The indications for chelation depend on the blood lead level and the patient's clinical state. A medical toxicologist or regional poison control center (1-800-222-1222) should be consulted for advice about selection and use of these antidotes.

1. Severe toxicity—Patients with severe intoxication (encephalopathy or levels > 70–100 mcg/dL) should receive edetate calcium disodium (ethylenediaminetetraacetic acid, EDTA), 1500 mg/m^2/kg/day (approximately 50 mg/kg/day) in four to six divided doses or as a continuous intravenous infusion. Some clinicians also add dimercaprol (BAL), 4–5 mg/kg intramuscularly every 4 hours for 5 days, for patients with encephalopathy.

2. Less severe toxicity—Patients with less severe symptoms and asymptomatic patients with blood lead levels between 45 and 69 mcg/dL may be treated with edetate calcium disodium alone in dosages as above. An oral chelator, succimer (DMSA), is available for use in patients with mild to moderate intoxication. The usual dose is 10 mg/kg orally every 8 hours for 5 days, then every 12 hours for 2 weeks.

Centers for Disease Control and Prevention (CDC). Childhood lead poisoning prevention. Recommended actions based on blood lead level. https://www.cdc.gov/lead-prevention/hcp/clinical-guidance/?CDC_AAref_Val=https://www.cdc.gov/nceh/lead/advisory/acclpp/actions-blls.htm, accessed September 23, 2025.

Lanphear B et al. Lead poisoning. N Engl J Med. 2024;391:1621. [PMID: 39476342]

LSD & OTHER HALLUCINOGENS

A variety of substances—ranging from naturally occurring plants and mushrooms to synthetic substances such as phencyclidine (PCP), toluene and other solvents, dextromethorphan, and lysergic acid diethylamide (LSD)—are used for their hallucinogenic properties. The mechanism of toxicity and the clinical effects vary for each substance.

Many hallucinogenic plants and mushrooms produce anticholinergic delirium, characterized by flushed skin, dry mucous membranes, dilated pupils, tachycardia, and urinary retention. Other plants and mushrooms may contain hallucinogenic indoles such as mescaline, psilocybin, and LSD, which typically cause marked visual hallucinations and perceptual distortion, widely dilated pupils, and mild tachycardia. PCP and ketamine are antagonists of NMDA receptors and produce an acute dissociative state often associated with vertical and horizontal nystagmus. Both ketamine and psilocybin increasingly are used to treat chronic pain, depression, and PTSD. Toluene and other hydrocarbon solvents (eg, butane, trichloroethylene, "chemo," etc.) cause euphoria and delirium and may sensitize the myocardium to the effects of catecholamines, leading to fatal dysrhythmias. Other drugs used for their psychostimulant effects include synthetic cannabinoid receptor agonists, *Salvia divinorum*, synthetic tryptamines, and phenylethylamines, and mephedrone and related cathinone derivatives. See https://www.erowid.org/psychoactives/psychoactives.shtml for descriptions of various hallucinogenic substances.

Treatment

A. Emergency and Supportive Measures

Maintain a patent airway and assist respirations if necessary. Treat coma, hyperthermia, hypertension, and seizures as outlined at the beginning of this chapter. For recent large ingestions, consider giving activated charcoal orally or by gastric tube.

B. Specific Treatment

Patients with anticholinergic delirium may benefit from a dose of physostigmine, 0.5–1 mg intravenously, not to exceed 1 mg/min. Dysphoria, agitation, and psychosis associated with LSD or mescaline intoxication may respond to benzodiazepines (eg, lorazepam, 1–2 mg orally or intravenously) or haloperidol (2–5 mg intramuscularly or intravenously) or another antipsychotic drug (eg, olanzapine or ziprasidone). Monitor patients who have sniffed solvents for cardiac dysrhythmias (most commonly premature ventricular contractions, ventricular tachycardia, ventricular fibrillation); treatment with β-blockers such as propranolol (1–5 mg intravenously) or esmolol (250–500 mcg/kg intravenously, then 50 mcg/kg/min by infusion) may be more effective than lidocaine or amiodarone.

Holze F et al. Pharmacological properties of psychedelics with a special focus on potential harms. Curr Top Behav Neurosci. 2026;77:25. [PMID: 39080236]

Johnston JN et al. Ketamine and serotonergic psychedelics: an update on the mechanisms and biosignatures underlying rapid-acting antidepressant treatment. Neuropharmacology. 2023;226:109422. [PMID: 36646310]

Simon MW et al. Clinical effects of psychedelic substances reported to United States Poison Centers: 2012 to 2022. Ann Emerg Med. 2024;84:605. [PMID: 39093248]

MARIJUANA & SYNTHETIC CANNABINOIDS

Marijuana refers to the crushed dried leaves and flowers of the *Cannabis* plant. These dried leaves and flowers contain the psychoactive cannabinoid Δ-9-tetrahydrocannabinal (THC), which binds to endogenous cannabinoid receptors. Marijuana is usually smoked in cigarettes or pipes but may also be vaporized or added to a variety of foods, beverages, and candies. Resin from the plant may be dried and pressed into blocks called hashish, and solvents may be used to extract THC into highly concentrated oils (butane hash oil). THC is used medically as an appetite stimulant, as an antiemetic, and in the treatment of a variety of medical conditions. It has now been legalized for both medical and recreational use in an increasing number of US states (https://disa.com/map-of-marijuana-legality-by-state). Toxicity is dose dependent but varies significantly by individual, prior experience, and degree of tolerance. Synthetic cannabinoids ("Spice," "K2," "Black Mamba") are laboratory designed analogs of THC. They have become increasingly popular and are associated with a variety of adverse side effects, including seizures, kidney dysfunction, and serious neuropsychiatric symptoms. Cannabidiol (CBD) is a constituent of *Cannabis* that does not produce THC-like intoxication. CBD extracts are available over the counter and via the internet for a variety of proposed effects (anti-inflammatory, antioxidant, anxiolysis) and by prescription for some pediatric seizure disorders. Overdoses are typically not dangerous.

Clinical Findings

Onset of symptoms after smoking is usually rapid (minutes) with a duration of effect of approximately 2 hours. Symptoms may be delayed after ingestion and can result in prolonged intoxication (up to 8 hours). Mild intoxication may result in euphoria, palpitations, heightened sensory awareness, altered time perception, and sedation. More severe intoxication may result in anxiety, visual hallucinations, and acute paranoid psychosis. Physical findings include tachycardia, orthostatic hypotension, conjunctival injection, incoordination, slurred speech, and ataxia. Long-term heavy marijuana use is associated with recurrent nausea, abdominal pain, and vomiting, termed the **cannabinoid hyperemesis syndrome**. Children may inadvertently be exposed to marijuana through the consumption of THC-containing candies or other foods. Children may experience more severe symptoms including stupor, coma, and seizures. **E-cigarette or vaping-associated acute lung injury** is a syndrome of diffuse lung injury associated with vaping THC adulterated with vitamin E acetate.

Treatment

A. Emergency and Supportive Measures

Treat anxiety and paranoia with simple reassurance and placement into a calming environment. Benzodiazepines such as lorazepam or diazepam may be used for more severe behavioral and psychomotor symptoms. Hypotension and sinus tachycardia should be treated with intravenous fluids.

B. Specific Treatment

There is no specific antidote available. Consider activated charcoal early after ingestion of large quantities. Topical capsaicin and haloperidol have been used with variable success for the treatment of acute vomiting in patients with cannabinoid hyperemesis syndrome.

Gorelick DA. Cannabis-related disorders and toxic effects. N Engl J Med. 2023;389:2267. [PMID: 38091532]
Prete MM et al. Adverse clinical effects associated with the use of synthetic cannabinoids: a systematic review. Drug Alcohol Depend. 2025;272:112698. [PMID: 40334326]

METHANOL & ETHYLENE GLYCOL

Methanol (wood alcohol) is commonly found in a variety of products, including solvents, duplicating fluids, record cleaning solutions, and paint removers. It is sometimes ingested intentionally by patients with alcohol use disorder as a substitute for ethanol and may also be found as a contaminant in home-brewed alcohols. *Ethylene glycol is the major constituent in most antifreeze compounds.* The toxicity of both agents is caused by metabolism to highly toxic organic acids—methanol to formic acid; ethylene glycol to glycolic and oxalic acids. Diethylene glycol is a nephrotoxic solvent that has been improperly substituted for glycerin in various liquid medications (cough syrup, teething medicine, acetaminophen), causing numerous deaths, including in Gambia in 2022.

Clinical Findings

Shortly after ingestion of methanol or ethylene glycol, patients usually appear "drunk." Serum osmolality (measured by freezing point depression) is usually increased, but acidosis is often absent early. After several hours, metabolism to toxic organic acids leads to a severe anion gap metabolic acidosis, tachypnea, confusion, convulsions, and coma. Methanol intoxication frequently causes visual disturbances, while ethylene glycol often produces oxalate crystalluria and AKI. **Note:** *Point-of-care analytical devices commonly used in the emergency department may falsely measure glycolic acid (a toxic metabolite of ethylene glycol) as lactic acid.*

Treatment

A. Emergency and Supportive Measures

For patients presenting within 30–60 minutes after ingestion, empty the stomach by aspiration through a nasogastric tube. Charcoal is not very effective but should be administered if other poisons or drugs have also been ingested.

B. Specific Treatment

Patients with significant toxicity (manifested by severe metabolic acidosis, altered mental status, markedly elevated osmol gap, or evidence of end-organ toxicity) should undergo hemodialysis as soon as possible to remove the parent compound and the toxic metabolites. Treatment with folic acid, thiamine, and pyridoxine may enhance the breakdown of toxic metabolites.

Ethanol blocks metabolism of the parent compounds by competing for the enzyme alcohol dehydrogenase. Fomepizole (4-methylpyrazole; Antizol) blocks alcohol dehydrogenase and is much easier to use than ethanol. If started before onset of acidosis, fomepizole may be used as the sole treatment for ethylene glycol ingestion in some cases. A regional poison control center (1-800-222-1222) should be contacted for indications and dosing.

Ghannoum M et al; EXTRIP Workgroup. Extracorporeal treatment for ethylene glycol poisoning: systematic review and recommendations from the EXTRIP workgroup. Crit Care. 2023;27:56. [PMID: 36765419]
Mousavi-Roknabadi RS et al. Methanol poisoning during COVID-19 pandemic; a systematic scoping review. Am J Emerg Med. 2022;52:69. [PMID: 34883289]
Ross JA et al. Toxic alcohol poisoning. Emerg Med Clin North Am. 2022;40:327. [PMID: 35461626]

METHEMOGLOBINEMIA-INDUCING AGENTS

A large number of chemical agents are capable of oxidizing ferrous hemoglobin to its ferric state (methemoglobin), a form that cannot carry oxygen. Drugs and chemicals known to cause methemoglobinemia include benzocaine (a local anesthetic found in some topical anesthetic sprays and a variety of nonprescription products), aniline, propanil (an herbicide), nitrites, nitrogen oxide gases, nitrobenzene, dapsone, phenazopyridine (Pyridium), and many others. Dapsone has a long elimination half-life and may produce prolonged or recurrent methemoglobinemia. Amyl nitrite and isobutyl nitrite ("poppers") are inhaled as sexual stimulants but can result in methemoglobinemia. Intentional ingestion of sodium nitrite is used increasingly as a method of suicide.

Clinical Findings

Methemoglobinemia reduces oxygen-carrying capacity and may cause dizziness, nausea, headache, dyspnea, confusion, seizures, and coma. The severity of symptoms depends on the percentage of hemoglobin oxidized to methemoglobin; severe poisoning is usually present when methemoglobin fractions are > 40–50%. Even at low levels (15–20%), patients appear cyanotic because of the "chocolate brown" color of methemoglobin, but they have normal PO_2 results on ABG determinations. *Conventional pulse oximetry gives inaccurate oxygen saturation measurements*; the reading is often between 85% and 90%. Severe metabolic acidosis may be present. Hemolysis may occur, especially in patients susceptible to oxidant stress (ie, those with glucose-6-phosphate dehydrogenase deficiency).

Treatment

A. Emergency and Supportive Measures

Administer high-flow oxygen. If the causative agent was recently ingested, administer activated charcoal. Repeat-dose activated charcoal may enhance dapsone elimination.

B. Specific Treatment

Methylene blue enhances the conversion of methemoglobin to hemoglobin by increasing the activity of the enzyme methemoglobin reductase. For symptomatic patients, administer 1–2 mg/kg (0.1–0.2 mL/kg of 1% solution) intravenously. The dose may be repeated once in 15–20 minutes if necessary. Patients with hereditary methemoglobin reductase deficiency or glucose-6-phosphate dehydrogenase deficiency may not respond to methylene blue treatment. In severe cases where methylene blue is not available or is not effective, exchange blood transfusion may be necessary.

Timmons P. Seizures and severe methaemoglobinaemia following accidental ingestion of amyl nitrite. BMJ Case Rep. 2024;17:e259384. [PMID: 38806397]

MUSHROOMS

There are thousands of mushroom species that cause a variety of toxic effects. The most dangerous species of mushrooms are *Amanita phalloides* and related species, which contain potent cytotoxins (amatoxins). Ingestion of even a portion of one amatoxin-containing mushroom may be sufficient to cause death.

The characteristic pathologic finding in fatalities from amatoxin-containing mushroom poisoning is acute massive necrosis of the liver.

Clinical Findings

Amatoxin-containing mushrooms typically cause a delayed onset (8–12 hours after ingestion) of severe abdominal cramps, vomiting, and profuse diarrhea, followed in 1–2 days by AKI, hepatic necrosis, and hepatic encephalopathy. *Cooking the mushrooms does not prevent poisoning.*

Monomethylhydrazine poisoning (*Gyromitra* and *Helvella* species) is more common following ingestion of uncooked mushrooms, as the toxin is water-soluble. Vomiting, diarrhea, hepatic necrosis, convulsions, coma, and hemolysis may occur after a latent period of 8–12 hours.

Treatment

A. Emergency Measures

After the onset of symptoms, efforts to remove the toxic agent are probably useless, especially in cases of amatoxin or gyromitrin poisoning, where there is usually a delay of 8–12 hours or more before symptoms occur and patients seek medical attention. However, activated charcoal is recommended for any recent ingestion of an unidentified or potentially toxic mushroom. Administer intravenous fluids liberally to replace massive losses from vomiting and diarrhea; monitor CVP, urinary output, and kidney function tests to help guide volume replacement.

B. Specific Treatment

A variety of purported antidotes (eg, thioctic acid, penicillin, corticosteroids) have been suggested for amatoxin-type mushroom poisoning, but controlled studies are lacking and experimental data in animals are equivocal. *Aggressive fluid replacement for diarrhea and intensive supportive care for hepatic failure are the mainstays of treatment.* Silymarin (silibinin), a derivative of milk thistle, is commonly used in Europe, but is commercially available in the United States only as an oral nutritional supplement. The European intravenous product (Legalon-SIL) can be obtained in the United States under an emergency IND provided by the FDA. Contact the regional poison control center (1-800-222-1222) for more information. *N*-Acetylcysteine has also been used and may provide some benefit. Liver transplant may be the only hope for survival in gravely ill patients—contact a liver transplant center early.

Tan JL et al. Amanitin intoxication: effects of therapies on clinical outcomes—a review of 40 years of reported cases. Clin Toxicol (Phila). 2022;60:1251. [PMID: 36129244]

OPIATES & OPIOIDS

Prescription and illicit opiates and opioids (eg, morphine, heroin, codeine, oxycodone, fentanyl, hydromorphone) are popular drugs of misuse and abuse and the cause of frequent hospitalizations for overdose. These drugs have widely varying potencies and durations of action; for example, *some of the illicit fentanyl derivatives are up to 2000 times more potent than morphine.* The opioid epidemic in the United States has become increasingly dangerous due to the presence of fentanyl as a replacement or adulterant in the heroin, cocaine, and other drugs sold illegally. *Users of illicit drugs are advised to assume there is fentanyl in any drug not sold by a pharmacy.* Overdose deaths involving synthetic opioids increased during the COVID-19 pandemic and pose a significant public health concern. All of these agents decrease CNS activity and sympathetic outflow by acting on opiate receptors in the brain. Tramadol is an analgesic that is unrelated chemically to opioids but acts on opioid receptors. Buprenorphine is a partial agonist-antagonist opioid used for the outpatient treatment of both chronic pain and opioid addiction (see Table 5–6). Kratom (*Mitragyna speciosa*) is an herbal supplement with agonist activity at mu opioid receptors. While it has been marketed as a "safe" and natural treatment for patients with opioid use disorder, overdose is associated with both agitation and drowsiness and in severe cases seizures, hallucinations, and respiratory depression.

Clinical Findings

Mild intoxication is characterized by euphoria, drowsiness, and constricted pupils. More severe intoxication may cause hypotension, bradycardia, hypothermia, coma, and respiratory arrest. Pulmonary edema may occur. Death is usually due to apnea or pulmonary aspiration of gastric contents. Methadone may cause QT interval prolongation and torsades de pointes. While the duration of effect for heroin is usually 3–5 hours, methadone intoxication may last for 48–72 hours or longer. Tramadol, dextromethorphan, and meperidine also occasionally cause seizures. With meperidine, the metabolite normeperidine is probably the cause of seizures and is most likely to accumulate with repeated dosing in patients with CKD. Wound botulism has been associated with skin-popping, especially involving "black tar" heroin. Buprenorphine added to an opioid regimen may precipitate acute withdrawal symptoms. Many opioids, including fentanyl, tramadol, oxycodone, and methadone, are not detected on routine urine toxicology "opiate" screening.

Treatment

A. Emergency and Supportive Measures

Protect the airway and assist ventilation. Administer activated charcoal for recent large ingestions.

B. Specific Treatment

***Naloxone** is a specific opioid antagonist, available without prescription in the United States, that can rapidly reverse signs of narcotic intoxication.* Although it is structurally related to opioids, it has no agonist effects of its own. If no intravenous access is available, administer naloxone, 4 mg intranasally, otherwise administer 0.2–2 mg intravenously and repeat as needed to awaken the patient and maintain airway protective reflexes and spontaneous breathing. Large doses (up to 10 mg) may be required for patients intoxicated by some opioids (eg, codeine, fentanyl derivatives). **Caution:** *The duration of effect of naloxone is only about 2–3 hours; repeated doses may be necessary for patients intoxicated by long-acting drugs such as methadone. Continuous observation for at least 3 hours after the last naloxone dose is mandatory.* The immediate post-overdose period is an important opportunity to discuss harm reduction measures (take-home naloxone, fentanyl testing strips, safe injection practices) and to consider initiation of medications for opioid use disorder (buprenorphine, methadone).

Duhart Clarke SE et al. Consuming illicit opioids during a drug overdose epidemic: illicit fentanyls, drug discernment, and the radical transformation of the illicit opioid market. Int J Drug Policy. 2022;99:103467. [PMID: 34662847]

Lima RA et al. Feasibility of emergency department-based fentanyl test strip distribution. J Addict Med. 2022;16:730. [PMID: 35972152]

Peterkin A et al. Current best practices for acute and chronic management of patients with opioid use disorder. Med Clin North Am. 2022;106:61. [PMID: 34823735]

PESTICIDES: CHOLINESTERASE INHIBITORS

Organophosphorus and carbamate insecticides (organophosphates: parathion, malathion, etc; carbamates: carbaryl, aldicarb, etc) are widely used in commercial agriculture and home gardening and have largely replaced older, more environmentally persistent organochlorine compounds such as DDT and chlordane. The organophosphates and carbamates—also called anticholinesterases because they inhibit the enzyme acetylcholinesterase—cause an increase in acetylcholine activity at nicotinic and muscarinic receptors and in the peripheral and CNS. There are a variety of chemical agents in this group, with widely varying potencies. Most of them are poorly water-soluble, are often formulated with an aromatic hydrocarbon solvent such as xylene, and are well absorbed through intact skin. Most chemical warfare "nerve agents" (such as GA [tabun], GB [sarin], GD [soman], and VX) are organophosphates.

Clinical Findings

Inhibition of cholinesterase results in abdominal cramps, diarrhea, vomiting, excessive salivation, sweating, lacrimation, miosis, wheezing and bronchorrhea, seizures, and skeletal muscle weakness. Initial tachycardia is usually followed by bradycardia. Profound skeletal muscle weakness, aggravated by excessive bronchial secretions and wheezing, may result in respiratory arrest and death. Symptoms and signs of poisoning may persist or recur over several days, especially with highly lipid-soluble agents such as fenthion or dimethoate.

The diagnosis should be suspected in patients who present with miosis, sweating, and diarrhea. Serum and RBC cholinesterase activity is usually depressed at least 50% below baseline in those patients who have severe intoxication.

Treatment

A. Emergency and Supportive Measures

If the agent was recently ingested, consider gut decontamination by aspiration of the liquid using a nasogastric tube followed by administration of activated charcoal. If the agent is on the person's skin or hair, wash repeatedly with soap or shampoo and water. Providers should take care to avoid skin exposure by wearing gloves and waterproof aprons. Dilute hypochlorite solution (eg, household bleach diluted 1:10) is reported to help break down organophosphate pesticides and nerve agents on equipment or clothing.

B. Specific Treatment

Atropine reverses excessive muscarinic stimulation and is effective for treatment of salivation, bronchial hypersecretion, wheezing, abdominal cramping, and sweating. However, it does not interact with nicotinic receptors at autonomic ganglia and at the neuromuscular junction and has no direct effect on muscle weakness. Administer 2 mg intravenously, and if there is no response after 5 minutes, give repeated boluses in rapidly escalating doses (eg, doubling the dose each time) as needed to dry bronchial secretions and decrease wheezing; as much as several hundred milligrams of atropine have been given to treat severe poisoning.

Pralidoxime (2-PAM, Protopam) is a more specific antidote that reverses organophosphate binding to the cholinesterase enzyme; therefore, it should be effective at the neuromuscular junction as well as other nicotinic and muscarinic sites. It is most likely to be clinically effective if started very soon after poisoning, to prevent permanent binding of the organophosphate to cholinesterase. However, clinical studies have yielded conflicting results regarding the effectiveness of pralidoxime in reducing mortality. Administer 1–2 g intravenously as a loading dose and begin a continuous infusion (200–500 mg/hour, titrated to clinical response). Continue to give pralidoxime as long as there is any evidence of acetylcholine excess. Pralidoxime is of questionable benefit for carbamate poisoning because carbamates have only a transitory effect on the cholinesterase enzyme. Other, unproven therapies for organophosphate poisoning include magnesium, sodium bicarbonate, clonidine, and extracorporeal removal.

Thiermann H et al. Approaches to the treatment of nerve agent poisoning with oximes–from experimental studies to the intensive care unit. Clin Toxicol (Phila). 2025;63:375. [PMID: 40421756]

SALICYLATES

Salicylates (aspirin, methyl salicylate, bismuth subsalicylate, etc) are found in a variety of over-the-counter and prescription medications. Salicylates uncouple cellular oxidative phosphorylation, resulting in anaerobic metabolism and excessive production of lactic acid and heat, and they also interfere with several Krebs cycle enzymes. A *single ingestion of > 200 mg/kg of salicylate is likely to produce significant acute intoxication.* Poisoning may also occur as a result of *chronic excessive dosing* over several days. Although the half-life of salicylate is 2–3 hours after small doses, it may increase to 20 hours or more in patients with intoxication.

Clinical Findings

Acute ingestion often causes nausea and vomiting, occasionally with gastritis. Moderate intoxication is characterized by hyperpnea (deep and rapid breathing), tachycardia, tinnitus, and elevated anion gap metabolic acidosis. (A normal anion gap sometimes occurs due to salicylate interference with the chemistry analyzer, falsely raising the measured chloride.) Serious intoxication may result in agitation, confusion, coma, seizures, cardiovascular collapse, pulmonary edema, hyperthermia, and death. The prothrombin time is often elevated owing to salicylate-induced hypoprothrombinemia. CNS intracellular glucose depletion can occur despite normal measured serum glucose levels.

Diagnosis of salicylate poisoning is suspected in any patient with metabolic acidosis and is confirmed by measuring the serum salicylate level. Patients with levels > 100 mg/dL (1000 mg/L or 7.2 mcmol/L) after an acute overdose are more likely to have severe poisoning. On the other hand, patients with subacute or chronic intoxication may suffer severe symptoms with levels of only 60–70 mg/dL (4.3–5 mcmol/L). The ABG typically reveals respiratory alkalosis with an underlying metabolic acidosis.

Treatment

A. Emergency and Supportive Measures

Administer activated charcoal orally. Gastric lavage followed by administration of extra doses of activated charcoal may be needed in patients who ingest > 10 g of aspirin. The desired ratio of charcoal to aspirin is about 10:1 by weight; while this cannot always be given as a single dose, it may be administered over the first 24 hours in divided doses every 2–4 hours along with whole bowel irrigation. Give glucose-containing fluids to reduce the risk of cerebral hypoglycemia. Treat metabolic acidosis with intravenous sodium bicarbonate. This is critical because acidosis (especially acidemia, pH < 7.40) promotes greater entry of salicylate into cells, worsening toxicity. **Warning:** *Sudden and severe deterioration can occur after rapid sequence intubation and controlled ventilation if the pH is allowed to fall due to hypercarbia during the apneic period.*

B. Specific Treatment

Alkalinization of the urine enhances renal salicylate excretion by trapping the salicylate anion in the urine. Add 100 mEq (two ampules) of sodium bicarbonate to 1 L of 5% dextrose in 0.2% saline and infuse this solution intravenously at a rate of about 150–200 mL/hour. Unless the patient is oliguric or hyperkalemic, add 20–30 mEq of potassium chloride to each liter of intravenous fluid. Patients who are volume-depleted often fail to produce an alkaline urine (paradoxical aciduria) unless potassium is given.

Hemodialysis may be lifesaving and is indicated for patients with severe metabolic acidosis, markedly altered mental status, or significantly elevated salicylate levels (eg, > 100 mg/dL [1000 mg/L or 7.2 mcmol/L] after acute overdose or > 60 mg/dL [600 mg/L or 4.3 mcmol/L] with subacute or chronic intoxication).

Oyekanmi O et al. Peri-mortem rigidity in a fatal case of severe salicylate poisoning. Clin Toxicol (Phila). 2024;62:267. [PMID: 38738682]

SEAFOOD POISONINGS

A variety of intoxications may occur after eating certain types of fish or other seafood. These include scombroid, ciguatera, paralytic shellfish, and puffer fish poisoning. The mechanisms of toxicity and clinical presentations are described in Table 42–7. In most cases, the seafood has a

Table 42–7. Common seafood poisonings (listed in alphabetical order).

Type of Poisoning	Mechanism	Clinical Presentation
Ciguatera	Reef fish ingest toxic dinoflagellates, whose toxins accumulate in fish meat. Commonly implicated fish in the United States are barracuda, jack, snapper, and grouper.	1–6 hours after ingestion, people develop abdominal pain, vomiting, and diarrhea accompanied by a variety of neurologic symptoms, including paresthesias, reversal of hot and cold sensation, vertigo, headache, and intense itching. Autonomic disturbances, including hypotension and bradycardia, may occur.
Paralytic shellfish poisoning	Dinoflagellates produce saxitoxin, which is concentrated by filter-feeding mussels and clams. Saxitoxin blocks sodium conductance and neuronal transmission in skeletal muscles.	Onset is usually within 30–60 minutes. Initial symptoms include perioral and intraoral paresthesias. Other symptoms include nausea and vomiting, headache, dizziness, dysphagia, dysarthria, ataxia, and rapidly progressive muscle weakness that may result in respiratory arrest.
Puffer fish poisoning	Tetrodotoxin is concentrated in liver, gonads, intestine, and skin. Toxic effects are similar to those of saxitoxin. Tetrodotoxin is also found in some North American newts and Central American frogs.	Onset is usually within 30–40 minutes but may be as short as 10 minutes. Initial perioral paresthesias are followed by headache, diaphoresis, nausea, vomiting, ataxia, and rapidly progressive muscle weakness that may result in respiratory arrest.
Scombroid	Improper preservation of large fish results in bacterial degradation of histidine to histamine. Commonly implicated fish include tuna, mahimahi, bonita, mackerel, and kingfish.	Allergic-like (anaphylactoid) symptoms are due to histamine, usually begin within 15–90 minutes, and include skin flushing, itching, urticaria, angioedema, bronchospasm, and hypotension as well as abdominal pain, vomiting, and diarrhea.

normal appearance and taste (scombroid may have a peppery taste).

Treatment

A. Emergency and Supportive Measures

Caution: *Abrupt respiratory arrest may occur in patients with acute paralytic shellfish and puffer fish poisoning.* Observe patients for at least 4–6 hours. Replace fluid and electrolyte losses from gastroenteritis with intravenous saline or other crystalloid solution.

For recent ingestions, it may be possible to adsorb residual toxin in the gut with activated charcoal, 50–60 g orally.

B. Specific Treatment

There is no specific antidote for paralytic shellfish or puffer fish poisoning.

1. Ciguatera—There are anecdotal reports of successful treatment of acute neurologic symptoms with mannitol, 1 g/kg intravenously, but this approach is not widely accepted. Gabapentin, 400 mg three times daily, may also relieve neuropathic symptoms.

2. Scombroid—Antihistamines such as diphenhydramine, 25–50 mg intravenously, and the H_2-blocker cimetidine, 300 mg intravenously, are usually effective.

Bengio M et al. An unusual presentation of severe ciguatera poisoning: case report. Am J Case Rep. 2024;25:e943149. [PMID: 38343128]

Huff A et al. Epidemiology of ciguatoxin poisoning outbreaks in the United States between 2001 and 2021. Foodborne Pathog Dis. 2025;22:445. [PMID: 39392108]

SNAKE BITES

The venom of poisonous snakes and lizards may be predominantly **neurotoxic** (coral snake) or predominantly **cytolytic** (rattlesnakes, other pit vipers). Neurotoxins cause respiratory paralysis; cytolytic venoms cause tissue destruction by digestion and hemorrhage due to hemolysis and destruction of the endothelial lining of the blood vessels. The manifestations of rattlesnake envenomation are mostly local pain, redness, swelling, and extravasation of blood. Perioral tingling, metallic taste, nausea and vomiting, hypotension, and coagulopathy may also occur. Thrombocytopenia can persist for several days after a rattlesnake bite. Neurotoxic envenomation may cause ptosis, dysphagia, diplopia, and respiratory arrest.

Treatment

A. Emergency and Supportive Measures

Immobilize the patient and the bitten part in a neutral position. *Avoid manipulation of the bitten area.* Transport the patient to a medical facility for definitive treatment. Do *not* give alcoholic beverages or stimulants; do *not* apply ice; do *not* apply a tourniquet. The potential trauma to underlying tissues resulting from incision and suction is not justified in view of the small amount of venom that can be recovered.

B. Specific Antidote and General Measures

1. Pit viper (eg, rattlesnake) envenomation—There are two commercially available antivenins for rattlesnake envenomation (CroFab and Anavip). Depending on the severity of symptoms CroFab is administered in increments of 4–6 vials by slow intravenous drip in 250–500 mL saline.

For more serious envenomation with marked local effects and systemic toxicity (eg, hypotension, coagulopathy), higher doses and additional vials may be required. The dosing of Anavip is 10 vials by slow intravenous infusion over 60 minutes initially followed by additional 10-vial increments as needed for more serious envenomations or for progression of symptoms. Monitor vital signs and the blood coagulation profile. Type and cross-match blood. The adequacy of venom neutralization is indicated by improvement in symptoms and signs, and the rate that swelling slows. Prophylactic antibiotics are not indicated after a rattlesnake bite.

2. Elapid (coral snake) envenomation—Give 3–5 vials of specific antivenom (Micuris Fulvis Antivenon) as soon as possible. To locate antisera for this or exotic snakes, call a regional poison control center (1-800-222-1222).

Seifert SA et al. Snake envenomation. N Engl J Med. 2022;386:68. [PMID: 34986287]
Velagapudi ME et al. Epidemiology and characteristics of coral snake bites reported to the National Poison Data System (2006–2022). J Am Coll Emerg Physicians Open. 2024;5:e13296. [PMID: 39371963]
Warpinski GP et al. North American envenomation syndromes. Emerg Med Clin North Am. 2022;40:313. [PMID: 35461625]

SPIDER BITES & SCORPION STINGS

Envenomation from most species of spiders in the United States causes only local pain, redness, and swelling. The more venomous black widow spiders (*Latrodectus mactans*) cause generalized muscular pains, muscle spasms, and rigidity. The brown recluse spider (*Loxosceles reclusa*) causes progressive local necrosis as well as hemolytic reactions (rare).

Stings by most scorpions in the United States cause only local pain. Stings by the more toxic *Centruroides* species (found in the southwestern United States) may cause muscle cramps, twitching and jerking, and occasionally hypertension, convulsions, and pulmonary edema. Stings by scorpions from other parts of the world are not discussed here.

Treatment

A. Black Widow Spider Bites

Pain may be relieved with parenteral opioids or muscle relaxants (eg, methocarbamol, 15 mg/kg). Calcium gluconate 10%, 0.1–0.2 mL/kg intravenously, may transiently relieve muscle rigidity, although its effectiveness is unproven. *Latrodectus* antivenom is possibly more effective, but because of concerns about acute hypersensitivity reactions (horse serum–derived), it is often reserved for very young persons, older adults, or those who do not respond promptly to the above measures. Horse serum sensitivity testing is required. (Instruction and testing materials are included in the antivenin kit.)

B. Brown Recluse Spider Bites

Because bites occasionally progress to extensive local necrosis, some authorities recommend early excision of the bite site, whereas others use oral corticosteroids. Anecdotal reports have claimed success with dapsone and colchicine. All of these treatments remain unproven.

C. Scorpion Stings

No specific treatment other than analgesics is required for envenomations by most scorpions found in the United States. An FDA-approved specific antivenom is available for *Centruroides* stings.

Herness J et al. Arthropod bites and stings. Am Fam Physician. 2022;106:137. [PMID: 35977137]
Kerns AF et al. Black widow spider exposures: a retrospective review of the National Poison Data System 2012-2022. Wilderness Environ Med. 2025;36:154. [PMID: 39670790]
Warpinski GP et al. North American envenomation syndromes. Emerg Med Clin North Am. 2022;40:313. [PMID: 35461625]

THEOPHYLLINE & CAFFEINE

Methylxanthines, including theophylline and caffeine, are nonselective adenosine receptor antagonists. In overdose, toxicity results from the release of endogenous catecholamines with β_1- and β_2-adrenergic stimulation. Theophylline may cause intoxication after an acute single overdose, or intoxication may occur as a result of chronic accidental repeated overmedication or reduced elimination resulting from hepatic dysfunction or interacting drug (eg, cimetidine, erythromycin). The usual serum half-life of theophylline is 4–6 hours, but this may increase to > 20 hours after overdose. Caffeine in energy drinks or herbal or dietary supplement products can produce similar toxicity.

Clinical Findings

Mild intoxication causes nausea, vomiting, tachycardia, and tremulousness. Severe intoxication is characterized by ventricular and supraventricular tachyarrhythmias, hypotension, and seizures. *Status epilepticus is common and often intractable to the usual anticonvulsants.* After acute overdose (but not chronic intoxication), hypokalemia, hyperglycemia, and metabolic acidosis are common. Seizures and other manifestations of toxicity may be delayed for several hours after acute ingestion, especially if a sustained-release preparation such as Theo-Dur was taken.

Diagnosis is based on measurement of the serum theophylline concentration. Seizures and hypotension are likely to develop in acute overdose patients with serum levels > 100 mg/L (555 mcmol/L). Serious toxicity may develop at lower levels (ie, 40–60 mg/L [222–333 mcmol/L]) in patients with chronic intoxication. Serum caffeine levels are not routinely available in clinical practice, but in a study of 51 fatal cases the median level was 180 mg/L (range, 33–567 mg/L).

Treatment

A. Emergency and Supportive Measures

After acute ingestion, administer activated charcoal. Repeated doses of activated charcoal may enhance theophylline and caffeine elimination by "gut dialysis." Addition of whole bowel irrigation should be considered for large ingestions involving sustained-release preparations.

Hemodialysis is effective in removing theophylline and is indicated for patients with status epilepticus or markedly elevated serum theophylline levels (eg, > 100 mg/L [555 mcmol/L] after acute overdose or > 60 mg/L [333 mcmol/L] with chronic intoxication). It has also been used in caffeine overdose. Extracorporeal membrane oxygenation (ECMO) has been used successfully in hemodynamic collapse after caffeine overdose.

B. Specific Treatment

Treat seizures with benzodiazepines (lorazepam, 2–3 mg intravenously, or diazepam, 5–10 mg intravenously) or phenobarbital (10–15 mg/kg intravenously). Phenytoin is not effective. Hypotension and tachycardia—which are mediated through excessive β-adrenergic stimulation—may respond to β-blocker therapy even in low doses. Administer esmolol, 25–50 mcg/kg/min by intravenous infusion, or propranolol, 0.5–1 mg intravenously.

Kobashi D et al. Severe caffeine poisoning successfully treated with high flow continuous hemodialysis. Am J Emerg Med. 2022;58:351.e3. [PMID: 35624048]

Mitsui D et al. Severe caffeine poisoning treated with intermittent hemodialysis under circulatory support. Am J Emerg Med. 2024;76:270.e5. [PMID: 38129271]

Ou HC et al. A successful experience using labetalol and hemodialysis to treat near-fatal caffeine poisoning: a case report with toxicodynamics. Am J Emerg Med. 2022;55:224.e1. [PMID: 34922795]

TRICYCLIC & OTHER ANTIDEPRESSANTS

Tricyclic and related cyclic antidepressants are among the most dangerous drugs involved in suicidal overdose. These drugs have anticholinergic and cardiac depressant properties ("quinidine-like" sodium channel blockade). Tricyclic antidepressants produce more marked membrane-depressant cardiotoxic effects than the phenothiazines.

Newer-generation antidepressants such as trazodone, fluoxetine, citalopram, paroxetine, sertraline, bupropion, venlafaxine, and fluvoxamine are not chemically related to the tricyclic antidepressant agents and, with the exception of bupropion, do not generally produce quinidine-like cardiotoxic effects. However, they may cause seizures in overdoses and serotonin syndrome.

Clinical Findings

Signs of severe intoxication may occur abruptly and without warning within 30–60 minutes after acute tricyclic overdose. Anticholinergic effects include dilated pupils, tachycardia, dry mouth, flushed skin, muscle twitching, and decreased peristalsis. Quinidine-like cardiotoxic effects include QRS interval widening (> 0.12 seconds; Figure 42–2), ventricular arrhythmias, AV block, and hypotension. Rightward-axis deviation of the terminal 40 milliseconds of the QRS has also been described.

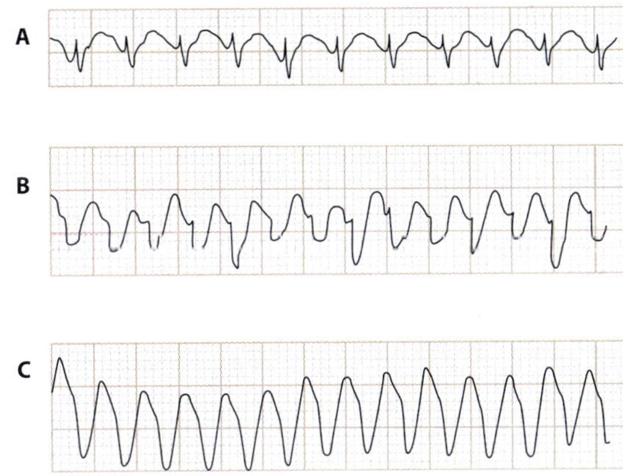

Figure 42–2. Cardiac arrhythmias resulting from tricyclic antidepressant overdose. **A:** Delayed intraventricular conduction results in prolonged QRS interval (0.18 seconds). **B** and **C:** Supraventricular tachycardia with progressive widening of QRS complexes mimics ventricular tachycardia. (Reproduced with permission from Benowitz NL, Goldschlager N. Cardiac disturbances in the toxicologic patient. In: Haddad LM, Winchester JF [editors], *Clinical Management of Poisoning and Drug Overdose*, 3rd edition. Saunders/Elsevier, 1998.)

Prolongation of the QT interval and torsades de pointes have been reported with several of the newer antidepressants. Seizures and coma are common with severe intoxication. Life-threatening hyperthermia may result from status epilepticus and anticholinergic-induced impairment of sweating. Among newer agents, bupropion and venlafaxine have been associated with a greater risk of seizures.

The diagnosis should be suspected in any overdose patient with anticholinergic side effects, especially if there is widening of the QRS interval or seizures. For intoxication by most tricyclic antidepressants, *the QRS interval correlates with the severity of intoxication more reliably than the serum drug level.*

Serotonin syndrome should be suspected if agitation, delirium, diaphoresis, tremor, hyperreflexia, clonus (spontaneous, inducible, or ocular), and fever develop in a patient taking serotonin reuptake inhibitors.

Treatment

A. Emergency and Supportive Measures

Observe patients for at least 6 hours and admit all patients with evidence of anticholinergic effects (eg, delirium, dilated pupils, tachycardia) or signs of cardiotoxicity.

Administer activated charcoal and consider gastric lavage after recent large ingestions. All of these drugs have large volumes of distribution and are not effectively removed by hemodialysis procedures.

B. Specific Treatment

Cardiotoxic sodium channel–depressant effects of tricyclic antidepressants may respond to boluses of sodium bicarbonate (50–100 mEq intravenously). Sodium bicarbonate provides a large sodium load that alleviates depression of the sodium-dependent channel. Reversal of acidosis may also have beneficial effects at this site. Maintain the pH between 7.45 and 7.50. Alkalinization does not promote excretion of tricyclic antidepressants. Prolongation of the QT interval or torsades de pointes is usually treated with intravenous magnesium or overdrive pacing. Severe cardiotoxicity in patients with overdoses of lipid-soluble drugs (eg, amitriptyline, bupropion) has reportedly responded to intravenous lipid emulsion (Intralipid), 1.5 mL/kg repeated one or two times if needed. Plasma exchange using albumin and ECMO have been reported to be successful in several cases.

Mild serotonin syndrome may be treated with benzodiazepines and withdrawal of the antidepressant. Moderate cases may respond to cyproheptadine (4 mg orally or via gastric tube hourly for three or four doses) or chlorpromazine (25 mg intravenously). Severe hyperthermia should be treated with neuromuscular paralysis and endotracheal intubation in addition to external cooling measures.

Mohammed T et al. Case report: management of an unknown TCA diagnosis: the importance of rapid diagnosis and the use of CVVHDF in toxin elimination. Toxicol Rep. 2023;11:307. [PMID: 37789950]

Pires KD et al. Successful treatment of confirmed severe bupropion cardiotoxicity with veno-arterial extracorporeal membrane oxygenation initiation prior to cardiac arrest. Cureus. 2024;16:e53768. [PMID: 38465186]

Cancer

43

Sunny Wang, MD
Tiffany O. Dea, PharmD, BCOP
Marc A. Dall'Era, MD
Andrew Ko, MD

INTRODUCTION TO CANCER

Etiology

Cancer is the second most common cause of death in the United States. In 2025, an estimated 2,041,910 cases of cancer were diagnosed, and 618,120 persons died of cancer. Table 43–1 lists the 10 leading cancer types in men and women by site. *However, death rates from cancers are declining.* Compared with the 1991 overall cancer death rate of 215 per 100,000 population, the 2019–2023 rate of 145.4 per 100,000 represents a 32% reduction in the overall cancer death rate. Importantly, death rates have declined in all four of the most common cancer types (prostate, breast, lung, and colorectum). Reductions in cancer mortality reflect successful implementation of a broad strategy of prevention, detection, and treatment. Due to these improvements, *the number of cancer survivors is increasing.* In 2025, an estimated 18.6 million people in the United States were alive in whom cancer had been previously diagnosed, approximately 5.4% of the population.

Modifiable Risk Factors

Tobacco use is the most common preventable cause of cancer death; at least 30% of all cancer deaths in the United States are directly linked to tobacco use. Clear evidence links tobacco use to at least 12 cancers. The most dramatic link is with lung cancer; > 80% of lung cancer deaths are attributable to smoking.

In 2023, the United States Department of Health and Human Services reported that 20% of adults in the United States were active tobacco users, a reduction from the 1955 peak of 57% for men and the 1965 peak of 34% for women. Cigarettes are the most common form of tobacco used in the United States, but among US youth, electronic cigarettes are the most popular form. From the Annual National Youth Tobacco Survey, the percent of middle and high school students in the United States who used e-cigarettes in 2024 was 5.9%, a decrease from 7.7% the year prior.

Tobacco cessation directed toward the individual should start with clinician counseling. *Simple, concise advice from a clinician can yield cessation rates of 10–20%.* Additive strategies include more intensive counseling; nicotine replacement therapy with patches, gum, lozenges, or inhalers; and prescription medication with bupropion or varenicline (see Chapter 1).

For those Americans who do not use tobacco, the most modifiable cancer risk factors are nutrition and physical activity. *Prudent recommendations to reduce cancer risk are to (1) avoid tobacco; (2) be physically active; (3) maintain a healthy weight; (4) consume a diet rich in fruits, vegetables, and whole grains; (5) lower consumption of saturated and trans dietary fats; (6) limit alcohol use; and (7) avoid excess sun exposure.*

Another modifiable cancer risk factor is radiation from radiographic studies. Both standardization of CT radiation doses and limiting testing have been important steps in minimizing this risk.

American Cancer Society. Cancer facts & figures 2025. https://www.cancer.org/research/cancer-facts-statistics/all-cancer-facts-figures/2025-cancer-facts-figures.html

Siegel RL et al. Cancer statistics, 2025. CA Cancer J Clin. 2025;75:10. [PMID: 39817679]

US Food and Drug Administration. Results from the Annual National Youth Tobacco Survey. https://www.fda.gov/tobacco-products/youth-and-tobacco/results-annual-national-youth-tobacco-survey-nyts

Staging

The Tumor, Node, Metastasis (TNM) system is the commonly used classification to stage cancer. Staging is important not only because it correlates with the patient's long-term survival but also because it is used to determine treatment strategies. Rules for staging for individual cancers are established and published by the *American Joint Committee on Cancer (AJCC).* The elements used for staging are tumor location, size, and level of invasion (T); absence or presence and extent of nodal metastases (N); and absence or presence of systemic metastases (M). Once the TNM designations have been determined, an overall stage (I, II, III, or IV) is assigned.

Certain characteristics of cancers, not reflected in the TNM stage, may be used to indicate prognosis and guide treatment. Pathologic features seen on routine histologic examination for some cancers are very important; examples include the Gleason score for prostate cancer, HPV

Table 43–1. Estimated 10 most common cancer cases in the United States in males and females (all races).

Rank	Males: Total Cases (%) [N] = 1,053,250	Females: Total Cases (%) [N] = 988,660
1	Prostate 313,780 (30)	Breast 316,950 (32)
2	Lung and bronchus 110,680 (11)	Lung and bronchus 115,970 (12)
3	Colon and rectum 82,460 (8)	Colon and rectum 71,810 (7)
4	Urinary bladder 65,080 (6)	Uterine corpus 69,120 (7)
5	Melanoma 60,550 (6)	Melanoma 44,410 (4)
6	Kidney and renal pelvis 52,410 (5)	Non-Hodgkin lymphoma 35,210 (4)
7	Non-Hodgkin lymphoma 45,410 (4)	Pancreas 32,490 (3)
8	Oral cavity and pharynx 42,500 (4)	Thyroid 31,350 (3)
9	Leukemia 38,720 (4)	Kidney and renal pelvis 28,570 (3)
10	Pancreas 34,950 (3)	Leukemia 28,170 (3)

Data from the American Cancer Society, 2025.

status of oropharyngeal cancer, and grade of sarcomas. Cancer specimens should also be sent for molecular diagnostic testing. Programmed death-ligand 1 (PD-L1) expression testing should be sent for certain cancers (including lung, head/neck, esophageal cancers).

Detterbeck FC et al. The proposed ninth edition TNM Classification of Lung Cancer. Chest. 2024;166:882. [PMID: 38885896]

Treatment

See Primary Cancer Treatment section below. Table 43–2 outlines treatment choices by cancer type for those responsive to systemic agents, and Tables 43–3, 43–4, 43–5, 43–6, 43–7, 43–8, and 43–9 provide lists of common chemotherapeutic agents.

TYPES OF CANCER

LUNG CANCER

BRONCHOGENIC CARCINOMA

ESSENTIALS OF DIAGNOSIS

- New cough or change in chronic cough.
- Dyspnea, hemoptysis, anorexia, weight loss.
- Enlarging lung nodule or mass; persistent opacity, atelectasis, or pleural effusion on chest radiograph or CT scan.
- Cytologic or histologic findings of lung cancer in sputum, pleural fluid, or biopsy specimen.

General Considerations

Lung cancer is the leading cause of cancer deaths in both men and women. The American Cancer Society (ACS) estimates 226,650 new diagnoses and 124,730 deaths from lung cancer in the United States in 2025, accounting for approximately 11% of new cancer diagnoses and 20% of all cancer deaths.

Cigarette smoking causes 85–90% of cases of lung cancer. Other environmental risk factors for the development of lung cancer include exposure to environmental tobacco smoke, radon, asbestos, diesel exhaust, ionizing radiation, metals (arsenic, chromium, nickel, iron oxide), and industrial carcinogens. A familial predisposition to lung cancer is recognized. Certain diseases are associated with an increased risk of lung cancer, including pulmonary fibrosis, COPD, and sarcoidosis.

The median age at diagnosis of lung cancer in the United States is 71 years; it is unusual under the age of 40 years. The combined relative 5-year survival rate for all stages of lung cancer is 28%.

There are five main histologic categories of bronchogenic carcinoma. **Squamous cell carcinomas** (29% of non–small-cell lung cancer [NSCLC] cases, based on US Surveillance, Epidemiology, and End Results National Program of Cancer Registries data, 2010–2017) arise from the bronchial epithelium and often present as intraluminal masses. They are usually centrally located and can present with hemoptysis. **Adenocarcinomas** (55% of NSCLC cases) arise from mucous glands or from any epithelial cell within or distal to the terminal bronchioles. They usually present as peripheral nodules or masses. **Adenocarcinomas in situ** (formerly **bronchioloalveolar cell carcinomas)** spread along preexisting alveolar structures (lepidic growth) without evidence of invasion. **Large cell carcinomas** (1.8% of cases) are a heterogeneous group of undifferentiated cancers that share large cells and do not fit into other categories. Large cell carcinomas are typically aggressive and have rapid doubling times. They present as central or peripheral masses. Cancers that are not better differentiated on pathologic review other than NSCLC or carcinomas not otherwise specified make up about 14% of cases. **Small cell carcinomas** (14% of all lung cancer cases) are tumors of bronchial origin that typically begin centrally, infiltrating submucosally to cause narrowing of the bronchus without a discrete luminal mass. They are aggressive cancers that often involve regional or distant metastasis on presentation.

For purposes of staging and treatment, bronchogenic carcinomas are divided into small-cell lung cancer (**SCLC**) and the other four types, labeled **NSCLC**. This practical classification reflects different natural histories and treatments. SCLC is prone to early hematogenous spread and has a more aggressive course with a median survival of 6–18 weeks if untreated.

Table 43–2. Treatment choices for selected cancers responsive to systemic agents (listed in alphabetical order by diagnosis).

Diagnosis	Initial Treatment
Acute lymphoblastic leukemia (ALL)	**Induction combination chemotherapy (Philadelphia chromosome–positive):** Cyclophosphamide, vincristine, doxorubicin/daunorubicin, dexamethasone (hyper-CVAD) alternating with cytarabine, methotrexate; or blinatumomab; add imatinib or dasatinib or nilotinib to either of the regimens **Induction combination chemotherapy (Philadelphia chromosome–negative):** Daunorubicin, vincristine, prednisone, pegaspargase, cyclophosphamide, cytarabine, mercaptopurine; or hyper-CVAD alternating with methotrexate and cytarabine
Acute myeloid leukemia (AML)	**Induction combination therapy:** Cytarabine with daunorubicin or idarubicin, with gemtuzumab ozogamicin (CD33-positive), or with midostaurin or quizartinib (*FLT3*-mutated) Liposomal encapsulation of cytarabine and daunorubicin (therapy-related or myelodysplasia-related changes for ≥ 60 y) **Alternative therapy for intensive induction ineligible:** Azacitidine or decitabine with venetoclax; or ivosidenib (*IDH1* mutation); or enasidenib (*IDH2* mutation)
Anal cancer	Mitomycin with 5-fluorouracil or capecitabine with radiation (localized cancer) Carboplatin and paclitaxel plus retifanlimab, with or without radiation therapy for control of the primary tumor (metastatic cancer) or FOLFOX
Biliary cancer	Gemcitabine and cisplatin plus durvalumab or pembrolizumab Pemigatinib or futibatinib (FGFR fusion) Ivosidenib (*IDH1* mutation) Zanidatamab or trastuzumab deruxtecan (*HER2* overexpression/amplification)
Bladder cancer	Mitomycin with 5-fluorouracil with radiation; or gemcitabine, cisplatin; or methotrexate, vinblastine, doxorubicin, cisplatin (MVAC), or pembrolizumab and enfortumab vedotin-ejfv (metastatic)
Breast cancer	**Adjuvant hormone therapy:** *Premenopausal:* Tamoxifen *Postmenopausal:* Aromatase inhibitors (anastrozole, letrozole, exemestane) **Adjuvant therapy (*HER2* negative):** Doxorubicin, cyclophosphamide, followed by paclitaxel, or Docetaxel, cyclophosphamide, or Olaparib if germline *BRCA1/2* pathogenic variants, or High-risk triple-negative—preoperative pembrolizumab/carboplatin/paclitaxel, followed by pembrolizumab/cyclophosphamide/doxorubicin or epirubicin, followed by adjuvant pembrolizumab **Adjuvant therapy (*HER2* positive):** Docetaxel, carboplatin, trastuzumab with or without pertuzumab, or Paclitaxel, trastuzumab
Carcinoid and other gastropancreatic neuroendocrine tumors	Octreotide LAR or lanreotide Well-differentiated tumors: Everolimus, sunitinib, cabozantinib Lutetium (Lu)-177 dotatate Capecitabine/temozolomide Poorly differentiated tumors are treated analogously to small cell carcinomas of the lung
Cervical cancer	**Early disease:** Surgery **Locally advanced:** Cisplatin (or carboplatin) with radiation; certain cases with cisplatin + pembrolizumab with radiation; certain cases with paclitaxel and carboplatin followed by cisplatin with radiation **Advanced:** Paclitaxel/cisplatin (or carboplatin), +/– bevacizumab + pembrolizumab with PD-L1-positive tumors, or atezolizumab
Chronic lymphocytic leukemia (CLL)	Venetoclax with obinutuzumab; or acalabrutinib with or without obinutuzumab, with or without venetoclax; or zanubrutinib
Chronic myeloid leukemia (CML)	Nilotinib or dasatinib or imatinib or bosutinib or asciminib

(*continued*)

Table 43–2. Treatment choices for selected cancers responsive to systemic agents (listed in alphabetical order by diagnosis). (continued)

Diagnosis	Initial Treatment
Colon cancer	5-fluorouracil, leucovorin, oxaliplatin (FOLFOX); or capecitabine, oxaliplatin (CAPEOX); or 5-fluorouracil, leucovorin, irinotecan (FOLFIRI); or 5-fluorouracil, leucovorin, oxaliplatin, irinotecan (FOLFIRINOX); or Capecitabine or 5-fluorouracil/leucovorin May add bevacizumab for advanced or metastatic disease May add cetuximab or panitumumab for *KRAS/NRAS/BRAF* wild-type and left-sided cancers with metastatic disease Pembrolizumab, dostarlimab-gxly; or nivolumab with or without ipilimumab (deficient mismatch repair [dMMR]/high-level microsatellite instability [MSI-H]) Encorafenib and cetuximab, +/– either FOLFOX or FOLFIRI (*BRAF* mutation) Trastuzumab deruxtecan or trastuzumab in combination with pertuzumab, lapatinib, or tucatinib (*HER2* overexpressing) (sotarasib or adagrasib) + (cetuximab or panitumumab) (*KRAS* G12C mutation) Salvage regimens: trifluridine/tipiracil plus bevacizumab; fruquintinib; regorafenib
Esophageal and esophagogastric junction cancer	5-fluorouracil, leucovorin, oxaliplatin, docetaxel (FLOT) plus durvalumab (perioperative) Carboplatin/paclitaxel + concurrent radiation (preoperative) plus nivolumab (postoperative for patients not achieving a compete pathologic response at the time of surgery) 5-fluorouracil/leucovorin + oxaliplatin (FOLFOX) or capecitabine + oxaliplatin with the addition of pembrolizumab, nivolumab, or zolbetuximab (depending on PD-L1 and Claudin 18.2 expression) (HER2-negative unresectable, recurrent, or metastatic disease) 5-fluorouracil/leucovorin + oxaliplatin (FOLFOX) or capecitabine + oxaliplatin + trastuzumab + pembrolizumab (*HER2*-positive, unresectable, recurrent, or metastatic disease; PD-L1 expression at least 1%) (Nivolumab +/– ipilimumab) or pembrolizumab (MSI-H/dMMR unresectable, recurrent, or metastatic disease) Salvage regimens: paclitaxel or irinotecan in combination with ramucirumab; trastuzumab deruxtecan for *HER2*-positive disease
Head and neck cancer (non-nasopharyngeal)	Cisplatin with radiation therapy, or Carboplatin with 5-fluorouracil with radiation therapy, or Docetaxel, cisplatin, 5-fluorouracil (induction) Pembrolizumab (PD-L1 ≥ 1%), or Pembrolizumab/cisplatin or carboplatin/5-fluorouracil (recurrent, unresectable, or metastatic disease)
Hepatocellular cancer	Atezolizumab with bevacizumab; or Tremelimumab-actl with durvalumab; or Lenvatinib or sorafenib Salvage regimens: cabozantinib, regorafenib, ramucirumab; immune checkpoint inhibitor (if patient did not previously receive)
Hodgkin lymphoma	Doxorubicin, bleomycin, vinblastine, dacarbazine (ABVD); or Brentuximab vedotin (BV) or nivolumab with doxorubicin, vinblastine, dacarbazine; or BV, etoposide, cyclophosphamide, doxorubicin, dacarbazine, dexamethasone (BrECADD)
Kidney (renal cell) cancer	**Clear cell histology:** Axitinib or lenvatinib plus pembrolizumab, or ipilimumab plus nivolumab, or cabozantinib plus nivolumab **Non–clear cell histology:** Cabozantinib with or without nivolumab or lenvatinib with pembrolizumab
Melanoma	Neoadjuvant: Nivolumab with ipilimumab or pembrolizumab Adjuvant: Nivolumab, pembrolizumab, or dabrafenib/trametinib (*BRAF* mutation) Metastatic: Nivolumab with ipilimumab or relatlimab-rmbw Dabrafenib/trametinib, vemurafenib/cobimetinib, or encorafenib/binimetinib (*BRAF* mutation)
Mesothelioma	Cisplatin or carboplatin/pemetrexed with or without bevacizumab or pembrolizumab, or Nivolumab with ipilimumab
Multiple myeloma	**(Transplant candidates):** Bortezomib, dexamethasone, lenalidomide, daratumumab or isatuximab-irfc followed by autologous or mini-allogeneic stem cell transplantation **(Non-transplant candidates):** Daratumumab, bortezomib, lenalidomide, dexamethasone; or Daratumumab, lenalidomide, dexamethasone; or Isatuximab-irfc, bortezomib, lenalidomide, dexamethasone

(*continued*)

Table 43–2. Treatment choices for selected cancers responsive to systemic agents (listed in alphabetical order by diagnosis). (continued)

Diagnosis	Initial Treatment
Non-Hodgkin lymphoma (intermediate and high-grade)	Cyclophosphamide, doxorubicin, vincristine, prednisone, rituximab[1] (CHOP-R); or Polatuzumab vedotin-piiq, rituximab, cyclophosphamide, doxorubicin, prednisone; or Etoposide, prednisone, vincristine, cyclophosphamide, doxorubicin, rituximab[1] (dose-adjusted R EPOCH) (for MYC and either BCL2 or BCL6 rearrangements)
Non-Hodgkin lymphoma (low-grade)	Bendamustine plus obinutuzumab or rituximab[1]; or CHOP with obinutuzumab or rituximab[1]; or Cyclophosphamide, vincristine, prednisone, with obinutuzumab or rituximab[1]; or Lenalidomide, rituximab[1]
Non–small cell lung cancer	**Neoadjuvant and adjuvant therapy:** Cisplatin, gemcitabine or docetaxel (squamous histology), or Cisplatin, pemetrexed (nonsquamous histology) Add nivolumab, pembrolizumab, or durvalumab to platinum-doublet chemotherapy if candidate for immune checkpoint inhibitor **Single-agent therapy for advanced or metastatic disease:** Erlotinib, gefitinib, osimertinib, afatinib, or dacomitinib (*EGFR* mutation positive) Sotorasib or adagrasib (*KRAS* G12C mutation positive) Alectinib, brigatinib, ceritinib, crizotinib, lorlatinib (*ALK* rearrangement) Crizotinib, entrectinib, or repotrectinib (*ROS1* rearrangement) Larotrectinib, entrectinib, or repotrectinib (*NTRK* gene fusion positive) Capmatinib, crizotinib, or tepotinib (*MET* amplification) Selpercatinib, or pralsetinib (*RET* rearrangement positive) Pembrolizumab, or atezolizumab, or cemiplimab-rwlc (PD-L1 ≥ 50%) **Combination therapy for advanced or metastatic disease:** Carboplatin or cisplatin/pemetrexed/pembrolizumab (nonsquamous); carboplatin/paclitaxel or albumin-bound paclitaxel/pembrolizumab (squamous)
Ovarian cancer	Paclitaxel, carboplatin, with or without bevacizumab, or 5-Fluorouracil/leucovorin or capecitabine, oxaliplatin
Pancreatic cancer	Combination chemotherapy: Gemcitabine, albumin-bound paclitaxel; or 5-fluorouracil, leucovorin, irinotecan, oxaliplatin (FOLFIRINOX); or Liposomal irinotecan, 5-fluorouracil, leucovorin, oxaliplatin (NALIRIFOX) FOLFIRINOX or gemcitabine plus cisplatin (for *BRCA1/2* or *PALB2* mutation), followed by maintenance olaparib Gemcitabine alone (poor performance status)
Prostate cancer	Androgen deprivation therapy (eg, leuprolide or degarelix) with or without abiraterone, enzalutamide, apalutamide, or docetaxel
Rectal cancer	5-fluorouracil or capecitabine with radiation (preoperative for localized disease); FOLFOX or capecitabine/oxaliplatin is sometimes included as part of induction or consolidation treatment in the preoperative setting or postoperatively as adjuvant treatment Refer to colon cancer for treatment of metastatic disease
Small cell lung cancer	Cisplatin, etoposide with radiation followed by durvalumab (limited stage) Cisplatin or carboplatin, etoposide, plus atezolizumab or durvalumab (extensive stage)
Soft tissue sarcomas	**Combination chemotherapy:** Doxorubicin, dacarbazine (AD), or Doxorubicin, ifosfamide, mesna (AIM), or Ifosfamide, epirubicin, mesna **Single-agent therapy:** Imatinib or avapritinib (GI stromal tumors) Doxorubicin or epirubicin or liposomal doxorubicin
Stomach (gastric) cancer	Same as esophageal/esophagogastric cancer
Testicular cancer	Carboplatin (stage I seminoma), Cisplatin, etoposide (EP), or Bleomycin, etoposide, cisplatin (BEP), or Etoposide, mesna, ifosfamide, cisplatin (VIP)

(continued)

Table 43–2. Treatment choices for selected cancers responsive to systemic agents (listed in alphabetical order by diagnosis). (continued)

Diagnosis	Initial Treatment
Thyroid cancer	**Single-agent therapy:** Radioiodine (^{131}I) lenvatinib (papillary), selpercatinib (medullary)
Uterine cancer	**Hormone therapy:** Progestins, tamoxifen, aromatase inhibitors **Chemotherapy:** Cisplatin with radiation followed by carboplatin/paclitaxel Carboplatin, paclitaxel with or without pembrolizumab or dostarlimab-gxly Carboplatin, paclitaxel, trastuzumab (*HER2* positive)
Waldenström macroglobulinemia/ lymphoplasmacytic lymphoma	**Plasmapheresis alone or followed by:** Bendamustine, rituximab[1]; or Zanubrutinib

[1]In patients with past hepatitis B virus (HBV) infection, rituximab should be used with anti-HBV agent (eg, entecavir) prophylaxis since HBV reactivation, fulminant hepatitis, and, rarely, death can occur otherwise.

Clinical Findings

Lung cancer is symptomatic at diagnosis in a majority of patients. The clinical presentation depends on the type and location of the primary tumor, the extent of local spread, and the presence of distant metastases and any paraneoplastic syndromes.

A. Symptoms and Signs

Anorexia, weight loss, or asthenia occurs in 55–90% of patients presenting with a new diagnosis of lung cancer. Up to 60% of patients have a new cough or a change in a chronic cough; 6–31% have hemoptysis; and 25–40% report pain, either nonspecific chest pain or pain from bony metastases to the vertebrae, ribs, or pelvis. Local spread may cause endobronchial obstruction with atelectasis and postobstructive pneumonia, pleural effusion (12–33%), change in voice (compromise of the recurrent laryngeal nerve), **superior vena cava syndrome** (obstruction of the superior vena cava with supraclavicular venous engorgement), and **Horner syndrome** (ipsilateral ptosis, miosis, and anhidrosis from involvement of the inferior cervical ganglion and the paravertebral sympathetic chain). Distant metastases to the liver are associated with asthenia and weight loss. Brain metastases (10% in NSCLC, more common in adenocarcinoma, and 20–30% in SCLC) may present with headache, nausea, vomiting, seizures, dizziness, or altered mental status.

Paraneoplastic syndromes are patterns of organ dysfunction related to immune-mediated or secretory effects of neoplasms. These syndromes occur in 10–20% of patients with lung cancer. In patients with small cell carcinoma, SIAD can develop in 10–15%; in those with squamous cell carcinoma, hypercalcemia can develop in 10%. Digital clubbing is seen in up to 20% of patients at diagnosis (see Figure 6–39). Other common paraneoplastic syndromes include increased ACTH production, anemia, hypercoagulability, peripheral neuropathy, and the Lambert-Eaton myasthenic syndrome.

B. Laboratory Findings

The diagnosis of lung cancer rests on examination of a tissue or cytology specimen. *Sputum cytology* is highly specific but insensitive; the yield is highest when there are lesions in the central airways. While the diagnostic yield of *CT-guided biopsy* of peripheral nodules approaches 80–90%, the rates of pneumothorax are significant (15–30%), especially in those with emphysema. *Thoracentesis*

Table 43–3. Common alkylating agents for cancer treatment (listed alphabetically within classes).

Agent	Usual Adult Dosage	Adverse Effects
Alkylating Agents—Nitrogen Mustards		
Cyclophosphamide (Cytoxan)	500–1000 mg/m² intravenously every 3 weeks; 100 mg/m²/day orally for 14 days every 4 weeks; various doses	Acute: nausea and vomiting Delayed: myelosuppression, alopecia, hemorrhagic cystitis, cardiotoxicity (high dose)
Alkylating Agents—Platinum Analogs		
Cisplatin (Platinol)	50–100 mg/m² intravenously every 3–4 weeks; 20 mg/m²/day intravenously for 5 days every 3 weeks; various doses	Acute: nausea and vomiting Delayed: nephrotoxicity, ototoxicity, neurotoxicity, myelosuppression, electrolyte disturbances

Table 43–4. Common antimetabolite agents for cancer treatment (listed alphabetically within classes).

Agent	Usual Adult Dosage	Adverse Effects
Antimetabolites—Folate Antagonists		
Pemetrexed (Alimta)	500 mg/m^2 intravenously every 3 weeks	Acute: nausea, vomiting, diarrhea, rash Delayed: myelosuppression, fatigue, mucositis
Antimetabolites—Pyrimidine Analogs		
Azacitidine (Vidaza)	75–100 mg/m^2 subcutaneously or intravenously for 7 days every 4 weeks	Acute: injection site reaction (subcutaneously), nausea, diarrhea, fever Delayed: myelosuppression, dyspnea, arthralgia
Capecitabine (Xeloda)	1000–1250 mg/m^2 orally twice a day for 14 days every 3 weeks	Acute: nausea, vomiting, diarrhea Delayed: hand-foot syndrome, mucositis, hyperbilirubinemia, myelosuppression
Fluorouracil (Adrucil)	400 mg/m^2 intravenous bolus followed by 2400 mg/m^2 intravenously over 46 hours every 2 weeks; 1000 mg/m^2 intravenously via continuous infusion for 4–5 days every 3–4 weeks; various doses	Acute: nausea, vomiting, diarrhea Delayed: myelosuppression, hand-foot syndrome, mucositis, photosensitivity, cardiotoxicity (rare)
Gemcitabine (Gemzar)	1000–1250 mg/m^2 intravenously on days 1 and 8 every 3 weeks or days 1, 8, 15 every 4 weeks; various doses	Acute: nausea, vomiting, rash, flu-like symptoms, fever, diarrhea Delayed: myelosuppression, edema, elevated transaminases

(sensitivity 50–65%) can be used to establish a diagnosis of lung cancer in patients with malignant pleural effusions. *Fine-needle aspiration (FNA)* of palpable supraclavicular or cervical lymph nodes is frequently diagnostic.

Fiberoptic bronchoscopy allows visualization of the major airways, cytology brushing of visible lesions or lavage of lung segments with cytologic evaluation of specimens, direct biopsy of endobronchial abnormalities, blind transbronchial biopsy of the pulmonary parenchyma or peripheral nodules, and FNA biopsy of mediastinal lymph nodes. *Electromagnetic navigational bronchoscopy* allows bronchoscopic approaches to small peripheral nodules. *Mediastinoscopy, video-assisted thoracoscopic surgery (VATS)*, and *thoracotomy* may be necessary in cases where less invasive techniques fail to yield a diagnosis.

C. Imaging

Nearly all patients with lung cancer have abnormal findings on CXR or CT scan (Figure 43–1). These findings are rarely specific for a particular diagnosis. Interpretation of characteristic findings in isolated nodules is described in Chapter 9.

D. Special Examinations

1. Staging—Accurate staging is crucial (1) to provide the clinician with information to guide treatment, (2) to provide the patient with accurate information regarding prognosis, and (3) to standardize entry criteria for clinical trials to allow interpretation of results.

Staging of NSCLC is based on the updated 9th edition of the *AJCC/Union for International Cancer Control* stage classification for lung cancer. The AJCC TNM international staging system attempts a physical description of the neoplasm: T describes the size and location of the primary tumor; N describes the presence and location of nodal metastases; and M refers to the presence or absence of distant metastases. These TNM stages are grouped into summary stages I–IV, and these are used to guide therapy (Table 43–10).

Table 43–5. Common antimicrotubules for cancer treatment (listed alphabetically within classes).

Agent	Usual Adult Dosage	Adverse Effects
Antimicrotubules—Vinca Alkaloids		
Vincristine (Oncovin)	0.5–1.4 mg/m^2 intravenously every 3 weeks; various doses; maximum single dose usually limited to 2 mg	Acute: constipation, nausea Delayed: peripheral neuropathy, alopecia
Antimicrotubules—Taxanes		
Paclitaxel (Taxol)	135–175 mg/m^2 intravenously every 3 weeks; 50–80 mg/m^2 intravenously weekly; various doses	Acute: diarrhea, nausea, vomiting, hypersensitivity Delayed: myelosuppression, peripheral neuropathy, alopecia, mucositis, arthralgia

Table 43–6. Common enzyme inhibitors for cancer treatment (listed alphabetically within classes).

Agent	Usual Adult Dosage	Adverse Effects
Enzyme Inhibitors—Anthracyclines		
Doxorubicin (Adriamycin)	45–75 mg/m² intravenously every 3 weeks; various doses	
Enzyme Inhibitors—Topoisomerase Inhibitors		
Etoposide (Vepesid)	50–100 mg/m² intravenously for 3–5 days every 3 weeks	Acute: nausea, vomiting, diarrhea, hypersensitivity, fever, hypotension Delayed: myelosuppression, alopecia, fatigue
Irinotecan (Camptosar)	180 mg/m² intravenously every other week; various doses	Acute: diarrhea, cholinergic syndrome, nausea, vomiting Delayed: myelosuppression, alopecia, asthenia

SCLC is traditionally divided into two categories: *limited disease* (30% of cases), when the tumor is limited to the unilateral hemithorax (including contralateral mediastinal nodes); or *extensive disease* (70% of cases), when the tumor extends beyond the hemithorax (including pleural effusion). It is also recommended to stage SCLC according to the TNM staging system (Table 43–10).

For both SCLC and NSCLC, a complete examination is essential to exclude obvious metastatic disease to lymph nodes, skin, and bone. A detailed history is essential because *the patient's performance status is a powerful predictor of disease course.* All patients should have measurement of a CBC, serum electrolytes, calcium, creatinine, liver biochemical tests, LD, and albumin.

NSCLC patients being considered for surgery require meticulous evaluation to identify those with resectable disease. CT imaging is key for staging candidates for resection. The sensitivity and specificity of CT imaging for identifying lung cancer metastatic to the mediastinal lymph nodes are 57% (49–66%) and 82% (77–86%), respectively. Therefore, *chest CT imaging alone does not provide definitive staging information.* CT imaging helps determine where to biopsy and how the mediastinum should be sampled.

The combination of PET using 2-[^{18}F] fluoro-2-deoxyglucose (FDG-PET) and CT is an important modality for identifying metastatic foci in the mediastinum or distant sites. The sensitivity and specificity of FDG-PET/CT for detecting mediastinal spread of primary lung cancer depend on the size of mediastinal nodes or masses. When mediastinal lymph nodes smaller than 1 cm are present, the sensitivity and specificity of FDG-PET/CT for tumor involvement of nodes are 74% and 96%, respectively. When CT shows

Table 43–7. Common hormonal agents for cancer treatment (listed alphabetically within classes).

Agent	Usual Adult Dosage	Adverse Effects
Hormonal—Antiandrogens		
Enzalutamide (Xtandi)	160 mg orally once daily	Acute: asthenia, diarrhea Delayed: hot flashes, arthralgia, peripheral edema, seizure (rare)
Hormonal—Aromatase Inhibitors		
Anastrozole (Arimidex)	1 mg orally once daily	Acute: nausea Delayed: hot flashes, peripheral edema, asthenia, hypercholesterolemia, arthralgia/myalgia, osteoporosis
Hormonal—LHRH Analogs		
Leuprolide (Lupron Depot, Eligard)	1 month: 7.5 mg intramuscularly or subcutaneously every month 3 month: 22.5 mg intramuscularly or subcutaneously every 3 months 4 month: 30 mg intramuscularly or subcutaneously every 4 months 6 month: 45 mg intramuscularly or subcutaneously every 6 months	
Hormonal—Selective Estrogen Receptor Modulators		
Tamoxifen (Nolvadex)	20–40 mg orally once daily	Acute: none Delayed: hot flashes, vaginal discharge, menstrual irregularities, arthralgia

Table 43–8. Common targeted therapies in cancer treatment (listed alphabetically within classes).

Agent	Usual Adult Dosage	Adverse Effects
Targeted Therapy—Monoclonal Antibodies		
Bevacizumab (Avastin)	5–15 mg/kg intravenously every 2–3 weeks	Acute: infusion-related reaction Delayed: hypertension, proteinuria, wound healing complications, GI perforation, hemorrhage
Cetuximab (Erbitux)	Loading dose 400 mg/m^2 intravenously; maintenance dose 250 mg/m^2 intravenously weekly	Acute: infusion-related reaction, nausea, diarrhea Delayed: acneiform skin rash, hypomagnesemia, asthenia, paronychial inflammation, dyspnea
Daratumumab/hyaluronidase, (Darzalex Faspro)	1800 mg subcutaneously over 3–5 minutes weekly for weeks 1–8, every 2 weeks for weeks 9–24, and every 4 weeks from week 25 until disease progression	Acute: infusion-related reaction, nausea Delayed: myelosuppression, fatigue, upper respiratory tract infection
Ipilimumab (Yervoy)	1–10 mg/kg intravenously every 3 weeks for a total of four doses	Acute: infusion-related reaction Delayed: immune-related reactions, fatigue, diarrhea, nausea, pruritus
Nivolumab (Opdivo)	240 mg intravenously every 2 weeks or 480 mg every 4 weeks; various doses	Acute: infusion-related reaction, vomiting Delayed: immune-mediated reactions, fatigue, nausea, decreased appetite
Pembrolizumab (Keytruda)	200 mg intravenously every 3 weeks or 400 mg every 6 weeks	Acute: infusion-related reaction, nausea Delayed: immune-mediated reactions, fatigue, cough
Rituximab (Rituxan)	375 mg/m^2 intravenously weekly for 4 weeks, or every 3–4 weeks; various doses	Acute: infusion-related reaction, TLS Delayed: lymphopenia, asthenia, rash, potential hepatitis B reactivation
Trastuzumab (Herceptin)	Initial dose 4 mg/kg intravenously, then 2 mg/kg intravenously weekly; or initial dose 8 mg/kg, then 6 mg/kg, intravenously every 3 weeks	Acute: headache, nausea, diarrhea, infusion-related reaction Delayed: myelosuppression, pyrexia, cardiomyopathy, pulmonary toxicity (rare)
Targeted Therapy—Kinase Inhibitors		
Acalabrutinib (Calquence)	100 mg orally every 12 hours	Acute: diarrhea Delayed: myelosuppression, upper respiratory infection, musculoskeletal pain
Imatinib (Gleevec)	100–800 mg orally once daily with food; various doses	Acute: nausea, vomiting, diarrhea Delayed: edema, muscle cramps, rash, myelosuppression, hepatotoxicity
Osimertinib (Tagrisso)	80 mg orally once daily	Acute: diarrhea Delayed: myelosuppression, rash, dry skin, nail toxicity, cardiomyopathy (rare), prolonged QT interval (rare)

Table 43–9. Common miscellaneous agents used in cancer treatment (listed alphabetically).

Agent	Usual Adult Dosage	Adverse Effects
Miscellaneous Agents		
Abiraterone (Zytiga)	1000 mg orally once daily	Acute: diarrhea, edema Delayed: adrenal insufficiency, hepatotoxicity, joint pain, hypokalemia
Bortezomib (Velcade)	1.3 mg/m^2 intravenous bolus or subcutaneously on days 1, 4, 8, 11 followed by a 10-day rest, or weekly for 4 weeks followed by 13-day rest; various doses	Acute: nausea, vomiting, diarrhea Delayed: peripheral neuropathy, fatigue, myelosuppression
Lenalidomide (Revlimid)	5–25 mg orally once daily on days 1–21 of 28-day cycle; or continuously	Acute: diarrhea, rash Delayed: myelosuppression, fatigue, VTE, potential for birth defects

AUC, area under the curve; AV, atrioventricular; CPK, creatine phosphokinase; LHRH, LH-releasing hormone; MCV, mean corpuscular volume; TLS, tumor lysis syndrome.

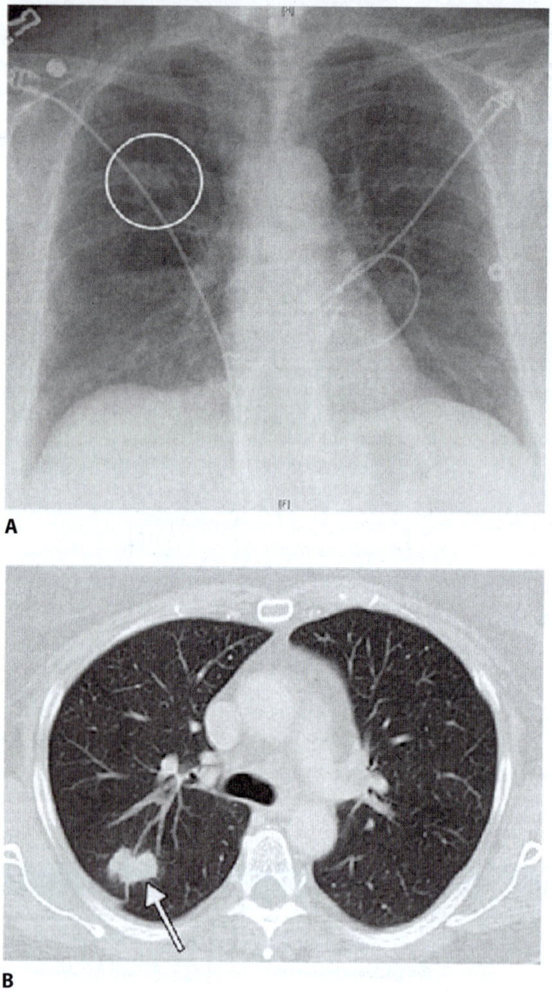

Figure 43–1. Squamous cell carcinoma of the right lung on CXR **(A)** and CT scan **(B)**. (Reproduced, with permission, from Elsayes KM, Oldham SA. *Introduction to Diagnostic Radiology*. McGraw-Hill, 2014.)

Table 43–10. Five-year survival rates for non–small cell lung cancer, based on Tumor, Node, Metastasis (TNM) staging, AJCC 9th edition staging manual, 9th edition database.

Stage	TNM Subset	5-Year Survival Rate for Clinical TNM	5-Year Survival Rate for Pathologic TNM
0	Carcinoma in situ		
1A1	T1aN0M0	82%	88%
1A2	T1bN0M0		
IA3	T1cN0M0		
IB	T2aN0M0	69%	78%
IIA	T2bN0M0	62%	68%
IIB	T1/T2, N1M0 T3N0M0	54%	61%
IIIA	T1/T2, N2M0 T3N1M0 T4, N0/N1, M0	44%	50%
IIIB	T1/T2, N3M0 T3/T4, N2M0	31%	35%
IIIC	T3/T4, N3M0	21%	21%
IVA	Any T, Any N, M1a/M1b	18%	—
IVB	Any T, Any N, M1c	7%	—

Data from Rami-Porta R et al. The International Association for the Study of Lung Cancer lung cancer staging project: proposals for revision of the TNM stage groups in the forthcoming (Ninth) edition of the TNM classification for lung cancer. J Thorac Oncol. 2024;19:1007.

lymph nodes larger than 1 cm, the sensitivity and specificity are 95% and 76%, respectively.

Obtaining an MRI of the brain is important to rule out brain metastases in all patients with SCLC and in patients with NSCLC with at least stage II disease or poorly differentiated histologies.

2. Preoperative assessment—See Chapter 3.

3. Pulmonary function testing—Many patients with NSCLC have moderate to severe chronic lung disease that increases the risk of perioperative complications as well as long-term pulmonary insufficiency following lung resection. *All patients considered for surgery require spirometry*. In the absence of other comorbidities, patients with good lung function (preoperative FEV_1 2 L or more) are at low risk for complications from lobectomy or pneumonectomy.

4. Screening—Screening with low-dose helical CT scans of the chest has been shown to improve lung cancer mortality rates. The National Lung Screening Trial, a multicenter randomized US trial involving over 53,000 current and former heavy smokers, showed that screening annually with low-dose helical CT for 3 years yielded a 20% relative reduction in lung cancer mortality and 6.7% reduction in all-cause mortality compared with chest radiography. Given these findings, US professional organizations have recommended annual screening with low-dose helical CT for lung cancer. The 2021 USPSTF recommendations specify *annual low-dose CT for smokers aged 50–80 years who have at least a 20 pack-year smoking history and who either currently smoke or have quit within the last 15 years.* Smoking cessation policies and efforts should be integrated with any screening program.

Treatment

A. Non–Small Cell Lung Carcinoma

Surgical resection offers the best chance for cure of NSCLC. Clinical features that preclude complete surgical resection include extrathoracic metastases or a malignant pleural effusion; or tumor involving the heart, pericardium, great vessels, esophagus, recurrent laryngeal or phrenic nerves, trachea, main carina, or contralateral mediastinal lymph nodes. Accordingly, stage I and stage II patients are treated with surgical resection where possible. Stage II and select cases of stage IB are additionally recommended to receive either neoadjuvant or adjuvant therapy. Stage IIIA patients have poor outcomes if treated with resection alone. They should undergo multimodality treatment that includes chemotherapy, immunotherapy, or radiotherapy. Inoperable stage IIIA and stage IIIB patients are treated with concurrent chemotherapy and radiation therapy followed by immunotherapy (checkpoint inhibitors) (Tables 43–2 and 43–8) and have improved survival. Stage IV patients are treated with systemic therapy (targeted therapy, chemotherapy, and/or immunotherapy) or symptom-based palliative therapy, or both.

Surgical approaches for early-stage cancers include lobectomy and sublobar resection. For patients who cannot tolerate lobectomy or have stage I primary tumors smaller than 2 cm, a sublobar resection (wedge resection or segmentectomy) may be considered. A phase 3 trial published in 2023 has shown that sublobar resection for patients with solitary primary tumors smaller than 2 cm achieves similar overall survival and disease-free survival compared to lobectomy.

Patients with clinical stage I primary NSCLC, who are not candidates for surgery because of significant comorbidity or other surgical contraindication, are candidates for *stereotactic body radiotherapy.* Stereotactic body radiotherapy, which is composed of multiple non-parallel radiation beams that converge, allows the delivery of a relatively large dose of radiation to a small, well-defined target.

Neoadjuvant therapy, in which antineoplastic medications are given *in advance* of surgery or radiation therapy, can also be considered. The Checkmate 816, Keynote 671, and Aegean trials showed that neoadjuvant treatment with a checkpoint inhibitor combined with chemotherapy prior to surgery and immunotherapy following surgery for patients with early-stage NSCLC leads to an improved event-free survival and pathologic complete response rates compared to neoadjuvant chemotherapy alone prior to surgery. Immune checkpoint inhibition (one form of immunotherapy) using programmed cell death 1 (PD-1) or programmed cell death–ligand 1 (PD-L1) inhibitors has an important role in the treatment of NSCLC (Tables 43–2 and 43–8). Checkpoint inhibitors release T cells from the inhibitory signals they receive from tumor cells via the PD-1 pathway, restoring antitumor immunity.

Adjuvant therapy consists of administering antineoplastic medications *following* surgery or radiation therapy. Cisplatin-containing regimens have shown an overall survival benefit in at least stage II disease and a subset of stage IB disease where primary tumor size exceeds 4 cm. Patients with epidermal growth factor receptor (*EGFR*) pathogenic variants (exon 19 del or L858R) and stage IB and higher are candidates for osimertinib to follow adjuvant chemotherapy per the ADAURA trial, which showed improved disease-free survival rates. For patients who did not receive neoadjuvant therapy, atezolizumab or pembrolizumab (checkpoint inhibitors) can be given for 1 year post–adjuvant chemotherapy to patients with resected stage IB–IIIB NSCLC and PD-L1 ≥ 1%, based on phase 3 trials showing improvement in disease-free survival compared with adjuvant chemotherapy without checkpoint inhibitor.

Patients with locally advanced disease (stages IIIA and IIIB) who are not surgical candidates have improved survival when treated with concurrent chemotherapy and radiation therapy followed by immunotherapy. The PACIFIC trial showed improved survival outcomes by adding durvalumab (PD-L1 inhibitor) as consolidation therapy post–definitive chemoradiation.

For stage IIIB and stage IV NSCLC, options for therapy include targeted therapy, cytotoxic chemotherapy, and immunotherapy. The approach to therapy is individualized based on molecular profiling and PD-L1 testing. Molecular profiling is offered as next-generation sequencing multigene assays. The key driver mutations in lung cancer include *EGFR, ALK, BRAF, ROS1, NTRK, MET, RET*, and *KRAS* pathogenic variants, but only a minority of all lung cancer cases harbor these mutations. Difficulties in testing may arise when only small fine-needle aspirate biopsies are obtained; to have sufficient tissue for analysis, it is recommended that clinicians obtain core biopsies. PD-L1 expression is a flawed but actively used biomarker to predict response to checkpoint inhibitor therapy (specifically, PD-1 and PD-L1 inhibitors).

Targeted therapy plays a pivotal role in NSCLC (Tables 43–2 and 43–8). Activating *EGFR* pathogenic variants are found in approximately 10–20% of the White population and 30–48% of the Asian population and are usually found among nonsmokers to light smokers, women, and persons with nonsquamous histologies (particularly adenocarcinomas). For patients with sensitizing *EGFR* variants, osimertinib (a third-generation EGFR tyrosine kinase inhibitor) with or without chemotherapy is recommended as first-line treatment. Response rates with third-generation EGFR tyrosine kinase inhibitors in patients with *EGFR* variants are at least 70%, and median overall survival is estimated to be 21–33 months. Amivantamab (an EGFR-MET bispecific antibody) with lazertininb (another third-generation EGFR tyrosine kinase inhibitor) is another FDA-approved option for first-line treatment for patients with sensitizing *EGFR* variants.

Approximately 5% of all patients with NSCLC carry translocations of *ALK* resulting in novel fusion gene products with oncogenic activity. For patients with *ALK*-rearranged lung cancers, ALK tyrosine kinase inhibitors are recommended therapeutic agents. Alectinib, brigatinib, ensartinib, and lorlatinib are recommended as first-line agents in *ALK*-rearranged lung cancer, with response rates ranging from 74–83%. Approximately 1–2% of NSCLC harbor *ROS1* rearrangements, and they are usually lung adenocarcinomas found among nonsmokers or light smokers. *ROS1*-rearranged lung cancers respond to crizotinib (*ALK, cMET*, and *ROS1* tyrosine kinase inhibitor) and entrectinib, repotrectinib, or taletrectinib (multikinase inhibitors, including ROS-1), with response rates > 70%. MET exon 14 (METex14) skipping mutations are found in 3% of lung adenocarcinomas. Capmatinib or tepotinib (MET inhibitors) is recommended as first-line treatment for patients with METex14 skipping mutation. *BRAF V600E* mutations have been found in 2% of NSCLC patients and first-line treatment includes the combination of dabrafenib (BRAF inhibitor) and trametinib (MEK inhibitor). This combination shows response rates > 60% in patients with *BRAF V600E*. Treatment with larotrectinib (TRKA/B/C inhibitor), entrectinib (multikinase inhibitor, including TRKA/B/C), or repotrectinib (TRKA/B/C and ROS1 inhibitor) is recommended for patients whose tumors reveal NTRK 1/2/3 gene fusion. Selpercatinib and pralsetinib (RET inhibitors) are recommended first-line treatments for RET fusion–positive NSCLC. Finally, *KRAS* pathogenic variants are found among 30% of patients with adenocarcinomas, are associated with smoking, and have a poor prognosis. Sotorasib and adagrasib (*KRAS* G12C inhibitors) are FDA-approved for treating *KRAS* G12C mutated lung cancers after progression on first-line treatment.

For patients with stage IV NSCLC, with no targetable pathogenic gene variants and regardless of PD-L1 status, phase 3 trials have shown improved survival outcomes with adding a checkpoint inhibitor to platinum-doublet chemotherapy as first-line therapy (Table 43–2). One-year survival for pembrolizumab with platinum-doublet chemotherapy was 69% compared with 49% with chemotherapy alone. For patients with metastatic NSCLC with tumors expressing PD-L1 ≥ 50%, PD-1 checkpoint inhibitors can be given alone or combined with chemotherapy. Significant side effects and toxicity, especially with combination immunotherapy, have been reported with checkpoint inhibitors, specifically autoimmune manifestations such as hepatitis, thyroiditis, hypophysitis, colitis, pneumonitis, and type 1 diabetes mellitus. Treatment with chemotherapy, immunotherapy, or both in the setting of stage IV NSCLC is not curative but can prolong survival and is palliative in intent, leading to improved quality of life and symptom control.

B. Small Cell Lung Carcinoma

Response rates of SCLC to chemotherapy (Table 43–2) are excellent with 80–90% response in limited-stage disease (50–60% complete response), and 60–80% response in extensive-stage disease (15–20% complete response). However, remissions tend to be short-lived with a median duration of 6–8 months. Once the disease has recurred, median survival is 3–4 months. Overall, 2-year survival is 20–40% in limited-stage disease and 5% in extensive-stage disease (Table 43–11). Modest improvement in survival has been achieved with the addition of a checkpoint inhibitor (atezolizumab or durvalumab) to cisplatin or carboplatin and etoposide therapy in extensive-stage disease. In limited SCLC, thoracic radiation therapy is given *concurrently* with chemotherapy, and adjuvant immunotherapy with durvalumab (PD-L1 inhibitor) for 2 years post-chemoradiation is recommended and improves survival outcomes. *There is a high rate of brain metastasis in patients with SCLC, even following a good response to chemotherapy.*

C. Palliative Therapy

Photoresection with the Nd:YAG laser is sometimes performed on central tumors to relieve endobronchial obstruction, improve dyspnea, and control hemoptysis. External beam radiation therapy is also used to control dyspnea, hemoptysis, endobronchial obstruction, pain from bony metastases, obstruction from superior vena cava syndrome, and symptomatic brain metastases. Resection of a solitary brain metastasis improves quality of life and survival when combined with radiation therapy if there is no evidence of other metastatic disease. Stereotactic radiation therapy is offered for limited brain metastases. Repeated thoracenteses, pleurodesis, and PleurX catheter tube placement are key interventions for palliation of symptomatic malignant pleural effusions. Pain is very common in advanced disease. Meticulous efforts at pain control are essential (see Chapter 5). In addition to standard oncologic care, early referral to specialty palliative care is recommended in advanced disease to aid in pain and other symptom management. Such palliative care can modestly improve survival.

Table 43–11. Median survival for small-cell lung carcinoma following treatment.

Stage	Mean 2-Year Survival	Median Survival
Limited	20–40%	15–20 months
Extensive	5%	8–13 months

Data from multiple sources, including Van Meerbeeck JP et al. Small-cell lung cancer. Lancet. 2011;378:1741 and Blackhall F et al. Treatment patterns and outcomes among patients with small-cell lung cancer in Europe: a retrospective study. BMJ Open. 2023;13(2):e052556.

Prognosis

The overall 5-year survival rate for lung cancer is approximately 28%. Predictors of survival include the tumor type (SCLC versus NSCLC), molecular profiling, and stage, and the patient's performance status and weight loss in the prior 6 months. *Patients with targetable mutations have better overall survival when compared with those without mutations due to superior efficacy of targeted drug therapy.*

When to Refer

- With abnormal chest imaging suspicious for cancer, refer to a pulmonologist, a thoracic surgeon, or both for further diagnostic steps, staging, and/or treatment.
- Once a diagnosis of lung cancer is established, also refer to an oncologist, a radiation oncologist, or both for treatment options, depending on stage.
- Locally extensive, regionally advanced, and metastatic disease often require multimodal treatment strategies.

When to Admit

- Hypoxemia, respiratory distress, or hemoptysis.
- Severe pain or new neurologic symptoms concerning for brain or spinal metastasis.
- For surgery or other interventions.

Cheng Y et al. Durvalumab after chemoradiotherapy in limited-stage small-cell lung cancer. N Engl J Med. 2024;391:1313. [PMID: 39268857]

Cho BC et al. Amivantamab plus lazertinib in previously untreated EGFR-mutated advanced NSCLC. N Engl J Med. 2024;391:1486. [PMID: 38924756]

Wakelee H et al. Perioperative pembrolizumab for early-stage non-small-cell lung cancer. N Engl J Med. 2023;389:491. [PMID: 37272513]

PULMONARY METASTASIS

Pulmonary metastasis results from the spread of an extrapulmonary malignant tumor through vascular or lymphatic channels or by direct extension. Metastases usually occur via the pulmonary artery and typically present as multiple nodules or masses on chest radiography. Metastases to the lungs are found in 20–55% of patients with various metastatic malignancies. Carcinomas of the kidney, breast, rectum, colon, cervix, and malignant melanoma are the most likely primary tumors.

Lymphangitic carcinomatosis denotes diffuse involvement of the pulmonary lymphatic network by primary or metastatic lung cancer, probably a result of extension of tumor from lung capillaries to the lymphatics. **Tumor embolization** from extrapulmonary cancer (renal cell carcinoma, HCC, choriocarcinoma) is an uncommon route for tumor spread to the lungs. Metastatic cancer may also present as a **malignant pleural effusion**.

Clinical Findings

A. Symptoms and Signs

Symptoms are uncommon but include cough, hemoptysis and, in advanced cases, dyspnea and hypoxemia. Symptoms are more often referable to the site of the primary tumor.

B. Laboratory Findings

The diagnosis of metastatic cancer involving the lungs is usually established by identifying a primary tumor. Appropriate studies should be ordered if there is a suspicion of any primary cancer, such as breast, thyroid, testis, colorectal, or prostate. If the history, physical examination, and initial studies fail to reveal the site of the primary tumor, attention is better focused on the lung, where tissue samples obtained by bronchoscopy, percutaneous needle biopsy, VATS, or thoracotomy may establish the histologic diagnosis and suggest the most likely primary cancer. Occasionally, cytologic studies of pleural fluid or pleural biopsy reveals the diagnosis.

C. Imaging

Chest radiographs usually show multiple spherical densities with sharp margins. The lesions are usually bilateral, pleural, or subpleural in location, and more common in lower lung zones. Lymphangitic spread and solitary pulmonary nodule are less common radiographic presentations of pulmonary metastasis. CT imaging of the chest, abdomen, and pelvis may reveal the site of a primary tumor and will help determine feasibility of surgical resection of the metastatic lung tumors. FDG-PET/CT scan is helpful in identifying the site of a primary cancer and identifying other areas of extrathoracic metastasis.

Treatment

Once the diagnosis has been established, management consists of treatment of the primary neoplasm, usually with systemic treatments, and treatment of any pulmonary complications. Surgical resection of a *solitary* pulmonary nodule (***metastasectomy***) can be considered in the patient with known current or previous extrapulmonary cancer. Local resection of one or more pulmonary metastases is feasible in a few carefully selected patients with various sarcomas and carcinomas (ie, testis, colorectal, and kidney). *About 15–25% of metastatic solid tumor patients have metastases limited to the lungs and are surgical candidates.* Unfavorable prognostic factors also include shorter disease-free interval from primary tumor treatment to presentation of metastases and a larger number of metastases. However, to date, there have been no randomized data confirming the benefit of metastasectomy for pulmonary metastasis. For patients with unresectable disease or primary neoplasms for which pulmonary metastasectomy should not be considered, systemic treatment tailored to the primary tumor can be offered. Diligent attention to palliative care is essential (see Chapter 5).

Ichinose J et al. Optimal timing for lung metastasectomy in patients with colorectal cancer. Interact Cardiovasc Thorac Surg. 2022;35:ivac224. [PMID: 35993901]

Mangiameli G et al. Lung metastases: current surgical indications and new perspectives. Front Surg. 2022;9:884915. [PMID: 35574534]

Woo W et al. The role of pulmonary metastasectomy for non-primary lung cancer: umbrella review of meta-analyses. J Surg Oncol. 2025;131:1035. [PMID: 39674949]

MESOTHELIOMA

ESSENTIALS OF DIAGNOSIS

- Unilateral, nonpleuritic chest pain and dyspnea.
- Distant (> 20 years earlier) history of exposure to asbestos.
- Pleural effusion or pleural thickening or both on CXR.
- Malignant cells in pleural fluid or tissue biopsy.

General Considerations

Mesotheliomas are primary tumors arising from the surface lining of the pleura (80% of cases) or peritoneum (20% of cases). *Numerous studies have confirmed the association of malignant pleural mesothelioma with exposure to asbestos.* The lifetime risk to asbestos workers of developing malignant pleural mesothelioma is as high as 10%. The latent period between exposure and onset of symptoms ranges from 20 to 40 years. The clinician should inquire about asbestos exposure through mining, milling, manufacturing, shipyard work, insulation, brake linings, building construction and demolition, roofing materials, and other asbestos products (pipes, textiles, paints, tiles, gaskets, panels).

Clinical Findings

A. Symptoms and Signs

The average interval between onset of symptoms and diagnosis is 2–3 months; the median age at diagnosis is 72–74 years in Western countries. Symptoms include the insidious onset of shortness of breath, nonpleuritic chest pain, and weight loss. Physical findings include dullness to percussion, diminished breath sounds and, in some cases, digital clubbing.

B. Laboratory Findings

Pleural fluid is exudative and often hemorrhagic. Cytologic tests of pleural fluid are often negative. *VATS biopsy is usually necessary to obtain an adequate specimen for histologic diagnosis.* The histologic variants of malignant pleural mesothelioma are epithelial (50–60%), sarcomatoid (10%), and biphasic (30–40%). Since distinction from benign inflammatory conditions and metastatic adenocarcinoma may be difficult, immunohistochemical stains are important to confirm the diagnosis.

C. Imaging

Radiographic abnormalities consist of nodular, irregular, unilateral pleural thickening and varying degrees of unilateral pleural effusion. *Sixty percent of patients have right-sided disease, while only 5% have bilateral involvement.* CT scans demonstrate the extent of pleural involvement. PET-CT is used to help differentiate benign from malignant pleural disease, improve staging accuracy, and identify candidates for aggressive surgical approaches.

Complications

Malignant pleural mesothelioma progresses rapidly as the tumor spreads along the pleural surface to involve the pericardium, mediastinum, and contralateral pleura. The tumor may eventually extend beyond the thorax to involve abdominal lymph nodes and organs. Progressive pain and dyspnea are characteristic. Local invasion of thoracic structures may cause superior vena cava syndrome, hoarseness, Horner syndrome, arrhythmias, and dysphagia.

Treatment

Chemotherapy and immunotherapy are the mainstay of treatment for pleural mesothelioma (Tables 43–2 and 43–8). Randomized trials have not shown a survival benefit for surgery, but these studies have limitations. Large-volume centers continue to consider surgery only for localized disease that is amenable to complete macroscopic surgical resection in a multimodal approach. For localized disease, surgical options include pleurectomy and decortication (surgical stripping of the pleura and pericardium from apex of the lung to diaphragm) or extrapleural pneumonectomy (a radical surgical procedure involving removal of the ipsilateral lung, parietal and visceral pleura, pericardium, and most of the hemidiaphragm). Surgical cytoreduction alone is not sufficient, and chemotherapy, radiation therapy, or both are included in a multimodality approach. In advanced unresectable disease, nivolumab and ipilimumab (checkpoint inhibitor therapy) or platinum therapy with pemetrexed can be offered first-line, with overall median survival rates ranging from 12–18 months in clinical trials.

Drainage of pleural effusions, pleurodesis, radiation therapy, and even surgical resection may offer palliative benefit to some patients.

Prognosis

Most patients die of respiratory failure and complications of local extension. Median survival time from diagnosis is 7–18 months. Five-year survival is 5–12%. Tumors that are predominantly sarcomatoid are more resistant to therapy and have a worse prognosis, with median survivals < 1 year. Poor prognostic features include poor performance status, non-epithelioid histology, male sex, nodal involvement, elevated LD, high WBC, low hemoglobin, and high platelet count.

When to Refer

- Upon diagnosis, refer to a pulmonologist, oncologist, or possibly a thoracic surgeon who can evaluate the patient for multidisciplinary treatment.

When to Admit

- For pleural fluid drainage (thoracenteses, placement of an indwelling drainage catheter).
- For severe dyspnea.

Kindler HL et al. Treatment of pleural mesothelioma: ASCO guideline update. J Clin Oncol. 2025;43:1006. [PMID: 39778125]

Popat S et al; ESMO Guideline Committee. Malignant pleural mesothelioma: ESMO clinical practice guidelines for diagnosis, treatment and follow-up. Ann Oncol. 2022;33:129. [PMID: 34861373]

Suraya R et al. Recent advances in mesothelioma treatment: immunotherapy, advanced cell therapy, and other innovative therapeutic modalities. Cancers (Basel). 2025;17:694. [PMID: 40002287]

HEPATOBILIARY CANCERS

HEPATOCELLULAR CARCINOMA

ESSENTIALS OF DIAGNOSIS

- Usually a complication of cirrhosis.
- Characteristic CT and MRI features may obviate the need for a confirmatory biopsy.

General Considerations

Malignant neoplasms of the liver that arise from parenchymal cells are called **HCCs** (accounting for 85% of liver cancers); those that originate in the ductular cells are called **cholangiocarcinomas** (15% or less). Uncommon tumors of the liver include mucinous cystic neoplasms of the liver (including biliary cystadenocarcinoma), angiosarcoma, lymphoma, and combined HCC-cholangiocarcinoma.

Worldwide, HCCs are the third most common cause of cancer-related deaths and the sixth most common in incidence. They are *associated with cirrhosis in 85% of cases.* The risk of HCC developing in a patient with cirrhosis is 3–5% a year. In Africa and most of Asia, *hepatitis B virus (HBV) infection* (including "occult" HBV infection; see Chapter 18) is a major etiologic factor, and a family history of HCC increases the risk synergistically. In the United States and other Western countries, cirrhosis caused by alcohol and **metabolic dysfunction-associated steatotic liver disease (MASLD)** has become the predominant cause. Incidence rates rose more than twofold after 1978, with a decrease in 35- to 49-year-olds after 2006 and in 55- to 64-year-olds after 2015 in White, Latina/Latino, and Asian/Pacific Islander persons and subsequently in Black, American Indian, and Alaskan native persons. Nevertheless, mortality rates have continued to increase in those over 65 years old. In Western countries, risk factors for HCC in patients known to have cirrhosis are male sex, age > 55 years (although there has been an increase in the number of younger cases), Latino/Latina or Asian ethnicity, family history in a first-degree relative, overweight, obesity (especially in early adulthood), alcohol use (especially in combination with obesity), tobacco use, diabetes mellitus, hypothyroidism (in women), a prolonged prothrombin time, a low platelet count, and an elevated serum transferrin saturation. The risk of HCC is higher in persons with a viral rather than nonviral cause of cirrhosis and may be lowest in persons with autoimmune diseases. Other associations include high levels of HBV replication, high hepatitis B surface antigen levels, HBV genotype C, hepatitis D coinfection, elevated serum ALT and bilirubin and low serum albumin levels, and increased liver stiffness in persons with chronic hepatitis B (in whom antiviral therapy to suppress HBV replication reduces the risk); hemochromatosis; aflatoxin exposure; α-1-antitrypsin deficiency; tyrosinemia; and radiation exposure. *In patients with the metabolic syndrome and MASLD, HCC may rarely arise from steatohepatitis in the absence of cirrhosis.* Hepatocellular adenoma may be a precursor to HCC (see Chapter 18).

The fibrolamellar variant of HCC generally occurs in young women with a second smaller peak in older persons; it is characterized by a distinctive histologic picture, absence of risk factors, unique genomic profiles, and an indolent course. Vinyl chloride exposure is associated with angiosarcoma of the liver.

Clinical Findings

A. Symptoms and Signs

The presence of HCC may be unsuspected until there is deterioration in the condition of a cirrhotic patient who was formerly stable. Cachexia, weakness, and weight loss are associated symptoms. The sudden appearance of ascites, which may be bloody, suggests *portal or hepatic vein thrombosis* by cancer or bleeding from a necrotic cancer.

Physical examination may show tender enlargement of the liver, occasionally with a palpable mass. In Africa, the typical presentation in young patients is a rapidly expanding abdominal mass. Auscultation may reveal a bruit over the tumor or a friction rub when the tumor has extended to the surface of the liver.

B. Laboratory Findings

Laboratory tests may reveal leukocytosis, as opposed to the leukopenia that is frequently encountered in cirrhotic patients. Anemia is common, but a normal or elevated hematocrit value may be found in up to one-third of patients owing to elaboration of erythropoietin by the tumor. Serum **α-fetoprotein (AFP)** levels are elevated in up to 70% of patients with HCC in Western countries; however, mild elevations (10–200 ng/mL [10–200 mcg/L]) are also often seen in patients with chronic hepatitis. Serum levels of **des-γ-carboxy prothrombin** are elevated in up to 90% of patients with HCC, but they may also be elevated in patients with vitamin K deficiency, chronic hepatitis, and metastatic cancer.

C. Imaging

Multiphasic helical CT and MRI with contrast enhancement are the preferred imaging studies for determining the location and vascularity of the tumor; MRI may be more sensitive than CT, and imaging with gadoxetic acid increases sensitivity. Lesions smaller than 1 cm may be difficult to characterize. Based on stringent criteria developed by the American College of Radiology through its Liver Imaging Reporting and Data System (LI-RADS), the Organ Procurement and Transplantation Network, and the American Association for the Study of Liver Diseases, arterial phase enhancement of *a lesion that is ≥ 1 cm in diameter followed by delayed hypointensity ("washout") (LI-RADS 5) has a 93% specificity, though only a 67% sensitivity, for HCC.*

Abbreviated MRI—shorter sequences of during the arterial phase of contrast—has shown promise in trials in Asia and is being explored in a large multicenter trial in the United States. PET may improve detection of extrahepatic metastases.

D. Liver Biopsy and Staging

Liver biopsy is diagnostic, although seeding of the needle tract by cancer represents a small but real potential risk (1–3%). For lesions smaller than 1 cm, ultrasonography may be repeated every 3 months followed by further investigation of enlarging lesions. For lesions 1 cm or larger, biopsy can be deferred when characteristic arterial hypervascularity and delayed washout are demonstrated on either multiphasic helical CT or MRI with contrast enhancement in a patient with cirrhosis or if surgical resection is planned.

HCC staging is important not only because it correlates with the patient's long-term survival but also because it is used to guide treatment decisions. The more widely used staging system is the **Barcelona Clinic Liver Cancer** classification, which takes into account the size and extent of the primary tumor(s), liver function (as measured by Child-Pugh score), and a patient's performance status. It has the advantage of linking overall stage with preferred treatment modalities and with an estimation of life expectancy.

Screening & Prevention

Screening for the development of HCC is recommended in patients with chronic hepatitis B (beginning as early as age 20 years in persons of African descent, age 40 years in Asian men or Asian persons with a family history of HCC, and age 50 years in persons of other ethnicities) or cirrhosis caused by hepatitis C virus (HCV), HBV, or alcohol. There is some evidence that screening for HCC leads to a survival advantage over clinical diagnosis, but only a minority of cases are detected by screening. The standard screening approach is performing ultrasonography and obtaining serum AFP level every 6 months, although AFP testing has low sensitivity. *A serum AFP level of ≥ 20 ng/mL (20 mcg/L) is generally the cutoff value that should trigger further evaluation by imaging.*

Ultrasonography is less sensitive and more operator-dependent but is used to screen for hepatic nodules in high-risk patients. The sensitivity of ultrasonography alone for detecting early HCC is only 63%. Among patients with cirrhosis, 25% of nodules < 2 cm in diameter detected on a screening ultrasonography prove to be HCC. Patients with cancers detected by surveillance have a less advanced stage on average and greater likelihood that treatment will prolong survival than those whose cancers were not detected by surveillance. However, controversy persists about whether surveillance reduces cancer-related mortality.

CT and MRI are considered too expensive for routine screening; however, "abbreviated" MRI in which the number of sequences acquired is limited is under study as a time- and cost-effective screening approach.

Treatment

If liver function is preserved (Child-Pugh class A or possibly B) and portal vein thrombosis is not present, surgical resection of a solitary HCC may result in cure. Laparoscopic and robotic liver resection can be performed in selected cases.

Liver transplantation may be appropriate for some patients with advanced cirrhosis, with reported 5-year survival rates of up to 75%. The recurrence-free survival may be better for liver transplantation than for resection in patients with well-compensated cirrhosis and small tumors (one tumor < 5 cm or three or fewer tumors each < 3 cm in diameter [**Milan criteria**]) and in those with expanded **University of California, San Francisco criteria** of one tumor ≤ 6.5 cm or three or fewer tumors ≤ 4.5 cm (or a combined tumor diameter of 8.5 cm) without vascular invasion. The **Extended Toronto criteria** include tumor differentiation, cancer-related symptoms, confinement of tumor to the liver, and absence of vascular invasion, without regard to tumor number or size, to determine candidacy for liver transplantation and appear to predict outcomes as well as the Milan criteria. After 6 months on the waiting list, patients with stage 2 HCC meeting the Milan criteria are awarded a fixed score of 3 points lower than the median Model for End-Stage Liver Disease (MELD) score (range, 6–40) for patients transplanted at the center where the candidate is listed (see Chapter 18), thereby increasing their chances of undergoing transplantation. However, orthotopic liver transplantation is often impractical because of the donor organ shortage, so living donor liver transplantation may be considered in these cases. Patients with larger tumors (3–5 cm), a serum AFP level of 1000 ng/mL (1000 mcg/L) or higher, or a MELD score of 20 or higher have poor posttransplantation survival. In patients with a serum AFP level > 1000 ng/mL (1000 mcg/L), downstaging by locoregional therapy to an AFP level < 500 ng/mL (500 mcg/L) improves survival following subsequent liver transplantation.

Treatment decisions are made based on tumor size, location, underlying liver function, and shared decision-making. Microwave ablation, radiofrequency ablation, cryotherapy, proton beam radiotherapy, histotripsy (a procedure that uses focused ultrasound), or ethanol injection of smaller tumors may prolong survival in patients who are not candidates for resection and have tumors that are accessible. Other liver-directed approaches, including stereotactic body radiation therapy, transarterial chemoembolization (TACE), and transarterial radioembolization (TARE), may be useful in patients with larger or multifocal tumors and are also often offered as a "bridge" to liver transplantation.

The combination of atezolizumab, an immune checkpoint inhibitor, and bevacizumab, an antibody to the vascular endothelial growth factor (VEGF) receptor, is the preferred first-line therapy for advanced HCC and has been shown to be superior to sorafenib (an oral multikinase inhibitor of Raf kinase, the VEGF receptor, and the platelet-derived growth factor receptor [and others]), which had previously represented the standard of care for patients with advanced HCC. The combination of immune checkpoint inhibitors tremelimumab and durvalumab was approved in 2022 as an alternative first-line (and second-line) therapy and may be preferable to atezolizumab and bevacizumab for patients in whom large or bleeding esophageal varices are present. Another dual immune checkpoint inhibitor combination, nivolumab plus ipilimumab, was also approved in 2025 as a frontline treatment option for this patient population. Nivolumab or pembrolizumab may be used for patients with advanced HCC in the second-line setting whose disease has progressed on prior oral multikinase inhibitor therapy.

Besides sorafenib, other oral multikinase inhibitors that are FDA-approved for the first- or second-line treatment of advanced HCC include lenvatinib, regorafenib, and cabozantinib. Ramucirumab, a monoclonal antibody targeting the VEGF receptor, is also an approved therapy for patients with an AFP level ≥ 400 ng/mL (400 mcg/L) who have previously been treated with sorafenib.

Various strategies combining the previously mentioned systemic agents and locoregional therapies (eg, embolization or radiation) have been or are being actively investigated for select patients with unresectable advanced HCC based on very specific eligibility criteria, including tumor size and portal vein involvement. For example, a large phase 3 trial evaluating TACE in combination with lenvatinib plus pembrolizumab has demonstrated a significant improvement in median progression-free survival compared with TACE plus placebo.

The **modified Response Evaluation Criteria in Solid Tumors** are used to assess treatment response based on tumor shrinkage and viability after locoregional and antiangiogenic treatment. Meticulous efforts at palliative care are essential for patients in whom disease progresses despite treatment or in whom advanced tumors, vascular invasion, or extrahepatic spread are present. Severe pain may develop in such patients due to expansion of the liver capsule by the tumor and requires concerted efforts at pain management, including the use of opioids (see Chapter 5).

Prognosis

In the United States, overall 1- and 5-year survival rates for patients with HCC are 23% and 5%, respectively. Five-year survival rates rise to 56% (and over 70% in those eligible for liver transplantation) for patients with localized resectable disease (T1, T2, selected T3 and T4; N0; M0) but are virtually nil for those with locally unresectable or advanced disease. In patients with HCV-related HCC, the serum AFP level at the time of diagnosis of cancer has been reported to be an independent predictor of mortality. A serum AFP level ≥ 200 ng/mL (200 mcg/L) or increases of > 15 ng/mL/month predict worse outcomes in patients awaiting liver transplantation. In patients who are not eligible for surgery, cachexia and an elevated serum CRP level are associated with reduced survival. The fibrolamellar variant has been reported to have a higher recurrence rate but better survival than conventional HCC.

When to Refer

All patients with HCC should be referred to a specialist.

When to Admit

- Complications of cirrhosis.
- Severe pain.
- For surgery and other interventions.

Brown ZJ et al. Management of hepatocellular carcinoma: a review. JAMA Surg. 2023;158:410. [PMID: 36790767]

Kudo M et al; LEAP-012 investigators. Transarterial chemoembolisation combined with lenvatinib plus pembrolizumab versus dual placebo for unresectable, non-metastatic hepatocellular carcinoma (LEAP-012): a multicentre, randomised, double-blind, phase 3 study. Lancet. 2025;405:203. Erratum in: Lancet. 2025;405:468. [PMID: 39798578]

Rimassa L et al. Combination immunotherapy for hepatocellular carcinoma. J Hepatol. 2023;79:506. [PMID: 36933770]

Ronot M et al. Screening of liver cancer with abbreviated MRI. Hepatology. 2023;78:670. [PMID: 36896975]

Shah PA et al. NAFLD-related hepatocellular carcinoma: the growing challenge. Hepatology. 2023;77:323. [PMID: 35478412]

Singal AG et al. AASLD Practice Guidance on prevention, diagnosis, and treatment of hepatocellular carcinoma. Hepatology. 2023;78:1922. [PMID: 37199193]

CARCINOMA OF THE BILIARY TRACT

ESSENTIALS OF DIAGNOSIS

- Presents with obstructive jaundice, usually painless, often with dilated biliary tract.
- Pain is more common in gallbladder carcinoma than cholangiocarcinoma.
- A dilated gallbladder may be palpable (Courvoisier sign).
- Diagnosis by cholangiography with biopsy and brushings for cytology.

General Considerations

Carcinoma of the gallbladder occurs in approximately 2% of all people operated on for biliary tract disease; the incidence, like that of carcinoma of the bile ducts, had been decreasing in the United States but may be increasing again in some Western countries because of lifestyle factors. The onset is notoriously insidious, and the diagnosis is often made incidentally in patients undergoing cholecystectomy for cholecystitis or cholelithiasis (often large, symptomatic stones). Risk factors include chronic infection of the gallbladder with *Salmonella typhi*, adenomatous gallbladder polyps over 1 cm in diameter (particularly with hypoechoic foci on endoscopic ultrasound), mucosal calcification of the gallbladder (**porcelain gallbladder**), anomalous pancreaticobiliary ductal junction, high parity in women, oral menopausal hormone therapy, increased BMI, and aflatoxin exposure. Spread of the cancer—by direct extension into the liver or to the peritoneal surface—may be seen on initial presentation.

Carcinoma of the bile ducts (cholangiocarcinoma) accounts for 10–15% of all hepatobiliary malignancies and 3% of all cancer deaths in the United States. It is more prevalent in persons aged 50–70 years, with a slight male predominance, and more common in Asia. About 50% arise at the confluence of the hepatic ducts (*perihilar*, or so-called **Klatskin tumors**), and 40% arise in the *distal extrahepatic bile duct* (the incidence of which has risen since 1990); the remainder are *intrahepatic* (the incidence of which rose dramatically from the 1970s to the early 2000s and has continued to increase, perhaps in part due to a greater recognition of this diagnosis, which previously had been classified as a cancer of unknown primary). Mortality from intrahepatic cholangiocarcinoma has been increasing at a higher rate than that for extrahepatic cholangiocarcinoma. The frequency of carcinoma in individuals with a choledochal cyst has been reported to be over 14% at 20 years, and surgical excision is recommended. Most cases of cholangiocarcinoma are sporadic. There is an increased incidence of cholangiocarcinoma in patients with bile duct adenoma; Caroli disease (a congenital disorder leading to multifocal areas of intrahepatic biliary duct dilation); a biliary-enteric anastomosis; ulcerative colitis, especially those with primary sclerosing cholangitis; biliary cirrhosis; diabetes mellitus; hyperthyroidism; chronic pancreatitis; heavy alcohol consumption; smoking; and past exposure to Thorotrast (a contrast agent). Premalignant lesions of the bile duct include biliary intraepithelial neoplasia and intraductal papillary neoplasia of the biliary system (biliary papillomatosis). In Southeast Asia, hepatolithiasis, chronic typhoid carriage, and infection of the bile ducts with helminths *(Clonorchis sinensis, Opisthorchis viverrini)* are associated with an increased risk of cholangiocarcinoma. HCV (and possibly HBV) infection, cirrhosis, HIV infection, MASLD, diabetes mellitus, obesity, and tobacco smoking are risk factors for intrahepatic cholangiocarcinoma.

Staging is important not only because it correlates with the patient's long-term survival but also because it is used to determine which patients should receive adjuvant or neoadjuvant therapy.

Clinical Findings

A. Symptoms and Signs

Progressive jaundice is the most common and usually the first sign of obstruction of the extrahepatic biliary system. Pain in the right upper abdomen with radiation into the back is usually present early in the course of gallbladder carcinoma but occurs later in the course of bile duct carcinoma. Anorexia and weight loss are common and may be associated with fever and chills due to cholangitis. Rarely, hematemesis or melena results from erosion of cancer into a blood vessel (*hemobilia*). Fistula formation between the biliary system and adjacent organs may also rarely occur. The course is usually one of rapid deterioration, with death occurring within a few months.

Physical examination reveals profound jaundice. Pruritus and skin excoriations are common. A palpable gallbladder with obstructive jaundice usually is said to signify malignant disease (**Courvoisier sign**); however, this clinical generalization has been proven to be accurate only about 50% of the time. Intrahepatic cholangiocarcinoma, however, rarely presents with obstructive symptoms. Hepatomegaly due to hypertrophy of the unobstructed liver lobe is usually present and is associated with liver tenderness. Ascites may occur with peritoneal implants.

B. Laboratory Findings

With biliary obstruction, laboratory examination reveals predominantly conjugated hyperbilirubinemia, with total serum bilirubin values ranging from 5 to 30 mg/dL. There is usually concomitant elevation of the alkaline phosphatase and serum cholesterol. AST is normal or minimally elevated. The serum CA 19-9 level is elevated in up to 85% of patients but does not distinguish cholangiocarcinoma from benign biliary stricture or obstruction.

C. Imaging

Ultrasonography and contrast-enhanced, triple-phase, helical CT may show a gallbladder mass in gallbladder carcinoma and intrahepatic mass or biliary dilatation in carcinoma of the bile ducts. However, oftentimes, biliary tract cancers are difficult to diagnose radiographically, as a discrete space-occupying lesion may not be readily visible. CT may sometimes show involved regional lymph nodes and atrophy of a hepatic lobe because of vascular encasement with compensatory hypertrophy of the unaffected lobe. MRI with *magnetic resonance cholangiopancreatography (MRCP)* and gadolinium enhancement permits visualization of the entire biliary tract and detection of vascular invasion and obviates the need for angiography and, in some cases, direct cholangiography; it is the imaging procedure of choice but may understage malignant hilar strictures. The features of intrahepatic cholangiocarcinoma on MRI appear to differ from those of HCC, with contrast washout in the latter but not the former. In indeterminate cases, PET can detect cholangiocarcinomas as small as 1 cm and lymph node and distant metastases, but false-positive results occur. *Endoscopic retrograde cholangiography* or *percutaneous transhepatic cholangiography* with biopsy and cytologic specimens can be helpful for ductular malignancies, although false-negative biopsy and cytology results are common. Digital image analysis and fluorescent in situ hybridization of cytologic specimens for polysomy improve sensitivity.

Treatment

In young and fit patients, curative surgery for gallbladder carcinoma may be attempted if the cancer is well localized. The 5-year survival rate for carcinoma of the gallbladder invading the lamina propria or muscularis (stage 1, T1a or 1b, N0, M0) is as high as 85% with laparoscopic cholecystectomy but drops to 60%, even with a more extended radical cholecystectomy (which involves removal of the gallbladder, gallbladder fossa in the liver, and regional lymph nodes) if there is perimuscular invasion (T2). The role of radical cholecystectomy for T3 and T4 tumors is debatable. If the cancer is unresectable at laparotomy, biliary-enteric bypass (eg, Roux-en-Y hepaticojejunostomy) can be performed.

Carcinoma of the bile ducts is curable by surgery in < 10% of cases. If resection margins are negative, the 5-year survival rate may be as high as 47% for intrahepatic cholangiocarcinomas, 41% for hilar cholangiocarcinoma, and 37% for distal cholangiocarcinomas, but the perioperative mortality rate may be as high as 10%. Factors predicting shorter survival for intrahepatic cholangiocarcinoma include large cancer size, multiple cancers, lymph node metastasis, and vascular invasion. Adjuvant chemotherapy with capecitabine has been shown to result in superior overall survival compared with no adjuvant therapy. Palliation can be achieved by placement of a self-expandable metal stent via an endoscopic or percutaneous transhepatic route. Covered metal stents may be more cost-effective than uncovered metal stents because of a longer duration of patency; however, they are associated with a higher rate of stent migration and cholecystitis due to occlusion of the cystic duct and are not associated with longer survival. For perihilar cancers, bilateral stents may be preferable to a unilateral stent when technically feasible. Plastic stents are less expensive initially, but not in the long term, because they are more prone to occlude than metal ones; they may be considered based on local expertise and physician preference. Photodynamic therapy in combination with stent placement prolongs survival when compared with stent placement alone in patients with nonresectable cholangiocarcinoma. Endoscopic retrograde cholangiopancreatography (ERCP)–directed radiofrequency ablation, TACE, and TARE are additional options. Radiotherapy may relieve pain and contribute to biliary decompression.

The combination of cisplatin and gemcitabine represents the standard chemotherapy backbone in patients with locally advanced or metastatic cholangiocarcinoma. Additionally, two phase 3 trials have demonstrated that the addition of an immune checkpoint inhibitor (either durvalumab or pembrolizumab) to chemotherapy improves overall survival in this patient population. Second-line therapy often consists of FOLFOX (folinic acid, fluorouracil, and oxaliplatin). Patients should also undergo comprehensive genomic profiling, as cholangiocarcinomas may harbor actionable molecular findings for which approved targeted therapies are currently available, typically in the second-line setting following immunochemotherapy. These include genetic alterations in the fibroblast growth factor receptor (FGFR) gene, for which oral small-molecule inhibitors (pemigatinib, futibatinib) have demonstrated clinical efficacy; However, even with targeted treatments, few patients survive for > 24 months.

Although cholangiocarcinoma is generally considered to be a contraindication to liver transplantation because of rapid cancer recurrence, a 5-year survival rate of 75% has been reported in select patients with stage I and II perihilar cholangiocarcinoma undergoing a combined-modality preoperative regimen, including chemoradiation and exploratory laparotomy followed by liver transplantation. A 5-year survival rate of 67% has been reported in those with intrahepatic cholangiocarcinoma.

For those patients whose disease progresses despite treatment, meticulous efforts at palliative care are essential (see Chapter 5).

When to Refer

All patients with carcinoma of the biliary tract should be referred to a specialist.

When to Admit

- Biliary obstruction.
- Cholangitis.

Cadamuro M et al. Advanced endoscopy meets molecular diagnosis of cholangiocarcinoma. J Hepatol. 2023;78:1063. [PMID: 36740048]

Eisenberg I et al. Drainage approach for malignant biliary obstruction: a changing paradigm. J Clin Gastroenterol. 2023;57:546. [PMID: 37079870]

European Association for the Study of the Liver. EASL-ILCA Clinical Practice Guidelines on the management of intrahepatic cholangiocarcinoma. J Hepatol. 2023;79:181. [PMID: 37084797]

Goyal L et al; FOENIX-CCA2 Study Investigators. Futibatinib for *FGFR2*-rearranged intrahepatic cholangiocarcinoma. N Engl J Med. 2023;388:228. [PMID: 36652354]

Kelley RK et al; KEYNOTE-966 Investigators. Pembrolizumab in combination with gemcitabine and cisplatin compared with gemcitabine and cisplatin alone for patients with advanced biliary tract cancer (KEYNOTE-966): a randomised, double-blind, placebo-controlled, phase 3 trial. Lancet. 2023;401:1853. Erratum in: Lancet. 2023;402:964. Erratum in: Lancet. 2024;403:1140. [PMID: 37075781]

Merters J et al. Integrating cytotoxic, targeted and immune therapies for cholangiocarcinoma. J Hepatol. 2023;78:652. [PMID: 36400328]

Rushbrook SM et al. British Society of Gastroenterology guidelines for the diagnosis and management of cholangiocarcinoma. Gut. 2023;73:16. [PMID: 37770126]

CARCINOMA OF THE PANCREAS & AMPULLA OF VATER

ESSENTIALS OF DIAGNOSIS

- Obstructive jaundice (may be painless).
- Enlarged gallbladder (may be painful).
- Upper abdominal pain with radiation to back, weight loss, and thrombophlebitis are usually late manifestations.

General Considerations

Adenocarcinomas are the most common cancers that arise in the pancreas and derive from ductal epithelial cells. Neuroendocrine tumors, which are discussed in this chapter, account for 1–2% of pancreatic neoplasms and may be functional (producing gastrin, insulin, glucagon, vasoactive intestinal peptide, somatostatin, growth hormone–releasing hormone, ACTH, and others) or nonfunctional. About 75% of pancreatic adenocarcinomas are located in the head and 25% in the body and tail of the organ. Pancreatic cancer accounts for 3% of all cancers and 7% of cancer deaths. The incidence is increasing, especially in women under age 55. **Ampullary carcinomas** are much less common. Risk factors for pancreatic cancer include age, tobacco use (which is thought to cause 20–25% of cases), heavy alcohol use, obesity, chronic pancreatitis, diabetes mellitus, prior abdominal radiation, family history, and possibly gallstones, gastric ulcer, and exposure to arsenic and cadmium. *New-onset diabetes mellitus after age 45 years occasionally heralds the onset of pancreatic cancer*, and weight loss may precede the diagnosis. Although there were signals of risk in older studies, among patients with diabetes, GLP-1–based therapy is not associated with increased risk up to 7 years later. About 7% of patients with pancreatic cancer have a family history of pancreatic cancer in a first-degree relative, compared with 0.6% of control patients. Most pancreatic cancers originate from pancreatic intraepithelial neoplasias, which are not readily visible on imaging studies.

In 10–15% of cases, pancreatic cancer occurs as part of a hereditary syndrome, including familial breast cancer (carriers of *BRCA2* have a 7% lifetime risk of pancreatic cancer), hereditary pancreatitis, familial atypical multiple mole melanoma, Peutz-Jeghers syndrome, ataxia-telangiectasia, and Lynch syndrome (hereditary nonpolyposis colorectal cancer [CRC]). All patients with a diagnosis of pancreatic cancer should undergo germline testing, irrespective of family history.

Cystic neoplasms account for < 10% of pancreatic neoplasms. *A cystic neoplasm should be suspected when a cystic lesion in the pancreas is found in the absence of a history of pancreatitis or trauma and has certain radiographic features such a solid component or associated pancreatic duct dilatation.* While pancreatic cysts are common (eg, pseudocysts) and do not usually pose any threat, at least 15% of all pancreatic cysts are neoplasms. Serous cystadenomas (which account for 32–39% of cystic pancreatic neoplasms) are benign. However, mucinous cystic neoplasms (defined by the presence of ovarian stroma and accounting for 10–45% of cystic pancreatic neoplasms), intraductal papillary mucinous neoplasms (21–33% of cystic pancreatic neoplasms), solid pseudopapillary tumors (< 5%, primarily in young women), and cystic islet cell tumors (3–5%) may have malignant potential. Their prognoses are generally better than that of typical pancreatic adenocarcinomas.

Clinical Findings

A. Symptoms and Signs

Pain is present in over 70% of cases and is often vague, diffuse, and located in the epigastrium or, when the lesion is in the tail, located in the left upper quadrant of the abdomen. Radiation of pain into the back is common and sometimes predominates. Sitting up and leaning forward may afford some relief, and this usually indicates that the lesion has spread beyond the pancreas and is inoperable. Diarrhea or steatorrhea (greasy, foul-smelling stools) due to malabsorption from pancreatic exocrine insufficiency is sometimes seen. Weight loss is a common finding and may be associated with depression. Hyperglycemia and decreases in subcutaneous abdominal fat and serum lipid levels have been reported to precede a diagnosis of pancreatic cancer. Occasional patients present with acute pancreatitis in the absence of an alternative cause. Jaundice is usually due to biliary obstruction by a cancer arising in the pancreatic head and infrequently can be accompanied by a palpable gallbladder (Courvoisier sign). The primary pancreatic tumor is rarely palpable on exam unless significantly enlarged. Ascites may be present if pancreatic cancer is diagnosed at an advanced stage, either due to peritoneal carcinomatosis or portal hypertension. Migratory thrombophlebitis is a rare sign.

B. Laboratory Findings

There may be mild anemia. The serum lipase or amylase level is occasionally elevated. Liver biochemical tests may suggest obstructive jaundice. Fecal elastase test may reveal pancreatic exocrine insufficiency in patients with symptoms of malabsorption. CA 19-9, with a sensitivity of 70% and a specificity of 87%, has generally not proven useful for early detection of pancreatic cancer; increased values are also found in acute and chronic pancreatitis and cholangitis. Plasma chromogranin A levels are elevated in 88–100% of patients with pancreatic neuroendocrine tumors (NETs) but this can be elevated among users of proton pump inhibitors (PPIs).

C. Imaging

Multiphase thin-cut helical (pancreatic protocol) CT generally is used for staging pancreatic cancers and detects a mass in 76–96% of cases. MRI is an alternative for patients who have a contraindication to CT. Ultrasonography is not reliable because of interference by intestinal gas. PET scan can sometimes help clarify equivocal findings on CT and identify small metastatic foci. Selective celiac and superior mesenteric arteriography may demonstrate vessel invasion by cancer, a finding that would preclude attempts at surgical resection, but it is used uncommonly since the advent of multiphase helical CT. Endoscopic ultrasound (EUS) can occasionally detect small pancreatic tumors not visible on CT scan and help determine nodal involvement and resectability; it is typically used to guide FNA or biopsy for tissue diagnosis. In some centers, pancreatoscopy or intraductal ultrasonography is used to evaluate filling defects in the pancreatic duct and assess resectability of intraductal papillary mucinous cancers. With obstruction of the splenic vein, splenomegaly or gastric varices are present, the latter detected by endoscopy, EUS, or angiography.

Cystic neoplasms can be distinguished by their appearance on CT, EUS, and ERCP and features of the cyst fluid on gross, cytologic, and genetic analysis. For example, serous cystadenomas may have a central scar or honeycomb appearance; mucinous cystadenomas are unilocular or multilocular and contain mucin-rich fluid with low glucose levels (< 25 mg/dL [1.4 mmol/L]), high carcinoembryonic antigen levels (> 192 ng/mL [192 mcg/L]), and *KRAS* and *GNAS* pathogenic variants; and intraductal papillary mucinous neoplasms are associated with a dilated pancreatic duct and extrusion of gelatinous material from the ampulla.

Staging

The TNM system is the commonly used classification to stage pancreatic cancer. Staging correlates with the patient's long-term survival and is used to determine which patients should receive adjuvant or neoadjuvant therapy. Localized (nonmetastatic) pancreatic cancer includes *resectable, borderline resectable,* and *locally advanced (unresectable)* disease based on the presence and extent of involvement of adjacent blood vessels, including the celiac artery, superior mesenteric artery and vein, and portal vein. Over 30% of patients present with locally advanced disease and over 50% with *metastatic disease.*

Treatment

In patients with localized pancreatic cancer, surgical resection consists of either a Whipple pancreaticoduodenectomy (for tumors located at the pancreatic head) or a distal pancreatectomy (for tumors in the pancreatic body or tail). Preoperative laparoscopy is sometimes performed to look for the presence of tiny peritoneal or liver metastases, in which case subsequent attempt at resection of the primary tumor would be contraindicated. The 5-year survival rate is

20–25% in patients who undergo successful resection and as high as 40% in those with negative surgical margins and without lymph node involvement. *The best surgical results are achieved at centers that specialize in the multidisciplinary treatment of pancreatic cancer.*

Adjuvant chemotherapy has demonstrated a disease-free and overall survival benefit in patients with resected pancreatic cancer. The best results to date have been reported with a modified FOLFIRINOX (5-fluorouracil, leucovorin, irinotecan, oxaliplatin) regimen, although this is only appropriate for fit patients who have recovered well following surgery. Other regimens that have shown a benefit include the combination of gemcitabine and capecitabine, gemcitabine alone, and, in Japan and other Asian countries, S-1, an oral fluoropyrimidine. The role of adjuvant chemoradiation is somewhat more controversial but may play a role in select patients, for example, those with microscopically positive surgical margins. Neoadjuvant chemotherapy with or without radiation is used to downstage patients with borderline resectable and locally advanced pancreatic cancer to increase the likelihood of a successful R0 (margin-negative resection) and is even used sometimes in patients with clearly resectable tumors. Common chemotherapy regimens for this purpose include FOLFIRINOX and gemcitabine with nanoparticle albumin-bound (nab)-paclitaxel.

For patients who present with obstructive jaundice due to a pancreatic head tumor, *endoscopic stenting of the bile duct is performed to relieve the jaundice.* A plastic stent has generally been preferred if the patient's anticipated survival is < 6 months (or if surgery is planned). A metal stent (or surgical biliary bypass) is preferred when anticipated survival is ≥ 6 months. Whether covered metal stents designed to prevent cancer ingrowth offer an advantage over uncovered stents is uncertain because covered stents are associated with higher rates of migration and acute cholecystitis due to occlusion of the cystic duct. Of note, preoperative endoscopic decompression of an obstructed bile duct can be achieved with either a plastic stent or short metal stent but does not reduce operative mortality and can be associated with perioperative complications. For patients with gastric outlet obstruction, endoscopic placement of a self-expandable duodenal stent or gastrojejunal bypass (either via endoscopic placement of a gastrojejunal stent or surgical creation of a gastrojejunostomy) may be performed. Celiac plexus nerve block (see Chapter 5) done under CT or EUS guidance or thoracoscopic splanchnicectomy may improve pain control. Chemoradiation or stereotactic radiation may also be used to treat unresectable cancers confined to the pancreas.

For patients with metastatic pancreatic cancer, the two most commonly used chemotherapy combinations are FOLFIRINOX and the doublet of gemcitabine plus nab-paclitaxel, both of which have been shown to confer improvements in progression-free and overall survival compared with gemcitabine alone. In patients who have received prior gemcitabine-based chemotherapy, the second-line regimen of 5-fluorouracil and leucovorin in combination with nanoliposomal irinotecan has resulted in improved survival compared with 5-fluorouracil and leucovorin alone. Targeted therapies (Daraxonrasib) for common genetic mutations show great promise.

There is a consensus that asymptomatic incidental pancreatic cysts 2 cm or smaller are at low risk for harboring invasive carcinoma. The cysts may be monitored by imaging tests (MRI) in 1 year and then every 2 years if no changes are observed, with EUS and FNA performed if a cyst enlarges to 2 cm or more. The development of a high-risk feature (dilated main pancreatic duct, presence of a solid component ≥ 5 mm, suspicious cytology) should prompt consideration of surgery. The optimal approach is uncertain, however, and the newest guidelines emphasize the importance of shared decision-making. Surgical resection is indicated for mucinous cystic neoplasms, symptomatic serous cystadenomas, solid pseudopapillary tumors (which have a 15% risk of malignant transformation), and cystic tumors larger than 2 cm in diameter that remain undefined after helical CT, EUS, and diagnostic aspiration. Intraductal papillary mucinous neoplasms involving the main pancreatic duct typically should be considered for resection, but those of branch ducts may be monitored with serial imaging if they (1) are asymptomatic and exhibit benign features; (2) have a diameter < 3 cm (some authorities recommend a diameter of 1.5 cm or smaller, but even lesions 3 cm or larger may be monitored in older adults with no other worrisome cyst features); and (3) lack nonenhancing mural nodules, a thick wall, or an abrupt change in the caliber of the pancreatic duct with distal pancreatic atrophy. Most lesions with such benign features remain stable on follow-up, but a risk of malignancy persists for > 10 years. Moreover, the risk of pancreatic ductal carcinoma and of nonpancreatic cancers is also increased in this group of patients. Endoscopic resection or ablation, with temporary placement of a pancreatic duct stent, may be feasible for ampullary adenomas, but patients must be followed for recurrence.

Prognosis

Carcinoma of the pancreas has a poor prognosis; 80–85% of patients present with advanced (unresectable or metastatic) disease, in whom the reported 5-year survival rate is 2–5%. From 1999 to 2020, mortality from pancreatic cancer in the United States has slowly increased to an age-adjusted mortality rate of 11.1 per 100,000. Obesity may adversely affect mortality in Western countries. Tumors of the ampulla have a better prognosis, with a reported 5-year survival rate of 20–40% after resection; jaundice and lymph node involvement are adverse prognostic factors. In persons with a family history of pancreatic cancer in at least two first-degree relatives, or with a genetic syndrome associated with an increased risk of pancreatic cancer, annual screening with EUS and alternating with MRI should be considered, generally beginning at age 50 years (age 40 years in *CKDN2A* or *PRSS1* pathogenic variant carriers and age 35 years in those with Peutz-Jeghers syndrome) or 10 years before the age at which pancreatic cancer was first diagnosed in a family member.

For those patients whose disease progresses despite treatment, meticulous efforts at palliative care are essential (see Chapter 5).

When to Refer

All patients with carcinoma involving the pancreas and the ampulla of Vater should be referred to a specialist.

When to Admit

Patients who require surgery and other interventions should be hospitalized.

Abboud Y et al. Increasing pancreatic cancer incidence in young women in the United States: a population-based time-trend analysis, 2001-2018. Gastroenterology. 2023;164:978. [PMID: 36775072]

Han Y et al. Optimal surveillance interval of branch duct intraductal papillary mucinous neoplasm of the pancreas. JAMA Surg. 2024:e237010. [PMID: 38231494]

Marchegiani G et al. Surveillance for presumed BD-IPMN of the pancreas: stability, size, and age identify targets for discontinuation. Gastroenterology. 2023;165:1016. [PMID: 37406887]

Redegalli M et al. Routine molecular profiling in both resectable and unresectable pancreatic adenocarcinoma: relevance of cytologic samples. Clin Gastroenterol Hepatol. 2023;21:2825. [PMID: 36280101]

Sawhney MS et al. ASGE guideline on screening for pancreatic cancer in individuals with genetic susceptibility: summary and recommendations. Gastrointest Endosc. 2022;95:817. [PMID: 35183358]

ALIMENTARY TRACT CANCERS

ESOPHAGEAL CANCER

ESSENTIALS OF DIAGNOSIS

- Progressive dysphagia to solid food.
- Weight loss common.
- Endoscopy with biopsy establishes diagnosis.

General Considerations

Esophageal cancer usually develops in persons 50–70 years of age. In the United States, there were an estimated 22,070 new cases of esophageal cancer, resulting in 16,250 deaths in 2025. The incidence of esophageal cancer is approximately four times higher in men than in women, as are the number of deaths attributable to esophageal cancer. There are two main histologic types: squamous cell carcinoma and adenocarcinoma, and their incidence has significant geographic variation. **Squamous cell carcinoma (SCC)** is associated with low socioeconomic status; consumption of tobacco, alcohol, hot beverages, and nitrosamines; and poor nutritional status. It accounts for over 90% of cases of esophageal cancer in Eastern and Southeast Asia and sub-Saharan Africa. **Adenocarcinoma** is associated with age; obesity; smoking; and chronic GERD with Barrett metaplasia. Adenocarcinomas make up most new cases of esophageal cancer in North America and Northern and Western Europe. Most (90%) squamous cell carcinomas occur in the upper and middle third of the esophagus, whereas adenocarcinomas are more common in the distal esophagus and gastroesophageal junction.

Clinical Findings

A. Symptoms and Signs

Approximately 30–40% of patients with esophageal cancer present with stage IV (metastatic) disease. While early symptoms are nonspecific and subtle, over 90% eventually have dysphagia to solid foods, which progresses over weeks to months. Odynophagia is sometimes present. Significant weight loss is common. Local tumor extension into the tracheobronchial tree may result in a tracheoesophageal fistula, characterized by aspirating, coughing, or both while eating.

B. Laboratory Findings

Laboratory findings are nonspecific. Anemia related to chronic disease or occult blood loss is common. Hypoalbuminemia may result from malnutrition.

C. Imaging

A barium esophagogram may be the first study obtained to evaluate dysphagia. The appearance of a polypoid, obstructive, or ulcerative lesion suggests carcinoma and requires endoscopic evaluation. Imaging typically consists of CT scans of the chest and abdomen, which may show abnormal wall thickening of the esophagus, regional lymphadenopathy, and, in cases of metastatic disease, the presence of metastatic lesions in the lungs, liver, distant lymph nodes, peritoneal cavity, or bones.

D. Upper Endoscopy

Endoscopy with biopsy establishes the diagnosis of esophageal carcinoma with a high degree of reliability. In some cases, significant submucosal spread of the tumor may yield nondiagnostic mucosal biopsies. Repeat biopsy may be necessary.

Staging

After confirmation of the diagnosis of esophageal carcinoma during upper endoscopy, the stage of the disease should be determined to guide therapy. If not yet performed, patients should undergo evaluation with contrast CT of the chest, abdomen, and pelvis, with or without concurrent PET, to look for local tumor extension, lymphadenopathy, and metastases. If there is no evidence of metastatic disease, then EUS represents a useful tool to more accurately assess the local extent of the esophageal tumor as well as the presence of lymph node involvement.

Differential Diagnosis

Esophageal carcinoma must be distinguished from other causes of progressive dysphagia, including peptic strictures and achalasia. Benign-appearing peptic strictures should be biopsied at presentation to exclude occult malignancy.

Treatment

The approach to esophageal cancer treatment depends on the cancer stage and anatomic location, patient comorbidities, age, and functional status, as well as the expertise of treating gastroenterologists, surgeons, oncologists, and radiation oncologists. Clinical trials evaluating the optimal treatment of esophageal cancer often have combined both SCCs and adenocarcinomas; however, their risk factors, pathobiology, and responses to treatment differ substantially. SCCs are the most common cancer of the cervical esophagus and typically more radiosensitive than adenocarcinomas. Because surgical resection of a cervical esophagus tumor often requires laryngectomy and neck dissection with attendant comorbidities, chemoradiation usually is preferred over surgery for curative intent treatment of SCC of the cervical esophagus. The discussion below applies to treatment of tumors arising in the thoracic esophagus and gastroesophageal junction.

A. Therapy for Resectable Disease

Superficial esophageal cancers confined to the epithelium (high-grade dysplasia or carcinoma in situ [Tis]), lamina propria (T1a), or submucosa (T1b) are increasingly recognized during endoscopic screening and surveillance programs. If performed by an experienced gastroenterologist, endoscopic mucosal resection of Tis and T1a cancers can achieve equivalent long-term survival as esophagectomy with less morbidity (see Barrett Esophagus, Chapter 17).

Esophagectomy is usually recommended for high-risk T1a tumors (eg, those with poor differentiation or lymphovascular invasion) and T1b tumors because of higher rates of lymph node metastasis, as well as for more locally advanced disease (stages IB–IIIB). Careful patient selection for surgery is critical since esophagectomy can be associated with considerable morbidity and even mortality (2%). Accepted surgical techniques include en bloc transthoracic excision of the esophagus with extended lymph node dissection, transhiatal esophagogastrectomy (entailing laparotomy with cervical anastomosis), and minimally invasive esophagectomy techniques. Meta-analysis data suggest equivalent oncologic outcomes between minimally invasive esophagectomy and conventional open techniques, with the former approach having the advantage of fewer postoperative complications and shorter hospital stays. Multiple meta-analyses have shown that, regardless of surgery type, surgery at a high-volume hospital is associated with decreased perioperative mortality and better outcomes.

Patients with stage I tumors have high cure rates with surgery alone and do not require multimodality therapy (eg, perioperative chemotherapy, radiation, or both). For patients with stage II and III tumors, where the risk of both locoregional and distant recurrence is higher, patients are typically recommended to receive additional therapy before or after their surgery or at both times to decrease the risk of relapse. The following represent the most common approaches in this context.

1. Surgery with perioperative chemotherapy—For esophageal and gastroesophageal junction adenocarcinomas, the phase 3 ESOPEC trial showed a survival benefit for perioperative FLOT (fluorouracil, leucovorin, oxaliplatin, and docetaxel) chemotherapy compared to neoadjuvant chemoradiotherapy. Based on this study, four cycles of preoperative plus four cycles of postoperative triplet FLOT chemotherapy is the standard of care; extrapolating from recently reported phase 3 data in gastric cancer, the immune checkpoint inhibitor durvalumab can confer additional disease-free and overall survival benefit when added to chemotherapy in this perioperative context.

2. Surgery with neoadjuvant chemoradiation therapy—Patients with stage II–III tumors who are not candidates for the more intensive perioperative FLOT chemotherapy regimen may receive neoadjuvant chemoradiation. The most commonly used regimen concurrent with radiation therapy consists of weekly carboplatin plus paclitaxel (administered at lower, radiosensitizing doses). FOLFOX represents an alternative regimen in select patients, though this may be associated with greater toxicity (Table 43–2). Radiation techniques that are less toxic, such as intensity-modulated radiation therapy or proton beam therapy, have been investigated. Following completion of neoadjuvant chemoradiation and surgical resection, patients who are found to have residual cancer at the time of surgery (and who have no contraindications to immunotherapy) should receive adjuvant therapy with the immune checkpoint inhibitor nivolumab for 1 year, as this strategy has shown to decrease the likelihood of disease relapse.

3. Chemotherapy plus radiation therapy without surgery—Concurrent chemotherapy plus radiation therapy achieves long-term survival in up to 25% of patients and is superior to radiation alone. Chemoradiation alone should be considered in patients with localized disease who are poor surgical candidates due to serious medical illness or poor functional status (Eastern Cooperative Oncology Group score > 2) or those who are concerned about the potential morbidity and long-term sequelae of an esophagectomy. Patients with cervical esophageal cancers, which appear similar biologically to head and neck cancers and in whom surgery is highly morbid and typically not recommended, also typically receive definitive chemoradiation.

4. Supportive care during treatment—Patients with significant tumor obstruction may require percutaneous gastric or jejunal tube placement to maintain adequate hydration and nutrition during neoadjuvant chemoradiation or chemotherapy. Multidisciplinary consultation is required to determine the optimal procedure and to optimize perioperative nutrition.

B. Therapy for Advanced Unresectable and Metastatic Disease

More than half of patients have either locally extensive tumor spread (T4b) that is unresectable or distant metastases (M1) at the time of diagnosis. Surgery is not warranted in these patients. The optimal treatment approach depends on the presence or absence of metastatic disease, expected survival, patient preference, and molecular characteristics of the tumor.

1. Chemotherapy or chemoradiation—Systemic therapy options are largely the same for metastatic esophageal, gastroesophageal junction, and gastric cancers, with the first line of chemotherapy typically consisting of a fluoropyrimidine/platinum combination such as FOLFOX (Table 43–2). Choice of treatment is also increasingly influenced by the results of molecular testing, including PD-L1 expression, mismatch repair/microsatellite instability (MMR/MSI) and, for adenocarcinomas, human epidermal growth factor receptor 2 (HER2) amplification and Claudin 18.2 expression testing. In patients with overexpression of HER2 (approximately 15% of cases), detected either by immunohistochemistry (IHC) or by amplification of the *HER2* gene via in situ hybridization or next-generation sequencing), the addition of the monoclonal antibody trastuzumab (see Chapter 19) to chemotherapy is associated with prolonged survival (Table 43–8). Moreover, in persons with PD-L1 expression, the immune checkpoint inhibitor pembrolizumab should be added as well. For patients without *HER2* amplification but who have increased PD-L1 expression, the addition of an immune checkpoint inhibitor to chemotherapy has been shown to improve progression-free and overall survival. Immunotherapy is also recommended for patients whose tumors harbor either microsatellite instability-high (MSI-H) or deficient mismatch repair (dMMR) protein expression; in such individuals, immunotherapy alone (ie, without chemotherapy) may be effective. For adenocarcinomas without *HER2* overexpression that do have Claudin 18.2 expression, the addition of zolbetuximab to chemotherapy prolongs survival. The optimal combination for tumors that express both PD-L1 and Claudin 18.2 is unknown.

Concurrent chemoradiation, either preceding or following chemotherapy, can be considered for select patients with locally advanced tumors (or with limited metastatic involvement) to try to achieve optimal local disease control.

2. Local therapy for esophageal obstruction—Patients with advanced esophageal cancer often have a poor functional and nutritional status. Radiation therapy alone to the area of esophageal obstruction may afford short-term relief of pain and dysphagia. Rapid palliation of dysphagia may be achieved by peroral placement of permanent expandable wire stents (alone or followed by radiation). However, placement of these stents is complicated by perforation, migration, or tumor ingrowth in up to 40% of cases.

Prognosis

The overall 5-year survival rate of esophageal carcinoma is < 20%. Apart from distant metastasis (M1b), the two most important predictors of poor survival are adjacent mediastinal spread (T4) and lymph node involvement. For those patients whose disease progresses despite chemotherapy, meticulous efforts at palliative care are essential (see Chapter 5).

When to Refer

- Patients should be referred to a gastroenterologist for evaluation and staging (endoscopy with biopsy, EUS) and palliative endoscopic stenting.
- Patients with curable and resectable disease for whom neoadjuvant therapy may be appropriate (stage IIB or IIIA) should be referred to medical, radiation, and surgical oncologists for consideration of neoadjuvant chemotherapy, chemoradiotherapy, and surgical resection.
- Patients with metastatic disease should be referred to medical and radiation oncologists for consideration of palliative chemotherapy or chemoradiation.
- Patients with metastatic disease and obstructive tumors not amenable to or refractory to palliative radiation or stenting may require referral to an interventional radiologist, gastroenterologist, or surgeon for gastric or jejunal tube placement for hydration and liquid artificial nutrition. Early referral to palliative care may improve symptom management in patients with advanced or metastatic disease.

When to Admit

Patients with high-grade esophageal obstruction with inability to manage oral secretions or maintain hydration should be admitted. Acute complications such as perforation, bleeding, aspiration, or fistula also may require admission.

Al-Haddad MA et al. American Society for Gastrointestinal Endoscopy guideline on endoscopic submucosal dissection for the management of early esophageal and gastric cancers: methodology and review of evidence. Gastrointest Endosc. 2023;98:285. [PMID: 37498265]

Kamboj AK et al. Clinical outcomes after endoscopic management of low-risk and high-risk T1a esophageal adenocarcinoma: a multicenter study. Am J Gastroenterol. 2024;119:662. [PMID: 37795907]

National Comprehensive Cancer Network. Esophageal and esophagogastric junction cancers, Version 2.2023, NCCN Clinical Practice Guidelines in Oncology. https://www.nccn.org/professionals/physician_gls/pdf/esophageal.pdf

Shitara K et al. Zolbetuximab in gastric or gastroesophageal junction adenocarcinoma. N Engl J Med. 2024;391:1159. [PMID: 39282934]

GASTRIC ADENOCARCINOMA

ESSENTIALS OF DIAGNOSIS

- Dyspeptic symptoms with weight loss, especially in patients > 40 years.
- Iron deficiency anemia: occult blood in stools.
- Abnormality detected on upper GI series, abdominal CT endoscopy; diagnosis established by endoscopic biopsy.

General Considerations

Gastric adenocarcinoma is the third most common cause of cancer death worldwide. Its main risk factors include increasing age, male sex, certain races (eg, Asian, Black, Lantinx), smoking, and *Helicobacter pylori* infection. Chronic *H pylori* gastritis is the strongest risk factor, increasing the relative risk 3.5- to 20-fold.

The incidence of gastric adenocarcinoma has declined significantly over the last 70 years, especially in Western countries, perhaps attributable to changes in diet (more fruits and vegetables), increased food refrigeration, reduced toxic environmental exposures, and effective treatment of *H pylori* infection.

In the United States in 2025, gastric cancer accounted for 1.3% of all new cancers (with an estimated 30,300 incident cases and an estimated 10,780 deaths). Globally, there is significant geographic variation in the incidence of gastric cancer, with particularly high rates in parts of eastern Asia, Eastern Europe, Chile, Colombia, and Central America.

There are two main histologic variants of gastric cancer: "intestinal-type" (which resembles intestinal cancers in forming glandular structures) and "diffuse" (which is poorly differentiated and lacks glandular formation).

The incidence of *intestinal-type gastric cancer* has declined significantly, but it is still the more common type (70–80%); it occurs twice as often in men as women and primarily affects older people (mean age 68 years). It is estimated that 60–90% of cases may be attributable to *H pylori*. Other risk factors for intestinal-type gastric cancer include pernicious anemia, a history of partial gastric resection > 15 years previously, smoking, and diets that are high in nitrates or salt and low in vitamin C.

Diffuse gastric cancer accounts for 20–30% of gastric cancer cases. In contrast to intestinal-type cancer, it affects men and women equally, occurs more commonly in young people, is not as strongly related to *H pylori* infection, and has a worse prognosis than intestinal-type cancer due to early metastasis. Diffuse gastric cancers are often attributable to acquired or hereditary pathogenic variants in the genes regulating the E-cadherin cell adhesion protein. Hereditary diffuse gastric cancer may arise at a young age, is often multifocal and infiltrating with signet ring cell histology and has a poor prognosis.

Most gastric cancers arise in the body and antrum. These may occur in a variety of morphologic types: (1) polypoid or fungating intraluminal masses; (2) ulcerating masses; (3) diffusely spreading (**linitis plastica**), in which the cancer spreads through the submucosa, resulting in a rigid, atonic stomach with thickened folds (prognosis is dismal); and (4) superficially spreading or "early" gastric cancer—confined to the mucosa or submucosa (with or without lymph node metastases) and associated with a more favorable prognosis.

In contrast to the dramatic decline in cancers of the distal stomach, a rise in incidence of tumors of the gastric cardia and gastroesophageal junction has been noted. These tumors have demographic and pathologic features that resemble Barrett-associated esophageal adenocarcinomas (see Esophageal Cancer, above).

Clinical Findings

A. Symptoms and Signs

Gastric carcinoma is generally asymptomatic until quite advanced. Symptoms are nonspecific and are determined in part by the location of the tumor. Dyspepsia, vague epigastric pain, anorexia, early satiety, and weight loss are the presenting symptoms in most patients. Patients may derive initial symptomatic relief from over-the-counter remedies, further delaying diagnosis. Ulcerating lesions can lead to acute GI bleeding with hematemesis or melena. Pyloric (gastric outlet) obstruction results in postprandial vomiting. Lower esophageal obstruction causes progressive dysphagia. Physical examination is rarely helpful.

B. Laboratory Findings

Iron deficiency anemia due to chronic blood loss or anemia of chronic disease is common. Stool tests may be positive for occult blood. Circulating tumor markers do not have established clinical validity in screening or diagnosis of gastric cancer.

C. Endoscopy

Upper endoscopy should be obtained in all patients over age 60 years with new onset of epigastric symptoms (dyspepsia) and young patients with "alarm" symptoms (dysphagia, recurrent vomiting, significant weight loss), especially in immigrants from countries with a high prevalence of gastric cancer. Endoscopy with biopsies of suspicious lesions is highly sensitive for detecting gastric carcinoma. However, it can be difficult to obtain adequate biopsy specimens in diffuse-type gastric cancer.

D. Imaging

Once a gastric cancer is diagnosed, staging evaluation by contrast CT of chest, abdomen, and pelvis and by EUS is indicated to delineate the local extent of the primary tumor as well as to evaluate for nodal or distant metastases. EUS is superior to CT in determining the depth of tumor penetration and is useful for evaluation of early gastric cancers that may be removed by endoscopic mucosal resection. PET or combined PET-CT imaging can be useful for detection of distant metastasis.

Screening

Due to the higher incidence of gastric cancer in East Asia, population-based nationwide screening by upper endoscopy has been implemented in South Korea and Japan. In the United States and other countries with a relatively low incidence of gastric cancer, routine screening for gastric cancer is not recommended but may be considered beginning at age 50 in people who are first-generation immigrants from high-incidence regions and people who belong to racial or ethnic groups who are at increased risk.

Because of its unproven efficacy and cost-effectiveness, screening and treating for *H pylori* infection are not recommended to prevent gastric cancer in asymptomatic US adults (but are recommended in patients who have immigrated from regions with a high incidence of gastric cancer or who have a family history of gastric cancer). However, a 2023 retrospective study of 716,567 patients with *H pylori* in a community-based population found a significant reduction after 8 years in the risk of gastric adenocarcinoma in those who were treated for *H pylori* versus who were untreated (HR 0.37).

Staging

The TNM system used to stage gastric adenocarcinoma correlates with the patient's long-term survival and is used to determine which patients should receive adjuvant or neoadjuvant therapy.

Pathologic review should include (1) grade of tumor, (2) histologic subtype, (3) depth of invasion, (4) whether lymphatic or vascular invasion is present, and (5) molecular testing for HER2 protein overexpression, dMMR proteins or MSI-H, PD-L1 expression, and Claudin 18.2 expression.

Differential Diagnosis

Ulcerating gastric adenocarcinomas are distinguished from benign gastric ulcers by biopsy. Approximately 3% of gastric ulcers initially believed to be benign later prove to be malignant. *All gastric ulcers identified at endoscopy should be biopsied to exclude malignancy.* Ulcers that are suspicious for malignancy to the endoscopist or that have atypia or dysplasia on histologic examination warrant repeat endoscopy in 2–3 months to verify healing and exclude malignancy. Nonhealing ulcers should be considered for resection. Infiltrative carcinoma with thickened gastric folds must be distinguished from lymphoma and other hypertrophic gastropathies.

Treatment

Surgical resection, systemic chemotherapy, radiotherapy, immunotherapy, and targeted therapy all have proven efficacy in gastric adenocarcinoma; therefore, multidisciplinary teamwork is paramount to treatment selection. The optimal role and sequencing of adjunctive therapies depends on the location and extent of the cancer, type of surgery, patient comorbidities and performance status, and institutional experience.

A. Curative Surgical Resection

Surgical resection is the primary treatment for nonmetastatic gastric adenocarcinoma and offers the potential for cure. Laparoscopic resection achieves similar outcomes as, and lower overall complication rates than, open gastrectomy. In Japan and in specialized US centers, endoscopic mucosal resection is performed in select patients with small (< 1–2 cm), early-stage (intramucosal or T1aN0) gastric cancers after careful staging with EUS. A staging laparoscopy prior to definitive surgery should be considered in patients with stage T1b or greater disease without radiographic evidence of distant metastases, as approximately 25% of patients undergoing surgery will be found to have locally unresectable tumors or peritoneal, hepatic, or distant lymph node metastases. The remaining patients with confirmed localized disease should undergo radical surgical resection. For adenocarcinoma localized to the distal two-thirds of the stomach, a partial or subtotal gastrectomy should be performed. For proximal gastric cancer or diffusely infiltrating disease, total gastrectomy is necessary. Vitamin B_{12} supplementation is required after gastrectomy.

B. Perioperative Chemotherapy, Chemoradiation, or Radiation Therapy

For patients with regional lymph node involvement, risk of recurrence with surgery alone is > 60%; therefore, further therapy is recommended. *Multidisciplinary treatment decision-making involving the surgeon, radiation oncologist, and medical oncologist is imperative.* The current gold standard, particularly in Western countries, consists of perioperative systemic therapy. Specifically, the perioperative triplet chemotherapy regimen FLOT (5-FU, leucovorin, oxaliplatin, docetaxel) was demonstrated in a phase 2/3 study to be superior to the previous standard of ECF. Recent evidence from the phase 3 MATTERHORN trial in patients with resectable (stage II–IVA) gastric and gastroesophageal junction cancer indicated that the addition of an immune checkpoint inhibitor (durvalumab) to FLOT chemotherapy further improves clinical outcomes, including a 2-year event-free survival of 67.4% compared with 58.5% with chemotherapy alone.

For patients with dMMR/MSI-H localized tumors (which represent 8–16% of gastric cancer cases), perioperative immunotherapy alone may represent an option, although further investigation is required. Hence, testing for either MMR or MSI status is recommended for all new gastric cancer diagnoses.

Pre- or postoperative (chemo)radiation therapy has been evaluated in multiple trials (ARTIST, CRITICS, TOPGEAR); overall, this modality has *not* demonstrated a clear benefit in the context of an appropriate gastric cancer operation and should not be routinely used. It may, however, be useful in select circumstances, particularly in patients who are at high risk for local recurrence (eg, those who do not achieve an R0 resection).

Tumors arising in the gastroesophageal junction are treated following algorithms for primary esophageal cancers (see Esophageal Cancer, above).

C. Treatment for Advanced and Metastatic Disease

Many patients will be found to have advanced or metastatic disease that is not amenable to curative intent surgery due to peritoneal or distant metastases or local invasion of other organs. In such patients, systemic therapy represents the mainstay of treatment. Systemic therapy regimens are generally the same as those used in esophageal adenocarcinomas (Table 43–2). Molecular testing for clinically actionable biomarkers (dMMR/MSI status; expression of PD-L1, HER2, Claudin 18.2) is critical to guide the use of targeted therapies, immunotherapy on top of chemotherapy, or both.

D. Palliative Modalities

For patients with unresectable disease and gastric outlet obstruction with good functional status, laparoscopic or endoscopic gastrojejunostomy may be indicated to prevent obstruction. In rare instances, palliative resection of the tumor may be appropriate to alleviate pain, bleeding, or obstruction. Duodenal stent placement, radiation therapy, or angiographic embolization can help relieve bleeding or obstruction.

Prognosis

The 5-year survival for gastric cancer varies greatly by stage, location, and histologic features. Following surgery, the 5-year survival rates for stage IA and IB cancers treated with curative intent are between 60% and 80%, but for stage IIIC cancers, they are as low as 18%. Proximal gastric tumors have a 5-year survival of < 15%, even with apparent localized disease. For those whose disease progresses despite therapy, palliative care is essential (see Chapter 5).

When to Refer

- Patients with dysphagia, weight loss, protracted vomiting, iron deficiency anemia, melena, or new-onset dyspepsia (especially if aged 60 years or older or associated with other alarm symptoms) in whom gastric cancer is suspected should be referred for endoscopy.
- Patients should be referred to a surgeon for attempt at curative resection of stage I, II, or III cancer, including staging laparoscopy if indicated.
- Prior to surgery, patients should be referred to an oncologist to determine the role for perioperative chemotherapy, immunotherapy, or both. Chemoradiation may play a role in select patients, typically following surgery.
- Patients who have undergone gastrectomy require consultation with a nutritionist due to propensity for malnutrition and complications, such as dumping syndrome and vitamin B_{12} deficiency, postoperatively.
- Patients with unresectable or metastatic disease should be referred to an oncologist for consideration of palliative chemotherapy or chemoradiation. Early referral to palliative care services may also be considered for symptom management in patients with advanced and metastatic disease.

When to Admit

Patients with acute bleeding, protracted vomiting, or inability to maintain hydration or nutrition should be admitted.

Al-Batran SE et al; FLOT4-AIO Investigators. Perioperative chemotherapy with fluorouracil plus leucovorin, oxaliplatin, and docetaxel versus fluorouracil or capecitabine plus cisplatin and epirubicin for locally advanced, resectable gastric or gastro-oesophageal junction adenocarcinoma (FLOT4): a randomised, phase 2/3 trial. Lancet. 2019;393:1948. [PMID: 30982686]

André T et al. Neoadjuvant nivolumab plus ipilimumab and adjuvant nivolumab in localized deficient mismatch repair/microsatellite instability-high gastric or esophagogastric junction adenocarcinoma: the GERCOR NEONIPIGA phase II study. J Clin Oncol. 2023;41:255. [PMID: 35969830]

Janjigian YY et al; MATTERHORN Investigators. Perioperative durvalumab in gastric and gastroesophageal junction cancer. N Engl J Med. 2025;393:217. [PMID: 40454643]

Li D et al. Effect of *Helicobacter pylori* eradication therapy on the incidence of noncardia gastric adenocarcinoma in a large diverse population in the United States. Gastroenterology. 2023;165:391. [PMID: 37142201]

GASTRIC LYMPHOMA

ESSENTIALS OF DIAGNOSIS

- Symptoms of dyspepsia, weight loss, or anemia.
- Distinguish primary gastric lymphoma with adjacent nodal spread from advanced systemic lymphoma with secondary gastric involvement.
- Upper GI series or endoscopy shows thickened folds, ulcer, mass, or infiltrating lesions; diagnosis established by endoscopic biopsy.
- Abdominal CT and EUS required for staging.

General Considerations

Gastric lymphomas may be primary (arising from the gastric mucosa) or may represent a site of secondary involvement in patients with nodal lymphomas. Distinguishing advanced **primary gastric lymphoma** with adjacent nodal spread from **secondary gastric lymphoma** spread from advanced nodal lymphoma is essential because the prognosis and treatment of primary and secondary gastric lymphomas are different. Primary gastric lymphoma is the second most common gastric malignancy, accounting for 3–5% of gastric cancers. More than 95% of these are non-Hodgkin B-cell lymphomas mainly consisting of either (1) **mucosa-associated lymphoid tissue (MALT)-type lymphoma** or (2) **diffuse large B-cell lymphoma**. Over 90% of low-grade primary gastric MALT-type lymphomas are associated with *H pylori* infection. *H pylori* leads to chronic inflammation, producing lymphoid tissue in the stomach mucosa (MALT) that can lead to malignant transformation.

Clinical Findings & Staging

The clinical presentation and endoscopic appearance of gastric lymphoma are like those of adenocarcinoma, which makes pathologic review imperative. Most patients have abdominal pain, weight loss, or bleeding. Patients with diffuse large B-cell lymphoma are more likely to have systemic symptoms.

At endoscopy, lymphoma may appear as an ulcer, mass, or diffusely infiltrating lesion. The diagnosis is established with endoscopic biopsy; FNA alone is not adequate. Since the disease can be multifocal, biopsies of both suspicious and normal-appearing areas are recommended. Biopsy specimens should be tested for *H pylori* and, if positive, for t(11;18) via PCR or fluorescence in situ hybridization (FISH). EUS is the most sensitive test for determining the depth of invasion and presence of perigastric lymphadenopathy. All patients should undergo staging with CT scanning of chest, abdomen, and pelvis.

1. MALT-type lymphomas—For gastric MALT lymphomas, the Lugano staging system is most frequently used. Stage I is confined to the GI tract, stage II involves local or regional lymph nodes, stage IIE has invasion of adjacent organs or tissues, and stage IV has distant metastases. There is no stage III.

2. Diffuse large B-cell lymphomas—For patients with diffuse large B-cell lymphomas involving the stomach, combination PET-CT imaging, bone marrow biopsy with aspirate, tumor lysis laboratory tests, and hepatitis B and HIV serologies may be required for staging and treatment planning (see Chapter 15).

Treatment

Treatment of primary gastric lymphomas depends on the tumor histology, grade, and stage.

A. MALT-Type Lymphomas

Those that are low-grade and localized to the stomach wall (stage I) or perigastric lymph nodes (stage IIE1) have an excellent prognosis. Patients with primary gastric MALT lymphoma should be tested for *H pylori* infection and treated if positive. Complete lymphoma regression after successful *H pylori* eradication occurs in approximately 75% of cases of stage I and approximately 55% of stage IIE low-grade lymphoma. Remission may take as long as a year, and relapse occurs in about 2% of cases per year.

Failure of antibiotic treatment to achieve lymphoma regression may be due to genetic factors. Rates of remission after *H pylori* eradication are lower in patients whose tumors harbor specific gene translocations, including t(11;18) (API2-MALT1), t(1;14), or t(14;18). Of cancers positive for t(11;18), 95% do not respond to antibiotics. Patients with localized marginal zone MALT-type lymphomas who are not infected with *H pylori* or do not respond to *H pylori* antibiotic therapy may be treated with radiation therapy.

Endoscopic surveillance after antibiotic or radiation treatment is recommended every 3–6 months for 5 years to evaluate for recurrence. The long-term survival of low-grade MALT stage I lymphoma is over 90% and for stage II is 35–65%. Surgical resection is *not* recommended.

B. Diffuse Large B-Cell Lymphoma

Diffuse large B-cell lymphomas (or other higher-grade lymphomas with secondary GI involvement) usually present at an advanced stage with widely disseminated disease and are treated according to stage and subtype of lymphoma (see Chapter 15).

Advanced-stage disease can be treated with chemoimmunotherapy or radiation therapy for GI bleeding, threatened end-organ function, bulky disease, or progression. Diffuse large B-cell lymphoma has been successfully treated with two chemotherapeutic options (cyclophosphamide-doxorubicin-vincristine-prednisone [CHOP] or rituximab-CHOP). The presence of perigastric lymph nodes and the degree of tumor infiltration of the gastric wall are indications to consider including radiotherapy in the treatment.

National Comprehensive Cancer Network. B-Cell Lymphomas, Version 3.2023, NCCN Clinical Practice Guidelines in Oncology. https://www.nccn.org/professionals/physician_gls/pdf/b-cell.pdf

GASTROINTESTINAL MESENCHYMAL TUMORS

Pathobiology & Diagnosis

GI mesenchymal tumors (stromal tumors, leiomyomas, and schwannomas) derive from mesenchymal stem cells. The most common are **GI stromal tumors (GISTs)**, which originate from interstitial cells of Cajal. GISTs occur most commonly in the stomach (60%). Most cases are sporadic, but about 5% of cases are part of familial genetic syndromes. GISTs are potentially malignant and have an unpredictable evolution. Determination of the GIST molecular subtype upon diagnosis is important because it informs therapeutic decisions in both the adjuvant and metastatic setting. Approximately 80–90% of GISTs have gain-of-function mutations in either *KIT*, a receptor tyrosine kinase, or in platelet-derived growth factor α (PDGFRα).

Mesenchymal tumors may cause symptoms (most commonly bleeding, pain, or obstruction) or may be discovered incidentally on imaging studies or endoscopy. At endoscopy, they appear as a submucosal mass that may have central umbilication or ulceration. EUS with guided FNA biopsy is the optimal study for diagnosing gastric mesenchymal tumors and distinguishing them from other submucosal lesions. Percutaneous biopsy is not recommended due to risk of bleeding or intra-abdominal seeding. CT of the abdomen and pelvis with contrast (or MRI) should be performed for staging purposes; additionally, PET scans offer complementary information and are particularly useful to monitor response to treatment.

It is difficult to distinguish benign from malignant tumors by EUS appearance. In general, lesions are more likely benign if they are smaller than 2 cm, have a smooth border, and have a homogeneous echo pattern on EUS. However, all GISTs have malignant potential, and the risk of developing metastasis increases with tumor size > 2 cm, nongastric location, and mitotic index > 5 mitoses per 50 HPF.

Treatment

A. Localized Treatment

Complete surgical resection, whether by laparotomy or laparoscopy, offers curative potential for localized GISTs. Surgical resection is recommended for tumors that are 2 cm or larger or are increasing in size, suspicious for malignancy on EUS, or symptomatic. The management of asymptomatic gastric lesions 2 cm or smaller depends on the EUS features. If no high-risk features are noted, endoscopic surveillance with serial EUS can be pursued. Because of the low but real long-term risk of malignancy, surgical resection should be considered in younger, otherwise healthy patients.

B. Systemic Treatment

The introduction of effective molecularly targeted therapies for GISTs has dramatically changed the clinical management and prognosis for patients with intermediate- and high-risk resected GISTs, as well as those with locally advanced and metastatic disease. *Molecular characterization is imperative in all cases being considered for systemic therapy.* The tyrosine kinase inhibitor imatinib is effective against the most common pathogenic mutations seen in GISTs, including *KIT* and some *PDGFRα* mutations. Neoadjuvant therapy with imatinib may be considered for patients with localized GIST tumors who are deemed to be at high risk for incomplete resection because of comorbidities, tumor size, or tumor location. Adjuvant therapy with imatinib improves both disease-free and overall survival for most mutations. Imatinib also represents the standard first-line treatment for patients with metastatic GIST, producing disease control in up to 80–85% of patients. Patients who subsequently experience disease progression on imatinib therapy may be treated with second-, third-, and fourth-line therapy with sunitinib, regorafenib, and ripretinib, respectively. Untreated metastatic GIST tumors are aggressive and carry a poor prognosis.

In the subset of tumors that have the *PDGFRα* D842V pathogenic variant, the KIT and PDGFRα inhibitor avapritinib results in an approximate 90% disease control rate. The role of immunotherapies for mesenchymal tumors is being investigated.

MALIGNANCIES OF THE SMALL INTESTINE

The frequency of different tumor types varies by location within the small intestine. Adenocarcinomas are most common in the duodenum and jejunum and NETs, in the ileum. Lymphomas and sarcomas each have similar incidences in the various segments of the small intestine.

1. Small Intestinal Adenocarcinomas

These cancers often present with abdominal pain and nausea. They are rare, with approximately 12,000 new diagnoses estimated for 2024 in the United States, and most often diagnosed at stage III or IV. The duodenum is the most common site of small bowel adenocarcinoma, specifically the periampullary region. **Ampullary carcinomas** may present with GI bleeding or jaundice due to bile duct obstruction. Surgical resection (Whipple pancreaticoduodenectomy) of localized lesions is curative in up to 40% of patients.

Most cases of **nonampullary adenocarcinomas** present with symptoms of obstruction, acute or chronic GI bleeding, or weight loss. Nonspecific findings on cross-sectional imaging and difficulty of endoscopic evaluation often delay diagnosis. For localized disease resection is potentially curative. The benefit of adjuvant therapy after resection of stage II or III tumors is unclear, but it is generally administered using CRC regimens. For advanced/unresectable disease, first-line doublet chemotherapy extrapolated from CRC regimens is standard. Small intestinal adenocarcinoma should be evaluated for MMR/MSI status. Pembrolizumab is an accepted treatment modality for mismatch repair-deficient tumors; more trials with immunotherapy are underway.

Huang J et al; NCD Global Health Research Group, Association of Pacific Rim Universities. Incidence, risk factors and temporal trends of small intestinal cancer: a global analysis of cancer registries. Gastroenterology. 2023;165:600. [PMID: 37277079]

National Comprehensive Cancer Network. Small Bowel Adenocarcinoma, Version 1.2026, NCCN Clinical Practice Guidelines in Oncology. https://www.nccn.org/professionals/physician_gls/pdf/small_bowel.pdf

2. Small Intestinal Lymphomas

Lymphomas may arise primarily in the GI tract (see Gastric Lymphoma above) or may involve it secondarily in patients with disseminated lymphoma. There is an increased incidence of small intestinal lymphomas in patients with AIDS, Crohn disease, and those receiving immunosuppressive therapy. The most common histologic subtypes are non-Hodgkin extranodal marginal zone (MALT) B-cell lymphomas and diffuse large B-cell lymphomas. However, enteropathy-associated T-cell lymphoma (sometimes associated with celiac disease) appears to be increasing in incidence in the United States. In the Middle East, lymphomas may arise in the setting of immunoproliferative small intestinal disease. Other types of intestinal lymphomas include primary intestinal follicular cell lymphoma, mantle cell lymphoma, post-transplant lymphoproliferative disorder, and Burkitt lymphoma (see Chapter 15).

Presenting symptoms or signs of primary small bowel lymphoma include abdominal pain, weight loss, nausea and vomiting, distention, anemia, and occult blood in the stool. Fevers are unusual. Protein-losing enteropathy may result in hypoalbuminemia. CT enterography helps localize the site of the lesion. Diagnosis requires endoscopic, percutaneous, or laparoscopic biopsy. Imaging and possibly bone marrow biopsy are required to determine stage.

Treatment depends on the tumor histologic subtype and stage of disease (see Chapter 15). If feasible, surgical resection of localized primary intestinal lymphoma may be appropriate. Following resection with negative margins, the role of adjuvant chemotherapy in patients with limited disease (stage IE) is unclear. Locoregional radiation should be considered if surgical margins are positive. Patients with more extensive disease generally are treated according to the tumor histology.

National Comprehensive Cancer Network. B-Cell Lymphomas, Version 3.2026, NCCN Clinical Practice Guidelines in Oncology. https://www.nccn.org/professionals/physician_gls/pdf/b-cell.pdf

3. Small Intestine Sarcoma

Sarcomas constitute approximately 10% of small bowel neoplasms and are commonly found in the jejunum and ileum. Most arise from stromal tumors (GISTs, see Gastrointestinal Mesenchymal Tumors, above); a minority arise from smooth muscle tumors (**leiomyosarcomas**). Common symptoms of small intestine sarcoma include pain, weight loss, bleeding, and perforation. As the lesions tend to enlarge extraluminally, obstruction is rare.

National Comprehensive Cancer Network. Soft Tissue Sarcoma, Version 3.2026 NCCN Clinical Practice Guidelines in Oncology. https://www.nccn.org/professionals/physician_gls/pdf/sarcoma.pdf

COLORECTAL CANCER

ESSENTIALS OF DIAGNOSIS

- Personal or family history of adenomatous or serrated polyps or colorectal cancer (CRC) is an important risk factor.
- Symptoms or signs depend on tumor location.
- Proximal colon: fecal occult blood, anemia.
- Distal colon: change in bowel habits, hematochezia.
- Diagnosis established by colonoscopy with biopsy.

General Considerations

CRC is the second leading cause of death due to malignancy in the United States. CRC will develop in approximately 4.1% of Americans and has a 5-year survival rate of 65%. In 2025 in the United States, there were estimated to be 107,320 new colon cancer cases (54,510 in men, 52,810 in women) and 46,950 new rectal cancer cases (27,950 in men, 19,000 in women), with an estimated 52,900 deaths. Over the last 10 years, CRC incidence has declined by 1.7% per year and mortality by 3.2% per year, which is attributed to population-based CRC screening. The percentage of US adults aged 50–75 years who were up-to-date with recommended CRC screening was 71.8% in 2021.

CRCs are almost all adenocarcinomas, which tend to form bulky exophytic masses or annular constricting lesions. Most are thought to arise from malignant transformation of an **adenomatous polyp** (tubular, tubulovillous, or villous adenoma) or **serrated polyp** (hyperplastic polyp, traditional serrated adenoma, or sessile serrated adenoma). Polyps that are "advanced" (ie, polyps at least 1 cm in size, adenomas with villous features or high-grade dysplasia, or serrated polyps with dysplasia) are associated with a greater risk of cancer.

Approximately 85% of sporadic CRC arise from adenomatous polyps. They have loss of function of one or more tumor suppressor genes (eg, p53, APC, or DCC) due to a combination of spontaneous pathologic variants of one allele combined with chromosomal instability and aneuploidy (abnormal DNA content) that leads to deletion and loss of heterozygosity of the other allele (eg, 5q, 17q, or 18p deletion). Activation of oncogenes such as *KRAS* and *BRAF* is present in a subset of cancers with prognostic and therapeutic implications discussed further below.

Another 10–20% of CRC arise from serrated polyps, most of which have hypermethylation of CpG-rich promoter regions. This leads to inactivation of the DNA mismatch repair (MMR) gene *MLH1*, resulting in microsatellite instability (MSI-high [or MSI-H]) (the presence of a high number of insertions or deletions at repetitive DNA units) and activation of pathogenic variants of the *BRAF* gene. The vast majority of MSI-H tumors are due to loss of a mismatch repair (MMR) protein, which can be assessed by IHC staining. Tumors lacking staining for an MMR protein are referred to as mismatch repair deficient (dMMR). MSI-H/dMMR CRCs are sensitive to immunotherapy. Serrated CRC have distinct clinical and pathologic characteristics, including diploid DNA content, predominance in the proximal colon, poor differentiation, and more favorable prognosis.

Finally, up to 5% of CRC are caused by inherited pathogenic germline variants resulting in **polyposis syndromes (eg, familial adenomatous polyposis)** or **Lynch syndrome**. These conditions are discussed further below and in Chapter 17.

Risk Factors

Several factors increase the risk of developing CRC, including smoking, consumption of red and processed meats, alcohol intake, diabetes mellitus, physical inactivity, obesity, and history of IBD or primary sclerosing cholangitis. However, *75% of all cases occur in people with no known predisposing factors.*

A. Age

The incidence of CRC rises sharply after age 45 years, and 88% of cases occur in persons over the age of 50 years. The median age at diagnosis is 66 years for men and 69 years for women. From the mid-1990s to the 2010s, CRC rates had been increasing in adults ages 20–50 while they decreased in adults over age 50, likely due to CRC screening programs. During the most recent period of analyzed data from 2012–2016, incidence rates have increased by 2.2% annually among those age < 50 years and decreased by 3.3% annually in those age 65 and older. The increase in **early-onset CRC** (younger than 50 years old) is characterized by more distal colon and rectal tumors and is evenly distributed between men and women. Germline variants are identified in approximately 15% of patients with early-onset CRC, of whom half have Lynch syndrome with MMR gene pathogenic variants; thus, 85% of early-onset CRC cases are considered to be sporadic. In the United States, the incidence of early-onset CRC is rising in all racial and ethnic groups. It is highest in Black adults, but the incidence is rising most quickly in non-Hispanic White adults. Epidemiologic studies suggest that the increase in sporadic (nonhereditary) early-onset CRC may be related to dietary changes (increased consumption of refined grains, red meats, and processed sugars), alcohol consumption, changes in the gut microbiome, sedentary lifestyle, obesity, and metabolic syndrome. It is estimated that by 2030, 10% of colon cancers and 20% of rectal cancers will occur in patients under age 50 years.

B. Family History of Neoplasia

A family history of CRC is present in approximately 20% of patients with colon cancer. Hereditary factors are believed to contribute to 20–30% of CRCs; however, the genes responsible for many of these cases have not yet been identified. Hereditary cancer syndromes (Lynch syndrome, polyposis syndromes, and other germline mutations) account for approximately 3–4% of CRC in patients 50 years or older but 15–20% of patients with early-onset CRC (see Chapter 17).

Lynch syndrome is the most common hereditary cancer syndrome responsible for CRC. Lynch syndrome is caused by pathogenic germline variants in one of four DNA mismatch repair genes or by a deletion in the *EPCAM* gene.

Approximately 6% of the Ashkenazi Jewish population has a missense pathologic variant in the *APC* gene *(APC I1307K)* that confers a modestly increased lifetime risk of developing CRC (OR 1.4–1.9) that phenotypically resembles sporadic CRC rather than familial adenomatous polyposis. Genetic screening is available, and patients harboring a variant in the *APC* gene merit more intensive colorectal screening.

A family history of CRC or adenomatous polyps is one of the most important risk factors for CRC. The risk of colon cancer is proportionate to the number and age of affected first-degree family members with colon neoplasia. Individuals with one first-degree family member diagnosed with CRC at age < 60 or two first-degree members diagnosed at any age have up to a 20% lifetime risk of developing CRC. First-degree relatives of patients with adenomatous polyps also have a twofold increased risk for colorectal neoplasia, especially if they were younger than 60 years when the polyp was detected or if the polyp was 10 mm or larger.

C. Inflammatory Bowel Disease

The risk of adenocarcinoma of the colon begins to rise 8 years after disease onset in patients with ulcerative colitis and Crohn colitis (see Chapter 17). For this reason, *initiation of surveillance with colonoscopy is recommended at 8–10 years after onset of IBD symptoms.*

D. Dietary and Lifestyle Factors and Chemoprevention

In epidemiologic studies, diets rich in fats and red meat are associated with an increased risk of colorectal adenomas and cancer, whereas diets high in fruits, vegetables, and fiber are associated with a decreased risk. However, prospective studies have *not* shown a reduction in colon cancer or recurrence of adenomatous polyps with diets that are low in fat; that are high in fiber, fruits, or vegetables; or that include calcium, folate, β-carotene, or vitamin A, C, D, or E supplements.

Meta-analyses suggest that individuals with increased physical activity are up to 27% less likely to develop colon cancer. There also is a correlation between increasing BMI and cancer risk, such that for each increase of 5 in BMI, there is a 5% increased cancer risk. Patients with higher levels of pre- and post-diagnosis physical activity experience reduced CRC-specific mortality and all-cause mortality. Maintaining a healthy body weight, a healthy diet, and a physically active lifestyle are recommended in CRC survivors.

E. Other Factors

The overall incidence of CRC is similar in men and women; however, similar incidence rates are reached in women about 4–6 years later than in men. A higher proportion of cancers are located in the proximal colon in women (46%) than men (37%). The incidence and mortality of colon adenocarcinoma are higher in Black and Native American persons than in White persons. It is unclear whether this is due to genetic or socioeconomic factors (eg, diet or reduced access to medical care).

Clinical Findings

A. Symptoms and Signs

Adenocarcinomas grow slowly and may be present for several years before symptoms appear. Many asymptomatic tumors may be detected by the presence of *fecal occult blood* (see Screening for Colorectal Neoplasms, below). Symptoms depend on the location of the carcinoma. Chronic blood loss from right-sided colonic cancers may cause iron deficiency anemia, manifested by fatigue and weakness. Obstruction, however, is uncommon because of the large diameter of the right colon and the liquid consistency of the fecal material. Lesions of the left colon often involve the bowel circumferentially. Because the left colon has a smaller diameter, and the fecal matter is solid, obstructive symptoms may develop with colicky abdominal pain and a change in bowel habits. Constipation may alternate with periods of increased frequency and loose stools. The stool may be streaked with blood, though marked bleeding is unusual. With rectal cancers, patients note tenesmus, urgency, and recurrent hematochezia. Physical examination is usually normal except in advanced disease. The liver should be examined for hepatomegaly, suggesting metastatic spread. For cancers of the distal rectum, digital examination is necessary to determine whether there is extension into the anal sphincter or fixation, suggesting extension to the pelvic floor.

B. Laboratory Findings

A CBC should be obtained to look for anemia. Elevated liver biochemical tests, particularly the serum alkaline phosphatase, raise suspicion of metastatic disease. The **serum carcinoembryonic antigen (CEA)** should be measured in all patients with proven CRC but is not appropriate for screening. The CEA is not elevated in many patients with confirmed CRC; conversely, the CEA may be elevated in active smokers and those with a variety of other nonmalignant conditions. That said, a preoperative CEA level > 5 ng/mL is a poor prognostic indicator. After complete surgical resection, CEA levels should normalize; persistently elevated levels suggest the presence of persistent disease and warrant further evaluation. CEA is routinely monitored at the time of adjuvant therapy and during postoperative surveillance for patients who had elevated levels before resection.

C. Colonoscopy

Colonoscopy is the required diagnostic procedure in patients with a clinical history suggestive of CRC or in patients with an abnormality suspicious for cancer detected on radiographic imaging. Colonoscopy and upper endoscopy should be considered in all adults with new-onset iron deficiency anemia. Colonoscopy permits biopsy for pathologic confirmation of malignancy. All new diagnoses of CRCs should be evaluated for MMR/MSI status.

D. Imaging

Chest, abdominal, and pelvic CT scans with intravenous contrast are required for preoperative staging of CRC. CT scans may demonstrate distant metastases but are less accurate in the determination of the level of local tumor extension (T stage) or lymphatic spread (N stage). Intraoperative assessment of the liver by direct palpation and ultrasonography can be performed to detect hepatic metastases (M stage). For ***rectal cancers*** (generally defined as tumors arising 12 cm or less proximal to the anal verge), pelvic MRI or endorectal ultrasonography is required to determine the depth of penetration of the cancer through the rectal wall (T stage) and perirectal lymph nodes (N stage), informing decisions about preoperative (neoadjuvant) chemoradiotherapy and operative management.

PET (with or without CT) is *not* routinely used for staging or surveillance since many CRCs are not highly PET avid and liver metastases may be inapparent amid high background liver activity.

Staging

The TNM system is the commonly used classification to stage CRC. Staging correlates with the patient's long-term survival and is used to determine which patients should receive neoadjuvant or adjuvant therapy.

Differential Diagnosis

The nonspecific symptoms of CRC may be confused with those of irritable bowel syndrome, diverticular disease, ischemic colitis, IBD, infectious colitis, and hemorrhoids. Neoplasm must be excluded in any patient who reports a change in bowel habits or hematochezia or who has an unexplained iron deficiency anemia or occult blood in stool samples.

Treatment

A. Colon Cancer

Surgical resection of the colonic tumor is the treatment of choice for almost all patients. Surgery may be curative in patients with stage I, II, and III disease and even some patients with metastatic (stage IV) disease. Multiple studies demonstrate that minimally invasive, laparoscopically assisted colectomy results in similar outcomes and rates of recurrence to open colectomy. Regional dissection of at least 12 lymph nodes should be performed to determine staging, which guides decisions about adjuvant therapy. Following complete endoscopic removal of an adenomatous polyp (polypectomy) that is found on pathologic review to contain a focus of cancer invasion into the submucosa (T1 disease; "malignant polyp"), observation is a reasonable alternative to further surgical resection in carefully selected patients. Pathology review of CRCs should include testing for mismatch repair proteins for all patients. Tumors of patients with metastatic CRC should also be sent for comprehensive molecular profiling to include mutational status of *KRAS, NRAS,* and *BRAF,* as well as *HER2* overexpression.

Following surgical resection, chemotherapy has been demonstrated to improve overall and tumor-free survival in select patients with colon cancer depending on stage (Table 43–2).

1. Stage I—Because of the excellent 5-year survival rate (approximately 92%), no adjuvant therapy is recommended for stage I colon cancer.

2. Stage II (node-negative disease)—The 5-year survival rate is approximately 87% for stage IIA disease and 63% for stage IIB disease. A significant survival benefit from adjuvant chemotherapy has not been demonstrated in most RCTs for stage II colon cancer (see discussion for stage III disease). However, otherwise healthy patients with stage II disease who are at higher risk for recurrence based on clinical or pathologic characteristics (perforation; obstruction; close or indeterminate margins; poorly differentiated histology; lymphatic, vascular, or perineural invasion; T4 tumors; or < 12 lymph nodes sampled) may benefit from adjuvant chemotherapy. Patients with MSI-H/dMMR tumors have a more favorable prognosis and do not benefit from 5-fluorouracil-based adjuvant therapy.

3. Stage III (node-positive disease)—With surgical resection alone, the expected 5-year survival rate is 30–50%. *Postoperative adjuvant chemotherapy significantly increases disease-free survival as well as overall survival by up to 30% and is recommended for all fit patients* (Table 43–2). Multiple large, well-designed studies of adjuvant therapy for stage III CRC have reported a higher rate of disease-free survival at 5 years for patients treated for 6 months postoperatively with a combination of FOLFOX than with 5-fluorouracil and leucovorin alone. Similar benefit was reported for patients treated with CAPOX (oxaliplatin plus capecitabine, an orally active fluoropyrimidine). The International Duration Evaluation of Adjuvant Therapy collaboration pooled data from six clinical trials of adjuvant therapy in patients with stage III colon cancer comparing 3 months with 6 months of adjuvant therapy for colon cancer. This analysis showed that 3 months of adjuvant therapy with CAPOX, but not FOLFOX, was noninferior to a 6-month treatment duration in the entire study cohort. In particular, in lower-risk patients (defined as T1–T3 N1 disease), 3 months of adjuvant therapy appears to be sufficient, whereas for those with high-risk disease (T4 or N2 tumors), 6 months of adjuvant chemotherapy remains the preferred treatment duration.

The addition of a biologic agent (bevacizumab or cetuximab) to adjuvant chemotherapy does not improve outcomes. However, patients with MSI-H/dMMR tumors benefit from the addition of the immune checkpoint inhibitor atezolizumab to standard adjuvant chemotherapy, with an improvement in 3-year disease-free survival rising from 76.6% to 86.4%. Compelling evidence suggests that even an abbreviated course of preoperative immunotherapy alone (nivolumab plus ipilimumab), without chemotherapy, may be an appropriate strategy for this subgroup.

4. Stage IV (metastatic disease)—Approximately 20% of patients have metastatic disease at the time of initial diagnosis, and another 25–30% eventually develop metastases when they recur following resection of earlier-stage disease. In the absence of cancer-directed treatment, the median survival is < 12 months; however, with effective therapy, median survival can be upwards of 30 months.

Moreover, a subset of patients have limited metastatic disease (termed oligometastatic) that is potentially curable with surgical resection. Resection of isolated liver metastases may result in long term (over 5 years) survival in 35–55% of cases. A subset of patients who have isolated pulmonary metastases may also undergo resection (or radiation) with potential cure. One recently published randomized controlled trial demonstrated that chemotherapy followed by liver transplantation could significantly improve survival in select patients with unresectable colorectal liver metastases compared with chemotherapy alone, but this does not represent standard practice. Surgical resection of the primary tumor may also be warranted to provide palliation of tumor bleeding or obstruction but otherwise has not been clearly demonstrated to improve survival in patients with unresectable metastatic disease.

Beyond surgical resection, radiation, and local ablative techniques for limited disease, the primary treatment for unresectable metastatic CRC is systemic therapy (cytotoxic chemotherapy, biologic therapy [eg, antibodies to cellular growth factors], immunotherapy, and combinations of these therapies). The goals of systemic therapy for patients with metastatic CRC are to slow tumor progression while maintaining a reasonable quality of life for as long as possible and, in select instances, to convert patients with initially unresectable metastatic disease to potentially resectable. **Tailoring treatment to the pathologic and molecular features of the cancer is critical.**

Two cytotoxic chemotherapeutic regimens—FOLFOX or FOLFIRI (the addition of irinotecan to 5-fluorouracil and folinic acid)—are the preferred first-line treatments for fit patients. For convenience, oral capecitabine (instead of intravenous 5-fluorouracil and leucovorin) can be used in combination with oxaliplatin since it has similar efficacy to 5-fluorouracil; however, combining capecitabine with irinotecan is less advisable due to increased toxicity (diarrhea).

Addition of biologic therapy to combination chemotherapy improves response rates and overall survival and is recommended in the first line of treatment in suitable patients. Genomic profiling and sidedness (whether the tumor is located in the left or right side of the colon) are used to help guide appropriate treatment decision-making. Multiple studies have shown that for patients with stage IV disease with KRAS/NRAS/BRAF wild-type, left-sided colon cancer, chemotherapy (FOLFOX or FOLFIRI) in combination with either cetuximab or panitumumab produces the best result. Conversely, patients with right-sided tumors, those whose tumors harbor a mutation in KRAS/NRAS/BRAF, or both should receive chemotherapy in combination with bevacizumab, a monoclonal antibody targeting VEGF.

Certain additional molecular subsets also warrant special attention. Approximately 10% of CRCs are *BRAF* mutant, with the most common of these being an activating V600E mutation. *BRAF*-mutated tumors are more commonly located in the right side of the colon and associated with more aggressive biology and poorer prognosis. A recent phase 3 study showed that in this group of patients, the addition of cetuximab plus encorafenib (an oral RAF inhibitor) to standard chemotherapy (FOLFOX) led to improvements in objective response rate, progression-free survival, and overall survival compared with standard treatment (FOLFOX with or without bevacizumab).

For the 3–5% of patients with metastatic MSI or dMMR CRC, immunotherapy alone with either a single (anti-PD1 monoclonal antibody) or doublet immune checkpoint inhibitor combination (anti-PD1 plus anti-CTLA4 monoclonal antibody) represents the preferred frontline therapy, as it has demonstrated improved progression-free survival, more durable responses, and fewer severe adverse events compared with standard chemotherapy.

Patients who show disease progression on first-line treatment should ideally continue with alternate therapy (ie, switch from FOLFOX to FOLFIRI or vice versa), as benefit has been shown for individuals who are exposed to all available cytotoxic therapies (fluoropyrimidine, oxaliplatin, irinotecan) during their disease course. The addition of the anti-VEGF monoclonal antibody ramucirumab to FOLFIRI has been shown to improve progression-free and overall survival (compared with FOLFIRI alone) in the second-line setting for patients previously treated with FOLFOX/bevacizumab.

Importantly, the selection of therapy depends on molecular phenotype and what regimen was used in the frontline setting. Anti-EGFR monoclonal antibodies for Ras wild-type tumors, combined RAF/EGFR inhibition for *BRAF*-mutated tumors, and immune checkpoint inhibitors (pembrolizumab, nivolumab) for MSI-H/dMMR tumors, were all originally tested and approved for use in the context of chemotherapy-pretreated patients (second-line and beyond), so patients who may not have been exposed to these agents in the frontline setting should ideally receive them as part of subsequent therapy unless there is a clear medical contraindication.

Because the list of potentially actionable pathogenic genetic variants continues to grow, extended molecular testing with a next-generation sequencing panel should be considered in all new diagnoses of metastatic CRC. Clinical trial participation should be considered for eligible patients who are intolerant of or ineligible for standard therapies or those in whom disease has progressed.

B. Rectal Cancer

The treatment approach to rectal cancer is guided by clinical staging as determined by colonoscopy and endorectal ultrasound or rectal MRI. In carefully selected patients with small (< 4 cm), mobile, well-differentiated T1 rectal cancers that are < 8 cm from the anal verge, transanal endoscopic or surgical excision may be considered. For rectal cancers that are any more locally advanced than this, surgery requires either a low anterior resection with a colorectal anastomosis or an abdominoperineal resection with a colostomy, depending on how far above the anal verge the cancer is located and the extent of local tumor spread.

The treatment approach for localized and locally advanced rectal cancers differs from that for colon cancers in that preoperative therapy, which historically has included radiation to reduce the risk of local relapse, is typically incorporated within a multimodal treatment plan. A commonly used treatment sequence for node-positive, T3/T4 tumors, or both includes preoperative chemoradiation or short-course radiation followed by surgical resection and then a period of adjuvant chemotherapy afterwards. However, there has been a gradual shift toward total neoadjuvant therapy, in which chemotherapy is moved from the postoperative to the preoperative setting (given either before or after radiation), with encouraging long-term results. Following neoadjuvant therapy, the operative approach (low anterior resection versus abdominoperineal resection with colostomy) depends on how far above the anal verge the cancer is located, its size and depth of penetration, and the patient's overall condition. Careful dissection of the entire mesorectum by either open or laparoscopic surgery reduces local recurrence to 5%. Although low anterior resections obviate a colostomy, they are associated with increased immediate postsurgical complications (eg, leak, dehiscence, stricture) and long-term defecatory complaints (eg, increased stool frequency and incontinence). With unresectable rectal cancer, the patient may be palliated with a diverting colostomy.

Treatment paradigms for rectal cancer continue to evolve. Given the potential acute- and long-term toxicities associated with radiation, studies have shown that it is safe and feasible to avoid radiation in patients with mid to high rectal cancers who exhibit a favorable clinical response to induction chemotherapy. Furthermore, select patients who achieve a complete clinical response to total neoadjuvant therapy may be candidates for nonoperative management, with close surveillance by endoscopy and cross-sectional imaging to ensure no local regrowth (or metastatic dissemination). Patients wishing to pursue this organ-preserving approach should be counseled on the potential for recurrence and the necessity of close follow-up. Finally, exciting data suggests that immunotherapy alone, without subsequent radiation or surgery, can produce durable complete responses in patients with locally advanced MSI-H/dMMR rectal cancer.

The treatment of metastatic rectal cancer parallels that for colon cancer, which was previously discussed.

Follow-Up After Surgery

Patients with CRC who have undergone resections for cure are monitored closely to look for evidence of symptomatic or asymptomatic tumor recurrence that may occasionally be amenable to curative resection. Patients should be evaluated every 3–6 months for 2 years and then every 6 months for a total of 5 years with history, physical examination, and laboratory surveillance, including serum CEA levels if baseline levels are elevated. The NCCN and American Society of Clinical Oncology guidelines recommend surveillance contrast CT scans of chest, abdomen, and pelvis up to every 6–12 months for up to 5 years post-resection in high-risk stage II and all stage III patients. Patients who had a complete preoperative colonoscopy should undergo another colonoscopy 1 year after surgical resection. Patients who did not undergo full colonoscopy preoperatively should undergo a full colonoscopy after completion of all adjuvant therapy to exclude other synchronous colorectal neoplasms. If a colonoscopy does not detect new adenomatous polyps 1 year postoperatively, surveillance colonoscopy should be performed every 3–5 years thereafter to look for metachronous polyps or cancer. Most CRC recurrences occur within 3 years of the conclusion of treatment, and almost all (> 90%) occur within 5 years.

Prognosis

The stage of disease at presentation remains the most important determinant of 5-year survival in CRC, which is estimated in older registries as: stage I, > 90%; stage II, 70–85%; stage III with fewer than four positive lymph nodes, 67%; stage III with more than four positive lymph nodes, 33%; and stage IV, 5–7%. Long-term registry follow-up data from the modern chemotherapy era are not yet available. For each stage, rectal cancers have a worse prognosis compared with colon cancers. For those patients whose disease progresses despite therapy, meticulous efforts at palliative care are essential (see Chapter 5).

Screening for Colorectal Neoplasms

CRC is ideal for screening because it is a common disease that is fatal in almost 50% of cases and yet is curable if detected at an earlier stage. Furthermore, *most cases arise from benign adenomatous or serrated polyps that progress over many years to cancer, and removal of these polyps has been shown to prevent the majority of cancers.* CRC screening is endorsed by the USPSTF, the ACS, the NCCN, and every professional gastroenterology and colorectal surgery society. Although there is continued debate about the optimal cost-effective means of providing population screening, there is now almost unanimous consent that screening of some kind should be offered to all adults ages 45–75 years. The 2018 ACS and 2021 USPSTF recommendations for screening are listed in Table 43–12. *Due to a rising incidence of CRC in adults younger than 50 years, the 2021 American College of Gastroenterology (ACG), 2021 USPSTF, 2018 ACS, and 2022 US Multi-society Task Force guidelines all endorse consideration of screening in asymptomatic, average-risk adults beginning at age 45 years, and at younger ages for high-risk adults (such as those with a history of IBD or primary sclerosing cholangitis, or those with a family history of a first-degree relative with colorectal neoplasia [*Table 43–12*]).*

The potential for harm from screening must be weighed against the likelihood of benefit, especially in older patients with comorbid illnesses and shorter life expectancy. Although routine screening is not recommended in adults above age 75 years, it may be considered on a case-by-case basis in adults aged 76–85 years, taking into account the patient's overall health and functional status and their prior screening history.

Patients with first-degree relatives with colorectal neoplasms (cancer or adenomatous polyps) are at increased risk. Therefore, most guidelines recommend initiating screening at age 40–50 years (or 10 years younger than the familial diagnosis) in individuals with first-degree relatives with CRC or with advanced adenomas. Recommendations for screening in families with inherited cancer syndromes or IBD are provided in Chapter 17.

Table 43–12. Recommendations for colorectal cancer screening,[1] based on 2021 USPSTF and 2018 American Cancer Society recommendations.[2]

Average-risk individuals aged ≥ 45 years[2]
Annual fecal occult blood testing using higher sensitivity tests (Hemoccult SENSA)
Annual fecal immunochemical test (FIT)
Fecal DNA test (with FIT every 1–3 years)
Flexible sigmoidoscopy every 5 years
Colonoscopy every 10 years
CT colonography every 5 years
Individuals with a family history of a first-degree relative with colorectal neoplasia
Single first-degree relative with colorectal cancer diagnosed at age 60 years or older: Begin screening at age 40 years. Screening guidelines same as average-risk individual; however, preferred method is colonoscopy every 10 years.
Single first-degree relative with colorectal cancer or advanced adenoma diagnosed before age 60 years, or two first-degree relatives: Begin screening at age 40 years or at age 10 years younger than age at diagnosis of the youngest affected relative, whichever is first in time. Recommended screening: colonoscopy every 5 years.

[1]For recommendations for families with inherited polyposis syndromes or hereditary nonpolyposis colon cancer, see Chapter 17.
[2]The USPSTF and American Cancer Society recommend screening of average-risk adults aged 45–75 years and screening of selected patients aged 76–85 years based on overall health, life expectancy, patient preferences, and prior screening results.

Screening tests may be classified into two broad categories: *stool-based tests* and *examinations that visualize the structure of the colon* by direct endoscopic inspection or radiographic imaging. The advantages and disadvantages of available tests are summarized below and should be discussed with patients prior to study selection. The US Multi-society Task Force and the 2021 ACG guidelines endorse the fecal immunochemical testing (FIT) and colonoscopy as the preferred stool-based and imaging-based screening modalities, respectively. However, the "best" test may be that which the patient agrees to do and then completes. Compliance with recommended testing can be increased significantly using a combination of automated reminders and personal outreach by health care providers.

A. Stool-Based Tests

1. Fecal occult blood test—Most CRCs and some large adenomas result in increased chronic blood loss. A variety of tests for fecal occult blood are commercially available that have varying sensitivities and specificities for colorectal neoplasia. These include *guaiac-based fecal occult blood testing* (***gFOBT***) (eg, Hemoccult SENSA) that detects the pseudoperoxidase activity of heme or hemoglobin and *testing that detects human globin* (***FIT***). In clinical trials, *FIT has proven superior to gFOBT in sensitivity for detection of CRC and advanced adenomas with similar specificity.*

Because FIT is not affected by diet or medications and has superior accuracy, its use is preferred by many health care plans instead of gFOBT. FIT is also a suitable option for patients seeking a noninvasive screening test who are willing to undertake annual fecal testing. *Patients with a positive FIT test must undergo further evaluation with colonoscopy.* In 14 clinical studies (n = 45,403), the pooled sensitivity and specificity of FIT for CRC in average-risk patients were 74% and 94%, respectively. FIT testing is also the preferred option for population-based screening in various European and Australian programs. For optimal neoplasia detection, FIT testing should be performed annually.

2. Multitarget stool DNA assay—*Stool DNA panel testing* measures gene variants and methylated gene markers from exfoliated tumor cells. Multitarget stool DNA testing (**mt-sDNA**) combines a fecal DNA panel with a FIT. In the United States, two commercially available mt-sDNA test (Cologuard and Cologuard Plus) are approved for colorectal screening in average-risk persons. Compared with other tests, the mt-sDNA tests are more expensive and require collection, preparation, and mailing of an entire stool specimen.

In a prospective comparative trial conducted in persons at average risk for CRC undergoing colonoscopy, the sensitivity for CRC for Cologuard was 92.3% versus 73.8% for FIT alone and the sensitivity for adenomas larger than 1 cm or serrated polyps for Cologuard was 42.4% versus 23.8% for FIT alone. Repeat testing is recommended in 3 years for persons with a negative test. A positive stool DNA panel test requires colonoscopy evaluation.

In 2024, the FDA approved a "next-generation" multitarget stool DNA test (Cologuard Plus) for patients at average risk for CRC. In a randomized prospective study of asymptomatic adults undergoing colonoscopy, the next-generation test had higher sensitivity than FIT for CRC (93.9% versus 67.3%) and advanced precancerous lesions (43.4% versus 23.3%) but lower specificity for advanced precancerous lesions (90.6% versus 94.8%).

B. Endoscopic Examinations of the Colon

1. Colonoscopy—Colonoscopy permits examination of the entire colon. In addition to detecting early cancers, colonoscopy allows removal of adenomatous polyps by biopsy or polypectomy, which is believed to reduce the risk of subsequent cancer. Over the past decade, there has been a dramatic increase in screening colonoscopy, with *over 60% of US adults screened in the past 10 years.* In asymptomatic individuals between 50 and 75 years of age undergoing screening colonoscopy, the prevalence of advanced colonic neoplasia is 4–11% and of colon cancer is 0.1–1%.

Although colonoscopy is believed to be the most sensitive test for detecting adenomas and cancer, it has several disadvantages. Adequate visualization of the entire colonic mucosa requires thorough bowel cleansing the evening and morning prior to the examination. To alleviate discomfort during the procedure, intravenous sedation is used for most patients, necessitating a companion to transport the patient home post-procedure. Serious complications occur uncommonly; they include perforation (0.1%), bleeding (0.25%), and death (2.9/100,000).

The skill of the operator has a major impact upon the quality of the colonoscopy examination. In several studies, the rate of CRC within 3 years of a screening colonoscopy was 0.7–0.9%, ie, approximately 1 in 110 patients. Population-based case-control and cohort studies suggest that colonoscopy is associated with greater reduction in CRC incidence and mortality in the distal colon (80%) than the proximal colon (40–60%). This may be attributable to incomplete examination of the proximal colon, and differences between the proximal and distal colon that include worse bowel preparation, suboptimal colonoscopic technique, and a higher prevalence of serrated polyps and flat adenomas, which are more difficult to identify than raised (sessile or pedunculated) polyps. To optimize diagnostic accuracy as well as patient safety and comfort, colonoscopy should be performed after optimal bowel preparation by a well-trained endoscopist who spends sufficient time (at least 7–9 minutes) carefully examining the colon (especially the proximal colon) while withdrawing the endoscope.

2. Flexible sigmoidoscopy—Use of a 60-cm flexible sigmoidoscope permits visualization of the rectosigmoid and descending colon. Patients with an adenomatous polyp of any size found during screening sigmoidoscopy should subsequently undergo colonoscopy to evaluate the proximal colon. In four RCTs, intention to screen with 1- or 2-time flexible sigmoidoscopy versus no screening was associated with a significant decrease in CRC-specific mortality.

The chief disadvantage of screening with flexible sigmoidoscopy is that it requires some bowel cleansing, it may be associated with some discomfort (since intravenous sedation is not used), and it does not examine the proximal colon. The prevalence of proximal versus distal neoplasia is higher in persons older than age 65 years, in Black adults, and in women.

C. Radiographic and Other Imaging of the Colon

1. CT colonography—CT colonography requires a similar bowel cleansing regimen as colonoscopy as well as insufflation of air into the colon through a rectal tube, which may be associated with discomfort.

Using imaging software with multidetector helical scanners, the sensitivity is > 95% for the detection of cancer and 86% for the detection of adenomatous polyps 6 mm or larger. CT colonography is less sensitive than colonoscopy for the detection of flat adenomas and serrated polyps.

The chief disadvantages of CT colonography are the need for a bowel preparation, limited availability in many health care systems, potential harms resulting from (repeated) low-dose ionizing radiation exposure, and the potential for finding incidental extracolonic findings that may lead to further evaluations. *CT colonography is an excellent screening option in patients who do not wish to undergo or are unsuitable for colonoscopy and in patients in whom colonoscopy could not be completed.*

2. Capsule colonoscopy—Imaging of the colon can be accomplished by oral ingestion of a capsule that captures video images of the colon. Compared with colonoscopy, the colon capsule has reduced sensitivity for polyps > 6 mm (64% versus 84%) and for CRCs (74% versus 100%). At present, it is approved by the FDA for evaluation in patients who are not suitable candidates for colonoscopy or in whom colonoscopy could not evaluate the proximal colon. In addition to its suboptimal sensitivity for neoplasia, the main disadvantages of capsule colonoscopy are its cost, need for extensive bowel preparation, varying reimbursement by insurance carriers, and small risk of small bowel obstruction.

When to Refer

- Patients with symptoms (change in bowel habits, hematochezia), signs (mass on abdominal examination or digital rectal examination [DRE]), or laboratory tests (iron deficiency anemia) suggestive of colorectal neoplasia should be referred for colonoscopy.
- Patients with suspected CRC or adenomatous polyps of any size should be referred for colonoscopy.
- Virtually all patients with proven CRC should be referred to a surgeon for resection. Patients with clinical stage T3 or node-positive rectal tumors (or both) also should be referred to medical and radiation oncologists preoperatively for neoadjuvant therapy. Patients with stage II, III, or IV colorectal tumors should be referred to a medical oncologist.

When to Admit

- Patients with complications of CRC (eg, obstruction, acute bleeding) requiring urgent evaluation and intervention.
- Patients with advanced metastatic disease requiring palliative care.

Adam R et al; Collaborative TransMet group. Liver transplantation plus chemotherapy versus chemotherapy alone in patients with permanently unresectable colorectal liver metastases (TransMet): results from a multicentre, open-label, prospective, randomised controlled trial. Lancet. 2024;404:1107. [PMID: 39306468]

Amatu A et al. Total neoadjuvant therapy followed by non-operative management or surgery in stage II-III rectal cancer (NO-CUT): a multicentre, single-arm, phase 2 trial. Lancet Oncol. 2025;26:1612. [PMID: 41308677]

Andre T et al; CheckMate 8HW Investigators. Nivolumab plus ipilimumab in microsatellite-instability-high metastatic colorectal cancer. N Engl J Med. 2024;391:2014. [PMID: 39602630]

Burke CA et al. AGA clinical practice update on approach to the use of noninvasive colorectal screening options: commentary. Gastroenterology. 2022;162:952. [PMID: 35094786]

Chalabi M et al. Neoadjuvant immunotherapy in locally advanced mismatch repair-deficient colon cancer. N Engl J Med. 2024;390:1949. [PMID: 38838311]

Courneya KS et al; CHALLENGE Investigators. Structured exercise after adjuvant chemotherapy for colon cancer. N Engl J Med. 2025;393:13. [PMID: 40450658]

Elez E et al; BREAKWATER Trial Investigators. Encorafenib, cetuximab, and mFOLFOX6 in *BRAF*-mutated colorectal cancer. N Engl J Med. 2025;392:2425. [PMID: 40444708]

Imperiale TF et al. Next-generation multitarget stool DNA test for colorectal cancer screening. N Engl J Med. 2024;390:984. [PMID: 38477986]

Issaka RB et al. AGA Clinical Practice update on risk stratification for colorectal cancer screening and post-polypectomy surveillance: expert review. Gastroenterology. 2023;165:1280. [PMID: 37737817]

National Comprehensive Cancer Network. Colon Cancer, Version 1.2026, NCCN Clinical Practice Guidelines in Oncology. https://www.nccn.org/professionals/physician_gls/pdf/colon.pdf

National Comprehensive Cancer Network. Rectal Cancer, Version 1.2026, NCCN Clinical Practice Guidelines in Oncology. https://www.nccn.org/professionals/physician_gls/pdf/rectal.pdf

Rahbari NN et al; SYNCHRONOUS and CCRe-IV Trial Groups. Primary tumor resection before systemic therapy in patients with colon cancer and unresectable metastases: combined results of the SYNCHRONOUS and CCRe-IV trials. J Clin Oncol. 2024;42:1531. [PMID: 38412408]

Sinicrope FA. Increasing incidence of early-onset colorectal cancer. N Engl J Med. 2022;386:1547. [PMID: 35443109]

CARCINOMA OF THE ANUS

Cancers arising from the mucosa of the anal canal are relatively rare, comprising only 2% of all GI malignancies. However, the incidence is increasing by about 2.7% per year. Anal carcinoma occurred in approximately 10,930 patients in the United States in 2025, more commonly in women than men (2:1 ratio). *Squamous cell carcinomas* (SCC) make up the majority of anal cancers; *adenocarcinomas* are relatively uncommon.

Over 90% of anal cancers are associated with HPV infections (most commonly, HPV-16 and -18). Anal cancer is increased among women with HPV-associated cervical, vulvar, or vaginal squamous intraepithelial lesions (CIN grade 3) or cancer, among men who are having sex with men, and among women and men who have HIV or have received a solid organ transplant.

Identification and screening of high-risk individuals with HPV testing and anal cytology facilitate detection of anal low- and high-grade squamous intraepithelial lesions (LSIL and HSIL, respectively) and early-stage cancers. Anoscopy (preferably high-resolution) with biopsy is warranted in patients with positive cytology. Early detection and treatment of HSIL with either topical treatment or surgical ablation may reduce progression to advanced cancer. In a 2022 phase 3 RCT of HIV-infected patients with anal HSIL, treatment with office ablation, excision, or topical therapies resulted in a lowering of progression to anal cancer at 48 months by 57% compared with those actively monitored without treatment.

The most common symptoms of anal carcinoma are bleeding, pain, and a palpable local mass. The lesion is often confused with hemorrhoids or other common anal disorders. These tumors tend to become annular, invade the sphincter, and spread upward via the lymphatics into the perirectal mesenteric lymphatic nodes. CT or MRI scans of the abdomen and pelvis and chest CT are required to identify regional lymphadenopathy or metastatic disease at diagnosis; PET imaging may be used in conjunction.

Treatment depends on the tumor location, histology, and stage. Well-differentiated and small (< 2 cm) superficial lesions of the perianal skin may be treated with wide local excision. The more common squamous cell carcinoma of the anal canal, as well as large perianal tumors invading the sphincter or rectum, are treated with combined-modality therapy consisting of external radiation with concurrent chemotherapy (5-fluorouracil or capecitabine plus mitomycin). Local control is achieved in approximately 80% of patients. Radical surgery (abdominoperineal resection) is reserved for patients whose disease recurs or persists following chemoradiation therapy.

The 5-year survival rate is 81% for localized anal cancer and 30% for metastatic disease. The combination of carboplatin and paclitaxel is the most commonly used regimen for the first-line treatment of metastatic anal squamous cell carcinoma, with the addition of retifanlimab (an immune checkpoint inhibitor) approved by the FDA in 2025. Checkpoint inhibitor therapy should be strongly considered in the second-line setting in all patients with good performance status who did not previously receive immunotherapy.

Treatment of anal adenocarcinoma is like that of rectal adenocarcinoma (previously mentioned), typically by trimodality therapy, including chemoradiotherapy, chemotherapy, and abdominoperineal resection.

National Cancer Institute. SEER cancer stat facts: anal cancer. https://seer.cancer.gov/statfacts/html/anus.html

National Comprehensive Cancer Network. Anal Carcinoma, Version 1.2026, NCCN Clinical Practice Guidelines in Oncology. https://www.nccn.org/professionals/physician_gls/pdf/anal.pdf

Palefsky JM et al; ANCHOR Investigators Group. Treatment of anal high-grade squamous intraepithelial lesions to prevent anal cancer. N Engl J Med. 2022;386:2273. [PMID: 35704479]

GASTROENTEROPANCREATIC NEUROENDOCRINE TUMORS (GEP-NETS)

ESSENTIALS OF DIAGNOSIS

- GEP-NETs are neuroendocrine tumors that originate in the GI tract, lungs, or pancreas.
- About 60% of GEP-NETs are nonsecretory or secretory without clinical manifestations; they may be detected incidentally or may present with weight loss, abdominal pain, or jaundice.
- Functioning pancreatic NETs (islet cell tumors) may secrete insulin, glucagon, gastrin, somatostatin, cholecystokinin, or vasoactive intestinal polypeptide (VIP).
- Gastrointestinal NETs (also called "carcinoids") may arise from the esophagus, stomach, small intestine, colon, or lungs; functioning NETs may secrete serotonin or gastrin.

General Considerations

Gastroenteropancreatic neuroendocrine tumors (GEP-NETs) occur in the gastrointestinal tract (65%), lungs (20%), or pancreas (15%). About 20% of cases present with metastases with unknown primary location. According to the 2022 WHO pathology classification system, GEP-NET are divided into **well-differentiated neuroendocrine tumors (NETs)** and **poorly differentiated neuroendocrine carcinomas (NECs)**. NETs can be grade 1, 2, or

3 based on proliferative index, while NECs are by definition all high-grade. *The treatment of NETs is entirely different than the treatment of NECs.* The reported incidence of GEP-NETs is about 37 per million annually in the United States. About 40% are functional, producing hormones that may cause symptoms and also serve as tumor markers for diagnosis and follow-up. At presentation, 65% of GEP-NETs are unresectable or metastatic. Up to 25% of GEP-NETs are associated with one of four different inherited disorders: multiple endocrine neoplasia type 1 (MEN1), Von Hippel-Lindau (VHL), neurofibromatosis type 1, and tuberous sclerosis complex. In MEN1, GEP-NETs are usually gastrinomas, carcinoids, or nonfunctioning tumors and are a common cause of morbidity and mortality. In VHL, GEP-NETs are usually multicentric and benign.

1. Gastrointestinal tract NETs (GI-NETs)—Frequently called "carcinoids," GI-NETs occur most commonly in the small intestine (45%), rectum (20%), appendix (17%), colon (11%), and stomach (< 10%). GI-NETs may secrete serotonin, gastrin, or substance P, although well-differentiated GI-NETs may not secrete any of these. Gastrin-secreting NETs (**gastrinomas**) are discussed further in Chapter 17 (see **Zollinger-Ellison syndrome**). *Additionally, most GI-NETs express somatostatin receptors on their cell surface, which aids in diagnostic imaging studies.* Multiple carcinoids are observed in about 28% of cases. Although tumors are usually indolent, metastatic spread, particularly to the liver, lymph nodes, and peritoneum, can occur.

Gastric NETs (gNETs) make up < 1% of gastric neoplasms. They may occur sporadically or secondary to chronic hypergastrinemia that results in hyperplasia and transformation of enterochromaffin cells in the gastric fundus. They are classified into three types. **Type 1 gNETs** are associated with chronic atrophic gastritis, gastric achlorhydria, and consequent secondary hypergastrinemia. **Type 2 gNETs** are associated with Zollinger-Ellison syndrome caused by a gastrin-secreting NET (gastrinoma) most commonly located in the pancreas or duodenum. Although 75% of gastrinomas are sporadic, gNETs caused by gastrinomas occur almost exclusively in patients with MEN1. **Type 3 gNETs** are most often solitary and larger than 2 cm. They have a strong propensity for hepatic or pulmonary metastases and may be associated with carcinoid syndrome at initial presentation.

Small intestinal NETs most commonly arise in the distal ileum within 60 cm of the ileocecal valve. Jejunal-ileal NETs are the second most frequent location. The risk of metastatic spread increases with increased tumor size and with invasion beyond the muscularis propria.

Appendiceal NETs are identified in 0.3% of appendectomies, usually as an incidental finding. Almost 80% of these tumors are smaller than 1 cm, and 90% are smaller than 2 cm. However, in patients with appendiceal NETs larger than 2 cm, approximately 90% develop nodal and distant metastases; therefore, right hemicolectomy is recommended in these cases.

Rectal NETs are usually detected incidentally as submucosal nodules during proctoscopic examination and often locally excised by biopsy or snare polypectomy before the histologic diagnosis is known. Rectal NETs smaller than 1 cm virtually never metastasize and are treated effectively with local endoscopic or transanal excision. Larger tumors are associated with the development of metastasis in 10% of patients. Hence, a more extensive cancer resection operation is warranted in otherwise healthy patients with rectal NETs larger than 1–2 cm, with high-risk features (such as invasion of muscularis propria or evidence of nodal involvement), or both.

2. Pancreatic NETs (pNETs)—Well-differentiated pancreatic NETs (pNETs) arise from islet cells and may (but often do not) secrete a variety of hormones, including gastrin, insulin, glucagon, somatostatin, and VIP. Nonfunctional pNETs produce no significant hormones but may secrete CgA or pancreatic polypeptide, which can be used as tumor markers.

Insulinomas are the most common functional type of pNET and are usually small, intrapancreatic, and benign (90%). Insulinomas are solitary in 95% of sporadic cases but are multiple in about 90% of cases arising in MEN 1 (see Chapter 28).

Gastrinomas are often malignant (about 50%) and metastasize to the liver. Sporadic gastrinoma is rarely suspected at the onset of symptoms; typically, there is an average of a 5-year delay in diagnosis. About 22% of gastrinomas arise in patients with MEN 1, who usually present at a younger age, often with multiple tumors; hyperparathyroidism can occur many years before or after the discovery of a gastrinoma (see Chapter 17, Zollinger-Ellison syndrome).

Glucagonomas are rare and usually malignant, despite their benign histologic appearance. They usually arise as a large intrapancreatic tumor with 60% having liver metastases apparent by the time of diagnosis. Besides glucagon, they usually secrete additional hormones, including gastrin.

Somatostatinomas are very rare and usually single. They arise in the pancreas (50%) or small intestine. They secrete somatostatin.

VIPomas are quite rare and are usually a single intrapancreatic tumor with metastases usually evident (80%) at diagnosis.

Cholecystokinin-producing tumors (CCKomas) are rare tumors of the endocrine pancreas.

Clinical Findings

A. Symptoms and Signs

Most **GI-NETs** < 1–2 cm are asymptomatic and can be difficult to detect by endoscopy or imaging studies or are found incidentally during workup for some other condition. Symptomatic GI-NETs may present with abdominal pain, weight loss, intestinal obstruction, intestinal bleeding, bowel infarction, or jaundice due to hepatic metastases.

Carcinoid syndrome, *which occurs in < 10% of patients with GI-NETs, is caused by tumor secretion of hormonal mediators, including serotonin.* Manifestations include facial flushing, abdominal cramps and diarrhea, bronchospasm, cardiac lesions (pulmonary or tricuspid stenosis or regurgitation in 10–30%), and telangiectasias. Dry skin and flushing typically affect the upper chest, neck, and face and can last from 30 seconds to 30 minutes, although flushing with bronchial carcinoids can persist for days. Flushing can be unprovoked or precipitated by exercise, anesthesia, emotional stimuli, or certain foods (eg, bananas, tomatoes, cheese, kiwi, eggplant, and alcohol). Tumor-induced fibrosis can also occur in the retroperitoneum, causing ureteral obstruction or Peyronie disease. Pellagra (glossitis, confusion, dry skin) from niacin deficiency may occur in patients with a heavy tumor burden. *More than 90% of patients with carcinoid syndrome have hepatic metastases, usually from NETs of small bowel origin.*

Foregut carcinoids secrete serotonin that is hepatically metabolized and therefore produce carcinoid syndrome only when they have metastasized to the liver. Ileal carcinoids often present with intestinal obstruction or intestinal bleeding. Hindgut carcinoids rarely produce serotonin and thus are not often associated with carcinoid syndrome. Bronchial carcinoids secrete serotonin and can produce carcinoid syndrome even in the absence of hepatic metastases.

Pancreatic pNETs may present with symptoms caused by local growth of the pancreatic tumor or hepatic metastases, including abdominal pain, vomiting, upper GI obstruction, jaundice, or hepatomegaly. Functioning pNETs may produce symptoms due to the hormones secreted. Insulinomas may present with symptoms of fasting hypoglycemia (see Chapter 29). Gastrinomas may be asymptomatic but usually present with manifestations of gastric acid hypersecretion (Zollinger-Ellison syndrome), including peptic ulcer disease and esophagitis. Symptoms include abdominal pain (75%), heartburn (44%), bleeding (25%), diarrhea, and weight loss (17%). (See Zollinger-Ellison syndrome in Chapter 17.)

Glucagonomas usually present with weight loss caused by glucagon-stimulated protein hepatic gluconeogenesis and related protein catabolism. Other common manifestations include diarrhea, nausea, peptic ulcers, hypoaminoacidemia, or necrolytic migratory erythema, known as "glucagonoma syndrome." Diabetes mellitus develops in about 35% of patients.

Somatostatinomas can present with a classic symptom triad: diabetes mellitus due to its inhibition of insulin and glucagon secretion, cholelithiasis due to its inhibition of gallbladder motility, and steatorrhea due to inhibition of pancreatic exocrine function. Diarrhea, hypochlorhydria, and anemia can also be seen.

VIPomas present with profuse unremitting *w*atery *d*iarrhea, *h*ypokalemia, and *a*chlorhydria ("WDHA"), the so-called *Verner-Morrison syndrome*.

CCKomas may present with liver metastases and symptoms of diarrhea, peptic ulcer disease, and weight loss.

B. Laboratory Findings

Serum chromogranin A is elevated in most NETs. Although its sensitivity for small, localized tumors is unknown, serum chromogranin A is elevated in almost 90% of patients with advanced small bowel NETs. However, an elevated chromogranin A level by itself is not diagnostic for a NET, as a variety of common medications, including PPIs, can cause falsely elevated serum levels. Although it is less sensitive than serum chromogranin A, the urinary 5-hydroxyindoleacetic acid (5-HIAA) level is also elevated in patients with metastatic GI-NETs and in carcinoid syndrome (symptomatic patients usually excrete > 25 mg of 5-HIAA per day in the urine). Because certain foods and medications can interfere with 5-HIAA levels, they should be withheld for 48 hours before the 24-hour urine collection.

For gNETs, initial diagnostic workup includes serum gastrin level (to distinguish types 1 and 2 from type 3), CBC, serum vitamin B_{12} level, and intrinsic factor antibody to diagnose pernicious anemia. For pancreatic NETs, functioning NETs are defined by the hormone secreted: insulinomas produce insulin, proinsulin, and C-peptide; gastrinomas secrete gastrin and CgA; glucagonomas secrete glucagon and other hormones, including gastrin; and CCKomas produce elevated serum levels of cholecystokinin and CgA.

C. Imaging

For gNETs, initial staging includes upper endoscopy and EUS. For other GI-NETs, abdominal CT or MRI may demonstrate a mesenteric mass with tethering of the bowel, lymphadenopathy, and hepatic metastasis. Most patients with carcinoid syndrome have liver metastasis on abdominal imaging. *Localization of other GEP-NETs and their metastases is best done with PET scanning using* ^{68}*Ga-DOTATATE, a radiolabeled somatostatin analog.* For localization of pancreatic insulinomas, preoperative localization studies have the following sensitivities: ultrasonography 25%, CT 25%, endoscopic ultrasonography 27%, transhepatic portal vein sampling 40%, and arteriography 45%. Nearly all insulinomas can be successfully located at surgery by the combination of intraoperative palpation (sensitivity 55%) and ultrasound (sensitivity 75%), together with ^{68}Ga-DOTATATE-PET (sensitivity 90%).

Treatment

For types 1 and 2 gNETs, small lesions may be successfully treated with endoscopic resection followed by endoscopic surveillance. Patients with tumors > 2 cm with high-grade histology should undergo surgical resection (see Small Intestinal Adenocarcinomas section). Type 2 gNETs with underlying gastrinoma and Zollinger-Ellison syndrome may be treated with *somatostatin analog (octreotide) therapy*. Localized sporadic type 3 gNETs should be treated with partial or total gastrectomy and regional lymphadenectomy.

Surgery is the primary initial treatment for most other GEP-NETs and is a reasonable option even for patients with stage IV disease. The aggressiveness of the surgery may vary from conservative debulking to radical resection and even liver transplantation. However, incidentally discovered nonfunctioning pNETs that are asymptomatic and smaller than 2 cm often can be monitored without surgery. Small intestinal carcinoids generally are indolent tumors with slow spread. There is no proven role for adjuvant therapy after complete resection. Five-year survival rates for patients with stage I and II disease are 96% and 87%, respectively. In patients with resectable disease who have lymph node involvement (stage III), the 5-year survival rate is 74%; however, by 25 years, < 25% remain disease-free. EUS-guided radiofrequency ablation is effective for most patients with pNETs up to 3 cm, even in those with multiple tumors.

Across stages, prognosis is strongly associated with histologic differentiation and grade. Patients with grade 1 disease may not require treatment for many years, even with metastatic disease. However, patients with grade 3 NETs may have a clinical course more like a NEC.

In patients with advanced disease, the decision to initiate therapy should be based on symptoms, burden of disease, rate of disease progression, and patient preference. Conventional cytotoxic chemotherapy agents do not achieve significant responses in NETs and have not been associated with improved outcomes. Tumor visualization of GEP-NETs on ^{64}Cu- or ^{68}Ga-DOTATATE-PET/CT imaging indicates that they may respond to long-acting preparations of somatostatin analogs, including octreotide (Sandostatin LAR Depot) and lanreotide. These agents, which inhibit hormone secretion from the tumor and can arrest tumor growth, represent the cornerstone of therapy for patients who are symptomatic from tumor bulk or carcinoid syndrome. In 90% of patients, this results in dramatic relief of carcinoid syndrome symptoms and may control tumor growth for a median of 1 year. Options at disease progression include octreotide dose escalation or the addition of oral agents such as everolimus (an mTOR inhibitor) or sunitinib (an anti-VEGF inhibitor). For patients with somatostatin receptor–positive disease on imaging, another option after progression is treatment with peptide receptor radionuclide therapy, which consists of a somatostatin analog conjugated to a radioactive isotope such as yttrium-90 or lutetium-177. In select patients with hepatic-dominant disease, resection of hepatic metastases or tumor debulking by liver-directed chemoembolization or radioembolization may provide longer-term disease control as well as dramatic improvement of carcinoid syndrome symptoms.

Patients with advanced, poorly differentiated intestinal NECs are treated in a similar fashion to those with small cell carcinomas. They have a poorer prognosis compared with NETs.

Prognosis

The prognosis for patients with GEP-NETs is variable, depending on the tumor grade and stage. Patients with well- or moderately well-differentiated GEP-NETs have a dramatically better survival than those with poorly differentiated tumors, with a median overall survival of 16.8 years across all stages of well-differentiated NETs. Primary anatomic location also affects prognosis, with rectal and appendiceal NETs having the longest median overall survival and pancreatic NETs having the shortest. Patients with localized NETs have an excellent prognosis, with an expected longevity of 1.5 to 3-plus decades depending on anatomic location; even patients with metastatic well-differentiated NETs have a median survival of > 6.5 years. In contrast, patients with poorly differentiated NETs have a median overall survival of < 1 year.

Chen Q et al. Impact of primary tumor resection and metastasectomy among gastroentero-pancreatic neuroendocrine tumors with liver metastases only on survival. HPB (Oxford). 2024;26:125. [PMID: 37806829]

Dasari A et al. Epidemiology of neuroendocrine neoplasms in the US. JAMA Netw Open. 2025;8:e2515798. Erratum in: JAMA Netw Open. 2025;8:e2547077. [PMID: 40553474]

Fernandes CJ et al. Gastroenteropancreatic neuroendocrine tumors. Gastroenterol Clin North Am. 2022;51:625. [PMID: 36153114]

Hofland J et al. European Neuroendocrine Tumor Society 2023 guidance paper for functioning pancreatic neuroendocrine tumour syndromes. J Neuroendocrinol. 2023;35:e13318. [PMID: 37578384]

CANCERS OF THE GENITOURINARY TRACT

PROSTATE CANCER

ESSENTIALS OF DIAGNOSIS

- Prostatic induration on DRE or elevation of PSA.
- Most often asymptomatic.
- Rarely: systemic symptoms (weight loss, bone pain).

General Considerations

Prostate cancer is the most common noncutaneous cancer and the second leading cause of cancer-related death in American men with an estimated 313,780 new prostate cancer diagnoses and 35,770 prostate cancer deaths in 2025. While prostate cancer incidence declined steadily up until 2014, it has since continued to rise. Most concerning is the rising incidence of advanced prostate cancer at diagnosis for men of all age groups. *The clinical incidence, however, does not match the prevalence of the disease.* Autopsy studies have demonstrated that > 40% of men over age 50 years have prostate cancer, and its prevalence increases with age with 30% of men aged 60–69 years and 67% of men aged 80–89 years harboring the disease at autopsy. Prostate cancer is an extremely heterogenous disease and most of these occult cancers are small, indolent, and organ-confined with little potential for regional or metastatic disease. Although the global prevalence of prostatic cancer at autopsy is relatively consistent, the clinical incidence varies considerably (highest in North America, Europe, the Caribbean, Australia/New Zealand, and Southern Africa, and lowest in Northern Africa and Asia). *Globally, prostate cancer is the second most common malignancy in men and the fifth leading cause of cancer mortality.*

Clinical Findings

A. Symptoms and Signs

Most prostate cancers are asymptomatic and are diagnosed because of elevations in serum PSA. However, some cases of prostate cancer are diagnosed based on discrete nodules or areas of induration within the prostate on a DRE.

Obstructive voiding symptoms are most often due to benign prostatic hyperplasia, which occurs in the same age group. Nevertheless, large or locally extensive prostatic cancers can cause obstructive voiding symptoms, including urinary retention. Lymph node metastases can lead to lower extremity lymphedema, though this is extremely unusual. Because the axial skeleton is the most common site of metastases, patients with advanced disease may present with back pain, pathologic fractures, or rarely neurologic symptoms from epidural metastases and cord compression.

B. Laboratory Findings

1. PSA serum tumor marker—PSA is a glycoprotein produced only by prostatic cells, either benign or malignant. The serum level is typically low in men without prostate cancer and correlates with the total volume of prostate tissue and tends to increase with age. Measurement of serum PSA is useful in detecting and staging prostate cancer, monitoring response to treatment, and identifying recurrence before it becomes clinically evident. *PSA is not specific for cancer, and there is considerable overlap of values with men with BPH.* It is important to realize that a PSA reference range of ≤ 4.0 ng/mL is not appropriate for all men and that *no PSA threshold excludes the diagnosis of prostate cancer* (Table 43–13). More recent data suggest that a man's baseline PSA in his 50s is associated with long-term prostate cancer risk. Median PSA levels for men aged 40–49 years and 50–59 years are 0.7 ng/mL and 0.9 ng/mL, respectively. Baseline PSA level may assist with patient counseling regarding long-term prostate cancer risk and set appropriate screening intervals. Prostate cancer will be diagnosed in approximately 18–30% of men with PSA 4.1–10 ng/mL (4.1–10 mcg/L) and 50–70% of men with PSA > 10 ng/mL (10 mcg/L).

In untreated patients with prostate cancer, the level of PSA correlates with the volume and stage of disease. Patients with PSA levels < 10 ng/mL (10 mcg/L) usually have localized and therefore potentially curable cancers with local therapy alone, while those with PSA levels > 40 ng/mL (40 mcg/L) are more likely to have advanced disease (seminal vesicle invasion, lymph node involvement, or occult distant metastases). Approximately 98% of patients with metastatic prostate cancer will have an elevated PSA level, yet treatment decisions cannot be made based on PSA testing alone. A rising PSA after therapy is usually consistent with progressive disease, either locally recurrent or metastatic, but does not always indicate that immediate additional therapy is necessary.

Table 43–13. Risk of prostate cancer in men with PSA ≤ 4.0 ng/mL (or mcg/L).

PSA Level (ng/mL [or mcg/L])	Percentage with Prostate Cancer	Percentage with High-Grade[1] Prostate Cancer
≤ 0.5	6.6	12.5
0.6–1.0	10.1	10.0
1.1–2.0	17.0	11.8
2.1–3.0	23.9	19.1
3.1–4.0	26.9	25.0

[1]High-grade cancer was defined as Gleason score ≥ 7.
Data from Thompson IM et al. Prevalence of prostate cancer among men with a PSA level ≤ 4.0 ng per milliliter. N Engl J Med. 2004;350:2239.

2. Miscellaneous laboratory testing—Patients with urinary retention or with ureteral obstruction due to locoregionally advanced prostate cancers may present with elevations in BUN or serum creatinine. Patients with bony metastases may have elevations in serum alkaline phosphatase or calcium. Laboratory and clinical evidence of disseminated intravascular coagulation can occur in patients with advanced prostate cancers.

3. Prostate biopsy—*Ultrasound-guided biopsy is the standard method for detection of prostate cancer.* A decision to recommend a prostate biopsy is generally not made on PSA levels alone but after careful prostate cancer risk assessment by utilizing either a multivariable clinical risk calculator or additional biomarker or imaging studies (Figure 43–2). The use of a spring-loaded, 18-gauge biopsy needle has allowed prostate biopsy to be performed with minimal patient discomfort and morbidity. Local anesthesia is standard and increases the tolerability of the procedure. While a transrectal approach is still most commonly practiced in the United States, rising rates of postbiopsy infection and sepsis have led to increasing utilization of a transperineal approach. This approach has very little risk for infection and often does not require prophylactic antibiotics. While extended-pattern biopsies, including a total of at least 10 biopsies, are associated with improved cancer detection and risk stratification of patients with newly diagnosed disease, suspicious hypoechoic prostatic lesions seen on transrectal ultrasound or pre-biopsy MRI may be targeted for biopsy. Patients with abnormalities of the seminal vesicles can have these structures specifically biopsied to identify local tumor invasion.

C. Imaging

Multiparametric MRI (mpMRI) has emerged as the imaging study of choice for localized prostate cancer detection and characterization. Prior to prostate cancer diagnosis, particularly among men with previous negative prostate biopsies, mpMRI is used to evaluate for suspicious prostatic lesions and to aid in the decision to undergo prostate biopsy. Such lesions may then be sampled via MRI-guided needle biopsy or via MR fusion (in which prostate MRI images are fused in real-time with images from an ultrasound-guided needle biopsy). It has clearly been shown that the use of mpMRI to guide the decision to undergo a prostate biopsy for a rising PSA can reduce unnecessary biopsies and limit detection of indolent disease. High-quality prostate MRI, however, is not universally available and there is considerable interobserver variability with interpretation.

Use of imaging for staging should be tailored to the likelihood of advanced disease in newly diagnosed cases. Asymptomatic patients with low- to intermediate-grade cancers, thought to be localized to the prostate on DRE and

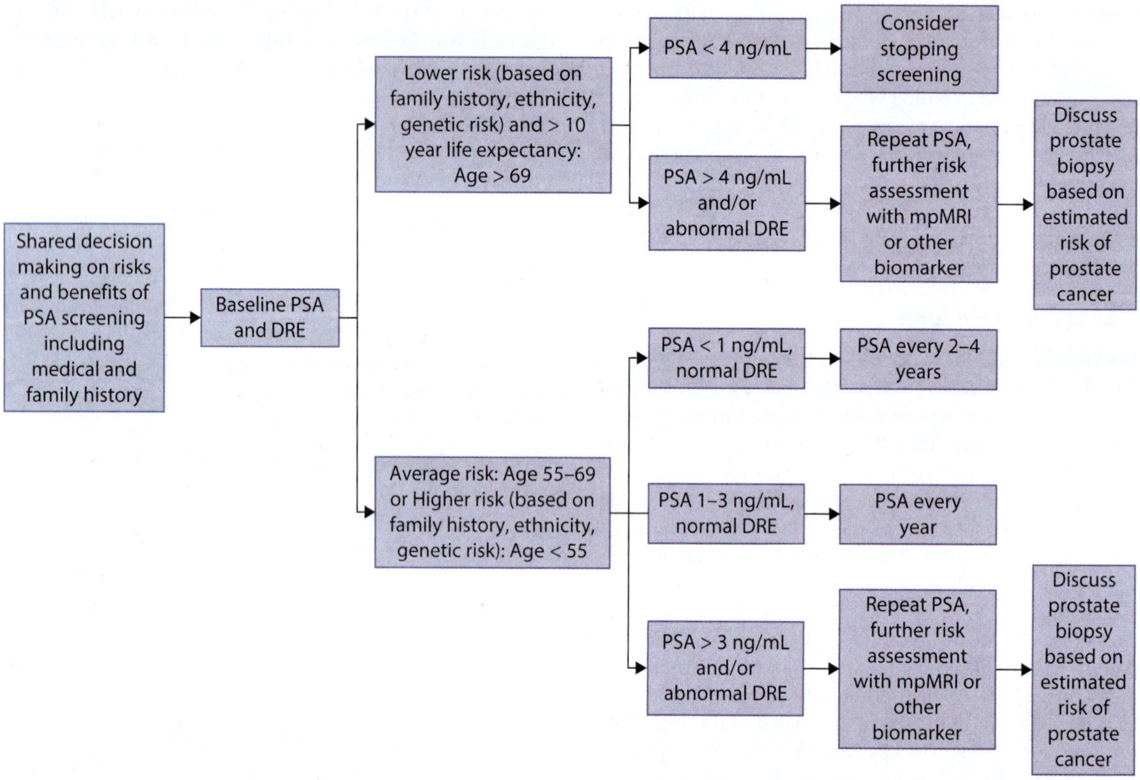

▲ **Figure 43–2.** An algorithm for prostate cancer early detection. DRE, digital rectal examination; mpMRI, multiparametric magnetic resonance imaging.

transrectal ultrasonography and associated with modest elevations of PSA (ie, < 10 ng/mL [10 mcg/L]), need no further imaging. Prostate cancer bony metastases tend to be multiple and most commonly occur in the axial skeleton. ^{18}**F-Fluciclovine (Axumin)** and **prostate-specific membrane antigen (PSMA) PET** *imaging* are approved and now available for initial staging of prostate cancer as well as to evaluate suspected cancer recurrence based on elevated PSA after prior treatment. The FDA has approved ^{68}**Ga PSMA-11**, **piflufolastat F 18 (Pylarify)**, and **flotufolastat F 18 (Posluma)** injections as PET imaging agents for prostate cancer, which have largely replaced standard nuclear medicine bone scans where available.

D. Genetic and Molecular Testing

The role of genetics and molecular testing in prostate cancer diagnosis and management is evolving. The American Society of Clinical Oncology (ASCO) published guidelines on the use of multigene panels for germline testing in men with prostate cancer. A family history of prostate cancer and certain other malignancies such as breast or ovarian cancer increases the risk of prostate cancer. Additionally, prostate cancer has been associated with several hereditary cancer syndromes (eg, Lynch syndrome, hereditary breast and ovarian cancer syndrome, etc.) with approximately 11% of patients with prostate cancer with at least one additional primary cancer carrying germline pathogenic variations. Consequently, some patients with prostate cancer and their families may have elevated risk for other cancers. Genetic variations, such as in *BRCA1/2*, are associated with lower PSA at diagnosis and increased risk of progression and death; approximately 12% of patients with metastatic prostate cancer have germline pathogenic variations in homologous DNA repair genes. Germline pathogenic genetic variations in DNA repair genes can have implications for treatment and, as a result, play a role in personalized treatment. Patients with prostate cancer should have a thorough review of their family history and those with any concern, referred for genetic counseling and possible testing. Additionally, patients with high-risk disease or metastatic disease should undergo genetic evaluation as well. NCCN guidelines recommend considering germline genetic testing in men presenting with localized high-risk, regionally advanced, or metastatic disease. Commercially available *cancer tissue RNA-based assays* are available for further risk assessment after prostate cancer diagnosis; these may help determine the need for and timing of prostate cancer treatment as well as treatment intensity.

Screening for Prostate Cancer

The impact of prostate cancer screening on mortality remains controversial. PSA-based screening can reduce the risk of prostate cancer–specific mortality, however, when performed in an organized fashion. Two large, randomized trials have evaluated the benefit of PSA screening for early detection of prostate cancer. In the US Prostate, Lung,

Colorectal, and Ovarian (PLCO) Cancer Screening Trial, no mortality benefit was observed after combined screening with PSA testing and DRE during 15-year follow-up. Although screening resulted in a 12% increase in prostate cancer detection, the cancer-specific mortality rate was similar in the screening and control arms (2.55 and 2.44 deaths per 10,000 person-years, respectively). However, an estimated 86% of control patients received at least one screening PSA test and 46% of control patients received yearly PSA screening (versus 99% and 84%, respectively, for the intervention arm) during the trial. This high degree of contamination in the control arm likely impacted the ability of this trial to detect meaningful differences in cancer detection.

Conversely, the European Randomized Study of Screening for Prostate Cancer trial demonstrated a significant reduction in prostate cancer mortality. The most recent update, with a median follow-up of 23 years, reports a 13% reduction in prostate cancer mortality with screening. The number of men needed to be invited for screening to prevent one prostate cancer death was 456 at 23 years compared with 570 at 16 years, while the number of prostate cancers needing to be diagnosed to prevent one prostate cancer death was reduced from 18 to 12, underscoring the importance of adequate long-term follow-up for prostate cancer.

Multiple practice guidelines recommend *discussion and shared decision-making* regarding the risks and benefits of PSA screening and prostate cancer early detection. While PSA measurement is the most widely performed method of screening, DRE is still recommended (Figure 43–2). PSA testing increases the detection rate of prostate cancers compared with DRE alone. PSA is not specific for cancer, and there is considerable overlap of values with men with BPH. PSA-detected cancers are more likely to be localized compared with those detected by DRE alone.

The frequency of PSA testing also remains a matter of debate. The traditional yearly screening approach may not be the most efficient; rather, earlier PSA testing at younger age may allow less frequent testing later and provide information regarding *PSA velocity* (changes in PSA over time). Men with PSA above the age-based median when tested between ages 40–60 years are at significantly increased risk for subsequent cancer detection over 25 years. Men aged 40–50 with PSA below 0.6 ng/mL (0.6 mcg/L) and those aged 50–60 years with PSA below 0.71 ng/mL (0.71 mcg/L) may require less frequent PSA testing. A secondary data analysis from the PLCO trial also demonstrated that baseline PSA for younger men in their 50s can predict long-term risk of prostate cancer and can be used to tailor PSA screening intervals. Men with a baseline PSA of < 1 ng/mL had a 1.5% incidence of prostate cancer at 13 years compared with 29.5% of men with baseline PSA levels > 4 ng/mL. The NCCN guidelines (https://www.nccn.org/professionals/physician_gls/pdf/prostate.pdf) for prostate cancer early detection incorporate many of these factors.

In 2018, the USPSTF issued a revised (Grade C) recommendation for men aged 55–69 years that the decision to undergo periodic PSA-based screening should be an individual one. Before deciding about screening, men should discuss its potential benefits and harms with their clinician, incorporating their own values and preferences in the decision. The revised recommendation acknowledges that, while screening offers some men a small potential benefit of reducing the chance of dying from prostate cancer, many other men will experience potential harms from screening. These include false-positive results that require additional testing and possible prostate biopsy; overdiagnosis and overtreatment of non–life-threatening disease; and treatment complications, such as incontinence and erectile dysfunction. In determining whether screening is appropriate in individual cases, the individual patient's family history, race/ethnicity, comorbid medical conditions, values about the benefits and harms of screening and treatment-specific outcomes, and other health needs should be considered. Clinicians should not screen men who do not express a preference for screening. For men aged 70 years or older, the USPSTF recommends against PSA-based screening (Grade D recommendation). The 2023 AUA/SUO guidelines on early detection of prostate cancer advise clinicians to engage in shared decision-making with men in whom prostate cancer screening would be appropriate, incorporating the patient's values and preferences. This update provides important information for clinicians on deciding when to start screening men and how often. (See https://www.auanet.org/guidelines-and-quality/guidelines/early-detection-of-prostate-cancer-guidelines.)

In general, *PSA levels in isolation should not be used to guide decisions regarding the need for prostate biopsies.* Additional biomarkers and imaging are now widely used to improve risk stratification for early detection of life-threatening prostate cancers. These also include establishment of age- and race-specific reference ranges, measurement of free serum and protein-bound levels of PSA (*percent free PSA*), and calculation of PSA velocity. Generally, men with PSA free fractions exceeding 25% are unlikely to have prostate cancer, whereas those with free fractions < 10% have an approximately 50% chance of having prostate cancer. Additional commercially available serum- and urine-based tests may better identify not only men at greater risk for prostate cancer but those with more aggressive disease. mpMRI is also frequently used in the screening setting after a concerning PSA level is found. Multiple studies suggest that incorporating mpMRI into a prostate cancer screening and early detection pathway can lead to fewer negative prostate biopsies while improving overall detection of higher-grade prostate cancers. However, not all prostate cancers are visualized on mpMRI with a negative predictive value of 0.75. There is also variability in MRI quality and interpretation that must be considered when using MRI as a screening test prior to referral to a urologist.

Staging

Most prostate cancers are adenocarcinomas. Most arise in the peripheral zone of the prostate, though a small percentage arise in the central (5–10%) and transition zones (20%) of the gland. Pathologists utilize the **Gleason grading system** whereby a "primary" grade is applied to the architectural pattern of malignant glands occupying the largest area of the specimen and a "secondary" grade is assigned to the next largest area of cancer. Grading is based on architectural rather than histologic criteria, and five "grades" are possible. Adding the score of the primary and secondary grades gives a Gleason score from 2 to 10. In current practice, however, Gleason scores of 2–5 are no longer assigned. Gleason score correlates with tumor volume, pathologic stage, and prognosis. A simplified five-grade group system has been introduced by the International Society of Urological Pathologists; it is based on Gleason score and is now widely utilized on pathology reports.

Treatment

A. General Measures

The optimal management of localized prostate cancer remains controversial owing to the plethora of treatment options, side effects of the various options, and indolent nature of many prostate cancers. These factors have contributed to uncertainty regarding a definitive survival benefit of treating localized prostate cancer. To help guide treatment decision-making, patients are risk stratified according to their PSA level at diagnosis, DRE, prostate cancer grade (Gleason score) and other clinical and pathological features. Multivariable instruments are available online for patients and clinicians to facilitate treatment decisions. Additionally, patients should have an assessment of life expectancy prior to treatment decision-making since all patients with low-risk disease and many with intermediate-risk disease with < 10-year life expectancy will not benefit from immediate treatment. Prognostic tissue-based risk biomarkers are also now available to help guide treatment decisions.

B. Active Surveillance

***Active surveillance** is now the preferred initial treatment recommendation for men with well-differentiated prostate cancer and low-risk clinical features.* The goal of active surveillance is to avoid treatment in men who may never require it while recognizing and definitively treating men harboring higher-risk disease in order to balance cancer risk with the morbidity of treatment. Active surveillance alone may be effective management for appropriately selected patients, typically those with low PSA, small volume, well-differentiated cancers, and life expectancy < 10–15 years. For such patients, active surveillance may involve serial PSA levels, DREs, periodic prostate mpMRI, and biopsies to reassess grade and extent of cancer. *Different than watchful waiting, the goal of active surveillance is to identify early changes in the cancer when curative intervention can still be applied.* Endpoints for intervention in patients on active surveillance, particularly PSA changes, have not been clearly defined and surveillance regimens remain an active area of research. *Most men are offered definitive treatment when cancer grade changes are noted on surveillance biopsy.* Contemporary series demonstrate freedom from definitive treatment in greater than half of patients at 5 years, and risk of developing metastases and suffering cancer-specific death in < 3% and 2%, respectively, at 10 years. Delayed therapy for clinical signs of progression seems to have no negative impact on survival.

Active surveillance is featured prominently in the AUA, NCCN, and EAU guidelines and is the preferred management in most men with low- and some intermediate-risk prostate cancer. This approach is increasingly accepted and incorporated in routine clinical practice.

***Watchful waiting** is the preferred treatment for men with limited life expectancy who can be followed with PSA alone in the absence of any symptoms or signs of metastatic disease.*

C. Radical Prostatectomy

During radical prostatectomy, the seminal vesicles, prostate, and ampullae of the vas deferens are removed. *Refinements in technique have allowed preservation of urinary continence in most patients and erectile function in selected patients.* Radical prostatectomy can be performed via open retropubic or laparoscopic (with or without robotic assistance) surgery. Organ-confined and lower-grade cancers rarely recur; however, cancers with adverse pathologic features (capsular penetration, seminal vesicle invasion, large cribriform or intraductal architecture) are associated with higher local (10–25%) and distant (20–50%) relapse rates.

Ideal candidates for radical prostatectomy include healthy patients with stages T1 and T2 prostate cancers. Patients with advanced local tumors (T4) or lymph node metastases are rarely candidates for prostatectomy alone, although surgery is sometimes used in combination with hormonal therapy and postoperative radiation therapy for select high-risk patients. Twenty-nine-year follow-up from the Scandinavian Prostate Cancer Group Study Number 4 randomized trial comparing radical prostatectomy to watchful waiting in men with localized prostate cancer demonstrated a prostate cancer survival advantage with surgery with an absolute difference in risk of 11.7%. The ProtecT trial randomized 1632 primarily low- and intermediate-risk men with clinically localized prostate cancer to either active monitoring, surgery, or radiotherapy. At 15 years follow-up, prostate cancer–specific mortality was low in all three groups and differences were not significant, though both surgery and radiotherapy were associated with lower rates of disease progression and metastases. An undetectable PSA (< 0.1 ng/mL) after surgery suggests no signs of residual or recurrent disease and no further imaging or treatment is required.

D. Radiation Therapy

Radiation can be delivered by a variety of techniques to the prostate and, when clinically indicated, to the pelvic lymph nodes. *Conformal techniques, including three-dimensional conformal radiation, intensity-modulated radiotherapy, and image-guided radiotherapy, have become the standard of care for external photon-based radiotherapy,* while *proton beam therapy* has gained acceptance as an alternative external beam therapy that theoretically may reduce toxicities. Additionally, hypofractionated and ultra-hypofractionated (ie, *stereotactic radiotherapy*) regimens have shown promising short- and intermediate-term outcomes versus conventionally dosed regimens. Low- and high-dose rate *brachytherapy*—the implantation of permanent or temporary radioactive sources (palladium, iodine, or iridium) into the prostate—can be used as monotherapy in those with low-grade or low-volume malignancies or combined with external beam radiation in patients with higher-grade or higher-volume disease. The PSA may initially rise after brachytherapy because of prostate inflammation and necrosis. This transient elevation ("PSA bounce") should not be mistaken for recurrence and may occur up to 20 months after treatment. Patients with intermediate and high-risk disease benefit from concomitant *androgen deprivation therapy (ADT)* for a specified period, which can be up to several years for men with high-grade, high-volume disease. As with surgery, the likelihood of local failure following radiation correlates with technique and cancer characteristics. The likelihood of a positive prostate biopsy > 18 months after radiation varies between 20% and 60%. Patients with local recurrence are at an increased risk of cancer progression and cancer death compared with those who have negative biopsies. Survival of patients with localized cancers (T1, T2, and selected T3) approaches 65% at 10 years. Ambiguous target definitions, inadequate radiation doses, and understaging of the cancer may be responsible for the failure noted in some series.

E. Focal Therapy

To reduce the morbidity of localized prostate cancer treatment, there has been a growing interest in focal therapy. Focal therapy delivers energy to the prostate, destroying the tumor(s) and a margin of normal prostate tissue while avoiding collateral damage to the neurovascular bundles, external urinary sphincter, bladder, and rectum. To date, several energy sources such as cryotherapy, high-intensity focused ultrasound, lasers, and irreversible electroporation have been evaluated and are in clinical use. Clinical practice guidelines recognize that the role for ablative therapies is largely unknown, but they can be offered to well-informed men with intermediate-risk disease, preferably in the setting of a clinical trial or registry.

F. Treatment for Locally and Regionally Advanced Disease

Those patients with high-risk or locally extensive cancers, including seminal vesicle and bladder neck invasion, are at increased risk for both local and distant relapse despite local therapy and often require multimodal approaches to treatment. Patients with advanced pathologic stage or positive surgical margins after prostatectomy are at an increased risk for local and distant tumor relapse. Due to these risks, such patients have been considered for *adjuvant therapy* (radiation for positive margins and seminal vesicle invasion, or androgen deprivation or radiation, or both, for lymph node metastases). Two RCTs demonstrated improved progression-free and metastasis-free survival with early radiotherapy in these men, and subsequent analysis showed improved overall survival in men receiving adjuvant radiation therapy. However, the publication of multiple trials comparing adjuvant radiotherapy with early-salvage therapy for detectable or rising PSA using contemporary radiotherapy techniques demonstrated no difference in 5-year biochemical progression-free survival, casting doubt on the benefit of adjuvant radiotherapy. The 2024 AUA/ASTRO/SUO Salvage Therapy for Prostate Cancer Guideline recommends PSA monitoring after treatment with early salvage therapy (PSA < 0.5) for recurrence. The EMBARK clinical trial demonstrated improved metastases free survival with enzalutamide with or without ADT over ADT alone for men with PSA recurrent, non-metastatic prostate cancer after primary therapy (radiation or prostatectomy) and rapid PSA doubling time of < 9 months. PSMA PET scans before salvage therapy are shown to induce changes in treatment in up to 34% of men and may lead to improved outcomes.

G. Metastatic Disease

Since death due to prostate carcinoma is almost invariably the result of failure to control metastatic disease, research has emphasized efforts to improve control of distant disease. Most prostate carcinomas are hormone dependent, and 70–80% of men with metastatic prostate carcinoma will respond to various forms of androgen deprivation. *Androgen deprivation therapy* may be effective at several levels along the pituitary–gonadal axis using a variety of methods or agents (Table 43–14). Use of LH-releasing hormone (LHRH) agonists (leuprolide, goserelin) achieves medical castration without orchiectomy and is the most common method of reducing testosterone levels. Both degarelix and relugolix are FDA-approved LHRH antagonists and have no short-term testosterone "flare" associated with LHRH agonists. Because of its rapid onset of action, *ketoconazole* should be considered in patients with advanced prostate cancer who present with spinal cord compression, bilateral ureteral obstruction, or disseminated intravascular coagulation. Although testosterone is the major circulating androgen, the adrenal gland secretes the androgens dehydroepiandrosterone, dehydroepiandrosterone sulfate, and androstenedione. In addition to immediate side effects of androgen deprivation (sexual dysfunction and hot flashes), the chronic suppression of testosterone leads to osteoporosis and risk of fractures, CVD and diabetes mellitus, and decreased muscle and increased fat. *Bisphosphonates* can prevent osteoporosis associated with androgen deprivation, decrease bone pain from metastases, and reduce skeletal-related events. *Denosumab*, a RANK ligand inhibitor, is approved for the prevention of skeletal-related events in patients with bone metastases from prostate cancer and also appears to delay the development of these metastases in patients with castration-resistant prostate cancer.

The management of advanced prostate cancer is rapidly evolving and is now initially based on the volume of metastatic disease at the time of diagnosis. Contemporary management consists of more than androgen deprivation therapy with orchiectomy, LHRH agonist, or LHRH antagonist alone and may even include radiation therapy to the primary tumor. Patients at risk for disease-related symptoms (bone pain, obstructive voiding symptoms) should receive *concurrent antiandrogens* due to the initial elevation of serum testosterone that accompanies LHRH agonists. For patients with hormone-naïve metastatic prostate cancer, the addition of systemic cytotoxic

Table 43–14. Androgen deprivation for prostate cancer (listed in alphabetical order, by level).

Level	Agent	Dose	Sequelae
Adrenal	Ketoconazole	400 mg three times orally daily	Adrenal insufficiency, nausea, rash, ataxia
	Corticosteroid		
	Prednisone	20–40 mg orally daily	GI bleeding, fluid retention
	CYP17a1 inhibitor		
	Abiraterone	1000 mg orally daily (with prednisone 5 mg orally twice daily)	Weight gain, fluid retention, hypokalemia, hypertension
Pituitary, hypothalamus	**LHRH agonists**		
	Leuprolide	Daily subcutaneous or depot injection	Erectile dysfunction, hot flushes, gynecomastia, rarely anemia
	Goserelin	Monthly to quarterly depot injection	
	Triptorelin	Monthly depot injection	
	Histrelin	Annual subcutaneous implant	
	LHRH antagonist		
	Degarelix	240 mg subcutaneously initial dose, then 80 mg subcutaneously monthly	Hot flushes, weight gain, erectile dysfunction, increased liver tests
Prostate	**Antiandrogens**		
	Flutamide	250 mg three times orally daily	No erectile dysfunction when used alone; nausea, diarrhea
	Bicalutamide	50 mg orally daily	Liver, cardiac, and pulmonary toxicity
	Enzalutamide	160 mg orally daily	Seizures, dizziness, asthenia
	Apalutamide	240 mg orally daily	Fatigue, leukopenia, hyperlipidemia, hyperglycemia, hyperkalemia, seizures (rare)
	Darolutamide	600 mg orally twice daily	Fatigue, extremity pain, rash
	Cytotoxic chemotherapeutic agents		
	Docetaxel	75 mg/m^2 intravenously once on day 1 of 21-day cycle (with prednisone 10 mg orally daily)	Bone marrow, skin, pulmonary, cardiac, GI, hepatic toxicities possible
	Cabazitaxel	20 mg/m^2 intravenously once on day 1 of 21-day cycle (with prednisone 10 mg orally daily)	
Testis	Orchiectomy		Gynecomastia, hot flushes, erectile dysfunction

LHRH, LH-releasing hormone.

chemotherapy with *docetaxel* to androgen deprivation therapy results in improved survival compared with androgen deprivation therapy alone in men with high-volume disease. Similarly, the addition of *abiraterone acetate plus prednisone* to androgen deprivation therapy results in superior survival compared with androgen deprivation therapy alone. Results from the PEACE-1 trial demonstrate that a three-drug regimen, with androgen deprivation therapy, docetaxel, and abiraterone acetate used together for men with high-volume metastatic prostate cancer, provides the best survival outcome for men with hormone-sensitive metastatic cancer. Other androgen receptor signaling inhibitors such as enzalutamide, apalutamide, or darolutamide are also used in this situation. With this *treatment intensification,* the median survival for men with de novo metastatic prostate cancer is now expected to be 5 years. A benefit of local external beam radiation therapy to the prostate gland was demonstrated by STAMPEDE in which patients with low-volume metastatic disease who received external radiotherapy plus standard systemic therapy had improved overall survival compared with those who received only standard systemic therapy. Data from the PEACE-1 study also demonstrated that adding radiation therapy in the setting of early metastatic disease improved radiographic progression-free but not overall survival. Although under investigation, radical prostatectomy is not performed in patients with metastatic disease. Guidelines recommend genomic testing for all men with metastatic prostate cancer, as men who are found to have specific germline or somatic pathogenic variants may benefit from personalized treatment strategies.

Poly(adenosine diphosphate-ribose) polymerase (PARP) inhibitors represent a class of anticancer agents with some activity against prostate cancer, particularly in patients harboring pathogenic variants in genes important for homologous recombination such as *BRCA1*, *BRCA2*, and *ATM*. Multiple PARP inhibitors are now approved for men with metastatic prostate cancer and may be given in combination with other hormonal agents. Based on data from the Amplitude trial, the FDA recently approved niraparib with abiraterone acetate as first-line therapy for men with *BRCA1/2*-mutated metastatic castrate-sensitive prostate cancer, which supports upfront genomic testing for all men presenting with metastatic disease. Patients with *castrate-resistant disease* or prostate cancer that demonstrates rising PSA or progression of disease despite castrate levels of serum testosterone (< 50 ng/dL) should continue their LHRH agonist/antagonist regimen. Additional treatment options are stratified based on the presence of metastatic disease. Patients with nonmetastatic castrate-resistant disease and long PSA doubling time (longer than 10 months) can simply be observed due to their relatively indolent disease. Conversely, nonmetastatic castrate-resistant patients with short doubling times (10 months or less) have demonstrated improved metastasis-free survival with the addition of one of the potent nonsteroidal androgen receptor antagonists, enzalutamide, apalutamide, or darolutamide, to androgen deprivation therapy. For patients with metastatic castrate-resistant prostate cancer, docetaxel was the first cytotoxic chemotherapy agent to improve survival. Enzalutamide and abiraterone improve overall survival in men with metastatic castrate-resistant prostate cancer in both the docetaxel-naïve and non-naïve setting. Cabazitaxel is a second-line taxane chemotherapy that improves overall survival in men who have received docetaxel. Sipuleucel-T, an autologous cellular immunotherapy, is FDA-approved in asymptomatic or minimally symptomatic men with metastatic castration-resistant prostate cancer. Radium-223 dichloride is approved for the treatment of men with castration-resistant, symptomatic bone metastases, with significant improvements in both overall survival and time to skeletal-related events (eg, fractures and spinal cord compression). Lutetium-177-PSMA-617 is the first theranostic radioligand agent for metastatic castration-resistant prostate cancer and is approved for use in men with PSMA-producing tumors who have progressed on other lines of therapy and is also now approved for earlier use before chemotherapy. Multiple PARP inhibitors are approved for use in men with homologous recombination repair, particularly *BRCA1/2*-mutated metastatic castration-resistant prostate cancer.

Prognosis

The likelihood of success of active surveillance or treatment can be predicted using risk assessment tools that usually combine stage, grade, PSA level, and number and extent of positive prostate biopsies. Several web-based tools are available (eg, https://www.mskcc.org/nomograms/prostate). Widely used nomograms include the *Kattan* nomogram and the *CAPRA* nomogram. CAPRA uses serum PSA, Gleason score, clinical stage, percent positive biopsies, and patient age in a point system to risk stratify and predict the likelihood of PSA recurrence 3 and 5 years after radical prostatectomy as well as metastasis and prostate cancer–specific and overall survival. The CAPRA nomogram has been validated on large multicenter and international radical prostatectomy and radiation-treated cohorts.

The patterns of prostate cancer progression have been well defined. Small and well-differentiated cancers (Gleason grade 3) are usually confined within the prostate, whereas large-volume (> 4 mL) or poorly differentiated (Gleason grades 4 and 5) cancers are more often locally extensive or metastatic to regional lymph nodes or bone. Penetration of the prostate capsule by cancer is common and occurs along perineural spaces. Seminal vesicle invasion is associated with a high likelihood of regional or distant disease and disease recurrence. The most common sites of lymph node metastases are the obturator and internal iliac lymph node chains and of distant metastases, the axial skeleton.

When to Refer

- Refer all patients to a urologist for management of localized disease or for active surveillance.
- For metastatic disease, medical oncology should be consulted for consideration of systemic treatments.
- Active surveillance may be appropriate in selected patients with very low-volume, low-grade prostate cancer.
- Localized disease may be managed by active surveillance, surgery, or radiation therapy.
- Locally extensive, regionally advanced, and metastatic disease often require multimodal treatment strategies.

Attard G et al. Niraparib and abiraterone acetate plus prednisone for HRR-deficient metastatic castration-sensitive prostate cancer: a randomized phase 3 trial. Nat Med. 2025;31:4109. [PMID: 41057655]

Morgan TM et al. Salvage therapy for prostate cancer: AUA/ASTRO/SUO guideline part I: introduction and treatment decision-making at the time of suspected biochemical recurrence after radical prostatectomy. J Urol. 2024;211:509. [PMID: 38421253]

Roobol MJ et al; ERSPC Investigators. European study of prostate cancer screening – 23-year follow-up. N Engl J Med. 2025;393:1669. [PMID: 41160819]

Shore ND et al. Improved survival with enzalutamide in biochemically recurrent prostate cancer. N Engl J Med. 2025 Oct 19. [Epub ahead of print] [PMID: 41124201]

Sushentsev N et al. Active monitoring, surgery, and radiotherapy for cribriform-positive and cribriform-negative prostate cancer: a secondary analysis of the PROTECT randomized clinical trial. JAMA Oncol. 2025;11:1512. [PMID: 41100113]

Tung N et al. Selection of germline genetic testing panels in patients with cancer: ASCO guideline. J Clin Oncol. 2024;42:2599. [PMID:38759122]

BLADDER CANCER

ESSENTIALS OF DIAGNOSIS

- Gross or microscopic hematuria.
- Irritative voiding symptoms.
- Positive urinary cytology in most patients.
- Filling defect within bladder noted on imaging.

General Considerations

Bladder cancer is the second most common urologic cancer; it occurs more commonly in men than women (3.1:1), and the mean age at diagnosis is 73 years. In 2024 in the United States, it is estimated that approximately 83,190 cases of bladder cancer will be diagnosed and 16,840 deaths will result. *Cigarette smoking and exposure to industrial dyes or solvents are risk factors for the disease and account for approximately 60% and 15% of new cases, respectively.* In the United States, almost all primary bladder cancers (98%) are epithelial malignancies, usually urothelial cell carcinomas (90%). Adenocarcinomas and squamous cell cancers account for approximately 2% and 7%, respectively. The latter is often associated with schistosomiasis, vesical calculi, or prolonged catheter use.

Clinical Findings

A. Symptoms and Signs

Hematuria—gross or microscopic, chronic or intermittent—is the presenting symptom in 85–90% of patients with bladder cancer (see Hematuria in Chapter 26). Irritative voiding symptoms (urinary frequency and urgency) occur in a small percentage of patients as a result of the location or size of the cancer. Most patients with bladder cancer do not have signs of the disease because of its superficial nature. Abdominal masses detected on bimanual examination may be present in patients with large-volume or deeply infiltrating cancers. Hepatomegaly or palpable lymphadenopathy may be present in patients with metastatic disease, and lymphedema of the lower extremities results from locally advanced cancers or metastases to pelvic lymph nodes.

B. Laboratory Findings

UA reveals microscopic or gross hematuria in the majority of cases. On occasion, hematuria is accompanied by pyuria. Azotemia may be present in a small number of cases associated with ureteral obstruction. Anemia may occasionally be due to chronic blood loss or to bone marrow metastases. Exfoliated cells from normal and abnormal urothelium can be readily detected in voided urine specimens. Cytology can be useful to detect the disease initially or to detect its recurrence. Cytology is sensitive in detecting cancers of higher grade and stage (80–90%), but less so in detecting noninvasive or well-differentiated lesions (50%). There are other novel urinary tumor markers under investigation for screening or assessing recurrence, progression, prognosis, or response to therapy.

C. Imaging

Bladder cancers may be identified as masses within the bladder using ultrasound, CT, or MRI. However, the presence of cancer is confirmed by cystoscopy and biopsy, with imaging primarily used to evaluate the upper urinary tract and to stage more advanced lesions.

D. Cystourethroscopy and Biopsy

The diagnosis and staging of bladder cancers are made by cystoscopy and transurethral resection. If cystoscopy—usually performed under local anesthesia—confirms the presence of a bladder tumor, the patient is scheduled for transurethral resection under general or regional anesthesia. Random bladder and transurethral prostate biopsies are occasionally performed to detect occult disease and potentially identify patients at greater risk for cancer recurrence and progression.

Pathology & Staging

Grading is based on cellular features: size, pleomorphism, mitotic rate, and hyperchromatism. Bladder cancer staging is based on the extent (depth) of bladder wall penetration and the presence of regional or distant metastases. Both cancer grade and stage influence the natural history of bladder cancer including local recurrence within the bladder and progression to higher-stage disease. Several bladder cancer variant histologies have been described and are important for both prognosis and treatment planning.

Treatment

Patients with non–muscle-invasive cancers (Tis, Ta, T1) are treated with complete *transurethral resection* with selective use of a *single dose intravesical chemotherapy* immediately following resection. Patients with carcinoma in situ (Tis) and those with high-grade, non–muscle-invasive lesions (Ta or T1) are good candidates for additional intravesical therapy after resection due to a high risk for cancer recurrence and progression with surveillance alone. Patients with high-risk noninvasive cancers are often also treated with re-resection to confirm stage and grade prior to adjuvant intravesical therapy. Some patients with high-grade T1 (particularly recurrent) bladder cancers are recommended for radical cystectomy.

Patients with muscle-invasive (T2+) but still localized cancers are at risk for both nodal metastases and progression and require more aggressive treatment. The gold standard treatment is *neoadjuvant chemotherapy* followed by *radical cystectomy*, which confers a survival advantage versus cystectomy alone. This is particularly important for higher-stage or bulky tumors to improve their surgical resectability. Trimodal bladder preservation therapy consisting of complete transurethral resection, sensitizing systemic chemotherapy, and external beam radiotherapy can offer similar outcomes in optimally selected patients.

A. Intravesical Therapy

Immunotherapeutic or chemotherapeutic agents delivered directly into the bladder via a urethral catheter can reduce the likelihood of recurrence in those who have undergone complete transurethral resection. Most agents are administered weekly for 6–12 weeks. Efficacy may be increased by prolonging contact time to 2 hours. The use of maintenance therapy after the initial induction regimen is beneficial.

Common agents include gemcitabine, mitomycin, docetaxel, valrubicin, and bacillus Calmette–Guérin (BCG), with the last being the only agent effective in reducing disease progression. *Induction intravesical BCG is the standard of care for patients with high-risk, non–muscle-invasive bladder cancer or carcinoma in situ after resection.* BCG recurrent or refractory disease may be particularly difficult to manage, and early cystectomy should be considered, as patients are at high risk for progression. In 2022, nadofaragene firadenovec-vncg was FDA-approved for patients with high-risk BCG unresponsive non-muscle-invasive bladder cancer. This is the first approved gene therapy for bladder cancer. Nogapendekin alfa inbakicept and, most recently, TAR-200, a novel intravesical gemcitabine-releasing system, have also been approved for use. Side effects of intravesical chemotherapy include irritative voiding symptoms and hemorrhagic cystitis. Patients in whom symptoms of infection develop from BCG may require antituberculosis therapy. Global BCG supply shortages have limited access to many patients with bladder cancer and novel agents are being tested in ongoing clinical trials.

B. Surgical Treatment

Although transurethral resection is the initial form of treatment for all bladder cancers (since it is diagnostic, it allows for proper staging, and it controls superficial cancers), muscle-invasive cancers require more aggressive treatment. *Partial cystectomy* can be considered in selected patients with solitary lesions at the bladder dome or those with cancer in a bladder diverticulum. *Radical cystectomy* in men entails removal of the bladder, prostate, seminal vesicles, and surrounding fat and peritoneal attachments and in women removal of the bladder, uterus, cervix, urethra, anterior vaginal vault, and usually the ovaries. In women with anterior cancers, vaginal and reproductive organ-sparing surgery can be considered. Bilateral pelvic lymph node dissection is performed in all patients. Randomized trials have demonstrated similar oncologic outcomes and risks of complications with both open and robot-assisted laparoscopic cystectomy; however, robot-assisted techniques result in significantly less blood loss, lower need for blood transfusion, and slightly shorter convalescence. The most common method for urinary diversion involves creating a *conduit of ileum or colon with a stoma that drains urine into an external appliance.* However, in highly selected patients, *continent forms of diversion* can be performed that avoid the necessity of an external appliance.

C. Radiotherapy

External beam radiotherapy delivered in fractions over a 6- to 8-week period is generally well tolerated, but approximately 10–15% of patients will develop bladder, bowel, or rectal complications. Local recurrence is common after radiotherapy alone (30–70%), and it is therefore combined with radiosensitizing systemic chemotherapy to improve complete response and to decrease recurrence rates. *Bladder-preserving chemoradiation* can be offered to those patients seeking to keep their bladder and is best suited for selected patients with solitary T2 or limited T3 tumors without ureteral obstruction. Radiation with or without chemotherapy can be offered to patients with localized cancers and to patients who are poor candidates for radical cystectomy or to patients with metastatic disease seeking palliation of local symptoms. Salvage cystectomy following primary bladder radiotherapy is more challenging with greater risk of complications.

D. Chemotherapy

Systemic chemotherapy is recommended for eligible patients with muscle-invasive or locally advanced bladder cancer (prior to cystectomy or radiation). *The antibody-drug conjugate enfortumab vedotin has replaced chemotherapy as the first-line agent in the metastatic setting (see Other Therapies section).* Cisplatin-based combination chemotherapy results in partial or complete responses in 15–45% of patients (Table 43–2) and is the preferred approach. Combination chemotherapy has been used to decrease recurrence rates in patients treated both with surgery and with radiotherapy. Patients who are not eligible for cisplatin should proceed with immediate cystectomy or consider enrollment in a clinical trial. Chemotherapy should also be considered before surgery in those with bulky lesions or those in whom regional metastases are suspected. A multicenter clinical trial showed improved 3-year progression-free survival with dose-dense methotrexate, vinblastine, doxorubicin, and cisplatin (MVAC) neoadjuvant chemotherapy versus a gemcitabine/cisplatin regimen. Alternatively, adjuvant chemotherapy has been used after cystectomy in patients at high risk for recurrence, such as those who have lymph node involvement or extravesical local invasion.

Metastatic disease is present in 15% of patients with newly diagnosed bladder cancer. Furthermore, metastases develop in up to 40% of patients within 2 years of cystectomy, including those patients who were believed to have localized disease at the time of treatment.

E. Immunotherapy

The FDA has approved several checkpoint inhibitors as immunotherapy for patients with urothelial cancer at various stages. Approved anti–PD-L1 inhibitors include atezolizumab, durvalumab, and avelumab (Table 43–2). Approved anti-PD1 inhibitors include nivolumab and pembrolizumab. All are approved for second-line treatment of locally advanced or metastatic urothelial cancer that progressed during or after platinum-based chemotherapy. Nivolumab is FDA-approved for use in combination with cisplatin and gemcitabine for the first-line treatment of adults with unresectable or metastatic urothelial carcinoma. Atezolizumab and pembrolizumab are approved as first-line therapy in cisplatin-ineligible patients whose tumors express PD-L1 or in patients ineligible for any platinum-based chemotherapy regardless of PD-L1 expression status. The KEYNOTE-361 randomized trial failed to show any benefit to adding pembrolizumab to chemotherapy in the first-line setting for patients with metastatic disease. Overall response rates of these agents are similar and range from 17% to 25% in locally advanced and metastatic urothelial bladder cancer. In many cases, responses to therapy are durable. Based on a single arm, phase 2 study, pembrolizumab is now FDA-approved for patients with high-risk, non–muscle-invasive bladder cancers who have failed intravesical BCG therapy. Nivolumab has also been approved in the adjuvant setting after radical cystectomy or nephroureterectomy for patients with urothelial carcinoma who are considered at high risk for recurrence. The phase 3 Niagara trial demonstrated improved event-free and overall survival with neoadjuvant chemotherapy and perioperative durvalumab compared to chemotherapy alone for patients with muscle-invasive bladder cancer undergoing cystectomy.

F. Other Therapies

Enfortumab vedotin is the first antibody-drug conjugate approved for advanced and metastatic urothelial carcinoma. The antibody targets Nectin-4 and demonstrates a 44% response rate (including 12% complete response) in patients who have progressed after multiple other lines of therapy. The EV302 trial showed dramatically improved survival rates with combination enfortumab vedotin and pembrolizumab over platinum-based chemotherapy alone and should be considered first-line therapy for metastatic urothelial carcinoma.

Activating pathogenic variants in the FGFR are common in urothelial carcinomas. The FGFR inhibitor erdafitinib is approved after initial therapy for patients with progressive metastatic urothelial carcinoma whose tumors harbor these mutations with expected response rates of up to 40%.

Prognosis

The frequency of recurrence and progression are correlated with grade. Whereas progression may be noted in few low-grade cancers (19–37%), it is common with poorly differentiated lesions (33–67%). Carcinoma in situ is most often found in association with papillary bladder cancers. Its presence identifies patients at increased risk for recurrence and progression.

At initial presentation, approximately 50–80% of bladder cancers are non–muscle-invasive: stage Ta, Tis, or T1. When properly treated, lymph node metastases and progression are uncommon in such patients and survival is excellent (81%). Five-year survival of patients with T2 and T3 disease ranges from 50% to 75% after radical cystectomy. Long-term survival for patients with metastatic disease at presentation is rare.

When to Refer

- Refer all patients to a urologist. Hematuria usually deserves evaluation with both upper urinary tract imaging and cystoscopy, particularly in a high-risk group (eg, older people).
- Refer when histologic diagnosis and staging require endoscopic resection of cancer.
- Muscle-invasive and locally advanced tumors should be referred to a urologist and medical oncologist since treatment requires multidisciplinary care.
- Metastatic urothelial cancer should be managed by a medical oncologist.

Daneshmand S et al; SunRISe-1 Study. TAR-200 for Bacillus Calmette-Guérin-unresponsive high-risk non-muscle-invasive bladder cancer: results from the phase IIb SunRISe-1 Study. J Clin Oncol. 2025;43:3578. [PMID: 40737582]

National Comprehensive Cancer Network. Bladder cancer, Version 1.2026, NCCN Clinical Practice Guidelines in Oncology. https://www.nccn.org/guidelines/guidelines-detail?category=1&id=1417

Powles T et al. Enfortumab vedotin and pembrolizumab in untreated advanced urothelial carcinoma. N Engl J Med. 2024;390:875. [PMID: 38446675]

Powles T et al. Perioperative durvalumab with neoadjuvant chemotherapy in operable bladder cancer. N Engl J Med. 2024;391:1773. [PMID: 39282910]

van der Heijden M et al. Nivolumab plus gemcitabine-cisplatin in advanced urothelial carcinoma. N Engl J Med. 2024;389:1778. [PMID: 37870949]

CANCERS OF THE URETER & RENAL PELVIS

Cancers of the ureter and renal pelvis are rare and occur more commonly in patients who have bladder cancer, Balkan nephropathy, or Lynch syndrome, patients who smoke, or those who have a long history of analgesic abuse. The majority are urothelial cell carcinomas. Gross or microscopic hematuria is present in most patients; flank pain secondary to bleeding and obstruction occurs less commonly. As with bladder cancers, urinary cytology is often positive in high-grade cancers. The most common signs identified at the time of CT or intravenous urography include an intraluminal filling defect, unilateral nonvisualization of the collecting system, and hydronephrosis. Ureteral and renal pelvic tumors must be differentiated from calculi, blood clots, papillary necrosis, or inflammatory and infectious lesions. Upper urinary tract lesions are accessible for diagnostic biopsy, fulguration, or resection using a ureteroscope. Treatment is based on the site, size, grade, depth of penetration, and number of cancers present. Endoscopic resection may be indicated in patients with limited renal function or focal, low-grade, cancers. Chemoablation with a mitomycin infused gel can be performed in very select patients with low-grade upper tract lesions. Most high-grade and high-volume cancers are excised with robotic, laparoscopic, or open nephroureterectomy (renal pelvic and upper ureteral lesions) or segmental excision of the ureter (distal ureteral lesions). A phase 3, randomized trial demonstrated significantly improved 3-year disease-free survival with dual agent adjuvant systemic chemotherapy after nephroureterectomy. Like with urothelial bladder cancers, use of chemotherapy prior to surgery may also improve outcomes and remains under investigation.

Masson-Lecomte A et al. European Association of Urology guidelines on upper urinary tract urothelial carcinoma: summary of the 2025 update. Eur Urol. 2025;87:697. [PMID: 40118741]
Pierorazio PM et al. Long-term outcomes of primary chemoablation of low-grade upper tract urothelial carcinoma with UGN-101, a mitomycin reverse thermal gel. J Urol. 2025;213:313. [PMID: 39561384]

RENAL CELL CARCINOMA

ESSENTIALS OF DIAGNOSIS

- Gross or microscopic hematuria.
- Flank pain or mass in some patients.
- Systemic symptoms such as fever, weight loss may be prominent.
- Solid renal mass on imaging.

General Considerations

Kidney (renal cell) and renal pelvis carcinomas account for 3.8% of all adult cancers. In 2025 in the United States, it is estimated that approximately 80,980 cases of renal cell carcinoma will be diagnosed and 14,510 deaths will result. Renal cell carcinoma has a peak incidence in the sixth decade of life and a male-to-female ratio of 2:1. It may be associated with several paraneoplastic syndromes.

Risk factors include physical inactivity, obesity, and diabetes mellitus. Cigarette smoking is the only known significant environmental risk factor. Renal cell carcinoma occurs in both sporadic and hereditary forms. There are several hereditary syndromes with autosomal dominant inheritance that can include renal cell carcinoma; these are important to consider when evaluating a patient with suspected kidney cancer (Table 43–15). There is an association with dialysis-related acquired cystic disease and specific genetic aberrations (eg, Xp11.2 translocation). Sporadic renal cell carcinoma is far more common than hereditary forms.

Renal cell carcinoma originates from the proximal tubule cells. Various histologic cell types are recognized (clear cell, papillary, chromophobe, collecting duct, and sarcomatoid). The WHO updated the pathologic classification of RCC types in 2022, which includes a group of molecularly defined subtypes. Histology, IHC, molecular signatures, and clinical aspects all vary by renal cell carcinoma type and assist with prognosis prediction and treatment decisions. Hereditary leiomyomatosis and renal cell carcinoma (HLRCC) is the most common hereditary syndrome.

Clinical Findings

A. Symptoms and Signs

Historically, 60% of patients presented with gross or microscopic hematuria. Flank pain or an abdominal mass was detected in approximately 30% of cases. The triad of flank pain, hematuria, and mass, found in only 10% of patients, is often a sign of advanced disease. Fever can occur as a paraneoplastic symptom. Symptoms of metastatic disease (cough, bone pain) occur in 20–30% of patients at presentation. Due to the widespread use of ultrasound and cross-sectional imaging, renal tumors are *frequently detected incidentally* in individuals with no urologic symptoms. Consequently, there has been profound stage migration toward lower stages of disease over the last 20 years with increased detection of small, indolent tumors. Population mortality rates have remained relatively stable.

B. Laboratory Findings

Contemporary studies suggest hematuria is present in < 50% of patients. Erythrocytosis from increased erythropoietin production occurs in 5%, though anemia is more common; hypercalcemia may be present in up to 10% of patients. *Stauffer syndrome* is a reversible syndrome of hepatic dysfunction (with elevated liver tests) in the absence of metastatic disease.

C. Imaging

Solid renal masses are often first identified by abdominal ultrasonography or CT. CT and MRI scanning are the most

Table 43–15. Hereditary syndromes with autosomal dominant inheritance that can include renal cell carcinoma (listed in alphabetical order).

Syndrome	Gene	Renal Tumor Histology	Associated Clinical Findings
Birt-Hogg-Dubé syndrome (BHD)	*FLCN 17p11.2*	HLRCC-associated RCC	Cutaneous fibrofolliculomas (facial), pulmonary cysts, spontaneous pneumothorax
Hereditary leiomyomatosis and renal cell carcinoma (HLRCC)	*FH 1q42.1*	Papillary	Cutaneous leiomyomas, uterine fibroids
Hereditary papillary renal carcinoma (HPRC)	*MET 7q34*	Chromophobe, oncocytoma, papillary, clear cell	None
von Hippel-Lindau disease (VHL)	*VHL 3p26*	Clear cell	CNS and retinal hemangioblastomas, pheochromocytoma, PNET, cystadenoma of pancreas, broad ligament, epididymis

Modified with permission from Haas NB, Nathanson KL. Hereditary kidney cancer syndromes. Adv Chronic Kidney Dis. 2014;21:81.

valuable imaging tests for renal cell carcinoma. These scans confirm the character of the mass and provide valuable staging information with respect to regional lymph nodes, renal vein or vena cava tumor thrombus, and adrenal or liver metastases. CT and MRI also provide valuable information regarding the contralateral kidney (function, bilaterality of neoplasm). CXR or CT excludes pulmonary metastases. Bone scans should be performed for large tumors and in patients with bone pain or elevated serum alkaline phosphatase levels. Brain imaging should be obtained in patients with high metastatic burden or in those with neurologic deficits.

Differential Diagnosis

Solid renal masses are renal cell carcinoma until proven otherwise. Other solid masses include renal angiomyolipomas (fat density usually detectable by CT), renal pelvis urothelial cancers (more central location, involvement of the collecting system, positive urinary cytology), renal oncocytomas (indistinguishable from renal cell carcinoma preoperatively with standard imaging), renal abscesses, and adrenal tumors (anterosuperior to the kidney).

Treatment

Surgical extirpation is the primary treatment for localized renal cell carcinoma. Patients with a single kidney, bilateral lesions, or significant medical renal disease should be considered for *partial nephrectomy.* Patients harboring a small cancer with a normal contralateral kidney and good kidney function are also candidates for partial nephrectomy, while *radical nephrectomy* is indicated in patients with cancers larger than 7 cm and those in whom partial nephrectomy is not technically feasible. Radiofrequency and cryosurgical ablation are alternative options instead of surgery in select patients with cancers < 3–4 cm with similar risk of metastatic progression but higher risk of local recurrence. Active surveillance is warranted in select patients (significant comorbidity, short life expectancy) and appears safe with low risk of 5-year systemic progression. Percutaneous biopsy can provide tumor histology and grade to help guide treatment decisions.

Cytotoxic chemotherapy has no role in the treatment of metastatic renal cell carcinoma. Historically, cytokine-based immunotherapies, such as interferon-α and interleukin-2, produced partial response rates of 15–20% and 15–35%, respectively (Table 43–2). Responders tended to have lower tumor burden, metastatic disease confined to the lung, and a high-performance status. Two randomized trials demonstrating a survival benefit of cytoreductive nephrectomy followed by systemic interferon-α compared with the use of systemic therapy alone led to the widespread adoption of cytoreductive nephrectomy. Patients most likely to benefit from cytoreduction were those with good performance status, lung only metastases, and good prognostic features.

The treatment of metastatic renal cell carcinoma has evolved rapidly over the last decade. Presently, management strategies are based on tumor histology (initial treatment choices are based on clear cell versus non–clear cell histology) and patient risk (favorable, intermediate, or poor). Risk is typically assessed according to the *International Metastatic RCC Database Consortium criteria* which includes the number of metastatic lesions at diagnosis. Targeted medications, specifically VEGF, Raf kinase, receptor tyrosine kinases, and mTOR inhibitors, are effective (40–60% response rates) in patients with advanced kidney cancer (Table 43–2). These oral agents, which include sunitinib, pazopanib, cabozantinib, axitinib, sorafenib, and lenvatinib, are generally well tolerated and particularly active for clear cell carcinoma. Sunitinib is approved for adjuvant use after complete surgical resection in patients with adverse pathologic features. The mTOR inhibitors everolimus and temsirolimus are approved for use in patients with prior anti-VEGF therapy, as is the combination of lenvatinib and everolimus. Immunotherapies have also dramatically improved the treatment landscape for patients with advanced kidney cancer. Nivolumab is an approved anti-PD-1 immunotherapy for treating metastatic disease that has progressed despite antiangiogenic therapy. Nivolumab in combination with the anti-CTLA4 immunotherapy ipilimumab (objective response rate 42%, complete response rate 9%) and pembrolizumab (anti-PD-1) in combination with the VEGF inhibitor axitinib (objective response rate 59%, complete response rate 5.8%) and lenvatinib in combination with pembrolizumab (objective response rate 71%, complete response rate 16.1%) have proved superior to sunitinib in previously untreated intermediate- and poor-risk metastatic clear cell renal cell carcinoma. Most recently, cabozantinib in combination with nivolumab and ipilimumab showed improved progression-free survival in patients with intermediate and poor prognostic risk advanced renal cell carcinoma over nivolumab or ipilimumab alone. Combination therapy with two or three agents is considered standard first-line treatment for metastatic RCC (Table 43–2). Pembrolizumab is also approved for adjuvant treatment after surgical resection of renal cell carcinoma in patients at high risk for disease recurrence. For patients with VHL disease and renal cell carcinoma, the novel HIF2α inhibitor, belzutifan, led to dramatic size reductions in both renal and non–renal neoplasms and offers a new treatment option. The LITESPARK-005 trial demonstrated superior progression-free survival with belzutifan over everolimus in non-VHL patients with progressive, previously treated advanced clear-cell RCC. Belzutifan is now FDA approved for patients with VHL or metastatic clear cell RCC following immunotherapy or VEGF tyrosine kinase inhibitor therapy. The utilization of *cytoreductive nephrectomy* in combination with contemporary agents has decreased in response to the results of the CARMENA trial in which patients with intermediate- and poor-risk clear cell renal carcinoma had similar survival following cytoreductive nephrectomy with or without sunitinib and adoption of combination immunotherapy regimens (nivolumab plus ipilimumab, pembrolizumab plus axitinib). Still, there remains a role for cytoreductive surgery in select patients with intermediate-risk disease. The SURTIME randomized trial compared immediate versus deferred cytoreductive nephrectomy in patients with metastatic renal cell carcinoma treated with sunitinib and showed an overall survival advantage with the deferred approach. This may serve to identify patients who respond the best to systemic therapy prior to undergoing removal of the primary tumor.

Prognosis

After radical or partial nephrectomy, tumors confined to the renal capsule (T1–T2) demonstrate 5-year disease free survival rate of 90–100%. Tumors extending beyond the renal capsule (T3 or T4) and node-positive tumors have 5-year disease-free survival rates of 50–60% and 0–15%, respectively. One subgroup of patients with nonlocalized disease has reasonable long-term survival, namely, those with solitary resectable metastases. In this setting, radical nephrectomy with resection of the solitary metastasis results in 5-year disease-free survival rate of 15–30%.

When to Refer

- Refer patients with solid renal masses or complex cysts to a urologist for further evaluation.
- Refer patients with renal cell carcinoma to a urologic surgeon for surgical excision.
- Refer patients with metastatic disease to an oncologist and urologist.

Choueiri TK et al; COSMIC-313 Investigators. Cabozantinib plus nivolumab and ipilimumab in renal cell carcinoma. N Engl J Med. 2023;388:1767. [PMID: 37163623]
Choueiri TK et al; LITESPARK-005 Investigators. Belzutifan versus everolimus for advanced renal-cell carcinoma. N Engl J Med. 2024;391:710. [PMID: 39167807]
Jonasch E et al; MK-6482-004 Investigators. Belzutifan for renal cell carcinoma in von Hippel-Lindau disease. N Engl J Med. 2021;385:2036. [PMID: 34818478]
Motzer RJ et al. Final analysis of nivolumab plus cabozantinib for advanced renal cell carcinoma from the randomized phase III CheckMate 9ER trial. Ann Oncol. 2026;37:33. [PMID: 40998092]
Rini BI et al. Pembrolizumab plus axitinib versus sunitinib for advanced clear cell renal cell carcinoma: 5-year survival and biomarker analyses of the phase 3 KEYNOTE-426 trial. Nat Med. 2025;31:3475. [PMID: 40750932]

OTHER PRIMARY TUMORS OF THE KIDNEY

Oncocytomas account for 3–5% of renal tumors, are usually benign, and are indistinguishable from renal cell carcinoma on preoperative imaging. These tumors are seen in other organs, including the adrenals, salivary glands, and thyroid and parathyroid glands.

Angiomyolipomas are rare benign tumors composed of fat, smooth muscle, and blood vessels. They are most commonly seen in patients with tuberous sclerosis (often multiple and bilateral) or in young to middle-aged women. CT scanning may identify the fat component, which is diagnostic for angiomyolipoma. Asymptomatic lesions < 5 cm in diameter usually do not require intervention; large lesions can spontaneously bleed. Acute bleeding can be treated by angiographic embolization or, in rare cases, nephrectomy. Lesions over 5 cm are often prophylactically treated with angioembolization or less commonly partial nephrectomy to reduce the risk of bleeding. **Epithelioid angiomyolipoma** is a very rare AML subtype with malignant potential.

SECONDARY CANCERS OF THE KIDNEY

The kidney is a not infrequent site for metastatic disease. Of the solid tumors, lung cancer is the most common (20%), followed by breast (10%), stomach (10%), and the contralateral kidney (10%). Lymphoma, both Hodgkin and non-Hodgkin, may also involve the kidney, although it tends to appear as a diffusely infiltrative process resulting in renal enlargement rather than a discrete mass.

TESTICULAR CANCERS (Germ Cell Tumors)

ESSENTIALS OF DIAGNOSIS

- Most common neoplasm in men aged 20–35 years.
- Patient typically discovers a painless nodule.
- Orchiectomy necessary for diagnosis.

General Considerations

Malignant tumors of the testis are rare, with approximately five to six cases per 100,000 males reported in the United States each year. Ninety to 95 percent of all primary testicular tumors are germ cell tumors and can be divided into two major categories: **nonseminomas**, including embryonal cell carcinoma (20%), teratoma (5%), choriocarcinoma (< 1%), and mixed cell types (40%); and **seminomas** (35%). The remainder of primary testicular tumors are non-germ cell neoplasms (Leydig cell, Sertoli cell, gonadoblastoma). The lifetime probability of developing testicular cancer is 0.3% for an American male.

Approximately 5% of testicular cancers develop in a patient with a history of cryptorchism, with seminoma being the most common. However, 5–10% of these tumors occur in the contralateral, normally descended testis. The relative risk of development of malignancy is higher for the intra-abdominal testis (1:20) and lower for the inguinal testis (1:80). Placement of the cryptorchid testis into the scrotum (orchidopexy) does not alter its malignant potential but does facilitate routine examination and cancer detection.

Testicular cancer is slightly more common on the right than the left, paralleling the increased incidence of cryptorchidism on the right side. One to 2 percent of primary testicular cancers are bilateral and up to 50% of these men have a history of unilateral or bilateral cryptorchidism. Primary bilateral testicular cancers may occur synchronously or asynchronously but tend to be of the same histology. Seminoma is the most common histologic finding in bilateral *primary* testicular cancers, while malignant lymphoma is the most common bilateral testicular tumor overall.

In animal models, exogenous estrogen administration during pregnancy has been associated with an increased development of testicular tumors with relative risk ranging from 2.8 to 5.3. Other acquired factors such as trauma and infection-related testicular atrophy have been associated with testicular tumors; however, a causal relationship has not been established.

Clinical Findings

A. Symptoms and Signs

The most common symptom of testicular cancer is painless enlargement of the testis. Sensations of heaviness are not unusual. Patients are usually the first to recognize an abnormality, yet often their delay in seeking medical attention ranges from 3 to 6 months. Acute testicular pain resulting from intratesticular hemorrhage occurs in approximately 10% of cases. Ten percent of patients are asymptomatic at presentation, and 10% manifest symptoms relating to metastatic disease such as back pain (retroperitoneal metastases), cough (pulmonary metastases), or lower extremity edema (vena cava obstruction).

A discrete mass or a diffuse testicular enlargement is noted in most cases. Secondary hydroceles may be present in 5–10% of cases. In advanced disease, supraclavicular adenopathy may be present, and abdominal examination may reveal a mass. Gynecomastia is seen in 5% of germ cell tumors.

B. Laboratory Findings

Several serum markers are important in the diagnosis and monitoring of testicular carcinoma, including human chorionic gonadotropin (hCG), α-fetoprotein, and LD. α-Fetoprotein is never elevated with pure seminomas, and while hCG is occasionally elevated in seminomas, levels tend to be lower than those seen with nonseminomas. LD may be elevated with either type of tumor and is a marker for disease burden. Liver tests may be elevated in the presence of hepatic metastases, and anemia may be present in advanced disease. As of 2025, a novel serum biomarker microRNA-371a-3p is emerging as new tool for surveillance of men with stage I testicular cancer after orchiectom.

C. Imaging

Scrotal ultrasound can readily determine whether a mass is intratesticular or extratesticular. Once the diagnosis of testicular cancer has been established by inguinal orchiectomy, clinical staging of the disease is accomplished by chest, abdominal, and pelvic CT scanning.

Staging

Testicular cancer is staged using the TNM system created based on extent of cancer in the testis, status of regional lymph nodes, the presence of metastases in distant lymph nodes or other viscera, and serum levels of tumor markers. Based on these features, germ cell tumors can be grouped to assign an overall stage: a stage I lesion is confined to the testis; a stage II lesion demonstrates regional lymph node involvement in the retroperitoneum; and a stage III lesion has distant metastasis.

Differential Diagnosis

An incorrect diagnosis is made at the initial examination in up to 25% of patients with testicular tumors. Scrotal ultrasonography should be performed if any uncertainty exists with respect to the diagnosis. Although most intratesticular masses are malignant, a benign lesion—epidermoid cyst—may rarely be seen. Epidermoid cysts are usually very small benign nodules located just underneath the tunica albuginea; occasionally, however, they can be large. Testicular lymphoma is discussed below.

Treatment

Inguinal exploration with early vascular control of the spermatic cord structures is the initial intervention. *If cancer cannot be excluded by examination of the testis, radical orchiectomy is warranted.* Scrotal approaches and open testicular biopsies should be avoided. Further therapy depends on the histology of the tumor as well as the clinical stage. Men treated for testis cancer are at risk for infertility and fertility preservation should be offered to all men with early referral to a specialist.

Patients with clinical stage I seminomas are candidates for surveillance (preferred), single-agent carboplatin, or adjuvant radiotherapy. Stage IIA and IIB seminomas (retroperitoneal disease < 2 cm diameter in IIA and 2–5 cm in IIB) are treated by radical orchiectomy plus retroperitoneal irradiation or primary systemic chemotherapy (etoposide and cisplatin or cisplatin, etoposide, and bleomycin) (Table 43–2). Seminomas of stage IIC (> 5-cm-diameter retroperitoneal nodes) and stage III receive primary systemic chemotherapy. After chemotherapy, surgical resection of residual retroperitoneal nodes is warranted if the node is > 3 cm in diameter and positive on PET scan, since 40% will harbor residual carcinoma.

Up to 75% of clinical stage I nonseminomas are cured by orchiectomy alone. Most patients without specific risk factors have low risk of recurrence and are generally offered surveillance after orchiectomy. These selection criteria include (1) cancer is confined within the tunica albuginea; (2) cancer does not demonstrate vascular invasion; (3) tumor markers normalize after orchiectomy; (4) radiographic imaging of the chest and abdomen shows no evidence of disease; and (5) the patient is reliable. Patients most likely to experience relapse on a surveillance regimen include those with predominantly embryonal cancer and those with vascular or lymphatic invasion identified in the orchiectomy specimen. Alternatives to surveillance for clinical stage I nonseminomas include adjuvant chemotherapy (bleomycin, etoposide, cisplatin) (Table 43–2) or retroperitoneal lymph node dissection.

Following orchiectomy, patients with metastatic disease are typically treated with combination chemotherapy (cisplatin and etoposide or cisplatin, etoposide, and bleomycin) (Table 43–2). Low-volume metastatic disease can be offered retroperitoneal lymph node dissection for seminomatous and non-seminomatous germ cell tumors. The Surgery in Early Metastatic Seminoma trial demonstrated an 81% 2-year recurrence-free survival with low morbidity in men with low-volume retroperitoneal metastatic seminoma treated with surgery alone. Low-volume, metastatic seminoma can also be offered radiation therapy. Nonseminomatous tumors are not sensitive to radiation therapy. With metastatic non-seminomatous germ cell cancers, if tumor markers normalize but a residual mass > 1 cm persists on imaging studies, it should be referred for surgical resection since 15–20% will harbor residual cancer and 40% will harbor teratomas. If tumor markers fail to normalize following primary chemotherapy, salvage chemotherapy is required (cisplatin, etoposide, and ifosfamide).

Postoperative active surveillance by the clinician and patient means patients are followed up every 2–6 months for the first 2 years and every 4–6 months in the third year. For nonseminomas, tumor markers are obtained at each visit, and CXRs and abdominal and pelvic CT scans are obtained every 4–6 months. For seminomas, serum tumor markers may be obtained (optional), chest imaging is obtained only as clinically indicated, and abdominal and pelvic CT scans are performed every 3–6 months. Follow-up continues beyond the initial 3 years; however, 80% of relapses will occur within the first 2 years. With rare exceptions, patients who relapse can be cured by chemotherapy or surgery.

Prognosis

The 5-year disease-free survival rates for stage I and IIA seminomas (retroperitoneal disease < 2 cm in diameter) treated by radical orchiectomy and retroperitoneal irradiation are 98% and 92–94%, respectively. Ninety-five percent of patients with stage III disease attain a complete response following orchiectomy and chemotherapy. The 5-year disease-free survival rate for patients with stage I nonseminomas (includes all treatments) ranges from 96–100%. For low-volume stage II disease, a 5-year disease-free survival of 90% is expected. Patients with bulky retroperitoneal or disseminated disease treated with primary chemotherapy followed by surgery have a 5-year disease-free survival rate of 55–80%.

When to Refer

Refer all patients with solid masses of the testis to a urologist and a medical oncologist if metastatic disease is suspected.

Belge G et al. Detection of recurrence through microRNA-371a-3p serum levels in a follow-up of stage I testicular germ cell tumors in the DRKS-00019223 study. Clin Cancer Res. 2024;30:404. [PMID: 37967143]

Daneshmand S et al. Surgery in early metastatic seminoma: a phase II trial of retroperitoneal lymph node dissection for testicular seminoma with limited retroperitoneal lymphadenopathy. J Clin Onc. 2023;41:3009. [PMID: 36913642]

SECONDARY CANCERS OF THE TESTIS

Secondary cancers of the testis are rare. In men over the age of 50 years, lymphoma is the most common. Overall, it is the most common secondary neoplasm of the testis, accounting for 5% of all testicular cancers. It may be seen in three clinical settings: (1) late manifestation of widespread lymphoma, (2) the initial presentation of clinically occult disease, and (3) primary extranodal disease. Radical orchiectomy is indicated to make the diagnosis. Prognosis is related to the stage of disease.

Metastasis to the testis is rare. The most common primary site of origin is the prostate, followed by the lung, GI tract, melanoma, and kidney.

CANCER COMPLICATIONS & EMERGENCIES

SPINAL CORD COMPRESSION

ESSENTIALS OF DIAGNOSIS

- Complication of metastatic solid tumor, lymphoma, or plasma cell myeloma.
- Back pain is the most common presenting symptom.
- Prompt diagnosis is essential because once a severe neurologic deficit develops, it is often irreversible.
- Emergent treatment may prevent or potentially reverse paresis and urinary and bowel incontinence.

General Considerations

Cancers that cause spinal cord compression most commonly metastasize to the vertebral bodies, resulting in physical damage to the spinal cord from edema, hemorrhage, and pressure-induced ischemia to its vasculature. Persistent compression can result in irreversible changes to the myelin sheaths resulting in permanent neurologic impairment.

Prompt diagnosis and therapeutic intervention are essential. Patients who are treated promptly after symptoms appear may have partial or complete return of function and, depending on tumor sensitivity to specific treatment, may respond favorably to subsequent anticancer therapy.

Clinical Findings

A. Symptoms and Signs

Back pain at the level of the tumor mass occurs in over 80% of cases and may be aggravated by lying down, weight bearing, sneezing, or coughing; it usually precedes the development of neurologic symptoms or signs. Since involvement is usually epidural, a mixture of nerve root and spinal cord symptoms often develops. Progressive weakness and sensory changes commonly occur. Bowel and bladder symptoms progressing to incontinence are late findings.

The initial findings of impending cord compression may be quite subtle, and there should be a high index of suspicion when back pain or weakness of the lower extremities develops in a patient with cancer.

B. Imaging

MRI is usually the initial imaging procedure of choice in a patient with cancer and new-onset back pain.

When neurologic findings suggest spinal cord compression, an emergent MRI should be obtained; the MRI should survey the entire spine to define all areas of tumor involvement for treatment planning purposes. MRI has a sensitivity of 93% and a specificity of 97% for diagnosis of metastatic spinal cord compression.

Treatment

Patients with a known cancer diagnosis found to have epidural impingement of the spinal cord should be given corticosteroids immediately. The initial dexamethasone dose is 10 mg intravenously followed by 4–6 mg every 6 hours intravenously or orally. Patients without a known diagnosis of cancer should have emergent surgery to relieve the impingement and obtain a pathologic specimen; preoperative corticosteroids should not be given since they might compromise the pathology results. Treatment planning requires consideration of spinal stability, radiosensitivity of tumor type, low- versus high-grade epidural spinal cord compression, and extent of multilevel involvement. *Patients with solid tumors who have a single area of compression and who are considered candidates for surgery are best treated first with surgical decompression followed by radiation therapy. If multiple vertebral body levels are involved with cancer, radiation therapy is the preferred treatment option.*

Hershkovich O et al. Acute metastatic spinal cord compression: urgent surgery versus radiotherapy and treatment result prediction versus actual results. Curr Oncol. 2022;29:7420. [PMID: 36290860]

Moreno DAV et al. Comprehensive guide to the diagnosis, management, and treatment of metastatic spinal cord compression syndrome. Surg Oncol. 2026:64:102341. [PMID: 41412011]

Vavourakis M et al. Comprehensive insights into metastasis-associated spinal cord compression: pathophysiology, diagnosis, treatment, and prognosis: a state-of-the-art systematic review. J Clin Med. 2024;13:3590. [PMID: 38930119]

MALIGNANT EFFUSIONS

ESSENTIALS OF DIAGNOSIS

- Occur in pleural, pericardial, and peritoneal spaces.
- Caused by direct neoplastic involvement of serous surface or obstruction of lymphatic drainage.
- Half of undiagnosed effusions in patients not known to have cancer are malignant.

General Considerations

The development of an effusion in the pleural, pericardial, or peritoneal space may be the initial finding in a patient with cancer, or an effusion may appear during the course of disease progression. Direct involvement of the serous surface with tumor is the most frequent initiating cause of the accumulation of fluid. The most common malignancies causing pleural and pericardial effusions are lung and breast cancers; the most common malignancies associated with malignant ascites are ovarian, colorectal, stomach, and pancreatic cancers.

Clinical Findings

A. Symptoms and Signs

Patients with pleural and pericardial effusions complain of shortness of breath and orthopnea. Patients with ascites complain of abdominal distention and discomfort. Cardiac tamponade causing pressure equalization in the chambers impairs both filling and cardiac output and can be life-threatening. Signs of tamponade include tachycardia, muffled heart sounds, pulsus paradoxus, and hypotension. Signs of pleural effusions include decreased breath sounds, egophony, and percussion dullness.

B. Laboratory Findings

Malignancy is confirmed as the cause of an effusion when analysis of the fluid specimen shows malignant cells in either the cytology or cell block specimen. However, the diagnostic sensitivity of fluid cytology is often low, depending on the cancer type.

C. Imaging

The presence of effusions can be confirmed with radiographic studies or ultrasonography.

Differential Diagnosis

The differential diagnosis of a malignant pleural or pericardial effusion includes nonmalignant processes, such as infection, PE, HF, and trauma. The differential diagnosis of malignant ascites includes similar benign processes, such as HF, cirrhosis, peritonitis, and pancreatic ascites. Bloody effusions are usually due to cancer, but a bloody pleural effusion can also be due to PE, trauma and, occasionally, infection. Chylous pleural or ascitic fluid is generally associated with obstruction of lymphatic drainage as might occur in lymphoma.

Treatment

The development of a malignant effusion is a late-stage manifestation of the cancer. Treatment is tailored to the underlying cancer, whether with targeted therapy, chemotherapy, or immunotherapy, depending on tumor testing results. Effective systemic treatment can lead to regression of the effusion. Acute symptoms related to the effusion often require urgent intervention with drainage of the effusion. Decisions regarding palliative management of malignant effusion are in large part dictated by the patient's symptoms and goals of care.

A. Pleural Effusion

A pleural effusion that is symptomatic may be managed initially with a *large-volume thoracentesis.* In some patients, the effusion slowly reaccumulates, which allows for periodic thoracentesis when the patient becomes symptomatic. However, in many patients, the effusion reaccumulates quickly, causing rapid return of shortness of breath. For those patients, two management options exist: *pleurodesis* or *indwelling pleural catheter* (eg, PleurX). In a meta-analysis of RCTs comparing indwelling pleural catheter with pleurodesis, indwelling pleural catheters resulted in shorter hospital stays and fewer repeat pleural interventions, but increased rates of cellulitis.

B. Pericardial Effusion

Fluid may be removed by needle aspiration or by placement of a catheter for more thorough drainage. As with pleural effusions, most pericardial effusions will reaccumulate. Management options for recurrent, symptomatic effusions include prolonged *catheter drainage* or surgical intervention such as a *pericardiotomy or pericardiectomy.*

C. Malignant Ascites

Patients with malignant ascites not responsive to chemotherapy are generally treated with *repeated large-volume paracenteses.* Since the frequency of drainage to maintain comfort can compromise the patient's quality of life, other alternatives include placement of a *catheter or port* so that the patient or caregiver can drain fluid as needed at home. For patients with portal hypertension from large hepatic masses, *diuretics may be useful to decrease the need for repeated paracentesis.*

Addala DN et al. Malignant pleural effusion: updates in diagnosis, management and current challenges. Front Oncol. 2022;12:1053574. [PMID: 36465336]
Martinez-Zayas G et al. Sensitivity and complications of thoracentesis and thoracoscopy: a meta-analysis. Eur Respir Rev. 2022;31:220053. [PMID: 36543349]
Westley R et al. Updates in the management of malignant pleural effusion: a clinical practice review. J Thorac Dis. 2025;17:6283. [PMID: 40950873]

HYPERCALCEMIA

ESSENTIALS OF DIAGNOSIS

- Most common paraneoplastic endocrine syndrome.
- Usually symptomatic and severe (≥ 15 mg/dL [3.75 mmol/L]); accounts for most inpatients with hypercalcemia.
- The neoplasm is clinically apparent in nearly all cases when hypercalcemia is detected.

General Considerations

Hypercalcemia affects 20–30% of patients with cancer at some point during their illness. The most common cancers causing hypercalcemia are myeloma, breast carcinoma, and NSCLC. Hypercalcemia is caused by one of three mechanisms: systemic effects of tumor-released proteins, direct osteolysis of bone by tumor, vitamin D–mediated osteoabsorption, or ectopic hyperparathyroidism.

Clinical Findings

A. Symptoms and Signs

Symptoms and signs of hypercalcemia can be subtle; more severe symptoms occur with higher levels of hypercalcemia and with a rapidly rising calcium level. Early symptoms typically include anorexia, nausea, fatigue, constipation, and polyuria; later findings may include muscular weakness and hyporeflexia, confusion, psychosis, tremor, and lethargy.

B. Laboratory Findings

Symptoms and signs are caused by free calcium; as calcium is bound by protein in the serum, *the measured serum calcium will underestimate the free or ionized calcium in patients with low albumin levels.* Free ionized calcium can be measured. When the corrected serum calcium rises above 12 mg/dL (3 mmol/L), especially if the rise occurs rapidly, sudden death due to cardiac arrhythmia or asystole may occur. Initial workup for hypercalcemia includes obtaining serum PTH, PTHrP, and calcitriol (1,25-dihydroxycholecalciferol) levels.

C. ECG

ECG in hypercalcemia often shows a shortening of the QT interval.

Treatment

Emergency management should begin with the initiation of *intravenous fluids* with 0.9% saline at 100–300 mL/h to ensure rehydration with brisk urinary output of the often volume-depleted patient. For moderate or severe hypercalcemia, treatment with *bisphosphonate* or *denosumab* (humanized monoclonal antibody to RANKL) is indicated. Bisphosphonates can be given if kidney function is normal or only marginally impaired. Choices include pamidronate or zoledronic acid. Denosumab is also the preferred choice for the management of bisphosphonate-refractory hypercalcemia or for patients with kidney dysfunction. Once hypercalcemia is controlled, treatment directed at the cancer should be initiated if possible. If hypercalcemia becomes refractory to bisphosphonates or denosumab, other agents include *calcitonin* or *corticosteroids.* Salmon calcitonin can be used in patients with severe, symptomatic hypercalcemia.

Fuleihan GE et al. Treatment of hypercalcemia of malignancy in adults: an Endocrine Society clinical practice guideline. Clin Endocrinol Metab. 2023;108:507. [PMID: 36545746]
Guise TA et al. Cancer-associated hypercalcemia. N Engl J Med. 2022;386:1443. Erratum in: N Engl J Med. 2022;387:96. [PMID: 35417639]
Walker MD et al. Hypercalcemia: a review. JAMA. 2022;328:1624. [PMID: 36282253]

HYPERURICEMIA & TUMOR LYSIS SYNDROME

ESSENTIALS OF DIAGNOSIS

- Complication of treatment-associated tumor lysis of hematologic and rapidly proliferating malignancies.
- May be worsened by thiazide diuretics.
- Rapid increase in serum uric acid can cause acute urate nephropathy from uric acid crystallization.
- Reducing pre-chemotherapy serum uric acid is fundamental to preventing urate nephropathy.

General Considerations

Tumor lysis syndrome (TLS) is seen most commonly following treatment of hematologic malignancies but can develop from any tumor highly sensitive to chemotherapy. TLS is caused by the massive release of cellular material including nucleic acids, proteins, phosphorus, and potassium. If both the metabolism and excretion of these breakdown products are impaired, hyperuricemia, hyperphosphatemia, and hyperkalemia will develop abruptly. AKI may then develop from the crystallization and deposition of uric acid and calcium phosphate within the renal tubules, further exacerbating the hyperphosphatemia and hyperkalemia.

Clinical Findings

A. Symptoms and Signs

Symptoms of hyperphosphatemia include nausea, vomiting, anorexia, muscle cramps, tetany, and seizures. High levels of phosphorus and co-precipitation with calcium can cause renal tubule blockage, further exacerbating the kidney injury. Hyperkalemia, due to release of intracellular potassium and impaired kidney excretion, can cause arrhythmias and sudden death.

B. Laboratory Findings

The laboratory diagnosis of TLS includes at least two of the following criteria observed within a 24-hour period: uric acid 8 mg/dL or higher (476 mcmol/L or higher), phosphate 4.5 mg/dL or higher (1.45 mmol/L or higher), potassium 6.0 mEq/L or more (6 mmol/L or more) (or a 25% increase from baseline for these parameters), and corrected serum calcium 7 mg/dL or lower (1.75 mmol/L or lower). A clinical diagnosis of TLS includes meeting the laboratory criteria and at least one clinical criterion: AKI (creatinine $\geq 1.5 \times$ upper limit of normal or increase > 0.3 g/dL or cardiac arrhythmia, sudden cardiac death, or seizure.

Treatment

Prevention is the most important factor in the management of TLS. Aggressive hydration at least 24 hours prior to chemotherapy as well as 24–48 hours after chemotherapy completion helps keep urine flowing and facilitates excretion of uric acid and phosphorus. It is recommended to maintain a urinary output of at least 100 mL/hour, and a daily urine volume of at least 3 L/day. For patients at moderate risk of developing TLS, eg, those with intermediate-grade lymphomas and acute leukemias, allopurinol should be given before starting chemotherapy with dose reductions for impaired kidney function. Rasburicase also is given intravenously to patients at high risk for developing TLS such as those with high-grade lymphomas or acute leukemias with markedly elevated WBC counts. Rasburicase cannot be given to patients with known glucose 6-phosphate dehydrogenase (G6PD) deficiency nor can it be given to pregnant or lactating women.

When to Refer

- Should urinary output drop, serum creatinine or potassium levels rise, or hyperphosphatemia persist, a nephrologist should be immediately consulted to evaluate the need for dialysis.

Bociek RG et al. Tumor lysis syndrome. N Engl J Med. 2025;393:1104. [PMID: 40961427]

Latcha S et al. Rescue therapies for AKI in onconephrology: rasburicase and glucarpidase. Semin Nephrol. 2022;42:151342. [PMID: 37167817]

Li D et al. Assessing the risk of tumor lysis syndrome associated with the use of antineoplastic agents: a real-world pharmacovigilance study based on the FDA Adverse Event Reporting System database. Ther Adv Drug Saf. 2024:15:20420986241274909. [PMID: 39247253]

INFECTIONS

Chapter 34 provide more detailed discussions of infections in the immunocompromised patient.

ESSENTIALS OF DIAGNOSIS

- In patients with neutropenia, infection is a medical emergency.
- Although sometimes attributable to other causes, the presence of fever, defined as a single temperature > 38.3°C (101°F) or a temperature of > 38°C (100.4°F) for > 1 hour, must be assumed to be due to an infection.

General Considerations

Many patients with disseminated neoplasms have increased susceptibility to infection. In some patients, this results from impaired defense mechanisms due to the underlying malignancy; in others, it results from the myelosuppressive and immunosuppressive effects of cancer chemotherapy or a combination of these factors. Patients with cancer are at higher risk for infection.

The source of a neutropenic febrile episode is determined in about 30% of cases through blood, urine, or sputum cultures. The bacterial organisms accounting for most infections in patients with cancer include gram-positive bacteria and gram-negative bacteria. Gram-positive organism infections are more common, but gram-negative infections are more serious and life-threatening. The risk of bacterial infections rises when the neutrophil count is below 500/mcL (0.5×10^9/L); the risk markedly increases when the count falls below 100/mcL (0.1×10^9/L) or when there is a prolonged duration of neutropenia, typically > 7 days.

Clinical Findings

A thorough physical examination should be performed. Appropriate cultures (eg, blood, sputum, urine and, if indicated, CSF) and COVID-19 testing should always be obtained. Two sets of blood cultures should be drawn before starting antibiotics; if the patient has an indwelling catheter, one of the cultures should be drawn from the line. A CXR should also be obtained.

Treatment

Empiric antibiotic therapy needs to be initiated within 1 hour of presentation and following the collection of blood cultures in the febrile neutropenic patient. The choice of antibiotics depends on a number of different factors including the patient's clinical status and any localizing source of infection. If the patient is clinically well, monotherapy with an intravenous β-lactam with anti-*Pseudomonas* activity (cefepime, ceftazidime, imipenem/cilastatin, piperacillin/tazobactam) should be started (see Infections in the Immunocompromised Patient, Chapter 34). If the patient is clinically ill with hypotension or hypoxia, an intravenous aminoglycoside or fluoroquinolone should be added for "double" gram-negative bacteria coverage. If there is a strong suspicion of a gram-positive organism, such as from a *S aureus* catheter infection, intravenous vancomycin can be given empirically. Low-risk patients may be treated with oral antibiotics in the outpatient setting.

Antibiotics should be continued until the neutrophil count is rising and > 500/mcL (0.5×10^9/L) for at least 1 day and the patient has been afebrile for 2 days. If an organism is identified through the cultures, the antibiotics should be adjusted to the antibiotic sensitivities of the isolate; treatment should be continued for the appropriate period of time and at least until the neutrophil count recovers and fever resolves.

Averbuch D et al. Empirical and targeted antimicrobial therapy in patients with febrile neutropenia and haematological malignancy or after haematopoietic cell transplantation: recommendations from the 10th European Conference on Infections in Leukaemia. Lancet Infect Dis. 2025 Nov 25:S1473. [Epub ahead of print] [PMID: 41314221]

Keck JM et al. Approach to fever in patients with neutropenia: a review of diagnosis and management. Ther Adv Infect Dis. 2022;9:20499361221138346. [PMID: 36451936]

Zimmer AJ et al. Bloodstream infections in hematologic malignancy patients with fever and neutropenia: are empirical antibiotic therapies in the United States still effective? Open Forum Infect Dis. 2022;9:ofac240. [PMID: 35854988]

PRIMARY CANCER TREATMENT

SYSTEMIC CANCER THERAPY

Detailed guidelines from the NCCN for cancer treatment can be found at www.nccn.org.

Use of cytotoxic medications, immunotherapy, hormones, antihormones, and biologic agents has become a highly specialized and increasingly effective means of treating cancer, with therapy administered and monitored by a medical oncologist or hematologist. Selection of specific medications or protocols for various types of cancer is based on results of clinical trials. Increasingly, agents are being identified that target specific molecular pathways or modulate the immune system. (See Table 43–2 for suggested agents for various cancers).

TOXICITY & DOSE MODIFICATION OF CHEMOTHERAPEUTIC AGENTS

Use of chemotherapy to treat cancer is generally guided by results from clinical trials in individual tumor types. Medication side effects and toxicities must be anticipated and carefully monitored. The short- and long-term toxicities of individual medications are listed in Tables 43–3 and 43–16.

A CBC including a differential count, with absolute neutrophil count and platelet count, and liver and kidney tests should be obtained before the initiation of chemotherapy and at regular intervals. *When the intent of chemotherapy is cure, including treatment in the adjuvant setting, every attempt should be made to schedule chemotherapy on time and at full dose.* A schema for dose modification is shown in Table 43–17.

1. Bone Marrow Toxicity

A. Neutropenia

Granulocyte colony-stimulating factor (G-CSF), given as either daily subcutaneous injections (eg, filgrastim, 300 mcg or 480 mcg) or as a one-time dose (pegfilgrastim, 6 mg) after cytotoxic chemotherapy is completed, reduces the duration and severity of granulocytopenia following cytotoxic chemotherapy (Table 43–16). The American Society of Clinical Oncology and NCCN guidelines recommend primary prophylaxis with G-CSF when there is at least a 20% risk of febrile neutropenia or when age, medical history, and disease characteristics put the patient at high risk for complications related to myelosuppression.

B. Anemia

Erythropoiesis-stimulating agents ameliorate the anemia and its associated symptoms caused by cancer chemotherapy but these medications have untoward effects, including an increased risk of thromboembolism, and possibly a decreased survival due to cancer-related deaths, as well as a shortened time to tumor progression. The FDA recommends that these medications should *not* be used when the intent of chemotherapy is curative. Administration of RBC transfusions is an alternative for managing symptomatic anemia in chemotherapy patients.

Table 43–16. Commonly used supportive care agents[1] (listed in alphabetical order, with categories).

Agent	Indication	Usual Dose	Adverse Effects
Bone-Modifying Agents			
Denosumab (Xgeva)	Osteolytic bone metastasis	120 mg subcutaneously every 4 weeks	Acute: nausea Delayed: hypocalcemia, hypophosphatemia, fatigue, osteonecrosis of the jaw
Zoledronic acid (Zometa)	Osteolytic bone metastasis, hypercalcemia of malignancy	4 mg intravenously every 3–4 weeks; 4 mg intravenously once, may repeat after 7 days	Acute: nausea Delayed: dyspnea, arthralgia, bone pain, osteonecrosis of the jaw, nephrotoxicity, hypocalcemia
Growth Factors			
Darbepoetin alfa (Aranesp)	Chemotherapy-induced anemia	2.25 mcg/kg subcutaneously weekly; 500 mcg subcutaneously every 3 weeks	Acute: injection site reaction Delayed: hypertension, thromboembolic events, increased risk of tumor progression or recurrence
Epoetin alfa (Epogen, Procrit)	Chemotherapy-induced anemia	40,000 U subcutaneously once weekly; 150 U/kg subcutaneously three times a week	Acute: injection site reaction Delayed: hypertension, thromboembolic events, increased risk of tumor progression or recurrence
Filgrastim (Neupogen)	Febrile neutropenia prophylaxis, mobilization of peripheral stem cells	5–10 mcg/kg/day subcutaneously or intravenously once daily, treat past nadir	Acute: injection site reaction Delayed: bone pain
Pegfilgrastim (Neulasta)	Febrile neutropenia prophylaxis	6 mg subcutaneously once per chemotherapy cycle	Acute: injection site reaction Delayed: bone pain
Miscellaneous Agents			
Allopurinol (Xyloprim)	Prevent hyperuricemia from tumor lysis syndrome	600–800 mg/day orally	Acute: none Delayed: rash
Leucovorin	Rescue after high-dose methotrexate; in combination with 5-fluorouracil for colon cancer	10 mg/m^2 intravenously or orally every 6 hours; 20 mg/m^2 or 200–500 mg/m^2 intravenously before 5-fluorouracil; various doses	Acute: nausea, vomiting, diarrhea Delayed: stomatitis, fatigue
Mesna (Mesnex)	Prevent ifosfamide-induced hemorrhagic cystitis	20% of ifosfamide dose intravenously at 0, 4, and 8 hours; various doses	Acute: nausea, vomiting Delayed: fatigue
Rasburicase (Elitek)	Prevent hyperuricemia from tumor lysis syndrome	3–6 mg intravenously once	Acute: hypersensitivity, nausea, vomiting, diarrhea, fever, headache Delayed: rash, peripheral edema

[1]For amifostine, levoleucovorin, pilocarpine, samarium, strontium, pamidronate, sargramostim, dexrazoxane, palifermin, radium, filgrastim-sndz, and tbo-filgrastim, see Table 43–16 in *CMDT Online* at www.accessmedicine.com.

Table 43–17. A common schema for dose modification of cancer chemotherapeutic agents.

Granulocyte Count	Platelet Count	Suggested Drug Dosage (% of Full Dose)
> 2000 cells/mcL (2 × 10^9/L)	> 100,000/mcL (100 × 10^9/L)	100%
1000–2000 cells/mcL (1–2 × 10^9/L)	75,000–100,000/mcL (75–100 × 10^9/L)	50%
< 1000 cells/mcL (1 × 10^9/L)	< 50,000/mcL (50 × 10^9/L)	0%

Erythropoiesis-stimulating agents can be an option in patients with cancer and symptomatic anemia undergoing palliative treatment; patient preference is important in determining when to use erythropoiesis-stimulating agents or transfusions. When using erythropoiesis-stimulating agents, treatment should not be initiated until the hemoglobin is < 10 g/dL (100 g/L) and the agent held when the hemoglobin is > 12 g/dL (120 g/L). To have maximum therapeutic effect, patients need to be iron replete.

C. Thrombocytopenia

Pharmacologic management of chemotherapy-induced thrombocytopenia is more limited. Two medications that activate the thrombopoietin receptor, romiplostim and eltrombopag, are

FDA-approved only for use in idiopathic thrombocytopenia, thrombocytopenia related to interferon therapy of hepatitis C, and thrombocytopenia in aplastic anemia.

2. Chemotherapy-Induced Nausea & Vomiting

Several cytotoxic anticancer medications can induce nausea and vomiting, which can be the most anticipated and stressful side effects for patients. Chemotherapy induced nausea and vomiting is mediated in part by the stimulation of at least two CNS receptors, 5-hydroxytryptamine subtype 3 ($5HT_3$) and neurokinin subtype 1 (NK_1). Chemotherapy-induced nausea and vomiting can be *anticipatory*, occurring even before chemotherapy administration; *acute*, occurring within minutes to hours of chemotherapy administration; or *delayed*, lasting up to 7 days. *Chemotherapy drugs are classified into high, moderate, low, and minimal likelihoods of causing emesis.* Highly emetogenic chemotherapy medications include cisplatin, cyclophosphamide, and anthracyclines. Moderately emetogenic chemotherapy drugs include azacitidine, carboplatin, cytarabine, and oxaliplatin. Low emetogenic medications include bortezomib, etoposide, gemcitabine, methotrexate, and paclitaxel. Medications with minimal risk of emesis include bevacizumab, cetuximab, rituximab, and trastuzumab.

Major advances have occurred in the development of highly effective antiemetic drugs. Antagonists to the $5HT_3$-receptor include alosetron, granisetron, ondansetron, and palonosetron. As a class of drugs, the $5HT_3$-receptor antagonists have the potential to cause ECG changes, including QT prolongation. Antagonists to the NK_1-receptor are aprepitant, fosaprepitant, and netupitant.

For highly emetogenic chemotherapy (eg, cisplatin), patients should be offered a four-drug regimen (a $5HT_3$-antagonist, dexamethasone, NK_1-receptor antagonist, and olanzapine), all given on the first day. For moderately emetogenic chemotherapy, standard regimens include both three-drug regimens (an NK_1-antagonist, a $5HT_3$-antagonist, and dexamethasone) or a two-drug combination ($5HT_3$-antagonist and dexamethasone). For low emetogenic chemotherapy drugs, a single agent such as a $5HT_3$-antagonist or prochlorperazine or dexamethasone can be given. Olanzapine is helpful for anticipatory or refractory nausea and vomiting.

The importance of treating chemotherapy-induced nausea and vomiting expectantly and aggressively beginning with the first course of chemotherapy cannot be overemphasized. Patients being treated in the clinic setting should always be given antiemetics for home use with written instructions as well as contact numbers to call for advice.

3. Gastrointestinal Toxicity

Untoward effects of cancer chemotherapy include damage to the more rapidly growing cells of the body such as the mucosal lining from the mouth through the GI tract. Oral symptoms range from mild mouth soreness to frank ulcerations. Not uncommonly, mouth ulcerations will have superimposed candida or herpes simplex infections. In addition to receiving cytotoxic chemotherapy, a significant risk factor for development of oral mucositis is poor oral hygiene and existing caries or periodontal disease. Patients undergoing treatment for head and neck cancer with concurrent chemotherapy and radiation therapy have a very high risk of developing severe mucositis. Toxicity in the GI tract usually manifests as diarrhea. GI symptoms can range from mild symptoms of loose stools to life-threatening diarrhea leading to dehydration and electrolyte imbalances. Medications most commonly associated with causing mucositis in the mouth and the GI tract are cytarabine, 5-fluorouracil, and methotrexate.

Preventive strategies for oral mucositis include pretreatment dental care, particularly for all patients with head and neck cancer and any patient with cancer and poor dental hygiene who will be receiving chemotherapy. Once mucositis is encountered, superimposed fungal infections should be treated with antifungal medications. Suspected herpetic infections can be treated with acyclovir or valacyclovir. Mucositis may also be managed with mouthwashes; it is also important to provide adequate pain medication.

Diarrhea is most associated with 5-fluorouracil, capecitabine, and irinotecan as well as the tyrosine kinase inhibitors (dasatinib, imatinib, sorafenib, sunitinib) and epithelial growth factor inhibitors (cetuximab, erlotinib). Mild to moderate diarrhea due to cytotoxic chemotherapy not related to immunotherapy, can be managed with oral antidiarrheal medication. Occasionally, severe diarrhea will cause dehydration, electrolyte imbalances, and AKI; these patients require inpatient management with aggressive intravenous hydration and electrolyte replacement. Diarrhea associated with checkpoint inhibitors is concerning for immune-related colitis and warrants workup to rule out infection. Consider a referral to a gastroenterologist for colonoscopy, an abdominal CT scan, and a trial of corticosteroids for grade 2 and higher diarrhea. Consider permanent discontinuation of the checkpoint inhibitor for grade 3 and higher diarrhea, especially any one of the CTLA-4 inhibitors.

4. Miscellaneous Drug-Specific Toxicities

The toxicities of individual drugs are summarized in Tables 43–3 and 43–16; however, several of these toxicities warrant additional mention, since they occur with frequently administered agents, and special measures are often indicated.

A. Neuropathy Due to Vinca Alkaloids and Other Chemotherapy Drugs

Neuropathy is caused by a number of different chemotherapy medications. The peripheral neuropathy can be sensory, motor, autonomic, or a combination of these types. In its mildest form, it consists of paresthesias of the fingers and toes. With continued therapy, the paresthesias can extend to the proximal interphalangeal joints, hyporeflexia appears in the lower extremities, and significant weakness can develop. Other drugs in the vinca alkaloid class as well as the taxane drugs (docetaxel and paclitaxel) and agents to treat myeloma (bortezomib and thalidomide) cause similar toxicity.

Constipation is the most common symptom of autonomic neuropathy associated with the vinca alkaloids.

Patients receiving these medications should be started on mild cathartics (eg, senna and polyethylene glycol [MiraLAX]) and other agents (see Table 17–4); otherwise, severe impaction may result from an atonic bowel.

B. Cardiotoxicity from Anthracyclines and Other Chemotherapy Drugs

A number of cancer medications are associated with cardiovascular complications, including (1) traditional chemotherapeutics (such as anthracyclines); (2) HER2 inhibitors (such as pertuzumab, trastuzumab); (3) VEGF signaling pathway inhibitors (eg, bevacizumab, lenvatinib, ramucirumab, sunitinib); (4) tyrosine kinase inhibitors (eg, dasatinib, nilotinib, osimertinib, lenvatinib, axitinib); (5) proteasome inhibitors (bortezomib, carfilzomib); and (6) immune checkpoint inhibitors (atezolizumab, ipilimumab, nivolumab, pembrolizumab).

The anthracycline medications can produce acute, subacute (days to months following administration), and delayed (years following administration) cardiac toxicity. *The most feared complication is the delayed development of HF. Patients receiving anthracyclines should have an assessment of LVEF.* If the LVEF is > 50%, anthracyclines can be administered; if the LVEF is < 30%, these medications should not be given. For patients with intermediate values, anthracyclines can be cautiously given, if necessary, at lower doses with LVEF monitoring between doses.

C. Cisplatin Nephrotoxicity and Neurotoxicity

Cisplatin is effective in treating testicular, bladder, head and neck, lung, and ovarian cancers. With cisplatin, the serious side effects of nephrotoxicity and neurotoxicity must be anticipated and aggressively managed. Patients must be vigorously hydrated prior to, during, and after cisplatin administration. Both kidney function and electrolytes must be monitored. The neurotoxicity is usually manifested as a peripheral neuropathy of mixed sensorimotor type and may be associated with painful paresthesias. Ototoxicity is a potentially serious manifestation of neurotoxicity and can progress to deafness. The second-generation platinum analog carboplatin is non-nephrotoxic, although it is myelosuppressive. In the setting of preexisting kidney disease or neuropathy, carboplatin can be substituted for cisplatin for some indications.

D. Immune Checkpoint Inhibitor–Associated Toxicity

Cancer immunotherapy has revolutionized cancer care. The modalities of cancer immunotherapeutics include checkpoint inhibition, adoptive cellular therapy, and cancer vaccines. As an example, consider checkpoint inhibition. Checkpoint inhibitors include PD-1 inhibitors such as pembrolizumab, nivolumab, cemiplimab and dostarlimab, and PD-L1 inhibitors such as atezolizumab, avelumab, and durvalumab. The PD-1 pathway limits the immune response through inhibitory intracellular signaling in effector and regulatory T cells and induces T-cell exhaustion. Thus, inhibitors of PD-1 or PD-L1 release T cells from the inhibitory signals they receive from tumor cells via the PD-1 pathway, restoring antitumor immunity. Cytotoxic T lymphocyte antigen 4 (CTLA4) is another negative regulator of T-cell activation. Ipilimumab is a recombinant human IgG1 immunoglobulin monoclonal antibody to CTLA4. CTLA4 blockade by ipilimumab results in T-cell activation and proliferation, and enhanced antitumor activity. Checkpoint inhibitors play key roles in multiple types of cancer, including melanoma, lung, bladder, kidney, esophageal, and triple-negative breast cancers.

Checkpoint inhibition, however, can lead to significant **immunotherapy-related adverse events (irAEs).** Autoimmune damage can occur in any organ or system of the body. *The most common irAEs include thyroiditis, dermatitis, colitis, hepatitis, and arthritis. Pneumonitis is an uncommon but serious irAE.* Grading of AEs is based on Common Terminology Criteria for Adverse Events (CTCAE). Mild grade 1 toxicities can be followed except for certain neurologic, hematologic, and cardiac toxicities. For grade 2 or higher irAEs, checkpoint inhibitors are held until resolution of the adverse event, and depending on the severity of the irAE, may need to be permanently discontinued. Rarely, fulminant and life-threatening toxicities can occur. *Glucocorticoids are the mainstay in management of irAEs, and if the event is refractory to steroids, infliximab and other immunosuppressive agents can be employed.*

PROGNOSIS

Patients receiving therapy for curative intent will often tolerate side effects with the knowledge that the treatment may result in eradication of their cancer. Patients receiving therapy for palliative intent often have their therapy tailored to improve quality of life while minimizing major side effects. A valuable sign of clinical improvement is the *general well-being* of the patient.

Naidoo J et al. Society for Immunotherapy of Cancer (SITC) consensus definitions for immune checkpoint inhibitor-associated immune-related adverse events (irAEs) terminology. J Immunother Cancer. 2023;11:e006398. [PMID: 37001909]

Shil S et al. Cancer therapy-induced cardiotoxicity: mechanisms and mitigations. Heart Fail Rev. 2025;30:1075. [PMID: 40481994]

Yan T et al. Achilles' heel of currently approved immune checkpoint inhibitors: immune related adverse events. Front Immunol. 2024:15:1292122. [PMID: 38410506]

Genetic & Genomic Disorders

44

Reed E. Pyeritz, MD, PhD

ACUTE INTERMITTENT PORPHYRIA

ESSENTIALS OF DIAGNOSIS

- Unexplained abdominal crisis, generally in young women.
- Acute peripheral or CNS dysfunction; recurrent psychiatric illnesses.
- Hyponatremia.
- Porphobilinogen in the urine during an attack.

General Considerations

Though there are several different types of porphyrias, the one with the most serious consequences and that usually presents in adulthood is **acute intermittent porphyria (AIP)**, which is inherited as an autosomal dominant condition, though it remains clinically silent in most patients who carry a pathogenic variant in *HMBS*. Clinical illness usually develops in women. Symptoms begin in the teens or 20s, but onset can begin after menopause in rare cases. The disorder is caused by partial deficiency of hydroxymethylbilane synthase activity, leading to increased excretion of aminolevulinic acid and porphobilinogen in the urine. The diagnosis may be elusive if not specifically considered. *The characteristic abdominal pain may be due to abnormalities in autonomic innervation in the gut.* In contrast to other forms of porphyria, cutaneous photosensitivity is absent in AIP. Attacks are precipitated by numerous factors, including drugs and intercurrent infections. Hyponatremia may occur, due in part to inappropriate release of ADH, although GI loss of sodium in some patients may be a contributing factor.

Clinical Findings

A. Symptoms and Signs

Patients show intermittent abdominal pain of varying severity, and in some instances, it may so simulate an acute abdomen as to lead to exploratory laparotomy. *Because the origin of the abdominal pain is neurologic, there is an absence of fever and leukocytosis.* Complete recovery between attacks is usual. Any part of the nervous system may be involved, with evidence for central, autonomic, and peripheral neuropathy. Peripheral neuropathy may be symmetric or asymmetric and mild or profound; in the latter instance, it can even lead to quadriplegia with respiratory paralysis. Other CNS manifestations include seizures, altered consciousness, psychosis, and abnormalities of the basal ganglia. Hyponatremia may further cause or exacerbate CNS manifestations.

B. Laboratory Findings

Often there is profound hyponatremia. *The diagnosis can be confirmed by demonstrating an increased amount of porphobilinogen in the urine during an acute attack.* Freshly voided urine is of normal color but may turn dark upon standing in light and air.

Most families have different pathogenic variants in *HMBS* causing AIP. These variants can be detected in about 90% of patients and used for presymptomatic and prenatal diagnosis.

Prevention

Avoidance of factors known to precipitate attacks of AIP—especially medications—can reduce morbidity. Sulfonamides and barbiturates are the most common culprits; others are listed in Table 44–1 and online at https://porphyriafoundation.org/for-patients/about-porphyria/treatment-options/. Starvation diets and prolonged fasting also cause attacks and so must be avoided. Hormonal changes during pregnancy can precipitate crises.

Treatment

Treatment with a high-carbohydrate diet diminishes the number of attacks in some patients and is a reasonable empiric gesture considering its benignity. A minimum of 300 g of carbohydrates per day should be provided orally or intravenously. Acute attacks may be life-threatening and require prompt diagnosis, withdrawal of the inciting agent (if possible), and treatment with analgesics and

Table 44–1. Some of the "unsafe" and "probably safe" medications used in the treatment of acute porphyrias (listed in alphabetical order, within categories).

Unsafe	Probably Safe
Alcohol	Acetaminophen
Alkylating agents	Amitriptyline
Barbiturates	Aspirin
Carbamazepine	Atropine
Chloroquine	β-Adrenergic blockers
Chlorpropamide	Chloral hydrate
Clonidine	Chlordiazepoxide
Dapsone	Corticosteroids
Ergots	Diazepam
Erythromycin	Digoxin
Estrogens, synthetic	Diphenhydramine
Food additives	Guanethidine
Glutethimide	Hyoscine
Griseofulvin	Ibuprofen
Hydralazine	Imipramine
Ketamine	Insulin
Meprobamate	Lithium
Methyldopa	Naproxen
Metoclopramide	Nitrofurantoin
Nortriptyline	Opioid analgesics
Pentazocine	Penicillamine
Phenytoin	Penicillin and derivatives
Progestins	Phenothiazines
Pyrazinamide	Procaine
Rifampin	Streptomycin
Spironolactone	Succinylcholine
Succinimides	Tetracycline
Sulfonamides	Thiouracil
Theophylline	
Tolazamide	
Tolbutamide	
Valproic acid	

intravenous glucose in saline. Electrolyte balance requires close attention. Hemin therapy has been used but with serious adverse effects, especially phlebitis and coagulopathy. Givosiran, a δ-aminolevulinic acid synthase-directed small interfering RNA, is standard of care. This medication reduces attacks and the need for hemin use; it requires monthly subcutaneous administration. Liver transplantation is an option for patients with disease poorly controlled by medical therapy.

When to Refer

- For management of severe abdominal pain, seizures, or psychosis.
- For preventive management when a patient with porphyria considers becoming pregnant.
- For genetic counseling and molecular diagnosis.

When to Admit

For an acute attack when accompanied by mental status changes, seizure, or hyponatremia.

Dickey AK et al. Givosiran: a targeted treatment for acute intermittent porphyria. Hematology Am Soc Hematol Educ Program. 2024;2024:426. [PMID: 39644007]

Stölzel U et al. High disease burden and healthcare resource usage in patients with acute porphyria—a population-based analysis. Liver Int. 2024;44:2639. [PMID: 39016183]

Takata T et al. Biomarkers that predict attacks of acute intermittent porphyria. Transl Gastroenterol Hepatol. 2022;7:44. [PMID: 36300151]

DOWN SYNDROME

ESSENTIALS OF DIAGNOSIS

- Typical craniofacial features (flat occiput, epicanthal folds, large tongue).
- Intellectual disability.
- Congenital heart disease (eg, atrioventricular canal defects) in 50% of patients.
- Three copies of chromosome 21 (trisomy 21) or a chromosome rearrangement that results in three copies of a region of the long arm of chromosome 21.

General Considerations

Nearly 0.5% of all human conceptions are trisomic for chromosome 21. Because of increased fetal mortality, birth incidence of Down syndrome is 1 per 700 but varies from 1 per 1000 in young mothers to more than three times as frequent in women of advanced maternal age. The presence of a fetus with Down syndrome can be detected in many pregnancies in the first or early second trimester through screening maternal serum for *α-fetoprotein* and other biomarkers ("multiple marker screening") and by detecting increased nuchal thickness and underdevelopment of the nasal bone on ultrasonography. Prenatal diagnosis with high sensitivity and specificity can be achieved by assaying fetal DNA that is circulating in maternal blood. *The chance of bearing a child with Down syndrome increases exponentially with the age of the mother at conception and begins a marked rise after age 35 years.* By age 45 years, the odds of having an affected child are as high as 1 in 40. The risk of other conditions associated with trisomy also increases, because of the predisposition of older oocytes to nondisjunction during meiosis. The risk of trisomy 21 is not increased in older fathers.

Clinical Findings

A. Symptoms and Signs

Down syndrome is usually diagnosed at birth on the basis of the typical craniofacial features, hypotonia, and single palmar crease. Several serious problems that may be evident at birth or may develop early in childhood include duodenal atresia, congenital heart disease (especially atrioventricular canal defects), and hematologic malignancy. The intestinal and cardiac anomalies usually are correctible by surgery. A transient neonatal leukemia generally responds to conservative management. The incidences of both acute lymphoblastic and especially myeloid leukemias are increased in childhood. Leukemia typically responds to reduced-dose chemotherapy, but if relapse occurs, outcome is poor. Intelligence varies across a wide spectrum. Other frequent complications include atlanto-axial instability, immune deficiency that predisposes to celiac disease, diabetes mellitus, frequent infections, and hypothyroidism. Many people with Down syndrome do well in sheltered workshops and group homes, but few achieve full independence in adulthood. An Alzheimer-like dementia usually becomes evident in the fourth or fifth decade of life. Patients with Down syndrome who survive childhood and who develop dementia have a reduced life expectancy; on average, they live to about age 55 years.

B. Laboratory Findings

Cytogenomic analysis should always be performed—even though most patients will have simple trisomy for chromosome 21—to detect unbalanced translocations; such patients may have a parent with a balanced translocation, and there will be a substantial recurrence risk of Down syndrome in future offspring of that parent and potentially that parent's relatives.

Treatment

Duodenal atresia should be treated surgically. Congenital heart disease should be treated as in any other patient. As yet, no medical treatment has been proven to affect the neurodevelopmental or the neurodegenerative aspects. Trials of supplementation with antioxidants have shown no benefit.

When to Refer

- For comprehensive evaluation of infants to investigate congenital heart disease, hematologic malignancy, and duodenal atresia.
- For genetic counseling of the parents.
- For signs of dementia in an adult patient.

When to Admit

A young patient should be hospitalized for failure to thrive, regurgitation, or breathlessness.

Costa ACS. On the therapeutic use of monoclonal antibodies against amyloid plaques in older adults with down syndrome: a narrative review and perspective. Brain Sci. 2024;14:1084. [PMID: 39595846]

Hamadelseed O et al. Stem cell-based therapeutic strategies for Down syndrome and Alzheimer's disease. Cell Res Ther. 2025;16:420. [PMID: 40760500]

Huang T et al. Chromosomal and cellular therapeutic approaches for Down syndrome: a research update. Biochem Biophys Res Commun. 2024;735:150664. [PMID: 39260337]

Jafri SK et al. Use of antioxidants supplementation of developmental outcomes in children with Down syndrome—a systematic review and meta-analysis. Child Care Health Dev. 2022;48:177. [PMID: 34644809]

Panchal K et al. Perspectives on the origin and therapeutic opportunities in Down syndrome-associated leukemia. Cancer Metastasis Rev. 2025;44:70. [PMID: 40965715]

Rana MS et al. The multifactorial causes of Down syndrome during pregnancy: a narrative review of genetic, environmental, and maternal influences. Health Sci Rep. 2025;8:e71615. [PMID: 41356612]

Shear MA et al. A systematic review and meta-analysis of cell-free DNA testing for detection of fetal sex chromosome aneuploidy. Prenat Diagn. 2023;43:133. [PMID: 36588186]

FAMILIAL HYPERCHOLESTEROLEMIA

ESSENTIALS OF DIAGNOSIS

- Elevated serum total cholesterol and LDL cholesterol.
- Autosomal dominant inheritance.
- Variation in *LDLR*, *PCSK9*, or *APOB*.

General Considerations

Familial hypercholesterolemia (FH) is a group of autosomal dominant and recessive conditions that result in elevated LDL levels in the blood. High LDL predisposes to atherosclerosis, which in turn leads to premature MI and stroke. The incidence of these serious complications increases with age and when associated with the other common predispositions to atherosclerosis, such as smoking and hypertension. About 1 in 500 people in the United States has FH; worldwide, the prevalence is about 10 million. Only about 15% of FH cases are diagnosed and even fewer are treated effectively. Individuals who inherit two copies of a mutant gene that causes FH have a more severe disease that typically presents in childhood with severe hypercholesterolemia and early-onset arterial disease.

Clinical Findings

A. Symptoms and Signs

Yellow lipid deposits appear on tendons, especially the Achilles (**tendon xanthoma**).

B. Laboratory Findings

Total serum cholesterol with the LDL component is particularly high. A detailed family history and genetic testing should be obtained when individuals are younger than 40 years with an LDL level > 200 mg/mL and for individuals older than 40 years with a level > 250 mg/mL.

Prevention

In most instances, the elevated LDL is inherited as an autosomal dominant trait. An affected individual in all likelihood inherited FH from one parent, and each of his or her children has a 50/50 chance of inheriting FH. In uncommon cases, both parents have a variation in the LDL receptor and one-quarter of their children, on average, will inherit two pathogenic variant alleles and have homozygous FH, which is a much more serious disease with manifestations in childhood.

Pathogenic variations in the following four genes can cause FH: (1) *LDLR*, which encodes the LDL receptor located on the surface of cells and responsible for moving LDL into the cell for metabolism is the most common variant gene in FH; (2) *APOB*, which encodes a component of LDL and pathogenic variants inhibit binding to LDL receptor; (3) *PCSK9*, which encodes a protein that normally reduces production of LDL receptors, so variants actually protect from hypercholesterolemia; and (4) *ARH*, a rare cause of FH that requires pathogenic variants in both alleles (autosomal recessive inheritance).

Treatment

Statins, usually at high doses, can reduce LDL levels, occasionally to acceptable levels (see Table 32–3). The earlier in life that treatment is begun, the better the outcome in reducing mortality from atherosclerosis. In homozygous FH, if high-dose statins do not reduce LDL sufficiently, treatment with a monoclonal antibody (eg, alirocumab and evolocumab) that blocks the action of the *PCSK9* enzyme (which inactivates hepatic receptors that transport LDL into the liver for metabolism) can be an expensive adjunct to standard therapy (see Chapter 32). If all else fails, then apheresis is needed to reduce LDL.

It is important to screen relatives who are at risk for FH by measuring LDL levels and by identifying the pathogenic genetic variant in the family and utilizing that for screening.

When to Refer

- For comprehensive evaluation of infants for their lipid profile.
- For genetic counseling of the patient, his or her parents, siblings, and offspring.
- For signs of atherosclerotic CVD.

When to Admit

For signs or symptoms of acute arterial occlusive events.

Santos RD et al. Recent advances in research and care of familial hypercholesterolaemia. Lancet Diabetes Endocrinol. 2025;13:1054. [PMID: 41138742]

Shakir A et al. Qualitative and quantitative effects of PCSK9 inhibitors in familial hypercholesterolemia: a synthetic review. Curr Probl Cardiol. 2023;48:101550. [PMID: 36529229]

FRAGILE X SYNDROME

ESSENTIALS OF DIAGNOSIS

- Expanded trinucleotide repeat (> 200) in the *FMR1* gene.
- Males: mental impairment and autism; large testes after puberty.
- Females: learning disabilities or mental impairment; premature ovarian failure.
- Late-onset tremor and ataxia in males and females with moderate trinucleotide repeat (55–200) expansion (premutation carriers).

Clinical Findings

A. Symptoms and Signs

This X-linked condition accounts for more cases of mental impairment in males than any condition except Down syndrome; about 1 in 4000 males is affected. The CNS phenotype includes autism spectrum, impulsivity and aggressiveness, and repetitive behaviors. The condition also affects intellectual function in females, although less severely and about 50% less frequently than in males. Affected (heterozygous) young women show no physical signs other than early menopause, but they may have learning difficulties, anxiety, sensory issues, or frank impairment. Affected males show macroorchidism (enlarged testes) after puberty, large ears and a prominent jaw, a high-pitched voice, autistic characteristics, and mental impairment. Some males show evidence of a mild connective tissue defect, with joint hypermobility and mitral valve prolapse.

Women who are premutation carriers (55–200 CGG repeats) are at increased risk for **premature ovarian insufficiency (FXPOI)** and mild cognitive abnormalities. Male and female premutation carriers are at risk for mood and anxiety disorders and the development of tremor and ataxia beyond middle age (**fragile X-associated tremor/ataxia syndrome, FXTAS**). Changes in the cerebellar white matter may be evident on MRI before symptoms appear. Because of the relatively high prevalence of premutation carriers in the general population (1/130–1/600), older people in whom any of these behavioral or neurologic problems develop should undergo testing of the *FMR1* locus.

B. Laboratory Findings

The first marker for this condition was a small gap, or fragile site, evident near the tip of the long arm of the X chromosome. Subsequently, the condition was found to be due to expansion of a trinucleotide repeat (CGG) near a gene called *FMR1*. All individuals have some CGG repeats in this location, but as the number increases beyond 52, the chances of further expansion during spermatogenesis or oogenesis increase.

Being born with one *FMR1* allele with 200 or more repeats results in mental impairment in most men and in about 60% of women. The more repeats, the greater the likelihood that further expansion will occur during gametogenesis; this results in anticipation, in which the disorder can worsen from one generation to the next.

Prevention

DNA diagnosis for the number of repeats has supplanted cytogenetic analysis for both clinical and prenatal diagnosis. This should be done on any male or female who has unexplained mental impairment. Newborn screening based on hypermethylation of the *FMR1* gene is being considered as a means of early detection and intervention.

Treatment

No treatment directly addresses the underlying genetic perturbation. Several treatments (lovastatin plus minocycline) that address the imbalances in neurotransmission have been developed based on the mouse model and show promise in early clinical trials. Valproic acid may reduce symptoms of hyperactivity and attention deficit, but standard therapies should be tried first. Delivery of normal copies of *FMR1* across the blood-brain barrier has shown promise in mice.

When to Refer

- For otherwise unexplained mental impairment or learning difficulties in boys and girls.
- For otherwise unexplained tremor or ataxia in middle-aged individuals.
- For premature ovarian failure.
- For genetic counseling.

Hagerman RJ et al. Fragile X syndrome: lessons learned and what new treatment avenues are on the horizon. Annu Rev Pharmacol Toxicol. 2022;62:365. [PMID: 34499526]
Morin-Parent F et al. Neurophysiological effects of a combined treatment of lovastatin and minocycline in patients with fragile X syndrome: ancillary results of the LOVAMIX randomized clinical trial. Autism Res. 2024;17:1944. [PMID: 39248107]
Protic DD et al. Fragile X syndrome: from molecular aspect to clinical treatment. Int J Mol Sci. 2022;23:1935. [PMID: 35216055]
Raspa M et al. Research gaps in fragile X syndrome: an updated literature review to inform clinical and public health practice. Dev Behav Pediatr. 2023;44:e56. [PMID: 36219479]
Vrelinov M Gene therapy for fragile X syndrome, challenges, and promises. Gene Med. 2025;27:e70049. [PMID: 41207793]

GAUCHER DISEASE

ESSENTIALS OF DIAGNOSIS

- Deficiency of β-glucocerebrosidase.
- Anemia and thrombocytopenia.
- Hepatosplenomegaly.
- Pathologic fractures.

Clinical Findings

A. Symptoms and Signs

Gaucher disease has an autosomal recessive pattern of inheritance. A deficiency of β-glucocerebrosidase causes an accumulation of sphingolipid within phagocytic cells throughout the body. Anemia and thrombocytopenia are common and may be symptomatic; both are due primarily to hypersplenism, but marrow infiltration with Gaucher cells may be a contributing factor. The abdomen can become painfully distended due to enlargement of the liver and spleen. Soft tissue masses, **Gaucheromas**, can occur anywhere in the body.

Cortical erosions of bones, especially the vertebrae and femur, are due to local infarctions, but the mechanism is unclear. Episodes of bone pain (termed "crises") are reminiscent of those in sickle cell disease. A hip fracture in a patient of any age with a palpable spleen—especially in a Jewish person of Eastern European origin—suggests the possibility of Gaucher disease. Peripheral neuropathy may develop in patients.

Patients with Gaucher disease and heterozygous carriers of a pathogenic variant in *GBA* are at increased risk for early-onset Parkinson disease and dementia with Lewy bodies.

Two uncommon forms of Gaucher disease, called **type II** and **type III**, involve neurologic accumulation of sphingolipid and a variety of neurologic problems. Type II is of infantile onset and has a poor prognosis. Heterozygotes for Gaucher disease are at increased risk for developing Parkinson disease.

B. Laboratory Findings

Bone marrow aspirates reveal typical Gaucher cells, which have an eccentric nucleus and periodic acid–Schiff (PAS)-positive inclusions, along with wrinkled cytoplasm and inclusion bodies of a fibrillar type. In addition, the serum acid phosphatase is elevated. Definitive diagnosis requires the demonstration of deficient glucocerebrosidase activity in leukocytes. Hundreds of pathogenic variants cause Gaucher disease and some are highly predictive of the neuronopathic forms. Thus, genetic testing, especially in a young person, is of potential value. Only four pathogenic variants in glucocerebrosidase account for > 90% of the disease among Ashkenazi Jews, in whom the carrier frequency is 1:15.

Prevention

Gaucher disease is the most common lysosomal storage disorder. *Most clinical complications can be prevented by early institution of enzyme replacement therapy.* Carrier screening, especially among those of Ashkenazi Jewish descent, detects those couples at 25% risk of having an affected child. Prenatal diagnosis through genetic variant analysis is feasible. Because of an increased risk of malignancy, especially plasma cell myeloma and other hematologic cancers, regular screening of adults with Gaucher disease is warranted.

Treatment

Several recombinant forms of the enzyme glucocerebrosidase for intravenous administration on a regular basis reduces total body stores of glycolipid and improves orthopedic and hematologic manifestations. *Unfortunately, the neurologic manifestations of types II and III have not improved with enzyme replacement therapy.* The major drawback is the exceptional cost of enzyme replacement therapy. Eliglustat tartrate is an oral inhibitor of glucosylceramide synthase and reduces the compound that accumulates; while still quite expensive, this approach eliminates the need for frequent intravenous infusions. Early treatment of affected children normalizes growth and bone mineral density and improves liver and spleen size, anemia, and thrombocytopenia. In adults with thrombocytopenia due to splenic sequestration, enzyme replacement often obviates the need for splenectomy.

Camou F et al. Gaucher disease, state of the art and perspectives. J Intern Med. 2025;298:155. [PMID: 40611398]

Stepien AM et al. Transition of patients with Gaucher disease type 1 from pediatric to adult care: results from two international surveys of patients and health care professionals. Front Pediatr. 2024;12:1439236. [PMID: 39346636]

Tenenbaum A et al. A machine learning model for early diagnosis of type 1 Gaucher disease using real-life data. J Clin Epidemiol. 2024;175:111517. [PMID: 39245415]

DISORDERS OF HOMOCYSTEINE METABOLISM

ESSENTIALS OF DIAGNOSIS

- **Hyperhomocysteinemia:** more vascular disease but lowering homocysteine levels is not helpful.
- **Homocystinuria:** Marfan-like habitus, ectopia lentis, mental impairment, thromboses.
- Elevated homocysteine in the urine or plasma.

General Considerations

Patients with clinical and angiographic evidence of CAD and cerebrovascular and peripheral vascular diseases and VTE tend to have higher levels of plasma homocysteine than persons without these vascular diseases. Elevated blood homocysteine also increases the risk of Alzheimer dementia in the older adults. Although these effects were initially thought to be due at least in part to heterozygotes for cystathionine β-synthase deficiency, there is little supporting evidence. *Rather, an important factor leading to hyperhomocysteinemia is folate deficiency.* Pyridoxine (vitamin B_6) and vitamin B_{12} are also important in the metabolism of methionine, and deficiency of any of these vitamins can lead to accumulation of homocysteine. *Several genes influence utilization of these vitamins and can predispose to deficiency.* For example, having one copy—and especially two copies—of an allele that causes thermolability of methylene tetrahydrofolate reductase predisposes people to elevated fasting homocysteine levels. Both nutritional and most genetic deficiencies of these vitamins can be corrected by dietary supplementation of folic acid and, if serum levels are low, vitamins B_6 and B_{12}. In the United States, cereal grains are fortified with folic acid. However, therapy with B vitamins and folate lowers homocysteine levels significantly but does not reduce the risk of either VTE or complications of CAD. Hyperhomocysteinemia occurs with ESKD. In the general population, elevated homocysteine correlates with cognitive impairment.

Clinical Findings

A. Symptoms and Signs

1. Hyperhomocysteinemia—Debate continues as to whether mild elevation of plasma homocysteine predisposes to occlusive arterial disease. Adults with hyperhomocysteinemia and associated vitamin deficiencies such as folate, pyridoxine, or vitamin B_{12} may have symptoms of the associated vitamin deficiencies.

2. Homocystinuria—In its classic form, homocystinuria is caused by cystathionine β-synthase deficiency and exhibits autosomal recessive inheritance with a prevalence of 1 per 100,000. This results in extreme elevations of plasma and urinary homocysteine levels, a basis for diagnosis of this disorder. Homocystinuria is similar in certain superficial aspects to Marfan syndrome, since patients may have a similar body habitus and ectopia lentis is almost always present. However, mental impairment is often present in homocystinuria, and the cardiovascular events are those of repeated venous and arterial thromboses whose precise cause remains obscure. Thus, the diagnosis should be suspected in patients in the second and third decades of life who have arterial or venous thromboses without other risk factors. Bone mineral density is reduced in untreated patients. Life expectancy is reduced, especially in untreated and pyridoxine-unresponsive patients; MI, stroke, and PE are the most common causes of death. This condition is diagnosed by newborn screening for hypermethioninemia; however, pyridoxine-responsive infants may not be detected. In addition, homozygotes for a common pathogenic allele, p.I278T, show marked clinical variability, with some unaffected as adults.

B. Laboratory Findings

Although many variations have been identified in the cystathionine β-synthase (*CBS*) gene, *amino acid analysis of plasma remains the most appropriate diagnostic test.* Patients should be studied after they have been off folate or pyridoxine supplementation for at least 1 week. Relatively few laboratories provide highly reliable assays for homocysteine. Processing of the specimen is crucial to obtain accurate results. The plasma must be separated within 30 minutes; otherwise, blood cells release the amino acid and the measurement will then be artificially elevated.

Prevention

Prenatal diagnosis and termination of the affected pregnancy are the only way to prevent the occurrence of *CBS*-deficient homocystinuria. Clinicians need to be aware of laws regarding the availability of emergency contraception and abortion in the jurisdiction of their practice.

Treatment

About 50% of patients have a form of *CBS* deficiency that improves biochemically and clinically through pharmacologic doses of pyridoxine (50–500 mg orally daily) and folate (5–10 mg orally daily). For these patients, treatment that begins in infancy can prevent neurologic impairment and the other clinical problems. Patients who do not respond to pyridoxine must be treated with a dietary reduction in methionine and supplementation of cysteine, again beginning in infancy. The vitamin betaine is also useful in reducing plasma methionine levels by facilitating a metabolic pathway that bypasses the defective enzyme.

Patients with classic homocystinuria who have suffered venous thrombosis receive anticoagulation therapy, but there are no studies to support prophylactic use of warfarin or antiplatelet agents.

Liu D et al. Association between homocysteine levels and mortality in CVD: a cohort study based on NHANES database. BMC Cardiovasc Disord. 2024;24:652. [PMID: 39548360]

Majtan T et al. Understanding the impact of mutations in the cystathionine beta-synthase gene: towards novel therapeutics for homocystinuria. Mol Cell Biol. 2025;45:327. [PMID: 40495464]

McCaddon A et al. Homocysteine-a retrospective and prospective appraisal. Front Nutr. 2023;10:1179807. [PMID: 37384104]

Prajjwal P et al. Association of Alzheimer's dementia with oral bacteria, vitamin B12, folate, homocysteine levels, and insulin resistance along with its pathophysiology, genetics, imaging, and biomarkers. Dis Mon. 2023;69:101546. [PMID: 36931946]

TURNER SYNDROME (Gonadal Dysgenesis)

ESSENTIALS OF DIAGNOSIS

- Short stature with normal GH levels.
- Primary amenorrhea or early ovarian failure.
- Epicanthal folds, webbed neck, short fourth metacarpals.
- Renal and cardiovascular anomalies.

Turner syndrome comprises a group of X chromosome disorders that are associated with spontaneous abortion, primary hypogonadism, short stature, and other phenotypic anomalies (Table 44–2). It affects 1–2% of fetuses, of which about 97% abort, accounting for about 10% of all spontaneous abortions. Nevertheless, it affects about 1 in every 2500 live female births. Patients with the classic syndrome (about 50% of cases) lack one of the two X chromosomes (45,XO karyotype). About 12% of patients harbor mosaicism for Y chromosome sequences. Other patients with Turner syndrome have X chromosome abnormalities, such as ring X or Xq (X/abnormal X) or X chromosome deletions affecting all or some somatic cells (mosaicism, XX/XO).

1. Classic Turner Syndrome (45,XO Gonadal Dysgenesis)

Clinical Findings

A. Symptoms and Signs

Features of Turner syndrome are variable and may be subtle in girls with mosaicism. Turner syndrome may be diagnosed in infant girls at birth, since they tend to be small and may exhibit severe lymphedema. Evaluation for childhood short stature often leads to the diagnosis. Girls and women with Turner syndrome have an increased risk of aortic coarctation and bicuspid aortic valves; these cardiac abnormalities are more common in patients with a webbed neck. Typical manifestations in adulthood include short stature, hypogonadism, webbed neck, high-arched palate, wide-spaced nipples, hypertension, and kidney abnormalities (Table 44–2). Emotional disorders are common. Affected women are also more prone to autoimmune disease, particularly thyroiditis, IBD, and celiac disease.

Hypogonadism presents as "delayed adolescence" (primary amenorrhea, 80%) or early ovarian failure (20%); girls with 45,XO Turner syndrome who enter puberty are typically found to have mosaicism if other tissues are karyotyped.

B. Laboratory Findings

Hypogonadism is confirmed in girls who have high serum levels of FSH and LH. GH and IGF-1 levels are normal. Karyotyping must employ at least 30 metaphase spreads to detect low-level mosaicism. *The classic monosomy X karyotype represents under 50% of cases.* Since X chromosomes are lost during normal aging, women over age 50 must have over 5% X mosaicism to qualify for the diagnosis of Turner mosaicism.

C. Imaging

A transthoracic ultrasound and MRI scan of the chest and abdomen should be done in all patients with Turner syndrome to determine whether cardiac, aortic, and renal abnormalities are present.

Treatment

For short stature, GH therapy should be started early, ideally by age 4–6 and before age 12 years. GH is given subcutaneously in doses of 50 mcg/kg/day or 4.5 IU/m^2/day; the GH dose is titrated to keep the serum IGF-1 levels within 3 SD above the mean for age. Rarely, GH treatment causes pseudotumor cerebri. The oral androgen oxandrolone (0.03–0.05 mg/kg/day) is added after age 10 for girls whose growth is inadequate with GH therapy alone. After age 12 years, estrogen therapy is begun with low doses of transdermal estradiol, with a gradual increase in dose over 2–3 years. Progesterone is added after 2 years of estrogen therapy or if menstrual bleeding occurs.

Complications & Surveillance

Women with Turner syndrome have a reduced life expectancy due in part to their increased risk of diabetes mellitus (types 1

Table 44–2. Manifestations of Turner syndrome (listed in alphabetical order by affected systems).

Affected Systems	Symptom, Sign, or Condition
Associated conditions	Autoimmune (Hashimoto) thyroiditis (37%) Diabetes mellitus (10%) or glucose intolerance (35%) Hyperlipidemia Hyperuricemia Neuroblastoma (1%) Obesity Rheumatoid arthritis
Cardiovascular anomalies	Aortic dilation or aneurysm (25% with bicuspid aortic valve) Bicuspid aortic valve (30%) with aortic stenosis or regurgitation Coarctation (14%) and cystic medial necrosis of aorta Hypertension (50%, idiopathic or due to coarctation or kidney disease) Partial anomalous pulmonary venous return (18%)
CNS disorders	Emotional immaturity (40%) Learning disabilities and ADHD (40%) Sensorineural hearing loss
Ear abnormalities	Conductive hearing loss (30%) and recurrent otitis media (60%) Low-set and posteriorly rotated ears
Eye abnormalities	Cataracts, corneal opacities Epicanthal folds (20%) Strabismus (15%) Ptosis (10%)
GI disorders	Achlorhydria Celiac disease (8%) Colon carcinoma Hepatic transaminases, elevated (65%) IBD (3%) Primary biliary cholangitis Telangiectasias with bleeding
Gonadal abnormalities	Gonadal dysgenesis (primary amenorrhea 80%) or early ovarian failure (20%)
Head and neck features	High-arched palate (35%) Low posterior hairline (40%) Micrognathia (60%) Pterygium colli (webbed neck 40%)
Kidney abnormalities (60%)	Horseshoe kidney (10%) Duplication or abnormal positioning of renal pelvis or ureters (15%)
Skeletal and extremity abnormalities	Short stature (98%) Broad (shield) chest (30%) with wide-spaced hypoplastic nipples Cubitus valgus of arms (50%) and knock knees (35%) Lymphedema of hands and feet (30%) Madelung wrist deformity (5%) Osteopenia (65%) Scoliosis (10%) Short fourth metacarpals (40%)
Skin and nail disorders	Hyperconvex nails Keloid formation Pigmented nevi

ADHD, attention-deficit/hyperactivity disorder.

and 2), hypertension, dyslipidemia, and osteoporosis. Annual surveillance should include a blood pressure determination and laboratory evaluations that include a serum TSH, liver enzymes, BUN, creatinine, and fasting serum lipids and glucose. Audiology exams are recommended every 1–5 years. Bone mineral densitometries should be measured periodically for women over age 18 years.

Bicuspid aortic valves are common and are associated with an increased risk of infective endocarditis, aortic valvular stenosis or regurgitation, and ascending aortic root dilation and dissection. The risk of aortic dissection is increased more than 100-fold in women with Turner syndrome.

Partial anomalous pulmonary vein connections can lead to left-to-right shunting of blood. Adults with Turner syndrome also have a high incidence of ECG abnormalities, such as long QT syndrome.

Patients with the classic 45,XO karyotype have a high risk of renal structural abnormalities, whereas those with 46,X/abnormal X are more prone to malformations of the urinary collecting system.

2. Turner Syndrome Variants

A. 46,X (Abnormal X) Karyotype

Patients with small distal short arm deletions of the X chromosome (Xp–) that include the *SHOX* gene often have short stature and skeletal abnormalities but have a low risk of ovarian failure.

B. 45,XO/46,XX and 45,XO/46,XY Mosaicism

45,XO/46,XX mosaicism results in a modified form of Turner syndrome. Such girls tend to be taller and may have more gonadal function and fewer other manifestations of Turner syndrome.

Patients may have ambiguous genitalia or male infertility with an otherwise normal phenotype.

Gravolt CH et al. Clinical practice guidelines for the care of girls and women with Turner syndrome. Eur J Endocrinol. 2024;190:G53. [PMID: 38748847]
Shankar RK et al. Evolution of health care in Turner syndrome. Am J Med Genet C Semin Med Genet. 2025;199:e32124. [PMID: 39610314]
Steiner M et al. Turner syndrome: an update. Adv Pediatr. 2022;69:177. [PMID: 35985709]
Yoon SH et al. Organ abnormalities caused by Turner syndrome. Cells. 2023;12:1365. [PMID: 37408200]

KLINEFELTER SYNDROME

ESSENTIALS OF DIAGNOSIS

- Males with hypergonadotropic hypogonadism and small testes.
- 47,XXY karyotype.

Clinical Findings

A. Symptoms and Signs

Boys with an extra X chromosome are normal in appearance before puberty; thereafter, they have disproportionately long legs and arms, sparse body hair, a female escutcheon (pattern of pubic hair), gynecomastia, and small testes. Infertility is due to azoospermia; the seminiferous tubules are hyalinized. The incidence is 1 in 660 newborn male infants, but the diagnosis is often not made until a man is evaluated for inability to conceive. Intellectual disability is somewhat more common than in the general population. Many men with Klinefelter syndrome have language-based learning problems. However, their intelligence usually tests within the broad range of normal. In adulthood, detailed psychometric testing may reveal a deficiency in executive skills. The risk of osteoporosis, breast cancer, DVT, and diabetes mellitus is much higher in men with Klinefelter syndrome than in 46,XY men.

B. Laboratory Findings

Low serum testosterone is common. The karyotype is typically 47,XXY, but other sex chromosome anomalies cause variations of Klinefelter syndrome.

Prevention

Screening for cancer (especially of the breast), DVT, and glucose intolerance is indicated.

Treatment

Treatment with testosterone after puberty is advisable but will not restore fertility. However, men with Klinefelter syndrome have had mature sperm aspirated from their testes and injected into oocytes, resulting in fertilization. After the blastocysts have been implanted into the uterus of a partner, conception has resulted. Men with Klinefelter syndrome, however, have an increased risk for aneuploidy in sperm, and therefore, genomic analysis of a blastocyst should be considered before implantation.

Berry ASF et al. Association of supernumerary sex chromosome aneuploidies with venous thromboembolism. JAMA. 2023; 329:235. [PMID: 36648468]
Cook B et al. The incidence of male breast cancer in Klinefelter syndrome and its proposed mechanisms. Breast. 2024;78:103827. [PMID: 39467394]

MARFAN SYNDROME

ESSENTIALS OF DIAGNOSIS

- Disproportionately tall stature, thoracic deformity, and joint laxity or contractures.
- Ectopia lentis and myopia.
- Aortic root dilation and dissection; mitral valve prolapse.
- Variation in *FBN1*, the gene encoding fibrillin-1.

General Considerations

Marfan syndrome, a systemic connective tissue disease, has an autosomal dominant pattern of inheritance. It is characterized by abnormalities of the skeletal, ocular, and cardiovascular systems; spontaneous pneumothorax; dural ectasia; and striae atrophicae. Of most concern is disease of the ascending aorta, which begins as a dilated aortic root. Histology of the aorta shows diffuse medial degeneration. Mitral valve prolapse is common and frequently leads to regurgitation.

Clinical Findings

A. Symptoms and Signs

Affected patients are typically tall, with particularly long arms, legs, and digits (**arachnodactyly**). However, there can be wide variability in the clinical presentation. Commonly, scoliosis and anterior chest deformity, such as pectus excavatum, are present. Ectopia lentis is present in about half of patients; severe myopia is common and retinal detachment can occur. Mitral valve prolapse is seen in more than half of patients. Aortic root dilation is common and leads to aortic regurgitation or dissection with rupture. Aneurysms of aortic branch arteries are more common than previously recognized. To diagnose Marfan syndrome, people with an affected relative need features in at least two systems. People with no family history need features in the skeletal system, two other systems, and one of the major criteria of ectopia lentis, dilation of the aortic root or aortic dissection or a pathogenic variant in the fibrillin gene (*FBN1*).

B. Laboratory Findings

Pathogenic variants in *FBN1* on chromosome 15 cause Marfan syndrome. Nonetheless, no simple laboratory test is available to support the diagnosis in questionable cases because related conditions may also be due to defects in fibrillin. The pathogenesis of Marfan syndrome involves aberrant regulation of transforming growth factor (TGF)-β activity. Pathogenic variants in either of two receptors for TGF-β (TGFBR1 and TGFBR2) can cause conditions that resemble Marfan syndrome in terms of aortic aneurysm and dissection and autosomal dominant inheritance. Variations in more than two dozen other genes can predispose adults to thoracic aortic aneurysm and dissection.

Prevention

There is prenatal and presymptomatic diagnosis for patients in whom the molecular defect in *FBN1* has been found.

Treatment

Children with Marfan syndrome require regular ophthalmologic surveillance to detect ectopia lentis, correct visual acuity and thus prevent amblyopia, and annual orthopedic consultation for diagnosis of scoliosis at an early enough stage so that bracing might delay progression. *Patients of all ages require echocardiography at least annually to monitor aortic root diameter and mitral valve function.* Long-term β-adrenergic blockade, titrated to individual tolerance but enough to produce a negative inotropic effect (eg, atenolol, 1–2 mg/kg orally daily), retards the rate of aortic dilation. Angiotensin receptor blockade is as effective as β-adrenergic blockade. Calcium channel blockers, once used as a substitute for β-blockade, are detrimental to the aorta. Restriction from vigorous physical exertion protects from aortic dissection; moderate exercise does not. *Prophylactic replacement of the aortic root when the diameter reaches 45–50 mm in an adult (normal: < 40 mm) prolongs life.* Earlier prophylactic surgery should be considered when there is a strong family history of aortic dissection or when the diameter of the aortic root increases > 3–4 mm per year. A valve-sparing procedure resuspends the patient's native aortic valve inside a graft that replaces the aneurysmal sinuses of Valsalva and ascending aorta, thus avoiding the need for lifelong anticoagulation. Women with Marfan syndrome are at heightened risk for aortic dissection in the peripartum and postpartum periods. Having an aortic root dimension > 40 mm should prompt consideration for prophylactic, valve-sparing aortic repair before undertaking a pregnancy.

Prognosis

People with Marfan syndrome who are untreated commonly die in the fourth or fifth decade from aortic dissection or HF secondary to aortic or mitral regurgitation. However, because of earlier diagnosis, lifestyle modifications, β-adrenergic or angiotensin receptor blockade, and prophylactic aortic and mitral valve surgery, life expectancy has increased by several decades. However, with the longer life expectancy, serious comorbidities that were previously infrequent are more common as a result. These comorbidities include obstructive sleep apnea, cardiomyopathy, aneurysms and dissections of the abdominal aorta and peripheral arteries, neurologic problems related to dural ectasia, and degenerative arthritis.

When to Refer

- For detailed ophthalmologic examination.
- For at least annual cardiologic evaluation.
- For moderate or more severe scoliosis.
- For pregnancy in a woman with Marfan syndrome.
- For genetic counseling.

When to Admit

Any patient with Marfan syndrome in whom severe or unusual chest pain develops should be hospitalized to exclude pneumothorax and aortic dissection.

Crafts LS et al. Family functioning and health-related quality of life in children and young adults with Marfan syndrome. Qual Life Res. 2025;34:1647. [PMID: 40100519]

Holmes KW et al. Cardiovascular outcomes in aortopathy: GenTAC registry of genetically triggered aortic aneurysms and related conditions. J Am Coll Cardiol. 2022;79:2069. [PMID: 35618343]

Pitcher A et al; Marfan Treatment Trialists' Collaboration. Angiotensin receptor blockers and β blockers in Marfan syndrome: an individual patient data meta-analysis of randomised trials. Lancet. 2022;400:822. [PMID: 36049495]

Whelan AR et al. Cardiovascular and obstetrical outcomes among delivering patients with Marfan or Loeys-Dietz syndrome: a retrospective analysis by hospital delivery setting. Am J Obstet Gynecol MFM. 2024;6:101340. [PMID: 38460826]

HEREDITARY HEMORRHAGIC TELANGIECTASIA

ESSENTIALS OF DIAGNOSIS

- Recurrent epistaxis.
- Mucocutaneous telangiectases.
- Visceral arteriovenous malformations (especially lung, liver, brain, bowel).

Clinical Findings

A. Symptoms and Signs

Hereditary hemorrhagic telangiectasia (HHT), formerly termed "Osler-Weber-Rendu syndrome," is an autosomal dominant disorder of development of the vasculature. Epistaxis may begin in childhood or later in adolescence. Punctate telangiectases of the lips, tongue, fingers, and skin generally appear in later childhood and adolescence. *Arteriovenous malformations (AVMs) can occur at any age in the brain, lungs, and liver.* Bleeding from the GI tract is due to mucosal vascular malformations and usually is not a problem until mid-adult years or later. Pulmonary AVMs can cause hypoxemia (with peripheral cyanosis, dyspnea, and clubbing) and right-to-left shunting (with embolic stroke or brain abscess). The criteria for diagnosis require presence of three of the following four features: (1) recurrent epistaxis, (2) visceral AVMs, (3) mucocutaneous telangiectases, and (4) being the near relative of a clearly affected individual. Variant analysis can be used for presymptomatic diagnosis or exclusion of the worry of HHT.

B. Laboratory Findings

MR or CT arteriography detects AVMs. Variants in at least five genes can cause HHT. Molecular analysis to identify three of these genes is available; variants in *ENG, ALK1*, and *SMAD4* account for about 87% of families with HHT. When the familial variant is known, molecular testing is far more cost-effective than repeated clinical screening of relatives who are at risk.

Prevention

Embolization of pulmonary AVMs with wire coils or other occlusive devices reduces the risk of stroke and brain abscess. Treatment of brain AVMs reduces the risk of hemorrhagic stroke. All patients with HHT with evidence of a pulmonary shunt should practice routine endocarditis prophylaxis. All intravenous lines (except those for transfusion of RBCs and radiographic contrast) should have an air-filter to prevent embolization of an air bubble. Prenatal diagnosis through variant detection is possible. All patients should be referred for genetic counseling.

Treatment

All patients in whom the diagnosis of HHT is considered should have an MRI of the brain with contrast. A contrast echocardiogram will detect most pulmonary AVMs when "bubbles" appear on the left side of the heart after 3–6 cardiac cycles. A positive contrast echocardiogram should be followed by an HRCT angiogram for localization of pulmonary AVMs. Patients who have AVMs with a feeding artery of 2 mm diameter or greater should undergo embolization. After successful embolization of all treatable pulmonary AVMs, the CT angiogram should be repeated in 6 months and 3 years. A person with a negative contrast echocardiogram should have the test repeated every 5 years. *Any person with a pulmonary AVM, even an embolized one, should utilize routine endocarditis prophylaxis.* Several studies suggest that treatment with anti-estrogenic agents (eg, tamoxifen), thalidomide or its relatives, or anti-vascular endothelial growth factor agents (eg, bevacizumab) can reduce epistaxis and GI bleeding and improve hepatic shunting. However, two randomized, controlled clinical trials of intranasal bevacizumab therapy failed to show an improvement in epistaxis.

Al-Samkari H. Systemic antiangiogenic therapies for bleeding in hereditary hemorrhagic telangiectasia: a practical, evidence-based guide for clinicians. Semin Thromb Hemost. 2022;48:514. [PMID: 35226946]

Anning R et al. Improvement in epistaxis management: the experience of a dedicated hereditary hemorrhagic telangiectasia clinic. ANZ J Surg. 2022;92:499. [PMID: 34724318]

Cerrone A et al. Hereditary hemorrhagic telangiectasia: on the brink of a new treatment era? Semin Thromb Hemost. 2025;51:91. [PMID: 39694043]

Kim AY et al. Hereditary hemorrhagic telangiectasia: a review of gene targets and emerging therapies. Cardiol Rev. 2025 Oct 13. [Epub ahead of print] [PMID: 41166505]

Pyeritz RE. Digital vascular lesions detected by transillumination. Am J Med Genet A. 2022;188:99. [PMID: 34529342]

45 Orthopedic Disorders & Sports Medicine

Anthony Luke, MD, MPH
C. Benjamin Ma, MD

GENERAL APPROACH TO MUSCULOSKELETAL INJURIES

Musculoskeletal problems account for about 10–20% of outpatient primary care clinical visits. Orthopedic problems can be classified as atraumatic (ie, degenerative or overuse syndromes) or traumatic (ie, injury-related) as well as acute or chronic. The history and physical examination are sufficient in most cases to establish the working diagnosis; the mechanism of injury is usually the most helpful part of the history in determining the diagnosis.

Treatment

For acute injuries in the outpatient setting, the initial treatment plan can follow the mnemonic PEACE and LOVE.

A. PEACE

For the first 24–72 hours, PEACE entails:

Protection of the injury by resting and avoiding activities that increase pain.

Elevation of the affected area to reduce soft tissue swelling.

Avoidance of anti-inflammatory agents because of concern that reducing acute inflammation may impair healing.

Compression to reduce acute swelling.

Education to provide the patient a clear and practical plan over the next few days, realistic expectations, and instructions for follow-up.

For an acute painful injury, immobilization by casting, slings, and braces is helpful for protection of an injured limb. Crutches are useful to reduce weight bearing. Rest, rehabilitation, and physical therapy are often needed. Other modalities commonly used by patients include ice or heat (or both), chiropractic manipulation, massage therapy, acupuncture, osteopathy, and other alternative treatments. Exercise instructions are more often delivered through telemedicine or via smartphone applications than in person. Controlling pain is an early concern for most patients. However, if possible, use of medications in the initial setting that may impair healing (eg, systemic NSAIDs) should be avoided or delayed in order to promote desired inflammation, though this practice is controversial. Acetaminophen or opioids, only if appropriate, can be used. Topical medications such as diclofenac cream, capsaicin cream or patch, lidocaine patches, and NSAID patches or gels can provide superficial local pain relief and are becoming first-line therapy due to their infrequent side effects. Other medications, such as muscle relaxants and co-analgesics for neuropathic pain, which include the $\alpha2\delta$ ligands (eg, gabapentin) or tricyclic antidepressants, are generally avoided in acute settings.

B. LOVE

This treatment plan is for the subacute and rehabilitation phase.

Load management entails gradual, progressive movement and loading to recover function but not overstress the healing tissues.

Optimism recognizes that a positive mindset is needed for successful recovery and is an encouraged part of guidance. Avoiding fear, catastrophizing, and poor expectations is important in the recovery process.

Vascularization involves cardiovascular exercise to maintain good blood flow to healing injured tissues.

Exercise includes rehabilitation to restore strength, mobility, and function.

Local injections can deliver treatments directly to the affected areas as well as create mechanical stimulation for healing. Common medications to inject include corticosteroid injections and hyaluronic acid (for osteoarthritis). Injections can be administered under ultrasonic guidance into an area of chronic tendinopathy, a partial tear, or arthritic joints. An additional procedure that can be performed alone or combined with an injection is percutaneous needle tenotomy, where a treatment needle is passed several times through the tendon (fenestration). There are limited clinical data about the benefits of percutaneous needle tenotomy. Hydrodissection techniques can also be added to musculoskeletal injections with the intent of separating soft tissue structures (commonly nerves) from surrounding scar tissue, fascia, or adjacent structures.

SHOULDER

1. Subacromial Impingement Syndrome

ESSENTIALS OF DIAGNOSIS

- Shoulder pain with overhead motion.
- Night pain with sleeping on shoulder.
- Numbness and pain radiation below the elbow are usually due to cervical spine disease.

General Considerations

The subacromial impingement syndrome is a collection of diagnoses that cause mechanical inflammation in the subacromial space, often occurring with shoulder flexion and/or internal rotation. Causes of impingement syndrome include rotator cuff tendinopathy (eg, biceps tendinitis and tears), superior labral anterior posterior tear, adhesive capsulitis, subacromial bursitis, osteoarthritis of the glenohumeral joint or acromioclavicular joint, shoulder instability, and calcific tendinitis. With any shoulder problem, it is important to establish the patient's hand dominance, occupation, and recreational activities because shoulder injuries may present differently depending on the demands placed on the shoulder joint. Baseball pitchers with impingement syndrome may report pain while throwing, while older adults with even full-thickness rotator cuff tears may not report any pain because the demands on the joint are lower.

Clinical Findings

A. Symptoms and Signs

Subacromial impingement syndrome classically presents with one or more of the following: anterior shoulder pain with overhead activities (arm flexion or abduction), nocturnal pain with sleeping on the shoulder, or pain on internal rotation (eg, putting on a jacket or bra). Internal impingement, a less common cause of shoulder pain but more specifically affecting overhead athletes, is characterized by posterior shoulder pain.

On inspection, there may be atrophy in the supraspinatus or infraspinatus fossa. The patient with impingement syndrome can have mild scapula winging or "dyskinesis." The patient often has a rolled-forward shoulder posture or head-forward posture. On palpation, there may be tenderness over the anterolateral shoulder at the edge of the greater tuberosity. The patient may lack full active range of motion but has preserved passive range of motion. Impingement symptoms can be elicited with the Neer and Hawkins impingement signs (Table 45–1). Most examination maneuvers, however, have low diagnostic accuracy and low quality of evidence; therefore the use of several maneuvers is recommended to confirm suspected pathologies.

B. Imaging

Four radiographic views should be ordered to evaluate subacromial impingement syndrome: (1) the anteroposterior (AP) scapula (to rule out glenohumeral joint arthritis); (2) the AP acromioclavicular joint (to evaluate the acromioclavicular joint for inferior spurs); (3) the lateral scapula (scapular Y) (to evaluate the acromial shape); and (4) the axillary lateral (to visualize the glenohumeral joint and show the presence of os acromiale). The presence of a subacromial spur does not correlate with shoulder function.

The gold standard for soft tissue imaging of the shoulder is MRI, which may demonstrate full- or partial-thickness tears or tendinosis. Ultrasound evaluation can demonstrate thickening of the rotator cuff tendons and tendinosis as well as tears and can usually differentiate partial tears from small full-thickness tears. However, an MRI may provide a definitive diagnosis. Ultrasound can also help in the evaluation of patients with previous hardware in the shoulder, making an MRI difficult to interpret, or for the early postoperative healing phase when the tendon has not healed completely. Ultrasound can be performed in a dynamic fashion to evaluate the function of the soft tissue.

Treatment

A. Conservative

The first-line treatment for impingement syndrome is usually a conservative approach with education, activity modification, and physical therapy exercises.

Impingement syndrome can be caused by muscle weakness or tear. Rotator cuff muscle strengthening can alleviate weakness or pain, unless the tendons are seriously compromised, in which case exercises may cause more symptoms. Physical therapy is directed at rotator cuff muscle strengthening, scapula stabilization, and postural exercises. There is no strong evidence supporting the effectiveness of ice and NSAIDs as prolonged therapy. In a Cochrane review, corticosteroid injections produced slightly better relief of symptoms in the short term when compared with placebo. Most patients respond well to conservative treatment.

B. Surgical

Procedures include arthroscopic acromioplasty with coracoacromial ligament release, bursectomy, or debridement or repair of rotator cuff tears. However, the value of acromioplasty alone for rotator cuff problems is not supported by evidence.

When to Refer

- Failure of conservative treatment over 3 months.
- Young and active patients with impingement due to full-thickness rotator cuff tears.

Akram MI et al. Traumatic versus atraumatic causes of shoulder impingement syndrome: a systematic review of pathophysiology and outcomes. Cureus. 2025;17:e93628. [PMID: 41181758]

Sidhar K et al. A simplified approach to evaluate and manage shoulder pain. J Am Board Fam Med. 2024;37:1156. [PMID: 40118541]

Table 45–1. Shoulder examination.

Maneuver	Description
Inspection	Check patient's posture and for "SEADS" (*s*welling, *e*rythema, *a*trophy, *d*eformity, *s*urgical scars).
Palpation	Include important landmarks: acromioclavicular (AC) joint, long head of biceps tendon, coracoid, and greater tuberosity (supraspinatus insertion).
Range of motion testing: Check range of motion actively (patient performs) and passively (clinician performs).	
Flexion 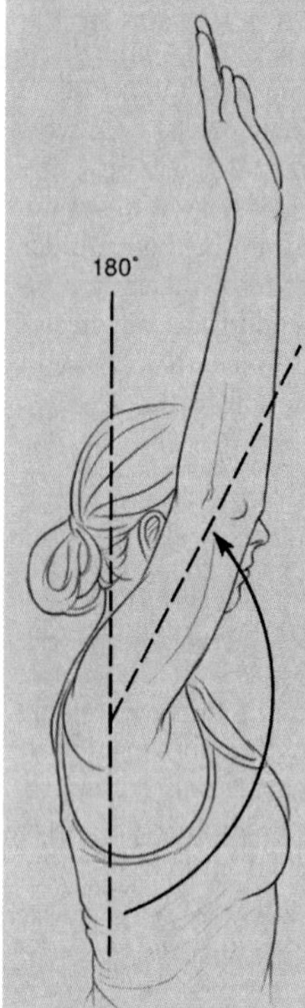 	Move the arm forward as high as possible in the sagittal plane.
External rotation 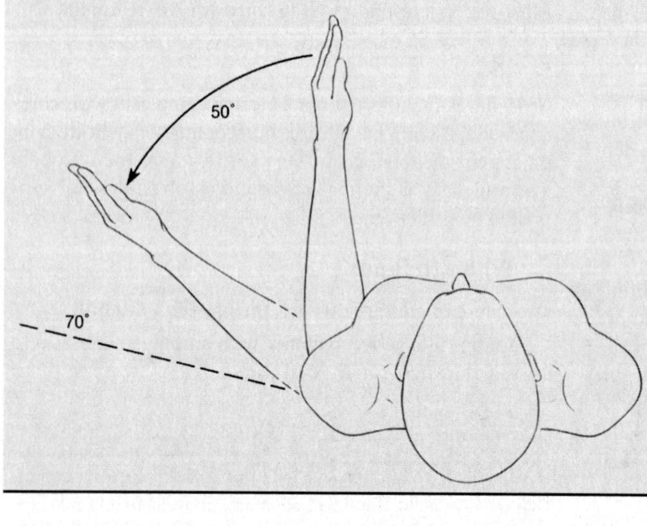 	Check with the patient's elbow touching their body so that external rotation occurs predominantly at the glenohumeral joint.

(*continued*)

Table 45–1. Shoulder examination. (continued)

Maneuver	Description
Internal rotation 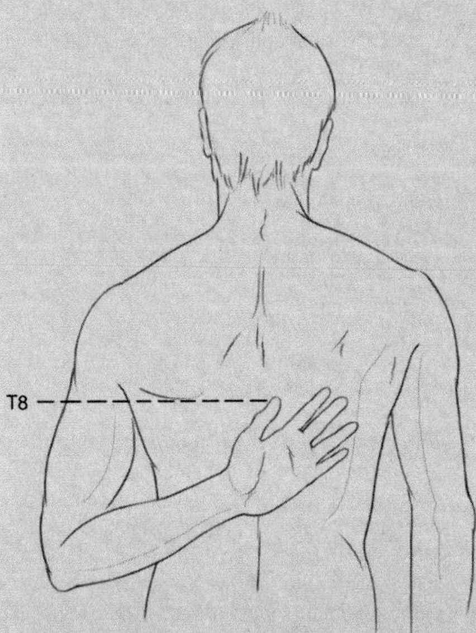	Patient reaches the thumbs as high as possible behind the spine on each side. The clinician records the highest spinous process that the individual can reach on each side (iliac crest = L4, inferior angle of scapula = T8).
Rotator Cuff Strength Testing	
Supraspinatus (open can) test 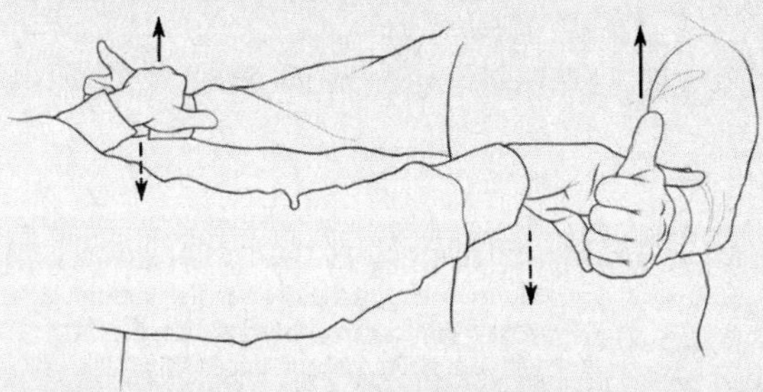	Perform resisted shoulder abduction at 90 degrees with slight forward flexion to around 45 degrees to test for supraspinatus tendon strength ("open can" test), or with shoulder abduction at 30 degrees and flexion to 30 degrees ("empty can" test).
External rotation 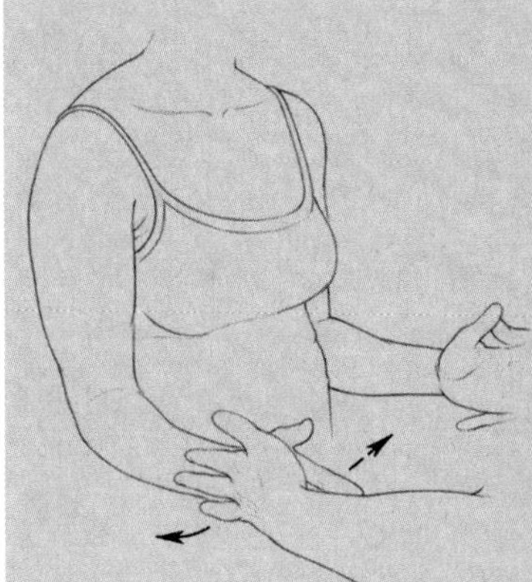	The patient resists by externally rotating the arms with elbows at their side.

(*continued*)

Table 45–1. Shoulder examination. (continued)

Maneuver	Description
Internal rotation (lift-off test) 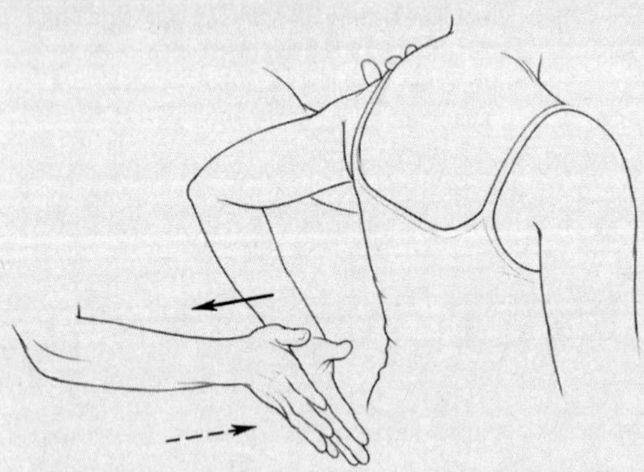	The clinician pushes the patient's hand toward the back while the patient resists. A positive lift-off indicates subscapularis tendon insufficiency. **Positive test:** Inability of the patient to hold their or the clinician's hand away from the body when reaching toward the small of the back.
Internal rotation (belly-press test) 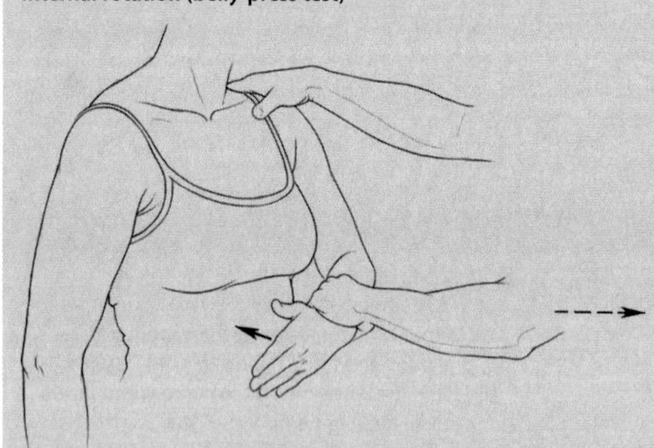	With the patient standing, the clinician puts the patient's forearm on the abdomen with the elbow flexed and the arm maximally internally rotated. The clinician places their hand between the patient's hand and abdomen to assess the patient's strength as the patient presses the arm against the abdomen with the elbow remaining forwardly flexed. A positive belly-press test indicates subscapularis tendon insufficiency. **Positive test:** Inability to hold the elbow in front of the trunk while pressing down with the hand on the abdomen.
Impingement Testing	
Neer impingement sign 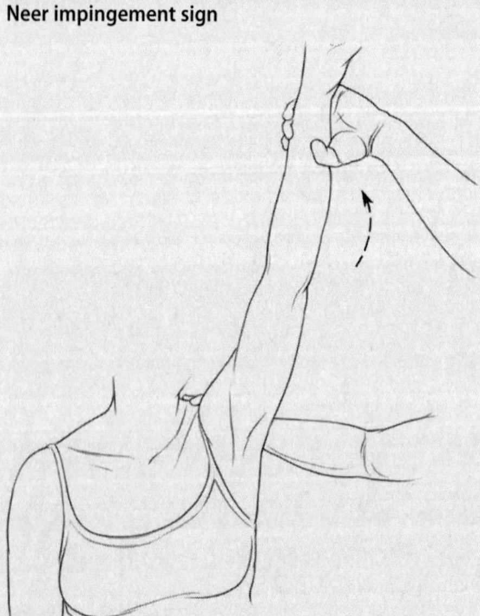	Perform by having the clinician flex the shoulder maximally in an overhead position. **Positive test:** Pain is reproduced with full passive shoulder flexion. Sensitivity is 79%; specificity is 53%.

(continued)

Table 45–1. Shoulder examination. (continued)

Maneuver	Description
Hawkins impingement sign 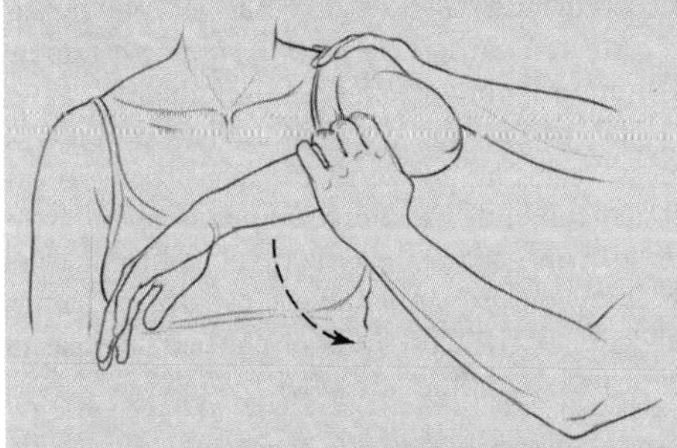	Perform with the shoulder forward flexed 90 degrees and the elbow flexed at 90 degrees. The shoulder is then maximally internally rotated to impinge the greater tuberosity on the undersurface of the acromion. **Positive test:** Pain is reproduced by this maneuver. Sensitivity is 79%; specificity is 59%.
Stability Testing	
Apprehension test 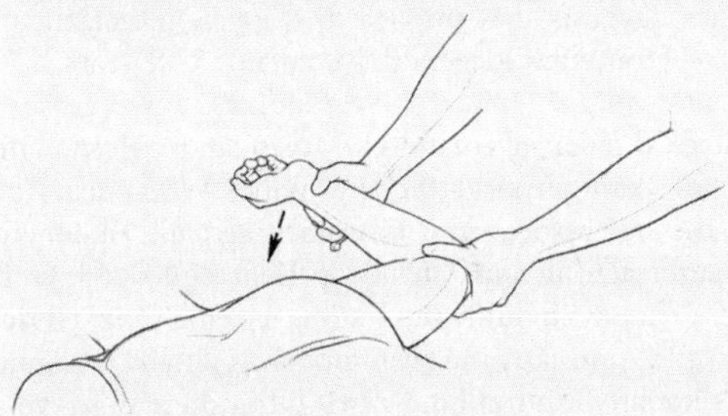	With persistent anterior instability or a recent dislocation, the patient feels pain or guards when the shoulder is abducted and externally rotated at 90 degrees. With posterior instability, the patient is apprehensive with the shoulder forward flexed and internally rotated to 90 degrees with a posteriorly directed force.
Load and shift test 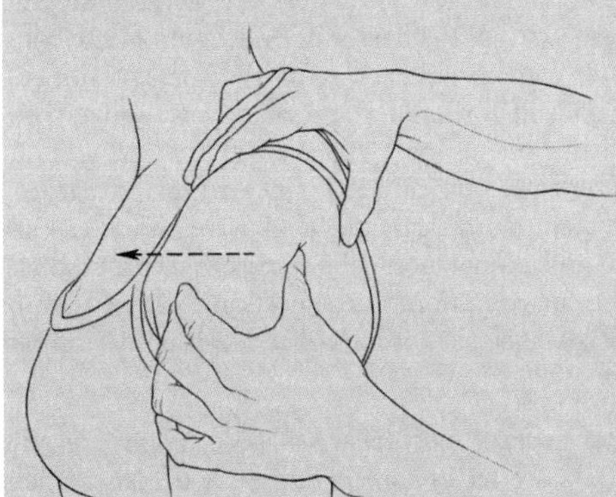	Perform to determine shoulder instability by manually moving the humeral head anteriorly and posteriorly in relation to the glenoid. However, this test can be difficult to perform when the patient is not relaxed.
O'Brien test 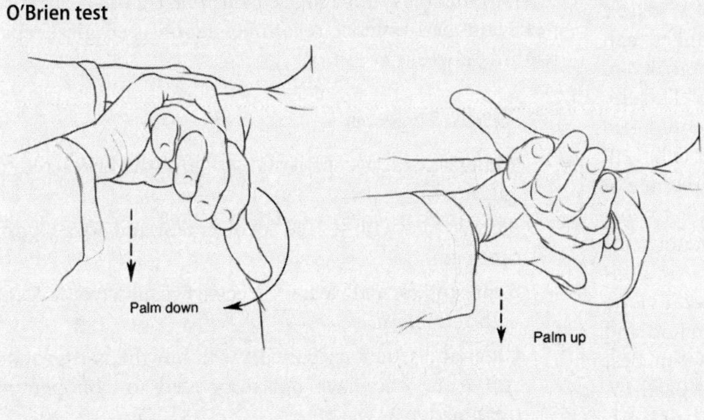	Performed to rule out labral cartilage tears that often occur following a shoulder subluxation or dislocation. The test involves flexing the patient's arm to 90 degrees, fully internally rotating the arm so the thumb is facing down (palm down), and adducting the arm to 10 degrees. Once positioned properly, the clinician applies downward force and asks the patient to resist. The test is then repeated in the same position except that the patient has his arm fully supinated (palm up). **Positive test:** There is pain deep in the shoulder with palm down more than the palm up. The O'Brien test can also be used to identify AC joint pathology. The patient would typically report pain equally directly over the AC joint with the palm down or up.

2. Rotator Cuff Tears

ESSENTIALS OF DIAGNOSIS

- A common cause of shoulder impingement syndrome after age 40 years.
- Difficulty lifting the arm with limited active range of motion.
- Weakness with resisted strength testing suggests full-thickness tears.
- Tears can occur following trauma or can be more degenerative.

General Considerations

Rotator cuff tears can be caused by acute injuries related to falls on an outstretched arm or to pulling on the shoulder. They may also develop from recurrent tendon strain from repetitive lifting or impingement from overhead movement. Partial rotator cuff tears often occur first. Full-thickness rotator cuff tears are usually more symptomatic and may require surgical treatment. The most commonly torn tendon of the shoulder is the supraspinatus.

Clinical Findings

A. Symptoms and Signs

Most patients report weakness, pain with overhead movement, or night pain. The clinical findings with rotator cuff tears include those of the impingement syndrome—but with full-thickness rotator cuff tears there may be more obvious weakness noted with light resistance testing of specific rotator cuff muscles. Table 45–1 demonstrates tests for supraspinatus tendon strength test ("open can" test), infraspinatus/teres minor strength and subscapularis strength, and the Neer and Hawkins impingement tests.

B. Imaging

Recommended radiographs are similar to impingement syndrome: AP scapula (glenohumeral), AP acromioclavicular joint views, lateral scapula (scapula Y), and axillary lateral. The AP scapula view is useful to visualize rotator cuff tears because degenerative changes can appear between the acromion and greater tuberosity of the shoulder, and to assess for arthritic changes. The elevation of the humeral head in relation to the glenoid also indicates large or "massive" rotator cuff tears. The AP acromioclavicular joint view evaluates for the presence of acromioclavicular joint arthritis, which can mimic rotator cuff tears, and for spurs that can cause rotator cuff impingement. Supraspinatus outlet views allow evaluation of the shape of the acromion. Axillary lateral views show the relationship of the humerus on the glenoid and can detect instability or dislocations. MRI is the best method for visualizing rotator cuff tears. The MR arthrogram can show partial or small (< 1 cm) rotator cuff tears. For patients who cannot undergo MRI testing or when postoperative artifacts limit MRI evaluations, ultrasonography can be helpful.

Treatment

1. Partial rotator cuff tears—Most partial rotator cuff tears can be treated conservatively with physical therapy and scapular and rotator cuff muscle strengthening. However, about 40% of the partial-thickness tears progress to full-thickness tears in 2 years. Physical therapy can strengthen the remaining muscles to compensate for loss of strength and can have high rate of success for chronic tears. Physical therapy is also an option for older sedentary patients. Injection of corticosteroids or platelet-rich plasma (PRP) may provide symptomatic relief.

2. Full-thickness rotator cuff tears—These tears do not heal well and have a tendency to increase in size with time; 49% of the tears get bigger over an average of 2.8 years. Evidence suggests that physical therapy is indicated initially for atraumatic degenerative rotator cuff tears, with success rates up to 70%. Ten-year studies, however, show that surgical repair of rotator cuff tears can result in better outcomes than physical therapy alone. When tears get larger, they are associated with worsening pain. Factors for good surgical outcome include patient age < 65 years, smaller tears with little retraction, a remaining tendon stump of 15 mm, early intervention for traumatic tears, and little or no fatty infiltration. Fatty infiltration is an irreversible degenerative process where muscle is replaced by fat following rotator cuff tear. Operative interventions are usually performed when the degree of infiltration is low. Most young active patients with acute, full-thickness rotator cuff tears can consult a shoulder specialist to optimize treatment. Full-thickness subscapularis tendon tears should be evaluated for early surgical repair since untreated tears can lead to premature osteoarthritis (OA) of the shoulder. Corticosteroid injections should be minimized, especially if surgery is a consideration, since injection within 6 months of surgery is associated with a higher surgical revision rate after 3 years.

3. Massive rotator cuff tears—These tears measure ≥ 5 cm. Data are limited, including poor evidence about the timing of surgical repair in order to optimize functional outcomes and reduce pain. For traumatic massive tears, the best practice recommendation is surgical repair within 12 weeks of injury.

When to Refer

- Young and active patients with full-thickness rotator cuff tears.
- Partial tears with ≥ 50% involvement and with significant pain.
- Acute rotator cuff tears, especially if massive (≥ 5 cm) with retraction.
- Older and sedentary patients with full-thickness rotator cuff tears who have not responded to nonoperative treatment.
- Full-thickness subscapularis tears.

Kuhn JE et al; Multicenter Orthopaedic Outcomes Network (MOON) Shoulder Group. 2024 Kappa Delta Ann Doner Vaughan Award: nonsurgical treatment of symptomatic, atraumatic full-thickness rotator cuff tears-a prospective multicenter cohort study with 10-year follow-up. J Am Acad Orthop Surg. 2024;32:1061. [PMID: 39325825]

3. Shoulder Dislocation & Instability

ESSENTIALS OF DIAGNOSIS

- Most dislocations (95%) are in the anterior direction.
- Pain and apprehension with an unstable shoulder that is abducted and externally rotated.
- Acute shoulder dislocations should be reduced as quickly as possible, using manual relocation techniques if necessary.

General Considerations

Stabilizing the shoulder joint relies heavily on rotator cuff muscle strength and also scapular control. In cases with poor scapular control or rotator cuff tears, shoulders may have more instability. Ninety-five percent of shoulder dislocations/instability occur in the anterior direction. Anterior dislocations usually are caused by stress on the arm in abduction, like a fall on an outstretched arm. Posterior dislocations are usually caused by falls from a height, epileptic seizures, or electric shocks. Traumatic shoulder dislocation can lead to ligamentous and bony injuries. The rate of repeated dislocation is directly related to the patient's age: patients age ≤ 21 have a 70–90% risk of redislocation, whereas patients age ≥ 40 have a much lower rate (20–30%). However, once the patient has a second dislocation, the recurrence rate is extremely high, up to 95%, regardless of age. Other risks include male sex and patients with hyperlaxity. Ninety percent of young active individuals who had traumatic shoulder dislocation have labral injuries. The labrum is the attachment site for the shoulder ligaments. Patients age > 55 are more likely to have rotator cuff tears or fractures following dislocation. Atraumatic shoulder dislocations are usually caused by intrinsic ligament laxity or repetitive microtrauma leading to joint instability. This is often seen in athletes involved in overhead and throwing sports (eg, in swimmers, gymnasts, and pitchers).

Clinical Findings

A. Symptoms and Signs

For acute traumatic anterior dislocation, patients have severe pain, with the humeral head dislocated anteriorly causing a deformity, with loss of the normal curve of the shoulder. The patient holds the shoulder and arm in an externally rotated position. Even after reduction, the patient will continue to have limited range of motion and pain for 4–6 weeks, especially following a first-time shoulder dislocation.

Posterior dislocations are harder to detect than anterior dislocations. The patient usually holds the shoulder and arm in an internally rotated position, which makes the shoulder deformity less obvious. There may be severe pain and muscle spasm, but the patient may still be able to move the joint.

Recurrent dislocations often are less painful with subsequent dislocations.

Atraumatic shoulder instability is usually well tolerated with activities of daily living. Patients usually describe a "sliding" sensation or "subluxation" during strenuous activities such as throwing or overhead lifting. Atraumatic dislocations may be less symptomatic and can often undergo spontaneous reduction of the shoulder with pain resolving within days after onset. The clinical examination for shoulder instability includes the apprehension test, the load and shift test, and the O'Brien test (Table 45–1). Most patients with persistent shoulder instability have preserved range of motion.

B. Imaging

Radiographs for acute dislocations should include a standard trauma series of AP and axillary lateral scapula (glenohumeral) views to determine the relationship of the humerus and the glenoid and to rule out fractures. Orthogonal views are used to identify a posterior shoulder dislocation, which can be missed with one AP view of the shoulder. An axillary lateral view of the shoulder can be safely performed even in the acute setting of a painful shoulder dislocation; a scapula Y view in the acute setting is insufficient to diagnose dislocation. For chronic injuries or symptomatic instability, these same recommended radiographic views are helpful to identify bony injuries and Hill-Sachs lesions (indented compression fractures at the posterior-superior part of the humeral head associated with anterior shoulder dislocation causing bone loss). MRI is commonly used to show soft tissue injuries to the labrum and to visualize associated rotator cuff tears. MRI arthrograms better identify labral tears and ligamentous structures. Three-dimensional CT scans are used to determine the significance of bone loss.

Treatment

1. Acute dislocation—Manual reduction is usually performed in the emergency department. The shoulder should be reduced as soon as possible. The FARES (Fast, Reliable, and Safe) method is the least painful method, with success rates > 88.7%. With the patient lying supine, the provider holds the patient's wrist with the arm extended. The provider applies gentle traction to the arm while making small oscillations with the joint in the horizontal plane to slowly abduct the arm to 90 degrees. When the arm reaches 90 degrees, the provider externally rotates the arm to achieve the joint reduction. Another traditional method is the gentle Stimson procedure: the patient lies prone with the dislocated arm hanging off the examination table with a weight (5–10 pounds) applied to the wrist to provide traction for 10–20 minutes. Afterward, gentle medial mobilization of the scapula is applied manually to assist the reduction.

Initial treatment of acute shoulder dislocations should include sling immobilization for 2–4 weeks along with pendulum exercises. Early physical therapy can be used to maintain range of motion and strengthening of rotator cuff muscles. Patients can also modify their activities to avoid active and risky sports. Patients with a traumatic incident and unilateral shoulder dislocation commonly have a Bankart lesion. (The dislocation tears part of the labrum of the glenohumeral joint.) Operative intervention is the only treatment that has been shown to decrease recurrence once a patient has a second dislocation. Even after arthroscopic stabilization surgery for a first or a subsequent dislocation, 5.9% can suffer another dislocation in the next 2 years. Repeated dislocations have been shown to increase the risk of arthritis and further bony deterioration. The more significant the bony deterioration, the less successful is the surgical outcome. Open and arthroscopic stabilization have similar outcomes.

2. Atraumatic shoulder instability—The treatment is different than that of traumatic shoulder instability. Patients with chronic, recurrent shoulder dislocations should be managed with physical therapy and a regular maintenance program, consisting of scapular stabilization and postural and rotator cuff strengthening exercises. Activities may need to be modified. Surgical reconstructions are less successful for atraumatic shoulder instability than for traumatic shoulder instability. However, patients with recurrent dislocations have much higher incidence of bone loss or biceps pathology when compared with patients with first-time dislocations. They are also more likely to require open surgery with bone augmentation rather than arthroscopic stabilization.

When to Refer

- Patients who are at risk for second dislocation, such as young patients and those with certain occupations (eg, police officers, firefighters, and rock climbers), to avoid recurrent dislocation or dislocation while at work.
- Patients who have not responded to a conservative approach or who have chronic instability.

Gonai S et al. An umbrella review of systematic reviews and meta-analyses for assessment and treatment of acute shoulder dislocation. Am J Emerg Med. 2025;87:16. [PMID: 39442380]

Wolf BR et al; MOON Shoulder Group. Recurrence after soft-tissue anterior shoulder stabilization: 2-year results from the MOON shoulder Cohort. J Shoulder Elbow Surg. 2025 Dec 29. [Epub ahead of print] [PMID: 41475470]

4. Adhesive Capsulitis ("Frozen Shoulder")

ESSENTIALS OF DIAGNOSIS

- Very painful shoulder triggered by minimal or no trauma.
- Pain out of proportion to clinical findings during the inflammatory phase.
- Stiffness during the "freezing" phase and resolution during the "thawing" phase.

General Considerations

Adhesive capsulitis ("frozen shoulder") is caused by acute inflammation of the shoulder capsule followed by scarring and remodeling. Injury to the shoulder likely triggers mast cell activation and release of growth factors and cytokines. Adhesive capsulitis is seen commonly in patients aged 40–65 years old, and it occurs more often in women than men, especially in perimenopausal women or in patients with endocrine disorders, such as diabetes mellitus or thyroid disease. There is a higher incidence of adhesive capsulitis following shoulder trauma (such as surgery) or breast cancer care (such as mastectomy), which may create a pro-inflammatory condition in the shoulder. Adhesive capsulitis is a self-limiting but very debilitating disease.

Clinical Findings

A. Symptoms and Signs

Patients usually have an extremely painful shoulder that has a limited range of motion with both passive and active movements. A useful clinical sign is limitation of movement of external rotation with the elbow by the side of the trunk (Table 45–1). Strength is usually normal but may appear diminished because of pain.

There are three phases: the inflammatory phase, the freezing phase, and the thawing phase. During the "inflammatory" phase, which usually lasts 4–6 months, patients report a very painful shoulder without obvious clinical findings to suggest trauma, fracture, or rotator cuff tear. During the "freezing" phase, which also usually lasts 4–6 months, the shoulder becomes stiffer even though the pain is improving. The "thawing" phase can take up to a year as the shoulder slowly regains its motion. The total duration of an idiopathic frozen shoulder is usually about 24 months; it can be much longer for patients who have trauma or an endocrinopathy.

B. Imaging

Standard AP, axillary, and lateral glenohumeral radiographs are useful to rule out glenohumeral arthritis, which can also present with limited active and passive range of motion. Imaging can also rule out calcific tendinitis, which is an acute inflammatory process in which calcifications are visible in the soft tissue. However, adhesive capsulitis is usually a clinical diagnosis, and it does not need an extensive diagnostic workup.

Treatment

During the "inflammatory" and "freezing" phases, NSAIDs and physical therapy help to maintain motion. There is also evidence of short-term benefit from an intra-articular corticosteroid injection or oral prednisone; a meta-analysis showed that intra-articular corticosteroid injection provided better pain relief than NSAIDs in the first 8 weeks. However, no difference was seen in range of motion or pain after 12 weeks, which is similar to other noncontrolled studies. One study demonstrated improvement at 6 weeks but not 12 weeks following 30 mg of daily prednisone for 3 weeks. During the "freezing" phase, the shoulder is less painful but remains stiff. Antiinflammatory medication is not as helpful during the "thawing" phase as it is during the "freezing" phase, and the shoulder symptoms usually resolve with time. Hydrodissection by intraarticular injection of large volumes of saline or anesthetic may improve symptoms. Intraarticular PRP injections show at least equal benefits to a corticosteroid injection and in one trial showed early gain in range of motion. Surgical treatments, which are rarely indicated, include manipulation under anesthesia and arthroscopic release.

When to Refer

- When the patient does not respond after > 6 months of conservative treatment.
- When there is no progress in or worsening of range of motion over 3 months.

Leafblad N et al. Adhesive capsulitis. Phys Med Rehabil Clin N Am. 2023;34:453. [PMID: 37003663]
Vita F et al. Retrospective analysis of ultrasound-guided hydrodistension in patients with post-traumatic adhesive capsulitis of the shoulder. Musculoskelet Surg. 2025 Dec 24. [Epub ahead of print] [PMID: 41444457]

SPINE PROBLEMS

1. Low Back Pain

ESSENTIALS OF DIAGNOSIS

- Nerve root impingement is suspected when pain is leg-dominant rather than back-dominant.
- Alarm symptoms (red flags) include unexplained weight loss, failure to improve with treatment, severe pain for > 6 weeks, and night or rest pain.
- Cauda equina syndrome is an emergency; it often presents with bowel or bladder symptoms (or both).
- Chronic management should address physical, emotional, cognitive and behavioral dimensions of back pain.

General Considerations

Low back pain remains the number one cause of disability globally and is the second most common cause for primary care visits. The three most attributable risk factors are occupational ergonomic factors, cigarette smoking, and high BMI. Approximately 80% of episodes of low back pain resolve within 2 weeks and 90% resolve within 6 weeks. Chronic low back pain is often defined as back pain for 12 weeks or more. The cause of low back pain is frequently difficult to diagnose; its cause is often multifactorial. The spine develops degenerative changes in the discs, facet joints, and vertebral endplates (Modic changes). Progressive osteoarthritis can narrow the neuroforamen and the spinal canal, resulting in stenosis and further compression of neural structures. The sacroiliac joints, muscles, and tendons also can cause pain.

Clinical Findings

A. Symptoms and Signs

Aggravating factors of flexion and prolonged sitting commonly suggest anterior spine disc problems, while extension pain suggests facet joint, stenosis, or sacroiliac joint problems. Serious causes for back pain include fracture, cancer, infection, cauda equina syndrome, and axial spondyloarthritis (Table 45–2). Red flags are concerning for serious spinal pathology while yellow flags are psychosocial factors in the absence of serious spinal pathology that may increase the likelihood of long-term chronicity and disability (Table 45–3).

1. Vertebral fracture—Risk factors for back pain due to vertebral fracture include use of corticosteroids, age > 70 years, osteoporosis, severe trauma, and presence of a contusion or abrasion.

Table 45–2. Risk factors and symptoms for serious spine pathology.

Fracture
Osteoporosis
Age
Pain worse when lying supine
Early menopause or late menarche
History of fracture
Malignancy
History of cancer
Requiring strong pain medication
Weight loss
Odd sensations in legs
Spinal infection
Immunosuppression
Corticosteroid use
History of tuberculosis
Fever
Neurologic dysfunction
Intravenous drug use
Night pain
Cauda equina syndrome
Bilateral radicular pain
Myotomal weakness
Changes to bladder function
Changes to bowel function
Saddle sensory disturbance
Inflammatory condition
Age
Past enthesitis, psoriasis, or arthritis
Uveitis
IBD
Nerve root condition
Myotomal weakness

Derived from Finucane LM. et al. International framework for red flags for potential serious spinal pathologies. J Orthop Sports Phys Ther 2020;50:350. [PMID: 32438853]

Table 45–3. Red and yellow flags for low back pain.[1]

Red Flags		
Patient history	**Medication history**	**Signs and symptoms**
Neoplasms Physical traumas Advanced age > 50 years (cancer risk) > 70 years (fracture risk) Weight loss Immunodeficiency Osteoporosis	Injection drug use Corticosteroid use or other immuno-suppressive drug use	High fever (≥ 38°C) Worst pain at night or rest Saddle anesthesia Weakness in lower limbs Bladder or bowel dysfunction (eg, overflow incontinence and urinary detention) Gait disturbance Abrupt, unexplained weight loss Night sweats Inflammatory back pain
Yellow Flags		
High baseline pain and disability Sleep problems Depression Anxiety Pain catastrophizing Work dissatisfaction Poor social support Low socioeconomic status General health-related (eg, opioid use and sedentary lifestyle) Fear-avoidance beliefs Irritability Toxic relationships Reduced perceived control over one's life		

[1]See text for definition of red flags and yellow flags. Derived from Finucane LM et al. International framework for red flags for potential serious spinal pathologies. J Orthop Sports Phys Ther 2020;50:350. [PMID: 32438853]

2. Malignancy—Alarm symptoms for back pain caused by cancer include unexplained weight loss, failure to improve with treatment, pain for > 6 weeks, and pain at night or rest. History of cancer and age older than 50 years are other risk factors for malignancy.

3. Infection—Alarm symptoms for infection include fever, rest pain, recent infection (UTI, cellulitis, pneumonia), or history of immunocompromise or injection drug use.

4. Cauda equina syndrome—Urinary retention or incontinence, saddle anesthesia, decreased anal sphincter tone or fecal incontinence, bilateral lower extremity weakness, and progressive neurologic deficits are symptoms suggestive of cauda equina syndrome.

5. Other serious causes of back pain—Psychosocial factors (yellow flags) and workplace factors should be assessed in cases where acute back pain becomes chronic (Table 45–3). The patient's previous response to treatments and the results of risk prediction tools can help guide management. Most patients with persistent low back pain have co-occurring areas of pain, especially axial pain (18–58%), extremity pain (6–50%), and multisite musculoskeletal pain (10–89%).

B. Physical Examination

The physical examination can be conducted with the patient in the standing, sitting, supine, and finally prone positions to avoid frequent repositioning of the patient.

1. Standing position—The patient's posture can be observed. Commonly encountered spinal asymmetries include scoliosis, thoracic kyphosis, and lumbar hyperlordosis. The active range of motion of the lumbar spine can be assessed while standing. The common directions include flexion, extension, rotation, and lateral bending. The one-leg standing extension test assesses for pain as the patient stands on one leg while extending the spine. A positive test can be caused by pars interarticularis fractures (spondylolysis or spondylolisthesis) or facet joint arthritis.

2. Sitting position—Motor strength, reflexes, and sensation can be tested (Table 45–4). The major muscles in the lower extremities are assessed for weakness by eliciting a resisted isometric contraction for about 5 seconds. Comparing the strength bilaterally to detect subtle muscle weakness is important. Similarly, sensory testing to light touch can be checked in specific dermatomes for corresponding nerve root function. Knee, ankle, and Babinski reflexes can be checked.

Table 45–4. Neurologic testing of lumbosacral nerve disorders.

Nerve Root	Motor	Reflex	Sensory Area
L1	Hip flexion	None	Groin
L2	Hip flexion	None	Thigh
L3	Extension of knee	Knee jerk	Knee
L4	Dorsiflexion of ankle	Knee jerk	Medial calf
L5	Dorsiflexion of first toe	Babinski reflex	First dorsal web space between first and second toes
S1	Plantar flexion of foot, knee flexors, or hamstrings	Ankle jerk	Lateral foot
S2	Knee flexors or hamstrings	Knee flexor	Back of the thigh
S2–S4	External anal sphincter	Anal reflex, rectal tone	Perianal area

3. Supine position—The hip should be evaluated for range of motion, particularly internal rotation. The straight leg raise test puts traction and compression forces on the lower lumbar nerve roots.

4. Prone position—The clinician can carefully palpate each vertebral level of the spine and sacroiliac joints for tenderness. A rectal examination is required if the cauda equina syndrome is suspected. Superficial skin tenderness to a light touch over the lumbar spine, overreaction to maneuvers in the regular back examination, low back pain on axial loading of spine in standing, and inconsistency in the straight leg raise test or on the neurologic examination suggest nonorthopedic causes for the pain or malingering (Waddell signs).

C. Imaging

In the absence of alarming "red flag" symptoms suggesting infection, malignancy, or cauda equina syndrome, most patients do not need diagnostic imaging, including radiographs, in the first 6 weeks. The Agency for Healthcare Research and Quality guidelines for obtaining lumbar radiographs are summarized in Table 45–5. Most clinicians obtain radiographs for new back pain in patients age > 50. If done, radiographs of the lumbar spine should include AP and lateral views. Oblique views can be useful if the neuroforamina or bone lesions need to be visualized. MRI is the method of choice in the evaluation of symptoms not responding to conservative treatment or in the presence of red flags of serious conditions.

D. Special Tests

Electromyography or nerve conduction studies may be useful in assessing patients with possible nerve root symptoms lasting longer than 6 weeks; back pain may or may not also be present. These tests are usually not necessary if the diagnosis of radiculopathy is clear.

Table 45–5. AHRQ criteria for lumbar radiographs in patients with acute low back pain even if < 6 weeks in duration.

Possible fracture
Major trauma
Minor trauma in patients > 50 years of age
Long-term corticosteroid use
Osteoporosis
> 70 years of age
Possible tumor or infection
> 50 years of age
< 20 years of age
History of cancer
Constitutional symptoms
Recent bacterial infection
Injection drug use
Immunosuppression
Supine pain
Nocturnal pain

AHRQ, Agency for Healthcare Research and Quality.
Adapted from Bigos S et al. Acute Low Back Problems in Adults. Clinical Practice Guideline Quick Reference Guide No. 14. AHCPR Publication No. 95-0643. Rockville, MD: Agency for Health Care Policy and Research, Public Health Service, U.S. Department of Health and Human Services. December 1994.

Treatment

A. Conservative

Nonpharmacologic treatments are key in the management of low back pain, including education, physical therapy, exercise therapy, and physical activity. A RCT showed that self-management strategies including pain education, exercises (postural strength, core stabilization, mobility, stretches), cognitive-behavioral strategies (relaxed breathing, progressive muscle relaxations, guided imagery, cognitive restructuring), and social strategies (pleasant activity scheduling, communication for navigating social roles) were better than medical care or spinal manipulation. Patients require information and reassurance, especially when serious pathology is absent. Discussion must include reviewing safe and effective methods of symptom control as well as how to decrease the risk of recurrence with proper lifting techniques, abdominal wall/core strengthening, weight loss, and cigarette smoking cessation. Tobacco may affect the small vessels by reducing the amount of water in the discs and increasing the rate of disc degeneration. Cognitive behavioral therapy and other psychological interventions of even < 10 hours duration produce better outcomes than active physical treatment alone, with post-treatment improvements in pain intensity in the short and long term.

1. Physical therapy—Exercise programs can be tailored to the patient's symptoms and pathology. An RCT demonstrated that individualized physical therapy was clinically more beneficial than advice alone with sustained improvements at 6 months and 12 months. Strengthening and stabilization exercises effectively reduce pain and functional limitation compared with usual care. Heat and cold therapies may be used for symptomatic treatment, with heat therapy showing short-term benefits for acute low back pain. The efficacy of transcutaneous electrical nerve stimulation (TENS), back braces, massage, and physical agents is unproven. There is good evidence that spinal manipulation and acupuncture provide short-term improvement compared with usual care. Improvements in posture, including chair ergonomics or standing desks, core stability strengthening, physical conditioning, and modifications of activities to decrease physical strain, are keys for ongoing management. A multidisciplinary approach to back pain care is beneficial to address the physical, psychological, and social aspects of low back pain, especially when pain is chronic. Opioids should be avoided, if possible.

2. Exercise therapy/physical activity—Systematic reviews of studies of low to moderate quality suggest that various exercises used for pain and disability have short-term benefit with no major difference between types of exercises. Complementary therapies, such as Tai Chi, Pilates, mindfulness-based stress reduction, core strengthening exercises, and yoga, have shown benefit for chronic low back pain. Compared with conventional rehabilitation and no intervention, yoga and core or stabilization exercises were statistically significant in improving physical function in patients with chronic low back pain. Digital apps that include exercise therapy, education, and behavioral support are useful for reducing pain intensity at long-term follow-up compared with rehabilitation alone.

3. Pharmacologic treatment—Medications, including oral and topical NSAIDs, and serotonin and norepinephrine reuptake inhibitors (duloxetine), were shown in a systematic review to produce a clinically meaningful reduction in pain. If medications are needed, NSAIDs are effective in the early treatment of low back pain (see Chapter 23 and Table 5–4). Topical capsicum is effective in the short term (≤ 3 months). Acetaminophen and oral corticosteroids are relatively ineffective for non-radicular chronic low back. There is limited evidence that muscle relaxants provide short-term relief; since these medications have addictive potential, they should be used with care. Muscle relaxants are best used if there is true muscle spasm that is painful rather than simply a protective response. Opioids alleviate pain in the short term but have the same side effects and concerns of long-term opioid use (see Chapter 5). Treatment of more chronic neuropathic pain with $\alpha 2\delta$ ligands (eg, gabapentin), serotonin-norepinephrine reuptake inhibitors (eg, duloxetine), or tricyclic antidepressants (eg, nortriptyline) may be useful (see Table 5–8). Antidepressants are not recommended for the treatment of general low back pain.

B. Nonsurgical Procedures

Procedural interventions include epidural injections of the spine, which may reduce pain in the short term and reduce the need for surgery in some patients within a 1-year period but not longer. Spinal injections are not recommended for initial care of patients with low back pain without radiculopathy. Studies are unclear and of limited quality regarding the effectiveness of PRP injections for low back pain. Intra-articular steroid injections and cooled radiofrequency ablation of the sacral lateral branch nerves and dorsal ramus of L5 can be considered for patients with persistent sacroiliac joint pain. There is fair evidence that thermal radiofrequency ablation of the facet joints improves pain for at least 6 months.

C. Surgical

Indications for back surgery include cauda equina syndrome, ongoing morbidity with minimal response to > 6 months of conservative treatment, cancer, infection, or severe spinal deformity. Prognosis is improved when there is an anatomic lesion that can be corrected and symptoms are neurologic. Spinal surgery has limitations. Patient selection is very important; the specific recommended surgery should have clear indications and expectations. Patients should understand that surgery can improve their pain but is unlikely to cure it. Surgery is not generally indicated for radiographic abnormalities alone when the patient is relatively asymptomatic. Depending on the surgery performed, possible complications include persistent pain; surgical site pain, especially if bone grafting is needed; infection; neurologic damage; non-union; cutaneous nerve damage; implant failure; DVT; and death.

When to Refer

- Patients with cancer, infection, fracture, or severe spinal deformity.
- Patients with severe symptoms affecting quality of life who have not responded to conservative treatment.

When to Admit

Patients with cauda equina syndrome, which requires emergent surgical intervention.

Bronfort G et al. Spinal manipulation and clinician-supported biopsychosocial self-management for acute back pain: the PACBACK randomized clinical trial. JAMA. 2026;335:497. [PMID: 41460638]

Earwood JS et al. Acute low back pain: diagnosis and management. Am Fam Physician. 2025;112:526. [PMID: 41252835]

2. Spinal Stenosis

ESSENTIALS OF DIAGNOSIS

- Pain is usually worse with back extension and relieved by sitting.
- Occurs in older patients.
- May present with neurogenic claudication symptoms with walking.

General Considerations

OA in the lumbar spine can cause narrowing of the spinal canal. A large disc herniation can also cause stenosis and compression of neural structures or the spinal artery resulting in "claudication" symptoms with ambulation. The condition usually affects patients age ≥ 50.

Clinical Findings

Patients report pain that worsens with extension. They describe reproducible single or bilateral leg symptoms that are worse after walking several minutes and that are relieved by sitting ("neurogenic claudication"). On examination, patients often exhibit limited extension of the lumbar spine, which may reproduce the symptoms radiating down the legs. A thorough neurovascular examination is recommended (Table 45–4). MRI and CT of the axial and sagittal lumbar planes enhance detection of lateral recess and central canal stenosis. Increased paraspinal fatty muscle infiltration seen on MRI is associated with increased disability and worse health-related quality of life.

Treatment

A. Conservative

Exercises, usually flexion-based as demonstrated by a physical therapist, can help relieve symptoms. Physical therapy showed similar results as surgical decompression in a randomized trial, though there was a 57% crossover rate from physical therapy to surgery. Facet joint corticosteroid injections can also reduce pain symptoms. The majority of studies found favorable short-term or intermediate-term benefits of lumbar epidural spinal injections. Lumbar epidural spinal injections are effective for immediate improvement in pain and function and provide short-term benefits in lumbar radiculopathy and some spinal stenosis cases. Optimal outcomes depend on the lumbar epidural spinal injection technique and patient stratification.

B. Surgical

The role of surgery for spinal stenosis is limited; surgery has not been shown to have clear benefit over nonsurgical treatment for lumbar spinal stenosis. However, if severe symptoms persist for 3 months despite conservative treatment, one can discuss the risks and benefits of surgery. Previous spinal surgery, duration of back pain > 12 months, and age > 70 years are predictors of failure and worsening of symptoms after surgery. Surgical treatments include spinal decompression (widening the spinal canal or laminectomy), nerve root decompression (freeing a single nerve), and spinal fusion (joining the vertebra to eliminate motion and diminish pain from the arthritic joints). Minimally invasive lumbar decompression does not leave hardware in the spine, and patients typically resume unrestricted normal activity within 24 hours. Percutaneous image-guided lumbar decompression uses minimally invasive techniques with instrumentation and image guidance to debulk a thickened ligamentum flavum. In one multicenter randomized trial, subgroups of patients with symptomatic spinal stenosis initially improved significantly more with surgery than with nonoperative treatment. However, long-term follow-up of the patients who received surgery showed less benefit of surgery between 4 and 8 years, suggesting that the advantage of surgery for spinal stenosis diminishes over time.

When to Refer

- If a patient exhibits radicular or claudication symptoms > 12 weeks.
- MRI or CT confirmation of significant, symptomatic spinal stenosis.

Alhaug OK et al. Predictors for failure after surgery for lumbar spinal stenosis: a prospective observational study. Spine J. 2023;23:261. [PMID: 36343913]

Anderson DB et al. Clinical assessment and management of lumbar spinal stenosis: clinical dilemmas and considerations for surgical referral. Lancet Rheumatol. 2024;6:e727. [PMID: 38723654]

Soin A et al. Lumbar epidural steroid injections for chronic spinal pain: a clinical review of efficacy and evidence. Cureus. 2025;17:e98348. [PMID: 41487815]

3. Lumbar Disc Herniation

ESSENTIALS OF DIAGNOSIS

- Pain with back flexion or prolonged sitting.
- Radicular pain into the leg due to compression of neural structures.
- Lower extremity numbness and weakness.

General Considerations

Lumbar disc herniation is usually due to bending or heavy loading (eg, lifting) with the back in flexion, causing herniation or extrusion of disc contents (nucleus pulposus) into the spinal cord area. However, there may not be an inciting incident. Disc herniations usually occur from degenerative disc disease (desiccation of the annulus fibrosis) in patients between 30 and 50 years old. The L5–S1 disc is affected in 90% of cases. Compression of neural structures, such as the sciatic nerve, causes radicular pain. Severe compression of the spinal cord can cause the cauda equina syndrome, a surgical emergency.

Clinical Findings

A. Symptoms and Signs

Discogenic pain typically is localized in the low back at the level of the affected disc and is worse with activity. "Sciatica" causes electric shock-like pain radiating down the posterior aspect of the leg often to below the knee. Symptoms usually worsen with back flexion such as bending or sitting for long periods (eg, driving). A significant disc herniation can cause numbness and weakness, including weakness of plantar flexion of the foot (L5/S1) or dorsiflexion of the toes (L4/L5). The cauda equina syndrome should be ruled out if the patient reports perianal numbness or bowel or bladder incontinence.

B. Imaging

Plain radiographs are helpful to assess spinal alignment (scoliosis, lordosis), disc space narrowing, and OA changes. MRI is the best method to assess the level and morphology of the herniation and is recommended if surgery is planned. Provocative lumbar discography (under fluoroscopic guidance, fluid is injected into a disc to pressurize it and a pain response is recorded) can be helpful for identifying the disc as the source of low back pain.

Treatment

For an acute exacerbation of pain symptoms, bed rest is appropriate for up to 48 hours. Otherwise, first-line therapy includes nonsteroidal anti-inflammatory drugs (NSAIDs) (Table 5–4), physical rehabilitation, activity modification, and functional exercise, including core stabilization and McKenzie back exercises (https://

sportsrehab.ucsf.edu/sites/g/files/tkssra10961/files/doc/McKenzie_Back_Program_Nov2025.pdf). The McKenzie exercises identify the mechanical direction of motion in the back that causes more or less pain, using careful history and physical examination to guide the treatment approach. An exercise protocol is designed to centralize or alleviate the pain.

Following nonsurgical treatment for a lumbar disc for > 1 year, the incidence of low back pain recurrence is ≥ 40% and is predicted by longer time to initial resolution of pain. In a randomized trial, oral prednisone caused a modest improvement in function at 3 weeks, but there was no significant improvement in pain in patients with acute radiculopathy who were monitored for 1 year. The initial dose for oral prednisone is approximately 1 mg/kg once daily with tapering doses over 10–15 days. Analgesics for neuropathic pain, such as the α2δ ligands (ie, gabapentin, pregabalin) or tricyclic antidepressants, may be helpful (Table 5–8). Epidural and transforaminal corticosteroid injections can be beneficial. There is moderate-quality evidence that epidural corticosteroid injections are effective, although the treatment effects are small (mean difference < 10%) and short-term for improving radicular pain for individuals. Epidural injections have not impacted long-term surgery rates for disc herniations. There is level I evidence for the use of transforaminal injections for radicular pain from disc herniation. PRP, bone marrow aspirate concentrate, and chemonucleolysis have demonstrated potential in delaying disc degeneration and enhancing tissue repair when injected alone or as an adjunct to surgical procedures. Intradiscal electrothermal therapy has limited success in 40–50% of patients with reduction of pain up to 2 years.

The severity of pain and disability as well as failure of conservative therapy are the most important reasons for surgery. A large trial has shown that patients who underwent surgery for a lumbar disc herniation achieved greater improvement than conservatively treated patients in all primary and secondary outcomes except return-to-work status after 8-year follow-up. Patients with sequestered fragments, symptom duration > 6 months, higher levels of low back pain, or who were neither working nor disabled at baseline showed greater surgical treatment effects. Microdiscectomy is the standard treatment with a low rate of complications and satisfactory results in > 90% in the largest series. It is performed by minimally invasive percutaneous endoscopic spine surgery, where an endoscope is used to remove fragments of disc herniation (interlaminar or transforaminal approaches) under local anesthesia for the treatment of primary and recurrent disc disease. The most commonly reported complications of endoscopic lumbar surgery include dural tear, infection, and epidural hematoma. A systematic review of 14 moderate quality studies suggests that percutaneous endoscopic discectomy and open microdiscectomy have similar results and complications. Patient-related risk factors for recurrent pain after percutaneous endoscopic discectomy include age ≥ 50 years, Modic changes, obesity (BMI ≥ 25), no college education, diabetes, heavy manual labor with poor ergonomics, cigarette smoking, the protrusion type of lumbar disc herniation, and a factor related to the surgical experience of spinal surgeons. Recurrent disc herniations are treated with decompression surgeries and spinal fusion surgeries. Disc replacement surgery has shown benefits in short-term pain relief, disability, and quality of life compared with spine fusion surgery.

When to Refer

- Progressive worsening of neurologic symptoms, especially leg dominant symptoms.
- Loss of motor function (sensory losses can be followed in the outpatient clinic).

When to Admit

Cauda equina syndrome requires urgent surgical intervention.

Tong Y et al. Recent advances and evolving strategies in the treatment of lumbar disc herniation. Front Neurol. 2025;16:1706784. [PMID: 41487424]

4. Neck Pain

ESSENTIALS OF DIAGNOSIS

- Chronic neck pain is mostly caused by degenerative joint disease.
- Whiplash often follows a traumatic neck injury.
- Poor posture is often a factor for persistent neck pain.

General Considerations

Most neck pain, especially in older patients, is due to mechanical degeneration involving cervical discs, facet joints, and ligamentous structure. Posture is a very important factor, especially in younger patients. Many work-related neck symptoms are due to poor posture and repetitive motions over time. Acute injuries can also occur secondary to trauma. Whiplash occurs from rapid flexion and extension of the neck and affects 15–40% of people in motor vehicle accidents; chronic pain develops in 5–7%. Neck fractures are serious traumatic injuries acutely and can lead to OA in the long term. Ultimately, degenerative conditions of the neck can result in cervical canal stenosis or neural foraminal stenosis, sometimes affecting underlying neural structures. Focal or multilevel cervical spinal cord compression can lead to cervical myelopathy. Cervical radiculopathy most commonly occurs at the C5–C7 disc levels and can cause neurologic symptoms in the upper extremities. Patients with neck pain may report associated headaches and shoulder pain. Both peripheral nerve entrapment and cervical radiculopathy, known as a "double crush" injury, may develop.

Clinical Findings

A. Symptoms and Signs

Neck pain may be limited to the posterior region or, depending on the level of the symptomatic joint, may radiate segmentally to the occiput, anterior chest, shoulder girdle, arm, forearm, and hand. It may be intensified by active or passive neck motions. The general distribution of pain and paresthesias corresponds roughly to the involved dermatome in the upper extremity. Progressive hand numbness, weakness, gait disturbance, and loss of fine motor skills are suggestive of cervical myelopathy.

The patient's posture should be assessed, checking for shoulder rolled-forward or head-forward posture as well as scoliosis in the thoracolumbar spine. Patients with discogenic neck pain often report pain with flexion, which causes cervical discs to herniate posteriorly. Extension of the neck usually affects the neural foraminal and facet joints of the neck. Rotation and lateral flexion of the cervical spine should be measured both to the left and the right. Limitation of cervical movements is the most common objective finding.

A detailed neurovascular examination of the upper extremities should be performed, including sensory input to light touch and temperature; motor strength testing, especially the hand intrinsic muscles (thumb extension strength [C6], opponens strength [thumb to pinky] [C7], and finger abductors and adductors strength [C8–T1]); and upper extremity reflexes (biceps, triceps, brachioradialis). Hyperreflexia and a positive Romberg test suggest the gait instability and hand weakness of cervical myelopathy. True cervical radiculopathy symptoms should match an expected dermatomal or myotomal distribution. The Spurling test involves asking the patient to rotate and extend the neck to one side. The clinician can apply a gentle axial load to the neck. Reproduction of the cervical radiculopathy symptoms is a positive sign of nerve root compression. Palpation of the neck is best performed with the patient in the supine position where the clinician can palpate each level of the cervical spine with the muscles of the neck relaxed. One study of patients with cervical radiculopathy, however, showed that only 62.6% of individuals had a concordant dermatomal pattern (where the radicular symptoms matched the involved root) and 67.3% had a standard muscle weakness pattern of the involved nerve.

B. Imaging and Special Tests

Standard radiographs of the cervical spine include the AP and lateral view. The odontoid view is usually added to rule out traumatic fractures and congenital abnormalities. Oblique views of the cervical spine can provide further information about arthritis changes and assess the neural foramina for narrowing. Plain radiographs can be normal in patients who have suffered an acute cervical strain. Comparative reduction in height of the involved disc space and osteophytes are frequent findings when there are degenerative changes in the cervical spine. Loss of cervical lordosis is commonly seen but is nonspecific.

MRI without intravenous contrast is the most sensitive method to assess the soft tissue structures of the cervical spine (such as the discs, spinal cord, and nerve roots). If the patient has signs of cervical radiculopathy or worsening chronic pain, an MRI may be appropriate, especially if there is any motor weakness. Intravenous contrast is considered if infection or tumor is suspected. CT scanning is the most useful method to evaluate bony abnormalities, such as fractures, cervical stenosis, or bone lesions.

Electromyography and nerve conduction studies are useful in differentiating peripheral nerve entrapment syndromes from cervical radiculopathy. However, sensitivity of electrodiagnostic testing for cervical radiculopathy ranges from only 50% to 71%, so a negative test does not rule out nerve root problems.

Treatment

Neck pain can usually be treated conservatively, in the absence of trauma or evidence of infection, malignancy, neurologic findings, or systemic inflammation. More frequent follow-up is recommended for patients when acute, severe symptoms are present early on after an injury. High pain-related disability is a predictor of poor outcome at 1 year even if individuals decline care. A course of specific neck exercises in physical therapy, including stretching, strengthening, and postural exercises, has been demonstrated to relieve symptoms with better short- to medium-term outcomes, although tailored programs were not clearly better than specific neck exercises. A soft cervical collar can be useful for short-term use (up to 1–2 weeks) in acute neck injuries. Ergonomics should be assessed at the workplace and at home. Chiropractic manual manipulation and mobilization can provide short-term benefit for mechanical neck pain. Although the rate of complications is low (5–10 million manipulations), care should be taken whenever there are neurologic symptoms present. Specific patients may respond to use of home cervical traction. NSAIDs are commonly used; opioids may be needed in cases of severe neck pain (Tables 5–5 and 5–6). Muscle relaxants (eg, cyclobenzaprine 5–10 mg orally three times daily) can be used short term if there is muscle spasm or as a sedative to aid in sleeping. Acute radicular symptoms can be treated with neuropathic medications (eg, gabapentin 300–1200 mg orally three times daily), and a short course (5–10 days) of oral prednisone can be considered (starting at 1 mg/kg). Cervical foraminal or facet joint corticosteroid injections can also reduce symptoms. Cervical branch radiofrequency ablation is a second line treatment for chronic neck pain. Surgeries are successful in reducing neurologic symptoms in 80–90% of cases but are still considered as treatments of last resort. Cervical myelopathy often requires surgery. Common surgeries for cervical degenerative disc disease include anterior cervical discectomy with fusion and cervical disc arthroplasty (replacing the degenerated disc with a prosthetic disc). A 2025 meta-analysis of 25 RCTs showed that cervical disc arthroplasty was superior to anterior discectomy and fusion for the treatment of symptomatic cervical disc disease, with better success, fewer secondary surgeries, and adverse events. Some results include more than 10 years of follow-up.

When to Refer

- Patients with severe symptoms with motor weakness.
- Surgical decompression surgery if the symptoms are severe and there is identifiable, correctable pathology.

Expert Panel on Neurological Imaging; Eldaya RW et al. ACR Appropriateness Criteria® Cervical Pain or Cervical Radiculopathy: 2024 Update. J Am Coll Radiol. 2025;22:S136. [PMID: 40409873]

UPPER EXTREMITY

1. Lateral & Medial Epicondylosis (Tendinopathy)

ESSENTIALS OF DIAGNOSIS

- Tenderness over the lateral or medial epicondyle.
- Pain with resisted strength testing and passive stretching of the affected tendon and muscle unit.
- Physical therapy and activity modification are more successful than anti-inflammatory treatments.

General Considerations

Tendinopathies involving the wrist extensors, flexors, and pronators are common concerns. The underlying mechanism of injury is repetitive overuse causing microtrauma at the tendon insertion, although acute strain injuries also can occur. The traditional term *epicondylitis* is a misnomer because histologically, tendinosis or degeneration in the tendon is seen rather than acute inflammation. Therefore, these entities should be referred to as *tendinopathy* or *tendinosis*. Lateral epicondylosis involves the wrist extensors, especially the extensor carpi radialis brevis. This is usually caused be lifting with the wrist and the elbow extended. Medial epicondylosis involves the wrist flexors and specifically the pronator teres tendon. Ulnar neuropathy and cervical radiculopathy should be considered in the differential diagnosis.

Clinical Findings

A. Symptoms and Signs

1. Lateral epicondylosis—The patient describes pain with the arm and wrist extended. For example, common concerns include pain while shaking hands, lifting objects, typing, or hitting a backhand in tennis ("tennis elbow").

2. Medial epicondylosis—Pain during motions in which the arm is repetitively pronated or the wrist is flexed is presenting symptom. This is also known as "golfer's elbow" due to the motion of turning the hands into pronation during the golf swing.

On examination, tenderness directly over the affected epicondyle is present, especially over the bony prominence where the tendon insertion occurs. The proximal tendon and musculotendinous junction also can be sore. Tendon pain can be reproduced over the epicondyle with resisted wrist extension and third digit extension for lateral epicondylosis and resisted wrist pronation and wrist flexion for medial epicondylosis. The pain is also often reproduced with passive stretching of the affected muscle groups, which can be performed with the arm in extension. It is useful to check the ulnar nerve (located in a groove at the posteromedial elbow) for tenderness as well as to perform a Spurling test for cervical radiculopathy (see Neck Pain, above).

B. Imaging

Radiographs are often normal, although a small traction spur may be present in chronic cases (enthesopathy). Diagnostic investigations are usually unnecessary, unless the patient does not improve after up to 3 months of conservative treatment. At that point, a patient who demonstrates significant disability due to the pain should be assessed with an MRI or ultrasound. Ultrasound and MRI can visualize the tendon and confirm tendinosis or tears.

Treatment

First-line treatment is usually conservative, including patient education regarding activity modification and management of symptoms. Ice and NSAIDs can help with pain (Table 5–4). The mainstay of treatment is physical therapy exercises. The most important steps are to begin a good stretching program followed by strengthening exercises, particularly eccentric ones. Counterforce elbow braces might provide some symptomatic relief, although there is no published evidence to support their use.

If the patient has severe or long-standing symptoms, corticosteroid injections can be considered. A randomized trial showed improvement with corticosteroid injection at 1 month and decreased tendon thickness but no improvement at 3 months. Percutaneous needle tenotomy showed some positive results as an alternative to surgery but lacks demonstrated efficacy in a randomized controlled study. PRP injections have been shown to be effective for lateral epicondylosis. Compared with prolotherapy, extracorporeal shock wave, and physiotherapy, PRP had better clinical and functional outcomes for chronic lateral epicondylosis over a 2-year follow-up, though all of these treatments have evidence of effectiveness. Study results have been inconsistent, though, about the use of PRP as a treatment for lateral epicondylitis, due to the varied methods of PRP preparations, varying postinjection recommendations, and improvement with placebo injections. Both leukocyte-rich and leukocyte-poor concentrations of PRP appeared to effectively treat lateral epicondylitis. Extracorporeal shock wave therapy has shown better efficacy for pain relief (as measured with visual analog scales) and better grip strength compared with ultrasound treatment. However, it is used less commonly than injection treatments of PRP and is still considered second-line therapy. While individual studies showed some benefits, a Canadian meta-analysis demonstrated that the highest-quality evidence did not support the use of exercise-based physical therapy, corticosteroid injections, PRP, or autologous blood injections, highlighting the challenge of treating these tendinopathies. There is preliminary suggestion of benefit with botulinum toxin injection.

When to Refer

Patients not responding to 6 months of conservative treatment should be referred for an injection procedure (PRP or tenotomy), surgical debridement, or repair of the tendon.

Lhee SH et al. Comparing the use of physiotherapy, shockwave therapy, prolotherapy, and platelet-rich plasma for chronic lateral epicondylosis: a prospective, randomized controlled trial with 2-year follow-up. Am J Sports Med. 2025; 53:2707. [PMID: 40815854]

2. Carpal Tunnel Syndrome

ESSENTIALS OF DIAGNOSIS

- Pain, burning, and tingling in the distribution of the median nerve.
- Initially, most bothersome during sleep.
- Later, weakness or atrophy of the thenar eminence.
- Can be caused by repetitive wrist activities.
- Commonly seen during pregnancy, diabetes mellitus, or rheumatoid arthritis.

General Considerations

An entrapment neuropathy, carpal tunnel syndrome is a painful disorder caused by compression of the median nerve between the carpal ligament and other structures within the carpal tunnel. Risk factors include repetitive hand use or previous wrist injury. The disorder is more common in women and may occur from fluid retention of pregnancy or hormonal changes. Patients with diabetes can get mononeuropathies. Carpal tunnel syndrome can be a feature of Charcot-Marie-Tooth disease; Ehlers-Danlos syndrome; rheumatic diseases, such as rheumatoid arthritis or inflammatory tenosynovitis; infiltrate disorders (myxedema, amyloidosis, sarcoidosis, leukemia, acromegaly); and hyperparathyroidism.

Clinical Findings

A. Symptoms and Signs

Carpal tunnel syndrome (CTS) presents with numbness, especially at night, waking the patient. Symptoms also are caused by manual activity involving wrist flexion. Aching pain may radiate proximally into the forearm and occasionally proximally to the shoulder and over the neck and chest. Impairment of sensation in the median nerve distribution may or may not be demonstrable. The **Phalen sign** is pain or paresthesia in the distribution of the median nerve when the patient flexes both wrists to 90 degrees for 60 seconds. A timed Phalen test is performed similarly, but the patient reports the time it takes to experience first symptoms up to 120 seconds. If the patient reports symptoms within 10 seconds, this test has a specificity of 96.8% and positive predictive value of 96.6% in predicting abnormal signs of nerve conduction. A **Tinel sign** is tingling or shock-like pain on volar wrist percussion (36–50% sensitive and 77% specific). The **carpal tunnel compression test** (Durkan test) induces numbness and tingling with direct application of pressure over the carpal tunnel for 30 seconds. Muscle weakness or atrophy, especially of the thenar eminence, can appear later than sensory disturbances as compression of the nerve worsens. **The CTS-6 tool** has good validity and reliability for diagnosing CTS. The six items are (1) numbness predominantly or exclusively over the medial nerve distribution (often the palmar surfaces of the thumb, the index and long fingers, and the radial half of the ring finger); (2) nocturnal numbness; (3) thenar hypotrophy; (4) loss of two-point discrimination < 5 mm; (5) a positive Phalen test; and (6) a positive Tinel sign.

B. Imaging

Ultrasound can demonstrate flattening of the median nerve beneath the flexor retinaculum. Sensitivity of ultrasound for carpal tunnel syndrome is variable but is estimated between 54% and 98%.

C. Special Tests

Electromyography and nerve conduction studies show evidence of sensory conduction delay before motor delay, which can occur in severe cases and is most helpful when the diagnosis is unclear. Electrodiagnosis can provide information on focal median mononeuropathy at the wrist and can classify carpal tunnel syndrome from mild to severe, which may help in worker's compensation cases.

Treatment

Treatment is directed toward relief of pressure on the median nerve. Patients with carpal tunnel syndrome should modify their hand activities if possible. The affected wrist can be splinted in the neutral position for periods up to 3 months, but a series of Cochrane reviews show limited evidence for splinting, exercises, and ergonomic positioning. Approximately 23% to 40% of individuals with CTS improve without specific treatment. Moderate evidence supports benefit from several physical therapy and electrophysical modalities (eg, ultrasound therapy and radial extracorporeal shockwave therapy). These modalities provide short-term and mid-term relief of carpal tunnel syndrome symptoms in different studies. Oral corticosteroids have shown benefit, though NSAIDs and acetaminophen have not shown much benefit. There is evidence that a corticosteroid injection to the carpal tunnel is more effective in the short term than surgery; however, a Dutch multicenter study suggested that surgery offers a higher chance of recovery after 18 months compared with starting with a corticosteroid injection. Methylprednisolone injections have been found to be more effective at 10 weeks than placebo, but the benefits diminish by 1 year. Knowledge of pertinent anatomy and consistent technique and ultrasound are helpful to ensure accurate needle placement during carpal tunnel injection. A systemic review and network meta-analysis examining different injections for CTS found that PRP injections to the carpal tunnel space had the best outcomes and longest results for symptom relief, followed by dextrose injections (prolotherapy), with corticosteroids providing only short-term benefits.

Carpal tunnel release surgery can be beneficial if the patient has a positive electrodiagnostic test, at least moderate symptoms, high clinical probability, unsuccessful non-operative treatment, and symptoms lasting > 12 months. An RCT showed both corticosteroid injection and surgery resolved symptoms, but only decompressive surgery led to resolution of neurophysiologic changes. Surgery can be done with an open approach or endoscopically, both yielding similar good improvements.

When to Refer

- If symptoms persist > 3 months despite conservative treatment, including the use of a wrist splint.
- If thenar muscle (eg, abductor pollicis brevis) weakness or atrophy develops.

Priya A et al. Correlating symptom severity index, clinical diagnostic criteria of CTS-6 and timed Phalen's test in clinical evaluation of carpal tunnel syndrome. J Family Med Prim Care. 2024;13:5047. [PMID: 39722997]

Shapiro LM et al; Management of Carpal Tunnel Syndrome Work Group; American Academy of Orthopaedic Surgeons. American Academy of Orthopaedic Surgeons/ASSH Clinical Practice Guideline Summary Management of Carpal Tunnel Syndrome. J Am Acad Orthop Surg. 2025;33:e356. [PMID: 39637428]

3. Dupuytren Contracture

ESSENTIALS OF DIAGNOSIS

- Benign fibrosing disorder of the palmar fascia.
- Contracture of one or more fingers can lead to limited hand function.

General Considerations

This relatively common disorder is characterized by hyperplasia of the palmar fascia and related structures, with nodule formation and contracture of the palmar fascia. The cause is unknown, but the condition has a genetic predisposition with an estimated heritability of 80% and occurs primarily in White men > 50 years of age, particularly in those of Celtic descent. The incidence is higher among patients with alcohol use disorder and those with chronic systemic disorders (especially cirrhosis). It is also associated with systemic fibrosing syndrome, which includes plantar fibromatosis (10% of patients), Peyronie disease (1–2%), mediastinal and retroperitoneal fibrosis, and Riedel struma. The onset may be acute, but slowly progressive chronic disease is more common. Younger age at treatment, cigarette smoking, dominantly affected PIP joint, and involvement of the little finger are associated with increased risk of progression or retreatment.

Clinical Findings

Dupuytren contracture manifests itself by nodular or cord-like thickening of one or both hands, with the fourth and fifth fingers most commonly affected. The patient may report tightness of the involved digits, with fixed flexion deformity at the metacarpophalangeal (MCP) joint, proximal interphalangeal (PIP) joint, or both with inability to extend the fingers. The contracture may be cosmetically unappealing, but in general it is well tolerated until the MCP fixed flexion deformity reaches 30 degrees or 15 degrees at the PIP joint; intervention is then considered.

Treatment

There are various nonsurgical treatments for Dupuytren contracture, including corticosteroids (oral, intramuscular, topical or intralesional); vitamin E; furazolidone; Aminosyn (an amino acid solution); tamoxifen; hyperbaric oxygen; radiotherapy; and physical therapies (ultrasound, splinting, frictional massage, or heat treatment with joint stretching). However, strong evidence for efficacy of these treatments is lacking. If the palmar nodule is growing rapidly, injections of triamcinolone or collagenase into the nodule may be of benefit, while collagenase *Clostridium histolyticum* (CCH) injections lyse collagen, thereby disrupting the contracted cords. Surgical options, including limited fasciectomy (LF) or percutaneous needle fasciotomy (PNF), are indicated for more severe flexion contractures. Splinting after surgery is beneficial. Recurrence and more adverse events are more likely to occur after surgery than with nonoperative treatments. Overall, surgical treatment is more successful for MCP joints than for PIP joints. Fasciectomies are more successful for severe conditions involving multiple fingers, while PNF is cost-effective and useful for milder cases and for single-digit involvement. A meta-analysis showed similar results in reducing long-term contracture among those treated with LF, PNF, and CCH. However, a multicenter RCT showed that LF performed better than CCH injections, with less contracture recurrence, but with more moderate and severe complications (complications were 5.1% with LF and 1.8% with CCH).

When to Refer

Referral can be considered when one or more digits are affected by severe contractures, which interfere with everyday activities and result in functional limitations.

Dias J et al. Collagenase injection versus limited fasciectomy for Dupuytren's contracture. N Engl J Med. 2024;24;391:1499. [PMID: 39383454]
Karjalainen VL et al. Progression of Dupuytren's contracture: a randomized controlled trial comparing surgery, needle fasciotomy, and collagenase injection. Plast Reconstr Surg. 2025 Dec 4. [Epub ahead of print] [PMID: 41334972]

4. Bursitis

ESSENTIALS OF DIAGNOSIS

- Often occurs around bony prominences where it is important to reduce friction.
- Typically presents with local swelling that is painful acutely.
- Septic bursitis can present without fever or systemic signs.

General Considerations

Inflammation of bursae can lead to fluid accumulation in the synovial membranes overlying bony prominences. Predisposing factors include trauma, infection, or conditions such as chronic rheumatologic diseases (rheumatoid arthritis, gout, pseudogout, SLE), HIV, chronic hygroma (micro-traumatic bursopathy), and diabetes. The two common sites are the olecranon and prepatellar bursae; however, others include subdeltoid, ischial, trochanteric, and semimembranosus-gastrocnemius (Baker cyst) bursae. Septic bursitis can result from infection, often preceded by direct trauma or posttraumatic acute bursopathy, or from preexisting conditions such as rheumatoid arthritis or gout.

Clinical Findings

A. Symptoms and Signs

Bursitis presents with focal tenderness and swelling and is less likely to affect range of motion of the adjacent joint. Olecranon or prepatellar bursitis, for example, causes an oval (or, if chronic, bulbous) swelling at the tip of the elbow or knee and does not affect joint motion. A bursa can also become symptomatic when it ruptures. Rupture of a Baker cyst, which occurs in the back of the knee and is usually related to degenerative changes, can cause calf pain and acute swelling that is often confused with DVT.

Tenderness, erythema and warmth, cellulitis, a report of trauma, and overlying skin lesion are more common in **septic bursitis** but can be present in aseptic bursitis as well. Patients with septic bursitis can be febrile but the absence of fever does not exclude infection; one-third of those with septic olecranon bursitis are afebrile.

B. Imaging

Imaging is unnecessary unless there is concern for osteomyelitis, trauma, or other underlying pathology. Baker cysts are best imaged by sonography but are also well imaged by MRI; imaging a presumed Baker cyst can exclude a DVT.

C. Special Tests

Acute swelling and redness at a bursal site call for aspiration to rule out infection especially if the patient either is febrile (temperature > 37.8°C) or has prebursal warmth (temperature difference > 2.2°C) or both (Figure 45–1). A bursal fluid WBC count of > 1000/mcL (1.0×10^9/L) indicates inflammation from infection, rheumatoid arthritis, or gout. The bursal fluid of septic bursitis characteristically contains a purulent aspirate, fluid-to-serum glucose ratio < 50%, WBC count > 3000 cells/mcL (3.0×10^9/L), and polymorphonuclear cells > 50%. Most cases are caused by *Staphylococcus aureus* (80–90%) or β-hemolytic streptococci; the Gram stain of bursal fluid is positive in two-thirds, but blood cultures are infrequently positive (0–19%). Elevated serum ESR and CRP can be seen but also occur with crystal-induced bursitis or rheumatoid bursitis.

Treatment

In general, aspiration and corticosteroid injections in mild, nonseptic bursitis should be avoided to reduce complications of iatrogenic infection and skin atrophy. Bursitis caused by trauma can be treated with local heat, rest, NSAIDs early on (Table 5–4), and if very painful or persistent, local corticosteroid injections. Repetitive minor trauma to the olecranon bursa should be eliminated by avoiding resting the elbow on a hard surface or by wearing an elbow pad. For chronic aseptic bursitis or when there are athletic or occupational demands, aspiration with intrabursal corticosteroid injection (methylprednisolone or triamcinolone 40 mg) can be performed. Ultrasound-guided aspiration and injection can improve the accuracy of the procedures. Treatment of a ruptured Baker cyst includes rest, leg elevation, and possibly injection of triamcinolone 40 mg into the knee anteriorly (the knee compartment communicates with the cyst).

Treatment for septic bursitis involves incision and drainage and antibiotics usually delivered intravenously, especially against *S aureus* and β-hemolytic streptococci (see Chapter 34). A clinical reassessment is suggested 3–5 days after the start of antibiotic therapy.

When to Refer

Elective surgical removal can be considered for chronic refractory cases with symptoms affecting activities of daily living.

When to Admit

Septic bursitis requires immediate treatment with intravenous antibiotics and usually incision and draining.

Darrieutort-Laffite C et al. 2023 French recommendations for diagnosing and managing prepatellar and olecranon septic bursitis. Joint Bone Spine. 2023;91:105664. [PMID: 37995861]
Zhang A et al. The immune pathology of bursitis in rheumatic inflammatory diseases, degenerative conditions and mechanical stress: a systematic review. Semin Arthritis Rheum. 2024; 68:152527. [PMID: 39146915]

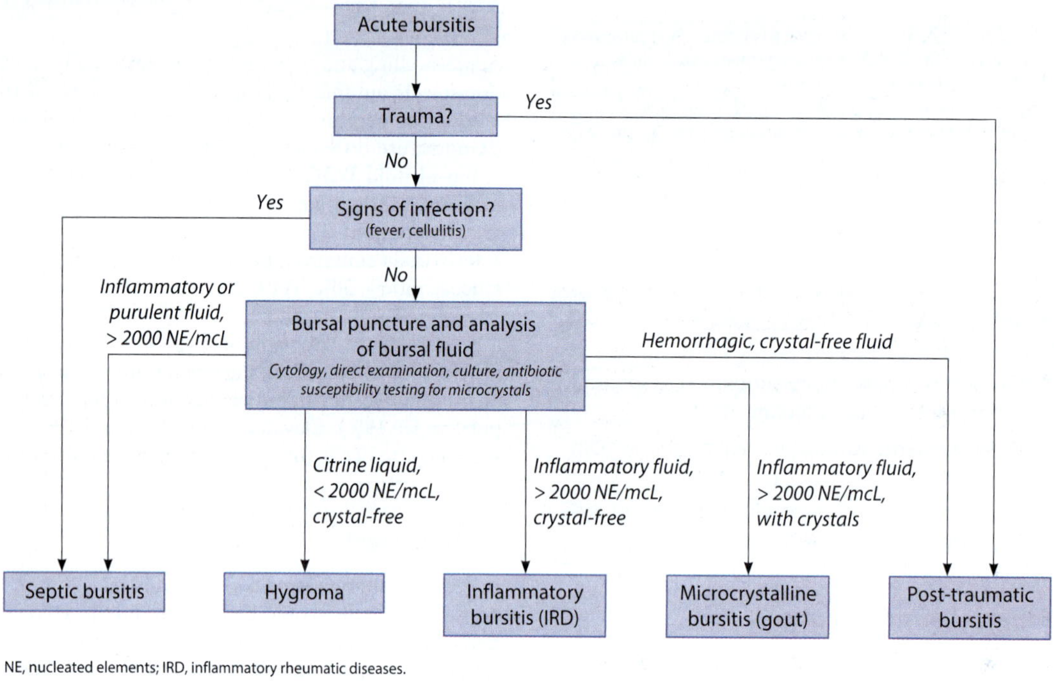

Figure 45–1. Diagnostic approach to bursitis. (Reproduced with permission from Darrieutort-Laffite C et al. 2023 French recommendations for diagnosing and managing prepatellar and olecranon septic bursitis. Joint Bone Spine. 2023;91(2):105664.)

HIP

1. Hip Fractures

ESSENTIALS OF DIAGNOSIS

- Internal rotation of the hip is the best provocative diagnostic maneuver.
- Hip fractures should be surgically repaired as soon as possible (within 24 hours).
- Delayed treatment of hip fractures in older adults leads to increased complications and mortality.

General Considerations

Approximately 10 million hip fractures occur globally each year. Hips fracture usually from a fall; high-velocity trauma is needed in younger patients. Stress fractures can occur in athletes or individuals with poor bone mineral density following repetitive loading activities. Osteoporosis, female sex, height > 68 inches, and age > 50 years are risk factors for hip fracture. There is a high mortality rate among older adult patients following hip fracture, with death occurring in 8–10% within 30 days and in approximately 22% within 1 year. Age > 90 years is a risk factor for mortality within 1 year, while male sex, frailty, general anesthesia, high BUN, and high preoperative neutrophil to lymphocyte ratio are risk factors for 90-day mortality.

Clinical Findings

A. Symptoms and Signs

Patients typically report pain in the groin, though pain radiating to the lateral hip, buttock, or knee also can commonly occur. If a displaced fracture is present, the patient will not be able to bear weight and the leg may be externally rotated. The ability to gently logroll the leg with the patient supine helps rule out a fracture. Examination of the hip demonstrates pain with deep palpation in the area of the femoral triangle (similar to palpating the femoral artery). Provided the patient can tolerate it, with the patient supine, the clinician flexes the hip to 90 degrees with the knee flexed to 90 degrees and tests internal and external rotation of the hips on each side. Pain with internal rotation of the hip is the most sensitive test to identify intra-articular hip pathology. Hip flexion, extension, abduction, and adduction strength can be tested.

Patients with hip stress fractures have less pain on physical examination than described previously but typically have pain with weight bearing. The Trendelenburg test can be performed to examine for weakness or instability of the hip abductors, primarily the gluteus medius muscle; the patient balances first on one leg, raising the non-standing knee toward the chest. The clinician can stand behind the patient and observe for dropping of the pelvis and buttock on the non-stance side. Another functional test is asking the patient to hop or jump during the examination. If the patient has a compatible clinical history of pain and is unable or unwilling to hop, then a stress fracture should be ruled out. The back should be carefully examined in patients who report hip discomfort, including examining for signs of sciatica.

Delay of operative intervention for displaced hip fractures leads to an increased risk of perioperative morbidity and mortality. A thorough medical evaluation and treatment should be done to maximize the patient's ability to undergo operative intervention. A patient unable to get up after a fall may have been immobile for hours or even days; rhabdomyolysis, hypothermia, DVT, PE, and other possible sequelae of prolonged immobilization must be excluded.

B. Imaging

Useful radiographic imaging of the hip includes AP views of the pelvis and bilateral hips and frog-leg-lateral views of the painful hip. A CT scan or MRI may be necessary to identify the hip fracture pattern or to exclude non-displaced fractures. Hip fractures are generally described by location, including femoral neck, intertrochanteric, or subtrochanteric.

Treatment

Almost all patients with a hip fracture will require surgery and may need to be admitted to the hospital for pain control while they await surgery. Surgery is recommended within the first 24 hours because studies have shown that delaying surgery 48 hours results in at least twice the rate of major and minor medical complications, including pneumonia, pressure injuries (formerly pressure ulcers), and DVT. High-volume centers with multidisciplinary teams (including orthopedic surgeons, internists, social workers, and specialized physical therapists) to comanage patients improve perioperative medical care and expedite preoperative evaluation, leading to reduced costs. Hip fractures can be treated with internal fixation or joint replacement surgery. Cemented total hip arthroplasty has clinically small to large improvements in health-related quality of life and lower mortality at 1 year compared with other hip replacement options. During the months of hip fracture recovery, prevention of pneumonia and functional decline and treatment of cardiac disease can reduce mortality.

Stress fractures in active patients require a period of protected weight bearing and a gradual return to activities, although it may take 4–6 months before a return to normal activities. Femoral neck fractures are commonly treated with hemiarthroplasty or total hip replacement. This allows the patient to begin weight bearing immediately postoperatively. Peritrochanteric hip fractures are treated with open reduction internal fixation, where plate and screw construct or intramedullary devices are used. The choice of implant will depend on the fracture pattern. Since fracture fixation requires the fracture to proceed to union, the patient may need to have protected weight bearing during the early postoperative period. Dislocation, periprosthetic fracture, and avascular necrosis of the hip are complications after surgery. Patients should be mobilized as soon as possible postoperatively to avoid pulmonary complications and pressure injuries. Supervised physical therapy and rehabilitation are important for the patient to regain as much function as possible. Unfortunately, most patients following hip fractures will lose some degree of independence. Patients with hip fracture surgery when compared with elective total hip replacement have been shown to have higher risk of in-hospital mortality.

Prevention

Bone density screening can identify patients at risk for osteopenia or osteoporosis, and treatment can be planned accordingly (see Chapter 30). Consensus is that there is benefit in using bisphosphonates, particularly during the third through fifth years of therapy, with considerations for drug holidays. After 5 years of bisphosphonate use, there is an increased risk for atypical femur fractures. Nutrition and bone health (bone densitometry) should be reviewed with the patient. However, there is no evidence that increasing calcium intake prevents hip fractures. For patients with decreased mobility, systemic anticoagulation should be considered to avoid DVT (see Table 16–14). Fall prevention exercise programs are available for older adult patients at risk for falls and hip fractures. Hip protectors are uncomfortable and have less use in preventing fractures. The World Health Organization recommends measuring health system performance for treatment of older adults with hip fractures with specific goals of surgery within 48 hours of fracture and postfracture pharmacologic treatment of osteoporosis.

When to Refer

- All patients in whom hip fracture is suspected since ideally, surgical intervention occurs within 48 hours of injury.
- All patients with hip fracture or in whom the diagnosis is uncertain after radiographs.
- Patients should receive osteoporosis screening and treatment in the event of hip fracture.

Chandran M et al. WHO benchmarks for equitable hip-fracture care and osteoporosis treatment in older people. Nat Rev Rheumatol. 2026;22:62. [PMID: 41198933]

Hong G et al. Trends in hip fracture surgery in the United States from 2016 to 2021: patient characteristics, clinical management, and outcomes. Br J Anaesth. 2024;133:955. [PMID: 39242278]

2. Hip Osteoarthritis

ESSENTIALS OF DIAGNOSIS

- Pain deep in the groin on the affected side.
- Swelling.
- Degeneration of joint cartilage.
- Loss of active and passive range of motion in severe OA; normal passive hip adduction makes OA unlikely.

General Considerations

In the United States, the prevalence of OA will grow as the number of persons age > 65 years doubles to > 70 million by 2030. The etiology of OA is often multifactorial, including previous trauma, prior high-impact activities, genetic factors, obesity, and rheumatologic or metabolic conditions. Femoroacetabular impingement, which affects younger active patients, is considered an early development of hip OA.

Clinical Findings

A. Symptoms and Signs

OA usually causes pain in the affected joint with joint loading or at the extremes of motion. Mechanical symptoms—such as swelling, grinding, catching, and locking—suggest internal derangement from damaged cartilage or bone fragments that affect smooth range of motion. Pain can also produce the sensation of "buckling" or "giving way" due to muscle inhibition. As the joint degeneration becomes more advanced, the patient loses active range of motion and may lose passive range of motion.

Patients report pain deep in the groin on the affected side and have problems with weight-bearing activities such as walking, climbing stairs, and getting up from a chair. They may limp and develop a lurch during their gait, leaning toward the unaffected side as they walk to reduce pressure on the arthritic hip. The most specific findings to identify hip osteoarthritis are squat causing posterior pain, groin pain on passive abduction or adduction, abductor weakness, and decreased passive hip adduction or less passive internal rotation compared with the contralateral leg. The presence of normal passive hip adduction is most useful for suggesting the absence of OA (–LR, 0.25).

B. Imaging

An AP weight-bearing radiograph of the pelvis with a lateral view of the symptomatic hip are preferred views for evaluation of hip OA. Joint space narrowing and sclerosis suggest early OA. Findings of femoroacetabular impingement are commonly reported on radiograph reports with arthritic changes and anatomic variations involving the acetabulum and femoral head neck junction. After age 35, MRI of the hips already shows labral changes in almost 70% of asymptomatic persons. Osteophytes near the femoral head or acetabulum and subchondral bone cysts (advanced Kellgren and Lawrence grade), superior or (supero) lateral femoral head migration, and subchondral sclerosis suggest the patient will more likely progress to total hip replacement. However, not all patients with radiographic hip OA have hip or groin pain; the converse is also true.

Treatment

A. Conservative

Changes in the articular cartilage are irreversible. Therefore, a cure for the diseased joint is not possible, although symptoms or structural issues can be managed to try to maintain activity level. Conservative treatment for patients with OA includes activity modification; physical therapy with hip-specific, lumbo-pelvic, and core strengthening therapeutic exercises (Table 45–6); weight loss; use of assistive devices (such as a cane); and proper footwear. There is strong evidence that NSAIDs are beneficial for osteoarthritis pain. Acetaminophen can also be used, while opioids are not recommended for conservative treatment of hip osteoarthritis. Corticosteroid injections have moderate evidence for short-term relief of pain. Hip injections are best performed under imaging to ensure accurate injection in the joint, typically using ultrasound, fluoroscopic, or CT guidance. The risk of rapidly progressive degenerative changes following a single low-dose (≤ 40 mg) triamcinolone injection is low; the risk is higher following a high-dose (≥ 80 mg) injection and multiple injections.

Table 45–6. Summary of physical activity for hip or knee osteoarthritis.

- The benefits of physical activity for patients with knee or hip OA include reduced pain and stiffness, increased mobility and physical function, and improvements in mental health, quality of life, and comorbid conditions.
- A prescription for physical activity should be personalized to a patient's physical abilities; affected joint/s; pain; comorbidities; preferences and goals; and access to facilities, programs, and equipment.
- Proven recommendations for a physical activity prescription include:
  - 150 minutes/week of moderate aerobic activity plus 2 days of strengthening exercises
  - As little as 45 minutes/week may be beneficial
  - 6000–10,000 steps/day
- Beneficial activities include walking, cycling, water aerobics or swimming, strength training, stretching, tai chi, yoga, gardening, household chores.
- Patients should be counseled to move more and reduce sedentary time.
- Supervised physical activity sessions, community-based physical activity programs, wearable activity monitors, goal setting, and peer support are techniques to increase adherence to and maintenance of a physical activity routine.

OA, osteoarthritis.

Reproduced with permission from Huffman KF et al. The critical role of physical activity and weight management in knee and hip osteoarthritis: A narrative review. J Rheumatol. 2024;51:224.

B. Surgical

Hip arthroscopy for early osteoarthritis, if there is femoroacetabular impingement, can provide symptom improvement for > 10 years. Unfortunately, when bilateral cartilage defects (acetabular and femoral) are present in more advanced stages of hip osteoarthritis (Tonnis stage 3), hip preservation surgery is contraindicated.

Joint replacement surgeries are effective and cost-effective for patients with significant symptoms, radiologic findings, and functional limitations, providing improvements in pain, function, and quality of life. In considering surgery, underrepresented populations are less willing to undergo total joint replacement, demonstrate worse surgical and functional outcomes, and have less access to hospital choices. Mental health issues including anxiety and depression do not appear to adversely affect a patient's benefit from total hip replacement, although patients with better mental health scores may note greater improvement in patient reported outcomes. There has not been clear clinical benefit of minimally invasive surgery compared with the standard invasive surgery for functional outcome; however, total blood loss is less, and the duration of surgery and length of hospital stay are shorter with minimally invasive surgery.

Hip resurfacing surgery is an alternative for younger patients. Rather than use a traditional artificial joint implant of the whole neck and femur, only the femoral head is removed and replaced. Evidence to date suggests that hip resurfacing is comparable to total hip replacement. The cumulative survival rate of this implant at 15 years is estimated to be 95.1%. Concerns following resurfacing surgery include the risk of femoral neck fracture and collapse of the head. Chromium metal ion release is elevated postoperatively for the first 6 months. The levels are not elevated past 1 year and do not appear to be a long-term concern. Dislocations were more frequent with total hip arthroplasty than metal-on-metal hip resurfacing: 4.4 versus 0.9 per 1000 person-years, respectively.

Guidelines recommend prophylaxis for venous thromboembolic disease for a minimum of 14 days after arthroplasty of the hip or knee using warfarin, low-molecular-weight heparin, fondaparinux, aspirin, rivaroxaban, dabigatran, apixaban, or portable mechanical compression (see Table 16–14). While bleeding risks are similar, patients taking warfarin are more likely to experience DVT and PE than patients taking rivaroxaban (see Chapter 16).

When to Refer

Patients with sufficient disability, limited benefit from conservative therapy, and evidence of severe OA on imaging can be referred for joint replacement surgery.

Hannon CP et al. Management of Osteoarthritis of the Hip Work Group; Staff of the American Academy of Orthopaedic Surgeons; Management of Osteoarthritis of the Hip Work Group and Staff of the American Academy of Orthopaedic Surgeons. American Academy of Orthopaedic Surgeons Clinical Practice Guideline Summary Management of Osteoarthritis of the Hip. J Am Acad Orthop Surg. 2024;15;32:e1027. [PMID: 3878135]

Saluja A et al. Hip resurfacing arthroplasty in men: a minimum 15-year follow-up study. J Arthroplasty. 2025;40:S72. [PMID: 40120657]

KNEE

1. Knee Pain

ESSENTIALS OF DIAGNOSIS

- Effusion can occur with intra-articular pathology (eg, OA, meniscus and cruciate ligament tears).
- Acute knee swelling (due to hemarthrosis) within 2 hours may indicate ligament injuries or patellar dislocation or fracture.

General Considerations

The knee is the largest joint in the body and is susceptible to injury from trauma, inflammation, infection, and degenerative changes. OA of the knees is common after 50 years of age and can develop due to previous trauma, aging, activities, alignment issues, and genetic predisposition.

Acute hemarthrosis represents bloody swelling that usually occurs within the first 1–2 hours following trauma. In situations where the trauma may be activity-related and not a result of a fall or collision, the causes of the hemarthrosis most commonly include anterior cruciate ligament (ACL) tear (responsible for > 70% in adults), fracture (patella, tibial plateau, femoral supracondylar, growth plate [physeal]), tendon ruptures (quadriceps and patella tendon), and patellar dislocation. Meniscal tears are unlikely to cause large hemarthrosis.

Clinical Findings

A. Symptoms and Signs

Duration and rapidity of symptom onset and the mechanism of injury or aggravating symptoms should be determined. Overuse or degenerative problems can occur with stress or compression from sports, hobbies, or occupation. A history of trauma or previous orthopedic problems with, or surgery to, the affected knee should also be specifically queried. Symptoms of infection (fever, recent bacterial infections, risk factors for STIs [such as gonorrhea] or other bacterial infections [such as staphylococcal infection]) should always be elicited.

Common symptoms include the following:

1. Grinding, clicking, or popping with bending may be indicative of OA or the patellofemoral syndrome.
2. "Locking" or "catching" when walking suggests an internal derangement, such as meniscal injury or a loose body in the knee.
3. Intra-articular swelling of the knee or an effusion indicates an internal derangement or a synovial pathology. Large swelling may cause a popliteal (Baker) cyst. Acute swelling within minutes to hours suggests a hemarthrosis, most likely due to an ACL injury, fracture, or patellar dislocation, especially if trauma is involved.
4. Lateral "snapping" with flexion and extension of the knee may indicate inflammation of the iliotibial band.
5. Pain that is worsened with bending and walking down stairs suggests a patellofemoral joint source, usually degenerative such as patellar chondromalacia or OA.
6. Pain that occurs when rising after prolonged sitting suggests a problem with tracking of the patella.

A knee joint effusion is characterized by swelling in the hollow or dimple around the patella and distention of the suprapatellar space.

The location of the knee pain combined with specific tests for anatomic structures are frequently sufficient to establish a diagnosis (Tables 45–7 and 45–8).

Table 45–7. Location of common causes of knee pain.

Medial knee pain
Medial compartment osteoarthritis
Medial collateral ligament strain
Medial meniscal injury
Anserine bursitis (pain over the proximal medial tibial plateau)
Anterior knee pain
Patellofemoral syndrome (often bilateral)
Osteoarthritis
Prepatellar bursitis (associated with swelling anterior to the patella)
"Jumper's knee" (pain at the inferior pole of the patella)
Septic arthritis
Gout or other inflammatory disorder
Lateral knee pain
Lateral meniscal injury
Iliotibial band syndrome (pain superficially along the distal iliotibial band near the lateral femoral condyle or lateral tibial insertion)
Lateral collateral ligament sprain (rare)
Posterior knee pain
Popliteal (Baker) cyst
Osteoarthritis
Meniscal tears
Hamstring or calf tendinopathy

B. Laboratory Findings

Laboratory testing of aspirated joint fluid, when indicated, can lead to a definitive diagnosis in most patients (see Tables 23–2 and 23–3).

C. Imaging

Knee pain is evaluated with plain (weight-bearing) radiographs and MRI most commonly, but CT and ultrasound are sometimes useful.

D. Treatment

Treatment of specific etiologies of knee pain is discussed below.

Duong V et al. Evaluation and treatment of knee pain: a review. JAMA. 2023;330:1568. [PMID: 37874571]

Hawker GA et al. OARSI Early-stage Symptomatic Knee Osteoarthritis Initiative. OARSI initiative to develop classification criteria for early-stage symptomatic knee OA (EsSKOA): what conditions should be considered in the differential diagnosis of EsSKOA? Osteoarthritis Cartilage. 2025;33:1141. [PMID: 40414550]

2. Anterior Cruciate Ligament Injury

ESSENTIALS OF DIAGNOSIS

- An injury involving an audible pop when the knee buckles.
- Acute swelling immediately (or within 2 hours).
- Instability occurs with lateral movement activities and going down stairs.

General Considerations

The ACL connects the posterior aspect of the lateral femoral condyle to the anterior aspect of the tibia. ACL tears are common with sporting injuries. They can result from both contact (valgus blow to the knee) and non-contact (jumping, pivoting, and deceleration) activities. The patient usually falls down following the injury and has acute swelling, difficulty with weight bearing, and instability. ACL injuries are common in skiing, soccer, football, and basketball among young adolescents and middle-aged patients. Prepubertal and older patients usually sustain fractures instead of ligamentous injuries.

Clinical Findings

A. Symptoms and Signs

Acute ACL injuries usually lead to acute swelling of the knee, causing difficulty with motion. After the swelling has resolved, the patient can walk with a "stiff-knee" gait or quadriceps avoidance gait because of the instability. Patients describe symptoms of instability while performing side-to-side maneuvers or descending stairs. Stability tests assess the amount of laxity of the knee while performing these maneuvers. The Lachman test is 84–87% sensitive and 93% specific, and the anterior drawer test is 48% sensitive and 87% specific for ACL laxity compared with the other side. The pivot shift test is 79% sensitive and 9% specific for rotational laxity of the knee (Table 45–8).

B. Imaging

Plain radiographs are usually negative in ACL tears but are useful to rule out fractures. A small avulsion injury can sometimes be seen over the lateral compartment of the knee ("Segond" fracture) and is pathognomonic of an ACL injury. An ACL injury that avulsed the tibial spine can be seen in radiographs. MRI is the best tool to diagnose ACL tears and associated articular and meniscal cartilage issues. It has > 95% sensitivity and specificity for ACL tears.

Treatment

Most young and active patients will require surgical reconstruction of the ACL. Some data suggest that reconstruction within 5 months of the tear has better outcomes. However, a small, randomized trial suggested that acute ACL injuries can be treated nonoperatively and delayed ACL reconstruction had similar outcomes to acute ACL reconstructions. Patients for whom the reconstruction is delayed, however, have more cartilage or meniscus problems at the time of surgery. Common surgical techniques use the patient's own tissue, usually the patellar, quadriceps, or hamstring tendons (autograft), or use a cadaver graft (allograft) to arthroscopically reconstruct the torn ACL; allografts have a higher failure rate compared with autografts, especially for younger patients. Primary ACL repair is being performed in a few centers for acute injuries (typically < 6 weeks) of a simple proximal ACL tear that has good tissue quality and vascularity, though ACL

Table 45–8. Knee examination.

Maneuver	Description
Inspection	Examine for the alignment of the lower extremities (varus, valgus, knee recurvatum), ankle eversion and foot pronation, gait, and "SEADS" (*s*welling, *e*rythema, *a*trophy, *d*eformity, *s*urgical scars).
Palpation	Include important landmarks: patellofemoral joint, medial and lateral joint lines (especially posterior aspects), pes anserine bursa, distal iliotibial band, and Gerdy tubercle (iliotibial band insertion).
Range of motion testing 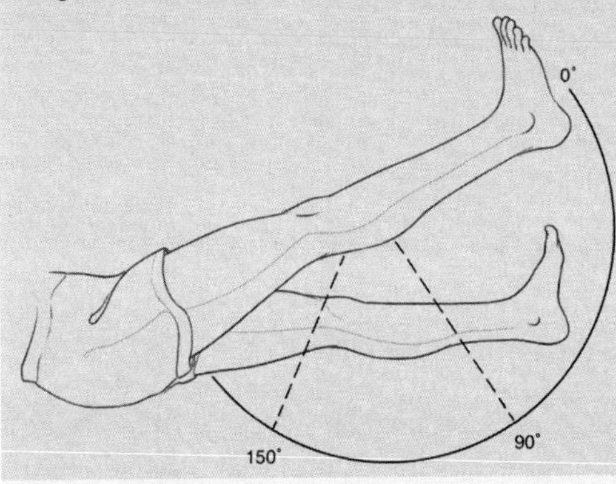	Check range of motion actively (patient performs) and passively (clinician performs), especially with flexion and extension of the knee normally 0–10 degrees of extension and 120–150 degrees of flexion.
Knee strength testing	Test resisted knee extension and knee flexion strength manually.
Ligament Stress Testing	
Lachman test 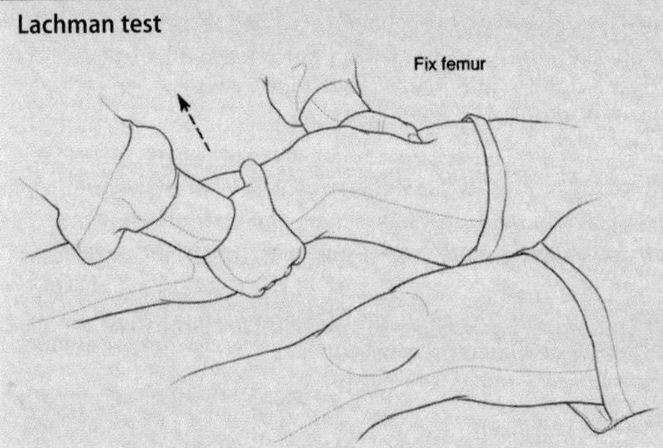	Performed with the patient lying supine and the knee flexed to 20–30 degrees. The examiner grasps the distal femur from the lateral side, and the proximal tibia with the other hand on the medial side. With the knee in neutral position, stabilize the femur, and pull the tibia anteriorly using a similar force to lift a 10- to 15-pound weight. **Positive test:** Excessive anterior translation of the tibia compared with the other side indicates injury to the anterior cruciate ligament.
Anterior drawer 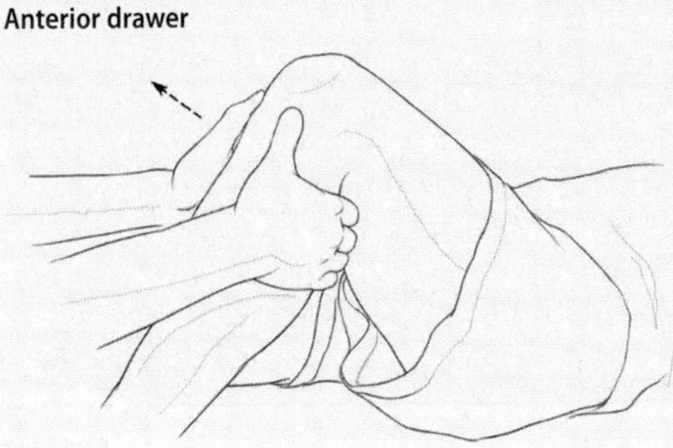	Performed with the patient lying supine and the knee flexed to 90 degrees. The clinician stabilizes the patient's foot by sitting on it and grasps the proximal tibia with both hands around the calf and pulls anteriorly. **Positive test:** There is anterior cruciate ligament laxity compared with the unaffected side.

(*continued*)

Table 45–8. Knee examination. (continued)

Maneuver	Description
Pivot shift 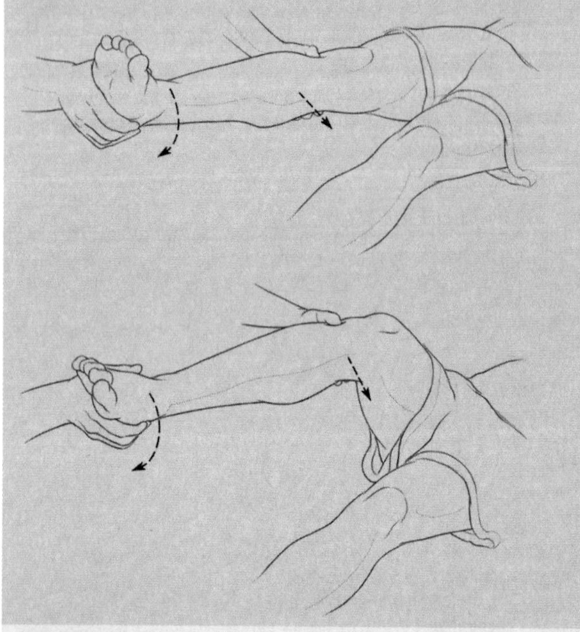	Used to determine the amount of rotational laxity of the knee. The patient is examined while lying supine with the knee in full extension. It is then slowly flexed while applying internal rotation and a valgus stress. **Positive test:** The clinician feels for a subluxation at 20–40 degrees of knee flexion. (The patient must remain very relaxed to have a positive test.)
Valgus stress 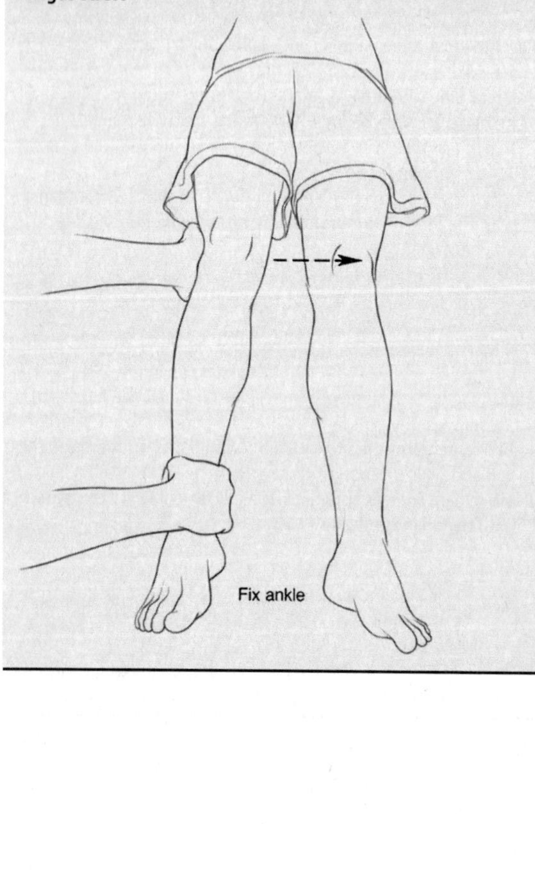	Performed with the patient lying supine. The clinician should stand on the outside of the patient's knee. With one hand, the clinician should hold the ankle while the other hand is supporting the leg at the level of the knee joint. A valgus stress is applied at the ankle to determine pain and laxity of the medial collateral ligament. The test should be performed at both 30 degrees and 0 degrees of knee extension. **Positive test:** Pain and laxity of the medial collateral ligament with valgus stress. The test results can be graded from 1 to 3. **Grade 1 injuries**: the patient has pain with the valgus stress test but no instability. **Grade 2 injuries**: the patient has pain, and the knee shows instability at 30 degrees of knee flexion. **Grade 3 injuries**: the patient has marked instability but not much pain.

(*continued*)

Table 45–8. Knee examination. (continued)

Maneuver	Description
Varus stress 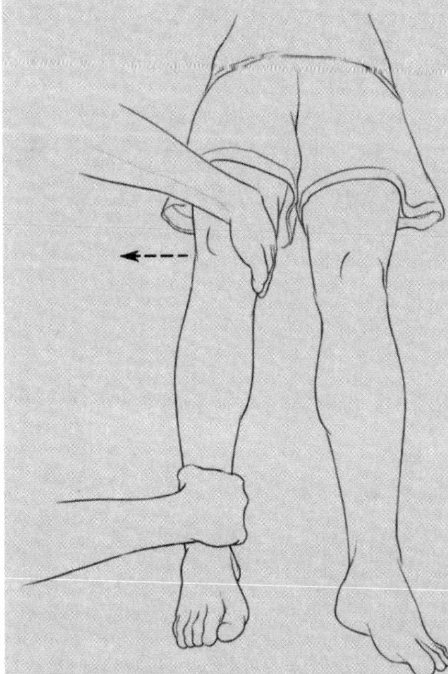	Performed with the patient lying supine. For the right knee, the clinician should be standing on the right side of the patient. The left hand of the examiner should be holding the ankle while the right hand is supporting the lateral thigh. A varus stress is applied at the ankle to determine pain and laxity of the lateral collateral ligament. The test should be performed at both 30 degrees and 0 degrees of knee flexion. **Positive test:** Pain and laxity of the lateral collateral ligament with varus stress. The test results can be graded from 1 to 3. **Grade 1 injuries:** the patient has pain with the varus stress test but no instability **Grade 2 injuries:** the patient has pain and the knee shows instability at 30 degrees of knee flexion **Grade 3 injuries:** the patient has marked instability but not much pain.
Meniscal Signs	
McMurray test	Performed with the patient lying supine. The clinician flexes the knee until the patient reports pain. For this test to be valid, it must be flexed pain-free beyond 90 degrees. **Positive test:** To test the medial meniscus, the clinician externally rotates the patient's foot and then extends the knee while palpating the medial knee for "click" in the medial compartment of the knee or pain reproducing pain from a meniscus injury. To test the lateral meniscus, the same maneuver is repeated while rotating the foot internally (53% sensitivity and 59–97% specificity).
Modified McMurray 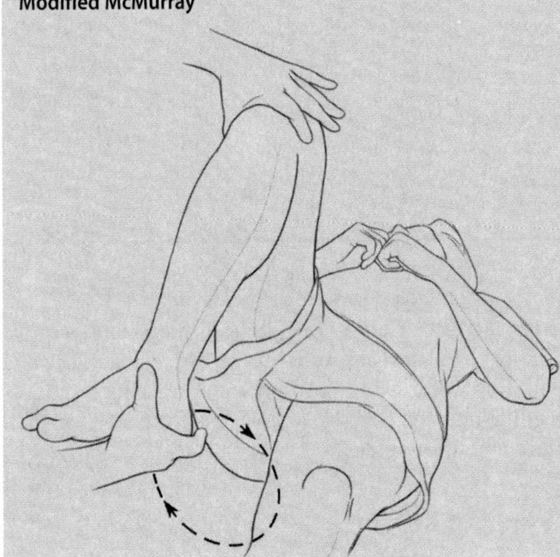	Performed with the patient lying supine and the hip flexed to 90 degrees. The knee is then flexed maximally with internal or external rotation of the lower leg. The knee can then be rotated with the lower leg in internal or external rotation to capture the torn meniscus underneath the condyles. **Positive test:** Pain over the joint line while the knee is being flexed and internally or externally rotated.

(*continued*)

Table 45–8. Knee examination. (continued)

Maneuver	Description
Modified McMurray (Cont.) 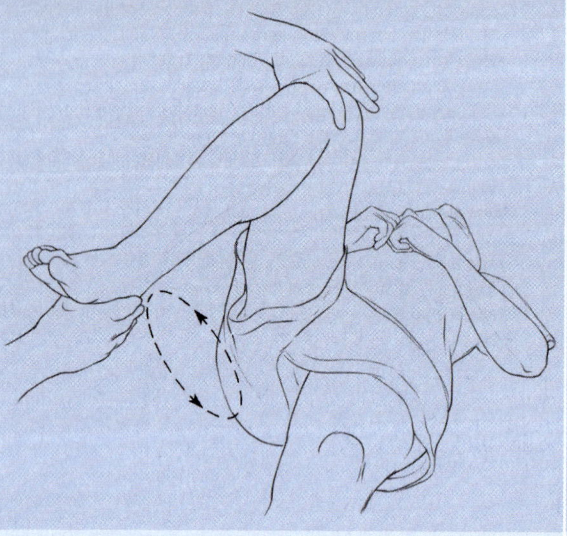	
Thessaly test 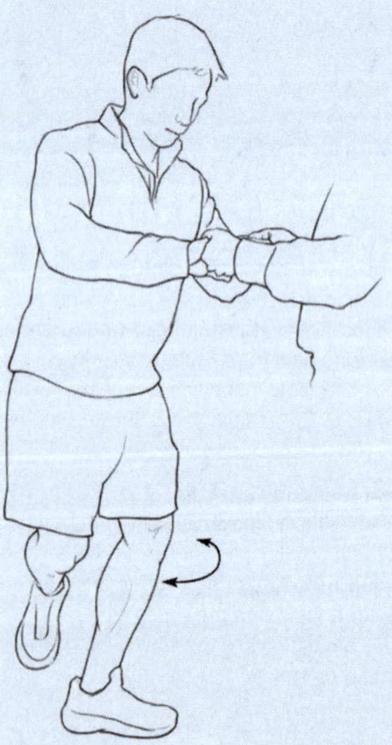	Performed with the patient standing on one leg with knee slightly flexed. The patient is asked to twist the knee while standing on one leg. **Positive test:** Pain is elicited during twisting motion.

reconstruction is the gold standard. Recovery from surgery usually requires 9–12 months before returning to competitive sports.

Nonoperative treatments are usually reserved for older patients or those with a very sedentary lifestyle. Physical therapy can focus on hamstring strengthening and core stability. An ACL brace can help stability. Longitudinal studies have demonstrated that nonoperative management of an ACL tear can lead to a higher incidence of meniscus tears. Cost-analysis studies have shown that early ACL reconstruction can be more beneficial than nonoperative treatment and delayed subsequent surgeries. There is strong support for using neuromuscular training programs to significantly reduce (by almost half) the risk of ACL rupture among athletes.

When to Refer

- Almost all ACL tears should be referred to an orthopedic surgeon for evaluation.

- Individuals with instability in the setting of a chronic ACL tear (> 6 months) should be considered for surgical reconstruction.
- Patients with an ACL tear and associated meniscus or articular injuries may benefit from surgery to address the other injuries.

Brophy RH et al. American Academy of Orthopaedic Surgeons Clinical Practice Guideline Summary: Management of anterior cruciate ligament injuries. J Am Acad Orthop Surg. 2023;31:531. [PMID: 36727995]

Watson S et al. A systematic review and meta-analysis of anterior cruciate ligament injury prevention programs: training to stay in the game. Am J Sports Med. 2026;54:733. [PMID: 41486737]

3. Collateral Ligament Injury

ESSENTIALS OF DIAGNOSIS

- Caused by a valgus or varus blow or stress to the knee.
- Pain and instability in the affected area.
- Limited range of motion.

General Considerations

The medial collateral ligament (MCL) is the most commonly injured ligament in the knee. It is usually injured with a valgus stress to the partially flexed knee. It can also occur with a blow to the lateral leg. The MCL is commonly injured with acute ACL injuries. The lateral collateral ligament (LCL) is less commonly injured, but this can occur with a medial blow to the knee. Since both collateral ligaments are extra-articular, injuries to these ligaments may not lead to any intra-articular effusion. Affected patients may have difficulty walking initially, but this can improve when the swelling decreases.

Clinical Findings

A. Symptoms and Signs

The main clinical findings for patients with collateral ligament injuries are pain along the course of the ligaments. The patient may have limited range of motion due to pain, especially during the first 2 weeks following the injury. The best tests to assess the collateral ligaments are the varus and valgus stress tests (Table 45–8). The knee is often unstable at both 30 degrees and 0 degrees of knee flexion. The overall sensitivity of the tests is 86–96%.

B. Imaging

Radiographs are usually nondiagnostic except for avulsion injuries. However, radiographs should be used to rule out fractures that can occur with collateral ligament injuries. MRI is usually not required for MCL injuries; however, it can be obtained to evaluate the location of the tear (proximal, midsubstance, and distal), as well as associated cruciate ligament injuries, menisci, or posterolateral corner injuries. However, lateral-sided injuries should have an MRI to evaluate the severity of injury and guide treatment.

Treatment

Most MCL injuries can be treated with protected weight bearing and physical therapy. For grade 1 and 2 injuries, the patient can usually bear weight as tolerated with full range of motion (see Table 45–8 for definitions of grade 1–3 injuries of the knee). A hinged knee brace can be given to patients with grade 2 MCL tears to provide stability. Early physical therapy is recommended to protect range of motion and muscle strength. Grade 3 MCL injuries require long leg braces to provide stability. Patients can weight-bear, but only with the knee locked in extension with a brace. The motion can then be increased with the brace unlocked. Grade 3 injuries can take up to 6–8 weeks to heal. MCL injuries do not usually require surgery. MCL repair or reconstruction is considered in higher-grade injuries, in large bone avulsions where the displaced fibers of the MCL prevent healing (Stener-like lesion), or in patients with chronic pain who fail nonoperative management. LCL injuries are less common but are usually associated with other ligament injuries (such as ACL and posterior cruciate ligament [PCL]). LCL injuries do not recover well with nonoperative treatment and usually require urgent surgical repair or reconstruction.

When to Refer

- Symptomatic instability with chronic MCL tears or acute MCL tears with other ligamentous injuries.
- LCL or posterolateral corner injuries require urgent surgical repair or reconstruction (within 1 week).

Mowers C et al. Medial collateral ligament reconstruction and repair show similar improvement in outcome scores, but repair shows higher rates of knee stiffness and failure: a systematic review. Arthroscopy. 2023;39:2231. [PMID: 36898592]

von Rehlingen-Prinz F et al. Location of medial collateral ligament tears: introduction to a magnetic resonance imaging-based classification. Skeletal Radiol. 2025;54:851. [PMID: 39083055]

4. Posterior Cruciate Ligament Injury

ESSENTIALS OF DIAGNOSIS

- Usually follows anterior trauma to the tibia, such as a dashboard injury from a motor vehicle accident.
- The knee may freely dislocate and reduce.
- One-third of multi-ligament injuries involving the PCL have neurovascular injuries.

General Considerations

The PCL is the strongest ligament in the knee. PCL injuries usually represent significant trauma and are highly associated with multi-ligament injuries and knee dislocations. More than 70–90% of PCL injuries have associated injuries to the posterolateral corner, MCL, and ACL. Neurovascular injuries occur in up to one-third of all knee dislocations or PCL injuries. There should be high suspicion for neurovascular injuries and a thorough neurovascular examination of the limb should be performed. Most acute PCL injuries should be evaluated by a specialist.

Clinical Findings

A. Symptoms and Signs

Most patients with acute injuries have difficulty with ambulation. Patients with chronic PCL injuries can ambulate without gross instability but may describe subjective "looseness" and often report pain and dysfunction, especially with bending or descending stairs. Clinical examinations of PCL injuries include the "sag sign"; the patient is placed supine and both hips and knees are flexed to 90 degrees. Because of gravity, the posterior cruciate ligament-injured knee will have an obvious set-off at the anterior tibia that is "sagging" posteriorly. The PCL ligament can also be examined using the posterior drawer test; the patient is placed supine with the knee flexed to 90 degrees. In a normal knee, the anterior tibia should be positioned about 10 mm anterior to the femoral condyle. The clinician can grasp the proximal tibia with both hands and push the tibia posteriorly. The movement, indicating laxity and possible tear of the PCL, is compared with the uninjured knee (90% sensitivity and 99% specificity). A PCL injury is sometimes mistaken for an ACL injury during the anterior drawer test since the tibia is subluxed posteriorly in a sagged position and can be abnormally translated forward, yielding a false-positive test for an ACL injury (Table 45–8). Pain, swelling, pallor, and numbness in the affected extremity may suggest a knee dislocation with possible injury to the popliteal artery. If the lateral knee is unstable with varus stress testing (Table 45–8), the patient should be assessed for a posterolateral corner injury, which consists of injuries to the LCL, popliteus tendon, and popliteofibular ligament. Injuries to the posterolateral corner usually require urgent surgical treatment.

B. Imaging

Radiographs are often nondiagnostic but are required to diagnose any fractures. MRI is used to diagnose PCL and other associated injuries.

Treatment

Most isolated PCL injuries can be treated nonoperatively. Acute injuries are usually immobilized using an extension knee brace; the patient uses crutches for ambulation. Physical therapy can help achieve increased range of motion and improved ambulation. Surgical reconstruction (or less commonly, repair) is usually reserved for high-grade tears in high-demand athletes, combined ligament injuries, or cases where nonoperative management has failed.

When to Refer

- The patient should be seen urgently within 1–2 weeks.
- Posterolateral corner injury requires urgent surgical reconstruction.
- Isolated PCL tears may require surgery if the tear is complete (grade 3) and the patient is symptomatic.

Knapik DM et al. Management of posterior cruciate ligament injury: a concise overview of current indications, techniques, and outcomes. J Am Acad Orthop Surg. 2026;34:e515. [PMID: 41202194]

5. Meniscus Injuries

ESSENTIALS OF DIAGNOSIS

- Patient may or may not report an injury.
- Joint line pain and pain with deep squatting are the most sensitive signs.
- Difficulty with knee extension suggests an internal derangement that should be evaluated urgently with MRI.

General Considerations

The menisci act as shock absorbers within the knee. Most meniscus injuries occur with acute injuries (usually in younger patients) or repeated microtrauma, such as squatting or twisting (usually in older patients).

Clinical Findings

A. Symptoms and Signs

Patients may have an antalgic (painful) gait and difficulty with squatting. They may report catching or locking of the meniscal fragment. Patients can usually point out the area of maximal tenderness along the joint line. Swelling usually occurs during the first 24 hours after the injury or later. Meniscus tears rarely lead to the immediate swelling that is commonly seen with fractures and ligament tears. Meniscus tears are commonly seen in arthritic knees. However, it is often unclear whether the pain is coming from the meniscus tear or the arthritis.

Physical findings may include effusion or joint line tenderness along the medial or lateral side of the knee (83% sensitivity; 83% specificity). Provocative tests, including the McMurray test, the modified McMurray test, and the Thessaly test, can be performed to confirm the diagnosis (Table 45–8). Most symptomatic meniscus tears cause pain with deep squatting and when waddling (performing a "duck walk").

B. Imaging

Radiographs are usually normal but may show joint space narrowing, early OA changes, or loose bodies. MRI of the knee is the best diagnostic tool for meniscal injuries (93% sensitivity and 95% specificity).

Treatment

Conservative treatment can be used for degenerative tears and some acute tears, especially in older patients. The treatment is similar as for patients with mild knee OA, including analgesics and physical therapy for strengthening and core stability. Neuromuscular exercises including lower extremity strengthening, balance, hip and core strengthening, and patient education are first-line nonoperative treatments. An RCT showed that physical therapy and home exercises were both helpful in cases of degenerative meniscus tears. An RCT showed that physical therapy compared with arthroscopic partial meniscectomy had similar outcomes at 6 months. However, 30% of the patients who were assigned to physical therapy alone underwent surgery within 6 months.

Randomized studies have shown that arthroscopic surgery has no benefit over sham operations in patients who have degenerative meniscal tears, especially with imaging showing signs of osteoarthritis. Another RCT found that patients with degenerative meniscus tears but no signs of arthritis on imaging treated conservatively with supervised exercise therapy had similar outcomes to those treated with arthroscopy at 2-year follow-up. Overall, patients can be treated with supervised exercise therapy first, and if they do not respond to nonoperative treatment, then meniscus surgery can be considered. Acute tears in young and active patients with clinical signs of internal derangement (catching and swelling) and without signs of arthritis on imaging or patients with acute mechanical locking with a displaced meniscus can be best treated arthroscopically with meniscus repair or debridement. There is also evidence that untreated meniscus root tears (tears where the meniscus attaches to the back or posterior aspect of the tibia) can lead to accelerated osteoarthritic changes. Surgical treatment is recommended for large displaced and/or bucket handle meniscus tears, and for acute meniscus root tears to restore knee function and reduce cartilage breakdown.

When to Refer

- If the patient has symptoms of internal derangement suspected as meniscus injury. The patient should receive an MRI to confirm the injury.
- If the patient cannot extend the knee due to a mechanical block, the patient should be evaluated as soon as possible. Certain shaped tears on MRI, such as bucket handle tears or meniscus root injuries, are amenable to meniscal repair surgery.
- If the patient has not responded to physical therapy and nonoperative treatment and continues to have symptoms related to the torn meniscus.

Katz JN et al. A randomized trial of physical therapy for meniscal tear and knee pain. N Engl J Med. 2025;393:1694. [PMID: 41160820].

Prill R, Ma CB, et al. The Formal EU-US Meniscus Rehabilitation 2024 Consensus: an ESSKA-AOSSM-AASPT Initiative Part II-Prevention, Nonoperative Treatment and Return to Sport. Orthop J Sports Med. 2025;13:23259671251349553. [PMID: 40519541]

Pujol N et al. The Formal EU-US Meniscus Rehabilitation 2024 Consensus: an ESSKA-AOSSM-AASPT Initiative: Part I-Rehabilitation Management After Meniscus Surgery (Meniscectomy, Repair and Reconstruction). Orthop J Sports Med. 2025;13:23259671251343088. [PMID: 40416991]

6. Patellofemoral Pain

ESSENTIALS OF DIAGNOSIS

- Pain experienced with bending activities (kneeling, squatting, climbing stairs).
- Lateral deviation or tilting of the patella in relation to the femoral groove.

General Considerations

Patellofemoral pain, also known as anterior knee pain, chondromalacia, or "runner's knee," describes any pain involving the patellofemoral joint. The pain affects any or all of the anterior knee structures, including the medial and lateral aspects of the patella as well as the quadriceps and patellar tendon insertions. Forces on the patellofemoral joint increase up to three times body weight as the knee flexes to 90 degrees (eg, climbing stairs), and five times body weight when going into full knee flexion (eg, squatting). Abnormal patellar tracking during flexion can lead to abnormal articular cartilage wear and pain. When the patient has ligamentous hyperlaxity, the patella can sublux out of the groove, usually laterally. Patellofemoral pain is also associated with muscle strength and flexibility imbalances as well as altered hip and ankle biomechanics.

Clinical Findings

A. Symptoms and Signs

Patients usually report pain in the anterior knee with bending and less commonly in full extension. Pain from this condition is localized under the patella but can sometimes be referred to the posterior knee or over the medial or lateral inferior patella. Symptoms may begin after trauma or after repetitive physical activity, such as running and jumping. With patellar maltracking, palpable and sometimes audible crepitus can occur.

Intra-articular swelling usually does not occur unless articular cartilage defects or OA changes develop. On physical examination, it is important to palpate the articular surfaces of the patella. The clinician can use one hand to move the patella laterally and use the fingertips of the other hand to palpate the lateral undersurface of the patella. Patellar mobility can be assessed by medially and laterally deviating the patella (deviation by one-quarter of the diameter of the patella is considered normal; more than one-half the diameter suggests excessive mobility). The apprehension sign suggests instability of the patellofemoral joint and is positive when the patient becomes apprehensive when the patella is deviated laterally. The patellar grind test is performed by grasping the knee superior to the patella and pushing it downward with the patient supine and the knee extended, pushing the patella inferiorly. The patient is asked to contract the quadriceps muscle to oppose this downward translation, with reproduction of pain or grinding being the positive sign for chondromalacia of the patella. There are two common presentations: (1) patients whose ligaments and patella are too loose (hypermobility); and (2) patients who have soft tissues that are too tight, leading to excessive pressure on the joint.

Quadriceps strength and hip stabilizers can be evaluated by having the patient perform a one-leg squat without support. Normally, with a one-leg squat, the knee should align over the second metatarsal ray of the foot. Patients who are weak may display poor balance, with dropping of the pelvis (similar to a positive hip Trendelenburg sign) or excessive internal rotation of the knee medially.

B. Imaging

Diagnostic imaging has limited use in younger patients and is more helpful in older patients to assess for OA or to evaluate patients who do not respond to conservative treatment. Radiographs may show lateral deviation or tilting of the patella in relation to the femoral groove. MRI may show thinning of the articular cartilage but is not clinically necessary, except prior to surgery or to exclude other pathology.

Treatment

A. Conservative

For symptomatic relief, use of local modalities such as ice and topical anti-inflammatory medications can be beneficial. Oral medications are reserved more for severe cases. If the patient has signs of patellar hypermobility, physical therapy exercises are useful to strengthen the quadriceps (especially the vastus medialis obliquus muscle) to help stabilize the patella and improve tracking (keeping the patella from shifting laterally or medially when the leg bends or straightens). There is good evidence that exercise therapy for patellofemoral pain syndrome may result in clinically important reduction in pain and improvement in functional ability. Lower quality research supports that hip and knee exercises are better than knee exercises alone. Strengthening the quadriceps and the posterolateral hip muscles such as the hip abductors that control rotation at the knee are recommended. Support for the patellofemoral joint can be provided by use of a patellar stabilizer brace or special taping techniques. Correcting lower extremity alignment (with appropriate footwear or over-the-counter orthotics) can help improve symptoms, especially if the patient has pronation or high-arched feet. If the patient demonstrates tight peripatellar soft tissues, special focus should be put on stretching the hamstrings, iliotibial band, quadriceps, calves, and hip flexors. The goal of conservative treatment is improvement in movement pattern to reduce load on the patellofemoral joint, focusing on hip and knee exercises and internal feedback.

B. Surgical

Surgery is rarely needed and is considered a last resort for patellofemoral pain. Procedures performed include lateral release or patellar realignment surgery. Surgery is indicated when patients have recurrent patella instability or dislocations.

When to Refer

Patients with persistent symptoms despite a course of conservative therapy.

Neal BS et al. Best practice guide for patellofemoral pain based on synthesis of a systematic review, the patient voice and expert clinical reasoning. Br J Sports Med. 2024;58:1486. [PMID: 39401870]

7. Knee Osteoarthritis

ESSENTIALS OF DIAGNOSIS

- Degeneration of joint cartilage.
- Pain with bending or twisting activities.
- Swelling.
- Loss of active and passive range of motion in severe OA.

General Considerations

It is estimated that > 32 million adults in the United States have knee OA and this will likely increase to 70 million persons by 2030 as the number of persons age > 65 increases. The etiology of OA is often multifactorial including previous trauma, repetitive microtrauma, prior high-impact activities, genetic factors, obesity, and rheumatologic or metabolic conditions.

Clinical Findings

A. Symptoms and Signs

OA usually causes pain in the affected joint with loading of the joint or at the extremes of motion. Mechanical symptoms—such as swelling, grinding, catching, and locking—suggest internal derangement, which is indicated by damaged cartilage or bone fragments that affect the smooth range of motion expected at an articular joint. Pain can also produce the sensation of "buckling" or "giving way" due to muscle inhibition (Table 45–4) (Table 45–5) (Table 45–6). As the joint degeneration becomes more advanced, the patient loses active range of motion and may lose passive range of motion as well.

As the condition worsens, patients with knee OA have an increasingly limited ability to walk. Symptoms include pain with bending or twisting activities and going up and down stairs. Swelling, limping, and pain while sleeping are common symptoms of OA, especially as it progresses.

B. Imaging

The most commonly recommended radiographs include bilateral weight-bearing 45-degree bent knee posteroanterior, lateral, and patellofemoral joint views (Merchant view). Radiographic findings include diminished width of the articular cartilage causing joint space narrowing, subchondral sclerosis, presence of osteophytes, and cystic changes in the subchondral bone. MRI of the knee is most likely unnecessary unless other pathology is suspected, such as ischemic osteonecrosis of the knee.

Treatment

A. Conservative

Changes in the articular cartilage are irreversible. Therefore, a cure for the diseased joint is not possible, although symptoms or structural issues can be addressed to try to maintain activity level. Conservative treatment for all patients with OA includes activity modification, therapeutic exercises, and weight loss. Lifestyle modifications also include proper footwear and avoidance of high-impact activities. Optimal exercise programs for knee OA should focus on improving aerobic capacity, quadriceps muscle strength, or lower extremity performance; ideally, the programs should occur three times a week and be supervised (Table 45–6).

Use of a cane in the hand opposite to the affected side is mechanically advantageous. Knee sleeves or braces provide some improvement in subjective pain symptoms most likely due to improvements in neuromuscular function. If patients have unicompartmental OA in the medial or lateral compartment, joint unloader braces are available to offload the degenerative compartment. Cushioning footwear and appropriate orthotics or shoe adjustments are useful for reducing impact to the lower extremities.

The first-line recommendation for pain management is topical nonsteroidal medication (eg, diclofenac gel) (Table 5–4). Alternatively, topical capsaicin may be effective. Oral medications that have been shown to significantly improve pain include ibuprofen, naproxen, diclofenac, and celecoxib. If a traditional NSAID is indicated, the choice should be based on cost, side-effect profile, and adherence (Table 5–4). For patients with increased risk of GI bleeding, a cyclooxygenase (COX)-2 inhibitor (ie, celecoxib) or adding a PPI to the NSAID is recommended. A COX-2 inhibitor is no more effective than traditional NSAIDs; it may offer short-term, but probably not long-term, advantage in preventing GI complications. Acetaminophen has been shown to be less effective than NSAIDs but can be used in patients when NSAID use is contraindicated. Tramadol can be used appropriately in patients with severe OA as alternative to NSAIDs, while opioid use is discouraged. Glucagon-like peptide-1 receptor agonists improve patient-reported outcomes in knee osteoarthritis, possibly due to disease-modifying effects that include lower blood glucose levels and weight loss. Supplements have shown some benefit for OA. Glucosamine and chondroitin sulfate are supplements that have been widely used and marketed for OA. Despite some initial promise, the best-controlled studies indicate these supplements are ineffective as analgesics in OA. However, they have minimal side effects and may be appropriate if the patient experiences subjective benefit. Genicular nerve block and radiofrequency ablation are effective for pain management over 24 months in some cases, although this is usually a later treatment after injection therapies.

Traditionally, knee joint corticosteroid injections are options to help reduce pain and inflammation and can provide short-term pain relief, usually lasting about 6–12 weeks. While intra-articular triamcinolone is still commonly used in knee arthritis, an RCT showed that 2 years of intra-articular triamcinolone every 3 months, compared with intra-articular saline, resulted in significantly greater quantitative cartilage volume loss by MRI and no significant difference in knee pain. In general, regular use of corticosteroid injections for long-term treatment of knee osteoarthritis should be avoided.

Viscosupplementation using injections of hyaluronic acid–based products is controversial. Because reviews suggested that viscosupplementation has a questionably clinically relevant effect size and an increased risk of non-threatening adverse events, the American Academy of Orthopedic Surgeons recommended that viscosupplementation should not be used in the treatment of knee OA.

PRP injections remain the most common orthobiologic treatment, as PRP contains high concentration of platelet-derived growth factors that regulate some biologic processes in tissue repair. There is a potential dose–response relationship between platelet dose and PRP effectiveness for knee OA treatment; the suggested optimal threshold is > 10 billion platelets for favorable clinical outcomes. Leukocyte-poor PRP is favored over leukocyte-rich PRP for most indications, though the use PRP for osteoarthritis is still not advocated by all medical organizations.

B. Surgical

Knee joint replacement surgery for advanced OA is very successful and cost-effective for patients with significant symptoms or functional limitations, providing improvements in pain, function, and quality of life. Practice guidelines from the American College of Rheumatology recommend joint replacement surgery for symptomatic moderate to severe osteoarthritis or advanced symptomatic osteonecrosis. They recommend delaying surgery for patients with diabetes until good glycemic control is achieved and for patients who smoke cigarettes until they adequately decrease or cease nicotine use. In patients with obesity, the ACR strongly encourages weight reduction before surgery, counseling on how to lose weight, and education on the increased risk of medical and surgical complications due to obesity. Long-term series describe a > 95% survival rate of the implant at 15 years. Minimally invasive surgeries and computer-assisted navigation during operation are being investigated as methods to improve techniques (eg, accurate placement of the hardware implant) and to reduce complication rates; however, major improvements have yet to be demonstrated. Two randomized trials demonstrated that arthroscopy does not improve outcomes at 1 year over placebo or routine conservative treatment of OA.

Knee realignment surgery, such as high tibial osteotomy or partial knee replacement surgery, is indicated in patients age < 60 with unicompartmental OA who would benefit from delaying total knee replacement.

When to Refer

Patients with sufficient disability, limited benefit from conservative therapy, and evidence of severe OA can be referred for joint replacement surgery.

Berrigan W et al. The effect of platelet dose on outcomes after platelet rich plasma injections for musculoskeletal conditions: a systematic review and meta-analysis. Curr Rev Musculoskelet Med. 2024;17:570. [PMID: 39331322]

Dell'Isola A et al. Osteoarthritis year in review 2025: epidemiology and therapy. Osteoarthritis Cartilage. 2025; 33:1300. [PMID: 40914550]

Kloppenburg M et al. Osteoarthritis. Lancet. 2025;405:71. Erratum in: Lancet. 2025;405:2278. [PMID: 39755397]

Zhu H et al. Glucagon-like peptide-1 receptor agonists as a disease-modifying therapy for knee osteoarthritis mediated by weight loss: findings from the Shanghai Osteoarthritis Cohort. Ann Rheum Dis 2023;82:1218. [PMID: 37258065]

ANKLE INJURIES

1. Inversion Ankle Sprains

ESSENTIALS OF DIAGNOSIS

- Most ankle injuries involve plantar flexion and inversion sprains affecting the lateral ligaments.
- The anterior drawer test and talar tilt test are the best tests to grade ligament injury severity.
- Consider chronic ankle instability or associated injuries if pain persists for > 3 months following an ankle sprain.

General Considerations

Ankle sprains (stretch or tear of ankle ligaments) are the most common sports injuries seen in outpatient clinics. While common, ankle sprains can negatively affect quality of life. One study found that respondents with a history of ankle sprain had higher BMI and overall pain, lower physical activity, and worse health-related quality of life scores than non-injured controls. The most common mechanism of injury is a plantar flexion and inversion sprain, which injures the anterior talofibular (ATF) ligament followed by the calcaneofibular (CF) ligament. Other injuries that can occur with inversion ankle injuries are listed in Table 45–9. Women appear to sustain an inversion injury more frequently than men. Chronic ankle instability is defined as persistent pain, swelling, and "giving way" in combination with recurrent sprains for at least 12 months after the initial ankle sprain. Chronic ankle instability can occur in up to 43% of ankle sprains despite physical therapy, which makes appropriate attention to acute ankle sprains important.

Table 45–9. Injuries associated with ankle sprains.

Ligaments
Subtalar joint sprain
Sinus tarsi syndrome (ongoing anterolateral posttraumatic ankle pain)
Syndesmotic (distal tibiofibular ligamentous) sprain
Deltoid sprain
Lisfranc (tarsometatarsal bony or ligamentous) injury
Tendons
Posterior tibial tendon strain
Peroneal tendon subluxation
Bones
Osteochondral talus injury
Lateral talar process fracture
Posterior impingement (os trigonum)
Fracture at the base of the fifth metatarsal
Jones fracture (between base and middle of fifth metatarsal)
Salter (growth plate) fracture (fibula)
Ankle fractures

Clinical Findings

A. Symptoms and Signs

Patients usually report "turning the ankle" during a fall or after landing on an irregular uneven surface such as a hole or an opponent's foot. Symptoms following a sprain include localized pain and swelling over the lateral aspect of the ankle, difficulty weight bearing, and limping. On examination, there may be swelling or bruising over the lateral aspect of the ankle. The anterior, inferior aspect below the lateral malleolus is most often the point of maximal tenderness consistent with ATF and CF ligament injuries. The swelling may limit motion of the ankle.

B. Stress Tests

1. Anterior drawer test—For this ankle stress test, the clinician keeps the foot and ankle in the neutral position with the patient sitting, then uses one hand to fix the tibia and the other to hold the patient's heel and draw the ankle forward. Normally, there may be approximately 3 mm of translation until an endpoint is felt. A positive test includes increased translation of one foot compared with the other with loss of the endpoint of the ATF ligament.

2. Subtalar tilt test—This stress test is performed with the foot in the neutral position with the patient sitting. The clinician uses one hand to fix the tibia and the other to hold and invert the calcaneus. Normal inversion at the subtalar joint is approximately 30 degrees. A positive test consists of increased subtalar joint inversion by > 10 degrees on the affected side with loss of endpoint for the CF ligament. To grade the severity of ankle sprains, no laxity on stress tests is considered a grade 1 injury, laxity of the ATF ligament on anterior drawer testing but a negative tilt test is a grade 2 injury, and both positive drawer and tilt tests signify a grade 3 injury. Difficulty jumping and landing 2 weeks after an acute ankle sprain, abnormal postural or hip muscle control, or ligamentous laxity 8 weeks after injury are poor prognostic signs.

C. Imaging

Routine ankle radiographic views include the AP, lateral, and oblique (mortise) views. Less common views requested include the calcaneal view and subtalar view. The **Ottawa Ankle Rules** remain the best clinical prediction rules to guide the need for radiographs and have an 86–99% sensitivity and a 97–99% negative predictive value for ankle pathology. If the patient is unable to bear weight immediately in the office setting or emergency department for four steps, then the clinician should check for (1) bony tenderness at the posterior edge of the medial or lateral malleolus and (2) bony tenderness over the navicular (medial midfoot) or at the base of the fifth metatarsal. If either malleolus demonstrates pain or deformity, then ankle radiographs should be obtained. If the foot has bony tenderness, obtain foot radiographs. An MRI is helpful when considering the associated injuries.

Treatment

Immediate treatment of an ankle sprain follows the PEACE and LOVE mnemonic (see General Approach to Musculoskeletal Injuries). NSAIDs are useful in reducing pain and swelling in the first 72 hours following the ankle sprain; notably, NSAIDs, paracetamol, and opioids have similar results in reducing early pain. Subsequent treatment involves protected weight bearing with crutches and an ankle stabilizer brace, especially for grade 2 and 3 injuries. Icing acutely after an ankle sprain can help with early pain and swelling; however, it does not appear to help with recovery from injury, so ice can be used with caution if it is more than 12 hours after injury. Early functional and dynamic rehabilitation exercises result in a shorter time to return to sport, increased functional performance, and decreased self-reported reinjury. Patients should be encouraged to do a program of exercises or physical therapy. Manual therapy with early ankle mobilization and stretching treatments is important to restore range of motion, especially ankle dorsiflexion. Proprioception and balance exercises (eg, "wobble board") can help restore function to the ankle, and there is moderate evidence that neuromuscular training can prevent future ankle sprains. There is strong evidence that bracing prevents ankle sprains; however, one study included in a meta-analysis made the effects of bracing nonsignificant. In general, an external ankle support (semirigid brace) is considered in the acute healing period (up to 8 to 12 weeks) and to avoid recurrent sprains. Chronic instability can develop after acute ankle sprain in 10–20% of people and may require surgical stabilization.

When to Refer

- Ankle fractures.
- Recurrent ankle sprains or signs of chronic ligamentous ankle instability.
- No response after > 3 months of conservative treatment.

Wang F et al. Preventive interventions for lateral ankle sprains: a systematic review and meta-analysis. Clin Rehabil. 2023;37:585. [PMID: 36630892]
Wu V et al. Management of acute ankle sprains: common questions and answers. Am Fam Physician. 2025;112:609. [PMID: 41533404]

2. Eversion ("High") Ankle Sprains

ESSENTIALS OF DIAGNOSIS

- Severe and prolonged pain.
- Limited range of motion.
- Mild swelling.
- Difficulty with weight bearing.

General Considerations

A syndesmotic injury or "high ankle" sprain involves the anterior *tibio*fibular ligament in the anterolateral aspect of the ankle, superior to the anterior *talo*fibular ligament. The injury mechanism often involves the foot being turned out or externally rotated and everted (eg, when being tackled). This injury is commonly missed or misdiagnosed as an ATF ligament sprain on initial visit.

Clinical Findings

A. Symptoms and Signs

Symptoms of a high ankle sprain include severe and prolonged pain over the anterior ankle at the anterior tibiofibular ligament, worse with weight bearing. This is often more painful than the typical ankle sprain. The point of maximal tenderness involves the anterior tibiofibular ligament, which is higher than the ATF ligament. It is also important to palpate the proximal fibula to rule out any proximal syndesmotic ligament injury and associated fracture known as a "Maisonneuve fracture." There is often some mild swelling in this area, with or without an ankle effusion. Range of motion is usually limited in all directions. To perform the **external rotation stress test**, the clinician fixes the tibia with one hand and grasps the foot in the other with the ankle in the neutral position. The ankle is then dorsiflexed and externally rotated, reproducing the patient's pain. (**Note:** The patient's foot should have an intact neurovascular examination before undertaking this test.)

B. Imaging

Radiographs of the ankle should include the AP, oblique (mortise), and lateral views. The mortise view may

…nonstrate loss of the normal overlap between the tibia and fibula, which should be at least 1–2 mm. Asymmetry in the joint space around the tibiotalar joint suggests disruption of the syndesmotic ligaments. If there is proximal tenderness in the lower leg especially around the fibula, an AP and lateral view of the tibia and fibula should be obtained to rule out a proximal fibula fracture. Radiographs during an external rotation stress test may visualize instability at the distal tibiofibular joint. MRI is the best method to visualize injury to the tibiofibular ligament and to assess status of the other ligaments and the articular cartilage.

Treatment

Whereas most ankle sprains are treated with early motion and weight bearing, treatment for a high ankle sprain should be conservative with a cast or walking boot with limited weight bearing for 4–6 weeks. Thereafter, protected weight bearing with crutches is recommended until the patient can walk pain-free. Physical therapy can start early to regain range of motion and maintain strength with limited weight bearing initially. Follow-up of athletes over 18 years showed that conservative treatment can be successful, although 27% of patients had radiographic signs of ankle arthritis, including some with heterotopic ossification.

When to Refer

If there is widening of the joint space and asymmetry at the tibiotalar joint, the patient should be referred urgently to a foot and ankle surgeon. Severe or prolonged persistent cases that do not heal may require internal fixation to avoid chronic instability at the tibiofibular joint.

Aiyer A et al. Advances in diagnosis and management of lateral ankle instability: a review of current literature. J Am Acad Orthop Surg Glob Res Rev. 2023;7:e23.00251. [PMID: 38149942]

Nussbaum ED et al. Nonoperative management of high ankle sprains: a case series with ≥18-year follow-up. Am J Sports Med. 2024;52:2807. [PMID: 39235770]

Ryan PM et al. Subtle syndesmotic instability. J Am Acad Orthop Surg. 2024;32:719. [PMID: 38295390]

Sexual & Gender Minority Health

46

Patricia A. Robertson, MD
Elaine Hsiang, MD
Kevin L. Ard, MD, MPH
Kenneth H. Mayer, MD
Mitzi Hawkins, MD

HEALTH CARE FOR SEXUAL & GENDER MINORITY PATIENTS

Definitions & Concepts

Gender identity is a person's internal sense of gender, which is independent from the sex assigned at birth. Gender is also independent from **sexual orientation**, which refers to a person's sexuality and encompasses three dimensions: *identity, behavior,* and *desire*. The term **sexual and gender minority (SGM)** refers to a broad group including lesbian, gay, bisexual, and queer people (**sexual minority [SM] people**), and transgender and gender nonbinary people (**gender minority [GM] people**). SGM populations are also commonly referred to as "**LGBTQ+**" or "**LGBTQIA+**"—the latter of which is inclusive of intersex people whose bodies do not fall within the male/female binary, and asexual individuals who experience varying ranges of sexual attraction or desire. The plus sign acknowledges that this acronym is nonexhaustive and includes additional identities such as genderqueer, Two-Spirit, pansexual, and fluid SGM identities.

Current population estimates of SGM adults in the United States range from 9.3–11%, depending on definitions, and differ across generations in the setting of evolving societal acceptance and safety, with approximately 23% in Generation Z (born 1997–2012) openly identifying as part of the community compared with 5.1% of Generation X (born 1965–1980). Reliable population estimates, however, are lacking because there are no consistently applied federal and other administrative survey methodologies.

Transgender people have a gender identity that differs from the sex that was assigned at birth, including those who identify as nonbinary and those who have a gender identity that is neither man nor woman. **Transmasculine** refers to those who have a male- or masculine-spectrum gender identity and were assigned female at birth, and **transfeminine** refers to those who have a female- or feminine-spectrum gender identity and were assigned male at birth. **Cisgender** refers to people whose gender identity and birth assigned sex are the same (ie, they are not transgender). *Transgender people may also be sexual minorities (eg, lesbian, gay, bisexual) or straight/heterosexual.* For the sake of expediency in this chapter, the sections on SM men and women do not consistently include gender identity descriptors. Readers should nonetheless recognize that, for example, SM transmasculine individuals who engage in vaginal receptive sex and cisgender SM women who have transfeminine partners with a penis may have potential contraception needs.

Sexual identities include **gay** (those who are predominantly attracted to or sexually active with people of the same gender), **bisexual** (those who are attracted to or sexually active with people of more than one sex or gender), and **heterosexual** or **straight** (someone who is attracted to or sexually active with people of another gender [historically the "opposite" gender]); however, other terms may be used, and terminology is continually evolving. A growing number of people identify as **pansexual**, which describes an attraction to people of any gender—man, woman, or throughout the gender spectrum. While historically used in a derogatory fashion, the term "**queer**" has been reclaimed by many SGM people to represent someone with a sexual orientation, gender identity, or **gender expression** (the external manifestation of gender) that differs from that of a cisgender, heterosexual person. *In addition, SGM people can have identities not covered above, multiple gender identities or sexual orientations, and identities that change over time or are situational (eg, during incarceration, in educational settings).*

The three dimensions of sexual orientation—identity, behavior, and attraction—do not necessarily overlap. Health risk factors (eg, substance use) and outcomes have been found to be different among different dimensions. For example, one study found that gay and lesbian individuals with sexual identity-behavior discordance reported poorer psychological functioning and higher rates of alcohol binge drinking and suicidal ideation compared with those with identity-behavior concordance. *The incomplete overlap of identity and behavior means that clinicians cannot rely upon self-reported identity to infer sexual behavior, and vice versa.*

It is best practice for clinicians to ask people for their name and pronouns by first offering the clinician's own name and pronouns. For example, the clinician may say "Hello, I'm Dr. (insert name). My pronouns are he/him. What name and pronouns would you like me to use for you?" Pronouns can also be included on ID badges and email signatures. To inquire about gender identity and sex assigned at birth, the following questions are recommended: "What is your gender identity?" and "What sex were you assigned at birth?" *The clinician must remember that name and pronouns may differ from what one thinks may "match" people's gender identity, sex assigned at birth, or gender expression, or what is on "official" documentation, but the clinician must always use the name and pronouns that people share at the time of the visit.*

People may also hide their SGM identities from others, including clinicians, to avoid stigma and discrimination. Revealing a person's sexual orientation, gender identity, or both is called "coming out." This process may occur at any point in life and is often repetitive and context-dependent (eg, being "out" to family but not to coworkers). **The health policy landscape is an important factor in the safety and visibility of SGM identities.** *Despite recent assertions by some governments, the binary concept of gender (that there are only girls and women or boys and men) is not evidence-based.* The dramatic rise in laws and policies affecting SGM health and the increase in state-level variability—particularly for younger SGM people needing gender-affirming care—all have important implications for the health and rights of SGM people and their willingness to seek care.

Clare C et al. Educational guidelines on sexual orientation, gender identity and expression, and sex characteristics: biases in medical education. Am J Ob Gyn. 2024;231:289. [PMID: 38432411]

Dawson L et al. LGBTQ+ Health Policy. KFF. October 8, 2025. https://www.kff.org/lgbtq/health-policy-101-lgbtq-health-policy. Accessed November 25, 2025.

Jones JM. LGBTQ+ Identification in U.S. Rises to 9.3%. Gallup. February 20, 2025. https://news.gallup.com/poll/656708/lgbtq-identification-rises.aspx. Accessed November 25, 2025.

Health Disparities & The Minority Stress Model

Providing compassionate and informed health care for SGM people involves acknowledging and addressing the negative effects of discrimination and stigma. *The theory of minority stress and resilience*, first published by Virginia Brooks in 1981, and later expanded by Ilan Meyer, proposes that *SGM individuals experience chronic, additive, and unique stresses that stem from living in discriminatory social conditions*; stressors include experiences of prejudice, expectations of rejection, the cognitive burden of deciding whether to come out in different circumstances, and internalized homophobia or transphobia.

SGM people also experience multiple social and structural barriers to equitable health. They are underserved by the medical community and understudied in medical research, with worse health outcomes compared with heterosexual and cisgender populations. These experiences also differ in those with additional marginalized identities ("*intersectionality*"); SGM people of color and those with disabilities, for example, face even greater health disparities. SGM people have higher rates of health care avoidance and delays compared to their non-SGM counterparts, which can lead to worse health outcomes. Among transgender people, health care avoidance and delays are associated with discrimination, refusal of care, and other negative experiences related to transgender identity, including in acute care settings. Other structural barriers to access to care among SGM people include financial issues, lack of anti-discrimination protections, and dramatic increases in legislation restricting gender-affirming care. SGM people have higher rates of poverty, lower rates of home ownership, and higher rates of homelessness than non-SGM people. These structural issues will take time to change. However, clinicians can impact the health outcomes of SGM people by ensuring that the clinical space is welcoming to people of all genders and sexual orientations (see below), obtaining comprehensive data on sexual orientation and gender identity, and being aware of the specific health needs of SGM people to advance the health of SGM patients. *A study from Norway found that affirming environments can counteract minority stress and support overall health.* There are significant numbers of SGM refugees from the increasing number of countries with anti-LGBTQ+ laws and policies, and clinicians need to be prepared to meet their health and legal needs with appropriate care and referrals.

The vast majority of SGM patients would like to come out to their clinician. Many clinicians, however, are concerned that their patients would be offended if asked about sexual orientation and gender identity. It is important that clinicians overcome any discomfort and ask appropriate questions of their patients in an inclusive and nonjudgmental way. There are multiple free online resources for clinicians, including the "Acknowledging Sex and Gender" module from the University of California, San Francisco Center of Excellence for Transgender Health, available at https://prevention.ucsf.edu/transhealth/education/acknowledging-gender-sex, and the "Teaching LGBTQ+ Health" course from the Stanford Teaching and Mentoring Academy, available at https://mededucation.stanford.edu/courses/teaching-lgbtq-health/. Specific populations have additional barriers to disclosure and thus shared decision making, such as those with non-English language preference; a study of Latino and Latina SGM patients and their clinicians found significant diversity among individuals and emphasized that providers need to be aware of patients' varying social support from family members and that professional interpreter services should be SGM competent. Patient–provider relationships are also influenced by country of practice; a 2024 study highlights the medical system's history of cruelty toward sexual and gender minorities in the United States, which helps to explain why many SGM individuals are reluctant to seek medical care across the country.

The number of adverse childhood experiences has been shown to be a predictor of future negative health outcomes. SGM individuals have higher adverse childhood experience scores than non-SGM individuals (18–60% versus 14% with four or more adverse childhood experiences). A study of transgender persons found that adverse childhood experiences were responsible for 18% of mental health variances. Additionally, the effect of neglect from being physically excluded from the family home due to sexual orientation or gender identity is a common experience that was not measured; many SGM youth are excluded from their home once they come out, which is strongly associated with future lack of housing, depression, and substance use.

SARS-CoV-2 disproportionately affected SGM populations. SGM individuals were more likely to work in sectors heavily disrupted by the pandemic and experienced higher rates of job loss, financial instability, and interruptions in medical care. Studies documented increases in depression, anxiety, and social isolation among SGM people, as well as disparities in access to housing and health care. While overall COVID-19 vaccination rates were relatively high among SGM adults, racial and ethnic disparities persisted. Emerging research also suggests greater risk of long COVID and related functional limitations among SGM populations.

Halem J et al. A legacy of cruelty to sexual and gender minority groups. N Engl J Med. 2024;391:385. [PMID: 39072484]
Liu M et al. Health care discrimination and care avoidance due to patient-clinician identity discordance among sexual and gender minority adults. Ann Fam Med. 2024;22:329. [PMID: 39038968]
Solberg MA et al. Adverse childhood experiences and health outcomes among sexual and gender minorities: a systematic review. J Child Adolesc Trauma. 2023;17:627. [PMID: 38938948]
Thomas SD et al. Health care avoidance and delay in the transgender population: a systematic review exploring associations with minority stress. Transgend Health. 2025;10:126. [PMID: 40309074]

Making Clinical Environments Welcoming to All SGM Patients

Part of serving SGM patients is to create a welcoming clinical space where each person is cared for and respected for all of who they are—including their sexual orientation, gender identity, and gender expression while considering other key aspects of their identities and lived experiences, such as race and ethnicity, age, educational level, geography, and geo-political context, ability, and primary language. The use of a patient's correct names and pronouns throughout encounters is critical. Implementation of comprehensive care, including acknowledging, respecting, and specifying care as needed for someone based on their sexual orientation, gender identity, gender expression, and correct names and pronouns, necessitates system change in many clinical settings. This includes making sure that (1) leadership is involved; (2) nondiscrimination policies are in place, followed, and prominently displayed; (3) open visitation policies are concordant with patients' choice of visitors; (4) outreach and engagement efforts are made for SGM patients; (5) staff receive culturally affirming training in the care of SGM people; (6) processes, forms, artwork, and reading materials reflect the diversity of SGM people; (7) data are collected about both sexual orientation and gender identity (including names and pronouns) in an open, inclusive, and nonjudgmental manner; (8) clinical care and services include prevention and wellness care with available family planning services and behavioral health services; (9) SGM staff are recruited and trained; (10) preventive care is concordant with clinical practice guidelines, where applicable; (11) if all gender bathrooms are not available, a posting states that patients are welcome to use the bathroom they are most comfortable with; and (12) SGM people are not seen as a monolith. One exercise is to look at clinic materials (ie, signs, posters, brochures, magazines, intake forms) and see if materials presume heterosexual behavior (*heteronormative*) or gender conformity (*cisnormative*). Often, materials discussing anatomy, sex, family planning, conception, pregnancy, and birth presume that everyone is cisgender, White, and primarily English-speaking. If so, find or create more broadly inclusive materials to replace them.

National LGBTQIA+ Health Education Center. https://www.lgbtqiahealtheducation.org. Accessed September 30, 2025.

Obtaining Gender & Sexual History from SGM Patients

The core history and physical examination are not different for SGM people in comparison to other patients. Clinicians should approach each patient as an individual, using correct pronouns and appropriate terminology, respecting gender and sexual diversity, and performing an appropriate physical examination for the clinical encounter.

It is important for the clinician to gather an accurate gender identity history and elicit any goals for gender-affirming care, especially for longitudinal patient care relationships. However, *patients should not be expected to discuss their gender identity or transition in detail unless it is relevant to the current visit.* In addition, it is crucial that clinicians understand that transgender patients may have physical appearances (gender expression), names, and pronouns that are not reflected in their legal names or sex marker, as listed on identity documents. Staff members must learn how to elicit patients' names and correct pronouns so that these can be used consistently. When relevant, anatomic changes from prior gender-affirming treatment should be noted.

As with all patients, a complete medical history should include a comprehensive sexual history. Clinicians may wish to preface discussion of the patient's sexual history with a statement indicating that this information is confidential. The Fenway Institute, which specializes in SGM health care, proposes using the following statement and follow-up questions: *"I am going to ask you some questions about your sexual health and sexuality that I ask all my patients. The answers to these questions are important for me to know how to help keep you healthy. Like the rest of this visit, this information is strictly confidential unless you tell me you are planning to harm yourself or someone else or describe someone else harming you."* Evidence suggests that most individuals are ready and willing to disclose to sensitive providers who make clear the intention behind their questions.

Key data to gather in a relevant sexual history include sexual function and satisfaction; number of partners if the

Table 46–1. Inclusive questions to elicit a comprehensive sexual history.

Are you currently having sex (or sexually active)? How many partners do you have?
When was the last time you had sex?
What is/are the gender(s) of your sexual partner(s)?
Do you or your partner(s) have other sex partners?
What body parts of yours touch which body parts of your partner(s)?
How many people have you had sex with during the last year?
Do you have any issues around sex that you would like to discuss?

patient is sexually active; the gender(s) of the patient's sexual partner(s); and the potential to conceive an unplanned pregnancy with the sexual partner(s) (Table 46–1). It should be noted that "sex" means different things to different people. Therefore, clinicians should determine the types of sexual practices the patient engages in (eg, oral sex, penile insertive anal sex, receptive anal sex, penis-in-vagina sex, fingers-in-anus sex) acknowledging these may not line up with clinicians' assumptions based on a person's sexual orientation. Clinicians must recognize that gender and sexual identity are distinct concepts (eg, transgender people should not be assumed to be heterosexual or straight). Additional key questions include how often barrier contraceptives are used, if at all, for the different sexual practices the patient engages in; and whether drugs or alcohol, or both, are consumed in conjunction with sex. Clinicians should also establish whether there is a history of STIs because a positive history may have implications for medical follow-up and sexual risk assessment (eg, frequency of screening, syphilis serologies, chlamydia and gonorrhea testing, and discussion about HIV preexposure prophylaxis [PrEP]).

Rather than a one-time intervention, gender and sexual history taking should be considered an ongoing process assessed over time and at critical junctures and changes in health status.

Centers for Disease Control and Prevention (CDC). A guide to taking a sexual history. https://www.cdc.gov/sti/hcp/clinical-guidance/taking-a-sexual-history.html. Accessed December 24, 2025.

The Electronic Health Record

Electronic health record (EHR) systems should include functionality for the recording of gender identity, and sex assigned at birth as well as chosen name and pronouns. Chosen name and pronoun should be displayed in all banners, schedules, and other viewing screens. Transgender persons can be identified within the EHR that supports the data collection of gender as separate from sex assigned at birth, by identifying those individuals whose entries for gender identity and assigned sex differ. *Collecting both gender identity and sex assigned at birth data is critical to understanding the population of people in care within a health system and their health needs*, such as age-appropriate cancer screening and appropriate interpretation of laboratory values, which may differ from EHR-labeled normative values for those using gender-affirming hormones.

In the United States, the assessment and documentation in the EHR of a patient's sexual orientation and gender identity have been advocated by the National Academy of Medicine, the Joint Commission, and the Health Resources and Services Administration as fundamental to improving access to and quality of care for SGM people. However, there are risks for SGM people with having their sexual orientation and gender identity documented in the EHR, particularly as federal and state efforts to restrict gender-affirming care and roll back nondiscrimination protections increase the possibility that health information may be used against patients, families, and clinicians. Examples of such risks include housing, child custody, and adoption discrimination. While Title VII of the Civil Rights Act of 1964 prohibits employment discrimination based on sexual orientation or gender identity, there remain no explicit, nationwide statutory protections in many domains, including housing, education, and credit. Further, SGM identities remain criminalized or heavily stigmatized in many countries, and cross-border data sharing or travel can expose SGM individuals to additional risk. Gender identity is likewise insufficiently protected. Therefore, *although sexual orientation and gender identity are critical to caring for the whole person, discussing with patients before documenting in the EHR is a best practice.* Much work remains to harmonize and integrate sexual orientation and gender identity data across EHR systems, strengthen privacy and data-sharing safeguards, and develop patient-centered consent and documentation workflows.

Davison K et al. Culturally competent gender, sex and sexual orientation information practices and electronic health records: rapid review. JMIR Med Inform. 2021;9:e25467. [PMID: 33455901]

Family Planning

A. Pregnancy Prevention

Comprehensive family planning for SGM people is important to address, so that all people can decide if, when, and how to build a family. Since a person's sexual orientation and gender identity do not determine sexual partners, all individuals should be asked about family-building intentions as well as contraception if pregnancy is undesired and their sexual activities that confer the possibility of pregnancy.

Cisgender SM women and other individuals assigned female at birth can and often have been sexually active with individuals with a penis. However, studies have shown that SM women receive fewer reproductive health services, including contraceptive counseling, compared to heterosexual women; SM women and GM individuals are less likely than their cisgender, heterosexual counterparts to use contraception; and that these disparities are especially prominent among certain racial and ethnic subgroups, specifically Black and Latina SM women. Barriers identified to adequate contraceptive care in these communities include lack of provider expertise with SGM health needs, stigma, and enacted or anticipatory discrimination.

SM adolescents, including those who identify as lesbian or bisexual, experience higher rates of unintended pregnancy than heterosexual peers. They are also more likely to have earlier and more frequent sexual activity with cisgender male partners and use less effective contraception. Unintended pregnancy risk continues into adulthood with one sample reporting 24% of SM women having had unintended pregnancies. SM people are also more likely to experience sexual assault, which can contribute to unintended pregnancy risk.

If a patient who is assigned female at birth is having penis-in-vagina sex, one suggested question might be, *"Are you planning to get pregnant this year?"* If the answer is no, this is an opportunity to explain effective contraception options. It is also a good time to talk about protection from STIs when having sex with a partner with a penis (ie, barrier methods). *As with any person engaging in penis-in-vagina sex, experts recommend additional contraceptives in addition to condoms.* Condoms are only 80% reliable in preventing pregnancy with typical use; the addition of contraceptive vaginal foam or film can increase the effectiveness to almost 100%. Long-acting reversible contraceptives are especially important to consider. Long-acting reversible contraceptives such as a subdermal implant in the arm (0.05% annual failure) or either the copper or levonorgestrel IUDs are highly effective. The use of emergency hormonal contraception should also be considered and can be prescribed to have at home. Levonorgestrel, a one-step emergency contraceptive tablet, is available over-the-counter and can be used within 72 hours of unprotected intercourse.

Importantly, *patients should be counseled that gender-affirming hormone therapy is not a reliable contraceptive method.* Anyone with a vagina, uterus, ovaries, and fallopian tubes can potentially become pregnant if they engage in penis-in-vagina sex. Transfeminine persons and nonbinary individuals who have a penis and testes may still produce sperm capable of fertilizing an oocyte even if using gender-affirming estrogen, testosterone blockers, or both. Transmasculine persons and nonbinary individuals who have a uterus and ovaries can become pregnant, even in the setting of testosterone-induced amenorrhea. *All patients capable of pregnancy should be counseled on the importance of contraceptive use if they do not desire pregnancy.* Any of the contraceptive methods available to cisgender people are appropriate for use by transgender people and those on hormone therapy. Little is known about the contraceptive preferences of transgender people and clinical recommendations rely on expert opinion. Since testosterone can be a teratogen, patients who become pregnant while using this therapy should be referred early in pregnancy to a specialist experienced in counseling patients about the risk of fetal exposure to exogenous hormones. There is also a national service (https://mothertobaby.org/) featuring current information on medications while pregnant or lactating.

The frequency of accessing abortion is the same between SGM persons and cisgender, straight persons. Termination of pregnancy can be considered in some situations or locations. A 2021 study evaluated pregnancy termination for transgender, nonbinary, and gender-expansive people and found that most preferred medication abortion, due to their belief that it was the least invasive, although most respondents had undergone a surgical abortion. Respondents most frequently recommended that clinics that provide abortions and other services adopt gender-neutral or gender-affirming intake forms, that providers use gender-neutral language, and that greater privacy be incorporated into the practice setting.

Since the 2022 *Dobbs v Jackson Women's Health Organization* decision to overturn *Roe v Wade* and return abortion regulation to individual states, access to abortion care has become highly heterogeneous across the United States, with many states enacting near-total bans or stringent gestational limits. This rapidly changing political landscape disproportionately affects SGM people, who already face barriers to reproductive and gender-affirming care. Thus, clinicians should be aware of laws, travel burdens, and safety considerations in the jurisdiction in which they practice when providing counseling about pregnancy options.

B. Family Building

Family building should be discussed with all patients, regardless of sexual orientation or gender identity. Options include foster-parenting or adoption (in some locations these options are not open to SGM persons), co-parenting a partner's child or children, becoming pregnant, contracting with a surrogate, or step-parenting. Some fertility practices refuse to assist SGM people with conception even if it is legal. In 2021, the American College of Obstetricians and Gynecologists reaffirmed Committee Opinion No. 749, stating, "No matter how a child comes into a family, all children and parents deserve equitable protections and access to available resources to maximize the health of that family unit." *All clinicians* "should recognize the diversity in parenting desires that exists in the lesbian, gay, bisexual, transgender, queer, intersex, asexual and gender nonconforming communities and should take steps to ensure that clinical spaces are affirming and open to all parties, such that equitable and comprehensive, reproductive health care can meet the needs of these communities."*

According to the Williams Institute, 18% of SGM people are parents to children under 18, including 35% of married adults. Approximately 5 million children in the US are being raised by an SGM parent. At some point in their lifetime, 32% of LGB people and 19% of transgender people report having a child.

*Reproduced with permission from ACOG Committee Opinion No. 749 Summary: Marriage and Family Building Equality for Lesbian, Gay, Bisexual, Transgender, Queer, Intersex, Asexual, and Gender Nonconforming Individuals. Obstetrics & Gynecology. 2018;132(2):539-540.

There are many paths to family building, and each is dependent on personal desires, reproductive capacity of the person and those of a partner(s) if any; any biologic/medical constraints; and legal/political options. Many options exist for conception and clinicians should be prepared to counsel patients, provide resources and refer as appropriate. Patients may decide to have inseminations with an unknown donor from a sperm bank (some unknown donors sign a release so that the child may contact the donor when the child reaches 18 years old), and some may decide to involve a known sperm donor. Most sperm banks are regulated regarding the administration of medical history forms, testing for STIs, and genetic screening. Known donors may have risk factors but are not routinely screened. It is important for future parents to be as informed as they can be about the legal implications of each option. In some states and countries, unless the insemination with known donor sperm takes place in the office of a physician, the known donor has full legal rights as well as financial responsibilities for the offspring. In one study of 129 lesbian mothers with 77 index offspring, 77.5% of the mothers were satisfied with the type of donor chosen (36% had chosen known sperm donors, 25% open-identity donors, and 39% unknown donors). Donor access and custody concerns were the primary themes mentioned by lesbian mothers regarding their satisfaction or dissatisfaction with the type of sperm donor they had selected. Donor siblings may connect through sites like "23andMe" and often choose to meet in person as adults.

Some SM women and couples in whom both partners have a uterus and ovaries decide to do "*co–in vitro fertilization (IVF)*," which is also known as "*reciprocal IVF*" in which one partner provides an egg, it is fertilized in the laboratory with sperm of a known or unknown donor, and then the other partner carries the pregnancy. A report in 2021 demonstrated significantly better reproductive outcomes after reciprocal IVF, with a clinical pregnancy rate of 60% compared with 40% after autologous IVF, and live birth rate of 57.1% in reciprocal IVF versus 29.8% in autologous IVF.

Lactation for the non-gestational parent can sometimes be induced by using a protocol that stemmed originally from the experiences of adoptive mothers who were motivated to breastfeed. Compared with straight women, infants born to lesbian-identified women have a lower chance of being breastfed or, if lactation is initiated, less chance of being breastfed for the first 6 months. The prevalence of a positive score on the Edinburgh Postnatal Depression screen was 35.6% in one study in SM postpartum women; higher concealment motivation was associated with depression symptoms via poor family and partner support.

Many SGM people delay childbearing until later in life, with resultant issues of age-related infertility, increased pregnancy loss, and fetal chromosomal abnormalities, as well as chronic health conditions such as hypertension that can affect obstetrical outcomes. A pre-conception visit that includes genetic counseling is often helpful with pregnancy planning, although there needs to be education of all genetic counselors about LGBTQA+ family constellations. Pregnancy outcomes of bisexual and lesbian women compared with women who identify as straight include increased risk of miscarriage and stillbirth, as well as very preterm birth.

There have been many studies on the overall outcomes of children of lesbian women, all of which have been favorable when comparing their children to children raised by straight parents. A 2020 study using administrative data from the Netherlands found that children of same-sex parents performed better in both primary and secondary education compared with children of different-sex parents.

Biologic options for pregnancy for cisgender gay men or transfeminine persons include conceiving with someone who may or may not be interested in co-parenting with them, or contracting with a friend, relative, or surrogate to carry the pregnancy after the sperm and a donor egg are fertilized and placed in the uterus of the surrogate. For transgender people, there are other options based on the organs they currently have. Prior to initiation of any gender-affirming hormones or gender-affirming surgical procedures, *a consultation with either an obstetrician/gynecologist or a reproductive endocrinologist to discuss fertility preservation and future genetic offspring is encouraged.* Reproductive planning is often not a priority for a transitioning youth but may become a desire in the future and may also be a priority for potential grandparents. Options are limited for transgender youth who have not undergone endogenous puberty before either starting gender-affirming hormones (with estrogen or testosterone) or puberty blockers and then going directly to estrogen or testosterone. *The only future fertility option is either testicular or ovarian tissue cryopreservation, which is considered experimental.* For transfeminine persons and gender nonbinary individuals who were assigned male sex at birth and who have reached adulthood after endogenous puberty, sperm can be stored, ideally prior to the initiation of estrogen. Of note, though some transfeminine persons still produce sperm even after long-term estrogen exposure, it is recommended that sperm cryopreservation occur prior to hormone start because the effect on fertility is hard to quantify and coming off hormones often can be dysphoric. For transmasculine persons and nonbinary individuals who were female sex assigned at birth and have gone through endogenous puberty, the next steps in genetic parentage will be based on the desire to carry a pregnancy and whether they have started gender-affirming hormones. Options include penis-in-vagina sex, intravaginal insemination, intrauterine insemination, and egg cryopreservation for the individual, a partner, or surrogate to carry. If a hysterectomy is planned as part of gender affirmation, discussion of whether ovaries are left in place should occur in light of consideration of future genetic parentage as well as future hormone regulation versus the risk of future ovarian cancer. In one study in Australia, however, only 7% of transgender and nonbinary adults had undertaken fertility preservation yet 95% said that fertility preservation should be offered to all transgender and nonbinary people. Participants who viewed genetic relatedness as important were more likely to have undertaken fertility preservation. Perinatal care providers should also ensure that all components of perinatal care are welcoming of SGM people.

All SGM persons planning a pregnancy should be encouraged to consult with a family attorney prior to conception, and if partnered, the partner needs to be aware of their rights and responsibilities. Parental and surrogacy laws in the United States and most other countries have *not* kept up with the variety of family constellations that are seen in SGM families.

Koh AS et al. Donor sibling relations among adult offspring conceived via insemination by lesbian parents. Hum Reprod. 2023;38:2166. [PMID: 37697711]
Leonard S et al. Sexual and/or gender minority disparities in obstetrical and birth outcomes. Am J Ob Gyn. 2022;226:846.e1. [PMID: 35358492]
Stein GL et al. Project Respect: experiences of seriously ill LGBTQ+ patients and partners with their health care providers. Health Aff Sch. 2023;1:qxad049. [PMID: 38756746]

HEALTH CARE FOR SEXUAL MINORITY WOMEN

SM women are addressed together in this section since most medical literature does not delineate clearly enough between various SM identities of cisgender women and focuses primarily on lesbian and bisexual women. The medical literature also does not sufficiently consider the intersection of sexual orientation and gender identity to evaluate the specific health needs and concerns of transgender SM women or gender diverse SM people assigned female at birth. In the United States, SM women are less likely to have primary care providers, get non-urgent medical care when needed, see a specialist, and feel that doctors spent enough time with them. Health care access is even more restricted at the intersection of sexual orientation, gender, race, and ethnicity. A 2021 study of Black and Latino/a SM gender-expansive women found that barriers to accessing care were linked to income and discrimination by providers. This is true worldwide with variability depending on the local sociopolitical climate. In countries with more restrictive laws and policies, health disparities are likely greater. Limited clinician training likely exacerbates the lack of preparedness to care for SM women. Given the increasing diversity of SGM identities, there is a critical need to expand research to include queer, pansexual, asexual, and other SM identities, and to examine how these and other intersecting minoritized identities shape health and health care access.

Cerezo A et al. Healthcare access and health-related cultural norms in a community sample of Black and Latinx sexual minority gender expansive women. J Homosex. 2023;70:782. [PMID: 34842502]
UCLA School of Law. Williams Institute. Health and socioeconomic well-being of LBQ women in the United States. March 2021. https://williamsinstitute.law.ucla.edu/publications/lbq-women-in-us/. Accessed September 30, 2025.

Health Disparities Affecting Sexual Minority Women

SM women experience significant health disparities compared with heterosexual women, including a higher prevalence of physical conditions (eg, asthma, arthritis, migraine, back pain, headaches, and CVD), disability, depression and other mental health conditions, substance use, intimate partner violence, and earlier all-cause mortality in large prospective cohorts. Sexual health and cancer-related care are also underrecognized and understudied among SM women. These disparities are linked to structural determinants of health, including a higher prevalence of adverse childhood experiences, discrimination in health care settings, and health care delays and avoidance.

Pulmonary disease has not been extensively studied in SM women, but data has consistently shown disproportionately higher rates of asthma and poorer lung health among SM women compared to heterosexual women. Emerging evidence suggests higher rates of COPD among SM women. However, smoking only partially explains these disparities, which raises concern for additional potential mediators of pulmonary health in SM populations, including access to screening and management of chronic respiratory disorders and lung cancer.

There is conflicting literature on whether SGM populations have a higher prevalence of diabetes and prediabetes. Further, many studies do not disaggregate by sexual orientation or gender identity, thus few remark specifically on SM women. In previous research, disparate rates of diabetes found among SM women were impacted by other sociodemographic factors such as race or ethnicity and weight. There are no intervention studies that focus on reducing diabetes and prediabetes among SM women.

As with other SGM populations, aging and advance care planning are priority issues. Qualitative work shows that SM older women frequently worry about stigma in long-term care, social isolation, and support, and whether staff will respect their partners and identities in residential facilities. Because many SM women have fewer or no children and may rely on "families of choice," *clinicians should explicitly identify and document health care decision makers and encourage completion of advance directives to ensure partners and chosen family are recognized.* This is especially important since same-sex/same-gender marriage is not legal in many countries and is still considered socially unacceptable in many areas of the United States. Elder mistreatment screening should also be incorporated into routine care as the scope of this problem is not yet well characterized.

Pinnamaneni M et al. Disparities in chronic physical health conditions in sexual and gender minority people using the United States Behavioral Risk Factor Surveillance System. Prev Med Rep. 2022;28:101881. Erratum in: Prev Med Rep. 2023;34:102191. [PMID: 35855927]
Tabor E et al. Sexuality and respiratory outcomes in the UK: disparities, development and mediators in multiple longitudinal studies. Public Health. 2025;247:105886. [PMID: 40768943]
Tran NK et al. Prevalence of 12 common health conditions in sexual and gender minority participants in the All of Us research program. JAMA Netw Open. 2023;6:e2324969. [PMID: 37523187]

Cardiovascular Disease

The risk of CVD, including MI and stroke, may be higher in SM women compared with heterosexual women.

Information on CVD outcomes is limited, however, with studies showing mixed results depending on methodology. Studies suggest that CVD risk is most influenced by psychosocial stress (ie, cumulative minority stress). Experimental and population-based studies have linked anti-SM contexts, high-stigma regions, and exposure to trauma to contribute to elevated blood pressure, reduced heart rate variability, and higher odds of diabetes, heart disease, and stroke. These issues are further compounded by race and ethnicity: in emerging research, Black lesbian and bisexual women exhibit particularly high burdens of cardiometabolic risk factors and CVD, underscoring the need for intersectional assessment and intervention.

Caceres BA… Rosendale N et al. Differences in ideal cardiovascular health between sexual minority and heterosexual adults. JAMA Cardiology. 2023;8:335. [PMID: 36811854]

Rosendale N et al. Differences in cardiovascular health at the intersection of race, ethnicity, and sexual identity. JAMA Netw Open. 2024;7:e249060. [PMID: 38691360]

Substance Use

A. Tobacco and Nicotine

Nicotine exposure (eg, cigarette smoking, vaping) is more common among SM women than in straight women, particularly among SM women of color, bisexual women, and queer youth. The tobacco industry's well-documented targeted marketing to SGM groups and the use of nicotine to cope with psychosocial stressors are contributing factors. Early initiation of nicotine use (before age 15) accounts for some of the disparities in adult rates. Protective factors against nicotine use for young SM women included connections with other SGM people and parental support.

Both traditional smoking cessation programs and targeted SGM programs are effective for SGM people, although research into SGM-specific interventions is limited. Studies have corroborated that both SGM-specific (such as relation to coming out, different norms and acceptability of smoking among SGM communities, or SGM-related minority stress) and previously identified factors seen in other populations (such as self-efficacy around quitting) are important to support SGM people in quitting smoking. Attention should be paid to youth-specific interventions and to messaging about cigarette smoking warnings. Patients should be encouraged to check with community or online resources for smoking cessation programs and encourage participation in SGM-tailored programs, if available.

Ganz O et al. Cigarette smoking behaviors and nicotine dependence at the intersection of sexual identity and sex in the United States: findings from the National Survey on Drug Use and Health. Prev Med Report. 2024;38:102593. [PMID: 38283968]

McQuoid J et al. Tobacco cessation and prevention interventions for sexual and/or gender minority-identified people and the theories that underpin them: a scoping review. Nic Tob Res. 2023;25:1065. [PMID: 36721977]

B. Alcohol and Other Substances

Substance use is more prevalent among SM women compared with straight women. This is especially well documented for alcohol use; however, it has been shown as well for use of sedatives, cannabis, hallucinogens, opiates, and stimulants. Higher rates of substance use emerge in adolescence and young adulthood and appear to have worsened during the COVID-19 pandemic, particularly for SM women of color and those in resource-limited or rural settings.

Substance use disparities among SM women are best understood in association with chronic minority stress and discrimination rather than solely individual level "risk-taking." Across multiple studies, substance use is consistently linked to psychosocial stressors such as enacted stigma and microaggressions, sexism, discrimination in health care and employment, housing insecurity, adverse childhood experiences, and co-occurring depression and anxiety. Qualitative and longitudinal data consistently find that substances are frequently used as coping strategies in the context of these structural and interpersonal harms. Heavier substance use (eg, alcohol) among Black and Latina SM women also suggests a complex, intersectional, syndemic relationship with racism.

Multiple interventions have been initiated to decrease alcohol and other substance use in SM women; however more research is needed. A 2020 study showed that greater LGBT supportive factors in a community (eg, Pride events) correlate with lower lifetime odds of marijuana use and smoking for youth. Community connectedness is protective against alcohol use in SGM people of color. Training in SGM cultural sensitivity is essential for treatment providers, as is organization-level interventions to ensure SGM-affirming care environments. Another approach studied in rural areas of the United States looked at training and deploying SGM peer advocates to support mental health and substance use and "bridge the gap in culturally competent care." SM women, compared with straight women, with lifetime alcohol use disorders are at heightened risk for concomitant psychiatric and drug use disorders, underscoring the need for substance abuse programs to address concurrent mental health concerns.

Greene N et al. Examining disparities in excessive alcohol use among Black and Hispanic lesbian and bisexual women in the United States: an intersectional analysis. J Stud Alcohol Drugs. 2020;81:462. [PMID: 32800082]

McCabe SE et al. Trends in binge drinking, marijuana use, illicit drug use, and polysubstance use by sexual identity in the United States (2006-2017). Subst Abus. 2022;43:194. [PMID: 34344281]

Noel JK Rosenthal SR et al. Sexual minority status, illicit drug use, and depressive symptoms. J LGBT Youth. 2024;21:490. [PMID: 38798775]

Body Weight and Disordered Eating

Issues regarding body weight and disordered eating among SM women are multifaceted and shaped by intersecting experiences of minority stress, structural inequities, and weight stigma rather than by individual behaviors alone.

Many cohort and survey studies report a higher prevalence of obesity and overweight among SM women than among heterosexual women, with some evidence that SM women of color are especially affected. Additional factors, such as poverty, identity-based microaggressions, and limited access to healthy food, also influence weight-related outcomes. SM women also report high levels of experienced and internalized weight stigma, often compounded by anti-fat bias in clinical encounters ("fat broken arm syndrome"), which can deter care-seeking and is associated with depression, disordered eating, and maladaptive coping strategies. Qualitative work highlights that many SM women value interventions to prioritize health, function, and acceptance of diverse body sizes over weight loss as a primary goal, while also recognizing that pain and other chronic conditions can be exacerbated for some at higher weights.

Disordered eating and body image concerns are also common among SM women. Although SM women are underrepresented compared to other SGM groups in the literature on disordered eating, existing cross-sectional and longitudinal cohort studies indicate that SM women have high rates of disordered eating behaviors, body dissatisfaction, and unhealthy weight-control practices, beginning in adolescence and continuing into adulthood. Previous studies have specifically tied internalized homophobia, SM identity concealment, and weight bias to binge eating and overeating behaviors. On the contrary, social support, resilience, and higher self-esteem appear to buffer against both disordered eating and poor mental health, highlighting the importance of SGM-affirming interventions and practitioners that address structural stigma and promote body diversity rather than reinforcing narrow weight ideals.

Devlin EA et al. Demographic and minority stress risk factors for obesity among sexual minority youth assigned female at birth. LGBT Health. 2024;11:103. [PMID: 37819720]

Leonard SI et al. Weight stigma and mental and emotional health among sexual and gender minority individuals: a scoping review. LGBT Health. 2024;11:496. [PMID: 37948558]

Sexually Transmitted Infections

STIs occur in SM women, but little epidemiologic data are available to delineate precise risks. Limited evidence suggests particularly high prevalence of bacterial vaginosis, HPV, and genital herpes (HSV) among SM women in the United States. Research on SM subpopulations, including Black SM women and SM women in China, suggest that sexual activity with men, multiple sex partners, unprotected sex, and partner power dynamics (including negotiating the use of protection) are individual risk behaviors associated with STI acquisition. SM women should not be presumed to be at no or low risk for STIs solely based on their sexual identity and should be asked about their sexual behaviors and screened per clinical guidelines.

1. Sexual practices—*Asking about sexual behaviors in addition to sexual identity is key to identifying STI risk and advising appropriate testing and prevention*, since risk may vary by specific sexual practice (eg, digital-vaginal, vaginal-vaginal, digital-anal, oral-vaginal, oral-anal contact) and specific pathogens. Often data are mixed and inconsistent with respect to whether sources speak to infection risk by identity group or behavior. Delineating behavior-based risk and identity-based risk are important for research, assessments, and interventions. While SM women have diverse sexual practices, the CDC categorizes STI risk by women who have sex with women (WSW) and women who have sex with women and men (WSWM) and has found that STI risk is particularly elevated among WSWM and adolescents. The CDC also noted that use of barrier protection in examined studies (eg, use of gloves, dental dams) was ubiquitously low. About 20–50% of SM women use sexual aids (eg, vibrators, dildos, or other sexual toys); these should not be shared with partners and should be cleaned after use. *Organisms, including HPV, can remain on these sexual aids for up to 24 hours after use, even after standard cleaning.*

2. Chlamydia, gonorrhea, and syphilis—Rates of *C trachomatis*, *N gonorrhoeae*, and *T pallidum* transmission between SM women are unknown. However, SM women can still transmit and contract these infections in relation to higher-sexual risk behaviors, barriers to health care access, and the misconception by patients, clinicians, or both that SM women are not at risk for STIs. Regardless of sexual orientation, the CDC recommends annual chlamydia and gonorrhea screening for all women from the age of first sexual activity to the age of 25 years and for higher-risk groups; as well as annual syphilis screening particularly for higher-risk groups.

3. HIV—Exchange of blood should be avoided as much as possible, especially between HIV-discordant partners, since viral genotype analysis has confirmed that *HIV can be transmitted sexually between women.* The clinician should encourage both new partners to have comprehensive STI and HIV screening prior to sexual contact and recommend barrier protection for 6 months until partners are again screened to verify that their HIV status is still negative. If a couple is consistently monogamous and HIV and other STI testing are negative, barrier precautions do not need to be continued. However, most SM women may not follow this advice if they feel they are at low risk for HIV. Some SM women are sex workers or have had sexual relationships with people with a penis and are at increased risk for STIs. CDC guidelines recommend that all women should be tested once in their lifetime for HIV, with testing repeated according to risk factors. If an SM woman is in a high-risk relationship for HIV transmission (eg, sex work, male partners, or a partner living with HIV), *they should be educated about PrEP for HIV prevention and prescribed the appropriate medication.*

4. Herpes simplex virus (HSV)—Both HSV-1 and HSV-2 can be transmitted sexually between SM women, especially given higher rates of orogenital sex. The same precautions regarding the transmission of HSV should be provided to women of all sexual identities; there should be no sexual contact during any prodromal symptoms that may precede a genital herpes outbreak or during the blister stage of the outbreak. Suppression of lesions can usually be accomplished with antiviral medications, such as acyclovir or valacyclovir, if the lesions are recurrent (see Chapter 6).

5. HPV—There is evidence of HPV transmission between female sexual partners. HPV antibodies and abnormal Papanicolaou smears have been seen in WSW who have never had sex with men. Thus, *all people with a cervix need cervical cancer screening*, which may include Papanicolaou smears, high-risk HPV strain testing, or both, according to timetables and risk factors provided by professional society guidelines (see Chapter 21). According to a systematic review and meta-analysis, SM women receive Papanicolaou testing at lower rates than heterosexual women, which may contribute to cervical cancer disparities. In addition to the need for increased office-based testing, home HPV testing kits are now available which hopefully will increase the testing and detection of cervical cancer.

The overall HPV vaccination rate is low in adult women regardless of sexual orientation, so improvement in all groups should be the goal. One study demonstrated that the 2010 Affordable Care Act did increase vaccination rates among SM women in the United States. *Administration of the HPV vaccine is critical to the prevention of cervical cancer.* The CDC recommends HPV vaccination for all persons through age 45 years.

6. Bacterial vaginosis, trichomonas, and vulvovaginal candidiasis—These infections, especially bacterial vaginosis, are common among women. According to the CDC, bacterial vaginosis is even more common among SM women. Sexual behaviors as having a new partner, having a partner with bacterial vaginosis, receptive oral sex, digital-vaginal sex, and digital-anal sex are associated with higher incidence of bacterial vaginosis. Routine asymptomatic screening for bacterial vaginosis, however, is not recommended and testing should be based on symptoms. For symptomatic bacterial vaginosis among SM women, one approach is to treat the symptomatic patient but not their female sexual partners. If symptoms recur, the female sexual partners should then be evaluated and treated with expedited partner therapy with consideration of re-treating the index patient. This strategy may also be used for treatment of recurrent or hard to treat vulvovaginal candidiasis, which technically is not considered to be sexually transmitted, but improvement has been detailed with treatment of index patients and their female partners. Trichomonas can be transmitted easily between female sexual partners and is relatively common among SM women, with prevalence rates in this population exceeding those of chlamydia or gonorrhea. Patient education including on avoiding shared sex toys, cleaning such toys, and barrier protection can help lower vaginitis incidence.

Various strategies for making reproductive and sexual health clinics and providers more amenable to serving SGM people were studied by a group in the United States, but the findings (such as ensuring counseling involves inclusive safe sex discussions) have broad face validity and relevance for other regional and medical focus settings as well.

Cancer

Little is known about the incidence and prevalence of various cancers in SM women, since sexual orientation has not been routinely included in cancer screening programs and cancer registries. However, *some data suggest that SM women may be at a higher risk for cancer-related mortality than heterosexual counterparts.* The National Health Interview Survey found bisexual women aged ≥ 65 years were 7.6% more likely to have a cancer diagnosis than a heterosexual woman of the same age, but the difference was not seen between lesbian and heterosexual women; the survey also found that lesbian and bisexual women have a higher prevalence of cancer risk factors, such as tobacco use, underscoring the need for vigilant screening. *Since SM women have barriers to accessing health care and may not see a clinician regularly, any visit to a health care provider is an opportunity to check on cancer screening status* (eg, colonoscopy, mammography, cervical cancer screening).

There is also recognition that upon receiving a cancer diagnosis, *SGM people face challenges in receiving equitable care throughout the cancer care continuum and may experience cancer differently and have different needs during their care.* One qualitative study with SGM breast cancer survivors underscored the challenges of disclosing sexual orientation during cancer care and the importance of provider recognition that varying social networks are critical to positive experiences of care provision. The National Health Interview Survey from 2013–2018 showed differences in the quality of life for lesbian and bisexual women surviving cancer compared with heterosexual women. Lesbian women reported higher odds of fair or poor self-rated health, COPD, and heart conditions. Bisexual women reported higher odds of severe psychological distress, heart conditions, and food insecurity than did heterosexual women. Bisexual women had lower odds of receiving a recent mammogram than did heterosexual women. The 2017 American Society for Clinical Oncology position statement recommends five action steps to enhance SGM cancer care and reduce disparities: (1) patient education and support, (2) workforce development and diversity, (3) quality improvement strategies, (4) policy solutions, and (5) research strategies. Information materials need to be changed and provider training enhanced to decrease heteronormative assumptions and the social isolation experienced by SGM cancer survivors. All providers need to consider whether their prevention, screening, diagnostic, treatment, and palliative approaches will be equitably experienced by SM women.

Jackson SS et al. Cancer disparities among sexual and gender minority populations. J Natl Med Assoc. 2023;115:S32. [PMID: 37202001]

A. Breast Cancer

The literature has been mixed on whether SM women have an increased risk of breast cancer compared with heterosexual women. SM women, however, do have an increased prevalence of *risk factors* predisposing to breast cancer, including nulliparity (and decreased breastfeeding), alcohol use, obesity, and cigarette smoking. Vulnerability to inadequate screening, the development of cancer, or delayed diagnosis may further correlate with certain experiences such as a masculine gender presentation or chest binding. The literature is also inconsistent regarding the rate of mammography screening in lesbian women; however, one study showed that bisexual women were less likely than heterosexual women and lesbian women to adhere to mammography screening guidelines. Resilience and recovery factors vary in some ways between heterosexual and SM women, and the latter may find that breast cancer support groups focus on heteronormative issues (eg, attractiveness to a male partner).

B. Cervical Cancer

Primary prevention of cervical cancer is essential. *All persons between the ages of 9 and 45 years (routine recommended age is 11 to 12 years old) should receive the HPV vaccine series.* HPV can be transmitted sexually between partners of any gender. Cervical cancer screening, with Papanicolaou smears, primary HPV testing, or both, should be part of SM women's health care at the same intervals as for heterosexual women according to national and international guidelines. SM women, however, receive Papanicolaou smears at a lower rate than sexually active heterosexual women, in part because many of the Papanicolaou smears are often done in reproductive health clinics; those who are not interested in becoming pregnant or do not have pregnancy-related needs may not access these clinical sites. In addition, some SM patients as well as their health care providers mistakenly think that SM women do not need Papanicolaou smears. *Any individual with a cervix needs cervical cancer screening starting at the age of 21 years, consistent with recommendations for cervical cancer screening for all cisgender women.* Cancer prevention and control strategies for SM women that target provider education and policy intervention are needed to improve SM women's relationships with their providers and increase cervical cancer screening rates.

C. Lung Cancer

Compared with heterosexual women, SM women are likely to have a higher rate of lung cancer due to their increased rate of cigarette smoking and associated social determinants of smoking. Research suggests that lung cancer screening with the use of low-dose helical CT is underutilized for SM populations. However, there are critical gaps in the literature regarding overall incidence and prevalence of lung cancer, screening and treatment utilization, barriers to screening initiation, and adherence among SM women.

D. Endometrial and Ovarian Cancer

Endometrial and ovarian cancers are increased among those with nulliparity, which is more likely in SM women. Obesity, a known risk factor for both cancers, appears to be more prevalent among SM women. Conversely, the use of oral contraceptives, which is protective against the development of both of these cancers, is lower in lesbian women than in heterosexual women. Vigilance toward and education about presenting signs and symptoms (eg, postmenopausal bleeding, early satiety, unintended weight loss) are important to detect cancers as early as possible. Neither incidence nor prevalence of endometrial or ovarian cancer has been determined in this SM population. Lesbian women are less likely than heterosexual women to have had bilateral salpingectomies or bilateral tubal ligations for sterilization; these procedures decrease the risk for ovarian cancer, since about 70% of ovarian cancers start in the fallopian tubes.

Violence

Compared with heterosexual women, SM women have higher exposures to violence throughout their lifetimes. Lifetime prevalence of sexual assault may be as high as 85%. One study concluded that sexual orientation clearly plays a role in victimization when they found that compared with heterosexual women, bisexual women had 3.7 times the odds of initial victimization and 7.3 times the odds of repeat victimization, and lesbian women had 3.2 times the odds of repeat victimization even after controlling for other sociodemographic factors. In a study of four countries in southern Africa, nearly one-third of lesbian and bisexual women experienced forced sex and assault including "corrective rape" by men as an attempt to change the women's sexual orientation.

SM women asylum applicants are frequently not granted asylum in the United States, despite being victims of severe violence in their home countries due to their sexual orientation. When studied, there are three possible mechanisms of erasure of violence in these cases: ruling that the violence experienced was not extreme, finding that the applicants' accounts of violence were unsubstantiated, or arguing that the violence experienced was unrelated to the applicants' sexual orientation.

The CDC reports that 61% of bisexual women and 44% of lesbian women experience rape, physical violence, and stalking by an intimate partner. These rates are higher than similar trauma in heterosexual women (35%). Additionally, approximately 20% of bisexual women compared with 10% of heterosexual women have been raped by an intimate partner in their lifetimes. The rate of stalking experienced by bisexual women is twice that of heterosexual women and a higher percentage of bisexual women report being afraid of an intimate partner. A study of United States veterans found that compared with heterosexual women veterans, SM women veterans were twice as likely to report emotional mistreatment and physical intimate partner violence and three times as likely to report sexual intimate partner violence.

SM women experience rates of intimate partner violence (IPV) that dramatically exceed those of heterosexual women. Bisexual and other non-monosexual women as well as SM women of color are at particularly high risk of physical, emotional, and sexual IPV. Compared to heterosexual women, bisexual women have a 3-4 times increased odds of lifetime reported IPV across some studies. SM women veterans have also been shown to have significantly higher odds of IPV victimization than heterosexual women veterans. Risk is shaped by many of the same factors seen in heterosexual populations (eg substance use, prior trauma), but is further amplified by SGM-specific stressors.

Despite alarming rates for women of any identity, SM women survivors of sexual assault and interpersonal violence may experience unique difficulties when seeking assistance. These problems include a limited understanding of interpersonal violence in the relationships of SM women, stigma, and systemic inequities (such as shelters unwelcome to this population, perpetrating partners being allowed into the same shelters as the survivor of the domestic violence, "outing" someone as a psychological threat, and staff lacking cultural sensitivity and appropriate training in working with SM women). Barriers to preventing SGM violence include stigma, systemic discrimination, and a lack of understanding of SGM IPV.

Porsch LM et al. Intimate partner violence among sexual minority women: a scoping review. Trauma Violence Abuse. 2023;24:3014. [PMID: 36154756]

Unmark E et al. Untangling the relationship between internalized heterosexism and psychological intimate partner violence perpetration: a comparative study of lesbian and bisexual women in Turkey and Denmark. J Interpers Violence. 2022;37:NP14337. [PMID: 33876984]

Mental Health

Mental health disparities among SM women are well documented. Compared with heterosexual women, SM women have higher rates of depression and anxiety, suicidality and self-harm behaviors, substance use disorders, disordered eating, and body image issues. Across numerous studies, bisexual women have been found to be at highest risk for adverse mental health outcomes. Research also suggests worse outcomes for SM women who identify as gender minorities or who are masculine-presenting. There is still a great need to expand research to include diverse SM women populations, as much of the extant literature focuses on white SM women.

Key associated risk factors include internalized homophobia, sexism, intimate partner violence, adverse childhood experiences. Additionally, many of the mental health disparities and health risks experienced by SM women have been attributed to *minority stress.* Therefore, rather than identifying these problems as synonymous with a SM identity or stemming from inborn association with minority sexual orientation, clinicians should recognize that *minority stress causes mental health challenges that stem from societal discrimination and stigma borne by individuals with minority identities (and behaviors).* Discrimination against SM women in health care settings has also been suggested as a deterrent of health care. Recent evidence has emerged that primary care providers may screen lesbian women less consistently than heterosexual women for depression. In addition, psychotherapists working with lesbian and transgender women have been shown to use microaggressive questioning, highlighting persistent heteronormative and cisnormative biases in mental health care and training.

The presence or absence of family support is a significant modifier of mental health outcomes for SGM youth, with significant implications for adulthood. Parental acceptance and family connectedness among SM youth have been shown to be protective factors against poor mental health outcomes in adulthood, including mood disorders and suicidality. On the contrary, parental rejection and forced sexual orientation and gender identity change efforts (conversion therapy) are strongly associated with substance use and suicidality. As of January 2026, conversion therapy for minors is banned in 25 countries; while there is no federal ban in the United States, conversion therapy is outlawed in 25 states as well as Puerto Rico and the District of Columbia, with variable laws across additional cities and regions (https://www.equaldex.com/issue/conversion-therapy).

Protective factors influencing the mental health of SM women include strong social support across four domains: family, friends, SGM communities, and intimate partners. For SM youth, school, peer, and family support, as well as efforts to build individual resilience, are associated with fewer depressive symptoms and suicidality, reinforcing the value of multilevel, identity-affirming interventions. Diverse social networks and access to multiple forms of support can promote resilience, although intersecting stressors related to race, class, and gender identity have not been well-researched and may very well mediate this relationship. Evidence from two decades of legal same-sex marriage within and across the United States further links legal recognition of relationships with improved mental health and reduces disparities between SM and heterosexual adults.

Gmelin JH et al. Increased risks for mental disorders among LGB individuals: cross national evidence from the world mental health surveys. Soc Psychiatry Psychiatr Epidemiol. 2022;57:2319. [PMID: 35851652]

Matouk K et al. Mental health disparities in sexual minority and transgender women: implications and considerations for treatment. Psychiatr Clin North Am. 2023;46:583. [PMID: 37500252]

HEALTH CARE FOR GAY & BISEXUAL MEN

This section is devoted to the primary care of cisgender gay, bisexual, and other men who have sex with men (**MSM**) regardless of their sexual identity. *Most health-related research that focuses on MSM categorizes men based on their sexual behavior as MSM, rather than their self-reported identification as gay, bisexual, or other identities.* Although sexual identity is not always congruent with sexual behavior, identity is important to recognize to optimize health and health care, especially when there is a difference based on sexual identity (eg, gay- versus bisexual-identified men).

Demographics

The size of the MSM population in the United States is not known with certainty due to variability in the definition of sexual orientation used in surveys and the possibility that some survey respondents do not disclose gay or bisexual orientations because of concerns about discrimination. Nevertheless, based on available data, it is estimated that at least 2.5% of American adult men identify as gay, and an additional 2.0% of men identify as bisexual. The prevalence of LGBT identification is higher among younger individuals, with approximately 21% of those born between 1997 and 2003 identifying as LGBT. The proportion of men who engage in sex with other men or experience sexual attraction to other men is estimated to be higher, with 7.3% and 6.2% of adult men reporting some same-sex attraction and sexual behavior, respectively, in one national survey.

Health Disparities

Gay, bisexual, and other MSM face health disparities stemming from the biologic aspects of their sexual behavior or from minority stress, or both. Because of these disparities, MSM have been identified as a priority population for health-related research and improvement in health care by both the National Academy of Medicine and the federal government's Healthy People 2030 initiative. These health disparities are exacerbated if MSM have experienced early life traumatic events, such as sexual abuse or familial rejection.

Office of Disease Prevention and Health Promotion (ODPHP). Healthy People 2030. Goal: improve the health, safety, and well-being of lesbian, gay, bisexual, and transgender people. https://odphp.health.gov/healthypeople/objectives-and-data/browse-objectives/lgbt. Accessed April 10, 2026.

A. HIV and Other STIs

1. HIV infections—*MSM account for approximately 71% of all new HIV infections in the United States,* despite representing a small proportion (<10% by any metric) of the country's male population. The high burden of HIV infection among MSM stems in part from the efficient transmission of the virus through receptive anal intercourse, which confers a higher risk of HIV infection than other sexual activities, such as penile-vaginal and oral intercourse. Role versatility can also uniquely potentiate HIV spread among MSM, since the same person can acquire HIV via receptive intercourse and then transmit by engaging in insertive anal intercourse with partners without HIV. The origin of disparate HIV rates between MSM and other populations is not solely biologic in origin, however, as societal stigma and psychosocial problems also contribute to sexual risk behavior among MSM. *MSM of color face an increased risk of HIV;* the CDC estimates that in the United States in 2022, 34% of new HIV diagnoses occurred among Black MSM, and 36% were among Latino MSM. Racial and ethnic disparities in HIV infections among MSM are not because of differences in sexual behavior or substance use but rather such factors as lack of access to medical care, lower rates of recent HIV testing among non-White MSM, and assortative mixing (ie, being more likely to have sex with partners from one's own racial or ethnic group).

2. Syphilis and gonococcal infection—Beyond HIV, *some STIs are more common among MSM.* In 2023, approximately 33% of primary and secondary syphilis diagnoses occurred in MSM. Syphilis is associated with a high likelihood of subsequent HIV acquisition in MSM and may serve as a marker for individuals who could benefit from intensive HIV prevention efforts, such as PrEP. Increased cases of ocular syphilis, occasionally resulting in blindness, have been reported, with most cases occurring in MSM. The incidence of gonorrhea among MSM exceeds that among men who have sex with women (MSW). MSM also are more likely than MSW to be infected with antibiotic-resistant gonorrhea. Most gonococcal infections in MSM occur at extragenital sites (ie, the pharynx or the rectum) where they may be asymptomatic, underscoring the importance of eliciting a comprehensive sexual history, including an inventory of potential anatomic exposures, to provide optimal STI screening for MSM. Recent studies demonstrate that doxycycline postexposure prophylaxis can significantly decrease bacterial STI incidence, an approach termed "doxy PEP."

3. Viral hepatitis—*MSM face increased risks of viral hepatitis.* Outbreaks of hepatitis A infection have been documented in MSM, likely due to anal sexual contact, including oral-anal exposure ("rimming") as well as insertive and receptive practices. Likewise, hepatitis B is more common among MSM than the general population; approximately 20% of MSM have evidence of either current or prior infection with hepatitis B by age 30 years. *This highlights the importance of universal hepatitis A and B vaccination for young gay and bisexual men, preferably prior to the initiation of sexual contact.* Finally, hepatitis C infection has been identified as prevalent among MSM with HIV and some MSM without HIV; although hepatitis C is generally not efficiently transmitted via sexual contact, it is associated with condomless receptive anal sex, group sex, manual insertion of fingers into the rectum ("fisting"), and recent STIs, which make the rectal mucosa more susceptible to hepatitis C acquisition and transmission. Screening for hepatitis C is crucial as the infection can be asymptomatic for years but may result in cirrhosis or hepatic cancer, and it is curable with currently available therapies.

4. Other infections—*HPV infection, which can cause anogenital warts, anal dysplasia, and anal cancer, is more common among MSM than MSW.* A meta-analysis estimated the prevalence of the oncogenic HPV type 16 in the anal canal to be 35.4% among MSM with HIV and 12.5% among MSM without HIV. Correspondingly, anal cancer incidence is higher among MSM with HIV than in MSM without HIV.

Enteric infections may be sexually transmitted among MSM engaging in anal sexual contact, especially oral-anal sexual contact, and should be considered in the differential diagnosis of GI concerns. These infections include giardiasis, amebiasis, and shigellosis. In addition, *Shigella* infections are more likely to be antibiotic-resistant among MSM than among other individuals.

Clusters of meningococcal disease among MSM in the United States and Europe have also been reported, particularly those frequenting saunas and bathhouses, prompting some jurisdictions to recommend meningococcal vaccination for MSM. Intimate contact with multiple partners has been identified as a risk factor for infection in some of these outbreaks.

The global clade II mpox outbreak beginning in 2022 predominantly affected MSM, who represented > 90% of all affected individuals. Before this outbreak, mpox was primarily reported in central and western Africa, outside of sporadic travel-related cases in other regions. Mpox causes a typically self-limited illness with rash and often fever, malaise, and lymphadenopathy. In the 2022 outbreak, anogenital lesions were identified in most affected people, suggesting sexual spread of the infection. While most people with mpox recover without the need for hospitalization or antiviral treatment, people who are immunocompromised, particularly those with advanced and untreated HIV infection, are at risk for severe disease, including disseminated infection and death. The optimal treatment for people with or at risk for severe disease from mpox is not known, as RCTs of tecovirimat have not shown benefit. Vaccination with a non-replicating vaccinia virus vaccine (MVA-BN, also called JYNNEOS) reduces the likelihood of acquiring mpox and renders the infection less severe if it occurs despite vaccination. The mpox outbreak had diminished substantially by late 2022, likely due to a combination of safer sex and immunity from infection and vaccination. However, clade II mpox transmission continues. In addition, a multinational outbreak of clade I mpox centered in Africa was identified; 10 cases of clade I mpox had been identified in the United States as of January 2026.

Centers for Disease Control and Prevention (CDC). Fast facts: HIV and gay and bisexual men. https://www.cdc.gov/hiv/data-research/facts-stats/gay-bisexual-men.html. Accessed September 30, 2025.

Centers for Disease Control and Prevention (CDC). First case of clade I mpox diagnosed in the United States. https://www.cdc.gov/han/2024/han00519.html. Accessed September 30, 2025.

Centers for Disease Control and Prevention (CDC). Increase in extensively drug-resistant shigellosis in the United States. https://www.cdc.gov/han/2023/han00486.html. Accessed September 30, 2025.

Centers for Disease Control and Prevention (CDC). Sexually transmitted infections surveillance. 2024. https://www.cdc.gov/sti-statistics/annual/index.html. Accessed September 30, 2025.

B. Behavioral Health

Likely due to minority stress (ie, growing up in non-affirming societies), MSM experience mental health disorders more commonly than other men. Whether defined by self-reported identity as gay or bisexual or behaviorally by report of sexual activity with other men, MSM have a higher lifetime prevalence of depression and anxiety disorders than men who identify as heterosexual or those who report sexual activity only with women. Behaviorally bisexual men experience a higher burden of both depression and anxiety disorders, compared with men who engage in only same-gender sexual behavior, in part because bisexual men may have less access to defined communities of choice, like self-identified gay men. The increased prevalence of mental health disorders among behaviorally bisexual men may also stem from dual stigmatization by both the straight and gay male communities, as well as internalized stigma. Among MSM overall, anti-gay violence, community alienation, and dissatisfaction with an idealized body image have all been associated with depression.

C. Substance Use

Compared with men who have only female sexual partners, MSM are more likely to report lifetime recreational drug use; they are specifically more likely to have used cocaine, hallucinogens, inhalants, analgesics, and tranquilizers. In addition, men who identify as gay or bisexual are more likely to smoke cigarettes than those who identify as straight. Although it is not clear that MSM are more likely than others to use methamphetamines, methamphetamine use in MSM communities has been linked to increased sexual risk behavior and transmission of hepatitis C, HIV, and other STIs. Consistent with the minority stress model, experiences of discrimination have been independently associated with substance use among MSM.

Blair CS et al. Examining the relative contributions of methamphetamine use, depression, and sexual risk behavior on rectal gonorrhea/chlamydia among a cohort of men who have sex with men in Los Angeles, California. Sex Transm Dis. 2022;49:216. [PMID: 34654768]

Preventive Care & Clinical Practice Guidelines

Clinicians can help address health disparities affecting MSM by following clinical practice guidelines that pertain to this population (Table 46–2). *The CDC recommends that sexually active MSM undergo screening for HIV, syphilis, gonorrhea, and chlamydia annually and more often if the sexual history warrants more frequent assessment.* An HIV antibody-antigen assay is preferred to HIV antibody alone for HIV screening because this test increases the sensitivity for detection of acute or recent HIV infection. Nucleic acid amplification testing (NAAT) provides optimal sensitivity for diagnosis of gonorrhea and chlamydia and can be performed on the oropharynx, rectum, urine, and urethra. MSM should be screened for these infections at any of the aforementioned sites that may have been exposed during sex, regardless of condom use. First-catch urine specimens for gonorrhea and chlamydia NAAT in men provide comparable accuracy to urethral swab; thus, there is no advantage to obtaining it for routine screening. Rectal and pharyngeal swabs for NAAT can be self-collected.

The CDC also recommends that MSM be screened for chronic hepatitis B infection at least once in their lives and that they be vaccinated against hepatitis A and B. Annual hepatitis C screening with a hepatitis C antibody test is recommended for MSM with HIV due to the elevated incidence of this infection in this population and the availability of well-tolerated, curative therapy. MSM without HIV who engage in sexual practices that may abrade the rectal mucosa (eg, group sex, fisting) may also benefit from annual hepatitis C screening.

The CDC, USPSTF, and the WHO recommend PrEP for HIV for MSM at high likelihood for HIV infection.

Table 46–2. Clinical practice guidelines pertaining to the care of men who have sex with men (MSM) (listed in alphabetical order, within categories).

Recommendation	Comments
Immunizations	
Hepatitis A and B	Consider prevaccination serologic testing if the immunization history is uncertain; vaccinate if seronegative
HPV	Recommended up to age 26 years; the vaccine may be offered to those aged 27–45 years
Meningococcal	Recommended by some jurisdictions due to outbreaks of meningococcal disease among MSM
Mpox	Recommended for people with HIV and MSM who, in the prior 6 months, have been diagnosed with an STI or had more than one sex partner
Medications	
Preexposure prophylaxis for HIV	For MSM at high, ongoing risk of HIV infection (eg, anal sex without a condom, recent STI diagnosis, sexual partner with HIV)
Postexposure prophylaxis for HIV	Consists of 28 days of antiretroviral medication following a discrete exposure to HIV
Postexposure prophylaxis for STIs with doxycycline	Consists of a single 200 mg dose of doxycycline taken within 72 hours after condomless sex for MSM with a history of a bacterial STI in the past year
Screening Tests	
Anal cytology	For MSM with HIV beginning at 35 years and for MSM without HIV beginning at 45 years
Behavioral health (depression, substance use)	At the first clinical encounter, with follow-up screening for those who report behavioral health concerns
Hepatitis C serology	Annually for MSM with HIV and MSM without HIV engaging in behaviors that might expose them to blood (eg, injection drug use or traumatic anal sexual practices)
HIV serology	At least annually, more often if indicated by the sexual history
Nucleic acid amplification test for gonorrhea and chlamydia	At least annually, more often if indicated by the sexual history; all potentially exposed sites (oropharynx, urethra, rectum) should be screened
Syphilis serology	At least annually, more often if indicated by the sexual history

FDA-approved options for MSM for PrEP include oral emtricitabine/tenofovir disoproxil fumarate, oral emtricitabine/tenofovir alafenamide, long-acting injectable cabotegravir, and long-acting injectable lenacapavir. Individuals with a high likelihood for HIV include those who engage in condomless anal sex outside of a monogamous relationship with a man without HIV; those who have a recent diagnosis of a bacterial STI; and those who have sexual partners with HIV who are not consistently virologically suppressed on antiretroviral therapy. PrEP has been shown in RCTs to prevent HIV infection in MSM and is addressed in more detail in Chapter 35. FDA-approved condoms can also decrease transmission of STIs during anal intercourse (One Male Condom); condomless anal intercourse carries the greatest sexual exposure risk of HIV transmission. These condoms can also be used to reduce the rate of pregnancy and the transmission of STIs during vaginal intercourse.

Clinicians who care for MSM should also be aware of antiretroviral postexposure prophylaxis (PEP) for HIV, which consists of antiretrovirals started within 72 hours of a discrete exposure to HIV and taken for 28 days, and either provide PEP themselves or be able to rapidly link patients to PEP care (see Chapter 35).

HPV immunization is recommended for all boys and young men up to age 26 years. For unvaccinated adults aged 27–45 years, shared decision making around HPV vaccination is recommended. *The HIV Medicine Association recommends routinely screening MSM with HIV for anal cancer and cancer precursors with anal cytology*; an RCT, the ANCHOR study, showed that treating anal cancer precursors significantly reduced the risk of anal cancer compared with monitoring alone. Patients with abnormal anal cytology are typically referred for high-resolution anoscopy with biopsy. Colonoscopy performed for colon cancer screening is not considered a substitute for anal cytology or high-resolution anoscopy because colonoscopy does not assess for cellular abnormalities in the anal canal. Anal cytology, high-risk HPV testing, or both for screening of MSM without HIV is recommended in international consensus guidelines, beginning at age 45. If a screening test is negative, it should be repeated in 12–24 months depending upon the screening strategy used (cytology, high-risk HPV testing, or both).

Mpox vaccination with MVA-BN (JYNNEOS) is recommended for MSM who have had recent exposure to or who anticipate risk for mpox. This includes men with a recent diagnosis of an STI, those with more than one recent sex partner, those who have had sex at a commercial sex venue or large public event, and those who anticipate any of these behaviors in the future (https://www.cdc.gov/monkeypox/vaccines/index.html).

Finally, clinicians should ensure that MSM are offered preventive care recommended for all individuals, including smoking cessation counseling and pharmacotherapy, screening for depression, and assessment for and counseling about alcohol misuse (see Health Care for Sexual Minority Women above). Some studies have found that behavioral health programs tailored specifically for MSM are more effective in promoting healthy behaviors than those that are not culturally sensitive.

Bachmann LH et al. CDC clinical guidelines on the use of doxycycline postexposure prophylaxis for bacterial sexually transmitted infection prevention, United States, 2024. MMWR Recomm Rep. 2024;73:1. [PMID: 38833414]

Kelley CF et al; PURPOSE 2 Study Team. Twice-yearly lenacapavir for HIV prevention in men and gender-diverse persons. N Engl J Med. 2024;392:1261. [PMID: 39602624]

Luetkemeyer AF et al; DoxyPEP Study Team. Postexposure doxycycline to prevent bacterial sexually transmitted infections. N Engl J Med. 2023;388:1296. [PMID: 37018493]

Stier EA et al. International Anal Neoplasia Society's consensus guidelines for anal cancer screening. Int J Cancer. 2024;154: 1694. [PMID: 38297406]

HEALTH CARE FOR TRANSGENDER & GENDER-DIVERSE PEOPLE

Terminology

This section addresses the unique health needs of transgender and gender-diverse persons. The terms **transgender** and **gender diverse** as used in this text are inclusive of those who identify with the terms **gender nonbinary**, **gender nonconforming**, **genderqueer**, and **transsexual**. The umbrella term "transgender" incorporates a range of identities and experiences of individuals whose gender identities or expression, or both, differ from those associated with the sex assigned to them at birth. In contrast, the gender of cisgender individuals is concordant with the sex assigned to them at birth. The term **transfeminine** as used in this text refers to persons who identify along a female or feminine spectrum and **transmasculine** refers to people who identify along a male or masculine spectrum. Despite this simplification, a significant proportion of transgender people do not identify with a binary conception of gender. Transgender people may use any pronoun, including the gender-neutral singular pronoun "they." It is also important to note that sexual orientation is distinct from gender and transgender people, like cisgender people, have a diversity of sexual attraction and activity.

Demographics

Few well-designed, long-term, large studies describe the population and well-being of transgender people. Additionally, methodological challenges exist in the description of the transgender population; these limitations include inconsistent or incomplete collection of sexual orientation and gender identity information in the medical record, population databases, and health studies, and variable case definition (self-identification, clinical diagnosis, or receipt of gender-affirming treatment). Survey-based studies that use self-identification report a prevalence of transgender and gender-diverse identities of 0.5–4.5% among adults and 2.5–8.4% among children and adolescents.

Herman J et al. How many adults and youth identify as transgender in the United States? The Williams Institute, UCLA School of Law. 2022. https://williamsinstitute.law.ucla.edu/publications/trans-adults-united-states/. Accessed September 30, 2025.

Disparities

Transgender people experience multiple structural barriers to health. High levels of societal stigma and discrimination, along with the lack of legal protections in education, the workplace, and housing, result in socioeconomic disadvantage and housing instability. Transgender people also face discrimination when seeking medical care. One in four transgender people reports delay in seeking medical care for fear of being mistreated based on their gender; among those who accessed a health care provider in the last year, 48% reported having a negative experience related to being transgender. These findings correlate with reports from health care professionals who state they lack the knowledge and skills necessary to provide care for transgender people.

James S et al. Early insights: a report of the 2022 US Transgender Survey. National Center for Transgender Equality. https://ustranssurvey.org/. Accessed September 30, 2025.

Gender-Affirming Medical & Surgical Interventions

Many, but not all, transgender people will seek gender-affirming medical or surgical treatments, or both, to align their physical appearance with their gender. Not all transgender people seek all interventions, and some may seek none; the standard of care is to provide transgender persons with adequate counseling and education on treatment options, expected outcomes, plan of care, and risks so that they can make an informed decision on which interventions they desire. When considering the risks of gender-affirming treatment, the clinician must also consider the significant risks of withholding such treatment on the well-being of transgender patients, including detrimental effects on mental health, increased suicidality, and increased substance use.

Even in the setting of political debate in the United States and elsewhere, particularly around transgender youth, there are guidelines and evidence supporting transgender health and gender-affirming treatments as medically necessary and essential services, shown to improve the well-being of transgender people in multiple psychosocial domains, including attendance at routine health maintenance. Gender-affirming care is delivered in diverse settings by health professionals of many disciplines and specialties. Many treatments, including hormone therapy, can be provided in an informed-consent model by appropriately trained specialty and primary care clinicians competent in making the diagnosis of gender incongruence. Mental health referral and treatment may be helpful for transgender people but is not a prerequisite for receiving gender-affirming treatments. Referral to experienced providers or a multidisciplinary team may often be appropriate.

Many gender-affirming treatments, including hormone therapy, impact the reproductive capacity of transgender people. Patients should be counseled on the reproductive implications of gender-affirming treatments along with options for family building and fertility preservation. *Gender-affirming hormone therapy is not a reliable form of contraception and all patients should be offered comprehensive family planning counseling.*

Guidance on the management of gender-affirming treatment is available from professional and specialty organizations along with publications from expert multidisciplinary clinics.

Coleman E et al. Standards of care for the health of transgender and gender diverse people, version 8. Int J Transgend Health. 2022;23:S1. [PMID: 36238954]

Deutsch MB. *Guidelines for the Primary and Gender-Affirming Care of Transgender and Gender Nonbinary People*, 2nd ed. 2016. https://transcare.ucsf.edu/guidelines. Accessed October 1, 2025.

Mann S et al. Public health and ethical risks of rollbacks on medicaid coverage for gender-affirming care. JAMA. 2025;334:853. [PMID: 40773192]

Rodriguez S et al. Making fertility preservation happen for the transgender community. Best Pract Res Clin Obstet Gynaecol. 2025;102:102652. [PMID: 40752317]

Yonko EA et al. US general election state-level ballot measures and legislative implications for LGBTQ+ health. JAMA Netw Open. 2026;9:e2552652. [PMID: 41505126]

A. Feminizing Hormone Therapy

The goals of feminizing hormone therapy include breast development, reduction of body hair, reduced muscle mass, and redistribution of body fat similar to that of cisgender women. The general approach of therapy is to obtain physiologic premenopausal cisgender female range estrogen and testosterone levels through the combined use of an estrogen with an androgen blocker and, in some cases, a progestin.

1. Estrogen—17-β-Estradiol is available in pill, patch, and injected formulation. The choice of route is based to some degree on patient preference (Table 46–3). Transdermal estradiol has a well-established safety profile based on studies in menopausal cisgender women. Injected estradiol is the least studied route and can be associated with both supratherapeutic levels as well as cyclical levels over the dosing interval. Estrogens should be continued after gonadectomy without reduction in dose. There is no direct evidence to guide decision making regarding the discontinuation of estrogen once a patient arrives at a menopausal age, though most experts believe initiating or continuing hormone therapy in transfeminine persons after age 50 is appropriate. Ethinyl-estradiol (found in hormonal contraceptives) and conjugated equine estrogens should *not* be used due to excess thrombogenicity.

The primary risk associated with estrogen therapy is VTE. The risk is minimal, however, when using 17-β-estradiol at physiologic estrogen dosing. Early studies showing 20- to 40-fold increased risk of VTE involved the use of ethinyl-estradiol at doses of up to 200 mcg daily and did not control for tobacco use. More recent studies found *no increased risk of VTE in transfeminine persons using transdermal 17-β-estradiol.* Thus, transdermal estradiol is the preferred route for those who use tobacco or with risk factors for or a personal history of VTE.

2. Anti-androgen—In the United States, the most commonly used anti-androgen is spironolactone, a potassium-sparing diuretic that is frequently used for female hirsutism or adult acne. Spironolactone inhibits both the synthesis of and action of testosterone. In higher doses (100–200 mg orally daily), spironolactone can lead to suppression of androgen levels into the female physiologic range. Common side effects include orthostasis and polyuria. Monitoring should include periodic assessment of kidney function and serum potassium. Other options for those who cannot tolerate spironolactone include a gonadotropin-releasing hormone (GnRH) analog, orchiectomy, or the use of a progestin. Finasteride and dutasteride (5-α-reductase inhibitors) are sometimes used as an alternative; however, they have limited effects. After gonadectomy, anti-androgens can be discontinued.

3. Progestins—Progestins may be an effective anti-androgen, particularly cyproterone acetate, which is used widely outside the United States as the primary androgen blocker in feminizing regimens. Although data are scant, some believe there is benefit to breast development, mood, sleep, and libido. In cisgender women, synthetic progestins have been associated with an excess thromboembolism and breast cancer risk. If used, micronized progesterone is recommended and should be initiated after at least several months of estrogen plus anti-androgen as to mirror breast development in cisgender women.

Iwamoto SJ et al. Approach to the patient: hormonal therapy in transgender adults with complex medical histories. J Clin Endocrinol Metab. 2024;109:592. [PMID: 37683089]

Szymczyk S et al. The potential health risks and benefits of progesterone in the transgender woman population-A narrative review. J Clin Med. 2024;13:6795. [PMID: 39597939]

B. Masculinizing Hormone Therapy

The goals of masculinizing hormone therapy include facial and body hair growth, deepening of the voice, increased muscle mass, clitoral growth, induction of amenorrhea, and redistribution of body fat similar to that of cisgender men. The mainstay of therapy is administration of testosterone to achieve physiologic cisgender male serum testosterone level (Table 46–4). Blockade of estrogen is *not* needed; however, ovulation and menstrual suppression may be warranted to eliminate moliminal symptoms or in those with ongoing menses.

Testosterone is available as a topical gel, patch, injected formulation, and subcutaneous pellet. The use of daily topical testosterone or using a weekly (versus biweekly)

Table 46–3. Feminizing hormone therapy (listed in alphabetical order, within categories).

Hormone Therapy	Dosage			Comments
	Initial, low[1]	Initial, Typical	Maximum, Typical[2]	
Anti-androgen				
Dutasteride			0.5 mg orally daily	
Finasteride	1 mg orally daily		5 mg orally daily	
Spironolactone	25 mg orally daily	50 mg orally twice daily	200 mg orally twice daily	
Estrogen				
Estradiol cypionate, intramuscularly	< 2 mg IM every 2 weeks	2 mg IM every 2 weeks	5 mg IM every 2 weeks	May divide dose into weekly injections for cyclical symptoms.
Estradiol oral/sublingual	1 mg orally/sublingually daily	2–4 mg orally/ sublingually daily	8 mg orally/sublingually daily	If > 2 mg, dose should be divided and taken twice daily.
Estradiol transdermal patch	Apply 0.05 mg/day patch topically weekly or twice weekly, depending on brand	Apply 0.1 mg/day patch topically weekly or twice weekly, depending on brand	Apply 0.1-0.4 mg/day patch topically weekly or twice weekly, depending on brand	Patches are applied weekly or twice weekly, depending on the brand. Maximum available single patch dose is 0.1 mg/day. Patients may find that > 2 patches at a time are cumbersome.
Estradiol valerate, intramuscularly[3]	< 20 mg IM every 2 weeks	20 mg IM every 2 weeks	40 mg IM every 2 weeks	May divide dose into weekly injections for cyclical symptoms.
Progestin				
Cyproterone acetate			10 mg orally daily	Used outside of the United States
Medroxyprogesterone acetate (Provera)	2.5 mg orally each night at bedtime		5–10 mg orally each night at bedtime	
Micronized progesterone	100 mg orally each night at bedtime		200 mg orally each night at bedtime	

[1]Initial low dosing for those who desire (or require due to medical history) a low dose or slow upward titration.
[2]Maximal effect does not necessarily require maximal dosing, as maximal doses do not necessarily represent a target or ideal dose. Dose increases should be based on patient response and monitored hormone levels.
[3]Available as standard US Pharmacopia (USP) as well as compounded products.

injection interval can help maintain even hormone levels in those with cyclical mood symptoms or pelvic cramping.

Prior concerns of testosterone-induced hepatotoxicity were based on the use of oral methyltestosterone. *There is no evidence to support a concern of hepatotoxicity in transmasculine persons using parenteral or topical testosterone.*

Common side effects of gender-affirming testosterone therapy include acne and male pattern baldness, both of which can be approached as in cisgender men. Hemoglobin and hematocrit should be monitored, and if the levels are elevated, consider reducing testosterone dose or changing to a transdermal form or weekly injections to maintain more even levels. It is important to use cisgender male reference ranges for hemoglobin and hematocrit due to the erythropoietic effects of testosterone and frequent oligo- or amenorrheic status of transmasculine people. Polycystic ovarian syndrome and obesity have been found to be at an increased prevalence in transmasculine persons prior to beginning testosterone therapy. Testosterone is not contraindicated in the presence of these conditions; instead, related metabolic disorders can be managed concurrently.

C. Monitoring Hormone Therapy

Hormone effects should be monitored both by clinical results as well as hormone levels, if available. *Patients should be reminded that results may vary and can take up to 5 years to reach maximal effect*; supraphysiologic hormone levels are not likely to enhance results but may incur excess risk. Note that reported laboratory reference range values may differ depending on the recorded sex of the patient; in general, clinicians should use the reference ranges driven by the current hormonal status of the patient. For example, female reference ranges will be included on automated laboratory reports of a transmasculine person taking

Table 46–4. Masculinizing hormone therapy (listed in alphabetical order).

Androgen	Dosage			Comments
	Initial, Low[1]	Initial, Typical	Maximum, Typical[2]	
Testosterone cream[3]	10 mg applied topically every morning	50 mg applied topically every morning	100 mg applied topically every morning	
Testosterone cypionate[4]	20 mg/week intramuscularly or subcutaneously	50 mg/week intramuscularly or subcutaneously	100 mg/week intramuscu larly or subcutaneously	If dosing every 2 weeks, double weekly dose.
Testosterone enthanate[4]	20 mg/week intramuscularly or subcutaneously	50 mg/week intramuscularly or subcutaneously	100 mg/week intramuscularly or subcutaneously	
Testosterone patch	Apply 1–2 mg/day patch topically every night	Apply 4 mg/day patch topically every night	Apply 8 mg/day patch topically every night	Patches come in 2-mg and 4-mg size. For lower doses, cut patch
Testosterone topical gel 1%	12.5–25 mg applied topically every morning	50 mg applied topically every morning	100 mg applied topically every morning	May come in pump or packet form. Each pump actuation delivers 12.5 mg of testosterone in 1.25 g of gel. Apply to upper arms/shoulders and/or right and left abdomen.
Testosterone topical gel 1.62%[5]	20.25 mg applied topically every morning	40.5–60.75 mg applied topically every morning	103.25 mg applied topically every morning	May come in pump or packet form. Each pump actuation delivers 20.25 mg of testosterone in 1.25 g of gel. Apply to upper arms/shoulders and/or right and left abdomen.
Testosterone topical solution 2%[5]	30 mg applied topically to the axilla every morning	60 mg applied topically to the axilla every morning	90–120 mg applied topically to the axilla every morning	Available as a metered-dose pump. One pump delivers 30 mg of testosterone. Apply to the axilla, preferably at the same time each morning.
Testosterone undecanoate[6]	N/A	750 mg intramuscularly, repeat in 4 weeks, then every 10 weeks	N/A	Requires participation in manufacturer-monitored program[6]

[1]Initial, low-dose regimen is recommended for genderqueer and nonbinary persons.
[2]Maximum dosing does not mean maximal effect. Furthermore, these dosage ranges do not necessarily represent a target or ideal dose. Dose increases or decreases should be based on patient response and monitored hormone levels.
[3]Testosterone creams are prepared by individual compounding pharmacies. Specific absorption and activity varies and consultation with the individual compounding pharmacist is recommended.
[4]Available as standard US Pharmacopia (USP) as well as compounded products.
[5]Doses < 20.25 mg with 1.62% gel or < 30 mg with 2% topical solution may be difficult, as these products are dispensed in fixed-dose pumps making partial dosing unreliable. Patients requiring lower doses and whose insurance does not cover 1% gel may require prior authorization or an appeal.
[6]Testosterone undecanoate has been associated with rare cases of pulmonary oil microembolism and anaphylaxis; in the United States, the drug is available only through the AVEED Risk Evaluation and Mitigation Strategy (REMS) Program (https://www.aveedrems.com/AveedUI/rems/preHome.action). All injections must be administered in an office or hospital setting by a trained and registered health care provider and monitored for 30 minutes afterward for adverse reactions.

testosterone if still registered as female. The interpreting clinician should use the male reference ranges for any tests run on this patient that have sexually dimorphic reference ranges. Tables 46–5 and 46–6 describe general monitoring recommendations, rationales, and "sex-specific" laboratory values that may require individualized interpretation.

D. Surgical Interventions

Gender-affirming surgeries, including facial, chest, genital, and other procedures (Table 46–7) are available to transgender people. Outcomes evaluation of gender-affirming surgeries demonstrate high level of patient satisfaction, an

Table 46–5. Laboratory monitoring for feminizing hormone therapy (listed in alphabetical order).

	Comments	Baseline	3 Months[1]	6 Months[1]	12 Months[1]	Yearly	As needed
Albumin[2]			X	X	X		X
BUN/creatinine/ potassium	Only if spironolactone is used	X	X	X	X	X	
Estradiol			X	X			X
Hemoglobin A_{1C}[3]		X					X
Lipids[3]		X					X
Prolactin	Only if symptomatic						X
Sex hormone binding globulin (SHBG)[2]							X
Total testosterone							X

[1]In first year of therapy only.
[2]Used to calculate bioavailable testosterone (http://www.issam.ch/freetesto.htm).
[3]Based on USPSTF guidelines.

increase in quality of life measures, and decrease in gender dysphoria. An increasing number of surgeries are being performed for gender affirmation; rates of complications and regrets are comparable to similar procedures performed for other indications.

Kloer C et al. Overview of gender affirming surgery for the gynecologic surgeon. J Gynecol Surg. 2021;37:269. http://doi.org/10.1089/gyn.2021.0042. Accessed October 1, 2025.

E. Long-Term Health Outcomes

The largest study of mortality among transgender people receiving gender-affirming hormone therapy is a 2011 Dutch cohort of 966 transfeminine persons and 365 transmasculine persons. Importantly, this study did not control for a number of risk factors, including tobacco use. All-cause as well as cardiovascular, cerebrovascular, and other disease-specific mortality among transmasculine persons did not differ from the general Dutch population of cisgender women. Among transfeminine persons, all-cause mortality was 51% higher than cisgender men in the general Dutch population, with the overwhelming majority of the difference due to HIV, drug overdose, and suicide; a 64% increased risk in cardiovascular mortality was seen; however, no significant difference was seen for cerebrovascular mortality.

Subsequent investigations, including those in European and United States cohorts, confirmed an increased risk of poor CVD outcomes among transgender and gender-diverse people. Data are conflicting on whether disparities in behavioral and social determinants of health contribute to poor cardiovascular outcomes. Transgender and gender-diverse people are more likely to experience health care and social discrimination, adverse childhood events, and psychological distress; the contribution of this excess minority stress to long-term health is unknown.

van Zijverden LM et al. Transgender persons receiving gender-affirming hormone therapy: risk of acute cardiovascular events in a Dutch cohort study. Eur Heart J. 2025:ehaf837. [Epub ahead of print] [PMID: 41187090]

Table 46–6. Laboratory monitoring for masculinizing hormone therapy (listed in alphabetical order).

	Baseline	3 Months[2]	6 Months[2]	12 Months[2]	Yearly	As Needed
Albumin[1]						X
Estradiol						X
Hemoglobin A_{1c}[3]						X
Hemoglobin and hematocrit	X	X	X	X	X	X
Lipids[3]						X
Sex hormone binding globulin (SHBG)[1]						X
Total testosterone		X	X	X		X

[1]Used to calculate bioavailable testosterone (http://www.issam.ch/freetesto.htm).
[2]In first year of therapy only.
[3]Based on USPSTF guidelines.

Table 46–7. Gender-affirming procedures (listed in alphabetical order, within categories).

Surgical interventions
Augmentation mammoplasty
Body contouring
Chest surgery (augmentation/mastectomy, also referred to as "top surgery")
Facial surgery (feminization/masculinization procedures)
Gonadectomy (orchiectomy, oophorectomy)
Hysterectomy, salpingectomy
Phalloplasty, scrotoplasty, metoidioplasty, vaginectomy (including placement of penile/testicular prostheses)
Thyrochondroplasty (tracheal cartilage shave/augmentation)
Voice surgery
Vulvoplasty, vaginoplasty
Other interventions
Chest binding
Facial and body hair removal (laser hair removal and electrolysis)
Genital tucking and packing
Hair implants
Voice therapy and modification

Cancer Risk & Screening

Several retrospective studies have not identified an increased risk of cancer in transgender people compared with assigned sex–matched controls. However, because of the numerous barriers to care as well as to identifying transgender people in clinical databases, underscreening and underreporting are likely. In general, an organ-based approach to screening should be taken, with attention to anatomic changes related to gender-affirming medical and surgical treatments. *There are no modifications to screening recommendations (or recommendations not to screen) for ovarian, uterine, or cervical cancer in transmasculine persons.* Breast cancer screening for transmasculine people who have not undergone mastectomy should be performed based on guidelines for cisgender women. The role of screening for breast cancer in transmasculine people who have undergone mastectomy is unknown and depends on the surgical technique used as well as technical limitations on screening small amounts of residual breast tissue. In transfeminine people, breast cancer screening using guidelines for cisgender women is recommended, with the modifications starting at age 50 years and only after a minimum of 5 years of lifetime estrogen exposure. Screening for prostate cancer in transfeminine people is complicated beyond the current debate over the utility of prostate cancer screening in cisgender men by the effects of feminizing hormones on prostatic hypertrophy and interpretation of tests of PSA.

Leone AG et al. Cancer in transgender and gender-diverse persons: a review. JAMA Oncol. 2023;9:556. [PMID: 36757703]

HIV

Disproportionately high rates of HIV infection among transgender people exist worldwide, and the largest burden of these infections is among transfeminine people and transgender people of color; the lack of targeted HIV prevention strategies for transgender communities may be one factor contributing to these disparities. Studies of pharmacologic PrEP, including daily oral medications and long-acting injectables, demonstrate acceptability and efficacy among transgender people; compared with cisgender MSM, however, adherence to PrEP was lower in transgender women and uptake and knowledge were lower among all transgender people. Disparities also exist in treatment of HIV, with transfeminine persons less likely to report receiving antiretroviral treatment and to remain in care. Modest interactions of unknown clinical significance may exist between antiretroviral medications and gender-affirming hormone therapy; clinical and laboratory response to therapy should be monitored. *Patients should be counseled that concurrent gender-affirming hormone therapy and antiretroviral therapy, including PrEP agents, are safe and effective.* Transgender people likely benefit from HIV prevention and treatment services integrated into other gender-affirming care.

47 Substance Use Disorders

J. Janet Ho, MD, MPH, FASAM
Jessica Ristau, MD
Soraya Azari, MD

SUBSTANCE USE DISORDERS (SUD)

ESSENTIALS OF DIAGNOSIS

- SUD are treatable, chronic health conditions that include periods of remission and activity.
- Not all non-prescribed substance use meets criteria for a SUD.
- SUD are characterized by ongoing use of substances despite harmful consequences and range from mild to severe *DSM-5* criteria.

General Considerations

SUD are a significant public health issue in the United States, with widespread implications for individual and societal well-being. Excessive alcohol use remains a leading preventable cause of death in the United States, with 178,000 people dying from acute and chronic complications related to excessive drinking each year. According to the 2024 National Survey on Drug Use and Health (NSDUH), approximately 46.6% of Americans ≥ age 12 reported using alcohol in the past month, while 25.5% had used any illicit drug in the same period. The same survey reports 9.7% of Americans over 12 years old met the criteria for an alcohol use disorder (AUD), and 9.8% had a diagnosable drug use disorder (including marijuana, prescription psychotherapeutic drugs, and illicit drugs).

With the increase in synthetic opioid use, the United States mortality rate related to opioid use has been climbing since 2010, rising sharply during the COVID-19 pandemic and resulting in 108,000 deaths in 2021. The first year that annual deaths have declined since 2018 was in 2023, with 105,000 drug-related overdose deaths, of which 76% involved opioids.

Addiction is a chronic, primary condition of the brain that manifests as a compulsive drive to use a substance despite harmful consequences. Similar to other chronic diseases, such as hypertension or diabetes, addiction is influenced by genetics and the environment, with cycles of relapse and remission. The model of neural changes underlying addiction is a three-stage recurring cycle. It begins with binges and intoxication (mediated by the basal ganglia), progresses to a withdrawal state and dysphoria (mediated by the extended amygdala), and then reaches a state of preoccupation and anxiety if the substance is not used (mediated by the pre-frontal cortex). Substances that cause use disorders share the ability to release dopamine in the basal ganglia (ventral striatum), but over time, dopamine release diminishes, requiring greater use for the same effect (tolerance).

SUD are treatable conditions but not easily curable. Sustained treatment can result in recovery of brain function, normalization of brain biochemistry, and the resolution of problematic behaviors. *Early* remission is defined as abstaining from drug use for at least 3 months, while *sustained* remission is defined as abstaining for 12 months or more. For some people who use drugs of addiction, remission is the goal. For others, a harm reduction approach with reduced or safer use is the goal. Some individuals may not be ready to make changes to their use of drugs of addiction. The approach to addiction treatment should be patient-centered, multipronged, nonjudgmental, and unbiased, using nonstigmatizing language, and keeping the patient's goals at the forefront in order to continue patient engagement in healthcare.

Clinical Findings

A. Screening for SUD

The 2020 USPSTF statement recommends screening for unhealthy drug use among adults ≥ 18 years in primary care settings, including those who are pregnant or postpartum (Grade B). An expert panel of the Substance Abuse and Mental Health Services Administration (SAMHSA) similarly recommends primary care clinicians periodically and routinely screen all patients for SUD to reduce bias and preclude missed opportunities for intervention.

Screening, Brief Intervention, and Referral to Treatment (SBIRT) is a comprehensive, universal, public health approach to the delivery of early intervention for persons with risky drug and alcohol use, and timely referral to more intensive treatment for persons with SUD. The SBIRT model includes **S**creening to assess the severity of substance use, **B**rief **I**ntervention (5–10 minutes) focused on increasing insight and awareness regarding substance use and motivation toward behavior change, and **R**eferral to **T**reatment, where appropriate. For hazardous drug use or mild SUD, brief interventions are often appropriate. For moderate to severe SUD, referral for treatment is indicated.

There are multiple validated screening tools to assess for substance use:

1. **National Institute on Drug Abuse (NIDA) Quick screen** (eg, Single-Question Screener) is adapted from a single-question screen validated in primary care settings to efficiently screen for drug use. It asks: *"In the past year, how often have you used illegal drugs or prescription opioids for non-medical reasons?"* If a patient asks what "non-medical reasons" means, one can clarify this to be use "differently from how it's prescribed" or use "for the feeling or experience it causes." A response other than zero is considered a positive screen that should be followed by identification of the substance(s) used and a more complete assessment through an in-depth history.
2. **NIDA TAPS** is a more comprehensive screening tool for SUD or risky substance use. This 4-item screening questionnaire asks about the use of tobacco, alcohol, prescription medications, and other substances in the past 12 months. This tool is validated in primary care settings for patients to self-administer or complete with interviewers (https://cde.nida.nih.gov/instrument/29b23e2e-e266-f095-e050-bb89ad43472f).
3. **CRAFFT** is a validated screening tool to identify substance use, risky use, and SUD among pregnant individuals and youths 12–21 years old. Its use is recommended by the American Academy of Pediatrics Bright Futures Guidelines for preventive care screenings and well-visits. A CRAFFT score ≥ 2 was found to be optimal in identifying substance-related problems. The screen starts by asking about the frequency of substance use in the past 12 months. This is followed by "Have you ever ridden in a car with someone (including yourself) who was 'high' or had been using alcohol or drugs?" "Do you ever use alcohol or drugs to relax, feel better about yourself, or fit in?" "Do you ever use alcohol or drugs while you are by yourself?" "Do you ever forget things you did while using alcohol or drugs?" "Do your family or friends ever tell you that you should cut down on your drinking or drug use?" "Have you ever gotten into trouble while you were using alcohol or drugs?" The CRAFFT screening questionnaire can be found at https://crafft.org/.

Screening should be nonjudgmental and prioritize patient privacy and trust to encourage honest responses and sustained engagement. Importantly, a positive result on a screening tool is not a diagnosis, but rather a gateway to further assessment, treatment, provision of harm reduction resources, and referral to evidence-based treatment options. Screening tools should be combined with other information, eg, toxicology testing, to provide a comprehensive assessment of a person's substance use risk. (See Urine Toxicology Testing, below.)

B. Diagnosis of SUD

The *DSM-5* criteria determine an SUD diagnosis and its severity. The diagnosis of SUD is made when at least 2 of 11 criteria are met over 12 months (Table 47–1). The Four Cs of addiction is a mnemonic to simplify recall of *DSM-5* criteria.

C. Urine Toxicology Testing

Toxicology testing is frequently used to augment the patient's self-report of disease activity by detecting and measuring substances used. The purpose of testing is to guide diagnosis and treatment and verify use of prescribed medications for SUD such as buprenorphine, a medication for opioid use disorder (MOUD). There is no clear evidence of benefit to routine toxicology testing when results will not change the treatment plan; rather, there may be potential harm in using testing for punitive reasons (such as dismissal from care).

Urine testing should involve patient informed consent unless the scenario is emergent and urine toxicology results will influence treatment, such as in evaluation of altered mental status or when the patient does not have capacity. Urine test results can have particularly significant implications in pregnant patients due to Child Protective Services involvement or management, and, as such, decisions to conduct testing should be taken only if results will meaningfully change care, and should be undertaken only after discussions with patients. Toxicology testing is available for various biologic samples including urine, oral fluid, hair, sweat, and meconium in newborns. The urine test is the preferred and most common source since it is easily collected, noninvasive, and has a wide variety of testing platforms available. Direct observation of urine sample collection is invasive and is not the standard of care. As of 2020, urine and oral fluid are the only sample source approved for federally mandated testing for substances.

There are two types of urine toxicology tests: immunoassays and liquid or gas chromatography with mass spectrometry. The specific substances identified and threshold cutoffs for each test vary by laboratory or institution. Urine toxicology results are frequently mis-interpreted by clinicians; reviewing results with a toxicology or laboratory science specialist is recommended when results differ from those expected. Many commercially available assays do not test for novel substances such as xylazine or isotonitazene.

1. Immunoassay screens—Antibody-based assays (eg, ELISA) are typically performed quickly, cost less than spectrometry-based methods, allow for same-day results, and therefore are often used for initial point-of-care testing. The tests produce qualitative results, showing only whether a substance was identified as present or not. Tested substances vary based on the laboratory, but most include amphetamines, cocaine, opiates, and benzodiazepines.

False positive results can occur with amphetamines, for example. In these cases, a follow-up (or "reflex") amphetamine confirmation testing will differentiate if the substance was an amphetamine, and if so, can further

Table 47–1. *DSM-5* criteria for diagnosing substance use disorders.

DSM-5 Criteria	Definition Including Four Cs	Example Phrases to Ask Diagnostic Criteria
Strong desire or urge to use	Craving	Are there people, places, things, emotions, or other triggers that make you feel a strong urge to use X? Do you find yourself using your opioid medication to treat symptoms other than pain (eg, anxiety)?
Use in increased amounts or longer than intended	Control (loss of)	Have you found yourself using larger amounts of X, or for longer periods, than you thought you would? Have you ever run out of prescribed medication before a refill was due?
Persistent wish or unsuccessful effort to cut down or control use		Have you tried to reduce or manage your use of X before?
Much time spent to obtain, use, or recover from use		Have you found yourself spending more time on using or getting X to use than you used to? How do you spend a typical day?
Failing to meet important obligations or fill roles	Consequences	Has use of X made it more challenging for you to do the things you need to do to maintain a job, housing, or take care of people you care about?
Continued use despite known or unknown problems socially and interpersonally (eg, interference with work, school, home)		Have you had conflict, stress, or lost connections with friends or family related to X use? Has use of X ever caused tension with work colleagues or health care providers?
Elimination or reduction of important activities because of opioid use		Are there activities or hobbies that you used to spend time on that you've given up or spent less time on due to X use?
Use in physically hazardous situations	Compulsive use	Have you ever driven a vehicle or operated any machinery while using X? Has use of X ever left you vulnerable, for instance using while in a public area?
Continued use despite known negative physical or psychological consequences		Have you ever been told by a medical provider that use of X was contributing to other physical or mental health issues that you've experienced?
Need for increased doses for effect, reduced effect per dose, or both[1]	Tolerance[1]	Have you found that you need to use larger amounts of X to get the same effect, as compared to when you first started using?
Withdrawal symptoms when use is decreased, or using to relieve withdrawal[1]	Dependence[1]	Do you notice uncomfortable symptoms when you stop using, such as…?

Severity of substance use disorder: **Mild**: 2–3 symptoms. **Moderate**: 4–5 symptoms. **Severe**: 6 or more symptoms.
X, substance being discussed.
[1]If a prescribed opioid is taken only as instructed, this item does not count toward a diagnosis of an opioid use disorder.

differentiate if it is a prescribed stimulant (such as prescription methylphenidate) or non-prescribed stimulant (such as methamphetamine). The detection of cocaine metabolites on immunoassay screens is specific, so the finding of cocaine is rarely a false positive. Only certain benzodiazepines are tested for by these assays, typically those with oxazepam as a metabolite such as alprazolam, diazepam and lorazepam, thus a confirmatory test using liquid/gas chromatography or mass spectrometry can help detect these benzodiazepines. The category called "opiates" refers to natural opiates derived from the opium poppy and detects morphine derivatives, including codeine, morphine, heroin, hydromorphone (depending on concentration), thebaine, and their metabolites. In contrast, the urine opiate screen does not test for semisynthetic and synthetic opioids with morphine-like activity, such as fentanyl, methadone, buprenorphine, or oxycodone. Specific testing for these opioids via immunoassay tests needs to be ordered separately.

2. Liquid/gas chromatography and mass spectrometry (LC/GC MS) tests—This specialized testing is most often used to confirm the presence of substances and it may take days to weeks to obtain results. LC/GC MS is a highly specific, quantitative test used to confirm unexpected test results from screens, confirm if there was a false-positive or false-negative immunoassay test, monitor therapeutic levels of drugs, or detect subversion of urine samples. Interpreting the results of mass spectrometry requires some knowledge of substance metabolism. For example, a patient may be prescribed morphine but has a mass spectrometry test that returns positive for hydromorphone. This finding is expected since hydromorphone is a metabolite of morphine. Opioid and benzodiazepine metabolism charts are accessible online (https://thepainsource.com/metabolism-of-opioids/ and https://thepainsource.com/metabolism-of-benzodiazepines/, respectively). *If a substance is present on the LC/GC MS testing, it is unlikely to be a false positive.*

Treatment

A. Nonpharmacologic and Behavioral Health Treatments

Nonpharmacologic treatments are a crucial component of comprehensive care for patients with SUD alongside medication. These treatments can help manage cravings and triggers and address underlying psychological and social drivers. Healthcare for SUD is considered an essential health benefit, meaning that insurance must provide coverage for treatment. The SAMHSA website has a treatment program locator (findtreatment.gov). Clinicians may see their patients assessed with the American Society of Addiction Medicine (ASAM) Level of Care Designation, which incorporates substance use, mental health, and medical comorbidities to determine the appropriate setting for care given that substance use treatment facilities offer different certified levels of care (such as inpatient or intensive outpatient treatment).

Key nonpharmacologic treatments include:

- **Behavioral therapies:** Techniques like cognitive-behavioral therapy equip individuals with skills to identify and manage triggers, cope with cravings, and develop healthy coping mechanisms.
- **Mutual help:** Belonging to peer support groups like Alcoholics Anonymous or Narcotics Anonymous provides a safe space for sharing experiences, gaining encouragement, and learning from others in recovery. This also includes peer support from recovery specialists and community health workers with lived experience.
- **Mindfulness and stress management:** Practices like meditation and yoga can help manage cravings, reduce anxiety, and promote self-awareness, fostering overall well-being.
- **Complementary and integrative therapies:** Acupuncture, massage therapy, and other approaches may offer holistic support by managing physical discomfort and promoting relaxation.
- **Vocational and social support:** Addressing employment, housing, and other social drivers of health can create a more stable environment conducive to recovery.

These forms of evidence-based treatment should be discussed and offered when they align with the patient's care goals. Integrating these approaches with medication treatment and addressing underlying social drivers of health help foster a holistic approach to address the complex issues surrounding SUDs and support long-term recovery.

Motivational interviewing is an evidence-based and patient-centered technique in clinical settings that uses supportive conversation to help individuals explore their ambivalence about change and build motivation to adopt healthier behaviors. Through reflective listening and open-ended questions, clinicians empower patients to identify their goals and develop a plan for positive change. Motivational interviewing can be used with SBIRT to collaborate with the patient to identify next steps in treatment. Skills training for motivational interviewing can be found online (https://motivationalinterviewing.org/).

B. Mental Health Treatment

Concurrent treatment of co-occurring mental health disorders through integrative or collaborative care is critical for treatment success. Multiple studies have shown that individuals with SUDs are at increased risk for suicide. Untreated mental health disorders can worsen medication adherence and program retention. Addressing both conditions simultaneously increases the chances of successful recovery and improved overall health.

Mental health disorders can contribute to the development or continuation of SUD, since drugs, including opioids, can be used to cope with conditions such as anxiety and depression. Addressing co-occurring conditions helps manage triggers, develop coping mechanisms, and build resilience, reducing the risk of returning to use. Individuals with co-occurring disorders often face greater stigma, health care disparities, and challenges accessing compassionate, evidence-based treatment, resulting in worse health outcomes.

C. Harm Reduction

Harm reduction is a powerful, evidence-based approach in SUD care, shifting the focus from solely achieving abstinence to minimizing the negative consequences associated with drug use. Harm reduction prioritizes patient health and well-being regardless of current usage and is an important approach to care for persons who may not be ready to change their substance use patterns. It recognizes that not everyone is ready or able to commit to complete abstinence and that a return to drug use may be part of the SUD disease course.

By meeting people "where they're at" and offering nonjudgmental support, harm reduction empowers individuals to take steps toward better health and improved quality of life despite ongoing use. It helps reduce the morbidity and mortality associated with drug use (eg, HIV, hepatitis C, and accidental overdose) and strives to address social and structural barriers that perpetuate SUD and limit access to care. Harm reduction includes advocating for policies that reduce stigma and criminalization of SUDs, while addressing social drivers of health by promoting housing and employment opportunities for individuals with SUD.

Key harm reduction interventions include:

- **Naloxone distribution:** Naloxone reverses opioid overdoses; equipping communities with access to naloxone can save lives.
- **Syringe service programs and safe supplies:** Syringe service programs and safe supply kits provide clean needles and syringes, along with other drug use equipment, to reduce the risk of bloodborne infections like HIV, hepatitis B, and hepatitis C associated with shared injecting equipment. These supplies can also include drug testing strips for fentanyl or xylazine.

- **Wound care and abscess management:** Addressing skin infections and other health complications arising from drug use promotes overall well-being.
- **Overdose safety planning:** Engaging the patient to identify higher-risk behaviors (eg, using alone or while intoxicated) and ways to mitigate their risks, such as identifying peer supports and treatment resources, helps reduce chances of opioid overdose. The Never Use Alone line is a resource for isolated patients intending to use opioids (877-696-1996).
- **Non-stigmatizing language:** Stigma towards addiction within healthcare settings is a significant barrier to effective treatment and recovery for individuals with SUD. Evidence shows that healthcare professionals may hold negative and often unconscious beliefs about people with opioid use disorder (OUD), viewing them as weak-willed, morally deficient, less likely to respond to treatment, or undeserving of care when patients are described as a "substance abuser" versus a "person with a substance use disorder." It is critical to role model and document with medically accurate, non-stigmatizing language with patients, families, and colleagues in conversation and documentation. Institutional stigma manifests itself in punitive policies or regulations that can further discourage patients from seeking timely care, disclosing drug use, remaining hospitalized until treatment is complete, or engaging in necessary upstream healthcare.

D. Racial Disparities and Culturally Informed Treatment

Documented racial disparities in medicine impact treatment recommendations and patient-provider communication. For OUD treatment, Black persons are 42% and 47%; American Indian or Alaskan Native, Asian, Hawaiian/Pacific Islander persons are 12% and 12%; and Latino/Latina persons are 22% and 20% less likely to receive buprenorphine or extended-release naltrexone, respectively, compared to White persons. Treatment receipt of buprenorphine has also been shown to increase in higher-income and White communities compared to lower-income communities of color. Furthermore, contingency management (see Stimulants: Amphetamines & Cocaine, below) the most effective evidence-based approach to stimulant use disorder, is less accessible in rural areas as compared to urban settings. Racism and inequity must be addressed on the individual, interpersonal and systemic levels, and clinical settings can work to provide equitable and culturally informed treatment. Culturally informed treatment is adapting treatment to meet the needs of the individuals served, and should not replace effective medication treatment, as evidenced by a study that demonstrated that MOUD was a key driver in treatment completion where culturally informed treatment was studied.

National Institute on Drug Abuse (NIDA). Drug Overdose Death Rates. https://nida.nih.gov/research-topics/trends-statistics/overdose-death-rates. Accessed February 01, 2024.

Schwenker R et al. Motivational interviewing for substance use reduction. Cochrane Database Syst Rev. 2023;12:CD008063. [PMID: 38084817]

Substance Abuse and Mental Health Services Administration. (2025). Key substance use and mental health indicators in the United States: Results from the 2024 National Survey on Drug Use and Health (HHS Publication No. PEP25-07-007, NSDUH Series H-60). Center for Behavioral Health Statistics and Quality, Substance Abuse and Mental Health Services Administration. https://www.samhsa.gov/data/data-we-collect/nsduh-national-surveydrug-use-and-health/national-releasesz

US Preventive Services Task Force; Krist AH et al. Screening for unhealthy drug use: US Preventive Services Task Force Recommendation Statement. JAMA. 2020;323:2301. [PMID: 32515821]

OPIOID USE DISORDER (OUD)

ESSENTIALS OF DIAGNOSIS

- OUD is diagnosed using *DSM-5* criteria, which also assess severity.
- In 2023, about 76% of all accidental drug overdose deaths involved an opioid, yet in 2024, only 17% of Americans ≥ age 12 with OUD received medication treatment.

General Consideration

OUD continues to be a major public health crisis in the United States, with a substantially increasing number of annual opioid-related deaths from 1999 to 2023, peaking in 2021 (111,079 people). The CDC's National Center for Health Statistics indicates that 2023 was the first year since 2018 with an annual decrease in drug overdose deaths (105,000 people). According to the 2024 NSDUH, an estimated 4.8 million Americans ≥ age 12 met criteria for an OUD; however, only < 20% received any medications treatment for OUD. In 2024, 8 million people < age 12 reported they misused prescription pain relievers in the past year. Rates of accidental overdose deaths have been driven in recent years by the introduction of potent synthetic opioids like nonpharmaceutical fentanyl into the drug supply.

While OUD prevalence rates vary across regions and demographics, certain groups are disproportionately affected. Risks of developing OUD are increased among (1) men, (2) persons of younger age (35–44 years old), and (3) persons who have adverse childhood experiences, another SUD, or psychiatric disease. From 1999 to 2022, opioid-related mortality rose for all racial and ethnic groups, with the most rapid increase being among Black, American Indian, and Latino/Latina Americans. In 2022, the highest death rates were amongst American Indian/Alaska Native and Black/African American people, at 46.9 and 36.6 deaths per 100,000, respectively, compared to 27.6 for White Americans. The myriad factors underlying these disparities include systematized stigma toward drugs and individuals who use drugs, racialized incarceration rates, a history of biased drug policies in the United States, structural racism, and racial segregation of health care. Access to MOUD is disproportionately low among Black and other historically marginalized persons compared to White persons, who are more likely to live in communities with access to buprenorphine prescribers and who are more likely to receive MOUD.

OUD can present in the context of opioid intoxication or withdrawal, neither of which is sufficient alone to make the diagnosis of OUD. Instead, OUD can be identified through *patterns* of ongoing opioid use despite harmful consequences, such as medical comorbidities related to drug use (eg, skin and soft tissue infections, endocarditis), and is diagnosed using the *DSM-5* criteria (see Table 47–1). Screening and history-taking may help diagnose OUD in patients with OUD without overt signs or symptoms of intoxication or withdrawal.

Clinical Findings

A. Diagnostic Criteria

The *DSM*-5 criteria can identify OUD and assess its severity. The diagnosis of OUD is made when at least 2 of the 11 *DSM-5* criteria are met over 12 months (see Table 47–1). Notably, the *DSM*-5 recognizes "tolerance" and "dependence" as natural physiologic adaptations for any person with consistent opioid exposure. Therefore, tolerance and dependence alone in a patient on prescribed long-term opioids taking their medication as directed do not satisfy the criteria for OUD.

B. Laboratory Findings

Comprehensive urine or oral fluid drug testing before treatment can help establish a baseline for drug testing, facilitate conversation about recent drug use (eg, a patient may be unaware the oxycodone they are taking contains fentanyl), inform treatment options (eg, presence of opioids is a contraindication to starting naltrexone), and help with monitoring treatment over time. However, the diagnosis of OUD is made by clinical assessment, and testing is not required for diagnosis or treatment initiation. Urine testing should be performed regularly after treatment is initiated to inform medical management based on detection of the treatment medication (ie, buprenorphine or methadone), and if other nonprescribed opioids are absent.

Consider screening for infectious diseases (eg, HIV, hepatitis B, and hepatitis C serologies), especially if a patient reports opioid use by injection route. Hepatitis test results can inform evaluation for treatment or preventive hepatitis A and hepatitis B vaccination. Positive HIV test results should trigger evaluation for treatment, and negative test results should inform discussion of preexposure prophylaxis and targeted education.

Liver biochemical tests can establish baseline levels before starting MOUD.

A pregnancy test can inform treatment options; it is not advisable to start naltrexone during pregnancy as this treatment has not been specifically studied in this population.

Complications

Infections from nonsterile injection drug use include cellulitis, abscesses at the injection site, endocarditis, or osteomyelitis. There is increased risk of infection with HIV, hepatitis B, and hepatitis C, especially if equipment is shared; there are reports of hepatitis C transmission from sharing equipment for intranasal insufflation. The risks are also increased for acquiring pneumonias and tuberculosis. The CDC recommends HIV preexposure prophylaxis for anyone with injection drug use and pneumococcal vaccination for anyone with any substance use.

Opioid-induced bowel syndrome with bloating, early satiety, and pain can occur since opioid agonists slow gut motility.

Opioid-induced hyperalgesia and co-occuring chronic pain from long-term use of opioid agonists, including MOUD, can result in hyperalgesia, an increased sensitivity to pain. Patients with OUD and those taking MOUD have been shown to have a lower pain threshold and higher opioid tolerance when compared to patients without OUD or those with OUD who have not taken methadone as MOUD. Chronic pain is common among people with OUD, and it is important to note that OUD and chronic pain are not mutually exclusive. In one study, up to 48–74% of patients with OUD reported having chronic pain, and in another study, 80% of patients at an opiate treatment program (OTP) reported having chronic pain.

Accidental overdose and mortality rates are vastly increased in persons with OUD. Studies have shown up to 63 times the all-cause mortality rate in those with OUD compared to those without OUD or with OUD on MOUD. In 2024, about 76% of all accidental drug overdose deaths involved an opioid.

Motor vehicle collisions and trauma are increased in persons with OUD.

Other complications from long-term opioid use include increased risk of hypogonadism and other hormonal disruptions, erectile dysfunction, fractures and bone density loss, delayed gastric emptying, and depression.

Treatment

OUD is a treatable medical condition with medications that have a robust evidence base to reduce morbidity and mortality. The three MOUDs approved by the FDA are buprenorphine, methadone, and extended-release naltrexone (Table 47–2). MOUD blocks or blunts the effects of nonprescribed opioids and reduces cravings to use opioids. These medications are effective in reducing mortality even without concurrent counseling or mental health support. Methadone and buprenorphine are also referred to as **opioid agonist treatment (OAT)**—in contrast to naltrexone, an opioid antagonist—and can therefore also be administered to reduce or eliminate opioid withdrawal symptoms.

Randomized clinical trials showed treatment with methadone, buprenorphine, or extended-release naltrexone significantly reduced nonmedical opioid use relative to no medication treatment. Studies have also found MOUD diminishes HIV and HCV transmission. *In contrast,*

Table 47–2. Comparison of MOUD.

	Buprenorphine (sublingual)	Buprenorphine (extended-release)	Methadone	Naltrexone (extended-release)
Mu-opioid receptor effect	Partial agonist	Partial agonist	Full agonist	Antagonist
Patient selection	Mild to severe OUD; patient preference	Moderate to severe OUD Sublocade[1]: Start after stable sublingual buprenorphine 8–24 mg dose daily for ≥ 7 days. Brixadi[1]: Adults who are currently treated with sublingual buprenorphine-naloxone or have tolerated a single 4-mg dose of sublingual buprenorphine-naloxone	Moderate to severe OUD; high opioid tolerance; patient preference	Long-term stability in OUD treatment; in a setting without access to opioid agonist treatment; patient preference after being counseled on risks and benefits May treat concurrent AUD
Initiation and stabilization	Traditional initiation: stop opioid use for 5–7 days (short acting) or 10–14 days (long acting or fentanyl) before initiation, confirm ≥ 3 withdrawal symptoms and urine toxicology. Low-dose initiation: continue full agonist during buprenorphine cross-titration (see Table 47–4).	Sublocade[1]: 300 mg subcutaneously monthly Brixadi[1]: If buprenorphine 4 mg sublingual dose is tolerated, give buprenorphine 16 mg subcutaneously weekly. Add additional buprenorphine 8 mg subcutaneously weekly after 3 days for a total of 24 mg subcutaneously weekly	Recommended initial dose is 30–50 mg orally, with reassessment after 4 hours for sedation. Can give additional 10 mg orally as needed once for a maximum total dose of 50 mg orally on day 1. Dose increases in 5–10 mg increments, no more frequently than every 3–7 days (depending on clinical response), are recommended to avoid over-sedation, toxicity, or iatrogenic overdose.	Tester dose: 25–50 mg orally daily for 1–3 days
Usual effective dose	16–24 mg sublingually	100–300 mg subcutaneously monthly in the abdomen (Sublocade) 8–32 mg subcutaneously weekly (buttock, thigh, abdomen, upper arm) (Brixadi) 64–128 mg subcutaneously monthly (buttock, thigh, abdomen, upper arm) (Brixadi)	60–200 mg orally daily	50 mg orally daily 380 mg intramuscularly every 3–4 weeks Intramuscular preferred over oral formulation
Half-life	Sublingual: 24–42 hours	43–60 days (Sublocade) 3–5 days (weekly Brixadi) 19–26 days (monthly Brixadi)	8–59 hours; takes 3–5 days to reach steady state	Oral: 4 hours Intramuscular: 5–10 days
Advantages	Can be prescribed in office-based settings and picked up in pharmacies More flexible dosing schedule Lower risk of respiratory depression or sedation Lower risk of accidental overdose Can treat pain	Same as sublingual buprenorphine with ease of weekly or monthly dosing No risk of diversion	Improved treatment retention Reduces accidental overdose mortality Improved OUD remission Effective in pregnancy No maximum dosage Can treat pain More structured delivery setting	Does not cause sedation or respiratory depression; lower stigma in some settings; no risk of diversion; no dependence.

(*continued*)

Table 47–2. Comparison of MOUD. (continued)

	Buprenorphine (sublingual)	Buprenorphine (extended-release)	Methadone	Naltrexone (extended-release)
Precautions	Severe liver impairment—CYP450 metabolism; risk of precipitated withdrawal during initiation; concurrent use of other CNS depressants (alcohol, benzodiazepines) can increase risk for respiratory depression (A); lower retention if doses < 16 mg sublingually daily	Injection-site reaction	Multiple drug-drug interactions with metabolism by cytochrome p450 Complex pharmacokinetics require careful monitoring Concurrent use of other CNS depressants (alcohol, benzodiazepines) can increase risk for respiratory depression (A)	Does not reduce cravings; can precipitate withdrawal if not adequate opioid abstinence; risk of fatal overdose if patient returns to use given loss of tolerance; inferior effect compared to opioid agonists treatment
Contraindications	Hypersensitivity; severe liver impairment	Hypersensitivity; patients with preexisting moderate to severe liver disease are not candidates	ECG QTc > 500 msecs; hypercapnia; respiratory depression (eg, severe COPD, severe OSA); hypersensitivity	Potential need for prescribed opioids (eg, upcoming surgeries, concurrent cancer pain)
Regulations and settings	Schedule III; can be prescribed by any clinician with a DEA license. Also used in OTP, inpatient settings	Schedule III; medication only available through REMS-certified pharmacies (ask for medication delivery) Provider must administer the injection.	Schedule II; can only be dispensed in OTP or acute hospital setting Not used in clinic settings Not visible on PDMP	Can be prescribed by any clinician with a DEA license Also used in OTP, inpatient settings

(A) The 2017 FDA Drug Safety Communication does not recommend holding opioid agonist treatment from patients solely on the basis of their benzodiazepine use, because untreated OUD can pose a greater risk of morbidity and mortality.
AUD, alcohol use disorder; DEA, Drug Enforcement Administration; ER, extended-release; OSA, obstructive sleep apnea; OTP, opioid treatment program; OUD, opioid use disorder; PDMP, prescription drug monitoring program; REMS, Risk Evaluation and Mitigation Strategies.
[1]Only Brixadi (and not Sublocade) is considered safe in pregnancy.

detoxification or medically supervised withdrawal alone (without subsequent medication treatment) is not an appropriate treatment for OUD; detoxification alone is associated with greater mortality and lower treatment retention compared to MOUD. Ideally, comprehensive treatment plans to support long-term remission include MOUD with behavioral therapy and access to harm reduction resources.

A. Pharmacotherapy

Buprenorphine as MOUD reduces opioid cravings and treats opioid withdrawal without producing euphoria and with a lower risk for adverse effects of full-agonist opioids. The combination sublingual product buprenorphine-naloxone or buprenorphine injection is generally recommended for MOUD and withdrawal treatment. The presence of naloxone in the combination product serves as a deterrent against nonprescribed injecting or intranasal opioid use; naloxone can induce withdrawal only if a person with opioid dependence injects or inhales buprenorphine-naloxone; if the buprenorphine-naloxone is taken sublingually as prescribed, a negligible amount of naloxone may be systemically absorbed and does not usually cause overt withdrawal. Nonetheless, naloxone frequently appears in urine toxicology results from patients taking buprenorphine-naloxone sublingually and some patients report mild withdrawal symptoms with use of the combination product.

Buprenorphine-naloxone as MOUD comes in three formulations: sublingual films and tablets and subcutaneous injection (extended-release). As of 2024, any clinician with a Drug Enforcement Administration (DEA) license can prescribe buprenorphine-naloxone for any indication; no X-waiver license is required.

There are two patient populations in which the mono-product buprenorphine is preferred. The first is in patients with decompensated cirrhosis, as the naloxone is not effectively eliminated by hepatic metabolism and can cause side effects such as nausea or headache. The other population is pregnant patients, as naloxone has not been formally studied in pregnancy. For patients with side effects to the combination product such as headache, a trial of the mono-product is a reasonable alternative. Extended-release buprenorphine comes in two formulations (Sublocade, dosed monthly, and Brixadi, dosed weekly or monthly). Only Brixadi is safe in pregnancy.

Buprenorphine has several unique properties: it (1) acts as a partial agonist at the mu-opioid receptor; (2) has a high affinity for the receptor with a long half-life of 24–44 hours; and (3) provides antagonism at the κ opioid receptor, facilitating its use as MOUD. The partial agonism means that, in contrast to full agonists, increasing beyond moderate doses of buprenorphine typically does not result in greater opioid effects on respiratory depression and sedation. High binding affinity of buprenorphine means it is more competitive than other opioids with lower mu-opioid agonist affinity (eg, heroin, oxycodone). Buprenorphine therefore blunts the effects of other full-agonist opioids on euphoria, can cause precipitated withdrawal if added to a system with full agonist opioids present, and also offers partial protection from accidental overdose. The minimum dose to provide overdose prevention is typically 8–16 mg sublingually based on ~10% mu-opioid receptor availability at this dose. Despite this high affinity, it is possible to effectively treat pain with short-acting full-agonist opioids (eg, oxycodone, hydromorphone) for patients receiving buprenorphine. κ-Opioid receptor antagonism is thought to reduce cravings, dysphoria, depression, hyperalgesia, and cravings. Buprenorphine has wide individual variation in pharmacokinetics, has an analgesic half-life of 6–8 hours in contrast to its pharmacologic half-life, is excreted primarily in the feces with 10–30% excretion in the urine, is extensively metabolized by the CYP450 system in the liver, and generally has fewer drug-drug interactions than methadone.

Buprenorphine-naloxone can be safely initiated in multiple settings: inpatient, office-based, or at home. Determining the appropriate initiation setting will rely on clinical judgment and may include consideration of a patient's experience with buprenorphine-naloxone and an assessment of their ability to manage initiation outside of clinical settings. Patients will need close monitoring during initiation and over the first few weeks. They should be educated on safe storage, administration with no food, tobacco smoking, or water until films/tablets are completely dissolved (can take up to 10 minutes). The decision to initiate buprenorphine-naloxone via traditional (Table 47–3) or low-dose initiation (Table 47–4) depends on patient preference and clinical scenario. High-dose buprenorphine-naloxone initiation has been described with some success in case series of patients treated in the emergency department who have severe opioid withdrawal and have had challenges initiating buprenorphine-naloxone with other methods in the past, such as in individuals with long-term use of nonprescribed fentanyl.

The 2022 FDA Drug Safety Communication regarding sublingual buprenorphine-naloxone and dental problems (tooth decay, cavities, oral infections, and loss of teeth) provides the following guidance: "After the medicine is completely dissolved, take a large sip of water, swish it gently around your teeth and gums, and swallow. You should wait at least 1 hour before brushing your teeth to avoid damage to your teeth and give your mouth a chance to return to its natural state." However, multiple commentaries have noted that the study informing this warning was problematic, including that sublingual buprenorphine-naloxone for OUD was compared to transdermal patches for chronic pain, and thus question the validity of the study. Buprenorphine-naloxone is still recommended as a first-line, effective treatment for OUD.

1. Traditional initiation method for buprenorphine-naloxone—To reduce the risk of precipitated withdrawal, an opioid-free period (eg, discontinuation of all full agonists for about 8–72 hours) with medically supervised withdrawal is traditionally required as the initiation method of buprenorphine-naloxone for OUD (Table 47–3). This may be intolerable or inappropriate for some patients,

Table 47–3. Protocol for traditional initiation of buprenorphine-naloxone for patients with OUD in withdrawal or patient preference. All doses are for sublingual buprenorphine-naloxone.

Preparation	Discontinue full mu-opioid agonists at least 8–12 hours for short-acting opioids, 24–48 hours for extended-release formulations, and at least 72 hours for methadone. Confirm that patient has been prescribed and picked up comfort meds (see Table 47–5). Start initiation of buprenorphine-naloxone only when there is mild-moderate opioid withdrawal (COWS ≥ 12) with at least three objective signs of withdrawal. Long-term non-pharmaceutical fentanyl use may require a lower starting trial dose of buprenorphine-naloxone or higher COWS score. Alternatively, consider high-dose buprenorphine-naloxone initiation (see text).
Day 1	Start buprenorphine (2–4 mg)-naloxone (0.5–1 mg) sublingually. The risk of precipitated withdrawal is reduced by starting buprenorphine at doses < 2 mg. Monitor over 60–90 minutes for precipitated withdrawal and treat if it develops. Reassess symptoms every 2–4 hours. If withdrawal persists, repeat doses of buprenorphine (2–4 mg)-naloxone (0.5–1 mg) sublingually every 2 hours to a maximum of 8 mg. Once it has been established that the initial dose of buprenorphine-naloxone is well tolerated, dose titration can be achieved fairly quickly.
Day 2	Give total buprenorphine-naloxone dose from Day 1. Give additional buprenorphine-naloxone 2–4 mg sublingually every 2–4 hours, up to 16 mg total.
Day 3–14	Ongoing titration. If the patient's therapeutic goals are met, the dose need not be adjusted. If continued cravings or withdrawal are present without sedation, increase dose of sublingual buprenorphine-naloxone by buprenorphine 2-1 to 4-2 mg daily to an effective dose of 16-4 to 24-6 mg daily. It can take 1–2 weeks to achieve a stable dose outpatient.

COWS, Clinical Opioid Withdrawal Scale.

Table 47–4. Two sample low-dose initiation protocols for sublingual buprenorphine or buprenorphine-naloxone.*

	For patients maintained on prescribed full agonist opioids, patients transitioning from very long-acting opioids (eg, moderate- to high-dose methadone, chronic nonprescribed fentanyl use) or based on patient preference.		
Options	Buprenorphine initiation with transdermal patch (A) and sublingual tab/film	Buprenorphine initiation with sublingual tab/film (B) only	Full agonist opioid plan
Patient selection	Less risk for precipitated withdrawal; does not require cutting films/ tablets	Transdermal formulation may not be available or may be cost prohibitive	
Day 1	Transdermal 40 mcg/hour (C)	0.5 mg sublingually once (D)	Continue baseline full-agonist dose in most cases until sublingual buprenorphine-naloxone dosing is at least buprenorphine 8–12 mg sublingually daily
Day 2	No changes	0.5 mg sublingually every 12 hours	
Day 3	1 mg sublingually every 12 hours	1 mg sublingually every 12 hours	
Day 4	1 mg sublingually every 8 hours	1 mg sublingually every 8 hours	
Day 5	2 mg sublingually every 12 hours	2 mg sublingually every 12 hours	
Day 6	4 mg sublingually every 12 hours	4 mg sublingually every 12 hours	
Day 7	12 mg sublingually in the morning	12 mg sublingually in the morning	Can discontinue or taper off full opioid agonist (E)
Day 8	Further adjustment by clinician[1]	Further adjustment by clinician[1]	

*Protocol applies to initiation of any **sublingual** buprenorphine formulation (the monoproduct or the combination buprenorphine-naloxone product). Only sublingual films and tablets for opioid use disorder (OUD) are available as monotherapy or in combination with naloxone. Formulations indicated for pain only do not contain naloxone (buccal films, transdermal patches, and intravenous injections). Extended-release subcutaneous buprenorphine injections for OUD do not contain naloxone.

[1]Continue to adjust buprenorphine dose to symptoms or indication by 2–4 mg sublingually daily (goal treatment for OUD is 24 mg sublingually daily). This protocol lists recommended titration steps. Protocol steps can be paused/continued without progression for several days as needed due to patient discomfort, clinical scenario, etc. Total daily dose can be consolidated once effective dose is reached. Return to a lower dosing level if a patient becomes sedate.

(A) The buprenorphine patch is FDA approved for pain. If the indication is OUD, the medication may not be covered by third-party payers for outpatients.

(B) Films may be preferred given they are easier to split.

(C) A 40 mcg/hour transdermal dose can be achieved by using two 20 mcg/hour transdermal patches. Continue wearing the transdermal patches until they expire in 7 days, then remove and do not replace. Note that it takes 3–4 days for a transdermal patch to reach steady state. Sublingual buprenorphine can be initiated while the patient is wearing transdermal patches.

(D) A 0.5 mg sublingual dose can be achieved by cutting a 2 mg buprenorphine film or tablet in quarters. If this is not permitted by inpatient pharmacies, use options for initiation by starting with transdermal or intravenous formulations, then rotating to sublingual.

(E) Short-acting full-opioid agonists may be appropriate to continue in some cases if clinically indicated (eg, treating concurrent acute pain like a traumatic fracture, terminal end-of-life pain).

such as (1) those who receive full opioid agonists as therapy for concurrent pain; (2) patients transitioning from very long-acting opioids (eg, methadone, fentanyl patches); and (3) patients who may have experienced precipitated withdrawal in the past or have significant fear of having this experience. For these patients, the low-dose initiation method (ie, "microdosing" or Bernese method) in which there is a period of concomitant buprenorphine-naloxone and full-agonist opioid cross-titration, may be more appropriate (Table 47–4).

2. Low dose initiation method for buprenorphine-naloxone—Low-dose initiation circumvents the need for stopping full-agonist opioids and going through a period of withdrawal before starting buprenorphine. Instead, small, and gradually increasing doses of buprenorphine-naloxone are administered with sufficient time between doses to establish equilibrium.

Full-agonist opioids are continued while buprenorphine-naloxone is started and titrated to a therapeutic dose (usually buprenorphine-naloxone 16 mg/4 mg to 24 mg/6 mg sublingually for OUD), via the low-dose method, at which time the full-agonist opioids may be stopped, tapered off, or continued depending on the clinical situation. Outpatient low-dose initiation is most effective when patients or caregivers can follow multi-step medication instructions and respond to telephone or nursing checks 1–2 days after initiation and then 3–7 days later, or with changes in the dosing regimen, to assess symptoms and triage adverse effects.

Low-dose initiation can be performed in any setting: inpatient or outpatient, and with any formulation of buprenorphine. Published protocols vary by timelines (eg, longer in outpatient settings or patients on moderate- to high-dose methadone, rapid for inpatient settings) and the buprenorphine-naloxone formulation used. Importantly, initiation protocols can be modified or paused if a patient experiences intolerable worry, withdrawal symptoms, or pain flares. See Table 47–4 for a sample of an initiation protocol using the buprenorphine patch and sublingual forms. Importantly, *the full-agonist opioid must be maintained during the initial phases of buprenorphine initiation to prevent a decrease in total opioid load resulting in iatrogenic withdrawal.* In the inpatient setting, non-MOUD opioid agonists can be administered. For example, hospitalized patients who use non-prescribed fentanyl long-term can be administered oxycodone immediate release 15–20 mg orally every 3 hours as needed for cravings or withdrawal symptoms as the non-MOUD opioid agonist until buprenorphine reaches steady state. In the outpatient setting, non-MOUD opioid agonists cannot legally be prescribed, and the patient should continue whichever opioid they have been using.

3. Withdrawal precipitated by the use of buprenorphine—If buprenorphine is introduced when opioid receptors are occupied by full agonists, buprenorphine will outcompete the full agonist to exert a partial opioid effect. The resulting shift from full opioid effect to partial opioid effect manifests as opioid withdrawal. This precipitated withdrawal can be treated by reducing the relative opioid deficit (ie, adding more buprenorphine or full agonist), or by pausing initiation and using nonopioid "comfort meds" to alleviate withdrawal symptoms (Table 47–5). Initiation can be reattempted in 24 hours.

4. Methadone—Despite widely documented effectiveness of methadone treatment, it remains a Schedule II drug with federal regulations limiting its use as MOUD to approved OTPs, which exacerbates a treatment gap of nearly 1 million people with OUD not receiving treatment. Methadone as MOUD is dosed to reduce opioid cravings and withdrawal symptoms, may blunt the euphoric effects of other opioids, and may be better at retaining patients in treatment compared to buprenorphine and extended-release naltrexone. About 1500 federally certified OTPs in the United States offer methadone treatment to patients who meet admission criteria. Historically, it has been difficult to get take-home bottles of methadone, but in 2024, federal regulations changed to allow a greater role for provider judgment in making decisions about take-home methadone. A patient now can be eligible for up to 7 take-home doses after only 14 days of treatment.

If a patient begins methadone treatment in the hospital, that patient needs to be connected to an OTP for ongoing medication. OTP connection should be facilitated in advance of discharge. For patients discharged to the community, discharge paperwork must include a "last dose letter" that includes the date, time, and dose of the last methadone administered so that the OTP can continue titration, rather than starting the patient from the standard initiation dose of up to 50 mg daily. If a patient is transferred to a facility that does not administer methadone, then an intake must be arranged at an OTP that will provide dosing. Either in-person or telehealth intakes are permitted, but coordination is needed between the hospital and the OTP. Ideally, there is ample lead-time (~1 week) to plan for logistical considerations. The average methadone half-life of 24 hours facilitates once daily dosing in methadone treatment, although the analgesic half-life is 6–8 hours. Methadone treatment initiation starts with doses of approximately 15–50 mg daily and are titrated to balance cravings with adverse effects, typically reaching stable doses of 80–200 mg in the era of fentanyl. Tapering off of methadone after a period of sustained stability may be considered, however longer lengths (even a lifetime) are associated with better outcomes.

5. Naltrexone—Naltrexone is an opioid antagonist at the mu-opioid receptor, so it blocks the euphoric and sedative effects of opioid agonists. Unlike buprenorphine and methadone, naltrexone does not treat physical dependence or withdrawal symptoms that may be associated with OUD. Because of its shorter half-life, it also does not infer the same protective effect against overdose as buprenorphine. *Naltrexone should only be initiated in a person who has completed opioid withdrawal, since it will otherwise precipitate withdrawal.* The SAMHSA generally recommends that a person wait 7 days after their last use of short-acting opioids or 10–14 days after their last use of long-acting opioids before starting naltrexone to reduce the risk of precipitated, acute opioid withdrawal. Naltrexone extended release is the preferred MOUD because the long-acting formulation improves adherence to the medication.

Table 47–5. Opioid withdrawal treatment with nonopioid adjuncts ("comfort meds").

Symptom	Medication	Dose (oral)	Frequency	Other
Nausea	Odansetron	4 mg	Every 6 hours, as needed	Can prolong QTc
Pain, headache	Acetaminophen Ibuprofen	650 mg 400–800 mg	Every 6 hours as needed Every 8 hours as needed	Avoid in liver failure Avoid in kidney failure
Diarrhea	Loperamide	4 mg	Every 6 hours, as needed	
Anxiety	Hydroxyzine	25–50 mg	Every 6 hours, as needed	Caution if patient is sedated or in older adults
Tremors, sweating	Clonidine	0.1 mg	Every 8 hours, as needed	Caution if blood pressure or heart rate is low

B. Monitoring Pharmacotherapy

After treatment initiation, regular follow-up should be continued for related medical issues. Additionally, provider engagement surrounding adherence to MOUD, overdose risk mitigation techniques, and discussion of triggers and recovery strategies should be continued. Behavioral treatments (eg, psychotherapy) should be offered if not already utilized.

For patients receiving methadone, the OTP will uptitrate and monitor the dosing, so best practice includes having the patient sign a release of information with the OTP. On urine toxicology testing, recent use of methadone is noted by a positive EDDP (2-ethylidene-1,5-dimethyl-3,3-diphenylpyrrolidine) test, a metabolite of methadone. Because methadone is long acting and lipophilic, EDDP may be present in the urine for weeks to months after last use for patients receiving methadone long-term.

For patients using sublingual buprenorphine, typical follow-up is every 1–2 weeks after initiation for monitoring and titration. Visits should remain frequent while titrating to an effective dose of at least 16 mg sublingually daily, and once stable, visits can be spaced out to every 1–3 months depending on the stability of remission. Urine toxicology tests should also be attained at regular intervals, with the goal of confirming the presence of buprenorphine metabolites (norbuprenorphine) and the absence of non-buprenorphine opioids. For patients taking subcutaneous, extended-release buprenorphine, the presence of buprenorphine does not need to be monitored as treatment is administered in clinic. However, urine toxicology testing can be administered to evaluate if other non-prescribed substances are present.

For patients using extended-release naltrexone, the monitoring is similar for extended-release buprenorphine, as the product is directly administered. Urine toxicology testing should be tailored to the patient scenario.

Amaducci A et al. Naloxone use in novel potent opioid and fentanyl overdoses in emergency department patients. JAMA Netw Open. 2023;6:e2331264. [PMID: 37642962]

American Society of Addiction Medicine (ASAM). The ASAM National Practice Guideline for the Treatment of Opioid Use Disorder: 2020 Focused Update. J Addict Med. 2020;14:267. [PMID: 32487948]

Barnett M et al. Racial inequality in receipt of medications for opioid use disorder. N Engl J Med. 2023;388:1779. [PMID: 37163624]

Cohen SM et al. Low dose initiation of buprenorphine: a narrative review and practical approach. J Addict Med. 2022;16:399. [PMID: 34954746]

Jones CM et al. Use of medication for opioid use disorder among adults with past-year opioid use disorder in the US, 2021. JAMA Network Open. 2023;6:e2327488. [PMID: 37548979]

Sokolski E et al. Rapid low-dose buprenorphine initiation for hospitalized patients with opioid use disorder. J Addict Med. 2023;17:e278. [PMID: 37579112]

Substance Abuse and Mental Health Services Administration (SAMHSA). Key Substance Use and Mental Health Indicators in the United States: Substance Abuse and Mental Health Services Administration. Medications for Opioid Use Disorder. Treatment Improvement Protocol (TIP) Series 63 Publication No. PEP21-02-01-002. Rockville, MD: Substance Abuse and Mental Health Services Administration, 2021. https://store.samhsa.gov/product/tip-63-medications-opioid-use-disorder/pep21-02-01-002. Accessed June 19, 2026.

OPIOID INTOXICATION & OVERDOSE

General Considerations

Opioid intoxication is the physiologic response to the acute effects of an opioid agonist through activation of the mu-opioid receptor in the CNS.

Opioid overdose is the most severe form of opioid intoxication syndrome. Overdose is a potentially fatal state in which opioids cause suppression of the respiratory centers in the brainstem and medulla. Opioid overdose is a medical emergency and requires immediate medical management. Of note, respiratory depression is preceded by the warning sign of sedation.

Mild to moderate intoxication, such as euphoria or sedation, is not life-threatening and occurs on a spectrum so that the presence of opioid intoxication is not always obvious on physical examination.

Tolerance, or the reduced responsiveness to a substance over time so that increased doses are needed to achieve the desired effect, is a critical concept in the context of opioid use. Tolerance is a predictor of overdose risk and severity; in patients with high tolerance, the required dose to cause respiratory depression may be lower than the dose required to produce the desired level of euphoria. Additionally, individuals who may lose tolerance (ie, post-hospitalization, post-incarceration, or a period of remission) are at higher risk for opioid overdose upon re-exposure to the doses of opioids that they used previously.

Clinical Findings

A. Symptoms and Signs

Opioid intoxication involves a spectrum of symptoms including the combination of altered mental status, respiratory depression, and miotic pupils. **Overdose** should be diagnosed when the respiratory rate is < 8 breaths per minute, signs of cyanosis are present, or if the patient is nonresponsive. Severe intoxication presents as overdose, which can be fatal if not intervened upon within the window of reversibility.

Physical examination findings of opioid intoxication include miosis with decreased blood pressure, heart rate, respiratory rate, or a combination of these. Other signs that suggest opioid use are dependent on the route of ingestion; oral, inhaled ("smoked"), intravenous, intranasal/insufflation ("snorting"), rectal ("booty bumping"), intramuscular, and subcutaneous ("skin popping"). For example, patients may have signs of skin irritation from frequent injections that resemble bruises with small dots ("track marks"), or skin and soft-tissue infections related to drug use.

Additional symptoms of opioid intoxication may include nausea, vomiting, confusion, constipation, depression, dry mouth (which can result in tooth decay), and pruritus.

B. Laboratory Findings

At the time of the opioid overdose, toxicology testing should be done to confirm which substances are present and to guide management. Not all substances (such as xylazine) will be found on basic urine toxicology testing. Consent for this testing requires consent from patients who are mentating with capacity but should be performed in nonresponsive patients without consent to inform treatment.

Treatment

A. General Measures

To manage an overdose, increasingly intensive measures are needed, initiated in the following order:

1. Verbal warning (ie, "Are you awake? I am going to administer naloxone because I am worried you are overdosing").
2. Sternal rub.
3. If no response, immediately administer naloxone 0.4–0.8 mg intravenously or intranasally.

B. Specific Measures

Naloxone can be administered intranasally or intravenously at 0.4–0.8 mg per dose. Naloxone will reverse CNS effects of opioids; onset of action is 2 minutes, and duration of action is 30–90 minutes. Naloxone can cause opioid withdrawal symptoms that are distressing but can be life-saving. Additional basic life support with frequent vital signs monitoring should be instituted while waiting for the naloxone to take effect; adequate intravenous access is required to administer supportive medications (such as fluids) and oxygen should be administered via nasal cannula. If cyanosis does not resolve, intubation may be necessary.

When a long-acting opioid has been used (eg, prolonged fentanyl use, methadone), the patient has responded to a bolus of naloxone, and respiratory depression and sedation persist after two initial boluses have been administered, a continuous naloxone infusion may be warranted. Infusion rates can start at two-thirds of the total effective bolus dose or 'wake-up dose' per hour (eg, 0.08 mg/hour for a patient requiring 0.12 mg of naloxone to 'wake up'). For patients receiving prescribed opioids for pain who may have respiratory depression and risk of accidental overdose, a lower tester dose of naloxone (0.04 mg intravenously) can be administered to test for reversal of opioid-related respiratory sedation and depression without entirely reversing opioid analgesia.

Of note, nonprescribed opioid overdoses commonly include other substances, including other cognitive and respiratory depressants, such as benzodiazepines, alcohol, and xylazine. Naloxone reverses only the opioid effects; it does not reverse respiratory sedation from nonopioid substances. In these instances, continued supportive care and advanced cardiopulmonary support is indicated if severe respiratory depression is present until the substance has metabolized.

National Institute on Drug Abuse (NIDA). Drugs and the brain. https://nida.nih.gov/publications/drugs-brains-behavior-science-addiction/drugs-brain. Accessed June 19, 2026.

OPIOID WITHDRAWAL

General Considerations

Opioid withdrawal can be agonizing; however, it is typically nonfatal in the absence of persistent and severe electrolyte imbalances due to severe diarrhea and vomiting. The duration and onset of the acute withdrawal phase depends on the opioid used. Opioids with longer half-lives result in later onset (eg, methadone, extended-release oxycodone) and typically have a longer duration of the acute withdrawal phase. The onset of non-pharmaceutical fentanyl withdrawal can be unpredictable and protracted as a result of a combination of various analogs of fentanyl in the substance used.

Clinical Findings

A. Symptoms and Signs

Opioid withdrawal is marked by nausea, vomiting, diarrhea, chills and sweating, tremors, muscle and bone pain, and anxiety. Clinically this can look similar to a severe case of influenza, or other viral or bacterial infections. As is the case with most SUDs, avoiding or minimizing the significant dysphoria and physical discomfort of the withdrawal state is often a primary trigger to continued use. The degree of opioid withdrawal is measured using the Clinical Opioid Withdrawal Scale (COWS) which incorporates subjective and objective findings (https://nida.nih.gov/sites/default/files/ClinicalOpiateWithdrawalScale.pdf). Moderate withdrawal is typically in the COWS 13–24 range. The COWS score is useful both to measure response to withdrawal management and to guide buprenorphine initiation.

B. Laboratory Findings

The immunoassay and the LC/GC MS tests generally demonstrate the presence of opioids within the past 1–3 days. Heroin is typically metabolized to morphine within 8 hours so it is only detectable within less than 1 day after use. In contrast, prolonged nonpharmaceutical fentanyl has been found to be present for up to 3 weeks after last use. Methadone typically can be detected for 7 days, and buprenorphine for 1–11 days after use.

Substances that can cause false-positive results include dextromethorphan, diphenhydramine, poppy seeds, quinine, quinolones, rifampin, and verapamil. False-negative results occur when the opioid is present at a level lower than the threshold for detection. Specimen contamination or tampering can be evaluated through the urine test results using temperature, creatinine concentration, pH, and specific gravity. Temperature strips should show urine is 90–100°F within 4 minutes of collection. Human urine has a pH level between 3 and 11, specific gravity between 1.002–1.020, urine creatinine > 20 mg/dL (< 5 mg/dL is inconsistent with human urine in cases of urine tampering by dilution), and creatinine concentration < 5 ng/mL. Oxidant tests can indicate the addition of bleach or another oxidant. Results outside these ranges suggest contamination or adulteration, in which case the testing should be repeated.

Treatment

Managing opioid withdrawal is important, as unmanaged opioid withdrawal is a well-described reason patients leave medical care before recommended by the medical team or use non-prescribed substances while hospitalized. The most effective method to manage opioid withdrawal is to initiate medication treatment like methadone or buprenorphine. Opioid withdrawal management incorporates both opioid (including MOUD) and nonopioid pharmacologic interventions (see Table 47–5). Options can vary by clinical site.

A. Treatment in the Emergency Department or Inpatient Setting

For patients who come to the emergency department or those who are hospitalized, any opioid can legally be administered to manage opioid withdrawal, including MOUD or other full-agonist opioids. Special hospital or provider DEA licensing is not required. MOUD should be offered as first-line treatment for opioid withdrawal and OUD. For the emergency department, the "Three Day Rule" is an emergency treatment clause that allows providers outside of an OTP to administer, but not dispense, narcotics for the treatment of opioid withdrawal. This law was expanded in 2020 to allow for the dispensing of narcotics with special permission. If MOUD initiation is declined, short-acting opioids or low-dose methadone (30–50 mg orally daily) can be administered while the patient is hospitalized to manage withdrawal symptoms. These opioids cannot legally be prescribed on discharge for OUD treatment outside of an OTP.

The titration of MOUD to an effective dose that quells cravings and opioid withdrawal symptoms can take time. For patients who report recent use of long-acting opioids such as non-pharmaceutical fentanyl or methadone, short-acting opioids can be administered as a bridge while the long-acting opioid is metabolized but before the buprenorphine can be initiated (using a traditional initiation protocol) (see Table 47–3) or while buprenorphine dosage is subtherapeutic (using a low dose bridging protocol) (see Table 47–4). Similarly, short-acting opioids can be administered as a bridge to ward off opioid withdrawal symptoms until methadone is titrated to therapeutic doses, which can take weeks.

B. Outpatient Treatment

Opioid prescribing is tightly regulated by the 1974 Narcotic Addict Treatment Act, which states that narcotics cannot be used to manage opioid withdrawal outside of federally designated OTPs (eg, official methadone clinics). Any clinician with a DEA license, however, can prescribe office-based buprenorphine treatment as MOUD and for management of withdrawal (see Table 47–3). Patients interested in outpatient management of OUD and opioid withdrawal with methadone need to seek care through an OTP that will administer methadone, as it cannot be prescribed.

American Society of Addiction Medicine (ASAM). The ASAM National Practice Guideline for the Treatment of Opioid Use Disorder: 2020 Focused Update. J Addict Med. 2020;14:267. [PMID: 32487948]

Kumar R et al. Buprenorphine. 2023 Nov 30. In: StatPearls [Internet]. Treasure Island (FL): StatPearls Publishing; 2024 Jan. [PMID: 29083570]

ALCOHOL USE DISORDER (AUD)

ESSENTIALS OF DIAGNOSIS

- Continued alcohol drinking despite medical and social contraindications, life disruptions, or impairment in social and occupational functioning.
- Physiologic dependence manifests by withdrawal when intake is interrupted; tolerance manifests by greater alcohol intake to maintain the same effect.
- Alcohol-associated illnesses include liver disease, cerebellar degeneration, pancreatitis, or alcohol-related injuries.

General Considerations

Alcohol use is a leading cause of morbidity and mortality, with potential harms resulting from both acute and chronic use. According to the 2023 National Survey on Drug Use and Health, 16.4 million people ≥ age 12 reported heavy alcohol use in the past month (≥ 5 drinks on any day or ≥ 15 per week for men, or ≥ 4 drinks on any day or ≥ 8 drinks per week for women). Ten percent of the American adult population over 12 years old, or 23.9 million people, reported AUD in the past year, making it the most common, non-nicotine SUD. Excessive alcohol use contributed to over 178,000 deaths each year.

Alcoholic beverages contain ethanol, a simple compound that is small and lipophilic, allowing it to easily cross the blood-brain barrier and interact with multiple neurotransmitter systems. Clinically, this can manifest acutely with decreased level of consciousness, slurred speech, and impaired balance and gait. The activation of γ-aminobutyric acid (GABA)-A receptors is believed to play a role in dopamine release in the mesolimbic dopamine system, the highly conserved pathway central to addictive disorders.

There is a spectrum of alcohol consumption. The majority of people are either abstinent or follow safe drinking limits; however, some persons have unhealthy use, defined as either exceeding safe limits or having an AUD. The National Institute on Alcohol Abuse and Alcoholism (NIAAA) defines safe drinking limits as ≤ 2 drinks in a day for men and ≤ 1 drink in a day for women (< 14 drinks/week in men, and < 7 drinks/week in women). Persons ≥ age 65 follow the same recommendations as women. A drink is defined by the CDC as 12-oz of beer, 8-oz of malt liquor, 5-oz of wine, or 1.5-oz or a "shot" of 80-proof distilled spirits or liquor. The NIAAA has an online drinking calculator that can be used to determine if the person is adhering to safe limits (https://rethinkingdrinking.niaaa.nih.gov/tools/calculators). Risky alcohol use is defined as people who drink > 4 drinks/day or 14 drinks/week for men (< age 65), and 3 drinks/day or 7 drinks/week for women (or men ≥ age 65), or engaging in binge drinking (≥ 4 for women, ≥ 5 for men in ~2 hours). A person may move bidirectionally through these classifiers throughout their lifespan.

AUD is a clinical diagnosis by *DSM-5* criteria, including loss of control with heavy and persistent use, drinking despite consequences, compulsion to use, cravings, tolerance, and withdrawal. There are no known safe drinking limits. A 2025 expert opinion article suggested that for those without AUD or comorbidities (including chronic illness, driving a vehicle, or pregnancy), drinking one standard drink equivalent per day with interspersed abstinent days may not constitute a meaningful risk to health.

As of 2024, the overall prevalence of AUD was 9.7% (higher rates in men than women [11.8% versus 7.6%]). Women often delay seeking help, and when they do, they tend to seek it in medical or mental health settings. Treatment completion rates are influenced by intersectional social factors, including gender, race, and ethnicity, so that 10–12% fewer minoritized women complete treatment compared to White men. Adoption and twin studies suggest some genetic influence. Ethnic distinctions are important—eg, 40% of Japanese individuals have aldehyde dehydrogenase deficiency, causing adverse side effects from alcohol, and a decreased risk of developing AUD. Patients with AUD have a higher prevalence of lifetime psychiatric disorders. Depression is often present and should be evaluated carefully and treated. Alcohol significantly increases the risk of death by suicide and has been associated with violent crimes and domestic assault.

There are several screening instruments that may help identify an AUD. One of the most useful is the **Alcohol Use Disorder Identification Test (AUDIT)** (see Table 1–6).

Clinical Findings

A. Symptoms and Signs

A distinction needs to be made between primary AUD (when there is no other major psychiatric diagnosis) and secondary AUD (when alcohol is used as self-medication for major underlying psychiatric disorders such as schizophrenia or affective disorder). This distinction is important, since the latter requires treatment for the specific psychiatric diagnosis. In primary and secondary AUD, at-risk drinking can be distinguished from AUD by taking a careful psychiatric history and evaluating the degree to which recurrent drinking impacts social role functioning and physical safety of the individual. The *DSM-5* criteria are useful in diagnosing AUD (see Table 47–1).

B. Laboratory Tests

1. Urine alcohol testing—Testing for alcohol consumption is mostly performed in the urine, either directly by measuring ethanol (which is quickly eliminated so a test can only detect use within 3 days) or measuring ethyl glucuronide, an ethanol metabolite that is typically positive for alcohol use in past 3 days.

2. Blood alcohol testing—For a 70-kg person, 1.5-oz of whiskey, a 5-oz glass of wine, or a 12-oz bottle of beer (roughly 15 g of alcohol) may raise the level of alcohol in the blood by 25 mg/dL. For a 50-kg person, the blood alcohol level would rise even higher (35 mg/dL) with the same consumption. Blood alcohol levels < 50 mg/dL rarely cause significant motor dysfunction (the legal limit for driving under the influence is commonly 80 mg/dL). Intoxication as manifested by ataxia, dysarthria, and nausea and vomiting often indicates a blood level > 150 mg/dL, and lethal blood levels range from 350 mg/dL to 900 mg/dL. Hazardous drinking can be measured by blood phosphatidylethanol levels, where a value of ≥ 0.22 mcmol/L is more sensitive and specific than urine alcohol testing.

Ethanol may contribute to the presence of an otherwise unexplained osmolar gap. There may also be increased serum liver biochemical tests, uric acid, and triglycerides and decreased serum potassium and magnesium. The most definitive biologic marker for chronic AUD is carbohydrate deficient transferrin, which can detect heavy use (60 g/day over 7–10 days) with high specificity. Other useful tests for diagnosing AUD are γ-glutamyl transpeptidase (GGT) measurement (levels > 30 U/L are suggestive of heavy drinking) and mean corpuscular volume (MCV) (> 95 fL in men and > 100 fL in women). If both are elevated, patients should be screened for unsafe alcohol use. Use of other recreational drugs with alcohol can interfere with the significance of these tests.

Complications

The medical, economic, and psychosocial problems of AUD are staggering. Alcohol use affects many organ systems, often in dose-dependent relationships, and contributes to over 200 conditions. A 2025 United States Surgeon General's report noted alcohol as the third leading preventable cause of cancer, and 25% of alcohol-related cancer cases were in those drinking < 2 drinks per day, noting risk even at safe dinking levels for men < age 65.

1. Liver disease—Ninety percent of alcohol is metabolized by the liver, thus exposing the liver to both alcohol and its toxic metabolites. Alcohol-related liver injury and disease (ALD) includes steatosis, steatohepatitis, alcohol-associated hepatitis, fibrosis and scarring, and HCC. In most ALD, not drinking alcohol can prevent further liver damage and improve survival rates.

2. Pancreatitis—Alcohol is the leading cause of chronic pancreatitis and the second leading cause of acute pancreatitis; cigarette smoking increases the risk of both types when used in combination with alcohol.

3. GI inflammation—GI mucosal inflammation, bleeding, and GERD can be due to damage of the epithelial lining by alcohol.

4. Heart disease and stroke—Heavy alcohol use causes > 37,000 deaths a year due to alcohol-related heart disease and stroke. Even low-level alcohol use contributes to increased risk for hypertension, arrhythmia (specifically atrial fibrillation), cardiomyopathy, and MI.

5. Cancer—Alcohol and its metabolites are recognized as carcinogens. Alcohol use has been associated with higher risk of head and neck cancers (oral cavity, larynx, pharynx, esophageal), GI cancer (liver, stomach, colorectal), and breast cancer in women.

6. Myopathy, fractures—Chronic, heavy alcohol use increases the risk of midline muscle atrophy and weakness. Daily drinking > 1.5–2 drinks can increase the risk of fractures due to disruption in bone remodeling and increase the risk of falls.

7. Gout—The risk of developing and flaring of gout increase in a dose-dependent manner with alcohol use.

8. Nervous system—Alcohol contributes to peripheral and central neuropathies through direct neurotoxicity and indirectly through inflammation and nutritional deficiencies. Peripheral neuropathies include symmetrical 'stocking-glove' sensory loss, postural hypotension, and erectile dysfunction. Cognitive effects include dementia, loss of memory and attention, and reduced brain volume.

9. Fetal alcohol syndrome—No amount of alcohol is known to be entirely safe in pregnancy. Fetal alcohol syndrome includes a spectrum of physical, behavioral, and cognitive impairments resulting from prenatal alcohol exposure.

Treatment

Only 2.5% of Americans aged 12 and older with AUD in 2024 received medication treatment. Treatment for AUD has been shown to increase rates of not drinking, reduce return to drinking, and reduce symptoms of protracted alcohol withdrawal.

Pharmacologic Treatments

The three FDA-approved medications to treat AUD are two first-line agents, naltrexone and acamprosate, and the second-line agent disulfiram (Table 47–6). Non-FDA approved treatments for patients intolerant to first-line agents or due to patient preference include gabapentin, topiramate, and baclofen.

Centers for Disease Control and Prevention. Alcohol Related Disease Impact (ARDI) application, 2024. Available at www.cdc.gov/ARDI.

Substance Abuse and Mental Health Services Administration. (2025). Key substance use and mental health indicators in the United States: Results from the 2024 National Survey on Drug Use and Health (HHS Publication No. PEP25-07-007, NSDUH Series H-60). Center for Behavioral Health Statistics and Quality, Substance Abuse and Mental Health Services Administration.

ACUTE ALCOHOL INTOXICATION

Clinical Findings

A. Symptoms and Signs

The signs of alcoholic intoxication depend on serum ethanol concentrations and can vary by person. Signs can include slurred speech, incoordination, drowsiness, psychomotor dysfunction, disinhibition, dysarthria, ataxia, and nystagmus. Hypotension and tachycardia may result from peripheral vasodilation from ethanol or due to vomiting and volume loss.

At serum alcohol concentrations from 20 mg/dL to 100 mg/dL, people may feel euphoria and have mild deficits in attention, cognition, and physical coordination. For concentrations 100–200 mg/dL, symptoms include greater deficits in coordination, motor skills, judgement, and speech, as well as mood variability. With severe intoxication at concentrations between 200 mg/dL and 300 mg/dL, patients may present with confusion, nausea, and vomiting. At concentrations > 300 mg/dL, symptoms can include loss of consciousness and respiratory depression. In very severe cases, intoxication can include seizures, shock syndrome, and death. Some individuals with high tolerance to ethanol from chronic use may show few signs of intoxication at concentrations > 300 mg/dL. Serious overdoses are frequently due to a combination of alcohol with other sedatives or drugs.

B. Laboratory Tests

Laboratory testing is usually not needed for patients with isolated mild alcohol intoxication. For more complicated or severe cases, acute intoxication can cause metabolic derangements such as hypoglycemia, hyperlactatemia, hypomagnesemia, hypokalemia, hypocalcemia, and hypophosphatemia. Generally, patients presenting with intoxication should be tested with a rapid bedside glucose, comprehensive urine toxicology screen, serum alcohol level, and metabolic panel. Patients with altered mental status require evaluation to rule out other serious conditions such as head trauma, infection, or hypoxia; alcohol intoxication should be a diagnosis of exclusion for altered mental status and coma.

Treatment

Management of acute intoxication is primarily supportive. Most patients only will require observation and serial examinations. Volume may be replaced with intravenous crystalloid fluids, if needed. Patients should be assessed for occult traumas and evaluated for ingestion and withdrawal of coexisting substances. Patients with intoxication may be agitated and aggressive; if they are a danger to self or others, they may require de-escalation techniques (eg, creating a calm environment, active listening, offering choices where possible) and medications such as benzodiazepines and first-generation antipsychotics (see below) to facilitate caregiving, if respiratory rate allows. Patients may need ICU higher level of care if vital signs are abnormal (eg, hypotension, tachycardia, fever, and hypothermia), hypoxia, hypoglycemia, or the need for parenteral sedation.

Table 47–6. FDA-approved medications for treatment of AUD.

Medication	First-Line Agents		Second-Line Agent
	Naltrexone	Acamprosate	Disulfiram
Effect	Reduces heavy alcohol use (NNT 12) and daily drinking; reduces return to any drinking (NNT 20); reduces cravings	Reduces return to any drinking (NNT 12); reduces drinking days overall; more effective than naltrexone at promoting abstinence; less effective than naltrexone at reducing cravings	Acts as a deterrent to drinking No better than placebo for return to any drinking or abstinence The disulfiram-alcohol reaction begins 10–30 minutes after drinking alcohol, can last several hours, and includes nausea, vomiting, facial flushing, headache, dizziness, sweating
Dosing	Goal dose: Daily: 50–100 mg orally Extended-release: 380 mg ventrogluteal intramuscularly monthly	666 mg orally three times daily	250–500 mg orally daily
Patient selection	Can be given to patients currently drinking	Consider for patients with OUD on MOUD (methadone, buprenorphine) or who require opioids High pill burden	Largest benefit with supervised dosing by a support person
Contraindications	Current or anticipated opioid use. Decompensated cirrhosis or acute liver failure Generally safe in Child-Pugh class A and B Caution in Child-Pugh class C Intramuscular naltrexone avoids first pass metabolism and may be safer if given for alcohol related liver disease and cirrhosis	Do not use if CrCl < 30 mL/minute. For CrCl 30–50 mL/minute, reduce dose to 333 mg orally three times daily No dose adjustment for liver impairment	Severe cardiac disease, psychosis, hypersensitivity Generally safe in Child-Pugh A; use caution in Child-Pugh class B
Side effects[1]	Nausea, vomiting, headache, dizziness	Diarrhea, vomiting, insomnia, anxiety	Headache, metallic taste in mouth
Mechanism of action	Nonselective opioid antagonist blocks indirect release of endogenous opioids due to the reduced rewarding effect of alcohol	Glutamate receptor modulator thought to restore balance between GABA and glutamate systems disrupted by alcohol	Inhibits the breakdown of aldehyde dehydrogenase resulting in buildup of acetaldehyde if alcohol ingested causing aversive symptoms of disulfiram-alcohol reaction
Management	If liver function studies are 3–5 times the upper limits of normal, pursue additional workup, but not a contraindication to initiation. Will cause precipitated opioid withdrawal if administered to a patient currently on opioids.	Most effective when started after completion of medically managed alcohol withdrawal	Should be taken at least 12 or more hours after last alcohol use. Avoid alcohol containing products (eg, mouthwash, sanitizer).

[1]Side effects tend to lessen with use for naltrexone and acamprosate.
AUD, alcohol use disorder; CrCl, creatinine clearance; GABA, γ-aminobutyric acid; MOUD, medication for opioid use disorder; NNT, number needed to treat; OUD, opioid use disorder.

All patients comatose from alcohol intoxication should be treated with intravenous thiamine to prevent or treat Wernicke encephalopathy (see below).

Ingestion of other alcohols (methanol or ethylene glycol) should be suspected in patients with severe metabolic acidosis and an increased anion gap (see Poisoning, Methanol & Ethylene Glycol). Isopropyl alcohol ingestion should be considered in a patient who has the appearance of alcohol intoxication, high levels of serum ketones or acetone yet without metabolic acidosis. All alcohol poisoning is associated with an increased osmolal gap if tested relatively close to time of ingestion.

ALCOHOL WITHDRAWAL

Clinical Findings

A. Symptoms and Signs

The differential diagnosis of alcohol withdrawal includes other sedative withdrawals and other causes of delirium. Acute alcoholic hallucinosis must be differentiated from other acute paranoid states such as amphetamine psychosis or paranoid schizophrenia.

The onset of withdrawal symptoms is usually 6–36 hours, and the peak intensity of symptoms is

48–72 hours after alcohol intake is stopped. The wide spectrum of manifestations of alcohol withdrawal ranges from anxiety, decreased cognition and tremulousness to increasing irritability and hyperreactivity to full-blown delirium tremens (DTs).

Alcohol withdrawal syndrome can be categorized as mild, moderate, or severe withdrawal, withdrawal seizures, and DTs (Table 47–7).

In addition to the symptoms of immediate withdrawal, longer-term symptoms include sleep disturbances, anxiety, depression, excitability, fatigue, and emotional volatility. These symptoms may persist for 3–12 months, and in some cases become chronic.

B. Laboratory Tests

Laboratory testing typically includes a CBC, serum electrolytes with potassium, magnesium and calcium, bedside blood glucose, serum creatinine, liver biochemical tests, amylase and lipase, comprehensive urine toxicology screen to rule out other co-ingested substances, and serum alcohol concentration. If there is a change from a patient's prior presentation (eg, new-onset seizure) or a change in consciousness, workup for occult trauma may include a head CT. An abdominal ultrasound may be considered for abdominal pain, or abnormal pancreatic or liver enzymes.

Complications

A. Alcoholic (Organic) Hallucinosis

This syndrome occurs either during heavy drinking or on withdrawal and is characterized by a paranoid psychosis without the tremulousness, confusion, and clouded sensorium seen in withdrawal syndromes. The patient appears normal except for the auditory hallucinations, which are frequently persecutory and may cause the patient to behave aggressively and in a paranoid fashion.

B. Chronic Alcoholic Brain Syndromes

These encephalopathies are characterized by increasing erratic behavior, memory and recall problems, and emotional instability—the usual signs of organic brain injury due to any cause. Wernicke-Korsakoff syndrome due to thiamine deficiency may develop with a series of episodes. **Wernicke encephalopathy** consists of the triad of confusion, ataxia, and ophthalmoplegia (typically sixth nerve palsy). Early recognition and treatment with thiamine can minimize damage. One of the possible sequelae is **Korsakoff psychosis**, characterized by both anterograde and retrograde amnesia, with confabulation early in the course. Early recognition and treatment with intravenous thiamine and B complex vitamins can minimize damage.

Table 47–7. Categories and presentations of alcohol withdrawal syndromes.

Category	Symptoms and Complications	Onset and Duration	Comment
Mild	**Symptoms:** Tremor, anxiety, tachycardia, nausea, vomiting, and insomnia	Within 6 hours after the last drink, often before the blood alcohol levels drop to zero Usually subside by day 2	
Moderate	Symptoms and signs fall between those of minor and major withdrawal		
Severe or major withdrawal	**Symptoms:** Disorientation, agitation, diaphoresis, whole body tremor, vomiting, hypertension, and hallucinations (visual more often than tactile, which is more often than auditory)	48–96 hours after the last drink	Usually preceded by prolonged heavy alcohol use
Withdrawal seizures (generalized nonfocal tonic-clonic)	**Symptoms:** Brief and resolve spontaneously More prevalent in persons who have a history of withdrawal syndromes	8 hours after the last drink but usually do not manifest > 48 hours after alcohol cessation	If left untreated, can recur in about 60% of patients
Delirium tremor (DT)	**Symptoms:** Extreme mental confusion, agitation, tremor, diaphoresis, sensory hyperacuity, visual hallucinations (often of snakes, bugs, etc), and autonomic hyperactivity (tachycardia and hypertension) **Complications (partial list):** Dehydration, electrolyte disturbances (hypokalemia, hypomagnesemia), arrhythmias and seizures, and even cardiovascular collapse and death	48–72 hours after the last drink but may occur up to 7–10 days later	Most severe form of alcohol withdrawal Develops in about 50% of patients who have had withdrawal seizures, but can develop in the absence of seizures When the patient has been hospitalized for an unrelated problem, the acute withdrawal syndrome is often unexpected, thus presenting as a diagnostic dilemma. Alcohol withdrawal should be suspected in every patient with unexplained delirium. Mortality rate has steadily decreased with early diagnosis and improved treatment

Treatment

Benzodiazepines (specifically diazepam) are the only proven method to prevent delirium tremens, however they also increase the risk of delirium. Long-acting benzodiazepines with active metabolites (such as diazepam or chlordiazepoxide) are preferred. For patients with advanced cirrhosis or acute alcohol-related hepatitis, lorazepam or oxazepam is preferred as the shorter half-life (lorazepam) and absence of active metabolizes (oxazepam) reduce risk if oversedation occurs. For this reason, chlordiazepoxide is avoided for patients with advanced cirrhosis due to its long half-life. Benzodiazepines can be administered via a fixed dose at fixed intervals regardless of Clinical Institute Withdrawal Assessment for Alcohol, Revised (CIWA-Ar) scores, or a "symptom-triggered" approach where they are administered only at CIWA scores above a certain cut-off, most commonly above 8–10. The CIWA-Ar is a validated tool that is widely used to determine severity of alcohol withdrawal. This survey assesses symptoms in 10 areas (both patient-reported and observable) and can be administered relatively quickly (Figure 47–1). One caveat is that patients must be able to communicate their symptoms to the provider. The maximum attainable score is 67. Clinical judgment should be used to determine final medication dosing, as dosing will vary between patients and degrees of withdrawal.

A small nonrandomized trail suggested that symptoms-triggered protocols were associated with lower readmission rates and reduced total dose of benzodiazepines, but with longer lengths of hospital stay. Phenobarbital, a barbiturate with similar properties to benzodiazepines but with a far longer half-life, has also been studied and is the treatment of choice in some institutions.

A. Assessing the Patient for Outpatient or Inpatient Treatment

All patients should be evaluated for their risk of complicated alcohol withdrawal with tools such as the Prediction of Alcohol Withdrawal Severity Scale (PAWSS) score (https://www.mdcalc.com/calc/10102/prediction-alcohol-withdrawal-severity-scale). While the PAWSS score was developed for use in the Emergency Department setting, it can be a useful decision point in the outpatient setting. For patients with low risk of withdrawal (PAWSS < 4), outpatient management is appropriate, with strict return precautions to the emergency department for worsening symptoms despite treatment. Reasons to escalate to inpatient level of care include active or worsening medical or psychiatric conditions, history of benzodiazepine use disorder, worsening withdrawal symptoms despite multiple doses of medication and the patient will not be monitored (eg, treatment setting is closing), patient appears over sedated, unstable vital signs or syncope, or a history of severe withdrawal within the past year.

B. Outpatient Management of Withdrawal

The standard treatment for alcohol withdrawal is with benzodiazepines; however, benzodiazepines are associated with risks including confusion, delirium and overdose particularly when combined with alcohol. In a 2022 review, only benzodiazepines prevented seizures, and only fixed dose diazepam prevented delirium tremens. There are emerging benzodiazepine-sparing protocols for inpatient use with close monitoring that involve oxcarbazepine, γ-hydroxybutyrate (GHB), carbamazepine, and gabapentin. A practical approach for outpatient management of alcohol withdrawal is first to assess the withdrawal severity risk using the PAWSS, then determine risks and benefits of treatments. A common outpatient management for those at low risk and (or) when use of benzodiazepines is deemed too high of a risk is with gabapentin (1200 mg orally daily for days 1–3, then 300–600 mg daily for days 4–7 with additional doses as needed); or in some cases if no contraindications exist, carbamazepine (600–800 mg orally daily tapered to 200–400 mg daily over 4–9 days). When benzodiazepines are appropriate, a single dose of chlordiazepoxide can be prescribed, 25–50 mg orally for mild withdrawal (CIWA-Ar < 10), 50–100 mg for moderate withdrawal (CIWA-Ar 10–18), or a 3–5 day fixed taper of diazepam 10–20 mg orally every 6–12 hours for the first 24 hours, then reduced to 5 mg every 6–12 hours.

C. Inpatient Management of Withdrawal

1. General management—When the history or presentation suggests that patients are actively in withdrawal or at significant risk for withdrawal including a PAWSS ≥ 4, they should be hospitalized. Risk factors for complex withdrawal include a recent drinking history; frequent alcohol consumption; prior withdrawal, seizures, hallucinosis, or DTs; a history of needing medication for detoxification; or a history of benzodiazepine or barbiturate use, abuse, or dependency.

For all hospitalized patients, general management includes ensuring adequate hydration, correction of electrolyte imbalances (particularly magnesium, calcium, and potassium), and administering the vitamins thiamine (100 mg intravenously daily for 3 days then orally daily for prevention), folic acid (1 mg orally daily), and a multivitamin orally daily. Thiamine should be given *prior* to any glucose-containing solutions to decrease the risk of precipitating Wernicke encephalopathy or Korsakoff syndrome. Providers should have a high index of suspicion for Wernicke encephalopathy if a patient exhibits any two of four Caine criteria: (1) malnourishment (eg, recent weight loss, peripheral neuropathy), (2) extra-ocular muscle movement abnormalities, (3) impaired gait, or (4) altered mental status, and should proceed with empiric Wernicke encephalopathy treatment (thiamine 500 mg intravenously three times daily for 3–5 days).

2. Assessing symptom severity—The severity of withdrawal will determine the patient's need for inpatient or intensive care. For those at risk for withdrawal and with mild withdrawal symptoms (eg, CIWA-Ar ≤ 10), admission to a medical unit is adequate. For those with moderate withdrawal (eg, CIWA-Ar 10–18), a higher acuity hospital environment is recommended. Those with severe withdrawal (eg, CIWA-Ar ≥ 19) should be admitted to the ICU.

3. Inpatient treatment of alcohol withdrawal symptoms—Alcohol withdrawal is most commonly treated with benzodiazepines. Studies of other treatment agents, such as phenobarbital

Patient: ____________ **Date:** __________ **Time:** __________ (24 hour clock, midnight = 00:00)

Pulse or heart rate, taken for 1 minute: ____________ **Blood pressure:** ______

NAUSEA AND VOMITING — Ask "Do you feel sick to your stomach? Have you vomited?" Observation.

0 no nausea and no vomiting
1 mild nausea with no vomiting
2
3
4 intermittent nausea with dry heaves
5
6
7 constant nausea, frequent dry heaves and vomiting

TACTILE DISTURBANCES — Ask "Have you any itching, pins and needles sensations, any burning, any numbness, or do you feel bugs crawling on or under your skin?" Observation.

0 none
1 very mild itching, pins and needles, burning, or numbness
2 mild itching, pins and needles, burning, or numbness
3 moderate itching, pins and needles, burning, or numbness
4 moderately severe hallucinations (formications)
5 severe hallucinations
6 extremely severe hallucinations
7 continuous hallucinations

TREMOR — Arms extended and fingers spread apart. Observation.

0 no tremor
1 not visible, but can be felt fingertip to fingertip
2
3
4 moderate, with patient's arms extended
5
6
7 severe, even with arms not extended

AUDITORY DISTURBANCES — Ask "Are you more aware of sounds around you? Are they harsh? Do they frighten you? Are you hearing anything that is disturbing to you? Are you hearing things you know are not there?" Observation.

0 not present
1 very mild harshness or ability to frighten
2 mild harshness or ability to frighten
3 moderate harshness or ability to frighten
4 moderately severe auditory hallucinations
5 severe hallucinations
6 extremely severe hallucinations
7 continuous hallucinations

PAROXYSMAL SWEATS — Observation.

0 no sweat visible
1 barely perceptible sweating, palms moist
2
3
4 beads of sweat obvious on forehead
5
6
7 drenching sweats

VISUAL DISTURBANCES — Ask "Does the light appear to be too bright? Is its color different? Does it hurt your eyes? Are you seeing anything that is disturbing to you? Are you seeing things you know are not there?" Observation.

0 not present
1 very mild photosensitivity
2 mild sensitivity
3 moderate sensitivity
4 moderately severe visual hallucinations
5 severe hallucinations
6 extremely severe hallucinations
7 continuous hallucinations

ANXIETY — Ask "Do you feel nervous?" Observation.

0 no anxiety, at ease
1 mildly anxious
2
3
4 moderately anxious, or guarded, so anxiety is inferred
5
6
7 severely anxious, equivalent...

HEADACHE, FULLNESS IN HEAD — Ask "Does your head feel different? Does it feel like there is a band around your head?" Do not rate for dizziness or lightheadedness. Otherwise, rate severity.

0 not present
1 very mild
2 mild
3 moderate
4 moderately severe
5 severe
6 very severe
7 extremely severe

AGITATION — Observation.

0 normal activity
1 somewhat more than normal activity
2
3
4 moderately fidgety and restless
5
6
7 paces back and forth during most of the interview, or constantly thrashes about

ORIENTATION AND CLOUDING OF SENSORIUM — Ask "What is today's date?... Who am I?". Serial additions: "Please count up by 5's — 0, 5, 10..."

0 oriented and can do serial additions
1 cannot do serial additions or is uncertain about date
2 disoriented for date by no more than 2 calendar days
3 disoriented for date by more than 2 calendar days
4 disoriented for date and place or person

Total **CIWA-Ar** Score ______

Rater's Initials ______

Maximum Possible Score 67

This assessment for monitoring withdrawal symptoms requires approximately 5 minutes to administer. The maximum score is 67 (see instrument). Patients scoring less than 8 (or 10, according to some experts) do not usually need additional medication for withdrawal.

▲ Figure 47–1. **Alcohol withdrawal assessment.** (Reproduced from Sullivan JT et al. Assessment of alcohol withdrawal: The revised clinical institute withdrawal assessment for alcohol scale [CIWA-Ar]. Br J Addict. 1989;84:1353. This scale is not copyrighted and may be used freely.)

and ketamine, have not demonstrated superiority to benzodiazepines. Continual assessment is recommended to determine the severity of withdrawal. Symptom-driven medication regimens are shown to prevent under- and oversedation and to reduce total benzodiazepine usage over fixed-dose schedules. Benzodiazepine-sparing order sets have successfully decreased usage of benzodiazepines through use of adjuncts such as gabapentin, valproic acid, clonidine, and dexmedetomidine.

4. Treating alcohol withdrawal symptoms based on CIWA-Ar score—

A. Minimal withdrawal symptoms (CIWA-Ar score < 8)—Patients who have a history of alcohol withdrawal with minimal withdrawal symptoms are suitable for withdrawal prophylaxis. The recommended benzodiazepine options include chlordiazepoxide or lorazepam orally, tapered over 3 days. The protocol calls for nursing assessment of sedation and withdrawal symptoms (CIWA-Ar) every 6 hours. If prophylactic medication is indicated, a sample tapering regimen may include lorazepam, 1 mg orally every 6 hours for 1 day, then 1 mg orally every 8 hours for 1 day, then 1 mg orally every 12 hours for 1 day, then discontinue; or chlordiazepoxide, 50 mg orally every 6 hours for 1 day, 25 mg orally every 6 hours for 2 days, then discontinue. Avoid chlordiazepoxide in older patients or in patients with liver disease. Lorazepam is preferred in patients with liver disease. Sedation is assessed 30–60 minutes after each medication dose. The benzodiazepine dose is held for oversedation or if the respiratory rate is < 10 breaths per minute. For CIWA-Ar score > 8, the provider must be notified, because this is suggestive of active withdrawal, and escalation of treatment must occur.

B. Mild withdrawal symptoms (CIWA-Ar score 8–15)—For patients in mild withdrawal, either chlordiazepoxide orally or lorazepam orally or intravenously can be as necessary to control symptoms without excessive sedation. After the first 2 hours, chlordiazepoxide or lorazepam is given every 4 hours and as needed. Typical dosing may include chlordiazepoxide 25–50 mg orally or lorazepam 0.5–1 mg orally or intravenously every 4 hours as needed. Additional doses of benzodiazepines should be given if the CIWA-Ar score remains between 8 and 15.

C. Moderate withdrawal (CIWA-Ar score 16–20)—For patients in moderate withdrawal, chlordiazepoxide 100 mg orally or lorazepam 3 or 4 mg orally or intravenously is given every hour for the first 2 hours. CIWA-Ar monitoring should occur every 2 hours. Dosing is adjusted to control symptoms without excessive sedation. After initial dosing, continued treatment could include chlordiazepoxide 50 mg orally or lorazepam 1–2 mg orally or intravenously every 2 hours as needed for CIWA-Ar score between 16 and 20, and chlordiazepoxide 25 mg orally or lorazepam 0.5–1 mg orally or intravenously every 2 hours for CIWA-Ar score between 8 and 15. The maximum dose of chlordiazepoxide is 600 mg in 24 hours. Patients should be monitored with continuous pulse oximetry and cardiac monitoring. The degree of sedation should be monitored 30–60 minutes after each oral dose of medication and for 15 minutes after each parenteral dose.

D. Severe withdrawal (CIWA-Ar score > 20)—Patients with severe withdrawal are at risk for the development of DTs and should be admitted to the ICU. Intravenous lorazepam can be used to treat severe withdrawal. A potential treatment protocol is to administer lorazepam 1–2 mg intravenously every 15 minutes until the patient is calm and sedated but awake. Initial CIWA-Ar monitoring should occur every 30 minutes. The patient can then receive lorazepam 2 mg orally or intravenously every hour as needed when the CIWA-Ar score is between 16 and 20, and lorazepam 1–2 mg orally or intravenously every hour as needed when the CIWA-Ar score is between 8 and 15. If the patient requires > 8 mg/hour of lorazepam as an initial dose or continues to demonstrate observable agitation, tremors, tachycardia, or hypertension despite high doses of lorazepam, consider adding dexmedetomidine, an α_2-agonist that produces sedation with minimal effect on respiratory drive. Dexmedetomidine is not recommended as a sole agent for the treatment of alcohol withdrawal but as an adjunctive therapy (along with benzodiazepines) to decrease the hyperadrenergic output in patients with severe alcohol withdrawal not controlled by benzodiazepines or in patients at risk for respiratory depression from high-dose benzodiazepine administration. The recommended dosing of dexmedetomidine is 0.2–0.7 mcg/kg/hour, with lorazepam 1–2 mg intravenously every 8 hours plus lorazepam 1–2 mg intravenously every hour as needed for agitation. In limited cases of severe withdrawal requiring frequent lorazepam boluses for at least 6 hours, continuous intravenous lorazepam infusion can be considered, but the patient must be monitored extremely carefully for signs of respiratory depression. Continuous pulse oximetry and close observance of the patient's respiratory status are required. Sedation is assessed 15 minutes after each intravenous dose. If withdrawal symptoms are refractory to escalating benzodiazepine usage, despite the addition of dexmedetomidine, adding phenobarbital or escalation to propofol should be considered. Patients receiving large doses of benzodiazepines often require intubation for airway protection, at which time initiation of propofol infusion for sedation, in addition to treatment of refractory alcohol withdrawal, is recommended. Phenobarbital monotherapy for alcohol withdrawal is used at some institutions, but sufficiently powered RCTs comparing the efficacy of phenobarbital to benzodiazepines are needed to inform adoption of new treatment regimens.

In all cases, benzodiazepines should be held if the patient is too sedated or has a respiratory rate < 10 breaths per minute. Do not bolus lorazepam in doses > 4 mg intravenously. Mixing benzodiazepines, eg, chlordiazepoxide orally every 8 hours with lorazepam, is not recommended. Instead, select a single agent and titrate as needed. Once a patient has been stable for 24 hours, the benzodiazepine dose can be reduced by 20% daily until withdrawal is complete.

Since the symptoms are primarily those of psychosis in the presence of a clear sensorium, they are handled like any other psychosis: hospitalization (when indicated) and adequate amounts of antipsychotic medications.

5. Managing other withdrawal-associated conditions— Meticulous examination for other medical problems is necessary. Alcoholic hypoglycemia can occur with low blood alcohol levels (see Chapter 31). Patients with severe AUD commonly have liver disease with associated clotting disorders and are also prone to injury—and the combination all too frequently leads to undiagnosed subdural hematoma.

Phenytoin does *not* appear to be useful in managing alcohol withdrawal seizures. Sedating doses of benzodiazepines are effective in treating alcohol withdrawal seizures. Thus, other anticonvulsants are not usually needed unless there is a preexisting seizure disorder.

Chronic brain syndromes secondary to a long history of alcohol intake are not clearly responsive to thiamine and vitamin replenishment. Attention to the social and environmental care for this type of patient is paramount.

6. Initiating psychological and social measures— Psychological and behavioral treatment become the primary considerations after successful treatment of alcoholic hallucinosis or withdrawal. Psychological and social measures should be initiated in the hospital prior to discharge. This increases the possibility of continued posthospitalization treatment.

Bahji A et al. Comparative efficacy and safety of pharmacotherapies for alcohol withdrawal: a systematic review and network meta-analysis. Addiction. 2022;117:2591. [PMID: 35194860]

Centers for Disease Control and Prevention. Alcohol Related Disease Impact (ARDI) application, 2024. Available at www.cdc.gov/ARDI

Malone D et al. Phenobarbital versus benzodiazepines in alcohol withdrawal syndrome. Neuropsychopharmacol Rep. 2023;43:532. [PMID: 37368937]

Substance Abuse and Mental Health Services Administration. (2025). Key substance use and mental health indicators in the United States: Results from the 2024 National Survey on Drug Use and Health (HHS Publication No. PEP25-07-007, NSDUH Series H-60). Center for Behavioral Health Statistics and Quality, Substance Abuse and Mental Health Services Administration. https://www.samhsa.gov/data/data-we-collect/nsduh-national-surveydrug-use-and-health/national-releases

The ASAM clinical practice guideline on alcohol withdrawal management. J Addict Med. 2020;14:1. [PMID: 32511109]

Tiglao SM et al. Alcohol withdrawal syndrome: outpatient management. Am Fam Physician. 2021;104:253. [PMID: 34523874]

Yang W et al. Alcohol use disorder: neurobiology and therapeutics. Biomedicines. 2022;10:1192. [PMID: 35625928]

STIMULANTS: AMPHETAMINES, AMPHETAMINE DERIVATIVES, & COCAINE

ESSENTIALS OF DIAGNOSIS

- Overdose death with synthetic opioids and stimulants is increasingly common.
- Stimulant use can cause irreversible neuropsychiatric and cardiovascular sequelae.
- Contingency management, a behavioral treatment using rewards for abstinence, is a highly effective treatment.

General Considerations

Commonly used stimulants include cocaine (in base form referred to as "crack"), methamphetamine ("speed", "crank", or "crystal meth"), and prescription stimulants (eg, dextroamphetamine/amphetamine [Adderall®], methlyphenidate [Ritalin]). Amphetamine derivatives and related drugs include MDMA ("ecstasy"), ephedrine ("herbal ecstasy"), and methcathinone ("cat" or "khat"). These drugs possess stimulant and hallucinogenic properties. Methcathinone derivatives such as methylenedioxypyrovalerone (MDPV), also known as "bath salts," are used as recreational drugs. While not classified as stimulants, amphetamine-like reactions have been reported after use of synthetic cannabinoids (eg, "Spice" and "K2"). Nonprescription medications and nutritional supplements may contain stimulant or sympathomimetic drugs such as ephedrine, yohimbine, or caffeine. *Increasingly, amphetamines and cocaine are adulterated with fentanyl or fentanyl analogs, or there is accidental exposure from shared smoking supplies,* resulting in unexpected coma, respiratory depression, and death (see also Opioid Use Disorders). National household surveys (NSDUH) from the United States of non-institutionalized populations from 2024 indicate that in the past year, 4.3 million adults have used cocaine (including crack cocaine), 3.9 million have used prescription stimulants, and 2.4 million have used methamphetamine. Applying *DSM-5* criteria, the estimated prevalence of stimulant use disorder is 4.3 million adults. Cocaine and prescription stimulant use is more common among persons 18–25 years old, while methamphetamine use predominates in those ≥ age 26. Geographically, methamphetamine use is concentrated in the western half of the United States, and risk factors for use include lower educational attainment, lower income, housing instability, criminal justice involvement, lack of insurance, comorbidities (eg, HIV, depression), and polysubstance use.

With illicit fentanyl and its analogs being the dominant non-prescription opioid that is consumed, co-use of stimulants is common. Overdose death involving psychostimulants and opioids have increased dramatically. Between 2021 and 2024, 59% of overdose deaths in the United States involved a stimulant (31% methamphetamine, 30% cocaine, and 3.8% involved both). Seventy-three percent of stimulant-involved overdose deaths co-involved opioids. Fourteen and one-half percent of deaths involved only stimulants. This has been termed the "fourth-wave" of overdose death in the United States. This unprecedented rise has revealed the need to rapidly improve and expand our treatments for stimulant use disorder. There is ongoing study to determine if individuals intentionally combine opioids and stimulants or primarily use stimulants and have unintended exposure to fentanyl (eg, drug contamination). The diagnosis of a stimulant use disorder is made using *DSM-5* criteria (see Table 47–1). Stimulants can be consumed by inhalation, intravenously, intramuscularly, intranasally, orally, or per rectum (eg, chemsex among men who have sex with men). Individuals may have a pattern of episodic, recreational use, and not progress to a use disorder. Alternatively, behavior dysregulation with cravings, tolerance, and potential withdrawal may develop; patients will use stimulants despite consequences of compulsiveness and loss of control over behavior.

Clinical Findings

A. Symptoms and Signs

Acute intoxication syndromes with stimulants are common in patients who come to emergency departments. Stimulants exert powerful effects on the cardiovascular and neuropsychiatric systems. Patients may have classic sympathomimetic overdose syndromes, including sweating, tachycardia, hypertension, mydriasis, psychomotor agitation, and/or an acute brain syndrome with confusion and disorientation. Patients may present with chest pain that may resemble a typical atherosclerotic acute coronary syndrome, or their ECG and biomarkers may be normal. Notably, in a study of patients with "cocaine chest pain", coronary artery disease was highly prevalent (17%). Additional presenting symptoms may include pulmonary hypertension, arrhythmias or cardiac arrest, stroke or TIAs, or acute psychosis. With severe intoxication, seizures and hyperthermia may occur. Methamphetamine is associated with psychosis, impacting 36% of patients who misuse the substance. Patients exhibit prominent delusions of persecution, ideas of reference, and hallucinations that may be auditory, tactile, or visual. Stimulant use may also be present in patients with accidents or injuries, unintentional overdose, and suicides or homicides. Acute obstetrical complications from stimulant use include spontaneous abortion, abruptio placentae, teratogenic effects, delayed fetal growth, and prematurity.

Chronic intoxication, or long-term use of stimulants, can have innumerable deleterious effects on the cardiovascular and neuropsychiatric systems. Stimulants exacerbate chronic illnesses such as hypertension, CAD, and atrial fibrillation. Stimulant-associated cardiomyopathy is a complication of long-term stimulant use, especially methamphetamine, and patients show high hospitalization rates and premature mortality. Long-term use of stimulants can cause neurocognitive impairment in the domains of executive function, memory, and planning. Longitudinal studies in Thailand of patients admitted for stimulant-induced psychosis suggest that even after abstaining, up to 38% of patients will have ongoing psychiatric disease. Chronic use of stimulants has several oral and skin manifestations, including dental caries and decay from decreased salivation and bruxism; ulceration and ischemia of the nasal turbinates; excoriation and ulcers from compulsive skin picking, particularly with delusional parasitosis which can cause significant psychological distress. Chorea or choreoathetosis (purposeless, irregular, and involuntary movements in the trunk and extremities) is a rare but striking complication. This syndrome typically resolves after cessation of use.

Sudden withdrawal of the drug is not life-threatening but usually produces craving, sleep disturbances, hyperphagia, lassitude, and severe depression (sometimes with suicidal ideation) lasting days to weeks.

B. Laboratory Tests

Immunoassays of urine samples to detect stimulant use are widely available. The cocaine immunoassay has high sensitivity and specificity, but the amphetamine assay has a high risk of false positive results (4–10%), with the following drugs commonly producing false positive results: trazodone, promethazine, bupropion, and labetalol (among others). It is recommended that a positive amphetamine screen be confirmed by gas chromatography mass spectrometry testing. Taking a medication review and checking a prescription activity report is also important for any positive test as the person may have had it prescribed (eg, mixed amphetamine salts or Adderall®). Other laboratory tests include a CBC, liver enzymes, glucose, electrolytes and kidney function, and markers of muscle breakdown (eg, CK) or cardiac injury (eg, troponin). HIV, STIs, and hepatitis screening is recommended. Cardiovascular risk assessment should be performed for patients with simulant use disorder via online calculators such as PREVENT, which includes cholesterol, GFR, and HbA_{1c}.

Complications

Hyperadrenergic syndromes from stimulant use can cause muscle hyperactivity, leading to rhabdomyolysis, acute kidney injury, and metabolic acidosis. Other medical complications include levamisole-related small vessel vasculitis in persons using cocaine or crack. Patients may have skin ulcerations (retiform purpura), including the nose and ear pinna, with neutropenia and abnormal ANA and p-ANCA (anti-MPO) tests. In patients with HIV, active stimulant use is a risk for a nonsuppressed viral load and HIV progression. Clinicians should be alert to possible stimulant use in patients with unexplained nasal bleeding or septal perforations, headaches, fatigue, insomnia, anxiety, depression, and chronic hoarseness.

Treatment

Treatment of acute intoxication syndromes is supportive and targets the dominant symptom while aiming to prevent end-organ damage. Acute agitation and paranoia may require use of sedatives (eg, benzodiazepines) and antipsychotics. Haloperidol, quetiapine, risperidone, aripiprazole, and olanzapine are effective at clinically relevant doses in stimulant-induced psychosis (see Table 28–3). Status epilepticus can be treated with phenobarbital 15 mg/kg intravenously. Sympathomimetic overdose syndromes may require cooling if hyperthermic (temperature > 39–40°C) (see Poisoning or Overdose-Related: Hyperthermia), fluid resuscitation (especially to prevent myoglobinuric kidney injury in patients who have rhabdomyolysis), and treatment of hypertension. Of note, the common teaching to avoid β-blockers in stimulant-induced chest pain due to unopposed α activity and vasoconstriction has been reconsidered. Numerous studies show that there is no conclusive evidence that unopposed α stimulation regularly occurs or that it predictably causes adverse outcomes. β-Blockers with mixed α- and β-blocking activity, such as labetalol and carvedilol, can effectively treat acute hypertension and tachycardia (eg, labetalol 20 mg intravenously over 2 minutes with repeat doses every 10 minutes, adding 10–20 mg up to 80 mg intravenously over one minute). Tachycardia or tachyarrhythmias can be treated with a short-acting β-blocker such as esmolol (25–100 mcg/kg/minute by intravenous infusion).

Treatment of stimulant withdrawal is supportive and may include medication to address symptoms such as sleep abnormalities and depressed mood.

Chronic treatment of stimulant use disorder can be behavioral or medical. The best behavioral treatment for stimulant use disorders recommended by the ASAM is contingency management. Contingency management uses operant conditioning, such that the patient gets a reward in response to doing a target behavior (eg, not using the drug), and if the reward is sufficiently large or salient, the target behavior continues. Contingency management programs are cost-effective, and increasingly available in some outpatient addiction programs, general medicine settings, or through online platforms, though broad access is still lacking. Other evidence-based behavioral treatments include cognitive behavioral therapy and the Matrix Model (a type of intensive outpatient treatment). Fellowship groups exist specifically for stimulants, including Crystal Meth Anonymous and Cocaine Anonymous. Harm reduction counseling should be provided to all patients, including offers of naloxone for any person at risk of unintentional overdose.

There are no FDA approved medications for treatment of stimulant use disorders. Off-label use of bupropion, bupropion and extended-release naltrexone, topiramate, or mirtazapine have been shown to decrease the frequency of methamphetamine use and are often trialed if the patient has a co-occurring disorder that also might benefit from the medication (eg, nicotine use disorder for bupropion). Modafinil or topiramate may be considered for cocaine use disorder.

Ciccarone D et al. Understanding stimulant use and use disorders in a new era. Med Clin North Am. 2022;106:81. [PMID: 34823736]

Clinical Guideline Committee (CGC) Members, ASAM Team, AAAP Team, IRETA Team. The ASAM/AAAP clinical practice guideline on the management of stimulant use disorder. J Addict Med. 2024;18:1. [PMID: 38669101]

National Institute on Drug Abuse website. https://nida.nih.gov/research-topics/mdma-ecstasy-molly. April 19, 2024. Accessed June 19, 2026.

Wagner K et al. Prevalence of fentanyl in methamphetamine and cocaine samples collected by community-based drug checking services. Drug and Alcohol Dependence. 2023;252:110985. [PMID: 3782698]

CANNABIS & CANNABINOIDS

ESSENTIALS OF DIAGNOSIS

- Cannabis use disorder (CUD) is the second most common SUD after AUD in the United States.
- Cannabis is a federal Schedule I illegal substance; state laws, however, shape legality of recreational or medicinal use and are the regulations most enforced.
- There are no FDA approved medications to treat CUD, however behavioral based treatments can be effective.

General Considerations

Cannabis is an umbrella term used to describe products such as cannabinoids, marijuana, and hemp derived from the *Cannabis sativa* plant. Cannabis activates endogenous brain cannabinoid (CB) receptors (CB1 receptors in the endocannabinoid system) and in other organs (such as CB2 receptors in the immune system). Cannabis has medicinal and non medicinal use, and CUD is the most common type of SUD (6.8%) after AUD. Worldwide, rates of CUD are near those of OUD. Cannabis is classified federally as a Schedule I drug due to its addictive potential so it cannot be prescribed. However, most states have legalized medical use of cannabis and federal law is generally not enforced in those states. Medicines with extracted or synthesized cannabinoids have shown small to modest benefits in treating chronic pain, muscle spasticity, chemotherapy-induced nausea and vomiting, and refractory epilepsy (specifically cannabidiol). With increasing legalization, the number of regular users who have used higher potency cannabis for medicinal or recreational purposes, as well as the rates of cannabis use complications, have risen. The most common routes of use are inhalation (via various modalities: pipe, rolled, or "vaping," etc.) or oral (ie, "edibles"). All cannabis formulations have become stronger, and delivery methods have been developed to further increase potency, such as vaping.

Synthetic cannabinoids (such as "K2," "Spice") have much higher potency and are associated with death, tachycardia, and seizures likely due to their higher toxicity and longer lasting effects. Adolescents are particularly impacted by cannabis, with use reported among 16.6%, and long-term complications of use include cognitive impairment, dependence, and reduced educational attainment.

Clinical Findings

A. Symptoms and Signs

1. Intoxication—The intoxication syndrome produces two phases: mild euphoria followed by sleepiness. In the acute state, the user has an altered time perception, less inhibited emotions, psychomotor problems, impaired immediate memory, and conjunctival injection. High doses produce transient psychotomimetic effects. Peak onset of action is reached within 3–10 minutes for inhaled cannabis versus 1–6 hours for oral formulations, which can have a half-life of 20–30 hours. Cannabis use frequently aggravates existing mental illness and adversely affects motor performance.

2. Withdrawal—Withdrawal produces insomnia, nausea, myalgia, and irritability. Cannabis withdrawal typically starts within 1–2 days after cessation, symptoms peak at 2–6 days and can take up to 3 weeks to resolve in more frequent cannabis users.

B. Laboratory Tests

Tetrahydrocannabinol (THC) can be detected in the urine up to 3 days after last use in most persons. However, it can be detected over a lengthier interval in those with long-term use as THC is absorbed in fat and can be eliminated over a longer time period. In one small high-quality study, the urine of persons with consistent use of high potency cannabis was positive for THC up to 24 days. In contrast, regular use of low dose THC containing hemp oil has not been shown to result in urine positive for THC. Almost all synthetic cannabinoids (other than "HU-210") do not cross react with THC immunoassays and are not included in confirmatory liquid chromatography and mass spectrometry testing; synthetic cannabinoids, therefore, do not appear on these urine drug tests.

Complications

Cannabis use can have significant medical complications. Acute use can be associated with cognitive impairment and acute psychosis, cardiac arrhythmias and car accidents, while long term use has been shown to worsen or increase the risk of serious mental illness including psychosis and impaired cognition in addition to other medical complications. Prolonged use can progress to CUD.

1. Acute intoxication—Cognitive impairments are common, including impaired verbal memory, increased disinhibition, reduced attention, and psychomotor disfunction that may recover within hours or days but can be prolonged with chronic use. Studies have shown that the reduced cognitive function may take up to 2–25 days to resolve with abstinence. Acute cannabis-associated psychotic symptoms can occur at rates of nearly 0.5% for lifetime occurrence and can manifest as hallucinations requiring emergency department level care. Cardiovascular complications include arrhythmias with acute use, and cardiovascular events with chronic and acute intoxication. From a public health perspective, acute cannabis consumption has been associated with a modest increase in traffic accidents (OR 1.25–1.97) that occurs most frequently 5–6 hours after use and is exacerbated with concomitant alcohol use when driving.

2. Long-term use—While many persons use cannabis regularly to treat mood or anxiety disorders, regular use has been associated with increased risk of major depression (two-fold for misuse and 3–5 times for those with CUD) and anxiety (two-fold for misuse, 3–4 times higher in those with CUD). Frequent cannabis use is associated with bipolar disorder (and greater symptom severity) and increased risk of psychosis (five-fold with daily use of high potency cannabis compared to non-users), versus a two-fold increased risk among daily users of low potency cannabis. Notably, infrequent use (< once per week) has not been associated with a psychotic disorder. Daily cannabis use is associated with MI and stroke, with increased use frequency associated with higher odds (25 and 42%, respectively).

3. Cannabis use disorder—The diagnosis is made using the *DSM-5* criteria, similar to the other substance use disorders (see Table 47–1). CUD is characterized by repeated use despite harm. Risks of developing CUD for those with chronic use are 22% (ever use) versus 33% (daily use), and risk factors are male gender, younger age, and high potency cannabis.

4. Hyperemesis syndrome—This syndrome is a unique complication categorized by cyclic episodes of nausea, vomiting and intense abdominal pain that occur with prolonged high potency cannabis use, and is relieved by hot baths, showers, capsaicin cream, and abstinence from cannabis.

5. Other symptoms—Pulmonary complications include non-specific symptoms such as cough, as well as specific pulmonary injury from contaminants ("e-cigarette" or vaping product use associated lung injury "EVALI"). Fertility can be impacted; long-term usage can depress plasma testosterone levels and reduce sperm counts, and cause abnormal menstruation and failure to ovulate. The intelligence quotient has been shown to decrease by 2 points per year after the start of frequent or dependent use of cannabis, and early onset of cannabis (< 25 years old) for those with frequent use are associated with lower educational achievement including early school drop-out and fewer academic degrees. During pregnancy, regular cannabis use increases the risk of maternal anemia and neonatal complications such as neonatal ICU stay and reduced birth weight.

Treatment

There is no specific pharmacologic treatment for intoxication, withdrawal, or ongoing CUD. A 2019 review of 12 trials that evaluated medications for CUD found that antidepressants (eg, SSRIs and serotonin-norepinephrine reuptake inhibitors) were less effective at achieving abstinence, overall cannabis use, or retention in treatment. Outcomes for antipsychotics, mood stabilizers, and atomoxetine were insufficient or not identified. Cannabinoids as treatment for CUD had no effect on abstinence compared to placebo, reducing cannabis use, or improving retention. For the acute intoxication phase, no specific treatment is necessary other than addressing acute complications as noted above. Cannabis withdrawal does not typically require hospitalization; however, for those with significant comorbid health disorders and with concurrent other substance use, inpatient management may be indicated. For CUD, motivational interviewing, cognitive behavioral therapy, and contingency management result in greater reductions in cannabis use.

Connor JP et al. Clinical management of cannabis withdrawal. Addiction. 2022;117:2075. [PMID: 34791767]
Hoch E et al. Cannabis, cannabinoids and health: a review of evidence on risks and medical benefits. Eur Arch Psychiatry Clin Neurosci. 2025;275:281. [PMID: 39299947]
Kondo K et al. Pharmacotherapy for the treatment of cannabis use disorder: a systematic review. 2020;172:398. [PMID: 32120384]

OTHER DRUG & SUBSTANCES

1. Psychedelics

Classic psychedelics include the semi-synthetic lysergic acid diethylamide (LSD) derived from the ergot fungus, mescaline, psilocybin, dimethyltryptamine (DMT), and other derivatives of phenylalanine and tryptophan, many of which have been used in myriad traditional sacramental and healing contexts worldwide. Lifetime classic psychedelic use has a prevalence of 13.6% in the US adult population. In contrast to most drug use, lifetime use of classic psychedelics has been found to significantly reduce odds of past month psychological distress and past year suicidal thinking, suicidal planning, and suicide attempt. A group of synthesized "novel psychedelics" (typically with names describing their chemical structures) remains understudied though increasingly used.

Clinical Findings

Psychedelic use can result in various responses. Generally, there is an initial feeling of tension that is followed by emotional release such as crying or laughing (1–2 hours after ingestion). Later and at higher doses, perceptual distortions occur, with visual illusions and hallucinations, and occasionally there is fear of ego disintegration (2–3 hours after ingestion). Major changes in time sense and mood lability then occur (3–4 hours after ingestion). A feeling of detachment and a sense of destiny and control follow (4–6 hours). Occasionally, the acute episode is terrifying (a "bad trip"), which may include panic, depression, confusion, or psychotic symptoms.

The most commonly affected organ systems include cardiovascular (tachycardia), neurologic (CNS depression, seizure, coma in severe cases), and GI (nausea or vomiting). Acute complications can include serotonin toxicity, which can include myoclonus, fever, hyperthermia, tachycardia, and agitation (see Poisonings, LSD & Other Hallucinogens).

Treatment

Treatment of the acute episode primarily involves reduction of harm to the individual from erratic behavior that may lead to injury or death. A structured environment is usually sufficient until the drug is metabolized. In severe cases, antipsychotic medications with minimal side effects (eg, haloperidol, 5 mg intramuscularly) may be given every several hours until the individual has regained control. In cases where "flashbacks" occur (mental imagery from a "bad trip" that is later triggered by mild stimuli such as marijuana, alcohol, or psychic trauma), a short course of an antipsychotic medication—eg, olanzapine, 5–10 mg daily orally, or risperidone, 2 mg daily orally, initially, and up to 20 mg daily and 6 mg daily, respectively—is usually sufficient. Lorazepam or clonazepam, 1–2 mg orally every 2 hours as needed for acute agitation, may be a useful adjunct. An occasional patient may have "flashbacks" for much longer periods and may require small doses of antipsychotic medications over the longer term.

2. Phencyclidine

Phencyclidine (PCP, angel dust, peace pill, hog) is simple to produce and mimics to some degree the traditional psychedelic drugs. PCP is a common deceptive substitute for LSD, tetrahydrocannabinol, and mescaline. It is available in crystals, capsules, and tablets to be inhaled, injected, swallowed, or smoked (it is commonly sprinkled on marijuana).

Clinical Findings

Absorption after smoking is rapid, with onset of symptoms in several minutes and peak symptoms in 15–30 minutes. Mild intoxication produces euphoria accompanied by a feeling of numbness. Moderate intoxication (5–10 mg ingestion) results in disorientation, detachment from surroundings, distortion of body image, combativeness, unusual feats of strength (partly due to its anesthetic activity), and loss of ability to integrate sensory input, especially touch and proprioception. Physical symptoms include dizziness, ataxia, dysarthria, nystagmus, retracted upper eyelid with blank stare, hyperreflexia, and tachycardia. There are increases in blood pressure, respiration, muscle tone, and urine production. Usage in the first trimester of pregnancy is associated with increased spontaneous pregnancy loss and congenital defects. Severe intoxication (≥ 20 mg ingestion) produces an increase in the moderate symptoms, with the addition of seizures, deepening coma, hypertensive crisis, and severe psychotic ideation. The drug is long-lasting (several days to several weeks) owing to high lipid solubility, gastroenteric recycling, and the production of active metabolites.

Overdose may be fatal, with the major causes of death being hypertensive crisis, respiratory arrest, and convulsions. Acute rhabdomyolysis has been reported and can result in myoglobinuric kidney failure (see Poisonings, LSD & Other Hallucinogens).

Differential diagnosis includes the use of the whole spectrum of "illicit" drugs, since in some ways phencyclidine mimics sedatives, psychedelics, and marijuana in its effects. Blood and urine testing can detect PCP use.

Treatment

GI decontamination is generally unnecessary in PCP ingestions; however, activated charcoal may be beneficial with massive ingestion of PCP or a dangerous co-ingestion if taken within one hour of ingestion. (see Poisonings, LSD & Other Hallucinogens). Treatment for agitation, violent behavior, and psychosis due to intoxication involves placing the patient in a calm and dark environment. Sedation and restraints (medication and physical) may be needed. Benzodiazepines (lorazepam 2–4 mg or diazepam 5–10 mg, both either intravenously or intramuscularly) are the preferred medication for chemical sedation. Repeated doses every 10 minutes may be required for adequate sedation. Benzodiazepines are also the first-line treatment for PCP-induced hypertension, seizures, and psychomotor agitation.

Additional treatment may include psychiatric evaluation if behavioral issues persist despite resolution of other complications. Otherwise, patients with mild symptoms can often be discharged 1–2 hours after symptoms resolve. Patients who present without symptoms to an emergency department after reporting PCP intake should be observed for at least 6 hours before discharge.

3. Sedatives (Anxiolytics)

See Anxiety Disorders, Chapter 28.

4. Caffeine

Caffeine is one of the most commonly used substances worldwide, with nearly 90% of adults reporting regular intake, although a caffeine use disorder is not described. Tea, cocoa, and cola drinks contribute to an intake of caffeine that is often high in many people. Low to moderate doses of caffeine (30–200 mg/day) may improve some aspects of performance (eg, vigilance). The approximate content of caffeine in a (180-mL) cup of beverage is as follows: brewed coffee, 80–140 mg; instant coffee, 60–100 mg; decaffeinated coffee, 1–6 mg; black leaf tea, 30–80 mg; tea bags, 25–75 mg; instant tea, 30–60 mg; cocoa, 10–50 mg; and 12-oz cola drinks, 30–65 mg. A 2-oz chocolate candy bar has about 20 mg. Some herbal teas (eg, "morning thunder") contain caffeine. Caffeine-containing analgesics usually contain approximately 30 mg per unit and have been used to treat post-operative headaches.

Symptoms of caffeinism (usually associated with ingestion > 500 mg daily) include anxiety, agitation, restlessness, insomnia, a feeling of being "wired," and somatic symptoms referable to the heart and GI tract. It is common for caffeinism to present as an anxiety disorder. It is also common for caffeine and other stimulants to precipitate severe symptoms in patients with compensated schizophrenia and bipolar disorder. Patients who are chronically depressed often use caffeine drinks as self-medication.

Caffeine intoxication from caffeine doses of 1 g (15 mg/kg) includes symptoms of tachycardia, insomnia, agitation, tachypnea, psychomotor agitation, GI irritation, and anxiety. Ingestion of caffeine in doses ≥ 5 g can lead to vomiting, seizures, arrhythmias and MI. Although rare, excessive consumption of caffeine can result in death. The fatal acute oral dose of caffeine is generally considered to be 5–10 g.

Caffeine withdrawal can occur after abrupt discontinuation of caffeine. The seven domains of caffeine withdrawal are drowsiness, difficulty concentrating, mood disturbances, low sociability and motivation, nausea or upset stomach, flu-like symptoms, and headache. Withdrawal may occur upon abstinence from chronic caffeine exposure at doses as low as 100 mg daily, and upon abstinence following only 3–7 days of caffeine exposure at higher doses. Caffeine withdrawal can occur in hospitalized patients who are not taking anything by mouth.

5. Miscellaneous Drugs & Solvents

MDMA/Molly/Ecstasy (3,4-methylenedioxymethamphetamine) is a synthetic drug that increases release of serotonin and dopamine, and is thus misused to increase energy, boost mood, and increase bonding with others. Use has been associated with panic attacks and anxiety, and chronic use can lead to insomnia, anxiety, paranoia, memory and attention problems. Complications of use include liver damage, extended depressed mood, sexual assault, hyponatremia, rhabdomyolysis, serotonin syndrome, multiorgan failure, cardiovascular events, arrhythmias, and death. Concurrent use with an SSRI can increase negative health effects.

Antihistaminic agents sold over the counter are frequently found in combination with a mild analgesic promoted as cold remedies. Medications containing phenylpropanolamine are banned from sale in the United States. Side effects of phenylpropanolamine relate to its effect as a stimulant, including precipitation of anxiety states, increased blood pressure effects, auditory and visual hallucinations, paranoid ideation, and occasionally delirium. Aggressiveness and some loss of impulse control were reported as well as sleep disturbances even with small doses.

Antihistamines, such as most over the counter sleep aids, usually produce some CNS depression. The mixture of antihistamines with alcohol often exacerbates the CNS effects. Scopolamine and bromides generally have been removed from over-the-counter products.

Anabolic steroid misuse includes nonprescribed use to increase muscle mass for appearance or strength. The practice is sometimes associated with significant mood swings, aggressiveness, and paranoid delusions in addition to medical problems such as cardiovascular (hyperlipidemia, hypertension, coronary artery disease, venous thromboembolism, arrhythmias, cardiomyopathy), GI (transaminitis, hepatic steatosis), genitourinary (testicular atrophy, sexual dysfunction, secondary hypogonadism), hematologic (erythrocytosis), infections (cellulitis), dermatologic (gynecomastia, acne, alopecia) and musculoskeletal (tendon ruptures), as well as an overall increased mortality. Alcohol and stimulant use may concomitantly occur more frequently in patients who misuse anabolic steroids. Withdrawal symptoms of steroid dependency include fatigue, depressed mood, restlessness, and insomnia.

Amyl nitrite can cause effects like changes in time perception, a "rush," and mild euphoria, and it has been used to enhance orgasms. Subjective effects last from 5 seconds to 15 minutes. Tolerance develops readily, but there are no known withdrawal symptoms. Abstinence for several days reestablishes the previous level of responsiveness. Long-term effects may include damage to the immune system and respiratory difficulties.

Nitrous oxide ("N_2O," "whippets") has partial agonist activity at the mu, κ, and σ opioid receptors. Intoxication is characterized by poor oxygenation (inhalants displace oxygen with other gasses), acute asphyxia, arrhythmia and sudden death. It can cause a transient state of excitation followed by sedation, ataxia, slurred speech, cognitive impairment, and slow reactivity. At high concentrations, hallucinations and psychosis can occur. Nitrous oxide typically clears in 5 minutes. Withdrawal syndromes have not been well documented. The most commonly noted complication is functional vitamin B_{12} deficiency marked by combined degeneration of the spinal cord with difficulty ambulating, and in rare cases altered mental status with CNS involvement. Treatment is with aggressive vitamin B_{12} supplementation (1000 mcg intramuscularly daily or every other day in the first week, followed by weekly for 4–8 weeks, then monthly). Concurrent megaloblastic anemia typically resolves in 6–8 weeks.

Inhalation of solvents and gases (including aerosols) can produce a form of inebriation similar to that of volatile anesthetics. Agents include gasoline, toluene, petroleum ether, lighter fluids, cleaning fluids, paint thinners, and solvents that are present in many household products (eg, nail polish). Typical intoxication states include euphoria, slurred speech, hallucinations, and confusion, and with high doses, acute manifestations are unconsciousness and cardiorespiratory depression or failure. Chronic exposure produces a variety of symptoms related to the liver, kidney, bone marrow, or heart. Lead encephalopathy can be associated with sniffing leaded gasoline. In addition, studies of workers chronically exposed to jet fuel showed significant increases in neurasthenic symptoms, including fatigue, anxiety, mood changes, memory difficulties, and somatic complaints. These same problems have been noted in long-term solvent use.

Journey JD et al. Phencyclidine toxicity. 2023 Sep 4. In: StatPearls [Internet]. Treasure Island (FL): StatPearls Publishing; 2025. [PMID: 29939642]
Simon MW et al. Clinical effects of psychedelic substances reported to United States poison centers: 2012 to 2022. Ann Emerg Med. 2024;84:605. [PMID: 39093248]
Windfeld-Mathiasen J et al. Mortality among users of anabolic steroids. JAMA. 2024;331:1229. [PMID: 38483396]

6. Newer Psychoactive Substances

Xylazine, an α_2-adrenergic agonist used in veterinary medicine as a sedative and muscle relaxant, depresses the CNS by reducing norepinephrine release. Xylazine is not approved for human use but increasingly has been found as an adulterant in illicit drugs, most commonly fentanyl in the United States. Complications of use include profound sedation, hypotension, bradycardia, and respiratory depression. As xylazine is not an opioid, it does not reverse with naloxone. Chronic use can cause ulcerative skin wounds that require intensive wound care and surgical debridement in some cases.

Medetomide, a compound related to xylazine but more potent, is replacing xylazine as an adulterant in the illicit drug supply in some parts of the United States; in Philadelphia in 2024, 87% of the drug supply contained medetomidine. Severe withdrawal syndromes include tachycardia, hypertension (> 180 mm Hg/100 mm Hg), uncontrolled nausea and vomiting, tremor, and diaphoresis, often requiring ICU management.

Kratom is derived from the *Mitragyna speciosa* tree (coffee plant) family, native to Southeast Asia. In the United States, kratom can be found in tea, capsules and packaged kratom drinks, extracts and gummies, and sold at herbal stores, smoke shops, and on the internet. Kratom is legal on the federal level; however, it is illegal in many states, cities or counties, and it has no FDA-approved uses. Low doses (1–5 g) have a stimulant effect (similar to coffee) and high doses (5–15 g) have opioid symptoms including analgesia and euphoria, while very high doses (≥ 15 g) are sedating. Acute side effects include nausea, constipation, vomiting, weight loss, insomnia, headache, irritability, dry mouth, decreased sex drive and hyperpigmentation. Withdrawal in some patients with chronic use of kratom can mimic opioid withdrawal; buprenorphine has been used for chronic treatment of kratom OUD.

Isotonitazene (aka "iso" or "nitazene"), a benzimidazole compound in the nitazene class, is a highly potent, full agonist at the mu opioid receptor that is chemically distinct from fentanyl and thus cannot be detected on fentanyl test strips. Isotonitazene was synthesized in the 1950s but has not been formally studied in humans. As a synthetic opioid mixed with heroin with or without fentanyl, it has been reported in unintentional overdose events, leading the DEA to name it as a Schedule I substance. Overdose involving nitazenes may require higher or repeated doses of naloxone. Extended testing for benzimidazole compounds may be indicated for opioid overdose syndromes that test negative for fentanyl.

GHB, an endogenous neurotransmitter and GABA analog, acts primarily as a CNS depressant by binding specific GHB receptors and by GABA-B receptor agonism. It also affects dopamine, serotonin, norepinephrine, and cholinergic systems. GHB is often used in club settings and "chemsex" for its euphoric, disinhibiting, and sedative effects. GHB has a narrow effect window; doses of 20–30 mg/kg produce euphoria and memory loss, while doses ≥ 40–60 mg/kg can cause coma. The drug is rapidly absorbed (peak levels at 20–40 minutes) and has a short half-life of 20–60 minutes, with effects typically lasting 2–6 hours. **GHB intoxication** is characterized by rapid onset of coma with characteristically sudden awakening. Other symptoms include CNS and respiratory depression, myoclonus and abnormal involuntary movements, bradycardia and hypothermia, nausea and vomiting, and respiratory arrest in severe cases. Management is primarily supportive as no specific antidote exists. Patients typically recover within 6 hours. **GHB withdrawal** can be severe and life-threatening, resembling alcohol withdrawal particularly after chronic multiple daily use. Clinical features include anxiety, tremors, agitation, and insomnia, autonomic dysfunction (tachycardia, hypertension, diaphoresis), auditory and visual hallucinations, delirium, disorientation, paranoid psychosis, and seizures in severe cases. Withdrawal typically lasts 3–12 days but can persist up to 21 days in severe cases. Benzodiazepines (eg, diazepam) are first-line treatment for GHB withdrawal, given in scheduled tapers and symptom triggered doses. Other adjuncts include baclofen (GABA-B agonist), barbiturates (pentobarbital, phenobarbital), propofol, or dexmedetomidine for severe cases, and antipsychotics for severe psychosis. Severe withdrawal may require ICU care with mechanical ventilation, sedative infusions (midazolam), and multimodal pharmacotherapy.

Borelli CM et al. Severe gamma-hydroxybutyrate withdrawal with delirium, hemodynamic lability, and rhabdomyolysis: a case series. Am J Addict. 2025;34:361. [PMID: 39953704]
Huo S et al. Notes from the field: suspected medetomidine withdrawal syndrome among fentanyl-exposed patients–Philadelphia, Pennsylvania, September 2024-January 2025. MMWR Morb Mortal Wkly Rep. 2025;74:266. [PMID: 40310762]
Karila L et al. Pharmacological treatment of GHB withdrawal syndrome. Current Addiction Reports. 2024;11:163. https://doi.org/10.1007/s40429-023-00531-1
Felmlee MA et al. γ-Hydroxybutyric acid: pharmacokinetics, pharmacodynamics, and toxicology. AAPS J. 2021;23:22. [PMID: 33417072]

Index

NOTE: Page numbers in **boldface** type indicate a major discussion. A *t* following a page number indicates tabular material, and *f* following a page number indicates a figure. Drugs are listed under their generic names.

Q

R

S